DUTTON'S ORTHOPAEDIC EXAMINATION, EVALUATION, AND INTERVENTION

NOTICE

DUTTON'S ORTHOPAEDIC EXAMINATION, EVALUATION, AND INTERVENTION

THIRD EDITION

Mark Dutton, PT
Allegheny General Hospital
West Penn Allegheny Health System (WPAHS)
Adjunct Clinical Instructor, Duquesne University
School of Health Sciences
Pittsburgh, Pennsylvania

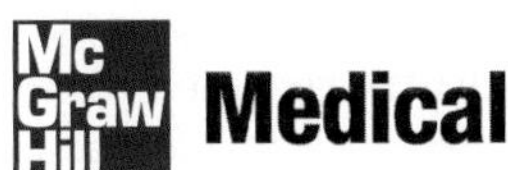

New York Chicago San Francisco Lisbon London Madrid Mexico City
Milan New Delhi San Juan Seoul Singapore Sydney Toronto

The McGraw·Hill Companies

Dutton's Orthopaedic Examination, Evaluation, and Intervention, Third Edition

1 2 3 4 5 6 7 8 9 0 CTP/CTP 17 16 15 14 13 12

Set ISBN 978-0-07-174404-1
Set MHID 0-07-174404-5
Book ISBN 978-0-07-174405-8
Book MHID 0-07-174405-3
DVD ISBN 978-0-07-174406-5
DVD MHID 0-07-174406-1

This book was set in Minion by Aptara, Inc.
The editors were Joe Morita and Brian Kearns.
The production supervisor was Catherine Saggese.
The illustration manager was Armen Ovsepyan.
Illustrations created by Dragonfly Media Group.
Project management was provided by Indu Jawwad, Aptara, Inc.
The designer was Alan Barnett; the cover designer was John Michael Graphics.
China Translation & Printing, Ltd. was printer and binder.

Library of Congress Cataloging-in-Publication Data

Dutton, Mark.
Dutton's Orthopaedic examination, evaluation, and intervention / Mark Dutton.
– 3rd ed.
p. ; cm.
Includes bibliographical references and index.
ISBN 978-0-07-174404-1 (set : hardcover : alk. paper) – ISBN
0-07-174404-5 (set : hardcover : alk. paper)
I. Title.
[DNLM: 1. Orthopedics—methods. 2. Musculoskeletal
Diseases—diagnosis. 3. Orthopedic Procedures—methods. 4. Physical
Examination—methods. WE 168]

616.7′075—dc23

2011053484

Please tell the author and publisher what you think of this book by sending your comments to pt@mcgraw-hill.com. Please put the author and title of the book in the subject line.

McGraw-Hill books are available at special quantity discounts to use as premiums and sales promotions, or for use in corporate training programs. To contact a representative please e-mail us at bulksales@mcgraw-hill.com.

For my parents,
Ron and Brenda, who have always helped, guided, and inspired me
and to my two daughters, Leah and Lauren who provide me with such joy.

Your Legacy

Will you have earned the respect of your peers and the admiration of your critics?

Will you have acted humbly during success and gracefully in the face of adversity?

Will you be remembered for how often you brought smiles to the hearts of others?

Will you have looked for the very best, and done your utmost to build worth, in others?

Will you have left this world a better place by the life you have lived?

Modified from *The Legacy You Leave ©2000 by Rick Beneteau*

Contents

Preface

The third edition of this book is an update of information provided in the second edition along with revisions to the various chapters. One of the most noticable changes in this edition are in the photos and illustrations, which are now in color.

The aim of the book is to continue to provide the reader with a systematic and logical approach to the examination and intervention of the orthopaedic patient. Such an approach must be eclectic, because no single approach works all of the time. Thus, this book attempts to incorporate the biomechanical concepts of the Norwegians and Australians; the mechanical diagnostic and classification approach of McKenzie; the selective tissue tension principles of Cyriax; the neurodynamic mobility tests of Butler; the muscle strength-length assessments of Janda, Jull, and Sahrmann; and the osteopathic approach of Mitchell.

For any intervention to be successful, an accurate diagnosis must be followed by a carefully planned and specific rehabilitation program to both the affected area and its related structures. This approach must take into consideration the structure involved and the stage of healing.

It is hoped that this book will be seen as the best available textbook, guide, review, and reference for health care students and clinicians involved in the care of the orthopaedic population.

Mark Dutton, PT

Comments about this book may be sent to me at pt@mcgraw-hill.com.

Acknowledgments

From inception to completion, the various editions span almost 12 years. Such an endeavor cannot be completed without the help of many. I would like to take this opportunity to thank the following:

- The faculty of the North American Institute of Manual and Manipulative Therapy (NAIOMT)—especially, Jim Meadows, Erl Pettman, Cliff Fowler, Diane Lee, and the late Dave Lamb.
- The exceptional team at McGraw-Hill, for their superb guidance throughout this object. Thank you especially to Joe Morita for his advice and support, and to other members of the initial lineup. Special thanks also to Brian Kearns.
- To the production crew of Aptara, especially Indu Jawwad.
- Bob Davis for his creative eye and the excellent photography.
- Leah for agreeing to be the photographic model.
- The staff of Human Motion Rehabilitation, Allegheny General Hospital including Dan Norkiewicz, Dave Hahn, Dean Hnaras, John Karp, Melissa Willis, Shawna Sutherland, Leslie Fisher, Joe Witt, Randi Marshak, Bruce Jacobs, Diane Ferianc, Keith Galloway, Dan McCool, Darcy Skrip, Renee Nacy, Mary Horton, Tara Stempfer, Andrea Parilak, Craig Castor, Eric Cardwell, Carrie Cochenour, Jodie Weiher, and Susan Berger.
- To the countless clinicians throughout the world who continually strive to improve their knowledge and clinical skills.

Introduction

"The very first step towards success in any occupation is to become interested in it."

—Sir William Osler (1849–1919)

Until the beginning of the last century, knowledge about the mechanism of healing and the methods to decrease pain and suffering were extremely limited. Although we may scoff at many of the interventions used in the distant past, many of the interventions we use today, albeit less radical, have still to demonstrate much more in the way of effectiveness. That may soon change with the recent emphasis within many health-care professions on evidence-based clinical practice. The process of evidence-based practice is presented in Table I-1. When combining clinical expertise with the best available external clinical evidence, clinicians can make informed decisions regarding patient management, including the selection and interpretation of the most appropriate evaluation procedures. In addition, intervention strategies that are based on the best available evidence will have a greater likelihood of success with the least associated risk.[1,2]

TABLE I-1 The Process of Evidence-Based Practice
1. Identify the patient problem. Derive a specific question.
2. Search the literature.
3. Appraise the literature.
4. Integrate the appraisal of literature with your clinical expertise, experience, patient values, and unique circumstances.
5. Implement the findings.
6. Assess outcome and reappraise.

Data from Sackett DL, Strauss SE, Richardson WS, et al.: *Evidence Based Medicine: How to Practice and Teach EBM*, 2nd edn. Edinburgh, Scotland: Churchill Livingstone, 2000.

The goal of every clinician should be to enhance patient/client satisfaction, increase efficiency, and decrease unwarranted treatment approaches.[2] The management of the patient/client is a complex process involving an intricate blend of experience, knowledge, and interpersonal skills. Obtaining an accurate diagnosis requires a systematic and logical approach. Such an approach should be eclectic, because no single approach works all of the time. For any intervention to be successful, accurate diagnosis must be followed by a carefully planned and specific rehabilitation program to both the affected area and its related structures. In this book, great emphasis is placed on the appropriate use of manual techniques and therapeutic exercise based on these considerations. Electrotherapeutic and thermal/cryotherapeutic modalities should be viewed as adjuncts to the rehabilitative process. The accompanying DVD to this book contains numerous video clips of manual techniques and therapeutic exercises, which the reader is encouraged to view. The following icon is used throughout the text to indicate when such clips are available. [VIDEO]

REFERENCES

1. Sackett DL, Rosenberg WM, Gray JA, et al.: Evidence based medicine: What it is and what it isn't. *BMJ* 312:71, 1996.
2. Schroder JA: Manual therapy and neural mobilization: Our approach and personal observations. *Orthopaedic Pract* 16:23, 2004.

SECTION I ANATOMY

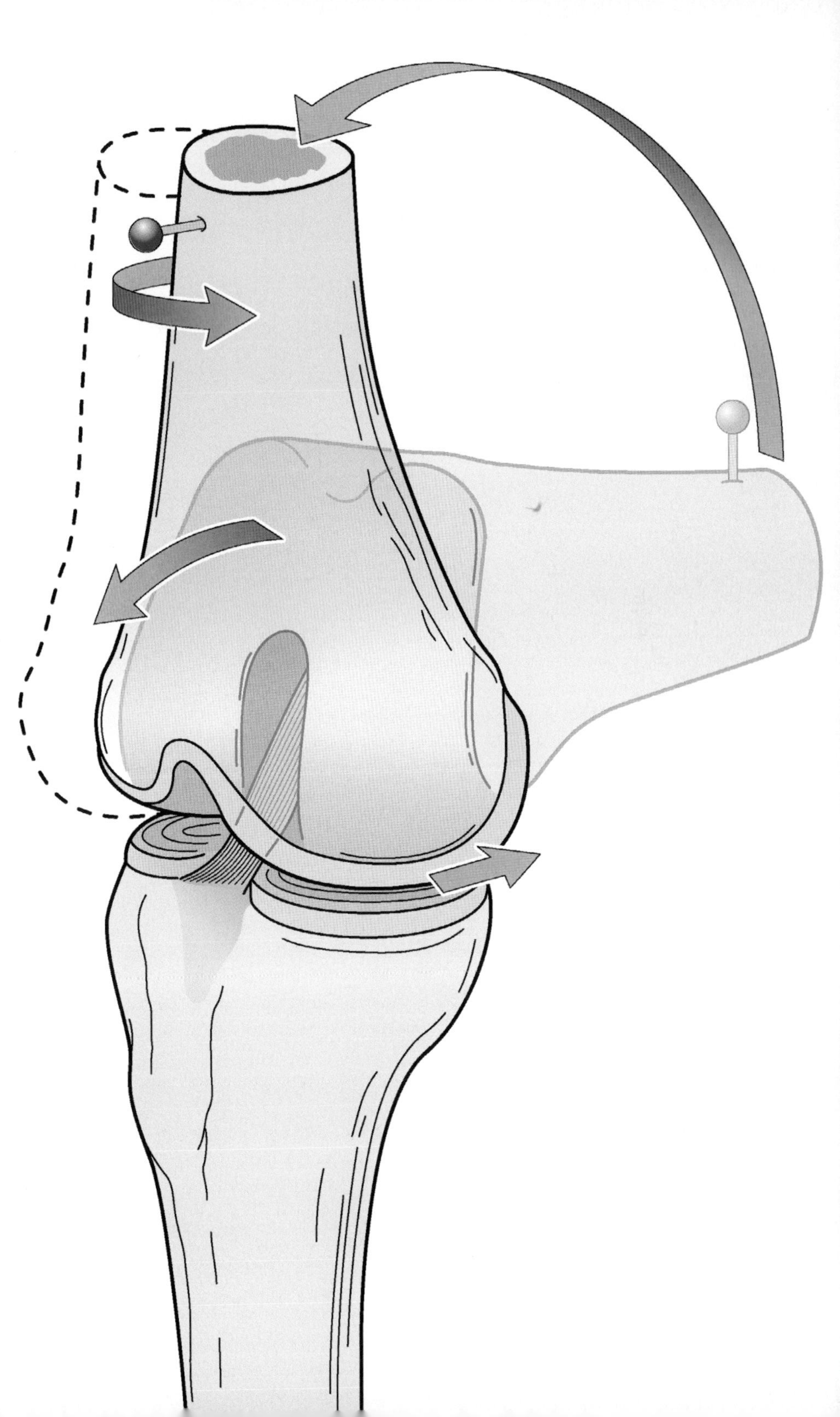

CHAPTER 1 The Musculoskeletal System

CHAPTER OBJECTIVES

At the completion of this chapter, the reader will be able to:

1. Describe the various types of biological tissue of the musculoskeletal system.
2. Describe the tissue mechanics and structural differences and similarities between muscle, tendons, fascia, and ligaments.
3. Define the various terminologies used to describe joint position, movements, and relationships.
4. Give definitions for commonly used biomechanical terms.
5. Describe the different planes of the body.
6. Describe the different axes of the body and the motions that occur around them.
7. Define the terms osteokinematic motion and arthrokinematic motion.
8. Differentiate between the different types of motion that can occur at the joint surfaces.
9. Describe the basic biomechanics of joint motion in terms of their concave–convex relationships.
10. Define the terms *closepacked* and *openpacked.*

OVERVIEW

Throughout the human body, there are four types of fundamental tissues:

- Epithelial. Covers all internal and external body surfaces and includes structures such as the skin and the inner lining of the blood vessels.
- Connective. Connective tissue (CT), which includes bone, cartilage, tendons, ligaments, and blood tissue, provides structural and metabolic support for other tissues and organs of the body.
- Muscle. Muscles are classified functionally as either voluntary or involuntary, and structurally as either smooth, striated (skeletal), or cardiac. There are approximately 430 skeletal muscles in the body, each of which can be considered anatomically as a separate organ. Of these 430 muscles, about 75 pairs provide the majority of body movements and postures.[1]
- Nervous. Nervous tissue provides a two-way communication system between the central nervous system (brain and spinal cord) and muscles, sensory organs, and various systems (see Chapter 3).

CONNECTIVE TISSUE

CT is divided into subtypes according to the matrix that binds the cells. CT proper has a loose flexible matrix, called *ground substance*. The most common cell within CT proper is the fibroblast. Fibroblasts produce collagen, elastin, and reticulin fibers. Collagen is a group of naturally occurring proteins. The collagens are a family of extracellular matrix (ECM) proteins that play a dominant role in maintaining the structural integrity of various tissues and in providing tensile strength to tissues. The ECM contains proteoglycans, lipids, water, and dissolved electrolytes. Proteoglycans, which are a major component of the ECM, are macromolecules that consist of a protein backbone to which are attached many extended polysaccharide units called *glycosaminoglycans (GAGs),* of which there are two types: chondroitin sulfate and keratin sulfate.[2,3] A simple way to visualize the proteoglycan molecule is to consider a test tube brush, with the stem representing the protein core and the GAGs representing the bristles.[4,5]

The various characteristics of collagen differ depending on whether it is loose or dense collagen. The anatomic and functional characteristics of loose and dense collagen are summarized in Table 1-1. Collagenous and elastic fibers are sparse and irregularly arranged in loose CT but are tightly packed in dense CT.[6] Elastic fibers are composed of a protein called *elastin*. As its name suggests, elastin provides elastic properties to the tissues in which it is situated.[7] Elastin fibers can stretch, but they normally return to their original shape when the tension is released. Thus, the elastic fibers of elastin determine the patterns of distention and recoil in most organs, including the skin and lungs, blood

TABLE 1-1 Loose and Dense Collagen

Joint Type	Anatomic Location	Fiber Orientation	Mechanical Specialization
Dense irregular connective tissue	Composes the external fibrous layer of the joint capsule, forms ligaments, bone, aponeuroses, and tendons	Parallel, tightly aligned fibers	Ligament: Binds bones together and restrains unwanted movement at the joints; resists tension in several directions Tendon: attaches muscle to bone
Loose irregular connective tissue	Found in capsules, muscles, nerves, fascia, and skin	Random fiber orientation	Provides structural support

vessels, and CT. Bundles of collagen and elastin combine to form a matrix of CT fascicles. This matrix is organized within the primary collagen bundles as well as between the bundles that surround them.[8]

The various types of CT as relate to the musculoskeletal system are described as follows:

Fascia

Fascia is viewed as a loose CT that provides support and protection to the joint, and acts as an interconnection between tendons, aponeuroses, ligaments, capsules, nerves, and the intrinsic components of muscle.[9,10] This type of CT may be categorized as fibrous or nonfibrous, with the fibrous components consisting mainly of collagen and elastin fibers, and the nonfibrous portion consisting of amorphous ground substance.[11]

Tendons

The function of tendons is to attach muscle to bone at each end of the muscle, and, when stretched, store elastic energy that contributes to movement.[12] In addition, tendons enable the muscle belly to be an optimal distance from the joint upon which it is acting.[12] The collagen fibers of tendons (95% of the collagen in tendons is type I, with the remaining 5% being type III and IV) are arranged in a quarter-stagger arrangement, which gives it a characteristic banding pattern and provides high strength and stability.[13] A loose CT matrix surrounds the bundles of collagen fibrils. The thickness of each tendon varies and is proportional to the size of the muscle from which it originates. Vascularity within the tendon is relatively sparse and corresponds with the lower metabolic/turnover rate of these tissues. Within the fascicles of tendons, which are held together by loose CT called *endotenon*, the collagen components are unidirectionally oriented. Endotenon contains blood vessels, lymphatics, and nerves and permits longitudinal movements of individual fascicles when tensile forces are applied to the structure. The CT surrounding groups of fascicles or the entire structure is called the *epitenon*. Tendons display viscoelastic mechanical properties that confer time-and rate-dependent effects on the tissue. Specifically, tendons are more elastic at lower strain rates and stiffer at higher rates of tensile loading. Tendons deform less than ligaments under an applied load and are able to transmit the load from muscle to bone.[8] The resting tendon has a slightly crimped or wave-like appearance. Total tendon strains (percentage deformity) of 1–2% result in the straightening of the crimp pattern of unloaded tendon collagen. Strains of 2–6% are well tolerated by most healthy tendons. However, with a strain higher than 6%, incomplete tears start to occur within the tendon, and complete structural failure typically occurs in the range of 8–10%.[14] As with all CT, tendons have a positive adaptive response to repeated physiologic mechanical loading, which results in biologic and mechanical changes. Although tendons withstand strong tensile forces well, they resist shear forces less well, and provide little resistance to compression force. A peritendinous connective-tissue sheath (paratenon) surrounds the entire tendon. This sheath consists of two layers: an inner (visceral) layer and an outer (parietal) layer with occasional connecting bridges (mesotenon). If there is synovial fluid between these two layers, the paratenon is called tenosynovium; if not, it is termed tenovagium.[8]

A tendon can be divided into three main sections:[12]

- The bone–tendon junction. At most tendon–bone interfaces, the collagen fibers insert directly into the bone in a gradual transition of material composition. The physical junction of tendon and bone is referred to as an enthesis,[15] and is an interface that is vulnerable to acute and chronic injury.[16] One role of the enthesis is to absorb and distribute the stress concentration that occurs at the junction over a broader area.
- The tendon midsubstance. Overuse tendon injuries can occur in the midsubstance of the tendon, but not as frequently as at the enthesis.
- The musculotendinous junction (MTJ). The MTJ is the site where the muscle and tendon meet. The MTJ comprises numerous interdigitations between muscle cells and tendon tissue, resembling interlocked fingers. Despite its viscoelastic mechanical characteristics, the MTJ is very vulnerable to tensile failure.[17,18]

CLINICAL PEARL

The MTJ is the location of most common muscle strains caused by tensile forces in a normal muscle–tendon unit.[8,19] In particular, a predilection for a tear near the MTJ has been reported in the biceps and triceps brachii, rotator cuff muscles, flexor pollicis longus, fibularis (peroneus) longus, medial head of the gastrocnemius, rectus femoris, adductor longus, iliopsoas, pectoralis major, semimembranosus, and the entire hamstring group.[20–22]

Ligaments

Skeletal ligaments are fibrous bands of dense CT that connect bones across joints. Ligaments can be named for the bones into which they insert (coracohumeral), their shape (deltoid), or their relationships to each other (cruciate).[23] The gross structure of a ligament varies according to location (intra-articular or extra-articular, capsular), and function.[24] Ligaments, which appear as dense white bands or cords of CT, are composed primarily of water (approximately 2/3), and of collagen (largely type I collagen (85%), but with small amounts of type III) making up most of the dry weight. The collagen in ligaments has a less unidirectional organization than it does in tendons, but its structural framework still provides stiffness (resistance to deformation—see Chapter 2).[25] Small amounts of elastin (1% of the dry weight) are present in ligaments, with the exception of the ligamentum flavum and the nuchal ligament of the spine, which contain more. The cellular organization of ligaments makes them ideal for sustaining tensile load, with many containing functional subunits that are capable of tightening or loosening in different joint positions.[26] At the microscopic level, closely spaced collagen fibers (fascicles) are aligned along the long axis of the ligament and are arranged into a series of bundles that are delineated by a cellular layer, the endoligament, and the entire ligament is encased in a neurovascular biocellular layer referred to as the epiligament.[23] Ligaments contribute to the stability of joint function by preventing excessive motion,[27] acting as guides or checkreins to direct motion, and providing proprioceptive information for joint function through sensory nerve endings (see Chapter 3) and the attachments of the ligament to the joint capsule.[28–30] Many ligaments share functions. For example while the anterior cruciate ligament of the knee is considered the primary restraint to anterior translation of the tibia relative to the femur, the collateral ligaments and the posterior capsule of the knee also help in this function.[23] The vascular and nerve distribution to ligaments is not homogenous. For example, the middle of the ligament is typically avascular, while the proximal and distal ends enjoy a rich blood supply. Similarly, the insertional ends of the ligaments are more highly innervated than the midsubstance.

Cartilage

Cartilage tissue exists in three forms: hyaline, elastic, and fibrocartilage.

- Hyaline cartilage, also referred to as articular cartilage, covers the ends of long bones and permits almost frictionless motion to occur between the articular surfaces of a diarthrodial (synovial) joint.[31] Articular cartilage is a highly organized viscoelastic material composed of cartilage cells called *chondrocytes*, water, and an ECM. Articular cartilage, the most abundant cartilage within the body, is devoid of any blood vessels, lymphatics, and nerves.[4,5] Most of the bones of the body form first as hyaline cartilage, and later become bone in a process called *endochondral ossification*. The normal thickness of articular cartilage is determined by the contact pressures across the joint—the higher the peak pressures, the thicker the cartilage.[24] Articular cartilage functions to distribute the joint forces over a large contact area, thereby dissipating the forces associated with the load. This distribution of forces allows the articular cartilage to remain healthy and fully functional throughout decades of life. The patellar has the thickest articular cartilage in the body.

CLINICAL PEARL

Chondrocytes are specialized cells that are responsible for the development of cartilage and the maintenance of the ECM.[32] Chondrocytes produce aggrecan, link protein, and hyaluronan, all of which are extruded into the ECM, where they aggregate spontaneously.[3] The aggrecans form a strong, porous-permeable, fiber-reinforced composite material with collagen. The chondrocytes sense mechanical changes in their surrounding matrix through intracytoplasmic filaments and short cilia on the surface of the cells.[24]

Articular cartilage may be grossly subdivided into four distinct zones with differing cellular morphology, biomechanical composition, collagen orientations, and structural properties, as follows:

  - *The superficial zone.* The superficial zone, which lies adjacent to the joint cavity, comprises approximately 10–20% of the articular cartilage thickness and functions to protect deeper layers from shear stresses. The collagen fibers within this zone are packed tightly and aligned parallel to the articular surface. This zone is in contact with synovial fluid and is responsible for most of the tensile properties of cartilage.
  - *The middle (transitional) zone.* In the middle zone, which provides an anatomic and functional bridge between the superficial and deep zones, the collagen fibril orientation is obliquely organized. This zone comprises 40–60% of the total cartilage volume. Functionally, the middle zone is the first line of resistance to compressive forces.
  - *The deep or radial layer.* The deep layer comprises 30% of the matrix volume. It is characterized by radially aligned collagen fibers that are perpendicular to the surface of the joint, and which have a high proteoglycan content. Functionally the deep zone is responsible for providing the greatest resistance to compressive forces.
  - *The tidemark.* The tidemark distinguishes the deep zone from the calcified cartilage, the area that prevents the diffusion of nutrients from the bone tissue into the cartilage.

- Elastic cartilage is a very specialized CT, primarily found in locations such as the outer ear and portions of the larynx.
- Fibrocartilage functions as a shock absorber in both weight-bearing and non–weight-bearing joints. Its large fiber content, reinforced with numerous collagen fibers, makes it ideal for bearing large stresses in all directions. Fibrocartilage is an avascular, alymphatic, and aneural tissue and derives its nutrition by a double-diffusion system.[33] Examples of fibrocartilage include the symphysis pubis, the intervertebral disk, and the menisci of the knee.

TABLE 1-2 General Structure of Bone[17]

Site	Comment	Conditions	Result
Epiphysis	Mainly develops under pressure Apophysis forms under traction Forms bone ends Supports articular surface	Epiphyseal dysplasias Joint surface trauma Overuse injury Damaged blood supply	Distorted joints Degenerative changes Fragmented development Avascular necrosis
Physis	Epiphyseal or growth plate Responsive to growth and sex hormones Vulnerable prior to growth spurt Mechanically weak	Physeal dysplasia Trauma Slipped epiphysis	Short stature Deformed or angulated growth or growth arrest
Metaphysis	Remodeling expanded bone end Cancellous bone heals rapidly Vulnerable to osteomyelitis Affords ligament attachment	Osteomyelitis Tumors Metaphyseal dysplasia	Sequestrum formation Altered bone shape Distorted growth
Diaphysis	Forms shaft of bone Large surface for muscle origin Significant compact cortical bone Strong in compression	Fractures Diaphyseal dysplasias Healing slower than at metaphysis	Able to remodel angulation Cannot remodel rotation Involucrum with infection Dysplasia gives altered density and shape

Bone

Bone is a highly vascular form of CT, composed of collagen, calcium phosphate, water, amorphous proteins, and cells. It is the most rigid of the CTs (Table 1-2). Despite its rigidity, bone is a dynamic tissue that undergoes constant metabolism and remodeling. The collagen of bone is produced in the same manner as that of ligament and tendon, but by a different cell, the osteoblast.[6] At the gross anatomical level, each bone has a distinct morphology comprising both cortical bone and cancellous bone. Cortical bone is found in the outer shell. Cancellous bone is found within the epiphyseal and metaphyseal regions of long bones as well as throughout the interior of short bones.[17] Skeletal development occurs in one of two ways:

- Intramembranous ossification. Mesenchymal stem cells within mesenchyme or the medullary cavity of a bone initiate the process of intramembranous ossification. This type of ossification occurs in the cranium and facial bones and, in part, the ribs, clavicle, and mandible.
- Endochondral ossification. The first site of ossification occurs in the primary center of ossification, which is in the middle of the diaphysis (shaft). About the time of birth, a secondary ossification center appears in each epiphysis (end) of long bones. Between the bone formed by the primary and secondary ossification centers, cartilage persists as the epiphyseal (growth) plates between the diaphysis and the epiphysis of a long bone. This type of ossification occurs in the appendicular and axial bones.

The periosteum is formed when the perichondrium, which surrounds the cartilage, becomes the periosteum. Chondrocytes in the primary center of ossification begin to grow (hypertrophy) and begin secreting alkaline phosphatase, an enzyme essential for mineral deposition. Calcification of the matrix follows and apoptosis (a type of cell death involving a programmed sequence of events that eliminates certain cells) of the hypertrophic chondrocytes occurs. This creates cavities within the bone. The exact mechanism of chondrocyte hypertrophy and apoptosis is currently unknown. The hypertrophic chondrocytes (before apoptosis) also secrete a substance called *vascular endothelial cell growth factor* that induces the sprouting of blood vessels from the perichondrium. Blood vessels forming the periosteal bud invade the cavity left by the chondrocytes and branch in opposite directions along the length of the shaft. The blood vessels carry osteoprogenitor cells and hemopoietic cells inside the cavity, the latter of which later form the bone marrow. Osteoblasts, differentiated from the osteoprogenitor cells that enter the cavity via the periosteal bud, use the calcified matrix as a scaffold and begin to secrete osteoid, which forms the bone trabecula. Osteoclasts, formed from macrophages, break down the spongy bone to form the medullary cavity (bone marrow). The function of bone is to provide support, enhance leverage, protect vital structures, provide attachments for both tendons and ligaments, and store minerals, particularly calcium. Bones also may serve as useful landmarks during the palpation phase of the examination. The strength of a bone is related directly to its density. Of importance to the clinician, is the difference between maturing bone and mature bone. The epiphyseal plate or growth plate of a maturing bone can be divided into four distinct zones:[34]

- Reserve zone: produces and stores matrix.
- Proliferative zone: produces matrix and is the site for longitudinal bone cell growth.
- Hypertrophic zone: subdivided into the maturation zone, degenerative zone, and zone of provisional calcification. It is within the hypertrophic zone that the matrix is prepared for calcification, and is here that the matrix is ultimately

calcified. The hypertrophic zone is the most susceptible of the zones to injury because of the low volume of bone matrix and the high amounts of developing immature cells in this region.[35]

- Bone metaphysis: the part of the bone that grows during childhood.

SKELETAL MUSCLE TISSUE

The microstructure and composition of skeletal muscle have been studied extensively. The class of tissue labeled *skeletal muscle* consists of individual muscle cells or fibers that work together to produce the movement of bony levers. A single muscle cell is called a *muscle fiber* or *myofiber*. Individual muscle fibers are wrapped in a CT envelope called *endomysium*. Bundles of myofibers, which form a whole muscle (fasciculus), are encased in the perimysium. The perimysium is continuous with the deep fascia. Groups of fasciculi are surrounded by a connective sheath called the epimysium. Under an electron microscope, it can be seen that each of the myofibers consists of thousands of *myofibrils*, which extend throughout its length. Myofibrils are composed of sarcomeres arranged in series.[36] All skeletal muscles exhibit four characteristics:[37]

1. Excitability, the ability to respond to stimulation from the nervous system.
2. Elasticity, the ability to change in length or stretch.
3. Extensibility, the ability to shorten and return to normal length.
4. Contractility, the ability to shorten and contract in response to some neural command. The tension developed in skeletal muscle can occur passively (stretch) or actively (contraction). When an activated muscle develops tension, the amount of tension present is constant throughout the length of the muscle, in the tendons, and at the sites of the musculotendinous attachments to bone.[1] The tensile force produced by the muscle pulls on the attached bones and creates torque at the joints crossed by the muscle. The magnitude of the tensile force is dependent on a number of factors.

One of the most important roles of CT is to mechanically transmit the forces generated by the skeletal muscle cells to provide movement. Each of the myofibrils contains many fibers called *myofilaments*, which run parallel to the myofibril axis. The myofilaments are made up of two different proteins: actin (thin myofilaments) and myosin (thick myofilaments) that give skeletal muscle fibers their striated (striped) appearance (Fig. 1-1).[36]

CLINICAL PEARL

The sarcomere is the contractile machinery of the muscle. The graded contractions of a whole muscle occur because the number of fibers participating in the contraction varies. Increasing the force of movement is achieved by recruiting more cells into cooperative action.

The striations are produced by alternating dark (A) and light (I) bands that appear to span the width of the muscle fiber. The A bands are composed of myosin filaments, whereas the I bands are composed of actin filaments. The actin filaments of the I band overlap into the A band, giving the edges of the A band a darker appearance than the central region (H band), which contains only myosin. At the center of each I band is a thin, dark Z line. A *sarcomere* represents the distance between each Z line. Each muscle fiber is limited by a cell membrane called a *sarcolemma*. The protein *dystrophin* plays an essential role in the mechanical strength and stability of the sarcolemma.[38] Dystrophin is lacking in patients with Duchenne muscular dystrophy.

Three types of contraction are commonly recognized: isometric, concentric, and eccentric (see Chapter 12).[39]

- ***Isometric contraction.*** Isometric contractions do not produce any appreciable change in muscle length.
- ***Concentric contraction.*** A concentric contraction produces a shortening of the muscle length. When a muscle contracts concentrically, the distance between the Z lines decreases, the I band and H bands disappear, but the width of the A band remains unchanged.[40] This shortening of the sarcomeres is not produced by a shortening of the actin and myosin filaments, but by a sliding of actin filaments over the myosin filaments, which pulls the Z lines together (sliding filament theory).
- ***Eccentric contraction.*** An eccentric contraction produces a "lengthening" of the muscle length. In reality, the muscle does not actually lengthen, it merely returns from its shortened position to its normal resting length.

CLINICAL PEARL

The sarcoplasm is the specialized cytoplasm of a muscle cell that contains the usual subcellular elements along with the Golgi apparatus, abundant myofibrils, a modified endoplasmic reticulum known as the sarcoplasmic reticulum (SR), myoglobin, and mitochondria. Transverse-tubules (T-tubules) invaginate the sarcolemma, allowing impulses to penetrate the cell and activate the SR.

Structures called *cross-bridges* serve to connect the actin and myosin filaments. The myosin filaments contain two flexible, hinge-like regions, which allow the cross-bridges to attach and detach from the actin filament. During contraction, the cross-bridges attach and undergo power strokes, which provide the contractile force. During relaxation, the cross-bridges detach. This attaching and detaching is asynchronous, so that some are attaching while others are detaching. Thus, at each moment, some of the cross-bridges are pulling, while others are releasing.

The regulation of cross-bridge attachment and detachment is a function of two proteins found in the actin filaments: tropomyosin and troponin (Fig. 1-2). Tropomyosin attaches directly to the actin filament, whereas troponin is attached to the tropomyosin rather than directly to the actin filament.

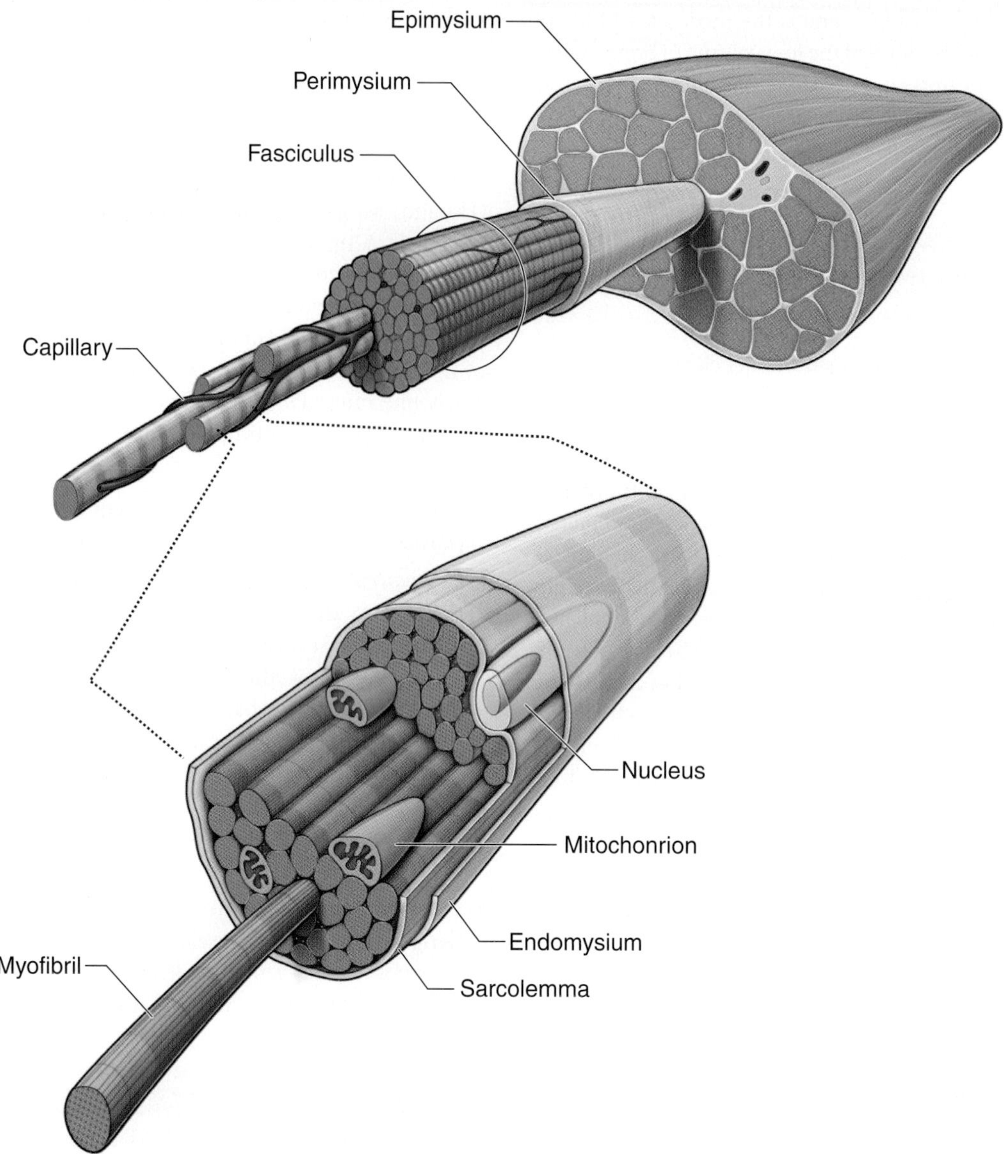

FIGURE 1-1 Microscopic structure of muscle.

CLINICAL PEARL

Tropomyosin and troponin function as the switch for muscle contraction and relaxation. In a relaxed state, the tropomyosin physically blocks the cross-bridges from binding to the actin. For contraction to take place, the tropomyosin must be moved.

Each muscle fiber is innervated by a somatic motor neuron. One neuron and the muscle fibers it innervates constitute a motor unit, or functional unit of the muscle. Each motor neuron branches as it enters the muscle to innervate a number of muscle fibers.

CLINICAL PEARL

The area of contact between a nerve and a muscle fiber is known as the motor end plate, or neuromuscular junction (NMJ).

The release of a chemical acetylcholine from the axon terminals at the NMJ causes electrical activation of the skeletal muscle fibers. When an action potential propagates into the transverse tubule system (narrow membranous tunnels formed from and continuous with the sarcolemma), the voltage sensors on the transverse tubule membrane signal the release of Ca^{2+} from the terminal cisternae portion of the SR (a series of interconnected sacs and tubes that surround each myofibril).[40] The released Ca^{2+} then diffuses into the sarcomeres and binds to troponin, displacing the tropomyosin, and allowing the actin to bind with the myosin cross-bridges (Fig. 1-2). Whenever a somatic motor neuron is activated, all of the muscle fibers that it innervates are stimulated and contract with *all-or-none* twitches. Although the muscle fibers produce all-or-none contractions, muscles are capable of a wide variety of responses, ranging from activities requiring a high level of precision, to activities requiring high tension.

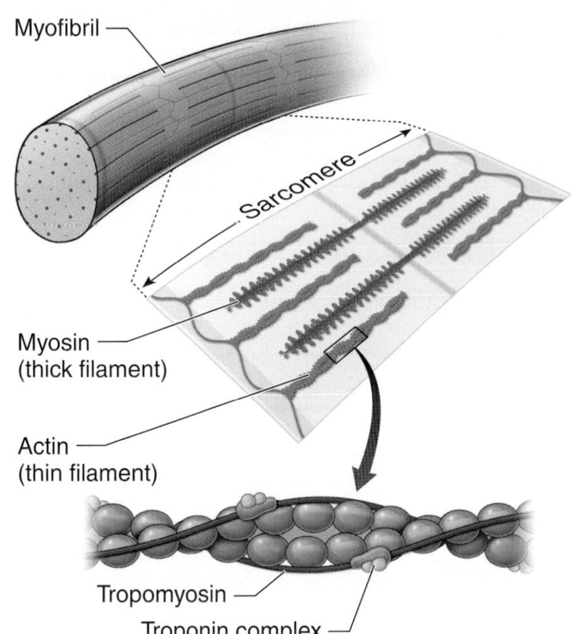

FIGURE 1-2 Troponin and tropomyosin action during a muscle contraction.

At the end of the contraction (the neural activity and action potentials cease), the SR actively accumulates Ca^{2+} and muscle relaxation occurs. The return of Ca^{2+} to the SR involves active transport, requiring the degradation of adenosine triphosphate (ATP) to adenosine diphosphate (ADP)*.[40] Because SR function is closely associated with both contraction and relaxation, changes in its ability to release or sequester Ca^{2+} markedly affect both the time course and magnitude of force output by the muscle fiber.[41]

CLINICAL PEARL

The SR forms a network around the myofibrils, storing and providing the Ca^{2+} that is required for muscle contraction.

On the basis of their contractile properties, two major types of muscle fiber have been recognized within skeletal muscle: type I (slow-twitch fibers), and type II (fast-twitch fibers) (Table 1-3).[42] Slow-twitch fibers are richly endowed with mitochondria and have a high capacity for oxygen uptake. They are, therefore, suitable for activities of long duration or endurance (aerobic), including the maintenance of posture. In contrast, fast-twitch fibers are suited to quick, explosive actions (anaerobic), including such activities as sprinting. A number of muscle subtypes have been recognized based on their qualities and aerobic to anaerobic (see Chapter 15) capabilities.

- Type A: possess good aerobic and anaerobic characteristics
- Type B: possess fair aerobic and poor anaerobic characteristics
- Type AB: possess aerobic and anaerobic characteristics somewhere between types A and B
- Type C: somewhat rare in humans

Based on the above, six fiber types can be distinguished: I, IC, IIA, IIB, IIAB, and IIC.[43] The type II (fast-twitch) fibers are separated based on mitochondria content into those that have a high complement of mitochondria (type IIA) and those that are mitochondria poor (type IIB). Type IIC fibers exhibit structural features of both red and white fibers and thus have fast contraction times and good fatigue resistance. Within this list, there appears to be a consistent order of recruitment based on fiber size: type I fibers first, followed by IC, IIC, IIA, IIAB, and, finally, IIB fibers.[43] The smaller type I fibers are the easiest to stimulate as they have the smaller motor units.

CLINICAL PEARL

In fast-twitch fibers, the SR embraces every individual myofibril. In slow-twitch fibers, it may contain multiple myofibrils.[44]

Theory dictates that a muscle with a large percentage of the total cross-sectional area occupied by slow-twitch type I fibers should be more fatigue resistant than one in which the fast-twitch type II fibers predominate.

Different activities place differing demands on a muscle (Table 1-4).[44] In humans, most limb muscles contain a relatively equal distribution of each muscle fiber type, whereas the back and trunk demonstrate a predominance of slow-twitch fibers. Although it would seem possible that physical training may cause fibers to convert from slow twitch to fast twitch or the reverse, this has not been shown to be the case.[45] However, fiber conversion from type IIB to type IIAB and IIA, and vice versa, has been found to occur with training.[46]

The effectiveness of a muscle to produce movement depends on a number of factors. These include the location and orientation of the muscle attachment relative to the joint, the limitations or laxity present in the musculotendinous unit, the type of contraction, the point of application, and the actions of other muscles that cross the joint.[1]

Muscles serve a variety of roles depending on the required movement:

- ***Prime agonist***. A muscle that is directly responsible for producing movement.
- ***Synergist (supporter)***. Performs a cooperative muscle function in relation to the agonist. Synergists can function as stabilizers or neutralizers.
  - ***Stabilizers (fixators)***. Muscles that contract statically to steady or support some part of the body against the pull of

*The most readily available energy for skeletal muscle cells is stored in the form of ATP and phosphocreatine (PCr). Through the activity of the enzyme ATPase, ATP promptly releases energy when required by the cell to perform any type of work, whether it is electrical, chemical, or mechanical.

TABLE 1-3 Comparison of Muscle Fiber Types				
Characteristics	**Type I**	**Type II A**	**Type II AB**	**Type II B**
Size (diameter)	Small	Intermediate	Large	Very large
Resistance to fatigue	High	Fairly high	Intermediate	Low
Glycogen content	Low	Intermediate	High	High
Twitch rate	Slow	Fast	Fast	Fast
Myosin ATPase content	Low	High	High	High
Major storage fuel	Triglycerides	Creatine phosphate glycogen	Creatine phosphate glycogen	Creatine phosphate glycogen

ATP, adenosine triphosphate.

the contracting muscles, against the pull of gravity, or against the effect of momentum and recoil in certain vigorous movements.

- ***Neutralizers.*** Muscles that act to prevent an undesired action of one of the movers.

- ***Antagonist.*** A muscle that has an effect opposite to that of the agonist.

CLINICAL PEARL

Following the stimulation of a muscle, a brief period elapses before the muscle begins to develop tension. This period is referred to as the *electromechanical delay* (EMD). The length of the EMD varies considerably among muscles. Fast-twitch fibers have shorter periods of EMD when compared with slow-twitch fibers.[47] It has been suggested that injury increases the EMD and, therefore, increases the susceptibility to injury.[48] One of the purposes of neuromuscular reeducation (see Chapter 14) is to return the EMD to a normal level.[49]

As previously mentioned, depending on the type of muscular contraction, the length of a muscle can remain the same (isometric), shorten (concentric), or "lengthen" (eccentric). The rate of muscle length change substantially affects the force that a muscle can develop during contraction.

- *Concentric contractions.* As the speed of a concentric contraction increases, the force it is capable of producing decreases.[50,51] The slower speed of contraction is thought to produce greater forces than can be produced by increasing the number of cross-bridges formed. This relationship can be viewed as a continuum, with the optimum velocity for the muscle somewhere between the slowest and fastest rates. At very slow speeds, the force that a muscle can resist or overcome rises rapidly up to 50% greater than the maximum isometric contraction.[50,51]

- *Eccentric contractions.* The following changes in force production occur during an eccentric contraction:

TABLE 1-4 Functional Division of Muscle Groups	
Movement Group	**Stabilization Group**
Primarily type IIa	Primarily type I
Prone to adaptive shortening	Prone to develop weakness
Prone to develop hypertonicity	Prone to muscle inhibition
Dominate in fatigue and new movement situations	Fatigue easily
Generally cross two joints	Primarily cross one joint
Examples	*Examples*
Gastrocnemius/Soleus	Peronei
Tibialis posterior	Tibialis anterior
Short hip adductors	Vastus medialis and lateralis
Hamstrings	Gluteus maximus, medius, and minimus
Rectus femoris	Serratus anterior
Tensor fascia lata	Rhomboids
Erector spinae	Lower portion of trapezius
Quadratus lumborum	Short/deep cervical flexors
Pectoralis major	Upper limb extensors
Upper portion of trapezius	Rectus abdominis
Levator scapulae	
Sternocleidomastoid	
Scalenes	
Upper limb flexors	

Data from Jull GA, Janda V: Muscle and motor control in low back pain. In: Twomey LT, Taylor JR, eds. *Physical Therapy of the Low Back: Clinics in Physical Therapy.* New York, NY: Churchill Livingstone, 1987:258.

- Rapid eccentric contractions generate more force than do slow ones (slower eccentric contractions).
- During slow eccentric muscle actions, the work produced approximates that of an isometric contraction.[50,51]

CLINICAL PEARL

The number of cross-bridges that can be formed is dependent on the extent of the overlap between the actin and myosin filaments.[52] Thus, the force a muscle is capable of exerting depends on its length. For each muscle cell, there is an optimum length, or range of lengths, at which the contractile force is strongest. At the optimum length of the muscle, there is near-optimal overlap of actin and myosin, allowing for the generation of maximum tension at this length.

- If the muscle is in a relatively shortened position, the overlap of actin and myosin reduces the number of sites available for cross-bridge formation. *Active insufficiency* of a muscle occurs when the agonist muscle is incapable of shortening to the extent required to simultaneously produce full range of motion at all of the joints it crosses.[1,53–55] For example, the finger flexors cannot produce a tight fist when the wrist is fully flexed, as they can when it is in neutral position.
- If the muscle producing the force is in a lengthened position compared with its optimum length, the actin filaments are pulled away from the myosin heads such that they cannot create as many cross-bridges.[56] *Passive insufficiency* of a muscle occurs when the muscle cannot lengthen to the extent required for full range of motion in the opposite direction.[1,53–55] For example, a larger range of hyperextension is possible at the wrist when the fingers are not fully extended.

The force and speed of a muscle contraction are based on the requirement of an activity and are dependent on the ability of the central nervous system to control the recruitment of motor units.[1] The motor units of slow-twitch fibers generally have lower thresholds and are relatively easier to activate than those of the fast-twitch motor units. Consequently, the slow-twitch fibers are the first to be recruited, even when the resulting limb movement is rapid.[57]

As the force requirement, speed requirement, or duration of an activity increases, motor units with higher thresholds are recruited.[58]

CLINICAL PEARL

The term *temporal summation* refers to the summation of individual contractile units. The summation can increase the muscular force by increasing the muscle activation frequency.[59]

Although each muscle contains the contractile machinery to produce the forces for movement, it is the tendon that transmits these forces to the bones in order to achieve movement or stability of the body in space.[8] The angle of insertion the tendon makes with a bone determines the line of pull, whereas the tension generated by a muscle is a function of its angle of insertion. A muscle generates the greatest amount of torque when its line of pull is oriented at a 90-degree angle to the bone, and it is attached anatomically as far from the joint center as possible.[1]

Just as there are optimal speeds of length change, and optimal muscle lengths, there are optimal insertion angles for each of the muscles. The angle of insertion of a muscle, and therefore its line of pull, can change during dynamic movements.[56] The *angle of pennation* is the angle created between the fiber direction and the line of pull. When the fibers of a muscle lie parallel to the long axis of the muscle, there is no angle of pennation. The number of fibers within a fixed volume of muscle increases with the angle of pennation.[56] Although maximum tension can be improved with pennation, the range of shortening of the muscle is reduced. Muscle fibers can contract to about 60% of their resting length. Since the muscle fibers in pennate muscles are shorter than the non-pennate equivalent, the amount of contraction is similarly reduced. Muscles that need to have large changes in length without the need for very high tension, such as the sartorius muscle, do not have pennate muscle fibers.[56] In contrast, pennate muscle fibers are found in those muscles in which the emphasis is on a high capacity for tension generation rather than range of motion (e.g., gluteus maximus).

CLINICAL PEARL

Skeletal muscle blood flow increases 20-fold during muscle contractions.[60] The muscle blood flow generally increases in proportion to the metabolic demands of the tissue, a relationship reflected by positive correlations between muscle blood flow and exercise. As body temperature elevates, the speeds of nerve and muscle functions increase, resulting in a higher value of maximum isometric tension and a higher maximum velocity of shortening possible with fewer motor units at any given load.[61] Muscle function is most efficient at 38.5°C (101°F).[62]

RESPIRATORY MUSCLES

Although the respiratory muscles share some mechanical similarities with skeletal muscles, they are distinct from other skeletal muscles in several aspects as follows[63,64]:

- Whereas skeletal muscles of the limbs overcome inertial loads, the respiratory muscles overcome primarily elastic and resistive loads.
- The respiratory muscles are under both voluntary and involuntary control.
- The respiratory muscles are similar to the heart muscles, in that they have to contract rhythmically and generate the required forces for ventilation throughout the entire life span of the individual. The respiratory muscles, however, do not contain pacemaker cells and are under the control of mechanical and chemical stimuli, requiring neural input from higher centers to initiate and coordinate contraction.

- The resting length of the respiratory muscles is a relationship between the inward recoil forces of the lung and the outward recoil forces of the chest wall. Changes in the balance of recoil forces will result in changes in the resting length of the respiratory muscles. Thus, simple and everyday life occurrences such as changes in posture may alter the operational length and the contractile strength of the respiratory muscles.[65] If uncompensated, these length changes can lead to decreases in the output of the muscles, and hence, a reduction in the ability to generate volume changes.[65] The skeletal muscles of the limbs, on the other hand, are not constrained to operate at a particular resting length.

CLINICAL PEARL

The primary respiratory muscles of the body include the diaphragm; the internal, external, and transverse intercostals; the levator costae; and the serratus posterior inferior and superior.

JOINTS

Arthrology is the study of the classification, structure, and function of joints. A joint represents the junction between two or more bones. Joints are regions where bones are capped and surrounded by CTs that hold the bones together and determine the type and degree of movement between them.[66] An understanding of the anatomy and biomechanics of the various joints is required to be able to assess and treat a patient thoroughly. When classified according to movement potential, joints may be classified as *synarthrosis or diarthrosis (synovial).*

Synarthrosis

There are three major types of synarthroses, based on the type of tissue uniting the bone surfaces[66]:

- Fibrous joints, which are joined by dense fibrous CT. Three types exist:
  - Suture (e.g., suture of the skull).
  - Gomphosis (e.g., tooth and mandible or maxilla articulation).
  - Syndesmosis (e.g., tibiofibular or radioulnar joints).
- Cartilaginous joints, originally referred to as amphiarthrosis joints, are stable joints that allow for minimal or little movement. These joints exist in humans in one of two ways: synchondrosis (e.g., manubriosternal joints) and symphysis (e.g., symphysis pubis)

Diarthrosis

This type of joint generally unites long bones and permits free bone movement and great mobility. These joints are characterized by a fibroelastic joint capsule, which is filled with a lubricating substance called *synovial fluid*. Consequently these joints are often referred to as synovial joints (see later). Examples include but are not limited to the hip, knee and shoulder, and elbow joints. Synovial joints are further classified based on complexity:

- Simple: a single pair of articular surfaces one male, or convex, surface and one female, or concave, surface.
- Compound: a single joint capsule containing more than a single pair of mating articulating surfaces.
- Complex: contain an intra-articular inclusion within the joint class such as a meniscus or disk that increases the number of joint surfaces.

Synovial joints have five distinguishing characteristics: joint cavity, articular cartilage, synovial fluid, synovial membrane, and a fibrous capsule. All synovial joints of the body are provided with an array of corpuscular (mechanoreceptors) and noncorpuscular (nociceptors) receptor endings imbedded in articular, muscular, and cutaneous structures with varying characteristic behaviors and distributions depending on the articular tissue (see Chapter 3). Synovial joints can be broadly classified according to structure or analogy (Fig. 1-3) into the following categories[67]:

- Spheroid. As the name suggests, a spheroid joint is a freely moving joint in which a sphere on the head of one bone fits into a rounded cavity in the other bone. Spheroid (ball and socket) joints allow motions in three planes (see later). Examples of a spheroid joint surface include the heads of the femur and humerus.
- Trochoid. The trochoid joint is characterized by a pivot-like process turning within a ring, or a ring on a pivot, the ring being formed partly of bone, partly of ligament. Trochoid joints permit only rotation. Examples of a trochoid joint include the humeroradial joint and the atlantoaxial joint.
- Condyloid. This type of joint is characterized by an ovoid articular surface, or condyle. One bone may articulate with another by one surface or by two, but never more than two. If two distinct surfaces are present, the joint is called condylar, or bicondylar. The elliptical cavity of the joint is designed in such a manner as to permit the motions of flexion, extension, adduction, abduction, and circumduction, but no axial rotation. The wrist-joint is an example of this form of articulation.
- Ginglymoid. A ginglymoid joint is a hinge joint. It is characterized by a spool-like surface and a concave surface. An example of a ginglymoid joint is the humeroulnar joint.
- Ellipsoid. Ellipsoid joints are similar to spheroid joints in that they allow the same type of movement albeit to a lesser magnitude. The ellipsoid joint allows movement in two planes (flexion, extension; abduction, adduction) and is biaxial. Examples of this joint can be found at the radiocarpal articulation at the wrist and the metacarpophalangeal articulation with the phalanges.
- Planar. As its name suggests, a planar joint is characterized by flat surfaces that slide over each other. Movement at this type of joint does not occur about an axis and is termed nonaxial. Examples of a planar joint include the intermetatarsal joints and some intercarpal joints.

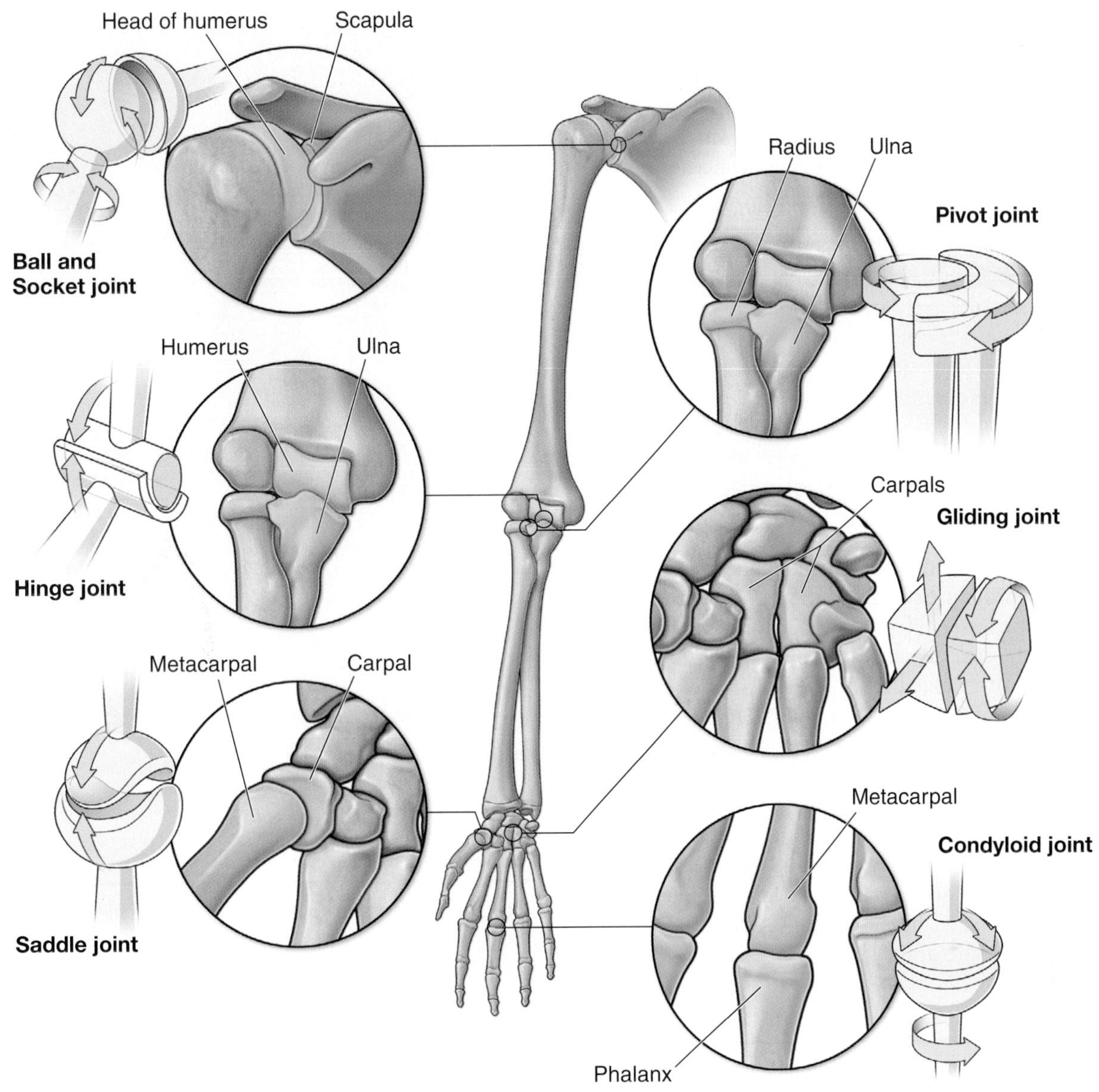

FIGURE 1-3 Types of diarthrotic or synovial joints.

In reality, no joint surface is planar or resembles a true geometric form. Instead, joint surfaces are either convex in all directions, or concave in all directions; that is they resemble either the outer or inner surface of a piece of eggshell.[68] Because the curve of an eggshell varies from point to point, these articular surfaces are called *ovoid*. The other major type of articular surface is the *sellar* joint.[68] Sellar joints are characterized by a convex surface in one cross-sectional plane, and a concave surface in the plane perpendicular to it (Fig. 1-3). Examples of a sellar joint include the interphalangeal joints, the carpometacarpal joint of the thumb, the humeroulnar joint, and the calcaneocuboid joints.

Physiological Range of Motion

The amount of available physiological joint motion is based on a number of factors, including

- the integrity of the joint surfaces and the amount of joint motion;
- the mobility and pliability of the soft tissues that surround a joint;
- the degree of soft-tissue approximation that occurs;
- the amount of scarring that is present[69]—interstitial scarring or fibrosis can occur in and around the joint capsules, within the muscles, and within the ligaments as a result of previous trauma;
- age—joint motion tends to decrease with increasing age;
- gender—in general, females have more joint motion than males.

Synovial Fluid

Articular cartilage is subject to a great variation of loading conditions, and joint lubrication through synovial fluid is necessary to minimize frictional resistance between the weight-bearing surfaces. Fortunately, synovial joints are blessed with a very superior lubricating system, which permits a remarkably frictionless interaction at the joint surfaces. A lubricated cartilaginous interface has a coefficient of friction* of 0.002.[70] By way of comparison, ice on ice has a higher coefficient of friction (0.03).[70] The composition of synovial fluid is nearly the same as blood plasma, but with a decreased total protein content and a higher concentration of hyaluronan.[71]

CLINICAL PEARL

Hyaluronan is a critical constituent component of normal synovial fluid and an important contributor to joint homeostasis.[72] Hyaluronan imparts anti-inflammatory and antinociceptive properties to normal synovial fluid and contributes to joint lubrication. It also is responsible for the viscoelastic properties of synovial fluid,[71] and contributes to the lubrication of articular cartilage surfaces.

Indeed, synovial fluid is essentially a dialysate of plasma to which hyaluronan has been added.[73] Hyaluronan is a GAG that is continually synthesized and released into synovial fluid by specialized synoviocytes.[73,74] The mechanical properties of synovial fluid permit it to act as both a cushion and a lubricant to the joint. Diseases such as osteoarthritis, affect the thixotropic properties (thixotropy is the property of various gels becoming fluid when disturbed, as by shaking) of synovial fluid, resulting in reduced lubrication and subsequent wear of the articular cartilage and joint surfaces.[75,76] It is well established that damaged articular cartilage in adults has a very limited potential for healing (see Chapter 2), because it possesses neither a blood supply nor lymphatic drainage.[77]

Bursae

Closely associated with some synovial joints are flattened, saclike structures called *bursae* that are lined with a synovial membrane and filled with synovial fluid. The bursa produces small amounts of fluid, allowing for smooth and almost frictionless motion between contiguous muscles, tendons, bones, ligaments, and skin.[78–80] A tendon sheath is a modified bursa. A bursa can be a source of pain if it becomes inflamed or infected.

KINESIOLOGY

When describing movements, it is necessary to have a starting position as the reference position. This starting position is referred to as the *anatomic reference position*. The anatomic reference position for the human body is described as the erect standing position with the feet just slightly separated and the arms hanging by the side, the elbows straight, and the palms of the hand facing forward (Fig. 1-4).

*Coefficient of friction is a ratio of the force needed to make a body glide across a surface compared with the weight or force holding the two surfaces in contact.

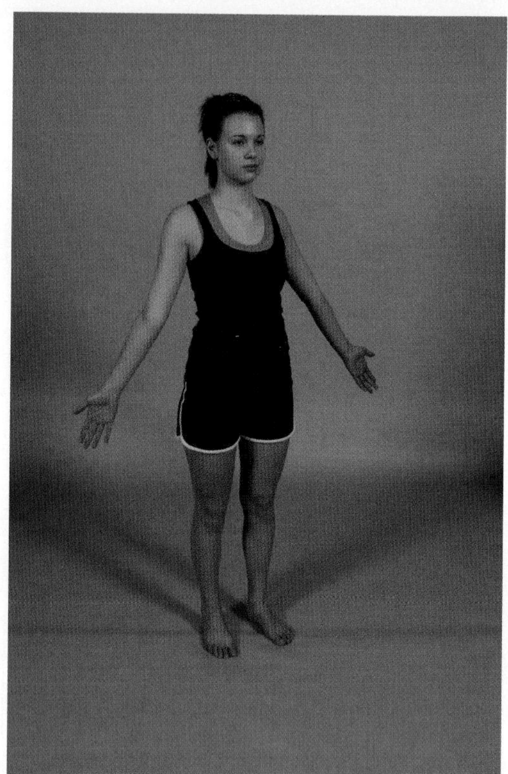

FIGURE 1-4 The anatomical position.

Directional Terms

Directional terms are used to describe the relationship of body parts or the location of an external object with respect to the body.[81] The following are commonly used directional terms:

- ***Superior or cranial.*** Closer to the head.
- ***Inferior or caudal.*** Closer to the feet.
- ***Anterior or ventral.*** Toward the front of the body.
- ***Posterior or dorsal.*** Toward the back of the body.
- ***Medial.*** Toward the midline of the body.
- ***Lateral.*** Away from the midline of the body.
- ***Proximal.*** Closer to the trunk.
- ***Distal.*** Away from the trunk.
- ***Superficial.*** Toward the surface of the body.
- ***Deep.*** Away from the surface of the body in the direction of the inside of the body.

MOVEMENTS OF THE BODY SEGMENTS

In general, there are two types of motions: translation, which occurs in either a straight or curved line, and rotation, which involves a circular motion around a pivot point. Movements of the body segments occur in three dimensions along imaginary *planes* and around various *axes* of the body.

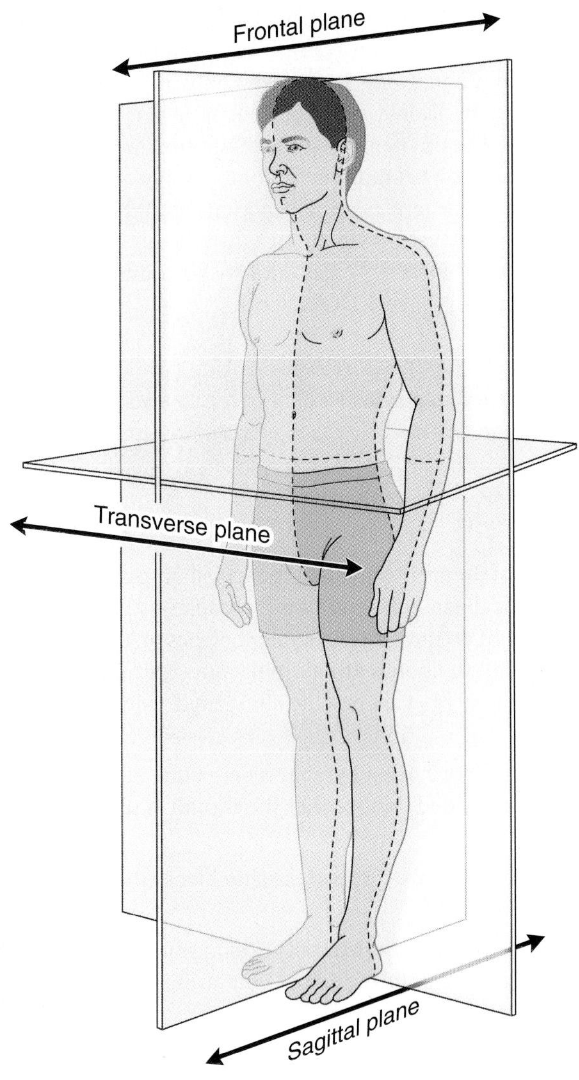

FIGURE 1-5 Planes of the body.

Planes of the Body

There are three traditional planes of the body corresponding to the three dimensions of space: sagittal, frontal, and transverse[81] (Fig. 1-5).

- ***Sagittal.*** The sagittal plane, also known as the *anterior-posterior or median plane,* divides the body vertically into left and right halves of equal size.
- ***Frontal.*** The frontal plane, also known as the *lateral* or *coronal plane,* divides the body equally into front and back halves.
- ***Transverse.*** The transverse plane, also known as the *horizontal plane,* divides the body equally into top and bottom halves.

Because each of these planes bisects the body, it follows that each plane must pass through the center of gravity.* If the movement described occurs in a plane that passes through the center of gravity, that movement is deemed to have occurred in a *cardinal* plane. An *arc of motion* represents the total number of degrees traced between the two extreme positions of movement in a specific plane of motion.[82] If a joint has more than one plane of motion, each type of motion is referred to as a *unit of motion.* For example, the wrist has two units of motion: flexion–extension (anterior–posterior plane) and ulnar–radial deviation (lateral plane).[82]

Few movements involved with functional activities occur in the cardinal planes. Instead, most movements occur in an infinite number of vertical and horizontal planes parallel to the cardinal planes (see discussion that follows).

Axes of the Body

Three reference axes are used to describe human motion: frontal, sagittal, and longitudinal (Fig. 1-6). The axis around which the movement takes place is always perpendicular to the plane in which it occurs.

- ***Frontal.*** The frontal axis, also known as the *transverse axis,* is perpendicular to the sagittal plane.
- ***Sagittal.*** The sagittal axis is perpendicular to the frontal plane.

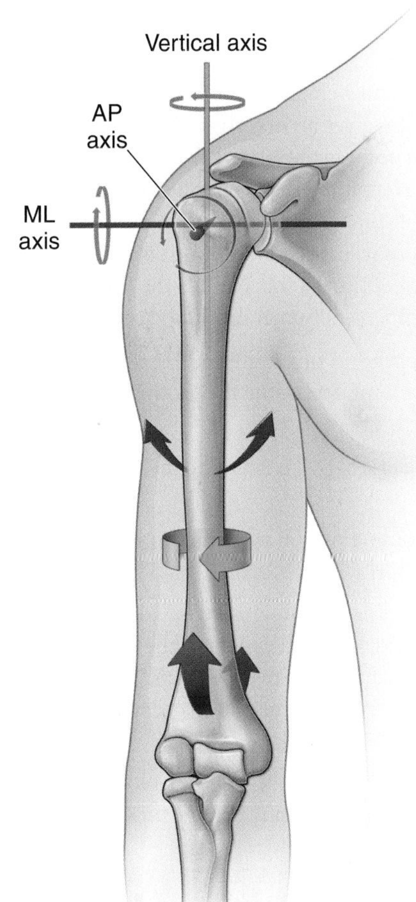

FIGURE 1-6 Axes of the body

*The center of gravity may be defined as the point at which the three planes of the body intersect each other. The line of gravity is defined as the vertical line at which the two vertical planes intersect each other.

- ***Longitudinal.*** The longitudinal axis, also known as the *vertical axis,* is perpendicular to the transverse plane.

Most movements occur *in* planes and *around* axes that are somewhere in between the traditional planes and axes. However, nominal identification of every plane and axis of movement is impractical. The structure of the joint determines the possible axes of motion that are available. For example, a hinge joint has only a frontal–horizontal axis. Condyloid (ovoid) joints have both a frontal–horizontal and a sagittal–horizontal axis. Ball-and-socket joints have frontal, sagittal–horizontal, and vertical axes. The axis of rotation remains stationary only if the convex member of a joint is a perfect sphere and articulates with a perfect reciprocally shaped concave member. The planes and axes for the more common planar movements (Fig. 1-7) are as follows:

- Flexion, extension, hyperextension, dorsiflexion, and plantar flexion occur in the sagittal plane around a frontal–horizontal axis.
- Abduction and adduction, side flexion of the trunk, elevation and depression of the shoulder girdle, radial and ulnar deviation of the wrist, and eversion and inversion of the foot occur in the frontal plane around a sagittal–horizontal axis.
- Rotation of the head, neck, and trunk; internal rotation and external rotation of the arm or leg; horizontal adduction and abduction of the arm or thigh; and pronation and supination of the forearm occur in the transverse plane around the longitudinal axis.
- Arm circling and trunk circling are examples of *circumduction.* Circumduction involves an orderly sequence of circular movements that occur in the sagittal, frontal, and intermediate oblique planes, so that the segment as a whole incorporates a combination of flexion, extension, abduction, and adduction. Circumduction movements can occur at biaxial and triaxial joints. Examples of these joints include the tibiofemoral, radiohumeral, hip, glenohumeral, and the spinal joints.

Both the configuration of a joint and the line of pull of the muscle acting at a joint determine the motion that occurs at a joint:

- A muscle whose line of pull is lateral to the joint is a potential abductor.
- A muscle whose line of pull is medial to the joint is a potential adductor.
- A muscle whose line of pull is anterior to a joint has the potential to extend or flex the joint. At the knee, an anterior line of pull may cause the knee to extend, whereas at the elbow joint, an anterior line of pull may cause flexion of the elbow.
- A muscle whose line of pull is posterior to the joint has the potential to extend or flex a joint (refer to preceding example).

DEGREES OF FREEDOM

The number of independent modes of motion at a joint is called the *degrees of freedom (DOF).* A joint can have up to 3 degrees of angular freedom, corresponding to the three dimensions of space.[83] If a joint can swing in one direction or can only spin, it is said to have 1 DOF.[84–87] The proximal interphalangeal joint is an example of a joint with 1 DOF. If a joint can spin and swing in one way only *or* it can swing in two completely distinct ways, but not spin, it is said to have 2 DOF.[84–87] The tibiofemoral joint, temporomandibular joint, proximal and distal radioulnar joints, subtalar joint, and talocalcaneal joint are examples of joints with 2 DOF. If the bone can spin and also swing in two distinct directions then it is said to have 3 DOF.[84–87] Ball-and-socket joints such as the shoulder and hip have 3 DOF.

CLINICAL PEARL

Joint motion that occurs only in one plane is designated as one degree of freedom; in two planes, two DOF; and in three planes, three DOF.

Because of the arrangement of the articulating surfaces—the surrounding ligaments and joint capsules—most motions around a joint do not occur in straight planes or along straight lines. Instead, the bones at any joint move through space in curved paths. This can best be illustrated using *Codman's paradox.*

1. Stand with your arms by your side, palms facing inward, thumbs extended. Notice that the thumb is pointing forward.
2. Flex one arm to 90 degrees at the shoulder so that the thumb is pointing up.
3. From this position, horizontally extend your arm so that the thumb remains pointing up but your arm is in a position of 90 degrees of glenohumeral abduction.
4. From this position, without rotating your arm, return the arm to your side and note that your thumb is now pointing away from your thigh.

Referring to the start position, and using the thumb as the reference, it can be seen that the arm has undergone an external rotation of 90 degrees. But where and when did the rotation take place? Undoubtedly, it occurred during the three separate, straight-plane motions or *swings* that etched a triangle in space. What you have just witnessed is an example of a conjunct rotation—a rotation that occurs as a result of joint surface shapes—and the effect of inert tissues rather than contractile tissues. Conjunct rotations can only occur in joints that can rotate internally or externally. Although not always apparent, most joints can so rotate. Consider the motions of elbow flexion and extension. While fully flexing and extending your elbow a number of times, watch the pisiform bone and forearm. If you watch carefully you should notice that the pisiform and the forearm move in a direction of supination during flexion, and pronation during extension of the elbow. The pronation and supination motions are examples of conjunct rotations.

Most habitual movements, or those movements that occur most frequently at a joint, involve a conjunct rotation. However, the conjunct rotations are not always under volitional control. In fact, the conjunct rotation is only under volitional control in joints with 3 DOF (glenohumeral and hip joints). In joints with fewer than 3 DOF (hinge

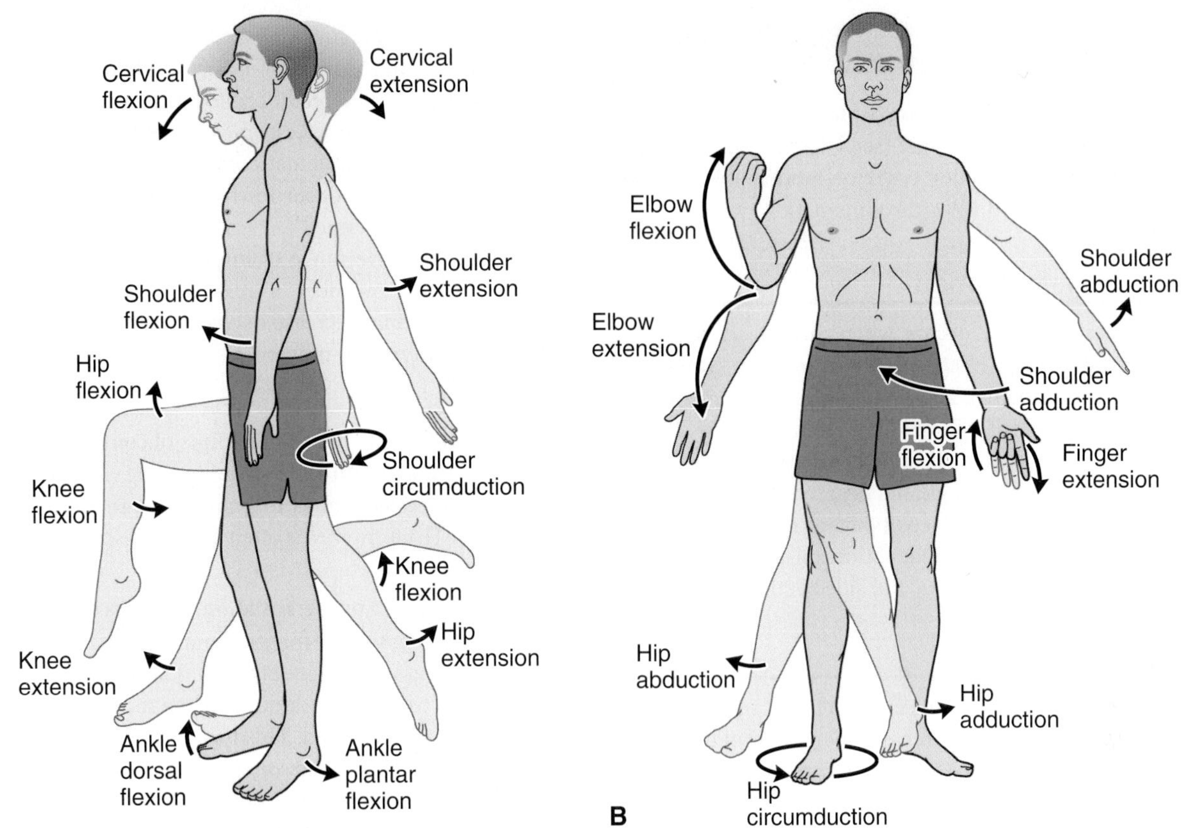

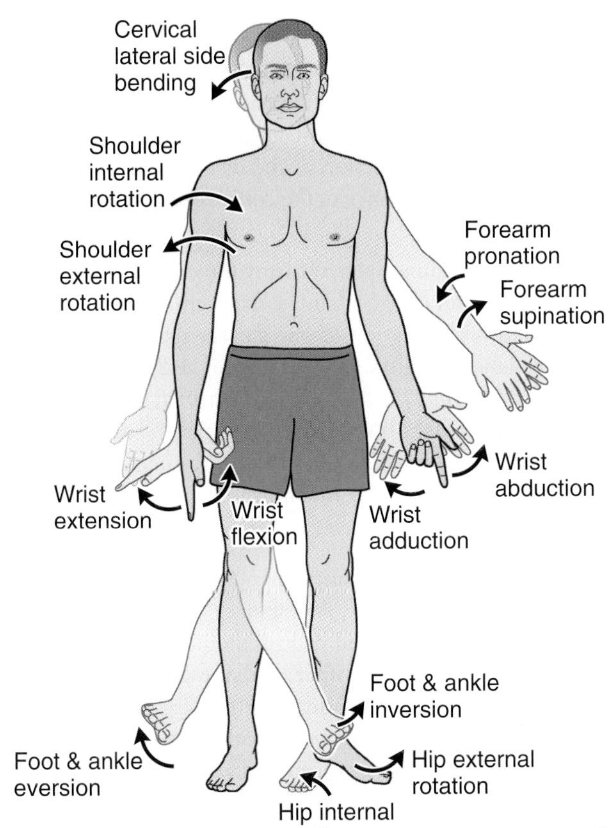

FIGURE 1-7 Movements of the body.

joints, such as the tibiofemoral and ulnohumeral joints), the conjunct rotation occurs as part of the movement but is not under voluntary control. The implications become important when attempting to restore motion at these joints: the mobilizing techniques must take into consideration both the relative shapes of the articulating surfaces as well as the conjunct rotation that is associated with a particular motion (see Chapter 10).

JOINT KINEMATICS

Kinematics is the study of motion. Kinetics is the term applied to the forces acting on the body (see Chapter 2). In studying joint kinematics, two major types of motion are involved: (1) osteokinematic and (2) arthrokinematic.

Osteokinematic Motion

Osteokinematic motion occurs when any object forms the radius of an imaginary circle about a fixed point. The axis of rotation for osteokinematic motions is oriented perpendicular to the plane in which the rotation occurs.[81] The distance traveled by the motion may be a small arc or a complete circle and is measured as an angle, in degrees. All human body segment motions involve osteokinematic motions. Examples of osteokinematic motion include abduction or adduction of the arm, flexion of the hip or knee, and side bending of the trunk.

Moment Arm

To understand the concept of a moment arm, an understanding of the anatomy and movement (kinematics) of the joint of interest is necessary. Although muscles produce linear forces, motions at joints are all rotary. For example, some joints can be considered to rotate about a fixed point. A good example of such a joint is the elbow. At the elbow joint, where the humerus and ulna articulate, the resulting rotation occurs primarily about a fixed point, referred to as the center of rotation (COR). In the case of the elbow joint, this COR is relatively constant throughout the joint range of motion. However, in other joints (for example the knee) the COR moves in space as the knee joint flexes and extends because the articulating surfaces are not perfect circles. In the case of the knee, it is not appropriate to discuss a single COR—rather we must speak of a COR corresponding to a particular joint angle, or, using the terminology of joint kinematics, we must speak of the instant center of rotation (ICR), that is, the COR at any "instant" in time or space. Thus, the moment arm is defined as the perpendicular distance from the line of force application to the axis of rotation.

Arthrokinematic Motion

The motions occurring at the joint surfaces are termed *arthrokinematic* movements. At each synovial articulation, the articulating surface of each bone moves relative to the shape of the other articulating surface. A normal joint has an available range of active, or physiologic, motion, which is limited by a physiologic barrier as tension develops within the surrounding tissues, such as the joint capsule, ligaments, and CT. At the physiologic barrier, there is an additional amount of passive, or accessory, range of motion. The small motion, which is available at the joint surfaces, is referred to as *accessory* motion, or *joint-play* motion. This motion can only occur when resistance to active motion is applied, or when the patient's muscles are completely relaxed.[88]

Beyond the available passive range of motion, the anatomic barrier is found. This barrier cannot be exceeded without disruption to the integrity of the joint.

Both the physiologic (osteokinematic) and accessory (arthrokinematic) motions occur simultaneously during movement and are directly proportional to each other, with a small increment of accessory motion resulting in a larger increment of osteokinematic motion. Normal arthrokinematic motions must occur for full-range physiologic motion to take place. Mennell[89,90] introduced the concept that full, painless, active range of motion is not possible without these motions and that a restriction of arthrokinematic motion results in a decrease in osteokinematic motion. Three fundamental types of movement exist between joint surfaces (Fig. 1-8):[91]

- ***Roll.*** A roll occurs when the points of contact on each joint surface are constantly changing (see Fig. 1-8). This type of movement is analogous to a tire on a car as the car rolls forward. The term *rock* is often used to describe small rolling motions.
- ***Slide.*** A slide is a pure translation. It occurs if only one point on the moving surface makes contact with varying points on the opposing surface (see Fig. 1-8). This type of movement is analogous to a car tire skidding when the brakes are applied suddenly on a wet road. This type of motion also is referred to as *translatory* or *accessory* motion. Although the roll of a joint always occurs in the same direction as the swing of a bone, the direction of the slide is determined by the shape of the articulating surface (Fig. 1-9). This rule is often referred to as the *concave–convex rule*: If the joint surface is convex relative to the other surface, the slide occurs in the opposite direction to the osteokinematic motion (see Fig. 1-9). If, on the other hand, the joint surface is concave, the slide occurs in the same direction as the osteokinematic motion. The clinical significance of the concave–convex rule is described in Chapter 10.
- ***Spin.*** A spin is defined as any movement in which the bone moves but the mechanical axis remains stationary. A spin involves a rotation of one surface on an opposing surface around a longitudinal axis (see Fig. 1-8). This type of motion is analogous to the pirouette performed in ballet. Spin motions in the body include internal and external rotation of the glenohumeral joint when the humerus is abducted to 90 degrees; and at the radial head during forearm pronation and supination.

Most anatomic joints demonstrate composite motions involving a roll, slide, and spin.

Osteokinematic and arthrokinematic motions are directly proportional to each other, and one cannot occur completely without the other. It therefore follows that if a joint is not functioning correctly, one or both of these motions may be at fault. When examining a patient with movement impairment, it is critical that the clinician determine whether the osteokinematic motion or the arthrokinematic motion is restricted so that the intervention can be made as specific as possible.

In the extremities, osteokinematic motion is controlled by the amount of flexibility of the surrounding soft tissues of the joint, where flexibility is defined as the amount of internal resistance to motion. In contrast, the arthrokinematic motion is controlled by the integrity of the joint surfaces and the supporting tissues of the joint. This characteristic can be noted

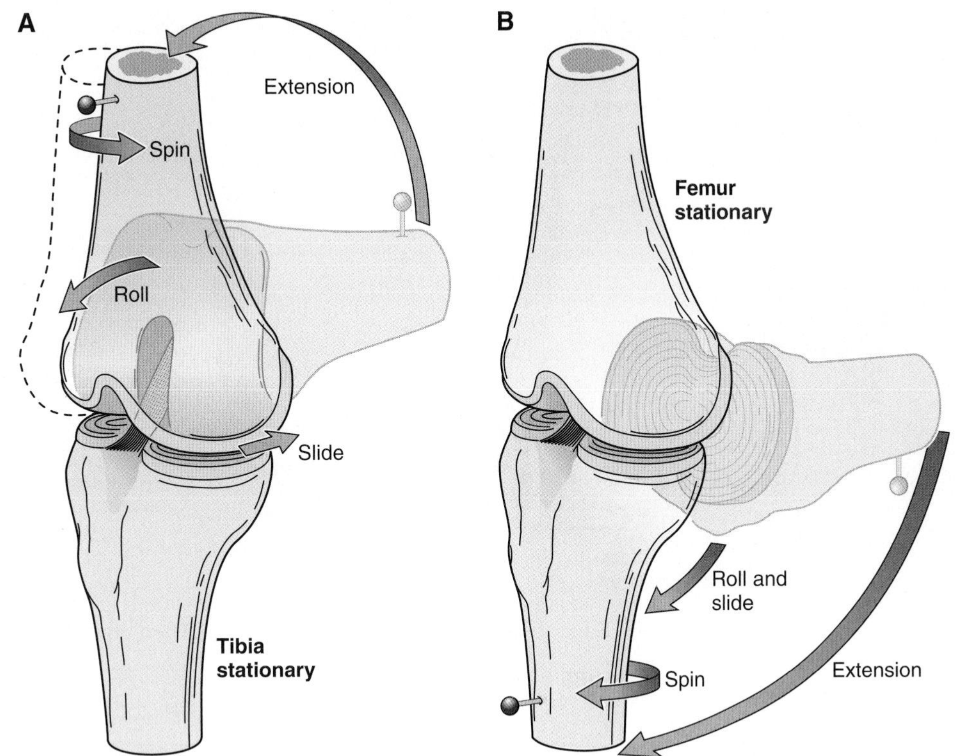

FIGURE 1-8 Arthrokinematics of motion.

clinically in a chronic rupture of the anterior cruciate ligament of the knee. Upon examination of that knee, the arthrokinematic motion (joint slide or glide) is found to be increased, illustrated by a positive Lachman's test, but the range of motion of the knee, its osteokinematic motion, is not affected (see Chapter 20).

In the spine, the osteokinematic motion is controlled by both the flexibility of the surrounding soft tissues *and* by the integrity of the joint surfaces and the supporting tissues of the joint. This characteristic can be noted clinically when examining the craniovertebral joint, where a restriction in the arthrokinematic motion (joint slide or glide) can be caused by either a joint restriction or an adaptively shortened suboccipital muscle (see Chapter 23).

The examination of these motions and their clinical implications are described in Chapter 4.

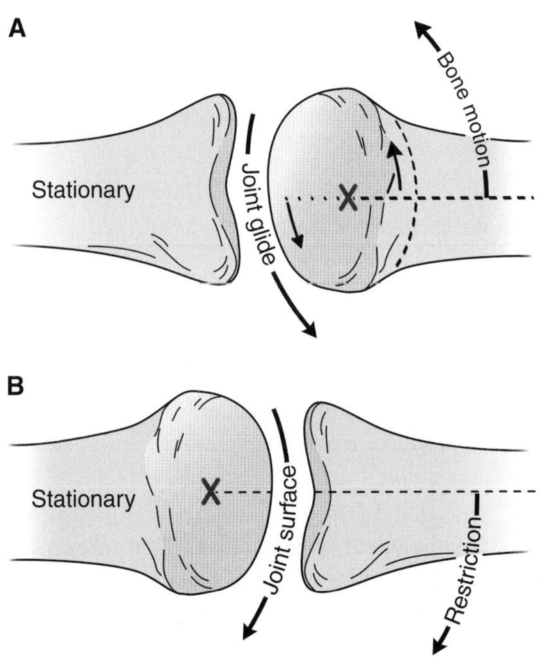

FIGURE 1-9 Gliding motions according to joint surfaces.

LEVERS

Biomechanical levers can be defined as rotations of a rigid surface about an axis. For simplicity sake, levers are usually described using a straight bar which is the lever, and the fulcrum, which is the point on which the bar is resting. The effort force attempts to cause movement of the load. That part of the lever between the fulcrum and the load is load arm. There are three types of levers:

- First-class: occurs when two forces are applied on either side of an axis and the fulcrum lies between the effort and the load (Fig. 1-10), like a seesaw. Examples in the human body include the contraction of the triceps at the elbow joint, or tipping of the head forwards and backwards.
- Second-class: occurs when the load (resistance) is applied between the fulcrum and the point where the effort is exerted (Fig. 1-10). This has the advantage of magnifying the effects of the effort so that it takes less force to move the resistance. Examples of 2nd class levers in everyday life include, the nutcracker, and the wheelbarrow—with the wheel acting as the fulcrum. Examples of second class levers in the human body include weight bearing plantarflexion

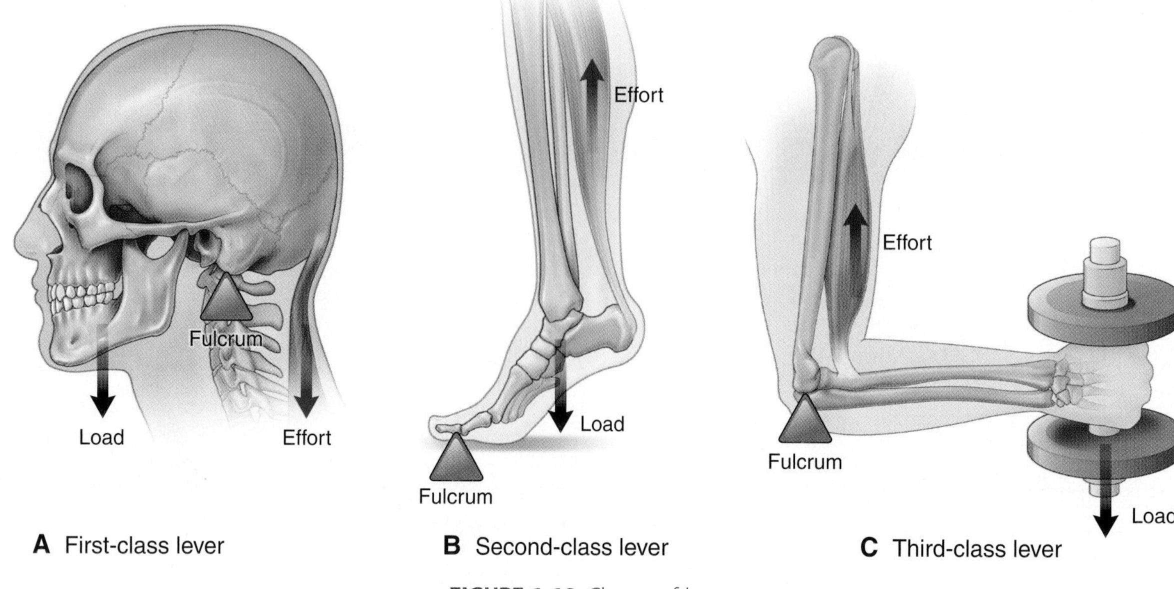

FIGURE 1-10 Classes of levers.

(rising up on the toes) (Fig. 1-10). Another would be an isolated contraction of the brachioradialis to flex the elbow, which could not occur without the other elbow flexors being paralyzed.

- Third class: occurs when the load is located at the end of the lever (Fig. 1-10) and the effort lies between the fulcrum and the load (resistance), like a drawbridge or a crane. The effort is exerted between the load and the fulcrum. The effort expended is greater than the load, but the load is moved a greater distance. Most movable joints in the human body function as third-class levers—flexion at the elbow.

When a machine puts out more force than is put in, the machine is said to have mechanical advantage (MA). The MA of the musculoskeletal lever is defined as the ratio of the internal moment arm to the external moment arm. Depending on the location of the axis of rotation, the first-class lever can have an MA equal to, less than, or greater than 1[83] Second-class levers always have an MA greater than 1. Third-class levers always have an MA less than 1. The majority of muscles throughout the musculoskeletal system function with an MA of much less than 1. Therefore, the muscles and underlying joints must 'pay the price' by generating and dispersing relative large forces, respectively, even for seemingly low-load activities.[83]

KINEMATIC CHAINS

When a body moves, it will do so in accordance with its kinematics, which in the human body takes place through arthrokinematic and osteokinematic movements. The expression *kinematic chain* is used in rehabilitation to describe the function or activity of an extremity or trunk in terms of a series of linked chains. A kinematic chain refers to a series of articulated segmented links, such as the connected pelvis, thigh, leg, and foot of the lower extremity.[83] According to kinematic chain theory, each of the joint segments of the body involved in a particular movement constitutes a link along the kinematic chain. Because each motion of a joint is often a function of other joint motions, the efficiency of an activity can be dependent on how well these chain-links work together.[92]

CLINICAL PEARL

The number of links within a particular kinematic chain varies, depending on the activity. In general, the longer kinematic chains are involved with the more strenuous activities.

Two types of kinematic chain systems are recognized: *closed kinematic chain* (CKC) systems, and the *open kinematic chain* (OKC) system (Table 1-5).[93]

Closed Kinematic Chain

A variety of definitions for a CKC activity have been proposed:

1. Palmitier[94] defined an activity as closed if both ends of the kinetic chain are connected to an immovable framework, thus preventing translation of either the proximal, or distal joint center, and creating a situation whereby movement at one joint produces a predictable movement at all other joints.
2. Gray[95] considered a closed-chain activity to involve fixation of the distal segment so that joint motion takes place in multiple planes, and the limb is supporting weight.
3. Dillman[96] described the characteristics of closed-chain activities to include relatively small joint movements, low joint accelerations, greater joint compressive forces, greater joint congruity, decreased shear, stimulation of joint

TABLE 1-5 Differential Features of OKC and CKC Exercises			
Exercise Mode	**Characteristics**	**Advantages**	**Disadvantages**
Open kinematic chain	1. Single muscle group 2. Single axis and plane 3. Emphasizes concentric contraction 4. Non–weight-bearing	1. Isolated recruitment 2. Simple movement pattern 3. Isolated recruitment 4. Minimal joint compression	1. Limited function 2. Limited function 3. Limited eccentrics 4. Less proprioception and joint stability with increased joint shear forces
Closed kinematic	1. Multiple muscle groups 2. Multiple axes and planes 3. Balance of concentric and eccentric contractions 4. Weight-bearing exercise	1. Functional recruitment 2. Functional movement patterns 3. Functional contractions 4. Increased proprioception and joint stability	1. Difficult to isolate 2. More complex 3. Loss of control of target joint 4. Compressive forces on articular surfaces

Data from Greenfield BH, Tovin BJ: The application of open and closed kinematic chain exercises in rehabilitation of the lower extremity. *J Back Musculoskel Rehabil* 2:38–51, 1992.

proprioception, and enhanced dynamic stabilization through muscle coactivation.[97]

4. Kibler[97] defines a closed-chain activity as a sequential combination of joint motions that have the following characteristics:
   a. The distal segment of the kinetic chain meets considerable resistance.
   b. The movement of the individual joints, and translation of their instant centers of rotation, occurs in a predictable manner that is secondary to the distribution of forces from each end of the chain.

Examples of closed kinematic chain exercises (CKCEs) involving the lower extremities include the squat and the leg press. The activities of walking, running, jumping, climbing, and rising from the floor all incorporate closed kinetic chain components. An example of a CKCE for the upper extremities is the push-up, or when using the arms to rise out of a chair.

CLINICAL PEARL

In most activities of daily living, the activation sequence of the links involves a closed chain whereby the activity is initiated from a firm base of support and transferred to a more mobile distal segment.

Open Kinematic Chain

It is generally accepted that the difference between OKC and CKC activities is determined by the movement of the end segment. The traditional definition for an open-chain activity included all activities that involved the end segment of an extremity moving freely through space, resulting in isolated movement of a joint.

Examples of an open-chain activity include lifting a drinking glass and kicking a soccer ball. Open kinematic chain exercises (OKCEs) involving the lower extremity include the seated knee extension and prone knee flexion. Upper extremity examples of OKCE include the biceps curl and the military press.

Many activities, such as swimming and cycling, traditionally viewed as OKC activities, include a load on the end segment; yet the end segment is not "fixed" and restricted from movement. This ambiguity of definitions for CKC and OKC activities has allowed some activities to be classified in opposing categories.[96] Thus, there has been a growing need for clarification of OKC and CKC terminology, especially when related to functional activities.

The work of Dillman and colleagues[96] and then Lephart and Henry[98] has attempted to address the confusion. Dillman and colleagues[96] proposed three classifications of activity because of the gray area between CKC and OKC activity. These classifications were based on the boundary condition, either moveable or fixed, and the presence or absence of a load on the end segment. An activity with a fixed boundary and no load does not exist, resulting in three classifications:

1. ***Moveable no load.*** These activities involve a moveable end with no load and closely resemble the extreme open-chain activity. An example of this type of activity is hitting a ball with a tennis racket.
2. ***Moveable external load.*** These activities involve a movable end with an external load and include a combination of open- and closed-chain actions, because they are characterized by cocontractions of the muscles around the joints. An example of this type of activity is the military press.
3. ***Fixed external load.*** These activities involve a fixed end with an external load, and closely resemble the extreme closed-chain activity. An example of this type of activity is the push-up.

Lephart and Henry suggested that a further definition could be made by analyzing the following characteristics of an activity:

- Direction of force.
- Magnitude of load.
- Muscle action.
- Joint motion.
- Neuromuscular function.

Under Lephart and Henry's classification, activities could be subdivided into four groups:

1. Activities that involve a fixed boundary with an external and axial load. An example of this type of activity is the use of a slide board.
2. Activities that involve a movable boundary with an external and axial load. An example of this type of activity is the bench press.
3. Activities that involve a movable boundary with an external and rotary load. An example of this type of activity is a resisted proprioceptive neuromuscular facilitation (PNF) motion pattern (see Chapter 10).
4. Activities that involve a moveable boundary with no load. An example of this type of activity is position training

Although both the Dillman and Lephart and Henry models appear to be describing the same concept, the Lephart and Henry model is distinct in that it incorporates diagonal or rotary components to the movements. These diagonal and rotary movements feature in the vast majority of functional activities.

CLOSE-PACKED AND OPEN-PACKED POSITIONS OF THE JOINT

Joint movements usually are accompanied by a relative compression (approximation) or distraction (separation) of the opposing joint surfaces. These relative compressions or distractions affect the level of *congruity* of the opposing surfaces. The position of maximum congruity of the opposing joint surfaces is termed the *close-packed* position of the joint. The position of least congruity is termed the *open-packed* position. Thus, movements toward the close-packed position of a joint involve an element of compression, whereas movements out of this position involve an element of distraction.

Close-Packed Position

The close-packed position of a joint is the joint position that results in:

- Maximal tautness of the major ligaments.
- Maximal surface congruity.
- Minimal joint volume.
- Maximal stability of the joint.

Once the close-packed position is achieved, no further motion in that direction is possible. This is the often-cited reason why most fractures and dislocations occur when an external force is applied to a joint that is in its close-packed position. In addition, many of the traumatic injuries of the upper extremities result from falling on a shoulder, elbow or wrist, which are in their close-packed position. This type of injury, a ***f***all ***o***n an ***o***utstretched ***h***and is often referred to as a FOOSH injury. The close-packed positions for the various joints are depicted in Table 1-6.

TABLE 1-6 Close-Packed Position of the Joints

Joint	Position
Zygapophyseal (spine)	Extension
Temporomandibular	Teeth clenched
Glenohumeral	Abduction and external rotation
Acromioclavicular	Arm abducted to 90 degrees
Sternoclavicular	Maximum shoulder elevation
Ulnohumeral	Extension
Radiohumeral	Elbow flexed 90 degrees; forearm supinated 5 degrees
Proximal radioulnar	5 degrees of supination
Distal radioulnar	5 degrees of supination
Radiocarpal (wrist)	Extension with radial deviation
Metacarpophalangeal	Full flexion
Carpometacarpal	Full opposition
Interphalangeal	Full extension
Hip	Full extension, internal rotation, and abduction
Tibiofemoral	Full extension and external rotation of tibia
Talocrural (ankle)	Maximum dorsiflexion
Subtalar	Supination
Midtarsal	Supination
Tarsometatarsal	Supination
Metatarsophalangeal	Full extension
Interphalangeal	Full extension

Open-Packed Position

In essence, any position of the joint, other than the close-packed position, could be considered as an open-packed position. The open-packed position, also referred to as the *loose-packed* position of a joint, is the joint position that results in:

- Slackening of the major ligaments of the joint.
- Minimal surface congruity.
- Minimal joint surface contact.
- Maximal joint volume.
- Minimal stability of the joint.

The open-packed position permits maximal distraction of the joint surfaces. Because the open-packed position causes

TABLE 1-7 Open-Packed (Resting) Position of the Joints	
Joint	**Position**
Zygapophyseal (spine)	Midway between flexion and extension
Temporomandibular	Mouth slightly open (freeway space)
Glenohumeral	55 degrees of abduction; 30 degrees of horizontal adduction
Acromioclavicular	Arm resting by side
Sternoclavicular	Arm resting by side
Ulnohumeral	70 degrees of flexion; 10 degrees of supination
Radiohumeral	Full extension; full supination
Proximal radioulnar	70 degrees of flexion; 35 degrees of supination
Distal radioulnar	10 degrees of supination
Radiocarpal (wrist)	Neutral with slight ulnar deviation
Carpometacarpal	Midway between abduction–adduction and flexion–extension
Metacarpophalangeal	Slight flexion
Interphalangeal	Slight flexion
Hip	30 degrees of flexion; 30 degrees of abduction; slight external rotation
Tibiofemoral	25 degrees of flexion
Talocrural (ankle)	10 degrees of plantar flexion; midway between maximum inversion and eversion
Subtalar	Midway between extremes of range of movement
Midtarsal	Midway between extremes of range of movement
Tarsometatarsal	Midway between extremes of range of movement
Metatarsophalangeal	Neutral
Interphalangeal	Slight flexion

the brunt of any external force to be borne by the joint capsule or surrounding ligaments, most capsular or ligamentous sprains occur when a joint is in its open-packed position. The open-packed positions for the various joints are depicted in Table 1-7.

CLINICAL PEARL

The open-packed position is commonly used during joint mobilization techniques (see Chapter 11).

REFERENCES

1. Hall SJ: The biomechanics of human skeletal muscle. In: Hall SJ, ed. *Basic Biomechanics.* New York, NY: McGraw-Hill, 1999:146–185.
2. Buckwalter JA, Mankin HJ: Articular cartilage. Part I: Tissue design and chondrocyte-matrix interactions. *J Bone Joint Surg* 79A:600–611, 1997.
3. Muir H: Proteoglycans as organizers of the extracellular matrix. *Biochem Soc Trans* 11:613–622, 1983.
4. Junqueira LC, Carneciro J, Kelley RO: *Basic Histology.* Norwalk, CT: Conn, Appleton and Lange, 1995.
5. Lundon K, Bolton K: Structure and function of the lumbar intervertebral disk in health, aging, and pathological conditions. *J Orthop Sports Phys Ther* 31:291–306, 2001.
6. Engles M: Tissue response. In: Donatelli R, Wooden MJ, eds. *Orthopaedic Physical Therapy (ed 3).* Philadelphia, PA: Churchill Livingstone, 2001:1 24.
7. Starcher BC: Lung elastin and matrix. *Chest* 117(5 Suppl 1):229S–234S, 2000.
8. Teitz CC, Garrett WE Jr, Miniaci A, et al: Tendon problems in athletic individuals. *J Bone and Joint Surg* 79-A:138–152, 1997.
9. Barnes J: *Myofascial Release: A Comprehensive Evaluatory and Treatment Approach.* Paoli, PA: MFR Seminars, 1990.
10. Smolders JJ: Myofascial pain and dysfunction syndromes. In: Hammer WI, ed. *Functional Soft Tissue Examination and Treatment by Manual Methods - The Extremities.* Gaithersburg, MD: Aspen, 1991:215–234.
11. Ellis JJ, Johnson GS: Myofascial considerations in somatic dysfunction of the thorax. In: Flynn TW, ed. *The Thoracic Spine and Rib Cage: Musculoskeletal Evaluation and Treatment.* Boston, MA: Butterworth-Heinemann, 1996:211–262.
12. Curwin SL: Tendon pathology and injuries: Pathophysiology, healing, and treatment considerations. In: Magee D, Zachazewski JE, Quillen WS, eds. *Scientific Foundations and Principles of Practice in Musculoskeletal Rehabilitation.* St. Louis, MI: WB Saunders, 2007:47–78.

13. Amiel D, Woo SL-Y, Harwood FL: The effect of immobilization on collagen turnover in connective tissue: A biochemical-biomechanical correlation. *Acta Orthop Scand* 53:325–332, 1982.
14. Jozsa L, Kannus P: Functional and mechanical behavior of tendons. In: Jozsa L, Kannus P, eds. *Human Tendons.* Champaign, IL: Human Kinetics, 1997:164–253.
15. Benjamin M, Toumi H, Ralphs JR, et al: Where tendons and ligaments meet bone: Attachment sites ('entheses') in relation to exercise and/or mechanical load. *J Anat* 208:471–490, 2006.
16. Maganaris CN, Narici MV, Almekinders LC, et al: Biomechanics and pathophysiology of overuse tendon injuries: Ideas on insertional tendinopathy. *Sports medicine* 34:1005–1017, 2004.
17. Reid DC: *Sports Injury Assessment and Rehabilitation.* New York, NY: Churchill Livingstone, 1992.
18. Garrett W, Tidball J: Myotendinous junction: Structure, function, and failure. In: Woo SL-Y, Buckwalter JA, eds. *Injury and Repair of the Musculoskeletal Soft Tissues.* Rosemont, IL: AAOS, 1988: 171–207.
19. Garrett WE Jr: Muscle strain injuries: clinical and basic aspects. *Med Sci Sports Exerc* 22:436–443, 1990.
20. Garrett WE: Muscle strain injuries. *Am J Sports Med* 24:S2–S8, 1996.
21. Safran MR, Seaber AV, Garrett WE: Warm-up and muscular injury prevention: An update. *Sports Med* 8:239–249, 1989.
22. Huijbregts PA: Muscle injury, regeneration, and repair. *J Man Manip Ther* 9:9–16, 2001.
23. Hildebrand KA, Hart DA, Rattner JB, et al: Ligament injuries: Pathophysiology, healing, and treatment considerations, In: Magee D, Zachazewski JE, Quillen WS, eds. *Scientific Foundations and Principles of Practice in Musculoskeletal Rehabilitation.* St. Louis, MI: WB Saunders, 2007:23–46.
24. Vereeke West R, Fu F: *Soft tissue physiology and repair, Orthopaedic Knowledge Update 8: Home Study Syllabus.* Rosemont, IL: American Academy of Orthopaedic Surgeons, 2005:15–27.
25. Amiel D, Kleiner JB: Biochemistry of tendon and ligament. In: Nimni ME ed. *Collagen.* Boca Raton, FL: CRC Press, 1988:223–251.
26. Woo SL-Y, An K-N, Arnoczky SP, et al: Anatomy, biology, and biomechanics of tendon, ligament, and meniscus. In: Simon S, ed. *Orthopaedic Basic Science.* Rosemont, IL: The American Academy of Orthopaedic Surgeons, 1994:45–87.
27. Safran MR, Benedetti RS, Bartolozzi AR, 3rd, et al: Lateral ankle sprains: A comprehensive review: Part 1: Etiology, pathoanatomy, histopathogenesis, and diagnosis. *Med Sci Sports Exerc* 31:S429–S437, 1999.
28. Smith RL, Brunolli J: Shoulder kinesthesia after anterior glenohumeral dislocation. *Phys Ther* 69:106–112, 1989.
29. McGaw WT: The effect of tension on collagen remodelling by fibroblasts: A stereological ultrastructural study. Connect. *Tissue Res* 14: 229, 1986.
30. Inman VT: Sprains of the ankle. In: Chapman MW, ed. *AAOS Instructional Course Lectures.* Illinois: Park Ridge, 1975:294–308.
31. Cohen NP, Foster RJ, Mow VC: Composition and dynamics of articular cartilage: Structure, function, and maintaining healthy state. *J Orthop Sports Phys Ther* 28:203–215, 1998.
32. Mankin HJ, Mow VC, Buckwalter JA, et al: Form and function of articular cartilage. In: Simon SR, ed. *Orthopaedic Basic Science.* Rosemont, IL: American Academy of Orthopaedic Surgeons, 1994:1–44.
33. Buchbinder D, Kaplan AS: Biology. In: Kaplan AS, Assael LA, eds. *Temporomandibular Disorders Diagnosis And Treatment.* Philadelphia, PA: WB Saunders, 1991:11–23.
34. Tippett SR: Considerations for the pediatric patient. In: Voight ML, Hoogenboom BJ, Prentice WE, eds. *Musculoskeletal Interventions: Techniques for Therapeutic Exercise.* New York, NY: McGraw-Hill, 2007:803–820.
35. Iannotti JP, Goldstein S, Kuhn J, et al: The formation and growth of skeletal tissues. In: Buckwalter JA, Einhorn TA, Simon SR, eds. *Orthopedic Basic Science.* Rosemont, IL: American Academy of Orthopedic Surgeons, 2000:77–109.
36. Jones D, Round D: *Skeletal Muscle in Health and Disease.* Manchester: Manchester University Press, 1990.
37. Loitz-Ramage B, Zernicke RF: Bone biology and mechanics, in Magee D, Zachazewski JE, Quillen WS, eds. *Scientific Foundations and Principles of Practice in Musculoskeletal Rehabilitation.* St. Louis, MI, WB Saunders, 2007:122-143.
38. Armstrong RB, Warren GL, Warren JA: Mechanisms of exercise-induced muscle fibre injury. *Med Sci Sports Exerc* 24:436–443, 1990.
39. Luttgens K, Hamilton K: The musculoskeletal system: The musculature. In: Luttgens K, Hamilton K, eds. *Kinesiology: Scientific Basis of Human Motion (ed 9).* Dubuque, IA: McGraw-Hill, 1997:49–75.
40. Van de Graaff KM, Fox SI: Muscle tissue and muscle physiology. In: Van de Graaff KM, Fox SI, eds. *Concepts of Human Anatomy and Physiology.* New York, NY: WCB/McGraw-Hill, 1999:280–305.
41. Williams JH, Klug GA: Calcium exchange hypothesis of skeletal muscle fatigue. A brief review. *Muscle Nerve* 18:421–434, 1995.
42. Brooke MH, Kaiser KK: The use and abuse of muscle histochemistry. *Ann N Y Acad Sci* 228:121–144, 1974.
43. Staron RS, Hikida RS: Histochemical, biochemical, and ultrastructural analyses of single human muscle fibers, with special reference to the C-fiber population. *J Histochem Cytochem* 40:563–568, 1992.
44. Jull GA, Janda V: Muscle and Motor control in low back pain. In: Twomey LT, Taylor JR, eds. *Physical Therapy of the Low Back: Clinics in Physical Therapy.* New York, NY: Churchill Livingstone, 1987:258–278.
45. Fitts RH, Widrick JJ: Muscle mechanics; adaptations with exercise training. *Exerc Sport Sci Rev* 24:427–473, 1996.
46. Allemeier CA, Fry AC, Johnson P, et al: Effects of spring cycle training on human skeletal muscle. *J Appl Physiol* 77:2385–2390, 1994.
47. Nilsson J, Tesch PA, Thorstensson A: Fatigue and EMG of repeated fast and voluntary contractions in man. *Acta Physiol Scand* 101:194–198, 1977.
48. Sell S, Zacher J, Lack S: Disorders of proprioception of arthrotic knee joint. *Z. Rheumatol* 52:150–155, 1993.
49. Mattacola CG, Lloyd JW: Effects of a 6 week strength and proprioception training program on measures of dynamic balance: A single case design. *J Athl Training* 32:127–135, 1997.
50. McArdle W, Katch FI, Katch VL: *Exercise Physiology: Energy, Nutrition, and Human Performance.* Philadelphia, PA: Lea and Febiger, 1991.
51. Astrand PO, Rodahl K: *The Muscle and its Contraction: Textbook of Work Physiology.* New York, NY: McGraw-Hill, 1986.
52. Edman KAP RC: The sarcomere length-tension relation determined in short segments of intact muscle fibres of the frog. *J Physiol* 385:729–732, 1987.
53. Boeckmann RR, Ellenbecker TS: Biomechanics. In: Ellenbecker TS, ed. *Knee Ligament Rehabilitation.* Philadelphia, PA: Churchill Livingstone, 2000:16–23.
54. Brownstein B, Noyes FR, Mangine RE, et al: Anatomy and biomechanics. In: Mangine RE, ed. *Physical Therapy of the Knee.* New York, NY: Churchill Livingstone, 1988:1–30.
55. Deudsinger RH: Biomechanics in clinical practice. *Phys Ther* 64:1860–1868, 1984.
56. Lakomy HKA: The biomechanics of human movement. In: Maughan RJ, ed. *Basic and Applied Sciences for Sports Medicine.* Woburn, MA: Mass, Butterworth-Heinemann, 1999:124–125.
57. Desmendt JE, Godaux E: Fast motor units are not preferentially activated in rapid voluntary contractions in man. *Nature* 267:717, 1977.
58. Gans C: Fiber architecture and muscle function. *Exerc Sport Sci Rev* 10:160, 1982.
59. Magee DJ, Zachazewski JE: Principles of stabilization training. In: Magee D, Zachazewski JE, Quillen WS, eds. *Scientific Foundations and Principles of Practice in Musculoskeletal Rehabilitation.* St. Louis, MI: WB Saunders, 2007:388–413.
60. Lash JM: Regulation of skeletal muscle blood flow during contractions. *Proc Soc Exp Biol Med* 211:218–235, 1996.
61. Rosenbaum D, Henning EM: The influence of stretching and warm-up exercises on Achilles tendon reflex activity. *J Sports Sci* 13:481–490, 1995.
62. Astrand PO, Rodahl K: *Physical Training: Textbook of Work Physiology.* New York, NY: McGraw-Hill, 1986.
63. Aubier M, Farkas G, Troyer AD, et al: Detection of diaphragmatic fatigue in man by phrenic stimulation. *J Appl Physiol* 50:538–544, 1981.
64. Fenn WO: A comparison of respiratory and skeletal muscles. In: Cori CF, Foglia VG, Leloir LF, et al eds. *Perspectives in Biology Houssay Memorial Papers.* Amsterdam: Elsevier, 1963:293–300.
65. Lewit K: Relation of faulty respiration to posture, with clinical implications. *J Amer Osteopath Assoc* 79:525–529, 1980.
66. Junqueira LC, Carneciro J: Bone. In: Junqueira LC, Carneciro J, eds. *Basic Histology (ed 10).* New York, NY: McGraw-Hill, 2003:141–159.
67. Van de Graaff KM, Fox SI: Histology. In: Van de Graaff KM, Fox SI, eds. *Concepts of Human Anatomy and Physiology.* New York, NY: WCB/McGraw-Hill, 1999:130–158.
68. Williams GR, Chmielewski T, Rudolph KS, et al: Dynamic knee stability: Current theory and implications for clinicians and scientists. *J Orthop Sports Phys Ther* 31:546–566, 2001.
69. Gleim GW, McHugh MP: Flexibility and its effects on sports injury and performance. *Sports Med* 24:289–299, 1997.

70. Chaffin D, Andersson G: *Occupational Biomechanics*. Wiley Interscience 53:103–107, 1985.
71. Dahl LB, Dahl IMS, Engstrom-Laurent A, et al: Concentration and molecular weight of sodium hyaluronate in synovial fluid from patients with rheumatoid arthritis and other arthropathies. *Ann Rheum Dis* 44:817–822, 1985.
72. Laurent TC, Fraser JRE: Hyaluronan. *FASEB J* 6:2397–2404, 1992.
73. Namba RS, Shuster S, Tucker P, et al: Localization of hyaluronan in pseudocapsule from total hip arthroplasty. *Clin Orthop Relat Res* 363: 158–162, 1999.
74. Marshall KW: Intra-articular hyaluronan therapy. *Curr Opin Rheumatol* 12:468–474, 2000.
75. O'Driscoll SW: The healing and regeneration of articular cartilage. *J Bone Joint Surg* 80A:1795–1812, 1998.
76. Dieppe P: The classification and diagnosis of osteoarthritis. In: Kuettner KE, Goldberg WM, eds. *Osteoarthritic Disorders*. Rosemont, IL: American Academy of Orthopaedic Surgeons, 1995:5–12.
77. Mankin HJ: Current concepts review. The response of articular cartilage to mechanical injury. *J Bone Joint Surg* 64A:460–466, 1982.
78. Ho G Jr, Tice AD, Kaplan SR: Septic bursitis in the prepatellar and olecranon bursae: An analysis of 25 cases. *Ann Intern Med* 89:21–27, 1978.
79. Buckingham RB: Bursitis and tendinitis. *Compr Ther* 7:52–57, 1981.
80. Reilly J, Nicholas JA: The chronically inflamed bursa. *Clin Sports Med* 6:345–370, 1987.
81. Hall SJ: Kinematic concepts for analyzing human motion. In: Hall SJ, ed. *Basic Biomechanics*. New York, NY: McGraw-Hill, 1999:28–89.
82. American Medical Association: *Guides to the Evaluation of Permanent Impairment (ed 5)*. Chicago, IL: American Medical Association, 2001.
83. Neumann DA: Getting started. In: Neumann DA, ed. *Kinesiology of the Musculoskeletal System: Foundations for Physical Rehabilitation*. St. Louis, MO: Mosby, 2002:3–24.
84. Lehmkuhl LD, Smith LK: *Brunnstrom's Clinical Kinesiology*. Philadelphia, PA: F.A. Davis Company, 1983:361–390.
85. MacConnail MA, Basmajian JV: *Muscles and Movements: A Basis for Human kinesiology*. New York, NY: Robert Krieger Pub Co, 1977.
86. Rasch PJ, Burke RK: *Kinesiology and Applied Anatomy*. Philadelphia, PA: Lea and Febiger, 1971.
87. Steindler A: *Kinesiology of the Human Body under Normal and Pathological Conditions*. Springfield, IL: Charles C Thomas, 1955.
88. Williams PL, Warwick R, Dyson M, et al: *Gray's Anatomy (ed 37)*. London: Churchill Livingstone, 1989.
89. Mennell JB: *The Science and Art of Joint Manipulation*. London: J & A Churchill, 1949.
90. Mennell JM: *Back Pain. Diagnosis and Treatment Using Manipulative Techniques*. Boston, MA: Little, Brown & Company, 1960.
91. MacConaill MA: Arthrology. In: Warwick R, Williams PL, eds. *Gray's Anatomy (ed 35)*. Philadelphia, PA: WB Saunders 388–398, 1975.
92. Marino M: Current concepts of rehabilitation in sports medicine. In: Nicholas JA, Herschman EB, eds. *The Lower Extremity And Spine In Sports Medicine*. St. Louis, MO: Mosby, 1986:117–195.
93. Blackard DO, Jensen RL, Ebben WP: Use of EMG analysis in challenging kinetic chain terminology. *Med Sci Sports Exerc* 31:443–448, 1999.
94. Palmitier RA, An KN, Scott SG, et al: Kinetic chain exercises in knee rehabilitation. *Sports Med* 11:402–413, 1991.
95. Gray GW: Closed chain sense. *Fitness Manage* 5:31–33, 1992.
96. Dillman CJ, Murray TA, Hintermeister RA: Biomechanical differences of open and closed chain exercises with respect to the shoulder. *J Sport Rehabil* 3:228–238, 1994.
97. Kibler WB: Closed kinetic chain rehabilitation for sports injuries. *Phys Med Rehabil Clin N Am* 11:369–384, 2000.
98. Lephart SM, Henry TJ: Functional rehabilitation for the upper and lower extremity. *Orthop Clin North Am* 26:579–592, 1995.

Tissue Behavior, Injury, Healing, and Treatment

CHAPTER 2

CHAPTER OBJECTIVES

At the completion of this chapter, the reader will be able to:

1. Describe the various types of stress that can be applied to the body.
2. Describe the various physiological processes by which the body adapts to stress.
3. Define the various common mechanisms of injury.
4. Describe the etiology and pathophysiology of musculoskeletal injuries associated with various types of body tissue.
5. Outline the pathophysiology of the healing process and the various stages of healing.
6. Describe the methods used to enhance healing and the factors that can impede the healing process.
7. Outline the more common surgical procedures available for musculoskeletal injuries.
8. Outline the principles behind postsurgical rehabilitation.
9. Describe the detrimental effects of immobilization.

OVERVIEW

Tissues in the body are designed to function while undergoing stresses of everyday living. This ability to respond to stress is due to the differing viscoelastic properties of musculoskeletal tissue, with each tissue responding to stress in an individual manner based on design. One of the contributing factors to maintaining musculoskeletal health is the ability of the biological tissues to withstand various stresses and strains that occur during activity—body weight, friction, and air or water resistance are all types of stresses that commonly act on the body. Maintaining this health is a delicate balance, because insufficient, excessive, or repetitive stresses can prove deleterious. The healing process is an intricate phenomenon that occurs following an injury or disease.

THE RESPONSE OF TISSUE TO STRESS

Kinetics is the term applied to the forces acting on the body. Posture and movement are both governed by the control of forces. The same forces that move and stabilize the body also have the potential to deform and injure the body.[1] A wide range of external and internal forces are either generated or resisted by the human body during the course of daily activities. Examples of these external forces include ground reaction force, gravity, and applied force through contact. Examples of internal forces include muscle contraction, joint contact, and joint shear forces (Fig. 2-1). Under the right circumstances, the body is able to respond to these stresses. The terms *stress* and *strain* have specific mechanical meanings. Stress or load is given in units of force per area, and is used to describe the type of force applied. Stress is independent of the amount of a material, but is directly related to the magnitude of force and inversely related to the unit area.[2] Strain is defined as the change in length of a material due to an imposed load divided by the original length.[2] The two basic types of strain are linear strain, which causes a change in the length of a structure, and shear strain, which causes a change in the angular relationships within a structure. It is the concentration of proteoglycans in solution (see Chap. 1) that is responsible for influencing the mechanical properties of the tissue, including compressive stiffness, sheer stiffness, osmotic pressure, and regulation of hydration.[3]

The inherent ability of a tissue to tolerate load can be observed experimentally in graphic form. When any stress is plotted on a graph against the resulting strain for a given material, the shape of the resulting load-deformation curve depends on the kind of material involved. The load-deformation curve, or stress–strain curve, of a structure (Fig. 2-2) depicts the relationship between the amount of force applied to a structure and the structure's response in terms of deformation or acceleration. The horizontal axis (deformation or strain) represents the ratio of the tissue's deformed length to its original length. The vertical axis of the graph (load or stress) denotes the internal resistance generated as a tissue resists its deformation, divided by its cross-sectional area. The

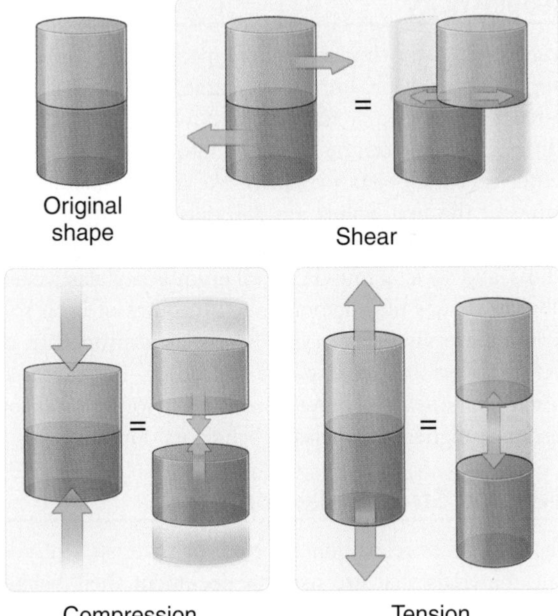

FIGURE 2-1 Internal forces acting on the body.

load-deformation curve can be divided into four regions, each region representing a biomechanical property of the tissue (Fig. 2-2):

- Toe region. Collagen fibers have a wavy, or folded, appearance at rest. When a force that lengthens the collagen fibers is initially applied to connective tissue, these folds are affected first. As the fibers unfold, the slack is taken up (see Crimp later). The toe region is an artifact caused by this take-up of slack, alignment and/or seating of the test specimen. The length of the toe region depends upon the type of material and the waviness of the collagen pattern.
- Elastic deformation region. Within the elastic deformation region, the structure imitates a spring—the geometric deformation in the structure increases linearly with increasing load, and after the load is released the structure returns to its original shape. The slope of the elastic region of the load-deformation curve from one point in the curve to another is called the modulus of elasticity or Young's modulus, and represents the extrinsic stiffness or rigidity of the structure—the stiffer the tissue, the steeper the slope. Young's modulus is a numerical description of the relationship between the amount of stress a tissue undergoes and the deformation that results. The ratio of stress to strain in an elastic material is a measure of its stiffness. Mathematically, the value for stiffness is found by dividing the load by the deformation at any point in the selected range. All normal tissues within the musculoskeletal system exhibit some degree of stiffness. Young's modulus is independent of specimen size and is, therefore, a measure of the intrinsic stiffness of the material. The greater the Young's modulus for a material, the better it can withstand greater forces. Larger structures will have greater rigidity than smaller structures of similar composition.
- Plastic deformation region. The end of the elastic deformation range and the beginning of the plastic deformation range represents the point where an increasing level of stress on the tissue results in progressive failure and microscopic tearing of the collagen fibers. Further increases in strain result in microscopic damage and in permanent deformation. The permanent change results from the breaking of bonds and their subsequent inability to contribute to the recovery of the tissue. Unlike the elastic region, removal of the load in this region will not result in a return of the tissue to its original length.
- Failure region. Deformations exceeding the ultimate failure point (Fig. 2-2) produce mechanical failure

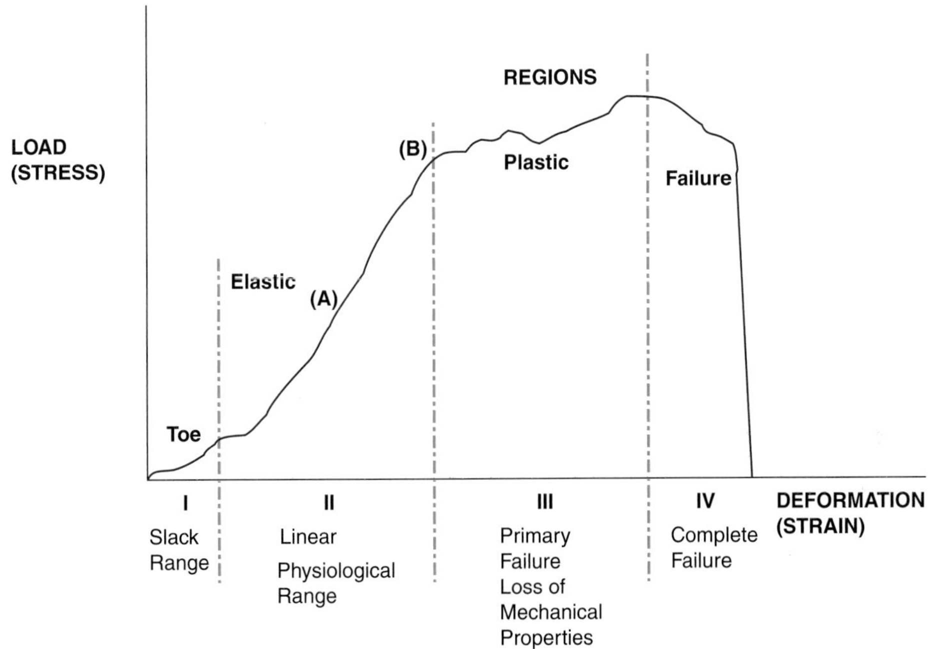

FIGURE 2-2 The stress–strain curve.

of the structure, which in the human body may be represented by the fracturing of bone or the rupturing of soft tissues.

CLINICAL PEARL

Stiffness = force/deformation. The gradient in the linear portion of the load-deformation curve immediately after the toe region represents the stiffness value. The load-deformation curve does not indicate the variable of time.

Elastic modulus = stress/strain. The larger the Young's modulus for a material, the greater the stress needed for a given strain.

Biological tissues are anisotropic, which means they can demonstrate differing mechanical behavior as a function of test direction. The properties of extensibility and elasticity are common to many biologic tissues. Extensibility is the ability to be stretched and elasticity is the ability to return to normal length after lengthening or shortening.[4]

A number of protective mechanisms exist in connective tissue to help respond to stress and strain including crimp, viscoelasticity, creep and stress relaxation, plastic deformation, and stress response.

CLINICAL PEARL

Protective tissue mechanisms include

- crimp
- viscoelasticity
- creep and stress relaxation
- plastic deformation
- stress response

Crimp

The crimp of collagen is one of the major factors behind the viscoelastic properties of connective tissue. Crimp, a collagen tissue's first line of response to stress, is different for each type of connective tissue, providing each with different viscoelastic properties. Collagen fibers are oriented obliquely when relaxed. However, when a load is applied, the fibers line up in the direction of the applied force as they uncrimp. Crimping is seen primarily in ligaments, tendons, and joint capsules. and occurs in the toe phase of the stress-strain curve (Fig. 2-2).

CLINICAL PEARL

If a load is applied to connective tissue and then removed immediately, the material recoils to its original size. If, however, the load is allowed to remain, the material continues to stretch. After a period of sustained stretch, the stretching tends to reach a steady-state value. Realignment of the collagen fibers in the direction of the stress occurs, and water and proteoglycans are displaced from between the fibers.

Viscoelasticity

Viscoelasticity is the time-dependent mechanical property of a material to stretch or shorten over time, and to return to its original shape when a force is removed. The mechanical qualities of a tissue can be separated into categories based on whether the tissue acts primarily like a solid, a fluid, or a mixture of the two. Solids are described according to their elasticity, strength, hardness, and stiffness. Bone, ligaments, tendons, and skeletal muscle are all examples of elastic solids. Biological tissues that demonstrate attributes of both solids and fluids are viscoelastic. The viscoelastic properties of a structure determine its response to loading. For example, a ligament demonstrates more viscous behavior at lower loads whereas, at higher loads, elastic behaviors dominate.[5]

Creep and Stress Relaxation

Creep and stress relaxation are two characteristics of viscoelastic materials that are used to document their behavior quantitatively.[4]

Creep is the gradual rearrangement of collagen fibers, proteoglycans, and water that occurs because of a constantly applied force after the initial lengthening caused by crimp has ceased. Creep is a time-dependent and transient biomechanical phenomenon. Short duration stresses (<15 minutes) do not have sufficient time to produce this displacement; however, longer times can produce it. Once creep occurs, the tissue has difficulty returning to its initial length (see below).

Stress relaxation is a phenomenon in which stress or force in a deformed structure decreases with time, while the deformation is held constant.[4] Unlike creep, stress relaxation responds with a high initial stress that decreases over time until equilibrium is reached and the stress equals zero, hence the label "relaxation". As a result, no change in length is produced.

Thus, stress to connective tissues can result in no change, a semipermanent change, or a permanent change to the microstructure of the collagenous tissue. The semipermanent or permanent changes may result in either *microfailure* or *macrofailure.*

Plastic Deformation

Plastic deformation of connective tissue occurs when a tissue remains deformed and does not recover its prestress length. Once all of the possible realignment has occurred, any further loading breaks the restraining bonds, resulting in microfailure. On average, collagen fibers are able to sustain a 3% increase in elongation (strain) before microscopic damage occurs.[6] Following a brief stretch, providing the chemical bonds remain intact, the collagen and proteoglycans gradually recover their original alignment. The recovery process occurs at a slower rate and often to a lesser extent. The loss of energy that occurs between the lengthening force and the recovery activity is referred to as *hysteresis.* The more chemical bonds that are broken with applied stress, the greater the hysteresis. If the stretch is of sufficient force and duration and a sufficient number of chemical bonds are broken, the tissue is unable to return to its original length until the bonds are re-formed. Instead, it returns to a new length and to a new level of strain resistance. Increased tissue excursion is now needed before tension develops in the structure. In essence, this has the effect of decreasing the stabilizing capabilities of the connective tissue.

Stress Response

Exercises may be used to change the physical properties of both muscles/tendons and ligaments, as both have demonstrated adaptability to external loads with an increase in strength: weight ratios.[7–9] The improved strength results from an increase in the proteoglycan content and collagen cross-links.[7–9]

> **CLINICAL PEARL**
>
> Three biomechanical attributes of connective tissue can have a clinical significance:
>
> - Structural behavior
> - Material behavior
> - Viscoelastic behavior

TISSUE INJURY

Soft-tissue injuries of all types are extremely common in the general population. Studies have shown that there is a linear relationship between soft-tissue injuries and aging, with fewer than 10% of individuals younger than 34 years being affected, in contrast to 32–49% of those older than 75 being affected.[10] Whether a stress proves to be beneficial or detrimental to a tissue is very much dependent on the physiologic capacity of the tissue to accept load. This capacity is dependent on a number of factors, among them:

- ***Health of the tissue.*** Healthy tissues are able to resist changes in their shape. Any tissue weakened by disease or trauma may not be able to adequately resist the application of force.
- ***Age.*** Increasing age reduces the capacity of the tissues to cope with stress loading.
- ***Proteoglycan and collagen content of the tissue.*** Both increasing age and exposure to trauma can result in unfavorable alterations in the proteoglycan and collagen content of the tissue.
- ***Ability of the tissue to undergo adaptive change.*** All musculoskeletal tissue has the capacity to adapt to change. This capacity to change is determined primarily by the viscoelastic property of the tissue.
- ***The speed at which the adaptive change occurs.*** This is dependent on the type and severity of the insult to the tissue. Insults of low force and longer duration may provide the tissue an opportunity to adapt. In contrast, insults of a higher force and shorter duration are less likely to provide the tissue time to adapt. The distinction between sudden and repetitive stress is important. An acute stress (loading) occurs when a single force is large enough to cause injury on biological tissues; the causative force is termed *macrotrauma*. A repetitive stress (loading) occurs when a single force itself is insufficient to cause injury on biological tissues. However, when repeated or chronic stress over a period of time causes an injury, the injury is called a *chronic injury*, and the causative mechanism is termed *microtrauma*. Etiologic factors for microtraumatic injuries are of two basic types: intrinsic or extrinsic. Intrinsic factors are physical characteristics that predispose an individual to microtrauma injuries and include muscle imbalances, leg length discrepancies, and anatomical anomalies.[11] Extrinsic factors, which are the most common cause of microtrauma injuries, are related to the external conditions under which the activity is performed. These include training errors, type of terrain, environmental temperature, and incorrect use of equipment.[11]

INJURY CLASSIFICATION

Injuries to the soft tissues can be classified as primary or secondary.

- Primary or macrotraumatic injuries can be self-inflicted, caused by another individual or entity, or caused by the environment.[12–15] These injuries include fractures and dislocations, which are outside the scope of practice for a physical therapist, and subluxations, sprains, and strains, which make up the majority of conditions seen in the physical therapy clinic. For the purposes on the intervention, primary injuries are generally classified into acute, subacute, or chronic.
  - Acute. This type of injury is usually caused by macrotrauma and indicates the early phase of injury and healing, which typically lasts approximately 7–10 days.
  - Subacute. This phase occurs after the acute phase and typically lasts from 5–10 days after the acute phase has ended.
  - Chronic. This type of injury can have several definitions. On the one hand it may indicate the final stage of healing that occurs 26–34 days after injury. On the other hand the term may be applied to an injury that lasts longer than normal and does not appear to be improving due to a persistent inflammatory state. The persistent inflammatory state results in an accumulation of repetitive scar adhesions, degenerative changes, and other harmful effects referred to as subclinical adaptations.

> **CLINICAL PEARL**
>
> An acute-on-chronic injury involves a reinjury of the tissue—an acute exacerbation of a chronic injury.
>
> - Secondary or microtraumatic injuries are essentially the inflammatory response that occurs with the primary injury.[16] Microtraumatic injuries include tendinitis, tenosynovitis, and bursitis.

TISSUE HEALING

Fortunately, the majority of tissue injuries heal without complication in a predictable series of events (Fig. 2-3). The most important factor regulating the regional time line of healing is sufficient blood flow.[17] Complications such as infection, compromised circulation, and neuropathy have an adverse effect on the healing process and can cause great physical and psychological stress to the involved patients and their families.

Stages of Tissue Healing

The general stages of soft tissue healing are described here, whereas the healing of specific structures is described later under the relevant headings. After microtrauma, macrotrauma, or disease, the body attempts to heal itself through a predictable series of overlapping events that include coagulation and inflammation (acute), which begins shortly after the initial injury; a migratory and proliferative process (subacute), which begins within days and includes the major processes of healing; and a remodeling process (chronic),

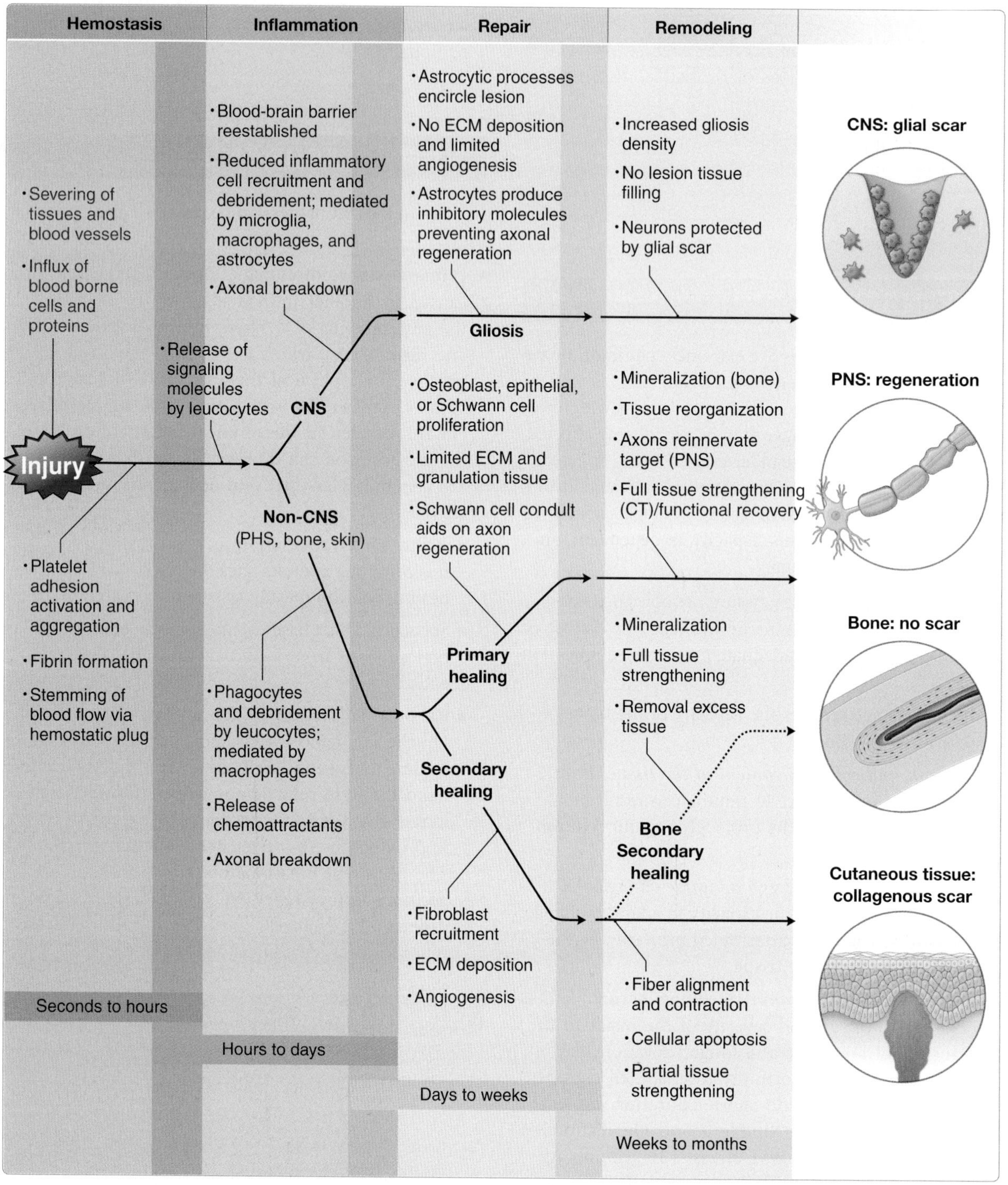

FIGURE 2-3 Stages of healing.

which may last for up to a year depending on the tissue type and is responsible for scar tissue formation and the development of new tissue.[12,17–21]

Whereas simplification of the complex events of healing into separate categories may facilitate understanding of the phenomenon, in reality these events occur as an amalgamation of different reactions, both spatially and temporally.[22]

Coagulation and Inflammation Stage

An injury to the soft tissue triggers a process that represents the body's immediate reaction to trauma.[17,23] The reaction that occurs immediately after a soft tissue injury includes a series of repair and defensive events. Following an injury to the tissues, the cellular and plasma components of blood and lymph enter the wound. Capillary blood flow is disrupted, causing hypoxia to the area. The blood congeals and, through several steps, a clot is formed. This initial period of vasoconstriction, which lasts 5–10 minutes, prompts a period of vasodilation, and the extravasation of blood constituents.[17] Extravasated blood contains platelets, which secrete substances that form a clot to prevent bleeding and infection, clean dead tissue and nourish white cells. These substances include macrophages and fibroblasts.[24] Coagulation and platelet release results in the excretion of platelet-derived growth factor (PDGF),[25] platelet factor 4,[26] transforming growth factor-alpha (TGF-α),[27] and transforming growth factor-beta (TGF-β).[28] The main functions of a cell-rich tissue exudate are to provide cells capable of producing the components and biological mediators necessary for the directed reconstruction of damaged tissue while diluting microbial toxins and removing contaminants present in the wound.[22]

Inflammation is mediated by chemotactic substances, including anaphylatoxins that attract neutrophils and monocytes.

- ***Neutrophils.*** Neutrophils are white blood cells of the polymorphonuclear (PMN) leukocyte subgroup (the others being eosinophils, and basophils) that are filled with granules of toxic chemicals (phagocytes) that enable them to bind to microorganisms, internalize them, and kill them.
- ***Monocytes.*** Monocytes are white blood cells of the mononuclear leukocyte subgroup (the other being lymphocytes). The monocytes migrate into tissues and develop into macrophages, providing immunological defenses against many infectious organisms. Macrophages serve to orchestrate a "long term" response to injured cells subsequent to the acute response.[29]

The white blood cells of the inflammatory stage serve to clean the wound debris of foreign substances, increase vascular permeability, and promote fibroblast activity.[29] Other cell participants include local immune accessory cells, such as endothelial cells, mast cells, and tissue fibroblasts. The PMN leukocytes, through their characteristic "respiratory burst" activity, produce superoxide anion radical, which is well known to be critical for defense against bacteria and other pathogens.[30] Superoxide is rapidly converted to a membrane permeable form, hydrogen peroxide (H_2O_2), by superoxide dismutase activity or even spontaneously.[29] Release of H_2O_2 may promote formation of other oxidants that are more stable (longer half-life) including hypochlorous acid, chloramines, and aldehydes.[29] The phagocytic cells that initiate the innate immune response produce a set of proinflammatory cytokines (e.g., TNF-α, IL-1, and IL-6) in the form of a cascade that amplifies the local inflammatory response, influences the adaptive immune response, and serves to signal the CNS of an inflammatory response. The extent and severity of this inflammatory response depend on the size and the type of the injury, the tissue involved, and the vascularity of that tissue.[15,20,31–33]

Local vasodilation is promoted by biologically active products of the complement and kinin cascades[22]:

- The complement cascade involves 20 or more proteins that circulate throughout the blood in an inactive form.[22] After tissue injury, activation of the complement cascade produces a variety of proteins with activities essential to healing.
- The kinin cascade is responsible for the transformation of the inactive enzyme kallikrein, which is present in both blood and tissue, to its active form, bradykinin. Bradykinin also contributes to the production of tissue exudate through the promotion of vasodilation and increased vessel-wall permeability.[34]

Because of the variety of vascular and other physiological responses occurring, this stage of healing is characterized by swelling, redness, heat, and impairment or loss of function. The edema is due to an increase in the permeability of the venules, plasma proteins, and leukocytes, which leak into the site of injury, resulting in edema.[35,36] New stroma, often called granulation tissue, begins to invade the wound space approximately 4 days after injury.[35,36] The complete removal of the wound debris marks the end of the inflammatory process.

Clinically, this stage is characterized by pain at rest or with active motion, or when specific stress is applied to the injured structure. The pain, if severe enough, can result in muscle guarding and a loss of function.

Two key types of inflammation are recognized: the normal acute inflammatory response and an abnormal, chronic, or persistent inflammatory response. Common causes for a persistent chronic inflammatory response include infectious agents, persistent viruses, hypertrophic scarring, poor blood supply, edema, repetitive mechanical trauma, excessive tension at the wound site, and hypersensitivity reactions.[37,38] The monocyte-predominant infiltration, angiogenesis, and fibrous change are the most characteristic morphologic features of chronic inflammation. This perpetuation of inflammation involves the binding of neutrophilic myeloperoxidase to the macrophage mannose receptor.[39]

Migratory and Proliferative Stage

The second stage of soft tissue healing, characterized by migration and proliferation, usually occurs from the time of the initial injury and overlaps the inflammation phase. Characteristic changes include capillary growth and granulation tissue formation, fibroblast proliferation with collagen synthesis, and increased macrophage and mast cell activity. This stage is responsible for the development of wound tensile strength.

After the wound base is free of necrotic tissue, the body begins to work to close the wound. The connective tissue in healing wounds is composed primarily of collagen, types I and III,[40] cells, vessels, and a matrix that contains glycoproteins and proteoglycans. Proliferation of collagen results from the actions of the fibroblasts that have been attracted to the area and stimulated to multiply by growth factors, such as PDGF, TGF-β, fibroblast growth factor (FGF), epidermal growth factor, and insulin-like growth factor-1, and tissue factors such as fibronectin.[22] This proliferation produces first fibrinogen and then fibrin, which eventually becomes organized into a honeycomb matrix and walls off the injured site.[41]

The wound matrix functions as a glue to hold the wound edges together, giving it some mechanical protection while also preventing the spread of infection. However, the wound matrix has a low tensile strength and is vulnerable to breakdown until the provisional extracellular matrix (ECM) is replaced with a collagenous matrix. The collagenous matrix facilitates angiogenesis by providing time and protection to new and friable vessels. Angiogenesis occurs in response to the hypoxic state created by tissue damage as well as to factors released from cells during injury.[22]

The process of neovascularization during this phase provides a granular appearance to the wound as a result of the formation of loops of capillaries and migration of macrophages, fibroblasts, and endothelial cells into the wound matrix. Once an abundant collagen matrix has been deposited in the wound, the fibroblasts stop producing collagen, and the fibroblast-rich granulation tissue is replaced by a relatively acellular scar, marking the end of this stage.

This fibrous tissue repair process occurs gradually and can last anywhere from 5 to 15 days to approximately 10 weeks, depending on the type of tissue and the extent of damage.[42] Upon progressing to this stage, the active effusion and local erythema of the inflammation stage are no longer present clinically. However, residual effusion may still be present at this time and resist resorption.[43,44]

Remodeling Stage

An optimal wound environment lessens the duration of the inflammatory and proliferative phases and protects fragile tissue from breakdown during early remodeling. The remodeling phase involves a conversion of the initial healing tissue to scar tissue. This lengthy phase of contraction, tissue remodeling, and increasing tensile strength in the wound can last for up to 1 year. Fibroblasts are responsible for the synthesis, deposition, and remodeling of the ECM. Following the deposition of granulation tissue, some fibroblasts are transformed into myofibroblasts, which congregate at the wound margins and start pulling the edges inward, reducing the size of the wound. Increases in collagen types I and III and other aspects of the remodeling process are responsible for wound contraction and visible scar formation. Epithelial cells migrate from the wound edges and continue to migrate until similar cells from the opposite side are met. This contracted tissue, or scar tissue, is functionally inferior to original tissue and is a barrier to diffused oxygen and nutrients.[45] Eventually, the new epidermis becomes toughened by the production of the protein keratin. The visible scar changes color from red or purple that blanches with slight pressure to nonblanchable white as the scar matures.

Imbalances in collagen synthesis and degradation during this phase of healing may result in hypertrophic scarring or keloid formation with superficial wounds. If the healing tissues are kept immobile, the fibrous repair is weak and there are no forces influencing the collagen—if left untreated, the scar formed is less than 20% of its original size.[46] Contraction of the scar results from cross-linking of the collagen fibers and bundles, and adhesions between the immature collagen and surrounding tissues, producing hypomobility. In areas where the skin is loose and mobile, this creates minimal effect. However, in areas such as the dorsum of the hand where there is no extra skin, wound contracture can have a significant effect on function. Consequently, controlled stresses must always be applied to new scar tissue to help prevent it from shortening.[17,33] Scarring that occurs parallel to the line of force of a structure is less vulnerable to reinjury than a scar that is perpendicular to those lines of force.[47]

CLINICAL PEARL

Despite the presence of an intact epithelium at 3–4 weeks after the injury, the tensile strength of the wound has been measured at approximately 25% of its normal value. Several months later, only 70–80% of the strength may be restored.[48] This would appear to demonstrate that the remodeling process may last many months or even years, making it extremely important to continue applying controlled stresses to the tissue long after healing appears to have occurred.[48]

Normally, the remodeling phase is characterized by a progression to pain-free function and activity. Clinically, the chronic inflammatory response is characterized by the signs and symptoms of acute inflammation (redness, heat, edema, and pain), but at a much less pronounced level. In the ideal world, the injured patient makes a smooth transition through the various stages of healing, and the sharp and burning acute pain is replaced by a duller ache, which then subsides to a point where no pain is felt. However, a persistent chronic inflammatory response results in the continued release of inflammatory products and a local proliferation of mononuclear cells. The macrophages remain in the inflamed tissue if the acute inflammation does not resolve, and begin to attract large numbers of fibroblasts, which invade and produce increased quantities of collagen.[11] This failure during the healing phase continuum can result in chronic pathologic changes in the tissue. Often, the increased collagen production results in decreased extensibility of a joint or soft tissue structure. Characteristics of this chronic inflammation include a physiologic response that is resistant to both physical and pharmacologic intervention, resulting in a failure to remodel adequately, an imperfect repair, and a persistence of symptoms.[37,49] In addition, fibrosis can occur in synovial structures, and in extra-articular tissues, including tendons and ligaments; in bursa; or in muscle.

FACTORS THAT IMPACT HEALING

Many factors can determine the outcome of the tissue injury, including those listed in Table 2-1. The focus of the rehabilitation should be to improve an individual's range of motion, flexibility, strength, and coordination to a level that approximate the demands of the desired activity (speed, agility, strength, power, endurance, etc.).

MUSCLE BEHAVIOR, INJURY, HEALING, AND TREATMENT

As outlined in Chapter 1, muscles primarily function to mechanically transmit the forces generated by the skeletal muscle cells to provide movement.

Behavior

There are approximately 430 skeletal muscles in the body, each of which can be considered anatomically as a separate organ. Of these 430 muscles, about 75 pairs provide the majority of body movements and postures.[50] Like any collagenous tissue, the musculotendinous unit exhibits viscoelastic properties (stress relaxation, creep, hysteresis, etc.) allowing it to respond to load and deformation appropriately, with the rate of deformation being directly proportional to the applied force when considering the viscous property. Three important factors can influence muscle performance:[51]

- Age. With aging, the cross-sectional area of muscle decline and the number of muscle fibers decreases by about 39% by age 80.[52] Type I muscle fibers are not affected much by aging, but type II fibers demonstrate a reduction in cross-sectional area of 26% from age 20 to 80, most likely a result of denervation.[53] These changes seem to be

TABLE 2-1 Factors Impacting Healing

Intrinsic (Local)	Systemic	Extrinsic
Extent of injury. Microtears involve only minor damage, whereas macrotears involve significantly greater destruction	Age. The ability to heal injuries decreases with age	Drugs. Nonsteroidal anti-inflammatory drugs and corticosteroids decrease inflammation and swelling, resulting in decreased pain
Edema. Swelling can cause increased pressure that can impede nutrition to the injured part, inhibit neuromuscular control, and retard the healing process	Obesity. Oxygen pressure in the tissues is lower in obese patients.	Absorbent dressings. The degree of humidity greatly affects the process of epithelialization—the epithelium regenerates twice as quickly in a moist environment
Hemorrhage. Bleeding produces the same negative effects on healing as does the accumulation of edema	Malnutrition. Wound healing places a higher than usual demand on a patient's energy resources. In every stage of wound healing, protein is needed. In addition adequate nutritional intake and body stores of all vitamins are essential.	Temperature, and oxygen tension. Hypothermia has a negative effect on healing. Oxygen tension relates to the neovascularization of the wound.
Poor vascular supply. Wounds heal poorly and at a slower rate when the blood supply is inadequate	Hormone levels. Hormones affect the composition and structure of a variety of tissues.	
Separation of tissue. A wound that has smooth edges and good apposition will tend to heal by primary intention with minimal scarring.	Infection. Infection can delay healing	Physical modalities. These can be used to promote an efficient healing environment for an injury when used individually, or in combination with other modalities or exercise
Muscle spasm. Spasm causes traction on the already torn tissue, preventing approximation.	General health. Comorbidity can play a significant role in the overall healing process. For example diabetes can impede tissue healing	Exercise. Exercise can help in the remodeling process of all connective tissues. Wolff's law states that tissue remodeling and the response to therapeutic exercise are determined by the specific adaptation of the tissue to the imposed level of demand.
Atrophy. Considered a secondary impairment to injury and subsequent disuse		
Degree of scarring. Scarring that occurs normally, but hypertrophic scarring produces keloids when the rate of collagen production exceeds the rate of collagen breakdown		

secondary to the declining demand of the muscle and lack of physical activity, and thus can be minimized or even reversed with adequate training.[52]

- Temperature. Collagenous tissues have an inverse temperature-elastic modulus relationship, especially at higher temperatures, which means that temperature elevation results in increased elasticity and decreased stiffness.[54] This would suggest that warming a muscle may confer a protective effect against muscle strain injury as warmer muscles must undergo greater deformation before failure. However, somewhat contradictory, a warm muscle may be prone to injury because it undergoes greater deformation to attain a given load.
- Immobilization or disuse. The effect of rigid immobilization on muscle has been well detailed (see Detrimental Effects of Immobilization later). However the results of restricted motion, in which joint and associated muscles are not allowed to move through the complete range, have not been well studied. Biomechanically, muscle immobilized in a shortened position develops less force and stretches to a shorter length before injury than does a nonimmobilized muscle. Muscle immobilized in a lengthened position responds differently; greater force and a greater change in length are required to cause a tear than in nonimmobilized muscle.

Injury

Muscle injury can result from excessive strain, excessive tension, contusions, lacerations, thermal stress, and myotoxic agents, such as some local anesthetics, excessive use of corticosteroids, and snake and bee venoms.[55] The majority of muscle injuries (>90%) are caused either by excessive strain of the muscle or by contusion.[56] Muscle strains may be graded by severity (Table 2-2). Muscle injuries are the most common injury in sports, with an incidence varying from 10 to 55% of all injuries sustained in sport events.[57,58] A number of factors contribute to muscle strain injury including[51]

- inadequate flexibility
- inadequate strength or endurance
- dyssynergistic muscle contraction
- insufficient warm-up
- inadequate rehabilitation from previous injury.

A distraction strain occurs in a muscle to which an excessive pulling force is applied, resulting in overstretching.[58] A contusion may occur if a muscle is injured by a heavy compressive force, such as a direct blow. At the site of the direct blow, a hematoma may develop. Two types of hematoma can be identified:[59]

1. ***Intramuscular.*** This type of hematoma is associated with a muscle strain or bruise. The size of the hematoma is limited by the muscle fascia. Clinical findings may include pain and loss of function.
2. ***Intermuscular.*** This type of hematoma develops if the muscle fascia is ruptured and the extravasated blood spreads into the interfascial and interstitial spaces. The pain is usually less severe with this type.

TABLE 2-2 Classification of Muscle Injury

Type	Related Factors
Exercise-induced muscle injury (delayed muscle soreness)	Increased activity Unaccustomed activity Excessive eccentric work Viral infections Secondary to muscle cell damage
Strains	
First degree (mild): minimal structural damage; minimal hemorrhage; early resolution	Onset at 24–48 hours after exercise Sudden overstretch Sudden contraction
Second degree (moderate): partial tear; large spectrum of injury; significant early functional loss	Decelerating limb Insufficient warm-up Lack of flexibility
Third degree (severe): complete tear; may require aspiration; may require surgery	Increasing severity of strain associated with greater muscle fiber death, more hemorrhage, and more eventual scarring Steroid use or abuse Previous muscle injury Collagen disease
Contusions Mild, moderate, severe Intramuscular vs. intermuscular	Direct blow, associated with increasing muscle trauma and tearing of fiber proportionate to severity

Data from: Reid DC: *Sports Injury Assessment and Rehabilitation*. New York, NY: Churchill Livingstone, 1992.

Healing

Skeletal muscle has considerable regenerative capabilities, and the process of skeletal muscle regeneration after injury is a well-studied cascade of events.[60–62] The essential process of muscle regeneration is similar, irrespective of the cause of injury, but the outcome and time course of regeneration vary according to the type, severity, and extent of the injury.[60,63,64] Broadly speaking, there are three phases in the healing process of an injured muscle: the destruction phase, the repair phase, and the remodeling phase.[59]

Destruction Phase

The muscle fibers and their connective tissue sheaths are totally disrupted, and a gap appears between the ends of the ruptured muscle fibers when the muscle fibers retract.[62] This phase is characterized by the necrosis of muscle tissue, degeneration, and an infiltration by PMN leukocytes as hematoma and edema form at the site of injury.

Repair Phase

The repair phase usually involves the following steps:

- ***Hematoma formation.*** The gap between the ruptured ends of the fibers is at first filled by a hematoma. During the first day, the hematoma is invaded by inflammatory cells, including phagocytes, which begin disposal of the blood clot.[62]

- *Matrix formation.* Blood-derived fibronectin and fibrin cross-link to form a primary matrix, which acts as a scaffold and anchorage site for the invading fibroblasts.[61,62] The matrix gives the initial strength for wound tissue to withstand the forces applied to it.[65] Fibroblasts begin to synthesize proteins of the ECM.
- *Collagen formation.* The production of type I collagen by fibroblasts increases the tensile strength of the injured muscle. An excessive proliferation of fibroblasts can rapidly lead to an excessive formation of dense scar tissue, which creates a mechanical barrier that restricts or considerably delays complete regeneration of the muscle fibers across the gap.[59,62]

During the first week of healing the injury site is the weakest point of the muscle–tendon unit. This phase also includes regeneration of the striated muscle, production of a connective-tissue scar, and capillary ingrowth. The regeneration of the myofibers begins with the activation of satellite cells, located between the basal lamina and the plasma membrane of each individual myofiber.[66]

Satellite cells, myoblastic precursor cells, proliferate to reconstitute the injured area.[64] During muscle regeneration, it is presumed that trophic substances released by the injured muscle activate the satellite cells.[67] Unlike the multinucleated myofibers, these mononuclear cells maintain mitotic potential and respond to cellular signals by entering the cell cycle to provide the substrate for muscle regeneration and growth.[66]

The satellite cells proliferate and differentiate into multinucleated myotubes and eventually into myofibers, which mature and increase in length and diameter to span the muscle injury. Many of these myoblasts are able to fuse with existing necrosed myofibers and may prevent the muscle fibers from completely degenerating.[66]

The final stage in the regenerative process involves the integration of the neural elements and the formation of a functional neuromuscular junction.[68,69] Provided that the continuity of the muscle fiber is not disrupted and the innervation, vascular supply, and ECM are left intact, muscle will regenerate without loss of normal tissue architecture and function.[70]

Remodeling Phase

In this phase, the regenerated muscle matures and contracts with reorganization of the scar tissue. There is often complete restoration of the functional capacity of the injured muscle.

The pathology of skeletal muscle damage varies, depending on the initiating cause. Muscle damage can occur during the prolonged immobility of hospitalization and from external sources such as mechanical injury.[71] One of the potential consequences of muscle injury is atrophy. The amount of muscle atrophy that occurs depends on the usage prior to bed rest and the function of the muscle.[71] Antigravity muscles (such as the quadriceps) tend to have greater potential for atrophy than antagonist muscles (such as the hamstrings). Research has shown that a single bout of exercise protects against muscle damage, with the effects lasting between 6 weeks[72] and 9 months.[73]

Muscle resistance to damage may result from an eccentric exercise-induced morphologic change in the number of sarcomeres connected in series.[74] This finding appears to support initiating a reconditioning program with gradual progression from lower intensity activities with minimal eccentric actions to protect against muscle damage.[71,75]

Treatment

The tensile strength of the healing muscle tissue increases over time. However, whereas normal intramuscular collagenous tissue has a greater proportion of type I collagen than type III collagen, initially after injury, type III collagen demonstrates a significant increase over type I collagen in the area of repair. Over time, the proportion of type I to type III collagen returns to normal. Controlled mobility and stress are key considerations in the post injury period to allow scar formation, muscle regeneration, correct orientation of new muscle fibers, and the normalization of the tensile properties of muscle. The following principles should guide the clinician when rehabilitating a muscle injury:[51]

- Prevention is easier than treatment.
- Intervention depends on the stage of healing.
- Controlled mobility and activity are best.
- Medications and modalities are important adjuncts to care.
- It is important to develop strong, flexible tissue using pain as the guiding factor.

Muscle and Aging

With age, there is a reduction in the ability to produce and sustain muscular power. This age-related phenomenon, termed *senescence sarcopenia*, can result in a 20–25% loss of skeletal muscle mass.[76]

CLINICAL PEARL

Sarcopenia (*sarco* = muscle, *penia* = lack of) is not a disease, but rather refers specifically to the universal, involuntary decline in lean body mass that occurs with age, primarily as a result of the loss of skeletal muscle.

Sarcopenia has important consequences. The loss of lean body mass reduces function, and loss of approximately 40% of lean body mass is fatal.[77,78] Sarcopenia is distinct from wasting—involuntary weight loss resulting from inadequate intake, which is seen in starvation, advanced cancer, or acquired immunodeficiency syndrome.

While a variety of studies have investigated the underlying mechanisms and treatments of age-related muscle loss, very few epidemiologic studies have looked at the prevalence, incidence, pathogenesis, and consequences of sarcopenia in elderly populations. It is likely that the determinants of sarcopenia are multifactorial and include genetic factors, environmental factors, and age-related changes in muscle tissue.[79]

The effects of aging on muscle morphology have been studied. Aging causes a decrease in muscle volume,[80] with type II fiber apparently being more affected by gradual atrophy.[81] Specifically, there is a disproportionate atrophy of type IIa muscle fibers with aging. These losses of muscular strength and muscle mass can have important health consequences, because they can predispose the elderly to disability, an increased risk of falls and hip fractures, and a decrease in bone mineral density.

CLINICAL PEARL

When older people maintain muscular activity, the losses in strength with age are reduced substantially. Age-related muscle fiber atrophy and weakness may be completely reversed in some individuals with resistance training.

TENDON BEHAVIOR, INJURY, HEALING, AND TREATMENT

As outlined in Chapter 1, tendons primarily function to transmit force between muscle and bone.[82]

Behavior

The organization of the tendon determines its mechanical behavior. Because tendons have more parallel collagen fibers than ligaments, and less realignment occurs during initial loading, the toe region of the load-deformation curve is smaller in tendons than in ligaments.[83] As force is applied to the tendon, a straightening of the crimp results in the toe region in the load-deformation curve, where little force is required to change tendon length.[82] As the load increases beyond the toe region, the collagen fibrils stretch, creating the linear region of the load-deformation curve.[82] Most tendons likely function in the toe and early linear regions under physiological loading conditions.[84] The total amount of load the tendon can resist and the amount it stretches during loading depend on its cross-sectional area, composition, and length. However, tendons can adapt structurally or materially to changes in the mechanical environment as a result of load conditions.[84] The compliance of tendons varies. Tendons of the digital flexors and extensors are very stiff, and their length changes very little when muscle forces are applied through them. In contrast, the tendons of some muscles, particularly those involved in locomotion and ballistic performance, are more elastic. For example, the Achilles tendon is stretched during the late stance phase in gait as the triceps surae is stretched as the ankle dorsiflexes. Near the beginning of the plantar flexion contraction, the muscle activation ceases and energy stored in the stretched tendon helps to initiate plantar flexion.

CLINICAL PEARL

As the amount of crimp in a tendon decreases with age, the toe region becomes smaller.

Injury

Tendons that transmit large loads under eccentric and elastic conditions are more subject to injury.[85] Most tendon injuries tend to occur from loading (sudden overload or repetitive), or rapid unloading. However, mechanical overload does not seem to be the only factor to explain a tendon injury and may even be merely a permissive factor, allowing the tendon problem to become symptomatic.[86]

CLINICAL PEARL

Tendons become weaker, stiffer, and less yielding as a result of the vascular, cellular, and collagen-related alterations that occur with aging.[83]

While it is easy to understand why a sudden overload could damage a tendon, it is not fully understood why the application of normal loads, repeated frequently, cause tendon damage. Repetitive loading can occur as a result of external factors, such as anatomic predisposition resulting from inflexibility, weakness, or malposition, excessive compression and friction.[87–89]

CLINICAL PEARL

Rapid force application or release is more likely to cause tendon damage than the same load applied gradually.[90]

Muscle physiology experiments have shown the force increases as the velocity of active muscle lengthening (eccentric) increases, while the opposite is true during concentric (shortening) muscle activations (see Chap. 1). Indeed, the tendon is exposed to larger loads during eccentric loading, especially if the movement occurs rapidly.[91,92] Almost all concentric contractions are preceded by a lengthening (eccentric) while the muscle is active. This activation pattern stretches the elastic elements in the muscle–tendon unit and contributes to movement *if* the muscle is allowed to immediately shorten after being lengthened.[84]

CLINICAL PEARL

Estimates of the Bureau of Labor Statistics[93] indicate that chronic tendon injuries account for 48% of reported occupational illnesses, whereas overuse injuries in sports account for 30–50% of all sports injuries.[94]

Terminology regarding tendon pathology has been somewhat confusing. Tendon injuries are typically classified as either acute or chronic.

- *Acute injuries.* Acute injuries include those in which the time and method of injury are known.[84] Acute injuries include tendon rupture and partial tendon tears. The term *tendinitis* implies an acute inflammatory reaction of the tendon, which is described as a microscopic tearing and inflammation of the tendon tissue, commonly resulting from tissue fatigue rather than direct trauma. Tendinitis can be graded according to severity:

- Grade I: Pain only after activity; does not interfere with performance; often generalized tenderness; disappears before the next exercise session.
- Grade II: Minimal pain with activity; does not interfere with intensity or distance; usually localized tenderness.
- Grade III: Pain interferes with activity; usually disappears between sessions; definite local tenderness.
- Grade IV: Pain does not disappear between activity sessions; seriously interferes with intensity of training; significant local signs of pain, tenderness, crepitus, and swelling.
- Grade V: Pain interferes with sport and activities of daily living; symptoms often chronic or recurrent; signs of tissue changes and altered associated muscle function.

- *Chronic injuries.* Chronic tendon injuries are not typically associated with a known onset or with inflammation, but involve repetitive loading that damages the tendon. Chronic injuries of the tendon can be separated into superficial and intratendon pathology. *Paratenonitis* is an inflammation of the outermost layer of the tendon, and may be accompanied by synovitis of the tendon sheath, referred to as *tenosynovitis. Tendinosis* is an intratendinous degenerative lesion without an inflammatory component (the suffix "-osis" is indicative of a degenerative process rather than an inflammatory disorder). Although these two pathologic processes can occur together, they are generally regarded as distinct independent conditions.[95]

CLINICAL PEARL

The term *tendinopathy* has been used to describe any abnormal condition of the tendon.

A tendinosis is characterized by the presence of dense populations of fibroblasts, vascular hyperplasia, and disorganized collagen.[96] The disorganized collagen is termed *angiofibroblastic hyperplasia*.[97] Degenerative tendinopathy occurs in approximately one-third of the population older than 35 years of age.[98] Although it is commonly presumed that pain results from an inflamed structure, it is not clear why tendinosis is painful, given the absence of acute inflammatory cells, nor is it known why the collagen fails to mature. Necropsy studies have shown that these degenerative changes also may be present in asymptomatic tendons.[99] The degree of degeneration increases with age and may represent part of the normal aging process.[100] The degeneration appears to be activity related, as well.[100]

The typical clinical finding for tendinopathy is a strong but painful response to resistance of the involved musculotendinous structure.

Healing

Acute tendon injuries that disrupt vascular tissues within the tendon result in a well studied healing process involving three overlapping phases:[101]

- Inflammation: this occurs as a hematoma forms within erythrocytes and activated platelets. This is followed by the infiltration of inflammatory cells, including neutrophils, monocytes, and macrophages that migrate to the injury site to remove debris. Shortly after, chemotactic signals induce fibroblasts to start synthesizing collagen.[95]
- Repair: this phase involves the deposition of collagen and tendon matrix components.
- Remodeling: during this phase the collagen becomes more structured and organized, although the injured site never achieves the original histologic or mechanical features of a healthy uninjured tendon.

Unlike most soft tissue healing, healing tendons pose a particular problem as they require both extensibility and flexibility at the site of attachment.[16,102–104] Following injury, the initial inflammatory stage triggers an increase in glycosaminoglycans (GAG) synthesis within days, rapidly followed by synthesis of types I and III collagen, such that the healing wound can be subjected to low levels of force within a matter of days.[84,102–105]

Treatment

While the treatment for tendinopathy is relatively straightforward, tendinopathies are difficult to grade in terms of providing guidance for treatment or prognosis. In either case, a judicious application of force must be used to encourage the new collagen fibrils to align in the direction of force application.[84] The major difference between the treatment of a tendinitis and a tendinosis is that controlling inflammation is the focus of the former, whereas loading based rehabilitation is the focus of the latter. Table 2-3 outlines some guidelines for treatment. Treatment of tendinosis involves a multifaceted approach, which includes[84]

- the identification and removal of all negative internal and/or external forces/factors
- the establishment of a stable baseline for treatment
- the determination of the tensile load starting point
- a progression of the loading program according to the patient's symptoms. Studies have shown that exercise, particularly eccentric-based exercise (Table 2-3), has positive effects on the mechanical and structural properties of tendons:
  - Nakamura and colleagues[106] demonstrated that eccentric exercises contributed to stable angiogenesis in early tendon injury whereas concentric exercises did not. Daily eccentric exercises were clinically beneficial and not harmful to tendon microcirculation.
  - Knobloch and colleagues[107] showed in a controlled study that in tendinosis lesions, an eccentric loading program resulted in a significant decrease in the paratenon vascularity and pain while not changing the oxygen saturation of the paratenon tissues.
  - Shalabi and colleagues[108] demonstrated decreased tendon volume, decreased MRI signal in the tendinosis lesions, and improved clinical pain scores in patients with Achilles tendinosis who were treated with eccentric training regimens.

TABLE 2-3 Eccentric-Based Treatment for Chronic Tendinopathy

Principles and Method	Description
1. Warm-up	A generalized exercise such as cycling or like jogging that does not cause local pain or discomfort Local heating modality, such as hot pack ultrasound
2. Stretching to improve flexibility	A minimum of two 30 second static stretches of the involved musculotendinous unit and its antagonist(s)
3. Completion of the specific eccentric exercise	Three sets of 10 repetitions, with a brief rest or stretch between each set. Symptoms should be felt after 20 repetitions (i.e., between 20 and 30 repetitions) at a level similar to that felt during activities. -If pain is felt before the 20th repetition, either the speed of movement is reduced, or the load is decreased -If no pain is experienced by 30 repetitions, the speed or load is increased. The intensity of subsequent treatments is based on the patient's response to the previous treatment
4. Repeat flexibility exercises	See step 2
5. Apply ice	Ice is applied for 10–15 min. to the painful to palpation area

Data from Curwin SL: Tendon pathology and injuries: Pathophysiology, healing, and treatment considerations. In: Magee D, Zachazewski JE, Quillen WS, eds. *Scientific Foundations and Principles of Practice in Musculoskeletal Rehabilitation*. St. Louis, MI: WB Saunders, 2007:47–78.

Conversely, immobilization adversely affects the biomechanical properties of a tendon, resulting in decreased tensile strength, increased stiffness, and a reduction in total weight.[83]

- The control of pain.
- Addressing the entire kinetic chain.

In addition, other modes of conservative treatment can be incorporated including:[95]

- Extracorporeal shockwave therapy (ESWT). Chen and colleagues[109] demonstrated that ESWT promoted tendon healing in a collagenase induced tendinopathy of a rat tendon. Rompe and colleagues[110] showed in a randomized controlled trial that eccentric exercise, combined with ESWT, was more effective than eccentric exercise alone. In contrast, Zwerver and colleagues[111] found that when ESWT was used as a solitary treatment during the competitive season it demonstrated no benefit over placebo treatment in the management of actively competing jumping athletes with patellar tendinopathy who had symptoms for less than 12 months.[112]
- Nonsteroidal anti-inflammatory agents (NSAIDs) and corticosteroids. Although steroids have been commonly used in the treatment of tendinosis, their benefit appears to be limited to short-term improvement in pain (i.e., <6 weeks), as there is no evidence to suggest long-term improvement.[113] This lack of efficacy is likely explained by the absence of inflammation as a significant factor in tendinosis pathology.
- Sclerosing treatments. Several studies have demonstrated that sclerosing treatment aids in the neovascularization of tendinosis lesions.[114,115]
- Platelet-rich plasma (PRP). PRP appears to be a promising intervention for tendinosis lesions.[116,117]
- Nitric oxide. Nitric oxide is an important cell signal molecule, and appears to be involved in numerous tissue types' responses to mechanical loading, modulating tendon healing, and collagen synthesis.[118]
- Matrix metalloproteinase inhibitors. This is a recent intervention for tendinosis. Matrix metalloproteinase inhibitors aim to decrease the catabolic enzymatic activity in tendinosis lesions.[119]

If the patient fails to improve completely within 6–14 weeks, the clinician must consider the following possibilities:[84]

- Incorrect loading magnitude or progression
- Incorrect diagnosis
- Noncompliance
- An unrecognized external factor.

LIGAMENT BEHAVIOR, INJURY, HEALING, AND TREATMENT

As outlined in Chapter 1, ligaments function to bind bones together at or near the margins of bony articulation.

Behavior

Because of their function as joint stabilizers, when a ligament is damaged, there is a loss of normal kinematic relationships between the connected bones, with the degree of loss based on severity. Structural changes occur in ligaments as a function of age. In middle-age, both ligaments and bone insertion sites begin to weaken, resulting in progressive losses in structural strength, and in the elderly ligaments lose mass, stiffness, strength, and viscosity.[5] Hormone levels can also affect ligaments producing gender-specific alterations. For example, it has been reported that joint and ligament laxity can change during pregnancy due to the presence of the hormone relaxin, and during different phases of the menstrual cycle.[120,121] Finally, ligament complexes are extremely sensitive to load and load history, such that load deprivation causes a rapid deterioration in ligament biochemical and mechanical properties, which results in a net loss in ligament strength and stiffness.[122–124] Conversely, movement has been shown to

TABLE 2-4 Ligament Injuries

Grade	Description	Signs and Symptoms	Implications
I (mild)	Some stretching or tearing of the ligamentous fibers	Mild pain Little or no swelling Some joint stiffness Minimal loss of structural integrity No abnormal motion Minimal bruising	Minimal functional loss Early return to training-some protection may be necessary
II (moderate)	Some tearing and separation of the ligamentous fibers	Moderate to severe pain Joint stiffness Significant structural weakening with abnormal motion Often associated hemarthrosis and effusion	Tendency to recurrence Need protection from risk of further injury May need modified immobilization May stretch out further with time
III (complete)	Total rupture of the ligament	Severe pain initially followed by little or no pain (total disruption of nerve fibers) Profuse swelling and bruising Loss of structural integrity with marked abnormal motion	Needs prolonged protection Surgery may be considered Often permanent functional instability

maintain normal ligament behavior, although it is not clear how much movement is required to maintain baseline ligament behaviors.[125] Exercise appears to increase ligament strength and stiffness.

Injury

In any particular position of a joint, several ligaments around the joints are likely to be in a taut state. If an external load is then applied to that joint, those ligaments that are taut will absorb the greatest amount of energy. If the load is sufficient to deform a taut ligament past its elastic (recovery) limit, the ligament will fail, and other ligaments, or structures will simultaneously become recruited into tension.[5] Depending on the size of the load, subsequent injury may also occur to these other ligaments, or structures. It is, therefore, unlikely for a truly *isolated* ligament injury ever to occur.[5] Point tenderness, joint effusion, and a history of trauma, are all characteristic of a ligamentous injury. Ligament injuries, referred to as sprains, may be graded by severity (Table 2-4). Stress tests applied perpendicular to the normal plane of joint motion can help distinguish between grade II and grade III ligament injuries. In grade III injuries, significant joint gapping occurs with the application of the stress test.[126] However, because of patient discomfort and guarding against possible pain, it is difficult to assess joint laxity by clinical examination alone. Currently, clinicians often use ancillary tests such as arthrometry or magnetic resonance imaging when diagnosing and grading soft tissue injuries.

Healing

The process of ligament healing follows the same course of repair as with other vascular tissues. However, intra-articular ligaments such as the anterior cruciate ligament (ACL) do not heal as well as extra-articular ligaments, because intra-articular ligaments have a limited blood supply and the synovial fluid may significantly hinder an inflammatory response.[83] The healing of extra-articular ligaments, however, occurs in four overlapping phases.

Phase I: Hemorrhagic

After disruption of the tissue, the gap is filled quickly with a blood clot (hematoma). PMN leukocytes and lymphocytes appear within several hours, triggered by cytokines released within the clot. The PMN leukocytes and lymphocytes respond to autocrine and paracrine signals to expand the inflammatory response and recruit other types of cells to the wound.[69]

Phase II: Inflammatory

Macrophages arrive within 24 –48 hours and are the predominant cell type within several days. Macrophages perform phagocytosis of necrotic tissues and also secrete multiple types of growth factors that induce neovascularization and the formation of granulation tissue. By the third day after injury, the wound contains macrophages, PMN leukocytes, lymphocytes, and multipotential mesenchymal cells, growth factors, and platelets. The growth factors are not only chemotactic for fibroblasts and other cells, but also stimulate fibroblast proliferation and the synthesis of collagen types I, III, and V, as well as noncollagenous proteins.[127,128]

Phase III: Proliferation

The last cell type to arrive within the wound is the fibroblast. Although debate continues, it currently is thought that fibroblasts are recruited from neighboring tissue and the systemic circulation.[129] These fibroblasts have abundant rough endoplastic reticulum and begin producing collagen and other matrix proteins within 1 week of injury. By the second week after disruption, the original blood clot becomes more organized because of cellular and matrix proliferation. Capillary buds begin to form. Total collagen content is greater than in the normal ligament or tendon, but collagen concentration is lower and the matrix remains disorganized.

Phase IV: Remodeling and Maturation

Phase IV is marked by a gradual decrease in the cellularity of the healed tissue. The matrix becomes denser and longitudinally oriented. Collagen turnover, water content, and the ratio of collagen types I to III begin to approach normal levels over several months.[130] An integrated sequence of biochemical and biomechanical signals are critical to ligament remodeling. These signals regulate the expression of structural and enzymatic proteins, including degradation enzymes such as collagenase, stromelysin, and plasminogen activator.[127] The healed tissue continues to mature but will never attain normal morphologic characteristics or mechanical properties. Ligament injuries can take as long as 3 years to heal to the point of regaining near-normal tensile strength,[131] although some tensile strength is regained by about the fifth week following injury, depending on the severity.[19,132–134] A ligament may have 50% of its normal tensile strength by 6 months after injury, 80% after 1 year, and 100% only after 1–3 years.[135–137]

Treatment

Immobilization and disuse dramatically compromise the structural material properties of ligaments, resulting in a significant decrease in the ability to resist strains and absorb energy.[83] Forces applied to the ligament during its recovery help it to develop strength in the direction that the force is applied.[135–139] Several studies have shown that actively exercised ligaments are stronger than those that are immobilized thus, it is important to minimize periods of immobilization and progressively stress the injured ligaments while exercising caution relative to biomechanical considerations for specific ligaments.[140] The current concept is that very low cyclical loads on ligaments promote scar proliferation and material remodeling, thus making the scar stronger and stiffer structurally[141,142] and, possibly, materially.[5] In conjunction with exercise it appears that the use of ice immediately after ligament injury decreases bleeding, swelling, and inflammation,[143] whereas heat, used after the first 48 hours appears to increase blood flow. However it is not known whether ice or heat have any effect on scar formation, or on the quality or quantity of ligament healing.

The surgical repair of torn ligament ends has been noted in the past to induce faster and stronger healing through a process that is likened to regeneration rather than scar formation.[5,144] However, although surgically repaired extra-articular ligaments heal with decreased scar formation and are generally stronger than unrepaired ligaments initially, this strength advantage might not be maintained as time progresses.[16]

Currently, a number of biological approaches are being used to improve ligament repair including the use of growth factors and gene therapy:[5]

- Growth factors. Growth factors are molecules that modify cell proliferation or the secretion of proteins. Thus far, the uses of growth factors in ligament healing have demonstrated variable results.
- Gene therapy. Gene therapy refers to the modification of the genetic expression of cells. Introduction of marker and therapeutic genes into ligaments using vectors has demonstrated initial success with evidence of functional alterations.[145] In addition, gene transfer has been used to manipulate the healing environment, opening the possibility of gene transfer to investigate ligament development.[145]

JOINT BEHAVIOR, INJURY, HEALING, AND TREATMENT

The amount of motion available at a joint is based on a number of factors, including the shape of the articulating surfaces, the health of the joint and the surrounding tissues, and the load-deformation history of the joint. In order to discuss these concepts, it is important to have an understanding of the normal barriers that can be felt during movement. Three distinct areas or zones are recognized:[146]

- Neutral zone: the zone in which there is little or no internal resistance offered by the tissues to movement and the range in which the crimp of the tissue is being taken up. Increases in the size of the neutral zone result in the feeling or perception that the crimp is taken up later in the range of motion. Such increases can occur because of injury, and joint instability, joint degeneration, muscle dysfunction (leading to loss of muscular control of the movement).[147] In contrast, the size of the neutral zone may be decreased by osteophyte formation, surgical fusion, muscle spasm, muscle strengthening, or adaptive tissue shortening.
- Elastic zone: the zone in which the first barrier or restriction of movement occurs. This zone occurs at the end of the neutral zone after the crimp has been taken up and tension starts to build within the tissues. The elastic zone extends from the crimp area through the physiological barrier (end of active movement) and toward the anatomic barrier (end of passive movement). The elastic zone can be increased by injury to the joint structures, mobilization techniques, and muscle lengthening, and be decreased by osteophyte formation, surgical fusion or repair, muscle hypertrophy, or immobilization.
- Plastic zone: the zone in which deformation of the tissues is extended beyond the tissues elastic recoil and the tissue begins to deform. If the deformation is sufficient, injury may occur.

Behavior

A door hinge and doorstop are a good analogy when describing joint motion behavior, in which the hinge represents the joint, and the doorstop represents the restriction imposed by the integrity of the joint and the surrounding tissues. Just as the doorstop prevents the door from swinging too far and damaging the wall, the integrity of the joint and its surrounding structures serve to prevent the joint moving past the normal range of motion and incurring injury.

Three descriptors are used to describe normal and abnormal joint motion:

- Hypomobile. If the movement of a joint is less than that considered normal, or when compared with the same joint on the opposite extremity, it may be deemed *hypomobile*. Hypomobility can be secondary to any of the following:[148]

- Joint fixation. This can occur when the joint is stuck at the extreme of range of motion secondary to a sudden macrotrauma, a prolonged or repeated microtrauma, or a microtrauma imposed on instability. Clinical findings associated with a joint fixation include limitation of gross motion or conjunct rotation toward the limitation. Also the clinician notes that the end feel in the direction opposite the fixation is abnormal and has a rather firm capsular end feel (see Chap. 4).
- Myofascial hypomobility. This is caused by muscle shortening (scars, contracture, or adaptive tissue changes). Clinical findings for myofascial hypomobility include an elastic end feel and a constant-length phenomenon. The constant length phenomenon occurs when the amount of movement available at one joint is dependent upon the position in which another joint is held. For example, during a supine straight leg raise, due to the anatomy (length) of the hamstrings, the amount of available hip flexion is decreased if the knee is maintained in a fully extended position as opposed to when the knee is allowed to flex.
- Articular hypomobility. This can be caused by intra-articular swelling or an intra-articular bleed. Clinical findings for an articular hypomobility include a spasm, or empty end feel, often accompanied with a capsular pattern (see Chap. 4).
- Pericapsular hypomobility. This is caused by capsular or ligamentous shortening, which creates a capsular pattern of restriction that does not demonstrate the constant length phenomenon. In addition a premature firm/hard capsular end feel exists if the joint is not inflamed, or possibly a spasm end feel if the joint is inflamed.

► Hypermobile. A joint that moves more than is considered normal, or when compared with the same joint on the opposite extremity may be deemed *hypermobile*. Laxity, a function of the ligament and joint capsule resistance, is a term used to imply that an individual has excessive joint range of motion, but has the ability to control the movement of the joint in that extra range. Hypermobility may occur as a generalized phenomenon or be localized to just one direction of movement, as follows:

- *Generalized hypermobility*. The more generalized form of hypermobility, as its name suggests, refers to the manifestations of multiple joint hyperlaxity, joint hypermobility, or articular hypermobility. This type of hypermobility can be seen in acrobats, gymnasts, and those individuals who are "double jointed." In addition, generalized hypermobility occurs with genetic diseases that include joint hypermobility as an associated finding, such as Ehlers–Danlos syndrome, osteogenesis imperfecta, and Marfan's syndrome.
- *Localized hypermobility*. Localized hypermobility is likely to occur as a reaction to neighboring stiffness. For example, a compensatory hypermobility may occur at a joint when a neighboring joint or segment is injured. The injury to the neighboring joint results in a decrease in motion at the injured joint. This decrease in movement of the neighboring joint is often the result of the body's initial response to trauma, which is a reflexive increase in tone of muscles in an attempt to stabilize the affected area. Over time, the prolonged increased tonus may result in a decreased blood supply and an increase in the buildup of lactic acid. In addition, the nociceptor's response in the muscle or the joint capsule may result in an inhibition of the segmental muscles, which, in turn, may lead to uncoordinated movements and produce myofascial trigger points.

CLINICAL PEARL

A distinction must be made between laxity, hypermobility, and flexibility.

- Laxity: a normal finding unless associated with symptoms.
- Hypermobility: a laxity associated with symptoms manifested by the patient's inability to control the joint during movement, especially at end range.[149]
- Flexibility is a function of contractile tissue resistance primarily, but is also a function of ligament and joint capsule resistance (see Chap. 13). Two types are recognized:[149]
  - Static: related to the available range of motion in one or more joints.
  - Dynamic: related to stiffness and ease of movement.

► Unstable. The term *instability*, specifically related to the joint, has been the subject of much research.[150–165] In contrast to a hypermobile joint, an unstable joint is associated with a potential or real pathologic state as it involves a disruption of the osseous and ligamentous structures of that joint as the result of some applied external load. Instability implies that an individual has increased joint range of motion but does not have the ability to stabilize the joint (loss of neuromuscular control). This loss of control results in pain, weakness, and transitory deformity. Joint stability may be viewed as a factor of joint integrity, elastic energy, passive stiffness, and muscle activation.

- *Joint integrity*. Joint integrity is enhanced in those ball-and-socket joints with deeper sockets or steeper sides, as opposed to those that are planar and shallower. Joint integrity is also dependent on the attributes of the supporting structures around the joint and the extent of any joint disease.
- *Muscle activation*. Muscles and tendons (see Chap. 1) can provide static stabilization (isometric contraction) and dynamic stabilization (agonist concentric and antagonist eccentric contractions—see Chap. 12). Passive stability can also be provided when the contractile unit is on stretch. Intrinsic muscle factors affecting stabilization include temporal summation, length tension relationships, force velocity relationships, and muscle architecture (see Chap. 1). Muscle activation can provide two forms of stabilization through the use of stabilizer and mobilizer muscles. The stabilizer muscles contract first to provide a

stable base from which the mobilizer muscles can function to position a joint for functional use. In the spine, the stabilizer muscles are divided into two groups: local stabilizers and global stabilizers (see Chap. 28).[146] From a rehabilitation standpoint, before retraining the mobilizer muscles, the clinician must ensure that the stabilizer muscles are performing correctly. This is the concept behind core stabilization or stabilization retraining progressions (see Chaps. 12 and 14).

- *Passive stiffness.* Passive stiffness is provided by the ligaments, capsules, skin, joints, bones, and other collagenous tissue. An injury to these passive structures causing inherent loss in the passive stiffness results in joint laxity.[166] Individual joints have passive stiffness that increases toward the joint end range. Dysfunction of the passive system is due most commonly to mechanical injury, overuse or repetitive stress, joint degeneration, or a disease process (e.g., rheumatoid arthritis).[146]
- *Muscle activation.* The central and peripheral nervous systems provide control through neural feedforward and feedback mechanisms from both active (muscle spindles, Golgi tendon organs) and passive systems (joint afferents) all of which help determine position, load, and joint demands while simultaneously controlling the contractile system to initiate conscious and unconscious movement (see Chap. 3).[146] Muscle activation increases stiffness, both within the muscle and within the joint(s) it crosses.[167] However, the synergist and antagonist muscles that cross the joint must be activated with the correct and appropriate activation in terms of magnitude or timing. A faulty motor control system may lead to inappropriate magnitudes of muscle force and stiffness, allowing a joint to buckle or undergo shear translation.[167]

Pathologic breakdown of the above factors may result in *clinical instability*. Instability is most obvious in movements that are executed too quickly or in cases where the loads placed on the joint are too great for the patient to control. For assessment purposes, instability can be divided into three types:

- Translational: refers to a loss of control of the small, arthrokinematic joint movements that occur when the patient attempts to stabilize the joint during movement.
- Anatomical: refers to excessive or gross physiological movement in the joint, which can lead to abnormal patterns of coupled and translational movements.[168]
- Functional: occurs when the severity of the instability adversely affects a patient's function and can include both translational and anatomical instability. Functional instability may result in[169–171] the following:
  - Long-term nonacute pain or short-term episodic pain;
  - Early morning stiffness;
  - Inconsistent function and dysfunction (e.g., full range of motion but abnormal movement, which may include angulation, hinging, or deviation);
  - A feeling of apprehension or giving way.

Methods to enhance joint stability are provided in Chapter 12.

Injury

Using the door hinge and stop analogy again, it can be seen that both too much motion (resulting in damage to the wall) and too little motion (resulting in an inability to get through the door opening) can be disadvantageous. Similar consequences can be seen at a joint: a hypermobile joint may have insufficient stability to prevent damage occurring, whereas a hypomobile joint may provide insufficient motion at the joint for it to be functional. Hypermobile joints usually preserve their stability under normal conditions, remaining functional in weight bearing, and within certain limits of motion.

Pathologic barriers, which can occur anywhere in the range of motion, are restrictions to movement that occur as a result of a pathologic process. The causes of pathologic barriers include microtrauma or macrotrauma, muscle spasm, edema, pain, and adaptive shortening or lengthening of the tissue. Three types of pathologic barriers are recognized:[146]

- Motion barrier. This type of barrier is related to muscle hypertonus, muscle spasm, adaptive muscle shortening, or muscle pain.
- Collagen barrier. This type of barrier results from a pathologic process affecting collagenous tissues, and usually results in adaptive shortening or pain, shifting the motion barrier to the left (earlier into the range of motion), resulting in a decrease in range of motion.
- Neurodynamic barrier. This type of barrier is the result of a pathologic process of neural tissues that must undergo lengthening and shortening in the course of range of motion and is manifested by the presence of neurological signs that commonly restrict movement (see Chap. 11).

Healing

The healing of the joint surfaces, or joint cartilage, is described in the next section (Cartilage Behavior, Injury, Healing, and Treatment).

Treatment

It is essential to distinguish patients who have greater mobility in all their joints (generalized hypermobility) from those who for some other reason have one or a few joints that are more mobile than the rest (localized hypermobility). While intervention is unlikely to be either warranted or of benefit with generalized hypermobility, the intervention for a localized hypermobility should address any neighboring *hypomobility*.

ARTICULAR CARTILAGE BEHAVIOR, INJURY, HEALING, AND TREATMENT

Behavior

In adults, the articular cartilage matrix is separated from the subchondral vascular spaces by the subchondral plate. Nutrition of the articular cartilage occurs by diffusion from the synovial fluid. Without a direct supply of nutrients from blood vessels or lymphatics, chondrocytes depend primarily on anaerobic metabolism. Chondrocytes are responsible for the development, maintenance, and repair of the ECM by a group with degradative enzymes (see Chap. 1). Chondrocytes in loaded joints experience hydrostatic compressive, tensile, and shear forces.

CLINICAL PEARL

Age determines the composition of the ECM as well as the organization of chondrocytes and their response to external factors such as cytokines.[172] With increasing age, there are zonal changes in the distribution of chondrocytes, although the total number of chondrocytes remains essentially unchanged. However, with increasing age, there is a decrease in the hydration of the matrix, with a corresponding increase in compressive stiffness resulting in increased forces for the underlying subchondral bone.[173]

Provided these forces are applied at an appropriate level, normal articular cartilage structure, and function will be maintained. Specifically, intermittent hydrostatic pressure is believed to maintain healthy cartilage in contrast to shear stresses, prolonged static loading, or the absence of loading.[174] In contrast, immobilization results in degenerative changes that are similar to those seen in osteoarthritis. The development of disease such as osteoarthritis is associated with dramatic changes in cartilage metabolism. This occurs when there is a physiological imbalance of degradation and synthesis by chondrocytes.[175]

The biomechanical behaviors of articular cartilage are best understood when the tissue is used as a biphasic medium.[173] Articular cartilage consists of two phases: a fluid phase and a solid phase. Water is the principal component of the fluid phase, contributing up to 80% of the wet weight of the tissue. The solid phase is characterized by the ECM, which is porous and permeable.[176] The relationship between proteoglycan aggregates and interstitial fluid provides compressive resistance to cartilage through negative electrostatic repulsion forces.[173] The initial and rapid application of articular contact forces during joint loading causes an immediate increase in interstitial fluid pressure, which causes the fluid to flow out of the ECM, generating a large frictional drag on the matrix.[177] This fluid pressure provides a significant component of total load support, thereby reducing the stress acting upon the solid collagen–proteoglycan matrix.[178] When the compressive load is removed, interstitial fluid flows back into the tissue. The low permeability of articular cartilage prevents fluid from being quickly squeezed out of the matrix, and the two opposing bones and surrounding cartilage confine the cartilage under the contact surface, which serves to restrict mechanical deformation.[173]

Articular cartilage is viscoelastic and exhibits time-dependent behavior when subjected to a constant local deformation.[54]

Injury

As articular cartilage is avascular, it is not capable of producing an inflammatory response, which is an important component of repair. Multiple factors are involved in cartilage breakdown including[174]

- an imbalance between ECM synthesis and degradation
- stress deprivation (immobilization, bed rest)
- developmental etiologies leading to abnormal force transmission (developmental hip dysplasia, coxa valgus, genu valgum)
- joint surface incongruously and joint instability
- disease (rheumatoid arthritis)

Injuries to articular cartilage can be divided into three distinct types:

- Type 1 injuries (superficial) involve microscopic damage to the chondrocytes and ECM (cell injury).
- Type 2 injuries (partial thickness) involve microscopic disruption of the articular cartilage surface (chondral fractures or fissuring).[83] This type of injury has traditionally had an extremely poor prognosis because the injury does not penetrate the subchondral bone and, therefore, does not provoke an inflammatory response.[83]
- Type 3 injuries (full-thickness) involve disruption of the articular cartilage with penetration into the subchondral bone, which produces a significant inflammatory process.[83]

Healing

The body's response to articular cartilage defects resulting from trauma upon impact loading depends on the lesion depth.[174] However, it is well known that the capacity of cartilage for repair is limited. The healing of articular cartilage is described here. Injuries of the articular cartilage that do not penetrate the subchondral bone become necrotic and do not heal. These lesions usually progress to the degeneration of the articular surface.[179] Although a short-lived tissue response may occur, it fails to provide sufficient cells and matrix to repair even small defects.[180,181]

Injuries that penetrate the subchondral bone undergo repair as a result of access to the blood supply of the bone. These repairs usually are characterized as fibrous, fibrocartilaginous, or hyaline-like cartilaginous, depending on the species, the age, and the location and size of the injury.[182] However, these reparative tissues, even those that resemble hyaline cartilage histologically, differ from normal hyaline cartilage both biochemically and biomechanically. Thus, by 6 months, fibrillation, fissuring, and extensive degenerative changes occur in the reparative tissues of approximately half of the full-thickness defects.[183,184] Similarly, the degenerated cartilage seen in osteoarthrosis does not usually undergo repair but instead progressively deteriorates.[179]

CLINICAL PEARL

Viscosupplementation, or intra-articular injections of hyaluronic acid, has been used to treat osteoarthritis. The proposed mechanisms of action results in the physical properties of the hyaluronic acid, as well as the anti-inflammatory, anabolic, local analgesic, and chondroprotective effects.[83] Numerous studies have supported the effectiveness of other potential chondroprotective agents including chondroitin sulfate and glucosamine sulfate for the relief of symptoms of osteoarthritis based on clinical trials and short-term follow-up.[83]

Current surgical options for full thickness cartilage defects are simple arthroscopic debridement, abrasion arthroplasty, microfracture, autologous chondrocyte cell implantation, mosaicplasty with either autologous tissue or fresh allograft.[83,185,186] Current research is focused on inducing the newly attracted or transplanted chondrocytes to become mature chondrocytes using growth factors. Bone morphogenic proteins (BMPs) are members of the TGF-superfamily and have a regulatory role in the differentiation of cartilage-forming and bone-forming cells.[83]

Treatment

Frequent exercise in animals has demonstrated hypertrophy of chondrocytes, an increase in the pericellular matrix, and an increase in the number of cells per chondron.

BONE BEHAVIOR, INJURY, HEALING, AND TREATMENT

Behavior

Bone matrix comprises three elements: organic, mineral, and fluid. It is the mineral content that distinguishes bone from other connective tissues, and provides the bone with its characteristic stiffness, while providing a mineral storage system. Collagen orientation in growing and mature bone has been linked to the mechanical behavior of individual layers of bone (lamellae), and the different types of bone. During normal activity, cortical bone sustains loads well within the linear region of the load-deformation curve, so that the bone bends but does not sustain permanent deformation (elastic deformation). However, even when maintained within the linear region, if loads are sustained repetitively over short period of time, changes to the bone may result (plastic deformation). For example, compressive forces shorten bone, and tensile forces elongate bone. Bone is strongest in compression and weakest in tension. Forces acting on bone include muscle contractions, gravity, and forces from outside the body, such as trauma.

When loads are sustained that exceed the linear region, microarchitectural damage can occur. Trabecular, or cancellous bone, is anisotropic in nature, which means its mechanical behavior differs in different directions or among various parts of the structure.

CLINICAL PEARL

Exercise related increases in cortical thickness and bone mineral content suggest that exercise can be a potent stimulus for bone remodeling.[187]

Injury

An injury to a bone is referred to as a fracture. A number of different types of fractures and fracture patterns are recognized (Fig. 2-4) (Table 2-5).

Healing

Bone healing is a complex physiologic process that follows an orderly cascade of events. The striking feature of bone healing, compared with healing in other tissues, is that repair is by the original tissue, not scar tissue. Regeneration is perhaps a better descriptor than repair. This is linked to the capacity for remodeling that intact bone possesses. Like other forms of healing, the repair of bone fracture includes the processes of inflammation, repair, and remodeling; however, the type of healing varies, depending on the method of treatment. In

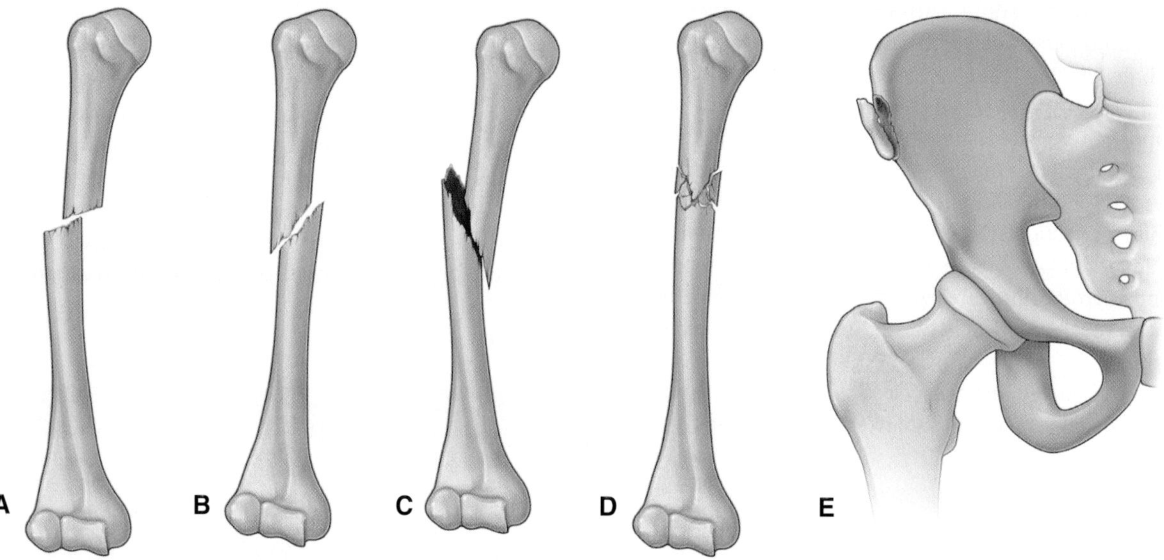

FIGURE 2-4 Fracture types. A. Transverse B. Oblique C. Spiral D. Comminuted E. Avulsion.

TABLE 2-5 Types of Fractures	
Types of Fracture	**Description**
Avulsion	An injury to the bone where a tendon or ligament pulls off a piece of the bone.
Closed	When there is a closed fracture; there is no broken skin—the fractured bone does not penetrate the skin (but may be seen under the skin) and there is no contusion from external trauma.
Comminuted	A fracture that has more than two fragments of bone which have broken off. It is a highly unstable type of bone fracture with many bone fragments.
Complete	A fracture in which the bone has been completely fractured through its own width.
Complex	This type of fractured bone severely damages the soft tissue which surrounds the bone
Compound (open)	The bone breaks and fragments of the bone penetrate through the internal soft tissue of the body and break through the skin from the inside. There is a high risk of infection if external pathogenic factors enter into the interior of the body.
Compression	Occurs when the bone is compressed beyond its limits of tolerance. These fractures generally occur in the vertebral bodies as a result of a flexion injury or without trauma in patients with osteoporosis. Compression fractures of the calcaneus are also common when patients fall from a height and land on their feet.
Epiphyseal	A fracture of the epiphysis and physis—growth plate. These injuries are classified using the Salter–Harris Classification.
Greenstick	The pathology of this type of fracture includes an incomplete fracture in which only one side of the bone breaks. The bone usually is "bent" and only fractured of the outside of the bend. It is mostly seen in children and is considered a stable fracture due to the fact that the whole bone has not been fractured. As long as the bone is kept rigid, healing is usually quick.
Hairline	This bone fracture has minimal trauma to the bone and surrounding soft tissues. It is a incomplete fracture with no significant bone displacement and is considered a stable fracture. In this type the fracture the crack only extends into the outer layer of the bone but not completely through the entire bone. It is also known as a Fissure Fracture.
Impaction	Occurs when one fragment is driven into another. This type of fracture is common in tibial plateau fractures in adults.
Oblique	A fracture which goes at an angle to the axis of the bone
Pathologic	A pathologic fracture occurs when a bone breaks in an area that is weakened by another disease process. Causes of weakened bone include tumors, infection, and certain inherited bone disorders.
Spiral	In this pattern, a bone has been broken due to a twisting type motion. It is highly unstable and may be diagnosed as an oblique fracture unless a correct X-ray has been taken. The spiral fracture resembles a corkscrew type which runs parallel with the axis of the broken bone.
Stress	These fractures may extend through all or only part of the way through the bone. These types of fractures are common in soldiers or runners and are far more common in women. They often occur in the spine, and lower extremity (most often in the fibula, tibia, or metatarsals). Stress fractures occur in a variety of age groups, ranging from young children to elderly persons. Stress fractures do not necessarily occur in association with a history of increased activity. Therefore, it is important to remember that the absence of a history of trauma or increased activity does not eliminate the possibility of stress or insufficiency fracture as a cause of musculoskeletal pain.

classic histologic terms, fracture healing has been divided into two broad phases: primary fracture healing and secondary fracture healing (Fig. 2-5).

- Primary osteonal (cortical) healing, involves a direct attempt by the cortex to reestablish itself once it has become interrupted. In primary cortical healing, bone on one side of the cortex must unite with bone on the other side of the cortex to reestablish mechanical continuity.
- Secondary callus healing involves responses in the periosteum and external soft tissues with the subsequent formation of a callus. The majority of fractures heal by secondary fracture healing.

Within these broader phases, the process of bone healing involves a combination of intramembranous and endochondral ossification (see Chap. 1). These two processes participate in the fracture repair sequence by at least four discrete stages of healing: the hematoma formation (inflammation or granulation) phase, the soft callus formation (reparative or revascularization) phase, the hard callus formation (maturing or modeling) phase, and the remodeling phase.[188]

- ***Hematoma formation (inflammatory) phase.*** Initially, the tissue volume in which new bone is to be formed is filled with the matrix, generally including a blood clot or hematoma (Fig. 2-5).[83] At this phase, the matrix within the injury site is bordered by local tissues, which also are often traumatized resulting in focal necrosis and reduced blood flow.[83] An effective bone healing response will include an initial inflammatory phase characterized by the release of a variety of products, including fibronectin, PDGF, and TGF,

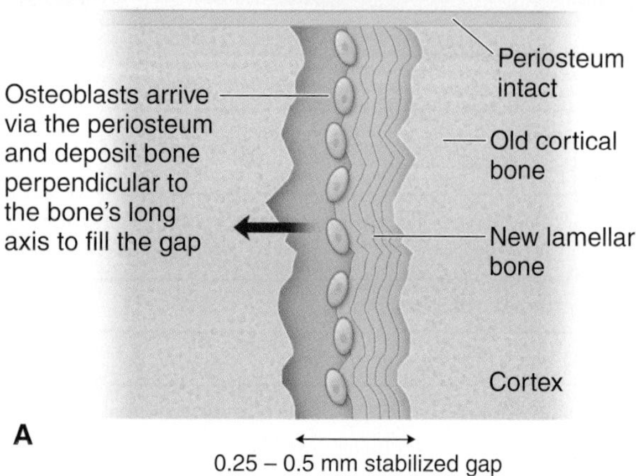

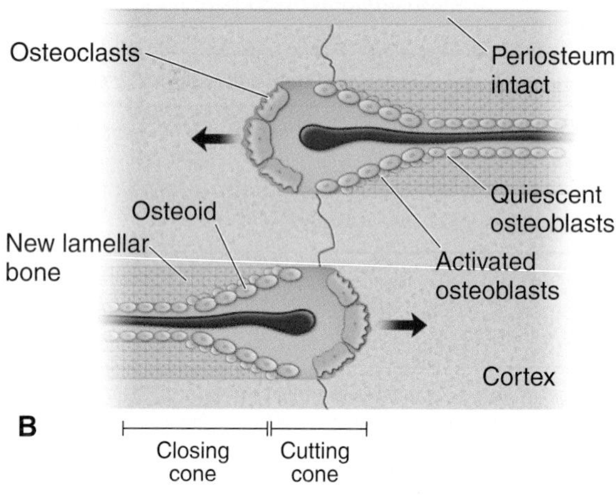

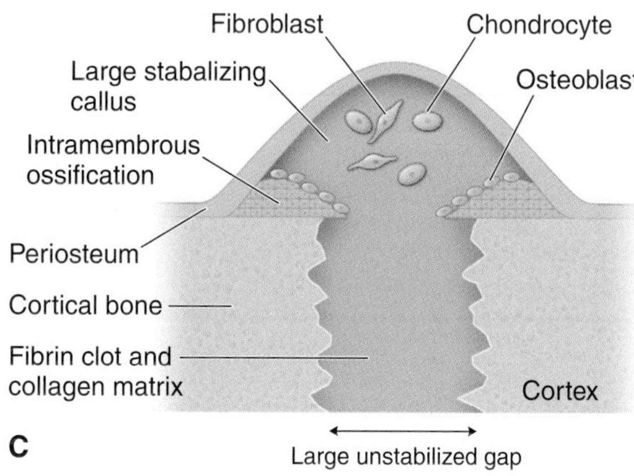

FIGURE 2-5 Fracture healing.

an increase in regional blood flow, invasion of neutrophils and monocytes, removal of cell debris, and degradation of the local fibrin clot.

- ***Soft callus formation (reparative or revascularization) phase.*** This phase is characterized by the formation of connective tissues, including cartilage, and formation of new capillaries from preexisting vessels (angiogenesis). During the first 7–10 days of fracture healing, the periosteum undergoes an intramembranous bone formation response, and histologic evidence shows formation of woven bone opposed to the cortex within a few millimeters of the site of the fracture. Differentiation is strongly influenced by the local oxygen tension and mechanical environment, as well as by signals from local growth factors.[83] By the middle of the second week, abundant cartilage overlies the fracture site, and this chondroid tissue initiates biochemical preparations to undergo calcification. Thus, the callus becomes a triple-layered structure consisting of an outer proliferating part, a middle cartilaginous layer, and an inner portion of new bony trabeculae (Fig. 2-5). The cartilage portion is usually replaced with bone as the healing progresses. During the period of casting, submaximal isometrics are initiated.
- ***Hard callus formation (modeling) phase.*** This phase is characterized by the systematic removal of the initial matrix and tissues that formed in the site, primarily through osteoclastic and chondroclastic resorption, and their replacement with more organized lamellar bone (woven bone) aligned in response to the local loading environment.[83] The calcification of fracture callus cartilage occurs by a mechanism almost identical to that which takes place in the growth plate. This calcification can occur either directly from mesenchymal tissue (intramembranous) or via an intermediate stage of cartilage (endochondral or chondroid routes). Osteoblasts can form woven bone rapidly, but the result is randomly arranged and mechanically weak. Nonetheless, bridging of a fracture by woven bone constitutes so-called clinical union. Once cartilage is calcified, it becomes a target for the ingrowth of blood vessels. Radiographically, a fracture is considered healed when there is progressive callus formation to the point where the fracture line is no longer visible. At this point, range of motion exercises are usually initiated.
- ***Remodeling phase.*** By replacing the cartilage with bone, and converting the cancellous bone into compact bone, the callus is gradually remodeled. During this phase, the woven bone is remodeled into stronger lamellar bone by the orchestrated action of osteoclast bone resorption and osteoblast bone formation (Fig. 2-5).

Radiologically or histologically, fracture gap bridging occurs by three mechanisms[188]:

1. ***Intercortical bridging (primary cortical union).*** This mechanism occurs when the fracture gap is reduced by normal cortical remodeling under conditions of rigid fixation. This mode of healing is the principle behind rigid internal fixation.[189]
2. ***External callus bridging by new bone arising from the periosteum and the soft tissues surrounding the fracture.*** Small degrees of movement at the fracture stimulate external callus formation.[190] This mode of healing is the aim in functional bracing[191] and intramedullary nailing.
3. ***Intramedullary bridging by endosteal callus.*** Normal periods of immobilization following a fracture range from as short as 3 weeks for small bones to about 8 weeks for the long bones of the extremities. Once the cast is removed, it is important that controlled stresses continue to be applied to the bone, because the period of bone healing continues for up to 1 year.[192,193]

TABLE 2-6 The Effect of Hormones on Healing		
Hormone	**Effect on Healing**	**Mechanism**
Calcitonin	Positive	Decreased osteoclastic activity
Thyroid hormone	Positive	Increases rate of bone remodeling
Parathyroid hormone	Positive	Increases rate of bone remodeling
Growth hormone	Positive	Increases amount of callus

Data from: Frenkel SR, Koval KJ: Fracture healing and bone grafting. In: Spivak JM, Di Cesare PE, Feldman DS, et al., eds. *Orthopaedics: A Study Guide*. New York, NY: McGraw-Hill, 1999:23–28.

The three key determinants of fracture healing are the blood supply and the degree of motion experienced by the fracture ends.

- Angiogenesis is the outgrowth of new capillaries from existing vessels. The degree of angiogenesis that occurs depends on well-vascularized tissue on either side of the gap and sufficient mechanical stability to allow new capillaries to survive. Angiogenesis leads to osteogenesis.
- The amount of movement that occurs between fracture ends can be stimulatory or inhibitory to the cascade of bone formation, depending on their magnitude. Excessive interfragmentary movement prevents the establishment of intramedullary blood vessel bridging. However, small degrees of micromotion have been shown to stimulate blood flow at the fracture site and stimulate periosteal callus.[194] Successful restoration of osseous morphology and internal architecture is conditional on the remodeling process. According to Wolff's law, bone remodels along lines of stress.[195] Bone is constantly being remodeled as the circumferential lamellar bone is resorbed by osteoclasts and replaced with dense osteonal bone by osteoblasts.[196]
- The environment is another factor, which modulates the repair process; hormones have impact on osteoblastic and osteoclastic activity (Table 2-6).

Augmented Healing

To date, a number of techniques have been developed to accomplish a quicker and more complete healing of fractures. These include the following:

- Pulsed electromagnetic fields (PEMF). A technique most commonly used for the treatment of nonunion fractures, failed fusions, and congenital pseudarthrosis. PEMF uses electrical energy to direct a series of magnetic pulses through injured tissue such that each magnetic pulse induces a tiny electrical signal that stimulates cellular repair.
- Ultrasound. There is some evidence that pulsed ultrasound may reduce fracture healing time for fractures by stimulating a local hyperemia, an increase in aggregate gene expression, increased mineralization, and more rapid endochondral ossification.[197]
- Direct current. Direct current stimulation surrounding the fracture site has been observed to decrease the oxygen tension with a concomitant rise in local pH in the region of the anode.[198,199]
- Demineralized bone matrix (DBM). DBM derived from human tissues has demonstrated the ability to aid in the stimulation of an osteoinductive and an osteoconductive response allowing for improved bone growth and fusion.[200–202] There are currently two types:
  - Osteoinductive: there are several commercially available DBM substances available, each with different amounts of DBM containing osteoinductive proteins.
  - Osteoconductive: osteoconductivity refers to the ability of some materials to serve as a scaffold on to which bone cells can attach, migrate, and grow and divide. In this way, the bone healing response is "conducted" through the graft site.

Treatment

Deciding the mode of fracture management requires a multifaceted approach. The initial medical approach involves stabilization of the fracture site, which prevents further blood loss and resets muscle tension. A decision is then made by the medical team as to whether surgery is required or whether a conservative approach would be more beneficial.

Surgical Options for Fractures

The advantage of operative treatment is the anatomical reduction of fracture fragments and early mobilization.

Percutaneous Pinning. Percutaneous pinning is a minimally invasive form of internal fixation in which fractures are pinned using Kirschner wires. The pins are driven through the skin and cortex of the bone, across the reduced fracture, and into the opposite cortex.[203] This mode is commonly used in fractures of the phalanges, metacarpals, distal radius, proximal humerus, and metatarsals. The disadvantage of this type of treatment is that the pins can bend or break within the bone, and no absolute stability is provided.

External Fixation. This mode of treatment maintains traction and alignment of the bone without the need to confine the patient to a bed. The threaded traction pins are inserted into the bone proximal and distal to the fracture site, and the fracture is manually reduced and fixed in position with carbon fiber bars spanning the fracture site outside the skin.[203] Using fine wires in a circular fixator, across the subchondral metaphysis, is least damaging to the medullary blood supply.[188] This type of fixation may provide enough stability to allow rapid endosteal healing without external callus.[204]

Open Reduction and Internal Fixation. The aim of this mode of treatment is to anatomically reduce and provide absolute stability to as many of the fracture fragments as possible.[203] A fracture that is rigidly internally fixed produces no periosteal callus and heals by a combination of endosteal callus and primary cortical union.[188]

Locking Plates. Locking plates are fracture fixation devices with threaded screw holes, which allow screws to thread to the plate and function as a fixed-angle scaffold.

Intramedullary Nailing. Fracture fixation with intramedullary nails provide relative stability—unless the nail is locked proximally and distally and has tight fixation at the fracture site, the fixation may have rotational and angular instability.[203] An intermedullary nail blocks endosteal healing but allows enough movement to trigger periosteal callus.[188] Early mobilization of patients after femoral and tibial rodding is a major advance compared to the prolonged immobilization in traction.[203]

Most fractures, especially upper extremity, can be managed without surgery if acceptable reduction can be achieved by closed means. Nonoperative treatment is usually reserved for nondisplaced fractures with a low risk of displacement, for displaced fractures that are stable after acceptable reduction is achieved, or for patients for whom anesthesia and surgery are contraindicated.[203] A variety of nonoperative devices can be used to treat fractures:[203]

- Splints and fracture braces: noncircumstantial coapted devices that lie along one or more surfaces of an extremity that are made of a prefabricated material (molded plastic) or plaster, and secured with elastic bandage. The aim of this type of splinting is to immobilize or passively correct stable fractures and their use is usually temporary, used for days to a few weeks.
- Casting: provides rigid circumferential support into which appropriate holes and three-point fixation can be incorporated. Casting more effectively immobilizes fracture fragments than either splinting or bracing. Particularly useful for maintaining reduction of ankle, tibia, pediatric forearm, and distal radius fractures.
- Skeletal traction: traction is applied either manually or via weights and pulleys to overcome the shortening force of muscles across the fracture site. The configuration of the skeletal traction varies according to the specific bone involved, but its use is dwindling due to the successful development of surgical reduction and internal fixation.

POSTSURGICAL REHABILITATION

Although many musculoskeletal conditions can be treated conservatively, surgical intervention is often indicated for cases in which a sufficient traumatic or degenerative injury has occurred. Over the years, the number of surgical procedures for orthopaedic conditions has increased considerably. However, although surgery can often correct the presenting problem, for the postsurgical patient to return to an appropriate level of function, some form of postsurgical rehabilitation is usually required. Indeed, a number of studies have reported that skilled intervention following most surgical procedures of the musculoskeletal system allows patients to achieve greater independence and control over their lives in a shorter timeframe than patients who do not receive these interventions.[205,206]

Postsurgical Complications

Although surgical procedures can offer many benefits, they are not without their complications. Some of the more serious of these complications include the following:

- ***Postsurgical infection.*** Postsurgical infections are perhaps the greatest challenge facing the modern-day surgeon. At any one time, 9% of hospitalized patients are being treated for an nosocomial infection.[207] *Staphylococcus aureus*, coagulase-negative staphylococci, *Enterococcus* spp., and *Escherichia coli* remain the most frequently isolated pathogens. An increasing proportion of infections are caused by antimicrobial-resistant pathogens, such as methicillin-resistant *S. aureus* (MRSA), or by *Candida albicans*.[208] Microorganisms may contain or produce toxins and other substances that increase their ability to invade a host, produce damage within the host, or survive on or in host tissue. For example, many gram-negative bacteria produce an endotoxin that stimulates cytokine production. In turn, cytokines can trigger the systemic inflammatory response syndrome that sometimes leads to multiple system organ failure.[208] In certain kinds of surgical procedures, some patient characteristics have been found to be possibly associated with an increased risk of an infection. These include coincident remote site infections or colonization, diabetes, cigarette smoking, systemic steroid use, obesity (>20% of ideal body weight), extremes of age, poor nutritional status, and perioperative transfusion of certain blood products.[208–210] Although physical therapists are not directly involved in surgical procedures, they are a potential mode of transmission for infections. Hand washing has been found to be an important infection control measure, although improving compliance with hand washing has been a challenge for most hospital infection control programs.[211]
- ***Venous thromboembolism.*** A thrombus, or blood clot, is an obstruction of the venous or arterial system. If a thrombus is located in one of the superficial veins, it is usually self-limiting. Venous thromboembolism is a vascular disease that manifests as deep vein thrombosis (DVT) or pulmonary embolism (PE). A DVT most commonly appears in the lower extremity and is typically classified as being either proximal (affecting the popliteal and thigh veins) or distal (affecting the calf veins). Proximal DVT is the more dangerous form of lower extremity DVT because it is more likely to cause life-threatening PE (see later).

CLINICAL PEARL

DVT is caused by an alteration in the normal coagulation system. This alteration in the fibrinolytic system, which acts as a system of checks and balances, results in a failure to dissolve the clot. If the clot becomes dislodged, it enters into the circulatory system through which it can travel to become lodged in the lungs (PE), obstructing the pulmonary artery or branches that supply the lungs with blood. If the clot is large and completely blocks a vessel, it can cause sudden death.

Certain patients are at increased risk for DVT[212–216]:

- Strong risk factors include fracture (pelvis, femur, and tibia), hip or knee replacement, major general surgery, major trauma, or spinal cord injury. A recent study indicated that up to 60% of patients undergoing total hip replacement surgery may develop a DVT without preventative treatment.[217,218]
- Moderate risk factors include arthroscopic knee surgery, central venous lines, chemotherapy, congestive heart or respiratory failure, hormone replacement therapy, malignancy, oral contraceptive therapy, cerebrovascular accident, pregnancy/postpartum, previous venous thromboembolism, and thrombophilia.
- Weak risk factors include bed rest greater than 3 days, immobility due to sitting (e.g., prolonged air travel), increasing age, laparoscopic surgery, obesity, pregnancy/antepartum, and varicose veins.

The association of DVT with venous stasis, vessel wall damage, and hypercoagulability was first proposed by Virchow in 1859.[219]

CLINICAL PEARL

Venous stasis: general anesthesia associated with a decrease in blood flow velocity, increased age, hypotension, varicosities, congestive heart failure, postsurgical immobility, and possibly obesity have been proposed as the major contributing factors that increase blood pooling in the lower extremities.

Vessel wall damage: several intraoperative factors during hip surgery, such as limb positioning, hip dislocation, local trauma, and retraction of local structures anterior to the hip have been demonstrated to lead to femoral vein injury and subsequent endothelial damage.[220]

Hypercoagulability: a variety of congenital and acquired conditions are associated with hypercoagulable states including abnormalities of fibrinogen and/or plasminogen, adenocarcinoma, pregnancy, systemic lupus erythematosus, and nephrotic syndrome.

Two-thirds of the fatalities resulting from DVT occur within 30 minutes of the initial symptoms.[221–223] Both DVT and PE can be symptomatic or asymptomatic. Clinical signs of a DVT have traditionally been described as including swelling of the extremity, tenderness or a feeling of cramping of the calf muscles that increases when the ankle is dorsiflexed (positive Homan's sign) or with weight bearing, vascular prominence, elevated temperature, tachycardia, and inflammation and discoloration or redness of the extremity. However, a purely clinical diagnosis is fraught with a high incidence of false positives and negatives. Musculoskeletal conditions that may mimic symptoms associated with DVT include hematoma, myositis, tendinitis, Baker's cyst, synovitis, osteomyelitis, and tumors.[224] The clinical decision rule described by Wells and colleagues[225–229] (Table 2-7) is being most commonly

TABLE 2-7 Clinical Decision Rule for Outpatients Suspected of Having a Proximal Deep Vein Thrombosis

Clinical Finding	Score[a]
Active cancer (within 6 months of diagnosis or palliative care)	1
Paralysis, paresis, or recent plaster immobilization of lower extremity	1
Recently bedridden >3 days or major surgery within 4 wks of application of clinical decision rule	1
Localized tenderness along distribution of the deep venous system (assessed by firm palpation in the center of the posterior calf, the popliteal space, and along the area of the femoral vein in the anterior thigh and groin.)	1
Entire lower extremity swelling	1
Calf swelling by >3 cm compared with asymptomatic lower extremity (measured 10 cm below tibial tuberosity)	1
Pitting edema (greater in the symptomatic lower extremity)	1
Collateral superficial veins (nonvaricose)	1
Alternative diagnosis as likely or greater than that of DVT (most common alternative diagnoses on cellulitis, calf strain, and postoperative swelling)	−2

[a]Score interpretation: ≤ 0 = probability of proximal lower extremity deep vein thrombosis (PDVT) of 3% (95% confidence interval = 1.7–5.9%), 1 or 2 = probability of PDVT of 17% (95% confidence interval = 12–23%), ≥ 3 = probability of PDVT of 75% (95% confidence interval = 63–84%).

Data from Wells PS, Anderson DR, Bormanis J, et al.: Value of assessment of pretest probability of deep-vein thrombosis in clinical management. *Lancet* 350: 1795–1798, 1997.

recommended for outpatients suspected of having DVT.[230,231] More accurate diagnostic procedures, outside the scope of physical therapy, include contrast venography, Doppler and B-mode ultrasound, venous duplex imaging, impedance plethysmography, and I-125 fibrinogen uptake.

- ***Prevention is the key with DVT.*** Methods of prevention may be classified as pharmacological and nonpharmacological. Pharmacological prevention includes anticoagulant drugs such as low-dose Coumadin (warfarin), low-molecular-weight heparin, adjusted-dose heparin, and heparin-antithrombin III combination. These drugs work by altering the body's normal blood-clotting process. Second tier drugs include dextran, aspirin, and low-dose subcutaneous heparin. Nonpharmacological prevention attempts to counteract the effects of immobility, including calf and foot/ankle exercises, and compression stockings. A recent study has shown that substantial hyperemia (a mean 22% increase in venous outflow) occurs after the performance of active ankle pumps for 1 minute, and venous outflow remains greater than the baseline level for 30 minutes reaching a maximum 12 minutes after these exercises.[218] Although this does not provide sufficient evidence that exercise alone prevents DVT, it suggests that the active ankle pump does influence venous hemodynamics. Finally, inferior vena caval (IVC) filters and Greenfield filters may be employed with a patient who has a contraindication to anticoagulation, previous complications with anticoagulants, or if anticoagulants have proved ineffective in the past.
- ***Pulmonary embolus.***[232] This is a part of the spectrum of diseases associated with venous thromboembolism. Under normal conditions, microthrombi (tiny aggregates of red cells, platelets, and fibrin) are formed and lysed continually within the venous circulatory system. This dynamic equilibrium ensures local hemostasis in response to injury without permitting uncontrolled propagation of a clot. Under pathological conditions, microthrombi may escape the normal fibrinolytic system to grow and propagate. PE occurs when these propagating clots break loose and embolize to block pulmonary blood vessels. PE most commonly results from DVT occurring in the deep veins of the lower extremities, proximal to and including the popliteal veins and in the axillary or subclavian veins (deep veins of the arm or shoulder). PE is an extremely common and highly lethal postsurgical condition that is a leading cause of death in all age groups. A good clinician actively seeks the diagnosis as soon as any suspicion of PE whatsoever is warranted, because prompt diagnosis and treatment can dramatically reduce the mortality rate and morbidity of the disease. Unfortunately, the diagnosis is missed more often than it is made because PE often causes only vague and nonspecific symptoms. Symptoms that should provoke a suspicion of PE must include chest pain, chest wall tenderness, back pain, shoulder pain, upper abdominal pain, syncope, hemoptysis, shortness of breath, painful respiration, new onset of wheezing, any new cardiac arrhythmia, or any other unexplained symptom referable to the thorax. It is important to remember that many patients with PE are initially completely asymptomatic and most of those who do have symptoms have an atypical presentation. Pulmonary angiography remains the criterion standard for the diagnosis of PE but is rapidly being replaced by multidetector computed tomographic angiography (MDCTA), since the latter modality is significantly less invasive, is easier to perform, and offers equal sensitivity and specificity.
- ***Poor wound healing.*** Wound-healing abnormalities cause great physical and psychological stress to the affected patients and are extremely expensive to treat. The rate of healing in acute surgical wounds is affected by both extrinsic factors (surgical technique, tension of wound suturing, maintenance of adequate oxygenation, cigarette smoking, prevention or eradication of infection, and types of wound dressing) and intrinsic factors (presence of shock or sepsis, control of diabetes mellitus, and the age, nutritional, and immune status of the patient).[233] Although many studies have documented relationships between malnutrition and poor wound healing, the optimal nutrient intake to promote wound healing is unknown. It is known, however, that vitamins A, C, and E, protein, arginine, zinc, and water play a role in the healing process.[234]
- ***Scars and adhesions.*** Surgery is a form of controlled macrotrauma to the musculoskeletal system. The tissues respond to this trauma in much the same way that they do to any other form of trauma or injury. As part of the postsurgical rehabilitation process, the involved structure is usually immobilized to protect the surgical site from injury. However, prolonged immobilization of a connective tissue can produce significant changes in its histochemical and biomechanical structure. These changes include a fibrofatty infiltration that can progress into fibrosis, creating adhesions around the healing site, and an increase in the microscopic cross-linking of collagen fibers resulting in an overall loss of extensibility of the connective tissues.[123,235–238] Unlike normal connective tissue, which is mature and stable with limited pliability, scar tissue is more vulnerable to breakdown.[19,41,239–241] Fortunately, controlled and skilled therapeutic interventions can reverse the detrimental effects of short-term immobilization. These include mobilization of the connective tissue with passive mobility techniques or active range of motion that help to restore the extensibility of the tissue. To assist with the overall healing of the incision, scar mobilization techniques may be performed to the patient's tolerance with lotion.

DETRIMENTAL EFFECTS OF IMMOBILIZATION

Continuous immobilization of connective and skeletal muscle tissues can cause some undesirable consequences. These include the following:

- ***Cartilage degeneration.***[241–245] Immobilization of a joint causes atrophic changes in articular cartilage through a reduction in the amount of matrix proteoglycans and cartilage softening.[242] Softened articular cartilage is vulnerable to damage during weight bearing. The reduction of the matrix proteoglycans concentration has been demonstrated to be highest in the superficial zone but also occurs throughout the uncalcified cartilage, diminishing with distance from the surface of articular cartilage.[246]

- ***Decreased mechanical and structural properties of ligaments.*** One study[9] showed that after 8 weeks of immobilization, the stiffness of a ligament decreased to 69% of control values, and even after 1 year of rehabilitation, the ligament did not return to its prior level of strength.

CLINICAL PEARL

Following a period of immobilization, connective tissues are more vulnerable to deformation and breakdown than normal tissues subjected to similar amounts of stress.[247]

- ***Decreased bone density.***[122,123,192,235,248] The interactions among systemic and local factors to maintain normal bone mass are complex. Bone mass is maintained because of a continuous coupling between bone resorption by osteoclasts and bone formation by osteoblasts, and this process is influenced by both systemic and local factors.[249] Mechanical forces acting on bone stimulate osteogenesis, and the absence of such forces inhibits osteogenesis. Marked osteopenia occurs in otherwise healthy patients in states of complete immobilization or weightlessness.[250,251] In children, bone has a high modeling rate and appears to be more sensitive to the absence of mechanical loading than bone in adults.[252]
- ***Weakness or atrophy of muscles*** (Table 2-8). Muscle atrophy is an imbalance between protein synthesis and degradation. After modest trauma, there is a decrease in whole body protein synthesis[253] rather than increased breakdown. With more severe trauma, major surgery, or multiple organ failure, both synthesis and degradation increase, the latter being more enhanced.[254,255]

CLINICAL PEARL

Disuse atrophy of muscle begins within 4 hours of the start of bed rest, resulting in decreases in muscle mass, muscle cell diameter, and the number of muscle fibers. However, strenuous exercise of atrophic muscle can lead to muscle damage, including sarcolemmal disruption, distortion of the contractile components of myofibrils, and cytoskeletal damage. Thus, a balance must be found.

TABLE 2-8 Structural Changes in the Various Types of Muscle Following Immobilization in a Shortened Position

Structural Characteristics	Muscle Fiber Type and Changes		
	Slow Oxidative	Fast Oxidative Glycolytic	Fast Glycolytic
Number of fibers	Moderate decrease	Minimal increase	Minimal increase
Diameter of fibers	Significant decrease	Moderate decrease	Moderate decrease
Fiber fragmentation	Minimal increase	Minimal increase	Significant increase
Myofibrils	Minimal decrease and disoriented	—	Wavy
Nuclei	Degenerated and rounded	Degenerated and rounded	Degenerated and rounded
Mitochondria	Moderate decrease, degenerated	Moderate decrease, degenerated	Minimal decrease, degenerated, swollen
Sarcoplasmic reticulum	Minimal decrease, orderly arrangement	Minimal decrease	Minimal decrease
Myofilaments	Minimal decrease, disorganized	Moderate decrease	Minimal decrease, wavy
Z band	Moderate decrease	—	Faint or absent
Vesicles	Abnormal configuration	—	—
Basement membrane	Minimal increase	—	—
Register of sarcomeres	Irregular projections, shifted with time	—	—
Fatty infiltration	Minimal increase	—	—
Collagen	Minimal increase between fibers	—	—
Macrophages	Minimal increased invasion	Minimal increased invasion	Minimal increased invasion
Satellite cells	Minimal increase	—	—
Target cells	Minimal increase	—	—

Data from Gossman MR, Sahrmann SA, Rose SJ: Review of length-associated changes in muscle. Experimental evidence and clinical implications. *Phys Ther* 62: 1799–1808, 1982. With permission from APTA.

The cause of muscle damage during exercised recovery from atrophy involves an altered ability of the muscle fibers to bear the mechanical stress of external loads (weight bearing) and movement associated with exercise. Strenuous exercise can result in primary or secondary sarcolemmal disruption, swelling or disruption of the sarcotubular system, distortion of the contractile components of myofibrils, cytoskeletal damage, and extracellular myofiber matrix abnormalities.[71] These pathologic changes are similar to those seen in healthy young adults after sprint running or resistance training.[71] It appears that the act of contracting while the muscle is in a stretched or lengthened position, known as an *eccentric contraction,* is responsible for these injuries.[256]

The clinician must remember that the restoration of full strength and range of motion may prove difficult if muscles are allowed to heal without early active motion, or in a shortened position, and that the patient may be prone to repeated strains.[131] Thus, range-of-motion exercises should be started once swelling and tenderness have subsided to the point that the exercises are not unduly painful.[131]

REVIEW QUESTIONS

1. Explain the difference between *primary* and *secondary* injuries.
2. Outline the differences between a *microtrauma* and a *macrotrauma*.
3. What are the three main stages of wound healing?
4. What are neutrophils?
5. What is the function of monocytes in the inflammation stage of wound healing?

REFERENCES

1. Neumann DA: Getting started. In: Neumann DA, ed. *Kinesiology of the Musculoskeletal System: Foundations for Physical Rehabilitation*. St. Louis, MO: Mosby, 2002:3–24.
2. Topoleski LD: Mechanical properties of materials. In: Oatis CA, ed. *Kinesiology: The Mechanics and Pathomechanics of Human Movement*. Philadelphia, PA: Lippincott Williams and Wilkins, 2004:21–35.
3. Woo SL-Y, Buckwalter JA: *Injury and Repair of the Musculoskeletal Tissue*. Park Ridge, IL: American Academy of Orthopaedic Surgeons, 1988.
4. Goel VK, Khandha A, Vadapalli S: *Musculoskeletal biomechanics, Orthopaedic Knowledge Update 8: Home Study Syllabus*. Rosemont, IL: American Academy of Orthopaedic Surgeons, 2005:39–56.
5. Hildebrand KA, Hart DA, Rattner JB, et al: Ligament injuries: Pathophysiology, healing, and treatment considerations. In: Magee D, Zachazewski JE, Quillen WS, eds. *Scientific Foundations and Principles of Practice in Musculoskeletal Rehabilitation*. St. Louis, MI: WB Saunders, 2007:23–46.
6. Noyes FR, Butler DL, Paulos LE, et al: Intra-articular cruciate reconstruction. I: Perspectives on graft strength, vascularization and immediate motion after replacement. *Clin Orthop* 172:71–77, 1983.
7. Laros GS, Tipton CM, Cooper R: Influence of physical activity on ligament insertions in the knees of dogs. *J Bone and Joint Surg* 53B:275–286, 1971.
8. Nimni ME: Collagen: Structure function and metabolism in normal and fibrotic tissue. *Semin Arthritis Rheum* 13:1–86, 1983.
9. Noyes FR, Torvik PJ, Hyde WB, et al: Biomechanics of ligament failure: II. An analysis of immobilization, exercise, and reconditioning effects in primates. *J Bone Joint Surg* 56A:1406–1418, 1974.
10. Bennett N, Jarvis L, Rowlands O, et al: *Results from the 1994 General Household Survey*. London: Office of Population Censuses and Surveys, HMSO, 1995.
11. Johanson MA: Contributing factors in microtrauma injuries of the lower extremity. *J Back Musculoskel Rehabil* 2:12–25, 1992.
12. Oakes BW: Acute soft tissue injuries: Nature and management. *Austr Family Physician* 10:3–16, 1982.
13. Garrick JG: The sports medicine patient. *Nurs Clin N Am* 16:759–766, 1981.
14. Muckle DS: Injuries in sport. *Royal S Health J* 102:93–94, 1982.
15. Kellett J: Acute soft tissue injuries: A review of the literature. *Med Sci Sports Exerc* 18:5, 1986.
16. Prentice WE: Understanding and managing the healing process through rehabilitation. In: Voight ML, Hoogenboom BJ, Prentice WE, eds. *Musculoskeletal Interventions: Techniques for Therapeutic Exercise*. New York, NY: McGraw-Hill, 2007, 19–46.
17. Singer AJ, Clark RAF: Cutaneous wound healing. *N Engl J Med* 341: 738–746, 1999.
18. Van der Mueulin JHC: Present state of knowledge on processes of healing in collagen structures. *Int J Sports Med* 3:4–8, 1982.
19. Clayton ML, Wier GJ: Experimental investigations of ligamentous healing. *Am J Surg* 98:373–378, 1959.
20. Hunt TK: *Wound Healing and Wound Infection: Theory and Surgical Practice*. New York, NY: Appleton-Century-Crofts, 1980.
21. Mason ML, Allen HS: The rate of healing of tendons. An experimental study of tensile strength. *Ann Surg* 113:424–459, 1941.
22. Wong MEK, Hollinger JO, Pinero GJ: Integrated processes responsible for soft tissue healing. *Oral Surg Oral Med Oral Pathol Oral Radiol Endod* 82:475–492, 1996.
23. Bryant MW: Wound healing. *CIBA Clin Symp* 29:2–36, 1977.
24. Heldin C-H, Westermark B: Role of platelet-derived growth factor in vivo. In: Clark RAF, ed. *The Molecular and Cellular Biology of Wound Repair*, 2nd ed. New York, NY: Plenum Press, 1996:249–273.
25. Katz MH, Kirsner RS, Eaglstein WH, et al: Human wound fluid from acute wounds stimulates fibroblast and endothelial cell growth. *J Am Acad Dermatol* 25:1054–1058, 1991.
26. Deuel TF, Senior RM, Chang D, et al: Platelet factor 4 is a chemotactic factor for neutrophils and monocytes. *Proc Natl Acad Sci* 74:4584–4587, 1981.
27. Schultz G, Rotatari DS, Clark W: EGF and TGF[alpha] in wound healing and repair. *J Cell Biochem* 45:346–352, 1991.
28. Sporn MB, Roberts AB: Transforming growth factor beta: Recent progress and new challenges. *J Cell Biol* 119:1017–1021, 1992.
29. Sen CK, Khanna S, Gordillo G, et al: Oxygen, oxidants, and antioxidants in wound healing: An emerging paradigm. *Ann N Y Acad Sci* 957:239–249, 2002.
30. Babior BM: Phagocytes and oxidative stress. *Am J Med* 109:33–44, 2000.
31. Amadio PC: Tendon and ligament. In: Cohen IK, Diegelman RF, Lindblad WJ, eds. *Wound Healing: Biomechanical and Clinical Aspects*. Philadelphia, PA: W. B. Saunders, 1992:384–395.
32. Peacock EE: *Wound Repair, 3rd ed.* Philadelphia, PA: WB Saunders, 1984.
33. Ross R: The fibroblast and wound repair. *Biol Rev* 43:51–96, 1968.
34. McAllister BS, Leeb-Lunberg LM, Javors MA, et al: Bradykinin receptors and signal transduction pathways in human fibroblasts: Integral role for extracellular calcium. *Arch Biochem Biophys* 304:294–301, 1993.
35. Evans RB: Clinical application of controlled stress to the healing extensor tendon: A review of 112 cases. *Phys Ther* 69:1041–1049, 1989.
36. Emwemeka CS: Inflammation, cellularity, and fibrillogenesis in regenerating tendon: Implications for tendon rehabilitation. *Phys Ther* 69:816–825, 1989.
37. Garrett WE, Lohnes J: Cellular and matrix response to mechanical injury at the myotendinous junction. In: Leadbetter WB, Buckwalter JA, Gordon SL, eds. *Sports-Induced Inflammation: Clinical and Basic Science Concepts*. Park Ridge. IL: American Academy of Orthopedic Surgeons, 1990:215–224.
38. Di Rosa F, Barnaba V: Persisting viruses and chronic inflammation: Understanding their relation to autoimmunity. *Immunol Rev* 164:17–27, 1998.
39. Lefkowitz DL, Mills K, Lefkowitz SS, et al: Neutrophil–macrophage interaction: A paradigm for chronic inflammation. *Med Hypotheses* 44:68–72, 1995.
40. Thomas DW, O'Neil ID, Harding KG, et al: Cutaneous wound healing: A current perspective. *J Oral Maxillofac Surg* 53:442–447, 1995.

41. Arem A, Madden J: Effects of stress on healing wounds: Intermittent non-cyclical tension. *J Surg Res* 42:528–543, 1971.
42. Merskey H, Bogduk N: *Classification of Chronic Pain: Descriptions of Chronic Pain Syndromes and Definition of Pain Terms. Report by the International Association for the Study of Pain Task Force on Taxonomy,* 2nd ed. Seattle, WA: IASP Press, 1994.
43. Safran MR, Zachazewski JE, Benedetti RS, et al: Lateral ankle sprains: A comprehensive review part 2: Treatment and rehabilitation with an emphasis on the athlete. *Med Sci Sports Exerc* 31:S438–S447, 1999.
44. Safran MR, Benedetti RS, Bartolozzi AR 3rd, et al: Lateral ankle sprains: A comprehensive review: Part 1: Etiology, pathoanatomy, histopathogenesis, and diagnosis. *Med Sci Sports Exerc* 31:S429–S437, 1999.
45. Chvapil M, Koopman CF: Scar formation: Physiology and pathological states. *Otolaryngol Clin North Am* 17:265–272, 1984.
46. Levenson SM, Geever EF, Crowley LV, et al: The healing of rat skin wounds. *Ann Surg* 161:293–308, 1965.
47. Farfan HF: The scientific basis of manipulative procedures. *Clin Rheum Dis* 6:159–177, 1980.
48. Orgill D, Demling RH: Current concepts and approaches to wound healing. *Crit Care Med* 16:899, 1988.
49. Stauber WT: Repair models and specific tissue responses in muscle injury. In: Leadbetter WB, Buckwalter JA, Gordon SL, eds. *Sports-Induced Inflammation: Clinical and Basic Science Concepts.* Park Ridge, IL: American Academy of Orthopedic Surgeons, 1990:205–213.
50. Hall SJ: The biomechanics of human skeletal muscle. In: Hall SJ, ed. *Basic Biomechanics.* New York, NY: McGraw-Hill, 1999:146–185.
51. Matzkin E, Zachazewski JE, Garrett WE, et al: Skeletal muscle: Deformation, injury, repair, and treatment considerations. In: Magee D, Zachazewski JE, Quillen WS, eds. *Scientific Foundations and Principles of Practice in Musculoskeletal Rehabilitation.* St. Louis, MI: WB Saunders, 2007:97–121.
52. Kirkendall DT, Garrett WE Jr: The effects of aging and training on skeletal muscle. *Am J Sports Med* 26:598–602, 1998.
53. Lexell J, Taylor CC, Sjostrom M: What is the cause of the ageing atrophy? Total number, size and proportion of different fiber types studied in whole vastus lateralis muscle from 15- to 83-year-old men. *J Neurol Sci* 84:275–294, 1988.
54. Woo SL, Lee TQ, Gomez MA, et al: Temperature dependent behavior of the canine medial collateral ligament. *J Biomech Eng* 109:68–71, 1987.
55. Huijbregts PA: Muscle injury, regeneration, and repair. *J Man Manip Ther* 9:9–16, 2001.
56. Jarvinen TA, Kaariainen M, Jarvinen M, et al: Muscle strain injuries. *Curr Opin Rheumatol* 12:155–161, 2000.
57. Garrett WE: Muscle strain injuries. *Am J Sports Med* 24:S2–S8, 1996.
58. Lehto MU, Jarvinen MJ: Muscle injuries, their healing process and treatment. *Ann Chir Gynaecol* 80:102–108, 1991.
59. Kalimo H, Rantanen J, Jarvinen M: Soft tissue injuries in sport. In: Jarvinen M, ed. *Balliere's Clinical Orthopaedics,* 1997:1–24.
60. Allbrook DB: Skeletal muscle regeneration. *Muscle Nerve* 4:234–245, 1981.
61. Hurme T, Kalimo H: Activation of myogenic precursor cells after muscle injury. *Med Sci Sports Exerc* 24:197–205, 1992.
62. Hurme T, Kalimo H, Lehto M, et al: Healing of skeletal muscle injury: An ultrastructural and immunohistochemical study. *Med Sci Sports Exerc* 23:801–810, 1991.
63. Zarins B: Soft tissue injury and repair: Biomechanical aspects. *Int J Sports Med* 3:9–11, 1982.
64. Kasemkijwattana C, Menetrey J, Bosch P, et al: Use of growth factors to improve muscle healing after strain injury. *Clin Orthop Relat Res* 370: 272–285, 2000.
65. Lehto M, Duance VJ, Restall D: Collagen and fibronectin in a healing skeletal muscle injury: An immunohistochemical study of the effects of physical activity on the repair of the injured gastrocnemius muscle in the rat. *J Bone Joint Surg* 67-B:820–828, 1985.
66. Menetrey J, Kasemkijwattana C, Day CS, et al: Growth factors improve muscle healing in vivo. *J Bone Joint Surg Br* 82B:131–137, 2000.
67. Alameddine HS, Dehaupas M, Fardeau M: Regeneration of skeletal muscle fibers from autologous satellite cells multiplied in vitro: an experimental model for testing cultured cell myogenicity. *Muscle Nerve* 12:544–555, 1989.
68. Barlow Y, Willoughby J: Pathophysiology of soft tissue repair. *Br Med Bull* 48:698–711, 1992.
69. Frank CB, Bray RC, Hart DA, et al: Soft Tissue Healing. In: Fu F, Harner CD, Vince KG, eds. *Knee Surgery.* Baltimore, MD: Williams and Wilkins, 1994:189–229.
70. Injeyan HS, Fraser IH, Peek WD: Pathology of musculoskeletal soft tissues. In: Hammer WI, ed. *Functional Soft Tissue Examination and Treatment by Manual Methods.* Gaithersburg, MD: Aspen, 1991: 9–23.
71. Kasper CE, Talbot LA, Gaines JM: Skeletal muscle damage and recovery. *AACN Clin Issues* 13:237–247, 2002.
72. Byrnes WC, Clarkson PM, White JS, et al: Delayed onset muscle soreness following repeated bouts of downhill running. *J Appl Physiol* 59:710, 1985.
73. Nosaka K, Sakamoto K, Newton M, et al: How long does the protective effect on eccentric exercise-induced muscle damage last. *Med Sci Sports Exerc* 33:1490–1495, 2001.
74. Lynn R, Talbot JA, Morgan DL: Differences in rat skeletal muscles after incline and decline running. *J Appl Physiol* 85:98–104, 1998.
75. Nosaka K, Clarkson P: Influence of previous concentric exercise on eccentric exercise-induced muscle damage. *J Sports Sci* 15:477, 1997.
76. Dutta C, Hadley EC: The significance of sarcopenia in old age. *J Gerontol Series A* 50A:1–4, 1995.
77. Kotler D, Tierney A, Pierson R: Magnitude of body cell mass depletion and the timing of death from wasting in AIDS. *Am J Clin Nutr* 50:444–447, 1989.
78. Roubenoff R, Castaneda C: Sarcopenia-understanding the dynamics of aging muscle. *JAMA* 286:1230–1231, 2001.
79. Castaneda C, Charnley J, Evans W, et al: Elderly women accommodate to a low-protein diet with losses of body cell mass, muscle function, and immune response. *Am J Clin Nutr* 62:30–39, 1995.
80. Jubrias SA, Odderson IR, Esselman PC, et al: Decline in isokinetic force with age: Muscle cross-sectional area and specific force. *Pflugers Arch* 434:246–253, 1997.
81. Larsson L, Sjodin B, Karlsson J: Histochemical and biochemical changes in human skeletal muscle with age in sedentary males, age 22–65 years. *Acta Physiol Scand* 103:31–39, 1978.
82. Butler DL, Grood ES, Noyes FR, et al: Biomechanics of ligaments and tendons. *Exerc Sport Sci Rev* 6:125–181, 1978.
83. Vereeke West R, Fu F: *Soft tissue physiology and repair, Orthopaedic Knowledge Update 8: Home Study Syllabus.* Rosemont, IL: American Academy of Orthopaedic Surgeons, 2005:15–27.
84. Curwin SL: Tendon pathology and injuries: Pathophysiology, healing, and treatment considerations. In: Magee D, Zachazewski JE, Quillen WS, eds. *Scientific Foundations and Principles of Practice in Musculoskeletal Rehabilitation.* St. Louis, MI: WB Saunders, 2007:47–78.
85. Woo SL-Y, An K-N, Arnoczky SP, et al: Anatomy, biology, and biomechanics of tendon, ligament, and meniscus. In: Simon S, ed. *Orthopaedic Basic Science.* Rosemont, IL: The American Academy of Orthopaedic Surgeons, 1994:45–87.
86. Almekinders LC, Temple JD: Etiology, diagnosis and treatment of tendonitis: An analysis of the literature. *Med Sci Sports Exerc* 30: 1183–1190, 1998.
87. Clement DB, Taunton JE, Smart GW: Achilles tendinitis and peritendinitis: Etiology and treatment. *Am J Sports Med* 12:179–183, 1984.
88. James SL, Bates BT, Osternig LR: Injuries to runners. *Am J Sports Med* 6:40–49, 1978.
89. Ilfeld FW: Can stroke modification relieve tennis elbow? *Clin Orthop Rel Res* 276:182–186, 1992.
90. Knorzer E, Folkhard W, Geercken W, et al: New aspects of the etiology of tendon rupture. An analysis of time-resolved dynamic-mechanical measurements using synchrotron radiation. *Arch Orthop Trauma Surg* 105:113–120, 1986.
91. Komi PV: *Strength and Power in Sport.* London: Blackwell Scientific Publications, 1992.
92. Komi PV, Buskirk E: Effects of eccentric and concentric muscle conditioning on tension and electrical activity of human muscle. *Ergonomics* 15:417, 1972.
93. Bureau of Labor Statistics: *Occupational injuries and illness in the United States by industry 1988.* Bulletin:2368, 1990.
94. Renstrom P: Sports traumatology today: A review of common current sports injury problems. *Ann Chir Gynaecol* 80:81–93, 1991.
95. Kaeding C, Best TM: Tendinosis: Pathophysiology and nonoperative treatment. *Sports Health* 1:284–292, 2009.
96. Leadbetter WB: Cell-matrix response in tendon injury. *Clin Sports Med* 11:533–578, 1992.

97. Nirschl RP: Tennis elbow tendinosis: Pathoanatomy, nonsurgical and surgical management. In: Gordon SL, Blair SJ, Fine LJ, eds. *Repetitive Motion Disorders of the Upper Extremity.* Rosemont, IL: American Academy of Orthopaedic Surgeons, 1995:467–479.
98. Jozsa LG, Kannus P: Overuse injuries of tendons. In: Jozsa LG, Kannus P, eds. *Human Tendons: Anatomy, Physiology, and Pathology.* Champaign, IL: Human Kinetics, 1997:164–253.
99. Kannus P, Jozsa L: Histopathological changes preceding spontaneous rupture of a tendon. A controlled study of 891 patients. *J Bone and Joint Surg* 73A:1507–1525, 1991.
100. Teitz CC, Garrett WE Jr, Miniaci A, et al: Tendon problems in athletic individuals. *J Bone Joint Surg* 79-A:138–152, 1997.
101. Kraushaar BS, Nirschl RP: Tendinosis of the elbow (tennis elbow). Clinical features and findings of histological, immunohistochemical, and electron microscopy studies. *J Bone Joint Surg (Am)* 81:259–278, 1999.
102. Hope M, Saxby TS: Tendon healing. *Foot Ankle Clin* 12:553–567, v, 2007.
103. Sharma P, Maffulli N: Basic biology of tendon injury and healing. *Surgeon* 3:309–316, 2005.
104. Platt MA: Tendon repair and healing. *Clin Podiatr Med Surg* 22:553–560, vi, 2005.
105. Abrahamsson SO, Lundborg G, Lohmander LS: Tendon healing in vivo. An experimental model. *Scand J Plast Reconstr Surg Hand Surg* 23:199–205, 1989.
106. Nakamura K, Kitaoka K, Tomita K: Effect of eccentric exercise on the healing process of injured patellar tendon in rats. *J Orthop Sci* 13:371–378, 2008.
107. Knobloch K, Kraemer R, Jagodzinski M, et al: Eccentric training decreases paratendon capillary blood flow and preserves paratendon oxygen saturation in chronic Achilles tendinopathy. *J Orthop Sports Phys Ther* 37:269–276, 2007.
108. Shalabi A, Kristoffersen-Wilberg M, Svensson L, et al: Eccentric training of the gastrocnemius-soleus complex in chronic Achilles tendinopathy results in decreased tendon volume and intratendinous signal as evaluated by MRI. *Am J Sports Med* 32:1286–1296, 2004.
109. Chen YJ, Wang CJ, Yang KD, et al: Extracorporeal shock waves promote healing of collagenase-induced Achilles tendinitis and increase TGF-beta1 and IGF-I expression. *J Orthop Res* 22:854–861, 2004.
110. Rompe JD, Furia J, Maffulli N: Eccentric loading versus eccentric loading plus shock-wave treatment for midportion Achilles tendinopathy: A randomized controlled trial. *Am J Sports Med* 37:463–470, 2009.
111. Zwerver J, Hartgens F, Verhagen E, et al: No effect of extracorporeal shockwave therapy on patellar tendinopathy in jumping athletes during the competitive season: A randomized clinical trial. *Am J Sports Med* 39:1191–1199, 2011.
112. van Leeuwen MT, Zwerver J, van den Akker-Scheek I: Extracorporeal shockwave therapy for patellar tendinopathy: a review of the literature. *Br J Sports Med* 43:163–168, 2009.
113. Andres BM, Murrell GA: Treatment of tendinopathy: What works, what does not, and what is on the horizon. *Clin Orthop Relat Res* 466:1539–1554, 2008.
114. Hoksrud A, Ohberg L, Alfredson H, et al: Ultrasound-guided sclerosis of neovessels in painful chronic patellar tendinopathy: A randomized controlled trial. *Am J Sports Med* 34:1738–1746, 2006.
115. Ohberg L, Alfredson H: Sclerosing therapy in chronic Achilles tendon insertional pain-results of a pilot study. *Knee Surg Sports Traumatol Arthrosc* 11:339–343, 2003.
116. Schnabel LV, Mohammed HO, Miller BJ, et al: Platelet rich plasma (PRP) enhances anabolic gene expression patterns in flexor digitorum superficialis tendons. *J Orthop Res* 25:230–240, 2007.
117. Mishra A, Pavelko T: Treatment of chronic elbow tendinosis with buffered platelet-rich plasma. *Am J Sports Med* 34:1774–1778, 2006.
118. Molloy TJ, Wang Y, Horner A, et al: Microarray analysis of healing rat Achilles tendon: Evidence for glutamate signaling mechanisms and embryonic gene expression in healing tendon tissue. *J Orthop Res* 24:842–855, 2006.
119. Arnoczky SP, Lavagnino M, Egerbacher M, et al: Matrix metalloproteinase inhibitors prevent a decrease in the mechanical properties of stress-deprived tendons: An in vitro experimental study. *Am J Sports Med* 35:763–769, 2007.
120. Ruedl G, Ploner P, Linortner I, et al: Are oral contraceptive use and menstrual cycle phase related to anterior cruciate ligament injury risk in female recreational skiers? *Knee Surg Sports Traumatol Arthrosc* 17:1065–1069, 2009.
121. Dragoo JL, Padrez K, Workman R, et al: The effect of relaxin on the female anterior cruciate ligament: Analysis of mechanical properties in an animal model. *Knee* 16:69–72, 2009.
122. Akeson WH, Amiel D, Abel MF, et al: Effects of immobilization on joints. *Clin Orthop* 219:28–37, 1987.
123. Akeson WH, Woo SL, Amiel D, et al: The connective tissue response to immobility: Biochemical changes in periarticular connective tissue of the immobilized rabbit knee. *Clin Orthop* 93:356–362, 1973.
124. Yasuda K, Hayashi K: Changes in biomechanical properties of tendons and ligaments from joint disuse. *Osteoarthritis Cartilage* 7:122–129, 1999.
125. Abramowitch SD, Woo SL: An improved method to analyze the stress relaxation of ligaments following a finite ramp time based on the quasi-linear viscoelastic theory. *J Biomech Eng* 126:92–97, 2004.
126. Frost HM: Does the ligament injury require surgery? *Clin Orthop* 49:72, 1966.
127. Murphy PG, Loitz BJ, Frank CB, et al: Influence of exogenous growth factors on the expression of plasminogen activators by explants of normal and healing rabbit ligaments. *Biochem Cell Biol* 71:522–529, 1993.
128. Pierce GF, Mustoe TA, Lingelbach J, et al: Platelet-derived growth factor and transforming growth factor-[beta] enhance tissue repair activities by unique mechanisms. *J Cell Biol* 109:429–440, 1989.
129. Woo SL-Y, Suh JK, Parsons IM, et al: Biological intervention in ligament healing effect of growth factors. *Sports Med Arthrosc Rev* 6:74–82, 1998.
130. Steenfos HH: Growth factors in wound healing. *Scand J Plast Hand Surg* 28:95–105, 1994.
131. Booher JM, Thibodeau GA: The body's response to trauma and environmental stress. In: Booher JM, Thibodeau GA, eds. *Athletic Injury Assessment,* 4th ed. New York, NY: McGraw-Hill, 2000:55–76.
132. Frank G, Woo SL-Y, Amiel D, et al: Medial collateral ligament healing. A multidisciplinary assessment in rabbits. *Am J Sports Med* 11:379, 1983.
133. Balduini FC, Vegso JJ, Torg JS, et al: Management and rehabilitation of ligamentous injuries to the ankle. *Sports Med* 4:364–380, 1987.
134. Gould N, Selingson D, Gassman J: Early and late repair of lateral ligaments of the ankle. *Foot Ankle* 1:84–89, 1980.
135. Vailas AC, Tipton CM, Mathes RD, et al: Physical activity and its influence on the repair process of medial collateral ligaments. *Connect Tissue Res* 9:25–31, 1981.
136. Tipton CM, Matthes RD, Maynard JA, et al: The influence of physical activity on ligaments and tendons. *Med Sci Sports Exerc* 7:165–175, 1975.
137. Tipton CM, James SL, Mergner W, et al: Influence of exercise in strength of medial collateral knee ligaments of dogs. *Am J Physiol* 218:894–902, 1970.
138. Laban MM: Collagen tissue: implications of its response to stress in vitro. *Arch Phys Med Rehab* 43:461, 1962.
139. McGaw WT: The effect of tension on collagen remodelling by fibroblasts: A stereological ultrastructural study. *Connect Tissue Res* 14:229, 1986.
140. Goodship AE, Birch HL, Wilson AM: The pathobiology and repair of tendon and ligament injury. *Vet Clin North Am Equine Pract* 10:323–349, 1994.
141. Hildebrand KA, Frank CB: Scar formation and ligament healing. *Can J Surg* 41:425–429, 1998.
142. van Grinsven S, van Cingel RE, Holla CJ, et al: Evidence-based rehabilitation following anterior cruciate ligament reconstruction. *Knee Surg Sports Traumatol Arthrosc* 18:1128–1144, 2010.
143. Bleakley C, McDonough S, MacAuley D: The use of ice in the treatment of acute soft-tissue injury: A systematic review of randomized controlled trials. *Am J Sports Med* 32:251–261, 2004.
144. Richter M, Bosch U, Wippermann B, et al: Comparison of surgical repair or reconstruction of the cruciate ligaments versus nonsurgical treatment in patients with traumatic knee dislocations. *Am J Sports Med* 30:718–727, 2002.
145. Hildebrand KA, Frank CB, Hart DA: Gene intervention in ligament and tendon: Current status, challenges, future directions. *Gene Ther* 11:368–378, 2004.
146. Magee DJ, Zachazewski JE: Principles of stabilization training. In: Magee D, Zachazewski JE, Quillen WS, eds. *Scientific Foundations and Principles of Practice in Musculoskeletal Rehabilitation.* St. Louis, MI: WB Saunders, 2007:388–413.

147. Behrsin JF, Andrews FJ: Lumbar segmental instability: Manual assessment findings supported by radiological measurement (a case study). *Austr J Physiol* 37:171–173, 1991.
148. Maffey LL: Arthrokinematics and mobilization of musculoskeletal tissue: The principles. In: Magee D, Zachazewski JE, Quillen WS, eds. *Scientific Foundations and Principles of Practice in Musculoskeletal Rehabilitation*. St. Louis, MI: WB Saunders, 2007:487–526.
149. Gleim GW, McHugh MP: Flexibility and its effects on sports injury and performance. *Sports Med* 24:289–299, 1997.
150. Answorth AA, Warner JJP: Shoulder instability in the athlete. *Orthop Clin North Am* 26:487–504, 1995.
151. Bergmark A: Stability of the lumbar spine. *Acta Orthop Scand* 60:1–54, 1989.
152. Boden BP, Pearsall AW, Garrett WE Jr, et al: Patellofemoral instability: Evaluation and management. *J Am Acad Orthop Surg* 5:47–57, 1997.
153. Callanan M, Tzannes A, Hayes KC, et al: Shoulder instability. Diagnosis and management. *Aust Fam Physician* 30:655–661, 2001.
154. Cass JR, Morrey BF: Ankle instability: Current concepts, diagnosis, and treatment. *Mayo Clin Proc* 59:165–170, 1984.
155. Clanton TO: Instability of the subtalar joint. *Orthop Clin N Am* 20:583–592, 1989.
156. Cox JS, Cooper PS: Patellofemoral Instability. In: Fu FH, Harner CD, Vince KG, eds. *Knee Surgery*. Baltimore, MD: Williams & Wilkins, 1994:959–962.
157. Freeman MAR, Dean MRE, Hanham IWF: The etiology and prevention of functional instability of the foot. *J Bone Joint Surg* 47B:678–685, 1965.
158. Friberg O: Lumbar instability: A dynamic approach by traction-compression radiography. *Spine* 12:119–129, 1987.
159. Grieve GP: Lumbar instability. *Physiotherapy* 68:2, 1982.
160. Hotchkiss RN, Weiland AJ: Valgus stability of the elbow. *J Orthop Res* 5:372–377, 1987.
161. Kaigle A, Holm S, Hansson T: Experimental instability in the lumbar spine. *Spine* 20:421–430, 1995.
162. Kuhlmann JN, Fahrer M, Kapandji AI, et al: Stability of the normal wrist. In: Tubiana R, ed. *The Hand*. Philadelphia, PA: WB Saunders, 1985:934–944.
163. Landeros O, Frost HM, Higgins CC: Post traumatic anterior ankle instability. *Clin Orthop* 56:169–178, 1968.
164. Luttgens K, Hamilton N: The Center of Gravity and Stability. In: Luttgens K, Hamilton N, eds. *Kinesiology: Scientific Basis of Human Motion,* 9th ed. Dubuque, IA: McGraw-Hill, 1997: 415–442.
165. Wilke H, Wolf S, Claes L, et al: Stability of the lumbar spine with different muscle groups: A biomechanical in vitro study. *Spine* 20:192–198, 1995.
166. Panjabi MM: The stabilizing system of the spine. Part 1. Function, dysfunction adaption and enhancement. *J Spinal Disord* 5:383–389, 1992.
167. McGill SM, Cholewicki J: Biomechanical basis for stability: An explanation to enhance clinical utility. *J Orthop Sports Phys Ther* 31:96–100, 2001.
168. Gertzbein SD, Seligman J, Holtby R, et al: Centrode patterns and segmental instability in degenerative disc disease. *Spine* 10:257–261, 1985.
169. Meadows JTS: *The Principles of the Canadian Approach to the Lumbar Dysfunction Patient, Management of Lumbar Spine Dysfunction – Independent Home Study Course*. La Crosse, WI: APTA, Orthopaedic Section, 1999.
170. Meadows J: *Orthopedic Differential Diagnosis in Physical Therapy*. New York, NY: McGraw-Hill, 1999.
171. Schneider G: Lumbar instability. In: Boyling JD, Palastanga N, eds. *Grieve's Modern Manual Therapy,* 2nd ed. Edinburgh: Churchill Livingstone, 1994.
172. Hardingham T, Bayliss M: Proteoglycans of articular cartilage: Changes in aging and in joint disease. *Semin Arthritis Rheum* 20:12–33, 1990.
173. Sophia Fox AJ, Bedi A, Rodeo SA: The basic science of articular cartilage: Structure, composition, and function. *Sports Health* 1:461–468, 2009.
174. Lundon K, Walker JM: Cartilage of human joints and related structures. In: Magee D, Zachazewski JE, Quillen WS, eds. *Scientific Foundations and Principles of Practice in Musculoskeletal Rehabilitation*. St. Louis, MI: WB Saunders, 2007:144–174.
175. Torzilli PA, Grigiene R, Borrelli J Jr, et al: Effect of impact load on articular cartilage: Cell metabolism and viability, and matrix water content. *J Biomech Eng* 121:433–441, 1999.
176. Pearle AD, Warren RF, Rodeo SA: Basic science of articular cartilage and osteoarthritis. *Clin Sports Med* 24:1–12, 2005.
177. Frank EH, Grodzinsky AJ: Cartilage electromechanics–I. Electrokinetic transduction and the effects of electrolyte pH and ionic strength. *J Biomech* 20:615–627, 1987.
178. Hayes WC, Bodine AJ: Flow-independent viscoelastic properties of articular cartilage matrix. *J Biomech* 11:407–419, 1978.
179. Wakitani S, Goto T, Pineda SJ, et al: Mesenchymal cell-based repair of large, full-thickness defects of articular cartilage. *J Bone Joint Surg* 76A:579–592, 1994.
180. Fuller JA, Ghadially FN: Ultrastructural observations on surgically produced partial-thickness defects in articular cartilage. *Clin Orthop* 86:193–205, 1972.
181. Ghadially FN, Thomas I, Oryschak AF, et al: Long-term results of superficial defects in articular cartilage: A scanning electron-microscope study. *J Pathol* 121:213–217, 1977.
182. Convery FR, Akeson WH, Keown GH: The repair of large osteochondral defects. An experimental study in horses. *Clin Orthop* 82:253–262, 1972.
183. Coletti JM Jr, Akeson WH, Woo SL-Y: A comparison of the physical behavior of normal articular cartilage and the arthroplasty surface. *J Bone and Joint Surg* 54-A:147–160, 1972.
184. Furukawa T, Eyre DR, Koide S, et al: Biochemical studies on repair cartilage resurfacing experimental defects in the rabbit knee. *J Bone and Joint Surg* 62-A:79–89, 1980.
185. Chu CR, Convery FR, Akeson WH, et al: Articular cartilage transplantation. Clinical results in the knee. *Clin Orthop Relat Res* 360:159–168, 1999.
186. Perka C, Sittinger M, Schultz O, et al: Tissue engineered cartilage repair using cryopreserved and noncryopreserved chondrocytes. *Clin Orthop Relat Res* 378:245–254, 2000.
187. Loitz-Ramage B, Zernicke RF: Bone biology and mechanics. In: Magee D, Zachazewski JE, Quillen WS, eds. *Scientific Foundations and Principles of Practice in Musculoskeletal Rehabilitation*. St. Louis, MI, WB Saunders, 2007:122–143.
188. Marsh DR, Li G: The biology of fracture healing: optimising outcome. *Br Med Bull* 55:856–869, 1999.
189. Muller ME: Internal fixation for fresh fractures and nonunion. *Proc R Soc Med* 56:455–460, 1963.
190. McKibbin B: The biology of fracture healing in long bones. *J Bone Joint Surg* 60B:150–161, 1978.
191. Sarmiento A, Mullis DL, Latta LL, et al: A quantitative comparative analysis of fracture healing under the influence of compression plating vs. closed weight-bearing treatment. *Clin Orthop* 149:232–239, 1980.
192. Bailey DA, Faulkner RA, McKay HA: Growth, physical activity, and bone mineral acquisition. In: Hollosky JO, ed. *Exercise and Sport Sciences Reviews*. Baltimore, MD: Williams and Wilkins, 1996: 233–266.
193. Stone MH: Implications for connective tissue and bone alterations resulting from rest and exercise training. *Med Sci Sports Exerc* 20: S162–S168, 1988.
194. Wallace AL, Draper ER, Strachan RK, et al: The vascular response to fracture micromovement. *Clin Orthop* 301:281–290, 1994.
195. Monteleone GP: Stress fractures in the athlete. *Orthop Clin North Am* 26:423, 1995.
196. Hockenbury RT: Forefoot problems in athletes. *Med Sci Sports Exerc* 31: S448–S458, 1999.
197. Busse JW, Bhandari M, Kulkarni AV, et al: The effect of low-intensity pulsed ultrasound therapy on time to fracture healing: A meta-analysis. *CMAJ* 166:437–441, 2002.
198. Brighton CT, Sennett BJ, Farmer JC, et al: The inositol phosphate pathway as a mediator in the proliferative response of rat calvarial bone cells to cyclical biaxial mechanical strain. *J Orthop Res* 10:385–393, 1992.
199. Kohavi D, Pollack SR, Brighton C: Short-term effect of guided bone regeneration and electrical stimulation on bone growth in a surgically modelled resorbed dog mandibular ridge. *Biomater Artif Cells Immobilization Biotechnol* 20:131–138, 1992.
200. Betz RR, Lavelle WF, Mulcahey MJ, et al: Histology of a fusion mass augmented with demineralized bone matrix for congenital scoliosis. *J Pediatr Orthop B* 20:37–40, 2011.
201. Kim YK, Kim SG, Lim SC, et al: A clinical study on bone formation using a demineralized bone matrix and resorbable membrane. *Oral Surg Oral Med Oral Pathol Oral Radiol Endod* 109:e6–e11, 2010.

202. Kinney RC, Ziran BH, Hirshorn K, et al: Demineralized bone matrix for fracture healing: Fact or fiction? *J Orthop Trauma* 24(Suppl 1):S52–S55, 2010.
203. Patel SK, Hick BH, Busconi BD: Fracture management. In: Magee D, Zachazewski JE, Quillen WS, eds. *Scientific Foundations and Principles of Practice in Musculoskeletal Rehabilitation*. St. Louis, MI, WB Saunders, 2007: 607–632.
204. Marsh D: Concepts of fracture union, delayed union, and nonunion. *Clin Orthop* 355:S22–S30, 1998.
205. Jennings JJ, Gerard F: Total hip replacement in patients with rheumatoid arthritis. *South Med J* 71:1112, 1978.
206. Opitz JL: Total joint arthroplasty: Principles and guidelines for postoperative physiatric management. *Mayo Clin Proc* 54:602, 1979.
207. Kmietowicz Z: Hospital infection rates in England out of control. *BMJ* 320:534, 2000.
208. Mangram AJ, Horan TC, Pearson ML, et al: Guideline for Prevention of Surgical Site Infection, 1999. Centers for Disease Control and Prevention (CDC) Hospital Infection Control Practices Advisory Committee. *Am J Infect Control* 27:97–132, 1999.
209. Nagachinta T, Stephens M, Reitz B, et al: Risk factors for surgical-wound infection following cardiac surgery. *J Infect Dis* 156:967–973, 1987.
210. Lilienfeld DE, Vlahov D, Tenney JH, et al: Obesity and diabetes as risk factors for postoperative wound infections after cardiac surgery. *Am J Infect Control* 16:3–6, 1988.
211. Boyce J: Is it time for action: Improving hand washing hygiene in hospitals. *Ann Intern Med* 130:153–155, 1999.
212. Gorman WP, Davis KR, Donnelly R: ABC of arterial and venous disease. Swollen lower limb-1: General assessment and deep vein thrombosis. *BMJ* 320:1453–1456, 2000.
213. Anderson FA, Wheeler HB: Natural history and epidemiology of venous thromboembolism. *Orthop Rev* 23:5–9, 1994.
214. Anderson FA Jr, Spencer FA: Risk factors for venous thromboembolism. *Circulation* 107:I9–16, 2003.
215. Anderson FA, Jr, Wheeler HB: Venous thromboembolism. Risk factors and prophylaxis. *Clin Chest Med* 16:235–251, 1995.
216. Anderson FA, Jr, Wheeler HB, Goldberg RJ, et al: The prevalence of risk factors for venous thromboembolism among hospital patients. *Arch Intern Med* 152:1660–1664, 1992.
217. McNally MA, Mollan RAB: Total hip replacement, lower limb blood flow and venous thrombogenesis. *J Bone and Joint Surg* 75B:640–644, 1993.
218. McNally MA, Mollan RAB: The effect of active movement of the foot on venous blood flow after total hip replacement. *J Bone and Joint Surg* 79A:1198–1201, 1997.
219. Virchow R: *Die Cellular Pathologie, Ihrer Begrundung Auf Physiologische Und Pathologische Gewebelehre,* 2nd ed. Berlin: Hirschwald, 1859.
220. Garmon RG: Pulmonary embolism: Incidence, diagnosis, prevention, and treatment. *J Am Osteopath Assoc* 85:176–185, 1985.
221. Skaf E, Stein PD, Beemath A, et al: Fatal pulmonary embolism and stroke. *Am J Cardiol* 97:1776–1777, 2006.
222. Perrier A, Bounameaux H: Accuracy or outcome in suspected pulmonary embolism. *N Engl J Med* 354:2383–2385, 2006.
223. McRae SJ, Ginsberg JS: Update in the diagnosis of deep-vein thrombosis and pulmonary embolism. *Curr Opin Anaesthesiol* 19:44–51, 2006.
224. Prandoni P, Mannucci PM: Deep-vein thrombosis of the lower limbs: Diagnosis and management. *Baillieres Best Pract Res Clin Haematol* 12:533–554, 1999.
225. Wells PS, Hirsh J, Anderson DR, et al: Accuracy of clinical assessment of deep-vein thrombosis. *Lancet* 345:1326–1330, 1995.
226. Wells PS, Anderson DR, Bormanis J, et al: Value of assessment of pretest probability of deep-vein thrombosis in clinical management. *Lancet* 350:1795–1798, 1997.
227. Wells PS, Anderson DR, Rodger M, et al: Excluding pulmonary embolism at the bedside without diagnostic imaging: Management of patients with suspected pulmonary embolism presenting to the emergency department by using a simple clinical model and d-dimer. *Ann Intern Med* 135:98–107, 2001.
228. Wells PS, Anderson DR, Rodger M, et al: Derivation of a simple clinical model to categorize patients probability of pulmonary embolism: Increasing the models utility with the SimpliRED D-dimer. *Thromb Haemost* 83:416–420, 2000.
229. Wells PS, Hirsh J, Anderson DR, et al: A simple clinical model for the diagnosis of deep-vein thrombosis combined with impedance plethysmography: Potential for an improvement in the diagnostic process. *J Intern Med* 243:15–23, 1998.
230. Riddle DL, Wells PS: Diagnosis of lower-extremity deep vein thrombosis in outpatients. *Phys Ther* 84:729–735, 2004.
231. Riddle DL, Hillner BE, Wells PS, et al: Diagnosis of lower-extremity deep vein thrombosis in outpatients with musculoskeletal disorders: A national survey study of physical therapists. *Phys Ther* 84:717–728, 2004.
232. Feied C, Handler JA: Pulmonary embolism, Available at: http://www.emedicine.com/EMERG/topic490.htm, 2006.
233. Thomas DR: Age-related changes in wound healing. *Drugs Aging* 18:607–620, 2001.
234. Scholl D, Langkamp-Henken B: Nutrient recommendations for wound healing. *J Intraven Nurs* 24:124–132, 2001.
235. Akeson WH, Amiel D, Woo SL-Y: Immobility effects on synovial joints: The pathomechanics of joint contracture. *Biorheology* 17:95–110, 1980.
236. Woo SL-Y, Matthews J, Akeson WH, et al: Connective tissue response to immobility: A correlative study of biochemical and biomechanical measurements of normal and immobilized rabbit knee. *Arthritis Rheum* 18:257–264, 1975.
237. Woo SL-Y, Gomez MA, Woo YK, et al: Mechanical properties of tendons and ligaments. II. The relationships of immobilization and exercise on tissue remodeling. *Biorheology* 19:397–408, 1982.
238. Akeson WH, Amiel D, Mechanic GL, et al: Collagen cross-linking alterations in the joint contractures: Changes in the reducible cross-links in periarticular connective tissue after 9 weeks immobilization. *Connect Tissue Res* 5:15, 1977.
239. Light KE, Nuzik S: Low-load prolonged stretch vs high-load brief stretch in treating knee contractures. *Phys Ther* 64:330–333, 1984.
240. Forrester JC, Zederfeldt BH, Hayes TL, et al: Wolff's law in relation to the healing skin wound. *J Trauma* 10:770–779, 1970.
241. Salter RB, Simmonds DF, Malcolm BW, et al: The biological effect of continuous passive motion on the healing of full-thickness defects in articular cartilage. *J Bone Joint Surg* 62A:1232–1251, 1980.
242. Jurvelin J, Kiviranta I, Tammi M, et al: Softening of canine articular cartilage after immobilization of the knee joint. *Clin Orthop* 207:246–252, 1986.
243. Behrens F, Kraft EL, Oegema TR Jr: Biochemical changes in articular cartilage after joint immobilization by casting or external fixation. *J Orthop Res* 7:335–343, 1989.
244. Salter RB, Field P: The effects of continuous compression on living articular cartilage. *J Bone Joint Surg* 42A:31–49, 1960.
245. O'Driscoll SW: The healing and regeneration of articular cartilage. *J Bone Joint Surg* 80A:1795–1812, 1998.
246. Haapala J, Arokoski JP, Hyttinen MM, et al: Remobilization does not fully restore immobilization induced articular cartilage atrophy. *Clin Orthop Relat Res* 362:218–229, 1999.
247. Deyo RA: Measuring functional outcomes in therapeutic trials for chronic disease. *Controlled Clin Trials* 5:223, 1984.
248. Lane JM, Riley EH, Wirganowicz PZ: Osteoporosis: Diagnosis and treatment. *J Bone Joint Surg* 78A:618–632, 1996.
249. Harris WH, Heaney RP: Skeletal renewal and metabolic bone disease. *N Engl J Med* 280:193–202, 253–259, 303–311, 1969.
250. Donaldson CL, Hulley SB, Vogel JM, et al: Effect of prolonged bed rest on bone mineral. *Metabolism* 19:1071–1084, 1970.
251. Mazess RB, Whedon GD: Immobilization and Bone. *Calcif Tiss Int* 35:265–267, 1983.
252. Rosen JF, Wolin DA, Finberg L: Immobilization hypercalcemia after single limb fractures in children and adolescents. *Am J Dis Child* 132:560–564, 1978.
253. Crane CW, Picou D, Smith R, et al: Protein turnover in patients before and after elective orthopaedic operations. *Br J Surg* 64:129–133, 1977.
254. Birkhahn RH, Long CL, Fitkin D, et al: Effects of major skeletal trauma on whole body protein turnover in man measured by L-(1,14C)-leucine. *Surgery* 88:294–300, 1980.
255. Arnold J, Campbell IT, Samuels TA, et al: Increased whole body protein breakdown predominates over increased whole body protein synthesis in multiple organ failure. *Clin Sci* 84:655–661, 1993.
256. McNeil PL, Khakee R: Disruptions of muscle fiber plasma membranes: Role in exercise-induced damage. *Am J Pathol* 140:1097–1109, 1992.

CHAPTER 3 The Nervous System

CHAPTER OBJECTIVES

At the completion of this chapter, the reader will be able to:

1. Describe the various components of the central and peripheral nervous systems.
2. Describe the anatomic and functional organization of the nervous system.
3. Describe the various components and distributions of the cervical, brachial, and lumbosacral plexuses.
4. Describe the difference between balance and proprioception.
5. Define proprioception and the role it plays in function.
6. Describe and differentiate among the various joint mechanoreceptors.
7. Recognize the characteristics of a lesion to the central nervous system (CNS).
8. List the findings and the impairments associated with the more common peripheral nerve lesions.
9. Perform a comprehensive examination of the neurologic system.
10. Describe some of the common pathologies of the nervous system.

OVERVIEW

In order to perform a comprehensive neuromusculoskeletal examination, the clinician must have a clear understanding of the signs and the symptoms indicating a compromise of the nervous system. The human nervous system can be subdivided into two anatomic divisions: the CNS, comprising the brain and the spinal cord, and the peripheral nervous system (PNS), formed by the cranial and the spinal nerves. The PNS is further subdivided into somatic and autonomic divisions. The somatic division innervates the skin, the muscles, and the joints, while the autonomic system innervates the glands and the smooth muscle of the viscera and the blood vessels.[1]

BASIC ANATOMY

The nerve cell, or neuron, which serves to store and process information, is the functional unit of the nervous system. The other cellular constituent is the neuroglial cell, or glia, which functions to provide structural and metabolic support for the neurons.[2]

Although neurons come in various sizes and shapes, there are four functional parts for each nerve fiber (Fig. 3-1):

- *Dendrite.* Dendrites serve a receptive function and receive information from other nerve cells or the environment.
- *Axon.* The axon cylinder, in which there is a bidirectional flow of axoplasm, conducts information and nutrition to other nerve cells and the tissues that the nerve innervates. Many axons are covered by myelin, a lipid-rich membrane. In myelinated fibers, there is a direct proportional relationship between fiber diameter and conduction velocity.[3] This membrane is divided into segments, approximately 1-mm long, by small gaps, called nodes of Ranvier, in which the myelin is absent.[4] Myelin has a high electrical resistance and low capacitance and serves to increase the nerve conduction velocity of neural transmissions through a process called *salutatory conduction*. The Schwann cell is responsible for laying down myelin around axons.
- *Cell body.* The cell body contains the nucleus of the cell and has important integrative functions.
- *Axon terminal.* The axon terminal is the transmission site for action potentials, the messengers of the nerve cell.

Peripheral nerves are enclosed in three layers of tissue of differing character. From the inside outward, these are the endoneurium, perineurium, and epineurium.[2] The nerve fibers embedded in endoneurium form a funiculus surrounded by perineurium, a thin but strong sheath of connective tissue. A fluid exists in the endoneurial spaces, which following nerve injury can produce intraneural edema, which in turn can play a major role in acute and chronic nerve lesions.[3] The nerve

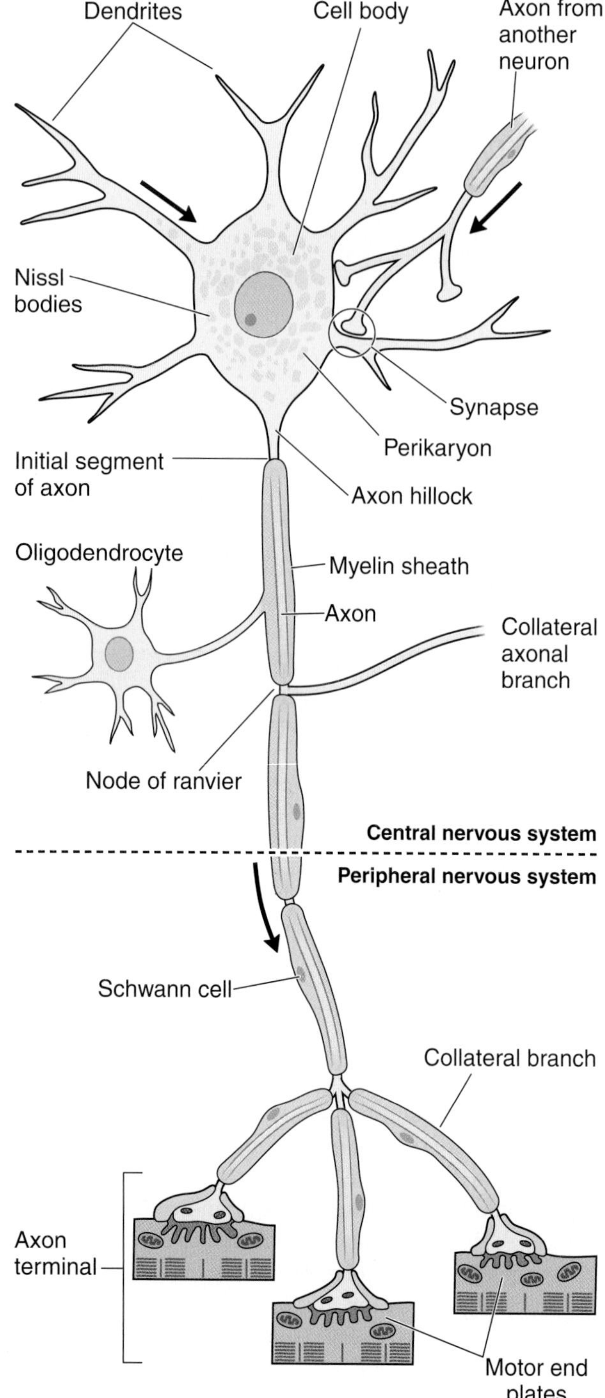

FIGURE 3-1 Schematic drawing of a neuron. (Reproduced, with permission, from Junqueira, LC, Carneiro, J: *Basic Histology Text and Atlas*, 11th ed, McGraw-Hill, 2005)

bundles are embedded in a loose areolar connective tissue framework, called the epineurium. The epineurium that extends between the fascicles is termed the inner or the interfascicular epineurium, whereas that surrounding the entire nerve trunk is called the epifascicular epineurium.[5] The connective tissue outside the epineurium is referred to as the adventitia of the nerve or the epineural tissue.[5] Although the epineurium is continuous with the surrounding connective tissue, its attachment is loose, so that nerve trunks are relatively mobile, except where tethered by entering vessels or exiting nerve branches (see Chap. 11).[6] There are no connective tissue components in the spinal nerves comparable to the epineurium and the perineurium of the peripheral nerve; at least they are not developed to the same degree.[7] As a result, the spinal nerve roots are more sensitive to both tension and compression. The spinal nerve roots also are devoid of lymphatics and, thus, are predisposed to prolonged inflammation.[8]

The communication of information from one nerve cell to another occurs at junctions called synapses, where a chemical is released in the form of a neurotransmitter. A difference in concentration exists across the cell membrane of potassium, sodium, and chloride ions. These ions can selectively permeate ion channels in the membrane so that an unequal distribution of net charge occurs. The resting membrane potential results from an internal negativity resulting from the active transport of sodium from inside to outside the cell, and potassium from outside to inside the cell.[3]

CLINICAL PEARL

Membrane potential ranges between −70 and −90 mv.

Central Nervous System

The CNS consists of the brain and an elongated spinal cord. The spinal cord participates directly in the control of body movements, the processing and transmission of sensory information from the trunk and the limbs, and the regulation of visceral functions.[1] The spinal cord also provides a conduit for the two-way transmission of messages between the brain and the body. These messages travel along the pathways, or tracts, that are fiber bundles of similar groups of neurons. Tracts may descend or ascend.

CLINICAL PEARL

Aggregates of tracts are referred to as columns or lemnisci.

The spinal cord is normally 42–45-cm long in adults and is continuous with the medulla and brain stem at its upper end (Fig. 3-2).[4] The conus medullaris serves as the distal end of the cord, and, in adults, the conus ends at the L1 or L2 level of the vertebral column. A series of specializations, the filum terminales and the coccygeal ligament, anchor the spinal cord and the dural sac inferiorly and ensure that the tensile forces applied to the spinal cord are distributed throughout its entire length.[9] The spinal cord has an external segmental organization. Each of the 31 pairs of spinal nerves that arise from the spinal cord has a anterior (ventral) root and a posterior (dorsal) root, with each root made up of one to eight rootlets and consisting of bundles of nerve fibers.[4] In the posterior (dorsal) root of a typical spinal nerve lies a spinal (sensory) ganglion (posterior (dorsal) root ganglion), a swelling that contains nerve cell bodies (Fig. 3-2).[4]

Three membranes, or meninges, envelop the structures of the CNS: dura mater, arachnoid, and pia mater (Fig. 3-3). The meninges, and related spaces, are important to both the nutrition and the protection of the spinal cord. The cerebrospinal fluid that flows through the meningeal spaces, and

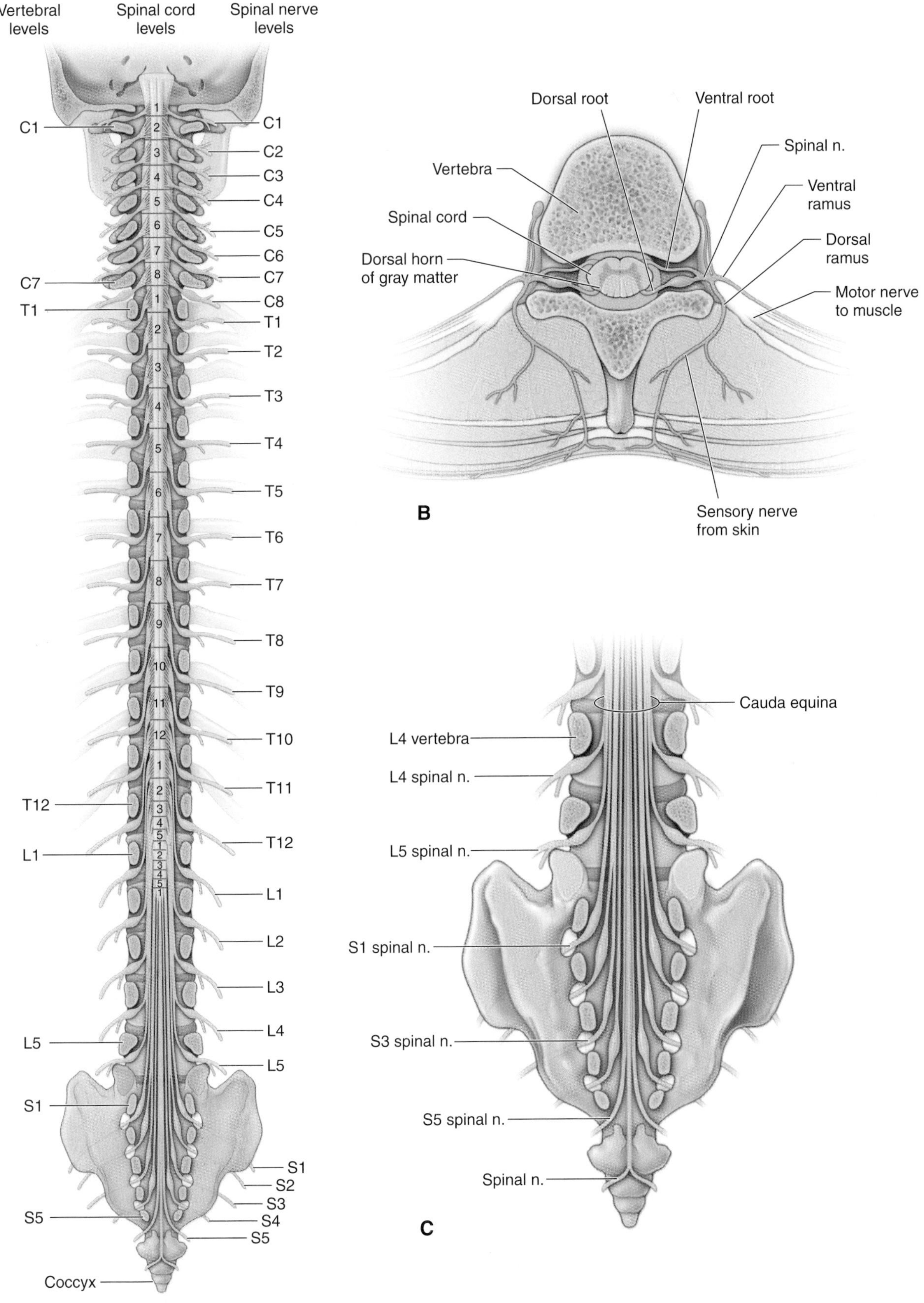

FIGURE 3-2 Schematic illustration of the spinal cord. (Reproduced, with permission, from Morton DA, Foreman KB, Albertine KH: *The Big Picture: Gross Anatomy*, McGraw-Hill, 2011)

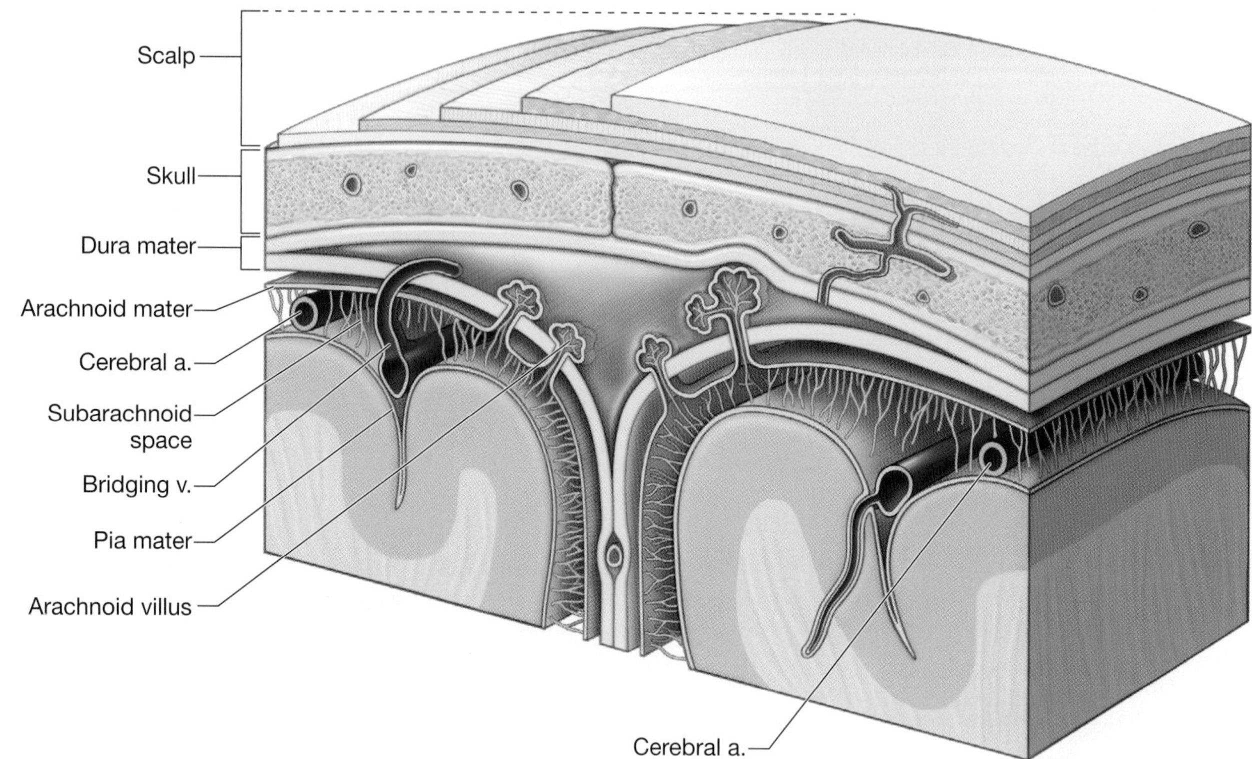

FIGURE 3-3 Schematic illustration of the relationship of the dura mater, arachnoid and pia mater. (Reproduced, with permission, from Morton DA, Foreman KB, Albertine KH: *The Big Picture: Gross Anatomy*, McGraw-Hill, 2011)

within the ventricles of the brain, provides a cushion for the spinal cord. The meninges also form barriers that resist the entrance of various noxious organisms.

Dura Mater

The dura mater (Latin, tough mother) is the outermost and the strongest of the membranes and is composed of an inner meningeal layer and an outermost periosteal layer. The dura runs uninterrupted from the interior of the cranium through the foramen magnum and surrounds the spinal cord throughout its distribution from the cranium to the coccyx at the second sacral level (S2).[9] The dura also is attached to the posterior surfaces of C2 and C3.[10]

The dura forms a vertical sac (dural sac) around the spinal cord, and its short lateral projections blend with the epineurium of the spinal nerves. The dura is separated from the bones and the ligaments that form the walls of the vertebral canal by an epidural space, which can become partly calcified or even ossified with age.[4]

Arachnoid

The arachnoid is a thin and delicate avascular layer, coextensive with the dura mater and the pia mater. Even though the arachnoid and the pia mater are interconnected by trabeculae, there is a space between them, called the subarachnoid space, which contains the cerebrospinal fluid. The supposedly rhythmic flow of this cerebrospinal fluid is the rationale used by craniosacral therapists to explain their techniques, although there is no evidence of this finding in the literature.

Pia Mater

The pia mater is the deepest of the layers. It is intimately related and firmly attached, via connective tissue investments, to the outer surface of the spinal cord and the nerve roots. The pia mater conveys the blood vessels that supply the spinal cord and has a series of lateral specializations, the denticulate (dentate) ligaments, which anchor the spinal cord to the dura mater.[9] These ligaments, which derive their name from their tooth-like appearance, extend the whole length of the spinal cord.

Peripheral Nervous System: Somatic Nerves

The PNS consists of the cranial nerves (CNs) and the spinal nerves.

Cranial Nerves

The CNs, typically, are described as comprising 12 pairs, which are referred to by the roman numerals I through XII (Fig. 3-4). The CN roots enter and exit the brain stem to provide sensory and motor innervation to the head and the muscles of the face. CN I (olfactory) and CN II (optic) are not true nerves but rather fiber tracts of the brain. The examination of the CN system is described later in this chapter (see section "Orthopaedic Neurologic Testing").

- **CN I (olfactory).** The olfactory tract arises from the olfactory bulb on the inferior aspect of the frontal lobe, just above the cribriform plate. From here it continues posteriorly as the olfactory tract and terminates just lateral to the optic chiasm. The olfactory nerve is responsible for the sense of smell.

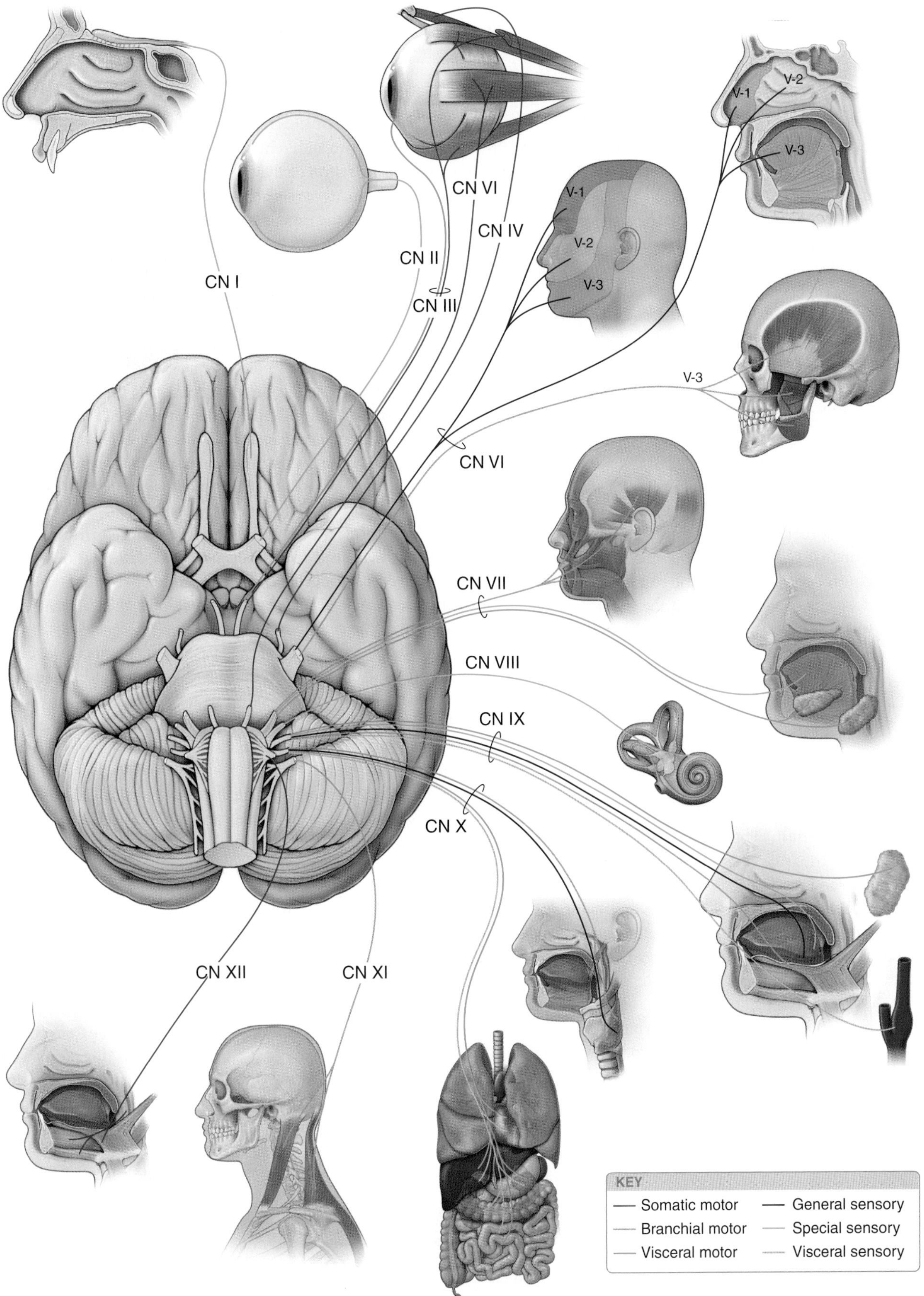

FIGURE 3-4 The CNs. (Reproduced, with permission, from Morton DA, Foreman KB, Albertine KH: *The Big Picture: Gross Anatomy,* McGraw-Hill, 2011)

- **CN II (optic).** The fibers of the optic nerve arise from the inner layer of the retina and proceed posteriorly to enter the cranial cavity via the optic foramen, to form the optic chiasm. The fibers from the nasal half of the retina decussate within the optic chiasm, whereas those from the lateral half do not. The optic nerve is responsible for vision.
- **CN III (oculomotor).** The oculomotor nerve arises in the oculomotor nucleus and leaves the brain on the medial aspect of the cerebral peduncle. It then extends from the interpeduncular fossa and runs between the posterior cerebral artery and the superior cerebellar artery, before leaving the cranial cavity and entering the cavernous sinus by way of the superior orbital fissure. The somatic portion of the oculomotor nerve supplies the levator palpebrae superioris muscle; the superior, medial, and inferior rectus muscles; and the inferior oblique muscles. These muscles are responsible for some eye movements. The visceral efferent portion of this nerve innervates two smooth intraocular muscles: the ciliary and the constrictor pupillae. These muscles are responsible for papillary constriction.
- **CN IV (trochlear).** The trochlear nerve arises from the trochlear nucleus, just caudal to the oculomotor nucleus at the anterior border of the periaqueductal gray (PAG) matter. The fibers cross within the midbrain and then emerge contralaterally on the posterior surface of the brain stem, before entering the orbit via the superior orbital fissure, to supply the superior oblique muscle.

Note: Because nerves III, IV, and VI are generally examined together, CN V is described after CN VI.

- **CN VI (abducens).** The abducens nerve originates from the abducens nucleus within the inferior aspect of the pons. Its long intracranial course to the superior orbital fissure makes it vulnerable to pathology in the posterior and middle cranial fossa. The nerve innervates the lateral rectus muscle.
- **CN V (trigeminal).** The trigeminal nerve is so named because of its tripartite division into the maxillary, ophthalmic, and mandibular branches. All three of these branches contain sensory cells, but the ophthalmic and the maxillary are exclusively sensory, the latter supplying the soft and hard palate, maxillary sinuses, upper teeth and upper lip, and mucous membrane of the pharynx. The mandibular branch carries sensory information but also represents the motor component of the nerve, supplying the muscles of mastication, both pterygoids, the anterior belly of digastric, tensor tympani, tensor veli palatini, and mylohyoid.

The spinal nucleus and the tract of the trigeminal nerve cannot be distinguished either histologically or on the basis of afferent reception from the cervical nerves. Consequently, the entire column can be viewed as a single nucleus and, legitimately, may be called the trigeminocervical nucleus.

- **CN VII (facial).** The facial nerve is made up of a sensory (intermediate) root, which conveys taste, and a motor root, the facial nerve proper, which supplies the muscles of facial expression, the platysma muscle, and the stapedius muscle of the inner ear. The intermediate root, together with the motor nerve and CN VIII, travels through the internal acoustic meatus to enter the facial canal of the temporal bone. From here, the intermediate nerve swells to form the geniculate ganglion and gives off the greater superficial petrosal nerve, which eventually innervates the lacrimal and salivary glands via the pterygopalatine ganglion and the chorda tympani nerve, respectively. The facial nerve proper exits the skull through the stylomastoid foramen.
- **CN VIII (vestibulocochlear).** The vestibulocochlear nerve subserves two different senses: balance and hearing. The cochlear portion of the nerve arises from spiral ganglia, and the vestibular portion arises from the vestibular ganglia in the labyrinth of the inner ear. The cochlear portion is concerned with the sense of hearing, whereas the vestibular portion is a part of the system of equilibrium, the vestibular system.

The vestibular system includes the vestibular apparatus of the inner ear, the vestibular nuclei and their neural projections, and the exteroreceptors throughout the body, especially in the upper cervical spine and the eyes.[11]

The apparatus of the inner ear consists of the static labyrinth, which comprises three semicircular canals (SCC) (Fig. 3-5), each orientated at right angles to the other. The labyrinth includes specialized sensory areas that are located in the utricle and the saccule (Fig. 3-5), within which otoliths are located (Fig. 3-5).

A series of filaments line the basement membrane of the SCC and project into endolymph, which deforms these filaments when head motion occurs. This deformation is registered by receptor cells, and when sudden perturbations occur, the frequency of nerve impulses along the afferent nerve supply of the cell body is altered.

Unlike the filaments of the SCC, the filaments of the utricle and saccule do not project into endolymph, but instead insert into a gelatinous mass, within which the otolith is embedded. Deformation of these filaments is produced by the weight of the otolith against the cilia, as the gelatinous mass is displaced during head movement.

The otoliths are responsible for providing information about gravitational forces, as well as vertical and horizontal motion. The filaments of the saccule also provide information about vertical motion. At rest, the endolymphatic fluid, or the gelatinous membrane, is stationary. When motion of the head occurs, the endolymphatic fluid, or the gelatinous membrane, initially remains stationary because of its inertia, while the canals move. This relative motion produces a dragging effect on the filaments and either increases or decreases the discharge rate, depending on the direction of shear. At the end of the head movement, the fluid and the membrane continue to move, and the cilia are now dragged in the opposite direction before coming to rest. In essence, the SCC receptors transmit a positive signal when movement begins, no signal when the motion has finished, and a normal level after the sensory cell has returned to its original position. As this occurs, other sensory cells orientated in the opposite direction react in the reverse fashion.

CLINICAL PEARL

The SCC detectors are so sensitive that they can detect angular accelerations as low as 0.2 degrees per second,[12] a rate of acceleration that would turn the head through 90 degrees in 30 seconds and produce a terminal velocity of 6 degrees per second: about as fast as the movement of the second hand of a watch.[13]

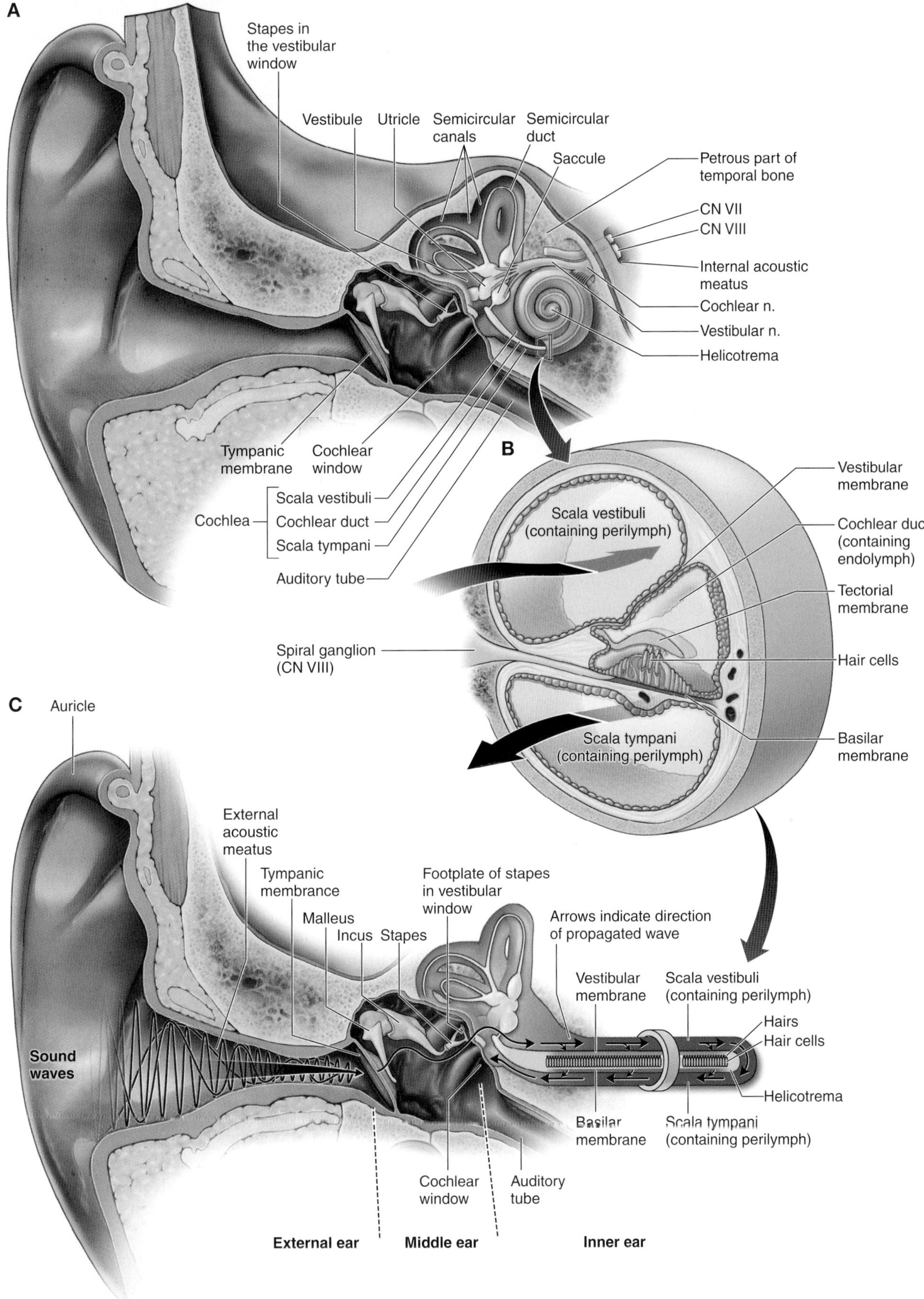

FIGURE 3-5 The apparatus of the inner ear. (Reproduced, with permission, from Morton DA, Foreman KB, Albertine KH: *The Big Picture: Gross Anatomy,* McGraw-Hill, 2011)

- **CN IX (glossopharyngeal).** The glossopharyngeal nerve contains somatic motor, visceral efferent, visceral sensory, and somatic sensory fibers. The motor fibers originate in the nucleus ambiguous, leaving the lateral medulla to join the sensory nerve, which arises from cells in the superior and petrous ganglia. The glossopharyngeal nerve exits the skull through the jugular foramen and serves a number of functions, including supplying taste fibers for the posterior third of the tongue.
- **CN X (vagus).** The functions of the vagus nerve are numerous and include the motor parasympathetic fibers to all the organs except the suprarenal (adrenal) glands, from its origin down to the second segment of the transverse colon. The vagus also controls some skeletal muscles, including:
  - Cricothyroid muscle
  - Levator veli palatini muscle
  - Salpingopharyngeus muscle
  - Palatoglossus muscle
  - Palatopharyngeus muscle
  - Superior, middle, and inferior pharyngeal constrictors
  - Muscles of the larynx.

The vagus nerve is thus responsible for such varied tasks as heart rate, gastrointestinal peristalsis, sweating, speech, and breathing. It also has some afferent fibers that innervate the inner (canal) portion of the outer ear.

- **CN XI (accessory).** The accessory nerve consists of a cranial component and a spinal component. The cranial root originates in the nucleus ambiguous and is often viewed as an aberrant portion of the vagus nerve. The spinal portion of the nerve arises from the lateral parts of the anterior horns of the first five or six cervical cord segments and ascends through the foramen magnum. The spinal portion of the accessory nerve supplies the sternocleidomastoid and the trapezius muscles.
- **CN XII (hypoglossal).** The hypoglossal nerve is the motor nerve of the tongue, innervating the ipsilateral side of the tongue as well as forming the descendens hypoglossi, which anastomoses with other cervical branches to form the ansa hypoglossi. The latter, in turn, innervates the infrahyoid muscles.

Spinal Nerves

There are a total of 31 symmetrically arranged pairs of spinal nerves, each derived from the spinal cord.[14] The spinal nerves are divided topographically into eight cervical pairs (C1–8), 12 thoracic pairs (T1–12), five lumbar pairs (L1–5), five sacral pairs (S1–5), and a coccygeal pair (Fig. 3-2).

The posterior (dorsal) and anterior (ventral) roots of the spinal nerves are located within the vertebral canal (Fig. 3-2). The portion of the spinal nerve that is not within the vertebral canal, and that usually occupies the intervertebral foramen, is referred to as a peripheral nerve. As the nerve roots begin to exit the vertebral canal, they must penetrate the dura mater before passing through dural sleeves within the intervertebral foramen. The dural sleeves are continuous with the epineurium of the nerves.

TABLE 3-1 Classification of Afferent, Cutaneous, and Efferents

Type	Conduction Velocity (m/s)	Function
Afferents		
I	70–120	Provide input from muscle and tendon receptors
II	36–72	Afferents from muscle spindles
III	27–68	Pressure/nociceptive afferents from joints and aponeuroses
IV	1–4	Pain
Cutaneous		
$A\alpha$, β	30–70	Tactile receptors
$A\delta$	12–30	Cold; fast nociception
C	0.5–1.0	Warmth; tissue damage nociception
Efferents		
α	60–100	Extrafusal muscle fibers
γ	10–30	Intrafusal muscle fibers
B	3–30	Preganglionic autonomic
C	0.5–2.0	Postganglionic autonomic

Essentially, there are four branches of spinal nerves[4]

- *Primary posterior (dorsal).* This type usually consists of a medial sensory branch and a lateral motor branch.
- *Primary anterior (ventral).* The primary anterior (ventral) division forms the cervical, brachial, and lumbosacral plexuses.
- *Communicating ramus.* The rami serve as a connection between the spinal nerves and the sympathetic trunk. Only the thoracic and upper lumbar nerves contain a white ramus communicans, but the gray ramus is present in all spinal nerves.
- *Meningeal or recurrent meningeal (also known as sinuvertebral).* These nerves carry sensory and vasomotor innervation to the meninges.

There are three functional types of nerve fibers in the major nerve trunks, which vary in quantity depending on the particular nerve: afferent (sensory), autonomic (visceral efferent), and motor (somatic efferent) (Table 3-1). The faster nerve fibers such as A delta fibers are more concerned with speed and quality of human movement whereas the C fibers conduct far more slowly and are more involved with nociception and, by the compounds they release, the health of surrounding tissue.[3]

Sensory Nerves

The sensory nerves carry afferents (a nerve conveying impulses from the periphery to the CNS) from a portion of the skin. They also carry efferents (a nerve conveying impulses from the CNS to the periphery) to the skin structures. When a sensory nerve is compressed, symptoms occur in the area of the nerve distribution. This area of distribution, called a dermatome, is a well-defined portion of the skin (Fig. 3-6)

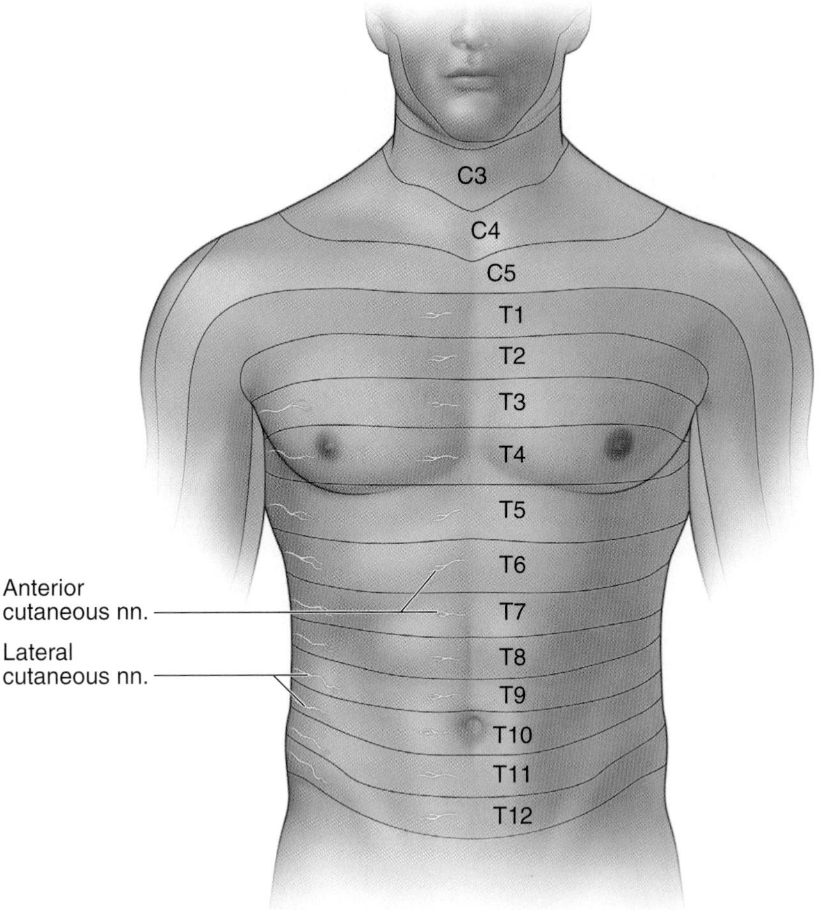

FIGURE 3-6 Segmental distribution of the body. (Reproduced, with permission, from Morton DA, Foreman KB, Albertine KH: *The Big Picture: Gross Anatomy*, McGraw-Hill, 2011)

and generally follows the segmental distribution of the underlying muscle innervation.[4]

CLINICAL PEARL

- A dermatome is the area of skin supplied by a single nerve root. Pain dermatomes have less overlap than light-touch dermatomes.[15]
- A myotome is a muscle or group of muscles supplied by a single nerve root.
- A sclerotome is an area of bone or fascia supplied by a single nerve root.

Examples of sensory nerves in the body are the lateral (femoral) cutaneous nerve (LCN) of the thigh (Fig. 3-7), the saphenous nerve, and the interdigital nerves (see later).

CLINICAL PEARL

Most individuals have no C1 posterior (dorsal) root; therefore, there is no C1 dermatome. When present, the C1 dermatome covers a small area in the central part of the neck close to the occiput.[4]

- *Motor nerves.* The motor nerves carry efferents to muscles and return sensation from muscles and associated ligamentous structures. Any nerve that innervates a muscle also mediates the sensation from the joint upon which that muscle acts. Examples of a motor nerve include the suprascapular nerve and the posterior (dorsal) scapular nerve. A hierarchical recruitment pattern exists in the nervous system for muscle recruitment called the *law of parsimony*.[16] The law of parsimony states that the nervous system tends to activate the fewest muscles or muscle fibers possible for the control of a given joint action. This hierarchical pattern of muscle recruitment makes practical sense from an energy perspective.[16]
- *Mixed nerves.* A mixed nerve is a combination of skin, sensory, and motor fibers to one trunk. Some examples of a mixed nerve are the median nerve, the ulnar nerve at the elbow as it enters the tunnel of Guyon, the fibular (peroneal) nerve at the knee, and the ilioinguinal nerve.

Cervical Nerves

The eight pairs of cervical nerves are derived from cord segments between the level of the foramen magnum and

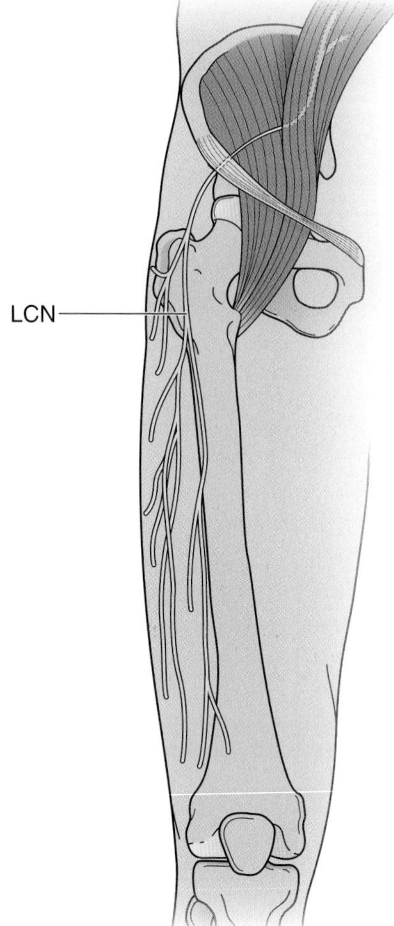

FIGURE 3-7 LCN of the thigh.

CLINICAL PEARL

Two studies[18,19] that analyzed magnetic resonance imaging (MRI) and computed tomography images of the cervical intervertebral foramens found that the cervical nerve root is located in the lower part of the interpedicular foramen and occupies the major inferior part of the intertransverse foramen. Anteriorly, compression of the nerve roots is likely caused by protruding discs and osteophytes of the uncovertebral region, whereas the superior articular process, the ligamentum flavum, and the periradicular fibrous tissues often affect the nerve posteriorly.[20–23]

the middle of the seventh cervical vertebra.[17] The spinal nerves from C3 to C7, exiting from the intervertebral foramen, divide into a larger anterior (ventral) ramus and a smaller posterior (dorsal) ramus. The anterior (ventral) ramus of the cervical spinal nerve travels on the transverse process in an anterior–lateral direction to form the cervical plexus and brachial plexus. The posterior (dorsal) ramus of the spinal nerve runs posteriorly around the superior articular process, supplying the facet (zygapophyseal) joint, ligaments, deep muscles, and skin of the posterior aspect of the neck.[9]

Each nerve joins with a gray communicating ramus from the sympathetic trunk and sends a small, recurrent meningeal branch back into the spinal canal to supply the dura with sensory and vasomotor innervation. It also branches into anterior and posterior primary divisions, which are mixed nerves that pass to their respective peripheral distributions. The motor branches carry a few sensory fibers that convey proprioceptive impulses from the neck muscles.

- *Posterior primary divisions.* The C1 (suboccipital) nerve is the only branch of the first posterior primary divisions. It is a motor nerve, serving the muscles of the suboccipital triangle, with very few, if any, sensory fibers.[17]
- *Anterior primary divisions.* The anterior primary divisions of the first four cervical nerves (C1–4) form the cervical plexus (Fig. 3-8).
  - *Cervical plexus (C1–4)*
  - *Sensory branches (see Fig. 3-6)*
- *Small occipital nerve (C2,3).* This nerve (Fig. 3-8) supplies the skin of the lateral occipital portion of the scalp, the upper median part of the auricle, and the area over the mastoid process.[17]
- *Great auricular nerve (C2,3).* This nerve (Fig. 3-8) supplies sensation to the ear and the face via the ascending ramus of the mandible. The nerve lies on or just below the deep layer of the investing fascia of the neck. It arises from the anterior rami of the second and third cervical nerves and emerges from behind the sternomastoid muscle, before ascending on it to cross over the parotid gland.
- *Cervical cutaneous nerve (cutaneous coli) (C2,3).* This nerve supplies the skin over the anterior portion of the neck.
- *Supraclavicular branches (C3,4).* These nerves supply the skin over the clavicle and the upper deltoid and pectoral regions, as low as the third rib.
- *Communicating branches.* The ansa cervicalis nerve (Fig. 3-8) is formed by the junction of two main nerve roots, derived entirely from anterior (ventral) cervical rami. A loop is formed at the point of their anastomosis, and sensory fibers are carried to the dura of the posterior fossa of the skull via the recurrent meningeal branch of the hypoglossal nerve. The communication with the vagus nerve from C1 is of undetermined function.
- *Muscular branches.* Communication with the hypoglossal nerve from C1 to C2 (Fig. 3-8) carries motor fibers to the geniohyoid and thyrohyoid muscles and to the sternohyoid and sternothyroid muscles by way of the superior root of the ansa cervicalis (Fig. 3-8). The nerve to the thyrohyoid branches from the hypoglossal nerve and runs obliquely across the hyoid bone to innervate the thyrohyoid. The nerve to the superior belly of the omohyoid branches from the superior root (Fig. 3-8) and enters the muscle at a level between the thyroid notch and a horizontal plane 2-cm

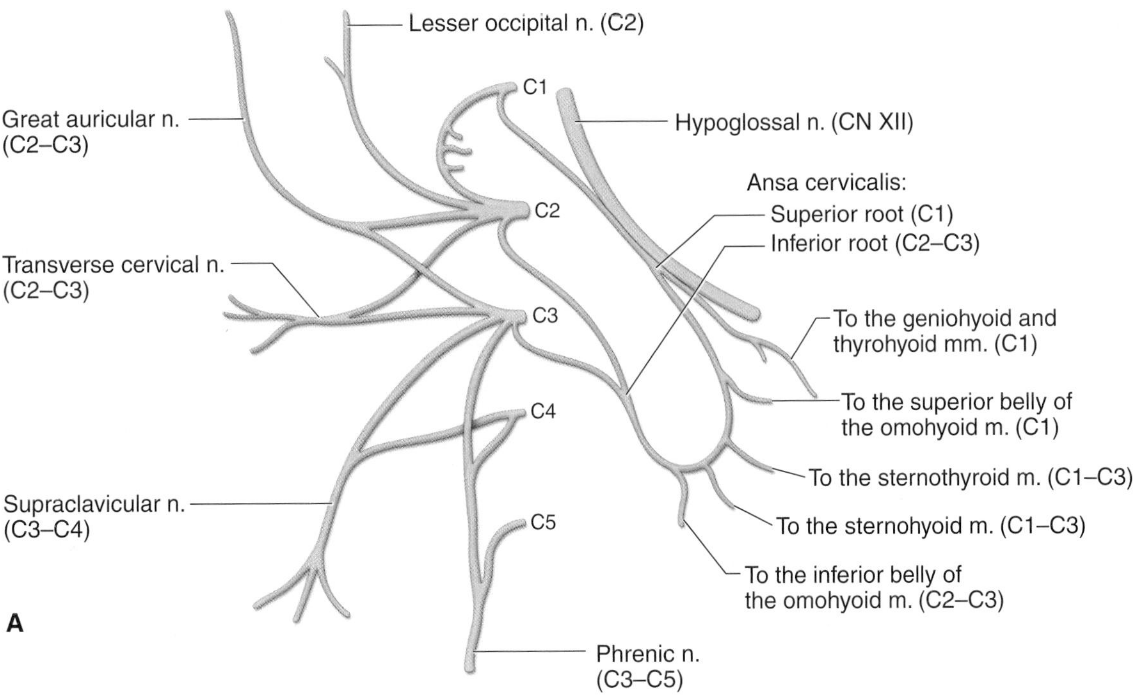

FIGURE 3-8 The cervical plexus. (Reproduced, with permission, from Morton DA, Foreman KB, Albertine KH: *The Big Picture: Gross Anatomy*, McGraw-Hill, 2011)

inferior to the notch. The nerves to the sternohyoid and sternothyroid share a common trunk, which branches from the loop (Fig. 3-8). The nerve to the inferior belly of the omohyoid also branches from the loop (Fig. 3-8). The loop is most frequently located just deep to the site where the superior belly (or tendon) of the omohyoid muscle crosses the internal jugular vein. There is a branch to the sternocleidomastoid muscle from C2, and there are branches to the trapezius muscle (C3–4) via the subtrapezial plexus.

Smaller branches to the adjacent vertebral musculature supply the rectus capitis lateralis and rectus capitis anterior (C1), the longus capitis (C2,4) and longus colli (C1–4), the scalenus medius (C3,4) and scalenus anterior (C4), and the levator scapulae (C3–5).

The phrenic nerve (C3–5) (see Fig. 3-8) passes obliquely over the scalenus anterior muscle and between the subclavian artery and the vein to enter the thorax behind the sternoclavicular joint, where it descends vertically through the superior and middle mediastinum to the diaphragm.[17] Motor branches supply the diaphragm. Sensory branches supply the pericardium, the diaphragm, and part of the costal and mediastinal pleurae.

CLINICAL PEARL

The phrenic nerve is the largest branch of the cervical plexus and plays a vital role in respiration.

Phrenic nerve involvement has been described in several neuropathies, including critical illness, polyneuropathy, Guillain–Barré syndrome, brachial neuritis, and hereditary motor and sensory neuropathy type 1.[24,25] The symptoms depend largely on the degree of involvement, and whether one or both of the nerves are involved.[17]

- Unilateral paralysis of the diaphragm causes few or no symptoms except with heavy exertion.
- Bilateral paralysis of the diaphragm is characterized by dyspnea upon the slightest exertion and difficulty with coughing and sneezing.[24,25]
- Phrenic neuralgia, which can result from neck tumors, aortic aneurysm, and pericardial or other mediastinal infections, is characterized by pain near the free border of the ribs, beneath the clavicle, and deep in the neck.[24,25]

Brachial Plexus

The brachial plexus (Fig. 3-9) arises from the anterior primary divisions of the fifth cervical through the first thoracic nerve roots, with occasional contributions from the fourth cervical and the second thoracic roots. The roots of the plexus, which consist of C5 and C6, join to form the superior (upper) trunk; C7 becomes the middle trunk, and C8 and T1 join to form the inferior (lower) trunks. Each of the trunks divides into anterior and posterior divisions, which then form cords (Fig. 3-9). The anterior divisions of the upper and middle trunk form the lateral cord, the anterior division of the inferior (lower) trunk forms the medial cord, and all three posterior divisions unite to form the posterior cord. The three cords, named for their relationship to the axillary artery, split to form the main branches of the plexus. These branches give rise to the peripheral nerves: musculocutaneous (lateral cord), axillary and radial (posterior cord), ulnar (medial cord), and median

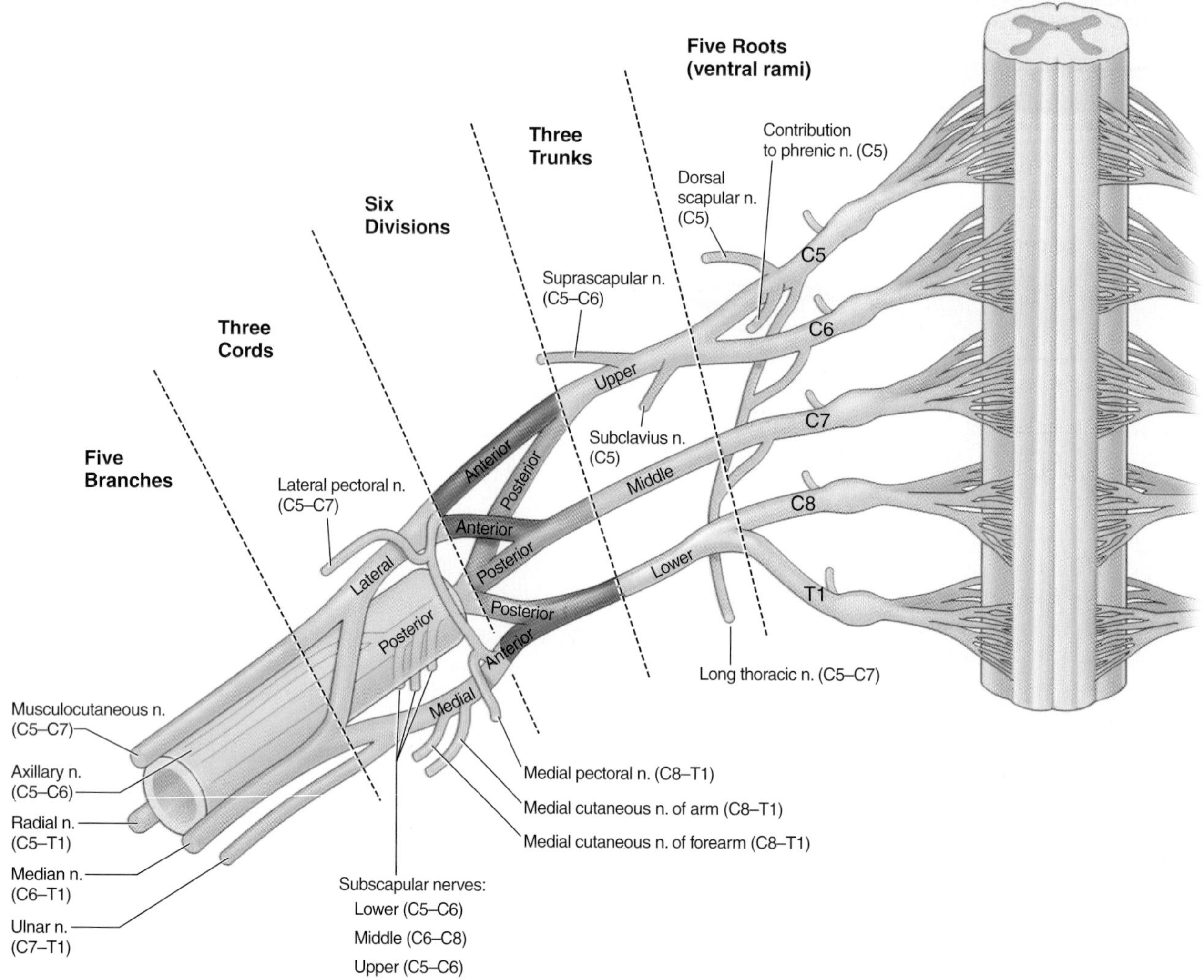

FIGURE 3-9 The brachial plexus. (Reproduced, with permission, from Morton DA, Foreman KB, Albertine KH: *The Big Picture: Gross Anatomy*, McGraw-Hill, 2011)

(medial and lateral cords).[26] Numerous smaller nerves arise from the roots, the trunks, and the cords of the plexus. Peripheral nerve injuries of the upper extremity and their respective clinical findings are listed in Table 3-2.

From the Roots

- The origin of the posterior (dorsal) scapular nerve (C5) frequently shares a common trunk with the long thoracic nerve (Fig. 3-9). The former passes through the scalenus medius anterior internally and posterior laterally, with the presence of some tendinous tissues. Leaving the long thoracic nerve, it often gives branches to the shoulder and the subaxillary region, before the branches join the long thoracic nerve again. The posterior (dorsal) scapular nerve supplies the rhomboids and the levator scapulae muscles. Posterior (dorsal) scapular nerve lesions can result from a forward posture of the head and the neck As this position increases tension in the anterior cervical spine, producing the potential for hypertonicity and hypertrophy of the medial scalene.[27] The chief complaint is usually one of scapular pain radiating to the lateral shoulder and arm.
- The long thoracic nerve (C5–7) is purely a motor nerve that originates from the anterior (ventral) rami of the fifth, the sixth, and the seventh cervical roots (Fig. 3-9). It is the sole innervation to the serratus anterior muscle. The fifth and the sixth cervical roots, along with the posterior (dorsal) scapular nerve, pass through the scalenus medius muscle, whereas the seventh cervical root passes anterior to it.[28] The nerve then travels beneath the brachial plexus and clavicle to pass over the first rib. From there, it descends along the lateral aspect of the chest wall, where it innervates the serratus anterior muscle. The long thoracic nerve extends as far inferior as the eighth or the ninth rib. Its long and relatively superficial course makes it susceptible to injury from any of the following causes:[10,29–31]
  - Entrapment of the fifth and the sixth cervical roots, as they pass through the scalenus medius muscle
  - Compression of the nerve during traction to the upper extremity by the undersurface of the scapula, as the nerve crosses over the second rib
  - Compression and traction to the nerve by the inferior angle of the scapula during general anesthesia or with vigorous passive abduction of the arm

TABLE 3-2 Peripheral Nerve Injury Related to the Cords of the Brachial Plexus			
Cord and Nerve	**Level of Injury**	**Motor Loss**	**Cutaneous Loss**
Posterior cord: radial (C5–T1)	Plexus—proximal to axillary nerve	All muscles innervated by radial nerve All muscles innervated by axillary nerve	Throughout radial and axillary distribution
	Axilla (brachioaxillary angle)	Triceps (medial and lateral heads) and anconeus	Posterior brachial cutaneous
	Spiral groove	All muscles innervated by radial nerve except medial head of triceps	Posterior antebrachial cutaneous
	Proximal to lateral epicondyle	Brachialis, brachioradialis, ECRL, and ECRB	
	Arcade of Frohse	Supinator, all muscles innervated by posterior interosseous nerve	Superficial radial (Wartenberg syndrome)
Posterior cord: axillary nerve (C5–6)	Axilla (quadrangular space)	Teres minor and deltoid	Lateral arm
Medial and lateral cord: median nerve (C5–T1)	Plexus (proximal to the joining of the medial and lateral cords)—thoracic outlet syndrome	All muscles innervated by median, musculocutaneous, and ulnar nerves	Throughout median, musculocutaneous, and ulnar distributions
	Ligament of Struthers—proximal to medial epicondyle	Pronator teres	
	Cubital fossa exit—between two heads of the pronator teres	Pronator teres, FCR, FDS, PL, and lumbricales I and II	
	Forearm	Anterior interosseous: FDP (I and II), FPL, and PQ median muscular branch: Thenar muscles (APB, FPB, and OP) and lumbricales I and II	Palmar branch: radial half of thumb Digital branch: posterior (dorsal) tips of thumb, index, and middle finger and radial half of ring finger
Lateral: musculocutaneous nerve (C5–7)	Coracobrachialis	Coracobrachialis Biceps Brachialis	
	Elbow		Lateral antebrachial cutaneous nerve: Lateral forearm
	Cubital tunnel	FCU, FDP, adductor pollicis, lumbricales, and interossei	Posterior and anterior aspects on the ulnar side of the hand
	Between the two heads of the FCU	FDP and FCU	
	Proximal to wrist	Deep branch: all hand muscles innervated by the ulnar nerve Superficial branch: Palmaris brevis	Medial: ulnar nerve (C8–T1)
	Guyon canal	Muscles of the hypothenar eminence (hand of benediction) and interossei	Ulnar aspect of the hand

ECRL, extensor carpi radialis longus; ECRB, extensor carpi radialis brevis; FCR, flexor carpi radialis; FDS, flexor digitorum superficials; PL, plamaris longus; FDP, flexor digitorum profundus; FPL, flexor pollicis longus; PQ, pronator quadratus; APB, abductor pollicis brevis; FPB, flexor pollicis brevis; OP, opponens pollicis; FCU, flexor carpi ulnaris; DIP, distal interphalangeal; PIP, proximal interphalangeal.

Lesions of the long thoracic nerve are common and are the single most common peripheral nerve lesion at the shoulder. The most common cause of long thoracic nerve injury results from carrying a heavy object on the shoulder. Other causes include postinfection, postinjection, postpartum, and postoperative.[32] Similar to other peripheral nerve injuries, trauma to the nerve can be caused by a direct blow or a traction force to the nerve. The traction injury can occur when concurrent head rotation away, side bending away, and neck flexion, are coupled with the arm positioned overhead.[33–35] Other mechanisms that have been attributed to long thoracic nerve dysfunction include lifting weights overhead, driving a golf ball, and serving a tennis ball.[36]

The typical clinical presentation includes the following:

- Vague pain in the neck and the scapula region
- An inability to fully elevate the arm overhead
- Shoulder flexion and abduction are weak and limited in AROM due to the loss of the trapezius–serratus

anterior force couple. The clinician should note winging of the scapula when testing the serratus anterior.

Conservative intervention includes protection of the serratus anterior with a brace or restraint,[32,35,37] galvanic stimulation to the serratus anterior, muscle taping,[38] strengthening exercises for the rhomboids, pectoralis, trapezius, and serratus anterior muscles.[33,36,39] The average rate of return ranges from 3–7 months[28,32] to 2 years.[36]

- A small branch from C5 passes to the phrenic nerve.
- Smaller branches from C6 to C8 extend to the scaleni and longus colli muscles.
- The first intercostal nerve extends from T1.

From the Trunks

A nerve extends to the subclavius muscle (C5–6) from the superior (upper) trunk, or fifth root. The subclavius muscle acts mainly on the stability of the sternoclavicular joint, with more or less intensity, according to the degree of the clavicular interaction with the movements of the peripheral parts of the superior limb, and seems to act as a substitute for the ligaments of the sternoclavicular joint.[40]

The suprascapular nerve originates from the superior (upper) trunk of the brachial plexus formed by the roots of C5 and C6 (see Fig. 3-9) at Erb's point.

From the Cords

- The medial and lateral pectoral nerves extend from the medial and lateral cords, respectively (see Fig. 3-9). They supply the pectoralis major and pectoralis minor muscles. The pectoralis major muscle has dual innervation.[41] The lateral pectoral nerve (C5–7) is actually more medial in the muscle, travels with the thoracoacromial vessels, and innervates the clavicular and sternal heads. The medial pectoral nerve (C8–T1) shares a course with the lateral thoracic vessels and provides innervation to the sternal and costal heads.[42] The main trunk of these nerves can be found near the origin of the vascular supply of the muscle.
- The three subscapular nerves from the posterior cord consist of:
  - The upper subscapular nerve (C5–6), which supplies the subscapularis muscle (see Fig. 3-9).
  - The thoracodorsal nerve, or middle subscapular nerve, which arises from the posterior cord of the brachial plexus with its motor fiber contributions from C6, C7, and C8 (see Fig. 3-9). This nerve courses along the posterior–lateral chest wall, along the surface of the serratus anterior, and deep to the subscapularis, giving rise to branches that supply the latissimus dorsi.
  - The lower subscapular nerve (C5–6) to the teres major and part of the subscapularis muscle (see Fig. 3-9).
- Sensory branches of the medial cord (C8–T1[43,44] or T1 alone[44]) comprise the medial cutaneous (antebrachial) nerve to the medial surface of the forearm and the medial cutaneous (brachial) nerve to the medial surface of the arm (see Fig. 3-9).

Obstetric Brachial Plexus Lesions

The pathomorphologic spectrum of traumatic brachial plexus impairments most often includes combinations of various types of injuries: compression of spinal nerves, traction injuries of spinal roots and nerves, and avulsions of spinal roots.[45] If the rootlets are traumatically disconnected from the spinal cord, they normally exit the intradural space; in rare cases, however, they may also remain within the dural space.

Brachial plexus injuries are most commonly seen in children and usually are caused by birth injuries. Stretch (neurapraxia or axonotmesis) and incomplete rupture are more common in obstetric brachial plexus palsy than complete rupture or avulsion.

Obstetrical brachial plexus palsy is classified into upper (involving C5, C6, and usually C7 roots), lower (predominantly C8 and T1), and total (C5–C8 and T1) plexus palsies.[46,47] Upper brachial plexus palsy, although described first by Duchenne,[48] bears the name Erb's palsy.[49] Most cases of obstetric brachial plexus palsy involve Erb's palsy, and the lesion is always supraclavicular. Lower brachial plexus palsy is extremely rare in birth injuries[44] and is referred to as Klumpke's palsy.[50]

The infant with Erb's palsy typically shows the classic "waiter's tip" posture of the paralyzed limb.[51,52] The arm lies internally rotated at the side of the chest, the elbow is extended (paralysis of C5,6) or slightly flexed (paralysis of C5–C7), the forearm is pronated, and the wrist and the fingers are flexed. This posture occurs because of paralysis and atrophy of the deltoid, biceps, brachialis, and brachioradialis muscles.[53]

Klumpke's paralysis is characterized by paralysis and atrophy of the small hand muscles and flexors of the wrist (the so-called claw hand). Prognosis of this type is more favorable. If the sympathetic rami of T1 are involved, Horner syndrome (ptosis, enophthalmos, facial reddening, and anhydrosis) may be present.

> **CLINICAL PEARL**
>
> - Mononeuropathy: injury to a single peripheral nerve (e.g., the radial nerve).
> - Polyneuropathy: involvement of more than one peripheral nerve. Occurs in such systemic diseases as diabetes.

Peripheral Nerves of the Upper Quadrant

Spinal Accessory Nerve

The spinal accessory, or simply the accessory, nerve is formed by the union of CN XI (see Cranial Nerves) and the spinal nerve roots of C3 and C4, and innervates the trapezius and the sternocleidomastoid (SCM) muscles. Thus dysfunction of the nerve causes paralysis of the SCM and the trapezius muscles.

Isolated lesions to this nerve result from forces acting across the glenohumeral (G-H) joint. Combined lesions of the axillary nerve result from forces acting broadly across the scapulothoracic joint. These lesions are associated with fractures of the clavicle and/or scapula and subclavian vascular lesions.[54]

The superficial course of the nerve makes it susceptible to injury during operative procedures or blunt trauma.[55] The accessory nerve is also vulnerable to stretch-type injuries,[56,57] such as during a manipulation of the shoulder under anesthesia.[58] However, stretch-type injuries do not always involve the SCM.[59] Accessory nerve paresis can also result from serious pathology such as a tumor at the base of the skull, or from surgery.[60]

Clinical findings for this condition include:

- neck, shoulder, and medial scapular pain;
- decreased cervical lordosis;
- a downwardly rotated scapula;
- winging of the scapula;
- trapezius weakness, especially with active arm elevation.

A confirmatory test includes resisted adduction of the scapula while the clinician applies counterpressure at the medial border of the inferior scapular angle. This will highlight weakness on the affected side.

Conservative intervention for this condition involves patient education to avoid traction to the nerve, specific upper, middle, and lower trapezius strengthening, neuromuscular electrical stimulation to the upper and lower trapezius, cervical proprioceptive neuromuscular facilitation (PNF) techniques, scapular PNF techniques, prone-on-elbows scapular stabilization exercises (see Chap. 25), and shoulder elevation strengthening. McConnell taping is also used to facilitate the middle and lower trapezius muscle.[58]

Suprascapular Nerve (C5–6)

The suprascapular nerve (Fig. 3-9) travels downward and laterally behind the brachial plexus and parallel to the omohyoid muscle beneath the trapezius to the superior edge of the scapula, through the suprascapular notch. The roof of the suprascapular notch is formed by the transverse scapular ligament. The suprascapular artery and vein initially run with the nerve and then run above the transverse suprascapular ligament over the notch. After passing through the notch, the nerve supplies the suprascapular muscle. It also provides articular branches to the G-H and acromioclavicular (A-C) joints and provides sensory and sympathetic fibers to two-thirds of the shoulder capsule and to the G-H and A-C joints. The nerve then turns around the lateral edge of the scapular spine to innervate the infraspinatus.

It is commonly taught that the suprascapular nerve provides the motor supply to the supraspinatus and infraspinatus muscles and sensory innervation to the shoulder joint but that it has no cutaneous representation. However, cutaneous branches are present in the proximal one-third of the arm,[61–63] and their distribution overlaps with that of the supraclavicular and axillary nerves.

CLINICAL PEARL

Pain related to suprascapular nerve entrapment may radiate to the lateral neck or posterior and lateral aspects of the G-H capsule area.

There are several ways the suprascapular nerve may be injured. These include compression traction and laceration.[64] A direct blow at Erb's point can cause a compression-type injury.[64] Compression neuropathy of the suprascapular nerve often occurs in the scapular notch under the transverse scapular ligament or at the spinoglenoid notch. This compression occurs through extraneural inflammation, lipoma or cyst development, scarring following distal clavicle resection, and ligament entrapment.[27,33,65,66]

Due to the location of this entrapment, entrapment of this nerve may be misdiagnosed as rotator cuff tendonitis, a tear of the rotator cuff, or cervical disk disease.[67,68]

The cause for this entrapment can be acute trauma resulting from a fall on an outstretched hand (FOOSH), scapular fracture, or overuse injuries involving repetitive overhead motions.[65,68,69]

As the suprascapular nerve is a mixed nerve, the patient presentation usually includes the following:

- A dull, deep ache at the posterior and lateral aspects of the shoulder, which may have a burning quality.
- Muscle atrophy and weakness of the supraspinatus and infraspinatus.
- Changes in G-H biomechanics with an increase of scapula elevation occurring during arm elevation. This may produce impingement-like findings and complicate the diagnosis.
- Full external rotation of the G-H joint and passive horizontal adduction are painful.[266] Electromyography (EMG) is the definitive test for suprascapular neuropathy.[70]

Conservative intervention includes rest, ice, analgesics, and a series of perineural injections of corticosteroid to help reduce neural inflammation. A home exercise program of scapular pivoter strengthening (see Chap. 16), scapulohumeral coordination exercises (see Chap. 16), and activity-specific training may be indicated.[33]

Surgical intervention, involving neurolysis, cyst removal, or the excision of the transverse scapular ligament is indicated if symptoms persist.

Musculocutaneous Nerve (C5–6)

The musculocutaneous nerve (Fig. 3-10) is the terminal branch of the lateral cord, which in turn is derived from the anterior division of the upper and middle trunks of the fifth through seventh cervical nerve roots.[71,72]

The nerve arises from the lateral cord of the brachial plexus at the level of the insertion of the pectoralis minor[72,73] and proceeds caudally and laterally, giving one or more branches

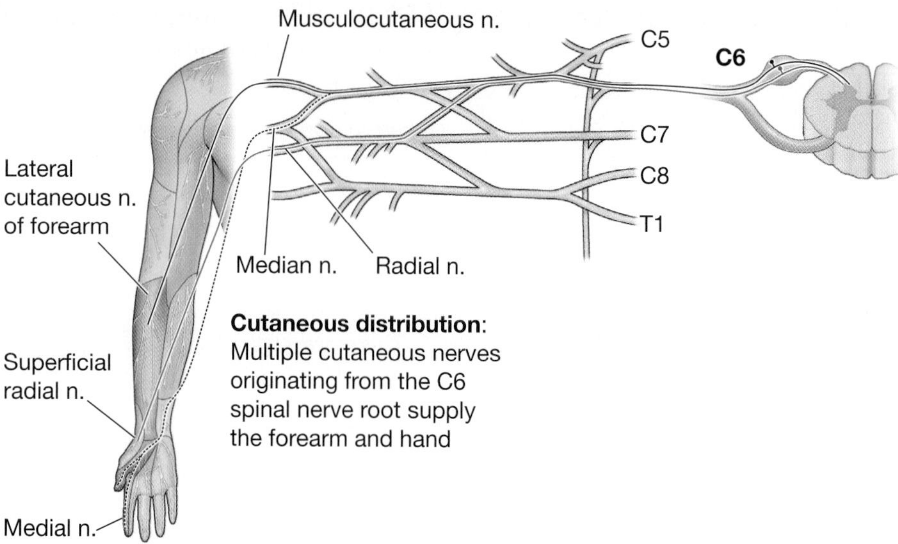

FIGURE 3-10 The musculocutaneous (C5–6) nerve. (Reproduced, with permission, from Morton DA, Foreman KB, Albertine KH: *The Big Picture: Gross Anatomy*, McGraw-Hill, 2011)

to the coracobrachialis, before penetrating this muscle 3–8 cm below the coracoid process.[72,74] The nerve then courses through, and supplies, the biceps brachii and brachialis muscles, before emerging between the biceps brachii and the brachioradialis muscles 2–5 cm above the elbow (see Fig. 3-11). At this level, now called the lateral cutaneous (antebrachial) nerve of the forearm, it divides into anterior and posterior divisions to innervate the anterior–lateral aspect of the forearm (Fig. 3-10).[72]

Atraumatic isolated musculocutaneous neuropathies are rare. Reported cases have been associated with positioning during general anesthesia,[75] peripheral nerve tumors, and strenuous upper extremity exercise without apparent underlying disease.[76–79] Mechanisms proposed for the exercise-related cases include entrapment within the coracobrachialis,[76–78] as well as traction between a proximal fixation point at the coracobrachialis and a distal fixation point at the deep fascia at the elbow.[72] Injury to this nerve can also result from demanding physical work involving shoulder flexion and repetitive elbow flexion with a pronated forearm.[76,79,81] Although rare, an isolated lesion to the musculocutaneous nerve can result in weakness of the biceps, coracobrachialis, and brachialis (Table 3-3). These muscles help stabilize the elbow and the G-H joint[50] and maintain the static position of the arm.[80]

The typical clinical presentation includes:

- reports or evidence of muscle wasting and sensory changes to the lateral side of the forearm;
- weakness of the biceps, brachialis, and coracobrachialis;
- diminished biceps reflex;
- decreased sensation at the lateral forearm; and
- positive EMG study.

Conservative intervention includes cessation of the strenuous activity and a gradual return to activity with resolution of symptoms.[79]

CLINICAL PEARL

Although a musculocutaneous nerve lesion would be expected to demonstrate weakness of elbow flexion, one would not expect to see weakness in all shoulder motions, with an injury isolated to the proximal musculocutaneous nerve.

Axillary Nerve (C5–6)

The axillary nerve is the last nerve of the posterior cord of the brachial plexus before the latter becomes the radial nerve (see Fig. 3-11). The axillary nerve arises as one of the terminal branches of the posterior cord of the brachial plexus, with its neural origin in the fifth and sixth cervical nerve roots. The axillary nerve crosses the anterior–inferior aspect of the subscapularis muscle, where it then crosses posteriorly through the quadrilateral space and divides into two major trunks. Along its course across the subscapular muscle, the axillary nerve releases its first articular branch to the inferior–anterior G-H joint capsule. The posterior trunk of the axillary nerve gives a branch to the teres minor muscle and the posterior deltoid muscle, before terminating as the superior lateral cutaneous (brachial) nerve of the arm (see Fig. 3-11). The anterior trunk continues, giving branches to supply the middle and anterior deltoid muscle.

The axillary nerve is susceptible to injury at several sites, including the origin of the nerve from the posterior cord, the anterior–inferior aspect of the subscapularis muscle and G-H joint capsule, the quadrilateral space, and within the subfascial surface of the deltoid muscle (Table 3-3).

Axillary nerve lesions may result from acute G-H dislocation, surgery to the G-H complex, blunt trauma to the axilla, secondary hematoma and fibrous formation, entrapment, and tractioning.[33,81–83]

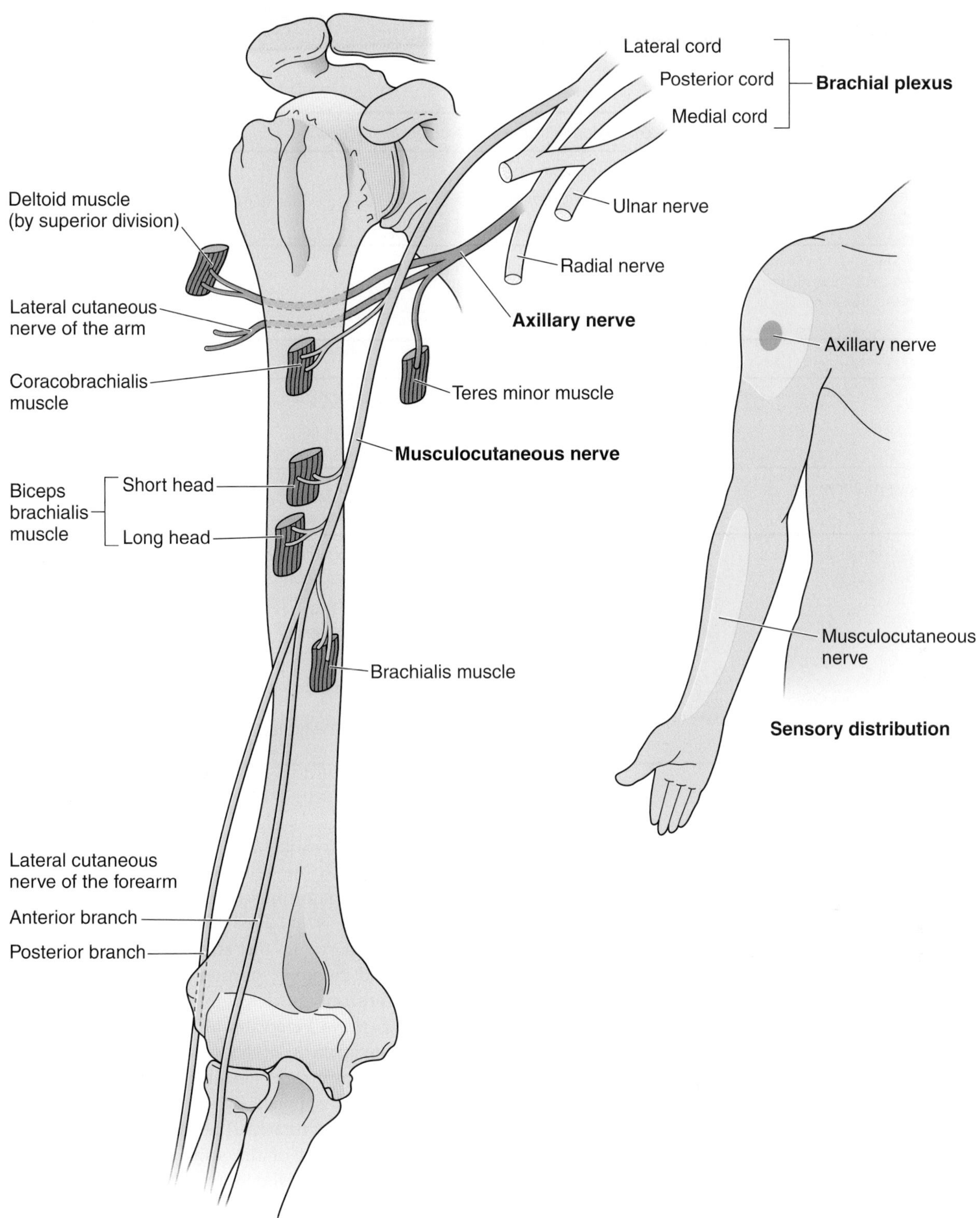

FIGURE 3-11 The musculocutaneous (C5–6) and axillary (C5–6) nerves. (Reproduced, with permission, from Waxman SG: *Clinical Neuroanatomy*, 26th ed, McGraw-Hill, 2010)

The typical clinical presentation includes:

- deep pain in the axilla, or in the anterior shoulder in the case of a G-H dislocation;
- tingling in the deltoid aspect of the shoulder;
- atrophy may be seen in the deltoid and teres minor;
- weakness when elevating the arm in flexion and abduction;[33]
- manual muscle testing will reveal weakness of the deltoid and teres minor; and
- sensory testing should highlight a loss of sensation at the lateral deltoid region.

The diagnostic test for this lesion is to ask the patient to abduct the arm to 90 degrees and to bring it back into

TABLE 3-3 Injury Findings Related to Nerves of the Brachial Plexus

Nerve	Findings
Spinal accessory nerve	Inability to abduct the arm beyond 90 degree Pain in shoulder with abduction
Musculocutaneous nerve	Weak elbow flexion with forearm supinated
Long thoracic nerve	Pain on flexing fully extended arm Inability to flex fully extended arm Winging of scapula at 90 degree of forward flexion
Suprascapular nerve	Increased pain on forward shoulder flexion Pain increased with scapular abduction Pain increased with cervical rotation to opposite side
Axillary nerve	Inability to abduct arm with neutral rotation
Suprascapular nerve compression or injury	Supraspinatus and infraspinatus weakness and atrophy (if compression prior to innervation of supraspinatus) Infraspinatus weakness and atrophy alone (if compression at the spinoglenoid notch)
Thoracic outlet syndrome	Symptoms reproduced by Roos test, Wright maneuver, Adson test, or hyperabduction test (variable) Diminution of pulse with Adson test, Wright maneuver, Halsted test, or hyperabduction test (variable)
Brachial plexus (stinger or burner)	History of traction force to neck rotation, neck side bending, shoulder abduction, or shoulder external rotation, with simultaneous scapula and clavicular depression Tenderness over brachial plexus Weakness in muscles innervated by involved portion of the plexus C5 (deltoid, supraspinatus, and infraspinatus) most commonly involved C6 (elbow flexors) second most commonly involved Sensory loss in involved nerve distribution Transient burning and pain

horizontal extension. A patient with an axillary lesion will demonstrate extreme difficulty with this.[84]

Intervention for this lesion is initially conservative and consists of thermal modalities, protection, and strengthening exercises.[33] Surgical exploration may be indicated in cases of complete denervation.

Radial Nerve (C6–8, T1)

The radial nerve (Fig. 3-12) is the largest branch of the brachial plexus. Originating at the lower border of the pectoralis minor as the direct continuation of the posterior cord, it derives fibers from the last three cervical and first thoracic segments of the spinal cord. During its descent in the arm, the radial nerve accompanies the profunda artery behind, and around, the humerus and in the musculospiral groove. It pierces the lateral intermuscular septum and reaches the lower anterior side of the forearm, where its terminal branches arise.

CLINICAL PEARL

The radial nerve is frequently entrapped at its bifurcation in the region of the elbow, where the common radial nerve becomes the sensory branch and a deep or posterior interosseous branch.

The radial nerve crosses the elbow immediately anterior to the radial head, just beneath the heads of the extensor origin of the extensor carpi radialis brevis (ECRB), and then divides, with the deep branch running through the body of the supinator muscle to the posterior aspect of the forearm.

The radial nerve in the arm supplies the triceps, the anconeus, and the upper portion of the extensor–supinator group of forearm muscles. In the forearm, the posterior interosseous nerve innervates all of the muscles of the six extensor compartments of the wrist, with the exception of the ECRB and extensor carpi radialis longus (ECRL).

The skin areas supplied by the radial nerve include the posterior cutaneous (brachial) nerve of the arm, to the posterior (dorsal) aspect of the arm; the posterior cutaneous (antebrachial) nerve of the forearm, to the posterior (dorsal) surface of the forearm; and the superficial radial nerve, to the posterior (dorsal) aspect of the radial half of the hand (see Fig. 3-12). The isolated area of supply is a small patch of skin over the posterior aspect of the first interosseous space (see Fig. 3-12).

Four radial nerve entrapments are commonly cited: high radial nerve palsy, posterior interosseous nerve palsy (PINS), radial tunnel syndrome, and superficial radial nerve palsy (see Chap. 17). The major disability associated with radial nerve injury is a weak grip, which is weakened because of poor stabilization of the wrist and the finger joints (Table 3-3). In addition, the patient demonstrates an inability to extend the thumb, the wrist, and the elbow, as well as the proximal phalanges. Pronation of the forearm

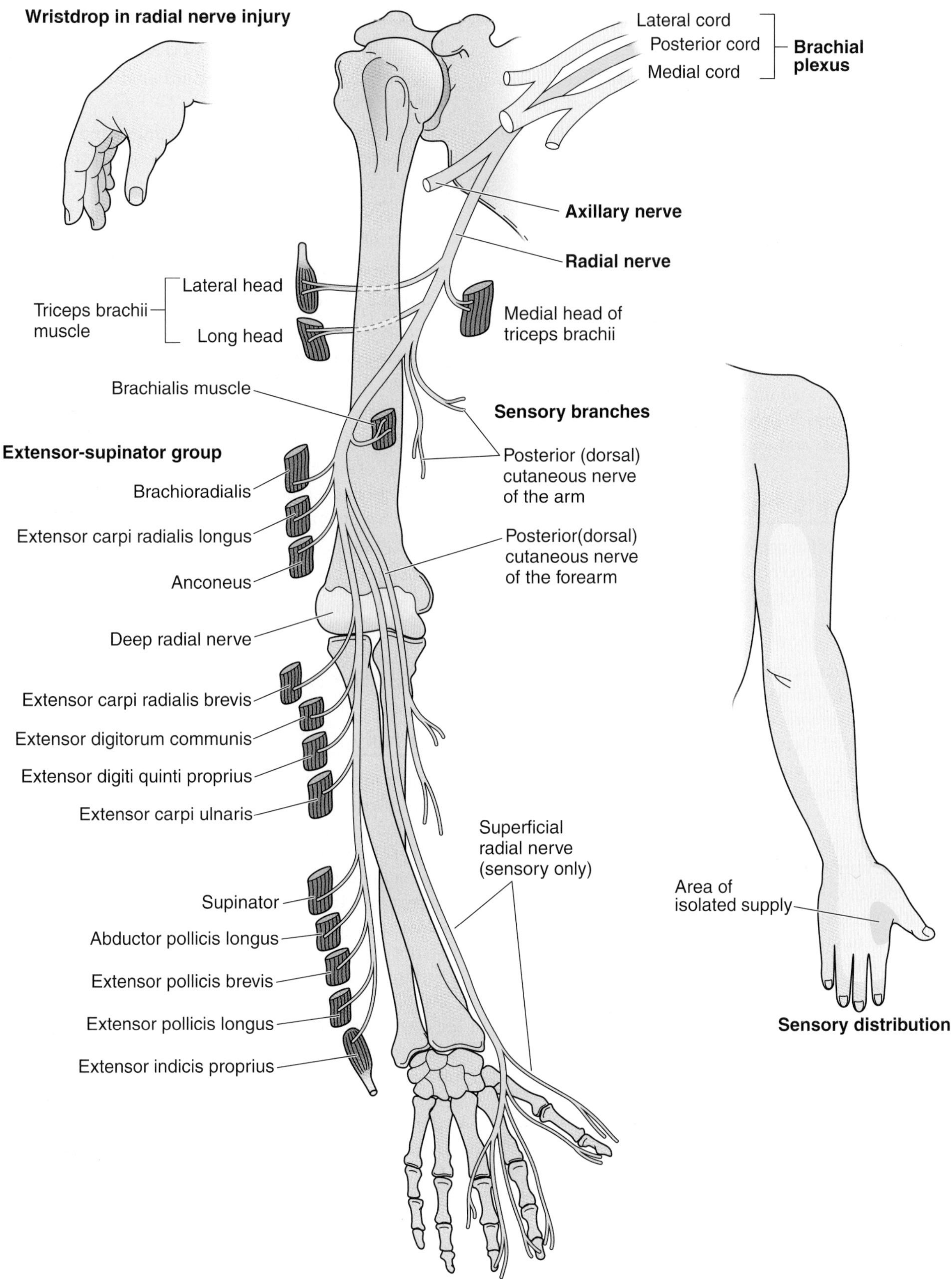

FIGURE 3-12 The radial nerve (C6–8, T1). (Reproduced, with permission, from Waxman SG: *Clinical Neuroanatomy*, 26th ed, McGraw-Hill, 2010)

and adduction of the thumb also are affected, and the wrist and the fingers adopt a position termed wrist drop. The triceps and other radial reflexes are absent, but the sensory loss is often slight, owing to overlapping innervation.

The site of the entrapment of the radial nerve can often be determined by the clinical findings, as follows:

- If the impairment occurs at a point below the triceps innervation, the strength of the triceps remains intact.

- If the impairment occurs at a point below the brachioradialis branch, some supination is retained.
- If the impairment occurs at a point in the forearm, the branches to the small muscle groups, extensors of the thumb, extensors of the index finger, extensors of the other fingers, and extensor carpi ulnaris may be affected.
- If the impairment occurs at a point on the posterior aspect of the wrist, only sensory loss on the hand is affected.

Conservative intervention for a radial nerve lesion depends on the location and the severity. As with all peripheral nerve injuries, every attempt must be made to maintain the appropriate range of the muscle or muscles innervated by the nerve, while helping to prevent contracture in those muscles antagonistic to the denervated muscle by using stretching techniques. In addition, muscle strengthening is prescribed for those uninvolved agonistic and synergistic muscles.

Median Nerve (C5–T1)

The trunk of the median nerve derives its fibers from the lower three (sometimes four) cervical and the first thoracic segment of the spinal cord. Although it has no branches in the upper arm, the nerve trunk descends along the course of the brachial artery and passes onto the anterior aspect of the forearm, where it gives off muscular branches, including the anterior interosseous nerve. It then enters the hand, where it terminates with both muscular and cutaneous branches (Fig. 3-13). The sensory branches of the median nerve supply the skin of the palmar aspect of the thumb and the lateral 2½ fingers as well as the distal ends of the same fingers (see Fig. 3-13).

The anterior interosseous nerve arises from the posterior aspect of the median nerve, approximately 5-cm distal to the medial humeral epicondyle, and passes with the main trunk of the median nerve between the two heads of the pronator teres.[26] It continues along the palmar aspect of the flexor digitorum profundus and then passes between the flexor digitorum profundus and the flexor pollicis longus, running in close proximity to the interosseous membrane, to enter the pronator quadratus.[26] It provides motor innervation to the flexor pollicis longus; the medial part of flexor digitorum profundus, involving the index and sometimes the middle finger; and to the pronator quadratus. It also sends sensory fibers to the distal radioulnar, radiocarpal, intercarpal, and carpometacarpal joints.[85] Variations in the distribution of the nerve have been noted; it may supply all or none of the flexor digitorum profundus and part of the flexor digitorum superficialis.[86]

The clinical features of median nerve impairment (Table 3-3), depending on the level of injury, include the following[17]:

- Paralysis is noted in the flexor–pronator muscles of the forearm (resulting in weakness or loss of pronation), all of the superficial palmar muscles, except the flexor carpi ulnaris, and all of the deep palmar muscles, except the ulnar half of the flexor digitorum profundus and the thenar muscles that lie superficial to the tendon of the flexor pollicis longus.
- At the wrist, there is weak flexion and radial deviation, and the hand inclines to the ulnar side.
- In the hand, an ape-hand deformity can be present (see Fig. 3-13). This deformity is associated with
  - an inability to oppose or flex the thumb or abduct it in its own plane;
  - a weakened grip, especially in the thumb and index finger, with a tendency for these digits to become hyperextended, and the thumb adducted;
  - an inability to flex the distal phalanx of the thumb and index finger;
  - weakness of middle finger flexion; and
  - atrophy of the thenar muscles.
- There is a loss of sensation to a variable degree over the cutaneous distribution of the median nerve, most constantly over the distal phalanges of the first two fingers.
- Pain is present in many median nerve impairments anywhere along its distribution.
- Atrophy of the thenar eminence is seen early. Atrophy of the flexor–pronator groups of muscles in the forearm is seen after a few months.
- The skin of the palm is frequently dry, cold, discolored, chapped, and at times keratotic.

The most common condition associated with median nerve entrapment is carpal tunnel syndrome (see Chap. 18). The various interventions for median nerve entrapment are discussed in Chapters 17 and 18.

Ulnar Nerve (C8, T1)

The ulnar nerve is the largest branch of the medial cord of the brachial plexus. It arises from the medial cord of the brachial plexus and contains fibers from the C8 and T1 nerve roots, although C7 may contribute some fibers (Fig. 3-14). The ulnar nerve continues along the anterior compartment of the arm, and it passes through the medial intermuscular septum at the level of the coracobrachialis insertion. As the ulnar nerve passes into the posterior compartment of the arm, it courses through the arcade of Struthers, which is a potential site for its compression.

At the level of the elbow, the ulnar nerve passes posterior to the medial epicondyle, where it passes through the cubital tunnel. From there, the ulnar nerve passes between the two heads of the flexor carpi ulnaris origin and traverses the deep flexor–pronator aponeurosis. This aponeurosis is superficial to the flexor digitorum profundus, but deep to the flexor carpi ulnaris and flexor digitorum superficialis muscles.[87,88]

CLINICAL PEARL

The intraneural topography of the ulnar nerve differs at various levels of the arm. At the medial epicondyle, the sensory fibers to the hand and the motor fibers to the intrinsic muscles are superficial, whereas the motor fibers to flexor carpi ulnaris and flexor digitorum profundus are deep.[89]. This may explain the common finding in "cubital tunnel syndrome" (see Chap. 17) of sensory loss and weakness of the ulnarly innervated intrinsic muscles, but relative sparing of flexor carpi ulnaris and flexor digitorum profundus strength.[90]

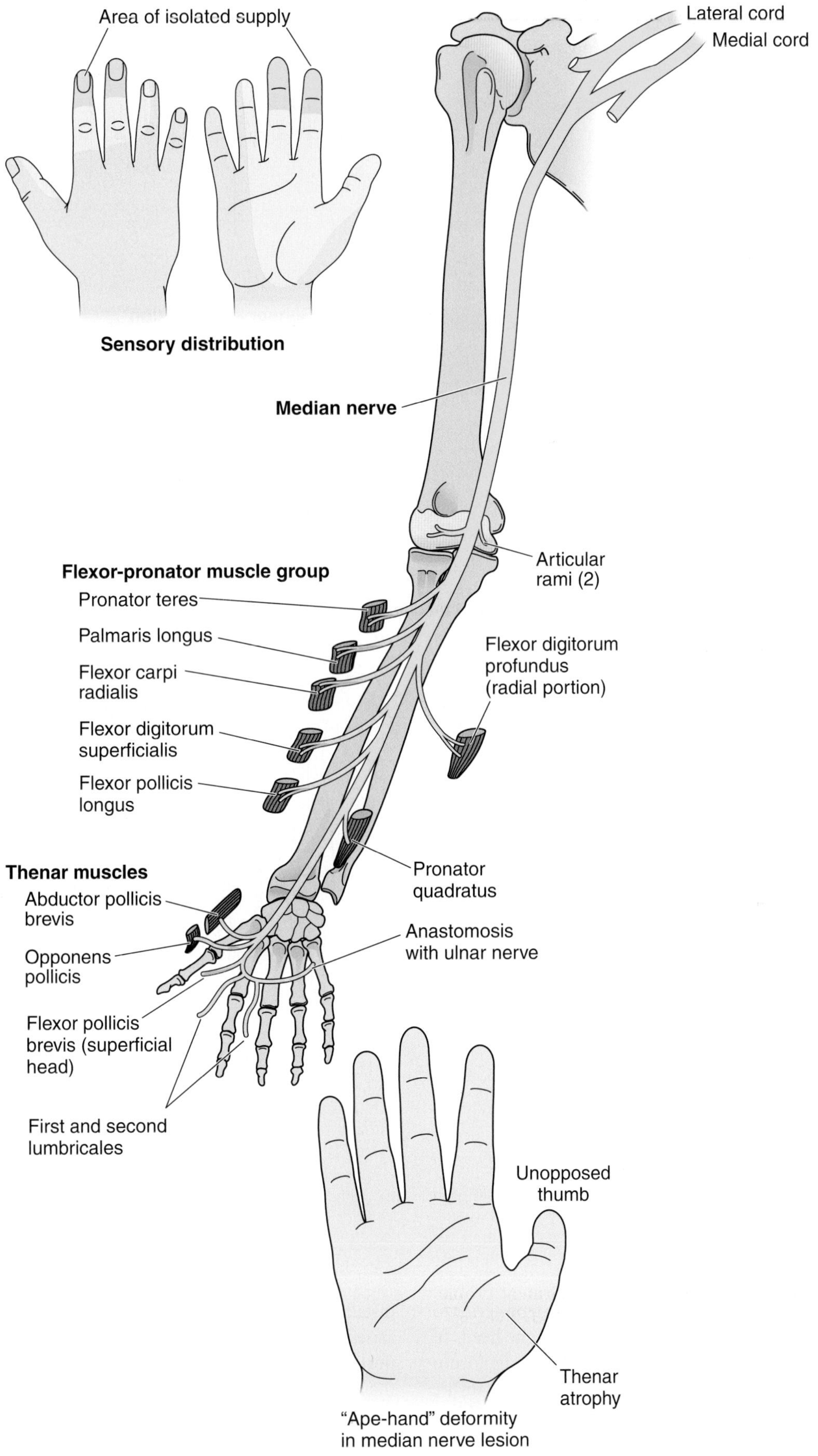

FIGURE 3-13 The median nerve (C6–8, T1). (Reproduced, with permission, from Waxman SG: *Clinical Neuroanatomy*, 26th ed, McGraw-Hill, 2010)

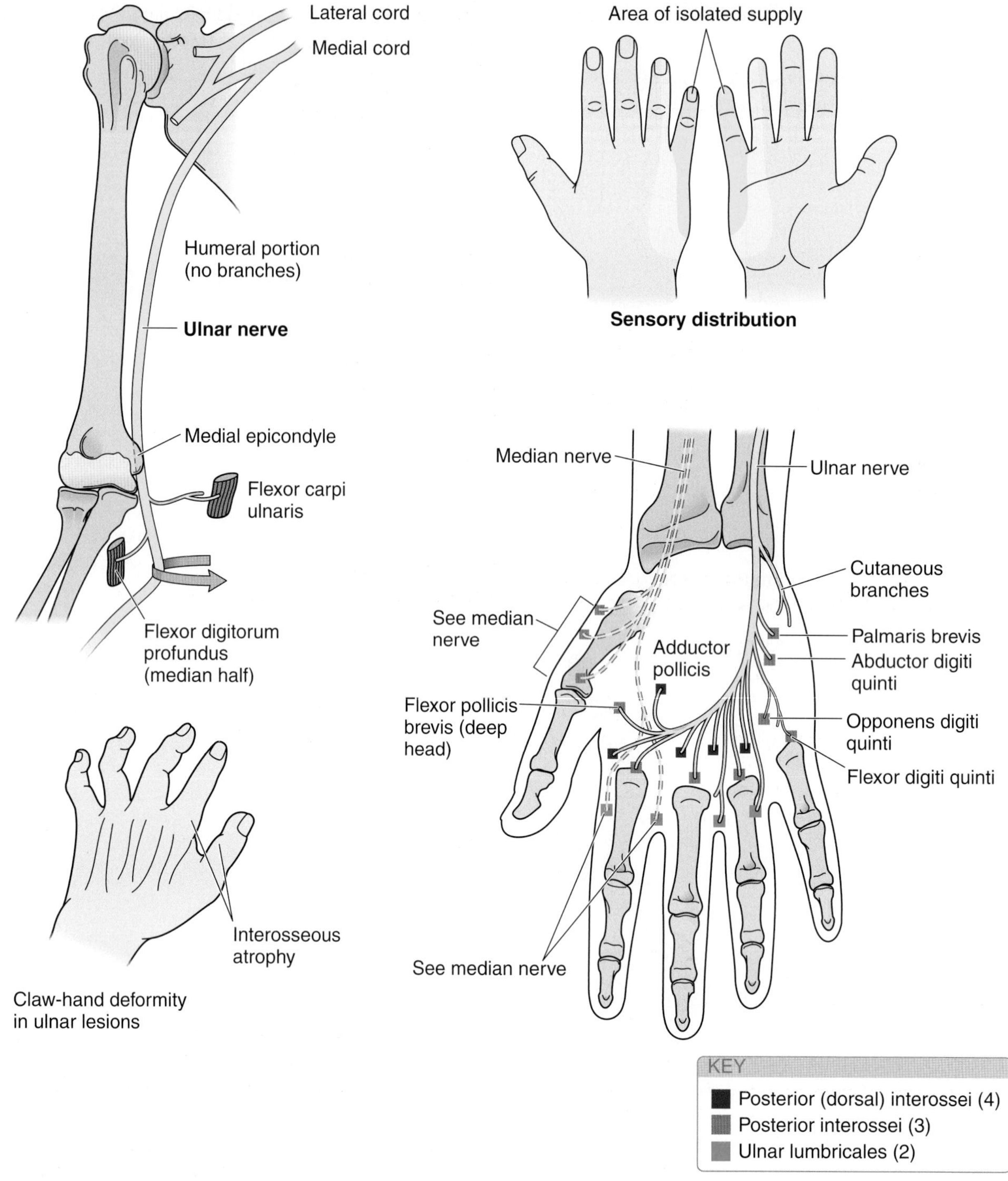

FIGURE 3-14 The ulnar nerve (C8, T1). (Reproduced, with permission, from Waxman SG: *Clinical Neuroanatomy*, 26th ed, McGraw-Hill, 2010)

The ulnar nerve enters the forearm by coursing posterior to the medial humeral condyle and passing between the heads of the flexor carpi ulnaris, before resting on the flexor digitorum profundus[91] (see Fig. 3-14). It then continues distally to the wrist passing between the flexor carpi ulnaris and the flexor digitorum profundus muscles, which it supplies. Proximal to the wrist, the palmar cutaneous branch of the ulnar nerve arises. This branch runs across the palmar aspect of the forearm and the wrist outside of the tunnel of Guyon to supply the proximal part of the ulnar side of the palm. A few centimeters more distally to the tunnel, a posterior (dorsal) cutaneous branch arises and supplies the ulnar side of the dorsum of the hand, the posterior (dorsal) aspect of the fifth finger, and the ulnar half of the forefinger. The ulnar nerve supplies the flexor carpi ulnaris, the ulnar head of the flexor digitorum profundus, and all of the small muscles deep and medial to the long flexor tendon of the thumb, except the first two lumbricales (see Fig. 3-14, indicated by terminal branches in hand). Its sensory distribution includes the skin of the little finger and the medial half of the hand and the ring finger (see Fig. 3-14).

The clinical features of ulnar nerve impairment (Table 3-3) include the following[17]:

- Claw hand (see Fig. 3-14), resulting from unopposed action of the extensor digitorum communis in the fourth and fifth digits.
- An inability to extend the second and distal phalanges of any of the fingers.
- An inability to adduct or abduct the fingers, or to oppose all the fingertips, as in making a cone with the fingers and the thumb.
- An inability to adduct the thumb.
- At the wrist, flexion is weak and ulnar deviation is lost. The ulnar reflex is absent.
- Atrophy of the interosseous spaces (especially the first) and of the hypothenar eminence.
- A loss of sensation on the ulnar side of the hand and ring finger and, most markedly, over the entire little finger.
- Partial lesions of the ulnar nerve may produce only motor weakness or paralysis of a few of the muscles supplied by the nerve. Lesions that occur in the distal forearm or at the wrist spare the deep flexors and the flexor carpi ulnaris.

The conservative interventions for the various ulnar nerve entrapments are discussed in Chapters 17 and 18.

Thoracic Nerves

In the thoracic region, there is great variability in the topography of the nerves and the structures that they serve.[92] Typically, the spinal root arises from the lateral end of the spinal nerve but, in 25% of cases, the spinal root is made up of two parts that arise from the superior border of the spinal nerve.[93] The thoracic spinal nerves are segmented into posterior (dorsal) primary and anterior (ventral) primary divisions. As elsewhere, the dermatomes of this region are considered to represent the cutaneous region innervated by one spinal nerve through both of its rami.[94]

Anterior (Ventral) Rami

There are 12 pairs of thoracic anterior (ventral) rami. The anterior (ventral) rami (anterior branches) from T2 through T11 become intercostal nerves. The 12th anterior (ventral) ramus, the subcostal nerve, is located below the last rib. The intercostal nerve has a lateral branch, providing sensory distribution to the skin of the lateral aspect of the trunk, and an anterior branch, supplying the intercostal muscles, parietal pleura, and the skin over the anterior aspect of the thorax and the abdomen. All of the intercostal nerves mainly supply the thoracic and the abdominal walls, with the upper two also supplying the upper limb. The thoracic anterior (ventral) rami of T3–6 supply only the thoracic wall, whereas the lower five rami supply both the thoracic and the abdominal walls. The subcostal nerve supplies both the abdominal wall and the gluteal skin.

Each anterior (ventral) ramus is connected with an adjacent sympathetic ganglion by gray and white rami communicantes (Fig. 3-15). The communicating rami are branches of the spinal nerves that transmit sympathetic autonomic fibers to and from the sympathetic chain of ganglia. The fibers pass from spinal nerve to chain ganglia through the white ramus and in the reverse direction through the gray. In the cervical, lower lumbar, and sacral levels, only gray rami are present and function to convey fibers from the sympathetic chain to the spinal nerves, a mechanism that ensures that all spinal nerves contain sympathetic fibers.

From each intercostal nerve, a collateral and lateral cutaneous branch leave before the main nerve reaches the costal angle. The intercostobrachial nerve arises from the lateral–collateral branch of the second intercostal nerve, pierces the intercostal muscles in the midaxillary line, and then traverses the central portion of the axilla, where a posterior axillary branch gives sensation to the posterior axillary fold. From here, the nerve passes into the upper arm along the posterior–medial border to supply the skin of this region[95] and to connect with the posterior cutaneous branch of the radial nerve.

Posterior (Dorsal) Rami

The distribution of all posterior (dorsal) rami is similar. The thoracic posterior (dorsal) rami travel posteriorly, close to the vertebral zygapophysial joints, before dividing into medial and lateral branches:

- The medial branches supply the short, medially placed back muscles (the iliocostalis thoracis, spinalis thoracis, semispinalis thoracis, thoracic multifidus rotatores thoracis, and intertransversarii muscles) and the skin of the back as far as the midscapular line. The medial branches of the upper six thoracic posterior (dorsal) rami pierce the rhomboids and trapezius, reaching the skin in close proximity to the vertebral spines, which they occasionally supply.
- The lateral branches supply smaller branches to the sacrospinalis muscles. The lateral branches increase in size the more inferior they are. They penetrate, or pass, the longissimus thoracis to the space between it and the iliocostalis cervicis, supplying both these muscles, as well as the levatores costarum. The 12th thoracic lateral branch sends a filament medially along the iliac crest, which then passes down to the anterior gluteal skin.

As mentioned previously, the recurrent meningeal or sinuvertebral nerve is functionally also a branch of the spinal nerve. This nerve passes back into the vertebral canal through the intervertebral foramen, supplying the anterior aspect of the dura mater, outer third of the annular fibers of the intervertebral disks, vertebral body, and the epidural blood vessel walls, as well as the posterior longitudinal ligament.[96]

The thoracic nerves may be involved in the same types of impairments that affect other peripheral nerves. A loss of function of one, or more, of the thoracic nerves may produce partial or complete paralysis of the abdominal muscles and a loss of the abdominal reflexes in the affected quadrants. With unilateral impairments of the nerve, the umbilicus usually is drawn toward the unaffected side when the abdomen is tensed (Beevor sign), indicating a paralysis of the lower abdominal muscles as a result of a lesion at the level of the 10th thoracic segment.

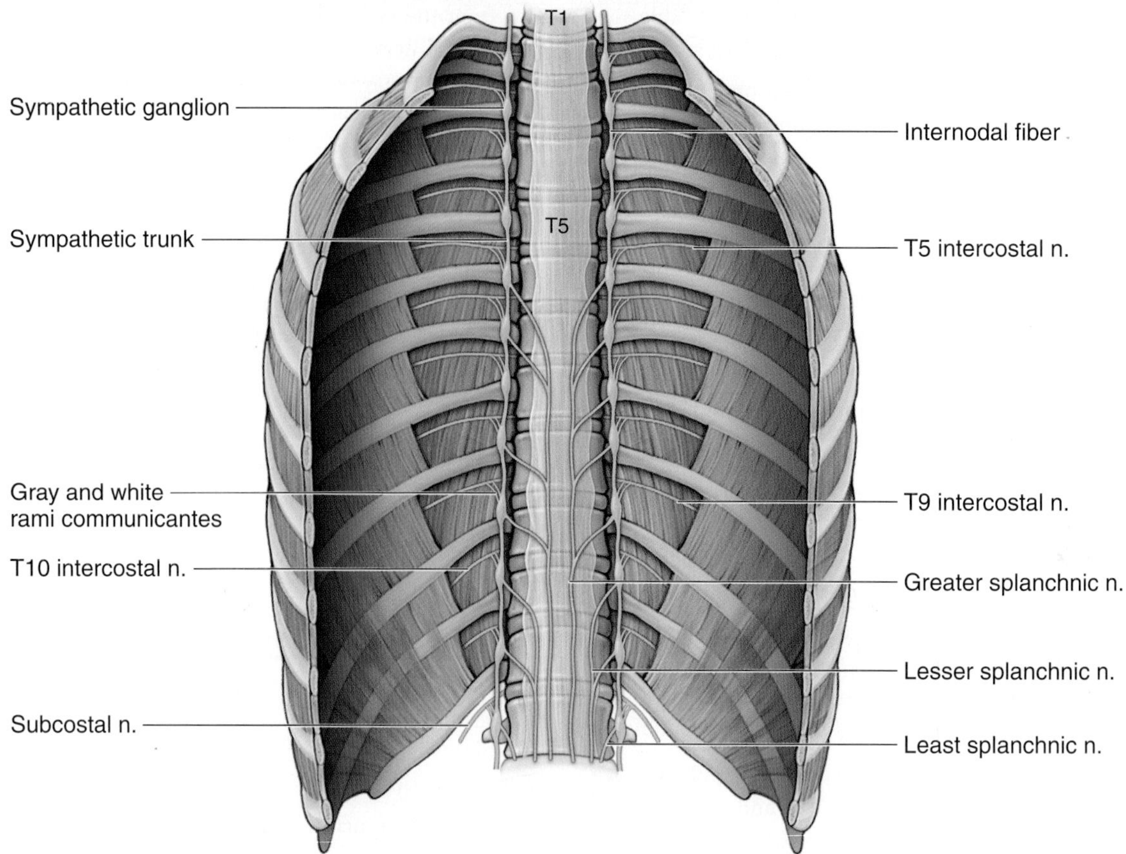

FIGURE 3-15 Thoracic spinal nerves. (Reproduced, with permission, from Morton DA, Foreman KB, Albertine KH: *The Big Picture: Gross Anatomy,* McGraw-Hill, 2011)

A specific syndrome, called the T4 syndrome,[97–99] has been shown to cause vague pain, numbness, and paresthesia in the upper extremity and generalized posterior head and neck pain.

Lumbar Plexus

The lumbar plexus (Fig. 3-16) is formed from the anterior (ventral) nerve roots of the second, third, and fourth lumbar nerves (in approximately 50% of cases, the plexus also receives a contribution from the last thoracic nerve), as they lie between the quadratus lumborum muscle and the psoas muscle. It then travels anteriorly into the body of the psoas muscle to form the LCN, femoral, and obturator nerves.

L1, L2, and L4 divide into upper and lower branches (see Fig. 3-16). The upper branch of L1 forms the iliohypogastric and ilioinguinal nerves. The lower branch of L1 joins the upper branch of L2 to form the genitofemoral nerve (see Fig. 3-16). The lower branch of L4 joins L5 to form the lumbosacral trunk. Peripheral nerve entrapment syndromes of the lower extremity are listed in Table 3-4.

- *Iliohypogastric nerve (T12, L1) (see Fig. 3-17).* This nerve emerges from the upper lateral border of the psoas major and then passes laterally around the iliac crest between the transversus abdominis and internal oblique muscles, before dividing into lateral and anterior cutaneous branches. The lateral (iliac) branch supplies the skin of the upper lateral part of the thigh, while the anterior (hypogastric) branch descends anteriorly to supply the skin over the symphysis.
- *Ilioinguinal nerve (L1) (see Fig. 3-17).* This nerve is smaller than the iliohypogastric nerve. It emerges from the lateral border of the psoas major to follow a course slightly inferior to that of the iliohypogastric, with which it may anastomose. It pierces the internal oblique, which it supplies before emerging from the superficial inguinal ring to supply the skin of the upper medial part of the thigh and the root of the penis and scrotum or mons pubis and labium majores. An entrapment of this nerve results in pain in the groin region, usually with radiation down to the proximal inner surface of the thigh, sometimes aggravated by increasing tension on the abdominal wall through standing erect.
- *Genitofemoral nerve (L1,2) (see Fig. 3-17).* This nerve descends obliquely and anteriorly through the psoas major before emerging from the anterior surface of the psoas and dividing into genital and femoral branches. The genital branch supplies the cremasteric muscle and the skin of the scrotum or labia, whereas the femoral branch supplies the skin of the middle upper part of the thigh and the femoral artery.

Collateral muscular branches supply the quadratus lumborum and intertransversarii from L1 and L4, and the psoas muscle from L2 and L3 (Fig. 3-17). The lower branch of L2, all of L3, and the upper branch of L4 split into a small anterior and a large posterior division (see Fig. 3-16). The three anterior divisions unite to form the obturator nerve; the three posterior divisions unite to form the femoral nerve, and the LCN (see Fig. 3-16).

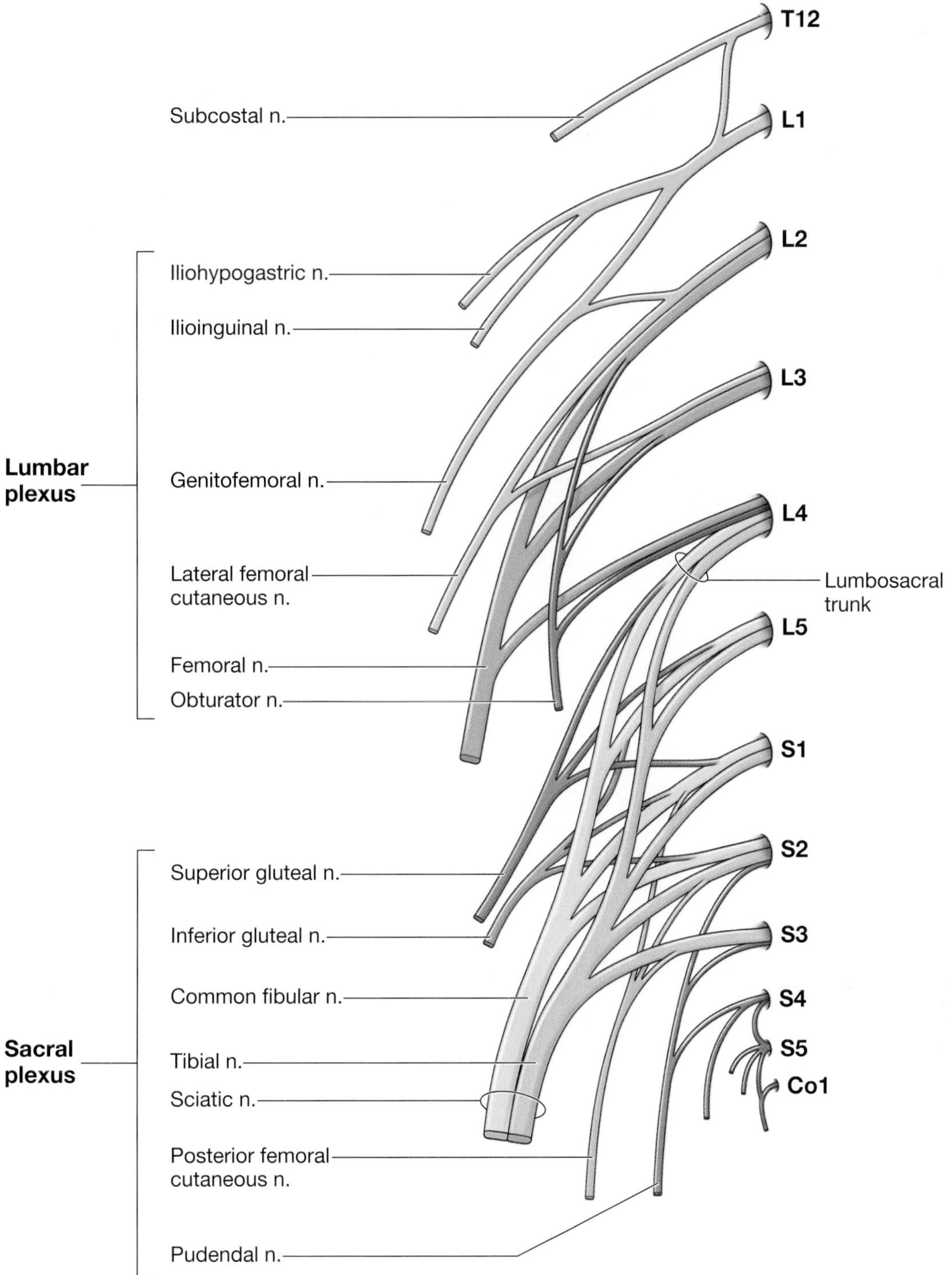

FIGURE 3-16 The lumbar plexus. (Reproduced, with permission, from Morton DA, Foreman KB, Albertine KH: *The Big Picture: Gross Anatomy,* McGraw-Hill, 2011)

Femoral Nerve (L2–4)

The femoral nerve, the largest branch of the lumbar plexus, arises from the lateral border of the psoas just above the inguinal ligament. The nerve descends beneath this ligament to enter the femoral triangle on the lateral side of the femoral artery, where it divides into terminal branches. Above the inguinal ligament, the femoral nerve supplies the iliopsoas muscle, and, in the thigh, it supplies the sartorius, pectineus, and quadriceps femoris muscles.

The sensory distribution of the femoral nerve includes the anterior and medial surfaces of the thigh via the anterior femoral cutaneous nerve and the medial aspect of the knee, the proximal leg, and articular branches to the knee via the saphenous nerve (Fig. 3-18), the largest cutaneous branch of the femoral nerve. The saphenous nerve exits from the adductor (Hunter's, or subsartorial) canal, descends under the sartorius muscle, and then winds around the posterior edge of the sartorius muscle at its tendon portion.

TABLE 3-4 Peripheral Nerve Entrapment Syndromes of the Lower Extremity

Lower Extremity		
Iliohypogastric nerve	The iliohypogastric nerve is rarely injured in isolation. The most common causes of injury are surgical procedures. These include transverse lower abdominal incisions, as in hysterectomies, or injuries from procedures such as inguinal herniorrhaphy and appendectomies. The injuries mainly occur if the incision extends beyond the lateral margin of the inferior rectus abdominis fibers. The damage can result from direct surgical trauma, such as passing a suture around the nerve and incorporating it into the fascial repair, or postoperative entrapment in scar tissue or neuroma formation. Sports injuries such as trauma or muscle tears of the lower abdominal muscles may also result in injury to the nerve. It may also occur during pregnancy due to the rapidly expanding abdomen in the third trimester. This is called the idiopathic iliohypogastric syndrome and is rare.	Symptoms include burning or lancinating pain immediately following the abdominal operation. The pain extends from the surgical incision laterally into the inguinal region and suprapubic region. Discomfort may occur immediately or up to several years after the procedure and may last for months to years. This discomfort is possibly because of the formation of scar tissue in the region. Occasionally, the pain may extend into the genitalia due to the significant overlap with other cutaneous nerves. Loss of sensation is usually minimal and not problematic. Iliohypogastric nerve entrapment causing symptoms similar to trochanteric bursitis refractory to conventional therapy has been reported. On examination, pain and tenderness are usually present in the area of scarring or entrapment. Hyperesthesia or hypoesthesia may occur in the area supplied by this nerve. Diagnosis is difficult due to the small area of cutaneous supply that this nerve provides. There may be overlap in sensory supply with the genitofemoral and ilioinguinal nerves Three major criteria are used to diagnose this nerve injury. The first is a history of surgical procedure in the lower abdominal area, although spontaneous entrapment can occur. Pain can usually be elicited by palpating laterally about the scar margin, and the pain usually radiates inferomedially toward the inguinal region and into the suprapubic and proximal genital area. Second, a definite area of hypoesthesia or hyperesthesia should be identified in the region of supply of the iliohypogastric nerve. Third, infiltration of a local anesthetic into the region where the iliohypogastric and ilioinguinal nerves depart the internal oblique muscle and where symptoms can be reproduced on physical examination by palpation should provide symptomatic relief. If no relief is obtained with injection, a different etiology should be sought for the discomfort. Alternate diagnoses include upper lumbar or lower thoracic nerve root pathology or discogenic etiology of the pain. If the iliohypogastric nerve is clearly identified as the source of pain and a favorable response is not obtained to local anesthetic injection, then

		surgical exploration and resection of the nerve should be considered. No reliable electrodiagnostic techniques are available to define the integrity of this nerve, although needle EMG of the lower abdominal musculature may serve as an adjunct in the diagnosis.
Ilioinguinal nerve	Causes of injury include lower abdominal incisions (Pfannenstiel), pregnancy, iliac bone harvesting, appendectomy, inguinal herniorrhaphy, inguinal lymph node dissection, femoral catheter placement, orchiectomy, total abdominal hysterectomy, and abdominoplasty. Nerve injury can also occur idiopathically. The prevalence of injury with surgery has declined due to the use of laparoscopic procedures. Tearing of the lower external oblique aponeurosis may also cause injury to this nerve. This injury has been reported in hockey players.	Symptoms could include hyperesthesia or hypoesthesia of the skin along the inguinal ligament. The sensation may radiate to the lower abdomen. Pain may be localized to the medial groin, labia majora or scrotum, and the inner thigh. The characteristics of the pain may vary considerably. Patients may be able to associate their pain clearly with a traumatic event or with the surgical procedure. Pain and tenderness may be present with application of pressure where the nerve exits the inguinal canal in up to 75% of patients. Sensory impairment is common in the distribution of the nerve supply noted above. Symptoms usually increase with hip extension (patients walk with a trunk in a forward-flexed posture). Pain may also be reproduced with palpation medial to the ASIS. The diagnosis can be made on the basis of local infiltration of anesthetic with or without steroid and should result in relief within 10 min. Unfortunately, no electrodiagnostic techniques are available to readily test this nerve. Abdominal needle EMG may be helpful in determining the severity of nerve injury, but EMG is not sensitive or specific.
Genitofemoral nerve	Nerve injury may result from hernia repair, appendectomy, biopsies, and cesarean delivery. Injury may also occur due to intrapelvic trauma to the posterior abdominal wall, retroperitoneal hematoma, pregnancy, or trauma to the inguinal ligament. Fortunately, injury to this nerve is rare, even with open herniorrhaphy.	Hypesthesia over the anterior thigh below the inguinal ligament, which is how it is distinguished from the iliohypogastric and ilioinguinal nerve. Groin pain is a common presentation of neuralgia from nerve injury or entrapment. The pain may be worse with internal or external rotation of the hip, prolonged walking, or even with light touch. Differential diagnoses include injury to the ilioinguinal and genitofemoral nerves as well as L1–2 radiculopathies. Some anatomic overlap may exist with the supply of the ilioinguinal and genitofemoral nerves, which makes the diagnosis somewhat difficult to establish.

(Continued)

TABLE 3-4 Peripheral Nerve Entrapment Syndromes of the Lower Extremity *(Continued)*

Lower Extremity		
Lateral cutaneous nerve (lateral femoral cutaneous) of the thigh LCN (meralgia paresthetica)	Entrapment usually occurs at the inguinal ligament. The peak incidence for this condition is in middle age. Differential diagnoses include lumbar radiculopathies and discogenic or nerve root problems at L2 and L3. The entrapment may be from intrapelvic causes, extrapelvic causes, or mechanical causes. Intrapelvic causes would include pregnancy, abdominal tumors, uterine fibroids, diverticulitis, or appendicitis. Injury has been described in cases of abdominal aortic aneurism. Examples of extrapelvic causes include trauma to the region of the ASIS (e.g., a seatbelt from a motor vehicle accident), tight garments, belts, girdles, or stretch from obesity and ascites. Mechanical factors include prolonged sitting or standing and pelvic tilt from leg length discrepancy. Diabetes can also cause this neuropathy in isolation or in the clinical setting of a polyneuropathy.	A protruding, pendulous abdomen, as seen in obesity and pregnancy, pushes the inguinal ligament forward and downward and drags the nerve with it over the kink. The angulation of the nerve is also exaggerated with extension of the thigh and relaxed with flexion. Extension also tenses the fascia lata and may add to the compression from the front. Therefore, it is common to encounter meralgia paresthetica in individuals who are obese and in women during their last trimester of pregnancy. The symptoms often are accentuated with walking down slopes and stairs, prolonged standing in the erect posture, and, sometimes, lying flat in bed. The patient learns to relieve symptoms by placing a pillow behind the thighs and assuming a slightly hunched posture while standing. The main symptoms are an uncomfortable numbness, tingling, and painful hypersensitivity in the distribution of the LCN, usually in the anterolateral thigh down to the upper patella region. Decreased appreciation of pinprick is elicited, together with a hyperpathic reaction to touch and even an after-discharge phenomenon of persistent, spontaneous tingling after the touch. Deep digital pressure medial to the ASIS may set off shooting paresthesia down the lateral thigh. The diagnosis is confirmed with a nerve block using 0.5% bupivacaine injected a finger's breadth medial to the ASIS. The resulting anesthesia over the sensory territory of the LCN should be concomitant with the complete cessation of pain and tingling. Differential diagnosis includes lumbar disc herniation at the L1–2 or L2–3 levels, which may require an MRI.
Piriformis syndrome	Multiple etiologies have been proposed to explain the compression or irritation of the sciatic nerve that occurs with the piriformis syndrome: ▸ ***Hypertrophy of the piriformis muscle.*** ▸ ***Trauma.*** Trauma, direct or indirect, to the sacroiliac or gluteal region can lead to piriformis syndrome and is a result of hematoma formation and subsequent scarring between the sciatic nerve and the short external rotators.	Six classic findings: 1. A history of trauma to the sacroiliac and gluteal regions 2. Pain in the region of the sacroiliac joint, greater sciatic notch, and piriformis muscle that usually causes difficulty with walking 3. Acute exacerbation of pain caused by stooping or lifting (and moderate relief of pain by traction on the affected extremity, with the patient in the supine position)

	▸ ***Hip flexion contracture.*** A flexion contracture at the hip has been associated with piriformis syndrome. This flexion contracture increases the lumbar lordosis, which increases the tension in the pelvic–femoral muscles, as these muscles try to stabilize the pelvis and spine in the new position. This increased tension causes the involved muscles to hypertrophy with no corresponding increase in the size of the bony foramina, resulting in neurological signs of sciatic compression. ▸ ***Gender.*** Females are more commonly affected by piriformis syndrome, with as much as a 6:1 female-to-male incidence. ▸ ***Ischial bursitis.*** ▸ ***Pseudoaneurysm of the inferior gluteal artery.*** ▸ ***Excessive exercise to the hamstring muscles.*** ▸ ***Inflammation and spasm of the piriformis muscle.*** This is often in association with trauma, infection, and anatomical variations of the muscle. ▸ ***Anatomical anomalies.*** Local anatomical anomalies may contribute to the likelihood that symptoms will develop.	4. A palpable sausage-shaped mass, tender to palpation, over the piriformis muscle on the affected side 5. A positive straight leg raise 6. Gluteal atrophy, depending on the duration of the condition. Other clinical signs include pain and weakness in association with resisted abduction and external rotation of the involved thigh, palpable and local muscle spasm (palpable in the obturatorinternus or, less commonly, in the piriformis muscle) The neurologic examination is usually normal. An examination of the hip and lower leg usually demonstrates restricted external rotation of the hip and lumbosacral muscle tightness.
Femoral nerve	Diabetic amyotrophy is the most common cause of femoral nerve neuropathy. Open injuries can occur from gunshots, knife wounds, glass shards, or needle puncture in some medical procedures. The most worrisome complication of major trauma to the femoral triangle region is an associated femoral artery injury. Most entrapment neuropathies occur below the inguinal ligament. Heat developed by methylmethacrylate in a total hip arthroplasty can injure the femoral nerve. Pelvic procedures that require the lower extremity to be positioned in an acutely flexed, abducted, and externally rotated position for long periods can cause compression by angling the femoral nerve beneath the inguinal ligament. The nerve may be compromised by pressure from a fetus in a difficult birth. Pelvic fractures and acute hyperextension of the thigh may also cause an isolated femoral nerve injury. Pelvic radiation, appendiceal or renal abscesses, and tumors can cause femoral nerve injuries as well. The nerve can also be injured by a compartment-like compression from a hemorrhage from hemorrhagic disorders or anticoagulant use.	The symptoms of a femoral neuropathy may include pain in the inguinal region that is partially relieved by flexion and external rotation of the hip and dysesthesia over the anterior thigh and anteromedial leg. Patients complain of difficulty, with walking and knee buckling depending on the severity of the injury. The nerve gives rise to the saphenous nerve in the thigh; therefore, numbness in this distribution can be present. Anterior knee pain may also be present due to the saphenous nerve supply to the patella. On examination, patients may present with weak hip flexion, knee extension, and impaired quadriceps tendon reflex and sensory deficit in the anteromedial aspect of the thigh. Pain may be increased with hip extension and relieved with external rotation of the hip. If compression occurs at the inguinal region, no hip flexion weakness is present. Sensory loss may occur along the medial aspect of the leg below the knee (saphenous distribution). Electrodiagnostic testing is typically performed for diagnosis but is also important to determine the extent of the injury and to determine prognosis of recovery. With electrodiagnostic testing, either surface or needle electrodes lateral to the femoral artery in the inguinal region

(Continued)

TABLE 3-4 Peripheral Nerve Entrapment Syndromes of the Lower Extremity *(Continued)*

Lower Extremity		
		is used for stimulation. The stimulation can be performed above and below the inguinal ligament. Disk electrodes from the vastus medialis are used to record stimulation. A saphenous nerve sensory study may also be performed (continuation of the sensory portion of the femoral nerve over the medial aspect of the leg and ankle). Needle examination should be completed for the paraspinal muscles as well as the iliopsoas (also L2–3) and hip adductors supplied by the obturator nerve to determine the presence of root or plexus injury versus peripheral nerve injury. The needle EMG is usually the most revealing portion of the electrodiagnostic test. The examiner must look not only for denervation potentials but also for any active motor units.
Saphenous nerve	The saphenous nerve can become entrapped where it pierces the connective tissue at the roof of Hunter canal, resulting in inflammation from a sharp angulation of the nerve through the structure and the dynamic forces of the muscles in this region. This results in contraction and relaxation of the fibrous tissue that impinges the nerve. The nerve can also be injured from an improperly protected knee or leg support during operation. It may be injured due to neurilemoma, entrapment by femoral vessels, direct trauma, pes anserine bursitis, varicose vein operations, and medial knee arthrotomies and meniscus repairs.	Symptoms of entrapment may include a deep aching sensation in the thigh, knee pain, and possibly paresthesias in the cutaneous distribution of the saphenous distribution in the leg and the foot. The infrapatellar branch may also become entrapped on its own. This is because it passes through a separate foramen in the sartorius muscle tendon, or it may course horizontally across the prominence of the medial femoral epicondyle, where it may be exposed to trauma. Patients report paresthesias and numbness about the infrapatellar region that is worse with flexion of the knee or compression from garments and braces. Saphenous nerve entrapment is a frequently overlooked cause of persistent medial knee pain that occurs in patients who experience trauma or direct blows to the medial aspect of the knee. As this is a purely sensory nerve, weakness should not be noted with an isolated injury of this nerve. If weakness is present, look for an injury of the femoral nerve or possibly an upper lumbar radiculopathy, particularly if thigh adduction is present (obturator nerve).

		Deep palpation proximal to the medial epicondyle of the femur may reproduce the pain and complaints. Some weakness may be present because of guarding or disuse atrophy from the pain, but no direct weakness will result from the nerve impingement. Sensory loss in the saphenous distribution may be present on examination. No weakness should be present in the quadriceps muscles or the hip adductors. The diagnosis may be made on the basis of injection of local anesthetic along the course of the nerve and proximal to the proposed site of entrapment. Nerve conduction techniques are available to assess neural conduction in the main branch of the saphenous nerve or the terminal branches. The routine tests may be disappointing with persons with subcutaneous adipose tissue or swelling. A side-to-side comparison of the nerve should be made and must demonstrate a lesion consistent with the patient's complaints. A somatosensory-evoked potential test can also be performed and the results compared with those of the contralateral side for diagnosis, although this test may be cumbersome and time-consuming. No findings should be present on needle examination of the muscle during EMG. Needle examination should include the quadriceps muscles and the adductor longus to assess for both femoral and obturator nerve injury. If findings are present in both of these muscles, then paraspinal muscles definitely should be examined to rule out radiculopathy.
Popliteal fossa (tibial nerve)	Compression of tibial nerve as it passes through the popliteal fossa. Usually caused by an enlarged Baker's cyst (which may also compress the common peroneal and sural nerves). Other causes include proliferation of the synovial tissue in patients with rheumatoid arthritis.	Pain behind the knee or in the calf muscles when the foot is dorsiflexed. Hypesthesia or anesthesia of the entire plantar surface of the foot. Incomplete flexion of the knee joint. Weakness of the gastrocnemius, tibialis posterior, flexor hallucis longus, flexor digitorum longus, and the intrinsic muscles of the foot (except for the extensor digitorum brevis).

(Continued)

TABLE 3-4 Peripheral Nerve Entrapment Syndromes of the Lower Extremity *(Continued)*

Lower Extremity		
Tarsal tunnel	Compression of the posterior tibial nerve behind the medial malleolus, or tarsal tunnel syndrome, is an uncommon entrapment neuropathy. The roof of the tunnel is formed by the flexor retinaculum stretched between the medial malleolus and the calcaneus. The tarsal bones are the floor. Numerous fibrous septae between the roof and the floor subdivide the tunnel into separate compartments at various points. The contents of the tarsal tunnel at its proximal end are, from front to back, (1) the flexor digitorum longus tendon, (2) the posterior tibialis tendon, (3) the posterior tibial artery and vein, (4) the posterior tibial nerve, and (5) the flexor hallucis longus tendon. The nerve has three terminal branches. It bifurcates into the medial and lateral plantar nerves within 1 cm of the malleolar–calcaneal axis in 90% of cases; the other 10% are 2–3 cm proximal to the malleolus. The calcaneal branch usually comes off the lateral plantar fascicles, but around 30% leave the main nerve trunk just proximal to the tunnel. Distally, the medial and lateral plantar nerves travel in separate fascial compartments. The medial branch supplies the intrinsic flexors of the great toe and the sensation over the medial plantar surface of the foot inclusive of at least the first three toes. The lateral branch supplies all of the intrinsics that cause extension of the interphalangeal joints, as well as sensation over the lateral plantar surface of the foot. The calcaneal branch provides sensation to the heel.	Early symptoms are burning, tingling, and dysesthetic pain over the plantar surface of the foot. Characteristically, the pain is set off by pressing or rubbing over the plantar skin, sometimes with after-discharge phenomenon. A Tinel sign often is evident over the course of the main nerve or its branches, and the pain may be aggravated by forced eversion and dorsiflexion of the ankle. In advanced cases, the intrinsic flexors of the great toe are weak and atrophied, producing hollowing of the instep. The lateral toes may also show clawing due to paralysis of the intrinsic toe flexors and the posterior (dorsal) digital extensors. The calcaneal branch often is spared because of its proximal takeoff.

EMG, electromyography; ASIS, anterosuperior iliac spine; LFCN, lateral cutaneous nerve of the thigh.

Modified from Hollis MH, Lemay DE: *Nerve Entrapment Syndromes of the Lower Extremity;* 2005. Available at: http:/www.emedicine.com/orthoped/topic422.htm.

Modified from Pang D. *Nerve Entrapment Syndromes*; 2004. Available at: http:/www.emedicine.com/med/topic2909.htm.

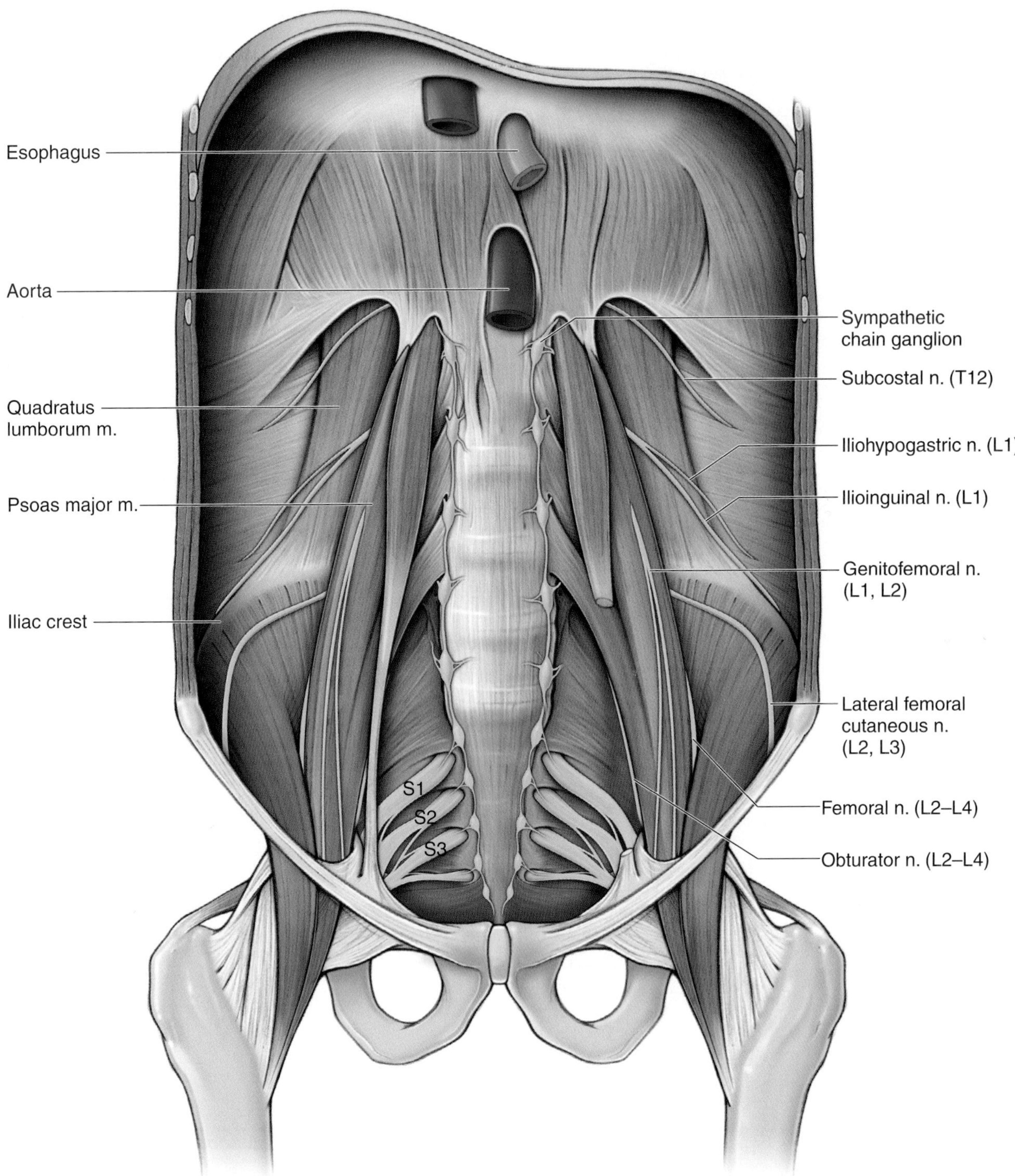

FIGURE 3-17 Branches of the lumbar plexus. (Reproduced, with permission, from Morton DA, Foreman KB, Albertine KH: *The Big Picture: Gross Anatomy,* McGraw-Hill, 2011)

- The infrapatellar branch pierces the sartorius muscle and courses anteriorly to the infrapatellar region.
- The descending branch passes down the medial aspect of the leg and, at the lower third of the leg, divides into two branches. One of the branches of the descending portion of the saphenous nerve courses along the medial border of the tibia and ends at the ankle, while the other branch passes anterior to the ankle and is distributed to the medial aspect of the foot, sometimes reaching as far as the metatarsophalangeal joint of the great toe.

Entrapment of the saphenous nerve often results in marked pain at the medial aspect of the knee.

Femoral nerve palsy has been reported after acetabular fracture, cardiac catheterization, total hip arthroplasty, or anterior lumbar spinal fusion, and spontaneously in hemophilia.[100–102]

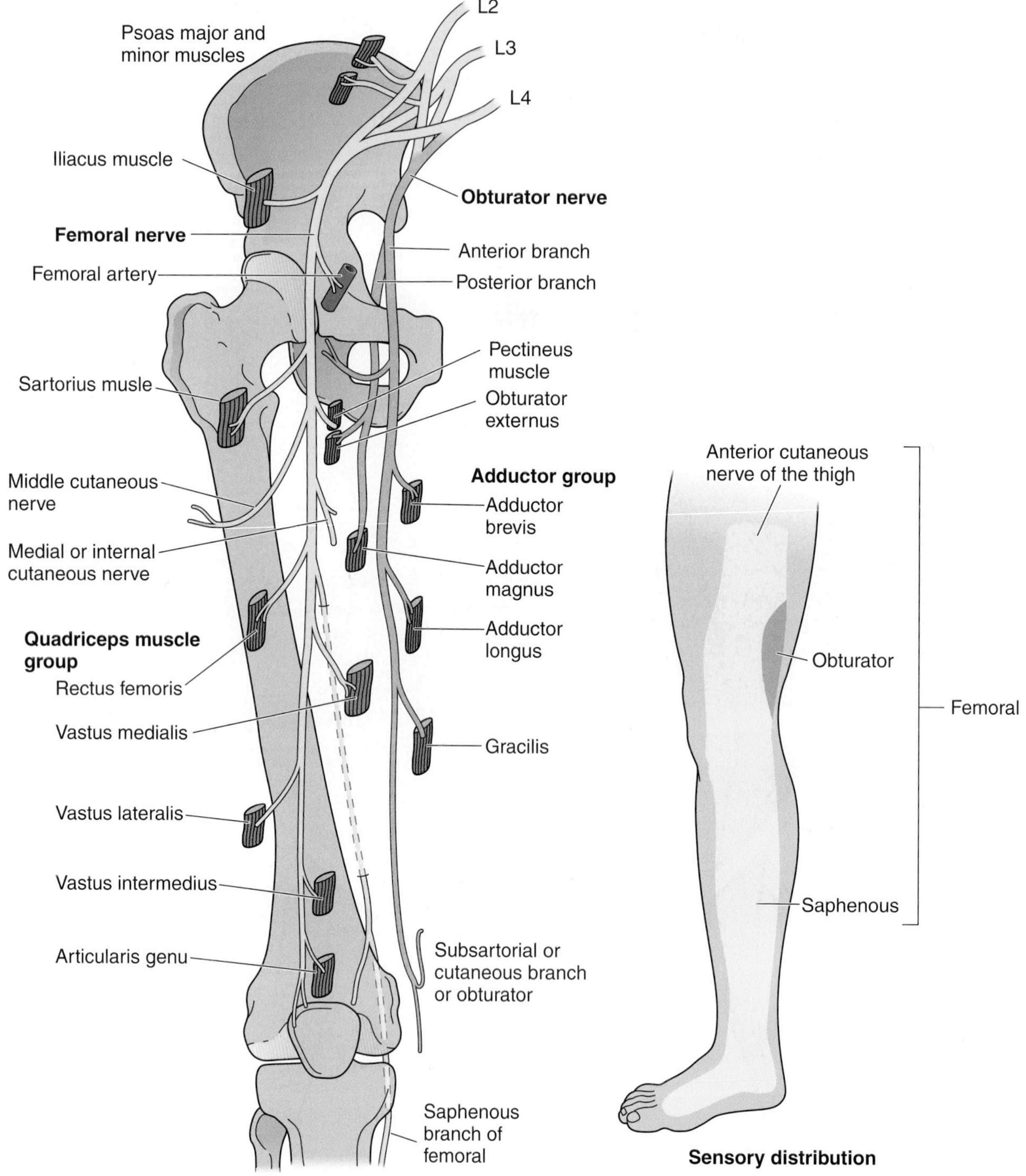

FIGURE 3-18 The femoral (L2–4) and obturator (L2–4) nerves. (Reproduced, with permission, from Waxman SG: *Clinical Neuroanatomy*, 26th ed, McGraw-Hill, 2010)

CLINICAL PEARL

An entrapment of the femoral nerve by an iliopsoas hematoma is the most likely cause of femoral nerve palsy.[103] Direct blows to the abdomen or a hyperextension moment at the hip that tears the iliacus muscle may produce an iliacus hematoma.

Obturator Nerve (L2–4)

The obturator nerve (see Fig. 3-18) arises from the second, third, and fourth lumbar anterior divisions of the lumbar plexus and emerges from the medial border of the psoas, near the brim of the pelvis. It then passes behind the common iliac vessels on the lateral side of the hypogastric vessels and the ureter and descends through the obturator canal in the upper part of the obturator foramen to the medial side of the thigh. While in the foramen, the obturator nerve splits into anterior and posterior branches.

- The anterior division of the obturator nerve gives an articular branch to the hip joint near its origin. It descends anterior to the obturator externus and adductor brevis deep to the pectineus and adductor longus and supplies muscular branches to the adductors longus and brevis, the gracilis, and, rarely, to the pectineus.[95] The anterior division divides into numerous named and unnamed branches, including the cutaneous branches to the subsartorial plexus and directly to a small area of skin on the middle internal part of the thigh, vascular branches to the femoral artery, and communicating branches to the femoral cutaneous and accessory obturator nerves.
- The posterior division of the obturator nerve pierces the anterior part of the obturator externus, which it supplies, and descends deep to the adductor brevis. It also supplies the adductors magnus and brevis (if it has not received supply from the anterior division) and gives an articular branch to the knee joint (see Fig. 3-18).

The obturator nerve may be involved by the same pathologic processes that affect the femoral nerve. Disability is usually minimal, although external rotation and adduction of the thigh are impaired, and crossing of the legs is difficult. The patient may also complain of severe pain, which radiates from the groin down the inner aspect of the thigh (see Fig. 3-18).[104,105]

LCN of the Thigh

The LCN of the thigh (Fig. 3-7) is purely sensory and is derived primarily from the second and third lumbar nerve roots, with occasional contributions from the first lumbar nerve root.[106,107] Sympathetic afferent and efferent fibers are also contained within the nerve.[108] The nerve leaves the lumbar plexus and normally appears at the lateral border of the psoas, just proximal to the crest of the ilium. From here, it courses laterally across the anterior surface of the iliacus (covered by iliac fascia) and approaches the lateral portion of the inguinal ligament posterior to the deep circumflex iliac artery. The nerve usually crosses beneath the inguinal ligament, just inferior–medial to the anterior superior iliac spine.[109] The site at which the LCN exits the pelvis varies. Meralgia paresthetica (see Table 3-4), the term used to describe LCN entrapment, has been reported with each of the five known variants as follows[110]:

- The split lateral attachment of the inguinal ligament. As the nerve curves medially and inferiorly around the anterior superior iliac spine, it may be subjected to repetitive trauma in this osteofibrous tunnel.[111]
- The nerve may pass posterior to the inguinal ligament and anterior to a sharp ridge of iliacus fascia, which can lead to a bowstring deformity of the nerve when the patient is supine.[112]
- Occasionally, the LCN enters the thigh within or beneath the substance of the sartorius muscle.[113]
- Several cases have been reported in which the LCN crosses over the iliac crest lateral and posterior to the anterior superior iliac spine. The nerve typically lies in a groove in the ilium and is subject to pressure from tight garments or belts.[112,113]
- The nerve may exit the pelvis in multiple branches, with entrapment of a single branch.[114]
- Alternatively, the nerve may be absent, with a branch from the femoral nerve arising below the inguinal ligament, or it may be replaced by the ilioinguinal nerve.[115]

Sacral Plexus

The lumbosacral trunk (L4,5) descends into the pelvis, where it enters the formation of the sacral plexus. The sacral plexus (Fig. 3-16) is formed by the anterior (ventral) rami of the L4 and L5 and the S1 through S4 nerves and lies on the posterior wall of the pelvis, anterior to the piriformis and posterior to the sigmoid colon, ureter, and hypogastric vessels in front. The L4 and L5 nerves join medial to the sacral promontory, becoming the lumbosacral trunk. The S1 through S4 nerves converge with the lumbosacral trunk in front of the piriformis muscle, forming the broad triangular band of the sacral plexus. The superior (upper) three nerves of the plexus divide into two sets of branches: the medial branches, which are distributed to the multifidi muscles, and the lateral branches, which become the medial cluneal nerves. The medial cluneal nerves supply the skin over the medial part of the gluteus maximus. The lower two posterior primary divisions, with the posterior division of the coccygeal nerve, supply the skin over the coccyx.

Collateral Branches of the Posterior Division

Superior Gluteal Nerve

The roots of the superior gluteal nerve (L4,5; S1) arise within the pelvis from the sacral plexus (see Fig. 3-16) and enter the buttock through the greater sciatic foramen, above the piriformis. The nerve runs laterally between gluteus medius and gluteus minimus, which it innervates before terminating in the tensor fascia lata, which it also supplies. Because the nerve passes between the gluteal muscles, it is at risk during surgery on the hip.[116]

Inferior Gluteal Nerve

The inferior gluteal nerve (L5; S1,2) passes below the piriformis muscle and through the greater sciatic foramen and travels to the gluteus maximus muscle (see Fig. 3-16). Nerves to the piriformis consist of short smaller branches from S1 and S2.

Superior Cluneal Nerve

The medial branch of the superior cluneal nerve passes superficially over the iliac crest, where it is covered by two layers of dense fibrous fascia. When the medial branch of the superior cluneal nerve passes through the fascia against the posterior iliac crest and the osteofibrous tunnel consisting of the two layers of the fascia and the superior rim of the iliac crest, the possibility of irritation or trauma to the nerve is increased, making this a potential site of nerve compression or constriction.[117]

Posterior Cutaneous (Femoral) Nerve of the Thigh

The posterior cutaneous (femoral) nerve (PCN) of the thigh constitutes a collateral branch, with roots from both the anterior and the posterior divisions of S1 and S2 and the anterior divisions of S2 and S3 (Fig. 3-16). Perineal branches pass to the skin of the upper medial aspect of the thigh and the skin of the scrotum or labium majores. Despite its close proximity to the sciatic nerve, however, injury to the PCN of the thigh is quite rare.

Collateral Branches of the Anterior Division

Collateral branches from the anterior divisions extend to the quadratus femoris and gemellus inferior muscles (from L4, L5, and S1) and to the obturator internus and gemellus superior muscles (from L5, S1, and S2).

Sciatic Nerve

The sciatic nerve (Fig. 3-19) is the largest nerve in the body. It arises from the L4, L5, and S1 through S3 nerve roots as a continuation of the lumbosacral plexus. The nerve is composed of the independent tibial (medial) and common fibular (peroneal) (lateral) divisions, which are usually united as a single nerve down to the lower portion of the thigh. The tibial division is the larger of the two divisions. Although grossly united, the funicular patterns of the tibial and common fibular (peroneal) divisions are distinct, and there is no exchange of bundles between them. The common fibular (peroneal) nerve is formed by the upper four posterior divisions (L4,5; S1,2) of the sacral plexus, and the tibial nerve is formed from all five anterior divisions (L4,5; S1–3).

The sciatic nerve usually exits the pelvis through the anterior third of the greater sciatic foramen.[118] Also running through the greater sciatic foramen is the superior gluteal artery, the largest branch of the internal iliac artery, and its accompanying vein.

Numerous variations have been described for the course of the sciatic nerve, including cases in which the sciatic nerve passes through the piriformis, and cases in which the tibial division passes below the piriformis while the common fibular (peroneal) division passes above or through the muscle. It seems that the tibial division always enters the gluteal region below the piriformis, and the variability is in the course of the common fibular (peroneal) division. Typically, the sciatic nerve descends along the posterior surface of the thigh to the popliteal space, where it usually terminates by dividing into the tibial and common fibular (peroneal) nerves (see Fig. 3-19). Innervation for the short head of the biceps femoris comes from the common fibular (peroneal) division, the only muscle innervated by this division above the knee. Rami from the tibial trunk pass to the semitendinosus and the semimembranosus muscles, the long head of the biceps femoris, and the adductor magnus muscle.

In most reports of sciatic nerve injury, regardless of the cause, the common fibular (peroneal) division is involved more frequently and often suffers a greater degree of damage than the tibial division; its susceptibility to injury being related to several anatomic features.

> **CLINICAL PEARL**
>
> Compared with the tibial division, the common fibular (peroneal) division is relatively tethered at the sciatic notch, and the neck of the fibula and may, therefore, be less able to tolerate or distribute tension, such as that occurs in acute stretching or with changes in limb position or length.

Injury to the sciatic nerve may result indirectly from a herniated intervertebral disk (protruded nucleus pulposus) or more directly from a hip dislocation, local aneurysm, or direct external trauma of the sciatic notch, the latter of which can be confused with a compressive radiculopathy of the lumbar or sacral nerve root.[119] Following are some useful clues to help distinguish the two conditions:

- Pain from an irritated lumbar spinal nerve root (radiculopathy) should not significantly change with the introduction of hip rotation during the straight leg raise test (Chap. 11), whereas if there is a sciatic nerve entrapment by the piriformis muscle, pain is likely to be accentuated by introducing hip internal rotation, which stretches the muscle fibers, and relieved by moving the hip into external rotation.
- Sciatic neuropathy produces sensory changes on the sole of the foot, whereas lumbosacral radiculopathy generally does not, unless there is a predominant S1 involvement.
- Compressive radiculopathy below the L4 level causes palpable atrophy of the gluteal muscles, whereas a sciatic entrapment spares these muscles.
- The sciatic trunk is frequently tender from root compression at the foraminal level, whereas it is not normally tender in a sciatic nerve entrapment.[120]

Individual case reports of bone and soft-tissue tumors along the course of the sciatic nerve have been described as a rare cause of sciatica.[121,122]

Tibial Nerve

The tibial nerve (L4,5; S1–3) is formed by all five of the anterior divisions of the sacral plexus, thus receiving fibers from the lower two lumbar and the upper three sacral cord segments. Inferiorly, the nerve begins its own course in the upper part of the popliteal space, before descending vertically through this space, and passing between the heads of the gastrocnemius muscle, to the dorsum of the leg. The portion of the tibial trunk below the popliteal space is called the *posterior tibial nerve*; the portion within the space is called the *internal popliteal nerve* (Fig. 3-20). The tibial nerve supplies the gastrocnemius, plantaris, soleus, popliteus, tibialis posterior, flexor digitorum longus, and flexor halluces longus muscles (see Fig. 3-20).

- **Sural Nerve.** The sural nerve (see Fig. 3-20) is a sensory branch of the tibial nerve. It is formed by the lateral sural cutaneous nerve from the common fibular (peroneal) nerve and the medial calcaneal nerve from the tibial nerve. The sural nerve supplies the skin on the posterior–lateral aspect of the lower one-third of the leg and the lateral side of the foot.

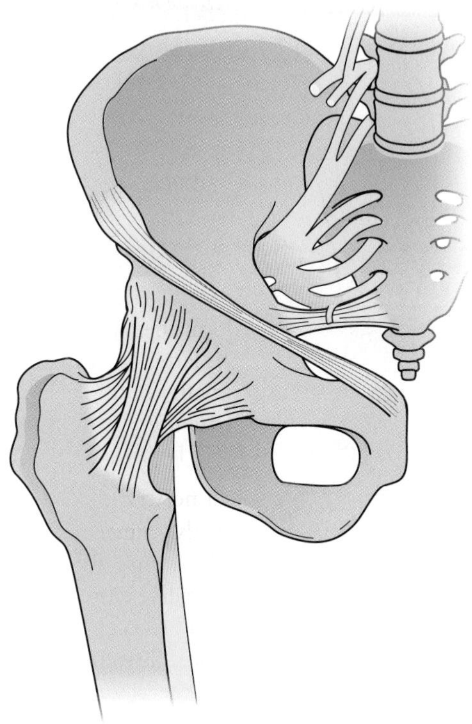

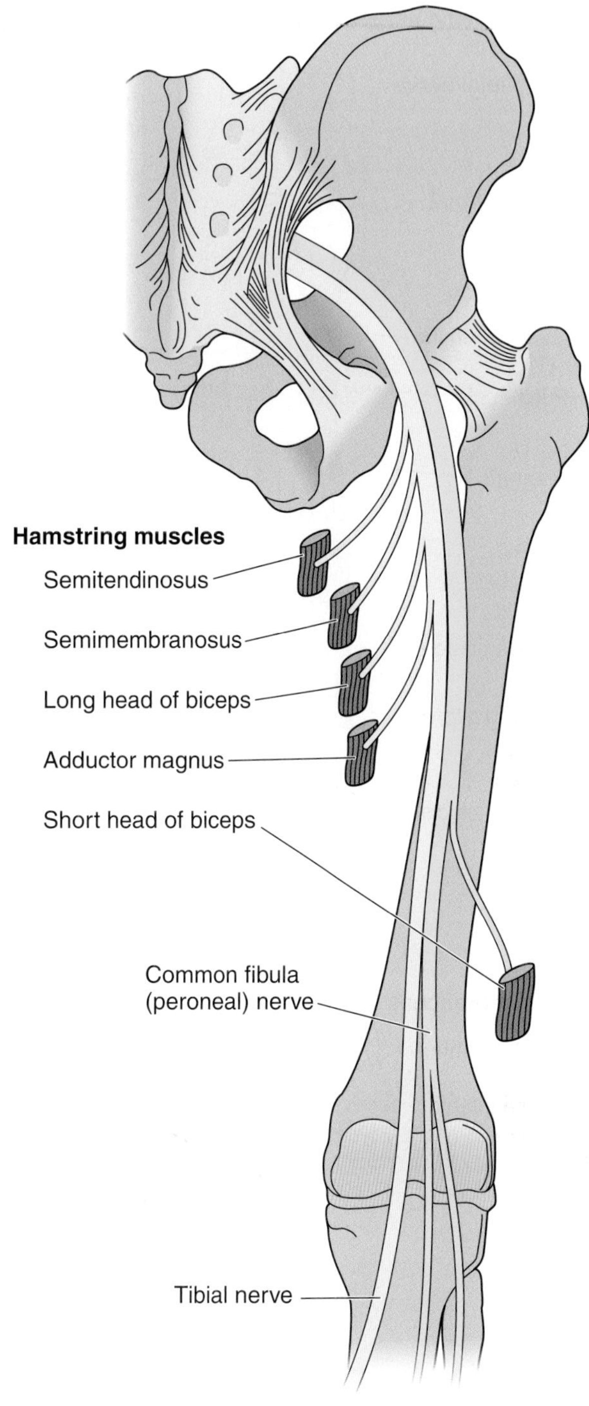

FIGURE 3-19 The sciatic nerve (L4, 5, S1–3). (Reproduced, with permission, from Waxman SG: *Clinical Neuroanatomy*, 26th ed, McGraw-Hill, 2010)

▸ **Terminal Branches of the Tibial Nerve.** In the distal leg, the tibial nerve lies laterally to the posterior tibial vessels, and it supplies articular branches to the ankle joint and to the posterior–medial aspect of the ankle. From this point, its terminal branches include the following:

- *Medial plantar nerve* (comparable to the median nerve in the hand). This nerve supplies the flexor digitorum brevis, abductor halluces, flexor halluces brevis, and first lumbrical muscles and sensory branches to the medial side of the sole, the plantar surfaces of the medial 3½ toes, and the terminal ends of the same toes (see Fig. 3-20).
- *Lateral plantar nerve* (comparable to the ulnar nerve in the hand). This nerve supplies the small muscles of the foot, except those innervated by the medial plantar nerve, and sensory branches to the lateral portions of the sole, the plantar surface of the lateral 1½ toes, and the distal phalanges of these toes (see Fig. 3-20). The interdigital nerves are most commonly entrapped between the second

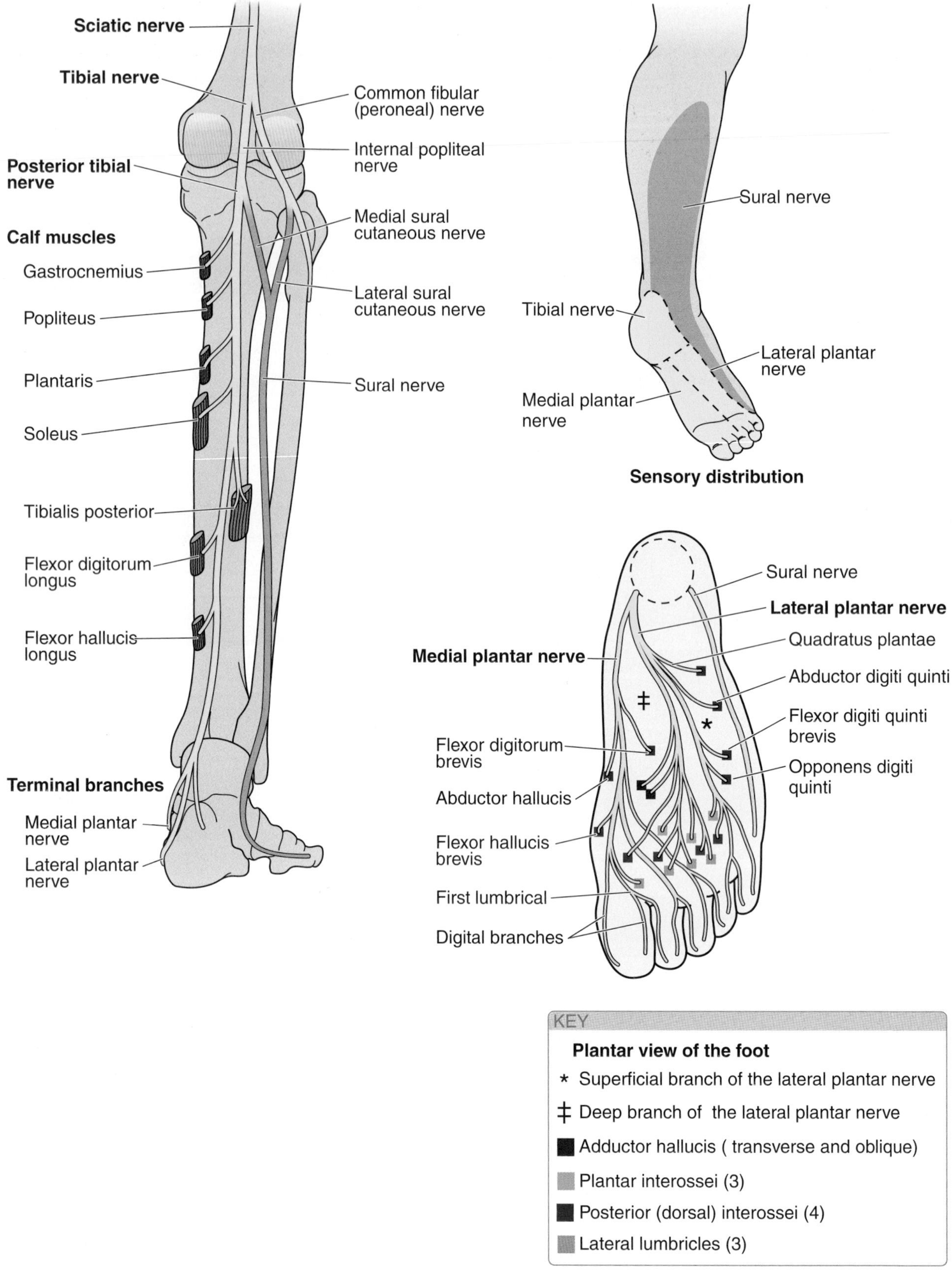

FIGURE 3-20 The tibial nerve (L4, 5, S1–3). (Reproduced, with permission, from Waxman SG: *Clinical Neuroanatomy*, 26th ed, McGraw-Hill, 2010)

and third and the third and fourth web spaces and the intermetatarsal ligaments as a result of a forced hyperextension of the toes, eventually resulting in an interdigital neuroma.

- *Medial calcaneal nerve.* As it passes beneath the flexor retinaculum, the tibial nerve gives off medial calcanean branches to the skin of the heel. An irritation of this nerve may result in heel pain.

Common Fibular (Peroneal) Nerve

The common fibular (peroneal) nerve (L4,5; S1–2) is formed by a fusion of the upper four posterior divisions of the sacral plexus, and thus derives its fibers from the lower two lumbar and the upper two sacral cord segments (see Fig. 3-21). In the thigh, it is a component of the sciatic nerve as far as the upper part of the popliteal space. The nerve gives off sensory branches in the popliteal space. These sensory branches include the superior and inferior articular branches to the knee joint and the lateral sural cutaneous nerve (see Fig. 3-20 and 3-21).

At the apex of the popliteal fossa, the common fibular (peroneal) nerve begins its independent descent along the posterior border of the biceps femoris and then crosses the dorsum of the knee joint to the upper external portion of the leg near the head of the fibula. The nerve curves around the lateral aspect of the fibula toward the anterior aspect of the bone, before passing deep to the two heads of the fibularis (peroneus) longus muscle, where it divides into three terminal rami: the recurrent articular, superficial, and deep fibular (peroneal) nerves.

- The recurrent articular nerve accompanies the anterior tibial recurrent artery, supplying the tibiofibular and knee joints, and a twig to the tibialis anterior muscle.

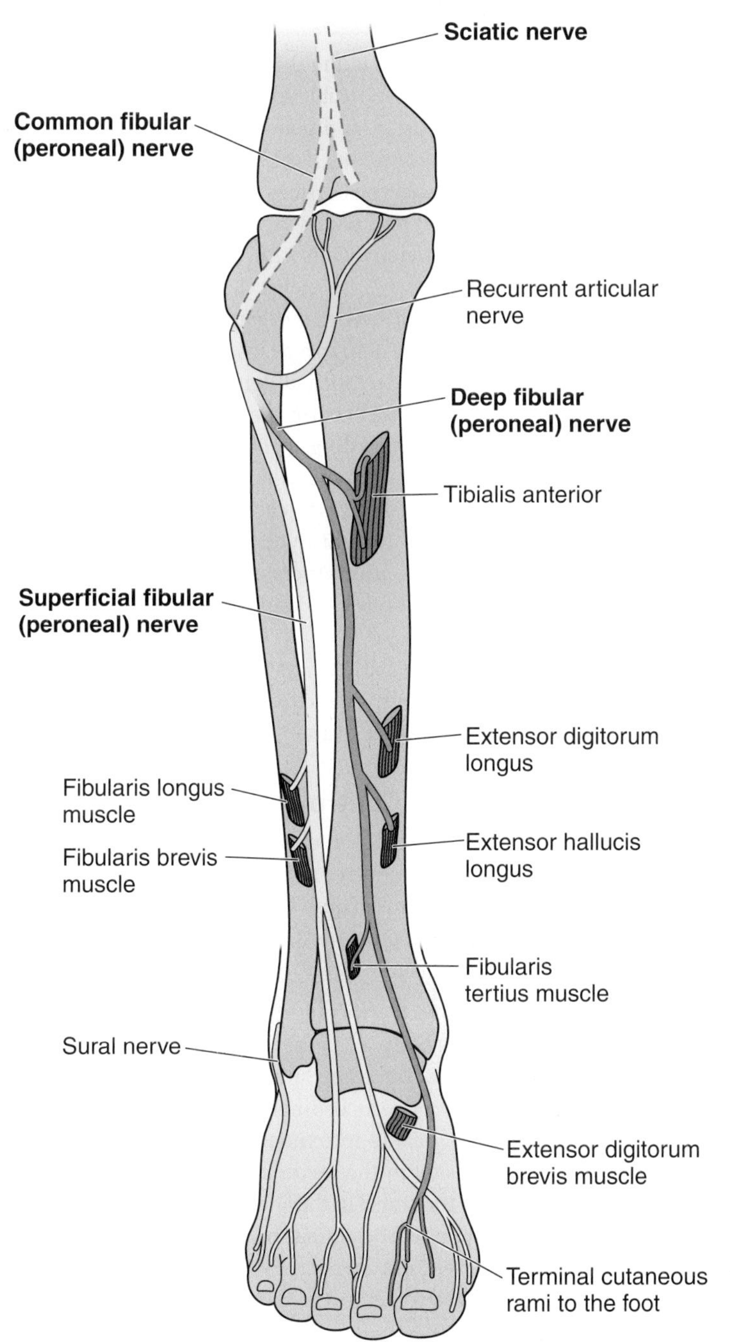

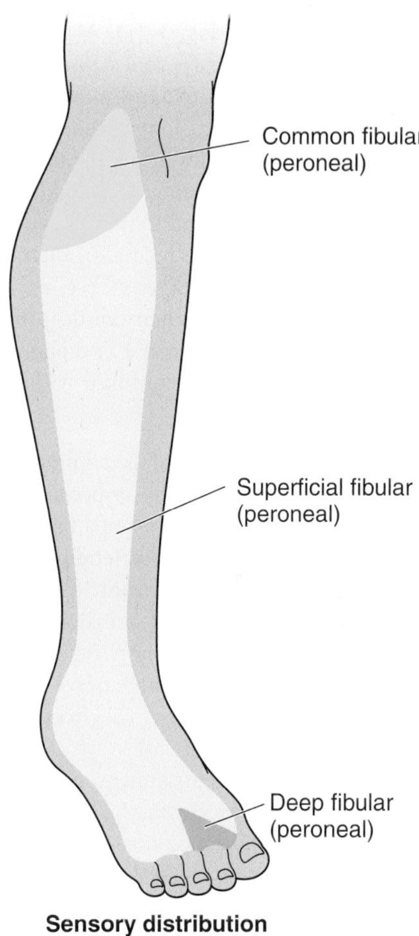

FIGURE 3-21 The common peroneal nerve (L4, 5, S1, 2). (Reproduced, with permission, from Waxman SG: *Clinical Neuroanatomy*, 26th ed, McGraw-Hill, 2010)

- The superficial fibular (peroneal) nerve arises deep to the fibularis (peroneus) longus (see Fig. 3-21). It then passes forward and downward between the peronei and the extensor digitorum longus muscles, to supply the fibularis (peroneus) longus and brevis muscles and provide sensory distribution to the lower front of the leg, the dorsum of the foot, part of the big toe, and adjacent sides of the second to fifth toes up to the second phalanges. When this nerve is entrapped, because it causes pain over the lateral distal aspect of the leg and the ankle, it is often confused with an intervertebral disk herniation involving the L5 nerve root.
- The deep fibular (peroneal) nerve passes anterior and lateral to the tibialis anterior muscle, between the fibularis (peroneus) longus and the extensor digitorum longus muscles, and to the front of the interosseous membrane and supplies the tibialis anterior, extensor digitorum longus, extensor halluces longus, and fibularis (peroneus) tertius muscles (see Fig. 3-21). At the level of the ankle joint, the deep fibular (peroneal) nerve passes behind the extensor halluces longus tendon and lies between it and the extensor digitorum longus tendon. The deep fibular (peroneal) nerve divides into a medial and lateral branch approximately 1.5 cm above the ankle joint. These terminal branches extend to the skin of the adjacent sides of the medial two toes (medial branch), to the extensor digitorum brevis muscle (lateral branch), and the adjacent joints (see Fig. 3-21). When the deep fibular (peroneal) nerve is entrapped, there is a complaint of pain in the great toe, which can be confused with a posttraumatic, sympathetic dystrophy.

An insidious entrapment of the common fibular (peroneal) nerve (and it is very vulnerable, especially at the fibula neck) can be confused with symptoms of a herniated intervertebral disk, tendonitis of the popliteus tendon, mononeuritis, idiopathic fibular (peroneal) palsy, intrinsic and extrinsic nerve tumors, and extraneural compression by a synovial cyst, ganglion cyst, soft-tissue tumor, osseous mass, or a large fabella.[123] Traumatic injury of the nerve may occur secondary to a fracture, dislocation, surgical procedure, application of skeletal traction, or a tight cast.[123]

The pain from an entrapment of the common fibular (peroneal) nerve is typically on the lateral surface of the knee, the leg, and the foot. Lateral knee pain is a common problem among patients seeking medical attention, and entrapment of the common fibular (peroneal) nerve is frequently overlooked in the differential diagnostic considerations, especially in the absence of trauma or the presence of a palpable mass at the neck of the fibula.

Pudendal and Coccygeal Plexuses

The pudendal and coccygeal plexuses are the most caudal portions of the lumbosacral plexus and supply nerves to the perineal structures (Fig. 3-22).

- The pudendal plexus supplies the coccygeus, levator ani, and sphincter ani externus muscles. The pudendal nerve is a mixed nerve, and a lesion that affects it or its ascending pathways can result in voiding and erectile dysfunctions.[124] A lesion in the afferent pathways of the pudendal nerve is often suspected clinically by suggestive patient histories, including organic neurologic disease or neurologic trauma. Lesions are also suspected when a neurologic physical examination to assess the function of signal segments S2, S3, and S4 is abnormal. The pudendal nerve divides into
  - the inferior hemorrhoidal nerves to the external anal sphincter and adjacent skin;
  - the perineal nerve; and
  - the posterior (dorsal) nerve of the penis.
- The nerves of the coccygeal plexus are the small sensory anococcygeal nerves derived from the last three segments (S4,5; C). They pierce the sacrotuberous ligament and supply the skin in the region of the coccyx.

Autonomic Nervous System

The autonomic system is the division of the peripheral nervous system that is responsible for the innervation of smooth muscle, cardiac muscle, and glands of the body. It functions primarily at a subconscious level.

The autonomic nervous system has two components, sympathetic (Fig. 3-23) and parasympathetic (Fig. 3-24), each of which is differentiated by its site of origin as well as the transmitters it releases.[125] In general, these two systems have antagonist effects on their end organs.

The sympathetic system can be involved in the modulation of pain, although under normal conditions, the sympathetic system has little or no effect on the activity of the peripheral afferent receptors. According to Blumberg and Janig,[126] the afferent neurons become hypersensitized as the result of direct trauma, producing allodynia, causalgia (complex regional pain syndrome type 1), and hyperalgesia.[127] Sensitized posterior (dorsal) horn neurons increase their receptive fields and begin to respond to both low- and high-threshold peripheral stimuli.[127,128]

A lesion to the sympathetic system has also been associated with Horner syndrome (see later discussion) and with Raynaud disease, a disorder of the peripheral vascular system.

Neuromuscular Control

Neuromuscular control involves the integration of motor learning and motor control which is controlled by the descending motor systems. These systems include the corticospinal tracts, the rubrospinal tract, the vestibulospinal tracts, and the reticulospinal tracts:

- Corticospinal tract: critical for skilled voluntary movement throughout the body.[129,130] There are two main divisions of the corticospinal tract, the lateral corticospinal tract and ventral (anterior) corticospinal tract. Most of the corticospinal fibers (approximately 80%) cross over to the contralateral side in the medulla oblongata (pyramidal decussation) and travel in the lateral corticospinal tract. 10% enter the lateral corticospinal tract on the same side. The remaining 10% cross over at the level that they exit the spinal cord, and these travel in the anterior corticospinal tract.

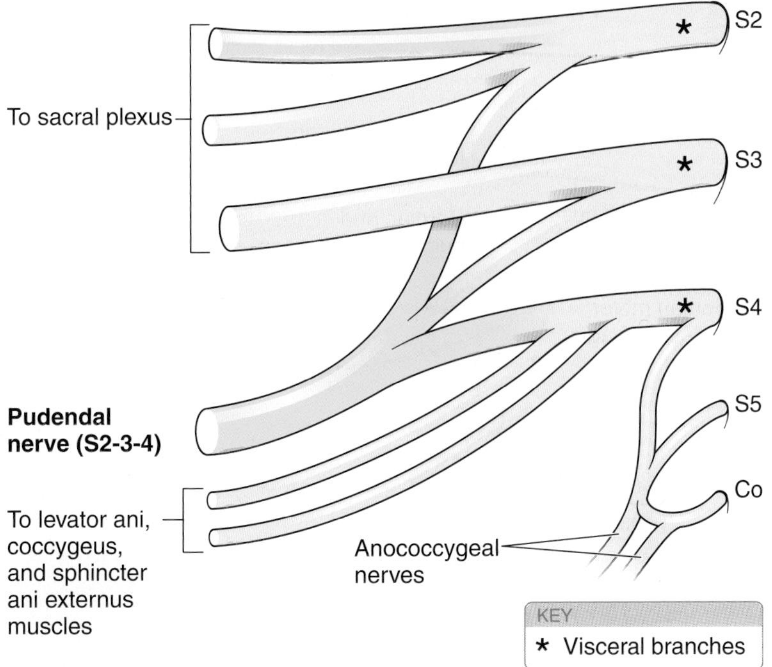

FIGURE 3-22 The pudendal and coccygeal plexuses. (Reproduced, with permission, from Waxman SG: *Clinical Neuroanatomy*, 26th ed, McGraw-Hill, 2010)

- Rubrospinal tract: important for rapid, coordinated movement of the entire limb, especially when the reach involves adapting the hand or foot to the shape of an object.[131]
- Vestibulospinal tracts: involved with integrating information from the vestibular system to control eye movements, head and neck movements, and postural reactions for balance.
- Reticulospinal tracts: activated in the early stages of movement, including movement planning, to help initiate the proper state in the postural control system and the proximal limb to support the distal movement that is to occur.[132]

Mobility and stability rely upon the combination of musculoskeletal properties and neural control. It is believed that there are certain programs for movement patterns that are inherent in the CNS and that these naturally develop during the maturation process of the CNS. For example, gait on a level surface is controlled by a set of neural circuits known as a central pattern generator (CPG). The locomotion-initiating systems in the brain stem rely upon the reticulospinal tracts as the principal route for initiation and regulation of locomotion.[133] The parameters of gait (e.g., cadence) depend on the environmental demands. When walking must occur on unusual surfaces, the CPG continues to operate but with input from the lateral corticospinal and rubrospinal systems to translate the visual perception and allow accurate placement of the foot.[134,135]

In much the same way as there is a CPG for locomotion, the nervous system has a number of built-in corrections for postural stability—the ability to maintain a stable upright stance against internal and external perturbations—that can occur rapidly and automatically to counteract these perturbations (see Balance, later). Once a CPG is formed, the individual no longer has to concentrate on performing the activity, but can do so with very little cortical involvement. The motor program for each of these activities is saved in an *engram* (a hypothetical means by which a patterned response has been stabilized at the level of unconscious competence) within the cerebral cortex.[136–138] Thousands of repetitions (practice) are required to begin the engram formation and millions are needed to perfect it.[138] Skilled performance is developed in proportion to the number of repetitions of an engram practiced just below the maximal level of ability to perform.[139,140]

The remaining motor responses rely on processing and planning at different levels: spinal cord, the brainstem and cerebellum, and the cerebral cortex. The complexity of the necessary processing affects the speed of motor responses, with spinal reflexes representing the shortest neuronal pathway and consequently the most rapid response to afferent stimuli. Certain actions, such as signing one's name, do not require sensory information for modification. These movements are said to be under open-loop control. Other movements, such as reflexively withdrawing the foot from a painful stimuli, rely on feedback from the sensory system. This type of control is referred to as closed-loop control. In a feedback (reactionary) control system, parameters are monitored and compared to a reference set point. If monitored parameters fall outside the boundaries of the set point, the controller triggers a response that will correct the system (e.g., a thermostat system that regulate room temperature).[141] In contrast, feedforward (anticipatory)

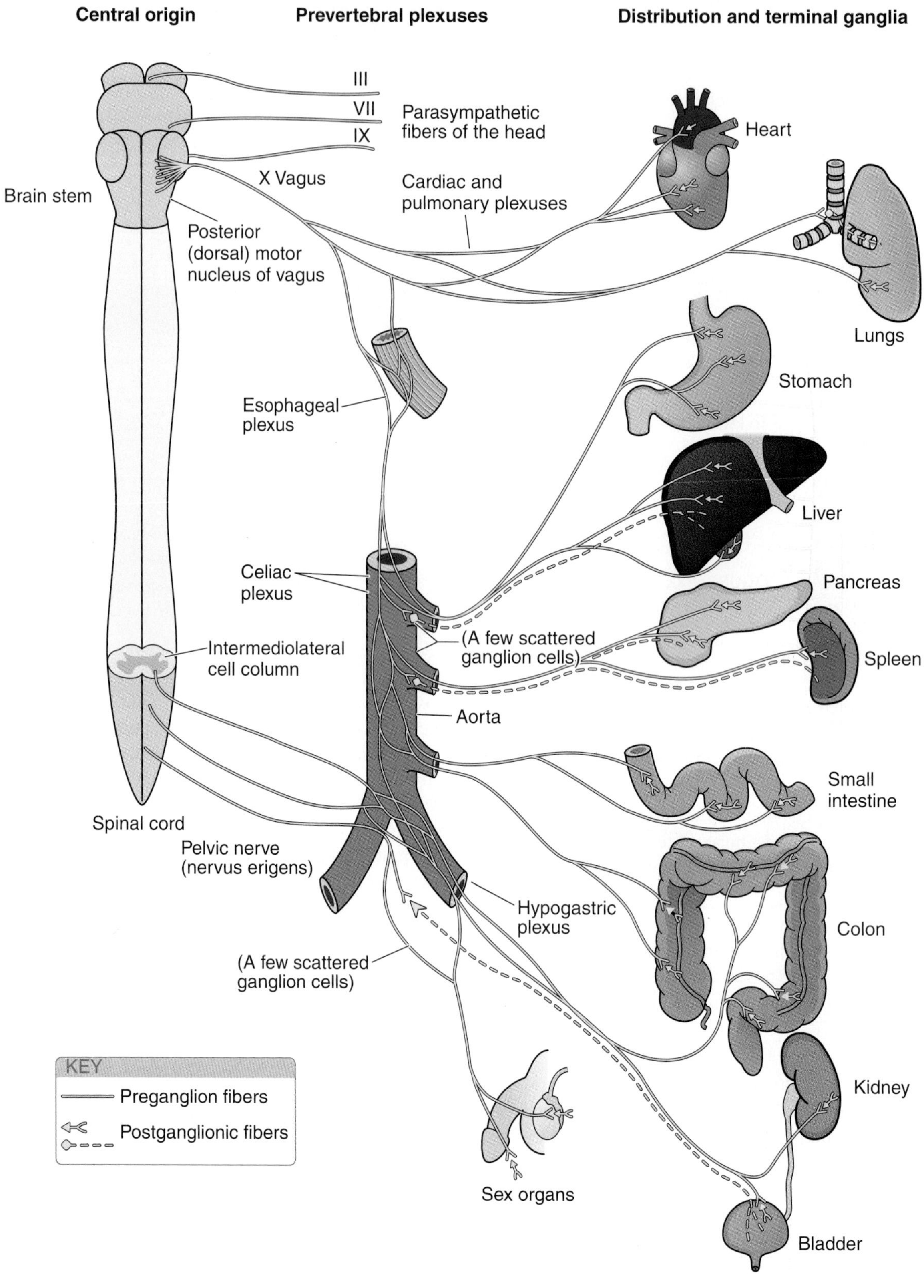

FIGURE 3-23 Sympathetic division of the autonomic nervous system (left half). (Reproduced, with permission, from Waxman SG: *Clinical Neuroanatomy*, 26th ed, McGraw-Hill, 2010)

actions differ in that they anticipate pending disturbances and act to prepare the system (e.g., an individual anticipates the need for new car and buys one before the existing car breaks down).[141] Feedforward actions are based on knowledge or previous experience. Evidence suggests that both feedforward and feedback control mechanisms contribute to dynamic stability.[142] Through feedforward and feedback controls, the sensorimotor system provides the direction that muscles require to achieve integrated multiplanar movements.[141]

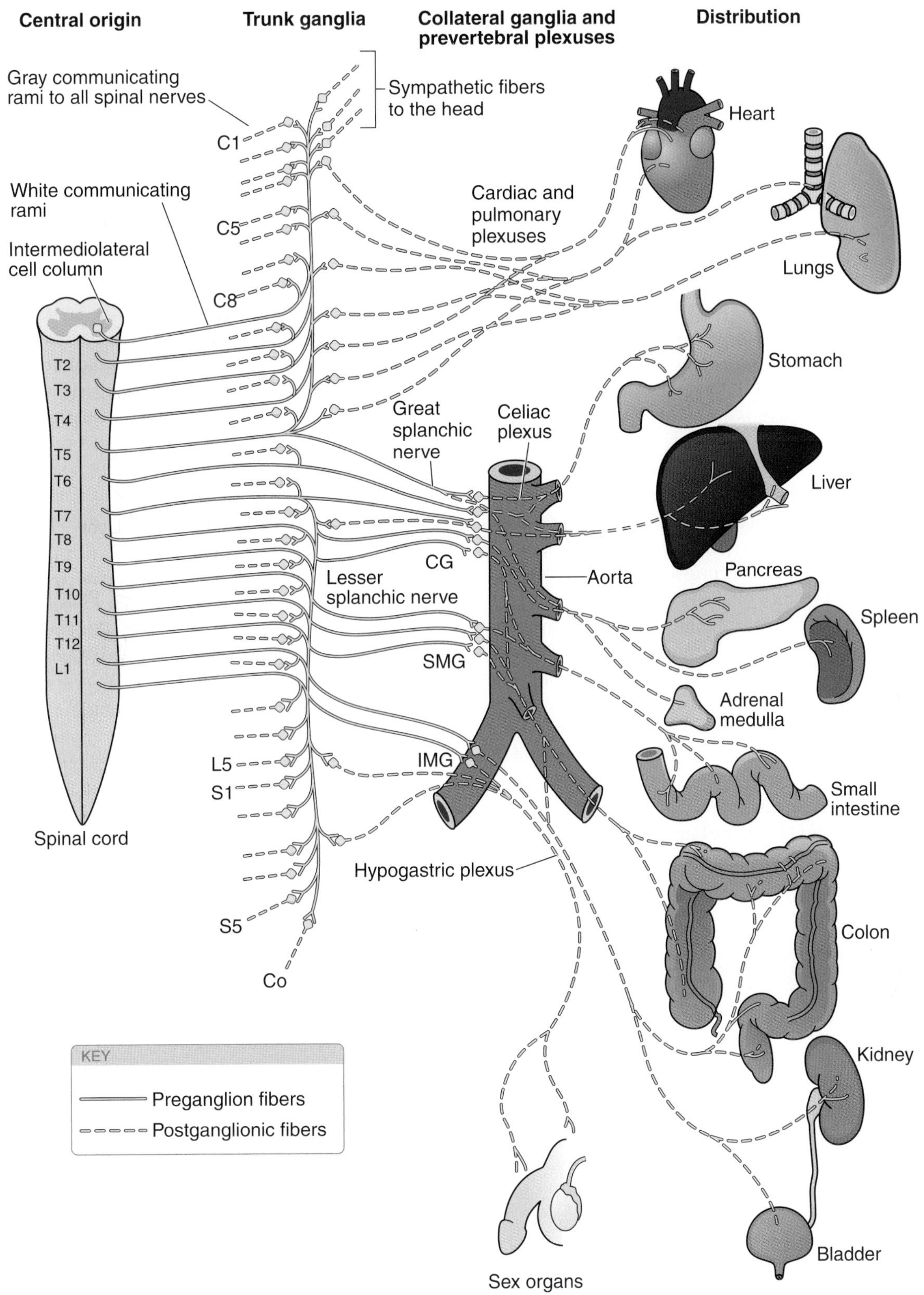

FIGURE 3-24 Parasympathetic division of the autonomic nervous system (left half). (Reproduced, with permission, from Waxman SG: *Clinical Neuroanatomy*, 26th ed, McGraw-Hill, 2010)

CLINICAL PEARL

Motor programs are codes within the nervous system that when initiated produce coordinated movement sequences.[143] These programs are usually under central control, the sensory input is used extensively in selecting the appropriate motor program, in monitoring whether or not movement is consistent with expectations and in reflexively modulating the movement so that it is specific to environmental variables.[143,144]

A patient cannot succeed in functional and recreational activities if his or her neuromuscular system is not prepared to meet the demands of the specific activities.[145] Two key components involved in neuromuscular control are proprioception and kinesthesia.

Proprioception

Proprioception is considered a specialized variation of the sensory modality of touch, which plays an important role in coordinating muscle activity and involves the integration of sensory input concerning static joint position (joint position sensibility), joint movement (kinesthetic sensibility), velocity of movement, and the force of muscular contraction from the skin, muscles, and joints.[146,147] Proprioception can be both conscious, as occurs in the accurate placement of a limb, and unconscious, as occurs in the modulation of muscle function.[147,148]

All synovial joints of the body are provided with an array of receptor endings (nociceptors, thermoreceptors, and mechanoreceptors) imbedded in articular, muscular, and cutaneous structures with varying characteristic behaviors and distributions (Table 3-1). These receptors provide information for the somatosensory system which mediates signals related to multiple sensory modalities (pain, temperature, and proprioception). The nociceptors provide information with regard to pain, while the thermoreceptors provide feedback related to temperature. The mechanoreceptors, which are stimulated by mechanical forces (soft-tissue elongation, relaxation, compression, and fluid tension), are usually classified into three groups based on receptor type: joint, muscle, or cutaneous. There is no evidence as yet that cutaneous receptors contribute to dynamic joint stability. There are four primary types of joint receptors that include Pacinian corpuscles, Ruffini endings, Golgi tendon organ (GTO)-like endings, and bare nerve endings.[17,149,150]

CLINICAL PEARL

The term *musculotendinous kinesthesia* refers to the capacity for musculotendinous structures to contribute proprioception information. Two types of muscle receptors are commonly described: muscle spindles and GTO (Box 3-1). It is most likely that the muscle and the joint receptors work complementary to one another in this complex afferent system, with each modifying the function of the other.[151] The muscle spindle functions as a stretch receptor, whereas the GTO functions as a monitor for the degree of tension within a muscle and tendon. Based on extensive work of Voss,[152] Peck et al.[153] proposed that in the extremities, smaller muscles with high muscle spindle concentrations, arranged in parallel with larger, less spindle-dense muscles, function primarily as kinesthetic monitors.[154]

- *Ruffini endings.* These slow-adapting, low-threshold stretch receptors are important postural mediators, signaling actual joint position or changes in joint positions.[155] They are primarily located on the *flexion* side (detect the stretch with extension of the joint) of the joint capsule, but are also found in ligaments, primarily near the origin and the insertion.[144,156] These slowly adapting receptors continue to discharge while the stimulus is present and contribute to reflex regulation of postural tone, to coordination of muscle activity, and to a perceptional awareness of joint position. An increase in joint capsule tension by active or passive motion, posture, mobilization, or manipulation causes these receptors to discharge at a higher frequency.[150,157]
- *Pacinian corpuscles.* These rapidly adapting, low-threshold receptors function primarily in sensing joint compression and increased hydrostatic pressure in the joint.[158] They are primarily located in the subcapsular fibroadipose tissue, the cruciate ligaments, the anulus fibrosus, ligaments, and the fibrous capsule. These receptors are entirely inactive in immobile joints but become active for brief periods at the onset of movement and during rapid changes in tension. They also fire during active or passive motion of a joint, or with the application of traction. This behavior suggests their role as a control mechanism to regulate motor unit activity of the prime movers of the joint.
- *GTO-like receptors.* These receptors, also referred to as Golgi ligament organs, are found in the joint capsule, ligaments, and menisci.[159] These slow-adapting and high-threshold receptors function to detect large amounts of tension. They only become active in the extremes of motion such as when strong manual techniques are applied to the joint. Their function is protective; to prevent further motion that would over displace the joint (a joint protective reflex), and their firing is inhibitory to those muscles that would contribute to excessive forces.
- *Bare nerve endings.* These high-threshold, nonadapting, free nerve ending receptors are inactive in normal circumstances but become active with marked mechanical deformation or tension.[160,161] They may also become active in response to direct mechanical or chemical irritation, and their sensitivity usually increases when joints are inflamed or swollen.[162]

Thus, the CNS is organized in a hierarchical and parallel fashion with the cortical centers of the brain being the location of the most complex processing, and the spinal cord being the location of the most basic processing.[144] At the upper end of the hierarchy, the motor cortex has a motor program, defined as an abstract plan of movement that, when initiated, results in the production of a coordinated movement sequence.[141,143] At the lower end of the hierarchy, specific motor units must contract to accomplish the movement. Rapid motor responses to somatosensory feedback mediated in the spinal cord are referred to as spinal reflexes.[144] These reflex actions include preparatory postural adjustments[163] and reaction movements. The former are preprogrammed neural mechanisms. The latter occur too fast for the long loop feedback of the CNS so that they are automatic and occur subconsciously (see Supraspinal reflexes later). Although the hierarchy is well established, research suggests these components also work in parallel so that any of the components may predominate in controlling some aspects of movement; the system is built for efficiency and redundancy.[141]

Box 3-1 Muscle Spindle and GTO

Muscle Spindle

Muscle spindles are encapsulated spindle-shaped structures lying in parallel with skeletal muscle fibers in the muscle belly. Essentially, the purpose of the muscle spindle is to compare the length of the spindle with the length of the muscle that surrounds the spindle. Spindles have three main components:[1]

- *Intrafusal muscle fibers.* 2–12 long, slender, and specialized skeletal muscle fibers. The central portion of the intrafusal fiber is devoid of actin or myosin and, thus, is incapable of contracting. As a result, these fibers are capable of putting tension on the spindle only. These intrafusal fibers are of two types: nuclear bag fibers and nuclear chain fibers. Nuclear bag fibers primarily serve as sensitivity meters for the changing lens of the muscle.[2,3] Nuclear chain fibers each contain a single row or chain of nuclei and are attached at their ends to the bag fibers.
- *Sensory neuron endings that wrap around the intrafusal fibers.* The sensory neurons are afferents structures (groups Ia and II afferents) that send information regarding static muscle length and changes in muscle length to the dorsal root ganglia of the spinal cord. The group Ia afferents relay information regarding rates of change, whereas the group II afferents relay information regarding steady-state muscle length.
- *Motor axons.* While muscles are innervated by alpha motor neurons, muscle spindles have their own motor supply, namely gamma motor neurons.

The muscle spindle can be stimulated in two different ways:

- By stretching the whole muscle, which stretches the mid portion of the spindle and depolarize the Ia afferents. Ia afferents depolarization can trigger two separate responses:[1]
  - A monosynaptic or disynaptic spinal reflex
  - A long loop transcortical reflex
- By contracting only the end portion of the intrafusal fibers, exciting the receptor (even if muscle length does not change).

If the length of the muscles surrounding the spindle is less than that of the spindle, a decrease in intrafusal fiber afferent activity occurs. For example, a quick stretch applied to a muscle reflexively produces a quick contraction of the agonistic and synergistic muscle (extrafusal) fibers. This has the effect of producing a smooth contraction and relaxation of muscle and eliminating any jerkiness during movement. The firing of the type Ia phasic nerve fibers is influenced by the rate of stretch: the faster and greater the stimulus, the greater the effect of the associated extrafusal fibers.[3,4]

Golgi Tendon Organs

GTOs are small, encapsulated structures spaced in series along the musculotendinous junction that become activated by stretch.[1] In contrast to the muscle spindle, GTOs function to protect muscle attachments from strain or avulsion, by using a postsynaptic inhibitory synapse of the muscle in which they are located.[5] The signals from the GTO may go both to local areas within the spinal cord and through the spinocerebellar tracts to the cerebellum.[6] The local signals result in excitation of interneurons, which in turn inhibit the anterior α motor neurons of the GTO's own muscle and synergist, while facilitating the antagonists.[6] This is theorized to prevent overcontraction, or stretch, of a muscle.[5]

1. Rose J: Dynamic lower extremity stability, in Hughes C, ed. *Movement disorders and neuromuscular interventions for the trunk and extremities – Independent Study Course* 18.2.5. La Crosse, WI: Orthopaedic Section, APTA, Inc., 2008, pp 1–34.
2. Grigg P: Peripheral neural mechanisms in proprioception. *J Sport Rehabil* 3: 1–17, 1994.
3. Swash M, Fox K: Muscle spindle innervation in man. *J Anat* 112:61–80, 1972.
4. Wilk KE, Voight ML, Keirns MA, et al.: Stretch-shortening drills for the upper extremities: theory and clinical application. *J Orthop Sports Phys Ther* 17: 225–239, 1993.
5. de Jarnette B: *Sacro-occipital technique.* Nebraska City, NE: Major Bertrand de Jarnette, DC, 1972.
6. Pollard H, Ward G: A study of two stretching techniques for improving hip flexion range of motion. *J Man Physiol Ther* 20:443–447, 1997.

CLINICAL PEARL

Proprioception can play a protective role in an acute injury through reflex muscle splinting via stimulation of the muscle spindles.[164]

Proprioceptive information is relayed to the cerebral cortex by one of the two major ascending systems, the dorsal column and the spinothalamic tract. Once processed and evaluated, the proprioceptive information is capable of influencing muscle tone, motor execution programs, and cognitive somatic perceptions or kinesthetic awareness.[151,165] All of this information helps generate a somatosensory image within the CNS.[151]

The ability of a joint to remain stable depends in part on its resistance to motion when subjected to external loads, referred to as its degree of stiffness. A joint's stiffness is the result of three components: passive factors associated with the material properties of the musculotendinous tissues; active intrinsic properties associated with the cross bridge attachment and length tension properties of the muscles that cross the joint (see Chap. 1); and reflexes associated with length feedback and force feedback from muscle spindles, tendon organs, and the influence of other somatosensory feedback on the fusimotor system.[144]

Following an injury, alterations occur with the stiffness of a joint and in the normal recruitment pattern and timing of muscular contractions.[166] These alterations are thought to result from an adjustment in the ratio of muscle spindles to GTO activity and a disruption of the proprioceptive pathway.[142,167,168] Any delay in response time to an unexpected load placed on the dynamic restraints can expose the static restraint structures to excessive forces, increasing the potential for injury.[169] Thus, the focus of neuromuscular rehabilitation must be directed toward creating an environment that promotes the restoration and development of motor responses and proprioception in the presence of altered sensory input.[170]

Fatigue may also play a part in injury, particularly if the fatigue produces a dominance of agonists or antagonists over the other.[168] Fatigue also reduces the capability of a muscle to absorb or dissipate loads. It seems plausible that some forms of muscle spindle desensitization, or perhaps ligament relaxation and Golgi tendon desensitization, occur with excessive fatigue.[171] This may then lead to a decreased efferent muscle response and reduced ability to maintain balance.

Proprioceptive deficits can also be found with aging,[172] arthrosis,[173] and joint instability.[148,164,166,167,174–177]

Kinesthesia

Kinesthesia, a sub-modality of proprioception, refers to the sense of movement of the body or one of the segments. Although the articular receptors quite clearly play a very active role, the stretch reflex controlled by two other sensors, the muscle spindle and the GTO, is also important. Information about movement sense travels up the spinocerebellar tract (Box 3-2).

CLINICAL PEARL

During a concentric muscle contraction, the muscle spindle output is reduced because the muscle fibers are either shortening or attempting to shorten, whereas during an eccentric contraction, the muscle stretch reflex generates more tension in the lengthening muscle.[154,178,179]

Motor Learning and Skill Acquisition

Motor learning is a complex set of internal processes that involve the relatively permanent acquisition and retention of a skill or task through practice.[180–182]

CLINICAL PEARL

Learning, unlike performance, is not something that can be directly measured. Rather, we measure behavior and infer learning when the change in behavior seems relatively permanent.[183] However, learning can be measured indirectly using retention tests or transfer tests:

- *Retention test*: involves allowing sufficient time between practice and testing to assess whether a relatively permanent change has occurred.
- *Transfer test*: involves the ability to transfer a skill used in one task to other situations.

Box 3-2 Spinocerebellar Tract

The spinocerebellar tract conducts impulses related to the position and movement of muscles to the cerebellum. This information enables the cerebellum to add smoothness and precision to patterns of movement initiated in the cerebral hemispheres. Spinocerebellar impulses do not reach the cerebrum directly and, therefore, have no conscious representation. Four tracts constitute the spinocerebellar pathway; they are the posterior spinocerebellar, cuneocerebellar, anterior spinocerebellar, and rostral spinocerebellar tracts.

The posterior spinocerebellar tract conveys muscle spindle or tendon organ-related impulses from the lower half of the body (below the level of the T6 spinal cord segment); the cuneocerebellar tract is concerned with such impulses from the body above T6. The *grain* of information carried in these two tracts is fine, often involving single muscle cells or portions of a muscle–tendon complex. A much broader representation is carried by the individual fibers of the anterior and rostral spinocerebellar tracts.

The axons conducting impulses from muscle spindles, tendon organs, and skin in the lower half of the body are large type Ia, type Ib, and type II fibers, the cell bodies of which are in the spinal ganglia of spinal nerves T6 and below.

Primary neurons below L3 send their central processes into the posterior columns. These processes then ascend in the columns to the L3 level. From L3 to T6, incoming central processes and those in the posterior columns project to the medial part of lamina VII, where there is a well-demarcated column of cells, called *Clarke's column*. Largely limited to the thoracic cord, Clarke's column can be seen from segments L3 to C8 of the cord. Here, the central processes of the primary neurons synapse with secondary neurons, the axons of which are directed to the lateral funiculi as the posterior spinocerebellar tracts.

- *Performance:* involves the acquisition of a skill. A change in performance is dependent upon practice or experience.
- *Learning:* involves both acquisition and retention of a skill. Two main types of learning are recognized:[183]
  - Declarative—the learning of facts.
  - Procedural—learning that is dependent on practice, association (associating a particular stimulus with another stimulus, or certain stimulus with a certain response, or certain response with a certain result), and adaptation (making adjustments based on previous results), habituation (filtering out irrelevant stimuli), and sensitization (integration of relevant stimuli).

For learning to occur there must be a goal. Inherent in the idea of the goal is motivation.[183]

- *Motor task.* There are three basic types of motor tasks or skills:[143,184]

- *Discrete:* involves a movement with a recognizable beginning and end. For example, throwing a ball, or opening a door.
- *Serial:* involves a series of discrete movements that are combined in a particular sequence. For example, the sequence of tasks that are involved in getting out of a chair when using crutches.
- *Continuous:* involves repetitive, uninterrupted movements that have no distinct beginning and ending. Examples include walking and cycling.

Stages of Motor Learning

There are three stages of motor learning:[185]

- *Cognitive.* This stage begins when the patient is first introduced to the motor task. This stage requires great concentration and variable performances filled with errors because the patient must determine the objective of the skill as well as the relational and environmental cues to control and regulate the movement. The patient is more concerned with what to do and how to do it. During this phase, the clinician should provide frequent and explicit positive feedback using various forms of feedback (verbal, tactile, visual), and allow trial and error to occur within safe limits.
- *Associative.* The patient is less concerned about every detail and more with performing and refining the skills. The important stimuli have been identified and their meaning is known. Conscious decisions about what to do become more automatic and the patient concentrates more on the task and appears less rushed. During this phase, the clinician should begin to increase the complexity of the task, emphasize problem solving, avoid manual guidance, and vary the sequence of tasks.
- *Autonomous.* This stage is characterized by an efficient and nearly automatic kind of performance. For example, when walking occurs automatically without conscious thought. During this phase, the clinician should set up a series of progressively more difficult activities the patient can do independently, such as increasing the speed, the distance, and the complexity of the task.

CLINICAL PEARL

Most patients in rehabilitation are often in the associated stage because they are familiar with the skills they need to perform, but the movement for a particular skill may be altered and need to be learned because of neuromuscular dysfunction.[170]

Practice

Practice, repeatedly performing a movement or series of movements in a task, is probably the single most important variable in learning a motor skill.[184,185] The various types of practice for motor learning are as follows:[184]

- Part versus whole.
  - *Part.* A task is broken down into separate components and the individual components (usually the more difficult ones) are practiced. After mastery of the individual components, the components are combined in a sequence so that the whole task can be practiced.
  - *Whole.* The entire task is performed from beginning to end and is not practiced in separate components.
- Blocked, random, and random blocked.
  - *Blocked.* The same task or series of tasks is performed repeatedly under the same conditions and in a predictable order. For example, consistently practicing walking in a straight line on a flat surface.
  - *Random.* Slight variations of the same task are carried out in an unpredictable order. For example, a patient could practice walking on various walking surfaces and in different directions.
  - *Random blocked.* Variations of the same task are performed in random order, but each variation of the task is performed more than once. For example, the patient walks on a particular surface and then repeats the same task a second time before moving on to a different surface.
- Massed versus distributed.
  - *Massed.* Involves participation in a long bout of practice, where substantially less time is spent in rest compared to practice during the practice period. The disadvantages of this type of practice are that the patient is not able to reflect on his or her performance between practices, there is more potential for fatigue and an increased likelihood of a slight detriment for learning.[143]
  - *Distributed.* This type of practice involves participation in a series of practices throughout the day. The advantage of this type of practice is that the patient is able to reflect on his or her performance between practices.
- Physical versus mental.
  - *Physical.* The movements of a task are actually performed.
  - *Mental.* A cognitive rehearsal of how a motor task is to be performed occurs prior to actually doing the task.
- Constant versus varied.
  - *Constant.* Occurs when the skill is practiced repeatedly without changing anything. For example, shooting hoops from only the foul line.
  - *Varied.* Occurs when a parameter is changed throughout the practice session. For example, shooting hoops from various areas of the court.

Feedback

Second only to practice, feedback is considered the next most important variable that influences learning. The various types of feedback associated with motor learning are as follows:[184]

- Intrinsic versus extrinsic (augmented).
  - *Intrinsic.* Intrinsic feedback is a natural part of task.[143] It can take the form of a sensory cue (proprioceptive, kinesthetic, tactile, visual, or auditory), or set of cues,

inherent in the execution of the motor task. The feedback can arise from within the learner and be derived from performance of the task. This type of feedback may immediately follow completion of a task or may occur even before the task has been completed.

- *Extrinsic.* Extrinsic feedback is supplemental feedback that is not normally an inherent part of the task. This type of feedback can include sensory cues from an external source (verbal, visual, or auditory). Unlike intrinsic feedback, the clinician can control the type, the timing, and the frequency of extrinsic feedback.

- Knowledge of results (KR) versus knowledge of performance (KP).
  - *KR:* immediate, posttask, extrinsic feedback about the outcome of a motor task. This type of feedback is primarily reserved for instances when individuals are unable to generate this type of information for themselves, or when the information may serve as a motivational tool.[143]
  - *KP:* feedback given about the nature or quality of the performance of the motor task. This type of feedback better facilitates motor skill learning than KR.

Feedback about performance can be provided at various times:

- Continuous versus Intermittent versus.
  - *Continuous:* is ongoing. This type of feedback improves skill acquisition more quickly during the initial stage of learning than intermittent feedback.
  - *Intermittent:* occurs irregularly, randomly. Intermittent feedback has been shown to promote learning more effectively than continuous feedback.
- Immediate, delayed, and summary.
  - *Immediate:* is given directly after a task is completed. This type of feedback is used most frequently during the cognitive (initial) stage of learning.
  - *Delayed:* is given after an interval of time elapses, allowing the learner to reflect on how well or poorly a task was done. This type of feedback promotes retention and generalizability of the learned skills.
  - *Summary:* is given about the average performance of several repetitions of the movement or task. This type of feedback is used most frequently during the associative stage of learning.

Skill Acquisition

A number of theories of skill acquisition have been proposed with respect to the predictability of the environment:

- Open (temporal and spatial factors in an unpredictable environment) versus closed skills (spatial factors only in a predictable environment), involving a single dimensional continuum. Using sports as an example, a closed skill could include shooting a foul shot in basketball. An everyday example of a closed skill is drinking from a cup. An example of an open skill in everyday life would be stepping onto a moving walkway, whereas in sport an open skill would involve throwing a touchdown pass. While closed skills allow an individual to evaluate the environment and perform the movement without much modification, open skills require more cognitive processing and decision making in choosing and adjusting the movement.[170] Open and closed skills can be viewed as a continuum, where the perceptual and habitual nature of a task determines whether the task is open or closed.
- *Gentile taxonomy of motor tasks.*[186] This is a two-dimensional classification system for teaching motor skills. Using the concept that motor skills range from simple to complex, Gentile expanded the popular one-dimensional classification system of open and closed skills to combine the environmental context together with the function of the action:[184,185]
  - The environmental (closed or open) context in which the task is performed. Regulatory conditions (other people, objects) in the environment may be either stationary (closed skills) or in motion (open skills).
  - The intertrial variability (absent or present) of the environment that is imposed on the task. When the environment in which a task is set is unchanging from one performance of a task to the next, intertrial variability is absent—the environmental conditions are predictable. For example, walking on a flat surface. Intertrial variability is present when the demands change from one attempt or repetition of the task to the next. For example, walking over varying terrain.
  - The need for a person's body to remain stationary (stable) or to move (transport) during the task. Skills that require body transport are more complex than skills that require no body transport as there are more variables to consider. For example, a body transport task could include walking in a crowded shopping mall.
  - The presence or absence of manipulation of objects during the task. When a person must manipulate an object, the skill increases in complexity because the person must do two things at once—manipulate the object correctly and adjust the body posture to fit the efficient movement of the object.

Balance

Balance, or postural control, is a complex motor control task involving the detection and integration of sensory information to assess the position and motion of the body in space and the execution of appropriate musculoskeletal responses to control body position within its stability limits, and within the context of the environment and task, whether stationary or moving.[187] Posture is the relative position of the various parts of the body with respect to one another, to the environment, and to gravity (see Chap. 6).[188]

Balance results from an integration of three components:[188]

- The nervous system, which provides sensory processing for perception of body orientation in space provided mainly by the visual, vestibular, and somatosensory systems. The sensory motor integration provides motor strategies for the planning, the programming, and the execution of balance responses.[189]

- Musculoskeletal contributions including postural alignment, flexibility, joint integrity, muscle performance, and mechanoreceptor sensation.
- Contextual effects that interact with the nervous and the musculoskeletal systems. These effects include whether the environment is closed (predictable) or open (unpredictable), the support surface, the amount of lighting, the effects of gravity and inertial forces on the body, and the characteristics of the task (new versus well learned, predictable versus unpredictable, single versus multiple).

Impaired balance can be caused by injury or disease to any of the structures involved in the stages of information processing.

CLINICAL PEARL

Proprioception and balance are not synonymous. Proprioception can be conscious or unconscious, whereas balance is typically conscious.

An individual's balance is greatest when the body's center of gravity (COG) is maintained over its base of support (BOS). Functional tasks require different types of balance control, including:[187]

- *Static balance:* involves maintaining a stable antigravity position while at rest, such as when standing and sitting.
- *Dynamic balance:* the ability to stabilize the body when the support surface is moving or when the body is moving on a stable surface, such as during sit to stand transfers or walking.
- *Automatic postural reactions:* the ability to maintain balance in response to unexpected external perturbations, such as standing on a bus that suddenly decelerates.

The maintenance of balance requires the integration of sensory information from a number of different systems: vision, vestibular, and somatosensory.[151] The vestibular system, with contributions from the inner ear (see Cranial Nerves), provides information about movement and spatial orientation. The visual system, which involves CN II, III, IV, and VI, assists in balance control by providing input about the position of the head or the body in space (see Supraspinal reflexes later). Through the vestibulo-ocular input, signals from the muscle spindles in the extraocular muscles, the position of the eyeball is controlled so that a visual image is maintained on the fovea. The coordination of eye movements during gaze is a complex affair and is controlled by efferent signals from the trochlear, the abducens, and the oculomotor nuclei via the fourth, the sixth, and the third CNs, respectively (refer to the discussion of cervico-ocular and vestibular reflexes later in this chapter).[12] Coordination of these nuclei is achieved by gaze centers in the reticular formation, the midbrain, and the cortex, and by the cerebellum, which have fibers that project into the three eye muscle nuclei and control the orbital movements concerned with slow and rapid eye movements.[12]

Automatic Postural Responses

To maintain balance, the body must continually adjust its position in space. A certain amount of anteroposterior and lateral sway normally occur while maintaining balance. For example, normal anteroposterior sway in adults is 12 degree from the most posterior to the most anterior position.[190] If the sway exceeds the limits of stability, some strategy must be employed to regain balance. Horak and Nashner[191] describes several different strategies used to maintain balance, including the ankle, the hip, and the stepping strategies, which are designed to adjust the body's COG so that the body is maintained within the BOS to prevent the loss of balance or falling:

- The ankle strategy, in which muscles around the ankles are used to provide postural stability in the anteroposterior plane, is employed with small perturbations.
- Weight-shift strategy is a movement strategy utilized to control medial–lateral perturbations involving shifting the bodyweight laterally from one leg to the other.
- Suspension strategy, which involves lowering the body's COG by flexing the knees, causing associated flexion of the ankles and the hips or a slight squatting motion.
- The hip strategy, in which muscles around the thigh, the hip, and the trunk are recruited, is employed with larger perturbations.
- The stepping strategy, in which a step is taken to maintain postural control, is employed if the two previous strategies are insufficient.

Most healthy individuals use combinations of the above strategies to maintain balance depending on the control demands.[188]

Anticipatory and Compensatory Postural Adjustments

Anticipatory postural adjustments occur in response to internal perturbations such as voluntary movements of the body by activating muscle synergies in advance of the actual perturbation. Research has shown that anticipatory postural adjustments are highly adaptable and vary according to the task demands.[192–194] For example, postural muscles in standing humans are activated prior to (and during) voluntary movement of an upper limb and are specific to this movement. Anticipatory postural adjustments have also been studied during leg movements,[195,196] trunk movements,[197,198] arm movements in standing subjects,[192,199] and during load release from extended arms.[200–202]

While anticipatory reactions are initiated by the subject, compensatory reactions, which occur later, are initiated by sensory feedback triggering signals. With anticipatory reactions, the CNS tries to predict postural perturbations associated with a planned movement and minimize them with anticipatory corrections in a feedforward manner, while compensatory reactions deal with actual perturbations of balance that occur because of the suboptimal efficacy of the anticipatory components.

The Neurophysiology of Pain

Pain, at some point or other, is felt by everyone and is considered an emotional experience that is highly individualized and extremely difficult to evaluate. Our knowledge of the pain system has greatly improved over the past few years with discoveries that have increased our understanding of the role of nociceptors and the processing of nociceptive information. Furthermore, new findings have illuminated our knowledge about the descending pathways that modulate nociceptive activity.

CLINICAL PEARL

Patients' attitudes, beliefs, and personalities may strongly affect their immediate experience of acute pain.

Types of Pain

Pain is the most common determinant for a patient to seek intervention. Pain is a broad and significant symptom that can be described using many descriptors. In addition, the pain perception and the response to the painful experience can be influenced by various cognitive processes, including anxiety, tension, depression, past pain experiences, and cultural influences.[203] Perhaps, the simplest descriptors for pain are acute and chronic.

Acute pain can be defined as "the normal, predicted physiological response to an adverse chemical, thermal, or mechanical stimulus . . . associated with surgery, trauma, and acute illness."[204] This type of pain usually precipitates a visit to a physician, because it has one or more of the following characteristics[205]:

- It is new and has not been experienced before.
- It is severe and disabling.
- It is continuous, lasting for more than several minutes, or recurs very frequently.
- The site of the pain may cause alarm (e.g., chest and eye).
- In addition to the sensory and affective components, acute pain is typically characterized by anxiety. This may produce a fight-or-flight autonomic response, which is normally used for survival needs. This autonomic reaction is also associated with an increase in systolic and diastolic blood pressure, a decrease in gut motility and salivatory flow, increased muscle tension, and papillary distention.[17,206]

CLINICAL PEARL

- Hyperalgesia is an increased response to noxious stimulus. Primary hyperalgesia occurs at the site of injury, whereas secondary hyperalgesia occurs outside the site of injury.
- Allodynia is defined as pain in response to a previously innocuous stimulus.
- Referred pain is a site adjacent to or at a distance from the site of an injury's origin. Referred pain can occur from muscle, joint, and viscera. For example, the pain felt during a myocardial infarction is often felt in the neck, shoulders, and back rather than in the chest, the site of the injury.

Acute pain following trauma, or the insidious onset of a musculoskeletal condition, is typically chemical in nature. Although motions aggravate the pain, they cannot be used to alleviate the symptoms. In contrast, cessation of movement (absolute rest) tends to alleviate the pain, although not necessarily immediately. The structures most sensitive to chemical irritation in order of sensitivity are:

- The periosteum and joint capsule
- Subchondral bone, tendon, and ligament
- Muscle and cortical bone
- The synovium and articular cartilage

CLINICAL PEARL

The aching type of pain, associated with degenerative arthritis and muscle disorders, is often accentuated by activity and lessened by rest. Pain that is not alleviated by rest, and that is not associated with acute trauma, may indicate the presence of a serious disorder such as a tumor or an aneurysm. This pain is often described as deep, constant, and boring and is apt to be more noticeable and more intense at night.[207]

Chronic pain is typically more aggravating than worrying, lasts for more than 6 months, and has the following characteristics[205]:

- It has been experienced before and has remitted spontaneously, or after simple measures.
- It is usually mild to moderate in intensity.
- It is usually of limited duration, although it can persist for long periods (persistent pain).
- The pain site does not cause alarm (e.g., knee and ankle).
- There are no alarming associated symptoms. However, patients with chronic pain may be more prone to depression and disrupted interpersonal relationships.[208–211]

The symptoms of chronic pain typically behave in a mechanical fashion, in that they are provoked by activity or repeated movements and reduced with rest or a movement in the opposite direction.

CLINICAL PEARL

Referred pain, which can be either acute or chronic, is pain perceived to be in an area that seems to have little or no relation to the existing pathology.

Transmission of Pain

A nociceptive neuron is the one that transmits pain signals. The nociceptive system is normally a quiescent system requiring strong, intense, potentially damaging stimulation before it becomes activated.[178] Any tissue that contains free nerve endings involved with nociception is capable of being a source of pain. Pain receptors (nociceptors), unlike other receptors, are nonadapting in nature; that is, they will continue to fire for as long as the stimulus is present. It is apparent that many peripheral nociceptors are polymodal. Nociceptor stimulation can only occur in one of the three ways[179]:

- Mechanical deformation resulting in the application of sufficient mechanical forces to stress, deform, or damage a structure.
- Excessive heat or cold.
- The presence of chemical irritants in sufficient quantities or concentrations. Key mediators that have been identified include bradykinin, serotonin, histamine, potassium ions, adenosine triphosphate, protons, prostaglandins, nitric oxide, leukotrienes, cytokines, and growth factors.[204] The effects of these mediators involve binding to specific receptors, activation of ion channels for depolarization, activation of intracellular second messenger systems, and release of a range of neuropeptides to promote neurogenic inflammation, and alteration of neuronal properties by modifying gene transcription.[178,204]

One of the most fundamental influences on nociceptor sensitivity is the pH of the surrounding tissue.[178] High local proton concentrations are known to occur in many inflammatory states and the consequent reduction in pH can contribute to sensitization and activation of polymodal nociceptors.[178,212]

The transmission of pain to the CNS occurs via two distinct pathways, which correspond to the two different types of pain: fast-conducting A delta and slow-conducting C fibers (Table 3-1), although not all the fibers are necessarily nociceptors. Each of these types of fibers has different pain characteristics: A delta fibers evoke a rapid, sharp, lancinating pain reaction; C fibers cause a slow, dull, crawling pain.

Rapid Pain

The fast, or dermatomal, pain signals are transmitted in the peripheral nerves by small, myelinated A fibers at velocities between 6 and 30 m (20 and 98 ft) per second. The fast pain impulse is a signal telling the subject that a threat is present and provoking an almost instantaneous and often reflexive response. This signal often is followed a second or more later by a duller pain that tells of either tissue damage or continuing stimulation.

Slow Pain

Slow, or sclerotomal, pain is transmitted in even smaller and unmyelinated C nerve fibers at much slower velocities, between 0.5 and 2 m (1.6 and 6.6 ft) per second. On entering the posterior (dorsal) horn of the spinal cord, the pain signals from both visceral and somatic tissues do one of the following three things:

- Synapse with interneurons that synapse directly with motor nerves and produce reflex movements.

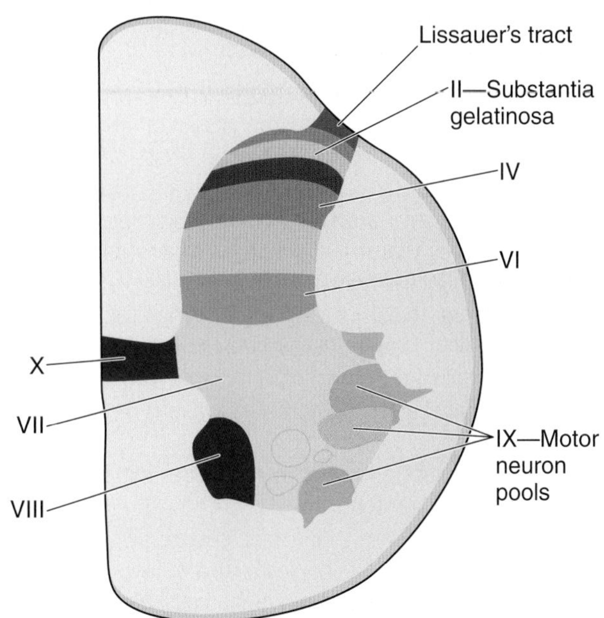

FIGURE 3-25 Laminas of the gray matter of the spinal cord. (Reproduced, with permission, from Waxman SG: *Clinical Neuroanatomy*, 26th ed, McGraw-Hill, 2010)

- Synapse with autonomic fibers from the sympathetic and parasympathetic systems and produce autonomic reflexes.
- Synapse with interneurons that travel to the higher centers in the brain.
  - The fast signals of the C fibers terminate in laminae I and V of the posterior (dorsal) horn (Fig. 3-25). Here they excite neurons (internuncial neurons, segmental motor neurons, and flexor reflex afferents) that send long fibers to the opposite side of the cord and then upward to the brain in the lateral division of the anterior–lateral sensory pathway (lateral spinothalamic tract (Box 3-3).
  - The slow signals of the C fibers terminate in laminae II and III of the posterior (dorsal) horn (Fig. 3-25). Most of the signal then passes through another short fiber neuron to terminate in lamina V. Here, the neuron gives off a long axon, most of which joins with the fast signal axons to cross the spinal cord and continue upward in the brain in the same spinal tract. Approximately 75–90% of all pain fibers terminate in the reticular formation of the medulla, pons, and mesencephalon. From here, other neurons transmit the signal to the thalamus, hypothalamus (pituitary), limbic system, and the cerebral cortex.

CLINICAL PEARL

Pain and nociceptive input can exert a strong influence on motor function and emotional state.[178]

The central pathways for processing nociceptive information begin at the level of the spinal cord (and medullary) posterior (dorsal) horn. As with the periphery, the posterior (dorsal) horn of the spinal cord contains many transmitters and receptors, both identified and accepted, including several neuroactive peptides (substance P, calcitonin gene-related

Box 3-3 Spinothalamic Tract

The spinothalamic tract helps mediate the sensations of pain, cold, warmth, and touch from receptors throughout the body (except the face) to the brain.[119,177–179] Laterally projecting spinothalamic neurons are more likely to be situated in laminae I and V. Medially projecting cells are more likely to be situated in the deep posterior (dorsal) horn and in the anterior (ventral) horn. Most of the cells project to the contralateral thalamus, although a small fraction projects ipsilaterally.[180] Spinothalamic axons in the anterior–lateral quadrant of the spinal cord are arranged somatotopically. At cervical levels, spinothalamic axons representing the lower extremity and caudal body are placed more laterally, and those representing the upper extremity and rostral body, more anterior medially.[181,182]

Most of the neurons show their best responses when the skin is stimulated mechanically at a noxious intensity. However, many spinothalamic tract cells also respond, although less effectively, to innocuous mechanical stimuli, and some respond best to innocuous mechanical stimuli.[183] A large fraction of spinothalamic tract cells also respond to a noxious heating of the skin, while others respond to stimulation of the receptors in muscle,[184] joints, or viscera.[118]

Spinothalamic tract cells can be inhibited effectively by repetitive electrical stimulation of peripheral nerves,[185] with the inhibition outlasting the stimulation by 20–30 minutes. Some inhibition can be evoked by stimulation of the large myelinated axons of a peripheral nerve, but the inhibition is much more powerful if small myelinated or unmyelinated afferents are included in the volleys.[186] The best inhibition is produced by stimulation of a peripheral nerve in the same limb as the excitatory receptive field, but some inhibition occurs when nerves in other limbs are stimulated. A similar inhibition results when high-intensity stimuli are applied to the skin, with a clinical transcutaneous electrical nerve stimulator (TENS) unit in place of direct stimulation of a peripheral nerve.[187]

As the spinothalamic tract ascends, it migrates from a lateral position to a posterior–lateral position. In the mid brain, the tract lies adjacent to the medial lemniscus. The axons of the secondary neurons terminate in one of a number of centers in the thalamus.

peptide, somatostatin, neuropeptide Y, and galanin), excitatory amino acids (aspartate and glutamate), inhibitory amino acids (γ-aminobutyric acid and glycine), nitric oxide, the arachidonic acid metabolites, the endogenous opioids, adenosine, and the monoamines (serotonin and noradrenaline).[213] This list indicates that there are diverse therapeutic possibilities for the control of the transmission of nociceptive information to the brain.

CLINICAL PEARL

Several compounds, classified as biogenic amine transmitters or neuroactive peptides, exist that can facilitate or inhibit synaptic activity.

Interneuronal networks in the posterior (dorsal) horn are responsible not only for the transmission of nociceptive information to neurons that project to the brain, but also for the modulation of that information. The information is passed to other spinal cord neurons, including the flexor motoneurons and the nociceptive projection neurons (e.g., certain patterns of stimulation can lead to enhanced reflex actions and the sensitization of projection neurons and increased nociceptive transmission). Other inputs result in the inhibition of projection neurons.

A small number of fast fibers are passed directly to the thalamus, and then to the cerebral cortex, bypassing the brain stem. It is believed that these signals are important for recognizing and localizing pain, but not for analyzing it. Of the slow signals, none, or at least very few, avoid the reticular system. Because most of the fast, and all of the slow, pain signals go through the reticular formation, they can have wide-ranging effects on almost the entire nervous system.

Lamina V (Fig. 3-25) is the area for convergence, summation, and projection. The response of the cells in lamina V depends largely on the intensity of the stimulus. High-intensity stimulation leads to facilitation of the cell, and relatively easy transmission across the cord to the other side and, from here, upward. More gentle stimulation inhibits this transmission. This inhibition is, according to theory, the result of pre- and postsynaptic effects produced by the cells of laminae II and III. Thus, the net effect at lamina V will determine whether the pain signal is relayed upward. If mild mechanoreceptor input dominates, the pain signal is stopped at this point. If, however, pain input dominates, or if the mechanoreceptor input is too strong, transmission of the pain signal occurs.

Over the last decade, researchers have begun to investigate the influence of pain on patterns of neuromuscular activation and control.[178] It has been suggested that the presence of pain leads to inhibition or delayed activation of muscles or muscle groups that perform key synergistic functions to limit unwanted motion.[214] This inhibition usually occurs in deep muscles, local to the involved joint, that perform a synergistic function in order to control joint stability.[215–217] It is now also becoming apparent that in addition to being influenced by pain, motor activity and emotional state can, in turn, influence pain perception.[178,218]

CLINICAL PEARL

It is important to assume that all reports of pain by the patient are serious in nature until proven otherwise with a thorough examination.[219] In general, the greater the degree of pain radiation, the greater the chance that the problem is acute or that it is occurring from a proximal structure, or both.

Although the pain intensity and the functional response to symptoms are subjective, patterns of pain response to stimulation of the pain generator are quite objective (e.g., antalgic gait).[220]

Referred pain can be generated by:[221]

- convergence of sensory input from separate parts of the body to the same posterior (dorsal) horn neuron via primary sensory fibers (convergence-projection theory)[208,222–224];

- secondary pain resulting from a myofascial trigger point (MTrP)[225];
- sympathetic activity elicited by a spinal reflex[226]; and
- pain-generating substances.[208]

Macnab[227] recommends the following classification for referred pain/symptoms:

- Viscerogenic
- Vasculogenic
- Neurogenic
- Psychogenic
- Spondylogenic

Viscerogenic Symptoms

The pain/symptoms in this category can be referred from any viscera in the trunk or abdomen. Visceral pain can be produced by chemical damage, ischemia, or spasm of the smooth muscles.

Viscerogenic pain may be produced when the nociceptive fibers from the viscera synapse in the spinal cord with some of the same neurons that receive pain from the skin. When the visceral nociceptors are stimulated, some are transmitted by the same neurons that conduct skin nociception and take on the same characteristics. Visceral pain has five important clinical characteristics:

- It is not evoked from all viscera.
- It is not always linked to visceral injury.
- It is diffuse and poorly localized.
- It is referred to other locations.
- It is often accompanied by autonomic reflexes, such as nausea and vomiting.

Viscerogenic pain tends to be diffuse because of the organization of visceral nociceptive pathways in the CNS. This organization demonstrates an absence of a separate pathway for visceral sensory information and a low proportion of visceral afferent nerve fibers compared with those of somatic origin.

Pain arising from problems in the peritoneum, pleura, or pericardium differs from that of other visceral impairments because of the innervation of these structures. The parietal walls of these structures are supplied extensively with both fast and slow pain fibers and, thus, can produce the sharp pain of superficial impairments.

CLINICAL PEARL

A visceral source of the symptoms should always be suspected if the symptoms are not altered with movement or position changes.

In general, symptoms from a musculoskeletal condition are provoked by certain postures, movements, or activities and relieved by others. However, this generalization must be viewed as such. It is also important to remember that musculoskeletal structures can refer symptoms (Table 3-5). Determining the mechanism often will clarify the cause of the symptoms. In

TABLE 3-5 Muscles Most Likely to Refer Pain to a Given Area

Location	Potential Muscles Involved
Chest pain	Pectoralis major Pectoralis minor Scaleni Sternocleidomastoid (sternal) Sternalis Iliocostalis cervicis Subclavius External abdominal oblique
Side of chest pain	Serratus anterior Latissimus
Abdominal pain	Rectus abdominis External abdominal oblique Transversus abdominis Iliocostalis thoracis Multifidi Quadratus lumborum Pyramidalis
Low thoracic back pain	Iliocostalis thoracis Multifidi Serratus posterior inferior Rectus abdominis Latissimus dorsi
Lumbar pain	Gluteus medius Multifidi Iliopsoas Longissimus thoracis Iliocostalis lumborum Iliocostalis thoracis Rectus abdominis
Pelvic pain	Coccygeus Levator ani Obturator internus Adductor magnus Piriformis Obliquus internus abdominis
Buttock pain	Gluteus medius Quadratus lumborum Gluteus maximus Iliocostalis lumborum Longissimus thoracis Semitendinosus Semimembranosus Piriformis Gluteus minimus Rectus abdominis

Data from Travell JG, Simons DG: *Myofascial Pain and Dysfunction—The Trigger Point Manual*. Baltimore, MD: Williams & Wilkins, 1983.

TABLE 3-6	Signs/Symptoms Suggestive of Back Pain due to Systemic Pathology
History	Insidious onset and progressive pattern of pain Sacral pain of nontraumatic origin Malignant disease Excessive fatigue Chronic immunosuppressive medication use Chronic corticosteroid or intravenous drug use Trauma related to physiological changes associated with aging (i.e., osteoporosis)
Age	Younger than 20 yr and older than 45 yr
Pain description	Nocturnal back pain that disrupts sleep Pain that causes constant movement or makes the patient curl up Pain that is unrelieved with rest or recumbency Pain that is unaffected by exertion or activity Severe, persistent back pain with full and painless movement of the spine Back pain accompanied by multiple joint pain or sustained morning stiffness Pain described as throbbing or pulsating sensation
Constitutional	Fever, sweats, nausea, or vomiting symptoms
Other	Palpable pulsating mass in the abdomen Severe/progressive bilateral weakness of lower extremities Neurological findings persisting longer than 1 mo Bowel or bladder incontinence Urinary retention Urinary-tract infection Constipation

Data from Stowell T, Cioffredi W, Greiner A, et al.: Abdominal differential diagnosis in a patient referred to a physical therapy clinic for low back pain. *J Orthop Sports Phys Ther* 35:755–764, 2005.

addition, what appears to be a musculoskeletal injury can actually be a systemic problem. For example, acute low back pain (LBP) can result in symptoms of varying intensity and distribution that can be caused by neuromuscular structures as well as underlying or coexisting systemic pathology (Table 3-6), such as a gastrointestinal pathology (Table 3-7).

Signs and symptoms that could increase suspicion for a gastrointestinal pathology include a report of pain that has no specific mechanism of injury, is unrelated to activity, and that occurs following eating. In addition, reports of night pain unrelated to movement, fever, unexpected weight loss, nausea/vomiting, bowel dysfunction, and food intolerance should also highlight the possibility of a gastrointestinal source. An abdominal palpation examination can be used to identify gross masses, pulsating masses, and/or pain.[228] Palpatory findings of tenderness, gross abnormal masses, or abnormal pulsations are indicative of a broad range of abdominal pathologies, including tumor, obstruction, and infection.

TABLE 3-7 Potential Areas of Cutaneous Referral from Various Viscera

Visceral Organ	Pain Referral
Heart (T1–5), bronchi, and lung (T2–4)	Under sternum, base of neck, over shoulders, over pectorals, and down one or both arms (L > R)
Esophagus (T5–6)	Pharynx, lower neck, arms, midline chest from upper to lower sternum
Gastric (T6–10)	Lower thoracic to upper abdomen
Gallbladder (T7–9)	Upper abdomen, lower scapular, and thoracolumbar
Pancreas	Upper lumbar or upper abdomen
Kidneys (T10–L1)	Upper lumbar, occasionally anterior abdomen approximately 4–5 cm lateral to umbilicus
Urinary bladder (T11–12)	Lower abdomen or low lumbar
Uterus	Lower abdomen or low lumbar

Data from Head H: *Studies in Neurology*. London: Oxford Medical Publications, 1920.

Vasculogenic Symptoms

Vasculogenic symptoms tend to result from venous congestion or arterial deprivation to the musculoskeletal areas. Vasculogenic pain may mimic a wide variety of musculoskeletal, neurologic, and arthritic disorders, because this type of pain is often worsened by activity. An example of a vasculogenic cause of symptoms occurs with an abdominal aortic aneurysm (Table 3-8).[228,229]

To help exclude a vasculogenic cause, it is important to review the cardiopulmonary, hematologic, and neurologic systems during the examination. Clinical evidence of arterial insufficiency includes lower extremity asymmetry, skin condition changes, skin temperature and color changes, and diminishing pulses.

Doppler examination, which is not within the scope of physical therapy practice, is the cornerstone of the vascular examination. This test examines blood flow in the major arteries and veins in the arms and the legs with the use of ultrasound. The ultrasound transducer produces high-frequency sound waves that echo off the blood vessels, resulting in a "swishing" noise during blood flow. A faster flow produces a higher pitch and a steeper waveform. In the lower extremity, segmental pressures are usually taken from six sites:

- High thigh
- Above the knee
- Below the knee
- Ankle
- Forefoot
- Digit

A pressure gradient of less than 20-mm Hg is normal, 20–30 mm Hg is borderline, and greater than 30 mm Hg is

TABLE 3-8 Common Signs and Symptoms of Pathologies Associated with Abdominal and Back Pain	
Pathology/Condition	**Signs/Symptoms**
AAA	Pain located in central lumbar region Palpable pulsating abdominal mass Pain described as pulsating or throbbing Patient unable to find comfortable position History of AAA or vascular claudication
Cancer (i.e., pancreatic, ovarian, and prostate metastasis to spine)	Night pain that disrupts sleep Pain that is unrelieved by rest Unexplained weight loss Fever and sweats Extreme fatigue Altered gastrointestinal or genitourinary function
Intestinal obstruction (i.e., volvulus, adhesions, tumor, and functional)	Colicky abdominal pain Abdominal distention Nausea/vomiting/sweating Constipation
Gastrointestinal infection/inflammation (i.e., peritonitis, appendicitis, and pancreatitis)	Abdominal pain and muscle guarding Rebound tenderness Any movement aggravates pain Fever, chills, sweating, and vomiting Pain relieved by sitting and leaning forward (pancreatitis)
Renal disorders (i.e., nephrolithiasis, urinary tract infection, and pyelonephritis)	Severe pain along upper urinary tract pain pattern Altered urinary tract function (frequency, urgency, and dysuria) Hematuria
Gynecological (i.e., endometriosis, pelvic inflammatory disease, and ovarian cysts)	Lumbopelvic and lower abdominal pain Cyclical pain, nausea, and vomiting Dysmenorrhea Abnormal uterine bleeding

AAA, abdominal aortic aneurysm.

Data from Stowell T, Cioffredi W, Greiner A, et al.: Abdominal differential diagnosis in a patient referred to a physical therapy clinic for low back pain. *J Orthop Sports Phys Ther* 35:755–764, 2005; Goodman CC, Boissonnault WG, Fuller KS: *Pathology: Implications for the Physical Therapist*, 2nd ed. Philadelphia, PA: WB Saunders, 2003.

considered abnormal. Pressure differences of less than 20 mm Hg between limbs are considered normal.

After the segmental pressures of the lower extremity are measured, brachial pressure on both sides is measured. Comparisons are made between ankle–arm, forefoot–arm, and digit–arm ratios. Normal values are >1 for the ankle–arm index, >0.75 for the forefoot–arm, and >0.65 for each digit–arm index.

Neurogenic Symptoms

The neurologic tissues comprise those tissues that are involved in nerve conduction. Neurogenic causes of symptoms may include:

- tumor compressing and irritating a neural structure of the spinal cord or the meninges;
- spinal nerve root irritation;
- peripheral nerve entrapment; and
- neuritis.

Psychogenic Symptoms

It is common to find emotional overtones in the presence of pain, particularly with lowback and neck pain. These overtones are thought to result from an inhibition of the pain control mechanisms of the CNS from such causes as grief, the side effects of medications, or fear of reinjury. Somatosensory amplification refers to the tendency to experience somatic sensation as intense, noxious, and disturbing. Barsky and colleagues[230] introduced the concept of somatosensory amplification as an important feature of hypochondriasis. Somatosensory amplification is observed in patients whose extreme anxiety leads to an increase in their perception of pain.

The term *nonorganic* was proposed by Waddell et al.[231] to define the abnormal illness behaviors exhibited by patients who have depression, emotional disturbance, or anxiety states. The presence of three of the following five Waddell signs has been correlated significantly with disability[232]:

- Superficial or nonanatomic tenderness to light touch that is widespread and refers pain to other areas.

- *Simulation tests.* These are a series of tests that should be comfortable to perform. Examples include axial loading of the spine through the patient's head with light pressure to the skull and passive hip and shoulder rotation with the patient positioned standing. Neither of these tests should produce LBP. If pain is reported with these tests, a nonorganic origin should be suspected.
- *Distraction test.*[233] This test involves checking a positive finding elicited during the examination on the distracted patient. For example, if a patient is unable to perform a seated trunk flexion maneuver, the same patient can be observed when asked to remove his or her shoes. A difference of 40–45 degrees is significant for inconsistency.
- *Regional disturbances.* These signs include sensory or motor disturbances that have no neurologic basis.
- *Overreaction.* This includes disproportionate verbalization, muscle tension, tremors, and grimacing during the examination.

The Somatosensory Amplification Rating Scale (SARS; Table 3-9) is a version of the Waddell's nonorganic physical signs, which has been modified to allow for a more accurate appraisal of the patient with exaggerated illness behavior.[230]

CLINICAL PEARL

It is important to remember that the Waddell and the SARS assessment tools are designed not to detect whether patients are malingering, but only to indicate whether they have symptoms of a nonorganic origin.

Spondylogenic Symptoms

A number of conditions can affect the musculoskeletal system, frequently producing pain. These include infections (e.g., osteomyelitis), inflammatory disorders, neoplasms, and metabolic disorders. Several findings are helpful in diagnosing such pathologic processes. These findings may include:

- severe and unrelenting pain;
- the presence of a fever;
- bone tenderness; and
- unexplained weight loss.

Pain Control Mechanisms

One of the earliest pain control mechanisms was proposed by Melzack and Wall[234] who postulated that interneurons in the substantia gelatinosa functioned like a gate to modulate sensory input. They proposed that the substantia gelatinosa interneuron projected to the second-order neuron of the pain–temperature pathway located in lamina V, which they called the transmission cell. It was reasoned that if the substantia gelatinosa interneuron were depolarized, it would inhibit the transmission of cell firing and, thus, decrease further transmission of input ascending in the spinothalamic tract. The degree of modulation appeared to depend on the proportion of input from the large A fibers and the small C fibers, so that the gate could be closed by either decreasing C fiber input or increasing A fiber or mechanoreceptive input. The gate theory was, and is, supported by practical evidence (e.g., rubbing a sore area appears to decrease the pain), although the experimental evidence for the theory is lacking. Researchers have identified many clinical pain states that cannot be fully explained by the gate control theory.[235] A problem with this theory is that there is an evidence to suggest that the A-beta fibers from the mechanoreceptor do not synapse in the substantia gelatinosa. In this case, the modulation at the spinal cord level must occur in lamina V, where there is a simple summation of signals from the pain fibers and the mechanoreceptor fibers. However, severe or prolonged pain tends to have the segment identifying all input as painful, and summation modulation has little, if any, effect.

Melzack and Wall expanded upon the gate theory and argued that the gate could be modified by a descending inhibitory pathway from the brain, or brain stem,[236] suggesting that the CNS apparently plays a part in this modulation in a mechanism called central biasing.

Numerous investigations have since been made of what is known as the descending analgesia systems. The thalamus represents the final link in the transmission of impulses to the cerebral cortex, processing almost all sensory and motor information prior to its transfer to cortical areas. The key brain sites involved in pain perception include the anterior cingulate cortex, anterior insular cortex, primary somatosensory cortex, secondary somatosensory cortex, a number of regions in the thalamus and cerebellum, and, interestingly, areas such as the premotor cortex that are normally linked to motor function.[178,237] Indeed, it is clear that both the basal ganglia (associated with planned action), the periaqueductal gray (PAG) of the midbrain region, and the raphe nucleus in the pons and the medulla receive nociceptive input as well as coordinating important aspects of movement and motor control.[178,238,239]

The PAG area of the upper pons sends signals to the raphe magnus nucleus in the lower pons and the upper medulla. This nucleus relays the signal down the cord to a pain-inhibitory complex located in the posterior (dorsal) horn of the cord. The nerve fibers derived from the PAG area secrete enkephalin and serotonin, whereas the raphe magnus releases enkephalin only. The PAG is also believed to be involved in complex behavioral responses to stressful or life-threatening situations or to promote recuperative behavior after a defense reaction.

Enkephalin is believed to produce presynaptic inhibition of the incoming pain signals to lamina I–V, thereby blocking pain signals at their entry point into the cord.[240] It is further believed that the chemical releases in the upper end of the pathway can inhibit pain signal transmission in the reticular formation and the thalamus. The inhibition from this system is effective on both fast and slow pains.

In the cortex, a negative-feedback loop, called the corticofugal system, originates at the termination point of the various sensory pathways.[241] Excessive stimulation of this feedback loop results in a signal being transmitted down from the sensory cortex to the posterior horn of the level from which the input arose. This response produces lateral or recurrent inhibition of the cells adjacent to the stimulated cell, thereby preventing the spread of the signal. This is an automatic gain control system to prevent overloading of the sensory system.

TABLE 3-9 Somatosensory Amplification Rating Scale		
Examination	**Percent**	**Score[a]**
Sensory examination		
1. No deficit or deficit well localized to dermatome		0
Deficit related to dermatome(s) but some inconsistency		1
Nondermatomal or very inconsistent deficit		2
Blatantly impossible (i.e., split down midline or entire body with positive tuning fork test)		3
2. Amount of body involved:		
Evaluate similar to burn (% of surface areas for an entire leg is 18%)	<15%	0
	15–35%	1
	36–60%	2
	>60%	3
Motor examination		
1. No deficit or deficit well localized to myotomes		0
Deficit related to myotome(s) but some inconsistency		1
Nonmyotomal or very inconsistent weakness, exhibits cogwheeling or giving way, weakness is coachable		2
Blatantly impossible, significant weakness that disappears when distracted		3
2. Amount of body involved	<15%	0
	15–35%	1
	36–60%	2
	>60%	3
Tenderness		
1. No tenderness or tenderness clearly localized to discrete, anatomically sensible structures		0
Tenderness not well localized, some inconsistency		1
Diffuse or very inconsistent tenderness, multiple anatomic structures involved (skin, muscle, bone, etc.)		2
Blatantly impossible, significant tenderness of multiple anatomic structures (skin, muscle, bone, etc.), which disappears when distracted		3
2. Amount of body involved	<15%	0
	15–35%	1
	36–60%	2
	>60%	3
Additional tests: distraction tests		
Distraction SLR rating determined by the difference in measurements between supine and seated	<20 degrees	0
	20–45 degrees	1
	>45 degrees	2
SLR supine at less than 45 degrees		3
Standing flexion versus long sit test		
Rating determined by two factors		1
Difference between hip ROM, standing versus supine	<20 degrees	0
	20–40 degrees	1
	41–50 degrees	2
	>50 degrees	3
Distance measurement from middle finger to toes, standing versus supine (long sit)	<5 cm	0
	6–10 cm	1
	11–18 cm	2
	>18 cm	3
Total score possible		27

SARS, Somatosensory Amplification Rating Scale; SLR, straight-leg raise; ROM, range of motion.

[a]SARS scores of 5 or greater are indicative of inappropriate illness behavior. The higher the score, the greater the exaggerated behavior.

Data from Barsky AJ, Goodson JD, Lane RS, et al.: The amplification of somatic symptoms. *Psychosom Med* 50:510–519, 1988.

Finally, two other neuroactive peptides, beta endorphin and dynorphin, have recently been discovered, both of which are theorized to be used as analgesics in the body to numb or dull pain in addition to promoting feelings of well-being and increasing relaxation.

Nonpharmacological Control of Pain

The pharmacological control of pain is discussed in Chapter 9. Clinicians can use several nonpharmacological therapeutic interventions to manage pain. These include:

- Transcutaneous electrical nerve stimulation (TENS). TENS is frequently used to treat a number of pain conditions including back pain, osteoarthritis, in fibromyalgia to name a few (see Chap. 8).
- Interferential current (see Chap. 8). Clinically, interferential current therapy is beneficial for treating painful conditions such as osteoarthritic pain. The potential mechanisms behind this pain control include an increase in blood flow, and the same mechanisms as TENS—segmental inhibition and activation of descending inhibitory pathways
- Thermal modalities (see Chap. 8).
- Cryotherapy (see Chap. 8).
- Manual therapy (see Chap. 10).
- Exercise (see Chaps. 12, 13, 14 and 15).
- Patient education. Patients can be educated on pain management techniques (relaxation, cognitive behavioral approaches, and biofeedback), positions and activities to avoid, and positions and activities to adopt.

Orthopaedic Neurologic Testing

An examination of the transmission capability of the nervous system can be performed as part of the orthopaedic examination to detect the presence of either an upper motor neuron (UMN/CNS) lesion or a lower motor neuron (LMN/PNS) lesion. In essence, neurological tissue is tested during active, passive, and resisted isometric movement, as well as those tests specific to the nervous system (e.g., reflex testing, sensory testing). Neurodynamic mobility testing is covered in Chapter 11.

UMNs are located in the white columns of the spinal cord and the cerebral hemispheres. A UMN lesion, also known as a central palsy, is a lesion of the neural pathway above the anterior horn cell or motor nuclei of the CNS. Signs and symptoms associated with a UMN lesion follow.

CLINICAL PEARL

A UMN lesion is characterized by spastic paralysis or paresis, little or no muscle atrophy, hyper-reflexive muscle stretch (deep tendon) reflexes in a nonsegmental distribution, and the presence of pathologic signs and reflexes.

- **Nystagmus.** Nystagmus is characterized by an involuntary loss of control of the conjugate movement of the eyes (approximately one or more axes) involved with smooth pursuit or saccadic movement. When the eyes oscillate like a sine wave, it is called *pendular nystagmus.* If the nystagmus consists of drifts in one direction with corrective fast phases, it is called *jerk nystagmus.* The more benign types of nystagmus include the proprioceptive causes of spontaneous nystagmus, postural nystagmus, and nystagmus that is elicited with head positioning or induced by movement (vestibular nystagmus). A unidirectional nystagmus is related to the geometric relationship of the semicircular canal, with a change in head position often exacerbating the nystagmus. On the other hand, a central vestibular nystagmus, which is caused by disease of the brain stem or the cerebellum, exhibits bidirectionality to the nystagmus (i.e., left beating on left gaze and right beating on right gaze).[242] The more serious causes of nystagmus include, but are not limited to, vertebrobasilar ischemia, tumors of the posterior cranial fossa, intracranial bleeding, craniocervical malformations, and autonomic dysfunction. Differentiation between the benign and serious causes of nystagmus is very important.
- Proprioceptive nystagmus occurs immediately upon turning the head (i.e., there is no latent period).
- The ischemic type of nystagmus has a latent period and is usually only evident when the patient's neck is turned to a position and maintained there for a period of a few seconds up to 3 minutes.[243,244]
- **Dysphasia.** Dysphasia is defined as a problem with vocabulary and results from a cerebral lesion in the speech areas of the frontal or temporal lobes. The temporal lobe receives most of its blood from the temporal branch of the cortical artery of the vertebrobasilar system and may become ischemic periodically, producing an inappropriate use of words.
- **Wallenberg Syndrome.** This is the result of a lateral medullary infarction.[245] Classically, sensory dysfunction in lateral medullary infarction is characterized by selective involvement of the spinothalamic sensory modalities with dissociated distribution (ipsilateral trigeminal and contralateral hemibody/limbs).[246] However, various patterns of sensory disturbance have been observed in lateral medullary infarction that includes contralateral or bilateral trigeminal sensory impairment, restricted sensory involvement, and a concomitant deficit of lemniscal sensations.[247,248]
- **Ataxia.** Ataxia is often most marked in the extremities. In the lower extremities, it is characterized by the so-called drunken-sailor gait pattern, with the patient veering from one side to the other and having a tendency to fall toward the side of the lesion. Ataxia of the upper extremities is characterized by a loss of accuracy in reaching for, or placing, objects. Although ataxia can have a number of causes, it generally suggests CNS disturbance, specifically a cerebellar disorder, or a lesion of the posterior columns.[249–251]
- **Spasticity.**[252–254] Spasticity is defined as a motor disorder characterized by a velocity-dependent increase (resistance increases with velocity) in tonic stretch reflexes with exaggerated tendon jerks, resulting from hyperexcitability of the stretch reflex. The spinal cord experiences spinal shock immediately following any

trauma causing tetraplegia or paraplegia, resulting in the loss of reflexes innervated by the portion of the cord below the site of the lesion. The direct result of this spinal shock is that the muscles innervated by the traumatized portion of the cord, the portion below the lesion, as well as the bladder, become flaccid. Spinal shock, which wears off between 24 hours and 3 months after injury, can be replaced by spasticity in some, or all of these muscles.

Spasticity occurs because the reflex arc to the muscle remains anatomically intact, despite the loss of cerebral innervation and control via the long tracts. During spinal shock, the arc does not function, but as the spine recovers from the shock, the reflex arc begins to function without the inhibitory or regulatory impulses from the brain, creating local spasticity and clonus.

CLINICAL PEARL

Medical etiologies for increased spasticity include a new or enlarged CNS lesion, genitourinary tract dysfunction (infection, obstruction, etc.), gastrointestinal disorders (bowel impaction, hemorrhoids, etc.), venous thrombosis, fracture, muscle strain, and pressure ulcers.

- **Drop Attack.** A drop attack is described as a loss of balance resulting in a fall, but with no loss of consciousness. Because it is the consequence of a loss of lower extremity control, it is never a good or benign sign. The patient, usually elderly, falls forward, with the precipitating factor being extension of the head. Recovery is usually immediate. Causes include:
  - a vestibular system impairment[255];
  - neoplastic and other impairments of the cerebellum[256];
  - vertebrobasilar compromise[257] (see Chap. 24);
  - sudden spinal cord compression;
  - third ventricle cysts;
  - epilepsy; and
  - type 1 Chiari malformation.[258]
- **Wernicke's encephalopathy.** This is an impairment, typically localized to the posterior (dorsal) part of the midbrain,[259] that produces the classic triad of abnormal mental state, ophthalmoplegia, and gait ataxia.[260]
- **Vertical diplopia.** A history of "double vision" should alert the clinician to this condition. Patients with vertical diplopia complain of seeing two images, one atop or diagonally displaced from the other.[261]
- **Dysphonia.** Dysphonia presents as a hoarseness of the voice. Usually, no pain is reported. Painless dysphonia is a common symptom of Wallenberg syndrome.[247]
- **Hemianopia.** This finding, defined as a loss in half of the visual field, is always bilateral. A visual field defect describes sensory loss restricted to the visual field and arises from damage to the primary visual pathways linking the optic tract and striate cortex (see section "Supraspinal Reflexes").
- **Ptosis.** Ptosis is defined as a pathologic depression of the superior eyelid such that it covers part of the pupil. It results from a palsy of the levator palpebrae and Müller's muscle.
- **Miosis.** Miosis is defined as the inability to dilate the pupil (damage to sympathetic ganglia). It is one of the symptoms of Horner syndrome.
- **Horner syndrome.** This syndrome is caused by interference to the cervicothoracic sympathetic outflow resulting from a lesion of (1) the reticular formation, (2) the descending sympathetic system, and (3) the oculomotor nerve caused by a sympathetic paralysis.[262] The other clinical signs of Horner syndrome are ptosis, enophthalmos, facial reddening, and anhydrosis. If Horner syndrome is suspected, the patient should immediately be returned or referred to a physician for further examination.
- **Dysarthria.** Dysarthria is defined as an undiagnosed change in articulation. Dominant or nondominant hemispheric ischemia, as well as brain stem and cerebellar impairments, may result in altered articulation.

The LMN begins at the α motor neuron and includes the posterior (dorsal) and anterior (ventral) roots, spinal nerve, peripheral nerve, neuromuscular junction, and muscle–fiber complex.[263] The LMN consists of a cell body located in the anterior gray column and its axon, which travels to a muscle by way of the cranial or peripheral nerve. Lesions to the LMN can occur in the cell body or anywhere along the axon. An LMN lesion is also known as a peripheral palsy. These lesions can be the result of direct trauma, toxins, infections, ischemia, or compression. The characteristics of an LMN lesion include muscle atrophy and hypotonus, diminished or absent muscle stretch (deep tendon) reflex of the areas served by a spinal nerve root or a peripheral nerve, and absence of pathologic signs or reflexes.

CLINICAL PEARL

The differing symptoms between a UMN lesion and an LMN lesion are the result of injuries to different parts of the nervous system. LMN impairment involves damage to a neurologic structure distal to the anterior horn cell, whereas UMN impairment involves damage to a neurologic structure proximal to the anterior horn cell, namely, the spinal cord or CNS.

Complaints of Dizziness

Although most causes of dizziness can be relatively benign, dizziness may signal a more serious problem, especially if it is associated with trauma to the neck or the head or with motions of cervical rotation and extension (e.g., vertebral artery compromise). The clinician must ascertain whether the symptoms result from vertigo, nausea, giddiness, unsteadiness, or fainting, among others. Nausea is an uneasiness of the stomach that often accompanies the urge to vomit but does not always lead to the forcible voluntary or involuntary emptying of stomach contents through the mouth (vomiting). If vertigo is suspected, the patient's physician should be informed, for further investigation. However, in and of itself, vertigo is not usually a contraindication to the continuation of the examination. Differential diagnosis includes primary CNS diseases, vestibular and ocular involvement, and, more rarely, metabolic disorders.[264] Patients complaining of dizziness can be classified into four subtypes (Table 3-10). Careful questioning can help in the differentiation of the cause. This differentiation is important, as certain types of dizziness are amenable to physical therapy interventions (Table 3-11); others produce contraindications to certain interventions, while still other causes of dizziness require medical referral.[265] The presence of presyncope would suggest compromise of the function of the cerebral hemispheres or the brainstem.[265] Different conditions can cause either a pancerebral hypoperfusion (Table 3-12) or a selective hypoperfusion of the brainstem, the latter of which includes vertebrobasilar insufficiency, vertebrobasilar infarction, and subclavian steal syndrome.[265] The presence of vertigo, nystagmus, hearing loss or tinnitus, and brainstem signs can help the clinician differentiate between a central or a peripheral vestibular lesion (Table 3-13).[265] Peripheral vertigo is manifested with general complaints such as unsteadiness and lightheadedness. Central vertigo is usually caused by a cerebellar disorder, an ischemic process, or a disturbance of the vestibular system (Table 3-14). Cervical vertigo, on the other hand, may be produced by localized muscle changes and receptor irritation.[244]

- Dizziness provoked by head movements or head positions could indicate an inner ear dysfunction. Dizziness provoked by certain cervical motions, particularly extension or rotation, also may indicate vertebral artery compromise. Dizziness resulting from vertebral artery compromise should be associated with other signs and symptoms, which could include neck pain and nausea. The pain associated with vertebral artery compromise develops on one side of the neck in one-fourth of patients and usually is confined to the upper anterolateral cervical region.[266] Persistent, isolated neck pain may mimic idiopathic carotidynia, especially if it is associated with local tenderness. Pain is also usually the initial manifestation of a carotid artery dissection, and the median time to the appearance of other symptoms is 4 days.[266]
- Dizziness associated with tinnitus or a hearing loss could indicate a tumor of CN VIII.
- Dizziness can occur if the calcareous deposits that lie on the vestibular receptors are displaced to new and sensitive regions of the ampulla of the posterior canal, evoking a hypersensitive response to stimulation with certain head positions or movements.[267,268] The Dix-Hallpike test can be used to help determine if the cause of the patient's dizziness is a vestibular impairment (benign paroxysmal positional vertigo, or BPPV), resulting from an accumulation of utricle debris (otoconia), which can move within the posterior SCC and stimulate the vestibular sense organ (cupula). This test usually is performed only if the vertebral artery test and instability tests do not provoke symptoms. The test involves having the clinician move the patient rapidly from a sitting to a supine position with the head turned so that the affected ear (provocative position) is 30–45 degree below the horizontal to stimulate the posterior SCC.[8] The endpoint of the test is when the patient's head overhangs the end of the table, so that the cervical spine is

TABLE 3-10 The Four Subtypes of Dizziness

Subtype	Description
Vertigo	A false sensation of movement of either the body or the environment, usually described as spinning, which suggests vestibular system dysfunction Usually episodic with an abrupt onset and often associated with nausea or vomiting The dysfunction can be located in the peripheral or central vestibular system Often accompanied by other signs and symptoms including impulsion (the sensation that the body is being hurled or pulled in space), oscillopsia (the visual illusion of moving back and forth or up and down), nystagmus, gait ataxia, nausea, and vomiting
Presyncope	Described as a sensation of an impending faint or loss of consciousness, which is not associated with an illusion of movement May begin with diminished vision or a roaring sensation in the ears May be accompanied by a transient neurological signs, e.g., dysarthria, visual disturbances, and extremity weakness Results from conditions that compromise the brain's supply of blood, oxygen, or glucose
Disequilibrium	A sense of imbalance without vertigo, or a sense that a fall is imminent, which is generally attributed to neuromuscular problems The unsteadiness or imbalance occurs only when erect and disappears when lying or sitting May result from visual impairment, peripheral neuropathy, musculoskeletal disturbances and may include ataxia
Other dizziness	Described as a vague or floating sensation with the patient having difficulty relating to specific feeling to the clinician Includes descriptions of a lightheadedness, heavy headedness, or wooziness that cannot be classified as any of the three previous subtypes The main causes of this subtype are psychiatric disorders including anxiety, depression, and hyperventilation

Data from Baloh RW: Approach to the dizzy patient. *Baillieres Clin Neurol* 3:453–465, 1994; Drachman DA, Hart CW: An approach to the dizzy patient. *Neurology.* 22:323–334, 1972; Hanson MR: The dizzy patient. A practical approach to management. *Postgrad Med* 85:99–102, 107–108, 1989; Eaton DA, Roland PS: Dizziness in the older adult, Part 2.

Treatments for causes of the four most common symptoms. *Geriatrics* 58:46, 49–52, 2003; Eaton DA, Roland PS: Dizziness in the older adult, Part 1. Evaluation and general treatment strategies. *Geriatrics* 58:28–30, 33–36, 2003; Huijbregts P, Vidal P: Dizziness in orthopaedic physical therapy practice: classification and pathophysiology. *J Man Manip Ther* 12:199–214, 2004; Simon RP, Aminoff MJ, Greenberg DA: *Clinical Neurology*, 4th ed. Stanford, CT: Appleton and Lange, 1999.

TABLE 3-11 Signs and Symptoms Indicative of Pathologies Amenable to Sole Physical Therapy Management

BPPV	Precipitated by positioning, movement, or other stimuli (see below) Short latency: 1–5 s Brief duration: <30 s Fatigable with repeated motion Associated signs and symptoms: nystagmus, nausea, and at times vomiting Occurs in people older than 40 yrs with peak incidence of onset in the sixth decade Rare in people under 20 yr Medical history of head trauma, labyrinthine infection, surgical stapedectomy, chronic suppurative otitis media, and degenerative changes to the inner ear may indicate nonidiopathic BPPV
Posterior SCC BPPV	Patients complain of dizziness when they quickly transfer to a supine position, especially when the head is turned to the affected side Positive response of vertigo and apogeotropic torsional nystagmus on ipsilateral Hallpike–Dix maneuver
Anterior SCC BPPV	Patients also complain of dizziness when they quickly transfer to a supine position, especially when the head is turned to the affected side, but there is less specificity as to the direction of head rotation Bilateral positive response on Hallpike–Dix maneuver with vertigo and geotropic torsional nystagmus on ipsilateral test Hallpike–Dix maneuver may also cause downbeating vertical nystagmus Positive response on straight head-hanging test
Horizontal SCC BPPV	Dizziness is brought on when rolling over in supine but can also occur with flexion and extension of the head or when transferring from supine to upright A bilaterally positive test with a purely horizontal nystagmus on Hallpike–Dix maneuver. The nystagmus will be geotropic beating in the direction of the face turn or downside ear. Nystagmus will occur in both directions but is generally stronger when the head is turned toward the affected side Positive roll test Positive walk–rotate–walk test to affected side
Cervicogenic dizziness	Intermittent positioning-type dizziness Precipitated by head and neck movement No latency period: onset of symptoms is immediate upon assuming the provoking position Brief duration but may last minutes to hours Fatigable with repeated motion Associated signs and symptoms: nystagmus, neck pain, suboccipital headaches, sometimes paresthesie in the trigeminal nerve distribution Possible lateral head tilt due to tightness of the sternocleidomastoid or upper trapezius Possible forward head posture Medical history of cervical spine trauma and degeneration Motion dysfunction in the upper cervical segments on AROM and PIVM testing Positive neck torsion test: nystagmus with reproduction of dizziness
Musculoskeletal impairments	Subjective complaints of weakness and unsteadiness Insidious onset Postural deviations negatively affecting the location of the COG in relation to the BOS: trunk flexion, hip flexion, knee flexion, and ankle plantar flexion contractures Decreased trunk extension, hip extension, knee extension, and ankle dorsiflexion on ROM testing Loss of strength and endurance in antigravity muscles Impaired joint position sense lower extremity

BPPV, benign paroxysmal positional vertigo; SCC, semicircular canal; PIVM, passive intervertebral motion.

Data from Huijbregts P, Vidal P: Dizziness in orthopaedic physical therapy practice: history and physical examination. *J Man Manip Ther* 13:221–250, 2005.

extended (Fig. 3-26). A positive test reproduces the patient's symptoms of vertigo and/or nystagmus.

- Dizziness associated with a recent change in medication is suggestive of an adverse drug reaction.[269]

Strength Testing

A myotome is defined as a muscle or group of muscles served by a single nerve root. *Key muscle* is perhaps a more accurate term. Manual muscle testing is traditionally used by the

TABLE 3-12 Characteristics of Pancerebral Hypoperfusion

Pancerebral Hypoperfusion	Description
Vasovagal presyncope	Parasympathetic hyperactivity causes a decrease in cardiac output with a subsequent decrease in cerebral blood flow Rarely occurs in the recumbent position
Cardiovascular presyncope	Should be suspected when syncope occurs with the patient in a recumbent position, during or after physical activity, or any patient with a known medical history of heart disease
Migraine	Characterized by a headache that is usually unilateral and of a pulsatile quality Nausea, photophobia, vomiting, and lassitude are frequently associated with migraine
Takayasu's disease	Most common in Asian-descent women. Can occur after exercise, standing, or head movement and is associated with impaired vision and confusion.
Carotid sinus syndrome	Pressure on the carotid sinus due to a tight collar or local neck tumor will cause vagal stimulation, leading to bradycardia and subsequent syncope.
Orthostatic hypotension	Syncope and presyncope happens when rapidly rising to a standing position, standing motionless for prolonged periods, and standing after prolonged recumbency.
Hyperventilation	Hyperventilation causes hypocapnia, which in turn results in cerebral vasoconstriction and CNS hypoperfusion.
Cough-related syncope	Syncope (and presyncope) may be caused by an increase in intracranial pressure due to coughing with resultant cerebral hypoperfusion.
Micturition syncope	Episodes occur mainly in men at night before, during, or after micturition. Peripheral blood pooling, vagus-induced bradycardia, and prolonged recumbency are likely responsible.
Glossopharyngeal neuralgia	The result of a glossopharyngeal–vagal reflex circuit causing transient brady-arrhythmia that results in cerebral hypoperfusion.
Hypoglycemia	Asking the patient whether the dizziness occurs mainly when he or she has not eaten may clue in the clinician to hypoglycemia as the cause for the dizziness.

Data from Huijbregts P, Vidal P: Dizziness in orthopaedic physical therapy practice: Classification and pathophysiology. *J Man Manip Ther* 12:199–214, 2004.

clinician to assess the strength of a muscle or muscle group that is representative of the supply from a particular nerve root. Valuable information can be gleaned from these tests, including:

TABLE 3-13 Differential Diagnostic Characteristics of Central Versus Peripheral Vertigo

	Central Lesions	Peripheral Lesions
Vertigo	Often constant Less severe	Often intermittent Severe
Nystagmus	Sometimes absent Uni- or multidirectional May be vertical	Always present Unidirectional Never vertical
Hearing loss or tinnitus	Rarely present	Often present
Brainstem signs	Typically present	Never present

Data from Simon RP, Aminoff MJ, Greenberg DA: *Clinical Neurology*, 4th ed. Stanford, CT: Appleton and Lange, 1999; Huijbregts P, Vidal P: Dizziness in orthopaedic physical therapy practice: Classification and pathophysiology. *J Man Manip Ther* 12:199–214, 2004.

- The amount of force the muscle is capable of producing and whether the amount of force produced varies with the joint angle.
- Whether any pain or weakness is produced with the contraction.
- The endurance of the muscle and how much substitution occurs during the test.

From the neurologic perspective, strength testing assesses the nerve supplying the muscle (Table 3-15, Table 3-16). Muscle weakness, if elicited, may be caused by a UMN lesion (along with spasticity, hyperactive reflexes, etc.), injury to a peripheral nerve, pathology at the neuromuscular junction, a nerve root lesion, or a lesion or disease (myopathy) of the muscle, its tendons, or the bony insertions themselves.[270] Pain, fatigue, and disuse atrophy can also cause weakness. For suspected nerve root lesions, key muscle testing is the method of choice, and the clinician attempts to determine if there are any specific patterns of muscle weakness (weakness in muscles served by the same nerve root). However, as manual muscle test was originally developed to examine motor function in patients with polio, an LMN syndrome, their use may be inappropriate for patients with a UMN syndrome. More information about strength testing is provided in Chapter 4.

Reflex Testing

As previously discussed, a reflex is a subconscious, programmed unit of behavior in which a certain type of stimulus from a receptor automatically leads to the response of an effector. The response can be a simple behavior, movement, or activity. Indeed, many somatic and visceral activities are essentially reflexive. The circuitry that generates these patterns varies greatly in complexity, depending on the nature of the reflex, with each influenced by a hierarchy of control mechanisms. The muscle stretch reflex (myotatic or deep tendon) is one of the simplest known reflexes, depending on just two neurons and one synapse,[271] which is influenced by cortical and subcortical input, and

TABLE 3-14	**Central Vestibular Disorders**
Disorder	**Description**
Drug intoxication	Many drug intoxication syndromes produce global cerebellar dysfunction including alcohol, sedative hypnotics, anticonvulsants, hallucinogens, and street drugs
Wernicke's encephalopathy	Comprises the diagnostic triad of ataxia, ophthalmoplegia (lateral rectus palsy), and confusion
Inflammatory disorders	Viral cerebellar infections can occur in patients with St. Louis encephalitis, AIDS dementia complex, and meningeal encephalitis
Multiple sclerosis	Rarely the first symptom of multiple sclerosis but is common during the course of the disease
Alcoholic cerebellar degeneration	Usually occurs in patients with a history of 10 or more years of binge drinking
Phenytoin-induced cerebellar degeneration	Long-term treatment with phenytoin (antiepileptic medication) may produce a global cerebellar degeneration
Hypothyroidism	Most common in middle-aged or elderly women Gait ataxia is the prominent finding
Paraneoplastic cerebellar degeneration	Appears to involve antibodies to tumor cell antigens cross-reacting with cerebellar Purkinje cells
Hereditary spinocerebellar degenerations	Autosomal-dominant spinocerebellar ataxias characterized by adult onset, slowly progressive cerebellar ataxia, e.g., Friedrich's ataxia
Ataxia telangiectasia	Autosomal-recessive disorder with an onset before age of 4 yr and global cerebellar involvement
Wilson's disease	A disorder of the copper metabolism with copper deposition in multiple body tissues
Creutzfeldt–Jakob disease	Characterized by dementia, cerebellar signs, and gait ataxia
Posterior fossa tumors	Present with headache, ataxia, nausea, vomiting, vertigo, and CN palsies
Posterior fossa malformations	Type 1 Arnold–Chiari malformation may have cerebellar involvement
Familial paroxysmal ataxia	A hereditary recurrent ataxia associated with nystagmus and dysarthria

Data from Huijbregts P, Vidal P: Dizziness in orthopaedic physical therapy practice: Classification and pathophysiology. *J Man Manip Ther* 12:199–214, 2004.

from the stimulation of two types of receptors: the GTO and the muscle spindle. Thus, tendon reflex activity depends on the status of the large motor neurons of the anterior horn (alpha motor neurons), the muscle spindles with the afferents fibers, and the small anterior horn cells (gamma neurons) whose axons terminate on the small intrafusal muscle fibers within the spindles.[272]

CLINICAL PEARL

Although used extensively, the term *deep tendon reflex* is a misnomer because tendons have little to do with the response other than being responsible for mechanically transmitting the sudden stretch from the reflex hammer to the muscle spindle. In addition some muscle stretch reflexes have no tendons.[272]

Muscle stretch reflexes are elicited by a short, sharp tap with the tendon hammer delivered to the tendon of a gently extended muscle. The physiology behind a muscle stretch reflex is described using the quadriceps reflex as an example. The tap of a reflex hammer on the tendon of the quadriceps femoris muscle, as it crosses the knee joint (Fig. 3-27), causes a brief stretch of the tendon and the muscle belly where the GTO and the muscle spindle are stimulated. Impulses are conducted along the axons of these motor neurons to the neuromuscular junctions, exciting the effectors (quadriceps femoris muscle), and producing a brief, weak contraction, which results in a momentary straightening of the leg (knee jerk).[271] The stretch reflex can be divided into the following two:

- Dynamic stretch reflex, in which the primary endings and type Ia fibers are excited by a rapid change in length. The speed of conduction along the type Ia fibers and the monosynaptic connection in the cord ensure that a very rapid contraction of the muscle occurs to control the sudden and potentially dangerous stretch of the muscle. The dynamic stretch reflex is over within a fraction of a second, but a secondary static reflex continues from the secondary afferent nerve fibers.
- Static stretch reflex. As long as a stretch is applied to the muscle, both the primary and the secondary endings in the nuclear chain continue to be stimulated, causing prolonged muscle contraction for as long as the excessive length of the muscle is maintained, thereby affording a mechanism for prolonged opposition to prolonged stretch.

The most important observation during reflex examination is the reflex's amplitude.[272] When a load is suddenly removed from a contracting muscle, shortening of the intrafusal fibers reverses both the dynamic and the static stretch reflexes, causing both sudden and prolonged inhibition of the muscle such that rebound does not occur.

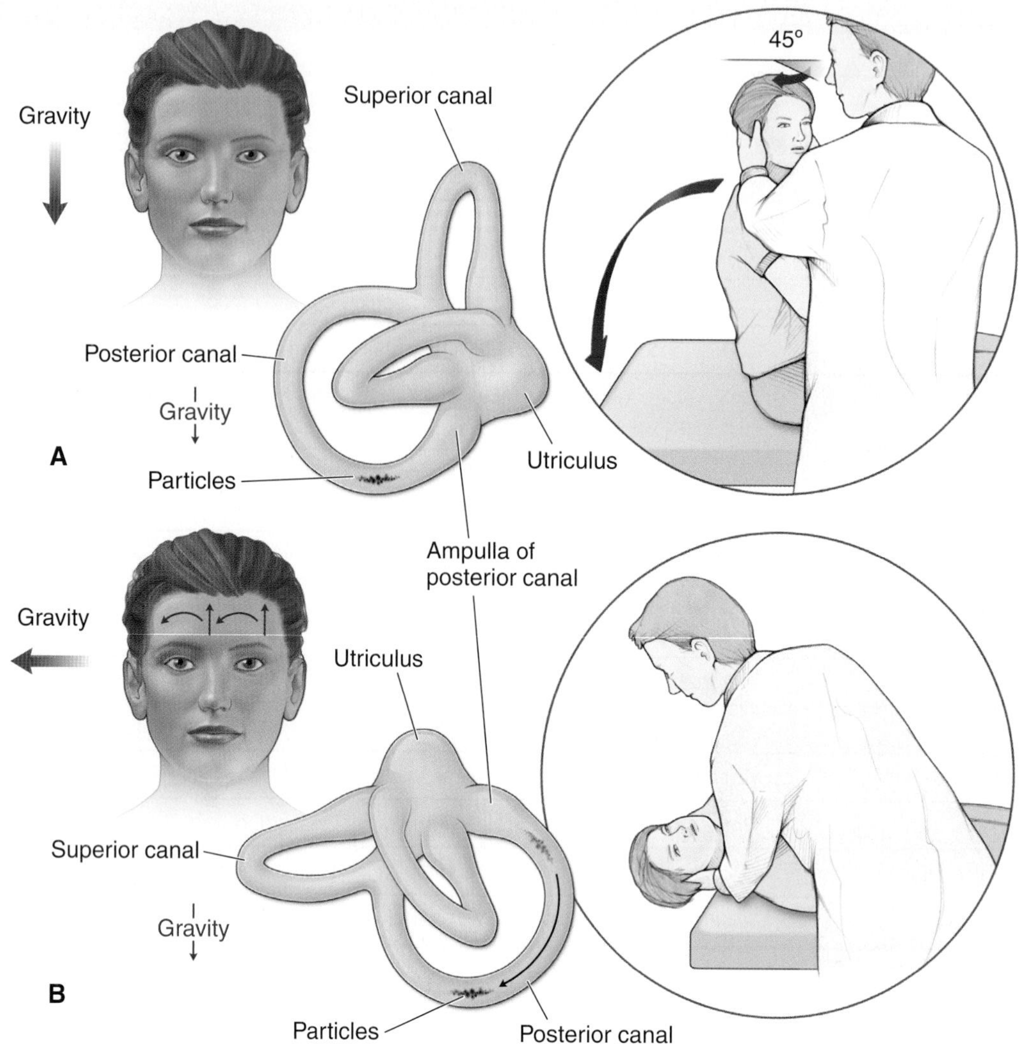

FIGURE 3-26 The dix-hallpike maneuver.

CLINICAL PEARL

Although several types of reflex hammers are popular today, no study has demonstrated any hammer to be superior to another.

Reflex integrity is defined as the intactness of the neural path involved in a reflex and the assessment of reflexes is extremely important in the diagnosis and localization of neurologic lesions.[2,273] The testing of the muscle stretch reflex provides the clinician with a direct way of assessing the peripheral nervous system and an indirect way of examining the CNS. Six of these are regularly tested (Table 3-17, Table 3-18): the biceps (C5), brachioradialis (C6), and triceps (C7) in the upper extremity, and the quadriceps (L4), extensor digitorum brevis (L5–S1) and Achilles (S1) in the lower extremities. It is worth noting that it is

TABLE 3-15 Evidence-Based Tests Using Manual Muscle Testing to Detect Cervical Radiculopathy

Manual Muscle Test	Reliability (kappa)	Sensitivity	Specificity	LR+	LR−	DOR	QUADAS Score
Deltoid	.62	24	89	2.18	0.85	2.55	10
Biceps	.69	24	94	4	0.8	4.84	10
Extensor carpi radialis	.63	12	90	1.2	0.97	1.23	10
Triceps	.29	12	94	2	0.93	2.13	10
Flexor carpi radialis	.23	6	89	0.54	1.05	0.51	10
Abductor pollicis brevis	.39	6	84	0.37	1.12	0.33	10

Data from: Wainner RS, Fritz JM, Irrgang JJ, et al.: Reliability and diagnostic accuracy of the clinical examination and patient self-report measures for cervical radiculopathy. *Spine* 28:52–62, 2003.

TABLE 3-16 Evidence-Based Tests Using Manual Muscle Testing to Detect Lumbar Radiculopathy								
Segmental Level	**Muscle or Muscle Group Tested**	**Reliability (kappa)**	**Sensitivity**	**Specificity**	**LR+**	**LR–**	**DOR**	**QUADAS Score**
L5-S1	Great toe extensors[a]	NT	48	50	0.95	1.1	0.9	3
	Great toe extensors[b]	NT	79	NT	NA	NA	NA	3
	Hip extensors[c]	NT	9	89	0.77	1.03	0.75	7
	Ankle plantar flexors[c]	NT	28	100	NA	NA	NA	7
L4–5	Great toe extensors[a]	NT	74	50	1.5	0.52	2.9	3
	Hip extensors[c]	NT	12	96	3	0.92	3.3	7
	Ankle plantar flexors[c]	NT	0	100	NA	NA	NA	7
L3–4	Great toe extensors[a]	NT	100	50	NA	NA	NA	3
	Ankle dorsiflexors[c]	NT	33	89	3.03	0.75	4.04	7
	Ankle plantar flexors[c]	NT	0	100	NA	NA	NA	7

[a]Knutsson B: Comparative value of electromyographic, myelographic and clinical-neurological examinations in diagnosis of lumbar root compression syndrome. *Acta Orthop Scand Supp* 49:1–135, 1961.

[b]Hakelius A, Hindmarsh J: The comparative reliability of preoperative diagnostic methods in lumbar disc surgery. *Acta Orthop Scand* 43:234, 1972.

[c]Kerr RS, Cadoux-Hudson TA, Adams CB: The value of accurate clinical assessment in the surgical management of the lumbar disc protrusion. *J Neuro Neurosurg Psychiatry* 51:169–173, 1988.

difficult to elicit a reflex response with the extensor digitorum brevis test, which is why it is not often performed.

CLINICAL PEARL

The abdominal and cremaster reflexes (superficial skin reflexes) are decreased or absent on the side affected by a corticospinal tract lesion and, thus, serve as adjuncts to the muscle stretch and plantar reflexes.[274]

Muscle Stretch Reflexes

To perform a muscle stretch reflex, the chosen tendon is normally struck directly and smartly with the reflex hammer. An exception is the biceps reflex, which is best tested by tapping the thumb, which has been placed over the tendon. The limb to be tested should be relaxed and in a flexed or semiflexed position. The Jendrassik maneuver can be used during testing to enhance a muscle reflex that is difficult to elicit:[275]

- For the upper extremity reflexes, the patient is asked to cross the ankles and then to isometrically attempt to abduct the legs.
- For the lower extremity reflexes, the patient is asked to interlock the fingers and then to isometrically attempt to pull the elbows apart (Fig. 3-28).

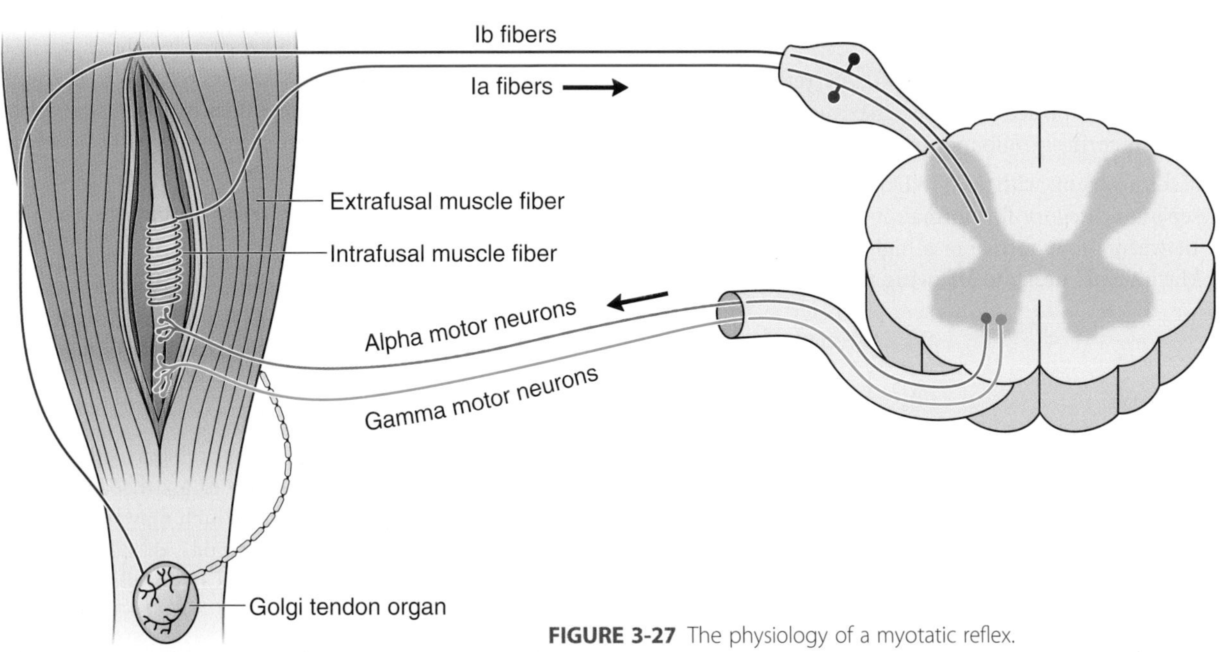

FIGURE 3-27 The physiology of a myotatic reflex.

TABLE 3-17 Common Deep Tendon Reflexes			
Reflex	**Site of Stimulus**	**Normal Response**	**Pertinent CNS Segment**
Jaw	Mandible	Mouth closes	CNV
Biceps	Biceps tendon	Biceps contraction	C5–6
Brachioradialis	Brachioradialis tendon or just distal to musculotendinous junction	Flexion of elbow and/or pronation of forearm	C5–6
Triceps	Distal triceps tendon above olecranon process	Elbow extension	C7–8
Patella	Patellar tendon	Leg extension	L3–4
Medial hamstrings	Semimembranosus tendon	Knee flexion	L5, S1
Lateral hamstrings	Biceps femoris tendon	Knee flexion	S1–2
Tibialis posterior	Tibialis posterior tendon behind medial malleolus	Plantar flexion of foot with inversion	L4–5
Achilles	Achilles tendon	Plantar flexion of foot	S1–2

CN, cranial nerve.

CLINICAL PEARL

In the elderly, up to 50% without neurologic disease lack an Achilles reflex bilaterally,[276] and small percentages (3–5 percent) of normal individuals have generalized hyperreflexia.[277]

Two muscle stretch reflex scales can be used to grade a reflex: National Institute of Neurological Disorders and Stroke (NINDS) scale and the Mayo Clinic scale. The NINDS scale uses the following five-point grading system:

- 0, absent (areflexia). The absence of a reflex signifies an interruption of the reflex arc.
- 1, slight and less than normal (hyporeflexia).
- 2, in the lower half of normal range.
- 3, in the upper half of normal range (brisk).
- 4, enhanced and more than normal (hyperreflexive). Includes clonus if present. A hyperreflexive reflex denotes a release from cortical inhibitory influences.

One of the problems with the NINDS scale is that it does not have a separate category for normal, making it necessary to choose between a low normal or a high normal.

The Mayo Clinic uses the following nine point scale:[278]

- Absent: −4
- Just elicitable: −3
- Low: −2
- Moderately low: −1
- Normal: 0
- Brisk: +1
- Very brisk: +2
- Exhaustible clonus: +3
- Continuous clonus: +4

An absent or exaggerated reflex is significant only when it is associated with one of the following:[279]

- The reflex is unusually brisk compared with reflexes from a higher spinal level.
- The exaggerated reflexes are associated with other findings of the UMN disease.
- The absent reflexes are associated with other findings of LMN disease.
- The reflex amplitude is asymmetric. Reflex asymmetry has more pathologic significance than the absolute activity of the reflex—a bilateral patella reflex of 3 is less significant than a 3 on the left and a 2 on the right. Additionally, in cases where the reflex findings are symmetrical, but either elevated or depressed, further investigation is required. For example, a patient presenting with symmetrically brisk patella tendon and Achilles stretch reflexes, while simultaneously having absent stretch reflexes in the upper extremity, requires further investigation (this is a typical finding with amyotrophic lateral sclerosis or Lou Gehrig disease, a mixed UMN and LMN pathology).[280]

The findings from the muscle reflex testing can occur as a generalized, or local, phenomenon:

- *Generalized hyporeflexia.* The causes of generalized hyporeflexia run the gamut from neurologic disease, chromosomal metabolic conditions, and hypothyroidism to schizophrenia and anxiety.[206]
- *Nongeneralized hyporeflexia.* Generally, an asymmetrically depressed or absent reflex is suggestive of pathology that is impacting the reflex arc directly, such as a LMN lesion or sensory paresis, which may be segmental (root), multisegmental (cauda equina), or nonsegmental (peripheral nerve). Nongeneralized hyporeflexia can result from peripheral neuropathy, spinal nerve root compression, and cauda equina syndrome. It is thus

TABLE 3-18 Evidence-based Neurologic Reflex Tests

Test	Study Description	Reliability	Sensitivity	Specificity	LR+	LR−	DOR	QUADAS Score
Hoffmann's	Retrospective study of 67 patients, seen during a 4-year period, with cervical pathology requiring surgical correction[a]	NT	0	0	0	0	0	6
	16 asymptomatic patients with a positive Hoffmann's reflex were prospectively studied with cervical radiographs and MRI[b]	NT	94	NT	NA	NA	NA	7
	36 patients with cervical myelopathy who had had MRI[c]	NT	82	NT	NA	NA	NA	3
	165 patients, of whom 124 had imaging of the spinal canal[d]	NT	58	74	2.23	0.57	3.93	8
Babinski	Two examiners independently assessed 100 patients receiving neck/shoulder physical examinations with a set of 66 clinical tests divided into nine categories[e]	98% agreement	NT	NT	NA	NA	NA	NA
	A prospective study of 144 patients with diagnosis of brain death[f]	NT	0	NT	NA	NA	NA	6
	Assessed the frequency of the Babinski response after planter stimulation by exposing the feet by removal of the bed sheet or socks in 10 patients with neurologic disease and 10 control subjects	NT	80	90	8	0.05	156	7
	81 children with spastic cerebral palsy were examined[g]	NT	76	NT	NA	NA	NA	11
Lhermitte sign	65 patients who underwent MRI of the cervical spine were prospectively evaluated[h]	NT	3	97	1	1	1	8
Biceps DTR for cervical radiculopathy	A blinded, prospective diagnostic test study of 82 patients with suspected cervical radiculopathy or carpal tunnel syndrome[i]	0.73 kappa	24	95	4.8	0.8	6	10
	Two examiners independently assessed 100 patients receiving neck/shoulder physical examinations with a set of 66 clinical tests divided into nine categories[e]	94%	NT	NT	NA	NA	NA	NA
Triceps DTR for cervical radiculopathy	A blinded, prospective diagnostic test study of 82 patients with suspected cervical radiculopathy or carpal tunnel syndrome[i]	NT	3	93	0.42	1.04	0.4	10
	Two examiners independently assessed 100 patients receiving neck/shoulder physical examinations with a set of 66 clinical tests divided into 9 categories[e]	88% agreement	NT	NT	NA	NA	NA	NA
	183 subjects prospectively analyzed (96 cervical radiculopathies, 45 normal studies, and 42 abnormal electrodiagnostic findings other than radiculopathy)[j]	NT	14	92	1.75	0.93	1.87	9

(Continued)

TABLE 3-18 Evidence-based Neurologic Reflex Tests *(Continued)*

Test	Study Description	Reliability	Sensitivity	Specificity	LR+	LR−	DOR	QUADAS Score
Brachioradialis DTR	A blinded, prospective diagnostic test study of 82 patients with suspected cervical radiculopathy or carpal tunnel syndrome[i]	NT	6	95	1.2	0.98	1.21	10
	Two examiners independently assessed 100 patients receiving neck/shoulder physical examinations with a set of 66 clinical tests divided into 9 categories[e]	92% agreement	NT	NT	NA	NA	NA	NA
	183 subjects prospectively analyzed (96 cervical radiculopathies, 45 normal studies, and 42 abnormal electrodiagnostic findings other than radiculopathy)[j]	NT	17	94	2.8	0.88	3.2	9
Quadriceps DTR (L3–4)	205 patients operated upon for herniated intervertebral discs[k]	NT	100	65	NA	NA	NA	3
Achilles DTR (L5-S1)	205 patients operated upon for herniated intervertebral discs[k]	NT	80	76	3.36	0.26	12.8	3
	100 patients with lumbar disc protrusions were studied to relate history and clinical signs to the myelograms and surgical findings[l]	NT	87	89	7.91	0.15	54.2	7
Extensor digitorum brevis DTR (L5-S1)	A prospective study of 88 subjects to evaluate the extensor digitorum brevis deep tendon reflex (EDBR) in a normal population and in patients with L-5 and S-1 radiculopathies[m]	NT	14	91	1.56	0.95	1.64	8

[a]Denno JJ, Meadows GR: Early diagnosis of cervical spondylotic myelopathy. A useful clinical sign. *Spine* 16:1353–5, 1991.

[b]Sung RD, Wang JC: Correlation between a positive Hoffmann's reflex and cervical pathology in asymptomatic individuals. *Spine* 26:67–70, 2001.

[c]Wong TM, Leung HB, Wong WC: Correlation between magnetic resonance imaging and radiographic measurement of cervical spine in cervical myelopathic patients. *J Orthop Surg* 12:239–242, 2004.

[d]Glaser J, Cure J, Bailey K, et al.: Cervical Spinal Cord Compression and the Hoffman Sign. *Iowa Orthop* J 21:49–52, 2001.

[e]Bertilson BC, Grunnesjo M, Strender LE: Reliability of clinical tests in the assessment of patients with neck/shoulder problems-impact of history. *Spine.* 28:2222–31, 2003.

[f]De Freitas G, Andre C: Absence of the Babinski sign in brain death. *J Neurol* 252:106–107, 2005.

[g]Ghosh D, Pradhan S: "Extensor toe sign" by various methods in spastic children with cerebral palsy. *J Child Nneurol* 13:216–20, 1998.

[h]Uchihara T, Furukawa T, Tsukagoshi H: Compression of brachial plexus as a diagnostic test of cervical cord lesion. *Spine* 19:2170–3, 1994.

[i]Wainner RS, Fritz JM, Irrgang JJ, et al.: Reliability and diagnostic accuracy of the clinical examination and patient self-report measures for cervical radiculopathy. *Spine.* 28:52–62, 2003.

[j]Lauder TD, Dillingham TR, Andary M, et al.: Predicting electrodiagnostic outcome in patients with upper limb symptoms: are the history and physical examination helpful? *Arch Phys Med Rehabil* 81:436–41, 2000.

[k]Knutsson B: Comparative value of electromyographic, myelographic and clinical-neurological examinations in diagnosis of lumbar root compression syndrome. *Acta Orthop Scand. Suppl* 49:1–135, 1961.

[l]Kerr RS, Cadoux-Hudson TA, Adams CB: The value of accurate clinical assessment in the surgical management of the lumbar disc protrusion. *JNeurol Neurosurg psychiatry* 51:169–73, 1988.

[m]Marin R, Dillingham TR, Chang A, et al.: Extensor digitorum brevis reflex in normals and patients with radiculopathies. *Muscle Nerve* 18:52–9, 1995.

important to test more than one reflex and to evaluate the information gleaned from the examination, before reaching a conclusion as to the relevance of the findings.

In those situations demonstrating an elevated or brisk reflex, the CNS's normal role of integrating reflexes may have been disrupted, indicating an UMN lesion, such as a brain stem or cerebral impairment, spinal cord compression, or a neurologic disease. However, the distinction has to be made between a brisk reflex and the one that is hyperreflexive. True neurological hyperreflexia contains a clonic component and is suggestive of CNS (UMN) impairment. The clinician also should note any additional recruitment that occurs during the reflex contraction of the target. A brisk reflex is a normal finding, provided that it is not masking a hyperreflexia caused by an incorrect testing technique. Unlike hyperreflexia, a brisk reflex does not have a clonic component. As with hyporeflexia, the clinician should assess more than one reflex before coming to a conclusion about a hyperreflexia. The presence of an UMN impairment can be confirmed by the presence of the pathologic reflexes (see next section).

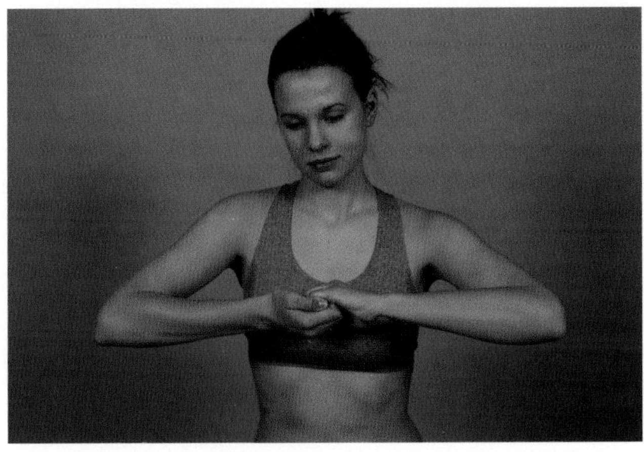

FIGURE 3-28 Jendrassik maneuver used during testing to enhance a muscle reflex.

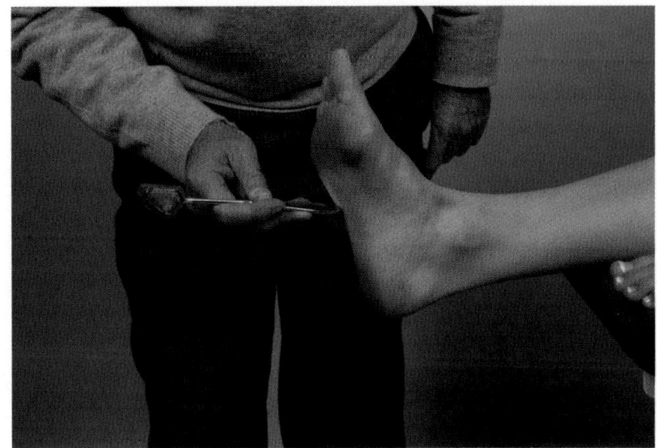

FIGURE 3-29 Babinski.

> **CLINICAL PEARL**
>
> Even though muscle stretch reflexes have long been assumed to be good objective signs, the interrater reliability of muscle stretch reflex grading for the same subject is quite variable and subjective due to both patient and clinician factors.[278,281]

Pathologic Reflexes

There are two basic pathologic reflexes: the Babinski and its variants (Chaddock, Oppenheim, Gordon, etc.) and the Hoffman and its variants (ankle and wrist clonus) (Table 3-19). A number of primitive reflexes are normally integrated by individuals as they develop. Pathologic reflexes occur when an injury or a disease process results in a loss of this normal suppression by the cerebrum on the segmental level of the brain stem or the spinal cord, resulting in a release of the primitive reflex.[282] Thus, the presence of pathologic reflexes is suggestive of CNS (UMN) impairment and requires an appropriate referral.

- **Babinski.** In this test, the clinician applies noxious stimuli to sole of the patient's foot by running a pointed object along the plantar aspect (Fig. 3-29).[283] A positive test, demonstrated by extension of the great toe (extensor toe sign) and a splaying (abduction) of the other toes, is indicative of an injury to the corticospinal tract.[284–286] A negative finding is slight toe flexion, smaller digits greater than the great toe. As Babinski observed,[284] the pyramidal tracts are not well developed in infants, and these signs, which are abnormal past the age of 3 years, are usually present.
- **Gonda-Allen.** The Gonda-Allen sign is a variant of the Babinski. The patient is positioned in supine. Grasping the patient's foot, the clinician provides a forceful downward stretch or snaps the distal phalanx of the second or fourth toe (Fig. 3-30). A positive response is the extensor toe sign.[287] The Gonda-Allen method is considered more sensitive than the classic Babinski method.[288]

TABLE 3-19 Pathologic Reflexes

Reflex	Eliciting Stimulus	Positive Response	Pathology
Babinski	Stroking of lateral aspect of side of foot	Extension of big toe and fanning of four small toes; normal reaction in newborns	Pyramidal tract lesion; organic hemiplegia
Chaddock	Stroking of lateral side of foot beneath lateral malleolus	Same response as above	Pyramidal tract lesion
Oppenheim	Stroking of anteromedial tibial surface	Same response as above	Pyramidal tract lesion
Gordon	Squeezing of calf muscles firmly	Same response as above	Pyramidal tract lesion
Brudzinski	Passive flexion of one lower limb	Similar movement occurs in opposite limb	Meningitis
Hoffmann	"Flicking" of terminal phalanx of the index, middle, or ring finger	Reflex flexion of distal phalanx of the thumb and of distal phalanx of the index or middle finger (whichever one was not "flicked")	Increased irritability of sensory nerves in tetany; pyramidal tract lesion
Lhermitte	Neck flexion	Electric shock-like sensation that radiates down spinal column into upper or lower limbs	Abnormalities (demyelination) in posterior part of cervical spinal cord

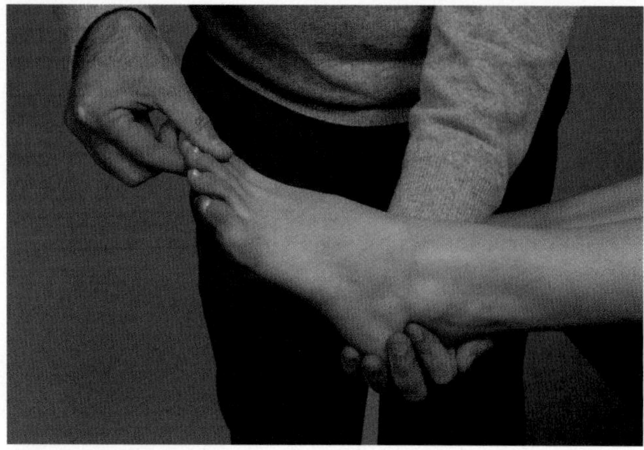

FIGURE 3-30 Gonda-Allen sign.

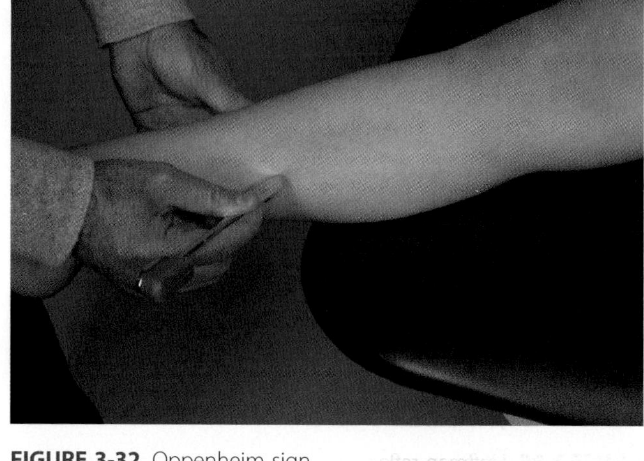

FIGURE 3-32 Oppenheim sign.

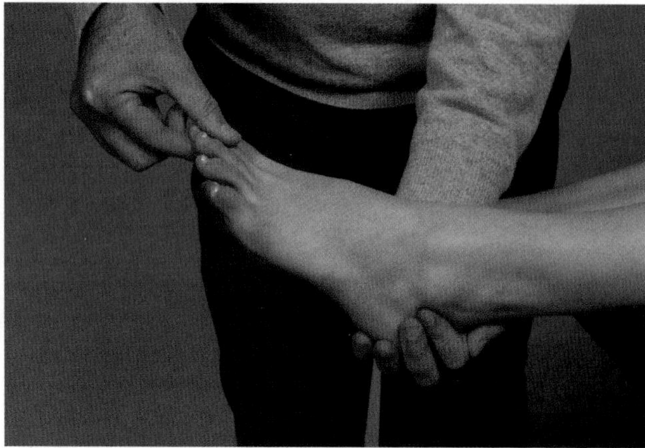

FIGURE 3-31 Allen-Cleckley sign.

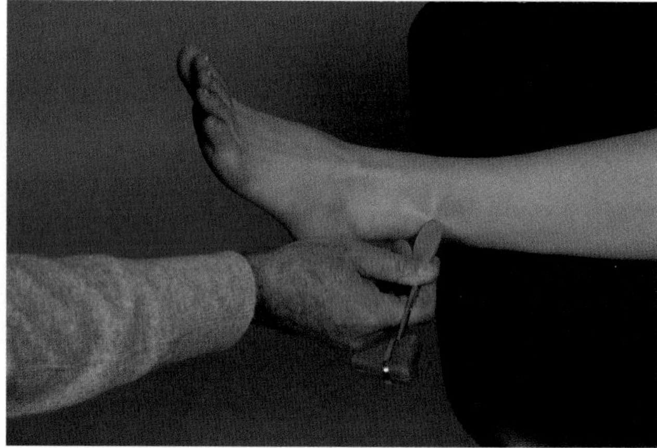

FIGURE 3-33 Chaddock sign.

- **Allen-Cleckley.** The Allen-Cleckley sign (Fig. 3-31) is another variant of the Babinski. The patient is positioned in supine. Grasping the patient's foot, the clinician provides a sharp upward flick of the second toe or pressure over the distal aspect or ball of the toe. A positive response is the extensor toe sign.[288]
- **Oppenheim sign.** The patient is positioned in supine. The clinician applies noxious stimuli along the shin of the patient's tibia by running a fingernail downward toward the foot (Fig. 3-32). A positive test, demonstrated by the extensor toe sign, is theoretically indicative of UMN impairment. However, the diagnostic value of this test is as yet unknown.[289]
- **Chaddock sign.** The patient is positioned in supine or sitting. The clinician strokes the lateral malleolus from proximal to distal with a solid, relatively sharp object (Fig. 3-33). A positive response is the extensor toe sign. The diagnostic value of this test is as yet unknown.[289]
- **Schaefer sign.** The patient is positioned in supine or sitting. The clinician provides a sharp, quick squeeze of the Achilles tendon (Fig. 3-34). A positive response is the extensor toe sign. This test remains unstudied for diagnostic value.
- **Hoffmann.** The Hoffmann sign, also referred to as the digital reflex, the snapping reflex, Tromner sign and

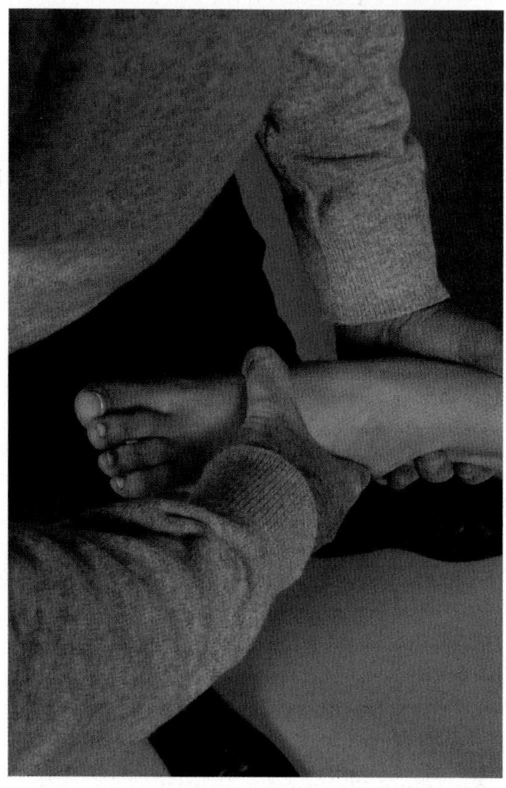

FIGURE 3-34 Schaefer sign.

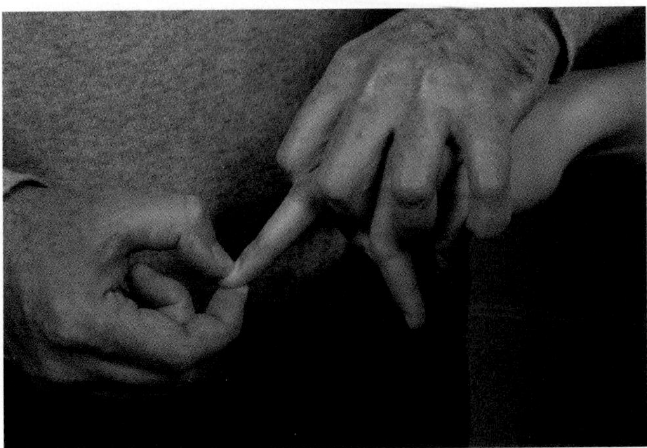

FIGURE 3-35 Hoffman reflex.

Jakobson sign, is the upper limb equivalent of the Babinski. However, unlike the Babinski, some normal individuals can exhibit a Hoffmann sign.[274] The clinician holds the patient's middle finger and briskly pinches the distal phalanx, thereby applying a noxious stimulus to the nail bed of the middle finger (Fig. 3-35).[274] A positive test is adduction and opposition of the thumb and slight flexion of the fingers. There are no known studies assessing the interexaminer reliability of this test (Table 3-18), and its significance remains disputed in the literature. Denno and Meadows[290] devised a dynamic version of this test to assist in the diagnosis of early spondylotic cervical myelopathy, which involved the patient performing repeated flexion and extension of the head before being tested for the Hoffmann sign.

- **Cross up going toe sign.** This is another variation of the Babinski. The patient is positioned in supine. The clinician passively raises the opposite limb into hip flexion and then instructs the patient to hold the leg in flexion while the clinician applies a downward force against the leg (Fig. 3-36). A positive test is associated with great toe extension of the opposite leg during resistance the hip flexion. Of the few studies of this test, Willoughby and Eason found the test to have little value as a sensitive indicator of a pyramidal tract lesion in 125 normal subjects and 192 patients with neurological disorders due to the high frequency of false positive signs in normal subjects and patients with other neurological disorders.[303]
- **Clonus.** The patient is positioned in supine or sitting. The technique can be applied to the wrist (sudden wrist extension) or to the ankle (sudden dorsiflexion) (Fig. 3-37). The stretch is then maintained. A positive response is more than three involuntary beats of the ankle or wrist (two to three twitches are considered normal). In some patients, there is a more sustained clonus; in others, there is only a very short-lived finding. During the testing, the patient should not flex the neck, as this can often increase the number of beats. A positive test is theoretically indicative of UMN impairment, but the diagnostic value of this test is as yet unknown.

Other pathological reflexes include:

- **Inverted radial (supinator) reflex.** The inverted radial reflex sign, introduced by Babinski, is commonly used in clinical practice to assess cervical myelopathy. There are two components of this abnormal reflex: (1) an absence of contraction of the brachioradialis muscle when the styloid process of the radius is tapped (Fig. 3-38), and (2) a hyperactive response of the finger flexor muscles; a response

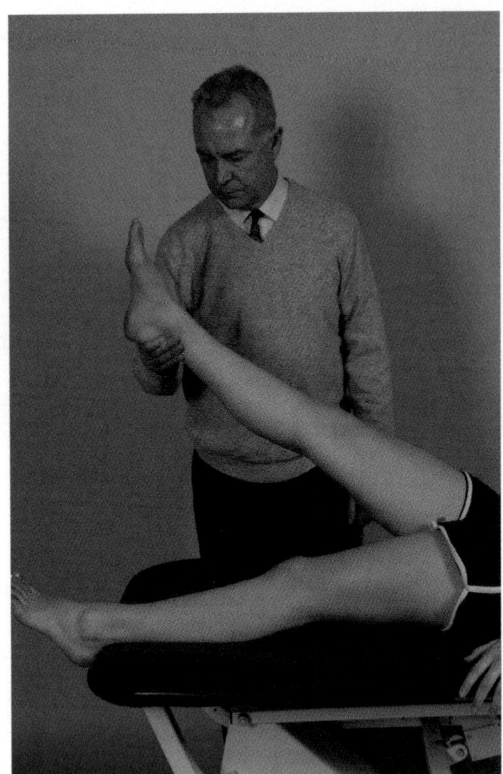

FIGURE 3-36 Cross up going toe sign.

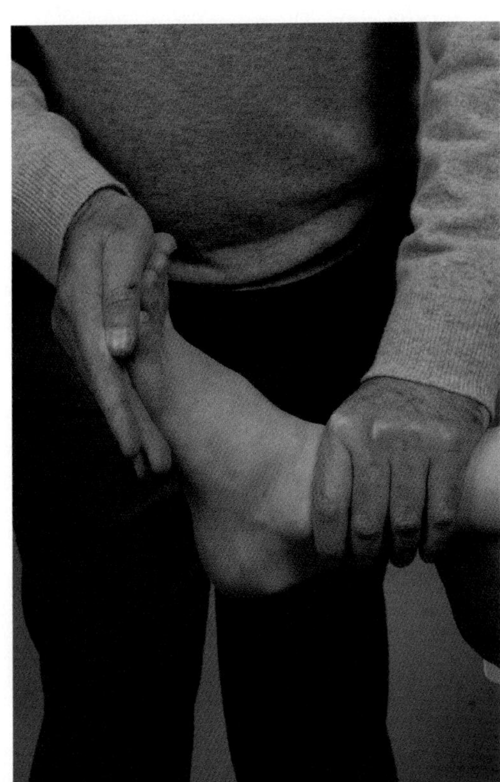

FIGURE 3-37 Clonus.

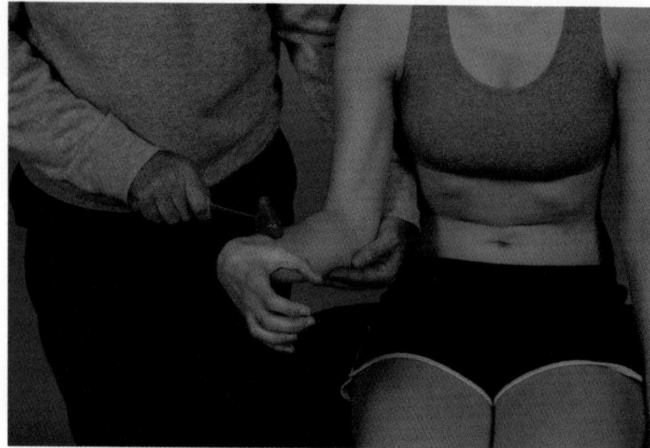

FIGURE 3-38 Inverted radial (supinator) reflex.

that is subserved by a lower spinal cord segment (C8).[291] To date, it is unknown whether the sign correlates with the presence or severity of myelopathy. Indeed, an isolated, inverted supinator reflex may be a variation of a normal clinical examination.[292] Theoretically, a true response is likely related to increased alpha motor neuron excitability below the level of the lesion; however, a possible contribution of the dynamic muscle spindles cannot be excluded.

- **Finger escape sign.** The patient is positioned in sitting. The clinician asks the patient to hold all of his/her fingers in extension. A positive sign involves the involuntary flexion and abduction within 1 minute of extended and adducted fingers when held statically. To date there has only been one study[293] that examined the sensitivity of the finger escape sign, which identified a sensitivity of 55% in a sample of 36 subjects with myelopathy.
- **Palmomental reflex.** The patient is positioned in supine or sitting. A number of methods to elicit this reflex have been advocated. The clinician may stroke the thenar eminence of the hand in a proximal to distal direction with a reflex hammer (Fig. 3-39) or may stroke the hypothenar eminence in a similar fashion. The procedure can be repeated up to five times to detect a continuous response. If the response diminishes, the test is considered negative. A positive test is contraction of the mentalis and orbicular oris muscles causing wrinkling of the skin of the chin and slight retraction (and occasionally elevation of the mouth). A study by Owen and Mulley[294] found that the reflex is often present in normal people and may be absent in disease states. The study concluded that testing merely for the presence or absence of the reflex lacks both specificity and sensitivity, but that a strong, sustained, and easily repeatable contraction of the mentalis muscle, which can be elicited by stimulation of areas other than the palm, is more likely to indicate cerebral damage. Another study[295] found diagnostic value in using combinations of two or three pathologic reflexes to distinguish between neurologically damaged patients and normal age-matched controls.
- **Beevor sign.** The patient is positioned supine, with the knees flexed and both feet flat on the bed. The patient is asked to raise the head against resistance, cough, or attempt to sit up with the hands resting behind the head.[296] The clinician observes for motion at the umbilicus, which should remain in a straight line. Beevor sign, an upward deflection of the umbilicus on flexion of the neck, is the result of paralysis of the inferior portion of the rectus abdominis muscle, so that the upper fibers predominate, pulling the umbilicus upwards. The condition may be caused by spinal cord injury at or below the level of T10.[253]

CLINICAL PEARL

Beevor sign is a common finding in patients with facioscapulohumeral dystrophy, even before functional weakness of abdominal wall muscles is apparent, but is absent in patients with other facioscapulohumeral disorders.[297]

- **Lhermitte symptom or "phenomenon".** This is not so much a pathologic reflex as it is a symptom, described as an electric shock-like sensation that radiates down the spinal column into the upper or the lower limbs with passive flexion of the neck with the patient in the long sit position (Fig. 3-40). It may also be precipitated by extending the head, coughing, sneezing, bending forward, or moving the

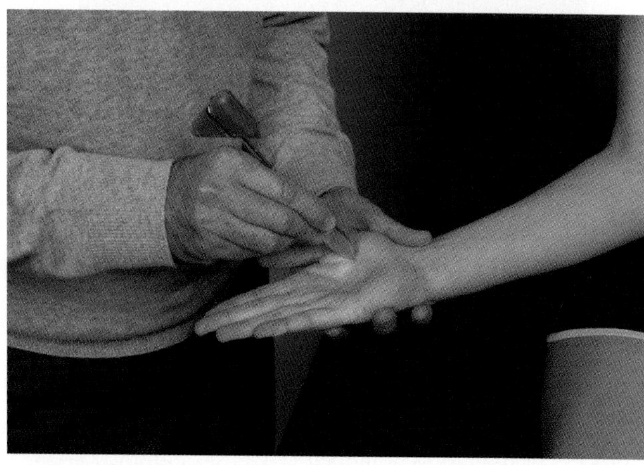

FIGURE 3-39 Palmomental reflex.

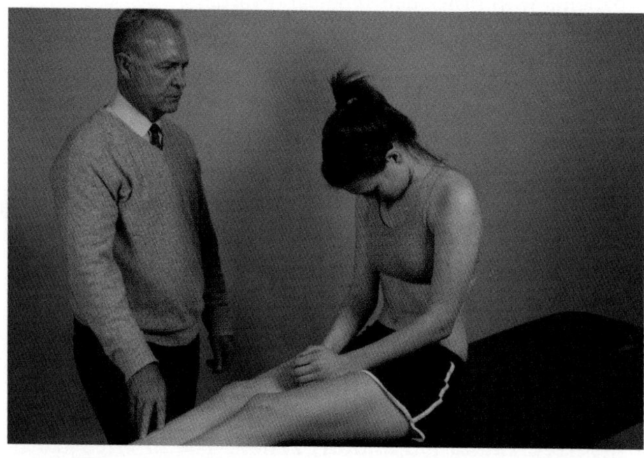

FIGURE 3-40 Lhermitte symptom.

limbs.[298] Lhermitte sign is most prevalent in patients with multiple sclerosis,[299] cervical spondylotic myelopathy, cervical radiation injury, and neck trauma.[300] Smith and McDonald[301] postulated that there is an increased mechanosensitivity to traction on the cervical cord of injured axons located within the posterior (dorsal) columns. Although a herniated disk is an anteriorly placed lesion and the spinothalamic tract is usually more affected than the posterior columns, flexion of the neck will produce stretching of the posterior aspects of the cord, but not the anterior part at the site of the impairment, and this may explain this particular symptom. To date, there are no reports investigating the interexaminer reliability of this test. One study[302] reported a sensitivity of 27%, specificity of 90%, positive predictive value of 55%, and negative predictive value of 75% for the active flexion and extension test, which partly resembles this test.

- **Mendel Bechtrew sign.** The patient is positioned in supine or sitting. The clinician taps on the dorsal aspect of the cuboid bone using the sharp end of a reflex hammer (Fig. 3-41). A positive response is flexion of the four lateral toes. This test remains unstudied for diagnostic value.

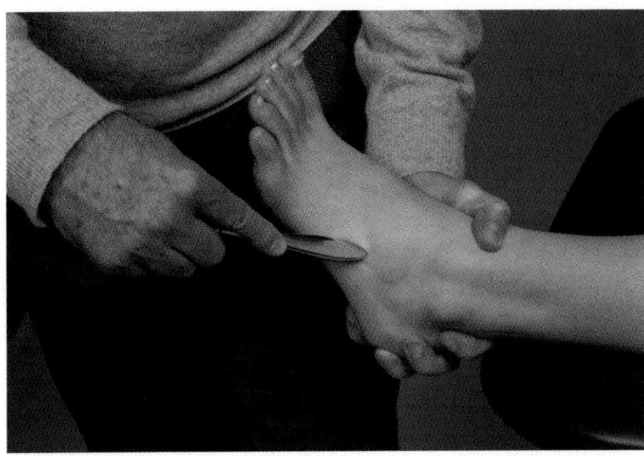

FIGURE 3-41 Mendel Bechtrew sign.

Supraspinal Reflexes

The supraspinal reflexes produce movement patterns that can be modulated by descending pathways and the cortex. A number of processes, which are involved in locomotor function, are oriented around these reflexes and are referred to as righting reflexes. Righting reflexes can be subcategorized as the following: visual righting reflexes, labyrinthine righting reflexes, neck righting reflexes, body on head righting reflexes, and body on body righting reflexes. The primary purpose of the righting reflexes is to maintain a constant position of the head in relation to a dynamic external environment.

The head and the neck are areas of intense reflex activity. Head movements, which occur almost constantly, must be regulated to maintain normal eye–head–neck–trunk relationships and to allow for visual fixation during head movements (Table 3-20). The visual field and pathway are important

TABLE 3-20 Reflex Activities Involving the Cervical Spine

Reflex	Eliciting Stimulus	Motor Response	Purpose
Tonic neck reflex	Neck movement that produces stretch to muscle spindles	Alteration of muscle tone in trunk and extremities	Assists with postural stability and enhances coordination
Cervicocollic reflex	Neck movement that produces stretch to muscle spindles	Eccentric contraction of the cervical muscles that oppose the initiating movement	Maintains smooth and controlled cervical movement
Cervicorespiratory reflex	Neck movement that produces stretch to muscle spindles	Alteration in respiratory rate	Assists in adjustments of respiration with changes in posture
Cervicosympathetic reflex	Neck movement that produces stretch to muscle spindles	Alteration in blood pressure	Assists in prevention of orthostatic hypotension with changes in posture
Trigeminocervical reflex	Touch stimulus to face	Head retraction	Protects against blows to face
Cervico-ocular reflex	Neck movement that produces stretch to muscle spindles	Movement of eyes in opposite direction of neck movement	Maintains gaze fixation during movements of head
Vestibulo-ocular reflex	Head movement stimulating semicircular canals	Movement of eyes in opposite direction of head movement	Maintains gaze fixation during movements of head
Smooth pursuit	Visual target moving across retinal field	Movement of eyes in the direction in which target is moving	Maintains gaze fixation on moving target
Saccades	New visual target in retinal field	Movement of eyes in the direction of new target	Fixates eyes on new target
Optokinetic reflex	Visual target moving across retinal field, causing perceived movement of head	Movement of eyes in opposite direction of perceived head movement	Maintains gaze fixation on moving target

Murphy DR: *Conservative Management of Cervical Spine Disorders.* New York: McGraw-Hill, 2000. With permission from McGraw-Hill.

regulators of postural control. Visual input for postural control helps fixate the position of the head and the upper trunk in space, primarily so that the center of mass of the trunk maintains its position over the well-defined limits of foot support. Aside from the visual field itself providing an important source of postural control, the extraocular muscles may also provide proprioceptive information through two distinct pathways into the oculomotor nuclei, one serving to generate eye rotations, while the other providing sensory information regarding eye alignment and stabilization.[304,305]

While the visual and vestibular systems are individually two of the most important providers of information, it is their constant interaction with each other and with cervical mechanoreceptors (particularly the short-range rotators, i.e., the obliquus capitis posterior inferior, rectus capitis posterior major, splenius capitis, and sternocleidomastoid) that makes the control of upright posture possible, especially when considering their combined role in the reflex modulation of muscular tone through various groups of postural muscles[306]:

- **Vestibulo-ocular reflex (VOR).** The VOR is stimulated by movement of the head in space and creates certain eye movements that compensate for head rotations or accelerations. The VOR may be subdivided into three major components:
  - The rotational VOR, which detects head rotation through the SCC.
  - The translational VOR, which detects linear acceleration of the head via the utricle and saccule.
  - The ocular counter-rolling response, or optokinetic reflex, which adapts eye position during head tilting and rotation.

  The VOR can be tested in a number of ways:
- **Dynamic visual acuity.[269]** After establishing baseline visual acuity with a Snellen chart, this test measures visual acuity with concurrent head movement. The patient's head is moved from side to side at a frequency of 1 Hz while the patient reads the Snellen chart. A decrease by two lines is suspicious and by three or more is indicative of an abnormal VOR.
- **Doll's head test.[269]** The clinician faces the patient, who fixes gaze on the clinician's nose. The clinician then oscillates the patient's head 30 degrees side to side at 0.5–1 Hz. Eye movements that are not smooth but interrupted by saccades toward the fixation target indicate bilateral vestibular lesions.
- **Head-shaking nystagmus test.[269]** The clinician holds the patient's head firmly, with the palms of the hands against the patient's cheeks, and produces a series of rapid but small horizontal head turns for approximately 30 seconds, with the patient's eyes closed. Upon opening the eyes, the nystagmus will beat away from the side of a unilateral peripheral vestibular lesion, or toward the lesioned side in patients with Ménière disease.
- **Head-thrust test.[269]** The patient fixates gaze on the clinician's nose. The clinician then moves the patient's head in a horizontal plane in a rapid, passive manner with unpredictable timing and direction. If the reflexive movement of the eyes is inappropriate (too big or too small), a corrective (saccadic) movement will occur. A patient with vestibular loss will have difficulty in maintaining gaze fixation, requiring a corrective saccade (fast eye movement) to maintain gaze fixation on the nose. Presence of this corrective action may indicate a lesion of the vestibular nerve.[307]
- **The cervico-ocular reflex.** The cervico-ocular reflex serves to orient eye movement to changes in neck and trunk position. Visual fixation at high speeds requires the contraction of the extraocular muscles to allow eye movements to counteract the effect of the head movements, even if the head is turning in the opposite direction. The ability to track and focus on a moving target that is moving across a visual field is termed smooth pursuit and requires a greater degree of voluntary control than the cervico-ocular and VORs can provide. The area in the brain stem where this integration of horizontal eye movements takes place is the paramedian pontine reticular formation. The ability to read a book or to scan a page requires saccadic eye movements. Unlike smooth pursuit, saccades can occur with a visual stimulus, by sound, verbal command, or tactile stimuli. However, like smooth pursuit, saccades are generated in the paramedian pontine reticular formation. The cervico-ocular reflex can be tested using three methods:
  - *Visual fixation.* The patient is seated and is asked to look straight ahead and focus on the tip of a pencil, which is held by the clinician at an arm's length from the patient. The test is repeated, with the patient's eyes turned to the extremes of horizontal and vertical gaze and the pencil tip positioned accordingly.
  - Smooth pursuit can be tested by having the patient fix his or her gaze on an object placed directly in front. The object is then moved to the right, while the patient follows it with the eyes. The clinician looks to see if the patient has any difficulty tracking the object. An abnormal response is observed if the patient's fixation on the target moving synchronously with the head is interrupted by rapid eye movements or saccades, which indicates that the pursuit is not holding the eye on the moving target. The object is moved back to the start position before being moved to the left, while the patient again follows it with the eyes. The object can then be moved in various directions, combining horizontal, vertical, and diagonal movements, to test if the patient can follow the object with the eyes without saccadic movements.
  - *Saccade test.* The patient is asked to rapidly move the eyes back and forth between two widely spaced targets while keeping the head still. An abnormal finding is if the patient takes multiple eye movements, rather than a single jump, to exactly fix on a target.

Difficulty with these tests may indicate a lesion of the cerebellum, reticular formation, cerebral cortex, or a CN lesion (oculomotor, trochlear, or abducens).[307]

- **The cervicocollic reflex (CCR).** The CCR serves to orient the position of the head and the neck in relation to disturbed trunk posture. Acting similarly to a stretch reflex, this reflex involves reflexive correction of cervical spine position through cocontraction of specific cervical muscles.

- **The vestibulocollic reflex (VCR).** The VCR maintains postural stability by actively stabilizing the head relative to space, through reflexive contraction of those cervical muscles opposite to the direction of cervical spine perturbation. It should be noted that this reflex is distinct and largely dissociated from the vestibulospinal reflex, which orients the extremities to the position of the head and the neck.[306]

The CCR and VCR reflexes appear perfectly suited through their dynamic and somatotopic characteristics to compensate for positional disturbances of the head and the neck with respect to the trunk.[308–310]

Sensation and Sensibility Testing

Sensation is the conscious perception of basic sensory input. Sensibility describes the neural events occurring at the periphery, nerve fibers, and nerve receptors. Sensation is what a clinician re-educates, whereas sensibility is what a clinician assesses.[311] The assessment of sensibility involves an understanding of the entire peripheral and central sensory pathways from the skin to the thalamus.

Altered sensory perceptions can result from injuries to peripheral nerves or from spinal nerve root compression. The posterior (dorsal) roots of the spinal nerves are represented by restricted peripheral sensory regions called dermatomes (Fig. 3-42). The peripheral sensory nerves are represented by more distinct and circumscribed areas (see Fig. 3-42). Paresthesia is a symptom of direct involvement of the nerve root. Paresthesia can be defined as an abnormal sensation of pins and needles, numbness, or prickling. Further irritation and destruction of the neural fibers interfere with conduction, resulting in a motor or sensory deficit, or a combination of both. It is, therefore, possible for a nerve root compression to cause pure motor paresis, a pure sensory deficit, or both, depending on which aspect of the nerve root is compressed. If pressure is exerted from above the nerve root, sensory impairment may result, whereas compression from below can induce motor paresis. Pain results if there is irritation of the neural fibers. In general, if a patient has a sensory deficit involving a peripheral nerve, he or she is able to accurately localize the area of anesthesia.[312] Sensory or sensibility testing examines the integrity and the intactness of cortical sensory processing, including proprioception, pallesthesia (the ability to sense mechanical vibration), stereognosis (the ability to perceive, recognize, and name familiar objects), and topognosis (the ability to localize exactly a cutaneous sensation).[273]

Two types of sensibility can be assessed[313]:

- *Protective.* This is evidenced by the ability to perceive pinprick, touch, and temperature.
- *Functional.* This is evidenced by a return of sensibility to a level that enables the hand to engage in full activities of daily living.

CLINICAL PEARL

There exists a hierarchy of sensibility capacity[313,314]:

- *Detection.* This is the simplest level of function and requires that the patient be able to distinguish a single-point stimulus from normally occurring atmospheric background stimulation.
- *Innervation density or discrimination.* This represents the ability to perceive that stimulus A differs from stimulus B.
- *Quantification.* This involves organizing tactile stimuli according to degree, texture, etc.
- *Recognition.* This is the most complicated level of function and involves the identification of objects with the vision occluded.

Based on the hierarchy of sensibility capacity, testing is classified neurophysiologically into four types: threshold tests, stress tests, innervation density tests, and sensory nerve conduction studies:[315]

- *Threshold tests.* Examples of threshold tests include vibratory testing and Semmes–Weinstein monofilament testing (see Specific Sensory Tests).
- *Stress tests.* Stress tests are those that combine the use of sensory tests with the activities that provoke the symptoms of nerve compression. These tests are helpful in cases of patient reports of mild nerve compression when no abnormalities are detected by baseline sensory testing. Examples of stress tests include the Phalen's test at the wrist (see Chap. 18).
- *Innervation density tests.* These are a class of sensory tests that test the ability to discriminate between two identical stimuli placed close together on the skin. These tests are helpful in assessing sensibility after nerve repair and during nerve regeneration (see Specific Sensory Tests).[316]
- *Sensory nerve conduction studies.* Sensory nerve conduction studies are electrophysiologic tests that assess the conduction of sensory action potentials along a nerve trunk.[315] These tests require only passive cooperation of the patient, not subjective interpretation of a stimulus. A slowing of nerve conduction velocity or an alteration in potential amplitudes indicates a compression or partial laceration of the nerve.[10]

A full examination of the sensory system involves specific testing of pain, temperature, pressure, vibration, position, and discriminative sensations. For patients with no apparent neurologic symptoms or signs, an abbreviated examination may be substituted.

Specific Sensory Tests

Sensation

- **Origin.** Lateral spinothalamic tract (see Box 3-2).

The segmental innervation of the skin has a high degree of overlap, especially in the thoracic spine, requiring that the clinician tests the full area of the dermatome. This is done to

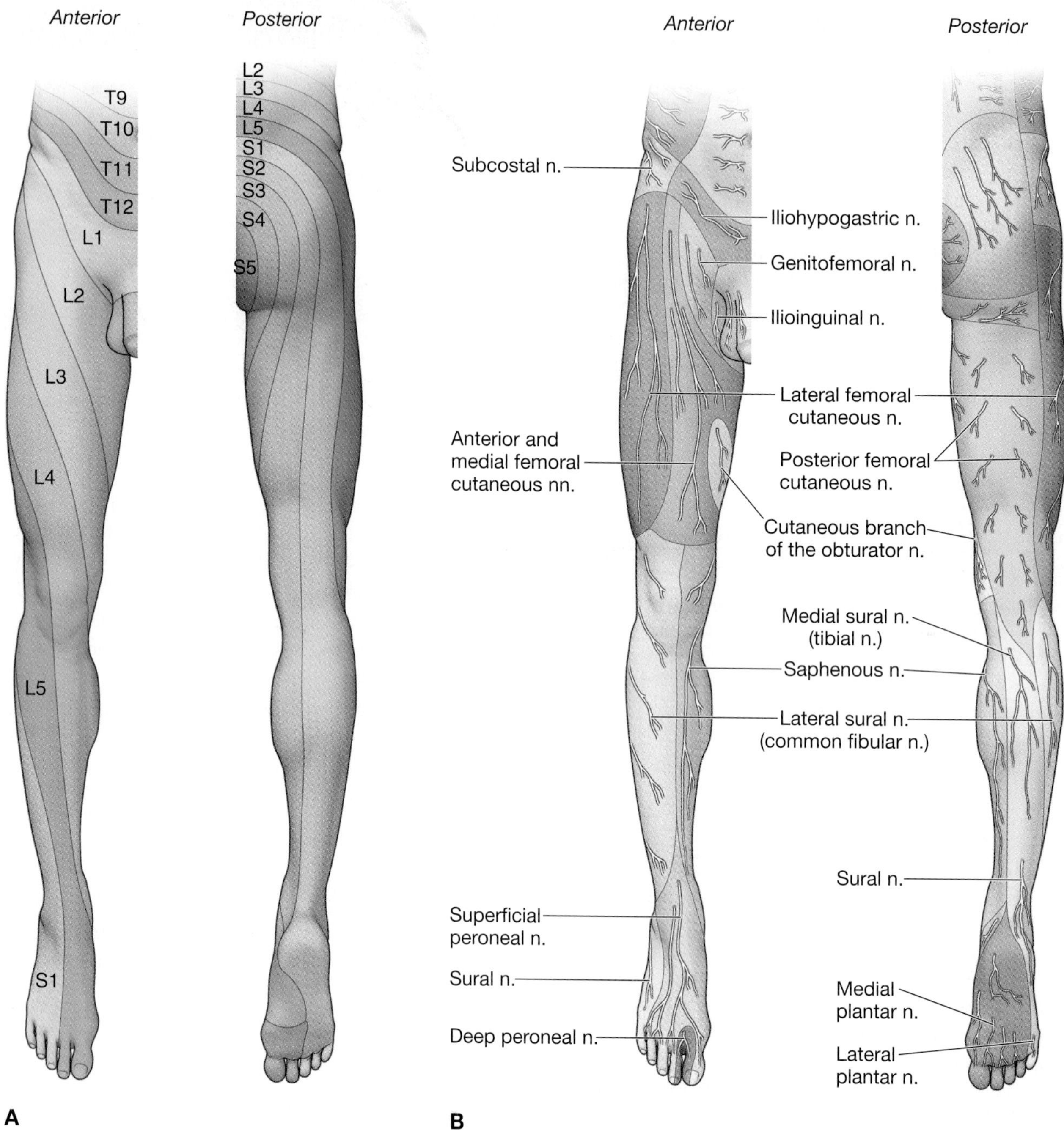

FIGURE 3-42 Lower extremity dermatomes. (Reproduced, with permission, from Morton DA, Foreman KB, Albertine KH: *The Big Picture: Gross Anatomy,* McGraw-Hill, 2011)

seek out the area of sensitivity, or autogenous area, which is a small region of the dermatome with no overlap, and the only area within a dermatome that is supplied exclusively by a single segmental level.[317] There are two components to the dermatome tests:

- *Light touch.* Information about light touch, two-point discrimination, vibration, and proprioception are carried by the posterior (dorsal) column–medial lemniscal tract. Light touch tests for hypoesthesia throughout the dermatome. In terms of sensation loss, light touch is the most sensitive and the first to be affected with palsy. If the light touch test is positive, the areas of reduced sensation are mapped out for the autogenous area, and then the pinprick test is performed to map out the whole of the autogenous area.[8] The use of a vibrating tuning fork has been found to be a valid and reliable test of the functional integrity of the large myelinated nerve fibers.[318]
- *Pinprick.* Information about pain is carried by the lateral spinothalamic tract (see Box 3-2). The pinprick test examines for near anesthesia in the autonomous, no-overlap area. This test is performed using a sharp safety pin, occasionally substituting the blunt end for the point as a stimulus. Pinprick testing is the most common way of determining the sensory "level" caused by a spinal cord lesion, because information about pain, temperature, and crude touch is carried by the spinothalamic tract.[275] When investigating an area of cutaneous sensory loss, it is recommended that the clinician begins the pinprick test in the area of anesthesia and works

TABLE 3-21 Sensibility Testing for Radiculopathy

Nerve or Dermatome Tested	Method	Reliability (kappa)	Sensitivity	Specificity	LR+	LR−	DOR	QUADAS Score
Axillary	Light touch[a]	.69	NT	NT	NA	NA	NA	NA
Musculocutaneous	Light touch[a]	.67	NT	NT	NA	NA	NA	NA
Radial	Light touch[a]	.31	NT	NT	NA	NA	NA	NA
Median	Light touch[a]	.73	NT	NT	NA	NA	NA	NA
Ulnar	Light touch[a]	.59	NT	NT	NA	NA	NA	NA
C5	Pinprick[b]	.67	29	86	2.07	0.82	2.51	10
C6	Pinprick[b]	.28	24	66	0.70	1.15	0.61	10
C7	Pinprick[b]	.40	28	77	1.21	0.93	1.30	10
C8	Pinprick[b]	.16	12	81	0.63	1.08	0.58	10
T1	Pinprick[b]	.46	18	79	0.85	1.03	0.82	

[a]Jepsen JR, Laursen LH, Hagert CG, et al.: Diagnostic accuracy of the neurological upper limb examination I: inter-rater reproducibility of selected findings and patterns. *BMC Neurol* 6:8, 2006.

[b]Wainner RS, Fritz JM, Irrgang JJ, et al.: Reliability and diagnostic accuracy of the clinical examination and patient self-report measures for cervical radiculopathy. *Spine.* 28:52–62, 2003.

outward until the border of normal sensation is located.[319] The clinician stimulates in the aforementioned patterns and asks the patient "Is this sharp or dull?" or, when making comparisons using the sharp stimulus, "Does this feel the same as this?" (*Note*: It is important that the clinician uses as light a touch as the patient can perceive and not, under any circumstances, presses hard enough to draw blood.)[319] Pinprick sensation is difficult to test because of the natural variations in the pressure put on the pin and the sensitivity of different parts of the skin.

Table 3-21 outlines some of the studies that have been performed to assess the reliability, sensitivity, and specificity of various sensibility tests in detecting radiculopathy.

Pain

Temperature

- *Origin.* Lateral spinothalamic tract.
- *Test.* Using two test tubes, filled with hot and cold water, the clinician touches the skin and asks the patient to identify "hot" or "cold." The impulses for temperature sensation travel together with pain sensation in the lateral spinothalamic tract. The testing of skin temperature can also help the clinician to differentiate between a venous and an arterial insufficiency.[319] With venous insufficiency, an increase in skin temperature is usually noted in the area of occlusion, and the area also appears bluish in color. Pitting edema, especially around the ankles, sacrum, and hands, also may be present. However, if pitting edema is present and the skin temperature is normal, the lymphatic system may be at fault. With arterial insufficiency, a decrease in skin temperature is usually noted in the area of occlusion, and the area appears whiter. It is also extremely painful.

Pressure

- *Origin.* Spinothalamic tract.
- *Test.* Firm pressure is applied to the patient's muscle belly.

Sensory Threshold

- *Origin.* Posterior (dorsal) column/medial lemniscal tract (Box 3-4).
- Threshold tests measure the intensity of the stimulus necessary to depolarize the cell membrane and produce an action potential—the ability to detect. Threshold tests are helpful in assessing diminished sensibility in nerve compressions and in monitoring nerve recovery after

Box 3-4 Posterior (Dorsal) Medial Lemniscus Tract

The posterior (dorsal) medial lemniscus tract conveys impulses concerned with well-localized touch and with the sense of movement and position (kinesthesia). It is important in moment-to-moment (temporal) and point-to-point (spatial) discrimination and makes it possible for a person to perform a task such as putting a key in a door lock without light or to visualize the position of any part of his or her body without looking. Lesions to the tract from destructive tumors, hemorrhage, scar tissue, swelling, infections, and direct trauma, among others, abolish or diminish tactile sensations and movement or position sense. The cell bodies of the primary neurons in the posterior (dorsal) column pathway are located in the spinal ganglion. The peripheral processes of these neurons begin at receptors in the joint capsule, muscles, and skin (tactile and pressure receptors).

surgical decompression.[315,320] Examples of threshold tests include vibratory testing and Semmes–Weinstein monofilament testing.

- *Test.* Vibration testing is performed using a 128-Hz tuning fork applied to a bony prominence such as the ulna or radius in the upper extremity, and the patella or tibia in the lower extremity. The patient is asked to report the perception of both the start of the vibration sensation and the cessation of vibration on dampening. The time difference (in seconds) is recorded and compared with the uninvolved side. Alternatively, a vibrometer, such as the Bio-Thesiometer can be used.[315] The Bio-Thesiometer is an electrically controlled testing instrument that produces vibration at a fixed frequency (120 Hz) with variable amplitude. The vibrating head is applied to the patient's fingertip and the amplitude is slowly and gradually increased. The threshold is recorded as the voltage required to perceive the vibratory stimulus.[315] The clinician applies a series of five trials to determine the cumulative ability of correct responses. A positive test is decreased ability to report when the vibration is applied and reports of vibration dampening while still being applied. If vibration sense is absent, the clinician should retest, moving proximally along the extremity.
- *Test.* The assessment of cutaneous sensibility was first described in 1899, using horse hairs of varying thickness.[321] In 1960, Semmes and Weinstein[322] made the testing procedure more exacting when they introduced the use of pressure-sensitive nylon monofilaments mounted onto Lucite rods (Fig. 3-43). These monofilaments, which are graded according to thickness, are calibrated to exert specific pressures. Each kit consists of 20 probes, each numbered from 1.65 to 6.65, a number that represents the logarithm of 10 multiplied by the force in milligrams required to bow the filaments.[323] The patient is blindfolded or turns away during the examination and the clinician applies each filament perpendicular to the skin until the filament bends, starting with the filament with the lowest number and gradually moving up the scale until the patient feels one before or just as it bends.[324,325] The test is repeated three times for confirmation.[326]

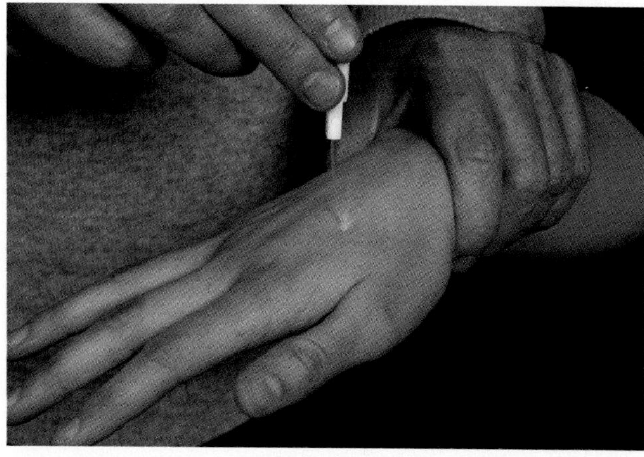

FIGURE 3-43 Semmes and Weinstein filament testing.

CLINICAL PEARL

A cross-sectional multi-group comparison study[327] that examined three screening sensory tests (the Semmes–Weinstein 10 g monofilament examination, superficial pain sensation, and vibration by the on-off method) found all three screening tests to be significantly and positively correlated with nerve conduction studies.

Position Sense (Proprioception)

- *Origin.* Posterior (dorsal) column/medial lemniscal tract (see Box 3-4).
- *Test.* Proprioception here refers to an awareness of the position of joints at rest. The patient is tested for his/her ability to perceive passive movements of the extremities, especially the distal portions. The clinician grasps the patient's big toe, holding it by its sides between the thumb and the index finger, and then pulls it away from the other toes to avoid friction and to prevent extraneous tactile stimulation from indicating a change of position.[319] "Down" and "up" are demonstrated to the patient as the clinician moves the patient's toe clearly upward and downward. Then, with his or her eyes closed, the patient is asked for an "up" or "down" response as the clinician moves the toe in a small arc. This movement is repeated several times on each side, avoiding simple alternation of the stimuli. If position sense is impaired, then the clinician should retest, moving proximally along the extremity. Alternatively, the patient is asked to duplicate the position with the opposite extremity. The joint position sense component of proprioception can also be assessed through the reproduction of both active and passive joint repositioning with the patient blindfolded. The clinician positions the limb to be tested at a preset target angle and holds it there for a minimum of 10 seconds to allow the patient to mentally process the target angle.[319] Following this, the limb is returned to the starting position. The patient is then asked to actively move the limb to the preset target angle. The angular displacement is recorded as the error in degrees from the preset target angle.

Movement Sense (Kinesthesia)

- *Origin.* Posterior (dorsal) column/medial lemniscal tract (see Box 3-4).
- *Test.* The patient is asked to indicate verbally the direction of movement while the extremity is in motion. The clinician must grip the patient's extremity over neutral borders.

Stereognosis

- *Origin.* Posterior (dorsal) column/medial lemniscal tract (see Box 3-4).
- *Test.* The patient is asked to recognize, through touch alone, various small objects such as comb, coins, pencils, and safety pins that are placed in his or her hand.

Graphesthesia

- *Origin.* Posterior (dorsal) column/medial lemniscal tract (see Box 3-4).

- *Test.* The patient is asked to recognize letters, numbers, or designs traced on the skin. Using a blunt object, the clinician draws an image on the patient's palm, asking the patient to identify the number, the letter, or the design.

Neuromuscular Control Testing

Assessment of neuromuscular control can be examined clinically by assessing balance and postural control using the following:[188]

- *Static balance tests.* This includes observation of the patient maintaining different postures. Standardized tests include the single leg balance stance test, Romberg test; sharpened (tandem) Romberg, stork stand test, and timed stance battery (Table 3-22).

CLINICAL PEARL

The Balance Error Scoring System (BESS) is commonly used to evaluate balance, particularly in patients with concussion and fatigue. The BESS consists of three stances: double-leg stance (hands on the hips and feet together), single-leg stance (standing on the nondominant leg with hands on hips), and a tandem stance (standing with the nondominant foot behind the dominant foot in a heel-to-toe fashion). The aforementioned stances are performed on a firm surface and on a foam surface with the eyes closed, with errors (opening the eyes, stumbling or falling out of the position, lifting the hands of the hips, lifting the forefoot or heel, stepping, abducting the hip by more than 30 degrees, or failing to return to the test position in more than 5 seconds) counted during each 20-second trial. The reliability of the BESS ranges from moderate (<0.75) to good (>0.75) while some studies report reliability coefficients below clinically acceptable levels. [Bell DR, Guskiewicz KM, Clark MA, et al: Systematic review of the balance error scoring system. *Sports Health* 3:287–295, 2011.]

- *Dynamic balance tests.* This includes observation of the patient standing or sitting on an unstable surface, or performing postural transitions and functional activities. Emery and colleagues[328] recently described a clinical balance measurement tool designed specifically for neurologically intact adolescents. Participants were timed as they balanced on a high density foam pad with eyes open and eyes closed. Easily reproduced clinically, this test may be used to assess the neuromuscular system's ability to maintain balance on a pliant surface.
- *Anticipatory postural control tests.* This includes observation of the patient catching a ball, opening doors, lifting objects of different weights. Standardized tests include the functional reach test, multidirectional reach test, and the star excursion balance test (Table 3-22).
- *Reactive postural control tests.* This includes observation of the patient's responses to pushes (small or large, slow or rapid, anticipated and unanticipated). Standardized tests include the pull test, backward release, and postural stress test (Table 3-22).
- *Sensory organization tests.* This can be tested using the clinical test of sensory integration on balance, also called the Foam and Dome test (Table 3-22).
- *Vestibular tests.* This includes observation for nystagmus and vertiginous positions. Standardized tests include the Dix–Hallpike maneuver (see Dizziness section), VOR testing (see Reflex Testing section), oculomotor tests (see CN Examination section), Fukuda stepping test (Table 3-22), and the dizziness handicap inventory (Table 3-22).
- *Balance during functional activities.* Functional tasks are observed to test the patient's ability to demonstrate mobility (the ability to move from one position to another independently and safely), static postural control (the ability to maintain postural stability and orientation with the center of mass over the base support and the body at rest), dynamic postural control (the ability to maintain stability and orientation with the center of mass over the BOS while parts of the body are in motion), and skill (the ability to consistently perform coordinated movement sequences for the purposes of investigation and interaction with the physical and social environment) during functional tasks.[329] Standardized tests for this include the Tinetti performance-oriented mobility assessment (Table 3-22), timed up and go test (Table 3-22), Berg balance scale (Table 3-22), gait abnormality rating scale (see Chap. 6), and the functional gait assessment (see Chap. 6).
- *Safety during gait, locomotion, or balance.* This includes documentation on the patient's fall history and a home assessment. Standardized tests for this include the activities-specific balance competence scale, and the fall efficacy scale.

Returning to demanding physical activity requires more advanced functional testing. Single-leg hop tests are commonly used for return to sport assessment as they mimic lower extremity functional demands that challenge stability: generation of power, acceleration and deceleration of body weight, dynamic control of triplanar forces, and maintenance of postural stability.[141] The most commonly used single-leg hop tests include:

- *Hop for distance.* The patient is asked to stand on one limb and to hop as far forward as possible, landing on the same limb and to maintain the landing for a minimum of 2 seconds while the toe measurement (to the nearest centimeter) is recorded.
- *6 m timed hop.* The patient is asked to perform large one-leg hops in series over the 6 m, which is timed to the nearest one-tenth of a second
- *Triple hop for distance.* The patient is asked to perform three hops as far as possible, landing on the same leg and maintaining the landing for a minimum of 2 seconds while the toe measurement (to the nearest centimeter) is recorded.
- *6 m timed crossover hop.* The patient is asked to perform three hops as far as possible crossing over a 15-cm wide strip marking on each hop and to maintain landing after the third hop for 2 seconds. The first of the three hops is lateral with respect to the direction of the crossover (measured to the nearest centimeter).

TABLE 3-22	Balance and Functional Assessment Tests
Test	**Description**
Romberg[a]	Assesses the patient's ability to stand with the feet parallel and together with the eyes open and then closed for 30 s. With the eyes open, the vision, proprioception, and vestibular systems provide input to the cerebellum to maintain truncal stability. If there is a mild lesion in the vestibular or proprioception systems, the patient is usually able to compensate with the eyes open. When the patient closes their eyes, however, visual input is removed and instability can be provoked (a positive Romberg sign). Patients with a vestibular lesion tend to fall in the direction of the lesion.[b] If there is a more severe proprioceptive or vestibular lesion, or if there is a midline cerebellar lesion causing truncal instability, the patient will be unable to maintain this position even with their eyes open.[b] Note that instability can also be seen with lesions in other parts of the nervous system such as the UMNs or LMNs or the basal ganglia, so these should be tested for separately in other parts of the exam. The Romberg test has predictive validity with regard to recurrent falls over a 6-month period in patients with Parkinson's disease: sensitivity was 65% and specificity greater than 90%.[c]
Sharpened (tandem) Romberg[a]	Assesses the patient's ability to stand with the feet in the heel-to-toe position with the arms folded across the chest and eyes closed for 1 min. The rationale for this test is the same as for the Romberg. The ataxic patient will prefer to stand with a wider BOS and will show reluctance when asked to stand with the feet close together.
Single-leg balance stance[d]	Assesses the patient's ability to stand on one leg without shoes and with the arms placed across the chest without letting the legs touch each other. Five 30-s trials are performed for each leg, with the maximum possible score of 150 s per leg. In the acute stage of vestibular loss, a patient will be unable to perform this test[e]; however, patients who have a compensated vestibular loss may test normal.[e] This screening test is not specific to vestibular loss, as patients with other balance disorders may have difficulty performing single leg stance[e]
Stork stand[f]	Assesses the patient's ability to stand on both feet with the hands on the hips, then lift one leg and place the toes of that foot against the knee of the other leg. On command from the tester, the patient then raises the heel to stand on the toes and try to balance as long as possible without letting either the heel touch the ground or the other foot move away from the knee. Normal adults should be able to balance for 20–30 s on each leg
Functional Reach[g] and the Multidirectional Reach[h]	Both of these tests require the patient to reach in different directions as far as possible without changing the BOS
Star Excursion Balance[9,10]	A test of lower extremity reach that challenges an individual's limits of stability. The patient balances on the involved leg while reaching as far as possible with the uninvolved leg in each of eight prescribed vectors or directions while maintaining balance on the contralateral leg. The vectors are named in reference to the stance leg. The test intends to demonstrate dynamic balance deficits by comparing the performance of the involved limb to the uninvolved limb as the ability to reach a distant point along a given vector requires a combination of postural stability, strength, and controlled motion on the stance leg
Pull test[k]	The clinician stands behind the patient and asks the patient to maintain their balance when pulled backwards. The clinician pulls back briskly to assess the patient's ability to recover, being careful to prevent the patient from falling
Backward release[l]	The patient is asked to stand with feet shoulder width apart. The clinician places their hand between the patient's scapulae and the patient is asked to lean back against the clinician's hand. Once the patient is leaning backwards into the clinician's hand, the clinician unexpectedly removes the support. The amount of force created by the patient's lean should be sufficient to invoke a loss of balance that requires a change in the BOS (i.e., at least one backward step)
Postural stress test (PST)[m]	The PST measures an individual's ability to withstand a series of destabilizing forces applied at the level of the subject's waist. Scoring of the postural responses is based on a nine-point ordinal scale, where a score of 9 represents the most efficient postural response and a score of 0 represents a complete failure to remain upright.
Clinical Test of Sensory Integration on Balance (foam and dome test)[n]	This test measures the patient's ability to balance under six different sensory conditions: 1. Standing on a firm surface with the eyes open 2. Standing on a firm surface with the eyes closed 3. Standing on a firm surface wearing a dome made from a modified Japanese lantern 4. Standing on a foam cushion with the eyes open 5. Standing on foam with the eyes closed 6. Standing on foam wearing the dome

(Continued)

TABLE 3-22 Balance and Functional Assessment Tests *(Continued)*

Test	Description
	For each of these conditions the patient stands with the feet parallel and the arms at the sides or the hands on the hips a minimum of three 30-s trials of each condition are performed. Patients with vestibulopathy will have difficulty maintaining an upright posture.[e] Individuals who rely heavily on visual input for balance will become unstable or fall in conditions 2, 3, 5, and 6, whereas those who rely heavily on somatosensory inputs show deficits with conditions 4, 5, and 6
Fukuda stepping test[o]	The test is performed by having the patient stand with the eyes closed and the arms extended forward to shoulder height. The patient is asked to march in place for 50 steps at the pace of a brisk walk. Progressive turning toward one side of 30 degrees or more is considered a positive test and indicates a unilateral peripheral vestibular deficit.
Dizziness handicap inventory[p]	This test assesses a person's perception of the effects of a balance problem and the emotional, physical, or functional adjustments that the person makes. Questionnaire consists of 25 items that are divided into functional (nine items), emotional (nine items), and physical (seven items) subscales. Each item is assigned a value of 4 for a *yes*, 2 points for a *sometimes*, and 0 points for a *no*.
The Berg Balance Scale (BBS)[q]	This 14-item scale was developed to measure balance among older people with impairment in balance function by assessing the performance of functional tasks.
Timed Up and Go (TUG) Test[r]	Patients are timed (in seconds) when performing the TUG under three conditions: 1. TUG alone—from sitting in a chair, stand up, walk 3 m, turn around, walk back, and sit down 2. TUG Cognitive—complete the task while counting backwards from a randomly selected number between 20 and 100 3. TUG manual—complete the task while carrying a full cup of water The time taken to complete the task is strongly correlated to level of functional mobility (i.e. the more time taken, the more dependent in activities of daily living)
Tinetti performance-oriented mobility assessment (POMA)[s]	Easily administered task-oriented test that measures an adult's gait and balance abilities. Rates the ability of an individual to maintain balance while performing activities of daily living-related tasks. Components include balance, lower and upper extremity strength

[a]Newton R: Review of tests of standing balance abilities. *Brain Injury*: [BI] 3: 335–43, 1989.

[b]Simon RP, Aminoff MJ, Greenberg DA: *Clinical Neurology*, 4th ed.). Stanford, CT, Appleton and Lange, 1999.

[c]Bloem BR, Grimbergen YA, Cramer M, et al.: Prospective assessment of falls in Parkinson's disease. *J Neurol*. 248:950–8, 2001.

[d]Vellas BJ, Wayne SJ, Romero L, et al.: One-leg balance is an important predictor of injurious falls in older persons. *JAm Geriatr Soc* 45:735–8, 1997.

[e]Herdman SJ, Whitney SL: Physical therapy assessment of vestibular hypofunction, in Herdman SJ (ed): Vestibular Rehabilitation. 2nd ed. Philadelphia, PA: Davis, 2000.

[f]Hungerford BA, Gilleard W, Moran M, et al.: Evaluation of the ability of physical therapists to palpate intrapelvic motion with the Stork test on the support side. *Phys Ther* 87:879–87, 2007.

[g]Duncan PW, Weiner DK, Chandler J, et al.: Functional reach: a new clinical measure of balance. *J Gerontol*. 45:M192–7, 1990.

[h]Newton RA: Validity of the multi-directional reach test: a practical measure for limits of stability in older adults. *J Gerontol A, Biol Sci Med Sci* 56:M248–52, 2001.

[i]Gray GW: *Lower Extremity Functional Profile*. Adrian, Michigan, MI: Win Marketing, Inc., 1995.

[j]Olmsted LC, Carcia CR, Hertel J, et al.: Efficacy of the Star Excursion Balance Tests in Detecting Reach Deficits in Subjects With Chronic Ankle Instability. *J Ath Train* 37:501–506, 2002.

[k]Munhoz RP, Li JY, Kurtinecz M, et al.: Evaluation of the pull test technique in assessing postural instability in Parkinson's disease. *Neurology* 62:125–7, 2004.

[l]Rose DJ: *Fallproof! A comprehensive balance and mobility program*. Champaign, IL:, Human Kinetics, 2003.

[m]Wolfson LI, Whipple R, Amerman P, et al.: Stressing the postural response. A quantitative method for testing balance. *J Am Geriatr Soc* 34:845–50, 1986.

[n]Shumway-Cook A, Horak FB: Assessing the influence of sensory interaction of balance. Suggestion from the field. *Phys Ther*. 66:1548–50, 1986.

[o]Fukuda T: The stepping test: two phases of the labyrinthine reflex. *Acta Otolaryngol* 50:95–108, 1959.

[p]Jacobson GP, Newman CW: The development of the Dizziness Handicap Inventory. *Arch Otolaryngol Head Neck Surg*. 116:424–7, 1990.

[q]Berg KO, Wood-Dauphinee SL, Williams JI, et al.: Measuring balance in the elderly: validation of an instrument. *Can J Public Health. Revue canadienne de sante publique 83 Suppl* 2:S7–11, 1992.

[r]Podsiadlo D, Richardson S: The timed "Up & Go": a test of basic functional mobility for frail elderly persons. *J Am Geriatr Soc*. 39:142–8, 1991.

[s]Tinetti ME: Performance-oriented assessment of mobility problems in elderly patients. *J Am Geriatr Soc* 34:119–26, 1986.

The average of each trial type is used to calculate a limb symmetry index (LSI). The LSI is calculated by comparing the performance of the involved and uninvolved limb (LSI=involved/uninvolved*100% for the distance measures and LSI=uninvolved/involved*100% for the timed hop).[330]

Coordination

Voluntary movement patterns involve functionally linked muscles or synergies that act cooperatively to produce an action and are defined by precise spatial and temporal organization. The movement patterns can be assessed using various simple coordination tasks.

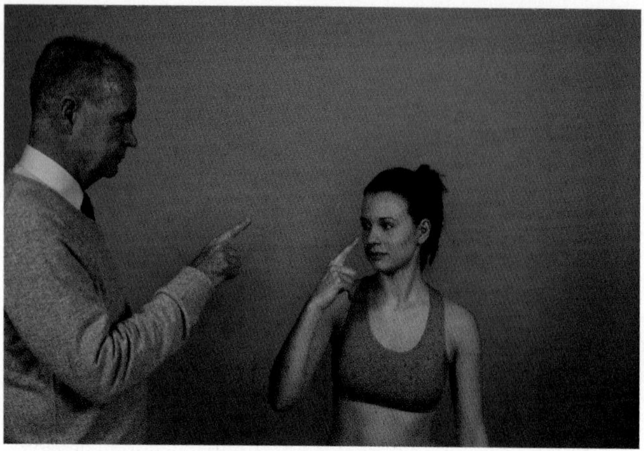

FIGURE 3-44 Finger-to-nose test.

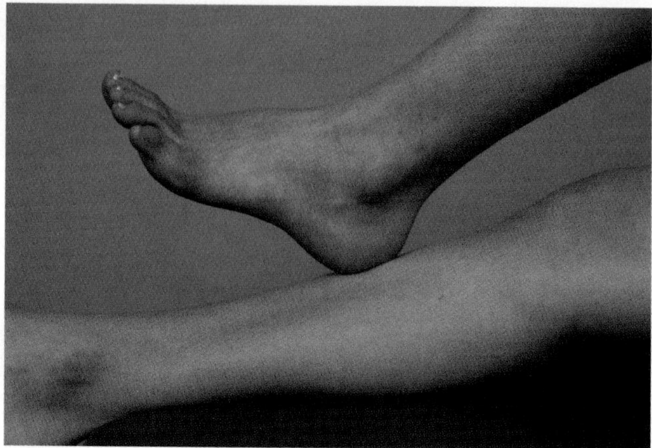

FIGURE 3-46 Heel-to-shin test.

- *Finger-to-nose test.*[269] In the finger-to-nose test, the patient is asked to move the index finger to the tip of the nose or the chin with the eyes open, while the clinician observes the quality of arm motion (Fig. 3-44). Closing the eyes eliminates visual substitution. Mild cerebellar ataxia results in an intention tremor near the beginning and the end of the movement with possible overshooting of the target.[331]
- *Finger-to-finger test.*[269] With the finger-to-finger test, the patient attempts to touch his or her finger to the clinician's finger (Fig. 3-45). Horizontal overshooting implicates a unilateral labyrinthine lesion; vertical overshooting occurs in patients with midline lesions to the medulla oblongata or the bilateral cerebellar flocculus.
- *Heel-to-shin test.*[269] The heel-to-shin test, which tests for leg ataxia, involves having the supine patient track the heel of the foot smoothly up and down the contralateral shin (Fig. 3-46). Alternatively, the patient can be positioned in sitting and can be asked to touch the great toe to the clinician's finger.

Tonal Abnormality

An examination of tone consists of initial observation of resting posture and palpation, and passive motion testing, and active motion testing while observing for any abnormalities.[319]

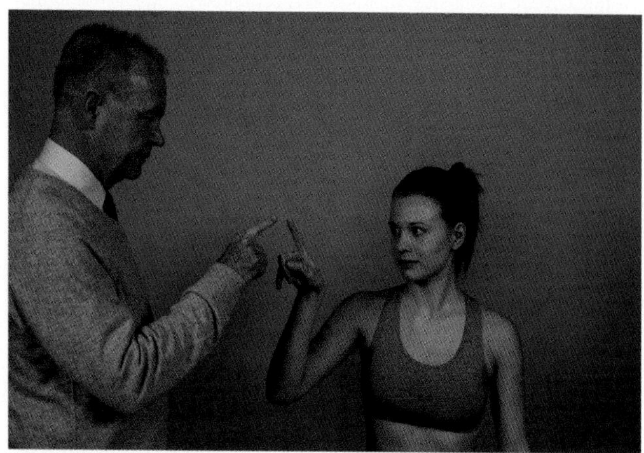

FIGURE 3-45 Finger-to-finger test.

Spasticity

Spasticity is defined as a velocity-dependent resistance to passive stretch. Larger and quicker stretches produce stronger resistance of the spastic muscle.

- *Clasped-knife phenomenon.* During rapid movement, initial high resistance (spastic catch) may be followed by a sudden inhibition or letting go of the limb (relaxation) in response to a stretch stimulus.
- *Clonus.* This is an exaggeration of the stretch reflex and is characterized by cyclical, spasmodic alternation of muscular contraction and relaxation in response to sustained stretch of the spastic muscle.

Rigidity

Rigidity is defined as an increased resistance to all motions, rendering body parts stiff and immovable.

- *Cogwheel phenomenon.* This is a ratchet-like response to passive movement, characterized by an alternate giving and increased resistance to movement.
- *Leadpipe rigidity.* Characterized by constant rigidity throughout the range of motion, this finding is common in patients with Parkinson disease.

Hypotonia

Hypotonia and flaccidity are the terms used to define decreased or absent muscular tone. This state is manifested by diminished resistance to passive movement, dampened or absent stretch reflexes, and limbs that are easily moved.

Dystonia

Dystonia is a hyperkinetic movement disorder characterized by disordered tone and involuntary movements involving large portions of the body. Dystonia typically results from a CNS lesion but can be inherited.

Posturing

In cases of significant brain lesions, the body can adopt two characteristic positions:

- *Decorticate positioning.* Upper extremities are held in flexion and the lower extremities, in extension.

- *Decerebrate positioning.* Upper and lower extremities are held in extension.

CN Examination

With practice, the entire CN examination can be performed in approximately 5 minutes (Table 3-23).[312] The following rhyme may be used to help remember the order and tests for the CN examination[332]:

Smell and see
And look around,
Pupils large and smaller.
Smile, hear!
Then say ah . . .

TABLE 3-23 CNs and Methods of Testing

Nerves	Function: Afferent (Sensory)	Function: Efferent (Motor)	Tests
I—Olfactory	Smell	—	Unilateral identification of familiar odors (e.g., chocolate and coffee)
II—Optic	Sight	—	Visual acuity, peripheral vision, and pupillary light reflex
III—Oculomotor	—	*Voluntary motor:* levator of eyelid; superior, medial, and inferior recti; and inferior oblique muscle of eyeball *Autonomic:* smooth muscle of eyeball	Upward, downward, and medial gaze; reaction to light
IV—Trochlear	—	*Voluntary motor:* superior oblique muscle of eyeball	Extraocular eye movements: downward and lateral gaze
V—Trigeminal	Touch, pain: skin of face, mucous membranes of nose, sinuses, mouth, and anterior tongue	*Voluntary motor:* muscles of mastication	Corneal reflex; sensation above eye, between eye and mouth, below mouth to angle of jaw; clench teeth, push down on chin to separate jaws
VI—Abducens	—	*Voluntary motor:* lateral rectus muscle of eyeball	Lateral gaze (eye abduction)
VII—Facial	Taste: anterior two-thirds of tongue	*Voluntary motor:* facial muscles *Autonomic:* lacrimal, submandibular, and sublingual glands	Facial expressions (close eyes tight, smile and show teeth, and whistle and puff cheeks) and identify familiar tastes (e.g., sweet and sour)
VIII—Vestibulocochlear (acoustic nerve)	Hearing/equilibrium	—	Hearing tests and balance and coordination tests
IX—Glossopharyngeal	Visceral sensibility (pharynx, tongue, and tonsils); taste	*Voluntary motor:* unimportant muscle of pharynx *Autonomic:* parotid gland	Gag reflex, ability to swallow, and phonation
X—Vagus	Touch, pain; pharynx, larynx, trachea, bronchi, and lungs Taste: tongue and epiglottis	*Voluntary motor:* muscles of palate, pharynx, and larynx *Autonomic:* involuntary muscle and gland control	Gag reflex, ability to swallow, and speech (phonation)
XI—Accessory	—	*Voluntary motor:* movement of head and shoulders—sternocleidomastoid and trapezius muscles	Resisted head and shoulder shrug
XII—Hypoglossal	—	*Voluntary motor:* movement of tongue	Tongue protrusion (if injured, tongue deviates toward injured side) and inspection of tongue for atrophy

And see if you can swallow.
If you're left in any doubt,
Shrug and stick your tongue right out.

CN I (Olfactory)

The sense of smell is tested by having the patient identify familiar odors (e.g., coffee, lavender, and vanilla) with each nostril. The clinician should avoid irritant odors that can stimulate the trigeminal nerve.

CN II (Optic)

The optic nerve is tested by examining visual acuity and confrontation. Although the formal testing of visual acuity is presented here, in reality, it is sufficient to test this aspect of CN II at the same time that CN III, IV, and VI are being tested.

Visual Acuity

This is a test of central vision. If possible, the clinician should use a well-lit Snellen eye chart. The patient is positioned 20 ft from the chart. Patients who use corrective lenses other than reading glasses should be instructed to use them. The patient is asked to cover one eye and to read the smallest line possible. A patient who cannot read the largest letter should be positioned closer to the chart and the new distance noted. The clinician determines the smallest line of print from which the patient can identify more than half the letters. The visual acuity designated at the side of this line, together with the use of glasses, if any, is recorded.

Visual acuity is expressed as a fraction (e.g., 20/20), in which the numerator indicates the distance of the patient from the chart and the denominator the distance at which a normal eye can read the letters.

Confrontation Test

This is a rough clinical test of peripheral vision that also highlights a loss of vision in one of the visual fields. The patient and the clinician sit facing each other, with their eyes level. Both the lateral and medial fields of vision are tested. The entire lateral field is tested with both eyes open, and the medial field is tested by covering one eye. When testing the medial field of vision, the clinician covers the patient's eye that is directly opposite to the clinician's own (not diagonally opposite).

With arms outstretched and hands holding a small object such as a pencil, the clinician slowly brings the object into the peripheral field of vision of the patient. This is performed from eight separate directions. Each time the patient is asked to say "now" as soon as he or she sees the object. During the examination, the clinician should keep the object equidistant between his or her own eye and the patient's so that the patient's visual field can be compared to the clinician's own.

CN III (Oculomotor), CN IV (Trochlear), and CN VI (Abducens)

These three CNs are tested together. The clinician:

- Inspects the size and the shape of each pupil for symmetry.

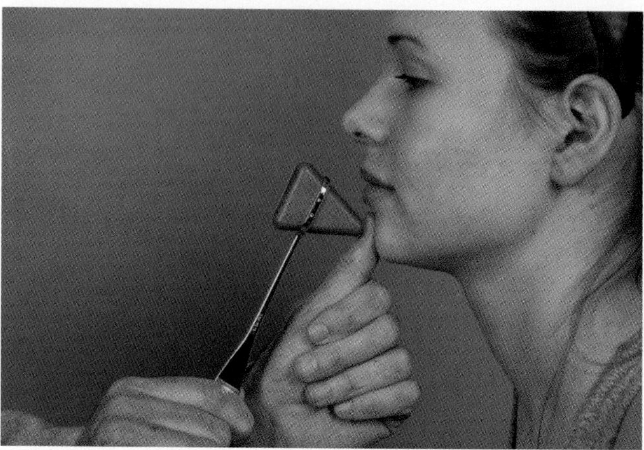

FIGURE 3-47 Jaw tendon reflex assessment.

- Tests the consensual pupillary response to light. This is tested by having the patient cover one eye, while the clinician observes the uncovered eye. The uncovered eye should undergo the same changes as the covered by first dilating, and then constricting, when the covered eye is uncovered.
- Looks for the ability of the eyes to track movement in the six fields of gaze. The standard test is to smoothly move a target in an "H" configuration and then in midline just above eye level toward the base of the nose (convergence).[8] The patient should be able to smoothly track a target at moderate speed, without evidence of nystagmus.
- Looks for ptosis of the upper eyelids.

CN V (Trigeminal)

The patient is asked to clench the teeth, and the clinician palpates the temporal and masseter muscles. The three sensory branches of the trigeminal nerve are tested with pinprick close to the mid-line of the face, because the skin that is more lateral is overlapped by the nerves of the face.[8] The jaw muscle stretch reflex is assessed for the presence of hyperreflexia (Fig. 3-47).

CN VII (Facial)

The clinician inspects the face at rest and in conversation with the patient and notes any asymmetry. The patient is asked to smile. If there is any asymmetry, the patient is asked to frown or wrinkle the forehead. Loss or reduced ability to smile and frown is caused by a peripheral palsy, whereas the loss of the smile, only, is caused by a supranuclear lesion.[8]

CN VIII (Vestibulocochlear)

The vestibular nerve can be tested in a number of ways, depending on the objective. Balance testing assesses the vestibulospinal reflex. Caloric stimulation can be used to assess the VOR. The VOR can also be assessed by testing the ability of the eyes to follow a moving object.

The clinician assesses the function of the cochlear component of the nerve—hearing—by gently rubbing two fingers equidistant from each of the patient's ears simultaneously or by using a 256-Hz tuning fork and asking the patient to identify in which ear the noise appears to be the loudest.

There are three basic types of hearing loss[332]:

- *Conductive.* This type of hearing loss applies to any disturbance in the conduction of the sound impulse as it passes through the ear canal, the tympanic membrane, the middle ear, and the ossicular chain to the footplate of the stapes, which is situated in the oval window. As a general rule, an individual with conductive hearing loss speaks softly, hears well on the telephone, and hears best in a noisy environment.
- *Sensorineural.* This type of hearing loss applies to a disturbance anywhere from the cochlea through the auditory nerve and on to the hearing center in the cerebral cortex. As a general rule, an individual with a perceptive hearing loss usually speaks loudly, hears better in a quiet environment, and hears poorly in a crowd and on the telephone.
- *Mixed.* This type of hearing loss is a combination of conductive and sensorineural.

If hearing loss is present, then the clinician should test for lateralization and compare air and bone conduction.

Lateralization

The clinician places a tuning fork over the vertex, middle of the forehead, or front teeth. The patient is asked whether the vibration is heard more in one ear (Weber test). Normal individuals cannot lateralize the vibration to either ear. In conduction deafness (e.g., that caused by middle ear disease), the vibration is heard more in the affected ear. In sensorineural deafness, the vibration is heard more in the normal ear.

Air and Bone Conduction

Air conduction is assessed by placing the tuning fork in front of the external auditory meatus, whereas bone conduction is assessed by placing the tuning fork on the mastoid process (Rinne test). In a normal individual, the tuning fork is heard louder and longer by air than by bone conduction. In conduction deafness, bone conduction hearing is better. In sensorineural deafness, both air and bone conduction are reduced, although air conduction is the better of the two.

CN IX (Glossopharyngeal)

The gag reflex is used to test this nerve, but this test is reserved for severely affected patients only.

CN X (Vagus)

The clinician listens to the patient's voice and notes any hoarseness or nasal quality. The patient is asked to open the mouth and say "Aah," while the clinician watches the movements of the soft palate and pharynx. The soft palate should rise symmetrically, the uvula should remain in the midline, and each side of the posterior pharynx should move medially.

CN XI (Spinal Accessory)

From behind the patient, the clinician notes any atrophy or fasciculation in the trapezius muscles and compares side to side. The patient is asked to shrug both shoulders upward against the clinician's hand. The strength of contraction should be noted.

The patient is asked to attempt to turn his or her head to each side against the clinician's hand. The contraction of the sternocleidomastoid and the force of contraction should be noted.

CN XII (Hypoglossal)

The clinician inspects the tongue, as it lies on the floor of the mouth, looking for fasciculation. The patient is then asked to stick out the tongue. The clinician looks for asymmetry, atrophy, or deviation from the midline. The patient is asked to move the tongue from side to side, as the clinician notes symmetry of movement.

REVIEW QUESTIONS*

1. Injury to the radial nerve in the spiral groove would result in:
   A. weakness of elbow flexion
   B. inability to initiate abduction
   C. inability to control rotation during abduction
   D. inability of the rotator cuff muscles to hold the humeral head in its socket
   E. none of the above
2. A patient with a musculocutaneous nerve injury is still able to flex the elbow. The major muscle causing elbow flexion is the
   A. brachioradialis
   B. flexor carpi ulnaris
   C. pronator quadratus
   D. extensor carpi ulnaris
   E. pectoralis major
3. Which of the following muscles is *not* innervated by the median nerve?
   A. abductor pollicis brevis
   B. flexor pollicis longus
   C. medial heads of flexor digitorum profundus
   D. superficial head of flexor pollicis brevis
   E. pronator quadratus
4. The nerve that innervates the first lumbrical muscle in the hand is the
   A. median nerve
   B. ulnar nerve
   C. radial nerve
   D. anterior interosseous nerve
   E. LCN of the hand

*Additional questions to test your understanding of this chapter can be found in the Online Learning Center for *Orthopaedic Assessment, Evaluation, and Intervention* at www.duttononline.net.

5. After a nerve injury, regeneration occurs proximally first and then progresses distally at a rate of approximately 1 mm per day.

Following a radial nerve injury in the axilla, which muscle would be the last to recover?

A. long head of the triceps

B. anconeus

C. extensor indicis

D. extensor digiti minimi

E. supinator

REFERENCES

1. Martin J: Introduction to the central nervous system. In: Martin J, ed. *Neuroanatomy: Text and Atlas*, 2nd ed. New York, NY: McGraw-Hill, 1996:1–32.
2. Waxman SG: *Correlative Neuroanatomy*, 24th ed. New York, NY: McGraw-Hill, 1996.
3. Butler DS, Tomberlin JP: Peripheral nerve: structure, function, and physiology. In: Magee D, Zachazewski JE, Quillen WS, eds. *Scientific Foundations and Principles of Practice in Musculoskeletal Rehabilitation*. St. Louis, MO: WB Saunders, 2007:175–189.
4. Pratt N: *Anatomy of the Cervical Spine*. La Crosse, WI: Orthopaedic Section, APTA, 1996.
5. Millesi H, Terzis JK: Nomenclature in peripheral nerve surgery. In: Terzis JK, ed. *Microreconstruction of Nerve Injuries*. Philadelphia, PA: WB Saunders, 1987:3–13.
6. Thomas PK, Olsson Y: Microscopic anatomy and function of the connective tissue components of peripheral nerve. In: Dyck PJ, Thomas PK, Lambert EH, et al., eds. *Peripheral Neuropathy*. Philadelphia, PA: WB Saunders, 1984:97–120.
7. Rydevik B, Garfin SR: Spinal nerve root compression. In: Szabo RM, ed. *Nerve Compression Syndromes: Diagnosis and Treatment*. Thorofare, NJ: Slack, 1989:247–261.
8. Meadows J: *Orthopedic Differential Diagnosis in Physical Therapy*. New York, NY: McGraw-Hill, 1999.
9. Sunderland S: Anatomical perivertebral influences on the intervertebral foramen. In: Goldstein MN, ed. *The Research Status of Spinal Manipulative Therapy*. Bethesda, MD: HEW Publication No (NIH), 1975:76–998.
10. Sunderland S: *Nerves and Nerve Injuries*. Edinburgh: E & S Livingstone, Ltd, 1968.
11. Durrant JD, Freeman AR: Concepts in vestibular physiology. In: Finestone AJ, ed. *Dizziness and Vertigo*. Boston, MA: John Wright PSG Inc., 1982:13–43.
12. Meadows J: *A Rationale and Complete Approach to the Sub-Acute Post-MVA Cervical Patient*. Calgary, AB: Swodeam Consulting, 1995.
13. Bogduk N: Innervation and pain patterns of the cervical spine. In: Grant R, ed. *Physical Therapy of the Cervical and Thoracic Spine*. New York, NY: Churchill Livingstone, 1988.
14. Neumann DA: Elbow and forearm complex. In: Neumann DA, ed. *Kinesiology of the Musculoskeletal System: Foundations for Physical Rehabilitation*. St. Louis, MO: Mosby, 2002:133–171.
15. Martin JH, Jessell TM: Anatomy of the somatic sensory system. In: Kandel ER, Schwartz JH, Jessell TM, eds. *Principles of Neural Science*. New York, NY: Elsevier, 1991:353–366.
16. Fawcett DW: The nervous tissue. In: Fawcett DW, ed. *Bloom and Fawcett: A Textbook of Histology*. New York, NY: Chapman & Hall, 1984:336–339.
17. Chusid JG: *Correlative Neuroanatomy & Functional Neurology*, 19th ed. Norwalk, CT: Appleton-Century-Crofts, 1985:144–148.
18. Daniels DL, Hyde JS, Kneeland JB, et al.: The cervical nerves and foramina: Local-coil MRI imaging. *AJNR* 7:129–133, 1986.
19. Pech P, Daniels DL, Williams AL, et al.: The cervical neural foramina: Correlation of microtomy and CT anatomy. *Radiology* 155:143–146, 1985.
20. Tanaka N, Fujimoto Y, An HS, et al.: The anatomic relation among the nerve roots, intervertebral foramina, and intervertebral discs of the cervical spine. *Spine* 25:286–291, 2000.
21. Goodman BW: Neck pain. *Prim Care* 15:689–707, 1988.
22. Brooker AEW, Barter RW: Cervical spondylosis: A clinical study with comparative radiology. *Brain* 88:925–936, 1965.
23. Gore DR, Sepic SB, Gardner GM, et al.: Roentgenographic findings in the cervical spine of asymptomatic people. *Spine* 6:521–526, 1987.
24. Carter GT, Kilmer DD, Bonekat HW, et al.: Evaluation of phrenic nerve and pulmonary function in hereditary motor and sensory neuropathy type 1. *Muscle Nerve* 15:459–456, 1992.
25. Bolton CF: Clinical neurophysiology of the respiratory system. *Muscle Nerve* 16:809–818, 1993.
26. Jenkins DB: *Hollinshead's Functional Anatomy of the Limbs and Back*, 7th ed. Philadelphia, PA: WB Saunders, 1998.
27. Koppell HP, Thompson WAL: *Peripheral Entrapment Neuropathies*, 2nd ed. New York, NY: R.E. Kreiger, 1976.
28. Dumestre G: Long thoracic nerve palsy. *J Man Manip Ther* 3:44–49, 1995.
29. Gozna ER, Harris WR: Traumatic winging of the scapula. *J Bone Joint Surg* 61A:1230–1233, 1979.
30. Kauppila LI: The long thoracic nerve: Possible mechanisms of injury based on autopsy study. *J Shoulder Elbow Surg* 2:244–248, 1993.
31. Kauppila LI, Vastamaki M: Iatrogenic serratus anterior paralysis: Long-term outcome in 26 patients. *Chest* 109:31–34, 1996.
32. Johnson JTH, Kendall HO: Isolated paralysis of the serratus anterior muscle. *J Bone Joint Surg* 37A:567–574, 1955.
33. Miller T: Peripheral nerve injuries at the shoulder. *J Man Manip Ther* 6:170–183, 1998.
34. Martin JT: Postoperative isolated dysfunction of the long thoracic nerve: A rare entity of uncertain etiology. *Anesth Analg* 69:614–619, 1989.
35. Gregg JR, Labosky D, Hearty M, et al.: Serratus anterior paralysis in the young athlete. *J Bone Joint Surg* 61A:825–832, 1979.
36. Schultz JS, Leonard JA: Long thoracic neuropathy from athletic activity. *Arch Phys Med Rehab* 73:87–90, 1992.
37. Warner JJ, Navarro RA: Serratus anterior dysfunction. Recognition and treatment. *Clin Orthop Relat Res* 349:139–148, 1998.
38. Brecker LR: Jenny McConnell offers new technique for problem shoulders. *Adv Phys Ther* 11–12, 1993.
39. Goodman CE, Kenrick MM, Blum MV: Long thoracic nerve palsy: A follow-up study. *Arch Phys Med Rehab* 56:352–355, 1975.
40. Reis FP, de Camargo AM, Vitti M, et al.: Electromyographic study of the subclavius muscle. *Acta Anat* 105:284–290, 1979.
41. Hoffman GW, Elliott LF: The anatomy of the pectoral nerves and its significance to the general and plastic surgeon. *Ann Surg* 205:504, 1987.
42. Strauch B, Yu HL: *Atlas of Microvascular Surgery: Anatomy and Operative Approaches*. New York, NY: Thieme Medical Publishers, 1993.
43. Kerr A: The brachial plexus of nerves in man, the variations in its formation and branches. *Am J Anat* 23:285–376, 1918.
44. Wichman R: Die Rückenmarksnerven und ihre segmentbezüge. In: Kerr A, ed. *The Brachial Plexus of Nerves in Man, the Variations in its Formation and Branches*. 23:285–376, 1918.
45. Beghi E, Kurland LT, Mulder DW, et al.: Brachial plexus neuropathy in the population of Rochester, Minnesota, 1970–1981. *Ann Neurol* 118; 320–323, 1985.
46. Terzis JK, Liberson WT, Levine R: Obstetric brachial plexus palsy. *Hand Clin* 2:773, 1986.
47. Terzis JK, Liberson WT, Levine R: Our experience in obstetrical brachial plexus palsy. In: Terzis JK, ed. *Microreconstruction of Nerve Injuries*. Philadelphia, PA: Saunders, 1987:513.
48. Duchenne GBA: *De l'Électrisation localisée et de son application à la pathologie et à la thérapeutique par courants induits et par courants galvaniques interrompus et continus*, 3rd ed. Paris: Librairie J. B. Baillière et fils, 1872.
49. Erb W: Uber eine eigenthümliche Localisation von Lahmungen im plexus brachialis. *Naturhist.-Med Ver Heidelberg Verh* 2:130, 1874.
50. Klumpke A: Contribution à l'étude des paralysies radiculaires du plexus brachial. *Rev Med* 5:739, 1885.
51. Brown KLB: Review of obstetrical palsies: Nonoperative treatment. In: Terzis JK, ed. *Microreconstruction of Nerve Injuries*. Philadelphia, PA: WB Saunders, 1987:499.
52. Brown KLB: Review of obstetrical palsies: Nonoperative treatment. *Clin Plast Surg* 11:181, 1984.
53. Gilbert A, Tassin J-L: Obstetrical palsy: A clinical, pathologic, and surgical review. In: Terzis JK, ed. *Microreconstruction of Nerve Injuries*. Philadelphia, PA: WB Saunders, 1987:529.
54. Bonnard C, Anastakis DJ, van Melle G, et al.: Isolated and combined lesions of the axillary nerve: A review of 146 cases. *J Bone Joint Surg* 81B:212–217, 1999.

55. Wright TA: Accessory spinal nerve injury. *Clin Orth Rel Res* 108:15–18, 1975.
56. Wright PE II, Jobe MT: Peripheral nerve injuries. In: Canale ST, Daugherty K, Jones L, eds. *Campbell's Operative Orthopaedics*, 9th ed. St Louis, MO: Mosby Year Book, 1998:3827–3894.
57. Cohn BT, Brahms MA, Cohn M: Injury to the eleventh cranial nerve in a high school wrestler. *Orthop Rev* 15:590–595, 1986.
58. Laska T, Hannig K: Physical therapy for spinal accessory nerve injury complicated by adhesive capsulitis. *Phys Ther* 81:936–944, 2001.
59. Petersen CM: Spinal accessory nerve palsy. *J Man Manip Ther* 4:65–69, 1996.
60. Winkel D, Matthijs O, Phelps V: *Pathology of the shoulder, Diagnosis and Treatment of the Upper Extremities*. Maryland, MD: Aspen, 1997:68–117.
61. Ajmani ML: The cutaneous branch of the human suprascapular nerve. *J Anat* 185:439–442, 1994.
62. Horiguchi M: The cutaneous branch of some human suprascapular nerves. *J Anat* 130:191–195, 1980.
63. Murakami T, Ohtani O, Outi H: Suprascapular nerve with cutaneous branch to the upper arm [in Japanese]. *Acta Anat Nippon* 52:96, 1977.
64. Drye C, Zachazewski JE: Peripheral nerve injuries. In: Zachazewski JE, Magee DJ, Quillen WS, eds. *Athletic Injuries and Rehabilitation*. Philadelphia, PA: WB Saunders, 1996:441–463.
65. Ringel SP, Treihaft M, Carry M, et al.: Suprascapular neuropathy in pitchers. *Am J Sports Med* 18:80–86, 1990.
66. Mallon WJ, Bronec PR, Spinner RJ, et al.: Suprascapular neuropathy after distal clavicle resection. *Clin Orthop* 329:207–211, 1996.
67. Fabre T, Piton C, Leclouerec G, et al.: Entrapment of the suprascapular nerve. *J Bone Joint Surg* 81B:414–419, 1999.
68. Drez DJ Jr: Suprascapular neuropathy in the differential diagnosis of rotator cuff injuries. *Am J Sports Med* 4:43–45, 1976.
69. Ferretti A, Cerullo G, Russo G: Suprascapular neuropathy in volleyball players. *J Bone Joint Surg* 69A:260–263, 1987.
70. Clein L: Suprascapular entrapment neuropathy. *J Neurosurg* 43:337–342, 1975.
71. Delagi EF, Perotto A: Arm. In: Delagi EF, Perotto A, eds. *Anatomic Guide for the Electromyographer*, 2nd ed. Springfield, IL: Charles C Thomas, 1981:66–71.
72. Sunderland S: The musculocutaneous nerve. In: Sunderland S, ed. *Nerves and Nerve Injuries*, 2nd ed. Edinburgh: Churchill Livingstone, 1978:796–801.
73. de Moura WG Jr: Surgical anatomy of the musculocutaneous nerve: A photographic essay. *J Reconstr Microsurg* 1:291–297, 1985.
74. Flatow EL, Bigliani LU, April EW: An anatomic study of the musculocutaneous nerve and its relationship to the coracoid process. *Clin Orthop* 244:166–171, 1989.
75. Dundore DE, DeLisa JA: Musculocutaneous nerve palsy: An isolated complication of surgery. *Arch Phys Med Rehabil* 60:130–133, 1979.
76. Braddom RL, Wolf C: Musculocutaneous nerve injury after heavy exercise. *Arch Phys Med Rehab* 59:290–293, 1978.
77. Sander HW, Quinto CM, Elinzano H, et al.: Carpet carrier's palsy: Musculocutaneous neuropathy. *Neurology* 48:1731–1732, 1997.
78. Mastaglia FL: Musculocutaneous neuropathy after strenuous physical activity. *Med J Aust* 145:153–154, 1986.
79. Kim SM, Goodrich JA: Isolated proximal musculocutaneous nerve palsy. *Arch Phys Med Rehab* 65:735–736, 1984.
80. Bierman W, Yamshon LJ: Electromyography in kinesiologic evaluations. *Arch Phys Med Rehabil* 29:206–211, 1948.
81. Mendoza FX, Main K: Peripheral nerve injuries of the shoulder in the athlete. *Clin Sports Med* 9:331–341, 1990.
82. Paladini D, Dellantonio R, Cinti A, et al.: Axillary neuropathy in volleyball players: report of two cases and literature review. *J Neurol Neurosurg Psychiatry* 60:345–347, 1996.
83. Loomer R, Graham B: Anatomy of the axillary nerve and its relation to inferior capsular shift. *Clin Orth Rel Res* 291:103–106, 1993.
84. Ombregt L, Bisschop P, et al.: Nerve lesions and entrapment neuropathies of the upper limb. In: Ombregt L, ed. *A System of Orthopaedic Medicine*. London: WB Saunders, 1995:378–401.
85. Stern PJ, Kutz JE: An unusual variant of the anterior interosseous nerve syndrome: A case report and review of the literature. *J Hand Surg* 5:32–34, 1980.
86. Hope PG: Anterior interosseous nerve palsy following internal fixation of the proximal radius. *J Bone Joint Surg* 70B:280–282, 1988.
87. Amadio PC, Beckenbaugh RD: Entrapment of the ulnar nerve by the deep flexor-pronator aponeurosis. *J Hand Surg Am* 11A:83–87, 1986.
88. Hirasawa Y, Sawamura H, Sakakida K: Entrapment neuropathy due to bilateral epitrochlearis muscles: A case report. *J Hand Surg Am* 4:181–184, 1979.
89. Sunderland S: *The Ulnar Nerve, Nerves and Nerve Injuries*. Edinburgh: Churchill Livingstone, 1968:816–828.
90. Apfelberg DB, Larson SJ: Dynamic anatomy of the ulnar nerve at the elbow. *Plast Reconstr Surg* 51:76–81, 1973.
91. Chen FS, Rokito AS, Jobe FW: Medial elbow problems in the overhead-throwing athlete. *J Am Acad Orthop Surg* 9:99–113, 2001.
92. Groen GJ, Stolker RJ: Thoracic neural anatomy. In: Giles LGF, Singer KP, eds. *Clinical Anatomy and Management of the Thoracic Spine*. Oxford: Butterworth-Heinemann, 2000:114–141.
93. Hovelacque A: *Anatoime des neufs craniens et radichiens et du sisteme grand sympathetique chez l'homme*. Paris: Gaston Doin et Cie, 1927.
94. Haymaker W, Woodhall B: *Peripheral Nerve Injuries. Principles of Diagnosis*. London: WB Saunders, 1953.
95. Williams PL, Warwick R, Dyson M, et al.: *Gray's Anatomy*, 37th ed. London: Churchill Livingstone, 1989.
96. Mannheimer JS, Lampe GN: *Clinical Transcutaneous Electrical Nerve Stimulation*. Philadelphia, PA: F. A. Davis, 1984:440–445.
97. McGuckin N: The T4 syndrome. In: Grieve GP, ed. *Modern Manual Therapy of the Vertebral Column*. New York, NY: Churchill Livingstone, 1986:370–6.
98. DeFranca GG, Levine LJ: The T4 syndrome. *J Manip Physiol Ther* 18:34–37, 1995.
99. Grieve GP: Thoracic musculoskeletal problems. In: Boyling JD, Palastanga N, eds. *Grieve's Modern Manual Therapy of the Vertebral Column*, 2nd ed. Edinburgh: Churchill Livingstone, 1994:401–428.
100. Warfel BS, Marini SG, Lachmann EA, et al.: Delayed femoral nerve palsy following femoral vessel catheterization. *Arch Phys Med Rehabil* 74:1211–1215, 1993.
101. Hardy SL: Femoral nerve palsy associated with an associated posterior wall transverse acetabular fracture. *J Orthop Trauma* 11:40–42, 1997.
102. Papastefanou SL, Stevens K, Mulholland RC: Femoral nerve palsy: An unusual complication of anterior lumbar interbody fusion. *Spine* 19:2842–2844, 1994.
103. Fealy S, Paletta GA Jr: Femoral nerve palsy secondary to traumatic iliacus muscle hematoma: course after nonoperative management. *J Trauma* 47:1150–1152, 1999.
104. Bradshaw C, McCrory P, Bell S, et al.: Obturator neuropathy a cause of chronic groin pain in athletes. *Am J Sports Med* 25:402–408, 1997.
105. Harvey G, Bell S: Obturator neuropathy. An anatomic perspective. *Clin Orthop Relat Res* 363:203–211, 1999.
106. Ecker AD, Woltman HW: Meralgia paresthetica: A report of one hundred and fifty cases. *J Am Med Assoc* 110:1650–1652, 1938.
107. Keegan JJ, Holyoke EA: Meralgia paresthetica: An anatomical and surgical study. *J Neurosurg* 19:341–345, 1962.
108. Reichert FL: Meralgia paresthetica; a form of causalgia relieved by interruption of the sympathetic fibers. *Surg Clin North Am* 13:1443, 1933.
109. Edelson JG, Nathan H: Meralgia paresthetica. *Clin Orthop* 122:255–262, 1977.
110. Ivins GK: Meralgia paresthetica, the elusive diagnosis: Clinical experience with 14 adult patients. *Ann Surg* 232:281–286, 2000.
111. Nathan H: Gangliform enlargement on the lateral cutaneous nerve of the thigh. *J Neurosurg* 17:843, 1960.
112. Ghent WR: Further studies on meralgia paresthetica. *Can Med J* 85:871, 1961.
113. Stookey B: Meralgia paresthetica: Etiology and surgical treatment. *JAMA* 90:1705, 1928.
114. Williams PH, Trzil KP: Management of meralgia paresthetica. *J Neurosurg* 74:76, 1991.
115. Sunderland S: Traumatized nerves, roots and ganglia: Musculoskeletal factors and neuropathological consequences. In: Knorr IM, Huntwork EH, eds. *The Neurobiologic Mechanisms in Manipulative Therapy*. New York, NY: Plenum Press, 1978:137–166.
116. Kenny P, O'Brien CP, Synnott K, et al.: Damage to the superior gluteal nerve after two different approaches to the hip. *J Bone Joint Surg* Br 81B:979–981, 1999.
117. Lu J, Ebraheim NA, Huntoon M, et al.: Anatomic considerations of superior cluneal nerve at posterior iliac crest region. *Clin Orthop Relat Res* 347:224–228, 1998.
118. Netter FH: *Lumbar, sacral, and coccygeal plexuses (The CIBA collection of medical illustrations), Nervous system, pt I*. West Caldwell, NJ: Ciba, 1991:122–123.

119. Sogaard I: Sciatic nerve entrapment: Case report. *J Neurosurg* 58:275–276, 1983.
120. Robinson DR: Pyriformis syndrome in relation to sciatic pain. *Am J Surg* 73:355–358, 1947.
121. Benyahya E, Etaouil N, Janani S, et al.: Sciatica as the first manifestation of leiomyosarcoma of the buttock. *Rev Rheum* 64:135–137, 1997.
122. Lamki N, Hutton L, Wall WJ, et al.: Computed tomography in pelvic liposarcoma: A case report. *J Comput Tomogr* 8:249–251, 1984.
123. Resnick D: *Diagnosis of bone and joint disorders.* Philadelphia, PA: Saunders, 1995.
124. Ohsawa K, Nishida T, Kurohmaru M, et al.: Distribution pattern of pudendal nerve plexus for the phallus retractor muscles in the cock. *Okajimas Folia Anat Jpn* 67:439–441, 1991.
125. Morgenlander JC: The autonomic nervous system. In: Gilman S, ed. *Clinical Examination of the Nervous System.* New York, NY: McGraw-Hill, 2000:213–225.
126. Blumberg H, Janig W: Clinic manifestations of reflex sympathetic dystrophy and sympathetically maintained pain. In: Wall PD, Melzack R, eds. *Textbook of Pain.* London: Churchill Livingstone, 1994: 685–698.
127. Woolf CJ: The dorsal horn: State-dependent sensory processing and the generation of pain. In: Wall PD, Melzack R, eds. *Textbook of Pain.* London: Churchill Livingstone, 1994:201–220.
128. Walker SM, Cousins MJ: Complex regional pain syndromes: including 'reflex sympathetic dystrophy' and 'causalgia'. *Anaesth Intensive Care* 25:113–125, 1997.
129. Linortner P, Fazekas F, Schmidt R, et al.: White matter hyperintensities alter functional organization of the motor system. *Neurobiol Aging*, 2010.
130. Lawrence DG, Kuypers HG: The functional organization of the motor system in the monkey. I. The effects of bilateral pyramidal lesions. *Brain* 91:1–14, 1968.
131. van Kan PL, McCurdy ML: Discharge of primate magnocellular red nucleus neurons during reaching to grasp in different spatial locations. Experimental brain research. Experimentelle Hirnforschung. *Experimentation Cerebrale* 142:151–157, 2002.
132. Buford JA, Davidson AG: Movement-related and preparatory activity in the reticulospinal system of the monkey. Experimental brain research. Experimentelle Hirnforschung. *Experimentation Cerebrale* 159:284–300, 2004.
133. Drew T, Prentice S, Schepens B: Cortical and brainstem control of locomotion. *Prog Brain Res* 143:251–261, 2004.
134. Drew T: Motor cortical activity during voluntary gait modifications in the cat. I. Cells related to the forelimbs. *J Neurophysiol* 70:179–199, 1993.
135. Drew T, Jiang W, Kably B, et al.: Role of the motor cortex in the control of visually triggered gait modifications. *Can J Physiol Pharmacol* 74:426–442, 1996.
136. Agnati LF, Franzen O, Ferre S, et al.: Possible role of intramembrane receptor-receptor interactions in memory and learning via formation of long-lived heteromeric complexes: focus on motor learning in the basal ganglia. *J Neural Transm Suppl* 65:1–28, 2003.
137. Agnati LF, Fuxe K, Ferri M, et al.: A new hypothesis on memory – a possible role of local circuits in the formation of the memory trace. *Med Biol.* 59:224–229, 1981.
138. Morris C, Chaitow L, Janda V: Functional examination for low back syndromes. In: Morris C, ed. *Low Back Syndromes: Integrated Clinical Management.* New York, NY: McGraw-Hill, 2006:333–416.
139. Kottke FJ: From reflex to skill: the training of coordination. *Arch Phys Med Rehabil* 61:551–561, 1980.
140. Kottke FJ, Halpern D, Easton JK, et al.: The training of coordination. *Arch Phys Med Rehabil* 59:567–572, 1978.
141. Rose J: Dynamic lower extremity stability. In: Hughes C, ed. *Movement Disorders and Neuromuscular Interventions for the Trunk and Extremities – Independent Study Course 18.2.5.* La Crosse, WI: Orthopaedic Section, APTA, Inc., 2008:1–34.
142. Williams GR, Chmielewski T, Rudolph KS, et al.: Dynamic knee stability: current theory and implications for clinicians and scientists. *J Orthop Sports Phys Ther* 31:546–566, 2001.
143. Schmidt R, Lee T: *Motor Control and Learning,* 4th ed. Champaign, IL: Human Kinetics, 2005.
144. Williams GN, Krishnan C: Articular neurophysiology and sensorimotor control. In: Magee D, Zachazewski JE, Quillen WS, eds. *Scientific Foundations and Principles of Practice in Musculoskeletal Rehabilitation.* St. Louis, MO: WB Saunders, 2007:190–216.
145. Voight ML, Cook G, Blackburn TA: Functional lower quarter exercises through reactive neuromuscular training. In: Bandy WD, ed. *Current Trends for the Rehabilitation of the Athlete – Home Study Course.* La Crosse, WI: Sports Physical Therapy Section, APTA, Inc., 1997.
146. McCloskey DI: Kinesthetic sensibility. *Physiol Rev* 58:763–820, 1978.
147. Borsa PA, Lephart SM, Kocher MS, et al.: Functional assessment and rehabilitation of shoulder proprioception for glenohumeral instability. *J Sport Rehabil* 3:84–104, 1994.
148. Lephart SM, Warner JJP, Borsa PA, et al.: Proprioception of the shoulder joint in healthy, unstable and surgically repaired shoulders. *J Shoulder Elbow Surg* 3:371–380, 1994.
149. Freeman MAR, Wyke BD: An experimental study of articular neurology. *J Bone Joint Surg* 49B:185, 1967.
150. Wyke BD: The neurology of joints: a review of general principles. *Clin Rheum Dis* 7:223–239, 1981.
151. Voight ML, Cook G: Impaired neuromuscular control: Reactive neuromuscular training. In: Voight ML, Hoogenboom BJ, Prentice WE, eds. *Musculoskeletal Interventions: Techniques for Therapeutic Exercise.* New York, NY: McGraw-Hill, 2007:181–212.
152. Voss H: Tabulation of the absolute and relative muscular spindle numbers in human skeletal musculature. *Anat Anz* 129:562–572, 1971.
153. Peck D, Buxton DF, Nitz A: A comparison of spindle concentrations in large and small muscles acting in parallel combinations. *J Morphol* 180:243–252, 1984.
154. Nyland J, Lachman N, Kocabey Y, et al.: Anatomy, function, and rehabilitation of the popliteus musculotendinous complex. *J Orthop Sports Phys Ther* 35:165–179, 2005.
155. Grigg P, Hoffmann AH: Properties of Ruffini afferents revealed by stress analysis of isolated sections of cat knee capsule. *J Neurophysiol* 47:41–54, 1982.
156. Zimny ML: Mechanoreceptors in articular tissues. *Am J Anat* 182:16–32, 1988.
157. Wyke BD: Articular neurology and manipulative therapy. In: Glasgow EF, Twomey LT, Scull ER, et al., eds. *Aspects of Manipulative Therapy,* 2nd ed. New York, NY: Churchill Livingstone: 72–77, 1985.
158. Grigg A, Hoffman AH, Fogarty KE: Properties of Golgi-Mazzoni afferents in cat knee joint capsule, as revealed by mechanical studies of isolated joint capsule. *J Neurophysiol* 47:31–40, 1982.
159. Schutte MJ, Happel RT: Joint innervation in joint injury. *Clin Sports Med* 9:511–517, 1990.
160. Milne RJ, Foreman RD, Giesler GJ, et al.: Convergence of cutaneous and pelvic visceral nociceptive inputs onto primate spinothalamic neurons. *Pain* 11:163–183, 1981.
161. Vierck CJ, Greenspan JD, Ritz LA: Long-term changes in purposive and reflexive responses to nociceptive stimulation following anterior-lateral chordotomy. *J Neurosci* 10:2077–2095, 1990.
162. Schaible HG, Schmidt RF: Discharge characteristics of receptors with fine afferents from normal and inflamed joints: influence of analgesics and prostaglandins. *Agents Actions Suppl* 19:99–117, 1986.
163. Lee WA: Anticipatory control of postural and task muscles during rapid arm flexion. *J Mot Behav* 12:185–196, 1980.
164. Lephart SM, Henry TJ: Functional rehabilitation for the upper and lower extremity. *Orthop Clin North Am* 26:579–592, 1995.
165. Phillips CG, Powell TP, Wiesendanger M: Projection from low-threshold muscle afferents of hand and forearm to area 3a of baboon's cortex. *J Physiol* 217:419–446, 1971.
166. Barrett DS: Proprioception and function after anterior cruciate ligament reconstruction. *J Bone Joint Surg* 73B:833–837, 1991.
167. Barrack RL, Skinner HB, Buckley SL: Proprioception in the anterior cruciate deficient knee. *Am J Sports Med* 17:1–6, 1989.
168. Skinner HB, Wyatt MP, Hodgdon JA, et al.: Effect of fatigue on joint position sense of the knee. *J Orthop Res* 4:112–118, 1986.
169. Voight ML, Cook G: Impaired neuromuscular control: Reactive neuromuscular training. In: Prentice WE, Voight ML, eds. *Techniques in Musculoskeletal Rehabilitation.* New York, NY: McGraw-Hill, 2001:93–124.
170. Chmielewski TL, Hewett TE, Hurd WJ, et al.: Principles of neuromuscular control for injury prevention and rehabilitation. In: Magee D, Zachazewski JE, Quillen WS, eds. *Scientific Foundations and Principles of Practice in Musculoskeletal Rehabilitation.* St. Louis, MO: WB Saunders, 2007:375–387.
171. Johnston RB III, Howard ME, Cawley PW, et al.: Effect of lower extremity muscular fatigue on motor control performance. *Med Sci Sports Exerc* 30:1703–1707, 1998.

172. Skinner HB, Barrack RL, Cook SD: Age-related decline in proprioception. *Clin Orthop* 184:208–211, 1984.
173. Barrett DS, Cobb AG, Bentley G: Joint proprioception in normal, osteoarthritic and replaced knees. *J Bone Joint Surg* 73-B:53–56, 1991.
174. Beard DJ, Kyberd PJ, Fergusson CM, et al.: Proprioception after rupture of the anterior cruciate ligament. An objective indication of the need for surgery? *J Bone Joint Surg* 75-B:311–315, 1993.
175. Corrigan JP, Cashman WF, Brady MP: Proprioception in the cruciate deficient knee. *J Bone Joint Surg* 74-B:247–250, 1992.
176. Fremerey RW, Lobenhoffer P, Zeichen J, et al.: Proprioception after rehabilitation and reconstruction in knees with deficiency of the anterior cruciate ligament: a prospective, longitudinal study. *J Bone Joint Surg Br* 82:801–806, 2000.
177. Voight M, Blackburn T: Proprioception and balance training and testing following injury. In: Ellenbecker TS, ed. *Knee Ligament Rehabilitation.* Philadelphia, PA: Churchill Livingstone, 2000:361–385.
178. Wright A, Zusman M: Neurophysiology of pain and pain modulation. In: Boyling JD, Jull GA, eds. *Grieve's Modern Manual Therapy: The Vertebral Column.* Philadelphia, PA: Churchill Livingstone, 2004: 155–171.
179. Bogduk N: The anatomy and physiology of nociception. In: Crosbie J, McConnell J, eds. *Key Issues in Physiotherapy.* Oxford: Butterworth-Heinemann, 1993:48–87.
180. Winstein CJ, Knecht HG: Movement science and its relevance to physical therapy. *Phys Ther* 70:759–762, 1990.
181. Winstein CJ: Knowledge of results and motor learning–implications for physical therapy. *Phys Ther* 71:140–149, 1991.
182. Winstein CJ: Motor learning considerations in stroke rehabilitation. In: Duncan PW, Badke MB, eds. *Stroke Rehabilitation: The Recovery of Motor Control.* Chicago, IL: Yearbook Medical Publishers, Inc., 1987:109–134.
183. Buford JA: Neuroscience of motor control and learning. In: Hughes C, ed. *Movement Disorders and Neuromuscular Interventions for the Trunk and Extremities – Independent Study Course 18.2.1.* La Crosse, WI: Orthopaedic Section, APTA, Inc., 2008:1–23.
184. Kisner C, Colby LA: Therapeutic exercise: Foundational concepts. In: Kisner C, Colby LA, eds. *Therapeutic Exercise. Foundations and Techniques,* 5th ed. Philadelphia, PA: FA Davis, 2002:1–36.
185. Magill RA: *Motor Learning and Control: Concepts and Applications,* 8th ed. New York, NY: McGraw-Hill, 2007.
186. Gentile AM: Skill acquisition: action, movement, and neuromotor processes. In: Carr J, Shepherd R, eds. *Movement Science: Foundations for Physical Therapy in Rehabilitation.* Gaithersburg, MD: Aspen, 2000:111–187.
187. Kloos AD, Givens-Heiss D: Exercise for impaired balance. In: Kisner C, Colby LA, eds. *Therapeutic Exercise. Foundations and Techniques,* 5th ed. Philadelphia, PA: FA Davis, 2002:251–272.
188. Kloos A: Mechanics and control of posture and balance. In: Hughes C, ed. *Movement Disorders and Neuromuscular Interventions for the Trunk and Extremities – Independent Study Course 18.2.2.* La Crosse, WI: Orthopaedic Section, APTA, Inc., 2008:1–26.
189. Horak FB: Postural orientation and equilibrium: what do we need to know about neural control of balance to prevent falls? *Age Ageing* 35 (Suppl 2):ii7–ii11, 2006.
190. Nashner LM: Sensory, neuromuscular, and biomechanical contributions to human balance., *Balance: Proceedings of the American Physical Therapy Association Forum.* Nashville, TN, June 13–15 1989.
191. Horak FB, Nashner LM: Central programming of postural movements: adaptation to altered support-surface configurations. *J Neurophysiol* 55:1369–1381, 1986.
192. Cordo PJ, Nashner LM: Properties of postural adjustments associated with rapid arm movements. *J Neurophysiol* 47:287–302, 1982.
193. Nashner LM, Forssberg H: Phase-dependent organization of postural adjustments associated with arm movements while walking. *J Neurophysiol* 55:1382–1394, 1986.
194. Krishnamoorthy V, Latash ML: Reversals of anticipatory postural adjustments during voluntary sway in humans. *J Physiol* 565:675–684, 2005.
195. Rogers MW, Pai YC: Dynamic transitions in stance support accompanying leg flexion movements in man. Experimental brain research. Experimentelle Hirnforschung. *Experimentation Cerebrale* 81:398–402, 1990.
196. Mouchnino L, Aurenty R, Massion J, et al.: Coordination between equilibrium and head-trunk orientation during leg movement: a new strategy build up by training. *J Neurophysiol* 67:1587–1598, 1992.
197. Oddsson L, Thorstensson A: Fast voluntary trunk flexion movements in standing: motor patterns. *Acta Physiol Scand* 129:93–106, 1987.
198. Pedotti A, Crenna P, Deat A, et al.: Postural synergies in axial movements: short and long-term adaptation. Experimental brain research. Experimentelle Hirnforschung. *Experimentation Cerebrale* 74:3–10, 1989.
199. Friedli WG, Hallett M, Simon SR: Postural adjustments associated with rapid voluntary arm movements 1. Electromyographic data. *J Neurol Neurosurg Psychiatry* 47:611–622, 1984.
200. Aruin AS, Latash ML: The role of motor action in anticipatory postural adjustments studied with self-induced and externally triggered perturbations. Experimental brain research. Experimentelle Hirnforschung. *Experimentation Cerebrale* 106:291–300, 1995.
201. De Wolf S, Slijper H, Latash ML: Anticipatory postural adjustments during self-paced and reaction-time movements. Experimental brain research. Experimentelle Hirnforschung. *Experimentation Cerebrale* 121:7–19, 1998.
202. Benvenuti F, Stanhope SJ, Thomas SL, et al.: Flexibility of anticipatory postural adjustments revealed by self-paced and reaction-time arm movements. *Brain Research* 761:59–70, 1997.
203. Denegar CR, Donley PB: Impairment due to pain: Managing pain during the rehabilitation process. In: Voight ML, Hoogenboom BJ, Prentice WE, eds. *Musculoskeletal Interventions: Techniques for Therapeutic Exercise.* New York, NY: McGraw-Hill, 2007:99–110.
204. Dray A: Inflammatory mediators of pain. *Br J Anaesth* 75:125–131, 1995.
205. Wiener SL: *Differential Diagnosis of Acute pain by Body Region.* New York, NY: McGraw-Hill, 1993:1–4.
206. Adams RD, Victor M: *Principles of Neurology,* 5th ed. New York, NY: McGraw-Hill, Health Professions Division, 1993.
207. Judge RD, Zuidema GD, Fitzgerald FT: Musculoskeletal system. In: Judge RD, Zuidema GD, Fitzgerald FT, eds. *Clinical Diagnosis,* 4th ed. Boston, MA: Little, Brown and Company, 1982:365–403.
208. Bonica JJ: Neurophysiological and pathological aspects of acute and chronic pain. *Arch Surg* 112:750–761, 1977.
209. Burkhardt CS: The use of the McGill Pain Questionnaire in assessing arthritis pain. *Pain* 19:305, 1984.
210. Chaturvedi SK: Prevalence of chronic pain in psychiatric patients. *Pain* 29:231–237, 1987.
211. Dunn D: Chronic regional pain syndrome, type 1: Part I. *AORN J* 72: 421–424,426,428–432,435,437–442,444–449,452–458, 2000.
212. Steen KH, Reeh PW, Anton F, et al.: Protons selectively induce lasting excitation and sensitization to mechanical stimulation of nociceptors in rat skin, in vitro. *J Neurosci* 12:86–95, 1992.
213. Besson JM: The neurobiology of pain. *Lancet* 353:1610–1615, 1999.
214. Sterling M, Jull G, Wright A: The effect of musculoskeletal pain on motor activity and control. *J Pain.* 2:135–145, 2001.
215. Hides JA, Richardson CA, Jull GA: Multifidus muscle recovery is not automatic after resolution of acute, first-episode low back pain. *Spine* 21:2763–2769, 1996.
216. Hodges P, Richardson C: Inefficient muscular stabilisation of the lumbar spine associated with low back pain: a motor control evaluation of transversus abdominis. *Spine* 21:2540–2650, 1996.
217. Voight M, Weider D: Comparative reflex response times of the vastus medialis and the vastus lateralis in normal subjects and subjects with extensor mechanism dysfunction. *Am J Sports Med* 10:131–137, 1991.
218. Dubner R, Ren K: Endogenous mechanisms of sensory modulation. *Pain Suppl* 6:S45–S53, 1999.
219. Grieve GP: The masqueraders. In: Boyling JD, Palastanga N, eds. *Grieve's Modern Manual Therapy,* 2nd ed. Edinburgh: Churchill Livingstone, 1994:841–856.
220. Donelson R, Aprill C, Medcalf R, et al.: A prospective study of centralization in lumbar referred pain. A predictor of symptomatic discs and anular competence. *Spine* 22:1115–1122, 1997.
221. Takahashi Y, Sato A, Nakamura SI, et al.: Regional correspondence between the ventral portion of the lumbar intervertebral disc and the groin mediated by a spinal reflex. A possible basis of discogenic referred pain. *Spine* 23:1853–1858; discussion 1859, 1998.
222. Akeyson EW, Schramm LP: Processing of splanchnic and somatic input in thoracic spinal cord of the rat. *Am J Physiol* 266:R257–R267, 1994.
223. Bryan RN, Trevino DL, Coulter JD, et al.: Location and somatotopic organization of the cells of origin of the spinocervical tract. *Exp Brain Res* 17:177–189, 1973.

224. Dawson NJ, Schmid H, Pierau F-K: Pre-spinal convergence between thoracic and visceral nerves of the rat. *Neurosci Lett* 138:149–152, 1992.
225. Schmidt RF: *Fundamentals of Sensory Physiology (in Japanese)*. Tokyo: Kinpodo, 1980:120–125.
226. Jinkins JR, Whittemore AR, Bradley WG: The anatomic basis of vertebrogenic pain and the autonomic syndrome associated with lumbar disc extrusion. *Am J Roentgenol* 152:1277–1289, 1989.
227. MacNab I: *Backache*. Baltimore, MD: Williams and Wilkins, 1978:98–100.
228. Stowell T, Cioffredi W, Greiner A, et al.: Abdominal differential diagnosis in a patient referred to a physical therapy clinic for low back pain. *J Orthop Sports Phys Ther* 35:755–764, 2005.
229. Goodman CC, Boissonnault WG, Fuller KS: *Pathology: Implications for the Physical Therapist*, 2nd ed. Philadelphia, PA: Saunders, 2003.
230. Barsky AJ, Goodson JD, Lane RS, et al.: The amplification of somatic symptoms. *Psychosom Med* 50:510–519, 1988.
231. Waddell G, Main CJ, Morris EW, et al.: Chronic low back pain, psychological distress and illness behavior. *Spine* 9:209–213, 1984.
232. Werneke MW, Harris DE, Lichter RL: Clinical effectiveness of behavioral signs for screening low-back pain patients in a work oriented physical rehabilitation program. *Spine* 18:2412, 1993.
233. Kenna O, Murtagh A: The physical examination of the back. *Aust Fam Physician* 14:1244–1256, 1985.
234. Melzack R, Wall PD: On the nature of cutaneous sensory mechanisms. *Brain* 85:331–356, 1962.
235. Nathan PW: The gate-control theory of pain—a critical review. *Brain* 99:123–158, 1976.
236. Melzack R: The gate theory revisited. In: LeRoy PL, ed. *Current Concepts in the Management of Chronic Pain*. Miami, FL: Symposia Specialists, 1977.
237. Casey KL: Forebrain mechanisms of nociception and pain: analysis through imaging. *Proc Natl Acad Sci U S A*. 96:7668–7674, 1999.
238. Chudler EH, Dong WK: The role of the basal ganglia in nociception and pain. *Pain* 60:3–38, 1995.
239. Lovick TA: The periaqueductal gray-rostral medulla connection in the defence reaction: efferent pathways and descending control mechanisms. *Behav Brain Res* 58:19–25, 1993.
240. Mayer DJ, Price DD: Central nervous system mechanisms of analgesia. *Pain* 2:379–404, 1976.
241. Fields HL, Anderson SD: Evidence that raphe-spinal neurons mediate opiate and midbrain stimulation-produced analgesias. *Pain* 5:333–349, 1978.
242. Abadi RV: Mechanisms underlying nystagmus. *J R Soc Med* 95:231–234, 2002.
243. Hulse M: *Die zervikalen Gleichgewichtsstorungen*. Berlin: Springer, 1983.
244. Dvorak J, Dvorak V: Differential diagnosis of vertigo. In: Gilliar WG, Greenman PE, eds. *Manual Medicine: Diagnostics*, 2nd ed. New York, NY: Thieme Medical Publishers, 1990:67–70.
245. Rigueiro-Veloso MT, et al.: Wallenberg's syndrome: a review of 25 cases. *Rev Neurol* 25:1561, 1997.
246. Norrving B, Cronqvist S: Lateral medullary infarction: prognosis in an unselected series. *Neurology* 41:244–248, 1991.
247. Chia L-G, Shen W-C: Wallenberg's lateral medullary syndrome with loss of pain and temperature sensation on the contralateral face: clinical, MRI and electrophysiological studies. *J Neurol* 240:462–467, 1993.
248. Kim JS, Lee JH, Suh DC, et al.: Spectrum of lateral medullary syndrome: correlation between clinical findings and magnetic resonance imaging in 33 subjects. *Stroke* 25:1405–1410, 1994.
249. Jenkins IH, Frackowiak RSJ: Functional studies of the human cerebellum with positron emission tomography. *Rev Neurol* 149:647–653, 1993.
250. Molinari M, Leggio MG, Solida A, et al.: Cerebellum and procedural learning: evidence from focal cerebellar lesions. *Brain* 120:1753–1762, 1997.
251. Kim SG, Ugurbil K, Strick PL: Activation of a cerebellar output nucleus during cognitive processing. *Science* 265:949–951, 1994.
252. Pierrot-Deseilligny E, Mazieres L: Spinal mechanisms underlying spasticity. In: Delwaide PJ, Young RR, eds. *Clinical Neurophysiology in Spasticity: Contribution to Assessment and Pathophysiology*. Amsterdam: Elsevier BV, 1985:63–76.
253. Hoppenfeld S: *Orthopedic Neurology – A Diagnostic Guide to Neurological Levels*. Philadelphia, PA: JB Lippincott, 1977.
254. Ashby P, McCrea D: Neurophysiology of spinal spasticity. In: Davidoff RA, ed. *Handbook of the Spinal Cord*. New York, NY: Marcel Decker, 1987:119–143.
255. Meissner I, Wiebers DO, Swanson JW, et al.: The natural history of drop attacks. *Neurology* 36:1029–1034, 1986.
256. Zeiler K, Zeitlhofer J: Syncopal consciousness disorders and drop attacks from the neurologic viewpoint. *Wiener Klinische Wochenschrift* 100: 93–99, 1988.
257. Kameyama M: Vertigo and drop attack. With special reference to cerebrovascular disorders and atherosclerosis of the vertebral-basilar system. *Geriatrics* 20:892–900, 1965.
258. Bardella L, Maleci A, Di Lorenzo N: Drop attack as the only symptom of type 1 Chiari malformation. Illustration by a case. (Italian). *Rivista di Patologia Nervosa e Mentale* 105:217–222, 1984.
259. Schochet SS, Jr: Intoxications and metabolic diseases of the central nervous system. In: Nelson JS, Parisi JE, Schochet SS Jr, eds. *Principles and Practice of Neuropathology*. St. Louis, MO: Mosby, 1993: 302–343.
260. Harper CG, Giles M, Finlay-Jones R: Clinical signs in the Wernicke-Korsakoff complex: a retrospective analysis of 131 cases diagnosed at necropsy. *J Neurol Neurosurg Psychiatry* 49:341–345, 1986.
261. Brazis PW, Lee AG: Binocular vertical diplopia. *Mayo Clin Proc* 73:55–66, 1998.
262. Giles CL, Henderson JW: Horner's syndrome: an analysis of 216 cases. *Am J Ophthalmol* 46:289–296, 1958.
263. Jermyn RT: A nonsurgical approach to low back pain. *J Am Osteopath Assoc* 101:(suppl):S6–S11, 2001.
264. Mohn A, di Ricco L, Magnelli A, et al.: Celiac disease–associated vertigo and nystagmus. *J Pediatr Gastroenterol Nutr* 34:317–318, 2002.
265. Huijbregts P, Vidal P: Dizziness in orthopedic physical therapy practice: classification and pathophysiology. *J Man Manip Ther* 12:199–214, 2004.
266. Silbert PL, Mokri B, Schievink WI: Headache and neck pain in spontaneous internal carotid and vertebral artery dissections. *Neurology* 45:1517–1522, 1995.
267. Bogduk N: Cervical causes of headache and dizziness. In: Grieve GP, ed. *Modern Manual Therapy of the Vertebral Column*. New York, NY: Churchill Livingstone, 1986:289–302.
268. Fast A, Zincola DF, Marin EL: Vertebral artery damage complicating cervical manipulation. *Spine* 12:840, 1987.
269. Huijbregts P, Vidal P: Dizziness in orthopedic physical therapy practice: history and physical examination. *J Man Manip Ther* 13:221–250, 2005.
270. Magee DJ: Principles and concepts. In: Magee DJ, ed. *Orthopedic Physical Assessment*, 5th ed. Philadelphia, PA: W.B. Saunders, 2008:1–70.
271. Diamond MC, Scheibel AB, Elson LM: *The Human Brain Coloring Book*. New York, NY: Harper & Row, 1985.
272. Nadler SF, Rigolosi L, Kim D, et al.: Sensory, motor, and reflex examination. In: Malanga GA, Nadler SF, eds. *Musculoskeletal Physical Examination – An Evidence-Based Approach*. Philadelphia, PA: Elsevier-Mosby, 2006:15–32.
273. Guide to physical therapist practice. *Phys Ther* 81:S13–S95, 2001.
274. Gilman S: The physical and neurologic examination. In: Gilman S, ed. *Clinical Examination of the Nervous System*. New York, NY: McGraw-Hill, 2000:15–34.
275. Currier RD, Fitzgerald FT: Nervous system. In: Judge RD, Zuidema GD, Fitzgerald FT, eds. *Clinical Diagnosis*, 4th ed. Boston, MA: Little, Brown and Company, 1982 :405–445.
276. van Adrichem JA, van der Korst JK: Assessment of the flexibility of the lumbar spine. A pilot study in children and adolescents. *Scand J Rheumatol* 2:87–91, 1973.
277. O'Keeffe ST, Smith T, Valacio R, et al.: A comparison of two techniques for ankle jerk assessment in elderly subjects. *Lancet* 344:1619–1620, 1994.
278. Manschot S, van Passel L, Buskens E, et al.: Mayo and NINDS scales for assessment of tendon reflexes: between observer agreement and implications for communication. *J Neurol Neurosurg Psychiatry* 64:253–255, 1998.
279. Soloman J, Nadler SF, Press J: Physical examination of the lumbar spine. In: Malanga GA, Nadler SF, eds. *Musculoskeletal Physical Examination – An Evidence-Based Approach*. Philadelphia, PA: Elsevier-Mosby, 2006: 189–226.
280. Halle JS: The neuromusculoskeletal scan examination. In: Voight ML, Hoogenboom BJ, Prentice WE, eds. *Musculoskeletal Interventions: Techniques for Therapeutic Exercise*. New York, NY: McGraw-Hill, 2007:47–80.
281. Vogel HP: Influence of additional information on interrater reliability in the neurologic examination. *Neurology* 42:2076–2081, 1992.
282. Halle JS: Neuromusculoskeletal scan examination with selected related topics. In: Flynn TW, ed. *The Thoracic Spine and Rib Cage:*

Musculoskeletal Evaluation and Treatment. Boston, MA: Butterworth-Heinemann, 1996:121–146.

283. Dommisse GF, Grobler L: Arteries and veins of the lumbar nerve roots and cauda equina. *Clin Orthop* 115:22–29, 1976.
284. Babinski J: Réflexes tendineux & réflexes osseux. Paris: Imprimerie Typographique R. Tancrede, 1912.
285. Babinski J: Du phénomène des orteils et de sa valeur sémiologique. *Semaine Méd* 18:321–322, 1898.
286. Babinski J: De l'abduction des orteils. *Rev Neurol* 11:728–729, 1903.
287. Gonda VE: A new tendon stretch reflex; its significance in disease of the pyramidal tract. Schweizer Archiv fur Neurologie und Psychiatrie. Archives suisses de neurologie et de psychiatrie. *Archivio svizzero di neurologia e psichiatria* 71:97–99, 1953.
288. Ghosh D, Pradhan S: "Extensor toe sign" by various methods in spastic children with cerebral palsy. *J Child Neurol* 13:216–220, 1998.
289. Kumar SP, Ramasubramanian D: The Babinski sign–a reappraisal. *Neuro India* 48:314–318, 2000.
290. Denno JJ, Meadows GR: Early diagnosis of cervical spondylotic myelopathy: a useful clinical sign. *Spine* 16:1353–1355, 1991.
291. Estanol BV, Marin OS: Mechanism of the inverted supinator reflex. A clinical and neurophysiological study. *J Neurol Neurosurg Psychiatry* 39:905–908, 1976.
292. Kiely P, Baker JF, O'HEireamhoin S, et al.: The evaluation of the inverted supinator reflex in asymptomatic patients. *Spine* 35:955–957, 2010.
293. Wong TM, Leung HB, Wong WC: Correlation between magnetic resonance imaging and radiographic measurement of cervical spine in cervical myelopathic patients. *J Orthop Surg* 12:239–242, 2004.
294. Owen G, Mulley GP: The palmomental reflex: a useful clinical sign? *J Neurol Neurosurg Psychiatry* 73:113–115, 2002.
295. Isakov E, Sazbon L, Costeff H, et al.: The diagnostic value of three common primitive reflexes. *Eur Neurol* 23:17–21, 1984.
296. Post M: *Physical Examination of the Musculoskeletal System*. Chicago, IL: Year Book Medical Publishers, 1987.
297. Awerbuch GI, Nigro MA, Wishnow R: Beevor's sign and facioscapulohumeral dystrophy. *Arch Neurol* 47:1208–1209, 1990.
298. Kanchandani R, Howe JG: Lhermitte's sign in multiple sclerosis: a clinical survey and review of the literature. *J Neurol Neurosurg Psychiatry* 45:308–312, 1982.
299. Al-Araji AH, Oger J: Reappraisal of Lhermitte's sign in multiple sclerosis. *Mult Scler* 11:398–402, 2005.
300. Newton HB, Rea GL: Lhermitte's sign as a presenting symptom of primary spinal cord tumor. *J Neurooncol* 29:183–188, 1996.
301. Smith KJ, McDonald WI: Spontaneous and mechanically evoked activity due to central demyelinating lesion. *Nature* 286:154–155, 1980.
302. Sandmark H, Nisell R: Validity of five common manual neck pain provoking tests. *Scand J Rehabil Med* 27:131–136, 1995.
303. Willoughby EW, Eason R: The crossed upgoing toe sign: a clinical study. *Ann Neurol* 14:480–482, 1983.
304. Buttner-Ennever JA, Horn AKE: The neuroanatomical basis of oculomotor disorders: the dual motor control of extraocular muscles and its possible role in proprioception. *Curr Opin Neurol* 15:35–43, 2002.
305. Buttner-Ennever JA, Cohen B, Horn AKE, et al.: Efferent pathways of the nucleus of the optic tract in monkey and their role in eye movements. *J Comp Neurol* 373:90–107, 1996.
306. Morningstar MW, Pettibon BR, Schlappi H, et al.: Reflex control of the spine and posture: a review of the literature from a chiropractic perspective. *Chiropr Osteopat* 13:16, 2005.
307. Kori AA, Leigh JL: The cranial nerve examination. In: Gilman S, ed. *Clinical Examination of the Nervous System*. New York, NY: McGraw-Hill, 2000:65–111.
308. Dutia MB: Interaction between vestibulocollic and cervicocollic reflexes: automatic compensation of reflex gain by muscle afferents. *Prog Brain Res* 76:173–180, 1988.
309. Dutia MB, Price RF: Interaction between the vestibulo-collic reflex and the cervico-collic stretch reflex in the decerebrate cat. *J Physiol* 387:19–30, 1987.
310. Keshner EA: Motor control of the cervical spine. In: Boyling JD, Jull GA, eds. *Grieve's Modern Manual Therapy: The Vertebral Column*. Philadelphia, PA: Churchill Livingstone, 2004:105–117.
311. Mackinnon SE, Dellon AL: Sensory rehabilitation after nerve injury. In: Mackinnon SE, Dellon AL, eds. *Surgery of the Peripheral Nerve*. New York, NY: Thieme Medical Publishers, 1988:521.
312. Goldberg S: *The Four Minute Neurological Examination*. Miami, FL: Medmaster Inc., 1992.
313. Anthony MS: Wounds. In: Clark GL, Shaw Wilgis EF, Aiello B, et al., eds. *Hand Rehabilitation: A Practical Guide*, 2nd ed. Philadelphia, PA: Churchill Livingstone, 1998:1–15.
314. Fess EE: Documentation: essential elements of an upper extremity assessment battery. In: Hunter JM, Mackin EJ, Callahan AD, eds. *Rehabilitation of the Hand: Surgery and Therapy*, 4th ed. St. Louis, MO: Mosby, 1995:185.
315. Tan AM: Sensibility testing. In: Stanley BG, Tribuzi SM, eds. *Concepts in Hand Rehabilitation*. Philadelphia, PA: FA Davis, 1992:92–112.
316. Moberg E: Objective methods for determining the functional value of sensibility in the hand. *J Bone Joint Surg* 40A:454–476, 1958.
317. Dutton M: *Manual Therapy of the Spine: An Integrated Approach*. New York, NY: McGraw-Hill, 2002.
318. Dellon AL: Clinical use of vibratory stimuli to evaluate peripheral nerve injury and compression neuropathy. *Plast Reconstr Surg* 65:466–476, 1980.
319. Meadows JTS: *Manual Therapy: Biomechanical Assessment and Treatment, Advanced Technique*. Calgary, AB: Swodeam Consulting, Inc., 1995.
320. Gelberman RH, Szabo RM, Williamson RV, et al.: Sensibility testing in perpheral nerve compression syndromes. An experimental study in humans. *J Bone Joint Surg* 65A:632–638, 1983.
321. von Frey M, Kiesow F: Uber die Function der Tastkorperchen Yeit. *Ztschr Psychol Physiol Sinnesorg* 20:126–163, 1899.
322. Semmes J, Weinstein S, Ghent L, et al.: *Somatosensory Changes after Penetrating Brain Wounds in Man*. Cambridge, MA: Harvard University Press, 1960.
323. Tubiana R, Thomine J-M, Mackin E: *Examination of the Hand and Wrist*. London: Mosby, 1996.
324. Blair SJ, McCormick E, Bear-Lehman J, et al.: Evaluation of impairment of the upper extremity. *Clin Orthop* 221:42–58, 1987.
325. Callahan AD: Sensibility testing. In: Hunter J, Schneider LH, Mackin E, et al., eds. *Rehabilitation of the Hand: Surgery and Therapy*. St Louis, MO: Mosby, 1990:605.
326. Omer GE: Report of committee for evaluation of the clinical result in peripheral nerve injury. *J Hand Surg* 8:754–759, 1983.
327. Olaleye D, Perkins BA, Bril V: Evaluation of three screening tests and a risk assessment model for diagnosing peripheral neuropathy in the diabetes clinic. *Diabetes Res Clin Pract* 54:115–128, 2001.
328. Emery CA, Cassidy JD, Klassen TP, et al.: Development of a clinical static and dynamic standing balance measurement tool appropriate for use in adolescents. *Phys Ther* 85:502–514, 2005.
329. O'Sullivan SB: Examination of motor function: motor control and motor learning. In: O'Sullivan SB, Schmitz TJ, eds. *Physical Rehabilitation*, 5th ed. Philadelphia, PA: FA Davis, 2007:227–271.
330. Barber SD, Noyes FR, Mangine RE, et al.: Quantitative assessment of functional limitations in normal and anterior cruciate ligament-deficient knees. *Clin Orthop Relat Res* 204–214, 1990.
331. Simon RP, Aminoff MJ, Greenberg DA: *Clinical Neurology*, 4th ed. Stanford, CT, Appleton and Lange, 1999.
332. Judge RD, Zuidema GD, Fitzgerald FT: Head. In: Judge RD, Zuidema GD, Fitzgerald FT, eds. *Clinical Diagnosis*, 4th ed. Boston, MA: Little, Brown and Company, 1982:123–151.

SECTION II

EXAMINATION AND EVALUATION

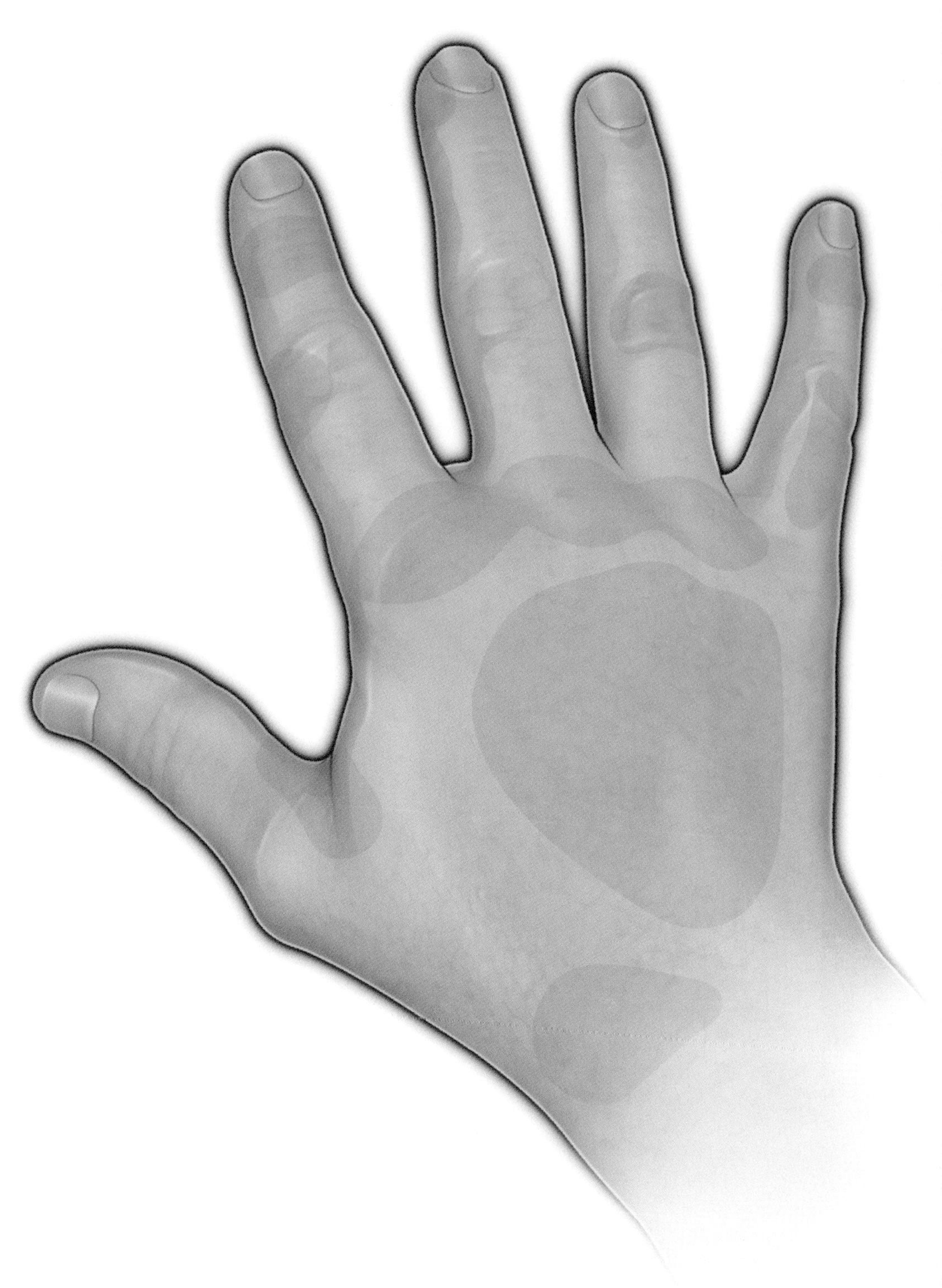

CHAPTER 4 Patient/Client Management

CHAPTER OBJECTIVES

At the completion of this chapter, the reader will be able to:

1. Understand the principles and considerations of a comprehensive examination.
2. List the components involved in the continuum of care.
3. Take a complete history.
4. Explain the importance of the systems review.
5. List the components of the tests and measures portion of the examination.
6. Understand the value of a complete observation of the patient and the information that can be gleaned from such an assessment.
7. Describe the differences between a traditional examination and a postsurgical examination.
8. Explain the differences between the examination and the evaluation.
9. Explain how to determine whether a technique is clinically useful.
10. Outline the components of clinical documentation.

OVERVIEW

Patient/client management comprises five elements:[1]

1. Examination of the patient
2. Evaluation of the data and the identification of problems
3. Determination of the diagnosis
4. Determination of the prognosis and the *plan of care* (POC)
5. Implementation of the POC (intervention)

The examination process involves a complex relationship between the clinician and the patient. The aims of the examination process are to provide an efficient and effective exchange and to develop a rapport between the clinician and the patient. The success of this interaction involves a myriad of factors. Successful clinicians are those who demonstrate effective communication, sound clinical reasoning, critical judgment, creative decision making, and competence.

The primary responsibility of a clinician is to make decisions in the best interest of the patient. Although the approach to the examination should vary with each patient, and from condition to condition, there are several fundamental components to the examination process. The principles outlined in this chapter, and integrated throughout this text, are based on the views of a number of experts,[2–12] as well as principles I have learned, and used, over the years.

All clinicians should commit to be lifelong students of their profession and should strive toward a process of continual self-education. Part of this process involves the utilization of the expertise of more experienced clinicians. This necessitates that the early years of practice are spent in an environment in which the novice is surrounded by a staff of varying levels of clinical and life experiences, both of which can serve as valuable resources. The clinician can also improve by investing time in reading relevant material, attending continuing education courses, completing home study courses, watching videos specializing in techniques, and observing exceptional clinicians. Exceptional clinicians are those who demonstrate excellent *technical* skills, combined with excellent *people* skills.

CLINICAL PEARL

From the patient's point of view, there is no substitute for interest, acceptance, and especially empathy on the part of the clinician.[13]

Finally, one must also never forget that the patient can serve as the most valuable resource. Each interaction with a patient is an opportunity to increase knowledge, skill, and understanding. Integral to this relationship is patient confidentiality. Patient confidentiality must always be strictly adhered to. Except when discussing the patient's condition with other clinicians with the object of teaching or learning, the clinician should not discuss the patient's condition with anyone without the patient's permission.

Much about becoming a clinician relates to an ability to communicate with the patient, the patient's family, and the other members of the health-care team. The nonverbal cues are especially important, because they often are performed subconsciously. Special attention needs to be paid to cultural diversity and to nonverbal communication such as voice volume, postures, gestures, and eye contact. The appearance of the clinician is also important, if a professional image is to be projected.

Communication between the clinician and the patient begins when the clinician first meets the patient and continues throughout any future sessions. Communication involves interacting with the patient using terms he or she can understand, and being sensitive to cultural diversity as appropriate. The introduction to the patient should be handled in a professional yet empathetic tone. Listening with empathy involves understanding the ideas being communicated and the emotion behind the ideas. In essence, empathy is seeing another person's viewpoint, so that a deep and true understanding of what the person is experiencing can be obtained.

At the end of the first visit and at subsequent visits, the clinician should ask if there are any questions. Each session should have closure, which may include a handshake, if appropriate.

Examination Considerations

An *examination* refers to the gathering of information from the chart, other caregivers, the patient, the patient's family, caretakers, and friends in order to identify and define the patient's problem(s) and to design an intervention plan.[14] In contrast, an *evaluation* is the level of judgment necessary to make sense of the findings in order to identify a relationship between the symptoms reported and the signs of disturbed function.[14]

The examination is an ongoing process that begins with the patient referral or initial entry and continues throughout the course of rehabilitation. During the examination phase, the clinician hypothesizes the clinical problem then chooses and implements measures to test the hypotheses. The examination must be performed with a scientific rigor that follows a predictable and strictly ordered thought process. The purpose of the examination is to obtain information that identifies and measures a change from normal. This is determined using information related by the patient, in conjunction with clinical signs and findings. The examination should not be viewed as an algorithm. Rather, it is a framework that has specific points that can be applied to various situations. The strength of an examination relies on the accuracy of the findings of the testing procedures. Diagnostic tests are divided into two main categories:[15]

1. Tests that result in a discrete outcome—they permit interpretations from the test as present/absent, disease/not disease, mild/moderate/severe.
2. Tests that result in a continuous outcome—they provide data on an interval or a scale of measurement such as degrees of range of motion.

For the clinician to formulate an appropriate interpretation and an accurate final diagnosis, the tests chosen must be useful. *Reliability*, *validity*, and *significance* are essential in determining the usefulness of a test (see Evaluation):

Reliability. A test is considered reliable if it produces precise, accurate, and reproducible information.[16]

Validity. Test validity is defined as the degree to which a test measures what it purports to be measuring, and how well it correctly classifies individuals with or without a particular disease.[17–19]

Significance. The term significance is used in statistics to describe the probability of something happening. A study generally will give a value of p for any conclusions they draw (see Evaluation).

The Examination

Examination tools can be divided into two categories:[20]

- *Performance-based or self-report measures.* Performance-based measures involve the clinician's performance of the test or observation of the patient's performance. Examples include assessment of joint mobility, muscle strength, or balance. Self-report measures involve the patient rating his or her performance during activities such as walking, stair climbing, or sporting activity based on the ability to perform a task, difficulty with the task, help needed for the task, and pain during performance of the task. For example, the *Fear Avoidance Beliefs Questionnaire* (FABQ),[21] which was originally designed to help measure how much fear and avoidance impacted a patient with low back pain thereby helping to identify those patients for whom psychosocial interventions may be beneficial (Table 4-1). However, the scale can be modified to apply to patients with other types of

TABLE 4-1 FABQ

Instructions: Here are some of the things that other patients have told us about their pain. For each statement, please circle the number from 0 to 6 to say how many physical activities such as bending, lifting, walking, or driving affect or would affect your back pain.

Statements

1. My pain is caused by physical activity.
2. Physical activity makes my pain worse.
3. Physical activity might harm my back.
4. I should not do physical activities that (might) make my pain worse.
5. I cannot do physical activities that (might) make my pain worse.

The following statements are about how your normal work affects or would affect your back pain:

6. My pain was caused by my work or by an accident at work.
7. My work aggravated my pain.
8. I have a claim for compensation for my pain.
9. My work is too heavy for me.
10. My work makes or would make my pain worse.
11. My work might harm my back.
12. I should not do my normal work with my present pain.
13. I cannot do my normal work with my present pain.
14. I cannot do my normal work till my pain is treated.
15. I do not think that I will be back to my normal work within 3 months.
16. I do not think that I will ever be able to go back to that work.

Data from Waddell G, Newton M, Henderson I, et al: A Fear-Avoidance Beliefs Questionnaire (FABQ) and the role of fear-avoidance beliefs in chronic low back pain and disability. *Pain.* 1993:52;157–1568.

chronic pain as only two items mention the word "back". The scoring for the FABQ is outlined in Table 4-2.

- Generic or disease-specific measures. A number of generic or disease-specific measures currently exist that examine the performance of functional activities. Disease-specific measures are questionnaires that concentrate on a region of primary interest that is generally relevant to the patient and clinician.[22] As a result of this focus on a regional disease state, the likelihood of increased responsiveness is higher. Some examples of the primary focus of these instruments include populations (rheumatoid arthritis), symptoms (back pain), and function (activities of daily living).[22] The disadvantage of a disease-specific outcome is that general information is lost, and therefore, it is generally recommended that when evaluating patient outcomes, both a disease-specific and generic outcome measure should be used.[22]

CLINICAL PEARL

The clinician must always remember that measurements may appear to be objective but that the interpretation of any measurement is always subjective.[23]

Patient discomfort should always be kept to a minimum. It is important that examination procedures only be performed to the point at which symptoms are provoked or begin to increase, if they are not present at rest.

The examination consists of three components of equal importance: (1) patient history, (2) systems review, and (3) tests and measures.[14] These three components are closely related, in that they often occur concurrently. One further element, observation, occurs throughout.

History

The history taking, specific to each joint, is detailed in each of the chapters. The history usually precedes the systems review and the tests and measures components of the examination, but it may also occur concurrently. Whenever it occurs, it should always be used in conjunction with the findings from the system review and the tests and measures rather than performed in a vacuum. One of the purposes of the history (Table 4-3) is to focus the examination, especially if the clinician has a good understanding of the underlying anatomy and biomechanics. There has been a recent trend to put less emphasis on the history and use the results from imaging studies to determine a clinical diagnosis, which is ironic given the fact that much of these diagnostic tests would be unnecessary if more attention was paid to the clinical examination.[24] Indeed, multiple studies have demonstrated the incidence of MRI abnormalities in the spine,[25] the shoulder,[26] the knee,[27] and other areas in *normal* subjects. Obviously, an improper diagnosis leads to an inappropriate treatment.

CLINICAL PEARL

A study by O'Shea and colleagues[28] found that the correct diagnosis of knee injuries was made in 83% of patients utilizing the history and the physical examination alone.

Ideally, the interview of a patient should be conducted in a quiet, well-lit room that offers a measure of privacy. To encourage good communication, the clinician and the patient should be at a similar eye level, facing each other, with a comfortable space between them (approximately 3 feet). The clinician must record the history in a systematic fashion so that every question has a purpose and no subject areas are neglected. Formal questioning using a questionnaire (Table 4-4) helps to ensure that all of the important questions are asked. Knowing the importance of each question is based on the didactic background of the clinician, as is the ability to convert the patient's responses into a working hypothesis. For example, if the patient reports that lumbar flexion relieves their low-back pain, but that lumbar extension aggravates it, the clinician needs to know which structures are stressed in lumbar extension, but unstressed in lumbar flexion.

The method of questioning should be altered from patient to patient, as the level of understanding and answering abilities varies between each individual. In general, the interview should flow as an active conversation, not a question-and-answer session. A transfer of accurate information must occur between the patient and the clinician. A successful learning process requires the clinician to have patience, focus, and self-criticism.[6]

TABLE 4-2 FABQ Scoring[a]

Response	Points
Completely disagree	0
	1
	2
Unsure	3
	4
	5
Completely agree	6

Fear-avoidance beliefs about work (scale 1) = (points for item 6) + (points for item 7) + (points for item 9) + (points for item 10) + (points for item 11) + (points for item 12) + (points for item 15)

Fear-avoidance beliefs about physical activity (scale 2) = (points for item 2) + (points for item 3) + (points for item 4) + (points for item 5)

Items not in scale 1 or 2: 1 8 13 14 16

Interpretation:

- minimal scale scores: 0
- maximum scale 1 score: 42 (7 items)
- maximum scale 2 score: 24 (4 items)
- The higher the scale scores the greater the degree of fear and avoidance beliefs shown by the patient.

Performance:

- Internal consistency (alpha) 0.88 for scale 1 and 0.77 for scale 2

[a]Data from Waddell G, Newton M, Henderson I, et al: A Fear-Avoidance Beliefs Questionnaire (FABQ) and the role of fear-avoidance beliefs in chronic low back pain and disability. *Pain.* 1993:52;157–168.

TABLE 4-3 Data Generated from a Patient History

General demographics	Includes information about the patient's age, height, weight, and marital status and primary language spoken by the patient.[a]
Social history and social habits	Includes information about the patient's social history, including support systems, family and caregiver resources, and cultural beliefs and behaviors.[1] An individual's response to pain and dysfunction is, in large part, determined by his or her cultural background, social standing, educational and economical status, and anticipation of functional compromise.[b]
Occupation/employment	Includes information about the patient's occupation, employment, and work environment, including current and previous community and work activities.[1] The clinician must determine the patient's work demands, the activities involved, and the activities or postures that appear to be aggravating the condition or determine the functional demands of a specific vocational or avocational activity to which the patient is planning to return. Work-related low back injuries and repetitive motion disorders of the upper extremities are common in patients whose workplaces involve physical labor. Habitual postures may be the source of the problem in those with sedentary occupations. Patients who have sedentary occupations may also be at increased risk of overuse injuries when they are not at work, as a result of recreational pursuits (the *weekend warrior*).
Growth and development	Includes information about the patient's developmental background and hand or foot dominance. Developmental or congenital disorders that the clinician should note include such conditions as Legg–Calvé–Perthes disease, cerebral palsy, Down syndrome, spina bifida, scoliosis, and congenital hip dysplasia.
Living environment	The clinician should be aware of the living situation of the patient, including entrances and exits to the house, the number of stairs, and the location of bathrooms within the house.
Functional status and activity level	Includes information about the patient's current and prior level of function, with particular reference to the type of activities performed and the percentage of time spent performing those activities.
Past history of current condition	It is important for the clinician to determine whether the patient has had successive onsets of similar symptoms in the past, because recurrent injury tends to have a detrimental effect on the potential for recovery. If the patient's history indicates a recurrent injury, the clinician should note how often, and how easily, the injury has recurred and the success or failure of previous interventions.
Past medical/surgical history	Includes information with regard to allergies, childhood illnesses, and previous trauma. In addition, information on any health conditions, such as cardiac problems, high blood pressure, or diabetes, should be elicited, as these may impact exercise tolerance (cardiac problems and high blood pressure) and speed of healing (diabetes). If the surgical history is related to the current problem, the clinician should obtain as much detail about the surgery as possible from the surgical report, including any complications, precautions, or postsurgical protocols. Although this information is not always related to the presenting condition, it does afford the clinician some insight as to the potential impact or response the planned intervention may have on the patient.
Family history and general health status	Certain diseases, such as rheumatoid arthritis, diabetes, cardiovascular disease, and cancer, have familial tendencies. The general health status refers to a review of the patient's health perception, physical and psychological function, as well as any specific questions related to a particular body region, or complaint.[1]

[a]Guide to physical therapist practice. *Phys Ther.* 2001:81;513–595.
[b]Judge RD, Zuidema GD, Fitzgerald FT, The medical history and physical, in Judge RD, Zuidema GD, Fitzgerald FT (eds): *Clinical Diagnosis* (4 ed). Boston, MA: Little, Brown and Company, 1982:9–19.

Open-ended questions or statements, such as "Tell me why you are here," are used initially to encourage the patient to provide narrative information, help determine the patient's chief complaint, and to decrease the opportunity for bias on the part of the clinician.[29] More specific questions, such as "How did this pain begin?" are asked as the examination proceeds (Table 4-5). The specific questions help to focus the examination and deter irrelevant information. The clinician should provide the patient with encouraging responses, such as a nod of the head, when the information is relevant and when needed to steer the patient into supplying necessary information. *Neutral* questions should be used whenever possible. These questions are structured in such a way so as to avoid leading the patient into giving a particular response. Leading questions, such as "Does it hurt more when you walk?" should be avoided. A more neutral question would be, "What activities make your symptoms worse?"

In addition to the details listed in Table 4-5, the history can help the clinician to:

- develop a working relationship with the patient and establish lines of communication with the patient. To help establish a rapport with the patient, the clinician should

TABLE 4-4 Sample Medical History Questionnaire

GENERAL MEDICAL HISTORY GENERAL INFORMATION

Physician Diagnosis:________________________ Date: ____________________

Last Name First Name

The information requested may be needed if you have a medical emergency.

________________________ __________ ____________

Person to be notified in emergency________________ Phone ____________ Relationship

Are you currently working? (Y) or (N) Type of work: If not, why?

GENERAL MEDICAL HISTORY:

Please check (√) if you have been treated for:

( ) Heart problems
( ) Fainting or dizziness
( ) Shortness of breath
( ) Calf pain with exercise
( ) Severe headaches
( ) Recent accident
( ) Head trauma/concussion
( ) Muscular weakness
( ) Cancer
( ) Joint dislocation(s)
( ) Broken bone
( ) Difficulty sleeping
( ) Frequent falls
( ) Unexplained weight loss
( ) Tremors
( ) High blood pressure (hypertension)
( ) Kidney disease
( ) Liver disease
( ) Weakness or fatigue
( ) Hernias
( ) Blurred vision
( ) Bowel/bladder problems
( ) Difficulty swallowing
( ) A wound that does not heal
( ) Unusual skin coloration
( ) Lung disease/problems
( ) Arthritis
( ) Swollen and painful joints
( ) Irregular heart beat
( ) Stomach pains or ulcers
( ) Pain with cough or sneeze
( ) Back or neck injuries
( ) Diabetes
( ) Stroke(s)
( ) Balance problems
( ) Muscular pain with activity
( ) Swollen ankles or legs
( ) Jaw problems
( ) Circulatory problems
( ) Epilepsy/seizures/convulsions
( ) Chest pain or pressure at rest
( ) Allergies (latex, medication, food)
( ) Constant pain unrelieved by rest
( ) Pregnancy
( ) Night pain (while sleeping)
( ) Nervous or emotional problems
( ) Any infectious disease (TB, AIDS, hepatitis)
( ) Tingling, numbness, or loss of feeling? If yes, where?
( ) Constant pain or pressure during activity

Do you use tobacco? (Y) or (N) If yes, how much?

Are you presently taking any medications or drugs? (Y) or (N)

If yes, what are you taking them for?

1. Pain

On the line provided, mark where your "pain status" is today.

|——————————————————————————|

No pain Most servere pain

2. Function. On a scale of 0 to 10 with 0 being able to perform all of your normal daily activities, and 10 being unable to perform any of your normal daily activities, give yourself a score for your *current ability* to perform your activities of daily living. __________

Please list any major surgery or hospitalization:

Hospital:__________________ Approx. Date:__________

Reasons:

Hospital:__________________ Approx. Date:__________

Reasons:

Have you recently had an X-ray, MRI, or CT scan for your condition? (Y) or (N)

Facility: ________________ Approx. date:__________

Findings: ________________

Please mention any additional problems or symptoms you feel are important: ____________________

____

Have you been evaluated and/or treated by another physician, physical therapist, chiropractor, osteopath or health care practitioner for this condition? (Y) or (N) If yes, please circle which one.

TABLE 4-5 Contents of the History

History of Current Condition
Did the condition begin insidiously or was trauma involved?
How long has the patient had the symptoms?
Where are the symptoms?
How does the patient describe the symptoms?
Reports about numbness and tingling suggest neurologic compromise. Reports of pain suggest a chemical or mechanical irritant. Pain needs to be carefully evaluated in terms of its site, distribution, quality, onset, frequency, nocturnal occurrence, aggravating factors, and relieving factors.

Past History of Current Condition
Has the patient had a similar injury in the past?
Was it treated or did it resolve on its own? If it was treated, how was it treated and did intervention help?
How long did the most recent episode last?

Past Medical/Surgery History
How is the patient's general health?
Does the patient have any allergies?

Medications Patient is Presently Taking

Other Tests and Measures
Has the patient had any imaging tests such as X-ray, MRI, CT scan, bone scan?
Has the patient had an EMG test, or a nerve conduction velocity test, which would suggest compromise to muscle tissue and/or neurologic system?

Social Habits (Past and Present)
Does the patient smoke? If so, how many packs per day?
Does the patient drink alcohol? If so, how often and how much?
Is the patient active or sedentary?

Social History
Is the patient married, living with a partner, single, divorced, or widowed?
Is the patient a parent or single parent?

Family History
Is there a family history of the present condition?

Growth and Development
Is the patient right- or left-handed?
Were there any congenital problems?

Living Environment
What type of home does the patient live in with reference to accessibility?
Is there any support at home?
Does the patient use any extra pillows or special chairs to sleep?

Occupation/Employment/School
What does the patient do for work?
How long has he or she worked there?
What does the job entail in terms of physical requirements?
What level of education did the patient achieve?

Functional Status/Activity Level
How does the present condition affect the patient's ability to perform activities of daily living?
How does the present condition affect the patient at work?
How does the patient's condition affect sleep?
Is the patient able to drive? If so, for how long?

CT, computed tomography; EMG, electromyogram; MRI, magnetic resonance imaging.
Data from Clarnette RG, Miniaci A: Clinical exam of the shoulder. *Med Sci Sports Exerc.* 1998:30;1–6.

discuss the information provided on the medical history form with the patient, at either the initial or the subsequent visits.

- determine the chief complaint, its mechanism of injury, its severity, and its impact on the patient's function. It is worth remembering that a patient's chief complaint can sometimes differ from the chief concern, but both should be addressed.
- ascertain the specific location and the nature of the symptoms.
- determine the irritability of the symptoms.
- establish a baseline of measurements.
- ascertain which medications the patient is currently taking and whether they are prescribed or over the counter (see Chap. 9).

- elicit information about the past history of the current condition.
- determine the goals and the expectations of the patient from the physical therapy intervention. It is important that the clinician and the patient discuss and determine mutually agreed-upon anticipated goals and expected outcomes. The discussion can help the clinician determine whether the patient has realistic expectations or will need further patient education concerning his or her condition and typical recovery time frames.

CLINICAL PEARL

It is important to remember that symptoms can be experienced without the presence of recognized clinical signs, and that signs can be present in the absence of symptoms. The former scenario is more common, but the latter can occur when a pathologic reflex or a positive cranial nerve test (see Chap. 3) is detected in the absence of any subjective complaints. In such a scenario, a positive finding could be a false-positive result, or it could be prognostic.[4]

- elicit reports of potentially life-threatening symptoms, or *red flags*, that require an immediate medical referral (see Chap. 5).

The components of the patient history described in this section are based on the *Guide to Physical Therapist Practice*.[14]

Age

Certain conditions are related to age, ethnicity, gender, morphology, and family history. For example,

- degenerative and overuse syndromes are more frequent in the over 40 age group.
- cervical spondylosis is often seen in persons 25 years of age or older, and it is present in 60% of those older than 45 years and 85% of those older than 65 years of age.[30–32]
- the onset of ankylosing spondylitis often occurs between the ages of 15 and 35 years.[33]
- both osteoporosis and osteoarthritis are more often associated with the older population.
- diseases such as Legg–Perthes disease or Scheuermann's are seen in adolescents or teenagers.
- prostate cancer has a higher incidence in men older than 50 years.[34]
- among African-Americans in the United States, 1 in 600 has sickle cell anemia.[35]
- Caucasians experience higher osteoporotic fracture rates than either Asians or African-Americans.[36]
- some diseases, such as hypertension and renal disease, are more prevalent in African-American populations than among Caucasians.[37,38]
  - basal cell carcinoma and melanoma are more common among Caucasians.
  - the male-to-female ratio of bladder cancer is 2:1 to 4:1, and the disease is twice as common in male Caucasians as in African-American men in the United States.[39,40]
  - breast cancer is the most frequently diagnosed cancer and the second leading cause of cancer-related deaths among women in the United States.[41]
  - melanoma is the leading cause of cancer death in women aged 25–36 years.[42]
  - anterior knee pain caused by patellofemoral syndrome is most common in young teenage girls and young men in their 20s.[43]
  - obesity has been linked to many diseases such as diabetes, cardiovascular disease, and degenerative joint disease.
  - many diseases can be linked to family history, including diabetes, cardiovascular disease, and Charcot Marie Tooth disease.

History of Current Condition

This portion of the history taking can prove to be the most challenging as it involves the gathering of both positive and negative findings, followed by the dissemination of the information into a working hypothesis. An understanding of the patient's history of the current condition can often help determine the prognosis and guide the intervention.

The clinician should determine the circumstances and manner in which the symptoms began and the progression of those symptoms.[6] The mode of onset, or the mechanism of injury, can be either traumatic (macrotraumatic) or atraumatic (microtraumatic) and can give clues as to the extent and nature of the damage caused.

If the injury is traumatic, the clinician should determine the specific mechanism, in terms of both the direction and the force, and relate the mechanism to the presenting symptoms. If the injury is recent, an inflammatory source of pain is likely. A sudden onset of pain, associated with trauma, could indicate the presence of an acute injury such as a soft tissue tear or even a fracture, whereas immediate pain and locking are most likely to result from an intra-articular block. Joint locking and twinges of pain may indicate a loose body moving within the joint. Reports of a joint "giving way" usually indicate joint instability or a reflex inhibition or weakness of muscles. An injury that is not recent but which the symptoms have persisted could indicate a biomechanical dysfunction. Oftentimes a particular motion or posture may continue to aggravate the condition.

If the onset is gradual or insidious, the clinician must determine if there are any predisposing factors, such as changes in the patient's daily routines or exercise programs. Symptoms of pain or limitations of movement, with no apparent reason, are usually a result of inflammation, early degeneration, repetitive activity (microtrauma), or sustained positioning and postures.[44] However, such symptoms may also be associated with something more serious, such as a vascular insufficiency, a tumor, or an infection.

If pain is present, the clinician's major focus should be to seek the cause and methods to control it. Pain may be constant, variable, or intermittent. Variable pain is pain that is perpetual, but that varies in intensity. Variable pain usually indicates the involvement of both a chemical and a mechanical source. The mechanical cause of constant pain is less understood but is thought to be the result of the deformation of collagen, which compresses or stretches the nociceptive-free nerve endings, with the excessive forces being perceived as pain.[45] Thus, specific movements or positions should influence pain of a mechanical nature.

Chemical, or inflammatory, pain is more constant and is less affected by movements or positions than mechanical pain. Intermittent pain is unlikely to be caused by a chemical irritant. Usually, this type of pain is caused by prolonged postures, a loose intra-articular body, or an impingement of a musculoskeletal structure.

CLINICAL PEARL

Constant pain following an injury continues until the healing process has sufficiently reduced the concentration of noxious irritants.

Unfortunately, the source of the pain is not always easy to identify, because most patients present with both mechanical and chemical pain.

Finally, the clinician should determine if a specific intervention has been used in the past for the same condition and, if so, the clinician should ask about the effectiveness of that intervention.

Location

The clinician should determine the location of the symptoms because this can indicate which areas need to be included in the physical examination. Information about how the location of the symptoms has changed since the onset can indicate whether a condition is worsening or improving. In general, as a condition worsens, the pain distribution becomes more widespread and distal (peripheralized). As the condition improves, the symptoms tend to become more localized (centralized). A body chart may be used to record the location of symptoms (see Fig. 4-1).

CLINICAL PEARL

Symptoms that are distal and superficial are easier for the patient to specifically localize than those that are proximal and deep.

It must be remembered that the location of symptoms for many musculoskeletal conditions is quite separate from the source, especially in those peripheral joints that are more proximal, such as the shoulder and the hip. For example, a cervical radiculopathy can produce symptoms throughout the upper extremity. The term *referred pain* is used to describe symptoms that have their origin at a site other than where the patient feels the pain. For example, pain due to osteoarthritis of the hip is often felt in the anterior groin and thigh along with the sclerotomes or the dermatomes for L2 and L3. The concept of referred pain is often difficult for patients to understand. An explanation of referred pain enables the patient to better understand and answer questions about symptoms they might otherwise have felt irrelevant. The major sources of referred pain are neurogenic, vasculogenic, viscerogenic, and spondylogenic (see Chap. 3). If the extremity appears to be the source of the symptoms, the clinician should attempt to reproduce the symptoms by loading the peripheral tissues. If this proves unsuccessful, a full investigation of the spinal structures must ensue.

Behavior of Symptoms

The presence of pain should not always be viewed negatively by the clinician. After all, its presence helps to determine the location of the injury, and its behavior aids the clinician in determining the stage of healing and the impact it has on the patient's function. For example, whether the pain is worsening, improving, or unchanging provides information on the effectiveness of an intervention. In addition, a gradual increase in the intensity of the symptoms over time may indicate to the clinician that the condition is worsening or that the condition is nonmusculoskeletal in nature (Table 4-6).[6,46]

Maitland[7] introduced the concept of the *degree of irritability*. An irritable structure has the following characteristics:

- *A progressive increase in the severity of the pain with movement or a specific posture.* An ability to reproduce constant pain with a specific motion or posture indicates an irritable structure.
- *Symptoms increased with minimal activity.* An irritable structure is one that requires very little to increase the symptoms.
- *Increased latent response of symptoms.* Symptoms that do not resolve within a few minutes following a movement or posture indicate an irritable structure.

According to McKenzie and May,[44] the intervention for the patient whose symptoms have a low degree of irritability and which are gradually resolving should focus only on education initially. However, if the improvement ceases, a mechanical intervention may then be necessary.[44]

The frequency and duration of the patient's symptoms can help the clinician to classify the injury according to its stage of healing: acute (inflammatory), sub-acute (migratory and proliferative), and chronic (remodeling) (Table 4-7) (see Chap. 2).

- Acute conditions: present for 7 to 10 days.
- Subacute conditions: present for 10 days to several weeks.
- Chronic conditions: present for more than several weeks.

In the case of a musculoskeletal injury that has been present without any formal intervention for a few months, there is a good possibility that adaptive shortening of the healing collagenous tissue has occurred, which may result in a failure to heal, and the persistence of symptoms.[44] The persistence of symptoms usually indicates a poorer prognosis, as it may indicate the presence of a chronic pain syndrome. Chronic pain syndromes have the potential to complicate the intervention process (see Chap. 5).[44]

Name:
Date: Signature:

Please use the diagram below to indicate where you feel symptoms right now.
Use the following key to indicate different types of symptoms.

KEY:
Pins and Needles= 000000 Stabbing= /////// Burning= XXXXX Deep Ache= ZZZZZZ

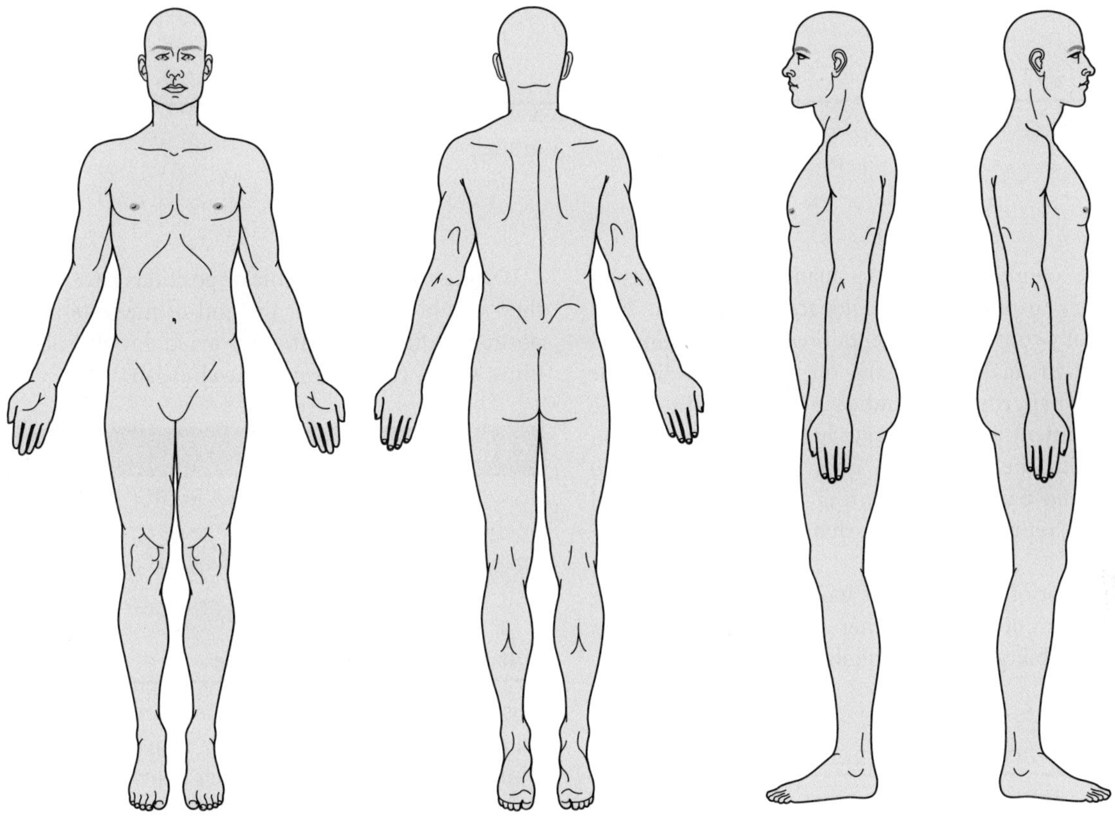

Please use the three scales below to rate your pain over the past 24 hours. Use the upper line to describe your pain level right now. Use the other scales to rate your pain at its worst and best over the past 24 hours.

RATE YOUR PAIN: 0= No Pain 10=Extremely Intense

1. Right now 0 1 2 3 4 5 6 7 8 9 10
2. At its worst 0 1 2 3 4 5 6 7 8 9 10
3. At its best 0 1 2 3 4 5 6 7 8 9 10

FIGURE 4-1 Body chart.

TABLE 4-6 Differentiation Between Musculoskeletal and Systemic Pain

Musculoskeletal Pain	Systemic Pain
Usually decreases with cessation of activity	Reduced by pressure
Generally lessens at night	Disturbs sleep
Aggravated with mechanical stress	Not aggravated by mechanical stress
Usually continuous or intermittent	Usually constant or in waves

Data from Meadows J: *Orthopaedic Differential Diagnosis in Physical Therapy*. New York, NY: McGraw-Hill, 1999.

If the frequency and duration of the patient's symptoms are reported to be increasing, it is likely the condition is worsening. Conversely, a decrease in the frequency and duration of the symptoms generally indicate that the condition is improving.

TABLE 4-7 Stages of Healing

Stage	General Characteristics
Acute or inflammatory	Area is red, warm, swollen, and painful. Pain is present without any motion of involved area
Subacute or tissue formation (neovascularization)	Pain usually occurs with activity or motion of involved area
Chronic or remodeling	Pain usually occurs after the activity

TABLE 4-8 Patient Pain Evaluation Form

Name: ______________________________

Date: ______________ Signature: ______________

Please use the three scales below to rate your pain over the past 24 hours. Use the upper line to describe your pain level right now. Use the other scales to rate your pain at its worst and best over the past 24 hours.

RATE YOUR PAIN: 0 = NO PAIN, 10 = EXTREMELY INTENSE

1.	Right now	0	1	2	3	4	5	6	7	8	9	10
2.	At its worst	0	1	2	3	4	5	6	7	8	9	10
3.	At its best	0	1	2	3	4	5	6	7	8	9	10

One of the simplest methods to quantify the intensity of pain is to use a 10-point *visual analog scale* (VAS). The VAS is a numerically continuous scale that requires the pain level be identified by making a mark on a 100-mm line, or by circling the appropriate number in a 1–10 series (Table 4-8).[47] The patient is asked to rate his or her present pain compared with the worst pain ever experienced, with 0 representing no pain, 1 representing minimally perceived pain, and 10 representing pain that requires immediate attention.[48]

If the behavior of the symptoms includes locking or giving way, the clinician must elicit further details about the causes of the hypomobility, the hypermobility, or the instability (see Chap. 2).

Aggravating and Easing Factors

Of particular importance are the patient's chief complaint and the relationship of that complaint to specific aggravating activities or postures. Questions must be asked to determine whether the pain is sufficient to prevent sleep or to wake the patient at night and the effect that activities of daily living, work, sex, and so forth, have on the pain.

Musculoskeletal conditions are typically aggravated with movement and alleviated with rest. If no activities or postures are reported to aggravate the symptoms, the clinician needs to probe for more information. For example, if a patient complains of back pain, the clinician needs to determine the effect that walking, bending, sleeping position, prolonged standing, and sitting have on the symptoms. Sitting or standing upright increases the lumbar lordosis and can aggravate symptoms in a patient with an anterior instability of the lumbar spine, spondylolisthesis, stenosis, or a lumbar zygapophyseal joint irritation. Sitting in a slouched posture typically aggravates symptoms of a lumbar disk protrusion or a sacroiliac joint dysfunction. Nonmechanical events that provoke the symptoms could indicate a nonmusculoskeletal source for the pain[46]:

- *Eating.* Pain that increases with eating may suggest *gastrointestinal* (GI) involvement.
- *Stress.* An increase in overall muscle tension prevents muscles from resting.
- *Cyclical Pain.* Cyclical pain can often be related to systemic events (e.g., menstrual pain).

If aggravating movements or positions have been reported, they should be tested at the end of the tests and measures portion of the examination to avoid any overflow of symptoms, which could confuse the clinician.

CLINICAL PEARL

Any relieving factors reported by the patient can often provide sufficient information to assist the clinician with the intervention plan.

Nature of the Symptoms

It is important to remember that pain perception is highly subjective and is determined by a number of factors. The clinician must determine whether pain is the only symptom, or whether there are other symptoms that accompany the pain, such as bowel and bladder changes, tingling (paresthesia), radicular pain or numbness, weakness, and increased sweating.

- *Bowel or bladder dysfunction.* This finding usually indicates a compromise (compression) of the cauda equina.
- *Paresthesia.* Peripheral neuropathies can manifest as abnormal, frequently unpleasant sensations, which are variously described by the patient as numbness, pins and needles, and tingling.[49] When these sensations occur spontaneously without an external sensory stimulus, they are called *paresthesias* (Table 4-9).[49] Patients with paresthesias typically demonstrate a reduction in the perception of cutaneous and proprioceptive sensations. The seriousness of the paresthesia depends on its distribution. Although complaints of paresthesia can be the result of a relatively benign impingement of a peripheral nerve (see Chap. 3), the reasons for its presence can vary in severity and seriousness.
- *Radicular pain.* This type of pain is produced by nerve root irritation and is typically described as sharp or shooting. Numbness that has a dermatomal pattern indicates spinal nerve root compression. Radiating pain refers to an increase in pain intensity and distribution. Radiating pain typically travels distally from the site of the injury.

TABLE 4-9 Causes of Paresthesia

Paresthesia Location	Probable Cause
Lip (perioral)	Vertebral artery occlusion
Bilateral lower or bilateral upper extremities	Central protrusion of disk impinging on spine
All extremities simultaneously	Spinal cord compression
One-half of body	Cerebral hemisphere
Segmental (in dermatomal pattern)	Disk or nerve root
Glove-and-stocking distribution	Diabetes mellitus neuropathy and lead or mercury poisoning
Half of face and opposite half of body	Brain stem impairment

- *Weakness.* Any weakness should be investigated by the clinician to determine whether it is the result of spinal nerve root compression, peripheral nerve lesion, disuse, inhibition resulting from pain or swelling, injury to the contractile or inert tissues (muscle, tendon, bursa, etc.), or a more serious pathology such as a fracture (see section "Muscle Performance: Strength, Power, and Endurance" in the later discussion of tests and measures).
- *Increased sweating.* This finding can have a myriad of causes, ranging from increased body temperature, as a result of exertion, fever, apprehension, and compromise, to the autonomic system. Night sweats are of particular concern, because they often indicate the presence of a systemic problem.[50]

Quality of Symptoms

The quality of the symptoms depends on the type of receptor being stimulated (see Chap. 3).

- Stimulation of the cutaneous A-δ nociceptors leads to pricking pain.[51]
- Stimulation of the cutaneous C nociceptors results in burning or dull pain.[52]
- Activation of the nociceptors in muscle by electrical stimulation produces aching pain.[53]
- Electrical stimulation of visceral nerves at low intensities results in vague sensations of fullness and nausea, but higher intensities cause a sensation of pain.[54]

CLINICAL PEARL

Because motor and sensory axons run in the same nerves, disorders of the peripheral nerves (neuropathies) usually affect both motor and sensory functions.

Motivational-affective circuits may also mimic pain states, most notably in patients with anxiety, neurotic depression, or hysteria.[55] The mnemonic MADISON outlines the behavioral indicators that suggest motivational-affective pain[56,57]:

1. *M*ultiple complaints, including complaints about unrelated body parts.
2. *A*uthenticity claims in an attempt to convince the clinician that the symptoms exist.
3. *D*enial of the negative effect the pain is having on function.
4. *I*nterpersonal variability, manifested by different complaints to different clinicians or support staff.
5. *S*ingularity of symptoms, wherein the patient requests special consideration because of his or her type and level of pain.
6. *O*nly you, whereby the clinician is placed at a special level of expertise.
7. *N*othing works.

A description of pain is commonly sought from the patient. Because pain is variable in its intensity and quality, describing pain is often difficult for the patient. The *McGill Pain Questionnaire* (MPQ)[58] was the first systematic attempt to use verbal descriptors to assess the quality of the patient's symptoms, and has been the most widely used instrument in pain research and practice (Table 4-10). The MPQ is a self-report inventory of 78 pain descriptors distributed across 20 subcategories (with six additional descriptors in the present pain index). The subcategories are further grouped into three broad categories, termed *sensory*, *affective*, and *evaluative*, respectively, in addition to a miscellaneous category. The implication is that each word reflects a particular sensory quality of pain.

The patient is asked to indicate on a body diagram the location of the pain and to rate his or her symptoms based on the 20 categories of verbal descriptors of pain.[59] The 20 categories are ranked according to severity.[60] The patient is then asked to describe how the pain changes with time (continuous, rhythmic, or brief) and how strong the pain is (mild, discomforting, distressing, horrible, or excruciating).

The most commonly reported measure from the MPQ instrument, the pain-rating index total, provides an estimate of overall pain intensity. This measure, obtained by summing all the descriptors selected from the 20 subclasses, has a possible range of 0–78. Separate scores for each class may be obtained by summing the values associated with the words selected from subclasses that comprise that dimension. Scores for each of these dimensions vary in range from 0 to 42 for the sensory class, 0 to 14 for the affective class, and 0 to 5 for the evaluative class.

The strength of the MPQ is its ability to distinguish patients with a sensory pain experience from those who have an affective pain experience. The MPQ has been found to be sensitive to intervention effects[61] and to have a high test–retest reliability[58] and good construct validity.[62]

Symptom magnification, an exaggerated subjective response to symptoms in the absence of adequate objective findings, is an increasingly common occurrence in the clinic. The patients who display this type of behavior are a difficult

TABLE 4-10 Modified McGill Pain Questionnaire

Patient's Name ______________________ Date __________

Directions: Many words can describe pain. Some of these words are listed below. If you are experiencing any pain, check (√) every word that describes your pain.

A.	Flickering Quivering Pulsing Throbbing Beating Pounding
B.	Jumping Flashing Shooting
C.	Pricking Boring Drilling Stabbing
D.	Sharp Cutting Lacerating
E.	Pinching Pressing Gnawing Cramping Crushing
F.	Tugging Pulling Wrenching
G.	Hot Burning Scalding Searing
H.	Tingling Itchy Smarting Stinging
I.	Dull Sore Hurting Aching Heavy
J.	Tender Taut Rasping Splitting
K.	Tiring Exhausting
L.	Sickening Suffocating
M.	Fearful Frightful Terrifying
N.	Punishing Grueling Cruel Vicious Killing
O.	Wretched Blinding
P.	Annoying Troublesome Intense Unbearable
Q.	Spreading Radiating Penetrating Piercing
R.	Tight Numb Drawing Squeezing Tearing
S.	Cool Cold Freezing
T.	Nagging Nauseating Agonizing Dreadful Torturing

KEY TO PAIN QUESTIONNAIRE

Group A: Suggests vascular disorder
Groups B–H: Suggests neurogenic disorder
Group I: Suggests musculoskeletal disorder
Groups J–T: Suggests emotional disorder

SCORING GUIDE: ADD UP TOTAL NUMBER OF CHECKS (√):

Total: 4–8 = NORMAL
8–10 = Focusing too much on pain
10–16 = May be helped more by a clinical psychologist than by a physical therapist
>16 = Unlikely to respond to therapy procedures

population to deal with. The causes of symptom magnification can be categorized into two main patient types:

1. Patients with a psychosomatic overlay and those whose symptoms have a psychogenic cause.
2. Patients who are involved in litigation.

The concept of malingering is discussed in Chapter 5.

Imaging Studies

It is important for the clinician to determine whether the patient has undergone any imaging studies and, if so, the results of those studies. The role that imaging studies play in the examination and evaluation processes is outlined in Chapter 7. It is important to remember that, in general, imaging tests have a high sensitivity (few false negatives) but low specificity (high false-positive rate), so are thus used in the clinical decision-making process to test a hypothesis but should not be used in isolation.

Based on the history, there may be times when the extent of the remainder of the examination may have to be limited. The decision to limit the examination is based on the presence of any subjective features that indicate the need for caution. These features include[63]

- an irritable or severe disorder;
- worsening symptoms;
- subjective evidence of potential involvement of vital structures, such as the vertebrobasilar system, the spinal cord or the *central nervous system* (CNS), or the spinal nerve roots;
- symptoms that do not behave in a predictable manner.

Observation

Observational information forms the basis of the early clinical impression. It is, in essence, the beginning of the clinical search for patient consistency and reliability. Observation of the patient begins when the patient enters the clinic. As the clinician greets the patient and takes him or her to the treatment room, an initial observation is made. This early observation can provide the clinician with information that includes, but is not limited to, how the patient holds the extremity, whether an antalgic gait is present, and how much discomfort appears to be present. Much can be learned from thorough observation[64]:

- How does the patient arise from a seated position to greet the clinician, easily or in a guarded manner?
- Does the patient look directly into the eyes of the clinician or look away? Is there a nervousness or fear present?
- Is there an exaggerated pain response, as demonstrated by facial expression and/or voiced complaints?
- Does the patient sit to the side with the majority of weight on one buttock while the opposite leg is extended, a position associated with a lumbar spinal nerve root syndrome?[65–67]
- In the case of an adult, is a spouse, or significant other, in attendance and does such a presence seem appropriate? If the presence appears inappropriate, some form of abuse occurring at home should be suspected.
- In the case of a child, is there any unexplained or excessive bruising, and does the parent or guardian appear to be answering for the child? These findings could indicate some form of abuse occurring at home.
- Does the patient require assistance in ambulation, transferring, or changing of clothing?
- Does the patient answer his or her own questions or have an overly attentive assistant (i.e., spouse, parent, friend, or relative)? An overly attentive assistant could indicate some form of abuse occurring at home.
- Do the observation findings match the findings from the history?

Throughout the history, systems review, and tests and measures, collective observations form the basis for diagnostic deductions. Some of the observations made may be very subtle. For example, hoarseness of the voice could suggest laryngeal cancer, whereas a weakened, thickened, and lowered voice may indicate hypothyroidism.[68] Warm, moist hands felt during a handshake may indicate hyperthyroidism.[68] Cold, moist hands may indicate an anxious patient. Patients react differently to injury. Some patients may exaggerate the symptoms through facial expressions and gestures, whereas others remain stoic. Patients may appear calm and pleasant, defensive, angry, apprehensive, or depressed. Anxious patients, or patients in severe pain, often appear restless. Clinicians must learn to adopt their approaches to these different reactions. For example, an anxious or apprehensive patient may require more reassurance than a calm and pleasant patient.

Much of the observation involves assessment of posture (see Chap. 6). Postural deviations negatively affecting the location of the center of gravity in relation to the base of support may result in a patient complaining of pain and/or dysfunction when in sustained positions. Changes in the contours of the body shape or posture can be so specific that it often is possible to isolate the single muscle involved, the movements affected, and the related joint dysfunction from observation alone.[69] For example, a change in a soft tissue contour as compared to the other side could indicate muscle atrophy. These deviations and changes prompt further musculoskeletal examination to determine the cause and potential management strategies. If there are any obvious deformities, the clinician must determine whether they are structural or functional:

- Structural: those deformities present at rest. For example, torticollis, and kyphosis.
- Functional: deformities that are the result of assumed postures and which disappear when the posture is changed. For example, a functional scoliosis due to a leg length discrepancy that disappears when the patient bends forward.

The patient's position of comfort can provide the clinician with valuable information. For example, patients with lateral recess spinal stenosis of the lumbar spine, congestive heart failure, or pulmonary disease often prefer the sitting position, whereas patients with pericarditis often sit and lean forward.[68] Patients with a posterior–lateral lumbar disk herniation often prefer to stand or lie rather than sit.

The more formal observation, which is included in each of the relevant chapters, includes, but is not limited to, an analysis of the presence of any asymmetry, scars, crepitus, color changes, and swelling.

Systems Review

The information from the history and the systems review serves as a guide for the clinician in determining which structures and systems require further investigation. The systems review is the part of the examination that identifies possible health problems that require consultation with, or referral to, another health-care provider (Table 4-11).[14] The systems review consists of a limited examination of the anatomic and physiologic status of all systems (i.e., musculoskeletal, neurological, cardiovascular, pulmonary, integumentary, GI, urinary system, and genitoreproductive).[14] The systems review includes the following components[14]:

- For the cardiovascular/pulmonary system, the assessment of heart rate, respiratory rate, blood pressure, and edema. There are four so-called *vital signs* that are standard in most medical settings: temperature, heart rate, blood pressure, and respiratory rate. Pain is considered by many to be a fifth vital sign.[70–79] The clinician should monitor at least heart rate and blood pressure in any person with a history of cardiovascular disease or pulmonary disease, or those at risk for heart disease.[80]
- *Temperature.* Body temperature is one indication of the metabolic state of an individual; measurements provide information concerning basal metabolic state, possible presence or absence of infection, and metabolic response to exercise.[81] "Normal" body temperature of the adult is 98.4°F

TABLE 4-11 Signs and Symptoms Requiring Immediate Medical Referral

Signs/Symptoms	Common Cause
Angina pain not relieved in 20 min	Myocardial infarction
Angina pain with nausea, sweating, and profuse sweating	Myocardial infarction
Bowel or bladder incontinence and/or saddle anesthesia	Cauda equina lesion
Anaphylactic shock	Immunological allergy or disorder
Signs/symptoms of inadequate ventilation	Cardiopulmonary failure
Patient with diabetes who is confused, is lethargic, or exhibits changes in mental function	Diabetic coma
Patient with positive McBurney's point or rebound tenderness	Appendicitis or peritonitis
Sudden worsening of intermittent claudication	Thromboembolism
Throbbing chest, back, or abdominal pain that increases with exertion accompanied by a sensation of a heartbeat when lying down and palpable pulsating abdominal mass	Aortic aneurysm or abdominal aortic aneurysm

Data from Goodman CC, Snyder TEK: Differential Diagnosis in Physical Therapy. Philadelphia, PA: WB Saunders, 1990; Stowell T, Cioffredi W, Greiner A, et al: Abdominal differential diagnosis in a patient referred to a physical therapy clinic for low back pain. *J Orthop Sports Phys Ther.* 2005:35;755–764.

(37°C). However, a temperature in the range of 96.5–99.4°F (35.8–37.4°C) is not at all uncommon. Fever or pyrexia is a temperature exceeding 100°F (37.7°C).[82] Hyperpyrexia refers to extreme elevation of temperature above 41.1°C (or 106°F).[81] Hypothermia refers to an abnormally low temperature (below 35°C or 95°F). The temperature is generally taken by placing the bulb of a thermometer under the patient's tongue for 1–3 minutes, depending on the device. In most individuals, there is a diurnal (occurring everyday) variation in body temperature of 0.5–2°F. The lowest ebb is reached during sleep. Menstruating women have a well-known temperature pattern that reflects the effects of ovulation, with the temperature dropping slightly before menstruation, and then dropping further 24–36 hours prior to ovulation.[82] Coincident with ovulation, the temperature rises and remains at a somewhat higher level until just before the next menses. It is also worth noting that in adults older than 75 years of age and in those who are immunocompromised (e.g., transplant recipients, corticosteroid users, persons with chronic renal insufficiency, or anyone taking excessive antipyretic medications), the fever response may be blunted or absent.[81]

- *Heart rate.* In most people, the pulse is an accurate measure of heart rate. The heart rate or pulse is taken to obtain information about the resting state of the cardiovascular system and the system's response to activity or exercise and recovery.[81] It is also used to assess patency of the specific arteries palpated and the presence of any irregularities in the rhythm.[81] When the heart muscle contracts, blood is ejected into the aorta and the aorta stretches. At this point, the wave of distention (pulse wave) is most pronounced, but relatively slow moving (3–5 m/s). As it travels toward the peripheral blood vessels, it gradually diminishes and becomes faster. In the large arterial branches, its velocity is 7–10 m/s; in the small arteries, it is 15–35 m/s. When taking a pulse, the fingers must be placed near the artery and pressed gently against a firm structure, usually a bone. The pulse can be taken at a number of points. The most accessible is usually the radial pulse, at the distal aspect of the radius. Sometimes, the pulse cannot be taken at the wrist and is taken at the elbow (brachial artery), at the neck against the carotid artery (carotid pulse), behind the knee (popliteal artery), or in the foot using the dorsalis pedis or posterior tibial arteries. The pulse rate can also be measured by listening directly to the heart beat, using a stethoscope. One should avoid using the thumb when taking a pulse, as it has its own pulse that can interfere with detecting the patient's pulse. The normal adult heart rate is 70 beats per minute (bpm), with a range of 60–80 bpm. A rate of greater than 100 bpm is referred to as tachycardia. Normal causes of tachycardia include anxiety, stress, pain, caffeine, dehydration, or exercise. A rate of less than 60 bpm is referred to as bradycardia. Athletes may normally have a resting heart rate lower than 60. The normal range of resting heart rate in children is between 80 and 120 bpm. The rate for a newborn is 120 bpm (normal range 70–170 bpm).

CLINICAL PEARL

There is normally a transient increase in pulse rate with inspiration, followed by a slowing down with expiration.[22]

- *Respiratory rate.* The normal chest expansion difference between the resting position and the fully inhaled position is 2–4 cm (females > males). The clinician should compare measurements of both the anterior–posterior diameter and the transverse diameter during rest and at full inhalation. Normal respiratory rate is between 8 and 14 per minute in adults and slightly quicker in children. The following breathing patterns are characteristic of disease[82]:
  - Cheyne–Stokes respiration, characterized by a periodic, regular, sequentially increasing depth of respiration, occurs with serious cardiopulmonary or cerebral disorders.

- Biot's respiration, characterized by irregular spasmodic breathing and periods of apnea, is almost always associated with hypoventilation due to CNS disease.
- Kussmaul's respiration, characterized by deep, slow breathing, indicates acidosis, as the body attempts to blow off carbon dioxide.
- Apneustic breathing is an abnormal pattern of breathing characterized by a postinspiratory pause. The usual cause of apneustic breathing is a pontine lesion.
- Paradoxical respiration is an abnormal pattern of breathing, in which the abdominal wall is sucked in during inspiration (it is usually pushed out). Paradoxical respiration is due to paralysis of the diaphragm.

▸ *Blood pressure.* Blood pressure is a measure of vascular resistance to blood flow.[81] The normal adult blood pressure can vary over a wide range. The assessment of blood pressure provides information about the effectiveness of the heart as a pump and the resistance to blood flow. It is measured in mm Hg and is recorded in two numbers. The systolic pressure is the pressure that is exerted on the brachial artery when the heart is contracting, and the diastolic pressure is the pressure exerted on the artery during the relaxation phase of the cardiac cycle.[81] The JNC 7 report released in May 2003 has added a new category of prehypertension and has established more aggressive guidelines for medical intervention of hypertension. The normal values for resting blood pressure in adults are:

- normal: systolic blood pressure <120 mm Hg and diastolic blood pressure <80 mm Hg;
- prehypertension: systolic blood pressure 120–139 mm Hg or diastolic blood pressure 80–90 mm Hg;
- stage 1 hypertension: systolic blood pressure 140–159 mm Hg or diastolic blood pressure 90–99 mm Hg;
- stage 2 hypertension: systolic blood pressure ≥160 mm Hg or diastolic blood pressure ≥100 mm Hg.

The normal values for resting blood pressure in children are:

- systolic: birth to 1 month, 60–90 mm Hg; up to 3 years of age, 75–130 mm Hg; and over 3 years of age, 90–140 mm Hg;
- diastolic: birth to 1 month, 30–60 mm Hg; up to 3 years of age, 45–90 mm Hg; and over 3 years of age, 50–80 mm Hg.

Orthostatic hypotension is defined as a drop in systolic blood pressure when assuming an upright position. Orthostatic hypotension can occur as a side effect of antihypertensive medications (see Chap. 9), and in cases of low blood volume in patients who are postoperative or dehydrated, and in those with dysfunction of the autonomic nervous system, such as that which occurs with a spinal cord injury or postcerebrovascular accident.[81] Activities that may increase the chance of orthostatic hypotension, such as application of heat modalities, hydrotherapy, pool therapy, moderate-to-vigorous exercise using the large muscles, sudden changes of position, and stationary standing, should be avoided in susceptible patients.[81] The normal systolic range generally increases with age. The pressure should be determined in both the arms. Causes of marked asymmetry in blood pressure of the arms include the following: errors in measurements, marked difference in arm size, thoracic outlet syndromes, embolic occlusion of an artery, dissection of an aorta, external arterial occlusion, coarctation of the aorta, and atheromatous occlusion.[82]

▸ *Edema.* Edema is an observable swelling from fluid accumulation in certain body tissues. Edema most commonly occurs in the feet and legs, where it is also referred to as peripheral edema. Swelling or edema may be localized at the site of the injury or diffused over a larger area. In general, the amount of swelling is related to the severity of the injury. However, in some cases, serious injuries produce very limited swelling, whereas, in others, minor injuries cause significant swelling. Edema occurs as a result of changes in the local circulation and an inability of the lymphatic system to maintain equilibrium. The swelling is the result of the accumulation of excess fluid under the skin, in the interstitial spaces or compartments within the tissues that are outside of the blood vessels. Most of the body's fluids that are found outside of the cells are normally stored in two spaces: the blood vessels (referred to as blood volume) and the interstitial spaces (referred to as interstitial fluid). Generally, the size of lymph nodes is dependent on the size of the drainage area. Usually, the closer the lymph node is to the spinal cord, the greater the size of the lymph node. The neck is the exception to the rule. In various diseases, excess fluid can accumulate in either one or both of the interstitial spaces or blood vessels. An edematous limb indicates poor venous return. Pitting edema is characterized by an indentation of the skin after the pressure has been removed. A report of rapid joint swelling (within 2–4 hours) following a traumatic event may indicate bleeding into the joint. Swelling of a joint that is more gradual, occurring 8–24 hours following the trauma, is likely caused by an inflammatory process or synovial swelling.

The more serious reasons for swelling include fracture, tumor, congestive heart failure, and deep vein thrombosis.

▸ For the integumentary system, the assessment of skin integrity, skin color, and presence of scar formation. The integumentary system includes the skin, the hair, and the nails. The examination of the integumentary system may reveal manifestations of systemic disorders. The overall color of the skin should be noted. Cyanosis in the nails, the hands, and the feet may be a sign of a central (advanced lung disease, pulmonary edema, congenital heart disease, or low hemoglobin level) or peripheral (pulmonary edema, venous obstruction, or congestive heart failure) dysfunction.[81] Palpation of the skin, in general, should include assessment of temperature, texture, moistness, mobility, and turgor.[81] Skin temperature is best felt over large areas using the back of the clinician's hand. An assessment should be made as to whether this is localized or generalized warmth[81]:

- *Localized.* May be seen in areas of the underlying inflammation or infection.
- *Generalized.* May indicate fever or hyperthyroidism.

Skin texture is described as smooth or rough (coarse). Skin mobility may be decreased in areas of edema or in scleroderma.

TABLE 4-12 Upper-Quarter-Quadrant Scanning Motor Examination			
Muscle Action	**Muscle Tested**	**Root Level**	**Peripheral Nerve**
Shoulder abduction	Deltoid	Primarily C5	Axillary
Elbow flexion	Biceps brachii	Primarily C6	Musculocutaneous
Elbow extension	Triceps brachii	Primarily C7	Radial
Wrist extension	Extensor carpi radialis longus, brevis, and extensor carpi ulnaris	Primarily C6	Radial
Wrist flexion	Flexor carpi radialis and flexor carpi ulnaris	Primarily C7	Median nerve for radialis and ulnar nerve for ulnaris
Finger flexion	Flexor digitorum superficialis, flexor digitorum profundus, and lumbricales	Primarily C8	Median nerve for superficialis and both median and ulnar nerves for profundus and lumbricales
Finger abduction	Posterior (dorsal) interossei	Primarily T1	Ulnar

- For the musculoskeletal system, the assessment of gross symmetry, gross range of motion, gross strength, weight, and height.
- For the neuromuscular system, a general assessment of gross coordinated movement (e.g., balance, locomotion, transfers, and transitions). In addition, the clinician observes for peripheral and cranial nerve integrity and notes any indication of neurological compromise such as tremors or facial tics.
- For communication ability, affect, cognition, language, and learning style, the clinician notes whether the patient's communication level is age appropriate; whether the patient is oriented to person, place, and time; and whether the emotional and behavioral responses appear to be appropriate to his or her circumstances. It is important to verify that the patient can communicate their needs. The clinician should determine whether the patient has a good understanding of his or her condition, the planned intervention, and the prognosis. The clinician should also determine the learning style that best suits the patient.

The Scanning Examination

Designed by Cyriax,[83] the scanning examination is based on sound anatomic and pathologic principles. The Cyriax scanning (screening) examination traditionally follows the history and is often incorporated as part of the systems review, especially if:

- there are symptoms when no history of trauma is present.
- there is no history to explain the signs and symptoms.
- the signs and symptoms are unexplainable.

The purpose of the scanning examination is to help rule out the possibility of symptom referral from other areas, to ensure that all possible causes of the symptoms are examined, and to ensure a correct diagnosis.

The scanning examination is typically applied to patients presenting with neuromusculoskeletal complaints and differs from the five elements of patient/client management from *The Guide* in that the latter can be used as a system to approach virtually any type of patient, ranging from a pediatric patient with a permanent neurological condition to a patient with a serious injury to the integument, such as a burn patient.[84] The other major difference between the two approaches is that the scanning examination is designed to identify a specific pathoanatomical dysfunction, while *The Guide* works within movement-based diagnostic categories known as practice patterns.[84] Thus, the tests used in the scanning examination may produce a medical diagnosis rather than a physical therapy diagnosis.[85] The scanning examination should be carried out until the clinician is confident that there is no serious pathology present and is routinely carried out unless there is some good reason for postponing it (e.g., recent trauma, in which case a modified differential diagnostic examination is used).[4] Often, the scanning examination does not generate enough signs and symptoms to formulate a working hypothesis or a diagnosis. In this case, further testing with the tests and measures outlined in *The Guide* are required in order to proceed. The clinician must choose which scanning examination to use, based on the presenting signs and symptoms. The upper quarter scanning examination (Table 4-12) is appropriate for upper thoracic, upper extremity, and cervical problems, whereas the lower quarter scanning examination (Table 4-13) is typically used for thoracic, lower extremity, and lumbosacral problems. The preferred sequence of the scanning examination is outlined in Table 4-14.

The tests of the Cyriax[83] upper or lower quarter scanning examination (Table 4-15) can be used to:

- examine the patient's neurologic status. The tests that comprise the scanning examination are designed to detect neurologic weakness, the patient's ability to perceive sensations, and the inhibition of the muscle stretch reflexes and other reflexes by the CNS, which would highlight the presence of a lesion to the central or peripheral nervous systems (see Chap. 3).
- help determine whether the symptoms are being referred.
- confirm or refute the physician's diagnosis.
- help rule out any serious pathology, such as a fracture or a tumor.
- assess the status of the contractile and inert tissues.[83]
  - *Contractile.* The term *contractile tissue*, as defined by Cyriax, is a bit of a misnomer, because the only true

TABLE 4-13 Lower-Quarter-Quadrant Scanning Motor Examination

Muscle Action	Muscle Tested	Root Level	Peripheral Nerve
Hip flexion	Iliopsoas	L1–2	Femoral to iliacus and lumbar plexus to psoas
Knee extension	Quadriceps	L2–4	Femoral
Hamstrings	Biceps femoris, semimembranosus, and semitendinosus	L4–S3	Sciatic
Dorsiflexion with inversion	Tibialis anterior	Primarily L4	Deep fibular (peroneal)
Great toe extension	Extensor hallicus longus	Primarily L5	Deep fibular (peroneal)
Ankle eversion	Fibularis (peroneus) longus and brevis	Primarily S1	Superficial fibular (peroneal) nerve
Ankle plantarflexion	Gastrocnemius and soleus	Primarily S1	Tibial
Hip extension	Gluteus maximus	L5–S2	Inferior gluteal nerve

contractile tissue in the body is the muscle fiber. However, included under this term are the muscle belly, tendon, tenoperiosteal junction, submuscular/tendinous bursa, and bone (tendo-osseous junction), because all are stressed to some degree with a muscle contraction.

- *Inert.* Inert tissue, according to Cyriax, includes the joint capsule, the ligaments, the bursa, the articular surfaces of the joint, the synovium, the dura, the bone, and the fascia.

NB: The tendo-osseous junction and the bursae are placed in each of the subdivisions, owing to their close proximity to contractile tissue and their capacity to be compressed or stretched during movement.

▸ Generate a working hypothesis.

TABLE 4-14 Typical Sequence of Upper- or Lower-Quarter Scanning Examinations

1. Initial observation: involves everything from initial entry of the patient, including gait, demeanor, standing and sitting postures, obvious deformities and postural defects, scars, radiation burns, creases, and birthmarks
2. Patient history
3. Scanning examination
4. Active range of motion
5. Passive overpressure
6. Resistive tests
7. Deep tendon reflexes
8. Sensation testing
9. Special tests

Negative scan

If, at the end of the scan, the clinician has determined that the patient's condition is appropriate for physical therapy but has not determined a diagnosis to treat the patient, the clinician needs to perform further testing

Positive scan (results in a diagnosis)

1. Specific interventions (traction, manual techniques, and specific exercises) can be given if the diagnosis is one that will benefit from physical therapy.
2. Patient is returned to physician for more tests if signs and symptoms are cause for concern.

The thoroughness of the scanning examination is influenced by both patient tolerance and professional judgment. A general guideline is that the examination must continue until the clinician is confident that the patient's symptoms are not the result of a serious condition that demands medical attention.

The tests included in the scanning examination are strength testing, sensation testing (light touch and pinprick), muscle stretch reflexes, and the pathological reflexes (see Chap. 3). The various tests of the scanning examinations specific to the cervical, thoracic, and lumbar spine are described in the relevant chapters.

At the end of each of the scanning examinations, either a medical diagnosis (e.g., disk protrusion, prolapse, or extrusion; acute arthritis; specific tendonitis; muscle belly tear; spondylolisthesis; or stenosis) can be made or the scanning examination is considered negative. A negative scanning examination does not imply that there were no findings;

TABLE 4-15 Components of the Scanning Examination and the Structures Tested

Component	Description
Active ROM	Willingness to move, ROM, integrity of contractile and inert tissues, pattern of restriction (capsular or noncapsular), quality of motion, and symptom reproduction
Passive ROM	Integrity of inert and contractile tissues, ROM, end-feel, and sensitivity
Resisted	Integrity of contractile tissues (strength and sensitivity)
Stress	Integrity of inert tissues (ligamentous-disk stability)
Dural	Dural mobility
Neurologic	Nerve conduction
Dermatome	Afferent (sensation)
Myotome	Efferent (strength and fatigability)
Reflexes	Afferent–efferent and CNSs

ROM, range of motion.

TABLE 4-16 Scan Findings and Interventions

Conditions	Findings	Protocol
Disk protrusion, prolapse, and extrusion	Severe pain	Gentle manual traction in progressive extension
All movements reduced		
Anterior–posterior instability	Flexion and extension reduction greater than rotation	Traction and/or traction manipulation in extension
Arthritis	Hot capsular pattern	PRICEMEM (protection, rest, ice, compression, elevation, medication, electrotherapeutics, and manual therapy)
Subluxation of segment	One direction restricted	Exercises in pain-free direction
Arthrosis of segment	All directions restricted	Exercises in pain-free direction

rather, the results of examination were insufficient to generate a diagnosis upon which an intervention could be based. In this case, further examination is required using the various tests and measures pertinent to the body region.

The entire scanning examination should take no more than a few minutes to complete.

If a diagnosis is rendered from the scan, an intervention may be initiated using the guidelines outlined in Table 4-16. The scan or the history, or both, also may have indicated to the clinician that the patient's condition is in the acute stage of healing. Although this is not a diagnosis in the true sense, it can be used for the purpose of the intervention plan.

Although two studies[86,87] questioned the validity of some aspects of the selective tissue tension examination, no definitive conclusions were drawn from these studies. The scarcity of research to refute the work of Cyriax would suggest that its principles are sound and that its use should be continued.

Tests and Measures

The tests and the measures (Table 4-17) component of the examination, which serves as an adjunct to the history and the systems review, involves the physical examination of the patient. The tests and the measures now currently used in physical therapy have been largely influenced by the work of a number of clinicians over the years, including Cyriax,[83,88–90] Maitland,[7,91] Grieve,[92] Kaltenborn,[5] Butler,[12] Sahrmann,[11] and McKenzie.[93,94]

CLINICAL PEARL

The physical examination must be modified based on the history; for example, the examination of an acutely injured patient differs greatly from that of a patient in less discomfort or distress. In addition, the examination of a child differs in some respects from that of an adult (see Chap. 30).

The traditional goals of the physical examination have been to determine the structure involved, reproduce the patient's symptoms, confirm or refute the working hypothesis, and establish an objective data baseline.[6,95] More recently, the focus of the examination has shifted to include the identification of impairments, functional limitations, disabilities, or changes in physical function and health status resulting from injury, disease, or other causes. This information is then used through the evaluation process to establish the diagnosis and the prognosis, and to determine the intervention.[14]

The physical examination must be supported by as much science as possible, so that the decision about which test(s) to use during the examination should be based on the best available research evidence. According to Sackett and colleagues,[96] *evidence-based practice* (EBP) involves the integration of best research evidence with clinical expertise and patient values. A good test must differentiate the target disorder from

TABLE 4-17 Tests and Measures

Aerobic capacity and endurance
Anthropometric characteristics
Arousal, attention, and cognition
Assistive and adaptive devices
Circulation (arterial, venous, and lymphatic)
Cranial and peripheral nerve integrity
Environmental, home, and work (job, school, and play) barriers
Ergonomics and body mechanics
Gait, locomotion, and balance
Integumentary integrity
Joint integrity and mobility
Motor function (motor control and learning)
Muscle performance (strength, power, and endurance)
Neuromotor development and sensory integration
Orthotic, protective, and supportive devices
Pain
Posture
Prosthetic requirements
Range of motion (including muscle length)
Reflex integrity
Self-care and home management (ADLs and IADLs)
Sensory integrity (including proprioception and kinesthesia)
Ventilation and respiration and gas exchange
Work, community, and leisure integration or reintegration

ADLs, activities of daily living; IADLs, instrumental activities of daily living.
Data from American Physical Therapy Association: Guide to physical therapist practice. *Phys Ther.* 2001:81;S13–S95.

other disorders, with which it might otherwise be confused.[97] The gathering of evidence must occur in a systematic, reproducible, and unbiased manner to select and interpret diagnostic tests and to assess potential interventions.[98] The EBP process generally occurs in five steps[99]:

- Formulating a clinical question including details about the patient type or problem, the intervention being considered, a comparison intervention, and the outcome measure to be used.
- Searching for the best evidence, which can include a literature search on Ovid, EMBASE, PubMed, PEDro, or other medical search engine database, using the keywords from the clinical question.
- Critical appraisal of the evidence. In general, there are two types of clinical studies—those that analyze primary data and those that analyze secondary data.[22] Studies that collect and analyze primary data include case reports and series and case-controls, cross-sectional, cohort (both prospective and retrospective), and randomized controlled trials.[22] Analysis of second-rate data occurs in systematic reviews or meta-analysis for the purpose of pooling or synthesizing data to answer a question that is perhaps not practical or answerable within an individual study.[22] Another way to broadly categorize studies is experimental, where an intervention is introduced to subjects, or observational, in which no active treatment is introduced to subjects.[22]
- Applying the evidence to the patient.
- Evaluation of the outcome.

The choice of which tests to use should be based on pretest probabilities, which are used to assess the diagnostic possibility of a disorder. The results from these tests are then combined with value judgments to arrive at the correct diagnosis. Unfortunately, many tests and procedures used in physical therapy practice are not, as yet, evidence based. This is particularly true with the so-called special tests (see "Special Tests"). Indeed, many of the purportedly effective special tests listed in many orthopaedic texts exhibit such poor diagnostic accuracy that only 50% of patients who have a positive test result are found to have the condition that the test is supposed to detect.[98,100] Without EBP, clinicians fail to provide the consumer with scientific evidence regarding clinically effective and cost-effective practice. Throughout this text, wherever possible, the sources of evidence will be identified for each of the examination and intervention techniques described. However, in an ever-changing profession, it is ultimately the reader's responsibility to remain updated with practice recommendations and decide the appropriateness of the evidence for each of their patients in their own unique clinical setting.

The neurologic tests of the orthopaedic examination are described in Chapter 3. Before proceeding with the tests and measures, the clinician must obtain a valid consent and a full explanation must be provided to the patient as to what procedures are to be performed and the reasons for these. The chosen tests used by the clinician must be based on the patient's history or the presentation. At times, a complete examination cannot be performed. For example, if the joint to be examined is too acutely inflamed, the clinician may defer some of the examinations to the subsequent visit.

Active Physiological Range of Motion of the Extremities

Active movements of the involved area are performed before passive movements. During the history, the clinician should have deduced the general motions that aggravate or provoke the pain. Any movements that are known to be painful are performed last. The range of motion examination should be used to confirm the exact directions of motion that elicit the symptoms. The diagnosis of restricted movement in the extremities can usually be simplified by comparing both sides, provided that at least one side is uninvolved. Under normal circumstances, the normal (uninvolved) side is tested first as this allows the clinician to establish a baseline, while also showing the patient what to expect. Active range of motion testing may be deferred if small and unguarded motions provoke intense pain, because this may indicate a high degree of joint irritability, or other serious condition. The normal active range of motion for each of the joints is depicted in Table 4-18.

Active range of motion testing gives the clinician information about the following:

- Quantity of available physiologic motion.
- Presence of muscle substitutions.
- Willingness of the patient to move.
- Integrity of the contractile and the inert tissues.

TABLE 4-18 Active Ranges of Joint Motions

Joint	Action	Degrees of Motion
Shoulder	Flexion	0–180
	Extension	0–40
	Abduction	0–180
	Internal rotation	0–80
	External rotation	0–90
Elbow	Flexion	0–150
Forearm	Pronation	0–75
	Supination	0–85
Wrist	Flexion	0–80
	Extension	0–60
	Radial deviation	0–20
	Ulnar deviation	0–30
Hip	Flexion	0–125
	Extension	0–30
	Abduction	0–40
	Adduction	0–20
	Internal rotation	0–40
	External rotation	0–50
Knee	Flexion	0–150
Ankle	Plantarflexion	0–40
	Dorsiflexion	0–20
Foot	Inversion	0–30
	Eversion	0–20

- Quality of motion. A painful arc during range of motion, with or without a painful limitation of movement, indicates the presence of a derangement.[101] For example, there may be an arc of pain between 60 and 120 degrees on shoulder abduction, indicating an impingement of the structures under the acromion process or the coracoacromial ligament.
- Symptom reproduction.
- Pattern of motion restriction (e.g., capsular or noncapsular, opening or closing restriction—see later).

Capsular and Noncapsular Patterns of Restriction

Cyriax[83] introduced the terms *capsular* and *noncapsular* patterns of restriction, which link impairment to pathology (Table 4-19). A capsular pattern of restriction is a limitation of pain and movement in a joint-specific ratio, which is usually present with arthritis, or following prolonged immobilization.[83] It is worth remembering that a consistent capsular pattern for a particular joint might not exist and that these

TABLE 4-19 Capsular Patterns of Restriction

Joint	Limitation of Motion (Passive Angular Motion)
Glenohumeral	External rotation > abduction > internal rotation (3:2:1)
Acromioclavicular	No true capsular pattern; possible loss of horizontal adduction and pain (and sometimes slight loss of end range) with each motion
Sternoclavicular	See acromioclavicular joint
Humeroulnar	Flexion > extension (±4:1)
Humeroradial	No true capsular pattern; possible equal limitation of pronation and supination
Superior radioulnar	No true capsular pattern; possible equal limitation of pronation and supination with pain at end ranges
Inferior radioulnar	No true capsular pattern; possible equal limitation of pronation and supination with pain at end ranges
Wrist (carpus)	Flexion = extension
Radiocarpal	See wrist (carpus)
Carpometacarpal	Flexion = extension
Midcarpal	Flexion = extension
Carpometacarpal 1	Retroposition
Carpometacarpals 2–5	Fan > fold
Metacarpophalangeal 2–5	Flexion > extension (±2:1)
Interphalangeal 2–5	
Proximal (PIP)	Flexion > extension (±2:1)
Distal (DIP)	Flexion > extension (±2:1)
Hip	Internal rotation > flexion > abduction = extension > other motions
Tibiofemoral	Flexion > extension (±5:1)
Superior tibiofibular	No capsular pattern; pain at end range of translatory movements
Talocrural	Plantar flexion > dorsiflexion
Talocalcaneal (subtalar)	Varus > valgus
Midtarsal	Inversion (plantar flexion, adduction, and supination)
Talonavicular calcaneocuboid	> Dorsiflexion
Metatarsophalangeal 1	Extension > flexion (±2:1)
Metatarsophalangeals 2–5	Flexion ≥ extension
Interphalangeals 2–5	
Proximal	Flexion ≥ extension
Distal	Flexion ≥ extension

Data from Cyriax J: Textbook of Orthopaedic Medicine, Diagnosis of Soft Tissue Lesions. 8th edn. London: Bailliere Tindall, 1982.

patterns are based on empirical findings and tradition, rather than on research.[86,102]

A noncapsular pattern of restriction is a limitation in a joint in any pattern other than a capsular one and may indicate the presence of a joint derangement, a restriction of one part of the joint capsule, or an extra-articular lesion that obstructs joint motion.[83]

A positive finding for joint hypomobility would be a reduced range in a capsular or noncapsular pattern. The hypomobility can be painful, suggesting an acute sprain of a structure, or painless, suggesting a contracture or an adhesion of the tested structure. Significant degeneration of the articular cartilage presents with crepitus (joint noise) on movement when compression of the joint surfaces is maintained.

While abnormal motion is typically described as being reduced, abnormal motion may also be excessive. Excessive motion is often missed and is erroneously classified as normal motion. To help determine whether the motion is normal or excessive, *passive range of motion* (PROM), in the form of passive overpressure, and the end-feel are assessed (see next section).

CLINICAL PEARL

Apprehension from the patient during active range of motion that limits a movement at near or full range suggests instability, whereas apprehension in the early part of the range suggests anxiety caused by pain.

Full and pain-free active range of motion suggests normalcy for that movement, although it is important to remember that normal *range* of motion is not synonymous with normal motion.[103] Normal motion implies that the control of motion must also be present. This control is a factor of muscle flexibility, joint stability, and central neurophysiologic mechanisms. These factors are highly specific in the body.[104] A loss of motion at one joint may not prevent the performance of a functional task, although it may result in the task being performed in an abnormal manner. For example, the act of walking can still be accomplished in the presence of a knee joint that has been fused into extension. Because the essential mechanisms of knee flexion in the stance period and foot clearance in the swing period are absent, the patient compensates for these losses by hiking the hip on the involved side, by side bending the lumbar spine to the uninvolved side, and through excessive motion of the foot.

Single motions in the cardinal planes are usually tested first. These tests are followed by dynamic and static testing. Dynamic testing involves repeated movements. Static testing involves sustaining a position. Sustained static positions may be used to help detect postural syndromes.[101] McKenzie advocates the use of repeated movements in specific directions in the spine and the extremities. Repeated movements can give the clinician some valuable insight into the patient's condition[101]:

- Internal derangements tend to worsen with repeated motions.
- Symptoms of a postural dysfunction remain unchanged with repeated motions.
- Pain from a dysfunction syndrome is increased with tissue loading but ceases at rest.
- Repeated motions can indicate the irritability of the condition.
- Repeated motions can indicate to the clinician the direction of motion to be used as part of the intervention. If pain increases during repeated motion in a particular direction, exercising in that direction is not indicated. If pain only worsens in part of the range, repeated motion exercises can be used for the part of the range that is pain free or that does not worsen the symptoms.
- Pain that is increased after the repeated motions may indicate a retriggering of the inflammatory response, and repeated motions in the opposite direction should be explored.

Combined motion testing may be used when the symptoms are not reproduced with the cardinal plane motions (flexion, extension, abduction, etc.), the repeated motions, or the sustained positions. Compression and distraction also may be added to all of the active motion tests in an attempt to reproduce the symptoms.

Active Physiological Range of Motion of the Spine

Active physiologic intervertebral mobility, or active mobility, tests of the spine were originally designed by osteopaths to assess the ability of each spinal joint to move actively through its normal range of motion, by palpating over the transverse processes of a joint during the motion (see also Position Testing of the Spine). Theoretically, by palpating over the transverse processes, the clinician can indirectly assess the motions occurring at the zygapophyseal joints at either side of the intervertebral disk. However, the clinician must remember that, although it is convenient to describe the various motions of the spine occurring in a certain direction, these involve the integration of movements of a multijoint complex.

The human zygapophyseal joints are capable of only two major motions: gliding upward and gliding downward. If these movements occur in the same direction, flexion or extension of the spine occurs, while if the movements occur in opposite directions, side flexion occurs.

Osteopaths use the terms *opening* and *closing* to describe flexion and extension motions, respectively, at the zygapophyseal joint. Under normal circumstances, an equal amount of gliding occurs at each zygapophyseal joint with these motions.

- During flexion, both zygapophyseal joints glide superiorly (open).
- During extension, both zygapophyseal joints glide inferiorly (close).
- During side flexion, one joint is gliding inferiorly (closing), while the other joint is gliding superiorly (opening). For example, during right side flexion, the right joint is gliding inferiorly (closing), while the left joint is gliding superiorly (opening).

By combining flexion or extension movements with side flexion, a joint can be "opened" or "closed" to its limits. Thus, flexion and right-side flexion of a segment assesses the ability of the left joint to maximally open (flex), whereas extension and left-side flexion of a segment assesses the ability of the left joint to maximally close (extend).

There is a point that may be considered as the center of segmental rotation, about which all segmental motion must occur. In the case of a zygapophyseal joint impairment (hypermobility or hypomobility), it is presumed that this center of rotation will be altered.

If one zygapophyseal joint is rendered hypomobile (i.e., the superior facet cannot move to the extreme of superior or inferior motion), then the pure motions of flexion and extension cannot occur. This results in a relative asymmetric motion of the two superior facets, as the end of range of flexion or extension is approached (i.e., a side-flexion motion will occur). However, this side-flexion motion will not be about the normal center of segmental rotation. The structure responsible for the loss of zygapophyseal joint motion, whether it is a muscle, disk protrusion, or the zygapophyseal joint itself, will become the new axis of vertebral motion, and a new component of rotation about a vertical axis, normally unattainable, will be introduced into the segmental motion. The degree of this rotational deviation is dependent on the distance of the impairment from the original center of rotation.

Because the zygapophyseal joints in the spine are posterior to the axis of rotation, an obvious rotational change occurring between full flexion and full extension (in the position of a vertebral segment) is indicative of zygapophyseal joint motion impairment.

By observing any marked and obvious rotation of a vertebral segment occurring between the positions of full flexion and full extension, one may deduce the probable pathologic impairment.

CLINICAL PEARL

Active motion induced by the contraction of the muscles determines the so-called physiologic range of motion,[105] whereas passively performed movement causes stretching of noncontractile elements, such as ligaments, and determines the anatomic range of motion.

Passive Physiological Range of Motion of the Extremities

Passive motions are movements performed by the clinician without the assistance of the patient. Passive movements are performed in the anatomic range of motion for the joint and normally demonstrate slightly greater range of motion than active motion—the barrier to active motion should occur earlier in the range than the barrier to passive motion.

If the patient can complete the active physiological range of motion easily, without presenting pain or other symptoms, then passive testing of that motion is usually unnecessary. However, if the active motions do not reproduce the patient's symptoms, because the patient avoids going into the painful part of the range, or the active range of motion appears incomplete, it is important to perform gentle passive overpressure. Pain during passive overpressure is often due to the movement, stretching, or pinching of noncontractile structures. Pain that occurs at the mid-end range of active and passive movement is suggestive of a capsular contraction or a scar tissue that has not been adequately remodeled.[101] Pain occurring at the end of PROM may be due to a stretching of the contractile structures, as well as noncontractile structures.[106] Thus, PROM testing gives the clinician information about the integrity of the contractile and inert tissues, and with gentle overpressure, the *end-feel*. Cyriax[83] introduced the concept of the end-feel, which is the quality of resistance at end range. To execute the end-feel, the point at which resistance is encountered is evaluated for quality and tenderness. Additional forces are needed as the end range of a joint is reached, and the elastic limits are challenged. This space termed the *end-play zone* requires a force of overpressure to be reached so that, when that force is released, the joint springs back from its elastic limits. The end-feel can indicate to the clinician the cause of the motion restriction (Tables 4-20 and 4-21).

CLINICAL PEARL

One study that looked at the intra- and inter-rater reliability of assessing end-feel, and pain and resistance sequence in subjects with painful shoulders and knees, found the end-feel to have good intrarater reliability, but unacceptable inter-rater reliability.[86]

Although some clinicians feel that overpressure should not be applied in the presence of pain, this is erroneous. Most, if not all, of the end-feels that suggest acute or serious pathology are to be found in the painful range, including spasm and the empty end-feel.

The end-feel is very important in joints that have only very small amounts of normal range, such as those of the spine. The type of end-feel can help the clinician determine the presence of dysfunction. For example, a hard, capsular end-feel indicates a pericapsular hypomobility, whereas a jammed or a pathomechanical end-feel indicates a pathomechanical hypomobility. A normal end-feel would indicate normal range, whereas an abnormal end-feel would suggest abnormal range, either hypomobile or hypermobile. An association between an increase in pain and abnormal pathologic end-feels compared with normal end-feels has been demonstrated.[107]

The planned intervention, and its intensity, is based on the type of tissue resistance to movement, demonstrated by the end-feel, and on the acuteness of the condition (Table 4-22).[83] This information may indicate whether the resistance is caused by pain, muscle, capsule ligament, disturbed mechanics of the joint, or a combination.

CLINICAL PEARL

According to Cyriax, if active and passive motions are limited or painful in the same direction, the lesion is in an inert tissue, whereas if the active and passive motions are limited or painful in the opposite direction, the lesion is in a contractile tissue.[83]

TABLE 4-20 Normal End-Feels

Type	Cause	Characteristics and Examples
Bony	Produced by bone-to-bone approximation	Abrupt and unyielding; gives impression that further forcing will break something *Examples:* Normal: elbow extension Abnormal: cervical rotation (may indicate osteophyte)
Elastic	Produced by muscle–tendon unit; may occur with adaptive shortening	Stretches with elastic recoil and exhibits constant-length phenomenon; further forcing feels as if it will snap something *Examples:* Normal: wrist flexion with finger flexion, the straight-leg raise, and ankle dorsiflexion with the knee extended Abnormal: decreased dorsiflexion of the ankle with the knee flexed
Soft-tissue approximation	Produced by contact of two muscle bulks on either side of a flexing joint where joint range exceeds other restraints	Very forgiving end-feel that gives impression that further normal motion is possible if enough force could be applied *Examples:* Normal: knee flexion and elbow flexion in extremely muscular subjects Abnormal: elbow flexion with obese subject
Capsular	Produced by capsule or ligaments	Various degrees of stretch without elasticity; stretch ability is dependent on thickness of tissue Strong capsular or extracapsular ligaments produce hard capsular end-feel, whereas thin capsule produces softer one Impression given to clinician is that if further force is applied, something will tear *Examples:* Normal: wrist flexion (soft), elbow flexion in supination (medium), and knee extension (hard) Abnormal: inappropriate stretch ability for specific joint; if too hard, may indicate hypomobility due to arthrosis; and if too soft, hypermobility

Data from Meadows JTS: Manual Therapy: Biomechanical Assessment and Treatment, Advanced Technique. Calgary: Swodeam Consulting, Inc., 1995.

The quantity and quality of movement refer to the ability to achieve end-range without deviation from the intended movement plane.

Both the passive and active physiological ranges of motion can be measured using a goniometer, which has been shown to have a satisfactory level of intraobserver reliability.[108–110] Visual observation in experienced clinicians has been found to be equal to measurements by goniometry.[111]

The recording of range of motion varies. The American Medical Association recommends recording the range of motion on the basis of the neutral position of the joint being zero, with the degrees of motion increasing in the direction the joint moves from the zero starting point.[112] A plus sign (+) is used to indicate joint hyperextension and a minus sign (–) to indicate an extension lag. The method of recording chosen is not important, provided the clinician chooses a recognized method and documents it consistently with the same patient.

Passive Physiological Range of Motion of the Spine

The passive physiologic intervertebral mobility, or passive mobility, tests use the same principles as the active physiologic intervertebral mobility tests to assess the ability of each joint in the spine to move passively through its normal range of motion, while the clinician palpates over the interspinous spaces. During extension, the spinous processes should approximate, whereas during flexion, they should separate.

If pain is reproduced, it is useful to associate the pain with the onset of tissue resistance to gain an appreciation of the acuteness of the problem. The passive mobility tests of the spine are described in the appropriate chapters.

Flexibility

The examination of flexibility is performed to determine if a particular structure, or group of structures, has sufficient extensibility to perform a desired activity. The extensibility

TABLE 4-21 Abnormal End-Feels

Type	Causes	Characteristics and Examples
Springy	Produced by articular surface rebounding from intra-articular meniscus or disk; impression is that if forced further, something will give way	Rebound sensation as if pushing off from a rubber pad *Examples:* Normal: axial compression of cervical spine Abnormal: knee flexion or extension with displaced meniscus
Boggy	Produced by viscous fluid (blood) within joint	"Squishy" sensation as joint is moved toward its end range; further forcing feels as if it will burst joint *Examples:* Normal: none Abnormal: hemarthrosis at knee
Spasm	Produced by reflex and reactive muscle contraction in response to irritation of nociceptor, predominantly in articular structures and muscle; forcing it further feels as if nothing will give	Abrupt and "twangy" end to movement that is unyielding while the structure is being threatened but disappears when threat is removed (kicks back) With joint inflammation, it occurs early in range, especially toward close-packed position, to prevent further stress With irritable joint hypermobility, it occurs at end of what should be normal range, as it prevents excessive motion from further stimulating the nociceptor Spasm in grade II muscle tears becomes apparent as muscle is passively lengthened and is accompanied by a painful weakness of that muscle *Note:* Muscle guarding is not a true end-feel, as it involves co-contraction *Examples:* Normal: none Abnormal: significant traumatic arthritis, recent traumatic hypermobility, and grade II muscle tears
Empty	Produced solely by pain; frequently caused by serious and severe pathologic changes that do not affect joint or muscle and so do not produce spasm; demonstration of this end-feel is, with exception of acute subdeltoid bursitis, de facto evidence of serious pathology; further forcing simply increases pain to unacceptable levels	Limitation of motion has no tissue resistance component, and resistance is from patient being unable to tolerate further motion due to severe pain; it is not same feeling as voluntary guarding, but rather it feels as if patient is both resisting and trying to allow movement simultaneously *Examples:* Normal: none Abnormal: acute subdeltoid bursitis and sign of the buttock
Facilitation	Not truly an end-feel, as facilitated hypertonicity does not restrict motion; it can, however, be perceived near end range	Light resistance as from constant light muscle contraction throughout latter half of range that does not prevent end of range being reached; resistance is unaffected by rate of movement *Examples:* Normal: none Abnormal: spinal facilitation at any level

Data from Meadows JTS: Manual Therapy: Biomechanical Assessment and Treatment, Advanced Technique. Calgary: Swodeam Consulting, Inc., 1995.

and habitual length of connective tissue are factors of the demands placed upon it. These demands produce changes in the viscoelastic properties and, thus, the length–tension relationship of a muscle or muscle group, resulting in an increase or a decrease in the length of those structures. A decrease in the length of the soft-tissue structures, or adaptive shortening, is very common in postural dysfunctions. Adaptive shortening also can be produced by

- restricted mobility;
- tissue damage secondary to trauma;
- prolonged immobilization;
- disease;
- hypertonia. Hypertonic muscles that are superficial can be identified through observation and palpation. Observation will reveal the muscle to be raised, and light palpation will

TABLE 4-22	Abnormal Barriers to Motion and Recommended Manual Techniques	
Barrier	**End-feel**	**Technique**
Pain	Empty	None
Pain	Spasm	None
Pain	Capsular	Oscillations (I, IV)
Joint adhesions	Early capsular	Passive articular motion stretch (I–V)
Muscle adhesions	Early elastic	Passive physiologic motion stretch
Hypertonicity	Facilitation	Muscle energy (Hold/relax, etc.)
Bone	Bony	None

provide information about tension, as the muscle will feel hard and may stand out from those around it.

Flexibility can be measured objectively using standardized tests, or a goniometer. A more subjective test for flexibility includes an examination of the end-feel, which can detect a loss of motion resulting from excessive tension of the agonist muscle. Visual observation, which has been found to have a variability of 30% in patients with low back pain and sciatica, may also be used.[113]

Joint Integrity and Mobility

Joint integrity and mobility testing can provide valuable information about the status and the mobility of each joint and its capsule. Kaltenborn[5] introduced the concept of motion restriction of a joint based on its arthrokinematics. In order for a joint to function completely, both the osteokinematic and arthrokinematic motions have to occur normally (see Chap. 1). It, therefore, follows that if a joint is not functioning completely, either the physiologic range of motion is limited compared with the expected norm or there is no PROM available between the physiologic barrier and the anatomic barrier. As previously mentioned, the assessment of the end-feel can help determine the cause of the restriction.[57] In general, the physiologic motion is controlled by the contractile tissues, whereas the accessory motion is controlled by the integrity of the joint surfaces and the noncontractile (inert) tissues. This guideline may change in the case of a joint that has undergone degenerative changes, which can result in a decrease in the physiologic motions (capsular pattern of restriction). It is important that the intervention to restore the complete function of the joint be aimed at the specific cause.

Joint pain and dysfunction do not occur in isolation.[114,115] Various measurement scales have been proposed for judging the amount of accessory joint motion present between two joint surfaces (see Chap. 10), most of which are based on a comparison with a comparable contralateral joint, using manually applied forces in a logical and precise manner.[116] In the extremities, these tests are referred to as passive articular mobility, or joint glide tests. In the spine, these tests are referred to as the passive physiologic accessory intervertebral motion testing.

CLINICAL PEARL

In general, if the concave-on-convex glide (see Chap. 1) is restricted, there is a contracture of the trailing portion of the capsule, whereas if the convex-on-concave glide is restricted, there is an inability of the moving surface to glide into the contracted portion of the capsule.

The passive articular mobility tests involve the clinician assessing the arthrokinematic, or accessory, motions using joint glides, and determining whether the glide is hypomobile, normal, or hypermobile (see Chap. 2).[5–7]

Accessory motions are involuntary motions. With few exceptions, muscles cannot restrict the glides of a joint, especially if the glides are tested in the open-packed position of a peripheral joint and, at the end of available range, in the spinal joints.

Thus, if the clinician assesses the accessory motion of the joint by performing a joint glide, information about the integrity of the inert structures will be given. There are two scenarios:

1. *The joint glide is unrestricted.* An unrestricted joint glide indicates two differing conclusions:
   a. The integrity of both the joint surface and the periarticular tissue is good. If the joint surface and the periarticular structures are intact, the patient's loss of motion must be the result of a contractile tissue. The intervention for this type involves soft-tissue mobilization techniques designed to change the length of a contractile tissue.
   b. The joint glide is unrestricted but excessive. The excessive motion may indicate a pathological hypermobility or instability, or it may be normal for the individual. In these cases, the end-feel can provide some useful information. The intervention for this type concentrates on stabilizing techniques designed to give secondary support to the joint through muscle action.
2. *The joint glide is restricted.* If the joint glide is restricted, the joint surface and the periarticular tissues are implicated as the cause of the patient's loss of motion, although as previously mentioned, the contractile tissues cannot definitively be ruled out. The intervention for this type of finding initially involves a specific joint mobilization to restore the glide. Once the joint glide is restored following these mobilizations, the osteokinematic motion can be assessed again. If it is still reduced, the contractile tissues are likely to be at fault. Distraction and compression can be used to help differentiate the cause of the restriction.
   a. *Distraction.* Traction is a force imparted passively by the clinician that results in a distraction of the joint surfaces. If the distraction is limited, a contracture of connective tissue should be suspected.

If the distraction increases the pain, it may indicate a tear of connective tissue and may be associated with increased range.

If the distraction eases the pain, it may indicate an involvement of the joint surface.

b. *Compression*. Compression is the opposite force to distraction, and involves an approximation of joint surfaces.

If the compression increases the pain, a loose body or an internal derangement of the joint may be present.

If the compression decreases the pain, it may implicate the joint capsule.

Thus, by assessing these joint motions, the clinician can determine the

- cause of a limitation in a joint's physiologic range of motion;
- end-feel response of the tissues;
- stage of healing;
- integrity of the support structures (e.g., ligaments) of a joint (for example, the integrity of the anterior cruciate ligament is tested with the Lachman test).

Based on the information gleaned from the joint glide assessment, the clinician makes clinical decisions as to which intervention to use. If the joint glide is felt to be restricted, and there is no indication of a bony end-feel or severe irritability, joint mobilization techniques are used. If the joint glide is found to be unrestricted, the clinician may decide to employ a technique that increases the extensibility of the surrounding connective tissues, such as muscle energy, because abnormal shortness of these connective tissues, including the ligaments, the joint capsule, and the periarticular tissues, can restrict joint mobility.

CLINICAL PEARL

Caution must be used when basing clinical judgments on the results of accessory motion testing, because few studies have examined the validity and reliability of accessory motion testing of the spine or extremities and little is known about the validity of these tests for most inferences.[116] A study of the predicted value of positive and negative test results in addition to the sensitivity and specificity of the various tests would be of value.[116]

Position Testing in the Spine

The position tests are screening tests designed by osteopaths to examine the relative position of a zygapophyseal joint, or joints, to the joint(s) below (see appropriate chapters). As with all screening tests, position testing is valuable in focusing the attention of the clinician to a specific area but is not appropriate for making a definitive statement concerning the movement status of the segment. However, when combined with the results of the passive and active movement testing, position tests help to form the working hypothesis.

Muscle Performance: Strength, Power, and Endurance

Strength measures the power with which musculotendinous units act across a bone-joint lever-arm system to actively generate motion, or passively resist movement against gravity and variable resistance.[112]

According to Cyriax, pain with a contraction generally indicates an injury to the muscle or a capsular structure.[83] This suspicion can be confirmed by combining the findings from the isometric test with the findings of the passive motion and the joint distraction and compression tests (Table 4-23). Cyriax reasoned that if you isolate and then apply tension to a structure, you can make a conclusion as to the integrity of that structure.[83] His work also introduced the concept of tissue reactivity. Tissue reactivity is the manner in which different stresses and movements can alter the clinical signs and symptoms. This knowledge can be used to gauge any subtle changes to the patient's condition.[117]

In addition to examining the integrity of the contractile and inert structures, strength testing may be used to examine the integrity of the key muscles (see Chap. 3). Pain with muscle testing may indicate a muscle injury, a joint injury, or a combination of both. Pain that occurs consistently with resistance, at whatever the length of the muscle, may indicate a tear of the muscle belly. Weakness with muscle testing must be differentiated between weakness throughout the range of motion (pathological weakness) and weakness that only occurs in certain positions (positional weakness). According to Cyriax,[83,89] strength testing can provide the clinician with the following findings:

- A weak and painless contraction may indicate palsy or a complete rupture of the muscle–tendon unit. The motor disorder associated with peripheral neuropathy is first

TABLE 4-23 Differential Diagnosis of Contractile, Inert, and Neural Tissue Injury

	Contractile Tissue	Inert Tissue	Neural Tissue
Pain	Cramping, dull, and ache	Dull–sharp	Burning and lancinating
Paresthesia	No	No	Yes
Duration	Intermittent	Intermittent	Intermittent–constant
Dermatomal distribution	No	No	Yes
Peripheral nerve sensory distribution	No	No	Yes (if peripheral nerve involved)
End-feel	Muscle spasm	Boggy and hard capsular	Stretch

manifested by weakness and a diminished or absent tendon reflex (see Chap. 3).[49]

- A strong and painless contraction indicates a normal finding.
- A weak and painful contraction. A study by Franklin and colleagues[87] indicated that the conditions related to this finding need to include not only serious pathology, such as a significant muscle tear or a tumor, but relatively minor muscle damage and inflammation such as that induced by eccentric isokinetic exercise.[106]
- A strong and painful contraction indicates a grade I contractile lesion.

Pain that does not occur during the test, but occurs upon the release of the contraction, is thought to have an articular source, produced by the joint glide that occurs following the release of tension.

CLINICAL PEARL

Pain that occurs with resistance, accompanied by pain at the opposite end of passive range, indicates muscle impairment.

The degree of certainty regarding the findings just described depends on a combination of the length of the muscle tested and the force applied. To fully test the integrity of the muscle–tendon unit, a maximum contraction must be performed in the fully lengthened position of the muscle–tendon unit. Although this position fully tests the muscle–tendon unit, there are some problems with testing in this manner:

- The joint and its surrounding inert tissues are in a more vulnerable position and could be the source of the pain.
- It is difficult to differentiate between damage to the contractile tissue of varying severity. The degree of significance with the findings in resistive testing depends on the position of the muscle and the force applied (Table 4-24). For example, pain reproduced with a minimal contraction in the rest position for the muscle is more strongly suggestive of a contractile lesion than pain reproduced with a maximal contraction in the lengthened position for the muscle.

TABLE 4-24 Strength Testing Related to Joint Position and Muscle Length

Muscle Length	Rationale
Fully lengthened	Muscle in position of passive insufficiency Tightens the inert component of the muscle Tests for muscle tears (tendoperiosteal tears) while using minimal force
Mid-range	Muscle in strongest position Tests overall power of muscle
Fully shortened	Muscle in its weakest position Used for the detection of palsies, especially if coupled with an eccentric contraction

- As a muscle lengthens, it reaches a point of passive insufficiency, where it is not capable of generating its maximum force output (see Chap. 1).

If the same muscle is tested on the opposite side, using the same testing procedure, the concern about the length of the muscle is removed, because the focus of the test is to provide a comparison with the same muscle on the opposite side, rather than to assess the absolute force output.

To assess strength, strength values using *manual muscle testing* (MMT) have traditionally been used between similar muscle groups on opposite extremities, or antagonistic ratios. This information is then used to determine whether a patient was fully rehabilitated. It should be noted that there is considerable variability in the amount of resistance that normal muscles can hold against. The application of resistance throughout the arc of motion (make test or active resistance test) in addition to resistance applied at only one point in the arc of motion (break test) can help in judging the strength of a muscle.[106] During all testing, stabilization of the body part on which the muscle originates in addition to careful avoidance of substitution by other muscle groups are emphasized. Substitutions by other muscle groups during testing indicate the presence of weakness. It does not, however, tell the clinician the cause of the weakness.

CLINICAL PEARL

MMT has been shown to be less sensitive in detecting strength deficits in stronger muscles than in weaker muscles.[106]

Several scales have been devised to assess muscle strength. For example, Janda[118] used a 0–5 scale with the following descriptions:

- *Grade 5: N (normal).* A normal, very strong muscle with a full range of movement and one that is able to overcome considerable resistance. This does not mean that the muscle is normal in all circumstances (e.g., when at the onset of fatigue or in a state of exhaustion). If the clinician is having difficulty differentiating between a grade 4 and a grade 5, the eccentric "break" method of muscle testing may be used. This procedure starts as an isometric contraction, but then the clinician applies sufficient force to cause an eccentric contraction or a "break" in the patient's isometric contraction.
- *Grade 4: G (good).* A muscle with good strength and full range of movement, and one that is able to overcome moderate resistance. The subjectivity involved in a grade 4 score is one of the major criticisms of MMT as the grading requires the clinician to assign an ordinal number to a subjective evaluation of resistance offered by the patient.
- *Grade 3: F (fair).* A muscle that can move through the complete range of movement against gravity only with no additional resistance applied. If the muscle strength is less than grade 3, then the methods advocated in muscle testing manuals must be used.[106]
- *Grade 2: P (poor).* A very weak muscle that is only able to move through the complete range of motion if the force of gravity is eliminated.

- *Grade 1: T (trace).* A muscle with evidence of slight contractility but demonstrates no effective movement.
- *Grade 0.* A muscle with no evidence of any contractility.

The grading systems for MMT produce ordinal data with unequal rankings between grades. For example, the grades 5 (normal) and 4 (good) typically encompass a large range of a muscle's strength, while the grades of 3 (fair), 2 (poor), and 1 (trace) include a much narrower range.[106] If the popular methods to grade muscles are analyzed, the frailties and similarities become obvious. If the muscle strength is less than grade 3, these testing grades are useful, but it is the grades of 3 and higher that produce the most confusion. Some of the confusion arises from the descriptions of maximal, moderate, and minimal, or considerable, which removes much of the objectivity from the tests.

CLINICAL PEARL

Studies have demonstrated that reliability in MMT is dependent on the specific muscle being examined. For example, Florence and colleagues[119] found high reliability in the proximal muscles as opposed to the distal muscles, and Barr and colleagues[120] found the upper body muscles to be more reliably tested than the lower body ones.[121]

To be a valid test, strength testing must elicit a maximum contraction of the muscle being tested. The following strategies ensure that this occurs:

1. *Placing the joint that the muscle to be tested crosses, in (or close to) its open-packed position.* This strategy helps protect the joint from excessive compressive forces, and the surrounding inert structures from excessive tension.
2. *Placing the muscle to be tested in a shortened position.* This puts the muscle in an ineffective physiologic position and has the effect of increasing motor neuron activity.
3. *Using gravity-minimized positions.* This strategy avoids the effect of the weight of the moving body segment on force measurements. For example, to test the strength of the hip abductors, the patient is positioned in supine so that the muscle action pulls in a horizontal plane relative to the ground.[106]
4. *Having the patient perform an eccentric muscle contraction by using the command "Don't let me move you."* Because the tension at each cross-bridge and the number of active cross-bridges is greater during an eccentric contraction, the maximum eccentric muscle tension developed is greater with an eccentric contraction than with a concentric one.
5. *Breaking the contraction.* It is important to break the patient's muscle contraction, in order to ensure that the patient is making a maximal effort and that the full power of the muscle is being tested. Although force values determined with *make* and *break* tests are highly correlated, break tests usually result in greater force values than make tests,[122,123] so they should not be used interchangeably.
6. *Holding the contraction for at least 5 seconds.* Weakness resulting from nerve palsy has a distinct fatigability. The muscle demonstrates poor endurance, because usually it is only able to sustain a maximum muscle contraction for about 2–3 seconds before complete failure occurs. This strategy is based on the theories behind muscle recruitment, wherein a normal muscle, while performing a maximum contraction, uses only a portion of its motor units, keeping the remainder in reserve to help maintain the contraction. A palsied muscle, with its fewer functioning motor units, has very few, if any, motor units in reserve. If a muscle appears to be weaker than normal, further investigation is required, as follows:
   a. The test is repeated three times. Muscle weakness resulting from disuse will be consistently weak and should not become weaker with several repeated contractions. In contrast, a palsied muscle becomes weaker with each contraction.
   b. Another muscle that shares the same innervation is tested. Knowledge of both spinal and peripheral nerve innervation will aid the clinician in determining which muscle to select (see Chap. 3).
7. *Comparing findings with uninvolved side.* One study found no statistically significant difference in force between the dominant and nondominant lower extremities, but did find the difference between the dominant and nondominant upper extremities.[124] Sapega[125] recommends that the difference in muscle force between sides of greater than 20% probably indicates abnormality, while the difference of 10 to 20% possibly indicates abnormality.

As always, these tests cannot be evaluated in isolation but have to be integrated into a total clinical profile, before drawing any conclusion about the patient's condition.

CLINICAL PEARL

MMT is an ordinal level of measurement[125] and has been found to have both inter- and intra-rater reliability, especially when the scale is expanded to include plus or minus a half or a full grade.[18,126,127] Training in standardized testing positions, stabilization, and grading criteria resulted in higher agreement and correlation coefficients between testers.

Although the grading of muscle strength has its role in the clinic, and the ability to isolate the various muscles is very important in determining the source of nerve palsy, specific grading of individual muscles does not give the clinician much information on the ability of the structure to perform functional tasks. In addition, measurements of isometric muscle force are specific to a point or small range in the joint range excursion and, thus, cannot be used to predict dynamic force capabilities.[128–130]

More recently, the use of *quantitative muscle testing* (QMT) has been recommended to assess strength, as it produces interval data that describe force production. QMT methods include:

- The use of handheld dynamometers. Although more costly and time consuming than MMT, handheld dynamometry can be used to improve objectivity and sensitivity. Patients are typically asked to push against the dynamometer with a maximal isometric contraction (make test), or hold a position until the clinician and the dynamometer overpower the muscle producing an eccentric contraction (break tests).[106] Normative force values for particular muscle groups by patient age and gender have been reported, with some authors including regression equations that take into account body weight and height.[131]

CLINICAL PEARL

Depending on the study, handheld dynamometers have demonstrated good to excellent intra-tester reliability and poor to excellent inter-tester reliability.[132–136]

- *The use of an isokinetic dynamometer.* This is a stationary, electromechanical device that controls the velocity of the moving body segment by resisting and measuring the patient's effort so that the body segment cannot accelerate beyond a preset angular velocity.[106] Isokinetic dynamometers measure torque and range of motion as a function of time, and can provide an analysis of the ratio between the eccentric contraction and concentric contraction of a muscle at various positions and speeds.[137] This ratio is aptly named the *eccentric/concentric ratio*.[138] The ratio is calculated by dividing the eccentric strength value by the concentric strength value. Various authors[139,140] have demonstrated that the upper limit of this ratio is 2.0 and that lower ratios indicate pathology.[138,141] Alternatively, the same recommendations for MMT advocated by Sapega[125] can be used: a difference in muscle force between sides of greater than 20% probably indicates abnormality, while the difference of 10–20% possibly indicates abnormality. To ensure the validity of isokinetic dynamometry measurements, calibration of equipment is necessary and should be performed each day of testing, at the same speed and damp setting during the testing.[142]

One of the major criticisms of muscle testing is the over estimation of strength when a muscle is weak as identified by QMT, compared to the same muscle being graded as normal by MMT, such that a theoretical percentage score based on MMT is likely to grossly overestimate the strength of a patient.[121] For example, Beasley[143] showed that 50% of knee extensor strength needed to be lost before MMT was able to identify weakness.

Studies that compare the reliability of MMT and QMT often come to the conclusion that MMT may be consistent and reliable, but it is unable to detect subtle differences in strength.[144,145] Thus, although MMT results are more consistent, the variation produced by QMT can appreciate differences in strength undetectable in MMT.[121]

Regardless of the type of muscle testing used, the procedure is innately subjective and depends on the subject's ability to exert a maximal contraction. This ability can be negatively impacted by such factors as pain, poor comprehension, motivation, cooperation, fatigue, and fear.

CLINICAL PEARL

Voluntary muscle strength testing will remain somewhat subjective until a precise way of measuring muscle contraction is generally available.[112] This is particularly true when determining normal and good values.

Motor Function

Motor function is the ability to demonstrate the skillful and efficient assumption, maintenance, modification, and control of voluntary postures and movement patterns.[14] The criteria for simple motor patterns are that the movement[69,118]

- is performed exactly in the desired direction;
- is smooth and of a constant speed;
- follows the shortest and most efficient path;
- is performed in its full range.

The criteria for complex motor patterns are as follows[69]:

- Synchronization between the primary movers in the distal regions with those more proximal.
- Smooth propagation of motion from one region of the body to another.
- Absence of inefficient movement patterns or muscle recruitment.
- Optimal relationships between the speed of motion initiated in one region and the speed of motion in other regions.

CLINICAL PEARL

Indications of a systemic neurologic compromise that has impacted motor function include abnormal movement patterns, movement synergies, or gait disturbances. Primitive movement patterns are those seen with compromise to the CNS, such as the flexor withdrawal pattern.[146]

The upper extremities can work together, when they are in direct or indirect contact with each other (clasping the hands together or holding an object with two hands), or separately. The lower extremities can work together off a stable base or separately. In the bilateral combinations, the two limbs are separated, but both are involved in the activity. The limbs may be moved in the same direction, termed *symmetric* (breaststroke swimming); in opposite directions, termed *reciprocal* (swimming the crawl); toward one side of the body (pulling on a rope above one side of the head), termed *asymmetric*; or toward opposite sides of the body (swimming side stroke), termed *cross-diagonal* or *reciprocal asymmetric*.[147]

Mass movement patterns involve combined motions of the joints within the kinetic chain, depending on the desired motion.[148] For example, a mass pattern of the lower extremity could involve hip, knee, and ankle dorsiflexion, with the rotation and abduction–adduction component varying. Advanced movement patterns involve such combinations as hip extension, knee flexion, and plantar flexion, or hip flexion, knee extension, and dorsiflexion—motions that occur with normal gait.[148]

Aerobic Capacity and Endurance

Aerobic capacity endurance is the ability to perform work or participate in activity over time, using the body's oxygen uptake, delivery, and energy-release mechanisms (see Chap. 15).[14] Clinical indications for the use of the tests and measures for this category are based on the findings from the history and systems review. These indications include, but are not limited to, pathology, pathophysiology, and impairment to[14]:

- cardiovascular system (e.g., abnormal heart rate, rhythm, and blood pressure);
- endocrine/metabolic system (e.g., osteoporosis);
- multiple systems (e.g., trauma and systemic disease);
- neuromuscular system (e.g., generalized muscle weakness and decreased endurance);
- pulmonary system (e.g., abnormal respiratory pattern, rate, and rhythm).

The aerobic capacity and endurance of a patient can be measured using standardized exercise test protocols (e.g., ergometry, step tests, time or distance walk or run tests, and treadmill tests) and the patient's response to such tests.[14]

Anthropometric Characteristics

Anthropometric characteristics are traits that describe body dimensions, such as height, weight, girth, and body fat composition.[14] The use of an anthropometric examination and the subsequent measurements varies. Clearly, if a noticeable amount of effusion or swelling is present, these measurements serve as an important baseline from which to judge the effectiveness of the intervention.

Circulation

Circulation is defined by *The Guide* as the movement of blood through organs and tissues to both deliver oxygen and remove carbon dioxide and cellular byproducts.[14] Circulation also involves the passive movement of lymph through channels. The examination of the circulation includes an examination of those cardiovascular signs not tested in the aerobic capacity and endurance portion, and the anthropometric characteristics portion of the examination, including the patient's physiologic response to position change, an inspection of the nail beds, capillary refill, and monitoring of the pulses of the extremities.

In general, the posterior (dorsal) pedis pulse is used in the lower extremities to assess the patency of the lower extremity vessels, whereas the radial pulse is used for the upper extremities.

Work, Environmental, and Home Barriers (Job, School, and Play)

Work, environmental, and home barriers are the physical impediments that keep patients from functioning optimally in their surroundings.[14]

Ergonomics and Body Mechanics

Ergonomics is the relationship among the worker; the work that is done; the actions, tasks, or activities inherent in that work (job, school, and play); and the environment in which the work (job, school, and play) is performed.[14] Body mechanics are the interrelationships of the muscles and joints, as they maintain or adjust posture in response to forces placed on or generated by the body.

It is not within the scope of this text to detail the scientific and engineering principles related to ergonomics and the numerous tests used to quantify these measures. Ergonomics as it relates to posture is discussed within the related chapters.

Gait, Locomotion, and Balance

Gait analysis is an important component of the examination process (see Chap. 6) and should not be reserved only for those patients with lower extremity dysfunction. Although the act of walking is often taken for granted, normal and reciprocal gait requires a finely tuned series of reflexes.[149] The examination of gait is performed to highlight any breakdown within these reflexes, including imbalances of flexibility or strength, or compensatory motions.[150]

Gait, like posture, varies between individuals, and a gait that differs from normal is not necessarily pathologic. The analysis of gait is described in Chapter 6.

Balance is an essential component for participation in sports and for activities of daily living (see Chap. 3). During the history, the patient may describe symptoms of dizziness, lightheadedness, a sense of impending faint, or poor balance. Ataxia is a discoordination or clumsiness of movement that is not associated with muscular weakness, but has very strong associations with CNS dysfunction (see Chap. 3).[151] A sudden onset of unilateral deafness may be due to labyrinth artery infarction, possibly indicating an infarction in the vertebrobasilar system,[152] Ménière's disease, acoustic neuroma, autoimmune disease of the inner ear, Friedrich's ataxia, vestibulocochlear nerve compression, diabetes mellitus, otosclerosis, or an adverse drug reaction.[153] Nausea and vomiting are common complaints in balance disorders. The assessment of balance is discussed in Chapter 3.

Orthotic, Adaptive, Protective, and Assistive Devices

These devices are implements and equipments used to support or protect weak or ineffective joints or muscles and serve to enhance performance.[14] Examples of such devices include canes, crutches, walkers, reachers, and ankle foot orthoses.

Posture

Posture describes the relative positions of different joints at any given moment.[46] The postural examination gives an overall view of the patient's muscle function in both chronic and acute pain states. The examination enables the clinician to differentiate between possible provocative causes, such as structural variations, altered joint mechanics, muscle imbalances, and the residual effects of pathology. The assessment of posture is detailed in Chapter 6 and in the relevant chapters.

Work (Job, School, and Play), Community, and Leisure Integration and Reintegration

In short, this category refers to the process of assuming or resuming roles and functions.

Self-care and Home Management (Including Activities of Daily Living and Instrumental Activities of Daily Living)

This portion of the examination addresses the patient's perception of his or her condition, namely issues regarding the patient's perception on their functional level and quality of life.

Palpation

Palpation is a fundamental skill used in a number of the tests and measures. Both Gerwin and colleagues[154] and Njoo and Van der Does[155] found that training and experience are essential in performing reliable palpation tests. Palpation, which can play a central role in the performance of several manual therapy techniques,[156] is performed to:[157,158]

- check for any vasomotor changes such as an increase in skin temperature that might suggest an inflammatory process;
- localize specific sites of swelling;
- determine the presence of muscle tremors, and/or fasciculations;
- identify specific anatomic structures and their relationship to one another;
- identify sites of point tenderness. Hyperalgic skin zones can be detected using skin drag, which consists of moving the pads of the fingertips over the surface of the skin and attempting to sense resistance or drag.
- identify soft-tissue texture changes or myofascial restriction. Normal tissue is soft and mobile and moves equally in all directions. Abnormal tissue may feel hard, sensitive, or somewhat crunchy or stringy.[159]
- locate changes in muscle tone resulting from trigger points, muscle spasm, hypertonicity, or hypotonicity. However, a study by Hsieh and colleagues[160] found that among non-expert physicians, physiatric or chiropractic, trigger point palpation is not reliable for detecting taut band and local twitch response, and only marginally reliable for referred pain after training. The most useful diagnostic test to detect these changes is to create a fold in the tissue, and to stretch it.[161] The tissue should be soft and supple, and there should be no resistance to the stretch.
- determine circulatory status by checking distal pulses.
- detect changes in the moisture of the skin.

The pertinent palpation areas for each of the joints are described, within the relevant chapters.

Function

Functional testing is a complex and multifactorial process in which the clinician makes a determination about the patient's level of functional independence based on principles of physiology, biomechanics, and motor behavior:[162]

- *Physiology.* Relevant physiological issues include the functions of body structures and systems, the extent of the injury, and the patient's healing status, energy systems, adaptation, and overall fitness level.
- *Biomechanics.* Biomechanical considerations include functional anatomy, direction/planes of motion and stress, kinematics (time, distance, position, displacement, velocity), and kinetics (force, torque, mass, acceleration, inertia, momentum).
- *Motor behavior.* Motor behavior issues include proprioception, perception, transfer, practice, learning, control, coordination, and performance.

It is important for the clinician to determine what functional factors are important to the patient, and what functions are necessary for the patient to perform work-related, recreational, or social activities. It is worth remembering that insurance companies reimburse based on intervention goals that improve work-related and functional abilities, and not on those goals that enhance a patient's ability to perform recreational pursuits.

A number of variables affect function. These include age, gender, physical capacity (strength, power, flexibility, dexterity, agility, speed, muscular endurance, cardiovascular endurance, coordination, and skill), healing status (phase of healing, weight-bearing status, precautions/contraindications, and comorbidities), and psychological profile (motivation, fear, and coping mechanisms).[162]

Throughout this text, functional testing methods are outlined in each of the appropriate chapters. Part of the functional assessment includes an assessment of those muscles that are prone to weakness, which can provide the clinician with the following information[163]:

- Strength of individual muscles or muscle groups that form a functional unit.
- Nature, range, and quality of simple movement patterns.
- Relationship between the strength and the flexibility of a muscle or muscle group.
- The ability of the whole body to perform a task.

Muscle function testing, therefore, should address the production and control of motion in functional activities. Although there is general agreement about the role of the trunk and the pelvic musculature in normal functioning of the vertebral column, protection against pain, and recurrence of low back disorders,[93,164,165] more research is needed to determine the role of functional strength in the extremities.

Special Tests

Special tests for each area are dependent on the special needs and structure of each joint. Numerous tests exist for each joint. With a few notable exceptions, the reliability of most orthopaedic testing is either poor or unproven. Therefore, the clinician is wise to avoid overreliance on labeling a specific test as positive or negative.[166] Rather, the patient's response to provocative maneuvers should be carefully noted and be used to provide a framework within which the clinician builds a complete picture of the clinical entity.[166] In addition, the clinician should use more than one examination maneuver to make the diagnosis. One study[167] reported improved sensitivity, specificity, and positive predictive value with the utilization of combinations of tests rather than using tests in isolation.

The special tests are only performed if there is some indication that they would be helpful in arriving at a diagnosis. The tests help confirm or implicate a particular structure and may also provide information as to the degree of tissue damage.

In the joints of the spine, examples of special tests include directional stress tests (posterior–anterior pressures and anterior, posterior, and rotational stressing), joint quadrant testing, vascular tests, and repeated movement testing. Examples of special tests in the peripheral joints include ligament stress tests (i.e., Lachman for the anterior cruciate ligament), articular stress testing (valgus stress applied at the elbow), and glenohumeral impingement tests. Special tests can be categorized according to intent:

- *Provocative tests.* Provocative tests include those that are designed to put pressure on an involved structure and reproduce the pain that has brought the patient into the clinic, while ruling out involvement of other structures. Although palpation fits the criteria as a provocative test, its importance to the examination warrants its own section. Examples for other provocative tests include the Spurling's test (cervical foraminal encroachment test) to detect a potential cervical radiculopathy, the thoracic outlet tests, the neurodynamic mobilizations tests (e.g., the straight leg raise—see Chap. 11) that assess for neural adhesions and nerve root problems, and the selective tissue tension tests designed by Cyriax.[90] These tests, which by their very nature are designed to reproduce the patient's symptoms, should be used judiciously, and only after consultation with the patient to describe the reasons for the testing.
- *Clearing tests.* The purpose of the clearing tests is to remove a structure or region as a potential source of the patient's problem. The clearing tests are typically used when a patient presents with symptoms in either the lower extremities or upper extremities. For example, in a patient complaining of shoulder pain, the clinician must determine if the symptoms are local, or are referred. To help in this decision-making process, the cervical spine must be "cleared" so it can be ruled out as a potential source. This can be done through a combination of neck side bending, rotation, and extension in an effort to reproduce the symptoms. If the symptoms are not reproduced with these maneuvers, the cervical spine can no longer be considered an obvious source of the symptoms. Because the cervical spine has the potential to refer pain throughout the entire upper extremity, it is always worth consideration as a cause of symptoms in the shoulder, the elbow, the wrist and the hand. Similarly, because the lumbar spine and the sacroiliac joint have the potential to refer symptoms into the lower extremities, they should always be considered in cases of hip, knee, and ankle and foot symptoms. In addition, neighboring joints should always be considered as potential causes of symptoms until cleared.

The special tests for each of the joints are described in the various chapters of this book, with emphasis placed on those that are evidence based. The interpretation of the findings from the special tests depends on the skill and experience of the clinician, as well as the degree of familiarity with the tests. While special tests are associated with false-positive and false-negative results, a positive test finding in conjunction with other aspects of the examination is highly suggestive of pathology.[106]

Reflex and Sensory Testing

Reflex and sensory testing is covered in Chapter 3. The neurological examination is only carried out if the clinician feels the nervous system is involved, or if the clinician is unsure as to whether there is any neurological involvement.

Neuromeningeal Mobility Tests

The neurodynamic mobility tests, described in Chapter 11, examine for the presence of any abnormalities of the dura, both centrally and peripherally. These tests are used if a dural adhesion or irritation is suspected. The tests employ a sequential and progressive stretch to the dura until the patient's symptoms are reproduced.[12] Theoretically, if the dura is scarred, or inflamed, a lack of extensibility with stretching occurs. Because the sinuvertebral nerve innervates the dural sleeve, the pain caused by an inflamed dura is felt by the patient at multisegmental levels and is described as having an ache-like quality. If the patient experiences sharp or stabbing pain during the test, a more serious underlying condition should be suspected.

Evaluation

Once the examination is complete, the clinician should be able to add and subtract the various findings, determine the accuracy of the working hypothesis, and make an evaluation, which involves developing the diagnosis, the prognosis, and the realistic POC.[168] According to Grieve,[92] an evaluation is the level of judgment necessary to make sense of the findings, in order to identify a relationship between the symptoms reported and the signs of disturbed function. Thus, while the evaluation is used to determine the diagnosis, the prognosis, and the POC, it is the diagnosis that guides the intervention.

CLINICAL PEARL

The diagnosis and the prognosis are critical to shaping the final POC. A physical therapy diagnosis refers to the cluster of signs and symptoms, syndromes, or categories and is used to guide the physical therapist in determining the most appropriate intervention strategy for each patient.[169]

Clinical Decision Making

Patients may be referred to physical therapy with a nonspecific diagnosis, an incorrect diagnosis, or no diagnosis at all.[170] Physical therapists are responsible for thoroughly examining each patient and then either treating the patient according to established guidelines, or referring the patient to a more appropriate healthcare provider.[171] A diagnosis can only be made when all potential causes for the signs and symptoms have been ruled out, so the clinician should resist the urge to categorize a condition based on a small number of findings. The best indicator for the correctness of a diagnosis is the quality of the hypothesis considered, because if the appropriate diagnosis is not considered from the start, any subsequent inquiries will be misdirected.[172] Ultimately, given the role of physical therapists as movement specialists, task analysis should form the basis of the diagnosis.[173] Once impairments have been highlighted, a determination can be made as to the reason for those impairments, and the relationship between the impairments and the patient's functional limitations or disabilities.

Decision making encompasses the selection of tests during the examination process, interpretation of data from the detailed history and examination, establishment of the diagnosis, estimation of the prognosis, determination of intervention strategies, sequence of therapeutic procedures, and establishment of discharge criteria.[169] The decision-making process is a multifaceted fluid process which combines tacit knowledge with accumulated clinical experience.[174] The experienced clinician is able to recognize patterns and extrapolate information from them using forward reasoning, to develop an accurate working hypothesis.[175] This is accomplished through an estimate of the proportional contribution of tissue pathology and *impairment clusters* to the patient's functional limitations.[20] Using this information, the clinician puts a value on examination findings, considering relevant environmental, social, cultural, psychological, medical, and physical findings and clusters the information into recognizable, understandable, or identifiable diagnoses, dysfunctions, or classification syndromes.[20] According to Kahney,[176] the expert seems to do less problem solving than the novice, because the former has already stored solutions to many of the clinical problems previously encountered.[177]

One of the problems for the clinician is how to attach relevance to all of the information gleaned from the examination. This judgment process can be viewed as a continuum. At one end of the continuum is the novice who uses very clear-cut signposts, while at the other end there is the experienced clinician who has a vast bank of clinical experiences from which to draw.[177] Experts are able to see meaningful relationships, possess enhanced memory, are skilled in qualitative analysis, and have well-developed reflection skills.[174] This combination of skills allows the expert to systematically organize the information to make efficient and effective clinical decisions.

What differentiates diagnosis by the physical therapist from diagnosis by the physician is not the process itself but the phenomena being observed and clarified.[178] Sackett et al.[98] proposed three strategies of clinical diagnosis:

- *Pattern recognition.* This is characterized by the clinician's instantaneous realization that the patient conforms to a previously learned pattern of disease.
- *History and physical examination.* This method requires the clinician to consider all hypotheses of the potential etiology.
- *Hypothetico-deductive method.* In this method, the clinician identifies early clues and formulates a short list of potential diagnoses.

The clinician's knowledge base is critical in the evaluation process.[172] Experienced clinicians appear to have a superior organization of knowledge, and they use a combination of hypothetico-deductive reasoning and pattern recognition to derive the correct diagnosis or working hypothesis.[172]

A number of frameworks have been applied to clinical practice for guiding clinical decision making and providing structure to the healthcare process.[179–185] While the early frameworks were based on disablement models, the more recent models have focused on enablement perspectives using algorithms. An algorithm is a systematic process involving a finite number of steps that produces the solution to a problem. Algorithms used in healthcare allow for clinical decisions and adjustments to be made during the clinical reasoning and decision-making process because they are not prescriptive or protocol driven.[174] The most commonly used algorithm in physical therapy is the *hypothesis-oriented algorithm for clinicians* (HOAC) designed by Rothstein and Echternach.[182] The HOAC is designed to guide the clinician from evaluation to intervention planning with a logical sequence of activities, and requires the clinician to generate working hypotheses early in the examination process, the latter of which is a strategy often used by expert clinicians.

When integrating evidence into clinical decision making, an understanding of how to appraise the quality of the evidence offered by clinical studies is important. One of the major problems in evaluating studies is that the volume of literature makes it difficult for the busy clinician to obtain and analyze all of the evidence necessary to guide the clinical decision-making process.[16] The other problem involves deciding whether the results from the literature are definite enough to indicate an effect other than chance. Judging the strength of the evidence becomes an important part of the decision-making process.

CLINICAL PEARL

Clinical prediction rules (CPRs) are tools designed to assist clinicians in decision making when caring for patients. However, although there is a growing trend toward producing a number of CPRs in the field of physical therapy, few CPRs presently exist (see Chap. 8).

The standard for the assessment of the efficacy and value of a test or intervention is the clinical trial, that is, a prospective study assessing the effect and value of a test or intervention against a control in human subjects.[186] Unfortunately, many of the experimental studies that deal with physical therapy topics are not clinical trials, because there is no control to judge the efficacy of the test or intervention, and there are no tests or interventions from which to draw comparisons.[187] The best evidence for making decisions about interventions comes from randomized controlled trials, systematic reviews, and evidence based clinical practice guidelines (Table 4-25).[188] The ideal clinical trial includes a blinded, randomized design and a control group. It may be possible to discriminate between high- and low-quality trials by asking three simple questions[188]:

1. Were subjects randomly allocated to conditions?
   Random allocation implies that a nonsystematic,

TABLE 4-25	Randomized Controlled Trials, Systematic Reviews, and Clinical Practice Guidelines
Randomized controlled trials (RCTs)	Involve experiments on people. Less exposed to bias. Ensures comparability of groups. Typically, volunteers agree to be randomly allocated to groups receiving one of the following: ▸ Treatment and no treatment ▸ Standard treatment and standard treatment plus a new treatment ▸ Two alternate treatments The common feature is that the experimental group receives the treatment of interest and the control group does not. At the end of the trial, outcomes of subjects in each group are determined—the difference in outcomes between groups provides an estimate of the size of the treatment effect.
Systematic reviews	Reviews of the literature conducted in a way that is designed to minimize bias. Can be used to assess the effects of health interventions, the accuracy of diagnostic tests, or the prognosis for a particular condition. Usually involve criteria to determine which studies will be considered, the search strategy used to locate studies, the methods for assessing the quality of the studies, and the process used to synthesize the findings of individual studies. Particularly useful for busy clinicians who may be unable to access all the relevant trials in an area and may otherwise need to rely upon their own incomplete surveys of relevant trials.
Clinical practice guidelines	Recommendations for management of a particular clinical condition. Involve compilation of evidence concerning needs and expectations of recipients of care, the accuracy of diagnostic tests, and effects of therapy and prognosis. Usually necessitates the conduct of one or sometimes several systematic reviews. May be presented as clinical decision algorithms. Can provide a useful framework upon which clinicians can build clinical practice.

Data from Maher CG, Herbert RD, Moseley AM, et al: Critical appraisal of randomized trials, systematic reviews of randomized trials and clinical practice guidelines. In: Boyling JD, Jull GA, (eds.) *Grieve's Modern Manual Therapy: The Vertebral Column*. Philadelphia, PA: Churchill Livingstone, 2004:603–614; Petticrew M: Systematic reviews from astronomy to zoology: myths and misconceptions. *BMJ*. 2001:322;98–101.

unpredictable procedure was used to allocate subjects to conditions.

2. Was there blinding of assessors and patients? Blinding of assessors and patients minimizes the risk of the placebo effect and the "Hawthorne effect," an experimental artifact that is of no clinical utility, where patients report better outcomes than they really experienced because they perceive that this is what is expected from them.[189]
3. Was there adequate follow-up? Ideally, all subjects who enter the trial should subsequently be followed up to avoid bias. In practice, this rarely happens. As a general rule, losses to follow-up of less than 10% avoid serious bias, but losses to follow-up of more than 20% cause potential for serious bias.

Numerous physical therapy tests exist that are designed to help the clinician rule out some of the many possible diagnoses. Regardless of which test is chosen, the test must be performed reliably by the clinician in order for the test to be a valuable guide. Reliability describes the extent to which test or measurement is free from error. A test is considered reliable if it produces precise, accurate, and reproducible information.[16] Two types of reliability are often described:

- *Interrater.* Determines whether the same single examiner can repeat the test consistently.
- *Intrarater.* Determines whether two or more examiners can repeat a test consistently.

Reliability is quantitatively expressed by way of an index of agreement, with the simplest index being the percentage agreement value. The statistical coefficients most commonly used to characterize the reliability of the tests and measures are the *intraclass correlation coefficient* (ICC) and the kappa statistic (κ), both of which are based on statistical models[190]:

- The ICC is a reliability coefficient calculated with variance estimates obtained through an *analysis of variance* (Table 4-26).[191] The advantage of the ICC over correlation

TABLE 4-26 Intraclass Correlation Coefficient Benchmark Values

Value	Description
<0.75	Poor-to-moderate agreement
>0.75	Good agreement
>90	Reasonable agreement for clinical measurements

Data from Portney L, Watkins MP: *Foundations of Clinical Research: Applications to Practice*. Norwalk, CT: Appleton & Lange, 1993.

coefficients is that it does not require the same number of raters per subject, and it can be used for two or more raters or ratings.[191]

- The κ statistic is a chance-corrected index of agreement that overcomes the problem of chance agreement when used with nominal and ordinal data.[192] With nominal data, the κ statistic is applied after the percentage agreement between testers has been determined. However, with higher scale data, it tends to underestimate reliability.[193] Theoretically, the κ statistic can be negative if agreement is worse than chance. Practically, in clinical reliability studies, the κ statistic usually varies between 0.00 and 1.00.[193] The κ statistic does not differentiate among disagreements; it assumes that all disagreements are of equal significance.[193]
- *Standard error of measurement* (SEM). The SEM reflects the reliability of the response when the test is performed many times and is an indication of how much change there might be when the test is repeated.[193] If the SEM is small, then the test is stable with minimal variability between tests.[193]

Test validity is defined as the degree to which a test measures what it purports to be measuring, and how well it correctly classifies individuals with or without a particular disease.[17–19] A test is considered to have diagnostic accuracy if it has the ability to discriminate between patients with and without a specific disorder.[194]

In order to determine if a test is both reliable and valid, the test must be examined in a research study and, preferably, multiple studies.

Validity is directly related to the notion of sensitivity and specificity. The sensitivity and specificity of any physical test to discriminate relevant dysfunction must be appreciated to make meaningful decisions.[195] Sensitivity is the ability of the test to pick up what it is testing for, and specificity is the ability of the test to reject what it is not testing for.

- Sensitivity represents the proportion of patients with a disorder who test positive. A test that can correctly identify every person who has the disorder has a sensitivity of 1.0. *SnNout* is an acronym for when *sen*sitivity of a symptom or sign is high, a *n*egative response rules *out* the target disorder. Thus, a so-called highly sensitive test helps rule out a disorder. The positive predictive value is the proportion of patients with positive test results who are correctly diagnosed.
- Specificity is the proportion of the study population without the disorder that test negative.[196] A test that can correctly identify every person who does not have the target disorder has a specificity of 1.0. *SpPin* is an acronym for when *sp*ecificity is extremely high, a *p*ositive test result rules *in* the target disorder. Thus, a so-called highly specific test helps rule in a disorder or condition. The negative predictive value is the proportion of patients with negative test results who are correctly diagnosed.

CLINICAL PEARL

Interpretation of sensitivity and specificity values is easiest when their values are high.[197] A test with a very high sensitivity, but low specificity, and vice versa, is of little value, and the acceptable levels are generally set at between 50% (unacceptable test) and 100% (perfect test), with an arbitrary cutoff at about 80%.[196]

Once the specificity and sensitivity of the test is established, the predictive value of a positive test versus a negative test can be determined if the prevalence of the disease/dysfunction is known. For example, when the prevalence of the disease increases, a patient with a positive test is more likely to have the disease (a false-negative is less likely). A negative result of a highly sensitive test will probably rule out a common disease, whereas if the disease is rare, the test must be much more specific for it to be clinically useful.

The *likelihood ratio* (LR) is the index measurement that combines sensitivity and specificity values and can be used to gauge the performance of a diagnostic test, as it indicates how much a given diagnostic test result will lower or raise the pretest probability of the target disorder.[97,196]

CLINICAL PEARL

Diagnostic tests are used for the purpose of discovery, confirmation, and exclusion.[198] Tests for discovery and exclusion must have high sensitivity for detection, whereas confirmation tests require high specificity.[199]

Four measures contribute to sensitivity and specificity (Table 4-27):

- *True positive.* The test indicates that the patient has the disease or the dysfunction, and this is confirmed by the gold standard test.
- *False positive.* The clinical test indicates that the disease or the dysfunction is present, but this is not confirmed by the gold standard test.
- *False negative.* The clinical test indicates absence of the disorder, but the gold standard test shows that the disease or dysfunction is present.
- *True negative.* The clinical and the gold standard test agree that the disease or dysfunction is absent.

These values are used to calculate the statistical measures of accuracy, sensitivity, specificity, negative and positive predictive values, and negative and positive LRs, as indicated in Table 4-28. Another way to summarize diagnostic test performance using Table 4-27 is via the *diagnostic odds ratio* (DOR): DOR = true/false = (a∗d)/(b∗c). The DOR of a test is the ratio of the odds of positivity in disease relative to the odds of positivity in the nondiseased. The value of a DOR ranges from 0 to infinity, with higher values indicating better discriminatory

TABLE 4-27 2 × 2 table

		Disease/outcome	
		Present	**Absent**
Test	Positive (+)	a (true +ve)	b (false +ve)
	Negative (−)	c (false −ve)	d (true −ve)

TABLE 4-28 Definition and Calculation of Statistical Measures		
Statistical Measure	**Definition**	**Calculation**
Accuracy	The proportion of people who were correctly identified as either having or not having the disease or dysfunction	(TP + TN)/(TP + FP + FN + TN)
Sensitivity	The proportion of people who have the disease or dysfunction and who test positive	TP/(TP + FN)
Specificity	The proportion of people who do not have the disease or dysfunction and who test negative	TN/(FP + TN)
Positive predictive value	The proportion of people who test positive and who have the disease or dysfunction	TP/(TP + FP)
Negative predictive value	The proportion of people who test negative and who do not have the disease or dysfunction	TN/(FN + TN)
Positive LR	How likely a positive test result is in people who have the disease or dysfunction as compared to how likely it is in those who do not have the disease or dysfunction	Sensitivity/(1−specificity)
Negative LR	How likely a negative test result is in people who have the disease or dysfunction as compared to how likely it is in those who do not have the disease or dysfunction	(1−sensitivity)/specificity

TP, true positive; TN, true negative; FP, false positive; FN false negative.
Data from Fritz JM, Wainner RS: Examining diagnostic tests: an evidence-based perspective. Phys Ther. 2001, 81:1546–1564; Powell JW, Huijbregts PA: Concurrent criterion-related validity of acromioclavicular joint physical examination tests: a systematic review. *J Man Manip Ther.* 2006:14;E19–E29.

test performance. A value of 1 means that a test does not discriminate between those patients with the disorder and those without.

CLINICAL PEARL

The DOR value rises steeply when sensitivity or specificity becomes near perfect.

The *quality assessment of studies of diagnostic accuracy* (QUADAS)[200] is an evidence-based quality assessment tool currently recommended for use in systematic reviews of *diagnostic accuracy studies* (DAS). The aim of DAS is to determine how good a particular test is at detecting the target condition. DAS allow the calculation of various statistics that provide an indication of "test performance"—how good the index test is at detecting the target condition. These statistics include sensitivity, specificity, positive and negative predictive values, positive and negative LRs, and diagnostics odds ratios. The QUADAS tool is a list of 14 questions which should each be answered "yes", "no", or "unclear" (Table 4-29). A score of 10 or greater of "yes" answers is indicative of a higher quality study, whereas a score of less than 10 "yes" answers suggests a poorly designed study. Throughout this text, the QUADAS score is used (if known) to evaluate the various physical therapy examination tests.

Prognosis

The prognosis is the predicted optimal level of function that the patient will attain within a certain time frame. The prognosis represents a synthesis, based on an understanding of the extent of pathology, premorbid conditions, the ability of surrounding tissue structures to compensate in the short or long term, the healing processes of the various tissues, the patient's age, foundational knowledge, theory, evidence, experience, and examination findings, and takes into account the patient's social, emotional, and motivational status.[20,173] This information helps guide the intensity, duration, and frequency of the intervention and aids in justifying the intervention.

The patient's aspirations and patient-identified problems, together with those problems identified by the clinician, determine the focus of the goals.[173] The patient and clinician should come to an agreement regarding the most important problems, around which care should be focused, and together establish relevant goals.[173] Patient education and patient responsibility become extremely important in determining the prognosis.

Plan of Care

The POC is organized around the patient's goals. The physical therapist's POC consists of consultation, education, and intervention. Intervention (see Chap. 8) is organized into three categories[173]:

1. *Remediation.* Consists of enhancing skills and resources or reversing impairments and assumes that the potential for change exists in the system and the person.
2. *Compensation or adaptation.* Refers to the alteration of the environment or the task and is the approach taken when it is determined that remediation is not possible.
3. *Prevention.* Refers to the management of anticipated problems.

TABLE 4-29	The QUADAS Tool[a]			
Item		**Yes**	**No**	**Unclear**
1.	Was the spectrum of patients representative of the patients who will receive the test?	( )	( )	( )
2.	Were selection criteria clearly described?	( )	( )	( )
3.	Is the reference standard likely to correctly classify the target condition?	( )	( )	( )
4.	Is the time period between reference standard and index test short enough to be reasonably sure that the target condition did not change between the two tests?	( )	( )	( )
5.	Did the whole sample or a random selection of the sample, receive verification using a reference standard of diagnosis?	( )	( )	( )
6.	Did patients receive the same reference standard regardless of the index test result?	( )	( )	( )
7.	Was the reference standard independent of the index test (i.e., the index test did not form part of the reference standard)?	( )	( )	( )
8.	Was the execution of the index test described in sufficient detail to permit replication of the test?	( )	( )	( )
9.	Was the execution of the reference standard described in sufficient detail to permit its replication?	( )	( )	( )
10.	Were the index test results interpreted without knowledge of the results of the reference standard?	( )	( )	( )
11.	Were the reference standard results interpreted without knowledge of the results of the index test?	( )	( )	( )
12.	Were the same clinical data available when test results were interpreted as would be available when the test is used in practice?	( )	( )	( )
13.	Were uninterpretable/ intermediate test results reported?	( )	( )	( )
14.	Were withdrawals from the study explained?	( )	( )	( )

[a]Data from: Whiting P, Rutjes AW, Reitsma JB, et al: The development of QUADAS: a tool for the quality assessment of studies of diagnostic accuracy included in systematic reviews. *BMC Med Res Methodol.* 2003, 3:25.

Progress, and Reexamine

The selection of intervention procedures, and the intervention progression, must be guided by continuous reexamination of the patient's response to a given procedure, making the reexamination of patient dysfunction before, during, and after each intervention essential.[201]

At each visit, the clinician must reexamine the patient's status. To evaluate progress, comparisons are made between the findings from the initial examination and subsequent visits. There are three possible scenarios following a reexamination:

1. *The patient's function has improved.* In this scenario, the intensity of the intervention may be incrementally increased.
2. *The patient's function has diminished.* In this scenario, the intensity and the focus of the intervention must be changed. Further review of the home exercise program may be needed. The patient may require further education on activity modification and the use of heat and ice at home. The working hypothesis must be reviewed. Further investigation is needed.
3. *There is no change in the patient's function.* Depending on the time that has elapsed since the last visit, there may be a reason for the lack of change. This finding may indicate the need for a change in the intensity of the intervention. If the patient is in the acute or subacute stage of healing, a decrease in the intensity may be warranted to allow the tissues more of an opportunity to heal. In the chronic stage, an increase in intensity may be warranted.

The developing health-care system of the last decade has dramatically limited patients' access to rehabilitation services and has increased the accountability of the health-care provider.[202] This development has placed a burden on the physical therapy profession to make the necessary changes to deal effectively with health-care reform, so that physical therapists become more accountable for their professional performance and more cost-effective in their provision of patient care.[202] It is important that examination and intervention techniques continue to be verified through peer-reviewed research, patient outcome databases, and an increased efficiency and effectiveness.[203,204]

Documentation

Documentation in health care includes any entry into the patient/client record. This documentation, considered a legal document, becomes a part of the patient's medical record. The SOAP (Subjective, Objective, Assessment, Plan) note format has traditionally been used to document the examination and intervention process.

- Subjective: information about the condition from patient or family member.
- Objective: measurement a clinician obtains during the physical examination.
- Assessment: analysis of problems including the long and short-term goals.
- Plan: a specific intervention plan for the identified problem(s).

The purposes of documentation are as follows:[205]

- To document what the clinician does to manage the individual patient's case.
- To record examination findings, patient status, intervention provided, and the patient's response to treatment.
- To communicate with all other members of the health-care team—this helps provide consistency among the services provided. This includes communication between the physical therapist and the physical therapist assistant.
- To provide information to third-party payers, such as Medicare and other insurance companies who make decisions about reimbursement based on the quality and completeness of the physical therapy note.
- To help the physical therapist organize his/her thought processes involved in patient care.
- To be used for quality assurance and improvement purposes and for issues such as discharge planning.
- To serve as a source of data for quality assurance, peer and utilization review, and research.

REVIEW QUESTIONS*

1. Give a definition of empathy.
2. Differentiate between the terms examination and evaluation.
3. What are the three components of the examination?
4. What is the difference between a leading question and a neutral question?
5. What is the purpose of the systems review?

*Additional questions to test your understanding of this chapter can be found in the Online Learning Center for *Orthopaedic Assessment, Evaluation, and Intervention* at www.duttononline.net.

REFERENCES

1. Guide to physical therapist practice: revisions. American Physical Therapy Association. *Phys Ther* 79, 2001.
2. Kibler WB: Shoulder rehabilitation: principles and practice. *Med Sci Sports Exerc* 30:40–50, 1998.
3. Nirschl RP, Sobel J: *Arm Care. A Complete Guide to Prevention and Treatment of Tennis Elbow*. Arlington, Virginia, VA: Medical Sports, 1996.
4. Meadows J: *Orthopedic Differential Diagnosis in Physical Therapy*. New York, NY: McGraw-Hill, 1999.
5. Kaltenborn FM: *Manual Mobilization of the Extremity Joints: Basic Examination and Treatment Techniques*, 4th ed. Oslo, Norway: Olaf Norlis Bokhandel, Universitetsgaten, 1989.
6. Maitland G: *Vertebral Manipulation*. Sydney: Butterworth, 1986.
7. Maitland G: *Peripheral Manipulation*, 3rd ed. London: Butterworth, 1991.
8. Evjenth O, Hamberg J: *Muscle Stretching in Manual Therapy, A Clinical Manual*. Alfta, Sweden :Alfta Rehab Forlag, 1984.
9. Lee DG: Biomechanics of the thorax. In: Grant R, ed. *Physical Therapy of the Cervical and Thoracic Spine*. New York, NY: Churchill Livingstone, 1988:47–76.
10. Lee DG: *The Pelvic Girdle: An Approach to the Examination and Treatment of the Lumbo-Pelvic-Hip Region*, 2nd ed. Edinburgh: Churchill Livingstone, 1999.
11. Sahrmann SA: *Diagnosis and Treatment of Movement Impairment Syndromes*. St Louis, MO: Mosby, 2001.
12. Butler DS: *Mobilization of the Nervous System*. New York, NY: Churchill Livingstone, 1992.
13. Judge RD, Zuidema GD, Fitzgerald FT: Introduction. In: Judge RD, Zuidema GD, Fitzgerald FT, eds. *Clinical Diagnosis*, 4th ed. Boston, MA: Little, Brown and Company, 1982:3–8.
14. *Guide to physical therapist practice*: Phys Ther 81:S13–S95, 2001.
15. Cipriani DJ, Noftz II JB: The utility of orthopedic clinical tests for diagnosis. In: Magee D, Zachazewski JE, Quillen WS, eds.. *Scientific Foundations and Principles of Practice in Musculoskeletal Rehabilitation*. St. Louis, MO: WB Saunders, 2007:557–567.
16. Cleland J: *Introduction, Orthopedic Clinical Examination: An Evidence-Based Approach for Physical Therapists*. Carlstadt, NJ: Icon Learning Systems, LLC, 2005:2–23.
17. Feinstein AR: *Clinimetrics*. Westford, MA: Murray Printing Company, 1987.
18. Marx RG, Bombardier C, Wright JG: What we know about the reliability and validity of physical examination tests used to examine the upper extremity. *J Hand Surg* 24A:185–193, 1999.
19. Roach KE, Brown MD, Albin RD, et al: The sensitivity and specificity of pain response to activity and position in categorizing patients with low back pain. *Phys Ther* 77:730–738, 1997.
20. Sullivan PE, Puniello MS, Pardasaney PK: Rehabilitation program development: clinical decision-making, prioritization, and program integration. In: Magee D, Zachazewski JE, Quillen WS, eds. *Scientific Foundations and Principles of Practice in Musculoskeletal Rehabilitation*. St. Louis, MO: WB Saunders, 2007:314–327.
21. Waddell G, Newton M, Henderson I, et al: A Fear-Avoidance Beliefs Questionnaire (FABQ) and the role of fear-avoidance beliefs in chronic low back pain and disability. *Pain* 52:157–168, 1993.
22. Fisher C, Dvorak M: *Orthopaedic research: What an orthopaedic surgeon needs to know, Orthopaedic Knowledge Update: Home Study Syllabus*. Rosemont, IL: American Academy of Orthopaedic Surgeons, 2005:3–13.
23. Delitto A: Subjective measures and clinical decision making. *Phys Ther* 69:580, 1989.
24. Simel DL, Rennie D: The clinical examination. An agenda to make it more rational. *JAMA* 277:572–574, 1997.
25. Jensen MC, Brant-Zawadzki MN, Obuchowski N, et al: Magnetic resonance imaging of the lumbar spine in people without back pain. *N Engl J Med* 331:69–73, 1994.
26. Miniaci A, Dowdy PA, Willits KR,et al: Magnetic resonance imaging evaluation of the rotator cuff tendons in the asymptomatic shoulder. *Am J Sports Med* 23:142–145, 1995.
27. LaPrade RF, Burnett QM, II, Veenstra MA, et al: The prevalence of abnormal magnetic resonance imaging findings in asymptomatic knees. With correlation of magnetic resonance imaging to arthroscopic findings in symptomatic knees. *Am J Sports Med* 22:739–745, 1994.

28. O'Shea KJ, Murphy KP, Heekin RD,et al: The diagnostic accuracy of history, physical examination, and radiographs in the evaluation of traumatic knee disorders. *Am J Sports Med* 24:164–167, 1996.
29. Goodman CC, Snyder TK: Introduction to the interviewing process. In: Goodman CC, Snyder TK, eds. *Differential Diagnosis in Physical Therapy*. Philadelphia, PA: Saunders, 1990:7–42.
30. Murphy DR, Coulis CM, Gerrard JK: Cervical spondylosis with spinal cord encroachment: should preventive surgery be recommended? *Chiropr Osteopat* 17:8, 2009.
31. Rao RD, Currier BL, Albert TJ, et al: Degenerative cervical spondylosis: clinical syndromes, pathogenesis, and management. *Instr Course Lect* 57:447–469, 2008.
32. Binder AI: Cervical spondylosis and neck pain. *BMJ* 334:527–531, 2007.
33. Haslock I: Ankylosing spondylitis. *Baillieres Clin Rheumatol* 7:99, 1993.
34. Potosky AL, Feuer EJ, Levin DL: Impact of screening on incidence and mortality of prostate cancer in the United States. *Epidemiol Rev* 23: 181–186, 2001.
35. Steinberg MH: Management of sickle cell disease. *N Engl J Med* 340:1021–1030, 1999.
36. Anderson JJ, Pollitzer WS: Ethnic and genetic differences in susceptibility to osteoporotic fractures. *Adv Nutr Res* 9:129–149, 1994.
37. Falkner B: Insulin resistance in African Americans. *Kidney Int Suppl*: S27–S30, 2003.
38. Fogo AB: Hypertensive risk factors in kidney disease in African Americans. *Kidney Int Suppl* S17–S21, 2003.
39. Wingo PA, Tong T, Bolden S: *Cancer statistics*, 1995. *CA Cancer J Clin* 45:8, 1995.
40. Parkin DM, Muir CS: Cancer incidence in five continents. Comparability and quality of data. *IARC Sci. Pub* 66:45, 1992.
41. Ries LAG, Eisner MP, Kosary CL,et al: *SEER cancer statistics review, 1973–1997*. Bethesda, MD: National Cancer Institute, 2000.
42. Martinez JC, Otley CC: The management of melanoma and nonmelanoma skin cancer: a review for the primary care physician. *Mayo Clin Proc* 76:1253–1265, 2001.
43. McKenzie R, May S: Mechanical Diagnosis. In: McKenzie R, May S, eds. *The Human Extremities: Mechanical Diagnosis and Therapy*. Waikanae, New Zealand: Spinal Publications New Zealand Ltd, 2000: 79–88.
44. McKenzie R, May S: History. In: McKenzie R, May S, eds.. *The Human Extremities: Mechanical Diagnosis and Therapy*. Waikanae, New Zealand: Spinal Publications New Zealand Ltd, 2000:89–103.
45. Bogduk N: The anatomy and physiology of nociception. In: Crosbie J, McConnell J, eds. *Key Issues in Physiotherapy*. Oxford: Butterworth-Heinemann, 1993:48–87.
46. Goodman CC, Snyder TEK: *Differential Diagnosis in Physical Therapy*. Philadelphia, PA: WB Saunders Company, 1990.
47. Huskisson EC: Measurement of pain. *Lancet* 2:127, 1974.
48. Halle JS: Neuromusculoskeletal scan examination with selected related topics. In: Flynn TW, ed. *The Thoracic Spine and Rib Cage: Musculoskeletal Evaluation and Treatment*. Boston, MA: Butterworth-Heinemann, 1996:121–146.
49. Rowland LP: Diseases of the motor unit. In: Kandel ER, Schwartz JH, Jessell TM, eds. *Principles of Neural Science*, 4th ed. New York, NY: McGraw-Hill, 2000:695–712.
50. D'Ambrosia R: *Musculoskeletal Disorders: Regional Examination and Differential Diagnosis*, 2nd ed. Philadelphia, PA: J.B. Lippincott, 1986.
51. Konietzny F, Perl ER, Trevino D, et al: Sensory experiences in man evoked by intraneural electrical stimulation of intact cutaneous afferent fibers. *Exp Brain Res* 42:219–222, 1981.
52. Ochoa J, Torebjörk E: Sensations evoked by intraneural microstimulation of C nociceptor fibres in human skin nerves. *J Physiol* 415:583–599, 1989.
53. Torebjörk HE, Ochoa JL, Schady W: Referred pain from intraneural stimulation of muscle fascicles in the median nerve. *Pain* 18:145–156, 1984.
54. Ness TJ, Gebhart GF: Visceral pain: a review of experimental studies. *Pain* 41:167–234, 1990.
55. Chaturvedi SK: Prevalence of chronic pain in psychiatric patients. *Pain* 29:231–7, 1987.
56. Goldstein R: Psychological evaluation of low back pain. *Spine: State of the Art Reviews* 1:103, 1986.
57. Norris TR: History and physical examination of the shoulder. In: Nicholas JA, Hershman EB, Posner MA, eds. *The Upper Extremity in Sports Medicine*, 2nd ed. St Louis, MO: Mosby Year-Book, Inc, 1995:39–83.
58. Melzack R: The McGill Pain Questionnaire: Major properties and scoring methods. *Pain* 1:277, 1975.
59. Melzack R, Torgerson WS: On the language of pain. *Anaesthesiology* 34:50, 1971.
60. Liebenson C: Pain and disability questionnaires in chiropractic rehabilitation. In: Liebenson C, ed. *Rehabilitation of the Spine: A Practitioner's Manual*. Baltimore, MD: Lippincott Williams & Wilkins, 1996:57–71.
61. Burkhardt CS: The use of the McGill Pain Questionnaire in assessing arthritis pain. *Pain* 19:305, 1984.
62. Pearce J, Morley S: An experimental investigation of the construct validity of the McGill Pain Questionnaire. *Pain* 115:115, 1989.
63. Magarey ME: Examination of the cervical and thoracic spine. In: Grant R, ed. *Physical Therapy of the Cervical and Thoracic Spine*, 2nd ed. New York, NY: Churchill Livingstone, 1994:109–144.
64. Morris C, Chaitow L, Janda V: Functional examination for low back syndromes. In: Morris C, ed. *Low Back Syndromes: Integrated Clinical Management*. New York, NY: McGraw-Hill, 2006:333–416.
65. Puranen J, Orava S: The hamstring syndrome—a new gluteal sciatica. *Ann Chir Gynaecol* 80:212–214, 1991.
66. Puranen J, Orava S: The hamstring syndrome. A new diagnosis of gluteal sciatic pain. *Am J Sports Med* 16:517–521, 1988.
67. Christie HJ, Kumar S, Warren SA: Postural aberrations in low back pain. *Arch Phys Med Rehabil* 76:218–224, 1995.
68. Judge RD, Zuidema GD, Fitzgerald FT: General Appearance. In: Judge RD, Zuidema GD, Fitzgerald FT, eds. *Clinical Diagnosis*, 4th ed. Boston, MA: Little, Brown and Company, 1982: 29–47.
69. Vasilyeva LF, Lewit K: Diagnosis of muscular dysfunction by inspection. In: Liebenson C, ed. *Rehabilitation of the Spine: A Practitioner's Manual*. Baltimore, MD: Lippincott Williams & Wilkins, 1996:113–142.
70. Davis MP, Walsh D: Cancer pain: how to measure the fifth vital sign. *Cleve Clin J Med* 71:625–632, 2004.
71. Salcido RS: Is pain a vital sign? *Adv Skin Wound Care* 16:214, 2003.
72. Sousa FA: [Pain: the fifth vital sign]. *Rev Lat Am Enfermagem* 10:446–447, 2002.
73. Lynch M: Pain: the fifth vital sign. Comprehensive assessment leads to proper treatment. *Adv Nurse Pract* 9:28–36, 2001.
74. Lynch M: Pain as the fifth vital sign. *J Intraven Nurs* 24:85–94, 2001.
75. Merboth MK, Barnason S: Managing pain: the fifth vital sign. *Nurs Clin North Am* 35:375–383, 2000.
76. Torma L: Pain—the fifth vital sign. *Pulse* 36:16, 1999.
77. Pain as the fifth vital sign. *J Am Optom Assoc* 70:619–620, 1999.
78. Joel LA: The fifth vital sign: pain. *Am J Nurs* 99:9, 1999.
79. McCaffery M, Pasero CL: Pain ratings: the fifth vital sign. *Am J Nurs* 97:15–16, 1997.
80. Frese EM, Richter RR, Burlis TV: Self-reported measurement of heart rate and blood pressure in patients by physical therapy clinical instructors. *Phys Ther* 82:1192–1200, 2002.
81. Bailey MK: Physical examination procedures to screen for serious disorders of the low back and lower quarter. In: Wilmarth MA, ed. *Medical Screening for the Physical Therapist. Orthopaedic Section Independent Study Course 14.1.1 La Crosse*. Wisconsin, WI: Orthopaedic Section, APTA, Inc, 2003:1–35.
82. Judge RD, Zuidema GD, Fitzgerald FT: Vital Signs. In: Judge RD, Zuidema GD, Fitzgerald FT, eds. *Clinical Diagnosis*, 4th ed. Boston, MA: Little, Brown and Company, 1982:49–58.
83. Cyriax J: *Textbook of Orthopaedic Medicine, Diagnosis of Soft Tissue Lesions* 8th ed. London: Bailliere Tindall, 1982.
84. Halle JS: The neuromusculoskeletal scan examination. In: Voight ML, Hoogenboom BJ, Prentice WE, eds. *Musculoskeletal Interventions: Techniques for Therapeutic Exercise*. New York, NY: McGraw-Hill, 2007:47–80.
85. Meadows JTS: *Manual Therapy: Biomechanical Assessment and Treatment, Advanced Technique*. Calgary, AB: Swodeam Consulting, Inc., 1995.
86. Hayes KW: An examination of Cyriax's passive motion tests with patients having osteoarthritis of the knee. *Phys Ther* 74:697, 1994.
87. Franklin ME: Assessment of exercise induced minor lesions: The accuracy of Cyriax's diagnosis by selective tissue tension paradigm. *J Orthop Sports Phys Ther* 24:122, 1996.
88. Cyriax J: *Examination of the Shoulder. Limited Range Diagnosis of Soft Tissue Lesions* 8th ed. London: Balliere Tindall, 1982.
89. Cyriax JH, Cyriax PJ: *Illustrated Manual of Orthopaedic Medicine*. London: Butterworth, 1983.

90. Cyriax J: *Diagnosis of Soft Tissue Lesions, Textbook of Orthopaedic Medicine* 7th ed. Baltimore, MD: Williams & Wilkins, 1980:682.
91. Maitland GD: The hypothesis of adding compression when examining and treating synovial joints. *J Orthop Sports Phys Ther* 2:7, 1980.
92. Grieve GP: *Common Vertebral Joint Problems.* New York, NY: Churchill Livingstone Inc, 1981.
93. McKenzie RA: *The Lumbar Spine: Mechanical Diagnosis and Therapy.* Waikanae, NZ: Spinal Publication, 1981.
94. McKenzie R, May S: Introduction. In: McKenzie R, May S, eds. *The Human Extremities: Mechanical Diagnosis and Therapy.* Waikanae, New Zealand: Spinal Publications New Zealand Ltd, 2000:1–5.
95. Stetts DM: Patient Examination. In: Wadsworth C, ed. *Current Concepts of Orthopaedic Physical Therapy — Home study Course 11.2.2.* La Crosse, WI: Orthopaedic Section, APTA, 2001.
96. Sackett DL, Strauss SE, Richardson WS, et al: *Evidence Based Medicine: How to Practice and Teach EBM,* 2nd ed. Edinburgh, Scotland: Churchill Livingstone, 2000.
97. Jaeschke R, Guyatt G, Sackett DL: Users guides to the medical literature. III. How to use an article about a diagnostic test. B. What are the results and will they help me in caring for my patients? *JAMA* 27:703–707, 1994.
98. Sackett DL, Haynes RB, Tugwell P: *Clinical Epidemiology: A Basic Science for Clinical Medicine.* Boston, MA: Mass, Little, brown and Co, 1985.
99. Straus SE, Richardson WS, Glasziou P, et al: Evidence-Based Medicine, University Health Network, http://www.cebm.utoronto.ca/, 2006.
100. Fess EE: The need for reliability and validity in hand assessment instruments. *J Hand Surg* 11A:621–623, (editorial), 1986.
101. McKenzie R, May S: Physical Examination. In: McKenzie R, May S, eds. *The Human Extremities: Mechanical Diagnosis and Therapy.* Waikanae, New Zealand: Spinal Publications New Zealand Ltd, 2000: 105–121.
102. Rothstein JM: Cyriax reexamined. *Phys Ther* 74:1073, 1994.
103. Farfan HF: The scientific basis of manipulative procedures. *Clin Rheum Dis* 6:159–177, 1980
104. Harris ML: Flexibility. *Phys Ther* 49:591–601, 1969.
105. Dvorak J, Antinnes JA, Panjabi M,et al: Age and gender related normal motion of the cervical spine. *Spine* 17:S393–S398, 1992.
106. White DJ: Musculoskeletal examination. In: O'Sullivan SB, Schmitz TJ, eds. *Physical Rehabilitation,* 5th ed. Philadelphia, FA Davis, 2007: 159–192.
107. Petersen CM, Hayes KW: Construct validity of Cyriax's selective tension examination: association of end-feels with pain at the knee and shoulder. *J Orthop Sports Phys Ther* 30:512–527, 2000.
108. Boone DC, Azen SP, Lin C-M,et al: Reliability of goniometric measurements. *Phys Ther* 58:1355–1360, 1978.
109. Mayerson NH, Milano RA: Goniometric measurement reliability in physical medicine. *Arch Phys Med Rehab* 65:92–94, 1984.
110. Riddle DL, Rothstein JM, Lamb RL: Goniometric reliability in a clinical setting: shoulder measurements. *Phys Ther* 67:668–673, 1987.
111. Williams JG, Callaghan M: Comparison of visual estimation and goniometry in determination of a shoulder joint angle. *Physiotherapy* 76:655–657, 1990.
112. American Medical Association: *Guides to the Evaluation of Permanent Impairment,* 5th ed. Chicago, IL: American Medical Association, 2001.
113. Nelson MA, Allen P, Clamp SE, et al: Reliability and reproducibility of clinical findings in low-back pain. *Spine* 4:97–101, 1979.
114. Stokes M, Young A: The contribution of reflex inhibition to arthrogenous muscle weakness. *Clin Sci* 67:7–14, 1984.
115. Watson D, Trott P: Cervical headache: an investigation of natural head posture and upper cervical flexor muscle performance. *Cephalalgia* 13:272–284, 1993.
116. Riddle DL: Measurement of accessory motion: Critical issues and related concepts. *Phys Ther* 72:865–874, 1992.
117. Tovin BJ, Greenfield BH: *Impairment-based diagnosis for the shoulder girdle, Evaluation and Treatment of the Shoulder: An Integration of the Guide to Physical Therapist Practice.* Philadelphia, PA: F.A. Davis, 2001:55–74.
118. Janda V: *Muscle Function Testing.* London: Butterworths, 1983.
119. Florence JM, Pandya S, King WM, et al: Intrarater reliability of manual muscle test (Medical Research Council scale) grades in Duchenne's muscular dystrophy. *Phys Ther* 72:115–122; discussion 122–126, 1992.
120. Barr AE, Diamond BE, Wade CK, et al: Reliability of testing measures in Duchenne or Becker muscular dystrophy. *Arch Phys Med Rehabil* 72:315–319, 1991.
121. Nadler SF, Rigolosi L, Kim D, et al: Sensory, motor, and reflex examination. In: Malanga GA, Nadler SF, eds. *Musculoskeletal Physical Examination – An Evidence-Based Approach.* Philadelphia, PA: Elsevier-Mosby, 2006:15–32.
122. Bohannon RW: Make Tests and Break Tests of Elbow Flexor Muscle Strength. *Phys Ther* 68:193–194, 1988.
123. Stratford PW, Balsor BE: A comparison of make and break tests using a hand-held dynamometer and the Kin-Com. *J Orthop Sports Phys ther* 19:28–32, 1994.
124. Andrews AW, Thomas MW, Bohannon RW: Normative values for isometric muscle force measurements obtained with hand-held dynamometers. *Phys Ther* 76:248–259, 1996.
125. Sapega AA: Muscle performance evaluation in orthopedic practice. *J Bone Joint Surg* 72A:1562–1574, 1990.
126. Iddings DM, Smith LK, Spencer WA: Muscle testing: part 2. Reliability in clinical use. *Phys Ther Rev* 41:249–256, 1961.
127. Silver M, McElroy A, Morrow L, et al: Further standardization of manual muscle test for clinical study: applied in chronic renal disease. *Phys Ther* 50:1456–1465, 1970.
128. Astrand PO, Rodahl K: *Textbook of Work Physiology.* New York, NY: McGraw-Hill, 1973.
129. Astrand PO, Rodahl K: *The Muscle and its Contraction: Textbook of Work Physiology.* New York, NY: McGraw-Hill, 1986.
130. Muller EA: Influences of training and inactivity of muscle strength. *Arch Phys Med Rehab* 51:449–462, 1970.
131. Phillips BA, Lo SK, Mastaglia FL: Muscle force measured using "break" testing with a hand-held myometer in normal subjects aged 20 to 69 years. *Arch Phys Med Rehabil* 81:653–661, 2000.
132. Beck M, Giess R, Wurffel W, et al: Comparison of maximal voluntary isometric contraction and Drachman's hand-held dynamometry in evaluating patients with amyotrophic lateral sclerosis. *Muscle Nerve* 22:1265–1270, 1999.
133. Roy MA, Doherty TJ: Reliability of hand-held dynamometry in assessment of knee extensor strength after hip fracture. *Am J Phys Med Rehabil* 83:813–818, 2004.
134. Hutten MM, Hermens HJ: Reliability of lumbar dynamometry measurements in patients with chronic low back pain with test-retest measurements on different days. *Eur Spine J* 6:54–62, 1997.
135. Stokes HM, Landrieu KW, Domangue B, et al: Identification of low effort patients through dynamometry. *J Hand Surg* 20A:1047–1056, 1995.
136. Bohannon RW: Hand-held compared with isokinetic dynamometry for measurement of static knee extension torque (parallel reliability of dynamometers). *Clin Phys Physiol Meas* 11:217–222, 1990.
137. Hartsell HD, Forwell L: Postoperative eccentric and concentric isokinetic strength for the shoulder rotators in the scapular and neutral planes. *J Orthop Sports Phys Ther* 25:19–25, 1997.
138. Hartsell HD, Spaulding SJ: Eccentric/concentric ratios at selected velocities for the invertor and evertor muscles of the chronically unstable ankle. *Br J Sports Med* 33:255–258, 1999.
139. Griffin JW: Differences in elbow flexion torque measured concentrically, eccentrically and isometrically. *Phys Ther* 67:1205–1208, 1987.
140. Hortobagyi T, Katch FI: Eccentric and concentric torque-velocity relationships during arm flexion and extension. *J Appl Physiol* 60:395–401, 1995.
141. Trudelle-Jackson E, Meske N, Highenboten C, et al: Eccentric/concentric torque deficits in the quadriceps muscle. *J Orthop Sports Phys Ther* 11:142–145, 1989.
142. Rothstein JM, Lamb RL, Mayhew TP: Clinical uses of isokinetic measurements. Critical issues. *Phys Ther* 67:1840–1844, 1987.
143. Beasley WC: Quantitative muscle testing: principles and applications to research and clinical services. *Arch Phys Med Rehabil* 42:398–425, 1961.
144. Bohannon RW: Manual muscle test scores and dynamometer test scores of knee extension strength. *Arch Phys Med Rehabil* 67:390–392, 1986.
145. Mulroy SJ, Lassen KD, Chambers SH, et al: The ability of male and female clinicians to effectively test knee extension strength using manual muscle testing. *J Orthop Sports Phys Ther* 26:192–199, 1997.
146. Brunnstrom S: *Movement Therapy in Hemiplegia.* New York, NY: Harper & Row Pub Inc, 1970.
147. Knott M, Voss DE: *Proprioceptive Neuromuscular Facilitation,* 2nd ed. New York, NY: Harper & Row Pub Inc., 1968.

148. Voss DE, Ionta MK, Myers DJ: *Proprioceptive Neuromuscular Facilitation: Patterns and Techniques*, 3rd ed. Philadelphia, PA: Harper and Row, 1985:1–342.
149. Mann RA: Biomechanics of the foot. *Instructional Course Lectures* 31:167–180, 1982.
150. Ayub E: Posture and the Upper Quarter. In: Donatelli RA, ed. *Physical Therapy of the Shoulder*, 2nd ed. New York, NY: Churchill Livingstone, 1991:81–90.
151. Simon RP, Aminoff MJ, Greenberg DA: *Clinical Neurology*, 4th ed. Stanford, CT: Appleton and Lange, 1999.
152. Baloh RW: Vertigo. *Lancet* 352:1841–1846, 1998.
153. Huijbregts P, Vidal P: Dizziness in orthopedic physical therapy practice: history and physical examination. *J Man Manip Ther* 13: 221–250, 2005.
154. Gerwin RD, Shannon S, Hong C, et al: Interrater reliability in myofascial trigger point examination. *Pain* 17:591–595, 1997.
155. Njoo KH, Van der Does E: The occurrence and inter-rater reliability of myofascial trigger points in the quadratus lumborum and gluteus medius: A prospective study in non-specific low back patients and controls in general practice. *Pain* 58:317–321, 1994.
156. Farrell JP: Cervical passive mobilization techniques: The Australian approach. *Physical Medicine and Rehabilitation: State-of-the-Art Reviews* 4:309–334, 1990.
157. Dyson M, Pond JB, Joseph J, et al: The stimulation of tissue regeneration by means of ultrasound. *Clin Sci* 35:273–285, 1968.
158. Dyson M, Suckling J: Stimulation of tissue repair by ultrasound: a survey of the mechanisms involved. *Physiotherapy* 64:105–108, 1978.
159. Ramsey SM: Holistic manual therapy techniques. *Prim Care* 24:759–785, 1997.
160. Hsieh CY, Hong CZ, Adams AH, et al: Interexaminer reliability of the palpation of trigger points in the trunk and lower limb muscles. *Arch Phys Med Rehabil* 81:258–264, 2000.
161. Dvorak J, Dvorak V: General Principles of Palpation. In: Gilliar WG, Greenman PE, eds. *Manual Medicine: Diagnostics*, 2nd ed. New York, NY: Thieme Medical Publishers, 1990:71–75.
162. Austin G: Functional testing and return to activity. In: Magee D, Zachazewski JE, Quillen WS, eds. *Scientific foundations and principles of practice in musculoskeletal rehabilitation*. St. Louis, MO: WB Saunders, 2007:633–664.
163. Jull GA, Janda V: Muscle and Motor control in low back pain. In: Twomey LT, Taylor JR, eds. *Physical Therapy of the Low Back: Clinics in Physical Therapy*. New York, NY: Churchill Livingstone, 1987:258–278.
164. Woolbright JL: Exercise protocol for patients with low back pain. *JAOA* 82:919, 1983.
165. Nachemson A: Work for all. For those with low back pain as well. *Clin Orthop* 179:77, 1982.
166. Resnick DN, Morris C: History and physical examination for low back syndromes. In: Morris C, ed. *Low Back Syndromes: Integrated Clinical Management*. New York, NY: McGraw-Hill, 2006:305–331.
167. Andersson GBJ, Deyo RA: History and physical examination in patients with herniated lumbar discs. *Spine* 21:10S–18S, 1996.
168. Cwynar DA, McNerney T: A primer on physical therapy. *Lippincott's Primary Care Practice* 3:451–459, 1999.
169. Guide to Physical Therapist Practice. 2nd ed. American Physical Therapy Association. *Phys Ther* 81:9–746, 2001.
170. Clawson AL, Domholdt E: Content of physician referrals to physical therapists at clinical education sites in Indiana. *Phys Ther* 74:356–360, 1994.
171. Leerar PJ: Differential diagnosis of tarsal coalition versus cuboid syndrome in an adolescent athlete. *J Orthop Sports Phys Ther* 31:702–707, 2001.
172. Jones MA: Clinical reasoning in manual therapy. *Phys Ther* 72:875–884, 1992.
173. Schenkman M, Deutsch JE, Gill-Body KM: An integrated framework for decision making in neurologic physical therapist practice. *Phys Ther* 86:1681–1702, 2006.
174. Hoogenboom BJ, Voight ML: Clinical reasoning: An algorithm-based approach to musculoskeletal rehabilitation. In: Voight ML, Hoogenboom BJ, Prentice WE, eds. *Musculoskeletal Interventions: Techniques for Therapeutic Exercise*. New York, NY: McGraw-Hill, 2007: 81–95.
175. Brooks LR, Norman GR, Allen SW: The role of specific similarity in a medical diagnostic task. *J Exp Psychol Gen* 120:278–287, 1991.
176. Kahney H: *Problem solving: current issues*. Buckingham: Open University Press, 1993.
177. Coutts F: Changes in the musculoskeletal system. In: Atkinson K, Coutts F, Hassenkamp A, eds. *Physiotherapy in Orthopedics*. London: Churchill Livingstone, 1999:19–43.
178. Jette AM: Diagnosis and classification by physical therapists: A special communication. *Phys Ther* 69:967, 1989.
179. Higgs J, Jones M: *Clinical Reasoning in the Health Professions*, 2nd ed. London: Butterworth-Heinemann, 2000:118–127.
180. Rothstein JM, Echternach JL, Riddle DL: The Hypothesis-Oriented Algorithm for Clinicians II (HOAC II): a guide for patient management. *Phys Ther* 83:455–470, 2003.
181. Echternach JL, Rothstein JM: Hypothesis-oriented algorithms. *Phys Ther* 69:559–564, 1989.
182. Rothstein JM, Echternach JL: Hypothesis-oriented algorithm for clinicians. A method for evaluation and treatment planning. *Phys Ther.* 66:1388–1394, 1986.
183. Schenkman M, Butler RB: A model for multisystem evaluation, interpretation, and treatment of individuals with neurologic dysfunction. *Phys Ther* 69:538–547, 1989.
184. Schenkman M, Butler RB: A model for multisystem evaluation treatment of individuals with Parkinson's disease. *Phys Ther* 69:932–943, 1989.
185. Schenkman M, Donovan J, Tsubota J, et al: Management of individuals with Parkinson's disease: rationale and case studies. *Phys Ther* 69:944–955, 1989.
186. Friedman LM, Furberg CD, DeMets DL: *Fundamentals of Clinical Trials*, 2nd ed. Chicago, IL: Mosby-Year Book, 1985:2, 51, 71.
187. Bloch R: Methodology in clinical back pain trials. *Spine* 12:430–432, 1987.
188. Maher CG, Herbert RD, Moseley AM, et al: Critical appraisal of randomized trials, systematic reviews of randomized trials and clinical practice guidelines. In: Boyling JD, Jull GA, eds. *Grieve's Modern Manual Therapy: The vertebral column*. Philadelphia, PA: Churchill Livingstone, 2004:603–614.
189. Wickstrom G, Bendix T: The "Hawthorne effect"—what did the original Hawthorne studies actually show? *Scand J Work Environ Health* 26:363–367, 2000.
190. Wainner RS: Reliability of the clinical examination: how close is "close enough"? *J Orthop Sports Phys Ther* 33:488–491, 2003.
191. Huijbregts PA: Spinal motion palpation: A review of reliability studies. *J Man & Manip Ther* 10:24–39, 2002.
192. Laslett M, Williams M: The reliability of selected pain provocation tests for sacroiliac joint pathology. *Spine* 19:1243–1249, 1994.
193. Portney L, Watkins MP: *Foundations of Clinical Research: Applications to Practice*. Norwalk, CT: Appleton & Lange, 1993.
194. Schwartz JS: Evaluating diagnostic tests: what is done—what needs to be done. *J Gen Intern Med* 1:266–267, 1986.
195. Jull GA: Physiotherapy management of neck pain of mechanical origin. In: Giles LGF, Singer KP, eds. *Clinical Anatomy and Management of Cervical Spine Pain. The Clinical Anatomy of Back Pain*. London, England: Butterworth-Heinemann, 1998:168–191.
196. Van der Wurff P, Meyne W, Hagmeijer RHM: Clinical tests of the sacroiliac joint, a systematic methodological review. part 2: validity. *Man Ther* 5:89–96, 2000.
197. Davidson M: The interpretation of diagnostic tests: A primer for physiotherapists. *Aust J Physiother* 48:227–233, 2002.
198. Feinstein AR: Clinical biostatistics XXXI: on the sensitivity, specificity & discrimination of diagnostic tests. *Clin Pharmacol Ther* 17:104–116, 1975.
199. Anderson MA, Foreman TL: Return to Competition: Functional Rehabilitation. In: Zachazewski JE, Magee DJ, Quillen WS, eds. *Athletic Injuries and Rehabilitation*. Philadelphia, PA: WB Saunders, 1996:229–261.
200. Whiting P, Rutjes AW, Reitsma JB, et al: The development of QUADAS: a tool for the quality assessment of studies of diagnostic accuracy included in systematic reviews. *BMC Med Res Methodol* 3:25, 2003.
201. Yoder E: Physical therapy management of nonsurgical hip problems in adults. In: Echternach JL, ed. *Physical Therapy of the Hip*. New York, NY: Churchill Livingstone, 1990:103–137.
202. DeCarlo MS, Sell KE: The effects of the number and frequency of physical therapy treatments on selected outcomes of treatment in patients with anterior cruciate ligament reconstructions. *J Orthop Sports Phys Ther* 26:332–339, 1997.
203. Coile RC: Forecasting the future-Part two. *Rehab Manage* 7:59–63, 1994.
204. Nugent J: Blaze your trails through managed care. *PT Mag* 2:19–20, 1994.
205. Kettenbach G: Background Information. In: Kettenbach G, ed. *Writing SOAP Notes with Patient/Client Management Formats*, 3rd ed. Philadelphia, PA: FA Davis, 2004:1–5.

Differential Diagnosis

CHAPTER 5

CHAPTER OBJECTIVES

At the completion of this chapter, the reader will be able to:

1. Understand the importance of differential diagnosis.
2. Recognize some of the signs and symptoms that indicate the presence of a serious pathology.
3. Discuss the concept of malingering.
4. Describe why certain signs and symptoms (red flags) require medical referral.
5. Describe the various infective diseases and inflammatory disorders that the orthopaedic clinician may encounter
6. Describe the various neoplastic and metabolic diseases that can impact the orthopaedic patient.
7. Discuss the differences between fibromyalgia and myofascial pain syndrome.
8. List the various systemic or medical pathologies that can mimic musculoskeletal pathology in various body regions.

OVERVIEW

An important component of the Vision 2020 statement set forth by the American Physical Therapy Association[1] is achieving direct access through independent, self-determined, professional judgment and action. With the majority of states now permitting direct access to physical therapists, many physical therapists now have the primary responsibility for being the gatekeepers of health care and for making medical referrals. In light of the APTA's movement toward realizing "Vision 2020," an operational definition of autonomous practice and the related term autonomous physical therapist practitioner is defined by the APTA's Board as follows:

- "Autonomous physical therapist practice is practice characterized by independent, self-determined professional judgment and action."
- "An autonomous physical therapist practitioner within the scope of practice defined by the 'Guide to Physical Therapist Practice' provides physical therapy services to patients who have direct and unrestricted access to their services, and may refer as appropriate to other health-care providers and other professionals and for diagnostic tests."[2]

Through the history and physical examination, physical therapists diagnose and classify different types of information for use in their clinical reasoning and intervention.[3] The Guide clearly articulates the physical therapist's responsibility to recognize when a consultation with, or referral to, another health-care provider is necessary.[4] This responsibility requires that the clinician have a high level of knowledge, including an understanding of the concepts of medical screening and differential diagnosis. The results of a number of studies have demonstrated that physical therapists can provide safe and effective care for patients with musculoskeletal conditions in a direct access setting.[5–7] Indeed, in a study by Childs et al.,[8] physical therapists demonstrated higher levels of knowledge in managing musculoskeletal conditions than medical students, physician interns and residents, and most physician specialists except for orthopedists. In addition, physical therapist students enrolled in educational programs conferring the doctoral degree achieved higher scores than their peers enrolled in programs conferring the master's degree.[8] Furthermore, licensed physical therapists who were board certified achieved higher scores and passing rates than their colleagues who were not board certified.[8]

In an effort to aid the differential diagnosis of musculoskeletal conditions commonly encountered by physical therapists, screening tools have been designed to help recognize potential serious disorders (red or yellow flags).[9]

- Red-flag findings are symptoms or conditions that may require immediate attention and supersede physical therapy being the primary provider of service (Table 5-1), as they are typically indicative of nonmechanical (non-neuromusculoskeletal) conditions or pathologies of visceral origin.
- Yellow-flag findings are potential confounding variables that may be cautionary warnings regarding the patient's condition and that require further investigation. Examples include dizziness, abnormal sensation patterns, fainting, progressive weakness, and circulatory or skin changes.

TABLE 5-1 Red-Flag Findings

History	Possible Condition
Constant and severe pain, especially at night	Neoplasm and acute neuromusculoskeletal injury
Unexplained weight loss	Neoplasm
Loss of appetite	Neoplasm
Unusual fatigue	Neoplasm and thyroid dysfunction
Visual disturbances (blurriness or loss of vision)	Neoplasm
Frequent or severe headaches	Neoplasm
Arm pain lasting > 2–3 mo	Neoplasm or neurologic dysfunction
Persistent root pain	Neoplasm or neurologic dysfunction
Radicular pain with coughing	Neoplasm or neurologic dysfunction
Pain worsening after 1 mo	Neoplasm
Paralysis	Neoplasm or neurologic dysfunction
Trunk and limb paresthesia	Neoplasm or neurologic dysfunction
Bilateral nerve root signs and symptoms	Neoplasm, spinal cord compression, and vertebrobasilar ischemia
Signs worse than symptoms	Neoplasm
Difficulty with balance and coordination	Spinal cord or CNS lesion
Fever or night sweats	Common findings in systemic infection and many diseases
Frequent nausea or vomiting	Common findings in many diseases, particularly of the gastrointestinal system
Dizziness	Upper cervical impairment, vertebrobasilar ischemia, craniovertebral ligament tear, inner ear dysfunction, CNS involvement, and cardiovascular dysfunction
Shortness of breath	Cardiovascular and/or pulmonary dysfunction and asthma
Quadrilateral paresthesia	Spinal cord compression (cervical myelopathy) and vertebrobasilar ischemia

CNS, central nervous system.
Data from Meadows J: *A Rationale and Complete Approach to the Sub-Acute Post-MVA Cervical Patient.* Calgary, AB: Swodeam Consulting, 1995.

Stith and colleagues[10] describe the red-flag findings found within the patient's history, which indicate a need for a referral to the physician. The presence of any of the following findings during the patient history, systems review, and/or scanning examination may indicate serious pathology requiring a medical referral:

- ***Fevers, chills, or night sweats.*** These signs and symptoms are almost always associated with a systemic disorder such as an infection.[11]
- ***Recent unexplained weight changes.*** An unexplained weight gain could be caused by congestive heart failure, hypothyroidism, or cancer.[12] An unexplained weight loss could be the result of a gastrointestinal disorder, hyperthyroidism, cancer, or diabetes.[12]
- ***Malaise or fatigue.*** These complaints, which can help determine the general health of the patient, may be associated with a systemic disease.[11]
- ***Unexplained nausea or vomiting.*** This is never a good symptom or sign.[11]
- ***Unilateral, bilateral, or quadrilateral paresthesias.*** The distribution of neurologic symptoms can give the clinician clues as to the structures involved. Quadrilateral paresthesia always indicates the presence of central nervous system (CNS) involvement.
- ***Shortness of breath.*** Shortness of breath can indicate a myriad of conditions. These can range from anxiety and asthma to a serious cardiac or pulmonary dysfunction.[11]
- ***Dizziness.*** The differential diagnosis of dizziness can be quite challenging. Patients often use the word "dizziness" to refer to feelings of lightheadedness, various sensations of body orientation, blurry vision, or weakness in the legs.
- ***Nystagmus.*** Nystagmus is characterized by a rhythmic movement of the eyes, with an abnormal shifting away from fixation and rapid return.[13] Failure of any one of the main control mechanisms for maintaining steady gaze fixation (the vestibuloocular reflex and a gaze-holding system) results in a disruption of steady fixation.
- ***Bowel or bladder dysfunction.*** Bowel and bladder dysfunction may indicate involvement of the cauda equina. *Cauda equina syndrome* is associated with compression of the spinal nerve roots that supply neurologic function to the bladder and bowel. A massive disk herniation may cause spinal cord or cauda equina compression. One of the early signs of cauda equina compromise is the inability to urinate while sitting down, because of the increased levels of pressure. The most common sensory deficit occurs over the buttocks, posterior–superior thighs, and perianal regions (the so-called saddle anesthesia), with a sensitivity of approximately 0.75.[14] Anal sphincter tone is diminished in 60–80% of cases.[14,15] Rapid diagnosis and surgical decompression of this abnormality is essential to prevent permanent neurologic dysfunction.
- ***Severe pain.*** An insidious onset of severe pain with no specific mechanism of injury.

- Pain at night that awakens the patient from a deep sleep, usually at the same time every night, and which is unrelated to a movement. This finding may indicate the presence of a tumor.
- Painful weakness. The presence of a painful weakness almost always indicates serious pathology, including but not limited to a complete rupture of contractile tissue or nerve palsy.
- A gradual increase in the intensity of the pain. This symptom typically indicates that the condition is worsening, especially if it continues with rest.

▸ ***Radiculopathy.*** Neurologic symptoms associated with more than two lumbar levels or more than one cervical level. With the exception of central protrusions or a disk lesion at L4 through L5, disk protrusions typically only affect one spinal nerve root. Multiple-level involvement could suggest the presence of a tumor or other growth, or it may indicate symptom magnification. The presence or absence of objective findings should help determine the cause.

Performing a medical screen is an inherent step in making a diagnosis for the purpose of deciding whether a patient referral is warranted, but the medical screen performed by the physical therapist is not synonymous with differential diagnosis. Differential diagnosis involves the ability to quickly differentiate problems of a serious nature from those that are not, using the history and physical examination. Problems of a serious nature include, but are not limited to, visceral diseases, cancer, infections, fractures, and vascular disorders. The purpose of the medical screen is to confirm (or rule out) the need for physical therapy intervention; the appropriateness of the referral; whether there are any red-flag findings, red-flag risk factors, or clusters of red-flag signs and/or symptoms; and whether the patient's condition falls into one of the categories of conditions outlined by the Guide.[16] Boissonnault and Bass[17] noted that screening for medical disease includes communicating with a physician regarding a list or pattern of signs and symptoms that have caused concern but not to suggest the presence of a specific disease.[3]

In clinical practice, physical therapists commonly use a combination of red-flag findings, the scanning examination, and the systems review to detect medical diseases. The combined results provide the physical therapist with a method to gather and evaluate examination data, pose and solve problems, infer, hypothesize, and make clinical judgments, such as the need for a patient/client referral.[16]

Systemic dysfunction or disease can present with seemingly bizarre symptoms. These symptoms can prove to be very confusing to the inexperienced clinician. Complicating the scenario is that certain patients who are pursuing litigation can also present with equally bizarre symptoms. These patients may be subdivided into two groups:

1. Those patients with a legitimate injury and cause for litigation who genuinely want to improve.
2. Those patients who are merely motivated by the lure of the litigation settlement and who have no intention of showing signs of improvement until their case is settled. Termed *malingerers*, these patients are a frustrating group for clinicians to deal with, because, like the nonorganic patient type, they display exaggerated complaints of pain, tenderness, and suffering.

Malingering is defined as the intentional production of false symptoms or the exaggeration of symptoms that truly exist.[18] These symptoms may be physical or psychological but have, in common, the intention of achieving a certain goal. Any individual involved in litigation, whether the result of a motor vehicle accident, work injury, or accident, has the potential for malingering.[19] Malingering can be thought of as synonymous with faking, lying, or fraud, and it represents a frequently unrecognized and mismanaged medical diagnosis.[18] Unfortunately, due to the similarity between malingerers and nonorganic patients, this deception often causes a significant, negative response from the clinician toward malingerers and nonorganic patients alike.

It is most important that the clinician addresses any suspected deception in a structured and unemotional manner and that interactions with the patient be performed in a problem-oriented, constructive, and helpful fashion.[18]

CLINICAL PEARL

The diagnosis of malingering should be made based on the production of actions in the attainment of a known goal, without elaboration of those actions based on the negative emotional response of the clinician.[18]

With very few exceptions, patients in significant pain look and feel miserable, move extremely slowly, and present with consistent findings during the examination. In contrast, malingerers present with severe symptoms and exaggerated responses during the examination but can often be observed to be in no apparent distress at other times. This is particularly true if the malingering patient is observed in an environment outside of the clinic.

However, it cannot be stressed enough that all patients should be given the benefit of the doubt until the clinician, with a high degree of confidence, can rule out an organic cause for the pain.

A number of clinical signs and symptoms can alert the clinician to the possibility of a patient who is malingering. These include:

▸ subjective complaints of paresthesia with only stocking-glove anesthesia (conditions including diabetic neuropathy and the T4 syndrome must be ruled out);

▸ inappropriate scoring on the Oswestry Low Back Disability Questionnaire (Table 5-2), Neck Disability Index (Table 5-3), and McGill Pain Questionnaire (see Chap. 4);

▸ muscle stretch reflexes inconsistent with the presenting problem or symptoms;

▸ cogwheel motion of muscles during strength testing for weakness;

▸ the ability of the patient to complete a straight-leg raise in a supine position, but difficulty in performing the equivalent range (knee extension) in a seated position.

TABLE 5-2 Oswestry Low Back Disability Questionnaire

PLEASE READ: This questionnaire is designed to enable us to understand how much your low back pain has affected your ability to manage your everyday activities. Please answer each section by marking the **ONE BOX** that most applies to you. We realize that you feel that more than one statement may relate to your problem, but please just mark the one box that most closely describes your problem at this point in time.

Name:

Date:

Section 1—Pain Intensity

☐ The pain comes and goes and is very mild
☐ The pain is mild and does not vary much
☐ The pain comes and goes and is moderate
☐ The pain is moderate and does not vary much
☐ The pain comes and goes and is severe
☐ The pain is severe and does not vary much

Section 2—Personal Care

☐ I have no pain when I wash or dress
☐ I do not normally change my way of washing and dressing even though it causes some pain
☐ I have had to change the way I wash and dress because these activities increase my pain
☐ Because of pain I am unable to do **some** washing and dressing without help
☐ Because of pain I am unable to do **most** washing and dressing without help
☐ Because of pain I am unable to do **any** washing and dressing without help

Section 3—Lifting (*Skip if you have not attempted lifting since the onset of your back pain.*)

☐ Can lift heavy weights without increasing my pain
☐ Can lift heavy weights but it increases my pain
☐ Pain prevents me from lifting heavy weights off the floor
☐ Pain prevents me from lifting heavy weights off the floor but I can manage if they are conveniently positioned, e.g., on a table
☐ Pain prevents me from lifting heavy weights but I can manage light to medium weights if they are conveniently positioned
☐ I can only lift very light weight at the most

Section 4—Walking

☐ I have **no** pain when I walk
☐ I have **some** pain when I walk but it does not prevent me from walking normal distances
☐ Pain prevents me from walking **long** distances
☐ Pain prevents me from walking **intermediate** distances
☐ Pain prevents me from walking **short** distances
☐ Pain prevents me from walking at all

Section 5—Sitting

☐ Sitting does not cause me any pain
☐ I can sit as long as I need to, provided I have my choice of chair
☐ Pain prevents me from sitting more than 1 h
☐ Pain prevents me from sitting more than $1/2$ h
☐ Pain prevents me from sitting more than 10 min
☐ Pain prevents me from sitting at all

Section 6—Standing

☐ Standing does not cause me any pain
☐ I have some pain when I stand but it does not increase with time
☐ Pain prevents me from standing more than 1 h
☐ Pain prevents me from standing more than $1/2$ h
☐ Pain prevents me from standing more than 10 min
☐ Pain prevents me from standing at all

Section 7—Sleeping

☐ I have no pain when I lie in bed
☐ I have some pain when I lie in bed but it does not prevent me from sleeping well
☐ Because of pain my sleep is reduced by 25%
☐ Because of pain my sleep is reduced by 50%
☐ Because of pain my sleep is reduced by 75%
☐ Pain prevents me from sleeping at all

Section 8—Sex Life (if applicable)

☐ My sex life is normal and causes no pain
☐ My sex life is normal but increases my pain
☐ My sex life is nearly normal but is very painful
☐ My sex life is severely restricted
☐ My sex life is nearly absent because of pain
☐ Pain prevents any sex life at all

Section 9—Social Life

☐ My social life is normal and causes no pain
☐ My social life is normal but increases my pain
☐ Pain has no significant effect on my social life, apart from limiting my more energetic interests (sports, etc.)
☐ Pain has restricted my social life and I do not go out often
☐ Pain has restricted social life to my home
☐ I have no social life because of pain

Section 10—Traveling

☐ I have no pain when I travel
☐ I have some pain when I travel but none of my usual forms of travel make it worse
☐ Traveling increases my pain but has not required that I seek alternative forms of travel
☐ I have had to change the way I travel because my usual form of travel increases my pain
☐ Pain has restricted all forms of travel
☐ I can only travel while lying down

CLINICAL PEARL

Whatever the reasoning or motivation behind the malingering patient, the success rate from the clinician's viewpoint will be low, and so it is well worth recognizing these individuals from the outset.

In contrast to symptoms related to malingering, is the patient with psychogenic symptoms. This type of patient tends to exhibit an exaggeration of the symptoms in the absence of objective findings. Psychogenic symptoms are common in patients with anxiety, depression, or hysteria, making it important for the clinician to determine the level of psychological stress in a patient who demonstrates symptom

TABLE 5-3 Neck Disability Index

This questionnaire has been designed to give the doctor information as to how your neck pain has affected your ability to manage in everyday life. Please answer every section and mark in each section only the **ONE BOX** that applies to you. We realize you may consider that two of the statements in any one section relate to you, but please just mark the box that most closely describes your problem.

Section 1—Pain Intensity

☐ I have no pain at the moment
☐ The pain is very mild at the moment
☐ The pain is moderate at the moment
☐ The pain is fairly severe at the moment
☐ The pain is the worst imaginable at the moment

Section 2—Personal Care (Washing, Dressing, etc.)

☐ I can look after myself normally without causing extra pain
☐ I can look after myself normally but it causes extra pain
☐ It is painful to look after myself and I am slow and careful
☐ I need some help but manage most of my personal care
☐ I need help every day in most aspects of self-care
☐ I do not get dressed, I wash with difficulty and stay in bed

Section 3—Lifting

☐ I can lift heavy weights without extra pain
☐ I can lift heavy weights but it gives extra pain
☐ Pain prevents me from lifting heavy weights off the floor, but I can manage if they are conveniently positioned, for example, on a table
☐ Pain prevents me from lifting heavy weights, but I can manage light to medium weights if they are conveniently positioned
☐ I can lift very light weights
☐ I cannot lift or carry anything at all

Section 4—Reading

☐ I can read as much as I want to with no pain in my neck
☐ I can read as much as I want to with slight pain in my neck
☐ I can read as much as I want with moderate pain in my neck
☐ I can't read as much as I want because of moderate pain in my neck
☐ I can hardly read at all because of severe pain in my neck
☐ I cannot read at all

Section 5—Headaches

☐ I have no headaches at all
☐ I have slight headaches which come infrequently
☐ I have moderate headaches which come infrequently
☐ I have moderate headaches which come frequently
☐ I have severe headaches which come frequently
☐ I have headaches almost all the time

Section 6—Concentration

☐ I can concentrate fully when I want to with no difficulty
☐ I can concentrate fully when I want to with slight difficulty
☐ I have a fair degree of difficulty in concentrating when I want to
☐ I have a lot of difficulty in concentrating when I want to
☐ I have a great deal of difficulty in concentrating when I want to
☐ I cannot concentrate at all

Section 7—Work

☐ I can do as much work as I want to
☐ I can only do my usual work, but no more
☐ I can do most of my usual work, but no more
☐ I cannot do my usual work
☐ I can hardly do any work at all
☐ I can't do any work at all

Section 8—Driving

☐ I can drive my car without any neck pain
☐ I can drive my car as long as I want with slight pain in my neck
☐ I can drive my car as long as I want because of moderate pain in my neck
☐ I can't drive my car as long as I want because of moderate pain in my neck
☐ I can hardly drive at all because of severe pain in my neck
☐ I can't drive my car at all

Section 9—Sleeping

☐ I have no trouble sleeping
☐ My sleep is slightly disturbed (less than 1 h sleepless)
☐ My sleep is mildly disturbed (1–2 h sleepless)
☐ My sleep is moderately disturbed (2–3 h sleepless)
☐ My sleep is greatly disturbed (3–5 h sleepless)
☐ My sleep is completely disturbed (5–7 h sleepless)

Section 10—Recreation

☐ I am able to engage in all my recreation activities with no neck pain at all
☐ I am able to engage in all my recreation activities, with some pain in my neck
☐ I am able to engage in most, but not all of my usual recreation activities because of pain in my neck
☐ I am able to engage in a few of my usual recreation activities because of pain in my neck
☐ I can hardly do any recreation activities because of pain in my neck
☐ I can't do any recreation activities at all

Data from Vernon H, Mior S: The neck disability index: A study of reliability and validity. *J Manip Physiol Ther* 14:409–415, 1991.

magnification. Waddell and Main[20] have proposed a number of characteristics of this illness behavior (Table 5-4).

INFECTIVE DISEASES

Osteomyelitis

Osteomyelitis is an acute or chronic inflammatory process of the bone and its marrow secondary to infection with pyogenic organisms or other sources of infection, such as tuberculosis, or specific fungal infections (mycotic osteomyelitis), parasitic infections (Hydatid disease), viral infections, or syphilitic infections (Charcot arthropathy). The following are the two primary categories of acute osteomyelitis:

- ***Hematogenous osteomyelitis.*** It is an infection caused by bacterial seeding from the blood. The most common site is the rapidly growing and highly vascular metaphysis of growing bones.

TABLE 5-4	Waddell Test for Nonorganic Physical Signs
Test	**Inappropriate Response**
Tenderness	Superficial, nonanatomic to light touch
Simulation	
Axial loading	Axial loading on standing patient's skull produces low back pain
Rotation	Passive, simultaneous rotation of shoulders and pelvis produces low back pain
Distraction	Discrepancy between findings on supine and seated straight leg raising
Regional disturbances	
Weakness	Giving way (Cogwheel) weakness
Sensory	Nondermatomal sensory loss
Overreaction	Disproportionate facial expression, verbalization, or tremor during examination

Data from Waddell G, McCulloch JA, Kummel E, et al.: Nonorganic physical signs in low-back pain. *Spine* 5:117–125, 1980.

- ***Direct or contiguous inoculation.*** This type of osteomyelitis is caused by direct contact of the tissue and bacteria during surgery, a penetrating wound, or as a result of poor dental hygiene.

Disease states known to predispose patients to osteomyelitis include diabetes mellitus, sickle-cell disease, acquired immune deficiency syndrome, IV drug abuse, alcoholism, chronic steroid use, immunosuppression, and chronic joint disease. Clinical signs and symptoms associated with osteomyelitis include fever (approximately 50% of cases), fatigue, edema, erythema, tenderness, and reduction in the use of the extremity.

CLINICAL PEARL

The most common clinical finding in patients with osteomyelitis is constant pain with marked tenderness over the involved bone.

INFLAMMATORY DISORDERS

Perhaps, the most common inflammatory disorders of the musculoskeletal system are the rheumatoid diseases.

Rheumatoid Arthritis

Rheumatoid arthritis (RA) can be defined as a chronic, progressive, systemic, inflammatory disease of connective tissue, characterized by spontaneous remissions and exacerbations (flare-ups). It is the second most common rheumatic disease after osteoarthritis (OA), but it is the most destructive to synovial joints. Unlike OA, RA involves primary tissue inflammation rather than joint degeneration. Although most individuals who develop RA do so in their early-to-middle adulthood, some experience a late onset RA in their older years.

Although the exact etiology of RA is unclear, it is considered one of many autoimmune disorders. Abnormal immunoglobulin (Ig) G and IgM antibodies develop in response to IgG antigens, to form circulating immune complexes. These complexes lodge in connective tissue, especially synovium, and create an inflammatory response. Inflammatory mediators, including cytokines (e.g., tumor necrosis factor), chemokines, and proteases, activate and attract neutrophils and other inflammatory cells. The synovium thickens, fluid accumulates in the joint space, and a pannus forms, eroding joint cartilage and bone. Bony ankylosis, calcifications, and loss of bone density follow.

Rheumatoid disease typically begins in the joints of the arm or hand. The individual complains of joint stiffness lasting longer than 30 minutes on awakening, pain, swelling, and heat (synovitis). Unlike with OA, the distal interphalangeal joints of the fingers usually are not involved in RA.

The signs and symptoms of RA vary among individuals, depending on the rate of progress of the disease. A complete musculoskeletal examination helps diagnose the disease. Clinical manifestations include both joint involvement and systemic problems; some are associated with the early stages of RA, whereas others are seen later in advanced disease.

Complaints of fatigue, anorexia, low-grade fever, and mild weight loss are commonly associated with RA. As the disease worsens, joints become deformed, and secondary osteoporosis (see "Metabolic Disease") can result in fractures, especially in older adults. Hand and finger deformities are typical in the advanced stages of the disease. Palpable subcutaneous nodules, often appearing on the ulnar surface of the arm, are associated with a severe, destructive disease pattern. As the disease progresses over years, systemic manifestations increase and potentially life-threatening organ involvement begins. Cardiac problems, such as pericarditis and myocarditis, and respiratory complications, such as pleurisy, pulmonary fibrosis, and pneumonitis, are common. RA can affect body image, self-esteem, and sexuality in older adults. The person with RA loses control over body changes, is chronically fatigued, and eventually may lose independence in activities of daily living (ADLs). As a reaction to these losses, individuals may display the phases of the grieving process, such as anger or denial. Some people become depressed, feeling helpless and hopeless because no cure presently exists for the condition. Chronic pain and suffering interfere with quality of life.

The physical therapy examination of the patient with RA involves

- measurement of independence with functional activities;
- measurement of joint inflammation;
- measurement of joint range of motion;
- determination of limiting factors including pain, weakness, and fatigue.

Because RA affects multiple body systems, lessens quality of life, and affects functional ability, the approach to managing the client with this condition must be interdisciplinary. Management typically includes drug therapy, physical or occupational therapy, and recreational therapy. Some clients also need psychologic counseling to help cope with the disease.

Rest and energy conservation are crucial for managing RA (Table 5-5). Pacing activities, obtaining assistance, and allowing rest periods help conserve energy. Positioning joints in their optimal functional position helps prevent deformities.

TABLE 5-5 Intervention Strategies for Rheumatoid Arthritis

Objective	Intervention	Example
Pain control	Therapeutic heat to decrease rigidity of joints, increase the flexibility of fibrous tissue, and decrease pain and muscle spasm Massage, usually applied with heat treatment and before stretching, can be used to relieve pain and prevent adhesions Therapeutic cold can be used for analgesic and vasoconstriction purposes in inflamed joints during the acute period. Care must be taken to avoid adverse effects	Heat applications: Aquatic therapy Instructions on the wearing of warm pajamas, sleeping bag, and electric blanket Paraffin for hands Ultrasound Heating pads—moist heat better than dry heat
Minimizing the effects of inflammation	Joint protection strategies Splinting Rest from abuse Body mechanics education	As needed—balance rest with activity by using splinting (articular resting) Resting splints are used to rest the joint in the appropriate position in the acute period Dynamic splints are used to exert adequate force that the tissue can tolerate and provide sufficient joint volume Functional splints are used to protect the joint in the course of activity Stabilizer splints are used in cases of permanent contractures. Gradual casting can be used to apply a stretch to the contracture
Preventing limitation and restoring ROM in affected joints	Range of motion and stretching exercises	Acute stage: passive and active assisted to avoid joint compression Subacute/chronic stages: active exercises, passive stretching or contract–relax techniques
Maintaining and improving strength	Resistive exercises Endurance exercises Electrical stimulation	Acute and subacute stages: isometric exercises progressing cautiously to resistive Subacute/chronic stages: strengthening exercises that avoid substitutions and minimize instability, atrophy, deformity, pain, and injury Chronic stage: judicious use of concentric exercise Provision of encouragement to exercise—fun and recreational activities of moderate intensity and 30 min duration per day Swimming Tai Chi Short-term electrical stimulation is useful in cases of excessive muscle atrophy and in those who cannot exercise
Ensuring normal growth and development	Posture and positioning Mobility and assistive devices	To maintain joint range of motion, patients should spend 20 min/d in prone to stretch the hip flexors and quadriceps; assess leg length discrepancy in standing and avoid scoliosis Extended comb handles, thicker spoons, shoehorns Clothes with easy openings and/or Velcro

Ambulatory and adaptive devices can help individuals maintain independence in ADLs. For example, a long-handled shoehorn may help in putting on shoes. Velcro attachments on shoes often are a better option than laces. Styrofoam or paper cups may collapse or bend, whereas a hard plastic or china cup may be easier to handle. The clinician should also review principles of joint protection with the patient and family and provide adaptive equipment as needed to perform ADLs independently.

Strengthening exercises and other pain-relief measures, such as the use of ice and heat, can be prescribed. Ice application is used for hot, inflamed joints. Heat is used for painful joints that are not acutely inflamed. Showers, hot packs (not too heavy), and paraffin dips are ideal for heat application.

Some RA patients have associated syndromes. Two such syndromes are Sjogren and Felty syndromes. Sjogren syndrome is characterized by dryness of the eyes (keratoconjunctivitis), mouth (xerostomia), and other mucous membranes. Felty syndrome is characterized by leukopenia and hepatosplenomegaly, often leading to recurrent infections. It encompasses a diverse group of pathogenic mechanisms in RA, all of which result in decreased levels of circulating neutrophils.

No single test or group of laboratory tests can confirm a diagnosis of RA, but they can support the findings from the patient's history and the physical findings. A number of immunologic tests, such as the rheumatoid factor and antinuclear antibody titer, are available to aid diagnosis. Normal values differ, depending on the precise laboratory technique used.

Juvenile Arthritis

The descriptive term *juvenile idiopathic arthritis* was adopted as an umbrella term to indicate disease of childhood onset, characterized primarily by arthritis of no known etiology persisting for at least 6 weeks. Juvenile RA (JRA) is the most prevalent pediatric rheumatic diagnosis among children in the United States. Substantial evidence points to an autoimmune pathogenesis.[21] JRA is not a single disease. Rather, it is a group of diseases of unknown etiology, which are manifested by chronic joint inflammation. JRA is classified as systemic, pauciarticular, or polyarticular disease, according to onset within the first 6 months. General history of JRA includes the following:

- Disease onset is either insidious or abrupt, with morning stiffness and arthralgia during the day.
- Individuals with JRA may have a school history of absences, and their abilities to participate in physical education classes may reflect severity of the disease. Typically, patients with JRA and their parents and/or caregivers are concerned about missing school; in contrast, when psychogenic factors predominate (e.g., pain syndromes), patients and their parents and/or caregivers are more worried about returning to school than about missing school.
- Limping may be observed in individuals with more severe JRA; however, the presence of limping also raises the possibility of trauma or another orthopaedic problem.
- Injury suggests the possibility of trauma to a joint (e.g., meniscal tear).
- A preceding illness raises the possibility of infectious trigger of JRA or postinfectious arthritis.
- Illness onsets with a history of enteritis raises the possibility of reactive arthritis.
- History of travel with exposure to ticks raises the possibility of arthritis caused by Lyme disease.
- Gastrointestinal symptoms raise the possibility of inflammatory bowel disease.
- Very severe joint pain raises the possibility of acute rheumatic fever (also suggested by migratory but not additive arthritis, with fevers), acute lymphocytic leukemia (with metaphyseal pain on examination and a decrease in two or more cell lines), septic arthritis, or osteomyelitis.
- Weight loss without diarrhea may be observed in individuals with active JRA and is sometimes associated with anorexia. This symptom is also observed in individuals with acute lymphocytic leukemia with other obvious findings (e.g., severe bone pain).
- Weight loss with diarrhea may be observed in persons with inflammatory bowel disease.
- Photophobia may be observed in persons with usually asymptomatic uveitis.
- Orthopnea suggests pericarditis in children with systemic JRA; the differential diagnosis includes systemic lupus erythematosus (SLE) and viral pericarditis.
- Systemic-onset JRA is characterized by spiking fevers, typically occurring several times each day, with temperature returning to the reference range or below the reference range.
- Systemic-onset JRA may be accompanied by an evanescent rash, which is typically linear, affecting the trunk and extremities.
- Arthralgia is often present. Frank joint swelling is atypical; arthritis may not occur for months following onset, making diagnosis difficult.
- Pauciarticular disease is characterized by arthritis affecting four or fewer joints.
  - Typically, larger joints (e.g., knees, ankles, and wrists) are affected.
  - Monoarticular arthritis in a hip is highly unusual.
  - When the knee is affected, limping may be noted, particularly in the mornings.
- Polyarticular disease affects at least five joints.
  - Both large and small joints can be involved, often in symmetric bilateral distribution.
  - Severe limitations in motion are usually accompanied by weakness and decreased physical function.
- Some children may have a generalized myalgia.
- Localization to proximal muscles raises the possibility of a myositis.
- Consider Legg–Calvé–Perthes disease, toxic synovitis of the hip, septic arthritis, osteomyelitis, or, in an older child, slipped capital femoral epiphysis or chondrolysis of the hip.

Chronic involvement can result in atrophy of extensor muscles in the thigh, tight hamstring muscles, and knee flexion contractures.

Gout

Gout is the most common form of inflammatory arthritis in men older than 40 years and appears to be on the increase.[22] High blood levels of uric acid lead to inflammation, joint swelling, and severe pain. Symptoms are caused by deposits of sodium urate or calcium pyrophosphate crystals in joints and periarticular tissues. Several factors have been identified as predisposing a person to gout, including lifestyle elements of obesity, high-purine diet, and habitual alcohol ingestion.

Onset is usually sudden, often during the night or early morning. The classic finding of gouty arthritis (gout) is warmth, swelling, cutaneous erythema, and severe pain of the first metatarsophalangeal (MTP) joint. However, other joints may also be involved. These include the shoulder, knee, wrist, ankle, elbow, or fingers. Fever, chills, and malaise accompany an episode of gout. As the condition becomes chronic, the patient may report morning stiffness and joint deformity, progressive loss of function, or disability. Chronic gouty nephropathy may occur.

In the United States, the self-reported prevalence of gout almost trebled in men aged 45–64 years between 1969 and 1981.[23] The rising prevalence of gout is thought to stem from dietary changes, environmental factors, increasing longevity, subclinical renal impairment, and the increased use of drugs causing hyperuricemia, particularly diuretics.[24]

Differential diagnosis includes cellulitis, septic arthritis, RA, bursitis related to bunion, sarcoidosis, multiple myeloma, and hyperparathyroidism.

Ankylosing Spondylitis

Ankylosing spondylitis (AS, also known as Bekhterev or Marie–Strümpell disease) is a chronic rheumatoid disorder that affects 1–3 per 1,000 people. Thoracic involvement in AS occurs almost universally. The patient is usually between 15 and 40 years. There is a 10–20% risk that offspring of patients with the disease will later develop it.[25] Although males are affected more frequently than females, mild courses of AS are more common in the latter.[26]

A human leukocyte antigen (HLA) haplotype association (HLA-B27) has been found with AS and remains one of the strongest known associations of disease with HLA-B27, but other diseases are also associated with the antigen. The disease includes involvement of the anterior longitudinal ligament and ossification of the intervertebral disk, thoracic zygapophyseal joints, costovertebral joints, and manubriosternal joint. This multijoint involvement of the thoracic spine makes the checking of chest expansion measurements a required test in this region.

In time, AS progresses to involve the whole spine and results in spinal deformities, including flattening of the lumbar lordosis, kyphosis of the thoracic spine, and hyperextension of the cervical spine. These changes, in turn, result in flexion contractures of the hips and knees, with significant morbidity and disability.[26]

The most characteristic feature of the back pain associated with AS is pain at night.[27] Patients often awaken in the early morning (between 2 and 5 AM) with back pain and stiffness and usually either take a shower or exercise before returning to sleep.[26] Back ache during the day is typically intermittent, irrespective of exertion or rest.[26]

Calin and colleagues[28] describe five screening questions for AS:

1. Is there morning stiffness?
2. Is there improvement in discomfort with exercise?
3. Was the onset of back pain before age 40 years?
4. Did the problem begin slowly?
5. Has the pain persisted for at least 3 months?

Using at least four positive answers to define a "positive" result, the sensitivity of these questions was 0.95 and specificity was 0.85.[28]

Peripheral arthritis is uncommon in AS, but when it occurs, it is usually late in the course of the arthritis.[29] Peripheral arthritis developing early in the course of the disease is a predictor of disease progression.[30] The arthritis usually occurs in the lower extremities in an asymmetric distribution, with involvement of the "axial" joints, including shoulders and hips, more common than involvement of more distal joints.[26,31]

Inspection usually reveals a flat lumbar spine and gross limitation of side bending in both directions. Mobility loss tends to be bilateral and symmetric. There is loss of spinal elongation on flexion (Schober test), although this can occur in patients with chronic low back pain (LBP) or spinal tumors and is thus not specific for inflammatory spondylopathies.[32] The patient may relate a history of costochondritis, and, upon examination, rib springing may give a hard end-feel. Basal rib expansion often is decreased. The glides of the costotransverse joints and distraction of the sternoclavicular joints are decreased, and the lumbar spine exhibits a capsular pattern.

As the disease progresses, the pain and stiffness can spread up the entire spine, pulling it into forward flexion, so that the patient adopts the typical stooped-over position. The patient gazes downward, the entire back is rounded, the hips and knees are semiflexed, and the arms cannot be raised beyond a limited amount at the shoulders.[33]

Longitudinal studies in patients with AS have revealed that deformities and disability occur within the first 10 years of disease.[30] Most of the loss of function occurs during the first 10 years and correlates significantly with the occurrence of peripheral arthritis, radiographic changes of AS in the spine, and the development of the so-called bamboo spine.

An exercise program is particularly important for these patients to maintain functional spinal outcomes.[34] The goal of exercise therapy is to maintain the mobility of the spine and involved joints for as long as possible and to prevent the spine from stiffening in an unacceptable kyphotic position. A strict regimen of daily exercises, which include positioning, and spinal extension exercises, breathing exercises, and exercises for the peripheral joints, must be followed. Several times a day, patients should lie prone for 5 minutes, and they should be encouraged to sleep on a hard mattress and avoid the side-lying position. Swimming is the best routine sport.

Psoriatic Arthritis

Psoriatic arthritis is an inflammatory arthritis associated with psoriasis. It affects men and women with equal frequency.[31] Its peak onset is in the fourth decade of life, although it may occur in children and in older adults. Psoriatic arthritis can manifest in one of a number of patterns, including distal joint disease (affecting the distal interphalangeal joints of the hands and feet), asymmetric oligoarthritis, polyarthritis (which tends to be asymmetric in half the cases), and arthritis mutilans (a severe destructive form of arthritis and the spondyloarthropathy that occurs in 40% of patients, but most commonly in the presence of one of the peripheral patterns).[31] Patients with psoriatic arthritis have less tenderness over both affected joints and tender points than patients with RA.[35]

The spondyloarthropathy of psoriatic arthritis may be distinguished from AS by the pattern of the sacroiliitis.[36] Whereas sacroiliitis in AS tends to be symmetric, affecting both sacroiliac joints to the same degree, it tends to be asymmetric in psoriatic arthritis,[31] and patients with psoriatic arthritis do not have as severe a spondyloarthropathy as patients with AS.[25]

Another articular feature of psoriatic arthritis is the presence of dactylitis, tenosynovitis (often digital, in flexor and extensor tendons and in the Achilles tendon), and enthesitis.[36] The presence of erosive disease in the distal interphalangeal joints is typical.[36]

Nail lesions occur in more than 80% of the patients with psoriatic arthritis and have been found to be the only clinical feature distinguishing patients with psoriatic arthritis from patients with uncomplicated psoriasis.[37] Other extra-articular features include iritis, urethritis, and cardiac impairments similar to those seen in AS, although less frequently.[36]

Psoriatic arthritis may result in significant joint damage and disability.

NEOPLASTIC DISEASE

Benign Tumors: Osteoblastoma and Osteoid Osteoma

Osteoblastoma and osteoid osteoma are benign bone-forming tumors with similar clinical findings.

- Osteoblastoma is a solitary bone neoplasm. It is most common in the vertebrae of children and young adults. Short and flat bones are more commonly affected than the long bones (76.5% vs. 23.5%).[38] In the vertebrae, the body is only rarely affected primarily; usually, it is involved only secondarily by tumors extending from other segments of the same or the nearest vertebra.[38]
- Osteoid osteoma is a benign osteoblastic tumor of unknown etiology. It occurs most often in the long bones, although the spine is the location of 10% of all osteoid osteomas.[39]

Painful scoliosis is a well-recognized presentation of spinal osteoid osteoma and osteoblastoma and is thought to be caused by pain-provoked muscle spasm on the side of the lesion.[38]

Malignant Tumors

Metastatic disease of the spine is the most frequent neoplastic disorder of the axial skeleton. Malignant tumors can be primary or secondary.

1. ***Primary.*** Primary tumors include the following
   a. ***Multiple myeloma.*** Myeloma is a plasma cell tumor. It is the most common malignant primary bone tumor. Early in its course, it can easily be overlooked as the cause of back pain. Common presentations of myeloma include bone pain, recurrent or persistent infection, anemia, renal impairment, or a combination of these. Some patients are asymptomatic. Presenting features, which require urgent specialist referral, include:
      (1) persistent, unexplained backache associated with loss of height and osteoporosis;
      (2) symptoms suggestive of spinal cord or nerve root compression.
   b. ***Chordoma.*** Chordomas are rare tumors of notochordal origin, representing approximately 5% of all malignant tumors of bone.[40] They typically are slow-growing, locally aggressive tumors. Chordomas usually are diagnosed in patients with pain or symptoms caused by compression of the surrounding structures. The clinical presentation initially may be mild in nature, leading to considerable delay in seeking medical attention. Vertebral chordomas involve the spinal cord and nerve roots progressively, resulting in pain, numbness, motor weakness, and, eventually, paralysis.
   c. ***Osteosarcoma.*** Osteosarcoma is a relatively uncommon malignancy. The peak incidence of osteosarcoma occurs in the second decade, with an additional smaller peak after age of 50 years.[41] These tumors typically arise in the metaphyseal regions of long bones, with the rib, distal femur, proximal tibia, and proximal humerus representing the four most common sites. The metaphysis of the vertebra is also predilected.[38] Osteosarcomas frequently penetrate and destroy the cortex of the bone and extend into the surrounding soft tissues.

   The initial clinical symptom of a malignant tumor is frequently pain in the affected area, which may also be associated with localized soft-tissue swelling or limitation of motion in the adjacent joint.[42]
2. ***Secondary.*** Metastases to the spine most commonly arise from breast and lung cancer and from lymphoma.[43,44] Lesions associated with primary tumors from the breast, prostate, kidney, and thyroid and lesions associated with lymphoma and myeloma account for 75% of all spinal metastases.[43,44] When lung cancer is included, the percentage is greater than 90.[45] The clinical findings for a secondary spinal tumor are similar to those of a primary tumor.

METABOLIC DISEASE

Osteoporosis

Osteoporosis can result from insufficient bone formation, excessive bone resorption, or a combination of these two phenomena (see Chap. 1). The result is decreased bone mineral density (BMD) and a progressive loss of trabecular connectivity that is irreversible and diminishes the bone quality in terms of its mechanical resistance to deformity underloading.[46] Osteoporosis causes fractures of the vertebrae and fractures of other bones such as the proximal humerus, distal forearm, proximal femur (hip), and pelvis.

Osteoporosis has been classified into two broad general types: type 1 (postmenopausal) and type 2 (involutional).[47] Type 2 osteoporosis generally is seen in the older age population and has been referred to as senile osteoporosis.[47]

CLINICAL PEARL

Women are more prone to develop osteoporosis because of the contribution of the loss of estrogen to accelerated bone loss in the postmenopausal female population.

It has been estimated that 15% of postmenopausal Caucasian women in the United States and 35% of women older than 65 years have osteoporosis.[47] Further, 50% of women older than 50 years have osteopenia of the femoral neck, and 20% have osteoporosis at this site.[48] The incidence of hip fracture rises dramatically with age to 3.4 per 100 in the 65–74-year-old age group and 9.4 per 100 in those older than 85 years.[46] The presence of a significant vertebral fracture (see "Vertebral Fracture") is associated with increased mortality.[49] Patients with these fractures have a relative risk of death that is nine times greater than healthy counterparts.[50] Approximately 20% of women with vertebral fractures have another fracture of a different bone within a year.[49]

Numerous risk factors have been identified as contributing to the likelihood that an individual will develop bone loss. Genetics plays a major role, and female gender, positive family history, and racial characteristics associated with Caucasian, Asian, or Hispanic background increase the risk of osteoporosis.[51] Low body weight (less than 85% ideal body weight, or less than 127 lb) has also been correlated with the development of osteoporosis.[47]

Modifiable risk factors associated with osteoporosis include early or iatrogenic menopause, pregnancy at an early age, smoking, sedentary lifestyle, alcoholism, low body fat, low calcium intake, high caffeine intake, prolonged bed rest, and anorexia.[47,52,53] Medications such as corticosteroids, some diuretics, and thyroid hormone preparations can also increase bone loss and the risk of osteoporosis significantly.[54,55]

In addition to risk factors for the disease, there are independent risk factors for fractures, including use of medications in elderly patients with adverse CNS side effects, balance problems, poor muscle strength, visual impairment, home environmental factors such as stairs, and medical comorbidities that increase the likelihood of falls.[46,52]

The diagnosis of osteoporosis often is first established by the presence of an osteoporotic fracture. However, a physical therapist may treat a patient with an undiagnosed low BMD. These patients have a lowered fracture threshold. It is important to be able to identify this patient type, so that safer choices can be made with regard to the types of intervention. At present, the only diagnostic tool available that is within the scope of practice of the physical therapist is the identification of those risk factors previously mentioned.[56]

The specific effects of physical activity on bone health have been investigated in several studies.[53,54,56–60] The conclusions drawn from these studies suggest that there is:

- strong evidence that physical activity early in life contributes to higher peak bone mass[59];
- some evidence that resistance and high-impact exercise are likely the most beneficial for prevention;
- some evidence that high-intensity aerobic exercise (70–90% of maximal heart rate) may reverse or attenuate BMD loss;
- some evidence that high-load low-repetition routines are more effective at increasing BMD than low-load high-repetition regimens.

Exercise during the middle years of life has numerous health benefits, but there are few studies on the effects of exercise on BMD.[59] Exercise during the later years, in the presence of adequate calcium and vitamin D intake, probably has a modest effect on slowing the decline in BMD, but it is clear that exercise late in life, even beyond age 90 years, can increase muscle mass and strength twofold or more in frail persons.[59]

Randomized clinical trials of exercise have been shown to reduce the risk of falls by approximately 25%,[61,62] but there is no experimental evidence that exercise affects fracture rates.[59] It also is possible that regular exercisers might fall differently, thereby reducing the risk of fracture caused by falls, but this hypothesis requires testing.[59]

The availability of new, effective drug therapies in the past decade has revolutionized the intervention for osteoporosis, and it is important that clinicians at least be aware of the intervention options. Many hormonal and hormone replacement therapies are also available. Experimental evidence indicates that slow-release sodium fluoride and low-dose parathyroid hormone are capable of increasing bone formation and thus preventing bone loss in women who are estrogen deficient.[63]

Diagnostic tools have focused on bone density. New minimally invasive procedures are finding a place among interventions for patients with osteoporotic fractures. For example, the use of injected hydroxyapatite cements into distal radius fractures for percutaneous stabilization has shown efficacy as an intervention for patients with these fractures.[64]

CLINICAL PEARL

It should be the responsibility of every health-care provider to educate their young female patients about the benefits of sufficient exercise and the recommended dietary calcium intake to build healthy bone.

What is known about prevention is that a key factor in the development of osteoporosis in later life is a deficient level of peak bone mass at physical maturity[65] and that physical activity and calcium intake play substantial roles in the development of bone mass during these developmental years.[66]

Osteomalacia

Osteomalacia is the least common of the traditional forms of metabolic bone disease. It is characterized by impairment of bone mineralization, leading to an accumulation of unmineralized matrix or osteoid in the skeleton.[67] Among the causes of osteomalacia, the most important are disorders of vitamin D availability, synthesis, or action.[68]

Clinically, osteomalacia is manifested by progressive generalized bone pain, muscle weakness, hypocalcemia, and pseudofractures. In its late stages, osteomalacia is characterized by a waddling gait.[69] Osteomalacia is believed to be rare in the United States because of the routine fortification of milk and a few other foods with vitamin D. However, patients with various gastrointestinal diseases are known to be at risk.[69]

Paget Disease

Paget disease (osteitis deformans) of the bone is an osteometabolic disorder. The disease is described as a focal disorder of accelerated skeletal remodeling that may affect one or more bones. This remodeling produces a slowly progressive enlargement and deformity of multiple bones.

Despite intensive studies and widespread interest, the etiology of Paget disease remains obscure. The pathologic process consists of three phases:

- *Phase I.* An osteolytic phase characterized by prominent bone resorption and hypervascularization.
- *Phase II.* A sclerotic phase, reflecting previously increased bone formation but currently decreased cellular activity and vascularity.
- *Phase III.* A mixed phase, with both active bone resorption and compensatory bone formation, resulting in a disorganized skeletal architecture. The bones become sponge-like, weakened, and deformed.

Complications include pathologic fractures, delayed union, progressive skeletal deformities, chronic bone pain, neurologic compromise of the peripheral and central nervous systems with facial or ocular nerve compression and spinal stenosis, and pagetic arthritis.

Involvement of the lumbar spine may produce symptoms of clinical spinal stenosis. Involvement of the cervical and thoracic spine may predispose patients to myelopathy.

Although this disorder may be asymptomatic, when symptoms do occur, they occur insidiously. Paget disease is managed either medically or surgically.

Spondylolisthesis

Spondylolisthesis usually occurs in the lumbar spine (see Chap. 28).

Clinically, these patients complain of LBP that is mechanical in nature. Mechanical pain is worsened with activity and alleviated with rest. Patients may also complain of leg pain, which can have a radicular-type pattern or, more commonly, will manifest as neurogenic claudication. If neurogenic claudication is present, the patient may complain of bilateral thigh and leg tiredness, aches, and fatigue.[70] Questions regarding bicycle use versus walking can help the clinician to differentiate neurogenic from vascular claudication. Both cycling and walking increase symptoms in vascular claudication due to the increased demand for blood supply. However, the symptoms of neurogenic claudication worsen with walking but are unaffected by cycling, due to the differing positions of the lumbar spine adopted in each of these activities. Patients with neurogenic claudication are far more comfortable leaning forward or sitting, which flexes the spine, than walking.[71] The position of forward flexion increases the anteroposterior diameter of the intervertebral canal, which allows a greater volume of the neural elements and improves the microcirculation.

Range of motion for flexion of the lumbar spine frequently is normal with both types of claudication. Some patients are able to touch their toes without difficulty. Strength is usually intact in the lower extremities. Sensation also is usually intact. A check of distal pulses is important to rule out any coexisting vascular insufficiency. Findings such as hairless lower extremities, coldness of the feet, or absent pulses are signs of peripheral vascular disease (PVD). Sensory defects in a stocking-glove distribution are more suggestive of diabetic neuropathy. The muscle stretch reflexes generally will be normal or diminished. If hyperreflexic symptoms and other upper motor neuron (UMN) signs, such as clonus or a positive Babinski test, are found, further investigation is necessary including examination of the cervical, thoracic, and lumbar spine to rule out a lesion of the spinal cord or cauda equina.

Differential diagnosis includes coexisting OA of the hip, myelopathy, spinal tumors, and infections.

Generalized Body Pain

When discussing the issue of differential diagnosis with generalized body pain, it is well worth mentioning two conditions: fibromyalgia (FM) and myofascial pain syndrome (MPS). Although these conditions share several features, they are distinct entities whose physical findings and interventions differ significantly.[72]

Fibromyalgia

Primary FM is a common form of nonneuropathic chronic neuromuscular pain, which is poorly understood. FM is characterized by widespread and generalized body aches of at least 3 months duration, which can cause pain or paresthesias, or both, in a nonradicular pattern.[73–75] FM is not a disease, but rather a syndrome with a common set of characteristic symptoms, including constitutional symptoms of fatigue, nonrestorative sleep, and the presence of a defined number of tender points.[76]

The relationship of tender points to FM has been the focus of much research,[77–80] and, according to the criteria of the American College of Rheumatology, a positive tender point is defined as a point that becomes painful (not merely tender) when approximately 4 kg of pressure is applied.[81] A positive tender point count of 11 or more of 18 standardized sites, when present in combination with the history of widespread pain, yields a sensitivity of 88.4% and a specificity of 81.1% in the diagnosis of FM.

The pathology and pathophysiology of the tender point remain elusive. Normally, small C-fibers in the skin are activated by chemical, mechanical, or thermal stimuli. The impulses are sent up the spinothalamic tract to the brain where they are processed. In FM, the constant bombardment of noxious inputs to C-fibers leads to central sensitization (allodynia).[82] As a consequence, large, myelinated A-delta fibers begin carrying some signals normally transmitted by the C-fibers. Central sensitization further expands to involve autonomically mediated B-fibers. It has also been hypothesized that the myalgias may result from neurohumoral changes rather than local metabolic or pathophysiologic features.[83] Prevalence of FM is about 10–20 times greater in women than in men, although the reason for this is unknown. Sleep studies show that stage 4 sleep is the most interrupted; however, sleep disturbances are common in the general population and not endemic to FM patients.[84]

The medical intervention for FM includes the prescription of drugs that influence chemicals in the ascending and descending pain tracts, chemicals that influence cerebral function, nonsteroidals, and muscle relaxants.[82] A multifaceted physical therapy approach involving cardiovascular fitness training, spray and stretch, strength and endurance training, massage, and electrotherapeutic and physical modalities, including microstimulation, may help to reduce some of the disease consequences.[85]

Myofascial Pain Syndrome

MPSs are closely associated with tender areas that have come to be known as myofascial trigger points (see Chap. 10).[75,86–89] Dysfunctional joints are also associated with trigger points and tender attachment points.[90] MPS often manifests with symptoms suggestive of neurologic disorders, including diffuse pain and tenderness, headache, vertigo, visual disturbances, paresthesias, incoordination, and referred pain that often can be clarified by the musculoskeletal and neurologic examination.[91] MPS should always be considered as a diagnosis in the presence of persistent pain.[88,92–96]

Differential Diagnosis within Specific Regions

The intent of the following sections is to provide the physical therapist with potential diagnoses based on the location of symptoms. It was Grieve who coined the term *masqueraders* to indicate those conditions that may not be musculoskeletal in origin and that may require skilled intervention elsewhere. To aid the clinician in the detection of these masqueraders, both neuromusculoskeletal disorders and serious underlying medical conditions are included in the following sections, according to the various body regions. Although not inclusive, these diagnoses should provide the clinician with a list of possibilities to encourage divergent thinking during each examination.

CAUSES OF HEAD, FACE, EYE, AND TEMPOROMANDIBULAR JOINT SYMPTOMS

The causes of head, face, and temporomandibular joint symptoms include, but are not limited to, those listed in Table 5-6.

TABLE 5-6 Potential Causes of Head and Facial Pain
Trauma
Headache
Occipital neuralgia
Osteoarthritis
Rheumatoid arthritis and related rheumatoid arthritis variants (dermatomyositis and temporal arteritis)
Lyme disease
Fibromyalgia
Arteriovenous malformation
Intracranial infection (meningitis)
Cerebrovascular disease
Tumor
Encephalitis
Systemic infections
Multiple sclerosis
Miscellaneous

Trauma

Head pain is common following trauma to the head and neck. The traumatic episodes that do not produce profound neurologic damage are termed *concussions* (contusions). Concussion is not always associated with some degree of loss of consciousness and typically involves a sudden acceleration (or deceleration) force, which causes the brain to move suddenly within the skull. For a loss of consciousness to occur, these forces must disconnect the alerting system in the brain stem, resulting in a temporary lack of activity in the reticular formation, probably secondary to hypoxia resulting from induced ischemia.[97] It is estimated that a velocity of only 20 mph can cause concussion from inertial loading (no head impact) in most healthy adults.[98]

Headache

Headaches are a common complaint. Approximately 85–95% of the adult population in the United States experience a headache during a given 1-year period,[99] although only 1.7–2.5% of patients visit the emergency department for a complaint of headache,[100] with most choosing to treat themselves with over-the-counter medications.[101,102]

Headaches, in general, can be grouped into two main divisions: benign or nonbenign and primary or secondary. Primary headaches are the result of some underlying structural abnormality or disease process, whereas secondary headaches are the result of an underlying pathologic process.[103] The origin of benign headaches can vary. Common causes include neurologic (trigeminal neuralgia (TN), cervical neuralgia, atypical facial pain, posttraumatic, and postlumbar puncture), musculoskeletal (tension headache, occipital headache, and cervicogenic headache), and vascular (migraine, cluster, and hypertension).[104,105] Other headaches, such as chronic daily and rebound, are thought to be related to a combination of neurologic and musculoskeletal causes. OA, RA and related RA variants (dermatomyositis and temporal arteritis), Lyme disease, FM, and complex regional pain syndrome (formerly known as reflex sympathetic dystrophy—see Chap. 18) have also been indicated as additional sources of head and neck pain.[105] Diseases of the sinus (maxillary sinusitis, frontal sinusitis, or malignancy), diseases of the eye (inflammation of the iris and glaucoma), and infection and inflammation of the ear apparatus may also cause headaches.[104,106] Sensitivity to tapping over the sinuses is fairly diagnostic for sinusitis, whereas diminished vision is characteristic of glaucoma.[104,106]

Migraine Headache

Migraines are equally distributed among the sexes in childhood, but two out of every three adults with migraine headaches are women.[105] According to the International Headache Society,[107] there are two types of migraine headaches: migraine without aura (common migraine) and migraine with aura. The migraine without aura type involves episodes lasting 4–72 hours, and symptoms are typically unilateral and with a pulsating quality of moderate or severe intensity, which is thought to result from a change in the blood vessels of the brain. This type of headache is aggravated by routine physical activity and is associated with nausea, auras, photophobia, and phonophobia.

The migraine with aura type is characterized by reversible aura symptoms, which typically develop gradually over more than 4 minutes but last no longer than 60 minutes.[107]

It is thought that migraine headaches are a different expression of a common underlying problem.[105] As with cluster headaches, it has long been recognized that migraine headaches are exacerbated by disturbances or irregularities in sleep patterns.[103]

Cluster Headache

Cluster headaches are severe, unilateral, retro-orbital headaches. This type of headache is more common in men than in women. As their name suggests, cluster headaches occur in groups or clusters, and they tend to occur at predictable times of day. Cluster headaches may also develop because of specific sleep disorders, such as sleep apnea, bruxism, or sleep deprivation.[103]

Cluster headaches are often accompanied by nasal congestion, eyelid edema, rhinorrhea, miosis, lacrimation, and ptosis (drooping eyelid) on the symptomatic side.[103] These headaches can last from 15 to 180 minutes if untreated.[107]

Unlike migraine sufferers, who feel obliged to lie down during a severe headache, individuals with cluster headaches feel better during a headache by remaining in an erect posture and moving about.[105] Cluster headaches are thought to result from vasodilation in branches of the external carotid artery, because they often are triggered by vasodilating substances, such as nitroglycerine and alcohol.[108]

Tension-Type Headache

The term *tension-type headache* is designated by the International Headache Society to describe what was previously called *tension headache*, muscle contraction headache, psychomyogenic headache, stress headache, ordinary headache, and psychogenic headache.[107] The International Headache Society distinguishes between the episodic and the chronic varieties of tension-type headaches and divides them into two groups: those associated with a disorder of the pericranial muscles and those not associated with this type of disorder.[107]

Tension headaches, which constitute up to 70% of headaches and which occur more often in women than in men, are thought to result from emotional stress.[105,109] They are characterized by a bilateral, nonthrobbing ache in the frontal or temporal areas and by spasm or hypertonus of the neck muscles.[108] Unlike migraine headaches, tension-type headache is typically relieved by physical activity and usually responds well to soft tissue and specific traction techniques.

Benign Exertional Headache

Benign exertional headache (BEH) has been recognized as a separate entity for more than 70 years.[110] Characteristic features of BEH include[111]

- headache that is specifically brought on by physical exercise, particularly with straining and Valsalva-type maneuvers, such as those seen in weightlifting;
- bilateral and throbbing at onset and may develop migrainous features in patients susceptible to migraine;
- duration of 5 minutes to 24 hours;
- prevented by avoiding excessive exertion;
- no association with any systemic or intracranial disorder.

Clearly, the major differential diagnosis to be considered in this situation would be a subarachnoid hemorrhage, which needs to be excluded by appropriate investigations.

Effort-Induced Headache

Effort headaches have been reported to be the most common type of headache in athletes.[112] These headaches differ from BEH in that they are not necessarily associated with a power or straining type of exercise. The clinical features of this effort headache syndrome include[111]

- an onset of mild-to-severe headache with aerobic-type exercise;
- more frequency in hot weather;
- vascular-type headache (i.e., throbbing);
- short duration of headache (4–6 hours);
- provoking exercise may be maximal or submaximal;
- patient may have prodromal "migrainous" symptoms;
- headache tends to recur in individuals with exercise;
- patient may have a past history of migraine;
- normal neurological examination and investigations.

Occipital Headache

The occipital headache is felt by many clinicians to be referred as pain from a cervical disorder,[113–115] especially when cervical traction temporarily decreases the headache.[105]

The underlying musculoskeletal mechanism for this type of headache is often structural, including cervical hypomobility or hypermobility, joint subluxation, and degenerative bony changes. Postures, movements, or activities that put strain on the neck have been associated with headaches.[116] In one study,[117] 51% of patients associated their headaches with sustained neck flexion during reading, studying, typing, or driving a car. Sixty-five percent of headache patients reported a chronic course lasting between 2 and 20 years, and only 7% reported pain of less than 1 week's duration.

The general misunderstanding is that there is no cervical sensory reference to the head area, because the posterior (dorsal) ramus of C1 has no sensory component and that only the trigeminal nerve has sensory input to the vertex and frontal regions. In fact, there is considerable sensory input into the root of C1 but not from a cutaneous source (see "Occipital Neuralgia").[118] Experiments have confirmed a close trigeminocervical relationship.[119,120] Because the head and neck comprise one functional unit, cervical musculoskeletal disorders can refer to headache or temporomandibular or facial pain—with or without neck pain.[121] Cervical headaches are described in more detail in Chapter 23.

Hypertension Headache

Hypertension headaches usually occur in individuals with diastolic readings above 120 mm Hg, although the intensity of these headaches does not necessarily parallel the height of the blood pressure levels.[122] Typically, the headache begins in the early morning, reaching a peak upon awakening, and then diminishes once the patient rises and begins daily activity.[104] The headache usually is described as a nonlocalized, dull, and throbbing ache that is aggravated by activities that increase blood pressure, such as bending, coughing, or exertion.[106] The distribution of the headache can vary and may extend over the entire cranium.[104]

External Compression Headache

This entity, formerly known as *swim-goggle headache*, manifests with pain in the facial and temporal areas that results from wearing excessively tight face masks or swimming goggles.[111,123] It is commonly seen in swimmers and divers. The etiology is believed to be related to continuous stimulation of cutaneous nerves by the application of pressure, although neuralgia of the supraorbital nerve has also been implicated.[111]

Idiopathic Carotidynia Headache[124]

Idiopathic carotidynia is associated with unilateral facial or orbital pain in half of the patients with this condition. The pain remains isolated in about 10% of patients, but usually there is an ipsilateral headache. The characteristic unilateral headache is most commonly located in the frontotemporal area, but it occasionally involves the entire hemicranium or the occipital area. The onset of headache is usually gradual, but it may be an instantaneous, excruciating, "thunderclap" headache that mimics a subarachnoid hemorrhage. The headache is most commonly described as a constant steady aching, but it may also be throbbing or steady and sharp. The median interval between the onset of neck pain and the appearance of other symptoms is 2 weeks, whereas other symptoms occur only approximately 15 hours after the onset of headache.

Chronic Daily Headache

Chronic daily headaches, following trauma to the head or neck, are a common occurrence,[125] with the duration of these headaches unrelated to the severity or type of trauma.[126,127] These headaches typically consist of a group of disorders that can be subclassified into primary and secondary types.[128]

- The primary chronic daily headache disorders include transformed migraine, chronic tension-type headache, new daily persistent headache, and hemicrania continua. This type of headache is defined as a constant tension headache with migrainous exacerbations.[129,130]
- The secondary chronic daily headaches include cervical spine disorders, headache associated with vascular disorders, and nonvascular intracranial disorders.

Chronic daily headache usually evolves over time from episodic migraine, but the cause is still controversial. Individuals suffering from chronic daily headache often suffer from rebound headache as well. Rebound headache is the worsening of head pain in chronic headache sufferers. It is caused by the frequent and excessive use of nonnarcotic analgesics.[131] Several studies have demonstrated that as many as three-quarters of patients with chronic daily headache suffer from drug-induced rebound headache.[132,133]

The role of trauma in chronic daily headaches, however, may be understated. Tension headaches may well initiate a headache in patients predisposed by some previous and forgotten traumatic incident.

Posttraumatic Headache

In addition to the immediate pain following a head injury, posttraumatic headache, a more prolonged and enduring headache, may develop.[134] This condition, resembling either migraine or tension-type headache, may last for weeks, months, or years. It may also be associated with posttraumatic syndrome, which includes a variety of symptoms, such as irritability, insomnia, anxiety, seizure, amnesia, depression, and reduced ability to concentrate.[134]

The more serious causes of headache associated with trauma include subdural hematoma, epidural hematoma, intracerebral hematoma, aneurysm, subarachnoid hemorrhage, or cerebral contusion.

The clinician should attempt to establish the overall health of the patient through a review of the systems[108]:

- ***Nervous system.*** The physical examination of the nervous system can include sensory and motor testing of the cranial and spinal nerves, reflex testing, and an examination of gait, balance, and coordination. The need for such testing often can be determined through the presence of the signs and symptoms.
- ***Cardiovascular system.*** Fluctuations in blood pressure are often associated with headaches.
- ***Endocrine system.*** Headaches may be associated with hormonal changes and hormonal replacement therapy.[135]
- ***Musculoskeletal system.*** An examination must be made of the middle and upper cervical segments and the temporomandibular joint. In addition, a thorough postural examination should be performed to assess for muscle imbalances and overall alignment. Relative flexibility and strength are assessed during upper limb movements. Finally, the clinician should examine for myofascial trigger points and the presence of adverse neural tension (see Chap. 11).

Occipital Neuralgia

Occipital neuralgia is a rare neuralgic disorder that involves the greater occipital nerve.[136] The greater occipital nerve originates from the second cervical root (C2). Occipital neuralgia is a headache syndrome that is characterized by occipital and suboccipital headache that may radiate to the frontal, periorbital, retroorbital, maxillary, and mandibular regions.[137] It may also be associated with neck pain, dizziness, paresthesias or hyperesthesia of the posterior scalp, and loss of the normal cervical lordosis. Occipital neuralgia is more common in women than in men.[138] The pain usually awakens the patient from sleep in the morning but may occur at any time of day.[138] The causes of occipital neuralgia include

- scalp trauma from a direct blow;
- compression neuropathy;
- sustained contraction (spasm) of the posterior neck muscles,[136] especially the semispinalis capitis, obliquus capitis inferior, and trapezius muscles[139];
- hyperextension injury and resultant compression of the ganglion and root of C2;
- fracture of the atlas or axis;
- gout;
- mastoiditis;
- OA of the craniovertebral joints.

Diagnosis is usually made using palpation over the greater occipital nerve as it passes the superior nuchal line. The intervention for patients with occipital neuralgia involves infiltrating the nerve with a mixture of local anesthetic and corticosteroid.[139]

Glossopharyngeal Neuralgia

The cause of glossopharyngeal neuralgia is at present unknown, although most authors place the site of disturbance in the region of the posterior root[140,141] or in the spinal tract of the nerve.[142] Glossopharyngeal neuralgia is characterized by intense unilateral attacks of pain in the retrolingual area, radiating to the depth of the ear.[106] The pain, typically, is aggravated by movement or contact with the pharynx, especially with swallowing.

Trigeminal Neuralgia

TN, or tic douloureux, is a severe chronic pain syndrome characterized by dramatic, brief stabbing or electric shock-like pain paroxysms felt in one or more divisions of the trigeminal distribution, either spontaneously or on gentle tactile stimulation of a trigger point on the face or in the oral cavity.[143] It is unclear whether TN is a neuropathic pain state of the central or peripheral nervous system.

Bell Palsy

Bell palsy is a lower motor neuron (LMN) disease of the facial nerve characterized by a wide range of facial muscle movement dysfunction from mild paresis to total paralysis. Individual patients display a spectrum of symptoms: some maintain only reduced movement throughout the course of the disorder while others rapidly become totally paralyzed over a 24-hour period. Bell palsy is the most common form of facial paralysis, with an incidence of 20–30 per 100,000 persons.[144] The diagnosis is established by the exclusion of several localized lesions, such as temporal bone fracture, acoustic neuroma, suppuration or tumor of the middle ear, and disorders of the parotid gland.[145]

Fundamental to management issues of this disorder is the question of its etiology, once thought to be idiopathic. Two recent independent studies[146,147] strongly support the concept that the facial paralysis associated with Bell palsy is the result of a viral inflammatory response that induces edema and ischemia of the facial nerve as it passes through its bony canal. The infectious agents associated with Bell palsy are herpes simplex virus type 1, varicella zoster virus, and the spirochete *Borrelia burgdorferi*, the causative organism of Lyme disease.[148]

The intervention for this condition is empiric, varying from observation alone to the use of corticosteroids, electric stimulation, surgical decompression, and antiviral agents. Transcranial magnetic stimulation of the facial nerve has also been reported to be useful.[149]

Healing is occasionally incomplete, resulting in residual nerve dysfunction, including partial palsy and motor synkinesis (involuntary movement accompanying a voluntary one) and autonomic synkinesis (involuntary lacrimation after a voluntary muscle movement). On the basis of the study of Peitersen,[150] all patients regain some function, and 85% of all patients will regain normal or very near-normal function within 6–8 weeks.

Surgical management of Bell palsy has been controversial since its inception because of the following points: issues of patient selection criteria based on electrodiagnostic studies, site of decompression, limited number of patients who require decompression at any single center, and the inability to transfer results from study to study because of the continued use of independent facial function grading systems.[151]

Ramsay Hunt Syndrome

Ramsay Hunt syndrome, a herpetic inflammation of the geniculate or facial nerve ganglia, or both, manifests as a peripheral facial nerve palsy accompanied by an erythematous vesicular rash on the ear (zoster oticus) or in the mouth.[152] It is the second most common cause of atraumatic peripheral facial paralysis. Other frequent symptoms and signs can include tinnitus, hearing loss, nausea, vomiting, vertigo, and nystagmus.

Compared with Bell palsy, patients with Ramsay Hunt syndrome often have more severe paralysis at onset and are less likely to recover completely. The intervention for Ramsay Hunt syndrome can involve medication. Prednisone and acyclovir may improve outcome, although a prospective randomized treatment trial remains to be undertaken.[152]

Arteriovenous Malformation

This congenital malformation may manifest with an abrupt onset of head and facial pain.

Meningitis

The brain is protected from infection by the skull, pia, arachnoid, and dural meninges covering its surface and by the blood–brain barrier. When any of these defenses are broached by a pathogen, infection of the meninges and subarachnoid space can occur, resulting in meningitis.[153] Rigidity of the neck can occur with neuralgia and other irritative lesions of the meninges, such as meningitis.[154]

Since the fifth century BC, the seriousness of infectious meningitis has been recognized.[155] In the twentieth century, the annual incidence of bacterial meningitis ranges from approximately 3 per 100,000 population in the United States[156] to 500 per 100,000 in the so-called meningitis belt of Africa.[157]

Predisposing factors for the development of community-acquired meningitis include preexisting diabetes mellitus, otitis media, pneumonia, sinusitis, and alcohol abuse.[158]

The clinical features of meningitis reflect the underlying pathophysiologic processes.[154] Once the blood–brain barrier is breached, an inflammatory response within the cerebrospinal fluid (CSF) occurs. The resultant meningeal inflammation and irritation elicit a protective reflex to prevent stretching of the inflamed and hypersensitive nerve roots, which is detectable clinically as neck stiffness (Kernig or Brudzinski signs).[159,160]

> **CLINICAL PEARL**
>
> Rigidity of the neck can occur with neuralgia and other irritative lesions of the meninges, such as meningitis.[154]

The meningeal inflammation may also cause a generalized headache, cranial nerve palsies, vomiting, and nausea.[161] If the inflammatory process progresses to cerebral vasculitis or causes cerebral edema and elevated intracranial pressure, alterations in mental status, headache, vomiting, seizures, and cranial nerve palsies may ensue.[153]

Despite classic descriptions of meningeal signs and sweeping statements about its clinical presentation, the signs and symptoms of meningitis have been inadequately studied.[154] Based on the limited studies, the following points should be remembered during the examination[154]:

- The absence of all three signs of the classic triad of fever, neck stiffness, and an altered mental status virtually eliminates a diagnosis of meningitis. Fever is the most sensitive of the classic triad of signs and occurs in a majority of patients, with neck stiffness being the next most sensitive sign. Alterations in mental status also have a relatively high sensitivity, indicating that normal mental status helps to exclude meningitis in low-risk patients. Changes in mental status are more common in bacterial than in viral meningitis.
- Among the signs of meningeal irritation, Kernig and Brudzinski signs appear to have low sensitivity but high specificity.

Cerebrovascular Disease

The frequency of headache with cerebrovascular disease is dependent on the size and location of the hemorrhage. Small hemorrhages may occur without an associated headache. Although a headache may be the presenting symptom of cerebrovascular disease, associated neurological changes are also likely and are more indicative of cerebrovascular disease. These could include, but are not limited to, loss of the ability to sit, stand, and walk; right- or left-sided weakness; visual disturbances; aphasia; apraxia; dysphasia; seizures; and mental status changes.

Intracranial Bleeding

Depending on the rate of arterial or venous bleeding, signs of intracranial bleeding may take minutes to days. A meningeal artery or branch laceration with an associated overlying skull fracture is a frequent source of delayed epidural bleeding.[162] However, venous bleeding is also associated with delayed and chronic hematomas by nature of the low pressure and slow rate of bleeding.[162] Other causes of low-tension hemorrhages are small dural lesions or diffuse cerebral contusion sites.

A subarachnoid hemorrhage can be the cause of head, facial, orbital, or neck pain. The pain, which is usually severe, may occur in one region or over all of the areas. Neck stiffness and pain on movement are common findings and often are associated with nausea and vomiting. Other possible findings include

- UMN signs and symptoms (Babinski, clonus, hyperreflexia, ataxia, and so on);
- photophobia;
- motor or sensory disturbances;
- syncope;
- somnolence and lethargy;
- seizures;
- visual disturbances;
- dysphasia.

Patients with intracranial bleeding usually prefer to remain still, with their eyes closed. They often become disoriented and demonstrate judgment and memory abnormalities.

Tumors

A complete discussion of each type of brain tumor is beyond the scope of this text. Tumors of the brain may be classified according to type as follows:

- ***Astrocytomas.*** Astrocytomas are benign brain tumors. Glioblastoma multiforme, a type of astrocytoma, is the most common adult brain neoplasm.
- ***Oligodendrogliomas.*** These are benign primary brain tumors that arise from oligodendrocytes.
- ***Meningiomas.*** These tumors are slow growing and benign and comprise about 20% of all intracranial tumors in adults.
- ***Metastatic tumors.*** These are tumors that originate from tissues outside of the brain. They can occur as single or multiple tumors.

The term *benign* is misleading when referring to brain tumors. Although benign may mean curable, this is not always true with brain tumors. Tumors, benign or otherwise, are space-occupying lesions that may increase to a size that compresses nearby structures or increases intracranial pressure. Patients with tumors of the brain may present acutely with the following symptoms:

- Abrupt onset of severe headache
- Facial pain
- Episodes of loss of consciousness
- Changes in mental status
- Nausea and vomiting
- Focal neurologic signs and symptoms
- Neck stiffness or pain

Encephalitis

Encephalitis is an inflammation of the brain. The inflammation may be caused by an arthropod-borne virus, or it may occur as a sequela of influenza, measles, German measles, chickenpox, herpes simplex, or other infectious diseases. Clinical findings include

- signs of meningeal irritation (Kernig or Brudzinski sign);
- changes in mental status;
- signs of increased intracranial pressure, including increased restlessness, vomiting, seizures, and pupil irregularities;
- behavioral changes.

Systemic Infections

Systemic infections that are capable of provoking head or facial pain include Rocky Mountain spotted fever, Lyme disease, pneumonia, and pyelonephritis.

Rocky Mountain Spotted Fever

This condition begins abruptly with a high fever and bilateral frontal or frontotemporal headache. The classic rash begins on the distal aspects of the extremities and spreads proximally. Serologic tests are required to confirm the diagnosis.

Lyme Disease

Lyme disease is a bacterial infection that is transmitted to humans by ticks that usually live on mice or deer. Most infections are acquired in three distinct sections of the United States: along the northeast coast, in areas of Wisconsin and Minnesota, and, to a lesser extent, in northern California and southern Oregon. People who hike, camp, or live in or near wooded areas in these locations during summer months are most at risk for Lyme disease. Following a bite from a deer tick, a red bump may occur at the site of the bite. If the tick is infected, a larger rash may form around the bite. The classic description of the rash is an enlarging area of redness with partial central clearing. However, it may take several days before the lesion expands enough to have the classic appearance.

The most common signs and symptoms associated with the rash are nonspecific flu-like symptoms, including myalgia, arthralgias, fever, joint pain and swelling, headache, fatigue, motor or sensory radiculoneuritis, mononeuritis multiplex, or neck stiffness.[163]

Cardiac symptoms can include fluctuating degrees of atrioventricular block, occasionally acute myopericarditis or mild left-ventricular dysfunction, and, rarely, cardiomegaly or fatal pancarditis.[163]

The initial diagnosis usually is based on the recognition of the characteristic clinical findings. The culture of *B. burgdorferi* from specimens in Barbour–Stoenner–Kelly medium permits a definitive diagnosis.[163]

Pneumonia

Pneumonia is an inflammation of the lungs, usually caused by an infection of the lung tissue by one of many different microorganisms. The presenting symptoms depend on how much of the lung is affected and the type of infection. Related to this body region, patients with pneumonia may present with fever and severe headache.

Pyelonephritis

Acute pyelonephritis is an inflammation of the kidney and renal pelvis. Clinical signs and symptoms of acute pyelonephritis include fever; shaking chills; thoracolumbar, interscapular, neck, and flank pain; nausea and vomiting; costovertebral angle tenderness; and, less commonly, symptoms of cystitis such as dysuria and increased frequency.[164] In addition, a bifrontal or generalized headache may accompany the neck pain and stiffness.

Multiple Sclerosis

Multiple sclerosis (MS) is a chronic demyelinating disorder with a wide range of clinical manifestations that reflects multifocal areas of CNS myelin destruction. In adults, the clinical presentation of MS at onset is characterized by motor system (26.5%), sensory system (25%), or optic nerve (21%) involvement or a combination of all three.[165] Cerebellar and sphincteric involvement are less frequent (14.1% each).[165]

Patients with motor weakness may develop paralysis affecting one or more, or all, limbs. Sensory dysfunction may occur in one modality (e.g., to light touch, temperature, or deep sensation) and may manifest as hypoesthesia/anesthesia or hypersensitivity with numbness, burning sensation, paresthesia, and dysesthesia in various parts of the body.[165] Optic neuritis is associated with a decrease in visual acuity, sometimes resulting in blindness, accompanied by orbital pain when the involved eye moves. Examples of acute or paroxysmal pain include head and facial pain, painful tonic spasms, radicular pain, and dysesthesia.[166] Other manifestations include fatigue, cognitive loss, and mood disturbance.

Most patients with MS (85%) have a relapsing–remitting course of disease, with each relapse being associated with new neurologic symptoms or worsening of existing ones. With additional relapses, the possibility of complete recovery is reduced and permanent disability may develop.[165] In the remaining 15% of patients, the disease course is primary progressive, with continuous neurologic deterioration.[165]

MS usually manifests between 20 and 40 years, with a peak onset at around 30 years and a female-to-male ratio of 2:1. At present, MS is regarded as being modifiable, but incurable.

Miscellaneous Causes

Temporal Arteritis

This condition, also known as giant cell arteritis, is an inflammatory condition affecting the medium-sized blood vessels that supply the head, eyes, and optic nerves. The disease usually affects those over 60 years and is characterized by severe headache, which can begin abruptly or gradually, and is usually throbbing in nature. Associated symptoms may include flu-like symptoms, swollen and tender temporal arteries, jaw weakness, scalp tenderness, and visual loss. Women are approximately four times more likely to suffer from this disease than men.[167]

Acute Sinusitis

Sinusitis is an infection or inflammation of the sinuses. Sinuses are hollow air spaces located within the skull or bones of the head surrounding the nose. Each sinus has an opening into the nose for the free exchange of air and mucus, and each is joined with the nasal passages by a continuous mucous membrane lining. Anything that causes a swelling in the nose, such as an infection, an allergic reaction, or an immune reaction, may affect the sinuses. Sinusitis involves an infection or inflammation of one or more of the following:

- *Frontal sinuses* over the eyes in the brow area
- *Maxillary sinuses* inside each cheekbone
- *Ethmoid sinuses* just behind the bridge of the nose and between the eyes
- *Sphenoid sinuses* behind the ethmoids in the upper region of the nose and behind the eyes

Air trapped within a blocked sinus, along with pus or other secretions, may cause pressure on the sinus wall and subsequent pain. Similarly, when air is prevented from entering a sinus by a swollen membrane at the opening, a vacuum may be created, which also causes pain. The location of the sinus pain depends on which sinus is affected. Symptoms can include

- headache upon awakening in the morning and tenderness to palpation over the frontal sinuses;
- upper jaw, cheek, and tooth pain (maxillary sinuses);
- pain and swelling of tear ducts in the corner of the eyes and pain between the eyes and sides of the nose (ethmoid sinuses);
- earaches, neck pain, and deep aching at the top of the head (sphenoid sinuses).

Other symptoms of sinusitis include

- fever;
- weakness;
- tiredness;
- cough that may be more severe at night;
- runny nose (rhinitis) or nasal congestion.

On rare occasions, acute sinusitis may result in brain infection and other serious complications.

Eclampsia

Eclampsia is the most commonly occurring hypertensive disease in pregnancy. Worldwide, preeclampsia and eclampsia contribute to the death of a pregnant woman every 3 minutes.[168] The classic clinical presentation consists of blurred vision, severe headaches, epileptic seizures or coma manifesting during the third trimester or early puerperium in women who already have the triad of preeclamptic symptoms: edema, proteinuria, and hypertension.[169] The diagnosis of eclampsia requires the exclusion of other medical or neurologic disorders underlying the symptomatology. The differential diagnostic considerations include sinus or cerebral vein thrombosis, subarachnoid hemorrhage from an aneurysm, infectious or autoimmune-inflammatory disorders, and sickle-cell crisis.

CSF Hypotension

This condition commonly occurs following a lumbar puncture, which can produce leakage of CSF through a dural tear. A lumbar puncture is a routine procedure performed for a variety of functions: spinal anesthesia, intrathecal administration of cytotoxic and antibiotic drugs, myelography, obtaining CSF samples, and pressure measurement.[170] The leak of CSF results in CSF hypovolemia and downward shifting of the brain, causing pressure on the pain-sensitive dural sinuses that is amplified in the upright posture and relieved with recumbence.[171] The clinical manifestations of CSF hypotension are headache and backache, which usually start within hours to a week following the lumbar puncture. More serious complications may include labyrinthine and ocular cranial nerve disturbances, meningitis, subdural hematomas, and fistulas.

Temporomandibular Joint Dysfunction

See Chapter 26.

Periodontal Disease

Periodontal disease may be associated with a small increased risk of coronary heart disease.[172] Clinically, periodontitis starts as an acute inflammation of the apical periodontal ligament and the neighboring spongiosa, accompanied by well-known imminent symptoms such as pain, tenderness to percussion, and swelling.

Thyroiditis

Acute bacterial thyroiditis (or pyogenic thyroiditis) is a rare, potentially life-threatening complication of bacterial infection elsewhere in the body, especially following an upper respiratory tract infection.[173] The condition occurs in all age groups, although women with preexisting thyroid disease constitute the group most likely to develop thyroid infection. In childhood, it is often linked to local anatomic defects. The ample blood supply and lymphatic drainage, high iodine content, and protective thyroid capsule contribute to the low incidence of infection.

Common pathogens include *Streptococcus pyogenes*, *Streptococcus pneumoniae*, and *Staphylococcus*. Less common organisms include *Salmonella*, *Bacteroides*, *Haemophilus influenzae*, *Streptococcus viridans*, and other streptococcal organisms.[173] Clinical signs and symptoms include fever

(92%), anterior neck pain (100%), tenderness (94%), warmth (70%), erythema (82%), dysphagia (91%), dysphonia (82%), and pharyngitis (69%).[173]

Fracture of the Facial Bones or Skull

The examination of the face for a fracture requires knowledge not only of normal anatomy but also of common fracture patterns in the face. Computed tomography (CT) is currently the imaging procedure of choice for most facial fractures, because it highlights the complex anatomy and fractures of the facial bones and their related soft-tissue complications extremely well. Approximately 60–70% of all facial fractures involve the orbit.[174] The exception to this is a local nasal bone fracture or a zygomatic arch fracture. The most common mechanism producing facial fractures is auto accidents. Other mechanisms include fights or assaults, falls, sports, industrial accidents, and gunshot wounds. Less than 10% of all facial fractures occur in children, perhaps because of the increased resiliency of a child's facial skeleton.[174] The nose is the most frequently injured facial structure, and the most commonly missed facial fracture of the face is a fracture of the nasal bone. Patients with a temporal bone fracture may present with a conductive hearing loss caused by dislocations in the ossicular chain. Facial nerve paralysis may also occur secondary to either transection or edema of the facial nerve.

Trochleitis[175]

Trochleitis is a local inflammatory process of the superior oblique tendon trochlea characterized by periocular pain. Eye movement in supraduction typically aggravates the pain. Physical examination demonstrates exquisite point tenderness over the trochlea of the superior oblique muscle. The cause often is unknown, but trochleitis can occur in RA, SLE, psoriasis, or enteropathic arthropathy. Rare causes include sinusitis, trauma, and metastasis.

CAUSES OF CERVICAL PAIN

The causes of cervical pain are numerous, as outlined in Table 5-7 and Fig. 5-1.

TABLE 5-7 Potential Causes of Cervical Pain
Thyroid disease
Subarachnoid hemorrhage
Retropharyngeal abscess
Carotodynia
Cardiac disease
Trauma
Myofascial pain syndrome
Tumors
Temporomandibular joint dysfunction
Meningitis
Epidural hematoma
Lyme disease
Cervical disk disease or herniation
Vertebral artery disorders
Torticollis
Rheumatoid arthritis
Ankylosing spondylitis
Gout
Osteoarthritis
Occipital neuralgia

Thyroid Disease

The thyroid gland synthesizes, stores, and secretes thyroid hormones, mainly L-thyroxine (T4). L-triiodothyronine (T3) is produced from T4 by deiodination, mainly in liver, kidney, and muscle. The thyroid gland controls the metabolic rate of many organs and tissues. The thyroid gland cannot function normally unless it is exposed to thyroid-stimulating hormone (TSH), which is produced by the thyrotrophs of the anterior pituitary.[176] Under-activity (hypothyroidism) and overactivity of thyroid function (hyperthyroidism), which represent the most common endocrine problems, have widespread manifestations, including cervical pain, and often require long-term treatment.

Hypothyroidism

Most patients with hypothyroidism have disease of the thyroid gland. Occasionally, hypothyroidism develops in patients with normal thyroid glands because of inadequate stimulation by TSH. Such individuals have disorders of the anterior pituitary or hypothalamus. Thyroid hormone deficiency affects practically all body functions. The complaints and physical findings vary widely from patient to patient, depending on the severity of the deficiency. Patients may present with weakness, fatigue, arthralgias and myalgias, muscle cramps, cold intolerance, constipation, lethargy, dryness of the skin, headache, neck pain, menorrhagia, hoarseness, edema, and weight gain.[176] Most patients have varying degrees of brittle nails and hair, pallor, delayed relaxation time of the muscle stretch reflexes, keratinic skin color, thickening of the tongue, mental status changes, and diastolic hypertension.[176] In some patients, severe hypothermia, edema, and even effusions into the pleura, and peritoneal and pericardial cavities may occur.[176]

Hyperthyroidism

Hyperthyroidism denotes clinical disorders associated with increased serum concentrations of free T4 estimate or free T3, or both. The most common causes of hyperthyroidism are Graves disease, nodular goiter, and thyroiditis. Excessive thyroid hormone concentrations affect many body functions. Such symptoms include[176]

- nervousness;
- restlessness;
- heat intolerance;
- increased and inappropriate perspiration;
- fatigue;
- muscle cramps;
- paratracheal neck pain;
- increased frequency of bowel movements;

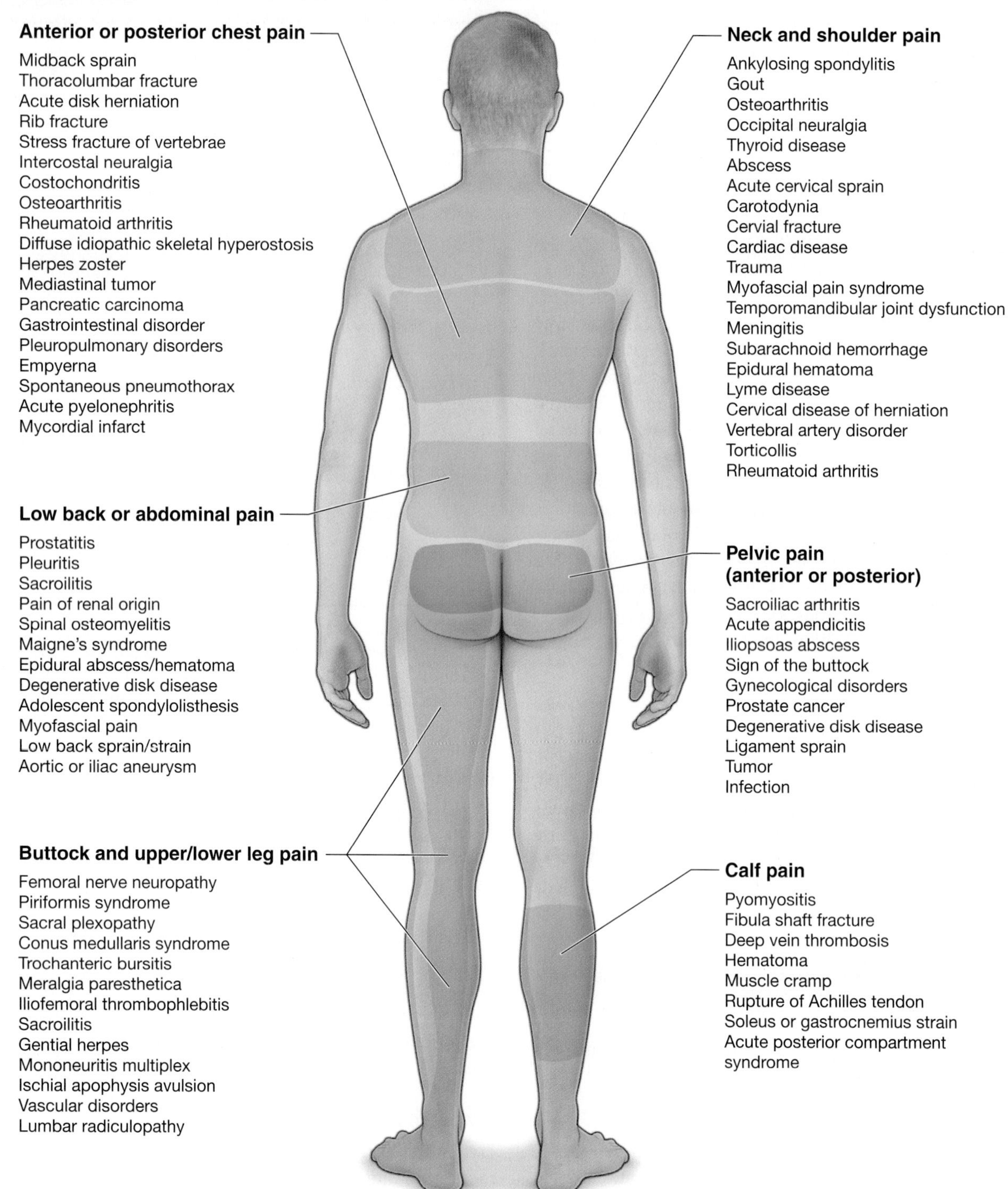

FIGURE 5-1 Potential causes of cervical, thoracic, lumbar, pelvic, and lower extremity pain.

- weight loss in association with unchanged or increased food ingestion;
- palpitations.

The clinical signs of hyperthyroidism, which vary widely among patients, may include exophthalmus, tachycardia, fine resting tremors, moist warm skin, heat radiation from the skin, hyperreflexia, onycholysis, an enlarged thyroid gland with or without a bruit, and diplopia.[176] Patients who are found to have relatively specific symptoms and signs (such as goiter, nodule, eye findings of Graves' disease, or tremor) should be referred to an endocrinologist for consideration of treatment.

Subarachnoid Hemorrhage

See the discussion of intracranial bleeding under "Causes of Head, Face, Eye, and Temporomandibular Joint Pain" earlier in the chapter.

Retropharyngeal Abscess

Retropharyngeal abscess (RPA) is a relatively uncommon infection of the space anterior to the prevertebral layer of the deep cervical fascia. This infection is most common in children younger than 3 or 4 years, because of the rich concentration of lymph nodes in this space.[177] The infection in children classically results from extension of oropharyngeal infections, including pharyngitis, tonsillitis, and adenitis.[178] Trauma, often caused by a fall while holding a pencil or stick in the mouth, and dental infections are the usual underlying causes of RPA in older children and adults.[178] The major causative organisms are *Strep. pyogenes*, *Staphylococcus aureus*, and oropharyngeal anaerobic bacteria.[179] The infection progresses through three stages: cellulitis, phlegmon (diffuse inflammation of the soft or connective tissue), and abscess.

RPA can produce posterior neck and shoulder pain and stiffness. These symptoms are also associated with hyperextension of the neck, torticollis, fever, irritability, muffled voice, stertor, and other signs of upper airway obstruction.[178] The pain often is worsened with swallowing. Swelling of the lateral or posterior aspect of the neck can be present.

The differential diagnosis includes acute epiglottitis, foreign body aspiration, vertebral osteomyelitis, hematoma (particularly in boys with hemophilia), and lymphoma.[178]

Carotodynia

In addition to sinus and dental abnormalities and stress, several different neurologic conditions can cause facial pain. These include various neuralgias (trigeminal, vagoglossopharyngeal, and cranial), carotodynia (a painful carotid artery), and optic neuritis. Pain characteristics and results of specific neurologic tests establish the diagnosis. Carotodynia is associated with neck pain, tenderness, and a unilateral headache.

Cardiac Disease

See the discussion of myocardial infarction under "Causes of Thoracic Pain" later.

Trauma or Whiplash

See Chapter 25.

Tumors

Tumors of the adult cervical spine may be primary, arising from the bone, or secondary (i.e., metastatic from a distant primary site.) Tumors of the cervical cord may cause neck pain. These tumors may be primary, metastatic, extramedullary, or intramedullary. Pain of insidious onset, with or without neurologic signs and symptoms (e.g., progressive leg weakness, bladder paralysis, and sensory loss), may occur.

Temporomandibular Joint Dysfunction

See Chapter 26.

Meningitis

See the discussion under "Causes of Head, Face, Eye, and Temporomandibular Joint Symptoms" earlier.

Epidural Hematoma

Most cervical epidural hematomas are spontaneous, with precipitating factors that include coagulopathy, vascular malformation, neoplasm, and pregnancy.[180] Cervical epidural hematoma can also be caused by trauma although this is uncommon. Traumatic causes of spontaneous epidural hematoma include vertebral trauma, epidural steroid injection, lumbar puncture, penetrating injuries, birth trauma, and spinal manipulation.[181] Excessive movement of the cervical spine, which may occur with a cervical manipulation, can injure the epidural veins, either by direct trauma or by a sudden increase in venous pressure, resulting in a cervical epidural hematoma.[180,182] The clinician must be particularly mindful of the risk factors for the complications of spinal manual therapy, such as misdiagnosis, unrecognized neurologic manifestations, improper technique, presence of coagulation disorder or disk herniation, and manipulation of the cervical spine.[183]

Presenting signs and symptoms vary. The onset of neck pain is often the first symptom, but epidural hematoma has been diagnosed in its absence. Compression of the spinal cord can also produce sensory deficits, motor deficits, and bowel or bladder incontinence.

Lyme Disease

See the discussion of systemic infections under "Causes of Head, Face, Eye, and Temporomandibular Joint Symptoms" earlier.

Cervical Disk Disease or Herniation

See Chapter 25.

Vertebral Artery Disorders

See Chapter 24.

Torticollis

As many as 80 different causes of torticollis have been documented in the literature.[235] Torticollis is not a specific diagnosis but, rather, a sign of an underlying disorder resulting in the characteristic tilting of the head to one side. Differential diagnosis of torticollis ranges from innocuous abnormalities that require no specific therapy (see Chap. 25) to potentially life-threatening tumors of the CNS. The neuromuscular causes of torticollis may be classified as congenital or acquired. Congenital muscular torticollis is the most common type of torticollis.[184] Several causes are implicated, including fetal positioning, difficult labor and delivery, cervical muscle abnormalities, Sprengel deformity, and Klippel-Feil syndrome.[185] In addition to torticollis, patients with Klippel–Feil syndrome have the classic clinical triad described by Klippel and Feil in 1912: short, broad necks; restricted movement; and low hairlines.[186,187] The restricted neck mobility is the result of the fusion of a variable number of cervical vertebrae, sometimes reducing their number, and cervical spina bifida.[188] Extraosseous changes, hemivertebra, vertebral body clefts, and thoracolumbar abnormalities sometimes are also seen.[189]

Acquired torticollis, which includes spasmodic torticollis, is clinically similar but has different etiologies (see Chap. 25).[190] Acquired torticollis in children may be related to trauma or infections, as in Grisel syndrome, which occurs after head, neck, and pharyngeal infections.[191] In this syndrome, the soft-tissue inflammation associated with pharyngitis, mastoiditis, or tonsillitis results in accumulation of fluid in the nearby cervical joints.[192] This edema may then lead to subluxation of the atlantoaxial joint.

Spasmodic torticollis is the involuntary hyperkinesis of neck musculature, causing turning of the head on the trunk, sometimes with additional forward flexion (anterocollis), backward extension (retrocollis), or lateral flexion (laterocollis).[190] It is also marked by abnormal head postures.[192] The sternocleidomastoid muscle is involved in 75% of cases and the trapezius in 50%.[192] Other muscles that might become involved include the rectus capitis, obliquus inferior, and splenius capitis.[193] In some cases, the spasm generalizes to the muscles of the shoulder, girdle, trunk, or limbs.[194]

Neck movements can vary from jerky to smooth[194,195] and are aggravated by standing, walking, or stressful situations but, usually, do not occur with sleep.[247]

Spontaneous remissions (partial or complete) have been reported in up to 60% of patients in some series[195]; others note full remission in 16%, with sustained remission for 12 months of 6–12%.[196,197]

Various treatments for torticollis have been described. Spencer and colleagues[198] described a single-subject study using behavioral therapies that consisted of progressive relaxation, positive practice, and visual feedback. Their patient had significant improvements in all areas, which were maintained at a 2-year follow-up examination.

Agras and Marshall[199] used massed negative practice (i.e., repeating the spasmodic positioning), 200–400 repetitions of the movement daily, which achieved full resolution of symptoms in one of two patients. Results persisted for 22 months.

Another single-case study used positive practice (exercising against the spasmodic muscle groups) in a bed-ridden woman who had symptoms of spasmodic torticollis for 8 years. After 3 months of positive practice, she was able to ambulate unassisted; her therapeutic gains were maintained at a 1-year follow-up examination.[198]

Biofeedback has also been used successfully as an intervention for torticollis.[200]

Rheumatoid Arthritis

Involvement of the cervical spine is common in RA, AS, and juvenile polyarthritis.[97] Fifty percent or more of patients with RA have evidence of neck involvement, especially at the atlantoaxial joint.[97] These patients are prone to a cervical derangement, of which an anterior subluxation of C1 on C2, during head flexion, is the most common.[201] Although most patients with anterior subluxation have no neurologic complications, the more advanced and unstable lesions may result in myelopathy.[97]

Patients can also experience severe bony erosions of one or both of the lateral zygapophyseal joints. This erosion can result in occipital pain with cervical rotation and a rotational head-tilt deformity if the lesion is unilateral.[201]

The symptoms of these spondyloarthropathies typically fall into two categories:

1. ***Pain resulting from the inflammatory process.*** RA of the cervical spine may cause generalized aching of the posterior neck and shoulder, and occipital pain. This pain is often worse with neck flexion.
2. ***Derangement or deformity.*** This finding results from joint damage, typically with a concomitant risk to the nearby neural structures. Radicular symptoms may be present in one or both upper extremities. With myelopathy, spastic weakness, hyperreflexia, and other UMN signs are present. Depending on the level of involvement within the cervical spine, signs and symptoms of vertebral artery compromise may also be present.

Ankylosing Spondylitis

AS commonly affects the C1–C2 segment, although this is usually a late manifestation of the disease process. Following ankylosing of the sacroiliac, lumbar, and thoracic segments, the atlantoaxial joint becomes painful initially, only to be less symptomatic as the joint begins to lose motion.[97]

Neurologic injury associated with AS is usually the result of cervical fracture of the syndesmophytes and resulting pseudoarticulation.[97,202] AS is described further under "Causes of Thoracic Pain".

Gout

Although the occurrence of gout in the neck is distinctly uncommon, the medications used to treat it can have serious side effects in this region. These complications include ligament laxity with resultant instability and neck pain.[203]

Osteoarthritis

Degenerative OA of the subaxial cervical spine is common in elderly patients[204] and is typically characterized by posterior neck, shoulder, and arm pain in a specific dermatomal pattern rather than occipitocervical pain.[205] Diffuse or focal trigger point tenderness may be present in the posterior neck on the involved side.

OA of the atlantoaxial joints may be overlooked when the patient has occipitocervical pain associated with degenerative changes in the subaxial spine.

Occipital Neuralgia

See the discussion under "Causes of Head, Face, Eye, and Temporomandibular Joint Symptoms" earlier.

CAUSES OF THORACIC PAIN

Thoracic pain has a wide differential diagnosis (Fig. 5-1). Pain may originate from structures within the thorax, such as the heart, lungs, or esophagus. However, musculoskeletal causes of chest pain must be considered. Musculoskeletal problems of the chest wall can occur in the ribs, sternum, articulations, or myofascial structures. The cause is usually evident in the case of direct trauma.

TABLE 5-8	Systemic Causes of Thoracic Pain
Systemic Origin	**Location**
Gallbladder disease	Mid-back between scapula
Acute cholecystitis	Right subscapular area
Peptic ulcer: stomach	5–10th thoracic vertebrae or duodenal ulcers
Pleuropulmonary disorders	
Basilar pneumonia	Right upper back
Empyema	Scapula
Pleurisy	Scapula
Spontaneous pneumothorax	Ipsilateral scapula
Pancreatic carcinoma	Middle thoracic or lumbar spine
Acute pyelonephritis	Costovertebral angle (posteriorly)
Esophagitis	Mid-back between scapula
Myocardial infarction	Mid-thoracic spine
Biliary colic	Right upper back, mid-back between scapula, right interscapular, or subscapular areas

Data from Goodman CC, Snyder TEK: *Differential Diagnosis in Physical Therapy*. Philadelphia. PA: WB Saunders, 1990.

TABLE 5-9 Potential Causes of Thoracic Pain
Mediastinal tumors
Pancreatic carcinoma
Gastrointestinal disorders
Pleuropulmonary conditions
Spontaneous pneumothorax
Myocardial infarction
Herpes zoster
Acute disk herniation
Vertebral fracture
Rib fracture
Stress fracture
Intercostal neuralgia
Costochondritis
Osteoarthritis
Rheumatoid arthritis
Diffuse idiopathic skeletal hyperostosis
Manubriosternal dislocations

Systemic origins of musculoskeletal pain in the thoracic spine (Table 5-8) are usually accompanied by constitutional symptoms affecting the whole body and by other associated symptoms that the patient may not relate to the pain and, therefore, may fail to mention to the clinician. These additional symptoms should be discovered during the subjective examination by the careful interviewer. When the patient (or the examination) indicates the presence of an associated fever (or night sweats), a referral to a physician is indicated.

The close proximity of the thoracic spine to the chest and respiratory organs may result in a correlation between respiratory movements and increased thoracic symptoms. When screening the patient through the subjective history, the clinician should remember that symptoms of pleural, intercostal muscular, costal, and dural origin all increase on coughing or deep inspiration; thus, only pain of a cardiac origin is ruled out when symptoms increase in association with respiratory movements.

The causes of thoracic pain include those listed in Table 5-9.

Gastrointestinal Conditions

The subjective history often provides several clues to a gastrointestinal cause of chest pain.

Colorectal Cancer

Colorectal cancer is the third most common cancer in both men and women in the United States. Risk factors include age, a diet rich in fat and cholesterol, inflammatory bowel disease (especially ulcerative colitis), and genetic predisposition.[206] The most common metastatic presentation of colon cancer is in the thoracic spine and rib cage.[3] The overall 5-year survival rate from colon cancer is approximately 60%, and nearly 60,000 people die of the disease each year in the United States.[206] The 5-year survival rate is different for each stage; the staging classification for colon cancer can predict prognosis well. The Dukes classification was traditionally used to predict prognosis but has since been replaced by the TNM staging (Table 5-10):

- Tumor (primary).
- Node (regional lymph)
- Metastasis (remote).

TABLE 5-10 TNM Staging of Cancer

Stage	Primary Tumor (T)	Regional Lymph Node (N)	Remote Metastasis (M)
Stage 0	Carcinoma in situ	N0	M0
Stage I	Tumor may invade submucosa (T1) or muscle (T2)	N0	M0
Stage II	Tumor invades muscle (T3) or perirectal tissues (T4)	N0	M0
Stage IIIA	T1–T4	N1	M0
Stage IIIB	T1–T4	N2–N3	M0
Stage IV	T1–T4	N1–N3	M1

An excellent correlation exists between the stage and the 5-year survival rate in patients with colon cancer[206]:

- For stage I or Dukes stage A, the 5-year survival rate following surgical resection exceeds 90%.
- For stage II or Dukes stage B, the 5-year survival rate is 70–85% following resection, with or without adjuvant therapy.
- For stage III or Dukes stage C, the 5-year survival rate is 30–60% following resection and adjuvant chemotherapy.
- For stage IV or Dukes stage D, the 5-year survival rate is poor (approximately 5%).

It is important for the physical therapist to assist other health-care professionals in stressing the importance of routine screening examinations for colorectal cancer (sigmoidoscopy and colonoscopy) for individuals with a family history of colon cancer, and for those patients over 50 years of age.[3] The information collected by a physical therapist during a history or physical examination that could serve as red flags for colon cancer are

1. age greater than 50 years;
2. history of colon cancer in an immediate family member;
3. bowel disturbances (e.g., rectal bleeding or black stools);
4. unexplained weight loss;
5. back or pelvic pain that is unchanged by positions or movement.[207]

Peptic Ulcer Disease

Peptic ulceration of the stomach or duodenum is often accompanied by abnormalities of the gastric mucosa, and the key to determining the cause of ulcer disease often lies in histologic diagnosis of the associated *gastritis* or *gastropathy*.

The terms *ulcer disease* and *peptic ulcer* are used synonymously to refer to erosions or ulcers of the stomach and duodenum.

Ulcer disease was long assumed to be idiopathic, caused by acid hypersecretion or psychologic stress, or a combination. *Helicobacter pylori* is now well recognized as a major risk factor for the development of peptic ulcer disease.[208]

The patient usually describes a typical history of ulcers characterized by periodic symptoms, relief with antacids, and the relationship of pain to certain foods and the timing of meals. For example, the patient may have relief from pain after eating initially, but the pain then returns and increases 1–2 hours after eating when the stomach is emptied. In the pediatric age group, abdominal pain is a very common reason for seeking medical advice. It is also the most common presenting symptom of peptic ulcer disease. However, peptic and other erosive or ulcerative gastritides and gastropathies of the stomach and duodenum are relatively uncommon in this age group.[209]

The pain of a peptic ulcer occasionally occurs only in the back between the 8th and 10th thoracic vertebrae. Duodenal ulcers may refer pain from the fifth thoracic vertebra, either at the midline or just at either side of the spine. This localization may accompany penetration through the viscera (organs). When questioned further, the patient may indicate that blood is present in the feces.

The differential diagnosis of ulcer disease includes esophagitis, gastritis, gastropathy, nonulcer dyspepsia, gallbladder or liver disease, pneumonia, and pancreatitis among others.[209]

Acute Cholecystitis

Acute cholecystitis is the result of cystic duct obstruction by gallstones or biliary sludge. In this condition, ductal obstruction is soon followed by chemical inflammation and a superimposed infection of the gallbladder. Acute cholecystitis may refer intense, sudden, paroxysmal pain to the right scapula, mid-back, or right shoulder. Pain intensity often increases with movement or respirations. Rebound tenderness and abdominal muscle guarding are often present. A low-grade fever also may be present. There may be reports of nausea and vomiting. Finally, mild jaundice, which is more apparent in fair-skinned patients, may be observed in those experiencing acute cholecystitis.[210] This finding is attributable to edema of the common bile duct, which causes bilirubin to diffuse across the inflamed gallbladder mucosa.[210]

Biliary Colic

Biliary colic is a common initial presentation of gallstone disease. The pain of biliary colic is referred to the right posterior upper quadrant, with pain in the right shoulder. There may be interscapular pain, with referred pain to the right side. Occasionally, the pain beneath the right costal margin may be confused with the shoulder girdle pain secondary to intracostal nerve compression. The pain is initially intermittent. Pain usually recurs, but the interval to the next attack of pain is quite variable.

Severe Esophagitis

Gastroesophageal reflux disease is defined as symptoms or mucosal damage (esophagitis) resulting from the exposure of the distal esophagus to refluxed gastric contents. Esophageal pain has many patterns. It is often described as burning, sometimes as gripping, and it can also be pressing, boring, or stabbing. It may be associated with a foul taste, morning pain, worsening pain after a meal, and epigastric tenderness. Severe esophagitis may refer pain to the anterior chest. It tends to be felt mainly in the throat or epigastrium. On occasion, it can radiate to the neck, back, or upper arms—all of which may equally apply to cardiac pain.

Pancreatic Carcinoma

The most frequent symptom of a pancreatic carcinoma is pain. It first may be noted as a paroxysmal (sudden, recurrent, or intensifying) or steady, dull pain, radiating from the epigastrium into the back. The pain is usually slowly progressive, is worse at night, and is unrelated to digestive activities. Other signs and symptoms may include jaundice, anorexia, severe weight loss, and gastrointestinal difficulties unrelated to meals. The disease is predominantly found in men (3:1) and occurs in the sixth and seventh decades.

Mediastinal Tumors

Most spinal tumors occur in the first half of life. Although primary tumors of the thoracic spine are rare, the thoracic spine is the most common site for metastases. Tumors occur in the thoracic spine because of its length and proximity to the mediastinum. The vascularization of the vertebrae in the mid-to-lower thoracic spine is generally through a watershed effect rather than by direct segmental arteries, which leaves the region susceptible to a secondary metastatic invasion from lymph nodes involved with lymphoma, breast, or lung cancer.[211,212]

Tumors of T12–L2 (typically, multiple myeloma) may compress the conus medullaris containing the S3–S5 nerve roots. This may lead to an impairment of the urinary or anal sphincter, which is sometimes associated with saddle anesthesia.

Myocardial Infarction

Pain of myocardial origin, resulting from a sudden and complete occlusion of the coronary artery, frequently radiates over the left pectoral region, left shoulder, medial left arm, right upper extremity, epigastrium, and jaw and can, therefore, mimic musculoskeletal pain. The pain typically has a crushing or gripping quality over the substernal region. Angina pectoris pain, which is a symptom that represents an imbalance between myocardial perfusion and demand, may be exertional or variant, making it difficult for the clinician to recognize. The distribution of symptoms for angina pectoris includes substernal and chest pressure, shoulder pain, and neck or jaw pain, which worsens with exertion and improves with rest. This condition constitutes a medical emergency.

Pleuropulmonary Conditions

Pneumothorax

Pneumothorax is defined as the entry of air into the pleural space with secondary lung collapse.[213] The pleura is a thin serous layer that covers the lungs (visceral pleura). The pleural space extends from 3 cm above the midpoint of the clavicle down to the 12th rib overlying the kidney. Three types of pneumothorax may cause thoracic pain: spontaneous, iatrogenic, and traumatic.

Spontaneous pneumothorax, in contrast to iatrogenic and traumatic pneumothorax, occurs without any precipitating event. Primary spontaneous pneumothorax, seen in otherwise healthy individuals, is rarely life threatening. Secondary spontaneous pneumothorax, seen in patients with underlying lung disease, is a more serious condition and is associated with substantial mortality.

Several findings in the examination of the respiratory and cardiovascular systems may help establish the diagnosis of pneumothorax. Patients with pneumothorax present with pleuritic pain or breathlessness. The pain is localized to the side of the pneumothorax. This pain may be referred to the ipsilateral scapula or shoulder, across the chest, or over the abdomen. Pneumothorax may also be associated with hemoptysis (blood in sputum), tachycardia (increased heart rate), tachypnea (rapid respirations), and cyanosis (blue lips and skin resulting from lack of oxygen).[12] The patient may be most comfortable sitting in an upright position.

A chest radiograph is usually sufficient to confirm the diagnosis. Intervention can range from simple aspiration, tube drainage, and chemical sclerosis of the pleura to thoracoscopy and thoracotomy.

Pleural Effusion

Pleural effusion describes fluid (transudative or exudative) within the pleural space. Pleural effusion usually results from an underlying disease, such as heart failure, or from medical disorders leading to hypoalbuminemia.[214] It may also be caused by infection (bacterial or mycobacterial), malignancy, collagen vascular disease, pancreatitis, or pulmonary embolism.[215]

Pleural effusions may be asymptomatic but, if large, produce breathlessness or pain, or both.[214] Breath sounds are reduced on the affected side, and the percussion note is stony dull.[214]

Intervention usually involves drainage of the fluid.

Acute Disk Herniation

Disk lesions account for a high percentage of the causes of anterior and posterior thoracic pain syndromes (see Chap. 27).[216] Thoracic disk herniations do not have a characteristic clinical presentation, and the symptomatology may be confused with other diagnoses. In a review of the literature, covering 280 cases of thoracic disk herniation,[217] only 23% had sensory symptoms, most commonly numbness, paresthesias, or dysesthesias. A thoracic disk herniation can produce posterior, anterior, or radicular (bilateral or unilateral) pain, which can be so severe as to mimic a myocardial infarction. All movements are severely limited and extremely painful and may reproduce radicular pain.

Vertebral Fracture

A high percentage of spinal fractures involve the thoracolumbar spine. Fractures of the thoracolumbar spine can be classified into four groups according to mechanism:

- *Flexion compression (wedge of compression fracture).* Compression fractures are relatively benign, because they involve only the anterior column, with varying degrees of middle and posterior column insult. They are thought to occur because of the relative stiffness of the thoracic spine compared with the greater mobility of the neighboring lumbar spine.[218] These fractures, which most commonly occur in the mid-thoracic and mid-lumbar spine, are typically stable, unless severe. Diagnosis is confirmed with a lateral radiograph, which demonstrates anterior wedging. Burst fractures involve both the anterior and the middle columns and also may involve ligamentous or bony injury of the posterior column. Although the mechanism for this type of fracture is the same as for compression fractures, the axial loading is of a greater magnitude and typically is combined with flexion. Consequently, the anterior body undergoes a bursting effect, with retropulsion of part of the posterior vertebral body wall (middle column) into the canal, decreasing the canal size.[219]
- *Axial compression.* This type usually results in a burst fracture involving failure of both the anterior and the middle columns. Both columns are compressed, and the result is a loss of height of the vertebral body.
- *Flexion distraction.* This type results in an injury called a Chance (or seatbelt) fracture, involving failure of the posterior column with injury to the ligamentous components, bony components, or both.

- Rotational fracture dislocation. This type results from a combination of side flexion and rotation with or without involvement of a posterior-anteriorly directed force. Osteoporosis causes fractures of the vertebrae.

Osteoporotic fractures are most common in the mid to low thoracic spine and result from the inability of the vertebral body to sustain the compression forces involved with everyday activities.[58] The prevalence rate for these fractures increases steadily with age, ranging from 20% for 50-year-old women to 65% for older women.[220] Most vertebral fractures do not have a history of an identifiable trauma (sensitivity, 0.30).[32] Many patients remain undiagnosed and present with symptoms such as back pain and increased kyphosis. Fractures that occur at the levels of T1–T10 can have associated damage to the spinal cord, whereas fractures at T11–T12 can manifest as mixed spinal cord, conus medullaris, or spinal nerve root injuries.[221]

Rib Fracture

Rib fractures are very common in the blunt trauma population, with one review demonstrating that 10% of patients admitted to a level 2 trauma center had evidence of rib fractures.[222] However, the true incidence of rib fractures is not known, because up to 50% of rib fractures may be missed on a standard chest X-ray film.[223] The primary symptom of a rib fracture is pain on inspiration, resulting in hypoventilation.[221] On physical examination, there is local tenderness, crepitation, and, on occasion, a palpable defect.

Stress Fracture of the Rib

There are more reports of stress fractures of the first rib than any other single rib.[224] A contraction of the anterior scalene muscle produces bending forces at the subclavian sulcus, which is the usual site of the fracture.[225] This mechanism usually occurs in overhead activities, such as pitching, basketball, tennis, or weightlifting.[226,227]

Pain occurs in the region of the shoulder, anterior cervical triangle, or clavicular region.[227] The pain may radiate to the sternum or pectoral region. The onset is usually insidious, although it may start with acute pain. Pain may occur with deep breathing.[228]

Tenderness to palpation may be present medial to the superior angle of the scapula, at the base of the neck, supraclavicular triangle, or deep in the axilla.[224] Shoulder movements may be painful or restricted.

The recommended treatment of a first rib stress fracture involves immobilization of the shoulder girdle on the affected side with a sling.[224] Pain resolves within 2–8 weeks of immobilization.[227]

Stress fractures of the other ribs may also occur. The most common cause is a change in technique or training load. Examination may reveal local tenderness to palpation. Rib springing is usually positive for pain.

Intercostal Neuralgia

Neurogenic pain of the thorax can be the result of infection, such as varicella zoster (shingles), mechanical compression of the nerve by a disk protrusion, an osteophyte, a neuroma, a fracture, or a condition called *postherpetic neuralgia*. Neuralgic pain, which typically has a burning quality, is unchanged by analgesics or rest.

Epidemic Myalgia

Epidemic myalgia, also known as epidemic pleurodynia or Bornholm disease, is characterized by the abrupt onset of chest or abdominal pain, usually accompanied by fever, and was first described in the late 1800s.[229] This acute viral illness is caused mainly by Coxsackie B virus, but other enteroviruses may be implicated.[224] The mode of transmission is via a shared water source,[230] and there is a 3–5-day incubation period. Peak incidence is during the soccer and American football seasons, and outbreaks involving athletic teams have been reported.[230]

Presentation usually follows a nonspecific prodromal illness (early set of symptoms), with sudden onset of sharp lateral chest or abdominal pains.[224] The intercostal and upper abdominal wall muscles are most commonly involved, with the pleura being involved rarely.[231] The pain is intermittent and exacerbated by movement, coughing, and deep inspiration.[224] It is accompanied by fever and malaise.

Diagnosis is made by isolation of the virus from the feces or on throat swab in the early stages of the disease. The condition is self-limiting and rarely requires any specific treatment.[224] Symptoms usually resolve after a few days but may recur.

Costochondritis

Costochondritis is a common but poorly understood condition that manifests as chest wall pain. It is usually characterized by pain and tenderness on the costochondral or chondrosternal joints in the absence of swelling. The second to fifth costal cartilages are the most commonly affected.[231]

Diagnosis is based on a history of chest pain with associated anterior chest wall tenderness that is localized to the costochondral junction of one or more ribs. Swelling, heat, and erythema usually are absent. The pain may be provoked by certain movements, such as adduction of the arm on the affected side, with accompanying rotation of the head to the same side.[224]

Costochondritis is a mostly benign, self-limiting condition. Symptoms usually resolve within 1 year.[232]

Osteoarthritis

OA of the thoracic spine affects three sites: the intervertebral disk, the zygapophyseal joints, and the articulations of the rib with the vertebral body and transverse process.[216]

Osteoarthritic changes in the zygapophyseal and costovertebral joints occur most commonly at T11 and L1, which coincides with those joints whose orientation is more sagittal, and the area that sustains the peak incidence of traumatic fractures in the thoracic spine.[218,233] OA of the costovertebral and costotransverse joints is a frequent source of chronic pain but is not typically associated with neurologic changes.[216] This condition is associated with local pain and tenderness at the site of degeneration. Rib joint pain typically is exacerbated by exaggerated respiratory movements.[234]

Spondylosis, disk degeneration, and Schmorl nodes are most frequently encountered within the T10–T12 vertebrae,[233] probably as a result of a reduced resistance to torsion in this area.[235]

The relationship between zygapophyseal joint orientation and OA suggests that repeated torsional trauma might well have a significant role in the development of OA in zygapophyseal joints that are sagittally oriented.[233]

Rheumatoid Arthritis

Thoracic pain related to RA is associated with pain and stiffness that is greatest in the morning and usually improves with movement.[216,236] Inspection usually shows a flat thoracolumbar spine, and a gross limitation of side flexion in both directions is demonstrated.

Ankylosing Spondylitis

See section "Ankylosing Spondylitis" earlier in the chapter.

Diffuse Idiopathic Skeletal Hyperostosis

Diffuse idiopathic skeletal hyperostosis, or Forestier disease, is a metabolic disease that typically affects men older than 40 years and does not usually result in severe disability.[237] The disease is characterized by an ossification of the anterior longitudinal ligaments and all related, anatomically similar ligaments,[216] without marked disk disease, which results in overall stiffness of the spine, particularly in the morning, and palpable tenderness.

Manubriosternal Dislocations

Traumatic disruption of the manubriosternal joint most often occur via one of two mechanisms.[238,239] The first and most common mechanism results from a direct compression injury to the anterior chest. The direction of applied force displaces the fragment posteriorly and downward. The second type of mechanism follows hyperflexion with compression injury to the upper thorax. The force is transmitted to the sternum through the clavicles, chin, or upper two ribs.

CAUSES OF LUMBAR PAIN

Numerous potential disorders may cause low back discomfort, as indicated in Fig. 5-1 and Table 5-11.

TABLE 5-11 Potential Causes of Lumbar Pain
Renal dysfunction
Colorectal cancer
Epidural abscess and epidural hematoma
Sacroiliitis
Metastasis
Maigne syndrome
Aortic or iliac aneurysm
Prostatitis
Pleural dysfunction
Ankylosing spondylitis
Stiff-person syndrome

Renal Origin

Pain of renal origin is associated with pelvic, flank, or LBP.

Acute Pyelonephritis

See the discussion of pyelonephritis under "Causes of Head, Face, Eye, and Temporomandibular Joint Symptoms" earlier.

Renal Cortical Abscess

Renal abscess has been described as an elusive diagnosis in patients with variable symptoms of insidious onset. This condition can cause flank pain, chills, and fever and may be associated with a history of recent infection.

Urologic management of renal abscesses includes surgical exploration, percutaneous drainage, intravenous antibiotic therapy, or nephrectomy.[240,241]

Acute Glomerulonephritis

This condition occasionally can manifest with bilateral flank pain, costovertebral angle tenderness, and fever. Malaise, fatigue, anorexia, and nausea frequently accompany this condition.

Ureteral Colic

Ureteral colic causes constant severe pain in the right lower abdomen. The pain is caused by passage of a calculus (kidney stone), blood clot, or tissue fragment in the lower half of the ureter. The pain, which may be intermittent, radiates down the course of the ureter into the urethra or groin area. Accompanying signs and symptoms include nausea, vomiting, sweating, and tachycardia.

Kidney stones are associated with conditions of hypercalcemia (excess calcium in the blood) such as hyperparathyroidism, metastatic carcinoma, multiple myeloma, senile osteoporosis, specific renal tubular disease, hyperthyroidism, and Cushing disease.[12] Other conditions associated with calculus formation are infection, urinary stasis, dehydration, and excessive ingestion or absorption of calcium.[12]

Urinary Tract Infection

A urinary tract infection (UTI) affecting the lower urinary tract is related directly to an irritation of the bladder and the urethra. The intensity of symptoms depends on the severity of the infection, and, although LBP may be the patient's chief complaint, further questioning usually elicits additional urologic symptoms, such as urinary frequency, urinary urgency, or hematuria. The diagnosis of UTI is based on symptoms and the presence of pathogens and white blood cells in urine.

Epidural Abscess

Most spinal epidural abscesses or infections are thought to result from the spread of bacteria, usually from a cutaneous or mucosal source. Infection in the spinal epidural space is an uncommon but potentially fatal condition that often constitutes a surgical emergency. The infectious agent may enter the epidural space by several routes[242]:

- Insertion of an epidural needle and catheter
- Migration along the outside of a catheter
- Local spread through soft tissue and bone
- Hematogenous spread
- Injection or infusion of contaminated fluid

Early diagnosis is essential for successful treatment.[243] The diagnosis of spinal abscess can be difficult because of its rarity and the insidious presentation. The signs and symptoms may develop slowly over days to several weeks. Fever is not always present.[244] Localized back pain or radicular pain is frequently the first sign of epidural infection.[244,245] This initial finding is followed by progressive radicular and cord compression signs.[244,245] Pain is the most consistent symptom and occurs in virtually all patients at some time during their illness.[243]

Intervention depends on the cause and ranges from antibiotic therapy to surgery.

Prostatitis

Prostatitis is an inflammation of the prostate gland. The cause of the inflammation is usually infection, which can be bacterial or nonbacterial. In acute bacterial prostatitis, patients complain of a sudden onset of fever, chills, and low back or perineal pain. Typically, dysuria, frequency, or hesitancy is present. Patients with chronic bacterial prostatitis may have no systemic symptoms; that is, they may not have fever or chills, although complaints of perineal or LBP usually are present. Patients with nonbacterial prostatitis have a variable presentation and lack systemic symptoms. These patients have mild pain and may have voiding symptoms.

Differential diagnosis includes prostatodynia, cystitis, urethritis, and benign prostatic hypertrophy.

Pleural Dysfunction

Although usually associated with thoracic pain, pleuritic pain can produce right lower abdomen pain. The cause is usually pneumonia or pulmonary embolism. The symptoms accompanying pneumonia include fever, coughing, rales, wheezes, chills, and purulent sputum. Pulmonary embolism is usually associated with dyspnea, fever, cough, rales, and wheezes. High-risk patients for pulmonary embolism include those with recent

- trauma;
- surgery;
- pregnancy;
- heart failure;
- malignancy;
- previous embolism;
- prolonged travel in automobile or airplane;
- prolonged immobilization.

Aortic Aneurysm

The anatomy of the aorta is segmentally described in three sections: ascending aorta, aortic arch, and descending aorta. The portion of the aorta above the diaphragm is designated as thoracic, and the abdominal aorta is that portion below the diaphragm. The aorta consists of three layers: adventitia (the outermost), media, and intima.

An acute aortic dissection is caused by a transverse disruption in the intima and media.[246] This disruption results in the formation of a hematoma within the media. Aortic aneurysms can be described as either fusiform (circumferential dilatation) or saccular (balloon-like).[247]

The underlying causes of aortic disease are associated with many factors, including atherosclerosis, hypertension, medial degeneration and aging, aortitis, congenital abnormalities, trauma, smoking, cellular enzyme dysfunction, and hyperlipidemia.[246]

Acute aortic dissection is characterized by the onset of intense pain, described as sharp, tearing, or stabbing. The pain occurs in the chest and spreads toward the back and into the abdomen. The pain associated with this condition is unaffected by position. Distal pulses frequently are decreased or absent. This is a potentially life-threatening condition, requiring immediate transport of the patient to an emergency department. The patient is admitted to the intensive care unit for further evaluation and to temporarily manage the crisis with antihypertensive medications.[246]

Metastasis

Malignant neoplasm (primary or metastatic) is the most common systemic disease affecting the spine, although it accounts for less than 1% of episodes of LBP.[32] Metastatic lesions affecting the lumbar spine occur most commonly from the ovary, breast, kidney, thyroid, lung, or prostate gland. According to a study by Deyo and Diehl[248] that reviewed 1,975 consecutive patients seeking medical care for LBP, the four clinical findings with the highest positive likelihood ratios for detecting the presence of cancer resulting in LBP were a previous history of cancer, failure to improve with conservative medical treatment during the past month, an age of at least 50 years or older, and unexplained weight loss of more than 4.5 kg (10 lb) in 6 months.[248] The absence of all four of these findings confidently rules out malignancy.[248,249]

Ankylosing Spondylitis

See section “Ankylosing Spondylitis” earlier in the chapter.

Stiff-Person Syndrome

Stiff-person syndrome (SPS), also known as Moersch–Woltmann syndrome, or stiff-man syndrome is a rare, disabling neurological disorder, which is often underdiagnosed because of a lack of awareness of its clinical manifestations. Variants of the syndrome may involve one limb only (stiff-leg syndrome) or a variety of additional neurological symptoms and signs such as eye movement disturbances, ataxia, or Babinski signs (progressive encephalomyelitis with rigidity and myoclonus) or be associated with malignant disease (paraneoplastic SPS).[250]

SPS has an insidious onset, usually in the fourth or fifth decades, with a slow progression over months or years, followed by long-lasting stabilization. SPS is characterized by fluctuating symmetrical muscle rigidity and back pain with superimposed painful episodic spasms of the axial and proximal limb muscles.[251]

- The muscle rigidity associated with SPS can lead to contractures, and simultaneous contraction of the thoracolumbar paraspinal and abdominal wall muscles causes lumbar hyperlordosis.
- The episodic spasms, which are often provoked by noise, touch, emotional upset, or sudden movement, may manifest as an excessive startle reaction. These spasms can be violent enough to cause excruciating pain and, in rare cases, generate forces capable of fracturing long bones. Patients with SPS may exhibit excessive fear and avoidance of circumscribed situations that are assumed by patients to be difficult to master because of an increase in stiffness, paroxysmal spasms, or sudden falls.[252] Such situations include crossing a street, climbing downstairs without banisters, or walking unaided. Patients may be incapacitated by the phobia to the same degree as the motor symptoms themselves. It has been suggested that the presence of this particular anxiety is one of the reasons for the frequent misdiagnosis of *psychogenic movement disorder* in these patients.[252]

The rigidity and spasms gradually impair voluntary movements and postural reflexes, resulting in slow, restricted movements and an increased risk of falls. Intellect is not affected, and motor and sensory nerve examination is also normal. However, almost all patients have an abnormal electromyographic (EMG) pattern, which shows continuous motor unit activity in affected muscles.

The cause of SPS is unknown, but an autoimmune-mediated chronic encephalomyelitis is suggested due to its frequent association with other autoimmune disorders such as type 1 diabetes or thyroiditis.

The mainstays of treatment for SPS are drugs that enhance GABA-mediated central inhibition (diazepam, baclofen, sodium valproate, and vigabatrin) and antispastic physical therapy. SPS should be considered in all patients with unexplained back pain, stiffness, and muscle spasms, as early recognition and therapeutic intervention can significantly decrease morbidity and improve quality of life. Stiffness and spasms resembling SPS may occur as dominant symptoms in a variety of recognized neurological diseases such as MS, brain stem or spinal cord tumors, and paraneoplastic or circulatory diseases of the spinal cord.[250]

CAUSES OF BUTTOCK AND UPPER AND LOWER LEG PAIN

The causes for buttock and upper and lower leg pain include those listed in Fig. 5-1 and Table 5-12.

TABLE 5-12 Potential Causes of Buttock and Upper- and Lower-Leg Pain
Femoral nerve neuropathy
Lumbar disk herniation
Piriformis syndrome
Intermittent claudication
Sacral plexopathy
Conus medullaris syndrome
Trochanteric bursitis
Meralgia paresthetica
Iliofemoral thrombophlebitis
Sacroiliitis
Mononeuritis multiplex
Ischial apophysis and avulsion
Gluteal compartment syndrome
Genital herpes
Vascular disorders

Lumbar Disk Herniation

See Chapter 28.

Femoral Nerve Neuropathy

Femoral neuropathy has been described as a complication of compression resulting from[253]

- hematoma;
- hemophilia;
- leukemia;
- hysterectomy and pelvic surgery;
- lithotomy position;
- blunt trauma;
- iliac artery aneurysm;
- inguinal herniorrhaphy;
- malignancy and radiation therapy;
- Epstein–Barr virus infection;
- diabetes mellitus.

Typical signs of femoral neuropathy are weakness of ipsilateral hip flexion, knee extension, and paresthesias of the anteromedial thigh. Symptoms may vary with both degree and location of injury. The more distal injuries may have either sensory or motor symptoms, whereas the proximal injuries tend to have both. A decreased or absent knee jerk is usually present. The differential diagnoses of upper lumbar nerve root symptoms include spondylolisthesis, disk prolapse, or an infective cause such as diskitis or an epidural abscess.

Piriformis Syndrome

The "piriformis syndrome," a fairly common but often undiagnosed cause of buttock and leg pain, has been described as an anatomic abnormality of the piriformis muscle and the sciatic nerve, which can result in irritation of the sciatic nerve by the piriformis muscle causing buttock and hamstring pain. Piriformis syndrome may also be described as a sensation in which the hamstring muscles feel "tight" or are "about to tear."[254]

Multiple etiologies have been proposed to explain the compression or irritation of the sciatic nerve that occurs with the piriformis syndrome[255]:

- ***Hypertrophy of the piriformis muscle.***[256,257]
- ***Overuse of the piriformis muscle.*** Although there is disagreement, overuse seems to be the most common cause of piriformis syndrome.[258] This suggests that patients must be effectively cautioned about returning too quickly to the type of activity that bought about the piriformis syndrome once recovered.
- ***Trauma.***[259–261] Trauma, direct or indirect, to the sacroiliac or gluteal region can lead to piriformis syndrome and is a result of hematoma formation and subsequent scarring between the sciatic nerve and the short external rotators.
- ***Hip flexion contracture.*** A flexion contracture at the hip has been associated with piriformis syndrome. This flexion contracture increases the lumbar lordosis, which increases the tension in the pelvic–femoral muscles, as these muscles try to stabilize the pelvis and spine in the new position. This increased tension causes the involved muscles to hypertrophy with no corresponding increase in the size of the bony foramina, resulting in neurological signs of sciatic compression.[262]
- ***Gender.*** Females are more commonly affected by piriformis syndrome, with as much as a 6:1 female-to-male incidence.[261,263–266]
- ***Ischial bursitis.***
- ***Pseudoaneurysm of the inferior gluteal artery.***[259]
- ***Excessive exercise to the hamstring muscles.***[267]
- ***Inflammation and spasm of the piriformis muscle.***[268] This is often in association with trauma,[256,269] infection, and anatomical variations of the muscle.[262,270,271]
- ***Anatomical anomalies.*** In 1938, anomalies of the piriformis muscle, with a subsequent alteration in the relationship between the piriformis muscle and the sciatic nerve, were implicated in sciatica.[270] Local anatomical anomalies may contribute to the likelihood that symptoms will develop. Patients with this condition report radicular pain that is much like the nerve-root pain associated with lumbar disk disease with movement of the hip.[272] These patients typically present with a history of gluteal trauma, symptoms of pain in the buttock and intolerance to sitting, tenderness to palpation of the greater sciatic notch, and pain with flexion, adduction, and internal rotation of the hip.

As early as 1937, two findings on physical examination were attributed to sciatic pain, with the piriformis as the cause[273]:

1. Positive straight-leg raise (pain in the vicinity of the greater sciatic notch on extension of the knee, with the hip flexed to 90 degrees and tenderness to palpation of the greater sciatic notch).
2. Freiberg sign (pain with passive internal rotation of the hip).

Robinson[269] has been credited with introducing the term *piriformis syndrome* and outlining its six classic findings:

1. A history of trauma to the sacroiliac and gluteal regions.
2. Pain in the region of the sacroiliac joint, greater sciatic notch, and piriformis muscle that usually causes difficulty with walking.
3. Acute exacerbation of pain caused by stooping or lifting (and moderate relief of pain by traction on the affected extremity with the patient in the supine position).
4. A palpable sausage-shaped mass, tender to palpation, over the piriformis muscle on the affected side.
5. A positive straight-leg raise.
6. Gluteal atrophy, depending on the duration of the condition.

Other clinical signs have since been introduced. Pace and Nagle[261] described a diagnostic maneuver that is now referred to as the Pace sign: pain and weakness in association with resisted abduction and external rotation of the involved thigh.

Local muscle spasm usually is palpable in the obturator internus or, less commonly, in the piriformis muscle. The neurologic examination is usually normal.[254] An examination of the hip and lower leg usually demonstrates restricted internal rotation of the hip and lumbosacral muscle tightness.[254]

Botulinum neurotoxins have been successfully used in clinical practice to reduce the strength of idiopathic muscular spasm and muscle tightness caused by overuse, trauma, or occupation in the piriformis muscle.[274,275] Currently, the use of botulinum neurotoxins in MPSs focuses on the myoneural junctions of intrafusal muscle fibers.[276] One study showed that this form of injection followed by physical therapy significantly shortens recovery time, thereby reducing both the patient's pain and treatment time.[276]

The physical therapy intervention for this condition is described in Chapter 19.

Sacral Plexopathy

The sciatic nerve is the most frequently injured lower extremity nerve. Sciatic nerve compression has been reported secondary to piriformis entrapment, heterotopic ossification around the hip,[277] a ruptured aneurysm, retroperitoneal bleeding, pelvic fracture, dislocation or fracture of the hip, tumor, misplaced intramuscular injections, myofascial bands in the distal thigh,[278] and myositis ossificans of the biceps femoris muscle.[279] Additional causes include post-traumatic or anticoagulant-induced extraneural hematomas[280] and compartment syndrome of the posterior thigh.[281] Entrapment sciatic neuropathy complicating total hip arthroplasty has been described secondary to escaped cement, subfascial hematoma, and nerve impingement during trochanteric wiring.[282]

In the usual situation, the patient complains of an immediate onset of painful paresthesia, radiating down the posterior and posterolateral thigh and calf, and into the foot. Differential diagnosis also includes an L5–S1 radiculopathy caused by a herniated disk or zygapophyseal joint disease with lateral recess or foramen stenosis.

Intermittent Claudication

The blood supply of the lumbar and sacral plexuses usually derives from branches of the internal iliac artery (iliolumbar artery, superior and inferior gluteal artery, and lateral sacral artery) and the deep iliac circumflex artery.[283] Acute ischemic impairments of the lumbosacral plexus are caused by high-grade stenosis and occlusion of the iliac arteries or of the distal abdominal aorta.

The most frequent cause of such acute ischemic impairments of the lumbosacral plexus is surgery of the aortic bifurcation and the pelvic arteries, or radiation therapy.[284] Finally, intraarterial injections into the iliac arteries or gluteal arteries may result in persistent ischemic plexopathy.[285]

Reduced perfusion within the area of the internal iliac artery can result in a temporary ischemic impairment of the lumbosacral plexus. This impairment occurs only during muscular activity of the legs. In this condition, the pain is mostly localized to the pelvis and is followed by paresthesia, a diminishing of the muscle stretch reflexes, with possible motor weakness. This special type of intermittent claudication is usually associated with stenosis of the pelvic arteries, including the internal iliac arteries.[285]

The diagnosis is confirmed by changes in the lumbar motor-evoked potentials after exertion. These changes exclude the diagnosis of ischemia of the lower spinal cord or conus medullaris.

Peripheral nerves have a high tolerance to ischemia because of collateral circulation.[286] However, during leg activity, the muscles supplied by branches of the external iliac arteries experience a steal phenomenon that privileges the leg muscles over the pelvic organs.[285]

Although the neurologic examination of the inactive patient usually discloses no abnormality, the clinical diagnosis of this type of intermittent claudication caused by exercise-induced ischemia of the lumbosacral plexus is based mainly on two specific features[285]:

1. The symptoms appear in correlation with the degree of muscle activity. In early stages of the disease, complaints only occur during walking uphill or riding a bicycle. This allows a distinction from the intermittent claudication caused by spinal stenosis. In the latter, symptoms predominantly appear during walking downhill. In addition, patients with spinal stenosis can ride a bicycle for a long distance without complaints.
2. In addition to pain, progressive sensorimotor deficits in the area of the lumbosacral plexus occur during exertion. This cannot be seen in patients with peripheral arterial occlusive disease.

Conus Medullaris Syndrome

Conus medullaris syndrome results from an injury to the spinal cord. The injury can be caused by trauma, such as bone or bullet fragments. It may also result from cyst formation, aortic surgery, and vascular disease.

The symptoms include severe low back and buttock pain, lower limb weakness, and saddle hyperesthesia or anesthesia. Bowel and bladder changes are also frequently reported.

Meralgia Paresthetica

The term *meralgia paresthetica* comes from the Greek words *meros* (thigh) and *algos* (pain). Meralgia paresthetica is a syndrome of pain and/or dysesthesia caused by entrapment or neurinoma formation of the lateral cutaneous (femoral) nerve (LCFN) of the thigh.[287–289] It is also known as Bernhardt–Roth syndrome. Although more commonly involving the LCFN, meralgia paresthetica can also occur to other nerves that traverse the hip, such as the ilioinguinal, genitofemoral, obturator, and anterior cutaneous nerves of the thigh.[290]

The LCFN is primarily a sensory nerve but also includes efferent sympathetic fibers carrying vasomotor, pilomotor, and sudomotor impulses.[291] It is quite variable and may be derived from several different combinations of lumbar nerves, including L2 and L3, L1 and L2, L2 alone, and L3 alone.[292] The LCFN may be associated with the femoral nerve as it passes through the inguinal ligament, or it may anastomose with the femoral nerve distal to the inguinal ligament.[289]

The compression of the nerve, which is most common in middle-aged men, may be at the level of the roots, but it may also be compressed along the retroperitoneal course.

Numerous direct and indirect causes for the disease have been suggested in the literature, including[293–297]

- obesity;
- ascites;
- direct trauma;
- abdominal distention, including pregnancy;
- abdominopelvic tumors or inflammations; it may occur as the first sign of a lumbar cord tumor;
- metastatic carcinoma in the iliac crest;
- anatomic variation at the site of passage[295];
- retroperitoneal tumors;
- leg-length discrepancy;
- idiopathic causes;
- tight clothing around the waist;
- complications after thoracoabdominal surgery;
- complications after iliac bone graft harvesting.

Toxic and metabolic disorders, such as diabetes mellitus, alcoholism, and lead poisoning, which have been reported to be causative in several cases, have all been described to increase susceptibility of individual peripheral nerves, including the LCFN, to mechanical insults.[298,299]

Neuropathy of this nerve may cause pain, numbness, and dysesthesia in the anterolateral aspect of the thigh, which is most marked on walking, standing, and sleeping in the prone position.[300] Sitting may relieve the symptoms in some patients but exacerbate them in others depending on the cause. Eventually, no position provides relief. Patients may have secondary hip, knee, and calf pain. Entrapment of the lateral cutaneous nerve of the thigh can also be the cause of chronic groin pain.[301–303]

Differential diagnosis includes back, hip, and groin pathology. Meralgia paresthetica symptoms may be confused with more frequently seen symptoms produced by entrapment of the upper lumbar nerve roots.[304,305]

Intervention is dependent on the cause.

Iliofemoral Thrombophlebitis

Thrombophlebitis of the superficial veins of the leg is usually regarded as a mild and uncomplicated disease. Although this is generally true in the case of acute thrombosis of the branches of the saphenous vein, the natural history of superficial venous thrombophlebitis involving the main trunk may not be as benign. The relationship between superficial venous thrombophlebitis and deep venous thrombosis (DVT) with attendant pulmonary embolus has become the focus of more recent studies. An association with DVT has been reported with frequencies of 12–44%,[306] and there have been several reports of pulmonary embolism in thrombophlebitis.[307]

The clinical signs and symptoms of iliofemoral thrombophlebitis include generalized leg pain, bluish discoloration, and swelling of the lower extremities. This condition may also be associated with acute lower abdominal, groin and flank pain, fever, chills, and localized tenderness.

Mononeuritis Multiplex

Mononeuritis multiplex can occur in association with a number of other medical conditions, including RA, vasculitis, polyarteritis nodosa, diabetes mellitus, sarcoidosis, and amyloidosis. An ischemic mechanism is the most likely cause of mononeuritis multiplex. It is generally accepted that mononeuritis multiplex in RA results from ischemia caused by vasa nervorum vasculitis. Involvement of peripheral nerves precedes involvement of the CNS. The classic symptoms for mononeuritis multiplex include a sudden onset of severe aching, burning or lancinating leg pain, paresthesias, sensory loss, and motor weakness.[308] The symptoms can involve one or more nerves in each leg, usually in an asymmetric pattern.[308]

Ischial Apophysitis and Avulsion

The ischial apophysis constitutes the insertion of the hamstrings and the adductor magnus muscles. Ischial tuberosity pain may be caused by several clinical entities, which include acute and old bony or periosteal avulsions and apophysitis. The clinical diagnostic criterion for ischial apophysitis consists of a gradual increase in functional and palpatory pain at the ischial tuberosity, without any major trauma at the beginning of the symptoms. Usually, there is asymmetry on plain radiographs of the ischial tuberosities in apophysitis. The radiograph demonstrates a sclerotic area and osteoporotic patches on the lower margin of the ischial tuberosity. Patients with an avulsion usually report an acute traumatic incident. An avulsion fragment may be visible on plain radiograph immediately after injury or later. The pain is usually local but may also radiate down the thigh. Active or resisted knee flexion increases the pain, unless the avulsion is complete. Complete avulsions can be painless.

The healing process of an avulsion may lead to heterotrophic bone formation.

Differential diagnosis includes intervertebral disk disease, piriformis syndrome, ischial bursitis, and pubic arch stress fracture.

Conservative intervention for apophysitis consists of modification of activities. Avulsions require at least 1 month of rest from training, depending on the displacement. Urgent surgical intervention is recommended in cases of a complete or nearly complete soft-tissue avulsion of the hamstring muscle.[309]

Gluteal Compartment Syndrome

The characteristic finding for a gluteal compartment syndrome is a tense, swollen buttock following a mechanism of severe contusion, such as a fall from a height.[310] The swelling in the buttock can result in necrosis of the gluteal muscles or sciatic neuropathy, or both. The patient should be referred immediately to an orthopaedic surgeon. A fasciotomy is typically performed if the pressure within the gluteal compartment is 30 mm Hg or higher for a duration of 6–8 hours.[311]

Genital Herpes

Genital herpes is a chronic, viral, sexually transmitted disease for which there is no cure. It affects over 30 million people in the United States and continues to increase worldwide.[312] The majority of individuals are asymptomatic; however, some present with painful and recurrent genital lesions and systemic complications. As a chronic illness, the individual's response to the disease may produce serious psychosocial morbidity.[313] Women are more likely to have genital herpes than men.[314]

Vascular Disorders

Gradual obstruction of the aortic bifurcation produces[12]

- bilateral buttock and leg pain;
- weakness and fatigue of the lower extremities;
- atrophy of the leg musculature;
- absent femoral pulses;
- color and temperature changes in the lower extremities;
- pain that is often aggravated with lumbar extension;
- a pulsing sensation in the abdomen. On occasion, an abdominal aortic aneurysm can cause severe back pain. Prompt medical attention is imperative because rupture can result in death. The patients are usually men in their sixth or seventh decade, who present with a deep, boring pain in the mid-lumbar region. Other historical clues of coronary disease or intermittent claudication of the lower extremities may be present. An examination may reveal a pulsing abdominal mass.
- peripheral pulses may be diminished or absent.[315]

Involvement of the femoral artery along its course, or at the femoral–popliteal junction, produces[12]

- thigh and calf pain;
- absent pulses below the femoral pulse.

Obstruction of the popliteal artery or its branches produces pain in the calf, ankle, or foot.

CAUSES OF PELVIC PAIN

The causes of pelvic pain include those listed in Fig. 5-1 and Table 5-13.

Sacroiliac Arthritis

Sacroiliac arthritis is characterized by pain in the posterior aspect of the sacrum, or by groin pain (uncommon), which can

TABLE 5-13 Potential Causes of Pelvic Pain
Sacroiliac arthritis
Acute appendicitis
Iliopsoas abscess
Iliopsoas hematoma
Sign of the buttock
Gynecologic disorders
Prostate cancer

radiate into the posterior thigh. The pain is usually increased with walking, either at heel strike or at midstance. Frequently the pain wakes the patient when turning in bed.

Lumbar extension is the most painful motion, ipsilateral side bending and rotation less so, and flexion least of all. If pain is increased with unilateral weight bearing or hopping but is reduced if a sacroiliac belt is worn, sacroiliac joint arthritis may be present.

The sacroiliac joint stress tests described in Chapter 27 are used to help with the clinical diagnosis. Imaging studies are used to confirm the diagnosis.

Acute Appendicitis

This condition frequently begins with dull and aching pain in the right lower abdomen. The pain is intensified with walking, coughing, and trunk movements. There is usually an associated low-grade fever. Dysuria, diarrhea, constipation, or increased urinary frequency also may be reported. The patient is often able to localize the pain to McBurney point, which is located by palpation at the midpoint between the anterior superior iliac spine and the umbilicus.

Less common signs include rectal or testicular tenderness and right lower abdominal skin hyperesthesia.

Iliopsoas Abscess

The pain associated with an iliopsoas abscess occurs in the right lower abdomen. The pain is usually mild to moderate and is increased with hip extension and palpation in the right iliac fossa. The abscess is caused by an infection of the thoracolumbar spine, such as tuberculosis, or is secondary to an intestinal disorder, such as Crohn disease.[316]

Iliopsoas Hematoma

Hematomas are more frequently seen in the iliacus muscle than the psoas.[317] The causes of these hematomas include

- heparin anticoagulation or DVT prophylaxis therapy;
- hemophilia;
- trauma from either a direct blow to the abdomen or a hyperextension moment at the hip, such as occurs in a slip or fall.

Nontraumatic hematomas often manifest insidiously with no obvious lesion or ecchymosis. Patients initially may complain of flank pain but frequently will develop motor and sensory deficits along the femoral nerve distribution of the affected side. Flank pain refers to pain in the side of the trunk between the right or left upper abdomen and the back. A palpable lower abdominal mass may be present, depending on the size and location of the hematoma.

Iliopsoas hematomas have been successfully managed with conservative treatment. This intervention involves bed rest for 24–48 hours, followed by gentle hip range of motion exercises. Progressive strengthening exercises are then initiated according to patient tolerance.

Surgical intervention involves evacuation of the clot.

Sign of the Buttock

The sign of the buttock is not technically a cause of pain but is, rather, a collection of signs indicating a serious pathology present posterior to the axis of flexion and extension in the hip.[318] Among the causes of the syndrome are osteomyelitis, infectious sacroiliitis, fracture of the sacrum or pelvis, septic bursitis, ischiorectal abscess, gluteal hematoma, gluteal tumor, and rheumatic bursitis.

The sign of the buttock typically includes almost all of the following:

- Limited straight-leg raising
- Limited hip flexion
- Limited trunk flexion
- Noncapsular pattern of restriction at the hip
- Painful and weak hip extension
- Gluteal swelling
- Empty end-feel on hip flexion

Greenwood and colleagues[319] have suggested that a noncapsular pattern of the hip in the presence of a positive sign of the buttock indicates that the pathology is not amenable to a physical therapy intervention.

Gynecologic Disorders

Gynecologic disorders have the potential to cause midpelvic or low back discomfort.

Pelvic Inflammatory Disease

Pelvic inflammatory disease (PID) is the general term describing endometritis, salpingitis, tuboovarian abscess, or pelvic peritonitis. The microbial etiology of PID is unclear but is assumed to occur by the ascending spread of microorganisms from the vagina or endocervix into the upper genital tract.[320] PID has been considered primarily a sexually transmitted disease, caused in large part by the sexually transmitted pathogens *Neisseria gonorrhoeae* and *Chlamydia trachomatis*.[320] However, endogenous microorganisms that are part of the lower genital tract flora can also be recovered from the endometrium, fallopian tubes, and peritoneal fluid of women with acute PID.[320]

The characteristic presentation of PID is one of suprapubic pain. The pain is usually constant or crampy and may be associated with fever, chills, and direct abdominal tenderness.[316] The use of an intrauterine device doubles the risk of endometritis.[316]

The onset of PID is usually within 7 days of the beginning of a menstrual cycle. There may be fever and vaginal discharge.

Tubal Pregnancy

In its early stages, this condition usually produces mild and colicky lower abdominal pain. The pain is caused by an ectopic pregnancy, in which the embryo locates itself in the fallopian tube instead of the uterus. Tubal pregnancy is usually associated with abnormal menstruation and irregular spotting or staining.

Endometriosis

Endometriosis is a common gynecological disorder that affects up to one in seven women and as many as 30–50% of all infertile women.[321] Endometriosis can be found anywhere in the pelvis, including the broad ligaments, uterosacral ligaments, and ovaries. The condition is linked to abdominal, midline, and pelvic pain. The incidence and prevalence of endometriosis are highest in the same age range as that of people with nonspecific LBP.[322] Associated signs and symptoms include pelvic pain, pain on defecation, diarrhea, dysmenorrhea, dyspareunia (difficult or painful coitus), and dysuria.[323] The severity of the pain is not dependent on the stage of the disorder.[324] The diagnosis of endometriosis can be elusive, because its most common symptoms are also symptoms of multiple disorders.[321] Although endometriosis is not considered a malignant disorder, it has characteristics in common with malignant cells. For instance, endometriosis, like cancer, can be both locally and distantly metastatic; it attaches to other tissues, invades, and damages them.[325] Given the associated symptoms with this disorder, it is imperative to include endometriosis as a differential diagnosis in women of reproductive age with pelvic, lower back, and lower extremity pain.[322]

Interstitial Cystitis

Interstitial cystitis is a clinical syndrome of urinary frequency or pelvic pain, or both, in a patient in whom no other pathology can be established. Interstitial cystitis has no single, definable presentation. The pain that occurs with this syndrome is not limited to pain on voiding (dysuria); it can refer to locations throughout the pelvis, including the urethra, vagina, suprapubic area, lower abdomen, lower back, medial aspect of the thigh, and inguinal area, in any combination.[326]

Prostate Cancer

Prostate cancer is the most common nonskin cancer and the second leading cause of male cancer deaths among U.S. men. Risk factors for prostate cancer include age, familial history of cancer, and ethnicity. Whether chronic or recurrent prostatic inflammation contributes to prostate cancer development has not been ascertained.

Prostate cancer is often diagnosed when a man seeks medical assistance because of urinary obstruction or sciatica. The sciatic (low back, hip, and leg) pain is caused by metastasis of the cancer to the bones of the pelvis, lumbar spine, or femur.

Prostate cancer screening or early detection has been accomplished using digital rectal examination, measurement of serum prostate-specific antigen (PSA) and its various forms, transrectal ultrasonography, and combinations of these tests.

- ***Digital rectal examination.*** The vast majority of prostatic carcinomas arise in the peripheral zone of the prostate, which comprises the posterior surface of the gland, including the apical, lateral, posterolateral, and anterolateral portions of the prostate. It is this part of the gland that is accessible by digital rectal examination.
- ***PSA.*** Measurement of PSA levels is regarded widely as the most clinically useful tool for the early diagnosis of prostate cancer. The routine use of serum PSA testing in men beginning at age 50 years has also led to a marked decrease in the age at diagnosis of prostate cancer patients.

CAUSES OF HIP, TROCHANTERIC, PUBIC, AND THIGH PAIN

Potential causes of trochanteric, pubic, and thigh pain include those listed in Fig. 5-2 and Table 5-14. Pain felt in the hip and pelvis may originate from hip structures or may be referred from structures in the torso or viscera.

Dislocation and Fracture-Dislocation of the Hip

A traumatic posterior dislocation of the hip usually occurs in a motor vehicle accident or fall. There is usually severe groin and lateral hip pain. The leg is shortened and held flexed, adducted, and internally rotated. Posterior dislocations are more common than anterior dislocations.

An anterior dislocation usually occurs as the result of forced abduction. Anterior dislocations cause groin pain and tenderness. In a superior–anterior (pubic) dislocation, the leg is held extended and externally rotated. In an inferior–anterior (obturator) dislocation, the thigh is abducted, externally rotated, and held in flexion.

The intervention for a hip dislocation is early closed reduction under spinal or general anesthesia. Congenital dislocations of the hip are described in Chapter 17.

Labral Tear

See Chapter 19.

Hip Fracture

A fracture of the proximal femur (femoral neck, intertrochanteric, or subtrochanteric) usually results from a fall but can occur spontaneously, especially in the elderly. The characteristic findings include severe groin, anterior thigh, and, sometimes, trochanteric pain and tenderness. Fracture of the femoral neck typically occurs in an elderly osteoporotic patient, with a female-to-male ratio of 4:1.[327] Depending on the severity and location of the fracture, there may be a shortening of the involved leg.

Pubic Stress Fracture

Pubic rami fractures are the most commonly seen pubic fractures, with the superior ramus more commonly involved than the inferior ramus. Pubic rami and pubic bone fractures account for more than 70% of all pelvic fractures.[328] Pubic stress fractures are associated with a gradual onset of groin

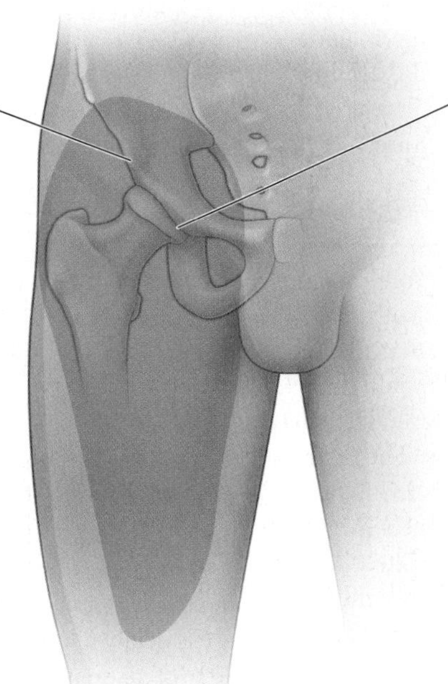

FIGURE 5-2 Potential causes of trochanteric, pubic, and thigh pain.

pain, which is intensified with weight bearing, walking, or abduction of the thigh.

Femoral Neck Stress Fracture

See Chapter 19.

Osteitis Pubis

See Chapter 29.

Adductor Muscle Strain

See Chapter 19.

TABLE 5-14 Potential Causes of Trochanteric, Pubic, and Thigh Pain

Dislocation and fracture dislocation of the hip
Labral tear
Hip or pelvis fracture
Pubic stress fracture
Femoral neck stress fracture
Osteoarthritis of the hip
Septic arthritis of the hip
Reiter syndrome
Transient synovitis of hip in children or adolescents
Avascular necrosis of femoral head
Iliopsoas abscess
Iliofemoral venous thrombosis
Obturator, femoral, or inguinal hernia
Osteomyelitis pubis
Compartment syndrome
Genital herpes

Reiter Syndrome

Reiter syndrome refers to the clinical triad of nongonococcal urethritis, conjunctivitis, and arthritis first described by Reiter in 1916.[329] This form of arthritis usually follows an infection of the genitourinary or gastrointestinal tract. It usually manifests at least one other extra-articular feature, with asymmetric involvement of the large weight-bearing joints.[31] The joints of the mid-foot and the MTP and interphalangeal joints of the toes are most commonly affected. Onset is usually between the ages of 20 and 40, with males predominantly affected.[31]

The association of Reiter syndrome with HLA-B27, occurring in 70–90% of patients, has been recognized for nearly as long as the association of HLA-B27 with AS.[330]

Transient Synovitis of the Hip in Children or Adolescents

Transient synovitis of the hip is one of the most common causes of hip pain and limp in young children. It is defined as an acute, self-limiting inflammation of the synovial lining of the hip joint. The cause of the inflammation is still a subject of great discussion. Proposed causes have included[331]

- virus;
- trauma;
- allergy.

The classic patient with transient synovitis of the hip is a 3–8-year-old boy with a history of acute unilateral hip pain associated with a limp. Anterior thigh or medial knee pain is occasionally the predominant complaint. Because of the pain and the reactive effusion, hip motion is limited. The hip is usually held in a position of flexion and external rotation, so that the hip capsule is lax as much as possible and the elevated intracapsular pressure is slightly relieved.[331]

Transient synovitis usually lasts 3–10 days. The intervention involves methods to alleviate the symptoms. This includes rest, avoidance of weight bearing on the involved extremity, and antiinflammatory therapy. Traction may be considered as a temporary means of relieving pressure on the joint.

OA of the Hip

OA of the hip is one of many causes of hip and groin pain in older patients. It is important to identify patients with symptomatic OA correctly and to exclude conditions that may be mistaken for, or coexist, with it.[332,333] Periarticular pain that is not reproduced by passive motion suggests an alternate etiology such as bursitis, tendonitis, or periostitis. The distribution of painful joints also helps to distinguish OA from other types of arthritis, because metacarpophalangeal (MCP), wrist, elbow, ankle, and shoulder arthritis are unlikely locations for OA, except after trauma. Symptoms that include prolonged morning stiffness (greater than 1 hour) should raise suspicion of an inflammatory arthritis, such as RA.

The primary goals of treatment are to relieve pain, maintain joint function and mobility, and reduce joint swelling. This intervention approach involves focusing on modifying risk factors, particularly obesity, and attempting specific treatments, such as moderate exercise and pharmacotherapy.[334]

Septic Arthritis of the Hip

The clinical presentation of septic arthritis of the hip is similar to that of synovitis of the hip. However, because delayed diagnosis of septic arthritis can be life threatening, correct and early differentiation of septic arthritis and transient synovitis is important.[331] Compared with patients who have transient synovitis, those with septic arthritis usually have more severe pain and spasm. The leg is rigid and is held in the standard flexed and externally rotated position to increase capsular capacity.[331]

Avascular Necrosis of the Femoral Head

Avascular necrosis of the femoral head is also known as aseptic necrosis or osteonecrosis. According to Kenzora and colleagues,[335,336] the term *avascular necrosis* should be reserved exclusively for posttraumatic causes, because they originate in ischemia as a result of blood flow interruption. When the etiology of the necroses has not been established clearly or is obscure, it is best to use the general term *idiopathic osteonecrosis*.

Several etiologic factors have been implicated in the development of nontraumatic avascular necrosis of the hip, but the precipitating event that is common to most, if not all, is a mechanical interruption of the circulation of the femoral head. If the affected area is sufficiently large and the collateral circulation is inadequate, avascular necrosis will develop. This may occur by direct external vascular occlusion without disruption of the vessels, as in marrow infiltrative diseases. Arterial thrombosis probably occurs in the vascular disorders, and emboli have been implicated in sickle-cell disease and caisson disease (dysbaric osteonecrosis). The systemic administration of steroids and an excessive intake of alcohol are the two factors most often associated with idiopathic osteonecrosis.[337] Overall, etiologic factors can be clearly identified in most patients; perhaps only 10–20% of patients have truly idiopathic osteonecrosis.

The symptoms of avascular necrosis and idiopathic osteonecrosis are nonspecific and usually insidious in onset. The pain, which is typically felt in the groin, proximal thigh, or buttock area, is usually exacerbated by weight bearing, but it is often present at rest. The clinical findings vary, and it is only when the femoral head becomes deformed that limitations of motion in a noncapsular pattern occur. Axial loading of the joint, as in the scour test, may reproduce the symptoms. A limp or an antalgic gait is typically a late finding, and the functional disability is proportionate to the level of pain.[337] Usually, the pain becomes more severe as fragmentation and collapse of the femoral head take place. Sometimes the pain will lessen if spontaneous improvement occurs, and small lesions may remain asymptomatic and resolve spontaneously.[337]

Clinically diagnosed avascular necrosis is progressive in 70–80% of patients who are managed nonoperatively, and this progression usually results in collapse of the femoral head.[337] Although conservative intervention is aimed at limiting the stresses through the hip joint, and utilizing a support, operative intervention generally is recommended.

A parallel condition that occurs in children (most common in boys aged 5–8 years) is Legg–Calvé–Perthes disease (see Chap. 30).

Iliopsoas Abscess

See the discussion under "Causes of Pelvis Pain" earlier.

Trochanteric Bursitis

See Chapter 19.

Obturator, Femoral, or Inguinal Hernia

The clinical diagnosis of inguinal and femoral hernias is usually straightforward. A few hernias, however, present a diagnostic problem. This diagnostic difficulty is usually encountered in obese patients or in patients with reducible hernias that are not protruding at the time of physical examination. False-positive findings include lipoma of the spermatic cord and preperitoneal lipoma. A cord lipoma appears as a smooth, finger-like projection of fat parallel to the cord vessels at rest. During straining, longitudinal sliding occurs. Unlike indirect inguinal hernias, the anteroposterior diameter of the inguinal canal does not increase during the Valsalva maneuver.

Osteomyelitis Pubis

Bony infection or inflammation of the pubic area is rare. Osteomyelitis pubis is an entity characterized by pelvic pain, a wide-based gait, and bony destruction of the margins of the pubic symphysis.[338] Delay in its diagnosis is common because the presentation is similar to that of osteitis pubis and urologic, gynecologic, and abdominal lesions. Osteomyelitis pubis should be considered when a patient presents with the following signs: pain or pubic tenderness, painful hip abduction, and fever.[338]

Antibiotic treatment is essential, with the specific drug therapy depending on identification of the causative agent.

Compartment Syndrome

Compartment syndrome is a condition in which myoneural anoxia results from a prolonged increase in tissue pressure within a closed osseofascial space. This compromises local blood flow of skeletal muscle, resulting in ischemia and necrosis.

Local blood flow may be impaired by

- an increase in the pressure of the compartment resulting from the application of a tight bandage or plaster cast;
- a decrease in arterial flow, as in PVD;
- an increase in venous pressure that can reduce the gradient for local blood flow.

False aneurysms of the profunda femoris artery are a rare but recognized complication following orthopaedic procedures in the upper thigh. Such procedures include internal fixation of intertrochanteric, subtrochanteric, and intracapsular femoral neck fractures; subtrochanteric osteotomy; and intramedullary nailing of the femur.[339]

A compartment syndrome of the thigh usually manifests as a pulsating, expanding swelling of the upper thigh with an audible bruit. Potential complications include expansion and extensive soft-tissue destruction and pressure to neighboring structures.[339] This can result in neuropathy or venous outflow obstruction and thrombosis. Rupture and severe hemorrhage, infection of the aneurysm, and sepsis of the nearby prosthesis, as well as fracture nonunion, also have been reported.[339]

Early recognition and repair of the aneurysm is of paramount importance to avoid life- and limb-threatening complications from delayed diagnosis.[339] Any unexplained thigh swelling encountered following a surgical procedure on the proximal femur and shaft should alert the clinician to a potential injury to the profunda femoris artery.[339]

Genital Herpes

See the discussion under "Causes of Buttock and Upper and Lower Leg Pain" earlier.

TABLE 5-15 Potential Causes of Shoulder Pain
Tendinous and capsular lesions
Traumatic synovitis
Subluxation
Dislocation
Spondyloarthropy
Acute arthritis
Infections
Tumor
Clay shoveler fracture
Degenerative conditions
Metabolic conditions
Cerebrovascular disease
Multiple sclerosis
Amyotrophic lateral sclerosis
Guillain–Barré syndrome
Syringomyelia
Cervical radicular pain
Elbow dysfunction
Peripheral nerve entrapment
Brachial plexopathy
Herpes zoster
Gallbladder dysfunction
Cardiac dysfunction
Pulmonary dysfunction
Diaphragm
Spleen

CAUSES OF SHOULDER AND UPPER ARM PAIN

The causes of shoulder and upper arm pain include those listed in Tables 5-15 and 5-16.

TABLE 5-16 Origin and Location of Shoulder Pain

Right Shoulder		Left Shoulder	
Systemic Origin	**Location**	**Systemic Origin**	**Location**
Peptic ulcer	Lateral border of right scapula	Ruptured spleen	Left shoulder
		Myocardial ischemia	Left pectoral/shoulder area
Myocardial ischemia	Right shoulder and down arm	Pancreas	Left shoulder
Hepatic/biliary			
Acute cholecystitis	Right shoulder, between scapulae, and right subscapular area		
Liver abscess	Right shoulder		
Gallbladder	Right upper trapezius		
Liver disease (hepatitis, cirrhosis, and metastatic tumors)	Right shoulder and right subscapular area		

Data from Goodman CC, Snyder TEK: *Differential Diagnosis in Physical Therapy*. Philadelphia, PA: WB Saunders Company, 1990.

Local Conditions

Tendinous and Capsular Lesions

See Chapter 16.

Synovitis

The shoulder joint is composed of two synovial cavities: the subacromial–subdeltoid bursa and the glenohumeral joint. In rotator cuff diseases, subacromial synovitis is responsible for the generation of shoulder pain, and its severity may correlate with the intensity of pain. During inflammation, the so-called hyperalgesia occurs, which is characterized by intensified pain with a reduced threshold to somatic stimulation.

Pigmented villonodular (PVN) synovitis is one of a group of benign, proliferative lesions arising from the synovium of joints, bursae, and tendon sheaths.[340] Traditionally, these lesions have been identified as a benign giant cell tumor of the tendon sheath, hemorrhagic villous synovitis, and proliferative synovitis.[341] PVN synovitis in the knee and hand has been described frequently, but its occurrence at the shoulder is rare.

The cause of PVN synovitis is unclear, but it may be related to inflammation or trauma. The lesions develop slowly, and patients usually present with a gradual onset of pain at the affected joint.[340] A palpable, tender, soft-tissue mass may be present. PVN synovitis is regarded as a locally aggressive but benign tumor. Early diagnosis and treatment are essential to preserve joint function and integrity. The treatment of choice is complete synovectomy or bursectomy, or arthroscopic synovectomy.[340]

Subluxation

Shoulder subluxation can be caused by trauma, overuse, or hemiplegia. The traumatic and overuse causes of shoulder subluxation, which can often be diagnosed on the basis of history and physical examination, are described in Chapter 16. The most common complaints are of instability, restricted activities, and pain. Strength and range of motion are usually normal. The most common significant finding on physical examination is apprehension.

Shoulder pain is a common complication of hemiplegia. One of the most commonly cited causes of shoulder pain in hemiplegia is shoulder subluxation. Shoulder subluxation occurs in hemiplegia because of the paralysis of active restraints, which play a critical role in maintaining glenohumeral joint integrity. In this population, glenohumeral joint subluxation may inhibit functional recovery by limiting glenohumeral range of motion.

Unfortunately, the available options for preventing and treating shoulder subluxation in the hemiplegic population are limited. Armboards and laptrays have not been shown to be effective and may lead to an overcorrection of inferior subluxation.[342] This overcorrection may predispose the involved shoulder to impingement syndromes. The use of slings remains controversial. Slings may cause lateral subluxation, contribute to the deleterious effects of joint immobilization, or promote undesirable synergistic patterns of muscle activation.[342] Intramuscular neuromuscular electrical stimulation (NMES) delivered via percutaneously placed electrodes may address the limitations of transcutaneous systems in the treatment of shoulder subluxation and pain.[342]

Dislocation

In contrast to the hip, in which the ball-and-socket joint is deep and well stabilized, the articular surface of the shoulder rests in the shallow glenoid cavity. Ninety-five percent of shoulder dislocations occur in the anterior direction and result in stretching and detachment of the anterior capsule and labrum.[343] Dislocation of the shoulder is a common and often disabling injury, resulting in damage to nerves, blood vessels, and the rotator cuff muscles. Most shoulder dislocations are traumatic in origin. The most common mechanisms are a fall on an outstretched hand, a blow against the anterior arm when the limb is extended and externally rotated, or, rarely, a blow to the back of the shoulder.

Traumatic shoulder dislocations are accompanied by extreme pain that worsens as the supporting musculature goes into spasm.[344] Generally, patients present with the arm somewhat abducted and externally rotated, often grasped tightly by the opposite hand to minimize movement.[344]

The examination of a patient who has recently dislocated the shoulder is often difficult because of associated pain and muscle guarding. It is important to attempt to examine for axillary nerve function (deltoid power and overlying sensation), supraspinatus power, and glenohumeral range of motion.[345] Axillary nerve palsy and avulsion of the supraspinatus are common complications of a dislocated shoulder. Associated fractures may be present. Vascular compromise is uncommon in this injury, but when it occurs, rapid surgical referral is necessary to save the limb.[344]

Spondyloarthropathy

RA affects the joints in a characteristic and symmetric fashion. In addition to the smaller joints, RA can affect the larger joints, including the shoulders. It results in pain and stiffness, which are usually greatest in the morning.[346–348] This condition should be considered when patients have symmetric involvement of the shoulder, morning stiffness, constitutional signs, and physical signs of joint inflammation.[349] Synovial inflammation of the subacromial–subdeltoid bursae can occur, resulting in pain on abduction to approximately 90 degrees in both shoulders.[349] Chronic inflammation or long-term corticosteroid use, or both, may also result in rotator cuff tearing, another viable cause of pain and function loss in the patient with RA. This should be suspected when significant weakness is noted on abduction or external rotation of the shoulder.[349] The clinician should also look for other signs of inflammatory arthritis, which include synovial thickening of the MCP joints and thickening at, and loss of range of motion of, the wrists. The rheumatoid factor is often negative in older patients with RA.[349]

CLINICAL PEARL

Polymyalgia rheumatica is another cause of shoulder pain in older individuals. These patients have pain in the shoulder and hip girdle muscles, profound morning stiffness, and malaise.[349] This condition can be difficult to distinguish from RA in older people.

Acute Arthritis

Septic arthritis of the shoulder is uncommon but can occur in patients who are debilitated from generalized disease,[350] in those taking immunosuppressive medications, or in combination with an underlying shoulder disease process, such as rotator cuff tearing[351] or RA.[352,353]

Diabetic patients are at higher risk of developing monoarticular steroid-sensitive arthritis.[354] A condition of unknown etiology, it can affect the rotator cuff and the glenohumeral joint capsule.[355] As the name suggests, the condition is provoked by the patient's reaction to hydrocortisone.

Diagnosis requires joint aspiration and bacteriological testing. Monoarticular arthritis, which usually resolves spontaneously in 2 years with medical intervention,[356] is an absolute contraindication to capsular stretching.[357]

Degenerative Conditions

Intrinsic glenohumeral arthritis is an infrequent cause of shoulder pain, but loss of glenohumeral motion is often seen in patients with periarticular syndromes (see Chap. 16).[349] Although the rotator cuff often is intact, the subscapularis muscle often is shortened, limiting external rotation.[358] X-ray findings include[358]

- flattening posterior erosion of the glenoid and an enlarged or deformed humeral head[359,360];
- inferiorly located osteophytes;
- acromioclavicular arthritic changes.[359]

Infections

Osteomyelitis

The most commonly involved bones with acute hematogenous osteomyelitis in order of frequency are femur, tibia, humerus, fibula, radius, phalanges, calcaneus, ulna, ischium, metatarsals, and vertebral bodies.[361] Patients with sickle-cell disease are at an increased risk of bacterial infections, and osteomyelitis is the second most common infection in these patients.[362]

Patients usually present with fever, malaise, irritability, pain, and localized tenderness at the site of infection. Muscle guarding may also be a feature, as well as decreased movement and pain of the affected limb and adjacent joints. These symptoms may be accompanied by edema and erythema over the involved area.

Cat-Scratch Disease

Cat-scratch disease is generally a benign, self-limited infectious disease in immunocompetent patients. It is caused by Bartonella *henselae*, a small, Gram-negative, argyrophilic, nonacid-fast, pleomorphic bacillus.[363] Domestic cats, especially kittens, serve as a reservoir for *B. henselae*.[363] In general, patients present with a history of a scratch, bite, or close contact with a kitten or cat. Often a red-brown nontender papule develops at the region of the inoculation within 3–10 days and may persist for several weeks. Most patients develop tender regional lymphadenopathy, particularly in the axilla, and many develop fever.

Tumors

The differential diagnosis of all painful shoulders includes tumors of a wide variety. Evaluation of a shoulder tumor has several areas in common with other musculoskeletal neoplasms. Thorough evaluation of patients requires not only routine radiography but also radionuclide imaging, CT scanning, magnetic resonance imaging (MRI), and angiography. The typical clinical features of a bone tumor include variable pain, which is often worse at night and markedly unresponsive to salicylates. Surgical treatment of shoulder tumors depends on the patient's age and the type, extent, and aggressiveness of the tumor.

Vascular Conditions

Nontraumatic avascular necrosis of the humeral head may be idiopathic or associated with the systemic use of corticosteroids, dysbaric conditions (blockage of the blood vessels by a bubble of nitrogen coming out of solution), transplantation, systemic illness, alcoholism, sickle-cell disease, hyperuricemia, pancreatitis, lymphoma, or Gaucher disease.[353,364–367]

Diagnosis is through imaging, particularly MRI, which detects the pathology at its earliest stage.

Metabolic Conditions

Gout is a metabolic disease characterized by recurrent episodes of acute arthritis that can manifest in the shoulder joints.

Fractures

See Chapter 16.

Referred Pain

Referred pain from the cervical region may be experienced in the shoulder or interpreted as a distal sensation.[368]

Referral sources for this region include the heart,[369] pleura, lung tissue, diaphragmatic pain,[370] lymph nodes of the neck, shoulder, chest, and breast tissue.[370]

Pain in the shoulder area can be caused by direct or referred pain from an underlying malignancy, such as a Pancoast tumor (see "Tumor").[370] The scapula and humerus are frequently sites of metastases in tumors of the kidney, breast, lung, and prostate.[349] These patients have persistent pain that is unaffected by movement but is associated with fatigue, weight loss, and other constitutional signs. A history of gradually progressive pain, starting as a mild ache but developing into persistent severe pain, should initiate a search for a malignancy.[349] Severe shoulder pain in a patient with a normal physical examination of the shoulder and cervical spine should increase the suspicion of a malignancy.

Intrinsic neck pathology can cause referred pain to the head, anterior and posterior chest wall, shoulder girdle, and upper limb.[368] In the case of radiculopathy, muscle function might be affected directly. Cervical spine symptoms are usually affected by head position, with neck extension causing an exacerbation and flexion producing some relief.[349]

Intracerebral and Intraspinal Conditions

Cerebrovascular Disease

See the discussion under "Causes of Head, Face, Eye, and Temporomandibular Joint Symptoms" earlier.

Subclavian Steal Syndrome

This condition (see Chap. 24) results in signs and symptoms of cerebral ischemia and upper arm pain. Ischemia is the result of subclavian artery stenosis proximal to the origin of the vertebral artery and, subsequently, "steals" of blood from the cerebral circulation of the Circle of Willis and basilar vessel (see Chap. 24).

The symptoms of subclavian steal syndrome are usually precipitated or aggravated by arm exercises.[371]

Multiple Sclerosis

Pain, either acute or chronic, occurs in more than 65% of patients with MS[372] during all stages of the disease. Chronic pain may be characterized by dysesthetic extremities, back and shoulder pain, and pain secondary to spasticity.[166] Complications of disuse, such as frozen shoulder and osteoporosis, are other painful syndromes that may develop.[166]

Amyotrophic Lateral Sclerosis

Amyotrophic lateral sclerosis (ALS), commonly referred to as Lou Gehrig's disease, is a neurodegenerative disorder that causes rapid loss of motor neurons in the brain and spinal cord, leading to paralysis and death. Diagnosis is based solely on clinical data. The diagnosis of ALS depends upon the recognition of a characteristic constellation of symptoms and signs and supportive electrophysiological findings. For clinically definite ALS diagnosis, UMN and LMN signs in bulbar and two spinal regions or in three spinal regions are required. The LMN weakness and muscle atrophy involves both peripheral nerve and myotomal distributions. The clinical hallmark of ALS is the coexistence of muscle atrophy, weakness, fasciculations, and cramps (caused by LMN degeneration), together with hyperactive or inappropriately brisk muscle stretch reflexes, pyramidal tract signs, and increased muscle tone (due to corticospinal tract involvement).[373] Muscle cramps are often already present before other symptoms develop. Most patients present with asymmetrical, distal weakness of the arm or leg. ALS is a progressive disease. The symptoms usually progress first in the affected extremity and then gradually spread to adjacent muscle groups and remote ipsilateral or contralateral regions. Although disability is usually limited in the early stages, ALS progresses relentlessly. Most patients are ultimately unable to walk, care for themselves, speak, and swallow.[373] However, there is usually no clinical involvement of parts of the CNS other than the motor pathways.[373]

Respiratory weakness due to high cervical (phrenic nerve, C4) and thoracic spinal cord involvement is the most common cause of death in ALS, often in conjunction with aspiration pneumonia.[373]

Guillain–Barré Syndrome

Guillain–Barré syndrome (GBS) is challenging to identify because of its multitude of presentations and manifestations. GBS may be defined as a postinfectious, acute, paralytic peripheral neuropathy. It can affect any age group, although there is a peak incidence in young adults. GBS appears to be an inflammatory or immune-mediated condition.

The majority of patients describe an antecedent febrile illness. Upper respiratory infections are seen in 50% of cases and are caused by a variety of viruses. The illness is usually an acute respiratory or gastrointestinal condition that lasts for several days and then resolves. This is followed in 1–2 weeks by the development of a progressive ascending weakness or paralysis, which is usually symmetric. The progression of the weakness or paralysis can be gradual (1–3 weeks) or rapid (1–2 days). The patient reports difficulty or instability with walking, arising from a chair, and ascending or descending stairs. Associated signs and symptoms include cranial nerve involvement (facial weakness), paresthesias, sensory deficits, difficulty in breathing, diminished muscle stretch reflexes, autonomic dysfunction (tachycardia and vasomotor symptoms), oropharyngeal weakness, and ocular involvement.[374]

The differential diagnosis for GBS is quite large and includes the spectrum of illnesses causing acute or subacute paralysis. These include spinal cord compression (myelopathy), UMN disorders, poliomyelitis, transverse myelitis, polyneuropathy, SLE, polyarteritis nodosa, myasthenia gravis, and sarcoidosis.[374]

All patients with suspected GBS should be hospitalized for vigilant monitoring because of the high risk of respiratory failure, which occurs in approximately one-third of patients.[374]

Syringomyelia

Syringomyelia is a disease that produces fluid-containing cysts (syrinx) within the spinal cord, often associated with stenosis of the foramen magnum. The syrinx can occur within the spinal cord (syringomyelia) or brain stem (syringobulbia). Syringomyelia has been found in association with various disorders, including spinal column or brain stem abnormalities (scoliosis, Klippel–Feil syndrome, Chiari I malformation), intramedullary tumors, and traumatic degeneration of the spinal cord. Chiari I malformation is the most common condition in patients with syringomyelia.

Painful dysesthesias, which have been described variously as burning pain, pins-and-needles sensations, and stretching or pressure of the skin, occur in up to 40% of patients with syringomyelia.[375] The pain tends to arise in a dermatomal pattern and is accompanied, in most cases, by hyperesthesia.

Radiologic features that suggest syringomyelia include an increase in the width and depth of the cervical canal, bony abnormalities at the craniovertebral junction, diastematomyelia, and occipitalization of the atlas.

Extraspinal Conditions

The extraspinal causes of shoulder pain include tumor, clay shoveler fracture, brachial plexopathy, and herpes zoster.

Tumor. Pancoast syndrome is a constellation of characteristic symptoms and signs that includes shoulder and arm pain along the distribution of the eighth cervical nerve trunk and first and second thoracic nerve trunks, Horner syndrome (see Chap. 3), and weakness and atrophy of the muscles of the hand, most commonly caused by local extension of an apical lung tumor at the superior thoracic inlet.[376,377] These tumors are called *superior pulmonary sulcus tumors* or *Pancoast tumors.*

The most common initial symptom is shoulder pain due to the localization of the Pancoast tumors in the superior pulmonary sulcus. Pain can radiate up to the head and neck or down to the medial aspect of the scapula, axilla, anterior part of the chest, or ipsilateral arm, often along the distribution of the ulnar nerve.[378] This radicular causalgic pain is often difficult to treat. Sensory loss and motor deficit in the upper extremity may also occur. Weakness and atrophy of the intrinsic muscles of the hand are not uncommon, along with pain and paresthesia of the medial aspect of the arm, forearm, and fourth and fifth digits along the distribution of the ulnar nerve, caused by extension of the tumor to the C8 and T1 nerve roots.[378]

The differential diagnosis of Pancoast syndrome includes other primary thoracic neoplasms, metastatic and hematologic conditions, infectious diseases, thoracic outlet syndromes, and pulmonary amyloid nodules.[378]

Clay Shoveler Fracture. Clay shoveler fracture is a rare condition. The condition was first described by McKellar[379] and was based on a few cases reported, found in English men, who spent long hours digging heavy clay. It has since been described in power lifters.[380] The condition is characterized by a traction fracture of the lower cervical or upper thoracic spine due to an excessive pull of the trapezius, rhomboid muscles during heavy work. Typically, the patient reports a sudden onset of sharp neck, shoulder, and arm pain and exhibits limited active bilateral elevation to around 150 degrees. Passive elevation remains unaffected. Other conditions that mimic these symptoms include a fracture of the first rib, mononeuritis of the long thoracic nerve, mononeuritis of the accessory nerve, a C5 root palsy, or a total rupture of the supraspinatus.[357]

Brachial Plexopathy.[381] Idiopathic brachial plexopathy (IBP) is a syndrome of shoulder pain and weakness. IBP has a number of pseudonyms, including neuralgic amyotrophy, Parsonage–Turner syndrome, and idiopathic brachial neuritis. The initial symptom typically seen with IBP is sudden, sharp, and throbbing pain in the shoulder girdle, followed by weakness in the scapular and proximal arm muscles. Sensory loss is usually not prominent. The pain usually subsides within 24 hours to 3 weeks, and the weakness and atrophy are recognized as the pain resolves. Weakness is maximal within 2–3 weeks of the onset of symptoms and often is accompanied by muscle wasting and scapular winging. Slow resolution of the weakness follows in nearly all patients, but recovery may be incomplete.

Herpes Zoster.[382] Herpes zoster is characterized by deep, boring, or stabbing thoracic and arm pain. Varicella zoster virus infection is unique because of its two clinical manifestations: varicella (chickenpox) and herpes zoster (shingles). After an individual has chickenpox, the virus lies dormant in the posterior (dorsal) root ganglia and sensory ganglia of cranial nerves. Herpes zoster occurs if the virus becomes reactivated, causing an acute, painful infection of a sensory nerve and its corresponding cutaneous area of innervation. Herpes zoster, therefore, occurs only in individuals previously infected with the chickenpox virus.

Postherpetic neuralgia is the most common complication of herpes zoster. It arises from inflammatory injury to sensory nerves, ganglia, and nerve roots and from maladaptive responses to pain signaling and the likely inability of pain receptors to return to normal after the inflammation subsides. The nerve dysfunction can result in hyperesthesia, hypoesthesia, dysesthesia, and allodynia (pain as the result of innocuous stimuli, such as clothing touching the affected skin).

The characteristic rash begins as erythematous macules and papules that progress to vesicles within 24 hours, then to pustules (3–4 days), and finally to crusts (7–10 days). The most common distribution of herpes zoster is unilateral involvement of the thoracic dermatome, followed by the cranial, cervical, and lumbar dermatomes. Involvement of the maxillary division of the trigeminal nerve causes vesicles of the uvula and tonsillar area. Involvement of the mandibular branch produces vesicles on the floor of the mouth, buccal membranes, and the anterior part of the tongue. Herpes zoster near or involving the eyes is considered an emergency, because this potentially serious development can lead to blindness.

In general, the diagnosis of herpes zoster is based on the history and the clinical examination, which shows the characteristic painful, grouped vesicular rash in a dermatomal distribution. Acute herpes-zoster infection is a self-limiting condition, and the primary treatment goals are to reduce and manage the acute pain and modify the duration of the rash and inflammation.

CAUSES OF ELBOW AND FOREARM PAIN

The causes of elbow and forearm pain include those listed in Table 5-17.

Fracture

See Chapter 17.

Dislocation

See Chapter 17.

TABLE 5-17 Potential Causes of Elbow and Forearm Pain
Fracture
Dislocation
Osteochondritis
Ligament sprain
Arthrosis
Peripheral nerve entrapment
Soft-tissue injury or tendonitis (lateral epicondylitis, medial epicondylitis, triceps tendonitis, bicipital tendonitis, brachialis tendonitis, and Little League elbow)
Infective arthritis
Polyarthritis
Gout
Bursitis
Vascular disorders
Referred pain

Osteochondritis Dissecans Capitellum

See Chapter 17.

Ligament Sprain

See Chapter 17.

Arthrosis

Arthrosis of the elbow is often the result of a previous micro- or macrotraumatic injury to the elbow. Unless the case is severe, the patient does not complain of much pain, except perhaps with vigorous activity. However, complaints of early morning stiffness and pain at the end of the day are common. Motion testing reveals a capsular pattern, with a bony end-feel, in both flexion and extension, and crepitus is felt during both motions. There is no specific treatment for this condition. Surgery may be necessary to remove loose bodies or for debridement in severe cases.

Peripheral Nerve Entrapment

See Chapters 3 and 17.

Soft-Tissue Injury or Tendonitis

See Chapter 17.

Infective Arthritis

The source of infective arthritis is commonly tooth decay or a pelvic disease. A history of a puncture wound of the skin also should arouse suspicion. The pain is described as a severe aching or throbbing. The involved joint feels hot and appears swollen. The involved elbow is usually held stiffly in slight flexion. Associated findings include fever and joint tenderness.

Polyarthritis

The polyarthritis that can affect the elbow include acute rheumatic fever, Reiter syndrome, and Lyme disease arthritis.

Gout

Gout at the elbow is characterized by acute pain, swelling, redness, and tenderness of the elbow joint.

Bursitis

See Chapter 17.

Vascular Disorders

Volkmann Ischemia (Anterior Compartment Syndrome)

This condition occurs as the result of increased tissue fluid pressure within a fascial muscle compartment that reduces capillary blood perfusion below a level necessary for tissue viability.[383] In the upper extremity, acute compartment syndrome that involves the forearm is the most common type of compartment syndrome. Nerve injury resulting from the compression produces a deformed limb known as *Volkmann ischemic contracture*.[384]

Acute compartment syndrome can be caused by constrictive casts or dressings, limb placement during surgery, blunt trauma, hematoma, burns, frostbite, snake bite, strenuous exercise, and fractures.[383] Clinical findings include[383]

- a swollen and tense tender compartment;
- severe pain, exacerbated with passive stretch of the forearm muscles;
- sensibility deficits;
- motor weakness or paralysis;
- no absence of radial and ulnar pulses at the wrist.

The clinical diagnosis is confirmed by measuring the intracompartmental tissue fluid pressure.

Conservative intervention involves the removal of the constricting splint, dressing, or cast. Surgical intervention, by performing a fasciotomy, is reserved for patients whose symptoms do not resolve quickly.[383]

Acute Axillary or Brachial Artery Occlusion

The causes of arterial occlusion include emboli from the heart or from an atheromatous plaque or aneurysm of the innominate or subclavian-axillary arteries.[385] Trauma to the chest, shoulder, or upper arm may also cause arterial obstruction. The five P's describe the signs and symptoms of this medical emergency:

- Pain
- Paralysis
- Paresthesias
- Pallor
- Pulses (absent)

The pain is usually severe and constant, involving the forearm, hand, and fingers. Paralysis and paresthesia indicate severe ischemia of the arm. Gangrene can begin to develop 6 hours after the onset of symptoms in such scenarios. The pallor occurs because of lack of blood flow and cutaneous vasoconstriction. The absence of pulses confirms occlusion.

Referred Pain

Referred pain to the elbow can have a number of causes, including coronary heart disease, polyarthritis, or an acute C8 radiculopathy.

CAUSES OF WRIST, HAND, AND FINGER PAIN

The causes of wrist, hand, and finger pain include, but are not limited to, those listed in Table 5-18 and shown in Fig. 5-3.

Fracture

See Chapter 18.

TABLE 5-18	Causes of Wrist, Hand, and Finger Pain
Fracture	
Sprains and dislocations	
Triangular fibrocartilage complex lesions	
Tenosynovitis	
Tendonitis	
Carpal instability	
Gout and pseudogout	
Rheumatoid arthritis	
Psoriatic arthritis	
Osteoarthritis	
Carpal tunnel syndrome	
Infection	
Kienböck disease	
Ganglia	
Tumors	
Peripheral nerve entrapment	
Reflex sympathetic dystrophy/complex regional pain syndrome	
Vascular occlusion	
Mononeuritis multiplex	
Referred pain	

Sprains and Dislocations

See Chapter 18.

Triangular Fibrocartilage Complex Lesions

See Chapter 18.

Tenosynovitis

See Chapter 18.

Tendonitis

See Chapter 18.

Carpal Instability

See Chapter 18.

Gout and Pseudogout

Gouty arthritis and pseudogout are metabolic joint diseases caused by the deposition of sodium urate or calcium pyrophosphate crystals in the joint, leading to arthritis (see also, earlier discussions). The wrists are the second most commonly affected joint in pseudogout, after the knees. Radiographs demonstrate crystal deposits in articular fibrocartilage of the wrist.[386] Septic arthritis of the wrist can cause destruction of joint cartilage and bony structures. Generally, the diagnosis of acute infection is not problematic, but differentiation between pure soft-tissue infection and infection involving the bony structures can be complicated.[387] Furthermore, identification of a chronic infection as the cause of chronic wrist pain may be difficult.[388,389] If there is a clinical suspicion, a (ultrasound-guided) needle aspiration or synovial biopsy should be taken.[387] The new generation of ultrasonography has proven to be a valuable technique, with a high success rate, for obtaining synovial fluid or membrane samples for pathologic and bacteriologic examinations.[390]

Rheumatoid Arthritis

In the hand, many common deformities can be seen, such as ulnar deviation of the MCP joints, boutonnière deformity, and swan neck deformities of the digits (see Chap. 18).

Psoriatic Arthritis

See section "Psoriatic Arthritis" earlier in the chapter.

Osteoarthritis

See Chapter 18.

Carpal Tunnel Syndrome

See Chapter 18.

Infection

Wrist

The most common infection of the wrist is infectious tenosynovitis of the flexor pollicis longus.

Hand

These infections include

- bursal infections;
- space infections;
- infected bites;
- ***Cellulitis.*** Cellulitis is an infection of the skin and underlying structures. With treatment, it usually follows a relatively benign course. However, in some cases, the same pathogens can cause other diseases, such as necrotizing fasciitis or toxic shock syndrome, and even death. The most common pathogens in cellulitis are *Staph. aureus* and β-hemolytic streptococci. Symptoms include localized redness, swelling, and pain. Associated symptoms include fever, chills, and nausea and vomiting. Cellulitis typically is treated with systemic antibiotics via either the oral or the intravenous route.

Fingers

Paronychia and Eponychia. Paronychia is an acute inflammation of the lateral or proximal nail folds that is usually caused by infection, producing a red, tender, throbbing, and intensely painful swelling of the proximal or lateral nail folds.[391] It is the most common infection of the hand. If the infection involves the eponychium as well as the lateral fold, it is called eponychia.

Mild cases of paronychia typically are treated with warm soaks two to four times daily and splinting with or without systemic antibiotics. The more severe cases require incision and drainage.[392]

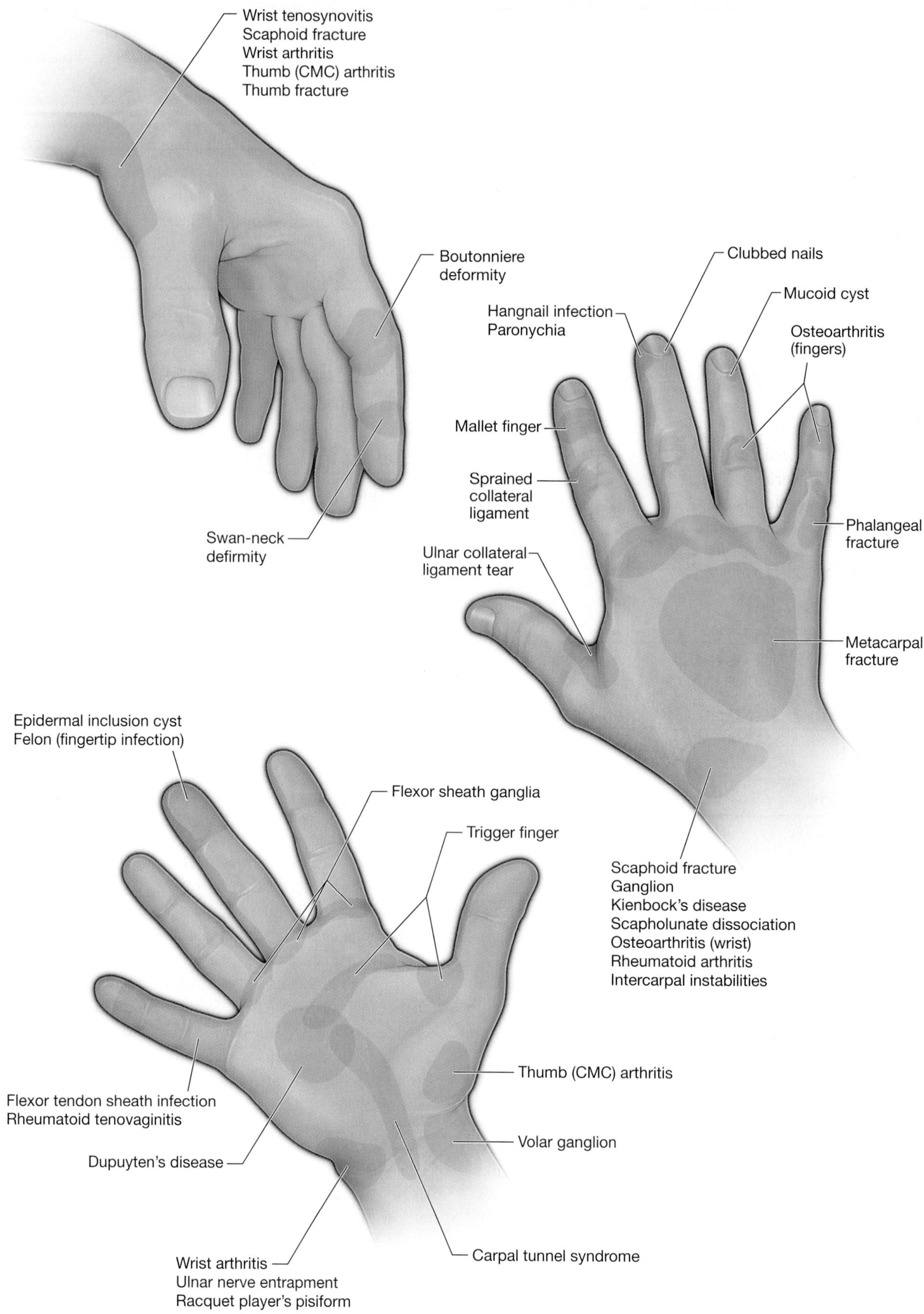

FIGURE 5-3 Potential causes of wrist and hand pain.

Differential diagnosis includes apical abscess, felon, and subungual infection.[393] A subungual infection may result from an extension of the paronychia under the nail.[393]

Felon

A felon is an abscess of the terminal phalanx pulp. The most common cause is a puncture wound. Initially, the condition is characterized by mild swelling, erythema, and tenderness. Over a period of a few days, the pulp becomes tense, red, and exquisitely tender.[393]

Mild cases are treated with antibiotics and elevation. Most cases, however, require a combination of incision and drainage, and systemic antibiotics.

Web Space Infections

A web space abscess usually is caused by a puncture in the skin between the fingers. It is characterized by its collar-button or dumbbell shape, as the expanding abscess penetrates the palmar fascia.[393] Swelling and tenderness are noted on the palmar and posterior (dorsal) aspects of the web space. The adjacent fingers adopt an abducted position. Intervention involves incision and drainage.

Herpetic Whitlow

Herpetic whitlow is a viral infection of the fingers. It is caused by contact with the herpes simplex virus.[393] The condition usually manifests with intense throbbing and erythema of the involved finger. The condition is self-limiting and typically lasts for 2–3 weeks. The intervention is conservative and symptomatic.[393]

Kienböck Disease

Kienböck disease, or lunatomalacia, is a complication of injury to the lunate. It is defined as an aseptic or avascular necrosis of the lunate. The etiology of this disease remains elusive, although it is thought that trauma plays a large part in disrupting the blood supply to the bone.[394] The disease occurs predominantly in males, with a 2:1 prevalence,[395] and the majority of patients are 20–40 years.[396]

Subjective complaints include pain on the central-posterior (dorsal) aspect of the wrist, especially during and after activities. Stiffness of the hand is another common complaint.[397] With time, the pain becomes severe and constant, with accompanying weakness of grip strength and loss of wrist motion, especially wrist extension.[397] Imaging techniques are needed to make a definitive diagnosis.

The intervention for Kienböck disease depends on the stage of the disease. Conservative measures involve immobilization during the acute phase. Surgical options include joint leveling by radial shortening or ulnar lengthening, intercarpal fusion, arthroplasty, and vascularized bone grafts.[398]

Ganglia

Ganglia are thin-walled cysts containing mucoid hyaluronic acid that develop spontaneously over a joint capsule or tendon sheath. Ganglia, seen primarily in 20–30-year olds, may also occur in association with such systemic diseases as arthritis or with trauma.[399–402] The exact cause of the ganglia is controversial. However, there is consensus that a one-way connection to the synovial sheath allows fluid to enter the cyst but not to flow freely back into the sheath.[399]

Upon examination, a ganglion is smooth, round, or multilobulated and tender with applied pressure. The key to distinguishing a ganglion from other soft-tissue tumors is the history of size variation (Table 5-19). Suspicious soft-tissue masses require evaluation and further diagnostic testing or excisional biopsy.[399]

Tumors

Benign tumors account for the majority of tumors of the wrist and hand, although malignancies can occur.[403] The clinical

TABLE 5-19 Differential Diagnosis of Wrist Ganglia

Non-Neoplastic Masses Extraskeletal	Neoplastic Masses Soft Tissue
Aneurysm/arteriovenous malformation	Benign tumor (chondroma, fibroma, giant cell tumor of tendon sheath, hemangioma, lipoma, and neuroma)
Anomalous muscle and other anomalous structure	Malignant tumor (epithelioid sarcoma, malignant fibrous histiocytoma, metastasis, and synovial sarcoma)
Bursa	*Skeletal*
Displaced tendon	Benign tumor (cyst, chondroma, giant cell tumor, collagen osteochondroma, and osteoid osteoma)
Foreign-body granulomas	Malignant tumor (chondrosarcoma, metastasis, and osteosarcoma)
Hypertrophic structure	*Infectious*
Nerve entrapment	Fungus, mycobacteria, pyogen, tuberculosis
Nerve ganglion	*Disease/metabolic*
Periarticular calcaneal	Rheumatoid arthritis and disease, rheumatoid nodule, synovial cyst, and tenosynovitis
Repetitive use fibrosis	Gout and pseudogout
Scar	Neuritis (PIN), vasculitis, and amyloidosis
Tendon entrapment	
Tuberous sclerosis	
Skeletal	
Arthritic residuum	
Pigmented villonodular synovitis	
Posttraumatic residuum: subluxed scaphoid	

Data from Kozin SH, Urban MA, Bishop AT, et al.: Wrist ganglia: Diagnosis and treatment. *J Musculo Med* 10:75–76, 1993.

presentation is variable and depends on the condition, location, size, and degree of soft-tissue involvement, although there are a number of scenarios that warrant suspicion of a possible occult lesion[404]:

- A young patient complaining of bone pain that is not related to any preceding trauma.
- Presence of swelling, or of a mass, in the absence of trauma.
- Pain or swelling that persists despite intervention.

Peripheral Nerve Entrapment

Pain of a neurogenic origin can be referred to the wrist and hand. These can include C5–T1 nerve-root lesions, peripheral nerve lesions, thoracic outlet syndrome, and brachial plexus tension syndromes. In addition, neurogenic causes can be secondary to adhesion formation or trauma.

Proximal Nerve Entrapment

Proximal causes of pain, paresthesias, and numbness in the lateral hand, thumb, and index and middle fingers include

- C6 or C7 radiculopathy (see Chap. 25);
- thoracic outlet syndrome (see Chap. 25);
- pronator teres syndrome (see Chap. 17).

Proximal causes of these symptoms in the medial hand and the fourth and fifth fingers include

- C8 radiculopathy;
- brachial plexus compression at the thoracic outlet;
- cubital tunnel syndrome (see Chap. 17).

Distal Nerve Entrapment (see Chap. 18)

Entrapment of the following nerves may occur:

- Median nerve (carpal tunnel syndrome)
- Ulnar nerve (Guyon canal entrapment)
- Radial nerve

Complex Regional Pain Syndrome (Reflex Sympathetic Dystrophy)

See Chapter 18.

Vascular Occlusion

An embolus or trauma may obstruct the brachial, ulnar, or radial artery. The amount of pain distal to the obstruction is dependent on the degree of collateral circulation. Prolonged restriction to the blood flow may result in gangrene.

Raynaud Phenomenon

Raynaud phenomenon is a vascular disorder that can affect one hand or both hands and the feet. Reversible vasospasm of the extremities occurs either as an isolated symptom without underlying disorder (primary Raynaud phenomenon) or in association with another disorder or condition (secondary Raynaud phenomenon). The clinical findings include digital pallor followed by cyanosis and then rubor.[405] Throbbing and tingling sensations usually accompany the rubor stage.

Raynaud phenomenon is usually managed with simple measures, such as using warm clothes, mittens (not gloves), hand warmers, and automatic car starters.[406] The most frequently used drugs are calcium-channel antagonists.

Scleroderma

Scleroderma means "hard skin." The term is used to describe two distinct diseases: localized scleroderma and systemic scleroderma. Localized scleroderma is primarily a cutaneous disease. Systemic sclerosis is a multisystem connective tissue disease. The etiology of both of these diseases is not known.

There are two main subsets of systemic sclerosis, limited scleroderma (formerly referred to as CREST syndrome) and diffuse scleroderma:

- ***Limited scleroderma.*** Patients generally have a long history of Raynaud phenomenon, in some cases 10–15 years, and mildly puffy or swollen fingers before they present to their physician with a digital ulcer, heartburn, or shortness of breath.
- ***Diffuse scleroderma.*** Patients have a much more acute onset of disease. They have arthralgias, carpal tunnel syndrome, swollen hands, swollen legs, and crepitus-like friction rubs over the tendon areas of hands, wrists, and ankles. These patients potentially have severe problems not only from skin thickening and contractures but also from other organ systems, including gastrointestinal, pulmonary, cardiovascular, and renal.

Raynaud phenomenon is present in almost all patients with scleroderma.

Mononeuritis Multiplex

This condition is associated with a sudden onset of severe aching or sharp forearm and hand pain, paresthesias, and dysesthesias in the distribution of the median, ulnar, or radial nerves.[405] Mononeuritis multiplex can occur in association with a number of other medical conditions, including RA, vasculitis, polyarteritis nodosa, diabetes mellitus, sarcoidosis, and amyloidosis. An ischemic mechanism is the most likely cause of mononeuritis multiplex. It is generally accepted that mononeuritis multiplex in RA results from ischemia caused by vasa nervorum vasculitis.

Referred Pain: Viscerogenic

The heart, apical lung, and bronchus are all capable of referring pain to the wrist and hand.

CAUSES OF KNEE PAIN

Generalized Knee Pain

Causes of generalized knee pain include

- fracture (supracondylar, patellar, and proximal tibia);
- acute dislocation of the tibiofemoral joint;
- acute dislocation of the patella;

- intra-articular ligament injury (see Chap. 20);
- monoarthritis;
- polyarthritis;
- reactive arthritis;
- complex regional pain syndrome (CRPS) (reflex sympathetic dystrophy);
- referred pain.

Anterior Knee Pain

Anterior knee pain is a common problem in active adolescents and young adults. The causes of anterior knee pain generally fall under three categories[407]:

- ***Focal musculoskeletal lesions.*** This group consists mainly of lesions that can be clinically and radiologically defined. Such lesions include Osgood–Schlatter disease, jumper's knee, bipartite patella, tumors, plical irritation, and ligamentous injuries (see Chap. 20). These lesions normally respond well to locally applied interventions.
- ***Traumatic lesions.*** This group includes all (see Chap. 20) the conditions with a specific mechanism of injury involving direct trauma. These conditions include osteochondritis dissecans and bone contusions.
- ***Miscellaneous lesions.*** This group includes the more obscure causes of anterior knee pain including dynamic problems, such as maltracking of the patella and the excessive lateral pressure syndrome (see Chap. 20), as well as idiopathic chondromalacia, referred pain, CRPS, and psychogenic pain.

Musculoskeletal Causes

Osgood–Schlatter Disease

See Chapter 30.

Bursitis

See Chapter 20.

Jumper's Knee

See Chapter 20.

Bipartite Patella

This condition is common in childhood. It is often bilateral and usually is regarded as a variation of normal ossification. Very rarely, in response to overuse or acute injury, the synchondrosis separating the two centers of ossification may become painful and the site of local tenderness. There are three sites at which bipartite patella is found and each has an important soft-tissue attachment[407]:

- Distal pole of the patella with attachment of the patellar tendon. This type may represent the end stage of Sinding–Larsen–Johansson syndrome.
- Lateral margin of the patella with attachment of the lateral retinaculum.
- Superior-lateral corner of the patella, the insertion of vastus lateralis. This is the most common site for symptoms.

Trauma-Related Causes

Osteochondritis Dissecans[420]

Osteochondritis dissecans (OCD) is a rare cause of anterior knee pain in young athletes. It involves the weight-bearing portions of the medial and lateral femoral condyles. Occasionally, pain may not be the most prominent symptom, but a catching sensation with knee flexion or an extensor weakness may be the primary complaint. Sometimes the lesion is associated with maltracking. If the lesion is small, a painful arc is produced as it passes over the articular surface of the femur during movement.

MRI, CT, and bone scans are often used to characterize these lesions.

Conservative intervention with rest is appropriate for intact lesions, which usually will show no sclerosis, and in patients younger than 13 or 14 years, in whom healing is the rule.[407]

Surgical techniques can be used to securely attach the loose osteochondral fragments to the underlying bone.

Bone Contusion

Bone contusions (bruises) are related to trauma and can occur in sites other than the knee. There is no unique mechanism of injury, but they seem to result from direct impact, axial overloading, and impingement. They pose a potential risk for chondrolysis and stress fracture, and mobilization and weight bearing should be increased gradually.

Miscellaneous Causes

Tumors

Neoplastic involvement of the knee is a less common cause of knee pain. Malignant primary tumors arising from the patella include hemangioendothelioma, hemangiosarcoma, lymphoma, fibrous histiocytoma, osteoblastoclastoma, and plasmacytoma.[408] Soft-tissue sarcomas are the most common malignant tumor of the knee, and these include osteosarcomas, Ewing sarcoma, rhabdomyosarcoma, and synovial sarcomas.[409,410] Metastasis to the patella is rare.[411]

Benign tumors are more prevalent at this site. In a published series of 42 patellar tumors,[412] 90% were benign, with the most common diagnosis being chondroblastoma. Other benign tumors of the knee may include osteochondromas, nonossifying fibromas, and osteoid osteomas. Very rarely, soft-tissue tumors may occur within the fat pad; in addition, synovial lesions, such as PVN synovitis, can cause anterior knee pain, clicking, and catching.[407]

A history of knee pain worsened by activity and relieved by rest suggests benign involvement. However, pain that is constant, unrelenting, severe, and that occurs at night suggests a malignant process.[413–415] In malignant tumors of the patella, pathologic fracture is often the presenting complaint.

Plicae

See Chapter 20.

Hoffa Syndrome

See Chapter 20.

Osteomyelitis of the Patella

Osteomyelitis of the patella usually affects children between the ages of 5 and 15 years. It is exceedingly rare in adults and in children younger than 5 years.[416]

The patient may present with complaints of an insidious onset of pain and swelling in the knee and calf. Pain localized to the patella may be mild or severe, causing a limp and restriction of motion. Motion is less severely affected than in patients with septic arthritis. Swelling may be minimal in the more indolent cases, or marked with distention of the prepatellar bursa or the knee, which may divert attention from the patella. Cellulitis overlying the patella may also be present. Isolated pinpoint tenderness over the patella is probably the single most useful clinical sign.[416]

Differential diagnosis of the swollen knee in an individual with sepsis includes septic arthritis; osteomyelitis of the distal femur, proximal tibia, or patella; and septic bursitis.[417] With more benign symptoms and the presence of a lytic lesion of the patella, neoplasm and Brodie abscess must be considered.[417]

Excessive Lateral Pressure Syndrome

See Chapter 20.

Maltracking of the Patella

See Chapter 20.

Iatrogenic Causes: Infrapatellar Contracture Syndrome

See Chapter 20.

Medial Knee Pain

The causes of medial knee pain include the following.

- Medial meniscus tear: see Chapter 20.
- Medial Collateral Ligament Sprain: see Chapter 20.
- Medial Collateral Ligament Bursitis: see Chapter 20.
- Hoffa's Disease: see Chapter 20.
- Pes Anserine Bursitis: see Chapter 20.
- Semimembranosus Tendonitis: see Chapter 20.

Lateral Knee Pain

The causes of lateral knee pain include the following.

- Iliotibial band friction syndrome: see Chapter 20.
- Popliteus tenosynovitis
- Popliteus tendon rupture
- Lateral meniscal tear: see Chapter 20.
- Lateral collateral ligament sprain
- Tibiofibular disorder: see Chapter 20.
- Biceps femoris tendonitis: see Chapter 20.
- Osteochondral fracture of the lateral femoral condyle

Posterior Knee Pain

The causes of posterior knee pain include the following.

- Gastrocnemius Muscle Strain or Rupture
- Plantaris Muscle Strain or Rupture
- Hamstring Muscle and Tendon Disorder
- Muscle Spasm or Cramp
- Posterior cruciate ligament or posterior capsule tear: see Chapter 20.
- Baker cyst: see Chapter 20.

CAUSES OF LOWER LEG PAIN

Anterolateral Lower Leg Pain

The causes of anterolateral lower leg pain include those listed in Table 5-20.

Anterior Compartment Syndrome

Compartment syndrome is a condition of pain associated with increased tissue pressure in the involved muscular compartment. This condition is suggested by lower leg muscular pain with running or other activity, and is relieved, very rapidly, by stopping the activity. The clinical signs of compartment syndrome can be remembered using the mnemonic of the five P's: pain, paralysis, paresthesia, pallor, and pulses. Pain, especially disproportionate pain, is often the earliest sign, but the loss of normal neurologic sensation is the most reliable sign.[418,419]

Palpation of the compartment in question may demonstrate swelling or a tense compartment.[420] A decrease or loss of two-point discrimination also can be an early finding of compartment syndrome.[418,419] Clinical findings may also include shiny, erythematous skin overlying the involved compartment (described as "woody") and excessive swelling. Intracompartmental tissue pressure is usually lower than arterial blood pressure, making peripheral pulses and capillary refill poor indicators of blood flow within the compartment.[420]

Compartment syndrome is confirmed by elevated compartment pressures. Normal tissue pressure ranges between 0 and 10 mm Hg.[420] Capillary blood flow within the compartment may be compromised at pressures greater than 20 mm Hg. Muscle and nerve fibers are at risk of ischemic necrosis at pressures greater than 30–40 mm Hg.

Differential diagnosis includes tibial stress fracture, anterior tibialis tendonitis, and the catch-all group of "shin splints." Acute compartment syndrome requires emergent surgical fasciotomy.

TABLE 5-20 Potential Causes of Anterolateral Leg Pain
Anterior compartment syndrome
Lateral compartment syndrome
Irritation of the superficial fibular (peroneal) nerve
Muscle strain of one or more of the fibularis (peroneal) muscles or of anterior tibialis

Lateral Compartment Syndrome

Lateral compartment syndrome is very rare. It is often misdiagnosed as tenosynovitis of the tibialis anterior and flexor hallucis longus, fibular stress fracture, or a lateral gastrocnemius strain. Characteristic findings include tenderness along the proximal half of the leg, with swelling and tightness over the lateral compartment. On occasion, there may be complaints of numbness over the posterior aspect of the foot caused by compression of the superficial fibular (peroneal) nerve.[419,420]

Intervention is based on the severity of the symptoms. In mild cases, treatment involves relative rest, education, and examination for underlying etiologies.[421] These include lower extremity malalignment, muscle imbalances, training errors, inadequate footwear, and poor technique.[421]

An acute compartment syndrome, or one that does not respond to conservative intervention, requires an open fasciotomy.

Irritation of the Superficial Peroneal Nerve

Compression of a peripheral nerve causes deformation of the nerve fibers, local ischemia, edema, and increased endoneurial pressure caused by accelerated vascular permeability, resulting in the loss of nerve fiber function (see Chap. 3).

Muscle Strain

See Chapter 20.

Calf Pain

The causes of calf pain include those listed in Table 5-21.

Pyomyositis

Pyomyositis is a term used to denote a spontaneous muscle abscess of skeletal muscle. It is predominantly a disease of tropical countries. The etiology of pyomyositis is poorly understood. Local mechanical trauma at the time of incidental bacteremia is frequently postulated as a mechanism. Underlying conditions, such as immunodeficiency, or chronic illness, such as diabetes mellitus, may predispose to pyomyositis.

The natural history of pyomyositis may be divided into three stages: invasive, purulent, and late.

1. ***Invasive stage:***[422] This stage occurs when the organism enters the muscle. It is characterized by an insidious onset of dull, cramping pain, with or without fever and anorexia. There is localized edema, sometimes described as indurated or woody, but usually little or no tenderness. This stage lasts from 10 to 21 days.
2. ***Purulent stage.*** This stage occurs when a deep collection of pus has developed in the muscle. The muscle usually but not always is tender, and fever and chills are common. The overlying skin may be normal or show mild erythema.
3. ***Late stage.*** This stage is characterized by exquisite tenderness of the site, which is red and fluctuant. The patient has high fever and occasionally may be in septic shock.

The iliopsoas is one of the most common sites of pyomyositis (see the discussion of iliopsoas abscess under "Causes of Pelvic Pain" earlier), but they can also occur in other leg muscles.

TABLE 5-21 Potential Causes of Calf Pain
Pyomyositis
Fibular shaft fracture
Deep vein thrombosis
Hematoma
Rupture of Achilles tendon
Soleus muscle strain
Acute posterior compartment syndrome
Muscle cramps

Fibular Shaft Fracture

Direct trauma is the most common cause of isolated fibular fractures.[423] Another cause is a forced muscle contraction of the soleus.[424] Fibular stress fractures are common in long-distance runners. Loading of the fibula occurs maximally during the initial period of stance and forces up to three times body weight are transmitted through the leg.[425] Thus, pain with this condition is typically reported with weight bearing during the initial period of stance. There also may be tenderness over the fracture site.

Deep Venous Thrombosis

Muscle veins drain into the deep veins of the lower extremity. Soleal muscle veins drain into the fibular and tibial posterior veins. The veins of the gastrocnemius drain into the popliteal vein. Thrombosis usually develops as a result of venous stasis or slow-flowing blood around venous valve sinuses (see Chap. 2). Extension of the primary thrombus occurs within or between the deep and superficial veins of the leg, and the propagating clot causes venous obstruction, damage to valves, and possible venous thromboembolism (VTE). Most episodes of VTE are clinically silent. The most common cause of leg swelling is edema, but expansion of all or part of a limb may result from an increase in any tissue component (muscle, fat, blood, etc.).[426]

The clinical features of a deep vein thrombosis (DVT) include[426]

- calf pain or tenderness, or both;
- swelling with pitting edema;
- swelling below the knee (distal deep vein thrombosis) or up to the groin (proximal deep vein thrombosis);
- increased skin temperature;
- superficial venous dilation;
- cyanosis, in patients with severe obstruction.

The intervention is aimed at reducing symptoms and preventing complications. The main complications of a DVT are pulmonary embolism (see Chap. 2), postthrombotic syndrome, and recurrence of thrombosis.[426] Proximal thrombi are a major source of morbidity and mortality. Distal thrombi are generally smaller and more difficult to detect noninvasively, and their prognosis and clinical importance are less clear.[426]

Hematoma

A strain of the gastrocnemius muscle may follow a trivial trauma. Complete or partial tears of the musculotendinous unit may result in a hematoma. Clinical manifestations of gastrocnemius hematoma may include local swelling, pain, and tenderness aggravated by passive dorsiflexion of the ankle joint. This condition can mimic a DVT. The subjective history may help with the diagnosis. A definite diagnosis is established by CT scanning examination, which will reveal a local soft-tissue mass within the gastrocnemius consistent with a hematoma.

Rupture of the Achilles Tendon

See Chapter 21.

Soleus Muscle Strain

See Chapter 21.

Acute Posterior Compartment Syndrome

Acute calf pain can occur as a result of a posterior compartment syndrome. Causes include a DVT, rupture of a Baker cyst, and spontaneous rupture of the medial head of the gastrocnemius. The diagnosis of posterior compartment syndrome is made by measuring the pressure in the posterior compartment. The intervention usually involves a fasciotomy.

Anteromedial Lower Leg Pain

The causes of anteromedial lower leg pain include those listed in Table 5-22.

Stress Fracture of the Tibia

Tibial stress fractures are a common cause of shin soreness and a very common cause of exertional leg pain. Simple muscle strains are probably the most common cause of acute exercise-induced leg pain, whereas more subacute or chronic pain may be caused by stress fractures or chronic (exertional) compartment syndrome.

Recognition of anterior tibial stress fractures is important because these fractures are prone to nonunion and avascular necrosis. They are also at greater risk of becoming displaced than are posterior tibial stress fractures. This increased susceptibility to complication has been attributed to a predominance of tensile forces along the anterior diaphysis rather than compressive forces along the posterior diaphysis.

Bone grafting, electrical stimulation, and internal localization are sometimes needed.

TABLE 5-22 Potential Causes of Anteromedial Lower-Leg Pain
Stress fracture of tibia
Medial tibial stress syndrome
Saphenous neuritis
Osteomyelitis of tibia
Soleus syndrome
Shin splints
Greater saphenous vein thrombosis

Medial Tibial Stress Syndrome

See Chapter 21.

Saphenous Neuritis

Saphenous neuritis, also known as *gonalgia paresthetica*, is a painful condition caused by either irritation or compression at the adductor canal or elsewhere along the course of the saphenous nerve.[427] The condition may also be associated with surgical or nonsurgical trauma to the nerve, especially at the medial or anterior aspect of the knee.

Saphenous neuritis can imitate other pathology around the knee or calf, particularly a medial meniscal tear, muscle injury, or OA. As an isolated entity, saphenous neuritis may appear in conjunction with other common problems, such as OA and patellofemoral pain syndrome. Its clinical appearance is characterized by a dull or achy pain along the course of the saphenous nerve on the medial side of the thigh, knee, or calf. Hyperesthesia of the nerve is common. There is usually tenderness to light palpation along the course of the nerve, especially at the exit of the nerve from the adductor canal, near the medial joint line, or along the nerve in the proximal third of the leg. The diagnosis is confirmed by relief of symptoms after injection of the affected area with local anesthetic.

Initial treatment can include nonsurgical symptomatic care, treatment of associated pathology, desensitization therapy, transcutaneous electrical nerve stimulation (TENS), and diagnostic or therapeutic injections of local anesthetic. In recalcitrant cases, surgical decompression and neurectomy are potential options. The key to treatment is prompt recognition; palpation of the saphenous nerve should be part of every routine examination of the knee.

Osteomyelitis of the Tibia

Osteomyelitis is a severe infection that can arise after operative treatment of bone and from acute penetrating trauma to the bone. The tibia is the most common site of posttraumatic osteomyelitis.[428] Posttraumatic tibial osteomyelitis results from trauma or nosocomial infection from the treatment of trauma that allows organisms to enter bone, proliferate in traumatized tissue, and cause subsequent bone infection.[428] The resulting infection is usually polymicrobial.

Patients with posttraumatic osteomyelitis of the tibia may present with localized bone and joint pain, erythema, swelling, and drainage around the area of trauma, surgery, or wound infection.[428] Signs of bacteremia, such as fever, chills, and night sweats, may be present in the acute phase of osteomyelitis, but not in the chronic phase.[428]

Radiographs are important for the diagnosis, staging, and evaluation of the progression of posttraumatic osteomyelitis.[428]

CAUSES OF ANKLE PAIN

The causes of generalized ankle pain include those shown in Fig. 5-4 and listed in Table 5-23.

Crystal-Induced Arthropathies

Two types of arthritis, gout and pseudogout, are quite common in the ankle joint. Episodes of acute arthritis in this

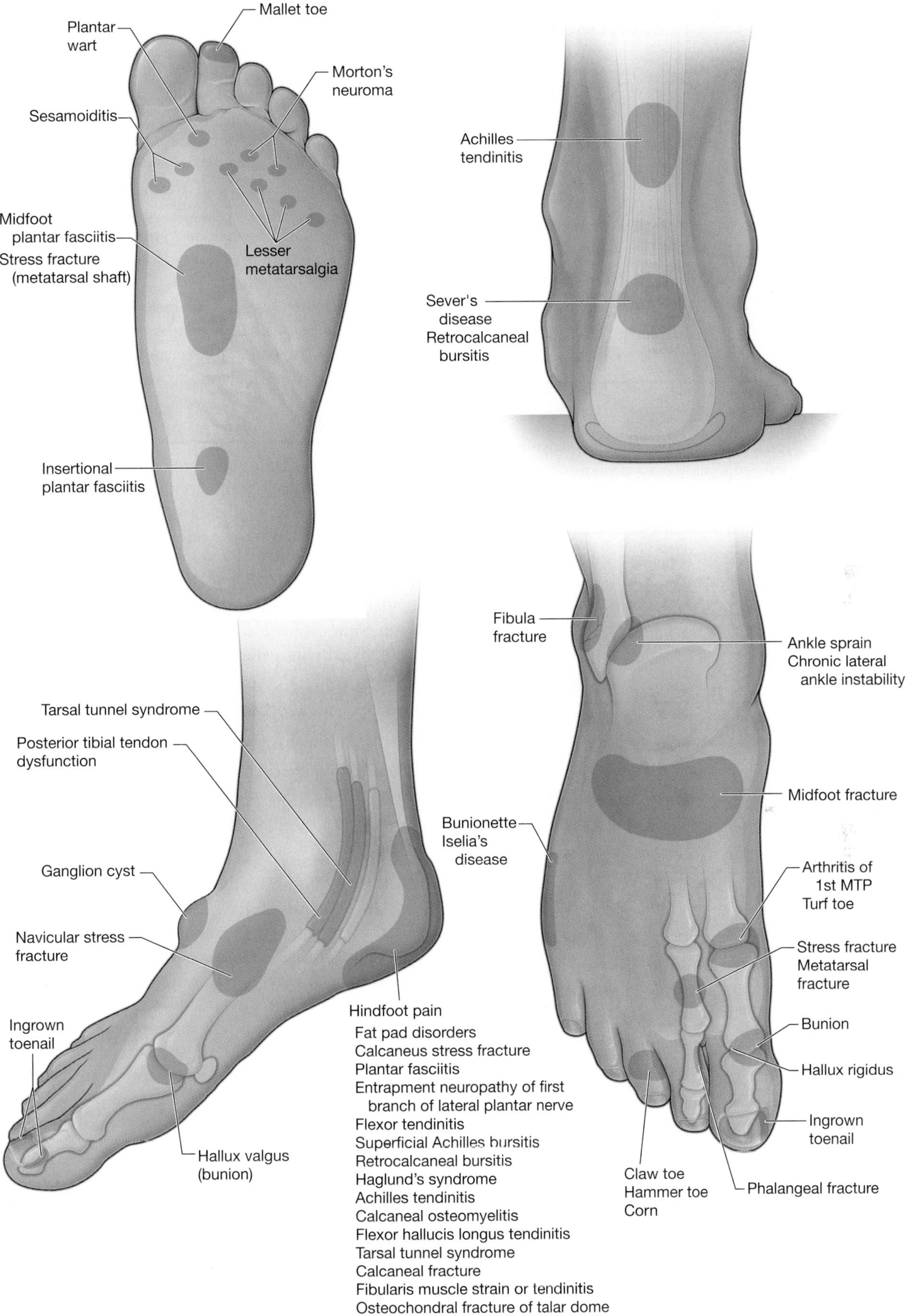

FIGURE 5-4 Potential causes of foot and ankle pain.

TABLE 5-23 Potential Causes of Generalized Ankle Pain
Crystal-induced arthropathies
Ligament sprain
Tendonitis
Fracture
Bursitis
Os trigonum
Osteochondritis dissecans of talus
Acute monarthritis
Transient migratory osteoporosis
Polyarthritis
Lyme arthritis
Reiter syndrome
Rheumatoid arthritis

region, without an apparent cause, should arouse suspicion of a gout attack, especially in a middle-aged man.

Ligament Sprain

See Chapter 21.

Tendonitis

See Chapter 21.

Fracture

See Chapter 21.

Bursitis

See Chapter 21.

Os Trigonum

The term *os trigonum* refers to a failure of the lateral tubercle of the posterior process to unite with the body of the talus during ossification, producing an impingement with extreme plantar flexion.[429] The posterior aspect of the talus often exhibits a separate ossification center, appearing at 8–10 years in girls and 11–13 years in boys. Fusion usually occurs 1 year after its appearance.[430,431] When fusion does not occur, an os trigonum is formed. It has been reported to be present in approximately 10% of the general population and is often unilateral.[430,432–434]

The origin of this ossicle may be congenital or acquired. Congenitally, it can be a persistent separation of the secondary center of the lateral tubercle from the remainder of the posterior talus secondary to repeated microtrauma during development.[430,434] The acquired form may be secondary to an actual fracture that has not united.[430,434,435] With either form, the os trigonum is usually asymptomatic in most cases.[429] However, it can become symptomatic in young athletes who actively plantar flex the ankle, such as ballet dancers, gymnasts, ice skaters, or, on occasion, soccer players.[430,432,434,436,437]

The pain, which is typically in the posterolateral ankle, results from the mechanical impingement of the posterior talus between the posterior tibia and the calcaneus.[429] Repetitive impingement of the soft tissues in this interval can also result in hypertrophic capsulitis.[430,433,438–440] Associated posteromedial pain[430,436,439] may indicate a concurrent flexor hallucis longus tendonitis. The diagnosis is confirmed with imaging studies.

Plain radiographs should include a lateral view of the ankle and a lateral view in plantarflexion. A bone scan may be used to determine the reactivity of the os trigonum,[430,441] but absence of uptake does not exclude impingement.[429]

Differential diagnosis includes posterior ankle impingement, Achilles tendonitis, fibularis tendonitis, and flexor hallucis longus tendonitis.[430]

Conservative intervention may include rest, antiinflammatory medications, avoidance of plantarflexion casting, and injection.[430,436] The pain, however, usually returns once the young athlete resumes their sports.

Osteochondritis Dissecans

OCD of the talus may result from an inversion stress to the ankle. This is actually a "transchondral fracture" secondary to trauma.[442] More commonly, onset of pain is insidious, and some prior macrotrauma is evident.[429] Young patients may present with pain over the anterolateral or posteromedial talus. They often report recurrent ankle effusions or weakness. Plain radiographs of the ankle usually show the lesion, but sometimes a bone scan or MRI is necessary for diagnosis.[443] The Berndt–Harty[444] classification of talus OCD is as follows:

- ***Type I.*** Small area of compression of subchondral bone.
- ***Type II.*** Partially detached osteochondral fragment.
- ***Type III.*** Completely detached osteochondral fragment but remaining in its crater.
- ***Type IV.*** Displaced osteochondral fragment.

Berndt and Harty[444] reported that 43% of OCD lesions involve the middle third of the lateral talus, with 57% involving the posterior third of the medial talus.[442] One study[445] reported that lateral OCD lesions rarely heal on their own, whereas most medial lesions do.[442]

The intervention for type I and II lesions begins with casting and orthotics.[429] The intervention for type III medial lesions starts off conservatively, as well, but may require arthroscopic or open debridement. Type III lateral lesions and type IV lesions all require arthroscopic removal or pinning for the best chance of healing.[446]

CAUSES OF FOOT PAIN

Generalized Foot Pain

The causes of generalized foot pain include those shown in Fig. 5-4 and listed in Table 5-24.

Infection

Infection of the foot includes such diagnoses as cellulitis, necrotizing fasciitis, and osteomyelitis.

TABLE 5-24	Potential Causes of Generalized Foot Pain
Trauma	
Infection	
Rheumatoid arthritis	
Gout	
Pseudogout	
Systemic lupus erythematosus	
Sickle-cell disease	
Reflex sympathetic dystrophy/complex regional pain syndrome	
Peripheral vascular disease	
Peripheral polyneuropathy	
Systemic disorders	
Nerve and root compression syndromes	
Foot cramps	
Cold injury	
Bites	
Cutaneous disorders	

Cellulitis. Cellulitis is common after foot and ankle surgery. It is important to distinguish a superficial infection from one that involves the deeper soft-tissue envelope and possibly the joint or bone.

- ***Superficial.*** With a superficial infection, the skin is warm, tender, and erythematous, but joint motion is painless. Occasionally, lymphangitis or lymphadenopathy is present. The area is tender to palpation. The most common causative organisms in uncompromised hosts are *Staph. aureus* and β-hemolytic streptococci.
- ***Deep.*** Deep infections with abscess formation are a serious complication. In patients with deep infections, the skin is warm, tender, swollen, and possibly fluctuant. White blood cell count and temperature may be increased. Plain radiographs, MRI, and needle aspiration are helpful in making the diagnosis.

Necrotizing Fasciitis. Necrotizing fasciitis is characterized by rapidly progressive necrosis and edema of the subcutaneous fat and fascia that can result in septic shock, end-organ failure, and loss of limb or life. Patients who are immunocompromised, such as those with human immunodeficiency virus (HIV) infections, diabetes mellitus, and alcoholism, are at increased risk of necrotizing fasciitis. Clinical signs of necrotizing fasciitis include tense edema and erythema that do not respond to antibiotics or elevation. Patients are usually febrile.

Osteomyelitis. Fever, local pain, edema, exudative drainage, and elevated leukocyte count and sedimentation rate are typical findings with osteomyelitis. Surgical treatment of patients with osteomyelitis consists of debridement of all necrotic and infected tissue and appropriate antibiotic therapy. Treatment may also include the use of antibiotic-impregnated methylmethacrylate beads, local or vascularized soft-tissue flaps, autogenous bone grafts, or vascularized bone grafts once the infection is eradicated.

Rheumatoid Arthritis

RA characteristically involves the synovial tissues of the small joints of the feet, rather than the talocrural or subtalar joint. Three times more women than men are affected. In 17% of cases, the disease first manifests in the foot.[447]

The early stage of the disease should be suspected in young women presenting with bilateral foot pain and a tendency for morning stiffness in the MTP joints of the feet.

Gout

About 60% of initial attacks of gout involve the great toe (podagra), which becomes swollen and excruciatingly painful.[447]

Pseudogout

Pseudogout involves joints in addition to the MTP joint, including the talonavicular or subtalar joints.[447]

Systemic Lupus Erythematosus

SLE is a systemic autoimmune disease with clinical features that include glomerulonephritis, rashes, serositis, hemolytic anemia, thrombocytopenia, and CNS involvement.[448] This disease occurs most commonly in women of childbearing age.

The variety of neurologic presentations of SLE can include cranial neuropathies, stroke syndromes, movement disorders, spinal cord lesions, seizure disorders, dementias, cognitive disturbances, psychoses, and mood disorders. Peripheral nervous system manifestations include symmetric polyneuropathies, mononeuritis multiplex, acute inflammatory demyelinating polyneuropathies, chronic relapsing inflammatory demyelinating polyneuropathies, and autonomic failure.

SLE is considered to be the prototypical human autoimmune disease mediated by pathogenic immune complexes.

Sickle-Cell Disease[449]

Sickle-cell disease is an inherited blood disorder that affects mostly African-Americans. It leaves patients vulnerable to repeated crises that can cause severe pain, multisystem organ damage, and early death. Sickle-cell crises typically begin during the preschool or early elementary school years. How often they recur and how long each attack lasts vary considerably.

The crisis begins when a trigger—such as an acute infection (especially viral), stress, dehydration, or extremely hot or cold temperatures—causes the red blood cells to release oxygen. People with sickle-cell disease have abnormal hemoglobin, called *hemoglobin S (HbS)*, which forms long polymers upon deoxygenation. The rod-like polymers change the normally round and pliable red blood cells into stiff cells with a crescent, or sickle, shape.

Bundles of these deformed cells plug up the capillaries throughout the body, reducing blood flow. This vasoocclusion causes localized tissue hypoxia, which, in turn, promotes further sickling. Tissue infarction and necrosis soon follow.

Pain is usually the main symptom. It may be localized or diffuse, constant or intermittent. About half of all patients also have fever, swelling in the joints of the hands or feet, long bone pain, tachypnea, hypertension, nausea, and vomiting. Hospitalization becomes necessary when these complications are severe. Acute chest syndrome and cerebrovascular accidents are life-threatening complications of sickle-cell disease. In addition, the patient may develop an infarct in a lung, causing acute chest syndrome, characterized by a combination of chest pain, dyspnea, fever, and leukocytosis.

Complex Regional Pain Syndrome

Complex Regional Pain Syndrome (CRPS) formerly known as reflex sympathetic dystrophy (RSD), is a regional, posttraumatic, neuropathic pain problem that most often affects one or more limbs (see Chap. 18 for CRPS of the upper extremity).[450]

Most patients with CRPS have an identifiable inciting or initiating injury, which may be trivial, such as a minor limb sprain, or severe, such as trauma involving a major nerve or nerves. Adults can present with CRPS after a fracture or trauma with immobilization. With children, CRPS occurs most often in athletic girls (1:6, boys to girls) with an average age of 12 years.[451]

Most of the cases of CRPS in the lower extremity, including the foot and ankle, have a history of minor trauma. The key features are pain, allodynia and hyperalgesia, abnormal vasomotor activity, and abnormal sudomotor activity persisting beyond the period of normal healing. Allodynia is defined as a disproportionately increased pain response to a nonnoxious stimulus. Hyperalgesia is defined as a disproportionately increased pain response to a mildly noxious stimulus.

Patients with CRPS often adopt a protective posture to protect the affected extremity from mechanical and thermal stimulation. They may wear a stocking to guard the involved extremity. Allodynia may be so severe that the patient will not allow the physician or therapist to examine or even touch the affected limb.

Successful treatment of CRPS depends on an aggressive and multidisciplinary approach. Because pain and limb dysfunction are the major clinical problems, physical rehabilitation and pain control are the main treatment objectives. Early referral to a pain clinic for possible sympathetic nerve blocks or neurosuppressive medications may be indicated.

Peripheral Vascular Disease

PVD is common in the western world. PVD, typically begins its progression in midlife (for men, at approximately 45 years, and for women, 55–60 years).[452] Arteries generally have smooth linings, which allow blood to flow unimpaired. Arteriosclerosis is a degenerative arterial disease that refers to the so-called hardening of the arteries. In this condition, muscle and elastic tissue are replaced with fibrous tissue, and calcification may occur.

Atherosclerosis is the most common type of arteriosclerosis. It is characterized by the formation of atheromatous plaques, which are deposits of fatty material in the lining of medium- and large-sized arteries. These arteries then become narrowed and rough as more fat is deposited. Blood clots form more easily because of the roughness of the vessel wall, further narrowing the artery and, thus, potentially limiting blood flow. A reduction of blood supply to the organs and tissues prevents them from performing adequately. In addition, the plaques are liable to break down and form ulcers. Thromboses may then develop as a result of the roughening and ulceration of the inner coat of the arteries.

Patients suffering from reduced blood supply to the lower limbs often experience effort-related cramp in the calves, thighs, and buttocks, which disappears at rest. This condition is known as *intermittent claudication.*

PVD with claudication can be confused with neurogenic claudication and spinal stenosis. The major difference is the response of the pain to rest or to the position of the spine. Unlike the pain from spinal stenosis, the pain from PVD is not relieved by trunk flexion or aggravated with sustained trunk extension (Table 5-25).

The site of claudication indicates the most likely site of the narrowing or blockage. When severe, claudication can become debilitating, can limit mobility, and sometimes is associated with a worsened quality of life and loss of functional independence. Pain may occur at more regular intervals, as the disease process continues to its end stage—critical limb ischemia—until finally it occurs when the patient is at rest (rest pain). At this stage, rest pain is usually worse when the legs are elevated and during sleep, with the patient gaining relief by hanging the foot over the side of the bed. The development of nonhealing wounds or gangrene (tissue death) may occur at this stage.

This disease process can lead to loss of limb and life; therefore, investigation and early diagnosis are important. The patient who presents with typical, reproducible, exertional discomfort in the buttocks, thighs, or calves that disappears with rest is likely to have claudication and symptomatic PVD.

Peripheral Polyneuropathy

Polyneuropathy is a syndrome with many different causes. Clinical features in painful neuropathies include sensory loss, paresthesia, paradox hyperalgesia, paroxysms, and increased pain on repetitive stimulation.

Systemic Disorders

The systemic disorders that can cause foot pain include

- carcinoma;
- leukemia;
- lymphoma;
- myeloma;
- amyloidosis;
- connective tissue diseases (polyarteritis nodosa and SLE);
- renal failure;
- acquired immunodeficiency syndrome;
- sarcoidosis;
- cutaneous disorders.

Nerve and Root Compression Syndromes

See Chapter 21.

Forefoot Pain

The causes of forefoot pain include those shown in Fig. 5-4 and listed in Table 5-26.

Metatarsalgia

Metatarsalgia, in its broadest definition, includes discomfort around the metatarsal heads or the plantar aspects of the metatarsal heads. Metatarsalgia is discussed in Chapter 21.

TABLE 5-25 Differentiating Causes of Claudication

Vascular Claudication	Neurogenic Claudication	Spinal Stenosis
Pain[a] is usually bilateral	Pain is usually bilateral but may be unilateral	Usually bilateral pain
Occurs in calf (foot, thigh, hip, or buttocks)	Occurs in back, buttocks, thighs, calves, and feet	Occurs in back, buttocks, thighs, calves, and feet
Pain consistent in all spinal positions	Pain is decreased in spinal flexion and increased in spinal extension and with walking	Pain is decreased in spinal flexion and increased in spinal extension and with walking
Pain is brought on by physical exertion (e.g., walking), relieved promptly by rest (1–5 min), and increased by walking uphill	Pain is decreased by recumbency	Pain is relieved with prolonged rest (may persist hours after resting) and decreased when walking uphill
No burning or dysesthesia	Burning and dysesthesia from back to buttocks and leg(s)	Burning and numbness present in lower extremities
Decreased or absent pulses in lower extremities	Normal pulses	Normal pulses
Color and skin changes in feet; cold, numb, dry, or scaly skin; and poor nail and hair growth	Good skin nutrition	Good skin nutrition
Affects ages of 40–60+ years	Affects ages of 40–60+ years	Peaks in the seventh decade, affects men primarily

[a]Pain associated with vascular claudication also may be described as an "aching," "cramping," or "tired" feeling.
Data from Goodman CC, Snyder TEK: *Differential Diagnosis in Physical Therapy*. Philadelphia, PA: WB Saunders, 1990.

Freiberg Disease

Freiberg disease, an avascular necrosis of the second metatarsal epiphysis, is a source of metatarsalgia.[429] The disease is an osteochondrosis of congenital, traumatic, or vascular etiology that leads to eventual collapse and deformity of a lesser metatarsal head. It is unlikely that an athletic injury is the sole cause of Freiberg disease, although a mechanical stress to the forefoot may exacerbate a previously subclinical condition. The condition is most common in the second metatarsal head, with a predilection of 68–82%.[453,454] Less commonly, it may occur at the third, fourth, or fifth metatarsal heads.

The female-to-male ratio in Freiberg disease is 5:1, and the typical patient is a female adolescent aged 11–17 years.[455] The condition may be asymptomatic early in its course and manifest in young adulthood to middle age.

Physical examination usually reveals unilateral pain over the second metatarsal head, that is worse with activity, limited range of motion, periarticular swelling, and, occasionally, a plantar callosity under the second metatarsal head.[456]

This condition is usually self-limiting and requires only conservative treatment in the form of rest from high-impact activities, an orthosis to correct pronation,[457] a range-of-motion walking boot, or a short leg cast for more severe acute pain. Patients with severe antalgia should use crutches. Hoskinson[454] reported success with conservative treatment in 11 of 28 patients, although all had restriction of joint motion.

The surgical intervention for Freiberg disease involves debridement of the joint, removal of loose bodies, and removal of metatarsal head osteophytes, with reshaping of the head.[458] A dorsiflexion osteotomy of the metatarsal head also has been advocated to rotate the healthy plantar cartilage up into articulation with the proximal phalanx.

TABLE 5-26 Potential Causes of Forefoot Pain

Metatarsalgia
Freiberg disease
Morton neuroma
Arthritis
Fracture
Forefoot sprain
Bursitis
Idiopathic synovitis
Arterial insufficiency

Morton Neuroma

An interdigital neuroma, or Morton neuroma, is a mechanical entrapment neuropathy of the interdigital nerve. The entrapment may occur as the nerve courses on the plantar side of the distal aspect of the transverse intermetatarsal ligament, where it is vulnerable to traction injury and compression during the toe-off phase of running or during repetitive positions of toe rise.[459]

The most commonly involved nerve is the third interdigital nerve, between the third and fourth metatarsal heads, followed in incidence by the second interdigital nerve and, rarely, the first and fourth interdigital nerves.[459,460]

The individual with an interdigital neuroma will complain of symptoms of forefoot burning, cramping, tingling, and numbness in the toes of the involved interspace, with occasional proximal radiation in the foot.[459]

Morton neuroma is described further in Chapter 21.

Arthritis

See Chapter 21.

Fracture

See Chapter 21.

Forefoot Sprain

See Chapter 21.

Bursitis

See Chapter 21.

Medial Forefoot and Great Toe Pain

The causes of medial forefoot and great toe pain include those shown in Fig. 5-4 and listed below.

Nail Lesions

See Chapter 21.

Hallux Valgus

See Chapter 21.

Hallux Rigidus

See Chapter 21.

Arthritis of the First MTP Joint

See Chapter 21.

Midfoot Pain

The causes of midfoot pain include those shown in Fig. 5-4 and listed below.

- Longitudinal arch strain
- Aseptic necrosis of the navicular
- Tendonitis of the flexor hallucis longus or fibularis (peroneal)

Tendonitis

See Chapter 21.

Subtalar Osteochondral Fracture

See Chapter 21.

Accessory Navicular

The accessory navicular is the most common accessory bone in the foot. It occurs on the medial plantar border of the navicular at the site of the tibialis posterior tendon insertion.[461] The incidence in the general population has been reported to be between 4% and 14%,[461,462] but few patients actually become symptomatic.[429] A histologic study by Grogan and colleagues in 1989[463] suggested that tensile failure in the cartilaginous synchondrosis was the cause of pain.

In the adolescent athletic population, symptoms may arise secondary to pressure over the bony prominence, a tear in the actual synchondrosis, or tibialis posterior tendonitis.[462]

The patient usually presents with pain and a prominence over the navicular in a pronated foot. There is usually local tenderness to palpation and pain with resisted foot inversion.[461] It has been hypothesized that when the tibialis posterior tendon inserts into the accessory navicular, a weaker insertion point, it contributes to a drop in the medial arch of the foot and a pes planus.[464] However, Sullivan and Miller[465] found no difference in the longitudinal arches of those with an accessory navicular and those without.[429]

Physical examination can be supplemented by radiographic assessment. The anteroposterior view or a 45-degree eversion oblique view is usually diagnostic.[461]

The intervention for this condition consists of orthotics, trial of casting, range of motion exercises, and eventual removal if symptoms continue.[461–463,465–468]

Köhler Bone Disease

Köhler bone disease is an aseptic necrosis of unknown etiology that typically affects the tarsal navicular bone.[429] The condition usually is caused by repetitive microtrauma to the maturing epiphysis.[429] It is largely found in active boys aged 4–7 years.

Köhler bone disease is typically self-limiting and should not require any type of surgery. Initial intervention involves decreased activity or a short leg cast for 3–6 weeks.[469] Orthotics may be necessary to maintain the longitudinal arch.

Stress Fracture of the Navicular

See Chapter 21.

Acquired Flatfoot

See Chapter 21.

Osteoarthritis

See Chapter 21.

Plantar Fascial Pain

See Chapter 21.

Cuboid Subluxation Syndrome

See Chapter 21.

Posterior (Dorsal) Foot Pain

Tendonitis of the Extensor Hallucis Longus, Extensor Digitorum Longus, or Tibialis Anterior

See Chapter 21.

Hindfoot Pain

The causes of generalized hindfoot pain include those shown in Fig. 5-4 and are as follows.

Intra-articular Calcaneal Fractures

The calcaneus is the most frequently fractured tarsal bone, with calcaneal fractures accounting for 65% of tarsal injuries and approximately 2% of all fractures.[470] Acute complications include swelling, fracture blisters, and compartment syndromes. Late complications include arthritis; malunion, including calcaneofibular abutment; and heel pad problems. Complications associated with operative treatment include wound dehiscence, infection, and iatrogenic nerve injury.

Fat Pad Disorders

Calcaneus Stress Fracture

See Chapter 21.

Plantar Fasciitis

See Chapter 21.

Entrapment Neuropathy of the First Branch of the Lateral Plantar Nerve

See Chapter 21.

Flexor Tendonitis

See Chapter 21.

Superficial Achilles Bursitis

See Chapter 21.

Retrocalcaneal Bursitis

See Chapter 21.

Haglund Syndrome

See Chapter 21.

Achilles Tendonitis

See Chapter 21.

Achilles Tendon Rupture

See Chapter 21.

Calcaneal Osteomyelitis

Primary hematogenous osteomyelitis of the calcaneus is uncommon and accounts for 3–10% of all acute bone infections in children.[471] The calcaneus has a so-called metaphyseal equivalent region that borders the apophysis and is susceptible to hematogenous infection, as in long bones.[472] *Staph. aureus* has been found to be the most common bacterial agent in hematogenous calcaneal osteomyelitis.

Clinical findings include fever, pain, and swelling around the foot and ankle. The differential diagnosis may include septic arthritis of the ankle, cellulitis, stress fracture, calcaneal apophysitis, Achilles enthesopathy, and subcutaneous abscess.

Tibialis Posterior Tendonitis

See Chapter 21.

Flexor Hallucis Longus Tendonitis

See Chapter 21.

Tarsal Tunnel Syndrome

Tarsal tunnel syndrome is a compressive neuropathy of the posterior tibial nerve, or one of its branches, which usually occurs at the level of the ankle. This relatively rare syndrome was first described by Keck[473] and Lam[474] in two separate reports in 1962.

The posterior tibial nerve often is entrapped as it courses through the tarsal tunnel, passing under the deep fascia, the flexor retinaculum, and within the abductor hallucis muscle.[475] The most common site of entrapment is at the anterior–inferior aspect of thc tunnel, where the nerves wind around the medial malleolus.[476]

The etiology is multifactorial and may be posttraumatic, neoplastic, inflammatory,[477] or a result of rapid weight gain,[478] fluid retention,[478] abnormal foot or ankle mechanics,[479–481] or a valgus foot deformity.[482–484]

The diagnosis is based on history and clinical examination. The typical patient reports a poorly localized burning sensation or pain and paresthesia at the medial plantar surface of the foot, with the distribution correlating with the level of entrapment of the medial or lateral plantar nerve as they join to form the posterior tibial nerve.[447] Discomfort is worse after activity and typically is accentuated during the end of a working day.[475] Some patients have cramps in the longitudinal foot arch. Resting pain is reported infrequently but can disturb sleep.[447] Plantar fasciitis has similar findings and must be ruled out.[485]

The physical examination can reveal any one, or all, of the following:

- Positive Tinel sign, sometimes with pain radiating distally toward the mid-sole, along the posterior branch of the nerve.[486] Percussion should be performed with and without weight bearing.[487]
- Pain with passive dorsiflexion[477] or eversion.[486]
- Decreased two-point discrimination on the plantar aspect of the foot.[486]
- Varus or valgus deformity of the heel.[478,482,484,486]
- Weakness of the foot intrinsics with sustained plantar flexion of the toes.
- Normal results from the neurologic examination.[488]

The most effective conservative interventions for tarsal tunnel syndrome are local corticosteroid injections, an orthoses for foot deformity,[484,489] strengthening of the foot intrinsics to restore the medial longitudinal arch,[481] weight loss for obese patients,[481] and a heel lift to decrease tension on the tibial nerve.[477]

Surgical intervention, which typically occurs after a trial course of conservative measures, involves decompression of the nerve.[482,483] The overall results from early surgical decompression are beneficial in most patients.[478]

Calcaneal Fracture

See Chapter 21.

Medial Ankle Sprain

See Chapter 21.

Peroneal Muscle Strain or Tendonitis

See Chapter 21.

Lateral Ankle Sprain

See Chapter 21.

Osteochondral Fracture of the Talar Dome

See Chapter 21.

Stress Fracture of the Lateral Malleolus

See Chapter 21.

CASE-STUDY

NECK PULSING

HISTORY

A 37-year-old woman presented to the office complaining that her head "wanted to go back." Her symptoms began approximately 6 months earlier, with painless "pulsing" on the left side of her neck that became worse with stressful situations and physical activity but was relieved by relaxationand sleep. She could briefly stop the pulsing by placing her hand on the right posterior aspect of the neck. Her symptoms had progressed to an extension of the neck with spasm, which caused her to lean forward to maintain eye contact with others. She also noted an occasional "eye tic," which seemed to come and go spontaneously. She denied any paresthesias, weakness, dysphasia, visual changes or hearing loss, or bowel or bladder changes. Although she had no family history of specific neurologic problems, the patient reported a maternal aunt who had "facial tics." The patient had a medical history notable for anxiety and several phobias for which she had received psychological counseling. Vascular studies had ruled out vascular disease and the presence of an aneurysm in the neck and trunk. Imaging studies had ruled out fracture or tumor.

Questions

1. What aspects of the history should alert the clinician to the possibility of a serious pathology?
2. What could be the significance of the pulsing?
3. Does this presentation/history warrant further investigation? Why or why not?

CASE-STUDY

GROIN PAIN IN A MIDDLE-AGED FEMALE

HISTORY

A 56-year-old moderately obese woman presents with a prescription that reads "hip OA, evaluate and treat."

Patient presented with left groin pain of an insidious onset that was worsening. The pain started approximately 3 months ago, when the patient commenced a walking program to lose some weight. The symptoms improve with rest, but worsen with activity, especially with walking and stair negotiation. The series of radiographs taken at the physician's office revealed slight degenerative changes at the hip joint.

Questions

1. What aspects of the history should alert the clinician to the possibility of a serious pathology?
2. What is the significance of an insidious onset?
3. Does this presentation/history warrant further investigation? Why or why not?

CASE-STUDY

BACK AND LEG PAIN

HISTORY

A 55-year-old man presented with complaints of an insidious onset of severe back and left leg pain. Progressively worsening symptoms of pain over the past few months were followed by left foot drop. An MRI examination was interpreted as mild lumbar spine degenerative disk disease without evidence of nerve-root compromise. The patient could report no specific aggravating or relieving activities but did report pain at night, not related to movement in bed. The patient's past medical history was significant for a renal transplantation approximately 20 years previously.

Questions

1. What aspects of the history should alert the clinician to the possibility of a serious pathology?
2. What is the significance of night pain that is unrelated to movement?
3. Does this presentation/history warrant further investigation? Why or why not?

CASE-STUDY

LEFT-SIDED LOW BACK AND LEG PAIN

HISTORY

A 45-year-old man presented with complaints of intermittent variable left-sided LBP that extended into his left posterior thigh and intermittent variable tingling along the anterolateral aspect of his left lower extremity.[249] This was the patient's first visit to a health-care facility for this condition; therefore, medical records were not available. The symptoms began about 2 months ago, with no specific mechanism of injury. The patient reported working as a quality control manager for a pharmaceutical lab. His job required sitting for approximately 50% of the day and occasional lifting of boxes weighing between 4.5 and 9.1 kg. Activities or positions that increased or aggravated all of the patient's symptoms included lying supine, coughing and sneezing, prolonged walking, and sitting for longer than an hour. Activities that decreased the patient's symptoms included applying a heating pad to his low back region and taking over-the-counter ibuprofen (200 mg) every four hours. The patient noted that his symptoms were most intense in the evening and into the night, with pain sometimes causing him difficulty with falling asleep. The patient also remarked that he would sometimes awaken because of pain but was able to fall asleep after finding a comfortable position. The patient's past medical history was unremarkable for cancer, bowel and bladder problems, hypertension, diabetes, or recent weight changes.

Questions

1. What aspects of the history should alert the clinician to the possibility of a serious pathology?
2. What types of conditions have an insidious onset?
3. Does this presentation/history sound like a neuromuscular problem or does this condition warrant further investigation? Why or why not?

CASE-STUDY

RIGHT BUTTOCK PAIN

HISTORY

A 55-year-old woman presented for physical therapy with a physician diagnosis of "right lumbosacral radiculitis." The patient had a 10-month history of right buttock pain with radiation to the posterolateral right lower limb, which was associated with intermittent numbness and tingling of the distal lower limb and foot. She denied any LBP or any radiation of pain down her left lower limb. The pain was exacerbated by walking uphill, by lying on her right side, and after exercise. It was not worse with bending or with Valsalva maneuver. Past medical history was significant for chronic LBP, lymphoma (diagnosed at age of 23 years and treated successfully with local radiation to the neck and axillae), status postmeningioma resection, status postbilateral modified radical mastectomy for carcinoma in situ, and hypothyroidism.[490] An MRI of the lumbosacral spine revealed multilevel degenerative disk disease from L3 and L4 through L5–S1, with mild foraminal narrowing bilaterally. There was no evidence of focal herniation or canal stenosis.

Questions

1. What structure(s) could be the cause of these symptoms?
2. Does the history of the symptoms follow a pattern associated with a musculoskeletal disorder? If not, why not?
3. What in the patient's past medical history needs to be noted?
4. What tests or questions would you use to help rule out the potentially serious causes of these symptoms such as cauda equina compression?
5. What impairment could cause an increase in these symptoms when walking uphill and lying on the right side?
6. Why would the patient's symptoms increase after exercise?
7. What is your working hypothesis at this stage based on the various diagnoses that could manifest with leg pain and paresthesia, and what tests you would use to rule out each one?
8. Does this presentation/history warrant a scanning examination? Why or why not?

CASE-STUDY

INTERMITTENT LEG NUMBNESS

HISTORY

A 46-year-old man presented to the clinic with a 10-year history of sensations that he described as a mixture both of pins and needles and of cotton wool around the second and third toes of his feet. The symptoms developed suddenly while at work and had progressed to intermittent numbness of both legs from the waist down. Over the following 10 years, the patient suffered momentarily from electric-type sensations radiating down into his legs, more so on the right than on the left. In addition, he noticed stiffness in his gait and reduced sensation on passing urine, and an aching sensation had developed in the buttocks. He had a history of infrequent LBP over a number of years. The patient's physician had given him a workup for MS, but the results were negative.

Questions

1. What aspects of the history should alert the clinician to the possibility of a serious pathology?
2. What is the significance of the gait stiffness?
3. What is the significance of the reduced sensation on passing urine?
4. Does this presentation/history warrant a scanning examination? Why or why not?

REVIEW QUESTIONS*

1. List five categories of referred pain.
2. Give a broad definition of malingering.
3. True or false: Osteoid osteomas are malignant tumors.
4. Degenerative spondylolisthesis occurs most commonly at which spinal levels?
5. Which type of headache is associated with auras?

*Additional questions to test your understanding of this chapter can be found in the Online Learning Center for *Orthopaedic Assessment, Evaluation, and Intervention* at www.duttononline.net.

REFERENCES

1. American Physical Therapy Association House of Delegates: Vision 2020, HOD 06-00-24-35. Alexandria, VA: American Physical Therapy Association, 2000.
2. Guide to Physical Therapist Practice, 2nd ed. American Physical Therapy Association. *Phys Ther* 81:9–746, 2001.
3. DuVall RE, Godges J: Introduction to physical therapy differential diagnosis: the clinical utility of subjective examination. In: Wilmarth MA, ed. *Medical Screening for the Physical Therapist. Orthopaedic Section Independent Study Course 14.1.1.* La Crosse, WI: Orthopaedic Section, APTA, Inc, 2003:1–44.
4. Guide to physical therapist practice. *Phys Ther* 81:S13–S95, 2001.
5. Overman SS, Larson JW, Dickstein DA, et al.: Physical therapy care for low back pain. Monitored program of first-contact nonphysician care. *Phys Ther* 68:199–207, 1988.
6. Weale AE, Bannister GC: Who should see orthopaedic outpatients–physiotherapists or surgeons? *Ann R Coll Surg Engl* 77:71–73, 1995.
7. Mitchell JM, de Lissovoy G: A comparison of resource use and cost in direct access versus physician referral episodes of physical therapy. *Phys Ther* 77:10–18, 1997.
8. Childs JD, Whitman JM, Sizer PS, et al.: A description of physical therapists' knowledge in managing musculoskeletal conditions. *BMC Musculoskelet Disord* 6:32, 2005.
9. Fritz J, Flynn TW: Autonomy in physical therapy: less is more. *J Orthop Sports Phys Ther* 35:696–968, 2005.
10. Stith JS, Sahrmann SA, Dixon KK, et al.: Curriculum to prepare diagnosticians in physical therapy. *J Phys Ther Educ* 9:50, 1995.
11. Stetts DM: Patient examination. In: Wadsworth C, ed. *Current Concepts of Orthopaedic Physical Therapy - Home Study Course 11.2.2.* La Crosse, WI: Orthopaedic Section, APTA, 2001.
12. Goodman CC, Snyder TEK: *Differential Diagnosis in Physical Therapy.* Philadelphia, PA: WB Saunders Company, 1990.
13. Magee DJ: Head and face. In: Magee DJ, ed. *Orthopedic Physical Assessment*, 4th ed. Philadelphia, PA: WB Saunders, 2002:67–120.
14. Kostuik JP, Harrington I, Alexander D, et al.: Cauda equina syndrome and lumbar disc herniation. *J Bone Joint Surg* 68A:386–391, 1986.
15. O'Laoire SA, Crockard HA, Thomas DG: Prognosis for sphincter recovery after operation for cauda equina compression owing to lumbar disc prolapse. *BMJ* 282:1852–1854, 1981.
16. Boissonnault W, Goodman C: Physical therapists as diagnosticians: drawing the line on diagnosing pathology. *J Orthop Sports Phys Ther* 36:351–353, 2006.
17. Boissonnault WG, Bass C: Medical screening examination: not optional for physical therapists. *J Orthop Sports Phys Ther* 14:241–242, 1991.
18. LoPiccolo CJ, Goodkin K, Baldewicz TT: Current issues in the diagnosis and management of malingering. *Ann Med* 31:166–174, 1999.
19. American Psychiatric Association: *Diagnostic and Statistical Manual of Mental Disorders*, 4th ed. Washington, DC: American Psychiatric Association, 1994.
20. Waddell G, Main CJ, Morris EW, et al.: Chronic low back pain, psychological distress and illness behavior. *Spine* 9:209–213, 1984.
21. Miller ML, Kress AM, Berry CA: Decreased physical function in juvenile rheumatoid arthritis. *Arthritis Care Res* 12:309–313, 1999.
22. Roubenoff R: Gout and hyperuricaemia. *Rheum Dis Clin North Am* 16:539–550, 1990.
23. Lawrence RC, Hochberg MC, Kelsey JL, et al.: Estimates of the prevalence of selected arthritic and musculoskeletal diseases in the United States. *J Rheumatol* 16:427–441, 1989.
24. Isomaki H, von Essen R, Ruutsalo H-M: Gout, particularly diuretics-induced, is on the increase in Finland. *Scand J Rheumatol* 6:213–216, 1977.
25. Gladman DD, Brubacher B, Buskila D, et al.: Differences in the expression of spondyloarthropathy: a comparison between ankylosing spondylitis and psoriatic arthritis: genetic and gender effects. *Clin Invest Med* 16:1–7, 1993.
26. Haslock I: Ankylosing spondylitis. *Baillieres Clin Rheumatol* 7:99, 1993.
27. Gran JT: An epidemiologic survey of the signs and symptoms of ankylosing spondylitis. *Clin Rheumatol* 4:161–169, 1985.
28. Calin A, Porta J, Fries JF, et al.: Clinical history as a screening test for ankylosing spondylitis. *JAMA* 237:2613–2614, 1977.

29. Cohen MD, Ginsurg WW: Late onset peripheral joint disease in ankylosing spondylitis. *Arthritis Rheum* 26:186–190, 1983.
30. Carrett S, Graham D, Little H, et al.: The natural disease course of ankylosing spondylitis. *Arthritis Rheum* 26:186–190, 1993.
31. Gladman DD: Clinical aspects of the spondyloarthropathies. *Am J Med Sci* 316:234–238, 1998.
32. Deyo RA, Rainville J, Kent DL: What can the history and physical examination tell us about low back pain? *JAMA* 268:760–765, 1992.
33. Turek SL: *Orthopaedics - Principles and Their Application*, 4th ed. Philadelphia, PA: JB Lippincott, 1984.
34. Kraag G, Stokes B, Groh J, et al.: The effects of comprehensive home physiotherapy and supervision on patients with ankylosing spondylitis: an 8-month follow-up. *J Rheumatol* 21:261–263, 1994.
35. Buskila D, Langevitz P, Gladman DD, et al.: Patients with rheumatoid arthritis are more tender than those with psoriatic arthritis. *J Rheumatol* 19:1115–1119, 1992.
36. Gladman DD: Psoriatic arthritis. In: Kelley WN, Harris ED, Ruddy S, et al., eds. *Textbook of Rheumatology*, 5th ed. Philadelphia, PA: WB Saunders, 1997:999–1005.
37. Gladman DD, Anhorn KB, Schachter RK, et al.: HLA antigens in psoriatic arthritis. *J Rheumatol* 13:586–592, 1986.
38. Della Rocca C, Huvos AG: Osteoblastoma: varied histological presentations with a benign clinical course. An analysis of 55 cases. *Am J Surg Pathol* 20:841–850, 1996.
39. Azouz EM, Kozlowski K, Marton D, et al.: Osteoid osteoma and osteoblastoma of the spine in children: Report of 22 cases with brief literature review. *Pediatr Radiol* 16:25–31, 1986.
40. Bjornsson J, Wold LE, Ebersold MJ, et al.: Chordoma of the mobile spine: a clinicopathologic analysis of 40 patients. *Cancer* 71:735–740, 1993.
41. Dorfman HD, Czerniak B: Bone cancers. *Cancer* 75:203–210, 1995.
42. Dahlin DC, Coventry MB: Osteogenic sarcoma: a study of six hundred cases. *J Bone Joint Surg Am* 49A:101–110, 1967.
43. Boland PJ, Lane JM, Sundaresan N: Metastatic disease of the spine. *Clin Orthop* 169:95–102, 1982.
44. Harrington KD: Metastatic disease of the spine. *J Bone Joint Surg* 68A:1110–1115, 1986.
45. Bell GR: Surgical treatment of spinal tumors. *Clin Orthop Related Res* 335:54–63, 1997.
46. Rosier RN: Expanding the role of the orthopaedic surgeon in the treatment of osteoporosis. *Clin Orthop Related Res* 385:57–67, 2001.
47. Lane JM, Russell L, Khan SN: Osteoporosis. *Clin Orthop* 372:139–150, 2000.
48. Praemer A, Furner S, Rice DP: Musculoskeletal Conditions in the United States. In: Praemer A, Furner S, Rice DP, eds. *Osteoporosis*. Rosemont, IL: American Academy of Orthopaedic Surgeons, 1999:40–47.
49. Silverman SL: The clinical consequences of vertebral compression fracture. *Bone* 13:S27–S31, 1992.
50. Erickson K, Baker S, Smith J: Kyphoplasty – minimally invasive vertebral compression fracture repair. *Aorn J* 78:766–773; quiz 777–780, 2003.
51. Eisman JA: Genetics of osteoporosis. *Endocrine Rev* 20:788–804, 1999.
52. Cummings SR, Nevitt MC, Browner WS, et al.: Risk factors for hip fracture in white women. *N Engl J Med* 332:767–773, 1995.
53. Scheiber LB, Torregrosa L: Early intervention for postmenopausal osteoporosis. *J Musculoskel Med* 16:146–157, 1999.
54. Lane JM, Riley EH, Wirganowicz PZ: Osteoporosis: diagnosis and treatment. *J Bone Joint Surg* 78A:618–632, 1996.
55. Bukata SV, Rosier RN: Diagnosis and treatment of osteoporosis. *Curr Opin Orthop* 11:336–340, 2000.
56. Huijbregts PA: Osteoporosis: diagnosis and conservative treatment. *J Man & Manip Ther* 9:143–153, 2001.
57. Block J, Smith R, Black D, et al.: Does exercise prevent osteoporosis. *JAMA* 257:345, 1987.
58. Cummings SR, Kelsey JL, Nevitt MD, et al.: Epidemiology of osteoporosis and osteoporotic fractures. *Epidemiol Rev* 7:178–208, 1985.
59. NIH Consensus Development Panel on Osteoporosis Prevention D, and Therapy: Osteoporosis prevention, diagnosis, and therapy. *JAMA* 285:785–795, 2001.
60. Snow-Harter C, Marcus R: Exercise, bone mineral density, and osteoporosis. *Exerc Sport Sci Rev* 19:351–388, 1991.
61. Buchner DM, Beresford SAA, Larson E, et al.: Effects of physical activity on health status in older adults. II: Intervention studies. *Annu Rev Public Health* 13:469–488, 1992.
62. Nelson ME, Fiatarone MA, Morganti CM, et al.: Effects of high intensity strength training on multiple risk factors for osteoporotic fractures. A randomized controlled trial. *JAMA* 272:1909–1914, 1994.
63. Compston J: Does parathyroid hormone treatment affect fracture risk or bone mineral density in patients with osteoporosis? *Nat Clin Pract Rheumatol* 1:1, 2007.
64. Jupiter JB, Winters S, Sigman S, et al.: Repair of five distal radius fractures with an investigational cancellous bone cement: a preliminary report. *J Orthop Trauma* 11:110–116, 1997.
65. Bailey DA, Faulkner RA, McKay HA: Growth, physical activity, and bone mineral acquisition. In: Hollosky JO, ed. *Exercise and Sport Sciences Reviews*. Baltimore, MD: Williams and Wilkins, 1996:233–266.
66. Recker R, Davies M, Hinders SH, et al.: Bone gain in young adult women. *JAMA* 268:2403–2408, 1992.
67. Frame B, Parfitt M: Osteomalacia: current concepts. *Ann Intern Med* 89:966–982, 1978.
68. Strewler GJ: Mineral metabolism and metabolic bone disease. In: Greenspan FS, Strewler GJ, eds. *Basic and Clinical Endocrinology*, 5th ed. Stamford, CT: Appleton & Lange, 1997:263–316.
69. Basha B, Rao DS, Han ZH, et al.: Osteomalacia due to vitamin D depletion: a neglected consequence of intestinal malabsorption. *Am J Med* 108:296–300, 2000.
70. Laus M, Tigani D, Alfonso C, et al.: Degenerative spondylolisthesis: lumbar stenosis and instability. *Chir Organi Mov* 77:39–49, 1992.
71. Postacchinia F, Perugia D: Degenerative lumbar spondylolisthesis. Part I: etiology, pathogenesis, pathomorphology, and clinical features. *Ital J Orthop Traumatol* 17:165–173, 1991.
72. Borg-Stein J, Stein J: Trigger points and tender points: one and the same? Does Injection treatment help? *Rheum Dis Clin North Am* 22:305–322, 1996.
73. Freundlich B, Leventhal L: The fibromyalgia syndrome. In: Schumacher HR, Klippel JH, Koopman WJ, eds. *Primer on the Rheumatic Diseases*. Atlanta, GA: Arthritis Foundation, 1993:227–230.
74. Stockman R: The courses, pathology and treatment of chronic rheumatism. *Edinb Med J* 15:107–116, 1904.
75. Grodin AJ, Cantu RI: Soft tissue mobilization. In: Basmajian JV, Nyberg R, eds. *Rational Manual Therapies*. Baltimore, MD: Williams & Wilkins, 1993:199–221.
76. Schneider MJ: Tender points/fibromyalgia vs. trigger points/myofascial pain syndrome: A need for clarity in terminology and differential diagnosis. *J Man Physiol Ther* 18:398–406, 1995.
77. Campbell SM: Is the tender point concept valid? *Am J Med* 81:33–37, 1986.
78. Campbell SM, Clark S, Tindall EA, et al.: Clinical characteristics of fibrositis: I. A "Blinded" controlled study of symptoms and tender points. *Arthritis Rheum* 26:817–824, 1983.
79. Cott A, Parkinson W, Bell J, et al.: Interrater reliability of the tender point criterion for fibromyalgia. *J Rheumatol* 19:1955–1959, 1992.
80. Croft P, Schollum J, Silman A: Population study of tender point counts and pain as evidence of fibromyalgia. *BMJ* 309:696–699, 1994.
81. Wolfe F, Smythe HA, Yunus MB, et al.: The American College of Rheumatology 1990 criteria for the classification of fibromyalgia. *Arthr Rheum* 33:160–172, 1990.
82. Wallace DJ: Is there a role for cytokine based therapies in fibromyalgia. *Curr Pharm Des* 12:17–22, 2006.
83. Simms RW: Muscle studies in fibromyalgia syndrome. *J Musculoske Pain* 2:117–123, 1994.
84. Farney RJ, Walker JM: Office management of common sleep/wake disorders. *Med Clin North Am* 79:391–414, 1995.
85. Offenbacher M, Stucki G: Physical therapy in the treatment of fibromyalgia. *Scand J Rheumatol* 29:78–85, 2000.
86. McClaflin RR: Myofascial pain syndrome: primary care strategies for early intervention. *Postgrad Med* 96:56–73, 1994.
87. Travell JG, Simons DG: *Myofascial Pain and Dysfunction – The Trigger Point Manual*. Baltimore, MD: Williams & Wilkins, 1983.
88. Fricton JR: Myofascial pain. *Baillieres Clin Rheumatol* 8:857–880, 1994.
89. Vecchiet L, Giamberardino MA, Saggini R: Myofascial pain syndromes: clinical and pathophysiological aspects. *Clin J Pain* 7(Suppl):16–22, 1991.
90. Liebenson C: Active muscular relaxation techniques (part 2). *J Manipulative Physiol Ther* 13:2–6, 1990.
91. Aronoff GM: Myofascial pain syndrome and fibromyalgia: a critical assessment and alternate view. *Clin J Pain* 14:74–85, 1998.
92. Chen S-H, Wu Y-C, Hong C-Z: Current management of myofascial pain syndrome. *Clin J Pain* 6:27–46, 1996.
93. Esenyel M, Caglar N, Aldemir T: Treatment of myofascial pain. *Am J Phys Med Rehabil* 79:48–52, 2000.

94. Fricton JR: Clinical care for myofascial pain. *Dental Clin N Am* 35:1–29, 1991.
95. Goldman LB, Rosenberg NL: Myofascial pain syndrome and fibromyalgia. *Semin Neurol* 11:274–280, 1991.
96. Krause H, Fischer AA: Diagnosis and treatment of myofascial pain. *Mt Sinai J Med* 58:235–239, 1991.
97. Hardin J Jr: Pain and the cervical spine. *Bull Rheum Dis* 50:1–4, 2001.
98. Nordhoff LS Jr: Cervical trauma following motor vehicle collisions. In: Murphy DR, ed. *Cervical Spine Syndromes.* New York, NY: McGraw-Hill, 2000:131–150.
99. Barton CW: Evaluation and treatment of headache patients in the emergency department: a survey. *Headache* 34:91–94, 1994.
100. Thomas SH, Stone CK: Emergency department treatment of migraine, tension and mixed-type headache. *J Emerg Med* 12:657–664, 1994.
101. Oates LN, Scholz MJ, Hoffert MJ: Polypharmacy in a headache centre population. *Headache* 33:436–438, 1993.
102. Robinson RG: Pain relief for headaches: is self-medication a problem? *Can Fam Physician* 39:867–872, 1993.
103. Biondi DM: Headaches and their relationship to sleep. *Dent Clin North Am* 45:685–700, 2001.
104. Esposito CJ, Crim GA, Binkley TK: Headaches: a differential diagnosis. *J Craniomand Pract* 4:318–322, 1986.
105. Friedman MH, Nelson AJ Jr: Head and neck pain review: traditional and new perspectives. *J Orthop Sports Phys Ther* 24:268–278, 1996.
106. Appenzeller O: *Pathogenesis and Treatment of Headache.* New York, NY: Spectrum Publications, Inc., 1976.
107. International Headache Society Headache Classification and Diagnostic Criteria for Headache Disorders: Cranial neuralgias, and facial pain. *Cephalalgia* 8:19–22, 71, 72, 1988.
108. Nicholson GG, Gaston J: Cervical headache. *J Orthop Sports Phys Ther* 31:184–193, 2001.
109. Cohen MJ, McArthur DL: Classification of migraine and tension headache from a survey of 10,000 headache diaries. *Headache* 21:25–29, 1981.
110. Tinel J: La cephelee a l'effort, syndrome de distension des vienes intracraniences. *La Med* 13:113–8, 1932.
111. McCrory P: Headaches and exercise. *Sports Med* 30:221–229, 2000.
112. Williams S, Nukada H: Sport and exercise headache. Part 2: diagnosis and classification. *Br J Sports Med* 28:96–100, 1994.
113. Fredriksen TA, Hovdal H, Sjaastad O: Cervicogenic headache: clinical manifestation. *Cephalalgia* 7:147–160, 1987.
114. Hunter CR, Mayfield FH: Role of the upper cervical roots in the production of pain in the head. *Am J Surg* 48:743–751, 1949.
115. Wilson PR: Chronic neck pain and cervicogenic headache. *Clin J Pain* 7:5–11, 1991.
116. Lewit K: Vertebral artery insufficiency and the cervical spine. *Br J Geriatr Pract* 6:37–42, 1969.
117. Jull GA: Headaches associated with cervical spine: a clinical review. In: Boyling JD, Palastanga N, eds. *Grieve's Modern Manual Therapy*, 2nd ed. Edinburgh: Churchill Livingstone, 1994.
118. Kimmel DL: The cervical sympathetic rami and the vertebral plexus in the human foetus. *J Comparative Neurol* 112:141–161, 1959.
119. Abrahams VC, Richmond FJR, Rose PK: Absence of monosynaptic reflex in dorsal neck muscles of the cat. *Brain Res* 92:130–131, 1975.
120. Kerr FWL, Olafsson RA: Trigeminal cervical volleys: convergency on single units in the spinal gray at C1 and C2. *Arch Neurol* 5:171–178, 1961.
121. Friedman MH, Weisberg J: *Temporomandibular Joint Disorders.* Chicago, IL: Quintessence Publishing Company, Inc., 1985.
122. Campbell CD, Loft GH, Davis H, et al.: TMJ symptoms and referred pain patterns. *J Prosthet Dent* 47:430–433, 1982.
123. Pestronk A, Pestronk S: Goggle migraine. *N Engl J Med* 308:226–227, 1983.
124. Silbert PL, Mokri B, Schievink WI: Headache and neck pain in spontaneous internal carotid and vertebral artery dissections. *Neurology* 45:1517–1522, 1995.
125. Appenzeller O: Post-traumatic headaches. In: Dalessio DJ, ed. *Wolff's Headache and Other Head Pain*, 5th ed. New York, NY: Oxford University Press, 1987:289–303.
126. Packard RC: Posttraumatic headache: permanency and relationship to legal settlement. *Headache* 32:496–500, 1992.
127. Yamaguchi M: Incidence of headache and severity of head injury. *Headache* 32:427–431, 1992.
128. Silberstein SD: Tension-type headaches. *Headache* 34:S2–S7, 1994.
129. Mathew NT, Subits E, Nigam M: Transformation of migraine into daily chronic headache. Analysis of factors. *Headache* 22:66–68, 1982.
130. Sheftell FD: Chronic daily headache. *Neurol Clin* 42:32–36, 1992.
131. Kudrow L: Paradoxical effects of frequent analgesic use. *Adv Neurol* 33:335–341, 1982.
132. Warner JS, Fenichel GM: Chronic post-traumatic headache often a myth? *Neurology* 46:915–916, 1996.
133. Mathew NT: Chronic refractory headache. *Neurology* 43:S26–S33, 1993.
134. Saper JR, Magee KR: *Freedom From Headaches.* New York, NY: Simon & Schuster, 1981.
135. Goodman CC, Boissonnault WG: *Pathology: Implications for the Physical Therapist.* Philadelphia, PA: WB Saunders, 1998.
136. Sulfaro MA, Gobetti JP: Occipital neuralgia manifesting as orofacial pain. *Oral Surg Oral Med Oral Pathol Oral Radiol Endod* 80:751–755, 1995.
137. Shankland W: Differential diagnosis of headaches. *J Craniomand Pract* 4:47–51, 1986.
138. Cox C, Cocks R: Occipital neuralgia. *J Med Assoc Alabama* 1:23–28, 1979.
139. Vital JM, Grenier F, Dautheribes M, et al.: An anatomic and dynamic study of the greater occipital nerve (n. of Arnold): applications to the treatment of Arnold's neuralgia. *Surg Radiol Anat* 11:205–210, 1989.
140. Wolff HG: *Headache and Other Head Pain,* 2nd ed. New York, NY: Oxford University Press, 1987:53–76.
141. Dandy WE: An operation for the cure of tic douloureux. Partial section of the sensory root at the pons. *Arch Surg* 18:687, 1929.
142. Sjoqvist O: *Surgical Section of Pain Tracts and Pathways in the Spinal Cord And Brain Stem, 4 Congr Neurol Internat.* Paris: Masson, 1949.
143. Devor M, Amir R, Rappaport ZH: Pathophysiology of trigeminal neuralgia: the ignition hypothesis. *Clin J Pain* 18:4–13, 2002.
144. Hadar T, Tovi F, Sidi J, et al.: Specific IgG and IgA antibodies to herpes simplex virus and varicella zoster virus in acute peripheral facial palsy patients. *J Med Virol* 12:237–245, 1983.
145. Morgan M, Nathwani D: Facial palsy and infection: the unfolding story. *Clin Infec Dis* 14:263–271, 1992.
146. Murakami S, Mizobuchi M, Nakashiro Y, et al.: Bell's palsy and herpes simplex virus: identification of viral DNA in endoneurial fluid and muscle. *Ann Intern Med* 124:27–30, 1996.
147. Burgess RC, Michaels L, Bales JF Jr, et al.: Polymerase chain reaction amplification of herpes simplex viral DNA from the geniculate ganglion of a patient with Bell's palsy. *Ann Otol Rhinol Laryngol* 103:775–779, 1994.
148. Nasatzky E, Katz J: Bell's palsy associated with herpes simplex gingivostomatitis. A case report. *Oral Surg Oral Med Oral Pathol Oral Radiol Endod* 86:293–296, 1998.
149. Maccabee PJ, Amassian VE, Cracco RQ, et al.: Intracranial stimulation of facial nerve in humans with magnetic coil. *Electroencephalogr Clin Neurophysiol* 70:350–354, 1988.
150. Peitersen E: The natural history of Bell's palsy. *Am J Otol* 4:107–111, 1982.
151. Gantz BJ, Rubinstein JT, Gidley P, et al.: Surgical management of Bell's palsy. *Laryngoscope* 109:1177–1188, 1999.
152. Sweeney CJ, Gilden DH: Ramsay Hunt syndrome. *J Neurol Neurosurg Psychiatry* 71:149–154, 2001.
153. Lindsay KW, Bone I, Callander R: *Neurology and Neurosurgery Illustrated.* New York, NY: Churchill Livingstone, 1991.
154. Attia J, Hatala R, Cook DJ, et al.: Does this adult patient have acute meningitis? *JAMA* 282:175–181, 1999.
155. Sprengell C: *The Aphorisms of Hippocrates, and the Sentences of Celsus,* 2nd ed. London: R Wilkin, 1735.
156. Tunkel AR, Scheld WM: Pathogenesis and pathophysiology of bacterial meningitis. *Clin Microbiol Rev* 6:118–136, 1993.
157. Scheld WM: Meningococcal diseases. In: Warren KS, Mahmoud AAF, eds. *Tropical and Geographical Medicine,* 2nd ed. New York, NY: McGraw-Hill, 1990:798–814.
158. Durand ML, Calderwood SB, Weber DJ, et al.: Acute bacterial meningitis in adults: a review of 493 episodes. *N Engl J Med* 328:21–28, 1993.
159. Brody IA, Wilkins RH: The signs of Kernig and Brudzinski. *Arch Neurol* 21:215–218, 1969.
160. O'Connell JEA: The clinical signs of meningeal irritation. *Brain* 69:9–21, 1946.
161. Harvey AM, Johns RJ, McKusick VA, et al.: *The Principles and Practice of Medicine.* Norwalk, CT: Appleton & Lange, 1988.
162. Pozzati E, Frank F, Frank G, et al.: Subacute and chronic extradural hematomas: a study of 30 cases. *J Trauma* 20:795–799, 1980.
163. Steere AC: Lyme disease. *N Engl J Med* 345:115–125, 2001.
164. Gilstrap LC 3rd, Cunningham FG, Whalley PJ: Acute pyelonephritis in pregnancy: an anterospective study. *Obstet Gynecol* 57:409–413, 1981.

165. Pinhas-Hamiel O, Sarova-Pinhas I, Achiron A: Multiple sclerosis in childhood and adolescence: clinical features and management. *Paediatric Drugs* 3:329–336, 2001.
166. Krupp LB, Rizvi SA: Symptomatic therapy for underrecognized manifestations of multiple sclerosis. *Neurology* 58:S32–S39, 2002.
167. Arunagiri G, Santhi S, Harrington T: Horner syndrome and ipsilateral abduction deficit attributed to giant cell arteritis. *J Neuroophthalmol* 26:231–232, 2006.
168. Myers JE, Baker PN: Hypertensive diseases and eclampsia. *Curr Opin Obstet Gynecol* 14:119–125, 2002.
169. Thomas SV: Neurological aspects of eclampsia. *J Neurol Sci* 155:37–43, 1998.
170. Carson D, Serpell M: Choosing the best needle for diagnostic lumbar puncture. *Neurology* 47:33–37, 1996.
171. Raymond JR, Raymond PA: Post lumbar puncture headache: etiology and management. *West J Med* 148:551–554, 1988.
172. DeStefano F, Anda RF, Kahn HS, et al.: Dental disease and risk of coronary heart disease and mortality. *BMJ* 306:688–691, 1993.
173. Andres JC, Nagalla R: Acute bacterial thyroiditis secondary to urosepsis. *J Am Board Fam Pract* 8:128–129, 1995.
174. Dolan KD, Jacoby C, Smoker WR: The radiology of facial fractures. *Radiographics* 4:575–663, 1984.
175. Yanguela J, Pareja JA, Lopez N, et al.: Trochleitis and migraine headache. *Neurology* 58:802–805, 2002.
176. Surks MI, Ocampo E: Subclinical thyroid disease. *Am J Med* 100:217–223, 1996.
177. Thompson JW, Cohen SR, Reddix P: Retropharyngeal abscess in children: a retrospective and historical analysis. *Laryngoscope* 98:589–592, 1988.
178. Lee SS, Schwartz RH, Bahadori RS: Retropharyngeal abscess: epiglottitis of the new millennium. *J Pediatr* 138:435–437, 2001.
179. Asmar BL: Bacteriology of retropharyngeal abscess in children. *Pediatr Infect Dis J* 9:595–596, 1990.
180. Segal DH, Lidov MW, Camins MB: Cervical epidural hematoma after chiropractic manipulation in a healthy young woman: case report. *Neurosurgery* 39:1043–1045, 1996.
181. Pan G, Kulkarni M, MacDougall DJ, et al.: Traumatic epidural hematoma of the cervical spine: Diagnosis with magnetic resonance imaging. *J Neurosurg* 68:798–801, 1988.
182. Tseng SH, Chen Y, Lin SM, et al.: Cervical epidural hematoma after spinal manipulation therapy: case report. *J Trauma* 52:585–586, 2002.
183. Powell F, Hanigan W, Olivero W: A risk/benefit analysis of spinal manipulation therapy for relief of lumbar or cervical pain. *Neurosurgery* 33:73–79, 1993.
184. Kiesewetter WB, Nelson PK, Pallandino VS, et al.: Neonatal torticollis. *JAMA* 157:1281–1285, 1955.
185. Gorlin RJ, Cohen MM, Levin LS: *Syndromes of the Head and Neck*, 3rd ed. New York, NY: Oxford University Press, 1990.
186. Klippel M, Feil A: Anomalie de la colonne vertebrale par absence des vertebres cervicale. *Bull Mem Soc Anat* 87:185–188, 1912.
187. Klippel M, Feil A: Un cas d'absence des vertebres cervicales avec cage thoracique remontant jusqu'a la base du crane. *Nouv Iconogr Salpetriere* 25:223–224, 1912.
188. Chaumien JP, Rigault P, Maroteaux P, et al.: Le soi-disant syndrome de Klippel-Feil et ses incidences orthopediques. *Rev Chir Orthop* 76:30–38, 1990.
189. Gonzalez-Reimers E, Mas-Pascual A, Arnay-De-La-Rosa M, et al.: Klippel-Feil syndrome in the prehispanic population of El Hierro (Canary Islands). *Ann Rheum Dis* 60:174, 2001.
190. Smith DL, DeMario MC: Spasmodic torticollis: a case report and review of therapies. *J Am Board Fam Pract* 9:435–441, 1996.
191. Wilson BC, Jarvis BL, Haydon RC: Nontraumatic subluxation of the atlantoaxial joint: Grisel's syndrome. *Larynoscope* 96:705–708, 1987.
192. Britton TC: Torticollis–what is straight ahead? *Lancet* 351:1223–1224, 1998.
193. Colbassani HJ Jr, Wood JH: Management of spastic torticollis. *Surg Neurol* 25:153–158, 1986.
194. Adams RD, Victor M: *Principles of Neurology*. 5th ed. New York, NY: McGraw-Hill, Health Professions Division, 1993.
195. Lowenstein DH, Aminoff MJ: The clinical course of spasmodic torticollis. *Neurology* 38:530–532, 1988.
196. Rondot P, Marchand MP, Dellatolas G: Spasmodic torticollis–review of 220 patients. *Can J Neurol Sci* 18:143–151, 1991.
197. Jahanshahi M, Marion MH, Marsden CD: Natural history of adult-onset idiopathic torticollis. *Arch Neurol* 47:548–552, 1990.
198. Spencer J, Goetsch VL, Brugnoli RJ, et al.: Behavior therapy for spasmodic torticollis: a case study suggesting a causal role for anxiety. *J Behav Ther Exp Psychiatry* 22:305–311, 1991.
199. Agras S, Marshall C: The application of negative practice to spasmodic torticollis. *Am J Psychiatry* 121:579–582, 1965.
200. Leplow B: Heterogeneity of biofeedback training effects in spasmodic torticollis: a single-case approach. *Behav Res Ther* 28:359–365, 1990.
201. Halla JT, Hardin JG: The spectrum of atlantoaxial (C1–2) facet joint involvement in rheumatoid arthritis. *Arthr Rheum* 22:325–329, 1990.
202. Murray G, Persellin R: Cervical fracture complicating ankylosing spondylitis. *Am J Med* 70:1033–1041, 1981.
203. Patte D, Goutallier D, Monpierre H, et al.: Over-extension lesions. *Rev Chir Orthop* 74:314–8, 1988.
204. Bohlman HH: Degenerative arthritis of the lower cervical spine. In: McEvarts C, ed. *Surgery of the Musculoskeletal System*, 2nd ed. New York, NY: Churchill Livingstone, 1990:1857–1886.
205. Emery SE, Bohlman HH: Osteoarthritis of the cervical spine. In: Moskowitz RW, Howell DS, Goldberg VM, et al., eds. *Osteoarthritis. Diagnosis and Medical/Surgical Management*. Philadelphia, PA: WB Saunders, 1992:651–668.
206. El-Deiry WS: Colon Cancer, Adenocarcinoma. Available at: http://www.emedicine.com/med/topic413.htm#target1, 2006.
207. Suadicani P, Hein HO, Gyntelberg F: Height, weight, and risk of colorectal cancer. An 18-year follow-up in a cohort of 5249 men. *Scand J Gastroenterol* 28:285–288, 1993.
208. Marshall BJ, Armstrong JA, McGechie DB, et al.: Attempt to fulfill Koch's postulates for pyloric campylobacter. *Med J Aust* 142:436–439, 1985.
209. Hassall E: Peptic ulcer disease and current approaches to Helicobacter pylori. *J Pediatr* 138:462–468, 2001.
210. Farrar JA: Emergency! Acute cholecystitis. *Am J Nurs* 101:35–36, 2001.
211. Sim FH: Metastatic bone disease and myeloma. In: Evarts CM, ed. *Surgery of the Musculoskeletal System*. Philadelphia, PA: Churchill Livingstone, 1983:320–393.
212. Chade HO: Metastatic tumours of the spine. In: Vinken PJ, Bruyn GW, eds. *Spinal Tumors*. Amsterdam: North Holland Publishers, 1976:415–433.
213. Light RW: Pneumothorax. In: Light RW, ed. *Pleural Diseases*, 3rd ed. Baltimore, MD: Williams & Wilkins, 1995:242–277.
214. Peek GJ, Morcos S, Cooper G: The pleural cavity. *BMJ* 320:1318–1321, 2000.
215. Jay SJ: Pleural effusions, 1: preliminary evaluation—recognition of the transudate. *Postgrad Med* 80:164–167, 1986.
216. Bland JH: Diagnosis of thoracic pain syndromes. In: Giles LGF, Singer KP, eds. *Clinical Anatomy and Management of the Thoracic Spine*. Oxford: Butterworth-Heinemann, 2000:145–156.
217. Acre CA, Dohrmann GJ: Thoracic disc herniation: improved diagnosis with computed tomographic scanning and a review of the literature. *Surg Neurol* 23:356–361, 1985.
218. Singer KP, Willen J, Breidahl PD, et al.: The influence of zygapophyseal joint orientation on spinal injuries at the thoracolumbar junction. *Surg Radiol Anat* 11:233–239, 1989.
219. O'Brien MF, Lenke LG: Fractures and dislocations of the spine. In: Dee R, Hurst L, Gruber M, et al., eds. *Principles of Orthopaedic Practice*, 2nd ed. New York, NY: McGraw-Hill, 1997:1237–1293.
220. Yacyshyn E, Evans JM: Case management study: osteoporotic vertebral compression fracture. *Bull Rheum Dis* 47:1–2, 1998.
221. Reid ME: Bone trauma and disease of the thoracic spine and ribs. In: Flynn TW, ed. *The Thoracic Spine and Rib Cage*. Boston, MA: Butterworth-Heinemann, 1996:87–105.
222. Ziegler DW, Agarwal NN: The morbidity and mortality of rib fractures. *J Trauma* 37:975–979, 1994.
223. Trunkey D: *Cervicothoracic Trauma*. New York, NY: Thieme, 1986.
224. Gregory PL, Biswas AC, Batt ME: Musculoskeletal problems of the chest wall in athletes. *Sports Med* 32:235–250, 2002.
225. Gupta A, Jamshidi M, Robin JR: Traumatic first rib fractures: is angiography necessary? A review of 73 cases. *Cardiovasc Surg* 5:48–53, 1997.
226. Jenkins SA: Spontaneous fractures of both first ribs. *J Bone Joint Surg* 34B:9–13, 1952.
227. Lankenner PAJ, Micheli LJ: Stress fractures of the first rib: a case report. *J Bone Joint Surg Am* 67:159–160, 1985.
228. Mintz AC, Albano A, Reisdorff EJ, et al.: Stress fracture of the first rib from serratus anterior tension: an unusual mechanism of injury. *Ann Emerg Med* 19:411–414, 1990.

229. Sylvest E: *Epidemic Myalgia: Bornholm Disease.* London: Oxford University Press, 1934.
230. Ikeda RM, Kondracki SF, Drabkin PD, et al.: Pleurodynia among football players at a high school. *JAMA* 270:2205–2206, 1993.
231. Fam AG, Smythe HA: Musculoskeletal chest wall pain. *Can Med Assoc J* 133:379–389, 1985.
232. Disla E, Rhim HR, Reddy A, et al.: Costochondritis: a prospective analysis in an emergency department setting. *Arch Int Med* 154:2466–2469, 1994.
233. Singer KP, Malmivaara A: Pathoanatomical characteristics of the thoracolumbar junctional region. In: Giles LGF, Singer KP, eds. *Clinical Anatomy and Management of the Thoracic Spine.* Oxford: Butterworth-Heinemann, 2000:100–113.
234. Lawrence DJ, Bakkum B: Chiropractic management of thoracic spine pain of mechanical origin. In: Giles LGF, Singer KP, eds. *Clinical Anatomy and Management of Thoracic Pain.* Oxford: Butterworth-Heinemann, 2000:244–256.
235. Markolf KL: Deformation of the thoracolumbar intervertebral joints in response to external loads. *J Bone Joint Surg* 54A:511–533, 1972.
236. Heywood AWB, Meyers OL: Rheumatoid arthritis of the thoracic and lumbar spine. *J Bone and Joint Surg* 68B:362–368, 1986.
237. Weinfeld RM, Olson PN, Maki DD, et al.: The prevalence of diffuse idiopathic skeletal hyperostosis (DISH) in two large metropolitan hospital populations. *Skel Radiol* 26:222–225, 1997.
238. Cameron HU: Traumatic disruption of the manubriosternal joint in the absence of rib fractures. *J Trauma* 20:892, 1980.
239. Thirupathi R, Husted C: Traumatic disruption of the manubriosternal joint. *Bull Hosp Jt Dis* 42:242–247, 1982.
240. Anderson KA, McAninch JW: Renal abscesses: classification and review of 40 cases. *Urology* 16:333, 1980.
241. Siegel JF, Smith A, Moldwin R: Minimally invasive treatment of renal abscess. *J Urol* 155:52–55, 1996.
242. Goucke CR, Graziotti P: Extradural abscess following local anaesthetic and steroid injection for chronic back pain. *Br J Anaesth* 65:427–429, 1990.
243. Mackenzie AR, Laing RB, Smith CC, et al.: Spinal epidural abscess: the importance of early diagnosis and treatment. *J Neurol Neurosurg Psychiatry* 65:209–212, 1998.
244. Baker AS, Ojemann RG, Swartz MN, et al.: Spinal epidural abscess. *N Engl J Med* 293:463–468, 1975.
245. Obrador GT, Levenson DJ: Spinal epidural abscess in hemodialysis patients: report of three cases and review of the literature. *Am J Kidney Dis* 27:75–83, 1996.
246. Nauer K A: Acute dissection of the aorta: a review for nurses. *Crit Care Nurs Q* 23:20–27, 2000.
247. Gruendemann BJ, Fernsebner B: *Comprehensive Perioperative Nursing.* Boston, MA: Jones & Bartlett Publishers, 1995.
248. Deyo RA, Diehl AK: Cancer as a cause of back pain: frequency, clinical presentation, and diagnostic strategies. *J Gen Intern Med* 3:230–238, 1988.
249. Ross MD, Bayer E: Cancer as a cause of low back pain in a patient seen in a direct access physical therapy setting. *J Orthop Sports Phys Ther* 35:651–658, 2005.
250. Meinck HM: Stiff man syndrome. *CNS Drugs* 15:515–526, 2001.
251. Bastin A, Gurmin V, Mediwake R, et al.: Stiff man syndrome presenting with low back pain. *Ann Rheum Dis [Letter]* 61:939–940, 2002.
252. Henningsen P, Meinck HM: Specific phobia is a frequent non-motor feature in stiff man syndrome. *J Neurol Neurosurg Psychiatry* 74:462–5, 2003.
253. Sharma KR, Cross J, Santiago F, et al.: Incidence of acute femoral neuropathy following renal transplantation. *Arch Neurol* 59:541–545, 2002.
254. McCrory P: The "piriformis syndrome" – myth or reality? *Br J Sports Med* 35:209–210, 2001.
255. Beauchesne RP, Schutzer SF: Myositis ossificans of the piriformis muscle: an unusual cause of piriformis syndrome. A case report. *J Bone Joint Surg Am* 79:906–910, 1997.
256. Jankiewicz JJ, Hennrikus WL, Houkom JA: The appearance of the piriformis muscle syndrome in computed tomography and magnetic resonance imaging. A case report and review of the literature. *Clin Orthop* 262:205–209, 1991.
257. Palliyath S, Buday J: Sciatic nerve compression: diagnostic value of electromyography and computerized tomography. *Electromyog Clin Neurophysiol* 29:9–11, 1989.
258. Fishman LM, Dombi GW, Michaelsen C, et al.: Piriformis syndrome: diagnosis, treatment, and outcome – a 10-year study. *Arch Phys Med Rehabil* 83:295–301., 2002.
259. Papadopoulos SM, McGillicuddy JE, Albers JW: Unusual cause of piriformis muscle syndrome. *Arch Neurol* 47:1144–1146, 1990.
260. Tesio L, Bassi L, Galardi G: Transient palsy of hip abductors after a fall on the buttocks. *Arch Orthop and Trauma Surg* 109:164–165, 1990.
261. Pace JB, Nagle D: Piriformis syndrome. *Western J Med* 124:435–439, 1976.
262. Pecina M: Contribution to the etiological explanation of the piriformis syndrome. *Acta Anat Nippon* 105:181–187, 1979.
263. Boyd KT, Pierce NS, Batt ME: Common hip injuries in sport. *Sports Med* 24:273–288, 1997.
264. Durrani Z, Winnie AP: Piriformis muscle syndrome: an underdiagnosed cause of sciatica. *J Pain Symptom Manage* 6:374–379, 1991.
265. Solheim LF, Siewers P, Paus B: The piriformis muscle syndrome. Sciatic nerve entrapment treated with section of the piriformis muscle. *Acta Orthop Scand* 52:73–75, 1981.
266. Steiner C, Staubs C, Ganon M, et al.: Piriformis syndrome: pathogenesis, diagnosis, and treatment. *J Am Osteopath Assn* 87:318–323, 1987.
267. Julsrud ME: Piriformis syndrome. *J Am Podiat Med Assn* 79:128–131, 1989.
268. Pfeifer T, Fitz WFK: Das Piriformis-Syndrom. *Zeitschr Orthop* 127:691–694, 1989.
269. Robinson DR: Pyriformis syndrome in relation to sciatic pain. *Am J Surg* 73:355–358, 1947.
270. Beaton LE, Anson BJ: The sciatic nerve and the piriformis muscle: their interrelation a possible cause of coccygodynia. *J Bone Joint Surg* 20:686–688, 1938.
271. Hughes SS, Goldstein MN, Hicks DG, et al.: Extrapelvic compression of the sciatic nerve. An unusual cause of pain about the hip: report of five cases. *J Bone Joint Surg* 74-A:1553–1559, 1992.
272. Benson ER, Schutzer SF: Posttraumatic piriformis syndrome: diagnosis and results of operative treatment. *J Bone Joint Surg* 81A:941–949, 1999.
273. Freiberg AH: Sciatic pain and its relief by operations on muscle and fascia. *Arch Surg* 34:337–350, 1937.
274. Lang AM: Botulinum toxin type B in piriformis syndrome. *Am J Phys Med Rehabil* 83:198–202, 2004.
275. Childers MK, Wilson DJ, Gnatz SM, et al.: Botulinum toxin type A use in piriformis muscle syndrome: a pilot study. *Am J Phys Med Rehabil* 81:751–759, 2002.
276. Fishman LM, Konnoth C, Rozner B: Botulinum neurotoxin type B and physical therapy in the treatment of piriformis syndrome: a dose-finding study. *Am J Phys Med Rehabil* 83:42–50; quiz 51–53, 2004.
277. Thakkar DH, Porter RW: Heterotopic ossification enveloping the sciatic nerve following posterior fracture-dislocation of the hip: a case report. *Injury* 13:207–209, 1981.
278. Banerjee T, Hall CD: Sciatic entrapment neuropathy. *Neurosurgery* 45:216–217, 1976.
279. Jones BV, Ward MW: Myositis ossificans in the biceps femoris muscles causing sciatic nerve palsy: a case report. *J Bone Joint Surg* 62B:506–507, 1980.
280. Richardson RR, Hahn YS, Siqueira EB: Intraneural hematoma of the sciatic nerve: case report. *J Neurosurg* 49:298–300, 1978.
281. Zimmerman JE, Afshar F, Friedman W, et al.: Posterior compartment syndrome of the thigh with a sciatic palsy. *J Neurosurg* 46:369–372, 1977.
282. Johanson NA, Pellicii PM, Tsairis P, et al.: Nerve injury in total hip arthroplasty. *Clin Orthop* 179:214–222, 1983.
283. Day MH: The blood supply of the lumbar and sacral plexuses in the human foetus. *J Anat* 98:104–116, 1964.
284. Wohlgemuth WA, Rottach KG, Stoehr M: Radiogene Amyotrophie: Cauda equina Läsion als Strahlenspätfolge. *Nervenarzt* 69:1061–1065, 1998.
285. Wohlgemuth WA, Rottach KG, Stoehr M: Intermittent claudication due to ischaemia of the lumbosacral plexus. *J Neurol Neurosurg Psychiatry* 67:793–795, 1999.
286. Roberts JT: The effect of occlusive arterial diseases of the extremities on the blood supply of nerves. Experimental and clinical studies on the role of the vasa nervorum. *Am Heart J* 35:369–392, 1948.
287. Hager W: Neuralgia femoris. Resection des Nerv. cutan. femoris anterior externus. *Heilung Dtsch Med Wochenschr* 11:218, 1885.
288. Roth VK: Meralgia paraesthetica. *Med Obozr Mosk* 43:678, 1895.
289. Ivins GK: Meralgia paresthetica, the elusive diagnosis: clinical experience with 14 adult patients. *Ann Surg* 232:281–286, 2000.

290. Lambert SD: Athletic injuries to the hip. In: Echternach J, ed. *Physical Therapy of the Hip*. New York, NY: Churchill Livingstone, 1990:143–164.
291. Reichert FL: Meralgia paresthetica; a form of causalgia relieved by interruption of the sympathetic fibers. *Surg Clin North Am* 13:1443, 1933.
292. Sunderland S: *Nerves and Nerve Injuries*. Edinburgh: E & S Livingstone, Ltd, 1968.
293. Yamamoto T, Nagira K, Kurosaka M: Meralgia paresthetica occurring 40 years after iliac bone graft harvesting: case report. *Neurosurgery* 49:1455–1457, 2001.
294. Nathan H: Gangliform enlargement on the lateral cutaneous nerve of the thigh. *J Neurosurg* 17:843, 1960.
295. Stookey B: Meralgia paresthetica: etiology and surgical treatment. *JAMA* 90:1705, 1928.
296. Bernhardt M: Ueber eine wenig bekannte Form der Beschäftigungsneuralgie. *Neurol Centralbl* 15:13–17, 1896.
297. Lorei MP, Hershman EB: Peripheral nerve injuries in athletes: treatment and prevention. *Sports Med* 16:130–147, 1993.
298. Dellon AL, Mackinnon SE, Seiler WA 4th: Susceptibility of the diabetic nerve to chronic compression. *Ann Plast Surg* 20:117, 1988.
299. Asbury AK: Focal and multifocal neuropathies of diabetes. In: Dyck PJ, Thomas PK, Winegrad AI, et al., eds. *Diabetic Neuropathy*. Philadelphia, PA: WB Saunders, 1987:45–55.
300. Edelson R, Stevens P: Meralgia paresthetica in children. *J Bone Joint Surg* 76A:993–999, 1994.
301. Ashby EC: Chronic obscure groin pain is commonly caused by enthesopathy: "Tennis elbow" of the groin. *Br J Surg* 81:1632–1634, 1994.
302. Martens MA, Hansen L, Mulier JC: Adductor tendinitis and musculus rectus abdominis tendonopathy. *Am J Sports Med* 15:353–356, 1987.
303. Zimmerman G: Groin pain in athletes. *Aust Fam Physician* 17:1046–1052, 1988.
304. Kallgren MA, Tingle LJ: Meralgia paresthetica mimicking lumbar radiculopathy. *Anesth Analg* 76:1367–1368, 1993.
305. Cubukcu S, Karsli B, Alimoglu MK: Meralgia paresthetica and low back pain. *J Back Musculoskel Rehabil* 17:135–139, 2004.
306. Bounameaux H, Reber-Wasem MA: Superficial thrombophlebitis and deep vein thrombosis: a controversial association. *Arch Intern Med* 157:1822–1824, 1997.
307. Markovic MD, Lotina SI, Davidovic LB, et al.: Acute superficial thrombophlebitis: modern diagnosis and therapy. *Srp Arch Celok Lek* 125:261–266, 1997.
308. Wiener SL: Unilateral and bilateral upper and lower leg pain references. In: Wiener SL, ed. *Differential Diagnosis of Acute Pain by Body Region*. New York, NY: McGraw-Hill, 1993:559–570.
309. Orava S, Kujala UM: Rupture of the ischial origin of the hamstring muscles. *Am J Sports Med* 23:702–705, 1995.
310. Owen CA: Gluteal compartment syndromes. *Clin Orthop* 132:57, 1978.
311. Schmalzried TP, Neal WC, Eckardt JJ: Gluteal compartment and crush syndromes. *Clin Orthop* 277:161, 1992.
312. Clark JL, Tatum NO, Noble SL: Management of genital herpes. *Am Fam Physician* 51:175–182, 187–188, 1995.
313. Tariq A, Ross JD: Viral sexually transmitted infections: current management strategies. *J Clin Pharm Ther* 24:409–414, 1999.
314. Swanson JM: The biopsychosocial burden of genital herpes: evidence-based and other approaches to care. *Dermatol Nurs* 11:257–268; quiz 269–270, 1999.
315. D'Ambrosia R: *Musculoskeletal Disorders: Regional Examination and Differential Diagnosis*, 2nd ed. Philadelphia, PA: J.B. Lippincott, 1986.
316. Wiener SL: *Differential Diagnosis of Acute pain by Body Region*. New York, NY: McGraw-Hill, 1993:1–4.
317. Fealy S, Paletta GA Jr: Femoral nerve palsy secondary to traumatic iliacus muscle hematoma: course after nonoperative management. *J Trauma* 47:1150–1152, 1999.
318. Cyriax J: *Textbook of Orthopaedic Medicine, Diagnosis of Soft Tissue Lesions*, 8th ed. London: Bailliere Tindall, 1982.
319. Greenwood MJ, Erhard R, Jones DL: Differential diagnosis of the hip vs. lumbar spine: five case reports. *J Orthop Sports Phys Ther* 27:308–315, 1998.
320. Hillier SL, Kiviat NB, Hawes SE, et al.: Role of bacterial vaginosis-associated microorganisms in endometritis. *Am J Obstet Gynecol* 175:435–441, 1996.
321. Rice VM: Conventional medical therapies for endometriosis. *Ann N Y Acad Sci* 955:343–352; discussion 389–393, 396–406, 2002.
322. Troyer MR: Differential diagnosis of endometriosis in a young adult woman with nonspecific low back pain. *Phys Ther* 18:801–810, 2007.
323. Murphy AA: Clinical aspects of endometriosis. *Ann N Y Acad Sci* 955:1–10; discussion 34–36, 396–406, 2002.
324. Vercellini P, Trespidi L, De Giorgi O, et al.: Endometriosis and pelvic pain: relation to disease stage and localization. *Fertil Steril* 65:299–304, 1996.
325. Swiersz LM: Role of endometriosis in cancer and tumor development. *Ann N Y Acad Sci* 955:281–292; discussion 293–295, 396–406, 2002.
326. Parsons CL, Zupkas P, Parsons JK: Intravesical potassium sensitivity in patients with interstitial cystitis and urethral syndrome. *Urology* 57:428–433, 2001.
327. Barnes R: Subcapital fractures of the femur. *J Bone Joint Surg* 58B:2, 1976.
328. Connolly WB, Hedburg EA: Observations on fractures of the pelvis. *J Trauma* 9:104, 1969.
329. Arnett FC: Reactive arthritis (Reiter's syndrome) and enteropathic arthritis. In: Klippel JH, ed. *Primer on the Rheumatic Diseases*, 11th ed. Atlanta, GA: Arthritis Foundation, 1997:184–188.
330. McClusky OE, Lordon RE, Arnett FC Jr: HL-A 27 in Reiter's syndrome and psoriatic arthritis: a genetic factor in disease susceptibility and expression. *J Rheumatol* 1:263–268, 1974.
331. Do TT: Transient synovitis as a cause of painful limps in children. *Curr Opin Pediatr* 12:48–51, 2000.
332. Spiera H: Osteoarthritis as a misdiagnosis in elderly patients. *Geriatrics* 42:37–42, 1987.
333. Schon L, Zuckerman JD: Hip pain in the elderly: evaluation and diagnosis. *Geriatrics* 43:48–62, 1988.
334. Puppione AA, Schumann L: Management strategies for older adults with osteoarthritis: how to promote and maintain function. *J Am Acad Nurse Pract* 11:167–171, 1999.
335. Kenzora JE: Symposium on idiopathic osteonecrosis: Foreword. *Orthop Clin North Am* 16:593–594, 1985.
336. Kenzora JE, Steele RE, Yosipovitch ZH, et al.: Experimental osteonecrosis of the femoral head in adult rabbits. *Clin Orthop* 130:8–46, 1978.
337. Guerra JJ, Steinberg ME: Distinguishing transient osteoporosis from avascular necrosis of the hip. *J Bone Joint Surg Am* 77:616–624, 1995.
338. Pauli S, Willemsen P, Declerck K, et al.: Osteomyelitis pubis versus osteitis pubis: a case presentation and review of the literature. *Br J Sports Med* 36:71–73, 2002.
339. Karkos CD, Hughes R, Prasad V, et al.: Thigh compartment syndrome as a result of a false aneurysm of the profunda femoris artery complicating fixation of an intertrochanteric fracture. *J Trauma* 47:393–395, 1999.
340. Sawmiller CJ, Turowski GA, Sterling AP, et al.: Extraarticular pigmented villonodular synovitis of the shoulder: a case report. *Clin Orthop Related Res* 335:262–267, 1997.
341. Schwartz H, Krishnan U, Pritchard D: Pigmented villonodular synovitis. *Clin Orthop* 247:243–255, 1989.
342. Chae J, Yu D, Walker M: Percutaneous, intramuscular neuromuscular electrical stimulation for the treatment of shoulder subluxation and pain in chronic hemiplegia: a case report. *Am J Phys Med Rehabil* 80:296–301, 2001.
343. Shearman CM, el-Khoury GY: Pitfalls in the radiologic evaluation of extremity trauma: Part I. The upper extremity. *Am Fam Physician* 57:995–1002, 1998.
344. Urquhart BS: Emergency: anterior shoulder dislocation. *Am J Nurs* 101:33–35, 2001.
345. Paxinos A, Walton J, Tzannes A, et al.: Advances in the management of traumatic anterior and atraumatic multidirectional shoulder instability. *Sports Med* 31:819–828, 2001.
346. Curran J, Ellman M, Brown N: Rheumatologic aspects of painful conditions of the shoulder. *Clin Orthop Rel Res* 173:27–37, 1983.
347. Corrigan AB, Robinson RG, Terenty T, et al.: Benign rheumatoid arthritis of the aged. *BMJ* 1:444–446, 1974.
348. Deal CL, Meenan RF, Goldenberg DL, et al.: The clinical features of elderly-onset rheumatoid arthritis. *Arthritis Rheum* 28:987–994, 1985.
349. Daigneault J, Cooney LM Jr: Shoulder pain in older people. *J Am Geriatr Soc* 46:1144–1151, 1998.
350. Baker GL, Oddis CV, Medsger TA Jr: Pasteurella multocida polyarticular septic arthritis. *J Rheumatol* 14:355–357, 1987.
351. Armbuster TG, Slivka J, Resnick D, et al.: Extraarticular manifestations of septic arthritis of the glenohumeral joint. *J Roentgenol* 129:667–672, 1977.

352. Kraft SM, Panush RS, Longley S: Unrecognized staphylococcal pyarthrosis with rheumatoid arthritis. *Semin Arthritis Rheum* 14:196–201, 1985.
353. Smith KL, Matsen FA: Total shoulder arthroplasty versus hemiarthroplasty: current trends. *Orthop Clin North Am* 29:491–506, 1998.
354. Bridgman JF: Periarthritis of the shoulder and diabetes mellitus. *Ann Rheum Dis* 31:69–71, 1972.
355. Balsund B, Thomsen S, Jensen E: Frozen shoulder: current concepts. *Scand J Rheumatol* 19:321–325, 1990.
356. Steinbrocker O, Argyros TG: Frozen shoulder: treatment by local injection of depot corticosteroids. *Arch Phys Med Rehabil* 55:209–213, 1974.
357. Ombregt L, Bisschop P, ter Veer HJ, et al.: The shoulder girdle: disorders of the inert structures. In: Ombregt L, ed. *A System of Orthopaedic Medicine*. London: WB Saunders, 1995:282–286.
358. Stralka SW, Head PL: Musculoskeletal pattern I: impaired joint mobility, motor function, muscle performance, and range of motion associated with joint arthroplasty. In: Tovin BJ, Greenfield BH, eds. *Evaluation and Treatment of the Shoulder: An Integration of the Guide to Physical Therapist Practice*. Philadelphia, PA: FA Davis, 2001:264–291.
359. Cofield RH: Degenerative and arthritic problems of the glenohumeral joint. In: Rockwood CA, Master R, eds. *The Shoulder*. Philadelphia, PA: WB Saunders, 1990:678–749.
360. Fenlin JM Jr: Total glenohumeral joint replacement. *Orthop Clin North Am* 6:525, 1975.
361. Dich VQ, Nelson JD, Haltalin KC: Osteomyelitis in infants and children: a review of 163 cases. *Am J Dis Child* 129:1273–1278, 1975.
362. Barrett-Connor E: Bacterial infection and sickle cell anemia: An analysis of 250 infections in 166 patients and review of the literature. *Medicine* 50:97–112, 1971.
363. Bass J, Vincent J, Person D: The expanding spectrum of Bartonella infections: II. Cat scratch disease. *Pediatr Infect Dis J* 16:163–179, 1997.
364. Bradford DS, Szalapski EWJ, Sutherland DER, et al.: Osteonecrosis in the transplant recipients. *Surg Gynecol Obstet* 159:328–334, 1984.
365. Cruess RL: Corticosteroid-induced osteonecrosis of the humeral head. *Orthop Clin North Am* 16:789–796, 1985.
366. Cruess RL: Steroid-induced avascular necrosis of the head of the humerus. *J Bone and Joint Surg* 58B:313–317, 1976.
367. Rossleigh MA, Smith J, Straus DJ, et al.: Osteonecrosis in patients with malignant lymphoma. *Cancer* 58:1112–1116, 1986.
368. Dwyer A, Aprill C, Bogduk N: Cervical zygapophyseal joint pain patterns: a study from normal volunteers. *Spine* 15:453, 1990.
369. Booth RE, Rothman RH: Cervical angina. *Spine* 1:28–32, 1976.
370. Boissonnault WG: Pathological origins of trunk and neck pain, part 1: pelvic and abdominal viscera disorders. *J Orthop Sports Phys Ther* 12:192–207, 1990.
371. Webster MW, Downs L, Yonas H, et al.: The effect of arm exercise on regional cerebral blood flow in the subclavian steal syndrome. *Am J Surg* 168:91–93, 1994.
372. Thompson AJ: Multiple sclerosis: symptomatic management. *J Neurol* 243:559–565, 1996.
373. Borasio GD, Miller RG: Clinical characteristics and management of ALS. *Semin Neurol* 21:155–166, 2001.
374. Pascuzzi RM, Fleck JD: Acute peripheral neuropathy in adults. *Neurol Clin* 15:529–547, 1997.
375. Levy WJ, Mason L, Hahn JF: Chiari malformation presenting in adults: a surgical experience in 127 cases. *Neurosurgery* 12:377–390, 1983.
376. Pancoast HK: Superior pulmonary sulcus tumor: tumor characterized by pain, Horner's syndrome, destruction of bone and atrophy of hand muscles. *JAMA* 99:1391–1396, 1932.
377. Pancoast HK: Importance of careful roentgen-ray investigations of apical chest tumors. *JAMA* 83:1407–1411, 1924.
378. Arcasoy SM, Jett JR: Superior pulmonary sulcus tumors and Pancoast's syndrome. *N Engl J Med* 337:1370–1376, 1997.
379. McKellar H: Clay shoveller's fracture. *J Bone and Joint Surg* 12:63–75, 1940.
380. Herrick R: Clay-shoveller's fracture in power lifting. *Am J Sports Med* 9:29–30, 1981.
381. Hyde GP, Postma GN, Caress JB: Laryngeal paresis as a presenting feature of idiopathic brachial plexopathy. *Otolaryngol Head Neck Surg* 124:575–576, 2001.
382. Lee VK, Simpkins L: Herpes zoster and postherpetic neuralgia in the elderly. *Geriatr Nurs* 21:132–135; quiz 136, 2000.
383. Botte MJ, Gelberman RH: Acute compartment syndrome of the forearm. *Hand Clin* 14:391–403, 1998.
384. Benjamin A: The relief of traumatic arterial spasm in threatened Volkmann's ischemic contracture. *J Bone Joint Surg* 39:711–713, 1957.
385. Wiener SL: Acute elbow and forearm pain. In: Wiener SL, ed. *Differential Diagnosis of Acute pain by Body Region*. New York, NY: McGraw-Hill, 1993:509–520.
386. Bijlsma JWJ, Breedveld FC, Dequeker J, et al.: *Leerboek Reumatologie*. Bohn: Stafleu VanLoghum, 1992.
387. van Vugt RM, Bijlsma JWJ, van Vugt AC: Chronic wrist pain: diagnosis and management. Development and use of a new algorithm. *Ann Rheum Dis* 58:665–674, 1999.
388. Hausman MR, Lisser SP: Hand infections. *Orthop Clin North Am* 23:171–186, 1992.
389. Viegas SF: Atypical causes of hand pain. *Am Fam Physician* 35:167–172, 1987.
390. van Vugt RM, van Dalen A, Bijlsma JWJ: Ultrasound guided synovial biopsy of the wrist. *Scand J Rheumatol* 26:212–214, 1997.
391. Mayeaux EJ Jr: Nail disorders. *Dermatology* 27:333–351, 2000.
392. Daniel CR: Paronychia. *Dermatology* 3:461, 1985.
393. Lee SJ, Cutcliffe DA, Hurst LC: Infections of the upper extremity. In: Dee R, Hurst LC, Gruber MA, et al., eds. *Principles of Orthopaedic Practice*, 2nd ed. New York, NY: McGraw-Hill, 1997:1193–1199.
394. Kienböck R: Concerning traumatic malacia of the lunate and its consequences: degeneration and compression fractures. *Clin Orth Rel Res* 149:4–5, 1980.
395. Waggy C: Disorders of the wrist. In: Wadsworth C, ed. *Orthopaedic Physical Therapy Home Study Course – The Elbow, Forearm, and Wrist*. La Crosse, WI: Orthopaedic Section, APTA, Inc., 1997.
396. Alexander AH, Lichtman DM: Kienbock's disease. In: Lichtman DM, ed. *The Wrist and its Disorders*. Philadelphia, PA: WB Saunders, 1988.
397. Beckenbaugh RD, Shives TC, Dobyns JH, et al.: Kienböck's disease: the natural history of Kienböck's disease and consideration of lunate fractures. *Clin Orthop* 149:98–106, 1980.
398. Salmon J, Stanley JK, Trail IA: Kienbock's disease: conservative management versus radial shortening. *J Bone Joint Surg* 82B:820–823, 2000.
399. Onieal M-E: *Essentials of Musculoskeletal Care*, 1st ed. Rosemont, IL: American Academy of Orthopaedic Surgeons, 1997.
400. Onieal M-E: *The Hand: Examination and Diagnosis, American Society for Surgery of the Hand*, 3rd ed. New York, NY: Churchill Livingstone, 1990.
401. Gunther SF: Dorsal wrist pain and the occult scapholunate ganglion. *J Hand Surg Am* 10A:697–703, 1985.
402. Tham S: Intraosseous ganglion cyst of the lunate: diagnosis and management. *J Hand Surg Am* 17A:429–432, 1992.
403. Bogumill GP, Sullivan DJ, Baker GI: Tumors of the hand. *Clin Orthop* 108:214–222, 1975.
404. Shaffer B, Bradley JP, Bogumill GP: Unusual problems of the athlete's elbow, forearm, and wrist. *Clin Sports Med* 15:425–438, 1996.
405. Wiener SL: Acute wrist, hand, and finger pain. In: Wiener SL, ed. *Differential Diagnosis of Acute Pain by Body Region*. New York, NY: McGraw-Hill, 1993:521–555.
406. Steen VD: Treatment of systemic sclerosis. *Am J Clin Dermatol* 2:315–325, 2001.
407. Jackson AM: Anterior knee pain. *J Bone Joint Surg* 83B:937–948, 2001.
408. Boyle A, Walton N: Malign anterior knee pain. *J R Soc Med* 93:639–640, 2000.
409. Jacobson JA, Lenchik L, Ruhoy MK, et al.: MR imaging of the infrapatellar fat pad of Hoffa. *Radiographics* 17:675–691, 1997.
410. Gebhardt MC, Ready JE, Mankin HJ: Tumors about the knee in children. *Clin Orthop Rel Res* 255:86–110, 1990.
411. Sadat-Ali M: Metachronous multicentric giant cell tumour: a case report. *Indian J Cancer* 34:169–176, 1997.
412. Kransdorf MJ: Primary tumours of the patella. A review of 42 cases. *Skeletal Radiol* 18:365–371, 1989.
413. Pavlovich RI, Day B: Anterior knee pain in the adolescent: an anatomical approach to etiology. *Am J Knee Surg* 10:176–180, 1997.
414. Mochida H, Kikuchi S: Injury to the infrapatellar branch of saphenous nerve in arthroscopic knee surgery. *Clin Orthop* 320:88–94, 1995.
415. Pinar H, Özkan M, Akseki D, et al.: Traumatic prepatellar neuroma: an unusual cause of anterior knee pain. *Knee Surg Sports Traumatol Arthrosc* 4:154–156, 1996.
416. Kankate RK, Selvan TP: Primary haematogenous osteomyelitis of the patella: a rare cause for anterior knee pain in an adult. *Postgrad Med J* 76:707–709, 2000.
417. Roy DR: Osteomyelitis of the patella. *Clin Orthop Related Res* 389:30–34, 2001.

418. Mars M, Hadley GP: Raised intracompartmental pressure and compartment syndromes. *Injury* 29:403–411, 1998.
419. Matsen FA, Winquist RA, Krugmire RB: Diagnosis and management of compartment syndromes. *J Bone Joint Surg* 62A:286–291, 1980.
420. Perron AD, Brady WJ, Keats TE: Orthopedic pitfalls in the ED: acute compartment syndrome. *Am J Emerg Med* 19:413–416, 2001.
421. Windsor RE, Chambers K: Overuse injuries of the leg. In: Kibler BW, Herring JA, Press JM, eds. *Functional Rehabilitation of Sports and Musculoskeletal Injuries*. Gaithersburg, MD: Aspen, 1998:265–272.
422. Gubbay AJ, Isaacs D: Pyomyositis in children. *Pediatr Infect Dis J* 19:1009–1012; quiz 1013, 2000.
423. Leach KL: Fractures of the tibia and fibular. In: Rockwood CA, Green DP, eds. *Fractures in Adults*. Philadelphia, PA: Lippincott, 1984:1652.
424. Warren DK, Wiss DA, Ting A: Isolated fibular shaft fracture in a sprinter. *Am J Sports Med* 18:209–210, 1990.
425. Mann RA, Hagy J: Biomechanics of walking, running, and sprinting. *Am J Sports Med* 8:345–350, 1980.
426. Gorman WP, Davis KR, Donnelly R: ABC of arterial and venous disease. Swollen lower limb-1: general assessment and deep vein thrombosis. *BMJ* 320:1453–1456, 2000.
427. Morganti CM, McFarland EG, Cosgarea AJ: Saphenous neuritis: a poorly understood cause of medial knee pain. *J Am Acad Orthop Surg* 10:130–137, 2002.
428. Mader JT, Cripps MW, Calhoun JH: Adult posttraumatic osteomyelitis of the tibia. *Clin Orthop Related Res* 360:14–21, 1999.
429. Omey ML, Micheli LJ: Foot and ankle problems in the young athlete. *Med Sci Sports Exerc* 31:S470–S486, 1999.
430. Brodsky AE, Khalil MA: Talar compression syndrome. *Am J Sports Med* 14:472–476, 1986.
431. McDougall A: The os trigonum. *J Bone Joint Surg* 37B:257–265, 1955.
432. Keene JS, Lange RH: Diagnostic dilemmas in foot and ankle injuries. *JAMA* 256:247–251, 1986.
433. Kelikian H, Kelikian AS: *Disorders of the Ankle*. Philadelphia, PA: WB Saunders, 1985.
434. Marotta JJ, Micheli LJ: Os trigonum impingement in dancers. *Am J Sports Med* 20:533–536, 1992.
435. Ihle CL, Cochran RM: Fracture of the fused os trigonum. *Am J Sports Med* 10:47–50, 1982.
436. Hedrick MR, McBryde AM: Posterior ankle impingement. *Foot Ankle* 15:2–8, 1994.
437. Wredmark T, Carlstedt CA, Bauer H, et al.: Os trigonum syndrome: a clinical entity in ballet dancers. *Foot Ankle* 11:404–406, 1991.
438. Ecker M, Rilter M: The symptomatic os trigonum. *JAMA* 201:204–206, 1967.
439. Hamilton WG, Geppert MJ, Thompson FM: Pain in the posterior aspect of the ankle in dancers. *J Bone Joint Surg* 78A:1491–1500, 1996.
440. Veazey BL, Heckman JD, Galindo MJ, et al.: Excision of ununited fractures of the posterior process of the talus: a treatment for chronic posterior ankle pain. *Foot Ankle* 13:453–457, 1992.
441. Burkus JK, Sella EJ, Southwick WD: Occult injuries of the talus diagnosed by bone scan and tomography. *Foot Ankle* 4:316–324, 1982.
442. McManama GB Jr: Ankle injuries in the young athlete. *Clin Sports Med* 7:547, 1988.
443. Sullivan JA: *Ankle and Foot Injuries in the Pediatric Athlete, Pediatric and Adolescent Sports Medicine*. Philadelphia, PA: WB Saunders, 1994:441–455.
444. Berndt AL, Harty M: Transchondral fractures (osteochondritis dissecans) of the talus. *J Bone Joint Surg* 41(A):988, 1959.
445. Roden S, Tillegard P, Unander-Scharin L: Osteochondritis dissecans and similar lesions of the talus. *Acta Orthop Scand* 23:51, 1953.
446. Gregg J, Das M: Foot and ankle problems in preadolescent and adolescent athletes. *Clin Sports Med* 1:131–147, 1982.
447. Mann RA: Pain in the foot. *Postgrad Med* 82:154–162, 1987.
448. Lahita RG: The clinical presentation of systemic lupus erythematosus. In: Lahita RG, ed. *Systemic Lupus Erythematosus*. San Diego, CA: Academic press, 1999:325–336.
449. Tigner R: Handling a sickle cell crisis. *RN* 61:32–35; quiz 36, 1998.
450. Rho RH, Brewer RP, Lamer TJ, et al.: Complex regional pain syndrome. *Mayo Clin Proc* 77:174–180, 2002.
451. Koman LA, Barden A, Smith BP, et al.: Reflex sympathetic dystrophy in an adolescent. *Foot Ankle* 14:273–277, 1993.
452. Goodall S: Peripheral vascular disease. *Nurs Stand* 14:48–52; quiz 53–54, 2000.
453. Gauthier G, Elbaz R: A subchondral bone fracture: a new surgical treatment. *Clin Orthop* 142:93–95, 1979.
454. Hoskinson J: Freiburg's disease: a review of long-term results. *Proc R Soc Med* 67:106–107, 1974.
455. Katcherian DA: Treatment of Freiburg's disease. *Orthop Clin North Am* 25:69–81, 1994.
456. Smillie IS: Freiburg's infraction (Koehler's second disease). *J Bone Joint Surg* 39B:580, 1955.
457. Harris RI, Beath T: Hypermobile flatfoot with short tendo Achilles. *J Bone Joint Surg* 30A:116, 1948.
458. Mann RA, Coughlin MJ: Keratotic disorders of the skin. In: Mann RA, Coughlin MJ, eds. *Surgery of the Foot and Ankle*. St. Louis, MO: Mosby-Yearbook, 1993:533–441.
459. Hockenbury RT: Forefoot problems in athletes. *Med Sci Sports Exerc* 31: S448–S458, 1999.
460. Wu KK: Morton's interdigital neuroma: a clinical review of its etiology, treatment, and results. *J Foot Ankle Surg* 35:112–119, 1996.
461. Sullivan JA: The child's foot. In: Morrissy RT, ed. *Lovell and Winter's Pediatric Orthopaedics*, 4th ed. Philadelphia, PA: Lippincott, 1996:1077–1135.
462. Chen YJ, Shih HN, Huang TJ, et al.: Posterior tibial tendon tear combined with a fracture of the accessory navicular: a new subclassification? *J Trauma* 39:993–996, 1995.
463. Grogan DP, Gasser SI, Ogden JA: The painful accessory navicular: a clinical and histopathological study. *Foot Ankle* 10:164, 1989.
464. Kidner FC: The prehallux in relation to flatfoot. *JAMA* 101:1539, 1933.
465. Sullivan JA, Miller WA: The relationship of the accessory navicular to the development of the flatfoot. *Clin Orthop* 144:233, 1979.
466. Bennett GL, Weiner DS, Leighley B: Surgical treatment of symptomatic accessory tarsal navicular. *J Pediatr Orthop* 10:445, 1990.
467. Hunter-Griffin LY: Injuries to the leg, ankle, and foot. In: Sullivan JA, Grana WA, eds. *The Pediatric Athlete*. Park Ridge, IL: American Academy of Orthopaedic Surgeons, 1990:187–198.
468. Veitch JM: Evaluation of the Kidner operation and treatment of symptomatic accessory tarsal scaphoid. *Clin Orthop* 131:210, 1978.
469. Manusov EG, Lillegard WA, Raspa RF, et al.: Evaluation of pediatric foot problems: part I. The forefoot and midfoot. *Am Fam Physician* 54:592–606, 1996.
470. Sanders R: Current concepts review: displaced intraarticular fractures of the calcaneus. *J Bone Joint Surg* 82A:225–250, 2000.
471. Antoniou D, Conner AN: Osteomyelitis of the calcaneus and talus. *J Bone Joint Surg* 56A:338–345, 1974.
472. Nixon GW: Hematogenous osteomyelitis of metaphyseal equivalent locations. *AJR Am J Roentgenol* 130:123–129, 1978.
473. Keck C: The tarsal tunnel syndrome. *J Bone Joint Surg* 44A:180–182, 1962.
474. Lam S: A tarsal tunnel syndrome. *Lancet* 2:1354–1355, 1962.
475. Turan I, Rivero-Melian C, Guntner P, et al.: Tarsal tunnel syndrome. Outcome of surgery in longstanding cases. *Clin Orthop Related Res* 343:151–156, 1997.
476. DeLisa JA, Saleed MA: The tarsal tunnel syndrome. *Muscle Nerve* 6:664–670, 1983.
477. Chater EH: Tarsal-tunnel syndrome in rheumatoid arthritis. *Br Med J* 3:406, 1970.
478. Cimino W: Tarsal tunnel syndrome. Review of the literature. *Foot Ankle* 11:47–52, 1990.
479. Francis H, March L, Terenty T, et al.: Benign joint hypermobility with neuropathy: documentation and mechanism of tarsal tunnel syndrome. *J Rheumatol* 14:577–581, 1987.
480. Joubert MJ: Tarsal tunnel syndrome. *S Afr Med J* 46:507–508, 1972.
481. Rask M: Medial plantar neurapraxia (Jogger's Foot). *Clin Orthop* 134:193–195, 1978.
482. DiStefano V, Sack J, Whittaker R, et al.: Tarsal tunnel syndrome: Review of the literature and two case reports. *Clin Orthop* 88:76–79, 1972.
483. Edwards W, Lincoln C, Bassett F, et al.: The tarsal tunnel syndrome: diagnosis and treatment. *JAMA* 207:716–720, 1969.
484. Radin E: Tarsal tunnel syndrome. *Clin Orthop* 181:167–170, 1983.
485. Jackson DL, Haglund BL: Tarsal tunnel syndrome in runners. *Sports Med* 13:146–149, 1992.
486. Lam SJS: Tarsal tunnel syndrome. *J Bone Joint Surg* 49B:87–92, 1967.
487. Van Wyngarden TM: The painful foot, part II: Common rearfoot deformities. *Am Fam Physician* 55:2207–2212, 1997.
488. Linscheid R, Burton R, Fredericks E: Tarsal tunnel syndrome. *South Med J* 63:1313–1323, 1970.
489. Stefko RM, Lauerman WC, Heckman JD: Tarsal tunnel syndrome caused by an unrecognized fracture of the posterior process of the talus. *J Bone Joint Surg* 76A:116–118, 1994.
490. Bodack MP, Cole JC, Nagler W: Sciatic neuropathy secondary to a uterine fibroid: a case report. *Am J Phys Med Rehabil* 78:157–159, 1999.

Gait and Posture Analysis

CHAPTER 6

CHAPTER OBJECTIVES

At the completion of this chapter, the reader will be able to:

1. Summarize the various components of the gait cycle.
2. Apply the knowledge of gait components to gait analysis.
3. Perform a comprehensive gait analysis.
4. Categorize the various compensations of the body and their influences on gait.
5. Recognize the manifestations of abnormal gait and develop strategies to counteract these abnormalities.
6. Describe and demonstrate a number of abnormal gait syndromes.
7. Make an accurate judgment when recommending an assistive device to improve gait and function.
8. Describe and demonstrate the various gait patterns used with assistive devices.
9. Evaluate the effectiveness of an intervention for a gait dysfunction.
10. Summarize the components of a postural assessment.
11. Perform a thorough posture assessment.
12. Recognize the most common manifestations of abnormal posture.
13. Make an accurate judgment when recommending postural adjustments.
14. Evaluate the effectiveness of a postural adjustment.

OVERVIEW

The assessment of symmetry within locomotion and posture is critical in the evaluation of neuromusculoskeletal dysfunction. For most individuals, gait or posture is an innate characteristic, as much a part of their personality as their smile. Indeed, many people can be recognized in a group by their gait or posture. The purpose of this chapter is to describe the various components of gait and posture and to provide the clinician with the necessary tools for the analysis of each.

Gait and the Gait Cycle

The lower kinetic chain has two main functions: to provide a stable base of support (BOS) in standing and to propel the body through space with gait. While maintaining a static equilibrium of forces, the objective with mobility is to create and control dynamic, unbalanced forces to produce movement.[1] Gait is thus an example of controlled instability. It is not clear whether gait is learned or is preprogrammed at the spinal cord level. However, once mastered, gait allows us to move around our environment in an efficient manner, requiring little in the way of conscious thought, at least in familiar surroundings. Bipedal gait has allowed the arms and hands to be free for exploration of the environment. Even though gait appears to be a simple process, it is prone to breakdown. Although individual gait patterns are characterized by significant variation, three essential requirements have been identified for locomotion: progression, postural control, and adaptation:[2]

- Progression. The fall that occurs at the initiation of gait so that an individual must take the first step is controlled by the central nervous system (CNS).[3] The CNS computes in advance the required size and direction of this fall toward the supporting foot. Progression of the head, arms, and trunk is initiated and terminated in the brain stem that maintains a central pattern generator (CPG) through the spinal cord (see Chapter 3). The locomotor CPG produces self-sustaining patterns of stereotype motor output resulting in gait-like movements. In addition, gait relies on the control of the limb movements by reflexes. Two such reflexes include the stretch reflex and the extensor thrust. The stretch reflex is involved in the extremes of joint motion, whereas the extensor thrust may facilitate the extensor muscles of the lower extremity during weight bearing.[4] Both the CPG and the reflexes that mediate afferent input to the spinal cord are under the control of the brainstem and are therefore subconscious.[5] This would tend to indicate that verbal coaching (i.e., feedback that is processed in the cortex) regarding an aberrant gait pattern might be less effective than a sensory input that will elicit a brain stem-mediated postural response.[1]

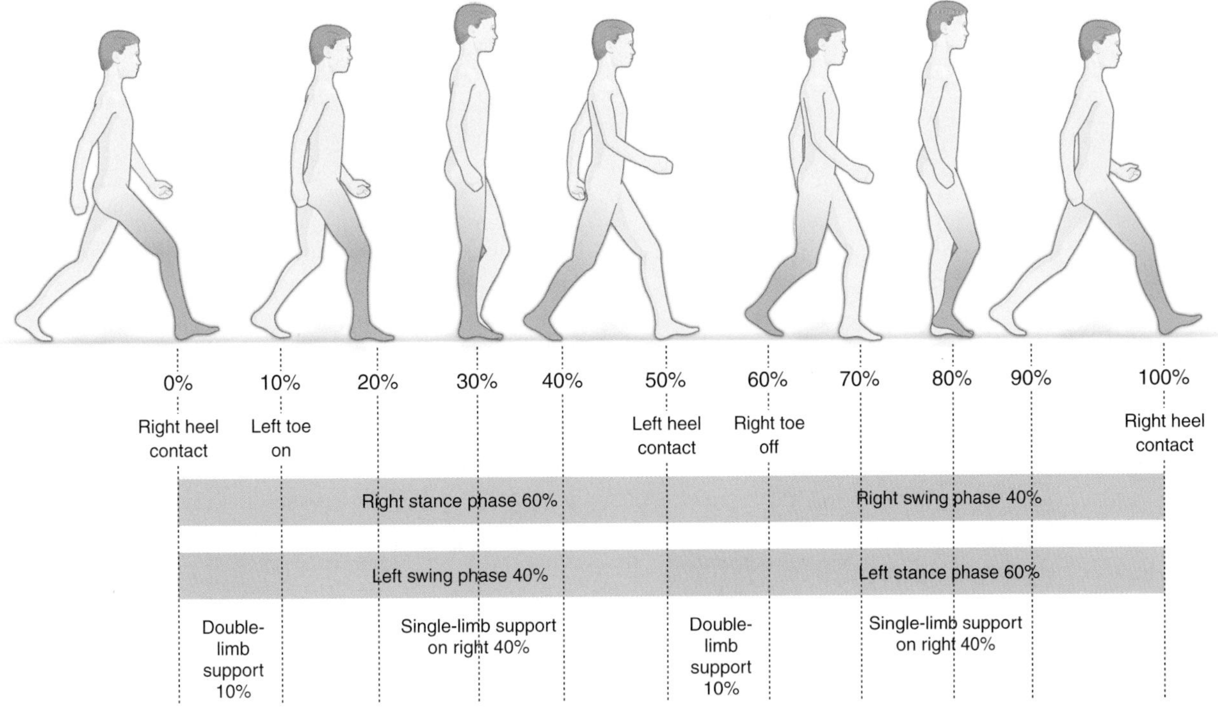

FIGURE 6-1 The two phases of gait.

- Postural control. Postural control is dynamically maintained to appropriately position the body for efficient gait.
- Adaptation. Although central pattern generation occurs independent of sensory input, afferent information from the periphery can influence the CPG. Adaptation is achieved by adjusting the central pattern generated to meet task demands and environmental demands.

Gait, therefore, is initiated grossly in the spinal cord and fine tuned by the higher brain centers.[1] In patients who have developed dysfunctional gait patterns, physical therapy can help to restore this exquisite evolutionary gift.[6] Pain, weakness, and disease can all cause a disturbance in the normal rhythm of gait. However, except in obvious cases, abnormal gait does not always equate with impairment.

In addition to neural input, normal human gait also involves a complex synchronization of the cardiopulmonary and muscular systems in which the cardiopulmonary system produces the energy required for gait.

Walking involves the alternating action of the two lower extremities. This walking pattern is studied as a gait cycle. The *gait cycle* is defined as the interval of time between any of the repetitive events of walking. Such an event could include the point when the foot first contacts the ground to the point when the same foot contacts the ground again.[7] The gait cycle consists of two phases (Fig. 6-1):

1. ***Stance.*** This phase constitutes approximately 60–65% of the gait cycle[8,9] and describes the entire time the foot is in contact with the ground and the limb is bearing weight. The stance phase begins when the foot makes contact with the ground and concludes when the ipsilateral foot leaves the ground. The stance phase takes about 0.6 seconds during an average walking speed.
2. ***Swing.*** The swing phase constitutes approximately 35–40% of the gait cycle[8,9] and describes the phase when the foot is not in contact with the ground. The swing phase begins as the foot is lifted from the ground and ends when the ipsilateral foot makes contact with the ground again.[7]

CLINICAL PEARL

In terms of energy expenditure, the swing phase requires relatively little, relying heavily on passive soft-tissue tension, gravity, and momentum to accelerate and decelerate individual segments.[1] In contrast, stance requires more dynamic activity, with muscles in the stance limb supporting the body and propelling it forward.

Stance Phase

Within the stance phase, two tasks and five intervals are recognized.[8,10,11] The two tasks are weight acceptance and single-limb support. The five intervals are initial contact, loading response, midstance, terminal stance, and preswing[11] (Fig. 6-2). Initial contact and toe-off are instantaneous events. The initial contact, which occurs when one foot makes contact with the ground, takes place at the beginning of the stance phase. As the initial contact of one foot is occurring, the contralateral foot is preparing to come off the floor.

Weight Acceptance

The weight acceptance task includes the intervals of initial contact and loading response. The initial contact interval accounts for the first 10% of the gait cycle and describes the phase when one foot is coming off the floor while the other foot

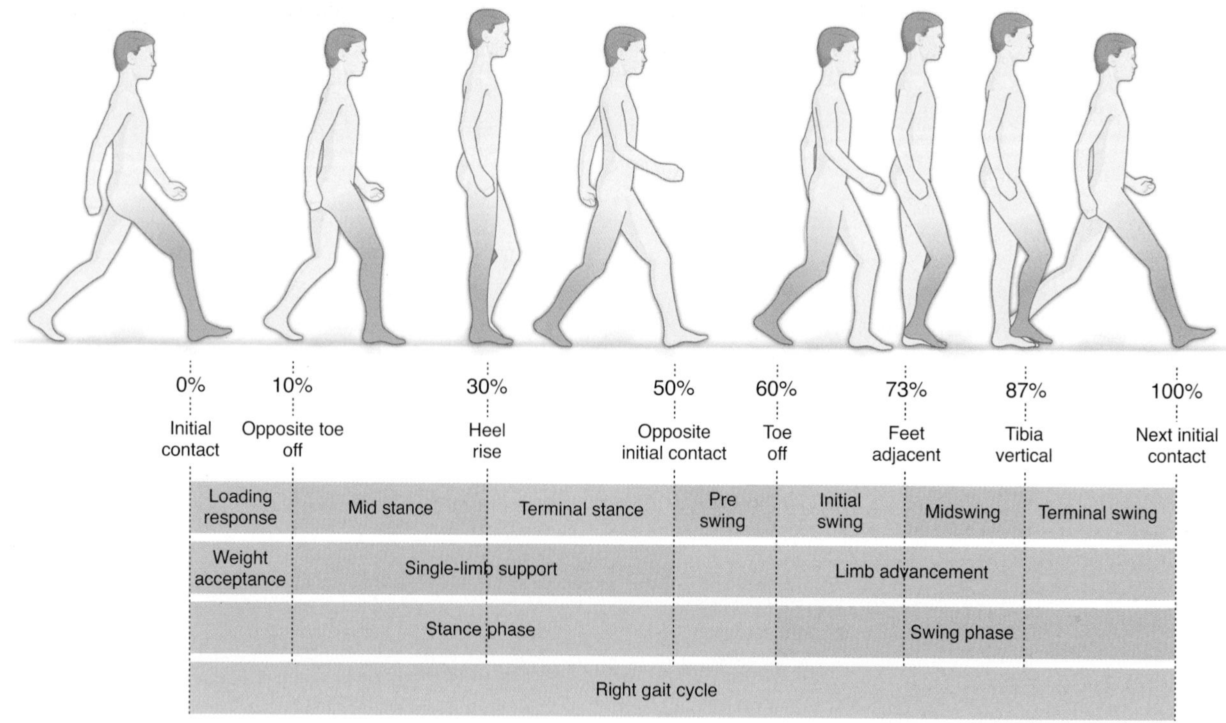

FIGURE 6-2 The intervals of gait.

is accepting body weight and absorbing the shock of initial contact. Because both feet are in contact with the floor, this phase is referred to as *double support* or the *initial double stance* phase.[11] The *loading response* interval begins as one limb bears weight while the other leg begins to go through its swing phase.

Single-Leg Support

The single-legged support task includes the three intervals of midstance, terminal stance, and preswing.

The *midstance* interval, representing the first half of the single-limb support task, begins as one foot is lifted and continues until the body weight is aligned over the forefoot.[11] The loading response and midstance intervals account for the next 40% of the gait cycle.[11]

The *terminal stance* interval is the second half of the single-limb support task. It begins when the heel of the weight-bearing foot lifts off the ground and continues until the contralateral foot strikes the ground.

The *preswing* interval begins with initial contact of the contralateral limb and ends with the ipsilateral toe-off. During this phase, the stance leg is unloading the body weight to the contralateral limb and preparing the leg for the swing phase. The terminal stance and preswing intervals account for the next 10% of the gait cycle.[11] Because both feet are on the floor at the same time during this interval, double support occurs for the second time in the gait cycle. This last portion of the stance phase is, therefore, referred to as the *terminal double stance*. The phase of single-limb support of one limb equals the phase of swing for the other.[11]

Swing Phase

Gravity and momentum are the primary sources of motion for the swing phase.[4] Within the swing phase, one task and three intervals are recognized.[8,10,11] The task involves limb advancement. The three intervals are initial swing, midswing, and terminal swing.[11]

Limb Advancement

The swing phase involves the forward motion of the non-weight-bearing (NWB) foot. The three intervals of the swing phase include the following:[11]

1. ***Initial swing.*** This interval begins with the lifting of the foot from the floor and ends when the swinging foot is opposite the stance foot. It represents the 60–73% phase of the gait cycle.[11]
2. ***Midswing.*** This interval begins as the swinging limb is opposite the stance limb and ends when the swinging limb is forward and the tibia is vertical. It represents the 73–87% phase of the gait cycle.[11]
3. ***Terminal swing.*** This interval begins with a vertical tibia of the swing leg with respect to the floor and ends the moment the foot strikes the floor. It represents the last 87–100% of the gait cycle.

The precise duration of the gait cycle intervals depends on a number of factors, including age, impairment, and the patient's walking velocity. Velocity is defined as the distance a body moves in a given time and is thus calculated by dividing the distance traveled by the time taken. Normal free gait velocity on a smooth and level surface averages about 62 m/min for adults, with men being about 5% faster than women.[12] As gait speed increases, it develops into jogging and then running, with changes in each of the intervals. For example, as speed increases, the stance phase decreases and the terminal double stance phase disappears altogether. This produces a double unsupported phase.[13] Although the motion occurring at each of the lower extremity joints is similar for walking and for running, the required range of motion increases with the speed of the activity.

GAIT PARAMETERS

A normal gait pattern is a factor of a number of parameters.

Step Width

The step width is the distance between both feet. The normal step width, which is considered to be between 5 and 10 cm (2–4 in.), forms the BOS during gait. The size of the BOS and its relation to the center of gravity (COG) are important factors in the maintenance of balance and, thus, the stability of an object. The COG must be maintained over the BOS, if equilibrium is to be maintained. The BOS includes the part of the body in contact with the supporting surface and the intervening area.[14] As the COG moves forward with each step, it briefly passes beyond the anterior margin of the BOS, resulting in a temporary loss of balance.[14] This temporary loss of equilibrium is counteracted by the advancing foot at initial contact, which establishes a new BOS. A larger than normal step width or BOS is observed in individuals who have muscle imbalances of the lower limbs and trunk, as well as those who have problems with overall static dynamic balance.[15] Assistive devices, such as crutches or walkers, can be prescribed to increase the BOS and, therefore, enhance stability. The step width should be seen to decrease to around zero with increased speed. If the step width decreases to a point below zero, crossover occurs, whereby one foot lands where the other should, and vice versa.[16]

Step Length

Step length is measured as the distance between the point of initial contact of one foot and the point of initial contact of the opposite foot. The average step length is about 72 cm (28 in.). The measurement should be equal for both legs.

Stride Length

Stride length is the distance between successive points of foot-to-floor contact of the same foot. A stride is one full lower extremity cycle. Two step lengths added together make the stride length. The average stride length for normal adults is 144 m (56 in.).[12]

Typically, the step and stride lengths do not vary more than a few centimeters between tall and short individuals. Men typically have longer step and stride lengths than women. Step and stride lengths decrease with age, pain, disease, and fatigue.[17,18] A decrease in step or stride length may also result from a forward head posture, a stiff hip, or a decrease in the availability of motion at the lumbar spine. The decrease in step and stride length that occurs with aging is thought to be the result of a number of factors including an overall decrease in joint range of motion, and the increased likelihood of falling during the swing phase of ambulation, caused by diminished control of the hip musculature.[19] This lack of control prevents the aged person from being able to intermittently lose and recover the same amount of balance that the younger adult can lose and recover.[19]

Cadence

Cadence is defined as the number of separate steps taken in a certain time. Normal cadence is between 90 and 120 steps per minute.[20,21] The cadence of women is usually six to nine steps per minute slower than that of men.[14] Cadence is also affected by age, decreasing from the age of 4 to the age of 7 years, and then again in advancing years.[22]

CLINICAL PEARL

Compared with men, women generally have narrower shoulders, greater valgus at the elbow, greater varus at the hip, and greater valgus at the knee.[23] Women also have a smaller Achilles tendon, a narrower heel in relationship to the forefoot, and a foot that is narrower than a man's in length. On average, women walk at a lower cadence than men (6–9 steps higher), and at lower speeds.[24–28] Because leg length in women is 51.2% of total body height compared with 56% in men, women have slightly shorter stride lengths,[24,25,27–31] although when normalized for height, women would tend to have the same or slightly greater stride lengths.[28–30]

Velocity

The primary determinants of gait velocity are the repetition rate (cadence), physical conditioning, and the length of the person's stride.[12]

CLINICAL PEARL

A mathematical relationship exists between cadence, stride length, and velocity, such that if two of them are directly measured, the third may be derived by calculation[7] (Table 6-1).

Vertical Ground Reaction Forces

Newton's third law states that for every action there is an equal and opposite reaction. During gait, vertical ground reaction forces are created by a combination of gravity, body weight, and the firmness of the ground. Under normal conditions, we are mostly unaware of these forces. However, in the presence of joint inflammation or tissue injury, the significance of these forces becomes apparent. Vertical ground reaction force begins with an impact peak of less than body weight and then

TABLE 6-1 Gait Parameters

Cadence (steps/min) = velocity (m/s) × 120/stride length (m)
Stride length (m) = velocity (m/s) × 120/cadence (steps/min)
Velocity (m/s) = cadence (steps/min) × stride length (m)/120

Data from Levine D, Whittle M: *Gait Analysis: The Lower Extremities.* La Crosse, WI: Orthopaedic Section, APTA, Inc., 1992.

exceeds body weight at the end of the initial contact interval, dropping during midstance and rising again to exceed the body weight, reaching its highest peak during the terminal stance interval. Thus, there are two peaks of ground reaction force during the gait cycle: the first at maximum limb loading during the loading response and the second during terminal stance.

The ground reaction force vector changes from anterior to the hip joint at initial contact to a progressively posterior position at late stance, when the ground reaction force is posterior to the hip.[32,33] Peak flexion torque occurs at initial contact but gradually declines, changing to an extension torque in midstance. The extension torque remains until terminal stance.[32,33]

During the gait cycle, the tibiofemoral joint reaction force has two peaks: the first immediately following initial contact (two to three times body weight) and the second during preswing (three to four times body weight).[34] Tibiofemoral joint reaction forces increase to five to six times body weight for running and stair climbing, and eight times body weight with downhill walking.[34–36]

It is well established that joint angles and ground reaction force components increase with walking speed.[37] This is not surprising, because the dynamic force components must increase as the body is subjected to increasing deceleration and acceleration forces when walking speed increases.

CLINICAL PEARL

Because leg length in women is 51.2% of total body height compared with 56% in men, women must strike the ground more often to cover the same distance.[38] Furthermore, because their feet are shorter, women complete the heel-to-toe gait in a shorter time than men do. Therefore, the cumulative ground reaction forces are likely to be greater in women.[23]

Mediolateral Shear Forces

Mediolateral shear in walking gait begins with an initial medial shear (occasionally lateral) after initial contact, followed by lateral shear for the remainder of the stance phase.[32,33] At the end of the stance phase, the shear shifts to a medial direction because of propulsion forces.

Anteroposterior Shear Forces

Anteroposterior shear forces in gait begin with an anterior shear force at initial contact and the loading response intervals, and a posterior shear at the end of the terminal stance interval.

CHARACTERISTICS OF NORMAL GAIT

Much has been written about the criteria for normal and abnormal gait.[7,9,24,32,39–44] Although the presence of symmetry in gait appears to be important, asymmetry in itself does not guarantee impairment. It must be remembered that the definition of what constitutes the so-called normal gait is elusive. Unlike posture, which is a static event, gait is dynamic and as such is protean.

CLINICAL PEARL

Good alignment of the weight-bearing segments of the body:

- Reduces the likelihood of strain and injury by reducing joint friction and tension in the soft tissues.
- Improves the stability of the weight-bearing limb and the balance of the trunk. The stability of the body is directly related to the size of the BOS. In order to be stable, the intersection of the line of gravity with the BOS should be close to the geometric center of the base.[45]
- Reduces excess energy expenditure.

Gait involves the displacement of body weight in a desired direction, utilizing a coordinated effort between the joints of the trunk and extremities and the muscles that control or produce these motions. Any interference that alters this relationship may result in a deviation or disturbance of the normal gait pattern. This, in turn, may result in increased energy expenditure or functional impairment.

Perry[20] lists four *priorities* of normal gait:

1. Stability of the weight-bearing foot throughout the stance phase.
2. Clearance of the NWB foot during the swing phase.
3. Appropriate prepositioning (during terminal swing) of the foot for the next gait cycle.
4. Adequate step length.

Gage[22] added a fifth priority, energy conservation. The typical energy expended in normal gait (2.5 kcal/min) is less than twice that spent while sitting or standing (1.5 kcal/min).[22] Two-dimensional kinetic data have revealed that approximately 85% of the energy for normal walking comes from the plantar flexors of the ankle, and 15% from the flexors of the hip.[46] It has been proposed that the type of gait selected is based on metabolic energy considerations.[47] Current commonly used parameters to measure walking efficiency include oxygen consumption, heart rate, and comfortable speed of walking.[48–50] Economy of mobility is a measurement of submaximal oxygen uptake (submax VO_2) for a given speed.[51,52] A decline in functional performance may be evidenced by an increase in submax VO_2 for walking.[53] This change in economy of mobility may be indicative of an abnormal gait pattern.[53] Some researchers have reported no gender differences for economy of mobility,[54–56] whereas others suggest that men are more economical or have lower energy costs than women at the same work.[57–59] Age-related declines in economy of mobility also have been reported in the literature, with differing results. Some researchers reported that older adults were less economical than younger adults while walking at various speeds.[51,60,61] Conversely, economy of mobility appears to be unaffected by aging for individuals who maintain higher levels of physical activity.[62–64]

Some authors have claimed that a limb-length discrepancy leads to mechanical and functional changes in gait[65] and

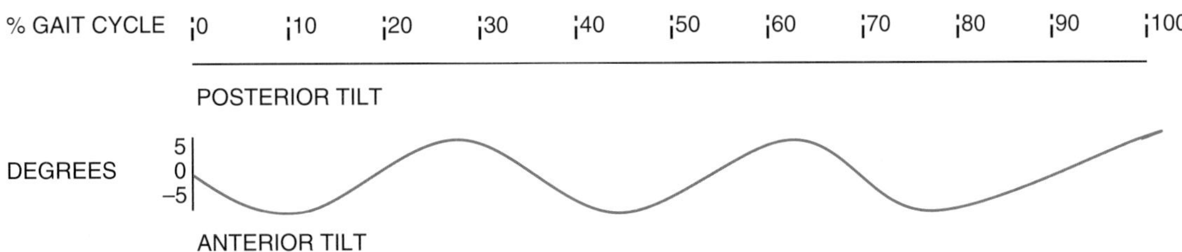

FIGURE 6-3 Pelvic motion during normal gait.

increased energy expenditure.[66] Intervention has been advocated for limb-length discrepancies of less than 1 cm to discrepancies greater than 5 cm,[65–67] but the rationale for these recommendations has not been well defined, and the literature contains little substantive information regarding the functional significance of these discrepancies.[68] For example, Gross found no noticeable functional or cosmetic problems in a study of 74 adults who had less than 2 cm of discrepancy and 35 marathon runners who had as much as 2.5 cm of discrepancy.[67]

CLINICAL PEARL

The cardiovascular benefits derived from increases in gait speed may be acceptable for a normal population or advanced rehabilitation but should be used cautiously with postsurgical patients.[69]

For gait to be efficient and to conserve energy, the COG* must undergo minimal displacement:

- Any displacement that elevates, depresses, or moves the COG beyond normal maximum excursion limits wastes energy.
- Any abrupt or irregular movement will waste energy even when that movement does not exceed the normal maximum displacement limits of the COG.

CLINICAL PEARL

The COG in men is at a point that corresponds to 56.18% of their height. In women, the COG is at a point that corresponds to 55.44% of their height.[70]

To minimize the energy costs of walking, the body uses a number of biomechanical mechanisms. In 1953, Saunders, Inman, and Eberhart[71] proposed that six kinematic features—the Six Determinants—have the potential to reduce the energetic cost of human walking. The six determinants are as follows:[72]

- Lateral displacement of the pelvis: To avoid significant muscular and balancing demands, the pelvis shifts side to side (approximately 2.5–5 cm or 1–2 in.) during the gait cycle in order to center the weight of the body over the stance leg. If the lower extremities dropped directly vertical from the hip joint, the center of mass would be required to shift 3–4 in. to each side to be positioned effectively over the supporting foot. The combination of femoral varus and anatomical valgum at the knee permits a vertical tibial posture with both tibias in close proximity to each other. This narrows the step width to 5–10 cm (2–4 in.) from heel center to heel center, thereby reducing the lateral shift required of the COG toward either side.
- Pelvic rotation: The rotation of the pelvis normally occurs about a vertical axis in the transverse plane toward the weight-bearing limb. The total pelvic rotation is approximately 4 degrees to each side.[22] Forward rotation of the pelvis on the swing side prevents an excessive drop in the body's COG. The pelvic rotation also results in a relative lengthening of the femur by lessening the angle of the femur with the floor, and thus step length, during the termination of the swing period.[11]
- Vertical displacement of the pelvis: Vertical pelvic shifting keeps the COG from moving superiorly and inferiorly more than 5 cm (2 in.) during normal gait (Fig. 6-3). Due to the shift, the high point occurs during midstance, and the low point occurs during initial contact. The amount of vertical displacement of the pelvis may be accentuated in the presence of a leg length discrepancy, fusion of the knee, or hip abductor weakness, the latter of which results in a Trendelenburg sign. The Trendelenburg sign is said to be positive if, when standing on one leg, the pelvis drops on the side opposite to the stance leg. The weakness is present on the side of the stance leg—the gluteus medius is not able to maintain the COG on the side of the stance leg.
- Knee flexion in stance: Knee motion is intrinsically associated with foot and ankle motion. At initial contact before the ankle moves into a plantarflexed position, and thus is relatively more elevated, the knee is in relative extension. Responding to a plantarflexed posture at loading response, the knee flexes. Midstance knee flexion prevents an excessive rise in the body's COG during that period of the

*The COG of the body is located approximately at midline in the frontal plane and slightly anterior (5 cm or 2 in.) to the second sacral vertebra in the sagittal plane.

gait cycle. If not for the midstance knee flexion, the COG's rise during midstance would be larger, as would its total vertical displacement. Passing through midstance as the ankle remains stationary with the foot flat on the floor, the knee again reverses its direction to one of extension. As the heel comes off the floor in terminal stance, the heel begins to rise as the ankle plantarflexes and the knee flexes. In preswing, as the forefoot rolls over the metatarsal heads, the heel elevates even more as further plantarflexion occurs and flexion of the knee increases.

- Ankle mechanism: For normal foot function and gait, the amount of ankle joint motion required is approximately 10 degrees of dorsiflexion (to complete midstance and begin terminal stance) and 20 degrees of plantarflexion (for full push off in preswing). At initial contact, the foot is in relative dorsiflexion due to the muscle action of the pretibial muscles and the triceps surae. This muscle action produces a relative lengthening of the leg, resulting in a smoothing of the pathway of the COG during stance phase.
- Foot mechanism: The controlled lever arm of the forefoot at preswing is particularly helpful as it rounds out the sharp downward reversal of the COG. Thus it does not reduce a peak displacement period of the COG as the earlier determinants did but rather smoothes the pathway. An adaptively shortened gastrocnemius muscle may produce movement impairment by restricting normal dorsiflexion of the ankle from occurring during the midstance to heel raise portion of the gait cycle. This motion is compensated for by increased pronation of the subtalar joint, increased internal rotation of the tibia, and resultant stresses to the knee joint complex.

CLINICAL PEARL

A decrease in flexibility or joint motion, or both, may result in an increase in both "internal resistance" and the energy expenditure required.

Joint Motions

During the gait cycle, the swing of the arms is out of phase with the legs. As the upper body moves forward, the trunk twists about a vertical axis. The thoracic spine and the pelvis rotate in opposite directions to each other to enhance stability and balance. In contrast, the lumbar spine tends to rotate with the pelvis. The shoulders and trunk rotate out of phase with each other during the gait cycle.[73] Unless they are restrained, the arms tend to swing in opposition to the legs, the left arm swinging forward as the right leg swings forward, and vice versa.[4] When the arm swing is prevented, the upper trunk tends to rotate in the same direction as the pelvis, producing an awkward gait.

CLINICAL PEARL

Different patterns of interlimb coordination between arms and legs have been observed within the human walking mode.[74,75] At lower walking speeds, the arms are synchronized to the stepping frequency (2:1 ratio of arm to leg), whereas at higher walking velocities, the arms are synchronized to the stride frequency (1:1 ratio of arm to leg). These results also suggest that at lower speeds, the resonant frequency of the arms dominates the interlimb coupling, whereas at higher speeds, the resonant frequency of the legs is dominant.[76]

Maximum flexion of both the elbow and the shoulder joints occurs at the initial contact interval of the opposite foot, and maximum extension occurs at the initial contact of the foot on the same side.[77]

Although the majority of the arm swing results from momentum, the pendular actions of the arms are also produced by gravity and muscle action.[4,78]

- The posterior deltoid and teres major appear to be involved during the backward swing.
- The posterior deltoid serves as a braking mechanism at the end of the forward swing.
- The middle deltoid is active in both the forward and the backward swing, perhaps to prevent the arms from brushing against the sides of the body during the swing.

The motions that occur at each of the lower extremity joints during the stance phase of the gait cycle are outlined in Table 6-2 and Fig. 6-4.

Hip

The function of the hip is to extend the leg during the stance phase and flex the leg during the swing phase (Table 6-2). Hip motion occurs in all three planes during the gait cycle.

- The hip rotates approximately 40–45 degrees in the sagittal plane during a normal stride, beginning in external rotation at initial contact.[33] The hip begins to internally rotate during the loading response. Maximum internal rotation is reached just before midstance. The hip externally rotates during the swing phase, with maximal external rotation occurring in terminal swing.[32]
- The hip flexes and extends once during the gait cycle, with the limit of flexion occurring at the middle of the swing phase, and the limit of extension being achieved before the end of the stance phase (Table 6-2). Maximum hip flexion of 30–35 degrees occurs in late swing phase at about 85% of the gait cycle; maximum extension of approximately 10 degrees is reached near toe-off at approximately 50% of the cycle.[32,33,79] The ligaments of the hip helps to stabilize the joint in extension.
- In the coronal plane, hip adduction occurs throughout early stance and reaches a maximum at 40% of the cycle[79] Hip adduction totaling 5–7 degrees occurs in early swing phase, which is followed by slight hip abduction at the end of the swing phase, especially if a long stride is taken.[32,33,79] Perry reports that the total transverse plane motion is 8 degrees.[33]

The greatest force on the hip occurs during midstance. Painful hip, knee, or ankle conditions cause this interval to be shortened to decrease the time spent in the painful position.

TABLE 6-2	Joint Motions in the Lower Extremities During Gait		
Phase	**Hip**	**Knee and Tibia**	**Ankle and Foot**
Initial contact	Hip begins to move toward extension from a position of 20–40 degrees of flexion; slight adduction and external rotation Reaction force anterior to hip joint creating flexion moment moving toward extension	Knee positioned in full extension before initial contact but flexes as heel makes contact Tibia positioned in slight external rotation Reaction force behind knee rapidly increases causing flexion moment	Foot positioned in supination (rigid) at heel contact, with the ankle moving into plantar flexion Reaction forces behind the joint axis; plantar flexion moment at heel strike
Loading response	Hip moves into extension, adduction, and internal rotation. Flexion moment	Knee in 20 degrees of knee flexion, moving toward extension Tibia into internal rotation Flexion moment	Foot positioned in pronation to adapt to support surface, with the ankle moving from plantar flexion to dorsiflexion over a fixed foot Maximum plantar flexion moment; reaction force is beginning to shift anteriorly, producing a dorsiflexion moment
Midstance	Hip moves through neutral position with the pelvis rotating posteriorly Reaction force now posterior to hip joint creating extension moment	Knee in 15 degrees of flexion, moving toward extension Tibia in neutral rotation Maximum flexion moment	Foot in neutral and ankle in 3 degrees of dorsiflexion Slight dorsiflexion moment
Terminal stance	Hip positioned in 10–15 degrees of hip extension, abduction, and external rotation Extension moment decreases after double-limb support begins	Knee in 4 degrees of flexion, moving toward extension Tibia in external rotation Reaction forces moving anterior to the joint; extension moment	Foot in supination becoming rigid for push off Ankle in 15 degrees dorsiflexion toward plantar flexion Maximum dorsiflexion moment
Preswing	Hip moving toward 10 degrees of extension, abduction, and external rotation Continued decrease of extension moment	Knee moving from near full extension to 40 degrees of flexion Tibia in external rotation Reaction forces moving posterior to knee as knee flexes; flexion moment	Foot in supination and ankle in 20 degrees of plantar flexion Dorsiflexion moment

Data from Giallonardo LM: Gait. In: Myers RS, ed. *Saunders Manual Physical Therapy Practice.* Philadelphia, PA, WB Saunders, 1995:1108–1109.

CLINICAL PEARL

The movements of the thigh and lower leg occur in conjunction with the rotation of the pelvis. The pelvis, thigh, and lower leg normally rotate toward the weight-bearing limb at the beginning of the swing phase.[73]

Knee

The knee flexes twice and extends twice during each gait cycle: once during weight bearing and once during NWB.

The knee flexes to about 20 degrees during the loading response interval, and this acts as a shock-absorbing mechanism. The knee then begins to extend, and as the heel rises during the terminal stance interval, it is almost fully extended, but flexes again as the swing phase begins. The flexion occurs so that the lower limb can be advanced during the swing phase with minimum vertical displacement of the COG. The knee then continues to flex as the leg moves into the swing phase, before extending again prior to initial contact.[7] In normal walking, about 60 degrees of knee motion is required for adequate clearance of the foot during the swing phase. This peak flexion is required immediately after toe-off because at that point in the gait cycle, the toe is still pointed toward the ground.[22]

CLINICAL PEARL

The common problem at the knee during the stance phase is excessive flexion. During the swing phase, the most common error results from inadequate motion.

If excessive flexion at the knee occurs in midstance, the ground reaction force moves posteriorly to the knee and generates a flexion rather than an extension moment of force. This change in the moment requires the quadriceps and, to some degree, the hip extensors to maintain stability.

Excessive flexion at the knee results in excessive flexion occurring at the hip. This, in turn, increases the magnitude of the load on both the hip and the knee joints.[80]

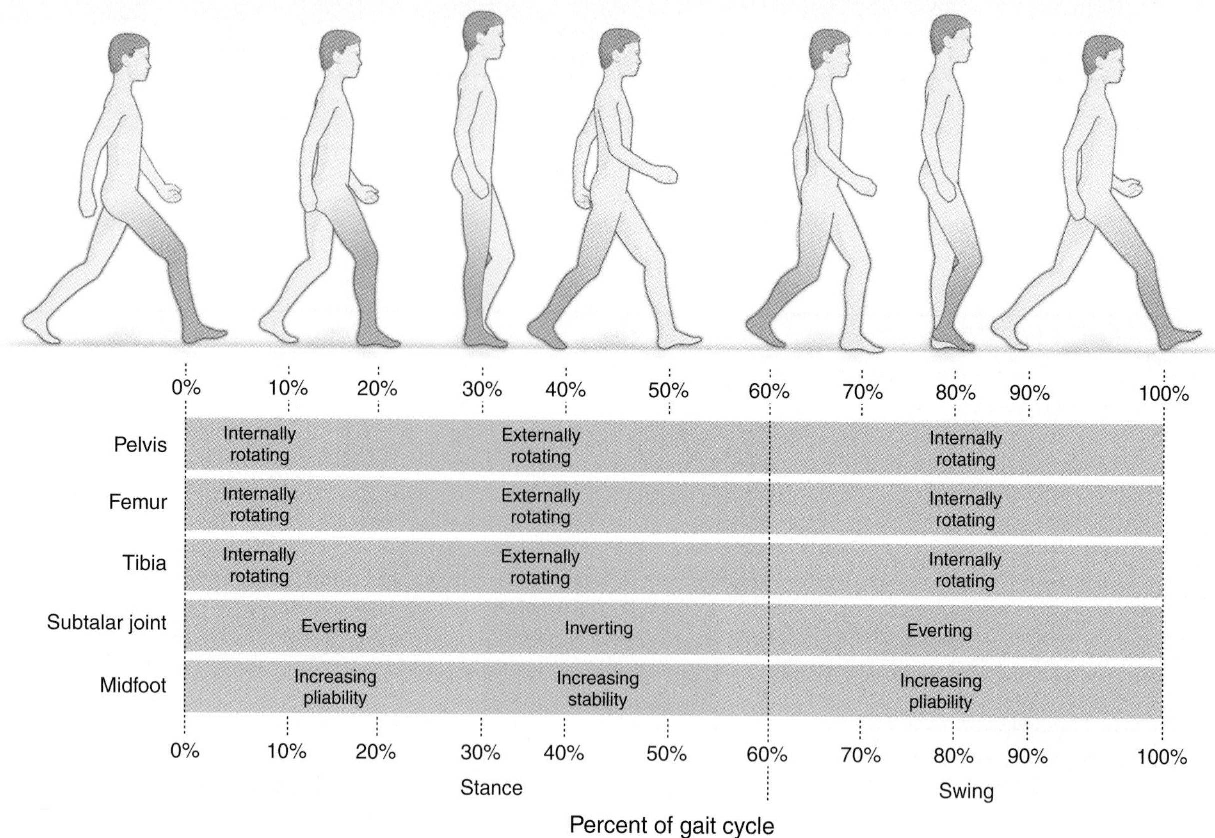

FIGURE 6-4 Joint kinematics in the horizontal plane during gait.

The arthrokinematics involved during the loading response include an anterior gliding of the femoral condyles, which serves to "unlock" the knee. This forward gliding is controlled by the passive restraint of the posterior cruciate ligament (PCL) and by the active contraction of the quadriceps muscles.

CLINICAL PEARL

Because anterior cruciate ligament (ACL)-reconstructed patients may experience patellofemoral pain, [81–83] especially those with patella tendon autografts, it is important to prescribe exercises that decrease ACL strain through increased flexion and minimize patellofemoral pain by exercising with the knee near full extension.[69] This has been recognized as a "paradox";[84,85] however, exercises performed between the two extremes, approximately 30–60 degrees of knee flexion, may avoid excessive ACL strain and limit patellofemoral pain.[69] However, patellofemoral contact pressures can increase dramatically with increased knee flexion.[86–88] As a result, patellofemoral pain is exacerbated but can be avoided and treated by strengthening the quadriceps in the 0–30 degrees knee flexion range.[89]

A loss of knee extension, which can occur with a flexion deformity, results in the hip being unable to extend fully, which can alter the gait mechanics. Patients with patellofemoral dysfunction demonstrate less knee flexion than normal in the stance phase of gait, combined with increased external rotation of the femur during the swing phase.[42] Excessive compensatory internal rotation of the femur of the weight-bearing leg during the stance phase may result in abnormal stresses being placed on the patellofemoral joint.[42]

Foot and Ankle

Ankle joint motion during the gait cycle occurs primarily in the sagittal plane. During normal gait, the initial contact with the ground is made by the heel. In individuals with poor control of dorsiflexion (e.g., hemiplegics), the initial contact is made with the lower part of the heel and forefoot simultaneously. This is usually accompanied by a toe drag during the swing phase. A knee flexion contracture or spasticity may cause the same alteration. Similarly, if the quadriceps are weak, the patient may extend the knee by using the hand or may hit the heel hard on the ground to whip the knee into extension. If heel pain occurs at initial contact, this pain may cause increased flexion of the knee, with early plantarflexion to relieve the stress or pressure on the painful tissues.[90]

The ankle is usually within a few degrees of the neutral position at the time of initial contact, with the heel slightly inverted and the subtalar joint slightly supinated.[91] The initial impact is taken through the lateral tubercle of the calcaneus, a structure unique to humans and designed to tolerate the shock of heel strike via the calcaneal fat pad. As the heel contacts the ground, its forward momentum comes to an abrupt halt. During the loading response interval, plantar flexion occurs at the talocrural joint, with pronation occurring at the subtalar joint.[91] The pronation of the subtalar joint unlocks the foot and allows maximal range of motion of the midtarsal joint, which brings the articulating surfaces of the cuboid and navicular to a position relatively parallel to the weight-bearing surface and allows the forefoot to become supple.[92,93] This increase in midtarsal joint mobility enhances the foot's ability to adapt to the support surface. Abnormal responses during this interval include excessive or no knee motion as a result of weak quadriceps, plantar flexor contractures, or spasticity.[90]

CLINICAL PEARL

There are two broad types of errors of the foot and ankle joints in the stance and swing phases:

1. Malrotation
2. Varus or valgus deformity

In the stance phase, these deviations may interfere with the first and fourth of Perry's priorities of gait (stability in stance and adequate step length). In the swing phase, these deviations may interfere with priorities 2 and 3 (clearance of the foot in swing and prepositioning of the foot in terminal swing).

The malrotation in stance rotates the plane of the foot outside of the plane of progression, resulting in the COG prematurely passing outside of the BOS. This alteration, in turn, results in a shortening of the contralateral step length. In addition, if the foot is malrotated significantly into external rotation, a valgus moment and an external rotation moment are introduced at the knee.

Varus and valgus deformities produce a loss of stability throughout the stance phase, because they introduce large external moments in the coronal plane that must be balanced by large muscle moments, if stability is to be maintained.

At the end of the midstance interval, the talocrural joint is maximally dorsiflexed, and the subtalar joint begins to supinate. During the latter part of the stance phase, the foot must become a rigid lever. However, if pain is elicited during this interval, the heel may lift off the floor early. From the midstance to the terminal stance interval, the foot is in supination.[92] Supination at the subtalar joint locks the foot into a rigid lever[91,94] by promoting supination at the midtarsal joint, which results in the articulating surfaces of the cuboid and calcaneus adopting a position that is perpendicular to one another, thus stabilizing their articulation.[93] The fixed cuboid acts as a fulcrum for the fibularis (peroneus) longus muscle, facilitating plantar flexion of the first metatarsal in pushing off.[92]

CLINICAL PEARL

An adaptively shortened gastrocnemius muscle may produce movement impairment by restricting normal dorsiflexion of the ankle from occurring during the midstance to heel raise portion of the gait cycle. This motion is compensated for by increased pronation of the subtalar joint, increased internal rotation of the tibia, and resultant stresses to the knee joint complex.

Once the ankle is fully close packed, the heel is lifted by a combination of passive force and contraction from the taut gastrocnemius and the soleus. The lifting of the heel accentuates the force applied to the mid- and forefoot and reinforces the close packing of this area, while simultaneously unclose packing the ankle joint.

As ankle plantar flexion reaches its peak at the end of the terminal stance interval, the first metatarsophalangeal (MTP) joint is passively extended. This extension of the first MTP places tension on the plantar fascia and helps to elevate the medial longitudinal arch through the windlass mechanism of the plantar fascia (see Chapter 21). This windlass mechanism creates a dynamic stable arch and, hence, a more rigid lever for push off.[92] However, if pain is elicited during this interval, the patient is unable to push off on the medial aspect of the foot and instead compensates by pushing off on the lateral aspect of the foot.

While the forefoot is on the ground and the heel is off, the heel is inverted and the foot is supinated.[91] The plantar flexion action helps to smooth the pathway of the COG. The heel rise coincides with the opposite leg swinging by the stance leg.[95] Approximately 40% of the body weight is borne by the toes in the final stages of foot contact.[96,97] Muscle activity during push off is designed to initiate propulsion.[92] However, if the plantar flexors are weak, the push off may be absent.

CLINICAL PEARL

Bojsen-Möller[98] describes the heel rise and the push off as taking place at the MTP joints around two primary axes: one oblique and one transverse. The heel rise occurs first around the oblique axis, which passes through the MTP joints of the second through the fifth toes. This is followed by the push off around the transverse axis passing through the MTP joints of the first and second toes. The resistance arm offered against the force arm of the triceps surae during the push off varies and is 20% longer when the push off is being performed along the transverse axis. Bojsen-Möller characterizes the motion around the oblique MTP joint axis as a low-gear motion and the motion around the transverse axis as a high-gear motion.[96,98,99] High-gear motion is used for sprinting and low-gear motion is used for uphill walking with loads and in the first step of a sprint.

From initial contact to early midstance, the tibia moves anteriorly, internally rotating within the ankle mortise, and producing talar adduction and plantar flexion, and calcaneal eversion (weight-bearing pronation of the subtalar joint).[92] The forward tibial advancement requires approximately 10 degrees of ankle joint dorsiflexion to prevent excessive pronation at the subtalar and oblique midtarsal joints.[9,93,100]

During the swing phase, the ankle must dorsiflex in order for the forefoot to clear the ground. However, if the ankle dorsiflexor muscles are weak, the patient must utilize a steppage gait, manifested by excessive flexion at the hip so that the toes can clear the ground. Prior to the next initial contact, the ankle

TABLE 6-3	Muscle Actions in the Lower Extremities During the Stance Phase of Gait		
Phase	**Hip**	**Knee and Tibia**	**Ankle and Foot**
Initial contact	Gluteus maximus and hamstrings work eccentrically to resist flexion moment and decelerate the leg	Quadriceps femoris contracts eccentrically to control rapid knee flexion and to prevent buckling	The dorsiflexors (tibialis anterior, extensor digitorum longus, and extensor hallucis longus) contract eccentrically to slow plantar flexion.
Loading response	Gluteus maximus and hamstrings contract concentrically to bring the hip into extension	After the foot is flat, quadriceps activity becomes concentric to bring the femur over the tibia	Dorsiflexion activity decreases; tibialis posterior, flexor hallucis longus, and flexor digitorum longus work eccentrically to control pronation
Midstance	Iliopsoas works eccentrically to resist extension; gluteus medius contracts in reverse action to stabilize opposite pelvis	Quadriceps activity decreases; gastrocnemius works eccentrically to control excessive knee extension	Plantar flexor muscles (gastrocsoleus and fibularis [peroneal] muscles) are activated to control dorsiflexion of the tibia and fibula over a fixed foot by contracting eccentrically
Terminal stance	Iliopsoas activity continues	Gastrocnemius begins to work concentrically to start knee flexion	Plantar flexor muscles begin to contract concentrically to prepare for push off
Preswing	Adductor magnus works eccentrically to control or stabilize the pelvis; iliopsoas activity continues	Quadriceps femoris contracts eccentrically	Plantar flexor muscles at peak activity but become inactive as the foot leaves the ground

Data from Giallonardo LM: Gait. In: Myers RS, ed. *Saunders Manual Physical Therapy Practice.* Philadelphia, PA, WB Saunders, 1995:1108–1109.

adopts a neutral position in terms of dorsiflexion and plantar flexion.

Muscle Actions During Gait

During the swing phase, the semispinalis, rotatores, multifidus, and external oblique muscles are active on the side toward which the pelvis rotates.[4] The erector spinae and internal oblique abdominal muscles are active on the opposite side. The psoas major and quadratus lumborum help to support the pelvis on the side of the swinging limb while the contralateral hip abductors also provide support.

The ankle and hip muscles are responsible for the majority of positive work performed during walking (54% of the hip and 36% of the ankle).[101] The knee contributes the majority of the negative work (56%).[101] The muscle actions that occur during the stance phase of gait are depicted in Table 6-3.[102]

Hip

During the early to midportion of the swing phase, the iliopsoas is the prime mover, with assistance from the rectus femoris, sartorius, gracilis, adductor longus, and possibly the tensor fascia latae, pectineus, and short head of the biceps femoris during the initial swing interval.[4] Perry notes the adductor longus muscle to be "the first and most persistent hip flexor."[40] In terminal swing, there is no appreciable action of the hip flexors when ambulating on level ground. Instead, the hamstrings and gluteus maximus are strongly active to decelerate hip flexion and knee extension.[33,79] Both these superficial muscles and their deeper counterparts, such as the hip adductors, gemelli, and short rotators, certainly contribute.[44] In rapid walking, there is increased activity of the sartorius and the rectus femoris during the swing phase.[4]

CLINICAL PEARL

- The hip flexors (primarily the iliopsoas muscle) contract to slow extension, whereas the hip extensors (primarily the hamstring muscles) contract to slow flexion.
- The hip abductor muscles provide stability during single-leg support, a critical event of the hip.[44]

During initial contact, the gluteal muscles and the hamstrings contract isometrically with moderate intensity. The passive hip extension moment at initial contact has been calculated to be approximately 60–100% of the total moment occurring during the stance phase, suggesting that passive elastic energy is stored and released during gait.[103] The loading response interval is accompanied by hamstring and gluteus maximus activity, which aids hip extension.[33,79,104] The adductor magnus muscle supports hip extension and also rotates the pelvis externally toward the forward leg. In midstance, coronal plane muscle activity is greatest, as the abductors stabilize the pelvis.[105–109] The muscle activity initially is eccentric, as the pelvis shifts laterally over the stance leg.

CLINICAL PEARL

The major problems that occur at the hip during gait are inadequate power, inadequate or inappropriate range of motion, and malrotation.

Weakness of the hip flexors is best seen during the preswing and initial swing intervals. Weakness of the hip abductors is noted during the single support phase of stance, because the hip abductors are required to prevent collapse of the pelvis toward the unsupported side (Trendelenburg sign). Weakness of the hip extensors is usually seen at initial contact and during loading response.

If the hamstrings are weak, the initial contact may be excessively harsh to lock the knee into extension.

As the flexors, adductors, and internal rotators of the hip are dominant over their antagonists, flexion, adduction, and internal rotation deformities tend to be the rule.

Malrotation of the hip usually results from conditions such as femoral anteversion.

The gluteus medius and minimus remain active in terminal stance for lateral pelvic stabilization. The iliacus and anterior fibers of the tensor fasciae latae are also active in the terminal stance and preswing intervals.[33,79] Notable, but inconsistent, muscle activity of the rectus femoris is described by several authors.[33,79,104] The only muscles of the hip that contract significantly during the last part of the stance phase are the adductor magnus, longus, and possibly brevis.[4]

Knee

The functions of the knee during gait are to absorb shock, reduce vertical displacement of the COG, maintain the stride length, bear weight, and allow the foot to move through its swing. During the swing phase, there is very little activity from the knee flexors. The knee extensors contract slightly at the end of the swing phase prior to initial contact. During level walking, the quadriceps achieve peak activity during the loading response interval (25% maximum voluntary contraction) and are relatively inactive by midstance as the leg reaches the vertical position and locks, making quadriceps contraction unnecessary.[39,110–112] In graded exercise, Brandell[113] examined the effect of speed and grade on electromyographic (EMG) activity of the quadriceps and calf musculature. The author concluded that increases in speed and grade resulted in a relative increase in EMG activity of the quadriceps compared with the calf musculature. Recently Ciccotti and colleagues[114] noted similar magnitudes and profiles of EMG activity in the quadriceps during level walking (1.5 m/s) and ascending a ramp of 10% grade at the same speed as level walking. Although minimal data were presented for comparison, the authors did note a decrease in vastus lateralis activity from 16% to less than 10% of maximum manual muscle test, with the addition of a grade. Therefore, it remains questionable whether graded walking actually facilitates quadriceps activity.[69]

CLINICAL PEARL

If the quadriceps muscles are weak, the trunk muscles thrust the pelvis forward to provide forward momentum to the leg.

Hamstring involvement is also important to normal knee function. The hamstrings provide dynamic stability to the knee by resisting both mediolateral and anterior translational forces on the tibia.[35] The coactivation of the antagonist muscles about the knee during the loading response aids the ligaments in maintaining joint stability by equalizing the articular surface pressure distribution and controlling tibial translation.[115,116] EMG activity of the hamstrings during level walking has shown that the hamstrings decelerate the leg prior to heel contact and then act synergistically with the quadriceps during the stance phase to stabilize the knee.[111,117] The hamstrings also demonstrate activity at the end of the stance phase. Hamstring activity during graded walking and increased speed demonstrates increased activity and for a longer duration.[4]

CLINICAL PEARL

Not only are quadriceps and hamstrings strengthening exercises important in knee rehabilitation, but proper range of motion must also be considered.[69]

Foot and Ankle

During the beginning of the swing phase, the tibialis anterior, extensor digitorum longus, extensor hallucis longus, and possibly the fibularis (peroneus) tertius contract concentrically with slight-to-moderate intensity, tapering off during the middle of the swing phase.[4,118,119] As the swing phase begins, the fibularis (peroneus) longus also contracts concentrically to evert the entire foot and bring the sole of the foot parallel with the substrate. At the point where the leg is perpendicular to the ground during the swing phase, the tibialis anterior, extensor digitorum longus, and extensor hallucis longus group of muscles contract concentrically to dorsiflex and invert the foot in preparation for the initial contact.[4,118,119] There is very little activity, if any, from the plantar flexors during the swing phase.

Following initial contact, the anterior tibialis works eccentrically to lower the foot to the ground during the loading response interval.[118,119] Loss of this plantar flexion control can result in an inability to transfer weight to the anterior foot, increased ankle dorsiflexion, and increased knee flexion. Calcaneal eversion is controlled by the eccentric activity of the posterior tibialis, and the anterior movement of the tibia and talus is limited by the eccentric action of the gastrocnemius and soleus muscle groups as the foot moves toward midstance.[102] Pronation occurs in the stance phase to allow for shock absorption, ground terrain changes, and equilibrium.[93,120] The triceps surae become active again from midstance to the late stance phase, contracting eccentrically to control ankle dorsiflexion, as the COG continues to move forward. In late stance phase, the Achilles tendon is stretched, as the triceps surae contracts and the ankle dorsiflexes.[121] At this point, the heel rises off the ground, and the action of the plantar flexors changes from one of eccentric contraction to one of concentric contraction. The energy stored in the stretched tendon helps to initiate plantar flexion and the initiation of propulsion.[121] The fibularis (peroneus) longus provides important stability to the forefoot during propulsion.

CLINICAL PEARL

During the stance phase, three ankle rocker phases are recognized:

1. The first rocker occurs between the initial contact and when the foot is flat on the floor. This rocker involves the ankle dorsiflexors, working eccentrically to gradually permit the foot to come into full contact with the ground.
2. During the second rocker, the foot remains flat on the ground, while the tibia advances. This motion results from the plantar flexors, working eccentrically to control the ankle dorsiflexion that occurs.
3. The third rocker is the push off required for advancement of the limb. This is the phase of power generation.

Thus, the first two rockers are deceleration rockers, in which the perspective muscles are working eccentrically by undergoing a lengthening contraction with energy absorption. The third rocker is an acceleration rocker and aids in propulsion. Abnormal muscle moments at the ankle during the stance phase can manifest as weakness of the tibialis anterior, resulting in a "foot slap" at initial contact during the first rocker. Weakness of the triceps surae allows the tibia to progress too rapidly during the second rocker, causing the ground reaction force to fall behind the knee and inducing knee flexion. Abnormal muscle moments during the swing phase include excessive activity of the plantar flexors and insufficient strength of the dorsiflexors, resulting in foot drop and poor foot clearance.

CLINICAL EXAMINATION OF GAIT

The clinical examination of gait can be performed using methods ranging from observation to computerized analysis (Table 6-4). Computerized gait analysis measures gait parameters more precisely than is possible with clinical observation alone,[122,123] and it is used in the evaluation and treatment planning for patients with gait abnormalities.[124] However, computerized gait analysis is often cost prohibitive and, thus, not practical for most clinicians, who must therefore rely on their powers of observation. The reliability and agreement both between and within raters for gait problems detected by observation alone has been reported. Krebs and colleagues[123] found moderate reliability within and between physical therapists observing children's gait from videotape. Eastlack and associates[125] found only slight to moderate reliability between raters in the assessment of deviations at a single joint from a videotape.[124]

Perhaps, the most commonly used gait analysis chart is the one designed by the Rancho Los Amigos Medical Center (Fig. 6-5), which allows the clinician to determine deviations and their effect on gait in a user-friendly format.

Several other examination tools are available. Some of these tools are specific to a particular population. For example, the modified version of the Gait Abnormality Rating Scale (Table 6-5) can be used with community-dwelling frail older persons to help predict individuals who are at high risk for falling.[126]

Dysfunction of the vestibular system may lead to gait abnormalities.[127,128] The Functional Gait Assessment (Table 6-6) is a 10-item test that comprises seven of the eight items from a previous test called the Dynamic Gait Index, which was developed to assess postural stability during gait tasks in the older adult (greater than 60 years of age) at risk for falling.[129] According to the designers of the Functional Gait Assessment, the tool demonstrates acceptable reliability, internal consistency, and concurrent validity with other balance measures used for patients with vestibular disorders.[128] Intervention strategies for vestibular dysfunction are described in Chapter 14.

Observational Analysis

Observational analysis of gait should focus on one gait interval at a time. For example, the clinician should observe the pattern of initial contact with the floor and then, in turn, study the actions throughout the initial contact at the ankle, knee, hip, pelvis, trunk, and upper extremities.

A paper walkway, approximately 25-ft long, on which the patient's footprints can be recorded, is very useful for gait analysis.[41,130] To assess gait, knowledge of what is deemed abnormal and the reasons for those abnormalities are prerequisite (Table 6-7).

Gait is assessed by having the patient walk barefoot and with footwear. Barefoot walking provides information about foot function without support and can highlight compensations, such as excessive pronation and foot deformities, such as claw toes.[131] Having the patient walk with footwear can provide information about the effectiveness of the footwear to counteract the compensations. The patient should be asked to walk on the toes and then on the heels. An inability to perform either of these actions could be the result of pain, weakness, or a motion restriction, or a combination of all. Metatarsalgia is indicated if the metatarsal heads are made more painful with barefoot walking. Pain at initial contact may indicate a heel spur, bone contusion, calcaneal fat pad injury, or bursitis.

The patient's footwear is examined for patterns of wear. The greatest amount of wear on the sole of the shoe should occur beneath the ball of the foot and in the area corresponding to the first, second, and third MTP joints, and slight wear to the lateral side of the heel. The upper portion of the shoe should demonstrate a transverse crease at the level of the MTP joints. A stiff first MTP joint can produce a crease line that runs obliquely, from forward and medial to backward and lateral.[132] Scuffing of the top of the shoe at its front might indicate tibialis anterior weakness or adaptively shortened heel cords.[131]

The patient's foot is also examined for callus formation, blisters, corns, and bunions. Callus formation on the sole of the foot is an indicator of dysfunction and provides the clinician with an index to the degree of shear stresses applied to the foot,

TABLE 6-4 Strengths and Limitations of Gait Analysis Methods		
Method	**Strengths**	**Limitations**
Observational analysis	1. Widely available 2. Can be enhanced by simple videotaping 3. Allows classification of gross gait patterns 4. Inexpensive	1. Subjective 2. Unable to measure more subtle phenomena
Stride analysis	1. Provides quantitative information regarding time–distance parameters 2. Easy and fast 3. Low space requirements 4. Relatively inexpensive	1. Does not permit angular kinematic and kinetic analysis 2. Requires that patients have distinct swing phase involving removal of floor contact.
Angular kinematic analysis	1. Permits precise measurement of joint angular excursions 2. Objective and quantitative	1. Requires technically trained personnel for measurement and interpretation of results 2. High space requirements 3. Limited portability 4. Expensive
Force plate and pressure plate analyses	1. Permits precise measurement of external loads 2. Permits analysis of inverse dynamics 3. Provides information regarding load patterns and distributions on stance limb	1. Limited usefulness in isolation 2. Typically requires permanent installation (gait lab) 3. Requires technically trained personnel for measurement and interpretation of results 4. Expensive
Electromyographic analysis	1. Provides measurement of motor performance and functional role of musculature 2. Enhances interpretation of kinematic and kinetic parameters	1. Requires technical expertise for measurement and interpretation 2. Subject to interference and artifact during sampling 3. Invasiveness of intramuscular technique poses risk to patients 4. Expensive

Data from: Spivak JM, DiCesare PE, Feldman DS, et al., eds. *Orthopaedics: A Comprehensive Study Guide*. New York: McGraw-Hill, 1999:209.

and a clear outline of abnormal weight-bearing areas.[133] Adequate amounts of calluses may provide protection, but in excess amounts they may cause pain. Callus formation under the second and third metatarsal heads could indicate excessive pronation in a flexible foot, or Morton neuroma, if just under the former. A callus under the fifth, and sometimes the fourth, metatarsal head may indicate an abnormally rigid foot.

The patient is asked to walk in his or her usual manner and at the usual speed. The clinician begins the gait assessment with an overall look at the patient while they walk and noting the cadence, stride length, step length, and velocity. The arm swing during gait should also be observed. If an individual has a problem with the foot or ankle on one side, the opposite arm swing is often decreased.[95]

The patient is observed from head to toe and then back again, from the side, from the front, and then from the back.

In addition to observing the patient walking at his or her normal pace, the clinician should also observe the patient walking at varying speeds. This can be achieved on a treadmill by adjusting the speed or by asking the patient to change the walking speed.

Once an overall assessment has been made of the patient's gait, the clinician can focus attention on the various segments of the kinetic chain of gait, including the trunk, pelvis, lumbar spine, hip, knee, and ankle and foot.

Attempts are made to determine the primary cause of any gait deviations or compensations (see Table 6-7).

Anterior View

When observing the patient from the front, the clinician can note the following:

- Head position—the subject's head should not move too much during gait in a lateral or vertical direction and should remain fairly stationary during the gait cycle. A "bouncing" gait is characteristic of adaptively shortened gastrocnemii or increased tone of the gastrocnemius and soleus.

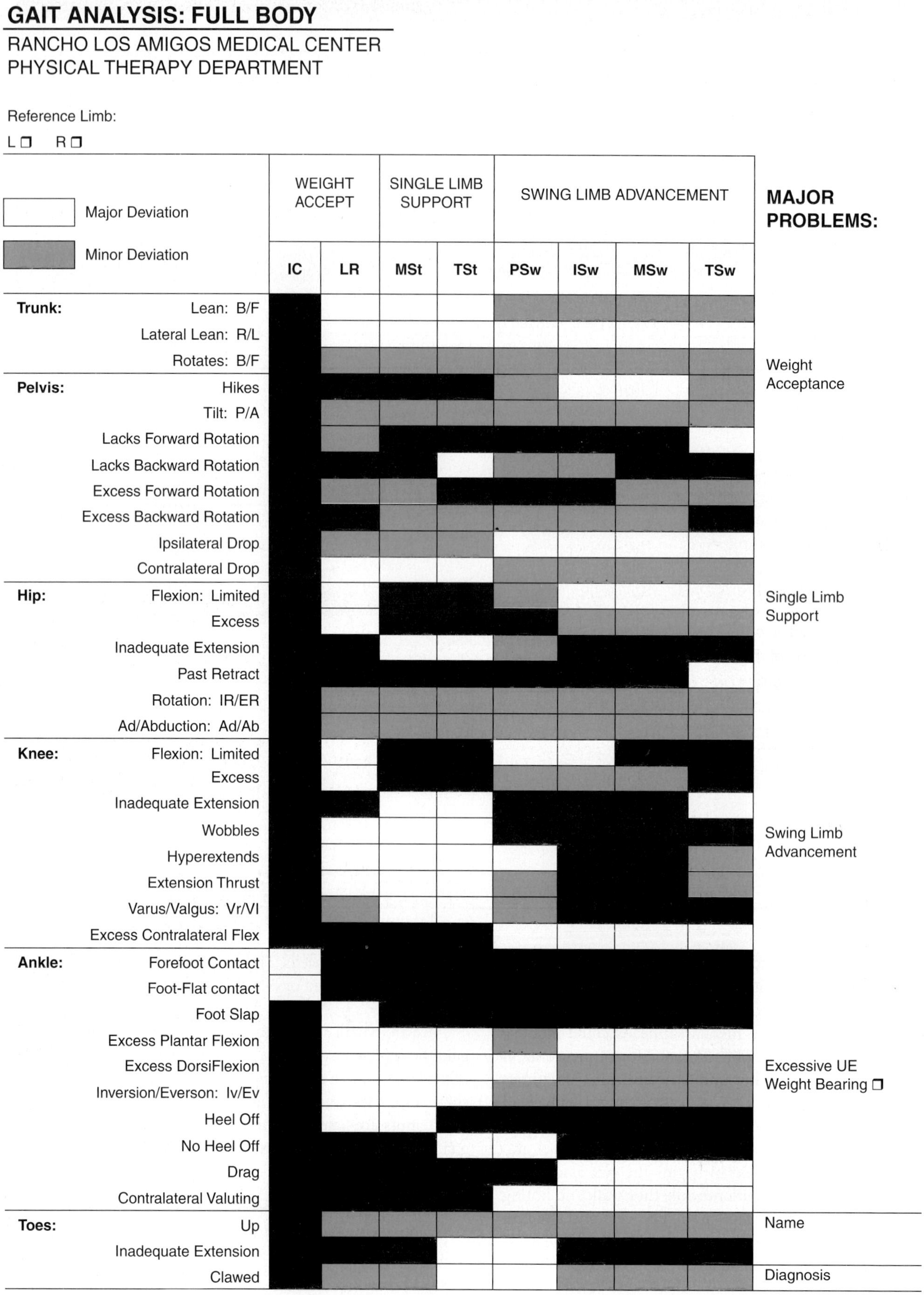

GAIT ANALYSIS: FULL BODY

RANCHO LOS AMIGOS MEDICAL CENTER
PHYSICAL THERAPY DEPARTMENT

Reference Limb:

L ❒ R ❒

Major Deviation (white) / Minor Deviation (gray)		WEIGHT ACCEPT		SINGLE LIMB SUPPORT		SWING LIMB ADVANCEMENT				**MAJOR PROBLEMS:**
		IC	LR	MSt	TSt	PSw	ISw	MSw	TSw	
Trunk:	Lean: B/F									
	Lateral Lean: R/L									
	Rotates: B/F									Weight Acceptance
Pelvis:	Hikes									
	Tilt: P/A									
	Lacks Forward Rotation									
	Lacks Backward Rotation									
	Excess Forward Rotation									
	Excess Backward Rotation									
	Ipsilateral Drop									
	Contralateral Drop									
Hip:	Flexion: Limited									Single Limb Support
	Excess									
	Inadequate Extension									
	Past Retract									
	Rotation: IR/ER									
	Ad/Abduction: Ad/Ab									
Knee:	Flexion: Limited									
	Excess									
	Inadequate Extension									
	Wobbles									Swing Limb Advancement
	Hyperextends									
	Extension Thrust									
	Varus/Valgus: Vr/Vl									
	Excess Contralateral Flex									
Ankle:	Forefoot Contact									
	Foot-Flat contact									
	Foot Slap									
	Excess Plantar Flexion									
	Excess DorsiFlexion									Excessive UE Weight Bearing ❒
	Inversion/Everson: Iv/Ev									
	Heel Off									
	No Heel Off									
	Drag									
	Contralateral Valuting									
Toes:	Up									Name
	Inadequate Extension									
	Clawed									Diagnosis

FIGURE 6-5 Rancho Los Amigos gait analysis chart.

TABLE 6-5 Modified Gait Abnormality Rating Scale

Name _____________ No._____________ Visit ___________ Date_____________

1. Variability—a measure of inconsistency and arrhythmicity of stepping and of arm movements

0 = fluid and predictably paced limb movements
1 = occasional interruptions (changes in velocity), approximately 25% of time
2 = unpredictability of rhythm approximately 25–75% of time
3 = random timing of limb movements

2. Guardedness—hesitancy, slowness, diminished propulsion, and lack of commitment in stepping and arm swing

0 = good forward momentum and lack of apprehension in propulsion
1 = center of gravity of head, arms, and trunk (HAT) projects only slightly in front of push off, but still good arm–leg coordination
2 = HAT held over anterior aspect of foot, and some moderate loss of smooth reciprocation
3 = HAT held over rear aspect of stance-phase foot, and great tentativity in stepping

3. Staggering—sudden and unexpected laterally directed partial losses of balance

0 = no losses of balance to side
1 = a single lurch to side
2 = two lurches to side
3 = three or more lurches to side

4. Foot Contact—the degree to which the heel strikes the ground before the forefoot

0 = very obvious angle of impact of heel on ground.
1 = barely visible contact of heel before forefoot.
2 = entire foot lands flat on ground.
3 = anterior aspect of foot strikes ground before heel

5. Hip ROM—the degree of loss of hip range of motion seen during a gait cycle

0 = obvious angulation of thigh backward during double support (10 degrees)
1 = just barely visible angulation backward from vertical
2 = thigh in line with vertical projection from ground
3 = thigh angled forward from vertical at maximum posterior excursion

6. Shoulder extension—a measure of the decrease of shoulder ROM

0 = clearly seen movement of upper arm anterior (15 degrees) and posterior (20 degrees) to vertical axis of trunk
1 = shoulder flexes slightly anterior to vertical axis
2 = shoulder comes only to vertical axis, or slightly posterior to it during flexion
3 = shoulder stays well behind vertical axis during entire excursion

7. Arm–heel strike synchrony—the extent to which the contralateral movements of an arm and leg are out of phase

0 = good temporal conjunction of arm and contralateral leg at apex of shoulder and hip excursions all of the time
1 = arm and leg slightly out of phase 25% of the time
2 = arm and leg moderately out of phase 25–50% of time
3 = little or no temporal coherence of arm and leg

ROM, range of motion.

TABLE 6-6 Functional Gait Assessment Requirements: A Marked 6 m (20 ft) Walkway That is Marked with a 13.48 cm (12 in) Width

1. Gait level surface

Instructions: Walk at your normal speed from here to the next mark (6 m/20 ft)

Grading: Mark the highest category that applies

(3) Normal: Walks 6 m/20 ft, in less than 5.5 s, no assistive devices, good speed, no evidence for imbalance, normal gait pattern, deviates no more than 15.24 cm (6 in.) outside of the 30.48 cm (12 in.) walkway width

(2) Mild impairment: Walks 6 m/20 ft, in less than 7 s but greater than 5.5 s, uses assistive device, slower speed, mild gait deviations, or deviates 15.24–25.4 cm (6–10 in.) outside of the 30.48 cm (12 in.) walkway width

(Continued)

TABLE 6-6	Functional Gait Assessment Requirements: A Marked 6 m (20 ft) Walkway That is Marked with a 13.48 cm (12 in) Width *(Continued)*

(1) Moderate impairment: Walks 6 m/20 ft, slow speed, abnormal gait pattern, evidence for imbalance, or deviates 25.4–38.1 cm (10–15 in.) outside of the 30.48 cm (12 in.) walkway width. Requires more than 7 s to ambulate 6 m (20 ft)

(0) Severe impairment: Cannot walk 6 m/20 ft without assistance, severe gait deviations or imbalance, deviates greater than 38.1 cm (15 in.) outside of the 30.48 cm (12 in.) walkway width, or reaches and touches the wall

---

2. Change in gait speed

Instructions: Begin walking at your normal pace (for 1.5 m/5 ft). When I tell you "go," walk as fast as you can (for 1.5 m/5 ft). When I tell you "slow," walk as slowly as you can (for 1.5 m/5 ft)

Grading: Mark the highest category that applies

(3) Normal: Able to smoothly change walking speed without loss of balance or gait deviation. Shows a significant difference in walking speeds between normal, fast, and slow speeds. Deviates no more than 15.24 cm (6 in.) outside of the 30.48 cm (12 in.) walkway width

(2) Mild impairment: Is able to change speed but demonstrates mild gait deviations, deviates 15.24–25.4 cm (6–10 in.) outside of the 30.48 cm (12 in.) walkway width, or no gait deviations but unable to achieve a significant change in velocity, or uses an assistive device

(1) Moderate impairment: Makes only minor adjustments to walking speed, or accomplishes a change in speed with significant gait deviations, or changes speed but has significant gait deviations, deviates 25.4–38.1 cm (10–15 in.) outside of the 30.48 cm (12 in.) walkway width, or changes speed but loses balance but is able to recover and continue walking

(0) Severe impairment: Cannot change speeds, deviates greater than 38.1 cm (15 in.) outside of the 30.48 cm (12 in.) walkway width, or loses balance and has to reach for wall or be caught

---

3. Gait with horizontal head turns

Instructions: Walk from here to the next mark (6 m/20 ft) away. Begin walking at your normal pace. Keep walking straight; after three steps, turn your head to the right and keep walking straight while looking to the right. After three more steps, turn your head to the left and keep walking straight while looking left. Continue alternating looking right and left every three steps until you have completed two repetitions in each direction

Grading: Mark the highest category that applies

(3) Normal: Performs head turns smoothly with no change in gait velocity. Deviates no more than 15.24 cm (6 in.) outside of the 30.48 cm (12 in.) walkway width

(2) Mild impairment: Performs head turns smoothly with slight change in gait velocity, i.e., minor disruption to smooth gait path, deviates 15.24–25.4 cm (6–10 in.) outside of the 30.48 cm (12 in.) walkway width, or uses assistive device

(1) Moderate impairment: Performs head turns with moderate change in gait velocity, slows down, deviates 25.4–38.1 cm (10–15 in.) outside of the 30.48 cm (12 in.) walkway width but recovers, can continue to walk

(0) Severe impairment: Performs task with severe disruption of gait, i.e., staggers outside of the 30.48 cm (12 in.) walkway width, loses balance, stops, or reaches for wall

---

4. Gait with vertical head turns

Instructions: Walk from here to the next mark (6 m/20 ft) away. Begin walking at your normal pace. Keep walking straight; after three steps, tip your head up and keep walking straight while looking up. After three more steps, tip your head down, keep walking straight while looking down. Continue alternating looking up and down every three steps until you have completed two repetitions in each direction

Grading: Mark the highest category that applies.

(3) Normal: Performs head turns smoothly with no change in gait. Deviates no more than 15.24 cm (6 in.) outside of the 30.48 cm (12 in.) walkway width

(2) Mild impairment: Performs task with slight change in gait velocity, i.e., minor disruption to smooth gait path, deviates 15.24–25.4 cm (6–10 in.) outside of the 30.48 cm (12 in.) walkway width, or uses assistive device

(1) Moderate impairment: Performs task with moderate change in gait velocity, slows down, deviates 25.4–38.1 cm (10–15 in.) outside of the 30.48 cm (12 in.) walkway width but recovers, can continue to walk

(0) Severe impairment: Performs task with severe disruption of gait, i.e., staggers outside of the 30.48 cm (12 in.) walkway width, loses balance, stops, or reaches for wall

---

5. Gait and pivot turn

Instructions: Begin with walking at your normal pace. When I tell you, "turn and stop," turn as quickly as you can to face the opposite direction and stop

Grading: Mark the highest category that applies

(3) Normal: Pivot turns safely within 3 s and stops quickly with no loss of balance

(2) Mild impairment: Pivot turns safely in >3 s and stops with no loss of balance, or pivot turns safely within 3 s and stops with mild imbalance, requires small steps to catch balance

(1) Moderate impairment: Turns slowly, requires verbal cueing, or requires several small steps to catch balance following turn and stop

(0) Severe impairment: Cannot turn safely, requires assistance to turn and stop

(Continued)

TABLE 6-6	Functional Gait Assessment Requirements: A Marked 6 m (20 ft) Walkway That is Marked with a 13.48 cm (12 in) Width *(Continued)*

6. Step over obstacle

Instructions: Begin walking at your normal speed. When you come to the shoebox, step over it, not around it, and keep walking

Grading: Mark the highest category that applies

(3) Normal: Is able to step over 2 stacked shoe boxes take together (22.86 cm/9 in. total height) without changing gait speed, no evidence of imbalance

(2) Mild impairment: Is able to step over one shoebox (11.43 cm/4.5 in. total height) without changing gait speed; no evidence of imbalance

(1) Moderate impairment: Is able to step over one shoe box (11.43 cm/4.5 in. total height) but must slow down and adjust steps to clear box safely. May require verbal cueing

(0) Severe impairment: Cannot perform without assistance

---

7. Gait with narrow base of support

Instructions: Walk on the floor with arms folded across the chest, feet aligned heel to toe in tandem for a distance of 3.6 m (12 ft). The number of steps taken in a straight line are counted for a maximum of 10 steps

Grading: Mark the highest category that applies

(3) Normal: Is able to ambulate for 10 steps heel to toe with no staggering

(2) Mild impairment: Ambulates 7–9 steps

(1) Moderate impairment: Ambulates 4–7 steps

(0) Severe impairment: Ambulates less than 4 steps heel to toe or cannot perform without assistance

---

8. Gait with eyes closed

Instructions: Walk at your normal speed from here to the next mark (6 m/120 ft) with your eyes closed

Grading: Mark the highest category that applies

(3) Normal: Walks 6 m/20 ft, no assistive devices, good speed, no evidence of imbalance, deviates no more than 15.24 cm (6 in.) outside of the 30.48 cm (12 in.) walkway width. Ambulate 6 m/20 ft in less than 7 s

(2) Mild impairment: Walks 6 m/20 ft, uses assistive devices, slower speed, mild gait deviations, deviates 15.24–25.4 cm (6–10 in.) outside of the 30.48 cm (12 in.) walkway width. Ambulate 6 m/20 ft in less than 9 s but greater than 7 s

(1) Moderate impairment: Walks 6 m/20 ft, slow speed, abnormal gait pattern, evidence for imbalance, deviates 25.4–38.1 cm (10–15 in.) outside of the 30.48 cm (12 in.) walkway width. Requires more than 9 s to ambulate 6 m/20 ft

(0) Severe impairment: Cannot walk 6 m/20 ft without assistance, severe gait deviations or imbalance, deviates greater than 38.1 cm (15 in.) outside 30.48 cm (12 in.) walkway width, or will not attempt task

---

9. Ambulating backward

Instructions: Walk backward until I tell you to stop

Grading: Mark the highest category that applies

(3) Normal: Walks 6 m/20 ft, no assistive devices, good speed, no evidence of imbalance, normal gait and, deviates no more than 15.24 cm (6 in.) outside of the 30.48 cm (12 in.) walkway width

(2) Mild impairment: Walks 6 m/20 ft, uses assistive devices, slower speed, mild gait deviations, deviates 15.24–25.4 cm (6–10 in.) outside of the 30.48 cm (12 in.) walkway width

(1) Moderate impairment: Walks 6 m/20 ft, slow speed, abnormal gait pattern, evidence for imbalance, deviates 25.4–38.1 cm (10–15 in.) outside of the 30.48 cm (12 in.) walkway width

(0) Severe impairment: Cannot walk 6 m/20 ft without assistance, severe gait deviations or imbalance, deviates greater than 38.1 cm (15 in.) outside 30.48 cm (12 in.) walkway width, or will not attempt task

---

10. Steps

Instructions: Walk up these stairs as you would at home, i.e., using the railing if necessary. At the top, turn around and walk down

Grading: Mark the highest category that applies

(3) Normal: Alternating feet, no rail

(2) Mild impairment: Alternating feet, must use rail

(1) Moderate impairment: Two feet to a stair, must use rail

(0) Severe impairment: Cannot do safely

TOTAL SCORE: ________/30

Data from Wrisley DM, Marchetti GF, Kuharsky DK, et al.: Reliability, internal consistency, and validity of data obtained with the functional gait assessment. *Phys Ther* 84:906–918, 2004.

- Amount of lateral tilt of the pelvis.
- Amount of lateral displacement of the trunk and pelvis.
- Whether there is excessive swaying of the trunk or pelvis.
- Amount of vertical displacement—vertical displacement can be assessed by observing the patient's head.
- Reciprocal arm swing—movements of the upper trunk and limbs usually occur in the opposite direction to the pelvis and the lower limbs.
- Whether the shoulders are depressed, retracted, or elevated.
- Whether the elbows are flexed or extended.
- Amount of hip adduction or abduction that occurs. Causes of excessive adduction include an excessive angle of the coxa vara, hip abductor weakness, hip adductor contracture or spasticity, and contralateral hip abduction contracture. Excessive hip abduction may be caused by an abduction contracture, a short leg, obesity, impaired balance, or hip flexor weakness.[134]
- Amount of valgus or varus at the knee—during gait, there may be an obvious varus-extension thrust. According to Noyes and colleagues, this gait pattern is characteristic of chronic injuries to the posterolateral structures of the knee.[135]
- Width of the BOS, or step width.
- Degree of "toe-out"—the term *toe-out* refers to the angle formed by the intersection of the line of progression of the foot and the line extending from the center of the heel through the second metatarsal. The normal toe-out angle is approximately 7 degrees, and this angle decreases as the speed of gait increases.[30]
- Whether any circumduction of the hip occurs. Hip circumduction can indicate a leg-length discrepancy, decreased ability of the knee to flex, or hip abductor shortening or overuse.
- Whether any hip hiking occurs. Hip hiking can indicate a leg-length discrepancy, hamstring weakness, or shortening of the quadratus lumborum.
- Evidence of thigh atrophy.
- Degree of rotation of the whole lower extremity. Because positioning the lower extremity in external rotation decreases the stress on the subtalar joint complex, an individual with a foot or ankle problem often adopts this position during gait.[95] Excessive internal or external rotation of the femur can indicate adaptive shortening of the medial or lateral hamstrings, respectively, resulting in anteversion or retroversion, respectively.

Lateral View

When observing the patient from the side, the clinician can note the following:

- Amount of thoracic and shoulder rotation. Each shoulder and arm should swing reciprocally, with equal motion.
- Orientation of trunk. The trunk should remain erect and level during the gait cycle, as it moves in the opposite direction to the pelvis. Compensation can occur in the lumbar spine for a loss of motion at the hip. A backward lean of the trunk may result from weak hip extensors or inadequate hip flexion. A forward lean of the trunk may result from pathology of the hip, knee, or ankle; abdominal muscle weakness; decreased spinal mobility; or hip flexion contracture. Forward leaning during the loading response and early midstance intervals may indicate hip extensor weakness.[136]
- Orientation of the pelvic tilt. An anterior pelvic tilt of >10 degrees is considered normal. Excessive anterior tilting can be caused by weak hip extensors, hip flexion contracture, or hip flexor spasticity. Excessive posterior pelvic tilting during gait usually occurs in the presence of hip flexor weakness.
- Degree of hip extension. Causes of inadequate hip extension and excessive hip flexion include hip flexion contracture, iliotibial band contracture, hip flexor spasticity, or pain.[134] Causes of inadequate hip flexion may include hip flexor weakness or hip joint arthrodesis.[134]
- Knee flexion and extension. The knee should be extended during the initial contact interval, followed by slight flexion during the loading response interval. During the swing phase, there must be sufficient knee flexion. Causes of excessive knee flexion and inadequate knee extension include inappropriate hamstring activity, knee flexion contracture, soleus weakness, and excessive ankle plantar flexion. Causes of inadequate flexion and excessive extension at the knee include quadriceps weakness, pain, quadriceps spasticity, excessive ankle plantar flexion, hip flexor weakness, and knee extension contractures.[137] Individuals with genu recurvatum may have a functional strength deficit in the quadriceps muscle or gastrocnemius that allows knee hyperextension.[138]
- Ankle dorsiflexion and plantar flexion. During midstance, the ankle dorsiflexes and the body pivots over the stationary foot. At the end of the stance phase, the ankle should be seen to plantar flex to raise the heel. At the beginning of the swing phase, the ankle is plantar flexed, moving into dorsiflexion as the swing phase progresses and reaches a neutral position at the time of heel contact at the termination of the swing. Excessive plantar flexion in midswing, initial contact, and loading response may be caused by pretibial (especially the anterior tibialis) weakness. Excessive plantar flexion also may be caused by plantar flexion contracture, soleus and gastrocnemius spasticity, or weak quadriceps.[90] Excessive dorsiflexion may be caused by soleus weakness, ankle fusion, or persistent knee flexion during the midstance phase.[136]
- Stride length of each limb.
- Cadence. The cadence should be normal for the patient's age (Table 6-7).
- Heel rise. An early heel rise indicates an adaptively shortened Achilles tendon.[95] Delayed heel rise may indicate a weak gastrocnemius–soleus complex.
- Heel contact. A low heel contact during initial contact may be caused by plantar flexion contracture, tibialis anterior weakness, or premature action by the calf muscles.[90]
- Preswing. An exaggerated preswing is manifested by the patient walking on the toes. Causes include pes equines

TABLE 6-7 Some Gait Deviations and Their Causes	
Gait Deviations	**Reasons**
Slower cadence than expected for person's age	Generalized weakness Pain Joint motion restrictions Poor voluntary motor control/weakness of lower limb muscles
Shorter stance phase on involved side and decreased swing phase on uninvolved side Shorter stride length on uninvolved side Decrease lateral sway over involved stance limb Decrease in velocity	Antalgic gait, resulting from painful injury to lower limb and pelvic region
Stance phase longer on one side	Pain Lack of trunk and pelvic rotation Restrictions in lower limb joints Increased muscle tone
Lateral trunk lean (purpose is to bring center of gravity of trunk nearer to hip joint)	Ipsilateral lean (toward the stance leg)—marked hip abductor weakness (compensated gluteus medius/Trendelenburg gait) Contralateral lean—decreased hip flexion in swing limb—mild hip abductor weakness (gluteus medius/Trendelenburg gait) Painful hip Abnormal hip joint (congenital dysplasia, coxa vara, etc.) Wide walking base Unequal leg length Adaptive shortening of quadratus lumborum on swing side Contralateral hip adductor spasticity
Anterior trunk leaning at initial contact (occurs to move line of gravity in front of axis of knee)	Weak or paralyzed knee extensors or gluteus maximus Hip pain
Anterior trunk leaning during mid and terminal stance, as the hip is moved over the foot	Hip flexion contracture Pes equinus deformity
Posterior trunk leaning during initial contact to loading response (occurs to bring line of external force behind axis of hip)	Weak or paralyzed hip extensors, especially gluteus maximus (gluteus maximus gait) Hip pain Hip flexion contracture Inadequate hip flexion in swing Decreased knee range of motion
Increased lumbar lordosis in terminal stance	Inability to extend hip, usually due to hip flexion contracture or ankylosis
Excessive posterior horizontal pelvic rotation	Adaptively shortened/spasticity of hip flexors on same side Limited hip joint flexion
Hip circumduction during swing (ground contact can be avoided by swinging leg if it is swung outward for natural walking to occur; leg that is in its stance phase needs to be longer than leg that is in its swing phase to allow toe clearance of swing foot)	Functional leg-length discrepancy(shortening of the swing leg secondary to reduced hip flexion, reduced knee flexion, and/or lack of ankle dorsiflexion) Arthrogenic stiff hip or knee
Hip hiking (pelvis is lifted on side of swinging leg, by contraction of spinal muscles and lateral abdominal wall)	Functional leg-length discrepancy (shortening of the swing leg secondary to reduced hip flexion, reduced knee flexion, and/or lack of ankle dorsiflexion) Functionally or anatomically short-stance leg Hamstring weakness Quadratus lumborum shortening
Vaulting (ground clearance of swinging leg will be increased if the patient goes up on toes of stance phase leg)	Functional leg-length discrepancy Vaulting occurs on shorter limb side

(Continued)

TABLE 6-7 Some Gait Deviations and Their Causes *(Continued)*

Gait Deviations	Reasons
Abnormal internal hip rotation (produces "toe-in" gait)	Adaptive shortening of iliotibial band Weakness of hip external rotators Femoral anteversion Adaptive shortening of hip internal rotators
Abnormal external hip rotation (produces "toe-out" gait)	Adaptive shortening of hip external rotators Femoral retroversion Weakness of hip internal rotators
Increased hip adduction (scissors gait), which results in excessive hip adduction during swing (scissoring), decreased base of support, and decreased progression of opposite foot	Spasticity or contracture of ipsilateral hip adductors Ipsilateral hip adductor weakness Coxa vara
Inadequate hip extension/excessive hip flexion, which results in loss of hip extension in midstance (forward leaning of trunk, increased lordosis, and increased knee flexion and ankle dorsiflexion) and late stance (anterior pelvic tilt), and increased hip flexion in swing	Hip flexion contracture Iliotibial band contracture Hip flexor spasticity Pain Arthrodesis (surgical or spontaneous ankylosis) Loss of ankle dorsiflexion
Inadequate hip flexion, which results in decreased limb advancement in swing, posterior pelvic tilt, circumduction, and excessive knee flexion to clear foot	Hip flexor weakness Hip joint arthrodesis
Decreased hip swing through (psoatic limp), which is manifested by exaggerated movements at pelvis and trunk to assist hip to move into flexion	Legg–Calvé–Perthes disease Weakness or reflex inhibition of psoas major muscle
Excessive knee extension/inadequate knee flexion, which results in decreased knee flexion at initial contact and loading response, increased knee extension during stance, and decreased knee flexion during swing	Pain Anterior trunk deviation/bending Weakness of quadriceps; hyperextension is a compensation and places body weight vector anterior to knee Spasticity of the quadriceps; noted more during the loading response and during initial swing intervals Joint deformity
Excessive hip and knee flexion during swing	Lack of ankle dorsiflexion of the swing leg Functionally or anatomically short contralateral stance leg
Excessive knee flexion/inadequate knee extension at initial contact or around midstance; results in increased knee flexion in early stance, decreased knee extension in midstance and terminal stance, and decreased knee extension during swing	Knee flexion contracture, resulting in decreased step length and decreased knee extension in stance Increased tone/spasticity of hamstrings or hip flexors Decreased range of motion of ankle dorsiflexion in swing phase Weakness of plantar flexors, resulting in increased dorsiflexion in stance Lengthened limb
Inadequate dorsiflexion control ("foot slap") during initial contact to midstance. Steppage gait during the acceleration through deceleration of the swing phase. The exaggerated knee and hip flexion are used to lift foot higher than usual, for increased ground clearance resulting from foot drop	Weak or paralyzed dorsiflexors Lack of lower limb proprioception Weak or paralyzed dorsiflexor muscles Functional leg-length discrepancy
Increased walking base/step width (>20 cm)	Deformity such as hip abductor muscle contracture Genu valgus Fear of losing balance Leg-length discrepancy
Decreased walking base/step width (<10 cm)	Hip adductor muscle contracture Genu varum

(Continued)

TABLE 6-7 Some Gait Deviations and Their Causes (Continued)	
Gait Deviations	**Reasons**
Excessive eversion of calcaneus during initial contact through midstance	Excessive tibia vara (refers to frontal plane position of the distal one-third of leg, as it relates to supporting surface) Forefoot varus Weakness of tibialis posterior Excessive lower extremity internal rotation (due to muscle imbalances and femoral anteversion)
Excessive pronation during midstance through terminal stance	Insufficient ankle dorsiflexion (<10 degrees) Increased tibial varum Compensated forefoot or rearfoot varus deformity Uncompensated forefoot valgus deformity Pes planus Long limb Uncompensated medial rotation of tibia or femur Weak tibialis anterior
Excessive inversion and plantar flexion of the foot and ankle during swing and at initial contact	Pes equinovarus (spasticity of the plantar flexors and invertors)
Excessive supination during initial contact through midstance	Limited calcaneal eversion Rigid forefoot valgus Pes cavus Uncompensated lateral rotation of tibia or femur Short limb Plantar flexed first ray Upper motor neuron muscle imbalance
Excessive dorsiflexion during initial contact through toe-off	Compensation for knee flexion contracture Inadequate plantar flexor strength Adaptive shortening of dorsiflexors Increased muscle tone of dorsiflexors Pes calcaneus deformity
Excessive plantar flexion during midstance through toe-off	Increased plantar flexor activity Plantar flexor contracture
Excessive varus during initial contact through toe-off	Contracture Overactivity of muscles on medial aspect of foot
Excessive valgus during initial contact through toe-off	Weak invertors Foot hypermobility
Decreased or absence of propulsion (plantar flexor gait) during mid-stance through toe-off	Inability of plantar flexors to perform function, resulting in a shorter step length on the involved side

Data from Giallonardo LM: Clinical evaluation of foot and ankle dysfunction. *Phys Ther* 68:1850–1856, 1988; Epler M: Gait. In: Richardson JK, Iglarsh ZA, eds. *Clinical Orthopaedic Physical Therapy*. Philadelphia, PA: WB Saunders, 1994:602–625; Hunt GC, Brocato RS: Gait and foot pathomechanics. In: Hunt GC, ed. *Physical Therapy of the Foot and Ankle*. Edinburgh: Churchill Livingstone, 1988; Krebs DE, Robbins CE, Lavine L, et al.: Hip biomechanics during gait. *J Orthop Sports Phys Ther* 28:51–59, 1998; Larish DD, Martin PE, Mungiole M: Characteristic patterns of gait in the healthy old. *Ann N Y Acad Sci* 515:18–32, 1987; Levine D, Whittle M: *Gait Analysis: The Lower Extremities*. La Crosse, WI: Orthopaedic Section, APTA, Inc., 1992; Perry J: *Gait Analysis: Normal and Pathological Function*. Thorofare, NJ: Slack Inc., 1992; Song KM, Halliday SE, Little DG: The effect of limb-length discrepancy on gait. *J Bone Joint Surg* 79A:1690–1698, 1997.

deformity, adaptive shortening or increased tone of the triceps surae, weakness of the dorsiflexors, and knee flexion occurring at midstance. A decreased preswing is often characterized by a lack of plantar flexion at terminal stance and preswing. Causes for this can include ankle or foot pain or weakness of the plantar flexor muscles.

Posterior View

When observing the patient from the back, the clinician can note the following:

- *Amount of subtalar inversion (varus) or eversion (valgus).* Excessive inversion and eversion usually relate to abnormal

TABLE 6-8	Some Causes of Antalgic Gait
Cause	**Examples**
Bone disease	Fracture Infection Tumor Avascular necrosis (Legg–Calvé–Perthes disease, Osgood Schlatter disease, and Köhler bone disease)
Muscle disorder	Traumatic rupture and contusion Cramp secondary to fatigue, strain, malposition, or claudication Inflammatory myositis
Joint disease	Traumatic arthritis Infectious arthritis Rheumatoid arthritis Crystalline arthritis (gout and pseudogout) Hemarthrosis Bursitis
Neurologic disease	Lumbar spine disease with nerve root irritation or compression
Other	Hip, knee, or foot trauma Corns, bunions, blisters, or ingrown toenails

Data from Judge RD, Zuidema GD, Fitzgerald FT: Musculoskeletal system. In: Judge RD, Zuidema GD, Fitzgerald FT, eds. *Clinical Diagnosis*, 4th edn. Boston: Little, Brown and Company, 1982:365–403.

muscular control. Generally speaking, varus tends to be the dominant dysfunction in spastic patients, whereas valgus tends to be more common with flaccid paralysis.[90]

- BOS/step width.
- Pelvic list.
- Degree of hip rotation—as in standing, excessive femoral internal rotation past the midstance of gait will accentuate genu recurvatum. Causes of excessive external hip rotation may include gluteus maximus overactivity and excessive ankle plantar flexion.[134] Causes of excessive internal hip rotation include medial hamstring overactivity, hip adductor overactivity, anterior abductor overactivity, and quadriceps weakness.[134]
- Amount of hip adduction or abduction.
- Amount of knee/tibial rotation.

ABNORMAL GAIT SYNDROMES

Each of the attributes of normal gait described earlier under "Characteristics of Normal Gait" are subject to compromise by disease states, particularly neuromuscular conditions.[101] In general, gait deviations fall under four headings: those caused by weakness, those caused by abnormal joint position or range of motion, those caused by muscle contracture, and those caused by pain.[22,139]

- Weakness implies that there is inadequate internal joint movement or loss of the natural force–couple relationship.
- Neuromuscular conditions may be associated with abnormalities of muscle tone, timing of muscle contractions, and proprioceptive and sensory disturbances, the latter of which can profoundly affect reflex postural balance.
- Abnormal joint position can be caused by an imbalance of flexibility and strength around a joint or by contracture.
- Contractures, changes in the connective tissue of muscles, ligaments, and the joint capsule, may produce changes in gait. If the contracture is elastic, the gait changes are apparent in the swing phase only. If the contractures are rigid, the gait changes are apparent during the swing and the stance phases.
- Pain can alter gait, as the patient attempts to use the position of minimal articular pressure (see "Antalgic Gait"). Pain may also produce muscle inhibition and eventual atrophy.

Antalgic Gait

The antalgic gait is characterized by a decrease in the stance phase on the involved side in an attempt to eliminate the weight from the involved leg and use of the injured body part as much as possible. The antalgic gait pattern can result from numerous causes (Table 6-8), including disease, joint inflammation (Table 6-9), or an injury to the muscles, tendons, and ligaments of the lower extremity. In the case of joint inflammation, attempts may be made to avoid positions of maximal intraarticular pressure and to seek the position of minimum articular pressure[140]:

- Minimum articular pressure occurs at the ankle at 15 degrees of plantar flexion.
- Minimum articular pressure occurs at the knee at 30 degrees of flexion. With a painful knee, the gait is characterized by a decrease in knee flexion at initial contact and the loading response interval, and an increase in knee extension during the remainder of the stance phase.
- Minimum articular pressure occurs at the hip at 30 degrees of flexion.

Perhaps surprisingly, recent studies have shown that the gait pattern is altered in individuals with low back pain.[141] These individuals exhibit a cautious gait exemplified by a reduction in cycle duration as well as hip flexion–extension excursion.[142] When compared to healthy controls, patients with back pain exhibit similar patterns of activation across the gait cycle, but with premature activity in the lumbar spine and hip extensor muscles, and prolonged activity of the gluteus maximus and spine extensors.[141] This raises the question as to what role the CNS plays in this alteration of gait.[143]

Equinus Gait

Spastic diplegia is the most common pattern of motor impairment in patients with cerebral palsy.[144] In these patients, motor impairment occurs as a result of a number of deficits, including poor muscle control, weakness, impaired balance,

TABLE 6-9 Gait Abnormalities in Arthritic Disease and Associated Conditions and Treatment Examples

Disorder	Gait Abnormalities: Observational	Time–Distance	Angular	Kinetic and EMG	Treatment
Osteoarthritis of the hip, unilateral involvement	Lateral lurch gait pattern	1. ↑ Stance time, uninvolved side 2. ↑ Double-limb support 3. ↑ Step time, involved side 4. ↓ Step length, involved side 5. ↓ Velocity	↓ Hip flexion–extension excursion, involved side	↓ Hip abductor moment	Assistive device (cane or crutches)
Rheumatoid arthritis with hindfoot pain and deformity	1. Antalgic gait pattern 2. Flat-foot gait pattern	1. ↓ Velocity 2. ↓ Single-limb support, involved side 3. ↓ Cadence 4. ↓ Stride length 5. Delayed heel rise	1. ↑ Knee flexion during stance 2. ↑ Dorsiflexion during stance 3. ↓ Plantar flexion during terminal stance 4. ↑ Subtalar eversion during terminal stance	↑ Tibialis anterior activation during terminal stance and preswing	Cane Rigid AFO or hindfoot orthoses Rocker bottom shoes
Total knee arthroplasty, unilateral		1. ↓ Single-limb support, involved side 2. ↓ Stride length	↓ Knee flexion during stance	↓ Knee extensor moment	N/A

EMG, electromyography.
Data from Spivak JM, DiCesare PE, Feldman DS, et al., eds. *Orthopaedics: A Comprehensive Study Guide.* New York: McGraw-Hill, 1999:213.

hypertonicity, and spasticity.[145] However, reduced joint motion as a consequence of spasticity is perhaps the most noticeable and recorded impairment. As a consequence, muscle–tendon units frequently become contracted over time, contributing to malalignment of the extremity during gait.

Equinus gait (toe-walking), one of the more common abnormal patterns of gait in patients with spastic diplegia (see also "Spastic Gait"), is characterized by forefoot strike to initiate the cycle and premature plantar flexion in early to midstance.[146] Toe-walking may be a primary gait deviation, which is the consequence of excessive myostatic contracture of the triceps surae, excessive dynamic contraction of the ankle plantar flexors, or a combination of both factors. Additionally, toe-walking may be a compensatory deviation for myostatic deformity or dynamic overactivity of the ipsilateral hamstring muscles, which directly limits knee alignment and secondarily compromises foot and ankle position during stance phase.

Associated gait deviations are frequently seen at the knees, hips, and pelvis in children with cerebral palsy who are walking on their toes[147]:

- Deviations seen at the knees include increased flexion in stance phase at initial contact and in midstance, and delayed and diminished peak knee flexion in swing phase.
- The hips often show diminished extension in the sagittal plane at terminal stance.
- A common deviation seen at the pelvis in children with cerebral palsy who are toe-walking is an increased anterior tilt.

Gluteus Maximus Gait

The gluteus maximus gait, which results from weakness of the gluteus maximus, is characterized by a posterior thrusting of the trunk at initial contact in an attempt to maintain hip extension of the stance leg. The hip extensor weakness also results in an anterior tilt of the pelvis, which eventually translates into hyperlordosis of the spine to maintain posture.

Quadriceps Gait

Quadriceps weakness can result from a peripheral nerve lesion (femoral), spinal nerve root lesion (L2–4), trauma, or disease (muscular dystrophy). Although often appearing to have a normal gait pattern when walking on a level surface, the patient with quadriceps weakness/paralysis often demonstrates difficulty walking on rough or inclined surfaces and stairs and is unable to run. In such instances forward motion is propagated by circumducting each leg. To compensate, the patient leans the body toward the uninvolved side to balance the COG and swings the involved leg like a pendulum.

TABLE 6-10 Gait Abnormalities Associated with Muscle Weakness and Treatment Examples					
	Gait Abnormalities				
Disorder	**Observational**	**Time–Distance**	**Angular**	**Kinetic and EMG**	**Treatment**
Dorsiflexor paresis or paralysis	1. Steppage gait pattern 2. Foot slap gait pattern	1. ↓ Time to foot flat 2. ↓ Step length	1. Ankle plantar flexion during swing 2. ↑ Hip and knee flexion during swing	↓ Dorsiflexor moment	AFO
Hip abductor weakness	1. Trendelenberg gait pattern 2. Lateral lurch gait pattern	1. ↑ Double-limb support 2. ↓ Step length 3. ↓ Velocity	1. ↑ Hip adduction during midstance, with Trendelenberg 2. ↑ Lateral trunk tilt with lateral lurch 3. ↓ Pelvic tilt during swing, involved side, with Trendelenberg	Hip abductor ↓ moment during stance with lateral lurch	Assistive device (cane and crutches)
Plantar flexor paresis or paralysis	No pattern discernible	1. Prolonged midstance 2. ↓ Step length, uninvolved side 3. ↓ Single-limb support, involved side	1. ↑ Stance phase knee flexion 2. ↑ Stance phase dorsiflexion	1. ↓ Plantar flexor power during late stance. 2. Prolonged stance phase quadriceps activation	AFO

EMG, electromyography; AFO, ankle–foot orthosis.
Data from Spivak JM, DiCesare PE, Feldman DS, et al., eds. *Orthopaedics: A Comprehensive Study Guide.* New York: McGraw-Hill, 1999:214.

Steppage Gait

This type of gait occurs in patients with a foot drop. A foot drop is the result of weakness or paralysis of the dorsiflexor muscles resulting from an injury to the muscles, their peripheral nerve supply, or the nerve roots supplying the muscles (Table 6-10).[148] The patient lifts the leg high enough to clear the flail foot off the floor, by flexing excessively at the hip and knee, and then slaps the foot on the floor.

Trendelenburg Gait

This type of gait results from weakness of the hip abductors (gluteus medius and minimus). The normal stabilizing effect of these muscles is lost, and the patient demonstrates an excessive lateral list, in which the trunk is thrust laterally in an attempt to keep the COG over the stance leg. A positive Trendelenburg sign is also present (Table 6-10).

Plantar Flexor Gait

This type of gait is characterized by walking on the toes (Table 6-10). The plantar flexor gait demonstrates premature firing of the calf muscle in the swing phase of gait with EMG.[149] A toe-walking gait pattern describes dynamic ankle deviations that include[147]

- a loss of heel strike at initial contact, with disruption of the first ankle rocker;
- disruption of the second rocker, with ankle plantar flexion (instead of dorsiflexion) occurring at midstance;
- variable disruption of the third rocker in terminal stance;
- variable ankle alignment during swing phase.

This is a common gait deviation in children with cerebral palsy. For the clinician, the challenge is to distinguish between changes that are the direct consequence of such an underlying neuromuscular disorder and are, therefore, primary, and those changes that result from biomechanical constraints of toe-walking and are, therefore, secondary or compensatory. It is not unusual for normal children to display intermittent tiptoe gait when they first begin to walk; however, a more mature heel-toe gait pattern should become consistent by the age of 2 years.[150] Older children with persistent tiptoe gait are often labeled idiopathic toe walkers. Toe-walking that begins after a mature heel-toe gait pattern has been established may signify muscular dystrophy, diastematomyelia, peroneal muscular atrophy, or spinal cord tumor. Toe-walking has been associated with premature birth, developmental delay, schizophrenia, autism, and various learning disorders.[151]

Spastic Gait

A spastic gait may result from either unilateral or bilateral upper motor neuron lesions. A number of types are recognized.

TABLE 6-11 Gait Abnormalities Associated with Neurologic Disorders and Treatment Examples					
	Gait Abnormalities				
Disorder	**Observational**	**Time–Distance**	**Angular**	**Kinetic and EMG**	**Treatment**
Ataxia	"Ataxic" gait pattern	Variable stride to stride	Variable stride to stride	Variable stride to stride	1. Orthotic stabilization to control movement variability 2. Walking aids (e.g., crutches and walker)
Hemiplegia from stroke	1. "Stiff-legged" gait pattern 2. Equinus or equinovarus gait pattern 3. Circumduction	1. ↑ Double-limb support 2. ↓ Step length, involved side 3. Delayed heel rise 4. ↓ Velocity 5. ↓ Stride length 6. ↓ Cadence 7. Absent heel contact 8. Toe drag during swing	1. ↑ Plantar flexion during swing 2. ↓ Knee flexion during stance and swing	1. ↑ Knee flexor moment during stance 2. ↓ Amplitude of joint powers 3. Abnormal timing of muscle activation (i.e., mass synergy patterns)	1. Ankle–foot orthosis 2. Rectus femoris release 3. Tendo-Achilles lengthening 4. Tendon transfer, foot and ankle 5. Functional electrical stimulation
Parkinson disease	1. "Shuffling" gait pattern 2. "Frozen" gait pattern	1. ↓ Stride length 2. ↓ Step length 3. ↓ Step width 4. ↓ Cadence 5. ↓ Velocity	↓ Angular excursions throughout	Agonist–antagonist coactivation with "frozen" pattern	Pharmaceutical/medical management

Data from Spivak JM, DiCesare PE, Feldman DS, et al. eds. *Orthopaedics: A Comprehensive Study Guide.* New York: McGraw-Hill, 1999:214.

Spastic Hemiplegic (Hemiparetic) Gait

This type of gait results from a unilateral upper motor neuron (UMN) lesion. Spastic hemiplegic gait is frequently seen following a completed stroke. Spasticity of all muscles on the involved side is noted, but it is more marked in some muscle groups. During gait, the leg tends to circumduct in a semicircle, rotating outward, or is pushed ahead, with the foot dragging and scraping the floor. The upper limb typically is carried across the trunk for balance (Table 6-11).

Spastic Paraparetic Gait

This type of gait results from bilateral UMN lesions (e.g., cervical myelopathy in adults and cerebral palsy in children). Spastic paraparetic gait is characterized by slow, stiff, and jerky movements. Spastic extension occurs at the knees, with adduction at the hips (scissors gait).

Ataxic Gait

The ataxic gait is seen in two principal disorders: cerebellar disease (cerebellar ataxic gait) and posterior column disease (sensory ataxic gait) (Table 6-11).

Cerebellar Ataxic Gait

The nature of the gait abnormality with a cerebellar lesion is determined by the site of the lesion. In vermal lesions, the gait is broad based, unsteady, and staggering, with an irregular sway. The patient is unable to walk in tandem or in a straight line. The ataxia of gait worsens when the patient attempts to stop suddenly or to turn sharply, resulting in a tendency to fall.

In hemispheral lesions, the ataxia tends to be less severe, but there is persistent lurching or deviation toward the involved side.

Sensory Ataxic Gait

With this type of ataxia, because the patient is unaware of the position of the limbs, the gait is broad based, and the patient tends to lift the feet too high and slap on the floor in an uncoordinated and abrupt manner. The patient tends to watch the floor and the feet to maximize attempts at visual correction and may have difficulty walking in the dark.

Parkinsonian Gait

The Parkinsonian gait is characterized by a flexed and stooped posture, with flexion of the neck, elbows, metacarpophalangeal joints, trunk, hips, and knees (Table 6-11). The patient has difficulty initiating movements and walks using short steps, with the feet barely clearing the ground. This results in a shuffling type of gait with rapid steps. As the patient gets going, he or she may lean forward and walk progressively faster, as though chasing the COG (propulsive or festinating gait). Less commonly, deviation of the COG backward may cause retropulsion. There is also a lack of associated arm movement during the gait, because the arms are held stiffly.

Hysterical Gait

The hysterical gait is nonspecific and bizarre. It does not conform to any specific organic pattern, with the abnormality varying from moment to moment and from one examination to another. There may be ataxia, spasticity, inability to move, or other types of abnormality. The abnormality is often minimal or absent when the patient is unaware of being watched or when distracted. However, although all hysterical gaits are bizarre, all bizarre gaits are not hysterical.

Pregnancy

Substantial hormonal and anatomic changes occur during pregnancy, which dramatically alter body mass, body mass distribution, and joint laxity. During pregnancy, musculoskeletal disorders are common and may cause problems ranging from mild discomfort to serious disability. It is widely presumed that pregnant women exhibit marked gait deviations. The results of a recent study appear to refute that notion.[152] The study concluded that velocity, stride length, and cadence during the third trimester of pregnancy were similar to those measured 1 year postpartum and that only small deviations in pelvic tilt and hip flexion, extension, and adduction were observed during pregnancy.[152] The study found significant increases ($p < 0.05$) in hip extensor, hip abductor, and ankle plantar flexor kinetic gait parameters, which suggests an increased use of hip extensor, hip abductor, and ankle plantar flexor muscles to compensate for increases in body mass and changes in body mass distribution during pregnancy. These increases keep speed, stride length, cadence, and joint angles relatively unchanged.[152] However, these compensations may result in overuse injuries to the muscle groups about the pelvis, hip, and ankle, including low back, pelvic, and hip pain; calf cramps; and other painful lower extremity musculoskeletal conditions associated with pregnancy.[152] It was unclear from this study whether the women examined had gained normal amounts of weight associated with pregnancy. It would seem obvious that obesity associated with pregnancy may have differing affects on gait.

Obesity

As obesity is reaching epidemic proportions in the United States and is a growing problem in developed countries, the clinician needs to be aware of its effects on the normal gait pattern to help discriminate compensatory patterns as opposed to pathologic manifestations. Obesity is associated with a number of comorbidities, such as coronary artery disease, type 2 diabetes, gall bladder disease, and sleep apnea. Given a normal body mass index (defined as the weight in kilograms divided by the square of the height in meters) ranging from 18.5 to 24.9, 34% of the adult population is overweight (body mass index of 25–29.9) and another 27% is obese (body mass index of 30 or more).[153]

The gait used by the obese patient is often described as a waddling gait. Depending on the degree of obesity, the waddling gait is characterized by increased lateral displacement, pelvic obliquity, hip circumduction, increased knee valgus, external foot progression angle, overpronation, and increases in the normalized dynamic BOS. Nantel and colleagues[154] compared the biomechanical parameters between obese and nonobese children during self-paced walking. Kinematics were captured with eight VICON optoelectronic cameras (Oxford Metrics Limited, Oxford, UK) recording at 60 Hz. Findings from the study revealed that obese children modified their hip motor pattern by shifting from extensor to flexor moment earlier in the gait cycle. This led obese children to significantly decrease the mechanical work done by the hip extensors during weight acceptance and significantly increase the mechanical work done by the hip flexors, compared with nonobese children. Finally, there was a significant decrease in the single support duration in the obese group compared with nonobese. Gushue and colleagues[155] attempted to quantify the three-dimensional knee joint kinematics and kinetics during walking in children of varying body mass and to identify effects associated with obesity. The study found that the overweight group walked with a significantly lower peak knee flexion angle during early stance, and no significant differences in peak internal knee extension moments were found between groups. However, the overweight group showed a significantly higher peak internal knee abduction moment during early stance. These data suggest that although overweight children may develop a gait adaptation to maintain a similar knee extensor load, they may not be able to compensate for alterations in the frontal plane, which may lead to increased medial compartment joint loads.[155] Finally, in a study by de Souza and colleagues,[156] an outpatient population (age 47.2 ± 12.9 years, 94.1% females, BMI 40.1 ± 6.0 kg/m^2, $n = 34$) had their gait analyzed by an experienced physical therapist. Variables included speed, cadence, stride, step width, and foot angle, which were compared to reference values. All variables were significantly lower in the obese patients, except for step width, which was increased. Speed was 73.3 ± 16.3 vs. 130 cm/s, cadence was 1.4 ± 0.2 vs. 1.8 steps/s, stride was 106.8 ± 13.1 vs. 132.0 cm, and step width was 12.5 ± 3.5 vs. 10.0 cm ($p < 0.05$). The authors concluded that these findings were consistent with poor skeletal muscle performance, high metabolic expenditure, and constant physical exhaustion.[156]

CLINICAL PEARL

Obese adults demonstrate a longer stance time, decreased stride length, a step width that is double that of the nonobese, an increased support period (double and single), altered hip abduction angles, and decreased gait velocity (1.09 m/s).[157]

Obesity also impacts other areas of mobility such as sit to stand transfers. In obese adults, sit to stand is performed by placing the feet further under the body and utilizing less hip flexion than in the nonobese.[143] While this results in a decrease torque at the hip, it also results in an increase torque demand and joint stress at the knee.[158] Perhaps more alarmingly is the finding that obese children have significant difficulty with the sit to stand task.[143] In one study, 69% of obese children required assistance to perform a sit to stand transfer.[159]

Although the functional comorbidities of excess body weight such as gait problems are perhaps clinically insignificant compared to those associated with certain metabolic sequelae, they may interfere with the quality of life and also act to increase muscle, bone, and joint stress. For example, the changes in the natural alignment of the weight-bearing segments may result in overuse injuries such as tendonitis and bursitis and eventual osteoarthritis of the hip or knee, or both.

JOINT REPLACEMENT SURGERY

Individuals undergoing knee replacement and hip replacement surgery demonstrate impaired gait patterns:[143]

- *Knee replacement.* The gait tends to present with slower preoperative and postoperative cadence than age-matched normals, as well as shorter step length both preoperatively and postoperatively.[160] These changes remain stable for 1–2 years after surgery.[160] Individuals with knee replacement surgery also continue to exhibit reduced knee excursion during gait before and after surgery at all time points.[160] Muscle activation also remains altered with a stiff knee gait pattern that involves coactivation during the stance phase predominating up to 2 years postoperatively.[161]
- *Hip replacement.* Individuals undergoing both the posterolateral and the anterolateral surgical approaches have demonstrated altered gait parameters at 6 months postoperative.[162] The anterolateral approach tends to lead to greater trunk forward inclination and a Trendelenburg gait pattern, whereas the posterolateral approach has a greater incidence of dislocation.[162]

ASSISTIVE DEVICES

The most common cause for the breakdown of the normal gait cycle is an injury to one or both of the lower extremities. Such an injury usually results in an antalgic gait. If the injury is severe enough, an assistive device is needed. Assistive devices are used to make ambulation as safe and as painless as possible. However, it must be remembered that there is an energy cost associated with the use of assistive devices. Energy expenditure during walking with assistive devices such as crutches or a walker has generally been examined only in younger people with contrasting results. One study[163] showed that walking with crutches resulted in lower VO2 compared with walking with a rollator or a standard walker. Compared with unassisted walking, walking with a wheeled walker resulted in more oxygen use. Another study[164] found that subjects 75 years of age or older, consumed an average of 2.8 METS when walking while using a wheeled walker; this corresponds to a moderate level of intensity according to the ACSM scale for the very old.[165–167]

In essence, an assistive device is an extension of the upper extremity, used to provide support, balance, and weight bearing normally provided by an intact functioning lower extremity.[168] Assistive devices function to reduce ground reaction forces, with the size of the BOS that they provide being proportional to the amount of reduction in these forces.

Assistive devices, in order of the stability they provide, include a walker, crutches, walker cane, quad cane, straight cane, and bent cane, with the walker providing the most stability.

The indications for using an assistive device include[169]

- decreased ability to bear weight through the lower extremities;
- muscle weakness or paralysis of the trunk or lower extremities;
- decreased balance and proprioception in the upright posture.

Correct fitting of an assistive device is important to ensure for the safety of the patient and to allow for minimal energy expenditure. Once fitted, the patient should be taught the correct walking technique with the device. The fitting depends on the device chosen:

- ***Walkers, hemiwalking canes, quad canes, and standard canes.*** The height of the device handle should be adjusted to the level of the greater trochanter of the patient's hip.
- ***Standard crutches.*** A number of methods can be used for determining the correct crutch length for axillary crutches. The crutch tip should be vertical to the ground and positioned approximately 15-cm (6 in.) lateral and 15-cm (6 in.) anterior to the patient's foot. The handgrips of the crutch are adjusted to the height of the greater trochanter of the hip of the patient. There should be a 5–8-cm (2–3 in.) gap between the top of the axillary pads and the patient's axilla. Bauer and colleagues[170] found that the best calculation of ideal crutch length was either 77% of the patient's height or the height minus 40.6 cm (16 in.).
- ***Forearm/loftstrand crutches.*** The crutch is adjusted so that the handgrip is level with the greater trochanter of the patient's hip and the top of the forearm cuff just distal to the elbow.
- ***Canes.*** Using a cane to aid walking is perhaps as old as the history of humankind. In ancient times, canes were used for support, defense, and the procurement of food.[171] Later, canes became a symbol of power and aristocracy.[172] Currently, canes are used to provide support and protection, to reduce pain in the lower extremities, and to improve balance during ambulation.[173] It is common practice to instruct patients with lower extremity pain to use the cane in the hand contralateral to the symptomatic side.[174] The use of a cane in the contralateral hand helps preserve reciprocal motion and a more normal pathway for the COG.[175] Use of a cane in this fashion also helps to decrease forces at the hip, as estimated by external kinematics and kinetics.[176–179] Use of a cane can transmit 20–25% of body weight away from the lower extremities.[180,181] The cane also allows the subject to increase the effective BOS, thereby decreasing the hip abductor force exerted.

GAIT TRAINING WITH ASSISTIVE DEVICES

The clinician must always provide adequate physical support and instruction while working with a patient using an assistive gait device. The clinician positions himself or herself on the involved side of the patient, to be able to assist the patient on the side where the patient will most likely have difficulty. In addition, a gait belt should be fitted around the patient's waist to enable the clinician to assist the patient. When ambulating with a patient, the clinician should be just behind the patient, standing toward the involved side.

The selection of the proper gait pattern to instruct the patient is dependent on the patient's balance, strength, cardiovascular status, coordination, functional needs, and weight-bearing status:

- ***NWB.*** Patient is not permitted to bear any weight through the injured limb.
- ***Partial weight-bearing (PWB).*** Patient is permitted to bear a portion (25%, 50%, etc.) of his or her weight through the injured limb.
- ***Touch down weight-bearing/toe touch weight-bearing.*** Patient is permitted minimal contact of the injured limb with the ground for balance. The expression "as though walking on eggshells" can be used to help the patient understand.
- ***Weight-bearing as tolerated.*** The patient is permitted to bear as much weight through the injured limb as is comfortable.
- ***Full weight-bearing.*** Patient no longer medically requires an assistive device.

Several gait patterns are recognized (Table 6-12).

TABLE 6-12 Gait Patterns when Using Assistive Devices

Pattern	Description
Two-point pattern	Closely approximates the normal gait pattern, but requires the use of an assistive gait device (canes or crutches) on each side of the body The patient moves the assistive gait device and the contralateral lower extremity at the same time Requires some coordination and is used when there are no weight-bearing restrictions in the presence of bilateral weakness or to enhance balance
Two-point modified	Is the same as the two-point except that it requires only one assistive device, positioned on the opposite side of the involved lower extremity This pattern cannot be used if there are any weight-bearing restrictions, i.e., PWB, NWB, but is appropriate for a patient with unilateral weakness or mild balance deficits The patient is instructed to move the cane and the involved leg simultaneously, and then the uninvolved leg
Four-point pattern	Requires the use of an assistive gait device (canes or crutches) on each side of the body, is used when the patient requires maximum assistance with balance and stability The pattern is initiated with the forward movement of one of the assistive gait devices, and then the contralateral lower extremity, the other assistive gait device, and finally the opposite lower extremity (e.g., right crutch, then left foot; left crutch, then right foot)
Four-point modified	Is the same as the four-point except that it requires only one assistive device, positioned on the opposite side of the involved lower extremity This pattern cannot be used if there are any weight-bearing restrictions, i.e., PWB, NWB, but are appropriate for a patient with unilateral weakness or mild balance deficits The patient is instructed to move the cane, then the involved leg, and then the uninvolved leg
Three-point	Used for nonweight-bearing—when the patient is permitted to bear weight through only one lower extremity. Involves the use of two crutches or a walker (cannot be used with a cane or one crutch) Requires good upper body strength, good balance, and good cardiovascular endurance The pattern is initiated with the forward movement of the assistive gait device(s). Next, the involved lower extremity is advanced, while staying NWB as the patient then presses down on the assistive gait device and advances the uninvolved lower extremity
Three-point modified or 3 point 1	A modification of the three-point gait pattern that requires two crutches or a walker This pattern is used when the patient can bear full weight with one lower extremity but is only allowed to partially bear weight on the involved lower extremity. In partial weight bearing, only part of the patient's weight is allowed to be transferred through the involved lower extremity The pattern is initiated with the forward movement of one of the assistive gait devices, and then the involved lower extremity is advanced forward, allowing only PWB (Fig. 23-7). The patient presses down on the assistive gait device and advances the uninvolved lower extremity, using either a "swing-to" or a "swing-through" pattern

Sit-to-Stand Transfers

Before the patient can begin ambulation, he or she must first learn to safely transfer from a sitting position to a standing position. The wheels of the bed or wheelchair are locked, and the patient is reminded of any weight-bearing restrictions. The patient is asked to slide to the front edge of the chair or bed, and the weight-bearing foot is placed underneath the body so that the COG is closer to the BOS, which will make it easier for the patient to stand.

The patient is then instructed to lean forward and push up with the hands from the bed or armrests.

- If the patient is being instructed on the use of a walker, he or she should grasp the handgrips of the walker only after becoming upright and should not be permitted to try to pull up to a standing position using the walker, because this can cause the walker to tip over and increase the potential for falls.
- If the patient is using crutches, he or she is instructed to hold both crutches with the hand on the same side as the involved lower extremity. The patient then presses down on the handgrips of the crutches, the armrest, or bed and with the uninvolved lower extremity, to stand. Once standing, and with adequate balance, the patient moves the crutches into position and begins to ambulate.
- If the patient is using one or two canes, he or she is instructed to push up with the hands from the bed or armrests. Once standing, the patient should grasp the handgrip(s) of the cane(s) with the appropriate hand and begin to ambulate.

Stand-to-Sit Transfers

The stand-to-sit transfer is essentially the reverse of the sit-to-stand transfer. In order to sit down using an assistive device, the patient must first back up against the front edge of the bed or chair. If the patient has difficulty bending the knee of the involved lower extremity, he or she is instructed to slowly advance this extremity forward. Once in position

- the patient using a walker reaches for the bed or armrest with both hands and slowly sits down;
- the patient using crutches moves both crutches to the hand on the side of the involved lower extremity. With that hand holding onto both handgrips of the crutches, the patient reaches back for the bed or armrest with the other hand before slowly sitting down;
- The patient using one or two canes places the handgrip of the cane(s) against the edge of the chair or bed. Next, the patient reaches back for the bed or armrest and slowly sits down.

Stair Negotiation

Ascending Stairs

To ascend steps, the patient must first move to the front edge of the step. The walker will have to be turned toward the opposite side of the handrail or wall. Ascending more than two to three stairs with a walker is not recommended.

- To ascend stairs using a walker, the patient is instructed to grasp the stair handrail with one hand and to turn the walker sideways so that the two front legs of the walker are placed on the first step. When ready, the patient pushes down on the walker handgrip and the handrail and advances the uninvolved lower extremity onto the first step. The patient then advances the uninvolved lower extremity to the first step and moves the legs of the walker to the next step. This process is repeated as the patient moves up the steps.
- To ascend steps or stairs with crutches, the patient should grasp the stair handrail with one hand and grasp both crutches by the handgrips with the other hand. If the patient is unable to grasp both crutches with one hand, or if the handrail is not stable, then the patient should use both crutches only, although this is not recommended if there are more than two to three steps. When in the correct position at the front edge of the step, the patient pushes down on the crutches and handrail, if applicable, and advances the uninvolved lower extremity to the first step. The patient then advances the involved lower extremity and finally the crutches. This process is repeated for the remaining steps.
- To ascend steps or stairs with one or two canes, the patient should use the handrail and the cane(s). If the handrail is not stable, then the patient should use the cane(s) only. The patient pushes down on the cane(s) or handrail, if applicable, and advances the uninvolved lower extremity to the first step. The patient then advances the involved lower extremity. This process is repeated for the remaining steps.

Descending Stairs

In order to descend steps, the patient must first move to the front edge of the top step. Descending more than two to three stairs with a walker is not recommended.

- To descend stairs using a walker, the walker is turned sideways so that the two front legs of the walker are placed on the lower step. One hand is placed on the rear handgrip, and the other hand grasps the stair handrail. When ready, the patient lowers the involved lower extremity down to the first step. Then the patient pushes down on the walker and handrail and advances the uninvolved lower extremity down the first step. This process is repeated as the patient moves down the steps.
- To descend steps or stairs with crutches, the patient should use one hand to grasp the stair handrail and the other to grasp both crutches and handrail. If the patient is unable to grasp both crutches with one hand, or if the handrail is not stable, then the patient should use both crutches only, although this is not recommended if there are more than two to three steps. When ready, the patient lowers the involved lower extremity down to the first step. Next, the patient pushes down on the crutches and handrail, if applicable, and advances the uninvolved lower extremity down to the first step. This process is repeated for the remaining steps.
- To descend steps or stairs with one or two canes, the patient should use the cane(s) and handrail. If the handrail is not stable, then the patient should use the cane(s) only. When ready, the patient lowers the involved lower extremity down to the first step. Next, the patient pushes down on the cane(s) and handrail, if applicable, and advances the uninvolved

lower extremity down to the first step. This process is repeated for the remaining steps.

Instructions

Whichever gait pattern is chosen, it is important that the patient receive verbal and illustrated instructions for use of the assistive gait device to negotiate stairs, curbs, ramps, doors, and transfers. These instructions should include any weight-bearing precautions pertinent to the patient, the appropriate gait sequence, and a contact number at which to reach the clinician if questions arise.

POSTURE

As with the so-called good movement, *good posture* is a subjective term reflecting what the clinician believes to be correct based on ideal models. Various attempts have been made to define and interpret posture.[79,182–185] Good posture may be defined as "the optimal alignment of the patient's body that allows the neuromuscular system to perform actions requiring the least amount of energy to achieve the desired effect."[184] Postural or skeletal alignment has important consequences as each joint has a direct effect on both its neighboring joint and on the joints further away. A syndrome is a characteristic pattern of symptoms or dysfunctions. Abnormal or *nonneutral* alignment is defined as "positioning that deviates from the midrange position of function."[186] To be classified as abnormal or dysfunctional, the alignment must produce physical functional limitations. These functional limitations can occur anywhere along the kinetic chain, at adjacent or distal joints through compensatory motions or postures.

The overall contour of the normal vertebral column in the coronal plane is straight. In contrast, the contour of the sagittal plane changes with development. At birth, a series of primary curves give a kyphotic posture to the whole spine. With development of the erect posture, secondary curves develop. For example, the cervical spine forms a lordotic curve that develops secondary to the response of an upright posture, which initially occurs when the child begins to lift the head at 3–4 months. The presence of the curve allows the head and eyes to remain oriented forward and provides a shock-absorbing mechanism to counteract the axial compressive force produced by the weight of the head.[35] The curves in the spinal column provide it with increased flexibility and shock-absorbing capabilities.[187]

Postural alignment is both static and dynamic. The postural control system, the mechanism by which the body maintains balance and equilibrium, has been divided into several subsystems, namely, the vestibular, visual, and somatosensory subsystems (see Chapter 3).[188,189] In a multisegmented organism such as the human body, many postures are adopted throughout the course of a day. Nonneutral alignment, whether maintained statically, or performed repetitively, appears to be a key precipitating factor in soft tissue and neurologic pain.[190] This may be the result of an alteration in joint load distribution or in the force transmission of the muscles. This alteration can result in a muscle imbalance.

The ability to maintain correct posture appears to be related to a number of factors:[191,192]

- ***Energy cost.***[192] The increase in metabolic rate over the basal rate when standing is so small, compared with a metabolic cost of moving and exercising, as to be negligible. The type of posture that involves a minimum of metabolic increase over the basal rate is one in which the knees are hyperextended, the hips are pushed forward to the limit of extension, the thoracic curve is increased, the head is projected forward, and the upper trunk is inclined backward in a posterior lean.
- ***Strength and flexibility.*** Pathological changes to the neuromuscular system (e.g., excessive wearing of the articular surfaces of joints, the development of osteophytes and traction spurs, and maladaptive changes in the length-tension development and angle of pull of muscles and tendons) may be the result of the cumulative effect of repeated small stresses (microtrauma) over a long phase of time or of constant abnormal stresses (macrotrauma) over a short phase of time (see Chapter 2). Strong, flexible muscles are able to resist the detrimental effects of faulty postures for longer phases and provide the ability to unload the structures through a change of position. However, these changes in position are not possible if the joints are stiff (hypomobile) or too mobile (hypermobile), or the muscles are weak, shortened, or lengthened.
- ***Age.*** As the human body develops from infancy to old age, several physical and neurological factors may affect posture. As discussed, at birth, a series of primary curves cause the entire vertebral column to be concave forward, or flexed, giving a kyphotic posture to the whole spine, although the overall contour in the coronal plane is straight. In contrast, the contour of the sagittal plane changes with development. At the other end of the lifespan, the aging adult tends to alter posture in several ways. A common function of aging, at least in women, is the development of a stooped posture associated with osteoporosis.
- ***Psychological aspects.***[192] Not all posture problems can be explained in terms of physical causes. Atypical postures may be symptoms of personality problems or emotional disturbances.
- ***Evolutionary and heredity influences.***[192] The transformation of the human race from arboreal quadrupeds to upright bipeds is likely related to the need to the male hominid to have the hands and arms available for carrying a wider variety of foods from fairly long distances.[193] This transformation was responsible not only for the changes in the weight-bearing parts of the musculoskeletal structure but also for changes in the upper extremities, which are now free for the development of a greater variety of manipulative skills. In attempting to correct an individual's posture, one must be realistic and accept the limits imposed by possible hereditary factors.
- ***Structural deformities.*** The normal coronal and sagittal alignment of the spine can be altered by many conditions, including leg-length inequality (see Chapter 29), congenital anomalies, developmental problems, trauma, or disease (Table 6-13).[194–196]

TABLE 6-13	Common Structural Deformities	
Deformity	**Description**	**Manifestation**
Lordosis	An excessive anterior curvature of the spine. Pathologically, it is an exaggeration of the normal curves found in the cervical and lumbar spines The pelvic angle, normally approximately 30 degrees, is increased with lordosis There are two types of exaggerated lordosis: pathological lordosis and swayback deformity *Pathological lordosis:* Involves scapulae protraction, internally rotated arms, internally rotated legs, and forward head, accompanied by weakness of the deep lumbar extensors and tightness of the hip flexors and tensor fasciae latae, combined with weak abdominals *Swayback deformity:* Increased pelvic inclination to approximately 40 degrees and kyphosis of the thoracolumbar spine. A swayback deformity results in the spine's bending back rather sharply at the lumbosacral angle. With this postural deformity, the entire pelvis shifts anteriorly, causing the hips to move into extension. To maintain the center of gravity in its normal position, the thoracic spine flexes on the lumbar spine. The result is an increase in the lumbar and thoracic curves. Such a deformity may be associated with tightness of the hip extensors, lower lumbar extensors, and upper abdominals, along with weakness of the hip flexors, lower abdominals, and lower thoracic extensors	Causes of increased lordosis include 1. postural deformity 2. lax muscles, especially the abdominal muscles, in combination with tight muscles, especially hip flexors or lumbar extensors 3. a heavy abdomen, resulting from excess weight or pregnancy 4. hip flexion contractures 5. spondylolisthesis 6. congenital problems, such as bilateral congenital dislocation of the hip 7. failure of segmentation of the neural arch 8. fashion (e.g., wearing high-heeled shoes)
Kyphosis	Excessive posterior curvature of the spine Pathologically, it is an exaggeration of the normal curve found in the thoracic spine There are four types of kyphosis: 1. Round back—a long, rounded curve with decreased pelvic inclination (<30 degrees) and thoracolumbar kyphosis. The patient often presents with the trunk flexed forward and a decreased lumbar curve. On examination, there are tight hip extensors and trunk flexors, with weak hip flexors and lumbar extensors 2. Humpback or gibbus—a localized, sharp posterior angulation in the thoracic spine 3. Flat back—decreased pelvic inclination to 20 degrees and a mobile lumbar spine 4. Dowager hump—often seen in older patients, especially women. The deformity commonly is caused by osteoporosis, in which the thoracic vertebral bodies begin to degenerate and wedge in an anterior direction, resulting in a kyphosis	There are several causes of kyphosis, including tuberculosis, vertebral compression fractures, Scheuermann disease, ankylosing spondylitis, senile osteoporosis, tumors, compensation in conjunction with lordosis, and congenital anomalies The congenital anomalies include a partial segmental defect, as seen in osseous metaplasia, or centrum hypoplasia and aplasia In addition, paralysis may lead to a kyphosis because of the loss of muscle action needed to maintain the correct posture, combined with the forces of gravity

Data from Magee DJ: Assessment of posture. In: Magee DJ, ed. *Orthopaedic Physical Assessment*. Philadelphia, PA: WB Saunders, 2002:873–903; Kendall FP, McCreary EK, Provance PG: *Muscles: Testing and Function*. Baltimore, MD: Williams & Wilkins, 1993.

▸ ***Disease.*** The normal coronal alignment of the spine can be altered by many conditions, including joint degeneration and scoliosis. *Scoliosis*, which is a descriptive term for lateral curvature, is usually accompanied by a rotational abnormality. Scoliosis can be idiopathic, a result of congenital deformity, pain, or degeneration, or be associated with numerous neuromuscular conditions, such as leg-length inequality (see Chapter 29). Sagittal plane alignment can also be altered by disease and injury. This alteration is manifested clinically with areas of excessive kyphosis or lordosis, or a loss of the normal curves. Respiratory conditions (e.g., emphysema), general weakness, excess weight, loss of proprioception, or muscle spasm (as seen in cerebral palsy or with trauma) may also lead to poor posture.[197]

- ***Pregnancy.*** Although never substantiated, postural changes have often been implicated as a major cause of back pain in pregnant women.[198,199] The relationship between posture and the back pain experienced during pregnancy is unclear. This may be because significant skeletal alignment changes that are related to back pain that are occurring at the pelvis during pregnancy but may not be directly measured by postural assessments, such as lumbar lordosis, sacral base angle, and pelvic tilt. Moore et al.[200] found a significant relationship ($r = 0.49$) between change in lordosis during 16–24 and 34–42 weeks of pregnancy and an increase in low back pain. Ostgaard et al.[201] found that abdominal sagittal diameter ($r = 0.15$), transverse diameter ($r = 0.13$), and depth of the lordosis ($r = 0.11$) were related to the development of back pain during pregnancy. Bullock et al.,[199] in the only study that used a validated and reliable posture assessment instrument, found no relationship between spinal posture (thoracic kyphosis, lumbar lordosis, and pelvic tilt) magnitude or changes during pregnancy, and back pain. The results from a study by Franklin and Conner-Kerr[202] suggest that from the first to the third trimester of pregnancy, lumbar lordosis, posterior head position, lumbar angle, and pelvic tilt increase; however, the magnitudes and the changes of these posture variables are not related to back pain.
- ***Habit.*** The most common postural problem is poor postural habit and its associated adaptive changes. Poor posture, and, in particular, poor sitting posture, is considered to be a major contributing factor in the development and perpetuation of shoulder, neck, and back pain. Muscles maintained in a shortened or lengthened position eventually will adapt to their new positions. Although these muscles initially are incapable of producing a maximal contraction in the newly acquired positions,[203] changes at the sarcomere level eventually allow the muscle to produce maximal tension at the new length.[204] Although this may appear to be a satisfactory adaptation, the changes in length produce changes in tension development, as well as changes in the angle of pull.[205] It is theorized that, if a muscle lengthens as part of a compensation, muscle spindle activity increases within that muscle, producing reciprocal inhibition of that muscle's functional antagonist and resulting in an alteration in the normal force–couple and arthrokinematic relationship, thereby effecting the efficient and ideal operation of the movement system.[204,206–209] For example, a passively insufficient muscle is activated earlier in a movement than a normal muscle and has a tendency to be more hypertonic, thereby producing a reflex inhibition of the antagonists.[206,207,210,211] It is difficult to determine why a particular posture becomes dysfunctional in one individual, yet not in another. Differing adaptive potentials of the tissues between individuals may be among the causes in addition to neurologic, neurodevelopmental, and neurophysiologic factors.

CLINICAL PEARL

The pain from any sustained position is thought to result from ischemia of the isometrically contracting muscles, localized fatigue, or an excessive mechanical strain on the structures. Intramuscular pressure can compress the blood vessels and prevent the removal of metabolites and the supply of oxygen, either of which can cause temporary pain.[212,213]

Postural development begins at a very early age. As the infant starts to activate the postural system, skeletal muscles develop according to their predetermined specific uses in various recurrent functions and movement strategies.[214] Jull and Janda[211 215] developed a system that characterized muscles based on common patterns of kinetic chain dysfunction into two functional divisions (see Table 1-4 in Chapter 1):

- ***Postural muscles.*** These relatively strong muscles are designed to counter gravitational forces and provide a stable base for other muscles to work from, although they are likely to be poorly recruited, lax in appearance, and show an inability to perform inner range contractions over time.
- ***Phasic muscles.*** These muscles tend to function in a dynamically antagonistic manner to the postural muscles. Phasic muscles tend to become relatively weak compared to the postural muscles, are more prone to atrophy and adaptive shortening, and show preferential recruitment in synergistic activities. In addition, these muscles will tend to dominate movements and may alter posture by restricting movement.

The work of Jull and Janda[211] also introduced the concept of postural patterns and described a lower quadrant syndrome called the *pelvic crossed syndrome*. In this syndrome, the erector spinae and iliopsoas are adaptively shortened (tight), and the abdominals and gluteus maximus are weak. This syndrome promotes an anterior pelvic tilt, an increased lumbar lordosis, and a slight flexion of the hip. The hamstrings frequently are adaptively shortened in this syndrome, and this may be a compensatory strategy to lessen the anterior tilt of the pelvis,[208] or because the glutei are weak. In addition to increasing the lumbar lordosis, an increased thoracic kyphosis and a compensatory increase in cervical lordosis to keep the head and eyes level occurs. Janda also described an upper quadrant syndrome called the *upper crossed syndrome*.[215] This syndrome involves adaptive shortening of the levator scapulae, upper trapezius, pectoralis major and minor, and sternocleidomastoid (SCM), and weakness of the deep neck flexors and lower scapular stabilizers. The syndrome produces elevation and protraction of the shoulder and rotation and abduction of the scapula, together with scapular winging. It also theoretically produces a forward head and hypermobility of the C4–C5 and T4 segments.

More recently, Sahrmann[204] has stressed the importance of the relationship of neighboring joints along both directions of the kinetic chain to determine the mechanical cause of the symptoms.

CLINICAL PEARL

Postural imbalances involve the entire body, as should any corrections. It is important to remember that an appropriate examination must take place prior to any intervention.

Many studies have evaluated the effect of injury to the neuromuscular system.[216–222] If muscle control is poor, joint strain and pain may result.[223,224] Trauma to tissues that contain mechanoreceptors may result in partial deafferentation, which can lead to proprioceptive deficits and alter joint function.[225,226] For example, in addition to the mechanical restraint provided by ligaments, it has been observed that ligaments provide neurologic feedback that directly mediates reflex muscle contractions about a joint.[225,227]

As the neuromuscular system declines, certain predictable and stereotypical changes tend to occur.[228] These include increased lumbar lordosis and thoracic kyphosis, decreased hip extension, decreased medial–lateral stability and increased hip flexed posture due to muscle imbalance and decreased anterior–posterior stability, decreased stride length, greater weight placed on the forefoot, increased double-foot stance time, decreased proprioception, and harder heel strike.[214] As the decline progresses, the locomotor system becomes less able to adapt to its environment, requiring greater attention to recruit more sensory information in order to maintain postural control. Many of the changes that occur in the developing neuromuscular system interestingly recur in some sort of reverse order during the degrading process.[214] These changes include a transition from an ankle strategy during gait back to a hip strategy, a broadened stance to combat increased medial–lateral instability, a shortened stride length to better maintain COG, decreased integration of upper body counter rotation, increased visual sensory input, and recruitment of additional afferentation for postural equilibrium, such as the use of a cane, the aid of a more posturally stable person, or both.[214]

Examination

The assessment of posture primarily involves information gleaned from the history in addition to visual and palpatory observations. A clear understanding of functional anatomy and topographical landmarks is vital.[214] As with gait analysis, various attempts have been made to objectively measure posture, including radiography, goniometry, inclinometry, flexible ruler measurement, photography, the Iowa anatomical position system, and plumb line assessment. Because there is an almost endless variety of activity postures and because these are extremely difficult to assess, a convenient custom has been to accept the standing posture as the individual's basic posture from which all other postures stem.[192] Under this concept, ideal postural alignment for standing (viewed from the side) was defined as a straight line (line of gravity) that passes through the ear lobe, the bodies of the cervical vertebrae, the tip of the shoulder, midway through the thorax, through the bodies of the lumbar vertebrae, slightly posterior to the hip joint, slightly anterior to the axis of the knee joint, and just anterior to the lateral malleolus (Fig. 6-5).

CLINICAL PEARL

A simple and commonly applied parameter of global balance is the plumbline offset taken from a full-length standing radiograph. The center of C2 (or C7) is drawn vertically downward, and the distance from the center of the sacrum is noted on the coronal projection, while the offset from the anterior–superior edge or posterior–-superior edge of S1 is noted on the lateral projection.

Although this measurement is simple, it may not accurately reflect the balance of the spine—the plumbline measurement is a radiographic value and not a representation of the applied forces.

Theoretically, this postural alignment results in minimum stress being applied to each joint, with minimal muscle activity being required to maintain the position.

To assess posture accurately, the patient must be adequately undressed. Standard protocols for patient attire vary with respect to, among other factors, regional, societal, religious, legal, health-care specialty, gender, and age-related issues.[214] Ideally, male patients should be in shorts, and female patients should be in a bra and shorts, and the patient should not wear shoes or stockings. However, if the patient uses walking aids, braces, collars, or orthoses, they should be noted and may be used after the patient has been assessed in the "natural" state to determine the effect of the appliances.[197] In addition, the floor on which the patient stands and is assessed, should be a level, hard surface. A slight degree of padded carpeting is acceptable, although a hard floor is preferable.[214]

The patient should assume a comfortable and relaxed posture, looking straight ahead, with feet approximately 4–6 in. apart. Often, it takes some time for the patient to adopt the usual posture because of tenseness, uneasiness, or uncertainty.[197] For the static examination, the clinician must be oriented to the patient so that the dominant eye (Table 6-14) is located in the midline between the landmarks being compared. The static assessment of posture is initially performed in a global fashion, with the patient in the standing, sitting, and lying (supine and prone) positions.[197] Although it may seem contrary, unassisted still, upright postural stance requires greater stability than unassisted walking, which is why walking occurs first in the toddler.[214] During mature still, upright stance, the hip joints account for the majority of medial–lateral stability, while the ankle joints account for a great deal of anterior–posterior stability.[229]

When observing a patient for abnormalities in posture, the clinician looks for asymmetry.[197] Regional asymmetry should trigger further evaluation of that area, but asymmetry alone does not confirm or rule out the presence of dysfunction. As some asymmetry between left and right sides is normal, the clinician must make the determination as to whether the apparent deviation is normal or caused by pathology. It must be remembered that postural adaptations can occur in a number of ways, including changes in gait, joint loading, neural function, muscle coordination, respiratory function, endurance, strength, and balance.[214] After the patient has been examined in the aforementioned positions, the examiner may decide to include other habitual, sustained, or repetitive

TABLE 6-14 Identifying the Dominant Eye

- Having made a circle with the first finger and thumb and, holding the arm out in front of the face, observe an object across the room, through that circle, with both eyes open
- Close one eye
- If the object is still in the circle, the dominant eye is open
- If, however, the image shifts out of the circle when only one eye is open, open the closed eye and close the open eye, and the image should shift back into clear view, inside the circle
- The eye that sees the same view when both eyes were open is the one to use in close observation of the body
- When attempting to assess by observation, a position should be adopted that allows the dominant eye to be closest to the center of what is being viewed

Data from Morris C, Chaitow L, Janda V: Functional examination for low back syndromes. In: Morris C, ed. *Low Back Syndromes: Integrated Clinical Management*. New York: McGraw-Hill, 2006:333–416; Dinnar U, Beal MC, Goodridge JP, et al.: Description of fifty diagnostic tests used with osteopathic manipulation. *J Am Osteopath Assoc* 81:314–321, 1982; Dinnar U, Beal MC, Goodridge JP, et al.: Classification of diagnostic tests used with osteopathic manipulation. *J Am Osteopath Assoc* 79:451–455, 1980.

postures assumed by the patient to see whether these postures increase or alter symptoms.[197]

Static Examination

The static postural examination, as it relates to each joint and the various postural syndromes that exist, is described in the relevant chapters. A summary of the most common findings and faults are listed in Table 6-13. Common lower limb skeletal malalignments and possible correlated and compensatory motions or postures are compiled in Table 6-15.

Due to the relationships between head, neck, thorax, lumbar spine, and pelvis, any deviation in one region can affect the other areas. A number of common postures are described here.

- ***Pelvic and lumbar region.*** The more common faulty postures of the pelvic and lumbar region include[230]
  - ***Lordotic posture.*** (Fig. 6-6) It is characterized by an increase in the lumbosacral angle, an increase in lumbar lordosis, and an increase in the anterior pelvic tilt and hip flexion.[231] This posture is commonly seen in pregnancy, obesity, and those individuals with weakened abdominal muscles. Potential muscle impairments include
    - decreased mobility in the hip flexor muscles (iliopsoas, tensor fascia latae, rectus femoris) and lumbar extensor muscles (erector spinae);
    - impaired muscle performance due to stretched and weakened abdominal muscles (rectus abdominis, internal and external obliques, and transversus abdominis).

This posture places stress throughout the lumbar spine on the anterior longitudinal ligament, the zygapophyseal (facet) joints, and narrows the posterior disk space and the intervertebral foramen, all of which are potential sources of symptoms.

- ***Slouched posture***: This posture, also referred to as the swayback,[182] is characterized by a shifting of the entire pelvic segment anteriorly, resulting in relative hip extension, and a shifting of the thoracic segment posteriorly, resulting in a relative flexion of the thorax on the upper lumbar spine (Fig. 6-6). As a result, there is an increased lordosis in the lower lumbar region, increased kyphosis in the thoracic region, and usually a forward (protracted) head. This posture is commonly seen throughout most age groups and is typically the result of fatigue or muscle weakness. Potential muscle impairments include the following:
  - Decreased mobility in the upper abdominal muscles (upper segments of the rectus abdominis and obliques), internal intercostal, hip extensor, and lower lumbar extensor muscles and related fascia.
  - Impaired muscle performance due to stretched and weakened lower abdominal muscles (lower segments of the rectus abdominis and obliques), extensor muscles of the lower thoracic region, and hip flexor muscles.

This posture places stress on the iliofemoral ligaments, the anterior longitudinal ligament of the lower lumbar spine, and the posterior longitudinal ligament of the upper lumbar and thoracic spine. In addition, there is narrowing of the intervertebral foramen in the lower lumbar spine and approximation of the zygapophyseal (facet) joints in the lower lumbar spine.

- ***Flat low back posture.*** This posture is characterized by a decreased lumbosacral angle, decreased lumbar lordosis/extension, and posterior tilting of the pelvis (Fig. 6-6). This posture is commonly seen in those individuals who spend long periods slouching or flexing in the sitting or standing positions. The potential muscle impairments include
  - decreased mobility in the trunk flexor (rectus abdominis, intercostals) and hip extensor muscles;
  - impaired muscle performance due to stretched and weak lumbar extensor and possibly hip flexor muscles.

This posture can apply stress on the posterior longitudinal ligament, the posterior disk space, and on the normal physiological lumbar curve, which reduces the shock-absorbing effects of the lumbar region and predisposes the patient to injury.

- ***Cervical and thoracic region.*** The more common faulty postures of the cervical and thoracic region include[230]
  - ***Round back with forward head.*** This posture is characterized by increased kyphotic thoracic curve, protracted scapulae (round shoulders), and forward head

TABLE 6-15 Skeletal Malalignment of the Lower Quarter and Correlated and Compensatory Motions or Postures

Malalignment	Possible Correlated Motions or Postures	Possible Compensatory Motions or Postures
Ankle and foot		
Ankle equinus		Hypermobile first ray Subtalar or midtarsal excessive pronation Hip or knee flexion Genu recurvatum
Rearfoot varus Excessive subtalar supination (calcaneal valgus)	Tibial; tibial and femoral; or tibial, femoral, and pelvic external rotation	Excessive internal rotation along the lower-quarter chain Hallux valgus Plantar-flexed first ray Functional forefoot valgus Excessive or prolonged midtarsal pronation
Rearfoot valgus Excessive subtalar pronation (calcaneal valgus)	Tibial; tibial and femoral; or tibial, femoral, and pelvic internal rotation Hallux valgus	Excessive external rotation along the lower-quarter chain Functional forefoot varus
Forefoot varus	Subtalar supination and related rotation along lower quarter	Plantar-flexed first ray Hallux valgus Excessive midtarsal or subtalar pronation or prolonged pronation Excessive tibial; tibial and femoral; or tibial, femoral, and pelvic internal rotation; or all with contralateral lumbar spine rotation
Forefoot valgus	Hallux valgus Subtalar pronation and related rotation along lower quarter	Excessive midtarsal or subtalar supination Excessive tibial; tibial and femoral; or tibial, femoral, and pelvic external rotation; or all with ipsilateral lumbar spine rotation
Metatarsus adductus	Hallux valgus Internal tibial torsion Flat foot In-toeing	
Hallux valgus	Forefoot valgus Subtalar pronation and related rotation along the lower quarter[33]	Excessive tibial; tibial and femoral; or tibial, femoral, and pelvic external rotation; or all with ipsilateral lumbar spine rotation
Knee and tibia		
Genu valgus	Pes planus Excessive subtalar pronation External tibial torsion Lateral patellar subluxation Excessive hip adduction Ipsilateral hip excessive internal rotation Lumbar spine contralateral rotation	Forefoot varus Excessive subtalar supination to allow lateral heel to contact ground In-toeing to decrease lateral pelvic sway during gait Ipsilateral pelvic external rotation
Genu varus	Excessive lateral angulation of tibia in frontal plane (tibial varum and tibia vara) Internal tibial torsion Ipsilateral hip external rotation Excessive hip abduction	Forefoot valgus Excessive subtalar pronation to allow medial heel to contact ground Ipsilateral pelvic internal rotation
Genu recurvatum	Ankle plantar flexion Excessive anterior pelvic tilt	Posterior pelvic tilt Flexed trunk posture Excessive thoracic kyphosis
External tibial torsion	Out-toeing Excessive subtalar supination with related rotation along lower quarter	Functional forefoot varus Excessive subtalar pronation with related rotation along lower quarter

(Continued)

TABLE 6-15 Skeletal Malalignment of the Lower Quarter and Correlated and Compensatory Motions or Postures *(Continued)*

Malalignment	Possible Correlated Motions or Postures	Possible Compensatory Motions or Postures
Internal tibial torsion	In-toeing Metatarsus adductus Excessive subtalar pronation with related rotation along lower quarter	Functional forefoot valgus Excessive subtalar supination with related rotation along lower quarter
Excessive tibial retroversion (posterior slant of tibial plateaus)	Genu recurvatum	
Inadequate tibial retrotorsion (posterior deflection of proximal tibia due to hamstrings pull)	Flexed knee posture	
Inadequate tibial retroflexion (bowing of the tibia)	Altered alignment of Achilles tendon, causing altered associated joint motion	
Bowleg deformity of tibia (tibia vara and tibial varum)	Internal tibial torsion	Forefoot valgus Excessive subtalar pronation
Hip and femur		
Excessive femoral anteversion anteversion)	In-toeing	Excessive external tibial torsion
	Excessive subtalar pronation	Excessive knee external rotation
	Lateral patellar subluxation	Excessive tibial; tibial and femoral; or tibial, femoral, and pelvic external rotation; or all with ipsilateral lumbar spine rotation
Femoral retrotorsion (retroversion)	Out-toeing	Excessive knee internal rotation
	Excessive subtalar supination	Excessive tibial; tibial and femoral; or tibial, femoral, and pelvic internal rotation; or all with contralateral lumbar spine rotation
Excessive femoral neck to shaft angle coxa valga)	Long ipsilateral lower limb and correlated motions or postures of a long limb	Excessive ipsilateral subtalar pronation Excessive contralateral subtalar supination Contralateral plantar flexion
	Posterior pelvic rotation	Ipsilateral genu recurvatum
	Supinated subtalar joint and related external rotation along the lower quarter	Ipsilateral hip or knee flexion Ipsilateral forward pelvis with contralateral lumbar spine rotation
Decreased femoral neck to shaft angle (coxa vara)	Pronated subtalar joint and related internal rotation along lower quarter	Excessive ipsilateral subtalar supination Excessive contralateral subtalar pronation
	Short ipsilateral lower limb and correlated motions or postures along lower quarter: anterior pelvic rotation	Ipsilateral plantar flexion Contralateral genu recurvatum Contralateral hip or knee flexion Ipsilateral backward pelvic rotation with ipsilateral lumbar spine rotation

Data from Riegger-Krugh C, Keysor JJ: Skeletal malalignments of the lower quarter: Correlated and compensatory motions and postures. *J Orthop Sports Phys Ther* 23:164–170, 1996.

(excessive flexion of the lower cervical spine and hyperextension of the upper cervical spine) (Fig. 6-7). The causes for this posture are similar to those found with the flat low back posture. The potential muscle impairments include the following:

- Decreased mobility in the muscles of the anterior thorax (intercostal muscles), muscles of the upper extremity originating on the thorax (pectoralis major and minor, latissimus dorsi, serratus anterior), muscles of the cervical spine and head that attach to the scapular and upper thorax (levator scapulae, SCM, scalene, upper trapezius), and muscles of the suboccipital region (rectus capitis posterior major and minor, obliquus capitis inferior and superior).
- Impaired muscle performance due to stretched and weak lower cervical and upper thoracic erector spinae and scapular retractor muscles (rhomboids, middle trapezius), anterior throat muscles (suprahyoid and

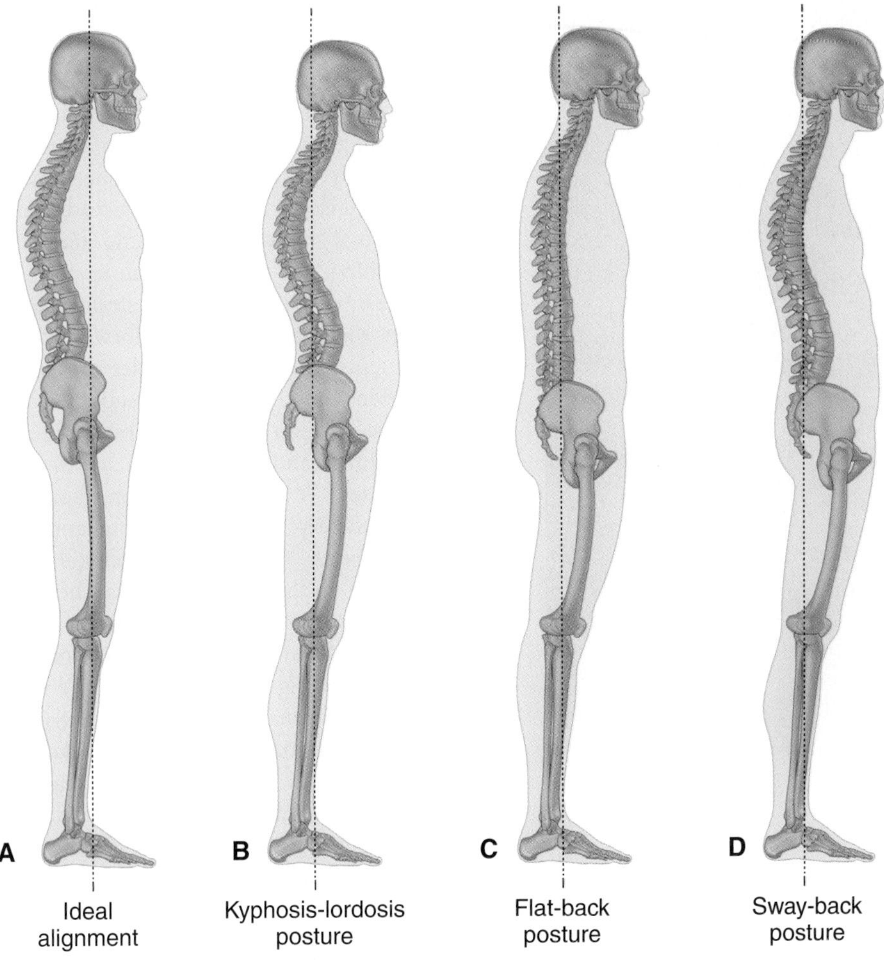

FIGURE 6-6 Common postural dysfunctions.

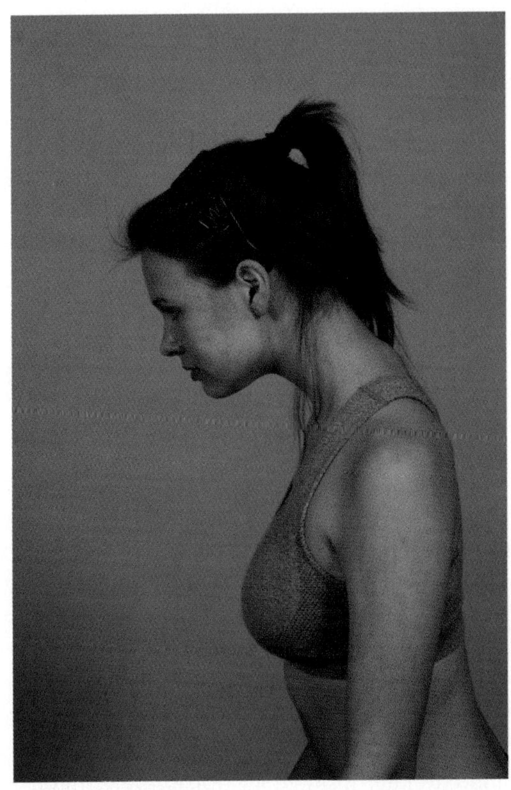

FIGURE 6-7 Forward-head posture.

infrahyoid), and capital flexors (rectus capitis anterior and lateralis, superior oblique longus colli, longus capitis).

This posture can place excessive stress on any or all of the following structures:

- Anterior longitudinal ligament in the upper cervical spine and posterior longitudinal ligament in the lower cervical and thoracic spine.
- Irritation of the zygapophyseal (facet) joints in the upper cervical spine.
- Impingement on the neurovascular bundle from anterior scalene or pectoralis minor muscle tightness (thoracic outlet syndrome).
- Impingement of the cervical plexus from levator scapulae muscle tightness.
- Temporomandibular joint dysfunction.
- Lower cervical disk lesions.
- Flat upper back and neck posture. This posture is characterized by a decrease in the thoracic curve, depressed scapulae, depressed clavicles, and decreased cervical lordosis with increased flexion of the occiput on the atlas. Although not common, this posture occurs primarily with

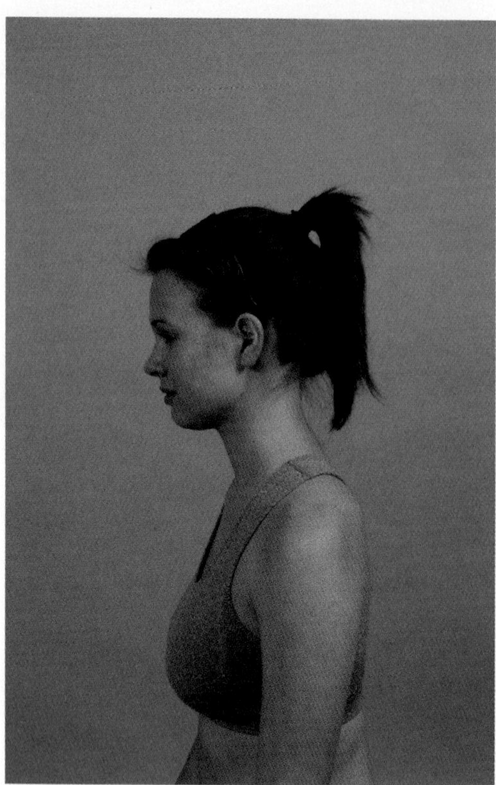

FIGURE 6-8 Flat Upper Back and Neck Posture.

exaggeration of the military posture (Fig. 6-8). The potential muscle impairments include the following:

- Decreased mobility in the anterior neck muscles, thoracic erector spinae, and scapular retractors, with potentially restricted scapular movement, which can interfere with shoulder elevation.
- Impaired muscle performance in the scapular protractor and intercostal muscles of the anterior thorax.

This posture can place stress on the neurovascular bundle in the thoracic outlet between the clavicle and ribs and can decrease the shock-absorbing function of the kyphotic curvature, thereby predisposing the neck to injury.

Forward Head. Forward head posture is described (in sitting or standing) as the excessive anterior positioning of the head, in relation to a vertical reference line, increased lower cervical spine lordosis, and rounded shoulders with thoracic kyphosis. Other postural adaptations associated with the forward head posture include protracted scapulae with tight anterior muscles and stretched posterior muscles and the development of a cervicothoracic kyphosis between C4 and T4.[207,232,233] For each inch that the head is anterior to the COG, the weight of the head is added to the load borne by the cervical structures.[234] For example, the average head weighs 10 lb. If the chin is 2 in. anterior to the manubrium, 20 lb is added to the load. If normal motion is undertaken in this poor postural environment, the result may be abnormal strain placed on the joint capsule, ligaments, intervertebral disks (IVDs), levator scapulae, upper trapezius, SCM, scalene, and suboccipital muscles.

Sustained forward head postures may cause a painful fatigue in the levator scapulae, rhomboids, and lower portion of the trapezius, a condition referred to as *tired neck syndrome*.[235] The traumatized muscles may cause pain, which in turn causes the patient to restrict motion. Patients with these postural abnormalities may experience myofascial pain that can cause referral zone pain.[195] This myofascial pain is thought to be caused by waste products produced by the muscles or from localized ischemia of those structures. An underlying cycle of abnormal relaxation in some muscles, with shortening, stretching, and a loss of tone in others, occurs during this process, with resultant joint strain and dysfunction.

As the head is brought forward by flexing the cervical segments, the scalene muscles are permitted to adaptively shorten, thus lessening the support of the upper ribs. The cervical flexion is followed by an increase of the thoracic curvature, and the tension of the spinal musculature increases.[236,237] In this position, capital extension must now occur to keep the eyes horizontal and allow the individual to look ahead.[182,238,239] This occipital hyperextension of the cranium on the cervical spine has been related to head, neck, and temporomandibular joint pain. A postural-pain relationship has been described by Willford and colleagues[240] in people wearing multifocal corrective lenses.

Under normal circumstances, the COG for the head falls slightly anterior to the ear. The habitual placement of the head anterior to the COG of the body places undue stress on the temporomandibular joint, the cervical and upper thoracic facet joints (especially at the cervicothoracic junction), and the supporting muscles.[183,184]

The abduction of the scapulae or protraction of the shoulders causes a lowering of the coracoid process, producing adaptive shortening of the pectoralis minor, which, in turn, may flatten the anterior chest wall and alter the motion of the scapula, producing a mechanical impairment of the shoulder.

Protraction of the shoulder girdles also limits extension of the upper thoracic spine, which, in turn, limits elevation and abduction of the shoulders. This alteration can lead to a hypermobility or instability of the glenohumeral joint and overuse syndromes of the shoulder elevators or abductors. Shoulder protraction also causes the humerus to rotate internally which stretches the posterior glenohumeral joint capsule; in addition, it increases the anterior force at the joint as a result of gravity. The former may lead to posterior instability and rotatory hypermobility, and the latter to anterior instability and a biceps tendonitis, as this muscle becomes overused in its attempt to stabilize the glenohumeral joint.

The anteriorly displaced line of gravity induced by the forward head posture has an effect on respiration. This change in posture is postulated to have the following consequences[241]:

1. ***Open-mouth breathing.***[242] Open-mouth breathing is the normal pattern of breathing for a newborn. This pattern of breathing becomes abnormal if it persists into the 5–7 years. A child with a long bout of sinus infections and blockages is forced to use mouth breathing as the primary method of breathing. With the development of the teeth and tongue, the oral passageway for air is gradually reduced, forcing the child to open the mouth further in order to breathe. It is postulated that this can result in[243–245]:
   - a failure to filter inspired air of pathogens and particles. These particles go directly into the alveoli, producing an

inflammatory reaction in the lungs that results in bronchospasm or asthma and stimulates a future hypersensitivity to any new particles;

- a failure to humidify inspired air, so that the air entering the lungs is dry;
- a failure to warm the inspired air. Cold or cool air entering the lungs stimulates an increased presence of white blood cells, increasing the hypersensitivity of the lungs. Early intervention with mouth breathers is essential, and it is recommended that the child be encouraged to keep the tongue against the roof of the mouth while breathing.

2. ***Thoracic hyperflexion.*** Although only theoretical, the thoracic compensation is necessary to counteract the backward tilting of the head and to return the eyes to a horizontal position. This compensation produces the following:
   - A reduction in thoracic extension.
   - A reduced ability of the ribs to elevate during inspiration, resulting from a reduced ability of the thoracic cavity to expand during inspiration.[243–245]
   - An increase in the respiratory rate.[243–245]
   - A shortening of the scalene muscles. Because of their newly acquired shortened position, the muscles have a reduced ability to contract, resulting in a reduced ability to elevate the first rib; a reduced ability to increase the vertical dimension of the thoracic cavity during inspiration[242–244]; and an increase in apical breathing.[243–245]

The forces from the cervical and thoracic regions of the spine can be transmitted to the lumbar spine, increasing the lordotic curve.[246,247] The exaggeration of the lumbar curve is accompanied by a shift of the weight to the posterior part of the vertebral bodies and to the articular processes, producing maximum joint strain of the lumbosacral junction and a forward inclination of the pelvis.

The increased forward inclination of the pelvis may produce a shortening of the erector spinae group and flexors of the hip, accompanied by a lengthening of the abdominal and hamstring muscles. These muscle imbalances serve to maintain the deformity.[248]

The intervention for forward head is outlined in Chapter 25.

Dynamic Examination

It should be apparent that any postural examination should include a dynamic assessment, as a static examination alone cannot demonstrate the effect of a particular posture on function. A dynamic examination that assesses functional movement patterns, such as the *Selective Functional Movement Assessment*[249,250], helps the clinician to ascertain whether the apparent postural abnormality is dysfunctional. The Selective Functional Movement Assessment assesses functional movement using four categories:

- Functional and nonpainful
- Functional and painful
- Dysfunctional and nonpainful
- Dysfunctional and painful

Within these categories, the term *functional* describes any unlimited or unrestricted movement, whereas the term *dysfunctional* is used to describe movements that are limited or restricted and which reproduce pain and/or demonstrate a lack of mobility, stability, or symmetry within a given functional movement. Although most clinicians can appreciate that repeated movement patterns performed in a therapeutic manner may be beneficial, it must also be remembered that repeated motions performed erroneously can produce changes in muscle tension, muscle strength, length, and stiffness.[204] It is quite normal for muscles to frequently change their lengths during movements. However, this change in resting length may become pathologic, when it is sustained through incorrect habituation or as a response to pain.

The dynamic postural examination can also be designed to assess each joint to its extremes of motion. The following should serve as a guideline:

- Joints of the extremities: active movements through the full range of each direction for each joint, with passive overpressure and a maximum isometric contraction applied at the end range. Combined motions should also be assessed, for example, elbow flexion and supination.
- Joints of the spine: flexion, extension, side bending, and rotation of the cervical, thoracic, and lumbar spine in sitting, standing, and lying as appropriate. Combined motion should also be assessed, for example, cervical flexion with rotation superimposed on the flexion.
- Functional movements: deep squatting (heels flat and shoulders flexed), Apley scratch test (fingertips touching behind the back).

During these various movements, the clinician is looking for symmetry, ease of movement, and the provocation of any symptoms.

Special Tests

The special tests used in the assessment of posture include all those that are related to the assessment of muscle length and strength. Examples include manual muscle testing, the Thomas test, and the Ober test. These tests are described in the relevant chapters. In addition, the clinician should examine neurodynamic mobility for the presence of adverse neural tension (see Chapter 11).

Intervention

The focus of therapeutic intervention for posture and movement impairment syndromes is to alleviate symptoms and to play a significant role in educating the patient against habitual abuse. Interestingly, despite the widespread inclusion of postural correction in therapeutic interventions, there is limited experimental data to support its effectiveness. Therapeutic exercise programs for the correction of muscle imbalances traditionally focus on regaining the normal length of a muscle, so that good movement patterns can be achieved. The intervention of any muscle imbalance is divided into three stages:

1. Restoration of normal length of the muscles. If the muscle activity is inhibited, the muscle should be stretched in the inhibitory phase. If the muscle is hypertonic, muscle energy

techniques may be used to produce minimal facilitation and a minimal stretch. With true adaptive shortening of the muscle, stronger resistance is used to activate the maximum number of motor units, followed by vigorous stretching of the muscle.

2. Strengthening of the muscles that have become inhibited and weak. Vigorous strengthening should be initially avoided to prevent substitutions and the reinforcement of poor patterns of movement.
3. Establishing optimal motor patterns to secure the best possible protection to the joints and the surrounding soft tissues.

In addition to using specific techniques to stretch and strengthen muscles, muscle energy (see Chapter 10), proprioceptive neuromuscular facilitation, and the incorporation of a more "wholistic" approach can often have a beneficial effect on postural dysfunction and movement impairment. There is a growing interest in the field of integrative care—the blending of complementary or *wholistic* therapies with conventional medical practice. Wholistic approaches provide whole-person care—addressing people rather than diseases, caring rather than curing, using all possible therapeutic modalities rather than a limited few, and empowering patients wherever possible to use self-care approaches and to be active participants in decisions regarding their health.

Examples of these "wholistic" approaches, currently used in association with physical therapy, include the Alexander technique, Feldenkrais method, Trager psychophysical integration (TPI), Pilates, Tai Chi Chuan (TCC), and yoga.

Alexander Technique

The Alexander technique[251] is commonly viewed as a series of breathing and posture techniques. However, the purpose of the technique is to make patients more aware of structural imbalances, different ways of moving, and the excessive tensions that can be produced in activities of daily living. Although it is not within the scope of this chapter to fully describe the Alexander technique, some of its principles are outlined here, and the reader is encouraged to learn more about this technique through further reading.

The Alexander technique uses reeducation to change the thought processes, as well as the postural and movement habits, that are theorized to provoke pain. According to this theory, the main reflex in the body, termed the *primary control*, which is situated in the area of the neck, controls all of the other reflexes of the body. Dysfunction of this main reflex, resulting from increased tension in the neck, causes a pulling back of the head and changes the relationship of the neck and back, eventually causing tensions in other parts of the body.

Based on these assumptions, Alexander devised three *directions*[251]:

1. ***Allow the neck to be free.*** The purpose of this direction is to eliminate any excess tension in the muscles of the neck.
2. ***Allow the head to go forward and upward.*** When the neck muscles are released, the head goes slightly forward and upward.
3. ***Allow the back to lengthen and widen.*** As the head moves slightly forward and upward, the spine lengthens. Because an increase in the spine length can also narrow the spine, widening of the back, through a retraction of the shoulders and broadening of the rib cage, is encouraged.

Feldenkrais Method

The Feldenkrais method of somatic education is a self-discovery process using movement. It was developed by Dr Moshe Feldenkrais, a physicist and electronics engineer. The aim of the Feldenkrais method is for an individual to move through relaxation and self-awareness, with minimum effort and maximum efficiency. The method teaches that many pains and movement restrictions are the result not of an actual physical defect or the inevitable deteriorations of age, but of habitual poor use.[252] Over time, this causes fatigue, disability, and pain.

The antidote, according to Feldenkrais, is to relearn certain functional movements and postures using the so-called organic learning style, based on the way humans learn to perform, as they develop during early childhood. During this growth phase, some of the movements are learned correctly, others are not. Incorrect movement patterns may result in inefficient movements or restrictions to movements. In humans, the premotor cortex relates to posture stability and the act of reaching. It is also the supplementary motor area for planning, programming, and initiating movement.[253] These latter components require correct sequencing and organization. The Feldenkrais method is seen as a way of reprogramming the nervous system and reteaching the body how to perform the functional movement patterns correctly.

Functional movement patterns involve the integration and sequencing of movement patterns while maintaining neuromuscular control. These patterns and postures are developed using the two aspects of the Feldenkrais method: awareness through movement (ATM) and functional integration (FI). Although closely related, ATM and FI have fundamental differences:

- ATM is usually done in a group, whereas FI involves one-on-one learning.
- ATM involves the performance of gentle exploratory movements using verbal guidance. In contrast, FI uses guidance into nonhabitual movements, with tactile cueing by a trained practitioner.

Both the aspects work toward changing old movement patterns or creating new movement patterns. Individuals are led through a series of movement sequences. All movements are performed slowly, without pause and short of the range of discomfort and pain. The proponents of the Feldenkrais method claim that these movements promote improved attention and awareness.[254] It is also claimed that these movements refine the ability to detect information and make perceptual discriminations.[254] Regular use of such attentive explorations and integration of the skills lead to an automatic use of these motor abilities. An example of a Feldenkrais exercise is to move one's head in one direction and one's shoulder and eyes in the other.[255] These movement sequences are usually repeated a number of times.

Five key principles are involved in the development of the Feldenkrais method:[254,256]

1. Self-organization: Dynamic systems theorists believe that behaviors are assembled in the moment and context of the current movement task.
2. Behavior is dynamic and plastic.
3. Perturbation is the instrument of change.
4. Choice is necessary.
5. Human development follows a logical sequence.

The Feldenkrais method is both educational and experimental. It is process-, not goal-, oriented and is entirely pragmatic.[257] With acute conditions, the patient is started in the position of maximum comfort. The lesson then uses any movement, however small, within the limit of comfort. The patient is encouraged to become aware of the smoothness and clarity of the movement. The movement is repeated and practiced. Further movements within this framework are investigated and practiced. These movements are simple initially, becoming more complex as the patient gains confidence.[257]

Trager Psychophysical Integration

TPI is a multifaceted intervention, consisting of light, gentle, and painless movements to facilitate the release of deep-seated physical (and mental) patterns.[258] TPI was designed at the beginning of the twentieth century by Dr Milton Trager and has been shown to be effective in promoting mobility and decreasing pain for patients with a wide variety of diagnoses, including cerebral palsy,[259] chronic spinal pain and dysfunction,[260] and arthritis.[258,261]

According to TPI philosophy, detrimental physical patterns are those developed by poor posture, trauma, stress, and poor movement habits.[262] Trager techniques serve to produce overall relaxation on the part of the patient, developing a sense of integration and effortless movement through a series of guided movements and mental gymnastics.[263,264]

The Trager approach is broken down into two components: *tablework* and *mentastics*.

Tablework

Tablework consists of a series of gentle and painless movements that resemble general mobilization techniques. The body of the patient is passively moved by the clinician who looks and feels for involvement of the tissue. The aim is to provoke a feeling of softness and freedom to motion throughout the body.[260] Using these movements, the entire body is mobilized. Rhythmic rocking motions are initiated during these movements to stimulate the vestibular and reticular activating systems of the patient. This is theorized to produce an overall sense of relaxation and well-being through an inhibition of the sympathetic system and the facilitation of the parasympathetic system.[265]

Mentastics

Mentastics is a system of active movements, designed to enhance the feeling of well-being provided by the tablework exercises. Mentastics encourage the patient *not* to control the movement, as in traditional exercise, but to *let go* of the control.[260] The patient is taught to listen to signals of pain and fatigue and to change the symptoms by altering the movement. Over time, the patient learns how to move comfortably and to release tension.[264]

Pilates

The Pilates method of body conditioning (Pilates Inc.) is a technique and apparatus developed in the 1940s by Joseph Pilates, who was prone to chronic illness as a child.

The Pilates method was first embraced by the dance community, but its inherent concept of core stabilization, mind–body awareness, and control of movement and posture has since been used successfully in rehabilitation, for the development of overall strength and fitness in patients with back pain, balance deficits, and urinary incontinence due to pelvic floor muscle weakness.

The Pilates method uses many of the concepts and techniques that physical therapists commonly employ, with an increased emphasis on neuromuscular control. As such, the Pilates method focuses on motor training, rather than on motor strength, using precise and controlled exercises. The Pilates method stresses the importance of the so-called powerhouse muscles of the body; deep, coordinated breathing; postural symmetry; and controlled movement. According to the Pilates method, the powerhouse muscles include the transversus abdominis, the lumbar multifidus, the pelvic floor muscles, and the diaphragm muscle. Approximately 10 repetitions are needed for each exercise.

The Pilates exercises emphasize the maintenance of a neutral spine throughout machine and mat exercises. Many of the Pilates exercises involve squeezing the inner thighs together in the Pilates stance, while simultaneously engaging the pelvic floor muscles, in an effort to increase trunk stability. The *Pilates stance* involves slight external rotation in both hips and lower extremities, while maintaining the thighs in firm contact. Other Pilates exercises include instructions on how to isolate a transversus abdominis contraction from the rest of the abdominal muscles. This is commonly achieved using the verbal cueing of "pull your belly button toward your spine." This contraction is then practiced in a variety of positions and techniques, in order to enhance spinal, or core, stability. Pelvic stability is encouraged with such verbal cueing as "pull your sitting bones together," thereby producing a contraction of the ischiococcygeal muscle that provides support for the pelvic contents, in addition to contributing to sacroiliac joint stability.

Although many of the Pilates exercises can be performed on mats, specially designed Pilates equipment may also be used. Four basic machines comprise the Pilates equipment line:

1. ***Reformer.*** This is the basic machine of the Pilates method. It resembles a twin bed in size and frame and is equipped with handholds, pulleys, and cables that exercisers push or pull with their hands or feet. The reformer usually is used in the rehabilitation of hamstring tears, stress fractures, and low back injuries.
2. ***Cadillac or trapeze table.*** This piece of equipment is equipped with multiple bars and straps and features a pull-down bar. It is used for overall conditioning.
3. ***Multichair.*** The multichair is the equipment of choice for footwork and for ankle rehabilitation. It can be adapted for such activities as one-arm pushes, lunges, and dips.

4. ***Ladder-barrel.*** This piece of equipment consists of a sliding base and five rungs and is used for a variety of strengthening and flexibility exercises.

The use of Pilates apparatus to train stabilization strategies during movement may enhance the effect of the more relatively static mat exercises.

Tai Chi Chuan

TCC is a Chinese low-speed and low-impact conditioning exercise and is well known for its slow and graceful movements. During the practice, diaphragmatic breathing is coordinated with graceful motions to achieve mind tranquility.

Classical Yang TCC includes 108 postures, with some repeated sequences. Each training session includes 20 minutes of warm-up, 24 minutes of TCC practice, and 10 minutes of cool down.[240] Warm-up exercise is very important, because it may enhance TCC performance and prevent injury. It usually includes 10 movements (ROM exercises, stretching, and balance training), with 10–20 repetitions.[266]

The exercise intensity of TCC depends on training style, posture, and duration.[267,268] A high-squat posture and short training duration are suited to those with low levels of fitness or elderly participants; a low-squat posture and longer durations are suited to healthy or younger participants.[266]

Recent investigations have found that TCC is beneficial to cardiorespiratory function,[269] strength,[270] balance,[270,271] flexibility,[271] microcirculation,[272] and psychological profile.[267] Hartman and colleagues[273] also reported that TCC could control fatigue and regulate pain during activities and could improve walking speed and self-care activities in patients with osteoarthritis.

Yoga

Yoga, a literal translation from the Sanskrit word for "union," is a 5000-year-old Indian practice. There are 40 main schools of yoga philosophy, of which Hatha (pronounced haht-ha) yoga is the most popular in the United States. According to Indian tradition, Hatha yoga is one of the four main traditions of Tantra yoga, a holistic approach to the study of the universe from the point of the individual. Hatha yoga is based on the practice of physical postures (asanas), breath control (pranayama), and meditation in order to energize subtle channels of the mind called nadis.

- ***Asanas.*** Physical postures that are performed using isometric contractions and held firmly from a time that ranges from seconds to minutes. There are 84 basic asanas in Hatha yoga, which are categorized in accordance with the movement they create in the body.
- ***Pranayama.*** Yoga breathing is performed slowly and without strain throughout the routine, with a brief pause of 1–2 seconds after each inhalation and exhalation.

The theoretical benefits associated with yoga encompass physiological, psychological, psychomotor, cognitive, and biochemical aspects. The physiological, psychological, psychomotor, and cognitive benefits include reduced stress; improved attention, memory, and learning efficiency; decreased pulse rate, respiratory rate, and blood pressure; and increased muscular strength and aerobic and muscular endurance.[274–281] The biochemical benefits include an increase in high-density lipoprotein cholesterol, a decrease in low-density lipoprotein cholesterol, and an increase in hematocrit levels.[274]

REVIEW QUESTIONS*

1. List the two phases and three tasks of the gait cycle.
2. List, in order of occurrence, the eight intervals of the gait cycle.
3. As speed increases, what effect is there on the stance phase and the double stance phase?
4. True or false: The thoracic spine and the pelvis rotate in opposite directions to each other during the gait cycle.
5. From midstance to terminal stance, in which direction should the ilium rotate?
6. Describe the characteristics of the *lower crossed syndrome*.
7. List five causes of postural dysfunction.
8. Describe the different characteristics of the two functional divisions of muscles outlined by Janda and Jull.

*Additional questions to test your understanding of this chapter can be found in the Online Learning Center for Orthopaedic Assessment, Evaluation, and Intervention at www.duttononline.net.

REFERENCES

1. Rose J: Dynamic lower extremity stability. In: Hughes C, ed. *Movement Disorders and Neuromuscular Interventions for the Trunk and Extremities – Independent Study Course 18.2.5.* La Crosse, WI: Orthopaedic Section, APTA, Inc., 2008:1–34.
2. Das P, McCollum G: Invariant structure in locomotion. *Neuroscience* 25:1023–1034, 1988.
3. Mann RA, Hagy JL, White V, et al: The initiation of gait. *J Bone Joint Surg Am* 61A:232–239, 1979.
4. Luttgens K, Hamilton N: Locomotion: Solid surface. In: Luttgens K, Hamilton N, eds. *Kinesiology: Scientific Basis of Human Motion*, 9th ed. Dubuque, IA: McGraw-Hill, 1997:519–549.
5. Dobkin BH, Harkema S, Requejo P, et al: Modulation of locomotor-like EMG activity in subjects with complete and incomplete spinal cord injury. *J Neurol Rehabil* 9:183–190, 1995.
6. Donatelli R, Wilkes R: Lower kinetic chain and human gait. *J Back Musculoskelet Rehabil* 2:1–11, 1992.
7. Levine D, Whittle M: *Gait Analysis: The Lower Extremities.* La Crosse, WI: Orthopaedic Section, APTA, Inc., 1992.
8. Mann RA, Hagy J: Biomechanics of walking, running, and sprinting. *Am J Sports Med* 8:345–350, 1980.
9. Murray MP: Gait as a total pattern of movement. *Am J Phys Med* 46:290, 1967.
10. Scranton PE, Rutkowski R, Brown TD: Support phase kinematics of the foot. In: Bateman JE, Trott AW, eds. *The Foot and Ankle.* New York, NY: BC Decker Inc., 1980:195–205.
11. Perry J: Gait cycle. In: Perry J, ed. *Gait Analysis: Normal and Pathological Function.* Thorofare, NJ: Slack Inc, 1992:3–7.
12. Perry J: Stride analysis. In: Perry J, ed. *Gait Analysis: Normal and Pathological Function.* Thorofare, NJ: Slack Inc, 1992:431–441.
13. Mann RA, Moran GT, Dougherty SE: Comparative electromyography of the lower extremity in jogging, running and sprinting. *Am J Sports Med* 14:501–510, 1986.
14. Luttgens K, Hamilton N: The center of gravity and stability. In: Luttgens K, Hamilton N, eds. *Kinesiology: Scientific Basis of Human Motion*, 9th ed. Dubuque, IA: McGraw-Hill, 1997:415–442.

15. Epler M: Gait. In: Richardson JK, Iglarsh ZA, eds. *Clinical Orthopaedic Physical Therapy*. Philadelphia, PA: WB Saunders, 1994:602–625.
16. Subotnick SI: Variations in angles of gait in running. *Phys Sportsmed* 7:110–114, 1979.
17. Ostrosky KM, Van Sweringen JM, Burdett RG, et al: A comparison of gait characteristics in young and old subjects. *Phys Ther* 74:637–646, 1994.
18. Adelaar RS: The practical biomechanics of running. *Am J Sports Med* 14:497–500, 1986.
19. Basmajian JVe: *Therapeutic Exercise*, 3rd ed. Baltimore, MD: Williams & Wilkins, 1979.
20. Perry J: *Gait Analysis: Normal and Pathological Function*. Thorofare, NJ: Slack Inc, 1992.
21. Rogers MM: Dynamic foot mechanics. *J Orthop Sports Phys Ther* 21:306–316, 1995.
22. Gage JR, Deluca PA, Renshaw TS: Gait analysis: Principles and applications with emphasis on its use with cerebral palsy. *Instr Course Lect* 45:491–507, 1996.
23. Frey C: Foot health and shoewear for women. *Clin Orthop Relat Res* 372:32–44, 2000.
24. Oberg T, Karsznia A, Oberg K: Basic gait parameters: Reference data for normal subjects, 10–79 years of age. *J Rehabil Res Dev* 30:210–223, 1993.
25. Molen NH, Rozendal RH, Boon W: Fundamental characteristics of human gait in relation to sex and location. Proceedings of the Koninklijke Nederlandse Akademie van Wetenschappen-Series C. *Biol Med Sci* 45:215–223, 1972.
26. Finley FR, Cody KA: Locomotive characteristics of urban pedestrians. *Arch Phys Med Rehabil* 51:423–426, 1970.
27. Sato H, Ishizu K: Gait patterns of Japanese pedestrians. *J Hum Ergol (Tokyo)* 19:13–22, 1990.
28. Richard R, Weber J, Mejjad O, et al: Spatiotemporal gait parameters measured using the Bessou gait analyzer in 79 healthy subjects: Influence of age, stature, and gender. *Rev Rhum Engl Ed* 62:105–114, 1995.
29. Murray MP, Kory RC, Sepic SB: Walking patterns of normal women. *Arch Phys Med Rehabil* 51:637–650, 1970.
30. Murray MP, Drought AB, Kory RC: Walking patterns of normal men. *J Bone Joint Surg Am* 46A:335–360, 1964.
31. Bhambhani Y, Singh M: Metabolic and cinematographic analysis of walking and running in men and women. *Med Sci Sports Exerc* 17:131–137, 1985.
32. Giannini S, Catani F, Benedetti MG, et al: *Terminology, Parameterization and Normalization in Gait Analysis, Gait Analysis: Methodologies and Clinical Applications*. Washington, DC: IOS Press, 1994:65–88.
33. Perry J: *The hip, Gait Analysis: Normal and Pathological Function*. Thorofare, NJ: Slack Inc, 1992:111–129.
34. Reinking MF: Knee anatomy and biomechanics. In: Wadsworth C, ed. *Disorders of the Knee – Home Study Course*. La Crosse, WI: Orthpaedic Section, APTA, Inc., 2001.
35. Norkin C, Levangie P: *Joint Structure and Function: A Comprehensive Analysis*. Philadelphia, PA: F.A. Davis Company, 1992.
36. Kuster MS, Wood GA, Stachowiak GW, et al: Joint load considerations in total knee replacement. *J Bone Joint Surg Br* 79B:109–113, 1997.
37. Andriacchi TP, Ogle JA, Galante JO: Walking speed as a basis for normal and abnormal gait measurements. *J Biomech* 10:261–268, 1977.
38. Corrigan J, Moore D, Stephens M: The effect of heel height on forefoot loading. *Foot Ankle* 11:418–422, 1991.
39. Arsenault AB, Winter DA, Marteniuk RG: Is there a 'normal' profile of EMG activity in gait? *Med Biol Eng Comput* 24:337–343, 1986.
40. Berchuck M, Andriacchi TP, Bach BR, et al: Gait adaptations by patients who have a deficient anterior cruciate ligament. *J Bone Joint Surg Am* 72-A:871–877, 1990.
41. Boeing DD: Evaluation of a clinical method of gait analysis. *Phys Ther* 57:795–798, 1977.
42. Dillon P, Updyke W, Allen W: Gait analysis with reference to chondromalacia patellae. *J Orthop Sports Phys Ther* 5:127–131, 1983.
43. Hunt GC, Brocato RS: Gait and foot pathomechanics. In: Hunt GC, ed. *Physical Therapy of the Foot and Ankle*. Edinburgh: Churchill Livingstone, 1988:39–57.
44. Krebs DE, Robbins CE, Lavine L, et al: Hip biomechanics during gait. *J Orthop Sports Phys Ther* 28:51–59, 1998.
45. Luttgens K, Hamilton N: The standing posture. In: Luttgens K, Hamilton N, eds. *Kinesiology: Scientific Basis of Human Motion*, 9th ed. Dubuque, IA: McGraw-Hill, 1997:445–459.
46. Winter DA: Biomechanical motor patterns in normal walking. *J Mot Behav* 15:302–329, 1983.
47. Hoyt DF, Taylor CF: Gait and the energetics of locomotion in horses. *Nature* 292:239–240, 1981.
48. Corcoran PJ, Brengelmann G: Oxygen uptake in normal and handicapped subjects in relation to the speed of walking beside a velocity-controlled cart. *Arch Phys Med Rehabil* 51:78–87, 1970.
49. Gonzalez EG, Corcoran PJ, Reyes RL: Energy expenditure in below-knee amputees: correlation with stump length. *Arch Phys Med Rehabil* 55:111–119, 1974.
50. Waters RL, Hislop HJ, Perry J, et al: Energetics: Application to the study and management of locomotor disabilities. *Orthop Clin North Am* 9:351–377, 1978.
51. Martin PE, Rothstein DE, Larish DD: Effects of age and physical activity status on the speed-aerobic demand relationship of walking. *J Appl Physiol* 73:200–206, 1992.
52. Prampero PE: The energy cost of human locomotion on land and in the water. *Int J Sports Med* 7:55–72, 1986.
53. Davies MJ, Dalsky GP: Economy of mobility in older adults. *J Orthop Sports Phys Ther* 26:69–72, 1997.
54. Daniels J, Krahenbuhl G, Foster C, et al: Aerobic responses of female distance runners to submaximal and maximal exercise. *Ann N Y Acad Sci* 301:726–733, 1977.
55. Pate RR, Barnes CG, Miller CA: A physiological comparison of performance-matched female and male distance runners. *Res Q Exerc Sport* 56:245–250, 1985.
56. Wells CL, Hecht LH, Krahenbuhl GS: Physical characteristics and oxygen utilization of male and female marathon runners. *Res Q Exerc Sport* 52:281–285, 1981.
57. Bransford DR, Howley ET: Oxygen cost of running in trained and untrained men and women. *Med Sci Sports Exerc* 9:41–44, 1977.
58. Daniels J, Daniels N: Running economy of elite male and females runners. *Med Sci Sports Exerc* 24:483–489, 1992.
59. Howley ET, Glover ME: The caloric costs of running and walking one mile for men and women. *Med Sci Sports Exerc* 6:235–237, 1974.
60. Larish DD, Martin PE, Mungiole M: Characteristic patterns of gait in the healthy old. *Ann N Y Acad Sci* 515:18–32, 1987.
61. Waters RL, Hislop HJ, Perry J, et al: Comparative cost of walking in young and old adults. *J Orthop Res* 1:73–76, 1983.
62. Allen W, Seals DR, Hurley BF, et al: Lactate threshold and distance running performance in young and older endurance athletes. *J Appl Physiol* 58:1281–1284, 1985.
63. Trappe SW, Costill DL, Vukovich MD, et al: Aging among elite distance runners: A 22-year longitudinal study. *J Appl Physiol* 80:285–290, 1996.
64. Wells CL, Boorman MA, Riggs DM: Effect of age and menopausal status on cardiorespiratory fitness in masters women runners. *Med Sci Sports Exerc* 24:1147–1154, 1992.
65. Moseley CF: Leg-length discrepancy. In: Morrissy RT, ed. *Lovell and Winter's Pediatric Orthopaedics*, 3rd ed. Philadelphia, PA: J. B. Lippincott, 1990:767–813.
66. Beaty JH: Congenital anomalies of lower extremity. In: Crenshaw AH, ed. *Campbell's Operative Orthopaedics*, 8th ed. St. Louis, MO: Mosby-Year Book, 1992:2126–2158.
67. Gross RH: Leg length discrepancy: How much is too much? *Orthopedics* 1:307–310, 1978.
68. Song KM, Halliday SE, Little DG: The effect of limb-length discrepancy on gait. *J Bone Joint Surg Am* 79A:1690–1698, 1997.
69. Lange GW, Hintermeister RA, Schlegel T, et al: Electromyographic and kinematic analysis of graded treadmill walking and the implications for knee rehabilitation. *J Orthop Sports Phys Ther* 23:294–301, 1996.
70. Croskey MI, Dawson PM, Luessen AC, et al: The height of the center of gravity in man. *Am J Physiol* 61:171–185, 1922.
71. Saunders JBD, Inman VT, Eberhart HD: The major determinants in normal and pathological gait. *J Bone Joint Surg Am* 35:543–558, 1953.
72. Whitehouse PA, Knight LA, Di Nicolantonio F, et al: Heterogeneity of chemosensitivity of colorectal adenocarcinoma determined by a modified ex vivo ATP-tumor chemosensitivity assay (ATP-TCA). *Anticancer Drugs* 14:369–75, 2003.
73. Richardson JK, Iglarsh ZA: Gait. In: Richardson JK, Iglarsh ZA, eds. *Clinical Orthopaedic Physical Therapy*. Philadelphia, PA: Saunders, 1994:602–625.
74. Craik R, Herman RM, Finley FR: The human solutions for locomotion: Interlimb coordination. In: Herman RM, Grillner S, Stein PS, eds. *Neural Control of Locomotion*. New York, NY: Plenum, 1976:51–63.
75. Wagenaar RC, Van Emmerik RE: Dynamics of pathological gait: Stability and adaptability of movement coordination. *Hum Mov Sci* 13:441–471, 1994.

76. Van Emmerik RE, Wagenaar RC, Van Wegen EE: Interlimb coupling patterns in human locomotion: Are we bipeds or quadrupeds? *Ann N Y Acad Sci* 860:539–542, 1998.
77. Murray MP, Sepic SB, Barnard EJ: Patterns of sagittal rotation of the upper limbs in walking. *Phys Ther* 47:272–284, 1967.
78. Hogue RE: Upper extremity muscular activity at different cadences and inclines during normal gait. *Phys Ther* 49:963–972, 1969.
79. Oatis CA: Role of the hip in posture and gait. In: Echternach J, ed. *Clinics in Physical Therapy: Physical Therapy of the Hip*. New York, NY: Churchill Livingstone, 1983:165–179.
80. Gage JR: *Gait Analysis in Cerebral Palsy*. London: MacKeith Press, 1991.
81. Hejgaard RJ, Sandberg H, Hede A, et al: The course of differently treated isolated ruptures of the anterior cruciate ligament as observed by prospective stress radiography. *Clin Orthop* 182:236–241, 1984.
82. Johnson RJ, Erickson E, Haggmark T, et al: Five to ten year follow-up evaluation after reconstruction of the anterior cruciate ligament. *Clin Orthop* 83:122–140, 1984.
83. Straub T, Hunter RE: Acute anterior cruciate ligament repair. *Clin Orthop* 227:238–250, 1988.
84. Palmitier RA, An KN, Scott SG, et al: Kinetic chain exercises in knee rehabilitation. *Sports Med* 11:402–413, 1991.
85. Paulos LE, Noyes FR, Grood ES: Knee rehabilitation after anterior cruciate ligament reconstruction and repair. *Am J Sports Med* 9:140–149, 1981.
86. Ahmed AM, Burke DL: In vitro measurement of static pressure distribution in synovial joints: I. Tibial surface of the knee. *J Biomed Eng* 105:216-225, 1983.
87. Huberti HH, Hayes WC: Contact pressures in chondromalacia patellae and the effects of capsular reconstructive procedures. *J Orthop Res* 6:499–508, 1988.
88. Matthews LS, Sonstegard DA, Henke JA: Load bearing characteristics of the patello-femoral joint. *Acta Orthop Scand* 48:511–516, 1977.
89. Bourne MH, Hazel WA, Scott SG, et al: Anterior knee pain. *Mayo Clin Proc* 63:482–491, 1988.
90. Perry J: Ankle and foot gait deviations. In: Perry J, ed. *Gait Analysis: Normal and Pathological Function*. Thorofare, NJ: Slack, Inc., 1992:185–220.
91. Hunt GC: *Functional biomechanics of the subtalar joint, Orthopaedic Physical Therapy Home Study Course 92-1: Lower Extremity*. La Crosse, WI: Orthopaedic Section, APTA, Inc., 1992.
92. Donatelli R: Normal anatomy and pathophysiology of the foot and ankle. In: Wadsworth C, ed. *Contemporary Topics on the Foot and Ankle*. La Crosse, WI: Orthopedic Section, APTA, Inc., 2000.
93. Root M, Orien W, Weed J: *Clinical biomechanics: normal and abnormal function of the foot*. Los Angeles, CA: Clinical Biomechanics Corp, 1977.
94. Inman VT, Ralston HJ, Todd F: *Human Walking*. Baltimore, MD: Williams & Wilkins, 1981.
95. Mann RA: Biomechanical approach to the treatment of foot problems. *Foot Ankle* 2:205–212, 1982.
96. Bojsen-Möller F, Lamoreux L: Significance of dorsiflexion of the toes in walking. *Acta Orthop Scand* 50:471–479, 1979.
97. Mann RA, Hagy JL: The function of the toes in walking, jogging and running. *Clin Orthop* 142:24, 1979.
98. Bojsen-Möller F: Normal and pathologic anatomy of metatarsals [German]. *Orthopade* 11:148–153, 1982.
99. Bojsen-Möller F: Calcaneocuboid joint and stability of the longitudinal arch of the foot at high and low gear push off. *J Anat* 129:165–176, 1979.
100. Perry J: The mechanics of walking: A clinical interpretation. In: Perry J, Hislop HJ, eds. *Principles of Lower Extremity Bracing*. New York, NY: American Physical Therapy Association, 1967:9–32.
101. Dee R: Normal and abnormal gait in the pediatric patient. In: Dee R, Hurst LC, Gruber MA, et al. eds. *Principles of Orthopaedic Practice*, 2nd ed. New York, NY: McGraw-Hill, 1997:685–692.
102. Donatelli RA: Normal anatomy and biomechanics. In: Donatelli RA, ed. *Biomechanics of the Foot and Ankle*. Philadelphia, PA: WB Saunders, 1990:3–31.
103. Yoon YS, Mansour JM: The passive elastic moment at the hip. *J Biomech* 15:905–910, 1982.
104. Lehmkuhl LD, Smith LK: *Brunnstrom's Clinical Kinesiology*. Philadelphia, PA: F.A. Davis Company, 1983:361–390.
105. Neumann DA, Cook TM: Effects of load and carry position on the electromyographic activity of the gluteus medius muscles during walking. *Phys Ther* 65:305–311, 1985.
106. Neumann DA, Cook TM, Sholty RL, et al: An electromyographic analysis of hip abductor activity when subjects are carrying loads in one or both hands. *Phys Ther* 72:207–217, 1992.
107. Neumann DA, Hase AD: An electromyographic analysis of the hip abductors during load carriage: Implications for joint protection. *J Orthop Sports Phys Ther* 19:296–304, 1994.
108. Neumann DA, Soderberg GL, Cook TM: Comparisons of maximal isometric hip abductor muscle torques between sides. *Phys Ther* 68:496–502, 1988.
109. Neumann DA, Soderberg GL, Cook TM: Electromyographic analysis of the hip abductor musculature in healthy right-handed persons. *Phys Ther* 69:431–440, 1989.
110. Adler N, Perry J, Kent B, et al: Electromyography of the vastus medialis oblique and vasti in normal subjects during gait. *Electromyogr Clin Neurophysiol* 23:643–649, 1983.
111. Battye CK, Joseph J: An investigation by telemetering of the activity of some muscles in walking. *Med Biol Eng Comput* 4:125–135, 1966.
112. Dubo HIC, Peat M, Winter DA, et al: Electromyographic temporal analysis of gait: Normal human locomotion. *Arch Phys Med Rehabil* 57:415–420, 1976.
113. Brandell BR: Functional roles of the calf and vastus muscles in locomotion. *Am J Phys Med Rehabil* 56:59–74, 1977.
114. Ciccotti MG, Kerlan RK, Perry J, et al: An electromyographical analysis of the knee during functional activities-I. The normal profile. *Am J Sports Med* 22:645–650, 1994.
115. Baratta R, Solomonow M, Zhou BH, et al: Muscular coactivation: The role of the antagonist musculature in maintaining knee stability. *Am J Sports Med* 16:113–122, 1988.
116. Draganich LF, Jaeger RJ, Fralj AR: Coactivation of the hamstrings and quadriceps during extension of the knee. *J Bone Joint Surg Am* 71A:1076–1081, 1989.
117. Molbech S: On the paradoxical effect of some two-joint muscles. *Acta Morphol Neerl Scand* 6:171, 1965.
118. Basmajian JV, Deluca CJ: *Muscles Alive: Their Functions Revealed by Electromyography*. Baltimore, MD, Williams & Wilkins, 1985.
119. Rose J, Gamble JG: *Human Walking*. Baltimore, MD: Williams & Wilkins, 1994.
120. Mann RA: *Biomechanics of running, AAOS Symposium on the Foot and Leg in Running Sports*. St. Louis, MO: CV Mosby Co, 1982:30–44.
121. Teitz CC, Garrett WE Jr, Miniaci A, et al: Tendon problems in athletic individuals. *J Bone Joint Surg* 79-A:138–152, 1997.
122. Kadaba MP, Ramakrishnan HK, Wootten ME, et al: Repeatability of kinematic, kinetic, and electromyographic data in normal adult gait. *J Orthop Res* 7:849–860, 1989.
123. Krebs DE, Edelstein JE, Fishman S: Reliability of observational kinematic gait analysis. *Phys Ther* 65:1027–1033, 1985.
124. Skaggs DL, Rethlefsen SA, Kay RM, et al: Variability in gait analysis interpretation. *J Pediatr Orthop* 20:759–764, 2000.
125. Eastlack ME, Arvidson J, Snyder-Mackler L, et al: Interrater reliability of videotaped observational gait-analysis assessments. *Phys Ther* 71:465–472, 1991.
126. VanSweringen JM, Paschal K, Bonino P, et al: The modified gait abnormality rating scale for recognizing the risk of recurrent falls in community-dwelling elderly adults. *Phys Ther* 76:994–1002, 1996.
127. Herdman SJ, Borello-France DF, Whitney SL: Treatment of vestibular hypofunction. In: Herdman SJ, ed. *Vestibular Rehabilitation*. Philadelphia, PA: FA Davis, 1994:287–315.
128. Wrisley DM, Marchetti GF, Kuharsky DK, et al: Reliability, internal consistency, and validity of data obtained with the functional gait assessment. *Phys Ther* 84:906–918, 2004.
129. Shumway-Cook A, Woollacott M: *Motor Control – Theory and Practical Applications*. Baltimore, MD: Williams & Wilkins, 1995.
130. McPoil TG, Schuit D, Knecht HG: A comparison of three positions used to evaluate tibial varum. *J Am Podiatr Med Assoc* 78:22–28, 1988.
131. Appling SA, Kasser RJ: Foot and ankle. In: Wadsworth C, ed. *Current Concepts of Orthopedic Physical Therapy – Home Study Course*. La Crosse, WI: Orthopaedic Section, APTA, 2001.
132. Hertling D, Kessler RM: *Management of Common Musculoskeletal Disorders: Physical Therapy principles and methods*, 3rd ed. Philadelphia, PA: Lippincott Williams & Wilkins, 1996.
133. Reid DC: *Sports Injury Assessment and Rehabilitation*. New York: Churchill Livingstone, 1992.
134. Perry J: Hip Gait Deviations. In: Perry J, ed. *Gait Analysis: Normal and Pathological Function*. Thorofare, NJ: Slack, Inc., 1992:245–263.

135. Noyes FR, Dunworth LA, Andriacchi TP, et al: Knee hyperextension gait abnormalities in unstable knees. *Am J Sports Med* 24:35–45, 1996.

136. Perry J: Pelvis and trunk pathological gait. In: Perry J, ed. *Gait Analysis: Normal and Pathological Function.* Thorofare, NJ: Slack, Inc., 1992:265–279.

137. Perry J: Knee Abnormal Gait. In: Perry J, ed. *Gait Analysis: Normal and Pathological Function.* Thorofare, NJ: Slack, Inc., 1992:223–243.

138. Stauffer RN, Chao EYS, Gyory AN: Biomechanical gait analysis of the diseased knee joint. *Clin Orthop* 126:246–255, 1977.

139. Rengachary SS: Gait and Station; examination of coordination. In: Wilkins RH, Rengachary SS, eds. *Neurosurgery*, 2nd ed. New York, NY: McGraw-Hill, 1996:133–137.

140. Eyring EJ, Murray W: The effect of joint position on the pressure of intra-articular effusion. *J Bone Joint Surg* 47A:313–322, 1965.

141. Vogt L, Pfeifer K, Banzer W: Neuromuscular control of walking with chronic low-back pain. *Man Ther* 8:21–28, 2003.

142. Childs JD, Sparto PJ, Fitzgerald GK, et al: Alterations in lower extremity movement and muscle activation patterns in individuals with knee osteoarthritis. *Clin Biomech* 19:44–49, 2004.

143. Kegelmeyer D: Stability of gait and fall prevention. In: Hughes C, ed. *Movement Disorders and Neuromuscular Interventions for the Trunk and Extremities – Independent Study Course 18.2.6.* La Crosse, WI: Orthopaedic Section, APTA, Inc., 2008:1–20.

144. Blair E, Stanley F: Issues in the classification and epidemiology of cerebral palsy. *Mental Retard Devel Disab Res Rev* 3:184–193, 1997.

145. Baddar A, Granata K, Damiano DL, et al: Ankle and knee coupling in patients with spastic diplegia: effects of gastrocnemius-soleus lengthening. *J Bone Joint Surg Am* 84A:736–744, 2002.

146. Abel MH, Damiano DL, Pannunzio M, et al: Muscle-tendon surgery in diplegic cerebral palsy: functional and mechanical changes. *J Pediatr Orthop* 19:366–375, 1999.

147. Davids JR, Foti T, Dabelstein J, et al: Voluntary (normal) versus obligatory (cerebral palsy) toe-walking in children: A kinematic, kinetic, and electromyographic analysis. *J Pediatr Orthop* 19:461–469, 1999.

148. Morag E, Hurwitz DE, Andriacchi TP, et al: Abnormalities in muscle function during gait in relation to the level of lumbar disc herniation. *Spine* 25:829–833, 2000.

149. Griffin PP, Walter WW, Shiavi R, et al: Habitual toe walkers: A clinical and EMG gait analysis. *J Bone Joint Surg Am* 59A:97–101, 1977.

150. Statham L, Murray MP: Early walking patterns of normal children. *Clin Orthop* 79:8–24, 1971.

151. Stricker SJ, Angulo JC: Idiopathic toe walking: A comparison of treatment methods. *J Pediatr Orthop* 18:289–293, 1998.

152. Foti T, Davids JR, Bagley A: A biomechanical analysis of gait during pregnancy. *J Bone Joint Surg Am* 82A:625–632, 2000.

153. National Center for Health Statistics: *Prevalence of Overweight and Obesity Among Adults: United States.* Hyattsville, MD, 2000.

154. Nantel J, Brochu M, Prince F: Locomotor strategies in obese and non-obese children. *Obesity (Silver Spring).* 14:1789–1794, 2006.

155. Gushue DL, Houck J, Lerner AL: Effects of childhood obesity on three-dimensional knee joint biomechanics during walking. *J Pediatr Orthop* 25:763–768, 2005.

156. de Souza SA, Faintuch J, Valezi AC, et al: Gait cinematic analysis in morbidly obese patients. *Obes Surg* 15:1238–1242, 2005.

157. Spyropoulos P, Pisciotta JC, Pavlou KN, et al: Biomechanical gait analysis in obese men. *Arch Phys Med Rehabil* 72:1065–1070, 1991.

158. Wearing SC, Hennig EM, Byrne NM, et al: The biomechanics of restricted movement in adult obesity. *Obes Rev* 7:13–24, 2006.

159. Hills AP, Hennig EM, Byrne NM, et al: The biomechanics of adiposity–structural and functional limitations of obesity and implications for movement. *Obes Rev* 3:35–43, 2002.

160. Solak AS, Kentel B, Ates Y: Does bilateral total knee arthroplasty affect gait in women? Comparison of gait analyses before and after total knee arthroplasty compared with normal knees. *J Arthroplasty* 20:745–750, 2005.

161. Benedetti MG, Catani F, Bilotta TW, et al: Muscle activation pattern and gait biomechanics after total knee replacement. *Clin Biomech (Bristol, Avon)* 18:871–876, 2003.

162. Madsen MS, Ritter MA, Morris HH, et al: The effect of total hip arthroplasty surgical approach on gait. *J Orthop Res* 22:44–50, 2004.

163. Holder CG, Haskvitz EM, Weltman A. The effects of assistive devices on the oxygen cost, cardiovascular stress, and perception of non-weight-bearing ambulation. *J Orthop Sports Phys Ther* 1993;18:537–542.

164. Eggermont LH, van Heuvelen MJ, van Keeken BL, et al: Walking with a rollator and the level of physical intensity in adults 75 years of age or older. *Arch Phys Med Rehabil* 87:733–736, 2006.

165. Garber CE, Blissmer B, Deschenes MR, et al: American College of Sports Medicine position stand. Quantity and quality of exercise for developing and maintaining cardiorespiratory, musculoskeletal, and neuromotor fitness in apparently healthy adults: Guidance for prescribing exercise. *Med Sci Sports Exerc* 43:1334–1359, 2011.

166. Chodzko-Zajko WJ, Proctor DN, Fiatarone Singh MA, et al: American College of Sports Medicine position stand. Exercise and physical activity for older adults. *Med Sci Sports Exerc* 41:1510–1530, 2009.

167. The recommended quantity and quality of exercise for developing and maintaining cardiorespiratory and muscular fitness in healthy adults. Position stand of the American College of Sports Medicine. *Schweiz Z Sportmed* 41:127–137, 1993.

168. Hoberman M: Crutch and cane exercises and use. In: Basmajian JV, ed. *Therapeutic Exercise*, 3rd ed. Baltimore, MD: Williams & Wilkins, 1979:228–255.

169. Duesterhaus MA, Duesterhaus S: *Patient Care Skills*, 2nd ed. East Norwalk, CT: Appleton and Lange, 1990.

170. Bauer DM, Finch DC, McGough KP, et al: A comparative analysis of several crutch-length-estimation techniques. *Phys Ther* 71:294–300, 1991.

171. Lyu SR, Ogata K, Hoshiko I: Effects of a cane on floor reaction force and center of force during gait. *Clin Orthop Relat Res* 375:313–319, 2000.

172. Blount WP: Don't throw away the cane. *J Bone Joint Surg Am* 38A:695–708, 1956.

173. Joyce BM, Kirby RL: Canes, crutches and walkers. *Am Fam Physician* 43:535–542, 1991.

174. Deaver GG: What every physician should know about the teaching of crutch walking. *JAMA* 142:470–472, 1950.

175. Baxter ML, Allington RO, Koepke GH: Weight-distribution variables in the use of crutches and canes. *Phys Ther* 49:360–365, 1969.

176. Edwards BG: Contralateral and ipsilateral cane usage by patients with total knee or hip replacement. *Arch Phys Med Rehabil* 67:734–740, 1986.

177. Oatis CA: Biomechanics of the hip. In: Echternach J, ed. *Clinics in Physical Therapy: Physical Therapy of the Hip.* New York: Churchill Livingstone, 1990:37–50.

178. Olsson EC, Smidt GL: Assistive devices. In: Smidt G, ed. *Gait in Rehabilitation.* New York: Churchill Livingstone, 1990:141–155.

179. Vargo MM, Robinson LR, Nicholas JJ: Contralateral vs. ipsilateral cane use: effects on muscles crossing the knee joint. *Am J Phys Med Rehabil* 71:170–176, 1992.

180. Jebsen RH: Use and abuse of ambulation aids. *JAMA* 199:5–10, 1967.

181. Kumar R, Roe MC, Scremin OU: Methods for estimating the proper length of a cane. *Arch Phys Med Rehabil* 76:1173–1175, 1995.

182. Kendall FP, McCreary EK, Provance PG: *Muscles: Testing and Function.* Baltimore, MD: Williams & Wilkins, 1993.

183. Turner M: Posture and pain. *Phys Ther* 37:294, 1957.

184. Ayub E: Posture and the upper quarter. In: Donatelli RA, ed. *Physical Therapy of the Shoulder*, 2nd ed. New York, Churchill Livingstone, 1991:81–90.

185. Greenfield B, Catlin P, Coats P, et al: Posture in patients with shoulder overuse injuries and healthy individuals. *J Orthop Sports Phys Ther* 21:287–295, 1995.

186. Putz-Anderson V: *Cumulative Trauma Disorders: A Manual for Musculoskeletal Diseases of the Upper Limbs.* Bristol, PA: Taylor & Francis, 1988.

187. White AA, Punjabi MM: *Clinical Biomechanics of the Spine*, 2nd ed. Philadelphia, PA: J.B. Lippincott Company, 1990.

188. Johansson R, Magnusson M: Human postural dynamics. *Crit Rev Biomed Eng* 18:413–437, 1991.

189. Johansson R, Magnusson M: Determination of characteristic parameters of human postural dynamics. *Acta Otolaryngol Suppl* 468:221–225, 1989.

190. Keller K, Corbett J, Nichols D: Repetitive strain injury in computer keyboard users: pathomechanics and treatment principles in individual and group intervention. *J Hand Ther* 11:9–26, 1998.

191. Darnell MW: A proposed chronology of events for forward head posture. *J Craniomandibular Pract* 1:49–54, 1983.

192. Hamilton N, Luttgens K: The Standing posture. In: Hamilton N, Luttgens K, eds. *Kinesiology: Scientific Basis of Human Motion*, 10th ed. New York, McGraw-Hill, 2002:399–411.

193. Lovejoy CO: Evolution of human walking. *Sci Am* 259:118–125, 1988.

194. Korr IM, Wright HM, Thomas PE: Effects of experimental myofascial insults on cutaneous patterns of sympathetic activity in man. *J Neural Transm* 23:330–355, 1962.
195. Travell JG, Simons DG: *Myofascial Pain and Dysfunction – The Trigger Point Manual.* Baltimore, MD: Williams & Wilkins, 1983.
196. Beal MC: The short leg problem. *J Am Osteopath Assoc* 76:745–751, 1977.
197. Magee DJ: Assessment of posture. In: Magee DJ, ed. *Orthopedic Physical Assessment.* Philadelphia, PA: W.B. Saunders, 2002:873–903.
198. Berg G, Hammar M, Moller-Nielsen J, et al: Low back pain during pregnancy. *Obstet Gynecol* 71:71–75, 1988.
199. Bullock JE, Jull GA, Bullock MI: The relationship of low back pain to postural changes during pregnancy. *Aust J Physiother* 33:10–17, 1987.
200. Moore K, Dumas GA, Reid JG: Postural changes associated with pregnancy and their relationship with low back pain. *Clin Biomech (Bristol, Avon)* 5:169–174, 1990.
201. Ostgaard HC, Andersson GBJ, Schultz AB, et al: Influence of some biomechanical factors on low back pain in pregnancy. *Spine* 18:61–65, 1993.
202. Franklin ME, Conner-Kerr T: An analysis of posture and back pain in the first and third trimesters of pregnancy. *J Orthop Sports Phys Ther* 28:133–138, 1998.
203. Tardieu C, Tabary JC, Tardieu G, et al: Adaptation of sarcomere numbers to the length imposed on muscle. In: Guba F, Marechal G, Takacs O, eds. *Mechanism of Muscle Adaptation to Functional Requirements.* Elmsford, NY: Pergamon Press, 1981:99–114.
204. Sahrmann SA: *Diagnosis and Treatment of Movement Impairment Syndromes.* St Louis, MO: Mosby, 2001.
205. Seidel-Cobb D, Cantu R: Myofascial treatment. In: Donatelli RA, ed. *Physical Therapy of the Shoulder,* 3rd ed. New York, NY: Churchill Livingstone, 1997:383–401.
206. Janda V: Muscle strength in relation to muscle length, pain and muscle imbalance. In: Harms-Ringdahl K, ed. *Muscle Strength.* New York, NY: Churchill Livingstone, 1993:83–91.
207. Janda V: *Muscle Function Testing.* London: Butterworths, 1983.
208. Lewit K: *Manipulative Therapy in Rehabilitation of the Motor System,* 3rd ed. London: Butterworths, 1999.
209. Lewit K, Simons DG: Myofascial pain: relief by post-isometric relaxation. *Arch Phys Med Rehabil* 65:452–456, 1984.
210. Janda V: Muscles, motor regulation and back problems. In: Korr IM, ed. *The Neurological Mechanisms in Manipulative Therapy.* New York, NY: Plenum, 1978:27–41.
211. Jull GA, Janda V: Muscle and Motor control in low back pain. In: Twomey LT, Taylor JR, eds. *Physical Therapy of the Low Back: Clinics in Physical Therapy.* New York, NY: Churchill Livingstone, 1987:258–278.
212. Smith A: Upper limb disorders – time to relax? *Physiotherapy* 82:31–38, 1996.
213. Wilder DG, Pope MH, Frymoyer JW: The biomechanics of lumbar disc herniation and the effect of overload and instability. *J Spinal Disord* 1:16, 1988.
214. Morris C, Chaitow L, Janda V: Functional examination for low back syndromes. In: Morris C, ed. *Low Back Syndromes: Integrated Clinical Management.* New York, NY: McGraw-Hill, 2006:333–416.
215. Janda V: Muscles and motor control in cervicogenic disorders: assessment and management. In: Grant R, ed. *Physical Therapy of the Cervical and Thoracic Spine.* New York, NY: Churchill Livingstone, 1994:195–216.
216. Barrack RL, Skinner HB, Cook SD, et al: Effect of articular disease and total knee arthroplasty on knee joint position sense. *J Neurophysiol* 50:684–687, 1983.
217. Barrack RL, Skinner HB, Buckley SL: Proprioception in the anterior cruciate deficient knee. *Am J Sports Med* 17:1–6, 1989.
218. Corrigan JP, Cashman WF, Brady MP: Proprioception in the cruciate deficient knee. *J Bone Joint Surg Br* 74-B:247–250, 1992.
219. Fremerey RW, Lobenhoffer P, Zeichen J, et al: Proprioception after rehabilitation and reconstruction in knees with deficiency of the anterior cruciate ligament: a prospective, longitudinal study. *J Bone Joint Surg Br* 82:801–806, 2000.
220. Payne KA, Berg K, Latin RW: Ankle injuries and ankle strength, flexibility and proprioception in college basketball players. *J Athl Train* 32:221–225, 1997.
221. Sell S, Zacher J, Lack S: Disorders of proprioception of arthrotic knee joint. *Z Rheumatol* 52:150–155, 1993.
222. Voight M, Blackburn T: Proprioception and balance training and testing following injury. In: Ellenbecker TS, ed. *Knee Ligament Rehabilitation.* Philadelphia, PA: Churchill Livingstone, 2000:361–385.
223. Panjabi MM: The stabilizing system of the spine. Part 1. Function, dysfunction adaption and enhancement. *J Spinal Disord* 5:383–389, 1992.
224. Panjabi M, Hult EJ, Crisco J III, et al: Biomechanical studies in cadaveric spines. In: Jayson MIV, ed. *The Lumbar Spine and Back Pain.* New York, NY: Churchill Livingstone, 1992:133–135.
225. Lephart SM, Pincivero DM, Giraldo JL, et al: The role of proprioception in the management and rehabilitation of athletic injuries. *Am J Sports Med* 25:130–137, 1997.
226. Schutte MJ, Happel RT: Joint innervation in joint injury. *Clin Sports Med* 9:511–517, 1990.
227. Kennedy JC, Alexander IJ, Hayes KC: Nerve supply of the human knee and its functional importance. *Am J Sports Med* 10:329–335, 1982.
228. Janda V: *Pain in the Locomotor System, Proceeding of the Second annual Interdisciplinary Symposium on Rehabilitation in Chronic Low Back Disorders.* Los Angeles, CA: College of Chiropractic Postgraduate Division, 1988.
229. Winter DA, MacKinnon CD, Ruder GK, et al: An integrated EMG/biomechanical model of upper body balance and posture during human gait. *Prog Brain Res* 97:359–367, 1993.
230. Kisner C, Colby LA: The spine and posture: structure, function, postural impairments, and management guidelines. In: Kisner C, Colby LA, eds. *Therapeutic Exercise. Foundations and Techniques,* 5th ed. Philadelphia, PA: FA Davis, 2002:383–406.
231. Cailliet R: *Low Back Pain Syndrome,* 4th ed. Philadelphia, PA: FA Davis Co, 1991:263–268.
232. Refshauge KM, Bolst L, Goodsell M: The relationship between cervicothoracic posture and the presence of pain. *J Man Manip Ther* 3:21–24, 1995.
233. Saunders H: *Evaluation, Treatment and Prevention of Musculoskeletal Disorders,* 2nd ed. Minneapolis, MN: Viking Press, 1985.
234. Cailliet R: *Neck and Arm Pain,* 3rd ed. Philadelphia, PA: FA Davis, 1990.
235. Maigne J-Y: Cervicothoracic and thoracolumbar spinal pain syndromes. In: Giles LGF, Singer KP, eds. *Clinical Anatomy and Management of the Thoracic Spine.* Oxford: Butterworth-Heinemann, 2000:157–168.
236. Goldberg ME, Eggers HM, Gouras P: The ocular motor system. In: Kandel ER, Schwartz JH, Jessell TM, eds. *Principles of Neural Science.* Norwalk, CT: Appleton & Lange, 1991:660–677.
237. Scariati P: Neurophysiology relevant to osteopathic manipulation. In: DiGiovanna EL, ed. *Osteopathic Approach to Diagnosis and Treatment.* Philadelphia, PA: Lippincott, 1991.
238. Grieve G: Common patterns of clinical presentation. In: Grieve GP, ed. *Common Vertebral Joint Problems,* 2nd ed. London: Churchill Livingstone, 1988:283–302.
239. Stratton SA, Bryan JM: Dysfunction, evaluation, and treatment of the cervical spine and thoracic inlet. In: Donatelli R, Wooden M, eds. *Orthopaedic Physical Therapy,* 2nd ed. New York, NY: Churchill Livingstone, 1993:77–122.
240. Willford CH, Kisner C, Glenn TM, et al: The interaction of wearing multifocal lenses with head posture and pain. *J Orthop Sports Phys Ther* 23:194–199, 1996.
241. Lewit K: Chain reactions in disturbed function of the motor system. *J Man Med* 3:27, 1987.
242. Vig PS, Sarver DM, Hall DJ, et al: Quantitative evaluation of nasal airflow in relation to facial morphology. *Am J Orthod* 79:263–272, 1981.
243. Lewit K: Relation of faulty respiration to posture, with clinical implications. *J Am Osteopath Assoc* 79:525–529, 1980.
244. Bolton PS: The somatosensory system of the neck and its effects on the central nervous system, *Proceedings of the Scientific Symposium,* World Federation of Chiropractic, 1997:32–49.
245. Chaitow L, Monro R, Hyman J, et al: Breathing dysfunction. *J Bodywork Mov Ther* 1:252–261, 1997.
246. Christie HJ, Kumar S, Warren SA: Postural aberrations in low back pain. *Arch Phys Med Rehabil* 76:218–224, 1995.
247. Nachemson A, Morris JM: In vivo measurements of intradiscal pressure. *J Bone Joint Surg Am* 46:1077, 1964.
248. Troyanovich SJ, Harrison DE, Harrison DD: Structural rehabilitation of the spine and posture: Rationale for treatment beyond the resolution of symptoms. *J Manipulative Physiol Ther* 21:37–50, 1998.
249. Cook G, Voight ML: Essentials of functional exercise: a four-step clinical model for therapeutic exercise prescription. In: Prentice WE, Voight ML, eds. *Techniques in Musculoskeletal Rehabilitation.* New York, NY: McGraw-Hill, 2001:387–407.
250. Cook EG, Kiesel KB: *Selective Functional Movement Assessment, Physical Therapy Course Manual.* Danville, VA: Functionalmovement.com, 2004.

251. Brennan R: *The Alexander Technique: Natural Poise for Health.* New York, NY: Barnes & Noble Books, Inc., 1991.
252. Wanning T: Healing and the mind/body arts. *AAOHN J* 41:349–351, 1993.
253. Ryverant J: *The Feldenkrais method: Teaching by Handling.* New York, NY: KS Gringer, 1983.
254. Buchanan PA, Ulrich BD: The Feldenkrais method: a dynamic approach to changing motor behavior. *Res Q Exerc Sport* 72:315–323, 2001.
255. Feldenkrais M: *The Elusive Obvious.* Cupertino, CA: Meta Publications, 1981.
256. Nelson SH: Playing with the entire self: The Feldenkrais method and musicians. *Semin Neurol* 9:97–104, 1989.
257. Lake B: Acute back pain: treatment by the application of Feldenkrais principles. *Aust Fam Physician* 14:1175–1178, 1985.
258. Ramsey SM: Holistic manual therapy techniques. *Prim Care* 24:759–785, 1997.
259. Witt P, Parr C: Effectiveness of Trager psychophysical integration in promoting trunk mobility in a child with cerebral palsy, a case report. *Phys Occup Ther Pediatr* 8:75–94, 1988.
260. Witt P: Trager psychophysical integration: an additional tool in the treatment of chronic spinal pain and dysfunction. *Trager J* 2:4–5, 1987.
261. Savage FL: *Osteoarthritis: A Step-By-Step Success Story to Show Others How They Can Help Themselves.* Barrytown, NY: Station Hill Press, 1988.
262. Juhan D: *Multiple Sclerosis: The Trager Approach.* Mill Valley, CA: Trager Institute, 1993.
263. Heidt P: Effects of therapeutic touch on the anxiety level of the hospital patient. *Nurs Res* 30:32–37, 1991.
264. Stone A: PT. The Trager Approach. In: Davis C, ed. *Complementary Therapies in Rehabilitation; Holistic Approaches for Prevention and Wellness.* Thorofare, NJ: SLACK, 1997.
265. Watrous I: The Trager approach: an effective tool for physical therapy. *Phys Ther For* 1:22–25, 1992.
266. Lan C, Lai JS, Chen SY: Tai Chi Chuan: an ancient wisdom on exercise and health promotion. *Sports Med* 32:217–224, 2002.
267. Brown DR, Wang Y, Ward A, et al: Chronic psychological effects of exercise and exercise plus cognitive strategies. *Med Sci Sports Exerc* 27:765–775, 1995.
268. Zhuo D, Shephard RJ, Plyley MJ, et al: Cardiorespiratory and metabolic responses during Tai Chi Chuan exercise. *Can J Appl Sport Sci* 9:7–10, 1984.
269. Lai JS, Wong MK, Lan C, et al: Cardiorespiratory responses of Tai Chi Chuan practitioners and sedentary subjects during cycle ergometry. *J Formos Med Assoc* 92:894–899, 1993.
270. Jacobson BH, Chen HC, Cashel C, et al: The effect of T'ai Chi Chuan training on balance, kinesthetic sense, and strength. *Percept Mot Skills* 84:27–33, 1997.
271. Hong Y, Li JX, Robinson PD: Balance control, flexibility, and cardiorespiratory fitness among older Tai Chi practitioners. *Br J Sports Med* 34:29–34, 2000.
272. Wang JS, Lan C, Wong MK: Tai Chi Chuan training to enhance microcirculatory function in healthy elderly men. *Arch Phys Med Rehabil* 82:1176–1180, 2001.
273. Hartman CA, Manos TM, Winter C, et al: Effects of T'ai Chi Training on function and quality of life indicators in older adults with osteoarthritis. *J Am Geriatr Soc* 48:1553–1559, 2000.
274. Jayasinghe SR: Yoga in cardiac health (a review). *Eur J Cardiovasc Prev Rehabil* 11:369–375, 2004.
275. Corliss R: The power of yoga. *Time* 157:54–63, 2001.
276. Chandler K: The emerging field of yoga therapy. *Hawaii Med J* 60:286–287, 2001.
277. Bhobe S: Integrated approach to yoga. *Nurs J India* 91:33, 42, 2000.
278. Bhatnagar OP, Anantharaman V: The effect of yoga training on neuromuscular excitability and muscular relaxation. *Neurol India* 25:230–232, 1977.
279. Bastille JV, Gill-Body KM: A yoga-based exercise program for people with chronic poststroke hemiparesis. *Phys Ther* 84:33–48, 2004.
280. Balasubramanian B, Pansare MS: Effect of yoga on aerobic and anaerobic power of muscles. *Indian J Physiol Pharmacol* 35:281–282, 1991.
281. Arambula P, Peper E, Kawakami M, et al: The physiological correlates of Kundalini Yoga meditation: a study of a yoga master. *Appl Psychophysiol Biofeedback* 26:147–153, 2001.

Imaging Studies in Orthopaedics

CHAPTER 7

CHAPTER OBJECTIVES

At the completion of this chapter, the reader will be able to:

1. List the various imaging studies available.
2. Discuss the advantages and disadvantages of each of the imaging studies.
3. Describe how the various musculoskeletal tissues are depicted in imaging studies.
4. Understand the strengths and weaknesses of each of the imaging studies.
5. Outline the rationale for the choice of one imaging technique versus another.
6. Describe how the results from imaging studies may help in the clinical decision-making process.

OVERVIEW

For health-care professionals involved in the primary management of neuromusculoskeletal disorders, diagnostic imaging is an essential tool. The availability of diagnostic images to physical therapists greatly depends on the practice setting. For example, physical therapists in the United States army, with primary-care physical therapy provided with credentials, have had privileges for ordering diagnostic imaging procedures since the early 1970s.[1] Although, outside of the United States military health system, the ordering of imaging studies is not within the scope of physical therapy practice, clinicians frequently request or receive imaging study reports. Although the interpretation of diagnostic images is always the responsibility of the radiologist, it is important for the clinician to know what importance to attach to these reports, and the strengths and weaknesses of the various techniques that image bone and soft tissues, such as muscle, fat, tendon, cartilage, and ligament. In general, imaging tests have a high sensitivity (few false negatives) but low specificity (high false-positive rate), so are thus used in the clinical decision-making process to test a hypothesis but should not be used in isolation. In addition, imaging studies are expensive and somewhat more invasive compared to a physical examination, so the clinician must weigh the relative value of recommending an imaging study in relation to the working hypothesis. For example, when there is little likelihood that imaging will reveal anything that will change the course of treatment, the tests should be considered unnecessary.[1] In addition, the clinician needs to understand that the results of an imaging study may not correlate with the results of the physical examination. Although imaging may provide evidence of pathology, the mere presence of the abnormality may or may not be relevant to the presenting signs and symptoms. In such situations, the clinician should place no more or less weight on the imaging than on other aspects of the decision-making process.

RADIOGRAPHY

In 1895, Wilhelm Conrad Röentgen was experimenting with a type of electrical tube that produced an electrical discharge when a high voltage current was passed through it.[2] When Röentgen shielded the tube with heavy black cardboard, he noticed that a fluorescent screen a few feet away lit up and glowed indicating that some form of energy was passing through the tube. Further experiments led Röentgen to discover that these energy waves could reliably reproduce images of the human skeleton on a glass photographic plate.[2] Röentgen named these energy waves *x-rays* because "x" was the unknown quantity in a mathematical equation, and he was unsure of what the rays were composed of.[2] In 1896, Henri Becquerel discovered the basic nature of radiation and almost immediately an article appeared in the *Journal of the American Medical Association* theorizing on the possible diagnostic and therapeutic uses of this new discovery.[2] X-rays were soon determined to be part of the electromagnetic spectrum with the ability to penetrate through body tissues of varying densities. It was also discovered that the amount of beam absorbed as it passed through the body depended on the density of the tissue. This allowed physicians to use the images to view a number of anatomical structures. Initially, only small segments of the body could be radiographed in a single exposure—studies of large, thick body parts such as the abdomen, and hip could not be adequately covered. Then, in 1912, Dr Gustav Bucky published his findings describing a stationary, cross-hatched or "honey-combed" lead grid, which helped absorb scatter radiation and thus enhanced image quality. The grid consisted of wide strips of lead arranged in two parallel series that intersected at right angles. One disadvantage of the stationary grid is that the lead strips left "blank" or white lines on the film ("grid lines"). A few years later, Dr Hollis Potter introduced a multileafed focused grid, which moved the grid sideways across the film during the exposure, thereby blurring out the shadows of the grid strips, and further enhancing the image quality. Over the years, various mechanisms have been utilized to achieve this movement. Two physical factors responsible for grid efficiency are the grid ratio and grid frequency.

- Grid ratio: The height of the lead strip in relationship to the distance between them. Example: A 10:1 grid has lead strips 10 mm tall and these strips are 1 mm apart. The strips are ten times as tall as the distance between them.
- Grid frequency: Defined as the number of lead strips per centimeter (or per inch). The greater the frequency, the thinner the strips, and the greater the likelihood of scattered photons passing through.

Grid selection involves a compromise between film quality and patient exposure. High-ratio grids produce films with better contrast at the cost of increased patient exposure; however, proper alignment is more critical.

CLINICAL PEARL

A number of pieces of radiology equipment are named after Doctor Gustav Bucky:

- Bucky factor: sometimes referred to as grid factor or grid conversion factor (GCF)—a ratio of patient dose with a grid and without a grid. It measures the penetration of primary and secondary radiation with and without a grid.
- Bucky slot cover: a cover that shields the opening under the radiology exam table that houses the bucky tray. This cover is engaged when the bucky tray is moved to the foot of the exam table and is used during fluoroscopy.
- Bucky tray: houses the image receptor

Conventional (plain film) radiography is generally considered to be the first order diagnostic imaging modality.[3] The basic process is fairly simple. The patient's body part of interest is oriented in a prescribed position and the film plate, receptor or, detector is positioned to capture the particles of the X-ray beam that are not absorbed by the tissues of the body. Both sides of the film are thinly coated with a fluorescent gel, and then the film is placed within a two layered hard plastic shell, which protects the film and allows easy portability. An X-ray machine then directs electromagnetic radiation upon the specified region of the body.

CLINICAL PEARL

The term *radiograph* refers to the image produced on the radiographic film. X-ray film, like any photographic film, initially produces a negative image. Once the brief exposure of the patient to X-rays has occurred, the X-ray film is placed into a mechanical or electronic film developer and the final image is produced.

Exposure to the X-ray particles causes the film to darken, whereas areas of absorption appear lighter on the film.

Tissues of greater density allow less penetration of the X-rays and, therefore, appear lighter on the film. A difference in radio density is necessary for two structures to appear different on resultant radiographs. The following structures are listed in order of descending density: metal, bone, soft tissue, water or body fluid, fat, and air. Because air is the least dense material in the body, it absorbs the least amount of X-ray particles, resulting in the darkest portion of the film. Bones can have varying densities within the body. For example, cancellous bone is less dense than cortical bone and thus appears lighter than the cortical bone on the radiograph. Soft tissues often cannot be separated because they have similar radio densities.

CLINICAL PEARL

An infection of the lung tissues like pneumonia has a great deal of water and cellular matter in it. This material absorbs a great deal of radiation and thus little of the film is exposed. Therefore, if pneumonia is present, it is easily diagnosed by the appearance of a large white shadow (or "infiltrate") in the middle of the normally homogenous black lung.

Numerous technical factors are manipulated and equilibrated in order to produce a high-quality diagnostic image, while keeping the radiation dose as low as possible. Long focal film distances, short object film distances, small focal spots, short exposure time, tight collimation, and optimal film/screen combinations can all be used to enhance the image.[4] Reducing radiation exposure to the lowest levels may be addressed by attention to details of patient centering, shielding, and collimation, reducing repeat films, and the timely calibration of X-ray equipment.[4]

Digital radiography exists in the form of computed radiography or direct radiography. Image processing and distribution is achieved through a picture archiving and communication system. However, the spatial resolution of digital radiography systems is not yet as great as that with film screen radiography.[5]

Plain-film, or conventional, radiographs are relatively inexpensive and give an excellent view of cortical bone (Figs. 7-1–7-7). Radiographs may be more specific than MRI in differentiating potential causes of bony lesions because of the proven ability to characterize specific calcification patterns and periosteal reactions.[1] Plain radiographs are not considered sensitive to the early changes associated with tumors, infections, and some fractures.[6] However, they can be very helpful in detecting fractures and subluxations in patients with

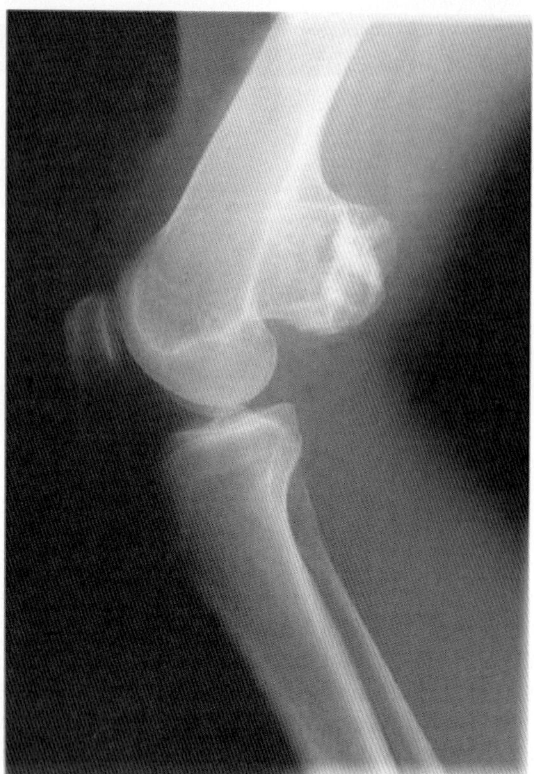

FIGURE 7-1 Radiograph showing abnormal bone growth of femur.

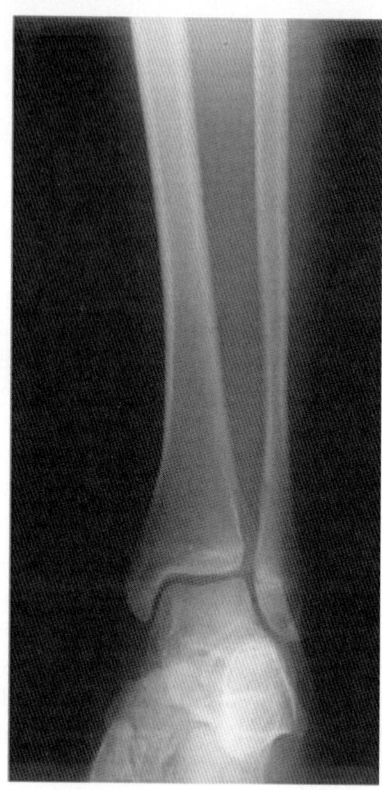

FIGURE 7-3 Radiograph showing grade I Salter-Harris fracture of fibula.

a history of trauma.[7] Radiographs may also be used to highlight the presence of degenerative joint disease, which is characterized by an approximation of the joint surfaces on the radiograph. However, radiographs do not provide the most accurate image of soft tissue structures, such as muscles, tendons, ligaments, and intervertebral disks.

Radiographs are a 2-D representation of a 3-D structure. During the initial exposure to reading radiographs, it is

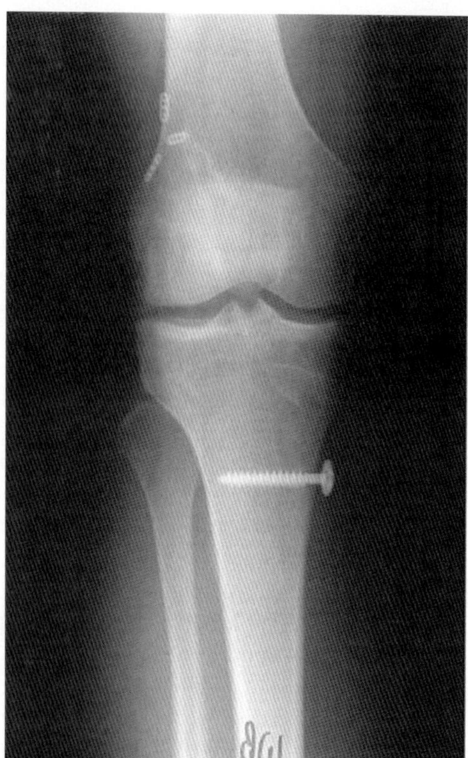

FIGURE 7-2 Radiograph showing extensive history of ACL reconstructions (3).

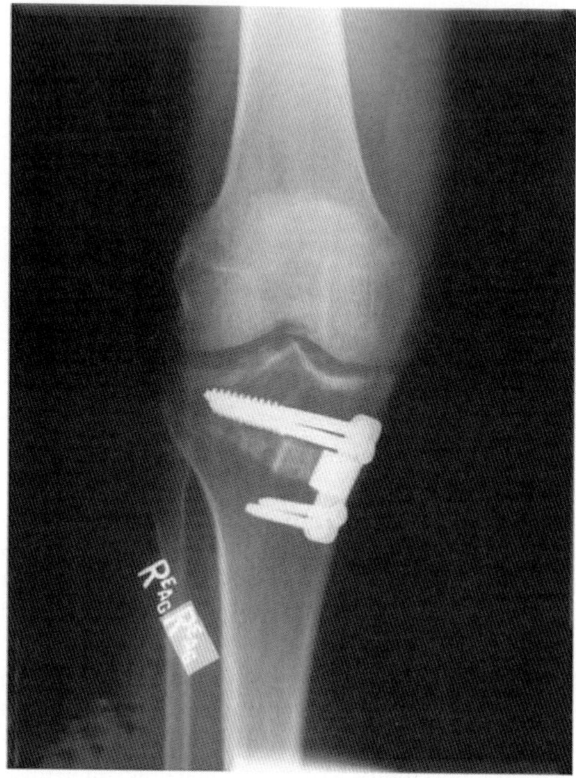

FIGURE 7-4 Radiograph following medial wedge osteotomy of right knee.

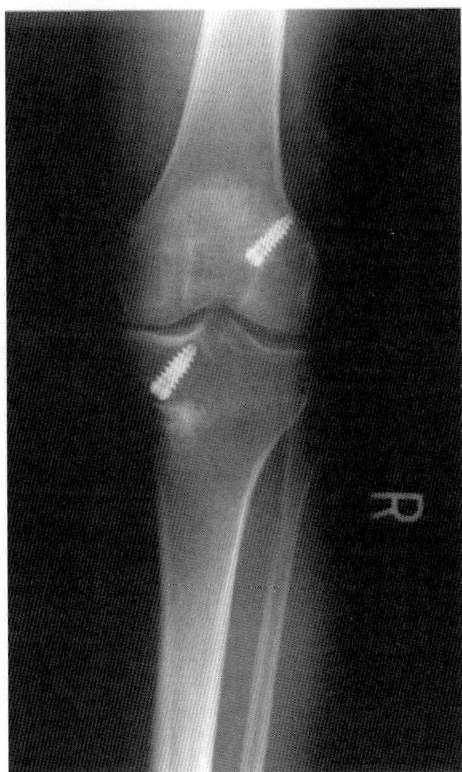

FIGURE 7-5 Radiograph following ACL reconstruction (allograft) of right knee.

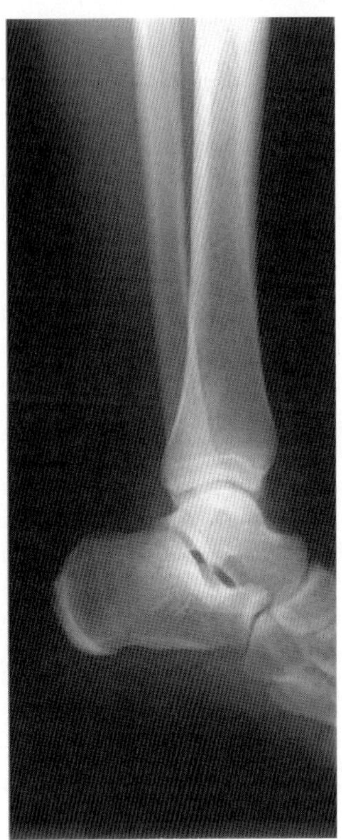

FIGURE 7-7 Radiograph showing right ankle avulsion fracture/deltoid sprain.

important that the clinician examines as many "normal" radiographs as possible. There is a great deal of variation in the human body and a great deal of variation in what is considered to be normal. When evaluating radiographs, a systematic approach such as the mnemonic ABCS is recommended[8]:

- ***A: Architecture or alignment.*** The entire radiograph is scanned from top to bottom, side to side, and in each corner to check for the normal shape and alignment of each bone. The outline of each bone should be smooth and continuous. Breaks in continuity usually represent fractures. Malalignments may indicate subluxations or dislocations, or in the case of the spine, scoliosis. Malalignment in a setting of trauma must be considered traumatic rather than degenerative until proven otherwise.[4]

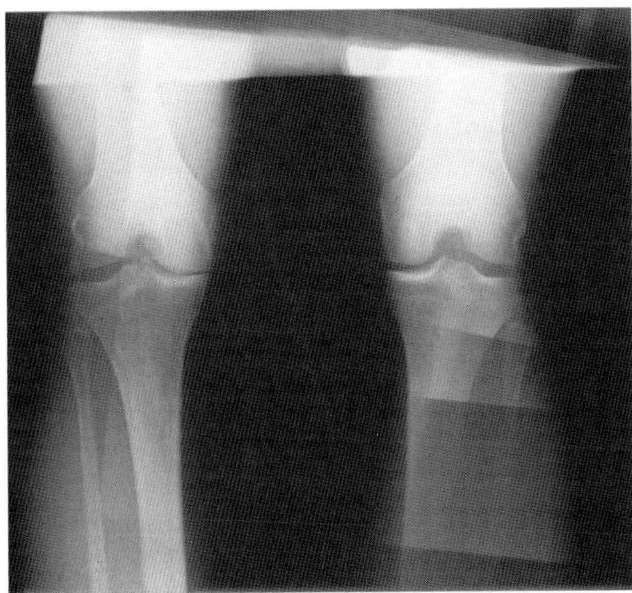

FIGURE 7-6 Radiograph showing end-stage medial compartment degeneration (Varus malalignment) of right knee.

- ***B: Bone density.*** The clinician should assess both general bone density and local bone density. The cortex of the bone should appear denser than the remainder of the bone. Subchondral bone becomes sclerosed in the presence of stress in accordance with Wolff's law[9] and increases its density. This is a radiographic hallmark of osteoarthritis.
- ***C: Cartilage spaces.*** Each joint should have a well-preserved joint space between the articulating surfaces. A decreased joint space typically indicates that the articular cartilage is thinned from a degenerative process such as osteoarthritis.
- ***S: Soft tissue evaluation.*** Trauma to soft tissues produces abnormal images resulting from effusion, bleeding, and distension.

For all joints and regions, there are standard, or routine, radiographic series that are typically obtained.[10] A radiographic series is a group of X-rays films, taken of one area of the body, from different angles. These groups of films have been standardized by long years of experience and standards of care to provide all the needed information about an area of interest. For example, a standard chest X-ray uses certain established angles and amounts of radiation to enhance the view of the soft tissues of the heart and lungs, whereas a rib series uses an entirely different set of angles and radiation to bring out the bony detail with more clarity. In addition to the standard series, there are also additional or special views that can be ordered to visualize a particular structure more effectively[10] (Table 7-1). For example, a patient presenting with pain in the "anatomic snuffbox" area of the wrist may have a fracture of the scaphoid bone, requiring a special view of the area rather than a standard wrist series. It is important that the clinician has an appreciation of various views and what each represents.

Radiographs, like all medical procedures, have risks and benefits. Ionizing radiation can increase the risk of cancer, and in sufficient doses can cause death.[11] In addition to the health risks, the overutilization of radiologic studies has become a significant economic problem in the United States.[12] For these reasons there has been an increased need for clinical prediction or decision rules indicating a need for radiography for specific types of injury at certain areas of the body. A clinical decision rule (CDR) is a tool that can quantify individual contributions from the components of the examination to determine the diagnosis, prognosis, or treatment for a given patient.[1]

Clinical Applications

Cervical Spine

CDRs for reevaluation of cervical spine injuries remain controversial, although consensus exists that cervical radiographic studies are over utilized in the emergency department.[13] In addition to the routine projections for the cervical spine, the anteroposterior (A-P) and lateral views, a number of other views can be used to aid in the evaluation of trauma and arthritis (Table 7-1). The A-P view provides information about the shape of the vertebra, the presence of any lateral wedging or osteophytes, and the disk space. In the lower cervical spine the A-P view can also provide information about the presence of a cervical rib. The lateral view provides information about the lordosis and general shape of the cervical curve and cervical vertebrae. This view also provides information about any anterior or posterior displacement of the vertebrae, the size of the disk space, the integrity of the vertebral edges (lipping), facet subluxation, soft tissue abnormalities, and the presence of any osteophytes. By measuring the prevertebral soft tissue width at the anteroinferior border of the C-3 vertebra, a determination can be made as to the presence of edema or hemorrhage if the width is wider than the normal 7 mm.[14]

> **CLINICAL PEARL**
>
> The normal ratio of spinal canal diameter to vertebral body diameter (Torg ratio) is 1. A Torg ratio that is less than 0.8 indicates possible cervical stenosis.[15]

Radiographic images are limited in their ability to detect instability of the craniovertebral region because of very incomplete image definition of soft tissues, but the disruption of normal skeletal relationships may indicate a loss of integrity of the interposed tissues. To measure the degree of atlantoaxial subluxation, the anterior atlantodens interval (AADI), which measures the spatial relationship between the odontoid process and the anterior arch of the atlas has been used. Before skeletal maturity, this value may be up to 4–5 mm. In adults and older children, a value of 3 mm is generally considered to be the upper limit of normal.[16] Roche and colleagues[17] have proposed that 3–6 mm suggests transverse ligament damage and greater than 6 mm implies alar ligament injury. However, AADI interpretations must be used with caution. The posterior atlantodens interval (PADI), which is the distance between the posterior surface of the odontoid and the anterior margin of the posterior ring of the atlas, may be a more valuable measurement, as it results in a more accurate reflection of canal size and potential for neurologic compromise. A PADI of 40 mm is considered the lower limit to avoid encroachment onto the spinal cord.[17]

Thoracic Spine

Standard views of the thoracic spine include the A-P view and lateral view (Table 7-1).

A-P view. This view is used to help the clinician determine if there is any wedging of the vertebrae (suggestive of structural kyphosis resulting from conditions such as Scheuermann's disease or a wedge fracture), whether the disk spaces appear normal, whether there is normal symmetry of the ribs, whether there is any malposition of the heart and lungs, whether any scoliosis is present, and whether the ring epiphysis, if present, is normal. From a disease perspective, in patients with suspected ankylosing spondylitis, the clinician is observing for a *bamboo spine*. The Cobb method is a technique used to measure spinal curvature in cases of suspected scoliosis. A line is drawn parallel to the superior cortical plate of the proximal end vertebra and to the inferior cortical plate of the distal end vertebra. A perpendicular line is then used to join each of these lines, and the angle of intersection of the perpendicular lines is the angle of spinal curvature resulting from scoliosis.

Lateral view. This view is to help the clinician determine if there is a normal kyphosis, whether the disk spaces appear normal, the angle of the ribs, the presence of any osteophytes, whether there is any wedging of the vertebrae, and whether there are any Schmorl's nodules, indicating herniation of the intervertebral disk into the vertebral body.

Lumbar Spine

Routine projections for the lumbar spine are the posteroanterior (P-A) or A-P, and lateral views (Table 7-1). Lower back radiographs have been described as the single most overprescribed diagnostic imaging procedure.[18,19] Specific guidelines have been developed by the Agency for Health Care Policy and Research to help reduce the ordering of lumbar plain films that are of minimal diagnostic value.[18] Imaging in the event of spinal trauma must be fully evaluated regarding the forces involved as well as the metabolic bone health of the patient.[1] Symptoms that are not relieved by rest or changes in position, symptoms that sharply increase with movement, unremitting paraspinal musculature spasm, and an unwillingness to move the spine all suggest a spinal fracture.[1]

Pelvis. Routine projections for the pelvis are outlined in Table 7-1. Additional views include the following:

TABLE 7-1 Standard and Special Radiographic Views

Region	Common Views/ Special Views	Patient Position	Purpose and Structures Imaged
Shoulder complex	A-P, external rotation	The patient is supine or erect, preferably erect, and slightly oblique, so the scapula is near parallel to the film. The forearm is supinated with a slight abduction of the shoulder for external rotation, and the elbow is slightly flexed. Central ray perpendicular to the coracoid process	Anatomic position of the shoulder girdle with the greater tuberosity seen in profile, laterally. The glenohumeral and acromioclavicular joints, proximal humerus, clavicle, and portions of scapula can all be viewed in this position
	A-P, internal rotation	The patient is positioned as for external rotation except that the back of the hand rests on the hip. Central ray is perpendicular to the coracoid process	Provides approximately 90-degree opposing view to anteroposterior, external rotation including a true lateral of the humerus with the lesser tuberosity seen in profile, medially
	Axillary	Has many variations but essentially consists of the X-ray beam passing through the axilla from inferior to superior . The West Point axillary view is obtained with the patient prone and the tube angled 25 degrees cranially and medial to the midline of the glenohumeral joint. The Stryker notch view is taken with the patient supine and the arm flexed (without abduction), and the cassette beneath the shoulder. The central ray is directed 10 degrees cranially	The glenohumeral joint, coracoid process, and the acromion process can be seen in addition to the humeral head position with respect to glenoid fossa West Point view maximizes visualization of the anterior inferior glenoid rim, enhancing the detection of bony Bankart lesions Stryker notch view: maximizes the visualization of the humeral head and Hill-Sachs lesions
	A-P, lateral scapula		Useful in identifying fractures of scapula
	Transscapular or Y view		Entire scapula; best view for comminuted and displaced fractures of the scapula
Acromioclavicular joints	A-P	The patient is erect with the arms hanging at the sides. The central ray is 15 degrees cranially at the level of the coracoid process.	A bilateral frontal projection of the AC joint
	Stress	As above except with 10–20-lb weight strapped (if the patient holds the weight, the resulting muscle contraction may produce a false-negative) to the patient's wrist	Helps differentiate incomplete from complete injuries
Sternoclavicular	P-A	The patient is positioned in prone. The central ray is perpendicular to the midpoint of the body at the level of the sternoclavicular joints	A frontal view of the sternoclavicular joints and medial aspects of the clavicles.
	Serendipity	The patient is supine or erect, facing the tube. A 40-degree cranial tilt of the central ray.	Allows for evaluation of anterior and posterior dislocation
Elbow	A-P	The elbow is extended with the forearm supinated and the patient leaning laterally until the anterior surface of the elbow is parallel with the plain X-ray cassette of the film. Central ray is perpendicular to the elbow joint	An A-P projection of the elbow joint including the distal end of the humerus, the humeroulnar and humeroradial joints, and the proximal end of the forearm
	Lateral	The elbow is flexed 90 degrees and the hand is in a lateral position. Central ray is perpendicular to the elbow joint	Integrity of olecranon articulation with olecranon fossa; look for fat pad signs

(Continued)

TABLE 7-1	Standard and Special Radiographic Views *(Continued)*		
Region	**Common Views/ Special Views**	**Patient Position**	**Purpose and Structures Imaged**
	Epicondylar groove (cubital tunnel)	This view is an axial view, modified by 15 degrees of external rotation	Used to determine whether there is bony encroachment on the cubital tunnel, contributing to ulnar nerve entrapment
	Radial head-capitellum	Obtained in the same position as a lateral view with the primary beam angled 45 degrees toward the shoulder and centered on the radial head	Best view of radial head, capitellum, and coronoid process
Forearm	A-P, lateral	Both views include the elbow and the wrist, and both views are centered on the midshaft of the forearm bones	Entire radius and ulna, wrist, elbow
Wrist	P-A	Forearm and hand on X-ray cassette with palmar surface down; the hand is slightly arched, placing the wrist in close contact with the film. Central ray perpendicular to the midcarpus	P-A projection of all carpals, the distal end of the radius and ulna, and the proximal ends of the metacarpals, carpal alignment
	Lateral	Elbow flexed 90 degrees, the forearm and arm on the X-ray cassette are ulnar side down. Central ray perpendicular to the carpus	Lateral view of the carpus, the proximal end of the metacarpals and the distal end of the radius and ulna highlighting posterior (dorsal)/volar relationships
	Posterior oblique	From the lateral position, the forearm is pronated until the wrist forms an angle of approximately 45 degrees with the plane of the film. The central ray is perpendicular to the scaphoid	Demonstrates the carpal bones on the lateral side of the wrist, in particular the scaphoid. In addition the first metacarpal, thumb carpometacarpal joint, and trapezium can be viewed
Hand	P-A	Forearm and hand on X-ray cassette with palmar surface down. Central ray perpendicular to the third metacarpophalangeal joint	P-A view of the carpals, metacarpals and phalanges (except the thumb), and the distal ends of the radius and ulna. This position yields an oblique view of the thumb. A true anterior–posterior projection of the thumb is obtained by turning the hand into a position of extreme internal rotation and holding the extended fingers back with the opposite hand, with the posterior (dorsal) surface of the thumb resting on the X-ray cassette
	Lateral	Forearm and hand on X-ray cassette, ulnar side down with fingers superimposed. Central ray perpendicular to the MCP joints	Lateral view of the bony and soft tissue structures highlighting the posterior (dorsal)/volar relationships so that anterior and posterior displacement of fracture fragments can be seen
	Posterior oblique	Forearm and hand on X-ray cassette, ulnar side down with the forearm pronated so that the fingers, which are slightly flexed, touch the cassette and the MCP joints form an angle of approximately 45 degrees. Central ray perpendicular to the third MCP joint.	Oblique view of the bone and soft tissue of the hand. With a slight adjustment of this position, a true lateral of the thumb can be obtained.
Hip	A-P pelvis	Patient supine with the feet internally rotated 15 degrees (to eliminate overlay of the greater trochanter). Central ray perpendicular to the midpoint of the film	Frontal projection of the entire pelvis, both hips and proximal femurs

(Continued)

TABLE 7-1	Standard and Special Radiographic Views *(Continued)*		
Region	**Common Views/ Special Views**	**Patient Position**	**Purpose and Structures Imaged**
	Lateral-oblique (frog leg)	The patient is turned to a near lateral position and toward the affected side with the hip and knee flexed. A straight tube is centered on the femoral head	Extremely valuable for examining the femoral head and neck, especially to exclude fractures and to assess the apophysis and femoral capital epiphysis in the immature patient
Knee	A-P	Patient supine with the knee extended. Central ray 5–7 degrees cranial to the knee joint	Frontal view of the tibiofemoral joint space and articular surfaces; distal femur; proximal tibia
	Lateral	Lateral with the affected side down and the knee flexed approximately 30 degrees. The central ray is 5 degrees cranial	Lateral view of the patellar position, distal femur; proximal tibia and fibula
	Sunrise axial	The patient is positioned in prone and the knee is flexed more than 90 degrees. The beam is angled perpendicular to the X-ray cassette	Patellofemoral joint and medial/lateral positioning of patellar; intercondylar groove
	Intercondylar	The patient is positioned kneeling on the table with the knee flexed to 70 degrees and the beam centered on the inferior pole of the patella.	Intercondylar fossa, notch of popliteal tendon, tibial spines, intercondylar eminence, posterior aspects of the distal femur and proximal tibia, intercondylar eminence of tibia
	Merchant	The patient is supine and the knees are flexed over the end of the X-ray cassette. The beam is directed toward the feet and the film cassette is held on the shins	Patellar, femoral condyles. Preferred view of articular surface of the patellar, subtle dissertations
Ankle	A-P	The patient is positioned in supine with the foot vertical. The central ray perpendicular to a point midway between the malleoli	Frontal projection of the ankle joint, the distal end of the tibia and fibula, and the proximal portion of the talus. Neither the syndesmosis nor the inferior portion of the lateral malleoli is well demonstrated in this projection
	Mortise	Supine with the leg and foot rotated internally approximately 15 degrees. The central ray perpendicular to the ankle joint	The syndesmosis is well seen without overlap of the anterior process of the distal tibia; best view of mortise and distal aspect of the lateral malleolus
	Lateral	Lateral side of the ankle down; the patient is supine and turned toward the affected side. The central ray is perpendicular to the lateral malleolus	A lateral view of the distal third of the tibia and fibula, the ankle joint, talus, calcaneus, and the hind foot
	Impingement	The ankle is positioned in extreme plantar flexion to detect posterior impingement, and weight-bearing and maximum dorsiflexion to detect and anterior impingement	To assess bony contribution to posterior or anterior impingement
	Oblique tarsal	The ankle is positioned to provide an oblique view of the foot	Best view to detect a fracture of the anterior process of the calcaneus, but can also demonstrate fractures of the base of the fifth metatarsal
	Inversion stress	Best performed with a calibrated standardized device needed to position and stress the ankle	Check for lateral instability
	Eversion stress	Best performed with a calibrated standardized device needed to position and stress the ankle	Check for medial instability

(Continued)

TABLE 7-1 Standard and Special Radiographic Views *(Continued)*

Region	Common Views/ Special Views	Patient Position	Purpose and Structures Imaged
Foot	Dorsoplantar	Patient supine with the knee flexed and the sole of the foot resting on the X-ray cassette. Central ray is perpendicular to the base of the third metatarsal	A frontal projection of the tarsals, metatarsals, and phalanges; tarsometatarsal, metatarsophalangeal, and interphalangeal joints.
	Lateral	Lateral side down with the patient supine. The central ray is perpendicular to the midfoot	A true lateral projection of the talocrural, subtalar, transverse, and tarsometatarsal joint; hind foot, midfoot, and forefoot relationships
	Medial oblique	Supine with the knee flexed and the leg rotated medially until the sole of the foot forms an angle of 30 degrees to the plane of the film. The central ray is perpendicular to the midfoot	The calcaneocuboid, cuboid-fourth and fifth metatarsal, cuboid cuneiform, and talonavicular articulations Less overlap of tarsals than anteroposterior Good view of sinus tarsi
	Harris Beath (axial) view of the hind foot	The patient is positioned in sitting on the X-ray table, leg extended, and the heel resting on the cassette. The ankle is extended and held in this position by the patient applying traction to the forefoot with a bandage or strap. A 45 degrees cranial tube angle is used with the primary beam entering the sole of the foot at the level of the base of the fifth metatarsal	Best shows the articular surfaces of both the posterior and medial subtalar joints, coalition at the medial facet, and avulsions fractures at the medial or lateral aspects of the calcaneal tuberosity
Cervical spine	A-P	The patient is placed either supine or erect. The central ray is 15–20 degrees cranial at the most prominent point of the thyroid cartilage	A frontal view of the C3–C7 vertebral bodies, and the upper two or three thoracic bodies, the interpedicular spaces, the superimposed transverse and articular processes, the uncinate processes, and the intervertebral disk spaces
	Lateral	The patient is lateral to the X-ray cassette, either seated or standing. The central ray is perpendicular to the midneck	A lateral view of the C1–C7 vertebral bodies, disk spaces, the articular pillars, spinous processes, and the lower five facet joints . Depending on how well the shoulders can be depressed, the seven cervical vertebrae and sometimes the upper one or two thoracic vertebrae can be seen; all seven cervical vertebrae, particularly in trauma cases, must be seen
	A-P Obliques	Obtained by rotating the entire patient 45 degrees one way and then the other, obtaining images in each position.	Provides information on the neural foramen and posterior elements of the cervical spine. Best view for detecting osteoarthritic encroachment of the intervertebral foramina
	A-P open mouth	The patient's head is positioned in slight extension to prevent the front teeth from being superimposed over the odontoid	Anteroposterior view of C1–C2 articulation. Fractures of C1 and arthritic changes at the C1–C2 facets may also be identified.
	Flexion/extension laterals	Obtained by asking the patient to flexed and then extend the neck, obtaining images in each position	Stress films to check for instability that may not be detected on routine neutral views

(Continued)

TABLE 7-1 Standard and Special Radiographic Views *(Continued)*			
Region	**Common Views/ Special Views**	**Patient Position**	**Purpose and Structures Imaged**
	Pillar	An A-P view taken with 20–30 degrees of caudal tube angulation, with a pad under the upper thoracic spine to elevate the shoulders and to allow extension of the cervical spine	Shows the articular pillars or lateral masses to advantage as the central beam is angulated parallel to their sloping course, caudad in the A-P projection, and cranial in the P-A projection. Occult fractures may be detected with this view
	Swimmers view	Obtained by positioning the patient so that one arm is raised above their head and the other is by their side like a freestyle swimmer	Best view of C7–T2, prevents obstruction by shoulders. Proximal humerus, lateral clavicle, AC joint, superior lateral aspect of the scapula
Thoracic spine	A-P	Obtained with the patient in the supine position, arms by the side and shoulders at the same level. The knees are slightly flexed to reduce the dorsal kyphosis and, using a straight to, the beam is sent to 10 cm below the sternal notch	T1–T12 vertebral end plates, pedicles, and spinous processes; intervertebral disk spaces; costovertebral joints; medial aspect posterior ribs
	Lateral	The patient is positioned standing side-on, with the shoulder just touching the Bucky for support. The arms are extended and the patient's balance is stabilized. The film is centered on T7	T1–T12 vertebral end plates, pedicles, spinous processes; intervertebral disk spaces and foramina
	Posterior oblique	The patient is positioned with their back against the bucky, and then rotated posteriorly so they are angled 45 degrees with the affected side touching the bucky. The arm on the affected side is positioned so that it is away from the area of interest (either out to the side, or over the patient's head)	Facet joints, pedicles, and the pars interarticularis
	Anterior oblique	The patient is positioned with their back against the bucky, and then rotated anteriorly so they are angled 45 degrees with the affected side touching the bucky. The arm on the affected side is positioned so that it is away from the area of interest (either out to the side, or over the patient's head)	Sternum, axillary portion of the ribs
Lumbar spine	A-P or posteroanterior	Either frontal projection is adequate and can be taken with the patient supine or erect with patient comfort dictating the position. If the patient is supine, the knees and hips should be flexed. The central ray is perpendicular to L3	A frontal view of the L1–L5 vertebral bodies, pedicles, disk spaces, the lamina, and the spinous and transverse processes. The Ferguson view in an A-P view with a cranial angulation, which essentially compensates for the normal lordosis of the lumbosacral region, and allows one to see the junction clearly
	Lateral	Supine or erect. If supine, the left side is down with the hips and knees flexed to a comfortable position. The central ray is perpendicular to L3	A lateral view of the lumbar vertebral bodies and their disk spaces, the spinous processes, the lumbosacral junction, sacrum and coccyx, the intervertebral foramina, and the pedicles

(Continued)

TABLE 7-1 Standard and Special Radiographic Views (Continued)			
Region	**Common Views/ Special Views**	**Patient Position**	**Purpose and Structures Imaged**
	Obliques	The patient is positioned in supine with their body angled 30 to 45 degrees	Not only shows the neural foramina but also demonstrates the pars interarticularis to aid in the detection of spondylolysis; best view of facet joints
	L5–S1 (coned down lateral) spot view	The patient is positioned standing in a lateral position with the arms across the chest	Lateral of L4–S1 vertebral bodies and disk spaces
	Flexion–extension	The patient is positioned standing side-on and is asked to flex and extend the lumbar spine. An image is taken at each position	Many enhance spondylolisthesis or retrolisthesis or demonstrate pivotal motion at a given disk
Sacroiliac joint	A-P axial, obliques	The patient is positioned in standing, with the affected side rotated 20–30 degrees away from the film.	A-P images bilateral sacroiliac joints; obliques image unilateral sacroiliac joint
Pelvis	A-P	Supine with the feet internally rotated approximately 15 degrees. Central ray perpendicular to the midpoint of the pubic symphysis	A frontal view of the pelvic girdle and proximal third of both femora
	Oblique	Also called the bilateral "frog leg" position, and the patient is positioned accordingly for a bilateral view	Detection of acetabular and pubic rami fractures
	Inlet	Patient supine and the beam angled 10 degrees cranially	
	Outlet	Patient supine and the beam angled 15 degrees caudad	
	Judet	Patient positioned so that the injured side is rotated 45 degrees internally and externally	Internally rotated: an anterior oblique view or obturator oblique view is obtained which demonstrates the iliopubic (anterior) column and the posterior lip of the acetabulum Externally rotated: a posterior oblique view or iliac oblique view is obtained which shows the ilioischial (posterior) and the anterior acetabular rim

A-P, anteroposterior; P-A, posteroanterior.

Data from Shankman S: Conventional radiography and tomography. In: Spivak JM, Di Cesare PE, Feldman DS, et al., eds. *Orthopaedics: A Study Guide.* New York, NY: McGraw-Hill, 1999:173–178; Barr JB: Medical screening for the physical therapist: Imaging principles. In: Wilmarth MA, ed. *Medical Screening for the Physical Therapist. Orthopaedic Section Independent Study Course 14.1.1.* La Crosse, WI: Orthopaedic Section, APTA, Inc., 2003:1–15; Deyle G: Diagnostic Imaging in Primary Care Physical Therapy. In: Boissonnault WG, ed. *Primary Care for the Physical Therapist: Examination and Triage.* St Louis, MD: Elsevier Saunders, 2005:323–347.

Prone view of the symphysis pubis. This view improves detail of the symphysis in patients with groin strain, as well as demonstrating the pubic rami. The view is taken with the patient lying prone to bring the symphysis close to the film and with 20–30 degrees of cranial tube angulation.

Obturator view. This view, which can be obtained supine or prone, provides the clinician with more detail of the pubic rami and ischial tuberosities. In the supine position, the cranial angulation of the tube is 25–30 degrees and, if the prone position is used, the angulation is caudal. The primary beam is centered just below the inferior margin of the symphysis.

Flamingo views. These views of the symphysis are used in the diagnosis of pelvic instability by demonstrating movement of the symphysis under weight-bearing stress. Two P-A views of the symphysis are obtained with weight bearing on each leg in turn. Any movement at the symphysis in excess of 2 mm is considered abnormal.

Cone P-A/A-P view. These views of the sacroiliac joints (SIJs) are used when an abnormality of the SIJ is suspected on a routine view of the pelvis. A tube angulation of about 30 degrees is used although this will vary depending upon the lumbar curve.

Shoulder. Radiographic examination of the shoulder girdle may be tailored to be given clinical situation. A trauma series consists of an A-P, axillary, and scapular lateral views (Table 7-1).

A-P view. A true A-P of the shoulder girdle is one in which the X-ray beam is perpendicular to the scapula. This requires obliquing the patient 45 degrees such that the scapula itself is parallel to the X-ray cassette. In this way, the glenohumeral (GH) joint is seen without overlap of the humeral head and glenoid fossa. One view that is helpful in the evaluation of impingement syndrome is the outlet view, which centers the beam at the coracoacromial arch. A standing bilateral A-P image is used to assess the clavicle and acromioclavicular (AC) joint.

Axillary. This view shows the relation of the humeral head to the glenoid and is used to diagnose anterior and posterior dislocations at the GH joint, AC joint dysfunctions, and to look for avulsion fractures of the glenoid or a Hill-Sachs lesion (see Chapter 16). The technique requires that the patient be able to abduct the arm 70–90 degrees.

Scapular-Y. The "scapular-Y" view, obtained by tilting the X-ray beam approximately 60 degrees relative to the A-P view, provides good visualization of the humerus relative to the glenoid and the acromion and coracoid process.[20]

Stryker notch view. The patient is positioned in supine with the arm forward flexed and the hand on top of the head. The beam is centered on the coracoid process. This view is used to assess a Hill Sachs lesion or a Bankart lesion (see Chapter 16).

West Point view. The patient is positioned in prone. This projection gives a good view of the glenoid to delineate glenoid fractures.

Arch view. The arch view is used to determine the width and height of the subacromial arch and helps to determine the type of acromial arch (see Chapter 16).

Elbow. The standard X-ray series of the elbow includes A-P and lateral views (Table 7-1).[21]

- *A-P view*. The A-P view is taken with the elbow extended and the forearm supinated, with the X-ray beam directed perpendicular to the anterior aspect of the elbow. The A-P view demonstrates the humeroradial, humeroulnar, as well as the medial and lateral epicondyles. The carrying angle of the elbow can also be measured from the A-P view.
- *Lateral view*. The lateral view is taken with the elbow flexed at 90 degrees and forearm in a neutral position, with the X-ray beam directed perpendicular to the lateral aspect of the elbow. The lateral view best demonstrates the coronoid process of the ulna and the tip of the olecranon. Fat pads are also best identified on the lateral view.

Special views can be ordered to help define specific symptomatic areas and include oblique, axial, radial head, and stress views.

Medial oblique views. This view is taken with the arm internally rotated, the elbow extended, and the forearm pronated. This view allows better visualization of the trochlea, olecranon, and coronoid process of the ulna.

Lateral oblique views. This view is taken with the arm externally rotated, the elbow extended, and the forearm supinated. The lateral oblique view provides good visualization of the radiocapitellar joint, proximal radioulnar joint, and medial epicondyle. Often nondisplaced or minimally displaced fractures and loose bodies not seen on the A-P or lateral views will be demonstrated on the oblique views.

Axial view. The axial view is obtained with the arm on the cassette, the elbow flexed to 110 degrees, and the X-ray beam directed perpendicular to the arm. The reverse axial view is obtained with the forearm on the cassette, the elbow completely flexed, and the beam projected perpendicular to the forearm. The axial and reverse axial views best demonstrate the olecranon fossa and the olecranon, respectively.

Radial head view: The radial head view will help identify occult radial head fractures. This view is obtained with the elbow flexed to 90 degrees and the beam angled at 45 degrees to the lateral elbow. A-P stress views demonstrate subtle changes in joint space and congruency with varus or valgus stress on the elbow. These changes are then compared to the nonstressed A-P view or to a stress view of the opposite side. Widening of the radiocapitellar joint with varus stress reflects injury to the lateral ligaments. Widening of the humeroulnar joint with valgus stress reflects injury to the medial ligaments.

The radiocapitellar view is especially helpful in demonstrating radial head and capitellum fractures. A line drawn through the mid portion of the radius normally passes through the center of the capitellum on the lateral view of the elbow. The lateral projection, angles the central beam cranially, projecting the radiocapitellar joint free of the ulnar trochlear articulation. Views of the cubital tunnel can be obtained with the elbow flexed approximately 45 degrees, and the forearm supinated with its posterior (dorsal) surface against the X-ray cassette. The central ray is angled approximately 20 degrees with respect to the olecranon process. This is particularly useful for looking at the bony aspect of the cubital tunnel where the ulnar nerve lies and can show osteophytes and loose bodies.

Wrist. In addition to the standard and special radiographic views depicted in Table 7-1, an anterior oblique position or semi-supinated oblique view may be obtained for the evaluation of arthritis. From the lateral position, the forearm is supinated until the wrist forms an angle of approximately 45 degrees with the plane of the film. The pisiform-triquetral joint compartment is only seen with such a view. Early erosions that are associated with inflammatory arthritis, especially rheumatoid arthritis, may occur at this joint. Stress views of the first carpometacarpal joints can be obtained by asking the patient to press the tips of the thumb together with the hands in a nearly lateral position. Radial subluxation of the first carpometacarpal joint is most commonly seen in basal joint osteoarthritis.

The carpal tunnel view is taken with the wrist hyperextended. The X-ray beam is angled along (parallel to) the volar aspect of the wrist showing the bony anatomy of the carpal tunnel. This view is helpful in detecting erosions in the carpal tunnel and may detect occult fractures of the hook of the hamate, which may be difficult to see on routine radiographs.

Motion series of the wrist may aid in the detection of ligamentous injuries that result in instability. This includes P-A radial and ulnar deviation views and lateral volar and dorsiflexion views. Such static views may be normal in the setting of ligamentous injury and dynamic video fluoroscopy of the wrist may be required. The clenched fist anterior–posterior view may demonstrate a scapholunate dissociation by driving the capitate proximally between the lunate and scaphoid. Specialized views of the scaphoid itself have been designed for the detection of occult fractures.

Hand. All significant hand injuries, including those with any degree of swelling, should be evaluated radiographically even if the likelihood of a fracture seems remote.[22] Chip or avulsion fractures may not be suspected on the basis of the clinical examination and yet if undetected and untreated may result in a significant disability.[22] Rotational deformity involving the metacarpal or proximal phalanx can result in a poorly functioning partially disabled hand. With a rotational alignment of the distal interphalangeal joint, the planes of the fingernails are not parallel when one compares the planes of the injured nail to the normal fingernail of the opposite hand.

In addition to the standard and special radiographic views depicted in Table 7-1, stress views of the first metacarpophalangeal joint may be required for evaluation of the ligamentous injuries. Specifically, abduction stress views of the injured and normal form may demonstrate widening of the ulnar aspect of the joint with radial subluxation of the proximal phalanx when the ulnar collateral ligament is disrupted, as with the "gamekeeper thumb" (see Chapter 18). Fractures of the fourth and fifth metacarpal are frequently undetected until a lateral view with 10 degrees of supination is obtained.[22] Second and third metacarpal injuries are often detected on a lateral view with 10 degrees of pronation.[22] Finger injuries require a true lateral view without superimposition of the other digits.[22]

Hip. There are two projections in the routine hip series (Table 7-1):

- ***A-P view.*** This view allows the clinician to:
  - compare the two hips for symmetry.
  - note the neck shaft angle (coxa vara or coxa valga), and the shape of the femoral head.
  - view the joint spaces (presence of osteophytes or arthritis), pelvic lines, and other landmarks.
  - note the presence of any bone disease (e.g., Legg–Calve–Perthes disease).
  - note any evidence of fracture, dislocation, or pelvic distortion.
- ***Lateral-oblique view.*** This view allows the clinician to look for any pelvic distortion or any slipping of the femoral head.

In addition to the standard and special radiographic views, cross-table lateral filming is the best approximation of a true lateral film of the hip and is particularly useful in assessing subtle subcapital fractures and as a postoperative evaluation of hip arthroplasty. The patient is positioned in supine with the film cassette centered at the greater trochanter. The knee and hip of the unaffected side are flexed. The central ray is perpendicular to the long axis of the femoral neck and the film cassette. The Judet view is used if there is a suspicion of a fracture in the region of the acetabulum. This view is taken by rolling the patient 40 degrees one way and then the other, acquiring images in both positions by using a straight tube centered on the femoral head.

CLINICAL PEARL

- Pistol grip deformity: abnormal head neck offset (i.e., flattening of the superior femoral head).
- Sagging rope sign: occurs with Legg–Calve–Perthes disease as a result of avascular necrosis of a developing femoral head, and indicates damage to the growth plate.
- Teardrop sign: results from superior migration of the femoral head in relation to the pelvis due to joint degeneration. The teardrop sign is visible at the base of the pubic bone, extending vertically inferiorly to terminate in a round teardrop, or head.

Tibiofemoral Joint. In addition to the standard and special radiographic views depicted in Table 7-1, weight-bearing views of the knees with and without flexion are particularly helpful in the evaluation of arthritis and the detection of joint space narrowing which may not be as obvious with nonweight-bearing or nonstanding views. Weight-bearing with flexion is particularly helpful in the detection of osteoarthritis when focal cartilage loss can be seen posteriorly. The Ottawa knee CDRs and the Pittsburgh CDRs are guidelines for the selective use of radiographs in knee trauma. Application of these rules may lead to a more efficient evaluation of knee injuries and a reduction in health costs without an increase in adverse outcomes.[12] The Ottawa knee CDRs, which have been demonstrated to have near 100% sensitivity for knee fractures and reduce the need for knee radiographs by 20% when used by emergency physicians,[3] is summarized in Table 7-2. The Pittsburgh CDR of the knee indicating the need for radiographic studies is summarized in Table 7-3.

TABLE 7-2 Ottawa Knee Rules for Radiography

Indications for Radiography, if Any	Exclusion Criteria
Patients older than 55 yr	Age younger than 18 yr
Tenderness at the head of the fibula	Isolated superficial skin injuries
Isolated tenderness of the patella	Injuries more than 7 d old
Inability to flex to 90 degrees	Recent injuries being reevaluated
Inability to weight bear four steps both immediately after the injury and in the emergency department	Patients with altered levels of consciousness
	Paraplegia or multiple injuries

Data from Seaberg DC, Yealy DM, Lukens T, et al: Multicenter comparison of two clinical decision rules for the use of radiography in acute, high-risk knee injuries. *Ann Emerg Med* 32:8–13, 1998.

TABLE 7-3 Pittsburgh Decision Rules for Radiography	
Indications for Radiography if the Mechanism of Injury Is blunt trauma or Fall and Either	Exclusion Criteria
The patient is younger than 12 or older than 50 yr	Knee injuries sustained more than 6 days before presentation
The injury causes an inability to walk more than Four weight-bearing steps in the emergency Department	Patients with only superficial lacerations and abrasions History of previous surgeries or fractures on the affected knee Patients being reassessed for the same injury

Data from Seaberg DC, Yealy DM, Lukens T, et al: Multicenter comparison of two clinical decision rules for the use of radiography in acute, high-risk knee injuries. *Ann Emerg Med* 32:8–13, 1998.

Patellofemoral Joint.

- ***Lateral radiographs.***[23] Radiographs should include a lateral view with posterior condyles approximated as closely as possible. The distance between the lateral femoral condyles and the trochlea is a measure of trochlear depth. The absence of the groove at any point along the trochlear arc is pathologic. The convergence of the bony trochlea and the lateral femoral condyles on a lateral radiograph is termed the crossing sign.
- ***Axial radiographs.***[23] The axial view should be obtained in the manner described by Merchant and colleagues but with the knee flexed 50 degrees rather than 45 degrees to better detect abnormal tilt and lateral displacement. Lateral displacement, in particular, is most pronounced in the early degrees of flexion, before the patella engages the trochlear groove.

Ankle. The Ottawa ankle CDR was developed to help predict fractures in patients with ankle injuries and has been shown to be 100% sensitive and 40% specific and to reduce the need for emergency department ankle radiographs by 36%.[3,24] Using this CDR, radiography is indicated if any of the following are present:

- Bone tenderness at the posterior edge or tip of the lateral malleolus.
- Bone tenderness at the posterior edge or tip of the medial malleolus.
- Inability to bear weight both immediately and in the emergency department.

Standard views of the ankle include the A-P, mortise, and lateral views (Table 7-1):

A-P view. This view provides the clinician with information about the shape, position, and texture of the bones, and helps determine whether there is any fractured or new subperiosteal bone.

Mortise view. This view provides information about the ankle mortise and the distal tibiofibular joint.

Lateral view. This view provides the clinician with information about the shape, position, and texture of bones, including the tibial tubercle, talus, and calcaneus.

Other nonroutine views include the following:

- *Dorsoplantar view of the foot.* This view provides information with regard to the forefoot.
- *Medial oblique view of the foot.* This view provides information about the tarsal bones and joints and the metatarsal shafts and bases. In addition this view can highlight any pathology in the calcaneocuboid joint.

Stress views of the ankles are routinely utilized for assessment of instability and injury to the lateral collateral ligament of structures (Table 7-1). Both the affected and normal side are examined for comparison. Complete tears of the deltoid ligament may be demonstrated with eversion stress. However, the value of stress roentgenograms of the ankle is a controversial topic.[25,26] The stress views include inversion to assess talar tilt and the anterior drawer stress. The accuracy of these tests increases with the use of local anesthesia and a comparison with the uninvolved ankle.

The anterior drawer test is performed with a lateral view of the ankle in neutral position, while attempting to manually translate the foot anteriorly with respect to the leg.[25,26] The sagittal plane translation of the talus with respect to the tibia is measured. When compared with the same foot unstressed, anterior subluxation of more than 3 mm is considered to indicate an anterior talofibular ligament (ATFL) injury.[27]

The talar tilt test is used more often and is felt to be more reliable. In this examination, a mortise or A-P view of the ankle held in neutral position to slight plantar flexion with an inversion stress applied to the foot is obtained.[25,26] The angle to be measured is that formed by a line parallel to subchondral bone of the distal tibia and proximal talus. It is the consensus that a talar tilt test is positive, when the injured ankle has a stressed tibiotalar angle of 5[28]–15 degrees[29] greater than the uninjured side. However, the absolute number of degrees is not as important as the functional instability of the patient, as laxity does not always mean instability.[25,26]

Stress Radiograph. A stress radiograph is a procedure using radiographs taken while a stress is applied to a joint. An unstable joint demonstrates widening of the joint space when the stress is applied. For example, spine flexion and extension views can be helpful in assessing spinal mobility and stability and are typically ordered in the acutely injured athlete when there is a high degree of suspicion of spine injury. Greater than 2 mm of motion beyond normal at any segmental level in the spine would suggest instability and warrant further examination.

Video Fluoroscopy. Fluoroscopic procedures involve the use of X-rays to evaluate the quality and quantity of joint motion. Because of the relatively high exposure of radiation with this technique, it is used mainly in the detection of joint instability.

Contrast-Enhanced Radiography. Contrast-enhanced radiography procedures involve the use of a contrasting agent to highlight different structures. These agents may be administered orally, rectally, or by injection. Different contrast media may be used and include radiopaque organic iodides and radiotranslucent gases. Contrast-enhanced radiography procedures include the following:

- ***Arthrography.*** Arthrography is the study of structures within an encapsulated joint using a contrast medium with or without air that is injected into the joint space. The contrast medium distends the joint capsule. This type of radiograph is called an *arthrogram.* An arthrogram outlines the soft tissue structures of a joint that would otherwise not be visible with a plain-film radiograph. This procedure is commonly performed on patients with injuries involving the shoulder or the knee. The primary general indications for performing a conventional arthrogram are[30]
  - to confirm intracapsular positioning of a needle or catheter following a joint aspiration or prior to an anesthetic joint injection
  - in place of an MR scan (see later) if it is not available, contraindicated, or if the patient is too obese for the gantry or is claustrophobic
  - for the diagnosis and treatment of adhesive capsulitis

  Arthrography can also be performed in conjunction with magnetic resonance imaging (MRI) or computed tomography (CT) (see later).
- ***Myelography.*** Myelography is the radiographic study of the spinal cord, nerve roots, dura mater, and spinal canal. The contrast medium is injected into the subarachnoid space, and a radiograph is taken. This type of radiograph is called a *myelogram.* Myelography is used frequently to diagnose intervertebral disk herniations, spinal cord compression, stenosis, nerve root injury, or tumors. The nerve root and its sleeve can be observed clearly on direct myelograms. When myelography is enhanced with CT scanning, the image is called a *CT myelogram* (see later).
- ***Diskography.*** Diskography is the radiographic study of the intervertebral disk. A radiopaque dye is injected into the disk space between two vertebrae. A radiograph is then taken. This type of radiograph is called a *diskogram.* An abnormal dye pattern between the intervertebral disks indicates a rupture of the disk. The indications for lumbar or cervical diskogram are[30]
  - severe or unremitting low back or neck pain with or without radicular symptoms in a patient with negative standard imaging studies or degenerative disk disease
  - for use in preoperative planning prior to spinal fusion to include only those painful disk levels
  - in the evaluation of neural foramina masses, which may represent an extruded disk herniation or nerve sheath tumor
  - to determine accurate needle placement prior to chymopapain injection
  - persistent pain in the postoperative period
- ***Angiography.*** Angiography is the radiographic study of the vascular system. A water-soluble radiopaque dye is injected either intra-arterially (arteriogram) or intravenously (venogram). A rapid series of radiographs is then taken to follow the course of the contrast medium as it travels through the blood vessels. Angiography is used to help detect injury to or partial blockage of blood vessels. The indications for angiography are[30]
  - as a diagnostic study, following possible vascular injury from trauma
  - embolization of active bleeding sites not amenable to surgical control, such as within the pelvis
  - evaluation of bone and soft tissue tumors (the findings will assess neovascularity of the lesion, the extent of the tumor, and invasion or impingement of major vessels)
  - preoperative or palliative intra-arterial embolization or chemotherapy
  - diagnosis and treatment of arteriovenous malformations
  - evaluation of the arterial anatomy prior to bone or soft tissue grafts
  - diagnosis of arteritis that is further complicating collagen vascular disease

Computed Tomography

The word "*tomography*" is derived from the Greek *tomos* (slice) and *graphia* (to write). CT images are useful to evaluate injured areas where the 3-D configuration of the structure make the plain radiographs difficult to interpret.[31] The CT image is not recorded in a conventional radiographic manner. A CT scanner system, also known as computerized axial tomography (CAT) and computerized transaxial tomography (CTI), consists of a scanning gantry, which holds the X-ray tube and detectors (moving parts), a moving table or couch for the patient, an X-ray generator, computer processing unit, and a display console or workstation.[32] Images are obtained in the transverse (axial) plane of the patient's body by rotating the X-ray tube 360 degrees.

The images are produced by rotating a thin collimated X-ray beam through a 180-degree arc around the patient such that structures of a certain depth will be stationary in the beam and appear with enhanced clarity, whereas tissues superficial and deep to this level will be relatively obscured by motion. The basic principle of any tomographic system is that all parts of the object that are perpendicular to the direction of the tube motion are maximally blurred, whereas those parts that are parallel to the direction of motion are not blurred but merely elongated.

Like conventional radiography, CT also uses radiation, but instead of a unidirectional beam, both the radiation source and detector systematically encircle the body. The X-rays are absorbed in part by the patient's body. The amount of X-rays transmitted through the body is detected on the opposite side of the gantry by an array of detectors. Each array detector responds to the amount of rays detected by downloading data to the system's computer, which assigns a numeric value based on the attenuation property of the various tissues of the body, and then forms an image based on the differential absorption of the X rays. These attenuation values, or relative attenuation coefficient (μ), are expressed in Hounsfield units (HU) and are normalized to water.[4] Hence, water measures 0 HU, bone (the highest absorption values) measures >400 HU, muscle measures 40 HU, fat measures −120 HU, and air (the lowest absorption values) measures −1000 HU.[32] In essence, the CT image is a map of the linear attenuation value of the tissue. By adjusting the level and the width of the displayed ranges of HU (window), the operator can study different tissues optimally. Software has been introduced through the years to allow for fast image reconstruction in any desired plane (2 D) or surface reconstruction (3 D).[32] The continuous movement offered by spiral CT, referred to as multislice or multidetector CT scanners, greatly reduces scan time. These newer multislice CT scanners represent a major improvement in helical CT scan technology, wherein simultaneous activation of multiple detector rows positioned along the longitudinal or z-axis (direction of table or gantry) allows acquisition of interweaving helical sections.[33] With this design, section thickness is determined by detector size and not by the collimator (a device that filters a stream of rays so that only those travelling parallel to a specified direction are allowed through) itself.[33]

Image quality in CT imaging depends on a variety of factors, which are mostly selected by the operator. Two parameters are used to define the image quality of a given system: spatial resolution and contrast resolution:[32]

- Spatial resolution: Spatial resolution is defined as the ability of the system to distinguish between two closely spaced objects. For improvement of spatial resolution, the operator selects a small matrix size (256 × 256), small field of view, and thin slices. Special reconstruction algorithms can also be chosen to improve spatial resolutions.
- Contrast resolution: Contrast resolution is defined as the ability of the system to discriminate between two adjacent areas with different attenuation values. The operator has several choices to improve contrast resolution: appropriate selection of reconstruction algorithm, tube current (measured in milliamperes), scanning time (measured in seconds), pixel size (matrix), and slice thickness. It must be remembered that increasing tube current or scanning time increases the radiation dose. Another strategy to increase contrast resolution is to use contrast material, either intra-articular or intravenous. The contrast resolution of CT is dramatically better than conventional radiography (approximately 100 times), and the images provide greater soft tissue detail than do plain films.[4]

Provided the patient remains motionless during the study, the CT scan provides good visualization of the shape, symmetry, and position of structures by delineating specific areas (Fig. 7-8). This information can be helpful in the examination of acute trauma, aneurysms, infections, hematomas, cysts, and tumors.

Clinical Applications

Cervical Spine

CT is most often utilized in the cervical spine examination in the assessment of potential fractures, but may not be the modality of choice when used in isolation for soft tissue imaging. For example, the accuracy of CT imaging ranges from 72% to 91% in the diagnosis of disk herniation, but approaches 96% when combining CT with myelography.[34,35] A CT myelogram (CTM) is a diagnostic tool that uses radiographic contrast media (dye) that is injected into the subarachnoid space (cerebrospinal fluid, CSF). After the dye is injected, the contrast medium serves to illuminate the spinal canal, cord, and nerve roots during imaging. The low viscosity of the water-soluble contrast permits filling of the nerve roots and better visualization.[4]

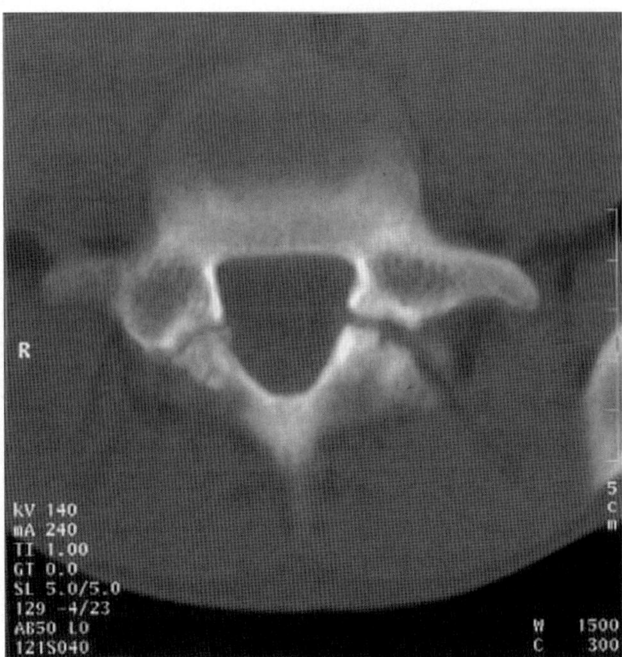

FIGURE 7-8 CT image of lumbar spine showing bilateral spondylolysis at the L5–S1 level.

CLINICAL PEARL

Multiple studies have indicated CT to be superior to radiography in detecting fractures of the cervical spine, even small fractures.[36]

Shoulder. CT is typically used for suspected fractures, particularly of the glenoid rim.

Elbow, Forearm, Wrist, and Hand. CT is preferred over radiography in cases of suspected ligamentous instability. In addition, fracture lines and fragment locations can best be delineated with the help of CT. CT has also been used to provide accurate assessment of the reorientation of the distal radius articular surface following fracture, which is critical in determining whether closed or open reduction is the preferred course of action.[37]

Pelvis and Hip. CT of the hip and pelvis is helpful with identifying the spatial relationships of fractures of the femoral head and acetabulum and any associated fragments, particularly in cases of complicated fractures.[38] CT is also recommended when considering congenital hip dysplasia, preoperative prosthesis planning, and the detection of neoplasms.[39]

Knee. CT scans often used to view soft tissues as well as bone of the knee joint complex.

Ankle and Foot. CT often enables delineation of cortical and trabecular orientations of bone, and the articular surfaces in the joints better than plain films. This is particularly true in cases such as a talar dome injury.

Magnetic Resonance Imaging

MRI has been a viable imaging technique since the early 1980s and has now become the standard modality for differentiating among soft tissues in the neuromusculoskeletal system.[40] Unlike CT, which depends upon multiple thin slices of radiation that are "backplotted" through Fourier transformers, MRI is the result of the interaction between magnetic fields, radiofrequency (RF) waves, and complex image reconstruction techniques. Normally, the axes of protons in the body have a random orientation. However, if the body or body part is placed within a high magnetic field, the protons align themselves parallel with, or perpendicular to, the direction of the magnetic field. Protons also have a natural spinning motion at a specific frequency (Lamor frequency). When an RF pulse of the same frequency as that of the spinning protons within the magnetic field is applied, the protons are deflected from their newly unlined axis by a specific angle with the degree of deflection being dependent on the strength of the applied RF wave pulse. The protons, now spinning synchronously or coherently at an angle with the magnetic field, induce a current in a nearby transmitter–receiver coil or antenna. This small nuclear signal is then recorded, amplified, measured, and localized (linked to the exact location in the body where the MRI signal is coming from), producing a high contrast, clinically useful MR image. The signal starts to decay as soon as the RF pulse is discontinued and the protons begin to relax back to a state of equilibrium. The decaying of the signal is intimately related to two factors:

- The realignment of the protons within the magnetic field (longitudinal relaxation).
- The loss of coherence or synchrony (dephasing) of the protons as they continue spinning at an angle to the magnetic field (transverse relaxation).

These two phenomena, called relaxation times T1 and T2 respectively, are biological parameters with tissue specific relaxation constants for different types of tissue and their molecular composition. For example, tissues such as water have very mobile protons that return very quickly to alignment in the magnetic field, whereas bone protons are largely immobile. T1 and T2 can be measured independently to create images that are dependent on different T1 values of the tissues (T1-weighted images, T1WI) or on different T2 values (T2-weighted images, T2WI). Images containing T1 and T2 information are called balanced images or proton density-weighted images (PDWI). Contrast between tissues is dependent on the differences between T1, T2, and PD values on T1WI, T2WI, or PDWI. For example, fat (including marrow fat) is bright on T1WI, while CSF is dark, and structures with high fibrous tissue content such as tendons, ligaments, and cortical bone are also dark. With T2WI, fluid including CSF, synovial fluid, and edema is bright, while the fat signal varies, and fibrous structures such as tendons, ligaments, and cortical bone are again dark.

The specific techniques for obtaining the MRI are called *pulsed sequences*. These pulse sequences result from changing imaging parameters such as the repetition time (TR), echo time (TE), or angle of deflection (RF or flip angle) (FA). By changing these parameters, the operator can control the rate of repetition of the RF pulses (TR), the time elapsed between an RF pulse and the production of the signal or echo (TE), and the intensity of the applied RF pulse which determines the FA. Images obtained using short TR and short TE will produce T1-weighted contrast. Images obtained with long TR and long TE will produce T2-weighted contrast, and images obtained with long TR and short TE will produce PD-weighted contrast. The latter sequences are termed spin echo (SE) and have been a mainstay of lumbar spine imaging. Table 7-4 itemizes the differences in signal intensities on T1-weighted and T2-weighted MR images.

Because of the unique properties of magnetic imaging, MRI is subject to a number of artifacts. The most important of these are metallic artifacts, specifically those produced by ferromagnetic objects, which distort the alignment of protons in the scanner's main magnetic field.[4] Such spatial distortion may produce grossly erroneous measurements. Somewhat less common artifacts include banding artifacts, "wraparound" (an adjacent area wrapping into the area of interest, seen on very small fields of view) and chemical shift artifact (seen when tissues and markedly different chemical structures lie directly adjacent to one another, for instance, at the discovertebral interface).[4]

Clinical Applications

The advantages of MRI include its excellent tissue contrast, ability to provide cross-sectional images, noninvasive nature, and complete lack of ionizing radiation. MRI provides an excellent view of anatomic and physiologic tissues (Figs. 7-9 and 7-10). It is commonly used to assess the CNS and soft tissue injuries. In addition, MRI has been shown to be sensitive in the detection of occult bone lesions, and it can also detect and help assess both occult and traumatic bone lesions, especially occult stress and posttraumatic fracture.[31] General contraindications for MRI include[4]

- intracranial aneurysm clips
- cardiac pacemakers
- some prosthetic heart valves
- implanted cardiac defibrillators
- carotid artery vascular clamp
- spinal cord stimulators (neuro stimulators)
- insulin infusion pump (implanted drug infusion device)
- bone growth stimulator
- metallic hardware, devices, fragments
- hearing aids and dentures (must be removed)
- cochlear implants, ocular implants, penile implants
- some shrapnel and bullets
- intraocular foreign bodies

TABLE 7-4 Differences in Signal Intensity on T1-Weighted (T1W) Versus T2-Weighted (T2W) Images		
Tissue	**T1W**	**T2W**
Cortical bone	Low	Low
Tendons and ligaments	Low	Low
Fibrocartilage	Low	Low
Muscle	Intermedia	Intermediate
Nonneoplastic tumor	Low intermediate	Low/intermediate/possible high
Neoplastic tumor	Low intermediate	Intermediate-high/possible low
Water, CSF	Low	High
Inflammation	Low	High
Proteinaceous fluid, abscess	Intermediate	High
Fat	High	High (slightly lower than on T1W)
Hemorrhage, acute	High	High
Hemorrhage, chronic	Low	High

Data from Morris C, ed. *Low Back Syndromes: Integrated Clinical Management*. New York: McGraw-Hill, 2006:495.

- tattooed eyeliner
- some types of makeup

Spine. The combination of multiplanar capabilities and high contrast resolution that MR images provide are ideal for spinal imaging. MRI has demonstrated excellent sensitivity in the diagnosis of lumbar disk herniation, and is considered the imaging study of choice for detection and staging of demyelinating disorders involving the spine (e.g., multiple sclerosis) and syringomyelia and for detecting nerve root impingement, although the latter use is tempered by the prevalence of abnormal findings in asymptomatic subjects.[41] It can, however, detect ligament and disk disruption, which cannot be demonstrated by other imaging studies.[42,43]

Shoulder. The main indications for MRI of the shoulder include rotator cuff pathology, GH joint instability, and shoulder pain of unknown etiology.

Elbow. The main indications for MRI at the elbow joint are to differentiate bone and soft tissues, study mass lesions, tendon and ligamentous lesions, osteochondral lesions, pediatric

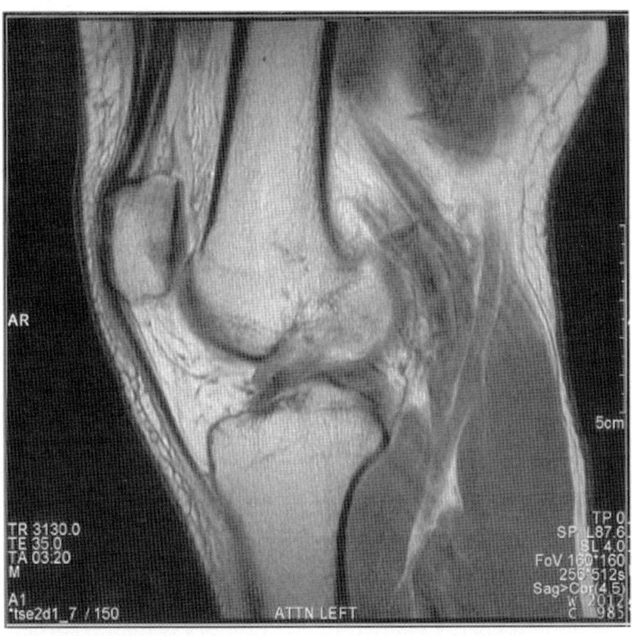

FIGURE 7-9 MRI showing ACL-deficient left knee.

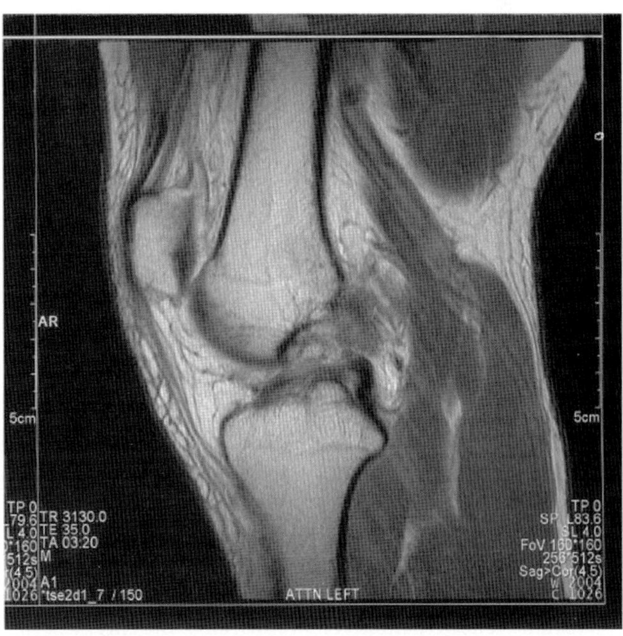

FIGURE 7-10 MRI showing ACL-deficient left knee—different view.

elbow fractures, compressive neuropathies, and miscellaneous conditions.[40]

Hand and Wrist. The most frequent indications for MRI of the hand and wrist include: the evaluation of palpable mass lesions, ligamentous tears, triangular fibrocartilage complex tears, posttraumatic avascular necrosis of the scaphoid, Kienböck's disease (avascular necrosis of the lunate), tendon tears, and compressive neuropathies.[40]

Hip. MRI is most commonly used in the hip to evaluate for the presence of avascular necrosis or osteonecrosis of the femoral head.[40] Other indications for MRI of the hip include transient osteoporosis of the hip, osteochondral lesions, tumors, synovial chondromatosis, and pigmented villonodular synovitis (PVNS).[40]

Knee. The knee is one of the areas of the musculoskeletal system most commonly imaged by MRI. Meniscal and ligamentous injuries (Figs. 7-9 and 7-10) can be diagnosed with an accuracy of almost 95%.[40]

Ankle and Foot. The most common indications for MRI of the ankle include: tendon lesions, osteochondritis dissecans, chronic ankle instability, and pain of unknown etiology.[40]

Diagnostic Ultrasound (Ultrasonography)

Ultrasonography evolved with the development of military sonar, the sending and recording of a certain frequency of sound wave as it is transmitted and then reflected off various objects. Although initially used primarily for abdominal imaging, ultrasound imaging is rapidly becoming appreciated for its musculoskeletal applications. Diagnostic and therapeutic ultrasounds are similar in that both produce frequencies greater than 20,000 Hz. Continuous or pulsed therapeutic ultrasound produces 1 MHz or 3 MHz thermal and nonthermal energy, whereas diagnostic ultrasound produces pulsed waves at 7.5–20 MHz that are processed to produce pulsed echo images. A diagnostic ultrasound system is composed of a set of transducers, a power system, and computer unit with a display screen. The transducer, which is the device that sends and receives the ultrasound waves, is composed of an array of quartz crystals that generate these waves. As ultrasound waves are transmitted through the body, they are reflected at tissue interfaces, and the time it takes for the waves to be reflected back to the transducing probe allows the computer to produce an image. The reflectivity of the sound wave is influenced by two factors as follows[44]:

- Acoustic impedance of the two tissues composing the interface. Acoustic impedance is the product of the density of the material and the speed of sound transmission within the substance. The reflectivity is greatest at the interfaces between tissues of dissimilar acoustic impedance.
- The angle of incidence of the sound beam. When the angle of incidence of the sound beam is at 90 degrees or perpendicular to the tissue interface, the reflectivity is highest and decreases with increasing angle.

At highly reflective interfaces, almost all of the energy of the sound beam is reflected, producing a sound void area beneath the interface. This occurs between soft tissues and air or calcium. The sound beam appears to be enhanced when it passes through tissue such as water or other fluids that do not absorb ultrasound, therefore, showing as sound void areas. Thus, different tissues transmit sound waves at different velocities and, therefore, create different images. More dense tissue such as bone and collagen reflects more waves than less dense tissue such as water or fat.

Ultrasonography is perhaps more operator dependent than any other imaging modality.[44] The ultrasound transducer must be held at a 90-degree angle to the scanning target tissue to prevent artifacts so that the maximal number of waves will be processed into an accurate image. Technical considerations are also important because it is necessary to operate with high resolution transducers to obtain images with sufficient diagnostic information. Despite its disadvantages, ultrasonography is a readily available technique, is less expensive than most other imaging modalities (with the exception of plain films), does not involve ionizing radiation, and is noninvasive.[44] In addition, it allows real-time imaging, a feature that is very useful to some conditions, such as snapping tendon syndrome or developmental dysplastic hip, where dynamic imaging provides additional information.[44] Some of the disadvantages of ultrasonography, including those already mentioned, are a small field of view and the presence of artifacts. Comet fail artifact is caused by deep echogenicity bands that cross tissue boundaries and is usually associated with metal or glass foreign bodies. Other artifacts are refraction and reverberation. Refraction occurs when the ultrasonography probe is not maintained at a 90-degree angle (perpendicular) to the examined tissues which can cause an incorrect depiction of structure or lesion. Reverberation occurs at highly reflective interfaces causing the appearance of phantom structures.

Ultrasonography can be used to diagnose any pathological condition that is located superficially enough to be detected by the transducer, and is currently used in orthopaedics to help detect soft tissue injuries, tumors, bone infections, and arthropathy and to evaluate bone mineral density. Tendons are well-suited because of the parallel fascicles of collagen and the ground substance which provide different receptivity, attenuation, and backscatter. Ultrasonography is particularly useful in staging muscle injuries, allowing for a more accurate estimate of when an athlete can return to sport. Ultrasound imaging may also be used to assess the degree and quality of fracture healing and in the detection of synovitis and wood and plastic foreign bodies. Finally, ultrasonography can be used to confirm proper placement of an injection and provide diagnostic information as well as to provide treatment for inflammatory conditions such as bursitis, intraarticular loose bodies, cysts, and nerve thickening. Future uses for ultrasound imaging will likely include the placement of tissue grafts (stem cells, platelets, matrixes) to aid in the healing of injuries because of its real-time imaging capabilities.

Radionucleotide Bone Scanning

Radionucleotide scanning studies involve the introduction of bone seeking isotopes, which are administered to the patient orally or intravenously and allowed to localize to the skeleton. The photon energy emitted by the isotopes is then recorded using a gamma camera 2–4 hours later. The pathophysiologic

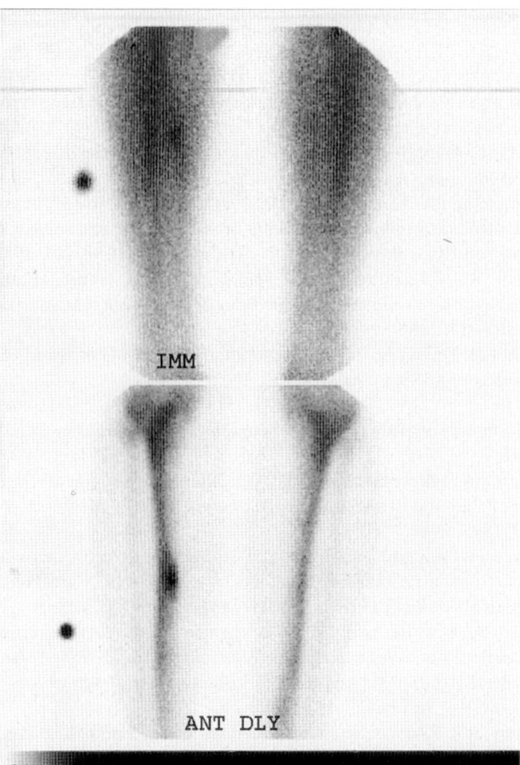

FIGURE 7-11 Bone scan showing stress fracture of right tibia.

basis of the technique is complex but depends on localized differences in blood flow, capillary permeability, and metabolic activity that accompany any injury, infection, repair process, or growth of bone tissue.[31] The most common radionuclide scanning test is the bone scan (Fig. 7-11). This test is used to detect particular areas of abnormal metabolic activity within a bone. The abnormality shows up as a so-called hot spot, which is darker in appearance than normal tissue. The bone scan is an extremely sensitive but fairly nonspecific tool for detecting a broad range of skeletal and soft tissue abnormalities. An abnormal bone scan may indicate tumor, avascular necrosis, bone infection (osteomyelitis), Paget's disease, or recent fracture. Comparison of the affected and unaffected side is generally used to detect differences in uptake. Whole body or spot views, patient positioning, and the number of views employed depend on the indication for the examination.

Three Phase Bone Scan

The three phase bone scan consists of the following image phases[45]:

1. Flow study. The injection is the same as for a routine bone scan, but imaging is begun immediately after the injection. Sequential images are obtained every 2–3 seconds for 60 seconds.
2. Blood pool. Immediately following the flow study, a blood pool image is obtained over the area of interest. This image serves as a marker of extravascular tissue activity.
3. Delayed static images. After a minimum of 2 hours, images are obtained over the area of interest. These images demonstrate radioisotope uptake in the osseous structures.

SPECT Scan[45]

Single photon emission computed tomography (SPECT) scanning improves both the detection and localization of an abnormality by permitting spatial separation of bone structures that overlap on standard planar images. After acquisition of the study, a computer is used to reconstruct images in axial, sagittal, and coronal planes. To date, bone SPECT has been found to be of particular clinical value in studies of the vertebral column and has been shown to be more sensitive than plain film radiology, with the majority of SPECT lesions corresponding to identifiable disease on CT. SPECT scanning is a highly sensitive means of detecting spondylolysis, a fracture of the pars interarticularis.

Clinical Applications

Radionucleotide bone scans are used throughout the body. Applications of the radionuclide bone scan can be divided into traumatic and nontraumatic categories as follows[31]:

- Traumatic.
  - Fractures.
  - Anatomically difficult locations. These include the scapula, sternum, sacrum, and portions of the pelvis.
  - Occult fractures (nondisplaced or stress fractures). Bone scans can reveal metabolic disturbance at a fracture site within 24 hours of the injury, long before a conventional radiograph shows any abnormality and often before they are symptomatic.[31] Such fractures include the tibia (Fig. 7-11), scaphoid, radial head, and the femoral neck. Stress fractures of the metatarsals and other bones are seen on bone scan up to 2 weeks before becoming visible on plain radiographs.
  - Traumatic osteonecrosis without fracture.
- Nontraumatic
  - Osteomyelitis. This condition causes localized increased uptake of the isotope which is visible on bone scan within 48 hours of the beginning of infection.
  - Tumor, primary or metastatic. These are usually detectable by bone scan by the time they cause symptoms. The ability of the scan to cover the whole skeleton is particularly useful for determining the presence and extent of metastatic disease.
  - Occult fractures.
  - Tendinitis and tenosynovitis.
  - Hip pain.
  - Adults: aseptic necrosis, arthritis, transient osteoporosis, occult femoral neck fracture. Aseptic necrosis appears either as a hotspot overlying the femoral head or as a cold central area surrounded by a ring of increased uptake. Transient osteoporosis, an entity mainly affecting young men, also demonstrates increased uptake of the femoral head when viewed under a bone scan. However, transient osteoporosis displays a decreased bone density when viewed on plain films. Arthritis causes increased uptake of isotope in periarticular bone on both sides of the joint. Occult femoral neck fractures resulting from normal stress

placed on bones weakened by osteoporosis are seen on bone scan as bands of increased uptake localized to the neck of the femur.

- Children: arthritis, Legg–Perthes disease. The bone scan in Legg–Perthes disease reveals decreased up-take at the femoral head early in the disease. Later, a ring of increased uptake may surround the cold spot.

REVIEW QUESTIONS*

1. Which imaging study is generally considered to be the first order diagnostic imaging modality?
2. List the following structures in order of descending density: air, water or body fluid, metal, bone, soft tissue, and fat.
3. Which imaging modality gives the best view of cortical bone?
4. What conditions are stress radiographs helpful in detecting?
5. Which of the imaging modalities relies on the use of a very powerful magnet to produce images?
6. Which of the imaging studies is used to study structures within an encapsulated joint using a contrast medium with or without air that is injected into the joint space?
7. What is the radiographic study of the vascular system called?
8. What are the two parameters used to define image quality of a CT scan?

*Additional questions to test your understanding of this chapter can be found in the Online Learning Center for *Orthopaedic Assessment, Evaluation, and Intervention* at www.duttononline.net. Answers for the above questions appear at the back of this book.

REFERENCES

1. Deyle G: Diagnostic imaging in primary care physical therapy. In: Boissonnault WG, ed. *Primary Care for the Physical Therapist: Examination and Triage*. St Louis, MO, Elsevier Saunders, 2005:323–347.
2. Agee OF: Roentgen. Early radiology, and subsequent development of diagnostic radiology. A history. *J Fla Med Assoc* 82:738–744, 1995.
3. Stiell IG, Greenberg GH, McKnight RD, et al: Decision rules for the use of radiography in acute ankle injuries: Refinement and prospective validation. *JAMA* 269:1127–1132, 1994.
4. Skogsbergh DR, Jones KM: Diagnostic imaging approaches to the evaluation of low back syndrome. In: Morris C, ed. *Low back syndromes: Integrated clinical management*. New York, NY: McGraw-Hill, 2006:477–509.
5. Mattoon JS: Digital radiography. *Vet Comp Orthop Traumatol* 19:123–132, 2006.
6. Sartoris DJ: Diagnosis of ankle injuries: The essentials. *J Foot Ankle Surg* 33:101–107, 1994.
7. Schutter H: *Intervertebral disc disorders, Clinical Neurology*. Philadelphia, PA: Lippincott-Raven, 1995:chap. 41.
8. Swain JH: An introduction to radiology of the lumbar spine. In: Wadsworth C, ed. *Orthopedic Physical Therapy Home Study Course*. La Crosse, WI: Orthopedic Section, APTA, 1994: 1–6.
9. Wolff J: *The Law of Remodeling (Maquet P, Furlong R, (trans))*. Berlin: Springer-Verlag, 1986 (1892)
10. Barr JB: Medical screening for the physical therapist: Imaging principles. In: Wilmarth MA, ed. *Medical screening for the physical therapist*. Orthopaedic Section Independent Study Course 14.1.1 La Crosse, Wisconsin, Orthopaedic Section, APTA, Inc, 2003:1–15.
11. Shankman S: Conventional radiography and tomography. In: Spivak JM, Di Cesare PE, Feldman DS, et al., eds. *Orthopaedics: A study guide*. New York, NY: McGraw-Hill, 1999:173–178.
12. Tandeter HB, Shvartzman P: Acute knee injuries: Use of decision rules for selective radiograph ordering. *Am Fam Physician* 60:2599–2608, 1999.
13. Stiell IG: Clinical decision rules in the emergency department. *CMAJ* 163:1465–1466, 2000.
14. Templeton PA, Young JW, Mirvis SE, et al: The value of retropharyngeal soft tissue measurements in trauma of the adult cervical spine. Cervical spine soft tissue measurements. *Skeletal radiology* 16:98–104, 1987.
15. Cantu RC: Functional cervical spinal stenosis: A contraindication to participation in contact sports. *Medicine and science in sports and exercise* 25:316–317, 1993.
16. Imhof H, Fuchsjager M: Traumatic injuries: Imaging of spinal injuries. *European radiology* 12:1262–1272, 2002.
17. Roche CJ, Eyes BE, Whitehouse GH: The rheumatoid cervical spine: Signs of instability on plain cervical radiographs. *Clinical radiology* 57:241–249, 2002.
18. Acute low back problems in adults: Guideline overview. Agency for Health Care Policy and Research Rockville, Maryland. *J Natl Med Assoc* 87:331–333, 1995.
19. Acute low back problems in adults: Assessment and treatment. Acute Low Back Problems Guideline Panel. Agency for Health Care Policy and Research. *Am Fam Physician* 51:469–484, 1995.
20. Rubin SA, Gray RL, Green WR: The scapular "Y" view: A diagnostic aid in shoulder trauma. A technical note. *Radiology* 110:725–726, 1974.
21. Wilder RP, Guidi E: Anatomy and examination of the elbow. *J Back Musculoskel Rehabil* 4:7–16, 1994.
22. Simon RR, Koenigsknecht SJ: Fractures of the hand. In: Simon RR, Koenigsknecht SJ, eds. *Emergency Orthopedics: The extremities*, 4th ed. New York: McGraw-Hill, 2001:98–133.
23. Grelsamer RP, Stein DA: Rotational malalignment of the patella. In: Fulkerson JP, ed. *Common patellofemoral problems*. Rosemont, IL, American Academy of Orthopaedic Surgeons, 2005:19–28.
24. Stiell IG, McKnight RD, Greenberg GH, et al: Implementation of the Ottawa Ankle Rules. *JAMA* 271:827–832, 1994.
25. Safran MR, Zachazewski JE, Benedetti RS, et al: Lateral ankle sprains: A comprehensive review part 2: Treatment and rehabilitation with an emphasis on the athlete. *Med Sci Sports Exerc* 31:S438–S447, 1999.
26. Safran MR, Benedetti RS, Bartolozzi AR III, et al: Lateral ankle sprains: A comprehensive review: Part 1: Etiology, pathoanatomy, histopathogenesis, and diagnosis. *Med Sci Sports Exerc* 31:S429–S437, 1999.
27. Anderson KJ, Lecocq JF, Lecocq EA: Recurrent anterior subluxation of the ankle joint: A report of two cases and an experimental study. *J. Bone Joint Surg* 34A:853–860, 1952.
28. Cass JR, Morrey BF: Ankle instability: Current concepts, diagnosis, and treatment. *Mayo Clinic Proceedings* 59:165–170, 1984.
29. Sedlin ED: A device for stress inversion or eversion roentgenograms of the ankle. *J. Bone Joint Surg* 42A:1184–1190, 1960.
30. Schoenberg NY: Interventional radiology and angiography. In: Spivak JM, Di Cesare PE, Feldman DS, et al., eds. *Orthopaedics: A study guide*. New York, McGraw-Hill, 1999:183–191.
31. Simon RR, Koenigsknecht SJ: Special imaging techniques. In: Simon RR, Koenigsknecht SJ, eds. *Emergency Orthopedics: The extremities*, 4th ed. New York: McGraw-Hill, 2001:73–76.
32. Beltran J, Rosenberg ZS: Computed tomography. In: Spivak JM, Di Cesare PE, Feldman DS, et al., eds. *Orthopaedics: A study guide*. New York, NY: McGraw-Hill, 1999:179–182.
33. Carrino JA, Morrison WB: *Musculoskeletal imaging, Orthopaedic Knowledge Update 8: Home Study Syllabus*. Rosemont, IL, American Academy of Orthopaedic Surgeons, 2005:119–136.
34. Jahnke RW, Hart BL: Cervical stenosis, spondylosis, and herniated disc disease. *Radiol Clin North Am* 29:777–791, 1991.
35. Modic MT, Ross JS, Masaryk TJ: Imaging of degenerative disease of the cervical spine. *Clin Orthop* 239:109–120, 1989.
36. Mintz DN: Magnetic resonance imaging of sports injuries to the cervical spine. *Semin Musculoskelet Radiol* 8:99–110, 2004.
37. Malone TR, Hazle C, Grey ML: Imaging of the forearm, wrist, and hand. In: Malone TR, Hazle C, Grey ML, eds. *Imaging in rehabilitation*. New York, NY: McGraw-Hill, 2008:158–195.
38. Malone TR, Hazle C, Grey ML: Imaging of the pelvis and hip. In: Malone TR, Hazle C, Grey ML, eds. *Imaging in rehabilitation*. New York, McGraw-Hill, 2008:196–229.
39. Erb RE: Current concepts in imaging the adult hip. *Clin Sports Med* 20:661–696, 2001.

40. Beltran J: Magnetic resonance imaging. In: Spivak JM, Di Cesare PE, Feldman DS, et al., eds. *Orthopaedics: A study guide*. New York, McGraw-Hill, 1999:193–201.
41. Forristall RM, Marsh HO, Pay NT: Magnetic resonance imaging and contrast CT of the lumbar spine: comparison of diagnostic methods and correlation with surgical findings. *Spine* 13:1049–1054, 1988.
42. Harris JH, Yeakley JW: Hyperextension-dislocation of the cervical spine: Ligament injuries demonstrated by magnetic resonance imaging. *J Bone Joint Surg* 74B:567, 1992.
43. Ellenberg MR, Honet JC, Treanor WJ: Cervical radiculopathy. *Arch Phys Med Rehabil* 75:342–352, 1994.
44. Grijseels S, Beltran J: Ultrasonography. In: Spivak JM, Di Cesare PE, Feldman DS, et al., eds. *Orthopaedics: A study guide*. New York, NY: McGraw-Hill, 1999:199–201.
45. Finkel JE: Musculoskeletal scintigraphy. In: Spivak JM, Di Cesare PE, Feldman DS, et al, eds. *Orthopaedics: A study guide*. New York, NY: McGraw-Hill, 1999:203–208.

SECTION III INTERVENTION

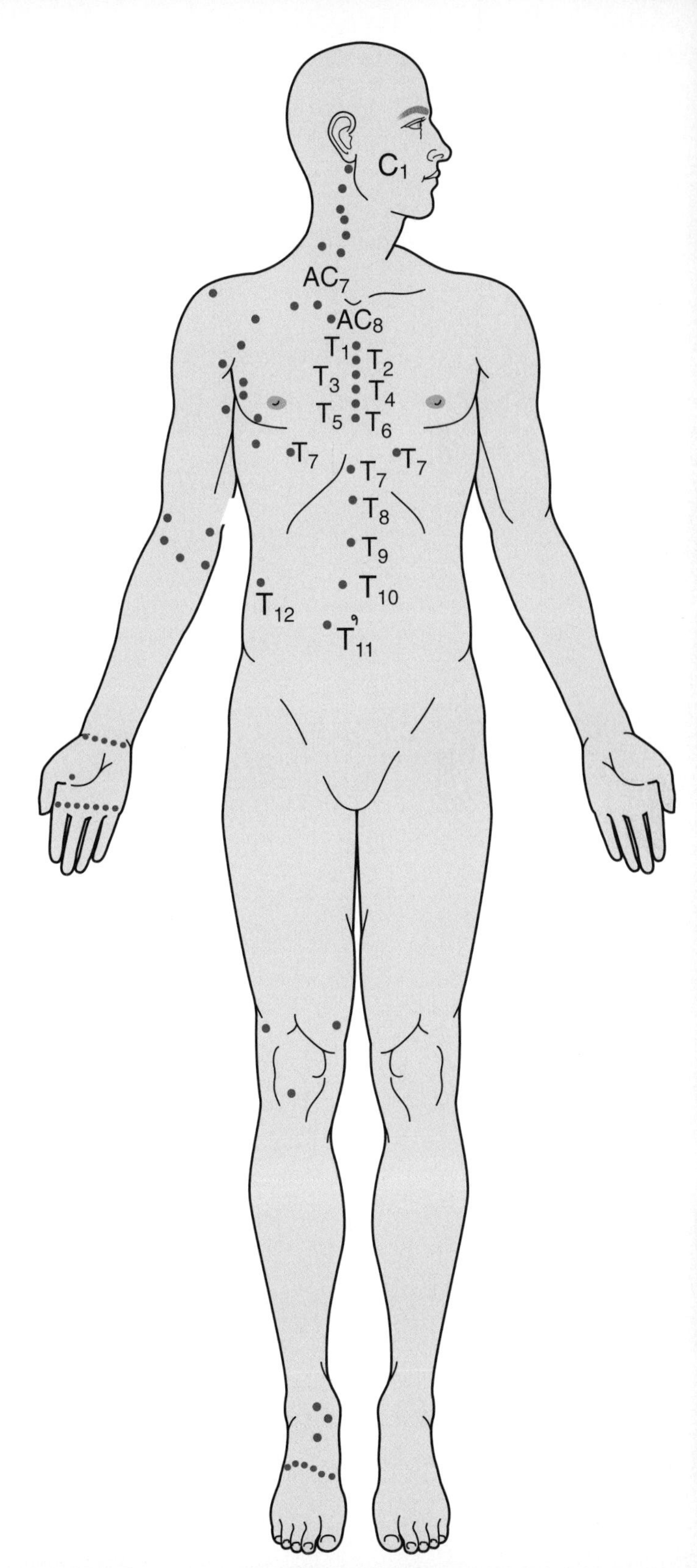

CHAPTER 8 The Intervention

CHAPTER OBJECTIVES

At the completion of this chapter, the reader will be able to:

1. Understand and describe the principles of a comprehensive rehabilitation program during the various phases of healing.
2. Discuss the various components of the intervention and their respective importance.
3. List the clinical tools that can be used to decrease pain and inflammation and promote healing.
4. Discuss the intrinsic and extrinsic stimuli that can be used to promote and progress healing.
5. Describe the benefits of each of the electrotherapeutic modalities.
6. Describe the benefits of each of the physical agents and mechanical modalities.
7. Understand the rationale for the therapeutic techniques used in each of the three stages of healing.
8. Understand the importance of patient education.

OVERVIEW

The purpose of the physical therapy intervention is to safely return a patient to his or her preinjury state, with as little risk of reinjury as possible and with the minimum amount of patient inconvenience. Normally, this is achieved with a gradual progression of strengthening and flexibility exercises, while avoiding further damage to an already compromised structure.[1] For the contractile tissues, such as the muscles, this is accomplished through measured rest, rehabilitative exercise, high-voltage electrical stimulation, central (cardiovascular) aerobics, general conditioning, and absence from abuse.[2] The inert structures, such as ligaments and menisci, rely more on the level of tension and force placed on them for their recovery, which stimulates the fibroblasts to produce fiber and glycosaminoglycans.[3] The progression to high-functional demands or sports-specific exercises may be made, depending on the patient's requirements. For the athlete, the criteria for return to play should include no pain, full pain-free ROM, normal flexibility/strength/balance, good general fitness, normal sports mechanics, and demonstration of sports-specific skills.[4]

According to the "Guide to Physical Therapist Practice,"[5] an intervention is "the purposeful and skilled interaction of the physical therapist and the patient/client and, when appropriate, with other individuals involved in the patient/client care, using various physical therapy procedures and techniques to produce changes in the condition consistent with the diagnosis and prognosis."

Three components comprise the physical therapy intervention: coordination, communication, and documentation; patient/client-related instruction; and direct interventions (Box 8-1).[5]

An intervention is most effectively addressed from a problem-oriented approach and is based on the patient's functional needs and on mutually agreed-upon goals.[5] Decisions about the intervention are made to improve the patient's ability to perform basic tasks and to restore functional homeostasis. The most successful intervention programs are those that are custom designed from a blend of clinical experience and scientific data, with the level of improvement achieved being related to goal setting and the attainment of those goals (Table 8-1). The necessary knowledge to perform an intervention includes[6]

- the temporal phases of tissue healing, common problems associated with each phase, and stresses that tissues can safely tolerate during each phase;
- movement characteristics including amount of range, control, and capacity required for various functional activities;
- the range of available intervention strategies and procedures to promote healing and corresponding outcomes in varied patient populations;
- sequencing of various interventions to challenge appropriately involved tissues and the whole patient. For example, being able to recognize the underlying tissue healing and balance disorders in a patient status posthip fracture with diabetes mellitus, the need for aerobic conditioning in assessing patients with low back dysfunction, and the importance of body mechanics education in prenatal and postnatal exercise classes; and

Box 8-1 Components of an Intervention

Coordination, Communication, and Documentation

These interventions may include case management, communication with other health-care providers or insurers, and the coordination of care with the patient/client or significant others involved in the care of the patient/client. This is to ensure a continuum of care among health-care providers. Other interventions may include documentation of care, discharge planning, education plans, patient-care conferences, record reviews, and referrals to other professionals or resources.

Patient-Related Instruction

Patient education can include, but is not limited to, verbal, written, or pictorial instructions, which may be part of a home program. Computer-assisted instruction and demonstrations by the patient/client or caregivers are also examples of instructions that may be given. Audiovisual aides and demonstrations of exercises or functional activities may be used. This enables the patient/client to continue with the program when out of the clinic, either independently or with assistance.

Direct Interventions

Direct interventions are selected on the basis of the findings in the evaluation and examination of the patient/client, diagnosis, prognosis, and anticipated outcomes and goals for the individual. The direct interventions are performed with or on the patient. This section encompasses the largest component of patient care. Examples of direct interventions include, but are not limited to, therapeutic exercise, aerobic exercise, functional training, manual therapy, and use of assistive devices and modalities.

- intervention strategies to promote overall health and well-being, and to prevent secondary dysfunction.

CLINICAL PEARL

The goal of the intervention process is to achieve the desired functional outcomes by reduction of existing impairments, prevention of secondary impairments, enhancement of functional ability, promotion of optimal health, and reduction of environmental challenges.[6,7]

Whether the identification of the specific structure or structures causing the dysfunction is necessary, in order to proceed with an intervention, remains controversial. Cyriax[8] designed his examination process to selectively stress specific tissues in order to identify the structure involved and its stage of pathology. In contrast, McKenzie[9] and Maitland[10,11] seldom identified the involved structure, believing that it is not always possible, or even necessary, for the prescription of appropriate therapeutic interventions. Indeed, based on the Maitland and McKenzie philosophy, the therapeutic strategy is determined solely from the

TABLE 8-1 Key Questions for Intervention Planning
What is the stage of healing: acute, subacute, or chronic?
How long do you have to treat the patient?
What does the patient do for activities?
How compliant is the patient?
How much *skilled* physical therapy is needed?
What needs to be taught to prevent recurrence?
Are any referrals needed?
What has worked for other patients with similar problems?
Are there any precautions?
What is your skill level?

Data from Guide to physical therapist practice. *Phys Ther* 81:S13–S95, 2001.

responses obtained from tissue loading and the effect that loading has on symptoms.[9] Once these responses have been determined, the focus of the intervention is to provide sound and effective self-management strategies for patients, which avoid harmful tissue loading.[9] However, although self-management must be encouraged whenever feasible, these strategies have their limitations. One cannot realistically expect the majority of patients to fully rehabilitate themselves with a condition that requires the integration of a multitude of decision-making processes such as occurs with a total joint replacement, or an anterior cruciate ligament reconstruction.

CLINICAL PREDICTION RULES

Many interventions for musculoskeletal disorders have shown small effects when tested in randomized controlled trials. Identifying patients who respond best to certain treatments has received increased interest in research activity. With a clinical prediction rule (CPR), a combination or cluster of patient characteristics is used to determine the diagnosis, prognosis, or likely response to treatment of that individual.[12] The development of a CPR involves the following stages: derivation (analyzing a data set to establish a rule with predictive power), narrow validation (evaluating the rule in a similar clinical setting and population), broad validation (evaluating the rule in multiple clinical settings), and impact analysis (determining whether the rule changes clinicians' behavior, improves patient outcomes, or reduces costs).[12] Thus far, however, all of the CPRs have been derived using single-arm study designs and, therefore, the results of these studies must be interpreted with caution, as these CPRs run a greater risk of identifying prognostic factors rather than factors that modify the effect of a treatment.[13] Other important limitations of many of the current CPRs are the use of short-term outcomes only, arguably trivial findings, and limited rule application potential.[13] To date, only one CPR on spinal manipulation for low back pain[14] underwent validation in a controlled trial and can be considered for clinical application (and only in a population similar to that tested).[13]

INTERVENTION BASED ON STAGE OF HEALING

The intervention is typically guided by short- and long-term goals, which are dynamic in nature, being altered as the patient's condition changes, and strategies with which to achieve those goals based on the stages of healing (Table 8-1). Intervention strategies can be subdivided into active (direct) or passive (indirect), with the goal being to make the intervention as active as possible at the earliest opportunity.

Many factors can contribute to the patient's resistance to improvement. In some cases, it may be an individual factor that, when eliminated, will allow the patient to respond well. In the majority of cases, the resistance to improvement is based on the interaction of multiple factors, which must be recognized and corrected.

Misjudgments are sometimes made with the intervention. In general, the patient's pain should not last more than a couple of hours after an intervention. Pain that lasts longer than 2 hours is usually an indication that the intensity of the intervention, rather than the intervention itself, has been inappropriate. The clinician has to remove the notion that all pain is bad. In many respects, a slight increase in pain following an intervention is a more desirable finding than no change in pain, because it indicates that the correct structure is being stressed, albeit too aggressively.

Acute Phase

Clinical findings during the acute stage are associated with inflammation and include pain, edema, redness, heat, and impairment or loss of function (see Chapter 2). Although the redness and heat are not necessarily problems that require a specific treatment goal, pain, edema, and loss of function certainly are. Given the number of pathologic entities that can be evoked by the repair process, such as complex regional pain syndrome (CRPS, previously referred to as reflex dystrophy) and myositis ossificans, it is clear that neurophysiologic processes are at work. Usually, during the acute phase, there is pain at rest or with active motion, or when specific stress is applied to the injured structure. The pain, if severe enough, can result in muscle guarding and loss of function. With passive mobility testing, pain is reported before tissue resistance is felt by the clinician.

Pain

A major focus of physical therapy is the control of pain. At the simplest level, the transmission of information relating to pain from the periphery to the cortex is critically dependent on integration at three levels within the central nervous system: the spinal cord, brain stem, and forebrain (see Chapter 3). Although pain serves as a protective mechanism, allowing an individual to be aware of a situation's potential for producing tissue damage and to minimize further damage, it can persist beyond its usefulness. In addition, the presence of pain can stimulate muscle spasm, which in turn can lead to circulatory deficiency, muscle atrophy, and loss of function. The challenge for the clinician during the various phases of healing is to control the pain while simultaneously progressing the patient. To control the pain, the source of pain must be first identified. Once identified, several different approaches can be used to provide pain relief as follows[15]:

- Encourage the body's central biasing mechanisms (see Chapter 3) through the use of cognitive processes (motivation, relaxation techniques, positive thinking, and mental focus).
- Minimize further tissue damage through the application of the principles of PRICEMEM (protection, rest, ice, compression, elevation, manual therapy, early motion, and medications—see later). Therapeutic modalities are probably the most frequently used tool in all of musculoskeletal rehabilitation. Physical agents, including therapeutic cold, heat, sound, light, diathermy, electrical current, massage, and compression can be used throughout the rehabilitation program at appropriate times. Clearly, an understanding of the physiological basis for using these agents is critical if clinicians are to use these agents effectively. During the acute phase, physical agent interventions (therapeutic cold and compression) should be applied as soon as possible after the injury to help control pain.
- Educate the patient as to the rationale of the treatment and what he or she can expect.
- Recognize that all pain, even psychosomatic pain, feels very real to the patient.

Inflammation and Edema

Inflammation and edema occur as part of the healing process (see Chapter 2). In addition to controlling pain, the goals during the initial phase of intervention for an acute lesion are to control the inflammation and edema and to protect the damaged structures from further damage, while attempting to promote and progress tissue healing and increase function.

CLINICAL PEARL

Several tools are at the clinician's disposal to help control inflammation and edema. These include elevation of the injured part as appropriate, compression, the application of electrotherapeutic and physical modalities (cryotherapy, and high-voltage electrical stimulation), gentle ROM exercises, and graded manual techniques.

Loss of Function

Neuromuscular inhibition can result from pain and joint effusion and should be addressed as early as possible. Function can be enhanced through the use of assistive and supportive devices (crutches, canes, sling, immobilizer, etc.).

PRICEMEM

- ***Protection*** Excessive tissue loading must be avoided. For example, in the lower extremity when ambulation is painful, crutches or other assistive devices are advocated until the patient can bear weight painlessly.[16]

- ***Rest.*** Rest is generally defined as absence from abuse, rather than a complete absence from activity.[2] Prolonged immobilization can have a detrimental effect on muscles, ligaments, bones, collagen, and joint surfaces. In response to the training stimulus, the involved components will undergo some breakdown at the subcellular, cellular, or tissue level, which will temporarily lower the functional ability of each. A rest period allows the body to adapt by resynthesizing the protein in these structures to a higher level than before the overload.[17–19] This process of synthesizing takes between 12 and 48 hours depending on the intensity (quality) of the exercise and the volume (total amount) of the load.[20] However, it is important to remember that if the training stimulus is stopped, reduced, or altered too much, the training effect will decline.
- ***Ice.*** The therapeutic application of cold or cryotherapy has been used as a healing modality since the days of the ancient Greeks.[21] Garrick[16] recommends that ice be used until the swelling has ceased. Limiting the effusion serves to hasten the healing process by minimizing the amount of extracellular fluid and hematoma to be reabsorbed.[22,23]
- ***Compression.*** The most common method of applying compression is via an elastic bandage.[24] Compression provided by a pneumatic device,[25,26] or by a felt pad incorporated into an elastic wrap or taping,[27] has also been demonstrated to be effective in decreasing effusion.
- ***Elevation.*** Elevation of an extremity aids in venous return and helps minimize swelling. Elevation and compression should be continued until the swelling has completely dissipated.[16]
- ***Manual Therapy.*** The controlled application of various manual techniques can have several therapeutic benefits (see Chap. 10). These benefits are theoretically achieved through[28,29]
  - stimulation of the large-fiber joint afferents of the joint capsule, soft tissue, and joint cartilage, which aids in pain reduction;
  - stimulation of endorphins, which aids in pain reduction;
  - decrease of intra-articular pressure, which aids in pain reduction;
  - mechanical effect, which increases joint mobility;
  - remodeling of local connective tissue;
  - increase of the gliding of tendons within their sheaths; and
  - increase in joint lubrication.

Manual techniques, which are discussed in Chapter 10, allow the clinician to choose the degree of specificity of an intervention. Although the goal is to be as specific as possible, there are many times when a general technique is appropriate. General techniques are typically less aggressive, are applied to the larger muscle groups or regions, and often can be performed by the patient as part of the home exercise program. General manual therapy techniques that can be used during this stage include *gentle* massage to increase blood flow. Specific manual techniques that can be used during this stage include passive joint distractions and glides (grade I or II).

- ***Early Motion.*** Early motion is advocated to[30]
  - reduce the muscle atrophy that occurs primarily in type I fibers[31–33];
  - maintain joint function;
  - prevent ligamentous "creeping";
  - reduce the chance of arthrofibrosis or excessive scarring[34–38]; and
  - enhance cartilage nutrition and vascularization, thereby permitting an early recovery and enhanced comfort.[33,39,40]

CLINICAL PEARL

The benefits of early mobilization are to prevent the detrimental physiologic effects of immobilization, including the loss of muscle, ligament, and bone strength[41,42]; formation of adhesions[43]; and the loss of proprioception.[44]

Therapeutic exercise is the foundation of physical therapy and a fundamental component of the vast majority of interventions. Prescribed accurately, therapeutic exercise can be used to restore, maintain, and improve a patient's functional status by increasing strength, endurance, and flexibility. Research has demonstrated that joint motion stimulates the healing of torn ligaments around a joint[45,46] and that early joint motion stimulates collagen bundle orientation along the lines of force, a kind of Wolff's law of ligaments.[45,47] When designing an exercise program, the clinician should create exercises that are safe yet challenging, progressive, systematic, proprioceptively enriched, activity-specific, and based on evidence-based science.[48] A typical exercise continuum includes a number of progressions, which includes the following[48]:

- Activities initially performed slowly before being progressed to a faster pace.
- The performance of familiar activities and then unfamiliar activities.
- Activities are initially performed on a stable base of support, and are then made progressively more challenging by increasing the amount of control required and with the introduction of activities that require dynamic control.
- The introduction of resistance during the movements. The initial resistance used is of low force and then incrementally increased.
- Correct performance of the activity with increasing levels of complexity.

CLINICAL PEARL

The goal of the functional exercise progression is to identify the motion, or motions, that the patient is able to exercise into, without eliciting symptoms other than postexercise soreness.[49]

- ***Medications.*** Pharmacologic intervention, which can play an important role in the management of the pain and inflammation associated with orthopaedic conditions is described in Chapter 9.

Tissue repair can be viewed as an adaptive life process in response to both intrinsic and extrinsic stimuli.[50] Physical therapy cannot accelerate the healing process, but with correct education and supervision, it can ensure that the healing process is not delayed or disrupted and that it occurs in an optimal environment.[9]

CLINICAL PEARL

The promotion and progression of tissue repair involves a delicate balance between protection and application of controlled functional stresses to the damaged structure.

The rehabilitation procedures used to assist with this repair process differ, depending on the type of tissue involved, the extent of the damage, and the stage of healing. Healing is related to the signs and symptoms present rather than the actual diagnosis. These signs and symptoms inform the clinician as to the stage of repair that the tissue is undergoing. Awareness of the various stages of healing is essential for determining the intensity of a particular intervention, if the clinician is to avoid doing any harm. Decisions to advance or change the rehabilitative process need to be based on the recognition of these signs and symptoms, and on an awareness of the time frames associated with each of the phases.[51,52]

Janda[53] introduced the concept of the direct and indirect effects of neural input on muscle activation, and noted the influence that pain and swelling can have on direct muscle inhibition.

CLINICAL PEARL

According to Janda,[53] muscular development cannot proceed in the presence of pain, because pain has the potential to create a high degree of muscle inhibition that can alter muscle-firing patterns.

In addition to, and in conjunction with, the principles of PRICEMEM, electrotherapeutic and physical modalities can be used during this stage to help control pain, swelling, and muscle guarding. Heat, continuous ultrasound, and phonophoresis are introduced once the acute stage is ebbing.

During the inflammatory stage, it is also important for the patient to function as independently as possible. The aims of this phase are to avoid painful positions, improve ROM, reduce muscle atrophy through gentle isometric muscle setting, and maintain aerobic fitness.[50,54,55]

The criteria for advancement from this phase include adequate pain control and tissue healing, near-normal ROM, and tolerance for strengthening.[4]

Subacute or Intermediate Phase

Clinically, this stage is characterized by a decrease in pain and swelling and an increase in pain-free active and passive ROM (see Chapter 2). During passive ROM, the occurrence of pain is synchronous with tissue resistance.

Although the pain-free ROM may be increased in this phase, it is still not within normal limits, and stress applied to the injured structures still produces pain, although the pain experienced is lessened.[56,57]

Therapeutic Exercise

The various types of therapeutic exercise are described in Chapters 12, 13, 14, and 15. The role of exercise during recovery is discussed in this chapter. The various characteristics of an exercise load include the following[20]:

- Intensity (i.e., speed, resistance). Intensity is the rate at performing work, or the load or resistance under which the patient exercises.
- Duration (amount of time of the exercise session).
- Frequency (number of sessions per week).
- Volume of training. This is calculated by multiplying the resistance (force × distance) by the total number of repetitions performed in a specified period of time. Volume may also be calculated by adding the frequency and duration of rehabilitation or training sessions.
- Length (number of weeks or months).
- Pattern (continuous versus interval).
- Mode (e.g., running, cycling, swimming).

Progressions in the total load of exercise can be achieved by increasing the intensity, time, or frequency, or a combination of the three (see Chapters 12, 13, 14, and 15).[20] During recovery from injury, it seems that the fibroblasts need to be guided so that the replaced collagen fibers are laid along the lines of stress.

CLINICAL PEARL

The intervention goals during this phase are to protect the healing collagen, direct its orientation to be parallel to the lines of force it must withstand, and prevent cross-linking and scar contracture. If these goals are achieved, the scar will be strong and extensible.

Gentle movements to the area provide natural tensions for the healing tissues and help produce a stronger repair,[58] so a progressive increase in movement should be encouraged. Each individual responds uniquely to exercise depending on a number of variables, including the following[20]:

- Genetic endowment. Each individual has a given genetic potential that will limit the extent to which the effects of physical training can be manifested. The farther an individual is from the genetic limit, the larger will be the improvement, but as the individual gets closer to the limit, less improvement will be elicited. Gender also plays an important role, as women tend to have less muscle mass and more body fat at a given training level.[20]
- Biological age. An individual's biological age has a greater impact than chronological age. Younger adults have a greater response to training than do older adults.[59]
- Training state. Individuals at lower levels of fitness will respond with a higher rate and magnitude of adaptation than when they possess higher levels of fitness.[60]

- Health status. During either sickness or injury, the amount of adaptive energy is reduced, along with the ability to perform at optimal intensities and volumes of work. This necessitates a reduction (or elimination) in the prescription of exercise during such times.
- Fatigue state. Fatigue limits one's ability to work at optimal intensities or durations.

Early motion exercises follow a predictable path: Passive ROM is progressed to active assistive and then to active ROM, based on tissue and patient responses. Strengthening exercises during this stage are initially restricted to submaximal isometrics (see Chapter 12). The submaximal isometrics are initially performed in the early part of the range, before being performed at multiple angles of the pain-free ROM. As ROM and joint play improve, concentric exercises (see Chapter 12) are initiated, with the resistance being increased as tolerated.

CLINICAL PEARL

The criteria for advancement to the chronic or advanced stage of rehabilitation include no complaints of pain; full, pain-free ROM; good flexibility and balance; and strength of 75–80%, or greater, compared with uninvolved side.[4]

Manual Therapy

As with therapeutic exercise, manual therapy (see Chapter 10) plays an integral role in the healing process by providing controlled stresses to the healing tissues. Manual therapies during this stage include joint mobilizations (grade II) to help restore normal joint play, transverse friction massage, and gentle contract–relax techniques. It is important to emphasize to the patient that an overly aggressive approach during this stage can result in a delay or disruption in the repair process through an increase in the stimulation of the inflammatory chemical irritants and exudates.

Chronic or Advanced Phase

During this stage, pain typically is felt at the end of range with passive ROM, after the tissue resistance has been encountered (see Chapter 2). The only intervention that consistently appears beneficial across a wide spectrum of spinal and nonspinal musculoskeletal problems is the continued application of controlled stresses.

Manual Therapy

Manual techniques may be required in this stage to emphasize the restoration of joint motion and to increase the extensibility of soft tissues. Techniques to increase joint motion may include joint mobilizations (grades III–V). Techniques to increase soft-tissue extensibility include a variety of techniques including passive stretching and myofascial release (see Chapter 10).

Therapeutic Exercise

The musculoskeletal tissues respond to the controlled stresses applied to them by adaptation. This response has been described as a specific adaptation to imposed demand (SAID) (see Chapter 12).[61]

CLINICAL PEARL

The SAID principle acknowledges that the human body responds to explicit demands placed upon it with a specific and predictable adaptation. Since each load demands a specific adaptation, various loads (cross-training) will stimulate various adaptations.[20]

The application of inappropriate stresses can lead to various forms of tissue dysfunction, such as contracture, laxity, fibrosis, adhesion, diminished function, repeated structural failure, and an alteration in neurophysiologic feedback.[62,63]

CLINICAL PEARL

If the ROM and joint play are restricted, the patient continues with isometrics at various angles in the range. Otherwise, the patient is progressed through the resisted exercises.

The hierarchy for the resistive exercise progression is based on patient tolerance and response to ensure that any progress made is done in a safe and controlled fashion. The typical sequence occurs in the following order[64]:

- Small arc submaximal concentric/eccentric
- Full ROM submaximal concentric/eccentric
- Full ROM submaximal eccentric
- Functional/activity-specific plane submaximal concentric
- Functional ROM submaximal eccentric
- Open- and closed-kinetic chain exercises performed concentrically and then eccentrically
- Full ROM submaximal concentric isokinetic
- Full ROM submaximal eccentric isokinetic
- Functional ROM submaximal eccentric isokinetic

In the instance of chronic conditions, a slight increase or worsening of symptoms is sometimes permissible with exercise,[53] because the desensitization of some of the structures may require a mechanical input via stimulation of the large A fibers (see Chapter 3). However, the increase in symptoms may also signal a retriggering of the inflammatory process.[65] To help prevent these pathologic changes, Liebenson[66] recommends the following:

- Patient education about how to identify and control external sources of biomechanical overload.
- Early identification of psychosocial factors of abnormal illness behavior.
- Identification and rehabilitation of the functional pathology.

What is considered to be "normal" flexibility, strength, speed, and aerobic or anaerobic endurance for most patients in rehabilitation is inadequate for those patients returning to sport.[67] As skill is associated with enhanced mechanical efficiency and reduced risk of injury, skill in exercise-specific action should be established before the training load is increased.[20]

Return to Function

In the modern, cost-conscious health-care environment, the stage at which the patient is ready to return to full function is not often played out in the clinic. Although patient education emphasizing a slow and gradual return to activity can, to some extent, prepare the subject for this phase, reinjury, or insufficient recovery, is a real possibility.

The terms *function* and *functional* have been used extensively within the field of rehabilitation. In the context of physical therapy, function has been defined as "those activities identified by an individual as essential to support physical, social, and psychological well-being and to create a personal sense of meaningful living."[68] Functional limitations have been described as the "limitation of performance at the level of the whole organism or person . . . and should not be confused with diseases, disorders, conditions, or impairments involving specific tissue, organ, or system abnormalities that result in signs or symptoms."[68]

Therefore, in order to restore function, the clinician must think beyond the level of impairments of specific tissues and structures resulting from injury, but instead focus on the functional limitations of the patient. Such focus requires knowledge of functional testing rather than the traditional clinical testing (e.g., range of motion, strength). Functional tasks can be designed to assess the balance, balance reach, excursion, speed and agility, endurance, strength, and power of the patient, which can then be equated with function.[69] Similarly, functional progression training should involve not merely the reproduction of an activity or task by an exercise. Instead, the ultimate goal of functional training is the restoration of the patient's confidence, which implies a return to normal of the neurovascular, neurosensory, and kinesthetic systems of the body, so that the reflex performance of a movement is not deliberate, hesitant, or dyskinetic.[70–72]

It should be obvious that the speed and extent by which the injured tissues heal determines both the speed and the extent of the progression toward an optimum functional outcome. While it is virtually impossible to hasten the healing process, it is possible to prescribe a controlled and safe continuum, in which the patient can improve his or her functional status, without harming the healing structures.

Functional progression training, as with exercise progressions, must be designed in a sequential, step-by-step manner, beginning with simple tasks and progressing to highly coordinated tasks, with each step in the process requiring greater skill than the last. The overriding principle of functional rehabilitation is to return patients to the functional level they desire, or at which they were previously functioning.[71]

Ideally, the functional progression should be based on the SAID principle (see Chapter 12) in order to prepare the patient to meet the specific demands of his or her vocation, activities of daily living, or recreation. A task-oriented approach requires the clinician to understand the specific requirements of an occupation, activity, or sport. The clinician should assume that the tasks involve motions or stresses in all three planes; multiple joints, segments, or limbs; contributions from uniarticular and multiarticular muscles; and the simultaneous need for the body to move and be stable.[73] Important specific considerations include the[73]

- common postures and movement patterns;
- amount of motion;
- speed of movement;
- nature and magnitude of forces/resistances;
- dominant directions/planes of motion;
- muscular activation patterns;
- joint-specific demands;
- symmetry or asymmetry of motion;
- unilateral or bilateral limb demands; and
- environmental demands.

Functional progressions that are specific to the lower or upper extremity are included in various chapters of this book. Functional progressions and their grading for the nonathlete are also included.[74] A number of functional progressions for athletes have been devised to guide the clinician. Most of these progressions originated from postsurgical protocols, in particular, from anterior cruciate ligament reconstructions and rotator cuff surgery, which deal with various functional levels.

Rehabilitation Modalities

Clinicians have at their disposal a battery of physical agents and electrotherapeutic modalities for use in the acute phase and once the acute stage of healing has subsided. The modalities used during the acute phase involve the application of cryotherapy, electrical stimulation, pulsed ultrasound, and iontophoresis. Modalities used during the later stages of healing include thermotherapy, phonophoresis, electrical stimulation, ultrasound, iontophoresis, and diathermy (Tables 8-2 and 8-3).

At present, with the exception of cryotherapy, there is insufficient evidence to support or reject the use of modalities.[75–77] However, the absence of evidence does not always mean that there is evidence of absence (of effect), and there is always the risk of rejecting therapeutic approaches that are valid.[78]

CLINICAL PEARL

It is important that the clinician should have an understanding of the principles that relate to a particular modality so that the modality is used when indicated, and the maximum therapeutic benefit may be derived from its use.

If modalities have a place in the clinic, it is during the acute phase of healing, when there is little the clinician can do in the form of manual techniques or therapeutic exercise. In the remodeling or functional phase, thermal modalities may be used to promote blood flow to the healing tissues and to prepare the tissues for exercise or manual techniques. However, at the earliest opportunity, the patient should be weaned away from these modalities, and the focus of the intervention should shift to the application of movement and the

TABLE 8-2 Clinical Decision Making on the Use of Various Therapeutic Modalities in Treatment of Acute Injury

Phase	Approximate Time Frame	Clinical Picture	Possible Modalities Used	Rationale for Use
Initial acute	Injury—day 3	Swelling, pain to touch, and pain on motion	CRYO	↓ Swelling, ↓ pain
			ESC	↓ Pain
			IC	↓ Swelling
			LPL	↓ Pain
			Rest	
Inflammatory response	Days 1–6	Swelling subsides, warm to touch, discoloration, pain to touch, and pain on motion	CRYO	↓ Swelling, ↓ pain
			ESC	↓ Pain
			IC	↓ Swelling
			LPL	↓ Pain
			Range of motion	
Fibroblastic repair	Days 4–10	Pain to touch, pain on motion, and swollen	THERMO	Mildly ↑ circulation
			ESC	↓ Pain–muscle pumping
			LPL	↓ Pain
			IC	Facilitate lymphatic flow
			Range of motion	
			Strengthening	
Maturation-remodeling	Day 7—recovery	Swollen, no more pain to touch, and decreasing pain on motion	ULTRA	Deep heating to ↑ circulation
			ESC	↑ Range of motion, ↑ strength
			LPL	↓ Pain
			SWD	↓ Pain
			MWD	Deep heating to ↑ circulation
			Range of motion	
			Strengthening	
			Functional activities	

CRYO, cryotherapy; ESC, electrical stimulating currents; IC, intermittent compression; LPL, low-power laser; MWD, microwave diathermy; SWD, shortwave diathermy; THERMO, thermotherapy; ULTRA, ultrasound; ↓, decrease; ↑, increase.
Data from Prentice WE: Using therapeutic modalities in rehabilitation. In: Prentice WE, Voight ML, eds. *Techniques in Musculoskeletal Rehabilitation*. New York: McGraw-Hill, 2001:299.

repeated and prolonged functional restoration of the involved structures.

Two categories of modalities are recognized:

1. Physical agents and mechanical modalities
2. Electrotherapeutic modalities

Physical Agents

- ***Cryotherapy.*** The use of ice, or cryotherapy, by itself[79] or in conjunction with compression,[25–27,80] has been demonstrated to be effective in minimizing the amount of exudate. Cryotherapy, which removes heat from the body, thereby decreasing the temperature of the body tissues, is the most commonly used modality for the intervention of acute musculoskeletal injuries.[57,59–61] Hocutt and colleagues[80] demonstrated that cryotherapy started within 36 hours of injury was statistically better than heat for complete and rapid recovery. Patients using cryotherapy within 36 hours of injury reached full activity in an average of 13.2 days compared with an average 30.4 days for those initiating cryotherapy more than 36 hours after injury. Individuals who used heat required 33.3 days for return to full activity.[80]

The physiologic effects of a local cold application are principally the result of vasoconstriction, reduced metabolic function,[62] and reduced motor and sensory conduction velocities.[63,64] These effects include the following:

- ***A decrease in muscle and intra-articular temperature.*** The decrease in muscle temperature[65] and intra-articular structures[66–68] occurs because of a decline in local blood flow[57,59,61,69,70] and appears to be most noticeable between the temperatures of 40°C and 25°C.[71] Temperatures below 25°C, which typically occur after 30 minutes of cryotherapy, actually result in an increase in blood flow (Hunting effect),[71] with a consequent unfavorable increase in hemorrhage and an exaggerated acute inflammatory response.[64] The reduction in muscle and intra-articular temperature is maintained for several hours after removal of the cooling agent.[72] A prolonged application of cold, however, can result in a sympathetically mediated reflex vasodilation in an attempt to rewarm the area, which may actually worsen the swelling.[72,73]
- ***Local analgesia.***[77,79,81–85] The stages of analgesia achieved by cryotherapy are outlined in Table 8-4.[80] It is worth

TABLE 8-3	Indications and Contraindications for Therapeutic Modalities	
Therapeutic Modality	**Physiologic Responses (Indications for Use)**	**Contraindications and Precautions**
Electrical stimulating currents High voltage	Pain modulation Muscle re-education Muscle pumping contractions Retard atrophy Muscle strengthening Increase ROM Fracture healing Acute injury	Pacemakers Thrombophlebitis Superficial skin lesions
Low voltage	Wound healing Fracture healing Iontophoresis	Malignancy Skin hypersensitivities Allergies to certain drugs
Interferential	Pain modulation Muscle re-education Muscle pumping contractions Fracture healing Increase ROM	Same as high voltage
Russian	Muscle strengthening	Pacemakers
Micro-electric nerve stimulation	Fracture healing Wound healing	Malignancy Infections
Shortwave diathermy and microwave diathermy	Increase deep circulation Increase metabolic activity Reduce muscle guarding and spasm Reduce inflammation Facilitate wound healing Analgesia Increase tissue temperatures over a large area	Metal implants Pacemakers Malignancy Wet dressings Anesthetized areas Pregnancy Acute injury and inflammation Near eyes Areas of reduced blood flow Anesthetized areas
Cryotherapy (cold packs and ice massage)	Acute injury Vasoconstriction and decreased blood flow Analgesia Reduce inflammation Reduce muscle guarding/spasm	Allergy to cold Circulatory impairments Wound healing Hypertension
Thermotherapy (hot whirlpool, paraffin, hydrocollator, and infrared lamps)	Vasodilation and increased blood flow Analgesia Reduce muscle guarding and spasm Reduce inflammation Increase metabolic activity Facilitate tissue healing	Acute and post–acute trauma Poor circulation Circulatory impairments Malignancy
Low-power laser	Pain modulation (trigger points) Facilitate wound healing	Pregnancy Near eyes
Ultraviolet	Acne Aseptic wounds Folliculitis Pityriasis rosea Tinea	Psoriasis Eczema Herpes Diabetes Pellagra

(Continued)

TABLE 8-3 Indications and Contraindications for Therapeutic Modalities (*Continued*)

Therapeutic Modality	Physiologic Responses (Indications for Use)	Contraindications and Precautions
	Septic wounds Sinusitis Increase calcium metabolism	Lupus erythematosus Hyperthyroidism Renal and hepatic insufficiency Generalized dermatitis Advanced atherosclerosis
Ultrasound	Increase connective tissue extensibility Deep heat Increased circulation Treatment of most soft-tissue injuries Reduce inflammation Reduce muscle spasm	Infection Acute and post–acute injury Epiphyseal areas Pregnancy Thrombophlebitis Impaired sensation Near eyes
Intermittent compression	Decrease acute bleeding Decrease edema	Circulatory impairment

ROM, range of motion.
Data from Prentice WE: Using therapeutic modalities in rehabilitation. In: Prentice WE, Voight ML, eds. *Techniques in Musculoskeletal Rehabilitation*. New York: McGraw-Hill, 2001:301.

remembering that the timing of the stages depends on the depth of penetration and the depth of the overlying adipose tissue.[86] The patient should be advised as to these various stages, especially in light of the fact that the burning or aching phase occurs before the therapeutic phases.

- ***Decreased muscle spasm.***[26,77,87–89]
- ***Decrease in edema.***[21,77,90]
- ***Decrease in nerve conduction velocity (NCV).***[91]

Several methods of applying cryotherapy have been examined in different studies. The use of ice chips in toweling has been shown to be more effective in decreasing skin temperature than ice chips in plastic bags, or cold gel packs.[92,93] Findings from another study[94] indicated that ice massage and ice bags are equally effective in decreasing intramuscular temperature and in maintaining the duration of temperature depression. That study also found that ice massage achieves maximal intramuscular temperature decrease sooner than the ice bag.[94]

TABLE 8-4 Stages of Analgesia Induced by Cryotherapy

Stage	Response	Time after Initiation of Cryotherapy (min)
1	Cold sensation	0–3
2	Burning or aching	2–7
3	Local numbness or analgesia	5–12
4	Deep tissue vasodilation without increase in metabolism	12–15

Data from Hocutt JE, Jaffee R, Rylander R, et al: Cryotherapy in ankle sprains. *Am J Sports Med* 10:316–319, 1982.

Ice massage is recommended in all of the phases when any inflammation is present, but particularly in the acute phase, because of its effectiveness in reducing both pain and edema.[85,94–97] Ice that has been frozen in a paper cup is applied to the area in small, circular motions for 10–15 minutes before and after activity, up to six times a day.

Cold packs applied directly to the joint area are useful in decreasing pain.[84] Current recommendations are to apply ice for 20–30 minutes every 2 hours.[98]

The application of cold to an area is contraindicated over superficial nerves or healing wounds in patients with Raynaud disease or cold sensitivity and in areas with poor circulation or sensation.[99]

- ***Thermotherapy.*** Thermotherapy involves the therapeutic application of heat, which involves the transfer of thermal energy. Five types of heat transfer exist:

1. *Convection* occurs when a liquid or gas moves past a body part. An example of this type of heat transfer is the whirlpool.
2. *Evaporation* occurs when there is a change in the state of a liquid to a gas and a resultant cooling takes place. An example of this type of heat transfer occurs during spray and stretch techniques.
3. *Conversion* occurs when one form of energy is converted into another form. Examples of this type of heat transfer include ultrasound, shortwave diathermy, and microwave diathermy.
4. *Radiation* occurs when there is a transmission and absorption of electromagnetic waves.
5. *Conduction* occurs when heat is transferred between two objects that are in contact with each other. An example of this type of heat transfer occurs with hydrocollator heating packs.

Thermotherapy is used in the subacute and chronic stages of healing, because the deep heating of structures during the acute inflammatory stage has the potential to destroy collagen fibers and accelerate the inflammatory process,[100] whereas in the later stages of healing, an increase in blood flow to the injured area is beneficial.

The physiologic effects of a local heat application include the following[101–105]:

- Dissipation of body heat through selective vasodilation and shunting of blood via reflexes in the microcirculation, and regional blood flow.[106]
- Decreased muscle spasm.[83,106–108] This probably results from a decrease in neural excitability of the sensory nerves.
- Increased capillary permeability, cell metabolism, and cellular activity, all of which have the potential to increase the delivery of oxygen and chemical nutrients to the area, while decreasing venous stagnation.[102,109]
- Increased analgesia through hyperstimulation of the cutaneous nerve receptors.
- Increased tissue extensibility,[106] which has obvious implications for the application of stretching techniques. The best results are obtained if heat is applied during the stretch and if the stretch is maintained until cooling occurs after the heat has been removed.

CLINICAL PEARL

For a heat application to have a therapeutic effect, the amount of thermal energy transferred to the tissue must be sufficient to stimulate normal function, without causing injury to the tissue.[110]

An applied temperature of 40°C and 45°C is considered effective for a heat intervention. Commercial hot packs, or electric heating pads, are a conductive type of superficial moist heat, and the temperature of the unit is set anywhere between 65°C and 90°C. The moist heat pack causes an increase in the local tissue temperature, reaching its highest point about 8 minutes after the application.[111] The depth of penetration for traditional heating pads (and cold packs) is about 1 cm, which results in changes in the cutaneous blood vessels and the cutaneous nerve receptors.[93]

Wet heat produces a greater rise in local tissue temperature compared with dry heat at a similar temperature.[112] However, at higher temperatures, wet heat is not tolerated as well as dry heat.

It is important to assess the patient's sensitivity to temperature, pain, and circulation status prior to the use of thermotherapy. Moist heat should not be applied to an area with decreased sensation, poor circulation, an open wound, or an acute injury.[99] The application of moist heat to an area of malignancy is also contraindicated, because it can increase the temperature of the tumor and increase the rate of growth.[99] Hemophiliacs are also at risk with thermotherapy because of the increased blood flow.

- ***Ultrasound.*** Ultrasound, which produces a high-frequency alternating current, is primarily used for its ability to deliver heat to deep musculoskeletal tissues such as tendon, muscle, and joint structures using ultrasonic waves. These sound waves are delivered through a transducer, which has a piezoelectric crystal, the latter of which vibrates very rapidly, converting electrical energy to acoustical energy. As the energy, which leaves the transducer in a straight line, travels further from the transducer, the waves begin to diverge. The depth of penetration of the sound waves depends on a number of factors including the absorption and scattering of the beam, the medium being used (gel or lotion), the contact quality of the transducer, the treatment surface, and the tissue type (muscle, skin, fat, etc.).[113,114] Scar tissue, tendon, and ligament demonstrate the highest absorption. Tissues that demonstrate poor absorption include bone, tendinous and aponeurotic attachments of skeletal muscle, cartilaginous covering of joint surfaces, and peripheral nerves lying close to bone.[115] The portion of the sound head that produces the sound wave is referred to as the effective radiating area (ERA). The ERA is always smaller than the transducer.

Clinical units typically deliver ultrasound of 0.75–3 MHz, with duty cycles ranging from 20% to 100%. The depth of penetration of the ultrasound is roughly inversely related to its frequency.[116,117] A frequency of 3 MHz is more superficial, reaching a depth of approximately 2 cm, whereas 1 MHz is effective to a depth of 4 or 5 cm.[118] Duty cycles less than 100% are usually termed *pulsed ultrasound*, whereas a 100% duty cycle is referred to as *continuous ultrasound*. Continuous-mode ultrasound produces a thermal effect. Pulsed ultrasound does not. The thermal effects of ultrasound are similar to those previously described for thermotherapy. The nonthermal or mechanical properties of ultrasound are less well defined but are believed to alter cellular permeability and metabolism and may be important in the promotion of wound healing by reducing edema, pain, and muscle spasms.[119–122]

The beam nonuniformity ratio of ultrasound is the maximal/average intensity (W/cm^2) found in the ultrasound field. Each transducer produces sound waves in response to the vibration of the crystal. This vibration has different intensities at points on the transducer head, having peaks and valleys of intensity. The greater the ratio difference in the beam nonuniformity ratio, the more likely the transducer will have *hot spots*. Hot spots are areas of high intensity. High intensities have been shown to cause unstable cavitational effects and to retard tissue repair.[122,123] Intensities of 0.1–0.3 W/cm^2 are recommended for acute lesions, whereas 0.4–0.8 W/cm^2 are recommended for chronic lesions.[124]

Treatment times for ultrasound are based on the principle of 1 minute of ultrasound per treatment head area, although account must be taken of the pulse ratio employed. The pulse ratio needs to be higher for more acute lesions (1:4) and lower for more chronic ones (1:1 or continuous).

One study[125] demonstrated that to achieve a tissue temperature of 4°C, using continuous ultrasound, the following parameters and application times are necessary:

- 1 MHz at 1.5 W/cm^2 for 13 minutes
- 3 MHz at 1.5 W/cm^2 for 4.5 minutes

It must be remembered that the effects of ultrasound are predominantly empirical and are based on reported biophysical effects within tissue,[123,126] and on anecdotal experience in clinical practice.[127–129] Despite the paucity of documented evidence in terms of randomized control studies,[130] many benefits have been ascribed to ultrasound. These include the following:

- Production of cellular excitation, enhancing cellular activity rather than dampening it, and enhancing the inflammatory cascade, thereby encouraging the tissues to move into their next phase.[115,131–133]
- Decreased swelling when applied in a pulsed format during the inflammatory stage of healing.[123,124,126,134–139]
- Stimulation of the active cells and a maximization of scar production activity and quality, if applied during the neurovascular phase.[139–141] During the latter phase, ultrasound appears to enhance the remodeling of tissue.[123,137,140]
- An alteration of the parameters of ultrasound, which changes the intent of the intervention.[56]

▸ ***Phonophoresis.*** Phonophoresis is a specific type of ultrasound application in which pharmacologic agents are introduced in an attempt to drive these drugs transdermally into subcutaneous tissues.[135,142–148] Theoretically, increases in cell permeability and local vasodilation may result in increased diffusion of the topical agent.[135,143,144]

The efficacy of phonophoresis has not been conclusively established. Some early studies have shown drug penetration as deep as 10 cm,[148–150] but a more recent study has cast doubt on these findings.[151] Other studies have examined the effects of phonophoresis with different corticosteroid concentrations, compared with ultrasound alone, in the intervention of various musculoskeletal conditions. Recent papers have argued that many of the commonly used cream-based preparations do not allow adequate transmission of the acoustic wave.[113,114,138] Gel-based preparations appear to be superior with respect to the transmissivity of ultrasound. Consequently, gel-based corticosteroid compounds might be expected to be superior for phonophoresis applications.

Mechanical Modalities

Traction. Mechanical or manual traction has been advocated throughout the spine despite the lack of evidence for its effectiveness. Traction has been advocated to distract the zygapophyseal joint, to increase the space between the vertebrae, to enlarge the intervertebral foramina, to stretch the joint capsule and ligaments, to improve blood supply (intermittent traction), and to reduce muscle spasms and pain.[152] Manual traction is usually the first form applied as it provides the clinician with information about the patient's reaction to traction. Ideally, the manual traction should be applied specifically by applying longitudinal traction to a segment while stabilizing the segments above and below using various locking techniques. The advantage of mechanical traction is that it allows the clinician to quantify the amount of force being used. The two most common modes employed with mechanical traction include the following:

▸ Sustained or static. This type of traction is applied continuously for a number of minutes and is recommended for patients with joint and/or nerve root irritability, those with reasonable developing neurological signs that have been associated with irritability, and those patients with severe arm pain combined with reduced neck movement toward the painful side.

▸ Intermittent. This type of traction is applied for short periods, with the rest period in between and as indicated for patients with an acute joint derangement, those requiring generalized joint mobilization, and pain coming from muscle spasm.

Contraindications to mechanical traction include impaired cognitive function, rheumatoid arthritis, osteoporosis, evidence of instability, claustrophobia, spinal tumors, spinal infections, spondylolisthesis, vascular compromise, and very old or young patients.

Two types of mechanical traction are described, cervical and lumbar.

- ***Cervical.*** Cervical traction is applied with the patient in sitting or supine position, although the supine position is generally preferred as it removes the weight of the patient' s head. With intermittent traction, a duty cycle of either 1:1 or 3:1 is used, and the treatment time varies according to the condition being treated—5–10 minutes is recommended for acute conditions and disk protrusion and 15–30 minutes is recommended for other conditions.[153–155] Weights of 25–45 lb appear necessary to produce vertebral separation with cervical traction.[156] Twenty to twenty-five pounds is necessary to straighten the lordotic curvature of the cervical spine. Approximately 8–10 lb or 7–10% of the patient's body weight is recommended initially to treat disk protrusions, muscle spasm, and to elongate soft tissue in acute conditions.[153–155] Less force appears to be necessary when treatment is directed to the upper cervical area.[156] It is possible to apply traction more specifically by varying the angle of neck flexion[153–155]:
  - To increase the intervertebral space at the C1–C5 levels, approximately 0–5 degrees should be used.
  - To increase the intervertebral space at the C5 through C7 levels, 25–30 degrees of flexion is recommended.
  - Twenty-four to thirty-five degrees of flexion is recommended for zygapophyseal joint separation.
  - Zero degree of flexion is recommended for disk dysfunction.

Lumbar. The total treatment times to be used in lumbar traction are only partially research based and can range from 5 minutes to 30 minutes.[157–159] The traction force necessary to cause effective vertebral separation varies (approximately 50% of the patient's body weight).[157–159]

▸ ***Hydrotherapy.***

- ***Whirlpool.*** A whirlpool may be used in an attempt to facilitate the resorption of effusion. A cold whirlpool is indicated in acute and subacute conditions, in which gentle exercise of the injured part is permitted. The temperature for a cold whirlpool is in the range of 50–60°F (10–16°C). A warm whirlpool is indicated in chronic conditions. During the treatment, the body part may be exercised. The temperature of a warm whirlpool is in the range of 100–110°F (39–45°C).

- ***Contrast bath.*** Contrast baths are an alternating cycle of warm and cold whirlpools that create a cycle of alternating vasoconstriction and vasodilation. Contrast baths are used most often in the management of extremity injuries.[160,161] In a study by Myrer and colleagues,[162] contrast therapy of 20 minutes' duration had no impact on the intramuscular temperature of the gastrocnemius of their subjects 1 cm below the subcutaneous fat, as measured by a microprobe.[162]
- ***Prolotherapy.*** Prolotherapy, also known as "proliferation therapy," is a relatively controversial injection-based pain management technique that may be used as an intervention for degenerative or chronic injury to ligaments, tendons, fascia, and joint capsular tissue. Prolotherapy involves the injection of a small volume of an irritant solution (e.g., dextrose 10%, sodium morrhuate, and phenol–glycerine–glucose) at multiple sites on painful ligament and tendon insertions and in adjacent joint spaces. Although prolotherapy is not administered by physical therapists, patients seen in the clinic may have received a course of prolotherapy from their physician and is thus included for completeness.

Prolotherapy is purported to allow rapid production of new collagen and cartilage through stimulation of the immune system's healing mechanism. The number of injections required per intervention are based on the type of injury. Rabago and colleagues[163] reviewed data from 34 case reports and case series and two nonrandomized control trials and suggested that prolotherapy was efficacious for many musculoskeletal conditions. However, they concluded that further investigation with high-quality randomized controlled trials was required before it would be possible to determine whether or not prolotherapy was effective.

- ***Sclerosing therapy.*** Sclerosing injections have been used on patients with various conditions, including chronic low back pain,[164–166] shoulder impingement,[167] tennis elbow,[168] Achilles tendinosis,[169,170] and patella tendinosis,[171] with good results. Sclerosing therapy involves the injecting of abnormal vessels that are associated with painful tendons with a sclerosing agent to decrease pain. High-resolution color Doppler ultrasound shows intratendinous Doppler activity in patients with chronic tendinopathy. The affected area is sclerosed with vascular ingrowth. The injected chemical (e.g., Polidocanol) irritates the vascular intima to cause a vessel thrombosis. In addition, it may also sclerose the nerves adjacent to the new vessels, either directly (by destruction) or indirectly (by ischemia), which could explain the reduction in pain following the procedure.

Electrotherapeutic Modalities

▶ ***Electrical Stimulation.*** Historically, many clinicians have advocated electrical stimulation as a means of edema and pain reduction and to enhance an individual's functional level and independence in the acute phase.[90,172–176] Electrical stimulation is traditionally used to[177]

- produce a muscle contraction;
- stimulate sensory nerves to help treat pain. For example, transcutaneous electrical nerve stimulation (TENS); and
- create an electrical field within the tissues to stimulate or alter the healing process.

In addition to its use in the acute phase, electrical stimulation can be used in the other stages of healing for the reduction of pain and for neuromuscular reeducation.

Electrical current that passes through tissue forces nerves to depolarize. The type of nerve influenced in this way and the rate at which the fiber is depolarized will determine the physiologic and, therefore, therapeutic effect achieved.[178,179] Recent reports in the literature using animal models have shown varied results, based on the type of waveform, polarity used, and frequency of intervention.[180–186]

The limited studies on postsurgical or acutely injured patients seem to indicate that electrical muscle stimulation is either as effective as or more effective than isometric exercises at increasing muscle strength and bulk[187–191] in both atrophied[192] and normal muscles.[193,194]

However, according to Taylor and colleagues,[186] the present regimens being used (i.e., one intervention per day or three times per week) may be insufficiently aggressive to provide benefit.

▶ ***Transdermal Iontophoresis.*** Transdermal iontophoresis is a method by which ionic therapeutic agents are administered through the skin by the application of a low-level electrical current. Iontophoresis has proved to be valuable in the intervention of musculoskeletal disorders. Iontophoresis causes an increased penetration of drugs and other compounds into tissues by the use of an applied current through the tissue. The principle behind iontophoresis is that an electrical potential difference actively causes ions in solution to transfer according to their electrical charge. Ionized medications do not ordinarily penetrate tissues, and, if they do, it is not normally at a rate rapid enough to achieve therapeutic levels.[195] This problem is overcome by providing a direct current energy source.[195,196]

CLINICAL PEARL

Negatively charged ions are repelled from a negative electrode and attracted toward the positive electrode. In contrast, the positive ions are repelled from the positive electrode and attracted toward the negative electrode.[195,196]

Iontophoresis has, therefore, been used for the transdermal delivery of systemic drugs in a controlled fashion.[197] The factors affecting the quality of the transdermal iontophoretic transport include pH; the intensity of the current, or current density, at the active electrode; ionic strength; concentration of drug; molecular size; and the duration of the current flow (continuous or pulse current).[198–200]

Iontophoresis can be performed using a wide range of chemicals (Table 8-5). If the ionic source is in an aqueous solution, it is recommended that a low concentration be used (2–4%) to aid in the dissociation.[201] Although electrons flow from negative to positive, regardless of electrode size, having a

TABLE 8-5 Various Ions Used in Iontophoresis

Ion	Polarity	Solution	Purpose/Condition
Acetate	–	2–5% acetic acid	Calcium deposits[171]
Atropine sulfate	+	0.001–0.01%	Hyperhidrosis
Calcium	+	2% calcium chloride	Myopathy and muscle spasm
Chlorine	–	2% sodium chloride	Scar tissue and adhesions
Copper	+	2% copper sulfate	Fungus infection
Dexamethasone	+	4 mg/mL dexamethasone Na–P	Tendonitis and bursitis[172]
Lidocaine	+	4% lidocaine	Trigeminal neuralgia[173]
Hyaluronidase	+	Wydase	Edema[174]
Iodine	–	Iodex ointment	Adhesions and scar tissue[175]
Magnesium	+	2% magnesium sulfate (Epsom salts)	Muscle relaxant[176] and bursitis
Mecholyl	+	0.25%	Muscle relaxant
Potassium iodide	–	10%	Scar tissue
Salicylate	–	2% sodium salicylate	Myalgia and scar tissue
Tap water	±	—	Hyperhidrosis

+, positive; –, negative.

larger negative pad than a positive one will help shape the direction of flow.

Current intensity is recommended to be at 5 mA or less. The duration of the treatment can vary from 10 to 20 minutes. Longer durations have been shown to produce a decrease in the skin impedance, thus increasing the likelihood of burns from an accumulation of ions under the electrodes.[202] An accumulation of negative ions under the positive electrode produces hydrochloric acid. An accumulation of positive ions under the negative electrode produces sodium hydroxide.

Other complications have included prolonged erythema that resolved in 24 hours, tingling, burning, and pulling sensations that were especially apparent at the start of the current or if the amperage was turned up too rapidly. The visible erythema demonstrates the clear increase of blood flow and the influence of the iontophoresis.

Currently, research has been focused on the development of iontophoretic patches for the systemic delivery of drugs as (1) they provide the option to monitor and control the power supplied during use, (2) can detect the number of times the patch has been used, and (3) the controller can be rendered unusable to avoid abuse, once the drug is exhausted.

Extracorporal Shock Wave Therapy. High-energy extracorporeal shock waves have been used in urology for the disintegration of stone concretion for almost 15 years. For the past 10 years, this technology has emerged as a treatment modality for managing pain caused by a broad range of musculoskeletal conditions. These conditions include tendinopathies and nonunion and delayed union of fractures.[203–205] Currently, the therapeutic mechanisms of shock waves in musculoskeletal problems or their specific biologic effects on the various musculoskeletal tissues (bone, cartilage, tendon, ligament) are not fully understood. [206] The extracorporeal shock wave is an acoustic wave characterized by high positive pressures of more than 1,000 bar (100 MPa), which can be developed within an extremely short rise time (10^{-9} seconds) and followed by a low-pressure phase of tensile stress equivalent to 100 bar (10 Mpa).[207] A clinically applicable shock wave represents nothing more than a controlled explosion, producing a sonic pulse in much the same way as a fast-flying aircraft may produce a sonic boom.[206] When the shock wave enters the tissue, it may be dissipated and reflected so that the kinetic energy is absorbed according to the integral structure of the tissues or structures that are exposed to the shock waves.[206] However, because the duration of the shock wave is so short (3–5 microseconds) and is generated at low frequencies, no thermal effect is generated. For shock waves to be effective in the clinical situation, the maximally beneficial pulse energy must be concentrated at the point at which treatment is to be provided. There are three mechanisms by which extracorporeal shock wave therapy (ESWT) units generate the shock waves: electromagnetic, electrohydraulic, and piezoelectric. The electromagnetic and piezoelectric units tend to generate lower energy shock waves than the electrohydraulic units.[208] Medically useful shock waves usually are generated through a fluid medium (water) and a coupling gel to facilitate transmission into biologic tissues. The energy flux density (ED) refers to the shock wave energy "flow" through an area perpendicular to the direction of propagation[208]; 1,000–2,000 shock waves of an ED from 0.01 to 0.4 mJ/mm^2 are usually applied two to three times at weekly intervals.[207] Pulse duration is usually fixed at 3–5 microseconds and the calculation of dose (total energy delivered) depends on the choice of energy level and the total number of shock wave impulses delivered.[208] Most patients report a sharp pain sensation during the application of ESWT, necessitating a skin sensation test prior to its use.

A meta-analysis by Ogden et al.[209] reported that, of various applications of ESWT on musculoskeletal conditions, the use of ESWT for treating chronic, recalcitrant heel pain syndrome was the most credible.

ESWT is contraindicated for use in patients suffering from hemophilia (because it may cause microvascular disruption) and malignancy, and ESWT should not be applied over growth plates or where exposure to lung tissue may occur (clavicle or first rib).[206,208]

Transcutaneous Electrical Nerve Stimulation. TENS was first introduced in the early 1950s to determine the suitability of patients with pain as candidates for the implantation of posterior (dorsal) column electrodes. TENS has since been shown to be effective in providing pain relief in the early stages of healing following surgery[188,210–214] and in the remodeling phase.[215–218]

The percentage of patients who benefit from short-term TENS pain intervention has been reported to range from 50% to 80%, and good long-term results with TENS have been observed in 6–44% of patients.[215,217,219,220]

TENS units typically deliver symmetric or balanced asymmetric biphasic waves of 100- to 500-millisecond pulse duration, with zero net current to minimize skin irritation,[221] and may be applied for extended periods.

Three modes of action are theorized for the efficacy of this modality (see Chapter 3):

1. ***Gate control mechanism.*** Spinal gating control through stimulation of the large, myelinated A-alpha fibers inhibits transmission of the smaller pain transmitting unmyelinated C fibers and myelinated A-delta fibers.[213,222]
2. ***Endogenous opiate control.*** When subjected to certain types of electrical stimulation of the sensory nerves, there may be a release of enkephalin from local sites within the central nervous system and the release of β-endorphin from the pituitary gland into the cerebrospinal fluid.[221,223,224] A successful application can produce an analgesic effect that lasts for several hours.
3. ***Central biasing.*** Intense electrical stimulation, approaching a noxious level, of the smaller C or pain fibers produces a stimulation of the descending neurons.

Hyperbaric Oxygen Therapy

Hyperbaric oxygen therapy (HBOT) is the medical use of oxygen at a level higher than atmospheric pressure, which produces an excess of oxygen in the body. This increased dissolved oxygen in the plasma has been shown to more effectively reach injured tissues than oxygen-bound hemoglobin.[225] The current literature includes studies of treatment of numerous different orthopaedic conditions using HBOT, including delayed onset muscle soreness, chronic wounds, fibromyalgia, complex regional pain syndrome, migraine and cluster headaches, and edema.[225] The only absolute contraindication to HBOT is untreated pneumothorax.

Aquatic Therapy

Current research shows aquatic therapy to be beneficial in the treatment of everything from orthopaedic injuries to spinal cord damage, chronic pain, cerebral palsy, multiple sclerosis, and many other conditions. Among the psychological aspects, water motivates movement because painful joints and muscles can be moved more easily and painlessly in water.

The indications for aquatic therapy include instances when partial weight-bearing ambulation is necessary, to increase range of motion, when standing balance needs to be improved, when endurance/aerobic capacity needs to be improved, or when the goal is to increase muscle strength via active-assisted, gravity-assisted, active or resisted exercise.

Contraindications to aquatic therapy include incontinence, urinary tract infections, unprotected open wounds, heat intolerance, severe epilepsy, uncontrolled diabetes, unstable blood pressure, or severe cardiac and/or pulmonary dysfunction. In general, pregnant women are quite sensitive to core temperature elevations and should therefore exercise in cool to neutral temperatures.

Physical Properties and Resisted Forces

There are several physical properties of water, which make exercising in water differ from that on land:

- Density. Although the human body is mostly water, the body's density is slightly less than that of water and averages a specific gravity of 0.974, with men averaging higher density than women. Any object with a specific gravity less than that of water will float. The buoyant values of different body parts vary according to a number of factors:
- Bone to muscle weight. Lean body mass, which includes bone, muscle, connective tissue, and organs, has a typical density near 1.1.
- The amount and distribution of fat. Fat mass, which includes both essential body fat plus fat in excess of essential needs, has a density of about 0.9.

Consequently, the human body displaces a volume of water weighing slightly more than the body, forcing the body upward by a force equal to the volume of the water displaced, as discovered by Archimedes.

- Hydrostatic pressure: Pressure is directly proportional to both the liquid density and to the immersion depth when the fluid is incompressible. Water exerts a pressure of 22.4 mm Hg/ft of water depth, which translates to 1 mm Hg/1.36 cm (0.54 inches) of water depth. Thus, a human body emerged to a depth of 48 inches is subjected to a force equal to 88.9 mm Hg, slightly greater than normal diastolic blood pressure.[226] The effects of hydrostatic pressure, which is the force that aids resolution of edema in an injured body part, begin immediately on the motion, causing plastic deformation of the body over a short period. This results in a cranial displacement of blood, a rise in right atrial pressure, increase in pleural surface pressure, compression of the chest wall, and a cranial displacement of the diaphragm.
- Buoyancy: As the body is gradually immersed, water is displaced, creating the force of buoyancy. A human with specific gravity of 0.97 reaches floating equilibrium when 97% of his or her total body volume is submerged:[226]
  - with neck depth immersion, only about 15 lb of compressive force is exerted on the spine, hips, and knees.
  - with immersion up to the symphysis pubis, 40% of the body weight is effectively offloaded.
  - with immersion up to the umbilicus, 50% of the body weight is effectively offloaded.
  - with immersion up to the xiphoid, 60% or more (depending on whether the arms are overhead or beside the trunk) of the body weight is effectively offloaded.
- Viscosity: refers to the magnitude of internal friction specific to a fluid during motion. A limb moving relative to water is

subjected to the resistive effects of the fluid called drag force and turbulence when present.[226]

- Drag force: It is a factor of the shape of an object and its speed of movement. Objects that are more streamlined (minimizing the surface area at the front of the object) produce less drag force.
- Turbulence: Under turbulent flow conditions, resistance increases as a log function of velocity.

Viscous resistance increases as more forces are exerted against it, but that resistance drops to zero almost immediately on cessation of force.

Thermodynamics

The heat capacity of water is 1,000 times greater than the equivalent volume of air. The therapeutic utility of water depends greatly on both its ability to retain heat and its ability to transfer heat energy. Heat transfer begins immediately on immersion, and as the heat capacity of the human body is less than that of water (0.83 versus 1.00), the body equilibrates faster than the water does.

CLINICAL PEARL

Water is an efficient conductor, transferring heat 25 times faster than air. This thermal conductive property, in combination with the high specific heat of water, makes the use of water in rehabilitation very versatile because water retains heat or cold while delivering either to the immersed body part.[226]

Design and Special Equipment

Certain characteristics of the pool should be taken into consideration if it is to be used for rehabilitation purposes:

- The pool should not be smaller than 10′ × 12′.
- The pool should have both a shallow (1.25 m/2.5 ft) and a deep (2.5 m/5 ft plus) area to allow for standing exercises and swimming or nonstanding exercise.
- The pool bottom should be flat and the depth gradations clearly marked.

Variable temperature control for the water should be available (water that is too warm can lead to fatigue or even heat exhaustion because evaporation of perspiration is not possible in water, whereas water that is too cool can cause shivering, increase muscular tension, or produce hypothermia):

- Cold plunge tanks are often used at temperatures of 10–15°C to produce a decrease in muscle pain and speed recovery from overuse injury.
- Most public and competitive pools operate in the range of 27–29°C.
- Typical therapy pools operate in the range of 33.5–35.5°C.
- Hot tubs are usually maintained at 37.5–41°C.

Rescue tubes, inner tubes, and wet vests should be purchased to assist in floatation activities. Hand paddles and pull buoys can be used for strengthening the upper extremity. Kick boards and fins are useful for strengthening the lower extremity.

Advantages

Aquatic therapy offers a number of advantages over traditional land-borne exercises:

- The buoyancy of the water allows active exercise while providing a sense of security and causing little discomfort. Deep water running drills, using a buoyancy vest, can be used to maintain fitness during recovery from lower limb injury and as a form of cross-training to reduce impact with the aim of reducing overuse injuries.
- Early in the rehabilitation process, aquatic therapy is useful in restoring range of motion and flexibility using a combination of the water's buoyancy, resistance, and warmth.
- The buoyancy provides support. An aquatic exercise program can be designed to vary the amount of gravity loading by using buoyancy as a counterforce. Shallow water vertical exercises generally approximate closed chain exercises, albeit with reduced joint loading because of the counterforce produced by buoyancy. Deepwater exercises more generally approximate open chain system, as do horizontal exercises. Paddles and other resistive equipment tend to close the kinetic chain.
- The slow-motion effect of moving in water provides extra time to control movement and to react. Aquatic exercise protocols have been successfully used to improve balance and coordination in older individuals, who face an increased risk of falling.[227]
- The water provides tactile stimulation and feedback.
- The buoyancy of water can be used to provide a gradual transition from non–weight-bearing to full–weight-bearing exercises by adjusting the amount the body is submerged. For acute injuries, programs typically start at non–weight-bearing depths, limiting activity below pain onset, and then progressing in weight-bearing exercise levels as symptoms permit.
- The intensity of exercise can be controlled by manipulating the body's position or through the addition of exercise equipment. During aquatic treadmill running, oxygen consumption is three times greater at a given speed of ambulation in water than on land, thus the training effect may be achieved at a significantly slower speed than on land.[228]

Disadvantages

The disadvantages of aquatic therapy include:

- Cost of building and maintenance.
- Difficulty in treating patients with inherent fear of water.
- Potential adverse effects on the cardiovascular system. Because an individual immersed in water is subjected to external water pressure in a gradient, which within a relatively small depth exceeds venous pressure, blood is displaced upward to the venous and lymphatic systems, first into the thighs, then into the abdominal cavity vessels, and finally into the great vessels of the chest cavity and into the

heart.[226] The following cardiovascular changes can occur with immersion of the body:

- An increase in central venous pressure.
- An increase in pulse pressure as a result of the increased cardiac filling and decreased heart rate during thermoneutral or cool immersion.
- An increase in central blood volume.
- An increase in cardiac volume, cardiac output, and stroke volume.
- A decrease in sympathetic vasoconstriction resulting in a reduction in both peripheral venous tone and systemic vascular resistance.

▸ Potential adverse effects on the pulmonary system. Immersion of the body to the level of the thorax causes a shifting of blood into the chest cavity and increased compression of the chest.[226] The combined effect is to alter pulmonary function, increase the work of breathing, and change respiratory dynamics. However, while care must be taken with patients who have inspiratory muscle weakness due to conditions such as congestive heart failure and chronic obstructive lung disease, respiratory strengthening can also be an important aspect of high-level athletic performance.

Postsurgical Rehabilitation

Traditional interventions for postsurgical patients have involved adhering to exercise protocols designed by the surgeon performing the operation in order to limit postsurgical stress. This has led to an emphasis on interventions based solely on exercises linked to time frames, a sort of "cookbook" approach, rather than a comprehensive approach designed in conjunction with the physical therapist based on clinical findings and individual consideration.

Among the key factors that must be considered in the postsurgical rehabilitation are[229]

- ▸ type of surgery;
- ▸ patient's age;
- ▸ patient's physical status, including weight, and other medical conditions, such as any history of cardiovascular or peripheral vascular disease (PVD), or diabetes;
- ▸ social lifestyle of the patient;
- ▸ preoperative joint contracture or muscle atrophy;
- ▸ method of fixation;
- ▸ surrounding soft tissues involved;
- ▸ degree of correction of biomechanical alignment;
- ▸ functional and recreational goals of the patient; and
- ▸ frequency of visits during the episode of care.

These factors may influence the rate at which the patient progresses through the rehabilitation process, as well as determine the extent of functional return that can be expected in the long term.

The stages of healing described in Chapter 2 should not be viewed as distinct entities or as rigid templates but as a continuum that must be modified on the basis of clinical findings and subjective responses. For example, responses to an intervention that indicate an overly aggressive approach include

- ▸ increased area of pain;
- ▸ pain at rest that lasts longer than 2 hours after exercising[230]; and
- ▸ pain that alters the performance of an activity or exercise in a detrimental manner.[230]

Obviously, each surgical procedure is different, as is the healing capacity of each individual. In addition, each surgeon has his or her opinion as to the intensity of the postsurgical intervention. These opinions must always be respected. The point at which the tools of intervention are used following surgery may vary, and although estimated timetables are provided with each of the protocols, the intention is to provide the clinician with intervention ideas rather than a regimented timescale.

Realistic goal setting is important following surgery. Postsurgical rehabilitation goals should be based on the status of the uninvolved extremity as long as the uninvolved extremity has no deficits. For cases in which the uninvolved extremity does have deficits, the clinician should use the guidelines from expected norms. The patient should be involved in the goal-setting process when possible.

Patient/Client-Related Instruction

Patient/client-related instruction forms the cornerstone of every intervention. During the physical therapy visits, the clinician and the patient work to alter the patient's perception of the functional capabilities. Together, the patient and clinician discuss the parts of the patient's life that he or she can and cannot control and then consider how to improve those parts that can be changed. It is imperative that the clinician spends time educating the patient about his or her condition, so that the patient can fully understand the importance of his or her role in the rehabilitation process and become an educated consumer. Educating the patient about strategies to adopt in order to prevent recurrences and to self-manage his or her condition is also very important. Discussions about intervention goals must continue throughout the rehabilitative process and must be mutually acceptable.

Oftentimes, the physician relies on the physical therapist to give a broader explanation about the condition and to answer questions and concerns related to the rehabilitative process. The aim of patient education is to create independence, not dependence, and to foster an atmosphere of learning in the clinic. A detailed explanation should be given to the patient in a language that he or she can understand. This explanation should include

- ▸ the name of the structure(s) involved, the cause of the problem, and the effect of the biomechanics on the area. Whenever possible, an illustration of the offending structure should be shown to the patient. Anatomic models can be used to explain biomechanical principles in layperson's terms.
- ▸ information about tests, diagnosis, and interventions that are planned.

- the prognosis of the problem and a discussion about the patient's functional goals. An estimation of healing time is useful for the patient, so that he or she does not become frustrated at a perceived lack of progress.
- what patients can do to help themselves. This includes the allowed use of the joint or area, a brief description about the relevant stage of healing, and the vulnerability of the various structures during the pertinent healing phase. This information makes the patient aware and more cautious when performing activities of daily living, recreational activities, and the home exercise program. Emphasis should be placed on dispelling the myth of "no pain, no gain," and patients should be encouraged to respect pain. Patients often have misconceptions about when to use heat and ice, and it is the role of the clinician to clarify such issues.
- home exercise program. Before prescribing a home exercise program, the clinician should take into consideration the time that will be needed to perform the program. In addition, the level of tolerance and motivation for exercise vary among individuals and are based on their diagnosis and stage of healing. A short series of exercises, performed more frequently during the day, should be prescribed for patients with poor endurance or when the emphasis is on functional reeducation. Longer programs, performed less frequently, are aimed at building strength or endurance. Each home exercise program needs to be individualized to meet the patient's specific needs. Although two patients may have the same diagnosis, the examination may reveal different positive findings and stages of healing, both of which may alter the intervention.

There are probably as many ways to teach as there are to learn. The clinician needs to be aware that people may have very different preferences for how, when, where, and how often to learn. It is not within the scope of this text to discuss all of the theories on learning, but an overview of the major concepts is merited.

Litzinger and Osif[231] organized individuals into four main types of learners, based on instructional strategies:

1. ***Accommodators.*** This type looks for the significance of the learning experience. These learners enjoy being active participants in their learning and will ask many questions, such as, "What if?" and "Why not?"
2. ***Divergers.*** This type is motivated to discover the relevancy of a given situation and prefers to have information presented in a detailed, systematic, and reasoned manner.
3. ***Assimilators.*** This type is motivated to answer the question, "What is there to know?" These learners like accurate, organized delivery of information, and they tend to respect the knowledge of the expert. They are perhaps less instructor intensive than some other types of learners and will carefully follow prescribed exercises, provided a resource person is clearly available and able to answer questions.
4. ***Convergers.*** This type is motivated to discover the relevancy, or "how," of a situation. The instructions given to this type of learner should be interactive, not passive.

Another way of classifying learners that is frequently used was devised by Taylor,[186] who proposed that there are three common learning styles:

1. ***Visual.*** As the name suggests, the visual learner assimilates information by observation, using visual cues and information such as pictures, anatomic models, and physical demonstrations.
2. ***Auditory.*** Auditory learners prefer to learn by having things explained to them verbally.
3. ***Tactile.*** Tactile learners, who learn through touch and interaction, are the most difficult of the three groups to teach. Close supervision is required with this group until they have demonstrated to the clinician that they can perform the exercises correctly and independently. Proprioceptive neuromuscular facilitation techniques, with the emphasis on physical and tactile cues, often work well with this group.

A patient's learning style can be identified by asking how he or she prefers to learn. Some patients will prefer a simple handout with pictures and instructions; others will prefer to see the exercises demonstrated and then be supervised while they perform the exercises. Some may want to know why they are doing the exercises, which muscles are involved, why they are doing three sets of a particular exercise, and so on. Others will require less explanation.

If the clinician is unsure about the patient's learning style, it is recommended that each exercise first be demonstrated by the clinician and then by the patient. The rationale and purpose behind each of the exercises must be given, as well as the frequency and intensity expected.

Compliance is vitally important in the healing process. Compliance can be defined as engaging in behavior as instructed or prescribed.[232] Another term "adherence," which can be defined as choosing to engage in behaviors, is similar in that both vary from patient to patient and both are related to motivation. Motivation, a psychological feature that drives an organism toward a desired goal, is considered vital to maintaining behavior. Motivation has been classified as either intrinsic (internal) or extrinsic (external). A number of motivational theories have been proposed (Table 8-6).

Anecdotally, unmotivated patients may progress more slowly. Much literature has conceptualized or reported poor motivation in rehabilitation as secondary to patient-related factors, including depression, apathy, cognitive impairment, low self-efficacy (e.g., low confidence in one's ability to successfully rehabilitate), fatigue, and personality factors.[233] Various studies have found that average compliance with medication regimens occurs only in 50–60% of patients, and compliance with physical therapy programs is approximately 40%.[234] Other reports have found that compliance was decreased if the physical therapists did not provide their patients with positive feedback.[235]

Several considerations should be made to increase compliance:

- The patient's age—older individuals tend to adhere to exercise programs more than younger individuals.[236]

TABLE 8-6 Motivational Theories

Theory	Proponents	Description
Social cognitive	Bandura[a]	Individuals act as contributors to the own motivation, behavior, and development. Behavior and characteristics are modified by environment. Primary mediators include self-efficacy and the ability to self-regulate. Mastery is the best way to create a strong sense of efficacy.
Self-determination	Lepper et al.[b]	Choices made are based on experiences, thoughts, contemplations, and interactions with others. Essential psychological needs include competence, relatedness, and autonomy. Comprised of five minitheories:[c] ► Cognitive Evaluation Theory (CET): intrinsic motivation is a lifelong creative wellspring. CET highlights the critical roles played by competence and autonomy in fostering intrinsic motivation. ► Organismic Integration Theory: extrinsic motivation is behavior that aims toward outcomes extrinsic to the behavior itself. Highlights supports for autonomy and relatedness as critical to internalization. ► Causality Orientations Theory: describes individual differences in people's tendencies to orient toward environments and regulate behavior in various ways based on rewards, gains, and approval. ► Basic Psychological Needs Theory: psychological well-being and optimal functioning is predicated on meeting the needs of autonomy, competence, and relatedness. ► Goal Contents Theory: Goals are seen as differentially affording basic need satisfactions and are thus differentially associated with well-being.
Health belief model	Ajzen[d] and Fishbein[e]	An individual's attitude, social norms, and perceived control are accurate predictors of behavioral intentions. Involves the TRA and the TPB: ► TRA is most successful when applied to behavior under an individual's voluntary control. ► TPB theorizes that if an individual's perceived control, self-efficacy, or self-esteem is low, the perception and belief that he or she can influence behavior in a positive manner is undermined.
Humanistic	Maslow[f]	Based on the concept that there is a hierarchy of biogenic and psychogenic needs that humans must progress through. Hypothesizes that the higher needs in this hierarchy only come into focus once all the needs that are lower down are mainly or entirely satisfied.
Transtheoretical model	Prochaska and DiClemente[g]	Describes five stages of change: ► Precontemplation: defined by a lack of intention to take action. ► Contemplation: defined by the individual thinking about engaging in a behavior or activity in the near future. ► Preparation: defined by the individual intending to take action in the immediate future. ► Action: defined by the individual actively engaged in the behavior or change. ► Maintenance: defined by an individual who has engaged in a behavior or change for longer than 6 mo.

TPB, theory of planned behavior; TRA, theory of reasoned action.

[a]Bandura A: Social foundations of thought and action: a social-cognitive theory. Upper Saddle River, NJ: Prentice Hall, 1986.

[b]Lepper MK, Greene D, Nisbett R: Undermining children's intrinsic interest with extrinsic reward: A test of the "overjustification" hypothesis. *J Personality Social Psychol* 28:129–137, 1973.

[c]University of Rochester: Self-determination theory: approach to human motivation and personality. Available at: http://www.psych.rochester.edu/SDT/theory.php.

[d]Ajzen I: From intentions to actions: a theory of planned behavior: In Kuhl J, Beckmann J, eds. *Action-Control: From Cognition to Behavior.* Heidelberg: Springer, 1985:11–39.

[e]Ajzen I, Fishbein M: *Understanding Attitudes and Predicting Social Behavior.* Englewood Cliffs, NJ: Prentice Hall, 1980.

[f]Maslow A: *The Farther Reaches of Human Nature.* New York: Viking Press, 1971.

[g]Prochaska JO, DiClemente CC: Stages and processes of self-change of smoking: toward an integrative model of change. *J Consult Clin Psychol* 51:390–395, 1983.

- The patient's marital status—singles tend to have lower rates of adherence to physical activity/exercise than married couples.[237]
- The patient's education—individuals with high levels of education show more compliance to exercise programs than those who are uneducated.[237]
- The patient's gender—males report greater levels of total and vigorous activity than females.[237]
- The patient's biomedical status—poorer health tends to lead to decreased adherence.[238]
- The patient's socioeconomic status—an individual's income bracket tends to influence the ability to access medical care, as well as exercise equipment and venues.[239–241]
- The patient's ethnicity—Caucasians appear to participate in more physical activities than other racial or ethnic groups, regardless of age.[237]

Finally, a number of factors have been outlined to improve compliance; including[242–244]

- involving the patient in the intervention planning and goal setting;
- realistic goal setting for both short- and long-term goals;
- promoting high expectations regarding final outcome;
- promoting perceived benefits;
- projecting a positive attitude;
- providing clear instructions and demonstrations with appropriate feedback;
- keeping the exercises pain free or with a low level of pain; and
- encouraging patient problem solving.

Health Promotion, Wellness, and Physical Fitness

In 1996, the Surgeon General's report on physical activity and health highlighted the importance of engaging in an active lifestyle to prevent the insidious onset of chronic disease and illness.[245] Healthy People 2010 established goals for promoting a healthy lifestyle for individuals in the United States.[246]

The World Health Organization has defined health promotion as "the process of enabling people to increase control over their health and its determinants, and thereby improve their health."*

The National Wellness Institute has delineated six components of wellness†:

- Social. This includes contributing to one's environment and community and emphasizing the interdependence between others and nature.
- Occupational. This includes satisfaction and enriching life through work.
- Spiritual. This includes an appreciation of the depth of an expansive life and having meaning in one's life.
- Physical. This includes awareness of the need for regular physical activity, good diet and nutrition, and avoiding habits that are harmful to wellness.
- Intellectual. This includes being able to solve problems, expand knowledge and skills, and have an openness to new ideas.
- Emotional. This includes awareness and acceptance of one's feelings and thinking of oneself positively.

*Available at http://w3.whosea.org/EN/Section1174/Section1458/Section2057.htm, accessed September 2005.

†Available at www.nationalwellness.org/index.php?id= 166&id_tier=81, accessed September 2005.

Physical therapists serve as major providers of health promotion, wellness, and fitness by making patients and clients more aware of lifestyle changes, particularly in the areas of physical activity, lifelong health promotion, and creating an environment that supports health practices leading to a healthy lifestyle.[247] Evidence exists that when healthcare professionals counsel patients about risk reduction, those patients are more likely to change poor health habits, thus enhancing a healthier lifestyle.*

The effects of physical activity and exercise on various physiological and psychological parameters across the lifespan for use of exercise prescriptions support their role in preventing disease and improving function and health. This is particularly relevant in promoting mobility and dependence of the elderly, the older old, and the frail elderly.[247]

REVIEW QUESTIONS

1. What are the three components that comprise the intervention?
2. What does the pneumonic PRICEMEM stand for?
3. Give five therapeutic benefits of the application of manual therapy in the early stages of healing.
4. With passive mobility testing, which stage of healing is indicated when pain is reported before tissue resistance is felt by the clinician?
5. What are the intervention goals during the inflammatory stage of healing?

*Available at www.healthwellness.org/archive/research/study5.htm, accessed November 2004.

REFERENCES

1. Hungerford DS, Lennox DW: Rehabilitation of the knee in disorders of the patellofemoral joint: Relevant biomechanics. *Orthop Clin North Am* 14:397–444, 1983.
2. Nirschl RP: Prevention and treatment of elbow and shoulder injuries in the tennis player. *Clin Sports Med* 7:289–308, 1988.
3. Grimsby O, Power B: Manual therapy approach to knee ligament rehabilitation. In: Ellenbecker TS, ed. *Knee Ligament Rehabilitation.* Philadelphia: Churchill Livingstone, 2000:236–251.
4. Herring SA, Kibler BW: A framework for rehabilitation. In: Kibler BW, Herring JA, Press JM, eds. *Functional Rehabilitation of Sports and Musculoskeletal Injuries.* Gaithersburg, MD: Aspen, 1998:1–8.
5. Guide to physical therapist practice. *Phys Ther* 81:S13–S95, 2001.

6. Sullivan PE, Puniello MS, Pardasaney PK: Rehabilitation program development: Clinical decision-making, prioritization, and program integration. In: Magee D, Zachazewski JE, Quillen WS, eds. *Scientific Foundations and Principles of Practice in Musculoskeletal Rehabilitation*. St. Louis, MI: WB Saunders, 2007:314–327.
7. Jette DU, Grover L, Keck CP: A qualitative study of clinical decision making in recommending discharge placement from the acute care setting. *Phys Ther* 83:224–236, 2003.
8. Cyriax J: *Textbook of Orthopaedic Medicine, Diagnosis of Soft Tissue Lesions*, 8th ed. London: Bailliere Tindall, 1982.
9. McKenzie R, May S: Introduction. In: McKenzie R, May S, eds. *The Human Extremities: Mechanical Diagnosis and Therapy*. Waikanae, New Zealand: Spinal Publications New Zealand Ltd, 2000:1–5.
10. Maitland GD: The hypothesis of adding compression when examining and treating synovial joints. *J Orthop Sports Phys Ther* 2:7, 1980.
11. Maitland G: *Peripheral Manipulation*, 3rd ed. London: Butterworth, 1991.
12. McGinn TG, Guyatt GH, Wyer PC, et al: Users' guides to the medical literature: XXII: How to use articles about clinical decision rules. Evidence-Based Medicine Working Group. *JAMA* 284:79–84, 2000.
13. Stanton TR, Hancock MJ, Maher CG, et al: Critical appraisal of clinical prediction rules that aim to optimize treatment selection for musculoskeletal conditions. *Phys Ther* 90:843–854, 2010.
14. Flynn T, Fritz J, Whitman J, et al: A clinical prediction rule for classifying patients with low back pain who demonstrate short-term improvement with spinal manipulation. *Spine* 27:2835–2843, 2002.
15. Denegar CR, Donley PB: Impairment due to pain: Managing pain during the rehabilitation process. In: Voight ML, Hoogenboom BJ, Prentice WE, eds. *Musculoskeletal Interventions: Techniques for Therapeutic Exercise*. New York: McGraw-Hill, 2007:99–110.
16. Garrick JG: A practical approach to rehabilitation. *Am J Sports Med* 9:67–68, 1981.
17. Thevenet D, Tardieu-Berger M, Berthoin S, et al: Influence of recovery mode (passive vs. active) on time spent at maximal oxygen uptake during an intermittent session in young and endurance-trained athletes. *Eur J Appl Physiol* 99:133–142, 2007.
18. Wigernaes I, Hostmark AT, Stromme SB, et al: Active recovery and post-exercise white blood cell count, free fatty acids, and hormones in endurance athletes. *Eur J Appl Physiol* 84:358–366, 2001.
19. Hakkinen K, Myllyla E: Acute effects of muscle fatigue and recovery on force production and relaxation in endurance, power and strength athletes. *J Sports Med Phys Fitness* 30:5–12, 1990.
20. Wenger HA, McFadyen PF, Middleton L, et al: Physiological principles of conditioning for the injured and disabled. In: Magee D, Zachazewski JE, Quillen WS, eds. *Scientific Foundations and Principles of Practice in Musculoskeletal Rehabilitation*. St. Louis, MI: WB Saunders, 2007:357–374.
21. McMaster WC: Cryotherapy. *Phys Sports Med* 10:112–119, 1982.
22. Hettinga DL: Inflammatory response of synovial joint structures. In: Gould JA, Davies GJ, eds. *Orthopaedic and Sports Physical Therapy*. St. Louis: C. V. Mosby, 1985:87–117.
23. Thorndike A: *Athletic Injuries: Prevention, Diagnosis and Treatment*. Philadelphia: Lea and Febiger, 1962.
24. Maadalo A, Waller JF: Rehabilitation of the foot and ankle linkage system. In: Nicholas JA, Hershman EB, eds. *The Lower Extremity and Spine in Sports Medicine*. St. Louis: C. V. Mosby, 1986:560–583.
25. Quillen WS, Rouillier LH: Initial management of acute ankle sprains with rapid pulsed pneumatic compression and cold. *J Orthop Sports Phys Ther* 4:39–43, 1981.
26. Starkey JA: Treatment of ankle sprains by simultaneous use of intermittent compression and ice packs. *Am J Sports Med* 4:142–143, 1976.
27. Wilkerson GB: Treatment of ankle sprains with external compression and early mobilization. *Phys Sports Med* 13:83–90, 1985.
28. Cole AJ, Farrell JP, Stratton SA: Functional rehabilitation of cervical spine athletic injuries. In: Kibler BW, Herring JA, Press JM, eds. *Functional Rehabilitation of Sports and Musculoskeletal Injuries*. Gaithersburg, MD: Aspen, 1998:127–148.
29. Farrell JP: Cervical passive mobilization techniques: The Australian approach. Physical Medicine and Rehabilitation: State-of-the-Art Reviews 4:309–334, 1990.
30. Hoogenboom BJ, Voight ML: Clinical reasoning: An algorithm-based approach to musculoskeletal rehabilitation. In: Voight ML, Hoogenboom BJ, Prentice WE, eds. *Musculoskeletal Interventions: Techniques for Therapeutic Exercise*. New York: McGraw-Hill, 2007: 81–95.
31. Booth FW: Physiologic and biochemical effects of immobilization on muscle. *Clin Orthop Relat Res* 219:15–21, 1987.
32. Booth FW, Kelso JR: The effect of hind-limb immobilization on contractile and histochemical properties of skeletal muscle. *Pflugers Arch* 342:231–238, 1973.
33. Haggmark T, Eriksson E: Cylinder or mobile cast brace after knee ligament surgery. *Am J Sports Med* 7:48–56, 1979.
34. Farmer JA, Pearl AC: Provocative issues. In: Leadbetter WB, Buckwalter JA, Gordon SL, eds. *Sports Induced Inflammation: Clinical and Basic Science Concepts*. Park Ridge, IL, American Academy of Orthopaedic Surgeons, 1990:781–791.
35. Helminen HJ, Jurvelin J, Kuusela T, et al: Effects of immobilization for 6 weeks on rabbit knee articular surfaces as assessed by the semi-quantitative stereomicroscopic method. *Acta Anat Nippon* 115:327–335, 1983.
36. Kibler WB: Concepts in exercise rehabilitation of athletic injury. In: Leadbetter WB, Buckwalter JA, Gordon SL, eds. *Sports-Induced Inflammation: Clinical and Basic Science Concepts*. Park Ridge, IL: American Academy of Orthopaedic Surgeons, 1990:759–769.
37. Salter RB, Field P: The effects of continuous compression on living articular cartilage. *J Bone Joint Surg* 42A:31–49, 1960.
38. Woo SL-Y, Tkach LV: The cellular and matrix response of ligaments and tendons to mechanical injury. In: Leadbetter WB, Buckwalter JA, Gordon SL, eds. *Sports-Induced Inflammation: Clinical and Basic Science Concepts*. Park Ridge, IL: American Academy of Orthopaedic Surgeons, 1990:189–202.
39. Cox JS: Surgical and nonsurgical treatment of acute ankle sprains. *Clin Orthop* 198:118–126, 1985.
40. Eiff MP, Smith AT, Smith GE: Early mobilization versus immobilization in the treatment of lateral ankle sprains. *Am J Sports Med* 22:83–88, 1994.
41. Astrand PO, Rodahl K: *Textbook of Work Physiology*. New York: McGraw-Hill, 1973.
42. Zarins B: Soft tissue injury and repair: Biomechanical aspects. *Int J Sports Med* 3:9–11, 1982.
43. Frank G, Woo SL-Y, Amiel D, et al: Medial collateral ligament healing. A multidisciplinary assessment in rabbits. *Am J Sports Med* 11:379, 1983.
44. Leach RE: The prevention and rehabilitation of soft tissue injuries. *Int J Sports Med* 3(Suppl 1):18–20, 1982.
45. Akeson WH, Woo SLY, Amiel D, et al: The chemical basis for tissue repair. In: Hunter LH, Funk FJ, eds. *Rehabilitation of the Injured Knee*. St. Louis: C. V. Mosby, 1984:93–147.
46. Tipton CM, James SL, Mergner W, et al: Influence of exercise in strength of medial collateral knee ligaments of dogs. *Am J Physiol* 218:894–902, 1970.
47. Noyes FR, Torvik PJ, Hyde WB, et al: Biomechanics of ligament failure: II. An analysis of immobilization, exercise, and reconditioning effects in primates. *J Bone Joint Surg* 56A:1406–1418, 1974.
48. Clark MA: Advanced core stabilization training for rehabilitation, reconditioning, and injury prevention. In: Wilmarth MA, ed. *Orthopaedic Physical Therapy: Topic - Strength and Conditioning - Independent Study Course 15.3*. La Crosse, WI: Orthopaedic Section, APTA, Inc., 2005.
49. Hyman J, Liebenson C: Spinal stabilization exercise program. In: Liebenson C, ed. *Rehabilitation of the Spine: A Practitioner's Manual*. Baltimore: Lippincott Williams & Wilkins, 1996:293–317.
50. Dehne E, Tory R: Treatment of joint injuries by immediate mobilization. Based upon the spiral adaptation concept. *Clin Orthop Relat Res* 77:218–232, 1971.
51. Hunt TK: *Wound Healing and Wound Infection: Theory and Surgical Practice*. New York: Appleton-Century-Crofts, 1980.
52. Singer AJ, Clark RAF: Cutaneous wound healing. *N Engl J Med* 341:738–746, 1999.
53. Janda V: Muscle strength in relation to muscle length, pain and muscle imbalance. In: Harms-Ringdahl K, ed. *Muscle Strength*. New York: Churchill Livingstone, 1993:83–91.
54. Bourne MH, Hazel WA, Scott SG, et al: Anterior knee pain. *Mayo Clinic Proc* 63:482–491, 1988.
55. Brody LT, Thein JM: Nonoperative treatment for patellofemoral pain. *J Orthop Sports Phys Ther* 28:336–344, 1998.
56. Safran MR, Zachazewski JE, Benedetti RS, et al: Lateral ankle sprains: A comprehensive review part 2: Treatment and rehabilitation with an emphasis on the athlete. *Med Sci Sports Exerc* 31:S438–S447, 1999.
57. Safran MR, Benedetti RS, Bartolozzi AR III, et al: Lateral ankle sprains: A comprehensive review: Part 1: Etiology, pathoanatomy, histopathogenesis, and diagnosis. *Med Sci Sports Exerc* 31:S429–S437, 1999.

58. Evans RB: Clinical application of controlled stress to the healing extensor tendon: A review of 112 cases. *Phys Ther* 69:1041–1049, 1989.
59. Lemmer JT, Hurlbut DE, Martel GF, et al: Age and gender responses to strength training and detraining. *Med Sci Sports Exerc* 32:1505–1512, 2000.
60. Wenger HA, Bell GJ: The interactions of intensity, frequency and duration of exercise training in altering cardiorespiratory fitness. *Sports Med* 3:346–56, 1986.
61. Klaffs CE, Arnheim DD: *Modern Principles of Athletic Training*. St. Louis: C. V. Mosby, 1989.
62. Porterfield JA, DeRosa C: *Mechanical Low Back Pain*, 2nd ed. Philadelphia: WB Saunders, 1998.
63. Barlow Y, Willoughby J: Pathophysiology of soft tissue repair. *Br Med Bull* 48:698–711, 1992.
64. Davies GJ: *Compendium of Isokinetics in Clinical Usage and Rehabilitation Techniques*, 4th ed. Onalaska, WI: S & S Publishers, 1992.
65. McKenzie R, May S: Physical examination. In: McKenzie R, May S, eds. *The Human Extremities: Mechanical Diagnosis and Therapy*. Waikanae, New Zealand: Spinal Publications New Zealand Ltd, 2000:105–121.
66. Liebenson C: Integrating rehabilitation into chiropractic practice. In: Liebenson C, ed. *Rehabilitation of the Spine: A Practitioner's Manual*. Baltimore: Lippincott Williams & Wilkins, 1996:13–43.
67. Keggereis S: The construction and implementation of functional progressions as a component of athletic rehabilitation. *J Orthop Sports Phys Ther* 5:14–19, 1985.
68. American Physical Therapy Association. Guide to physical therapist practice. Second edition. American Physical Therapy Association. *Phys Ther* 81:9–746, 2001.
69. Tippett SR, Voight ML: *Functional Progressions for Sports Rehabilitation*. Champaign, IL: Human Kinetics, 1995.
70. Markey KL: Rehabilitation of the anterior cruciate deficient knee. *Clin Sports Med* 4:513–526, 1985.
71. Markey KL: Functional rehabilitation of the anterior cruciate deficient knee. *Sports Med* 12:407–417, 1991.
72. DeLorme TL: Restoration of muscle power by heavy resistance exercise. *J Bone and Joint Surg* 27:645–667, 1945.
73. Austin G: Functional testing and return to activity. In: Magee D, Zachazewski JE, Quillen WS, eds. *Scientific Foundations and Principles of Practice in Musculoskeletal Rehabilitation*. St. Louis, MI: WB Saunders, 2007:633–664.
74. Palmer ML, Epler M: *Clinical Assessment Procedures in Physical Therapy*. Philadelphia: JB Lippincott, 1990.
75. Chapman CE: Can the use of physical modalities for pain control be rationalized by the research evidence? *Can J Physiol Pharmacol* 69:704–712, 1991.
76. Feine JS, Lund JP: An assessment of the efficacy of physical therapy and physical modalities for the control of chronic musculoskeletal pain. *Pain* 71:5–23, 1997.
77. McMaster WC, Liddle S, Waugh TR: Laboratory evaluation of various cold therapy modalities. *Am J Sports Med* 6:291–294, 1978.
78. Watson T: The role of electrotherapy in contemporary physiotherapy practice. *Man Ther* 5:132–141, 2000.
79. Knight KL: *Cryotherapy: Theory, Technique, and Physiology*. Chattanooga, TN: Chattanooga Corp, 1985.
80. Hocutt JE, Jaffee R, Rylander R, et al: Cryotherapy in ankle sprains. *Am J Sports Med* 10:316–319, 1982.
81. Daniel DM, Stone ML, Arendt DL: The effect of cold therapy on pain, swelling, and range of motion after anterior cruciate ligament reconstructive surgery. *Arthroscopy* 10:530–533, 1994.
82. Konrath GA, Lock T, Goitz HT, et al: The use of cold therapy after anterior cruciate ligament reconstruction. A prospective randomized study and literature review. *Am J Sports Med* 24:629–633, 1996.
83. Michlovitz SL: The use of heat and cold in the management of rheumatic diseases. In: Michlovitz SL, ed. *Thermal Agents in Rehabilitation*. Philadelphia: FA Davis, 1990:158–174.
84. Speer KP, Warren RF, Horowitz L: The efficacy of cryotherapy in the postoperative shoulder. *J Shoulder Elbow Surg* 5:62–68, 1996.
85. Knight KL: *Cryotherapy in Sports Injury Management*. Champaign, IL: Human Kinetics, 1995.
86. Kellett J: Acute soft tissue injuries: A review of the literature. *Med Sci Sports Exerc* 18:5, 1986.
87. McMaster WC: A literary review on ice therapy in injuries. *Am J Sports Med* 5:124–126, 1977.
88. Hartviksen K: Ice therapy in spasticity. *Acta Neurol Scand* 3(Suppl):79–84, 1962.
89. Basset SW, Lake BM: Use of cold applications in the management of spasticity. *Phys Ther Rev* 38:333–334, 1958.
90. Lamboni P, Harris B: The use of ice, air splints, and high voltage galvanic stimulation in effusion reduction. *Athl Training* 18:23–25, 1983.
91. Waylonis GW: The physiological effects of ice massage. *Arch Phys Med Rehab* 48:42–47, 1967.
92. Belitsky RB, Odam SJ, Hubley-Kozey C: Evaluation of the effectiveness of wet ice, dry ice, and cryogen packs in reducing skin temperature. *Phys Ther* 67:1080–1084, 1987.
93. Oosterveld FGJ, Rasker JJ, Jacobs JWG, et al: The effect of local heat and cold therapy on the intraarticular and skin surface temperature of the knee. *Arthritis Rheum* 35:146–151, 1992.
94. Zemke JE, Andersen JC, Guion WK, et al: Intramuscular temperature responses in the human leg to two forms of cryotherapy: Ice massage and ice bag. *J Orthop Sports Phys Ther* 27:301–307, 1998.
95. Doucette SA, Goble EM: The effect of exercise on patellar tracking in lateral patellar compression syndrome. *Am J Sports Med* 20:434–440, 1992.
96. Fisher RL: Conservative treatment of patellofemoral pain. *Orthop Clin North Am* 17:269–272, 1986.
97. Meeusen R, Lievens P: The use of cryotherapy in sports injuries. *Sports Med* 3:398–414, 1986.
98. Adamson C, Cymet T: Ankle sprains: Evaluation, treatment, rehabilitation. *Maryland Med J* 46:530–537, 1997.
99. Cwynar DA, McNerney T: A primer on physical therapy. *Lippincott's Prim Care Pract* 3:451–459, 1999.
100. Feibel A, Fast A: Deep heating of joints: A reconsideration. *Arch Phys Med Rehab* 57:513–514, 1976.
101. Clark D, Stelmach G: Muscle fatigue and recovery curve parameters at various temperatures. *Res Q* 37:468–479, 1966.
102. Baker R, Bell G: The effect of therapeutic modalities on blood flow in the human calf. *J Orthop Sports Phys Ther* 13:23, 1991.
103. Knight KL, Aquino J, Johannes SM, et al: A re-examination of Lewis' cold induced vasodilation in the finger and ankle. *Athl Training* 15:248–250, 1980.
104. Zankel H: Effect of physical agents on motor conduction velocity of the ulnar nerve. *Arch Phys Med Rehab* 47:197–199, 1994.
105. Abramson DI, Bell B, Tuck S: Changes in blood flow, oxygen uptake and tissue temperatures produced by therapeutic physical agents: Effect of indirect or reflex vasodilation. *Am J Phys Med* 40:5–13, 1961.
106. Frizzell LA, Dunn F: Biophysics of ultrasound. In: Lehman JF, ed. *Therapeutic Heat and Cold*, 3rd ed. Baltimore: Williams & Wilkins, 1982:353–385.
107. Lehman JF, Masock AJ, Warren CG, et al: Effect of therapeutic temperatures on tendon extensibility. *Arch Phys Med Rehabil* 51:481–487, 1970.
108. Kalenak A, Medlar CE, Fleagle SB, et al: Athletic injuries: Heat vs cold. *Am Fam Phys* 12:131–134, 1975.
109. Barcroft H, Edholm OS: The effect of temperature on blood flow and deep temperature in the human forearm. *J Physiol* 102:5–20, 1943.
110. Griffin JG: Physiological effects of ultrasonic energy as it is used clinically. *J Am Phys Ther Assoc* 46:18, 1966.
111. Lehmann JF, Silverman DR, Baum BA, et al: Temperature distributions in the human thigh, produced by infrared, hot pack and microwave applications. *Arch Phys Med Rehabil* 47:291, 1966 [AQ1].
112. Abramson DI, Tuck S, Lee SW, et al: Comparison of wet and dry heat in raising temperature of tissues. *Arch Phys Med Rehabil* 48:654, 1967.
113. Benson HAE, McElnay JC: Transmission of ultrasound energy through topical pharmaceutical products. *Physiotherapy* 74:587–589, 1988.
114. Cameron MH, Monroe LG: Relative transmission of ultrasound by media customarily used for phonophoresis. *Phys Ther* 72:142–148, 1992.
115. Dyson M: Mechanisms involved in therapeutic ultrasound. *Physiotherapy* 73:116–120, 1987.
116. Lehman JF, deLateur BJ, Stonebridge JB, et al: Therapeutic temperature distribution produced by ultrasound as modified by dosage and volume of tissue exposed. *Arch Phys Med Rehabil* 48:662–666, 1967.
117. Lehman JF, deLateur BJ, Warren CG, et al: Heating of joint structures by ultrasound. *Arch Phys Med Rehabil* 49:28–30, 1968.
118. Goldman DE, Heuter TF: Tabulator data on velocity and absorption of high frequency sound in mammalian tissues. *J Acoust Soc Am* 28:35, 1956.
119. Dyson M: Non-thermal cellular effects of ultrasound. *Br J Cancer* 45:165–71, 1982.
120. Paaske WP, Hovind H, Sejrsen P: Influence of therapeutic ultrasound irradiation on blood flow in human cutaneous, subcutaneous and muscular tissue. *Scand J Clin Invest* 31:388, 1973.

121. Warren CG, Koblanski JN, Sigelmann RA: Ultrasound coupling media: Their relative transmissivity. *Arch Phys Med Rehab* 57:218–222, 1976.
122. Dyson M, Pond JB: The effect of pulsed ultrasound on tissue regeneration. *Physiotherapy* 56:136, 1970.
123. Dyson M, Suckling J: Stimulation of tissue repair by ultrasound: A survey of the mechanisms involved. *Physiotherapy* 64:105–108, 1978.
124. Binder A, Hodge G, Greenwood AM, et al: Is therapeutic ultrasound effective in treating soft tissue lesions? *BMJ* 290:512–514, 1985.
125. Draper DO, Castel JC, Castel D: Rate of temperature increase in human muscle during 1-MHz and 3-MHz continuous ultrasound. *J Orthop Sports Phys Ther* 22:142–150, 1995.
126. Dyson M, Pond JB, Joseph J, et al: The stimulation of tissue regeneration by means of ultrasound. *Clin Sci* 35:273–285, 1968.
127. Ebenbichler GR, Resch KL, Graninger WB: Resolution of calcium deposits after therapeutic ultrasound of the shoulder. *J Rheumatol* 24:235–236, 1997.
128. Aldes JH, Klaras T: Use of ultrasonic radiation in the treatment of subdeltoid bursitis with and without calcareous deposits. *West J Surg* 62:369–376, 1954.
129. Flax HJ: Ultrasound treatment for peritendinitis calcarea of the shoulder. *Am J Phys Med Rehabil* 43:117–124, 1964.
130. Robertson VJ, Baker KG: A review of therapeutic ultrasound: Effectiveness studies. *Phys Ther* 81:1339–1350, 2001.
131. Nussbaum EL, Biemann I, Mustard B: Comparison of ultrasound, ultraviolet C and laser for treatment of pressure ulcers in patients with spinal cord injury. *Phys Ther* 74:812–823, 1994.
132. Dyson M, Luke DA: Induction of mast cell degranulation in skin by ultrasound. *IEEE Trans Ultrason Ferroelectr Freq Control* 33:194–201, 1986 [AQ1].
133. Nussbaum EL: Ultrasound: To heat or not to heat - that is the question. *Phys Ther Rev* 2:59–72, 1997.
134. Makulolowe RTB, Mouzos GL: Ultrasound in the treatment of sprained ankles. *Practitioner* 218:586–588, 1977.
135. Dinno MA, Crum LA, Wu J: The effect of therapeutic ultrasound on the electrophysiologic parameters of frog skin. *Med. Biol* 25:461–470, 1989.
136. Falconer J, Hayes KW, Chang RW: Therapeutic ultrasound in the treatment of musculoskeletal conditions. *Arthritis Care Res* 3:85–91, 1990.
137. Maxwell L: Therapeutic ultrasound. Its effects on the cellular & molecular mechanisms of inflammation and repair. *Physiotherapy* 78:421–426, 1992.
138. Ter Haar GR, Stratford IJ: Evidence for a non-thermal effect of ultrasound. *Br J Cancer* 45:172–175, 1982.
139. Young SR, Dyson M: The effect of therapeutic ultrasound on angiogenesis. *Ultrasound Med Biol* 16:261–269, 1990.
140. Dyson M, Niinikoski J: Stimulation of tissue repair by therapeutic ultrasound. *Infect Surg* 16:37–44, 1982.
141. Young SR, Dyson M: Effect of therapeutic ultrasound on the healing of full-thickness excised skin lesions. *Ultrasonics* 28:175–180, 1990.
142. Antich TJ: Phonophoresis: The principles of the ultrasonic driving force and efficacy in treatment of common orthopedic diagnoses. *J Orthop Sports Phys Ther* 4:99–102, 1982.
143. Bommannan D, Menon GK, Okuyama H, et al: Sonophoresis II: Examination of the mechanism(s) of ultrasound-enhanced transdermal drug delivery. *Pharm Res* 9:1043–1047, 1992.
144. Bommannan D, Okuyama H, Stauffer P, et al: Sonophoresis. I: The use of high-frequency ultrasound to enhance transdermal drug delivery. *Pharm Res* 9:559–564, 1992.
145. Byl NN: The use of ultrasound as an enhancer for transcutaneous drug delivery: Phonophoresis. *Phys Ther* 75:539–553, 1995.
146. Byl NN, Mckenzie A, Haliday B, et al: The effects of phonophoresis with corticosteroids: A controlled pilot study. *J Orthop Sports Phys Ther* 18:590–600, 1993.
147. Ciccone CD, Leggin BG, Callamaro JJ: Effects of ultrasound and trolamine salicylate phonophoresis on delayed onset muscle soreness. *Phys Ther* 71:39–51, 1991.
148. Davick JP, Martin RK, Albright JP: Distribution and deposition of tritiated cortisol using phonophoresis. *Phys Ther* 68:1672–1675, 1988.
149. Griffin JE, Touchstone JC: Effects of ultrasonic frequency on phonophoresis of cortisol into swine tissues. *Am J Phys Med* 51:62–78, 1972.
150. Griffin JE, Touchstone JC, Liu AC-Y: Ultrasonic movement of cortisol into pig tissue: Movement into paravertebral nerve. *Am J Phys Med* 44:20–25, 1965.
151. Munting E: Ultrasonic therapy for painful shoulders. *Physiotherapy* 64:180–181, 1978.
152. Bradnam L, Rochester L, Vujnovich A: Manual cervical traction reduces alpha-motoneuron excitability in normal subjects. *Electromyogr Clin Neurophysiol* 40:259–266, 2000.
153. Colachis SC, Strohm BR: Cervical traction: Relationship of traction time to varied tractive force with constant angle of pull. *Arch Phys Med Rehabil* 46:815–819, 1965.
154. Deets D, Hands KL, Hopp SS: Cervical traction: A comparison of sitting and supine positions. *Phys Ther* 57:255–261, 1977.
155. Harris PR: Cervical traction: Review of literature and treatment guidelines. *Phys Ther* 57:910–914, 1977.
156. Saunders HD, Ryan RS: Spinal traction. In: Placzek JD, Boyce DA, eds. *Orthopaedic Physical Therapy Secrets*. Philadelphia: Hanley & Belfus, Inc., 2001:93–98.
157. Austin R: Lumbar traction a valid option. *Aust J Physiother* 44:280, 1998.
158. Lee RY, Evans JH: Loads in the lumbar spine during traction therapy. *Aust J Physiother* 47:102–108, 2001.
159. Pellecchia GL: Lumbar traction: A review of the literature. *J Orthop Sports Phys Ther* 20:262–267, 1994.
160. Cox JS: The diagnosis and management of ankle ligament injuries in the athlete. *Athl Training* 18:192–196, 1982.
161. Marino M: Principles of therapeutic modalities: Implications for sports medicine. In: Nicholas JA, Hershman EB, eds. *The Lower Extremity and Spine in Sports Medicine*. St. Louis: C. V. Mosby, 1986:195–244.
162. Myrer JW, Draper DO, Durrant E: Contrast therapy and intramuscular temperature in the human leg. *J Athl Train* 29:318–325, 1994.
163. Rabago D, Best TM, Beamsley M, et al: A systematic review of prolotherapy for chronic musculoskeletal pain. *Clin J Sport Med* 15:376–380, 2005.
164. Dechow E, Davies RK, Carr AJ, et al: A randomized, double-blind, placebo-controlled trial of sclerosing injections in patients with chronic low back pain. *Rheumatology (Oxford)* 38:1255–1259, 1999.
165. Hurst NP: Sclerosing injections in patients with chronic low back pain. *Rheumatology (Oxford)* 39:925, 2000.
166. Sweetman BJ: Sclerosing injections for chronic low back pain. *Rheumatology (Oxford)* 39:924–925, 2000.
167. Alfredson H, Harstad H, Haugen S, et al: Sclerosing polidocanol injections to treat chronic painful shoulder impingement syndrome-results of a two-centre collaborative pilot study. *Knee Surg Sports Traumatol Arthrosc* 7:7, 2006.
168. Zeisig E, Ohberg L, Alfredson H: Sclerosing polidocanol injections in chronic painful tennis elbow-promising results in a pilot study. *Knee Surg Sports Traumatol Arthrosc* 8:8, 2006.
169. Ohberg L, Alfredson H: Ultrasound guided sclerosis of neovessels in painful chronic Achilles tendinosis: Pilot study of a new treatment. *Br J Sports Med* 36:173–175; discussion 176–177, 2002.
170. Alfredson H, Ohberg L: Sclerosing injections to areas of neo-vascularisation reduce pain in chronic Achilles tendinopathy: A double-blind randomised controlled trial [published online ahead of print February 2, 2005]. *Knee Surg Sports Traumatol Arthrosc* 13:338–344, 2005.
171. Hoksrud A, Ohberg L, Alfredson H, et al: Ultrasound-guided sclerosis of neovessels in painful chronic patellar tendinopathy: A randomized controlled trial [published online ahead of print July 10, 2006]. *Am J Sports Med* 34:1738–1746, 2006.
172. Brown S: Ankle edema and galvanic muscle stimulation. *Physician Sportsmed* 9:137, 1981.
173. Frank C, Schachar N, Dittrich D, et al: Electromagnetic stimulation of ligament healing in rabbits. *Clin Orthop* 175:263–272, 1983.
174. Ralston DJ: High voltage galvanic stimulation: Can there be a state of the art? *Athl Training* 21:291–293, 1985.
175. Tropp H: *Functional Instability of the Ankle Joint*. Linkoping, Sweden: Linkoping University, 1985.
176. Voight ML: Reduction of post-traumatic ankle edema with high voltage pulsed galvanic stimulation. *Athl Training* 20:278–279, 1984.
177. Prentice WE: Using therapeutic modalities in rehabilitation. In: Prentice WE, Voight ML, eds. *Techniques in Musculoskeletal Rehabilitation*. New York: McGraw-Hill, 2001:289–303.
178. Scott O: Stimulative effects. In: Kitchen S, Bazin S, eds. *Clayton's Electrotherapy*. London: WB Saunders, 1996:61–80.
179. Low J, Reed A: *Electrotherapy Explained: Principles and Practice*. Oxford: Butterworth-Heinemann, 2000.

180. Bettany JA, Fish DR, Mendel FC: Influence of high voltage pulsed direct current on edema formation following impact. *Phys Ther* 70:219–224, 1990.
181. Bettany JA, Fish DR, Mendel FC: High voltage pulsed direct current effect on edema formation following hyperflexion injury. *Arch Phys Med Rehabil* 71:877–881, 1991.
182. Bettany JA, Fish DR, Mendel FC: Influence of cathodal high voltage pulsed current on acute edema. *J Clin Electrophysiol* 2:5–8, 1990.
183. Fish DR, Mendel FC, Schultz AM, et al: Effect on anodal high voltage pulsed current on edema formation in frog hind limbs. *Phys Ther* 71:724–733, 1991.
184. Karnes JL, Mendel FC, Fish DR: Effects of low voltage pulsed current non edema formation in frog hind limbs following impact injury. *Phys Ther* 72:273–278, 1992.
185. Reed BV: Effect of high voltage pulsed electrical stimulation on microvascular permeability to plasma proteins: A possible mechanism of minimizing edema. *Phys Ther* 68:491–495, 1988.
186. Taylor K, Fish DR, Mendel FR, et al: Effect of a single 30 minute treatment of high voltage pulsed current on edema formation in frog hind limbs. *Phys Ther* 72:63–68, 1992.
187. Delitto A, Rose SJ, McKowen JM, et al: Electrical stimulation versus voluntary exercise in strengthening thigh musculature after anterior cruciate ligament surgery. *Phys Ther* 68:660–663, 1988.
188. Gotlin RS, Hershkowitz S, Juris PM, et al: Electrical stimulation effect on extensor lag and length of hospital stay after total knee arthroplasty. *Arch Phys Med Rehabil* 75:957, 1994.
189. Laughman RK, Youdas JW, Garrett TR, et al: Strength changes in the normal quadriceps femoris muscle as a result of electrical stimulation. *Phys Ther* 63:494–499, 1983.
190. McMiken DF, Todd-Smith M, Thompson C: Strengthening of human quadriceps muscles by cutaneous electrical stimulation. *Scand J Rehabil Med* 15:25–28, 1983.
191. Snyder-Mackler L, Delitto A, Bailey SL, et al: Strength of the quadriceps femoris muscle and functional recovery after reconstruction of the anterior cruciate ligament. A prospective, randomized clinical trial of electrical stimulation. *J Bone Joint Surg Am* 77:1166–1173, 1995.
192. Gould N, Donnermeyer BS, Pope M, et al: Transcutaneous muscle stimulation as a method to retard disuse atrophy. *Clin Orthop* 164:215–220, 1982.
193. Selkowitz DM: Improvement in isometric strength of quadriceps femoris muscle after training with electrical stimulation. *Phys Ther* 65:186–196, 1985.
194. Currier DP, Mann R: Muscular strength development by electrical stimulation in healthy individuals. *Phys Ther* 63:915–921, 1983.
195. Gangarosa LP: *Iontophoresis in Dental Practice.* Chicago: Quintessence Publishing, 1982.
196. Coy RE: *Anthology of Craniomandibular Orthopedics.* Seattle: International College Of Craniomandibular Orthopedics, 1993.
197. Burnette RR: Iontophoresis. In: Hadgraft J, Guy RH, eds. *Transdermal Drug Delivery: Developmental Issues and Research Initiatives.* New York: Marcel Dekker, 1989:247–291.
198. Chien YW, Siddiqui O, Shi M, et al: Direct current iontophoretic transdermal delivery of peptide and protein drugs. *J Pharm Sci* 78:376–384, 1989.
199. Grimnes S: Pathways of ionic flow through human skin in vivo. *Acta Dermatol Venereol* 64:93–98, 1984.
200. Lee RD, White HS, Scott ER: Visualization of iontophoretic transport paths in cultured and animal skin models. *J Pharm Sci* 85:1186–1190, 1996.
201. O'Malley E, Oester Y: Influence of some physical chemical factors on iontophoresis using radioisotopes. *Arch Phys Med Rehabil* 36:310–313, 1955.
202. Zeltzer L, Regalado M, Nichter LS, et al: Iontophoresis versus subcutaneous injection: A comparison of two methods of local anesthesia delivery in children. *Pain* 44:73–78, 1991.
203. Krischek O, Hopf C, Nafe B, et al: Shock-wave therapy for tennis and golfer's elbow–1 year follow-up. *Arch Orthop Trauma Surg* 119:62–66, 1999.
204. Rossouw P: Tennis elbow - is extracorporeal shock wave therapy (ESWT) an alternative to surgery? *J Bone Joint Surg Br* 81-B:306, 1999.
205. Rompe JD, Riedel C, Betz U, et al: Chronic lateral epicondylitis of the elbow: A prospective study of low-energy shockwave therapy and low-energy shockwave therapy plus manual therapy of the cervical spine. *Arch Phys Med Rehab* 82:578–582, 2001.
206. Ogden JA, Toth-Kischkat A, Schultheiss R: Principles of shock wave therapy. *Clin Orthop Relat Res* 387:8–17, 2001.
207. Rompe JD: Differenzierte Anwendung extrakorporaler Stosswellen bei Tendopathien der Schulter und des Ellenbogens. *Electromedica* 65:20, 1997.
208. Cheing GLY, Chang H: Extracorporeal shock wave therapy. *J Orthop Sports Phys Ther* 33:337–343, 2003.
209. Ogden JA, Alvarez RG, Marlow M: Shockwave therapy for chronic proximal plantar fasciitis: A meta-analysis. *Foot Ankle Int* 23:301–308, 2002.
210. Smith MJ: Electrical stimulation for the relief of musculoskeletal pain. *Phys Sports Med* 11:47–55, 1983.
211. Magora F, Aladjemoff L, Tannenbaum J, et al: Treatment of pain by transcutaneous electrical stimulation. *Acta Anaesthesiol Scand* 22:589–592, 1978.
212. Mannheimer JS, Lampe GN: *Clinical Transcutaneous Electrical Nerve Stimulation.* Philadelphia: F. A. Davis, 1984:440–445.
213. Woolf CF: Segmental afferent fiber-induced analgesia: Transcutaneous electrical nerve stimulation (TENS) and vibration. In: Wall PD, Melzack R, eds. *Textbook of Pain.* New York: Churchill Livingstone, 1989:884–896.
214. Smith MJ, Hutchins RC, Hehenberger D: Transcutaneous neural stimulation use in post-operative knee rehabilitation. *Am J Sports Med* 11:75–82, 1983.
215. Long DM: Fifteen years of transcutaneous electrical stimulation for pain control. *Stereotact Funct Neurosurg* 56:2–19, 1991.
216. Fried T, Johnson R, McCracken W: Transcutaneous electrical nerve stimulation: Its role in the control of chronic pain. *Arch Phys Med Rehabil* 65:228–231, 1984.
217. Eriksson MBE, Sjölund BH, Nielzen S: Long-term results of peripheral conditioning stimulation as an analgesic measure in chronic pain. *Pain* 6:335–347, 1979.
218. Fishbain DA, Chabal C, Abbott A, et al: Transcutaneous electrical nerve stimulation (TENS) treatment outcome in long term users. *Clin J Pain* 12:201–214, 1996.
219. Ishimaru K, Kawakita K, Sakita M: Analgesic effects induced by TENS and electroacupuncture with different types of stimulating electrodes on deep tissues in human subjects. *Pain* 63:181–187, 1995.
220. Eriksson MBE, Sjölund BH, Sundbärg G: Pain relief from peripheral conditioning stimulation in patients with chronic facial pain. *J Neurosurg* 61:149–155, 1984.
221. Murphy GJ: Utilization of transcutaneous electrical nerve stimulation in managing craniofacial pain. *Clin J Pain* 6:64–69, 1990.
222. Melzack R: The gate theory revisited. In: LeRoy PL, ed. *Current Concepts in the Management of Chronic Pain.* Miami: Symposia Specialists, 1977.
223. Salar G: Effect of transcutaneous electrotherapy on CSF b-endorphin content in patients without pain problems. *Pain* 10:169–172, 1981.
224. Clement-Jones V: Increased b endorphin but not metenkephalin levels in human cerebrospinal fluid after acupuncture for recurrent pain. *Lancet* 8:946–948, 1980.
225. Wang J, Li F, Calhoun JH, et al: The role and effectiveness of adjunctive hyperbaric oxygen therapy in the management of musculoskeletal disorders. *J Postgrad Med* 48:226–231, 2002.
226. Becker BE: Aquatic therapy: Scientific foundations and clinical rehabilitation applications. *PM R* 1:859–872, 2009.
227. Kaneda K, Sato D, Wakabayashi H, et al: A comparison of the effects of different water exercise programs on balance ability in elderly people. *J Aging Phys Act* 16:381–392, 2008.
228. Gleim GW, Nicholas JA: Metabolic costs and heart rate responses to treadmill walking in water at different depths and temperatures. *Am J Sports Med* 17:248–252, 1989.
229. Auberger SS, Mangine RE: *Innovative Approaches to Surgery and Rehabilitation, Physical Therapy of the Knee.* New York: Churchill Livingstone, 1988:233–262.
230. O'Connor FG, Sobel JR, Nirschl RP: Five step treatment for overuse injuries. *Phys Sports Med* 20:128, 1992.
231. Litzinger ME, Osif B: Accommodating diverse learning styles: Designing instruction for electronic information sources. In: Shirato L, ed. *What is Good Instruction Now? Library Instruction for the 90s.* Ann Arbor, MI: Pierian Press, 1993:26–50.
232. Brawley LR, Culos-Reed SN: Studying adherence to therapeutic regimens: Overview, theories, recommendations. *Control Clin Trials* 21:156S–163S, 2000.

233. Lenze EJ, Munin MC, Quear T, et al: The Pittsburgh Rehabilitation Participation Scale: Reliability and validity of a clinician-rated measure of participation in acute rehabilitation. *Arch Phys Med Rehabil* 85:380–384, 2004.
234. Deyo RA: Compliance with therapeutic regimens in arthritis: Issues, current status, and a future agenda. *Sem Arthritis Rheum* 12:233–244, 1982.
235. Sluijs EM, Kok GJ, van der Zee J: Correlates of exercise compliance in physical therapy. *Phys Ther* 73:771–782; discussion 783–786, 1993.
236. Lee JY, Jensen BE, Oberman A, et al: Adherence in the training levels comparison trial. *Med Sci Sports Exerc* 28:47–52, 1996.
237. Keele-Smith R, Leon T: Evaluation of individually tailored interventions on exercise adherence. *West J Nurs Res* 25:623–640; discussion 641–651, 2003.
238. Boyette LW, Lloyd A, Boyette JE, et al: Personal characteristics that influence exercise behavior of older adults. *J Rehab Res Dev* 39:95–103, 2002.
239. Cohen B, Vittinghoff E, Whooley M: Association of socioeconomic status and exercise capacity in adults with coronary heart disease (from the Heart and Soul Study). *Am J Cardiol* 101:462–466, 2008.
240. Wister AV: The effects of socioeconomic status on exercise and smoking: Age-related differences. *J Aging Health* 8:467–488, 1996.
241. Clark DO: Age, socioeconomic status, and exercise self-efficacy. *Gerontologist* 36:157–164, 1996.
242. Blanpied P: Why won't patients do their home exercise programs? *J Orthop Sports Phys Ther* 25:101–102, 1997.
243. Chen CY, Neufeld PS, Feely CA, et al: Factors influencing compliance with home exercise programs among patients with upper extremity impairment. *Am J Occup Ther* 53:171–180, 1999.
244. Friedrich M, Cermak T, Madebacher P: The effect of brochure use versus therapist teaching on patients performing therapeutic exercise and on changes in impairment status. *Phys Ther* 76:1082–1088, 1996.
245. U.S. Department of Health & Human Services: *Physical Activity and Health: A Report of the Surgeon General.* Atlanta: National Center for Chronic Disease Prevention and Health Promotion, 1996.
246. U.S. Department of Health & Human Services: Office of Disease Prevention and Health Promotion—Healthy People 2010. *Nasnewsletter* 15:3, 2000.
247. Moffat M: Clinicians' roles in health promotion, wellness, and physical fitness. In: Magee D, Zachazewski JE, Quillen WS, eds. *Scientific Foundations and Principles of Practice in Musculoskeletal Rehabilitation.* St. Louis, MI: WB Saunders, 2007:328–356.

Pharmacology for the Orthopaedic Physical Therapist

CHAPTER 9

CHAPTER OBJECTIVES

At the completion of this chapter, the reader will be able to:

1. Differentiate between pharmacokinetics and pharmacodynamics.
2. Describe the process behind drug development, regulation, and distribution.
3. Describe controlled substances and their potential for abuse.
4. Recognize the three different names used for drugs.
5. Describe the various modes of action of drugs.
6. Describe the various drug receptor sites within the body.
7. Outline the different administration routes used for drug delivery.
8. Understand the potential effects of physical agents and exercise on drug delivery.

OVERVIEW

Physical therapists in many states are now positioned to provide care for patients prior to physician intervention. Although the dispensing of medications is out of the scope of practice for a physical therapist, questioning the patient about prescribed medication use can reveal medical conditions that the patient might not consider related to his or her present problem.[1] As physical therapists attempt to account for the effects of their interventions, it becomes apparent that they must also understand the effect and potential interactions of all available and reasonable resources, including pharmacological interventions, offered by other members of the health-care team.[1] Drug therapy is one of the mainstays of modern treatments and physical therapists often encounter patients who are taking various medications. These medications may be administered to treat preexisting conditions that are not directly related to the condition being treated with physical therapy but can nonetheless have an impact on the patient's response to rehabilitation.[2] Medications also can have an impact on clinical findings and on the success of an intervention.[3] For example:

- Pain medications, muscle relaxants, and nonsteroidal anti-inflammatory drugs (NSAIDs) can mask signs and symptoms, thereby affecting examination findings and increasing the potential for injury during the performance of prescribed exercises.[4] However, if the patient has a significant amount of pain, appropriate use of these medications may enhance treatment, allowing a more rapid progression than would otherwise be possible. However, as the patient improves, the need for this medication should lessen.
- Certain medications can produce changes in musculoskeletal structures. For example, prolonged use of corticosteroids may produce osteoporosis and weakening of connective tissues.[5]
- A patient undergoing anticoagulant therapy has a reduced clotting ability and is more susceptible to bruising or hemarthrosis. It is worth remembering that aspirin and aspirin-based products have an anticoagulant effect.

Pharmacology is the broad area of study that deals with how chemical substances affect living tissue on a molecular level and how drugs affect specific patient populations (Table 9-1). The Guide to Physical Therapist Practice[6] identifies clinical pharmacology as an essential component of appropriate patient monitoring, modality delivery, and communication among medical professionals. It is important for the physical therapist to have a working knowledge of pharmacology because of the number of drugs currently on the market and the number of physical therapy patients that are likely to have been prescribed medications. The prescription-drug-writing privileges exercised by select military therapists and the evolution of the physical therapy profession promote consideration of an expanded pharmacological role in physical therapy practice.[7] While the importance of a pharmacologically integrated approach to comprehensive patient management cannot be over emphasized, it is worth remembering that while some drugs can enhance physical therapy interventions, many can have negative consequences.

TABLE 9-1	Pharmacology Terms and Definitions
Term	**Definition**
Drug	Any substance that can be used to modify a chemical process or processes in the body, for example, to treat an illness, relieve a symptom, enhance a performance or ability, or to alter states of mind. The word "drug" is etymologically derived from the Dutch/Low German word "droog," which means "dry," since in the past, most drugs were dried plant parts.
Pharmacology	The science of studying both the mechanisms and the actions of drugs, usually in animal models of disease, to evaluate their potential therapeutic value.
Pharmacy	The mixing and dispensing of drugs. The monitoring of drug prescriptions for appropriateness and the monitoring of patients for adverse drug interactions.
Pharmacotherapeutics	The use of chemical agents to prevent, diagnose, and cure disease.
Pharmacokinetics	The study of how the body absorbs, distributes, metabolizes, and eliminates a drug.
Pharmacodynamics	The study of the biochemical and physiologic effects of drugs and their mechanisms of action at the cellular or organ level.
Pharmacotherapy	The treatment of a disease or condition with drugs.
Pharmacogenetics	The study of how variation in human genes leads to variations in our response to drugs and helps direct therapeutics according to a person's genotype.
Toxicology	A study of the negative effects of chemicals on living things, including cells, plants, animals, and humans.

PHARMACOKINETICS

Pharmacokinetics is the study of the physicochemical factors involved as the body absorbs, distributes, metabolizes, and eliminates a drug. To have a desirable effect, drugs must have the appropriate concentration at the site of action. Absorption is the process by which a drug is made available to the body fluids that distribute the drug to the organ systems. A prerequisite to absorption is drug dissolution.[8] For those drugs administered other than directly into the bloodstream, an absorbed drug must cross at least two layers of cells.[8] The physicochemical properties of drugs, their dosage formulations, and routes of administration determine the level of drug absorption and the response that occurs. The primary routes of administration include oral, buccal, sublingual, rectal, parenteral, topical, and inhalational (Table 9-2). As the target cells become exposed to increasing concentrations of the drug, increasing numbers of receptors become activated, and the magnitude of the response increases until there is a maximal response. In pharmacology, the term *bioavailability* is used to describe the rate and extent of a therapeutically active drug that reaches the systemic circulation and is available at the site of action. Bioavailability is one of the essential tools in pharmacokinetics, as bioavailability must be considered when calculating dosages. The concept of equivalence among drug products is also important in making clinical decisions:

- Chemical equivalence refers to drug products that contain the same compound in the same amount and that meet current official standards; however, inactive ingredients in drug products may differ.
- Bioequivalence refers to chemical equivalents that, when administered to the same person in the same dosage regimen, result in equivalent concentrations of drug in the blood and tissues.
- Therapeutic equivalence refers to drug products that, when administered to the same person in the same dosage regimen, provide essentially the same therapeutic effect or toxicity. Bioequivalent products are expected to be therapeutically equivalent.

TABLE 9-2	Methods for Drug Administration
Method	**Description**
Enteral	
Oral	Chewed, sucked, or swallowed
Sublingual or buccal	Placed under the tongue or in the cheek
Rectal	Placed in the rectum as a suppository or enema
Parenteral	
Intravenous	Direct placement of a drug into the bloodstream
Intramuscular	Injected into the muscle
Intra-articular	Administered directly into the synovial fluid of a joint
Subcutaneous	Administered below the dermis
Intrathecal	Injected into the subarachnoid or subdural spaces to bypass the blood–brain barrier
Epidural	Administered into the epidural space
Other	
Inhalational	
Topical	
Transdermal	

Thus, the physicochemical properties of a drug govern its absorptive potential, but the properties of the dosage form (which partly depend on its design and manufacture) and the mode of administration can largely determine drug bioavailability.

The *volume of distribution* is used to indicate how a systemic dose of the medication is ultimately dispersed throughout the body. Volume of distribution represents how much of the drug appears in the plasma relative to the total amount of drug administered, thus having important implications as to the amount of drug that reaches the target tissue. Because of high levels of blood flow, well-perfused organs such as the heart, liver, kidney, and brain rapidly receive most of the drug during the first few minutes after absorption.[9] Tissues with less vascular perfusion such as muscle, skin, and fat require several minutes longer to achieve a steady state. The process of absorption, distribution, biotransformation, and excretion of a drug as related to passage across cell membranes is dependent upon the characteristics of the drug's molecular size, shape, solubility, site of absorption, degree of ionization, and relative lipid solubility of its ionized and nonionized forms.[9] *Clearance* is the rate at which the active form of the drug is removed or eliminated from the body. It is the time taken to clear the drug from blood plasma. The rate of the process to inactivate a drug or eliminate it from the circulation is referred to as the elimination half-life (see later).

Transport Across Cell Membranes

When given by most routes (excluding intravenously), a drug must traverse semipermeable cell membranes at several locations before reaching the systemic circulation (Fig. 9-1). These membranes are biologic barriers that selectively inhibit the passage of drug molecules and are composed primarily of a bimolecular lipid matrix, containing mostly cholesterol and phospholipids. The lipids provide stability to the membrane and determine its permeability characteristics. Globular proteins of various sizes and composition are embedded in the matrix; they are involved in transport and function as receptors for cellular regulation. Drugs may cross a biologic barrier by diffusion through the water-filled channels or specialized ion channels, passive diffusion through the lipid membrane, carrier-mediated processes that include a facilitated diffusion, active transport, or pinocytosis.

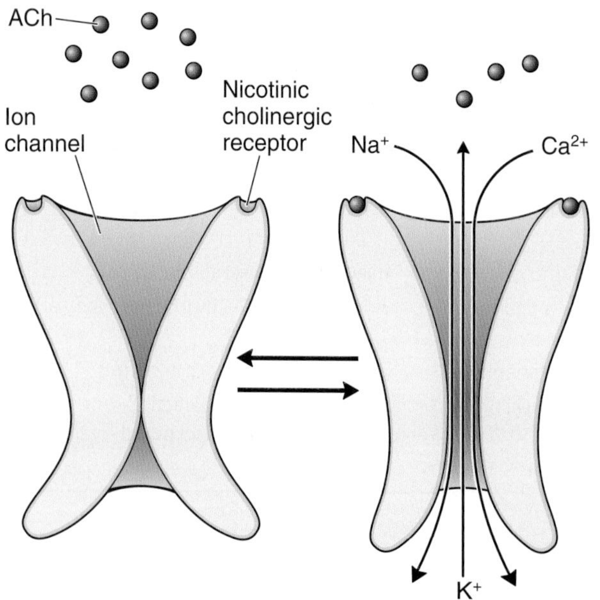

FIGURE 9-1 Drug transfer across a cell membrane.

Diffusion

Most drugs are weak organic acids or bases, existing in nonionized and ionized forms in an aqueous environment. The nonionized form is usually lipid soluble and diffuses readily across cell membranes. The ionized form cannot penetrate the cell membrane easily because of its low lipid solubility and the high electrical resistance provided by the lipid portion of the membrane. Steroids are nonionized (lipid soluble), the receptors for which are located inside the cell rather than on the external surface of the cell. Distribution of an ionizable drug across a membrane at equilibrium is determined by the drug's p*K*a (the pH at which concentrations of nonionized and ionized forms of the drug are equal) and the pH gradient, when present. For a weak acid, the higher the pH, the lower the ratio of nonionized to ionized forms. In plasma (pH, 7.4), the ratio of nonionized to ionized forms for a weak acid (e.g., with a p*K*a of 4.4) is 1:1000; in gastric fluid (pH, 1.4), the ratio is reversed (1000:1). When the weak acid is given orally, the concentration gradient for nonionized drug between stomach and plasma tends to be large, favoring diffusion through the gastric mucosa. At equilibrium, the concentrations of nonionized drug in the stomach and in the plasma are equal because only the nonionized drug can penetrate the membranes; the concentration of ionized drug in the plasma would then be about 1000 times greater than that in the stomach. For a weak base with a p*K*a of 4.4, the outcome is reversed. Thus theoretically, weakly acidic drugs (e.g., aspirin) are more readily absorbed from an acid medium (stomach) than are weak bases (e.g., quinidine).

Passive Diffusion. In this process, transport across a cell membrane depends on the concentration gradient of the solute. Most drug molecules are transported across a membrane by simple diffusion from a region of high concentration (e.g., gastrointestinal [GI] fluids) to one of low concentration (e.g., blood). Because drug molecules are rapidly removed by the systemic circulation and distributed into a large volume of body fluids and tissues, drug concentration in blood is initially low compared with that at the administration site, producing a large gradient. The diffusion rate is not only directly proportional to the gradient but also depends on the molecule's lipid solubility, degree of ionization, and size and the area of the absorptive surface. Because the cell membrane is composed of lipids, lipid-soluble drugs diffuse across the membrane more rapidly than relatively lipid-insoluble drugs. Small molecules tend to penetrate membranes more rapidly than large ones.

Facilitated Passive Diffusion. For certain molecules (e.g., glucose), the rate of membrane penetration is greater than predicted due to their low lipid solubility. One theory is that a carrier component combines reversibly with the substrate molecule at the cell membrane exterior, and the carrier–substrate complex diffuses rapidly across the membrane, releasing the substrate at the interior surface. Carrier-mediated diffusion is characterized by selectivity and saturability: The carrier transports only those substrates with a relatively specific molecular configuration, and the process is limited by the availability of carriers. The process does not require energy expenditure, and transport against a concentration gradient does not occur.

Active Transport. This process is characterized by selectivity and saturability and requires energy expenditure by the cell. Substrates may accumulate intracellularly against a concentration gradient. Active transport appears to be limited to drugs structurally similar to endogenous substances. These drugs are usually absorbed from sites in the small intestine. Active transport processes have been identified for various ions, vitamins, sugars, and amino acids.

Pinocytosis. A cell engulfs fluid or particles. The cell membrane invaginates (encloses) the fluid or particles, then fuses again, forming a vesicle that later detaches and moves to the cell interior. This mechanism requires energy expenditure. Pinocytosis probably plays a minor role in drug transport, except for protein drugs.

Distribution of Drugs

The distribution of a drug refers to the movement or transport of a drug to the site of action. Once a drug enters the systemic circulation, it is distributed to different parts of the body including the interstitial and intracellular fluid, and extravascular tissues. The rate at which this occurs depends on a variety of factors including the following[10]:

- The rate of organ blood flow.
- The degree of drug ionization in different compartments.
- The binding of a percentage of the drug molecules to serum protein. The primary protein that binds drug molecules is serum albumin. Binding prevents the drug from exerting any pharmacologic action. The unbound molecules are the portions of the drug that can penetrate capillary walls to reach the site of action.
- The number of competing drugs within the system. Some drugs compete for the same binding sites. This competition may result in higher levels of the unbound drug acting on the body.
- Molecular weight.
- Blood–brain barrier. Many drugs that easily penetrate other body organs do not appreciably enter the brain because of the sieve-like action of the blood–brain barrier.
- Lipid solubility.
  - Lipid soluble drugs are more likely to penetrate the blood–brain barrier than other drugs because they pass through the cell membrane.
  - Lipid soluble drugs may be stored in adipose tissue, which acts as a drug repository.
- Any local metabolism that occurs at any tissue other than the target organ.

Metabolism of Drugs

Metabolism refers to the process of transforming a drug into a compound that can be excreted. Metabolism occurs primarily in the liver, which reduces the drugs pharmacological activity and lipid solubility. Drug metabolism involves two processes or phases:

- ***Phase I.*** These reactions are catabolic and involve oxidation, reduction, full hydrolysis reactions, with oxidation occurring most frequently.
- ***Phase II.*** During this phase the drug undergoes conjugation reactions.

Drug Elimination

Drugs are eliminated from the body by a variety of routes including elimination in fluids (urine, breast milk, saliva, tears, and sweat), through the GI tract in the feces, and expelled in exhaled air through the lungs. The kidney is the primary organ for the excretion of drugs that have been inactivated by the liver into water-soluble metabolites.[11] Excretion of a drug by the kidneys occurs by two processes[10]:

- ***Glomerular filtration.*** The process in which drugs are filtered through the glomerulus and then carried through the tubule into the urine. The rate of drug excretion depends upon renal blood flow. Renal blood flow may be diminished with kidney pathology and the aging process.[8]
- Active secretion of the drug by the tubule into the urine.

Drug Half-Life

The rate at which a drug disappears from the body, through metabolism, excretion, or a combination is called the half-life. It is the amount of time required for half of the drug that is in the body to be eliminated. Two terms are used to describe half-life:

- Elimination half-life.
  - The time in which the concentration of the drug in the plasma falls to one-half of its original amount.
  - A drug's rate of disappearance from the body, whether by metabolism, excretion or a combination of both.
- Biological half-life.
  - The time in which the duration of action falls to one-half of its original duration.
  - The time of the drug's response rather than its plasma concentration.

Knowing the half-life of a drug is critical in determining how often and in what dosage a drug must be administered to achieve and maintain therapeutic levels of concentration. The dosage interval (time between administrations of the drug) is equal to the half-life of a particular drug. The shorter the half-life, the more often the patient must take the medication. Theoretically a steady state will be reached when the amount of the drug taken will equal the amount that is excreted. A steady state is usually reached after five half-lives of the drug have occurred. Thus, drugs with long half-lives may take several days to weeks to reach a steady state.

Drug Allergy and Drug-Induced Illnesses

Drug allergies or hypersensitivities range from mild presentations to very severe life-threatening events. For a drug to produce a reaction, it must have antigenic effects and stimulate antibody formation or the formation of sensitized T-lymphocytes, which is immune-related. Drug allergies are generally classified into four types:

- *Type I (anaphylactic reactions).* Anaphylaxis is the most severe allergic reaction and involves the skin and pulmonary and cardiovascular systems, producing cardiovascular and respiratory collapse. The signs and symptoms associated with anaphylactic shock, which usually occur within minutes after antigen exposure, but may still occur up to 1 hour later, include:
  - Neurological: dizziness, weakness, and seizures.
  - Ocular: pruritus, lacrimation, edema around the eyes.
  - Respiratory: nasal congestion, hoarseness, stridor, cough, dyspnea, tachypnea, bronchospasm, and respiratory arrest.
  - Cardiac: tachycardia, hypotension, arrhythmias, myocardial infarction.
  - Integumentary: flushing, erythema, urticaria.
  - Gastrointestinal (GI): nausea, vomiting, and diarrhea.
- *Type II (cytotoxic reaction).* The antigens adhere to the target cell and begin to destroy the target tissue. The clinical manifestations include:
  - Fever
  - Arthralgia
  - Rash
  - Splenomegaly
  - Lymph node enlargement.
- *Type III (autoimmune reaction).* A complex mediated hypersensitivity reaction in which the body has difficulty in eliminating antigen–antibody complexes. Manifestations include serum sickness, glomerulonephritis, vasculitis, and pulmonary disorders.
- *Type IV (cell-mediated hypersensitivity).* This type of reaction is mediated through T-lymphocytes as opposed to antibodies. Manifestations include local or tissue reaction.

The Effects of Exercise on Pharmacokinetics

The bioavailability of drugs can be altered with exercise, primarily because of the influence upon the drug's absorption site caused by exercise.[12] The effects of exercise on drug distribution are complex and are dependent on factors that pertain to the characteristics of each drug as well as exercise-related factors such as exercise intensity, mode, and duration.[2] According to the limited information available, the effects of exercise on bioavailability following oral drug administration have produced conflicting results. Exercise increases muscular blood flow and temperature and the subsequent enhancement of absorption through molecular diffusion across biological membranes. For example, there is an increased binding of digoxin (a heart medication that reduces the ventricular rate) in working skeletal muscle.[12] On the other hand, exercise may sequester some drugs such as propranolol (a medication used to treat hypertension) in muscle and reduce the availability of the drug for elimination. In addition, exercise decreases the clearance of highly extracted drugs and increases their plasma concentration. Hepatic blood flow has been found to be reduced as much as 50% with an exercise intensity level of 70% of maximal oxygen uptake.[13] Decreasing hepatic blood flow could potentially decrease the clearance of drugs that are metabolized as a function of blood through the liver. In a similar fashion, since exercise reduces renal blood flow, the plasma concentrations of those drugs that are primarily eliminated by the kidneys may increase.[13]

However, exercise does appear to enhance absorption from intramuscular, subcutaneous, transdermal (iontophoresis, phonophoresis), and inhalation sites. However, exercise at the site of administration also increases cutaneous blood flow which, in the case of iontophoresis and phonophoresis, could be therapeutically unfavorable as the target site of drug administration could become diluted below therapeutic levels.[8]

The Effects of Physical Agents on Pharmacokinetics

Similar to exercise, physical therapy modalities have the potential to alter the pharmacokinetics of locally and systemically administered drugs, primarily by affecting blood flow and tissue kinetic and metabolic activity.[8,14] Thermal agents that increase regional blood flow can potentially increase delivery of a drug to a specific tissue site, although there are a few studies that have documented whether these changes have any clinical relevance. However, application of local heat to the site of the drug administration will almost certainly increase dispersion of the drug away from the delivery site.[2] Theoretically, cold can restrict drug delivery by causing vasoconstriction at the cryotherapy site.[2]

The Effects of Manual Techniques on Pharmacokinetics

Manual techniques that increase blood flow to an area, such as massage, increase drug absorption from local subcutaneous injection sites.[15] Whether massage has an effect on the delivery of systemically administered drugs is not known at present.

In conclusion, because some physical therapy interventions are capable of producing complex changes in the pharmacokinetics of certain drugs, any variation in the clinical response that is observed during or after a physical therapy session, should raise the suspicion about the potential pharmacokinetic affect of a drug.[8] In addition, if maintaining the plasma concentration of a drug at a certain level is important, consideration should be given to alternative drugs if the patient is to receive a treatment that may affect the absorption, distribution, and metabolism of a drug.[14]

PHARMACOTHERAPY

An understanding of the potential effects of certain types of drugs commonly encountered during the rehabilitation process is essential.[15]

Musculoskeletal Pharmacology

Drugs are widely used in the management of both acute and chronic pain and inflammation. By far the most frequently encountered and/or prescribed drug agents in physical therapy practice are those that are prescribed to control pain and/or inflammation.

Opioid Analgesics

Most of the narcotics used in medicine are referred to as opioids, as they are derived directly from opium or are synthetic opiates.[16] Examples of these opioids include codeine, Darvon (propoxyphene hydrochloride), morphine, and Demerol (meperidine) (see "Narcotic Analgesics"). Opioid analgesics are more effective in controlling pain of a constant duration versus sharp intermittent pain.[17]

Nonopioid Analgesics

Nonopioid analgesics comprise a heterogeneous class of drugs including the salicylates (aspirin and diflunisal), para-aminophenol derivatives (primarily acetaminophen), and the NSAIDs, such as ibuprofen, Voltaren, Relafen, Naprosyn, Motrin, Indocin, Feldene, Lodine, Celebrex, and many others. Despite their diverse structures, nonopioid analgesics have similar therapeutic effects, oral efficacy, and similar side effect profiles. Nonopioid analgesics are better tolerated compared to opioids by ambulatory patients, have less sedative effects, and are much less likely to produce tolerance or dependence. Conversely, the hazards of long-term administration of these drugs are recognized.

Salicylates[7]. Aspirin, an acetylsalicylic acid, has been recognized for its pharmaceutical properties for centuries. The pharmacology of aspirin is quite consistent with that of other NSAIDs and it remains the prototype for comparisons of the efficacy and safety of new medications in its class. Aspirin continues to be the first-line drug for a variety of conditions, including mild pain, fever, osteoarthritis, rheumatoid arthritis, stroke prevention therapy, and potential reduction of prostate cancer incidence.[18] Other NSAIDs differ from aspirin in kinetics, duration of action, and patient tolerance, but the overall efficacy is very similar.

Para-Aminophenol Derivatives. Of the para-aminophenol derivatives, only acetaminophen (Tylenol) is widely used. Acetaminophen is not typically classified as an NSAID because of its lack of an anti-inflammatory effect (it does not inhibit prostaglandin synthesis in peripheral tissues). Acetaminophen is primarily centrally-acting yet exerts its analgesic and antipyretic effects peripherally by weak inhibition of both isoforms of cyclooxygenase through an unknown mechanism.[19]

Nonsteroidal Anti-inflammatory Drugs. NSAIDs are distinguished from true steroid agents such as cortisone (cortisol), prednisone (see later), and from the opiate derived analgesics.

NSAIDs have antipyretic, anticlotting (nonselective NSAIDs only), analgesic, and anti-inflammatory effects and are by far the most frequently encountered form of drug in physical therapy practice. NSAIDs are the first-line drug choice for the treatment of mild to moderate pain, soft tissue injury, osteoarthritis, gout, and inflammatory rheumatic disorders.[7] Of those patients seeing physical therapists, 25–40% are taking prescription anti-inflammatory agents, with about 40% of those using multiple NSAIDs concomitantly.[7,20,21] While it has been shown that NSAIDs may be of benefit in muscle and tendon healing, there is growing evidence of impairment of bone and cartilage healing due to NSAIDs.[7]

The analgesic and anti-inflammatory activity of NSAIDs is primarily due to the inhibition of arachidonic acid metabolism.[22] Arachidonic acid is present on cell membranes throughout the body and acts as a substrate for prostaglandin, prostacyclin, and thromboxane synthesis.[7] Arachidonic acid is released from cell membranes in response to physical, chemical, hormonal, and bacterial or other stimuli.[7]

NSAIDs also seem to promote the inhibition of the release of cyclooxygenase-1 (COX-1) and cyclooxygenase-2 (COX-2) and the synthesis of prostaglandins at an injury site.[22]

- ***COX-1 inhibitors.*** COX-1 is constitutively present in virtually all tissues under normal conditions.[7] The inhibition of COX-1 by NSAIDs has a tendency to produce a number of adverse effects on multiple organ systems, including GI inflammation, ulceration, bleeding, and increased potential for perforation. [23] Other possible side effects include an alteration of normal function in the GI mucosa and kidney blood flow, delayed wound healing, edema, nausea, dyspepsia, and fluid retention. NSAIDs may also alter kidney blood flow by interfering with the synthesis of prostaglandins in the kidney involved in the autoregulation of blood flow and glomerular filtration.[24]
- ***COX-2 inhibitors.*** Much attention has been given to the selective COX-2 inhibitors, such as celecoxib (Celebrex), which were developed to provide NSAID benefits without affecting the GI mucosa, renal tissue, or platelet aggregation.[7] COX 2 is typically not found on cell membranes under baseline conditions but is induced and upregulated by cytokines, such as interleukin-1 in the presence of cell stress or injury.[7] Because COX-2 inhibitors do not produce the same GI effects as COX-1 inhibitors, they are safer to use in patients who are predisposed to gastric or kidney malfunctions. COX-2 drugs block only the COX-2 enzyme, which is responsible for triggering pain and inflammation.[22] Because COX 1 is not affected, the patient's stomach lining is protected and bleeding tendencies are avoided. However, the enthusiasm for the coxibs have been somewhat tempered by data suggesting they are associated with a higher risk of cardiovascular events than the nonselective NSAIDs, which led to the withdrawal from the market of two widely distributed drugs: Vioxx and Bextra.[25]

The pharmacokinetics of NSAIDs have been studied extensively[7]:

- ***Absorption.*** NSAIDs are typically lipid-soluble weak acids and are ideally suited for rapid absorption from the acidic stomach and duodenum. After ingestion, most NSAIDs will exhibit an effect within 15–30 minutes. The time interval to perceive symptom relief varies with the rate of enzymatic breakdown of previously synthesized prostaglandins and the time required for the ingested drug agent to inhibit replacement. Once in the bloodstream NSAIDs, except for aspirin, are heavily bound to plasma proteins. Despite the high level of NSAID protein binding, a therapeutic effect is exerted by the constant dissociation of the drug from its binding protein and release as free or active fraction within the serum. Because of NSAIDs' high-protein affinity they may displace other more weakly protein-bound drugs unintentionally, such as warfarin (Coumadin), sulfonylurea hypoglycemic agents (Diabinese, Glucotrol, Micronase, etc.), and methotrexate (Folex, Mexate, and Rheumatrex).

- ***Distribution.*** NSAIDs are widely distributed throughout most body tissues.
- ***Metabolism.*** The liver is responsible for metabolism and bioconversion of NSAIDs. Integration of NSAID half-life data into modality selection permits its planning for maximal drug benefit and minimized adverse impact on therapy. It is worth noting that drugs with longer half-lives are associated with the highest risk for adverse effect. The effect of a given NSAID will vary among individual patients, sometimes leading to a trial of several different agents in an effort to obtain the best therapeutic effect. In clinical practice, 7–10 days are generally long enough to ascertain the effect of a given drug.
- ***Elimination.*** NSAIDs are eliminated by renal excretion. Alterations in urine pH can affect the level of ionized or nonionized drug residue and, therefore, rates of elimination.

Local Anesthetics. Local anesthetics decrease sensation in a body part without a loss of consciousness or impairments of vital functions that are associated with the use of a general anesthetic.[17] All local anesthetics are membrane stabilizing drugs that act by reversibly decreasing the rate of depolarization and repolarization of nociceptor membranes by inhibiting sodium influx through sodium-specific ion channels in the neuronal cell membrane. When the influx of sodium is interrupted, an action potential cannot arise and signal conduction is inhibited. The local adverse effects of anesthetic agents include neurovascular manifestations such as prolonged anesthesia and paresthesia, which are symptoms of localized nerve impairment. Depending on the local tissue concentrations of local anesthetics, there may be excitatory or depressant effects on the central nervous system, which can include generalized convulsions, coma, respiratory arrest, and death.

Corticosteroids. Corticosteroids can be classified as natural or synthetic. The natural form (mineralocorticoids) is produced by the adrenal glands, under the control of the hypothalamus, and is involved in maintaining fluid and electrolyte balance. Glucocorticoids (cortisol, and drugs such as prednisone), are used primarily for the treatment of a range of immunological and inflammatory musculoskeletal conditions. Although glucocorticoids affect nearly every major organ system in the body, their primary role is to regulate blood glucose. Corticosteroids exert their anti-inflammatory effects by binding to a high-affinity intracellular cytoplasmic receptor present in all human cells,[26] which in turn interact with discrete nucleotide sequences to alter gene expression. Because most steroid receptors in target cells are located in the cytoplasm, they need to get into the nucleus to alter gene expression. The side effects from excess corticosteroids are associated with a number of negative side effects, including a catabolic effect on all types of supportive joint tissue. Exogenous steroid use leads to Cushing's syndrome[27]:

- ***Cutaneous manifestations.*** Cutaneous manifestations of hypercortisolism include delayed wound healing, acanthosis nigricans (a velvety, thickened, hyperpigmented plaque that usually occurs on the neck or in the axillary region), acne, ecchymoses after minor trauma, hyperpigmentation, hirsutism, petechia, and striae.
- ***Hypokalemia.*** Hypokalemia (a potentially fatal condition in which the body fails to retain sufficient potassium to maintain health) is a well-recognized side effect of corticosteroid therapy and is probably related to the mineralocorticoid effect of hydrocortisone, prednisone, and prednisolone. Dexamethasone has no mineralocorticoid effect.
- ***Myopathy.*** There are two recognized forms of corticosteroid-induced myopathy: acute and chronic. Acute myopathy may in part be caused by hypokalemia, although corticosteroids (especially massive dosages) may have a direct effect on skeletal muscle. Both proximal and distal muscle weakness occur acutely, usually with an associated and significant elevation in serum creatinine phosphokinase, which is indicative of focal and diffuse muscle necrosis. In the more chronic form of myopathy, weakness is more insidious in onset and primarily involves proximal muscle groups.
- ***Hyperglycemia.*** Hyperglycemia is a condition in which an excessive amount of glucose circulates in the blood plasma. When hyperglycemia is combined with the immunosuppressive effect of corticosteroids, there is a significant increase in the risk for infection.
- ***Neurological impairments.*** These can include vertigo, headache, convulsions, and benign intracranial hypertension.
- ***Osteoporosis.*** Corticosteroids inhibit bone formation directly via inhibition of osteoblast differentiation and type I collagen synthesis and indirectly by inhibition of calcium absorption and enhancement of urinary calcium excretion.
- ***Ophthalmologic side effects.*** Corticosteroids increase the risk of glaucoma by increasing intraocular pressure, regardless of whether administered intranasally, topically, periocularly, or systemically.
- ***Growth suppression.*** Corticosteroids interfere with bone formation, nitrogen retention, and collagen formation, all of which are necessary for anabolism and growth.

Disease Modifying Antirheumatic Drugs. Disease modifying antirheumatic drugs (DMARDs), sometimes referred to as slow acting antirheumatic drugs (SAARDs), are a group of drugs that appear to decrease inflammation, though they are not categorized as anti-inflammatory drugs. DMARDs differ from NSAIDs since they do not decrease prostaglandin production, do not directly relieve pain, nor reduce fever. In effect, DMARDs slow the disease process by modifying the immune system. DMARDs are most commonly used in the treatment of rheumatoid arthritis, when combined with anti-inflammatory agents, and corticosteroids, but some are also used for ankylosing spondylitis, psoriatic arthritis, and lupus. Studies throughout the years have shown DMARDs to be very effective drugs, with uncommonly observed serious side effects.

The newest DMARDs are biological agents that specifically target and block interleukin-1 or tumor necrosis factor, both of which are cytokines that play a role in the inflammatory process in diseases such as rheumatoid arthritis.

Skeletal Muscle Relaxants. Skeletal muscle relaxants, such as Flexeril, Robaxin, and Soma, are thought to act by decreasing muscle tone without causing an impairment in motor function, and by acting centrally to depress polysynaptic reflexes. As muscle guarding and spasm accompany many musculoskeletal injuries, it was originally thought that these drugs, by eliminating the spasm and guarding, would facilitate the progression of a rehabilitation program. However, other drugs with sedative properties, such as barbiturates, also depress polysynaptic reflexes, making it difficult to assess if centrally acting skeletal muscle relaxants are actually muscle relaxants as opposed to nonspecific sedatives.[28] There presently exists a discrepancy between the common clinical use of skeletal muscle relaxants and the results of controlled clinical trials evaluating their efficacy in comparison with placebo. Supporting evidence does not exist for their efficacy in pain of myogenic origin nor is it clear if they provide an additive effect with exercises aimed at muscle relaxation.

Because nearly all of the oral skeletal muscle relaxants have the potential to produce drowsiness, sedation, or muscle weakness, these agents can have an effect on the patient's ability to perform motor-related tasks or participate in therapy programs.[17]

Examples of Disease-Specific Drugs

Musculoskeletal System Pharmacology

Osteoporosis. While estrogen therapy is still used in the treatment of osteoporosis, there are a number of medication options presently being used. The current drug options for osteoporosis fall into four categories:[17]

1. Bisphosphonates (alendronate [Fosamax] and risedronate sodium [Actonel]). These are antiresorptive agents that decrease osteoclastic bone resorption. The results are decreased bone remodeling, indirectly increased bone mass, and a reduced risk of fractures.
2. Calcitonin (Miacalcin). This is a calcium lowering hormone secreted by the thyroid gland that exerts its effects by direct inhibition of osteoclast activity, and promotion of renal excretion of calcium and other minerals.
3. Selected receptor molecules (raloxifene hydrochloride [Evista]). This is a nonhormonal medication that acts as an estrogen agonist in bone to suppress bone remodeling without unfavorable stimulation of the estrogen receptors located on the breast tissue or the uterus.
4. Strontium Ranelate. A drug that offers the dual mechanisms of action of combining the antiresorptive effect with the anabolic effect of new bone formation.

Gout. The medications prescribed to treat gout usually depend on whether the patient produces too much uric acid or does not excrete uric acid properly. If the body produces too much uric acid, a drug such as allopurinol (Lopurin, Zyloprim) is used to slow uric acid production. In the case where the body does not excrete uric acid well, another drug such as probenecid (Benemid, Probalan) can be used.

Neurologic System Pharmacology.

Antianxiety Medications

Selective Serotonin Reuptake Inhibitors. Selective serotonin reuptake inhibitors (SSRIs) are commonly prescribed psychotherapeutic agents. Serotonin is a neurotransmitter synthesized from the amino acid L-tryptophan. Synthesis is necessary in both the central and peripheral nervous systems because serotonin cannot cross the blood–brain barrier. Once synthesized, serotonin is either stored in neuronal vesicles or metabolized by monamine oxidase (MAO) to 5-hydroxyindoleacetic acid. The most serious drug-related adverse effect of SSRIs is the potential to produce serotonin syndrome (SS). SS, characterized by mental status changes, neuromuscular dysfunction, and autonomic instability, is thought to be secondary to excessive serotonin activity in the spinal cord and brain. Symptoms attributed to serotonin excess may include

- restlessness
- hallucinations
- shivering
- diaphoresis
- nausea
- diarrhea
- headache

Commonly prescribed SSRIs include sertraline (Zoloft), fluoxetine (Prozac), paroxetine (Paxil), and fluvoxamine (Luvox).

Monoamine Oxidase Inhibitors (MAOIs)[29]. Neurotransmitters are generally monoamines. When released into the synaptic space, neurotransmitters are either reabsorbed into the proximal nerve or destroyed by monoamine oxidase (MAO) in the synaptic cleft. The two types of MAO are MAO-A and MAO-B. MAO-A is found primarily in the liver and GI tract with some found in the monoaminergic neurons. MAO-A present in the liver is involved in the elimination of ingested monoamines, such as dietary tyramine. Circulating monoamines such as epinephrine, norepinephrine, and dopamine are inactivated when they pass through a liver rich in MAO-A. MAO-B, on the other hand, is found primarily in the brain and in platelets.

MAOIs act by inhibiting the activity of MAO preventing the breakdown of monoamine neurotransmitters (norepinephrine, serotonin, and dopamine) thereby increasing the available monamines available within the central nervous system (CNS).

The MAOI agents currently available in the United States include phenelzine sulfate (Nardil), tranylcypromine sulfate (Parnate), isocarboxazid (Marplan), and selegiline (specific for the MAO-B enzyme), all of which irreversibly bind to MAO.

Benzodiazepines[30]. Benzodiazepines (BZDs) are sedative/hypnotic agents that are used for a variety of situations, including seizure control, anxiety, alcohol withdrawal, insomnia, control of drug-associated agitation, as muscle relaxants (antispasticity agents), and as preanesthetic agents. They also are combined frequently with other medications for conscious sedation before procedures or interventions.

γ-Aminobutyric acid (GABA) is the major inhibitory neurotransmitter in the CNS. BZDs exert their action by potentiating the activity of GABA. They bind to a specific receptor on the $GABA_A$ receptor complex, which facilitates the binding of GABA to its specific receptor site. BZD binding causes increased frequency of opening of the chloride channel complexes with the $GABA_A$ receptor. The reversal potential for $GABA_A$/chloride complexes is negative to threshold for generating an action potential. In this way, activation of the $GABA_A$ receptor/chloride pore is inhibitory.

Enhanced GABA neurotransmission results in sedation, striated muscle relaxation, anxiolysis, and anticonvulsant effects. Stimulation of peripheral nervous system (PNS) GABA receptors may cause decreased cardiac contractility, vasodilation, and enhanced perfusion.

Beta-blockers. Beta-blockers, for example, Propranolol, are a class of drugs used for various indications, including the management of cardiac arrhythmias, hypertension, cardioprotection after myocardial infarction, and to block the autonomic response in persons with social phobia.

Sedatives/Hypnotics. Sedative/hypnotics are a group of drugs that cause CNS depression and are mainly used in the treatment of insomnia, but can also be used to treat anxiety, depression, and psychosis. BZDs, which are non-barbiturates (see above) are the most commonly used agents in this class.[31] Although barbiturates produce a sedative-hypnotic effect, the associated rapid development of tolerance carries with it a high risk of physical and psychological dependence, withdrawal syndromes, and fatalities by overdose. For these reasons, barbiturates are not routinely prescribed. BZDs induce sleep by decreasing the number of arousals between the different stages of sleep thereby allowing for more continuous total sleep time. Most sedative/hypnotics stimulate the activity of GABA, the principal inhibitory neurotransmitter in the CNS. γ-Hydroxybutyric acid (GHB) is a sedative/hypnotic recently banned for sale to the public because of frequent abuse and serious adverse toxic effects. GHB is a neuroinhibitory neurotransmitter or neuromodulator in the CNS. It also appears to increase $GABA_B$ receptor activity and dopamine levels in the CNS. Three other types of medications act on the same receptor as BZDs and, therefore, share some of the same pharmacological properties. These include the following:

- Zolpidem. Zolpidem is used to treat insomnia, and is particularly effective in initiating sleep. Zolpidem can also be used as an anticonvulsant and muscle relaxant.
- Zaleplon. Zaleplon is effective in the treatment of insomnia where difficulty in falling asleep is the primary complaint. The side effects of zaleplon are similar to the side effects of BZDs, although with less next-day sedation.
- Zopiclone. Zopiclone is a non-BZD hypnotic agent used in the treatment of insomnia. In the United States, zopiclone is not commercially available, although its active stereoisomer, eszopiclone, is sold under the names Lunesta.

Mild toxicity of sedative/hypnotics resembles ethanol intoxication and can include excessive drowsiness, impaired psychomotor coordination, decreased concentration, and cognitive deficits.[31] Moderate poisoning leads to respiratory depression and hyporeflexia. Severe poisoning leads to flaccid areflexic coma, apnea, and hypotension.

Occasionally, hyperreflexia, rigidity, clonus, and Babinski signs are present. Miosis is common, but mydriasis may be present with certain agents. The nonbarbiturates, such as methyprylon and glutethimide, more commonly present with mydriasis. Hypotension is usually secondary to vasodilation and negative cardiac inotropic effects.

Narcotic Analgesics. The term narcotic specifically refers to any substance that induces sleep. In current practice, narcotic refers to any of the many opioids or opioid derivatives.

Activation of the opiate receptors results in the inhibition of synaptic neurotransmission in the CNS and PNS. Opioids bind to opiate receptors thereby inducing a postsynaptic response. The physiological effects of opioids are mediated principally through μ and κ receptors in the CNS and periphery. μ receptor effects include analgesia, euphoria, respiratory depression, and miosis. κ receptor effects include analgesia, miosis, respiratory depression, and sedation. Two other opiate receptors that mediate the effects of certain opiates include σ and δ sites. σ receptors mediate dysphoria, hallucinations, and psychosis; δ receptor agonism results in euphoria, analgesia, and seizures. The opiate antagonists (e.g., naloxone, nalmefene, naltrexone) antagonize the effects at all four opiate receptors.

Common classifications divide the opioids into agonist, partial agonist, or agonist–antagonist agents and natural, semisynthetic, or synthetic. Opioids decrease the perception of pain, rather than eliminate or reduce the painful stimulus. Inducing slight euphoria, opioid agonists reduce the sensitivity to exogenous stimuli. The GI tract and the respiratory mucosa provide easy absorption for most opioids.

Peak effects are generally reached in 10 minutes with the IV route, 10–15 minutes after nasal insufflation (e.g., butorphanol, heroin), 30–45 minutes with the IM (intramuscular) route, 90 minutes with the PO (by mouth) route, and 2–4 hours after dermal application (i.e., fentanyl). Following therapeutic doses, most absorption occurs in the small intestine. Toxic doses may delay absorption because of delayed gastric emptying and slowed gut motility.

Most opioids are metabolized by hepatic conjugation to inactive compounds that are excreted readily in the urine. Certain opiates (e.g., propoxyphene, fentanyl, and buprenorphine) are more lipid soluble and can be stored in the fatty tissues of the body. All opioids have a prolonged duration of action in patients with liver disease (e.g., cirrhosis) because of impaired hepatic metabolism. This may lead to drug accumulation and opioid toxicity. Renal failure also leads to toxic effects from accumulated drug or active metabolites (e.g., normeperidine).

Opioid toxicity characteristically presents with a depressed level of consciousness. Opiate toxicity should be suspected when the clinical triad of CNS depression, respiratory depression, and pupillary miosis are present. Drowsiness, conjunctival injection (redness of the white sclera of the eye), and euphoria are seen frequently. Other important presenting signs are ventricular arrhythmias, acute mental status changes, and seizures.

Examples of commonly prescribed opioids include codeine phosphate, Demerol, Dilaudid, Empirin with codeine,

Subli-maze, Synalgos-DC, Talwin 50, propoxyphene, morphine, Hydrocodone, Lorcet, Lortab, Zydone, Hydrocet, Oxycontin (Oxycodone), Percodan (Percocet), Darvon (Darvocet), and Vicodin (Vicoprofen).

Antidepressants

Tricyclic Antidepressants.[32] Tricyclic antidepressants (TCAs) are used in the treatment of depression, chronic pain, and enuresis (involuntary discharge of urine, especially while asleep). Patients with depression and those with chronic pain are at high risk for abuse, misuse, and overdosing of these drugs.

TCAs affect the cardiovascular, pulmonary, and GI systems, and the CNS. The toxic effects on the myocardium are related to the blocking of fast sodium channels, which involves the same mechanism as type IA antiarrhythmics (e.g., quinidine). The result is a slowing myocardium depolarization that leads to arrhythmia, myocardial depression, and hypotension. Hypotension also results from peripheral α-adrenergic blockade, which causes vascular dilatation. Inhibition of norepinephrine reuptake and subsequent depletion causes further hypotension. The effects on the pulmonary system include pulmonary edema, adult respiratory distress syndrome, and aspiration pneumonitis. The etiologies of the first two remain unclear, but the third, aspiration pneumonitis, is secondary to an altered mental status.

The anticholinergic effects of TCAs cause a slowing of the GI system, which results in delayed gastric emptying, decreased motility, and prolonged transit time.

CNS toxicity results from the anticholinergic effects and direct inhibition of biogenic amine reuptake. An excitation syndrome is the initial result and manifests as confusion, hallucinations, ataxia, seizures, and coma.

Examples of commonly prescribed TCAs include Amitriptyline, Clomipramine, Doxepin, Trimipramine, Desipramine, Nortriptyline, Protriptyline, Imipramine, Amoxapine (dibenzoxazepine), and Maprotiline (tetracyclic antidepressant).

Parkinson Disease and Parkinsonian Syndrome.[32]

Parkinson disease (PD) is a progressive neurodegenerative disease affecting every 100–150 per hundred thousand individuals, or about 1% of those over 60 years of age, in the US population.[33–35] PD is characterized clinically by tremor, bradykinesia, rigidity, and postural instability. The basal ganglia motor circuit modulates cortical output necessary for normal movement.

Levodopa, coupled with a peripheral decarboxylase inhibitor (PDI), remains the criterion standard of symptomatic treatment for PD. It provides the greatest antiparkinsonian benefit with the fewest adverse effects.

Dopamine agonists provide symptomatic benefit comparable to levodopa/PDI in early disease, but lack sufficient efficacy to control signs and symptoms by themselves in later disease.

Medications for PD usually provide good symptomatic control for 4–6 years. Whether levodopa has a toxic or protective effect in the brain with PD is unknown. As PD progresses, fewer dopamine neurons are available to store and release levodopa-derived dopamine. The patient's clinical status begins to fluctuate more and more closely in concert with plasma levodopa levels. Fluctuating levodopa-derived dopamine concentrations in association with advancing disease, therefore, may be responsible for development of motor fluctuations and dyskinesia.

In contrast to levodopa, the long-acting dopamine agonists (i.e., bromocriptine, pergolide, pramipexole, ropinirole, cabergoline) provide relatively smooth and sustained receptor stimulation.

The selection of medication depends in part on the nature and cause of the disability. If disability is due solely to tremor, a tremor-specific medication, such as an anticholinergic agent, is often used. Anticholinergic medications provide good tremor relief in approximately 50% of patients, but do not improve bradykinesia or rigidity. Because tremor may respond to one anticholinergic medication and not another, a second anticholinergic usually is tried if the first is not successful. These medications are usually introduced at a low dose and escalated slowly to minimize adverse effects, which include memory difficulty, confusion, and hallucinations. Adverse cognitive effects are relatively common, especially in the elderly.

If disability is due to a dopamine-responsive symptom such as bradykinesia, rigidity, decreased dexterity, slow speech, or shuffling gait, a dopaminergic medication (dopamine agonist or levodopa/PDI) are typically introduced. Symptomatic medications are started at a low dose, escalated slowly, and titrated to control symptoms. Most patients require symptomatic dopaminergic therapy to ameliorate bradykinesia and rigidity within 1–2 years after diagnosis.

For patients younger than 65 years, symptomatic therapy is normally initiated with a dopamine agonist and then add levodopa/PDI when the dopamine agonist alone no longer controls symptoms adequately. Dopamine agonists provide antiparkinsonian efficacy comparable to levodopa/PDI for 6–18 months or longer and may control symptoms adequately for several years.

For patients who are demented or those older than 70 years, who may be prone to adverse effects from dopamine agonists, and for those likely to require treatment for only a few years, physicians may elect not to use a dopamine agonist but depend on levodopa/PDI as the primary symptomatic therapy. For patients aged 65–70 years, a judgment is made based on general health and cognitive status.

Medications for Cerebrovascular Accidents. The ischemic cascade is a series of biochemical reactions that take place in the brain and other aerobic tissues after seconds to minutes of ischemia (inadequate blood supply; Table 9-3).[36] Since the ischemic cascade is a dynamic process, the efficacy of interventions to protect the ischemic cascade also may prove to be time dependent.

Theoretically, calcium channel blockers (e.g., nimodipine) should have the narrowest window of therapeutic opportunity, since calcium influx is one of the earliest events in the ischemic cascade.

Neuroprotectants affecting later events in the ischemic cascade include free-radical scavengers (e.g., tirilazad, citicoline) and neuronal membrane stabilizers (e.g., citicoline). Monoclonal antibodies against leukocyte adhesion molecules also are being evaluated as late neuroprotectants (e.g., enlimomab).

Anticoagulants are considered as potential treatments for cerebrovascular accidents (CVA). However, although heparin

TABLE 9-3	The Ischemic Cascade
Lack of oxygen causes the neuron's normal process for making ATP for energy to fail.	
The cell switches to anaerobic metabolism, producing lactic acid.	
ATP-reliant ion transport pumps fail, causing the cell to become depolarized, allowing ions, including calcium (Ca^{++}), to flow into the cell.	
The ion pumps can no longer transport calcium out of the cell, and intracellular calcium levels get too high.	
The presence of calcium triggers the release of the excitatory amino acid neurotransmitter glutamate.	
Glutamate stimulates AMPA receptors and Ca^{++}-permeable NMDA receptors, which open to allow more calcium into cells.	
Excess calcium overexcites cells and causes the generation of harmful chemicals like free radicals, reactive oxygen species, and calcium-dependent enzymes such as calpain, endonucleases, ATPases, and phospholipases. Calcium can also cause the release of more glutamate.	
As the cell's membrane is broken down by phospholipases, it becomes more permeable, and more ions and harmful chemicals flow into the cell.	
Mitochondria break down, releasing toxins, and apoptotic factors into the cell.	
The caspase-dependent apoptosis cascade is initiated, causing cells to "commit suicide."	
If the cell dies through necrosis, it releases glutamate and toxic chemicals into the environment around it.	
Toxins poison nearby neurons, and glutamate can overexcite them.	
If and when the brain is reperfused, a number of factors lead to reperfusion injury.	
An inflammatory response is mounted, and phagocytic cells engulf damaged but still viable tissue.	
Harmful chemicals damage the blood–brain barrier.	
Cerebral edema occurs because of leakage of large molecules like albumin from blood vessels through the damaged blood–brain barrier. These large molecules pull water into the brain tissue after them by osmosis. This "vasogenic edema" causes compression of and damage to brain tissue.	

AMPA = α-amino-5-hydroxy-3-methyl-4-isoxazole propionic acid; NMDA = *N*-methyl-D-aspartate.

prevents recurrent cardioembolic strokes and may help inhibit ongoing cerebrovascular thrombosis, no definitive evidence exists to show that initiating anticoagulation reduces brain injury in acute ischemic stroke.

Anticoagulation drug treatment is not without risk. Overall, intracranial hemorrhage occurs in 1–4% of patients who receive an anticoagulant for TIA or acute stroke. Accordingly, uncontrolled hypertension, intracranial hemorrhage, and uncontrolled bleeding at another site are contraindications to anticoagulation.

Several new oral anticoagulant medications, including ximelagatran, are in the final stages of clinical trials for use in the prophylaxis of ischemic thromboembolic stroke. Once approved for use, the potential of such drugs in the arena of stroke treatment may be significant.

Antiepileptic Drugs. Many structures and processes are involved in the development of a seizure, including neurons, ion channels, receptors, glia, and inhibitory and excitatory synapses.[37] The antiepileptic drugs (AEDs) are designed to modify these processes to favor inhibition over excitation in order to stop or prevent seizure activity. The AEDs can be grouped according to their main mechanism of action, although many of them have several actions and others have unknown mechanisms of action. The main groups are as follows.

Sodium Channel Blockers. The sodium channel blockade is the most common and the most well-characterized mechanism of currently available AEDs. AEDs that target these sodium channels prevent the return of the channels to the active state by stabilizing their inactive form. In doing so, repetitive firing of the axons is prevented. The presynaptic and postsynaptic blockade of sodium channels of the axons causes stabilization of the neuronal membranes, blocks and prevents posttetanic potentiation, limits the development of maximal seizure activity, and reduces the spread of seizures. AED examples include carbamazepine, oxcarbazepine, lamotrigine, zonisamide, and the hydantoins: phenytoin, fosphenytoin.

CLINICAL PEARL

Anticonvulsants in mood disorders have four major effects:

- Increasing of the seizure threshold
- Decreasing the seizure duration
- Decreasing the neurometabolic response to an episode
- Decreasing the phenomena of amygdaloid kindling

Side effects and toxicity. AEDs can produce dose-related adverse effects, which include dizziness, diplopia, nausea, ataxia, and blurred vision. Rare idiosyncratic adverse effects include aplastic anemia, agranulocytosis, thrombocytopenia, and Stevens–Johnson syndrome. Asymptomatic elevation of liver enzymes is observed commonly during the course of therapy in 5–10% of patients. Rarely, severe hepatotoxic effects can occur.

GABA receptor agonists. GABA has two types of receptors:

- ***$GABA_A$.*** $GABA_A$ receptor is stimulated and chloride channels open to allow the influx of negative ions (i.e., chloride). The $GABA_A$ receptors have multiple binding sites for BZDs, barbiturates, and others substances such as picrotoxins, bicuculline, and neurosteroids.
- ***$GABA_B$.*** The $GABA_B$ receptor is linked to a potassium channel.

Direct binding to $GABA_A$ receptors can enhance the GABA system by blocking presynaptic GABA uptake, by inhibiting the metabolism of GABA by GABA transaminase, and by increasing the synthesis of GABA. The BZDs most commonly used for treatment of epilepsy are lorazepam, diazepam, clonazepam, and clobazam. The two barbiturates mostly commonly used in the treatment of epilepsy are phenobarbital and primidone.

Side effects and toxicity. The most common effect is sedation. Other adverse effects include dizziness, ataxia, blurred vision, diplopia, irritability, depression, muscle fatigue, and weakness.

ABA reuptake inhibitors. At least four specific GABA-transporting compounds help in the reuptake of GABA; these carry GABA from the synaptic space into neurons and glial cells, where it is metabolized. Nipecotic acid and tiagabine (TGB) are inhibitors of these transporters; this inhibition makes increased amounts of GABA available in the synaptic cleft, which serves to prolong GABA-mediated inhibitory postsynaptic potentials (IPSPs).

Side effects and toxicity. The most common adverse effects include dizziness, asthenia, nervousness, tremor, depressed mood, and emotional lability. Diarrhea also was significantly more frequent among TGB-treated patients than placebo-treated patients. Other adverse effects included somnolence, headaches, abnormal thinking, abdominal pain, pharyngitis, ataxia, confusion, psychosis, and skin rash.

GABA transaminase inhibitor. GABA is metabolized by transamination in the extracellular compartment by GABA-transaminase (GABA-T). Inhibition of this enzymatic process leads to an increase in the extracellular concentration of GABA. Vigabatrin (VGB) inhibits the enzyme GABA-T.

Side effects and toxicity. The most common adverse effect is drowsiness. Other important adverse effects include neuropsychiatric symptoms, such as depression (5%), agitation (7%), confusion, and, rarely, psychosis. Minor adverse effects, usually at the onset of therapy, include fatigue, headache, dizziness, increase in weight, tremor, double vision, and abnormal vision.

Glutamate blockers. Glutamate and aspartate are the most two important excitatory neurotransmitters in the brain. The glutamate system is a complex system with macromolecular receptors with different binding sites (i.e., AMPA, kainate, NMDA, glycine, metabotropic site).

Examples of glutamate blockers include topiramate and felbamate.

Side effects and toxicity. Common adverse effects include insomnia, weight loss, nausea, decreased appetite, dizziness, fatigue, ataxia, and lethargy. Polytherapy is associated with increases in adverse effects.

Neuroleptics (Antipsychotics). The term neuroleptic refers to the effects on cognition and behavior of antipsychotic drugs that reduce confusion, delusions, hallucinations, and psychomotor agitation in patients with psychoses.[38] Also known as major tranquilizers and antipsychotic drugs, neuroleptic agents comprise a group of the following classes of drugs:

- Phenothiazines
- Aliphatics
- Piperidines
- Piperazines
- Thioxanthenes (e.g., droperidol)
- Butyrophenones (e.g., haloperidol)
- Dibenzoxazepines (e.g., loxapine)
- Dihydroindolone (e.g., molindone)
- Diphenylbutylpiperidine (e.g., pimozide)
- Benzisoxazole (e.g., risperidone)

The adverse effects of neuroleptics are not confined to psychiatric patients. Neuroleptics also are used as sedatives, for their antiemetic properties, to control hiccups, to treat migraine headaches, as antidotes for drug-induced psychosis, and in conjunction with opioid analgesia.

The major tranquilizers have complex CNS actions that are incompletely defined. Their therapeutic action is thought to be primarily antagonism of central dopaminergic (D-2 receptor) neurotransmission, although they also have antagonist effects at muscarinic, serotonergic, α_1-adrenergic, and H1-histaminergic receptors.

Although all antipsychotic preparations share some toxic characteristics, the relative intensity of these effects varies greatly, depending on the individual drug. Generally, all neuroleptic medications are capable of causing the following symptoms:

- ***Hypotension:*** Phenothiazines are potent α-adrenergic blockers that result in significant orthostatic hypotension, even in therapeutic doses for some patients. In overdose, the hypotension may be severe.
- ***Anticholinergic effects:*** Neuroleptic agent toxicity can result in tachycardia, hyperthermia, urinary retention, toxic psychosis, and hot dry flushed skin.
- ***Extrapyramidal symptoms:*** Alteration in the normal balance between central acetylcholine and dopamine transmission can produce dystonia, oculogyric crisis, torticollis, acute parkinsonism, akathisia, and other movement disorders. Chronic use of major tranquilizers is associated with buccolingual dysplasia (tardive dyskinesia, TD), parkinsonism, and akathisia.
- ***Neuroleptic malignant syndrome:*** All of the major tranquilizers have been implicated in the development of neuroleptic malignant syndrome (NMS)—a life-threatening derangement that affects multiple organ systems and results in significant mortality.
- ***Seizures:*** Most major tranquilizers lower the seizure threshold and can result in seizures at high doses and in susceptible individuals.
- ***Hypothermia:*** Certain major tranquilizers prevent shivering, limiting the body's ability to generate heat.
- ***Cardiac effects:*** Prolongation of the QT interval and QRS can result in arrhythmias.
- ***Respiratory depression:*** Hypoxia and aspiration of gastric contents can occur in children and in mixed overdose.

Spasticity. Spasticity is a motor disorder characterized by a velocity-dependent increase in tonic stretch reflexes with exaggerated tendon jerks, resulting from hyperexcitability of the stretch reflex, as one component of the upper motor neuron syndrome (see Chapter 3).[39,40]

Two types of GABA receptors, called A and B types, are found on neurons in the brain and spinal cord (see "Antiepileptic Drugs"). The drugs used to reduce spasticity work as agonists or antagonists at these receptors.

BZDs—diazepam and clonazepam. The BZDs bind $GABA_A$ receptor complexes on neurons located in the brainstem and at the spinal cord level and increase the affinity of GABA for the $GABA_A$ receptor complex. This results in an increase in presynaptic inhibition and the reduction of monosynaptic and polysynaptic reflexes. These drugs may improve passive range of motion and reduce hyperreflexia, painful spasms, and anxiety. Diazepam has a half-life of 20–80 hours and forms active metabolites that prolong its effectiveness. The half-life of clonazepam ranges from 18 to 28 hours.

Sedation, weakness, hypotension, adverse GI effects, memory impairment, incoordination, confusion, depression, and ataxia may occur. Tolerance and dependency can occur, and withdrawal phenomena, notably seizures, have been associated with abrupt cessation of therapy.

Baclofen—oral and intrathecal pump. Baclofen is a GABA agonist, and its primary site of action is the spinal cord, where it reduces the release of excitatory neurotransmitters and substance P by binding to the $GABA_B$ receptor. Studies show that baclofen improves clonus, flexor spasm frequency, and joint range of motion, resulting in improved functional status.

Adverse effects include sedation, ataxia, weakness, and fatigue.

Intrathecal baclofen is approved in the United States for the treatment of spasticity of spinal or cerebral origin. In children, intrathecal baclofen is particularly effective for the treatment of spasticity of the lower extremities. Complications of the procedure are relatively few and usually are limited to mechanical failures of the pump or the catheter. Adverse drug effects are usually temporary and can be managed by reducing the rate of infusion.

Oral Agents.

- ***Dantrolene sodium:*** Dantrolene sodium is useful for spasticity of supraspinal origin, particularly in patients with cerebral palsy or traumatic brain injury. It decreases muscle tone, clonus, and muscle spasm by acting at the level of the muscle fiber, affecting the release of calcium from the sarcoplasmic reticulum of skeletal muscle and thus reducing muscle contraction. It is, therefore, less likely than the other agents to cause adverse cognitive effects. Its peak effect is at 4–6 hours, with a half-life of 6–9 hours.

  Adverse effects include generalized weakness, including weakness of the respiratory muscles, drowsiness, dizziness, weakness, fatigue, and diarrhea.

- ***Tizanidine.*** Tizanidine (Zanaflex) is a new and effective therapeutic option for the management of spasticity due to cerebral or spinal damage. The antispasticity effects of tizanidine are the probable result of inhibition of the H-reflex. It may also facilitate inhibitory actions of glycine and reduce the release of excitatory amino acids and substance P, and may have analgesic effects. When combined with baclofen, tizanidine presents the opportunity to maximize therapeutic effects and minimize adverse effects by reducing the dosages of both drugs.

Tizanidine hydrochloride is a short-acting drug with extensive first-pass hepatic metabolism to inactive compounds following an oral dose. The half-life is 2.5 hours with peak plasma level at 1–2 hours, and therapeutic and side effects dissipate within 3–6 hours. Therefore, use must be directed to those activities and times when relief of spasticity is most important.

Dry mouth, somnolence, asthenia, and dizziness are the most common adverse events associated with tizanidine. Liver function problems (5%), orthostasis, and hallucinations (3%) are rare tizanidine-related adverse events.

Cardiovascular System Pharmacology

Many cardiovascular medications have the potential to alter responses to both acute and chronic exercise in a predictable manner. Knowledge of how common drugs alter these responses can assist the clinician in assessing the safety and appropriateness of exercise and in determining the effectiveness of exercise training.[41] Most medications that are prescribed for cardiovascular disease have either a direct or indirect effect on the heart or vascular system, including alteration of the myocardial oxygen consumption, peripheral blood flow, and cardiac preload or afterload.[41] Medications may either increase or decrease exercise capacity, or alter the expected changes in heart rate and blood pressure that normally occur with an increase in activity or at rest (Table 9-4).[41]

α-Adrenergic Blocking Drugs (α_1-Antagonists/Alpha-Blockers). These drugs work through the autonomic nervous system (ANS) by blocking alpha-receptors. Alpha-receptors normally promote constriction of the arterioles. Blocking constriction promotes dilation of vessels and lowers blood pressure as well as reducing the work of the heart in some situations. Alpha-blocking drugs also inhibit the actions of norepinephrine that raises blood pressure as part of the fight-or-flight response. Alpha-blockers are usually prescribed along with other blood-pressure-lowering drugs, such as a beta-blocking drug and/or a diuretic. There are now several medications available that combine the effects of blocking both the beta- and alpha-receptors (Labetalol [Normo-dyne, Trandate]).

Examples of alpha-blockers include doxazosin (Cardura), prazosin (Minipress), and terazosin (Hytrin).

Possible adverse side effects. Nausea and indigestion; these usually subside with long-term use. Less frequent effects are cold hands and feet, temporary impotence, and nightmares. Dizziness may occur initially or as the dosage is increased.

Angiotensin-Converting Enzyme Inhibitors. These drugs act to prevent production of a hormone, angiotensin II, which constricts blood vessels. They belong to the class of drugs called vasodilators—drugs that dilate blood vessels, an effective way to lower blood pressure and increase the supply of blood and oxygen to the heart and various other organs. In addition to dilating blood vessels, angiotensin-converting enzyme (ACE)-inhibiting medications may produce some beneficial effects indirectly by preventing the abnormal rise in hormones associated with heart disease, such as

TABLE 9-4 Effects of Medications on the Cardiovascular and Metabolic Responses to Exercise

Physiological Response	Specific Example	Medications That Could Alter Response
Cardiac output	Contractility Initiation/conduction of cardiac action potential	Increase by digitalis Decreased by β-blockers
Effects on peripheral circulation	Venodilation or constriction: preload Arterial vasoconstriction or dilation: afterload Blood volume	Decrease by nitrates Decrease by α_1-antagonists Decreased by diuretics
Myocardial oxygen consumption	Heart rate	Decreased by beta-blockers
	Blood pressure Systolic wall tension	Decreased by nitrates
Distribution of cardiac output	Blood flow to active skeletal muscles Blood flow to cutaneous vessels	Decreased by α_1-antagonists Decreased by α_1-antagonists
Metabolism	Fatty acid mobilization and oxidation Glycogenolysis	Decreased by beta-blockers Decreased by beta-blockers

Data from Peel C, Mossberg KA: Effects of cardiovascular medications on exercise responses. *Phys Ther* 75:387–396, 1995.

aldosterone. ACE inhibitors are widely used to treat high blood pressure, or hypertension, a major risk factor for cardiovascular disease. Used alone or in combination with other drugs, ACE inhibitors have also proved effective in the treatment of congestive heart failure.

Examples include benazepril (Lotensin), captopril (Capoten), enalapril (Vasotec, Vasotec I.V.), fosinopril (Monopril), lisinopril (Prinivil, Zestril), moexipril (Univasc), perindopril erbumine (Aceon), quinapril (Accupril), ramipril (Altace), spirapril (no brand names listed), and trandolapril (Mavik).

Possible Adverse Side Effects. Common side effects are dizziness or weakness, loss of appetite, a rash, itching, a hacking, unpredictable cough, and swelling.

Antiarrhythmic Drugs. These drugs, which are potent medications, correct an irregular heartbeat (arrhythmia) and slow a heart that is beating too fast (tachycardia).

Examples of antiarrhythmic drugs include amiodarone (Cordarone), digoxin (Lanoxin), disopyramide phosphate (Nor-pace), flecainide (Tambocor), propafenone (Rhythmol), lidocaine (Xylocaine), mexiletine (Mexitil), procainamide (Procan SR, Pronestyl, Pronestyl SR), quinidine gluconate (Duraquin, Quinaglute Dura-Tabs, Quinalan Sustained-Release), quinidine sulfate (Quinidex Extentabs), and tocainide (Tonocard).

Possible side effects. The most significant common side effects are weakening of heart contractions, worsening of some arrhythmias, weight loss, nausea, and tremors. Other less common effects are fever, rash, dry mouth, depressed white blood cell count, liver inflammation, confusion, loss of concentration, dizziness, and disturbances in vision. About 0.1–0.2% of patients suffer lung inflammation, a potentially serious side effect.

Anticoagulants, Antiplatelets, and Thrombolytics. These drugs are sometimes referred to as "blood thinners," but this term is not truly accurate, as they inhibit the ability of the blood to clot—preventing clots from forming in blood vessels and from getting bigger. Anticoagulants, antiplatelet agents, and thrombolytics each have specific indications and uses. Any patient who has had a heart valve replaced with a mechanical valve requires lifelong oral anticoagulants in order to prevent clots from forming on the valve. Patients who develop atrial fibrillation may require anticoagulants; clot formation in the left atrium is a potential hazard of this rhythmic disturbance. Oral anticoagulants are prescribed for patients who develop thrombophlebitis, an inflammation of the veins in the legs or pelvis. One of the dangers of this condition is the development of blood clots that may travel to the lungs and cause pulmonary emboli. Lastly, some patients who have a serious heart attack involving the anterior surface of the heart are prescribed an anticoagulant to prevent clots from forming on the inner lining of the scar.

Heparin is an anticoagulant that is administered intravenously when rapid anticoagulation is necessary. All patients undergoing open-heart surgery are treated with heparin while their blood is being oxygenated by the heart–lung machine. At the end of the operation, medication is given to reverse the effects of heparin.

Aspirin is not an anticoagulant but has a profound effect on platelets—blood cells that stick together and cause clots to form. Because of aspirin's ability to inhibit the clotting action of platelets, it is designated as an antiplatelet and is frequently prescribed in patients who have recovered from a heart attack, in order to prevent clots from forming in the veins used for coronary bypass surgery.

The most recent and exciting classes of drugs that are useful for people with heart attacks are the thrombolytic drugs. These agents are given intravenously as soon as possible with the goal of dissolving the offending clot within a coronary artery before it causes permanent, debilitating damage. The three most commonly used thrombolytics are t-PA, streptokinase, and APSAC.

Examples of these drugs are acetylsalicylic acid or aspirin (Alka-Seltzer, Anacin, Ascriptin, Bayer, Bufferin, Easprin, Ecotrin, St. Josephs, Zorprin), dipyridamole (Persantine), and warfarin (Coumadin, Panwarfin).

Possible side effects. Adverse effects are rare, but may include nausea, headache, flushing, dizziness or faintness, or rash.

β-Adrenergic Blockers. These drugs probably reduce blood pressure by reducing cardiac output (or perhaps by blocking the production of angiotensin). Beta-blockers are also used to treat hypertension. Specifically, they block responses from the beta nerve receptors. This serves to slow down the heart rate and to lower blood pressure. Beta-blockers also block the effects of some of the hormones that regulate blood pressure. During exercise or emotional stress, adrenaline and norepinephrine are released and normally stimulate the beta-receptors—sensors that transmit messages to the heart to speed up and pump harder. By blocking the receptors, beta-blockers act to reduce heart muscle oxygen demands during physical activity or excitement, thus reducing the possibility of angina caused by oxygen deprivation.

Examples of these drugs are acebutolol (Sectral), atenolol (Tenormin), betaxolol (Betoptic, Betoptic S, Kerlone), bisoprolol (Zebeta), metoprolol (Lopressor), carteolol (Cartrol Oral, Ocupress Ophthalmic), labetalol (Normodyne, Trandate), levobetaxolol, levobunolol, metoprolol (Lopressor, Toprol XL), nadolol (Corgard), penbutolol (Levatol), pindolol (Visken), propranolol (Inderal), sotalol (Betapace AF, Betapace), timolol (Betimol, Blocadren, Timoptic-XE, Timoptic, Timoptic, OcuDose).

Possible side effects. Lethargy and cold hands and feet because of reduced circulation may occur. These drugs may also cause nausea, nightmares or vivid dreams, and impotence.

Calcium Channel Blockers. Calcium plays a central role in the electrical stimulation of cardiac cells and in the mechanical contraction of smooth muscle cells in the walls of arteries. Calcium channel blockers are relatively new synthetic drugs that work by blocking the passage of calcium into the muscle cells that control the size of blood vessels. All muscles need calcium in order to contract; by preventing the muscles of the arteries from contracting, blood vessels dilate, allowing blood to flow through them more easily, and reducing blood pressure.

Examples of these drugs are diltiazem (Cardizem), nicardipine (Cardene), nifedipine (Procardia, Procardia XL), nimodipine (Nimotop), and verapamil (Calan, Isoptin, Verelan).

Possible side effects. Excessively slow heart rate, low blood pressure, headache, swelling of ankle/feet, constipation, nausea, tiredness, dizziness, redness of face and neck, palpitations, and rash.

Digitalis Drugs. Like many drugs, digitalis was originally derived from a plant, in this case the foxglove. Digitalis has the primary effect of strengthening the force of contractions in weakened hearts and is also used in the control of atrial fibrillation. The most commonly used digitalis products are digoxin and digitoxin. The drug penetrates all body tissues and reaches a high concentration in the muscle of the heart. Its molecules bind with cell receptors that regulate the concentration of sodium and potassium in the spaces between tissue cells and in the bloodstream. These two minerals determine the level of calcium. Digitalis preparations act by increasing the amount of calcium supplied to the heart muscle and thus enhancing its contractions. Digitalis drugs also affect electrical activity in cardiac tissues. They control the rate at which electric impulses are released and the speed of their conduction through the chamber walls. These two actions determine the two major uses of digitalis drugs in heart disease—treatment of heart failure and control of abnormal heart rhythms. Digitalis may be given on a short-term basis in acute heart failure or over a long period of time to treat chronic heart failure. Digitalis drugs can be used to treat disturbances of the heartbeat, particularly the abnormally rapid contractions of the atria referred to as atrial or supraventricular arrhythmias (especially atrial fibrillation). The drugs restore the normal heartbeat either by interrupting the abnormal rhythm or by slowing down the rapid beats to a rate at which effective and coordinated heart contractions are possible.

Example of these drugs are digoxin (Lanoxicaps, Lanoxin).

Possible side effects. Some side effects include tiredness, nausea, loss of appetite, and disturbances in vision.

Diuretics. Diuretics, commonly referred to as water pills, lower blood pressure by increasing the kidney's excretion of sodium and water, which in turn reduces the volume of blood. There are several types of diuretics, which are classified according to their site of action in the kidney.

- *Thiazide diuretics* work in the tubules (the structures that transport urine in the kidneys).
- *Loop diuretics* are more potent than the thiazide diuretics. They are so named because they work in the area of the kidney called the loop of Henle. They are usually prescribed when a thiazide diuretic proves insufficient or for patients with heart failure or compromised kidney function.
- *Potassium-sparing diuretics* work in the area of the kidney or distal tubule of the nephrons in the kidney where potassium is excreted. They prevent the excessive loss of potassium that sometimes occurs with the thiazides. They are most often given in conjunction with a thiazide or loop diuretics.

Examples of diuretics are chlorthalidone (Hygroton) and hydrochlorothiazide (Esidrix, Hydrodiuril, Oretic), and examples of potassium-sparing diuretics are amiloride (Midamor), spironolactone (Aldactone), and triamterene (Dyrenium).

Possible side effects. Although uncommon, lethargy, cramps, rash, or impotence may occur. Some of these effects may be caused by a loss of potassium and may be avoided by including a potassium supplement or potassium-sparing agent in the regimen.

Nitrates. The oldest and most frequently used coronary artery medications are the nitrates. Nitrates are potent vein and artery dilators, causing blood to pool in the veins and the arteries to open up, thus reducing the amount of blood returning to the heart. This decreases the work of the left ventricle and lowers the blood pressure. Nitrates may also increase the supply of oxygenated blood by causing the coronary arteries to open more fully, thus improving coronary blood flow. Nitrates effectively relieve coronary artery spasm. They do not, however, appear to affect the heart's contractions.

Example of nitrates are nitroglycerin (Deponit NTG, Minitran, Nitro-Bid, Nitrogard, Nitroglyn, Nitrol, Nitrolingual, Nitrong, Nitrostat, Transderm-Nitro, Tridil) and isosorbide dinitrate (Dilatrate-SR, Iso-Bid, Isordil, Sorbitrate, Sorbitrate SA).

Possible side effects. Headaches, flushing, and dizziness may occur.

Pulmonary System Pharmacology

The delivery of a drug to the lungs allows the medication to interact directly with the diseased tissue and reduce the risk of adverse effects, specifically systemic reactions, while also allowing for the reduction of dose compared to oral administration. The prescription of any pulmonary medication is founded on four basic goals[42]:

- Promotion of bronchodilation or relief of bronchoconstriction.
- Facilitation of the removal of secretions from the lungs.
- Improvement of alveolar ventilation or oxygenation.
- Optimization of the breathing pattern.

The relative importance of each of these goals depends on the specific disease process and the resultant respiratory problem.[42]

Most inhaled drugs are administered through a pressurized metered-dose inhaler. Dry pounder inhalers or breath-activated devices are delivery devices that scatter a fine powder into the lungs by means of a brisk inhalation. The other major drug delivery system for pulmonary problems is the nebulizer, a device that dispenses liquid medications as a mist of extremely fine particles in oxygen or room air so that is inhaled.

Bronchodilator Agents. Bronchodilator agents are a group of medications that produce an expansion of the lumina of the airway passages of the lungs. The primary goal of bronchodilator therapy is to influence the ANS via two opposing nucleotides: cyclic adenosine monophosphate (cAMP) and cyclic guanosine monophosphate (cGMP).[42] cAMP facilitates smooth muscle relaxation and inhibits mast cell degranulation, resulting in bronchodilation.[42] cGMP facilitates smooth muscle contraction and may enhance mast cell release of histamine and other mediators, resulting in bronchoconstriction.[42] Bronchodilator agents, which either stimulate (sympathomimetics) or inhibit (sympatholytics) adrenergic receptors, are central to the symptomatic management of chronic obstructive pulmonary disease (COPD) and asthma (Table 9-5).

Ancillary Pulmonary Medications. In addition to bronchodilators, several other drug groups are frequently used in the treatment of respiratory disorders, including decongestants, antihistamines, antitussives, mucokinetics, respiratory stimulants and depressants, and paralyzing and antimicrobial agents.[42]

Antitussives. Antitussives are drugs that suppress an ineffective, dry, hacking cough by decreasing the activity of the afferent nerves or decreasing the sensitivity of the cough center. The stimulus to cough is relayed to the cough center in the medulla and then to the respiratory muscles via the phrenic nerve. The primary adverse effect of antitussive agents is sedation, although GI distress and dizziness may also occur.[42]

Decongestants. Decongestants are used to treat upper airway mucosal edema and discharge by binding with the alpha-1 receptors in the blood vessels of the mucosal lining of the upper airways thereby stimulating vasoconstriction.[42] Primary side effects include headache, dizziness, nausea, nervousness, hypertension, and cardiac irregularities.[42]

Antihistamines. Histamines play a role in the modulation of neural activity within the CNS and the regulation of gastric secretion by means of two types of receptors:

- ***H_1-receptors.*** These are primarily located in vascular, respiratory, and GI smooth muscles and are specifically targeted for blockade by antihistamines in the treatment of asthma. H_1-antagonist drugs decrease the mucosal congestion, irritation, and discharge caused by inhaled allergens. The adverse effects most often attributable to antihistamines include sedation, fatigue, dizziness, blurred vision, loss of coordination, and GI distress.
- ***H_2-receptors.*** These act via G-proteins (guanine nucleotide binding proteins) to stimulate adenylate cyclase, the enzyme that synthesizes cAMP from adenosine triphosphate (ATP). Among the many responses mediated by these receptors are gastric acid secretion, smooth muscle relaxation, inotropic and chronotropic effects on heart muscle, and inhibition of lymphocyte function.

Mucokinetics. This class of drugs is responsible for promoting the mobilization and removal of secretions from the respiratory tract.[42] There are four basic types of mucokinetics agents[42]:

- Mucolytics act by disrupting the chemical bonds in mucoid and purulent secretions, decreasing the viscosity of the mucus and promoting expectoration. The primary adverse effects of these drugs include mucosal irritation, coughing, bronchospasm, and nausea.
- Expectorants increase the production of respiratory secretions, thus facilitating their ejection from the respiratory tract.
- Wetting agents make expectoration easier for the patient and are delivered by either continuous aerosol or intermittent ultrasonic nebulization.
- Surface active agents (surfactant) lower the surface tension of the medium in which these are dissolved. They are primarily used to stabilize aerosol droplets thereby enhancing their efficacy as carrier vehicles for nebulized drugs.

Antimicrobial Agents/Antibiotics. Penicillins are the mainstay in the treatment of respiratory infections.[42] First, second, and third generation cephalosporins are generally considered as alternatives to the penicillins, when penicillins are not tolerated by the patient or when they are ineffective.[42]

Oxygen.[42] Oxygen should be considered a drug when it is breathed in concentrations higher than those found in the atmospheric air. The therapeutic administration of oxygen can elevate the arterial oxygen tension and increase the arterial oxygen content, improving peripheral tissue oxygenation. When used judiciously, oxygen therapy has few side effects.

TABLE 9-5 Drugs That Have a Positive Influence on Bronchial Intralumenal Diameter			
Group	**Action**	**Mechanism of Action**	**Side Effects**
Beta-sympathomimetics	Bronchodilation	Increases cyclic AMP, decreases intracellular calcium concentrations, thus relaxing smooth muscle	Tremor, palpitations, tachycardia, headache, nervousness, dizziness, nausea, hypertension
Methylxanthines (a substance found in coffee, tea, and chocolate)	Bronchodilation	Blocks the degradation of cyclic AMP. Used for patients who do not respond to the standard asthma agents, and is occasionally used in the treatment of spinal cord injury	Agitation, tachycardia, headache, palpitations, dizziness, hypotension, chest pain, nausea, possibly diuresis
Alpha-sympatholytics	Bronchodilation	Blocks the decrease of cyclic AMP	Agitation, tachycardia, headache, palpitations, dizziness, hypotension, chest pain, nausea, possibly diuresis
Parasympatholytics	Prevents bronchoconstriction	Blocks parasympathetic stimulation, which prevents an increase in cyclic GMP, allowing cyclic AMP to increase; blocks the activity of the enzyme hosphodiesterase, which prevents the degradation of cyclic AMP	Central nervous system stimulation with low doses, depression with high doses; delirium, hallucinations, decreased gastrointestinal activity
Glucocorticoids	Bronchodilation	Administered systemically or topically. Blocks the release of arachidonic acid from airway epithelial cells, which in turn blocks production of prostaglandins and leukotrienes. Decreases inflammatory response	Cushingoid appearance; obesity; growth suppression; hyperglycemia and diabetes, mood changes, irritability, or depression; thinning of skin; muscle wasting; osteoporosis; hypertension; and immunosuppression
Cromolyn sodium (extract of a Mediterranean plant)	Bronchodilation	Prevents influx of calcium ions into the mast cell, thus blocking the release of mediators responsible for bronchoconstriction Used prophylactically to prevent exercise-induced bronchospasm and severe bronchial asthma via oral inhalation	Throat irritation, hoarseness, dry mouth, cough, chest tightness, bronchospasm

AMP = adenosine monophosphate; GMP = guanosine monophosphate.
Data from Cahalin LP, Sadowsky HS: Pulmonary medications. *Phys Ther* 75:397–414, 1995.

Metabolic and Endocrine System

Physical therapists routinely treat patients who are diagnosed with diabetes mellitus (DM). People with DM are at increased risk of developing chronic complications related to ophthalmic, renal, neurological, cerebrovascular, cardiovascular, and peripheral vascular disease.[43,44] The major classes of DM are insulin-dependent diabetes mellitus (IDDM), also known as type 1 DM, and noninsulin-dependent diabetes mellitus (NIDDM), also known as type 2 DM, and subclassed as obese or nonobese.[45] Type 1 DM results from autoimmune beta cell destruction, whereas type 2 DM is related to deficiency in insulin production or a condition of insulin resistance. Malnutrition-related DM, gestational DM, and other types of DM associated with specific conditions complete the classification. By its action on carbohydrate, protein, and lipid metabolism, insulin exerts a dominant effect on the regulation of glucose homeostasis.[45] Through various actions, insulin, a hormone which is secreted by the beta cells of the pancreas, lowers blood glucose by either suppressing glucose release from the liver, or by promoting uptake of glucose into peripheral tissues, especially muscle. Insulin also affects adipose tissue by activating lipogenesis (conversion of glucose into triglyceride).[45]

Glucagon, catecholamines, glucocorticoids, and growth hormone act in opposition to insulin by increasing blood glucose.

The classic intervention approach to DM is the triad of diet (weight management), exercise, and drug therapy.[45] Patients with IDDM require insulin replacement, with diet and exercise completing the treatment plan, whereas patients with NIDDM are often managed by diet and exercise prior to any use of pharmacological agents.

Drugs for Diabetes. Because patients with type 2 (NIDDM) diabetes have both insulin resistance and beta cell dysfunction, oral medication to increase insulin sensitivity is often given with an intermediate-acting insulin at bedtime or a long-acting insulin given in the morning or evening. The medications prescribed for DM have a variety of actions:

- Exenatide (Byetta) is an incretin-mimetic agent that mimics glucose-dependent insulin secretion and several other antihyperglycemic actions of incretins.
- Chlorpropamide (Diabinese) may increase insulin secretion from pancreatic beta cells.
- Tolbutamide (Orinase) increases insulin secretion from pancreatic beta cells.
- Tolazamide (Tolinase) increases insulin secretion from pancreatic beta cells.
- Acetohexamide (Dymelor) increases insulin secretion from pancreatic beta cells.
- Glyburide (DiaBeta, Micronase, PresTab, Glynase) increases insulin secretion from pancreatic beta cells.
- Glipizide (Glucotrol, Glucotrol XL) is second-generation sulfonylurea; stimulates insulin release from pancreatic beta cells.
- Repaglinide (Prandin) stimulates insulin release from pancreatic beta cells.
- Acarbose (Precose) delays hydrolysis of ingested complex carbohydrates and disaccharides and absorption of glucose; inhibits metabolism of sucrose to glucose and fructose.
- Miglitol (Glyset) delays glucose absorption in small intestine; lowers after-dinner hyperglycemia.
- Pioglitazone (Actos) improves target cell response to insulin without increasing insulin secretion from pancreas.
- Rosiglitazone (Avandia) is an insulin sensitizer; major effect in stimulating glucose uptake in skeletal muscle and adipose tissue.
- Pramlintide acetate (Symlin) is a synthetic analog of human amylin, a hormone made in beta cells; slows gastric emptying, suppresses after-dinner glucagon secretion, and regulates food intake.

Exercise has the effect of increasing glucose uptake of insulin-sensitive tissues by two mechanisms[45]:

- Increasing blood flow and thus enhancing glucose and insulin delivery to muscle.
- Stimulation of glucose transport by muscle contraction.

In a nondiabetic person, insulin levels fall during acute exercise and hepatic glucose production rises to meet the demands of the exercising muscle. In a diabetic patient, exercise lowers blood glucose concentration and transiently improves glucose tolerance during acute exercise. The metabolic response to exercise is based on the fitness level of the individual, the intensity and duration of the exercise, and timing of exercise in relation to insulin administration and meals.[45]

Additional benefits of exercise in a diabetic population include improved whole-body insulin sensitivity, improved glycemic control, reduction of certain cardiovascular risk factors, and an increase in psychological well-being.

Ergogenic Aids

Ergogenic aids is a term used to describe a broad category of topics including physiologic, pharmacologic, psychologic, and nutritional enhancement.[46] The most common pharmacologic enhancement used by athletes are anabolic–androgenic steroids, a synthetic derivative of the male hormone testosterone. The more appropriate term “anabolic–androgenic steroids” is frequently shortened to anabolic steroids.

Anabolic–Androgenic Steroids. The use of anabolic steroids for nonmedical purposes has been in existence for over 50 years. These synthetic agents have a core steroid structure that gives them both anabolic (tissue building) and androgenic (masculinizing) effects, although physiologically these effects are inseparable.[47] Anabolic steroids may be taken orally or parenterally. Orally ingested steroids are well absorbed from the stomach, excreted fairly rapidly from the body because of their short half-lives, are more toxic to the liver than injectable steroids, and are highly potent.[46,48–50] Injectable steroids are characterized by delayed uptake from the body, slower excretion, increased detectability in drug tests for longer periods of time, less liver toxicity, and have less potency than oral steroids.[46,48–50]

Studies on the effects of anabolic steroids on muscle strength provide inconsistent results.[46] Muscle strength increases will result from anabolic steroid use only if the following criteria are met[46,51]:

- The athlete must have been intensively trained in weightlifting immediately prior to the steroid regimen and must continue with intense weightlifting during the steroid regimen.
- The athlete must maintain a high protein, high calorie diet.
- Strength must be assessed with a single repetition, maximal-weight technique using the specific exercises with which the athlete trains, as opposed to single-joint, isolation-testing techniques.

Weight gain is commonly associated with anabolic steroid use. Whether these gains reflect muscle mass increases or fluid retention remains unclear.[46]

Although the potential benefits associated with anabolic steroid use remain questionable, the immediate and long-term side effects are well-established and include[46]

- increased risk of myocardial infarction and stroke;
- liver toxicity;
- significant decreases in plasma testosterone, testicular atrophy, impotence, prostate enlargement, decreased sperm counts, and a decrease in testosterone production from the testes;

- gynecomastia, characterized by a subareolar, button-like unilateral or bilateral plaque of tissue, and/or the development of breast tissue;
- increased musculotendinous injury;
- premature closure of the epiphysis in children, resulting in decreased adult height;
- alterations in lipid profiles—a significant rise in total serum cholesterol level and a decrease in high density lipoprotein (HDL); and
- alterations in mental status including, euphoria, aggressiveness, irritability, nervous tension, changes in libido, mania, depression (with withdrawal from steroids), and psychosis.

Amphetamines

The phenylethylamine structure of amphetamines is similar to catecholaminergic, dopaminergic, and serotonergic agonists (biogenic amines), which may explain their actions, with the clinical presentation being dependent on the type of amphetamine used. For example, methamphetamine lacks much of the peripheral stimulant properties of amphetamine while still offering euphoric and hallucinogenic properties. These actions are similar to those of cocaine; however, while effects of cocaine last for 10–20 minutes, duration of amphetamine action is much longer, lasting as long as 10–12 hours.

The routes of amphetamine administration may be oral (ingestion), inhalation (smoke), or injection (IV). Oral use is associated with an approximate one-hour lag time before onset of symptoms, whereas inhaled and IV methods yield effects within a few minutes. Peak plasma concentrations occur within 5 minutes with IV use, 30 minutes with nasal or IM use, and 2–3 hours postingestion.

Central Nervous System. Amphetamine compounds cause a general efflux of biogenic amines from neuronal synaptic terminals (indirect sympathomimetics). They inhibit specific transporters responsible for the reuptake of biogenic amines from the synaptic nerve ending and presynaptic vesicles. Amphetamines also inhibit MAO, which degrades biogenic amine neurotransmitters intracellularly. The net effect is an increase of monoamine neurotransmitter release into the synapse. Physiological adaptation occurs through receptor or coupling down regulation; this tolerance and an accompanying psychological tolerance can lead to escalating use of the drug and increased toxicity. Chronic use can lead to a depletion of biogenic amine stores and a paradoxical reverse effect of the drug—a wash out.

Elevated catecholamine levels usually lead to a state of increased arousal and decreased fatigue. Increased dopamine levels at synapses in the CNS may be responsible for movement disorders, schizophrenia, and euphoria. Serotonergic signals may play a role in the hallucinogenic and anorexic aspects of these drugs.

Other serotonergic and dopaminergic effects may include resetting the thermal regulatory circuits upward in the hypothalamus and causing hyperthermia. The hyperthermia produced by amphetamines is similar to that of the SS.

Peripheral Nervous System. Catecholaminergic (sympathomimetic) effects of amphetamines include inotropic and chronotropic effects on the heart, which can lead to tachycardia and other dysrhythmias. The vasoconstrictive properties of the drugs can lead to hypertension and/or coronary vasospasm.

The serotonergic action of amphetamines on peripheral vasculature can lead to vasoconstriction, which is especially problematic in placental vessels. Animal studies have shown that serotonergic actions of amphetamines effect changes in plasma levels of oxytocin, somatostatin, gastrin, and cholecystokinin.

Patients with amphetamine intoxication often are identified by a change of mental status alone or associated with another injury and/or illness. These changes include disorientation, headache, dyskinesias, agitation, symptoms of stroke, cardiovascular signs and symptoms (chest pain, palpitations), GI problems (dry mouth, nausea and vomiting, diarrhea), genitourinary dysfunction (difficult micturition), and skin changes (diaphoresis, erythematous painful rashes, needle marks, infected deep ulcerations (ecthyma)).

REVIEW QUESTIONS*

1. Describe the differences between pharmacodynamics and pharmacokinetics?
2. In relation to pharmacology and the ANS, what is the dominant tone?
3. Which two organs are primarily responsible for metabolizing drugs?
4. What effects do exercise and thermal physical agents have on drug metabolism?

*Additional questions to test your understanding of this chapter can be found in the Online Learning Center for *Orthopaedic Assessment, Evaluation, and Intervention at* www.duttononline.net.

REFERENCES

1. Boissonnault WG: *Examination in Physical Therapy Practice: Screening for Medical Disease.* New York, NY: Churchill Livingstone, 1991.
2. Ciccone CD: Basic pharmacokinetics and the potential effect of physical therapy interventions on pharmacokinetic variables. *Phys Ther* 75:343–351, 1995.
3. Magarey ME: Examination of the cervical and thoracic spine. In: Grant R, ed. *Physical Therapy of the Cervical and Thoracic Spine*, 2nd ed. New York, NY: Churchill Livingstone, 1994: 109–144.
4. Stetts DM: Patient Examination. In: Wadsworth C, ed. *Current Concepts of Orthopaedic Physical Therapy–Home Study Course 11.2.2.* La Crosse, WI: Orthopaedic Section, APTA, 2001.
5. Hertling D, Kessler RM: *Management of Common Musculoskeletal Disorders: Physical Therapy Principles and Methods*, 3rd ed. Philadelphia, PA: Lippincott Williams & Wilkins, 1996.
6. *Guide to physical therapist practice*: *Phys Ther* 81:S13–S95, 2001.
7. Biederman RE: Pharmacology in rehabilitation: Nonsteroidal anti-inflammatory agents. *J Orthop Sports Phys Ther* 35:356–367, 2005.
8. DuVall RE: Pharmacological competencies for effective medical screening. In: Wilmarth MA, ed. *Medical Screening for the Physical Therapist.* Orthopaedic Section Independent Study Course 14.1.1 La Crosse, Wisconsin, Orthopaedic Section, APTA, Inc, 2003: 1–14.
9. Benet LZ, Kroetz DL, Sheiner LB: Pharmacokinetics: The dynamics of drug absorption, distribution, and elimination. In: Hardman JG, Gilman AG, Limbrid LE, eds. *Goodman and Gilman's the Pharmacologic Basis of Therapeutics*, 9th ed. New York, McGraw-Hill, 1996: 3–27.

10. Brookfield WP: Pharmacologic Considerations for the Physical therapist. In: Boissonnault WG, ed. *Primary Care for the Physical Therapist: Examination and Triage*. St Louis, Elsevier Saunders, 2005: 309–322.
11. Eddy LJ: Introduction to Pharmacology. In: Wadsworth C, ed. *Orthopedic Physical Therapy Pharmacology Home Study Course 98-2*. La Crosse, WI: Orthopaedic Section, APTA, 1998.
12. van Baak MA: Influence of exercise on the pharmacokinetics of drugs. *Clin Pharmacokinet* 19:32–43, 1990.
13. Dossing M: Effect of acute and chronic exercise on hepatic drug metabolism. *Clin Pharmacokinet* 10:426–431, 1985.
14. Ciccone CD: Basic pharmacokinetics and the potential effect of physical therapy interventions on pharmacokinetic variables. In: Rothstein JR, ed. *Pharmacology: An American Physical Therapy Association Monograph*. Alexandria, VA: American Physical Therapy Association, 1995: 9–17.
15. Dionne RA: Pharmacologic treatments for temporomandibular disorders. *Oral Surg Oral Med Oral Pathol Oral Radiol Endod* 83:134–142, 1997.
16. Stephens E: Toxicity, Narcotics. Available at: http://www.emedicine.com/emerg/topic330.htm, 2010.
17. Schelhase EM, Chen JT, Jordan J, et al: Pharmacology and its impact on the rehabilitation process. In: Magee D, Zachazewski JE, Quillen WS, eds. *Scientific foundations and principles of practice in musculoskeletal rehabilitation*. St. Louis, MI: WB Saunders, 2007: 255–281.
18. Lichtenstein DR, Wolfe MM: COX-2-Selective NSAIDs: New and improved? *JAMA* 284:1297–1299, 2000.
19. Crofford LJ: Rational use of analgesic and antiinflammatory drugs. *N Engl J Med* 345:1844–1846, 2001.
20. Boissonnault WG: Prevalence of comorbid conditions, surgeries, and medication use in a physical therapy outpatient population: A multicentered study. *J Orthop Sports Phys Ther* 29:506–519; discussion 520–525, 1999.
21. Boissonnault WG, Koopmeiners MB: Medical history profile: Orthopaedic physical therapy outpatients. *J Orthop Sports Phys Ther* 20:2–10, 1994.
22. Sperling RL: NSAIDs. *Home Healthc Nurse* 19:687–689, 2001.
23. Holvoet J, Terriere L, Van Hee W, et al: Relation of upper gastrointestinal bleeding to non-steroidal anti-inflammatory drugs and aspirin: A case-control study. *Gut* 32:730–734, 1991.
24. Clive DM, Stoff JS: Renal syndromes associated with nonsteroidal anti-inflammatory drugs. *N Engl J Med* 310:563–572, 1984.
25. Spiegel BM, Targownik L, Dulai GS, et al: The cost-effectiveness of cyclooxygenase-2 selective inhibitors in the management of chronic arthritis. *Ann Intern Med* 138:795–806, 2003.
26. Brattsand R, Linden M: Cytokine modulation by glucocorticoids: Mechanisms and actions in cellular studies. *Aliment Pharmacol Ther* 10(Suppl. 2):81–90; Discussion 1–2, 1996.
27. Buchman AL: Side effects of corticosteroid therapy. *J Clin Gastroenterol* 33:289–294, 2001.
28. Elenbaas JK: Centrally acting oral skeletal muscle relaxants. *Am J Hosp Pharm* 37:1313–1323, 1980.
29. Marcus S: Toxicity, Monoamine Oxidase Inhibitor. Available at: http://www.emedicine.com/emerg/topic318.htm, 2010.
30. Mantooth R: Toxicity, Benzodiazepine. Available at: http://www.emedicine.com/emerg/topic58.htm, 2010.
31. Cooper J: Toxicity, Sedative-Hypnotics. Available at: http://www.emedicine.com/EMERG/topic525.htm, 2010.
32. Soghoian S, Doty CI: Toxicity, Tricyclic Antidepressant. Available at: http://www.emedicine.com/ped/topic2714.htm, 2006.
33. Henchcliffe C, Schumacher HC, Burgut FT: Recent advances in Parkinson's disease therapy: Use of monoamine oxidase inhibitors. *Expert Rev Neurother* 5:811–821, 2005.
34. Jankovic J: Parkinson's disease: Recent advances in therapy. *South Med J* 81:1021–1027, 1988.
35. Riederer P, Lange KW, Youdim MB: Recent advances in pharmacological therapy of Parkinson's disease. *Adv Neurol* 60:626–635, 1993.
36. Becker JU, Wira CR: Stroke, Ischemic. Available at: http://www.emedicine.com/EMERG/topic558.htm, 2010.
37. Ochoa JG, Riche W: Antiepileptic Drugs: An Overview. Available at: http://www.emedicine.com/neuro/topic692.htm, 2010.
38. Challoner K, Newton E: Toxicity, Neuroleptic Agents. Available at: http://www.emedicine.com/emerg/topic338.htm, 2010.
39. Vanek ZF, Menkes JH: Spasticity, Available at: http://www.emedicine.com/neuro/topic706.htm, 2010
40. Lance JW: Symposium synopsis. In: Feldman RG, Young RR, Koella WP, eds. *Spasticity: Disordered Motor Control*. Chicago, IL: Year Book Medical Publishers, 1980: 485–494.
41. Peel C, Mossberg KA: Effects of cardiovascular medications on exercise responses. *Phys Ther* 75:387–396, 1995.
42. Cahalin LP, Sadowsky HS: Pulmonary medications. *Phys Ther* 75:397–414, 1995.
43. Nathan DM: Prevention of long-term complications of non-insulin-dependent diabetes mellitus. *Clin Invest Med* 18:332–339, 1995.
44. Nathan DM: Long-term complications of diabetes mellitus. *N Engl J Med* 328:1676–1685, 1993.
45. Betts EF, Betts JJ, Betts CJ: Pharmacologic management of hyperglycemia in diabetes mellitus: Implications for physical therapy. *Phys Ther* 75:415–425, 1995.
46. Thein LA, Thein JM, Landry GL: Ergogenic aids. *Phys Ther* 75:426–439, 1995.
47. Landry GL, Primos WA Jr: Anabolic steroid abuse. *Adv Pediatr* 37:185–205, 1990.
48. Stephens MB: Ergogenic aids: powders, pills and potions to enhance performance. *Am Fam Physician* 63:842–843, 2001.
49. Silver MD: Use of ergogenic aids by athletes. *J Am Acad Orthop Surg* 9:61–70, 2001.
50. Kern A: Ergogenic aids. *Int J Sport Nutr Exerc Metab* 10:vi–vii, 2000.
51. Haupt HA, Rovere GD: Anabolic steroids: A review of the literature. *Am J Sports Med* 12:469–484, 1984.

CHAPTER 10

Manual Techniques

CHAPTER OBJECTIVES

At the completion of this chapter, the reader will be able to:

1. Give definitions for commonly used biomechanical terms used in manual therapy (MT).
2. List the criteria that are important for the correct application of a manual technique.
3. Summarize the various types of MT.
4. Apply the knowledge of the various MTs in the planning of a comprehensive rehabilitation program.
5. Recognize the manifestations of abnormal tissue and develop strategies using manual techniques to treat these abnormalities.
6. Categorize the various effects of MT on the soft tissues.
7. Make an accurate judgment when recommending an MT technique to improve joint or muscle function.

OVERVIEW

Touch has always been and continues to be a primary healing modality. The first written records of massage go back to Ancient China, and wall paintings in Egypt depict hands-on healing techniques that go back 15,000 years.[1] From this early "laying on of hands" evolved many of the techniques used today.

The techniques of MT fall under the umbrella of therapeutic touch. MT has become such an important component of the intervention for orthopaedic and neurologic disorders that it is considered by many as an area of specialization within physical therapy.[2–5]

Several MT approaches or techniques have evolved over the years. By their nature, many of these techniques have not been developed with the same scientific rigor as fields such as anatomy and physiology, and much of their use is based on clinical outcomes, rather than evidence-based proof. However, an absence of evidence does not always mean that there is evidence of absence (of effect), and there is always the risk of rejecting therapeutic approaches that are valid.[6]

Of the approaches commonly applied, the Cyriax,[7] Mennell,[8] and osteopathic techniques[9,10] (Table 10-1) originated from physicians, whereas the Maitland,[11,12] Kaltenborn,[13] and McKenzie[14] approaches (Table 10-2) were derived by physical therapists.[5,15,16]

Within these major philosophies, a number of subsets have also emerged, including myofascial release (MFR), positional release techniques, neurodynamic mobilization techniques (see Chap. 11), manually resisted exercise, proprioceptive neuromuscular facilitation (PNF), joint mobilization, and manipulation.

MT techniques have traditionally been used to produce a number of therapeutic alterations in pain and soft-tissue extensibility through the application of specific external forces.[11,13,17,18] Although it is generally agreed that manual techniques are beneficial for specific impairments, such as a restricted joint glide and adaptively shortened connective tissue, there is less agreement on which technique is the most effective. The decision about which approach or technique to use has traditionally been based on the clinician's belief, level of expertise, and decision-making processes. This has led to widespread opinions on which tools to use to measure outcome; how to apply a particular technique in terms of patient setup, intensity, and duration; and how to gauge an individual's response to a technique.

Unfortunately, the therapeutic efficacy of many MT techniques remains undetermined, although a number of theories exist. There are numerous concerns with determining the validity of studies addressing the efficacy of manual techniques:

- The selection of a particular technique is typically made on an ad hoc basis.
- The strong placebo effect associated with the laying on of hands.
- Many musculoskeletal conditions are self-limiting so that patients may improve with time regardless of the intervention.
- The difficulty of blinding clinicians and subjects to the intervention the subjects are receiving.
- Clear-cut definitions as to when one technique is more efficacious than another are lacking.
- Overreliance on MT techniques to improve a patient's status is a passive approach in an era when patient independence is stressed.

TABLE 10-1 Manual Therapy Approach—Physician Generated

	Cyriax (Orthopaedic Medicine) Assertions	Mennell Assertions	Osteopathic Assertions
Philosophy	All pain has an anatomic source and, therefore, all treatment must reach that anatomic source If the diagnosis is correct, the treatment will be of benefit to the source	Dysfunction indicates a serious pathologic process or joint disease Loss of normal joint movement or joint play can lead to dysfunction Joint manipulation can restore normal joint-play movements	Neuromusculoskeletal system is connected with other systems; therefore, disease processes can be evident in musculoskeletal system An abnormality in structure (somatic dysfunction) can lead to abnormal function of related components Manipulative therapy can restore and maintain normal structure and function relationships
Key concepts	Diagnosis of soft-tissue lesions Categorization of referred pain Differentiation between contractile and noncontractile lesions	Assessment of joint play	Diagnosis of somatic dysfunction Examination focuses on presence of asymmetry, restriction of movement, and palpation of soft-tissue texture changes (i. e., palpation of skin, muscle, and other connective tissue for feeling of thickness, swelling, tightness, or temperature change)
History	Observation and history Age and occupation Symptoms (site and spread, onset and duration, and behavior) Medical considerations Inspection	Present complaint Onset Nature of pain Localization of pain Loss of movement Past history Family history Medical systems review	History Knowledge of physical trauma, past history of visceral, and soft-tissue problems Present complaint Establish relationship from patient's history between time and mechanism to adaptation, and decompensation
Physical examination	Active movements Passive movements Resisted movements Neurologic examination Palpation Inspection	Inspection Palpation Examination of voluntary movements Muscle examination Special tests (e.g., roentgenography) Examination of joint-play movements	Postural analysis Regional screening functional units Pelvic girdle Foot Vertebral column Shoulder girdle Hand
Interpretation of evaluation	Identification of anatomic structure associated with lesion	Joint dysfunction	Determination of dysfunction: -Positional fault -Restriction fault Segmental or multisegmental
Treatment strategies	Injection Friction massage Manipulation Mobilization Physical therapy (e.g., exercise and modalities) Patient education	Manipulation Mobilization Physical therapy (e. g., exercise and modalities) Patient education	Manipulation Mobilization Muscle energy Myofascial techniques Counterstrain Exercise therapy Patient education

Data from Di Fabio RP: Efficacy of manual therapy. *Phys Ther* 72:853–864, 1992.

Indeed, research studies seem to agree and suggest that the most efficacious approach is a combination of manual techniques with other interventions, such as progressive exercises, the use of therapeutic modalities, and patient education about proper body mechanics, positions, and postures.[19–21] Regardless of which MT technique is used, all patients should undergo a full examination/evaluation before any technique is performed.

TABLE 10-2 Manual Therapy Approach—Physical Therapist Generated			
	Maitland (Australian) Assertions	**Kaltenborn (Norwegian) Assertions**	**McKenzie Assertions**
Philosophy	Personal commitment to understand patient Consideration and application of theoretical (e.g., pathology and anatomy) and clinical thinking (e.g., signs and symptoms) Continual assessment and reassessment of data	Biomechanical assessment of joint movements Pain, joint dysfunction, and soft tissue changes are found in combination	Predisposing factors of sitting posture, loss of extension range, and frequency of flexion contribute to spinal pain Patients should be involved in self-treatment
Key concepts	Examination, technique, and assessment are interrelated and interdependent Grades of movement (I–V) Strong emphasis on use of passive movement testing (testing accessory and physiologic joint movements) Differential assessment to prove or disprove clinical working hypothesis	Application of principles from arthrokinematics (e.g., concave–convex rule and close- and loose-packed positions) to determine existence of somatic dysfunction Grades of movement (I–III)	During movements of spine, positional change to nucleus pulposus takes place Strong emphasis on use of active motions Flexed lifestyle leads to a more posterior position of nucleus Intervertebral disk is common source of back pain
Evaluation framework	Subjective examination (as defined by Maitland)[14,15] Establish kind of disorder Area of symptoms Behavior of symptoms Irritability Nature Special questions Planning objective examination (as defined by Maitland)[14,15] Physical examination Observation Functional tests Active movements Isometric tests Other structures in plan Passive movements (e.g., special tests, physiologic and accessory joint movements, and relevant adverse neural tissue tension tests) Palpation Neurologic examination Highlight main findings	History ("five-by-five scheme") Immediate case history (e.g., assess symptoms for localization, time, character, etc.) Previous history (e.g., assess for kind of treatment, relief of symptoms, presence of similar symptoms or related symptoms) Social background Medical history Family history Patient's assessment of cause of complaint Physical examination Inspection Function (active and passive movements; testing with traction, compression, and gliding; and resisted tests) Palpation Neurologic tests Additional tests	History Interrogation (e.g., where did pain begin, how, constant or intermittent, what makes it better or worse, previous episodes, and further questions) Posture (sitting and standing) Examination of movement (flexion, extension, and side gliding) Movements in relation to pain Repeated movements Test movements Other tests (e.g., neurologic and other joints)
Evaluation	Initial assessment relates examination findings Behavior of patient's symptoms—pain or stiffness (somewhat analogous to McKenzie's derangement and dysfunction syndrome, respectively) Diagnosis, although no specific structure designated Stage of disorder Stability of disorder Irritability of disorder	Biomechanical assessment (i.e., restriction of joint mobility) and assessment of soft-tissue changes	Diagnosis according to syndrome, as opposed to specific structure Postural syndrome (end range strain on normal tissues) Dysfunction syndrome (adaptive shortening of structure) Derangement syndrome (disturbance of normal anatomic relationship)
Intervention strategies		Mobilization	Patient self-treatment using repeated active movements

(Continued)

TABLE 10-2 Manual Therapy Approach—Physical Therapist Generated *(Continued)*

	Maitland (Australian) Assertions	Kaltenborn (Norwegian) Assertions	McKenzie Assertions
	Based on continual assessment of subjective and objective findings Focus on treating pain or stiffness Mobilization Manipulation Adverse neural tissue mobilization Traction Exercise using movements that have positive influence on symptoms Patient education	Exercise (emphasis on proprioceptive neuromuscular facilitation) Traction/distraction Soft-tissue mobilization Manipulation Patient education	Exercise using movements that have positive influence on symptoms Mobilization or manipulation (if needed) Strong emphasis on patient education and self-treatment

Data from Di Fabio RP: Efficacy of manual therapy. *Phys Ther* 72:853–864, 1992.

CORRECT APPLICATION OF MANUAL TECHNIQUES

Despite the varied approaches and rationales, there is general agreement concerning criteria that are important for the correct application of a manual technique. These include[22]:

- ***Knowledge of the relative shapes of the joint surfaces (concave or convex).***[11–13,23] If the joint surface is convex relative to the other surface, the joint glide occurs in the direction opposite to the osteokinematic movement (angular motion). If, on the other hand, the joint surface is concave, the joint glide occurs in the same direction as osteokinematic movement.
- ***Duration, type, and irritability of symptoms***[11,12] (Table 10-3). This information can provide the clinician with some general guidelines in determining the intensity of the application of a selected technique (see "Indications for MT" later in this chapter).
- ***Patient and clinician position.*** Correct positioning of the patient is essential both to help the patient relax and to ensure safe body mechanics from the clinician. When patients feel relaxed, their muscle activity is decreased, reducing the amount of resistance encountered during the technique.
- ***Position of joint to be treated.*** The position of the joint to be treated must be appropriate for the stage of healing and the skill of the clinician. It is recommended that the resting position of the joint be used when the patient has an acute condition or the clinician is inexperienced. The resting position in this case refers to the position that the injured joint adopts, rather than the classic resting (open-packed) position for a normal joint. Other positions for starting the mobilization may be used by a skilled clinician in patients with nonacute conditions.
- ***Hand placement.*** Wherever possible, contact with the patient should be maximized. The hand should conform to the area being treated, so that the forces are spread over a larger area. A gentle and confident touch inspires confidence in the patient. Accurate hand placement is essential for efficient stabilization and for the accurate transmission of force.
- ***Specificity.*** Specificity refers to the exactness of the procedure, and is based on its intent. Whenever possible, the forces imparted by a technique should occur at the point where they are needed. Check one joint at a time, one movement at a time.

TABLE 10-3 Indications for Selection of Manual Technique Based on Duration of Symptoms

	Acute	Subacute	Chronic
Muscle energy	Strongly indicated	Strongly indicated	Use to prepare tissue for joint manipulation and prevent recurrence of dysfunction
Joint mobilization	Grades I and II	Grades II and III	Grades III and IV
Joint manipulation	Rarely indicated	Moderate-to-strong indication if muscle energy technique unsuccessful	Strong indication if muscle energy technique ineffective

Data from Ellis JJ, Johnson GS: Myofascial considerations in somatic dysfunction of the thorax. In: Flynn TW, ed. *The Thoracic Spine and Rib Cage: Musculoskeletal Evaluation and Treatment.* Boston, MA: Butterworth-Heinemann, 1996:211–262.

- ***Direction and type of force.*** When possible work with the force of gravity rather than against it. The direction of the force can be either *direct,* which is toward the motion barrier or restriction,[24] or *indirect*, which is away from the motion barrier or restriction.[25,26] Although the rationale for a direct technique is easy to understand, the rationale for using an indirect technique is more confusing. A good analogy is the stuck drawer that cannot be opened. Often the movement that eventually frees the drawer is an inward motion, followed by a pull.[22]
- ***Amount of force.*** The amount of force used depends on the intent of the manual procedure and a number of other factors, including but not limited to
  - age, sex, and general health status of the patient;
  - barrier to motion and end-feel (stage of healing) (Table 10-4);
  - type and severity of the movement disorder.
- ***Reinforcement of any gains made.*** It has been demonstrated that movement gained by a specific manual technique performed in isolation will be lost within 48 hours, if the motions gained are not reinforced.[27] Thus, the motions gained by a manual technique must be reinforced by both the mechanical and the neurophysiologic benefits of active movement.[28] These active movements must be as local and precise as possible to the involved segment or myofascial structure.

Reassessment is an integral part of any intervention. The clinician must be able to gauge how effective a technique has been so that necessary modifications can be made. Measurement procedures used by the clinician to determine the effectiveness of a manual intervention must adequately reflect changes in pain level, impairments, and functional ability. Although measurements of range of motion (ROM), pain, and strength are valid and reliable,[29–31] the functional measurement selected should be related to the particular functional limitation that the clinician is expecting to change with the intervention.[32] Complicating the measurement of outcome and the effectiveness of a technique is the placebo effect (a response resulting from the suggestion that something is beneficial, even though it may be inert). Although MT is not alone in its use of the placebo effect, it is increasingly important that clinicians determine the specific effects of everything they do.[33]

TABLE 10-4 Appropriate Technique Based on Barrier to Motion and End-Feel

Barrier	End-Feel	Technique
Pain	Empty	None
Pain	Spasm	None
Pain	Capsular	Oscillations
Joint adhesions	Early capsular	Passive articular motion stretch
Muscle adhesions	Early elastic	Passive physiologic motion stretch
Hypertonicity	Facilitation	Hold–relax
Bone	Bony	None

INDICATIONS FOR MT

MT is indicated in the following cases:

- Mild musculoskeletal pain
- A nonirritable musculoskeletal condition, demonstrated by pain that is provoked by motion but that disappears very quickly
- Intermittent musculoskeletal pain
- Pain reported by the patient that is relieved by rest
- Pain reported by the patient that is relieved or provoked by particular motions or positions
- Pain that is altered by changes related to sitting or standing posture

CONTRAINDICATIONS TO MT

Contraindications to MT include those that are absolute contraindications and those that are relative.[34,35]

Absolute

- Systemic or localized infection (e.g., osteomyelitis), febrile state
- Acute circulatory condition
- Malignancy
- An open wound at the treatment site, or sutures over the treatment site
- Recent fracture
- Hematoma
- Hypersensitivity of the skin
- Inappropriate end-feel (spasm, empty, and bony), or evidence of joint ankylosis, or joint hypermobility
- Advanced diabetes
- Rheumatoid arthritis (in a state of an exacerbation)
- Cellulitis
- Constant, severe pain, including pain at rest or that disturbs sleep, indicating that the condition is likely to be very irritable or in the acute stage of healing
- Extensive radiation of pain
- Any condition that has not been fully evaluated

Relative

- Joint effusion or inflammation
- Rheumatoid arthritis (not in a state of an exacerbation)
- Presence of neurologic signs
- Osteoporosis

- Pregnancy, if a technique is to be applied to the spine
- Dizziness
- Steroid or anticoagulant therapy

SOFT-TISSUE TECHNIQUES

Transverse Friction Massage

Transverse friction massage (TFM) is a technique devised by Cyriax, whereby repeated cross-grain massage is applied to muscle, tendons, tendon sheaths, and ligaments. TFM has long been used by physical therapists to increase the mobility and extensibility of individual musculoskeletal tissues, and to help prevent and treat inflammatory scar tissue.[7,36–41]

> **CLINICAL PEARL**
>
> TFM is indicated for acute or subacute ligament, tendon, or muscle injuries; chronically inflamed bursae; and adhesions in ligament or muscle, or between tissues. TFM also can be applied before performing a manipulation or a strong stretch to desensitize and soften the tissues.

TFM is contraindicated for acute inflammation, hematomas, debilitated or open skin, and peripheral nerves, and in patients who have diminished sensation in the area.

TFM is purported to have the following therapeutic effects:

- ***Traumatic hyperemia.***[7] According to Cyriax, longitudinal friction to an area increases the flow of blood and lymph, which, in turn, removes the chemical irritant by-products of inflammation. In addition, the increased blood flow reduces venous congestion, thereby decreasing edema and hydrostatic pressure on pain-sensitive structures.
- ***Pain relief.*** The application of TFM stimulates type I and II mechanoreceptors, producing presynaptic anesthesia. This presynaptic anesthesia is based on the gate theory of pain control (see Chaps. 3 and 8). However, if the frictions are too vigorous in the acute stage, the stimulation of nociceptors will override the effect of the mechanoreceptors, causing the pain to increase. Occasionally, the patient may feel an exacerbation of symptoms following the first two or three sessions of the massage, especially in the case of a chronically inflamed bursa.[42] In these cases, it is important to forewarn the patient.
- ***Decreasing scar tissue.*** The transverse nature of the friction assists with the orientation of the collagen in the appropriate lines of stress and also helps produce hypertrophy of the new collagen. Given the stages of healing for soft tissue (see Chap. 2), light TFM should only be applied in the early stages of a subacute lesion, so as not to damage the granulation tissue. These gentle movements theoretically serve to minimize cross-linking and so enhance the extensibility of the new tissue. Following a ligament sprain, Cyriax recommends immediate use of gentle TFM to prevent adhesion formation between the tissue and its neighbors, by moving the ligamentous tissue over the underlying bone.[7]

The application of the correct amount of tension to a healing structure is very important. The tissue undergoing TFM should, whenever possible, be positioned in a moderate but not painful stretch. The exception to this rule is when applying TFM to a muscle belly, which is usually positioned in its relaxed position.[7,43] Lubricant is not typically used with the application of TFM. However, ultrasound can be applied to a tissue before TFM.

Beginning with light pressure, and using a reinforced finger (i.e., middle finger over the index finger), or thumb, the clinician moves the skin over the site of the identified lesion back and forth, in a direction perpendicular to the normal orientation of its fibers. It is important that the patient's skin move with the clinician's finger to prevent blistering.

> **CLINICAL PEARL**
>
> The application of TFM is condition and patient dependent. The intensity of the application is based on the stage of healing. The pain induced by TFM should be kept within the patient's tolerance. Light pressure should be used in the early stages, before building up the pressure over a few minutes to allow for accommodation.

The amplitude of the massage should be sufficient to cover all of the affected tissue, and the rate should be at two to three cycles per second, applied in a rhythmical manner.

The duration of the friction massage is usually gauged by when desensitization occurs (normally within 3–5 minutes). Tissues that do not desensitize within 3–5 minutes should be treated using some other form of intervention. If the condition is chronic or in the remodeling stage of healing, then the frictions are continued for a further 5 minutes after the desensitization, in an effort to enhance the mechanical effect on the cross-links and adhesions. Following the application of TFM, the involved tissue is either passively stretched or actively exercised, taking care not to cause pain.

Most conditions amenable to TFM should resolve in 6–10 sessions over 2–8 weeks. When possible, patients should be taught how to apply TFM on themselves so that treatments can be continued at home. Tissues that do not show signs of improvement after three treatment sessions should be treated using some other form of intervention.

Myofascial Release

MFR is a series of techniques designed to release restrictions in the myofascial tissue and is used for the treatment of soft-tissue dysfunction. The development of a holistic and comprehensive approach for the evaluation and treatment of the myofascial system of the body is credited to John Barnes, who was strongly influenced by the teachings of Mennell[44] and Upledger.[45]

> **CLINICAL PEARL**
>
> Fascia is a tough connective tissue, composed of collagen, elastin, and a viscous gel, that exists in the body in the form of a continuous three-dimensional web of connective tissue, organized along the lines of tension imposed on the body (see Chap. 1).[46]

According to myofascial theory, the collagen provides strength to the fascia, the elastin gives it its elastic properties, and the gel functions to absorb the compressive forces of movement.[35] Three types of fascia are considered to exist[35,46]:

1. Superficial, lying directly below the dermis.
2. Deep, surrounding and infusing with muscle, bone, nerve, blood vessels, and organs to the cellular level.
3. Deepest, comprising the dura of the craniosacral system, which encases the central nervous system and brain (see Chap. 3).

The theory of MFR is based on the principle that trauma or structural abnormalities may create inappropriate fascial strain, because of an inability of the fascia to absorb or distribute the forces.[46] These strains to the fascia can result in a slow tightening of the fascia, causing the body to lose its physiologic adaptive capacity.[46] Over time, the fascial restrictions begin to pull the body out of its three-dimensional alignment, causing biomechanically inefficient movement and posture.[46] In addition, because of the association of fascia at the cellular level, it is theorized that trauma to or malfunction of the fascia can lead to poor cellular efficiency, disease, and pain throughout the body.[35,46] Three theoretical models for the manifestation of myofascial dysfunction are contraction, contracture, and cohesion–congestion (Table 10-5).

Thus, the purpose of MFR techniques is to apply a gentle sustained pressure to the fascia, in order to release fascial restrictions, thereby restoring normal pain-free function.[35] MFR relies entirely on the feedback received from the patient's tissues, with the clinician interpreting and responding to the feedback. This feedback is based on the Upledger concept of the natural body rhythm, called the craniosacral rhythm.[45] It is this rhythm that is theorized to guide the clinician as to the direction, force, and the duration of the technique.

It is not unusual for a patient to experience muscle soreness following MFR techniques. This soreness is thought to result from postural and alignment changes or from the techniques themselves.

Myofascial Stroking

The soft-tissue techniques used in MFR are purported to break up cross-restrictions of the collagen of the fascia. Three of the more commonly used techniques involve stroking maneuvers[35]:

- ***J stroke.*** This technique is used to increase skin mobility. Counterpressure is applied with the heel of the hand, while a stroke in the shape of the letter J is applied in the direction of the restriction, with two or three fingers, which creates some torque at the end of the stroke.
- ***Vertical stroke.*** The purpose of vertical stroking is to open up the length of vertically oriented superficial fascia. As in the J stroke, counterpressure is applied with one hand, while the stroking is performed with the other.
- ***Transverse stroke.*** As its name suggests, the transverse stroke is applied in a transverse direction to the body. Force is applied downward into the muscle with the fingertips of both hands, and the force is applied slowly and perpendicular to the muscle fibers.
- ***Cross-hands technique.*** The cross-hands technique is used for the release of deep fascial tissues. The clinician places crossed hands over the site of restriction. The elastic component of the fascia is then stretched until the barrier is met. At this point, the clinician maintains consistent gentle pressure at the barrier for approximately 90–120 seconds. Once the release is felt, the clinician reduces the pressure.

It is important to remember that the claimed benefits and effectiveness of MFR techniques are largely anecdotal, because at the time of writing there is no scientific experimental research to validate these claims.[47]

Soft-Tissue Mobilization

Soft-tissue mobilizations (STMs) are used in many of the manual techniques described within this chapter, including MFR, muscle energy (ME), and PNF. The techniques of STM described in this section are based on the concept that tissue restrictions occur at different layers, ranging from superficial to deep.

The general principles behind STM are that the superficial layers are treated before deep layers, with the force used applied in the direction of the maximum restriction, and where the choice of technique is dependent on the extent of the restriction, amount of discomfort, and degree of irritability. Deep tissue massage is recommended to reduce spasm[48] and promote pain reduction.[49] Several well-recognized STM techniques are described next.[50]

Sustained Pressure

This technique is applied to the center of the restricted tissue at the exact depth, direction, and angle of the maximal restriction. The sustained pressure technique can be modified by applying a force in either a clockwise or a counterclockwise

TABLE 10-5 Theoretical Models for the Manifestation of Myofascial Disorders

Model	Manifestation	End-Feel
Contraction	Muscle hypertonicity or spasm	Reactive, firm, and painful end-Feel
Contracture	Inert or noncontractile tissues that have undergone fibrotic alteration	Abrupt, firm, stiff, or hard end-Feel
Cohesion–congestion	Fluidochemical changes in microcellular transport systems, resulting in impairment	Boggy, stiff, or reactive end-Feel lymphatic flow, vascular stasis, or ischemia

Data from Ellis JJ, Johnson GS: Myofascial considerations in somatic dysfunction of the thorax. In: Flynn TW, ed. *The Thoracic Spine and Rib Cage: Musculoskeletal Evaluation and Treatment*. Boston, MA: Butterworth-Heinemann, 1996:211–262.

direction, while maintaining the sustained pressure. This spiral motion increases the tissue tension in one direction, while easing it in the other. Sustained pressure can also be applied perpendicular or parallel to the restriction.

Ischemic Compression

Ischemic compression, a similar technique to sustained pressure, can be used on both active and inactive trigger points. It is believed that the ischemic compression deprives the trigger points of oxygen, rendering them inactive and breaking the cycle of pain–spasm–pain. Usually, the pressure is applied for 8–12 seconds. If the patient reports a lessening of local and referred pain, the clinician can repeat the treatment. However, if the pain does not lessen, the clinician may need to adjust the pressure or choose an alternative technique.

General Massage

Massage can be defined as the systematic, therapeutic, and functional stroking and kneading of the body.[51] The French are credited with the introduction of massage into Europe, and many of the terms associated with massage still bear French names.[52] Massage has long been a central part of the physical therapy curriculum. Studies have demonstrated that deep massage increases the circulation and skin temperature of the massaged area, as a result of dilation of the capillaries.[53–56] A number of traditional massage techniques are used, including:

- ***Effleurage.*** This is a general stroking technique applied to the muscles and soft tissues in a centripetal direction (from distal to proximal), to enhance relaxation and increase venous and lymphatic drainage. The clinician applies a firm contact with the patient using the palms of the hand and, at the end of the stroke, lifts the hands from the patient's skin and replaces them at the starting position.[57] Oil or cream can be used to aid the stroking.
- ***Stroking.*** Stroking techniques are applied superficially along the whole length of a surface. These techniques are typically applied before the deeper techniques of massage to enhance relaxation.[56]
- ***Petrissage.*** This term is used to describe a group of techniques that involve the compression of soft-tissue structures and include kneading, wringing, rolling, and picking-up techniques, to release areas of muscle fibrosis and to "milk" the muscles of waste products that collect from trauma or abnormal inactivity.[58]
- ***Strumming.*** The technique of perpendicular strumming involves the application of repeated, rhythmic deformations of a muscle belly in a strumming fashion.

Acupressure

Acupressure is based on the ancient arts of shiatsu and acupuncture, involving manual pressure over the acupuncture points of the body, to improve the flow of the body's energy, known as *Qi*. This energy is thought to circulate throughout the body along a series of channels, called *meridians*. Traditional Eastern medicine is based on the concept that all disorders are reflected at specific points, either on the skin surface or just beneath it, along these channels. By careful manipulation of these points, the clinician can theoretically strengthen, disperse, or calm the Qi, enabling it to flow smoothly.[59] Modern acupressurists use traditional meridian acupuncture points; nonmeridian or extrameridian acupuncture points, which are fixed points not necessarily associated with meridians; and trigger points, which have no fixed locations and are found by eliciting tenderness at the site of most pain.[60] When acupressure is applied successfully, the patient is supposed to experience a sensation known as *teh chi*, defined as a subjective feeling of fullness, numbness, tingling, and warmth with some local soreness and a feeling of distention around the acupuncture point.[60] Western scientific research has proposed a number of mechanisms for the effect of acupressure in relieving pain, as follows:

- The gate control theory of pain.[61,62]
- Diffuse noxious inhibitory control. This theory implies that noxious stimulation of heterotopic body areas modulates the pain sensation originating in areas where a subject feels pain.[60]
- Stimulation of the production of endorphins, serotonin, and acetylcholine in the central nervous system, which enhances analgesia.[63–71]

Muscle Energy

The origin of ME techniques is credited to Fred Mitchell, Sr.[72] ME techniques combine the precision of passive mobilization, with the effectiveness, safety, and specificity of reeducation therapies and therapeutic exercise.[73]

CLINICAL PEARL

ME techniques require the active participation of the patient and are thus viewed as mobilization techniques, which utilize muscular facilitation and inhibition.[74]

ME techniques, which involve positioning a restricted muscle–joint complex at its restricted barrier, can be used to mobilize joints, strengthen weakened muscles, and stretch adaptively shortened muscles and fascia.[75] Optimal success with these techniques is more likely in the acute or subacute stages of healing, before prolonged joint changes have had the opportunity to occur.

According to the teachings of ME, muscles function as flexors, extensors, rotators, and side benders of joints, as well as being restrictors or barriers to movement. In other words, muscles both produce and control motion. Although it is obvious that muscles produce motion, it is easy to forget that they also resist motion. This resistance to motion is related to muscle tone, a complex neurophysiologic state governed by both cortical and spinal reflexes and by the afferent activity from the articular and muscle systems. Afferent input from types I and II mechanoreceptors located in the superficial and deep aspects of the joint capsule is projected to the motor neurons (see Chap. 3).[76,77] Exaggerated spindle responses are provoked by any motions that attempt to lengthen the muscle, creating an increase in resistance to those motions. Stretching or lengthening of the muscle also stimulates the Golgi tendon organs, which have an inhibitory influence on muscle tension, leading to muscle relaxation. In addition, it has been demonstrated that cutaneous stimulation of certain areas of the body can produce inhibition or excitation of specific motor neuron pools.[78]

It is theorized that the neuromuscular system is "scarred" by pain and impairment, producing asymmetry in the musculoskeletal system and resulting in a disruption of the harmony and rhythm of the body, referred to as somatic dysfunction.[73] Somatic dysfunctions can be described or named in one of three ways[24]:

1. The direction of increased freedom of motion
2. The position of the lesion
3. The direction of limitation of motion

In the presence of a somatic dysfunction, there is usually an asymmetric pattern of motion, with restriction in one direction and increased freedom in the opposite direction.[24] The triad of ART (*a*symmetry, *r*ange of motion restriction or barrier, and *t*issue texture)[26] helps to describe the characteristics of somatic dysfunction. Primary somatic dysfunctions, which may result from trauma, are reversible, as long as they are treated correctly and do not become chronic in terms of abnormal fibrosis or adhesions. Secondary somatic dysfunctions result from the consequences of visceral pathology, or from the adaptations made by somatic structures in response to forces or stresses imposed on them.

The consequence of a somatic dysfunction can be a change in the length of the tissues that surround a joint. Some of these tissues adaptively shorten, whereas others adaptively lengthen. These changes in length are theorized to produce changes in the neurophysiologic makeup of the muscle, affecting tension development, as well as changes in the angle of pull.

There is some commonality between ME and several procedures used in orthopaedic MT, such as PNF.[79] Greenman[26] summarizes the requirements for the correct application of ME techniques to be control, balance, and localization.

- The technique, which involves a controlled effort in a controlled direction, commences from a controlled position. Eccentric, concentric, and isometric contractions, at varying levels of effort, are used in ME, within a range of movement controlled by the clinician.
- The clinician balances the degree of force used, depending on the intention.
- The force used is localized as much as possible to the joint in question. The localization of force is more important than the intensity of the force.

The intent of ME is to treat somatic dysfunctions by restoring the muscles around a joint to their normal neurophysiologic state, through either stretching or strengthening the agonist and antagonist. Somatic dysfunctions include those in which the motion barrier is encountered before the physiologic barrier is reached.[73] The type of motion barrier is determined by the end-feel.

A normal end-feel would indicate normal range, whereas an abnormal end-feel would suggest abnormal range, either hypomobile or hypermobile, with the latter characterized by a loss of end-feel resiliency and an abrupt approach to the anatomic barrier. All ME techniques are classed as direct techniques because they engage the barrier.[25] Indirect techniques form the basis for the strain–counterstrain (positional release) techniques,[80] and the functional techniques,[81–83] both of which are discussed later.

The position of the clinician during the performance of the technique must allow easy access to the structures involved, while maintaining proper body mechanics. In each of the following recognized methods of ME, the setup is identical. The clinician positions the bone or joint so that the muscle group to be used is at its resting length. The patient is then given specific instructions about the direction in which to move, the intensity of the contraction, and the duration of the contraction.[75,79,84,85] The amounts of force and counterforce are governed by the length and strength of the muscle group involved, as well as by the patient's symptoms.[75] The clinician's force can match the effort of the patient, thus producing an isometric contraction and allowing no movement to occur, or it may overcome the patient's effort, thus moving the area or joint in the direction opposite to that in which the patient is attempting to move it, thereby incorporating an eccentric or isolytic contraction.[79] There appears to be no consensus as to whether to use the relaxation of the agonist or the antagonist to gain motion.[26,74,86–88]

Strain–Counterstrain (Positional Release)

Strain–counterstrain is a passive positional technique used in the treatment of musculoskeletal pain and related somatic dysfunction. According to strain–counterstrain theory, myofascial tender points (Fig. 10-1) are located and then monitored while a position of comfort, or ease, is established to evoke a therapeutic effect.[80,89,90] It is worth noting that to date no experimental studies have been published to confirm the existence of these tender points or the effectiveness of strain–counterstrain.

A possible neurophysiologic explanation of how and why these techniques work was first suggested by Korr,[91] who postulated that an injured joint and its related tissues behaved differently from those of an uninjured joint in that the γ motor neuron activity in the former became increased. Bailey[92] later refined the theory by suggesting that an inappropriate high "gainset" of the muscle spindle (see Chap. 3) resulted in changes characteristic of somatic dysfunction.[93] Thus, the techniques of strain–counterstrain appear to serve to effect the muscle spindle–γ loop, by allowing the extrafusal muscle fibers to lengthen to their normal relaxed state, thereby decreasing spindle output and interrupting the pain–spasm cycle.[93–95] Strain–counterstrain is also thought to improve blood flow to the area through a circulatory flushing of previously ischemic tissues.[94,96]

CLINICAL PEARL

The skill and success of strain–counterstrain techniques relies on the ability of the clinician to find the tender point and then to position, or move, the patient in such a way as to release muscular tension as well as relieve pain.[94]

When treating the spine, the first step in the examination procedure is modification of the sagittal posture of the patient to produce a flattening of the lordosis–kyphosis in the region to be examined.[93] In the extremities, the body part is placed in

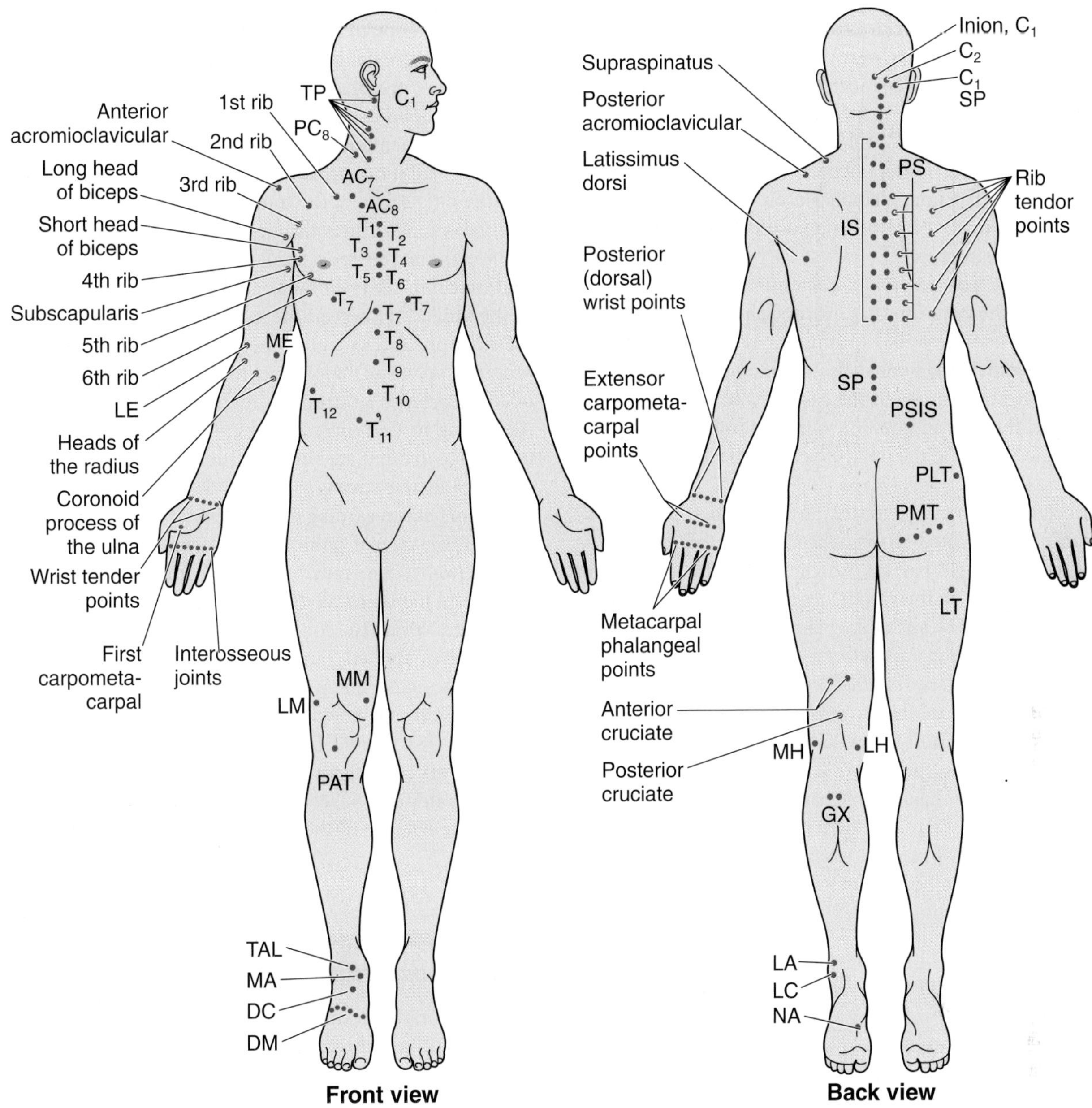

FIGURE 10-1 Strain–counterstrain tender points of the body. AC, anterior cervical; PC, posterior cervical; LH, lateral hamstring; MH, medial hamstring; GX, gastrocnemius; LA, lateral ankle; LC, lateral calcaneal; NA, navicular; LT, lateral trochanter; SP, spinous process; TP, transverse process; PS, paraspinal; LE, lateral epicondyle; ME, medial epicondyle; LM, lateral meniscus; MM, medial meniscus; PAT, patella; TAL, talus; MA, medial ankle; DC, posterior (dorsal) cuboid; DM, posterior (dorsal) metatarsal; IS, interspinal; PSIS, posterior superior iliac spine; PLT, posterolateral trochanteric; PMT, posteromedial trochanteric.

a position of relaxation. This *position of ease* (mobile point), which involves a shortening or folding of the tissues around the myofascial tender point, usually corresponds to the point of maximum relaxation. Any movement from this position produces an increase in tissue tension under the monitoring hand at the selected tender point site.[80,89,90] Tissue texture abnormalities and areas of tenderness are then sought. The position of greatest resistance and pain is usually the position that is directly related to that of the original mechanism of injury; thus, the position of ease is usually opposite to that direction. For example, if an ankle sustained an inversion injury, the position of comfort is likely to be in eversion. In most cases, the tender point will be in, or near, the area of discomfort. Once the correct position is achieved, it is then maintained for 90–120 seconds before the patient returns slowly to the normal position.[80] For example, if the biceps are being treated, the tender point is monitored, while the elbow is flexed and the forearm is simultaneously pronated. If the muscle is being moved in the correct direction, the tenderness should lessen. Slight adjustments from the recommended positions in this text may be needed. If there is more than one tender point, the clinician treats each one at a time, until the dominant one is found.

Once the tender point has been successfully removed, the clinician should focus on lengthening and/or strengthening the involved muscle.

Functional Techniques

Functional techniques are indirect techniques that use positional placement away from the restrictive barrier, similar to the techniques previously described for strain–counterstrain. The functional techniques were developed in the osteopathic profession in the 1950s, and much credit is given to Dr Andrew Taylor Still[97] for identifying the dysfunctions that are treated with these techniques.[81,98] Still considered the somatic lesion to be a mechanical involvement of the structure, and his teachings placed primary emphasis on pertinent anatomy, with palpation used to identify the position and arrangement of a particular structure.[82]

Although the term *functional technique* is itself somewhat of a misnomer, the criterion that distinguishes functional techniques from most manual techniques is the emphasis on moving the joint being treated away from, rather than toward, the restrictive barrier. As in the case of strain–counterstrain techniques, the joint in question is moved toward the normal physiologic barrier, at the opposite end of the ROM to that of the restriction.

According to functional technique theory, there is a dynamic balance point located between the restrictive barrier and the opposite physiologic barrier, which is the joint position in which the tensions in the soft tissues around the joint become balanced equally in all three planes.[99] If this balance is achieved, the clinician can detect a sense of "ease" under his or her palpating fingers. It is the deep segmental tissues, which support and position the bones of a segment, and their reaction to normal motion demands, that are at the heart of functional technique specificity.[100] If motion in any plane is initiated away from the dynamic balance point, the soft tissue tension around the treated segment increases, and there will be an increased sense of palpatory tension, or "bind."[101]

Two theories have been proposed to explain the beneficial effects of these techniques[101]:

1. The afferent input from the proprioceptors is inhibited, which, in turn, suppresses the local protective cord reflexes.
2. The techniques stimulate the mechanoreceptors sufficiently to inhibit the pain receptors, allowing the tissues to relax.

Once the patient has been positioned correctly, the clinician can use one of two intervention options:

1. ***Active.*** In this method, the clinician initiates movement along the path of least resistance through the sequential release of any soft-tissue tension that occurs, until the restrictive barrier is no longer detectable and normal motion is regained.
2. ***Passive.*** In this method, the clinician follows the articular unwinding through sequential releases of the treated joint to the point of full soft-tissue release, until the restrictive barrier is no longer detectable and normal motion is regained.

Craniosacral Therapy

Craniosacral therapy (CST) is an alternative, complementary therapy practiced throughout the United States and around the world by osteopathic and chiropractic physicians; physical, occupational, and massage therapists; and dentists.[102] CST is based around the assumption that cranial bone movement occurs through a respiratory mechanism comprising the brain, cerebrospinal fluid (CSF), intracranial and intraspinal membranes, cranial bones, spinal cord, and sacrum.[103] CST practitioners are of the opinion that restrictions, misalignments, immobility of the cranial sutures and tension of the intracranial meninges directly impact the health of an individual. In addition, practitioners of CST claim that they can identify alterations in the movement patterns of the sacrum and the cranial sutures through manual palpation. Palpation of the cranium theoretically allows the clinician to perceive the rhythmic impulse resulting from the widening and narrowing of the skull.[102] However, the reliability reports of identifying the rhythmic movement of the sutures using palpation have ranged from worse than chance to fair.[102,104] CST is also based on the existence of articular mobility at the cranial bones. According to CST practitioners, 5–10 g of force is recommended to manipulate human sutures. Despite the number of studies and the strong claims made by researchers from a variety of fields regarding the mobility of the cranial bones the research on cranial bone motion done to date is far from conclusive.[102] In a study by Downey et al.,[102] a rabbit model underwent incrementally increasing forces through the skull. Movement within the coronal suture did not occur until 500 g of force was applied. Furthermore, forces up to 22 kg were required to cause 1 mm of movement.[102]

It has been suggested that based on the lack of credible evidence, CST should be abandoned as a viable rehabilitative theory (i.e., that cranial sutures move), until such time that the advocates of CST contribute well-designed studies evaluating the efficacy of these techniques to the peer-reviewed literature.[104]

JOINT MOBILIZATIONS

Joint mobilization techniques include a broad spectrum, from the general passive motions performed in the physiologic cardinal planes at any point in the joint range to the semi-specific and specific accessory (arthrokinematic) joint glides, or joint distractions, initiated from the open-packed position of the joint.

These techniques form the cornerstone of most rehabilitative programs and involve low–high velocity passive movements within or at the limit of joint ROM, to restore any loss of accessory joint motion as the consequence of joint injury.[2] Although, theoretically, the joint capsule and articular surfaces are the structures affected by joint mobilizations, other periarticular tissues, such as tendons, muscles, and fascia are also likely affected. However, there are still no studies that identify histological joint changes resulting from joint mobilizations. There is also no conclusive research providing information regarding the optimal type of mobilization, the amount of time a joint should be mobilized, or the optimal amount of force required to treat any of the so-called joint impairments.

The indications for joint mobilizations include those already mentioned for MT techniques, but the evidence-based indications include the following:

- Increasing joint ROM. A number of studies addressing the effect of joint mobilizations on ROM provide evidence of an association.[105,106]

- Decrease pain. A number of studies have shown that hypoalgesia occurs as a result of joint mobilizations,[107–109] although the effect seems to occur regardless of the technique being used, the joint being treated, or the impairment being addressed.
- Promote muscle relaxation. Although there is some evidence that joint mobilizations can reduce muscle activity in muscles, the specific mechanism is unknown.[107]
- Improve muscle performance. Evidence suggests that joint mobilization can improve muscle performance, regardless of the presence or nature of the muscle impairment.[110]

CLINICAL PEARL

Mobilization techniques that utilize accessory movements and distractions are used primarily on inert tissues, and physiologic movements are used to mobilize both contractile and noncontractile tissues.[111]

Joint mobilizations are applied in a direction that is either parallel or perpendicular to the treatment plane, to restore the physiologic articular relationship within a joint and to decrease pain.[99] Additional benefits attributed to joint mobilizations include decreasing muscle guarding, lengthening the tissue around a joint, neuromuscular influences on muscle tone, and increased proprioceptive awareness.[112,113]

Three types of mobilizations are recognized, based on the level of participation by the clinician and patient:

1. Active, in which the patient exerts the force
2. Passive, in which the clinician exerts the force
3. Combined, in which the clinician and patient work together

To apply joint mobilizations, the components can be utilized in a variety of ways, depending on the method employed:

- ***Direct method.*** An engagement is made against a barrier in several planes.
- ***Indirect method.*** Maigne[114] postulated "the concept of painless and opposite motion," in which disengagement from the barrier occurs, and a balance of ligamentous tension is sought.
- ***Combined method.*** Disengagement is followed by direct retracing of the motion.

Several other schools of thought have been put forward to address the concepts of increasing joint ROM. Kaltenborn[13] introduced the Nordic program of MT, which utilizes Cyriax's[7] method to evaluate, and the specific osteopathic techniques of Mennell[8] for intervention. Further influence from Stoddard,[9] an osteopath, cemented the foundations of the Nordic system of MT. Evjenth,[115] who joined Kaltenborn's group, brought a greater emphasis on muscle stretching, strengthening, and coordination training.

Kaltenborn Techniques

Kaltenborn refers to the amount of joint play at a joint as *slack*. Each joint interface has a plane of motion, an imaginary line lying across the joint surfaces. According to Kaltenborn, all joint mobilizations, when performed correctly, should be made parallel or at right angles to this plane of motion, and are based on the concave–convex rule (Table 10-6).[13] For example, if extension of the tibiofemoral joint is restricted, either the femur (convex) can be stabilized and the tibia (concave) glided anteriorly or the tibia can be stabilized and the femur glided posteriorly. The concave–convex rule cannot be applied to every situation. Exceptions include movements at plane joints, movements for which the axis of rotation passes through the articulating surfaces, and movements at joints in which the concave side of the joint forms a deep socket.[116]

Kaltenborn's techniques use a combination of traction and mobilization to reduce pain and mobilize hypomobile joints. Three grades of traction are defined:

- ***Grade I—piccolo (loosen).*** This grade involves a traction force that neutralizes pressure in the joint, without producing any actual separation of the joint surfaces. Grade I traction is used to reduce the compressive forces on the articular surfaces, both in the initial intervention session and with all of the mobilization grades.
- ***Grade II—slack (take up the slack).*** This grade of traction separates the articulating surfaces and eliminates the play in the joint capsule.
- ***Grade III—stretch.*** This grade of traction actually stretches the joint capsule and the soft tissues surrounding the joint to increase mobility. Grade III traction is used in conjunction with mobilization glides according to the convex–concave rules to treat joint hypomobility in the remodeling stage of healing.[13]

Australian Techniques

The Australian approach was introduced primarily by Maitland,[12] whose grading system is used throughout this text. Under this system, the ROM is defined as the available range, not the full range, and is usually in one direction only (Fig. 10-2). Each joint has an anatomic limit, which is determined by the configuration of the joint surfaces and the surrounding soft tissues. The point of limitation is that point in the range that is short of the anatomic limit and is reduced by either pain or tissue resistance.

Maitland advocated five grades of joint mobilization or oscillations, each of which falls within the available ROM that exists at the joint—a point somewhere between the beginning point and the anatomic limit (see Fig. 10-2). Although the relationship that exists between the five grades in terms of their positions within the ROM is always constant, the point of limitation shifts further to the left, as the severity of the motion limitation increases:[11]

- Grade I: a small amplitude technique (about 25%) performed at the beginning of the available ROM
- Grade II: a large amplitude movement in the middle of the ROM (i.e., the middle 50%).
- Grade III: a large amplitude movement at the end of the ROM (i.e., the last 50%).
- Grade IV: a small amplitude movement at the end of ROM (the last 25%)

TABLE 10-6 Shape, Resting Position and Treatment Planes of the Joints

Joint	Convex Surface	Concave Surface	Resting Position	Treatment Plane and Relationship of the Osteokinematic motion (OM) and Arthrokinematic glide (AG)
Sternoclavicular	For elevation/depression, the sternum is concave, the clavicle is convex For protraction/retraction, the sternum is convex, the clavicle is concave		Arm resting by side	For elevation/depression the OM and AG are in opposite directions For protraction/retraction the OM and AG are in the same directions
Acromioclavicular	Clavicle	Acromion	Arm resting by side	OM and AG are in opposite directions
Glenohumeral	Humerus	Glenoid	55 degrees of abduction, 30 degrees of horizontal adduction	In scapular plane: OM and AG are in opposite directions
Humeroradial	Humerus	Radius	Elbow extended, forearm supinated	Perpendicular to long axis of radius: OM and AG are in the same directions
Humeroulnar	Humerus	Ulna	70 degrees of elbow flexion, 10 degrees of forearm supination	45° to long axis of ulna: OM and AG are in the same directions
Radioulnar (proximal)	Radius	Ulna	70 degrees of elbow flexion, 35 degrees of forearm supination	Parallel to long axis of ulna: OM and AG are in the opposite directions
Radioulnar (distal)	Ulnar	Radius	Supinated 10°	Parallel to long axis of radius: OM and AG are in the same directions
Radiocarpal	Proximal carpal bones	Radius	Line through radius and third metacarpal	Perpendicular to long axis of radius: OM and AG are in opposite directions
Intercarpal	Scaphoid	Trapezium and trapezoid	Midposition	Parallel to joint surfaces: OM and AG are in the same directions
Carpometacarpal joint of the thumb	For flexion/extension, the carpal is convex, the metacarpal is concave For abduction/adduction the carpal is concave, the metacarpal is convex		Midposition	For flexion/extension: OM and AG are in the same directions. For abduction/adduction: OM and AG are in opposite directions
Metacarpophalangeal (2–5)	Metacarpal	Proximal phalanx	Slight flexion	Parallel to joint: OM and AG are in the same directions

(Continued)

Interphalangeal	Proximal phalanx	Distal phalanx	Slight flexion	Parallel to joint: OM and AG are in the same directions
Hip	Femur	Acetabulum	Hip flexed 30 degrees, abducted 30 degrees, slight external rotation	OM and AG are in opposite directions
Tibiofemoral	Femur	Tibia	Flexed 25 degrees	On surface of tibial plateau: OM and AG are in the same directions
Patellofemoral	Patella	Femur	Knee in full extension	Along femoral groove: OM and AG are in opposite directions
Talocrural	Talus	Mortise	Plantarflexed 10 degree	In the mortise in anterior/posterior direction: OM and AG are in opposite directions
Subtalar	Calcaneus	Talus	Subtalar neutral between inversion/eversion	In talus, parallel to foot surface: OM and AG are in the same directions
Talonavicular	Talus	Navicular	Midposition	OM and AG are in the same directions
Calcaneocuboid	For flexion/extension the calcaneus is convex, the cuboid is concave. For abduction/adduction, the calcaneus is concave, the cuboid is convex			For flexion/extension: OM and AG are in the same directions. For abduction/adduction: OM and AG are in opposite directions
Metatarsophalangeal	Tarsal bone	Proximal phalanx	Slight extension	Parallel to joint: OM and AG are in the same directions
Interphalangeal	Proximal phalanx	Distal phalanx	Slight flexion	Parallel to joint: OM and AG are in the same directions

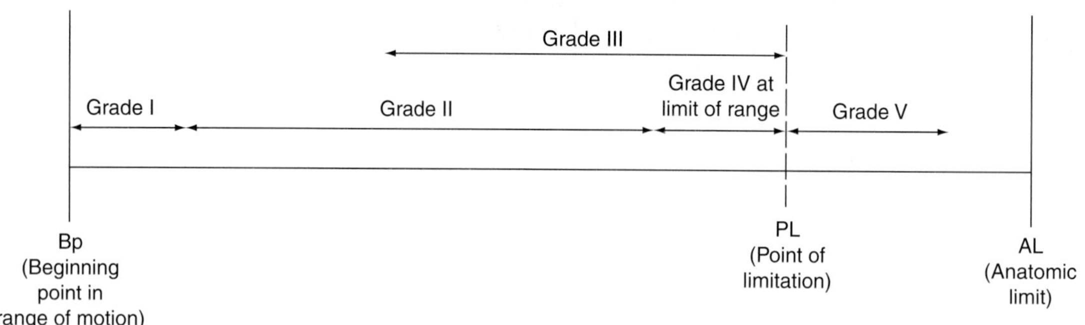

FIGURE 10-2 Maitland's five grades of motion.

- Grade V: a movement that exceeds the resistance barrier, commonly referred to as a high-velocity thrust technique or manipulation.

As with the Kaltenborn philosophy, the direction of the glide incorporated is determined by the concave–convex rule, and the joint to be mobilized is initially placed in its open-packed position. Many clinicians use a combination of Kaltenborn's grade III traction with Maitland's grade IV oscillations to decrease pain and increase joint mobility.

Maitland's grades I and II are used solely for pain relief and have no direct mechanical effect on the restricting barrier, although they do have a hydrodynamic effect. Mobilization-induced analgesia has been demonstrated in a number of studies in humans,[117–119] and is characterized by a rapid onset and a specific influence on mechanical nociception. Grade I and II joint mobilizations are theoretically effective in pain reduction, by improving joint lubrication and circulation in tissues related to the joint.[111,120] Rhythmic joint oscillations also possibly activate articular and skin mechanoreceptors that play a role in pain reduction.[77,121]

Maitland's grades III and IV have a mechanical, as well as a neurophysiologic, effect. Grade III and IV joint distractions and stretching mobilizations may, in addition to the above-stated effects, activate inhibitory joint and muscle spindle receptors, which aid in reducing restriction to movement.[77,111,120,121]

When joint motion is less than 50% but joint resistance to movement is the dominant dysfunction, a progression from the use of physiologic movements (grade IV; see Fig. 10-2) to stretch the joint limitation, and the use of accessory movements at the limit of the joint, is advocated.[12,111] Grades III and IV have been further subdivided into III+ (+ +) and IV+ (+ +), indicating that once the end of the range has been reached, a further stretch to impart a mechanical force to the movement restriction is given. [122] A grade V mobilization, defined as the skilled passive movement of a joint, is a short-duration, small-amplitude, high-velocity thrust that is applied at the physiologic limit of joint range (see Fig. 10-2).

CLINICAL PEARL

If the joint surface is convex relative to the other surface, the slide occurs in the opposite direction to the bone movement (angular motion). If, on the other hand, the joint surface is concave, the slide occurs in the same direction as the bone movement (angular motion).

In the spine, the convex rule applies at the occipitoatlantal joint, but below the second vertebra, as the zygapophyseal joint surfaces are relatively planar, the concave rule applies.

This rule is very important to remember for joint mobility testing and for joint mobilizations.

If during mobility testing, there is a limited glide:

- If the limitation occurs when the concave surface is moving, the restriction is likely due to a contracture of the trailing portion of the capsule.
- If the limitation occurs when the convex surface is moving, the restriction is likely due to an inability of the moving surface to move into the contracted portion of the capsule (may be due to adhesions between redundant folds of the capsule).

It is worth remembering that adhesions between collateral ligaments and the underlying tissue plane may limit movement in more than one direction.

If mobilizing in the appropriate direction according to the convex–concave rule appears to exacerbate the patient's symptoms, the clinician should apply the technique in the opposite direction until the patient can tolerate the appropriate direction.[123]

CLINICAL PEARL

Although sellar surfaces follow the same rules as ovoid surfaces, because of the nature of the curvature of their joint surfaces, the direction of the swing and the glide varies. For example, at the first carpometacarpal joint, the following biomechanics are involved:

Flexion/extension of metacarpal: the moving surface is concave.

1. The swing of the bone occurs in an anteromedial/posterolateral direction.
2. The base glides and rolls in an anteromedial/posterolateral direction.

Abduction/adduction of metacarpal: the moving surface is convex.

1. The swing of the bone occurs in an anterolateral/posteromedial direction.
2. The base glides in the opposite direction to the swing and rolls in the same direction as the swing.

Physiologic movement mobilizations and accessory and distraction mobilizations may be performed at any grade indicated. The mobilizations are performed both at the site of pain and to joints proximal to the site of pain to produce analgesia.[124]

The selection of the mobilization technique will depend on the barrier to movement felt by the clinician (the end-feel) and the acuteness of the condition (see Table 10-4). Muscle is usually the first barrier and is treated with light hold–relax techniques. Often some pain follows this initial mobilization, which is treated with grade III or IV oscillations.[122] As the pain is reduced, the real barrier to movement is approached. If this barrier is periarticular tissue, then grade IV+ rhythmical oscillations are used to stretch the tissue; if the joint is subluxed, erratic, jerky grade III+ are applied.[122]

Whichever technique or grade is employed, a number of further considerations help guide the clinician in addition to those mentioned under Correct Application of Manual Techniques:

- The position of the joint to be treated must be appropriate for the stage of healing and the skill of the clinician:
  - The resting or open pack position is used for the acute stage and/or inexperienced clinician.
  - Other starting positions may be employed by a skilled clinician in the nonacute stages.
- One half of the joint should be stabilized, while the other half is mobilized. Both the stabilizing and mobilizing hands should be placed as close as possible to the joint line. The other parts of the clinician involved in the mobilization should make maximum contact with the patient's body, to spread the forces over a larger area and reduce pain from contact of bony prominences. The maximum contact also results in more stability and increased confidence from the patient. An alternative technique, which produces the desired results, must be sought if the contact between opposite sexes is uncomfortable to either the patient or the clinician.
- The direction of the mobilization is almost always parallel or perpendicular to a tangent across adjoining joint surfaces and is appropriate for the arthrokinematics of the joint being treated.
- The mobilization should not move into or through the point of pain throughout the duration of the technique.
- The velocity and amplitude of movement is carefully considered and is based on the goal of the intervention, to restore the joint motion or to alleviate the pain, or both.
  - Slow stretches are used for large capsular restrictions.
  - Fast oscillations are used for minor restrictions.
- One movement is performed at a time, at one joint at a time.
- The patient is reassessed after a few movements if the joint is in the acute stage of healing, less frequently for other stages of healing.
- The intervention should be discontinued for the day when a large improvement has been obtained or when the improvement ceases.

Muscle reeducation is essential after mobilization or high-velocity thrust techniques and often produces a noticeable reduction in posttreatment soreness. While the joint is maintained in the new range, five to six gentle isometric contractions are asked for from the agonists and antagonists of the motion mobilized.[122] Recently, the emphasis has shifted from mobilization of the joint in straight planes to mobilizations that incorporate the combined or congruent rotations that occur with normal motion, in order to take up all of the slack in the capsule.

Mobilizations with Movements

The concept of mobilizations with movements (MWMs) was introduced by Mulligan.[125,126] MWMs are based on the principles of joint mobilization originated by Kaltenborn.[13]

CLINICAL PEARL

The techniques of MWM combine a sustained manual gliding force to a joint with concurrent physiologic motion of the joint, either actively performed by the patient or passively performed by the clinician, with the intent of causing a repositioning of so-called bony positional faults.[125,126]

With few exceptions, Mulligan's mobilization techniques are applied parallel to the plane of motion and are sustained throughout the movement until the joint returns to its starting position, with the intention of producing no pain when applied.[126] Indeed, the golden rule of MWMs is that if pain is produced with an MWM, the techniques are contraindicated. The most common cause of pain with these techniques occurs when the mobilization is not sustained throughout the whole motion.[126]

The movements used with MWMs are patient dependent and can include active, passive, and resisted movements. Their success is based on the theory that bony positional faults can contribute substantially to painful joint restrictions, which is similar to the theory behind the success of joint mobilizations.[126]

Mulligan's MWM techniques were originally designed for the cervical spine but have since been expanded to include virtually every joint in the body. Several studies[125 127–130] that looked at the effects of MWM concluded that MWM is a promising intervention.

Mulligan has devised a number of guidelines when applying these techniques[125,126]:

- The patient is placed in a weight-bearing position.
- Other interventions should be used in conjunction with these techniques.
- When treating hinge joints, the sustained glide or mobilization should be at right angles to the glide that usually occurs with the desired movement. For example, in the case of finger flexion, the glide-mobilization of the distal joint surface is applied in a medial or lateral direction.
- When joint movements involve adjacent long bones, as in the case at the wrist or ankle, it is often necessary for the clinician to adjust the relative positions of the long bones to enable pain-free joint movement to occur.

- ▸ The glide-mobilization is always successful in one direction only. The successful glide-mobilization is applied 10 times before reassessing the joint motion.
- ▸ Overpressure should be applied at the end range of the available active range of motion (AROM).

Mulligan techniques are described in detail in the relevant chapters of this text.

HIGH-VELOCITY THRUST TECHNIQUES

The earliest physicians to use high-velocity thrust techniques (joint manipulations) were English, and books on the subject were published in the early 1900s.[44,131–133]

Compared with the four grades of joint mobilization (grades I–IV), high-velocity thrust techniques are given the designation grade V. Recently, manipulative therapy has been broadly defined to include all procedures, in which the hands are used to massage, stretch, mobilize, adjust, or manipulate musculoskeletal tissues for therapeutic reasons.[134] However, in this text, high-velocity thrust techniques refer to grade V techniques. Although the grade V technique shares similarities with the grade IV mobilization in terms of amplitude and position in the joint range, grade V differs in the velocity of delivery. Applied at the barrier or point of joint restriction, a grade V technique involves the application of a fast impulse of small amplitude to restore joint play. The terms *velocity* and *amplitude* are used to describe the nature of the final activating force or thrust used. Most grades I–IV joint mobilizations use varying degrees of velocity and amplitude, whereas grade V techniques generally employ a high-velocity (quick) and low-amplitude (short-distance) thrust. Unlike mobilizations, which are applied singularly or repetitively within or at the physiologic range of joint motion,[135] high-velocity thrust techniques involve a thrust to a joint so that the joint is briefly forced beyond the restricted ROM.[2] The speed, force, and correct application of a high-velocity thrust technique are critical if serious injury is to be avoided. This is particularly true in the craniovertebral region, where an overzealous technique can result in serious consequences. At the time of writing, there is much discussion as to whether or not a patient should be required to sign an informed consent prior to receiving a high-velocity thrust technique. At the very least, the clinician has an ethical duty to obtain at least verbal consent or agreement after explaining the rationale for the technique and the possible side effects.[136]

CLINICAL PEARL

When performed correctly, a high-velocity thrust may actually be safer than many other repetitive, low-velocity, or prolonged stretch techniques. Theoretically, a high-velocity thrust technique minimizes the risk of creep and fatigue failure in normal collagen tissues. If damage does occur to tissues, it is more likely due to excessive amplitude of the thrust, excessive magnitude of the force used, or the fact that the thrusting force is passing through a mechanically unsound joint.[136]

High-velocity thrust techniques may consist of long-lever techniques that exert forces on a point on the body some distance from the treatment area, or short-lever techniques that comprise forces directed specifically at an isolated joint.[137] A lesion that might benefit from a high-velocity thrust technique may be defined by movement restriction and pain, especially a joint restriction that elicits pain on provocation. The decision to use a high-velocity thrust technique is made after first identifying the restriction through the end-feel. For example, when significant excessive collagen density (e.g., chronic capsular fibrosis) is thought to be the cause of the motion barrier, the use of a high-velocity thrust technique is deemed inappropriate.[136] In such cases, the technique utilizing a slow, prolonged stretch would be more appropriate. The plane or direction of joint restriction determines the type and direction of the high-velocity thrust technique to be used. The direction of the technique can be delivered either perpendicular to, or parallel to the joint surface to question:[136]

- ▸ Perpendicular: These techniques, more commonly known as distraction (gapping) techniques, aim to separate the joint surfaces and are usually delivered within the joint's pathological position of ease. This type of technique is only appropriate if the biomechanical assessment suggests an intra-articular inclusion or unstable joint which has become *locked up* or fixated beyond its neutral zone.
- ▸ Parallel: These techniques, aimed at improving the joint glide, are performed at the end of available range

Engaging the barrier, which requires a high level of skill, localizes the force, ensuring it will be applied to the restriction, thereby minimizing the magnitude and amplitude of the force. To successfully engage the barrier, a series of maneuvers called joint locking techniques are utilized. Excessive force or failure to localize the force of a technique results in a dissipation of physical forces, and unless the patient is able to absorb these forces, they may prove to be harmful, especially in the spinal regions.[24] These harmful effects can include fracture, spinal cord compression, vertebral artery compromise (see Chap. 24), cerebral ischemia, and even death.[138]

CLINICAL PEARL

Cervical manipulations have been linked to vertebrobasilar complications. In a review of the 58 cases in the English language literature of vertebrobasilar complications following cervical manipulation, Grant found the average age to be 37.3 years with a range of 7–3 years.[139] It was estimated from a study by Hosek.[140] that one in one million cervical manipulations will result in a serious vertebrobasilar effect, whereas Dvorak and Orelli[141] estimated a much higher incidence of one in 400,000. This latter figure would indicate that a clinician performing cervical manipulations on 15 patients each day for 30 years (allowing for vacations) stands a little better than one in four chance of causing a serious stroke in the course of a career. Put another way, one in four clinicians, manipulating at the same rate, will run into a serious problem from the vertebral artery.

LOCKING TECHNIQUES

The following two methods of locking are commonly cited for the lumbar spine (see Chap. 28):[136]

1. ***Locking from above.*** This technique places the lumbar spine into rotation and side bending to tighten the ligaments and capsule, thus stabilizing the joint, and can be performed in flexion, neutral, or extension of the lumbar spine. Because the clinician can only adequately control rotation motion when this is away from the edge of the bed, whichever side the patient is lying on the dictates the rotation that can be used—in the opposite direction from the patient side lying position (e.g., left side lying will permit right rotation). The side-bending motion is achieved by using the patient's lower arm to pull the shoulder girdle in either an inferior or a superior direction. For example, if the patient is lying on the left side, pulling the left shoulder girdle superiorly will produce right side bending of the trunk, whereas pulling the patient's left shoulder girdle inferiorly will produce left side bending. Flexion and extension can only be produced unilaterally in combination with the rotation. For example, with the patient in right side lying, flexion can be produced with left rotation by asking the patient to hold onto the edge of the table with their left hand (keeping the left shoulder girdle stationary), while the clinician pulls the patient's right arm horizontally forwards. Extension can be produced with left rotation by placing the patient's left hand onto their waist so that the weight of the patient's arm creates a left rotation with a backward displacement. This can be further enhanced by pulling the patient's right arm as vertical as possible while maintaining the right shoulder in a relatively stationary position. Neutral rotation (i.e., involving either flexion or extension) can be achieved by pulling the patient's right arm forward at a 45 degree angle. These patient positions enable the clinician to combine up to three components in the locking techniques simultaneously.
2. ***Locking from below.*** As with locking from above, the direction of the rotation is dictated by whichever side the patient lies on (e.g., the spine is rotated to the right if the patient is then left side lying). The rotation can be enhanced by bringing the nonweightbearing side of the pelvis anteriorly. Flexion and extension of the lumbar segments are produced through motions of the hip and pelvis as is performed with passive intervertebral joint motion (PIVM) testing. The following sequence is recommended:

- Produce the necessary flexion or extension motion to the appropriate level:
  - Flexion is facilitated by keeping the knees away from full flexion, thus utilizing tension in the hamstrings to rotate the pelvis posteriorly.
  - Extension is facilitated by keeping the patient's knees as flexed as possible, thereby utilizing the tension in the rectus femoris to rotate the pelvis anteriorly.
- Introduce the necessary side bending using the legs. Side bending is achieved by asking the patient to actively side tilt the pelvis by using commands such as "Push your lower leg down", or "Make your lower leg longer."

The clinician then carefully adjusts the position of the hips and knees without moving the pelvis until the upper needed in front of the lower to use rotation for a more secure lock. As with the locking techniques from above, the clinician has seven possible combinations:

- Neutral rotation, flexion, or extension.
- Ipsilateral extension (lower leg extending) or contralateral extension (upper leg extending)
- Ipsilateral flexion (lower leg extending), or contralateral flexion (upper leg extending)

With both locking techniques, the adjacent joints are positioned at the end of the available ROM for flexion/extension, side bending, or rotation. This positioning prevents further movement at these joints because either the ligaments are taut or the articular surfaces are contacting one another so that any further motion induced by a manual technique is likely to occur at the motion segment with the most slack—the motion segment targeted for treatment.

In the cervical spine, two types of locking techniques are also commonly advocated (see Chap. 25): craniovertebral locking and locking through segmental translation. Because of the potential for vertebral artery compromise in the craniovertebral region, the craniovertebral joints are often "locked" first before continuing motion into the middle and/or lower cervical spine joints. In the following example, a left side-bending technique is used. Although this locking technique may be used with the patient positioned in sitting or supine, if it is used in supine it is important to apply a small amount of compression to compensate for the loss of the spinal loading due to the weight of the head.

While palpating the C2 spinous process, the clinician slowly side-bends the patient's head to the left. If the side bending is performed around a sagittal craniovertebral axis, the C2 spinous process should be felt to move to the right, indicating left rotation of the C2 on the C3. Maintaining the left side-bent position, the head is now rotated to the right until the C2 spinous process regains a central position. The head is again side bent slightly to the left, and the C2 spinous process de-rotated back to midline. These motions are continued until a firm end-feel is reached. At this point, motion in the craniovertebral joints has now been exhausted, while the rest of the cervical joints remain in neutral. Being careful to maintain the position of the head, especially the right rotation, the side bending is continued left to the middle or the lower cervical level required. As the cervical joints are prevented from rotating to the left, the middle cervical side bending motion is exhausted very quickly.

When a specific force is applied to the bodily joints, clicking or popping sounds, called *cavitations,* may be heard. Distraction techniques are undoubtedly the easiest way to get the joint sound, especially from a normal joint. The actual causes of these cavitations or clicks is unknown, but are thought to result from a sudden release of synovial gas during the techniques. The gas is then reabsorbed by the joint over a period of about 30 minutes, which may explain why joints can only be "recracked" every 20–30 minutes. It is quite possible that these cavitations might produce a neuromuscular or neurochemical effect that will lead to temporary generalized changes, including the relief of pain. The mechanism behind the pain relief provided by a high-velocity thrust technique is not yet understood, although attempts have been made to explain the possible effects, including the freeing of an entrapped meniscoid or discal element,[142] an alteration in muscle tone,[143] and a mechanical disruption of intra-articular adhesions.[144–146] Certainly, it is known that restriction of motion at a joint produces joint adhesions, soft tissue contracture, and degenerative joint disease.[147–149] Therefore, by increasing the motion at a joint, a manipulation is thought to reverse the aforementioned detrimental effects. It is also possible that a high—velocity thrust technique may produce outcomes directly associated with a variety of psychological influences.[150] The only true test of a successful technique is by the determination of an objective change in the patient's articular function, as confirmed by active and passive motion tests.[136]

Prior to performing a high-velocity thrust technique, the clinician must attempt to determine the natural history of the joint through a subjective assessment or reaction to previous treatments. Ideally, the clinician should initially attempt to regain the lost motion utilizing other techniques such as joint mobilizations, ME, and ROM exercises prior to giving consideration to a high-velocity thrust technique. Unfortunately, a high-velocity thrust technique often becomes the procedure of choice because it carries a certain aura and is, therefore, often erroneously thought of as a panacea.[151] The indications and contraindications for high-velocity thrust techniques are the same as those outlined at the beginning of the chapter. Additional contraindications include the following:[136]

- Inability of the patient to relax.
- A past medical history that includes any condition that can weaken bone or collagen (e.g., rheumatoid arthritis, osteoporosis), any condition that may create abnormal hypomobility (e.g., Marfan syndrome, Ehlers–Danlos syndrome), any condition involving a joint fusion (surgical or otherwise), or any condition involving chemotherapy or radiotherapy for the treatment of cancer.
- Pediatric patient. The risk of damage to developing growth epiphyses and the question of whether the pretreatment explanation is understood, make children very precarious candidates for manipulation.

Once the determination is made to perform a high-velocity thrust technique, the clinician should place the joint into a premanipulative position for approximately 10 seconds and assess any change in the symptoms, the patient's reaction, and any localized or distal vascular or neurological signs or symptoms. These include vertebrobasilar artery or spinal cord signs or symptoms. Theoretically, the premanipulative position takes the target joint and its surrounding soft tissues slightly beyond the range through which a high-velocity thrust technique is to be performed. At the end of this hold, the patient is questioned as to the continued willingness of the technique to be performed, and whether this position is comfortable and nonirritating. Under no circumstance should a thrust technique be repeated, if the patient's symptoms are reported to worsen or if the first technique did not succeed with little force.

The evaluation of the effectiveness of high-velocity thrust interventions is difficult because the number of scientific studies on the subject is extremely limited.[152] It appears evident that these techniques can cause an immediate relief of low back pain in patients with acute low back pain,[153] although the degree of improvement varies between individuals. Some patients respond immediately to a high-velocity thrust technique; however, this population cannot be identified in advance, and there are no strong reasons for recommending high-velocity thrust techniques instead of mobilizations.[152]

NEUROPHYSIOLOGIC TECHNIQUES

Proprioceptive Neuromuscular Facilitation

PNF, a manual technique that promotes the response of the neuromuscular mechanism through stimulation of the proprioceptor, was developed at the Kabat Kaiser Institute by Herman Kabat and Margaret Knott during the late 1940s and early 1950s.[154] Initially, the approach was developed as a method of treatment for neurologically weak muscles due to anterior poliomyelitis. The techniques were later expanded for use in general muscle strengthening, joint mobilizations, and the stretching of adaptively shortened muscles.[155] The PNF stretching techniques are described in Chapter 13.

PNF techniques provide the clinician with an efficient means for examining and treating structural and neuromuscular dysfunctions.[156–158] Structural dysfunctions (myofascial and articular hypermobilities and hypomobilities) affect the body's capacity to assume and perform optimal postures and motions.[159] Neuromuscular dysfunctions (an inability to coordinate and efficiently perform purposeful movements) cause repetitive, abnormal, and stressful usage of the articular and myofascial systems, often precipitating structural dysfunctions and symptoms.[159–161] The theory behind PNF is that the human muscular system consists of muscle groups that are classified as agonists, antagonists, neutralizers, supporters, and fixators:[162]

- Agonists: work to produce a movement
- Antagonists: relax to allow movement
- Neutralizers: inhibit a muscle from performing more than one action
- Supporters: stabilize the trunk and proximal extremities
- Fixators: hold bones steady

Within specific movement patterns, these muscle groups must contract in the proper sequence for optimal effectiveness. Muscle contractions are classified as static or dynamic. Static contractions are those in which no motion occurs. Dynamic contractions are concentric, eccentric, or *maintained isotonic* (a PNF term), the latter of which involves the intention to move, but no motion occurs. Theoretically, the facilitation of total patterns of movement will promote

TABLE 10-7 Lower Extremity Proprioceptive Neuromuscular Facilitation Patterns

Start Position for D1 Pattern	
D1 Extension	**D1 Flexion**
Hip flexed, adducted, and externally rotated	Hip extended, abducted, and internally rotated
Knee flexed	Knee extended
Tibia internally rotated	Tibia externally rotated
Ankle and foot dorsiflexed and inverted	Ankle and foot plantarflexed and everted
Toes extended	Toes flexed
Movement into hip extension, abduction and internal rotation; ankle plantarflexion; foot eversion; toe flexion	Movement into hip flexion, adduction and external rotation; ankle dorsiflexion; foot inversion; toe extension
Start Position for D2 Pattern	
D2 Flexion	**D2 Extension**
Hip extended, adducted, and externally rotated	Hip flexed, abducted, and internally rotated
Knee extended	Knee flexed
Tibia externally rotated	Tibia internally rotated
Ankle and foot plantarflexed and inverted	Ankle and foot dorsiflexed and everted
Toes flexed	Toes extended
Movement into hip flexion, abduction and internal rotation; ankle dorsiflexion; foot eversion; toe extension	Movement into hip extension, adduction and external rotation; ankle plantarflexion; foot inversion; toe flexion

D1, diagonal 1; D2, diagonal 2.

motor learning in synergistic muscle patterns and these total patterns of movement and posture are important preparatory patterns for advanced functional skills. These patterns are designed to encourage the stronger synergistic muscle groups to assist the weaker ones during functional movements, and are concerned with gross motions as opposed to specific motions.

According to PNF theory, muscle function occurs three dimensionally around three planes of movement, with each movement associated with an antagonistic motion:

- Flexion or extension
- Adduction or abduction in the extremities and lateral movement in the trunk
- Internal or external rotation.

Combinations of these movements work together in spiral and diagonal patterns. The patterns, which integrate the motions of sport and daily living, are based on the infant developmental sequences such as rolling, crawling, and walking. There are two diagonal patterns for the lower extremity (Table 10-7), and two diagonal patterns for the upper extremity and scapula (Table 10-8), which are referred to as the diagonal 1 (D1) and diagonal 2 (D2) patterns. These D1 and D2 patterns are subdivided into those that move into flexion and those that move into extension. In addition to the upper and lower extremity patterns, patterns exist for the upper trunk, lower trunk, and cervical spine.

CLINICAL PEARL

PNF patterns can be performed unilaterally or bilaterally. For example, the chop and lift patterns used frequently in recruiting the stabilizing musculature of the trunk (see Chap. 28), are applications of the upper extremity diagonal that involve the use of both upper extremities in which one upper extremity is performing the D1 pattern while the other upper extremity is performing the D2 pattern (Figs. 10-3 and 10-4) with both upper extremities moving into flexion, or extension while using spiral and diagonal movements that cross the midline.

Knowledge of the normal functional movement patterns of the body allows the clinician to identify altered patterns of motion. Once the clinician has diagnosed impairments or functional limitation, the clinician makes a decision as to which pattern will be used and the goal of the technique. Basic procedures of facilitation include body positioning the mechanics, manual contacts, manual and maximal resistance, irradiation, verbal and visual cueing, traction and approximation, stretch, and timing.[163] The position of the patient, which often uses developmental positions, allows for consistency of measurement and plays a major role in influencing postural tone. The exercise pattern is initiated after positioning the patient so that the muscle groups are in the lengthened position. The muscle groups are then moved through their full range to their shortened position. The key to the success of PNF is the ability of the clinician to apply manual contact with appropriate pressure and exact positioning, which allows for a smooth, coordinated motion throughout the pattern. Manual contacts are used to isolate muscle groups, provide tactile cues, and influence the strength of the contraction. Appropriate pressure is described as the amount of resistance that facilitates the desired motor response of a smooth, coordinated, and optimal muscle contraction.[157,162] For example, the clinician can apply maximal resistance at specific points in the range to promote overflow to the weaker components of the movement pattern.

TABLE 10-8 Upper Extremity and Scapular Proprioceptive Neuromuscular Facilitation Patterns

D1 Flexion **Start Position for D1 Pattern**	**D1 Extension**
Scapula depressed and adducted	Scapula elevated and abducted
Shoulder extended, abducted, and internally rotated	Shoulder flexed, adducted, and externally rotated
Elbow extended	Elbow extended
Forearm pronated	Forearm supinated
Wrist extended and ulnarly deviated	Wrist flexed and radially deviated
Fingers abducted and extended	Fingers adducted and flexed
Thumb extended and abducted	Thumb flexed and adducted
Movement into shoulder flexion, adduction and internal rotation; scapular elevation and abduction; forearm supination; wrist flexion and radial deviation; finger flexion	Movement into shoulder extension, abduction and internal rotation; scapular depression and adduction; forearm pronation; wrist extension and ulnar deviation; finger extension
D2 Extension **Start Position for D2 Pattern**	**D2 Flexion**
Scapula elevated and adducted	Scapula depressed and abducted
Shoulder flexed, abducted, and externally rotated	Shoulder extended, adducted, and internally rotated
Elbow extended	Elbow extended
Forearm supinated	Forearm pronated
Wrist extended and radially deviated	Wrist flexed and ulnarly deviated
Fingers extended and abducted	Fingers adducted and flexed
Thumb extended and adducted	Thumb flexed and abducted
Movement into shoulder extension, adduction and internal rotation; scapular depression and abduction; forearm pronation; wrist flexion and ulnar deviation; finger flexion	Movement into shoulder flexion, abduction and external rotation; scapular elevation and adduction; forearm supination; wrist extension and radial deviation; finger extension

D1, diagonal 1; D2, diagonal 2.

The patient is first taught the diagonal PNF pattern from the starting position to the terminal position, using brief and simple verbal cues, such as "push," "pull," and "hold," as well as visual and tactile input while being careful to avoid exceeding the extensibility limits of the musculotendinous unit.

If a dysfunctional movement is identified in any of the diagonals of motion, the clinician can apply appropriate resistance in conjunction with various PNF techniques (Table 10-9) to facilitate the relearning and rehabilitative process.[156–159,162] For example, a quick stretch applied to a muscle before contraction facilitates a muscular response of greater force.

The following PNF techniques can be used for the development of muscular strength, endurance, and coordination.

Rhythmic Initiation

The rhythmic initiation technique is used to teach a patient a specific movement pattern, or with patients who are unable to initiate a movement, or those who have a limited ROM because of increased muscle tone.

The application of the technique involves a progression through the agonist pattern of passive, then active and assistive, then active movement. This technique is applied slowly against resistance through the available ROM, while avoiding activation of a quick stretch.

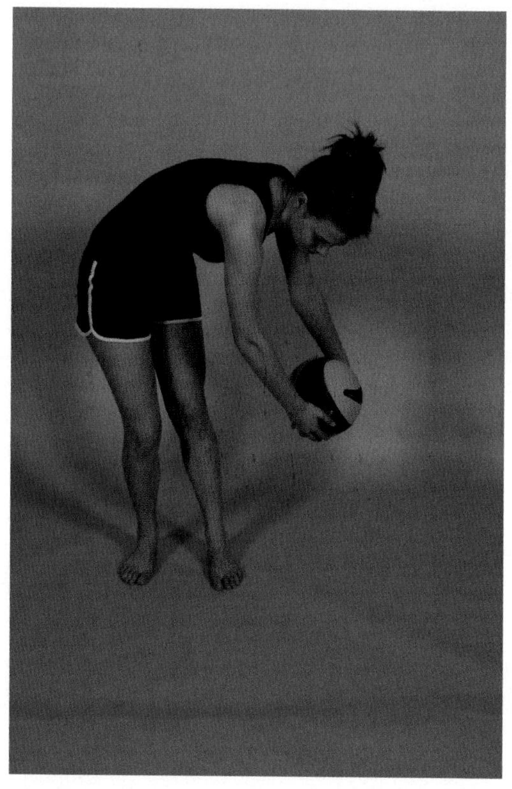

FIGURE 10-3 Chop PNF pattern.

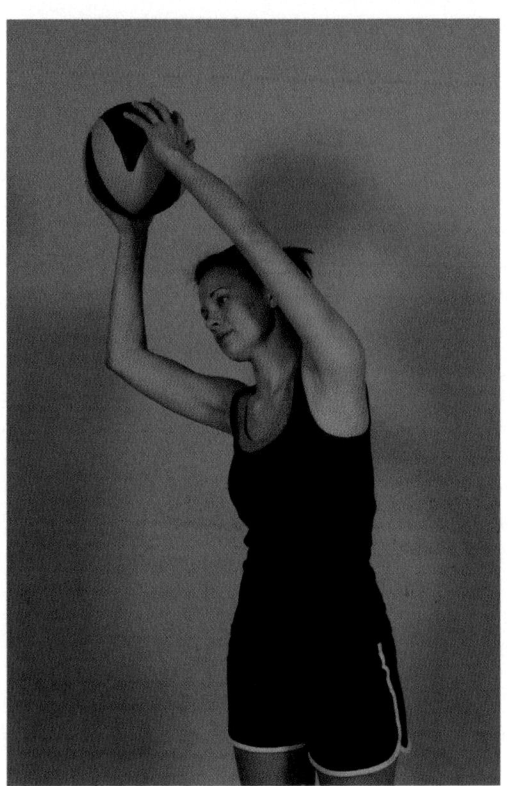

FIGURE 10-4 Lift PNF pattern.

Repeated Contraction

Repeated contraction is a useful technique for patients who have weakness, either at a specific point or throughout the entire range, and to correct imbalances that occur within the range. The patient is asked to push repeatedly by using the agonist concentrically and eccentrically against maximal resistance, until fatigue occurs in the weaker ranges of the motion. The amount of resistance to motion given by the clinician is modified to accommodate the strength of the muscle group. A stretch can be applied at the weakest point in the range to facilitate the weaker muscles and promote a smoother, more coordinated motion.

Stabilizing Reversal

This technique, also known as an *isotonic reversal*, can be used for developing AROM of the agonists, while also developing the normal reciprocal timing between the antagonists and agonists that occurs during functional movements. The technique involves a concentric contraction of the agonist followed immediately by a concentric contraction of the antagonist, with the initial agonist push contraction facilitating the pull contraction of the antagonist muscles.

Rhythmic Stabilization

The techniques of rhythmic stabilization, also called *stabilizing reversals*, emphasize the cocontraction of agonists and antagonists, which results in an increase in the holding power to a point where the position cannot be broken. This effect is achieved by alternating isometric contraction of the agonist with isometric contraction of the antagonist, to produce cocontraction of the two opposing muscle groups. The command "hold" is always given before movement is resisted in each direction. The goals of this technique are to improve stability around a joint, increase positional neuromuscular awareness, improve posture and balance, and enhance strength or stretch sensitivity of the tonic muscles in their functional range.[159]

The final step is to integrate the gains from the technique into function.

TABLE 10-9 PNF Techniques of Facilitation

Techniques of facilitation	Rhythmic initiation	Designed to improve the ability of the target agonist to direct and begin movement. Technique starts with passive movement in a chosen direction or pattern that encourages gradual patient participation before resisting the patient as performance improves
	Repeated contractions	Designed to repeatedly elongate the agonist muscle groups to reintroduce reflex output and initiate movement. If the clinician stretch occurs in the fully lengthened range, the technique is called repeated stretch. If the re-stretch occurs within the active range of motion, it is called repeated contractions.
	Reversals of antagonists	Designed to facilitate contraction of the agonist after contraction of the antagonist thereby improving static and dynamic posterolateral, and reciprocal movements.
	Dynamic reversals of antagonists	Designed to facilitate dynamic contractions of the antagonistic movements reciprocally in a range appropriate to the goal of the exercise. This technique can be used to increase active range of motion, strength in the available range of motion, and improve balance and coordination of the antagonists
	Stabilizing reversals	Designed to enhance balance and stability by applying alternating resistance to agonist–antagonist muscle pairs.
	Rhythmic stabilization	Designed to enhance cocontraction of the antagonists at any point in a given range of motion.
	Combination of isotonics	Designed to integrate movement by varying the type of agonist contraction (concentric, eccentric, and maintained dynamic) required for the function.

Box 10-1 Classification of Trigger Points

- *Active trigger points* are those that are symptomatic with respect to pain and refer a pattern of pain at rest or during motion (or both) that is specific for that muscle. An active trigger point usually produces restricted range of motion and a visible or palpable local twitch response during mechanical stimulation of the MTrP, but failure to elicit this response does not exclude MPS. MTrPs are always tender and cause muscle weakness.
- *Latent trigger points*, which represent the majority of trigger points, are usually asymptomatic but may have all the other clinical characteristics of active trigger points. Latent trigger points can persist for years after a patient recovers from an injury and may become active and create acute pain in response to minor overstretching, overuse, or chilling of the muscle.
- *Associated trigger points* develop in response to compensatory overload, shortened range of motion, or referred phenomena caused by trigger point activity in another muscle. There are two kinds of such trigger points:
  - *Satellite trigger points* are in the zone of referral of another muscle.
  - *Secondary trigger points* are activated because the muscle was overloaded as a synergist or an antagonist of a muscle harboring a primary trigger point.

Myofascial Trigger Point Therapy

The term *myofascial trigger point* is a bit of a misnomer, because trigger points can also be cutaneous, ligamentous, periosteal, and fascial.[164]

An MTrP is a hyperirritable location, approximately 2–5 cm in diameter,[165] within a taut band of muscle fibers that is painful when compressed and that can give rise to characteristic referred pain, autonomic phenomena, tenderness, and tightness. MTrPs, are classified as either active or latent (Box 10-1).[166] The patient's reaction to firm palpation of the MTrP is a distinguishing characteristic of myofascial pain syndrome (MPS) (given later) and is termed a *positive jump sign*.[167] This reaction may include withdrawal, wrinkling of the face, or a verbal response. This hyperirritability appears to be a result of sensitization of the chemonociceptors and mechanonociceptors located within the muscle.

CLINICAL PEARL

Some confusion exists as to the difference between trigger points and tender points. Although MTrPs can occur in the same sites as the tender points of fibromyalgia (FM) (see Chap. 5), MTrPs can cause referral of pain in a distinct and characteristic area, remote from the trigger point site, not necessarily in a dermatomal distribution.[168] Referred pain is, by definition, absent in the tender points of FM.[70,169]

Healthy tissues do not contain trigger points, are not tender to firm palpation, and do not refer pain. Several possible mechanisms can lead to development of MTrPs, including low-level muscle contractions, an uneven intramuscular pressure distribution, direct trauma, unaccustomed eccentric contractions, eccentric contractions in an unconditioned muscle, and maximal or submaximal concentric contractions.[170] Thus, MTrPs are typically located in areas that are prone to increased mechanical strain or impaired circulation (e.g., upper trapezius, levator scapulae, infraspinatus, quadratus lumborum, and gluteus minimus). As with all chronic pain conditions, concomitant social, behavioral, and psychological disturbances often precede or follow their development.[171,172]

Whatever the etiologic factors, it would appear that the development of MTrPs may be a progressive process, with a stage of neuromuscular dysfunction of muscle hyperactivity and irritability that is sustained by numerous perpetuating factors and then followed by a stage of organic dystrophic changes in the muscle bands with MTrPs.[167]

According to Simons,[173] the diagnosis of MPS can be made if five major criteria and at least one out of three minor criteria are met. The major criteria are

1. localized spontaneous pain;
2. spontaneous pain or altered sensations in the expected referred pain area for a given trigger point;
3. presence of a taut palpable band in an accessible muscle;
4. exquisite localized tenderness in a precise point along the taut band;
5. some degree of reduced range of movement when measurable.

Minor criteria include

1. reproduction of spontaneously perceived pain and altered sensations by pressure on the trigger point;
2. elicitation of a local twitch response of muscular fibers by " transverse" snapping palpation or by needle insertion into the trigger point;
3. pain relieved by muscle stretching or injection of the trigger point.

The major goals of MTrP therapy are to relieve pain and tightness of the involved muscles, improve joint motion, improve circulation, and eliminate perpetuating factors. When treating a patient for a specific muscle syndrome, it is important to explain the function of the involved muscle and to describe or demonstrate a few of the activities or postures that might overstress it, so that the patient can avoid such activities or postures.

A number of manual interventions for MTrPs are available; these include the following.[68,174–176]

Stretch and Spray or Stretch and Ice[69,164]

Although not technically a manual technique, the spray-and-stretch technique involves a manual stretch during its application.

The patient is placed in a position of maximum comfort to enhance muscle relaxation. The part of the body affected is then positioned so that a mild stretch is exerted specifically on the taut band. Parallel sweeps of the vapocoolant spray or ice are applied unidirectionally; then, while one of the clinician's hands anchors the base of the muscle, the other stretches the muscle to its full length.[173] The spray is held approximately 18 inches away from the skin, to allow for sufficient cooling of the spray. One or two sweeps of coolant are sprayed over the area of the involved muscle to reduce any pain. As the muscle is passively stretched, successive parallel sweeps of the spray are applied over the skin from the MTrP to the area of referred pain, covering as much of the referred pain pattern as possible. After each application of the spray-and-stretch technique, the muscle is selectively moved through as full a ROM as possible to normalize proprioceptive input to the central nervous system.[164] Intense cold stimulates cold receptors in the skin, which tends to inhibit pain. This technique is supposed to help block reflex spasm and pain, allowing for a gradual passive stretch of the muscle, which decreases muscle tension. Several treatments may be needed to eliminate the pain syndrome; results should be seen after four to six treatments.[164] If vaporized coolants are not available, ice may be used in their place, taking care to prevent chilling of the underlying muscles, which is less likely with the use of vaporized coolants.[164]

Muscle Stripping. Muscle stripping is used after first applying a lubricant to the skin. The technique involves the slow sliding of the thumb, knuckle, or elbow along the edge of a taut band with firm pressure, while at the same time attempting to bow it out.[164] This technique has the effect of applying brief ischemic compression, as the thumb slowly slides over the MTrPs, and of passively lengthening the taut band. Muscle stripping is as effective as the spray-and-stretch technique, although it is somewhat more painful.[164]

Massage Therapy. Deep massage mechanically helps break up the fibrous bands of MTrPs. The application of deep pressure produces local ischemia. When the pressure is released, a reactive hyperemia occurs, improving circulation and releasing energy to the area.[177]

Myofascial Release. These techniques, discussed in a previous section, combine massage with deep stretch techniques to relax muscle and break up the MTrPs.[46,69]

Ischemic Compression.[164] Compression can be applied with a thumb, knuckle, or elbow. The compression serves as the hyperstimulant, and the pain is usually relieved within 20–60 seconds. The technique involves the application of pressure directly on the trigger point, within the patient's tolerance. As the pain subsides, the clinician slowly increases the pressure until, ideally, the painful stimulus is eliminated and a softening of the area is felt.

Stretching. Lengthening of the taut band is an effective form of intervention. It is theorized to disengage the actin and myosin filaments of the skeletal muscle (see Chap. 1), allowing more normal muscle length and increased ROM, and results in normal, patterned proprioceptive input to the central nervous system, which may prevent the resumption of pain.[164] Lengthening can be accomplished with gentle stretching of the involved muscles.

Joint Mobilizations. Typically, treatment of a dysfunctional joint leads to spontaneous resolution of soft-tissue tension and the restoration of normal muscle lengths around the joint, thereby allowing the hypertonic muscles to relax.[44,84,88,178]

Nonmanual Interventions. The nonmanual interventions for MTrPs are included here for completeness.[68,174–176]

- ***Thermotherapy.*** Moist heat, ultrasound, or a hot-tub session of 5–15 minutes' duration helps relax underlying muscles and increase circulation, thereby improving the supply of nutrients and decreasing tension on the MTrPs.[69] Pain relief is theorized to be related to a washout of pain mediators by increased blood flow, changes in nerve conduction, or alterations in cell membrane permeability that decrease inflammation.[166,179]
- ***Cryotherapy.*** Brief, intense cold stimulation of the skin overlying the trigger point and its pain referral area is effective in releasing taut bands and inactivating trigger points, particularly when done in combination with a passive stretch.[164]
- ***Trigger point injections.*** Trigger point injections using various techniques have been widely used to inactivate MTrPs by disrupting the fibrous banding, although the injected local anesthetic agent seems less important for inactivation of the trigger point than the needling itself.[66,180,181] Trigger point injections should be followed by stretching and the application of heat.[69] The effectiveness of ultrasound therapy is comparable to trigger point injections and should be offered as a noninvasive treatment of choice to those patients who want to avoid injections.[166]
- ***Elimination of causative or perpetuating factors, if any.*** Mechanical and metabolic disorders need to be corrected to prevent further stress and strain on the muscles. Although many people have some degree of imbalanced body structure, structural imbalance is an extremely common contributing factor to myofascial constrictions and trigger points.[65,174,175,182,183] In addition, patients should be encouraged to limit caffeine intake to less than two caffeinated beverages per day and avoid smoking, both of which directly and indirectly aggravate MTrPs.[69] Nutrition deficiencies may require correction, and supplements of vitamins C, B1, B6, B12, and folic acid have been advocated because of their essential role in normal muscle metabolism.[164]
- ***Biofeedback and muscle relaxation.*** Biofeedback and muscle relaxation techniques can be used to avoid chronic muscle tension.
- ***Exercise.*** Exercise is important in limiting recurrences of MTrPs.[183]
- ***Counterirritation.*** This very old method of controlling pain has been used for centuries. Its success relates to the fact that it breaks the pain–spasm–pain cycle that so often perpetuates a painful condition through the gate control mechanism of pain control (see Chap. 3).
- ***Combination therapy.*** One study,[166] which looked at the combined intervention of ultrasound, trigger point injections, and stretching, found that the combination of these three interventions were effective in the reduction

of pain, and improving ROM, independent of the severity or duration of pain present before the treatment. Another study, which examined a combined intervention of ultrasound, massage, and exercise, found that patients who had massage and exercise had a reduction in the number and intensity of MTrPs, whereas ultrasound alone gave no pain reduction.[184]

- ***Electrotherapy.*** Electrotherapy has also been found to be an effective therapeutic modality to relieve pain from MTrPs,[64,175,185] although electrotherapy alone is reported not as effective as thermotherapy or intermittent cold with stretching.[175] Electrotherapy is thought to work by producing muscle contractions, which squeeze out the edema from needling, increase blood flow to the area, and relax the muscles.[65] Two major types of electrical stimulation therapy used for soft-tissue lesions are electrical nerve stimulation (ENS) and electrical muscle stimulation (EMS).
  - ENS is the application of a low-intensity electrical current on the peripheral nerve . In general, ENS, such as transcutaneous nerve stimulation, is used in reducing pain intensity and increasing the pain threshold of MTrPs (no matter how severe the initial pain).[186,187]
  - EMS is the application of electrical current with stronger intensity directly to the involved muscle. EMS can be used to enhance muscle circulation, reduce muscle spasm, eliminate muscle pain, and increase muscle strength.[182,185,187]

According to one study, ENS was found to be more effective than EMS for immediate pain relief, whereas EMS was more effective than ENS for improving ROM.[187]

REVIEW QUESTIONS*

1. Give five indications for the use of MT.
2. Give five absolute contraindications to MT.
3. Give the three purported benefits of TFM.
4. Which manual technique uses the passive positioning of the body in a position of ease (rather than motion restriction) to evoke a therapeutic effect?
5. Which manual techniques involve low-velocity passive movements within or at the limit of joint ROM, to restore any loss of accessory joint motion as the consequence of joint injury?

*Additional questions to test your understanding of this chapter can be found in the Online Learning Center for *Orthopaedic Assessment, Evaluation, and Intervention* at www. duttononline. net.

REFERENCES

1. Sucher BM: Myofascial release of carpal tunnel syndrome. *J Am Osteopath Assoc* 93:92–101, 1993.
2. Di Fabio RP: Efficacy of manual therapy. *Phys Ther* 72:853–864, 1992.
3. Cochrane CG: Joint mobilization principles: considerations for use in the child with central nervous dysfunction. *Phys Ther* 67:1105–1109, 1987.
4. Brooks SC: Coma. In: Payton OD, Di Fabio RP, Paris SV, et al., eds. *Manual of Physical Therapy.* New York, NY: Churchill Livingstone, 1989:215–238.
5. Farrell JP, Jensen GM: Manual therapy: a critical assessment of role in the profession of physical therapy. *Phys Ther* 72:843–852, 1992.
6. Watson T: The role of electrotherapy in contemporary physiotherapy practice. *Man Ther* 5:132–141, 2000.
7. Cyriax J: *Textbook of Orthopaedic Medicine, Diagnosis of Soft Tissue Lesions*, 8th ed. London: Bailliere Tindall, 1982.
8. Mennell JM: *Back Pain. Diagnosis and Treatment Using Manipulative Techniques.* Boston, MA: Little, Brown & Company, 1960.
9. Stoddard A: *Manual of Osteopathic Practice.* New York, NY: Harper & Row, 1969.
10. DiGiovanna EL, Schiowitz S: *An Osteopathic Approach to Diagnosis and Treatment.* Philadelphia, PA: JB Lippincott, 1991.
11. Maitland G: *Vertebral Manipulation.* Sydney: Butterworth, 1986.
12. Maitland G: *Peripheral Manipulation*, 3rd ed. London: Butterworth, 1991.
13. Kaltenborn FM: *Manual Mobilization of the Extremity Joints: Basic Examination and Treatment Techniques*, 4th ed. Oslo, Norway: Olaf Norlis Bokhandel, Universitetsgaten, 1989.
14. McKenzie RA: *The Lumbar Spine: Mechanical Diagnosis and Therapy.* Waikanae, NZ: Spinal Publication, 1981.
15. Cookson JC: Orthopedic manual therapy – an overview. Part 2: the spine. *Phys Ther* 59:259–267, 1979.
16. Cookson JC, Kent B: Orthopedic manual therapy – an overview. Part 1: the extremities. *Phys Ther* 59:136–146, 1979.
17. Threlkeld AJ: The effects of manual therapy on connective tissue. *Phys Ther* 72:893–902, 1992.
18. Jull GA, Janda V: Muscle and motor control in low back pain. In: Twomey LT, Taylor JR, eds. *Physical Therapy of the Low Back: Clinics in Physical Therapy.* New York, NY: Churchill Livingstone, 1987:258–278.
19. Nwuga VCB: Relative therapeutic efficacy of vertebral manipulation and conventional treatment in back pain management. *Am J Phys Med* 61:273–278, 1982.
20. Nicholson GG: The effects of passive joint mobilization on pain and hypomobility associated with adhesive capsulitis of the shoulder. *J Orthop Sports Phys Ther* 6:238–246, 1985.
21. Anderson M, Tichenor CJ: A patient with de Quervain's tenosynovitis: a case report using an Australian approach to manual therapy. *Phys Ther* 74:314–326, 1994.
22. Nyberg R: Manipulation: definition, types, application. In: Basmajian JV, Nyberg R, eds. *Rational Manual Therapies.* Baltimore, MD: Williams & Wilkins, 1993:21–47.
23. Nitz AJ: Physical therapy management of the shoulder. *Phys Ther* 66:1912–1919, 1986.
24. Kappler RE: Direction action techniques. *J Am Osteopath Assoc* 81:239–243, 1981.
25. Mitchell FL, Moran PS, Pruzzo NA: *An Evaluation and Treatment Manual of Osteopathic Muscle Energy Procedures.* Manchester, MO: Mitchell, Moran and Pruzzo Associates, 1979.
26. Greenman PE: *Principles of Manual Medicine*, 2nd ed. Baltimore, MD: Williams & Wilkins, 1996.
27. Nansel D, Peneff A, Cremata E, et al.: Time course considerations for the effects of unilateral cervical adjustments with respect to the amelioration of cervical lateral flexion passive end-range asymmetry. *J Manipulative Physiol Ther* 13:297–304, 1990.
28. Jull GA: Physiotherapy management of neck pain of mechanical origin. In: Giles LGF, Singer KP, eds. *Clinical Anatomy and Management of Cervical Spine Pain. The Clinical Anatomy of Back Pain.* London: Butterworth-Heinemann, 1998:168–191.
29. Riddle DL, Rothstein JM, Lamb RL: Goniometric reliability in a clinical setting: shoulder measurements. *Phys Ther* 67:668–673, 1987.
30. Price DD, McGrath PA, Rafii A, et al.: The validation of visual analogue scales as ratio scale measures for chronic and experimental pain. *Pain* 17:46–56, 1983.
31. Youdas JW, Carey JR, Garrett TR: Reliability of measurements of cervical spine range of motion: comparison of three methods. *Phys Ther* 71:98–104, 1991.
32. Fitzgerald GK, McClure PW, Beattie P, et al.: Issues in determining treatment effectiveness of manual therapy. *Phys Ther* 74:227–233, 1994.
33. Basmajian JV: Introduction: a plea for research validation. In: Basmajian JV, Nyberg R, eds. *Rational Manual Therapies.* Baltimore, MD: Williams & Wilkins, 1993:1–6.

34. Kessler RM, Hertling D: *Management of Common Musculoskeletal Disorders*, 2nd ed. Philadelphia, PA: Harper and Row, 1983.
35. Ramsey SM: Holistic manual therapy techniques. *Prim Care* 24:759–785, 1997.
36. Johnson GS: Soft tissue mobilization. In: Donatelli RA, Wooden MJ, eds. *Orthopaedic Physical Therapy*. New York, NY: Churchill Livingstone, 1994.
37. Cyriax JH, Cyriax PJ: *Illustrated Manual of Orthopaedic Medicine*. London: Butterworth, 1983.
38. Gersten JW: Effect of ultrasound on tendon extensibility. *Am J Phys Med* 34:662, 1955.
39. Hunter SC, Poole RM: The chronically inflamed tendon. *Clin Sports Med* 6:371, 1987.
40. Palastanga N: The use of transverse frictions for soft tissue lesions. In: Grieve GP, ed. *Modern Manual Therapy of the Vertebral Column*. London: Churchill Livingstone, 1986:819–826.
41. Walker JM: Deep transverse friction in ligament healing. *J Orthop Sports Phys Ther* 6:89–94, 1984.
42. Hammer WI: The use of transverse friction massage in the management of chronic bursitis of the hip or shoulder. *J Manipulative Physiol Ther* 16:107–111, 1993.
43. Forrester JC, Zederfeldt BH, Hayes TL, et al.: Wolff's law in relation to the healing skin wound. *J Trauma* 10:770–779, 1970.
44. Mennell JB: *The Science and Art of Joint Manipulation*. London: J & A Churchill, 1949.
45. Upledger JE, Vredevoogd JD: *Craniosacral Therapy*. Chicago, IL: Eastland Press, 1983.
46. Barnes J: *Myofascial Release: A Comprehensive Evaluatory and Treatment Approach*. Paoli, PA: MFR Seminars, 1990.
47. Morton T: Panel debates the pros and cons of myofascial release approach, APTA Progress Report, 10–12, 1988.
48. Sullivan SJ, Williams LRT, Seaborne DE, et al.: Effects of massage on alpha motorneuron excitability. *Phys Ther* 71:555–560, 1991.
49. Roy S, Irvin R: *Sports Medicine – Prevention, Evaluation, Management, and Rehabilitation*. Englewood Cliffs, NJ: Prentice-Hall, 1983.
50. Johnson GS: Soft tissue mobilization. In: Donatelli RA, Wooden MJ, eds. *Orthopaedic Physical Therapy*. Philadelphia, PA: Churchill Livingstone, 2001:578–617.
51. Grodin AJ, Cantu RI: Soft tissue mobilization. In: Basmajian JV, Nyberg R, eds. *Rational Manual Therapies*. Baltimore, MD: Williams & Wilkins, 1993:199–221.
52. Licht S: *Massage, Manipulation and Traction*. Connecticut, CT: E. Licht, 1960.
53. Kamenetz HL: History of massage. In: Basmajian JV, ed. *Manipulation, Traction and Massage*, 3rd ed. Baltimore, MD: Williams & Wilkins, 1985.
54. Wakim KG: The effects of massage on the circulation of normal and paralyzed extremities. *Arch Phys Med Rehabil* 30:135, 1949.
55. Crosman LJ, Chateauvert SR, Weisberg J: The effects of massage to the hamstring muscle group on range of motion. *J Orthop Sports Phys Ther* 6:168, 1984.
56. Beard G, Wood E: *Massage Principles and Techniques*. Philadelphia, PA: WB Saunders, 1965.
57. Palastanga N: Soft-tissue manipulative techniques. In: Palastanga N, Boyling JD, eds. *Grieve's Modern Manual Therapy: The Vertebral Column*, 2nd ed. Edinburgh: Churchill Livingstone, 1994: 809–822.
58. Hollis M: *Massage for Therapists*. Oxford: Blackwell, 1987.
59. Jarmey C, Tindall J: *Acupressure for Common Ailments*. New York, NY: Simon & Schuster Inc., 1991.
60. van Tulder MW: The effectiveness of acupuncture in the management of acute and chronic low back pain: a systematic review within the framework of the Cochrane Collaboration Back Review Group. *Spine* 24:1113, 1999.
61. Melzack R: The gate theory revisited. In: LeRoy PL, ed. *Current Concepts in the Management of Chronic Pain*. Miami, FL: Symposia Specialists, 1977:43–65.
62. Melzack R, Wall PD: On the nature of cutaneous sensory mechanisms. *Brain* 85:331–356, 1962.
63. Haldeman S: Manipulation and massage for the relief of pain. In: Wall PD, Melzack R, eds. *Textbook of Pain*, 2nd ed. Edinburgh: Churchill Livingstone, 1989:942–951.
64. Kahn J: Electrical modalities in the treatment of myofascial conditions. In: Rachlin ES, ed. *Myofascial Pain and Fibromyalgia, Trigger Point Management*. St. Louis, MO: Mosby, 1994:473–485.
65. Krause H, Fischer AA: Diagnosis and treatment of myofascial pain. *Mt Sinai J Med* 58:235–239, 1991.
66. Lewit K: The needle effect in the relief of myofascial pain. *Pain* 6:83–90, 1979.
67. Magora F, Aladjemoff L, Tannenbaum J, et al.: Treatment of pain by transcutaneous electrical stimulation. *Acta Anaesthesiol Scand* 22:589–592, 1978.
68. Sola AE, Bonica JJ: Myofascial pain syndromes. In: Bonica JJ, Loeser JD, Chapman CR, et al., eds. *The Management of Pain*. Philadelphia, PA: Lea & Febiger, 1990:352–367.
69. Travell JG, Simons DG: *Myofascial Pain and Dysfunction – The Trigger Point Manual*. Baltimore, MD: Williams & Wilkins, 1983.
70. Vecchiet L, Giamberardino MA, Saggini R: Myofascial pain syndromes: clinical and pathophysiological aspects. *Clin J Pain* 7(Suppl):16–22, 1991.
71. Stux G, Pomeranz B: *Basics of Acupuncture*. Berlin, Heidelberg: Springer-Verlag, 1988.
72. Mitchell FL Sr: *Structural Pelvic Function*. Indianapolis, IN: AAO Yearbook, 1958:71–89.
73. Mitchell FL Jr: Elements of muscle energy techniques. In: Basmajian JV, Nyberg R, eds. *Rational Manual Therapies*. Baltimore, MD: Williams & Wilkins, 1993:285–321.
74. Lewit K, Simons DG: Myofascial pain: relief by post-isometric relaxation. *Arch Phys Med Rehabili* 65:452–456, 1984.
75. Goodridge JP: Muscle energy technique: definition, explanation, methods of procedure. *J Am Osteopath Assoc* 81:249–254, 1981.
76. Wyke BD: The neurology of joints: a review of general principles. *Clin Rheum Dis* 7:223–239, 1981.
77. Wyke BD: The neurology of joints. *Ann R Coll Surg Engl* 41:25–50, 1967.
78. Hagbarth K: Excitatory inhibitory skin areas for flexor and extensor motoneurons. *Acta Physiol Scand* 94:1–58, 1952.
79. Chaitow L: An introduction to muscle energy techniques. In: Chaitow L, ed. *Muscle Energy Techniques*, 2nd ed. London: Churchill Livingstone, 2001:1–18.
80. Jones LH: *Strain and Counterstrain*. Colorado Springs, CO: American Academy of Osteopathy, 1981.
81. Bowles CH: *Musculo-Skeletal Segment as a Problem Solving Machine*. Indianapolis, IN: Yearbook of the Academy of Applied Osteopathy, 1964.
82. Johnston WL: Segmental behavior during motion. I. A palpatory study of somatic relations. II. Somatic dysfunction, the clinical distortion. *J Am Osteopath Assoc* 72:352–361, 1972.
83. Johnston WL: Segmental behavior during motion. III. Extending behavioral boundaries. *J Am Osteopath Assoc* 72:462–475, 1973.
84. Liebenson C: Active muscular relaxation techniques (part 2). *J Manipulative Physiol Ther* 13:2–6, 1990.
85. Liebenson C: Active muscular relaxation techniques (part 1). *J Manipulative Physiol Ther* 12:446–451, 1989.
86. Janda V: Muscles, motor regulation and back problems. In: Korr IM, ed. *The Neurological Mechanisms in Manipulative Therapy*. New York, NY: Plenum, 1978:27–41.
87. Janda V: *Muscle Function Testing*. London: Butterworths, 1983.
88. Janda V: Muscle strength in relation to muscle length, pain and muscle imbalance. In: Harms-Ringdahl K, ed. *Muscle Strength*. New York, NY: Churchill Livingstone, 1993:83–91.
89. Lewis C, Flynn TW: The use of strain-counterstrain in the treatment of patients with low back pain. *J Man Manip Ther* 9:92–98, 2001.
90. Kusunose R: Strain and counterstrain. In: Basmajian JV, Nyberg R, eds: *Rationale Manual Therapies*. Baltimore, MD: Williams & Wilkins, 1993: Chap 13.
91. Korr IM: Proprioceptors and somatic dysfunction. *J Am Osteopath Assoc* 74:638–650, 1975.
92. Bailey HW: Some problems in making osteopathic spinal manipulative therapy appropriate and specific. *J Am Osteopath Assoc* 75:486–499, 1976.
93. Schiowitz S: Facilitated positional release. *J Am Osteopath Assoc* 90:145–155, 1990.
94. Chaitow L: Associated techniques. In: Chaitow L, ed. *Modern Neuromuscular Techniques*. New York, NY: Churchill Livingstone, 1996:109–135.
95. Carew TJ: The control of reflex action. In: Kandel ER, Schwartz JH, eds. *Principles of Neural Science*. New York, NY: Elsevier Science Publishing, 1985:464.
96. Rathburn JB, Macnab I: The microvascular pattern of the rotator cuff. *J Bone Joint Surg Br* 52:540–553, 1970.

97. Still AT: *Osteopathy. Research and Practice*. Kirksville, MO: A.T. Still, 1910.
98. Hoover HV: Collected Papers, 1969 [MD1].
99. Mennel J: *Joint Pain and Diagnosis using Manipulative Techniques*. New York, NY: Little, Brown, 1964.
100. Bowles CH: Functional technique: a modern perspective. *J Am Osteopath Assoc* 80:326–331, 1981.
101. Bourdillon JF: *Spinal Manipulation*, 3rd ed. London: Heinemann Medical Books, 1982.
102. Downey PA, Barbano T, Kapur-Wadhwa R, et al.: Craniosacral therapy: the effects of cranial manipulation on intracranial pressure and cranial bone movement. *J Orthop Sports Phys Ther* 36:845–853, 2006.
103. Kimberly PE: Osteopathic cranial lesions. 1948. *J Am Osteopath Assoc* 100:575–578, 2000.
104. Flynn TW, Cleland JA, Schaible P: Craniosacral therapy and professional responsibility. *J Orthop Sports Phys Ther* 36:134–836, 2006.
105. Draper DO: Ultrasound and joint mobilizations for achieving normal wrist range of motion after injury or surgery: a case series. *J Athl Train* 45:486–491, 2010.
106. Kluding PM, Santos M: Effects of ankle joint mobilizations in adults poststroke: a pilot study. *Arch Phys Med Rehabil* 89:449–456, 2008.
107. Courtney CA, Witte PO, Chmell SJ, et al.: Heightened flexor withdrawal response in individuals with knee osteoarthritis is modulated by joint compression and joint mobilization. *J Pain* 11:179–185, 2010.
109. Moss P, Sluka K, Wright A: The initial effects of knee joint mobilization on osteoarthritic hyperalgesia. *Man Ther* 12:109–118, 2007.
109. Schomacher J: The effect of an analgesic mobilization technique when applied at symptomatic or asymptomatic levels of the cervical spine in subjects with neck pain: a randomized controlled trial. *J Man Manip Ther* 17:101–108, 2009.
110. Makofsky H, Panicker S, Abbruzzese J, et al.: Immediate effect of grade IV inferior hip joint mobilization on hip abductor torque: a pilot study. *J Man Manip Ther* 15:103–110, 2007.
111. Yoder E: Physical therapy management of nonsurgical hip problems in adults. In: Echternach JL, ed. *Physical Therapy of the Hip*. New York, NY: Churchill Livingstone, 1990:103–137.
112. Tanigawa MC: Comparison of hold-relax procedure and passive mobilization on increasing muscle length. *Phys Ther* 52:725–735, 1972.
113. Barak T, Rosen E, Sofer R: Mobility: passive orthopedic manual therapy. In: Gould J, Davies G, eds. *Orthopedic and Sports Physical Therapy*. St Louis, MO: CV Mosby, 1990:195–211.
114. Maigne R: *Orthopedic Medicine*. Springfield, IL: Charles C Thomas, 1972.
115. Evjenth O, Hamberg J: *Muscle Stretching in Manual Therapy, A Clinical Manual*. Alfta, Sweden: Alfta Rehab Forlag, 1984.
116. Loubert P: A qualitative biomechanical analysis of the concave-convex rule. Proceedings, 5th International Conference of the International Federation of Orthopaedic Manipulative Therapists. Vail, CO, 1992:255–256.
117. Vicenzino B, Collins D, Benson H, et al.: An investigation of the interrelationship between manipulative therapy-induced hypoalgesia and sympathoexcitation. *J Manipulative Physiol Ther* 21:448–453, 1998.
118. Vicenzino B, Collins D, Wright A: The initial effects of a cervical spine manipulative physiotherapy treatment on the pain and dysfunction of lateral epicondylalgia. *Pain* 68:69–74, 1996.
119. Vicenzino B, Gutschlag F, Collins D, et al.: An investigation of the effects of spinal manual therapy on forequarter pressure and thermal pain thresholds and sympathetic nervous system activity in asymptomatic subjects. In: Schachloch MO, ed. *Moving in on Pain*. Adelaide: Butterworth-Heinemann, 1995:64–173.
120. Grieve GP: Manual mobilizing techniques in degenerative arthrosis of the hip. *Bull Orthop Section APTA* 2:7, 1977.
121. Freeman MAR, Wyke BD: An experimental study of articular neurology. *J Bone Joint Surg* 49B:185, 1967.
122. Meadows JTS: The principles of the Canadian approach to the lumbar dysfunction patient. In: Wadsworth C, ed. *Management of Lumbar Spine Dysfunction – Independent Home Study Course 9.3*. La Crosse, WI: APTA, Orthopaedic Section, 1999:1–5.
123. Wadsworth C: *Manual Examination and Treatment of the Spine and Extremities*. Baltimore, MD: Williams & Wilkins, 1988.
124. Sluka KA, Wright A: Knee joint mobilization reduces secondary mechanical hyperalgesia induced by capsaicin injection into the ankle joint. *Eur J Pain* 5:81–87, 2001.
125. Mulligan BR: *Manual Therapy: "NAGS", "SNAGS", "PRP'S" etc*. Wellington: Plane View Series, 1992.
126. Mulligan BR: Manual therapy rounds: mobilisations with movement (MWM's). *J Man Man Ther* 1:154–156, 1993.
127. Abbott JH, Patla CE, Jensen RH: The initial effects of an elbow mobilization with movement technique on grip strength in subjects with lateral epicondylalgia. *Man Ther* 6:163–169, 2001.
128. Vicenzino B, Wright A: Effects of a novel manipulative physiotherapy technique on tennis elbow: a single case study. *Man Ther* 1:30–35, 1995.
129. Stephens G: Lateral epicondylitis. *J Man Manip Ther* 3:50–58, 1995.
130. Miller J: Mulligan concept – management of tennis elbow. *Ortho Div Rev* May–June:45–46, 2000.
131. Fisher AGT: *Treatment by Manipulation*, 5th ed. New York, NY: Paul B Hoeber, 1948.
132. Marlin T: Manipulative Treatment for the General Practitioner. London: Edward Arnold & Co, 1934.
133. Mixter WJ, Barr JS Jr: Rupture of the intervertebral disc with involvement of the spinal canal. *N Engl J Med* 211:210–215, 1934.
134. Haldeman S: Spinal manipulative therapy in sports medicine. *Clin Sports Med* 5:277–293, 1986.
135. Gatterman MI: Glossary. In: Gatterman MI, ed. *Foundations of Chiropractic*. St. Louis, MO: Mosby, 1995:474.
136. Pettman E: Principles and practices. In: Pettman E, ed. *Manipulative Thrust Techniques – An Evidence-Based Approach*. Abbotsford, BC: Aphema Publishing, 2006:12–26.
137. Gatterman MI: Introduction. In: Gatterman MI, ed. *Chiropractic Management of Spine Related Disorders*. Baltimore, MD: Williams & Wilkins, 1990:xv–xx.
138. Kleynhans AM: Complications of and contraindications to spinal manipulative therapy. In: Haldeman S, ed. *Modern Developments in the Principles and Practice of Chiropractic*. New York, NY: Appleton-Century-Crofts, 1980:359–384.
139. Grant ER: Clinical testing before cervical manipulation – can we recognise the patient at risk? *Proceedings of the Tenth International Congress of the World Confederation for Physical Therapy*. Sydney, 1987; 192.
140. Hosek RS, Schram SB, Silverman H: Cervical manipulation. *JAMA* 245:922, 1981.
141. Dvorak J, von Orelli F: [The frequency of complications after manipulation of the cervical spine (case report and epidemiology (author's transl)]. [German]. *Schweizerische Rundschau fur Medizin Praxis* 71:64–69, 1982.
142. Bogduk N, Engel R: The menisci of the lumbar zygapophyseal joints: a review of their anatomy and clinical significance. *Spine* 9:454–460, 1984.
143. Lantz CA: The vertebral subluxation complex. In: Gatterman MI, ed. *Foundations of Chiropractic: Subluxation*. St. Louis, MO: Mosby, 1995:149–174.
144. Enneking WF, Horowitz M: The intra-articular effects of immobilization on the human knee. *J Bone Joint Surg* 54-A:973–985, 1972.
145. Terrett ACJ, Vernon H: Manipulation and pain tolerance: a controlled study of the effects of spinal manipulation on paraspinal cutaneous pain tolerance levels. *Am J Phys Med* 63:217–225, 1980.
146. Vernon HT, Dhami MSI, Annett R: Abstract from symposium on low back pain, Canadian Foundation for Spinal Research. Vancouver, 1985.
147. Akeson WH, Woo SL, Amiel D, et al.: The connective tissue response to immobility: biochemical changes in periarticular connective tissue of the immobilized rabbit knee. *Clin Orthop* 93:356–362, 1973.
148. Akeson WH, Amiel D, Woo SL-Y: Immobility effects on synovial joints: the pathomechanics of joint contracture. *Biorheology* 17:95–110, 1980.
149. Akeson WH, Amiel D, Abel MF, et al.: Effects of immobilization on joints. *Clin Orthop* 219:28–37, 1987.
150. Gross AR, Aker PD, Quartly C: Manual therapy in the treatment of neck pain. *Rheum Dis Clin North Am* 22:579–598, 1996.
151. Assendelft W, Morton S, Yu E, et al.: Spinal manipulative therapy for low back pain: a meta-analysis of effectiveness relative to other therapies. *Ann Intern Med* 138:871–881, 2003.
152. Moritz U: Evaluation of manipulation and other manual therapy: criteria for measuring the effect of treatment. *Scand J Rehabil Med* 11:173–179, 1979.
153. Glover JR, Morris JG, Khosla T: A randomized clinical trial of rotational manipulation of the trunk. *Br J Indust Med* 31:59–64, 1974.
154. Voss DE, Ionta MK, Myers DJ: *Proprioceptive Neuromuscular Facilitation: Patterns and Techniques*, 3rd ed. Philadelphia, PA: Harper and Row, 1985:1–342.

155. Pollard H, Ward G: A study of two stretching techniques for improving hip flexion range of motion. *J Man Physiol Ther* 20:443–447, 1997.
156. Kabat H: *Proprioceptive Facilitation in Therapeutic Exercises, Therapeutic Exercises.* Baltimore, MD: Waverly Press, 1965:327–343.
157. Knott M, Voss DE: *Proprioceptive Neuromuscular Facilitation*, 2nd ed. New York, NY: Harper & Row Pub Inc., 1968.
158. Sullivan PE, Markos PD, Minor MAD: *An Integrated Approach to Therapeutic Exercise.* Reston, VA: Reston Publishing Company, 1982.
159. Johnson GS, Johnson VS: The application of the principles and procedures of PNF for the care of lumbar spinal instabilities. *J Man Manip Ther* 10:83–105, 2002.
160. Janda V: Muscle weakness and inhibition (pseudoparesis) in back pain syndromes. In: Grieve G, ed. *Modern Manual therapy of the Vertebral Column.* London: Churchill Livingstone, 1986:197–201.
161. Lewit K: The contribution of clinical observation to neurobiological mechanisms in manipulative therapy. In: Korr IM, ed. *The Neurobiological Mechanisms in Manipulative Therapy.* New York, NY: Plenum Press, 1977:3–25.
162. Saliba V, Johnson G, Wardlaw C: Proprioceptive neuromuscular facilitation. In: Basmajian JV, Nyberg R, eds. *Rational Manual Therapies.* Baltimore, MD: Williams & Wilkins, 1993:243–284.
163. Hanson C: Proprioceptive neuromuscular facilitation. In: Hall C, Thein-Brody L, eds. *Therapeutic Exercise: Moving Toward Function*, 2nd ed. Baltimore, MD: Lippincott Williams & Wilkins, 2005:309–329.
164. Smolders JJ: Myofascial pain and dysfunction syndromes. In: Hammer WI, ed. *Functional Soft Tissue Examination and Treatment by Manual Methods - The Extremities.* Gaithersburg, MD: Aspen, 1991:215–234.
165. Fricton JR: Management of masticatory myofascial pain. *Semin Orthod* 1:229–243, 1995.
166. Esenyel M, Caglar N, Aldemir T: Treatment of myofascial pain. *Am J Phys Med Rehabil* 79:48–52, 2000.
167. Fricton JR: Clinical care for myofascial pain. *Dent Clin North Am* 35:1–29, 1991.
168. McClaflin RR: Myofascial pain syndrome: primary care strategies for early intervention. *Postgrad Med* 96:56–73, 1994.
169. Wolfe F, Smythe HA, Yunus MB, et al.: The American College of Rheumatology 1990 criteria for the classification of fibromyalgia. *Arthritis Rheum* 33:160–172, 1990.
170. Dommerholt J, Bron C, Franssen E: Myofascial trigger points: and evidence-informed review. *J Manual Manipulative Ther* 14:203–221, 2006.
171. Fricton JR, Kroening R, Haley D, et al.: Myofascial pain syndrome of the head and neck: a review of clinical characteristics of 164 patients. *Oral Surg Oral Med Oral Pathol* 60:615–623, 1985.
172. Fricton JR: Behavioral and psychosocial factors in chronic craniofacial pain. *Anesthes Prog* 32:7–12, 1985.
173. Simons DG: Muscular pain syndromes. In: Fricton JR, Awad E, eds. *Advances in Pain Research and Therapy.* New York, NY: Raven Press, 1990:1–41.
174. Rosen NB: The myofascial pain syndrome. *Phys Med Rehabil Clin North Am* 4:41–63, 1993.
175. Simons DG: Myofascial pain syndromes. In: Foley KM, Payne RM, eds. *Current Therapy of Pain.* New York, NY: Churchill Livingstone, 1989:368–385.
176. Meisekothen-Auleciems L: Myofascial pain syndrome: A multidisciplinary approach. *Nurse Pract* 20:18–31, 1995.
177. Goldman LB, Rosenberg NL: Myofascial pain syndrome and fibromyalgia. *Semin Neurol* 11:274–280, 1991.
178. Lewit K: *Manipulative Therapy in Rehabilitation of the Motor System*, 3rd ed. London: Butterworths, 1999.
179. Falconer J, Hayes KW, Chang RW: Therapeutic ultrasound in the treatment of musculoskeletal conditions. *Arthritis Care Res* 3:85–91, 1990.
180. Hong C-Z: Lidocaine injection versus dry needling to myofascial trigger point: the importance of the local twitch response. *Am J Phys Med Rehabil* 73:256–263, 1994.
181. Wreje U, Brorsson B: A multi-center randomized controlled trial of sterile water and saline for chronic myofascial pain syndromes. *Pain* 61:441–444, 1995.
182. Chen S-H, Wu Y-C, Hong C-Z: Current management of myofascial pain syndrome. *Clin J Pain* 6:27–46, 1996.
183. Kine GD, Warfiend CA: Myofascial pain syndrome. *Hosp Pract* 9:194–196, 1986.
184. Gam AN, Warming S, Larsen LH, et al.: Treatment of myofascial trigger-points with ultrasound combined with massage and exercise – a randomised controlled trial. *Pain* 77:73–79, 1998.
185. Lee JC, Lin DT, Hong C-Z: The effectiveness of simultaneous thermotherapy with ultrasound and electrotherapy with combined AC and DC current on the immediate pain relief of myofascial trigger point. *J Musculoske Pain* 5:81–90, 1997.
186. Woolf CF: Segmental afferent fiber-induced analgesia: transcutaneous electrical nerve stimulation (TENS) and vibration. In: Wall PD, Melzack R, eds. *Textbook of Pain.* New York, NY: Churchill Livingstone, 1989:884–896.
187. Hsueh TC, Cheng PT, Kuan TS, et al.: The immediate effectiveness of electrical nerve stimulation and electrical muscle stimulation on myofascial trigger points. *Am J Phys Med Rehabil* 76:471–476, 1997.

Neurodynamic Mobility and Mobilizations

CHAPTER 11

CHAPTER OBJECTIVES

At the completion of this chapter, the reader will be able to:

1. Summarize the various types of neurodynamic examination and mobilization techniques.
2. Describe the proposed mechanisms behind the neurodynamic examination and mobilization techniques.
3. Apply knowledge of the various neurodynamic mobilization techniques in the planning of a comprehensive rehabilitation program.
4. Recognize the manifestations of abnormal nervous tissue tension and develop strategies using neurodynamic mobilization techniques to treat these abnormalities.
5. Evaluate the effectiveness of a neurodynamic mobilization technique when used as a direct intervention.

OVERVIEW

Neurodynamics is the study of the mechanics and physiology of the nervous system. The nervous system is an electrical, chemical, and mechanical structure with continuity between its two subdivisions: the central and peripheral nervous systems (see Chapter 3). In addition to permitting inter- and intraneural communication throughout the entire network, the nervous system is capable of withstanding mechanical stress as a result of its unique mechanical characteristics. Nervous tissue, a form of connective tissue, is viscoelastic. This viscoelasticity allows for the transfer of mechanical stress throughout the nervous system during trunk or limb movements. This adaptation results from changes in the length of the spinal cord[1] and the capacity of the peripheral nerves to adapt to different positions. The peripheral nerves adapt through a process of passive movement relative to the surrounding tissue via a gliding apparatus around the nerve trunk.[2,3] Three mechanisms appear to play an important role in this adaptability[3]:

- Elongation of the nerve against elastic forces. In normal daily movement, nerves may slide up to 2 cm in relation to surrounding tissues and contend with a strain of 10%.[4]
- Longitudinal movement of the nerve trunk in the longitudinal direction.
- An increase and decrease of tissue relaxation at the level of the nerve trunk.

According to Millesi,[3] the efficiency of this mechanism partially depends on the capacity of the loose connective tissue around the nerve (adventitia, conjunctiva nervorum, perineurium) to allow any traction forces to be distributed over the whole length of the nerve.[3] If this distribution of forces is compromised, an unfavorable rise in traction forces can occur at certain segments, depending on the anatomic site (see next section).[3]

The role that tension on the neural tissue plays in pain and dysfunction has been studied for over a century. During this time, a number of specific tests have been designed to examine the neurological structures for the presence of adaptive shortening and inflammation.[5–7] The more common of these neurodynamic mobility tests are described in this chapter.

PROPOSED MECHANISMS FOR NEURODYNAMIC DYSFUNCTION

The spinal dura (see Chapter 3) forms a loose sheath around the spinal cord from the foramen magnum to the level of the second sacral tubercle. From there it continues as the filum terminale to the end at the coccyx. Laterally, the dura surrounds the exiting spinal nerve roots at the level of the intervertebral foramen. There are three areas called *tension sites*, in which the dura is tethered to the bony canal, providing stability to the spinal cord. These tension sites are found at the segmental levels of C6, T6, and L4; the elbow; the shoulder; and the knee have similar sites.[5,8] As a result of these sites of tension, the neurologic tissues move in different directions, depending on where the stress is applied and in which order it is applied.[7]

During movement, neural tissue takes its lead from the movement of joints and muscles, with the physical loading of the nerve dependent on the location of the nerve in relation to the joint axis.[4] Various studies have demonstrated excursion of the nerve complex during movements of the extremity.[1,8–12] Under normal circumstances, the tension sites are not adversely affected by motion of the extremities. However, if the dura becomes adherent, excessive stress may be produced in the areas of adhesion, increasing the length of the dura

TABLE 11-1 Sites of Peripheral Nerve and Nerve Root Vulnerability

Site	Description
Tunnels	Hard sided tunnels, such as the carpal tunnel, increase the probability of spatial compromise of the nerve. Within a tunnel, the contained nervous system always has the potential to rub on the tunnel structure, creating friction, and any trauma or alteration to the tunnel structure can mechanically or chemically compromise the neural structures
Branches	It is more difficult for the nerve to move away from forces at those points where a nerve branches (e.g., radial nerve at the elbow)
Hard interfaces	A nerve is more readily compressed if it lies on a bone or passes through fascia (e.g., radial nerve in the spiral groove of the humerus)
Proximity to the surface	Superficial nerves, such as the sensory radial nerve in the forearm, are more vulnerable to external compression
Adherence to interfacing structures	Some areas of nerve are more firmly adherent to interfacing tissues than others (e.g., the common fibular (peroneal) nerve at the head of the fibula)

Data from: Butler DS, Tomberlin JP: Peripheral nerve: structure, function, and physiology. In: Magee D, Zachazewski JE, Quillen WS, eds. *Scientific Foundations and Principles of Practice in Musculoskeletal Rehabilitation*. St. Louis, MI: WB Saunders, 2007:175–189.

beyond its normal limit of tension (Table 11-1).[13] Theoretically, increased dural tension may be felt throughout the neuromeningeal system and, potentially, it may affect the range of motion available to the trunk and to an extremity. Pathomechanically, a decrease in the mobility of a nerve along its entire length makes the nerve more vulnerable to additional injuries during repetitive movements.[13,14]

CLINICAL PEARL

Neural tissue responds to trauma in the same way that a ligament or tendon does, by evoking the cascade of the inflammatory process, resulting in pain when stressed.[15,16] In addition to the effect that the inflammatory process can have on the nerve tissue, fibrous tissue formation can develop within the nerve root sheath causing adhesions between the sheath and the nerve root.[16,17]

The nerves and their microcirculation are vulnerable to tension, friction, and compressive forces at multiple sites along their routes.[14] A number of mechanisms (excluding diseases such as diabetes mellitus, hypothyroidism, immune deficiency syndromes, rheumatoid arthritis, and alcoholism) are hypothesized to contribute to an injury of the peripheral nerve trunk. These include the following[18]:

- ***Posture.*** Sustained postures that produce changes in the natural curves of the spine can result in a shortening of the distance traveled by the peripheral nerve trunk and eventual adaptive shortening of these structures. Correction of this posture, after sufficient time has elapsed for it to have taken place, may produce a stretching of the neural tissues.
- ***Direct trauma.*** Orthopaedic injuries account for some of the injuries to peripheral nerves. For example, the radial nerve is injured through orthopaedic trauma more than any other major nerve.[19] Nerve injuries can occur as the result of a direct blow to the nerve or secondary to damage of an adjacent structure such as a fracture,[20,21] joint dislocation,[22] or tendon rupture.[23] Other causes of direct nerve trauma have included injections,[24] joint manipulation,[25] and surgical procedures.[26] Neurological injury is one of the more serious complications of fracture and dislocation, both in the short and long term. For example, the prevalence of injury to the sciatic nerve after acetabular fracture or fracture-dislocation of the hip has been reported to be between 10–25%.[27]
- ***Extremes of motion.*** Given the course of many of the peripheral nerve trunks, it is not difficult to envision movements of the extremities that could place a traction force on these trunks. Indeed, those very same movements are exploited in some of the neurodynamic mobility tests.
- ***Electrical injury.*** In a 17-year review of burn unit admissions, permanent nerve injuries were found in 22% of electrocuted patients.[28] The upper limb was most commonly involved with the median and ulnar nerves most commonly injured.[28] Postneurologic symptoms in such cases can vary from neuropathy to complex regional pain syndrome (CRPS).
- ***Compression.*** Compression to a nerve can occur during muscle contraction and as a result of tight fascia, osteochondroma, ganglia, lipomas and other benign neoplasms, and bony protuberances.

CLINICAL PEARL

The sympathetic nervous system is part of the peripheral nervous system, and sympathetic neurons in peripheral nerves are subject to the same deformation and injury potential during movement as somatic neurons.[4]

Double-Crush Injuries

The double-crush syndrome (DCS) is a general term referring to the coexistence of dual neuropathies along the course of a peripheral nerve. The concept was proposed by Upton and McComas in 1973[29] who suggested that proximal compression of a nerve may decrease the ability of the nerve to withstand a more distal compression.

From the pathophysiological viewpoint, impairment of neural excursion, loss of elasticity, underlying abnormality of the connective tissue as well as direct pressure on the nerve may lead to disruption of axons, impairment of axonal transport, endoneural edema, or ischemic changes in nerves.[29] For example, according to this theory, a cervical radiculopathy, manifesting as little more than neck pain and stiffness, could precipitate a distal focal entrapment neuropathy.[29] The term *double-crush syndrome* is used to describe this mechanism of nerve injury: serial compromise of axonal transport along the same nerve fiber causing a subclinical lesion at the distal site to become symptomatic.

At least eight other etiologic mechanisms have been proposed to explain the relationship between the proximal and distal nerve fiber lesions[29–33]:

1. A proximal nerve lesion renders the distal nerve segment more vulnerable to compression because of serial constraints of axoplasmic flow.
2. The peripheral nerves possess an underlying susceptibility to pressure.
3. Interruption of lymphatic and venous drainage at the proximal nerve lesion site renders the distal nerve segment more vulnerable.
4. Endoneurial edema at one lesion site compromises neural circulation, rendering nerve fibers at the other site more vulnerable.
5. A connective tissue abnormality common to both sites along the nerve fibers.
6. Tethering of the nerve at one site causes injurious shear forces at the other site.
7. Entrapment of the nerve at one site causes decreased use of the muscle pump, which creates a slight, generalized edema of the limb. This increases tissue pressure in certain anatomic passages, which causes an additional entrapment nerve lesion.
8. The initial nerve lesion releases a metabolite that passes through the free intraneural circulation and increases the vulnerability of other segments of the nerve.

Since its introduction, the double-crush hypothesis has been invoked to explain a great number of coexisting proximal and distal nerve impairments. In fact, it has been expanded in various ways (i.e., to triple-crush, quadruple-crush, and multiple-crush syndromes, as well as the reversed DCS).[31,34,35] Despite its acceptance, there are situations where the double-crush hypothesis has anatomic and pathophysiologic restrictions that render it inapplicable in some clinical situations.[36] For the DCS to occur, there must be anatomic continuity of nerve fibers between the two (or more) lesions sites. If this is lacking, then sequential impairment of axoplasmic flow obviously cannot occur. Consequently, two focal nerve disorders along the same neural pathway (e.g., cervical root lesions and carpal tunnel syndrome) do not automatically fulfil this anatomic criterion of DCS unless the same axons are compromised at both sites.[36]

Although, experimental studies of the double-crush hypothesis have shown that successive lesions along a peripheral nerve can summate,[32,37,38] studies that have attempted to demonstrate the existence of DCS have proved inconclusive.[39–41]

Neurophysiological examination is critical in distinguishing between a single or a double lesion as well as determining the comparative severity of the two lesions.

NEURODYNAMIC MOBILITY EXAMINATIONS

Both Elvey[42] and Butler[13] have been credited with the development of the examination techniques for neurodynamic mobility. Elvey[42] developed what he named the *brachioplexus tension test,* which was later called the *upper limb tension test* (ULTT). Similar tests, such as the straight leg raise (SLR) and prone knee flexion tests, have been designed for the lower extremity. The slump test is considered to be a general test of neurodynamic mobility. The tension tests are designed to apply controlled mechanical and compressive stresses to the dura and other neurologic tissues, both centrally and peripherally.[43] These neurodynamic tests are designed to assess the contribution of the spinal nerve roots and peripheral nerves to extremity pain by employing a sequential and progressive stretch to the dura. The tests place tensile stresses on the dura of spinal nerve roots and peripheral nerves using a longitudinal traction force of the nerve until the patient's symptoms are reproduced.[6]

The examination of neural adhesions is by no means an exact science, but the principles are based on sound anatomic theory. Knowledge of the course of each of the peripheral nerves is thus essential in order to put a sequential and adequate tension through each of them (see Chapter 3).

Breig's tissue-borrowing phenomenon offers a plausible explanation for the neurodynamic tests.[44] Breig observed that tension produced in a lumbosacral nerve root results in displacement of the neighboring dura, nerve roots, and lumbosacral plexus toward the site of tension.[13,44–46] In effect, a borrowing of the resting slack in neighboring meningeal tissues occurs as neural structures are pulled toward the site of increased tension. This results in a decrease in the available slack and potential mobility of the neural tissues throughout the region.[7,44–48] This stretching and displacement of the nerve roots plexi reduces the available mobility of the peripheral nerves.[7,44–48]

Positive symptoms for the presence of neuropathic dysfunction include pain, paresthesia, and spasm.[18] Unfortunately, these signs and symptoms are also associated with a host of musculoskeletal injuries. Asbury and Fields[49] hypothesized that the type of pain that results from an injury to a peripheral nerve is characteristic and has two varieties:

1. ***Dysesthetic pain.*** This type of pain is felt in the peripheral sensory distribution of a sensory or mixed nerve and results from nociceptive afferent fibers.
2. ***Nerve trunk pain.*** This type of pain results from the nociceptors within the nerve sheaths and exhibits a pain distribution following the course of the nerve trunk.[18]

However, relying on the reproduction of a type of pain (a subjective issue at the best of times) is not sufficient to make the diagnosis of neural tissue dysfunction.

Because the subject of neural provocation tests and the intervention of neurodynamic mobilization remain controversial, the clinician should ensure that the results of these tests are always used in conjunction with findings from a complete neuromusculoskeletal examination, including the following:[18,43,50,51]

- ***Observation.*** An injury to a peripheral nerve trunk may result in visible atrophy within its motor distribution.
- ***Palpation.*** The clinician should carefully palpate along each of the nerve trunks in the region where they are superficial. Physical deformation of an irritated nerve should reproduce pain with palpation.
- ***Range of motion.*** In areas of decreased neural mobility, both active and passive range of motion may be diminished in the same direction. However, a lesion to the musculotendinous unit would also reproduce pain with the same maneuver, particularly in muscles that cross two joints.
- ***Resistive testing.*** Resistive tests can be used to examine for the presence of weakness in the distribution of a peripheral nerve and to help differentiate between pain reproduced with active or passive range of motion that indicates damage to the musculotendinous unit and pain that results from neural tension. For example, pain reproduced in the posterior thigh with the SLR may indicate a lesion of the hamstring muscle belly or a lesion to the sciatic nerve. If resisted knee flexion does not reproduce pain, the musculotendinous unit is unlikely to be at fault, leaving the sciatic nerve as the likely cause.

The purpose of the physical examination is to determine which tissue is at fault. This is accomplished by isolating (where possible) each tissue that has the potential to produce those symptoms and selectively stressing that tissue. Part of the problem with this approach lies in the fact that a positive finding for many of the techniques designed to assess the integrity of a neural structure may just be the result of a sensitive movement, rather than a stretch of the dura.[52] For example, when wrist extension is performed with the elbow in extension and the shoulder abducted, in addition to placing stress through the elbow and wrist joints, wrist flexors, and elbow flexors, the loading of the nervous system is continued proximally, at least up to the level of the axilla.[53]

Some of the so-called dural symptoms could also result from the imparted stretch on the dura during the various maneuvers, producing changes in the axoplasmic flow inside the nerves, provoking the firing of abnormal impulses, and decreasing the vascular supply to the nerve.[54–56]

SLUMP TEST

A neural tension test performed in a sitting position is necessary to simulate the extremes of spinal motion associated with symptom-provoking activities such as slouched sitting or entering and exiting a car.[57–59]

The slump test, popularized by Maitland,[59] is a combination of other neuromeningeal tests, namely, the seated SLR, neck flexion, and lumbar slumping. In the slump test, the patient is seated in full flexion of the thoracic and lumbar regions of the spine.[60] Sensitizing maneuvers are then systematically applied and released to the cervical spine and lower extremities while the tester maintains the patient's trunk position. The slump test assesses the excursion of neural tissues within the vertebral canal and intervertebral foramen[58] and detects impairments to neural tissue mobility from a number of sources as identified by Macnab[61] and Fahrni.[62] Maitland asserted that the slump test enables the tester to detect adverse nerve root tension caused by spinal stenosis, extraforaminal lateral disk herniation, disk sequestration, nerve root adhesions, and vertebral impingement.[57,58]

CLINICAL PEARL

The slump test has been shown to induce sympathetic responses in humans, so clinicians are urged to consider the possibility that the structure and function of sympathetic neurons, either in the trunk or in the peripheral nerve, may be adversely affected, particularly when injuries are longstanding or recurrent in nature.[4]

Several studies[44,48,63,64] have demonstrated the effects of trunk and head position on neural structures within the vertebral canal and intervertebral foramen during slump testing. These studies reported that full spinal flexion or flexion of the cervical, thoracic, and lumbar regions of the spine produces lengthening of the vertebral canal. This elongation of the vertebral canal stretches the spinal dura and transmits tension to the spinal cord, lumbosacral nerve root sleeves, and nerve roots.[44,48,63–65] During full spinal flexion, the cauda equina becomes taut and the lumbosacral nerve roots and root sleeves are pulled into contact with the pedicle of the superior vertebra.[44,63,64,66]

CLINICAL PEARL

One study[67] found that a positive slump test was recorded in 57% of subjects with apparent repetitive grade I hamstring strains suggesting some form of relationship between the hamstrings and the sciatic nerve.

When extension of the cervical spine is introduced, the dura and the nerve roots slacken as the vertebral canal begins to shorten.[44,63–66,68] Extending the thoracic and lumbar spines increases the slack in the neural tissues as the vertebral canal continues to shorten.[44,63–66,68]

Because the slump test is a combination of other tests, a choice as to its use needs to be made. Either the classic SLR test or its variations should be performed; or the slump test should be used.[69] The only advantage of the slump test over the SLR test is that it increases the compression forces through the intervertebral disks and will highlight the presence of dural adhesions.[69] Depending on which text is read, there is a wide variety of progressive steps to the slump test; particularly when the lumbar kyphosis stage is introduced. Although the specific order of implementation remains controversial, it is important that the clinician consistently use the same sequence with each patient.

CLINICAL PEARL

- *Bechterew's test.* Bechterew's test is an abbreviated slump test, performed by asking the seated patient to actively extend his or her uninvolved leg at the knee, to lower that leg and then subsequently extend the involved leg. If symptoms are not produced, the patient is asked to extend both legs at the knee simultaneously. A positive finding includes the reproduction of radicular pain below the knee, inability to attain full knee extension, leaning backward and bracing oneself on the table (tripod sign), or any combination thereof.
- *Sitting root test.* This is another test similar to the slump test. With the patient seated and his or her neck flexed to the chest, the clinician places one hand on the distal thigh of the tested leg to prevent hip flexion and uses the other hand to extend the lower leg at the knee. Any of the typical SLR responses is considered a positive finding. If the test is negative, the clinician may increase tension placed on neural elements by adding trunk flexion.

As soon as symptoms are reproduced during these tests, the test should be terminated. It is worth remembering that during a dural tension test, the dura itself does not move. It is merely stressed; hence, the name for the tests. One such method of sequencing is described next.

The patient is positioned sitting with the hands behind the back, the popliteal creases just off the edge of the bed and a slight arch in the back (Fig. 11-1), and the head flexed and then placed in neutral. This initial position is then followed by a slump of the lumbar and thoracic spine with a posterior pelvic tilt as the clinician maintains the patient's neck in neutral (Fig. 11-2).

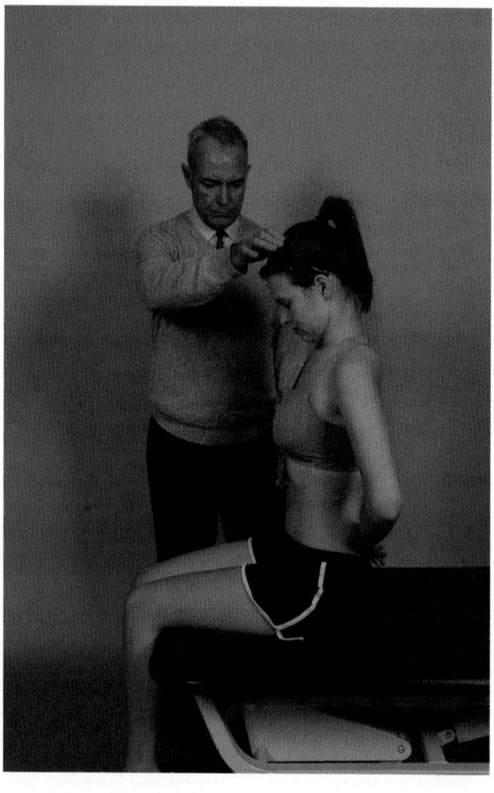

FIGURE 11-1 The slump test 1.

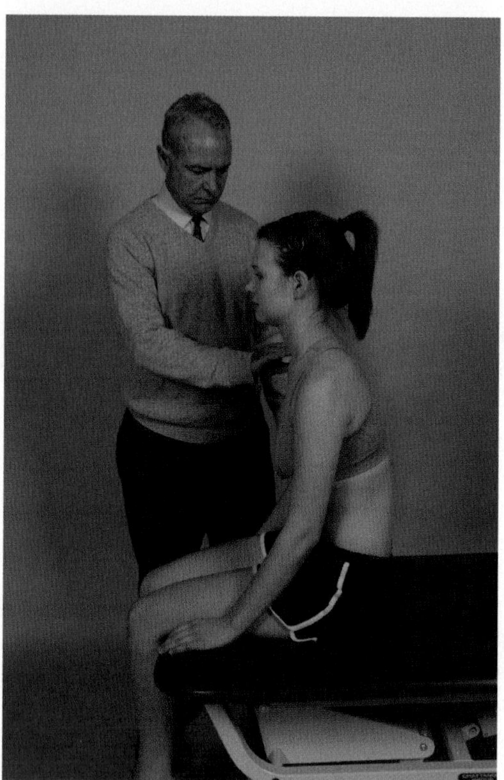

FIGURE 11-2 The slump test 2.

This maneuver has the effect of tightening the entire dura including the thorax dura. If the test is still negative, the patient is asked to flex the neck by first applying a chin tuck and placing the chin on the chest and then to straighten the knee as much as possible. Overpressure is then gently applied to the upper thoracic and the lower cervical spine and maintained throughout the examination (Fig. 11-3). The subject's ankle is then passively dorsiflexed to the point of slight resistance, while the knee is slowly passively extended to full extension or to the point when the subject reports an onset of neural mediated symptoms (Fig. 11-4). If the patient is unable to straighten the knee because of a reproduction of symptoms, he or she is asked to actively extend the neck. Following extension of the neck, if the patient cannot straighten the knee further, the test can be considered positive.

The test can also be performed in reverse because a positive response may occur in one direction but not the other.

It is important to note that no diagnostic accuracy studies have been performed to determine the sensitivity and specificity of the slump test. A recent study by Davis and colleagues[70] found the slump test had a high false positive rate in asymptomatic individuals and recommended that the current criteria for determining a positive test should be examined using new range of motion cutoff scores. The study also recommended that the test should be considered positive only when peripheral symptoms are reproduced before 22 degrees of knee extension.[70]

LOWER EXTREMITY TENSION TESTS

Sciatica is defined as pain along the course of the sciatic nerve or its branches and is most commonly caused by a herniated disk or by spinal stenosis.[71] Characteristically, patients with sciatica

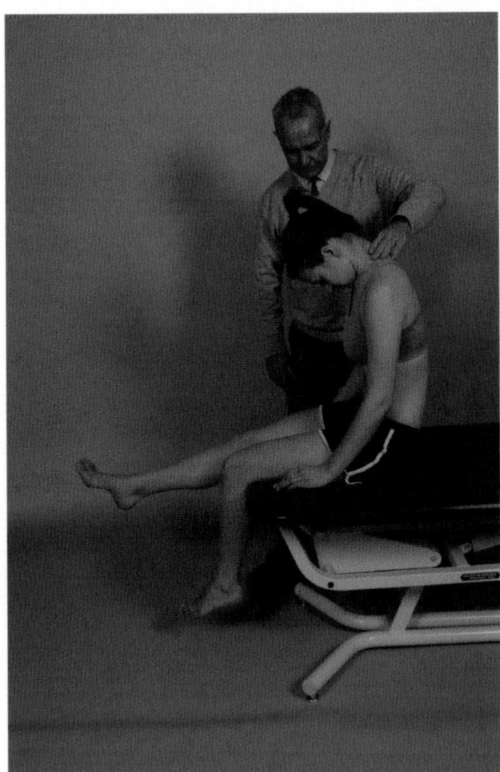

FIGURE 11-3 The slump test 3.

report gluteal pain radiating down the posterior thigh and leg, paresthesia in the calf or foot, and varying degrees of motor weakness. Extraspinal entrapment of the sciatic nerve (i.e., along its course within the pelvis or the lower extremity), although infrequent, is difficult to diagnose because its

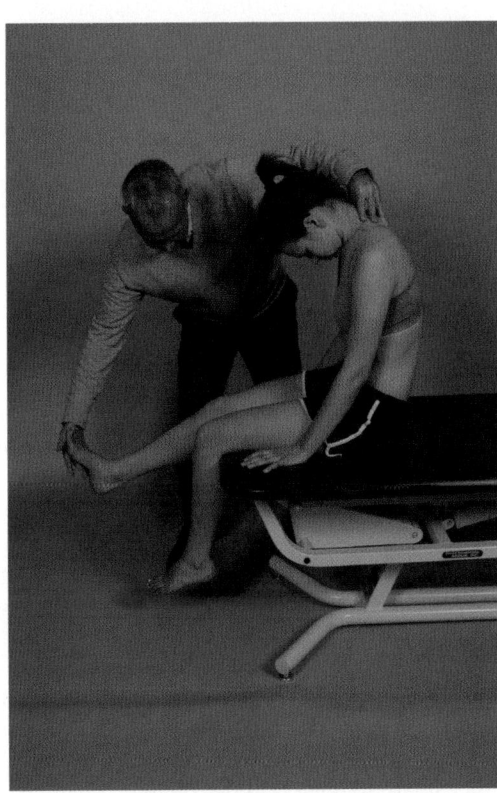

FIGURE 11-4 The slump test 4.

symptoms are similar to those of the more frequent causes of sciatica.[72–74]

Straight Leg Raise

The SLR test is recognized as the first neural tissue tension test to appear in the literature. It was first described by Lasègue well over 100 years ago.[75]

CLINICAL PEARL

The SLR test should be a routine test during the examination of the lumbar spine among patients with sciatica or pseudoclaudication. However, the test is often negative in patients with spinal stenosis.[76]

The patient is positioned supine with no pillow under the head. The patient's trunk and hip should remain neutral, avoiding internal or external rotation, and excessive adduction or abduction. Each leg is raised individually (uninvolved side first). To ensure that there is no undue stress on the dura, the tested leg is placed in slight internal rotation and adduction of the hip and extension of the knee. The clinician holds the patient's heel, maintaining the extension and neutral dorsiflexion at the ankle, and raises the straight leg (Fig. 11-5) until complaints of pain or tightness in the posterior thigh are elicited.[13] At this point, the range of motion is noted and the clinician then lowers the straight leg slightly until the patient reports a decrease in symptoms.

The evaluation of the findings from the SLR test requires that the range of motion measured and the symptoms produced are compared with the contralateral side and with expected norms.[7,77–80] Because sitting knee extension and the SLR culminate in essentially identical positions, symptomatic responses to the two types of maneuvers should be similar, although the angle at which pain is elicited may vary.[81]

CLINICAL PEARL

Confounding the results from the SLR test are the non-neural structures such as the sacroiliac joint, lumbar zygapophyseal joints, hip joint, muscles (hamstrings), and connective tissue. These structures may limit leg elevation and provoke patient discomfort during testing.[7,78–80,82]

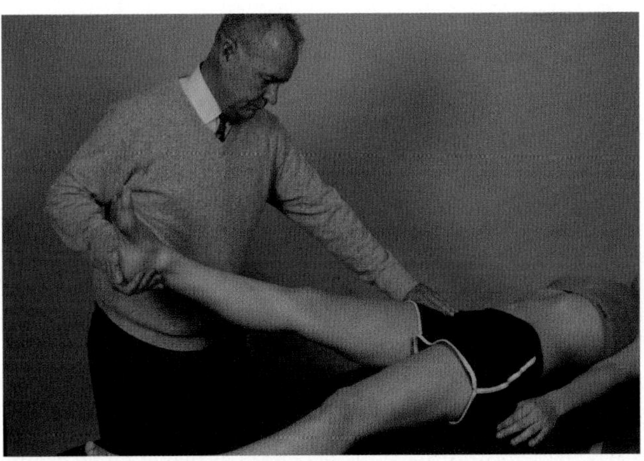

FIGURE 11-5 The straight leg raise.

It is generally agreed that the first 30 degrees of the SLR serves to take up the slack or crimp in the sciatic nerve and its continuations. Using symptom reproduction below 40 degrees as a criterion for a positive SLR test result has been found to increase the sensitivity to 72%.[83]

Pain in the 0- to 30-degree range may indicate the presence of

- acute spondylolisthesis
- tumor of the buttock
- gluteal abscess
- very large disk protrusion or extrusion[84]
- acute inflammation of the dura
- malingering patient
- the sign of the buttock

Between 30 and 70 degrees, the spinal nerves, their dural sleeves, and the roots of the L4, L5, S1, and S2 segments are stretched with an excursion of 2–6 mm.[85] After 70 degrees, although these structures undergo further tension, other structures also become involved. These additional structures include the hamstrings, gluteus maximus, hip, lumbar, and sacroiliac joints. An SLR test is positive if

- the range is limited by spasm to less than 70 degrees, suggesting compression or irritation of the nerve roots. A positive test reproduces the symptoms of sciatica, with pain that radiates below the knee, not merely back or hamstring pain.[76] When the SLR is severely limited, it is considered diagnostic for a disk herniation.[86]
- the pain reproduced is neurologic in nature. This pain should be accompanied by other signs and symptoms such as pain with coughing, tying of shoe laces and so on but not necessarily by muscle weakness.

CLINICAL PEARL

The SLR test places a tensile stress on the sciatic nerve and exerts a caudal traction on the lumbosacral nerve roots from L4 to S2.[7,9,62,66,80] During the SLR, the L4–L5 and S1–S2 nerve roots are tracked inferiorly and anteriorly, pulling the dura mater caudally, laterally, and anteriorly. Tension in the sciatic nerve, and its continuations, occurs in a sequential manner developing first in the greater sciatic foramen, then over the ala of the sacrum, next in the area where the nerve crosses over the pedicle, and finally in the intervertebral foramen.

The inferior and anterior pull on the nerve root, and the relative fixation of the dural investment at the anterior wall, produces a displacement that pulls the root against the posterior-lateral aspect of the disk and vertebra. In addition, any space-occupying lesions situated at the anterior wall of the vertebral canal at the fourth and fifth lumbar and first and second sacral segments may interfere with the dura mater or nerve root structures.

The following caveats are important for accurate assessment of the SLR:

- The patient must have the necessary available range of hip flexion (30–70 degrees).

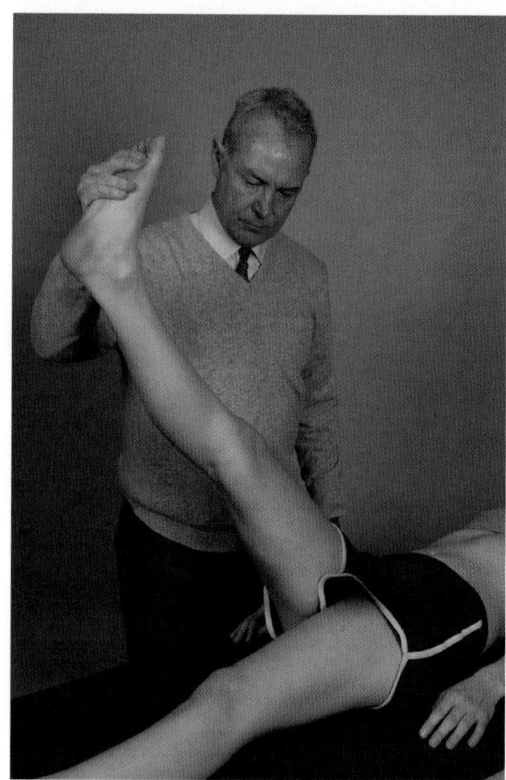

FIGURE 11-6 The straight leg raise with ankle dorsiflexion.

- The SLR produces a posterior shear and some degree of rotation in the lumbar spine (a region not well suited to shearing or rotational forces). Thus, back pain alone with the SLR is not a positive test.[81]

CLINICAL PEARL

Ipsilateral SLR has sensitivity but not specificity for a herniated IVD. For example, Deyo and colleagues[87] noted a sensitivity of 80% and a specificity of 40% for the SLR in the diagnosis of low lumbar disk herniation and Van den Hoogen and colleagues[88] reported a sensitivity of 88–100% and a specificity of 11–44% for the SLR in the diagnosis of lumbar disk herniation.

Sensitizers

Passive dorsiflexion of the ankle (Braggard's test) (Fig. 11-6) and/or passive cervical flexion (Soto-Hall test) may be used as sensitizers for the SLR test. The cervical flexion can also be performed actively (Fig. 11-7). In addition, further internal rotation or extreme adduction of the hip may also be added to the SLR. These additional maneuvers increase the tension exerted on the spinal cord, spinal dura, and lumbosacral nerve roots.[7,13,44–46,48,89] Research studies[44–47,63,89] have demonstrated that cervical flexion lengthens the spinal cord and dura. This action may provoke radicular symptoms without stressing nonneural tissues in the lower extremity.[13,58,90]

Thus, the dura can be pulled from below, using dorsiflexion, or from above, using cervical flexion. Further modifications can be incorporated to place stress through different branches of the sciatic and common fibular (peroneal) nerves by adjusting the ankle and foot position. Coppieters and colleagues[91] evaluated

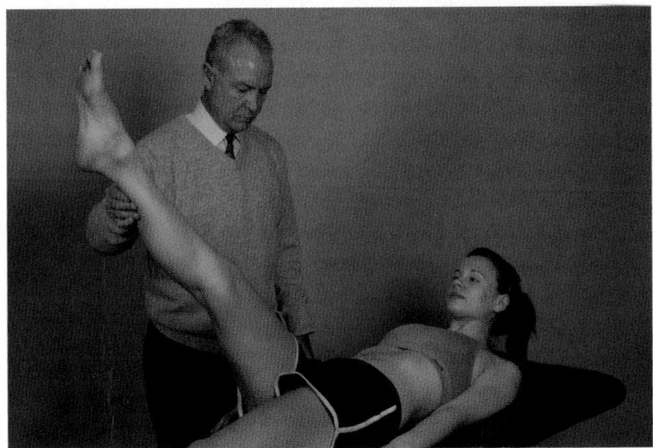

FIGURE 11-7 The straight leg raise with active cervical flexion.

the clinical hypothesis that strain in the nerves around the ankle and foot caused by ankle dorsiflexion can be further increased with hip flexion. Linear displacement transducers were inserted into the sciatic, tibial, and plantar nerves and plantar fascia of eight embalmed cadavers to measure strain during the modified SLR. Nerve excursion was measured with a digital caliper. Ankle dorsiflexion resulted in a significant strain and distal excursion of the tibial nerve. With the ankle in dorsiflexion, the proximal excursion and tension increases in the sciatic nerve associated with hip flexion were transmitted distally along the nerve from the hip to beyond the ankle. As hip flexion has an impact on the nerves around the ankle and foot but not on the plantar fascia, the modified SLR may be a useful test to differentially diagnose plantar heel pain. Although the modified SLR caused the greatest increase in nerve strain nearest to the moving joint, mechanical forces acting on peripheral nerves are transmitted well beyond the moving joint. Based on these findings, the following ankle and foot adjustments can be made:

- Dorsiflexion, foot eversion, and toe extension stress the tibial branch.
- Dorsiflexion and inversion stress the sural nerve.
- Plantar flexion and inversion stress the common fibular (peroneal) nerve (deep and superficial).

If symptoms are not reproduced with the SLR but the slump test is positive, numerous reasons have been proposed, and the following are few among them[69]:

- The presence of a soft disk protrusion, particularly a central soft protrusion. Soft central protrusions need loading through weight bearing and are often negative in a non–weight-bearing position.
- Acute spondylolisthesis.
- Posterior instability.
- Malingering patient/nonorganic symptoms.

CLINICAL PEARL

Kemp's test uses the patient's trunk as both a lever to induce tension and as a compressive force. The test may be performed with the patient in either the seated or standing position.

- *Seated.* With the patient seated and arms crossed over the chest, the clinician uses one hand to stabilize the patient's lumbosacral region on the side to be tested and the other arm to control the patient's upper body movement. The patient is passively directed into trunk flexion, rotation, sidebending, and finally extension. Depending on the patient's response, axial compression may be applied in the fully extended and rotated position to increase stress on the posterior joints. Radiating pain down the leg provoked anywhere along the arc of movement should be noted and the test should be discontinued at that point. Often patients will report dull or achy pain stemming from the lumbar spine that may be due to facet or extraspinal soft tissue irritation.
- *Standing.* The standing version of Kemp's test is performed by asking the patient to place the back of his or her hand on the ipsilateral gluteal region and then slide the hand distally down the posterior thigh. Axial compression may be applied by pressing downward on the patient's shoulders. For clinicians desiring either more control over patient positioning or less muscle activation, the seated version of Kemp's test may be preferable.

Crossed Straight Leg Raise Sign

The crossed SLR sign, or Well leg raising test of Fajersztajn,[80] is associated with the SLR test. There are three recognized types:

1. SLR that produces pain in the contralateral leg but not when the contralateral leg is raised.
2. SLR that produces pain in both legs.
3. SLR of either leg that produces pain in the contralateral limb. For example, SLR of the right leg produces pain in the left leg and SLR of the left leg produces pain in the right leg.

There are many theories as to the cause and significance of the crossover sign. One theory suggests that the neuromeninges are pulled caudally, resulting in compression of the dural sleeve against a large or medially displaced disk herniation. The crossed SLR is considered relatively insensitive but highly specific and is thought to be more significant than the SLR test in terms of its diagnostic powers to indicate the presence of a large disk protrusion.[92] For example, Kosteljanetz and colleagues [93] found the test to have 24% sensitivity and 100% specificity, and Kerr and colleagues[94] found the test to have a sensitivity of 25% and a specificity of 95%. One study goes so far as to recommend using the combined results from the SLR and crossed SLR for a more accurate diagnosis.[88]

The following findings are strongly predictive of disk herniation[84,92,95]:

- Severely limited SLR.
- Positive crossover SLR.
- Severely restricted and painful trunk movements.

Bilateral Straight Leg Raise

Once the unilateral SLR test is completed, the clinician should test both legs simultaneously (Fig. 11-8). A limitation of the

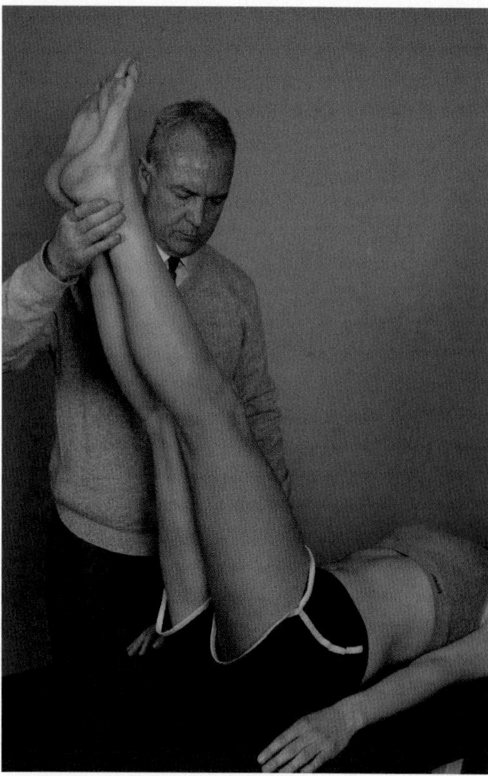

FIGURE 11-8 The bilateral straight leg raise.

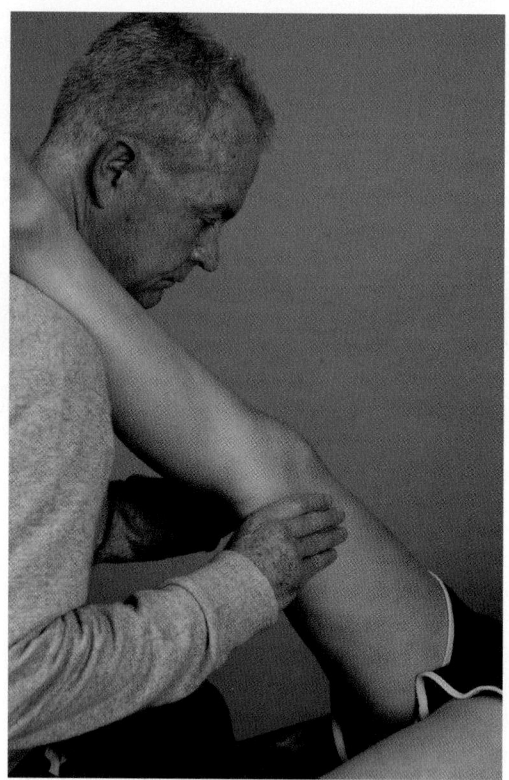

FIGURE 11-9 SLR bowstring (popliteal space pressure).

unilateral SLR is that it may not highlight the presence of a central disk protrusion, particularly a soft disk protrusion.[78] By performing a bilateral SLR and incorporating both neck flexion and dorsiflexion, central protrusions may be detected.[69]

Because a central protrusion may mimic a lateral recess stenosis, a differentiation test is needed. The bicycle test of van Gelderen[96] is advocated. The patient is appropriately positioned on a bicycle and asked to pedal against resistance.

- A patient with lateral spinal stenosis tolerates this position well.
- A patient with intermittent claudication of the lower extremities typically experiences an increase in symptoms with continued exercise, regardless of the position of the spine.
- A patient with intermittent cauda equina compression typically has an increase of symptoms with an increase in lumbar lordosis.
- A patient with a disk herniation usually fairs well if the lumbar spine remains extended.

Bowstring Tests

The bowstring tests are named after the technique applied to the nerve under examination. Both the tibial and the common fibular (peroneal) nerves can be tested and although the tests impart an insufficient stretch of the dura to detect chronic adhesions, they can be used to make a prognosis about acute disk herniations. A positive bowstring test is a strong indicator for surgery but it need only be performed if the SLR is positive with the addition of dorsiflexion.[69]

Sciatic Tension Test

The sciatic tension test, also referred to as the Deyerle and May test, reproduces the mechanics of the Bowstring test in a seated position. The tibial nerve travels down the middle of the posterior thigh between the femoral condyles and down the back and middle of the calf entering the foot under the medial malleolus of the ankle (see Chapter 3). The involved extremity is extended at the knee to the point of pain and then lowered slightly to decrease pain. The clinician supports the patient's leg on his or her shoulder and then applies finger pressure to the popliteal fossa in an attempt to tension the sciatic nerve (Fig. 11-9). If the symptoms return with this maneuver, the test is considered positive.

Common Fibular (Peroneal) Test

Typically, the common fibular (peroneal) nerve travels with the tibial branch to the posterior distal thigh region (see Chapter 3). It then wraps itself around the fibular head and has strong attachments to the tendon of the biceps femoris. The procedure for this test is similar to that of the tibial version of the test except that after the knee is slightly flexed, the clinician pulls the biceps femoris tendon at the fibular head medially and laterally (Fig. 11-10). If this maneuver reproduces the symptoms, it is considered a positive test.

Prone Knee Bending Test

The prone knee bending (PKB) test stretches the femoral nerve using hip extension and knee flexion to stretch the nerve termination in the quadriceps muscle.[69] This test has been used to indicate the presence of upper lumbar disk

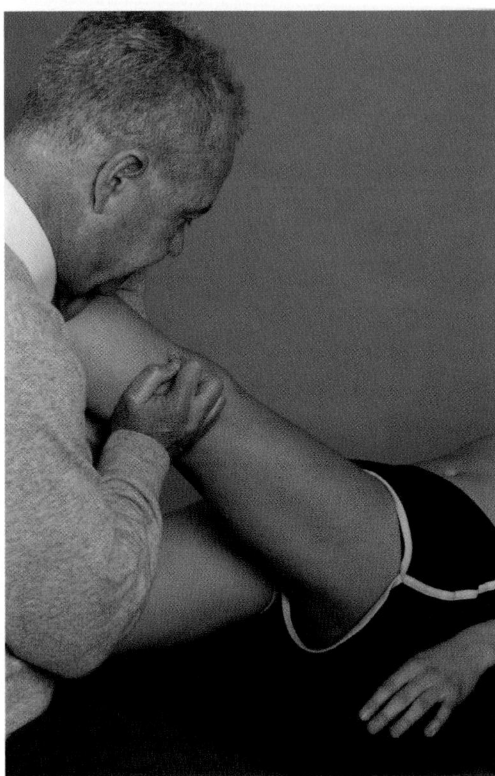

FIGURE 11-10 SLR bowstring (fibular head).

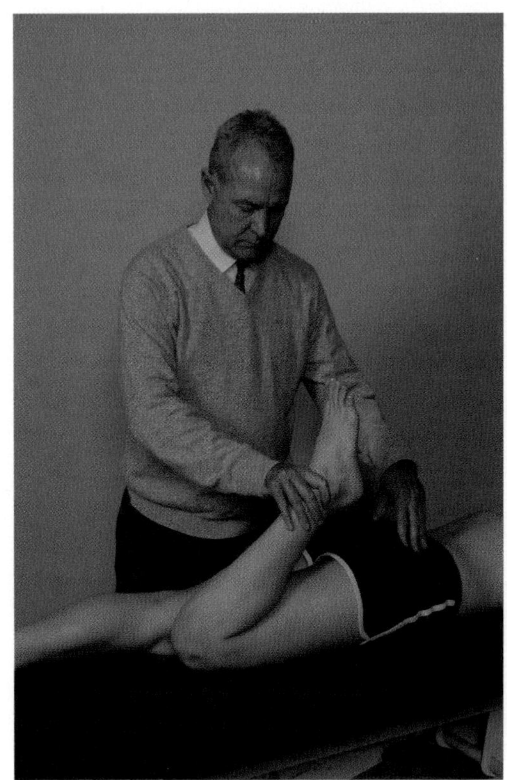

FIGURE 11-11 Prone knee bend.

herniations,[97] particularly when hip extension is added.[98] The femoral nerve travels anteriorly to both the hip and the knee (as does the rectus femoris). Therefore, the nerve roots and the rectus femoris are stretched with a combination of knee flexion and hip extension. The lateral cutaneous nerve of the thigh and the hip flexors travel anterior to the thigh and may be stressed with the hip extension component of this maneuver.

Some clinicians recommend performing a PKB test before executing a sacroiliac "upslip" correction because there is a small potential to avulse the L2–L3 nerve roots with this maneuver.

The PKB test is performed as follows: the patient is positioned prone, and the clinician stabilizes the ischium to prevent an anterior rotation of the pelvis. The clinician then gently moves the lower extremity into knee flexion, bending the knee until the onset of symptoms (Fig. 11-11). This maneuver is likely to produce a stretching sensation on the anterior aspect of the patient's thigh. The zone at which the dura is stretched is 80–100 degrees of knee flexion. Knee flexion greater than 100% introduces both a rectus femoris stretch and lumbar spine motion into the findings. A number of sensitizing maneuvers can be used including hip extension, plantar flexion, dorsiflexion, or head movements.

The test is positive if there is a reproduction of unilateral pain in the lumbar area, buttock, posterior thigh, or a combination in the 80–100 degree range of knee flexion which could indicate an L2, L3, or L4 nerve root impairment although an acute L4–S1 disk protrusion may also produce positive findings.[99]

The reliability and validity of the PKB is not known.[87] Porchet and colleagues[100] found the test to have a sensitivity of 84% but the positive findings were associated with severe lateral disk herniations.

Crossed Prone Knee Bending Test

This is a variation of the PKB test except that the uninvolved lower extremity is moved into knee flexion. A positive test is the reproduction of the patient's symptoms in the untested (opposite) leg. No diagnostic accuracy studies have been performed to determine the sensitivity and specificity of this test.

UPPER LIMB TENSION TESTS[13]

The role of adverse neuromechanics in the upper limb and trunk has received much attention over the past three decades,[42,101,102] and has been linked to chronic neck and arm pain and upper limb disorders.[16,29,103,104]

Upton and McComas[29] demonstrated that the peripheral nerve and its cervical roots may manifest irritation at simultaneous sites. A further study, which investigated adverse tension in the neural system in 20 subjects suffering from unilateral symptoms of tennis elbow, appeared to suggest that the adverse tension could be a factor.[103]

The relative mobility between the nerve root and its investing sheath, which occurs in the lumbar spine,[8] also has been demonstrated in the cervical spine.[42] This mobility is produced with certain movements of the arm and occurs maximally at C5 and C6, to a lesser degree at C7, and to an even lesser degree at C8 and T1.[16]

The ULTTs, or brachial plexus tension tests, involve an ordered sequence of movement of the shoulder girdle, arm, elbow, forearm, wrist, and hand. Because there are a number of tissues in the cervicobrachial region that could be stressed by these maneuvers, cervical side bending or cervical flexion,

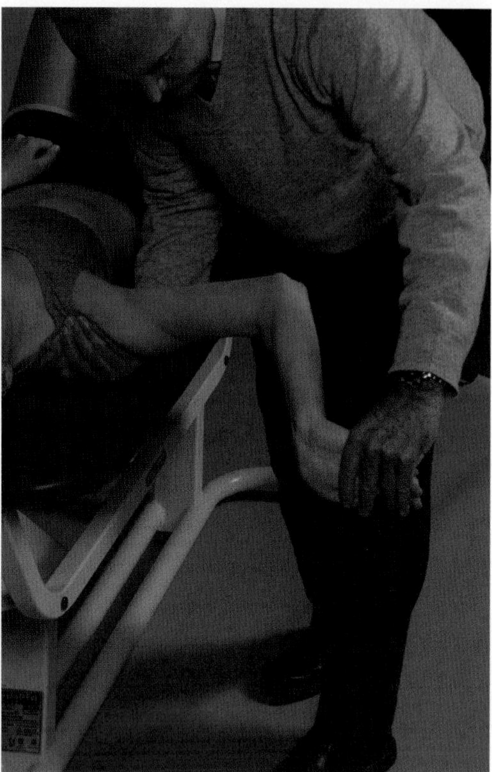

FIGURE 11-12 ULTT 1 (median nerve).

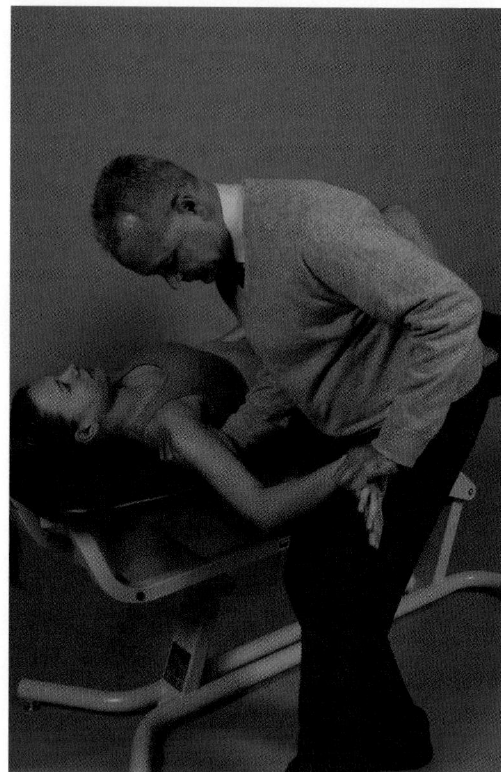

FIGURE 11-13 ULTT 2 (radial nerve).

which are thought to be more selective to the nervous system, are added.[105,106]

The principles behind the ULTT are the same as those described for the lower extremity tension tests. Therefore, only the procedures themselves are described here. During these procedures, care must be taken to maintain the cervical spine in neutral flexion–extension, side bending, and rotation.

ULTT 1 (Median Nerve Dominant)

The patient is positioned supine. The clinician depresses the shoulder girdle, abducts the humerus to approximately 110 degrees, supinates the forearm, and extends the elbow, wrist, and fingers (Fig. 11-12). The sensitizers for this test are cervical spine side flexions either toward or away from the involved side. The test is repeated on the contralateral extremity and the results are compared.

Several studies have shown that the longitudinal motion of the median nerve is affected by motion of the fingers and wrist, with digital flexion resulting in a proximal slide into the forearm, and wrist and finger extension both producing a distal slide of the nerve toward the hand.[10,12] Hyperextension of the wrist has been shown to cause the median nerve to slide 10–15 mm distally relative to a fixed bony landmark in the carpal tunnel whereas flexion of the wrist and fingers moves the nerve 4 mm proximally.[10]

ULTT 2 (Radial Nerve Dominant)

The patient is positioned supine. The clinician depresses, abducts, and internally rotates the shoulder, pronates the forearm, extends the elbow, and flexes the wrist and thumb (Fig. 11-13). The sensitizers for this test are cervical spine side flexions either toward or away from the involved side. The test is repeated on the contralateral extremity and the results are compared.

ULTT 3 (Ulnar Nerve Dominant)

The patient is positioned supine. The clinician extends the wrist, supinates the forearm, fully flexes the elbow, and depresses and abducts the shoulder. The sensitizers for this test are side flexion of the head and neck, both toward and away from the test side. The test is repeated on the contralateral extremity and the results are compared.

Evans[107] described a modification of the basic ULTT 3. The patient actively abducts the humerus with the elbow straight, stopping just short of the onset of symptoms. The patient then externally rotates the shoulder just short of symptoms and the clinician holds this position. Finally, the patient flexes the elbows so that the hand is placed behind the head. Reproduction of the symptoms with elbow flexion is considered a positive test.

Musculocutaneous Nerve

The patient is positioned supine with the head unsupported by a pillow. The clinician, facing the patient's feet, supports the patient's arm in about 80 degrees of elbow flexion. The shoulder is placed in full external rotation and approximately 10 degrees of abduction. Shoulder depression is then applied followed by glenohumeral extension (the "sensitizer"), elbow extension, and wrist ulnar deviation.

Axillary Nerve

The patient is positioned supine with the head unsupported by a pillow. The clinician places one hand on top of the patient's shoulder and depresses the shoulder. The glenohumeral joint is then externally rotated and the patient side flexes the head away from the tested side. The shoulder is then abducted to approximately 40 degrees.

Suprascapular Nerve

The patient is positioned supine with the head unsupported by a pillow. The clinician places a hand on top of the patient's shoulder. The patient's arm is placed in internal rotation and shoulder girdle protraction. The arm is then moved into horizontal adduction followed by the patient side bending the head away from the test side. The clinician now depresses the shoulder.

NEURODYNAMIC MOBILITY INTERVENTIONS

Adverse neural tension is an abnormal response to mechanical stimuli of neural tissue. The genesis of this abnormal tissue response can be from a variety of factors to include injuries (compression, vibration, and postsurgical), intraneural, extraneural, and anatomic.[108] A factor that receives a significant amount of attention involves that of repetitive strain injuries specifically with the upper extremities.

The detrimental effects of immobilization on musculoskeletal structures are well documented as are the benefits of early mobilization protocols.[109–118] The rationale behind the use of neural mobilization techniques is to attempt to restore the dynamic balance between the relative movement of neural tissues and surrounding mechanical interfaces, thereby allowing reduced intrinsic pressures on the neural tissue and improving nerve conduction velocity.[13,43] By applying early mobilization to the neural system, it seems possible that similar benefits should occur. The hypothesized benefits from such techniques include facilitation of nerve gliding, reduction of nerve adherence, dispersion of noxious fluids, increased neural vascularity, and improvement of axoplasmic flow.[43,119,120] However, an important distinction needs to be made between techniques that lengthen or stretch the dura and techniques that stretch the anatomic structures that surround the involved neural tissue.

Elvey[18] recommends an initial intervention of passive, gentle, and controlled oscillatory movements to the anatomic structures that surround the neural tissue before progressing to the techniques that stretch both the surrounding tissues and the neural tissues together. Using this approach, the treatment barrier is represented by the onset of muscle activity.[102] For example, in the cervical spine, the sequence of neurodynamic mobilizations is initiated with shoulder depression with the neck in neutral and the arm by the side followed by shoulder depression with fixation of the cervical spine, then shoulder depression, cervical fixation, and arm traction with the arm by the side. Once this progression has been performed without any adverse effects, the more specific movements used to isolate the nerve are employed.

Evidence for the efficacy of this gradual approach has been demonstrated in subjects with low back pain and radiculopathy,[58,59,121] lateral epicondylalgia,[122] and chronic cervicobrachial pain.[18,123] Cleland and colleagues[124] performed a pilot clinical trial to determine if slump stretching resulted in improvements in pain, centralization of symptoms, and disability in 30 patients with nonradicular low back pain with suspected mild to moderate neural mechanosensitivity. Patients were randomized to receive lumbar spine mobilization and exercise ($n = 14$) or lumbar spine mobilization, exercise, and slump stretching ($n = 16$). All patients were treated in physical therapy twice weekly for 3 weeks for a total of six visits. Upon discharge, outcome measures were reassessed. Independent *t*-tests were used to assess differences between groups at baseline and discharge. No baseline differences existed between the groups ($P > 0.05$). At discharge, patients who received slump stretching demonstrated significantly greater improvements in disability (9.7 points on the Oswestry Disability Index, $P > 0.01$), pain (0.93 points on the numeric pain rating scale, $P > 0.001$), and centralization of symptoms ($P > 0.01$) than patients who did not. The authors suggested that slump stretching is beneficial for improving short-term disability, pain, and centralization of symptoms and also recommended that future studies should examine whether these benefits are maintained at a long-term follow-up.[124]

A recent systematic review of randomized controlled trials with an analysis of therapeutic efficacy of neural mobilizations found only limited evidence to support its use.[120] However, choosing the right technique for the right patient based on causal mechanism is fraught with difficulty when it comes to heterogenous groups.[125]

Stretching Program for the Sciatic Nerve

The home stretching exercise to improve tissue mobility and neural extensibility is performed in three phases or positions as follows:[117]

1. The patient is positioned supine with the hips and knees are flexed at a comfortable range. Using the uninvolved leg, the patient lifts the heel of the involved side up until he or she experiences a stretch (Fig. 11-14). This position is maintained for approximately 1 minute (can be performed up a wall to provide additional support).
2. From the position in step 1, the patient slides the heel further up. If this maneuver provokes any paresthesias, the patient allows the heel back down. Progress is measured by timing the period during which the patient is able to keep the knee straight.
3. The patient performs the same maneuver as in step 2 but with a pillow under the head. This stretch is performed 3–5 times a day for 3–5 minutes at a time.

Stretches for the Upper Extremity Nerves

The recommended home stretching exercise to improve tissue mobility and neural extensibility of the peripheral nerves throughout the upper extremity is performed in four phases or positions as follows:[117]

1. The patient is seated with the cervical spine in neutral sidebending and the arm abducted to 90 degrees. The patient is asked to extend the fingers and to begin flexing

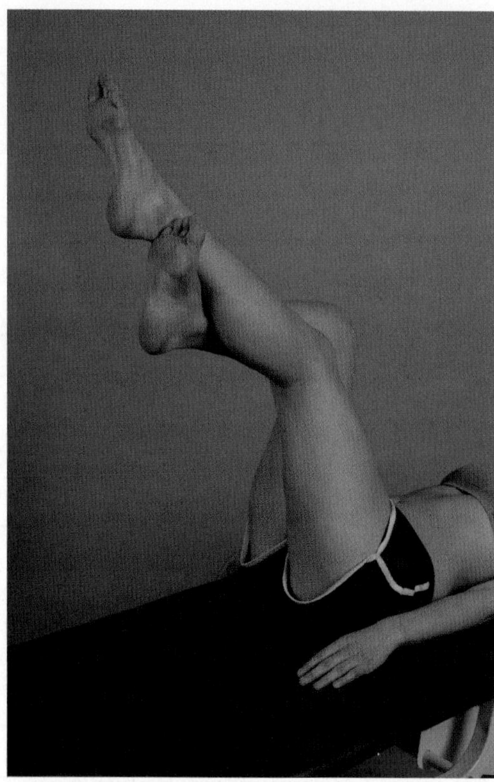

FIGURE 11-14 Sciatic nerve stretch.

the elbow while sidebending toward the elevated arm (Fig. 11-15A).

2. Keeping the upper extremity in the same position, the patient is asked to side bend the head away from the elevated arm (Fig. 11-15B). When a gentle stretch is felt, the position is held for 10–15 seconds.
3. When the patient is able to maintain the previous stretch for 30–60 seconds, trunk rotation away from the involved side is added.
4. Once full trunk rotation is achieved, various positions of cervical side bending and elbow flexion/extension can be attempted (Fig. 11-15C). For example, elbow extension combined with contralateral cervical side bending. To increase tension, forearm supination or pronation can be superimposed on the elbow motions.

Each position is held for 7 seconds and is repeated five times per session.

A series of home stretching exercise to improve tissue mobility and neural extensibility of the median nerve in cases of carpal tunnel syndrome have been advocated. Theoretically, stretching exercises of the median nerve affect symptom resolution in a carpal tunnel syndrome by[126]

- stretching the adhesions
- broadening the longitudinal area of contact between the median nerve and the transverse carpal ligament
- reducing tenosynovial edema by a milking action

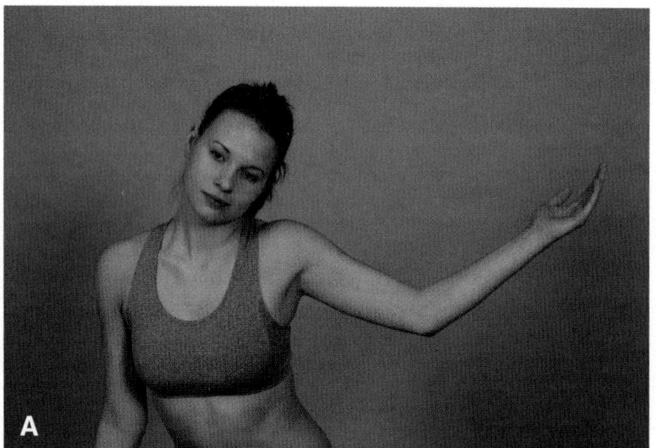

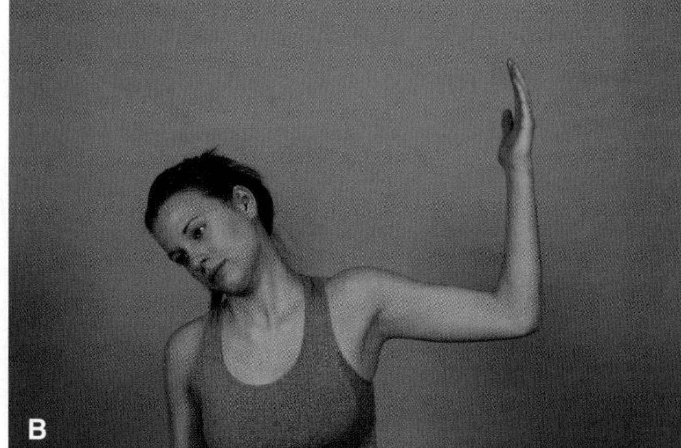

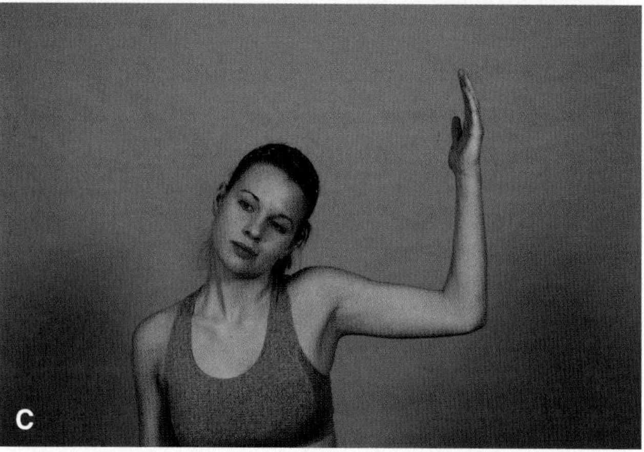

FIGURE 11-15 Upper extremity nerve stretches.

- improving venous return from the nerve bundles
- reducing pressure inside the carpal tunnel

Six positions are used for mobilization of the median nerve at the wrist:

1. The wrist in neutral, with the fingers and thumb in flexion
2. The wrist in neutral, with the fingers and thumb extended
3. The wrist and fingers extended, with the thumb in neutral
4. The wrist, fingers, and thumb extended
5. The wrist, fingers, and thumb extended, with the forearm supinated
6. The wrist, fingers, and thumb extended, with the forearm supinated and the other hand gently stretching the thumb

Each position is held for 7 seconds and is repeated five times per session.[126] All of the exercises performed in the clinic should be performed by the patient at home whenever possible.

REVIEW QUESTIONS*

1. List the number of mechanisms that are hypothesized to contribute to an injury of the peripheral nerve trunk.
2. Which term is used to describe a serial compromise of axonal transport along the same nerve fiber, causing a subclinical lesion at the distal site to become symptomatic?
3. In addition to complaints of pain, what other signs and symptoms are likely to be present with a diagnosis of neurodynamic tension?
4. The SLR test exerts a caudal traction on which of the lumbosacral nerve roots?
5. Within which range of the SLR are positive findings more significant for a decrease in neurodynamic mobility?

*Additional questions to test your understanding of this chapter can be found in the Online Learning Center for *Orthopaedic Assessment, Evaluation, and Intervention* at www.duttononline.net. Answers for the above questions appear at the back of this book.

REFERENCES

1. Inman V, Saunders J: The clinico-anatomical aspects of the lumbosacral region. *Radiology* 38:669–678, 1942.
2. Millesi H, Zoch G, Rath T: The gliding apparatus of peripheral nerve and its clinical significance. *Ann Chir Main Memb Super* 9:87–97, 1990.
3. Millesi H: The nerve gap. Theory and clinical practice. *Hand Clin* 2:651–263, 1986.
4. Butler DS, Tomberlin JP: Peripheral nerve: structure, function, and physiology. In: Magee D, Zachazewski JE, Quillen WS, eds. *Scientific Foundations and Principles of Practice in Musculoskeletal Rehabilitation.* St. Louis, MI: WB Saunders, 2007:175–189.
5. Butler DL, Gifford L: The concept of adverse mechanical tension in the nervous system: part 1: testing for "dural tension". *Physiotherapy* 75:622–629, 1989.
6. Butler DS: The upper limb tension test revisited. In: Grant R, ed. *Physical Therapy of the Cervical and Thoracic Spine.* Edinburgh: Scotland, Churchill Livingstone, 1994:217–244.
7. Slater H, Butler DS, Shacklock MD: The dynamic central nervous system: examination and assessment using tension tests. In: Boyling JD, Palastanga N, eds. *Grieve's Modern Manual Therapy*, 2nd ed. Edinburgh: Churchill Livingstone, 1994.
8. Brieg A, Troup J: Biomechanical considerations in the straight leg raising test. *Spine* 4:242–250, 1979.
9. Goddard MD, Reid JD: Movements induced by straight leg raising in the lumbosacral roots, nerves and plexus and in the intrapelvic section of the sciatic nerve. *J Neurol Neurosurg Psychiatry* 28:12–17, 1965.
10. McLellan DL, Swash M: Longitudinal sliding of the median nerve during movements of the upper limb. *J Neurol Neurosurg Psychiatry* 39:566–570, 1976.
11. Elvey RL: Peripheral neuropathic disorders and neuromusculoskeletal pain. In: Schachloch MO, ed. *Moving in on Pain.* Oxford: Butterworth-Heinmann, 1995.
12. Wilgis EF, Murphy R: The significance of longitudinal excursion in peripheral nerves. *Hand Clin* 2:761–766, 1986.
13. Butler DS: *Mobilization of the Nervous Sysytem.* New York, NY: Churchill Livingstone, 1992.
14. Keller K, Corbett J, Nichols D: Repetitive strain injury in computer keyboard users: pathomechanics and treatment principles in individual and group intervention. *J Hand Ther* 11:9–26, 1998.
15. Smyth MJ, Wright V: Sciatica and the intervertebral disc. An experimental study. *J Bone Joint Surg* 40A:1401–1418, 1958.
16. Elvey RL: Treatment of arm pain associated with abnormal brachial plexus tension. *Aust J Physiother* 32:225–230, 1986.
17. Murphy RW: Nerve roots and spinal nerves in degenerative disc disease. *Clin Orth Rel Res* 129:46–60, 1977.
18. Elvey RL, Hall TM: Nerve trunk pain: physical diagnosis and treatment. *Manual Therapy* 4:63–73, 1999.
19. Omer G Jr: Results of untreated peripheral nerve injuries. *Clin Orthop* 163:15, 1982.
20. Boerger TO, Limb D: Suprascapular nerve injury at the spinoglenoid notch after glenoid neck fracture. *J Shoulder Elbow Surg* 9:236–237, 2000.
21. Shim JS, Lee YS: Treatment of completely displaced supracondylar fracture of the humerus in children by cross-fixation with three Kirschner wires. *J Pediatr Orthop* 22:12–6, 2002.
22. Cornwall R, Radomisli TE: Nerve injury in traumatic dislocation of the hip. *Clin Orthop Relat Res* 377:84–91, 2000.
23. Fletcher MD, Warren PJ: Sural nerve injury associated with neglected tendo Achilles ruptures. *Br J Sports Med* 35:131–132, 2001.
24. Choi HR, Kondo S, Mishima S, et al: Axillary nerve injury caused by intradeltoid muscular injection: a case report. *J Shoulder Elbow Surg* 10:493–495, 2001.
25. Schram DJ, Vosik W, Cantral D: Diaphragmatic paralysis following cervical chiropractic manipulation: case report and review. *Chest* 119: 638–640, 2001.
26. Yavuzer G, Tuncer S: Accessory nerve injury as a complication of cervical lymph node biopsy. *J Phys Med Rehabil* 80A:622–623, 2001.
27. Jacob JR, Rao JP, Ciccarelli C: Traumatic dislocation and fracture dislocation of the hip. A long-term follow-up study. *Clin Orthop Relat Res* 214:249–263, 1987.
28. Moran KT, Kotowski MP, Munster AM: Long-term disability following high-voltage electric hand injuries. *J Burn Care Rehabil* 7:526, 1986.
29. Upton RM, McComas AJ: The double crush in nerve entrapment syndromes. *Lancet* 2:359–362, 1973.
30. Massey EW, Riley TL, Pleet AB: Coexistent carpal tunnel syndrome and cervical radiculopathy (double crush syndrome). *South Med J* 74:957–959, 1981.
31. Dahlin LB, Lundborg G: The neurone and its response to peripheral nerve compression. *J Hand Surg* 15B:5–10, 1990.
32. Dellon Al, Mackinnon SE: Chronic nerve compression model for the double crush hypothesis. *Ann Plast Surg* 26B:259–264, 1991.
33. Saplys R, Mackinnon SE, Dellon LA: The relationship between nerve entrapment versus neuroma complications and the misdiagnosis of de Quervain's disease. *Contemp Orthop* 15:51, 1987.
34. Narakas AO: The role of thoracic outlet syndrome in double crush syndrome. *Ann Chir Main Memb Super* 9:331–340, 1990.
35. Wood VE, Biondi J: Double-crush nerve compression in thoracic-outlet syndrome. *J Bone Joint Surg* 72A:85–88, 1990.
36. Wilbourn AJ, Gilliatt RW: Double-crush syndrome: a critical analysis. *Neurology* 49:21–29, 1997.
37. Nemoto K, Matsumoto N, Tazaki K-I, et al: An experimental study on the 'double crush' hypothesis. *J Hand Surg* 12B:552–559, 1987.
38. Baba M, Fowler CJ, Jacobs JM, et al: Changes in peripheral nerve fibres distal to a constriction. *J Neurol Sci* 54:197–208, 1982.

39. Swensen RS: The 'double crush' syndrome. *Neurology Chronicle* 4:1–6, 1994.
40. Russell BS: Carpal tunnel syndrome and the "double crush" hypothesis: a review and implications for chiropractic. *Chiropr Osteopat* 16:2, 2008.
41. Lo SF, Chou LW, Meng NH, et al: Clinical characteristics and electrodiagnostic features in patients with carpal tunnel syndrome, double crush syndrome, and cervical radiculopathy. *Rheumatol Int* 2011.
42. Elvey RL: Brachial plexus tension tests and the pathoanatomical origin of arm pain. In: Glasgow EF, Twomey LT, eds. *Aspects of Manipulative Therapy.* Melbourne, Victoria: Australia, Lincoln Institute of Health Sciences, 1979:105–110.
43. Shacklock M: Neurodynamics. *Physiotherapy* 81:9–16, 1995.
44. Breig A: *Adverse Mechanical Tension in the Central Nervous System.* Stockholm: Sweden, Almqvist & Wiskell, 1978.
45. Breig A, Troup JDG: Biomechanical considerations in the straight leg raising test. *Spine* 4:242–250, 1979.
46. Breig A, Marions O: Biomechanics of the lumbosacral nerve roots. *Acta Radiol* 1:1141–1160, 1963.
47. Reid JD: Effects of flexion-extension. Movements of the head and spine upon the spinal cord and nerve roots. *J Neurol Neurosurg Psychiatry* 23:214–221, 1960.
48. Smith CG: Changes in length and posture of the segments of the spinal cord with changes in posture in the monkey. *Radiology* 66:259–265, 1956.
49. Asbury AK, Fields HL: Pain due to peripheral nerve damage: an hypothesis. *Neurology* 34:1587–1590, 1984.
50. Coppieters MW, Stappaerts KH: The immediate effects of manual therapy in patients with cervicobrachial pain of neural origin: a pilot study. In: Singer K, ed. *Proceedings of the Seventh Scientific Conference of the International Federation of Orthopaedic Manipulative Therapists.* Perth: Australia, 2000:113–117.
51. Di Fabio RP: Neural mobilization: the impossible [editorial]. *J Orthop Sports Phys Ther* 31:224–225, 2001.
52. Butler DS: Commentary-adverse mechanical tension in the nervous system: a model for assessment and treatment. In: Maher C, ed. *Adverse Neural Tension Reconsidered.* Melbourne: Australian Physiotherapy Association, 1999:33–35.
53. Kleinrensink GJ, Stoeckart R, Vleeming A, et al: Mechanical tension in the median nerve. The effects of joint positions. *Clin Biomech* 10:240–244, 1995.
54. Devor M, Seltzer Z: Pathophysiology of damaged nerves in relation to chronic pain. In: Wall PD, Melzack R, eds. *Textbook of Pain*, 4th ed. Edinburgh: Churchill Livingstone, 1999:129–161.
55. Lundborg G, Rydevik B: Effects of stretching the tibial nerve of the rabbit. *J Bone Joint Surg* 55-B:390–401, 1973.
56. Ogato K, Naito M: Blood flow of peripheral nerves: effects of dissection, stretching and compression. *J Hand Surg* 11:10, 1986.
57. Maitland GD: Negative disc exploration: Positive canal signs. *Aust J Physiother* 25:129–134, 1979.
58. Maitland GD: Movement of pain sensitive structures in the vertebral canal and intervertebral foramina in a group of physiotherapy students. *S Afr J Physiother* 36:4–12, 1980.
59. Maitland GD: The slump test: examination and treatment. *Aust J Physiother* 31:215–219, 1985.
60. Maitland G: *Vertebral Manipulation.* Sydney: Butterworth, 1986.
61. Macnab I: Negative disc exploration. *J Bone Joint Surg* 53A:891–903, 1971.
62. Fahrni WH: Observations on straight leg raising with special reference to nerve root adhesions. *Can J Surg* 9:44–48, 1966.
63. Louis R: Vertebroradicular and vertebromedullar dynamics. *Anat Clin* 3:1–11, 1981.
64. Breig A: *Biomechanics of the Central Nervous System.* Stockholm: Sweden, Almqvist & Wiskell, 1960.
65. Penning L, Wilmink JT: Biomechanics of lumbosacral dural sac. A study of flexion-extension myelography. *Spine* 6:398–408, 1981.
66. Inman VT, Saunders JB: The clinicoanatomical aspects of the lumbosacral region. *Radiology* 38:669–678, 1941.
67. Turl SE, George KP: Adverse neural tension: A factor in repetitive hamstring strain? *J Orthop Sports Phys Ther* 27:16–20, 1998.
68. White AA, Punjabi MM: *Clinical Biomechanics of the Spine*, 2nd ed. Philadelphia, PA: J.B. Lippincott Company, 1990.
69. Meadows J: *Orthopedic Differential Diagnosis in Physical Therapy.* New York: McGraw-Hill, 1999.
70. Davis DS, Anderson IB, Carson MG, et al: Upper Limb Neural Tension and Seated Slump Tests: The False Positive Rate Among Healthy Young Adults Without Cervical or Lumbar Symptoms. *J Man Manip Ther* 16:136–141, 2008.
71. Bianco AJ: Low back pain and sciatica. Diagnosis and indications for treatment. *J Bone Joint Surg* 50A:170, 1968.
72. Bickels J, Kahanovitz N, Rubert CK, et al: Extraspinal bone and soft-tissue tumors as a cause of sciatica. Clinical diagnosis and recommendations: analysis of 32 cases. *Spine* 24:1611–1616, 1999.
73. Odell RT, Key JA: Lumbar disc syndrome caused by malignant tumors of bone. *JAMA* 157:213–216, 1955.
74. Paulson EC: Neoplasms of the bony pelvis producing the sciatic syndrome. *Minn Med* 11:1069–1074, 1951.
75. Lasègue C: Considérations sur la sciatique. *Arch Gen Med Paris* 2:258, 1864.
76. Deyo RA, Weinstein JN: Low back pain. *N Engl J Med* 344:363–370, 2001.
77. Cyriax J: *Textbook of Orthopaedic Medicine, Diagnosis of Soft Tissue Lesions*, 8th ed. London, Bailliere Tindall, 1982.
78. Smith C: Analytical literature review of the passive straight leg raise test. *S Afr J Physiother* 45:104–107, 1989.
79. Urban LM: The straight leg raising test: a review. In: Grieve GP, ed. *Modern Manual Therapy of the Vertebral Column.* Edinburgh: Churchill Livingstone, 1986:567–575.
80. Woodhall B, Hayes GJ: The well leg raising test of Fajersztajn in the diagnosis of ruptured lumbar intervertebral disc. *J Bone Joint Surg* 32A:786–792, 1950.
81. American Medical Association: *Guides to the Evaluation of Permanent Impairment*, 5th ed. Chicago, IL: American Medical Association, 2001.
82. Gajdosik RL, Barney FL, Bohannon RW: Effects of ankle dorsiflexion on active and passive unilateral straight leg raising. *Phys Ther* 65:1478–1482, 1985.
83. Andersson GBJ, Deyo RA: History and physical examination in patients with herniated lumbar discs. *Spine* 21:10S–18S, 1996.
84. Vucetic N, Svensson O: Physical signs in lumbar disc herniation. *Clin Orthop* 333:192, 1996.
85. Scham SM, Taylor TKF: Tension signs in lumbar disc prolapse. *Clin Orthop* 75:195–204, 1971.
86. Harada Y, Nakahara S: A pathologic study of lumbar disc herniation in the elderly. *Spine* 14:1020, 1989.
87. Deyo RA, Rainville J, Kent DL: What can the history and physical examination tell us about low back pain? *JAMA* 268:760–765, 1992.
88. van der Hoogen HJ, Koes BW, van Eijk JT, et al: On the course of low back pain in general practice: a one year follow up study. *Ann Rheum Dis* 57:13–19, 1998.
89. Lew PC, Morrow CJ, Lew MA: The effect of neck and leg flexion and their sequence on the lumbar spinal cord. *Spine* 19:2421–2424, 1994.
90. Cyriax J: Perineuritis. *Br Med J* 1:578–580, 1942.
91. Coppieters MW, Alshami AM, Babri AS, et al: Strain and excursion of the sciatic, tibial, and plantar nerves during a modified straight leg raising test. *J Orthop Res* 24:1883–1889, 2006.
92. Supic LF, Broom MJ: Sciatic tension signs and lumbar disc herniation. *Spine* 19:1066, 1994.
93. Kosteljanetz M, Bang F, Schmidt-Olsen S: The clinical significance of straight-leg raising (Lasegue's sign) in the diagnosis of prolapsed lumbar disc. Interobserver variation and correlation with surgical finding. *Spine* 13:393–395, 1988.
94. Kerr RS, Cadoux-Hudson TA, Adams CB: The value of accurate clinical assessment in the surgical management of the lumbar disc protrusion. *J Neurol Neurosurg Psychiatry* 51:169–173, 1988.
95. Hakelius A, Hindmarsh J: The comparative reliability of preoperative diagnostic methods in lumbar disc surgery. *Acta Orthop Scand* 43:234, 1972.
96. Dyck P, Doyle JB: "Bicycle test" of van Gelderen in diagnosis of intermittent cauda equina compression syndrome. *J Neurosurg* 46:667–670, 1977.
97. Dyck P: The femoral nerve traction test with lumbar disc protrusions. *Surg Neurol* 6:136, 1976.
98. Estridge MN, Rouhe SA, Johnson NG: The femoral nerve stretching test. *J Neurosurg* 57:813, 1982.
99. Christodoulide AN: Ipsilateral sciatica on femoral nerve stretch test is pathognomic of an L 4–5 disc protrusion. *J Bone Joint Surg* 21:1584, 1989.
100. Porchet F, Frankhauser H, de Tribolet N: Extreme lateral lumbar disc herniation: a clinical presentation of 178 patients. *Acta Neurochir (Wien)* 127:203–209, 1994.
101. Kenneally M, Rubenach H, Elvey R: The upper limb tension test: the SLR of the arm. In: Grant R, ed. *Physical Therapy of the Cervical and Thoracic Spine.* New York, NY: Churchill Livingstone, 1988.

102. Elvey RL, Hall T: Neural tissue evaluation and treatment. In: Donatelli RA, ed. *Physical Therapy of the Shoulder*, 3rd ed. New York: Churchill Livingstone, 1997:131–152.
103. Yaxley GA, Jull GA: Adverse tension in the neural system. A preliminary study of tennis elbow. *Aust J Physiother* 39:15–22, 1993.
104. Quintner J: Stretch-induced cervicobrachial pain syndrome. *Aust J Physiother* 36:99–104, 1990.
105. Selvaratnam PJ, Matyas TA, Glasgow EF: Non-invasive discrimination of brachial plexus involvement in upper limb pain. *Spine* 19:26–33, 1994.
106. Hack GD, Koritzer RT, Robinson WL, et al: Anatomic relation between the rectus capitis posterior minor muscle and the dura mater. *Spine* 20:2484–2486, 1995.
107. Evans RC: *Illustrated Essentials in Orthopedic Physical Assessment*. St. Louis, MO: Mosby-Year book Inc, 1994.
108. Schroder JA: Manual therapy and neural mobilization: Our approach and personal observations. *Orthopaedic Practice* 16:23–27, 2004.
109. Akeson WH, Amiel D, Abel MF, et al: Effects of immobilization on joints. *Clin Orthop* 219:28–37, 1987.
110. Amiel D, Woo SL-Y, Harwood FL: The effect of immobilization on collagen turnover in connective tissue: a biochemical-biomechanical correlation. *Acta Orthop Scand* 53:325–332, 1982.
111. Behrens F, Kraft EL, Oegema TR Jr: Biochemical changes in articular cartilage after joint immobilization by casting or external fixation. *J Orthop Res* 7:335–343, 1989.
112. Booth FW, Kelso JR: The effect of hind limb immobilization on contractile and histochemical properties of skeletal muscle. *Pflugers Arch* 342:231–238, 1973.
113. Eiff MP, Smith AT, Smith GE: Early mobilization versus immobilization in the treatment of lateral ankle sprains. *Am J Sports Med* 22:83–88, 1994.
114. Enneking WF, Horowitz M: The intra-articular effects of immobilization on the human knee. *J Bone Joint Surg* 54-A:973–985, 1972.
115. Giebel GD, Edelmann M, Huser R: Sprain of the cervical spine: early functional vs. immobilization treatment (in German). *Zentralbl Chir* 122:512–521, 1997.
116. Jurvelin J, Kiviranta I, Tammi M, et al: Softening of canine articular cartilage after immobilization of the knee joint. *Clin Orthop* 207:246–252, 1986.
117. Olson VL: Connective tissue response to injury, immobilization, and mobilization. In: Wadsworth C, ed. *Current Concepts in Orthopedic Physical Therapy—Home Study Course*. La Crosse, WI: Orthopaedic Section, APTA, Inc., 2001.
118. Woo SL-Y, Gomez MA, Woo YK, et al: Mechanical properties of tendons and ligaments. II. The relationships of immobilization and exercise on tissue remodeling. *Biorheology* 19:397–408, 1982.
119. Coppieters MW, Stappaerts KH, Wouters LL, et al: The immediate effects of a cervical lateral glide treatment technique in patients with neurogenic cervicobrachial pain. *J Orthop Sports Phys Ther* 33:369–378, 2003.
120. Ellis RF, Hing WA: Neural mobilization: a systematic review of randomized controlled trials with an analysis of therapeutic efficacy. *J Man Manip Ther* 16:8–22, 2008.
121. Stoddard A: *Manual of Osteopathic Practice*. New York, NY: Harper & Row, 1969.
122. Vicenzino B, Collins D, Wright A: The initial effects of a cervical spine manipulative physiotherapy treatment on the pain and dysfunction of lateral epicondylalgia. *Pain* 68:69–74, 1996.
123. Hall T, Elvey RL, Davies N, et al: *Efficacy of Manipulative Physiotherapy for the Treatment of Cervicobrachial Pain, Tenth Biennial Conference of the MPAA*. Melbourne: Manipulative Physiotherapists Association of Australia, 1997:73–74.
124. Cleland JA, Childs JD, Palmer JA, et al: Slump stretching in the management of non-radicular low back pain: a pilot clinical trial. *Man Ther* 11:279–286, 2006.
125. Shacklock M: Neural mobilization: a systematic review of randomized controlled trials with an analysis of therapeutic efficacy. *J Man Manip Ther* 16:23–24, 2008.
126. Rozmaryn LM, Dovelle S, Rothman K, et al: Nerve and tendon gliding exercises and the conservative management of carpal tunnel syndrome. *J Hand Ther* 11:171–179, 1998.

Improving Muscle Performance

CHAPTER 12

CHAPTER OBJECTIVES

At the completion of this chapter, the reader will be able to:

1. Outline the various roles of human skeletal muscle.
2. List the various roles of muscle in the human body.
3. Differentiate among muscle strength, endurance, and power.
4. Describe strategies to increase muscle strength.
5. List the different types of resistance that can be used to strengthen muscles.
6. List the different types of muscle contractions and the advantages and disadvantages of each.
7. Outline the various types of exercise progression and the components of each.
8. Describe strategies to increase muscle endurance.
9. Describe strategies to increase muscle power.
10. Explain the basic principles behind plyometrics.
11. Define delayed onset muscle soreness (DOMS) and explain why it occurs.
12. Define senescence sarcopenia.
13. List the changes that can occur with muscles during aging.
14. Describe the concept of specificity of training.

OVERVIEW

Movement of the body or any of its parts involves considerable activity from those muscles directly responsible. Muscle is the only biological tissue capable of actively generating tension. This characteristic enables human skeletal muscle to perform the important functions of maintaining upright body posture, moving body parts, and absorbing shock. For body motions to take place, the muscles producing movement must have a stable base from which to work from. Muscles serve a variety of roles depending on the required movement:

- ***Prime agonist.*** A muscle that is directly responsible for producing movement.
- ***Synergist (supporter).*** Performs a cooperative muscle function in relation to the agonist. Synergists can function as stabilizers or neutralizers.
  - ***Stabilizers (fixators).*** Muscles that contract statically to steady or support some part of the body against the pull of the contracting muscles, against the pull of gravity, or against the effect of momentum and recoil in certain vigorous movements.
  - ***Neutralizers.*** Muscles that act to prevent an undesired action of one of the movers.
- ***Antagonist.*** A muscle that has an effect opposite to that of the agonist.

Types of Muscle Contraction

The basic function of a muscle is to contract. The word *contraction*, used to describe the generation of tension within muscle fibers, conjures up an image of shortening of muscle fibers. However, a contraction can produce shortening or lengthening of the muscle, or no change in the muscle length. Thus, three types of contraction are commonly recognized (see Chap. 1): isometric, concentric, and eccentric.

- ***Isometric contraction.*** Isometric exercises provide a static contraction with a variable and accommodating resistance without producing any appreciable change in muscle length.[1]
- ***Concentric contraction.*** A concentric contraction (Fig. 12-1) produces a shortening of the muscle. This occurs when the tension generated by the agonist muscle is sufficient to overcome an external resistance and to move the body segment of one attachment toward the segment of its other attachment.[1]
- ***Eccentric contraction.*** An eccentric contraction (Fig. 12-2) occurs when a muscle slowly lengthens as it gives in to an external force that is greater than the contractile force it is exerting.[1] In reality, the muscle does not actually lengthen, it merely returns from its shortened position to its normal resting length. Eccentric muscle contractions, which are capable of generating greater forces than either isometric or concentric contractions,[2–4] are involved in activities that

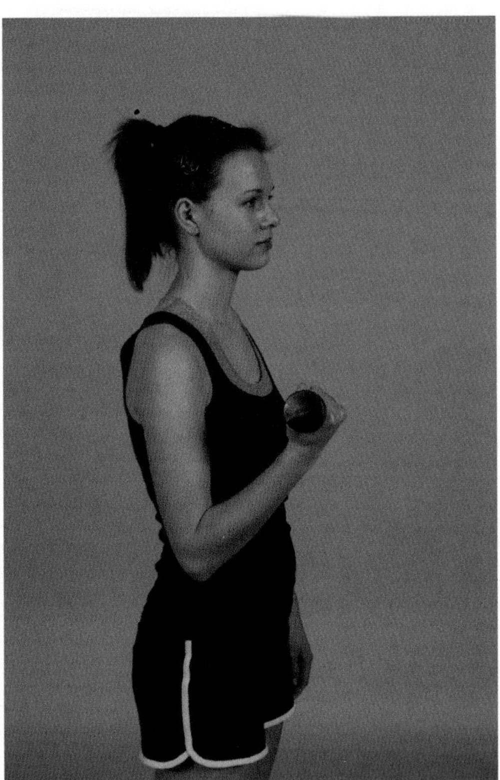

FIGURE 12-1 Concentric contraction.

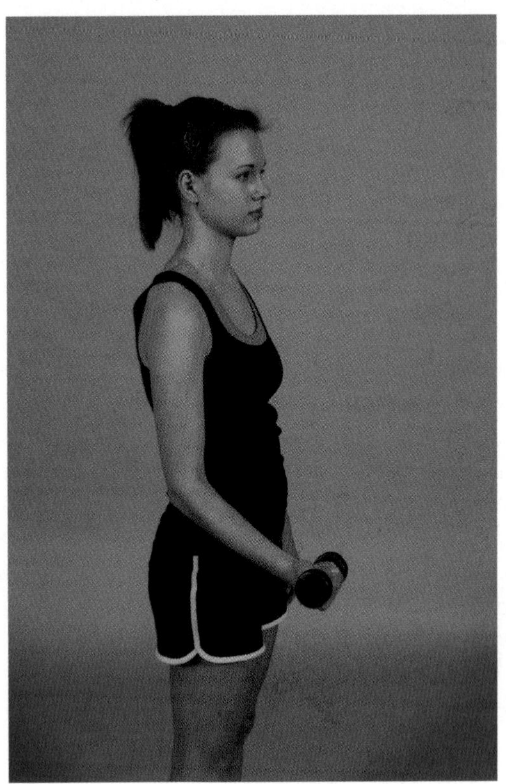

FIGURE 12-2 Eccentric contraction.

require a deceleration to occur. Such activities include slowing to a stop when running, lowering an object, or sitting down. Because the load exceeds the bond between the actin and myosin filaments during an eccentric contraction, some of the myosin filaments probably are torn from the binding sites on the actin filament while the remainder are completing the contraction cycle.[5] The resulting force is substantially larger for a torn cross-bridge than for one being created during a normal cycle of muscle contraction. Consequently, the combined increase in force per cross-bridge and the number of active cross-bridges results in a maximum lengthening muscle tension that is greater than the tension that could be created during a shortening muscle action.[5,6]

CLINICAL PEARL

An *isotonic* contraction is a contraction in which the tension within the muscle remains constant as the muscle shortens or lengthens.[1] This state is very difficult to produce and measure. Although the term *isotonic* is used in many texts to describe concentric and eccentric contractions alike, its use in this context is erroneous because in most exercise forms the muscle tension during exercise varies based upon the weight used, joint velocity, muscle length, and type of muscle contraction.[1]

Four other contractions are worth mentioning:

- ***Isokinetic contraction.*** An isokinetic contraction occurs when a muscle is maximally contracting at the same speed throughout the whole range of its related lever.[1] Isokinetic contractions require the use of special equipment that produces an accommodating resistance. Both high-speed/low-resistance and low-speed/high-resistance regimens result in excellent strength gains.[7–10] The major disadvantage of this type of exercise is its expense. In addition, there is the potential for impact loading and incorrect joint axis alignment.[11] Isokinetic exercises may also have questionable functional carryover.[12]
- ***Econcentric contraction.*** This type of contraction combines both a controlled concentric and a simultaneous eccentric contraction of the same muscle over two separate joints.[13] Examples of an econcentric contraction include the standing hamstring curl, in which the hamstrings work concentrically to flex the knee while the hip tends to flex eccentrically, lengthening the hamstrings. When rising from a squat, the hamstrings work concentrically as the hip extends and work eccentrically as the knee extends. Conversely, the rectus femoris work eccentrically as the hip extends and work concentrically as the knee extends.
- ***Isolytic contraction.*** An isolytic contraction is an osteopathic term used to describe a type of eccentric contraction that makes use of a greater force than the patient can overcome. The difference between an eccentric contraction and an isolytic contraction is that, in the former the contraction is voluntary, whereas in the latter it is involuntary. The isolytic contraction can be used in certain manual techniques to stretch fibrotic tissue (see Chap. 10).

Muscle Performance

The ability of a muscle to carry out its various roles is a measure of muscle performance. Muscle performance can be measured using a number of parameters. These include strength, endurance, and power.

- ***Strength.*** Strength may be defined as the amount of force that may be exerted by an individual in a single maximum muscular contraction against a specific resistance, or the ability to produce torque at a joint. Dynamometry is the process of measuring forces that are doing work. Muscle strength can be measured as follows (see Chap. 4):
  - Manual muscle testing (MMT): MMT is an acceptable standardized process utilized to find gross strength deficits and to isolate muscle groups and actions.
  - Using a dynamometer: A dynamometer is a device that measures strength by using a load cell or spring-loaded gauge. These measurements are more objective than MMT. Examples of a dynamometer include the following:
    - Handheld: This is used to assess the grip strength of a patient, or to measure muscle group strength by having the patient exert maximal force against the dynamometer.
  - Isometric: This measures the static strength of the muscle group by stabilizing the extremity using stabilization straps or verbal instruction.
  - Isokinetic: This measures the strength of a muscle group during a movement with constant, predetermined speed.
- ***Endurance.*** Muscular endurance is the ability of a muscle, or group of muscles, to continue to perform without fatigue. The nature of muscular endurance encourages the body to work aerobically. This phenomenon, called *steady state*, occurs after some 5–6 minutes of exercise at a constant intensity level.[14] During steady state, the rate of mitochondrial adenosine triphosphate (ATP) production is closely matched to the rate of ATP hydrolysis and demonstrates the existence of efficient cellular mechanisms to control mitochondrial ATP synthesis in a wide dynamic range.[15] Endurance exercise training produces an increase in mitochondrial volume density in all three muscle fiber types[16] and thus muscle aerobic power. With a higher mitochondrial density in trained muscle, the rate of substrate flux per individual mitochondrion will be less at any given rate of ATP hydrolysis.[15] Therefore, the required activation of mitochondrial respiration by adenosine diphosphate (ADP) to achieve a given rate of ATP formation will be less, resulting in increased ADP sensitivity of muscle oxidative phosphorylation.[15]
- ***Power.*** Mechanical power is the product of force and velocity. *Muscular power*, the maximum amount of work an individual can perform in a given unit of time, is the product of muscular force and velocity of muscle shortening. Muscular power is an important contributor to activities requiring both strength and speed. Maximum power occurs at approximately one-third of maximum velocity.[17] Muscles with a predominance of fast-twitch fibers generate more power at a given load than those with a high composition of slow-twitch fibers.[18] The ratio for mean peak power production by type IIb, type IIa, and type I fibers in skeletal tissue (see Chap 1) is 10:5:1.[19]

These three components of muscle performance are important in functional activities as they can allow the patient to interact with their environment in a more efficient and pain-free way through increased movement control and capacity.

CLINICAL PEARL

The ultimate source of energy for muscular contraction is the ATP molecule. The catabolic breakdown of the chemical bonds of the ATP molecule provides the energy necessary to allow myosin cross-bridges to pull the actin filaments across the myosin filaments, which results in muscle contraction (see Chap. 1).

Exercise Prescriptions

Before initiating an exercise program, it is necessary to conduct a needs analysis to evaluate the physical requirements and physical attributes of the patient. Determining the selection of exercise is dependent upon the goals and objectives and the needs analysis. As with prescriptions for medications, a successful exercise prescription requires the correct balance between the dose (exercise variables) and the response (specific health or fitness adaptations).[20] The dosage of an exercise refers to each particular patient's exercise capability, and is determined by a number of variables (Table 12-1).[21] For these variables to be effective, the patient must be compliant and be able to train without exacerbating the condition.[22]

CLINICAL PEARL

The training volume describes the total amount of resistance lifted during a strength training session, and is therefore dependent upon the weight lifted, the repetitions (reps), and sets.
Training volume = number of sets × number of reps × weight lifted per rep

Depending on the specific program design, resistance training is known to enhance muscular strength, power, or endurance and can provide a potent stimulus to the neuromuscular system. Other variables such as speed, balance, coordination, jumping ability, flexibility, and other measures of motor performance have also been positively enhanced by resistance training.[23]

TABLE 12-1 Resistive Exercise Variables
Resistance (load or weight)
Duration
Training frequency (weekly, daily)
Point of application
Bouts (timed sessions of exercise)
Sets and repetitions
Training volume
Mode (type of contraction)
Rests

CLINICAL PEARL

- If pain is present before resistance or the end-feel, the patient's symptoms are considered irritable. The intervention in the presence of irritability should not be aggressive, particularly inclusive of exercise[24]
- If pain occurs after resistance, then the patient's symptoms are not considered irritable and exercise, particularly stretching, can be more aggressive.

It is worth remembering that when the individual trains for two different types of adaptations (e.g., aerobic fitness versus strength), the training stimuli can interfere with one another and result in less improvement in one or both of the effects. For example when strength loads are combined with aerobic training, the aerobic adaptation is not detrimentally affected, but there is a negative impact on strength development.[25,26]

CLINICAL PEARL

Contraindications to muscle performance training:

- ***Inflammation.*** Exercise can increase swelling and cause damage to muscles or joints.
- ***Pain.*** Severe joint or muscle pain during exercise, or for more than 24 hours after exercise, requires an elimination or reduction of the exercise.

Each exercise session should include a 5–15 minute warm-up and a 5–15 minute cool-down period.

- Warm-up
  - includes low-intensity cardiorespiratory activities.
  - prevents the heart and circulatory system from being suddenly overloaded.
- Cool-down
  - includes low-intensity cardiorespiratory activities and flexibility exercises.
  - helps prevent abrupt physiological alterations that can occur with sudden cessation of strenuous exercise.

The length of the warm-up and cool-down sessions may need to be longer for deconditioned or older individuals. The type of exercise prescribed determines the type of warm-up.[27] The possible benefits of a warm-up prior to physical activity are listed in Table 12-2. The most effective warm-up consists of both general (walking, biking, jogging, and gentle resistive exercises) and specific (movements that are appropriate for the particular activity to be undertaken) exercises.[27]

Once the warm-up is completed, it is recommended that a flexibility program be incorporated to increase joint movement and muscle extensibility (see Chap. 13).

The initial exercise is prescribed at a level that the patient can perform, before progressing in difficulty. The early goals of exercise are concerned with increasing circulation, preventing atrophy, increasing protein synthesis, and reducing the level of metabolites.[22]

TABLE 12-2 Possible Benefits of a Warm-Up Prior to Physical Activity

Increased blood flow to muscles.
Increased oxyhemoglobin breakdown, with increased oxygen delivery to muscles.
Increased circulation leading to decreased vascular resistance.
Increased release of oxygen from myoglobin.
Enhanced cellular metabolism.
Reduced muscle viscosity leading to smoother muscle contraction and increased mechanical efficiency.
Increased speed of nerve impulses.
Increased sensitivity of nerve receptors.
Decreased activity of alpha fibers and sensitivity of muscles to stretch.
Decreased number of injuries due to increased range of motion.
Decreased stiffness of connective tissue leading to decreased likelihood of tears.
Increased cardiovascular response to sudden strenuous exercise.
Increased relaxation and concentration.

Data from Bahr R: Principles of injury prevention. In: Brukner P, Khan K, eds. *Clinical Sports Medicine,* 3rd edn. Sydney: McGraw-Hill, 2007:78–101; Stewart IB, Sleivert GG: The effect of warm-up intensity on range of motion and anaerobic performance. *J Orthop Sports Phys Ther* 27:154–161, 1998; Rosenbaum D, Hennig EM: The influence of stretching and warm-up exercises on Achilles tendon reflex activity. *J Sports Sci* 13:481–490, 1995; Green JP, Grenier SG, McGill SM: Low-back stiffness is altered with warm-up and bench rest: Implications for athletes. *Med Sci Sports Exerc* 34:1076–1081, 2002.

CLINICAL PEARL

Resistance training, particularly when incorporated into a comprehensive fitness program, reduces the risk factors associated with coronary heart disease, non–insulin-dependent diabetes, and colon cancer; prevents osteoporosis; promotes weight loss and maintenance; improves dynamic stability and preserves functional capacity; and fosters psychological well-being.[23]

The following factors should be considered with exercise prescriptions.

Frequency. Training frequency refers to the number of times strength-training sessions are completed in a given period (e.g., the number of work-outs per week). Optimal training frequency depends on several factors such as experience, training volume and status, intensity (see later), exercise selection, level of conditioning, recovery ability, and the number of muscle groups trained per workout session. Strength is most effectively enhanced by a program featuring high resistance and few reps. More training sessions can be accomplished and provide adequate rest if a *split routine* is used. A split routine divides the training session into groupings, split between the upper body and lower body exercises. Another alternative is to perform a push and pull exercise program, in which the strength training is divided into exercises in which the individual pushes a weight (e.g., triceps extension, bench press), then pulls a weight (e.g., biceps curl, latissimus dorsi pull down).

Based on the studies of isokinetic and eccentric/concentric exercise,[28,29] muscle strength recovery follows a steady, nonlinear, and predictable increase over time.[21] In the rehabilitation population, strengthening exercises are typically performed on a daily basis initially, with the weight and frequency governed by the individual's response to the exercise. As healing progresses, evidenced by a decrease in pain and swelling and an increase in range of motion, the exercises should be performed every other day. If the training loads are near the maximum capacity, more time for recovery will be required to minimize soreness and provide adequate rest.

Once sufficient strength is attained, even if the patient only performs the strength training at a minimum of once per week, the strength can be fairly well maintained over a 3-month period.[30]

Repetitions. Initial selection of a starting weight may require some trial and error to find the correct number of reps. For any given exercise, the amount of weight selected should be sufficient to allow 8–12 reps per exercise for three sets with a recovery period between sets of 60–90 seconds to elicit improvements in muscular strength and endurance as well as muscle hypertrophy.[31]

Duration. Duration refers to the length of the exercise session. Physical conditioning occurs over a period of 15–60 minutes depending on the level of intensity. Average conditioning time is 20–30 minutes for moderate intensity exercise. However, individuals who are severely compromised are more likely to benefit from a series of short exercise sessions (3–10 minutes) spaced throughout the day.

Rest periods. In most functional exercises, fatigue of the muscle being exercised is the goal. However, fatigue may also occur due to lack of coordination, insufficient balance, poor motivation, or the addition of compensatory movements. In addition, fatigue may also be associated with specific clinical diseases, e.g., multiple sclerosis, cardiac disease, peripheral vascular dysfunction, and pulmonary diseases. Because fatigue is detrimental to performance, rest is an important component of any exercise progression. The rest period must be sufficient to allow for muscular recuperation and development while alleviating the potential for overtraining.[32] In general, the heavier loads lifted, the longer the rest period between sets. The rest period between sets can be determined by the time the breathing rate, or pulse, of the patient returns to the steady state, or by using the following guidelines:

- muscular endurance: less than 30 seconds rest
- muscular hypertrophy: 60–90 seconds
- muscular strength: 2–5 minutes
- muscle power: 2–5 minutes

A 48-hour rest period between concurrent training sessions is generally recommended.[23]

CLINICAL PEARL

In the rehabilitation population, fatigue should be achieved without exceeding the patient's tolerance and while protecting the injury site. It is now clear that the development of fatigue probably involves several factors that influence force production in a manner dependent on muscle fiber type and activation pattern, and that one of these factors may be the regulation of Ca^{2+} by the sarcoplasmic reticulum.[33] Characteristics of muscle fatigue include reduction in muscle force production capability and shortening velocity, a reduction in the release and uptake of intracellular calcium by the sarcoplasmic reticulum, as well as prolonged relaxation of motor units between recruitment.[33,34]

One of the biggest challenges for a clinician is to find a balance between achieving a maximum training effect while alleviating fatigue. Fortunately, fatigue has a much faster decay time than the training effect. Thus, to remove the fatigue, the volume of training should be reduced while maintaining the training effect by holding the intensity of the training load constant.[35]

Intensity. Intensity refers to the power output (rate of performing work) or how much effort is required to perform the exercise. In clinical terms, intensity refers to the weight or resistance lifted by the patient. It is now recognized that an individual's perception of effort (rated perceived exertion or RPE) is closely related to the level of physiological effort.[36,37] The Borg Scale is commonly used to help determine a patient's RPE, as an individual's perception of effort is closely related to the level of physiological effort—a high correlation exists between a person's RPE multiplied by 10, and their actual heart rate.[36,37] For example, if a person's RPE is 15, then $15 \times 10 = 150$; so the heart rate should be approximately 150 beats per minute. A cardiorespiratory training effect can be achieved at a rating of "somewhat hard" or "hard" (13–16). Note that this calculation is only an approximation of heart rate, and the actual heart rate can vary quite a bit depending on age and physical condition. The original scale introduced by Borg[37] rated exertion on a scale of 6–20, but a more recent one designed by Borg included a category (C) ratio (R) scale, the Borg CR10 Scale® (Table 12-3).

TABLE 12-3 Rating of Perceived Exertion[a]

Traditional Scale	Verbal rating	Revised 10-Grade Scale	Verbal Rating
6		0	Nothing at all
7	Very, very light	0.5	Very, very weak
8		1.0	Very weak
9	Very light	2.0	Weak (light)
10		3.0	Moderate
11	Fairly light	4.0	Somewhat strong
12		5.0	Strong (heavy)
13	Somewhat hard	6.0	
14		7.0	Very strong
15	Hard	8.0	
16		9.0	
17	Very hard	10.0	Very, very strong (almost maximum) maximal
18			
19	Very, very hard		

[a]Data from Borg GAV: Psychophysical basis of perceived exertion. *Med Sci Sports Exerc* 14:377–381, 1992.

Patient responses that can modify the intensity include increases in pain level, muscle fatigue, time taken to recover from fatigue, cardiovascular response, compensatory movements, level of motivation, and degree of comprehension.

Speed of Exercise. The speed of the exercise should depend on the imposed demands of an individual. In some cases, increasing the speed of an exercise following the initial phase of learning a particular exercise and developing proficiency in the performance of the exercise is beneficial.[38] In addition, higher velocity training appears to improve peak power measures.[23]

Variation. Variation in training is a fundamental principle that supports the need for alterations in one or more program variables over time to allow for the training stimulus to remain optimal (Table 12-4).[23] The concept of variation has been rooted in program design universally for many years. The most commonly examined resistance training theory is periodization. Periodization is the systematic process of planned variations in a resistance-training program over a specified training cycle to prevent overtraining and to perform at peak or optimum levels at the right time.[39] Two models of periodization are classic (linear) and undulating (nonlinear)[23]:

- ***Classic.*** This model is characterized by high initial training volume and low intensity. As training progresses, volume decreases and intensity increases in order to maximize strength, power, or both.
- ***Undulating.*** The nonlinear program enables variation in intensity and volume within each 7- to 10-day cycle by rotating different protocols over the course of the training program. Nonlinear methods attempt to train the various components of the neuromuscular system within the same 7- to 10-day cycle. During a single workout, only one characteristic is trained in a given day (e.g., strength, power, or muscular endurance).

It has been shown that systematically varying volume and intensity is most effective for long-term progression.[23,39] Periodization consists of several phases including the macrocycle, mesocycle, and microcycle. The macrocycle for an athlete can, for example, last for 1 year ending with the end of a competitive season. The macrocycle is divided into several mesocycles. A mesocycle defines distinct variations in the resistance and exercise program. For example, a mesocycle for an athlete can be divided into three distinct phases[27]:

- ***Conditioning.*** This phase emphasizes developing aerobic and anaerobic fitness, strength, and power.
- ***Precompetition.*** This phase emphasizes correct technique.
- ***Competition.*** During this phase, the emphasis is on competitive performance while maintaining basic conditioning.

The final breakdown of periodization is the microcycle, which involves changes in training parameters such as intensity, work–rest ratios, sets, reps, exercise order, and specific exercises, and generally lasts for 1–2 weeks. A common format is a 4-week mesocycle that consists of three microcycles of 1 week each, in which the loads are progressively increased, followed by a 1-week microcycle of reduced volume and intensity.

When prescribing a progressive resistive exercise (PRE) regimen, the clinician should consider the individual's current health and fitness status, goals, access to appropriate equipment, and time available for training.[40] Training programs prescribed for competitive athletes, which often include exercises designed specifically to improve the development of explosive power, are generally inappropriate for children, untrained adults, elderly persons, or patients with chronic disease(s). Exercise progression in the orthopaedic population, including the post surgical population, is determined by the stage of healing and the degree of irritability of the structure, which are factors of patient response, as healing relates to signs and symptoms.

TABLE 12-4 Types of Training That Incorporate Variation

Circuit training	Circuit training or cross-training incorporates a wide variety of modes of training and uses high repetitions and low weight to provide a more general conditioning program aimed at improving body composition, muscular strength, and some cardiovascular fitness.
Interval training	Interval training includes an exercise period followed by a prescribed rest interval. It is perceived to be less demanding than continuous training and tends to improve strength and power more than endurance. With appropriate spacing of work and rest intervals, a significant amount of high-intensity work can be achieved and is greater than the amount of work accomplished with continuous training. The longer the work interval, the more the anaerobic system is stressed and the duration of the rest period is not important. In a short work interval, a work recovery ratio of 1:1 or 1:5 is appropriate to stress the aerobic system.

CLINICAL PEARL

Three terms are commonly used with resistance training prescriptions:

- **Repetitions.** The number of times a specific movement or exercise is repeated.
- **Repetition maximum (RM).** The RM is the maximum number of reps an individual can perform at a given weight. For example, a 10 RM is the weight the patient can lift a maximum of 10 times.
- **Set.** A particular number of reps. Whatever exercise progression is used to achieve an increase in the total number of reps while maintaining a sufficient effort, the number of sets must also be increased. This increase in sets must occur in conjunction with a reduction in the number of reps per set by 10–20%[22] or a reduction in the amount of resistance. Generally speaking, no more than three to five sets are used.

Specificity of Training

It appears that the muscle response to resistance training for people who have a broad range of conditions and who might consult a physical therapist is similar to muscle responses reported in young people without impairment.[41] Resistance training can have a beneficial effect in populations where pain is a particular problem, such as people with low back pain and people with osteoarthritis. In addition, resistance training can have a beneficial effect on conditions such as high blood pressure, fracture rehabilitation, and cardiovascular disease. The effect of resistance training on other impairment parameters, such as bone mineral density, fat mass, and aerobic capacity, remains inconclusive.[41] There is also evidence to suggest that improvements in the ability to generate muscle force can carry over into an improved ability to do everyday tasks. However, the effects are generally quite modest, and there are a number of examples in the literature where significant improvements in activity were not demonstrated after resistance training.[41] Part of the problem with drawing conclusions from the literature is the lack of details provided as to the specifics of the exercises prescribed. Specificity of training is an accepted concept in physical therapy rehabilitation. This concept involves the principle of the specific adaptation to imposed demand (SAID). Thus, the focus of the exercise prescription should be to improve the strength and coordination of functional or sports-specific movements with exercises that approximate the demands of the desired activity (speed, agility, strength, power, endurance, etc.).

CLINICAL PEARL

The principle of overload states that a greater than normal stress or load on the body is required for training adaptation to take place. To increase strength, the muscle must be challenged at a greater level than it is accustomed to. High levels of tension will produce adaptations in the form of hypertrophy and recruitment of more muscle fibers.

Three important concepts are related to the SAID principle:[26]

- Overload. When cells, tissues, and organs are loaded beyond what they normally are required to do, they will adapt to permit them to deal with these new loads more effectively. These training effects are specific to the energy supply systems that have been utilized, the locale of the stimulus, the specific muscle groups, the joint action(s), the type of contraction, and the speed of contraction. When loads are applied they should be specific to the desired effect (SAID), and be appropriate to the individual in terms of frequency, intensity, and duration. It is important to remember that once an adaptation has taken place to a specific load, this load is no longer an "overload" and the load must be progressively increased to get further improvements.
- Underload. When cells, tissues, and organs are loaded at a level below what is normally performed, the body will adapt by decreasing its ability in the underloaded component (detraining). Detraining occurs quickly after the cessation of training—a reduction in the VO_2 max can be detected within four weeks of detraining.

CLINICAL PEARL

An overprescription of resistance training exercise may result in overstress injuries, whereas underprescription will result in a failure to achieve the necessary or desired strength improvement.

- Overtraining. Overtraining occurs because of an inappropriate amount of rest, recovery, and unloading. It is manifested as an inability to recover from exercise, lowered resistance to injury, and chronic fatigue or exhaustion, and is caused by a loss in the body's adaptive capability after chronic high-volume loading or in response to a too large increase in either duration or intensity of training. The signs and symptoms of overtraining include loss of appetite, inability to sleep, lethargy, muscle soreness, chronic fatigue, declining performance, and altered metabolism.[42–44]

The SAID principle can be applied by exercising the muscles along each extremity and within the trunk in functional patterns.[45] The exercise component of the intervention should be as specific as the manual technique used in the clinic. Muscles can be classified into tonic and phasic groups according to how muscles develop from the myotomes[46] (Table 12-5).

CLINICAL PEARL

In general, tonic muscles function as endurance (postural) muscles, whereas phasic muscles function as the power muscles.[47,48]

Speed-strength training applies the principles of specificity of training and is typically used with highly conditioned

TABLE 12-5 The Various Muscle Types and Their Primary Innervation

Muscle Type	Characteristics	Primary Innervation	Examples
Type I	Tonic	Type 1a phasic nerve endings	Extensors
	Slow twitch		External rotators
	Small neuron		Abductors
Types IIa and IIb	Phasic	Anterior divisions of the nerve plexus	Flexors
	Fast twitch		Adductors
	Large neuron		Two-joint muscles

Data from Wilk KE, Voight ML, Keirns MA, et al.: Stretch-shortening drills for the upper extremities: theory and clinical application. *J Orthop Sports Phys Ther* 17:225–239, 1993.

athletes who want to take their performance to the next level. Speed-strength training involves taking some of the basic movements of a task and increasing the resistance. For sports, such as baseball and golf, athletes can use devices, such as an oversized ball or weighted golf club, to train the arms and trunk to work against a greater resistance. Sprinters have long benefited from the use of a small parachute to increase wind resistance, or by dragging a tire fastened by a rope. The theory behind speed-strength training is that once the higher resistance is removed the athlete's speed is improved when they perform the activity under normal resistance. Wherever possible, strength testing by the clinician should assess the function of a muscle. If a power muscle is assessed, its ability to produce power should be assessed. In contrast, an endurance muscle should be tested for its ability to sustain a contraction for a prolonged period, such as occurs with sustained postures.

In addition to speed-strength training, agility drills, rapid reflex, and specific skill training should form the core of many sport-specific exercise programs.

CLINICAL PEARL

The principles of resistance training can be easily remembered by the acronym PROS—progression, regularity, overload, and specificity.

Delayed Onset Muscle Soreness

Familiar to most individuals at some time, muscular soreness is one of the drawbacks to participating in an exercise program involving activity beyond what one usually experiences. The purpose of the recovery phase is to restore the muscles in the body to preexercise levels through promotion of venous turn and removal of metabolites from muscle, reestablishment of fluid balance, replacement of depleted fuel energy reserves, and relaxation in muscles that were active.[26] The recovery period is also necessary to replenish muscle glycogen following prolonged exercise of the continuous or integral nature. If the recovery period is insufficient, acute or DOMS can result. Acute soreness is apparent during the later stages of an exercise bout and during the immediate recovery period.[38] This results from an accumulation of end products that occurs with exercise, H+ ions, and lactate, but generally disappears between 2 minutes and 1 hour after cessation of exercise.[38] DOMS, on the other hand, appears 24–56 hours after the exercise bout.[49] DOMS can exhibit as anything, from minor muscle soreness to debilitating pain and swelling, but is most commonly described as causing a reduction in joint range of motion, shock attenuation, and peak torque.[50] A recent review of DOMS confirms that the mechanisms, treatment strategies, and impact on athletic performance remain uncertain.[51] Recognized mechanisms include lactic acid and potassium accumulation, muscle spasms, mechanical damage to the connective tissues, inflammation, enzyme efflux secondary to muscle cell damage, and edema.[51] There is certainly a marked increase in the proportion of disrupted muscle fibers after eccentric as compared with concentric exercise, which has been roughly correlated to the degree of DOMS.[52] Eccentric exercise is also linked to morphologic and metabolic signs of muscle alteration: myofibrillar damage along the Z-band,[53,54] mitochondrial swelling,[53,54] increased intramuscular pressure,[53,54] and impaired glycogen resynthesis.

Given the role of eccentric exercise in DOMS, prevention of DOMS involves the careful design of any eccentric program, which should include preparatory techniques, accurate training variables, and appropriate aftercare, including a cool-down period of low-intensity exercise to facilitate the return of oxygen to the muscle. It is a widely held belief among athletes and coaches that massage is an effective therapeutic modality that can enhance muscle recovery and reduce soreness following intense physical activity.[55] However, the actual scientific literature does not tend to support the positive efficacy of manual massage as a postexercise therapeutic modality in the athletic setting.[55–57]

To help prevent DOMS, there is some controversy as to whether a cool-down or warm-up should be used. A number of studies advocate a short (5–10 minutes) low-intensity warm-up (30–65% of VO_2 max) to assist in maintaining venous return and removal of metabolites above levels in passive rest.[58,59] However, one randomized controlled trial found that whereas a 10 minute warm-up reduced perceived muscle soreness (measured on a 100-mm visual analogue scale) 48 hours after exercise (mean effect of 13 mm, 95% CI 2 to 24 mm), a 10 minute cool-down had no apparent effect (mean effect of 0 mm, 95% CI 11 to 11 mm).[60]

If the prevention of DOMS is unsuccessful, the intervention should include, as appropriate, rest, local measures to reduce edema (e.g., cryotherapy, elevation of the involved limb(s)), drug therapy (typically nonsteroidal anti-inflammatory agents), or further exercise (aerobic submaximal exercise with no eccentric component, e.g., swimming, biking, or stepper machine, pain-free flexibility exercises, and high-speed [300 degrees per second] concentric-only isokinetic training).[21,61]

Types of Resistance Used in Exercise Programs

Resistance-training programs have the potential for many positive benefits provided the training is appropriately progressed to meet the needs of a person as his or her strength increases. Resistance can be applied to a muscle by any external force or mass, including any of the following.

Gravity

Gravity alone can supply sufficient resistance for a weakened muscle. With respect to gravity, muscle actions may occur

- in the same direction as gravity (downward);
- in the opposite direction to gravity (upward);
- in a direction perpendicular to gravity (horizontal);
- in the same or opposite direction to gravity, but at an angle.

The direction in which the muscle is working determines the role that gravity plays and the role that the muscle must play in order to counteract the forces of gravity. For example, if an arm muscle is working to lower a book to a table, the biceps muscle works eccentrically against the force of gravity to control the speed of the lowering. If the muscle works to lift the book from the table, the biceps muscle must work concentrically against the force of gravity.

CLINICAL PEARL

Active range of motion exercises are designed to work against gravity, whereas active assisted exercises are typically performed perpendicular to gravity.

Body Weight

A wide variety of exercises have been developed that do not require any equipment but rely solely on the patient's body weight for the resistance (e.g., push-up).

Small Weights

Cuff weights, dumbbells, and surgical tubing (elastic resistance) are economical ways of applying resistance. Small weights are typically used to strengthen the smaller muscles or to increase the endurance of larger muscles by increasing the number of reps. Free weights also provide more versatility than exercise machines, especially for three-dimensional exercises, as the movements do not occur in a straight line or plane. The disadvantage of free weights is that they offer no variable resistance throughout the range of motion and so the weakest point along the length–tension curve of each muscle limits the amount of weight lifted. According to a recent study, 96% of rehabilitation professionals use elastic resistance with their patients, and 85% of home exercise programs prescribed by rehabilitation professionals require elastic-resistance bands or tubing.[9,32,62–67] Elastic resistance offers a unique type of resistance that cannot be classified within the traditional subcategories of strengthening. The amount of variable resistance offered by elastic bands or tubing is a factor of the internal tension produced by the material. This internal tension is a factor of the elastic material's coefficient of elasticity, the surface area of the elastic material, and how much the elastic material is stretched.[32] It is commonly believed that the resistance provided by these bands or tubing increases exponentially at the end range of motion. However, the forces produced by elastic resistance are linear until approximately 500% elongation, at which point the forces increase exponentially.[32] As the elastic resistance is not stretched more than 300% in prescribed exercises, the exponential increase should not be attained. In addition, the torque production of elastic-resistance exercises is similar to that produced by a concentric/eccentric dumbbell exercise: a bell-shaped curve.[68]

Medicine Balls

Medicine balls provide the opportunities to improve strength, balance, and coordination through dynamic movements by training the body as a functional unit and strengthening the core and trunk musculature. Both upper and lower body medicine ball exercises can be performed using a variety of speeds, and medicine ball weights and sizes.

Exercise Machines

In situations where the larger muscle groups require strengthening, and where exercises need to be performed in straight and supported lines, a multitude of specific exercise machines can be used. These machines are most often used in the more advanced stages of a rehabilitation program when more resistance can be tolerated, but can also be used in the earlier stages depending on the size of the muscle undergoing rehabilitation. Examples of these machines include the multi-hip, the lat pull-down, the leg extension, and the leg curl machine. Exercise machines are often fitted with an oval-shaped cam or wheel that mimics the length of tension curve of the muscle (Nautilus, Cybex). Although these machines are a more expensive alternative to dumbbell or elastic resistance, they do offer some advantages:

- They provide more adequate resistance for the large muscle groups that cannot be achieved with free weights/cuff weights, or manual resistance.
- They are typically safer than free weights as control/support throughout the range is provided.
- They provide the clinician with the ability to quantify and measure the amount of resistance that the patient can tolerate over time (as compared with elastic resistance).

The disadvantages of exercise machines are as follows:

- the inability to modify the exercise to be more functional or three-dimensional and
- the inability to modify the amount of resistance at particular points of the range.

Manual Resistance

Manual resistance is a type of active exercise in which another person provides resistance manually. An example of manual resistance is proprioceptive neuromuscular facilitation (PNF) (see Chap. 10).

The advantages of manual resistance, when applied by a skilled clinician, are as follows[69]:

- Control of the extremity position and force applied. This is especially useful in the early stages of an exercise program when the muscle is weak.
- More effective reeducation of the muscle or extremity, using diagonal or functional patterns of movement.
- Critical sensory input to the patient through tactile stimulation and appropriate facilitation techniques (e.g., quick stretch).
- Accurate accommodation and alterations in the resistance applied throughout the range. For example, an exercise can be modified to avoid a painful arc in the range.
- Ability to limit the range. This is particularly important when the amount of range of motion needs to be carefully controlled (postsurgical restrictions).

The disadvantages of manual resistance include the following:

- The amount of resistance applied cannot be measured quantitatively.
- The amount of resistance is limited by the strength of the clinician/caregiver or family member.

- Difficulty with consistency of the applied force throughout the range, and with each rep.

Improving Muscle Performance

Progression is defined as "the act of moving forward or advancing toward a specific goal over time until the target goal has been achieved."[23] A progressive program is recommended to condition the patient for a return to activity and to prevent overload injuries. Such a program should address the following areas:[70–74]

- ***Flexibility.*** Attempts should be made to improve general body flexibility, with an emphasis on the specific activity or exercise. The general flexibility exercises should address the entire kinematic chain and not just the joint in question (e.g., shoulder rotation and elbow motion in the arm, low back, hip rotation, and hamstrings in the legs).
- ***Strengthening.*** The exercises to improve strength should be applied in appropriate amounts and locations to address sport- or functional-specific activities.
- ***Power.*** Power is incorporated through the use of rapid movements in appropriate planes with weights and ballistic activities.
- ***Endurance.*** Endurance can be built up with aerobic exercises.

Optimal resistance training progressions should always be based on sound rationale and should always be individualized to meet specific training goals. Each progression is made more challenging by altering one of the parameters of exercise including the intensity, duration, and frequency which are modified according to patient response.

Increasing Strength

Strengthening of a muscle occurs when the muscle is forced to work at a higher level than that to which it is accustomed. The extent of the functional and health benefits from exercise training depends on several factors including initial performance and health status, along with the exercise prescription variables previously discussed such as frequency, duration, intensity, variation, and rest intervals.[75]

To increase muscle strength most effectively, a muscle must work with increasing effort against progressively increasing resistance.[3,76] In a strength training program, the term *load* refers to the amount of weight used in a specific exercise. Most strength and conditioning programs describe the load as a percentage of a RM. The RM can be expressed as the greatest amount of load lifted one time (1 RM). As the load becomes heavier, the number of times an individual can lift (perform a rep) the load decreases, whereas if the load becomes lighter, more reps can be accomplished. If resistance is applied to a muscle as it contracts so that the metabolic capabilities of the muscle are progressively overloaded, adaptive changes occur within the muscle, which make it stronger over time.[4,77] These adaptive changes include the following[2,3,78–82]:

- ***An increase in the size of the muscle (hypertrophy).*** In normal individuals, an increase in strength after a resisted exercise program is thought to initially occur as a result of neural adaptation, followed by hypertrophy of muscle fibers if the exercise program is continued for a longer period. *Mitochondria* are the main subcellular structures that determine the oxygen demand of muscle. There is consensus that there is a dilution of mitochondrial volume density through an increase in myofibrillar (i.e., contractile protein) volume density as a consequence of strength-type exercise training.[14,83] This increase in myofibrillar volume density, or hypertrophy that occurs with strength training is regarded as the main cause for the overall increase in the anatomical cross-sectional area (CSA) of an entire muscle group. The fiber hypertrophy is typically greater for fast- than for slow-twitch muscle fibers.[84]
- ***An increase in the force per unit area.*** Strength training has also been shown to lead to an increase in the force per unit CSA of the muscle. This effect has been attributed either to an increase in neural drive[85] or to an actual increase in muscle specific tension due to a denser packing of muscle filaments.[86] A denser packing of contractile tissue along the tendon could theoretically increase the angle of pennation of muscle fibers.[87]
- ***A reduction in the time to peak force.***[88] This can be defined as the time from the onset of muscle activation until peak force is attained.
- ***An increase in the efficiency of the neuromuscular system.*** This increased efficiency results in
  - an increase in the number of motor units recruited,
  - an increase in the firing rate of each motor unit,
  - an increase in the synchronization of motor unit firing, and
  - an improvement in the endurance of the muscle.
- ***Stimulation of slow-twitch fibers (when performing workloads of low intensity) and stimulation of fast-twitch IIa fibers (when performing workloads of high intensity and short duration).***
- ***Rhythmic activities increase blood flow to the exercising muscles via contraction and relaxation.***
- ***The power of the muscle improves.***
- ***Improved bone mass (Wolff's Law).***
- ***Increase in metabolism/calorie burning/weight control.***
- ***Increased intramuscular pressure results from a muscle contraction of about 60% of its force generating capacity.***
- ***Cardiovascular benefits when using large muscle groups.*** Strength training of specific muscles has a brief activation period and uses a relatively small muscle mass, producing less cardiovascular metabolic demands than vigorous walking, swimming, etc.
- ***An increase in the rate of force development.***[88]
- Conversely, a muscle can become weak or atrophied through:
  - *Disease.*
  - *Neurologic compromise.*
  - *Immobilization.* Continuous immobilization of skeletal muscle tissues can cause some undesirable consequences.

These include weakness or atrophy of muscles. Muscle atrophy is an imbalance between protein synthesis and degradation. After modest trauma, there is a decrease in whole body protein synthesis rather than increased breakdown. With more severe trauma, major surgery, or multiple organ failure, both synthesis and degradation increase, the latter being more enhanced.

- *Disuse.*

Strengthening Exercises Based on Contraction Type

As outlined earlier in the chapter, a muscle can contract in a variety of ways. Each type of contraction has its advantages and disadvantages.

Isometric Exercises. Studies have demonstrated that a 6-second hold of 75% of maximal resistance is sufficient to increase strength when performed repetitively.[89,90] Isometric exercises have an obvious role when joint movement is restricted, either by pain or by bracing and casting. The primary role in this regard is to prevent atrophy and a subsequent decrease of ligament, bone, and muscle strength. Isometric exercises have the following disadvantages:

- Strength gains are not increased throughout the range (unless performed at multiple angles).
- They do not activate all of the muscle fibers (primary activation is of slow-twitch fibers).
- There are no flexibility or cardiovascular fitness benefits.
- Peak effort can be injurious to the tissues because of vasoconstriction and joint compression forces.
- There is limited functional carryover.[12]
- Considerable internal pressure can be generated, especially if the breath is held during contraction. This can prove injurious to patients with weakness in the abdominal wall (hernia) or cardiovascular impairment (increase in blood pressure through the Valsalva maneuver)[91] even if performed correctly.

Concentric Exercises. These contractions are commonly used in the rehabilitation process and in activities of daily living. The biceps curl and the lifting of a cup to the mouth are examples, respectively. Concentric exercises are dynamic and allow the clinician to vary the load from constant, using free weights, to variable, using an exercise machine. The speed of contraction can also be manipulated depending on the goal of the intervention. A number of programs have been designed for the progression of concentric exercise programs. Some of these PRE programs are summarized in Tables 12-6 and 12-7. Determining the RM is dependent upon the goals of the individual and his or her functional demands. A 10 RM testing load is often recommended to estimate the 1 RM. The rehabilitation program designed by DeLorme is based on a rep maximum of 10 (10 RM).[79] The Oxford technique[92] reverses the percentage of maximum in the three sets (Table 12-6), whereas the MacQueen technique[93,94] differentiates between beginning, intermediate, and advanced levels. In contrast, the program designed by Sanders is based on a formula that uses a percentage of body weight to determine starting weights.[95] The daily adjusted progressive resistive exercise (DAPRE) program, designed by Knight, allows for individual differences in the rates at which patients progress in

TABLE 12-6 Exercise Progressions

	Set(s) of 10	Amount of Weight	Repetitions
DeLorme program	1	50% of 10 RM	10
	2	75% of 10 RM	10
	3	100% of 10 RM	10
Oxford technique	1	100% of 10 RM	10
	2	75% of 10 RM	10
	3	50% of 10 RM	10
MacQueen technique	3 (beginning/intermediate)	100% of 10 RM	10
	4–5 (advanced)	100% of 2–3 RM	2–3
Sander program	Total of 4 sets (3 times per week)	100% of 5 RM	5
	Day 1: 4 sets	100% of 5 RM	5
	Day 2: 4 sets	100% of 3 RM	5
	Day 3: 1 set	100% of 5 RM	5
	2 sets	100% of 3 RM	5
	2 sets	100% of 2 RM	5
Knight DAPRE program	1	50% of RM	10
	2	75% of RM	6
	3	100% of RM	Maximum
	4	Adjusted working weight	Maximum
Berger's adjustment technique	3	100% of 10 RM	6–8

DAPRE, daily adjustable progressive resistive exercise; RM, repetition maximum.

TABLE 12-7	Adjustment Sequence for DAPRE Program	
Number of Repetitions Performed During Set	**Adjusted Working Weight for Fourth Set (lb)**	**Next Exercise Session (lb)**
0–2	−5–10	−5–10
3–4	0–5	Same weight
5–6	Same weight	+5–10
7–10	+5–10	+5–15
11	+10–20	+10–20

DAPRE, daily adjustable progressive resistive exercise.

their rehabilitation programs.[96] (Table 12-7) Finally, the Berger technique[97] selects an amount of weight that is sufficient to allow 6–8 RM in each of the three sets (the initial selection of a starting weight typically requires some trial and error), with a recovery period of 60 to 90 seconds between sets. If at least three sets of 6 RM cannot be completed, the weight is considered too heavy and is reduced. Conversely, if it is possible to do more than three sets of 8 RM, the weight is considered too light and is increased.

CLINICAL PEARL

The *1 RM equivalent* is a formula that takes into account the weight lifted and reps multiplied by a numeric equivalent.

1 RM = (weight lifted × number of reps × 0.03) + weight lifted.

For example, a patient who has lifted 100 pounds for a bench press a total of 12 reps, his or her RM equivalent will be equal to (100 × 12 × 0.03) + 100 = 136

A typical exercise prescription for high school, collegiate, and professional athletes includes three or more sets of a 6–12 RM per exercise performed 3 days/week.[40] For others, a 10–15 RM is generally recommended.[23] Initially, the strengthening exercises are performed on a daily basis, with the variables dependent on the patient's response to the exercise. This is progressed to every other day, and then to at least three times per week, but no more than four times per week.

CLINICAL PEARL

To determine how much weight should be increased for a particular exercise the *2 for 2 rule* method is recommended as it is relatively conservative. The rule states that the load should increase, if the individual can perform two or more reps over the assigned reps for that particular exercise over two consecutive workouts.

Eccentric Exercises. The clinical indications for the use of eccentric exercise are numerous[21] (Table 12-8).

CLINICAL PEARL

Functional strength is the ability of the neuromuscular system to perform combinations of concentric and eccentric contractions in the performance of activities that relate to a patient's needs and requirements in a multiplanar environment (see section "Specificity of Training").[98] Effective rehabilitation targets specific muscles with regard to functional muscle activity patterns and overall conditioning and uses a progression of increased activity, while preventing further trauma.[99] Incremental gains in function should be seen as strength increases.

TABLE 12-8 Clinical Indications for Eccentric-Biased Exercise
Mechanical, reproducible joint pain
Joint pain resistant to modality intervention
Unidirectional joint crepitus or pain arc
Deconditioned or low endurance patients
Plateaus in strength gains
Tendonitis presentations
Late-stage rehabilitation and performance training

Data from Albert M: Concepts of muscle training. In: Wadsworth C, ed. *Orthopaedic Physical Therapy. Topic—Strength and Conditioning Applications in Orthopaedics: Home Study Course 98a*. La Crosse, WI: Orthopaedic Section, APTA, Inc., 1998; Albert MS: Principles of exercise progression. In: Greenfield B, ed. *Rehabilitation of the Knee: A Problem Solving Approach*. Philadelphia, PA: FA Davis, 1993; Albert MS: *Eccentric Muscle Training in Sports and Orthopaedics*, 2nd edn. New York, NY: Churchill Livingstone, 1995.

Isokinetic Exercises. An isokinetic exercise is one in which the length of the muscle is changing while the contraction is performed at a constant velocity.[100] Isokinetic exercise requires special equipment that produces an accommodating and variable resistance. The main principle behind isokinetic exercise is that peak torque (the maximum force generated through the range of motion) is inversely related to angular velocity, the speed that a body segment moves through its range of motion. Put more simply, the resistance provided by an isokinetic machine moves at some pre-set speed, regardless of the torque applied to it by the individual, thus, the key to isokinetic exercise is not the resistance but the speed at which the resistance can be moved.[101]

Advantages for this type of exercise:

- Both high-speed/low-resistance and low-speed/high-resistance regimens result in excellent strength gains.[7–10]
- Both concentric and eccentric resistance exercises can be performed on the machines.
- Provides objective and quantifiable measurements of muscular strength.
- The machines provide maximum resistance at all points in the range of motion as a muscle contracts.
- The gravity-produced torque created by the machine adds to the force generated by the muscle when it contracts resulting in a higher torque output than it actually created by the muscle.

Disadvantages of this type of exercise:

- Expense. Isokinetic machines, which rely on hydraulic, pneumatic, and mechanical pressure systems, are very expensive, with purchase prices ranging between $50,000 and $80,000.

- Requires maximal effort to work effectively.
- The increased potential for impact loading and incorrect joint axis alignment.[11]
- Questionable functional carryover.[12]

Increasing Muscle Endurance

It is well established that endurance training results in enhanced performance and delayed onset of fatigue during endurance exercise. Endurance exercise training also leads to a shift of skeletal muscle mitochondria toward an increased use of lipids as a substrate source both at the same absolute and at the same relative exercise intensity.[14,102]

Muscular endurance training is typically prescribed during the general preparation phase of training to prepare the body for the increased work demands that will be required, and to program the body's neuromuscular coordination systems. It is worth remembering that working at a level to which the muscle is accustomed improves the endurance of that muscle but does not increase its strength.

To increase muscle endurance, exercises are performed against light resistance for many reps (no fewer than 20 per set) so that the amount of energy expended is equal to the amount of energy supplied. The amount of weight used during muscular endurance training can be determined by using a RPE scale, in which 1 is very light exertion and 10 is intense exertion. Using the example of a bench press, if an athlete plans to work at around level 3 and his maximum weight for the bench press is 220 pounds, he should reduce his workout weight by 70% (154 pounds) and increase the number of reps.

The number of reps used is a factor of the speed of one rep, and how many reps the athlete can complete in 60 seconds. For example, if under normal training conditions the athlete takes 3 seconds to raise the weight during a biceps curl and 3 seconds to lower it, the muscle is under tension for 6 seconds and the athlete is working at a speed of 10 reps per minute. By increasing the speed of the rep to 4 seconds (the time the muscle is under tension), the athlete must achieve at least 15 reps in order to build muscular endurance.

The major drawback of muscular endurance training is the increased potential for overuse injuries. This can be offset by manipulating one or more of the training variables, such as sets, loads, tempo, rest periods between sets, number of exercises, hand position, and grip width.

Increasing Muscle Power

Power is increased by having a muscle work dynamically against resistance within a specified period. In the context of rehabilitation, plyometric training can be viewed as the bridge between pure strength and sports-related exercises.[103]

Plyometrics. It has been demonstrated that when a concentric contraction is preceded by a phase of active or passive stretching, elastic energy is stored in the muscle. This stored energy is then used in the subsequent contractile phase. For example, during some functional activities, such as jumping, the movement involves an eccentric loading of a muscle or muscle group, followed immediately by a concentric muscle action, as part of a stretch-shortening cycle.[81] The eccentric/concentric actions utilize the stretch reflex or stretch-shortening cycle in which the muscle is preloaded with energy during the eccentric phase (much like stretching a rubber band apart) and the release of that stored energy for subsequent muscular actions (releasing the rubber band).[104] The stored elastic energy within the muscle is used to produce more force than can be provided by a concentric contraction alone (see later).[105–107]

The goal of plyometric training is to decrease the amount of time required between the yielding eccentric muscle contraction and the initiation of the overcoming concentric contraction.[108]

The training system of plyometrics is credited to Yuri Verhoshanski,[109] the renowned Soviet jump coach of the late 1960s, although the actual term *plyometrics* was first introduced in the mid-1970s by an American track coach Fred Wilt.[110] The term *plyometrics*, when broken down to the roots of the words, is a little confusing. *Plyo* comes from the Greek word *pleythein*, which means to increase, and *metric*, which means to measure. Plyometrics is associated with an enhancement of the ability of the muscle–tendon unit to produce maximal force in the shortest amount of time through activation of the myotatic reflex.[106,111–113] The tendon portion of the muscle–tendon unit has been found to be the main contributor to muscle–tendon unit length changes and the storage of elastic potential energy.[114]

Movement patterns in both athletics and activities of daily living involve repeated stretch-shortening cycles, in which an eccentric movement must be stopped and converted into a concentric movement in the opposite direction. When a muscle contracts in a concentric fashion, most of the force produced comes from the muscle fiber filaments sliding past one another. Force is registered externally by being transferred through the series elastic component of the muscle, and as the muscle lengthens like a spring during the eccentric contraction, the series elastic component is also stretched and contributes to the overall force production.[108]

Acceleration and deceleration are the most important components of all task-specific activities.[22] These activities use variable speed and resistance throughout the range of contraction, stimulating neurologic receptors and increasing their excitability. The nerve receptors involved in plyometrics are the muscle spindle, the Golgi tendon organ, and the joint capsule/ligamentous receptors (see Chap. 3). These neurologic receptors play an important role in fiber recruitment and physiologic coordination. Plyometric activities serve to improve the reactivity of these receptors. Two other reflex mechanisms, which result from neural signals generated by muscle receptors that project back to the muscle of origin as well as other muscles, can be initiated during plyometric exercise and may assist with motor coordination and joint stability:[115]

- ***Length feedback.*** These signals, generated by muscle stretch, occur around the same time frame as the stretch reflex, and serve to link muscles that are synergists through excitatory feedback and those with opposite actions by reciprocal inhibition.[116] Length feedback also links monoarticular muscles with excitatory feedback and contributes to joint stiffness.[116]

- *Force feedback*. These are signals generated by muscle force, which are provided by stimulation of the Golgi tendon organ, and which connect muscles that cross different joints and exert torque in different directions through inhibitory feedback. Force feedback regulates coupling between joints.[116]

Together, length and force feedback induced during the loading phase of a plyometric activity have the potential to improve neuromuscular control.[115]

The physiology of plyometrics can be broken down into a number of phases:

1. A loading phase (eccentric, deceleration, setting, yielding, or cocking phase), in which the muscle–tendon units of the prime movers and synergists are stretched as a result of kinetic energy or loading applied to the joint and begin to perform negative work.[115] Stretching of the muscle–tendon unit during this phase elicits the stretch-shortening cycle, which results in enhanced force production and performance when compared to the absence of stretch.[46] Stretch of active muscle during the loading phase elicits two mechanisms associated with the stretch-shortening cycle: muscle "potentiation" and activation of the muscle spindle[115]:
   - *Muscle potentiation*. An alteration of the muscle contractile properties that leads to higher force production through an increase in the proportion of cross-bridges attached to actin and a decrease in the cross-bridge detachment rate.
   - *Muscle spindle activation*. Sensory information from the muscle spindle is passed through a monosynaptic reflex loop to provide excitatory feedback to the same muscle (see Chap. 3). This results in short-latency reflex muscle activity (myotatic or stretch reflex). However, the stretch reflex may not be elicited in all muscles that are stretched during a plyometric activity. Monoarticular muscles are consistently activated, but biarticular muscles are not. Differences in reflex muscle activity between monoarticular and biarticular muscles may be explained by differences in muscle length changes during loading. In certain activities, some of the fascicles of biarticular muscles undergo lengthening (eccentric action), while the other muscle fascicles act nearly isometrically. This suggests that monoarticular muscles may benefit more than biarticular muscles from stretch reflex force augmentation for enhanced work output.
2. A coupling (amortization, transmission, pay-off, or reversal) phase: This phase marks the transition between the loading phase and the unloading phase.[46] The coupling phase, the definitive phase of plyometric exercise, is generally a period of quasi-isometric muscle action.[115] If this transition phase is not continuous, the activity will no longer be considered plyometric because the benefits of the stretch-shortening cycle will be lost.[115]
3. An unloading phase: The unloading (rebound, shortening, push-off, or propulsion) phase of a plyometric exercise occurs immediately after the coupling phase and involves shortening of the muscle–tendon unit. In the biphasic analysis of plyometric jumps, the unloading phase begins at the start of upward movement of the center of mass and ends when ground contact ceases.[117] Most plyometric activities terminate in a momentum phase, during which body segments continue to move as a result of the forces generated in the unloading phase.[115]

By reproducing these stretch-shortening cycles at positions of physiologic function, plyometric activities stimulate proprioceptive feedback to fine-tune muscle activity patterns. Stretch-shortening exercise trains the neuromuscular system by exposing it to increased strength loads and improving the stretch reflex[46] (see Chap. 3). The degree of performance enhancement during the momentum phase is dependent on the magnitude of the forces and quickness of movement during the plyometric activity.[115] In particular, higher forces are associated with a shorter coupling phase[118] and greater energy storage in the series elastic component.[119] Performance is also a consequence of the total contact duration (loading through unloading phases), because as the contact duration becomes shorter, higher forces and joint moments are generated[120] and the tendon contribution to work is increased.[115,121]

The mechanisms by which performance is enhanced during plyometric exercise depend on a number of factors:

- The activity must impart higher forces and faster speeds of movement.
- Prolonged contact times should be avoided. The goal of plyometric training is to decrease the amount of time required between the loading phase and the initiation of the overcoming concentric contraction. Prolonged contact times may result when the intensity is too high during the loading phase or when the transition between the loading and unloading phases is not continuous.[115]
- Plyometric exercises must be initiated at a lower intensity and progressed to more difficult, higher-intensity levels according to tolerance. Before initiating plyometric exercises, the clinician must ensure that the patient has an adequate strength and physical condition base.[46] Initially, the patient is instructed to perform fewer sets and reps. Later, the patient is permitted to do more sets, but not more reps.

Plyometric exercises were traditionally designed to enable lower extremity muscles—primarily the thighs, quadriceps, hamstrings, and calves—to attain maximal power using high-intensity workouts in short spurts of hops, leaps, or bounds. Therefore, care should be taken when applying the physiological principles derived from lower extremity investigations to upper-body and trunk applications, as it is unknown whether the upper extremity and trunk will respond in similar manner.[115] Plyometrics are typically introduced into the rehabilitation program in the later stages as many plyometric exercises, even at low intensities, expose joints to substantial forces and movement speeds.[115] Plyometric exercise is indicated for those patients who desire to return to activities that include explosive movements. Contraindications for initiating plyometric exercise are acute inflammation or pain, immediate postoperative status, and joint instability.[46] Joint pathologies such as arthritis, bone contusion, or chondral injury are relative contraindications, depending on the ability of the tissue to tolerate the high forces and joint loading required in many plyometric activities.[115] Musculotendinous injury is also a relative contraindication until the tissue is able to handle the rapid and high forces of a plyometric exercise.[115]

Guidelines for initiating plyometric exercise in rehabilitation are poorly developed. Most of the criteria have been established for high-intensity exercise in uninjured athletes and are grounded in opinion rather than research.[115] For example, it has been suggested that plyometric exercise should be initiated only after achieving the ability to perform one rep of a parallel squat with a load of 1.5–2.5 times body mass on the back and/or squat 60% of body mass 5 times within 5 seconds (lower extremity), and a bench press with one-third of body weight and/or perform five hand clap pushups (upper extremity).[103] In addition, success in the static stability tests[91] (Table 12-9) and dynamic stability tests (vertical jump for the lower extremities and medicine ball throw for the upper extremities) have also been used as a measure of preparation.[21]

Many different activities and devices can be used in plyometric exercises. Plyometric exercises may include diagonal and multiplanar motions with tubing or isokinetic machines. These exercises may be used to mimic any of the needed motions and can be performed in the standing, sitting, or supine positions. Generally, 48–72 hours of rest is recommended for recovery between plyometric training sessions.[122]

Lower Extremity Plyometric Exercises. Lower extremity plyometric exercises involve the manipulation of the role of gravity to vary the intensity of the exercise (Table 12-10). Thus, plyometric exercises can be performed horizontally or vertically.

- Horizontal plyometrics are performed perpendicular to the line of gravity. These exercises are preferable for most initial clinical rehabilitation plans because the concentric force is reduced and the eccentric phase is not facilitated.[21] Examples of these types of exercises include pushing a sled against resistance, and a modified leg press that allows the subject to push off and land on the foot plate.
- Vertical plyometric exercises (against or with gravitational forces) are more advanced. These exercises require a greater

TABLE 12-9 Static Stability Tests for Performance of Plyometrics

1. Single-leg stance: 30 sec
   Eyes open
   Eyes closed
2. Single-leg quarter squat: 30 sec
   Eyes open
   Eyes closed
3. Single-leg half squat: 30 sec
   Eyes open
   Eyes closed

Data from Voight ML, Tippert SR: Plyometric exercise in rehabilitation. In: Voight ML, Hoogenboom BJ, Prentice WE, eds. *Musculoskeletal Interventions: Techniques for Therapeutic Exercise.* New York, NY: McGraw-Hill, 2007:231–242.

TABLE 12-10 Lower Extremity Plyometric Drills

Warm-up drills
- Double-leg squats
- Double-leg leg press
- Double-leg squat-jumps
- Jumping jacks

Entry-level drills—two legged

Two-legged drills
- Side-to-side (floor/line)
- Diagonal jumps (floor/4 corners)
- Diagonal jumps (4 spots)
- Diagonal zig-zag (6 spots)
- Plyometric leg press
- Plyometric leg press (4 corners)

Intermediate-level drills

Two-legged box jumps
- One-box side jump
- Two-box side jumps
- Two-box side jumps with foam
- Four-box diagonal jumps
- Two-box with rotation
- One/two-box with catch
- One/two-box with catch (foam)

Single-leg movements
- Single-leg plyometric leg press
- Single-leg side jumps (floor)
- Single-leg side-to-side jumps (floor/4 corners)
- Single-leg diagonal jumps (floor/4 corners)

Advanced-level drills

Single-leg box jumps
- One-box side jumps
- Two-box side jumps
- Single-leg plyometric leg press (4 corners)
- Two-box side jumps with foam
- Four-box diagonal jumps
- One-box side jumps with rotation
- Two-box side jumps with rotation
- One-box side jump with catch
- One-box side jump rotation with catch
- Two-box side jump with catch
- Two-box side jump rotation with catch

Endurance/agility plyometrics
- Side-to-side bounding (20 ft)
- Side jump lunges (cone)
- Side jump lunges (cone with foam)
- Altering rapid step-up (forward)
- Lateral step-overs
- High stepping (forward)
- High stepping (backward)
- Depth jump with rebound jump
- Depth jump with catch
- Jump and catch (plyoball)

Data from Voight ML, Draovitch P, Tippett SR: Plyometrics. In: Albert MS, ed. *Eccentric Muscle Training in Sports and Orthopaedics.* New York, NY: Churchill Livingstone, 1995.

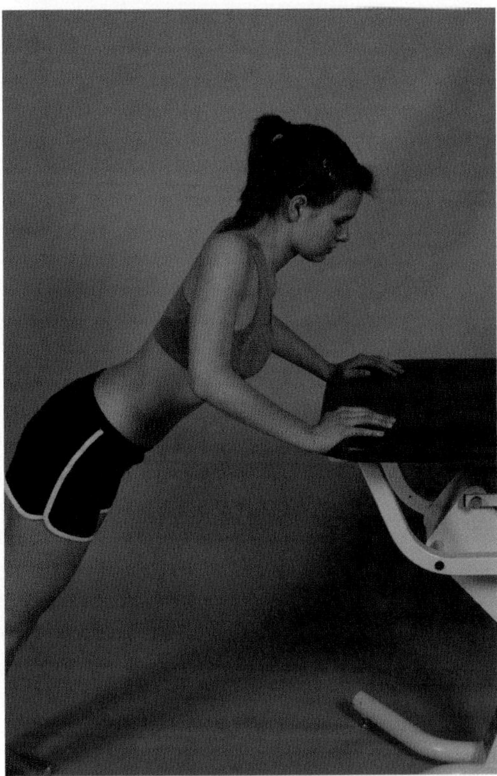

FIGURE 12-3 Push-off from table.

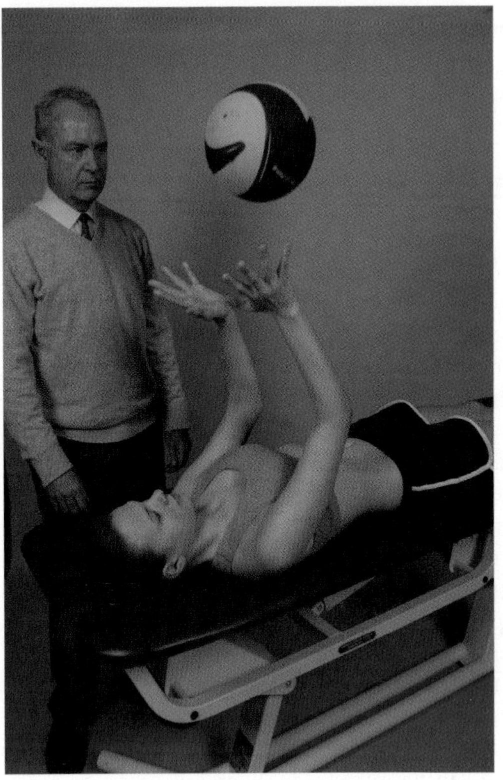

FIGURE 12-4 Medicine ball toss.

level of control.[21] The drop jump is an example—the subject steps off a box, lands, and immediately executes a vertical jump.

The footwear and landing surfaces used in plyometric drills must have shock-absorbing qualities, and the protocol should allow sufficient recovery time between sets to prevent fatigue of the muscle groups being trained.[123]

Upper Extremity Plyometric Exercises. Plyometric exercises for the upper extremity involve relatively rapid movements in planes that approximate normal joint function. For example, at the shoulder this would include flexion or abduction at the shoulder, trunk rotation and diagonal arm motions, and rapid external and internal rotation exercises.

Plyometrics should be performed for all body segments involved in the activity. Hip rotation, knee flexion and extension, and trunk rotation are power activities that require plyometric activation. Plyometric exercises for the upper extremity include push-offs (Fig. 12-3), corner push-ups, and weighted ball throws (Fig. 12-4). Medicine and other weighted balls are very effective plyometric devices. The weight of the ball creates a prestretch and an eccentric load when it is caught. This combination creates resistance and demands a powerful agonist contraction to propel it forward again. The exercises can be performed using one arm or both arms at the same time. The former emphasizes trunk rotation and the latter emphasizes trunk extension and flexion, as well as shoulder motion.

A variety of positive changes in athletic performance and neuromuscular function have been attributed to plyometric training, predominantly in the lower extremity:[115]

- Increased maximal vertical jump height.[124]
- Increased leg strength, especially when combined with weight training.[124]
- A faster rate of force development during jumping.[125]
- Delayed onset of muscle fatigue during jumping.[126]
- Correction of neuromuscular imbalances.[127]

Due to the scarcity of research on upper extremity performance plyometric training, the improvements in upper extremity performance remain largely anecdotal. It is also unknown whether patients recovering from injury will respond to plyometric exercise in a manner similar to uninjured subjects.[115]

Contraindications to Strengthening, Endurance, and Power Exercises

Absolute contraindications to exercise include unstable angina, uncontrolled hypertension, uncontrolled dysrhythmias, hypertrophic cardiomyopathy, and certain stages of retinopathy. Patients with congestive heart failure, myocardial ischemia, poor left ventricular function, or autonomic neuropathies must be carefully evaluated before initiating an exercise program.

A number of precautions need to be taken when exercising patients who have a compromised cardiovascular or pulmonary system (see Chap. 15):

- An appropriate level of intensity must be chosen.
- Too high a level can overload the cardiorespiratory and muscular systems and potentially cause injuries.
- Exercising at the level it is too high causes the cardiorespiratory system to work anaerobically, not aerobically.

- ▸ A sufficient period of time should be allowed for warm-up and cool-down to permit adequate cardiorespiratory and muscular adaptation.

Increasing Joint Stabilization

According to Voight,[128,129] the standard progression for stabilization exercises involves:

- ▸ Static stabilization exercises with closed chain loading and unloading (weight shifting). This phase initially employs isometric exercises around the involved joint on solid and even surfaces, before progressing to unstable surfaces. The early training involves balance training and joint repositioning exercises, and is usually initiated (in the lower extremities according to weight-bearing restrictions) by having the patient placing the involved extremity on a 6–8 inch stool, so that the amount of weight bearing can be controlled more easily. The proprioceptive awareness of a joint can also be enhanced by using an elastic bandage, orthotic, or through taping.[130–135] As full weight bearing through the extremity is restored, a number of devices such as a mini-trampoline, balance board, stability ball, and wobble board can be introduced. Exercises on these devices are progressed from double limb support, to single leg support, to support while performing sports-specific skills.

CLINICAL PEARL

A stability ball creates an unstable base, which challenges the postural stabilizer muscles more than using a stable base. It is important to choose the correct and appropriate size of stability ball, which is dependent upon patient size

45 cm ball: shorter than 5′

55 cm ball: 5′ to 5′ 8″

65 cm ball: 5′ 9″ to 6′3″

75 cm ball: taller than 6′3″

With the patient sitting on the ball with both feet firmly planted on the ground, the patient's thigh should be parallel to the floor (the knee may be slightly above the hips).

- ▸ Pumping up the ball to increase firmness increases the level of difficulty in any given exercise.
- ▸ The further away the ball is from the support points, the greater the demand for core stability.
- ▸ Decreasing the number of support points increases the difficulty of the exercise.

- ▸ Transitional stabilization exercises. The exercises during this phase involve conscious control of motion without impact, and replace isometric activity with controlled concentric and eccentric exercises throughout a progressively larger range of functional motion. The physiological rationale behind the exercises in this phase is to stimulate dynamic postural responses, and to increase muscle stiffness. Muscle stiffness (see Chap. 2) has a significant role in improving dynamic stabilization around the joint, by resisting and absorbing joint loads.[136]
- ▸ Dynamic stabilization exercises. These exercises involve the unconscious control and loading of the joint, and introduce both *ballistic* and *impact* exercises to the patient.

A delicate balance between stability and mobility is achieved by coordination between muscle strength, endurance, flexibility, and neuromuscular control.[137]

The neuromuscular mechanism that contributes to joint stability is mediated by the articular mechanoreceptors (see Chap. 3). These receptors provide information about joint position sense and kinesthesia.[134,135,138,139] Initially, closed-chain exercises are performed within the pain-free ranges or positions. Open chain exercises may be built upon the base of the closed chain stabilization to allow normal control of joint mobility.

The emphasis during these exercises is to concentrate on functional positioning during exercise rather than isolating open and closed chain activities.[137] The activities should involve sudden alterations in joint positioning that necessitate reflex muscular stabilization coupled with an axial load.[135,137] Such activities include rhythmic stabilization (an isometric contraction of the agonist followed by an isometric contraction of the antagonist) performed in both a closed and an open chain position,[140] and in the functional position of the joint.[137] The use of a stable, and then unstable, base during closed chain exercises encourages co-contraction of the agonists and antagonists.[140]

Weight shifting exercises are ideal for this. For example, the following weight shifting exercises may be used for the upper extremity:

- ▸ Standing and leaning against a treatment table or object.
- ▸ In the quadruped position, rocking forward and backward with the hands on the floor or on an unstable object.
- ▸ Kneeling forward in the three-point position (with one hand on the floor). A Body Blade® can be added to this exercise to increase the difficulty (Fig. 12-5).
- ▸ Kneeling in the two-point position (high-kneeling) (Fig. 12-6).
- ▸ Weight shifting on a Fitter® while in a kneeling position (Fig. 12-7).
- ▸ Weight shifting on a Swiss ball with the feet elevated on a support, and both hands on the Swiss ball in the push-up position (Fig. 12-8). The exercise can be made more difficult by raising the height of elevation of the feet, such as placing the feet on a chair.
- ▸ Slide board exercises in the quadruped position moving hands forwards and backwards, in opposite diagonals and in opposite directions.

Integration of the Entire Kinematic Chain

Although force-dependent motor firing patterns should be reestablished, special care must be taken to completely integrate all of the components of the kinetic chain to generate and funnel the proper forces to the appropriate joint. It should be

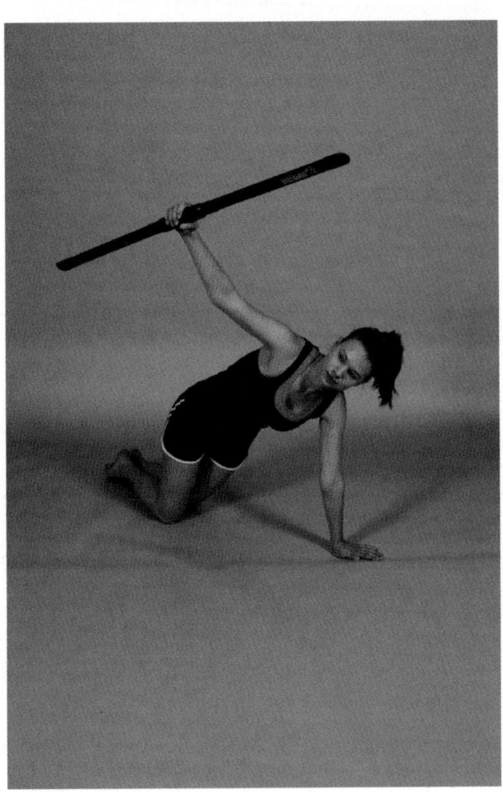

FIGURE 12-5 Three point kneeling with Bodyblade.

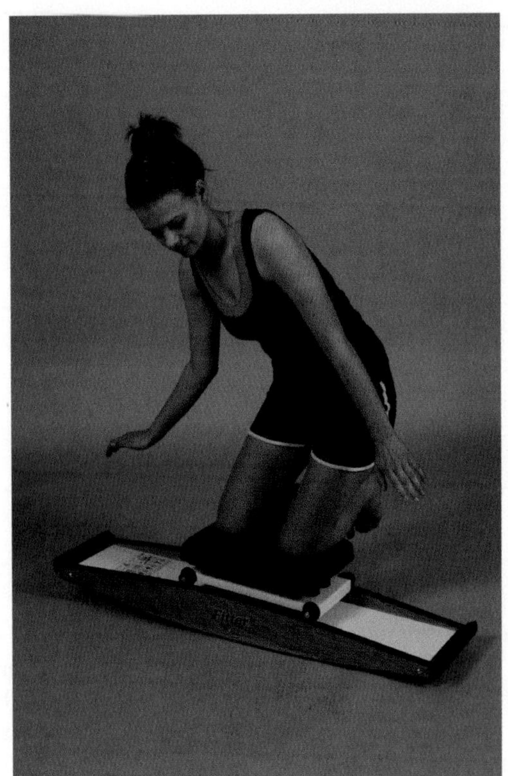

FIGURE 12-7 Weight shifting on a Fitter® while in a kneeling position.

clear that for a kinematic chain to operate efficiently, there must be an optimal sequential activation of the limb segments involved. This then allows for an efficient generation and transfer of force along the kinematic chain.[141] When choosing a mode of kinematic exercise, the variables of each type of exercise must be considered. The clinician should understand the principles of exercise application and the differences between open kinematic chain (OKC) and closed kinematic chain (CKC) movements, in order to accomplish a specific intervention goal (Table 12-11). A number of studies have

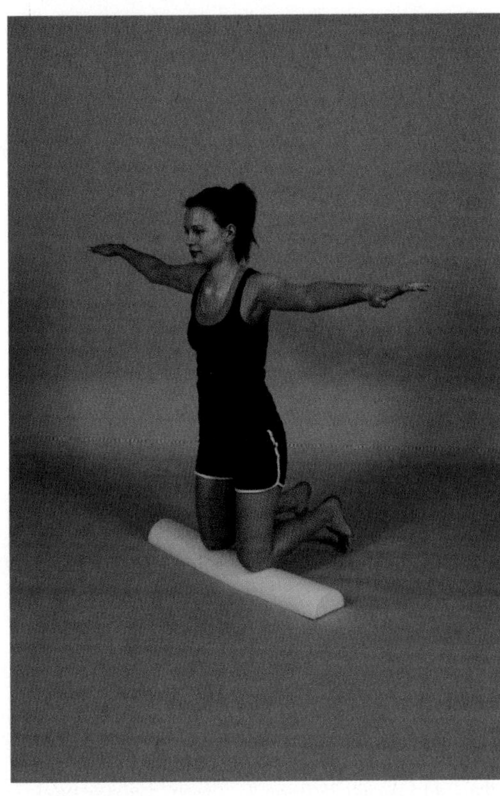

FIGURE 12-6 Hi-kneeling.

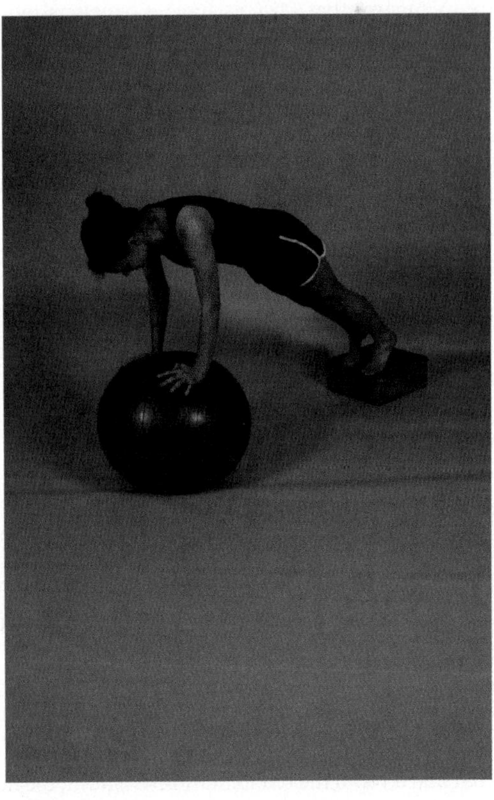

FIGURE 12-8 Weight shifting on a Swiss ball.

TABLE 12-11 Differential Features of OKC and CKC Exercises

Exercise Mode	Characteristics	Advantages	Disadvantages
Open kinematic chain	1. Single muscle group 2. Single axis and plane 3. Emphasizes concentric contraction 4. Non–weight-bearing	1. Isolated recruitment 2. Simple movement pattern 3. Isolated recruitment 4. Minimal joint compression	1. Limited function 2. Limited function 3. Limited eccentrics 4. Less proprioception and joint stability with increased joint shear forces
Closed kinematic	1. Multiple muscle groups 2. Multiple axes and planes 3. Balance of concentric and eccentric contractions 4. Weight-bearing exercise	1. Functional recruitment 2. Functional movement patterns 3. Functional contractions 4. Increase proprioception and joint stability	1. Difficult to isolate 2. More complex 3. Loss of control of target joint 4. Compressive forces on articular surfaces

Data from Greenfield BH, Tovin BJ: The application of open and closed kinematic chain exercises in rehabilitation of the lower extremity. *J Back Musculoskel Rehabil* 2:38–51, 1992.

illustrated the importance of the sequential activation of these links.[142,143] The benefit of closed kinematic chain exercises (CKCE) over open kinematic chain exercises (OKCE) is based on the premise that CKCEs, particularly in the lower extremities, appear to replicate functional tasks better than OCKEs. This is because the CKCEs appear to allow the entire linkage system of the kinematic chain to be exercised together.[45,74,144–150] In addition, CKCEs have been shown to enhance joint congruency, decrease the shearing forces, and stimulate the articular mechanoreceptors using axial loading and increased compressive forces.[147,151–155] Thus, CKC activities are purported to help reinforce the synchronization of the necessary muscle-firing patterns for both antagonist and agonist muscle groups used during stabilization and ambulation.[45] However, there also appears to be much in the literature to suggest that OKCEs have a beneficial effect on function,[8,156,157] especially when combined with specific closed chain exercises or when used to strengthen individual muscles.[144]

A comprehensive rehabilitation program thus should integrate the entire kinematic chain, using a blend of OKCEs and CKCEs. This integration must occur during functional exercises, with the emphasis determined by the activity to be restored.

CLINICAL PEARL

The rehabilitation of the kinematic chain should address the strength and flexibility of the entire kinematic chain, using the principle of specificity, with the specific elements of the rehabilitation program being determined by both the existing pathology and the functional goals of the patient.[144,158]

In addition, under the concept of specificity, rather than isolating OKCEs or CKCEs, it may be wise to emphasize functional positioning during the exercise training, while striking a balance between mobility and stability.[144,159]

Several objectives must be met if the rehabilitation of the functional kinematic chain is to be comprehensive.[144]:

1. The first objective in the rehabilitation program, the healing phase, is the restoration of functional stability, which is the ability to control the translation of the joint during dynamic functional activities, through the integration of both the primary and the secondary stabilizers.[160]
2. The second objective, the functional phase, is to restore sports- or functional-specific movement patterns. The functional phase begins once the patient has near-full, pain-free ROM.
3. The final objective is assessing the readiness of the patient to return to his or her prior level of function or level of athletic performance.

REVIEW QUESTIONS*

1. What are the four biomechanical properties of skeletal muscle?
2. Give three examples of a muscle that cross two or more joints.
3. What are the three main types of muscle contraction?
4. Define the characteristics of an isotonic contraction.
5. True/false: Rapid lengthening contractions generate more force than do slower lengthening contractions.

*Additional questions to test your understanding of this chapter can be found in the Online Learning Center for Orthopaedic Assessment, Evaluation, and Intervention at www.duttononline.net.

REFERENCES

1. Luttgens K, Hamilton K: The musculoskeletal system: the musculature. In: Luttgens K, Hamilton K, eds. *Kinesiology: Scientific Basis of Human Motion*, 9th ed. Dubuque, IA: McGraw-Hill, 1997:49–75.
2. Astrand PO, Rodahl K: *The Muscle and its Contraction: Textbook of Work Physiology*. New York, NY: McGraw-Hill, 1986.
3. Komi PV: *Strength and Power in Sport*. London: Blackwell Scientific Publications, 1992.
4. McArdle W, Katch FI, Katch VL: *Exercise Physiology: Energy, Nutrition, and Human Performance*. Philadelphia, PA: Lea and Febiger, 1991.
5. Lakomy HKA: The biomechanics of human movement. In: Maughan RJ, ed. *Basic and Applied Sciences for Sports Medicine*. Woburn, MA: Butterworth-Heinemann, 1999:124–125.

6. Verrall GM, Slavotinek JP, Barnes PG, et al.: Clinical risk factors for hamstring muscle strain injury: a prospective study with correlation of injury by magnetic resonance imaging. *Br J Sports Med* 35:435–439, 2001.
7. Worrell TW, Perrin DH, Gansneder B, et al.: Comparison of isokinetic strength and flexibility measures between hamstring injured and non-injured athletes. *J Orthop Sports Phys Ther* 13:118–125, 1991.
8. Anderson MA, Gieck JH, Perrin D, et al.: The relationship among isokinetic, isotonic, and isokinetic concentric and eccentric quadriceps and hamstrings force and three components of athletic performance. *J Orthop Sports Phys Ther* 14:114–120, 1991.
9. Steadman JR, Forster RS, Silfverskold JP: Rehabilitation of the knee. *Clin Sports Med* 8:605–627, 1989.
10. Montgomery JB, Steadman JR: Rehabilitation of the injured knee. *Clin Sports Med* 4:333–343, 1985.
11. Delsman PA, Losee GM: Isokinetic shear forces and their effect on the quadriceps active drawer. *Med Sci Sports Exerc* 16:151, 1984.
12. Albert MS: Principles of exercise progression. In: Greenfield B, ed. *Rehabilitation of the Knee: A Problem Solving Approach*. Philadelphia, PA: FA Davis, 1993:110–136.
13. Deudsinger RH: Biomechanics in clinical practice. *Phys Ther* 64: 1860–1868, 1984.
14. Hoppeler H, Fluck M: Plasticity of skeletal muscle mitochondria: structure and function. *Med Sci Sports Exerc* 35:95–104, 2003.
15. Tonkonogi M, Sahlin K: Physical exercise and mitochondrial function in human skeletal muscle. *Exerc Sport Sci Rev* 30:129–137, 2002.
16. Howald H, Hoppeler H, Claassen H, et al.: Influences of endurance training on the ultrastructural composition of the different muscle fiber types in humans. *Pflugers Arch* 403:369–376, 1985.
17. Hill AV: The heat and shortening and the dynamic constants of muscle. *Proc R Soc Lond B* 126;136–195, 1938.
18. Tihanyi J, Apor P, Fekete GY: Force-velocity – power characteristics and fiber composition in human knee extensor muscles. *Eur J Appl Physiol* 48:331–343, 1982.
19. Fitts RH, Widrick JJ: Muscle mechanics; adaptations with exercise training. *Exerc Sport Sci Rev* 24:427–473, 1996.
20. Rhea MR, Alvar BA, Burkett LN, et al.: A meta-analysis to determine the dose response for strength development. *Med Sci Sports Exerc* 35:456–464, 2003.
21. Albert M: Concepts of muscle training. In: Wadsworth C, ed. *Orthopaedic Physical Therapy: Topic – Strength and Conditioning Applications in Orthopaedics – Home Study Course 98A*. La Crosse, WI: Orthopaedic Section, APTA, Inc., 1998:1–5.
22. Grimsby O, Power B: Manual therapy approach to knee ligament rehabilitation. In: Ellenbecker TS, ed. *Knee Ligament Rehabilitation*. Philadelphia, PA: Churchill Livingstone, 2000:236–251.
23. Pollock ML, Gaesser GA, Butcher JD, et al.: The recommended quantity and quality of exercise for developing and maintaining cardiorespiratory and muscular fitness, and flexibility in healthy adults: American College of Sports Medicine Position Stand. *Med Sci Sports Exerc* 30:975–991, 1998.
24. Cyriax J: *Textbook of Orthopaedic Medicine, Diagnosis of Soft Tissue Lesions*, 8th ed. London: Bailliere Tindall, 1982.
25. Sporer BC, Wenger HA: Effects of aerobic exercise on strength performance following various periods of recovery. *J Strength Cond Res* 17:638–644, 2003.
26. Wenger HA, McFadyen PF, Middleton L, et al.: Physiological principles of conditioning for the injured and disabled. In: Magee D, Zachazewski JE, Quillen WS, eds. *Scientific Foundations and Principles of Practice in Musculoskeletal Rehabilitation*. St. Louis, MI: WB Saunders, 2007:357–374.
27. Bahr R: Principles of injury prevention. In: Brukner P, Khan K, eds. *Clinical Sports Medicine*, 3rd ed. Sydney: McGraw-Hill, 2007:78–101.
28. Grimby G, Thomee R: Principles of rehabilitation after injuries. In: Dirix A, Knuttgen HG, Tittel K, eds. *The Olympic Book of Sports Medicine*. Oxford: Blackwell Scientific Publications, 1984.
29. Thomee R, Renstrom P, Grimby G, et al.: Slow or fast isokinetic training after surgery. *J Orthop Sports Phys Ther* 8:476, 1987.
30. Graves JE, Pollock SH, Leggett SH, et al.: Effect of reduced training frequency on muscular strength. *Sports Med* 9:316–319, 1988.
31. Fleck SJ, Kraemer WJ: *Designing Resistance Training Programs*, 2nd ed. Champaign, IL: Human Kinetics Books, 1997.
32. Simoneau GG, Bereda SM, Sobush DC, et al.: Biomechanics of elastic resistance in therapeutic exercise programs. *J Orthop Sports Phys Ther* 31:16–24, 2001.
33. Williams JH, Klug GA: Calcium exchange hypothesis of skeletal muscle fatigue. A brief review. *Muscle Nerve* 18:421, 1995.
34. Allen DG, Lannergren J, Westerblad H: Muscle cell function during prolonged activity: cellular mechanisms of fatigue. *Exp Physiol* 80:497, 1995.
35. Shepley B, MacDougall JD, Cipriano N, et al.: Physiological effects of tapering in highly trained athletes. *J Appl Physiol* 72:706–711, 1992.
36. Borg GAV: Psychophysical basis of perceived exertion. *Med Sci Sports Exerc* 14:377–381, 1992.
37. Borg GAV: Perceived exertion as an indicator of somatic stress. *Scand J Rehabil Med* 2:92–98, 1970.
38. Canavan PK: Designing a rehabilitation program related to strength and conditioning. In: Wilmarth MA, ed. *Orthopaedic Physical Therapy: Topic – Strength and Conditioning – Independent Study Course 15.3*. La Crosse, WI: Orthopaedic Section, APTA, Inc., 2005.
39. Pearson D, Faigenbaum A, Conley M, et al.: The National Strength and Conditioning Association's basic guidelines for resistance training of athletes. *Strength Cond* 22:14–27, 2000.
40. Hass CJ, Feigenbaum MS, Franklin BA: Prescription of resistance training for healthy populations. *Sports Med* 31:953–964, 2001.
41. Taylor NF, Dodd KJ, Damiano DL: Progressive resistance exercise in physical therapy: a summary of systematic reviews. *Phys Ther* 85:1208–1223, 2005.
42. Kellmann M: Preventing overtraining in athletes in high-intensity sports and stress/recovery monitoring. *Scand J Med Sci Sports* 20(Suppl 2):95–102, 2010.
43. Manchester RA: Fatigue, performance, and overtraining. *Med Probl Perform Art* 25:47–48, 2010.
44. Roose J, de Vries WR, Schmikli SL, et al.: Evaluation and opportunities in overtraining approaches. *Res Q Exerc Sport* 80:756–764, 2009.
45. Palmitier RA, An KN, Scott SG, et al.: Kinetic chain exercises in knee rehabilitation. *Sports Med* 11:402–413, 1991.
46. Wilk KE, Voight ML, Keirns MA, et al.: Stretch-shortening drills for the upper extremities: theory and clinical application. *J Orthop Sports Phys Ther* 17:225–239, 1993.
47. Janda V: *Muscle Function Testing*. London: Butterworths, 1983.
48. Jull GA, Janda V: Muscle and Motor control in low back pain. In: Twomey LT, Taylor JR, eds. *Physical Therapy of the Low Back: Clinics in Physical Therapy*. New York, NY: Churchill Livingstone, 1987:258–278.
49. Byrnes WC, Clarkson PM, White JS, et al.: Delayed onset muscle soreness following repeated bouts of downhill running. *J Appl Physiol* 59:710, 1985.
50. Bennett M, Best TM, Babul S, et al.: Hyperbaric oxygen therapy for delayed onset muscle soreness and closed soft tissue injury. *Cochrane Database Syst Rev* CD004713, 2005.
51. Cheung K, Hume P, Maxwell L: Delayed onset muscle soreness : treatment strategies and performance factors. *Sports Med* 33:145–164, 2003.
52. Nureberg P, Giddings CJ, Stray-Gundersen J, et al.: MR imaging-guided muscle biopsy for correlation of increased signal intensity with ultrastructural change and delayed-onset muscle soreness after exercise. *Radiology* 184:865–869, 1992.
53. Friden J: Delayed onset muscle soreness. *Scand J Med Sci Sports* 12:327–328, 2002.
54. Friden J, Sjostrom M, Ekblom B: Myofibrillar damage following intense eccentric exercise in man. *Int J Sports Med* 4:170–176, 1983.
55. Cafarelli E, Flint F: The role of massage in preparation for and recovery from exercise. *Sports Med* 14:1–9, 1992.
56. Callaghan MJ: The role of massage in the management of the athlete: a review. *Br J Sports Med* 27:28–33, 1993.
57. Tiidus PM, Shoemaker JK: Effleurage massage, muscle blood flow and long-term post-exercise strength recovery. *Int J Sports Med* 16:475–483, 1995.
58. Belcastro AN, Bonen A: Lactic acid removal rates during controlled and uncontrolled recovery exercise. *J Appl Physiol* 39:932–936, 1975.
59. McMaster WC, Stoddard T, Duncan W: Enhancement of blood lactate clearance following maximal swimming. Effect of velocity of recovery swimming. *Am J Sports Med* 17:472–477, 1989.
60. Law RY, Herbert RD: Warm-up reduces delayed onset muscle soreness but cool-down does not: a randomised controlled trial. *Aust J Physiother* 53:91–95, 2007.
61. Hasson S, Barnes W, Hunter M, et al.: Therapeutic effect of high speed voluntary muscle contractions on muscle soreness and muscle performance. *J Orthop Sports Phys Ther* 10:499, 1989.

62. Antich TJ, Brewster CE: Rehabilitation of the nonreconstructed anterior cruciate ligament-deficient knee. *Clin Sports Med* 7:813–826, 1988.
63. Bynum EB, Barrack RL, Alexander AH: Open versus closed kinetic chain exercises in rehabilitation after anterior cruciate ligament reconstruction: a prospective randomized study, *Am J Sports Med* 23(4):401–406, 1995.
64. Mangine RE, Noyes FR, DeMaio M: Minimal protection program: advanced weight bearing and range of motion after ACL reconstruction-weeks 1 to 5. *Orthopedics* 15:504–515, 1992.
65. Steadman JR: Rehabilitation of acute injuries of the anterior cruciate ligament. *Clin Orthop* 172:129–132, 1983.
66. Steadman JR, Sterett WI: The surgical treatment of knee injuries in skiers. *Med Sci Sports Exerc* 27:328–333, 1995.
67. Zappala FG, Taffel CB, Scuderi GR: Rehabilitation of patellofemoral joint disorders. *Orthop Clin North Am* 23:555–565, 1992.
68. Rogers ME, Sherwood HS, Rogers NL, et al.: Effects of dumbbell and elastic band training on physical function in older inner-city African-American women. *Women Health* 36:33–41, 2002.
69. Engle RP, Canner GC: Proprioceptive neuromuscular facilitation (PNF) and modified procedures for anterior cruciate ligament (ACL) instability. *J Orthop Sports Phys Ther* 11:230, 1989.
70. Kibler WB: Concepts in exercise rehabilitation of athletic injury. In: Leadbetter WB, Buckwalter JA, Gordon SL, eds. *Sports-Induced Inflammation: Clinical and Basic Science Concepts.* Park Ridge, IL: American Academy of Orthopaedic Surgeons, 1990:759–769.
71. Kibler WB, Livingston B, Bruce R: Current concepts in shoulder rehabilitation. *Adv Op Orthop* 3:249–301, 1996.
72. Kibler WB, Livingston B, Chandler TJ: Shoulder rehabilitation: clinical application, evaluation, and rehabilitation protocols. *Instr Course Lect* 46:43–53, 1997.
73. Kibler WB: Shoulder rehabilitation: principles and practice. *Med Sci Sports Exerc* 30:40–50, 1998.
74. Kibler BW: Closed kinetic chain rehabilitation for sports injuries. *Phys Med Rehabil Clin N Am* 11:369–384, 2000.
75. Deschenes MR, Kraemer WJ: Performance and physiologic adaptations to resistance training. *Am J Phys Med Rehabil* 81:S3–S16, 2002.
76. Matsen FA III, Lippitt SB, Sidles JA, et al.: Strength. In: Matsen FA III, Lippitt SB, Sidles JA, et al., eds. *Practical Evaluation and Management of the Shoulder.* Philadelphia, PA: WB Saunders Company, 1994: 111–150.
77. Kisner C, Colby LA: *Therapeutic Exercise. Foundations and Techniques.* Philadelphia, PA: FA Davis, 1997.
78. Astrand PO, Rodahl K: *Physical Training: Textbook of Work Physiology.* New York, PA: McGraw-Hill, 1986.
79. DeLorme T, Watkins A: *Techniques of Progressive Resistance Exercise.* New York, PA: Appleton-Century, 1951.
80. Soest A, Bobbert M: The role of muscle properties in control of explosive movements. *Biol Cybern* 69:195–204, 1993.
81. Komi PV: The stretch-shortening cycle and human power output. In: Jones NL, McCartney N, McComas AJ, eds. *Human Muscle Power.* Champlain, IL: Human Kinetics, 1986:27–39.
82. Bandy W, Lovelace-Chandler V, Bandy B, et al.: Adaptation of skeletal muscle to resistance training. *J Orthop Sports Phys Ther* 12:248–255, 1990.
83. Luethi JM, Howald H, Claassen H, et al.: Structural changes in skeletal muscle tissue with heavy-resistance exercise. *Int J Sports Med* 7:123–127, 1986.
84. Yasuda T, Ogasawara R, Sakamaki M, et al.: Relationship between limb and trunk muscle hypertrophy following high-intensity resistance training and blood flow-restricted low-intensity resistance training. *Clin Physiol Funct Imaging* 31:347–51, 2011
85. Moritani T, de Vries HA: Neural factors vs. hypertrophy in the time course of muscle strength gain. *Am J Phys Med* 58:115–130, 1979.
86. Jones DA, Rutherford OM: Human muscle strength training: the effects of three different regimes and the nature of the resultant changes. *J Physiol* 391:1–11, 1987.
87. Gollinck PD, Timson BF, Moore RL, et al.: Muscular enlargement and number of muscle fibers in skeletal muscles of rats. *J Appl Physiol* 50: 936–943, 1981.
88. Hakkinen K, Alen M, Komi PV: Changes in isometric force and relaxation time, electromyographic and muscle fibre characteristics of human skeletal muscle during strength training and detraining. *Acta Physiol Scand* 125:573–585, 1985.
89. Hettinger T: *Isometrisches Muskeltraining.* Stuttgart, Germany: M.Thun, 1964.
90. Mueller K: *Statische und Dynamische Muskelkraft.* Frankfurt, Germany: M. Thun, 1987.
91. Green DJ, O'Driscoll G, Blankly BA, et al.: Control of skeletal blood flow during dynamic exercise. Contribution of endothelial derived nitric oxide. *Sports Med* 21:119–146, 1996.
92. Zinovieff AN: Heavy-resistance exercises the "Oxford technique". *Br J Phys Med* 14:129–132, 1951.
93. Macqueen IJ: The application of progressive resistance exercise in physiotherapy. *Physiotherapy* 42:83–93, 1956.
94. Macqueen IJ: Recent advances in the technique of progressive resistance exercise. *Br Med J* 2:1193–1198, 1954.
95. Sanders M: Weight training and conditioning. In: Sanders B, ed. *Sports Physical Therapy.* Norwalk, CT: Appleton & Lange, 1997:235–250.
96. Knight KL: Knee rehabilitation by the daily adjustable progressive resistive exercise technique. *Am J Sports Med* 7:336–337, 1979.
97. Berger R: *Conditioning for Men.* Boston, MA: Allyn & Bacon, 1973.
98. Clark MA: *Integrated Training for the New Millenium.* Thousand Oaks, CA: National Academy of Sports Medicine, 2001.
99. Lange GW, Hintermeister RA, Schlegel T, et al.: Electromyographic and kinematic analysis of graded treadmill walking and the implications for knee rehabilitation. *J Orthop Sports Phys Ther* 23:294–301, 1996.
100. Dvir Z: *Isokinetics: Muscle Testing, Interpretation and Clinical Applications.* New York, NY: Churchill Livingstone, 1995.
101. Prentice WE: Impaired muscle performance: regaining muscular strength and endurance. In: Voight ML, Hoogenboom BJ, Prentice WE, eds. *Musculoskeletal Interventions: Techniques for Therapeutic Exercise.* New York, NY: McGraw-Hill, 2007:135–151.
102. Holloszy JO, Coyle EF: Adaptations of skeletal muscle to endurance exercise and their metabolic consequences. *J Appl Physiol* 56:831–838, 1984.
103. Voight ML, Draovitch P, Tippett SR: Plyometrics. In: Albert MS, ed. *Eccentric Muscle Training in Sports and Orthopedics.* New York, NY: Churchill Livingstone, 1995.
104. Malone T, Nitz AJ, Kuperstein J, et al.: Neuromuscular concepts. In: Ellenbecker TS, ed. *Knee Ligament Rehabilitation.* Philadelphia, PA: Churchill Livingstone, 2000:399–411.
105. Asmussen E, Bonde-Petersen F: Apparent efficiency and storage of elastic energy in human muscles during exercise. *Acta Physiol Scand* 92:537–545, 1974.
106. Asmussen E, Bonde-Petersen F: Storage of elastic energy in skeletal muscles in man. *Acta Physiol Scand* 91:385–392, 1974.
107. Herrero AJ, Martin J, Martin T, et al.: Short-term effect of plyometrics and strength training with and without superimposed electrical stimulation on muscle strength and anaerobic performance: a randomized controlled trial. Part II. *J Strength Cond Res* 24:1616–1622, 2010.
108. Voight ML, Tippert SR: Plyometric exercise in rehabilitation. In: Voight ML, Hoogenboom BJ, Prentice WE, eds. *Musculoskeletal Interventions: Techniques for Therapeutic Exercise.* New York, NY: McGraw-Hill, 2007:231–242.
109. Verhoshanski Y, Chornonson G: Jump exercises in sprint training. *Track and Field Quarterly* 9:1909, 1967.
110. Wilt F: Plyometrics – what it is and how it works. *Athletic J* 55b:76, 1975.
111. Bosco C, Komi PV: Potentiation of the mechanical behavior of the human skeletal muscle through prestretching. *Acta Physiol Scand* 106:467–472, 1979.
112. Cavagna GA, Saibene FP, Margaria R: Effect of negative work on the amount of positive work performed by an isolated muscle. *J Appl Physiol* 20:157, 1965.
113. Cavagna GA, Disman B, Margarai R: Positive work done by a previously stretched muscle. *J Appl Physiol* 24:21–32, 1968.
114. Roberts TJ: The integrated function of muscles and tendons during locomotion. *Comp Biochem Physiol A Mol Integr Physiol* 133:1087–1099, 2002.
115. Chmielewski TL, Myer GD, Kauffman D, et al.: Plyometric exercise in the rehabilitation of athletes: physiological responses and clinical application. *J Orthop Sports Phys Ther* 36:308–319, 2006.
116. Nichols TR: A biomechanical perspective on spinal mechanisms of coordinated muscular action: an architecture principle. *Acta Anat (Basel)* 151:1–13, 1994.
117. Bobbert MF, Huijing PA, van Ingen Schenau GJ: Drop jumping. II. The influence of dropping height on the biomechanics of drop jumping. *Med Sci Sports Exerc* 19:339–346, 1987.
118. Bosco C, Komi PV, Ito A: Prestretch potentiation of human skeletal muscle during ballistic movement. *Acta Physiol Scand* 111:135–140, 1981.

119. Bobbert MF, Gerritsen KG, Litjens MC, et al.: Why is countermovement jump height greater than squat jump height? *Med Sci Sports Exerc* 28:1402–1412, 1996.
120. Bobbert MF, Huijing PA, van Ingen Schenau GJ: Drop jumping. I. The influence of jumping technique on the biomechanics of jumping. *Med Sci Sports Exerc* 19:332–338, 1987.
121. Kubo K, Kanehisa H, Takeshita D, et al.: In vivo dynamics of human medial gastrocnemius muscle-tendon complex during stretch-shortening cycle exercise. *Acta Physiol Scand* 170:127–135, 2000.
122. Chu DA: Rehabilitation of the lower extremity. *Clin Sports Med* 14: 205–222, 1995.
123. Wathen D: Literature review: explosive/plyometric exercises. *NSCA J* 15:16–19, 1993.
124. Robinson LE, Devor ST, Merrick MA, et al.: The effects of land vs. aquatic plyometrics on power, torque, velocity, and muscle soreness in women. *J Strength Cond Res* 18:84–91, 2004.
125. Jensen RL, Ebben WP: Kinetic analysis of complex training rest interval effect on vertical jump performance. *J Strength Cond Res* 17:345–349, 2003.
126. McLaughlin EJ: A comparison between two training programs and their effects on fatigue rates in women. *J Strength Cond Res* 15:25–29, 2001.
127. Myer GD, Ford KR, Palumbo JP, et al.: Neuromuscular training improves performance and lower-extremity biomechanics in female athletes. *J Strength Cond Res* 19:51–60, 2005.
128. Voight M, Blackburn T: Proprioception and balance training and testing following injury. In: Ellenbecker TS, ed. *Knee Ligament Rehabilitation.* Philadelphia, PA: Churchill Livingstone, 2000:361–385.
129. Voight ML, Cook G: Impaired neuromuscular control: reactive neuromuscular training. In: Prentice WE, Voight ML, eds. *Techniques in Musculoskeletal Rehabilitation.* New York, NY: McGraw-Hill, 2001: 93–124.
130. Jerosch J, Prymka M: Propriozeptive Fahigkeiten des gesunden Kniegelenks: Beeinflussung durch eine elastische Bandage. *Sportverletz Sportsch* 9:72–76, 1995.
131. Jerosch J, Hoffstetter I, Bork H, et al.: The influence of orthoses on the proprioception of the ankle joint. *Knee Surg Sports Traumatol Arthrosc* 3:39–46, 1995.
132. Perlau R, Frank C, Fick G: The effect of elastic bandages on human knee proprioception in the uninjured population. *Am J Sports Med* 23:251–255, 1995.
133. Robbins S, Waked E, Rappel R: Ankle taping improves proprioception before and after exercise in young men. *Br J Sports Med* 29:242–247, 1995.
134. Barrett DS: Proprioception and function after anterior cruciate ligament reconstruction. *J Bone Joint Surg Br* 73B:833–837, 1991.
135. Lephart SM, Pincivero DM, Giraldo JL, et al.: The role of proprioception in the management and rehabilitation of athletic injuries. *Am J Sports Med* 25:130–137, 1997.
136. McNair PJ, Wood GA, Marshall RN: Stiffness of the hamstring muscles and its relationship to function in ACL deficient individuals. *Clin Biomech* 7:131–137, 1992.
137. Borsa PA, Lephart SM, Kocher MS, et al.: Functional assessment and rehabilitation of shoulder proprioception for glenohumeral instability. *J Sport Rehabil* 3:84–104, 1994.
138. Lephart SM, Warner JJP, Borsa PA, et al.: Proprioception of the shoulder joint in healthy, unstable and surgically repaired shoulders. *J Shoulder Elbow Surg* 3:371–380, 1994.
139. Fremerey RW, Lobenhoffer P, Zeichen J, et al.: Proprioception after rehabilitation and reconstruction in knees with deficiency of the anterior cruciate ligament: a prospective, longitudinal study. *J Bone Joint Surg Br* 82:801–806, 2000.
140. Irrgang JJ, Whitney SL, Harner C: Nonoperative treatment of rotator cuff injuries in throwing athletes. *J Sport Rehabil* 1:197–222, 1992.
141. Kibler WB: Kinetic chain concept. In: Ellenbecker TS, ed. *Knee Ligament Rehabilitation.* Philadelphia, PA: Churchill Livingstone, 2000:301–306.
142. Putnam CA: Sequential motions of body segments in stroking and throwing skills: descriptions and explanations. *J Biomech* 26:125–135, 1993.
143. Van Gheluwe B, Hebbelinck M: The kinematics of the serve movement in tennis. In: Winter D, ed. *Biomechanics.* Champaign, IL: Human Kinetics, 1985:521–526.
144. Lephart SM, Henry TJ: Functional rehabilitation for the upper and lower extremity. *Orthop Clin North Am* 26:579–592, 1995.
145. Yack HJ, Collins CE, Whieldon TJ: Comparison of closed and open kinetic chain exercise in the anterior cruciate ligament-deficient knee. *Am J Sports Med* 21:49–54, 1993.
146. Witvrouw E, Lysens R, Bellemans J, et al.: Open versus closed kinetic chain exercises for patellofemoral pain. A prospective, randomized study. *Am J Sports Med* 28:687–694, 2000.
147. Meglan D, Lutz G, Stuart M: Effects of closed chain exercises for ACL rehabilitation upon the load in the capsule and ligamentous structures of the knee. *Orthop Trans* 17:719–720, 1993.
148. Lutz GE, Palmitier RA, An KN, et al.: Comparison of tibiofemoral joint forces during open-kinetic-chain and closed-kinetic-chain exercises. *J Bone Joint Surg Am* 75:732–739, 1993.
149. Irrgang JJ, Rivera J: *Closed Kinetic Chain Exercises for the Lower Extremity: Theory and Application. Home Study Course: Current Concepts in Rehabilitation of the Knee.* Indianapolis, IN: Sports Physical Therapy Section, 1994.
150. Blackburn JR, Morrissey MC: The relationship between open and closed kinetic chain strength of the lower limb and jumping performance. *J Orthop Sports Phys Ther* 27:430–435, 1998.
151. Voight ML, Bell S, Rhodes D: Instrumented testing of tibial translation during a positive Lachman's test and selected closed chain activities in anterior cruciate deficient knees. *J Orthop Sports Phys Ther* 15:49, 1992.
152. Clark FJ, Burgess RC, Chapin JW, et al.: Role of intramuscular receptors in the awareness of limb position. *J Neurophysiol* 54:1529–1540, 1985.
153. Grigg P: Peripheral neural mechanisms in proprioception. *J Sport Rehabil* 3:1–17, 1994.
154. Dillman CJ, Murray TA, Hintermeister RA: Biomechanical differences of open and closed chain exercises with respect to the shoulder. *J Sport Rehabil* 3:228–238, 1994.
155. Doucette SA, Child DP: The effect of open and closed chain exercise and knee joint position on patellar tracking in lateral patellar compression syndrome. *J Orthop Sports Phys Ther* 23:104–110, 1996.
156. Genuario SE, Dolgener FA: The relationship of isokinetic torque at two speeds to the vertical jump. *Res Q* 51:593–598, 1980.
157. Pincivero DM, Lephart SM, Karunakara RG: Relation between open and closed kinematic chain assessment of knee strength and functional performance. *Clin J Sports Med* 7:11–16, 1997.
158. Lephart SM, Borsa PA: Functional rehabilitation of knee injuries. In: Fu FH, Harner C, eds. *Knee Surgery.* Baltimore, MD: Williams & Wilkins, 1993.
159. Litchfield R, Hawkins R, Dillman CJ, et al.: Rehabilitation of the overhead athlete. *J Orthop Sports Phys Ther* 2:433–441, 1993.
160. Youmans W: The so-called "isolated" ACL syndrome: a report of 32 cases with some observation on treatment and its effect on results. *Am J Sports Med* 6:26–30, 1978.

Improving Range of Motion and Flexibility

CHAPTER 13

CHAPTER OBJECTIVES

At the completion of this chapter, the reader will be able to:

1. Define the different types of range of motion (ROM).
2. Describe strategies to increase ROM.
3. Describe the indications and contraindications for the various types of ROM exercises.
4. Define active insufficiency and passive insufficiency of a muscle.
5. Outline the indications and contraindications for continuous passive motion (CPM).
6. Define flexibility and describe its importance in rehabilitation.
7. List and describe two types of flexibility.
8. Describe strategies to increase flexibility using different techniques.

OVERVIEW

The terms *range of motion* and *flexibility* are often used synonymously by clinicians, yet they are not the same.

- Range of motion (ROM) refers to the distance and direction a joint can move. Each specific joint has a normal ROM that is expressed in degrees. Within the field of physical therapy, goniometry is commonly used to measure the total amount of available motion at a specific joint. ROM of a joint may be limited by the shape of the articulating surfaces and by capsular and ligamentous structures surrounding that joint.
- Flexibility refers to the ability to move a joint or series of joints through a full, nonrestricted, injury, and pain-free ROM. Flexibility is dependent on a combination of joint ROM, muscle flexibility, and neuromuscular control. When injury occurs, there is almost always some associated loss of the ability to move normally due to the pain, swelling, muscle guarding, or spasm. The subsequent inactivity results in a shortening of connective tissue and muscle, loss of neuromuscular control, or a combination of these factors.[1]

A decrease in ROM and/or in the flexibility of one joint can affect the entire kinetic chain. For example, a decreased ROM or flexibility in the shoulder can impact the function of the entire arm. In order to provide a treatment for a loss of movement, the clinician must make the determination as to the specific cause i.e., loss of ROM or decreased flexibility. For example, is the specific cause due to joint effusion, adaptive shortening of connective tissue structures, changes in bony architecture, or alignment of the articular surfaces?

RANGE OF MOTION AND FLEXIBILITY

Normal flexibility and ROM are necessary for efficient movement. Joint movement may be viewed as the amount of joint ROM, the arthrokinematic glide that occurs at the joint surfaces, termed *joint play*, whereas flexibility is determined by the degree of extensibility of the periarticular and connective tissues that cross the joint. A number of anatomic factors can limit the ability of a joint to move through a full, unrestricted ROM. These include

- muscles and their tendons
- connective tissue
- bone
- adipose tissue
- skin
- neural tissue

When referring to ROM, three major movements are recognized:[1]

- Active range of motion (AROM). AROM, also called dynamic flexibility, refers to the degree to which a joint can be moved by a single muscle contraction, usually through the mid range of movement. Active ROM does not maintain or increase strength, or develop skill or coordination except in the movement patterns used.

- Active assisted range of motion (AAROM). AAROM is AROM where the effect of gravity has been removed. For example, performing shoulder abduction while lying supine.
- Passive range of motion (PROM). PROM refers to the degree to which a joint can be passively moved to the endpoint in the ROM. PROM is important for injury prevention. Passive ROM does not prevent muscle atrophy, increase strength or endurance, or assist circulation to the same extent that active, voluntary muscle contraction does.

When referring to flexibility, two types are recognized, static and dynamic.

CLINICAL PEARL

In the early stages of the rehabilitation process, ROM exercises are performed in the following sequence: PROM→AAROM→AROM. It is important to remember when making the transition from PROM to AAROM or AROM, that gravity has a significant impact especially in individuals with weak musculature. These individuals may require assistance when the segment moves up against gravity, or moves downward, with gravity.

- Static flexibility. Static flexibility is defined as the range or motion available to a joint or series of joints.[2,3] Increased static flexibility should not be confused with joint hypermobility, or laxity, which is a function of the joint capsule and ligaments. Decreased static flexibility indicates a loss of motion. The end-feel encountered may help the clinician differentiate the cause among adaptive shortening of the muscle (muscle stretch), a tight joint capsule (capsular), and an arthritic joint (hard). Static flexibility can be measured by a number of tests, such as the toe touch and the sit and reach, both of which have been found to be valid and reliable.[4,5]
- Dynamic flexibility. Dynamic flexibility refers to the ease of movement within the obtainable ROM. Dynamic flexibility is measured actively. The important measurement in dynamic flexibility is *stiffness*, a mechanical term defined as the resistance of a structure to deformation.[6,7] An increase in ROM around a joint does not necessarily equate to a decrease in the passive stiffness of a muscle.[8–10] However, strength training, immobilization, and aging have been shown to increase stiffness.[11–14] The converse of stiffness is pliability. When a soft tissue demonstrates a decrease in pliability, it has usually undergone an adaptive shortening, or an increase in tone, termed *hypertonus*. There is a growing research to suggest that the limiting factors to preventing increases in ROM are not only the connective tissues but are also the result of neurophysiological phenomena controlled by the higher centers of the central nervous system (CNS).[15]

ENHANCING RANGE OF MOTION AND FLEXIBILITY

A number of factors influence connective tissue deformation:

- Sensory receptors. Two sensory receptors that monitor muscle activity, the muscle spindle and Golgi tendon organs (GTOs) (see Chapter 3), play an important role when attempting to increase flexibility through stretching. These two receptors can activate both spinal reflexes and long-loop pathways involving supraspinal centers. When a muscle is stretched, both the muscle spindles and the GTOs immediately begin sending a stream of sensory impulses to the spinal cord. Initially, impulses coming from the muscle spindles notify the CNS that the muscle is being stretched. Impulses return to the muscle from the spinal cord, causing the muscle to reflexively contract, thus resisting the stretch.[1] The GTOs respond to the change in length and the increasing tension by firing off sensory impulses of their own to the spinal cord and, if the stretch of the muscle continues for an extended period of time (at least 6 seconds), impulses from the GTOs begin to override muscle spindle impulses and cause a reflex relaxation of the antagonist muscle (autogenic inhibition).[1]

CLINICAL PEARL

In any synergistic muscle group, a contraction of the agonist causes a reflex relaxation in the antagonist muscle, allowing it to stretch and protect it from injury—this phenomenon is referred to as reciprocal inhibition.[1]

- Tissue temperature. At temperatures above 37°C (98.6°F), the cross-links between collagen fibrils are broken more easily and more rapidly, with the most profound changes occurring between 40–45°C (104–113°F).[16,17] A number of key points must be remembered by the clinician in order to effectively manipulate temperature:[18]
  - The amount of force required to attain/maintain a desired deformation decreases as temperature increases.
  - The time required to deform collagen to the point of failure is inversely related to temperature.
  - The higher the temperature, the greater the load collagen is able to tolerate before failure.
  - The higher the temperature, the greater the amount of deformation possible before failure.

It is important to make a distinction between stretching and warm-up as the two are not synonymous but often confused by the layman. While stretching places neuromusculotendinous units and their fascia under tension, a warm-up requires the performance of an activity that raises total body and muscle temperatures to prepare the body for exercise.[19] Research has shown that warm-up prior to stretching results in significant changes in joint ROM.[20] Anecdotally, it would make sense not to perform stretching at the beginning of the warm-up routine because the tissue temperatures are too low for optimal muscle–tendon function, and are less compliant and less prepared for activity. Some advocate stretching after an exercise session, citing that the increased musculotendinous extensibility leads to the potential for improved joint flexibility.[21] In one study, static stretching was done before, after, and both before and after each workout. All produced significant increases in ROM.[22]

- The amount of force used. Viscoelastic changes are not permanent, whereas plasticity changes, which are more difficult to achieve, result in a residual or permanent change in length. The key factor for any change in connective tissue length is the deforming force, in particular the magnitude and velocity applied. The application of low-load, long duration forces is recommended. A muscle usually requires a greater stretching force initially, possibly to break up adhesions or cross-linkages, and to allow for viscoelastic and plastic changes to occur in the collagen and elastin fibers.[23] Frequent stretching ensures that the lengthening is maintained before the muscle has the opportunity to recoil to its shortened state.[24]
- The direction of the stretch. To stretch a muscle appropriately, the stretch must be applied parallel to the muscle fibers. The orientation of the fibers can be determined by palpation. Typically, in the extremities, the muscle fibers run parallel to the bone.

A variety of stretching techniques can be used to increase the extensibility of the soft tissues.

Static Stretching. Static stretching involves the application of a steady force for a sustained period (Table 13-1). The stretch should be performed at the point just shy of the pain, although some discomfort may be necessary to achieve results.[23] Small loads applied for long periods produce greater residual lengthening than heavy loads applied for short periods.[25] Restoration of normal length of the muscles may be accomplished using the guidelines outlined in Table 13-1. Weighted traction or pulley systems may be used for this type of stretching. It is important for the patient to realize that the initial session of stretching may increase symptoms.[26] However, this increase in symptoms should be temporary, lasting for a couple of hours, at most.[24,27]

TABLE 13-1 Static Stretching Guidelines

- Heat should be applied to increase intramuscular temperature prior to, and during, stretching[1–4] This heat can be achieved with either through low-intensity warm-up exercise, or through the use of thermal modalities. The application of a cold pack following the stretch is used to take advantage of the thermal characteristics of connective tissue, by lowering its temperature and thereby theoretically prolonging the length changes—the elasticity of a muscle diminishes with cooling.[1–4]
- Effective stretching, in the early phase, should be performed every hour, but with each session lasting only a few minutes.
- With true muscle shortness, stronger resistance is used to activate the maximum number of motor units, followed by vigorous stretching of the muscle.
- Stretching should be performed at least three times a week using:
  - Low force, avoiding pain
  - Prolonged duration.
  - Rapid cooling of the muscle while it is maintained in the stretched position

Data from:
1. Assmussen E, Bonde-Peterson F: Storage of elastic energy in skeletal muscle in man. *Acta Physiol Scand* 91:385–392, 1974.
2. Bosco C, Komi PV: Potentiation of the mechanical behavior of the human skeletal muscle through prestretching. *Acta Physiol Scand* 106:467–472, 1979.
3. Cavagna GA, Saibene FP, Margaria R: Effect of negative work on the amount of positive work performed by an isolated muscle. *J Appl Physiol* 20:157, 1965.
4. Cavagna GA, Disman B, Margarai R: Positive work done by a previously stretched muscle. *J Appl Physiol* 24:21–32, 1968.

Dynamic Stretching. Dynamic stretching involves stretching by a muscular contraction to increase or decrease the joint angle where the muscle crosses, thereby elongating the musculotendinous unit as the end ROM is obtained[21] Dynamic stretching is a specific warm-up using activity-specific movements to prepare the muscles by taking them through the movements used in a particular sport.[21] Dynamic stretching does not incorporate end-range ballistic movements but rather the use of controlled movements through a normal ROM.[21]

There is some debate as to whether the static or dynamic method is better to stretch a muscle. Static stretching is considered the gold standard in flexibility training.[28] However, recent studies have found that static stretching is not an effective way to reduce injury rates,[29,30] and may actually inhibit athletic performance.[31] This is likely because the nature of static stretching is passive and does nothing to warm a muscle.[32] More dynamic methods of stretching involve either a contraction of the antagonist muscle group thus allowing the agonist to elongate naturally in a relaxed state, or eccentrically training a muscle through its full ROM.[28] The latter method would appear to address the problem that most injuries occur in the eccentric phase of activity.[29] A study by Nelson[28] that compared the immediate effect of static stretching, eccentric training, and no stretching/training on hamstring flexibility in high school and college athletes (75 subjects) found the flexibility gains in the eccentric training group to be significantly greater than the static stretch group.

Proprioceptive Neuromuscular Facilitation. The proprioceptive neuromuscular facilitation (PNF) techniques of contract–relax (CR), an agonist contraction (AC), or a contract-relax-agonist contraction sequence (CRAC) can be used to actively stretch the soft tissues:[1]

- CR. CR stretching begins as does static stretching in that the clinician supports the patient and brings a limb to the end of ROM until gentle stretching is felt. At that point, the clinician asks the patient to provide an isometric contraction of the muscle being stretched (the antagonist) for approximately 2 to 5 seconds after which the patient is asked to relax the muscle. The clinician moves the limb passively into the new range until a limitation is again felt and repeats the procedure two to four times.
- AC. AC stretching uses the principle of reciprocal inhibition. The clinician moves the limb to the position of gentle stretch and asks the patient for a contraction of the

muscle opposite the muscle being stretched (the antagonist). For example, when stretching the hamstring muscles, a simultaneous contraction of the quadriceps muscles can facilitate the stretch of the hamstrings. The contraction is held for 2 to 5 seconds and the technique is repeated 2 to 4 times.

- CRAC. This technique combines the CR and AC stretches. The clinician takes the limb to the point of gentle stretch and performs a CR sequence (i.e., resistance applied against the muscle being stretched). After contracting the muscle being stretched, the patient is asked to relax this muscle while contracting the opposing muscle group (antagonist), thus facilitating the stretch. For example, when stretching the hamstring muscles, the hamstrings are brought to a position stretch, the hamstrings are then contracted against resistance, and then relaxed, and then the quadriceps are contracted.

The majority of studies have shown the PNF techniques to be the most effective for increasing ROM through muscle lengthening when compared to the static or slow sustained, and the ballistic or bounce techniques,[33–37] although one study found it to be not necessarily better.[38]

Other techniques that can assist in lengthening of contractile tissue through relaxation include the following:

- The application of heat, which increases the extensibility of the shortened tissues, will allow the muscles to relax in length and more easily, reducing the discomfort of stretching. Heat without stretching has little or no effect on long-term improvement in muscle flexibility, whereas the combination of heat and stretching produces greater long-term gains in tissue length than stretching alone.
- Massage, which increases local circulation to the muscle and reduces muscle spasm and stiffness.
- Biofeedback, which teaches the patient to reduce the amount of tension in a muscle.

Ballistic Stretching. This technique of stretching uses bouncing movements to stretch a particular muscle. The muscle is stretched by momentum created from the bouncing movement of the body supplying the tensile force used for the stretch.[21] The patient quickly relaxes the muscle when reaching the end of ROM. This is performed in a cyclical bouncing motion and repeated several times, thus engaging a neurological component called active resistance—the contraction of muscles that resist elongation in the form of muscle reflex activity.[21,39] In comparisons of the ballistic and static methods, two studies[40,41] have found that both produce similar improvements in flexibility. However, the ballistic method appears to cause more residual muscle soreness or muscle strain, than those techniques that incorporate relaxation into the technique.[42–44]

Further research is needed to determine the appropriate stretching frequency and duration for long-lasting changes in flexibility. Researchers have reported that techniques utilizing cyclic and sustained stretching for 15 minutes on five consecutive days increased hamstring muscle length, and that a significant percentage of the increased length was retained 1 week posttreatment.[45] Other researchers have reported that after using four consecutive knee flexor static stretches of 30 seconds, the new knee ROM was maintained for 3 minutes but had returned to prestretch levels after 6 minutes.[46] A similar study using a sequence of five modified hold–relax stretches reported producing significantly increased hamstring flexibility that lasted 6 minutes after the stretching protocol ended.[47] The specific duration, frequency, and number of stretching repetitions vary in the literature. Evidence to date has shown that stretches are generally held anywhere from 10 to 60 seconds, with the research recommending that stretches be held between 15 and 30 seconds.[21,48,49] In contrast, little research has been conducted on the number of repetitions of a stretch in exercise session, although it has been determined that 80% of the length changes occur in the first four stretches of 30 seconds each.[21,50] Current American College of Sports Medicine Guidelines recommend three to five repetitions for each stretching exercise.[51]

SELF-STRETCHING

Self-stretching techniques include any stretching exercise that is carried out independently by the patient after instruction and supervision. Self-stretching techniques are included at the end of each of the joint chapters.

CONTINUOUS PASSIVE MOTION

CPM refers to passive motion performed by a mechanical device that moves the joint slowly and continuously through a controlled ROM.[52] CPM machines have been designed for use on many body parts, including the hip, knee (most common), ankle, shoulder, elbow, wrist, and hand. The subject of CPM device use following surgery has been debated for years, with some surgeons advocating, and others opposing its use.

CLINICAL PEARL

CPM protocols vary significantly, ranging from 24 hours a day for as long as 1 month, to as little as 6 hours a day after surgery.

The CPM machine is calibrated in degrees of motion and cycles per minute.

The use of a CPM device has been promoted as a means to facilitate a more rapid recovery by improving ROM, decreasing length of hospital stay, and lowering the amount of narcotic use.[53–63] However, studies have shown that the effect of CPM devices on analgesia consumption, ROM, hospital stay, and complications has been variable:

- Data support the use of CPM to decrease the rate of manipulation for poor ROM after total knee arthroplasty (TKA).
- The use of CPM has not been shown to result in more long-term increases in ROM than other methods of early movement and positioning.

- Although it appears that the use of a CPM device does help regain knee flexion quicker post TKA, it is not as effective in the enhancement of knee extension.
- Knee impairments or disability are not reduced with the use of a CPM at discharge from hospital.
- Because of standardized inpatient hospital clinical pathways, the length of hospital stay is not decreased by the use of a CPM device but, depending on the hospital involved, the overall cost is not increased.
- Wound complications probably are not increased with the use of CPM, provided good technique is used in wound closure.

CLINICAL PEARL

- It is still not clear whether ROM is achieved faster and whether the prevalence of deep vein thrombosis (DVT) and analgesics use are decreased with CPM.

Indications

- Decrease soft tissue stiffness
- Increase short-term ROM, which may result in early discharge from the hospital
- Promote healing of the joint surfaces (promotes cartilage growth) and soft tissue.
- Prevention of adhesions and contractures and thus joint stiffness
- Decrease postoperative pain

Contraindications

- Nonstable fracture sites
- Excessive edema
- Patient intolerance

Application and Patient Preparation

The procedure is explained to the patient. Any wound area must be covered. The clinician adjusts the unit so that the patient's anatomical joint is aligned with the mechanical hinge joint of the machine. The patient's limb is secured in the machine using the safety straps. The clinician sets the beginning and end ROM degrees, and then turns the unit on. Typically a low arc of 20–30 degrees is used initially and is progressed 10–15 degrees per day as tolerated. The rate of motion is typically one cycle per 45 seconds to two minutes. The patient is monitored during the first few minutes to ensure correct fit and patient comfort. Treatment duration varies from one hour three times a day to 24 hours a day.

REFERENCES

1. Prentice WE: Impaired mobility: restoring range of motion and improving flexibility. In: Voight ML, Hoogenboom BJ, Prentice WE, eds. *Musculoskeletal Interventions: Techniques for Therapeutic Exercise*. New York, NY: McGraw-Hill, 2007:165–180.
2. The American Orthopaedic Society for Sports Medicine: *Flexibility*. Chicago, IL: The American Orthopaedic Society for Sports Medicine, 1988.
3. Gleim GW, McHugh MP: Flexibility and its effects on sports injury and performance. *Sports Med* 24:289–299, 1997.
4. Kippers V, Parker AW: Toe-touch test: a measure of validity. *Phys Ther* 67:1680–1684, 1987.
5. Jackson AW, Baker AA: The relationship of the sit and reach test to criterion measures of hamstring and back flexibility in young females. *Res Q Exerc Sport* 57:183–186, 1986.
6. Litsky AS, Spector M: Biomaterials. In: Simon SR, ed. *Orthopaedic Basic Science*. Chicago, IL: The American Orthopaedic Society for Sports Medicine, 1994:447–486.
7. Johns R, Wright V: Relative importance of various tissues in joint stiffness. *J Appl Physiol* 17:824–830, 1962.
8. Toft E, Espersen GT, Kalund S, et al: Passive tension of the ankle before and after stretching. *Am J Sports Med* 17:489–494, 1989.
9. Halbertsma JPK, Goeken LNH: Stretching exercises: effect of passive extensibility and stiffness in short hamstrings of healthy subjects. *Arch Phys Med Rehabil* 75:976–981, 1994.
10. Magnusson SP, Simonsen EB, Aagaard P, et al: A mechanism for altered flexibility in human skeletal muscle. *J Physiol* 497:291–298, 1996.
11. Klinge K, Magnusson SP, Simonsen EB, et al: The effect of strength and flexibility on skeletal muscle EMG activity, stiffness and viscoelastic stress relaxation response. *Am J Sports Med* 25:710–716, 1997.
12. Lapier TK, Burton HW, Almon RF: Alterations in intramuscular connective tissue after limb casting affect contraction-induced muscle injury. *J Appl Physiol* 78:1065–1069, 1995.
13. McNair PJ, Wood GA, Marshall RN: Stiffness of the hamstring muscles and its relationship to function in ACL deficient individuals. *Clin Biomech* 7:131–137, 1992.
14. McHugh MP, Magnusson SP, Gleim GW, et al: A cross-sectional study of age-related musculoskeletal and physiological changes in soccer players. *Med Exerc Nutr Health* 2:261–268, 1993.
15. Hutton RS: Neuromuscular basis of stretching exercise. In: Komi PV, ed. *Strength and Power in Sports*. Oxford: Blackwell Science Publications, 1993:29–38.
16. Lehmann JF, Masock AJ, Warren CG, et al: Effect of therapeutic temperatures on tendon extensibility. *Arch Phys Med Rehabil* 51:481–487, 1970.
17. Kottke FJ, Pauley DL, Ptak RA: The rationale for prolonged stretching for correction of shortening of connective tissue. *Arch Phys Med Rehabil* 47:345–352, 1966.
18. Zachazewski JE: Range of motion and flexibility. In: Magee D, Zachazewski JE, Quillen WS, eds. *Scientific Foundations and Principles of Practice in Musculoskeletal Rehabilitation*. St. Louis, MI: WB Saunders, 2007:527–556.
19. Anderson B, Burke ER: Scientific, medical, and practical aspects of stretching. *Clin Sports Med* 10:63–86, 1991.
20. Wiktorsson-Moller M, Oberg B, Ekstrand J, et al: Effects of warming up, massage, and stretching on range of motion and muscle strength in the lower extremity. *Am J Sports Med* 11:249–252, 1983.
21. Wallman HW: Stretching and flexibility. In: Wilmarth MA, ed. *Orthopaedic Physical Therapy: Topic – Strength and Conditioning – Independent Study Course 15.3*. La Crosse, WI: Orthopaedic Section, APTA, Inc., 2005.
22. Cornelius WL, Hagemann RW Jr, Jackson AW: A study on placement of stretching within a workout. *J Sports Med Phys Fitness* 28:234–236, 1988.
23. Joynt RL: Therapeutic exercise. In: DeLisa JA, ed. *Rehabilitation Medicine: Principles and Practice*. Philadelphia, PA: JB Lippincott, 1988:346–371.
24. Kottke FJ: Therapeutic exercise to maintain mobility. In: Kottke FJ, Stillwell GK, Lehman JF, eds. *Krusen's Handbook of Physical Medicine and Rehabilitation*. Baltimore: WB Saunders, 1982:389–402.
25. Yoder E: Physical therapy management of nonsurgical hip problems in adults. In: Echternach JL, ed. *Physical Therapy of the Hip*. New York, NY: Churchill Livingstone, 1990:103–137.
26. Travell JG, Simons DG: *Myofascial Pain and Dysfunction – The Trigger Point Manual*. Baltimore: Williams & Wilkins, 1983.
27. Swezey RL: Arthrosis. In: Basmajian JV, Kirby RL, eds. *Medical Rehabilitation*. Baltimore: Williams & Wilkins, 1984:216–218.
28. Nelson RT: A comparison of the immediate effects of eccentric training vs. static stretch on hamstring flexibility in high school and college athletes. *N Am J Sports Phys Ther* 1:56–61, 2006.
29. Thacker SB, Gilchrist J, Stroup DF, et al: The impact of stretching on sports injury risk: a systematic review of the literature. *Med Sci Sports Exerc* 36:371–378, 2004.

30. Herbert RD, Gabriel M: Effects of stretching before and after exercising on muscle soreness and risk of injury: systematic review. *Br Med J* 325:468, 2002.
31. Shrier I: Does stretching improve performance? A systematic and critical review of the literature. *Clin J Sport Med* 14:267–273, 2004.
32. Murphy DR: A critical look at static stretching: are we doing our patient harm? *Chiropract Sports Med* 5:67–70, 1991.
33. Markos PD: Ipsilateral and contralateral effects of proprioceptive neuromuscular facilitation techniques on hip motion and electromyographic activity. *Phys Ther* 59:1366, 1979.
34. Holt LE, Travis TM, Okita T: Comparative study of three stretching techniques. *Percept Mot Skills* 31:611–616, 1970.
35. Tanigawa MC: Comparison of hold-relax procedure and passive mobilization on increasing muscle length. *Phys Ther* 52:725–735, 1972.
36. Sady SP, Wortman MA, Blanke D: Flexibility training: ballistic, static or proprioceptive neuromuscular facilitation? *Arch Phys Med Rehabil* 63:261–263, 1982.
37. Prentice WE: A comparison of static stretching and PNF stretching for improving hip joint flexibility. *J Athl Train* 18:56–59, 1983.
38. Hartley-O'Brien SJ: Six mobilization exercises for active range of hip flexion. *Res Q Exerc Sport* 51:625–635, 1980.
39. Muir IW, Chesworth BM, Vandervoort AA: Effect of a static calf-stretching exercise on the resistive torque during passive ankle dorsiflexion in healthy subjects. *J Orthop Sports Phys Ther* 29:106-13; discussion 114–5, 1999.
40. DeVries HA: Evaluation of static stretching procedures for improvement of flexibility. *Res Q* 33:222–229, 1962.
41. Logan GA, Egstrom GH: Effects of slow and fast stretching on sacrofemoral angle. *J Assoc Phys Ment Rehabil* 15:85–89, 1961.
42. Davies CT, White MJ: Muscle weakness following eccentric work in man. *Pflugers Arch* 392:168–171, 1981.
43. Friden J, Sjostrom M, Ekblom B: A morphological study of delayed muscle soreness. *Experientia* 37:506–507, 1981.
44. Hardy L: Improving active range of hip flexion. *Res Q Exerc Sport* 56: 111–114, 1985.
45. Starring DT, Gossman MR, Nicholson GG Jr, et al: Comparison of cyclic and sustained passive stretching using a mechanical device to increase resting length of hamstring muscles. *Phys Ther* 68:314–320, 1988.
46. Depino GM, Webright WG, Arnold BL: Duration of maintained hamstring flexibility after cessation of an acute static stretching protocol. *J Athl Train* 35:56–59, 2000.
47. Spernoga SG, Uhl TL, Arnold BL, et al: Duration of maintained hamstring flexibility after a one-time, modified hold-relax stretching protocol. *J Athl Train* 36:44–48, 2001.
48. Bandy WD, Irion JM, Briggler M: The effect of time and frequency of static stretching on flexibility of the hamstring muscles. *Phys Ther* 77: 1090–1096, 1997.
49. Roberts JM, Wilson K: Effect of stretching duration on active and passive range of motion in the lower extremity. *Br J Sports Med* 33:259–263, 1999.
50. Taylor DC, Dalton JD Jr, Seaber AV, et al: Viscoelastic properties of muscle-tendon units. The biomechanical effects of stretching. *Am J Sports Med* 18:300–309, 1990.
51. American College of Sports Medicine Position Stand. The recommended quantity and quality of exercise for developing and maintaining cardiorespiratory and muscular fitness, and flexibility in healthy adults. *Med Sci Sports Exerc* 30:975–991, 1998.
52. Kisner C, Colby LA: Range of motion. In: Kisner C, Colby LA, eds. *Therapeutic Exercise. Foundations and Techniques*, 5th edn. Philadelphia, PA: FA Davis, 2002:43–64.
53. Johnson DP: The effect of continuous passive motion on wound-healing and joint mobility after knee arthroplasty. *J Bone Joint Surg Am* 72A:421–426, 1990.
54. Basso M, Knapp L: Comparison of two continuous passive motion protocols for patients with total knee implants. *Phys Ther* 67:360–363, 1987.
55. Colwell CW, Morris BA: The influence of continuous passive motion on the results of total knee arthroplasty. *Clin Orthop* 276:225–228, 1992.
56. Coutts RD: Continuous passive motion in the rehabilitation of the total knee patient. It's role and effect. *Orthop Rev* 15:27, 1986.
57. Coutts RD, Toth C, Kaita JH: The Role of continuous passive motion in the postoperative rehabilitation of the total knee patient. In: Hungerford DS, ed. *Total Knee Arthroplasty: A Comprehensive Approach*. Baltimore, MD: Williams & Williams, 1984:126–132.
58. Jordan LR, Siegel JL, Olivo JL: Early flexion routine, an alternative method of continuous passive motion. *Clin Orthop* 315:231–233, 1995.
59. Maloney WJ, Schurman DJ, Hangen D, et al: The influence of continuous passive motion on outcome in total knee arthroplasty. *Clin Orthop* 256:162–168, 1990.
60. Vince KG, Kelly MA, Beck J, et al: Continuous passive motion after total knee arthroplasty. *J Arthroplasty* 2:281–284, 1987.
61. Wasilewski SA, Woods LC, Torgerson WR Jr, et al: Value of continuous passive motion in total knee arthroplasty. *Orthopedics* 13:291–295, 1990.
62. Walker RH, Morris BA, Angulo DL, et al: Postoperative use of continuous passive motion, transcutaneous electrical nerve stimulation, and continuous cooling pad following total knee arthroplasty. *J Arthroplasty* 6: 151–156, 1991.
63. McInnes J, Larson MG, Daltroy LH, et al: A controlled evaluation of continuous passive motion in patients undergoing total knee arthroplasty. *JAMA* 268:1423–1428, 1992.

Improving Neuromuscular Control

CHAPTER 14

CHAPTER OBJECTIVES

At the completion of this chapter, the reader will be able to:

1. Define the components of neuromuscular control.
2. Describe ways in which neuromuscular control can be improved through physical therapy.
3. Describe a number of exercises that can be used to improve neuromuscular control.
4. Provide examples to enhance balance retraining.
5. Explain the concepts related to stabilization retraining.

OVERVIEW

The entire rehabilitation process is focused on restoring function as quickly and as safely as possible. An important component of function is neuromuscular control. Neuromuscular control involves the detection, perception, and utilization of relevant sensory information in order to perform specific tasks. Successful performance of a task requires the intricate coordination of various body parts using information provided by peripheral receptors located in and around the articular structures (see chap. 3). This feedback provides information that assists with proprioception, balance, and neuromuscular control. It is now well accepted that neuromuscular control impairment can change movement patterns and increase the risk of musculoskeletal injury.

Neuromuscular rehabilitation (NMR) is a method of training the enhancement of these unconscious motor responses, by stimulating both the afferent signals and the central mechanisms responsible for dynamic joint control.[1] The aims of NMR are to improve the ability of the nervous system to generate a fast and optimal muscle-firing pattern, to increase joint stability, to decrease joint forces, and to relearn movement patterns and skills.[1] Before developing a neuromuscular training program, the faulty movement pattern or absent motor skill must be identified.[2] In addition, before initiating a neuromuscular training program, individuals must have adequate muscle strength to perform training exercises correctly. If weaknesses are present, training activities must begin at a more baseline level that includes weight training, technique instruction, and performing single plane versus multiplanar movements.[2] The three major components of NMR are proprioceptive retraining, balance retraining, and stabilization retraining.

PROPRIOCEPTIVE RETRAINING

Because afferent input is altered after joint injury, proprioceptive training must focus on the restoration of proprioceptive sensibility to retrain these altered afferent pathways and enhance the sensation of joint movement.[3] In designing exercises to improve three-dimensional dynamic lower extremity postural stability, the clinician should consider the following: [4]

- Postural differences between patients
- Lower extremity loading pathomechanics
- Hip, knee, and ankle joint positions for optimal muscle moment arm lengths
- The interplay between global and local proprioceptive mechanisms
- The concept of rehabilitating movements that facilitate the development of synergistic lower extremity muscle function

Although ROM and progressive resistance exercises (PREs) help reestablish joint proprioception, they are not as effective in restoring function as exercises that involve technique or task training. Technique or task training involves the performance of specific movements with an emphasis on proper technique, with the primary chosen movement being one that results in a large percentage of injuries, such as changing direction, transferring from sit to stand, or more advanced techniques such as performing a cut maneuver.[2] According to Voight,[3,5] the standard progression for proprioceptive retraining involves:

1. ***Static stabilization exercises with closed-chain loading and unloading (weight shifting).*** This phase initially employs isometric exercises around the involved joint on solid and even surfaces, before progressing to unstable surfaces. The early training involves balance training and joint repositioning exercises and usually is initiated (in the

lower extremities) by having the patient place the involved extremity on a 6–8-inch-high stool, so that the amount of weight bearing can be controlled more easily. The proprioceptive awareness of a joint can also be enhanced by using an elastic bandage or orthotic, or through taping.[6–11] As full-weight-bearing through the extremity is restored, a number of devices, such as a minitrampoline, balance board, Swiss ball, and wobble board, can be introduced. Exercises on these devices are progressed from double-limb support to single-leg support to full support while performing sports-specific skills.

2. ***Transitional stabilization exercises.*** The exercises during this phase involve conscious control of motion without impact and replace isometric activity with controlled concentric and eccentric exercises throughout a progressively larger range of functional motion. The physiologic rationale behind the exercises in this phase is to stimulate dynamic postural responses and increase muscle stiffness. Muscle stiffness has a significant role in improving dynamic stabilization around the joint, by resisting and absorbing joint loads.[12]
3. ***Dynamic stabilization exercises.*** These exercises involve the unconscious control and loading of the joint and introduce both ballistic and impact exercises to the patient.

A delicate balance between stability and mobility is achieved by coordination among muscle strength, endurance, flexibility, and neuromuscular control.[13] The neuromuscular mechanism that contributes to joint stability is mediated by the articular mechanoreceptors (see Chap. 3). These receptors provide information about joint position sense and kinesthesia.[10,11,14,15] The objective in NMR is to restore proximal stability, muscle control, and flexibility through a balance of proprioceptive retraining and strengthening.

Initially, closed kinetic chain exercises (CKCEs) are performed within the pain-free ranges or positions. Open kinetic chain exercises (OKCEs), including mild plyometric exercises, may be built upon the base of the closed-chain stabilization to allow normal control of joint mobility (see Chap. 12).

The neuromuscular emphasis during these exercises is on functional positioning during exercise rather than isolating open- and closed-chain activities.[13] The activities should involve sudden alterations in joint positioning that necessitate reflex muscular stabilization coupled with an axial load.[11,13] Such activities include rhythmic stabilization performed in both a closed- and an open-chain position[16] and in the functional position of the joint (see Chap. 12).[13] The use of a stable, and then an unstable, base during CKCEs encourages co-contraction of the agonists and antagonists.[16]

Following treatment of any joint, retraining of the muscles must be carried out to reestablish coordination. Proprioceptive neuromuscular facilitation (PNF) techniques are especially useful in this regard. PNF techniques require motions of the extremities in all three planes.[17] PNF techniques that use combinations of spiral and diagonal patterns are designed to enhance coordination and strength.[18] The diagonal patterns 1 and 2 (see Chap. 10) are appropriate, with resistance being added as appropriate.

BALANCE RETRAINING

Balance retraining focuses on the ability to maintain a position through both conscious and subconscious motor control. There are many factors to consider when developing an intervention program for balance impairment. As outlined in Chapter 3, impaired balance can be caused by injury or disease to any structures involved in the stages of information processing: somatosensory input, visual and vestibular input, sensory motor integration, and motor output generation.[19] The clinician needs to consider the patient's impairments across all systems and decide which impairments can be rehabilitated and which require compensation or substitution.

It is also important to determine the cause of the impairment—whether the problem results from musculoskeletal, neuromuscular, sensory, or cognitive (e.g., fear of falling) impairment.[20] The key elements of a comprehensive evaluation of individuals with balance problems include the following:[21]

- A thorough history of falls, including whether the onset of falls are sudden versus gradual; the frequency and direction of the falls; the environmental conditions, activities, presence of dizziness, vertigo, and lightheadedness at time of falls; current and past medications, and the presence of a fear of falling.
- Assessments to identify sensory input and/or sensory processing deficits, abnormal biomechanical and motor alignment, poor muscle strength and/or endurance, and decreased range of motion and/or flexibility. Of particular importance is core strength.[20]
- Assessment of coordination, and awareness of posture and the position of the body in space.
- Tests and observations to determine the impact of balance control system deficits on functional performance.
- Environmental assessments to determine full-risk hazards in a person's home.

Studies have shown that proprioception and kinesthesia do improve following rehabilitation.[10,11] For example, habituation exercises have proven beneficial for patients with acute unilateral vestibular loss, and adaptation and balance exercises have produced positive outcomes in patients with chronic bilateral vestibular deficits.[22] The type of intervention will depend on the deficits found during the clinical examination, and typically involves improving one or more of the following categories:[21]

- Static balance control
- Dynamic balance control
- Anticipatory balance control
- Reactive balance control
- Sensory reorganization
- Vestibular rehabilitation

Because balance training often involves activities that challenge the patient's limits of stability, it is important that the clinician takes steps to ensure the patient's safety. This includes the use of a gait belt, performing the exercises near

TABLE 14-1 Agility and Perturbation Training Examples

Activity	Progression
Sidestepping: the patient steps sideways, moving right to left and then left to right, approximately 10–20 feet, repeating two times in each direction for a total of four times.	The width of steps and the speed of steps are progressed every 1 to 2 sessions. The activity is initiated on a level surface and progressed to sidestepping over low obstacles when the patient is able to sidestep on level surfaces without difficulty.
Braiding activities: the patient combines front and back crossover steps while moving laterally (walking carioca). During each activity, the patient moves right to left and then left to right, approximately 10–20 feet, repeating two times in each direction for a total of four times.	The activity is progressed by increasing the width of steps and the speed of steps every 1 to 2 sessions.
Front and back crossover steps during forward ambulation: the patient crosses one leg in front of the other, alternating legs with each step, while walking forward approximately 10–20 feet. The patient then walks backwards to the start position while crossing one leg behind the other, alternating legs with each step.	Two repetitions are performed, beginning with partial crossover steps and progressing to full crossover steps when the patient's performance improves. The width of steps and the speed of steps can be progressed every 1 to 2 sessions.
Shuttle walking: plastic pylon markers are placed at distances of 5, 10, and 15 feet. The patient walks forward to the first marker, then returns to the start by walking backward. The patient then walks forward to the 10-foot marker, then returns to the 5-foot marker walking backward. The patient then walks to the 15-foot marker, returns to the 10-foot marker walking backward, then finishes by walking to the 15-foot marker.	The activity is progressed by increasing the width of steps and the speed of steps every 1 to 2 sessions.
Multiple changes in direction on command during walking: the clinician directs the patient to either walk forward, backwards, sideways, or on a diagonal by cueing the patient randomly with hand signals.	The duration of the exercise bout is approximately 30 seconds.
Double leg foam balance activity: the patient stands on a soft firm surface with both feet on the ground and the clinician attempts to perturb the patient's balance in a random fashion.	The duration of the activity is approximately 30 seconds. The difficulty is progressed as the patient improves by progressing to ball catching with the clinician perturbing the patient's balance while standing on foam and progressing to single-leg support if tolerated.
Tilt board balance training: the patient stands on a tilt board with both feet on the board. The clinician perturbs the tilt board in forward and backward and side to side directions for approximately 30 seconds each.	The difficulty of the activity is progressed by adding ball catching during the perturbations and progressing to single limb support perturbations based on patient tolerance.
Rollerboard and platform perturbations: the patient stands with one limb on a stationary platform and the other limb on a rollerboard. The clinician perturbs the rollerboard in multiple directions, at random, and the patient attempts to resist the perturbations. The activity lasts approximately 30 seconds and is then repeated by changing the limbs on the platform and the rollerboard.	If the patient has difficulty doing the activity in full standing, the activity may begin with the patient in a semi-seated position, with the hips resting on the bed. The activity is progressed to the full standing position as tolerated.

Data from: Fitzgerald GK, Piva SR, Gil AB, et al: Agility and Perturbation Training Techniques in Exercise Therapy for Reducing Pain and Improving Function in People With Knee Osteoarthritis: A Randomized Clinical Trial. Physical therapy, 2011.

a railing, and closely guarding the patient. Examples of agility and perturbations activities are outlined in Table 14-1. Balance training to promote static balance control involves changing the base of support of the patient while performing various tasks, first with their eyes open and then with the eyes closed. The lower the center of gravity, the more stable the patient feels. Thus, the prone or supine positions provide the lowest center of gravity and the most support, sitting the next, with standing providing the highest center of gravity and the least support. The usual progression employed in balance retraining involves a narrowing of the base of support while increasing the perturbation and changing the weight-bearing surface from hard to soft or from flat to uneven.

CLINICAL PEARL

It is important for the clinician to be aware of a number of factors that can affect balance and increase the risk of fall:

- Medications: the risk of falling can be increased when the patient is prescribed sedatives and antidepressants.

- Low vision: patients with balance issues should be advised to have regular eye examinations and to avoid areas with poor lighting.
- Sensory loss: sensory loss in the lower extremities can result in difficulties when walking on soft or uneven surfaces.

- Balance training for adults usually begins in the short sitting position, which allows the feet to provide anterior support. This position can be made more challenging by placing a wobble board or Swiss ball under the patient's buttocks. The patient is then progressed to quadruped, through tall kneeling, and finally to the standing position.
- Balance training for the pediatric population usually begins in the "W" sitting position, then to "Indian-style sitting," then to quadruped, through tall kneeling, and finally to the standing position.

Once the patient is able to stand, the structured sequence such as the one that follows is recommended.

- Static control of the trunk without extremity movement. These exercises involve closed chain loading/unloading. The patient is positioned in standing, with the feet positioned approximately shoulder-width apart. The purpose of the starting position is to provide a stable base from the proximal segments and trunk onto which challenges can be superimposed. For example:
  - Manual perturbations to a stable trunk. The clinician applies gentle perturbations to the patient's trunk in different directions.
  - Weight shifting while maintaining postural equilibrium. Initially, the patient, with the feet positioned approximately shoulder-width apart, is instructed to alternate transferring weight through one lower extremity then the other. Then the patient is asked to put one foot in front of the other and to transfer the weight from the rear foot to the front foot and back again.
- Dynamic control of trunk without extremity movement. For example, maintaining both feet on the ground while bending at the waist. As indicated, the range of motion is increased from a small range to a larger range.

Once this is mastered, the progression moves to exercises that incorporate static control of the trunk with extremity movement(s) superimposed using the following progression:

- Standing with the feet positioned approximately shoulder-width apart, the patient is asked to flex the hip and knee, so that the foot is approximately 6–8 inches off the floor. The exercise is repeated using the other leg. To add a challenge to the exercise, the patient can be trained with the eyes closed, or the patient can stand on an unstable surface.
- Standing with the feet positioned approximately shoulder-width apart, the patient grasps resistive-tubing with one hand and pulls the tubing toward the body using a smooth, comfortable motion (Fig. 14-1). This produces a forward weight shift that is stabilized with an isometric counterforce consisting of hip extension, knee extension, and ankle plantarflexion.[23]

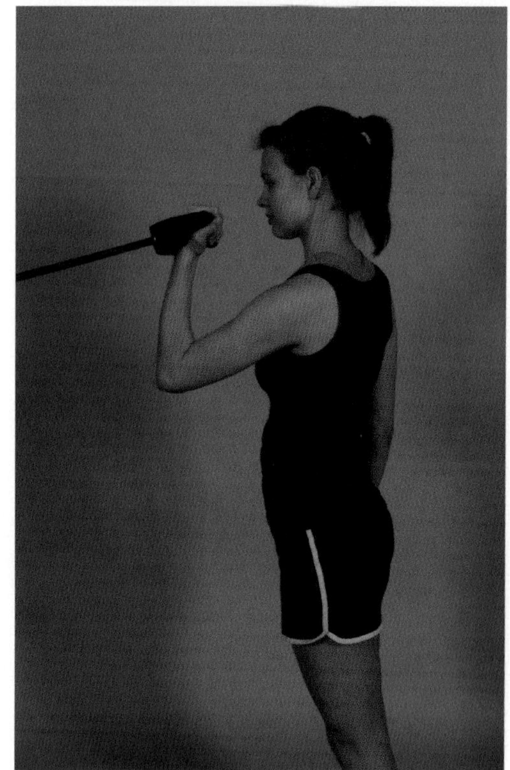

FIGURE 14-1 Forward weight shift exercise.

- The patient stands sideways to the resistive-tubing. The tubing is pulled by one hand in front of the body and the other hand behind the body to equalize the force and minimize the rotation (Fig. 14-2). This causes a lateral weight shift, which is stabilized with an isometric

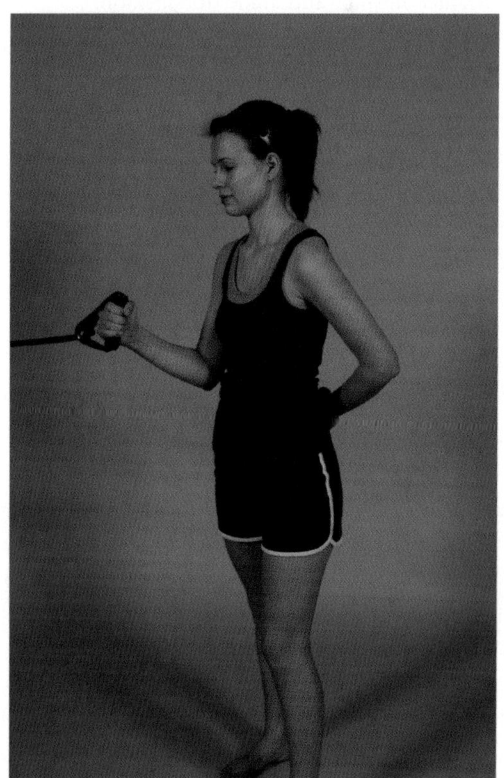

FIGURE 14-2 Lateral weight shift exercise.

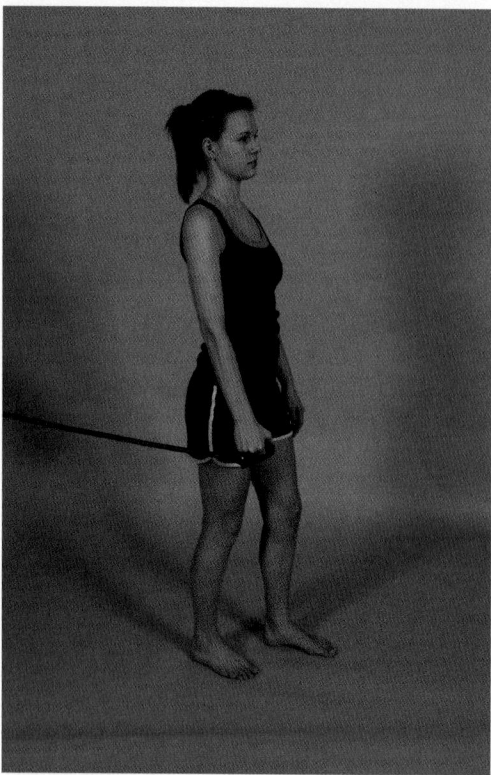

FIGURE 14-3 Posterior weight shift exercise.

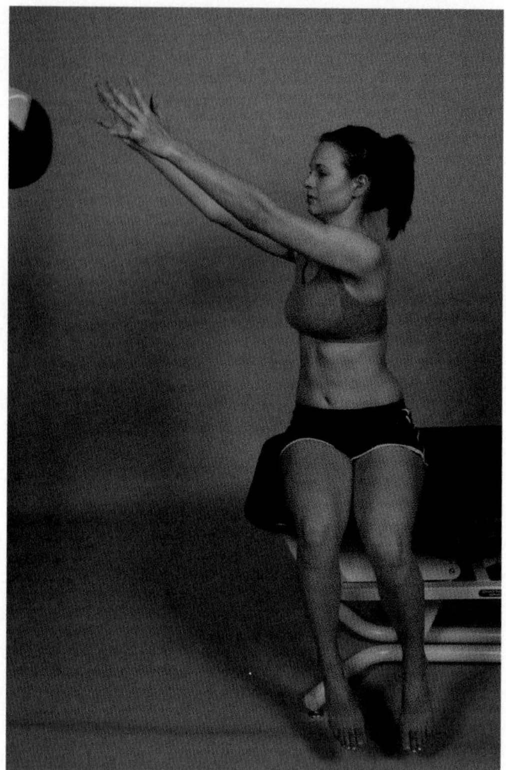

FIGURE 14-4 Medicine ball throw in sitting.

counterforce consisting of hip abduction, knee cocontraction, and ankle eversion.[23]

- The patient stands with his/her back to the tubing in the frontal plane (Fig. 14-3). The tubing is pulled to the body from behind, causing a posterior weight shift, which is stabilized by an isometric counterforce consisting of hip flexion, knee flexion, and ankle dorsiflexion.[23]

The aforementioned single plane exercises are progressed to multiplanar exercises in the following manner:

- PNF movement patterns are initiated using resistive-tubing. Initially the patient stands with both feet shoulder-width apart, and then the exercises are progressed so that the patient is standing on one leg. In addition to using resistive-tubing, medicine balls can be used.
- Ballistic extremity movements while maintaining trunk stability are introduced, first in sitting and then in standing. For example, maintain the sitting position while throwing a medicine ball (Fig. 14-4).

At the earliest opportunity functional tasks must be incorporated. A typical functional activity progression includes:

- Closed-chain activities (squats, lunges) initially, then open-chain activities superimposed on the closed chain by adding extremity motions to the squats and lunges (Fig. 14-5).
- Sit–stand–sit activities focusing on moving the body mass forward over the base of support, extending the lower extremities and raising the body mass over the feet, and then reversing the procedure.
- Stand–to–sit transitions focusing on balance control while pivoting and changing direction.
- Floor to standing raises using progression of side-sit to quadruped to kneeling to half kneeling to standing.
- Gait activities: ambulating forwards, backwards, sideward at varying speeds and base of support widths (narrow to wide). Resisted walking and/or running can also be used.

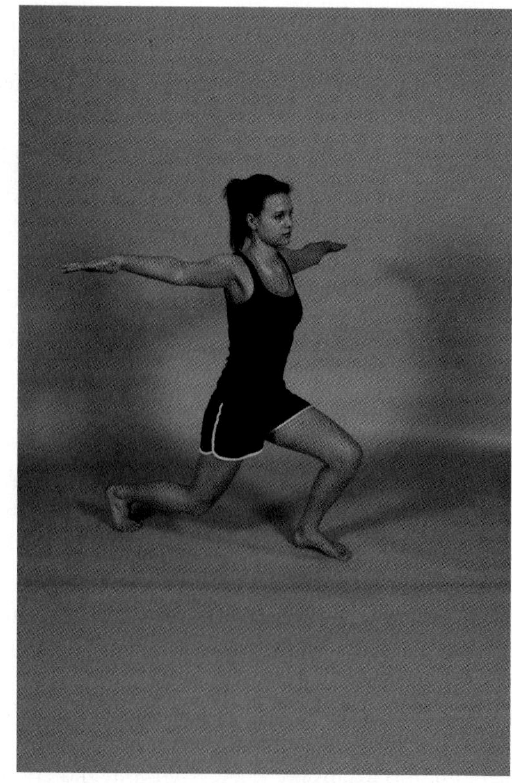

FIGURE 14-5 Lunge with arms raised out to sides.

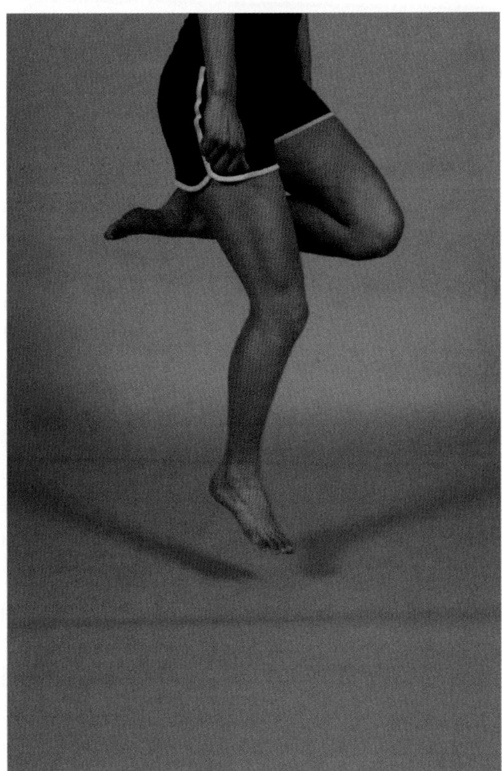

FIGURE 14-6 Hopping on one leg.

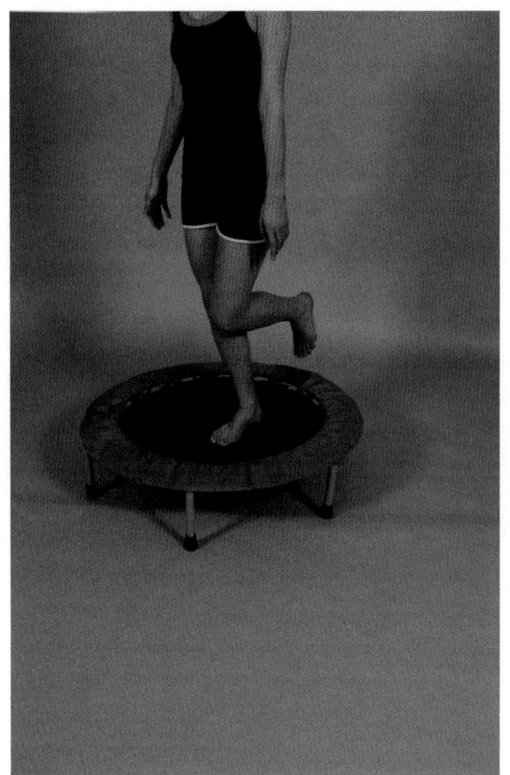

FIGURE 14-7 Minitrampoline standing on one leg.

- As appropriate, multidirectional drills including jumping (two-foot takeoff followed by two-foot landing), hopping (one-foot takeoff followed by landing on the same foot) (Fig. 14-6), and bounding (one-foot takeoff followed by an opposite-foot landing).[23]

CLINICAL PEARL

Various clinical devices have been designed to assist with proprioceptive training for the upper and lower extremity. These include, but are not limited to:

- Minitrampoline (Fig. 14-7)
- Biomechanical ankle platform system (BAPS)®
- Foam rollers
- Wobble board
- Kinesthetic ability training device (KAT)®
- Fitter®, Rocker boards, or foam balance mats

STABILIZATION RETRAINING

Stability normally involves the interaction of three systems—the neurological or central control system, the passive or inert tissues (e.g., ligaments, capsule), and the contractile (muscular) or active system (see Chap. 3).[24]

The *neutral zone* is a term used to define a region of laxity around the neutral resting position of a joint (see Chap. 2).[25] The neutral zone refers to the position of a joint in which minimal loading is occurring in the passive structures (all of the noncontractile elements of the joint including the ligaments, fascia, joint capsules, and non-contractile components of muscle), and the contribution of the active system (the muscles and tendons which surround and control joint motion) is most critical.[26,27]

CLINICAL PEARL

The size of the neutral zone is determined by the integrity of the passive restraint and active control systems, which in turn are controlled by the neural system.[25] Studies have demonstrated that a larger than normal neutral zone caused by injury or microtrauma is related to a lack of segmental muscle control, and is associated with injury.[25,28–31] Unfortunately, there is as yet no *clinical* method to measure the size of the neutral zone.

In both the spine and the extremities, certain muscles work as either mobilizers or stabilizers. The peripheral stabilizers rely on stabilization of the two primary dynamic bases or core structures—the pelvis and the scapula. The pelvis acts as a base for the whole body, especially for the spine and the lower limbs, whereas the scapula acts as a base for its respective upper limb.[24] During peripheral joint movement, the peripheral stabilizer muscles normally contract first to stabilize the core structures from which the mobilizers work.[24,32] The mobilizers then contract, resulting in a controlled movement pattern. For example, during upper extremity activity, the scapular stabilizers contract first to stabilize the scapula before the other shoulder muscles move the upper extremity into a functional position. However, with injury, a pathologic process, or other abnormality, an abnormal stabilizer recruitment pattern can develop, resulting in a dominance of the mobilizer muscles and eventual weakening of the local stabilizers.[24,32]

For stabilization retraining to be effective, the clinician must, therefore, ensure that a stable base is present from which the mobilizers can act. Once the stabilizer muscles are functioning efficiently, training of the mobilizer muscles can begin using the following sequence: isometric to concentric, to eccentric, and ecocentric (pseudo-isometric) contractions, and finally to functional movement (see Chap. 12).[24]

CLINICAL PEARL

An ecocentric contraction occurs when a two-joint muscle shortens at one end, while lengthening at the other end. An example involves the hamstrings when moving from standing to sitting.

The body has several natural stabilization methods including muscle contraction, muscle spasm, osteophyte formation, scar tissue formation, and adaptive shortening of inert tissue or muscle.[24] While the clinician cannot impact some of these natural stabilization methods such as muscle spasm, osteophyte and scar tissue formation, the clinician can use muscle contraction and adaptive shortening to the patient's advantage.

Stabilization retraining involves approximately 6 stages with 12 steps:[24,32,33]

- Stage 1. This stage typically occurs in the acute phase of healing.
  Step 1: Decrease pain. This can be accomplished through muscle relaxation techniques, patient education on joint resting positions and proper body mechanics, the use of electro physical agents, working in the pain-free range, and the use of medication.[34]
  Step 2: Allow freedom of movement and proper arthrokinematic movement of the joint. This can be accomplished through joint mobilization (joint capsule), prolonged passive stretch (inert tissue and muscle), muscle energy techniques (muscle), active release techniques (muscle), manipulation (joint), and neurodynamic techniques (nerve), depending on the tissue causing the restriction.[24]
- Stage 2. This stage is initiated once pain is under control and normal arthrokinematics are restored.
  Step 1: Ensure that the individual muscles will contract when and how they should, starting with an isometric contraction of the isolated muscle (stabilizers first). The initial emphasis is directed toward strengthening any weak stabilizer muscles using the inner range or muscle test position.
  Step 2: Ensure proper muscle recruitment and reeducation so that the muscles contract in the correct order—stabilizers first, then mobilizers. Once the patient can contract the muscle isometrically, concentric movement within the range that the patient has control using the mobilizers can be initiated, but only if the stabilizer muscles function properly.[24] Finally, training progresses to the use of eccentric contractions which allow the patient to maintain control of the base while lengthening during functional movements or slowing down a particular motion.[24]
  Step 3: Ensure muscle imbalance between muscle groups to ensure that the various force couples work together correctly and function to enable control and eliminate incoordination. In general, to correct muscle length, one should exercise lengthened muscles in the inner range to shorten them, and stretch short muscles to lengthen them.[24]
- Stage 3. This stage should only be initiated when the patient has learned to statically control the core structures.
  Step 1: Correct endurance and strength discrepancies. Exercises for stabilizer muscles may involve high-load, low-repetition training, although the focus should be on lower loads and high repetitions to build up resistance to fatigue.
- Stage 4. This stage is typically initiated at the same time the stage 3, provided the patient has successfully completed stages one and two and can demonstrate control of the core.
  Step 1: Retrain proprioception. Proprioceptive retraining is outlined at the beginning of the chapter.
- Stage 5. This stage involves the integration of five different steps into the program.[35]
  Step 1: Reeducate stabilizing muscle statically. This is achieved by ensuring proximal stabilization of the core while allowing distal movement through the extremities. Short arc movements are performed initially while the clinician observes for the expected proper sequence of muscle contractions (stabilizers then mobilizers), correct force-couple action, and good muscle cocontraction (static stabilization).
  Step 2: Teach advanced static stabilization exercises. This involves taking the patient into the mechanism of injury position and asking him or her to hold the position statically against resistance.
  Step 3: Teach dynamic stabilization exercises. This involves the use of controlled movement patterns to ensure the development of proper movement patterns (engrams—see Chap. 3) and voluntary control. Exercises during this step involve movement of the core, with the control muscles acting eccentrically while distal joints are moved concentrically through the full range of movement.
  Step 4: Teach advanced dynamic stabilization exercises. Exercises during this step include multidirectional stability training that require control of functional speeds, progressive eccentric exercises at functional speeds, and stressing of functional diagonal patterns used in the activities to which the person plans to return.
  Step 5: Teach functional stabilization. Functional activities are initially broken down into their component parts before performing the whole movement.
- Stage 6
  Step 1: Maintain or restore fitness throughout. Depending on the location of the injury, endurance exercises are prescribed for the upper extremities or lower extremities to improve or maintain cardiovascular fitness (see Chap. 15).
  Step 2: Return to sport or heavy manual labor as appropriate. In order to return to sport or heavy manual labor, there should be:[24]
  - Complete resolution of acute signs and symptoms
  - Sufficient dynamic, functional range of motion of all joints involved in the activity

- Adequate strength, endurance, and proprioceptive/kinesthetic sense to perform the expected skills successfully
- No alteration of the patient's normal mechanics that could predispose him or her to reinjury

REFERENCES

1. Risberg MA, Mork M, Krogstad-Jenssen H, et al: Design and implementation of a neuromuscular training program following anterior cruciate ligament reconstruction. *J Orthop Sports Phys Ther* 31:620–631, 2001.
2. Chmielewski TL, Hewett TE, Hurd WJ, et al: Principles of neuromuscular control for injury prevention and rehabilitation. In: Magee D, Zachazewski JE, Quillen WS, eds. *Scientific Foundations and Principles of Practice in Musculoskeletal Rehabilitation*. St. Louis, MI: WB Saunders, 2007:375–387.
3. Voight M, Blackburn T: Proprioception and balance training and testing following injury. In: Ellenbecker TS, ed. *Knee Ligament Rehabilitation*. Philadelphia, PA: Churchill Livingstone, 2000:361–385.
4. Nyland J, Lachman N, Kocabey Y, et al: Anatomy, function, and rehabilitation of the popliteus musculotendinous complex. *J Orthop Sports Phys Ther* 35:165–179, 2005.
5. Voight ML, Cook G: Impaired neuromuscular control: reactive neuromuscular training. In: Prentice WE, Voight ML, eds. *Techniques in Musculoskeletal Rehabilitation*. New York, NY: McGraw-Hill, 2001:93–124.
6. Jerosch J, Prymka M: Propriozeptive Fahigkeiten des gesunden Kniegelenks: Beeinflussung durch eine elastische Bandage. Sportverletz. *Sportsch* 9:72–76, 1995.
7. Jerosch J, Hoffstetter I, Bork H, et al: The influence of orthoses on the proprioception of the ankle joint. *Knee Surg Sports Traumatol Arthrosc* 3:39–46, 1995.
8. Perlau R, Frank C, Fick G: The effect of elastic bandages on human knee proprioception in the uninjured population. *Am J Sports Med* 23:251–255, 1995.
9. Robbins S, Waked E, Rappel R: Ankle taping improves proprioception before and after exercise in young men. *Br J Sports Med* 29:242–247, 1995.
10. Barrett DS: Proprioception and function after anterior cruciate ligament reconstruction. *J Bone Joint Surg Br* 73B:833–837, 1991.
11. Lephart SM, Pincivero DM, Giraldo JL, et al: The role of proprioception in the management and rehabilitation of athletic injuries. *Am J Sports Med* 25:130–137, 1997.
12. McNair PJ, Wood GA, Marshall RN: Stiffness of the hamstring muscles and its relationship to function in ACL deficient individuals. *Clin Biomech* 7:131–137, 1992.
13. Borsa PA, Lephart SM, Kocher MS, et al: Functional assessment and rehabilitation of shoulder proprioception for glenohumeral instability. *J Sport Rehabil* 3:84–104, 1994.
14. Lephart SM, Warner JJP, Borsa PA, et al: Proprioception of the shoulder joint in healthy, unstable and surgically repaired shoulders. *J Shoulder Elbow Surg* 3:371–380, 1994.
15. Fremerey RW, Lobenhoffer P, Zeichen J, et al: Proprioception after rehabilitation and reconstruction in knees with deficiency of the anterior cruciate ligament: a prospective, longitudinal study. *J Bone Joint Surg Br* 82:801–806, 2000.
16. Irrgang JJ, Whitney SL, Harner C: Nonoperative treatment of rotator cuff injuries in throwing athletes. *J Sport Rehabil* 1:197–222, 1992.
17. Voss DE, Ionta MK, Myers DJ: *Proprioceptive Neuromuscular Facilitation: Patterns and Techniques*, 3rd ed. Philadelphia, PA: Harper and Row, 1985:1–342.
18. Janda DH, Loubert P: A preventative program focussing on the glenohumeral joint. *Clin Sports Med* 10:955–971, 1991.
19. Kloos AD, Givens-Heiss D: Exercise for impaired balance. In: Kisner C, Colby LA, eds. *Therapeutic Exercise. Foundations and Techniques*, 5th ed. Philadelphia, PA: FA Davis, 2002:251–272.
20. Thein-Brody L, Dewane J: Impaired balance. In: Hall C, Thein-Brody L, eds. *Therapeutic Exercise: Moving Toward Function*, 2nd ed. Baltimore, MD: Lippincott Williams & Wilkins, 2005:149–166.
21. Kloos A: Mechanics and control of posture and balance. In: Hughes C, ed. *Movement Disorders and Neuromuscular Interventions for the Trunk and Extremities – Independent Study Course 18.2.2.* La Crosse, WI: Orthopaedic Section, APTA, Inc., 2008:1–26.
22. Herdman SJ, Blatt PJ, Schubert MC: Vestibular rehabilitation of patients with vestibular hypofunction or with benign paroxysmal positional vertigo. *Curr Opin Neurol* 13:39–43, 2000.
23. Voight ML, Cook G: Impaired neuromuscular control: Reactive neuromuscular training. In: Voight ML, Hoogenboom BJ, Prentice WE, eds. *Musculoskeletal Interventions: Techniques for Therapeutic Exercise*. New York, NY: McGraw-Hill, 2007:181–212.
24. Magee DJ, Zachazewski JE: Principles of stabilization training. In: Magee D, Zachazewski JE, Quillen WS, eds. *Scientific Foundations and Principles of Practice in Musculoskeletal Rehabilitation*. St. Louis, MI: WB Saunders, 2007:388–413.
25. Panjabi MM: The stabilizing system of the spine. Part 1. Function, dysfunction adaption and enhancement. *J Spinal Disord* 5:383–389, 1992.
26. Panjabi MM: The stabilizing system of the spine. Part II. Neutral zone and instability hypothesis. *J Spinal Disord* 5:390–396; discussion 397, 1992.
27. O'Sullivan PB: 'Clinical instability' of the lumbar spine: Its pathological basis, diagnosis and conservative management. In: Boyling JD, Jull GA, eds. *Grieve's Modern Manual Therapy: The vertebral column*. Philadelphia, PA: Churchill Livingstone, 2004:311–331.
28. Mimura M, Panjabi M, Oxland T, et al: Disc degeneration affects the multidirectional flexibility of the lumbar spine. *Spine* 19:1371–1380, 1994.
29. Kaigle A, Holm S, Hansson T: Experimental instability in the lumbar spine. *Spine* 20:421–430, 1995.
30. Wilke H, Wolf S, Claes L, et al: Stability of the lumbar spine with different muscle groups: A biomechanical In Vitro study. *Spine* 20:192–198, 1995.
31. Panjabi M, Abumi K, Duranceau J, et al: Spinal stability and intersegmental muscle forces. A biomechanical model. *Spine* 14:194–199, 1989.
32. Comerford MJ, Mottram SL: Movement and stability dysfunction—contemporary developments. *Man Ther* 6:15–26, 2001.
33. Biedert RM: Contribution of the three levels of nervous system motor control, spinal cord, lower brain, cerebral cortex. In: Lephart SM, Fu FH, eds. *Proprioception and Neuromuscular Control in Joint Stability*. Champaign, IL: Human Kinetics, 2000:23–36.
34. Hides J: Joint injury. In: Richardson C, Hodges P, Hides J, eds. *Therapeutic Exercise for Lumbopelvic Stabilization*. Edinburgh: Churchill-Livingstone, 2004:119–128.
35. Norris CM: Spinal stabilization. 1: Active lumbar stabilization—concepts. *Physiotherapy* 81:61–64, 1995.

Improving Cardiovascular Endurance

CHAPTER 15

CHAPTER OBJECTIVES

At the completion of this chapter, the reader will be able to:

1. Explain the importance of cardiovascular endurance in the overall health of an individual.
2. Describe the physiology of the cardiovascular system.
3. Describe the various types of energy and how each is generated.
4. Explain how the various muscle types are involved with endurance and aerobic activities.
5. Outline the precautions with aerobic conditioning.
6. Discuss the various methods by which aerobic conditioning can be enhanced through a rehabilitation program.

OVERVIEW

Physical activity has been defined as "any bodily movement produced by skeletal muscles that results in energy expenditure."[1] When a person undertakes work or exercise, a number of body systems adapt to the demands of the required tasks, particularly the cardiorespiratory and neuromuscular systems.[2] The maximum work capacity of the cardiorespiratory system is a factor of the maximal amount of oxygen that can be taken in and used by the body, or VO_{2max}, whereas the capacity of the neuromuscular system is a factor of the maximum tension that can be developed by the working muscle, or muscles—the maximal voluntary contraction. Assessment of the cardiovascular system provides the clinician with the justification for monitoring or not monitoring activities during a patient's rehabilitation or providing modifications in the exercise prescription.[3]

Whenever possible, the clinician should address the impact on the patient resulting from the loss of physical activity. This loss of activity affects both the cardiovascular and the musculoskeletal systems and can occur very rapidly. Thus, it is important that the rehabilitation program includes exercises that maintain, or improve, the patient's cardiovascular endurance, while monitoring safety concerns. If our sedentary society is to change to one that is more physically active, clinicians must play their role in communicating to their patients the amounts and types of physical activity that are needed to prevent disease and promote health, because patients respect their advice.[4,5] Patients should be routinely counseled to adopt and maintain regular physical activity. Inadequate reimbursement, limited knowledge of the benefits of physical activity, and a lack of training in community physical activity counseling are barriers to achieving these goals. While policy makers work to improve reimbursement for preventive services, clinicians should develop effective ways to teach physical activity counseling.[5] The personal physical activity practices of health professionals should not be overlooked. Health professionals should be physically active, not only to benefit their own health but also to make more credible their endorsement of an active lifestyle.[5]

PHYSICAL FITNESS

According to the Department of Health and Human Services, physical fitness is a set of attributes a person has in regards to his/her ability to perform physical activities that require aerobic fitness, endurance, strength, or flexibility and is determined by a combination of regular activity and genetically inherited ability.[6] Although commonly associated with the state of the cardiorespiratory system, which includes the ability to perform work or participate in activity over time using the body's oxygen uptake, delivery, and energy release mechanisms,[7] physical fitness also encompasses a number of attributes including:[8]

- Muscle strength, which is the ability of muscles to exert or resist a force.
- Muscle endurance, which is the ability of the muscle to perform work.
- Muscle power, which is the ability of a muscle to exert high force at high speed.
- Balance, which is the ability to maintain equilibrium when the body is static or moving.
- Agility, which is the ability to perform functional or powerful movements in opposite directions.
- Flexibility, which is the ability to stretch, easily bend, or be pliable.

PHYSICAL ACTIVITY

Physical activity is closely related to, but distinct from, the subsets of exercise and physical fitness. Exercise is defined as "planned, structured, and repetitive bodily movement done to improve or maintain one or more components of physical fitness."[1] This differs from the definition of physical fitness, which is "a set of attributes that people have or achieve that relates to the ability to perform physical activity."[1] Regular physical activity has long been regarded as an important component of a healthy lifestyle, and it is well established from controlled experimental trials that active individuals have high levels of cardiorespiratory fitness. Intermittent activity, provided it is continued, also confers substantial benefits.[9–11] Studies have demonstrated that within a few weeks of discontinuing an endurance training program, the positive effects of exercise are almost completely lost, with approximately half of that loss occurring within the first 2 weeks.[12,13]

Clinical experience and limited studies suggest that people who maintain or improve their levels of physical activity may be better able to perform daily activities, may be less likely to develop pain, and may be better able to avoid disability, especially as they advance into older age.[5] Regular physical activity may also contribute to better balance, coordination, and agility, which in turn may help prevent falls in the elderly.[14] Epidemiologic research has demonstrated protective effects of physical activity and risk for several chronic diseases, including coronary heart disease,[9,15,16] hypertension,[17,18] non–insulin-dependent diabetes mellitus,[19,20] osteoporosis,[21,22] colon cancer,[23] and anxiety and depression.[24] Patterns of physical activity appear to vary with demographic characteristics. Men are more likely than women to engage in regular activity,[25] vigorous exercise, and sports.[26] The total amount of time spent engaging in physical activity normally declines with age.[27,28] Adults at retirement age (65 years) show some increased participation in activities of light to moderate intensity, but, overall, physical activity declines continuously as age increases.[27,29] Elderly African Americans, and other ethnic minority populations, are less active than white Americans,[25,29,30] and this disparity is more pronounced for women.[30] People with higher levels of education participate in more leisure-time physical activity than do people with less education.[25] Differences in education and socioeconomic status account for most, if not all, of the differences in leisure-time physical activity associated with race and ethnicity.[31]

CARDIOVASCULAR PHYSIOLOGY

Oxygen is a vital component for life and the cardiovascular system provides a means by which oxygen is supplied to the various tissues of the body via the heart, blood vessels, blood, and lungs.

CLINICAL PEARL

The basal metabolic rate (BMR) is the amount of energy required to sustain the body at rest in a supine position. Thus, physical activity is measured as a ratio between the BMR and the rate required to perform a particular task. This ratio is measured as a metabolic equivalent (MET) of the task. Moderate physical activity is activity performed at an intensity of 3–6 METs and is the equivalent of brisk walking at 3–4 mph for most healthy adults.[5]

By definition, cardiorespiratory endurance is the ability to perform whole body activities (walking, jogging, swimming, etc.) for extended periods of time without unwarranted fatigue. The maximal amount of oxygen that can be used during exercise is referred to as maximal aerobic capacity (VO_{2max}). It is also common to see aerobic capacity expressed in METs.

A number of adaptations occur within the circulatory system in response to exercise:

- Heart rate. As the body begins to exercise, the working tissues require an increased supply of oxygen to meet increased demand. Monitoring heart rate (HR) is an indirect method of estimating oxygen consumption as, normally, these two factors have a linear relationship (this relationship is consistent at very low and very high intensity exercise). If a physical therapy intervention requires an increase in systemic oxygen consumption expressed as either an increase in MET levels, kcal, or VO_2, then HR should also be seen to increase.[32] Increases in HR produced by exercise are met by a decrease in diastolic filling time. The extent at which the HR increases with escalating workloads is influenced by many factors including age, fitness level, type of activity being performed, body position, presence of disease, medications, blood volume, and environmental factors such as temperature, humidity, and altitude. Failure of the HR to increase with increasing workloads, referred to as chronotropic incompetence, should be of concern, even if the patient is taking beta blockers—beta blockers slow the HR, which can prevent the increase in HR that typically occurs with exercise.[32]
- Stroke volume. Stroke Volume (SV) is the amount of blood pumped out by the left ventricle of the heart with each beat (the difference between end-diastolic volume and end-systolic volume). The volume of blood being pumped out with each beat increases with exercise, but only to the point when there is enough time between beats for the heart to fill up (approximately 110–120 beats per minute). In the normal heart, as workload increases, SV increases linearly up to 40–50% of aerobic capacity, after which it increases only slightly. Factors that influence the magnitude of change in SV include exercise intensity, body position, and ventricular function.
- Cardiac output. Cardiac output (CO) is the amount of blood (approximately 5L) discharged by each ventricle (not both ventricles combined) per minute, usually expressed as liters per minute. CO, the product of HR and SV, increases linearly with workload because of the increases in HR and SV in response to increasing exercise intensity. During exercise, CO increases to approximately 4 times than that experienced during rest. Factors that influence the magnitude of change in CO include age, posture, body size, presence of disease, and level of physical conditioning. A long-term beneficial training effect that occurs with regard

to HR is a reduced resting HR and reduced HR at a standard exercise load. This occurs because the heart becomes more efficient—the SV increases, brought about by increased venous return, and increased contractile conditions in the myocardium.

- Blood flow. The amount of blood flowing to the various organs increases during exercise, but there is a change in overall distribution of the CO—it is increased to active skeletal muscle, but decreased to nonessential organs. Total peripheral resistance, the sum of all forces that resist blood flow within the circulatory system, decreases during exercise primarily because of the vessel vasodilation in the active skeletal muscles.[33]
- Blood pressure. Blood pressure (BP) is defined as the pressure exerted by the blood on the walls of the blood vessels, specifically *arterial blood pressure* (the pressure in the large arteries). Systolic BP normally increases in proportion to oxygen consumption and CO, while diastolic BP normally shows little or no increase, or may decrease. Long-term aerobic training can result in reduced systolic and diastolic BP. Failure of the systolic BP to rise with an increase in intensity, referred to as exertional hypotension, is considered abnormal, and may occur in patients with cardiovascular problems. The minimal change in diastolic BP is due primarily to the vasodilation of the arteries from the exercise bout. Thus, the expansion in artery size may lower BP during the diastolic phase.[32]
- Oxygen consumption rises rapidly during the first minutes of exercise and levels off as the aerobic metabolism supplies the energy required by the working muscles.
- Mitochondria: An increase in size and number of the mitochondria.
- Hemoglobin concentration. Oxygen is transported throughout the system attached to hemoglobin, an iron containing protein that has the capability of easily accepting or giving up molecules of oxygen as needed.[33] The concentration of hemoglobin in circulating blood does not change with training; it may actually decrease slightly.[33] However, because training for improving cardiovascular endurance produces an increase in total blood volume, there is a corresponding increase in the amount of hemoglobin.
- Myoglobin: Increased myoglobin content.
- The use of fat and carbohydrates: Improved mobilization and use of fat and carbohydrates.
- Lung changes that occur due to exercise.
  - An increase in the volume of air that can be inspired in a single maximal ventilation. Ventilation is the process of air exchange in the lungs.
  - An increase in the diffusing capacity of the lungs.

THE ENERGY FOR MOVEMENT

During physical exercise, energy turnover in skeletal muscle may increase by 400 times compared with muscle at rest and muscle oxygen consumption may increase by more than 100 times.[34] The energy required to power muscular activity is derived from the hydrolysis of ATP to ADP and inorganic phosphate (P_i). Despite the large fluctuations in energy demand just mentioned, muscle ATP remains practically constant and demonstrates a remarkable precision of the system in adjusting the rate of the ATP generating processes to the demand.[35] There are three energy systems that contribute to the resynthesis of ATP via ADP rephosphorylation. These energy systems are as follows:

- ***Phosphagen system.*** The phosphagen system is an anaerobic process—can proceed without oxygen (O_2). Within the skeletal muscle cell at the onset of muscular contraction, phosphocreatine (PCr) represents the most immediate reserve for the rephosphorylation of ATP. The phosphagen system provides ATP primarily for short-term, high-intensity activities (i.e., sprinting) but is active at the start of all exercises regardless of intensity.[36] One disadvantage of the phosphagen system is that because of its significant contribution to the energy yield at the onset of near maximal exercise, the concentration of PCr can be reduced to less than 40% of resting levels within 10 seconds of the start of intense exercise.[37]
- ***Glycolysis system.*** The glycolysis system is an anaerobic process that involves the breakdown of carbohydrates—either glycogen stored in the muscle or glucose delivered through the blood—into pyruvate to produce ATP. Pyruvate is then transformed into lactic acid. Because this system relies upon a series of nine different chemical reactions, it is slower to become fully active. However, glycogenolysis has a greater capacity to provide energy than does PCr, and therefore it supplements PCr during maximal exercise and continues to rephosphorylate ADP during maximal exercise after PCr reserves have become essentially depleted.[36] The process of glycolysis can be in one of the two ways, termed fast glycolysis and slow glycolysis, depending on the energy demands within the cell. If energy must be supplied at a high rate, fast glycolysis is used primarily. If the energy demand is not so high, slow glycolysis is activated. The main disadvantage of the fast glycolysis system is that during very high-intensity exercise, hydrogen ions dissociate from the glycogenolytic end product of lactic acid.[35] The accumulation of lactic acid in the contracting muscle is recognized in sports and resistance training circles. An increase in hydrogen ion concentration is believed to inhibit glycolytic reactions and directly interfere with muscle excitation–contraction and coupling, which can potentially impair contractile force during exercise.[36] This inhibition occurs once the muscle pH drops below a certain level, prompting the appearance of phosphofructokinase (PFK), resulting in local energy production ceasing until replenished by oxygen stores.

CLINICAL PEARL

Lactic acid is the major energy source for providing the muscle with ATP during exercise bouts that last 1 to 3 minutes (e.g., running 400 to 800 m).

- ***Oxidative system.*** As its name suggests, the oxidative system requires O_2 and is consequently termed the "aerobic" system. The oxidative system is the primary source of ATP at rest and during low-intensity activities. It is worth noting that at no time during either rest or exercise does any single energy system provide the complete supply of energy. While being unable to produce ATP at an equivalent rate to that produced by PCr breakdown and glycogenolysis, the oxidative system is capable of sustaining low-intensity exercise for several hours.[36] However, because of an increased complexity, the time between the onset of exercise and when this system is operating at its full potential is around 45 seconds.[38]

The relative contribution of these energy systems to ATP resynthesis has been shown to depend upon the intensity and duration of exercise, with the primary system used being based on the duration of the event:[39]

- 0–10 seconds: ATP–PCr
- 10–30 seconds: ATP–PCr plus anaerobic glycolysis
- 30 seconds–2 minutes: anaerobic glycolysis
- 2–3 minutes: anaerobic glycolysis plus oxidative system
- >3 minutes and rest: oxidative system

RECOVERY

The performance of any activity requires a certain rate of oxygen consumption, so that an individual's ability to perform an activity is limited by the maximal amount of oxygen the person is capable of delivering into the lungs.[33] Fatigue and recovery from fatigue are complex processes that depend on physiologic and psychological factors. The physiologic factors include the adequacy of the blood supply to the working muscle and the maintenance of a viable chemical environment, whereas the psychological factors include motivation and incentive.[2] After an intense exercise session, anaerobic energy sources must be replenished before they can be called on again to provide energy for muscular contraction. The anaerobic energy sources of ATP–PCr and lactic acid are ultimately replenished by the oxidative energy system. The extra oxygen that is taken and used to replenish the anaerobic energy sources after cessation of the exercise effort was previously referred to as the *oxygen debt*, but is now more accurately referred to as *excess postexercise oxygen consumption* (EPOC).

The patient who is injured while performing an activity or exercise is likely to return to that activity once the symptoms subside.[5] Thus, the body needs to be prepared for a resumption of the stresses and demands that the activity or exercise will place upon it. If not, when the patient returns to competitive sports or functional and work activities, fatigue may result in alterations in efficient movements making the individual susceptible to injury.

PRECAUTIONS WITH AEROBIC CONDITIONING

Before beginning any exercise program, the clinician should perform a health screening check or risk factor assessment as part of the initial assessment to identify individuals who should consult a physician before initiating an exercise program. The following are considered risk factors for cardiovascular disease:[40]

- High BP: >140 mm Hg systolic or >90 mm Hg
- Smoking
- Elevated serum cholesterol: a total serum level >200, LDL >160 (individuals without heart disease, >100 in individuals with heart disease), or HDL <40 in men or <50 in women
- Lack of regular exercise (three or more times per week of regular exercise or moderate physical activity)
- Family history (mother or father with heart disease or stroke before age 60)
- Stress (particularly personality factors of anger and hostility)
- Diabetes
- Obesity
- Sex: men are at greater risk than women until women reach menopause, then equal risk
- Age: increasing age increases risk

CLINICAL PEARL

In cases of severe pulmonary disease, the cost of breathing can reach 40% of the total exercise oxygen consumption, thereby decreasing the amount of oxygen available for the exercising muscles.

Obese individuals should exercise at longer durations and lower intensities—they should be able to exercise while maintaining a conversation (talk test). In addition, to reduce stresses on weight-bearing joints, these individuals should perform exercises where their weight is supported (e.g., recumbent bike, swimming, etc.)

All patients should be monitored (i.e., HR, BP, and symptoms) during the initial assessment if they have been determined unsafe to exercise based on any risk factor or healthy lifestyle assessment.

During exercise, the clinician should note normal clinical responses to progressively increasing aerobic exercise. The magnitude of the change in cardiovascular responses during aerobic exercise is related to the physical activity status of the patient. For example, a patient whose HR takes longer than 5 minutes to return to resting levels after 2 minutes of exercise has poor cardiovascular function.[41] Once the individual has demonstrated normal vital signs and lack of symptoms with the activities, it may not be necessary to monitor further activities.

A number of precautions need to be taken when exercising patients who have been determined unsafe to exercise. These include:

- An appropriate level of intensity must be chosen:
  - Too high a level can overload the cardiorespiratory and muscular systems and potentially cause injuries or severe complications.
  - Exercising at a level which is too high causes the cardiorespiratory system to work anaerobically, not

aerobically. Initially the patient should be exercising at a level with the HR at 60% of his or her maximum (220–age of patient). If the patient is exercising within their target HR, they should be able to carry on a conversation.

- A sufficient period of time should be allowed for warm-up and cool-down to permit adequate cardiorespiratory and muscular adaptation.

CLINICAL PEARL

Conditioned individuals have a cardiovascular and pulmonary system that is more capable of delivering oxygen to sustain aerobic energy production at increasingly higher levels of intensity.

A rapid decline in cardiorespiratory fitness occurs during the first few weeks of deconditioning; for example, one study reported that 20 days of bed rest was associated with a 28% decrease in aerobic capacity.[42] The aforementioned decline in aerobic capacity after 20 days of bed rest was greater than that found after three decades of aging in the same subjects.[43]

Signs and symptoms of exercise intolerance include, but are not limited to:

- BP:
  - Systolic BP >200 to 210 mm Hg
  - Drop in systolic BP >20 mm Hg
  - Diastolic BP >110 mm Hg
- HR:
  - Increase in HR >50 bpm with low level activity
  - Significant arrhythmias
- Chest pain
- Nausea, vomiting
- Unusual or severe fatigue
- Syncope or moderate dizziness
- Marked dyspnea (2 +/4+)
- Severe claudication (grade III/IV)
- Cyanosis or severe pallor

CLINICAL PEARL

Currently, only a few studies have examined the acute effect of resistance exercise on cardiovascular function.[44,45] From these studies it has been found that the magnitude and directional change in cardiac volume and function during resistance exercise are, for the most part, opposite to those that occur during aerobic exercise.

TECHNIQUES FOR IMPROVING, MAINTAINING, AND MONITORING CARDIORESPIRATORY ENDURANCE

Aerobic conditioning is especially valuable for those who participate in sports that involve endurance.[46] Nirschl[47,48] recommends general body conditioning for patients, which provides the following benefits:

- Increased regional perfusion
- Neurophysiologic synergy and overflow
- Neurologic stimulation
- Minimization of the domino effect of weakness of adjacent structures
- Minimization of negative psychological effects
- Obesity control

A number of different training factors must be considered when attempting to maintain or improve cardiorespiratory endurance:

- Continuous training—the F.I.T.T. (Frequency, Intensity, Time, and Type) principle:
  - Frequency: to see at least minimal improvement in cardiorespiratory endurance, it is necessary for the average person to engage in no less than three sessions per week.
    - If the intensity is kept constant, there appears to be no additional benefit from twice a week versus four times or three times a week versus five times per week.
    - If the goal is weight loss, 5 to 7 days per week increases the caloric expenditure more than 2 days per week.
  - Intensity: the recommendations regarding training intensity (overload) vary. Relative intensity for an individual is calculated as a percentage of the maximum function, using $VO_{2\ max}$ or maximum HR (HR max). It is now recognized that an individual's perception of effort (relative perceived exertion or RPE) is closely related to the level of physiological effort (see Chap. 12).[49,50] For aerobic activities, the exercise intensity should be at a level that is 40–85% maximal aerobic power ($VO_{2\ max}$) or 55–90% of maximal HR.[51]

CLINICAL PEARL

If an individual is taking medications that may affect HR and BP responses (e.g., beta blockers), the Borg rating of perceived exertion is the only method for prescribing exercise intensity.

Two other common methods of monitoring intensity are employed:

- Monitoring HR—two formulas are commonly used:
  - Maximum heart rate reserve (MHRR): this method uses the difference between the maximum heart rate (MHR) and the resting heart rate (RHR), referred to as the maximum heart rate reserve (MHRR). When using this formula, the recommended intensity level range is 50–85% of $VO_{2\ max}$. For example, for a 40-year-old with a RHR of 65 bpm who wants to train at an intensity of 70%:
  - 220–40 = 180 bpm (MHR)
  - 180–65 = 115 bpm (MHRR)
  - (115 × 0.7) + 65 = 145 bpm

TABLE 15-1 Comparison of Physiologic Adaptations to Resistance Training and Aerobic Training		
Variable	**Result Following Resistance Training**	**Result Following Endurance Training**
Performance		
Muscle strength	Increases	No change
Muscle endurance	Increases for high-power output	Increases for low-power output
Aerobic power	No change or increases slightly	Increases
Maximal rate of force production	Increases	No change or decreases
Vertical jump	Ability increases	Ability unchanged
Anaerobic power	Increases	No change
Sprint speed	Improves	No change or improves slightly
Muscle fibers		
Fiber size	Increases	No change or increases slightly
Capillary density	No change or decreases	Increases
Mitochondrial density	Decreases	Increases
Fast heavy-chain myosin	Increases in amount	No change or decreases in amount
Enzyme activity		
Creatine phosphokinase	Increases	Increases
Myokinase	Increases	Increases
Phosphofructokinase	Increases	Variable
Lactate dehydrogenase	No change or variable	Variable
Metabolic energy stores		
Stored ATP	Increases	Increases
Stored creatine phosphate	Increases	Increases
Stored glycogen	Increases	Increases
Stored triglycerides	May increase	Increases
Connective tissue		
Ligament strength	May increase	Increases
Tendon strength	May increase	Increases
Collagen content	May increase	Variable
Bone density	No change or increase	Increases
Bone composition		
Percentage body fat	Decreases	Decreases
Fat-free mass	Decreases	No change

ATP, adenosine triphosphate.
Data from Clancy WG: Specific rehabilitation for the injured recreational runner. *Instr Course Lect* 38:483-486, 1989.

- The age-adjusted maximum heart rate (AAMHR)[52]: MHR = 220 – patient's age. For example, for a 40-year-old, the MHR is 220–40 = 180. The recommended level of intensity when using this formula is a range between 60–90% of an individual's MHR Therefore, the target heart range (60–90%) for a MHR of 180 is between 180 × 60% and 180 × 90% = 108 to 162 bpm.

CLINICAL PEARL

Tanaka and colleagues recently revealed that the AAMHR equation underestimates the actual maximal HR by 6 to 15 bpm for individuals between 60 and 90 years of age.[53] Based on these findings a new formula has been derived to estimate the age-predicted maximal HR: 208 – (0.7 × age).[54]

Regardless of which formula is used, the clinician should keep in mind that formulas are merely estimations (and highly inaccurate when used with patients taking prescribed medications that may affect HR and BP responses), and therefore, it is more important to be conservative in prescribing exercise intensity for any sedentary individual, elderly individual, or someone at moderate to high risk for cardiovascular disease.[3]

- Type of exercise: the type of activity chosen in continuous training must be aerobic—involving large muscle groups activated in a repetitive and rhythmic manner. Examples of aerobic activities are running, cycling, swimming, and cross-country skiing. Aerobic exercises allow the individual to speed up or slow down the pace to maintain the HR at a specified or target level.[33] Cross-training exercises, including cycling, upper body ergometer (UBE), and water running, increase cardiovascular endurance.

However, it must be remembered that although cross training can produce a similar cardiovascular effort as the original sport, it does not necessarily produce the same musculoskeletal effects (Table 15-1).

- Time (duration): duration is increased when intensity is limited, e.g., by initial fitness level. For minimal improvement to occur, the patient must participate in continuous activity for at least 20 minutes with a HR elevated to its working level. Three to five minutes per day produces a training effect in poorly conditioned individuals, whereas 20 to 60 minutes, 3 to 5 times a week is optimal for conditioned people. Generally, the greater the duration of the workout, the greater the improvement in cardiovascular endurance.[33] A number of pieces of exercise equipment can be used with continuous training:
  - Treadmill walking: progressing from slow to fast and short distances to longer distances with or without an incline.
  - Ergometers: these come in a variety of forms for both the upper extremities and the lower extremities. The pace progression is from slow to fast and the goal is to increase the time spent exercising.
  - Free weights and elastic resistance: the use of low resistance and high repetitions can produce an aerobic effect.

CLINICAL PEARL

Discontinuous training, also known as interval training, involves the use of repeated high-intensity exercise bouts that are interspersed with rest intervals. Although endurance levels can be improved with this method, more benefits are seen in the development of strength and power.

REFERENCES

1. Caspersen CJ, Powell KE, Christenson GM: Physical activity, exercise and physical fitness. *Public Health Rep* 100:125–131, 1985.
2. Kiser DM: Physiological and biomechanical factors for understanding repetitive motion injuries. *Semin Occup Med* 2:11–17, 1987.
3. Haykowsky MJ, Hillegass EA: Integration of the cardiovascular system in assessment and interventions in musculoskeletal rehabilitation. In: Magee D, Zachazewski JE, Quillen WS, eds. *Scientific Foundations and Principles of Practice in Musculoskeletal Rehabilitation.* St. Louis, MO: WB Saunders, 2007:414–431.
4. Lewis BS, Lynch WD: The effect of physician advice on exercise behavior. *Prev Med* 22:110–121, 1993.
5. Pate RR, Pratt M, Blair SN, et al: Physical activity and public health: a recommendation from the Centers for Disease Control and Prevention and the American College of Sports Medicine. *JAMA* 273:402–407, 1995.
6. U.S. Department of Health and Human Services: *Physical Activity and Health: A Report of the Surgeon General.* Atlanta, GA: National Center for Chronic Disease Prevention and Health Promotion, 1996.
7. *Guide to Physical Therapist Practice*: Second Edition. American Physical Therapy Association. *Phys Ther* 81:9–746, 2001.
8. Moffat M: Clinicians' roles in health promotion, wellness, and physical fitness. In: Magee D, Zachazewski JE, Quillen WS, eds. *Scientific Foundations and Principles of Practice in Musculoskeletal Rehabilitation.* St. Louis, MO: WB Saunders, 2007:328–356.
9. Paffenbarger RS, Hyde RT, Wing AL, et al: Physical activity, all-cause mortality, and longevity of college alumni. *N Engl J Med* 314:605–613, 1986.
10. Leon AS, Connett J, Jacobs DR Jr, et al: Leisure-time physical activity levels and risk of coronary heart disease and death: the Multiple Risk Factor Intervention trial. *JAMA* 258:2388–2395, 1987.
11. DeBusk RF, Stenestrand U, Sheehan M, et al: Training effects of long versus short bouts of exercise in healthy subjects. *Am J Cardiol* 65:1010–1013, 1990.
12. Winter DA: Moments of force and mechanical power in jogging. *J Biomech* 16:91–7, 1983.
13. Orlander J, Kiessling KH, Karlsson J, et al: Low intensity training, inactivity and resumed training in sedentary men. *Acta Physiol Scand* 101:351–362, 1977.
14. Parsons D, Foster V, Harman F, et al: Balance and strength changes in elderly subjects after heavy-resistance strength training. *Med Sci Sports Exerc* 24(suppl):S21, 1992.
15. Powell KE, Thompson PD, Caspersen CJ, et al: Physical activity and the incidence of coronary heart disease. *Annu Rev Public Health* 8:253–287, 1987.
16. Morris JN, Kagan A, Pattison DC, et al: Incidence and prediction of ischemic heart disease in London busman. *Lancet* 2:533–559, 1966.
17. Hagberg JM: Exercise, fitness, and hypertension. In: Bouchard C, Shephard RJ, Stephens T, et al, eds. *Exercise, Fitness, and Health.* Champaign, IL: Human Kinetics Publishers, 1990:455–566.
18. Paffenbarger RS, Wing AL, Hyde RT, et al: Physical activity and incidence of hypertension in college alumni. *Am J Epidemiol* 117:245–257, 1983.
19. Helmrich SP, Ragland DR, Leung RW, et al: Physical activity and reduced occurrence of non-insulin-dependent diabetes mellitus. *N Engl J Med* 325:147–152, 1991.
20. Manson JE, Rimm EB, Stampfer MJ, et al: Physical activity and incidence of non-insulin-dependent diabetes mellitus in women. *Lancet* 338:774–778, 1991.
21. Cummings SR, Kelsey JL, Nevitt MD, et al: Epidemiology of osteoporosis and osteoporotic fractures. *Epidemiol Rev* 7:178–208, 1985.
22. Snow-Harter C, Marcus R: Exercise, bone mineral density, and osteoporosis. *Exerc Sport Sci Rev* 19:351–388, 1991.
23. Lee I, Paffenbarger RS, Hsieh C: Physical activity and risk of developing colorectal cancer among college alumni. *J Natl Cancer Inst* 83:1324–1329, 1991.
24. Taylor CB, Sallis JF, Needle R: The relationship of physical activity and exercise to mental health. *Public Health Rep* 100:195–201, 1985.
25. Caspersen CJ, Christenson GM, Pollard RA: The status of the 1990 Physical Fitness Objectives—Evidence from NHIS 85. *Public Health Rep* 101:587–592, 1986.
26. Stephens T, Jacobs DR, White CC: A descriptive epidemiology of leisure-time physical activity. *Public Health Rep* 100:147–158, 1985.
27. Caspersen CJ, Pollard RA, Pratt SO: Scoring physical activity data with special consideration for elderly population. *Proceedings of the 21st National Meeting of the Public Health Conference on Records and Statistics: Data for an Aging Population.* Washington, DC: DHHS Publication, 1987:30–34.
28. Schoenborn CA: Health habits of US adults, 1985: the 'Alameda 7' revisited. *Public Health Rep* 101:571–580, 1986.
29. Caspersen CJ, Merritt RK: Trends in physical activity patterns among older adults: the Behavioral Risk Factor Surveillance System, 1986–1990. *Med Sci Sports Exerc* 24:S26, 1992.
30. DiPietro L, Caspersen C: National estimates of physical activity among white and black Americans. *Med Sci Sports Exerc* 23(suppl):S105, 1991.
31. White CC, Powell KE, Goelin GC, et al: The behavioral risk factor surveys, IV: the descriptive epidemiology of exercise. *Am J Prev Med* 3:304–310, 1987.
32. Grimes K: Heart disease. In: O'Sullivan SB, Schmitz TJ, eds. *Physical Rehabilitation*, 5th ed. Philadelphia, PA: FA Davis, 2007:589–641.
33. Sells P, Prentice WE: Impaired endurance: Maintaining aerobic capacity and endurance. In: Voight ML, Hoogenboom BJ, Prentice WE, eds. *Musculoskeletal Interventions: Techniques for Therapeutic Exercise.* New York, NY: McGraw-Hill, 2007:153–164.
34. Tonkonogi M, Sahlin K: Physical exercise and mitochondrial function in human skeletal muscle. *Exerc Sport Sci Rev* 30:129–137, 2002.
35. Sahlin K, Tonkonogi M, Soderlund K: Energy supply and muscle fatigue in humans. *Acta Physiol Scand* 162:261–266, 1998.
36. McMahon S, Jenkins D: Factors affecting the rate of phosphocreatine resynthesis following intense exercise. *Sports Med* 32:761–784, 2002.
37. Walter G, Vandenborne K, McCully KK, et al: Noninvasive measurement of phosphocreatine recovery kinetics in single human muscles. *Am J Physiol* 272:C525–C534, 1997.

38. Bangsbo J: Muscle oxygen uptake in humans at onset and during intense exercise. *Acta Physiol Scand* 168:457–464, 2000.
39. Sahlin K, Ren JM: Relationship of contraction capacity to metabolic changes during recovery from a fatiguing contraction. *J Appl Physiol* 67: 648–654, 1989.
40. Yusuf S, Hawken S, Ounpuu S, et al: Effect of potentially modifiable risk factors associated with myocardial infarction in 52 countries (the INTERHEART study): case-control study. *Lancet* 364:937–952, 2004.
41. Nutter P: Aerobic exercise in the treatment and prevention of low back pain. *Occup Med* 3:137–145, 1988.
42. Saltin B, Blomqvist G, Mitchell JH, et al: Response to exercise after bed rest and after training. *Circulation* 38:VII1–78, 1968.
43. McGuire DK, Levine BD, Williamson JW, et al: A 30-year follow-up of the Dallas Bedrest and Training Study: I. Effect of age on the cardiovascular response to exercise. *Circulation* 104:1350–1357, 2001.
44. Haykowsky M, Taylor D, Teo K, et al: Left ventricular wall stress during leg-press exercise performed with a brief Valsalva maneuver. *Chest* 119:150–154, 2001.
45. Lentini AC, McKelvie RS, McCartney N, et al: Left ventricular response in healthy young men during heavy-intensity weight-lifting exercise. *J Appl Physiol* 75:2703–2710, 1993.
46. Kibler WB: *Clinical Implications of Exercise: Injury and Performance, Instructional Course Lectures, American Academy of Orthopaedic Surgeons*. Rosemont, IL: American Academy of Orthopaedic Surgeons, 1994: 17–24.
47. Nirschl RP: Elbow tendinosis: tennis elbow. *Clin Sports Med* 11:851–870, 1992.
48. Nirschl RP: Prevention and treatment of elbow and shoulder injuries in the tennis player. *Clin Sports Med* 7:289–308, 1988.
49. Borg GAV: Psychophysical basis of perceived exertion. *Med Sci Sports Exerc* 14:377–381, 1992.
50. Borg GAV: Perceived exertion as an indicator of somatic stress. *Scand J Rehabil Med* 2:92–98, 1970.
51. American College of Sports Medicine: *Guidelines for Exercise Testing and Prescription*, 4th ed. Philadelphia, PA: Lea & Febiger, 1991.
52. Artalejo AR, Garcia-Sancho J: Mobilization of intracellular calcium by extracellular ATP and by calcium ionophores in the Ehrlich ascites-tumour cell. *Biochim Biophys Acta* 941:48–54, 1988.
53. Tanaka H, Monahan KD, Seals DR: Age-predicted maximal heart rate revisited. *J Am Coll Cardiol* 37:153–156, 2001.
54. Taylor RS, Brown A, Ebrahim S, et al: Exercise-based rehabilitation for patients with coronary heart disease: systematic review and meta-analysis of randomized controlled trials. *Am J Med* 116:682–692, 2004.

SECTION IV THE EXTREMITIES

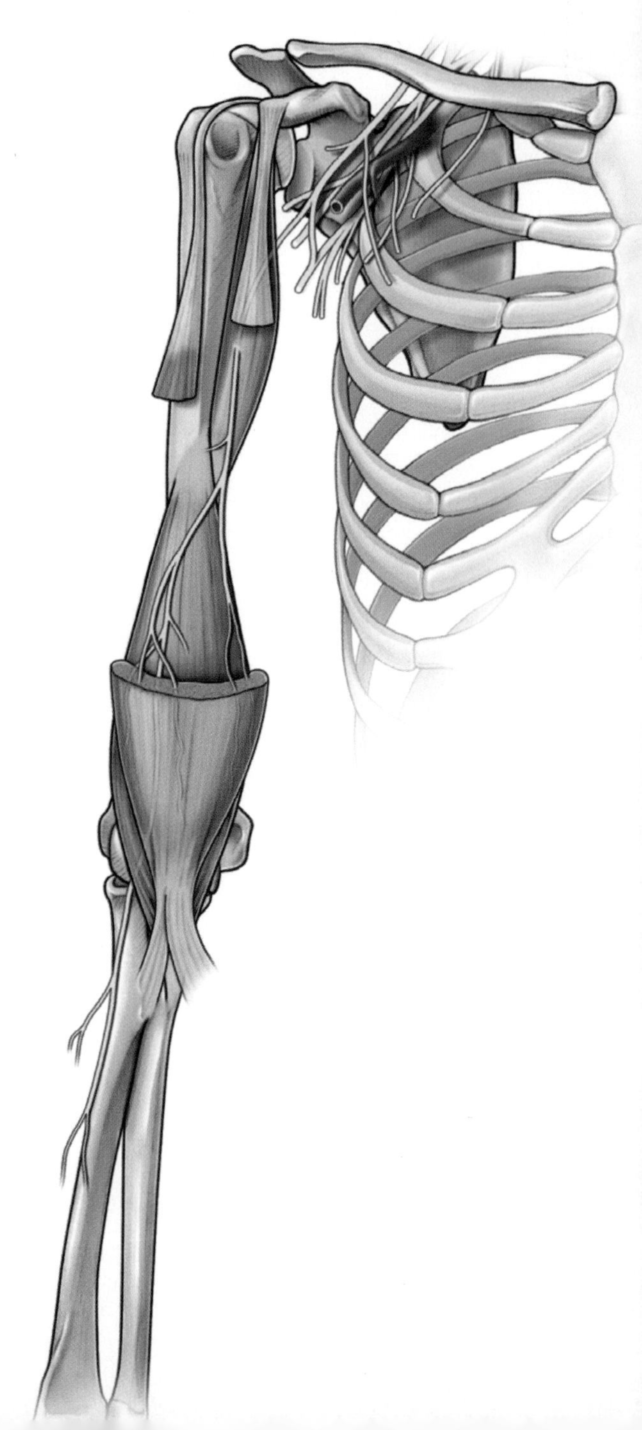

CHAPTER 16 The Shoulder

CHAPTER OBJECTIVES

At the completion of this chapter, the reader will be able to:

1. Describe the anatomy of the joints, ligaments, muscles, blood, and nerve supply that comprise the shoulder complex.
2. Describe the biomechanics of the shoulder complex, including the open- and close-packed positions, muscle force couples, and the static and dynamic stabilizers.
3. Describe the relationship between muscle imbalance and functional performance of the shoulder.
4. Describe the purpose and components of the tests and measures for the shoulder complex.
5. Perform a comprehensive examination of the shoulder complex, including history, systems review, palpation of the articular and soft tissue structures, specific passive mobility tests, passive articular mobility tests, and special tests.
6. Evaluate the key findings from the examination data to establish a physical therapy diagnosis and prognosis.
7. Summarize the various causes of shoulder dysfunction.
8. Describe and demonstrate intervention strategies and techniques based on the clinical findings and any established goals.
9. Evaluate the intervention effectiveness to determine progress and modify an intervention as needed.
10. Plan an effective home program and instruct the patient in its use.

OVERVIEW

The shoulder is the most rewarding joint in the body because when a limited or painful movement is found, the finding is seldom ambiguous and often implicates the offending structure.

—*James Cyriax, MD (1904–1985)*

The primary function of the shoulder complex is to position the hand in space, thereby allowing an individual to interact with his or her environment and to perform fine motor functions. An inability to position the hand results in profound impairment of the entire upper extremity.[1]

Secondary functions of the shoulder complex include the following:

- Suspending the upper limb.
- Providing sufficient fixation so that motion of the upper extremity or trunk can occur.
- Serving as a fulcrum for arm elevation. Three types of arm elevation are recognized: an upward motion of the upper extremity in the scapular plane (*scaption*) and the motions in either the coronal plane (*abduction*) or in the sagittal plane (*flexion*).

The shoulder is endowed with a unique blend of mobility and stability. The degree of mobility is contingent on a healthy articular surface, intact muscle–tendon units, and supple capsuloligamentous restraints. The degree of stability is dependent on intact capsuloligamentous structures, proper function of the muscles, and the integrity of the osseous articular structures.[1] Optimal functioning of the shoulder and arm can only take place if a delicate balance between mobility and stability is maintained.

ANATOMY

The shoulder complex functions as an integrated unit, involving a complex relationship between its various components. The components of the shoulder joint complex consist of (Fig. 16-1):

- three bones (the humerus, the clavicle, and the scapula);
- three joints (the sternoclavicular (S-C), the acromioclavicular (A-C), and the glenohumeral (G-H) joints);
- one "pseudojoint" (the articulation between the scapula and the thorax);
- one physiological area (the suprahumeral or subacromial space).

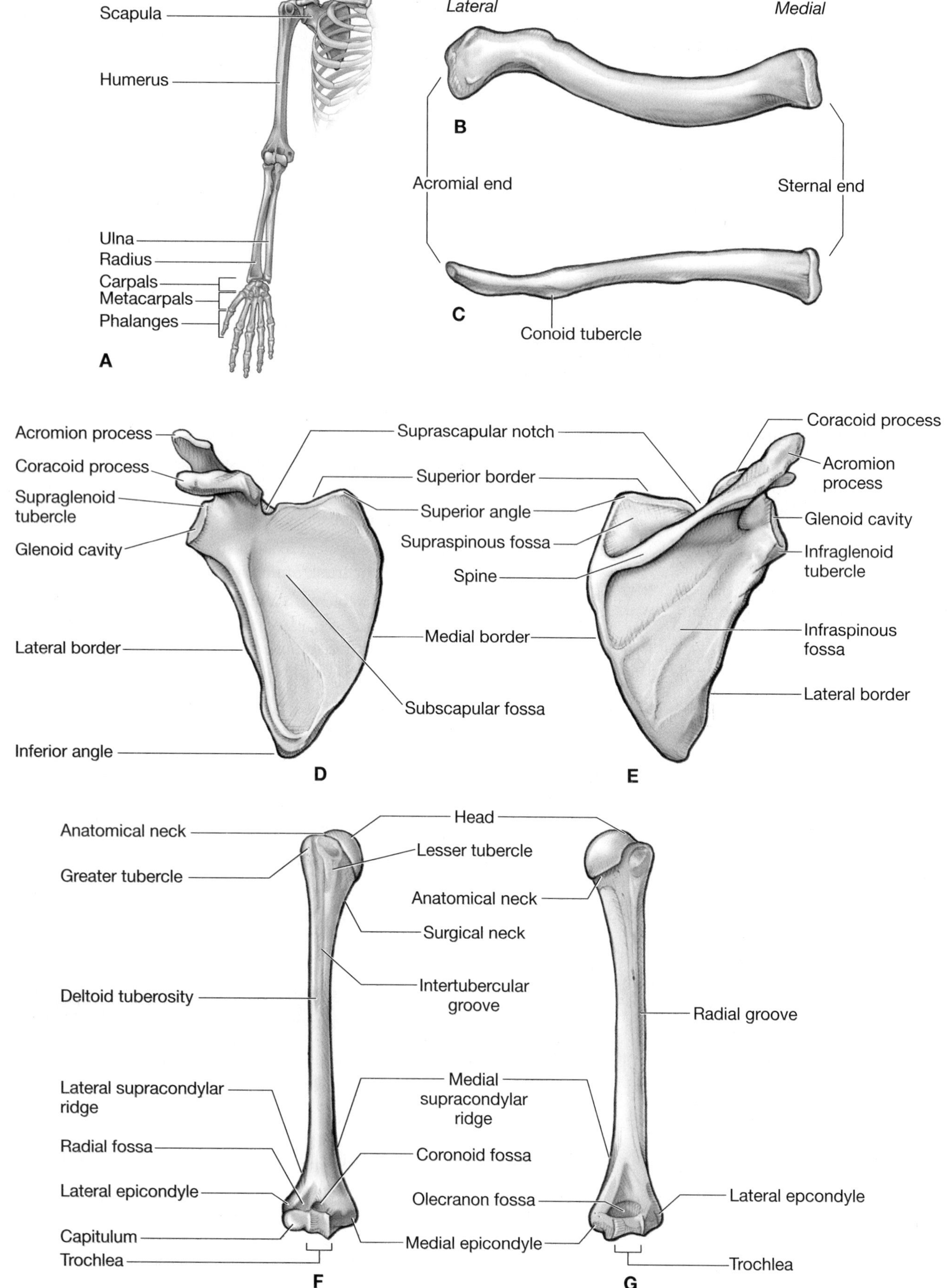

FIGURE 16-1 Bony anatomy of the shoulder. (Reproduced with permission from Morton DA, Foreman KB, Albertine KH: *The Big Picture: Gross Anatomy*. McGraw-Hill, 2011)

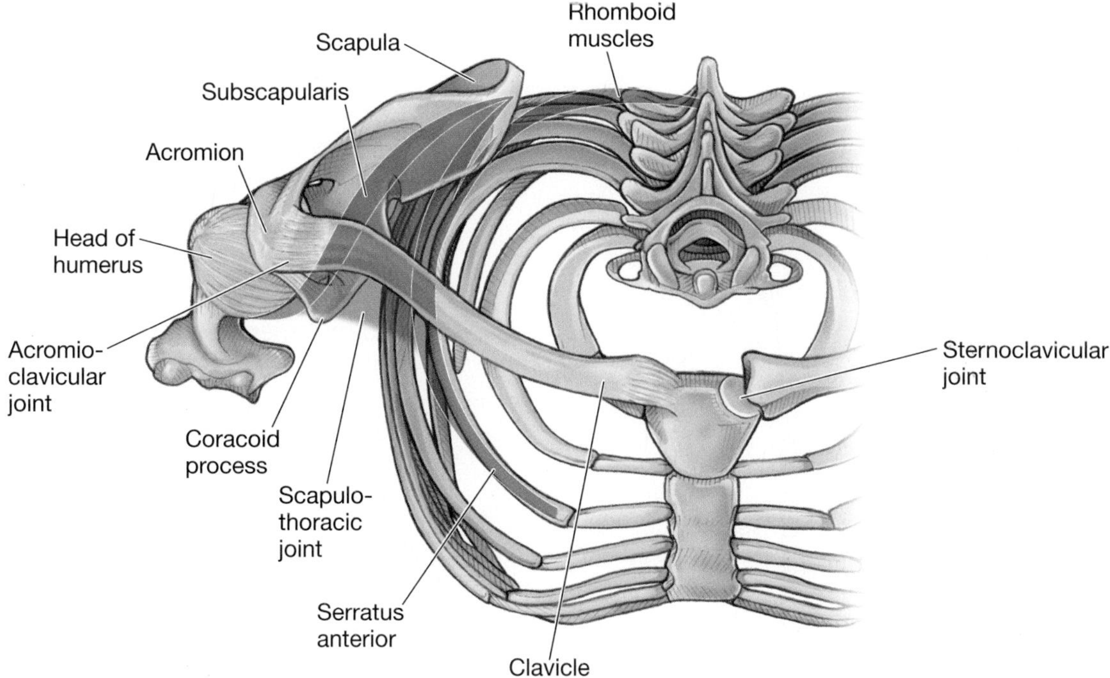

FIGURE 16-2 Superior aspect of shoulder showing angle of scapula. (Reproduced with permission from Morton DA, Foreman KB, Albertine KH: *The Big Picture: Gross Anatomy*. McGraw-Hill, 2011)

For optimal function to occur at the shoulder, motion also has to be available at the cervicothoracic junction and at the connections between the first three ribs and the sternum and spine.

GLENOHUMERAL JOINT

The G-H joint is a true synovial-lined diarthrodial joint that connects the upper extremity to the trunk, as part of the upper kinetic chain. The G-H joint is described as a ball and socket joint—the humeral head forms roughly half a ball or sphere (Fig. 16-1), whereas the glenoid fossa forms the socket.

The head of the humerus faces medially, posteriorly, and superiorly with the axis of the head forming an angle of 130–150 degrees with the long axis of the humerus.[2] In the frontal plane, the head of the humerus is angled posteriorly (retroverted) by 30–40 degrees.[3,4] The joint capsule of the G-H joint is lax inferiorly to permit full elevation of the arm.

The glenoid fossa of the scapula faces laterally, superiorly, and anteriorly at rest and inferiorly and posteriorly when the arm is in the dependent position (Fig. 16-2).[5] The glenoid fossa is flat and covers only one-third to one-fourth of the surface area of the humeral head. This arrangement allows for a great deal of mobility but little in the way of articular stability (Fig. 16-3). However, the glenoid fossa is made approximately 50% deeper (doubling the depth of the glenoid fossa across its equatorial line)[6] and more concave by a ring of fibrous cartilage[7] and dense fibrous collagen[8] called a labrum. The labrum forms a part of the articular surface and is attached to the margin of the glenoid cavity and the joint capsule.[9] It is also attached to the lateral portion of the biceps anchor superiorly.[10] In addition, approximately 50% of the fibers of the long head of the biceps (LHB) brachii originate from the superior labrum (the remainder originates from the superior glenoid tubercle),[8] with four different variations identified,[11] and continue posteriorly to become a periarticular fiber bundle, making up the bulk of the labrum.[10,12] The labrum enhances joint stability by increasing the humeral head contact areas to 75% vertically and 56% transversely.[5,9] The humeral–glenoid contact area provides two primary functions[13]: it spreads the joint loading over a broad area, and it permits movement of opposing joint surfaces with minimal friction and wear.[14] However, because the humeral head is larger than the glenoid, at any point during elevation, only 25–30% of the humeral

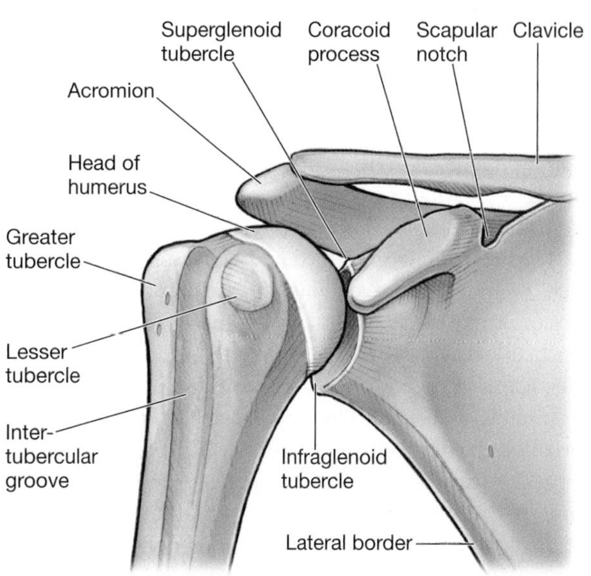

FIGURE 16-3 Glenohumeral joint. (Reproduced with permission from Morton DA, Foreman KB, Albertine KH: *The Big Picture: Gross Anatomy*. McGraw-Hill, 2011)

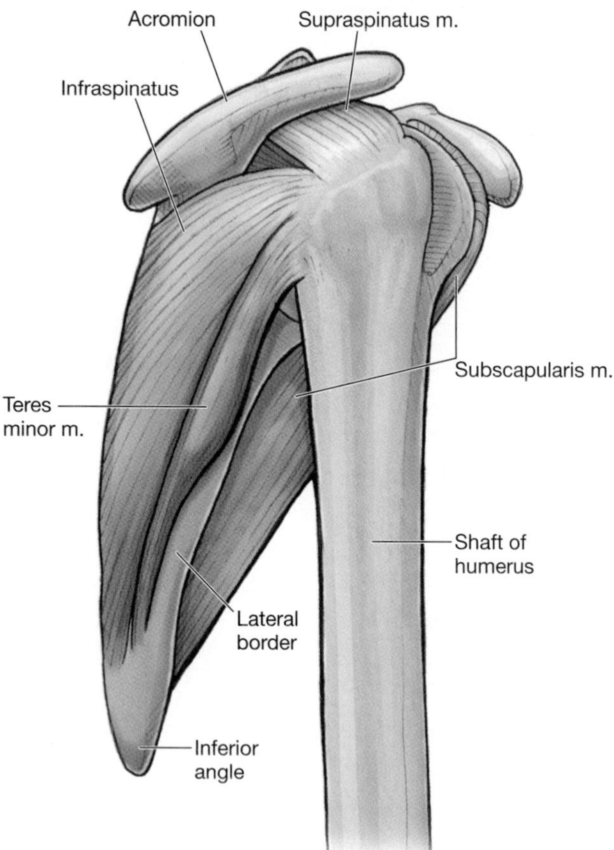

FIGURE 16-4 Rotator cuff muscles. (Reproduced with permission from Morton DA, Foreman KB, Albertine KH: *The Big Picture: Gross Anatomy*. McGraw-Hill, 2011)

head is in contact with the glenoid, with the greatest contact occurring during elevation rather than at the extremes. Contact between the humeral head and glenoid fossa is significantly reduced when the humerus is positioned in[15–17]

- adduction, flexion, and internal rotation (IR);
- abduction and elevation;
- adducted at the side, with the scapula rotated downward.

Although the labrum provides some stability for the G-H joint, additional support is provided by both dynamic and static mechanisms. The dynamic mechanisms include the muscles of the rotator cuff (supraspinatus, infraspinatus, teres minor, and subscapularis muscles) (Fig. 16-4) and a number of muscle force couples described later. The static mechanisms, which include reinforcements of the joint capsule, joint cohesion and geometry, and ligamentous support, are also described later.

The scapula (Fig. 16-1) functions as a stable base from which G-H mobility can occur. The scapula is a flat blade of bone that is oriented to contribute to stability: it lies along the thoracic cage at 30 degrees to the frontal plane, 3 degrees superiorly relative to the transverse plane to augment functional reaching motions above shoulder height,[18] and 20 degrees forward in the sagittal plane.[19–21] This orientation results in arm elevation occurring in a plane that is 30–45 degrees anterior to the frontal plane. When elevation of the arm occurs in this plane, the motion is referred to as *scapular plane abduction* or *scaption*.

CLINICAL PEARL

It has been recommended that many strengthening exercises for the shoulder joint complex be performed in the scapular plane. Reasons for this include the following:

- When the limb is positioned in the plane of the scapula, the mechanical axis of the G-H joint is in line with the mechanical axis of the scapula and movement of the humerus in this plane is less limiting than in the frontal or sagittal planes because the G-H capsule is not twisted.[22,23]
- Since the rotator cuff muscles originate on the scapula and attach to the humerus, the length–tension relationship of these muscles is enhanced in this position.

The scapula's wide and thin configuration allows for its smooth gliding along the thoracic wall and provides a large surface area for muscle attachments both distally and proximally.[24] In all, 16 muscles gain attachment to the scapula (Table 16-1). Six of these muscles, including the trapezius, rhomboids, levator scapulae, and serratus anterior, support and move the scapula, while nine of the others are concerned with G-H motion.[25–27]

Posteriorly, the scapula is divided by the elevated scapula spine into two unequally sized muscle compartments. The supraspinous fossa is small and serves as the site of origin for the supraspinatus muscle (see Fig. 16-4). The infraspinous fossa gives attachment for the downward-acting infraspinatus and teres minor muscles, important muscles for the stabilization of the humeral head (see "Muscles of the Shoulder Complex" section). The spine of the scapula (see Fig. 16-1) provides a continuous line of attachments for the supporting trapezius muscle along its upper border, whereas the deltoid muscle, which suspends the humerus, gains origin from its lower border. The undersurface of the scapula is covered by the subscapularis muscle, which also assists in stabilizing the humeral head against the glenoid fossa.

A prominent feature of the scapula is the large overhanging acromion (see Fig. 16-3), which, along with the coracoacromial ligament and the previously mentioned labrum, functionally enlarges the G-H socket. The position of the acromion also places the deltoid muscle in a dominant position to provide muscular support during elevation of the arm. Bigliani et al.[21,28] introduced the following acromion types:

TABLE 16-1 Muscles of the Scapula

Trapezius	Subscapularis
Levator scapulae	Coracobrachialis
Long and short head of the biceps	Pectoralis minor
Rhomboid major	Serratus anterior
Rhomboid minor	Long head of triceps
Supraspinatus	Teres major
Infraspinatus	Teres minor
Deltoid	Omohyoid

- Type I has a relatively flat undersurface
- Type II is slightly convex
- Type III is hooked

CLINICAL PEARL

Acromial morphology and the mechanical effect of the acromion is a strong predictor of rotator cuff impingement.[21] Cadaveric studies have confirmed a 70% incidence of rotator cuff tears in patients with a Type III acromial shape and only a 3% incidence in patients with a Type I acromion.[28,29]

The distance, or angle, between the scapula and the clavicle is variable and depends on function. While the shoulder is protracted, the angle is 50 degrees. At rest, the angle is approximately 60 degrees, and with retraction the angle increases to 70 degrees.[3]

Along the medial border of the scapula arise three muscles: the two rhomboid muscles and the serratus anterior (Fig. 16-5), all of which aid with scapular stability during arm elevation (see later). The coracoid process (see Fig. 16-3) projects forward like a crow's beak, for which it is named. This forward position provides an efficient lever whereby the small pectoralis muscle can help to stabilize the scapula. In addition, the process serves as a point of origin for the coracobrachialis and the short head of the biceps muscle.

The lateral attachment of the voluminous joint capsule of the G-H joint attaches to the anatomical neck of the humerus (Fig. 16-6).[6] Medially, the capsule is attached to the periphery of the glenoid and its labrum. The overall strength of the joint capsule bears an inverse relationship with the patient's age; the older the patient, the weaker the joint capsule. The fibrous portion of the capsule is very lax and has several recesses, depending on the position of the arm. At its inferior aspect, the capsule forms an axillary recess, which is both loose and redundant. The recess permits normal elevation of the arm, although it can also be the site of adhesions when the shoulder is immobilized in adduction. The anterior aspect of the joint capsule is reinforced by three ligaments (Z ligaments), which are described in the next section. The tendons of the rotator cuff (supraspinatus, infraspinatus, teres minor, and subscapularis) reinforce the superior, posterior, and anterior aspects of the capsule, as does the LHB tendon.

An inner synovial membrane lines the fibrous capsule and secretes synovial fluid into the joint cavity. The synovium typically lines the joint capsule and extends from the glenoid labrum down to the neck of the humerus. It also forms variously sized bursae, the largest of which, the subacromial or subdeltoid bursa, lies on the superior aspect of the joint (see later).

The greater and lesser tuberosities (see Fig. 16-1), which serve as attachment sites for the tendons of the rotator cuff muscles, are located on the lateral aspect of the anatomical neck of the humerus, an imaginary line that separates the humeral head from the rest of the humerus. The lesser tuberosity serves as the attachment for the subscapularis. The greater tuberosity serves as the attachment for the

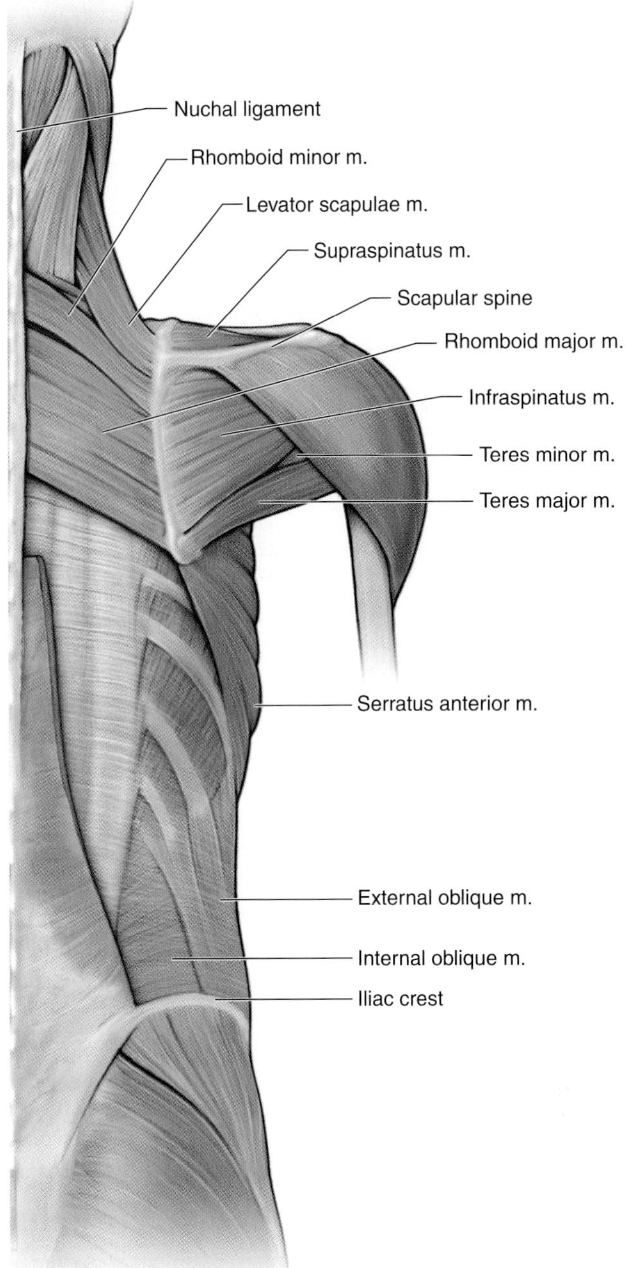

FIGURE 16-5 Rhomboid muscles and serratus anterior. (Reproduced with permission from Morton DA, Foreman KB, Albertine KH: *The Big Picture: Gross Anatomy*. McGraw-Hill, 2011)

supraspinatus, infraspinatus, and teres minor. The greater and lesser tuberosities are separated by the intertubercular groove (see Fig. 16-1), through which passes the tendon of the LHB on its route to attach to the superior rim of the glenoid fossa. This groove has wide variance in the angle of its walls, but 70% fall within a 60–75-degree range.[30] Certain shoulder disorders, including rotator cuff and bicipital tendinitis, have been associated with anomalies of this groove.[31] As the tendon of the LHB (Fig. 16-7) passes over the humeral head from its origin, it makes a right-angle turn to lie in the anterior aspect of the humerus. This abrupt turn may permit abnormal wearing of the tendon at this point.

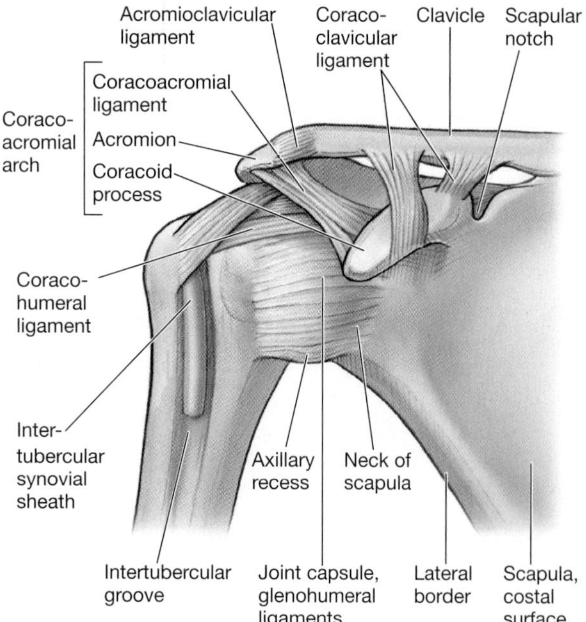

FIGURE 16-6 Glenohumeral joint and ligaments. (Reproduced with permission from Morton DA, Foreman KB, Albertine KH: *The Big Picture: Gross Anatomy.* McGraw-Hill, 2011)

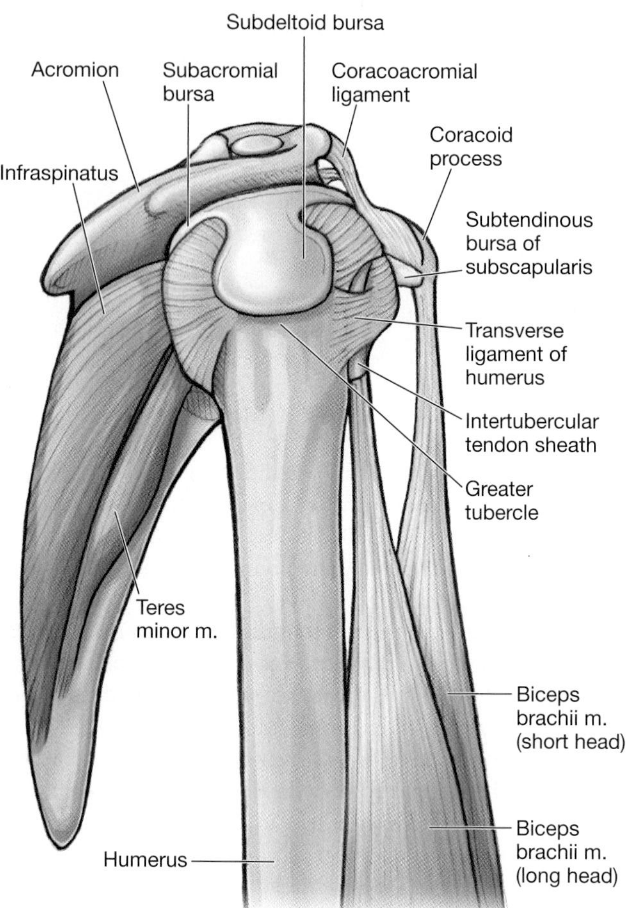

FIGURE 16-7 Soft tissue structures of the shoulder. (Reproduced with permission from Morton DA, Foreman KB, Albertine KH: *The Big Picture: Gross Anatomy.*McGraw-Hill, 2011)

The roof of this groove is formed by the transverse ligament. The transverse humeral ligament (Fig. 16-7), which runs perpendicular over the biceps tendon, was once thought to function as a restraint to the biceps tendon within the intertubercular groove. However, this appears to be the role of the coracohumeral ligament.[31]

The region below the greater and lesser tuberosities, where the upper margin of the humerus joins the shaft of the humerus, is referred to as the surgical neck (Fig. 16-1). The axillary nerve and posterior humeral circumflex artery lie in close proximity to the medial aspect of the surgical neck.

CLINICAL PEARL

Fractures of the surgical neck of the humerus occur more frequently than fractures of the anatomical neck, and they are most likely to cause damage to the axillary nerve.

Ligaments

A number of structures function as static stabilizers during motion of the arm to reciprocally tighten and loosen, thereby limiting translation and rotation of the G-H joint surfaces in a load-sharing fashion.[32] These include the G-H ligaments and the posterior capsule. Further static stabilization is provided by the glenoid labrum. The posterior capsule is under tension when the shoulder is in flexion, abduction, IR (in particular, the superior and middle segments), or in any combination of these.

At the anterior portion of the outer fibers of the joint capsule, three local reinforcements are present: the superior, middle, and inferior G-H ligaments (Fig. 16-6). Together with the coracohumeral ligament, these ligaments form a Z-pattern on the anterior aspect of the shoulder (Fig. 16-6).[33] In the midrange of rotation, the G-H ligaments are relatively lax and stability is maintained primarily by the action of the rotator cuff muscle group compressing the humeral head into the conforming glenoid articulation.[32] The G-H ligaments appear to produce a major restraint during shoulder flexion, extension, and rotation[34]:

- The anterior G-H ligament is under tension when the shoulder is in extension, abduction, and/or external rotation (ER).
- The posterior G-H ligament is under tension in flexion and ER.
- The inferior G-H ligament is the most important of the G-H ligaments. It is under tension when the shoulder is abducted, extended, and/or externally rotated. In addition, this ligament is a primary restraint against both anterior and posterior dislocations of the humeral head, and is the most important stabilizing structure of the shoulder in the overhead athlete.[35] At 0-degree abduction, the subscapularis muscle, the labrum, and the superior G-H ligament are the

primary restraints against anterior translation. At 45-degree abduction, the subscapularis muscle and the middle and inferior G-H ligaments, along with labrum, prevent anterior translation. When the arm is abducted more than 90 degrees, which is the most common position of anterior dislocation, the anterior fibers of the inferior G-H ligament are the primary restraint anterior movement.[9,36]

- The middle G-H ligament is under tension when the shoulder is flexed and externally rotated. In addition, the middle G-H ligament and the subscapularis tendon limit ER from 45 to 75 degrees of abduction, and are important anterior stabilizers.

Other ligaments (Fig. 16-6) help provide stability to the G-H joint. These include the following:

- ***The coracohumeral ligament.*** The coracohumeral ligament (see Fig. 16-6) arises from the lateral end of the coracoid process and runs laterally, where it is split into two bands by the presence of the biceps tendon. The posterior band blends with the supraspinatus tendon to insert near the greater tuberosity, and the anterior band blends with the subscapularis tendon to insert near the lesser tuberosity. The coracohumeral ligament covers the superior GH ligament anterosuperiorly and fills the space between the tendons of the supraspinatus and subscapularis muscles, uniting these tendons to complete the rotator cuff in this area. Tears of the cuff usually extend longitudinally between the supraspinatus and coracohumeral ligament so that the hood action of the cuff is lost. It is generally agreed that the posterior band of the coracohumeral ligament limits flexion, whereas the anterior band limits extension of the G-H joint.[37] Both the bands also limit inferior and posterior translation of the humeral head, strengthening the superoanterior aspect of the capsule.[37,38]
- ***The coracoacromial ligament.*** The coracoacromial ligament (see Fig. 16-6) is often described as the roof of the shoulder. It is a very thick structure that runs from the coracoid process to the anteroinferior aspect of the acromion, with some of its fibers extending to the A-C joint. The ligament consists of two bands that join near the acromion, and it is ideally suited, both anatomically and morphologically, to prevent separation of the A-C joint surfaces. The coracoclavicular ligaments and the costoclavicular ligament are described in the A-C joint section and the S-C joint section, respectively.

Coracoacromial Arch

The coracoacromial arch (Fig. 16-6) is formed by the anteroinferior aspect of the acromion process, and the coracoacromial ligament, which connects the coracoid to the acromion and the inferior surface of the A-C joint.[39–41] A number of structures are located in the subacromial space (Fig. 16-7) between the coracoacromial arch superiorly and the humeral head inferiorly, and the coracoid process, anteromedially. These include (from inferior to superior) the following:

- the head of the humerus,
- the long head of biceps tendon (intra-articular portion),
- the superior aspect of the joint capsule,
- the supraspinatus and upper margins of subscapularis and infraspinatus,
- the subdeltoid–subacromial bursae,
- the inferior surface of coracoacromial arch.

In normal individuals, the suprahumeral space averages 10–11 mm in height with the arm adducted to the side.[42,43] Elevating the arm decreases this space, and the space is at its narrowest between 60 and 120 degrees of scaption.[44] During overhead motion in the plane of the scapula, the supraspinatus tendon, the region of the cuff most involved in overuse syndromes of the shoulder, can pass directly underneath the coracoacromial arch. If the arm is elevated while internally rotated, the supraspinatus tendon passes under the coracoacromial ligament, whereas if the arm is externally rotated, the tendon passes under the acromion itself.[45]

Muscle imbalances or capsular contractures can cause an increase in superior translation of the humeral head, narrowing the subacromial space. For example, if the rotator cuff muscles are weak or injured, increased translation occurs between the humeral head and the glenoid labrum.[46] This increase in translation may lead to increased wear on the labrum, increased reliance on the static restraints (e.g., ligaments, capsule), and eccentric overloading of the dynamic (muscle) restraints, which in turn can result in instability and/or a condition termed "subacromial impingement syndrome (SIS)."[47,48]

Bursae

Approximately eight bursae are distributed throughout the shoulder complex. The subdeltoid–subacromial bursae (see Fig. 16-7) are collectively referred to as the subacromial bursa because they are often continuous in nature. The subacromial bursa is one of the largest bursae in the body and provides two smooth serosal layers, one of which adheres to the overlying deltoid muscle and the other to the rotator cuff lying beneath. This bursa is also connected to the acromion, greater tuberosity, and coracoacromial ligament. As the humerus elevates, it permits the rotator cuff to slide easily beneath the deltoid muscle. There are also smaller bursae interposed between most of the muscles in contact with the joint capsule:

- ***The subcoracoid bursa.*** This bursa is located under the coracoid process.
- ***The subscapular bursa.*** This bursa is located between the subscapular muscle tendon and the anterior neck of the scapula and protects the tendon as it passes under the coracoid process.

Neurology

The shoulder complex is embryologically derived from C5 to C8, except the A-C joint, which is derived from C4 (Fig. 16-8). The sympathetic nerve supply to the shoulder originates primarily in the thoracic region from T2 down as far as T8.[49]

One study[50] attempted to determine the variability of the course and the pattern of these nerves and found that the peripheral nerves contributing to the anterior shoulder joint included the axillary (C5–6), subscapular (C5–6), and lateral pectoral (C5–6). The same study found that the nerves

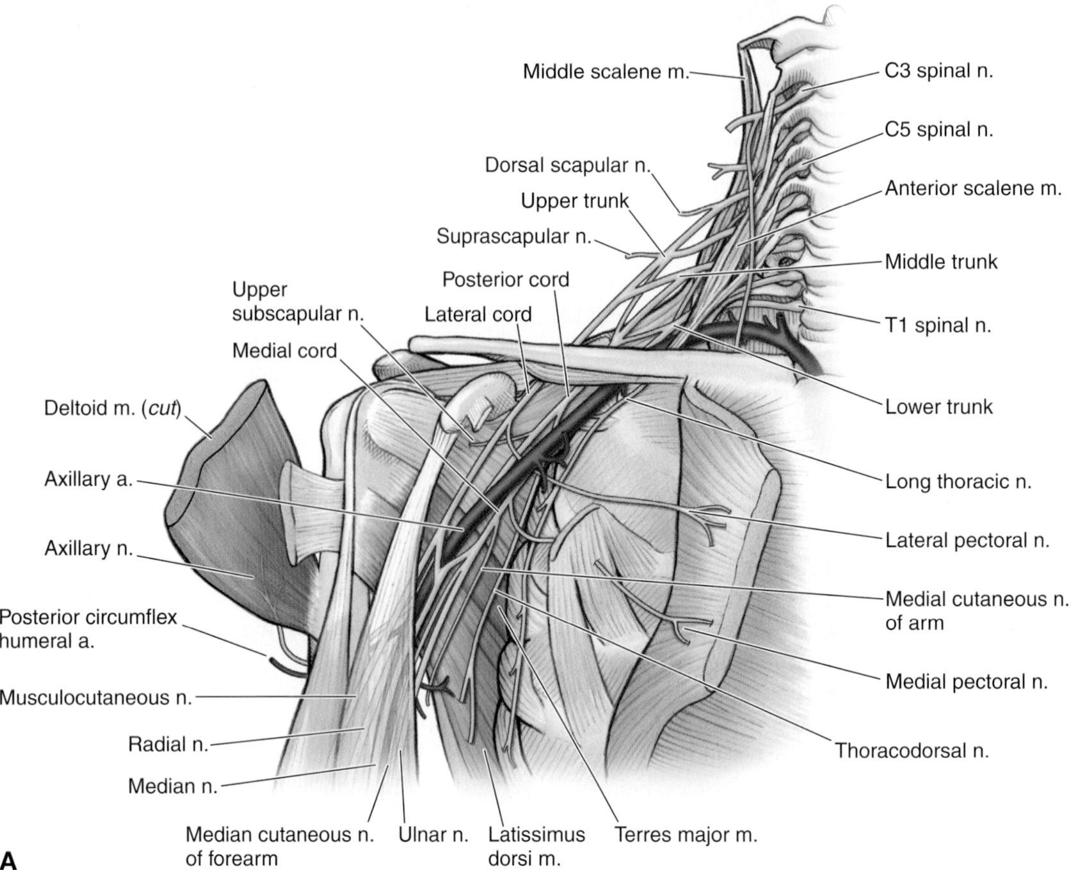

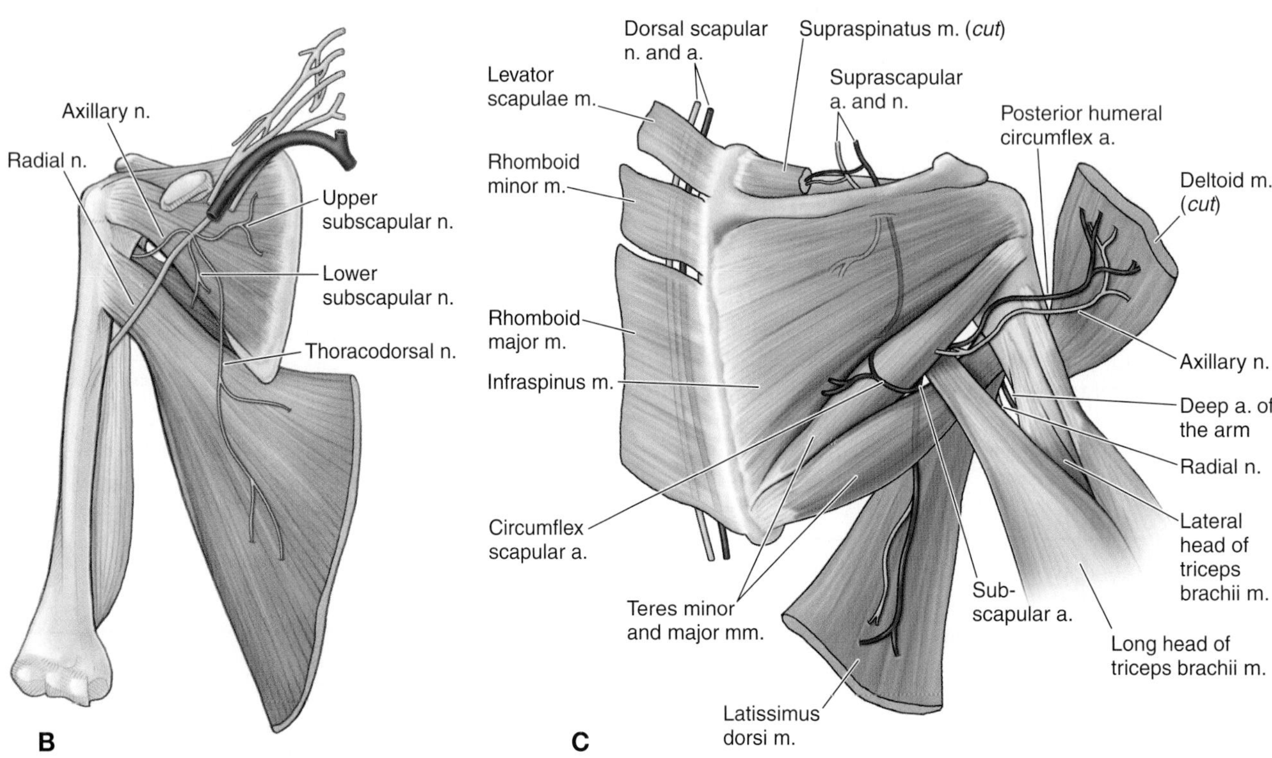

FIGURE 16-8 Neurological and vascular structures of the shoulder. (Reproduced with permission from Morton DA, Foreman KB, Albertine KH: *The Big Picture: Gross Anatomy*. McGraw-Hill, 2011)

contributing articular branches to the posterior joint structures are the suprascapular nerve (C5–6) and small branches of the axillary nerve.[50] The pathways of these nerves are described in Chapter 3.

Other nerves innervate the muscles that act upon the shoulder. These include the long thoracic nerve (C5–7), which innervates the serratus anterior, the spinal accessory nerve (cranial nerve XI and C3–4), which innervates the sternocleidomastoid (SCM) and trapezius muscles, and the musculocutaneous nerve (C5–7), which innervates the coracobrachialis, biceps brachii, and brachialis, before dividing into its cutaneous branches.

CLINICAL PEARL

Shoulder pain that persists despite extensive conservative approaches could be of neural origin, as the peripheral nerves that innervate the ligaments, capsule, and bursae of the shoulder joint may have been subject to damage, either at the time of initial trauma or through subsequent surgical intervention.[50–52]

Vascularization

The vascular supply to the shoulder complex is primarily provided by branches off the axillary artery (Fig. 16-9), which begins at the outer border of the first rib as a continuation of the subclavian artery. The axillary artery is commonly divided into three parts: above, behind, and below the pectoralis minor muscle. The axillary artery meets the more deeply placed brachial plexus in the neck, and here they are encased in the axillary sheath, together with the axillary vein.[53] The lateral, posterior, and medial cords of the brachial plexus descend behind the first portion of the artery and then take up their respective locations at the second portion of the artery (behind the pectoralis minor muscle). The branches off these cords also maintain their respective positions. Compression of the axillary artery (or, to a lesser degree, the axillary vein) can result in shoulder dysfunction and most commonly occurs in the posterior fossa around the shoulder and against the humerus with shoulder elevation.[53] The G-H joint receives its blood supply from the anterior and posterior circumflex humeral as well as the suprascapular and circumflex scapular vessels.[54] The vascular supply to the labrum arises mostly from its peripheral attachment to the capsule and is from a combination of the suprascapular circumflex scapular branch of the subscapular and posterior circumflex humeral arteries.[8]

The brachial artery provides the dominant arterial supply to each of the two heads of the biceps brachii. The artery travels in the medial intermuscular septum and is bordered by the biceps muscle anteriorly, the brachialis muscle medially, and the medial head of the triceps muscle posteriorly.[55]

The microvasculature of the rotator cuff has been the subject of much discussion and consists of three main sources: the thoracoacromial, suprahumeral, and subscapular arteries.[54] The supraspinatus receives its primary supply from the thoracoacromial arteries. The subscapularis receives its supply from the anterior humeral circumflex and the thoracoacromial arteries. The posterior rotator cuff muscles, the infraspinatus and teres minor, receive their blood supply from the posterior humeral circumflex and suprascapular artery. The circulation of the rotator cuff is unidirectional with no flow traversing the tide mark at the insertion of the supraspinatus.[56] The supraspinatus and biceps tendons appear to be particularly vulnerable to areas of relative avascularity, referred to as *critical zones*. The vascular compromise of the supraspinatus is thought to be due to a number of factors:

- It can be directly compressed by the subacromial structures. With the arm adducted to the side, the vessels within the supraspinatus tendon are poorly perfused.[57] Other arm positions, such as raising the arm above 30 degrees, have been shown to increase intramuscular pressure in the supraspinatus muscle to an extent that may impair normal blood perfusion.[57,58]
- Its blood vessels travel parallel to the tendon fibers, which make them vulnerable to stretch.[59] Avascularity appears to increase with age beginning as early as 20 years.[60]
- The presence of a critical zone just proximal to the supraspinatus insertion point.[57] Two early studies noted a critical zone that lies slightly proximal to the supraspinatus insertion point.[61,62] Since then, it has been determined that the critical zone is more likely a zone of anastomoses between the vessels supplying the bone and the tendon and is not less vascular except in certain positions.[57,63,64]

Although it is possible that sustained isometric contractions, prolonged adduction of the arm or increase in subacromial pressure[65] may reduce the microcirculation, it is unlikely that frequent abduction or elevation of the arm would produce selective avascularity of the supraspinatus or biceps tendon.

Close-Packed Position

The close-packed position for the G-H joint is 90 degrees of G-H abduction and full ER or full abduction and ER, depending on the source.

Open-Packed Position

Without IR or ER occurring, the open-packed position of the G-H joint has traditionally been cited as 55 degrees of semi-abduction and 30 degrees of horizontal adduction.[66] More recently, a cadaver study, which examined the point in the range at which maximal capsular laxity occurred in seven subjects, determined the open-packed position to be 39 degrees of abduction in the scapular plane or at the point which is 45% of the maximal available abduction range of motion (ROM).[67] This finding suggests that the open-packed position may be closer to neutral and that joint mobility testing and joint mobilizations of the G-H joint should be initiated according to a smaller angle of abduction than the traditionally cited open-packed position.[67]

The zero position for the G-H joint is the arm relaxed by the side, which, relative to the scapula, averages approximately 0 degree of abduction, 12 degrees of flexion, and 10 degrees of ER.[68]

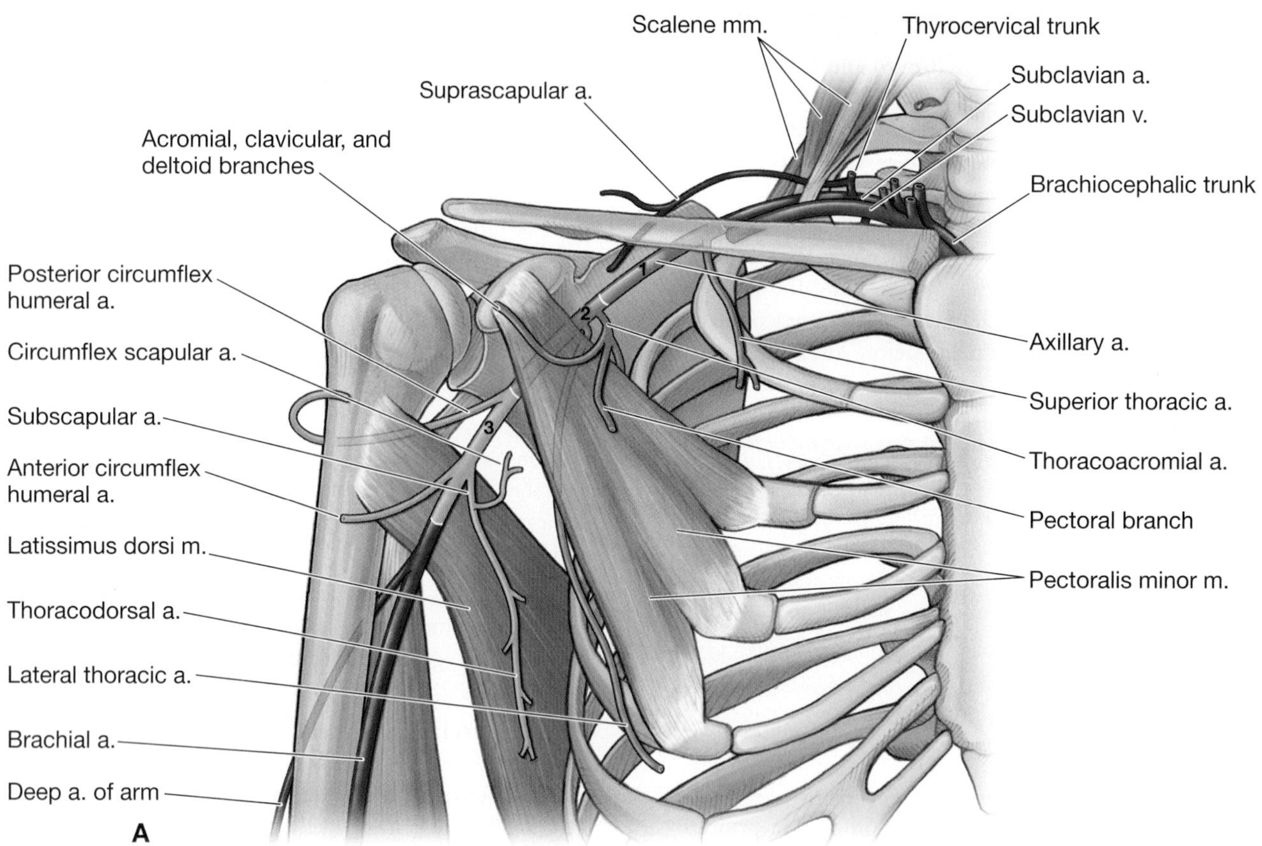

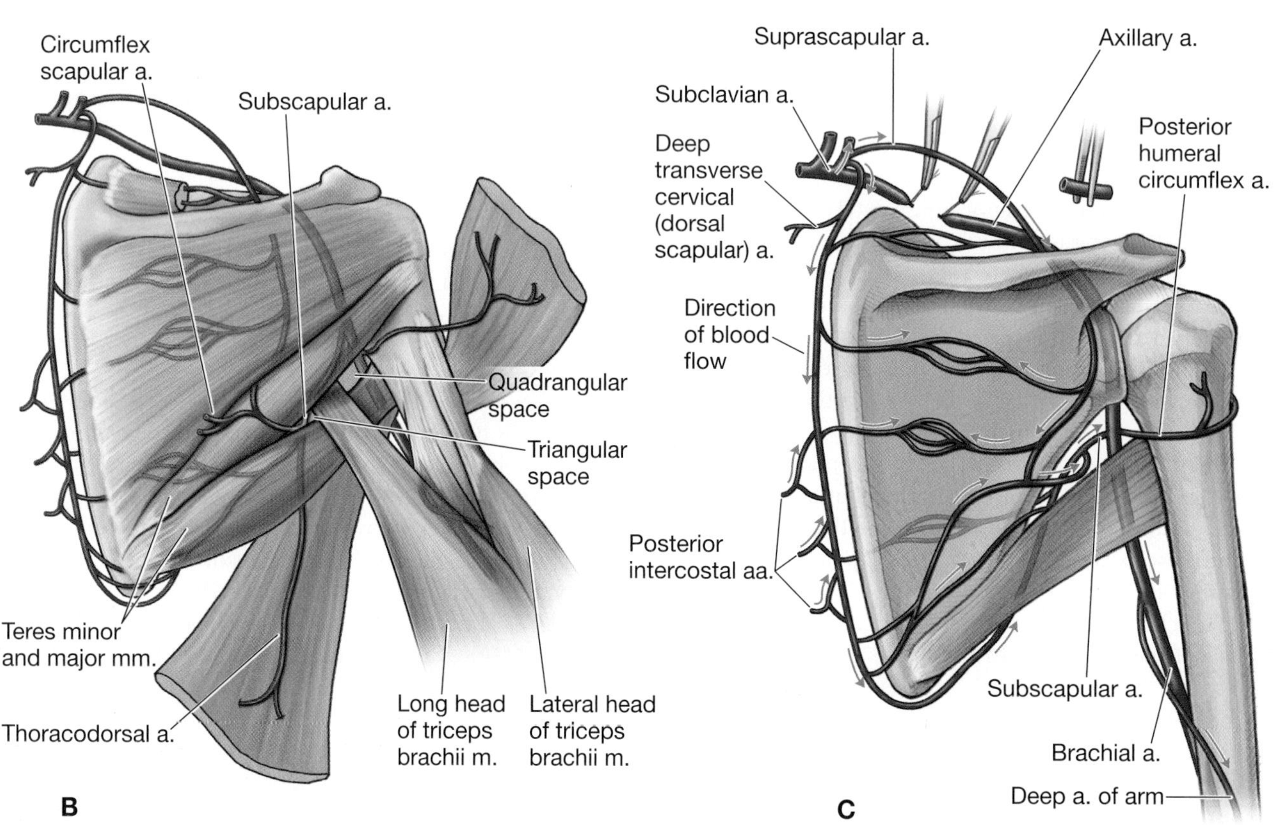

FIGURE 16-9 Vascularization of the shoulder. (Reproduced with permission from Morton DA, Foreman KB, Albertine KH: *The Big Picture: Gross Anatomy*. McGraw-Hill, 2011)

Capsular Pattern

According to Cyriax,[69] the capsular pattern for the G-H joint is that ER is the most limited, abduction the next most limited, and IR the least limited in a 3:2:1 ratio, respectively. However, this pattern only appears to be consistent with adhesive capsulitis of the shoulder. IR, rather than ER or abduction, appears to be the most limited motion in conditions with selected capsular hypomobility.[70]

THE ACROMIOCLAVICULAR JOINT

The A-C joint is a diarthrodial joint, formed by the medial margin of the acromion and the lateral end of the clavicle. The A-C joint is most often described as a gliding or plane joint, but the joint surfaces can vary from flat to slightly convex or concave, corresponding with the articulating surface of the acromion. In the early stages of development, the articular surfaces of the A-C joint are lined with hyaline cartilage, which changes to fibrocartilage at approximately 17 years of age on the acromial side of the joint, and until approximately 24 years of age on the clavicular side.[71] Within the A-C joint, there is variable presence of a thumbtack-shaped intra-articular fibrous disk that projects superiorly into, and incompletely divides, the A-C joint. This disk is subject to tearing.[71] When viewed from above, the clavicle is convex anteriorly in the medial two-thirds and convex posteriorly in the lateral one-third (see Fig. 16-1). Variability in the inclination of the joint is common and can be anywhere from 10 to 50 degrees, but the anteromedial border of the acromion usually faces anteriorly, medially, and superiorly.[72] This variability may account for the differences in vulnerability to separation seen among people.[73]

The A-C joint serves as the main articulation that suspends the upper extremity from the trunk, and it is at this joint about which the scapula moves. The clavicle serves as the lever by which the upper extremity acts on the torso and as an attachment site for many soft tissues.[71,74] The joint has a thin capsule lined with synovium, which is strengthened anteriorly, posteriorly, inferiorly and superiorly by A-C ligaments (see Fig. 16-6). The superior A-C ligament (see Fig. 16-6) gives support to the capsule and serves as the primary restraint to posterior translation and posterior axial rotation at the joint.[71] Other support structures for the joint include the costoclavicular, coracoclavicular (conoid and trapezoid) ligament, the pectoralis major, SCM, deltoid, and trapezius muscles (see Fig. 16-10).[74,75]

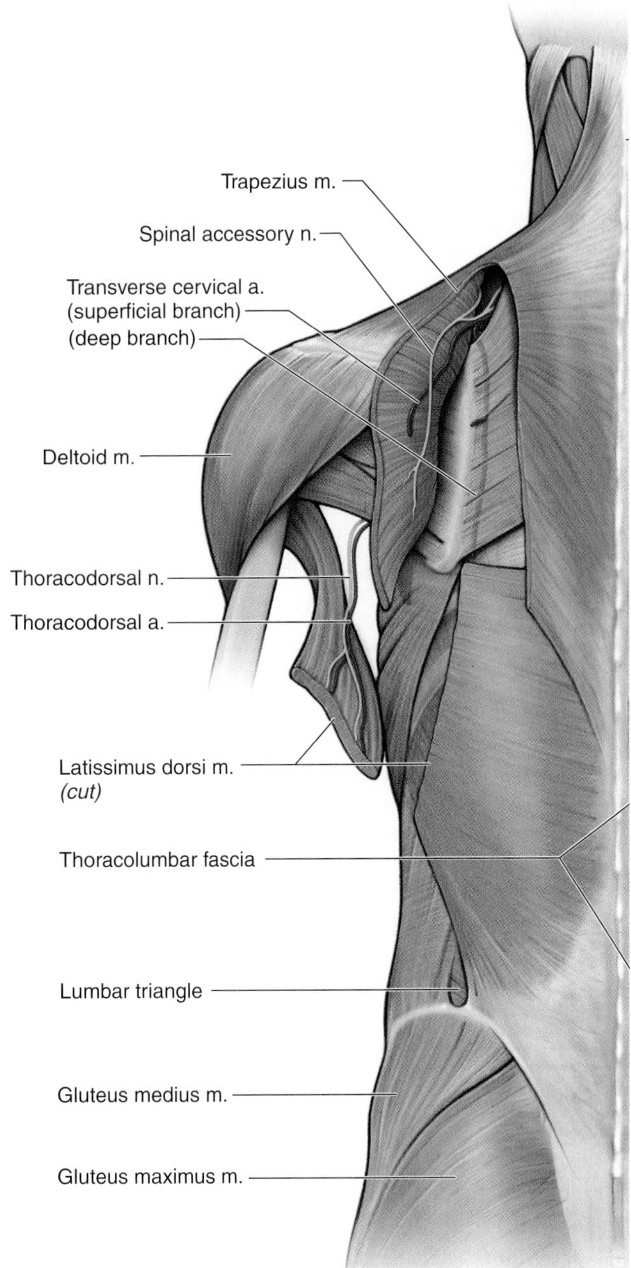

FIGURE 16-10 Muscles of the shoulder. (Reproduced with permission from Morton DA, Foreman KB, Albertine KH: *The Big Picture: Gross Anatomy*. McGraw-Hill, 2011)

CLINICAL PEARL

Degenerative changes of the A-C joint, including narrowing of the joint space and the formation of inferior osteophytes, can predispose an individual to SIS.[41,76,77]

Ligaments

The coracoclavicular ligament (conoid and trapezoid portions) (see Fig. 16-6) is the primary support for the A-C joint and runs from the coracoid process to the inferior surface of the clavicle. The conoid ligament (see Fig. 16-6) is fan shaped with its apex pointing inferiorly. It lies in the frontal plane and is the more medial of the two ligaments. This ligament functions to block coracoid movement away from the clavicle inferiorly.[78] The trapezoid ligament arises from the medial border of the upper surface of the coracoid process and runs superiorly and laterally to insert into the inferior surface of the clavicle. It is larger, longer, and stronger than the conoid and forms a quadrilateral sheet that lies in a plane that is at right angles to the plane formed by the conoid ligament. The function of this ligament is unclear, although its orientation suggests that it may block medial movement of the coracoid[78] or act as a restraint to superior or posterior displacement of the clavicle.[79] In addition, as the clavicle rotates upward, the coracoclavicular ligament dictates scapulothoracic rotation by virtue of its attachment to the scapula.[80]

> **CLINICAL PEARL**
>
> The conoid and trapezoid ligaments provide mainly vertical stability, with control of superior and anterior translation as well as anterior axial rotation.[71,78,81]

Neurology

Innervation to this joint is provided by the suprascapular, lateral pectoral, and axillary nerves (Fig. 16-8).[82]

Vascularization

The A-C joint receives its blood supply from branches of the suprascapular and thoracoacromial arteries (Fig. 16-9).

Capsular Pattern

Joints such as the A-C joint, which are not controlled by muscles, lack true capsular patterns. However, anecdotal clinical evidence suggests that the capsular pattern for the A-C joint is pain at the extremes of ROM, especially horizontal adduction and full elevation.

Close-Packed Position

The close-packed position for this joint is probably only achievable in the below-30 age group and clinically seems to correspond to 90 degrees of G-H joint abduction.

Open-Packed Position

The open-packed position for this joint is undetermined, although it is likely to be when the arm is by the side. This positions the clavicle in approximately 15–20 degrees of retraction relative to the coronal plane and elevated approximately 2 degrees from the horizontal plane.[83]

The motions available at the A-C joint occur around three axes:

- Rotation in an anteroposterior (A-P) direction around a longitudinal axis that projects through the A-C and S-C joints, and rotation in a superoinferior (vertical) direction. The A-P rotation occurs during arm elevation. The superoinferior rotation, which occurs around the costoclavicular ligament, is involved during protraction (anterior movement of the acromial end of the clavicle) and retraction (posterior motion of the acromial end). The A-P rotation of the clavicle on the scapula is three times greater than that of the superoinferior rotation. The clavicle can rotate approximately 30–50 degrees in the A-P direction, most of which is contributed by the mobile S-C joint. The A-C joint only contributes approximately 5–8 degrees to the rotation.[84] The type of glide and rotation that occurs with clavicular motion depends on the shoulder motion and the shape of the articular surfaces. If the lateral end of the clavicle presents a concave surface, an anterior glide is combined with an anterior rotation. If the lateral end presents a convex surface, an anterior glide is combined with a posterior rotation.

> **CLINICAL PEARL**
>
> The clavicle must rotate approximately 40–50 degrees for full elevation to occur; otherwise elevation would be limited to approximately 110 degrees.[84]

- Pure spin/rotation. A pure spin occurs during abduction/adduction (lateral and medial rotation of inferior scapula angle) motions.
- Glides. Glides of the clavicle can occur in an A-P and superoinferior direction.

The A-C joint is predisposed to chronic stress injury, especially in the situations in which it is subjected to repetitive high demand.[71,85] The joint can also be affected by direct trauma and by nontraumatic factors such as degenerative arthritis and inflammatory arthropathies.[74] Table 16-2 contains the pathologies and dysfunctions that may affect the A-C joint.

STERNOCLAVICULAR JOINT

The S-C joint represents the articulation between the enlarged medial end of the clavicle, the clavicular notch of the manubrium of the sternum, and the cartilage of the first rib, which forms the floor of the joint. The articulating surfaces of the S-C joint are covered with fibrocartilage. The S-C joint is angulated slightly upward approximately 20 degrees in a posterior and lateral direction. The clavicle presents with an irregularly shaped surface to the meniscus, and this lateral part of the joint acts as an ovoid. If held vertically, the proximal end of the clavicle is convex whereas the manubrium surface is concave (see Fig. 16-1). If held

TABLE 16-2	Pathologies and Dysfunctions that May Affect the A-C Joint
Traumatic conditions	Separation/dislocation (types I–VI) fracture
Infectious conditions	Septic arthritis
Inflammatory conditions	Rheumatoid arthritis Systemic lupus erythematosus Ankylosing spondylitis Subacromial bursitis Rotator cuff pathology
Degenerative joint disease	Osteoarthritis Osteolysis
Metabolic conditions	Gout

Data from Powell JW, Huijbregts PA: Concurrent criterion-related validity of acromioclavicular joint physical examination tests: A systematic review. *J Man Manip Ther* 14:E19–E29, 2006.

anteroposteriorly, the proximal end of the clavicle is concave and the manubrium is convex. A very thick meniscus is the key to the joint curvature. The disk is attached to the upper and posterior margin of the clavicle, and to the cartilage of the first rib by an intra-articular disk ligament, which functions to help prevent medial displacement of the clavicle, and completely divides the joint into two cavities: a larger one that is above and lateral to the disk, and a smaller one that is medial and below the disk. Greater movement occurs between the clavicle and the disk than between the disk and the manubrium. The S-C joint has very little bony stability and relies heavily on support from the surrounding capsule and ligaments.

Some confusion seems to exist about classification of the S-C joint—it has been classified as a ball and socket joint,[82] a plane joint,[86] and as a saddle joint.[82] These classifications depend on whether anatomy or function is being considered. For example, when its function is considered, the S-C joint acts similar to a ball and socket joint, allowing for motion in almost all planes, including rotation.

CLINICAL PEARL

During normal shoulder motion, the S-C joint permits 30–35 degrees of upward elevation, 35 degrees of combined forward and backward movement, and 45–50 degrees of rotation about the long axis of the clavicle.[3,87]

Ligaments

Because of its bony arrangement, the S-C joint itself is extremely weak, but is held securely by strong ligaments that hold the sternal end of the clavicle downward and toward the sternum. These ligaments include the following:

Capsular-Ligamentous Structures

Capsular Ligament. This ligament represents the inner aspect of the joint capsule. The anterior portion is heavier and stronger, and it covers the anterior aspect of the joint running obliquely from the proximal end of the clavicle to the sternum in an inferior and medial direction. The posterior component, which covers the posterior aspect of the joint, also runs obliquely from the proximal end of the clavicle to the sternum in an inferior and medial direction. The capsular ligament is considered the most important and strongest ligaments of the S-C joint and is most responsible for preventing upward displacement of the medial clavicle in the presence of a downward force on the distal end of the shoulder.[88]

Interclavicular. This ligament connects the superomedial sternal ends of each clavicle with the capsular ligaments and the upper sternum. Together, these structures help to hold up the shoulder. This function can be demonstrated by placing a finger in the superior sternal notch; the ligament is lax with elevation of the arm but becomes taut when both arms are hanging by the sides.

Costoclavicular (rhomboid ligament). This short and strong ligament, which runs from the upper border of the first rib to the inferior surface of the clavicle, consists of two laminae: fibers of the anterior lamina run superiorly and laterally and check elevation and lateral movement (upward rotation) of the clavicle.[88] The posterior lamina fibers run superiorly and medially and check downward rotation of the clavicle.[88]

Due to the support provided by the ligaments, the S-C joint is very stable and trauma to the clavicle usually results in a fracture rather than a joint dislocation.[89] Gross motions occur here as with the A-C joint. The SCM, which can be seen clearly with rotation of the head, has a tendinous sternal and clavicular insertion. The subclavius (C5–6) has a questionable function but may function as a dynamic ligament, which contracts and pulls the clavicle toward the manubrium.

Two types of translation also occur at this joint: anterior to posterior and superior to inferior, with the former exceeding the latter motion by 2:1.[90] These translations allow for three degrees of freedom (DOF): the movements of elevation, depression; protraction, retraction; and upward (backward) and downward (forward) motion.

- ***Protraction/retraction.*** Approximately 15–20 degrees of protraction and retraction of the clavicle are available. With protraction, the concave surface of the medial clavicle moves on the convex sternum, producing an anterior glide of the clavicle, and an anterior rotation of the lateral clavicle.[90] With retraction to the neutral position, the medial clavicle articulates with a flat surface and tilts/swings, causing an anterolateral gapping, and a posterior rotation at the lateral end.[90]
- ***Elevation/depression of the clavicle.*** There are 35–40 degrees of elevation and approximately 15 degrees of depression available,[3,87,90] involving the convex clavicle gliding on the concave sternum.

As the clavicle elevates and rolls upward on the manubrium, an inferior glide is produced, with the reverse occurring with depression. Elevation and depression movements at the S-C joint are associated with reciprocal motions of the scapula because of the lateral attachment of the clavicle to the scapula at the A-C joint.[75]

Rotation around the long axis produces a spin of the clavicle on the manubrium. Approximately 40 degrees of upward rotation and 5 degrees of downward rotation are available and are necessary to allow upward scapular rotation.[3,87]

CLINICAL PEARL

For the scapular to abduct and upwardly rotate throughout 180 degrees of humeral abduction, clavicular movement must occur at both the S-C and A-C joints.

Close-Packed Position

The close-packed position for the S-C joint is maximum arm elevation and protraction.

Open-Packed Position

The open-packed position for the S-C joint has yet to be determined, but is likely to be when the arm is by the side.

Capsular Pattern

Similar to the A-C joint, the S-C joint is not controlled by muscles and therefore lacks a specific capsular pattern. One possibility, seen clinically, is pain at the extreme ranges of motion, especially full arm elevation and horizontal adduction.

Neurology

Pain can be referred from this joint to the throat, anterior chest, and axillae. The neural supply to this joint is primarily from the following[91]:

- The anterior supraclavicular nerve
- The nerve to the subclavius (medial accessory phrenic) C5–6
- The T1 spinal nerve root

Vascularization

The S-C joint receives its blood supply from the internal thoracic and suprascapular arteries.[92]

SCAPULOTHORACIC JOINT

This articulation is functionally a joint, but it lacks the anatomic characteristics of a true synovial joint. However, the movement of the scapula on the wall of the thoracic cage is critical to shoulder joint motion. A lack of ligamentous support at this "joint" delegates the function of stability fully to the muscles that attach the scapula to the thorax.

An altered position of the scapula or an abnormal motion at this joint due to muscle imbalances have both been linked with shoulder complex dysfunction.[24,93,94] Motions at this joint are described according to the movement of the scapula relative to the thorax. Available motion consists of approximately 60 degrees of upward rotation of the scapula, 40–60 degrees of IR/ER, and 30–40 degrees of anterior and posterior tipping of the scapula.[95] Other motions occurring here include elevation and depression and adduction and abduction of the scapula (Fig. 16-11).

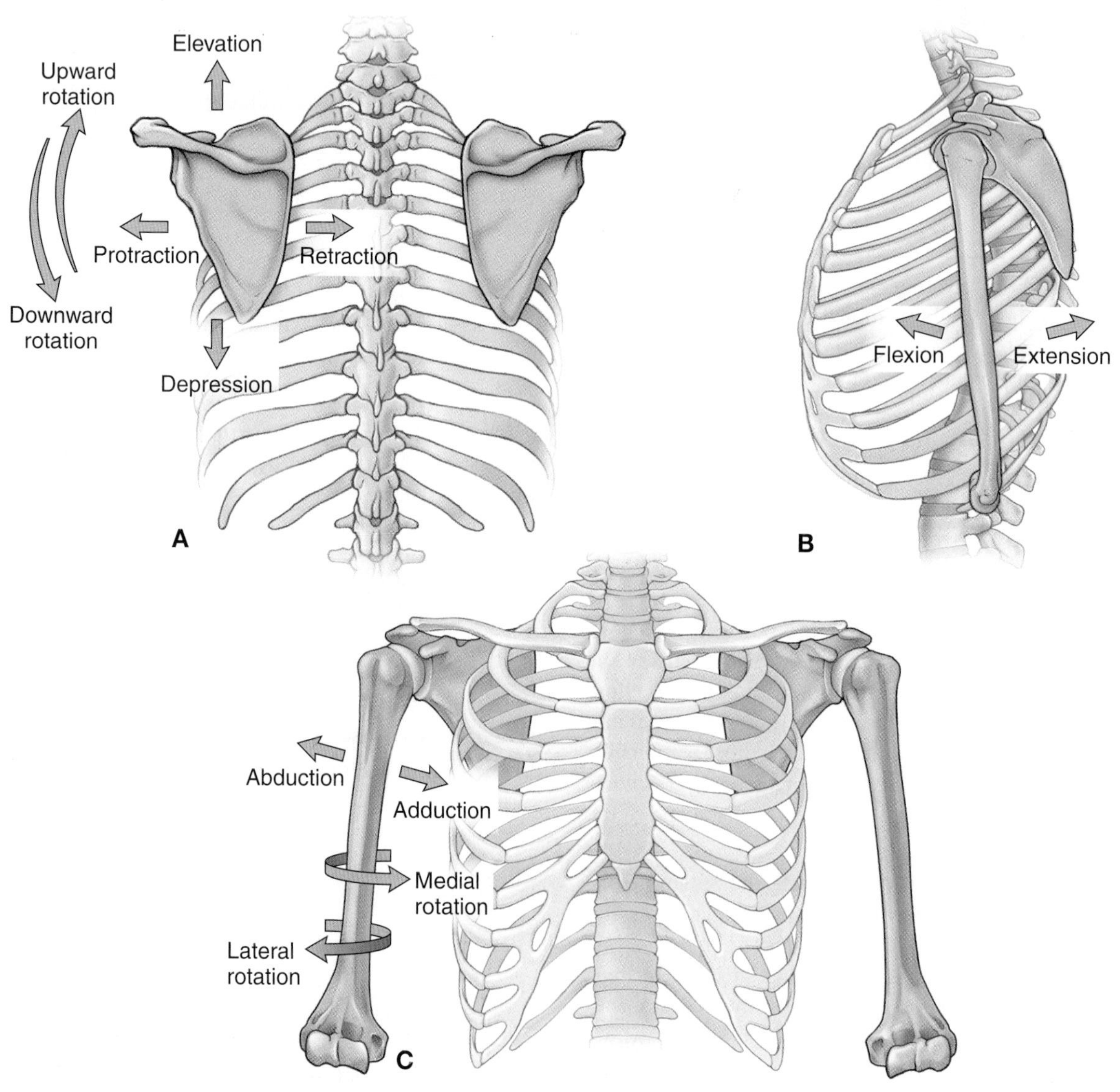

FIGURE 16-11 Movements of the scapula and upper extremity. (Reproduced with permission from Morton DA, Foreman KB, Albertine KH: *The Big Picture: Gross Anatomy*. McGraw-Hill, 2011)

Close-Packed and Capsular Pattern

Since the scapulothoracic joint is not a true joint, it does not have a close-packed position or a capsular pattern.

Open-Packed Position

Relative to the thorax, when the arm is by the side, the scapula is in an average of 30–45 degrees of IR, and slight upward rotation, and approximately 5–20 degrees of anterior tipping.[68,95]

Bursae

There are a number of bursae located in and around the scapulothoracic articulation. The scapulothoracic bursa is located between the thoracic cage and the deep surface of the serratus anterior.[96] The subscapular bursa is most often located between the superficial surface of the serratus anterior and the subscapularis.[96]

The scapulotrapezial bursa lies between the middle and lower trapezius fibers and the superomedial scapula.[96] The purpose and clinical significance of the scapulotrapezial bursa are not known. It may encourage smooth gliding of the superomedial angle of the scapula against the undersurface of the trapezius during scapular rotation in the same manner that the scapulothoracic bursa (between the serratus attachment at the anteromedial surface of the superior angle) encourages smooth gliding against the underlying ribs.[96] It is possible that inflammation of either of these bursae, directly or as a consequence of injury, may result in painful clicking at the superomedial angle of the scapula.[96]

The relationship of the spinal accessory nerve to the scapulotrapezial bursa may also have clinical importance, especially as it is closely applied to the superficial wall of the scapulotrapezial bursa.[96] The spinal accessory nerve receives afferent fibers from C3 and C4, which are thought to be proprioceptive, before reaching the deep surface of the trapezius.[96,97] As a consequence of their proximity, inflammation and fibrosis within the bursa may cause irritation and pain of the nerve, or interference with the normal proprioceptive feedback mechanism provided by the nerve.[96]

MUSCLES OF THE SHOULDER COMPLEX

A number of significant muscles control motion at the shoulder and provide dynamic stabilization. Rarely does a single muscle act in isolation at the shoulder. For simplicity, the muscles acting at the shoulder may be described in terms of their functional roles: scapular pivoters, humeral propellers, humeral positioners, and shoulder protectors (Table 16-3).[98]

Scapular Pivoters

The scapular pivoters comprise the trapezius, serratus anterior, levator scapulae, rhomboid major, and rhomboid minor.[98] As a group, these muscles are involved with motions at the scapulothoracic articulation, and their proper function is vital to the normal biomechanics of the whole shoulder complex. The scapular muscles can contract isometrically, concentric, or eccentrically, depending on the desired action and whether the action involves stabilization, acceleration, or deceleration. To varying degrees, the serratus anterior and all parts of the trapezius cooperate during the upward rotation of the scapula.

TABLE 16-3 Muscles of the Shoulder Complex
Scapular pivoters
Trapezius
Serratus anterior
Levator scapulae
Rhomboid major
Rhomboid minor
Humeral propellers
Latissimus dorsi
Teres major
Pectoralis major
Pectoralis minor
Humeral positioners
Deltoid
Shoulder protectors
Rotator cuff (supraspinatus, infraspinatus, teres minor, and subscapularis)
Long head of the biceps brachii

Trapezius

The trapezius muscle (Fig. 16-10) originates from the medial third of the superior nuchal line, the external occipital protuberance, the ligamentum nuchae, the apices of the seventh cervical vertebra, all the thoracic spinous processes, and the supraspinous ligaments of the cervical and thoracic vertebrae. The upper fibers descend to attach to the lateral third of the posterior border of the clavicle. The middle fibers of the trapezius run horizontally to the medial acromial margin and superior lip of the spine of the scapula. The inferior fibers ascend to attach to an aponeurosis gliding over a smooth triangular surface at the medial end of the spine of the scapula to a tubercle at the scapular lateral apex.

It has been suggested that the upper fibers of this muscle have a different motor supply than that to the middle and lower portions.[99,100] Recent clinical and anatomical evidence seems to suggest that the spinal accessory nerve provides the most important and consistent motor supply to all portions of the trapezius muscle, and although the C2–4 branches of the cervical plexus are present, no particular elements of innervation within the trapezius have been determined.[101]

One of the functions of the trapezius is to produce shoulder girdle elevation on a fixed cervical spine. For the trapezius to perform its actions, the cervical spine must first be stabilized by the anterior neck flexors to prevent simultaneous occipital extension from occurring. Failure to prevent this occipital extension would allow the head to translate anteriorly, resulting in a decrease in the length, and therefore the efficiency, of the trapezius[102] and an increase in the cervical lordosis.

CLINICAL PEARL

Complete paralysis of the trapezius usually causes moderate-to-marked difficulty in elevating the arm over the head. The task, however, can usually be completed through full range as long as the serratus anterior remains totally innervated.[103]

Serratus Anterior

The muscular digitations of the serratus anterior (see Fig. 16-5) originate from the upper eight to ten ribs and fascia over the intercostals. The muscle is composed of three functional components[104,105]:

- The upper component originates from the first and second ribs and inserts into the superior angle of the scapula.
- The middle component arises from the second, third, and fourth ribs and inserts into the anterior aspect of the medial scapular border.
- The lower component is the largest and most powerful, originating from the fifth through ninth ribs. It runs anterior to the scapula and inserts into the medial border of the scapula.

The serratus anterior is activated with all shoulder movements, but especially during shoulder flexion and abduction.[105] Working in synergy with the trapezius, as part of a force couple (see later), the main function of the serratus anterior is to protract and upwardly rotate the scapula,[106,107] while providing a strong, mobile base of support to position the glenoid optimally for maximum efficiency of the upper extremity.[108] Its lower fibers draw the lower angle of the scapula forward to rotate the scapula upward while maintaining the scapula on the thorax during arm elevation.[109] This moves the coracoacromial arch out of the path of the advancing greater tuberosity and opposes the excessive elevation of the scapula by the levator scapulae and trapezius muscles.[110] Without upward rotation and protraction of the scapula by the serratus anterior, full G-H elevation is not possible. In fact, in patients with complete paralysis of the serratus anterior, Gregg et al.[108] reported that abduction is limited to 110 degrees.

Dysfunction of the serratus anterior muscle causes winging of the scapula as the patient attempts to elevate the arm.[4,111] Scapulothoracic dysfunction can also contribute to G-H instability, as the normal stable base of the scapula is destabilized during abduction or flexion.[4,112,113]

The serratus anterior muscle is innervated by the long thoracic nerve (C5–7).

CLINICAL PEARL

Paralysis or weakness of the serratus anterior muscle results in disruption of normal shoulder kinesiology. The disability may be slight with partial paralysis or profound with complete paralysis. As a rule, persons with complete or marked paralysis of the serratus anterior cannot elevate the arms above 90 degrees of abduction.[103]

Levator Scapulae

The levator scapulae muscle (see Fig. 16-10) originates by tendonous strips from the transverse processes of the atlas, axis, and C3 and C4 vertebrae, and descends diagonally to insert into the medial superior angle of the scapula.

The levator scapulae can act on the cervical spine (see Chap. 23) and on the scapula. If it acts on the cervical spine, it can produce extension, side flexion, and rotation of the cervical spine to the same side.[114] When acting on the scapula during upper extremity flexion or abduction, the levator scapula muscle acts as an antagonist to the trapezius muscle, and provides eccentric control of scapular upward rotation in the higher ranges of motion.[115]

Both the trapezius and levator scapulae muscles are activated with increased upper extremity loads.[102,105,116]

The levator scapulae muscle is innervated by the posterior (dorsal) scapular nerve (C3–5).

Rhomboids

The rhomboid major muscle (Fig. 16-10) originates from the second to fifth thoracic spinous processes and the overlying supraspinous ligaments. The fibers descend to insert into the medial scapular border between the root of the scapular spine and the inferior angle of the scapula.

The rhomboid minor muscle (see Fig. 16-10) originates from the lower ligamentum nuchae, and the seventh cervical and first thoracic spinous processes, and attaches to the medial border of the scapula at the root of the spine of the scapula.

The rhomboid muscles help control scapular positioning, particularly with horizontal flexion and extension of the shoulder complex.[115]

The rhomboid muscles are innervated by the posterior (dorsal) scapular nerve (C4–5).

Humeral Propellers

The total muscle mass of the shoulder's internal rotators (subscapularis, anterior deltoid, pectoralis major, latissimus dorsi, and teres major) is much greater than that of the external rotators (infraspinatus, teres minor, and posterior deltoid).[103] This fact explains why the shoulder internal rotators produce approximately 1.75 times greater isometric torque than the external rotators.[117] Peak torques of the internal rotators also exceed the external rotators when measured isokinetically, under both concentric and eccentric conditions.[103,118]

Latissimus Dorsi

The latissimus dorsi muscle (see Fig. 16-12) originates from the spinous processes of the last six thoracic vertebrae, the lower three or four ribs, the lumbar and sacral spinous processes through the thoracolumbar fascia, the posterior third of the external lip of the iliac crest, and a slip from the inferior scapular angle. The scapular slip allows the latissimus dorsi to act at the scapulothoracic articulation. The latissimus dorsi inserts into the intertubercular sulcus of the humerus. The muscle functions as an extensor, adductor, and powerful internal rotator of the shoulder, and also assists in scapular depression, retraction, and downward rotation.[119] It is innervated by the thoracodorsal nerve (C6–8).

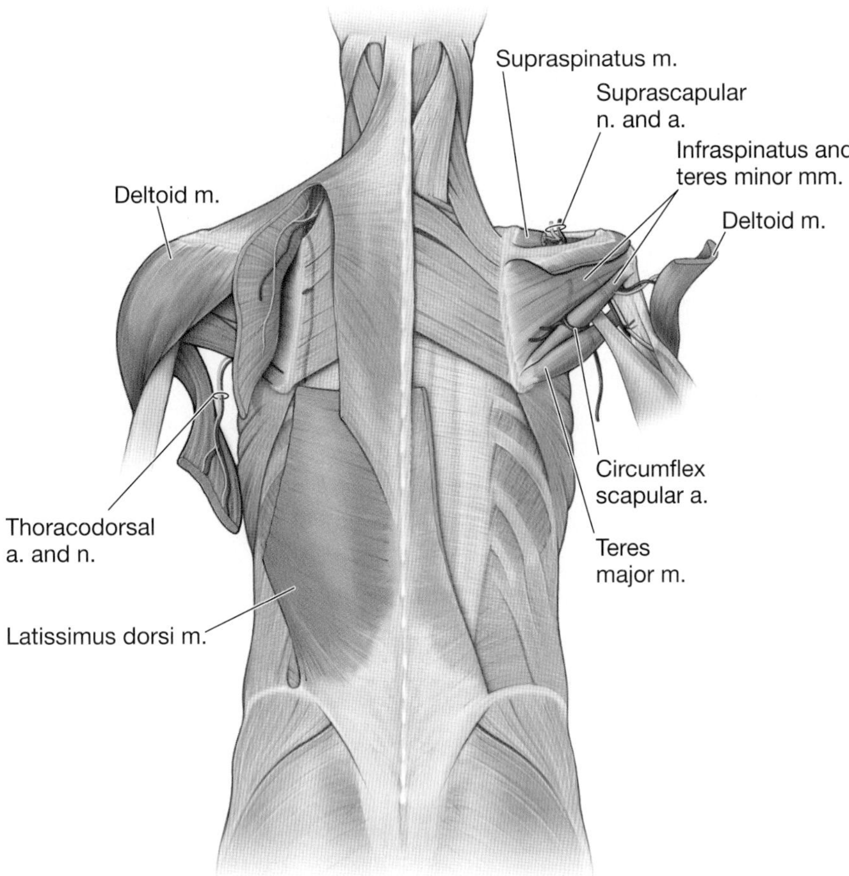

FIGURE 16-12 Latissimus dorsi. (Reproduced with permission from Morton DA, Foreman KB, Albertine KH: *The Big Picture: Gross Anatomy*. McGraw-Hill, 2011)

Teres Major

The teres major (see Fig. 16-12) originates from the inferior third of the lateral border of the scapula and just superior to the inferior angle. The teres major tendon inserts into the medial lip of the intertubercular groove of the humerus. The teres major functions to complement the actions of the latissimus dorsi in that it extends, adducts, and internally rotates the G-H joint. It is innervated by the lower subscapular nerve (C5, C6).

Pectoralis Major

The pectoralis major (see Fig. 16-13) originates from the sternal half of the clavicle, half of the anterior surface of the sternum to the level of the sixth or seventh costal cartilage, the sternal end of the sixth rib, and the aponeurosis of the obliquus externus abdominis. The fibers of the pectoralis major converge to form a tendon that inserts into the lateral lip of the intertubercular sulcus of the humerus. Although this muscle does not insert into the scapula, it does act upon the scapulothoracic articulation through its insertion on the humerus. The function of the pectoralis muscle depends on which fibers are activated:

- Upper fibers (clavicular head)—IR, horizontal adduction, flexion, abduction (once the humerus is abducted 90 degrees, the upper fibers assist in further abduction), and adduction (with the humerus below 90 degrees of abduction) of the G-H joint.
- Lower fibers (sternal head)—IR, horizontal adduction, extension, and adduction of the G-H joint.

The pectoralis major is innervated by the medial (lower fibers) and lateral (upper fibers) pectoral nerves (C8–T1 and C5–7, respectively).

CLINICAL PEARL

The pectoralis major and latissimus dorsi muscles are referred to as *humeral propeller* muscles as they have been shown to be the only muscles in the upper extremity to have a positive correlation between peak torque and velocity during the propulsive phase of the swim stroke.

Pectoralis Minor

The pectoralis minor (see Fig. 16-9) originates from the outer surface of the upper margins of the third to fifth ribs near their cartilage. The fibers of the pectoralis minor ascend laterally, converging to a tendon that inserts into the coracoid process of the scapula.

The pectoralis minor muscle is innervated by the medial pectoral nerve (C6–8).

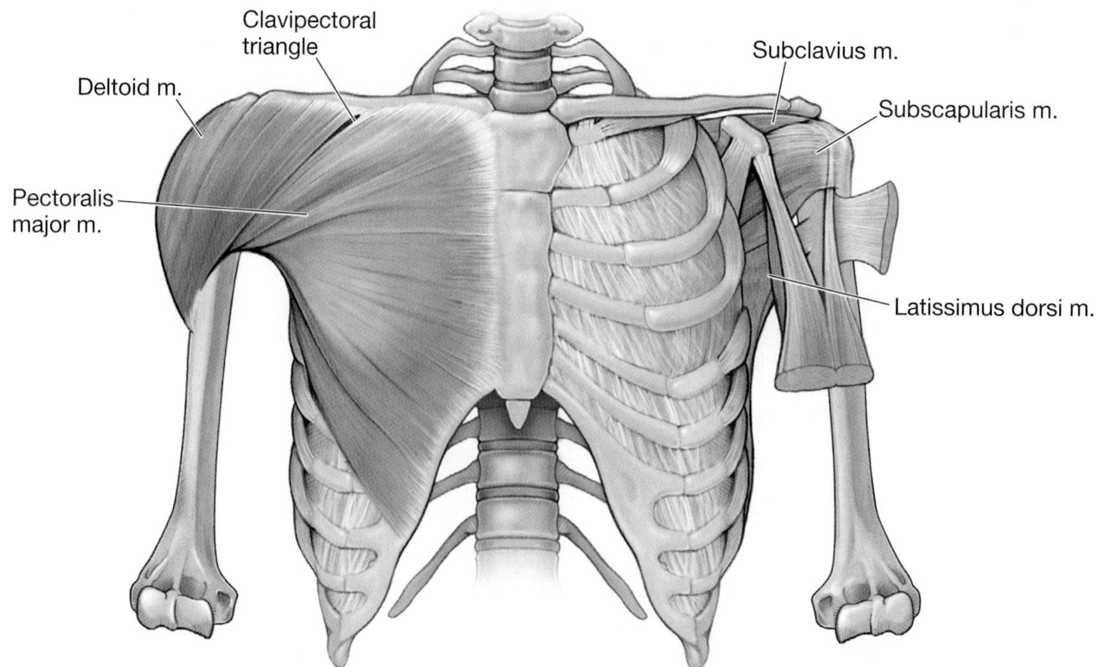

FIGURE 16-13 Pectoralis major muscle. (Reproduced with permission from Morton DA, Foreman KB, Albertine KH: *The Big Picture: Gross Anatomy.* McGraw-Hill, 2011)

Humeral Positioners

Deltoid

The deltoid muscle originates from the lateral third of the clavicle, the superior surface of the acromion, and the spine of the scapula (Fig. 16-13). It inserts into the deltoid tuberosity of the humerus. The deltoid can be described as three separate muscles—anterior, middle, and posterior—all of which function as humeral positioners, positioning the humerus in space.[98]

The deltoid muscle is innervated by the axillary nerve (C5–6).

Shoulder Protectors

Rotator Cuff

The rotator cuff muscles (Fig. 16-4), which consist of the supraspinatus, infraspinatus, teres minor, and subscapularis, are commonly involved with shoulder pathology. The anatomy of these muscles was described previously (see "Glenohumeral Joint" section). These muscles are referred to as the protectors of the shoulder since, in addition to actively moving the humerus, they fine-tune the humeral head position during arm elevation.[98] Compared with most joints that have a single axis on which torques are generated, the shoulder is very different, because it has no fixed axis. As a result, each muscle activation creates a unique set of rotational moments, which necessitates precise coordination in the timing and magnitude of muscle contractions.[73] Jenp et al.[120] used electromyography (EMG) to detect the most specific positions of highest activation for the individual rotator cuff muscles. The greatest activation of the subscapularis was with the arm in the scapular plane at 90 degrees of elevation and neutral humeral rotation. The subscapularis has also been shown to be an effective humeral head depressor in ER, whereas it produces almost no A-P translation in abduction and ER. The infraspinatus–teres minor muscles are very effective humeral head depressors with the arm in the sagittal plane and the humerus elevated to 90 degrees in the midrange of external/IR (the so-called "hornblower's" position). The supraspinatus could not be effectively isolated.

The rotator cuff muscles have an important role in the function of the shoulder and serve the following:

- *Assist in the rotation of the shoulder and arm.* At the G-H joint, elevation through abduction of the arm (Table 16-4) requires that the greater tuberosity of the humerus pass under the coracoacromial arch. For this to occur, the humerus must externally rotate, and the acromion must elevate.[121] ER of the humerus is produced actively by a contraction of the infraspinatus and teres minor, and by a twisting of the joint capsule. A force couple exists in the transverse plane between the subscapularis anteriorly and the infraspinatus and teres minor posteriorly in which cocontraction of the infraspinatus, teres minor, and subscapularis muscles both depresses and compresses the humeral head during overhead movements.

CLINICAL PEARL

The importance of the ER during humeral elevation (Table 16-5) can be demonstrated clinically. If the humerus is held in full IR, only approximately 60 degrees of G-H abduction is passively possible before the greater tuberosity impinges against the coracoacromial arch and blocks further abduction. This helps explain why individuals with marked IR contractures cannot abduct fully, but can elevate the arm in the forward plane.

TABLE 16-4	Contributors to Glenohumeral Abduction
Degree of Abduction	**Biomechanics Involved**
0–90	The concerted action of the active stabilizers (deltoid, biceps, and rotator cuff muscles) and the passive restraints (articular surfaces, osseous structures, and ligaments) is necessary for purposeful function. The supraspinatus contracts to initiate abduction of the glenohumeral joint.[a] The remaining rotator cuff muscles also contract to pull the humeral head into the glenoid fossa. At approximately 20 degrees of humeral abduction, scapular upward rotation begins with concurrent clavicular elevation and axial rotation.[b,c] At approximately 90 degrees, or a little more in females, the upper extreme of G-H abduction is reached, and clavicular elevation ceases due to tension of the costoclavicular ligament.[d] Continued abduction of the humerus requires continued upward rotation of the scapula, which by this point has rotated through a range of approximately 30 degrees.[e]
90–150	As the scapula continues to upwardly rotate, the glenoid fossa faces superiorly and laterally, and its inferior angle moves laterally through approximately 60 degrees. The scapular contribution peaks between 90 and 140 degrees.[f] The scapular upward rotation is accommodated at both the S-C and A-C joints by a posterior axial rotation of the clavicle of 30–40 degrees and a clavicular elevation of approximately 30–36 degrees.[c] The muscles producing this movement are the serratus anterior and trapezius, acting as a force couple on the scapulothoracic joint. The movement is limited by the acromion and S-C joint, and by the scapular and humeral adductors (notably the latissimus dorsi and pectoralis major).
150–180	Abduction beyond 150 degrees requires adequate motion at the vertebral joints of the upper thorax and cervical spine.[g] Bilateral abduction demands that the thoracic spine extends and the lumbar lordosis increases.

[a]Data from Poppen NK, Walker PS: Forces at the glenohumeral joint in abduction. *Clin Orthop* 135:165–170, 1978.
[b]Data from Poppen NK, Walker PS: Normal and abnormal motion of the shoulder. *J Bone Joint Surg* 58A:195–201, 1976.
[c]Data from Saha AK: Mechanisms of shoulder movements and a plea for the recognition of "Zero Position" of the glenohumeral joint. *Clin Orthop* 173:3–10, 1983.
[d]Data from Freedman L, Munro RR: Abduction of the arm in the scapular plane: Scapular and glenohumeral movements. *J Bone Joint Surg* 48A:1503–1510, 1966.
[e]Data from Abelew T: Kinesiology of the shoulder. In: Tovin BJ, Greenfield B, eds. *Evaluation and Treatment of the Shoulder—An Integration of the Guide to Physical Therapist Practice.* Philadelphia, PA: F.A. Davis, 2001:25–44.
[f]Data from Doody SG, Freedman L, Waterland JC: Shoulder movements during abduction in the scapular plane. *Arch Phys Med Rehabil* 51:595–604, 1970.
[g]Data from Kapandji IA: *The Physiology of the Joints, Upper Limb.* New York: Churchill Livingstone, 1991.

However, in clinical practice, shoulders having large rotator cuff tears and good function are frequently encountered. In the coronal plane, there is another force couple between the deltoid and the inferior rotator cuff muscles (infraspinatus, subscapularis, and teres minor). With the arm fully adducted, contraction of the deltoid produces a vertical force in a superior direction, resulting in an upward translation of the humeral head relative to the glenoid. Cocontraction of the inferior rotator cuff muscles produces both a compressive force and a downward translation of the humerus that counterbalances the force of the deltoid, thereby stabilizing the humeral head.

EMG studies have shown that during casual elevation of the arm in normal shoulders, the deltoid and the rotator cuff act continuously throughout the motion of abduction, each

TABLE 16-5	Contributors to Glenohumeral Elevation
Degree of Elevation and Main Contributor	**Biomechanics Involved**
0–60 degrees: glenohumeral elevation	A combined motion of flexion, abduction, and external rotation occurs at the glenohumeral joint, produced by the anterior deltoid, coracobrachialis, and the clavicular fibers of pectoralis major. Motion is limited by the increasing tension in the posterior coracohumeral ligament and the stretching of the shoulder extensors, adductors, and external rotators.[a]
60–120 degrees: sternoclavicular and acromioclavicular elevation	The scapula depresses, protracts, and abducts on the posterior thoracic wall, such that the glenoid fossa faces anteriorly and superiorly and its inferior angle faces laterally and anteriorly. This motion is accommodated by the S-C and A-C joints. The scapulothoracic motion is produced in the same manner as with abduction, by the serratus anterior and trapezius, and is limited by the ligaments of the two joints, and the tension in the shoulder extensor and adductor musculature.[a]
120–180 degrees—costospinal elevation	Kapandji[b] states that the extreme of flexion is the same as the extreme of abduction. That is, during unilateral elevation, the lateral displacement is produced by the contralateral spinal muscles while bilateral abduction requires an exaggeration of the lumbar lordosis to bring the arms vertical. In addition, the medial attachments of the first and second ribs descend while those of the fourth to sixth ascend and the third acts as the axis. Bilateral abduction demands that the thoracic spine extends and the lumbar lordosis increases.

[a]Data from Pettman E: Level III course notes. Berrien Springs, Michigan, North American Institute of Manual Therapy, Inc., 2003.
[b]Data from Kapandji IA: *The Physiology of the Joints, Upper Limb.* New York, Churchill Livingstone, 1991.

reaching a peak of activity between 120 and 140 degrees of abduction.[13,122] However, during more rapid and precise movements, such as those involved with throwing, a more selective pattern emerges with specific periods of great intensity.[123] Weakening of the rotator cuff appears to allow the deltoid to elevate the proximal part of the humerus in the absence of an adequate depressor effect from the rotator cuff, resulting in a decrease in the subacromial space and impingement of the rotator cuff on the anterior aspect of the acromion.[124,125]

- *Reinforce the G-H capsule.* The rotator cuff muscles, together with the coracohumeral ligament, and the LHB (often referred to as the fifth rotator cuff muscle) function as contractile ligaments. For example, firing of the rotator cuff muscles increases the tension of the middle G-H ligament when the arm is abducted to 45 degrees and externally rotated.[37]
- *Control much of the active arthrokinematics of the GH joint.* Contraction of the horizontally oriented supraspinatus produces a compression force directly into the glenoid fossa.[124] This compression force holds the humeral head securely in the glenoid cavity during its superior roll, which provides stability to the joint and also maintains a mechanically efficient fulcrum for elevation of the arm.[124] In the shoulder midrange position, when all of the passive restraints are lax, joint stability is achieved almost entirely by the rotator cuff. In addition, as previously mentioned, without adequate supraspinatus force, the near vertical line of force of a contracting deltoid tends to jam or impinge the humeral head superiorly against the coracoacomial arch.[103]

Long Head of the Biceps Brachii

The biceps brachii muscle is a large fusiform muscle in the anterior compartment of the upper extremity, which has two tendinous origins from the scapula (Fig. 16-7). The medial head and LHB normally originate from the coracoid process and supraglenoid tubercle of the scapula, respectively. However, a great deal of research has noted that the origin of the biceps tendon varies, not only in the type of insertion (single, bifurcated, or trifurcated), but also in the specific anatomical location where it inserts.[11,73] The proximal LHB tendon receives an arterial supply from labral branches of the suprascapular artery.[126] As it leaves its origin, the LHB tendon is surrounded by a synovial sheath, which ends at the distal end of the bicipital groove, making the tendon an intra-articular but extrasynovial structure.[73] As the LHB tendon moves between the greater and lesser tuberosities, it is stabilized in position by the tendoligamentous sling comprising the coracohumeral ligament, superior G-H ligament, and fibers from the supraspinatus and the subscapularis.[73,127] Once in the bicipital groove, the LHB tendon passes under the transverse humeral ligament, which bridges the groove.[128] After coursing through the groove, the two heads join to form the biceps muscle belly at the level of the deltoid insertion.[129] The medial tendon is interarticular, lying inside the G-H capsule.[39–41] This tendon is not as common a source of shoulder pain as the long tendon, and it rarely ruptures.[39–41]

The function of the biceps as a forearm supinator and secondarily as an elbow flexor is well known.[130] At the shoulder joint, however, the function of the LHB tendon is less clear, with most references regarding it as a week flexor of the shoulder.[131] Cadaveric studies have suggested that the LHB tendon functions as a humeral head depressor (in full ER), an anterior stabilizer, a posterior stabilizer, a limiter of ER, a lifter of the glenoid labrum, and a humeral head compressor of the shoulder.[132–135] The muscle has also been described as having an important role in decelerating the rapidly moving arm during activities such as forceful overhand throwing.[73] In the anatomical position, the biceps has no ability to elevate the humerus. If the arm is rotated 90 degrees externally, the tendon of the long head lines up with the muscle belly to form a straight line across the humeral head. As the biceps contracts in this position, the humeral head rotates beneath the tendon, resisting ER of the humeral head and increasing the anterior stability of the G-H joint.[86,136,137] Contraction of the LHB in this position fixes the humeral head snugly against the glenoid cavity, as the resultant force passes obliquely through the center of rotation of the humeral head and at right angles to the glenoid.[136] The humeral head is prevented from moving upwards by the hood-like action of the biceps tendon (Fig. 16-7), which exerts a downward force and assists the depressor function of the cuff.[138–140] Interestingly, the biceps tendon was found to be wider in cuff-deficient shoulders in one study.[141]

The biceps brachii muscle is innervated by the musculocutaneous nerve.

CLINICAL PEARL

A number of pathological conditions have been associated with the LHB tendon including LHB tendon degeneration, superior labrum anterior and posterior (SLAP) lesions, LHB tendon anchor abnormalities, and LHB tendon instability.[128]

Biomechanics

The G-H joint has three DOF: flexion/extension, abduction/adduction, and internal/ER. Available ranges of motion *at the G-H joint* are approximately as follows:

- ***Flexion and abduction.*** Approximately 100–120 degrees are available, with females demonstrating slightly more motion than males.
- ***External rotation.*** Approximately 60–80 degrees are available, with females demonstrating slightly more motion than males.
- ***Internal rotation.*** Approximately 80–90 degrees are available, with females demonstrating slightly more motion than males.
- ***Extension.*** Great variability exists with extension, with ranges existing from 10 to 90 degrees.

G-H motions (Table 16-11) consist of a combination of glides and rolls based on the concave–convex rule (see Chap. 10). At the G-H joint, the concave–convex rule dictates that the articulating surface moves in the opposite direction of the shoulder motion (Table 16-6). Motions at this joint do not occur in isolation, but rather as coupled motions.[142] For

TABLE 16-6	Glenohumeral Joint Motions and Their Appropriate Axis and Accessory Motions	
Plane/Axis of Motion	**Physiologic Motion**	**Accessory Motion**
Sagittal/mediolateral	Flexion/extension	Spin
Coronal/anteroposterior	Abduction	Inferior glide
Transverse/longitudinal	Adduction Internal rotation External rotation	Superior glide Posterior glide Anterior glide

example, ER and abduction occur with flexion, and ER and adduction accompany extension.[75]

Complete movement at the shoulder girdle involves a complex interaction between the G-H, A-C, S-C, scapulothoracic, upper thoracic, costal, and sternomanubrial joints, the upper thorax, and the lower cervical spine. Within the joints of the shoulder complex, there appear to be no well-defined points within the range where one joint's motion ends and another begins. Rather, they all blend into a smooth harmonious movement during arm raising (see Tables 16-4 and 16-5).

During shoulder rotation and arm activities, the scapula invariably acts as a platform upon which the activities are based. It is worth noting that the supporting structures of the G-H joint are only effective if the scapula can maintain its ROM with the humerus (see "The Dynamic Scapula" section).

The G-H joint has been described as being similar to a golf ball on a tee due to the size relationships. A more accurate biomechanical description is that the G-H joint is like a ball on a seal's nose.[143] As the ball or humeral socket moves, the seal's nose, or the scapula, needs to move to maintain the position of the ball on the glenoid. The orientation of the G-H joint causes motions at this joint to occur in the scapular plane. The shoulder has the greatest ROM of any joint, with a vast array of muscles producing those motions.[1] The correct function of these muscles is dependent on length–tension relationships and coordinated activation.[48] Over 1,600 different positions in three-dimensional space can be assumed by the shoulder.[144,145] Due to this wide ROM, the G-H joint is faced with the task of maintaining equilibrium between functional mobility and adequate stability during normal activities of daily living.[146] When sport is added to the equation, extremely high forces can be generated at the shoulder. For example, the angular velocity of an overhead throw reaches over 7,000 degrees per second, which is the fastest recorded human movement.[147]

CLINICAL PEARL

It has been estimated that the anterior translation forces generated with pitching are equal to one-half body weight during the late cocking phase, and there is a distraction force equal to body weight during the deceleration phase.[148]

The complex kinematics of this region probably account for the fact that strains and sprains may remain symptomatic for much longer than in other joints.[1]

TABLE 16-7	Static Restraints to Inferior Translation (Dependent on the Position of the Arm)
Degrees of Glenohumeral Abduction	**Restraining Structures**
0	Superior G-H and coracohumeral ligaments
90	Inferior G-H ligament (posterior band in external rotation, anterior band in internal rotation)

Data from Warner JJP, Deng XH, Warren RF, et al: Static capsuloligamentous restraints to superior-inferior translation of the glenohumeral joint. *Am J Sports Med* 20:675–685, 1992; Turkel SJ, Panio MW, Marshall JL, et al: Stabilizing mechanisms preventing anterior dislocation of the glenohumeral joint. *J Bone Joint Surg Am* 63:1208–1217, 1981.

Full elevation of the arm occurs through an arc of approximately 180 degrees and can occur in an infinite number of body planes.[149] Locally, this motion is a result of abduction of the G-H joint and upward rotation of the scapulothoracic joint. During abduction of the shoulder, the G-H joint is reported to contribute up to 120 degrees of the total arc of motion, with the remaining 60 degrees occurring at the scapulothoracic joint (see "The Dynamic Scapula" section). Arm elevation beyond 90 degrees requires motion in other, more distal joints such as the A-C and S-C joints (see "The Dynamic Scapula" section) and the vertebral joints of the upper thorax and lower cervical spine (Tables 16-8 and 16-9).

Glenohumeral Joint Arthrokinematics

Flexion at the G-H joint involves a pure spin if it occurs strictly in the sagittal plane; no roll or slide is necessary. Tension within the surrounding capsular structures, particularly the posterior structures, may cause a slight anterior translation of the humerus at the extremes of flexion.[46] However, although flexion in the sagittal plane involves a pure spin, elevation of the arm in the scapular plane involves a combination of flexion, abduction, and ER. Thus, at the joint surface of the G-H joint during arm elevation in the scapular plane, the head of the humerus spins (flexion component), glides inferiorly

TABLE 16-8	Static Restraints to Internal Rotation (Dependent on the Position of the Arm)
Degrees of Glenohumeral Abduction	**Restraining Structures**
0	Posterior band of inferior G-H ligament, teres minor, posterior capsule (superior)
45	Anterior and posterior bands of the inferior G-H ligament
90	Posterior band of the inferior G-H ligament, posterior capsule (inferior)

Data from Warner JJP, Deng XH, Warren RF, et al: Static capsuloligamentous restraints to superior-inferior translation of the glenohumeral joint. *Am J Sports Med* 20:675–685, 1992; Turkel SJ, Panio MW, Marshall JL, et al: Stabilizing mechanisms preventing anterior dislocation of the glenohumeral joint. *J Bone Joint Surg Am* 63:1208–1217, 1981.

TABLE 16-9	Dynamic and Static Restraints to External Rotation (Dependent on the Position of the Arm)
Degrees of Glenohumeral Abduction	**Restraining Structures**
0	Subscapularis, superior G-H, and coracohumeral ligaments
45	Subscapularis, middle G-H ligament, superior fibers of the inferior G-H ligament
90	Inferior G-H ligament

Data from Warner JJP, Caborn DNM, Berger RA, et al: Dynamic capsuloligamentous anatomy of the glenohumeral joint. *J Shoulder Elbow Surg* 2:115–133, 1993; Turkel SJ, Panio MW, Marshall JL, et al: Stabilizing mechanisms preventing anterior dislocation of the glenohumeral joint. *J Bone Joint Surg Am* 63:1208–1217, 1981.

(abduction component), and glides anteriorly (ER component) (Table 16-6).

Functional Movements

Depending on the type of function performed, motions of the shoulder complex involve both local motions and motions at other joints.

Kibler[150] labels the motions that occur in other joints of the body during an activity such as throwing (i.e., trunk and hip rotation) as *distant functions.* In contrast, those motions occurring at the shoulder during the same activity (i.e., G-H ER) are termed *local functions.*

Distant Functions

The majority of shoulder motions involve a series of sequentially activated links in a kinetic chain of body segments.[145,150] For those motions requiring more force, the number of links in the kinetic chain increases—the sequence of activation starts as a ground reaction force (GRF) and moves up through the knees and hips to the trunk, and into the shoulder. Approximately 50% of the total kinetic energy and force occurring at the G-H joint originate from a combination of the GRF and the forces from the legs and hips.[145,150,151] At the shoulder, G-H, A-C, S-C, and scapulothoracic joints, motion occurs simultaneously as a result of muscle action and ligamentous tension in these joints. The specific sequence of muscle activation in the upper extremity depends on the activity, although the direction of activation is usually from proximal to distal as this is the most efficient method for producing large forces and accelerations to the arm. As part of this activation sequence, specific muscle activation patterns and joint positions are developed depending on the activity. Any changes to this sequence of activation can produce an abnormal movement pattern, involving substitution or compensation from the more distal links.[47,152] For example, a throwing athlete with decreased trunk rotation due to stiffness has to rely more on the shoulder to provide the force for the throw. These adaptive patterns eventually result in either decreased performance or increased injury risk.

Local Functions

The G-H joint accounts for approximately two-thirds of all shoulder motions, with the remainder provided by the scapulothoracic joint.[87] For full motion to occur, a complex interaction between the deltoid, rotator cuff, LHB, G-H capsule, glenoid articulating cartilage, and scapular pivoters (trapezius, serratus anterior, levator scapulae, and rhomboids) is required.[153]

Stabilization of the Static Shoulder

The dependent shoulder requires very little muscular support. Its vertical stability is a result of the inferior lateral projection and upward inclination of the glenoid fossa, which is maintained by a mild contraction of the fibers of the trapezius. It was traditionally theorized that the humeral head was prevented from rolling off of this lateral projection by a moderate contraction of the supraspinatus and the deltoid.[134,154] More recent studies have demonstrated that the muscle tone of the rotator cuff is not a significant contributor to the static inferior stability of the dependent shoulder with light loads, but that maintenance of the intra-articular pressure and the adhesion and cohesion properties of the articular surfaces are far more significant.[155,156] However, the rotator cuff does provide a passive restraint to translation, especially to posterior translation, during the early-to-midranges of elevation.[157]

During the mid and end ranges of motion, a combination of several different static restraints create a vector that keeps the humeral head securely seated in the glenoid, through concavity compression—negative articular pressure (see Tables 16-7–16-9).[144,153,155,158–160] Static restraint is also provided by the anatomic curvature of the humerus and glenoid, the extra depth of the labrum, and ligamentous restraints (see Tables 16-7 and 16-8).[161] The ligamentous restraints contribute especially at the end ranges of motion[162] and are assisted with concomitant muscle activity (see Table 16-9).

Stabilization of the Dynamic Shoulder

Dynamic stability of the shoulder complex is dependent on a variety of mechanisms including the optimal alignment of the scapula, correct G-H orientation, and the quality of the length–tension relationship of the involved muscles, and correct functioning of the static restraints (Table 16-9).

The deltoid, pectoralis major, latissimus dorsi, and teres major muscles are prime movers of the G-H joint. EMG studies have shown that these muscles function along the line of pull, creating the potential for infinite lines of pull that may allow an almost 360 degrees arc of motion.[13,163] Indeed, like the temporomandibular joint, the G-H joint enjoys the benefit that all of its prime movers compress the joint surface, thus optimizing joint stability. The secondary movers of the G-H joint are the LHB, and the triceps.

CLINICAL PEARL

The LHB and the triceps muscles are major dynamic stabilizers of the G-H joint, predominately functioning as "shunt" muscles (muscles that produce a compression at the joint surfaces of the joints they cross) during high-velocity activities.

As motion occurs at the G-H joint, the glenoid cavity of the scapular adopts a diverse number of reciprocal positions. It is likely that these scapular positions are based on both the functional task and the placement of the hand. The scapular stabilizers include the serratus anterior, latissimus dorsi, trapezius, rhomboids, levator scapulae, and the pectoralis minor. Dysfunction or inhibition of any of these muscles can alter the position of the glenoid significantly, resulting in abnormal centering of the humeral head within the glenoid.[24,164,165]

The function of the rotator cuff in normal and pathologic conditions has been the subject of several studies.[12,99,138–141] Until recently, EMG or cadaver studies have been the primary method of evaluating the contribution of each rotator cuff and shoulder muscle to a particular motion or exercise.[12,99,138,142–145] For example, using cadavers, Keating et al.[146] determined that the subscapularis contributes 53% of the cuff moment and believed it to be the most important muscle in humeral head stabilization.

Magnetic resonance imaging (MRI) is now being used to show increases in muscle signal intensity detected immediately following exercise.[147–149] On the basis of the level of signal intensity, this so-called exercise-induced enhancement seen on MRI can determine which muscles are used for a given exercise.[140,147,148,150–152] For example, one study of the shoulder[149] demonstrated that side-lying abduction produced the greatest signal intensity in the supraspinatus, infraspinatus, and subscapularis muscles. Surprisingly, scaption with internal rotation (SIR), previously associated with isolation of the supraspinatus muscle, did not provide the highest increase in any muscle of the rotator cuff.[149] However, caution must be used in drawing conclusions from single studies, and further research is certainly warranted in this area.

As previously mentioned, the role of the capsuloligamentous complex in stabilizing the G-H joint during dynamic activities is complex and varies with both shoulder position and the direction of the translation force.[166] The posterior capsule is the main restraint against posterior translation of the humerus on the glenoid fossa with the arm below 90 degrees of abduction.[167] With the arm at 90 degrees of abduction, the inferior G-H ligament and the posteroinferior capsule become the main restraint.[167] The posterior band of the inferior G-H ligament resists inferior translation when the arm is at 90 degrees of abduction.

The Dynamic Scapula

The synchronized motions that occur between the scapula and the humerus during elevation are a combination of scapulothoracic motion and scapulohumeral motion.

Scapulohumeral Motion. The angle between the glenoid and the moving humeral head has to be maintained within a safe zone of 30 degrees of angulation during activities to decrease shear and translatory forces.[168] For this to occur, the scapula must be positioned muscularly in relation to the moving humerus and must also act as a stable base of muscle origin for the rotator cuff muscles. If the scapula cannot be controlled, the glenoid cannot be positioned correctly to allow for the optimal length–tension relationships within the shoulder complex.[110,112,161,169] This synchronized motion between the glenoid cavity and the humerus is referred to as *scapulohumeral rhythm* (Fig. 16-14). Proper rhythm involves a rotation of the scapula during arm elevation. By allowing the glenoid to stay centered under the humeral head, the strong tendency for a downward dislocation of the humerus is resisted and the glenoid is maintained within a physiologically tolerable range (Fig. 16-14). At full abduction, the glenoid completely supports the humerus.

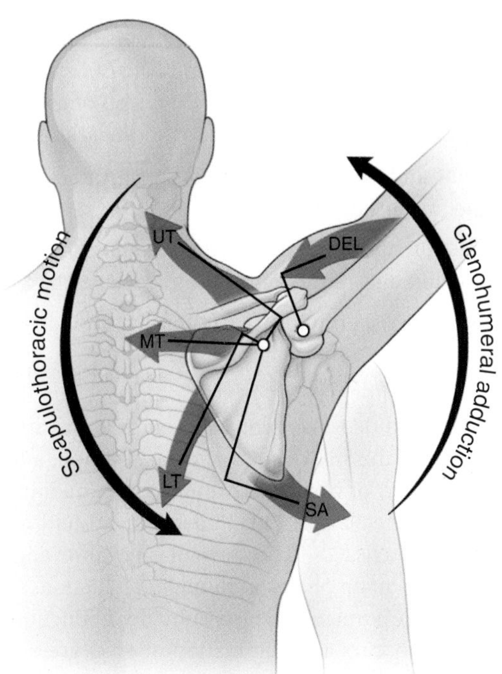

FIGURE 16-14 The scapulohumeral rhythm.

Several studies have examined the scapulohumeral rhythm three dimensionally.[25,26,87,170,171] An early study by Inman[87] determined that a 2:1 ratio existed between the motion occurring at the G-H joint and scapula, respectively. However, more recent studies have shown that this ratio is not consistent throughout the ROM.[21,107,153] As the humerus elevates to 30 degrees (setting phase), there is minimal movement of the scapula. In this initial portion of abduction, G-H motion predominates and the ratio has been found to be 4.4 degrees of G-H motion for every degree of scapular motion (4.4:1 ratio). From 30 to 90 degrees, the scapula abducts and upwardly rotates, and the ratio becomes 5 degrees of G-H motion to 4 degrees of scapular motion (5:4 ratio). As the shoulder moves above 90 degrees of abduction to full abduction, the scapula abducts and upwardly rotates 1 degree for every 1 degree of humeral elevation (1:1 ratio).[25,115,170] However, it must be kept in mind that these ratios are based on two-dimensional radiographic projections of angular rotations taken at discrete positions of elevation, whereas in reality, the arm moves in three dimensions, and that the scapulohumeral rhythm has also been found to change with external loading of the arm.[171]

CLINICAL PEARL

A reverse scapulohumeral rhythm, in which the scapula moves more than the humerus, occurs in conditions such as adhesive capsulitis.

Scapulothoracic Motion. Scapulothoracic motion is a vital component of shoulder function and consists of rotation and translation around approximately three axes of motion. These axes are considered to be embedded in the scapula.[172]

- Anterior and posterior tipping occurs around an axis parallel to the scapula.
- Protraction and retraction of the scapula occur through protraction and retraction of the clavicle at the S-C joint.
- IR and ER occur around an axis running through the scapula from superior to inferior.
- Elevation and depression of the scapula occurs through elevation and depression of the clavicle at the S-C joint. Throughout the 180 degrees of arm elevation, a total of 30–35 degrees of clavicle elevation occurs, in addition to rotation of the clavicle (30–35 degrees) around its longitudinal axis.[74,173] This clavicular elevation and rotation occur in two main phases of shoulder abduction. Assuming a 2:1 scapulohumeral rhythm, shoulder abduction up to 90 degrees occurs as a summation of 60 degrees of G-H abduction, and 30 degrees of scapulothoracic upward rotation. The 30 degrees of upward rotation occurs predominantly through a synchronous 20–25 degrees of clavicular elevation at the S-C joint and 5–10 degrees of upward rotation at the A-C joint.[103] The elevation of the clavicle raises the acromion during arm elevation allowing for the subacromial structures to pass under the coracoacromial arch.[24] Shoulder abduction from 90 to 180 degrees occurs as a summation of an additional 60 degrees of G-H joint abduction and an additional 30 degrees of scapulothoracic upward rotation.[103] During this late phase, the clavicle elevates only an additional 5 degrees at the S-C joint, whereas, at the A-C joint, the scapula upwardly rotates 20–25 degrees. Thus, by the end of 180 degrees of abduction, the 60 degrees of scapulothoracic upward rotation can be accounted for by 30 degrees of elevation at the S-C joint and 30 degrees of upward rotation at the A-C joint.[103] The motion at the A-C joint is controlled by tension in the coracoclavicular ligaments. Finally, the clavicle has been demonstrated in vivo to posteriorly rotate around its long axis during the late phase of shoulder abduction.[24] It is, as yet, unclear whether this posterior rotation occurs at the S-C or at the A-C joint. The rotation of the clavicle, though, is controlled by tension in the coracoclavicular ligaments and the clavipectoral fascia.

  Elevation of the arm in the scapular plane in healthy subjects is accompanied by posterior tipping and upward rotation of the scapula.[172] The upward rotation of the scapula occurs about an axis that passes through the base of the spine of the scapula and occurs in various phases (see Tables 16-4 and 16-5). Rotation of the scapula about the vertical axis shows a somewhat more variable pattern,[172] with some studies showing ER occurring predominantly at higher elevation angles,[68,174,175] whereas others demonstrate IR.[176–178]

- Upward and downward rotation occurs around an axis perpendicular to the plane of the scapula that travels through the A-C joint and S-C joint.[71] The upward rotation of the scapula during shoulder abduction helps to maintain an effective length–tension relationship between the three groups (force couples) of muscles that attach to the scapula. A *force couple* is defined as two forces that act in opposite directions to rotate a segment around its axis of motion.[86,179]

During the first 30 degrees of upward rotation of the scapula, the serratus anterior muscle and the upper and lower divisions of the trapezius muscle are considered the principal upward rotators of the scapula. Together these muscles form two force couples; one formed by the upper trapezius and the upper serratus anterior muscles (Fig. 16-14) and the other by the lower trapezius and lower serratus anterior muscles.[6,87,180]

The prime muscles that abduct the G-H joint are the middle deltoid and the supraspinatus muscles.[103] Elevation of the arm through flexion is performed primarily by the anterior deltoid, coracobrachialis, and LHB brachii.[103] The trapezius appears to be more critical for controlling the scapula during the initial phases of abduction, whereas the serratus has been found to be the most effective upward rotator of the scapula.[87,181] The lower trapezius contributes during the later phase of shoulder abduction by preventing tipping of the scapula and assisting in the stabilization of the scapula through eccentric control of the scapula during scapular upward rotation.[115,170]

CLINICAL PEARL

During approximately the first 150 degrees of arm elevation through flexion

- the upper and lower fibers of the trapezius contract concentrically,
- the fibers of the lower serratus anterior contract concentrically,
- the levator scapulae contracts eccentrically,
- the rhomboids contract eccentrically.

Approximately from 150 to 180 degrees

- the lower fibers of the serratus anterior contract isometrically,
- the lower fibers of the trapezius contract concentrically,
- the pectoralis minor contracts eccentrically,
- the upper fibers of the serratus anterior contract eccentrically.

The middle trapezius and rhomboids may also contribute to the scapular motions involved during arm elevation.[182] The antagonists are the pectoralis major, teres major, latissimus dorsi, and coracobrachialis, all working eccentrically. Normal motion of the scapula on the thorax is believed to include consistent contact between the thoracic wall, the medial border, and inferior angle of the scapula.[180,182] Loss of this contact has been clinically implicated as evidence of abnormal scapular kinematics. These abnormal scapular kinematics may result in additional stress on the anterior shoulder stabilizers.[183–185]

The appropriate force couples for the acromial elevation that occurs during G-H abduction are the lower trapezius and serratus muscles working together, paired with the upper trapezius and rhomboid muscles (Fig. 16-14).[24]

The EMG activity of the levator scapula muscle, upper and lower trapezius muscles, and serratus anterior muscle during arm elevation increases progressively as the humeral angle increases.[68] Activities that maintain an upwardly rotated scapula while accentuating scapular protraction, such as a push-up plus, elicit the greatest serratus anterior EMG activity.[75]

The last few degrees of shoulder elevation consist of upper thoracic movement once full G-H joint and shoulder girdle motion have been completed.[186] As the arm continues to elevate beyond the 150-degree mark, the thorax begins to extend and ipsilaterally rotate and side flex.

The scapula also functions during retraction and protraction along the thoracic wall (see Fig. 16-11).[24] Protraction occurs as the serratus anterior at the scapula and the pectoralis major at the humerus contract simultaneously. Retraction is produced by the combined action of the trapezius and rhomboids.[187] A 15–18-cm translation of the scapula around the thoracic wall occurs during retraction and protraction, depending on the size of the individual and the vigorousness of the activity.[24,151] This retraction and protraction is used during activities such as reaching and pulling, respectively.[24]

Lastly, the scapula functions to transfer the large forces and energy from the legs, hips, back, and trunk to the actual delivery mechanism, the arm and hand.[24,150,188,189]

EXAMINATION

The intervention strategies for the common pathologies of the shoulder complex are detailed after the examination section. An understanding of both is necessary. As mention of the various pathologies occurs with reference to the examination and vice versa, the reader is encouraged to alternate between the two. Shoulder complex conditions are often multifaceted, and patients with the same shoulder condition often present with diverse physical findings. It is critical that the clinician consider the shoulder girdle as a whole, rather than as a series of isolated articulations, and as a part of the whole kinetic chain. In the presence of shoulder complex dysfunction (assuming systemic or serious causes have been ruled out) there are three likely causes:

- Compromise of the passive restraint components of the shoulder girdle.
- Compromise of the neuromuscular system's production or control of shoulder girdle motion.
- Compromise to one or more of the neighboring joints that contribute to shoulder girdle motion, including
  - the A-C joint,
  - the S-C joint,
  - the joints of the upper thoracic spine and ribs,
  - the joints of the lower cervical spine.

Due to this complexity, all of the above-mentioned joints must be selectively tested in a specific sequence before proceeding with a more detailed examination of the suspected joint or joints.

HISTORY

A good history is the cornerstone of proper diagnosis, especially since shoulder pain has a broad spectrum of patterns and characteristics. A body chart can be used to record the patient's symptom distribution (see Chap. 4). The body chart is a symptomatic representation of a patient's complaints and can be an important element in guiding both the history and the tests and measures.

The history should begin with a brief outline of the patient's profile including age, occupation, hand dominance, recreational pursuits, work requirements, and activities of daily living (ADL).[190] Age is occasionally significant[191]:

- Children and adolescents may have an epiphysitis of the humerus, or an osteogenic sarcoma.
- Calcific deposits in the shoulder are more common between 20 and 40 years of age.
- Chondrosarcomas usually occur after age 30.
- Rotator cuff degeneration usually occurs in the 40s and 50s.
- A frozen shoulder is more common in those aged 45–60 years and is associated with medical conditions such as diabetes mellitus and ischemic heart disease.[190]

The exact mechanism of injury should be determined as it can help with a preliminary diagnosis[192]:

- Overhead exertion involving repetitive motions is a common mechanism for subacromial pathology, encompassing subacromial bursitis,[61] SIS,[40] rotator cuff tendinitis,[40,193] and rotator cuff tear.[194] It is also a common cause of bicipital tendinitis.
- A fall on an outstretched hand ("FOOSH" injury) can result in a sprain or strain injury to the wrist, elbow, and shoulder. More serious injuries from such a fall include fractures of the wrist and elbow, A-C separations, clavicular fractures, and G-H fractures and dislocations.
- A fall on the tip of the shoulder is a common mechanism for A-C separation. In addition, this mechanism can result in a compression periostitis (bone contusion) or a cervical spine injury, both of which appear remarkably similar to an A-C separation especially in the early stages.
- Forced horizontal extension of the abducted, externally rotated arm is a common mechanism for anterior dislocation.

It is important to establish the patient's chief presenting complaint (which is not always pain) as well as defining their other symptoms. The most common complaints associated with shoulder pathology include pain, instability, stiffness, deformity, locking, and swelling.[190] Patients sometimes complain of catching, clunking, grinding, or popping of the shoulder with various movements. These sounds and sensations may be asymptomatic and nonpathologic. However, they may also indicate pathology including labral disorders, rotator cuff tears, snapping scapular, subacromial bursitis, or biceps tendon disorders, especially if the sound or sensation is associated with pain or instability.[190] Periscapular pain is often associated with local muscle strain but may be referred.[1]

The quality of the pain is also important. Radicular pain tends to be sharp, burning, and radiating. Bone pain is deep, boring, and localized. Muscle pain can be dull, aching, and hard to localize. Tendon pain tends to be hot and burning. Vascular pain can be diffused, aching, and poorly localized and may be referred to other areas of the body. The intensity of pain may wax and wane with particular motions associated with specific activities. Common complaints with a rotator cuff tear include difficulty with elevation of the arm in abduction, as well as ER, and when patients attempt to put their hand behind their head or back.[195] Patients who report difficulty tucking in their shirts may have limited IR from posterior capsular stiffness.[196] The hallmark of posterior capsular contracture is symmetric loss of active and passive IR. Posterior capsular stiffness may occur independent of rotator cuff disease. Stiffness or loss of motion at the shoulder may be the chief complaint in conditions such as adhesive capsulitis.[190] A-C joint pain tends to occur with arm motion above 90 degrees of abduction and with horizontal abduction. Pain associated with an idiopathic frozen shoulder tends to be constant, but is particularly bad at night and frequently awakens the patient.[53]

Weakness may be the chief complaint, leading to some diagnostic confusion. It is important to distinguish true weakness from weakness secondary to pain, both in terms of history and examination findings.[197] Painless weakness is usually due to neurological problems or myopathies, although peripheral nerve injuries can be painful (Table 16-10). Shoulder weakness may be caused by a rotator cuff tear or nerve injury (suprascapular, axillary, long thoracic, or thoracodorsal nerves, or cervical nerve root injury) (see Table 16-10).[111]

TABLE 16-10 Peripheral Nerve Lesions

Nerve	Findings
Spinal accessory nerve	Inability to abduct the arm beyond 90 degrees Pain in the shoulder with abduction
Musculocutaneous nerve	Weak elbow flexion with forearm supinated
Long thoracic nerve	Pain on flexing a fully extended arm Inability to fully flex an extended arm Winging of the scapula at 90 degrees of forward shoulder flexion
Suprascapular nerve	Increased pain on forward shoulder flexion Pain increased with scapular abduction Pain increased with cervical rotation to the opposite side
Axillary nerve	Inability to abduct the arm with neutral rotation
Thoracodorsal nerve	Marked difficulty to resist shoulder extension Marked difficulty to resist shoulder internal rotation
Cervical spinal nerve root	Varies according to the level involved, so can include various combinations of the above

Symptoms that are not associated with movement should alert the clinician to a more serious condition (see "Systems Review" section). Pain that is worse at night, but increased when rolling onto the shoulder, points to a periarticular mechanical problem.[195]

Determining the location of pain is important. Anterior shoulder pain suggests bicipital tendinitis, whereas posterior shoulder pain might be due to a posterior labral tear.[53] Posterior neck pain may be indicative of a cervical radiculopathy, as neither the A-C joint nor a subacromial irritation refers pain to this area.[74,198]

CLINICAL PEARL

Pain due to rotator cuff pathology and impingement is usually felt over the anterior or lateral part of the shoulder, is characterized by radiation down the upper arm, and is aggravated with overhead activities.[190,199] Pain that radiates beyond the elbow is far less likely to be due to shoulder pathology, particularly if it is associated with any sensory disturbance in the limb such as distal radiation of pain, numbness, or paresthesias.[190] In such cases, the clinician should rule out thoracic outlet syndrome (TOS), cervical radiculopathy, or referred pain from neighboring areas.

Pain due to A-C joint pathology is usually located at the superior region of the shoulder or well localized at the A-C joint itself, and there is often a clear history of injury to this region. Severe pain on top of the shoulder with an associated deformity could indicate an A-C joint sprain.

The clinician should determine which positions or movements relieve the pain, as these can provide helpful information[192]:

- Pain relieved with arm elevation overhead could indicate a cervicogenic cause.[200]
- Pain relieved with the elbow supported is suggestive of A-C separation and rotator cuff tears.
- Pain relieved by circumduction of the shoulder with an accompanying click or clunk could indicate an internal derangement or subluxation.
- Pain relieved with arm distraction is suggestive of bursitis or rotator cuff tendinitis.
- Pain relieved when the arms are held in a dependent position suggests TOS.

An inquiry about general health, any existing medical conditions, medications, and allergies should be made. Corticosteroid use can cause osteoporosis and tendon atrophy and affects wound healing; therefore a history of its use may alter the differential diagnosis.[190,195] The use of anticoagulant medication should be noted. Patients who are undergoing renal dialysis are at increased risk for tendon tears, as are patients who are 80 years of age or older.[195] Bilateral shoulder involvement is not uncommon in these groups.

Past physical therapy interventions, previous injections, and previous surgery are important to document, as are previous shoulder injuries and what relationship, if any, they have with the present symptomatology.[190]

Systems Review

The clinician should be able to determine the suitability of the patient for physical therapy. If the clinician is concerned with any signs or symptoms of a visceral, vascular, neurogenic, psychogenic, spondylogenic, or systemic disorder (see Chap. 5) that is out of the scope of physical therapy, the patient should be referred back to his or her physician or another appropriate healthcare provider.

Scenarios related to the shoulder that may warrant further investigation by the clinician include an insidious onset of symptoms and complaints of numbness or paresthesia in the upper extremity.

The most common causes of numbness in the shoulder and arm are due to cervical or upper thoracic involvement, with either the segmental roots involved or the brachial plexus. The patient should be questioned about recent changes in work requirements or environment, and the presence of neck pain.[39–41,201] In studies where normal cervical ligaments and muscles,[202] cervical zygapophyseal joints,[203] and disks[204] have been stimulated, subjects have reported pain in the head, anterior and posterior chest wall, shoulder girdle, and upper limb depending on the cervical level stimulated.[115]

The Cyriax scanning examination (see Chap. 4) may demonstrate subtle weakness of the cervical root innervated muscles. Depressed or absent upper extremity reflexes are also frequently noted. Finally, reproduction of the patient's pain with cervical motion and not with shoulder movement is a strong indicator of cervical origin.

In addition to the cervical and upper thoracic spine, the related joints referring symptoms to the shoulder require clearing. These include the temporomandibular joint, costosternal joint, costovertebral and costotransverse joint, thoracic spine, and the elbow and forearm.[70,199]

Systemic causes of insidious shoulder pain include rheumatoid arthritis. Rheumatoid arthritis often affects the shoulders and hips in older individuals and can be difficult to distinguish from polymyalgia rheumatica. Morning stiffness lasting for more than 1 hour, constitutional signs, and physical signs of joint inflammation are all indicative of an inflammatory disease.[195] Other systemic sources of shoulder pain include lupus erythematosus and gallbladder and liver disease.[70] These latter conditions are associated with other signs and symptoms that are not related to movement and are systemic in nature. Chronic respiratory and cardiovascular conditions must also come into consideration.[190] The shoulder is very close to the chest and its viscera; therefore reference of symptoms to the shoulder from these structures is common (see Chap. 5). It is vital that questions be asked that would reveal a relationship between the onset of symptoms and local movements versus general exercise, the latter of which could implicate the lung, heart, or diaphragm.

CLINICAL PEARL

Severe progressive pain not affected by movement, which is persistent throughout the day and night, and is associated with systemic signs, may indicate referred pain from a malignancy. The exception to this may be adhesive capsulitis (frozen shoulder), which is often characterized by boring, unrelenting, aching pain, even at rest.[205]

Finally, a vascular examination should be performed and should include an assessment of general skin texture, color, temperature, hair growth, and alteration of sensation about and distal to the shoulder.[53] Autonomic signs and symptoms are suggestive of complex regional pain syndrome (CRPS) (refer to Chap. 18). Neurovascular compression or TOS tests are described in "Special Test" section in Chapter 25.

TESTS AND MEASURES

The physical examination of the shoulder complex should be focused and thorough, using the clinical impression gleaned from the history and systems review as a guide.

Observation

Observation of the patient begins when the patient enters the clinic. The clinician observes how the patient holds the arm, the overall position of the upper extremity, and the willingness of the patient to move the arm. During gait, an upper extremity should swing in tandem with its opposite lower extremity. Once in the examination room, the patient is appropriately disrobed and the shoulder is systematically inspected from anterior, lateral, and posterior positions. Total body alignment is examined for overall posture, the relative rotation of the humerus, structural malalignment such as kyphosis, the presence of scars, color changes, and swelling.[190] For example, a hollowed infraspinatus fossa is a hallmark of a rotator cuff tear, although a suprascapular nerve lesion should also be considered.[53] Anterior prominence of the humeral head or a high-riding outer clavicle suggest G-H dislocation or A-C separation, respectively.[53] The relative heights of the shoulder girdles should be assessed. The height of the shoulder may or may not be significant. If the shoulders are elevated, the neck appears short. If they are depressed, the A-C joint is seen to be lower than the S-C joint.[206] Elevation of the clavicle can be due to shortness of the upper trapezius such that the lateral end of the clavicle appears appreciably higher than its medial aspect.[206] A low shoulder can result from[192]

- adaptive laxity of the shoulder,
- leg length discrepancy,
- scoliosis,
- soft-tissue hypertonicity,
- mechanical dysfunction of the pelvis,
- hand dominance—the shoulder on the dominant side may be slightly lower and more muscular than the nondominant side; this is a normal finding.

Deformity is a common complaint with injuries of the A-C joint and fractures of the clavicle. For example, a second-degree sprain or severe first-degree sprain of the A-C joint can be seen as a high-riding lateral clavicle (elevation of the distal end) causing a step-off to form between the clavicle and acromion.[17,207] It is frequently referred to as a tent-pole deformity. The fountain sign describes swelling that is anterior to the A-C joint that is indicative of degeneration that has caused communication between the AC joint and a swollen subacromial bursa underneath. Other causes of deformity include an anterior dislocation of the shoulder, which may produce a squaring of the shoulder, as the deltoid is no longer rounded out over the humeral head.

Observation of muscle symmetry should be noted. Specific atrophy can imply certain diagnoses. For example, muscle weakness or atrophy, especially posttraumatic, might indicate peripheral nerve damage[208]:

- Atrophy of the deltoid from axillary nerve neuropathy can result in a squared appearance of the lateral shoulder,[207,208] which is best observed from the front.[17]
- Atrophy of the posterior deltoid can occur in patients with multidirectional instability.[208]
- Atrophy at the infraspinatus or supraspinatus fossa is a hallmark of a rotator cuff tear[16] or suprascapular nerve entrapment. Wasting of the supraspinati and infraspinati can be determined by pushing the examining finger into the respective muscle bellies.
- Atrophy of the trapezius may indicate compromise of the spinal accessory nerve. Atrophy of the trapezius is characterized by the appearance of a shoulder girdle that droops in association with a protracted inferior border of the scapula and an elevated acromion.[24,110,209]
- Atrophy of the serratus anterior muscle can create a prominent superior medial border of the scapula and a depressed acromion.

A balled-up muscle may indicate a muscle rupture, the most common of which are of the biceps and infraspinatus. Rupture of the LHB can be noticed by the change in contour of the anterior arm with bunching of the muscle (the "Popeye" appearance).[190]

Observable swelling in the shoulder may indicate a serious problem or damage.

The position and attitude of the scapula, both statically and dynamically, should be noted (see later). In standing, with their arms by the sides, the patients' medial (vertebral) border of the scapula should be 5–8 cm lateral to the thoracic spinous processes,[191,210] the medial end of the spine of the scapula should be level with the T3 spinous process, and the inferior angle of the scapula should be level with the T7 spinous process. The superior aspect of the medial border of the scapula begins at the level of the spinous process of T2 and extends to the level of the spinous process of T7. Excessive prominence of the scapular spine may indicate atrophy of the infraspinatus and supraspinatus.[208] Two conditions, which may present with deformity of the scapula as their main symptom, are Sprengel's deformity and winging of the scapula.[190]

Sprengel's deformity is the most common congenital abnormality affecting the shoulder. It is characterized by the presence of a hypoplastic, incorrectly rotated scapula, which sits abnormally high on the posterior chest wall. The condition results from a failure of the normal descent of the scapula, which occurs in utero, and is commonly associated with other significant musculoskeletal and visceral congenital abnormalities.[190]

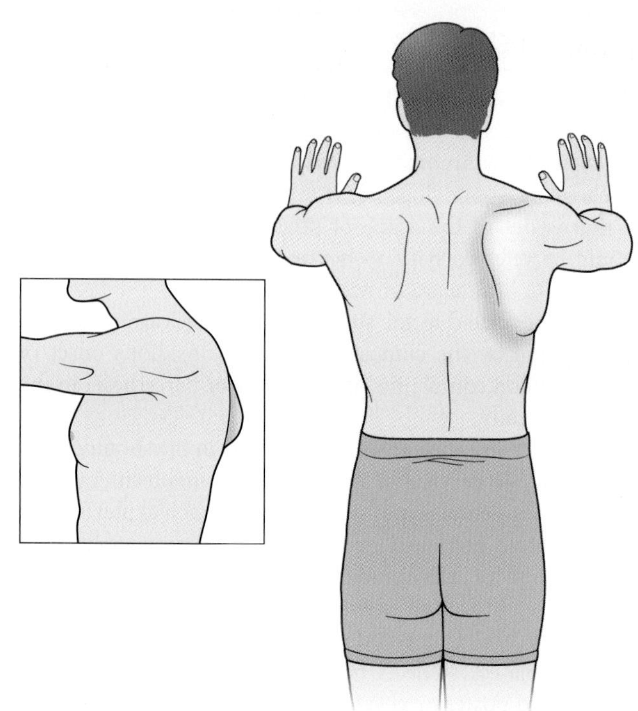

FIGURE 16-15 Scapular winging.

Winging of the scapula (Fig. 16-15) is due to a loss of the normal scapular stability. Subtle forms of scapular winging, usually evident at the inferior border, occur commonly with many shoulder disorders such as G-H joint stiffness and shoulder instability.[112] In cases of G-H joint stiffness, there is passive limitation of G-H motion, while with instability there is evidence of excessive movements or positive apprehension signs. Scapular winging may occur as the result of serratus anterior weakness, trapezius palsy,[209] excessive shortening of the pectoralis minor muscle,[2] or myopathies.[190,211–213] Scapular winging may also be caused by G-H joint stiffness, shoulder instability, and rotator cuff disease (see "Analysis of the Static Shoulder" section).

Gait

Gait is evaluated to observe freedom of the arm swing, reciprocal upper extremity movement, position of the arms and scapulae, and motion of the trunk and lower extremities (see Chap. 6).[70,199]

Posture

An analysis of posture prompts the clinician as to the area of movement disturbance or excessive stresses. Postural dysfunctions of the upper quarter are a common cause of shoulder pain. A wide variety of structural changes can produce shoulder pain.[183,214,215] Poor positioning of the cervical or thoracic spine may alter the position of the shoulder girdle.[216,217] For example, thoracic kyphosis, scoliosis, or neck lordosis can result in excessive protraction of the scapula, producing interscapular pain.[24,218] In the older patient (aged over 50 years), an increased thoracic kyphosis may be related to a decrease in shoulder elevation.[219]

The relationship of the humeral head to the acromion should be observed. One-third of the humeral head should be anterior to the acromion. A finding of less than one-third

TABLE 16-11 Common Muscle Imbalances of the Shoulder Complex	
Muscles Prone to Tightness	**Muscles Prone to Inactivity or Lengthening**
Upper trapezius	Middle and lower trapezius
Levator scapulae	Rhomboids
Pectoralis major and minor	Serratus anterior
Upper cervical extensors	Deep neck flexors
Sternocleidomastoid	Supraspinatus
Scalenes	Infraspinatus
Teres major and minor	
Subscapularis	

may indicate a tight posterior capsule or adaptive shortening of the external rotators.[220]

The patient's hands and arms should also be observed. Normally, the thumb faces anterior or slightly medial. If the posterior aspect of the hand faces anteriorly, there may be excessive adaptive shortening of the internal rotators.[220]

Muscle balances in the upper quadrant can cause a characteristic postural pattern of the forward head position.[221] The most common muscle imbalances are outlined in Table 16-11. The clinician should observe the trunk and neck positions in sitting and standing, as well as the relationship of the scapulae relative to the trunk and the humerus relative to the acromion. Any change in the scapular position has an impact on the A-C and S-C joint and can also alter the length–tension relationship of the scapular muscles.

The forward head and rounded shoulder posture include an abducted and elevated position of the scapula and an internally rotated humerus,[24,102,217,222] and is more common in patients presenting with shoulder pain[223] and interscapular pain.[223] Forward head posture (FHP) in the presence of abducted scapulae and protracted shoulders results in a decrease in the size of the subacromial space, which may predispose the patient to rotator cuff disorders.[224] This posture results in an adaptive shortening of the upper trapezius, levator scapulae, and pectoralis, with weakening and lengthening of the deep neck flexors and lower scapular stabilizers.[102,223,225]

If the pectoralis major is tight or strong, the muscle will be prominent. If there is an imbalance present, it will lead to rounded and protracted shoulders and a slight IR of the humerus.[226,227] The altered position of the scapulae can distort the course of the suprascapular nerve, placing it at risk for a traction injury during upper extremity movements.[228–230]

Normally, the insertion of the SCM is barely visible. If the clavicular insertion is prominent, it may indicate adaptive shortening of the SCM.[226] A groove along the SCM is an early sign of weakness of the deep neck flexors. A weakening and atrophy of the deep neck flexors has been proposed as a sign to estimate biological age.[231] The change in the anatomical relationship of the clavicle associated with this weakness and atrophy, decreases the width of the thoracic inlet, rendering the brachial plexus vulnerable to compression (refer to Chap. 25).[228,232,233]

A loss of bulk in the interscapular muscles may indicate tightness in the trapezius and levator scapula.

Analysis of the Static Scapula

An abnormal position of the scapula at rest is common in patients with shoulder overuse injuries.[102,206,223,225] The scapular position is initially examined with the arms by the side. The clinician notes any signs of winging, elevation, depression, adduction, abduction, and rotation of the scapula. Abnormalities in alignment include a flattening of the interscapular area and an increase in the distance between the thoracic spinous processes and the medial border of the scapula. When the scapula is abducted (more than 8 cm from the midline of the thorax), it is also rotated more than 30 degrees anterior to the frontal plane and produces a medial rotation of the humerus.[206]

Tipping of the scapula, in which the inferior angle protrudes away from the rib cage, often results from a weakness of the lower trapezius and positions the glenoid fossa so that it faces a more inferior direction.[115] This alignment is often associated with shortness of the pectoralis minor muscle or biceps brachii muscle.[206]

Adaptive shortening of the rhomboids and levator scapulae muscles, in the presence of a lengthened upper trapezius and serratus anterior, results in an elevation of the scapulae at the superior angle, and a downward rotation of the scapula. This causes the G-H joint to move into a position of abduction.[206,234] In addition, if the levator scapula adaptively shortens, both cervical and shoulder motions occur sooner than normal because the starting position of the scapula is changed. This modification to the starting position of the scapula for shoulder-elevated tasks presumably has an effect on the timing of the scapular muscles responsible for upward rotation. This results in an end position of arm elevation that is lower than usual (see "Examination of the Dynamic Scapula" section).[115]

Extremity dominance can affect the orientation of the scapula, with the greater degree of unilateral activity producing the greater changes. A bilateral comparison should be made and allowances made for the dominance. Bilateral comparisons do not always highlight dysfunctions. For example, the symmetrical effects of an adaptive shortening of the anterior chest and shoulder musculature, and lengthening of the posterior musculature that occurs in the forward head and rounded shoulder posture, will not be confirmed until during the mobility tests.

A number of static tests for the scapular position exist. The amount of scapular protraction available can be measured clinically using the method described by Diveta et al.,[235] who advocate two linear measurements with a piece of string. The distance in centimeters between the root of the scapular spine and the inferior angle of the acromion (scapular width) is divided into the distance from the third thoracic spinous process to the inferior angle of the acromion (scapular protraction). The resulting ratio provides a measurement of scapular protraction corrected for scapular size (normalized scapular protraction). This method of measurement of scapular protraction has been found to be both reliable and valid when compared with radiographic measurements.[223,235,236]

Palpation

Palpation must be performed in a systematic manner and must focus on specific anatomical structures (refer to

Figs. 16-1 through 16-13). The degree and location of tenderness is often a reliable physical sign leading to an accurate diagnosis.[53] For example, tenderness over the anterior acromion and greater tuberosity is suggestive of impingement, whereas tenderness over the posterior joint line could indicate joint pathology such as G-H arthritis or a torn posterior labrum.[53] Traditionally, palpation has been viewed as a static process. However, palpation is a dynamic process and should be performed along with other aspects of the examination. The optimal methods of palpating the shoulder tendons occur in regions where there is the least amount of overlying soft tissue.[237]

It is best to divide the shoulder complex into compartments for palpation as symptoms reproduced by palpation in these compartments are frequently associated with a specific underlying pathology.

Anterior and Superior Compartment

The clinician should begin anteriorly, with palpation of the contours of the clavicle. The anterior and superior aspects of the clavicle are covered by the platysma muscle. The sternal end of the clavicle, which projects cranially over the border of the manubrium, is covered by the SCM. The following areas related to the clavicle should be palpated for tenderness, swelling, or symptom reproduction:

- The supraclavicular fossa, bordered medially by the SCM and laterally by the omohyoid.
- The infraclavicular fossa, between the pectoralis major, deltoid, and clavicle. The coracoid process is located in the infraclavicular fossa, especially if the arm is placed in extension. Several palpable ligaments and muscles attach here including the coracoclavicular, on the conoid tubercle, the coracoacromial ligament, the pectoralis minor, the coracobrachialis, and the short head of the biceps. A prominent coracoid could indicate a posterior dislocation of the shoulder.
- The subclavius and costoclavicular ligament.
- The suprasternal (jugular) notch—this indentation on the superior border of the sternal manubrium is an important reference point. Three centimeters above the notch is the inferior border of the larynx, while the sternal bellies of the SCM form the sides of the notch. The interclavicular ligament is located within the notch. Disruption of the normal contours of the notch is associated with S-C dislocations.
- The S-C joint and joint line—arthrotic changes of the S-C joint are evidenced by crepitus at the joint during IR/ER of the humerus with the arm abducted to 90 degrees. The contours of the S-C joint are palpated and a comparison should be made with the contralateral side. Thickening of the S-C, or an S-C dislocation, produces an inability to abduct the arm.
- The A-C joint—injuries and arthritis of this joint are common, and focal tenderness is an important sign of A-C pathology.[190] Changes in the size and shape of the joint may indicate past or present separation, fracture, or osteoarthritis.

With the arm hanging by the side and the palm facing the body, the greater tuberosity lies laterally, and the lesser tuberosity lies anteriorly with respect to each other. They are separated by a bicipital groove. The bicipital groove is made more accessible for palpation with IR of the arm to 15–20 degrees.[237,238] Within this groove lies the biceps tendon, which should be palpated for tenderness. If the arm at rest appears slightly abducted and externally rotated, an anterior dislocation might be present. An adducted and internally rotated arm suggests many shoulder conditions, including a posterior dislocation.

The lesser tuberosity (shaped like an inverted teardrop) is palpated during passive IR and ER of the humerus at a point lateral to the coracoid process. The subscapularis can be palpated deep in the deltopectoral triangle at its insertion into the lesser tuberosity. This is accomplished by positioning the arm by the side in neutral rotation, and palpating just lateral to the coracoid.[237]

The greater tuberosity is located directly anterior to the acromion. It is best located with the patient in side-lying, facing the clinician, with the upper arm in front in approximately 60 degrees of shoulder flexion. The clinician palpates laterally along the spine of the scapula until contact is made with the superior facet of the greater tuberosity. The supraspinatus and posterior coracohumeral ligament insert into the superior facet, the infraspinatus on its middle facet, and the teres minor on its inferior facet. The supraspinatus, located just distal to the anterolateral corner of the acromion, can be made more discernible by positioning the patient's arm behind the back in slight extension.[237,239]

The subacromial–subdeltoid bursa can be palpated by putting the the patient in the prone position, and passively stretching the arm into extension before palpating anterior to the A-C joint. Tenderness reported with shoulder extension and relieved with shoulder flexion is indicative of an inflammation of this bursa.

The anterior joint capsule can be located by palpating one fingerbreadth lateral to the coracoid process with the arm by the side. Persistent tenderness at this point with IR and ER of the arm suggests capsular involvement.[240]

The muscle bellies, origins, and insertions of the upper trapezius, supraspinatus, and levator scapula should be palpated for tenderness or asymmetries.

Lateral Compartment

The deltoid muscle belly and insertion should be palpated for tenderness or atrophy.

Posterior Compartment

The spine of the scapula should be located. The clinician should be able to locate the inferior pole of the scapula, the medial border of the scapula, and the posterior angle of the acromion. The superior angle of the scapula should be level with the second rib, the spine of the scapula with the level of T3, and the inferior border with the level of T7.

The infraspinatus can be palpated just distal to the posterolateral acromion with the arm at 90-degree flexion and 10-degree adduction.[237] The teres minor is isolated and palpated using the same patient position.[237] To help locate the teres minor, the long head of the triceps is palpated by placing the patient's arm at 90 degrees of abduction followed by extension.

Once the long head of the triceps is located, the patient is repositioned and the teres minor, now superior to the long head of the triceps, can be palpated. Tenderness of the posterior capsule suggests capsular laxity.

Inferior Compartment

The lymph nodes in the axilla are palpated for swelling or tenderness. Also located in the inferior compartment are the anterior coracohumeral ligament, G-H ligament, transverse humeral ligament, and pectoralis major. The latissimus dorsi tendon can be palpated deep in the axilla.

The teres major tendon is palpated medial to the supeior part of the latissimus dorsi tendon insertion. It can be differentiated from the latissimus dorsi by using a combination of isometric IR and adduction with the patient's shoulder positioned at 90 degrees of abduction and maximum ER.

The subscapularis tendon is palpable between the serratus anterior and the latissimus dorsi while the patient's arm is elevated.

Active and Passive Range of Motion

Due to the complex nature of the arthrokinematics, osteokinematics, and myokinetics of this region, the results from the active and passive movements can be misleading; therefore care must be taken with interpretation of the findings. Passive testing should be performed when active motion is incomplete. Pain with end-range stress is an important clinical finding. Crepitus can be soft with rotator cuff pathology or harsh with G-H arthritis. Active motion testing provides the clinician with information regarding the following:

- Overall functional capacity of the shoulder.
- Painful or hesitant initiation or termination of movement. Such a hesitation may be a subtle sign of instability or rotator cuff dysfunction.[241]
- Quantity of movement (Table 16-12). Estimation of true G-H motion is performed by fixing the scapula at its inferior border.
- Developed trick movements or modifications to the movement, such as an altered plane, the use of trunk movements, or abnormal recruitment of muscles.
- Associated signs and symptoms not reproduced with nonfunctional motion testing.
- Presence of a capsular pattern (Table 16-13).
- Detection of a "painful arc."
- End-feels (see Table 16-12), if passive overpressure is applied.

McClure and Flowers[242] classify limited shoulder motion into two categories:

- Decreased ROM secondary to changes in the periarticular structures, including shortening of the capsule, ligaments, or muscles, as well as adhesion formation. Clinical findings for this category include a history of trauma,[243–245] immobilization,[243–245] presence of a capsular pattern,[246] capsular end-feel,[246] and no pain with the isometric testing.[246]
- Decreased ROM due to nonstructural problems, including the presence of pain, protective muscle spasm, or a loose body within the joint space.[247] Clinical findings for this

TABLE 16-12 Normal Ranges for Movements of the Shoulder Complex and Potential Causes of Pain

Motion	Range Norms (Degrees)	End-Feel	Potential Source of Pain
Elevation–flexion	170–180	Tissue stretch	▸ Suprahumeral impingement ▸ Stretching of G-H, A-C, S-C joint capsule ▸ Triceps tendon if elbow flexed
Extension	50–60	Tissue stretch	▸ Stretching of G-H I joint capsule ▸ Severe suprahumeral impingement ▸ Biceps tendon if elbow extended
Elevation–abduction	170–180	Tissue stretch	▸ Suprahumeral impingement ▸ A-C joint arthritis at terminal abduction
External rotation	80–90	Tissue stretch	▸ Anterior G-H instability
Internal rotation	60–100	Tissue stretch	▸ Suprahumeral impingement ▸ Posterior G-H instability

Data from Warner JJP, Caborn DNM, Berger RA, et al: Dynamic capsuloligamentous anatomy of the glenohumeral joint. *J Shoulder Elbow Surg* 2:115–133, 1993; Turkel SJ, Panio MW, Marshall JL, et al: Stabilizing mechanisms preventing anterior dislocation of the glenohumeral joint. *J Bone Joint Surg Am* 63:1208–1217, 1981; Data from Pagnani MJ, Warren RF: Stabilizers of the glenohumeral joint. *J Shoulder Elbow Surg* 3:173–190, 1994; O'Connell PW, Nuber GW, Mileski RA, et al: The contribution of the glenohumeral ligaments to anterior stability of the shoulder joint. *Am J Sports Med* 18:579–584, 1990; Karduna AR, Williams GR, Williams JL, et al: Kinematics of the glenohumeral joint: Influences of muscle forces, ligamentous constraints, and articular geometry. *J Orthop Res* 14:986–993, 1996; Davies GJ, DeCarlo MS: Examination of the shoulder complex. In Bandy WD, ed. *Current Concepts in the Rehabilitation of the Shoulder, Sports Physical Therapy Section—Home Study Course*, 1995.

TABLE 16-13	Close Packed, Open Packed, and Capsular Patterns of the Shoulder Complex		
	Close Packed	**Open Packed**	**Capsular Pattern**
Glenohumeral	90 degrees of G-H abduction and full external rotation; or full abduction	55-degree abduction, 30-degree horizontal adduction external rotation	External rotation, abduction, internal rotation
Acromioclavicular	90-degree abduction	Arm resting by side	Pain at extremes of range, especially horizontal adduction and full elevation
Sternoclavicular	Full arm elevation and shoulder protraction	Arm resting by side	Pain at extremes of range, especially horizontal adduction and full elevation

patient include a history of trauma or overuse, and the presence of a noncapsular pattern of motion restriction.

Riddle et al.[248] examined the intratester and intertester reliabilities for clinical goniometric measurements of shoulder passive ROM (PROM) using two different sizes of universal goniometers. Patients were measured without controlling therapist goniometric placement technique or patient position during measurements. Repeated PROM measurements of shoulder flexions VIDEO, extension VIDEO, abduction VIDEO, shoulder horizontal abduction, horizontal adduction, external rotation VIDEO, and internal rotation VIDEO were taken for two groups of 50 subjects each. The intratester intraclass correlation coefficients (ICCs) for all motions ranged from 0.87 to 0.99. The ICCs for the intertester reliability of PROM measurements of horizontal abduction, horizontal adduction, extension, and internal rotation ranged from 0.26 to 0.55. The intertester ICCs for PROM measurements of flexion, abduction, and external rotation ranged from 0.84 to 0.90. Goniometric PROM measurements for the shoulder appear to be highly reliable when taken by the same physical therapist, regardless of the size of the goniometer used.

The patient is asked to bring the arm actively through the ranges of motion. These motions include flexion, extension, abduction, IR (Fig. 16-43), ER, horizontal adduction, and shrugging of the shoulders.

Arm Elevation

The clinician should view the patient carefully as he or she attempts arm elevation. Elevation in the frontal plane (Fig. 16-16) and scapular plane is assessed. Typically, 170–180 degrees of elevation is possible in both of these planes, with the upper portion of the arm being able to be placed adjacent to the head. If the patient is unable to achieve 170–180 degrees, the clinician must determine where and why movement is not occurring. The presence of pain with arm elevation can provide the clinician with valuable information (Fig. 16-17). A common cause of pain with arm elevation is rotator cuff tendinopathy. If there is an arc of pain, the point in the range where the arc of pain occurs can be diagnostic in implicating the cause.

- Pain that occurs between 70 and 110 degrees of abduction is deemed a "painful arc" and may indicate rotator cuff impingement, or tearing, or subacromial bursitis.[76]
- Pain which occurs in the 120–160/160–180-degree range may indicate involvement of the A-C joint.[76]

CLINICAL PEARL

One study[76] attempted to differentiate various types of painful arcs and proposed that adding ER to the painful range indicated subscapularis involvement, or possibly supraspinatus and/or infraspinatus involvement when the pain was increased. Adding IR to the painful range, the supraspinatus and/or infraspinatus was more likely the source of involvement.[76]

Kibler[24] advocates the use of the "muscle assistance" or "scapular assistance" test (SAT) to assess scapular motion and position during elevation and lowering of the arm to see if the impingement may be due to a lack of acromial elevation (Fig. 16-18). As the patient elevates the arm, the clinician pushes laterally and superiorly on the inferior medial border of the scapula to simulate the serratus anterior/lower trapezius force couple. The test is considered positive if the manual

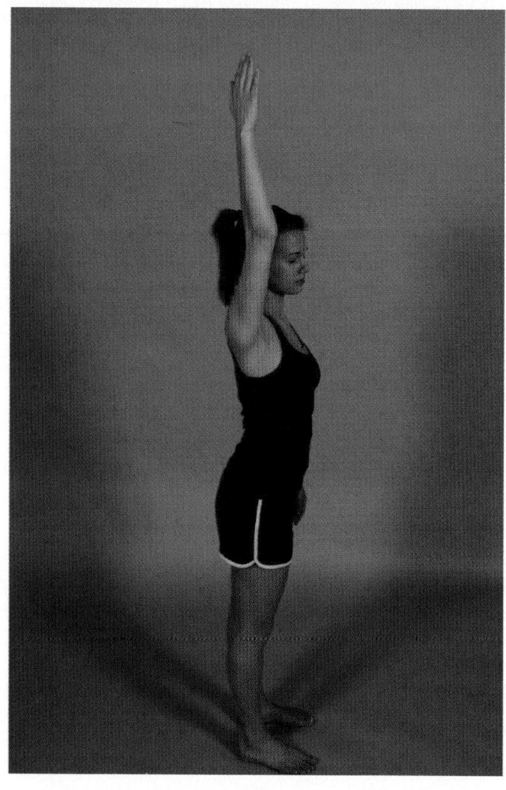

FIGURE 16-16 Elevation in the frontal plane.

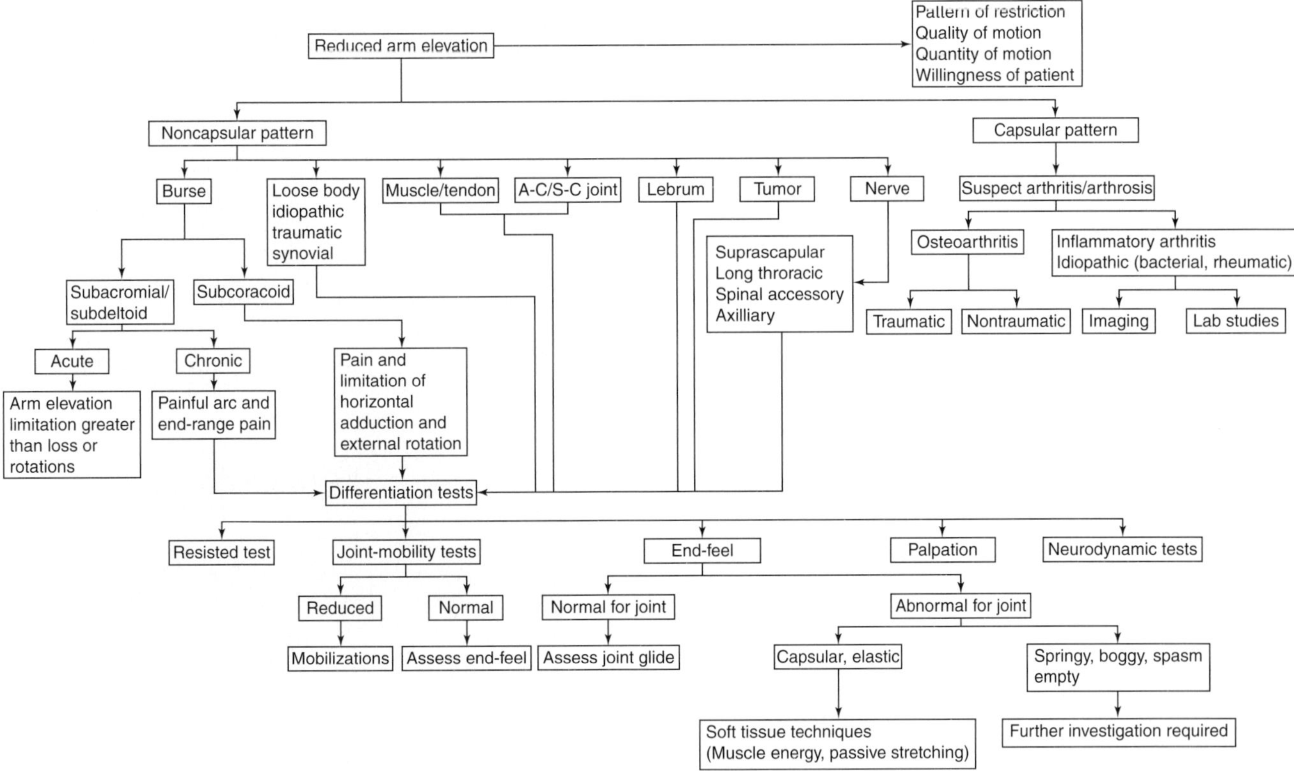

FIGURE 16-17 Causes of painful arm elevation.

assistance diminishes or abolishes the impingement symptoms.[24] The SAT is presumed to indirectly measure the function of the scapula rotators; however, other factors, such as thoracic posture and pectoralis minor length, have also been hypothesized to affect scapular rotation, and it is possible that these could be affected by the manual pressure provided during the SAT.[172,249,250] More importantly, the SAT is used to directly assess the influence of scapular motion on shoulder pain. In a study by Rabin et al.,[172] a modified version of the SAT, which included assisting posterior tipping of the scapula in addition to assisting upward rotation of the scapula, was found to possess acceptable interrater reliability for clinical use to assess the contribution of scapular motion to shoulder pain. The κ coefficient and percent agreement were 0.53 and 77%, respectively, when the test was performed in the scapular plane, and 0.62 and 91%, respectively, when the test was performed in the sagittal plane. In the modified version, the clinician places one hand on the superior aspect of the involved scapula, with the fingers over the clavicle. The other hand is placed over the inferior angle of the scapular so that the heel of the hand is just over the inferior angle and the fingers are wrapped around the lateral aspect of the thorax. The patient is asked to actively elevate his or her arm in the scapular plane, and during the movement the clinician facilitates upward rotation of the scapula by pushing upward and laterally on the inferior angle, as well as tilting the scapula posteriorly by pulling backwards on the superior aspect of the scapula.

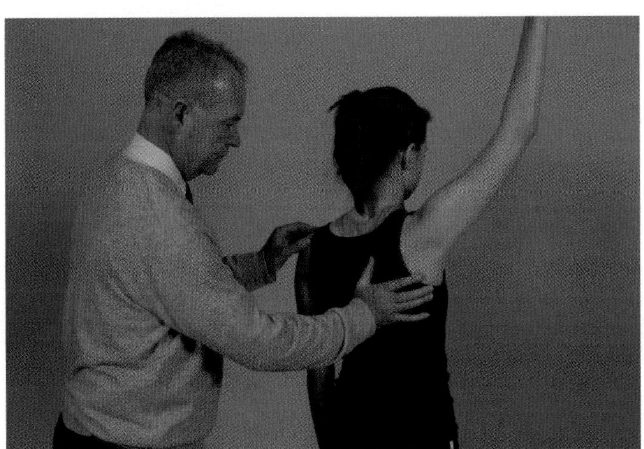

FIGURE 16-18 Scapular assist.

Weakness of the serratus anterior muscle, due to palsy or disuse, produces winging of the scapula as the patient attempts to elevate the arm.[4,111,113] In addition to winging, serratus anterior dysfunction presents with loss of scapular protraction during attempted shoulder elevation and the inferior tip of the scapula becomes prominent.[110]

Abduction of the shoulder requires a greater use of the upper and lower trapezius muscles, whereas shoulder flexion is more likely to recruit the serratus anterior muscle.[87,181]

Although lesions to the deltoid are rare, imbalances of the deltoid and the rotator cuff are common. When the deltoid becomes dominant, the humeral head is seen to glide superiorly during arm elevation because the downward pull of the rotator cuff muscles is insufficient to counterbalance the upward pull of the deltoid (*humeral superior glide syndrome*).[206] This alteration in the G-H force couple usually occurs during the middle phase of elevation[170] (between 80 and 140 degrees), because the upward translation force of the deltoid peaks during this phase, requiring more compressive and depressive forces from the rotator cuff muscles.[251,252]

An anterior glide of the humeral head, which occurs during arm elevation (*humeral anterior glide syndrome*)[206] suggests that the posterior deltoid has become the dominant external rotator.[206] This syndrome should be suspected if the pain is located in the anterior or anterior medial aspect of the shoulder and is increased by G-H IR, shoulder hyperextension, and horizontal abduction, and is decreased when the humeral head is prevented from moving anteriorly during shoulder rotation and flexion movements.[206]

When compared, the range achieved for unilateral elevation should be greater than that achieved when bilateral arm elevation is attempted. This is because the joints of the cervicothoracic junction have to be permitted to rotate toward the elevating arm. The clinician should observe the smoothness of the scapulohumeral rhythm during elevation and the ratio between the scapular upward rotation and G-H elevation (see "Examination of the Dynamic Scapula" section).

Compressive forces across the A-C joint occur mainly in the terminal 60 degrees of abduction. This often causes pain during this range if pathology exists at this joint.[190]

Extension

Active extension (Fig. 16-19) is normally 50–60 degrees. Care must be taken when measuring this motion as substitutions can occur to seemingly increase extension by bending forward at the waist or by retracting the scapula. Asymmetry of shoulder extension can indicate weakness of the posterior deltoid in one arm (swallowtail sign).

Rotation

The following arm positions can be used to assess IR and ER:

- The arm at shoulder level (at 90 degrees of shoulder abduction, 90 degrees of elbow flexion and with the palm parallel to the floor). Normal ER (Fig. 16-20), which is performed by rotating the hand toward the floor, is 90 degrees or beyond. Assessing ER in this position is helpful in determining the presence of a fracture of the greater tuberosity, or a decrement in the performance of a throwing athlete. IR is then carried out (Fig. 16-21), rotating the hand toward the hip, as if positioning it behind the body. Normal IR approaches 90 degrees. However, this test position is often uncomfortable and not very functional, except for pitchers.

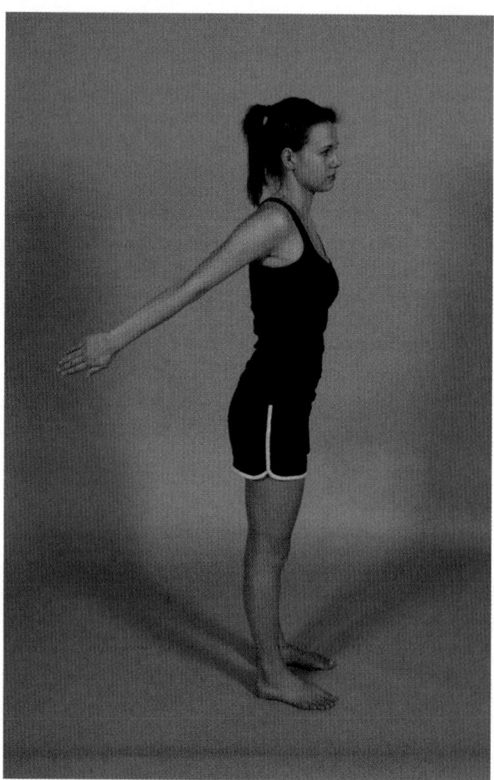

FIGURE 16-19 Shoulder extension AROM.

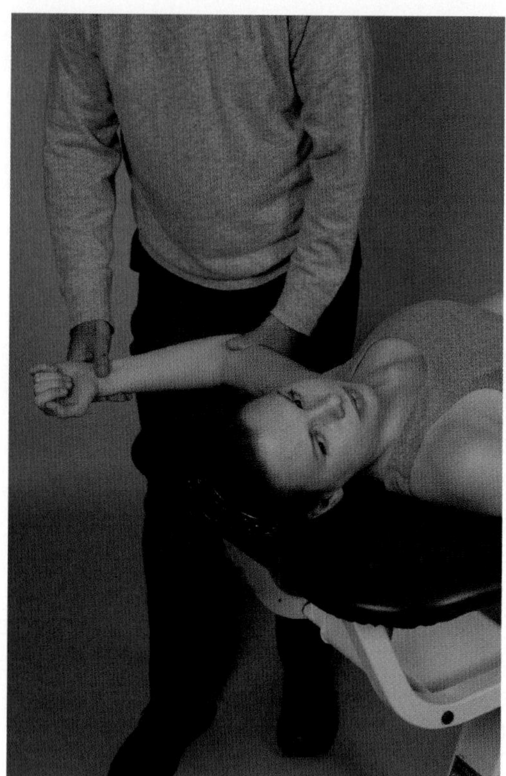

FIGURE 16-20 Shoulder external rotation in supine.

- The arm to the side and the elbow flexed to 90 degrees. ER is performed by moving the hand away from midline (Fig. 16-22), and IR is performed by moving the hand toward the abdomen (Fig. 16-23). Again, it is important to assess active and passive range, because a loss of active motion alone may indicate muscular weakness.
- The arm at the side and the forearm behind the back (Apley scratch test). This measurement for IR is assessed by the position reached with the extended thumb up the posterior (dorsal) aspect of the spine using the spinous processes as landmarks (Fig. 16-24).[253] This is more of a functional test, and the thumb tip of normal subjects will reach the T5–T10 level.[190] Loss of motion with this test affects the patient's ability to perform toileting duties, hook bras behind the back, reach into a back pocket, and tuck in shirts.[254] The examination is made relative to the opposite side, as there is quite a large variation in range among normal subjects. In a study by Hoving et al.,[255] which assessed the intrarater and interrater reliability among rheumatologists of a

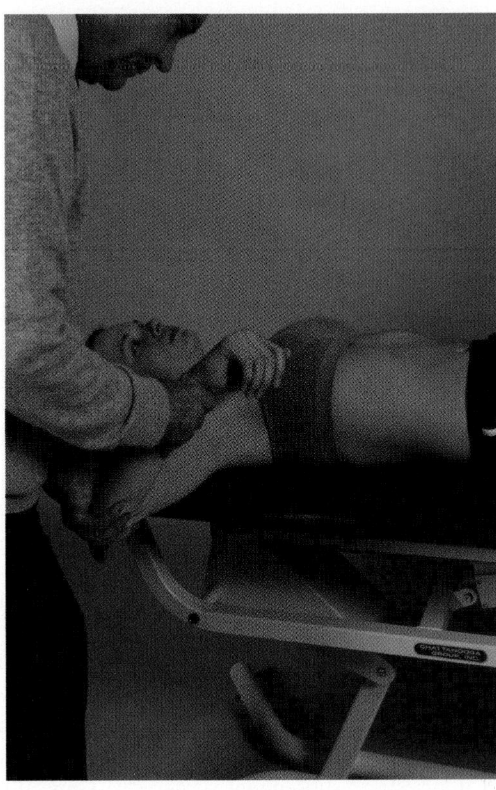

FIGURE 16-21 Shoulder internal rotation in supine.

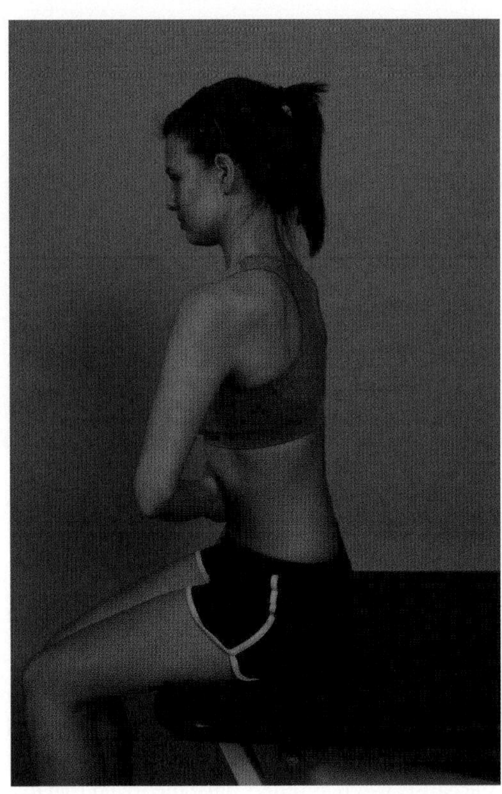

FIGURE 16-23 Shoulder internal rotation in sitting.

standardized protocol for measurement of shoulder movements, the movement of the hand behind the back (and total shoulder flexion) yielded the highest ICC scores for both intrarater reliability (0.91 and 0.83, respectively) and interrater reliability (0.80 and 0.72, respectively). However, in a study by Edwards et al.,[256] measurement of IR by vertebral level was not readily reproducible between observers.

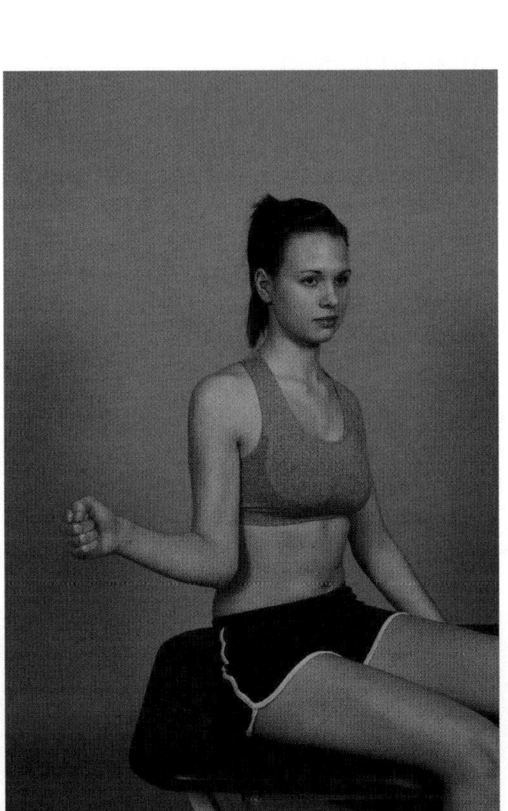

FIGURE 16-22 Shoulder external rotation in the upright position.

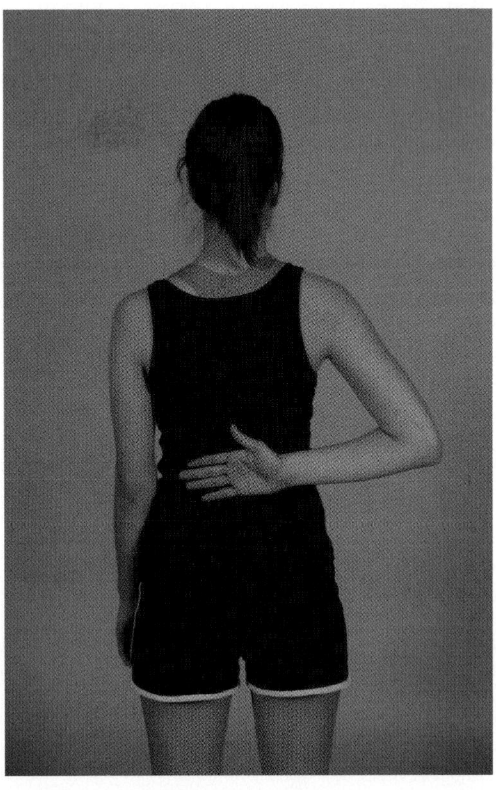

FIGURE 16-24 Apley scratch test.

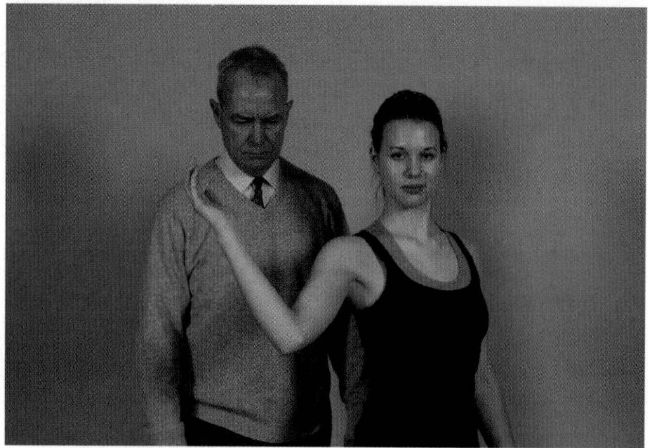

FIGURE 16-25 Shoulder ER at 45-degree abduction.

- The arm at 45-degree abduction in the scapular plane (Fig. 16-25). This position is used to assess ER for overhead athletes.

Most overhead athletes exhibit excessive ER and decreased IR. The cause of this adaptation has not been established, with some authors[257–260] documenting humeral osseous retroversion as the cause, whereas others have theorized that excessive ER and limited IR are due to anterior capsular laxity and posterior capsule tightness,[261] although no clinical studies have confirmed these findings to date. G-H IR deficit (GIRD) and posterior shoulder tightness (PST) have been linked to shoulder dysfunction based on a study series by Burkhart et al.[261–263] In cadaveric studies, tightening the posterior capsule by plication has been shown to increase anterior G-H translation during flexion and cross-body adduction, cause superior G-H translation with flexion and ER of the G-H joint, and markedly decrease IR.[46,264,265] Similarly, GIRD and PST have been demonstrated in throwing athletes with internal impingement[266] and in patients with secondary impingement.[267] However, the theory of posterior capsule tightness has come into question from other researchers who have determined that ROM in baseball pitchers—specifically, a loss of IR—does not correlate with an alteration in posterior G-H translation.[268,269]

CLINICAL PEARL

Three terms can be used to describe the relationship between IR and ER of the G-H joint[261]:

- GIRD: defined as the difference in IR between the two shoulders. Normally the difference should be within 20 degrees. GIRD results from posterior capsule shortening and has been shown to predispose baseball pitchers to a higher potential for shoulder injury.
- Glenohumeral ER gain (GERG): defined as the difference in ER between two shoulders.
  - If the GIRD/GERG ratio is greater than one, the patient will likely develop shoulder problems.[262]
- Total rotational motion (TRM): determined by adding the amount of ER and IR at 90 degrees of abduction to determine the TRM arc.

It is important not to disregard the effect of muscle forces on these biomechanical changes. Reinold et al.[270] recently examined the PROM of the shoulder in 31 professional baseball pitchers, before and immediately after pitching. The researchers reported that rotational range of G-H motion was immediately affected by overhead throwing and that mean IR ROM after pitching significantly decreased (73 ± 16 degrees before, 65 ± 11 degrees after) and total rotational motion decreased (average, 9 degrees). Mean ER before throwing (133 ± 11 degrees) did not significantly change after throwing (131 ± 10 degrees). The researchers hypothesized that this decrease in IR ROM was due to large eccentric forces being generated in the external rotators during the follow-through phase of throwing that caused microscopic muscle damage in the posterior shoulder musculature. Previous studies examining the effect of repetitive eccentric contractions have shown a subsequent loss of joint ROM in the upper and lower extremities following testing.[271–273]

Wilk et al.[274] proposed the TRM concept, where the amount of ER and IR at 90 degrees of abduction are added and a TRM arc is determined. The authors reported that the TRM in the throwing shoulders of professional baseball pitchers is within 5 degrees of the nonthrowing shoulder[274] and that a TRM arc outside the 5-degree range may be a contributing factor to shoulder injuries and subsequent surgery.[275] Thus, although the dominant shoulder has greater ER and less IR, the combined total motion should be equal bilaterally.[270]

CLINICAL PEARL

It is likely that bilateral comparisons of ER and IR are not useful in the assessment of the overhead athlete.

Horizontal Adduction

Horizontal adduction is performed by bringing the arm across in front of the body (Fig. 16-26). Pain with horizontal adduction may indicate A-C joint pathology (see "Crossover Impingement/Horizontal Adduction Test" section). Horizontal adduction is normally 130 degrees compared with 50–75 degrees if the arm is brought in front of the body.

The patient then completes the motions of shoulder girdle elevation (shrug) and depression and shoulder protraction

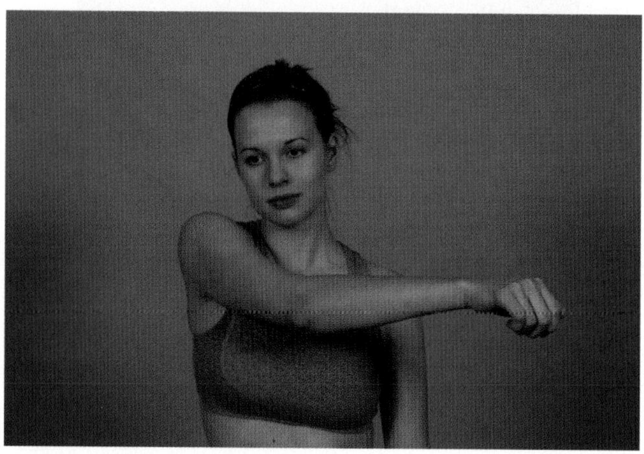

FIGURE 16-26 Horizontal adduction.

and retraction. An inability to shrug the shoulder may indicate a trapezius palsy.[110] Hiking of the shoulder and the scapular during arm elevation is often seen in patients with large rotator cuff tears.[195]

Movement combinations are assessed.

CLINICAL PEARL

If pain is reproduced when IR and extension are combined from a position of 90-degree abduction, the A-C joint, subcoracoid bursa, or subscapularis tendon may be implicated.

If the pain is reproduced with extension with the humerus at 90 degrees of flexion, the shoulder abductors, external rotators, and suprascapular nerve may be implicated. A jammed end-feel with this maneuver may indicate a thoracic dysfunction.

An isolated limitation of passive ER may indicate subcoracoid bursitis, which is aggravated by the pectoralis major muscle being stretched over it.[251]

PROM is performed if there is a deficiency in active motion to determine the end-feel.[246] Traditionally, PROM has been performed with the patient positioned in supine Given the importance of scapular motion during humeral elevation, care must be taken to not prevent the scapula from rotating during these tests.

A discrepancy between active and passive motion may indicate a painful periarticular condition.[227] Loss of active motion with preservation of passive motion is likely caused by a rotator cuff tear,[61] or rarely, suprascapular nerve injury.[201,276] A severely restricted active abduction pattern with no pain is suggestive of a rupture of the supraspinatus or deltoid. Loss of both active and passive motion is usually caused by adhesive capsulitis.[205]

A loss of PROM or active ROM (AROM) may be associated with a loss of flexibility in the passive restraints to motion. This can occur with both single plane motions and combined motions.[37,277–280] For example, if both IR and ER are restricted and muscle tightness has been ruled out as a cause, an adhesion of the middle G-H ligament is implicated.[280]

Examination of the Dynamic Scapula

Given the importance of the scapulothoracic joint to overall shoulder function, it is important to examine the scapulothoracic joint arthrokinematics and muscle power.[281]

A number of muscles play an important role in the kinematics of the scapula, including the trapezius and serratus anterior. Increased activity of the upper trapezius muscle, or imbalances between the upper and the lower trapezius muscle, during shoulder elevation may have adverse effects on the kinematics of the scapula.[93,115,183,282]

According to Sahrmann,[206] four abnormal clinical findings exist for the scapula:

- The scapular alignment is correct but its movement is impaired.
- The scapular alignment is impaired and its movement is impaired.
- The scapular alignment is impaired and its movement is of normal range, but does not correct or compensate for the impaired start position.
- The scapular alignment is impaired but its movement is sufficient to compensate for the impaired start position.

Kibler[24] recommends the use of the isometric "scapular pinch" test to examine the strength of the medial scapular muscles. This involves the patient squeezing his or her shoulder blades together (Fig. 16-27). Normally, the scapula can be held in this position for 15–20 seconds without difficulty. If a burning pain occurs in less than 15 seconds, Kibler suggests that scapular muscle weakness may be the cause.[24]

Observation of the scapulohumeral rhythm and scapulothoracic motion should reveal that the scapula stops its rotation when the arm has been elevated to approximately 140 degrees. Upon completion of the elevation, the inferior angle of the scapula should be in close proximity to the midline of the thorax, and the vertebral border of the scapular should be rotated 60 degrees. Movement beyond these points may indicate excessive scapular abduction.[206] At the end range of elevation, the scapula should slightly depress, posteriorly tilt, and adduct.[206] The motion of the scapula should be assessed carefully in patients with suspected multidirectional instability. A scapulothoracic dyskinesia (decrease in scapular abduction and ER with progressive arm abduction) is often observed in patients with anteroinferior instability.[283] Posteroinferior instability is characterized by excessive scapular retraction.[238] An inferior instability is characterized by a drooping of the lateral scapula or "scapular dumping."[238]

After positioning the patient in prone with his or her arm abducted to 90 degrees, ER is carried out to test the ability of the scapula to remain in its correct position rather than

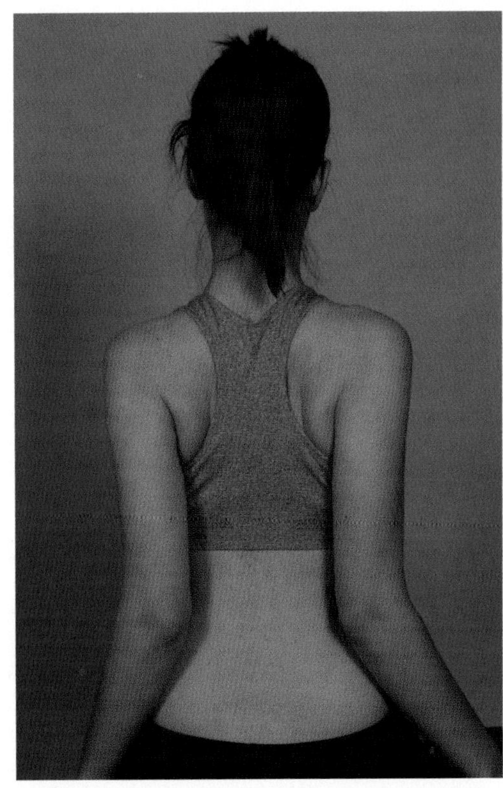

FIGURE 16-27 Scapular pinch.

abducting due to excessive lengthening of the thoracoscapular muscles (trapezius and rhomboids) and shortening of the scapulohumeral muscles.[206]

Resistive Tests

In addition to pain, shoulder dysfunction is often caused or exacerbated by a loss of motion or weakness. The resistive tests assess function in the important muscle groups of the upper kinetic chain (Tables 16-14 and 16-15).

Localized, individual isometric muscle tests around the shoulder girdle can give the clinician information about patterns of pain and weakness and with information regarding weakness resulting from a spinal nerve root or peripheral nerve palsy. A general assessment of shoulder strength is initially performed, testing flexion, extension, abduction, adduction, IR, and ER. Weakness on isometric testing needs to be analyzed for the type—increasing weakness with repeated contractions of the same resistance indicating a palsy versus consistent weakness with repeated contractions, which could suggest a deconditioned muscle or a significant muscle tear—and the pattern (spinal nerve root, nerve trunk, or peripheral nerve). A painful weakness (see Chap. 5) is invariably a sign of serious pathology and, depending on the pattern, could indicate a fracture or a tumor. However, if a single motion is painfully weak, this could indicate muscle inhibition due to pain. The various motions of shoulder can be assessed through their arcs of motion both concentrically and eccentrically against resistance, as appropriate.

TABLE 16-14 Muscle Groups Tested in the Shoulder Examination
Trunk flexors, extensors, and obliques
Scapulothoracic elevators
Scapulothoracic depressors
Scapulothoracic protractors
Scapulothoracic retractors
Scapulothoracic upward rotators
Scapulothoracic downward rotators
Glenohumeral flexors
Glenohumeral extensors
Glenohumeral abductors
Glenohumeral adductors
Glenohumeral internal rotators
Glenohumeral external rotators
Glenohumeral horizontal flexors
Glenohumeral horizontal extensors
Elbow flexors
Elbow extensors
Forearm supinators
Forearm pronators
Wrist flexors
Wrist extensors
Hand intrinsics

Data from Davies GJ, DeCarlo MS: Examination of the shoulder complex. In: Bandy WD, ed. *Current Concepts in the Rehabilitation of the Shoulder, Sports Physical Therapy Section—Home Study Course*, 1995.

CLINICAL PEARL

Pain with isometric muscle testing is generally considered a sign of first- or second-degree musculotendinous lesion (see Chap. 4). According to Cyriax,[246] pain that occurs during a muscle contraction is more likely to indicate a lesion within a muscle belly, whereas pain that occurs on release of the contraction is more likely to indicate a lesion within a tendon.[251] However, because of the large amount of accessory joint gliding that occurs in the shoulder girdle joints with isometric contraction, the tests for inert tissue involvement must be negative before coming to the conclusion that only the musculotendinous structure is at fault.

TABLE 16-15 Shoulder Girdle Muscle Function and Innervation

Muscles	Peripheral Nerve	Nerve Root	Motions
Pectoralis major	Pectoral	C5–C8	Adduction, horizontal adduction, and internal rotation Clavicular fibers: forward flexion Sternocostal fibers: extension
Latissimus dorsi	Thoracodorsal	C7 (C6, C8)	Adduction, extension, and internal rotation
Teres major	Subscapular	C5–C8	Adduction, extension, horizontal abduction, and internal rotation
Teres minor	Axillary	C5(6)	Horizontal abduction (also a weak external rotator)
Deltoid	Axillary	C5(6)	Anterior: forward flexion, horizontal adduction Middle: abduction Posterior: extension, horizontal abduction
Supraspinatus	Suprascapular	C5(6)	Abduction
Subscapularis	Subscapular	C5–C8	Adduction, and internal rotation
Infraspinatus	Suprascapular	C5(C6)	Abduction, horizontal abduction, and external rotation

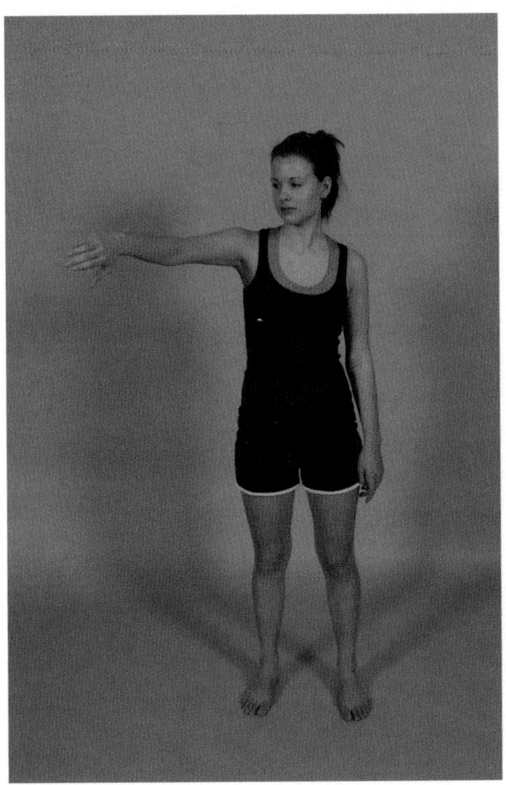

FIGURE 16-28 Jobe or empty-can test for supraspinatus.

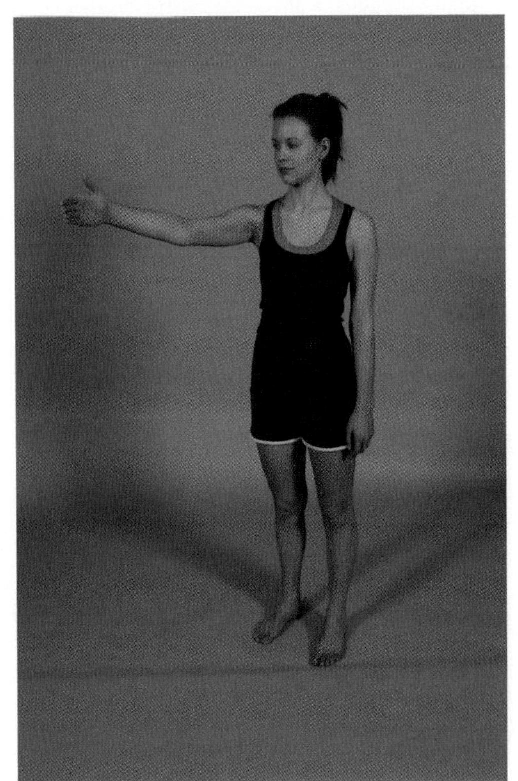

FIGURE 16-29 Full-can test.

A number of resistive tests have been designed to isolate the muscles of the shoulder complex. Cyriax[275] believed that supraspinatus tendinitis is the most common cause of a painful arc. The supraspinatus can be tested using the Jobe test or empty-can position (Fig. 16-28) **VIDEO**. The patient's arm is positioned in IR within the scaption plane, at approximately 90 degrees of shoulder flexion. Manual resistance is then applied by the clinician in a direction toward the floor. The Jobe test can be performed similarly with the humerus externally rotated (full-can test) (Fig. 16-29) **VIDEO**. One study[284] found the empty-can test to have a high sensitivity of 86% and a low specificity of 50% in diagnosing supraspinatus tendon tears in a series of 55 patients. However, in another study,[285] the full-can test had higher specificity (74% vs. 68%) and an equal sensitivity of 77% when compared with the empty-can test in a series of 136 patients.

A partial rupture of the supraspinatus tendon will result in abduction that is both weak and painful.[69] A painless weakness with abduction could indicate a complete rupture of the supraspinatus tendon, although the deltoid cannot be ruled out. The tendon of the supraspinatus can be passively stretched by positioning it in adduction and IR to see if this increases the pain.[286]

It has been documented that if coracohumeral pain decreases with the addition of arm traction during resisted abduction, subacromial–subdeltoid bursitis or an A-C joint lesion should be suspected.[287] However, this was not found to be the case with ultrasonography.[288]

The test position for the *infraspinatus* and *teres minor* muscles is 90 degrees of G-H flexion and one-half full ER (Fig. 16-30).[120] If the pain is isolated to ER, then the infraspinatus is at fault. If ER and resisted adduction are painful, the teres minor is at fault, although isolated involvement of the teres minor is not common. To test the teres minor further, the muscle is placed on stretch by putting the patient in prone position with his or her upper arms vertical, adducted, and externally rotated to approximately 20 degrees. The patient is asked to lean toward the tested side to increase the adduction.

The *teres major* muscle can be tested by putting the patient in the prone position with his or her hand resting on his or her lower back (Fig. 16-31) **VIDEO**. The patient is asked to adduct and extend the humerus while the clinician applies resistance at the elbow into shoulder abduction.

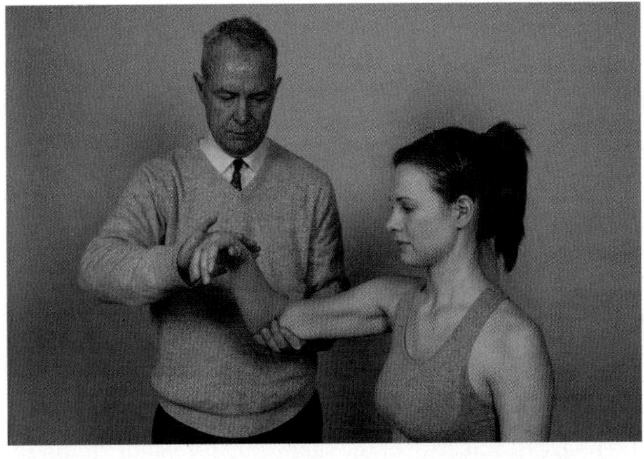

FIGURE 16-30 Resisted test for infraspinatus and teres minor.

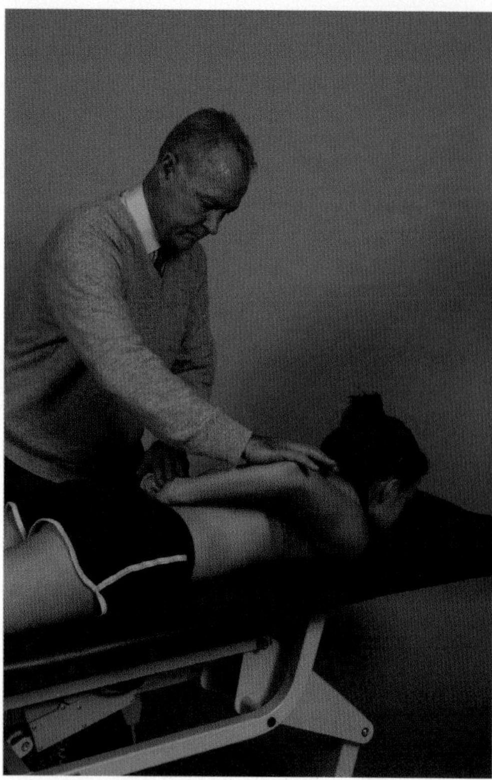

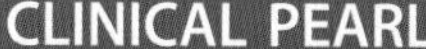

FIGURE 16-31 Resisted test for teres major.

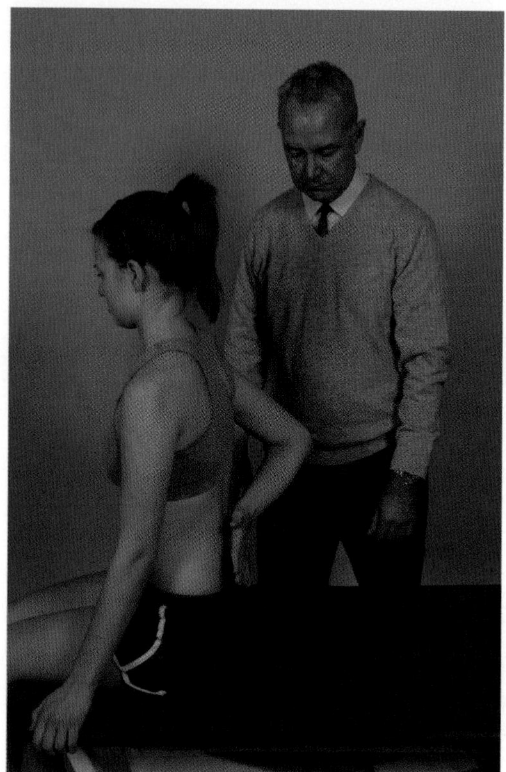

FIGURE 16-32 Lift-off test.

CLINICAL PEARL

A proper balance between agonist and antagonist muscle groups is necessary to provide dynamic stabilization to the shoulder joint.[289] For example to provide proper muscle balance, the G-H joint external rotator muscles should be at least 65% of the strength of the internal rotator muscles.[290] Ideally though, the ER–IR muscle strength ratio should be 66–75%.[290]

To assess for *rhomboid* dominance, the patient positions their arms by their side with their elbow flexed to approximately 90 degrees. Resisted ER in this position should not result in any scapular adduction, unless there is rhomboid dominance and poor control of G-H ER.[206] There should also be no superior or anterior gliding of the humerus during this test, unless deltoid dominance is occurring.[206]

Conditions to be ruled out if there is a painless weakness of ER include, but are not limited to, the following:

- A complete rupture of the infraspinatus tendon
- A C5 nerve root palsy
- A suprascapular nerve palsy
- Neuralgic amyotrophy

The *subscapularis* is best assessed using the lift-off test as described by Gerber and Krushell. The lift-off test is performed with the arm internally rotated so that the posterior surface of the hand rests on the lower back. Actively lifting the hand away from the back (Fig. 16-32) against a resisting force suggest integrity of the subscapularis. Failure to do so indicates a subscapularis tear. The test has been found to have a sensitivity of 80% and a specificity of 100% for a tear of the subscapularis.[291] A similar test is the IR lag sign test (see "Special Tests" section).

Resisted adduction is tested with the arm at 0 degree of abduction so that the subscapularis is not facilitated.[291] Pain with resisted adduction tends to be fairly rare, but could implicate the pectoralis major, latissimus dorsi, teres major, and teres minor.

CLINICAL PEARL

A patient with subacromial–subdeltoid bursitis, in the absence of a rotator cuff tear, will often demonstrate weakness of the rotator cuff secondary to pain if tested with the arm positioned in the arc of impingement. It will, however, show good strength if tested with the arm out of abduction. A patient with a significant cuff tear usually demonstrates profound weakness of the rotator cuff throughout various arm positions.

Testing of *deltoid* function is best done with resisted abduction with the arm at 90 degrees of abduction and neutral rotation (Fig. 16-33) **VIDEO**.[190] A painful arc cannot be produced by a lesion to the deltoid muscle due to its anatomical position.

Differential diagnosis will be needed to rule out several neurological disorders, which may provoke painless weakness on resisted abduction. These include an axillary nerve palsy, a suprascapular nerve palsy, or a fifth cervical root palsy.

The three components of the *trapezius* are assessed as follows:

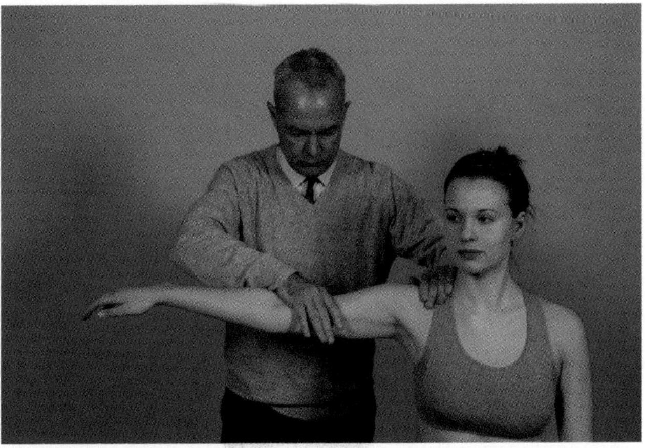

FIGURE 16-33 Resisted deltoid.

- *Upper trapezius (and levator scapulae).* Usually both sides are tested simultaneously. The patient is asked to shrug the shoulders to the ears. If the patient is unable to perform this action, he or she lies in the supine position to eliminate the effect of gravity and asked to repeat the test. Resistance is applied by the clinician in an attempt to depress the shoulders VIDEO. Unilateral resistance can be applied to the posterior lateral aspect of the head while stabilizing the shoulder.
- *Middle trapezius.* The patient lies in the prone position with the shoulder joint abducted to 90 degrees, elbow extended, and the forearm in maximum supination so that the thumb is pointing to the ceiling (Fig. 16-34) VIDEO. The clinician applies pressure on the humerus by pushing toward the floor.
- *Lower trapezius.* The patient lies in the prone position, with the upper limb supported in the elevated position and aligned in the direction of the lower trapezius muscle fibers (Fig. 16-35) VIDEO. Grades 0–2 are determined by the firmness of the muscle contraction. Grades 2+ and 3− are based on how far the limb is lifted from the table. Grades 3–5 require the application of resistance by the clinician.

As discussed in the biomechanics section, proper scapular movement and stability are imperative for asymptomatic

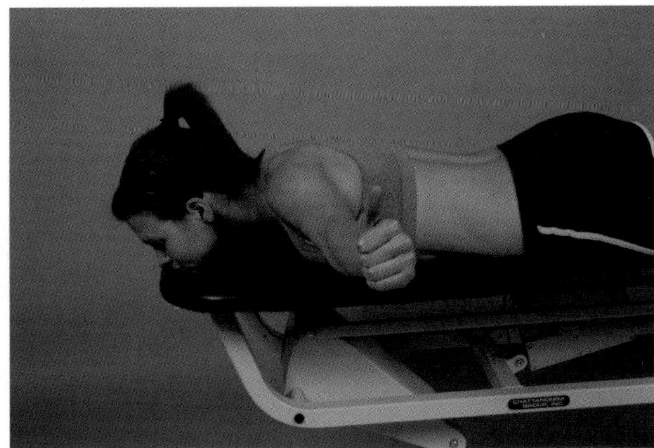

FIGURE 16-34 Middle trapezius test.

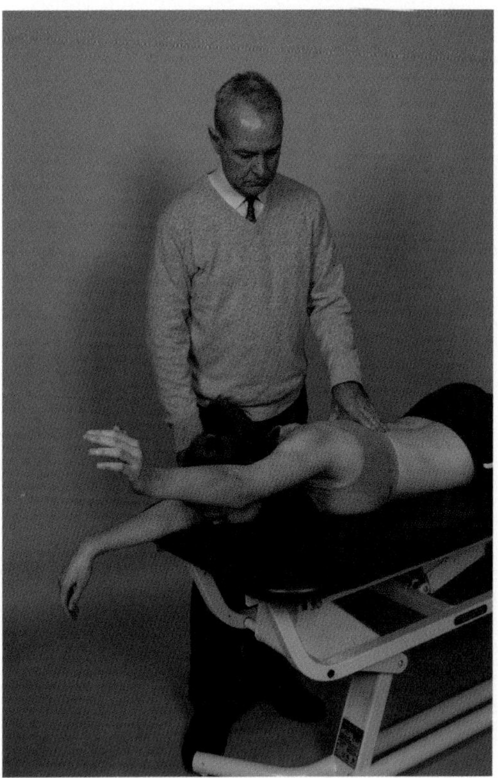

FIGURE 16-35 Lower trapezius test.

shoulder function.[24] The *serratus anterior* can be assessed in a number of ways VIDEO, including using the wall push-up. A more sensitive test involves putting the patient in the supine position with his or her shoulder flexed to 90 degrees and their elbow flexed. The patient is asked to protract the shoulder by lifting the elbow to the ceiling. Resistance is applied by the clinician at the hand, pushing downward (Fig. 16-36). Given that the serratus anterior functions to control upward rotation of the scapula during arm elevation, this ability should also be assessed.

Finally, resisted elbow flexion and extension, as well as forearm supination (see Chap. 17), are examined to assess the *biceps* VIDEO, *brachialis* VIDEO, and *triceps* function VIDEO. Isometric elbow extension and flexion with the muscles in a stretched position will help exclude the biceps and triceps muscles. Pain reproduced with resisted elbow flexion could indicate a lesion to one or more of the elbow flexors, such as an intra-articular lesion of the LHB or a lesion in the sulcus of the LHB. The sulcus lesion can be tested with the patient side-lying, facing away from the clinician, and their arm hanging behind them. The clinician stabilizes the scapula and applies a longitudinal force along the humerus in a superior direction to drive the humerus superiorly. A positive sign is pain reproduced with this maneuver.

A painless weakness of elbow flexion can result from a fifth cervical root palsy, or a sixth cervical root palsy (a complete rupture of all of the elbow flexors is an extremely unlikely event.)

The wrist and hand are also evaluated for motor function as appropriate (see Chap. 18).

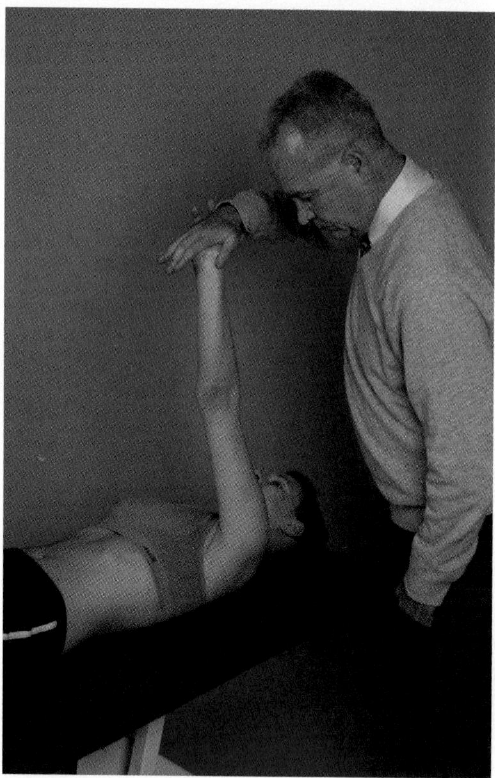

FIGURE 16-36 Serratus anterior test.

Examination of Movement Patterns

These tests are concerned with the coordination, timing, or sequence of activation of the muscles during movement.[206]

Serratus Anterior

The patient lies in the prone position and is asked to perform a push-up and then return to the start position extremely slowly. The clinician checks for the quality of scapula stabilization. If the stabilizers are weak, the scapula on the side of impairment will shift outward and upward with a resultant winging of the scapula.

Shoulder Abduction

The patient sits with his or her elbow flexed to control the humeral rotation. The patient is asked to slowly abduct the arm. Three components are evaluated:

- Abduction at the G-H joint
- Rotation of the scapula
- Elevation of the whole shoulder girdle—the abduction movement is stopped at the point at which the shoulder begins to elevate; this typically occurs at approximately 60 degrees of G-H abduction

Functional Testing

The assessment of shoulder function is an integral part of the examination of the shoulder complex. Functional testing of the shoulder complex can include tests designed to detect a biomechanical dysfunction or tests designed to assess the patient's ability to perform the basic functions of ADL. Given the number of different shoulder conditions that exist, it is important to remember that each of the following functional tests may have specific limited applications.

Biomechanical Function

There are only two functional motions within the shoulder girdle: arm elevation using a combination of flexion and abduction and arm extension with adduction. All other motions of the shoulder are parts or composites of these two basic functional sets.

Basic Function Testing

By referring to Table 16-16, the clinician can determine the functional status of the shoulder for basic functions simply by measuring the amount of available ROM. For example, humeral motions necessary for eating and drinking have been reported at 5–45 degrees of flexion, 5–35 degrees of abduction, and 5–25 degrees of IR relative to the trunk.[292] Combing hair has been found to require 112 degrees of arm elevation.[162]

Mannerkorpi[293] used three functional tests (hand-to-neck, hand-to-scapula, and hand-to-opposite scapula) to assess shoulder dysfunction in patients with fibromyalgia (Table 16-17). Yang and Lin[294] assessed the intertester and intratester reliability of these functional tests and found them to be reliable for documenting reduced function of the shoulder.

TABLE 16-16 Range of Motion Necessary at the Shoulder for Functional Activities

Activity	Necessary Range of Motion
Eating	70–100-degrees horizontal adduction 45–60-degrees abduction
Combing hair	30–70-degrees horizontal adduction 105–120-degrees abduction 90-degrees external rotation
Reach perineum	75–90-degrees horizontal abduction 30–45-degrees abduction 90-degrees or greater internal rotation
Tuck in shirt	50–60-degrees horizontal abduction 55–65-degrees abduction 90-degrees internal rotation
Position hand behind head	10–15-degrees horizontal adduction 110–125-degrees forward flexion 90-degrees external rotation
Put an item on a shelf	70–80-degrees horizontal adduction 70–80-degrees forward flexion 45-degrees external rotation
Wash opposite shoulder	60–90-degrees forward flexion 60–120-degrees horizontal adduction

Data from Matsen FH III, Lippitt SB, Sidles JA, et al: *Practical Evaluation of Management of the Shoulder.* Philadelphia, PA: WB Saunders, 1994:19–150; Magee DJ: *Shoulder, Orthopaedic Physical Assessment.* Philadelphia, PA: WB Saunders, 1992:90–142.

TABLE 16-17 Function-Related Tests

Hand to back of neck (shoulder flexion and external rotation)[a]	0	The fingers reach the posterior median line of the neck with the shoulder in full abduction and external rotation without wrist extension
	1	The fingers reach the median line of the neck but do not have full abduction and/or external rotation
	2	The fingers reach the median line of the neck, but with compensation by adduction in the horizontal plane or by shoulder elevation
	3	The fingers touch the neck
	4	The fingers do not reach the neck
Hand to scapula (shoulder extension and internal rotation)[b]	0	The hand reaches behind the trunk to the opposite scapula or 5 cm beneath it in full internal rotation. The wrist is not laterally deviated
	1	The hand almost reaches the opposite scapula, 6–15 cm beneath it
	2	The hand reaches the opposite iliac crest
	3	The hand reaches the buttock
	4	Subject cannot move the hand behind the trunk
Hand to opposite scapula (shoulder horizontal adduction)[c]	0	The hand reaches to the spine of opposite scapula in full adduction without wrist flexion
	1	The hand reaches to the spine of the opposite scapula in full adduction
	2	The hand passes the midline of the trunk
	3	The hand cannot pass the midline of the trunk

[a]This test measures an action essential for daily activities, such as using the arm to reach, pull, or hang an object overhead or using the arm to pick up and drink a cup of water.

[b]This test measures an action essential for daily activities, such as using the arm to pull an object out of a back pocket or tasks related to personal care.

[c]This test measures an action important for daily activities, such as using the arm to reach across the body to get a car's seat belt or using the arm to turn a steering wheel.

Data from Mannerkorpi K, Svantesson U, Carlsson J, et al: Tests of functional limitations in fibromyalgia syndrome: A reliability study. *Arthritis Care Res* 12:193–199, 1999.

The assessment tool outlined in Table 16-18 can also be used as a functional test of the shoulder. Several generic and region-specific outcome tools have been developed and used to document outcomes of patients with shoulder pathologies.

Shoulder Outcome Scales

A number of shoulder scales have been developed. Five of the most commonly used shoulder outcome scales are the University of California–Los Angeles (UCLA) shoulder scale, the simple shoulder test (SST), the shoulder pain and disability index (SPADI), the disabilities of the arm, shoulder, and hand (DASH), and the Penn Shoulder Score (PSS).

University of California–Los Angeles (UCLA) Shoulder Scale. The self-report section of the UCLA Shoulder Scale consists of two single-item subscales, one for pain and the other for functional level (Table 16-19). The items are Likert-type (a psychometric scale) and scored from 1 to 10, with higher scores indicating less pain and greater function.[295]

The Simple Shoulder Test. Lippitt et al.[296] advocate the use of the SST (Table 16-20). The SST is a standardized self-assessment of shoulder function consisting of 12 yes/no questions. The SST has high test and retest reproducibility and is sensitive to a wide variety of shoulder disorders.[296] In addition, the SST has been shown to be a practical tool for documenting the efficacy of treatment for shoulder conditions. Patients without rotator cuff disease or other shoulder disorders are able to do all 12 functions of the SST.[196,297–299]

When compared with other available shoulder self-assessment questionnaires, the SST has the highest test/retest reliability, takes the shortest amount of time for a patient to complete, is the easiest to score, and has satisfactory responsiveness.[300,301] The questions can be asked at the initial visit and then at subsequent visits to track progress.

Shoulder Pain and Disability Index.[302]. The SPADI consists of two self-report subscales of pain and disability. The items of both the subscales are visual analog scales (VASs). The five-item pain subscale asks people about their pain during ADL, and each item is anchored by the descriptors "no pain" (left anchor) and "worst pain imaginable" (right anchor). The eight disability items ask people about their difficulty performing ADL. These items are anchored with the descriptors "no difficulty" (left anchor) and "so difficult it required help" (right anchor). Each item is scored by measuring the distance from the left anchor to the mark made by the person. Subscales are scored in a three-part process. First, item scores within the subscale are summed. Second, this sum is divided by the summed distance possible across all items of the subscale to which the person responded. Third, this ratio is multiplied by 100 to obtain a percentage. Higher scores on the subscale indicate greater pain and greater disability. To obtain the SPADI total score, the pain and disability subscales scores are averaged.[302]

Disabilities of the Arm, Shoulder, and Hand. The acronym DASH was chosen to describe an outcome measure that reflects the impact on function of a variety of musculoskeletal

TABLE 16-18 Functional Testing of the Shoulder

Starting Position	Action	Functional Test
Sitting, cuff weight attached to wrist	Forward flex arm to 90 degrees, elbow extended	Raise 1–3-lb weight: functionally fair Raise arm without weight: functionally poor Cannot raise arm: nonfunctional
Sitting, cuff weight attached to wrist	Extend shoulder, elbow extended	Raise 4–5-lb weight: functional Raise 3–4-lb weight: functional fair Raise arm without weight: functionally poor Cannot extend arm: nonfunctional
Sitting with hand behind low back	Shoulder internal rotation	Raise 5-lb weight: functional Raise 1–3-lb weight: functional fair Raise arm without weight: functionally poor Cannot raise arm: nonfunctional
Side-lying, cuff weight attached to wrist	Shoulder external rotation	Raise 5-lb weight: functional Raise 3–4-lb weight: functional fair Raise arm without weight: functionally poor Cannot raise arm: nonfunctional
Sitting, cuff weight attached to wrist	Shoulder abduction to 90 degrees	Raise 5-lb weight: functional Raise 3–4-lb weight: functional fair Raise arm without weight: functionally poor Cannot raise arm: nonfunctional
Sitting, arm abducted to 145 degrees	Shoulder adduction	Pull 5-lb weight: functional Pull 3–4-lb weight: functional fair Pull 1–2-lb weight: functionally poor Cannot pull 1 lb: nonfunctional
Sitting	Shoulder elevation (shoulder shrug)	Five repetitions: functional Three to four repetitions: functional fair One to two repetitions: functionally poor Zero repetitions: nonfunctional
Sitting	Scapular depression	Five repetitions: functional Three to four repetitions: functional fair One to two repetitions: functionally poor Zero repetitions: nonfunctional

Data from Matsen FH III, Lippitt SB, Sidles JA, et al: *Practical Evaluation of Management of the Shoulder*. Philadelphia, PA: WB Saunders, 1994:19–150; Magee DJ: *Shoulder, Orthopaedic Physical Assessment*. Philadelphia, PA: WB Saunders, 1992:90–142; Palmer ML, Epler M: *Clinical Assessment Procedures in Physical Therapy*. Philadelphia, PA: JB Lippincott, 1990.

diseases and injuries in the upper extremity.[303] Items covered by the DASH questionnaire are symptoms and functional status. The components included under the concept of symptoms are pain, weakness, stiffness, and tingling/numbness.[303] There are three dimensions under functional status: physical, social, and psychological status. Two versions of the DASH are available: a 30-item questionnaire that has optional three-question modules for sport/music and heavy work activities (Table 16-21), and a 15–20-item questionnaire suitable for office use.

Penn shoulder score

PSS is a condition-specific self-report measure that uses a 100-point scale consisting of three subscales, including pain, satisfaction, and function. The pain subscale consists of three pain items that address pain at rest, with no activities, and with strenuous activities (Table 16-22).[304] All are based on a 10-point numeric rating scale with end points of "no pain" and "worst possible pain." Points are awarded for each item by subtracting the number circled from the maximum of 10. Therefore a patient is awarded 30 points for complete absence of pain. If a patient is not able to use the arm for normal or strenuous activities, zero points are awarded for that item. Patient satisfaction with shoulder function is also assessed with a 10-point numeric rating scale (Table 16-23). The end points are "not satisfied" and "very satisfied." A maximum of 10 points for this section indicates that the patient is "very satisfied" with the current level of function of his or her shoulder. The total PSS maximum score of 100 indicates high

TABLE 16-19 UCLA Shoulder Rating Scale

Pain	Rating
Always/unbearable/strong medication	1
Always/bearable/occasional medication	2
Little at rest/present with light activity	4
Present with heavy activity	6
Occasional and slight	8
None	10
Function	
Unable to use	1
Light activities	2
ADLs/light housework	4
Housework/shopping/driving	6
Slight restriction/over shoulder level OK	8
Normal	10
Active forward flexion	
>150	5
150	4
120	3
90	2
45	1
<30	0
Strength of forward flexion	
Normal grade	5
Good/grade	4
Fair/grade	3
Poor/grade	2
Contraction/grade	1
Nothing/grade 0	0
Patient satisfaction	
Satisfied	5
Not satisfied	0
TOTAL ______	

function, low pain, and high satisfaction with the function of the shoulder. The PSS has been found to be a reliable and valid measure for reporting outcome of patients with various shoulder disorders.[304]

Other tests, which are designed to assess shoulder function, include the following:

One-Arm Hop Test

The one-arm hop test is a functional performance test for athletes, which can be used in preseason screens or to assist in return-to-play decisions. The test requires the patient to be in a one-arm push-up position on the floor (Fig. 16-37). The patient uses his arm to hop onto a 10.2-cm (4-inch) step and back to the floor. The time required to perform five repetitions of this movement as quickly as possible is recorded and compared with the uninvolved arm. With sufficient training, a time of under 10 seconds is considered normal.[305]

The one-arm hop test requires concentric and eccentric muscle strength and coordination while the distal portion of the upper extremity has a significant load placed upon it.[305]

TABLE 16-20 The Simple Shoulder Test

1. Is your shoulder comfortable with your arm at rest by your side?
2. Does your shoulder allow you to sleep comfortably?
3. Can you reach the small of your back to tuck in your shirt with your hand?
4. Can you place your hand behind your head with the elbow straight out to the side?
5. Can you place a coin on a shelf at the level of your shoulder without bending your elbow?
6. Can you lift 1 lb (a full-pint container) to the level of your shoulder without bending your elbow?
7. Can you lift 8 lb (a full gallon container) to the level of the top of your head without bending your elbow?
8. Can you carry 20 lb at your side with the affected extremity?
9. Do you think you can toss a softball underhand 10 yards with the affected extremity?
10. Do you think you can throw a softball overhand 20 yards with the affected extremity?
11. Can you wash the back of your opposite shoulder with the affected extremity?
12. Would your shoulder allow you to work full time at your usual job?

Data from Matsen FA, Lippitt SB, Sidles JA, et al: Evaluating the shoulder. In: Matsen FA, Lippitt SB, Sidles JA, et al., eds. *Practical Evaluation and Management of the Shoulder.* Philadelphia, PA: WB Saunders, 1994:1–17.

Muscle Length Tests

Pectoralis Major

The patient lies in the supine position with the trunk stabilized. The clinician passively abducts the patient's arm and differentiates between the different bands of the pectoralis major.

Clavicular Portion. The patient's arm hangs loosely down over the edge of the table. The clinician moves the patient's shoulder down toward the floor. A slight barrier to the motion is normal, whereas a hard barrier is abnormal.

Sternal Portion. With the patient supine on a mat table, they actively abduct their arm fully. Their arm should maintain contact with the table throughout the range.

Pectoralis Minor

The patient lies in the supine position with the trunk stabilized. Adaptive shortening of the pectoralis minor is demonstrated if the lateral border of the spine of the scapula is more than 1 inch off the table.[206]

Latissimus Dorsi. The patient lies in the supine position with the trunk stabilized. The patient is asked to perform bilateral shoulder flexion. Under normal circumstances, the patient should be able to perform complete shoulder flexion without any increase in lumbar lordosis occurring.[206] Shoulder flexion that requires an increase in lumbar lordosis to complete is indicative of an adaptively shortened latissimus dorsi.

External Rotators

The patient lies in the supine position with the trunk stabilized. The shoulder is positioned at 90 degrees of abduction with the

TABLE 16-21 The DASH Questionnaire

Please rate your ability to do the following activities in the last week by circling the number below the appropriate response

	No Difficulty	Mild Difficulty	Moderate Difficulty	Severe Difficulty	Unable
1. Open a tight or new jar	1	2	3	4	5
2. Write	1	2	3	4	5
3. Turn a key	1	2	3	4	5
4. Prepare a meal	1	2	3	4	5
5. Push open a heavy door	1	2	3	4	5
6. Place an object on a shelf above your head	1	2	3	4	5
7. Do heavy household chores (e.g., wash walls, wash floors)	1	2	3	4	5
8. Garden or do yard work	1	2	3	4	5
9. Make a bed	1	2	3	4	5
10. Carry a shopping bag or briefcase	1	2	3	4	5
11. Carry a heavy object (over 10 lb)	1	2	3	4	5
12. Change a light bulb overhead	1	2	3	4	5
13. Wash or blow dry your hair	1	2	3	4	5
14. Wash your back	1	2	3	4	5
15. Put on a pullover sweater	1	2	3	4	5
16. Use a knife to cut food	1	2	3	4	5
17. Recreational activities which require little effort (e.g., cardplaying, knitting, etc.)	1	2	3	4	5
18. Recreational activities in which you take some force or impact through your arm, shoulder, or hand (e.g., golf, hammering, tennis, etc.)	1	2	3	4	5
19. Recreational activities in which you move your arm freely (e.g., playing frisbee, badminton, etc.)	1	2	3	4	5
20. Manage transportation needs (getting from one place to another)	1	2	3	4	5
21. Sexual activities	1	2	3	4	5

Disabilities of the arm, shoulder, and hand

	Not at all	Slightly	Moderately	Quite a Bit	Extremely
22. During the past week, to what extent has your arm, shoulder, or hand problem interfered with your normal social activities with family, friends, neighbors, or groups? (circle number)	1	2	3	4	5

	Not Limited at All	Slightly Limited	Moderately Limited	Very Limited	Unable
23. During the past week, were you limited in your work or other regular daily activities as a result of your arm, shoulder, or hand problem? (circle number)	1	2	3	4	5

Please rate the severity of the following symptoms in the last week (circle number)

	None	Mild	Moderate	Severe	Extreme
24. Arm, shoulder, or hand pain	1	2	3	4	5
25. Arm, shoulder, or hand pain when you performed any specific activity	1	2	3	4	5
26. Tingling (pins and needles) in your arm, shoulder, or hand	1	2	3	4	5
27. Weakness in your arm, shoulder, or hand	1	2	3	4	5
28. Stiffness in your arm, shoulder, or hand	1	2	3	4	5
29. During the past week, how much difficulty have you had sleeping because of the pain in your arm, shoulder or hand? (circle number)	1	2	3	4	5

(Continued)

TABLE 16-21 The DASH Questionnaire *(Continued)*

	Strongly Disagree	Disagree	Neither Agree nor Disagree	Agree	Strongly Agree
30. I feel less capable, less confident, or less useful because of my arm, shoulder, or hand problem (circle number)	1	2	3	4	5

Scoring DASH function/symptoms: Add up circled responses (items 1–30); subtract 30; divide by 1.20 = DASH score.

Sports/performing arts module (optional)

The following questions relate to the impact of your arm, shoulder, or hand problem on playing your musical instrument or sport. If you play more than one sport or instrument (or play both), please answer with respect to that activity which is most important.

Please indicate the sport or instrument which is most important to you: ______________________

I do not play a sport or an instrument. (You may skip this section.)

Please circle the number that best describes your physical ability in the past week. Did you have any difficulty

	No Difficulty	Mild Difficulty	Moderate Difficulty	Severe Difficulty	Unable
1. Using your usual technique for playing your instrument or sport?	1	2	3	4	5
2. Playing your musical instrument or sport because of arm, shoulder, or hand pain?	1	2	3	4	5
3. Playing your musical instrument or sport as well as you would like?	1	2	3	4	5
4. Spending your usual amount of time practicing or playing your instrument or sport?	1	2	3	4	5

Work module (optional)

The following questions ask about the impact of your arm, shoulder, or hand problem on your ability to work (including homemakers if that is your main work role).

I do not work. (You may skip this section.)

Please circle the number that best describes your physical ability in the past week. Did you have any difficulty

	No Difficulty	Mild Difficulty	Moderate Difficulty	Severe Difficulty	Unable
1. Using your usual technique for your work?	1	2	3	4	5
2. Doing your usual work because of arm, shoulder, or hand pain?	1	2	3	4	5
3. Doing your work as well as you would like?	1	2	3	4	5
4. Spending your usual amount of time doing your work?	1	2	3	4	5

TABLE 16-22 The Penn Shoulder Score, Part 1: Pain and Satisfaction Subscales

Please Circle the Number Closest to Your Level of Pain or Satisfaction	Office Use Only
Pain at rest with your arm by your side: 0 1 2 3 4 5 6 7 8 9 10 No pain — Worst pain possible	(10 —# circled)
Pain with normal activities (eating, dressing, bathing): 0 1 2 3 4 5 6 7 8 9 10 No pain — Worst pain possible	(10 —# circled) (Score 0 if not applicable)
Pain with strenuous activities (reaching, lifting, pushing, pulling, throwing): 0 1 2 3 4 5 6 7 8 9 10 No pain — Worst pain possible	(10 —# circled) (Score 0 if not applicable)
Pain score: =`30 How satisfied are you with the current level of function of your shoulder? 0 1 2 3 4 5 6 7 8 9 10 No pain — Worst pain possible	/10 (# circled)

Data from Leggin BG, Michener LA, Shaffer MA, et al: The Penn shoulder score: Reliability and validity. *J Orthop Sports Phys Ther* 36:138–151, 2006.

TABLE 16-23 The Penn Shoulder Score: Function Subscale

Please Circle the Number that Best Describes the Level of Difficulty You Might Have Performing Each Activity	No Difficulty	Some Difficulty	Much Difficulty	Can't Do At All	Did Not Do Before Injury
1. Reach the small of your back to tuck in your shirt with your hand	3	2	1	0	X
2. Wash the middle of your back/hook bra	3	2	1	0	X
3. Perform necessary toileting activities	3	2	1	0	X
4. Wash the back of opposite shoulder	3	2	1	0	X
5. Comb hair	3	2	1	0	X
6. Place hand behind head with elbow held straight out to the side	3	2	1	0	X
7. Dress self (including put on coat and pull shirt off overhead)	3	2	1	0	X
8. Sleep on affected side	3	2	1	0	X
9. Open a door with affected arm	3	2	1	0	X
10. Carry a bag of groceries with affected arm	3	2	1	0	X
11. Carry a briefcase/small suitcase with affected arm	3	2	1	0	X
12. Place a soup can (1–2 lb) on a shelf at shoulder level without bending elbow	3	2	1	0	X
13. Place a one gallon container (8–10 lb) on a shelf at shoulder level without bending elbow	3	2	1	0	X
14. Reach a shelf above your head without bending your elbow	3	2	1	0	X
15. Place a soup can (1–2 lb) on a shelf overhead without bending your elbow	3	2	1	0	X
16. Place a one gallon container (8–10 lb) on a shelf overhead without bending your elbow	3	2	1	0	X
17. Perform usual sport/hobby	3	2	1	0	X
18. Perform household chores (cleaning, laundry, cooking)	3	2	1	0	X
19. Throw overhand/swim/overhead racquet sports (circle all that apply to you)	3	2	1	0	X
20. Work full time at your regular job	3	2	1	0	X

SCORING
Total of columns = ___(a)
Number of *X*s × 3 = ___(b), 60–___(b) = ___(c) (if no *X*s are circled, function score = total of columns)
Function score = ___(a) ± ___(c) = ___ × 60 ___/60

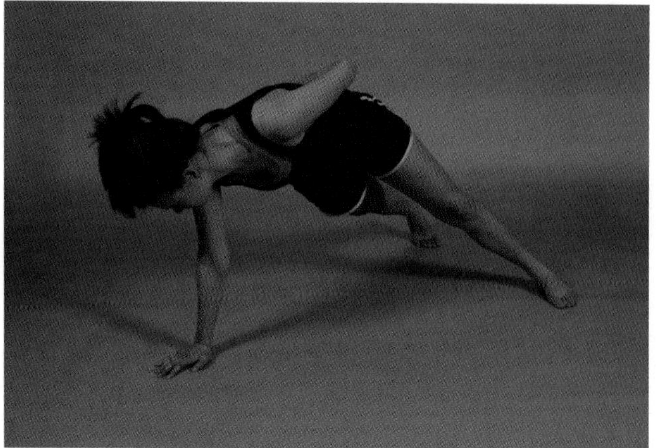

FIGURE 16-37 One arm push-up position.

elbow flexed to approximately 90 degrees. The patient is then asked to allow the shoulder to passively internally rotate. IR accompanied by an anterior tilt of the scapula, rather than the range of IR increasing, is indicative of adaptive shortness of the external rotators.[206] This is confirmed by having the patient perform the maneuver again while the clinician prevents the anterior tilt of the scapula from occurring. With the second test, there should be a decrease in the amount of passive IR available.

Passive Accessory Motion Tests

The passive accessory motion tests are performed at the end of the patient's available range to determine if the joint itself is responsible for the loss of motion. For all of these tests, the

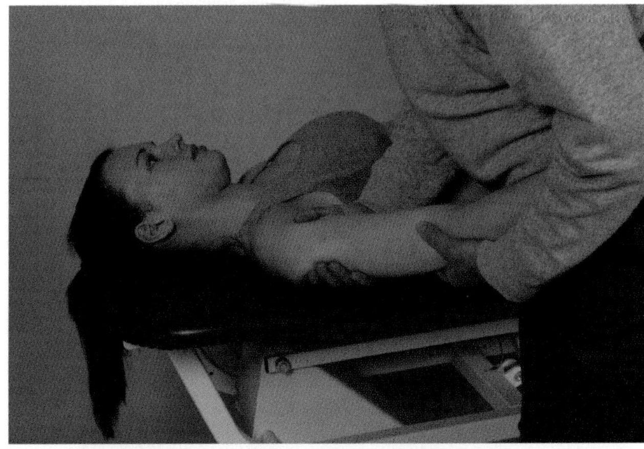

FIGURE 16-38 Glenohumeral distraction.

joint is initially positioned in the resting or open-packed position, the patient lies in the supine position with their head supported on a pillow if required, while the clinician stands facing the patient.

Distraction of the G-H Joint

The clinician palpates and stabilizes the shoulder girdle and the anterior thorax. With one hand, the clinician gently grasps the proximal third of the humerus. The clinician distracts the G-H joint perpendicular to the plane of the glenoid fossa in a lateral, anterior, and inferior direction (30 degrees off the sagittal plane) (Fig. 16-38). The quantity of motion is noted and compared with the other side. Alternatively, if the arm is positioned so that the long axis of the humerus is perpendicular to the flattened concave surface of the glenoid, the technique can be performed by pulling on the upper arm (Fig. 16-39).

Inferior Glide of the G-H Joint

The clinician palpates and stabilizes the coracoid process of the scapula and the lateral clavicle. With the other hand, the clinician gently grasps proximal to the patient's elbow. The humerus is glided inferiorly at the G-H joint, parallel to the superoinferior plane of the glenoid fossa (Fig. 16-40). The quantity of motion is noted and compared with the other side.

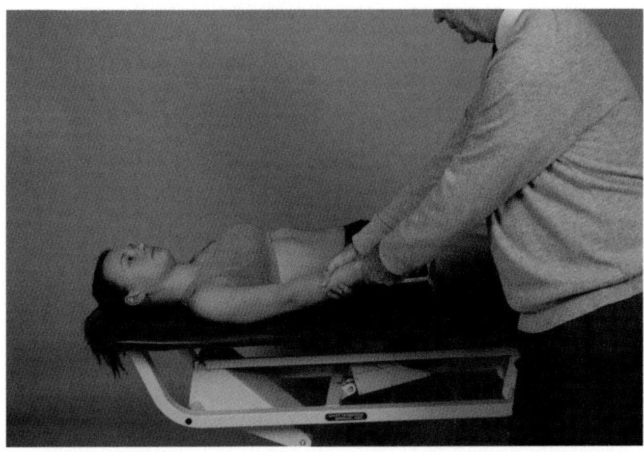

FIGURE 16-39 Glenohumeral distraction using arm pull.

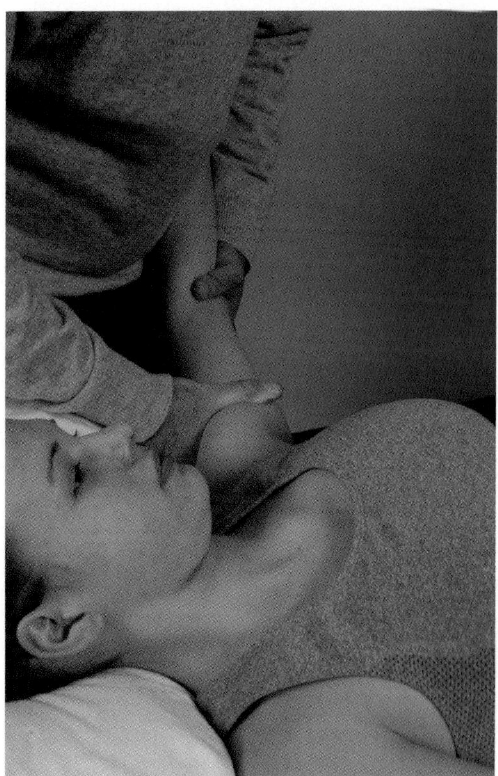

FIGURE 16-40 Inferior glide.

Posterior Glide of the G-H Joint

The clinician palpates and stabilizes the coracoid process and the lateral third of the clavicle. With the thenar eminence of the same hand, the clinician palpates the anterior aspect of the humeral head (Fig. 16-41). With the other hand, the clinician gently grasps the distal end of the humerus. From this position, the clinician glides the humerus posteriorly at the G-H joint, parallel to the A-P plane of the glenoid fossa. The quantity of motion is noted and compared with the other side.

Anterior Glide of the G-H Joint

There are two common variations for this technique, one with the patient in the supine position, and the other where the patient lies in the prone position:

- Patient supine. The clinician palpates the posterior aspect of the humeral head with one hand (Fig. 16-42). With the other hand, the clinician gently grasps the distal end of the humerus. From this position, the clinician glides the humerus anteriorly at the G-H joint, parallel to the A-P plane of the glenoid fossa. The quantity of motion is noted and compared with the other side.
- Patient prone. The clinician palpates the posterior aspect of the humeral head with one hand (Fig. 16-43). With the other hand, the clinician gently grasps the distal end of the humerus. From this position, the clinician glides the humerus toward the floor in an anterior direction, parallel to the A-P plane of the glenoid fossa. The quantity of motion is noted and compared with the other side.

The intervention for joint glide restrictions uses similar techniques and positioning as for the assessment except that the following:

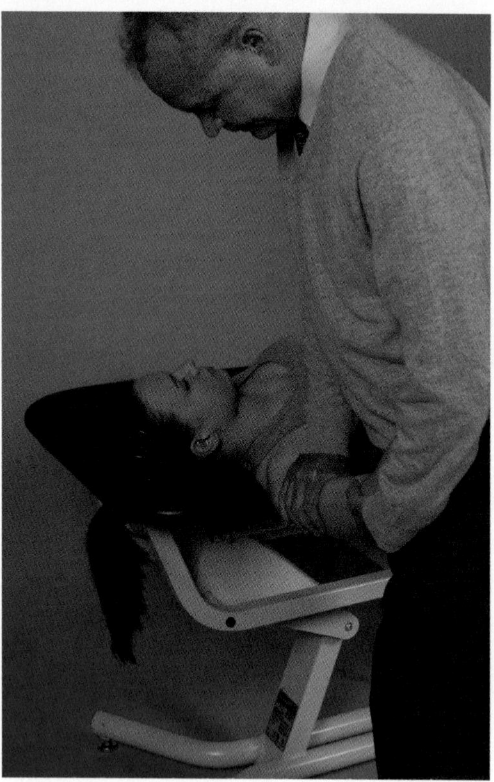
FIGURE 16-41 Posterior glide.

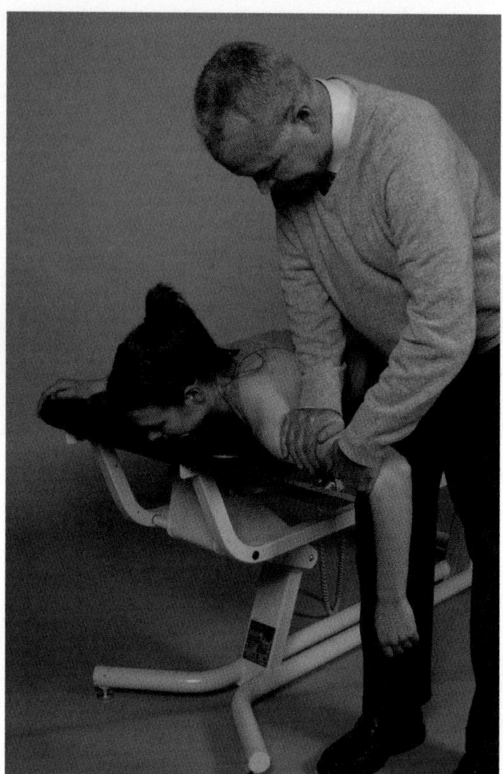
FIGURE 16-43 Anterior glide with patient prone.

- Grade I and II oscillations are used for pain and graded depending on the stage of healing.
- Grade III–V techniques are used to increase range.

Passive Accessory Motion Testing of the Scapulothoracic Joint

Distraction

The patient lies in the side-lying position. The patient's uppermost arm is placed in IR so that the posterior surface of the hand is positioned on the sacrum, if shoulder ROM allows. The clinician stands in front of the patient. The clinician places one hand over the acromion and the mobilizing hand is positioned adjacent to the inferior angle of the scapula. The clinician moves the scapula medially and inferiorly and then lifts the scapula away from the ribs (Fig. 16-44). The quantity and quality of motion is noted.

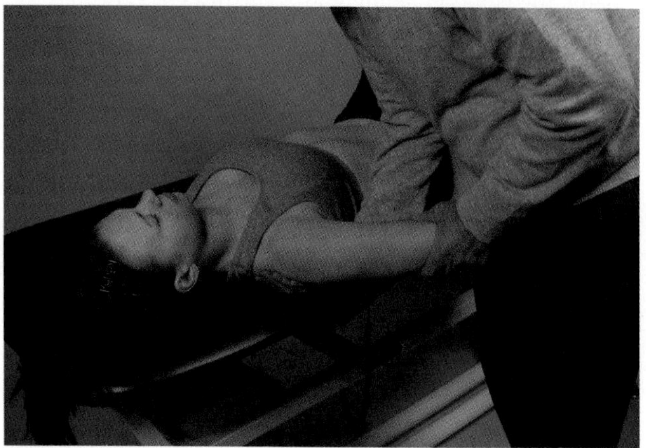
FIGURE 16-42 Anterior glide with patient supine.

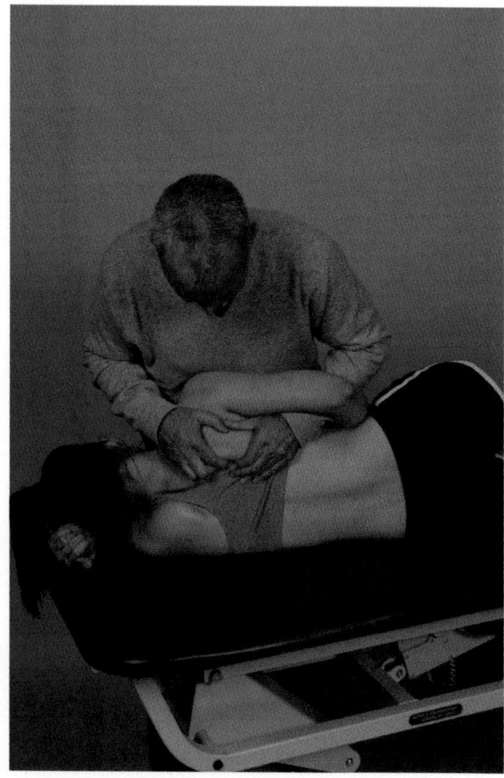
FIGURE 16-44 Distraction of scapulothoracic joint.

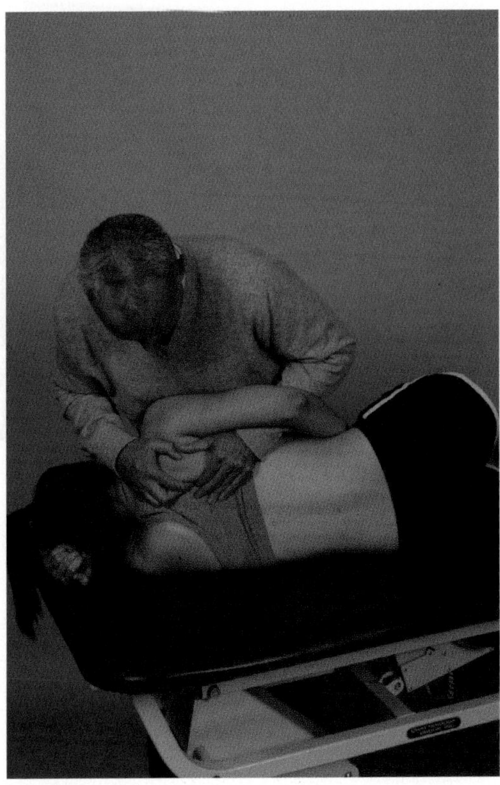

FIGURE 16-45 Superior glide of scapulothoracic joint.

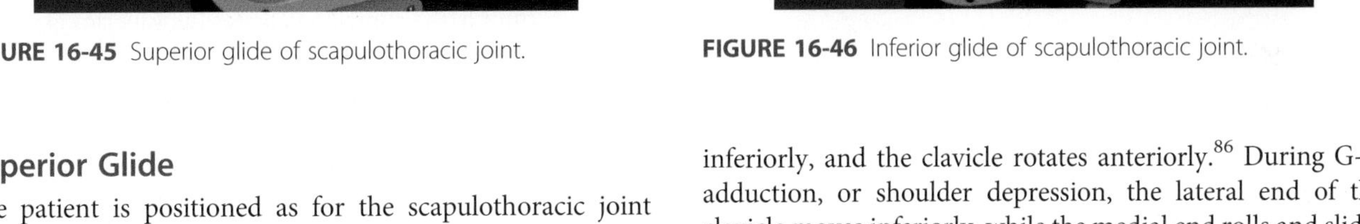

FIGURE 16-46 Inferior glide of scapulothoracic joint.

Superior Glide

The patient is positioned as for the scapulothoracic joint distraction technique, except the uppermost arm is positioned in neutral. Using the mobilizing hand, the clinician glides the scapula in a superior direction (Fig. 16-45).

Inferior Glide

The patient is positioned as for the scapulothoracic joint superior glide. Using the mobilizing hand, the clinician glides the scapula in an inferior direction (Fig. 16-46).

Medial Glide

The patient is positioned as for the superior glide of the scapulothoracic joint. The clinician positions both hands over the lateral surface of the scapula, with one hand over the axillary border and the other hand over the acromion. Using both hands the clinician glides the scapula in a medial direction (Fig. 16-47).

Lateral Glide

The patient is positioned as for the the medial glide of the scapulothoracic joint. The clinician places both hands and the fingertips over the vertebral border of the scapula and the scapula is glided in a lateral direction (Fig. 16-48).

Passive Accessory Motion Testing of the Acromioclavicular Joint

Anterior and Posterior Rotation of the Clavicle

During G-H abduction, or shoulder elevation, the lateral end of the clavicle moves superiorly, the medial end slides and rolls inferiorly, and the clavicle rotates anteriorly.[86] During G-H adduction, or shoulder depression, the lateral end of the clavicle moves inferiorly, while the medial end rolls and slides superiorly.[86] During this motion, the clavicle rotates posteriorly (see Table 16-24).[86]

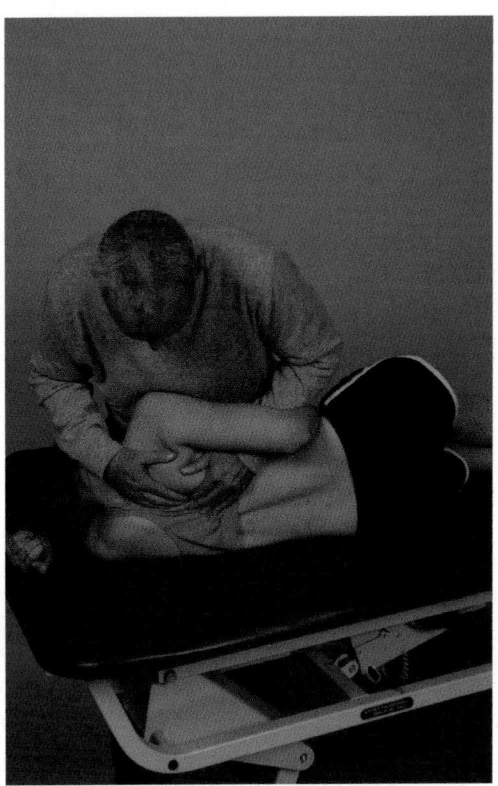

FIGURE 16-47 Medial glide of scapulothoracic joint.

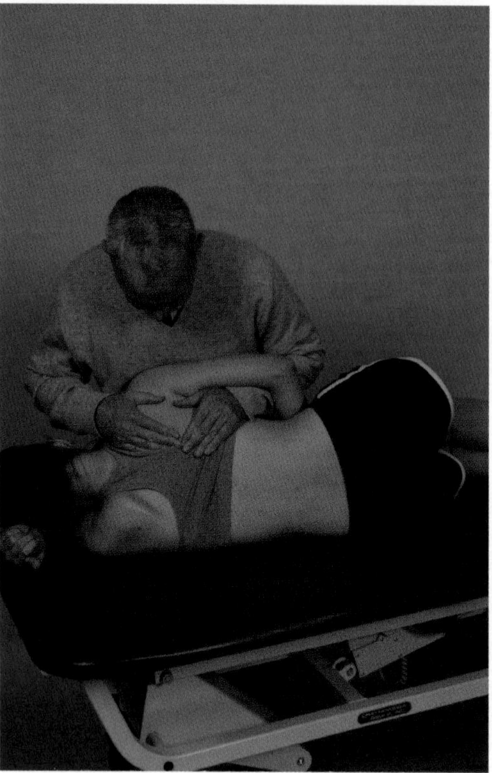

FIGURE 16-48 Lateral glide of scapulothoracic joint.

The patient lies in the side-lying or supine position. The clinician stabilizes the humerus with one hand and grasps the anterior and posterior aspects of the clavicle with the other hand, using the thumb, index, and middle fingers so that the fingers are hooked around the lateral aspect of the clavicle (Fig. 16-49). The clinician passively pulls the clavicle into the limit of anterior rotation and assesses the end-feel (see Fig. 16-49). The clinician then passively pushes the clavicle into the limit of posterior rotation and assesses the end-feel (see Fig. 16-49).

TABLE 16-24 Clavicle Motions in Relation to Other Motions

Moving Bone	Motion	Rotation
Ribs	Inspiration	Posterior
	Expiration	Anterior
Scapula	Protraction	Anterior
	Retraction	Posterior
	Elevation	Anterior
	Depression	Posterior
Head/neck	Ipsilateral rotation	Posterior
	Contralateral rotation	Anterior
	Ipsilateral flexion	Posterior
	Contralateral flexion	Anterior
	Flexion	Anterior
	Extension	Posterior

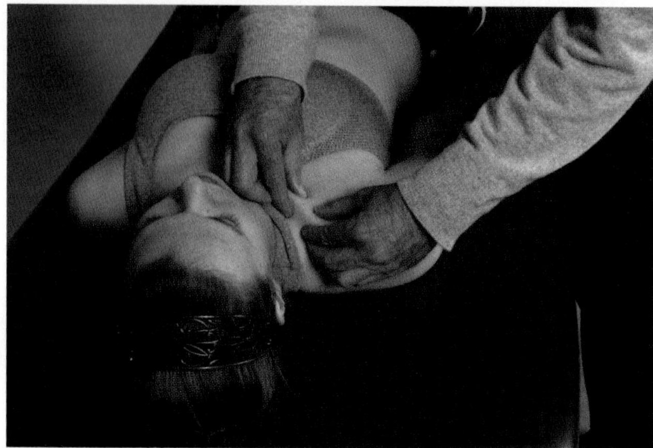

FIGURE 16-49 Anterior and posterior rotation of the clavicle.

Passive Accessory Motion Testing of the Sternoclavicular Joint

The patient lies in the supine position. It is assumed that the techniques are performed on the patient's right side.

Inferior Glide

Using one thumb, the clinician palpates the superior aspect of the medial end of the clavicle and the S-C joint and applies an inferior glide to the S-C joint (Fig. 16-50). The quantity and quality of motion is noted.

Superior Glide

Using the thumb and fingers of one hand, the clinician palpates the inferior aspect of the medial end of the clavicle and the S-C joint and applies a posterosuperior glide to the S-C joint (Fig. 16-51). The quantity and quality of motion is noted.

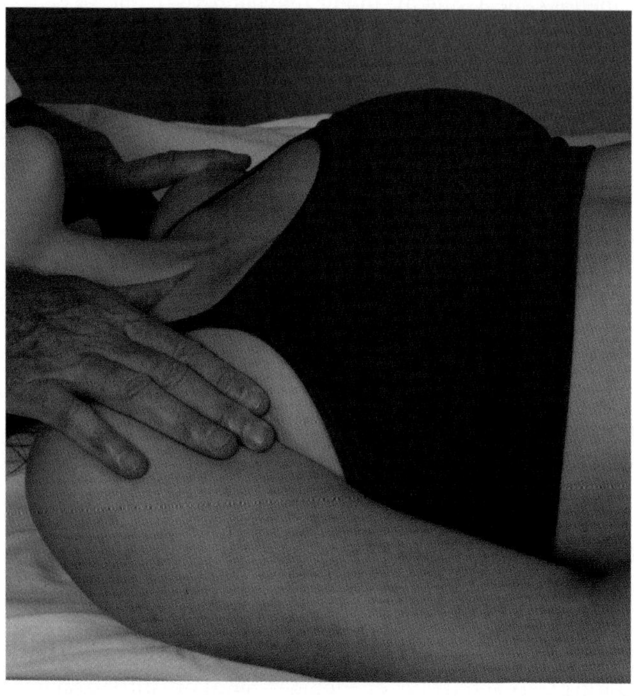

FIGURE 16-50 Inferior glide of S-C joint.

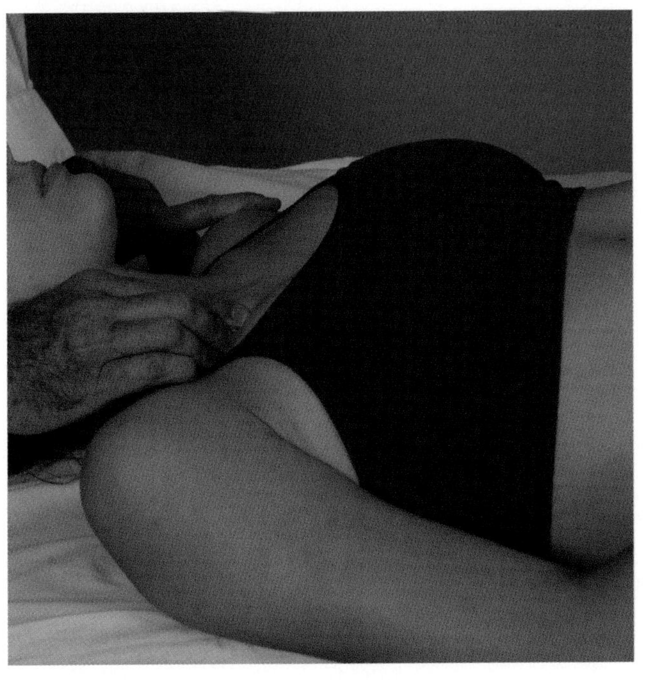

FIGURE 16-51 Superior glide of S-C joint.

Although some texts advocate assessing the anterior and posterior glides of this joint, both of these techniques can be uncomfortable for the patient, and provide little information for the clinician.

Special Tests

The special tests for the shoulder are divided into diagnostic categories. Selection for their use is at the discretion of the clinician and is based on a complete patient history and the findings from the physical examination. It is important to remember that rarely is a diagnostic test sensitive and specific enough to be used as the sole determinant, and multiple test may provide more diagnostic confidence.

Rotator Cuff Integrity and Subacromial Impingement Tests

The following tests have been described in the literature to assess rotator cuff integrity and the presence of SIS (Tables 16-24 and 16-25). Patients with SIS usually perceive pain when a compressing force is applied on the greater tuberosity and rotator cuff region.[306] Pain may also be elicited with shoulder

TABLE 16-25 Diagnostic Test Properties for Impingement and Rotator Cuff Tears

Diagnostic Test or Maneuver	Study Population	Sensitivity	Specificity	Positive Likelihood Ratio	Negative Likelihood Ratio
Hornblower's sign	54 patients aged 47–80 yr, mean age of 66 yr, operated on for combined supraspinatus and infraspinatus tears[a]	1.0	0.93	14.29	0.00
Empty-can test for supraspinatus tendon tears	143 shoulders with various symptoms, patients' age 13–80 yr, mean age 43 yr[b]	Pain 0.63 Weak 0.77 Both 0.89	0.55 0.68 0.50	1.40 2.41 1.78	0.67 0.34 0.22
Full-can test for supraspinatus tendon tears	143 shoulders with various symptoms, patients' age 13–80 yr, mean age 43 yr[b]	Pain 0.66 Weak 0.77 Both 0.86	0.64 0.74 0.57	1.83 2.96 2.00	0.53 0.31 0.25
Dropping sign for infraspinatus degeneration	54 patients aged 47–80 yr, operated on for combined supraspinatus and infraspinatus tears[a]	1.00	1.00	Not applicable	0.00
Palm-up test (Speed test) for biceps tendon tear	55 patients with impingement, mean age 51 yr, range 24–77 yr[c]	0.63	0.35	0.97	1.06
Combined tests: supraspinatus and external rotator weakness, and impingement sign	400 patients with shoulder injury that warranted arthroscopy, age range tests[d]	Not applicable	0.00	(3) 48.00 (2) 7.60 (1) 1.90	(3) 0.76 (2) 0.42 (1) 0.01
Transdeltoid palpation (Rent test)	109 patients for arthroscopy, aged 29–66 yr, mean age 51 yr[e]	0.957	0.968	29.91	0.04
Lift-off test for subscapularis tendon	16 patients, aged 39–66 yr, mean age 51 yr[f] 45 patients with shoulder symptomatology, aged 17–64 yr, mean age 41.5 yr[g]	0.89 0.89	1.00 0.36	Not applicable 1.39	0.11 0.31
Internal rotation lag sign (subscapularis tear)	A prospective study of 100 consecutive painful shoulders with impingement syndrome, stages 1 to 3. Lag signs were compared with the Jobe and lift-off signs.[h]	0.97	0.96	24.25	0.03

(Continued)

TABLE 16-25 Diagnostic Test Properties for Impingement and Rotator Cuff Tears *(Continued)*					
Diagnostic Test or Maneuver	**Study Population**	**Sensitivity**	**Specificity**	**Positive Likelihood Ratio**	**Negative Likelihood Ratio**
External rotation lag sign (subscapularis tear)	A prospective study of 100 consecutive painful shoulders with impingement syndrome, stages 1 to 3. Lag signs were compared with the Jobe and lift-off signs.[h]	0.70	1.00	NA	NA
Supraspinatus test	45 patients with shoulder symptomatology, aged 17–64 yr, mean age 41.5 yr[g]	1.00	0.53	2.13	0.00
Combined tests: supraspinatus and infraspinatus manual muscle test, and palpation	42 patients with rotator cuff tears seen for surgery, no age reported[i]	0.91	0.75	3.64	0.12
Neer impingement sign for rotator cuff tear	85 surgical patients aged 16–72 yr, mean age 40 yr[j]	0.84	0.51	1.71	0.31
	45 patients with shoulder symptomatology, aged 17–64 yr, mean age 41.5 yr[g]	0.33	0.61	0.85	1.10
Hawkins impingement sign for rotator cuff tear	85 surgical patients ages 16 to 72 yr, mean age of 40 yr[j]	0.88	0.43	1.54	0.28
	45 patients with shoulder symptomatology, aged 17–64 yr, mean age 41.5 yr[g]	0.44	0.53	0.94	1.06
Lift-off test for determining location of rotator cuff tear	55 patients with impingement, aged 24–77 yr, mean age 51 yr[c]	0.00	0.61	0.00	1.64
Supine impingement test (RC tear)	448 consecutive patients with suspected RCT referred for arthrography over a 4-year period[k]	0.97	0.09	1.07	0.33
The posterior impingement sign (RC tear or posterior labral tear)	69 athletes presented with posterior shoulder pain that developed during overhand athletics[l]	0.76	0.85	5.06	0.28
Infraspinatus test (RC disease)	8 physical examination tests were evaluated to determine their diagnostic values for three degrees of severity in rotator cuff disease: bursitis, partial-thickness rotator cuff tears, and full-thickness rotator cuff tears.[m]	0.42	0.90	4.20	0.65

[a]Data from Walch G, Boulahia A, Calderone S, et al: The 'dropping' and 'hornblower's' signs in evaluation of rotator-cuff tears. *J Bone Joint Surg Br* 80:624–628, 1998.

[b]Data from Itoi E, Tadato K, Sano A, et al: Which is more useful, the "full-can test" or the "empty-can test" in detecting the torn supraspinatus tendon? *Am J Sports Med* 27:65–68, 1999.

[c]Data from Leroux JL, Thomas E, Bonnel F, et al: Diagnostic value of clinical tests for shoulder impingement. *Rev Rheum* 62:423–428, 1995.

[d]Data from Murrell GA, Walton JR: Diagnosis of rotator cuff tears. *Lancet* 357:769–770, 2001.

[e]Data from Wolf EM, Agrawal V: Transdeltoid palpation (the rent test) in the diagnosis of rotator cuff tears. *J Shoulder Elbow Surg* 10:470–473, 2001.

[f]Data from Gerber C, Krushell RJ: Isolated rupture of the tendon of the subscapularis muscle: Clinical features in 16 cases. *J Bone Joint Surg* 73B:389–394, 1991.

[g]Data from Ure BM, Tiling T, Kirschner R, et al: The value of clinical shoulder examination in comparison with arthroscopy. A prospective study. *Unfallchirurg* 96:382–386, 1993.

[h]Data from Hertel R, Ballmer FT, Lombert SM, et al: Lag signs in the diagnosis of rotator cuff rupture. *J Elbow Shoulder Surg Am* 5:307–313, 1996.

[i]Data from Lyons AR, Tomlinson JE: Clinical diagnosis of tears of the rotator cuff. *J Bone Joint Surg Br* 74:414–415, 1992.

[j]Data from MacDonald PB, Clark P, Sutherland K: An analysis of the diagnostic accuracy of the Hawkins and Neer subacromial impingement signs. *J Shoulder Elbow Surg* 9:299–301, 2000.

[k]Data from Litaker D, Pioro M, El Bilbeisi H, et al: Returning to the bedside: Using the history and physical examination to identify rotator cuff tears. *J Am Geriatr Soc* 48:1633–1637, 2000.

[l]Data from Meister K, Buckley B, Batts J: The posterior impingement sign: Diagnosis of rotator cuff and posterior labral tears secondary to internal impingement in overhand athletes. *Am J Orthop* 33:412–415, 2004.

[m]Data from Park HB, Yokota A, Gill HS, et al: Diagnostic accuracy of clinical tests for the different degrees of subacromial impingement syndrome. *J Bone Joint Surg Am* 87:1446–1455, 2005.

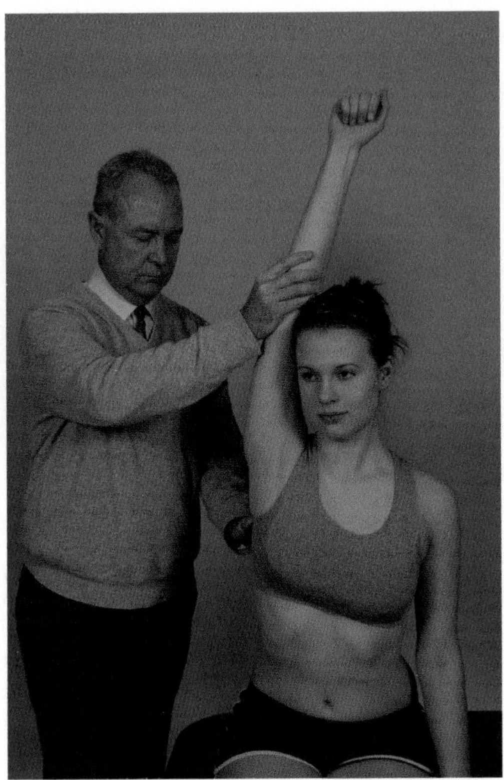

FIGURE 16-52 Neer impingement test.

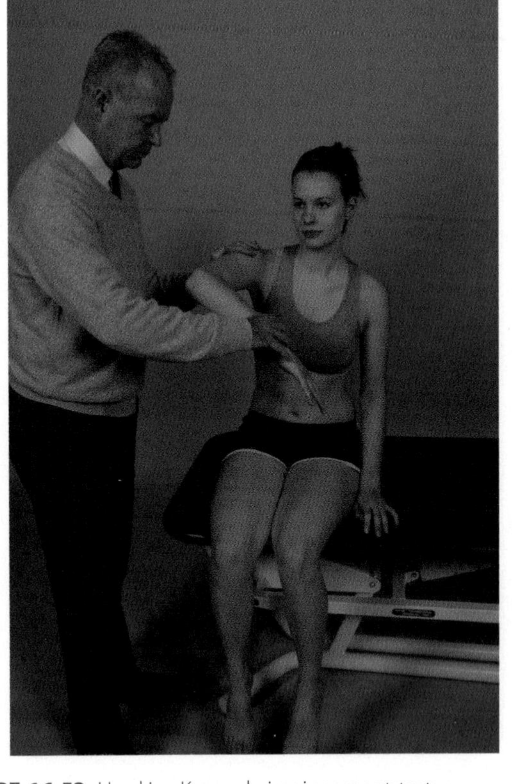

FIGURE 16-53 Hawkins Kennedy impingement test.

abduction in IR or ER.[306] It is important to remember that "impingement" is a broad diagnosis that encompasses a broad range of pathologies, making its diagnostic value questionable.

Neer Impingement Test. While scapular rotation is prevented by one hand of the clinician, the arm of the patient is passively forced into elevation at an angle between flexion and abduction by the clinician's other hand. Overpressure is applied with the G-H joint in neutral, IR, and then ER (Fig. 16-52). A positive Neer impingement test result is thought to represent impingement of the rotator cuff on the anterosuperior glenoid rim or coracoacromial ligament.[307] Post and Cohen[308] found the Neer test to have a sensitivity of 93% in the confirmation of subacromial impingement.

Hawkins–Kennedy Impingement Test.[309] The arm of the patient is passively flexed up to 90 degrees in the plane of the scapula. The arm is stabilized and the forearm is forced into IR (Fig. 16-53). In a cadaver study, Pink and Jobe[307] found that rotator cuff tendons were impinged under the acromion with the Hawkins–Kennedy test.

Ure et al.[310] found that the sensitivity of the Hawkins–Kennedy test was 62% and the sensitivity of thc Neer test was 46% in 45 patients with stage II SIS, as determined using arthroscopy.

McDonald et al.[311] assessed the diagnostic accuracy of the Neer and Hawkins impingement signs for the diagnosis of subacromial bursitis or rotator cuff pathology in 85 consecutive patients undergoing shoulder arthroscopy by a single surgeon. The Neer sign was found to have a sensitivity of 75% for the appearance suggestive of subacromial bursitis; this compared with 92% for the Hawkins sign.[311] For rotator cuff tearing, the sensitivity of the Neer sign was 85% and that of the Hawkins sign was 88%. Specificity and positive predictive values for the two tests were low, being not much higher than pretest probability. The two tests had a high negative predictive value (96% for bursitis, 90% for rotator cuff tearing) when they were combined.[311]

Another study[312] found that the Hawkins–Kennedy test was more accurate than the Neer test in a series of 44 shoulders, with the former having a sensitivity of 78% and the latter a 0%.

Supine Impingement Test. The patient lies in the supine position with the clinician standing to the side of the patient's involved shoulder. The clinician grasps the patient's wrist and distal humerus and elevates the patient's arm to end range (170 degrees or greater). The clinician then moves the patient's arm into ER and then adducts the arm toward the patient's ear (Fig. 16-54). The clinician now internally rotates the patient's arm (Fig. 16-55). The test is considered positive if the patient reports a significant increase in shoulder pain. This test does not appear to be diagnostic but may have value as a screening test since a negative finding may rule out a rotator cuff tear (Table 16-25).

Internal Rotation Lag Sign (subscapularis tear). The patient sits or stands with the involved arm behind the back and the palm facing outward. The clinician grasps the patient's shoulder with one hand and the wrist with the other and then lifts the patient's arm off the back (Fig. 16-56). The clinician then asks the patient to maintain this position as the wrist is released (Fig. 16-57). A positive test, which is manifested with an inability of the patient to maintain his or her arm off of the back, indicates a subscapularis tear. A study by Hertel et al.[313] reported high sensitivity (97%) and specificity (96%) with this test (Table 16-25), but the study had a potential for bias.

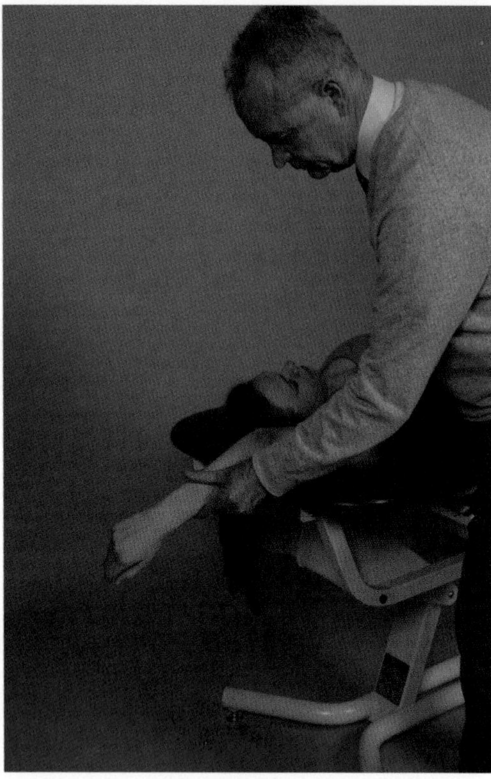

FIGURE 16-54 Supine impingement test—first position.

External Rotation Lag Sign (subscapularis tear). The patient sits with the clinician standing behind. The clinician grasps the patient's wrist and then places the elbow at 90 degrees of flexion and the shoulder at 20 degrees of elevation in the

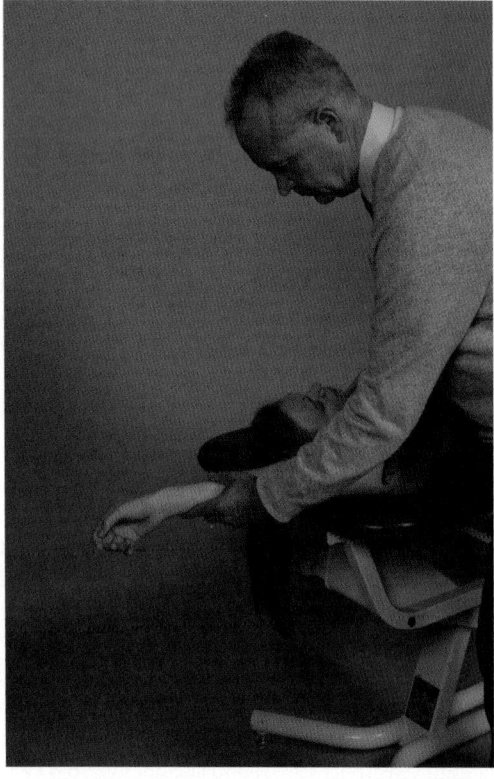

FIGURE 16-55 Supine impingement test—second position.

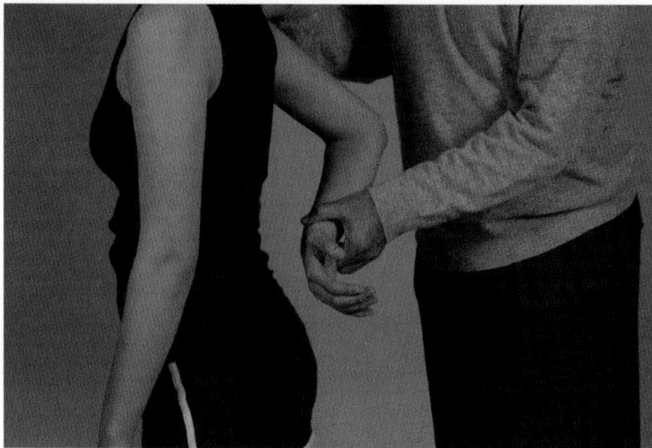

FIGURE 16-56 Internal rotation lag sign (subscapularis tear)—First position.

scapular plane. The clinician passively externally rotates the shoulder and, at the end range, asks the patient to maintain this position (Fig. 16-58) as the patient's wrist is released. A positive test, which is indicated by lag that occurs with the inability of the patient to maintain his or her arm near full ER (Fig. 16-59), indicates a supraspinatus/infraspinatus tear. A study by Hertel et al.[313] reported 70% sensitivity and 100% specificity with this test (Table 16-25), but the study had a potential for bias.

Belly Press Test.[291] The patient sits or stands with the elbow flexed to 90 degrees. The patient is asked to internally rotate the shoulder, causing the palm of the hand to be pressed into the stomach (Fig. 16-60). A positive test, which results in the elbow dropping behind the body into extension, indicates a subscapularis tear. The diagnostic value of this test, which was originally described as an alternative to the Lift-off test in those patients without adequate IR of the shoulder is as yet unknown.

The Posterior Impingement Sign. The patient lies in the supine position with the shoulder placed at 90–110 degrees of abduction and maximum ER (Fig. 16-61). A positive test is indicated by complaints of pain in the deep posterior shoulder and is indicative of a rotator cuff tear and/or a posterior labral tear (Table 16-25).

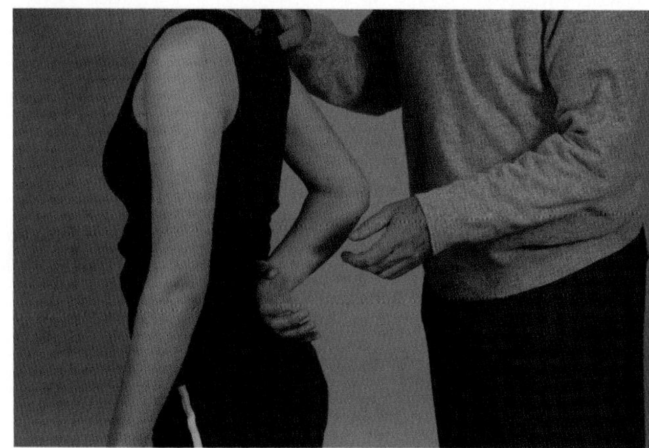

FIGURE 16-57 Internal rotation lag sign (subscapularis tear)—second position.

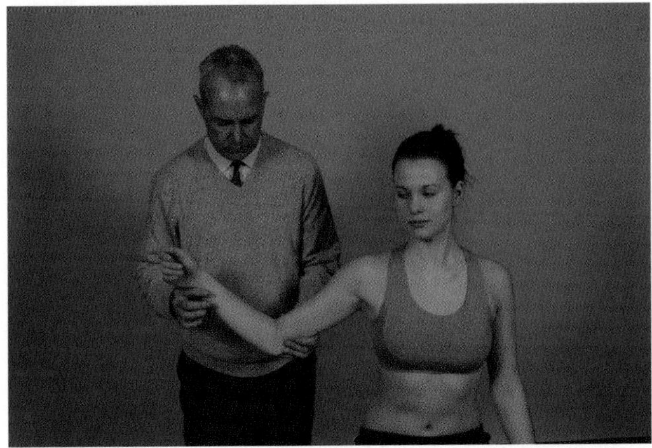

FIGURE 16-58 External rotation lag sign (subscapularis tear)—first position.

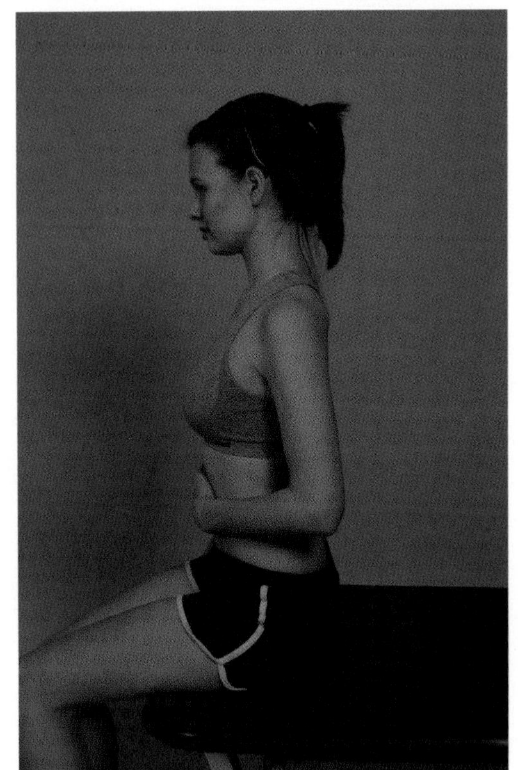

FIGURE 16-60 Belly press test.

Internal Rotation Resisted Strength Test.[314] The patient lies in the supine position with the clinician standing behind the patient. The clinician places the patient's shoulder at 90 degrees of abduction and 80 degrees of ER, with the elbow at 90 degrees of flexion. The clinician first applies a manual resistance to the wrist to assess isometric ER, and then applies manual resistance to the wrist to assess isometric IR. A comparison is made of the two results. The IR-resisted strength test can be used to differentiate between outlet impingement (Fig. 16-62) and nonoutlet or internal impingement based on the apparent weakness of IR versus ER of the arm: if the IR strength is weaker than the ER, the test is considered positive and the patient has internal impingement, whereas a negative test (more weakness in ER) would suggest classic outlet impingement. A study by Zaslav[314] reported 88% sensitivity and 96% specificity with this test (Table 16-26), but the study had a potential for bias. (Table 16-24).[314]

Infraspinatus Test. The patient sits with the elbow at 90 degrees of flexion, neutral forearm rotation, the elbow adducted against the body, and the shoulder at end-range ER. The clinician stands to the side of the patient and provides an IR force against the patient's isometric resistance. A study by Park et al.[315] reported that a positive test, which indicates subacromial impingement (all stages), occurs if the patient gives way due to either pain or weakness, or if there is a positive ER lag sign. However, even when combining the results of two tests, the study demonstrated only a small effect on posttest probability (Table 16-25).

Cross-body Adduction Test.[316] The patient sits and the clinician stands to the involved side of the patient. The patient is asked to elevate the arm to 90 degrees of shoulder flexion. The clinician then horizontally adducts the patient's arm to end range. A positive test for subacromial impingement or an A-C joint injury is indicated if shoulder pain is present (Table 16-25).

Painful Arc Test.[76] The patient stands and, while being observed by the clinician, is asked to actively abduct the involved shoulder. A positive test for subacromial

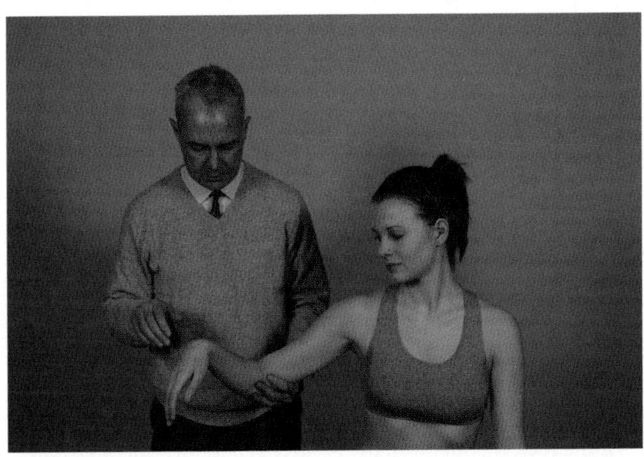

FIGURE 16-59 External rotation lag sign (subscapularis tear)—second position.

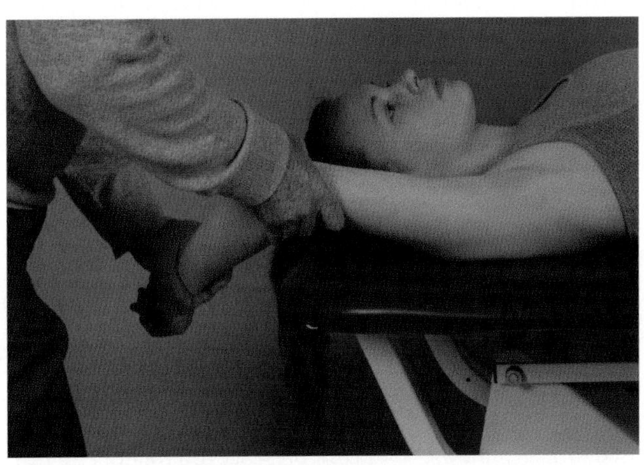

FIGURE 16-61 The posterior impingement sign.

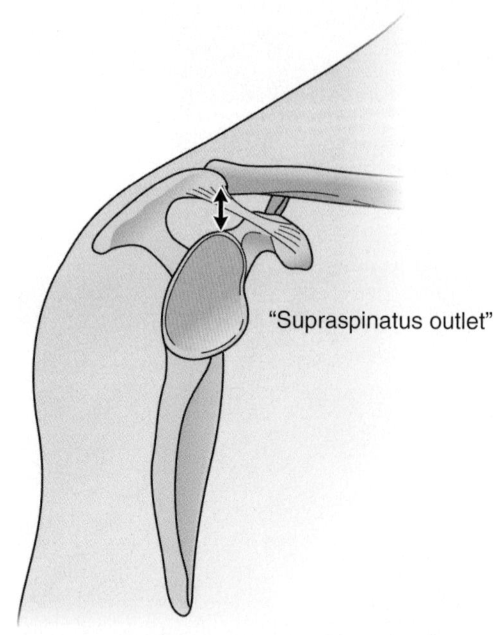

FIGURE 16-62 Supraspinatus outlet.

impingement is indicated if the patient reports shoulder pain in the 60–120-degree range. Pain outside this range is considered a negative test, and pain that increases in severity as the arm reaches 180 degrees is indicative of "a disorder of the A-C joint." Hermann et al.[317] found that the painful arc test was positive in 48.9% of 50 patients with degenerative impingement. Akgün et al.[318] observed 57.5% positive results with the test in stage II SIS patients. Although this test is good at detecting subacromial impingement, a positive finding is unlikely to aid the clinician in determining a specific diagnosis as there are a number of conditions that can be provoked with arm elevation (Table 16-25).

Transdeltoid Palpation (Rent Test).[319] The patient sits or stands with the involved arm relaxed and hanging on the side. The clinician stands behind the patient and holds the patient's distal arm with the patient's elbow flexed to 90 degrees (Fig. 16-63). The clinician then passively moves the patient's G-H joint into full extension, which allows greater palpation of the humeral head and tendons inserting into the greater tuberosity.[319] Palpation is performed at the anterior margin of the acromion. While palpating this area with the shoulder in the fully relaxed and extended position, the clinician moves the patient's arm into internal and external shoulder rotation to allow further palpation of the rotator cuff tendons (Fig. 16 64). In the presence of a complete rotator cuff tear, the eminence of the greater tuberosity appears quite prominent to palpation, and the torn area feels like a "sulcus," "rent," or soft-tissue defect (depression of approximately 1 finger-width) that has avulsed from the tuberosity.[319] Palpating the anterior and posterior margins of the cuff tear may elicit an avulsed edge.[319] It is recommended that this test be used to determine the absence or presence of a rotator cuff tear rather than the size of the tear (Table 16-25).

Yocum Test. The Yocum test is performed by having the patient lift the elbow to shoulder height while resting the hand on the opposite shoulder (Fig. 16-65). A study[284] comparing the Neer, Hawkins–Kennedy, and Yocum tests found all three to demonstrate a high sensitivity for diagnosing subacromial impingement.

Patte Test.[320,321] The Patte test, also known as the "hornblower's sign" (Fig. 16-30), is performed with the patient in the sitting or standing position. The patient's arm is supported at 90 degrees of abduction in the scapular plane, with the elbow flexed to 90 degrees. The patient is then asked to rotate the forearm externally against the resistance of the clinician's hand. If the patient is unable to externally rotate the shoulder in this position, the hornblower's sign is said to be present.

This test was found to have 100% sensitivity and 93% specificity in the diagnosis of irreparable degeneration of the teres minor muscle when compared with CT arthrography findings in a series of 54 shoulders scheduled for rotator cuff repair (Table 16-25).[322] The loss of integrity of the teres minor was confirmed at the time of surgery.

One study[284] attempted to determine the diagnostic value of three impingement tests (Yocum, Neer, and Hawkins–Kennedy), and four tests were used to determine the location of the specific rotator cuff lesion (Jobe empty can [see Resistive Tests], Gerber lift-off [see resisted tests], Patte test, and Speed's test [see later]) by comparing the clinical findings from the tests with the operative findings in a series of 55 patients with chronic shoulder pain and functional impairment.[323] The Neer test (89%), the Hawkins–Kennedy test (87%), and the Yocum test (78%), all demonstrated a high sensitivity for diagnosing subacromial impingement. Both the Jobe empty-can test (86%) and the Patte test (92%) demonstrated high sensitivity, but poor specificity (50 and 30%, respectively). Both the Gerber liftoff and the Speed's test demonstrated poor sensitivity (0 and 63%, respectively) and poor specificity (61 and 35%, respectively).[323]

Lock Test.[324,325] The Lock test is used to help differentiate the cause of symptoms when the patient complains of localized catching shoulder pain, and pain or restricted movement, when attempting to place the hand behind the back. Since the clinician controls the motion, this test can be a very sensitive test to help confirm the presence of an impingement of the supraspinatus tendon. It is assumed that the techniques are performed on the patient's right side.

The patient lies in the supine position with the right shoulder at the edge of the table, and the elbow positioned 10 degrees posterior to the frontal plane (Fig. 16-66). The clinician places his or her left hand under the scapula. The clinician's right hand is placed near the patient's right elbow.

After assessing the resting symptoms, the clinician slowly glides the patient's elbow anteriorly, noting the location of onset of resistance and/or pain in the available range. The end position for the test is achieved when the patient's right shoulder is in maximal humeral flexion with overpressure, and neither the patient nor the clinician can externally rotate the arm further while at this end range.

In the locking position, the greater tuberosity and its rotator cuff attachments are caught within the subacromial space. Further motion into ER, flexion, or abduction is not possible,

TABLE 16-26 Diagnostic Test Properties for Subacromial Impingement

Diagnostic Test or Maneuver	Study Population	Sensitivity	Specificity	Positive Likelihood Ratio	Negative Likelihood Ratio
Infraspinatus test (RC disease)	Eight physical examination tests were evaluated to determine their diagnostic values for three degrees of severity in rotator cuff disease: bursitis, partial-thickness rotator cuff tears, and full-thickness rotator cuff tears.[a]	0.42	0.90	4.20	0.65
Hawkins–Kennedy test	49 painful shoulders, 36 were swimmers; aged 12–23 yr, mean age 17 yr[b]	0.80	0.76	3.33	0.26
	44 subjects, 22 were swimmers; aged 14–26, mean age 17.7 yr[c]	0.78	1.00	Not applicable	0.21
	45 patients with shoulder symptomatology; aged 17–64 yr, mean age 41.5 yr[d]	0.62	0.69	2.00	0.55
	55 patients with impingement; mean age 51 yr, range 24–77 yr[e]	0.87	—	—	—
	125 painful shoulders; aged 18–70 yr, mean age 51.6 yr[f]	0.92	0.25	1.20	0.32
Neer test	49 painful shoulders, 36 were swimmers; aged 12–23 yr, mean age 17 yr[b]	0.39	1.0	Not applicable	0.61
	45 patients with shoulder symptomatology; aged 17–64 yr, mean age 41.5 yr[d]	0.46	0.66	1.35	0.82
	72 patients; aged 23–61 yr, mean age 42 yr[g]	0.93	—	—	—
	44 subjects, 22 were swimmers; aged 14–26, mean age 17.7 yr[c]	0.00	—	—	—
	55 patients with impingement; mean age 51 yr, range 24–77 yr[e]	0.89	—	—	—
	125 painful shoulders; aged 18–70 yr, mean age 51.6 yr[f]	0.89	0.31	1.30	0.37
Neer impingement sign for subacromial bursitis	85 surgical patients; aged 16–72 yr, mean age 40 yr[h]	0.75	0.48	1.44	0.52
Hawkins impingement sign for subacromial bursitis	85 surgical patients; aged 16–72 yr, mean age 40 yr[h]	0.92	0.44	1.64	0.18
Horizontal adduction	125 painful shoulders; aged 18–70 yr, mean age 51.6 yr[f]	0.82	0.28	1.10	0.65
Speed test	125 painful shoulders; aged 18–70 yr, mean age 51.6 yr[f]	0.69	0.56	1.50	0.57
Speed test for biceps or superior labrum anterior and posterior	45 patients with shoulder pain; age range 16–80 yr[i]	0.90	0.14	1.05	0.11
Yergason test	125 painful shoulders; aged 18–70 yr, mean age 51.6 yr[f]	0.37	0.86	2.70	0.73
Painful arc	125 painful shoulders; aged 18–70 yr, mean age 51.6 yr[f]	0.33	0.81	1.70	0.84
Internal rotation resisted strength test	115 surgical patients with a (+) Neer impingement sign; aged 17–76 yr, mean age 44 yr[j]	0.88	0.96	22.00	0.13

(Continued)

TABLE 16-26 Diagnostic Test Properties for Subacromial Impingement *(Continued)*

Diagnostic Test or Maneuver	Study Population	Sensitivity	Specificity	Positive Likelihood Ratio	Negative Likelihood Ratio
Gilcreest test: Palm up test for biceps long-head	55 patients with impingement; mean age 51 yr, range 24–77 yr[e]	0.63	0.35	0.97	1.06
Lift-off test	45 patients with shoulder symptomatology; aged 17–64 yr, mean age 41.5 yr[d]	0.92	0.59	2.24	0.14
Yocum test	55 patients with impingement; mean age 51 yr, range 24–77 yr[e]	0.78	—	—	—
Jobe test for supraspinatus	55 patients with impingement; mean age 51 yr, range 24–77 yr[e]	0.86	0.50	1.72	0.28
	45 patients with shoulder symptomatology; aged 17–64 yr, mean age 41.5 yr[d]	0.85	0.72	3.04	0.21
Patte test for infraspinatus	55 patients with impingement; mean age 51 yr, range 24–77 yr[e]	0.92	0.3	1.31	0.27
Drop-arm test	125 painful shoulders; aged 18–70 yr, mean age 51.6 yr[f]	0.08	0.97	2.80	0.95
Modified relocation test at 90, 110, and 120 degrees for internal impingement	14 overhand-throwing athletes failing 3 mo of rehabilitation; aged 21–31 yr, mean age 24 yr[k]	100% hard articular surface damage; 11 had frayed under surface of rotator cuff; 10 had frayed posterior superior labrum; at 90 degrees only eight patients had rotator cuff contact with labrum, all at 110 degrees, 12 at 120 degrees			

[a]Data from Park HB, Yokota A, Gill HS, et al: Diagnostic accuracy of clinical tests for the different degrees of subacromial impingement syndrome. *J Bone Joint Surg Am* 87:1446–1455, 2005.

[b]Data from Bak K, Faunl P: Clinical findings in competitive swimmers with shoulder pain. *Am J Sports Med* 25:254–260, 1997.

[c]Data from Rupp S, Berninger K, Hopf T: Shoulder problems in high level swimmers—impingement, anterior instability, muscular imbalance. *Int J Sports Med* 16:557–562, 1995.

[d]Data from Ure BM, Tiling T, Kirschner R, et al: The value of clinical shoulder examination in comparison with arthroscopy. A prospective study. *Unfallchirurg* 96:382–386, 1993.

[e]Data from Leroux JL, Thomas E, Bonnel F, et al: Diagnostic value of clinical tests for shoulder impingement. *Rev Rheum* 62:423–428, 1995.

[f]Data from Calis M, Akgun K, Birtane M, et al: Diagnostic values of clinical diagnostic tests in subacromial impingement syndrome. *Ann Rheum Dis* 59:44–47, 2000.

[g]Data from Post M, Cohen J: Impingement syndrome: A review of late stage II and early stage III lesions. *Clin Orth Rel Res* 207:127–132, 1986.

[h]Data from MacDonald PB, Clark P, Sutherland K: An analysis of the diagnostic accuracy of the Hawkins and Neer subacromial impingement signs. *J Shoulder Elbow Surg* 9:299–301, 2000.

[i]Data from Bennett WF: Specificity of the Speed's test: Arthroscopic technique for evaluating the biceps tendon at the level of the bicipital groove. *Arthroscopy* 14:789–796, 1998.

[j]Data from Zaslav KR: Internal rotation resistance strength test: A new diagnostic test to differentiate intra-articular pathology from outlet (Neer) impingement syndrome in the shoulder. *J Shoulder Elbow Surg* 10:23–27, 2001.

[k]Data from Hamner DL, Pink MM, Jobe FW: A modification of the relocation test: Arthroscopic findings associated with a positive test. *J Shoulder Elbow Surg* 9:263–267, 2000.

unless the arm is allowed to move into less flexion. Positive findings for this test include reproduction of the patient's symptoms and a decrease in ROM compared with the uninvolved shoulder.

Dropping Sign.[326] The "dropping sign" is performed with the patient sitting or standing. The clinician places the patient's elbow and shoulder at 90 degrees of flexion. The shoulder is then externally rotated to near end range and the patient is then asked to maintain this position as the wrist is released. A positive test for an infraspinatus tear is indicated by a lag that occurs with an inability to maintain the position, and the arm drops to a neutral position of shoulder rotation. This is called the dropping sign. This test was found to have a 100% sensitivity and a 100% specificity for irreparable degeneration of the infraspinatus muscle (confirmed at the time of surgery), although the test was performed with the arm at the patient's side, which is not the original description (Table 16-25).[322]

Rotator Cuff Rupture Tests

Drop-arm (Codman's) Test. The clinician passively raises the patient's arm to 90 degrees of abduction. The patient is asked to lower their arm with their palm down (Fig. 16-67). If at any point in the descent, the patient's arm drops, it is indicative of a rotator cuff injury (Table 16-27).

Supraspinatus Tests

Two techniques described in the literature can be used to test the supraspinatus muscle. In a 1982 report, Jobe and Moynes[327] suggested that the best position for isolating the supraspinatus was the empty-can position—the elbow extended, the shoulder in full IR, and the arm in the scapular plane (thumbs-down

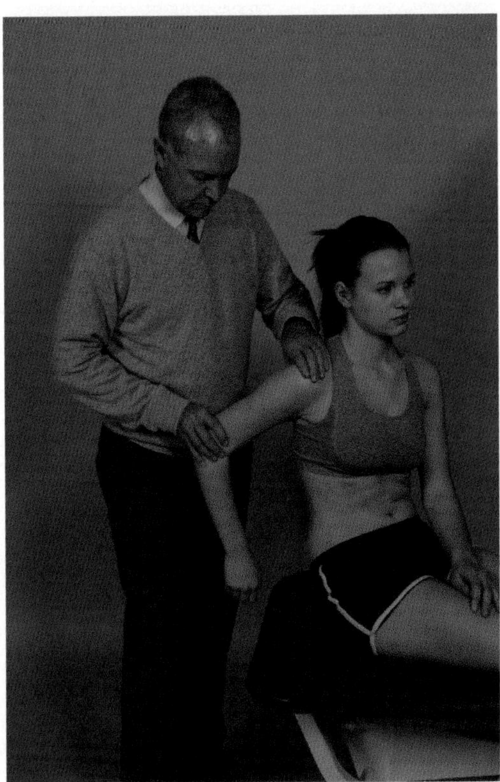

FIGURE 16-63 Transdeltoid palpation (Rent test)—first position.

position) (Fig. 16-28) (Table 16-25). In a 1990 article, Blackburn et al.[122] recommended testing in the prone position, in the full-can position—the elbow extended and the shoulder abducted to 100 degrees and externally rotated while the patient lifts the arm into abduction (thumbs-up position) (Fig. 16-29) (Table 16-25). Malanga et al.[328] noted that although both techniques significantly activate the supraspinatus muscle, neither truly isolates this muscle for testing because other muscles are active in both positions. However, dropping of the arm in either position usually indicates a significant supraspinatus muscle tear. More subtle weakness may represent early degeneration of the rotator cuff.

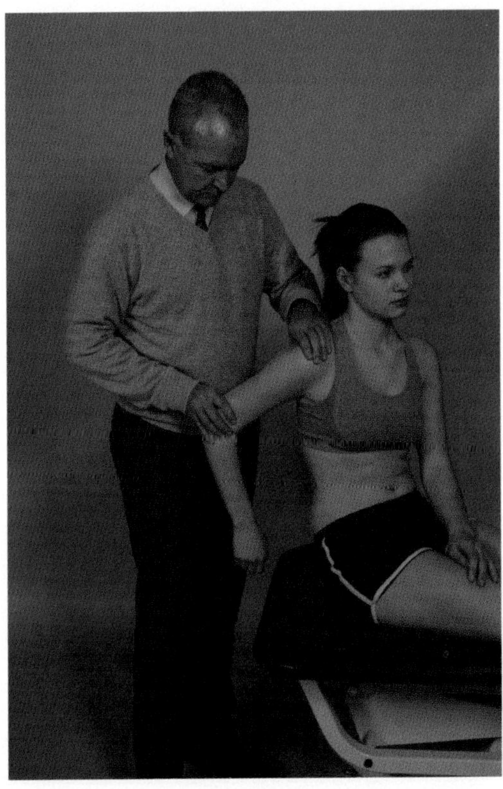

FIGURE 16-64 Transdeltoid palpation (Rent test)—second position.

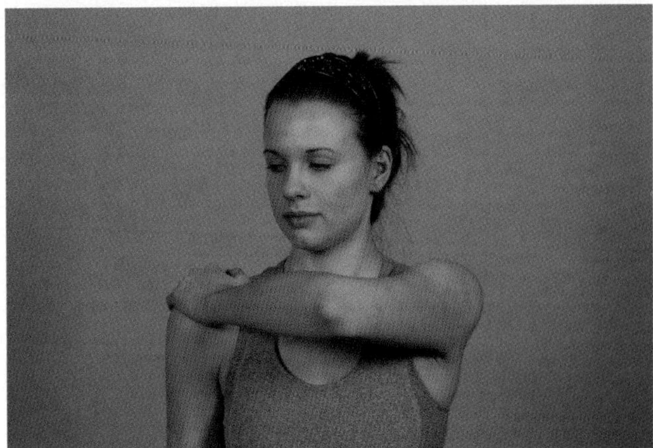

FIGURE 16-65 Yocum test.

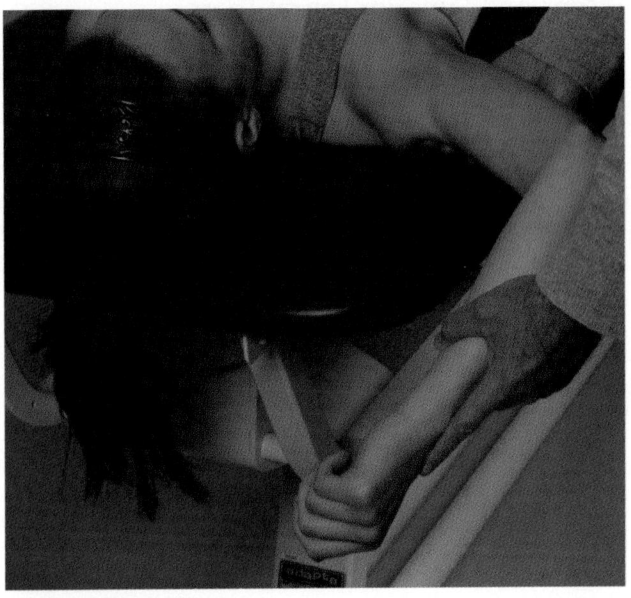

FIGURE 16-66 Lock test.

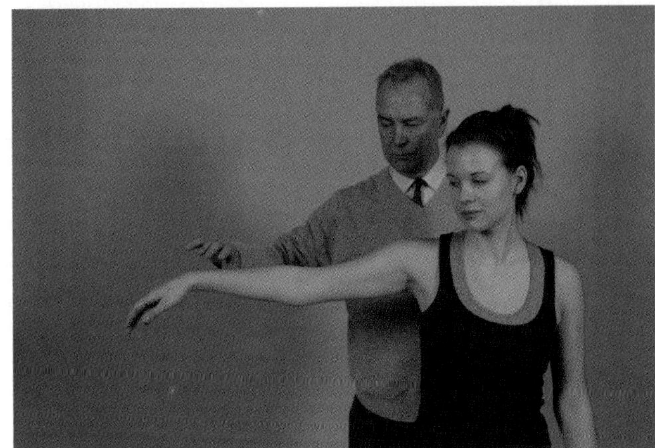

FIGURE 16-67 Drop-arm (Codman) test.

TABLE 16-27 Diagnostic Test Properties for Drop-Arm Test

Test for	Reliability	Sensitivity	Specificity	LR+	LR−	DOR	QUADAS Score
Supraspinatus tear[a]	NT	15	100	NA	NA	NA	8
RC tear[b]	NT	10	98	5.00	.92	5.43	5
Impingement or RC disease[c]	NT	27	88	2.25	.83	2.71	10
Supraspinatus tear[d]	0.28–0.66 kappa	NT	NT	NA	NA	NA	NA

[a]Data from Calis M, Akgun K, Birtane M, et al: Diagnostic values of clinical diagnostic tests in subacromial impingement syndrome. *Ann Rheum Dis* 59:44–47, 2000.
[b]Data from Murrell GA, Walton JR: Diagnosis of rotator cuff tears. *Lancet* 357:769–770, 2001.
[c]Data from Park HB, Yokota A, Gill HS, et al: Diagnostic accuracy of clinical tests for the different degrees of subacromial impingement syndrome. *J Bone Joint Surg Am* 87:1446–1455, 2005.
[d]Data from Ostor AJ, Richards CA, Prevost AT, et al: Interrater reproducibility of clinical tests for rotator cuff lesions. *Ann Rheum Dis* 63:1288–1292, 2004.

Biceps and Superior Labral Tears

The biceps tendon and superior labrum can be involved in various pathological processes including bicipital tendinitis, biceps rupture, biceps tendon subluxation or dislocation, and tears of the superior labrum (Table 16-28).[190]

Clunk Test. The Clunk test is the traditional test for diagnosing labral tears. The patient lies in the supine position. One hand of the clinician is placed on the posterior aspect of the shoulder over the humeral head, while the other hand grasps the humerus above the elbow (Fig. 16-68). The clinician fully

TABLE 16-28 Diagnostic Test Properties for Labral Injuries[a]

Diagnostic Test or Maneuver	Study Population	Sensitivity	Specificity	Positive Likelihood Ratio	Negative Likelihood Ratio
SLAPprehension test	66 consecutive arthroscopically confirmed SLAP lesions (no ages given)[b]	0.88	—	—	—
MRI vs. clinical test/physical examination (PE) (apprehension, relocation, load and shift, sulcus, crank)	54 patients with shoulder pain that was refractory to 6 mo conservative management; aged 17–57 yr, mean age 34 yr[c]	MRI 0.59 PE 0.90	MRI 0.85 PE 0.85	MRI 3.93 PE 6.00	MRI 0.48 PE 0.12
Crank test	62 patients with shoulder pain that was refractory to 3 mo conservative management; aged 18–57, mean age 28 yr[d]	0.91	0.93	13.00	0.10
Biceps load test for SLAP lesions in dislocators	75 patients with history of anterior dislocation; aged 16–41 yr, mean age 24.8 yr[e]	0.91	0.97	30.00	0.09
Biceps load test II	127 patients with shoulder pain; aged 15–52, mean age 30.6 yr[f]	0.90	0.97	30.00	0.10
Anterior slide test	Athletes with isolated superior label test, rotator cuff tears and instabilities, as well as asymptomatic athletes with rotational deficits; aged 18–32 yr, mean age 24.6 yr[g]	0.78	0.92	9.75	0.24
Active compression test	318 patients, 50 controls; no ages reported[h]	1.00	0.985	66.70	0.00
New provocation test for superior labrum	32 patients with throwing injuries; ages 17–29 yr, mean age 20.9 yr[i]	1.00	0.90	10.00	0.00
Speed test for biceps or SLAP	45 patients with shoulder pain; age range 16 80 yr[j]	0.90	0.14	1.05	0.11
Jobe test for anterior SLAP	102 type II SLAP lesions (53 throwers, aged 15 36 yr, mean age 24 yr; 49 nonthrowers with single event trauma, aged 27–72 yr, mean age 40 yr; total group age range from 15 to 72 yr, mean age 33 yr[k]	0.04	0.27	0.05	3.56
Jobe test for posterior SLAP		0.85	0.68	2.66	0.22

(Continued)

TABLE 16-28 Diagnostic Test Properties for Labral Injuries[a] *(Continued)*

Diagnostic Test or Maneuver	Study Population	Sensitivity	Specificity	Positive Likelihood Ratio	Negative Likelihood Ratio
Jobe test for combined SLAP lesions		0.59	0.54	1.28	0.76
Speed test for anterior SLAP		1.00	0.70	3.33	0.00
Speed test for posterior SLAP		0.29	0.11	0.33	6.45
Speed test for combined SLAP lesions		0.78	0.37	1.24	0.59
O'Brien test for anterior SLAP		0.88	0.42	1.52	0.29
O'Brien test for posterior SLAP		0.32	0.13	0.37	5.23
O'Brien test for combined SLAP lesions		0.85	0.41	1.44	0.37
Bicipital groove pain for anterior SLAP		1.00	0.47	1.89	0.00
Bicipital groove pain for posterior SLAP		0.32	0.13	0.37	5.23
Bicipital groove pain for combined SLAP lesions		0.74	0.35	1.14	0.74
Hawkins test	A series of 132 consecutive patients scheduled for diagnostic arthroscopy, examined preoperatively[l]	0.68	0.30	0.97	1.07
Active compression		0.63	0.50	1.26	0.74
Neer test		0.50	0.52	1.04	0.96
Relocation		0.50	0.53	1.06	0.94
Speed test		0.40	0.67	1.21	0.90
Anterior slide		0.10	0.82	0.56	1.10
Crank test		0.13	0.83	0.76	1.05
Pain provocation		0.15	0.90	1.50	0.94
Yergason test		0.13	0.94	2.17	0.93
Jerk test	In 172 painful shoulders, the Kim test was compared with the jerk test and was verified by arthroscopic examination.[m]	0.73	0.98	36.5	0.27
Kim test	In 172 painful shoulders, the Kim test was compared with the jerk test and was verified by arthroscopic examination.[m]	0.80	0.94	13.33	0.21

[a]Data from Deyle GD, Bang MD, Kane E: Evidence-based practice for the shoulder. In: Wilmarth MA, ed. *Evidence-Based Practice for the Upper and Lower Quarter*. La Crosse, WI: Orthopaedic Physical Therapy Home Study Course 13.2.1, Orthopaedic Section, APTA, Inc., 2003:14.

[b]Data from Berg EE, Ciullo JV: A clinical test for superior glenoid labral or 'SLAP' lesions. *Clin J Sport Med* 8:121–123, 1998.

[c]Data from Liu SH, Henry MH, Nuccion S, et al: Diagnosis of glenoid labral tears: A comparison between magnetic resonance imaging and clinical examinations. *Am J Sports Med* 24:149–154, 1996.

[d]Data from Liu SH, Henry MH, Nuccion SL: A prospective evaluation of a new physical examination in predicting glenoid labral tears. *Am J Sports Med* 24:721–725, 1996.

[e]Data from Kim SH, Ha KI, Han KY: Biceps load test: A clinical test for superior labrum anterior and posterior lesions (SLAP) in shoulders with recurrent anterior dislocations. *Am J Sports Med* 27:300–303, 1999.

[f]Data from Kim SH, Ha KI, Ahn JH, et al: Biceps load test II: A clinical test for slap lesions of the shoulder. *Arthroscopy* 17:160–164, 2001.

[g]Data from Kibler WB: Specificity and sensitivity of the anterior slide test in throwing athletes with superior glenoid labral tears. *Arthroscopy* 11:296–300, 1995.

[h]Data from O'Brien SJ, Pagnani MJ, Fealy S, et al: The active compression test; a new and effective test for diagnosing labral tears and acromioclavicular abnormality. *Am J Sports Med* 26:610–613, 1998.

[i]Data from Mimori K, Muneta T, Nakagawa T, et al: A new pain provocation test for superior labral tears of the shoulder. *Am J Sports Med* 27:137–142, 1999.

[j]Data from Bennett WF: Specificity of the speed's test: Arthroscopic technique for evaluating the biceps tendon at the level of the bicipital groove. *Arthroscopy* 14:789–796, 1998.

[k]Data from Morgan CD, Burkhart SS, Palmeri M, et al: Type II SLAP lesions: Three subtypes and their relationship to superior instability and rotator cuff tears. *Arthroscopy* 14:553–565, 1998.

[l]Data from Parentis MA, Mohr KJ, ElAttrache NS: Disorders of the superior labrum: Review and treatment guidelines. *Clin Orthop Relat Res* 77–87, 2002.

[m]Data from Kim SH, Park JS, Jeong WK, et al: The Kim test: A novel test for posteroinferior labral lesion of the shoulder—a comparison to the jerk test. The American journal of sports medicine 33:1188–92, 2005

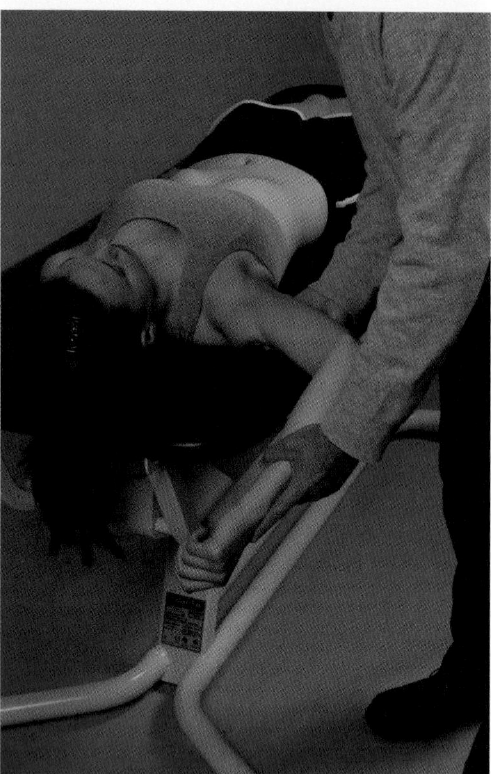

FIGURE 16-68 Clunk test.

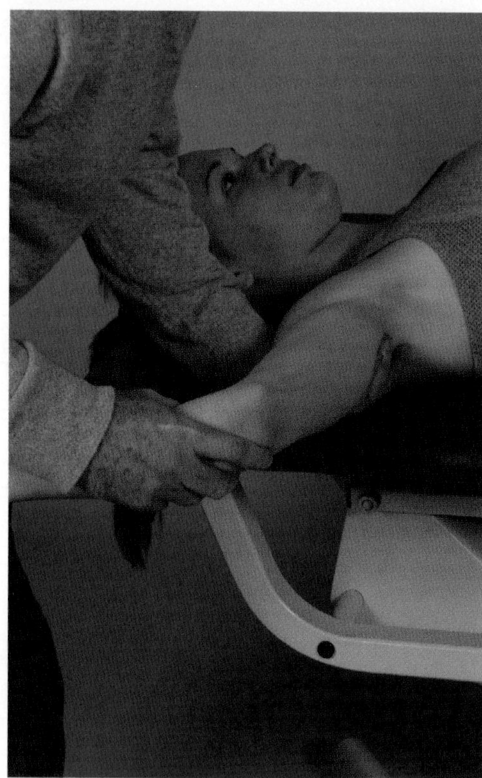

FIGURE 16-69 Crank Test.

abducts the arm over the patient's head. By placing the hand posterior to the humeral head, the clinician pushes anteriorly while the other hand externally rotates the humerus. A clunk-like sensation may be felt if a free labral fragment is caught in the joint.[190] Clinical studies have found that a click on manipulation of the G-H joint was a common finding in patients with labral tears, even in the absence of joint instability.[329,330]

The sensitivity of this test was found to be low (15%) in one study[331] when it was used to detect labral tears in a series of 96 arthroscopic surgery patients.

Crank Test. The crank test[332] is performed with the patient in the supine position. Their arm is elevated to 160 degrees in the scapular plane of the body and is positioned in maximal internal or ER. The clinician then applies an axial load along the humerus (Fig. 16-69). A positive test is indicated by the reproduction of a painful click in the shoulder during the maneuver. This test was found to have a high sensitivity (91%) and specificity (93%) for diagnosing labral tears in a series of 62 patients who presented with shoulder pain that was refractory to 3 months of conservative management.[332]

The crank test has been found to have a higher sensitivity (90%) than MRI (59%) and equal specificity (85%) to MRI in diagnosing labral tears (Table 16-28).[330]

Jerk Test. This test is used to detect a posteroinferior labral lesion.[333] The patient sits, with the clinician standing to the side and slightly behind the patient. The clinician grasps the patient's elbow with one hand and the scapula with the other, and then positions the patient's arm at 90 degrees of abduction and IR (Fig. 16-70). The clinician then provides an axial compression-based load to the humerus through the elbow while maintaining the horizontally abducted arm. The axial compression is maintained as the patient's arm is moved into horizontal adduction. A positive test is indicated by sharp shoulder pain with or without a clunk or click (Table 16-28).

Kim Test. This test is used to detect a posteroinferior labral lesion. The patient sits, with the clinician standing on the involved side. The clinician grasps the elbow with one hand and the midhumeral region with the other hand, then elevates the patient's arm to 90 degrees of abduction (Fig. 16-71). Simultaneously, the clinician provides an axial load to the humerus and a 45-degree diagonal elevation to the distal humerus concurrent with a posteroinferior glide to the proximal humerus (Fig. 16-72). A positive test is indicated by a sudden onset of posterior shoulder pain. A study by Kim

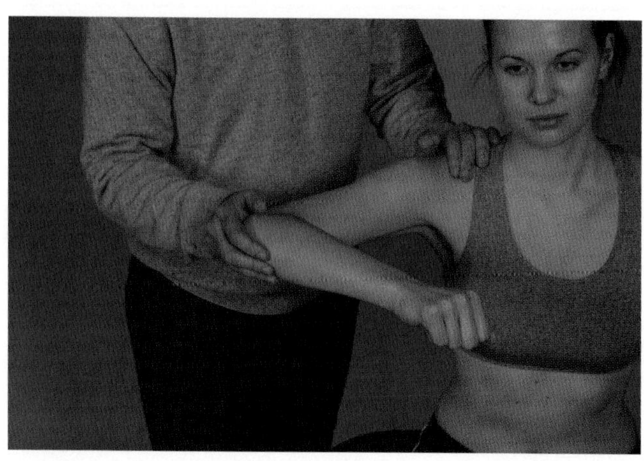

FIGURE 16-70 Jerk test.

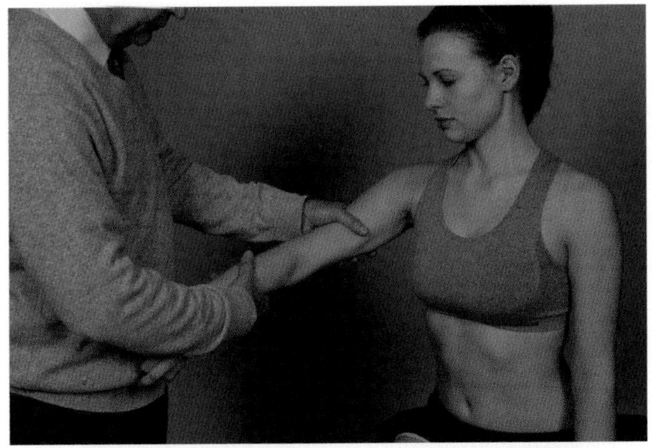

FIGURE 16-71 Kim test—first position.

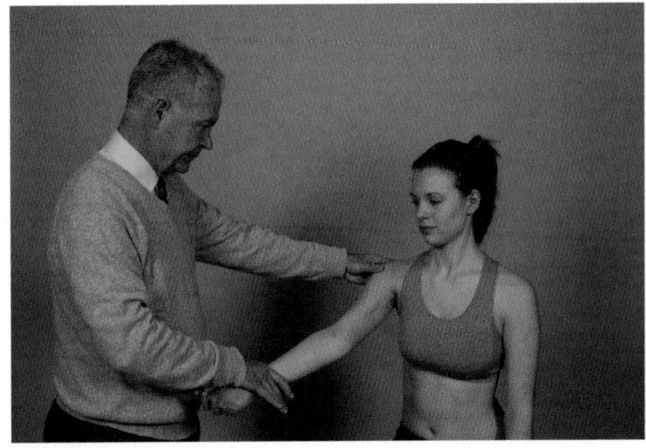

FIGURE 16-73 Speed's test.

et al.[333] found this test to have a sensitivity of 80% and a specificity of 94%, but more strict methodology needs to be followed to corroborate these statistics (Table 16-28).

Speed's Test. The patient's arm is positioned in shoulder flexion, full ER, full elbow extension, and full forearm supination (Fig. 16-73). Manual resistance is applied by the clinician. The test is positive if localized pain at the bicipital groove is reproduced. Wilk et al.[10] have introduced a dynamic version of the Speed's test. During this maneuver, the examiner provides resistance against both shoulder elevation and elbow flexion simultaneously as the patient elevates the arm overhead.

A positive Speed's test suggests a superior labral tear when resisted forward flexion of the shoulder causes bicipital groove pain or deep pain within the shoulder.[1,334] Speed's test is also used to detect bicipital tendinitis (Table 16-28) (see "Yergason's Test" section).[317,335]

Yergason's Test.[336] The patient sits or stands, and the upper arm is positioned with the elbow at 90 degrees of flexion and the forearm pronated. The patient is asked to supinate his or her forearm against the manual resistance of the clinician (Fig. 16-74).

Speed's and Yergason's tests probably discriminate bicipital tendon disorders .[300] However, irritation and edema may also occur in the long head of biceps in any stage of SIS. Biceps tendons may be thickened by fibrinoid degeneration in the SIS.[318,337] This may lead to an inappropriate diagnosis of primary bicipital tendinitis and subsequent tenodesis.[306] In a number of studies, the sensitivity of the Speed's test in biceps tendon disorders was found to be higher than that of the Yergason's test.[306,335,338]

O'Brien (active compression) Test. The O'Brien test (see also "Acromioclavicular Tests" section) is a two-part test. The patient stands with his or her involved shoulder at 90 degrees of flexion, 10 degrees of horizontal adduction, and maximum IR with the elbow in extension. In this position, the patient then resists a downward force applied by the clinician to the distal arm (Fig. 16-75). The patient is asked to report any pain as either "on top of the shoulder" (A-C joint) or "inside the shoulder" (SLAP lesion). The test is then repeated in the same manner except that the arm is positioned in maximum ER. The test is positive for a glenoid labral tear if the patient reports pain for clicking or pain "inside the shoulder" with resisted forward flexion in IR of the shoulder that is relieved by ER of the shoulder (Table 16-28).[1] O'Brien et al.[339] reported a sensitivity of 100% and a specificity of 98.5% for detecting a labral abnormality for this test although the test demonstrated poor study design. For example, the authors provided no data on the amount of force used for the test.

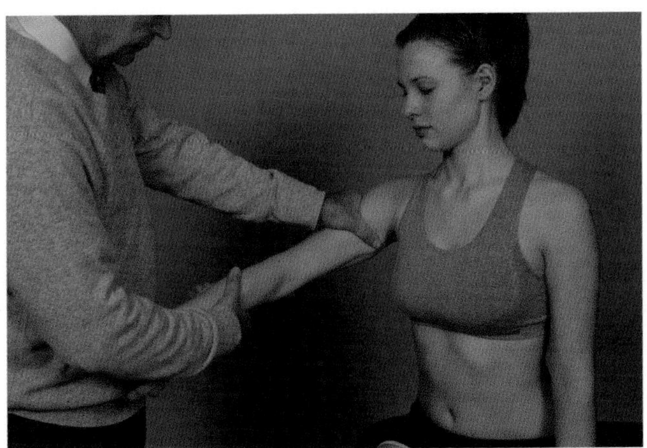

FIGURE 16-72 Kim test—second position.

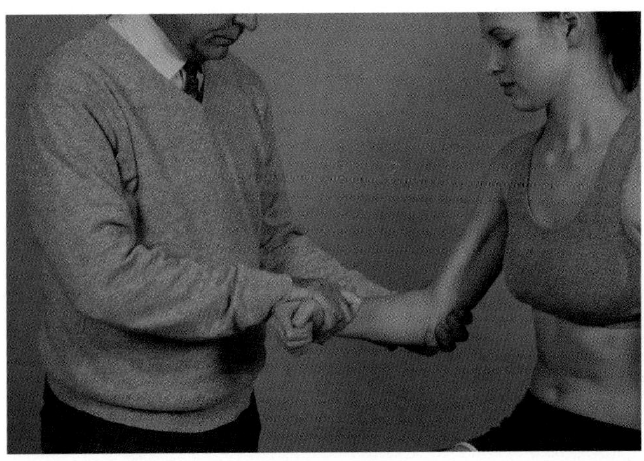

FIGURE 16-74 Yergason's test.

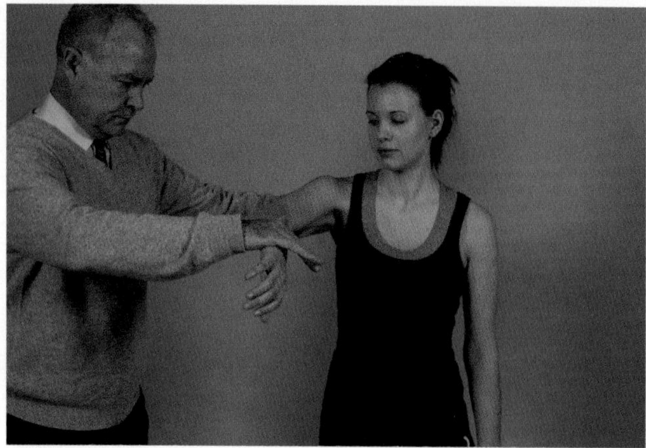

FIGURE 16-75 O'Brien (active compression) test.

Anterior Slide Test. The "anterior slide test"[340] is another clinical test designed to stress the superior labrum.[190] The patient stands or sits with one hand on the hip such that the thumb is positioned posteriorly. One of the clinicians' hands is placed over the patient's shoulder and the other hand behind the elbow (Fig. 16-76). A force is then applied anteriorly and superiorly at the patient's elbow, and the patient is asked to push back against the force. The test is considered positive if pain is localized to the anterosuperior aspect of the shoulder, if there is a pop or a click in the anterosuperior region, or if the maneuver reproduces the symptoms.[190]

The anterior slide test has demonstrated good sensitivity (78%) and high specificity (92%) when used to detect glenoid labrum tears.[340] However, other research[341–343] found the test to have very low sensitivity, indicating that there is little use for this test in the clinic to detect SLAP lesions.

Compression–Rotation Test. This test is performed with the patient in the supine position and the clinician standing on the involved side of the patient. The clinician passively positions the patient's shoulder at 90 degrees of abduction and the elbow at 90 degrees of flexion. The clinician first applies a compression force to the humerus and rotates the humerus back and forth from IR to ER in an attempt to trap the labrum within the joint (Fig. 16-77). When performing this maneuver, it is recommended that a variety of small and large circles are used, while providing joint compression, in an attempt to grind the labrum between the glenoid and the humeral head. A positive test is indicated by the production of a catching or snapping in the shoulder and McFarland et al.[341] found the test to have a sensitivity of 24% and specificity of 76%. However, another study by Snyder et al. concluded that SLAP [344] lesions can only be diagnosed arthroscopically.

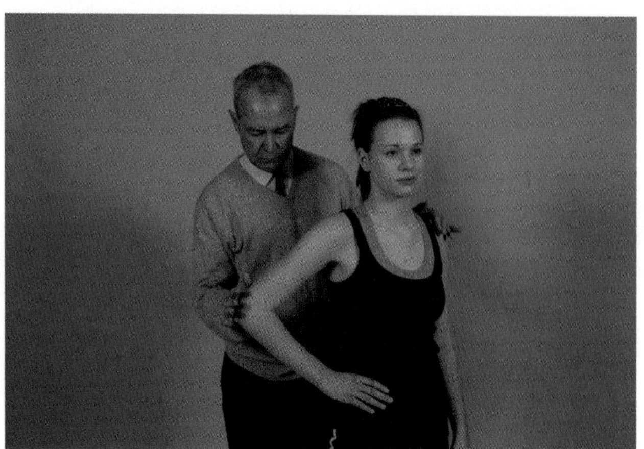

FIGURE 16-76 Anterior slide test.

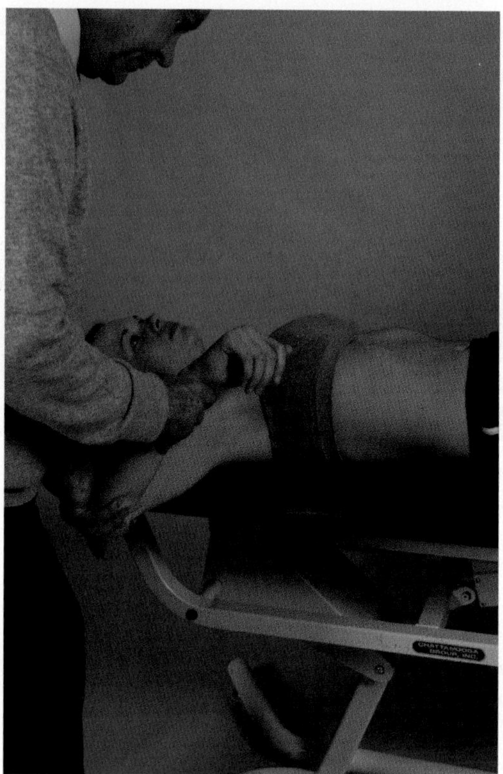

FIGURE 16-77 Compression–rotation test.

Biceps Load Test. The biceps load test was originally described by Kim et al.[345] During this test, the shoulder is placed at 90 degrees of abduction and maximally externally rotated (Fig. 16-78). At maximal ER and with the forearm in a supinated position, the patient is instructed to perform a biceps contraction against resistance.[10] Deep pain within the shoulder during his contraction is indicative of a SLAP lesion. Due to many design faults in the original study, this test has since been refined (biceps load II) with the shoulder being placed in the position of 120 degrees of abduction rather than the originally described 90 degrees, as this position was found to add greater sensitivity to the test (Table 16-28).[346]

Pronated Load Test. The pronated load test[10] is performed with the patient in a supine or seated position with the shoulder abducted to 90 degrees and externally rotated, and the forearm in a fully pronated position (to increase tension on the biceps and subsequently the labral attachment). When maximal ER is achieved, the patient is instructed to perform a resisted isometric contraction of the bicep against the clinician's resistance (Fig. 16-79). This test combines the active bicipital contraction of the biceps load test with the passive ER in the pronated position similar to the pain provocation test (see next).

Pain Provocation Test.[347] The patient is seated and the clinician stands behind the involved shoulder. The clinician

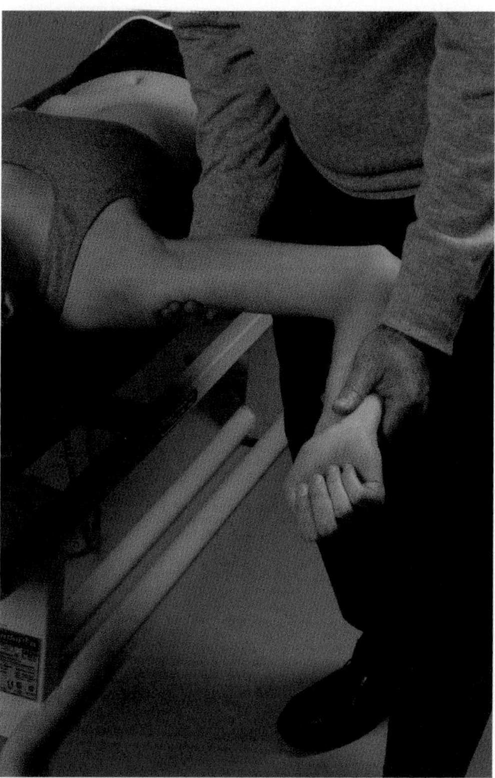

FIGURE 16-78 Biceps load test.

places the patient's shoulder at 90 degrees of abduction and toward end-range ER, the elbow at 90 degrees of flexion and the forearm in maximum supination (Fig. 16-80). The patient is asked to rate his or her pain in this position. The clinician

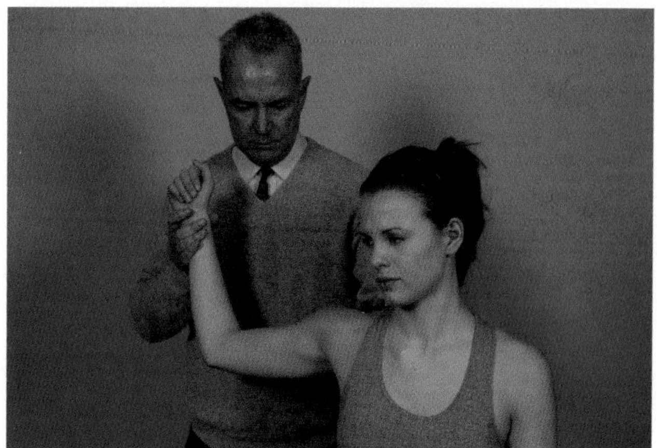

FIGURE 16-80 Pain provocation test.

then fully pronates the patient's forearm and asks the patient to again rate his or her pain. A positive test for a SLAP lesion is indicated if pain is produced with shoulder ER with the forearm in the pronated position or if the severity of the symptoms is greater in the pronated position. A study by Mimori et al.[347] found this test to have high sensitivity (100%) and high specificity (90%), although the study had many design faults.

Resisted Supination External Rotation Test.[348] During this test, the patient lies in the supine position with the clinician standing on the side of the involved shoulder. Supporting the patient's elbow with one hand, the clinician places the patient's shoulder at 90 degrees of shoulder abduction, 80–90 degrees of elbow flexion, and the forearm in neutral pronation/supination (Fig. 16-81). The patient is

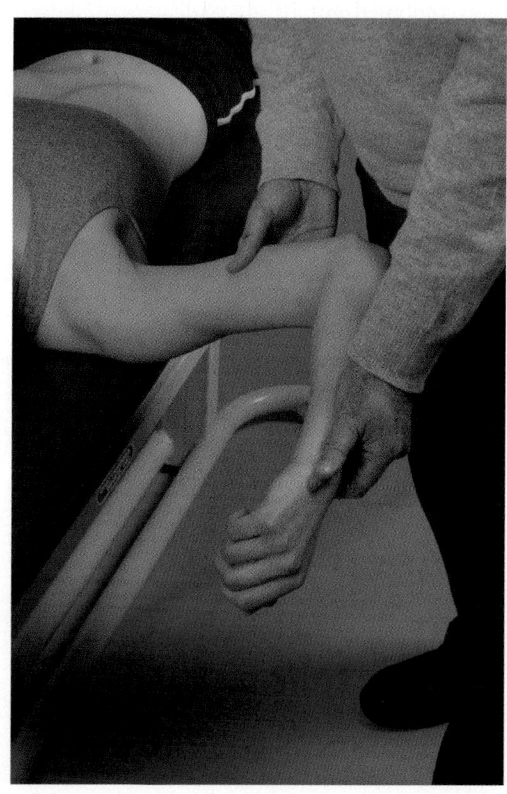

FIGURE 16-79 Pronated load test.

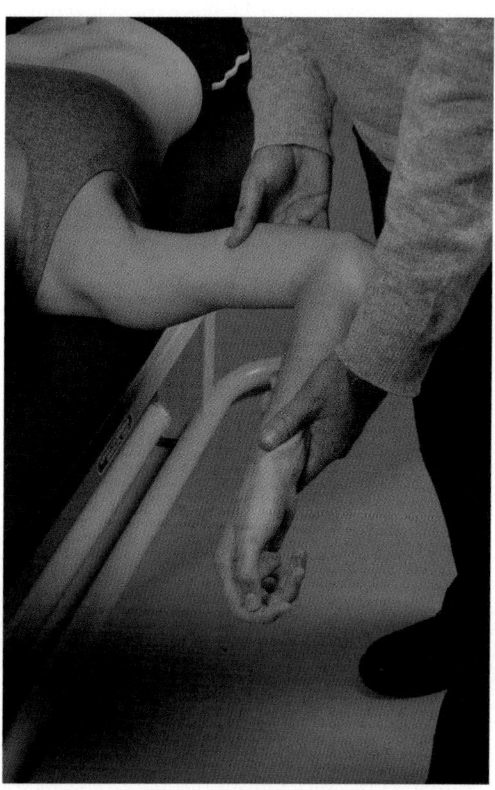

FIGURE 16-81 Resisted supination external rotation test.

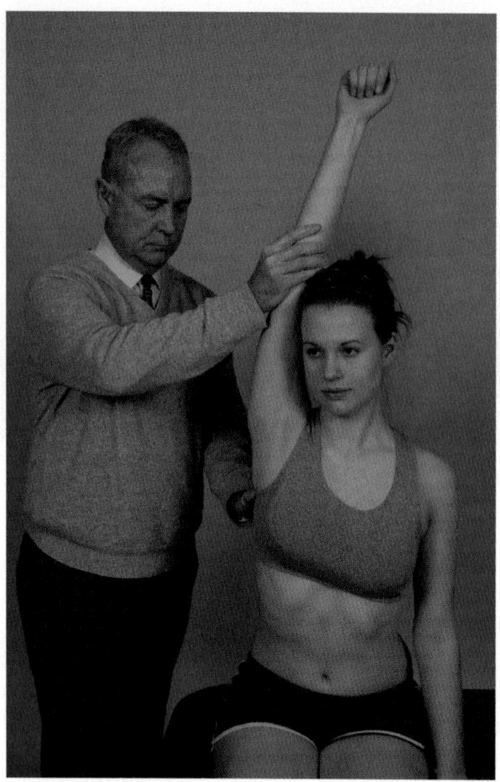

FIGURE 16-82 Forced shoulder abduction and elbow flexion test.

asked to attempt to supinate his or her arm The clinician resists against a maximal supination effort while gradually passively externally rotating the shoulder. A positive test for a torn labrum/instability is indicated by the production of pain in the anterior or deep shoulder, clicking or catching in the shoulder, or by reproduction of the patient's symptoms. A preliminary study of 40 patients revealed that this test had better sensitivity (82.8%), specificity (81.8%), positive predictive value (92.3%), negative predictive value (64.3%), and diagnostic accuracy (82.5%), compared with the crank test and O'Brien test.[348]

Forced Shoulder Abduction and Elbow Flexion Test. The patient sits, with the clinician standing behind and to the side of the involved shoulder. The clinician positions the patient's shoulder in maximum abduction with full elbow extension and notes any reports of pain in the posterior superior aspect of the shoulder (Fig. 16-82). The clinician then flexes the patient's elbow. A positive test for a superior labral tear is indicated by the production of pain in the posterior superior aspect of the shoulder during shoulder abduction with elbow extension that is diminished or relieved by the elbow flexion. In a study by Nakagawa et al.,[343] this test was found to have a sensitivity of 67% and a specificity of 67%. However, there were some design flaws with this study. For example, all of the subjects were young throwing athletes, and only two of the 54 subjects were female, leading to spectrum bias.

Wilk et al.[10] recommend that the selection of specific SLAP tests to perform should be based on the symptomatic complaints as well as the mechanism of injury described by the patient (Table 16-29).

TABLE 16-29 Selection of SLAP Tests Based on Mechanism of Injury

Mechanism	Test
Compressive injury	Active compression (O'Brien) Compression–rotation Clunk Anterior slide
Traction injury	Speed's Dynamic speed's Active compression
Overhead injury	Pronated load Resisted supination external rotation Biceps load I and II Pain provocation Crank

Data from Wilk KE, Reinold MM, Dugas JR, et al: Current concepts in the recognition and treatment of superior labral (SLAP) lesions. *J Orthop Sports Phys Ther* 35:273–291, 2005.

Acromioclavicular Tests

O'Brien Test. This is the same test described in the section "Biceps and Superior Labral Tears." The test has been found to be both highly sensitive and specific for diagnosing A-C joint abnormalities.[339] The test is considered positive for A-C joint dysfunction if the pain is localized to the AC joint on the first position and relieved or eliminated on the second position.[339,349]

Acromioclavicular Resisted Extension Test. This test is performed with the patient's shoulder positioned at 90 degrees of elevation combined with IR and 90 degrees of elbow flexion. The patient is then asked to horizontally abduct the arm against resistance (Fig. 16-83). This test is considered positive if it causes pain at the A-C joint.[350] Chronopoulos et al.[350] reported sensitivity of 72% and specificity of 85% with this test, but this study had some design flaws such as lack of blinding and not reporting patient inclusion/exclusion criteria.

Crossover Impingement/Horizontal Adduction Test. The patient's arm is positioned at 90 degrees of G-H flexion.

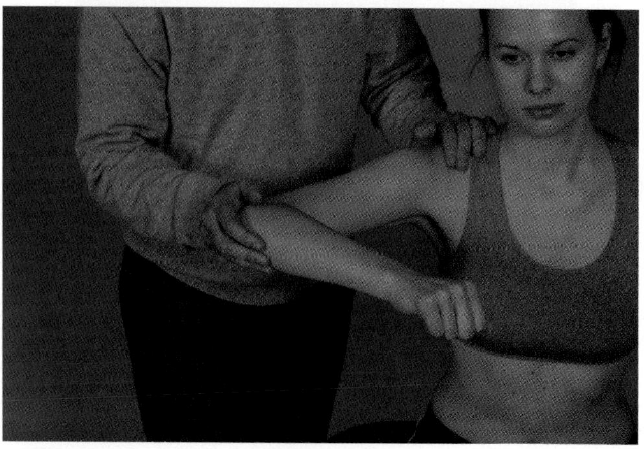

FIGURE 16-83 Acromioclavicular-resisted extension test.

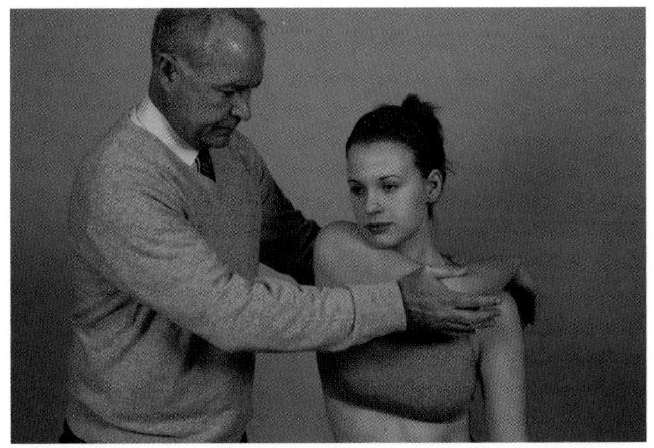

FIGURE 16-84 Cross-over impingement/horizontal adduction test.

The clinician passively moves the patient's arm into horizontal adduction and applies overpressure (Fig. 16-84). Although the crossover impingement/horizontal adduction test provokes compressive forces on the rotator cuff tendons that are localized under the A-C joint, it is a test more likely to be used to investigate A-C joint dysfunction.[318,337] Chronopoulos et al.[350] evaluated the crossover impingement test, the active compression test, and the A-C resisted extension test for the isolated and combined diagnostic utility with regard to chronic isolated A-C joint lesions. The study was a retrospective case–control study that used 35 patients diagnosed with chronic isolated A-C joint lesions and 580 control subjects who had undergone surgical procedures for other shoulder conditions. The authors concluded that the three tests studied had isolated clinical utility. They also analyzed the diagnostic utility of multitest regimens based on these three tests (Table 16-30) and suggested that the clinician should use a criterion of one positive test when high sensitivity is required, whereas a criterion of three positive tests is appropriate when high specificity is necessary.[349,350]

Examination of the Passive Restraint System

If following the ROM, strength, and functional movement tests, the clinician is unable to determine a working hypothesis from which to treat the patient, further examination is required. This more detailed examination involves the assessment of the mobility and stability of the passive restraint systems of the shoulder girdle (Table 16-31).

Stability Testing. It is important to remember that there is no correlation between the amount of joint laxity/mobility and joint instability at the shoulder.[351] Joint stability is more likely a function of connective tissue support and an intact neuromuscular system.[234]

Many provocative maneuvers including the anterior and posterior apprehension tests, the sulcus test,[352–354] and the load and shift test have been described previously. The reproduction of symptoms is important because laxity alone does not indicate instability. Side-to-side translational asymmetry often has been taken as being representative of disease, but healthy shoulders may also have asymmetry up to grade II laxity.[355,356]

Pain and muscle spasm can make the examination challenging. Rarely is examination with the patient under anesthesia useful for anything other than fine-tuning the amount of capsular shift required at surgery.[357]

Glenohumeral: Load and Shift Test. The patient lies in the supine position. The clinician is beside the patient with the inside of the hand over the patient's shoulder and forearm, stabilizing the scapula to the thorax. The clinician places his or her hand across the G-H joint line and humeral head, so that clinician's little finger is positioned across the anterior G-H joint line and humeral head (Fig. 16-85). The clinician then applies a "load and shift" of the humeral head across the stabilized scapula in an anteromedial direction to assess anterior stability, and in a posterolateral direction, to assess posterior instability. The normal motion anteriorly is half of the distance of the humeral head. Although attempts have been made to grade or quantify the degree of instability more specifically, the literature supports no consistency in the grading to date.[168,358–361] This test has been reported to be 100% sensitive for the detection of instability in patients with recurrent dislocation, but not in cases of recurrent subluxation.[359]

Apprehension Test. The patient lies in the supine position with the arm at 90 degrees of abduction and full ER. The

TABLE 16-30 Diagnostic Utility Multitest Regimens Consisting of Cross-Body Adduction Stress, Active Compression, and Acromioclavicular Resisted Extension Test

	Accuracy	Sensitivity	Specificity	Positive Predictive Value	Negative Predictive Value	Positive Likelihood Ratio	Negative Likelihood Ratio
≥1 Positive test	0.75 (237/315)	0.00 (16/16)	0.74 (221/299)	0.17 (16/94)	1.00 (221/221)	0.00	1.4
≥2 Positive tests	0.89 (279/315)	0.81 (13/16)	0.89 (266/299)	0.28 (13/46)	0.99 (266/269)	7.4	0.2
3 Positive tests	93 (294/315)	0.25 (4/16)	0.97 (290/299)	0.31 (4/13)	0.96 (290/302)	8.3	0.8

Data from Chronopoulos E, Kim TK, Park HB, et al: Diagnostic value of physical tests for isolated chronic acromioclavicular lesions. *Am J Sports Med* 32:655–661, 2004; Powell JW, Huijbregts PA: Concurrent criterion-related validity of acromioclavicular joint physical examination tests: A systematic review. *J Man Manip Ther* 14:E19–E29, 2006.

TABLE 16-31 Diagnostic Test Properties for Shoulder Laxity[a]

Diagnostic Test or Maneuver	Study Population	Sensitivity	Specificity	Positive Likelihood Ratio	Negative Likelihood Ratio
Shoulder relocation test (no force on humerus at start position)	100 surgical patient; ages not reported[b]	0.30 for pain 0.57 for apprehension	0.58 for pain 1.0 for apprehension	0.71 Not applicable	1.21 0.43
Shoulder relocation test (anterior-directed force on humerus at start position)	100 surgical patients' ages not reported[b]	0.54 for pain 0.68 for apprehension	0.44 for pain 1.0 for apprehension	0.96 Not applicable	1.05 0.32
Relocation test for posterosuperior glenoid rotator cuff lesions	20 throwing athletes; aged 19–35 yr, mean age 24.9 yr[c]	0.95 for pain	—	—	—
Anterior release test for anterior instability	100 athletes; aged 15–61, mean age 37 yr[d]	0.92	0.89	8.36	0.09
Load and shift[e]	Anterior Posterior Inferior	0.5 0.14 0.08	1.00 1.00 1.00	Not applicable Not applicable Not applicable	0.50 0.86 0.92
Grading translation anterior, posterior, and inferior	43 asymptomatic college athlete; mean age 19.2 yr[f]		Intraobserver reproducibility 46%, 73% when grades 0 and 1 equalized Interobserver 47% and 73% when equalized		
Hyperabduction test for stability; inferior glenohumeral ligament >105 degrees indicate laxity; normal 85–90 degrees	100 normals; aged 24–38 yr, mean age 28 yr[g] 90 patients with shoulder instability; aged 18–40 yr, mean age 24.3 yr 100 cadavers; aged 61–82 yr, mean age 76 yr	0.84	0.95	16.89	0.16

[a]Data from Deyle GD, Bang MD, Kane E: Evidence-based practice for the shoulder. In: Wilmarth MA, ed. *Evidence-Based Practice for the Upper and Lower Quarter*. La Crosse, WI: Orthopaedic Physical Therapy Home Study Course 13.2.1, Orthopaedic Section, APTA, Inc., 2003:15, Table 6. Permission from Orthopaedic Section, APTA.
[b]Data from Speer KP, Hannafin JA, Altchek DW, et al: An evaluation of the shoulder relocation test. *Am J Sports Med* 22:177–183, 1994.
[c]Data from Riand N, Levigne C, Renaud E, et al: Results of derotational humeral osteotomy in posterosuperior glenoid impingement. *Am J Sports Med* 26:453–459, 1998.
[d]Data from Gross ML, Distefano MC: Anterior release test: A new test for occult shoulder instability. *Clin Orth Rel Res* 339:105–108, 1997.
[e]Data from Tzannes A, Murrell GA: Clinical examination of the unstable shoulder. *Sports Med* 32:447–457, 2002.
[f]Data from Levy AS, Lintner S, Kenter K, et al: Intra- and interobserver reproducibility of the shoulder laxity examination. *Am J Sports Med* 27:460–463, 1999.
[g]Data from Gagey OJ, Gagey N: The Hyperabduction test. *J Bone Joint Surg Br* 83:69–74, 2001.

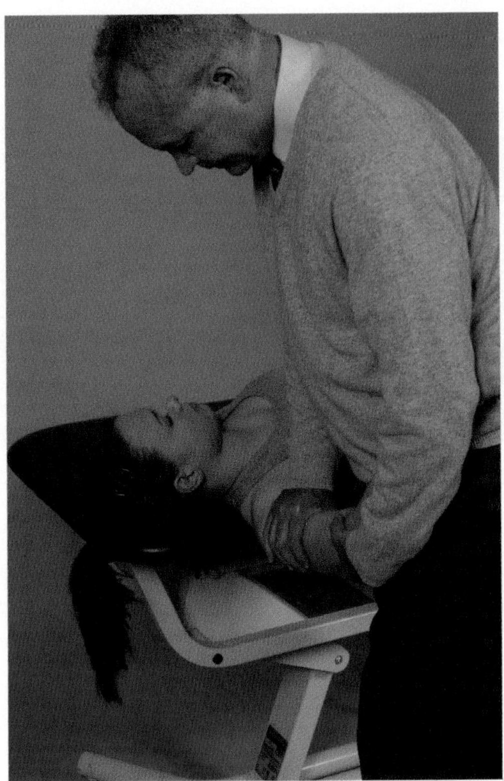

FIGURE 16-85 Load and shift test.

clinician holds the patient's wrist with one hand, while the other hand stabilizes the patient's elbow (Fig. 16-86). The clinician applies overpressure into ER. Patient's apprehension from this maneuver, rather than his/her pain, is considered a positive test for anterior instability. Pain with this maneuver, but without apprehension, may indicate pathology other than instability, such as posterior impingement of the rotator cuff.[75] In a study by Mok et al., [362] this test demonstrated a specificity of 61% and a sensitivity of 63%.

Sulcus Sign for Inferior Instability. The sulcus sign was described by Neer and Foster[353] and is used to detect inferior instability due to a laxity of the superior G-H and coraco-humeral ligaments. The patient's arm is positioned at 20–50 degrees of abduction and neutral rotation.[149,363] A positive test results in the presence of a sulcus sign (a depression greater than a fingerbreadth between the lateral acromion and the head of the humerus) (Fig. 16-87) when longitudinal traction is applied to the dependent arm in more than one position.[364]

The sulcus sign can be graded by measuring the distance from the inferior margin of the acromion to the humeral head. A distance of less than 1 cm is graded as 1+ sulcus, 1–2 cm as a 2+ sulcus, and greater than 2 cm as a grade 3+ sulcus.[353] A study by Levy et al.[365] evaluated the inter- and intraobserver reproducibility of the clinical examination of G-H laxity in the unanesthetized shoulder. Forty-three asymptomatic division I collegiate athletes underwent bilateral shoulder laxity examination initially and again after 3 months. Overall intraobserver reproducibility of examination was 46%. When grades 0 and 1 were equalized, overall intraobserver reproducibility improved to 74%. For both the equalized and nonequalized reproducibility values reported by all examiners, the κ values for intraobserver correlation were less than 0.5, which suggests that correlations were not better than those achieved by chance alone. Overall interobserver reproducibility was 47%. When grades 0 and 1 were equalized, interobserver reproducibility improved to 78%.

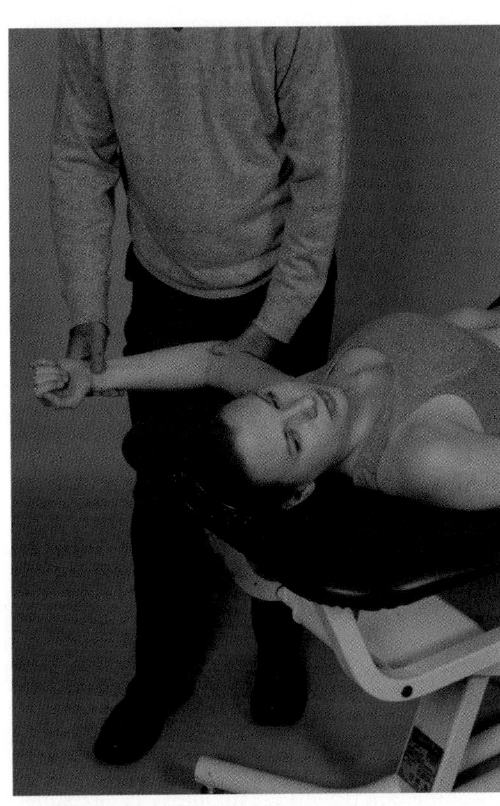

FIGURE 16-86 Apprehension test.

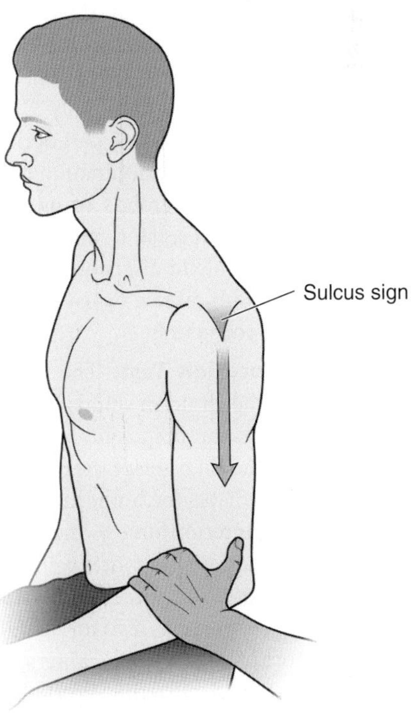

FIGURE 16-87 Sulcus sign.

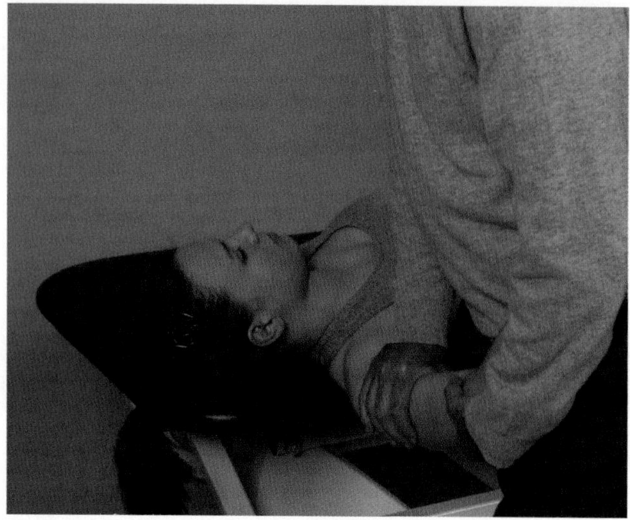

FIGURE 16-88 Subluxation/relocation test.

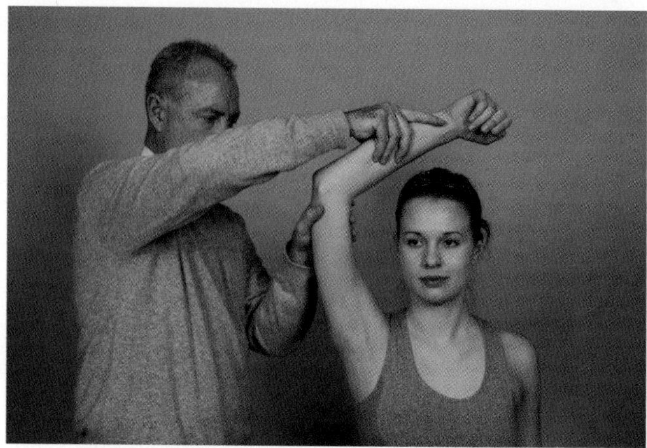

FIGURE 16-89 Rockwood test for anterior instability.

Jobe Subluxation/Relocation Test. This test is similar to the load and shift test, except that manual pressure is applied anteriorly by the clinician in an attempt to provoke a subluxation, before using manual pressure in the opposite direction to relocate the subluxation. The patient lies in the supine position with their arm at 90 degrees of abduction and full ER. The clinician grasps the patient's elbow with one hand to maintain the testing position and grasps the humeral head with the other hand (Fig. 16-88). The clinician gently applies an anterior pull on the humerus. Pain and apprehension from the patient indicate a positive test for a superior labral tear or anterior instability.[1] After pulling the humeral head anteriorly and demonstrating pain and apprehension, the clinician should then push the humeral head posteriorly while maintaining the shoulder in the same position (the relocation part of the test). Reduction of pain and apprehension further substantiates the clinical finding of anterior instability. The sensitivity and specificity of the relocation test is reported to be low when assessing pain response only, but very high when assessing the apprehension response only.[366]

The performance of the relocation part of the test (based on operative findings and manual examination under anesthesia) was compared between two groups of patients: those with anterior instability and with rotator cuff disease.[366] The study found that it is not possible to discriminate between anterior instability and rotator cuff disease by using the relocation test for assessing pain response only.

Modified Jobe Relocation Test. The patient lies in the supine position, and the clinician stands on the involved side of the patient. The clinician prepositions the shoulder at 120 degrees of abduction and then grasps the patient's forearm and maximally externally rotates the humerus. The clinician then applies a posterior to anterior force to the posterior aspect of the humeral head. If the patient reports pain with this maneuver, an anterior-to-posterior force is then applied to the proximal humerus. A positive test for labral pathology is indicated by a report of pain with the anterior-directed force and release of pain with the posterior directed force. In a small study of 14 overhead throwing athletes, aged 21–31 years, Hamner et al.[367] found the test to have high sensitivity (92%) and high specificity (100%). However, there were a number of design faults in the study that led to potential bias and further research is required.

Rockwood Test for Anterior Instability.[368] The patient is seated with the clinician standing. With the arm by the patient' s side, the clinician passively externally rotates the shoulder. The patient then abducts the arm to approximately 45 degrees and the test is repeated. The same maneuver is again repeated with the arm abducted to 90 degrees, and then 120 degrees (Fig. 16-89) to assess the different stabilizing structures. A positive test is indicated when apprehension is noted in the latter three positions (45, 90, and 120 degrees).

Anterior Release Test/Surprise Test.[369] The patient lies in the supine position with the shoulder at 90 degrees of abduction and the elbow flexed to 90 degrees. The clinician passively moves the patient's shoulder into ER while applying a posteriorly directed force to the head of the humerus. At the point of end-range ER, the clinician quickly releases the posterior force (Fig. 16-90) and notes whether the patient displays any sign of apprehension. In a study by Lo et al.,[370] which assessed the validity of the apprehension, relocation, and surprise tests as predictors of anterior shoulder instability, for those subjects who had a feeling of apprehension on all three tests, the mean positive and negative predictive values were 93.6% and 71.9%, respectively. The surprise test was the single most accurate test (sensitivity 63.89%; specificity 98.91%). An improvement in the feeling of apprehension or pain with the relocation test added little to the value of the tests. The results of this study would suggest that a positive instability examination on all three tests is highly specific and predictive of traumatic anterior G-H instability.[370]

Anterior Fulcrum Test.[371] The patient lies in the supine position with the shoulder positioned at approximately 90 degrees of abduction and ER. The clinician moves the arm into horizontal abduction while applying an anterior force to the G-H joint in a fulcrum maneuver (Fig. 16-91). The clinician notes the amount of translation and end feel in comparison with the opposite extremity. The test can be repeated at 45 degrees of abduction (to test the middle G-H ligament) and in adduction (to assess the superior G-H ligament).

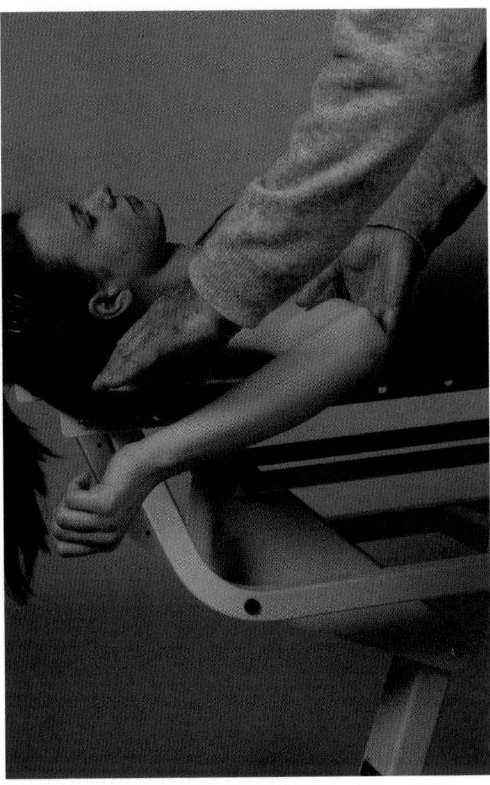

FIGURE 16-90 Anterior release test.

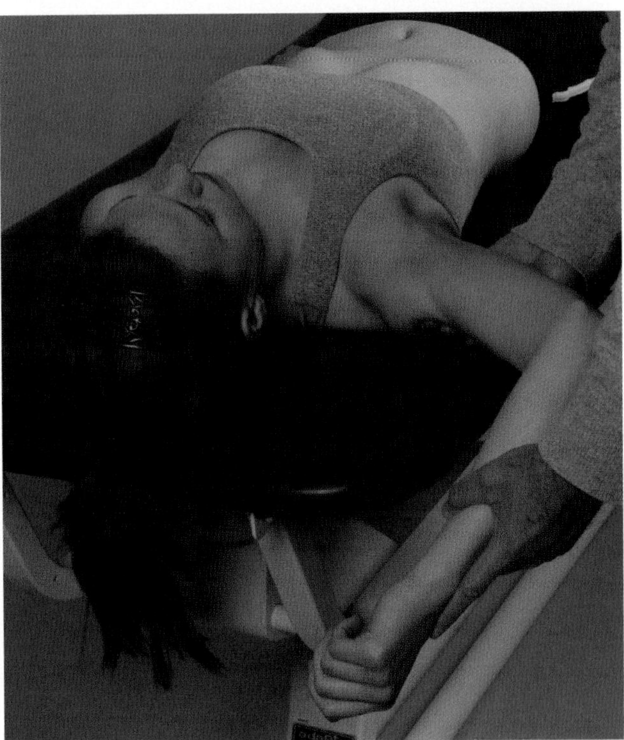

FIGURE 16-92 Lachman test of the shoulder.

Lachman Test of the Shoulder.[372] The patient lies in the supine position and the shoulder is abducted overhead to approximately 120–135 degrees of abduction and full ER (Fig. 16-92). The clinician then translates the G-H joint anteriorly and notes the amount of humeral translation as well as the endpoint of translation, in comparison with the uninvolved shoulder. Theoretically in this position, the integrity of the inferior G-H ligament and the anterior–inferior capsule is tested.

Thoracic Outlet Syndrome Tests

These tests are described in "Special Tests" section in Chapter 25.

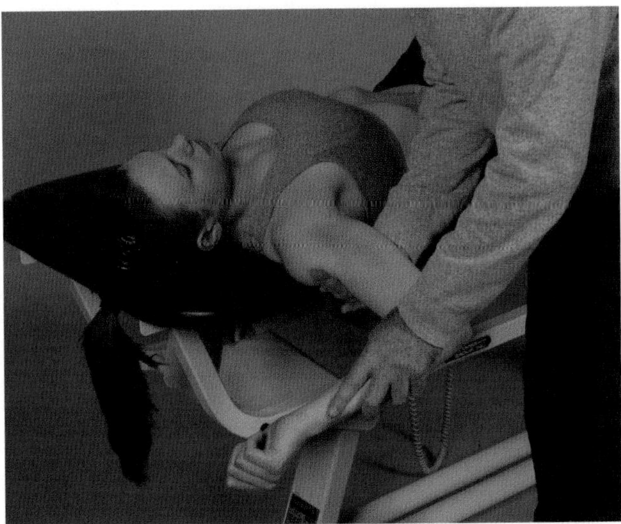

FIGURE 16-91 Anterior fulcrum test.

Diagnostic Studies

The conclusions on the radiology reports concerning single-plane views, which include an A-P view with the humerus in IR, and a second A-P view with the humerus in ER (see Chap. 7), should be treated with caution as they have been well documented to result in misdiagnosis.[373]

If A-C separation is suspected, a weighted view is performed with a weight suspended from the wrist on the involved side. Alternative or specialized views are sometimes used in an attempt to better define specific structures. For example, with a suspected shoulder dislocation, the West Point or Lawrence view (inferior–superior axial projection) is used to help display the inferior glenoid fossa and its relationship to the humeral head, in addition to the lateral perspective of the proximal humerus.

Arthrography aids in the diagnosis of full thickness rotator cuff tears.[374] Bone scans are rarely used in the diagnosis of shoulder pain, but a CT scan report can be useful in confirming the clinical findings in some cases.[1] The MRI is very reliable in detecting lesions of the capsule and labrum, as well as associated rotator cuff tears. It can generally indicate the approximate size of a rotator cuff tear and may also indicate whether the critically important subscapularis tendon is torn.[1,375,376]

In a limited number of studies, a comparison has been made as to the accuracy of physical diagnostic tests versus arthroscopic examination. One such study found that the physical therapists were unable to differentiate between a partial and complete tear of the rotator cuff tendons.[377] However, a later study showed that physical therapists were able to discern subacromial disorders and passive restraint disorders with an agreement of 85 and 67%, respectively.[378]

Evaluation

Following the examination, and once the clinical findings have been recorded, the clinician must attempt to determine a specific diagnosis or a working hypothesis, based on a summary of all of the findings. This diagnosis can be structure related (medical diagnosis) (Table 16-32), or a diagnosis based on the preferred practice patterns as described in the *Guide to Physical Therapist Practice*. Further details on the specific conditions listed in Table 16-30 is provided in the following sections.

INTERVENTION STRATEGIES

With the possible exceptions of acute traumatic shoulder dislocation and acute traumatic inability to raise the arm (acute massive rotator cuff tear), a minimum 6-week period of conservative empiric intervention is typically indicated for shoulder injuries. A number of guiding principles can be used in the conservative rehabilitation of the shoulder[379]:

- The shoulder must be rehabilitated according to the stage of healing and degree of irritability. The degree of irritability can be determined by inquiring about the vigor, duration, and intensity of the pain. Greater irritability is associated with very acutely inflamed conditions. The characteristic sign for an acute inflammation of the shoulder is pain at rest, which is diffuse in its distribution and often referred from the site of the primary condition.[324] Pain above the elbow indicates less severity than pain below the elbow. Chronic conditions usually have a low irritability, but can have an associated loss of AROM and PROM. The degree of movement and the speed of progression are both guided by the signs and symptoms.
- Rehabilitate the shoulder using scapular planes rather than the straight planes of flexion, extension, and abduction as the scapular planes are more functional.
- Short lever arms should initially be used with exercises as they decrease the torque at the shoulder. Short levers can be achieved by flexing the elbow or by exercising with the arm closer to the body.
- Obtain a stable scapular platform as early as possible.
- Achieve the closed-pack position of the G-H joint at the earliest opportunity. All ROM exercises for the shoulder have traditionally been initiated in the early ranges of flexion with the goal of achieving full elevation. Given the protection afforded the joint by the passive restraint system, thought should be given to providing ROM exercises initiated at the end ranges of elevation according to patient tolerance. Exceptions to this would be the patient whose condition precluded such exercises, that is, following shoulder surgery, adhesive capsulitis, or instability.
- Reproduce the forces and loading rates that will mimic the patient's functional demands as the rehabilitation progresses.

The manual techniques to increase joint mobility and the techniques to increase soft tissue extensibility are described in "Therapeutic Techniques" section.

ACUTE PHASE

The goals of the acute phase include the following:

- Protection of the healing site.
- Restoration of pain-free ROM throughout the remainder of the kinetic chain.
- Enhance patient comfort by decreasing pain and inflammation.
- Retard muscle atrophy.
- Minimize the detrimental effects of immobilization and activity restriction.[243,244,380–383]
- Maintain general cardiovascular fitness using lower extremity aerobic exercises such as walking.
- Independence with a home exercise program.

The principles of PRICEMEM (protection, rest, ice, compression, elevation, manual therapy, early motion, and medication) are applied as appropriate during the early stages of the acute phase,. Icing for 20–30 minutes three to four times a day, concurrent with nonsteroidal anti-inflammatory drugs (NSAIDs) or aspirin, can assist in reducing pain and swelling.

Early active-assisted and passive exercises are performed to nourish the articular cartilage and assist in collagen tissue synthesis and organization.[384–388] These exercises are initiated in pain-free arcs, below 90 degrees of abduction/flexion. Recommended ROM exercises for the acute phase include the following:

- Codman's or other pendulum exercises (Fig. 16-93) **VIDEO**. Codman's pendulum exercise is commonly prescribed after shoulder surgery or injury to provide grade I and grade II distraction and oscillations resulting in decreased pain and early joint mobilization.[389] One study,[389] which measured EMG activity of the shoulder muscles, found that the pendulum exercise did not have a significant effect on shoulder EMG activity. Generally, the supraspinatus/upper trapezius muscle activity was significantly higher than the deltoid and infraspinatus activity—especially in the patients with shoulder pathology. Many shoulder protocols suggest holding a weight while performing the pendulum exercises as rehabilitation progresses. Ellsworth et al.[389] found that performing the pendulum exercise with added weight did not result in significant increased shoulder EMG activity for the deltoid and infraspinatus muscles in subjects with or without shoulder pathology. However, patients with shoulder pathology had more difficulty relaxing their supraspinatus/upper trapezius muscles than did the healthy subjects.[389] Other PROM exercises can also be introduced. These include passive shoulder flexion (Fig. 16-94) **VIDEO**, abduction **VIDEO**, ER **VIDEO**, and IR and elbow flexion and extension **VIDEO**.
- Active assisted ROM (AAROM) exercises. AAROM may include wand or cane exercises that move the arm into functional planes while incorporating combinations of forward flexion (Fig. 16-95) **VIDEO**, extension, abduction, IR, and ER. Over-the-door pulley exercises are performed later in the acute phase as tolerated. However, care must be taken with these exercises in the presence of impingement or

TABLE 16-32 Differential Diagnosis for Common Causes of Shoulder Pain

Condition	Approximate Patient's Age	Mechanism of Injury	Area of Symptoms	Symptoms Aggravated by	Observation	AROM	PROM	End-Feel	Pain with Resisted	Tenderness Palpation
Rotator cuff tendinitis										
Acute	20–40	Microtrauma/ macrotrauma	Anterior and lateral shoulder	Overhead motions	Swelling—anterior shoulder	Limited abduction	Limited abduction	ER	Abduction	Pain below anterior acromial rim
Chronic	30–70	Microtrauma/ macrotrauma	Anterior and lateral shoulder	Overhead motions Atrophy of shoulder area	Atrophy of scapular area	Limited abduction and flexion	Pain on IR and ER at 90-degree abduction	ER IR	Abduction Pain below anterior acromial rim	Anterior shoulder
Bicipital tendinitis	20–45	Microtrauma	Anterior shoulder	Overhead motions May see signs of concomitant rotator cuff pathology	Possible swelling—anterior shoulder Pain on full flexion from full extension	Limited ER when arm at 90-degree abduction Biceps stability test may be abnormal (if tendon unstable)	Pain on combined extension of shoulder and elbow	Speed test painful, Yergason test occasionally painful	Elbow flexion	Of biceps tendon over bicipital groove
Rotator cuff rupture	40+	Macrotrauma	Posterior/ superior shoulder	Arm elevation	Atrophy of scapular area	Limited abduction Pain with or without restriction	Full and pain free	ER	Abduction	Pain below anterolateral acromial rim

(Continued)

TABLE 16-32 Differential Diagnosis for Common Causes of Shoulder Pain *(Continued)*

Condition	Approximate Patient's Age	Mechanism of Injury	Area of Symptoms	Symptoms Aggravated by	Observation	AROM	PROM	End-Feel	Pain with Resisted	Tenderness Palpation
Adhesive capsulitis	35–70	Microtrauma/ macrotrauma	Shoulder and upper arm—poorly localized	All motions	Atrophy of shoulder area	All motions limited especially ER and abduction	All motions limited especially ER and abduction	Capsular	Most/all	Varies
A-C joint sprain	Varies	Macrotrauma	Point of shoulder	Horizontal adduction	Step/bump at point of shoulder	Limited abduction Limited horizontal adduction	Limited abduction Pain with horizontal adduction	Flexion Flexion	ER Soft tissue thickening at point of shoulder	Point of shoulder
Subacromial bursitis	Varies	Microtrauma	Anterior and lateral shoulder	Overhead motions	Often unremarkable	Limited abduction and IR May have full range but pain in midrange of flexion/ abduction	Pain on IR at 90-degree abduction Pain only in midrange abduction and flexion		Most/all	Pain below anterolateral acromial rim
Glenohumeral arthritis	50+	Gradual onset, but can be traumatic	Poorly localized	Arm activity	Possible posterior positioning of humeral head	Capsular pattern (ER> abduction>IR)	Pain	Capsular	Weakness of rotator cuff, rather than pain	Poorly localized

SICK Scapula	20–40	Microtrauma	Anterior/superior shoulder Posterosuperior scapular Arm, forearm, hand	Overhead activities	Scapular malposition Inferior medial border prominence Dyskinesia of scapular movement	Decreased forward flexion which diminishes when clinician manually repositions the scapula into retraction and posterior tilt	Normal		Weakness rather than pain	Medial coracoid Superomedial angle cf scapula
Cervical radiculopathy	Varies	Typically none but can be traumatic	Upper back, below shoulder	Cervical extension, cervical side bending and rotation to ipsilateral side, full arm elevation	May have lateral deviation of head away from painful side	Decreased cervical flexion, cervical side bending and rotation to ipsilateral side; decreased arm elevation on involved side	Painful into restricted active range of motions Positive Spurling's test	Empty	Weakness rather than pain Other neurological changes	Varies; may have numbness over dermatomal area

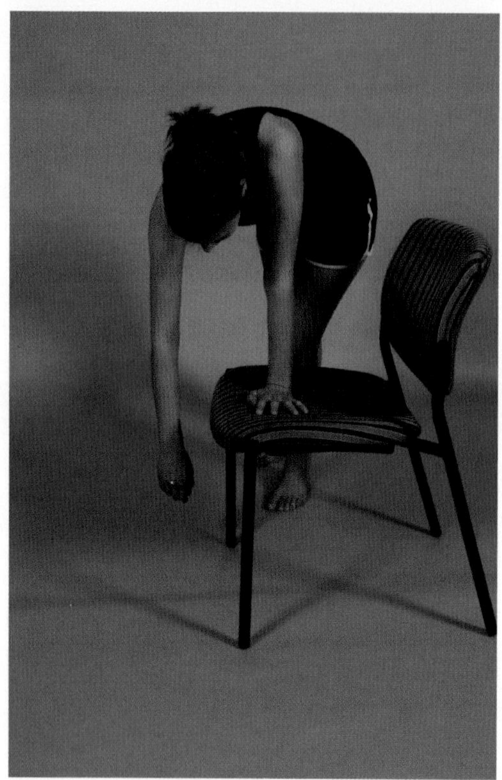

FIGURE 16-93 Codman's pendulum.

adhesive capsulitis as these exercises can reinforce poor scapulohumeral motion.

- Active exercises. These can be performed in a variety of positions including standing, sitting, or lying (Figs. 16-16 and 16-19).

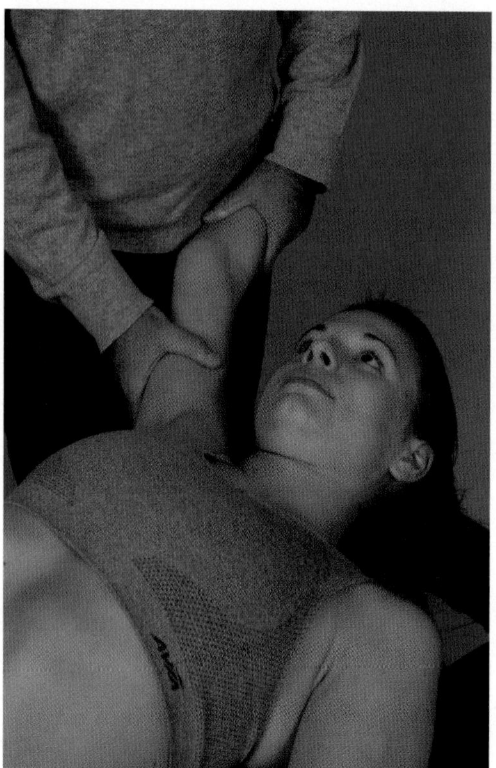

FIGURE 16-94 Passive shoulder flexion.

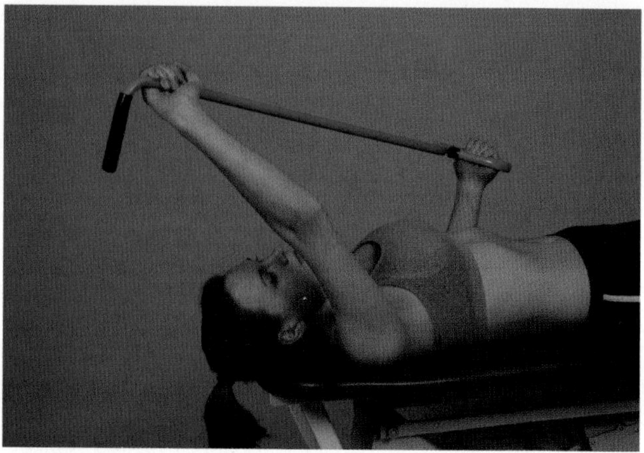

FIGURE 16-95 Active assisted shoulder flexion.

Strengthening exercises for the shoulder are introduced as early as tolerated, initially using isometric exercises, with the arm positioned below 90 degrees of abduction and 90 degrees of flexion. Elbow flexion (Fig. 16-96) and extension progressive-resistive exercises (PREs) are introduced as appropriate VIDEO. Specific scapular rehabilitation PREs are typically initiated with the isometric exercises, such as the scapular setting exercise VIDEO. Patterns of scapular retraction and protraction are initiated in single planes and then progressed to elevation and depression of the entire scapula. To improve backward reaching, the patient must first learn correct retraction procedures.

Jobe and Pink[98] believe that the order of strengthening in the rehabilitation process should follow a progression based on muscle function. They advocate strengthening the *G-H protectors* (rotator cuff muscles) and scapular *pivoters* (levator scapulae, serratus anterior, middle trapezius, and rhomboids

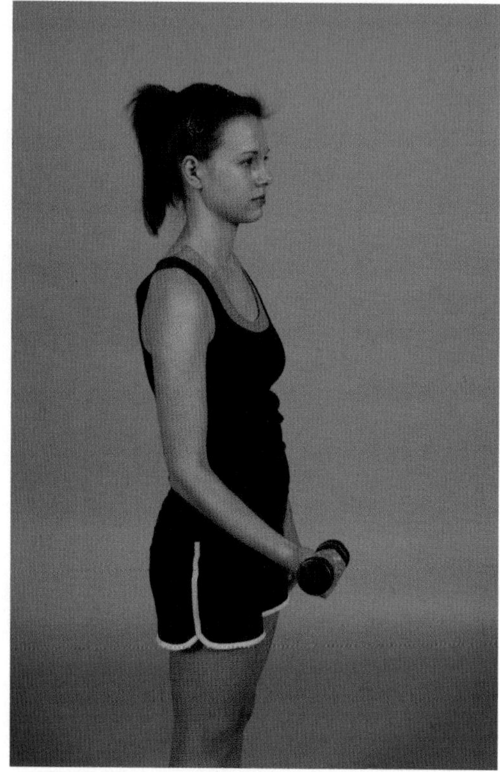

FIGURE 16-96 Elbow flexion PRE.

VIDEO) initially because of the role they play in providing stability. In contrast, exercises for the humeral "positioners" (deltoid) and the humeral "propellers" (latissimus dorsi and pectoralis major) are introduced in the "Functional Phase" section. Exercises for the *G-H protectors* include the AAROM wand exercises, progressing to AROM in the pain-free ranges throughout the functional planes. In addition, the incorporation of scapular retraction and scapular elevation exercises with G-H movements help stimulate a cocontraction of the G-H protectors and allow for a more normal physiologic sequence to redevelop. Scapular *pivoter* exercises include the *scapular pinch*, which is an isometric activity involving scapula retraction toward the midline (Fig. 16-27), and the YTWL exercise (the letters describe the shape the arms adopt) VIDEO.[152,153] Other resisted exercises for the scapular can be introduced at this stage to promote proximal stability. Examples include wall push-ups and isometric chair push-ups at varying degrees of elbow flexion (Fig. 16-97).

Once the arm can be safely elevated and held in the position of 90-degree abduction while standing or sitting, the patient lies in the supine position and the arm is actively raised as high as the pain-free range will allow (from 90 to 180 degrees, depending on tolerance), first without resistance and then with resistance VIDEO. From this position, the patient performs a serratus punch with a "plus." If applicable, the patient is progressed to full push-ups VIDEO. At the end of each push-up as the arm is fully straightened, an extra push is applied. This extra push with the push-up is termed as push-up plus (Fig. 16-98). This exercise strengthens the pectoralis minor, and the lower and middle serratus anterior.[13,122]

The application of joint compression with contraction through the application of closed-chain exercises is important, as closed-chain activities help to balance compression and

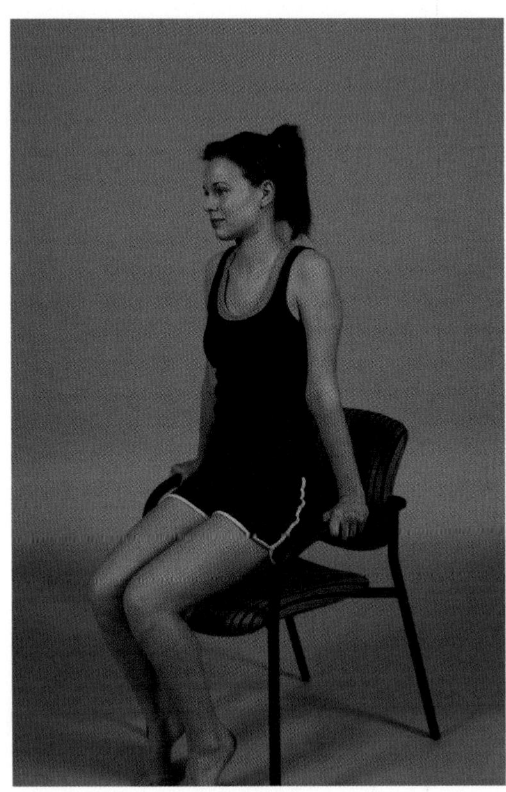

FIGURE 16-97 Isometric chair push-ups.

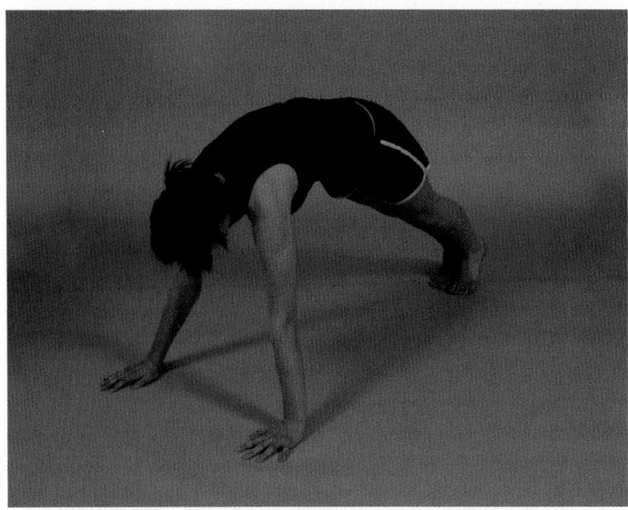

FIGURE 16-98 Push-up plus.

shear forces at the shoulder. These activities also encourage the correct sequencing of muscle contraction around the shoulder girdle and emphasize the cocontraction of force couples at the scapulothoracic and G-H joints.[87] This results in a correct scapular position and stabilization.[153] Closed-chain exercises may be done early in the rehabilitation phase as they do not put shear on the joint. They also allow the rotator cuff muscles to be activated without being inhibited by pain or deltoid overactivity. The closed-chain exercises can be initiated in the lower ranges using a table (Fig. 16-99), and then progressed to having the hands stabilized in the quadruped position, using a ball (Fig. 16-100). These exercises are started at elevations of 60 degrees or less and are moved up to 90 degrees of flexion, and then abduction, as tolerated to allow for healing of the tissues.[24,144,152,153]

Other closed-chain exercises can be performed by placing both hands on a table and flexing the shoulder to less than 60 degrees and abducting to 45 degrees. Progression is made to weight bearing on a tilt board or a circular board (Fig. 16-101) within tolerance. Other exercises that provide joint compression include the following:

- *Side-lying to sitting transfers* (Fig. 16-102).
- *Elbow rest.* The patient supine in a semireclined position, leaning on the elbows, with the humerus in a neutral or extended position (Fig. 16-103). This exercise can also be performed with the patient in prone (Fig. 16-104). Manual resistance can be applied by the clinician to make the exercise more challenging.
- *Table press-up.* The patient is seated on a chair or bed. The patient then raises and lowers the buttocks off the surface by straightening the elbow (Fig. 16-105). This works the triceps muscles, the pectoralis major and minor, and the latissimus dorsi muscles.[13] This exercise can be progressed to include pushing and pulling exercises and quadruped and tripod balancing (Fig. 16-106).

Flexibility exercises to stretch both the joint capsule and the shoulder girdle muscles are a vital component of the rehabilitation process. These include the sleeper stretch (Fig. 16-107) performed in side-lying VIDEO and then with the arm abducted to 90 degrees VIDEO. Gentle grade I or II oscillations are

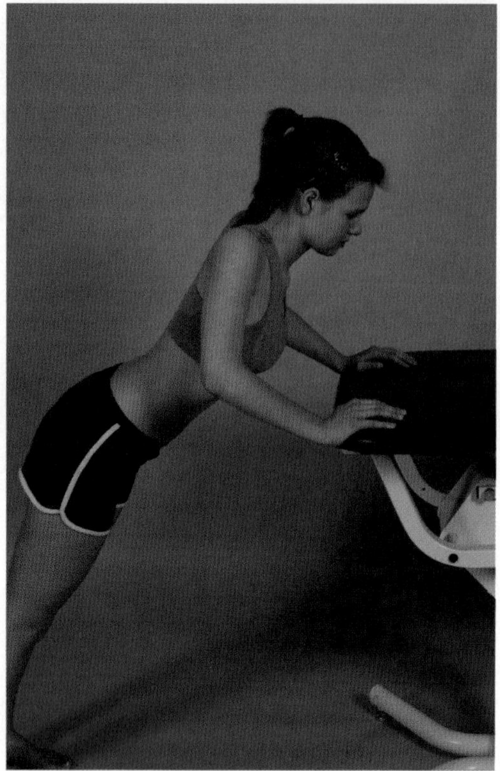

FIGURE 16-99 Closed-chain exercise using upper extremity compression.

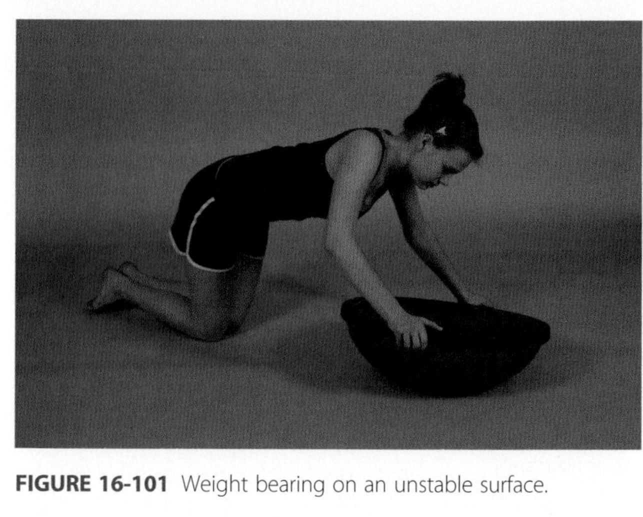

FIGURE 16-101 Weight bearing on an unstable surface.

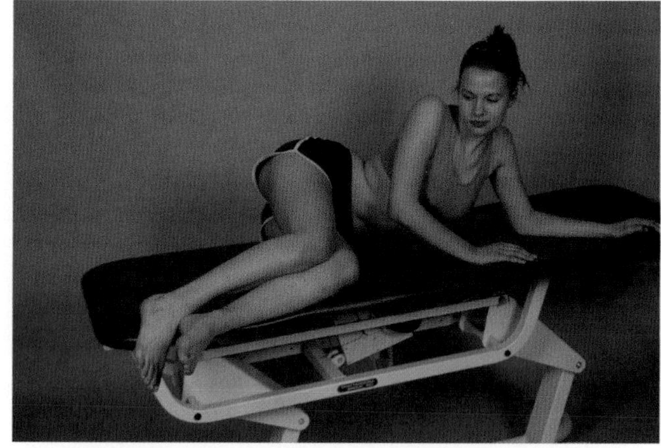

FIGURE 16-102 Side-lying to sitting transfer.

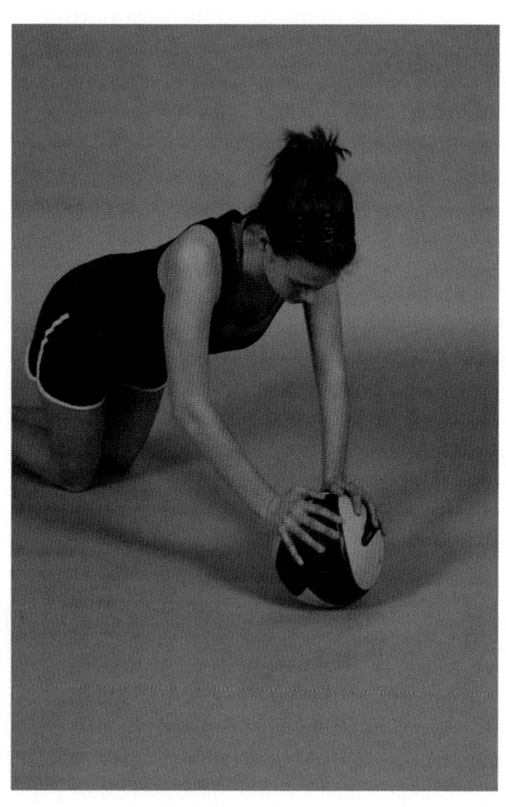

FIGURE 16-100 Joint compression in the quadruped position.

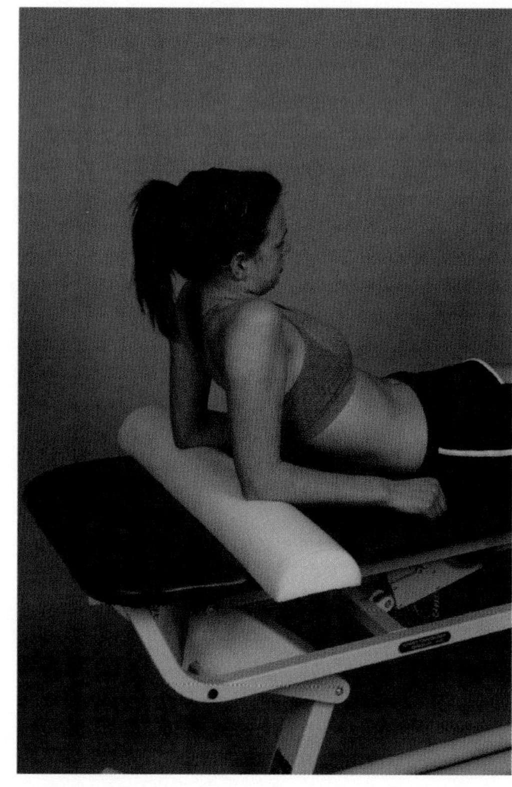

FIGURE 16-103 Elbow recline.

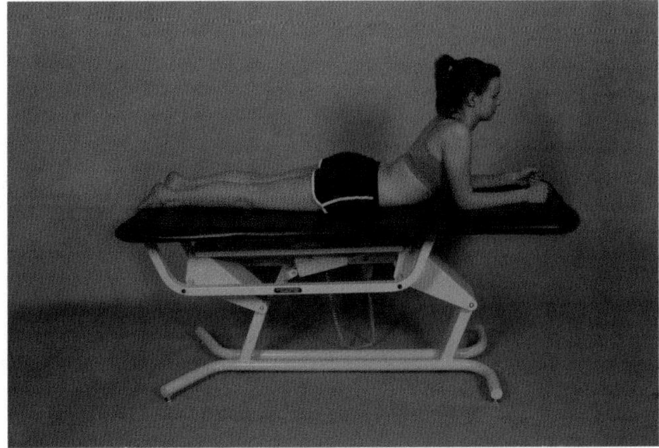

FIGURE 16-104 Prone on elbows with shoulder compression.

performed by the clinician as tolerated by the patient. Another stretch that can be performed is the supine horizontal adduction with IR stretch. To perform the stretch, the patient lies in the supine position with the shoulder flexed to 90 degrees. The clinician applies a stabilizing force to the lateral border of the scapula while the arm is horizontally adducted. At this point, the clinician applies a gentle force into IR. To supplement the stretches applied by the clinician, a number of techniques can be used by the patient to maintain and improve the ROM gains achieved in the clinic (see "Therapeutic Techniques" section).

Kinetic chain preparation can begin in the early stages while the shoulder is recovering from the injury or surgery. The length of the kinetic chain required depends on the needs of the patient and the goals of the rehabilitative process. Longer kinetic chains are associated with the more active patients, and may include the entire lower kinetic chain and the trunk in addition to the upper extremity (see "Biomechanics" section). Kinetic chain preparation will allow for the normal sequencing of velocity and force when the patient returns to their normal activities or athletic pursuits.[152,153]

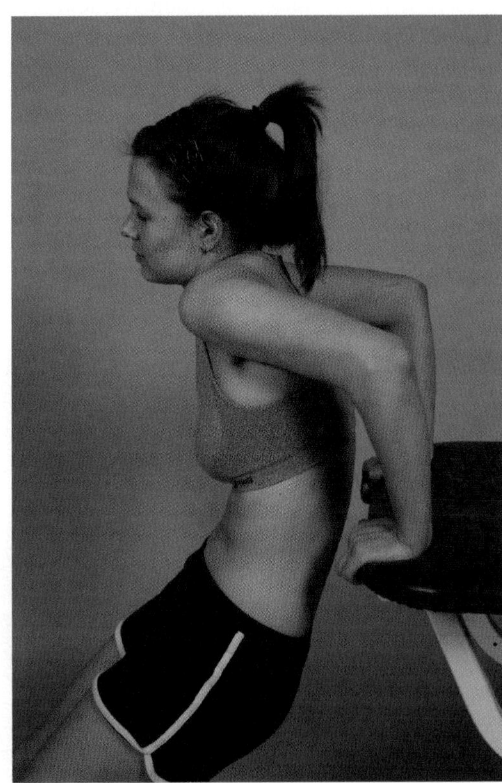

FIGURE 16-105 Table push-up.

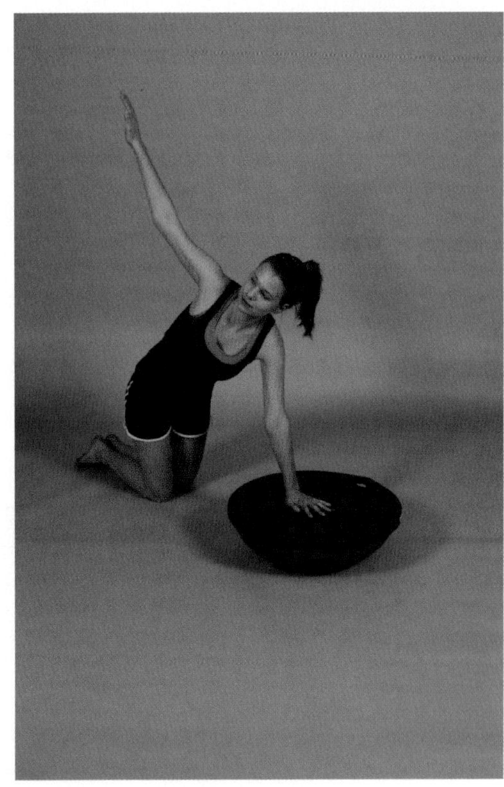

FIGURE 16-106 Quadriceps balancing.

According to Kibler,[153] progression to the functional phase of the rehabilitative process requires that the following criteria be met:

- Progression of tissue healing (healed or sufficiently stabilized for active motion and tissue loading)
- Pain-free ROM of at least 120-degree elevation
- Manual muscle strength in nonpathologic areas 4+/5

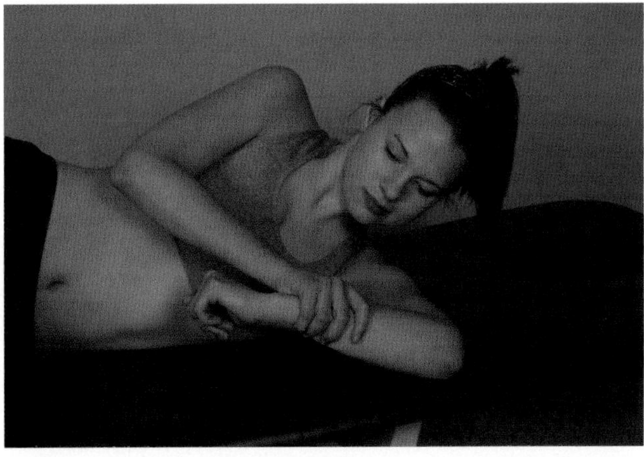

FIGURE 16-107 Sleeper stretch.

- Scapular control, with dominant side/nondominant side scapular asymmetry less than 1.5 cm with lateral slide test

Functional Phase

The functional phase is designed to address any tissue overload problems and/or functional biomechanical deficits. The goals of the functional phase include the following:

- Attain full range of pain-free motion with normal joint kinematics.
- Improve muscle strength to within normal limits.
- Improve neuromuscular control.
- Restore normal muscle force couples.

CLINICAL PEARL

The number of repetitions the patient is asked to perform should be based on the number the patient can do correctly with control, not a predetermined number.

CLINICAL PEARL

Generally speaking, exercise machines are not functional, emphasize the anterior muscle groups rather than posterior muscle groups (often opposite of the desired effect), and use long lever arms, making controlling the motion difficult and increasing the risk of a joint shear.

The exercises during this phase are performed slowly at first and are then progressed to higher functional speeds. Isolated muscle contractions can be achieved by placing the patient in the muscle test position for that muscle. Three sets of the strengthening exercises should be performed daily using weights of 1–10 lb. The number of repetitions is determined by tissue response (pain, fatigue, and compensatory patterns).

Correct activation and functioning of the scapula pivoters is essential. Proper strengthening of the scapular pivoters assures that the scapula follows the humerus, providing dynamic stability and assuring synchrony of the scapulohumeral rhythm. As the scapulothoracic muscles are not required to contract powerfully over short periods, or produce large amounts of force, it could be hypothesized that the scapulothoracic muscles serve a primarily postural function. Thus, in the rehabilitation of the scapulothoracic muscles, their postural function should be addressed and retrained. This can be accomplished in the form of endurance exercises by training the muscles with low weights and high repetitions, or sustained positions.[251]

CLINICAL PEARL

While the patient is performing exercises for the scapulohumeral rhythm, the clinician should note the following[390]:

- In the first phase of arm abduction (0–30 degrees), no or minimal scapula movement should occur.
- In the second phase (30–90 degrees), the scapula should rotate but show minimal protraction or elevation.
- In the third phase (90–180 degrees), ER of the humerus is necessary.

In scaption, the scapulohumeral rhythm is slightly different, with more individual variation in the movement, and more scapular rotation and protraction are common.[390]

Exercises for the scapular pivoters include the following:

- Shoulder shrugs (periscapular—trapezius, levator scapula). Resistance can be added to this exercise by having the patient hold dumbbells in the hands.
- Prone rowing. The patient lies prone on the table with a weight in the hand. With the elbow flexed to approximately 90 degrees, the patient raises the elbow to the ceiling (Fig. 16-108). This exercise strengthens the upper trapezius, levator scapulae, lower trapezius, posterior deltoid, and to a lesser extent, the middle trapezius, rhomboids, and middle deltoid.[13,122,391]
- Modified push-ups (see Fig. 16-109).
- Side-lying abduction exercises VIDEO are performed with the subject lying on his or her side and moving into

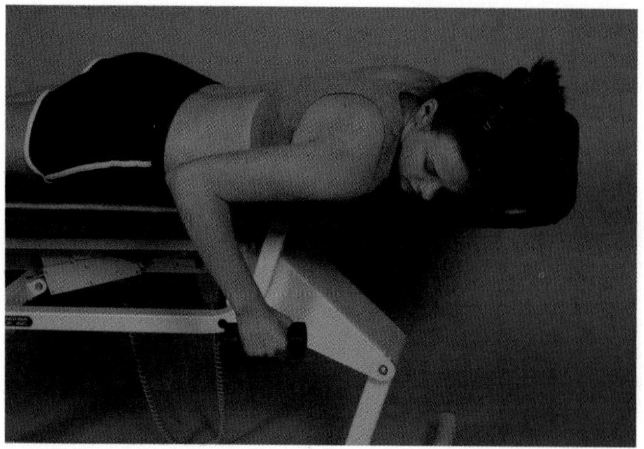

FIGURE 16-108 Prone rowing.

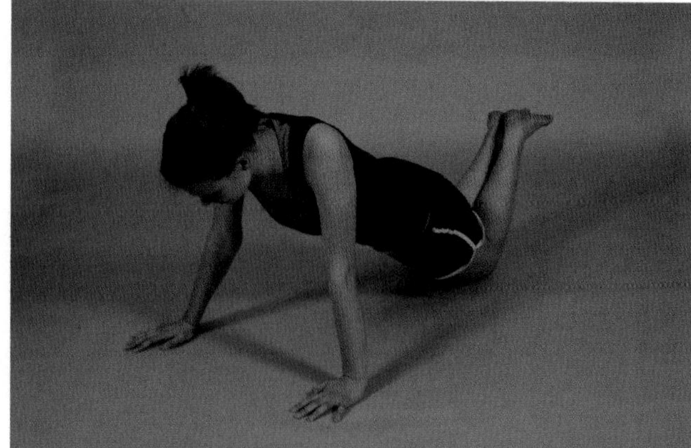

FIGURE 16-109 Modified push-ups.

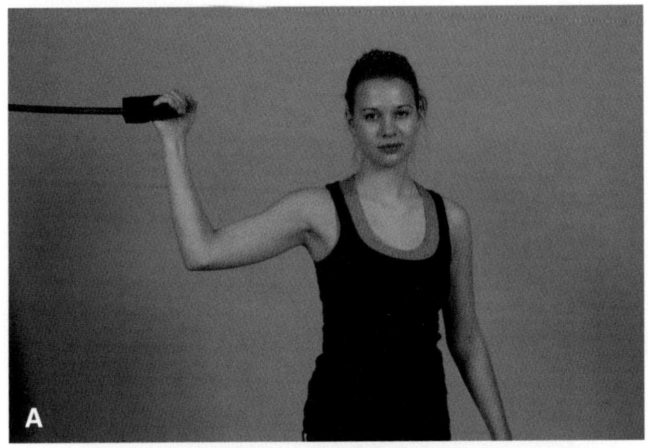

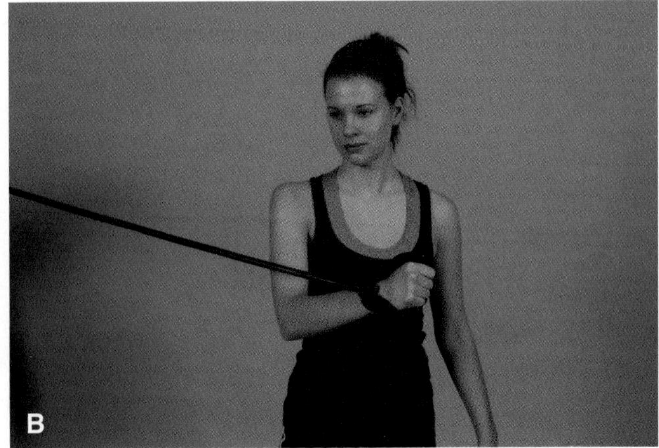

FIGURE 16-110 Diagonal exercise for the upper extremity. (A) Start position. (B) End position.

45-degree abduction in a neutral rotation position from a neutral or adducted position. Using MRI, side-lying abduction has been shown to produce the greatest signal intensity increase in three muscles of the rotator cuff: supraspinatus, infraspinatus, and subscapularis, as well as the deltoid.[392] A number of other exercises have been reported to demonstrate high subscapularis activity. These include IR at 90 degrees of abduction, the push-up plus, the diagonal exercise (Fig. 16-110A and 110B), and the dynamic hug exercise (Fig. 16-111).

Three exercises that are specific for the middle and lower trapezius include the following:

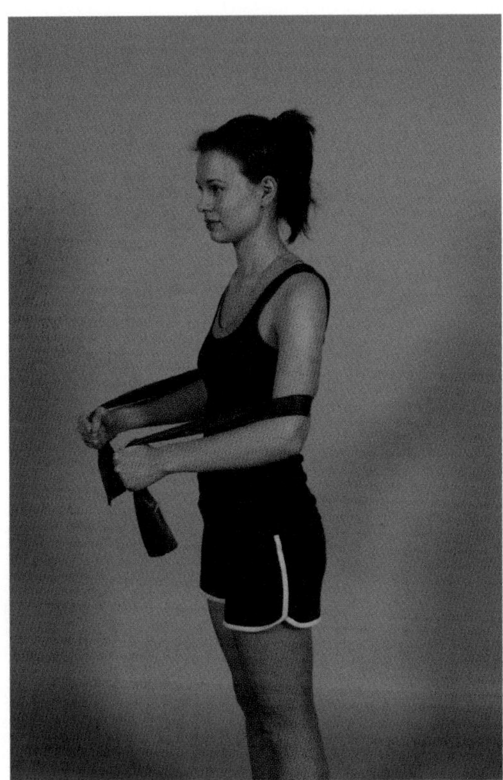

FIGURE 16-111 Dynamic hug exercise.

- Scapular pinches or squeezes.
- Thumb tubes. These are performed with the elbow extended and the thumb pointing posteriorly while grasping resistive tubing. The patient then performs a series of shoulder extension and/or horizontal abduction motions at various degrees of elevation.
- Power square patterns. These are performed by having the patient elevate the shoulders, pull back (retract) the shoulders while maintaining the elevation, depressing the shoulders while maintaining the retraction, and then moving the shoulders forward (protracting) while maintaining the depression.

Once scapular control has been achieved, exercises for the humeral positioners (the rotator cuff and deltoid) can be initiated to prevent humeral head migration, and to restore voluntary arthrokinematic control of the humeral head through rotator cuff coactivation and stabilization, as well as activation of the biceps and pectoralis major.[390] For example, by strengthening the infraspinatus, teres minor, and subscapularis muscles (relative to the supraspinatus and the deltoid), it may be possible to reestablish the normal balance and force couple during elevation of the G-H joint.[4,39,393]

Open-chain exercises designed to further strengthen the rotator cuff muscles are emphasized. These exercises may include the following:

- Elevation in the plane of the scapula (scaption)—also known as "empty the can," "supraspinatus exercise," "supraspinatus fly," and "Jobe's exercise"—is defined to be abduction in the plane of the scapula (90 degrees combined with 30 degrees of flexion) and IR.[327] Although useful as a special test, this motion does not help to reestablish scapulohumeral rhythm and can be counterproductive as it is often painful early in the rehabilitation process.
- Elevation in the plane of the scapula (scaption) in ER (full-can position). This exercise strengthens the scapula pivoters and may be preferable in the presence of impingement.[13,122,391]
- Military press. This exercise, which is performed by raising both the hands from shoulder height straight up toward the ceiling, strengthens the supraspinatus, subscapularis, upper

TABLE 16-33 Scapular and Humeral Control Exercises

Scapular Control	Humeral Control
Bent-over rowing	Prone horizontal abduction
Push-ups with a plus (maximum shoulder protraction)	Scaption in internal rotation (thumbs down)
Press-ups	Scaption with external rotation (thumbs up)
Forward punch-outs	Prone extension
Scapular squeezes	Side-lying internal and external rotation Prone 90 degrees/90 degrees (90-degree abduction, 90-degree elbow flexion) external rotation

trapezius,[392] anterior deltoid, middle serratus anterior, lower serratus anterior, and middle deltoid.[13,122] As the military press can cause impingement, care must be taken with its use. This exercise is probably better used in a prevention program.

- Scapula retraction with horizontal abduction of the externally rotated shoulder, done in prone. Blackburn et al.[122] demonstrated that externally rotating the humerus during prone exercise increased EMG activity to the highest levels. Horizontal abduction (90 degrees or 100 degrees) in ER strengthens the middle trapezius, infraspinatus and to a lesser extent, the teres minor and posterior deltoid (Table 16-33).[13,122,251,391] The patient lies prone on the table with both arms abducted to 90 degrees (Fig. 16-34) or 100 degrees and thumbs pointing toward the ceiling. With or without a weight in the hand, the patient then raises his/her thumbs toward the ceiling. If the arm is abducted to 100 degrees in the frontal plane, the lower trapezius is exercised.[122]
- Scapular retraction with horizontal abduction of the internally rotated shoulder, performed in prone (Fig. 16-112); this is similar to the previous exercise, but the patient now has the thumbs pointing down toward the ground. He or she is again prone and his or her arms are abducted to approximately 90 degrees. He or she then raises his or her hypothenar eminence toward the ceiling. This exercise strengthens, in order of effectiveness, the posterior deltoid, middle trapezius, rhomboids, middle deltoid, levator scapulae, infraspinatus, teres minor, upper trapezius, and lower trapezius.[13,122,391] This exercise can also be done in standing by using elastic resistance.
- Scapular dump (as though trying to empty things out of a can) exercises that incorporate arm, scapular, and trunk movements.
- Short-arc (pain-free) exercises into scaption, abduction, and forward flexion to 30 degrees initially and then to 90 degrees. These exercises should be performed in ER to facilitate clearance of the greater tuberosity under the coracoacromial ligament.

The open-chain exercises should also include resisted shoulder external VIDEO (Fig. 16-113) and internal VIDEO (Fig. 16-114) rotation with the arm in increasing amounts of abduction VIDEO

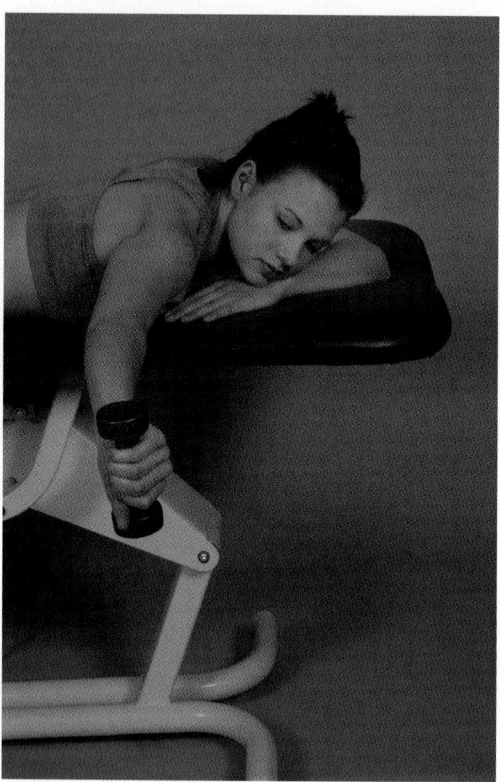

FIGURE 16-112 Prone shoulder retraction with glenohumeral joint in internal rotation.

to strengthen the infraspinatus/teres minor and subscapularis muscles, respectively. To avoid concurrent strengthening of the deltoid during the earlier phases of strengthening, the patient is instructed to hold a magazine or towel roll between the extremity and the trunk while strengthening the rotator cuff

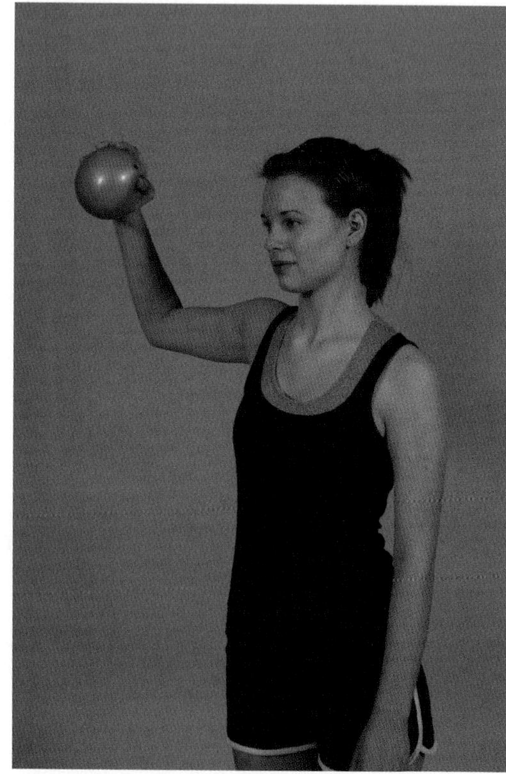

FIGURE 16-113 Resisted external rotation.

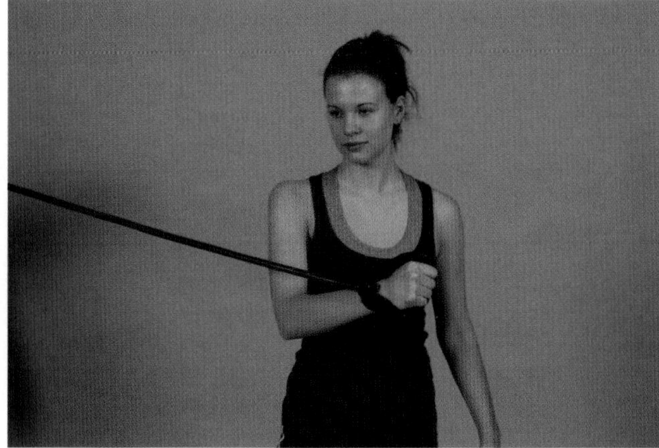

FIGURE 16-114 Resisted internal rotation.

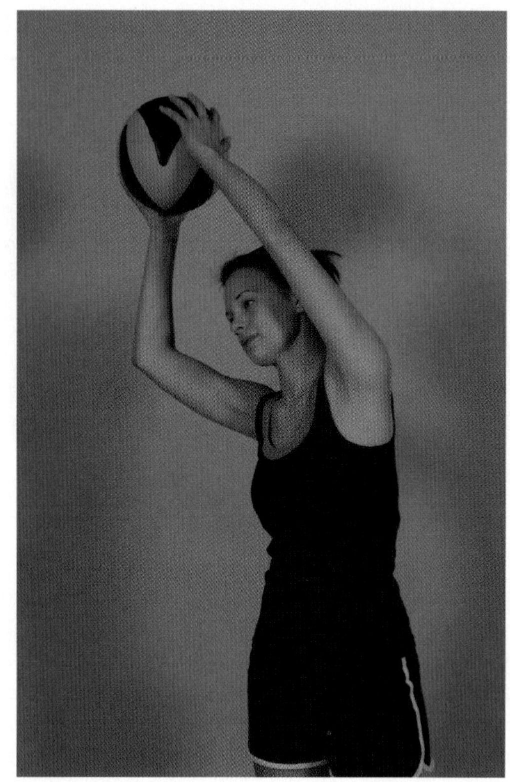

FIGURE 16-115 Trunk rotation exercises with medicine ball.

muscles. This forced adduction relaxes the deltoid and isolates the oblique muscles of the rotator cuff.

Once control in most of the range has been achieved, diagonal proprioceptive neuromuscular facilitation (PNF) exercises can be used to teach control and stabilization throughout the whole range. The shoulder D2 pattern (flexion, abduction, and ER) is especially useful for instability.[390]

Once the muscles can contract in the correct sequence, the humeral *propellers* (i.e., the latissimus dorsi, teres major, pectoralis minor and pectoralis major) are trained concentrically, while the humeral *positioners* and *protectors* (i.e., infraspinatus, teres minor, supraspinatus, posterior deltoid, and biceps) and scapula pivoters are trained eccentrically.

In addition to addressing the musculature of the shoulder complex, the clinician must address the whole kinetic chain involved in an activity to which the patient is planning to return. This may include rehabilitation of the legs and hips to focus on the generation of appropriate activity-specific force and velocity from the lower extremity.[152,153] Examples include exercises that develop normal agonist–antagonist force couples in the legs such as squats, plyometric depth jumps, lunges, and hip extensions. Most shoulder activities involve rotation and diagonal patterns.[144,152] Thus the exercises must incorporate trunk rotation exercises (using medicine ball or tubing), which integrate leg and trunk stabilization and incorporate diagonal patterns (Fig. 16-115). These exercises are progressed to incorporate combined patterns of hip and trunk rotation in both directions, and hip and shoulder diagonal patterns from the left hip to the right shoulder and from the right hip to the left shoulder.[144,152]

Endurance activities in the legs should also be emphasized. Both aerobic endurance for recovery from exercise bouts and anaerobic endurance for agility and power work are advocated. These can be done using mini-trampoline exercises, agility drills with running and jumping, jumping jacks, and slider or Fitter boards.[153]

The arthrokinematic movements of the joints in the entire kinetic chain must be addressed for hypomobility and hypermobility, as appropriate. These joints include the A-C joint, the S-C joint, the scapulothoracic joint, the cervical and upper thoracic spine, and the upper ribs. For example, the clinician should check for GIRD, restriction of the inferior G-H ligament, and any loss of range in the pectoralis major and pectoralis minor.

CLINICAL PEARL

The *circle concept of instability*[36,142] relates to the fact that injury to structures on one side of the joint sufficient to result in instability can, simultaneously, cause injury to structures on the other side or other parts of the joint, particularly in the presence of trauma. For example, a traumatic anterior instability of the shoulder can lead to injury of the posterior structures. Thus, the clinician must always be aware of potential injuries on the opposite side of the joint even if symptoms are predominantly on one side. In addition, if a joint is hypermobile in one direction, it may be hypomobile in the opposite direction. For example, with anterior instability, the posteroinferior capsule tends to be tight and therefore requires mobilization, whereas the anterior capsule is hypermobile and requires protection.[390]

Proprioception exercises can be introduced as soon as the patient has gained scapular control. These exercises can include the aforementioned closed-chain activities for the upper extremity. Open kinetic chain activities may also be used, but they are not as effective, and they do not require the same level of stability.[390]

Activity-specific progressions must be completed before full return to function is allowed. This is done to test all of the working components involved in the activity. Very few deviations from the normal parameters of arm motion, arm position, force generation, smoothness of all of the kinetic chain, and from preinjury form should be allowed as most of these adaptations will be biomechanically inefficient.[144,152,153,394,395]

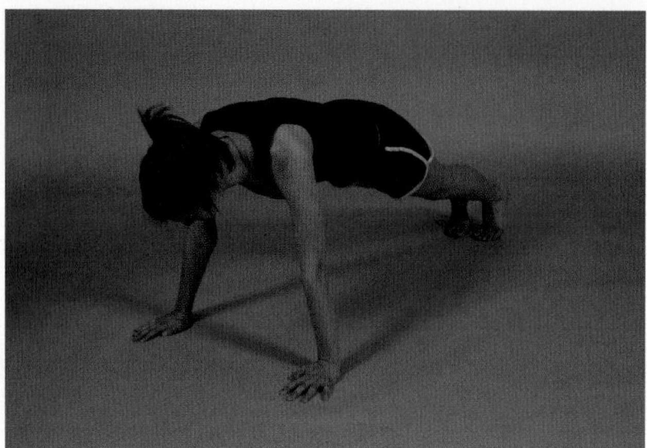

FIGURE 16-116 Regular push-up.

Advanced stabilization exercises are designed to test the ability of the patient to stabilize the scapula statically in positions above 30 degrees, most commonly in an open kinetic chain. The patient is asked to perform isometric hold or eccentric break activities of the internal and external rotators in various positions of G-H abduction, scaption, and forward flexion. Closed-chain exercises include wall falls, table falls, and balancing on different balance devices. Closed-chain exercises in this phase may also include the following:

- Regular push-ups (Fig. 16-116) are progressed as tolerated.
- Medicine ball catch-and-throw (Fig. 16-117) **VIDEO**.

Dynamic weight-shifting exercises are introduced during this phase. With the patient weight bearing on all fours in the quadruped position, and while keeping their hands stationary in the same position, the patient can rock the body forward and backward, and side to side. A similar exercise can be performed on an unsteady surface by using equipment such as the BOSU trainer **VIDEO**. Alternatively, the patient can slide their hands, or one hand, forward, backwards, and side to side while maintaining their trunk still. Resistance can be added using a Fitter board (Fig. 16-118).

Finally, dynamic stabilization exercises that involve controlled eccentric movement of the scapula while the arm moves are introduced.[153] Eccentric exercises are particularly important for those patients where tensile overloading is suspected to be the cause, and for the overhead athlete population.[379,396] Exercises such as bent over rows, and lunges with dumbbells are good examples.

The criteria for return to activity include the following[153]:

- Little or no pain
- Functional ROM with involvement of the whole kinetic chain
- Normal movement patterns and functional ability
- Appropriate levels of fitness
- Near-normal strength
- Ability to perform the necessary skills

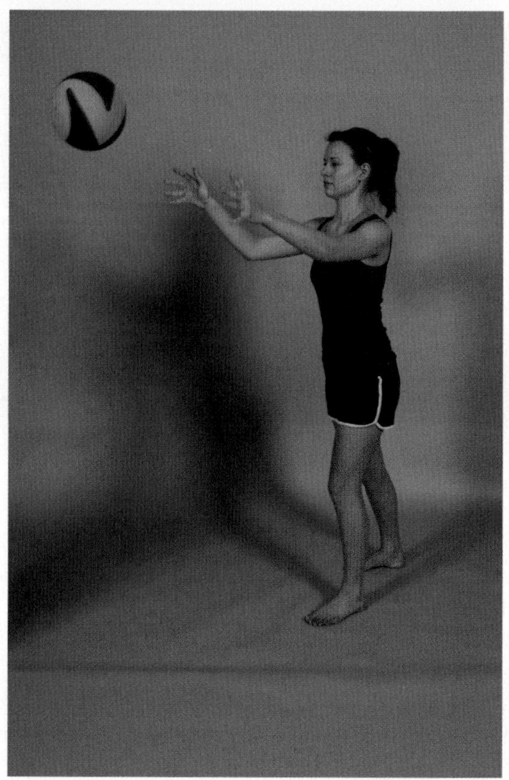

FIGURE 16-117 Medicine ball throw and catch.

Table 16-34 may be referred to for a typical program given for a pitcher returning to full function. This program can and should be modified as needed by the clinician. Each phase may take a longer or shorter time than that listed, and the program should be monitored closely.

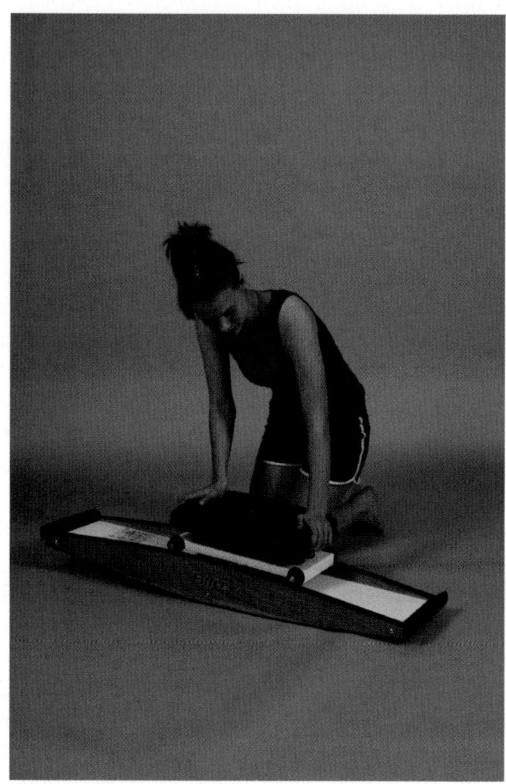

FIGURE 16-118 Fitter board exercise using upper extremities.

TABLE 16-34 Thrower's Ten Program
Dumbbell exercises for the deltoid and supraspinatus muscles
Prone horizontal shoulder abduction
Prone shoulder extension
Internal rotation at 90-degree abduction of the shoulder with elastic tubing
External rotation at 90-degree abduction of the shoulder with elastic tubing
Elbow flexion/extension exercises with elastic tubing
Serratus anterior strengthening: progressive push-ups
Diagonal *D2* pattern for shoulder flexion and extension with elastic tubing
Press-ups
Dumbbell wrist extension/flexion and pronation/supination

Data from Wilk KE, Arrigo C, Andrews JR: Rehabilitation of the elbow in the throwing athlete. *J Orthop Sports Phys Ther* 17:305–317, 1993.

PRACTICE PATTERN 4D: IMPAIRED JOINT MOBILITY, MOTOR FUNCTION, MUSCLE PERFORMANCE, RANGE OF MOTION WITH CONNECTIVE TISSUE DYSFUNCTION

The primary impairment in pattern 4D, when applied to the shoulder, is hypomobility due to capsular restriction. In addition to limited joint movement and decreased ROM associated with pain, the impairments in this pattern include decreased motor control and muscle performance.

The clinical findings in this pattern include, but are not limited to, pain, limited ROM in a capsular pattern of restriction, an alteration in the scapulohumeral rhythm, crepitus, and a positive impingement sign.

Arthritis

Traumatic Arthritis of the G-H Joint

Traumatic or primary G-H arthritis is an entity that has been well described and documented by Neer et al.,[326,397] who highlighted the presence of significant posterior glenoid erosion causing static posterior subluxation of the humeral head. Traumatic arthritis of the G-H joint rarely occurs in individuals under the age of 45. The condition is characterized by pain, progressive functional impairment, and reports of instability.[398] Passive horizontal adduction is usually the most limited and painful motion.

Conservative intervention consists of rest, modification of activity, and NSAIDs. Electrotherapeutic modalities and physical agents may be used to control pain and the active inflammation. Joint mobilizations of grade I or grade II may also be used to decrease pain. Once pain and inflammation is under control, the rehabilitation progresses to strengthening of the shoulder protectors and scapular pivoters, as described in the "Intervention Strategies" section.

Immobilization

Postsurgical immobilization occurs at any age, although it is more common in the elderly. The clinical progression is similar to that of traumatic arthritis. This condition should ideally be treated by prophylaxis.

Rheumatoid Arthritis

Rheumatoid arthritis is described in Chapter 5. Conservative intervention for this population includes patient education on how they can influence their disease process by alleviating the impairments, functional limitations, and disability. Electrotherapeutic modalities and cryotherapy can be used to help control pain and inflammation. Thermal modalities may also be used in the nonacute phases. Therapeutic exercise can be beneficial for the patients who are weak and stiff prior to the onset of end-stage arthritis, where the ROM and strength can be regained, or at least maintained.[399] However, caution must be used with those patients with end-stage arthritis who have stiffness secondary to joint incongruity, as they may actually have their symptoms exacerbated with aggressive stretching exercises.[399]

When pain becomes too severe and conservative intervention is unable to relieve this pain and restore function, surgical measures are considered. These measures may include synovectomy, G-H arthrodesis, or total joint arthroplasty.

Septic Arthritis

See Chapter 5.

Avascular Necrosis of the Humeral Head

Avascular necrosis of the humeral head is described in Chapter 5.

Hemorrhagic Shoulder (Milwaukee Shoulder)

L'épaule sénile hémorragique (the hemorrhagic shoulder of the elderly) was first described in 1968. It consisted of recurrent, blood-streaked effusions of the shoulder along with radiographic findings of severe degenerative G-H arthritis and a chronic tear of the rotator cuff.[400] The term *Milwaukee shoulder* was not introduced until 1981.[401–403]

The condition generally affects a subset of the elderly population who have G-H arthritis in conjunction with a complete rotator cuff tear.

One theory to explain the Milwaukee shoulder describes a hydroxyapatite-mineral phase that develops in the altered capsule, synovial tissue, or degenerative articular cartilage. This releases basic calcium phosphate crystals into the synovial fluid.[401–403] These crystals are phagocytized by synovial cells and form calcium phosphate crystal microspheroids. These induce the release of activated enzymes from these cells, causing destruction of the periarticular tissues and articular surfaces.[404]

Another theory is the cuff tear theory. In 1983, Neer et al.[405] postulated that untreated chronic, massive tears would lead to a degenerated G-H joint. The mechanism of destruction of the articular cartilage was said to include mechanical and nutritional alterations in the shoulder.[405] The mechanical factors include A-P instability of the humeral head resulting from a massive tear of the rotator cuff, and rupture or dislocation of the LHB that leads to proximal migration of the humeral head and acromial impingement.[404] G-H articular wear was thought to occur as a result of repetitive trauma from the altered biomechanics associated with the loss of the primary and secondary stabilizers of the G-H joint.[404] Changes in the composition of the articular cartilage follows because of inadequate diffusion of nutrients and the diminished quantity of synovial fluid.[404] Degenerative arthritis and subchondral collapse eventually develops.[404]

If the resultant rotator cuff tear arthropathy causes relatively mild symptoms, intervention should consist of mild anti-inflammatory medication and gentle stretching exercises to maintain or regain a functional ROM.[404] A strengthening program should follow to improve the active use of the arm for ADL. If conservative management fails, a humeral hemiarthroplasty is the procedure of choice to provide reliable relief of pain and functional improvement.[404]

Frozen Shoulder/Adhesive Capsulitis

Since this condition also involves an inflammation of the capsule, a patient with this condition could also be classified under preferred practice pattern 4E.

The frozen shoulder syndrome was first described by Duplay in 1872,[406] who used the term *periarthritis scapulohumerale*. It was not until 1934 that Codman[61] used the term *frozen shoulder* to describe this condition. In 1945, Neviaser introduced the term *adhesive capsulitis* to reflect his findings of a chronic inflammatory process at surgery and autopsy.[407]

Although the etiology of frozen shoulder remains elusive, the understanding of the pathophysiology has recently improved. Factors associated with adhesive capsulitis include female gender,[408] age older than 40 years,[409] trauma,[409] diabetes,[222,242,410–413] prolonged immobilization,[414] thyroid disease,[415–417] stroke or myocardial infarction,[411,418] certain psychiatric conditions,[419,420] and the presence of autoimmune diseases.[421,422]

The prevalence of frozen shoulder in the general population is slightly greater than 2%,[408,423] and 11% of the adult diabetic population.[410] Approximately 70% of patients with adhesive capsulitis are women, and 20–30% of those affected subsequently will have adhesive capsulitis develop in the opposite shoulder.[424] Complicating the diagnosis is the fact that there are many conditions that can cause shoulder stiffness (Tables 16-35 and 16-36).

Nash and Hazelman[425] have described the concept of primary and secondary frozen shoulders, with the former idiopathic in origin, and the latter either traumatic in origin or related to a disease process, neurologic, or cardiac condition.

TABLE 16-35 Intrinsic Causes of Shoulder Stiffness

Cause	Example
Bursitis	Subacromial Calcific tendinitis Snapping scapula
Biceps tendon	Tenosynovitis Partial or complete tears SLAP lesions
Rotator cuff	Impingement syndrome Partial rotator cuff tears Complete rotator cuff tears
Trauma	Fractures Glenoid Proximal humerus Surgery Postoperative shoulder, breast, head, neck, chest Gastrointestinal disorders Esophagitis Ulcer Cholecystitis
Instability—glenohumeral	Recurrent dislocation anterior and posterior Chronic dislocation
Arthritides	Glenohumeral and acromioclavicular Osteoarthritis Rheumatoid Psoriatic Infectious Neuropathic
Miscellaneous	Avascular necrosis Hemarthrasis Osteochondromatosis Suprascapular nerve palsy

Data from Cohen BS, Romeo AA, Bach BR: Shoulder injuries. In: Brotzman SB, Wilk KE, eds. *Clinical Orthopaedic Rehabilitation*. Philadelphia, PA: Mosby, 2003:125–250.

Primary Adhesive Capsulitis

Primary adhesive capsulitis is characterized by an idiopathic, progressive, and painful loss of active and passive shoulder motion, particularly ER, which causes the individual to gradually limit the use of the arm. Difficulty is reported with putting on a jacket or coat, putting objects into back pockets, or hooking garments in the back.[195,426–428] Inflammation and pain can cause muscle guarding of the shoulder muscles, without true fixed contracture of the joint capsule. Disuse of the arm results in a loss of shoulder mobility, whereas continued use of the arm through pain can result in development of subacromial impingement.[424] Over a period of weeks, compensatory movements of the shoulder girdle develop to minimize pain.[424] With time, there is resolution of pain and the individual is left with a stiff shoulder and with severe limitation of function.

Secondary or Idiopathic Adhesive Capsulitis

Zuckerman and Cuomo[429] defined idiopathic adhesive capsulitis as a condition characterized by substantial restriction of both active and passive shoulder motion that occurs in the absence of a known intrinsic shoulder disorder. Two clinical forms are recognized:

TABLE 16-36 Extrinsic Causes of Shoulder Stiffness

Cause	Example
Neurologic	Parkinson's disease Automatic dystrophy (CRPS) Intradural lesions Neural compression Cervical disk disease Neurofibromata Foraminal stenosis Neurologic amyotrophy Hemiplegia Head trauma
Muscular	Poliomyositis
Cardiovascular	Myocardial infarction Thoracic outlet syndrome Cerebral hemorrhage
Infections	Chronic bronchitis Pulmonary tuberculosis
Metabolic	Diabetes mellitus Progressive systemic sclerosis (scleroderma) Paget's disease Thyroid disease
Inflammatory	Rheumatologic disorders Polymyalgia rheumatica
Trauma	Surgery Axillary node dissection, sternotomy, thoracotomy Fractures Cervical spine, ribs, elbow, hand, etc.
Medications	Isoniazid, phenobarbitone
Congenital	Klippel–Feil Sprengel's deformity Glenoid dysplasia Atresia Contractures Pectoralis major Axillary fold
Behavioral	Depression Hysterical paralysis
Referred pain	Diaphragmatic irritation
Neoplastic	Pancoast tumor Lung carcinoma Metastatic disease

Data from Cohen BS, Romeo AA, Bach BR: Shoulder injuries. In: Brotzman SB, Wilk KE, eds. *Clinical Orthopaedic Rehabilitation*. Philadelphia, PA: Mosby, 2003:125–250.

1. One form is defined as when the pain is more noticeable than the motion restriction. This condition is self-limiting, and the patient spontaneously recovers within 6 months to a year. Two studies[430,431] of patients with idiopathic adhesive capsulitis found that the vast majority of patients with this condition were successfully treated with a specific shoulder-stretching exercise program.
2. The other form is defined as when the pain, which can radiate below the elbow, is as noticeable as the restriction. The patient complains of pain at rest and is unable to sleep on the involved side. ER of the G-H joint is usually affected more than abduction or flexion.[195] The initial phase of this condition is characterized by pain and progressive loss of motion lasting 2–6 months. This form responds well to a series of corticosteroid injections or local anesthetic (distension therapy).

To formulate a logical approach to the intervention of patients with adhesive capsulitis, the clinician needs to determine the degree of inflammation and irritability. To help in this determination, it is necessary to have a better understanding of the underlying cellular and biochemical pathophysiology of this disease.

There is disagreement as to whether the underlying pathologic process is an inflammatory condition,[432–434] or a fibrosing condition.[435] Significant evidence exists[421,422,434,436] in support of the hypothesis that the underlying pathologic changes in adhesive capsulitis are synovial inflammation with subsequent reactive capsular fibrosis, making adhesive capsulitis an inflammatory and a fibrosing condition, depending on the stage of the disease. The initial biologic trigger in this cascade of inflammation and subsequent fibrosis is unknown, although it is likely to involve multiple factors. In some areas, there seems to be a seasonal variation in patients presenting with adhesive capsulitis, suggesting that a virus is responsible.[424]

Stages of Progression

Adhesive capsulitis is suggested by Neviaser[407] to pass through four stages based on pathologic changes in the synovium and the subsynovium, with each stage having an individual intervention strategy, although there is controversy about this idea.[75]

Stage I. In stage I, patients present with mild signs and symptoms of less than 3 months' duration, which are often described as achy at rest and sharp at extremes of ROM. The symptoms often mimic those of an impingement syndrome, where restriction of motion is minimal and pain that appears to be due to a rotator cuff tendinitis has been present for less than 3 months. However, the patient reports a progressive loss of motion and intervention protocols for rotator cuff tendinitis fail. A capsular pattern of motion (loss of ER and abduction) is present, and a more subtle loss of IR in adduction. In adhesive capsulitis due to type 1 diabetes mellitus, the capsular pattern is typically equal to the limitation of ER and IR, which is greater than the limitation of abduction.

In this early stage, the majority of motion loss is secondary to the painful synovitis, rather than a true capsular contraction.

Stage II. Patients presenting with stage I and stage II adhesive capsulitis have pain on palpation of the anterior and posterior capsules and describe pain radiating to the deltoid insertion. An intra-articular injection of steroid and local analgesic given by a physician can be extremely useful in the diagnosis and intervention of adhesive capsulitis.[424] After the injection, passive G-H ROM is reevaluated. If the patient has significant improvement in pain and normalization of motion, the diagnosis of stage I adhesive capsulitis is confirmed.[424] If the patient has a significant improvement in pain but no significant improvement in ROM, then by definition he or she has stage II adhesive capsulitis, although it must be emphasized that these stages represent a continuum of the inflammatory and scarring processes.[432]

In stage II, symptoms have been present for 3–9 months with progressive loss of ROM and persistence of the pain pattern described above. The motion loss in stage II adhesive capsulitis reflects a loss of capsular volume and a response to the painful synovitis. The patient demonstrates a loss of motion in all planes, as well as pain in all parts of the range. Evaluation of AROM and PROM should be performed because documenting the initial ROM, especially passive motion, is critical in determining the efficacy of the intervention plan. The causes of the restricted PROM need to be assessed and a differentiation must be made between protective muscle guarding, adaptive changes in musculotendinous structures, or capsular adhesions and contracture.

CLINICAL PEARL

It is important to note that the restricted ROM seen in patients with adhesive capsulitis occurs both actively and passively, which is in contrast to a number of other shoulder conditions in which a loss of AROM of the G-H joint occurs, but reasonably good, if not full, PROM is maintained.[73]

Stage III. In stage III, patients present with a history of painful stiffening of the shoulder and a significant loss of ROM. Symptoms have been present for 9–14 months and have been observed to change with time. Patients often report a history of an extremely painful phase that has resolved, resulting in a relatively pain-free but stiff shoulder.

Poor scapulohumeral rhythm is observed during elevation of the arm. There is a dominance of the upper trapezius resulting in hiking of the shoulder girdle. This is attributed to a decreased inferior glide of the G-H joint, which prevents G-H abduction.[437]

Stage IV. Stage IV, also known as the "thawing stage" for adhesive capsulitis, is characterized by the slow, steady recovery of some of the lost ROM resulting from capsular remodeling in response to use of the arm and shoulder. Although many people feel less restricted in this phase, objective measurements show only minor improvement.[438] No arthroscopic or histologic data are available for patients with stage IV adhesive capsulitis because these patients rarely undergo surgery. Patients who present with stages III and IV adhesive capsulitis often report a history of long-standing pain at rest and pain at night that have resolved spontaneously.[439] The objective findings typically include a stiff shoulder, with striking alteration of scapulohumeral mechanics and limited use of the arm during ADL. A capsular pattern of motion is a characteristic finding. Resistance in the form of a capsular end-feel is felt before pain is reached as the G-H joint is taken through PROM.

Other pathologic conditions that can create a painful restriction of G-H motion should be ruled out. Typically, the physician uses a routine radiographic evaluation to rule out other causes for a stiff, painful shoulder including G-H arthritis, calcific tendinitis, or long-standing rotator cuff disease.[424] Radiographs usually are negative in patients with frozen shoulder, although there may be evidence of disuse osteopenia.[424] MRI has been used for investigative purposes in patients with adhesive capsulitis and has shown an increased blood flow to the synovium in frozen shoulder.[440]

Intervention

The conventional management for adhesive capsulitis incorporates patient advice, analgesics, NSAIDs, steroid injection, and a wide array of physical therapy methods.[441] The primary goal of conservative intervention is the restoration of the ROM and focuses on the application of controlled tensile stresses to produce elongation of the restricting tissues.[242,243,424,442–444] Once this has been established, strengthening of the rotator cuff and the three parts of the deltoid muscle is important. Systematic reviews concerning physical therapy interventions with adhesive capsulitis have traditionally compared the efficacy of one component of physical therapy. For example, comparing the effect of ultrasound alone or mobilization alone. The outcomes from these studies have been, perhaps not surprisingly, poor. However, when combined physical therapy methods are analyzed, the results have been more encouraging. Pajareya et al.[441] performed a randomized control trial of 122 patients to study the effectiveness of ibuprofen and a combination of physical therapy (PT) techniques versus ibuprofen alone. The PT intervention (three times a week for 3 weeks) included short-wave diathermy, joint mobilizations, and passive G-H stretching exercises up to the patient's tolerance. At 3 weeks it was concluded that the PT group demonstrated more beneficial effects than the group using ibuprofen alone.[441]

These results must be taken in the context of earlier studies that have indicated that a gradual return of full mobility occurs within 18 months to 3 years in most patients, even without specific intervention.[445–447] In a study by Diercks et al.,[448] 77 patients with idiopathic frozen shoulder syndrome were included in a prospective study to compare the effect of intensive physical rehabilitation treatment, including passive stretching and manual mobilization (stretching group) versus supportive therapy and exercises within pain limits (supervised neglect group). All patients were followed up within 24 months after the start of treatment. The study concluded that supervised neglect yields better outcomes than intensive physical therapy and passive stretching in patients with frozen shoulder with regard to the functional end result and the speed of recovery.

These conflicting findings may be the result of an incorrect treatment approach. As a general guideline, the patient with capsular restriction and low irritability may require aggressive soft tissue and joint mobilization, whereas patients with high irritability may require pain-easing manual therapy techniques.[449] In contrast, the emphasis on intervention for limited ROM due to nonstructural changes is aimed at addressing the cause of the pain.[247,423,429,436,446,450–452] The trust and confidence of the patient is essential, and it is important to ensure that no harm is caused, or that the clinician does not indicate any frustration. During the acute phase, pendulum exercises and low-grade joint mobilization techniques are recommended to relieve pain and apply a gentle stretch to the capsule. In addition, passive stretching of the upper trapezius and levator scapulae muscles can be performed by the clinician and then taught to the patient as part of a home exercise program. During the subacute phase, more aggressive ROM exercises can be incorporated using PNF techniques, wall climbing, and wall/corner stretches. As ROM returns, strengthening becomes the focus, initiating with isometrics, and then progressive strengthening of the shoulder complex during the chronic phase.

A number of questions are often raised by the patient with regard to corticosteroid injections. Although these questions are best answered by the appropriate physician, there is extensive information regarding the efficacy of intra-articular corticosteroid in the intervention of patients with adhesive capsulitis.[453–457] Hazelman[458] summarized numerous studies on the use of intra-articular corticosteroid and reported that the success of intervention is dependent on the duration of symptoms.

- Patients treated within 1 month of onset of symptoms recovered in an average of 1.5 months.
- Patients treated within 3 months of the onset of symptoms reported a significant improvement in symptoms.
- Patients treated within 2–5 months of onset of symptoms recovered within 8.1 months of onset of symptoms.
- Patients treated after 5 or more months of onset of symptoms had a more delayed recovery, with the time necessary for full recovery reported to be dependent on the duration of symptoms.
- Patients treated 6–12 months after onset of symptoms required an average of 14 months for full recovery.

These data, along with others, support the hypothesis that adhesive capsulitis is an inflammatory and fibrotic condition.[432,434,435,453,459] Early intervention with intra-articular corticosteroid may provide a chemical ablation of the synovitis, thus limiting the subsequent development of fibrosis and shortening the natural history of the disease.[432] With resolution of the synovitis and loss of the cytokine stimulus to the capsular fibroblasts, capsular remodeling and recovery of ROM take place.[432]

Surgical intervention is reserved for those patients who do not respond to conservative intervention. Historically, arthroscopy has been of little diagnostic and therapeutic value in patients with adhesive capsulitis of the shoulder,[409] and closed manipulation appears to be the operation of choice if conservative methods fail. However, closed manipulation is contraindicated in patients with significant osteopenia, recent surgical repair of soft tissues about the shoulder, or in the presence of fractures, neurologic injury and instability.[424]

Selective Hypomobility

A generalized decrease in shoulder ROM may be due to a number of reasons such as arthritis or adhesive capsulitis. Selective hypomobility is usually the result of a restriction of the joint capsule. An asymmetrical restriction of the capsule causes an obligate translation away from the side of the joint where the tightness is located. For example, a posterior capsule restriction causes an increase in anterior translation of the humeral head during cross-arm adduction and with flexion of the G-H joint.[46] The posterior capsule restriction also results in a superior translation of the humeral head with flexion of the G-H joint.

Passive movement testing may be used to detect the direction of the hypomobility by examining the end-feel, and the amount of translation that occurs. Such tests include the load and shift test, the anterior release test, and the sulcus sign test. ROM tests are used to determine the amount of internal and ER. There is a close association between the amount of IR at the G-H joint and the posterior shoulder capsule tightness.[460]

The intervention for this impairment includes a warm-up phase using a moist heating pad or upper-body ergometer. The patient is then taught the position to adopt to stretch the restricted portion of the capsule. The maximum stretch position is then maintained for approximately 20 minutes, or as long as the patient can tolerate, whichever occurs first. The patient is instructed to perform the warm-up and stretch at home. The duration of the stretch is gradually increased until the patient is able to tolerate the stretch position for 60 minutes per day.

The patient performs multiple angle isometrics or short-arc exercises in the newly acquired range to improve neuromuscular dynamic control. When full ROM has been restored, the patient performs full range resistive exercises and combinations of arm and trunk exercises, such as PNF.

According to Sahrmann, correction of resting scapular malalignment is always indicated in this patient population, particularly when the PROM is not restricted by more than 20 degrees.[206]

Downwardly Rotated Scapula[206]

The G-H joint becomes the site of compensation because the scapula does not fully rotate upwardly. The scapula should be constantly supported in its correct position by providing support for the arm. Exercise intervention should include strengthening for the serratus anterior and the trapezius. Stretching exercises are prescribed for those muscles found to be adaptively shortened in the examination. Those muscles usually include the rhomboid and levator scapulae.

Scapular Depression[206]

This syndrome is characterized by weakness and lengthening of the upper trapezius. It is often accompanied by adaptive shortness of the latissimus dorsi, pectoralis major, and pectoralis minor. When the scapula fails to elevate sufficiently during G-H flexion or abduction, the lower trapezius becomes more dominant than its upper counterpart. The intervention should focus on providing support for the shoulder so that it does not become depressed. The patient is instructed to perform shoulder shrugs with the G-H joint in its anatomic position and also with the shoulder flexed above 120 degrees. A mirror can be used to teach the patient to correct the depression of the shoulder girdle during arm elevation.

Stretching exercises are prescribed for those muscles found to be shortened in the examination.

Scapular Abduction Syndrome[206]

This syndrome is characterized by excessive scapular abduction during G-H flexion or abduction. It is also associated with a lengthening of the trapezius and possible lengthening of the rhomboid muscles and adaptive shortening of the serratus anterior, resulting in poor control of the scapula. Adaptive shortness of the deltoid or supraspinatus muscles can also indirectly hold the scapula in an abducted position. Intervention should focus on stretching the short G-H and thoracohumeral muscles and improving the performance of the adductor components of the lower and middle trapezius muscles.

Scapular Winging Syndrome

This syndrome is characterized by an inability to elevate and/or lower the arm without the scapula winging or its inferior angle tilting. This syndrome results from a weakness and adaptive shortness of the serratus anterior, with accompanying shortness of the pectoralis minor and scapulohumeral muscles.

Intervention should focus on stretching the pectoralis minor to correct the tilting and serratus anterior for strengthening and retraining.

Humeral Anterior Glide Syndrome[206]

This syndrome is characterized by a humeral head that is positioned more than one-third anteriorly to the acromion, and which moves anteriorly during G-H abduction. Other findings typically include relative tightness of the posterior capsule when compared with the anterior, weak or lengthened subscapularis, adaptive shortness of the scapulohumeral external rotators, and the pectoralis major.

Intervention should shorten and strengthen the subscapularis, and stretch the humeral external rotators and the pectoralis major.

Humeral Superior Glide Syndrome[206]

This syndrome is characterized by an excessive movement of the humeral head in a superior direction during G-H flexion, abduction, or elevation. Clinical findings usually include adaptive shortness of the deltoid, weakness of the rotator cuff muscles, and adaptive shortness of the humeral internal and/or external rotators. Intervention focuses on the deltoid; increasing its length if shortened, and diminishing its activity if dominant. The patient should be instructed to avoid performing activities that involve ER in adduction as well as abduction exercises and resisted shoulder flexion with the elbow extended, as these can exacerbate the condition.

Glenohumeral Instability

The structures involved in the maintenance of the static and dynamic stability of the shoulder, also provide neurologic feedback that mediates reflex stabilization around the joint.[461,462] Laxity is the physiologic motion and a necessary attribute of the G-H joint that allows normal ROM, which is normally asymptomatic.[357] Laxity is not always synonymous with instability.[463] In contrast, instability is the abnormal symptomatic motion of the G-H joint that affects normal joint kinematics and results in pain, subluxation, or dislocation of the shoulder.[143,461,464,465]

In the early years of life, the G-H joint is fairly stable due to the active mechanisms stabilizing the joint. However, if an individual becomes deconditioned, the dynamic mechanisms become unable to provide support and the joint becomes involved in a self-perpetuating cycle of instability, less use, more shoulder dysfunction, and further instability. In addition to redundance of the shoulder capsule, underlying causes of G-H instability can include genetic, collagen, and biomechanical factors.[357]

There is considerable variation in the amount of translation normally elicited in an asymptomatic shoulder.[355,356,360,466] Shoulder laxity tests show that translations in the asymptomatic shoulder as compared with the contralateral symptomatic shoulder can be as large as 11 mm in one direction.[356,467] Although it has been shown that healthy shoulders can have asymmetric translation in at least one direction, no healthy shoulder is asymmetric in all three directions.[356]

Characteristic of G-H instability is the complaint of the shoulder "slipping" or "popping out" during overhead activities. Instability of the shoulder can be classified by frequency (acute or chronic), magnitude, direction, and origin.[75] Acute traumatic instability with dislocation of the shoulder is the most dramatic variety, and often requires manipulative reduction. Shoulder instability may also be classified according to the direction of the subluxation as either unidirectional (anterior, posterior, or inferior), bidirectional, or multidirectional. Posterior instability, which results either from avulsion of the posterior glenoid labrum from the posterior glenoid, or stretching of the posterior capsuloligamentous structures, is often difficult to diagnose with no single test having high sensitivity and specificity. Recently, both multidirectional instability and its hallmark, inferior G-H instability, have been scrutinized much more closely.[134,156,468]

Most patients presenting with hypermobility or instability of the anterior G-H joint are athletic adolescents or young adults with joint laxity.[357,469] Anterior instability occurs when the abducted shoulder is repetitively placed in the anterior apprehension position of ER and horizontal abduction. Such individuals may have pain with overhead movements due to an inability to control the laxity through muscle support. They may develop enough instability directed superiorly that they present with impingement-like symptoms (instability–impingement overlap), especially in positions of abduction and ER.[470] In general, the patients have had normal asymptomatic shoulder function until some event precipitates symptoms. The event usually involves only relatively minor trauma when compared with the traumatic causes of unidirectional instability, or repetitive microtrauma as occurs in patients who participate in swimming and gymnastics.[278] The most common presenting complaint is pain.[471,472]

Unilateral dislocations occurring from acute traumatic events include the Bankart lesion or Hill-Sachs lesion. The Bankart lesion is an avulsion of the anterior inferior labrum from the glenoid rim and requires surgical stabilization (*t*raumatic, *u*nidirectional instability with *B*ankart lesion requiring *s*urgery or TUBS), using the Bankart procedure, which addresses the lesion without significant loss of ER,[473] or a capsular reconstruction procedure.

CLINICAL PEARL

Multidirectional instability (see later) is often described using the abbreviation AMBRII (*a*traumatic onset of *m*ultidirectional instability that is accompanied by *b*ilateral laxity or hypermobility. *R*ehabilitation is the primary course of intervention to restore G-H stability. However, if an operation is necessary, a procedure such as a capsulorrhaphy is performed to tighten the *i*nferior capsule and the rotator *i*nterval).[474]

The Hill-Sachs lesion is a compression fracture of the posterior humeral head at the site where the humeral head impacted the inferior glenoid rim. Dislocation of the G-H joint is not uncommon in older people, although the incidence is less after 50 years of age.[195] Chronic recurrent dislocations of the shoulder can lead to degenerative arthritis. An older person who dislocates a shoulder is likely to have concurrently torn the rotator cuff and should be examined with this idea in mind.[475–477] Lesser traumatic injuries can cause subluxation of the shoulder to such a degree that recurrent subluxation rather than dislocation becomes the source of dysfunction.[143]

The predominant pattern of instability is best determined from the patient's medical history and provocative maneuvers on physical examination.[357] The mechanism for a subluxation or recurrent dislocation usually involves a FOOSH injury, whereby the arm is forced into abduction, extension, and ER. Due to the potential for nerve injury with these dislocations, a thorough neurovascular examination is essential.[75]

Anterior Instability

Anterior instability of the G-H joint is the most common direction of instability. Repetitive overhead activities such as throwing can lead to microtrauma at the shoulder, leading to eventual breakdown of both the static and dynamic stabilizers of the joint, or G-H instability. Once the stability of the G-H joint has been compromised, the structures of the rotator cuff can become injured, resulting in a tear of one or more of the muscles. Patients who describe symptoms occurring in the abducted and externally rotated position have chronic anteroinferior instability.

The mechanism for an anterior dislocation is abduction, ER, and extension and is common in throwing and racquet sports, gymnastics, and swimming. Following an acute trauma, the patient typically complains of severe pain and a sense that the shoulder is "out." Radiographs confirm the dislocation, and reduction is often necessary. Frank anterior subluxation and dislocation of the G-H joint is rare in children but common in adolescents.[478] Severe pain causes the patient to immobilize the involved arm, in a slightly abducted and externally rotated position with the other hand. Spasm will typically occur to stabilize the joint. The humeral head will be palpable anteriorly and the posterior shoulder will exhibit a hollow beneath the acromion (see "Special Tests" section). In younger age groups (approximately 25 years and younger), the chance of recurrent anterior dislocation after the initial event is greater than 95%.[479] Recurrences are rare in patients older than 50 years of age.[465]

When anterior instability is suspected, the clinician should assess for tightness of the posterior capsule. Posterior capsule tightness has been shown to accentuate anterior translation and superior migration.[361] Loss of IR in young patients may be an important finding suggestive of posterior capsular contracture that is often associated with subtle instability.[197] The posterior joint glide is also restricted. Symptoms also include varying degrees of instability, transient neurologic symptoms, and easy fatigability.[472] Warner et al.[480] reported a lower IR-to-ER ratio for peak torque and total work in the dominant shoulder of patients with instability as compared with healthy controls. This suggests that an association exists between relative IR weakness and anterior instability.[357]

SLAP Lesions

Athletes performing overhead movements, particularly baseball pitchers, may develop a "dead arm" syndrome[481] in which they have a painful shoulder with throwing and can no longer throw a baseball with their preinjury velocity. The main problem is usually a tear of the superior labrum, the so-called SLAP lesion.[1] SLAP lesions are described as *s*uperior *l*abral lesions that are both *a*nterior and *p*osterior.[482] There are several injury mechanisms that are speculated to be responsible for creating SLAP lesions ranging from single traumatic events to repetitive microtraumatic injuries.[10] During a dislocation, tears to the glenoid labrum occur in isolation or in combination. The superior aspect of the labrum is more mobile and prone to injury due to its close attachment to the LHB tendon.[75] The lesion typically results from a FOOSH injury, sudden deceleration or traction forces such as catching a falling heavy object, or chronic anterior and posterior instability.[482,483]

Traumatic SLAP lesions can also develop in the nonathletic population.[483] This occurs as the result of a fall or motor vehicle accident (e.g., drivers who have their hands on the wheel and sustain a rear-end impact).

SLAP lesions have traditionally been classified into four main types[483] by signs and symptoms:

- ***Type I.*** This type involves a fraying and degeneration of the edge of the superior labrum. The patient loses the ability to horizontally abduct or externally rotate with the forearm pronated without pain.[484]
- ***Type II.*** This type involves a pathologic detachment of the labrum and biceps tendon anchor, resulting in a loss of the stabilizing effect of the labrum and the biceps.[485]
- ***Type III.*** This type involves a vertical tear of the labrum, similar to the bucket-handle tear of the knee meniscus, although the remaining portions of the labrum and biceps are intact.[75]
- ***Type IV.*** This type involves an extension of the bucket-handle tear into the biceps tendon, with portions of the labral flap and biceps tendon displaceable into the G-H joint.[75]

Maffet et al.[486] have suggested expanding the classification scale to a total of seven categories, adding descriptions for types V through VII.

- *Type V.* This type is characterized by the presence of a Bankart lesion of the anterior capsule that extends into the anterior superior labrum.
- *Type VI.* This type involves a disruption of the biceps tendon anchor with an anterior or posterior superior labral flap tear.
- *Type VII.* This is described as the extension of a SLAP lesion anteriorly to involve the area inferior to the middle G-H ligament.

Diagnosis of a SLAP lesion can often be difficult as the symptoms are very similar to those of instability and rotator cuff disease. No findings on physical examination have been found to be specific for identifying patients with a SLAP lesion. The patient typically complains of pain with overhead activities and symptoms of catching or locking.[487]

Several special tests can be used to help identify the presence of a SLAP lesion (see "Special Tests" section), including the O' Brien (active-compression) test, the clunk test,[329,330] the crank test,[332] the Speed's test,[483] the Jobe relocation test, the biceps load test,[345] and the anterior slide test.[340]

Conservative intervention should address the underlying hypermobility or instability of the shoulder using dynamic stabilization exercises of the G-H joint to effectively return function and symptomatic relief to the patient (see "Intervention Strategies" section).

Arthroscopic labral debridement is not an effective long-term solution for labral pathology.[488]

Studies of surgical labral repairs are generally good to excellent in terms of returning patients to their prior level of activity, whether sports or work.[75,487,489,490]

Posterior Instability

Posterior instabilities, which are rare and only comprise approximately 2% of all shoulder dislocations,[159] are often associated with seizure, electric shock, diving into a shallow pool, or motor vehicle accidents. Patients who have a posterior instability pattern typically report symptoms with the arm in a forward flexed, adducted position, such as when pushing open heavy doors. Posterior dislocations are classified as subacromial (posterior and inferior to the acromion process—the most common), subglenoid (posterior and inferior to the glenoid rim), and subspinous (medial to the acromion and inferior to the scapular spine).[75]

The most characteristic sign for a posterior dislocation is a loud clunk as the shoulder is moved from a forward flexed position into abduction and external rotation, a positive finding that is often misdiagnosed as an anterior dislocation. The findings for a posterior dislocation are usually severe pain, limited ER, often to less than 0 degree, and limited elevation to less than 90 degrees. There is usually a posterior prominence and rounding of the shoulder as compared to the opposite side, and a flattening of the anterior aspects of the shoulder. Looking down at the patient's shoulders from behind can best assess these asymmetries.

Inferior Instability

Inferior dislocations are very uncommon and are typically elicited by carrying heavy objects at one's side (i.e., grocery bags or a suitcase), or by hyperabduction forces that cause a levering of the humeral neck against the acromion.[464,488]

The diagnosis for this type of dislocation is relatively straightforward, as the patient's arm is typically locked in abduction.[75] The sulcus sign can be used to assess inferior stability.

Multidirectional Instability

Multidirectional instability is a symptomatic G-H instability that is present in more than one direction.[464] It is commonly believed that females have more joint laxity than males, a fact propagated by the medical literature and medical training.[357] In describing multidirectional instability of the shoulder, a typical patient is presented, as "an adolescent female who can habitually and reproducibly sublux one or both shoulders."[468] However, with the exception of a few articles, there is inadequate evidence to confirm this view. One of the exceptions was a recent study by Borsa et al., [491] which demonstrated that healthy women have significantly more anterior joint laxity and less anterior joint stiffness than do men. Another study by Huston and Wojtys[492] used an instrumented arthrometer to assess knee joint laxity in athletic and nonathletic men and women. Overall, they found women to have significantly more knee joint laxity than men. Interestingly, they found that athletic women had significantly less knee joint laxity than nonathletic women did, and athletic men had significantly less knee joint laxity than nonathletic men. These findings imply that physical training and conditioning may decrease joint laxity.[491]

The patient with a multidirectional instability is difficult to diagnose as there is usually no associated traumatic event or mechanism of injury. Rotator cuff pain is often the first presenting symptom. Patients with multidirectional instability typically have scapulothoracic dyskinesia that contributes to the instability.[283]

Lephart et al.[493] showed that patients with multidirectional instability also have deficits in shoulder proprioception. Therefore the intervention for patients with instability should begin with a rehabilitation program aimed at improving the dynamic stabilizers, neuromuscular coordination, and proprioception of the G-H and scapulothoracic joints.[24,357,494]

Intervention

Intervention goals for G-H instability or hypermobility are similar regardless of the instability classification. The goal is to restore dynamic stability and control to the shoulder using the dynamic stabilizers to contain the humeral head within the glenoid.[19,119,159,470,494]

A brief period of sling immobilization is usually necessary for comfort. Prolonged immobilization should be avoided because of the tendency of the shoulder to stiffen quickly, especially in the elderly population.[195] For patients with an anterior instability, ROM exercises for the G-H joint should emphasize posterior capsule stretching to decrease the accentuation of the anterior translation and superior migration. The positions and exercises to modify or avoid based on the direction of instability are illustrated in Table 16-37.[495]

The general approach for all forms of G-H instability includes the following:

TABLE 16-37 Exercise Modification According to the Direction of Glenohumeral Instability		
Direction of Instability	**Position to Avoid**	**Exercises to Modify or Avoid**
Anterior	Combined position of external rotation, extension, and abduction	Chest press, pull-down, push-up, bench press, military press, flyes
Posterior	Combined position of horizontal adduction, internal rotation, and flexion	Chest press, push-up, bench press, flyes, weight-bearing exercises
Inferior	Full elevation, dependent arm	Shrugs, elbow curls, incline press, military press

- ***Scapular stability exercises.*** These can be started early and include the scapular pinch (see Fig. 16-27) and shoulder shrug exercises.[24] In this early stage, the control of the scapula position can be aided by taping the scapular in a retracted or elevated position, or by the use of a figure-8 collar, both of which help to normalize the scapular muscle firing pattern.[24]
- ***Closed-chain exercises.*** These are normally performed with the hand stabilized on a wall or object, simulate normal functional patterns, and reorganize and reestablish normal motor firing patterns.[24,144,145,281] All of the movements of the scapula and shoulder are coupled and are predictable based on arm position.[170,496] Similar to the lower extremity, closed-chain exercises should involve integration of all the joints in the appropriate kinetic chain with the specific scapular maneuvers of elevation, depression, retraction, and protraction.[24]
- ***Early exercises to rehabilitate scapular dyskinesis.*** These include modified push-ups, and progress to facilitation patterns that include hip extension, trunk extension, and scapular retraction.[395] Clock exercises, in which the hand is placed on a wall and the scapula is rotated in elevation/depression and retraction/protraction, also develop coordinated patterns for scapular control.[395]

Open-chain exercises follow the isometric and closed-chain activities as these exercises are more strenuous.[24] Open-chain exercises include PNF patterns, diagonals, upright rows, and ER and scapular retraction activities, as well as machine exercises consisting of lat pull-downs.[24]

Progression of the scapular rehabilitation can be evaluated using the scapular slide measurements, and once the lateral slide asymmetry is less than 1 cm, specific strengthening for the rotator cuff can commence.[24]

Besides rehabilitation, activity modifications to avoid any arm positions that provoke symptoms can be helpful.[357]

Sprained Conoid and Trapezoid Ligaments

A sprain of these ligaments can result from a clavicular fracture, but it can also occur in sports that require the arm to be pulled into the extremes of extension or ER. Pain is felt at the extremes of all passive arm and scapula movements. Forced ER with the arm in horizontal abduction will usually be the most painful test, and differentiation between the two structures is made by palpation of the coracoid process. No limitation of active shoulder range is usually found and resistive movements are painless.

Interventions for these ligament sprains include electrotherapeutic modalities and physical agents, transverse friction massage (TFM), and progression of ROM of the shoulder complex and strengthening of the G-H muscles and scapular pivoters.

Acromioclavicular Joint Sprain

An injury to the A-C joint, which is one of the most frequently injured joints in the body, can be categorized as either acute traumatic or chronic.[71] The majority of acute traumatic injuries occur from a fall onto the shoulder with the arm adducted at the side. The ground reaction force produces displacement of the scapula in relation to the distal clavicle.[71] The chronic disorder may be atraumatic or posttraumatic, with the former being attributed to generalized osteoarthritis, inflammatory arthritis, or mechanical problems of the meniscus of this joint.[195] Injuries to the A-C joint were originally classified by Tossy et al.[497] and Allman[89] as incomplete (grades I and II) and complete (grade III). This classification has been expanded to include six types of injuries based on the direction and amount of displacement (Table 16-38).[80,498–500] As with the S-C joint, A-C joint injuries are classified according to ligamentous injury rather than injury to the joint itself:

- ***Type I.*** Tenderness and mild pain at the A-C joint. Sometimes there is a high, painful arc (160–180 degrees), and resisted adduction is painful. Passive A-P joint gliding is painful, especially in patients over 50 years of age.[501]
- ***Type II.*** Moderate to severe local pain with tenderness in the coracoclavicular space. The clavicle may appear to be slightly higher than the acromion, although in reality the opposite is true. All passive motions are painful at the end of ROM, and usually both resisted adduction and abduction are painful. Passive posteroanterior translation at the A-C joint is greater than that of the opposite joint.
- ***Type III.*** The patient usually holds the arm against the body in a slightly adducted position and exerts an upward axial pressure through the humerus. An obvious gap is visible between the acromion and the clavicle. All active motions are painful, especially abduction. The piano key phenomenon is present; after pushing the clavicle inferiorly, it springs back to its original position.
- ***Type IV.*** Similar findings as those of type III, except the pain is severe and the clavicle is displaced posteriorly.
- ***Type V.*** There is a large distance between the clavicle and coracoid process and there is tenderness to palpation over the entire lateral half of the clavicle.

TABLE 16-38	Classification of A-C Injuries and Clinical Findings
Type I	Isolated sprain of acromioclavicular ligaments Coracoclavicular ligaments intact Deltoid and trapezoid muscles intact Tenderness and mild pain at A-C joint High (160–180 degrees) painful arc Resisted adduction is often painful Intervention is with TFM, ice, and pain-free AROM
Type II	A-C ligament is disrupted Sprain of coracoclavicular ligament A-C joint is wider; may be a slight vertical separation when compared to the normal shoulder Coracoclavicular interspace may be slightly increased Deltoid and trapezoid muscles intact Moderate-to-severe local pain Tenderness in coracoclavicular space PROM all painful at end range with horizontal adduction being the most painful Resisted abduction and abduction are often painful Intervention initiated with ice and pain-free AROM/PROM; TFM introduced on day 4
Type III	A-C ligament is disrupted A-C joint dislocated and the shoulder complex displaced inferiorly Coracoclavicular interspace 25–100% greater than normal shoulder Coracoclavicular ligament is disrupted Deltoid and trapezoid muscles are usually detached from the distal end of the clavicle A fracture of the clavicle is usually present in patients under 13 yr of age Arm held by patient in adducted position Obvious gap visible between acromion and clavicle AROM all painful; PROM painless if done carefully Piano key phenomenon (clavicle springs back after being pushed inferiorly) present
Type IV	A-C ligament is disrupted A-C joint dislocated and the clavicle anatomically displaced posteriorly into or through the trapezius muscle Coracoclavicular ligaments completely disrupted Coracoclavicular interspace may be displaced but may appear normal Deltoid and trapezoid muscles are detached from the distal end of the clavicle Clavicle displaced posteriorly; Surgery indicated for types IV–VI
Type V	A-C ligaments disrupted Coracoclavicular ligaments completely disrupted A-C joint dislocated and gross disparity between the clavicle and the scapula (300–500% greater than normal) Deltoid and trapezoid muscles are detached from the distal end of the clavicle Tenderness over entire lateral half of the clavicle
Type VI	A-C ligaments disrupted Coracoclavicular ligaments completely disrupted A-C joint dislocated and the clavicle anatomically displaced inferiorly to the clavicle or the coracoid process Coracoclavicular interspace reversed with the clavicle being inferior to the acromion or the coracoid process Deltoid and trapezoid muscles are detached from the distal end of the clavicle Cranial aspect of shoulder is flatter than opposite side; Often accompanied with clavicle or upper rib fracture and/or brachial plexus injury

AROM, active range of motion; PROM, passive range of motion; TFM, transverse friction massage.
Data from Allman FL. Fractures and ligamentous injuries of the clavicle and its articulation. *J Bone Joint Surg Am* 1967;49:774–784; Rockwood CA Jr, Young DC. Disorders of the acromioclavicular joint. In: Rockwood CA Jr, Matsen FA III, eds. *The Shoulder*. Philadelphia, PA: WB Saunders, 1990:413–468.

- *Type VI.* The superior aspect of the affected shoulder is flatter than the noninvolved side. Often there are associated fractures of the clavicle and upper ribs, as well as injury to the brachial plexus.

Types I–III and V all involve inferior displacement of the acromion with respect to the clavicle. They differ according to the severity of ligamentous injury and the amount of resultant displacement.[173]

Types I and II typically result from a fall or a blow to the point on the lateral aspect of the shoulder, or a FOOSH injury.

Types III and IV usually involve a dislocation (commonly referred to as an A-C separation) and a distal clavicle fracture, both of which commonly disrupt the coracoclavicular ligaments.[71] In addition, damage to the deltoid and trapezius fascia, and rarely the skin, can occur.[71] Type IV injuries are characterized by posterior displacement of the clavicle.

Type VI injuries have a clavicle inferiorly displaced into either a subacromial or subcoracoid position. These types (IV, V, VI) also have complete rupture of all the ligament complexes and are much rarer injuries than types I through III.[71]

In the pediatric patient, A-C sprains are usually grade I or II and may occur without clavicular fracture.[478] Grade III sprains in this population commonly rupture the posterior (dorsal) clavicular periosteum. However, the coracoclavicular ligaments and A-C ligaments remain intact.[478]

The clinical findings are based on injury severity (Table 16-38). Patients who have suffered an injury to the joint typically present with a history of either a distinctive, traumatic mechanism of injury or a more insidious type of onset that began with pain and dysfunction.[73] The joint is quite superficial and direct palpation is accomplished easily. The patient may report that the arm feels better with a superiorly directed support on the arm, such as a sling. Pain is typically reproduced at the end range of passive elevation, passive ER and IR, and especially with passive horizontal adduction, across the chest. This cross-arm test compresses the A-C joint and is highly sensitive for A-C joint pathology.[71,74,80,502] The ROM available depends on the stage of healing and severity. In the very acute stage, range may be limited by pain, whereas the less acute stage will be painful at the end of range in full elevation or horizontal adduction. Pain, crepitus, or hypermobility may be encountered with mobility testing. Resistive movements are usually painless. It is important to assess for secondary injury to the surrounding soft tissues and to the other three articulations of the shoulder complex when there is a history of trauma to the A-C joint.

A complete radiographic examination including a 15-degree-superior A-P view, a lateral Y view, and an axillary film should confirm the diagnosis.[71]

The intervention for A-C joint sprains depends on the severity of the injury and the physical requirements of the patient.

- ***Types I and II.*** These patients will usually recover full and painless function with conservative intervention.[74] Although adhesive taping devices and orthotics have been used in the early phase after injury to attempt reduction of the clavicle in the type II injury, they have not demonstrated efficacy in any good experimental trials.[71] Ice, nonsteroidal anti-inflammatories, and analgesics should be used judiciously. Most physicians prescribe a sling for 1–2 weeks. Gentle ROM exercises and functional rehabilitation are started immediately following immobilization, and then isometric exercises are prescribed for those muscles with clavicular attachments. The exercises are progressed to PREs for the muscles that attach to the clavicle and the scapular pivoters. A graduated return to full activity is very important. Most patients will be back to full sport/occupation participation within 12 weeks, although they may have a slight cosmetic deformity.[71]
- ***Type III.*** The intervention for type III injuries is controversial.[71] A survey of orthopaedic residency programs in 1992 revealed that 86.4% preferred conservative intervention.[503] The natural history of this injury with conservative intervention suggests that patients have no long-term difficulty with pain or loss of function.[504–508] A more recent study[509] found no strength deficits at follow-up, although discomfort at higher levels of activity was more pronounced. There is a reported high complication rate with attempts at surgical stabilization.[510,511] Citing the concern regarding greater displacement, some authors have proposed surgical intervention, but there have been several controlled comparative studies[502,510,511] that suggest that conservative intervention gave results comparable to those of surgically treated patients, but without surgical complications.[71]

  A reasonable approach would be to initially treat all types conservatively with sling immobilization, followed by supervised rehabilitation.[71] Once the sling is removed, pendulum exercises can be initiated. PROM in the extremes of motion are avoided for the first 7 days, but the goal should be for full PROM after 2–3 weeks. A graduated resistance exercise program is initiated once pain is improved and AROM is full. These exercises should emphasize strengthening of the deltoid and upper trapezius muscles and promote dynamic stabilization of the shoulder complex.[198] Full return to sport is expected by 6–12 weeks.[71] If patients are still functionally limited after more than 3 months, a secondary reconstructive procedure may be necessary.[71]
- ***Types IV, V, and VI.*** These types of displacement all require surgical intervention.[74] Care should be taken to accurately identify these injuries and refer them early to a surgical specialist.[71] The greater displacement and injury includes damage to the deltoid and trapezius muscle and fascia. Failure to reduce these and repair them may lead to chronic pain and dysfunction.[71] The postsurgical progression involves gaining pain-free ROM prior to advancing to exercises to regain strength, manual techniques to normalize arthrokinematics, and functional training to improve neuromuscular control of the shoulder complex.

Late complications, including degenerative changes of the distal clavicle, can develop with a subluxed clavicle.[71] Symptoms may be treated with the selective use of modalities and steroid injections. If this conservative approach fails, then the patient should be considered as a surgical candidate.[71]

Acromioclavicular Joint Arthrosis

A-C joint arthrosis may be degenerative or posttraumatic. It is most commonly seen in middle-aged patients, either as an isolated entity or in combination with rotator cuff tendinitis and impingement syndrome.[71,74]

A-C joint arthrosis is diagnosed by the history and physical examination. Patients typically complain of pain locally or distributed to the anterolateral neck, the trapezius–supraspinatus region, and the anterolateral deltoid.[512] This pain is usually exacerbated with overhead and/or flexed and adducted positions of the arm.[71] Direct palpation to the A-C joint will sometimes reproduce the patient's pain. Impingement of the rotator cuff must be ruled out. The selective use of cortisone injections into the A-C joint or the subacromial space can be applied to help differentiate A-C pain from rotator cuff tendinitis and treat both of these conditions.[71,74]

Conservative intervention consists of rest, modification of activity, and NSAIDs. Electrotherapeutic modalities and cryotherapy may be used to control pain and the active inflammation. Joint mobilizations of grade I or II may also be used to decrease pain. Once pain and inflammation are under control, the rehabilitation progresses to strengthening of the dynamic restraints of the A-C joint (primarily the deltoid, trapezius, and pectorals).[74,198] Any activities involving raising the arm above the level of the shoulder or reaching across the chest should be avoided as these will tend to aggravate the A-C joint.[195]

Sternoclavicular Joint Sprain

The S-C joint can sustain sprains, dislocations, or other injuries, but is less involved than the A-C joint with osteoarthritis or mechanical conditions.[195] Posterior S-C dislocations, although rare, are frequently delayed in their diagnosis, and can even be life-threatening due to the pressure placed on many vital structures lying between the sternum and the cervical spine such as the trachea, esophagus, and major blood vessels. However, most of these dislocations occur anteriorly and are more obvious.[190]

Any trauma to the shoulder girdle may cause an S-C dislocation, although the joint is most commonly injured through motor vehicle accidents, followed by sports.[91] In sports, the mechanism of injury is usually secondary to a FOOSH with the arm in either a flexed and adducted position, or extended and adducted position.[470] The well-developed interarticular meniscus can be torn and can lead secondarily to degenerative changes. Irritation of this joint may also occur in inflammatory conditions, such as rheumatoid arthritis or repetitive microtrauma.[192] Infection of this joint usually indicates a systemic source, such as bacterial endocarditis.[195]

An injury to the S-C joint can be significant because the joint plays an integral role in scapular motion through the clavicle's articulation with the scapula. Subjectively, the patient reports discomfort with end-range movement of the shoulder. S-C injuries are graded according to severity of injury to the ligament supporting the joints rather than injury to the joint itself.[66]

- ***Type I.*** Sprain of S-C ligament.
- ***Type II.*** Subluxation, partial tear of capsular ligaments, disk, or costoclavicular ligaments.
- ***Type IIA.*** Anterior subluxation; this is the most common grade.
- ***Type IIB.*** Posterior subluxation.[192]
- ***Type IIIA.*** Anterior dislocation.
- ***Type IIIB.*** Posterior dislocation.
- ***Type IV.*** Habitual dislocation (rare).

The clinical presentation for S-C sprains are characterized by deformity, local pain or tenderness, and subsequent ecchymosis. With a posterior dislocation or subluxation, some shortness of breath or even venous congestion in the neck may be seen, with decreased circulation sometimes evident in the arm.[73]

Chronic subluxation or damage to the intra-articular disk can produce long-term discomfort with repetitive strong movements of the upper limb and therefore may require surgical stabilization of the S-C joint.[73]

The conservative intervention for first- or second-degree sprains (providing that the joint is deemed stable) is aimed at addressing the function of the shoulder complex, particularly the end ranges, and is dependent on the cause. Typically the shoulder is immobilized for 3–4 days, as pain dictates. In more severe sprains (second- or third-degree sprain with instability following reduction), a shoulder sling or figure-8 strap is worn for 2–3 weeks to minimize stress on the joint, and then the arm may be protected for a further 2 weeks.

- Appropriate modalities are used to control pain and the inflammatory process.
- ROM exercises are initiated early, and care is taken to avoid excessive movement at the S-C joint. Initially, until the pain and inflammation is under control, activities should be limited to midrange. ROM is increased based on patient tolerance.
- Any hypomobilities of the neighboring joints are addressed using specific mobilizations of an appropriate grade.
- In cases with residual ligamentous laxity, stabilization exercises should focus on strengthening those muscles that attach to the clavicle (pectoralis minor, sternal fibers of the pectoralis major and upper trapezius), performed within ranges that do not stress the joint. Exercises include incline bench, shoulder shrugs, and the seated push-up.[513] The scapular pivoters should also be strengthened. For example, exercises such as Superman, bent over row, rhomboids, and push-ups with a plus should be included.[513]
- Return to normal activity is permitted when the patient no longer has associated pain with movements of the shoulder complex, and the rehabilitation program has been progressed to the appropriate level of stress for the specific demands of the patient's activity.

Complications of anterior S-C dislocation include cosmetic deformity, recurrent instability, and late osteoarthrosis.[73] Complications of posterior dislocation include all of these plus pressure or rupture of the trachea, pneumothorax, rupture of the esophagus, pressure on the subclavian artery of brachial plexus, voice changes, and dysphagia.[73]

Total Shoulder Arthroplasty

A total shoulder arthroplasty (TSA) is a surgical option typically reserved for elderly patients with cuff-deficient arthritic shoulders.[514] Other patients who may require a TSA include those with bone tumors, rheumatoid arthritis, Paget's disease, osteonecrosis of the humeral head, fracture dislocations, and those who incur recurrent dislocations.[515,516]

The primary indication for surgical intervention is complaints of unremitting pain, rather than decreased motion, and a failure of conservative measures. Additional considerations include patient age, activity level, job requirements, and general health.[514]

A course of preoperative intervention is recommended. This should include an assessment of ROM, scapular mobility, muscle imbalances, and pain. The key muscles to examine preoperatively for strength include the rotator cuff, deltoid, trapezius, rhomboids, serratus anterior, latissimus dorsi, teres major, and pectoralis major and minor.[254] The patient should be provided with exercise instruction and patient education on postsurgical precautions. A course of shoulder stretching before a prosthetic arthroplasty may improve postsurgical function.[517]

The TSA is a very difficult procedure, and the outcome depends on the skill of the reconstruction, the soft tissue repair, the orientation of the implants, and the success of the rehabilitation.[405,515,518,519] The total shoulder replacement provides significantly greater pain relief than hemiarthroplasty, with approximately 80% of patients reporting pain relief after hemiarthroplasty versus more than 90% after shoulder replacement.[519]

Four types of replacement components have traditionally been used:

1. ***Unconstrained.*** This is the most widely used component and consists of a humeral component that exists with a scapular component.
2. ***Constrained.*** This type, in which the glenoid and humeral components are coupled and fixed to bone, was designed for patients who had severe deterioration of the rotator cuff but with a functioning deltoid. However, due to the high rate of associated complications, it is rarely used nowadays.
3. ***Reversed ball and socket.*** This design consists of a small humeral socket that slides on a larger ball-shaped glenoid component.
4. ***Semiconstrained.*** This type involves the use of a smaller and spherical humeral head with a head–neck angle of 60 degrees, which reportedly permits increased ROM.

The unconstrained technique and the postsurgical rehabilitation that follows this procedure are described in this section.

Although surgical techniques vary, most involve the dissection of the subscapularis or a rotator cuff repair, or a combination of both. The patient is usually placed in a sling or an elastic shoulder immobilizer following the operation that positions the humerus in adduction, IR, and slight forward flexion. An abduction splint may be issued if a rotator cuff repair is performed and is worn for 4–6 weeks, according to the surgeon's instructions.

The long-term outcome following shoulder arthroplasty depends on many factors including the quality of the soft tissue (especially the integrity of the rotator cuff), the quality of the bone, the type of implant and fixation used, the patient's expectations, and the quality of the rehabilitation program.[254]

Most surgeons have their own postsurgical rehabilitation protocols—only the surgeon knows the extent of soft tissue damage and repair, and any guidelines communicated to the clinician must be strongly adhered to. Typically, the only motions not allowed in the early weeks are active IR and active and passive ER beyond 35–40 degrees.

PATTERN 4E: IMPAIRED JOINT MOBILITY, MOTOR FUNCTION, MUSCLE PERFORMANCE, RANGE OF MOTION WITH LOCALIZED INFLAMMATION

In addition to those conditions producing impaired ROM, motor function, and muscle performance attributed to inflammation, this pattern includes conditions that cause pain and muscle guarding without the presence of structural changes. Such conditions include rotator cuff tears, tendinitis, bursitis, capsulitis, and tenosynovitis.

Rotator Cuff Pathology

Fifty to seventy percent of shoulder issues seen by clinicians are related to conditions of the rotator cuff (RC).[520,521] The frequency of RC problems is not surprising as these structures play an essential role in supporting the shoulder capsule and holding the humeral head in proper alignment in the glenoid cavity. Problems can occur from a number of sources including trauma, attrition, and the anatomical structure of the subacromial space. The supraspinatus is the tendon most often affected because of its location beneath the anterior acromion, and its extensions into the infraspinatus tendon that may also become involved.[522,523] Significant tears of the RC rarely involve the subscapularis tendon.[522,523]

A number of mechanisms are recognized and include compression, tensile overload, and macrotrauma.

- ***Compression.*** Compression of the RC can either be primary or secondary. Primary compression is due to a reduction in the size of the subacromial space (e.g., a type III hooked acromion process or a congenitally thick coracoacromial ligament in younger patients, or an osteophyte on the undersurface of the acromion process in the older patient). Secondary compression occurs as a result of a decrease in G-H joint stability that allows the humeral head to compress the RC.
- ***Tensile overload.*** Tension overload can also be either primary or secondary. Primary tensile overload occurs when the RC attempts to resist horizontal adduction, IR, anterior translation, and distraction forces during such activities as throwing (the deceleration phase) and hammering. Secondary tensile overload occurs as a result of G-H instability that places greater distractive and tensile forces on the RC, and eventual failure of the tendon.
- ***Macrotrauma.*** Macrotrauma and subsequent tearing of the tendon results when the forces generated by the trauma

exceed the tensile strength of the tendon. RC tears are not as common in the skeletally immature athlete as in the older athlete. Indeed, the incidences of RC tear increases with age. Approximately 50% of individuals older than 55 years demonstrated an arthrographically detectable RC tear.[524] Although cadaver studies of individuals older than 40 years have generally shown a prevalence of full-thickness RC tears between 5% and 20%,[525] the prevalence of partial-thickness RC tears has been shown to be in the 30–40% range in adult cadavers.[525]

A detailed history is important to diagnose a RC injury and the cause, and it can help to determine whether the patient's symptoms are related to a specific injury or event, or to a repetitive motion, or are of a more insidious onset (e.g., referred pain from the cervical spine, more serious referred symptoms of cardiac origin). Activities and arm positions that increase or decrease symptoms are also helpful in diagnosing and guiding treatment. Prior episodes of similar symptoms may give a useful clue to the patient's present condition. A social history should include the patient's occupation and sport (including position), and level of athletic participation. Repetitive motion can be associated with the symptoms. The presence of associated symptoms (e.g., instability, weakness, swelling, numbness, loss of motion, catching or popping of the shoulder) also provides helpful information.

Pain, weakness, and loss of shoulder motion are common symptoms reported with RC pathology. The patient complains initially of a dull ache radiating into the upper and lower arm. This ache is worse after activity, at night when the patient lies on the affected shoulder, and with actions such as reaching above the head or putting on a coat. The characteristic physical finding is the painful arc. The pain may begin around 50–60 degrees of abduction in patients with shoulder immobility. The symptoms may be relatively acute, either following an injury or associated with a known repetitive overuse activity.

In elderly patients, symptoms are often insidious and with no specific injury.

The clinician can often determine the involved tendon by resisting the AROM of each tendon.

Palpable anterior tenderness over the coracoacromial ligament is common with impingement.[28,526] Tenderness of the biceps tendon and at the supraspinatus insertion is also commonly found.

Patients with a painful arc and the above history, but no pain to resisted shoulder movements, are likely to have subacromial–subdeltoid bursitis.[195]

A study by Park et al.[527] evaluated eight physical examination tests for RC pathology (the Neer impingement sign, Hawkins–Kennedy impingement sign, painful arc sign, supraspinatus muscle strength test, Speed test, cross-body adduction test, drop-arm sign, and infraspinatus muscle strength test) to determine their diagnostic values, including likelihood ratios and posttest probabilities, for three degrees of severity in RC disease: bursitis, partial-thickness RC tears, and full-thickness RC tears. The sensitivity, specificity, positive predictive value, negative predictive value, and overall accuracy of the eight tests varied considerably—the combination of the Hawkins–Kennedy impingement sign, the painful arc sign, and the infraspinatus muscle test yielded the best posttest probability (95%) for any degree of impingement syndrome. The combination of the painful arc sign, drop-arm sign, and infraspinatus muscle test produced the best posttest probability (91%) for full-thickness RC tears.[527] The study concluded that the severity of the impingement syndrome affects the diagnostic values of the commonly used clinical tests and that the variable accuracy of these tests should be taken into consideration when evaluating patients with symptoms of RC disease.[527]

RC tears are described by size, location, direction, and depth.

Weakness to some extent always accompanies RC tears. The amount of weakness is directly related to the size of the tear.[1] For example, with small tears, the weakness may not be detected and the patient may have full ROM, although there may be a painful arc. Massive tears of the RC present with sudden profound weakness with an inability to raise the arm overhead, and exhibit a positive "drop-arm" sign (see "Special Tests" section).[528] In this situation, infiltration of the subacromial space with a local anesthetic may eliminate the pain and allow more accurate testing of the muscle–tendon unit. The use of corticosteroid injections for RC tears to promote healing is controversial because of their association with weakening the integrity of tendons with repeated use. Some studies have supported this belief,[39,529–531] although only one case of RC rupture following steroid injection has been reported in the literature.[529] Two recent studies have demonstrated that corticosteroid injections are more effective than anti-inflammatory drugs in the management of RC problems.[532,533] However, if the patient has not responded to 1–2 well-placed injections, either other intervention modalities should be considered or the diagnosis questioned.

Acute massive tears require prompt evaluation for surgical repair because little is known about the efficacy of conservative intervention.[1,295,534–541] However, the patient may decide against surgery for various reasons, including concerns about a successful repair, surgical risks, or lack of functional improvement.[542] The conservative program for full-thickness RC tears is directed toward stretching and strengthening the remaining RC, deltoid, pectoralis major, and trapezius muscles.[521,543] The postsurgical approach is initiated with some form of immobilization that restricts positions based on the surgical repair, and promotes pain control. For example in open repairs, flexion, and abduction might be restricted for as long as 4 weeks, or if the capsulolabral complex has been repaired the patient might spend up to 2 weeks in an airplane or ablation splint.[513] Exercises in the early phase include shoulder shrugs, isometrics, and then AAROM exercises. Once the subacute stage of healing has been achieved, the focus of the rehabilitation program is to regain full ROM and to gradually increase the stress to healing tissue. At this stage, AROM exercises are initiated before progressing to gradual resistance using surgical tubing with a focus on the restoration of normal arthrokinematics and a normal scapulothoracic rhythm.[513] The rehabilitation during the final stage of healing mirrors that of conservative management.

The conservative intervention for patients with a partial tear varies. If the symptomatic tear is partial, then a period of conservative intervention should be attempted.[501,521,544,545]

TABLE 16-39	Specific Strengthening Exercises for the Shoulder Girdle
Muscle	**Exercise**
Middle trapezius	Prone row Prone horizontal abduction with the arm and 90-degree abduction with ER
Lower trapezius	Prone horizontal at 90-degree abduction with ER Prone full can Prone ER at 90-degree abduction Bilateral ER
Upper trapezius	Shoulder shrugs Prone row Prone horizontal abduction at 90-degree abduction with ER
Supraspinatus	Full can Prone full can
Infraspinatus and teres minor	Sitting, external rotation of the arm with a towel roll Side-lying external rotation Prone ER at 90-degree abduction
Rhomboids and levator scapulae	Prone row Prone horizontal abduction at 90-degree abduction hip ER Prone extension with ER
Serratus anterior	Dynamic hug Push-up with plus Serratus punch 120°
Subscapularis	Lift-off (Gerber) IR at 0-degree abduction IR at 90-degree abduction IR diagonal exercise Shoulder dumps
Deltoid	Side-lying, 45-degree abduction

Data from Reinold MM, Escamilla RF, Wilk KE: Current concepts in the scientific and clinical rationale behind exercises for glenohumeral and scapulothoracic musculature. *J Orthop Sports Phys Ther* 39:105–117, 2009.

- Stage I. The focus of early rehabilitation is the reduction of pain and inflammation through modalities, activity modifications, and NSAIDs prescribed by the physician. Jobe and Nuber[184] describe a program of kinesiologic repair that strengthens the RC (to increase the depressor effect on the humeral head) and the scapular pivoters, but avoids any increase in the elevating effect of the deltoid. The mainstays of this strengthening program are the IR and ER exercises (Table 16-39).[251] These are initially performed as isometric exercises at various parts of the range. Once these are tolerated well, concentric exercises of the scapular pivoters are introduced beginning with manual resistance and progressing to free weights (see "Intervention Strategies" section). Care should be taken with exercises that involve the use of weights with the arm flexed or abducted away, or overhead, as these may exacerbate supraspinatus impingement and tendinitis symptoms if performed in the early stages of rehabilitation. The exercises prescribed should be as specific as possible, and tailored to the patient's functional and athletic goals. The lower extremity and trunk muscles that provide core stability should also be strengthened. Deficits in strength, strength imbalances, and flexibility in the legs, hips, and trunk should be addressed. This is particularly so in throwing athletes, where restrictions of the hip and back motion are common.[35,48,144,151]

  Manual techniques can be used to address any tightness in the capsule (usually the posterior and inferior aspects) or motion restrictions of the S-C or A-C joints (see "Therapeutic Techniques" section). The patient should be instructed on how to perform an isolated posterior capsule stretch.
- Stage II. Restoration of ROM using exercises, stretching techniques, and self-mobilization. During this stage, the patient should be exercising with free weights, with an emphasis on eccentric exercises of the RC. Concentric exercises for the upper trapezius and deltoid are added. These include shoulder flexion, and reverse flys. The serratus anterior is strengthened using push-ups and the push-up plus. Neuromuscular retraining exercises for the shoulder complex include rocking on all fours, and the Fitter board, as appropriate. Plyometric exercises using small medicine balls and push-ups with a hand clap are also included during this stage as appropriate. Neuromuscular techniques can also be applied manually and include quick reversals during PNF patterns. Other manual techniques include stretching of the capsule and any other pericapsular structures that appear tight.
- Stage III. PNF diagonal patterns are initiated in this stage in addition to eccentric exercises of the RC. Typical exercises performed in this stage include the military press, reverse flies, and push-ups.
- Stage IV. Plyometric strengthening and sport/activity specific training with a gradual return to normal activity.

Subacromial Impingement Syndrome

SIS is a recurrent and troublesome condition closely related to RC disease.[546] In the presence of a normal RC, normal scapular pivoters, and no capsular contractures, the humeral head translates less than 3 mm superiorly during the midranges of active elevation, whereas at the end ranges, A-P and superoinferior translations of 4–10 mm do occur, all of which are coupled with specific motions of IR or ER.[19,48,153,252,280,547–550] An increase in superior translation with active elevation may result in encroachment of the coracoacromial arch.[40,547] This encroachment produces a compression of the suprahumeral structures against the anteroinferior aspect of the acromion and coracoacromial ligament. Repetitive compression of these structures, coupled with other predisposing factors, results in a condition called SIS. SIS was first recognized by Jarjavay[551] in 1867, and the term *impingement syndrome* was popularized by Neer[40] in the 1970s.

Both intrinsic and extrinsic factors have been implicated as etiologies of the impingement process, and a number of impingement types have evolved. Two of those types include the outlet (intrinsic/internal) impingement and the nonoutlet (extrinsic/external) impingement (Fig. 16-64).

Outlet (Intrinsic or Internal) Impingement

This type of impingement occurs as a result of abnormal contact between the RC undersurface and the posterosuperior glenoid rim (Fig. 16-64). The etiology of posterosuperior glenoid impingement has been a source of much debate. Neer[40] proposed that a tight or crowded subacromial space (e.g., one in which the space is compromised by an anterior acromial osteophyte) could cause a mechanical abrasion of the RC against the acromion with abduction above 80–90 degrees without concomitant ER. Others have attributed internal impingement secondary to anterior microinstability and tightness of the capsule posteriorly.

Whatever the underlying cause, the abrasion of the soft tissue structures located between the head of the humerus and the roof of the shoulder during elevation of the arm produces an irritation, inflammation, and tearing of the RC muscles, an irritation of the LHB, and subacromial bursitis.[58,552,553]

This type of impingement is known as an *outlet impingement*, because it occurs at the supraspinatus outlet formed by the coracoid process, the anterior acromion, the A-C joint, and the coracoacromial ligament. It clinically manifests as a "painful arc." A painful arc describes a region of pain in a particular motion, which has pain-free areas on either side of it.[317] For example, during abduction the patient may feel an onset of pain at 80 degrees, which then disappears at 100 degrees. The general cause of a painful arc is impingement of a tender subacromial structure during motion, although loose bodies and instabilities may also cause a painful arc.

Although Neer and Poppen[554] reported that 90–95% of RC tears were the result of the outlet subacromial impingement, the role of age-related or senescent degeneration and tensile overload has been emphasized more recently (see later).[552,553,555–559]

Nonoutlet (Extrinsic/External) Impingement

Nonoutlet impingement, sometimes referred to as posterior internal impingement, in which the subacromial space appears to be normal, occurs in the younger patient performing repetitive overhead motions. The mechanism in this condition appears to be an impingement of the RC against the posterior superior glenoid labrum and the humeral head during forced humeral elevation and IR. This can eventually result in posterior superior tears in the glenoid labrum, and lesions in the posterior humeral head (Bankart lesion).

Primary and Secondary Impingement

Two other types of impingement, which relate to chronic disorders of the RC, have been proposed with four subclassifications (Table 16-40):[98,560]

- Primary (anterior) impingement refers to an intrinsic degenerative process in the structures occupying the subacromial space, which occurs when the superior aspect of the RC is compressed and abraded by the surrounding bony and soft tissues due to anatomical crowding, posterior capsular tightness, and/or excessive superior migration of the humeral head.[561] Patients with primary impingement are typically over the age of 40 and present with limited horizontal abduction (as compared with the uninvolved side), and limited IR (<50 degrees). This condition, commonly treated operatively, often is the result of cyclical repetitive abduction, forward flexion, and IR motion at the G-H joint.
- Secondary (coracoid) impingement occurs when the lesser tuberosity of the humerus encroaches on the coracoid process. The primary cause is G-H instability and/or tensile overload of the RC resulting in poor control of the humeral head during overhead activities involving forward flexion, IR, and abduction.[98,560,562] Secondary impingement is a condition found in both older and younger individuals with varying levels of activity, although patients in this group are usually younger than 35 years, have a history of traumatic anterior instability, a posterior defect of the humeral head, and damage to the posterior glenoid labrum. These individuals typically present with limited IR, excessive ER, and anterosuperior humeral head migration.[166]

TABLE 16-40 Jobe and Kvnite Classification of Shoulder Dysfunction in the Overhead Athlete[511]

- *Group IA*. This group, typically found in the older population, encompasses those patients with pure and isolated impingement and no instability
- *Group IB*. This group, typically found in the older population, encompasses those patients with instability secondary to mechanical trauma
- *Group II*. Patients in this group, who are usually young (<35 yr old) overhead athletes, demonstrate instability with impingement secondary to microtrauma that comes from overuse
- *Group III*. Patients in this group, who are also typically young overhead athletes, demonstrate atraumatic, generalized ligamentous laxity
- *Group IV*. Patients in this group are young (<35 yr old) who have experienced a traumatic event, resulting in instability in the absence of impingement

CLINICAL PEARL

It is recognized that primary impingement syndrome conditions can lead to secondary impingement if not managed appropriately.[563,564]

Thus the pathophysiology of SIS and RC disorders may have both intrinsic and extrinsic factors. In addition to the shape and form of the acromion, the amount of vascularization to the RC, the correct functioning of the dynamic stabilizers, and the condition of the A-C joint, a number of other intrinsic and extrinsic factors have been found to predispose an individual to SIS, including the following[39,41,56,63,565]:

1. ***Age.*** The age of the patient appears to be an important etiologic factor in the development of subacromial impingement in association with repetitive motion.[566–570] In the absence of repetitive motion as a causative factor, SIS is more common after the third decade of life and is

uncommon in individuals younger than 30 years.[39,40] In addition, there is a normal age-related increase in asymptomatic RC defects.[566–568,570,571] Constant and Murley[572] have also shown that there is an age-related decrease in shoulder function in healthy volunteers.

2. ***Position of the arm during activities.*** The arm position adopted during activities may contribute to the development of subacromial impingement significantly.[201] Because of the tangential vector of deltoid contraction, the tendency for superior translation of the humeral head is greatest between 60 and 90 degrees of elevation[44,547,573] Thus repetitive activities in this range of elevation place a high demand on the RC to counteract this tendency. In addition, repetitive activities that occur during higher levels of elevation of the arm bring the greater tuberosity and supraspinatus insertion into close proximity to the coracoacromial arch.[44,547,573]
3. ***Muscle imbalances.*** Sustained or repetitive overhead activity requires the scapular pivoters to constantly maintain appropriate scapular rotation.[39,112,125] Fatigue of the scapular pivoters may lead or contribute to relative subacromial impingement because of poor or asymmetric scapular rotation.[39,112,125] Secondary impingement can occur because of serratus anterior dysfunction, resulting in the anterior and inferior movement of the coracoacromial arch, which reduces available clearance for the RC and greater tuberosity as the shoulder is flexed forward.[4,112] Scapular lag from dysrhythmic scapulothoracic motion can also contribute to subacromial impingement because the acromion fails to rotate with the humerus, thereby producing a relative decrease in the acromiohumeral interval.[4,112] Defects in proprioception and motor coordination of the RC and the deltoid muscle were recently discussed as playing a major role in the development of SIS.[574,575]
4. ***Capsular tightness.***[576] Capsular tightness is a common mechanical problem related to primary impingement syndrome and has been reported to occur at the posterior,[112] anterior,[44] and inferior[437,535] portions of the capsule. Individuals who avoid painful overhead activity, or who are predisposed to motion imbalances because of their work or sport, can develop capsular tightness.[577] During the period of pain avoidance or unbalanced movement, the capsular connective tissue may lose the ability to lengthen due to decreased critical fiber distance and abnormal collagen fiber cross-linking. This in turn can lead to capsular tightness, joint stiffness, painful or limited function, and to an earlier onset or greater degree of subacromial compression, particularly in elevated planes of movement.[39,243,393,578] This is particularly true with a posterior capsular contracture, which commonly coexists with SIS and RC disease. Posterior capsular contracture may add to the abnormal subacromial contact by producing an anterosuperior translation during active elevation.[38,39] Tightness of the posterior capsule can also cause a decrease in IR of the G-H joint, which leads to an increase in the anterior and superior migration of the humeral head. In contrast, tightness of the anteroinferior capsule results in limited ER, preventing the greater tuberosity from sufficient ER to "clear" the coracoacromial arch.[121] Thus, the restoration of capsular mobility is an important component in the rehabilitation process.
5. ***Postural imbalance.*** Postural imbalance, particularly scapulothoracic dysfunction in relation to the FHP, has been implicated as an etiologic factor in secondary impingement syndrome.[39,282] The FHP, which is associated with an increase in the thoracic kyphosis angle, a forward shoulder posture, and a scapula that is positioned in relatively more elevation, protraction, downward rotation, and anterior tilt has been cited as a potential etiologic factor in the pathogenesis of SIS.[579] The effect of these changes leads to a loss of G-H flexion and abduction range, compression and irritation of the uppermost (bursal) surface of the supraspinatus tendon, resultant changes in the activation patterns of the length-dependent force couples, and a reduction in the range of G-H elevation.[579] However, the evidence for this is limited, with research studies reporting equivocal findings.[250,580–583] Postural imbalance can also occur as a secondary development in primary SIS.[576]
6. ***Repetitive overhead activities.*** Repetitive activities that involve humeral flexion have been reported to predispose individuals to RC disorders.[41,252] In fact, any repetitive elevation beyond 90 degrees has the potential to provoke RC disorders.[44]
7. ***Structural asymmetry.*** Scapular asymmetry and its role in impingement have been widely reported by investigators of upper extremity pathology.[112,223,480,584] Warner et al.[480] determined that 57% of their subjects with impingement syndrome demonstrated static scapular postural asymmetry, and all demonstrated weakness of the scapular pivoters (rhomboids, serratus anterior, lower trapezius, deltoid, and RC).
8. ***The position of the humerus at rest.*** This can affect the healing process of patients with primary shoulder impingement syndrome. The work of Rathburn and Macnab[57] illustrated the deleterious "wringing out" effect on RC tendon vascularity with an adducted dependent posture of the humerus.
9. ***Impaired scapular kinematics.*** Many researchers have studied the scapular kinematics in patients with SIS, but results of these studies to date have been largely variable, because often control subjects were included who were not matched to the subjects with SIS, or because the studies compared shoulder motion of the affected shoulder with the asymptomatic side only.[585]

A study by McClure et al.[586] included a matched control group as well as measurements of several physical characteristics of patients with SIS, including kinematics of the scapula, shoulder ROM, shoulder muscle force, and both upper thoracic spine and shoulder resting posture. All subjects were examined with the following tests and measures: (1) goniometric measurement of shoulder ROM, (2) assessment of upper thoracic spine and scapular resting posture, (3) measurement of shoulder isometric muscle force with a handheld dynamometer, and (4) assessment of shoulder kinematics with an electromagnetic motion analysis system during three active shoulder motions (shoulder flexion, scapular plane elevation, and ER at 90 degrees of abduction). The study had the following findings[585,586]:

- There were no differences in resting posture between the subjects with and without SIS.
- The SIS group demonstrated less ROM of the shoulder in all directions assessed, and less isometric muscle force for shoulder ER and scapular plane elevation.
- The subjects with SIS demonstrated slightly greater upward rotation of the scapula and elevation of the clavicle with shoulder flexion and slightly more posterior tilt and retraction of the clavicle with scapular plane elevation compared with those who did not have SIS.

Given the limited mobility and decreased shoulder muscle force identified in the SIS group and the kinematic differences identified between the two groups, it is tempting to conclude that the weakness of the shoulder musculature, or loss of mobility of the shoulder, or both, cause compensatory scapulothoracic movement strategies. However, further research is needed to determine whether a management strategy that specifically addresses the identified impairments of reduced muscle force, ROM, and altered kinematics results in greater improvements in pain, activity, and participation than competing noninvasive management strategies.[585,586]

If SIS is allowed to progress, the patient moves the shoulder less frequently due to the pain. The lack of movement increases the potential of developing adhesive capsulitis (frozen shoulder), particularly in the older patient. Neer[41] divided the impingement process into three stages, although the condition is a continuum of symptoms with overlap at the margins of each stage.[75] Each impingement stage is managed based on the specific findings and the intrinsic or extrinsic factors contributing to the problem, whether they result from compression, tensile overload, or macrotrauma.

Stage I. This stage consists of localized inflammation, slight bleeding, and edema of the RC. This stage is typically observed in patients under 25 years of age, although it can also be seen in older populations due to overuse. The patient reports pain in the shoulder and a history of acute trauma or repetitive microtrauma.

The physical examination during this stage reveals tenderness at the supraspinatus insertion and anterior acromion, a painful arc, and weakness of the RC secondary to pain, particularly when tested at 90-degree abduction or flexion. Acromial elevation and scapular stabilization are often jeopardized early in the injury process due to pain-based inhibition of the serratus anterior and lower trapezius, and due to subclinical adaptations altering the position of the scapula to accommodate injury patterns in subluxation or impingement.[152,153] Stage I is a reversible condition.

The subacromial space can be identified as a source of impingement by using the Neer impingement test supplemented with the Hawkins–Kennedy impingement test (see "Special Tests" sections).

The emphasis during the intervention of this phase is to control the pain and inflammation. The pain from subacromial impingement usually resolves with a period of rest and activity modification. Rest is advocated to prevent further trauma to the area and reduce excessive scar formation.[587] In addition to the rest and modification of activities, pain and inflammation may be controlled with the use of electrotherapeutic modalities, cryotherapy, and NSAIDs prescribed by the physician.

Stage II. Stage II represents a progressive process in the deterioration of the tissues of the RC. This stage is generally seen in the 26–40-year-old age group. Irritation of the subacromial structures continues as a result of the abnormal contact with the acromion. The subacromial bursa loses its ability to lubricate and protect the underlying RC, and tendinitis of the cuff develops. The patient often reports that a specific activity brings on their symptoms, especially an overhead activity. Pain is generally located on the top of the shoulder and will radiate to the midbrachium in the region of the deltoid insertion. The physical examination reveals crepitus or catching at approximately 100 degrees and restriction of PROM (due to fibrosis). This stage is no longer reversible with just rest. Although this stage often responds to long-term conservative care, it can progress to a partial thickness tear. If the level of symptoms is severe enough, surgery is often required. Conservative intervention during this stage involves a progressive strengthening program as described in the "Intervention Strategies" section.[588,589]

CLINICAL PEARL

A study by Bang and Deyle[590] determined that a combination of manual therapy applied by experienced clinicians and supervised exercise was better than exercise alone to increase strength, decrease pain, and improve function in patients with SIS.

Fifteen to twenty-eight percent of those patients diagnosed with SIS may eventually require surgery.[393,538] Surgical intervention is usually reserved for those who have failed to make satisfactory improvement over a period of 6 months. However, at least two randomized controlled clinical trials that examined the efficacy of conservative intervention with SIS have found that exercise supervised by a physical therapist was superior to placebo and was as effective as surgical subacromial decompression combined with postoperative rehabilitation in the intervention of patients with stage II primary impingement.[590,591] Another randomized controlled study[592] reported improved ROM, decreased pain, and increased function in patients with shoulder pain who underwent a program of individualized muscle stretching, strengthening, and retraining versus surgery.[590]

Stage III. Stage III is the end stage, common in the over-40 age group, where destruction of the soft tissue and rupture, or macrotrauma of the RC, is seen (see "Rotator Cuff Pathology" section). Localized atrophy can occur with this stage. Osteophytes of the acromion and A-C joint develop. The wear of the anterior aspect of the acromion on the greater tuberosity and the supraspinatus tendon eventually results in a full-thickness tear of the RC. The physical examination reveals atrophy of the infraspinatus and supraspinatus, and more limitation in AROM and PROM than the other stages.

Many protocols exist for patients with SIS. A progression from isometric exercises to close chain, and finally to open-chain activities beginning with scapulothoracic strengthening and scaption retraining, and then proceeding to RC strengthening, is generally recommended (see "-Intervention Strategies" section).

- Scapulothoracic strengthening and scaption retraining exercises include isometric scapular pinches and shrug exercises, rowing, press ups, and the push-up plus. Exercises to improve the scapulohumeral rhythm include the PNF D2 pattern, alternating serratus punches with tubing, and latissimus dorsi pull downs.
- Rotator cuff strengthening exercises include the empty can, biceps curl, IR and ER of the shoulder against resistive tubing, elbow extension, prone ER of the shoulder, and shoulder flexion and abduction (performed below 90 degrees).

Posterior Superior Glenoid Impingement

Posterior superior glenoid impingement is newly recognized as a source of RC pathology in athletes. This type of impingement is thought to result from an impingement of the RC between the greater tuberosity and the posterior superior glenoid labrum, although the actual cause has yet to be determined.[593,594]

Periarticular Syndromes

The historical features of all these syndromes are similar. Pain is increased after exercise and is usually worse at night, often waking the patient from sleep. Certain movements, such as reaching above the head or putting on a coat, will produce pain. ER and IR motions are usually within normal limits when compared with the uninvolved side, but abduction and flexion are painful between 70 and 110 degrees. Disorders of the periarticular inert structures, such as the bursae, are characterized by a noncapsular pattern. These can be divided into two subgroups. One group has a restricted range of passive movement, and the other has an unrestricted range. Two common periarticular syndromes that affect the shoulder in older patients are subacromial–subdeltoid bursitis and bicipital tendinitis.

According to Nevasier,[595] primary shoulder bursitis is seen only in gout, rheumatoid arthritis, pyogenic infections, and tuberculosis.[596] Secondary bursitis, due to the proximity of the bursae to an inflamed tendon, is far more common.

Calcified Bursitis

Etiology of this condition is a result of decreased vascularization, cuff degeneration, and/or increased levels of the HLA-1 antigen. There are three recognized stages:

- ***Precalcific***—calcium deposits in the matrix of vesicles
- ***Calcific***—continued calcium deposition and increased pressure
- ***Postcalcific***—the body decreases its blood supply to the area in an attempt to get rid of the calcium, producing severe pain (comparable to kidney stones)

The condition produces a limitation of ROM in all directions, and the area is very tender to touch or compression.

Conservative intervention consists of an intramuscular steroid injection to decrease pain and inflammation, ice applications, and Codman's exercises to relieve pressure. Typically, the pain decreases with an increase in ROM in 48–72 hours. After 72 hours, the bursitis is treated as a traumatic bursitis (see next).

Traumatic Bursitis and Hemorrhagic Bursitis

Traumatic bursitis is the result of direct trauma. But it can also be secondary to a degenerative rotator cuff. The patient often complains of pain at night. Pain is typically felt over the deltoid and its insertion, with the arm in extension. The patient demonstrates limited AROM and PROM in a noncapsular pattern, and an empty end-feel at approximately 70–80 degrees with G-H abduction.

The condition responds well to a conservative regimen of pain and inflammation control, capsular stretching (especially posteriorly), Codman's exercises, manual techniques to increase the acromiohumeral interval (scapula down and back, inferior glide), postural reeducation, restoration of normal synergy patterns for the G-H depressors, and functional restoration.

Calcific Tendinitis

Calcific tendinitis or, more accurately termed calcific tendinopathy, is characterized by a reactive calcification that affects the rotator cuff tendons. It is a common cause of shoulder pain.[597] Frequently, such calcifications are incidental radiographic findings in asymptomatic patients.[598] Approximately 50% of patients with calcific tendinitis have shoulder pain,[599,600] with associated acute or chronic painful restrictions of shoulder ROM, impacting ADLs.

The cause and pathogenesis of calcifications of the rotator cuff are unclear.[57,601] Ischemia as a result of hypovascularization in the so-called critical zone of the rotator cuff,[57] degeneration of the tendons,[601] and metabolic disturbances[602] have all been suggested as possible causes. According to Uhthoff et al.,[603,604] fibrocartilaginous transformation of the tendon tissue leads to calcium deposits. The course of the disease may be cyclic, with spontaneous resorption and reconstitution of the tendon.[603,604] The factor that triggers metaplasia has not yet been determined, although tissue hypoxia is thought to be the primary factor.[602] Clearly, degeneration of the rotator cuff tendons is a precursor for calcification.[195] Both shoulders are involved at 20–30% of patients with calcific tendinitis of the shoulder.[599,600] Calcific tendinitis is observed infrequently in people under age 40.[195] The prevalence of calcific tendinitis has been reported to be between 3% [599] and 7%.[605] Calcific tendinitis can be acute or chronic.[604] In general, the condition is found more frequently in women than men.[599] A relationship to occupation must be considered because there is a high incidence among clerical workers.[604]

The course of calcific tendinopathy is variable. In most cases, the deposits are located 1–2 cm from the insertion of the supraspinatus tendon on the greater tuberosity.[598] In some patients, the deposits are absorbed spontaneously with limited pain. Chronic calcific tendinitis generally presents with impingement symptoms of pain with overhead motion. Other patients have persistent and recurring episodes of severe pain.

Uhthoff[604] suggests dividing calcific tendinitis into a formative phase and a resorptive phase. In the formative phase, calcium deposits crystallize with minimal inflammation. Pain is usually mild and self-limiting during this phase. In the later, resorptive phase, the calcific material changes consistency from a solid to a paste or liquid. Shoulder pain is seen more often in this phase. This pain can be severe and develop abruptly. During these acute episodes of shoulder pain, the physical examination is often difficult due to pain limiting AROM and PROM.

Management of calcific tendinitis is often conservative, consisting of ice applications and pendulum exercises (prescribed in the acute phase) to prevent the development of adhesive capsulitis.[75]

Promising results have been reported for shock-wave therapy.[606,607] Ultrasound therapy, using a wide intensity range is commonly used as an intervention for painful musculoskeletal disorders.[608] The way in which ultrasound stimulates resorption of calcium deposits has not been established.[598] It may stimulate the accumulation of peripheral-blood mononuclear cells by activating endothelial cells. It may also act indirectly by increasing the intracellular calcium levels.[609] At higher intensities, ultrasound may trigger or accelerate the disruption of apatite-like microcrystals. The appearance of these smaller calcium crystals may then stimulate macrophages to remove calcifications by phagocytosis.[610,611] Finally, the increases in the temperature of tissue exposed to ultrasound may increase blood flow (i.e., induce hyperemia) and metabolism, thus facilitating the disintegration of calcium deposits.[598]

Invasive interventions directed at the calcium deposits, such as open surgical removal of the deposits, percutaneous needle aspiration and closed lavage of the deposits with lidocaine reduce pain and restore shoulder function in some patients, but not in all.[195,600,612–614]

Acute Subacromial–Subdeltoid Bursitis

This is an extremely uncomfortable condition. Active elevation is very painful and greatly restricted, and can be accompanied by a painful arc. While most patients with subacromial–subdeltoid bursitis describe a mechanical mechanism, bilateral bursitis is often seen in patients with inflammatory arthritis.[195] A differential diagnosis should be made between gouty arthritis, septic arthritis, a pathologic fracture, or a dislocation of the shoulder, and these can be differentiated from one another by their accompanying symptoms. Regardless of the severity of the pain, other conditions need to be ruled out. These include subscapular tendinitis, a pectoralis major lesion, a sprain of the conoid–trapezoid ligament, or early G-H arthritis. The pain of bursitis is usually reproduced with passive abduction at 180 degrees, passive IR, and passive horizontal adduction. Resistive testing may also produce pain. Associated and predisposing findings may also be noted. These include winging of the scapula, and forward head and rounded shoulder posture.

With the shoulder positioned in extension to expose more of the bursa, palpation of the shoulder region can elicit tenderness of the rotator cuff tendons and tenderness of the subacromial–subdeltoid bursa over the anterior humeral head.

Conservative intervention for this condition involves the use of modalities to help control the pain and inflammation, and patient education to avoid exacerbation.

Primary Chronic Subacromial–Subdeltoid Bursitis

Two types of primary chronic bursitis are defined:

1. The type caused by degenerative changes, especially of the supraspinatus and A-C joint. This can produce a reduced space for the bursa and cause an inflammatory reaction of the bursa.
2. The type caused by a systemic disease such as rheumatoid arthritis.

With primary chronic bursitis, pain develops gradually. The pain is usually localized to the shoulder and lateral deltoid area, but it can spread into the upper arm. Findings from the objective examination include a positive painful arc into abduction or forward flexion, but full movement in other directions. One or more resisted tests are often painful, but may be negative if repeated with an inferior pull on the arm.

The intervention of choice is a course of local anesthetic injections.

Secondary Chronic Subacromial–Subdeltoid Bursitis

Secondary chronic bursitis is more common than the primary type and results from other shoulder pathologies, including a rupture of the medial coracohumeral ligament. Similar to primary chronic bursitis, the pain develops gradually in the shoulder and lateral deltoid region, but can radiate into the upper arm.

The objective findings are the same as those for the primary chronic bursitis. However, the exception is that other pathologies are present and make a specific diagnosis more difficult.

The intervention of choice is similar to primary chronic bursitis, although the primary lesion should be sought and treated.

Bicipital Tendinitis

Tendinitis of the LHB occurs more often as a secondary condition related to an impingement syndrome.[427,595] Slatis and Aalto[615] described a three-part classification for biceps lesions:

- Type A: Impingement tendinitis, which occurs secondary to impingement syndrome and rotator cuff disease. Since the tendon passes beneath the anterior edge of the acromion, impingement can cause biceps tendinopathy as well as rotator cuff problems.
- Type B: A subluxation of the biceps tendon.
- Type C: Attrition tendinitis, commonly associated with spurring and fraying.

In addition, the biceps tendon sheath is a direct extension of the G-H joint, and inflammatory conditions such as rheumatoid arthritis can involve the biceps tendon.

Other researchers[616] have proposed two main categories related to age with younger patients developing problems due to repetitive trauma and anomalies of the bicipital groove, and the older age group developing problems associated with degenerative changes in the tendon.

The pain associated with inflammation of the LHB is typically felt along the anterior lateral aspect of the shoulder with radiation into the biceps muscle, and tenderness is noted directly over the bicipital groove.

Objective findings for this condition include the following:

- Full AROM and PROM, although pain is often reported at the end range of flexion and abduction.
- Normal accessory glides at the G-H joint (negating the need to use joint mobilizations).[427,595]
- Pain on palpation of the bicipital groove while the arm is positioned at 10 degrees of IR.
- Pain with resisted elbow flexion or resisted forward flexion of the shoulder.
- Pain on passive stretch of the biceps tendon.
- Positive Speed's test.

Every attempt must be made to identify associated lesions (e.g., those affecting the glenoid labrum and rotator cuff) or to note any contributing factors (e.g., a poorly stabilized scapular, the hypomobile cervical and/or thoracic spine, or altered muscle recruitment patterns).[73]

The conservative intervention for biceps tendinitis secondary to chronic impingement is similar to that described for rotator cuff tendinitis. These include electrotherapeutic modalities, physical agents, NSAIDs, TFM, and gentle stretching of the contractile tissues. Care must be taken with the TFM so as to not exacerbate the acutely or chronically inflamed tissue. Once the pain and inflammation are under control, the patient is progressed through ROM exercises within the pain-free ranges. Intensive strengthening is initiated when full pain-free AROM has been restored.

Subluxing Biceps Tendon

The LHB tendon, with its proximal point of exit at a 30–40-degree angle from the straight line of the tendon and the tunnel, swings from one side of the groove to the other during the motions of IR and ER of the humerus.[30] If the groove is shallow, the tendon may force its way over the lesser or greater tuberosity, tearing the transverse humeral ligament in the process. Repeated subluxation wears down the tuberosity and increases the frequency of the subluxation.

If the groove is narrow and tight, the constant pressure of the tendon has the potential to cause tendinitis or even rupture of the tendon.[30]

The pain, not often severe, has the same referral pattern as that of bicipital tendinitis. A click is typically felt during abduction and ER motions, with reduction of the tendon occurring with adduction and IR. There is tenderness over the bicipital groove, which follows the groove as the arm is rotated. On IR, the groove is under the coracoid, and during ER it is at the anteromedial line.[30]

The intervention depends largely on how important athletics is to the participant. Conservative intervention involves the temporary avoidance of the pain and click-provoking movements, and the application of TFM. In severe cases, surgical intervention may be indicated, which offers excellent results.[30]

Rupture of the Long Head of Biceps

A total rupture of the LHB is usually seen in middle-aged patients, resulting from repeated injections of steroid into the bicipital groove or in cases of chronic impingement.[195] The tendon is avascular, and as it weakens, it tears with a minimal amount of force.

Patients usually report hearing or feeling a "snap" at the time of the injury. Typically, rupture is followed by a few weeks of mild-to-moderate pain, followed by resolution of the pain and restoration of normal function.[195] When attempts are made to contract the biceps, the muscle belly rolls down over the distal humerus, producing a swelling close to the elbow instead of in the middle of the arm: the so-called "Popeye" sign. Functional limitations are unusual after this rupture, especially in the older population, because the short head of the biceps remains intact.[617] Typically, there is a negligible loss of elbow flexion and supination strength.

Surgical repair is rarely indicated except in the younger, active population (<50 years). With or without surgery, a rupture of the LHB increases the risk of developing an SIS. This results from the short head of the biceps pulling the humeral head upward, without the presence of the long head to hold the humeral head downward.

PATTERN 4G: IMPAIRED JOINT MOBILITY, MOTOR FUNCTION, MUSCLE PERFORMANCE, RANGE OF MOTION WITH FRACTURES

Atraumatic Osteolysis of the Distal Clavicle

Atraumatic osteolysis of the distal clavicle[71] (AODC) was first described in 1959 by Ehricht.[618]

The etiology is thought to be a stress failure of the distal clavicle due to an initial stress fracture, followed by cystic and erosive changes secondary to bone resorption. Subsequent bone formation and remodeling cannot occur because of continued stress on the joint.

It is most common in athletes involved in prolonged weight training and appears to be on the increase. The recent increase in incidence may be due to the emphasis on strength training regimens in sport. In a group of Danish weightlifters, the prevalence was found to be 27% compared with a normal (non–weight-lifting) control group.[619]

The symptoms usually begin insidiously. They are usually described as a painful, dull ache localized to the A-C joint. The ache, which tends to be worse at the beginning of exercise, may radiate into the deltoid and trapezius. Bench presses, dips, and push-ups are usually the most painful exercises. Abduction of the arm beyond 90 degrees causes pain. Throwing is also painful. On examination, there is point tenderness at the A-C joint and forced arm adduction across the chest increases the symptoms. Symptoms are bilateral in 20% of cases.

The most common differential diagnoses to be considered are cervical spondylosis and rotator cuff disease. AODC can be distinguished from rotator cuff tendinitis by selective injection of anesthetic into the A-C joint. An abolishment of the pain with the provocative maneuvers subsequent to the injection helps confirm the diagnosis.

The majority of patients with this condition respond to conservative management and activity modification, with most improving by reducing or eliminating their strength training activities.[619] However, even after several years' layoff, if strength training is reinstituted at the same level, the symptoms will commonly recur.[620,621] Other aspects of conservative intervention involve heat, NSAIDs, ROM, and stretching and strengthening exercises. The exercises should be performed below 90 degrees of abduction. Ultrasound has also been advocated.[619] Although a consideration, intra-articular injection of steroid does not provide long-lasting success. It is more helpful to aid in the diagnosis and predicting surgical success.

Conservative intervention failure is an indication for surgical management. This consists of resection of the distal clavicle, either open or arthroscopic.

Clavicle Fractures

Fractures of the clavicle account for 5 to 10% of all fractures and 35 to 40% of shoulder girdle injuries in adults. The clavicle is the most commonly fractured bone in childhood.[89] Fractures of the clavicle usually result from a FOOSH, a fall or blow to the point of the shoulder, or less commonly from a direct blow.

The classic presentation following a clavicular fracture is guarded shoulder motions and difficulty elevating the arm beyond 60 degrees. A clavicular deformity may also be observable. There is also exquisite tenderness to palpation or percussion (bony tap) over the fracture site. Horizontal adduction is painful. The diagnosis is confirmed by radiograph.

The conservative intervention for clavicle fractures includes approximation of the fracture ends followed by immobilization with a sling and figure-8 strap for 3–6 weeks. AAROM and then AROM exercises for the shoulder can be initiated once clinical union has been established (in 2–3 weeks). Due to the importance of the clavicle in shoulder function, joint mobilizations are started immediately after the period of immobilization, and strengthening exercises for the deltoid, pectoralis major, and upper trapezius muscles are prescribed when appropriate. As with all shoulder injuries, the clinician should ensure that the scapulohumeral rhythm is normal and symmetrical and that the essential stabilizing musculature of the G-H joint is intact. Normal healing times for clavicular fracture are 6 weeks in young children in 8 weeks in adults.[622] Surgical intervention is reserved for those cases involving neurovascular compression, an open fracture, associated fractures, and marked displacement.

Proximal Humeral Fractures

A proximal humeral fracture, involving the proximal third of the humerus, is the most common fracture of the humerus in the young and the elderly. In the skeletally immature patient, the fracture frequently presents as an epiphyseal fracture of the proximal humeral growth plate as the result from a direct blow to the anterior, lateral, or posterolateral aspect of the humerus, or a FOOSH injury.[623] In the elderly, the fractures usually occur through osteopenic bone following minimal trauma.

The majority of proximal humeral fractures are stable with no significant displacement of the fracture. This type is typically treated conservatively, with an emphasis on controlling distal edema and stiffness, and early motion at the shoulder to prevent the development of arthrofibrosis secondary to prolonged immobilization.[624]

The arm is usually immobilized in a sling until pain and discomfort subsides, often after 2 weeks if the fracture is classified as nondisplaced and stable. If the fracture is classified as nondisplaced it is considered unstable and the immobilization period is typically approximately 4 weeks. AROM exercises for the wrist and hand are initiated immediately following immobilization. Typically, passive and active assisted exercises for the shoulder can be initiated approximately 1 week after injury. Clinical unity of the fracture usually occurs after 1–4 weeks. This can be tested by having the patient stand with the involved arm at their side with the elbow flexed. The clinician places one hand on the humeral head, and then gently rotates the humerus with the other. Clinical unity is established when the fracture fragments move in unison and the movement is free of crepitation. At this point, gentle AROM exercises are initiated for the shoulder and elbow. Once clinical union is confirmed by radiograph (usually at around 6 weeks), full PROM exercises to the shoulder and elbow are performed, with progressive resistive exercises typically initiated at 6–8 weeks.

Scapular Fractures

Scapular fractures are not common, accounting for only 1% of all fractures, 3% of all shoulder injuries and 5% of fractures involving the entire shoulder.[625] The anatomic features of the scapula provide insight into the mechanisms of injury and offer a convenient classification system (Table 16-41):

- Injuries to the body or the spine of the scapula typically result from a direct blow with significant force, such as from a motor vehicle accident or a fall.
- Acromion injuries usually result from a direct downward force to the shoulder.
- Scapular neck fractures most frequently result from an anterior or posterior force applied to the shoulder.

TABLE 16-41 Classification of Glenoid Cavity Fractures

Type	Description
IA	Anterior rim fracture
IB	Posterior rim fracture
II	Fracture line through the glenoid fossa exiting at the lateral border of the scapula
III	Fracture line through the glenoid fossa exiting at the superior border of the scapula
IV	Fracture line through the glenoid fossa exiting at the medial border of the scapula
VA	Combination of types II and IV
VB	Combination of types III and IV
VC	Combination of types II, III, and IV
VI	Comminuted fracture

- Glenoid rim fractures most often result from force transmitted along the humerus after a fall onto a flexed elbow.
- Stellate glenoid fractures usually follow a direct blow to the lateral shoulder.
- Coracoid process fractures may result from either a direct blow to the superior aspect of the shoulder or a forceful muscular contraction that causes an avulsion fracture.

In addition to a history of trauma, the most common findings are tenderness, edema, and ecchymosis over the affected area. In addition, the upper extremity is held in adduction and any attempt to abduct the extremity increases pain.

Most scapular fractures, depending on location and classification, can be treated successfully without surgical intervention. Conservative intervention consists of approximately 7–10 days of sling immobilization, followed by a progressing regimen of pendular and gentle PROM exercises as comfort and control allow.[73] Once sufficient healing has been demonstrated radiographically, the patient is encouraged to discontinue immobilization and proceed with AAROM and AROM exercises. Exercises that strengthen the muscles that attach to the scapula and those that arise from the scapula must be introduced at the earliest opportunity.

TABLE 16-42 Potential Causes of Scapular Dyskinesis

Potential Causes	Examples
Abnormality in bony posture or injury	Excessive scapular protraction and acromial depression in all stages of motion which increases the risk for impingement Excessive resting kyphosis Forward head posture creates tightness to the anterior neck musculature, which again in turn facilitates the abnormal scapula position
AC joint injuries or instabilities	Can alter the center of rotation of the scapula, leading to faulty mechanics
Muscle function alterations	Alterations involving the serratus anterior and lower trapezius are a common source of dysfunction, especially in cases of secondary impingement Microtrauma due to excessive strain in the muscles, fatigue, and inhibition due to pain
Nerve damage	A rare cause
Contractures	Especially of the anterior musculature that attaches to the coracoid process (pectoralis minor and short biceps head) can create an anterior tilt and forward lean to the scapula, as can tightness to the posterior capsule and latissimus

Data from Kibler WB, McMullen J: Scapular dyskinesis and its relation to shoulder pain. *J Am Acad Orthop Surg* 11:142–151, 2003.

INTEGRATION OF PATTERNS 4B AND 4D: IMPAIRED JOINT MOBILITY, MOTOR FUNCTION, MUSCLE PERFORMANCE, RANGE OF MOTION SECONDARY TO IMPAIRED POSTURE, AND CONNECTIVE TISSUE DYSFUNCTION

Scapular Dyskinesis

Strengthening and stretching exercises for scapular muscles are a common part of rehabilitation programs designed for people with shoulder dysfunctions. Scapular dyskinesis is an alteration in the normal position or motion of the scapula that occurs during coupled scapulohumeral movements as a response to shoulder dysfunction.[626] The causes are many (Table 16-42). It should be suspected in patients with shoulder injury and can be identified and classified by specific physical examination. There are three types of scapular dyskinesis:

- Type I is characterized by prominence of the inferior medial scapular border. In throwers, this type may be referred to as a SICK scapula (malposition of the Scapula, prominence of the Inferior medial border of the scapula, Coracoid pain and malposition, and scapular dysKinesia).[262] A thrower with this syndrome presents with an apparent "dropped" scapula in the symptomatic shoulder compared with the contralateral shoulder's scapular position. Viewed from behind, the inferior medial scapular border appears very prominent, with the superior medial border and acromion less prominent. When viewed from the front, this tilting (protraction) of the scapula makes the shoulder appear to be lower than the opposite side. The pectoralis minor tightens as the coracoid tilts inferiorly and shifts laterally away from the midline, and its insertion at the coracoid becomes very tender.[262]
- Type II is characterized by protrusion of the entire medial border.
- Type III involves superior translation of the entire scapula and prominence of the superior medial border.

Evaluation of the patient should include the trunk segments, hip and lower extremity function, and scapular position and movement analysis. There may be pain at the coracoid process, and the entire medial border may be tender with trigger points found in the upper trapezius. There may even be painful scar tissue found in the musculature due to long-standing dyskinesis. Motion about the scapulothoracic joint should be smooth with no catching or rapid movements, which are more often seen during the lowering phase of the arm. Strength testing can include the isometric scapular pinch, the SAT, the scapular retraction test, and the lateral slide test (LST). Once all the factors involved in the dysfunction of the shoulder are identified, treatment can begin on restoring normal scapular position and movement. More extensive therapy, including strengthening, should not occur until this step is accomplished; otherwise the shoulder is being worked in a faulty position.

The intervention of scapular dyskinesis is directed at managing underlying causes and restoring normal scapular muscle activation patterns by kinetic chain-based rehabilitation protocols. Leg, back, and trunk flexibility and strength should be normalized, and exercises that emphasize kinetic chain activation of the leg, trunk, and scapula should be instituted. Useful combinations of movements to allow activation include trunk extension and scapular retraction, trunk rotation and scapular retraction, and one-legged stance and diagonal trunk rotation and scapular retraction. All of these exercises facilitate lower trapezius muscle activation.

Snapping Scapular

The term *snapping scapula* has been used to describe the clinical scenario of tenderness at the superomedial angle of the scapula, painful scapulothoracic motion, and scapulothoracic crepitus.[96,627–630] Infrequently, an underlying cause for the scapulothoracic dyskinesia is identified. The uncommon etiologies of snapping scapula include scapular exostoses, malunited scapular or rib fractures, and Sprengel's deformity.[628,631–633] Pain is usually reported at the superomedial angle of the scapula, with or without scapulothoracic crepitus.

The intervention for this condition is based on the cause. Common causes for this condition are an inflammation of the bursa between the scapula and thorax (scapulothoracic bursitis), prominence of the superomedial angle of the scapula, and muscular imbalance of the scapular pivoters.[96,628–630,634–637]

INTEGRATION OF PATTERNS 4B, 4C, 4F, AND 5F: IMPAIRED JOINT MOBILITY, MOTOR FUNCTION, MUSCLE PERFORMANCE, RANGE OF MOTION SECONDARY TO IMPAIRED POSTURE, SPINAL DISORDERS, MYOFASCIAL PAIN DYSFUNCTION, THORACIC OUTLET SYNDROME, COMPLEX REGIONAL PAIN SYNDROME, PERIPHERAL NERVE ENTRAPMENT

Impaired Posture

Patients with impaired posture have functional limitations associated with muscle imbalances, repetitive altered joint mobility, and pain. Impaired posture is commonly associated with referred pain to the shoulder. The most common posture referring pain to the shoulder is a forward head posture (FHP) with rounded shoulders. This posture is characterized by hypertrophy of the anterior chest and cervical musculature (including the pectoralis minor muscle and the anterior and medial scalene muscles). The position adopted in the FHP can compromise the space in the scalene triangle and cause compression of the neurovascular structures, resulting in a condition called TOS (see Chap. 23).[449]

This posture can also lead to soft tissue restrictions of the anterior shoulder muscles, suboccipital muscles, and shoulder rotators.[449]

The intervention includes a conservative regime of postural reeducation and exercises to restore the normal synergy patterns for G-H depressors, to increase shoulder stability, and facilitate functional restoration (see Chap. 25). Cervical and thoracic stabilization exercises may be introduced in addition to the correction of any muscle imbalances.

Referred Pain

See Chapter 5.

Scapulocostal Syndrome

Although this syndrome has been documented,[638–640] it is poorly understood. Scapulocostal syndrome (SCS) is an enthesopathy (a disorder of the attachment of a ligament, tendon, joint capsule, or muscle to bone) of the origin of the serratus posterior superior muscle. Clinically, it appears that SCS is a distinct variety of fibromyalgia.[640]

SCS has been postulated to have many causes including[640]

- ischemia[641]
- trigger point[638]
- postural degeneration[642,643]
- physical sloth[644]

Clinical findings for this syndrome include the following[640]:

- Pain of a cervicobrachial nature, described as burning and aching, is the most common presenting symptom.
- Active and passive motions of the shoulder girdle are usually full and pain free.
- Poor overall physical conditioning.

Conservative intervention, which includes intralesional injections and physical rehabilitation involving ROM, strengthening, and conditioning exercises, was shown in one study[640] to be successful in 95.9% of 201 patients.

Subclavian Steal Syndrome

See Chapter 5.

Myofascial Pain Syndrome

Shoulder pain can often be caused by myofascial dysfunction. The following muscles are most commonly involved. The intervention strategies for myofascial trigger points are described in Chapter 10.

Infraspinatus

The infraspinatus is a frequent cause of myofascial shoulder pain, with the trigger points in this muscle commonly referring pain deep into the shoulder joint. Due to the severity of the referred pain from this muscle's trigger points, it is often misdiagnosed as subdeltoid bursitis or supraspinatus tendinitis.

Pain can also be felt in the anterior shoulder and anterior upper arm. In extreme cases, the pain may refer to the extensor area of the forearm and into the hand.

Clinical findings can include the following[645]:

- A history of sleeping difficulty on the involved side because of pressure on trigger points. Sleeping on the uninvolved side can also produce pain because of stretching of the muscle. Supporting the involved arm on a pillow while sleeping on the uninvolved side is a significant help.

- Limited IR and adduction of the shoulder, including horizontal adduction in severe cases.
- Shoulder girdle muscle fatigue rather than weakness. Pain is elicited on resisted testing of the infraspinatus and middle and posterior deltoid muscles.
- Decreased grip strength.
- Positive signs of subacromial impingement due to dysfunction of the infraspinatus.

Anterior Deltoid

Anterior deltoid trigger points typically refer pain and tenderness in the area of the muscle itself. Clinical findings include decreased ER and extension of the shoulder.

Posterior Deltoid

Trigger points in this muscle (located posterior to the humeral head) and in the levator scapulae are the most frequent cause of myogenic posterior shoulder pain.[645] Pain is elicited on resisted testing, reaching across to the opposite shoulder anteriorly and toward the end of ER while the arm is abducted at 90 degrees because of the shortening action in the muscle.[645]

Levator Scapulae

This muscle is one of the most frequent myofascial sources of shoulder and neck pain. Pain reference is to the base of the neck, the posterior shoulder joint over the area of the humeral head, and along the medial scapular border.

Clinical findings include the following:

- painful ipsilateral rotation of the neck,
- a limitation of full shoulder abduction accompanied by reproduction of posterior shoulder pain.[645]

These trigger points are activated by holding a telephone receiver between the shoulder and ear; sleeping on a sofa with the head on the armrest, which causes prolonged stretching deformation of the muscle; postural stress due to shoulder girdle asymmetry; and psychologic distress.[645]

Scalenes

The pain pattern is similar for all three scalenes and can include the anterior chest, the upper arm both anterolaterally and posteriorly, the thumb and index finger, and the medial scapular area.[645] Tenderness is referred to the infraclavicular fossa and disappears immediately after inactivation of the trigger points.

Supraspinatus

Rarely occurring in isolation, supraspinatus trigger points refer pain around the shoulder area, particularly to the mid-deltoid region, and the lateral epicondyle of the humerus. When the muscle is less severely involved, the patient will have difficulty fully abducting the shoulder.

As described previously, supraspinatus dysfunction can have wide-ranging consequences in shoulder biomechanics.

Subscapularis

Pain from subscapularis trigger points is felt at rest or on motion over the posterior shoulder. The pain may also extend over the scapula and posteromedial arm as far as the wrist.

Clinical findings include the following:

- painful and limited shoulder abduction, especially if ER of the arm is added to the movement,
- painful resisted shoulder adduction and IR,
- decreased posterior glide of the G-H joint,
- positive subacromial impingement signs.

Trapezius

The trigger points of the trapezius are usually found in the upper trapezius near the distal clavicle and in the lower border of the lower trapezius near the medial scapular border. Both areas refer pain and tenderness to the top of the shoulder over the acromion.[645] These trigger points may cause tenderness of the A-C joint ligaments. Trigger points in the lower trapezius can refer pain into the ipsilateral posterior neck and suboccipital region.[645]

Thoracic Outlet Syndrome

The chief complaint of TOS is one of diffuse arm and shoulder pain, especially when the arm is elevated beyond 90 degrees. Potential symptoms include pain localized in the neck, face, head, upper extremity, chest, shoulder, or axilla; and upper extremity paresthesias, numbness, weakness, heaviness, fatigability, swelling, discoloration, ulceration, or Raynaud's phenomenon. TOS is described in Chapter 25.

Crutch Palsy

Brachial plexus compressive neuropathy following the use of axillary crutches is rare but well recognized. There are a number of documented reports of compressive neuropathies stemming from the incorrect use of axillary crutches, the so-called "crutch palsy."[646–648] The diagnosis of crutch palsy is usually made clinically by taking a careful history and performing a physical examination. This includes observation of the patient during ambulation using crutches and looking at the axilla for such signs of chronic irritation as hyperpigmentation and skin hypertrophy. A detailed neurologic examination is usually sufficient to determine the cord or terminal branch(es) involved and the level of the involvement.[646]

The incorrect use of axillary crutches, with excessive weight bearing on the axillary bar, leads to a sevenfold increase in force on the axilla.[649]

Complex Regional Pain (Shoulder/Hand) Syndrome

This condition is described in detail in Chapter 18.

Cervical Radiculitis

The onset of cervical radiculitis (see Chap. 25) can be insidious or traumatic, or secondary to shoulder disease such as adhesive capsulitis.[207,650]

The patient reports a wide range of symptoms. These range from mild discomfort to severe pain that is associated with neck motion restrictions, particularly hyperextension and rotation.[72,651]

Objectively, there may be a loss of cervical lordosis with associated paravertebral muscle spasm. Palpation may reveal tenderness over the posterior aspect of the neck, which can exacerbate the radicular symptoms in the arm.[652] The testing of muscle strength, sensation, and muscle stretch reflexes should help confirm the diagnosis.

Conservative intervention consists of the control of pain and inflammation through rest and activity modification. The patient is educated on positions to avoid, including rotation toward the involved side and neck extension. Once the pain is controlled, the program is progressed to cervical ROM and strengthening exercises, postural education, and general strengthening and conditioning of the upper extremities.

Peripheral Nerve Entrapment

There are a number of common peripheral nerve neuropathies in the shoulder region (see Chap. 3), which are being recognized with increasing frequency. The nerves that can be injured in the region include the suprascapular, accessory, long thoracic, axillary, posterior (dorsal) scapular, and musculocutaneous.

Quadrilateral Space Syndrome

Idiopathic quadrilateral space syndrome, a compression of the axillary nerve as it passes with the posterior circumflex artery through the quadrilateral space, is rare.

The typical clinical presentation includes[640]

- vague, poorly localized shoulder discomfort,
- pain with fatigue when the patient attempts to maintain the arm above shoulder level,
- paresthesias in a nondermatomal pattern,
- tenderness to palpation in the quadrilateral space can occur.[653]

The initial intervention is conservative and includes rest, muscle relaxants, and NSAIDs. Surgery may be required if there is no improvement in 3–6 months.[653]

Adverse Neural Tension

An abnormal response to mechanical stimuli of neural tissue is termed *adverse neural tension* (see Chap. 11).[654,655] The G-H joint can be the source of neurologic tension due to multidirectional instability, direct trauma, or poor posture and resultant tension on the brachial plexus.[207,656] The movements of shoulder ER and depression stretch the brachial plexus. Side flexion of the cervical spine away from the tested side also stretches the brachial plexus. Often the patient adopts postures to compensate for tight neurologic structures and relieve the tension on the brachial plexus. One of the most common of these adaptive postures is elevation of the shoulder girdle.

Adhesions of the brachial plexus can be detected using the upper limb tension tests 1 and 2 (refer to Chap. 11).[655]

THERAPEUTIC TECHNIQUES

Techniques to Increase Joint Mobility

With some slight variations, the same techniques that are used to examine the joint glides of the shoulder complex (see "Passive Accessory Motion Tests" section) can be used to mobilize the joints, with the clinician varying the intensity of the mobilizations based on the intent of the treatment, patient response, and the stage of tissue healing. Unlike the testing positions, where the joint is placed in the resting position, the joint position for mobilization techniques varies:

- The resting position is used if gentle techniques are to be used.
- The restricted ROM is approximated if more aggressive techniques are to be used.

The purposes of joint mobilization include the following:

- to increase accessory motion;
- to increase ROM;
- to decrease pain;
- to improve periarticular muscle performance.

Joint mobilization may be preferable to stretching at the shoulder because it provides a precise stretch to a specific part of the capsule. It also can be performed with less pain, reduced load on other periarticular structures, and less compressive force on articular structures[423,657] as compared with physiologic stretching.[1] A number of studies[282,658,659] have examined the efficacy of passive joint mobilization and/or PROM. They found this mode of intervention to be effective for enhancing ROM in the patient with SIS. Investigators have suggested that joint mobilization, especially posterior gliding, may have an important role in restoring capsular extensibility in primary SIS[437,480] by preventing or stretching abnormal collagen cross-linkage,[244] rupturing adhesions,[660] reducing edema,[661] or reducing pain.[662] In addition to the G-H joint, the clinician should also ensure that the mobility at the A-C, S-C, and scapulothoracic joints are normal.

Kaltenborn[286] stressed the importance of promoting joint glides for increasing capsular mobility and prevention of joint compression and periarticular soft tissue injury that may occur with long lever angular mobilizations.[432] Sustained manual capsule stretches are particularly effective in regaining motion.[1,663,664] Low load, prolonged stretching produces plastic elongation of tissues as opposed to the high tensile resistance seen in high load, brief stretching.[444,665] (i.e., the arm is brought to end range, pushed slightly beyond that range, and held in that position for 10–20 seconds).

Glenohumeral Joint

Distraction of the G-H Joint

This is a general technique to stretch G-H capsule.

Inferior Glide of the G-H Joint

This technique can be used to increase G-H abduction

Posterior Glide of the G-H Joint

This technique can be used to increase G-H IR, flexion, and horizontal adduction.

Anterior Glide of the G-H Joint

This technique can be used to increase G-H ER, extension, and horizontal abduction. Caution must be used when using this technique in patients with a history of G-H subluxation/dislocation.

Scapulothoracic Joint

Distraction

This technique is a general technique to apply a stretch to the serratus anterior and to break up adhesions at the scapulothoracic joint.

Superior Glide

This technique is applied to increase ROM into scapulothoracic joint elevation and ER.

Inferior Glide

This technique is applied to increase ROM into scapulothoracic joint depression and IR.

Medial Glide

This technique can be used for increasing ROM into scapulothoracic joint retraction, depression, and IR.

Lateral Glide

Although this technique can be used for increasing ROM into scapulothoracic joint protraction, elevation, and ER, it should be used with caution in patients with posture impairments involving shoulder as this motion might already be hypermobile.

Sternoclavicular Joint

The S-C joint rarely needs mobilizing as it is often hypermobile.

Acromioclavicular Joint

Anterior and Posterior Rotation of the Clavicle

This technique can be used to help with the overall motion of the clavicle, although these motions may already be hypermobile.

Superior Glide of the Acromion on the Clavicle

This technique can be used as a general mobilization technique and is particularly useful if the patient's A-C joint is tender to palpation.

SPECIFIC PASSIVE PHYSIOLOGIC MOBILIZATION: HUMERUS AND SCAPULA

Quadrant Technique

The quadrant technique previously described as the Lock test (special tests of the shoulder) can also be used as a mobilization technique. This is done by adjusting the intensity according to the irritability of the condition. If the pain is severe, grade IV (small oscillatory techniques just into the tissue resistance) are used. If this technique decreases the pain, the technique is reapplied and reassessed. If the intervention produces no change in the symptoms, the clinician increases the grade slightly or increases the vigor and reassesses. If the intervention produces an increase in pain, the clinician continues with the same intervention but at a lesser grade.

Scapular Assist

The clinician stands behind the patient. The scapula is stabilized with one hand and, as the patient raises the arm, the scapula motion is assisted by applying a compressive force over the scapula with one hand while stabilizing the A-C joint with the other hand (Fig. 16-18). A similar technique may be used for increasing motion at the end range of arm elevation. This is a good technique to gain ROM during the period when the scapular controllers are being strengthened but have not reached the point when they are able to work independently.

Posterior Capsule (Sleeper) Stretch

The patient is in side-lying with the affected shoulder toward the table and the arm at 90 degrees of forward flexion.[166] The patient is asked to roll forward to approximately 45-degree angle. At this point scapular winging should be noticeable. The clinician stands behind the patient and applies pressure with the palm of the hand onto the medial border of the scapular. The scapula is then depressed down toward the posterior thorax reversing the scapular winging, with the amount of scapula pressure gauged by the clinician's position in relation to the patient. The amount of forward roll and the degree of forward flexion of the involved extremity are important variables in adjusting the technique.

SPECIFIC PASSIVE/ACTIVE PHYSIOLOGIC MOBILIZATION OF THE SHOULDER

Elevation through Abduction

The patient lies in the supine position with his or her head supported. The patient's upper extremity is adducted across his or her abdomen. The clinician palpates the posterior aspect of the patient's wrist with one hand and the proximal forearm with the other. The motion barrier is localized by instructing the patient to elevate the arm in the scaption plane to the limit of the physiologic ROM.[666] From this position, the patient is instructed to hold still while the clinician applies a gentle resistance into further elevation. The contraction is held for 3–5 seconds, after which the patient is instructed to relax completely. The new barrier of elevation/abduction is located and the mobilization is repeated.

Elevation through Adduction

The technique is identical to the one already described with the exception that the abduction component is replaced by one of adduction so that the patient performs a combination of elevation and adduction.

MOBILIZATIONS WITH MOVEMENT

Decreased Elevation

The patient is seated and the clinician stands on his or her uninvolved side. The clinician places one hand over the scapula of the involved side. Using the other hand, the clinician reaches around the front of the patient to place the thenar eminence or a belt (Fig. 16-119) on the anterior aspect of the head of the humerus of the involved shoulder. The patient is asked to elevate his or her arm while the clinician applies a posterior glide to the humeral head (avoiding pressure over the sensitive coracoid process).[667] If this technique is successful, the patient is asked to hold a weight while elevating the arm (Fig. 16-119).

Decreased Internal Rotation

The patient is seated with his or her hands as far behind the back as possible. The clinician stands facing the patient on the involved side. The clinician places one hand in the crease of the patient's elbow and the web space of other hand in the patient's axilla to stabilize the scapula by using a lumbrical grip (Fig. 16-120). While maintaining the stabilization of the scapula, the clinician glides the humerus inferiorly in the glenoid fossa using the hand at the elbow and applies an adduction force by pressing their abdomen against the patient (see Fig. 16-120) as the patient internally rotates the shoulder (using their other hand to help if necessary). The technique can also be performed using a belt (Fig. 16-121).

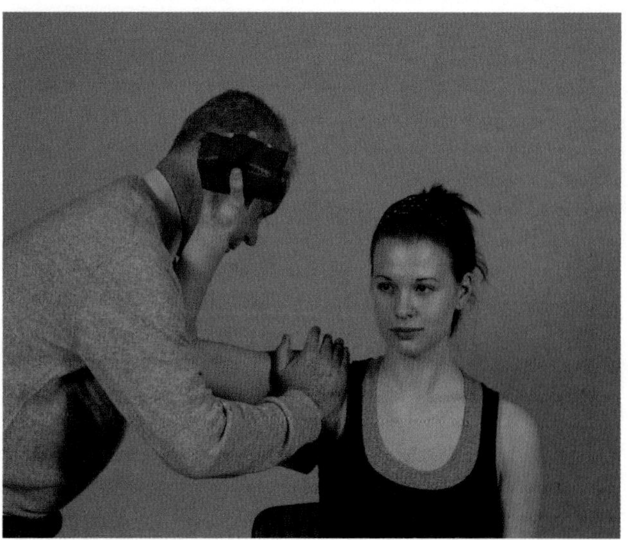

FIGURE 16-119 Mobilization with movement to increase elevation.

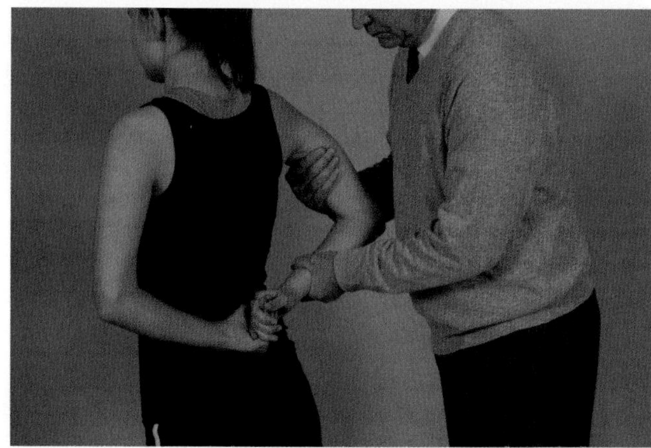

FIGURE 16-120 Mobilization with movement to increase internal rotation.

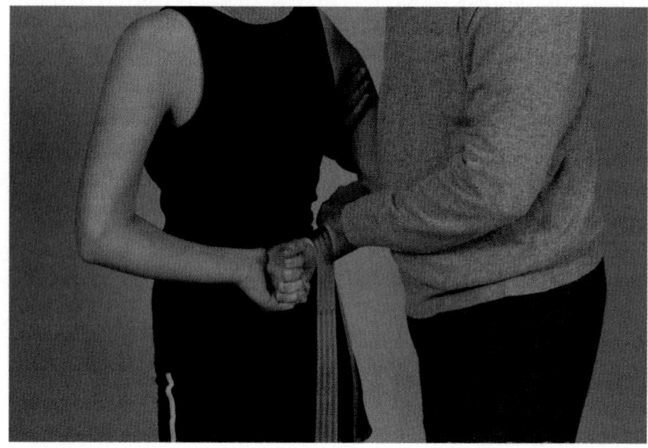

FIGURE 16-121 Mobilization with movement to increase internal rotation using belt.

Transverse Friction Massage

Deep TFM is a good treatment adjunct for tendon and ligament injuries of the shoulder. Since the procedure needs to be performed at a specific area, the examination must accurately determine which structure is involved.

Biceps

The patient is positioned with the shoulder abducted to 30 degrees and the elbow flexed. The clinician stands at the patient's side and supports the arm (Fig. 16-122). The clinician places his or her fingers on the biceps tendon and alternately applies a medial and lateral glide motion to the tendon to create gentle friction.

Supraspinatus

The supraspinatus tendon is located just distal to the anterolateral corner of the acromion. It can become more discernible by positioning the patient's arm in slight extension

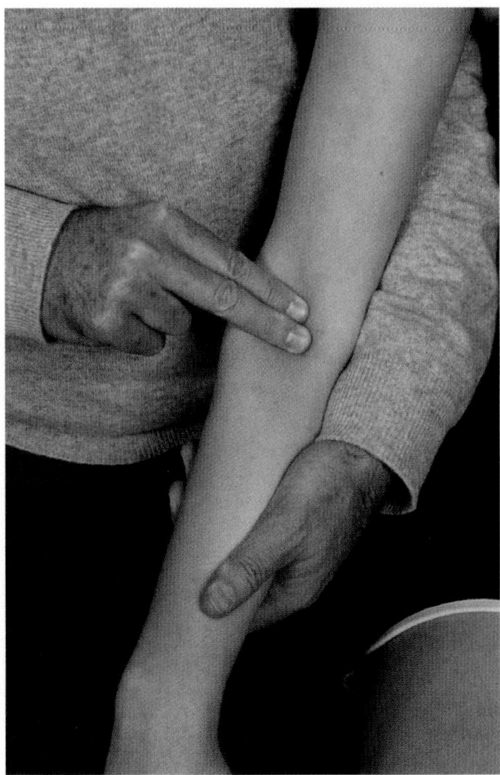
FIGURE 16-122 Transverse friction massage of biceps tendon.

behind the back (Fig. 16-123). The massage is applied perpendicular to the tendon at the point of relative hypovascularity, which is located approximately 1 cm proximal to its insertion into the greater tuberosity of the humerus.[61]

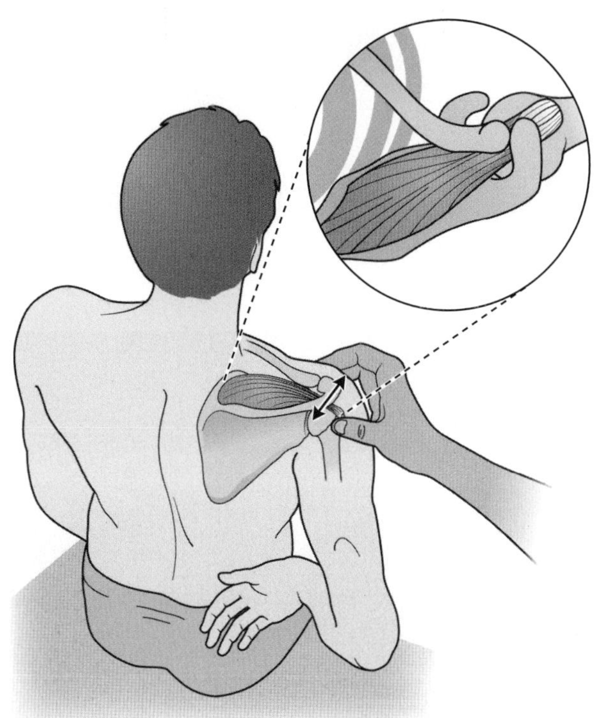
FIGURE 16-123 Transverse friction massage of the supraspinatus tendon.

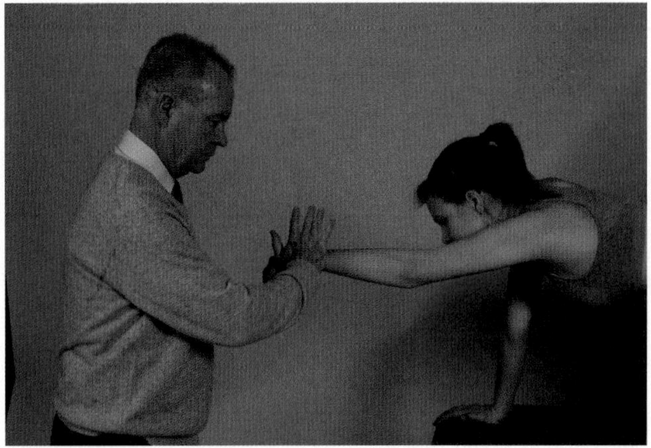
FIGURE 16-124 Rhythmic stabilization in quadruped.

Rhythmic Stabilization

The patient is positioned on all four limbs. The patient raises the involved arm to approximately 90 degrees of flexion and is asked to hold this position (Fig. 16-124) while the clinician applies a series of controlled alternating isometric contractions of the agonist and antagonist muscles to stimulate movement of the agonist, and develop stability, while monitoring scapular muscle activity.

The same exercise can be performed in a variety of positions.

Self-Stretches

The "Saw"

This exercise can be used to stretch the anterior capsule when motion above 90 degrees is restricted. The patient can be in the standing or sitting position. Maintaining his or her arm in approximately 90 degrees of elbow flexion, the patient is asked to perform a sawing motion as though cutting through wood.

Wall Walking

Wall walking can be used when attempting to regain full-range elevation. Clock exercises are a variation of wall walking. The hand is moved to the various positions on an imaginary clock face on the wall, ranging from 8 o'clock, through 12 o'clock, to 4 o'clock. This allows for rotation of the humerus throughout varying degrees of flexion or abduction to replicate rotator cuff activity. This exercise is first performed against a fixed resistance such as a wall or a countertop, and then can be moved to moveable resistance such as a ball or some other moveable implement.

Pulleys

Pulley exercises are commonly used as an active assisted exercise to help regain full overhead motion. However, it is recommended that pulley exercises not be used until the patient has at least 120 degrees of elevation, and then only used in a pain-free arc to decrease the potential for impingement.

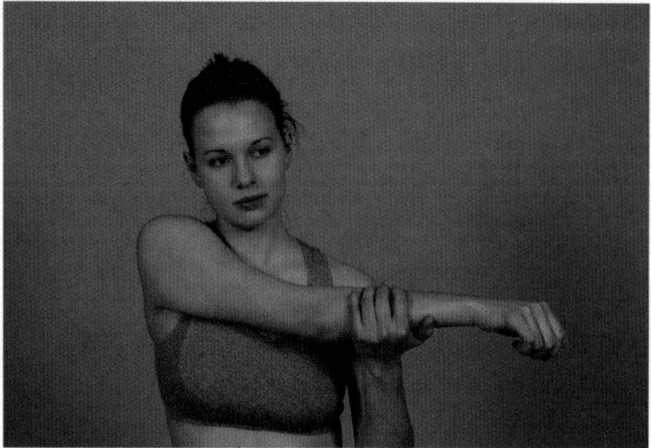

FIGURE 16-125 Horizontal adduction stretch.

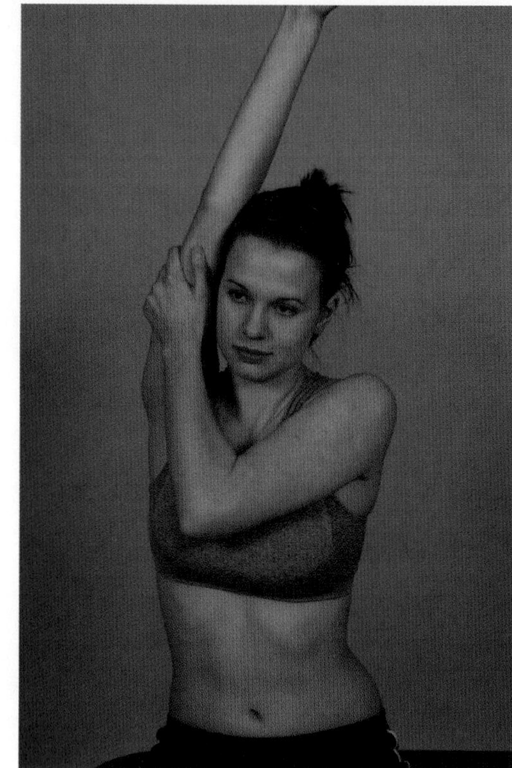

FIGURE 16-126 Inferior capsule stretch.

Wall Corner Stretch

This stretch is used to increase the flexibility of the anterior joint capsule, pectoralis major and minor, anterior deltoid, and coracobrachialis. The patient stands in a corner and places both hands and forearms on the wall, so that the upper arms are level with the shoulders. The stretch is applied by moving the trunk toward the wall, while keeping it perpendicular to the floor. The exercise can be modified to stretch one shoulder by performing the exercise in a doorway.

Horizontal Abductors and Posterior Capsule

The horizontal abductors (posterior deltoid, infraspinatus, teres minor, rhomboids, and middle trapezius) and the posterior joint capsule are stretched by having the patient pull the arm across the front of their body (Fig. 16-125). This exercise should be used with caution for those patients with an impingement syndrome or A-C dysfunction.

Inferior Capsule

The inferior capsule stretch is performed by placing the arm in the fully elevated overhead position (Fig. 16-126).

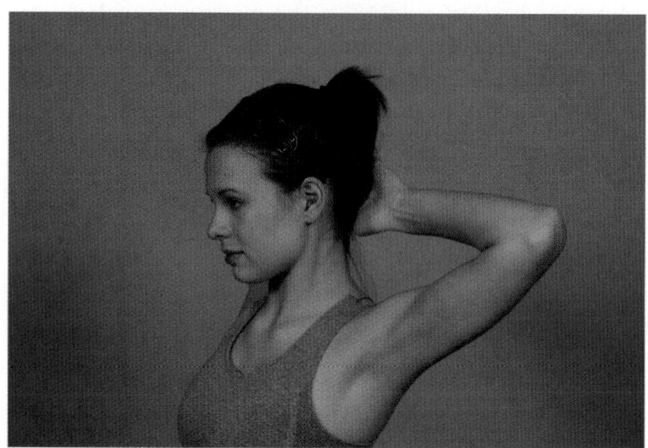

FIGURE 16-127 Pectoralis minor stretch.

Pectoralis Minor

The pectoralis minor can be stretched by asking the patient to clasp his or her hands behind the head (Fig. 16-127). From this position, the patient attempts to move the elbows in a posterior direction. Initially, the clinician can monitor the exercise to ensure that the stretch is occurring in the correct region.

Shoulder Flexors

A T-bar or L-bar is used for this exercise. Two positions are used depending on the intent of the stretch.

To stretch the latissimus dorsi, teres major and minor, the posterior deltoid, triceps, and inferior joint capsule, the patient lies in supine position with the arm overhead (Fig. 16-128). Overpressure can be applied with the bar.

To stretch the anterior deltoid, coracobrachialis, pectoralis major, biceps, and anterior joint capsule, the patient's arm is positioned out to the side in approximately 90 degrees of abduction. The patient extends the arm as far as is comfortable (Fig. 16-129). The bar can be used to apply overpressure into further shoulder extension.

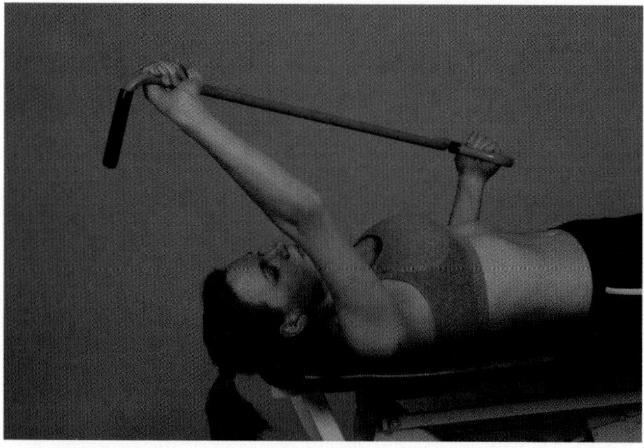

FIGURE 16-128 T-bar exercise for flexion.

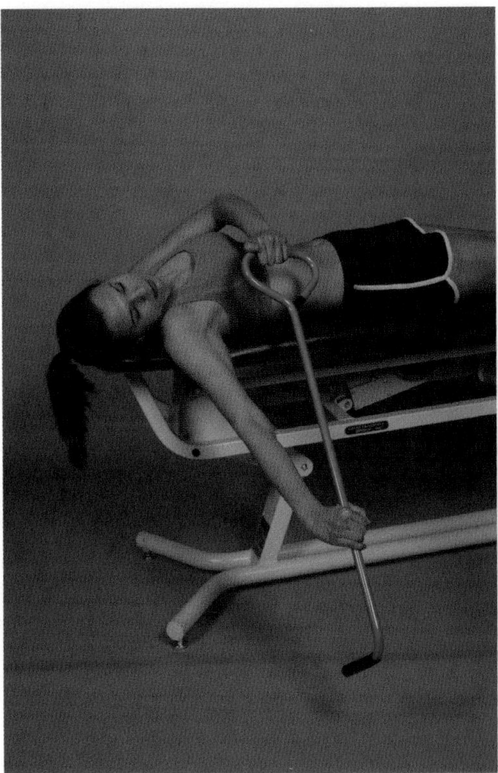

FIGURE 16-129 T-bar exercise for extension.

Shoulder Internal Rotators

A T-bar or L-bar is used for this exercise. The patient lies in supine position. The arm is flexed at the elbow and in one of the three positions of abduction at the shoulder: 0 degrees, 90 degrees (see Fig. 16-130), and 130 degrees. For each of the three positions, the shoulder is externally rotated as far as is comfortable. Overpressure is then applied by the bar to stretch the subscapularis, pectoralis major, anterior deltoid, latissimus dorsi, and the anterior joint capsule.

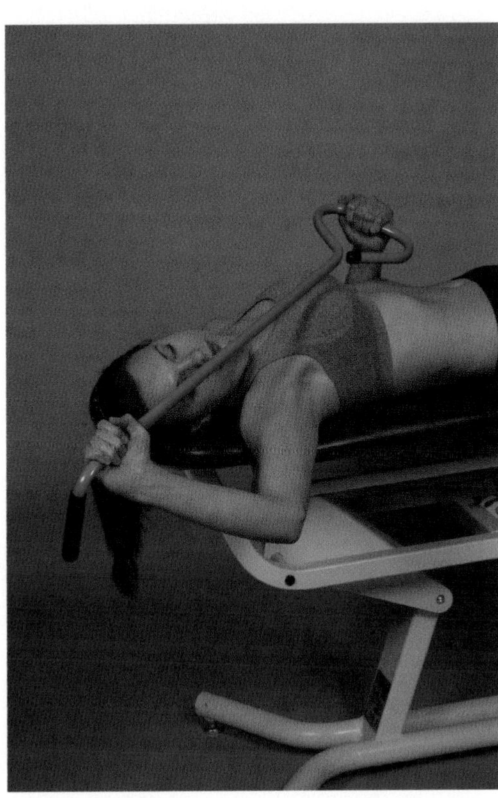

FIGURE 16-130 T-bar exercise into external rotation.

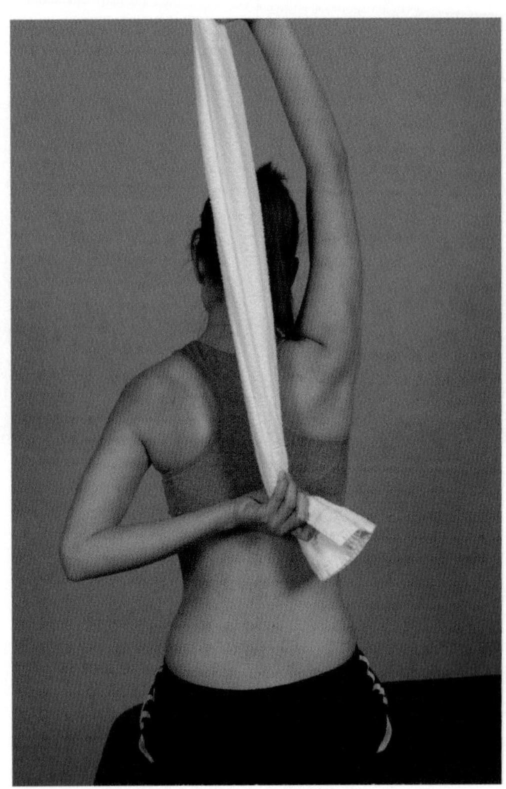

FIGURE 16-131 Towel stretch.

Shoulder External Rotators

A T-bar or L-bar is used for this exercise. The patient lies in supine position. The elbow is flexed and the arm is abducted into one of the three positions at the shoulder: 0 degrees, 90 degrees, and 130 degrees. For each of the three positions, the shoulder is internally rotated as far as is comfortable. Overpressure can then be applied using the bar to stretch the infraspinatus, teres minor, posterior deltoid, and posterior joint capsule.

Alternatively, the patient can sit sideways to a table. The entire upper arm is placed on the table top, bending the trunk as necessary. The elbow is flexed to approximately 90 degrees. Using the other arm, the patient grasps the forearm of the involved arm and moves it into IR as far as is comfortable. Rhythmic oscillations, or hold–relax techniques, can be applied at the end of range.

Towel Stretch

The towel-stretch exercise (Fig. 16-131) combines the motions of ER and IR and stretches the capsule accordingly.

AUTOMOBILIZATION TECHNIQUES

Inferior Distraction

The patient sits with a towel draped over his or her arm (Fig. 16-132). Using the opposite hand, the patient grasps the

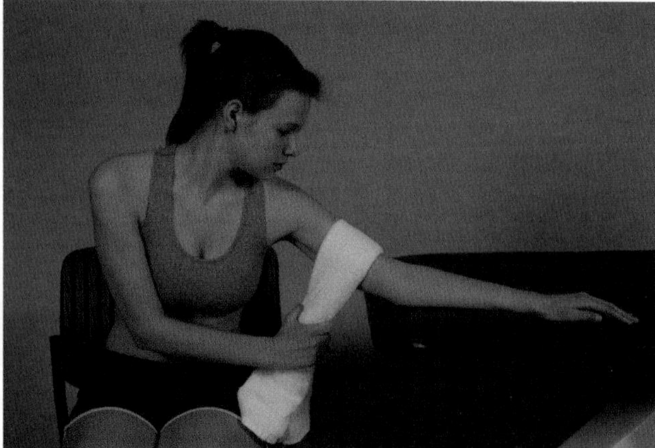

FIGURE 16-132 Self-inferior distraction.

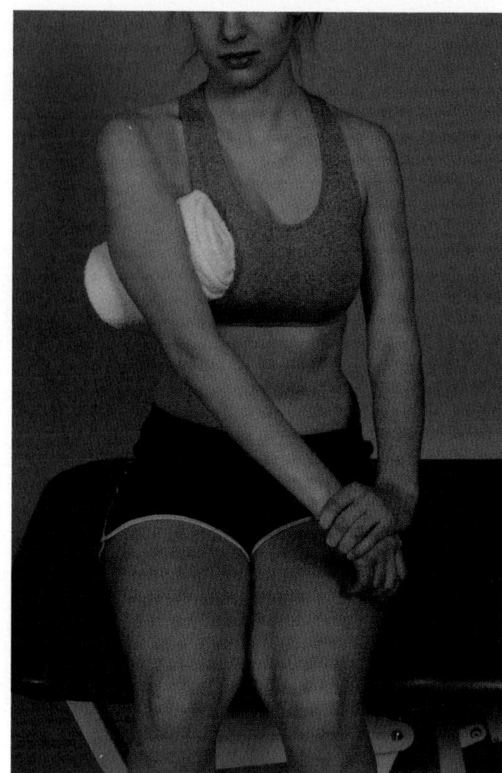

FIGURE 16-133 Inferior distraction with adduction.

involved arm either just proximal to the humeral epicondyles or by the forearm. From this position, the patient applies an inferior glide to the G-H joint as he or she pulls the involved arm downward toward the floor and uses rhythmic oscillations (see Fig. 16-132). For a sustained inferior distraction, a weight or bag can be placed in the hand.

Inferior Distraction with Adduction

The patient stands or sits on a stool. A towel roll is placed under the axilla, and the arm to be mobilized is positioned across the chest. Using the uninvolved hand, the patient grasps the involved forearm just above the styloid processes and pulls the arm rhythmically across the chest into G-H adduction, and downward toward the floor (Fig. 16-133).

Inferior Glide

This is a good technique if the patient's shoulder abduction range is limited to below 90 degrees. The patient sits sideways next to a table. The involved arm is comfortably positioned using a towel roll or pillow in as much abduction as can be tolerated painlessly. The elbow is in full extension (Fig. 16-134). Using the uninvolved hand, or a towel wrapped around the humerus, the patient grasps the superoanterior aspect of the proximal humerus of the involved arm (see Fig. 16-134). From this position, an inferior glide is produced by pushing the humerus directly downward, or pulling the towel toward the floor. Rhythmic oscillations can be used.

If the patient has more than 90 degrees of abduction, another technique is preferable. The patient stands against a wall with the involved shoulder positioned comfortably into abduction. The elbow is flexed to approximately 90 degrees and the fleshy part of the forearm rests against a wall. The other hand grasps the superoanterior aspect of the proximal humerus of the involved arm and applies an inferior glide by pushing the humerus downward toward the floor.

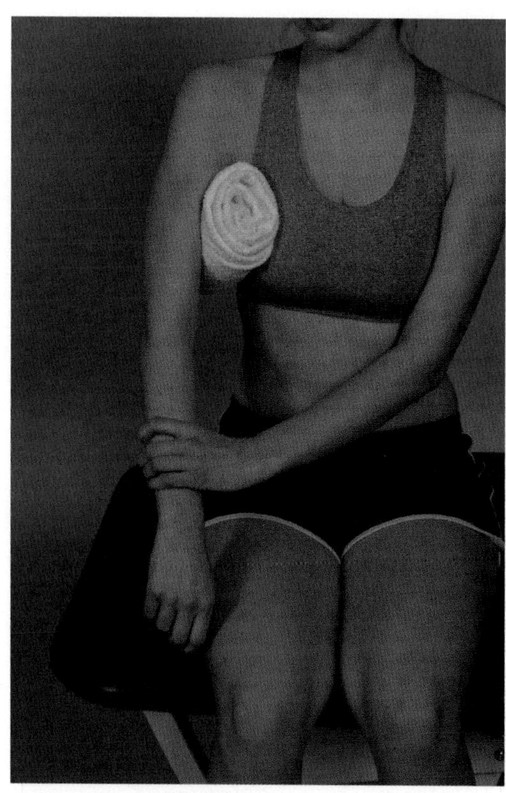

FIGURE 16-134 Inferior glide.

CASE STUDY

SHOULDER PAIN WITH CERTAIN MOTIONS

HISTORY AND SYSTEMS REVIEW

General Demographics

The patient is a 22-year-old male who lives at home with his parents.

History of Current Condition

Insidious onset of intermittent left shoulder pain began 2 weeks ago, with a report of occasional referral of pain into the upper left arm. The patient denies numbness or tingling into the left upper extremity. Pain increased sufficiently the past week to prompt the patient to see a physician, who diagnosed the condition as rotator cuff impingement and prescribed physical therapy and NSAIDs. The patient was also placed on work restrictions; maximum lift limited to 10 lb.

History of Current Condition

No history of left shoulder pain.

Medical and Surgical History

Unremarkable.

Medications

Ibuprofen, 800 mg daily.

Functional Status and Activity Level

The patient reported stiffness and soreness of the left shoulder on arising in the morning and again at the end of the day after working. Difficulty was also reported with putting on a jacket, driving to work which takes 45 minutes, and the use of a hedge trimmer. The patient reported that the shoulder pain interrupts his sleep two to three times every night and that he was having difficulty combing his hair, brushing his teeth, or lifting his arm without pain. He also reported that he enjoyed swimming but cannot swim the crawl or backstroke because of the pain. The patient described "cracking" and "popping" of the shoulder with activity.

Health Status (Self-Report)

Generally in good health but pain interferes with tasks at home and at work.

Questions

1. What structure(s) do you suspect to be involved in this patient?
2. What could the history of pain with certain overhead movements indicate?
3. Why do you think the patient's symptoms are worsened with certain functional and recreational activities?
4. What additional questions would you ask to help rule out cervical involvement or pain referred from a visceral structure?
5. What is your working hypothesis at this stage? List the various diagnoses that could present with these signs and symptoms, and the tests you would use to rule out each one.
6. Does this presentation/history warrant a Cyriax upper quarter/quadrant scanning examination? Why or why not?

CASE STUDY

STIFF AND PAINFUL SHOULDER

History and Systems Review

General Demographics

The patient is a 55-year-old female who lives alone.

History of Current Condition

The patient reports a 7-month history of unilateral shoulder girdle stiffness, pain, and weakness with a diagnosis from the physician of "right frozen shoulder." There was no history of trauma, but the patient reported an abrupt onset of very severe pain 7 months prior. Within several days, she also had right forearm and thumb pain of lesser severity, and weakness of the right shoulder.

The forearm and thumb pain had since resolved, and although there was some restricted motion of the shoulder, the more marked painful stiffness of the shoulder did not occur until 2 or 3 months after the onset of symptoms. After 3 months, she was having difficulties performing her job functions and sought medical attention. Thus far, she had been treated with a series of two corticosteroid injections, both of which had given her short-term relief.

History of Current Condition

Non-work-related right shoulder injury 5 years ago, which resolved in 2 months with a course of physical therapy, including ROM and strengthening exercises, which she followed for 1 month after discharge from physical therapy.

Medical and Surgical History

Unremarkable. Gall bladder surgery 2 years ago.

Medications

Daily 800 mg ibuprofen and high blood pressure medication.

Other Tests and Measures

None.

Occupational, Employment, and School

Patient was a mail reception clerk for the postal service, and her job involved monitoring incoming mail, which required repeated opening and lifting of mail packages.

Functional Status and Activity Level

Stiffness/soreness occurs at the first hour in the morning, and again at the end of the day after working. Pain interferes with sleep two times per night, especially with rolling in bed or driving to work, which takes 30 minutes. The patient discontinued her normal three-times-a-week aerobic workout and upper and lower body resistance exercises approximately 3 months ago.

Health Status (Self-Report)

In general, the patient is in good health, except for a minor heart problem (congestive heart failure) and high blood pressure.

Questions

1. At this point in the examination, is it possible to determine the patient's diagnosis? Why or why not?
2. What does the history of pain with sleeping on the shoulder and pain/stiffness in the morning tell the clinician?
3. Why do you think the patient's symptoms are related to time of day?
4. What additional questions would you ask to help rule out pain referred from a visceral structure given the patient's medical history?
5. Do you have a working hypothesis at this stage? List the various diagnoses that could present with these signs and symptoms, and the tests you would use to rule out each one.
6. Does this presentation/history warrant a scan? Why or why not?
7. Do you think the patient's age is a factor?

REVIEW QUESTIONS*

1. What is the capsular pattern of the G-H joint?
2. The shoulder joint is capable of much motion, but sacrifices some stability to achieve this degree of motion. The weakest portion of the shoulder joint capsule is located:
   A. anteriorly
   B. posteriorly
   C. laterally
   D. inferiorly
   E. superiorly
3. Name four muscles that internally rotate the shoulder.
4. Name three muscles that externally rotate the shoulder.
5. Name four muscles that attach to the greater tuberosity of the humerus.

*Additional questions to test your understanding of this chapter can be found in the Online Learning Center for *Orthopaedic Assessment, Evaluation, and Intervention* at www.duttononline.net.

REFERENCES

1. Burkhart SS: A 26-year-old woman with shoulder pain. *JAMA* 284:1559–1567, 2000.
2. Kapandji IA: *The Physiology of the Joints, Upper Limb*. New York: Churchill Livingstone, 1991.
3. Inman VT, Saunders JB: Observations on the function of the clavicle. *Calif Med* 65:158, 1946.
4. Perry J: Biomechanics of the shoulder. In: Rowe CR, ed. *The Shoulder*. New York: Churchill Livingstone, 1988:1–15.
5. Saha AK: Dynamic stability of the glenohumeral joint. *Acta Orthop Scand* 42:491–505, 1971.
6. Perry J: Normal upper extremity kinesiology. *Phys Ther* 58:265–278, 1978.
7. Bost F, Inman V: The pathological changes in recurrent dislocation of the shoulder. A report of Bankart's operative procedures. *J Bone Joint Surg* 24:595–613, 1942.
8. Cooper DE, Arnoczky SP, O'Brien SJ, et al: Anatomy, histology, and vascularity of the glenoid labrum. An anatomical study. *J Bone Joint Surg Am* 74:46–52, 1992.
9. Howell SM, Galinat BJ: The glenoid-labral socket: a constrained articular surface. *Clin Orthop* 243:122–125, 1989.
10. Wilk KE, Reinold MM, Dugas JR, et al: Current concepts in the recognition and treatment of superior labral (SLAP) lesions. *J Orthop Sports Phys Ther* 35:273–291, 2005.
11. Vangsness CT Jr, Jorgenson SS, Watson T, et al: The origin of the long head of the biceps from the scapula and glenoid labrum. An anatomical study of 100 shoulders. *J Bone Joint Surg Br* 76:951–954, 1994.
12. Huber WP, Putz RV: Periarticular fiber system of the shoulder joint. *Arthroscopy* 13:680–691, 1997.
13. Bradley JP, Tibone JE: Electromyographic analysis of muscle action about the shoulder. *Clin Sports Med* 4:789–805, 1991.
14. Bradley JP, Perry J, Jobe FW: The biomechanics of the throwing shoulder. *Perspect Orthop* 1:49–59, 1990.
15. Answorth AA, Warner JJP: Shoulder instability in the athlete. *Orthop Clin North Am* 26:487–504, 1995.
16. Alcheck DW, Dines DM: Shoulder injuries in the throwing athlete. *J Am Acad Orthop Surg* 3:159–165, 1995.
17. Boublik M, Hawkins RJ: Clinical examination of the shoulder complex. *J Orthop Sports Phys Ther* 18:379–385, 1993.

18. Mallon WJ, Brown HR, Vogler JB III et al: Radiographic and geometric anatomy of the scapula. *Clin Orthop Relat Res* 142–154, 1992.
19. Poppen NK, Walker PS: Normal and abnormal motion of the shoulder. *J Bone Joint Surg* 58A:195–201, 1976.
20. Saha AK: Mechanisms of shoulder movements and a plea for the recognition of "Zero Position" of the glenohumeral joint. *Clin Orthop* 173:3–10, 1983.
21. Warner JJP: The gross anatomy of the joint surfaces, ligaments, labrum, and capsule. In: Matsen FA, Fu FH, Hawkins RJ, eds. *The Shoulder: A Balance of Mobility and Stability*. Rosemont, IL: American Academy of Orthopedic Surgeons, 1993:7–29.
22. Yasojima T, Kizuka T, Noguchi H, et al: Differences in EMG activity in scapular plane abduction under variable arm positions and loading conditions. *Med Sci Sports Exerc* 40:716–721, 2008.
23. Makhsous M, Hogfors C, Siemienski A, et al: Total shoulder and relative muscle strength in the scapular plane. *J Biomech* 32:1213–1220, 1999.
24. Kibler BW: The role of the scapula in athletic shoulder function. *Am J Sports Med* 26:325–337, 1998.
25. Doody SG, Freedman L, Waterland JC: Shoulder movements during abduction in the scapular plane. *Arch Phys Med Rehabil* 51:595–604, 1970.
26. Freedman L, Munro RR: Abduction of the arm in the scapular plane: Scapular and glenohumeral movements. *J Bone Joint Surg* 48A:1503–1510, 1966.
27. Jobe FW, Moynes DR, Brewster CE: Rehabilitation of shoulder joint instabilities. *Orthop Clin North Am* 18:473–482, 1987.
28. Bigliani LU, Morrison D, April EW: The morphology of the acromion and its relationship to rotator cuff tears. *Orthop Trans* 10:228, 1986.
29. Bigliani LU, Ticker JB, Flatow EL, et al: The relationship of acromial architecture to rotator cuff disease. *Clin Sports Med* 4:823–838, 1991.
30. O'Donoghue DH: Subluxing biceps tendon in the athlete. *Clin Orthop* 164:26–29, 1982.
31. Petersson CJ: Spontaneous medial dislocation of the long head of the biceps brachii in its causation. *Clin Orthop* 211:224, 1986.
32. Gerber A, Warner JJ: Thermal capsulorrhaphy to treat shoulder instability. *Clin Orthop Relat Res* 400:105–116, 2002.
33. Ferrari DA: Capsular ligaments of the shoulder. *Am J Sports Med* 18:20–24, 1990.
34. O'Brien SJ, Neves MC, Armoczky SP, et al: The anatomy and histology of the inferior glenohumeral complex of the shoulder. *Am J Sports Med* 18:449, 1990.
35. Wilk KE, Arrigo C, Andrews JR: Current concepts in rehabilitation of the athlete's shoulder. *J South Orthop Assoc* 3:216–231, 1994.
36. Bowen MK, Warren RF: Ligamentous control of shoulder stability based on selective cutting and static translation experiments. *Clin Sports Med* 10:757–782, 1991.
37. Turkel SJ, Panio MW, Marshall JL, et al: Stabilizing mechanisms preventing anterior dislocation of the glenohumeral joint. *J Bone Joint Surg [Am]* 63:1208–1217, 1981.
38. Harryman DT III, Sidles JA, Harris SL, et al: The role of the rotator interval capsule in passive motion and stability of the shoulder. *J Bone Joint Surg* 74A:53–66, 1992.
39. Matsen FA III, Arntz CT: Subacromial impingement. In: Rockwood CA Jr, Matsen FA III, eds. *The Shoulder*. Philadelphia, PA: WB Saunders, 1990:623–648.
40. Neer CS II. Anterior acromioplasty for the chronic impingement syndrome in the shoulder: a preliminary report. *J Bone Joint Surg Am* 54:41–50, 1972.
41. Neer C: Impingement lesions. *Clin Orthop* 173:71–77, 1983.
42. Petersson CJ, Redlund-Johnell I: The subacromial space in normal shoulder radiographs. *Acta Orthop Scand* 55:57–58, 1984.
43. Weiner DS, Macnab I: Superior migration of the humeral head: a radiological aid in the diagnosis of the tears of the rotator cuff. *J Bone Joint Surg [Br]* 52:524–527, 1970.
44. Flatow EL, Soslowsky LJ, Ticker JB, et al: Excursion of the rotator cuff under the acromion. Patterns of subacromial contact. *Am J Sports Med* 22:779–788, 1994.
45. Wickiewicz TL: The impingement syndrome. *Postgraduate Advances in Sports Medicine—NATA Home Study Course*, 1986.
46. Harryman DT III, Sidles JA, Clark JM: Translation of the humeral head on the glenoid with passive glenohumeral motion. *J Bone Joint Surg* 72A:1334–1343, 1990.
47. Nichols TR: A biomechanical perspective on spinal mechanisms of coordinated muscular action. *Acta Anat Nippon* 15:1–13, 1994.
48. Kibler BW: Normal shoulder mechanics and function. *Instr Course Lect* 46:39–42, 1997.
49. Keele CA, Neil E: *Samson Wright's Applied Physiology*, 12th ed. London: Oxford University Press, 1971.
50. Aszmann OC, Dellon AL, Birely BT, et al: Innervation of the human shoulder joint and its implications for surgery. *Clin Orthop Relat Res* 330:202–207, 1996.
51. Bosley RC: Total acromionectomy. A twenty-year review. *J Bone Joint Surg* 73A:961–968, 1991.
52. Ellman H, Kay SP: Arthroscopic subacromial decompression for chronic impingement: 2- to 5-year results. *J Bone Joint Surg Br* 73:395–401, 1991.
53. Cole AJ, Reid MD: Clinical assessment of the shoulder. *J Back Musculoskel Rehabil* 2:7–15, 1992.
54. de La Garza O, Lierse W, Steiner W: Anatomical study of the blood supply in the human shoulder region. *Acta Anat* 145:412–415, 1992.
55. Willcox TM, Teotia SS, Smith AA, et al: The biceps brachii muscle flap for axillary wound coverage. *Plast Reconstr Surg* 110:822–826, 2002.
56. Rothman RH, Parke WW: The vascular anatomy of the rotator cuff. *Clin Orthop* 41:176–186, 1965.
57. Rathburn JB, Macnab I: The microvascular pattern of the rotator cuff. *J Bone Joint Surg Br* 52:540–553, 1970.
58. Jarvholm U, Styf J, Suurkula M, et al: Intramuscular pressure and muscle blood flow in the supraspinatus. *Eur J Appl Physiol* 58:219–224, 1988.
59. Taylor GI, Palmer JH: The vascular territories (angiosomes) of the body: experimental study and clinical implications. *Br J Plast Surg* 40:113, 1987.
60. Ling SC, Chen SF, Wan RX: A study of the vascular supply of the supraspinatus tendon. *Surg Radiol Anat* 12:161, 1990.
61. Codman EA: *The Shoulder, Rupture of the Supraspinatus Tendon and Other Lesions in or About the Subacromial Bursa*. Boston, MA: Thomas Todd, 1934.
62. Lindblom K: On pathogenesis of ruptures of the tendon aponeurosis of the shoulder joint. *Acta Radiol* 20:563, 1939.
63. Moseley HF, Goldie I: The arterial pattern of the rotator cuff of the shoulder. *J Bone Joint Surg* 45-B:780–789, 1963.
64. Iannotti JP, Swiontkowski M, Esterhafi J, et al: *Intraoperative Assessment of Rotator Cuff Vascularity Using Laser Doppler Flowmetry*. Las Vegas: American Academy of Orthopaedic Surgeons, 1989.
65. Sigholm G, Styf J, Korner L, et al: Pressure recording in the subacromial bursa. *J Orthop Res* 6:123–128, 1988.
66. Winkel D, Matthijs O, Phelps V: *Pathology of the shoulder, Diagnosis and Treatment of the Upper Extremities*. Maryland, MD: Aspen, 1997:68–117.
67. Hsu A-T, Chang J-H, Chang CH: Determining the resting position of the glenohumeral joint: A cadaver study. *J Orthop Sports Phys Ther* 32:605–612, 2002.
68. Ludewig PM: *Alterations in Shoulder Kinematics and Associated Muscle Activity in Persons with Shoulder Impingement Symptoms*. Iowa City: The University of Iowa, 1998.
69. Cyriax J: *Examination of the Shoulder. Limited Range Diagnosis of Soft Tissue Lesions*, 8th ed. London: Balliere Tindall, 1982.
70. Davies GJ, DeCarlo MS: Examination of the shoulder complex. In: Bandy WD, ed. *Current Concepts in the Rehabilitation of the Shoulder, Sports Physical Therapy Section— Home Study Course*, 1995.
71. Turnbull JR: Acromioclavicular joint disorders. *Med Sci Sports Exerc* 30: S26–S32, 1998.
72. DePalma AF: *Surgery of the Shoulder*, 2nd ed. Philadelphia, PA: Lippincott, 1973.
73. Chepeha JC: Shoulder trauma and hypomobility. In: Magee DJ, Zachazewski JE, Quillen WS, eds. *Pathology and Intervention in Musculoskeletal Rehabilitation*. St. Louis, MI: Saunders, 2009:92–124.
74. Gladstone JN, Rosen AL: Disorders of the acromioclavicular joint. *Curr Opin Orthop* 10:316–321, 1999.
75. Brody LT: Shoulder. In: Wadsworth C, ed. *Current Concepts of Orthopedic Physical Therapy—Home Study Course*. La Crosse, WI: Orthopaedic Section, APTA, 2001.
76. Kessel L, Watson M: The painful arc syndrome: Clinical classification as a guide to management. *J Bone Joint Surg Br* 59:166–172, 1977.
77. Neer CS II, Bigliani LU, Hawkins RJ: Rupture of the long head of the biceps related to subacromial impingement. *Orthop Trans* 1:70–77, 1977.
78. Fukuda K, Craig EV, Kai-Nan AN, et al: Biomechanical study of the ligamentous system of the acromioclavicular joint. *J. Bone Joint Surg* 68A:434–439, 1986.
79. Lee K, Debski RE, Chen C, et al: Functional evaluation of the ligaments at the acromioclavicular joint during anteroposterior and superoinferior translation. *Am J Sports Med* 25:858–862, 1997.

80. Rockwood CA Jr, Young DC: *Disorders of the Acromioclavicular Joint.* In: Rockwood CA Jr, Matsen FA III, eds. *The Shoulder.* Philadelphia, PA: WB Saunders, 1990:413–468.
81. Urist MR: Complete dislocation of the acromioclavicular joint: the nature of the traumatic lesion and effective methods of treatment with an analysis of 41 cases. *J Bone Joint Surg* 28:813–837, 1946.
82. Moore KL, Dalley AF: Upper limb. In: Moore KL, Dalley AF, eds. *Clinically Oriented Anatomy.* Philadelphia, PA: Williams & Wilkins, 1999:664–830.
83. Karduna AR, McClure PW, Michener LA, et al: Dynamic measurements of three-dimensional scapular kinematics: a validation study. *J Biomech Eng* 123:184–190, 2001.
84. Butters KP: Fractures of the clavicle. In: Rockwood CA, Matsen FA, eds. *The Shoulder*, 2nd ed. Philadelphia, PA: WB Saunders, 1990:432.
85. Norfray JF, Tremaine MJ, Groves HC, et al: The clavicle in hockey. *Am J Sports Med* 5:275–280, 1977.
86. Norkin C, Levangie P: *Joint Structure and Function: A Comprehensive Analysis.* Philadelphia, PA: F.A. Davis Company, 1992.
87. Inman T, Saunders JR, Abbott LC: Observations on the function of the shoulder joint. *J Bone Joint Surg* 26:1–18, 1944.
88. Bearn JG: Direct observations on the function of the capsule of the sternoclavicular joint in clavicular support. *J Anat* 101:159–170, 1967.
89. Allman FL Jr: Fractures and ligamentous injuries of the clavicle and its articulation. *J Bone Joint Surg* 49A:774–784, 1967.
90. Conway AM: Movements at the sternoclavicular and acromioclavicular joints. *Phys Ther Rev* 41:421–432, 1961.
91. Omer GE: Osteotomy of the clavicle in surgical reduction of anterior sternoclavicular dislocations. *J Trauma* 7:584–590, 1967.
92. Gray H: *Gray's Anatomy.* Philadelphia, PA: Lea & Febiger, 1995.
93. Paine RM, Voight M: The role of the scapula. *J Orthop Sports Phys Ther* 18:386–391, 1993.
94. Kibler WB, Chandler TJ, Livingston BP: Correlation of lateral scapular slide measurements with x-ray measurements. *Med Sci Sports Exerc* 31:237–248, 1999.
95. Ludewig PM: *Functional Shoulder Anatomy and Biomechanics.* La Crosse, WI: Orthopaedic Section, APTA, Inc., 2001.
96. Williams GR Jr, Shakil M, Klimkiewicz J, et al: Anatomy of the scapulothoracic articulation. *Clin Orthop Relat Res* 359:237–246, 1999.
97. Hollinshead WH: *Anatomy for Surgeons-The Back and Limbs*, 3rd ed. Philadelphia, PA: Harper and Row, 1982:300–308.
98. Jobe FW, Pink M: Classification and treatment of shoulder dysfunction in the overhead athlete. *J Orthop Sports Phys Ther* 18:427–431, 1993.
99. Haymaker W, Woodhall B: *Peripheral Nerve Injuries. Principles of Diagnosis.* London: WB Saunders, 1953.
100. Brodal A: *Neurological Anatomy.* London: Oxford University Press, 1981.
101. Mercer S, Campbell AH: Motor innervation of the trapezius. *J Man Manip Ther* 8:18–20, 2000.
102. Ayub E: Posture and the upper quarter. In: Donatelli RA, ed. *Physical Therapy of the Shoulder*, 2nd ed. New York: Churchill Livingstone, 1991:81–90.
103. Neumann DA: Shoulder complex. In: Neumann DA, ed. *Kinesiology of the Musculoskeletal System: Foundations for Physical Rehabilitation.* St. Louis, MA: Mosby, 2002:91–132.
104. White SM, Witten CM: Long thoracic nerve palsy in a professional ballet dancer. *Am J Sports Med* 21:626–629, 1993.
105. Jobe CM: Gross anatomy of the shoulder. In: Rockwood CA, Matsen FA, eds. *The Shoulder*, 2nd ed. Philadelphia, PA: WB Saunders, 1998:35–97.
106. Connor PM, Yamaguchi K, Manifold SG, et al: Split pectoralis major transfer for serratus anterior palsy. *Clin Orthop* 341:134–142, 1997.
107. Schultz JS, Leonard JA: Long thoracic neuropathy from athletic activity. *Arch Phys Med Rehabil* 73:87–90, 1992.
108. Gregg JR, Labosky D, Hearty M, et al: Serratus anterior paralysis in the young athlete. *J Bone Joint Surg* 61A:825–832, 1979.
109. Marks PH, Warner JJP, Irrgang JJ: Rotator cuff disorders of the shoulder. *J Hand Ther* 7:90–98, 1994.
110. Warner JJ, Navarro RA: Serratus anterior dysfunction. Recognition and treatment. *Clin Orthop Relat Res* 349:139–148, 1998.
111. Leffert RD: Neurological problems. In: Rockwood CA Jr, Matsen FR III, eds. *The Shoulder.* Philadelphia, PA: WB Saunders, 1990:750–773.
112. Warner JJP, Micheli LJ, Arslanian LE, et al: Scapulothoracic motion in normal shoulders and shoulders with glenohumeral instability and impingement syndrome. A study using Moire topographic analysis. *Clin Orthop* 285:191–199, 1992.
113. Post M: Pectoralis major transfer for winging of the scapula. *J Shoulder Elbow Surg* 4:1–9, 1995.
114. Kapandji IA: *The Physiology of Joints.* New York: Churchill Livingstone, 1974.
115. Dunleavy K: *Relationship Between the Shoulder and the Cervicothoracic Spine.* La Crosse, WI, Orthopedic Section, APTA, 2001.
116. Porterfield J, De Rosa C: *Mechanical Neck Pain: Perspectives in Functional Anatomy.* Philadelphia, PA: WB Saunders, 1995.
117. Murray MP, Gore DR, Gardner GM, et al: Shoulder motion and muscle strength of normal men and women in two age groups. *Clin Orthop Relat Res* 268–273, 1985.
118. Mikesky AE, Edwards JE, Wigglesworth JK, et al: Eccentric and concentric strength of the shoulder and arm musculature in collegiate baseball pitchers. *Am J Sports Med* 23:638–642, 1995.
119. Perry J: Muscle control of the shoulder. In: Rowe CR, ed: *The Shoulder.* New York, Churchill Livingstone, 1988:17–34.
120. Jenp Y, Malanga GA, Growney ES, et al: Activation of the rotator cuff in generating isometric shoulder rotation torque. *Am J Sports Med* 24:477–485, 1996.
121. Culham E, Peat M: Functional anatomy of the shoulder complex. *J Orthop Sports Phys Ther* 18:342–350, 1993.
122. Blackburn TA, McLeod WD, White B, et al: EMG analysis of posterior rotator cuff exercises. *Athl Train* 25:40–45, 1990.
123. Perry J, Glousman RE: Biomechanics of throwing. In: Nicholas JA, Hershman EB, eds. *The Upper Extremity in Sports Medicine.* St Louis, MO: CV Mosby, 1990:727–751.
124. Sharkey NA, Marder RA: The rotator cuff opposes superior translation of the humeral head. *Am J Sports Med* 23:270–275, 1995.
125. Sharkey NA, Marder RA, Hanson PB: The role of the rotator cuff in elevation of the arm. *Trans Orthop Res Soc* 18:137, 1993.
126. Altchek D, Wolf B: Disorders of the biceps tendon. In: Krishnan S, Hawkins R, Warren R, eds. *The Shoulder and the Overhead athlete.* Philadelphia, PA: Lippincott, Williams & Wilkins, 2004: 196–208.
127. Habermeyer P, Magosch P, Pritsch M, et al: Anterosuperior impingement of the shoulder as a result of pulley lesions: a prospective arthroscopic study. *J Shoulder Elbow Surg* 13:5–12, 2004.
128. Krupp RJ, Kevern MA, Gaines MD, et al: Long head of the biceps tendon pain: differential diagnosis and treatment. *J Orthop Sports Phys Ther* 39:55–70, 2009.
129. Mathes SJ, Nahai F: Biceps brachii. In: Mathes SJ, Nahai F, eds. *Clinical Atlas of Muscle and Musculocutaneous Flaps.* St. Louis, MO: Mosby, 1979:426–432.
130. Lucas DB: Biomechanics of the shoulder joint. *Arch Surg* 107:425–432, 1973.
131. Levy AS, Kelly BT, Lintner SA, et al: Function of the long head of the biceps at the shoulder: electromyographic analysis. *J Shoulder Elbow Surg* 10:250–255, 2001.
132. Andrews JR, Carson WG, McLeod WD: Glenoid labrum tears related to the long head of the biceps. *Am J Sports Med* 13:337–341, 1985.
133. Basmajian JV, Deluca CJ: *Muscles Alive: Their Functions Revealed by Electromyography.* Baltimore,MD: Williams & Wilkins, 1985.
134. Basmajian JV, Bazant FJ: Factors preventing downward dislocation of the adducted shoulder joint: an electromyographic and morphological study. *J Bone and Joint Surg* 41A:1182–1186, 1959.
135. Itoi E, Kuechle DK, Newman SR, et al: Stabilising function of the biceps in stable and unstable shoulders. *J Bone and Joint Surg [Am]* 75B:546–550, 1993.
136. Rodosky MW, Harner CD, Fu FH: The role of the long head of the biceps muscle and superior glenoid labrum in anterior stability of the shoulder. *Am J Sports Med* 22:121–130, 1994.
137. Pagnani M, Deng X-H, Warren RF, et al: Effect of lesions of the superior portion of the glenoid labrum on glenohumeral translation. *J Bone and Joint Surg* 77A:1002–1010, 1995.
138. Payne LZ, Deng X, Craig EV, et al: The combined dynamic and static contributions to subacromial impingement. *Am J Sports Med* 25:801–808, 1997.
139. Warner JJP, McMahon PJ: The role of the long head of the biceps brachii in superior stability of the glenohumeral joint. *J Bone and Joint Surg* 77A:366–372, 1995.
140. Kido T, Itoi E, Konno N, et al: The depressor function of biceps on the head of the humerus in shoulders with tears of the rotator cuff. *J Bone and Joint Surg* 82B:416–419, 2000.
141. Itoi E, Hsu HC, Carmichael SW, et al: Morphology of the torn rotator cuff. *J Anat* 186:429–434, 1995.

142. Terry GC, Hammon D, France P, et al: The stabilizing function of passive shoulder restraints. *Am J Sports Med* 19:26–34, 1991.
143. Rowe CR, Zarins B: Recurrent transient subluxation of the shoulder. *J Bone Joint Surg Am* 63:863–872, 1981.
144. Kibler WB, Livingston B, Bruce R: Current concepts in shoulder rehabilitation. *Adv Op Orthop* 3:249–301, 1996.
145. Pink MM, Screnar PM, Tollefson KD: Injury prevention and rehabilitation in the upper extremity. In: Jobe FW, ed: *Operative Techniques in Upper Extremity Sports Injuries*. St. Louis, MO: Mosby, 1996:3–15.
146. Jobe FW, Tibone JE, Moynes DR, et al: An EMG analysis of the shoulder in pitching and throwing: A preliminary report. *Am J Sports Med* 11:3–5, 1983.
147. Fleisig GS, Andrews JR, Dillman CJ, et al: Kinetics of baseball pitching with implications about injury mechanisms. *Am J Sports Med* 23:233–239, 1995.
148. Fleisig GS, Barrentine SW, Zheng N, et al: Kinematic and kinetic comparison of baseball pitching among various levels of development. *J Biomech* 32:1371–1375, 1999.
149. Pagnani MJ, Galinat BJ, Warren RF: Glenohumeral instability. In: DeLee JC, Drez D, eds. *Orthopaedic Sports Medicine: Principles and Practice*. Philadelphia, PA: WB Saunders, 1993.
150. Kibler WB: Biomechanical analysis of the shoulder during tennis activities. *Clin Sports Med* 14:79–85, 1995.
151. Kibler WB: Evaluation of sports demands as a diagnostic tool in shoulder disorders. In: Matsen FA, Fu F, Hawkins RJ, eds. *The Shoulder: A Balance of Mobility and Stability*. Rosemont, IL: Am. Acad. Orthop. Surgeons, 1994:379–399.
152. Kibler WB, Livingston B, Chandler TJ: Shoulder rehabilitation: clinical application, evaluation, and rehabilitation protocols. *Instruct Course Lect* 46:43–53, 1997.
153. Kibler WB: Shoulder rehabilitation: principles and practice. *Med Sci Sports Exerc* 30:40–50, 1998.
154. Ovesen J, Nielsen S: Experimental distal subluxation in the glenohumeral joint. *Arch Orthop and Trauma Surg* 104:78–81, 1985.
155. Gibb TD, Sidles JA, Harryman DT, et al: The effect of capsular venting on glenohumeral laxity. *Clin Orthop* 268:120–127, 1991.
156. Itoi E, Motzkin NE, Morrey BF, et al: The static rotator cuff does not affect inferior translation of the humerus at the glenohumeral joint. *J Trauma* 47:55–59, 1999.
157. Debski RE, Sakone M, Woo SL, et al: Contribution of the passive properties of the rotator cuff to glenohumeral stability during anterior-posterior loading. *J Shoulder Elbow Surg* 8:324–329, 1999.
158. Lee S-B, Kim K-J, O'Driscoll SW, et al: Dynamic glenohumeral stability provided by the rotator cuff muscles in the mid-range and end-range of motion. *J Bone and Joint Surg* 82A:849–857, 2000.
159. Matsen FA, Harryman DT, Sidles JA: Mechanics of glenohumeral instability. *Clin Sports Med* 10:783–788, 1991.
160. Habermeyer P, Schuller U, Wiedemann E: The intra-articular pressure of the shoulder: an experimental study on the role of the glenoid labrum in stabilizing the joint. *J Arthrosc* 8:166–172, 1992.
161. Warner JJP, Schulte KR, Imhoff AB: *Current concepts in shoulder instability*. In: *Advances in Operative Orthopedics*. St Louis, MO: CV Mosby, 1995:217–248.
162. Pearl ML, Harris SL, Lippitt SB, et al: A system for describing positions of the humerus relative to the thorax and its use in the presentation of several functionally important arm positions. *J Shoulder Elbow Surg* 1:113–118, 1992.
163. Freedman L, Munro RR: Abduction of the arm in the scapular plane: scapular and glenohumeral movements. A roentgenographic study. *J Bone Joint Surg Am* 48:1503–1510, 1966.
164. Abboud JA, Soslowsky LJ: Interplay of the static and dynamic restraints in glenohumeral instability. *Clin Orthop Relat Res* 48–57, 2002.
165. Mell AG, LaScalza S, Guffey P, et al: Effect of rotator cuff pathology on shoulder rhythm. *J Shoulder Elbow Surg* 14:58S–64S, 2005.
166. d'Hespeel CG: Current concepts: Rehabilitation of patients with shoulder impingement and tight posterior capsule. *Orthop Pract* 16:9–13, 2004.
167. Grood ES, Noyes FR, Butler DL, et al: Ligamentous and capsular restraints preventing medial and lateral laxity in intact human cadaver knees. *J Bone Joint Surg* 63A:1257–1269, 1981.
168. Glousman R, Jobe FW, Tibone JE: Dynamic EMG analysis of the throwing shoulder with glenohumeral instability. *J Bone Joint Surg* 70:220–226, 1988.
169. Babyar SR: Excessive scapular motion in individuals recovering from painful and stiff shoulders: causes and treatment strategies. *Phys Ther* 76:226–247, 1996.
170. Bagg SD, Forrest WJ: A biomechanical analysis of scapular rotation during arm abduction in the scapular plane. *Am J Phys Med* 67:238–245, 1988.
171. McQuade KJ, Smidt GL: Dynamic scapulohumeral rhythm: the effects of external resistance during elevation of the arm in the scapular plane. *J Orthop Sports Phys Ther* 27:125–133, 1998.
172. Rabin A, Irrgang JJ, Fitzgerald GK, et al: The intertester reliability of the Scapular Assistance Test. *J Orthop Sports Phys Ther* 36:653–660, 2006.
173. Rockwood CA: *Rockwood and Green's Fractures in Adults*. Philadelphia, PA: Lippincott, 1991:1181–1239.
174. Lukasiewicz AC, McClure P, Michener L, et al: Comparison of 3-dimensional scapular position and orientation between subjects with and without shoulder impingement. *J Orthop Sports Phys Ther* 29:574–583; discussion 584–586, 1999.
175. McClure PW, Michener LA, Sennett BJ, et al: Direct 3-dimensional measurement of scapular kinematics during dynamic movements in vivo. *J Shoulder Elbow Surg* 10:269–277, 2001.
176. Borstad JD, Ludewig PM: Comparison of scapular kinematics between elevation and lowering of the arm in the scapular plane. *Clin Biomech (Bristol, Avon)* 17:650–659, 2002.
177. Dayanidhi S, Orlin M, Kozin S, et al: Scapular kinematics during humeral elevation in adults and children. *Clin Biomech (Bristol, Avon)* 20:600–606, 2005.
178. McQuade KJ, Hwa Wei S, Smidt GL: Effects of local muscle fatigue on three-dimensional scapulohumeral rhythm. *Clin Biomech (Bristol, Avon)* 10:144–148, 1995.
179. Schenkman M, De Cartaya VR: Kinesiology of the shoulder complex. In: Andrews J, Wilk KE, eds. The Athlete's Shoulder. New York: Churchill Livingstone, 1994:15–35.
180. Dvir Z, Berme N: The shoulder complex in elevation of the arm: a mechanism approach. *J Biomech* 11:219–225, 1978.
181. Laumann U: Kinesiology of the shoulder: electromyographic and sterophotogrammetric studies. In: *Surgery of the Shoulder*. Philadelphia, PA: BC Decker Co, 1984.
182. Van Der Helm FCT: Analysis of the kinematic and dynamic behavior of the shoulder mechanism. *J Biomech* 27:527–550, 1994.
183. Kuhn JE, Plancher KD, Hawkins RJ: Scapular winging. *J Am Acad Orthop Surg* 3:319–325, 1995.
184. Jobe FW, Nuber G: Throwing injuries of the elbow. *Clin Sports Med* 5:621, 1986.
185. Jobe FW, Bradley JP, Pink M: Treatment of impingement syndrome in overhand athletes: A philosophical basis: I. *Surg Rounds Orthop* 4:19–24, 1990.
186. Lee DG: Biomechanics of the thorax. In: Grant R, ed. *Physical Therapy of the Cervical and Thoracic Spine*. New York: Churchill Livingstone, 1988:47–76.
187. Campos GER, Freitas VD, Vitti M: Electromyographic study of the trapezius and deltoideus in elevation, lowering, retraction and protraction of the shoulders. *Electromyogr Clin Neurophysiol* 34:243–247, 1994.
188. Elliott BC, Marshall R, Noffal G: Contributions of upper limb segment rotations during the power serve in tennis. *J Appl Biomech* 11:433–442, 1995.
189. Kennedy K: Rehabilitation of the unstable shoulder. *Oper Tech Sports Med* 1:311–324, 1993.
190. Clarnette RG, Miniaci A: Clinical exam of the shoulder. *Med Sci Sports Exerc* 30:1–6, 1998.
191. Magee DJ: *Orthopedic Physical Assessment*, 2nd ed. Philadelphia, PA: WB Saunders, 1992.
192. Souza TA: History and examination of the shoulder. In: Souza TA, ed. *Sports Injuries of the Shoulder—Conservative Management*. New York: Churchill Livingstone, 1994:167–219.
193. Burkhart SS: A stepwise approach to arthroscopic rotator cuff repair based on biomechanical principles. *Arthroscopy* 16:82–90, 2000.
194. Buckle P: Musculoskeletal disorders of the upper extremities: the use of epidemiological approaches in industrial settings. *J Hand Surg Am* 12:885–889, 1987.
195. Daigneault J, Cooney LM Jr: Shoulder pain in older people. *J Am Geriatr Soc* 46:1144–1151, 1998.
196. Matsen FA III, Lippitt SB, Sidles JA, et al: Shoulder motion. In: Matsen FA III, Lippitt SB, Sidles JA, et al, eds. *Practical Evaluation and Management of the Shoulder*. Philadelphia, PA: WB Saunders, 1994:19–58.

197. Miniaci A, Salonen D: Rotator cuff evaluation: imaging and diagnosis. *Orthop Clin North Am* 28:43–58, 1997.
198. Gladstone J, Wilk KE, Andrews J: Nonoperative treatment of acromioclavicular joint injuries. *Op Tech Sports Med* 5:78–87, 1998.
199. Cappel K, Clark MA, Davies GJ, et al: Clinical examination of the shoulder. In: Tovin BJ, Greenfield B, eds. *Evaluation and Treatment of the Shoulder—An Integration of The Guide to Physical Therapist Practice.* Philadelphia, PA: F.A. Davis, 2001:75–131.
200. Foreman SM, Croft AC: *Whiplash Injuries: The Cervical Acceleration/Deceleration Syndrome.* Baltimore, MD: Williams & Wilkins, 1988.
201. Cohen RB, Williams GR Jr: Impingement syndrome and rotator cuff disease as repetitive motion disorders. *Clin Orthop Relat Res* 351:95–101, 1998.
202. Feinstein B, Langton JBK, Jameson RF, et al: Experiments on referred pain from deep somatic tissues. *J Bone and Joint Surg [Am]* 36:981–997, 1954.
203. Dwyer A, Aprill C, Bogduk N: Cervical zygapophyseal joint pain patterns: a study from normal volunteers. *Spine* 15:453, 1990.
204. Cloward RB: Cervical discography: a contribution to the etiology and mechanism of neck, shoulder and arm pain. *Ann Surg* 150:1052–1064, 1959.
205. Cuomo F: Diagnosis, classification, and management of the stiff shoulder. In: Iannotti JP, Williams GR, eds. *Disorders of the Shoulder: Diagnosis and Management.* Philadelphia, PA: Lippincott Williams & Wilkins, 1999:397–417.
206. Sahrmann SA: Movement impairment syndromes of the shoulder girdle. In: Sahrmann SA, ed. *Movement Impairment Syndromes.* St Louis, MO: Mosby, 2001:193–261.
207. Hawkins RJ, Bokor DJ: Clinical evaluation of shoulder problems. In: Rockwood CA, Matsen FA, eds. *The Shoulder.* Philadelphia, PA: WB Saunders, 1990.
208. Silliman FJ, Hawkins RJ: Clinical examination of the shoulder complex. In: Andrews JR, Wilk KE, eds. *The Athlete's Shoulder.* New York: Churchill Livingstone, 1994.
209. Barron OA, Levine WN, Bigliani LU: Surgical management of chronic trapezius dysfunction. In: Warner JJP, Iannotti JP, Gerber C, eds. *Complex and Revision Problems in Shoulder Surgery.* Philadelphia, PA: Lippincott-Raven, 1997:377–384.
210. Hoppenfeld S: *Physical Examination of the Spine and Extremities.* East Norwalk, CT: Appleton-Century-Crofts, 1976.
211. Miniaci A, Fowler PJ: Impingement in the athlete. *Clin Sports Med* 12:91–110, 1993.
212. Miniaci A, Froese WG: Rotator cuff pathology and excessive laxity or instability of the glenohumeral joint. *Sports Med Arthrosc Rev* 3:26–29, 1995.
213. Ketenjian AY: Scapulocostal stabilization for scapular winging in fascioscapulohumeral muscular dystrophy. *J Bone Joint Surg* 60A:476–480, 1978.
214. Bagg SD, Forrest WJ: Electromyographic study of the scapular rotators during arm abduction in the scapular plane. *Am J Phys Med* 65:111–124, 1986.
215. Moseley JB, Jobe FW, Pink MM, et al: EMG analysis of the scapular muscles during a shoulder rehabilitation program. *Am J Sports Med* 20:128–134, 1992.
216. Bowling RW, Rockar PA, Erhard R: Examination of the shoulder complex. *Phys Ther* 66:1886–1893, 1986.
217. Kendall FP, McCreary EK, Provance PG: *Muscles: Testing and Function.* Baltimore, MD: Williams & Wilkins, 1993.
218. Griegel-Morris P, Larson K, Mueller-Klaus K, et al: Incidence of common postural abnormalities in the cervical, shoulder, and thoracic regions and their association with pain in two age groups of healthy subjects. *Phys Ther* 72:426–430, 1992.
219. Crawford HJ, Jull GA: The influence of thoracic posture and movement on range of arm elevation. *Physiother Theory Pract* 9:143–148, 1993.
220. Sahrmann SA: *Diagnosis and Treatment of Movement Impairment Syndromes.* St Louis, MO: Mosby, 2001.
221. Lewit K: *Manipulative Therapy in Rehabilitation of the Motor System,* 3rd ed. London: Butterworths, 1999.
222. Janda DH, Hawkins RJ: Shoulder manipulation in patients with adhesive capsulitis and diabetes mellitus. A clinical note. *J Shoulder Elbow Surg* 2:36–38, 1993.
223. Greenfield B, Catlin P, Coats P, et al: Posture in patients with shoulder overuse injuries and healthy individuals. *J Orthop Sports Phys Ther* 21:287–295, 1995.
224. Solem-Bertoft E, Thuomas KA, Westerberg CE: The influence of scapular retraction and protraction on the width of the subacromial space. *Clin Orthop* 296:99–103, 1993.
225. Turner M: Posture and pain. *Phys Ther* 37:294, 1957.
226. Jull GA, Janda V: Muscle and Motor control in low back pain. In: Twomey LT, Taylor JR, eds. *Physical Therapy of the Low Back: Clinics in Physical Therapy.* New York: Churchill Livingstone, 1987:258–278.
227. Greenfield B: Upper quarter evaluation: structural relationships and interindependence. In: Donatelli R, Wooden M, eds. *Orthopedic Physical Therapy.* New York: Churchill Livingstone, 1989:43–58.
228. Keller K, Corbett J, Nichols D: Repetitive strain injury in computer keyboard users: pathomechanics and treatment principles in individual and group intervention. *J Hand Ther* 11:9–26, 1998.
229. Pratt NE: Neurovascular entrapment in the regions of the shoulder and posterior triangle of the neck. *Phys Ther* 66:1894–1899, 1986.
230. Pecina M, Krmpotic-Nemanic J, Markiewitz A: *Tunnel Syndromes.* Boca Raton, FL: CRC, 1991.
231. Bourliere F: *The Assessment of Biological Age in Man.* Geneva: WHO, 1979.
232. Rayan GM, Jensen C: Thoracic outlet syndrome: provocative examination maneuvers in a typical population. *J Shoulder Elbow Surg* 4:113–117, 1995.
233. Sucher BM: Thoracic outlet syndrome—A myofascial variant: Part 2. Treatment. *J Am Osteopath Assoc* 90:810–823, 1990.
234. Jenkins WL: *Relationship of Overuse Impingement with Subtle Hypomobility or Hypermobility.* La Crosse, WI: Orthopaedic Section, APTA, Inc, 2001.
235. Diveta J, Walker ML, Skibinski B: Relationship between performance of selected scapular muscles and scapular abduction in standing subjects. *Phys Ther* 70:470–479, 1990.
236. Gibson MH, Goebel GV, Jordan TM, et al: A reliability study of measurement techniques to determine static scapular position. *J Orthop Sports Phys Ther* 21:100–106, 1995.
237. Mattingly GE, Mackarey PJ: Optimal methods for shoulder tendon palpation: A cadaver study. *Phys Ther* 76:166–174, 1996.
238. Matsen FA, Lippitt SB, Sidles JA, et al: *Practical Evaluation and Management of the Shoulder.* Philadelphia, PA: WB Saunders, 1994.
239. Jackson D, Einhorn A: Rehabilitation of the shoulder. In: Jackson DW, ed. *Shoulder Surgery in the Athlete.* Rockville, MD: Aspen, 1985.
240. Kulund DN: *The Injured Athlete.* Philadelphia, PA: JB Lippincott, 1982.
241. Andrews JR, Gillogly S: Physical examination of the shoulder in throwing athletes. In: Zarin B, Andrews JR, Carson WG, eds. *Injuries to the Throwing Arm.* Philadelphia, PA: WB Saunders, 1985.
242. McClure PW, Flowers KR: Treatment of limited shoulder motion: A case study based on biomechanical considerations. *Phys Ther* 72:929–936, 1992.
243. Akeson WH, Amiel D, Woo SL-Y: Immobility effects on synovial joints: The pathomechanics of joint contracture. *Biorheology* 17:95–110, 1980.
244. Woo SL-Y, Matthews J, Akeson WH, et al: Connective tissue response to immobility: A correlative study of biochemical and biomechanical measurements of normal and immobilized rabbit knee. *Arthritis Rheum* 18:257–264, 1975.
245. Akeson WH, Woo SL, Amiel D, et al: The connective tissue response to immobility: biochemical changes in periarticular connective tissue of the immobilized rabbit knee. *Clin Orthop* 93:356–362, 1973.
246. Cyriax J: *Textbook of Orthopaedic Medicine, Diagnosis of Soft Tissue Lesions,* 8th ed. London: Bailliere Tindall, 1982.
247. Neviaser RJ, Neviaser TJ: The frozen shoulder. Diagnosis and management. *Clin Orthop* 223:59–64, 1987.
248. Riddle DL, Rothstein JM, Lamb RL: Goniometric reliability in a clinical setting. Shoulder measurements. *Phys Ther* 67:668–673, 1987.
249. Borstad JD, Ludewig PM: The effect of long versus short pectoralis minor resting length on scapular kinematics in healthy individuals. *J Orthop Sports Phys Ther* 35:227–238, 2005.
250. Lewis JS, Wright C, Green A: Subacromial impingement syndrome: the effect of changing posture on shoulder range of movement. *J Orthop Sports Phys Ther* 35:72–87, 2005.
251. Johanson MA: *Solutions to Shoulder Disorders.* La Crosse, WI: Orthopaedic Section, APTA, 2001.
252. Poppen NK, Walker PS: Forces at the glenohumeral joint in abduction. *Clin Orthop* 135:165–170, 1978.
253. Brems JJ: Rehabilitation following shoulder arthroplasty. In: Friedman RJ, ed. *Arthroplasty of the Shoulder.* New York: Thieme, 1994:99–112.
254. Brown DD, Friedman RJ: Postoperative rehabilitation following total shoulder arthroplasty. *Orthop Clin North Am* 29:535–547, 1998.

255. Hoving JL, Buchbinder R, Green S, et al: How reliably do rheumatologists measure shoulder movement? *Ann Rheum Dis* 61:612–616, 2002.
256. Edwards TB, Bostick RD, Greene CC, et al: Interobserver and intraobserver reliability of the measurement of shoulder internal rotation by vertebral level. *J Shoulder Elbow Surg* 11:40–42, 2002.
257. Osbahr DC, Cannon DL, Speer KP: Retroversion of the humerus in the throwing shoulder of college baseball pitchers. *Am J Sports Med* 30:347–353, 2002.
258. Chant CB, Litchfield R, Griffin S, et al: Humeral head retroversion in competitive baseball players and its relationship to glenohumeral rotation range of motion. *J Orthop Sports Phys Ther* 37:514–520, 2007.
259. Reagan KM, Meister K, Horodyski MB, et al: Humeral retroversion and its relationship to glenohumeral rotation in the shoulder of college baseball players. *Am J Sports Med* 30:354–360, 2002.
260. Kronberg M, Brostrom LA, Soderlund V: Retroversion of the humeral head in the normal shoulder and its relationship to the normal range of motion. *Clin Orthop Relat Res* 113–117, 1990.
261. Burkhart SS, Morgan CD, Kibler WB: The disabled throwing shoulder: spectrum of pathology Part I: pathoanatomy and biomechanics. *Arthroscopy* 19:404–420, 2003.
262. Burkhart SS, Morgan CD, Kibler WB: The disabled throwing shoulder: spectrum of pathology Part III: The SICK scapula, scapular dyskinesis, the kinetic chain, and rehabilitation. *Arthroscopy* 19:641–661, 2003.
263. Burkhart SS, Morgan CD, Kibler WB: The disabled throwing shoulder: spectrum of pathology. Part II: evaluation and treatment of SLAP lesions in throwers. *Arthroscopy* 19:531–539, 2003.
264. Clabbers KM, Kelly JD, Bader D, et al: Effect of posterior capsule tightness on glenohumeral translation in the late-cocking phase of pitching. *J Sport Rehabil* 16:41–49, 2007.
265. Grossman MG, Tibone JE, McGarry MH, et al: A cadaveric model of the throwing shoulder: a possible etiology of superior labrum anterior-to-posterior lesions. *J Bone Joint Surg Am* 87:824–831, 2005.
266. Myers JB, Laudner KG, Pasquale MR, et al: Glenohumeral range of motion deficits and posterior shoulder tightness in throwers with pathologic internal impingement. *Am J Sports Med.* 34:385–91. Epub 2005 Nov 22, 2006.
267. Tyler TF, Nicholas SJ, Roy T, et al: Quantification of posterior capsule tightness and motion loss in patients with shoulder impingement. *Am J Sports Med* 28:668–673, 2000.
268. Borsa PA, Dover GC, Wilk KE, et al: Glenohumeral range of motion and stiffness in professional baseball pitchers. *Med Sci Sports Exerc* 38:21–26, 2006.
269. Borsa PA, Wilk KE, Jacobson JA, et al: Correlation of range of motion and glenohumeral translation in professional baseball pitchers. *Am J Sports Med* 33:1392–1399, 2005.
270. Reinold MM, Wilk KE, Macrina LC, et al: Changes in shoulder and elbow passive range of motion after pitching in professional baseball players. *Am J Sports Med* 36:523–527, 2008.
271. Jamurtas AZ, Theocharis V, Tofas T, et al: Comparison between leg and arm eccentric exercises of the same relative intensity on indices of muscle damage. *Eur J Appl Physiol* 95:179–185, 2005.
272. Prasartwuth O, Taylor JL, Gandevia SC: Maximal force, voluntary activation and muscle soreness after eccentric damage to human elbow flexor muscles. *J Physiol* 567:337–348, 2005.
273. Reisman S, Walsh LD, Proske U: Warm-up stretches reduce sensations of stiffness and soreness after eccentric exercise. *Med Sci Sports Exerc* 37:929–936, 2005.
274. Wilk KE, Meister K, Andrews JR: Current concepts in the rehabilitation of the overhead throwing athlete. *Am J Sports Med* 30:136–151, 2002.
275. Wilk KE, Macrina LC, Fleisig GS, et al: Correlation of glenohumeral internal rotation deficit and total rotational motion to shoulder injuries in professional baseball pitchers. *Am J Sports Med* 39:329–335, 2011.
276. Post M, Mayer J: Suprascapular nerve entrapment: diagnosis and treatment. *Clin Orthop* 223:126–130, 1987.
277. Warner JJP, Caborn DNM, Berger RA, et al: Dynamic capsuloligamentous anatomy of the glenohumeral joint. *J Shoulder Elbow Surg* 2:115–133, 1993.
278. Pagnani MJ, Warren RF: Stabilizers of the glenohumeral joint. *J Shoulder Elbow Surg* 3:173–190, 1994.
279. O'Connell PW, Nuber GW, Mileski RA, et al: The contribution of the glenohumeral ligaments to anterior stability of the shoulder joint. *Am J Sports Med* 18:579–584, 1990.
280. Karduna AR, Williams GR, Williams JL, et al: Kinematics of the glenohumeral joint: Influences of muscle forces, ligamentous constraints, and articular geometry. *J Orthop Res* 14:986–993, 1996.
281. Davies GJ, Dickhoff-Hoffman S: Neuromuscular testing and rehabilitation of the shoulder complex. *J Orthop Sports Phys Ther* 18:449–458, 1993.
282. Kamkar A, Irrgang JJ, Whitney S: Non-operative management of secondary shoulder impingement syndrome. *J Orthop Sports Phys Ther* 17:212–224, 1993.
283. Ozaki J: Glenohumeral movements of the involuntary inferior and multidirectional instability. *Clin Orthop* 238:107–111, 1989.
284. Leroux JL, Thomas E, Bonnel F, et al: Diagnostic value of clinical tests for shoulder impingement. *Rev Rheum* 62:423–428, 1995.
285. Itoi E, Tadato K, Sano A, et al: Which is more useful, the "full can test" or the "empty can test" in detecting the torn supraspinatus tendon? *Am J Sports Med* 27:65–68, 1999.
286. Kaltenborn FM: *Manual Mobilization of the Extremity Joints: Basic Examination and Treatment Techniques*, 4th ed. Oslo, Norway: Olaf Norlis Bokhandel, Universitetsgaten, 1989.
287. Winkel D, Matthijs O, Phelps V: *Examination of the Shoulder, Diagnosis and Treatment of the Upper Extremities*. Maryland: Aspen, 1997:42–67.
288. Pfund R, Jones MA, Magarey ME, et al: Manual test for specific structural differentiation in the subacromial space: correlation between specific manual testing and ultrasonography. *Proceedings of the Tenth Biennial Conference*, Melbourne, Manipulative Physiotherapists Association of Australia, 1997:146.
289. Wilk KE, Obma P, Simpson CD, et al: Shoulder injuries in the overhead athlete. *J Orthop Sports Phys Ther* 39:38–54, 2009.
290. Wilk KE, Arrigo CA, Andrews JR: Current concepts: the stabilizing structures of the glenohumeral joint. *J Orthop Sports Phys Ther* 25:364–379, 1997.
291. Gerber C, Krushell RJ: Isolated rupture of the tendon of the subscapularis muscle: clinical features in 16 cases. *J Bone Joint Surg* 73B:389–394, 1991.
292. Safee-Rad R, Shwedyk E, Quanbury AO, et al: Normal functional range of motion of upper limb joints during performance of three feeding activities. *Arch Phys Med Rehabil* 71:505–509, 1990.
293. Mannerkorpi K, Svantesson U, Carlsson J, et al: Tests of functional limitations in fibromyalgia syndrome: a reliability study. *Arthritis Care Res* 12:193–199, 1999.
294. Yang JL, Lin JJ: Reliability of function-related tests in patients with shoulder pathologies. *J Orthop Sports Phys Ther.* 36:572–576, 2006.
295. Ellman H, Hanker G, Bayer M: Repair of the rotator cuff: End results of factors influencing reconstruction. *J Bone Joint Surg* 68A:1136–1142, 1986.
296. Lippitt SB, Harryman DT III, Matsen FA III. A practical tool for evaluating function. The simple shoulder test. In: Matsen FA III, Fu FH, Hawkins RJ, eds. *The Shoulder: A Balance of Mobility and Stability*. Rosemont, IL: American Academy of Orthopaedic Surgeons, 1993:501–518.
297. Fuchs B, Jost B, Gerber C: Posterior-inferior capsular shift for the treatment of recurrent, voluntary posterior subluxation of the shoulder. *J Bone Joint Surg* 82A:16–25, 2000.
298. Harryman DT II, Matsen FA III, Sidles JA: Arthroscopic management of refractory shoulder stiffness. *Arthroscopy* 13:133–147, 1997.
299. Matsen FA, Lippitt SB, Sidles JA, et al: Evaluating the shoulder. In: Matsen FA, Lippitt SB, Sidles JA, et al, eds. *Practical Evaluation and Management of the Shoulder*. Philadelphia, PA: WB Saunders, 1994:1–17.
300. Beaton DE, Richards RR: Measuring function of the shoulder. A cross-sectional comparison of five questionnaires. *J Bone and Joint Surg* 78A:882–890, 1996.
301. Beaton DE, Richards RR: Assessing the reliability and responsiveness of five shoulder questionnaires. *J Shoulder Elbow Surg* 7:565–572, 1998.
302. Roach KE, Budiman-Mak E, Songsiridej N, et al: Development of a shoulder pain and disability index. *Arthritis Care Res* 4:143–149, 1991.
303. Hudak PL, Amadio PC, Bombardier C, et al: Development of an upper extremity outcome measure: the DASH (Disabilities of the Arm, Shoulder, and Hand). *Am J Ind Med* 29:602–608, 1995.
304. Leggin BG, Michener LA, Shaffer MA, et al: The Penn shoulder score: reliability and validity. *J Orthop Sports Phys Ther* 36:138–151, 2006.
305. Falsone SA, Gross MT, Guskiewicz KM, et al: One-arm hop test: reliability and effects of arm dominance. *J Orthop Sports Phys Ther* 32:98–103, 2002.
306. Calis M, Akgun K, Birtane M, et al: Diagnostic values of clinical diagnostic tests in subacromial impingement syndrome. *Ann Rheum Dis* 59:44–47, 2000.

307. Pink MM, Jobe FW: Biomechanics of swimming. In: Zachazewski JE, Magee DJ, Quillen WS, eds. *Athletic Injuries and Rehabilitation.* Philadelphia, PA: WB Saunders, 1996:317–331.
308. Post M, Cohen J: Impingement syndrome: a review of late stage II and early stage III lesions. *Clin Orthop Relat Res* 207:127–132, 1986.
309. Hawkins RJ, Kennedy JC: Impingement syndrome in athletics. *Am J Sports Med* 8:151–163, 1980.
310. Ure BM, Tiling T, Kirchner R, et al: Zuverlassigkeit der klinischen untersuchung der schulter im vergleich zur arthroskopie. *Unfallchirurg* 96:382–386, 1993.
311. MacDonald PB, Clark P, Sutherland K: An analysis of the diagnostic accuracy of the Hawkins and Neer subacromial impingement signs. *J Shoulder Elbow Surg* 9:299–301, 2000.
312. Rupp S, Berninger K, Hopf T: Shoulder problems in high level swimmers—impingement, anterior instability, muscular imbalance. *Int J Sports Med* 16:557–562, 1995.
313. Hertel R, Ballmer FT, Lombert SM, et al: Lag signs in the diagnosis of rotator cuff rupture. *J Elbow Shoulder Surg Am* 5:307–313, 1996.
314. Zaslav KR: Internal rotation resistance strength test: a new diagnostic test to differentiate intra-articular pathology from outlet (Neer) impingement syndrome in the shoulder. *J Shoulder Elbow Surg* 10:23–27, 2001.
315. Park IIB, Yokota A, Gill HS, et al: Diagnostic accuracy of clinical tests for the different degrees of subacromial impingement syndrome. *J Bone Joint Surg Am* 87:1446–1455, 2005.
316. McLaughlin H: On the frozen shoulder. *Bull Hosp Joint Dis* 12:383–393, 1951.
317. Hermann B, Rose DW: Stellenwert von Anamnese und klinischer Untersuchung beim degenerativen Impingement Syndrom im Vergleich zu operativen Befunden-eine prospektive Studie. *Z Orthop Ihre Grenzgeb* 134:166–170, 1996.
318. Akgün K, Karamehmetoglu SS, Sahin Ü, et al: Subakromiyal sikisma sendromu klinik tanisinda sikisma (Neer) testinin önemi. *Fizik Tedavi ve Rehabilitasyon Dergisi* 22:5–7, 1997.
319. Wolf EM, Agrawal V: Transdeltoid palpation (the Rent test) in the diagnosis of rotator cuff tears. *J Shoulder Elbow Surg* 10:470–473, 2001.
320. Patte D, Goutallier D, Monpierre H, et al: Over-extension lesions. *Rev Chir Orthop* 74:314–318, 1988.
321. Arthuis M: Obstetrical paralysis of the brachial plexus I. diagnosis: clinical study of the initial period. *Rev Chir Orthop Reparatrice Appar Mot* 58:124–136, 1972.
322. Walch G, Boulahia A, Calderone S, et al: The 'dropping' and 'hornblower's' signs in evaluation of rotator-cuff tears. *J Bone Joint Surg Br* 80:624–628, 1998.
323. Tomberlin J: *Physical Diagnostic Tests of the Shoulder: An Evidence-Based Perspective.* La Crosse, WI: Orthopedic Section, APTA, Inc., 2001.
324. Maitland G: *Peripheral Manipulation*, 3rd ed. London: Butterworth, 1991.
325. Mullen F: Locking and quadrant of the shoulder:relationships of the humerus and scapula during locking and quadrant, *Proceedings of the Sixth Biennial Conference, Manipulative Therapist Association of Australia*, Adelaide, Australia, 1989:130–137.
326. Neer CS: Anatomy of shoulder reconstruction. In: Neer CS, ed. *Shoulder Reconstruction.* Philadelphia, PA: WB Saunders, 1990:1–39.
327. Jobe FW, Moynes DR: Delineation of diagnostic criteria and a rehabilitation program for rotator cuff injuries. *Am J Sports Med* 10:336–339, 1982.
328. Malanga GA, Jenp YN, Growney ES, et al: EMG analysis of shoulder positioning in testing and strengthening the supraspinatus. *Med Sci Sports Exerc* 28:661–664, 1996.
329. Glascow S, Bruce RA, Yacobucci GN, et al: Arthroscopic resection of glenoid labral tears in the athlete. *Arthroscopy* 8:48–54, 1992.
330. Liu SH, Henry MH, Nuccion S, et al: Diagnosis of glenoid labral tears: a comparison between magnetic resonance imaging and clinical examinations. *Am J Sports Med* 24:149–154, 1996.
331. Hurley JA, Andersen TE: Shoulder arthroscopy: its role in evaluating shoulder disorders in the athlete. *Am J Sports Med* 18:480–483, 1990.
332. Liu SH, Henry MH, Nuccion SL: A prospective evaluation of a new physical examination in predicting glenoid labral tears. *Am J Sports Med* 24:721–725, 1996.
333. Kim SH, Park JS, Jeong WK, et al: The Kim test: a novel test for posteroinferior labral lesion of the shoulder – a comparison to the jerk test. *Am J Sports Med* 33:1188–1192, 2005.
334. Field LD, Savoie FH: Arthroscopic suture repair of superior labral detachment lesions of the shoulder. *Am J Sports Med* 21:783–791, 1993.
335. Magee DJ: *Shoulder, Orthopedic Physical Assessment.* Philadelphia, PA: WB Saunders, 1992:90–142.
336. Yergason RM: Rupture of biceps. *J Bone Joint Surg* 13:160, 1931.
337. Akgün K: *Kronik subakromiyal sikisma sendromunun konservatif tedavisinde ultrasonun etkinligi. [Proficiency Thesis].* Istanbul: University of Istanbul, 1993.
338. Bak K, Faunl P: Clinical findings in competitive swimmers with shoulder pain. *Am J Sports Med* 25:254–260, 1997.
339. O'Brien SJ, Pagnani MJ, Fealy S, et al: The active compression test; a new and effective test for diagnosing labral tears and acromioclavicular abnormality. *Am J Sports Med* 26:610–613, 1998.
340. Kibler WB: Specificity and sensitivity of the anterior slide test in throwing athletes with superior glenoid labral tears. *Arthroscopy* 11:296–300, 1995.
341. McFarland EG, Kim TK, Savino RM: Clinical assessment of three common tests for superior labral anterior-posterior lesions. *Am J Sports Med* 30:810–815, 2002.
342. Parentis MA, Mohr KJ, ElAttrache NS: Disorders of the superior labrum: review and treatment guidelines. *Clin Orthop Relat Res* 77–87, 2002.
343. Nakagawa S, Yoneda M, Hayashida K, et al: Forced shoulder abduction and elbow flexion test: a new simple clinical test to detect superior labral injury in the throwing shoulder. *Arthroscopy* 21:1290–1295, 2005.
344. Snyder SJ, Karzel RP, Del Pizzo W, et al: SLAP lesions of the shoulder. *Arthroscopy* 6:274–279, 1990.
345. Kim SH, Ha KI, Han KY: Biceps load test: A clinical test for superior labrum anterior and posterior lesions (SLAP) in shoulders with recurrent anterior dislocations. *Am J Sports Med* 27:300–303, 1999.
346. Kim SH, Ha KI, Ahn JH, et al: Biceps load test II: A clinical test for SLAP lesions of the shoulder. *Arthroscopy* 17:160–164, 2001.
347. Mimori K, Muneta T, Nakagawa T, et al: A new pain provocation test for superior labral tears of the shoulder. *Am J Sports Med* 27:137–142, 1999.
348. Myers TH, Zemanovic JR, Andrews JR: The resisted supination external rotation test: a new test for the diagnosis of superior labral anterior posterior lesions [published online ahead of print July 7, 2005]. *Am J Sports Med* 33:1315–1320.
349. Powell JW, Huijbregts PA: Concurrent criterion-related validity of acromioclavicular joint physical examination tests: A systematic review. *J Man Manip Ther* 14:E19–E29, 2006.
350. Chronopoulos E, Kim TK, Park HB, et al: Diagnostic value of physical tests for isolated chronic acromioclavicular lesions. *Am J Sports Med* 32:655–661, 2004.
351. Engebretsen L, Craig EV: Radiographic features of shoulder instability. *Clin Orthop* 291:29–44, 1993.
352. Neer CSI: Involuntary inferior and multidirectional instability of the shoulder: Etiology, recognition, and treatment. *Instr Course Lect* 34:232–238, 1985.
353. Neer CSI, Foster CR: Inferior capsular shift for involuntary inferior and multidirectional instability of the shoulder. *J Bone Joint Surg* 62A:897–908, 1980.
354. Pollock RG: Multidirectional and posterior instability of the shoulder. In: Norris TR, ed. *Orthopaedic Knowledge Update: Shoulder and Elbow.* Rosemont, IL: American Academy of Orthopaedic Surgeons, 1997: 85–94.
355. Emery RJH, Mullaji AB: Glenohumeral joint instability in normal adolescents: Incidence and significance. *J Bone Joint Surg* 73B:406–408, 1991.
356. Lintner SA, Levy A, Kenter K, et al: Glenohumeral translation in the asymptomatic athlete's shoulder and its relationship to other clinically measurable anthropometric variables. *Am J Sports Med* 24:716–720, 1996.
357. Brown GA, Tan JL, Kirkley A: The lax shoulder in females. Issues, answers, but many more questions. *Clin Orthop Relat Res* 372:110–122, 2000.
358. Bigliani LU: *The Unstable Shoulder.* Rosemont, IL: American Academy Orthopaedic Surgeons, 1995.
359. Gerber C, Ganz R: Clinical assessment of instability of the shoulder. *J Bone Joint Surg* 66B:551, 1984.
360. Hawkins RJ, Schutte JP, Janda DH, et al: Translation of the glenohumeral joint with the patient under anesthesia. *J Shoulder Elbow Surg* 5:286–292, 1996.
361. Hanyman DT, et al. Translation of the humeral head on the glenoid with passive glenohumeral motion. *J Bone Joint Surg* 72A:1334–1342, 1990.
362. Mok DWH, Fogg AJB, Hokan R, et al: The diagnostic value of arthroscopy in glenohumeral instability. *J Bone Joint Surg* 72B:698–700, 1990.
363. Callanan M, Tzannes A, Hayes KC, et al: Shoulder instability. Diagnosis and management. *Aust Fam Physician* 30:655–661, 2001.

364. Jobe FW, Bradley JP: The diagnosis and nonoperative treatment of shoulder injuries in athletes. *Clin Sports Med* 8:419–439, 1989.
365. Levy AS, Lintner S, Kenter K, et al: Intra- and interobserver reproducibility of the shoulder laxity examination. *Am J Sports Med* 27:460–463, 1999.
366. Speer KP, Hannafin JA, Altchek DW, et al: An evaluation of the shoulder relocation test. *Am J Sports Med* 22:177–183, 1994.
367. Hamner DL, Pink MM, Jobe FW: A modification of the relocation test: arthroscopic findings associated with a positive test. *J Shoulder Elbow Surg* 9:263–267, 2000.
368. Rockwood CA: Subluxations and dislocations about the shoulder. In: Rockwood CA, Green DP, eds. *Fractures in Adults—I.* Philadelphia, PA: JB Lippincott, 1984.
369. Gross ML, Distefano MC: Anterior release test: A new test for occult shoulder instability. *Clin Orthop Relat Res* 339:105–108, 1997.
370. Lo IK, Nonweiler B, Woolfrey M, et al: An evaluation of the apprehension, relocation, and surprise tests for anterior shoulder instability. *Am J Sports Med* 32:301–307, 2004.
371. Wilk KE, Andrews JR, Arrigo CA: The physical examination of the glenohumeral joint: Emphasis on the stabilizing structures. *J Orthop Sports Phys Ther* 25:380–389, 1997.
372. Andrews JR, Timmerman LA, Wilk KE: Baseball. In: Pettrone FA, ed. *Athletic Injuries of the Shoulder.* New York: McGraw-Hill, 1995:323–331.
373. Rockwood CA Jr, Szalay EA, Curtis RJ et al: X-ray evaluation of shoulder problems. In: Rockwood CA Jr, Matsen FA III, eds. *The Shoulder.* Philadelphia, PA: WB Saunders, 1990:178–207.
374. Swen WA, Jacobs WG, Neve WC, et al: Is sonography performed by the rheumatologist as useful as arthrography executed by the radiologist for the assessment of full thickness rotator cuff tears? *J Rheum* 25:1800–1806, 1998.
375. Kneeland JB: Magnetic resonance imaging: general principles and techniques. In: Iannotti JP, Williams GR, eds. *Disorders of the Shoulder: Diagnosis and Management.* Philadelphia, PA: Lippincott Williams & Wilkins, 1999:911–925.
376. Tirman PF, Feller JF, Janzen DL, et al: Association of glenoid labral cysts with labral tears and glenohumeral instability: radiologic findings and clinical significance. *Radiology* 190:653–658, 1994.
377. Magarey ME, Hayes MG, Trott PH: The accuracy of manipulative physiotherapy diagnosis of shoulder complex dysfunction: a pilot study. *Proceedings of the Sixth Niennial Conference.* Adelaide, Manipulative Physiotherapists Association of Australia, 1989:119–129.
378. Magarey ME, Hayes MG, Frick RA, et al: The shoulder complex: A preliminary analysis of diagnostic agreement reached from a physiotherapy clinical examination and an arthroscopic evaluation. In: Jull GA, ed. *Clinical Solutions: Proceedings of the Ninth Biennial Conference.* Gold Coast: Manipulative Physiotherapists Association of Australia, 1995:92–94.
379. Litchfield R, Hawkins R, Dillman CJ, et al: Rehabilitation of the overhead athlete. *J Orthop Sports Phys Ther* 2:433–441, 1993.
380. Booth FW: Physiologic and biochemical effects of immobilization on muscle. *Clin Orthop Relat Res* 219:15–21, 1987.
381. Eiff MP, Smith AT, Smith GE: Early mobilization versus immobilization in the treatment of lateral ankle sprains. *Am J Sports Med* 22:83–88, 1994.
382. Akeson WH, et al.: Collagen cross-linking alterations in the joint contractures: changes in the reducible cross-links in periarticular connective tissue after 9 weeks immobilization. *Connect Tissue Res* 5:15–21, 1977.
383. Akeson WH, Amiel D, Abel MF, et al: Effects of immobilization on joints. *Clin Orthop* 219:28–37, 1987.
384. Wilk KE, Arrigo C, Andrews JR: Rehabilitation of the elbow in the throwing athlete. *J Orthop Sports Phys Ther* 17:305–317, 1993.
385. Coutts RD: Continuous passive motion in the rehabilitation of the total knee patient. Its role and effect. *Orthop Rev* 15:27, 1986.
386. Dehne E, Tory R: Treatment of joint injuries by immediate mobilization based upon the spiral adaption concept. *Clin Orthop* 77:218–232, 1971.
387. Haggmark T, Eriksson E: Cylinder or mobile cast brace after knee ligament surgery. *Am J Sports Med* 7:48–56, 1979.
388. Noyes FR, Mangine RE, Barber S: Early knee motion after open and arthroscopic anterior cruciate ligament reconstruction. *Am J Sports Med* 15:149–160, 1987.
389. Ellsworth AA, Mullaney M, Tyler TF, et al: Electromyography of selected shoulder musculature during unweighted and weighted pendulum exercises. *N Am J Sports Phys Ther* 1:73–79, 2006.
390. Magee DJ, Mattison R, Reid DC: Shoulder instability and impingement syndrome. In: Magee DJ, Zachazewski JE, Quillen WS, eds. *Pathology and Intervention in Musculoskeletal Rehabilitation.* St. Louis, MI: Saunders, 2009:125–160.
391. Townsend J, Jobe FW, Pink M, et al: Electromyographic analysis of the glenohumeral muscles during a baseball rehabilitation program. *Am J Sports Med* 3:264–272, 1991.
392. Horrigan JM, Shellock FG, Mink JH, et al: Magnetic resonance imaging evaluation of muscle usage associated with three exercises for rotator cuff rehabilitation. *Med Sci Sports Exerc* 31:1361, 1999.
393. Morrison DS, Frogameni AD, Woodworth P: Nonoperative treatment of subacromial impingement syndrome. *J Bone Joint Surg Am* 79:732–737, 1997.
394. Kibler WB: Concepts in exercise rehabilitation of athletic injury. In: Leadbetter WB, Buckwalter JA, Gordon SL, eds. *Sports-Induced Inflammation: Clinical and Basic Science Concepts.* Park Ridge, IL: American Academy of Orthopaedic Surgeons, 1990:759–769.
395. Kibler BW: Closed kinetic chain rehabilitation for sports injuries. *Phys Med Rehabil Clin N Am* 11:369–384, 2000.
396. Dillman CJ, Murray TA, Hintermeister RA: Biomechanical differences of open and closed chain exercises with respect to the shoulder. *J Sport Rehabil* 3:228–238, 1994.
397. Neer CSI, Watson KC, Stanton FJ: Recent experience in total shoulder replacement. *J Bone and Joint Surg* 64:319–337, 1982.
398. Walch G, Ascani C, Boulahia A, et al: Static posterior subluxation of the humeral head: an unrecognized entity responsible for glenohumeral osteoarthritis in the young adult. *J Shoulder Elbow Surg* 11:309–314, 2002.
399. Hayes PRL, Flatow EL: Total shoulder arthroplasty in the young patient. *Instr Course Lect* 50:73–88, 2001.
400. DeSeze M: *L'épaule sénile hémorragique. L'actualité rhumatologique.* Paris: Expansion Scientifique Française, 1968:107–115.
401. Garancis JC, Cheung HS, Halverson PB, et al: "Milwaukee shoulder"—Association of microspheroids containing hydroxyapatite crystals, active collagenase, and neutral protease with rotator cuff defects. III. Morphologic and biochemical studies of an excised synovium showing chondromatosis. *Arthritis Rheum* 24:484–491, 1981.
402. Halverson PB, Cheung HS, McCarty DJ, et al: "Milwaukee shoulder"—Association of microspheroids containing hydroxyapatite crystals, active collagenase, and neutral protease with rotator cuff defects. II. Synovial fluid studies. *Arthritis Rheum* 24:474–483, 1981.
403. McCarty DJ, Halverson PB, Carrera GF, et al: "Milwaukee shoulder"—Association of microspheroids containing hydroxyapatite crystals, active collagenase, and neutral protease with rotator cuff defects. I. Clinical aspects. *Arthritis Rheum* 24:464–473, 1981.
404. Jensen KL, Williams GR, Russell IJ, et al: Rotator cuff tear arthropathy. *J Bone Joint Surg Am* 81-A:1312–1324, 1999.
405. Neer CS II, Craig EV, Fukuda H: Cuff-tear arthropathy. *J Bone Joint Surg* 65-A:1232–1244, 1983.
406. Duplay S: De la péri-arthrite scapulo-humérale et des raideurs de l'épaule qui en sont la consequénce. *Arch Gen Méd* 20:513–542, 1872.
407. Neviaser JS: Adhesive capsulitis of the shoulder. Study of pathological findings in periarthritis of the shoulder. *J Bone Joint Surg* 27:211–222, 1945.
408. Binder AI, Bulgen DY, Hazleman BL, et al: Frozen shoulder: A long-term prospective study. *Ann Rheum Dis* 43:361–364, 1984.
409. Lloyd-Roberts GG, French PR: Periarthritis of the shoulder: A study of the disease and its treatment. *Br Med J* 1:1569–1574, 1959.
410. Bridgman JF: Periarthritis of the shoulder and diabetes mellitus. *Ann Rheum Dis* 31:69–71, 1972.
411. Miller MD, Rockwood CA Jr: Thawing the frozen shoulder: The "patient" patient. *Orthopedics* 19:849–853, 1997.
412. Pal B, Anderson JJ, Dick WC: Limitations of joint mobility and shoulder capsulitis in insulin and noninsulin dependent diabetes mellitus. *Br J Rheumatol* 25:147–151, 1986.
413. Fisher L, Kurtz A, Shipley M: Relationship of cheiroarthropathy and frozen shoulder in patients with insulin dependent diabetes mellitus. *Br J Rheum* 25:141, 1986.
414. DePalma AF: Loss of scapulohumeral motion (frozen shoulder). *Ann Surg* 135:193–197, 1952.
415. Bowman CA, Jeffcoate WJ, Patrick M: Bilateral adhesive capsulitis, oligoarthritis and proximal myopathy as presentation of hypothyroidism. *Br J Rheumatol* 27:62–64, 1988.
416. Speer KP, Cavanaugh JT, Warren RF, et al: A role for hydrotherapy in shoulder rehabilitation. *Am J Sports Med* 21:850–853, 1993.
417. Wohlgethan JR: Frozen shoulder in hyperthyroidism. *Arthritis Rheum* 30:936–939, 1987.

418. Mintner WT: The shoulder-hand syndrome in coronary disease. *J Med Assoc Ga* 56:45–49, 1967.
419. Coventry MB: Problem of the painful shoulder. *JAMA* 151:177, 1953.
420. Tyber MA: Treatment of the painful shoulder syndrome with amitriptyline and lithium carbonate. *Can Med Assoc J* 111:137, 1974.
421. Bulgen DY, Binder A, Hazelman BL: Immunological studies in frozen shoulder. *J Rheumatol* 9:893–898, 1982.
422. Rizk TE, Pinals RS: Histocompatibility type and racial incidence in frozen shoulder. *Arch Phys Med Rehabil* 65:33–34, 1984.
423. Lundberg BJ: The frozen shoulder. *Acta Orthop Scand* 119(Suppl.):1–5, 1969.
424. Hannafin JA, Chiaia TA: Adhesive capsulitis. A treatment approach. *Clin Orthop Relat Res* 372:95–109, 2000.
425. Nash P, Hazelman BD: Frozen Shoulder. *Baillieres Clin Rheumatol* 3:551–566, 1989.
426. Neviaser JS: Adhesive capsulitis and the stiff and painful shoulder. *Orthop Clin North Am* 11:327–331, 1980.
427. Neviaser RJ: Painful conditions affecting the shoulder. *Clin Orthop* 173:63–69, 1983.
428. Reeves B: The natural history of the frozen shoulder syndrome. *Scand J Rheumatol* 4:193–196, 1975.
429. Zuckerman JD, Cuomo F: Frozen shoulder. In: Matsen FA III, Fu FH, Hawkins RJ, eds. *The Shoulder: A Balance of Mobility and Stability*. Rosemont, IL: American Academy of Orthopaedic Surgeons, 1993:253–267.
430. Shaffer B, Tibone JE, Kerlan RK: Frozen shoulder: A long-term follow-up. *J Bone Joint Surg Am* 74:738–746, 1992.
431. Griggs SM, Ahn A, Green A: Idiopathic adhesive capsulitis: a prospective functional outcome study of nonoperative treatment. *J Bone Joint Surg Am* 82-A:1398–1407, 2000.
432. Hannafin JA, DiCarlo EF, Wickiewicz TL, et al: Adhesive capsulitis: Capsular fibroplasia of the glenohumeral joint. *J Shoulder Elbow Surg* 3 (Suppl.):66–74, 1994.
433. Rodeo SA, Hannafin JA, Tom J, et al: Immunolocalization of cytokines and their receptors in adhesive capsulitis of the shoulder. *J Orthop Res* 15:427–436, 1997.
434. Wiley AM: Arthroscopic appearance of frozen shoulder. *Arthroscopy* 7:138–143, 1991.
435. Bunker TD, Anthony PP: The pathology of frozen shoulder. A Dupuytren-like disease. *J Bone Joint Surg* 77B:677–683, 1995.
436. Grubbs N: Frozen shoulder syndrome: A review of literature. *J Orthop Sports Phys Ther* 18:479–487, 1993.
437. Hjelm R, Draper C, Spencer S: Anterior-superior capsular length insufficiency in the painful shoulder. *J Orthop Sports Phys Ther* 23:216–222, 1996.
438. Uhthoff HK, Sarkar K: An algorithm for shoulder pain caused by soft tissue disorders. *Clin Orthop* 254:121, 1990.
439. Boyle-Walker KL, Gabard DL, Bietsch E, et al: A profile of patients with adhesive capsulitis. *J Hand Ther* 10:222–228, 1997.
440. Tamai K, Yamato M: Abnormal synovium in the frozen shoulder: A preliminary report with dynamic magnetic resonance imaging. *J Shoulder Elbow Surg* 6:534–543, 1997.
441. Pajareya K, Chadchavalpanichaya N, Painmanakit S, et al: Effectiveness of physical therapy for patients with adhesive capsulitis: a randomized controlled trial. *J Med Assoc Thai* 87:473–480, 2004.
442. McClure PW, Flowers KR: Treatment of limited shoulder motion using an elevation splint. *Phys Ther* 72:57, 1992.
443. Laska T, Hannig K: Physical Therapy for spinal accessory nerve injury complicated by adhesive capsulitis. *Phys Ther* 81:936–944, 2001.
444. Rizk TE, Christopher RP, Pinals RS, et al: Adhesive capsulitis (frozen shoulder): A new approach to its management and treatment. *Arch Phys Med Rehabil* 64:29–33, 1983.
445. Grey RG: The natural history of "idiopathic" frozen shoulder. *J Bone Joint Surg Am* 60:564, 1978.
446. Haggart GE, Digman RJ, Sullivan TS: Management of the "frozen" shoulder. *JAMA* 161:1219–1222, 1956.
447. Withers RJW: The painful shoulder: Review of one hundred personal cases with remarks on the pathology. *J Bone Joint Surg* 31:414–417, 1949.
448. Diercks RL, Stevens M: Gentle thawing of the frozen shoulder: a prospective study of supervised neglect versus intensive physical therapy in seventy-seven patients with frozen shoulder syndrome followed up for two years. *J Shoulder Elbow Surg* 13:499–502, 2004.
449. Tovin BJ, Greenfield BH: Impairment-based diagnosis for the shoulder girdle. In: *Evaluation and Treatment of the Shoulder: An Integration of the Guide to Physical Therapist Practice*. Philadelphia, PA: F.A. Davis, 2001:55–74.
450. Leffert RD: The frozen shoulder. *Instr Course Lect* 34:199–203, 1985.
451. Owens-Burkhart H: Management of frozen shoulder. In: Donatelli RA, ed. *Physical Therapy of the Shoulder*. New York: Churchill Livingstone, 1991:91–116.
452. Wadsworth CT: Frozen shoulder. *Phys Ther* 1878–1883, 1986.
453. Bulgen DY, Binder A, Hazelman BL, et al: Frozen shoulder: Prospective clinical study with an evaluation of three treatment regimens. *Ann Rheum Dis* 43:353–360, 1984.
454. D'Acre JE, Beeney N, Scott DL: Injections and physiotherapy for the painful stiff shoulder. *Ann Rheum Dis* 48:322–325, 1989.
455. DeJong BA, Dahmen R, Hogeweg JA, et al: Intraarticular triamcinolone acetonide injection in patients with capsulitis of the shoulder: A comparative study of two dose regimes. *Clin Rehabil* 12:211–215, 1998.
456. Quigley TB: Indications for manipulation and corticosteroids in the treatment of stiff shoulder. *Surg Clin North Am* 43:1715–1720, 1975.
457. Steinbrocker O, Argyros TG: Frozen shoulder: Treatment by local injection of depot corticosteroids. *Arch Phys Med Rehabil* 55:209–213, 1974.
458. Hazelman BD: The painful stiff shoulder. *Rheumatol Phys Med* 11:413–421, 1972.
459. Binder A, Hazelman BL, Parr G, et al: A controlled study of oral prednisone in frozen shoulder. *Br J Rheumatol* 25:288–292, 1986.
460. Tyler TF, Roy T, Nicholas SJ, et al: Reliability and validity of a new method of measuring posterior shoulder tightness. *J Orthop Sports Phys Ther* 29:262–274, 1999.
461. Kennedy JC, Alexander IJ, Hayes KC: Nerve supply of the human knee and its functional importance. *Am J Sports Med* 10:329–335, 1982.
462. Baxendale RA, Ferrell WR, Wood L: Responses of quadriceps motor units to mechanical stimulation of knee joint receptors in decerebate cat. *Brain Res* 453:150–156, 1988.
463. Lippitt SB, Harris SL, Harryman DT II, et al: In vivo quantification of the laxity of normal and unstable glenohumeral joints. *J Shoulder Elbow Surg* 3:215–223, 1994.
464. Flatow EL, Warner JJP: Instability of the shoulder: Complex problems and failed repairs: Part I. Relevant biomechanics, multidirectional instability, and severe glenoid loss. *Instr Course Lect* 47:97–112, 1998.
465. Rowe CR, Sakellarides HT: Factors related to recurrences of anterior dislocations of the shoulder. *Clin Orthop* 20:40, 1961.
466. Maki NJ: Cineradiographic studies with shoulder instabilities. *Am J Sports Med* 16:362–364, 1988.
467. Sidles JA, Harryman DT, Harris SL, et al: In vivo quantification of glenohumeral stability. *Trans Orthop Res Soc* 16:646, 1991.
468. Arendt EA: Multidirectional shoulder instability. *Orthopedics* 11:113–120, 1988.
469. Garth WP, Allman FL, Armstrong WS: Occult anterior subluxations of the shoulder in noncontact sports. *Am J Sports Med* 15:579–585, 1987.
470. Jobe FW, Tibone JE, Jobe CM, et al: The shoulder in sports. In: Rockwood CA Jr, Matsen FA III, eds. *The Shoulder*. Philadelphia, PA: WB Saunders, 1990:963–967.
471. Schenk TJ, Brems JJ: Multidirectional instability of the shoulder: Pathophysiology, diagnosis, and management. *J Am Acad Orthop Surg* 6:65–72, 1998.
472. Hawkins RJ, Abrams JS, Schutte J: Multidirectional instability of the shoulder-An approach to diagnosis. *Orthop Trans* 11:246, 1987.
473. Gill TD, Micheli LJ, Gebhard F, et al: Bankhart repair for anterior instability of the shoulder: long term outcomes. *J Bone and Joint Surg* 79A:850–857, 1997.
474. Lippitt SB, et al. Diagnosis and management of AMBRII syndrome. *Tech Orthop* 6:61–69, 1991.
475. Berbig R, Weishaupt D, Prim J, et al: Primary anterior shoulder dislocation and rotator cuff tears. *J Shoulder Elbow Surg* 8:220–225, 1999.
476. Sonnabend DH: Treatment of primary anterior shoulder dislocation in patients older than 40 years of age. *Clin Orthop* 304:74–77, 1994.
477. Tijimes J, Loyd HM, Tullos HS: Arthrography in acute shoulder dislocations. *South Med J* 72:564–567, 1979.
478. Ireland ML, Andrews JR: Shoulder and elbow injuries in the young athlete. *Clin Sports Med* 7:473–494, 1988.
479. Hovelius L, Eriksson K, Fredin H, et al: Recurrences after initial dislocation of the shoulder. *J Bone Joint Surg [Am]* 65:343–349, 1983.
480. Warner JJP, Micheli LJ, Arslanian LE, et al: Patterns of flexibility, laxity, and strength in normal shoulders and shoulders with instability and impingement. *Am J Sports Med* 18:366–375, 1990.

481. Burkhart SS, Morgan CD, Kibler WB: Shoulder injuries in overhead athletes: the "dead arm" revisited. *Clin Sports Med* 19:125–158, 2000.
482. Snyder SJ, Karzel RP, Del Pizzo W, et al: SLAP lesions of the shoulder. *Arthoscopy* 6:274–279, 1990.
483. Morgan CD, Burkhart SS, Palmeri M, et al: Type II SLAP lesions: three subtypes and their relationship to superior instability and rotator cuff tears. *Arthroscopy* 14:553–565, 1998.
484. Berg EE, DeHoll D: Radiography of the medial elbow ligaments. *J Shoulder Elbow Surg* 6:528–533, 1997.
485. Urban WP, Babom DNM: Management of superior labral anterior posterior lesions. *Oper Tech Orthop* 5:223, 1995.
486. Maffet MW, Gartsman GM, Moseley B: Superior labrum-biceps tendon complex lesions of the shoulder. *Am J Sports Med* 23:93–98, 1995.
487. Mileski RA, Snyder SJ: Superior labral lesions in the shoulder: Pathoanatomy and surgical management. *J Am Acad Orthop Surg* 6:121–131, 1998.
488. Cordasco FA, Bigliani LU: Multidirectional shoulder instability: open surgical treatment. In: Warren RF, Craig EV, Altchek DW, eds. *The Unstable Shoulder*. Philadelphia, PA: Lippincott-Raven Publishers, 1999:249–261.
489. Snyder SJ, Banas MP, Karzel RP: An analysis of 140 injuries to the superior glenoid labrum. *J Shoulder Elbow Surg* 4:243–248, 1995.
490. Berg EE, Ciullo JV: The SLAP lesion: a cause of failure after distal clavicle resection. *Arthroscopy* 13:85–89, 1997.
491. Borsa PA, Sauers EL, Herling DE: Patterns of glenohumeral joint laxity and stiffness in healthy men and women. *Med Sci Sports Exerc* 32:1685–1690, 2000.
492. Huston LJ, Wojtys EM: Neuromuscular performance characteristics in elite female athletes. *Am J Sports Med* 24:427–436, 1996.
493. Lephart SM, Warner JJP, Borsa PA, et al: Proprioception of the shoulder joint in healthy, unstable and surgically repaired shoulders. *J Shoulder Elbow Surg* 3:371–380, 1994.
494. Burkhead WZ Jr, Rockwood CA Jr: Treatment of instability of the shoulder with an exercise program. *J Bone Joint Surg* 74A:890–896, 1992.
495. Schneider R, Prentice WE: Rehabilitation of the shoulder. In: Prentice WE, Voight ML, eds. *Techniques in Musculoskeletal Rehabilitation*. New York: McGraw-Hill, 2001:411–456.
496. Happee R, Van Der Helm FCT: The control of shoulder muscles during goal directed movements. *J Biomech* 28:1179–1191, 1995.
497. Tossy JD, Mead MC, Simond HM: Acromioclavicular separations: Useful and practical classification for treatment. *Clin Orthop* 28:111–119, 1963.
498. Rockwood CA Jr: Injuries to the acromioclavicular joint. In: Rockwood CA Jr, Green DP, eds. *Fractures in Adults*, 2nd ed. Philadelphia, PA: JB Lippincott, 1984:860–910.
499. Williams GR, Nguyen VD, Rockwood CA Jr: Classification and radiographic analysis of acromioclavicular dislocations. *Appl Radiol* 7:29–34, 1989.
500. Wirth MA, Rockwood CA Jr: Chronic conditions of the acromioclavicular and sternoclavicular joints. In: Chapman MW, ed. *Operative Orthopaedics*, 2nd ed. Philadelphia, PA: JB Lippincott, 1993:1673–1683.
501. Gordon EJ: Diagnosis and treatment of common shoulder disorders. *Med Trial Tech Q* 28:25–73, 1981.
502. Bannister GC, Wallace WA, Stableforth PG, et al: The management of acute acromioclavicular dislocation: a randomized prospective controlled trial. *J Bone Joint Surg* 71B:848–850, 1989.
503. Cox JS: Current method of treatment of acromioclavicular joint dislocations. *Orthopedics* 15:1041–1044, 1992.
504. Bjerneld H, Hovelius L, Thorling J: Acromioclavicular separations treated conservatively: a five year follow-up study. *Acta Orthop Scand* 54:743–745, 1983.
505. Dias JJ, Steingold RF, Richardson RA, et al: The conservative treatment of acromioclavicular dislocation: review after five years. *J Bone Joint Surg* 69B:719–722, 1987.
506. Glick JM, Milburn LJ, Haggerty JF, et al: Dislocated acromioclavicular joint: follow-up study of thirty-five unreduced acromioclavicular dislocations. *Am J Sports Med* 5:264–270, 1977.
507. Rawes ML, Dias JJ: Long-term results of conservative treatment for acromioclavicular dislocation. *J Bone Joint Surg* 78B:410–412, 1996.
508. Sleeswijk-Viser SV, Haarsma SM, Speeckaert MTC: Conservative treatment of acromioclavicular dislocation: Jones strap versus mitella. *Acta Orthop. Scand* 55:483, 1984.
509. Tibone J, Sellers R, Tonino P: Strength testing after third-degree acromioclavicular dislocations. *Am J Sports Med* 20:328–331, 1992.
510. Larsen E, Bjerg-Nielsen A, Christensen P: Conservative or surgical treatment of acromioclavicular dislocation: a prospective, controlled randomized study. *J Bone Joint Surg* 68A:552–555, 1986.
511. Taft TN, Wilson FC, Oglesby JW: Dislocation of the acromioclavicular joint: an end-result study. *J Bone Joint Surg* 69A:1045–1051, 1987.
512. Gerber C, Galantay R, Hersche O: The pattern of pain produced by irritation of the acromioclavicular joint and the subacromial space. *J Shoulder Elbow Surg* 7:352–355, 1998.
513. Schneider R, Prentice WE, Blackburn TA: Rehabilitation of shoulder injuries. In: Voight ML, Hoogenboom BJ, Prentice WE, eds. *Musculoskeletal Interventions: Techniques for Therapeutic Exercise*. New York: McGraw-Hill, 2007:467–513.
514. Zeman CA, Arcand MA, Cantrell JS, et al: The rotator cuff-deficient arthritic shoulder: Diagnosis and surgical management. *J Am Acad Orthop Surg* 6:337–348, 1998.
515. Sisk TD, Wright PE: Arthroplasty of the shoulder and elbow. In: Crenshaw AH, ed. *Campbell's Operative Orthopaedics*, 8th ed. St Louis, MO: Mosby, 1992.
516. Bergmann G: Biomechanics and pathomechanics of the shoulder joint with reference to prosthetic joint replacement. In: Koelbel R, et al, eds. *Shoulder Replacement*. Berlin: Spring-Verlag, 1987:33.
517. Williams GR Jr, Rockwood CA Jr: Massive rotator cuff defects and glenohumeral arthritis. In: Friedman RJ, ed. *Arthroplasty of the Shoulder*. New York: Thieme Medical Publishers, 1994:204–214.
518. Cofield RH: Degenerative and arthritic problems of the glenohumeral joint. In: Rockwood CA, Master R, eds. *The Shoulder*. Philadelphia, PA: WB Saunders, 1990:678–749.
519. Gartsman GM, Roddey TS, Hammerman SM: Shoulder arthroplasty with or without resurfacing of the glenoid in patients who have osteoarthritis. *J Bone Joint Surg Am* 82:26–34, 2000.
520. Van der Windt DA, Koes BW, de Jong BA, et al: Shoulder disorders in general practice: Incidence, patient characteristics, and management. *Ann Rheum Dis* 54:959–964, 1995.
521. Goldberg BA, Nowinski RJ, Matsen FA III: Outcome of nonoperative management of full-thickness rotator cuff tears. *Clin Orthop Relat Res* 1:99–107, 2001.
522. Kunkel SS, Hawkins RJ: Open repair of the rotator cuff. In: Andrews JR, Wilk KE, eds. *The Athlete's Shoulder*. New York: Churchill Livingstone, 1994:141–151.
523. Leffert RD, Rowe CR: Tendon ruptures. In: Rowe CR, ed. *The Shoulder*. New York: Churchill Livingstone, 1988:131–154.
524. Pettersson G: Rupture of the tendon aponeurosis of the shoulder joint in anterior inferior dislocation. *Acta Chir Scand* 77(Suppl.):1–184, 1942.
525. Yamanaka K, Fukuda H, Hamada K, et al: Incomplete thickness tears of the rotator cuff. *Orthop Traumatol Surg [Tokyo]* 26:713–717, 1983.
526. Cuillo J: Swimmer's shoulder. *Clin Sports Med* 5:115, 1984.
527. Park HB, Yokota A, Gill HS, et al: Diagnostic accuracy of clinical tests for the different degrees of subacromial impingement syndrome. *J Bone Joint Surg Am* 87:1446–1455, 2005.
528. Norwood LA, Barrack RL, Jacobson KE: Clinical presentation of complete tears of the rotator cuff. *J Bone Joint Surg Am* 71:499–505, 1989.
529. Ford LT, DeBender J: Tendon rupture after local steroid injection. *South Med J* 72:827–830, 1979.
530. Watson M: Major ruptures of the rotator cuff: The results of surgical repair in 89 patients. *J Bone Joint Surg Br* 67:618–624, 1985.
531. Kennedy JD, Willis RB: The effects of local steroid injections on tendons: A biomechanical and microscopic correlative study. *Am J Sports Med* 4:11–21, 1976.
532. Adebago A, Nash P, Hazleman BL: A prospective double-blind dummy placebo controlled study comparing triamcinolone hexacetomide injection with oral diclofenic 50 mg TDS in patients with rotator cuff tendinitis. *J Rheum* 17:1207–1209, 1990.
533. Hollingworth GR, Ellis RM, Hattersley TS: Comparison of injection techniques for shoulder pain: Results of a double-blind, randomized study. *BMJ* 287:1339–1341, 1983.
534. Bateman JE: Diagnosis and treatment of rupture of the rotator cuff. *Surg Clin North Am* 43:1523–1530, 1963.
535. Cofield RH: Current concepts review: Rotator cuff disease of the shoulder. *J Bone Joint Surg* 67A:974–979, 1985.
536. Essman JA, Bell RH, Askew M: Full-thickness rotator-cuff tear. Analysis of results. *Clin Orthop* 265:170–177, 1991.
537. Hawkins RJ: Surgical management of rotator cuff tears in surgery of the shoulder. In: Bateman JE, Welsh RP, eds. *Surgery of the Shoulder*. New York: Dekker, 1984:161–175.

538. Bartolozzi A, Andreychik D, Ahmad S: Determinants of outcome in the treatment of rotator cuff disease. *Clin Orthop* 308:90–97, 1994.
539. Bokor DJ, Hawkins RJ, Huckell GH, et al: Results of nonoperative management of full-thickness tears of the rotator cuff. *Clin Orthop* 294:103–110, 1993.
540. Hawkins RH, Dunlop R: Nonoperative treatment of rotator cuff tears. *Clin Orthop* 321:178–188, 1995.
541. Itoi E, Tabata S: Conservative treatment of rotator cuff tears. *Clin Orthop* 275:165–173, 1992.
542. Matsen FA III, Arntz CT, Lippitt SB: Rotator cuff. In: Rockwood CA, Matsen FA III, eds. *The Shoulder*. Philadelphia, PA: WB Saunders, 1998:810–813.
543. Matsen FH III, Lippitt SB, Sidles JA, et al: *Practical Evaluation of Management of the Shoulder*. Philadelphia, PA: WB Saunders, 1994:19–150.
544. Nixon JE, DiStefano V: Ruptures of the rotator cuff. *Orthop Clin North Am* 6:423–445, 1975.
545. Ellman H: Diagnosis and treatment of incomplete rotator cuff tears. *Clin Orthop* 254:64–74, 1990.
546. Chard M, Sattele L, Hazleman B: The long-term outcome of rotator cuff tendinitis—A review study. *Br J Rheum* 27:385–389, 1988.
547. Deutsch A, Altchek DW, Schwartz E, et al: Radiologic measurement of superior displacement of the humeral head in the impingement syndrome. *J Shoulder Elbow Surg* 5:186–193, 1996.
548. Kelkar R, Flatow EL, Bigliani LU, et al: The effects of articular congruence and humeral head rotation on glenohumeral kinematics. *Adv Bioeng* 28:19–20, 1994.
549. Kelkar R, Newton PM, Armengol J, et al: Glenohumeral kinematics. *J Shoulder Elbow Surg* 2(Suppl.):S28, 1993.
550. Howell SM: Normal and abnormal mechanics of the glenohumeral joint in the horizontal plane. *J Bone Joint Surg* 70:227–235, 1988.
551. Jarjavay JF: Sur la luxation du tendon de la longue portion du muscle biceps humeral; sur la luxation des tendons des muscles peroniers latercux. *Gaz hebd med chir* 21:325, 1867.
552. Stenlund B, Goldie I, Hagberg M, et al: Shoulder tendinitis and its relation to heavy manual work and exposure to vibration. *Scand J Work Environ Health* 19:43–49, 1993.
553. Andersen JH, Gaardboe O: Musculoskeletal disorders of the neck and upper limb among sewing machine operators: a clinical investigation. *Am J Ind Med* 24:689–700, 1993.
554. Neer CS, Poppen NK: Supraspinatus outlet. *Orthop Trans* 11:234, 1987.
555. Brewer BJ: Aging of the rotator cuff. *Am J Sports Med* 17:102–110, 1979.
556. Ogata S, Uhthoff HK: Acromial enthesopathy and rotator cuff tears: A radiographic and histologic postmortem investigation of the coracoacromial arc. *Clin Orthop* 254:39–48, 1990.
557. Uhthoff HK, Loehr J: The effect of aging on the soft tissues of the shoulder. In: Matsen FA, Fu FA, Hawkins R, eds. *The Shoulder: A Balance of Mobility and Stability*. Rosemont, IL: American Academy of Orthopaedic Surgeons, 1993:269–278.
558. Ohlsson K, Hansson G-A, Balogh I, et al: Disorders or the neck and upper limbs in women in the fish processing industry. *Occup Environ Med* 51:826–832, 1994.
559. Checkoway H, Pearce N, Dement JM: Design and conduct of occupational epidemiology studies: I. design aspects of cohort studies. *Am J Ind Med* 15:363–373, 1989.
560. Jobe FW, Kvitne RS, Giangarra CE: Shoulder pain in the overhand and throwing athlete: the relationship of anterior instability and rotator cuff impingement. *Orthop Rev* 18:963–975, 1989.
561. Mohr KJ, Moynes Schwab DR, Tovin BJ: Musculoskeletal pattern F: impaired joint mobility, motor function, muscle performance, and range of motion associated with localized inflammation. In: Tovin BJ, Greenfield B, eds. *Evaluation and Treatment of the Shoulder: An Integration of the Guide to Physical Therapist Practice*. Philadelphia, PA: F.A. Davis, 2001:210–230.
562. Jobe CM, et al: Anterior shoulder instability, impingement and rotator cuff tear. In: Jobe FW, ed. *Operative Techniques in Upper Extremity Sports Injuries*. St Louis, MO: Mosby-Year Book, 1996.
563. Cools AM, Witvrouw EE, Declercq GA, et al: Scapular muscle recruitment patterns: trapezius muscle latency with and without impingement symptoms. *Am J Sports Med* 31:542–549, 2003.
564. Thigpen CA, Padua DA, Morgan N, et al: Scapular kinematics during supraspinatus rehabilitation exercise: a comparison of full-can versus empty-can techniques. *Am J Sports Med* 34:644–652, 2006.
565. Neer CS II, Welsh RP: The shoulder in sports. *Orthop Clin North Am* 8:583–591, 1977.
566. DePalma AF, Gallery G, Bennett CA: Variational anatomy and degenerative lesions of the shoulder joint. In: Blount W, ed. *American Academy of Orthopaedic Surgeons Instructional Course Lectures*. Ann Arbor, MI: JW Edwards, 1949:255–281.
567. DePalma AF, Gallery G, Bennett CA: Degenerative lesions of the shoulder joint at various age groups which are compatible with good function. In: Blount W, ed. *American Academy of Orthopaedic Surgeons Instructional Course Lectures*. Ann Arbor, MI: JW Edwards, 1950:168.
568. Ozaki J, Fujimoto S, Nakagawa Y, et al: Tears of the rotator cuff on the shoulder associated with pathological changes in the acromion: A study in cadavera. *J Bone Joint Surg [Am]* 70-A:1224–1230, 1988.
569. Petterson G: Rupture of the tendon aponeurosis of the shoulder joint in anterior inferior dislocation. *Acta Chir Scand* 99(Suppl.):1–184, 1942.
570. Sher J, Uribe J, Posada A, et al: Abnormal findings on magnetic resonance images of symptomatic shoulders. *J Bone Joint Surg* 77A:10–15, 1995.
571. Cotton RE, Rideout DF: Tears of the humeral rotator cuff: A radiological and pathological necropsy survey. *J Bone Joint Surg* 46B:314–328, 1964.
572. Constant CR, Murley AHG: A clinical method of functional assessment of the shoulder. *Clin Orthop* 214:160–164, 1987.
573. Soslowsky LJ, et al. Subacromial contact (impingement) on the rotator cuff in the shoulder. *Trans Orthop Res Soc* 17: 424, 1992.
574. Carpenter E, Blasier RB, Pellizzon GG: The effects of muscle fatigue on shoulder joint position sense. *Am J Sports Med* 26:262–265, 1998.
575. Halder AM, Zhau KD, O'Driscoll SW, et al: Dynamic contributions to superior shoulder instability. *J Orthop Res* 19:206–212, 2001.
576. Conroy DE, Hayes KW: The effect of joint mobilization as a component of comprehensive treatment for primary shoulder impingement syndrome. *J Orthop Sports Phys Ther* 28:3–14, 1998.
577. Donatelli RA: Mobilization of the shoulder. In: Donatelli RA, ed. *Physical Therapy of the Shoulder*. New York: Churchill Livingstone, 1991:271–292.
578. Cofield RH, Simonet WT: Symposium on sports medicine: part 2. The shoulder in sports. *Mayo Clin Proc* 59:157–164, 1984.
579. Grimsby O, Gray JC: Interrelationship of the spine to the shoulder girdle. In: Donatelli RA, ed. *Clinics in Physical Therapy: Physical Therapy of the Shoulder*, 3rd ed. New York: Churchill Livingstone, 1997:95–129.
580. Culham E, Peat M: Spinal and shoulder complex posture. II: Thoracic alignment and shoulder complex position in normal and osteoporotic women. *Clin Rehabil* 8:27–35, 1994.
581. DiVeta J, Walker ML, Skibinski B: Relationship between performance of selected scapular muscles and scapular abduction in standing subjects. *Phys Ther* 70:470–476, 1990.
582. Greenfield B, Catlin PA, Coats PW, et al: Posture in patients with shoulder overuse injuries and healthy individuals. *J Orthop Sports Phys Ther* 21:287–295, 1995.
583. Griegal-Morris P, Larson K, Mueller-Klaus K, et al: Incidence of common postural abnormalities in the cervical, shoulder and thoracic regions and their association with pain in two age groups of healthy subjects. *Phys Ther* 72:425–431, 1992.
584. Ruwe P, Pink M, Jobe FW, et al: The normal and the painful shoulders during the breast stroke: Electromyographic and cinematographic analysis of twelve muscles. *Am J Sports Med* 22:789–796, 1994.
585. Whitman JM: Research Reports : http://www.ptjournal.org/cgi/content/full/86/8/1076, The Bottom Line. *Phys Ther* 2006.
586. McClure PW, Michener LA, Karduna AR: Shoulder function and 3-dimensional scapular kinematics in people with and without shoulder impingement syndrome. *Phys Ther* 86:1075–1090, 2006.
587. Evans P: The healing process at cellular level: A review. *Physiotherapy* 66:256–260, 1980.
588. Davies GJ: *Compendium of Isokinetics in Clinical Usage and Rehabilitation Techniques*, 4th ed. Onalaska, WI: S & S Publishers, 1992.
589. Dvir Z: *Isokinetics: Muscle Testing, Interpretation and Clinical Applications*. New York: Churchill Livingstone, 1995.
590. Bang MD, Deyle GD: Comparison of supervised exercise with and without manual physical therapy for patients with shoulder impingement syndrome. *J Orthop Sports Phys Ther* 30:126–137, 2000.
591. Brox JI, Staff PH, Ljunggren AE, et al: Arthroscopic surgery compared with supervised exercises in patients with rotator cuff disease (stage II impingement syndrome). *Br Med J* 307:899–903, 1993.
592. Ginn KA, Herbert RD, Khouw W, et al: A randomized controlled clinical trial of a treatment for shoulder pain. *Phys Ther* 77:802–811, 1997.
593. Jobe CM: Posterior superior glenoid impingement: Expanded spectrum. *Arthroscopy* 11:530–539, 1995.

594. Paley KJ, Jobe FW, Pink MM, et al: Arthroscopic findings in the overhand throwing athletes: Evidence of posterior internal impingement of the rotator cuff. *Arthoscopy* 16:35–40, 2000.
595. Neviaser TJ: The role of the biceps tendon in the impingement syndrome. *Orthop Clin North Am* 18:383–386, 1987.
596. Hammer WI: The use of transverse friction massage in the management of chronic bursitis of the hip or shoulder. *J Man Physiol Ther* 16:107–111, 1993.
597. Uhthoff HK, Sarkar K: Calcifying tendinitis. In: Rockwood CA Jr, Matsen FA III, eds. *The Shoulder*. Philadelphia, PA: WB Saunders, 1990:774–788.
598. Ebenbichler GR, Erdogmus CB, Resch K, et al: Ultrasound therapy for calcific tendinitis of the shoulder. *N Engl J Med* 340:1533–1538, 1999.
599. Bosworth BM: Calcium deposits in the shoulder and subacromial bursitis: A survey of 12,122 shoulders. *JAMA* 116:2477–2482, 1941.
600. McKendry RJR, Uhthoff HK, Sarkar K, et al: Calcifying tendinitis of the shoulder: Prognostic value of clinical, histologic, and radiologic features in 57 surgically treated cases. *J Rheumatol* 9:75–80, 1982.
601. Booth RE Jr, Marvel JR Jr: Differential diagnosis of shoulder pain. *Orthop Clin North Am* 6:353–379, 1975.
602. Chard MD et al: Rotator cuff degeneration and lateral epicondylitis: A comparative histological study. *Ann Rheum Dis* 53:30–34, 1994.
603. Uhthoff HK: Calcifying tendinitis. *Ann Chir Gynaecol* 85:111–115, 1996.
604. Uhtoff HK, Sarkar K, Maynard JA: Calcifying tendinitis. *Clin Orthop* 118:164–168, 1976.
605. Wefling J, Kahn MF, Desroy M: Les calcifications de l'epaule, II: la maladie des calcifications tendineuses multiples. *Rev Rheum* 32:325–334, 1965.
606. Loew M, Jurgowski W, Mau HC, et al: Treatment of calcifying tendinitis of rotator cuff by extracorporeal shock waves: A preliminary report. *J Shoulder Elbow Surg* 4:101–106, 1995.
607. Rompe JD, Rumler F, Hopf C, et al: Extracorporal shock wave therapy for calcifying tendinitis of the shoulder. *Clin Orthop* 321:196–201, 1995.
608. Ter Haar G, Dyson M, Oakley EM: The use of ultrasound by physiotherapists in Britain, 1985. *Ultrasound Med Biol* 13:659–663, 1987.
609. Mortimer AJ, Dyson M: The effect of therapeutic ultrasound on calcium uptake in fibroblasts. *Ultrasound Med Biol* 14:499–506, 1988.
610. Naccache PH, Grimard M, Roberge C, et al: Crystal-induced neutrophil activation. I. Initiation and modulation of calcium mobilization and superoxide production by microcrystals. *Arthritis Rheum* 34:333–342, 1991.
611. Terkeltaub R, Zachariae C, Santoro D, et al: Monocyte-derived neutrophil chemotactic factor/interleukin-8 is a potential mediator of crystal-induced inflammation. *Arthritis Rheum* 34:894–903, 1991.
612. Ark JW, Flock TJ, Flatow EL, et al: Arthroscopic treatment of calcific tendinitis of the shoulder. *Arthroscopy* 8:183–188, 1992.
613. Klein W, Gassen A, Laufenberg B: Endoskopische subacromiale Dekompression und Tendinitis calcarea. *Arthoskopie* 5:247–251, 1992.
614. Gartner J: Tendinosis calcarea—Rehandlungsergebnisse mit dem needling. *Z Orthop Ihre Grenzgeb* 131:461–469, 1993.
615. Slatis P, Aalto K: Medial dislocation of the tendon of the long head of the biceps brachii. *Acta orthopaedica Scandinavica* 50:73–77, 1979.
616. De Palma AF: Bicipital tenosynovitis. *Surg Clin North Am* 22:1693–1702, 1953.
617. Warren RF: Lesions of the long head of the biceps tendon. *Instr Course Lect* 34:204–209, 1985.
618. Ehricht HG: Die osteolyse im lateralen claviculaende nach pressluftschaden. *Arch Orthop Unfallchir* 50:576 582, 1959.
619. Scavenius M, Iverson BF: Nontraumatic clavicular osteolysis in weight lifters. *Am J Sports Med* 20:463–467, 1992.
620. Cahill BR: Atraumatic osteolysis of the distal clavicle: A review. *Sports Med* 13:214–222, 1992.
621. Cahill BR: Osteolysis of the distal part of the clavicle in male athletes. *J Bone Joint Surg* 64A:1053–1058, 1982.
622. Bahk MS, Kuhn JE, Galatz LM, et al: Acromioclavicular and sternoclavicular injuries and clavicular, glenoid, and scapular fractures. *Instr Course Lect* 59:209–226, 2010.
623. Bigliani LU, Craig EV, Butters KP: Fractures of the shoulder. In: Rockwood CA, Green DP, Bucholz RW, eds. *Fractures in Adults*. Philadelphia, PA: Lippincott, 1991.
624. Cornell CN, Schneider K: Proximal humerus fractures. In: Koval KJ, Zuckerman JD, eds. *Fractures in the Elderly*. Philadelphia, PA: Lippincott-Raven, 1998.
625. Ideberg R, Grevsten S, Larsson S: Epidemiology of scapular fractures. Incidence and classification of 338 fractures. *Acta Orthop Scand* 66:395–397, 1995.
626. Kibler WB, McMullen J: Scapular dyskinesis and its relation to shoulder pain. *J Am Acad Orthop Surg* 11:142–151, 2003.
627. Boinet J: Snapping scapula. *Societe Imperiale de Chirurgie (2nd series)* 8:458, 1867.
628. Butters KP: The scapula. In: Rockwood CA, Matsen FA, eds. *The Shoulder*. Philadelphia, PA: WB Saunders Company, 1990:335–336.
629. Milch H: Partial scapulectomy for snapping in the scapula. *J Bone Joint Surg* 32A:561–566, 1950.
630. Milch H: Snapping scapula. *Clin Orthop* 20:139–150, 1961.
631. Alvik I: Snapping scapula and Sprengel's deformity. *Acta Orthop Scand* 29:10–15, 1959.
632. Cooley LH, Torg JS: Pseudowinging of the scapula secondary to subscapular osteochondroma. *Clin Orthop* 162:119–124, 1982.
633. Parsons TA: The snapping scapula and subscapular exostoses. *J Bone Joint Surg* 55B:345–349, 1973.
634. Bristow WR: A case of snapping shoulder. *J Bone Joint Surg* 6:53–55, 1924.
635. Cameron HU: Snapping scapulae: A report of three cases. *Eur J Rheum Inflam* 7:66–67, 1984.
636. Cobey MC: The rolling scapula. *Clin Orthop* 60:193–194, 1968.
637. Edelson JG: Variations in the anatomy of the scapula with reference to the snapping scapula. *Clin Orthop* 322:111–115, 1996.
638. Travell J, Rinzler S, Herman M: Shoulder pain: Pain and disability of the shoulder and arm. *JAMA* 120:417–422, 1942.
639. Michele AA, Davies JJ, Krueger FJ, et al: Scapulocostal syndrome (fatigue-postural paradox). *N Y State J Med* 50:1353–1356, 1950.
640. Fourie LJ: The scapulocostal syndrome. *S Afr Med J* 79:721–724, 1991.
641. Bazett HC, McGlone B: Note on the pain sensations which accompany deep punctures. *Brain* 51:18–23, 1928.
642. Todd TW: Posture and the cervical rib syndrome. *Ann Surg* 75:105–109, 1922.
643. Naffziger HC, Grant WC: Neuritis of the brachial plexus, mechanical in origin: The scalenus syndrome. *Surg Gynecol Obstet* 67:722–730, 1938.
644. Halliday JL: Psychosomatic medicine and the rheumatism problem. *Practitioner* 152:6–15, 1944.
645. Smolders JJ: Myofascial pain and dysfunction syndromes. In: Hammer WI, ed. *Functional Soft Tissue Examination and Treatment by Manual Methods—The Extremities*. Gaithersburg, MD: Aspen, 1991: 215–234.
646. Raikin S, Froimson MI: Bilateral brachial plexus compressive neuropathy (crutch palsy). *J Orthop Trauma* 11:136–138, 1997.
647. Rudin LN: Bilateral compression of radial nerve (crutch paralysis). *Phys Ther* 31:229, 1951.
648. Poddar SB, Gitelis S, Heydemann PT, et al: Bilateral predominant radial nerve crutch palsy: A case report. *Clin Orthop* 297:245–246, 1993.
649. Ang EJ, Goh JC, Bose K: A biofeedback device for patients on axillary crutches. *Arch Phys Med Rehabil* 70:644–647, 1989.
650. Hawkins RJ, Bilco T, Bonutti P: Cervical spine and shoulder pain. *Clin Orthop* 258:142–146, 1990.
651. Manifold SG, McCann PD: Cervical radiculitis and shoulder disorders. *Clin Orth Rel Res* 368:105–113, 1999.
652. DePalma AF: Shoulder-arm-pain of mesodermal, neurogenic, and vascular origin. In: DePalma AF, ed. *Surgery of the Shoulder*, 3rd ed. Philadelphia, PA: JB Lippincott, 1983:571–580.
653. Lubahn JD, Cermak MB: Uncommon nerve compression syndromes of the upper extremity. *J Am Acad Orthop Surg* 6:378–386, 1998.
654. Butler DL, Gifford L: The concept of adverse mechanical tension in the nervous system: Part 1: Testing for "dural tension". *Physiotherapy* 75:622–629, 1989.
655. Butler DS: *Mobilization of the Nervous Sysytem*. New York: Churchill Livingstone, 1992.
656. Brown JT: Nerve injuries complicating dislocation of the shoulder. *J Bone and Joint Surg [Br]* 34:562, 1952.
657. Johns R, Wright V: Relative importance of various tissues in joint stiffness. *J Appl Physiol* 17:824–830, 1962.
658. Nitz AJ: Physical therapy management of the shoulder. *Phys Ther* 66:1912–1919, 1986.
659. Nicholson GG: The effects of passive joint mobilization on pain and hypomobility associated with adhesive capsulitis of the shoulder. *J Orthop Sports Phys Ther* 6:238–246, 1985.

660. Enneking WF, Horowitz M: The intra-articular effects of immobilization on the human knee. *J Bone Joint Surg* 54-A:973–985, 1972.
661. Randall T, Portney L, Harris B: Effects of joint mobilization on joint stiffness and active motion of the metacarpophalangeal joint. *J Orthop Sports Phys Ther* 16:30–36, 1992.
662. Wyke BD: The neurology of joints. *Ann R Coll Surg Engl* 41:25–50, 1967.
663. Arem A, Madden J: Effects of stress on healing wounds: Intermittent non-cyclical tension. *J Surg Res* 42:528–543, 1971.
664. Warren CG, Lehmann JF, Koblanski JN: Elongation of rat tail: Effect of load and temperature. *Arch Phys Med Rehabil* 52:465–474, 1971.
665. Light KE, Nuzik S: Low-load prolonged stretch vs high-load brief stretch in treating knee contractures. *Phys Ther* 64:330–333, 1984.
666. Lee DG: *A Workbook of Manual Therapy Techniques for the Upper Extremity* 2nd ed. Delta, BC: DOPC, 1991.
667. Mulligan BR: *Manual Therapy: "NAGS", "SNAGS", "PRP'S" etc.* Wellington: Plane View Series, 1992.

CHAPTER 17 Elbow

CHAPTER OBJECTIVES

At the completion of this chapter, the reader will be able to:

1. Describe the anatomy of the joints, ligaments, muscles, and blood and nerve supply comprising the elbow complex.
2. Describe the biomechanics of the elbow complex, including open- and close-packed positions, normal and abnormal joint barriers, force couples, and stabilizers.
3. Describe the purpose and components of the tests and measures for the elbow complex.
4. Perform a comprehensive examination of the elbow complex, including palpation of the articular and soft-tissue structures, specific passive mobility and passive articular mobility tests, and stability tests.
5. Evaluate the total examination data to establish a prognosis.
6. Describe the relationship between muscle imbalance and functional performance of the elbow.
7. Outline the significance of the key findings from the tests and measures and establish a diagnosis or working hypothesis.
8. Summarize the various causes of elbow dysfunction.
9. Develop self-reliant intervention strategies based on clinical findings and established goals.
10. Describe and demonstrate intervention strategies and techniques based on clinical findings and established goals.
11. Evaluate the intervention effectiveness in order to progress or modify an intervention.
12. Plan an effective home program and instruct the patient in same.

OVERVIEW

The elbow serves an important linkage function that enables proper positioning of the hand and the transmission of power from the shoulder to the hand, thus augmenting the versatility and agility of the upper extremity. Unlike the shoulder, the elbow complex is an inherently strong and stable joint, because of the interrelationship of its articular surfaces and ligamentous constraints. However, the stability of the elbow complex allows little in the way of compensatory adjustments, making it particularly vulnerable to overuse injury from repetitious muscle activity and sudden movements of acceleration and deceleration. Appropriate diagnosis and treatment require a detailed understanding of the normal anatomy of the elbow.

ANATOMY

The elbow complex, enclosed within the capsule of the cubital articulation, is composed of three distinct articulations: the humeroulnar joint, the humeroradial joint, and the proximal radioulnar joint. The anterior joint capsule of the elbow originates from the distal humerus proximal to the radial and coronoid fossa, from where it then inserts distally into the rim of the coronoid and the annular ligament (AL).[1] Posteriorly, the capsule incorporates the area proximal to the olecranon process; it attaches distally along the articular margin of the sigmoid notch and the proximal aspect of the olecranon fossa.[2]

CLINICAL PEARL

The joint capsule of the elbow complex is thin but strong, and is reinforced medially and laterally by ligaments. Anteriorly, the capsule contributes 38% of the resistance to valgus force and 32% of the resistance to varus force in full extension.[3] The capsule of the joint does not respond well to injury or prolonged immobilization, and often forms thick scar tissue, which may result in flexion contractures of the elbow.[4–6]

HUMEROULNAR JOINT

The humeroulnar (trochlear) joint is a uniaxial hinge joint formed between the incongruent saddle-shaped joint surfaces of the spool-shaped trochlea of the humerus and the trochlear notch of the proximal ulna (Fig. 17-1). Anteriorly, the humeral

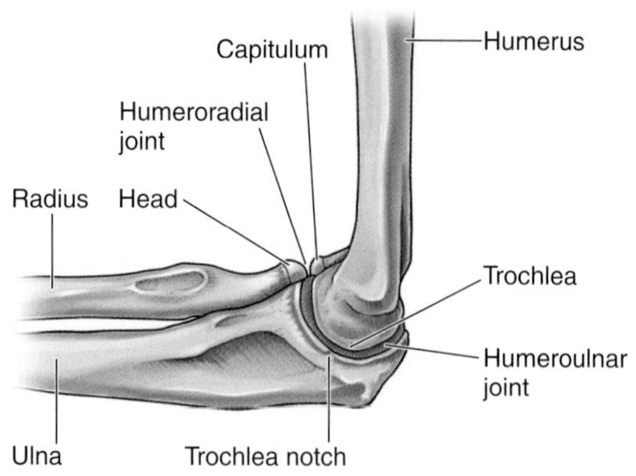

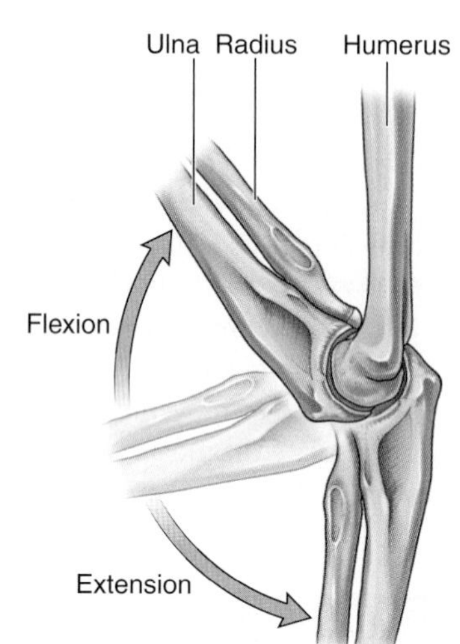

FIGURE 17-1 The bony structures of the elbow complex. (Reproduced with permission from Morton DA, Foreman KB, Albertine KH: *Gross Anatomy: The Big Picture.* McGraw-Hill, 2011)

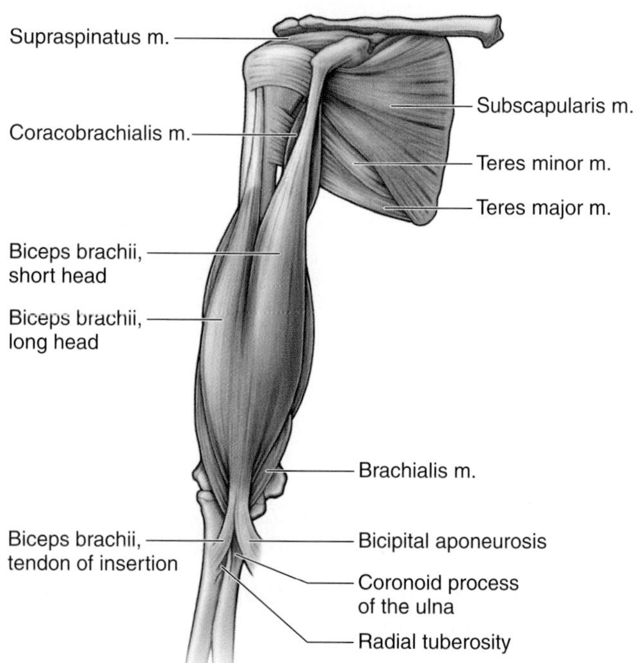

FIGURE 17-2 The biceps. (Reproduced with permission from Morton DA, Foreman KB, Albertine KH: *Gross Anatomy: The Big Picture.* McGraw-Hill, 2011)

trochlear groove is vertical and parallel to the longitudinal groove, while, posteriorly, the groove runs obliquely lateral and distal, forming an acute angle of about 15 degrees with the longitudinal axis of the humerus.[7] This valgus angulation is referred to as the "carrying angle" of the elbow. Three hundred degrees of the articular surface of the trochlea is covered with hyaline cartilage, compared with only 180 degrees on the trochlear notch.[8]

CLINICAL PEARL

The carrying angle serves to direct the ulna laterally during extension and increase the potential for elbow flexion motion, as the offset allows room anteriorly for approximation of the muscles of the arm and the forearm. The carrying angle is approximately 11–14 degrees in males and 13–16 degrees in females.[9–11]

The resting, or open-packed position for the humeroulnar joint is 70 degrees of flexion with 10 degrees of forearm supination. The close-packed position is full extension and maximum forearm supination. For the part of the joint between the coronoid process and the humerus, the close-packed position is maximum flexion. The capsular pattern is much more limitation of flexion than extension.[12]

HUMERORADIAL JOINT

The humeroradial (radiocapitellar) joint is a uniaxial hinge joint formed between the spherical capitellum of the humerus and the concave fovea of the radial head (see Fig. 17-1). The design of this joint allows the elbow to flex and extend and for the radius to rotate. The superior surface of the proximal end of the radius is biconcave, while the head of the radius is slightly oval. The radial tuberosity (see Fig. 17-2) serves as a site of attachment for the biceps brachii (see Fig. 17-2). The humerus widens at the elbow and forms the medial and lateral epicondyles.

CLINICAL PEARL

The resting, or open-packed position of the humeroradial joint is extension and forearm supination. The close-packed position is approximately 90 degrees of elbow flexion and 5 degrees of supination. There is no true capsular pattern at this joint, although clinically an equal limitation of pronation and supination is observed.

PROXIMAL RADIOULNAR JOINT

The radius and the ulna lie side by side, with the radius being the shorter and more lateral of the two forearm bones. The proximal or superior radioulnar joint is a uniaxial pivot joint. It is formed between the periphery of the convex radial head, and the fibrous osseous ring formed by the concave radial notch of the ulna (see Fig. 17-3), which lies distal to the trochlear notch, and the AL. The AL (Fig. 17-4) forms 80% of the articular surface of the proximal radioulnar joint (see Annular Ligament later).

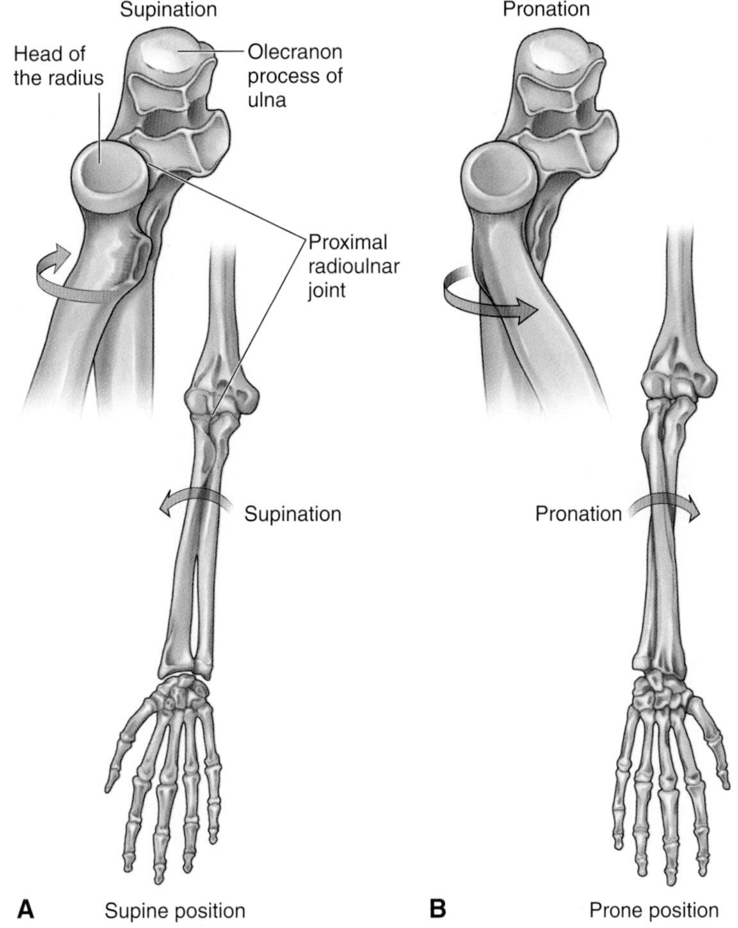

FIGURE 17-3 The proximal radioulnar joint. (Reproduced with permission, from Morton DA, Foreman KB, Albertine KH: *Gross Anatomy: The Big Picture*. McGraw-Hill, 2011)

CLINICAL PEARL

The resting, or open-packed position for the proximal radioulnar joint is 70 degrees of flexion and 35 degrees of forearm supination. The close-packed position is 5 degrees of forearm supination. The capsular pattern is minimal loss of motion, with pain at the end ranges of pronation and supination.[12]

The proximal and distal radioulnar joints together form a bicondylar joint. An interosseous membrane, sometimes

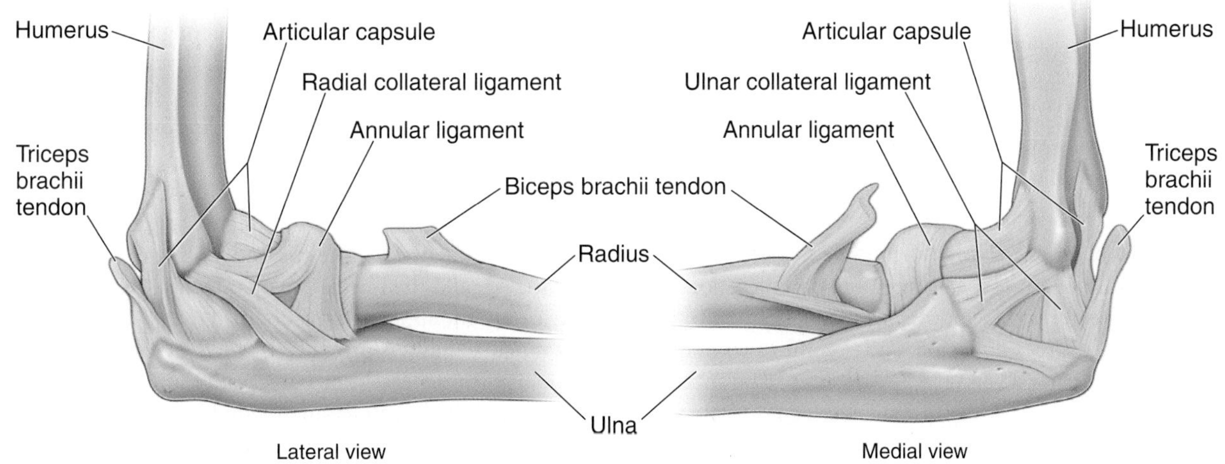

FIGURE 17-4 Elbow joint with ligaments detailed. (Reproduced with permission from Morton DA, Foreman KB, Albertine KH: *Gross Anatomy: The Big Picture*. McGraw-Hill, 2011)

referred to as the middle radioulnar articulation and located between the radius and the ulna, serves to help distribute forces throughout the forearm, and provide muscle attachment. Most of the fibers of the interosseous membrane of the forearm are directed away from the radius in an oblique medial and distal direction.[8] Approximately 8% of the compression force due to bearing weight to the forearm crosses the wrist between the lateral side of the carpus and the radius.[8] The remaining 20% of the compression force passes across the medial side of the carpal bones and the ulna.[8] Because of the fiber orientation of the interosseous membrane, some of the proximal directed force through the radius is transferred across the membrane to the ulna.[13]

LIGAMENTS

Support for the elbow complex is provided through strong ligaments (Fig. 17-4).

Medial Ligament Complex

The ulna collateral ligament (UCL) or medial collateral ligament (MCL) extends from the central two-thirds of the anteroinferior surface of the medial epicondyle to the proximal medial ulna, from just posterior to the axis of the elbow medial epicondyle,[14–16] to just distal to the tip of the coronoid (see Fig. 17-4).[17,18]

The fan-shaped MCL is the most important ligament in the elbow for providing stability against valgus stress, particularly in the range of 20–130 degrees of flexion and extension,[19] with the humeroradial joint functioning as a secondary stabilizer to valgus loads.[20,21] The MCL achieves this stability through almost the total range of flexion and extension due to its eccentric location with respect to the axis of elbow motion.[22–25] In full elbow extension, valgus stability of the elbow is provided equally by the MCL, the joint capsule, and the joint interactions.[5]

There are three distinct components of the MCL[14,17,26,27]: the anterior bundle, the transverse bundle, and the posterior bundle (Fig. 17-4).

Anterior Bundle

The anterior bundle of the MCL is the strongest and stiffest of the elbow collateral ligaments, with an average load to failure of 260 newtons (N).[19] The anterior bundle of the MCL inserts an average of 18 mm distal to the coronoid tip, and is composed of two other components, the anterior band and the posterior band, which perform reciprocal functions[17,22,26]:

- The anterior band of the anterior bundle is the most important component of the ligamentous complex, because it primarily stabilizes the elbow against valgus stress in the ranges of 0–60 degrees of flexion, and becomes a secondary restraint with further flexion.[3,14,17,20–22,24,26,28] The anterior band is primarily responsible for stability against valgus stresses at 30, 60, and 90 degrees of flexion, making it the most important component in resisting the valgus forces associated with overhead sports activities.[1] Recently, Ochi and colleagues[15] determined that the deep middle portion of the anterior band, previously described as the "guiding bundle,"[27] is a prime limiting factor in humeroulnar motion.[22,29]
- The posterior band is taut from 60 degrees to 120 degrees of elbow flexion, and is a secondary restraint to valgus stress at 30 degrees and 90 degrees of flexion, but a primary restraint to valgus at 120 degrees of elbow flexion.[26] The posterior band functions as an equal co-restraint with the anterior band at terminal elbow flexion,[3,19,22,26,28] and also acts as a primary restraint to passive elbow extension. In the higher degrees of flexion, the posterior band is nearly isometric and is thus functionally important in the overhead athlete in counteracting valgus stresses.[30]

Oblique (Transverse) Bundle

The oblique bundle, also known as Cooper's ligament, is variably present.[14,17,31] It does not cross the elbow joint and comprises fibers running along the medial joint capsule from the tip of the olecranon to the medial ulna, just distal to the coronoid.[14,32] The transverse fibers have little role in elbow stability due to the fact that they both originate and insert on the ulna.

Posterior Oblique Bundle

The posterior bundle of the MCL originates from the medial epicondyle and inserts onto the medial margin of the semilunar notch, forming the floor of the cubital tunnel and a thickening of the posterior elbow capsule.[32,33] Being thinner and weaker than the anterior bundle, the posterior bundle becomes taut at 60 degrees of elbow flexion, but provides only secondary restraint to valgus stress at flexion beyond 90 degrees.[22,23]

Lateral Ligament Complex

Unlike the medial ligament complex, the lateral ligamentous complex (see Fig. 17-4) is less discrete and individual variation is common. The lateral complex consists of the AL, the lateral-radial collateral ligament (LCL), and the lateral ulnar collateral ligament (LUCL).[19] The LCL courses distally and forms a broad conjoint insertion onto the proximal ulna.[34,35] The proximal margin of this conjoined insertion begins at the proximal aspect of the radial head, just inferior to the radial notch. From here, it progresses along a rough ridge in line with the supinator crest of the ulna.[19] The LCL is closely associated with the insertions of the extensor carpi radialis brevis (ECRB) and the supinator, with the latter muscle crossing this ligament complex obliquely from distal to proximal at its ulnar attachment and becoming confluent with the underlying AL and LCL more proximally at its humeral origin.[19] The LUCL originates from the lateral epicondyle from where it passes over the AL and then begins to blend with it distally where it inserts onto the supinator crest of the ulna.[14] It is unclear as to how much stability is provided by the LUCL, but it may help prevent posterolateral rotary instability.[36]

As a unit, the lateral ligament complex functions to maintain the ulnohumeral and radiohumeral joints in a reduced position when the elbow is loaded in supination. More specifically, the anterior portion of the LCL stabilizes the proximal radioulnar joint during full supination; the posterior portion stabilizes the joint during pronation. As the axis of rotation passes through the origin of the LCL, the various fibers of this ligament maintain consistent patterns of tension whether varus, valgus, or no force is applied to the elbow throughout the arc of flexion.[14,28] The LCL contributes only 9% of the restraint to varus stress at 90 degrees of flexion. In extension the LCL contributes 14% of this restraint.[28]

Insufficient lateral support of the elbow complex results in lateral gapping at the ulnohumeral joint and posterior translation of the radial head in relation to the capitellum.[19] However, the proximal radioulnar relationship remains undisturbed.

CLINICAL PEARL

As much as 50% of elbow stability is the result of the joint capsule, MCL and the lateral ligament complex. The remaining 50% is associated with the bony structure of the joint. Other structures also provide passive support to the elbow complex. Secondary restraints of the lateral elbow consist of the bony articulations, and the extensor muscles with their fascial bands and intermuscular septa (see "Force Couples of the Elbow"). Secondary restraints of the lateral elbow consist of the bony articulations, the joint capsule (see Fig. 17-4), and the extensor muscles with their fascial bands and intermuscular septa. These independently support the forearm unit from laterally rotating away from the humerus by virtue of their anatomic arrangement, and provide a secondary static and dynamic vector supporting the lateral joint.[35]

Annular Ligament

The AL (Fig. 17-4), which is wider proximally and distally, runs around the radial head from the anterior and the posterior margin of the radial notch, to approximate the radial head to the radial notch and enclose the radial circumference. The AL forms a band that encircles 80% of the radial head and functions to maintain the relationship between the head of the radius and the humerus and ulna. The internal circumference of the AL is lined with cartilage to reduce the friction against the radial head during pronation and supination.[8] The external surface of the ligament receives attachments from the elbow capsule, the radial collateral ligament, and the supinator muscle.

Quadrate Ligament

The quadrate ligament is a short, stout ligament that arises just below the radial notch of the ulna and attaches to the medial surface of the neck of the radius.[8] This ligament lends structural support to the capsule of the proximal radioulnar joint.[8]

BURSAE

There are numerous bursae in the elbow region.[23] The olecranon bursa is the main bursa of the elbow complex and lies posteriorly between the skin and the olecranon process. Under normal conditions, the bursa does not communicate with the elbow joint, although its superficial location puts it at high risk of injury from direct trauma to the elbow.

Other bursae in the posterior elbow region include the deep intratendinous bursa and a deep subtendinous bursa, which are present between the triceps tendon and olecranon. Anteriorly, the bicipitoradial bursa separates the biceps tendon from the radial tuberosity. Along the medial and lateral aspects of the elbow are the subcutaneous medial epicondylar bursa and the subcutaneous lateral epicondylar bursa.[37]

MUSCLES

A summary of the muscles of the elbow is outlined in Table 17-1. The muscles of the forearm are contained within three major fascial compartments, the anterior forearm, the posterior forearm, and the compartment referred to as the mobile wad (Table 17-2).

Elbow Flexors

Anatomic, biomechanic, and electromyographic (EMG) analyses have demonstrated that the prime movers of elbow flexion are the biceps, brachialis, and brachioradialis (see Table 17-1).[38] The pronator teres, flexor carpi radialis (FCR), flexor carpi ulnaris (FCU) (Fig. 17-5), and the extensor carpi radialis longus (ECRL) muscles are considered to be weak flexors of the elbow.[37] Most elbow flexors, and essentially all the major supinator and pronator muscles, have their distal attachments on the radius.[8] Contraction of these muscles, therefore, pulls the radius proximally against the humeroradial joint.[39,40] The combined efforts of all the elbow flexors can create large amounts of elbow flexion torque. The interosseous membrane transfers and dissipates a portion of this muscle force to the radius and to the ulna.[8] The reverse action of the elbow flexors can be used in a closed chain activity by bringing the upper arm closer to the forearm such as when performing a pull-up.[41]

Biceps Brachii

The biceps is a two-headed muscle that spans two joints. The short head of the biceps arises from the tip of the coracoid process of the scapula, whereas the long head arises from the supraglenoid tuberosity of the scapula (Fig. 17-2). The biceps has two insertions: the radial tuberosity and by the lacertus fibrosus (see Fig. 17-2).

At the elbow, the biceps is a dominant flexor, but its secondary function is supination of the forearm.[42] The supination action of the biceps increases the more the elbow is flexed and is maximal at 90 degrees. It diminishes again when the elbow is fully flexed. No,[43] or limited,[44] biceps muscle activity has been demonstrated during elbow flexion, with the forearm pronated.[37] The biceps, via its long head, also functions as a shoulder flexor (see Chap. 16).

Brachialis

The brachialis (Fig. 17-6) originates from the lower two-thirds of the anterior surface of the humerus and inserts on the ulnar tuberosity and the coronoid process. The brachialis is the workhorse of the elbow and functions to flex the elbow regardless of the degree of pronation and supination of the forearm.[44] It is the most powerful flexor of the elbow when the forearm is pronated.[45]

TABLE 17-1 Muscles of the Elbow, Forearm, Wrist, and Hand: Their Actions, Nerve Supply, and Nerve Root Derivation			
Muscles	**Nerve Supply**	**Nerve Root Derivation**	**Action**
Triceps	Radial	C7–C8	Elbow extension
Anconeus	Radial	C7–C8, (T1)	
Brachialis	Musculocutaneous	C5–C6, (C7)	Elbow Flexion
Biceps brachii	Musculocutaneous radial	C5–C6	
Brachioradialis		C5–C6, (C7)	
Biceps brachii	Musculocutaneous	C5–C6	Supination of the forearm
Supinator	Posterior interosseous (radial)	C5–C6	
Pronator quadratus	Anterior interosseous (median)	C8, T1	Pronation of the forearm
Pronator teres	Median	C6–C7	
Flexor carpi radialis	Median	C6–C7	
Extensor carpi radialis longus	Radial	C6–C7	Extension of the wrist
Extensor carpi radialis brevis	Posterior interosseous (radial)	C7–C8	
Extensor carpi ulnaris	Posterior interosseous (radial)	C7–C8	
Flexor carpi radialis	Median	C6–C7	Flexion of the wrist
Flexor carpi ulnaris	Ulnar	C7–C8	
Flexor carpi ulnaris	Ulnar	C7–C8	Ulnar deviation of the wrist
Extensor carpi ulnaris	Posterior interosseous (radial)	C7–C8	
Flexor carpi radialis	Median	C6–C7	Radial deviation of the wrist
Extensor carpi radialis longus	Radial	C6–C7	
Abductor pollicis longus	Posterior interosseous (radial)	C7–C8	
Extensor pollicis brevis	Posterior interosseous (radial)	C7–C8	
Extensor digitorum communis	Posterior interosseous (radial)	C7–C8	Extension of the fingers
Extensor indicis	Posterior interosseous (radial)	C7–C8	
Extensor digiti minimi	Posterior interosseous (radial)	C7–C8	
Flexor digitorum profundus	Lateral: Anterior interosseous (median) Medial: Ulnar	C8, T1 C8, T1	Flexion of the fingers (lateral aspect flexes the second and third digits; medial aspect flexes the fourth and fifth digits
Flexor digitorum superficialis	Median	C7–C8, T1	Flexion of the fingers

Brachioradialis

The brachioradialis (Fig. 17-5) arises from the proximal two-thirds of the lateral supracondylar ridge of the humerus and the lateral intermuscular septum. It travels down the forearm and inserts on the lateral border of the styloid process on the distal aspect of the radius.

The brachioradialis appears to have a number of functions, two of which occur with rapid movements of elbow flexion. Initially it functions as a shunt muscle, overcoming centrifugal forces acting on the elbow, and then by adding power to increase the speed of flexion.[42]

The brachioradialis also functions to bring a pronated or supinated forearm back into the neutral position of pronation and supination. In the neutral or pronated position, the muscle acts as a flexor of the elbow, an action that diminishes when the forearm is held in supination.[44,46]

Pronator Teres

The pronator teres (see Fig. 17-5) has two heads of origin: a humeral head and an ulnar head. The humeral head arises from the medial epicondylar ridge of the humerus and common flexor tendon, whereas the ulnar head arises from the medial aspect of the coronoid process of the ulna. The pronator teres inserts on the anterolateral surface of the midpoint of the radius. The muscle functions predominantly to pronate the forearm, but can also assist with elbow flexion.[5,45,46]

TABLE 17-2 Muscle Compartments of the Forearm	
Compartment	**Principal Muscles**
Anterior	Pronator teres Flexor carpi radialis Palmaris longus Flexor digitorum superficialis Flexor digitorum profundus Flexor pollicis longus Flexor carpi ulnaris Pronator quadratus
Posterior	Abductor pollicis longus Extensor pollicis brevis Extensor pollicis longus Extensor digitorum communis Extensor digitorum proprius Extensor digiti quinti Extensor carpi ulnaris
Mobile wad	Brachioradialis Extensor carpi radialis longus Extensor carpi radialis brevis

Extensor Carpi Radialis Longus

The ECRL arises from a point superior to the lateral epicondyle of the humerus on the lower third of the supracondylar ridge, just distal to the brachioradialis. It travels down the forearm to insert on the posterior surface of the base of the second metacarpal. The muscle functions as a weak flexor of the elbow, as well as assisting with wrist extension and radial deviation.

Flexor Carpi Radialis

The FCR (see Fig. 17-5) arises from the common flexor tendon on the medial epicondyle of the humerus and inserts on the base of the second and third metacarpal bones. The FCR functions to flex the elbow and wrist but also assists in pronation and radial deviation of the wrist.

Flexor Carpi Ulnaris

The FCU (see Fig. 17-5) has two heads of origin. The humeral head arises from the common flexor tendon on the medial epicondyle of the humerus. It inserts on the pisiform, hamate, and fifth metacarpal bones. The FCU functions to assist with elbow flexion in addition to flexion and ulnar deviation of the wrist.

Forearm Pronators

Pronator Teres

See above.

Pronator Quadratus

The fibers of the pronator quadratus run perpendicular to the direction of the arm, running from the most distal quarter of

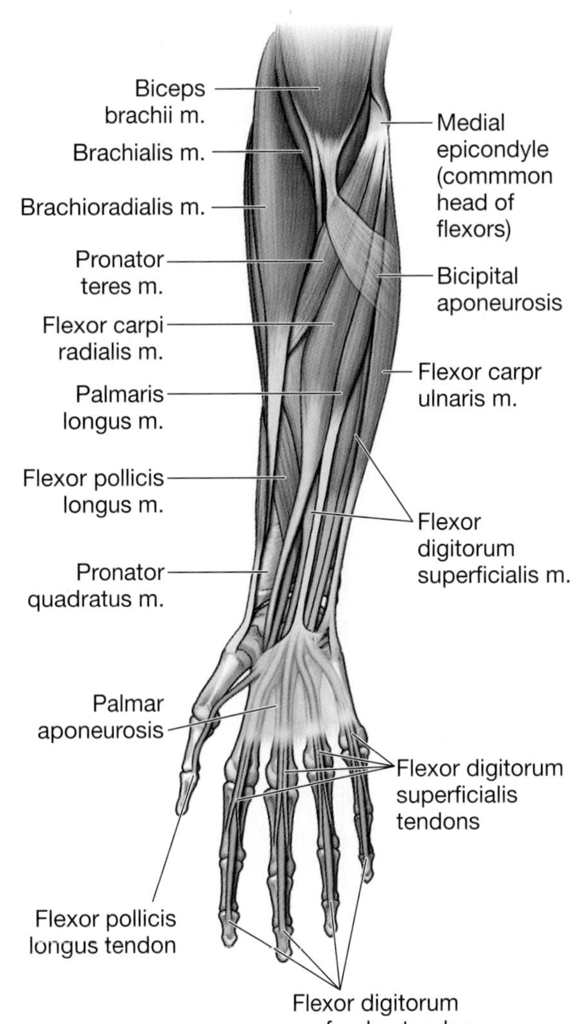

FIGURE 17-5 Muscles of the anterior forearm. (Reproduced with permission from Morton DA, Foreman KB, Albertine KH: *Gross Anatomy: The Big Picture.* McGraw-Hill, 2011)

the anterior ulna to the distal quarter of the anterior radius (see Fig. 17-5). It is the only muscle that attaches only to the ulna at one end and the radius at the other end.

The pronator quadratus is the main pronator of the hand.

Flexor Carpi Radialis

See above.

Forearm Supinators

Biceps

The effectiveness of the biceps as a supinator is greatest when the elbow is flexed to 90 degrees, placing the biceps tendon at a 90-degree angle to the radius. In contrast, with the elbow flexed only 30 degrees, much of the rotational efficiency of the biceps is lost.[41]

Supinator

The supinator originates from the lateral epicondyle of the humerus, LCL, the AL, the supinator crest, and the ulnar fossa. It inserts on the superior third of the anterior and lateral surface of the radius. The supinator muscle is a relentless

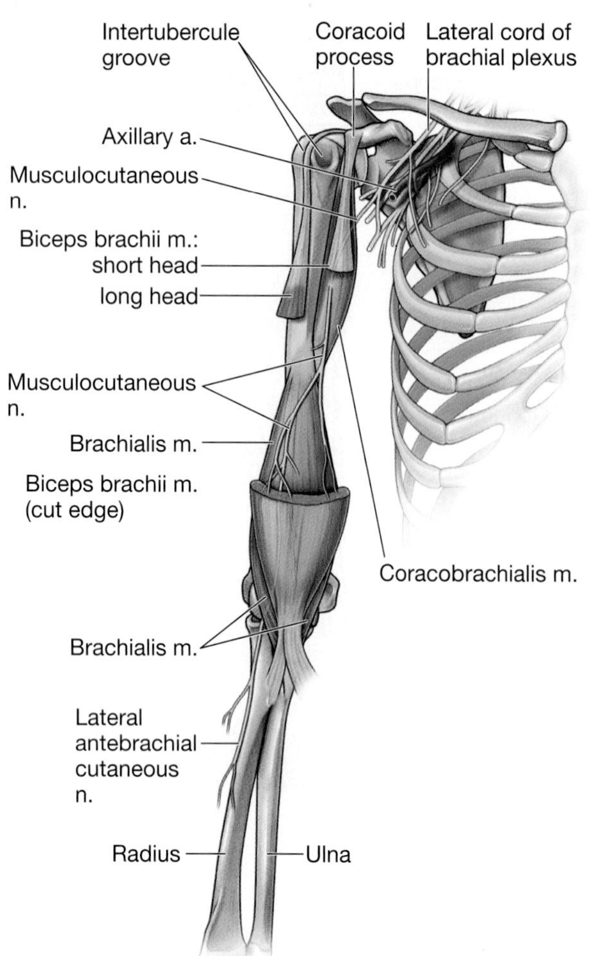

FIGURE 17-6 The brachialis muscle. (Reproduced with permission from Morton DA, Foreman KB, Albertine KH: *Gross Anatomy: The Big Picture.* McGraw-Hill, 2011)

forearm supinator, similar to the brachialis during elbow flexion. The supinator functions to supinate the forearm in any elbow position, while the previously mentioned ECRL and brevis work as supinators during fast movements, and against resistance.

The nervous system usually recruits the supinator muscle for low-power tasks that require a supination motion only, while the biceps remains relatively inactive—a fine example of the law of parsimony (see Chap. 3).[8]

CLINICAL PEARL

The muscles about the elbow help provide stability by compressing the joint surfaces through muscular contraction.[47] The flexor and pronator muscles, which originate at the medial epicondyle, provide additional static and dynamic support to the medial elbow,[5] with the FCU and flexor digitorum superficialis (FDS) being the most effective in this regard.[48]

Elbow Extensors

There are two muscles that extend the elbow: the triceps and the anconeus (see Table 17-1).

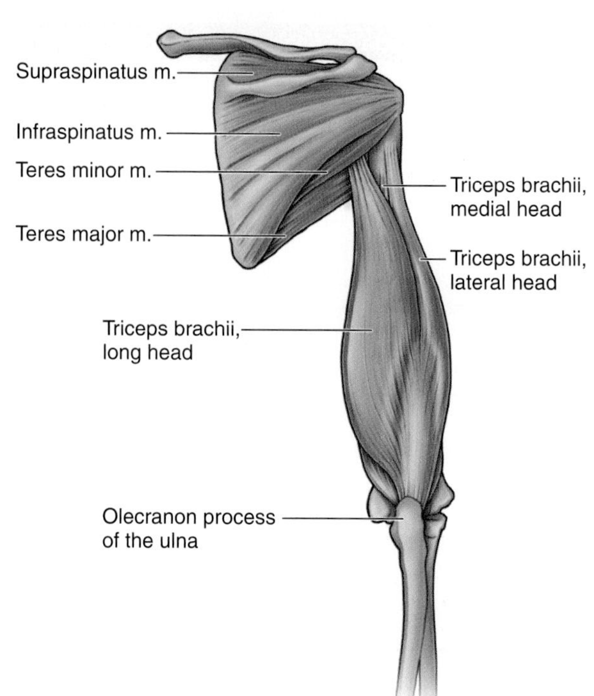

FIGURE 17-7 The triceps. (Reproduced with permission from Morton DA, Foreman KB, Albertine KH: *Gross Anatomy: The Big Picture.* McGraw-Hill, 2011)

Triceps Brachii

The triceps brachii (Fig. 17-7) has three heads of origin. The long head arises from the infraglenoid tuberosity of the scapula, the lateral head from the posterior and lateral surface of the humerus, and the medial head from the lower posterior surface of the humerus. The muscle inserts on the superoposterior surface of the olecranon and deep fascia of the forearm. The triceps has its maximal force in movements that combine both elbow extension and shoulder extension. Like the biceps, it is a two-joint muscle. The medial head of the triceps is the workhorse of elbow extension, with the lateral and long heads recruited during heavier loads.[49] During strong contractions of the triceps, for example a push-up, which involves a combination of elbow extension and shoulder flexion, as the triceps strongly contracts to extend the elbow, the shoulder simultaneously flexes by the action of the anterior deltoid, which overpowers the shoulder extension torque of the long head of the triceps.[41]

Anconeus

The anconeus arises from the lateral epicondyle of the humerus and inserts on the lateral aspect of the olecranon and posterior surface of the ulna. The exact function of the anconcus in humans has yet to be determined, although it appears to be a fourth head of the elbow extension mechanism, similar to the quadriceps of the knee.[8] It has been suggested that in addition to assisting with elbow extension, forearm pronation and supination, the anconeus functions to stabilize the ulnar head in all positions (except radial deviation) and to pull the subanconeus bursa and the joint capsule out of the way during extension, thus avoiding impingement.[5,44,50]

CLINICAL PEARL

Tendinitis of the anconeus can mimic tennis elbow, while hypertrophy of the anconeus muscle can compress the ulnar nerve.[51]

CUBITAL TUNNEL

The cubital tunnel, a fibro-osseous canal, was originally described by Feindel and Stratford.[52] The ulnar nerve passes through this tunnel. The floor of the tunnel is formed by the MCL, whereas the roof is formed by an aponeurosis, the arcuate ligament, or Osborne's band, which extends from the medial epicondyle to the olecranon and arises from the origin of the two heads of the FCU.[53–56] The medial head of the triceps constitutes the posterior border of the tunnel, and its anterior and lateral borders are formed by the medial epicondyle and olecranon, respectively.[30]

The volume of the cubital tunnel is greatest with the elbow held in extension.[57] As the elbow is brought into full flexion, there is a 55% decrease in canal volume.[53] Vanderpool and colleagues[58] reported that with each 45 degrees of flexion of the elbow, there was a concomitant 5-mm increase in distance between the ulnar and humeral attachments of the arcuate ligament. At full elbow flexion, there was a 40% elongation of the ligament and a decrease in canal height of approximately 2.5 mm.

A few other factors have been associated with a decrease in the size of the cubital tunnel. These include space-occupying lesions, osteoarthritis, rheumatoid arthritis, heterotopic bone formation, or trauma to the nerve.[57] Patients with systemic conditions such as diabetes mellitus, hypothyroidism, alcoholism, and renal failure also may have a predisposition.[59]

Bulging of the MCL has also been described as a factor.[58] More than 40% of athletes with valgus instability develop ulnar neuritis secondary to irritation from inflammation of the MCL.[60,61]

O'Driscoll and coworkers[56] reported that the groove on the inferior aspect of the medial epicondyle was not as deep as the groove posteriorly, and the floor of the canal seems to rise with elbow flexion.[56] These changes lead to an alteration of the cross-sectional area of the cubital tunnel from a rounded surface to a triangular or elliptic surface with elbow flexion.[53,57]

CLINICAL PEARL

The volume of the cubital tunnel is greatest with the elbow held in extension.

CUBITAL FOSSA

The cubital fossa (Fig. 17-8) represents a triangular space, or depression that is located over the anterior surface of the elbow joint, and which serves as an "entry way" to the forearm, or antebrachium. The boundaries of the fossa are

- ***lateral.*** Brachioradialis and ECRL muscles;
- ***medial.*** Pronator teres muscle;
- ***proximal.*** An imaginary line that passes through the humeral condyles;

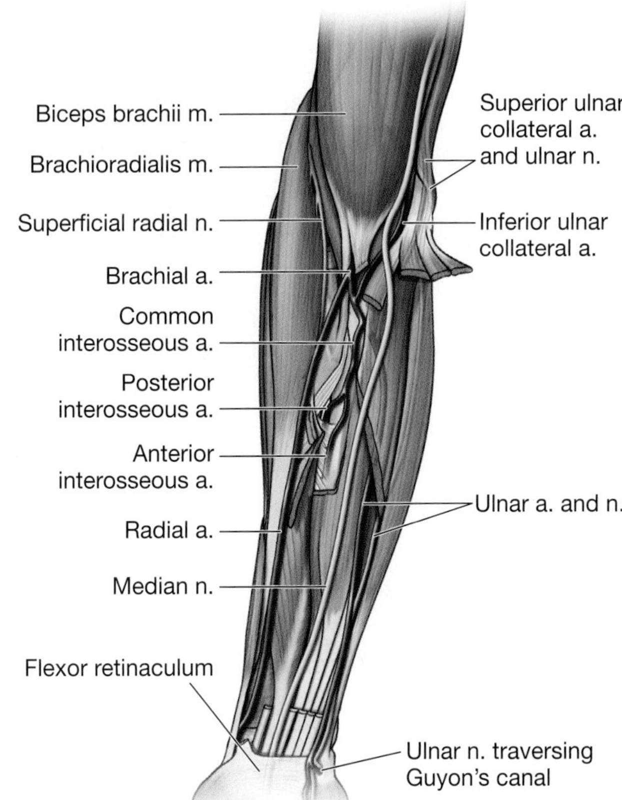

FIGURE 17-8 The cubital fossa. (Reproduced with permission from Morton DA, Foreman KB, Albertine KH: *Gross Anatomy: The Big Picture.* McGraw-Hill, 2011)

- ***floor.*** Brachialis muscle.

The contents of the fossa include (see Fig. 17-8)

- the tendon of the biceps brachii, which lies as the central structure in the fossa;
- the median nerve, which runs along the lateral edge of the pronator teres muscle;
- the brachial artery, which enters the fossa just lateral to the median nerve and just medial to the biceps brachii tendon;
- the radial nerve (not shown), which runs along the medial edge of the brachioradialis and ECRL muscles and is vulnerable to injury here;
- the median cubital or intermediate cubital cutaneous vein, which crosses the surface of the fossa.

NERVES

The neurologic supply of the bones, joints, muscles, and skin of the elbow and forearm is derived from the C5 through C8 nerve roots, which exit from the intervertebral foramina of C4–5 through C7–T1 (Fig. 17-6 and Fig. 17-9).[62]

Ulnar Nerve (C8–T1)

From its origin as the largest branch of the medial cord of the brachial plexus, the ulnar nerve continues along the anterior compartment of the arm, before passing through the medial intermuscular septum at the level of the coracobrachialis insertion.

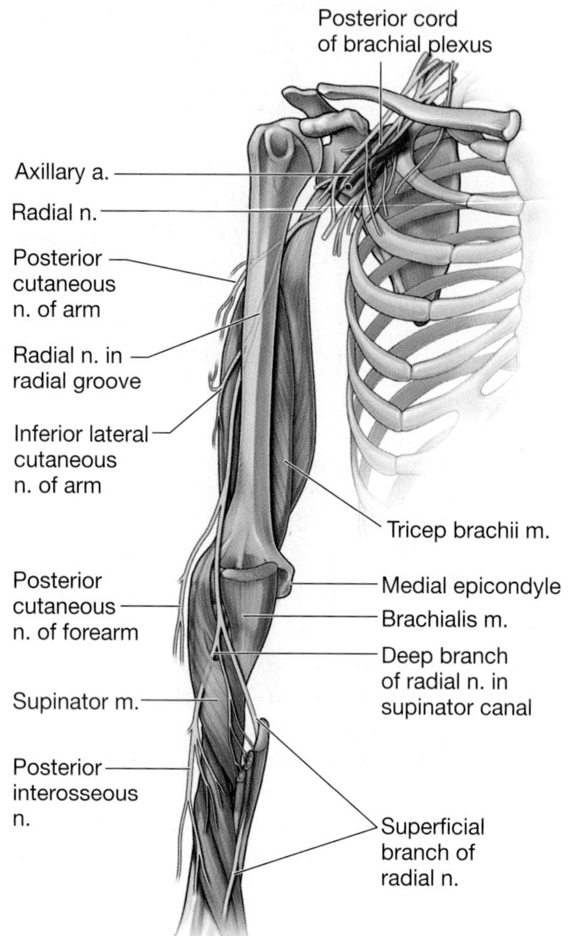

FIGURE 17-9 Nerve supply of the elbow and forearm. (Reproduced with permission from Morton DA, Foreman KB, Albertine KH: *Gross Anatomy: The Big Picture*. McGraw-Hill, 2011)

At the level of the elbow, the ulnar nerve passes posterior to the medial epicondyle, where it enters the cubital tunnel. Ulnar nerve compression in the cubital tunnel is a common entrapment neuropathy of the upper extremity, second only to carpal tunnel syndrome (CTS).[63] After leaving the cubital tunnel, the ulnar nerve passes between the two heads of the FCU origin and traverses the deep flexor–pronator aponeurosis.[64,65]

Median Nerve (C5–T1)

The median nerve extends medially down the upper arm across the anterior aspect of elbow joint. The ligament of Struthers arises from an abnormal spur on the shaft of the humerus and runs to the medial supracondylar process.[55] The supracondylar process with its ligamentous extension encloses a foramen, bounded medially by the medial intermuscular septum, and the distal anterior surface of the medial epicondyle, through which the brachial artery and median nerve pass.[66]

As the median nerve passes through the cubital fossa, the anterior interosseous nerve (AIN) branches off it, as it passes through the two heads of the pronator teres muscle. The AIN supplies the motor innervation to the index and middle flexor digitorum profundus (FDP), the flexor pollicis longus (FPL), and the pronator quadratus.

Radial Nerve (C5–T1)

The radial nerve sits superiorly and medially in the upper arm, and winds around humeral shaft. At a point approximately 10–12 cm proximal to the elbow joint, the radial nerve passes from the posterior compartment of the arm by piercing the lateral intermuscular septum.[67] The nerve travels in the anterior forearm between the brachialis muscle and the biceps tendon medially, and the brachioradialis, ECRL, and ECRB muscles laterally.[67] Within an area approximately 3 cm proximal or distal to the elbow joint, the radial nerve branches into a deep mixed nerve, the posterior interosseous nerve (PIN), and a superficial sensory branch.[68,69] After dividing, the two terminal divisions usually follow the same course, sharing a single epineurium for several centimeters, before the superficial radial nerve moves anteriorly to lie on the undersurface of the brachioradialis, and the deep branch travels posteriorly to enter the radial tunnel/supinator canal, distal to the origin of the ECRB, at the level of the radiohumeral joint.[67] Entering the canal, the deep branch supplies the ECRB then passes deep to the superficial head of the supinator, where the arcade of Fröhse* can impinge on the nerve.[70,71]

The nerve continues between the two heads of the supinator and innervates this muscle during its passage to the posterolateral aspect of the radius. On emerging from the supinator, a motor division (supplying the abductor pollicis longus, extensor pollicis brevis, extensor indicis proprius, and extensor pollicis longus muscles) and a mixed lateral branch (supplying the extensor carpi ulnaris, extensor digitorum communis, and extensor digiti minimi muscles) are recognized. The lateral branch continues along the posterior-radial border of the radius to the wrist as the sensory branch of the PIN, which innervates the posterior (dorsal) capsule of the wrist and intercarpal joints (see Chap. 18).[67,71]

The Radial Tunnel/Supinator Canal

The radial tunnel lies on the anterior aspect of the radius and is approximately three to four fingerbreadths long, beginning just proximal to the radiohumeral joint and ending at the site where the PIN passes deep to the superficial part of the supinator muscle.[72] The lateral wall of the tunnel is formed by the brachioradialis, ECRL, and ECRB. These muscles cross over the nerve to form the anterior wall of the radial tunnel as well, while the floor of the tunnel is formed by the capsule of the humeroradial joint, and the medial wall is composed of the brachialis and biceps tendon.[67]

VASCULAR SUPPLY

The vascular supply to the elbow (Fig. 17-10) includes the brachial artery, the radial and ulnar arteries, the middle and radial collateral artery laterally, and the superior and inferior ulnar collateral arteries.[37]

*The arcade of Fröhse is an inverted arched structure that lies within 1 cm distal of the fibrous edge of the ECRB and approximately 2–4 cm distal to the radiohumeral joint. It represents the proximal border of the superficial head of the supinator, through which the radial nerve passes.

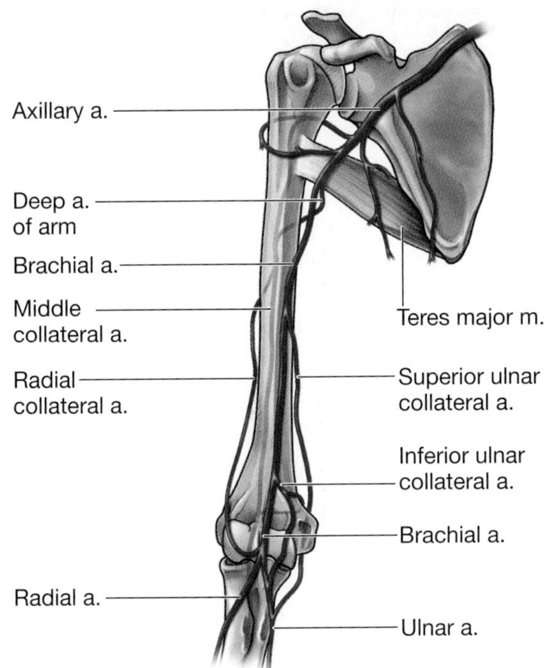

FIGURE 17-10 Vascular supply of the elbow and forearm. (Reproduced with permission from Morton DA, Foreman KB, Albertine KH: *Gross Anatomy: The Big Picture.* McGraw-Hill, 2011)

BIOMECHANICS

There is still controversy in the literature as to the precise biomechanics of the elbow,[73] and how the axes of motion relate to the anatomy of the joint. Biomechanically, the elbow predominantly functions as an important central link in the upper extremity kinetic chain, allowing for the generation and transfer of forces that occur in the upper extremity. The common stresses that occur at the elbow include valgus stress, which results in medial tension and lateral compression loading; varus stress, which results in lateral tension loading; extension stress; and multiple combinations of these stresses. These forces produce repetitive tensile loads on the ligamentous and muscular support systems around the elbow, and compressive and shear loads on the bony constraints.[74] Truly impressive loads can be placed through the elbow during activities such as throwing or pitching.

It is important that the elbow is able to move freely and painlessly throughout its available motion. These motions include elbow flexion and extension, and forearm pronation and supination.

Flexion–Extension

Flexion–extension of the elbow complex occurs about a relatively fixed axis of rotation passing through the center of arcs formed by the trochlea and the capitellum (Fig. 17-1). The maximal range of passive motion generally available to the elbow is from 5 degrees of hyperextension to 145 degrees of flexion. Full active extension in the normal elbow is some 5–10 degrees short of that obtainable by forced extension, due to passive muscular restraints (biceps, brachialis, and supinator).[75,76] Passive extension is limited by the impact of the olecranon process on the olecranon fossa, tension in the dermis, the fibers of the MCL, and the anterior capsule.[77] Excessive ectopic bone formation around the olecranon fossa can also limit full passive extension. Passive flexion is limited by bony structures (the head of the radius against the radial fossa and the coronoid process against the coronoid fossa), tension of the posterior capsular ligament, soft-tissue approximation, and passive tension in the triceps.[77]

TABLE 17-3 Structures that can Restrict Supination and Pronation

Limit Supination	Limit Pronation
Pronator teres, pronator quadratus	Biceps or supinator muscles
Palmar capsular ligament at the distal radioulnar joint	Posterior (dorsal) capsular ligament at the distal radioulnar joint
Oblique cord, interosseous membrane, and quadrate ligament	
Ulnocarpal complex	Ulnocarpal complex

Data from Neumann DA: Elbow and forearm complex. In: Neumann DA, ed. *Kinesiology of the Musculoskeletal System: Foundations for Physical Rehabilitation*. St. Louis, MO: Mosby, 2002:133–171.

Data from Kleinman WB, Graham TJ: The distal radioulnar joint capsule: Clinical anatomy and role in posttraumatic limitation of forearm rotation. *J Hand Surg [Am]* 23:588–599, 1998.

Data from Bert JM, Linscheid RL, McElfresh EC: Rotatory contracture of the forearm. *J Bone Joint Surg Am* 62:1163–1168, 1980.

Supination–Pronation

Pronation and supination require simultaneous joint movement at the proximal and distal radioulnar joints (Fig. 17-3).[8] The longitudinal axis of rotation about which supination and pronation occur is considered to pass from the center of the head of the radius to the convex articular surface of the ulnar at the distal radioulnar joint. Supination at the proximal radioulnar joint occurs as a spinning of the radial head within the fibro-osseous ring formed by the AL and radial notch of the ulna.[8] The arthrokinematics of pronation at the proximal radioulnar joint occurs by similar mechanisms.

Restrictions in the passive range of pronation and supination motions can occur from tightness in muscle and/or connective tissues (Table 17-3).[78,79]

HUMEROULNAR JOINT

The motions that occur at the humeroulnar joint involve impure flexion and extension, which are primarily the result of rotation of the concave trochlear notch of the ulna about the convex trochlea of the humerus. From a sagittal section, the firm mechanical link between the trochlear and the trochlear notch, however, limits the motion to essentially a sagittal plane.[8]

HUMERORADIAL JOINT

Any motion at the elbow and forearm complex involves motion at the humeroradial joint. Thus, any limitation of motion at the humeroradial joint can disrupt both flexion and extension, and pronation and supination.[8]

During flexion and extension of the elbow, the humeroradial joint follows the pathway dictated by the anatomy of the ulnohumeral joint to which it is firmly attached by the annular and interosseous ligaments.[62] At rest in full extension, little if any physical contact exists at the humeroradial joint.[8,80] During active flexion, however, muscle contraction pulls the radial fovea against the capitulum.[81,82]

Some supination and pronation also occur at this joint due to a spinning of the radial head.

Although the humeroradial joint provides minimal structural stability to the elbow complex, it does provide an important bony resistance against a valgus force.[8,21]

PROXIMAL RADIOULNAR JOINT

At the proximal radioulnar joint, one degree of freedom exists, permitting pronation and supination (Fig. 17-3). Both the fascia and the musculature of the forearm depend on the integrity of the interosseous radioulnar relationship for their mechanical efficiency.[62]

The proximal radioulnar joint is structurally an ovoid, with very little swing available to it due to its ligamentous constraints. As a consequence, its movement is confined to accommodating the osteokinematic spin of the radius. As the radial head forms the convex partner, there is a tendency for the radial head to move posterolaterally during pronation and anteromedially during supination, but these movements are strongly curtailed by the annular and interosseous ligaments.

COUPLED MOTIONS

Conjunct rotations occur at the elbow complex with all motions. In addition, the elbow motions of flexion and extension are associated with adduction and abduction motions. The ability to abduct and adduct can easily be observed during pronation and supination. In the fully supinated position, the ulna is much nearer the midline of the body than it is in full pronation. Therefore, abduction occurs with pronation, and adduction occurs with supination.

The abduction that occurs with extension occurs at the humeroulnar joint and is more apparent than real. An increase in the carrying angle of the forearm during extension must not be confused with the abduction of the ulna, which occurs because of the unequal ranges of extension between the ulna and the humerus, and the radius and the humerus (the capitellum being oriented more anteriorly than the trochlear). This inequity produces a conjunct humeral adduction with flexion and a conjunct humeroulnar abduction with extension, both of which are controlled by the lateral and medial collateral ligaments.[62]

Thus, it is apparent that pronation–supination and flexion–extension are interdependent, and each is a conjunct motion of the other, at least at the extremes of range. Since pronation and supination involve the proximal and distal radioulnar joints and the humeroulnar, humeroradial, and radiocarpal joints, mechanical dysfunction of any of these joints may become apparent, especially in the extremes of elbow flexion or extension.[62]

FORCE COUPLES OF THE ELBOW

The role of the elbow musculature as dynamic joint stabilizers is still somewhat unclear. Both varus and valgus forces are produced by muscles during elbow motions. The valgus forces are produced by the extensor carpi ulnaris (ECU), EDC, ECRL, and brachioradialis, while varus forces are produced by the FCR, FDS, pronator teres, and FCU. Forces transmitted across the articulating surfaces include the forces created by muscles working together to produce the desired activity. The important force couples of the elbow include[83]:

- the triceps/biceps during elbow extension and flexion;
- pronator teres and pronator quadratus/supinator during forearm pronation and supination;
- FCR, FCU, flexor digitorum communis/ECRL, ECRB, and extensor communis during wrist flexion and extension;
- triceps/biceps and brachioradialis; pronator teres/supinator; and FCR, FCU/ECRB, and ECRL during activities requiring elbow stabilization.

EXAMINATION

Since the elbow is one of the multiple links of the upper extremity kinetic chain, a thorough static and dynamic examination of the entire upper extremity and cervical spine as well as the trunk should be performed in addition to examination of the elbow proper. The physical examination must include at least inspection, range-of-motion testing, palpation, provocative testing, and neuromuscular testing. The interventions for the common pathologies of the elbow complex and their interventions are detailed after the examination is described. An understanding of both is obviously necessary. As mention of the various pathologies occurs with reference to the tests and measures and vice versa, the reader is encouraged to switch between the two.

HISTORY

During the history, the clinician must determine the chief complaint and location of symptoms. In addition to the questions listed under history in Chapter 4, answers to the following questions must be obtained:

- What is the patient's chief complaint? The patient's chief complaint can often afford clues as to the underlying pathology. For example, a chief complaint of pain upon leaning on the point of the elbow is usually associated with olecranon bursitis.
- How old is the patient? There are a number of age-related elbow conditions. For example, pain in a young child would be suggestive of nursemaid's elbow (dislocation of the head of the radius), elbow pain between the ages of 15 and 20 could be osteochondritis dissecans, and tennis elbow (lateral epicondylitis) typically occurs in individuals 35 years of age or older.
- Was there a mechanism of injury or any antecedent trauma? Traumatic elbow injuries often occur with a fall on the

outstretched hand (FOOSH) injury. This type of fall can result in a number of upper extremity and neck injuries. At the elbow, the FOOSH injury can result in a hyperextension injury of the joint. If the fall was on the tip of the elbow, or there was blunt trauma to the olecranon process, this may indicate an olecranon bursitis, ulnar nerve lesion, or olecranon fracture.[84] If the patient reports an insidious onset of symptoms, especially if the patient has complained of weakness and pain, the clinician should consider performing an examination of the cervical spine, and an upper quarter screening examination as part of the overall examination.

- Is the patient right- or left-hand dominant? This may have an impact on the ability of the elbow to rest or on the functional status of the patient.
- Is there a history of pain following overuse or repetitive activities? Elbow injuries are common in sports as well as from cumulative overuse in the athlete and nonathlete. For example, repetitive hyperextension, accompanied by pronation of the elbow, can stress the distal biceps and lacertus fibrosus in the cubital fossa.[85]
- Are the symptoms related to the patient's occupation? The improper use or unaccustomed use of tools such as hammers, saws, and screwdrivers can cause lateral or medial elbow pain.
- Is there any history of locking or catching of the elbow with movement? Twinges of pain, or locking of the elbow, could indicate a loose body within the joint. An inability to fully extend the elbow may indicate a number of conditions including synovitis of the elbow,[84] especially if it is accompanied by pain and fullness of the paraolecranon grooves.[86]
- Is the patient an athlete? A history of a "pop" followed by pain and swelling on the medial aspect of the elbow in a throwing athlete may indicate an MCL sprain.[87] Individuals involved in racquet sports commonly develop lateral elbow pain suggesting lateral epicondylitis (tennis elbow). In these situations, it is well worth investigating recent changes in equipment (e.g., tennis racquet head size, string tension, grip size). In a throwing athlete, the clinician should seek out details, including[88]
  - acute versus progressive injury;
  - intensity of symptoms;
  - duration of symptoms;
  - throwing schedule;
    - frequency of throwing;
    - intensity;
    - duration;
    - types and proportion of pitches delivered;
    - delivery style (sidearm versus overhead—the former is more injurious to the elbow);
    - types and proportions of throws delivered (e.g., curve balls are more deleterious than fastballs);
    - rest periods employed;
    - warm-up and cool-down regimens employed;
    - phase the pain manifests in (e.g., early cocking, acceleration, and follow-through);
  - restriction of motion;
  - locking or checkrein-type symptoms.
- How long has the patient had the symptoms and are the symptoms improving or worsening? Such information can give clues as to the stage of healing or seriousness of the condition.
- Where are the symptoms located? Determining the details can help the clinician determine whether the symptoms are from a local source, or whether they are referred, or the result of compromise to a peripheral nerve, or cervical spine nerve root (radiculopathy). With few exceptions, pain in a particular area of the elbow is caused by the surrounding or underlying physical structures (Table 17-4).

TABLE 17-4 Differential Diagnosis of Elbow Pain According to Symptom Location

Location	Possible Disorders
Anterior	Anterior capsular strain Distal biceps tendon rupture/tendinitis Dislocation of the elbow Pronator syndrome (throwers)
Medial	Medial epicondylitis Ulnar collateral ligament injury (MCL) Ulna neuritis or ulnar nerve subluxation Flexor–pronator muscle strain Fracture Little league elbow in skeletally immature throwers Valgus extension overload overuse symptoms
Posteromedial	Olecranon tip stress fracture Posterior impingement in throwers Trochlear chondromalacia
Posterior	Olecranon bursitis Olecranon process stress fracture Triceps tendinitis
Lateral	Capitellum fracture Cervical radiculopathy—referred pain Lateral epicondylitis Lateral collateral injury Osteochondral degenerative changes Osteochondritis dissecans (Panner's disease) Posterior interosseous nerve syndrome Radial head fracture Radial tunnel syndrome Synovitis

MCL, medial collateral ligament.

Data from Conway JE: Clinical evaluation of elbow injuries in the athlete. *J Musculoskeletal Med* 10:20–28, 1988; Wilk KE, Andrews JR: Elbow injuries. In: Brotzman SB, Wilk KE, eds. *Clinical Orthopaedic Rehabilitation*. Philadelphia, PA: Mosby, 2003:85–123.

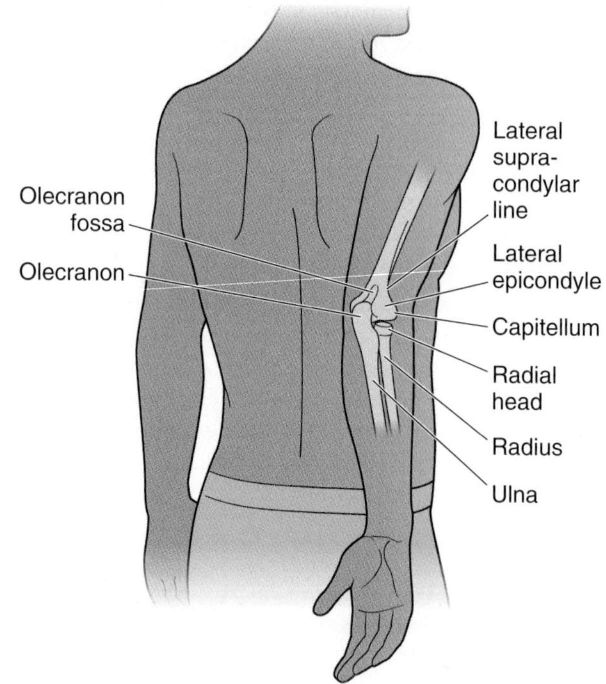

FIGURE 17-11 Lateral view of the elbow.

- ***Lateral elbow pain.*** Epicondylitis should be suspected if there is tenderness over a bony prominence (Fig. 17-11).
- ***Medial elbow pain.*** This is usually due to a tendinopathy at the site of the attachment of the superficial forearm flexors and the pronator teres muscle to the medial epicondyle (Fig. 17-12).[87] However, it may also indicate an MCL sprain, or an ulnar nerve compression.

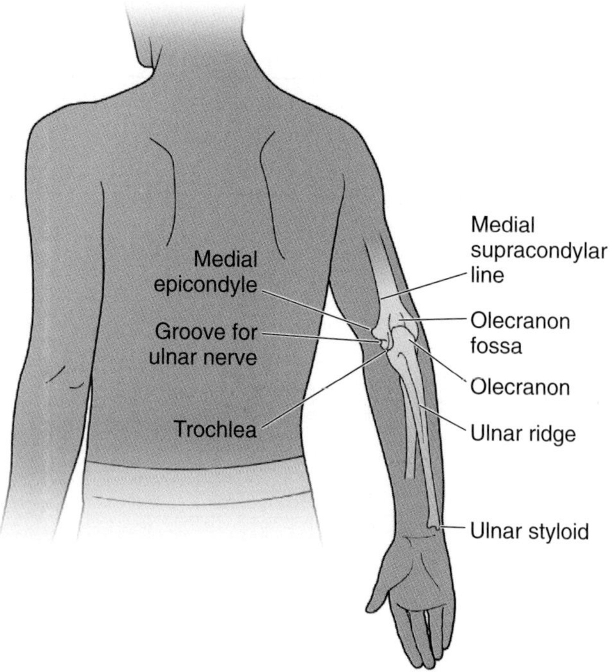

FIGURE 17-12 Medial view of the elbow.

- ***Posterior elbow pain.*** This suggests olecranon bursitis, triceps tendinosis, or a valgus extension overload.[89]
- ***Cubital fossa pain.*** This is most likely to result from a tear of the brachialis muscle at the musculotendinous junction and is a common injury in rock climbers,[90] or a biceps brachii lesion. Cubital fossa pain may also be associated with a compression of the PIN or a capsular injury.[91]
- ***Left-arm and elbow pain.*** This, when precipitated by physical exertion and relieved by rest, should suggest angina.[87]

- Are there any associated joint noises or crepitus? A snapping elbow is synonymous with the relatively common recurrent dislocation of the ulnar nerve. However, the medial head of the triceps muscle or tendon may also dislocate over the medial epicondyle and result in snapping either as the elbow is flexed or as it is extended from a flexed position.[84] Dislocation of the medial head of the triceps can occur in combination with dislocation of the ulnar nerve, producing the clinical finding of at least two snaps at the elbow, with or without discomfort on the medial side of the elbow and with or without ulnar neuropathy. Joint crepitus may also indicate the presence of a loose body or synovitis. Catching or locking sensations are suggestive of joint instability or a loose joint body.
- Which activities or arm positions appear to aggravate the condition? Grasping and twisting activities tend to stress the elbow structures.
- Is the pain constant or intermittent? A visual analog scale can be used to record the patient's pain level.
- Is there any associated pain in the neck or shoulder? Intrinsic pain of the elbow structures is exacerbated by movement of the elbow joint, whereas referred pain is usually independent of elbow activity (see "Systems Review," later).[84,92]
- Are there any other joints that appear to be painful? This finding may suggest a systemic or infectious component.
- Are the symptoms better or worse at particular times of day or night?
- Are there any sensory changes, paresthesia, and muscle weakness in the ipsilateral limb? Such neurological findings are suggestive of a spinal nerve root or peripheral nerve lesion.
- Is there any underlying joint disease? Several types of arthritides or osteochondrosis dissecans develop in the elbow region without a known cause.[89]
- How is the condition affecting the patient's function in activities of daily living and recreational pursuits?
- Has the patient had this condition before and, if so, how was it treated and what was the outcome?
- Is the patient taking any medications? What conditions in addition to the present condition are the medications for?
- How is the patient's general health?

SYSTEMS REVIEW

Signs or symptoms of a visceral, vascular, neurogenic, psychogenic, spondylogenic, or systemic disorder that may be local or referred are described in Chapter 5. Conditions that are out of the scope of physical therapy require that the patient be referred to an appropriate health-care provider. Scenarios related to the elbow that warrant further investigation include an insidious onset of symptoms and complaints of numbness or paresthesia in the upper extremity. The Cyriax scanning examination (see Chap. 4) can help highlight the presence or absence of neurological complications including spinal nerve root and peripheral nerve palsies. The scanning examination includes strength testing of the key muscles (see "Resistive Testing"), sensation testing, and reflex testing (see "Neurologic Examination").

Reproduction of the patient's elbow or other symptoms with cervical motion, rather than elbow movement, is a strong indicator of a cervical and upper thoracic source (ligaments, muscles, zygapophysial joints, and disks) for the symptoms, with either the segmental roots or the brachial plexus being involved.[19]

In addition to the cervical and upper thoracic spine, the related joints referring symptoms to the elbow require clearing, especially the shoulder.

Systemic causes of insidious elbow pain include gout, infective arthritis, polyarthritis, and vascular disorders, such as Volkmann's ischemia (see Chap. 5). Morning stiffness lasting for more than 1 hour, constitutional signs, and physical signs of joint inflammation are all indicative of an inflammatory disease. Systemic conditions are typically associated with other signs and symptoms that are not related to movement and that are systemic in nature (fever, chills, etc.). Respiratory and cardiovascular conditions must also come into consideration when examining the elbow.[84] The upper arm is very close to the chest and its viscera, so reference of pain to the elbow from these structures can occur.

CLINICAL PEARL

Severe progressive pain not affected by movement, persistent throughout the day and night, and associated with systemic signs may indicate referred pain from a malignancy.

Following the history and systems review, the clinician should be able to determine the suitability of the patient for physical therapy.

TESTS AND MEASURES

Observation

For an accurate and thorough examination of the elbow, the clinician must be able to visualize both arms. The involved elbow should be inspected for scars, deformities, and swelling. Any asymmetry in size or positioning between the extremities should be noted. The earliest sign of elbow effusion is a loss of the elbow dimples. Most swelling appears beneath the lateral epicondyle. Even minor swelling or effusion prevents full extension of the elbow. Anterior joint effusion is evidence of significant swelling. Gradual swelling over the posterior tip of the elbow, which can be golf ball sized and is often not tender to palpation, is usually olecranon bursitis. The clinician should observe for normal soft-tissue and bony contours. Hypertrophy of the dominant forearm is common in tennis players and pitchers.

CLINICAL PEARL

Sudden swelling in the absence of trauma suggests infection, inflammation, or gout.

The clinician should observe the "carrying angle" of the involved elbow (the angle formed between the arm and the forearm) and compare it to the other side. The carrying angle varies from 13 to 16 degrees for females, and 11 to 14 degrees for males.[5,11] Any difference in the carrying angle of the elbow is obvious when the elbow is in extension. An increased carrying angle (>15 degrees) is called *cubitus valgus*. Cubitus varus, or "gunstock deformity," is the term used to describe a decreased carrying angle (<10 degrees). The most common causes of an altered carrying angle are past trauma or epiphyseal growth disturbances. For example, a cubitus valgus can be caused by a lateral epicondylar fracture, whereas a cubitus varus is frequently the result of a supracondylar fracture.

The triangular relationship of the epicondyles and the olecranon at 90 degrees of elbow flexion and at full extension is often disrupted in the presence of a fracture, dislocation, or degeneration. At 90 degrees of flexion, the three bony landmarks form an isosceles triangle, and when the arm is extended they form a straight line.[89,93]

Excessive tension at the elbow can be produced in occupations that place the elbows in sustained positions of flexion and adduction (e.g., keyboard operators). The tension increases resistance to movement and joint play at the elbow.[94,95] Elbow flexion also increases tension at the fibrous arch that connects the two heads of the FCU, which can lead to compression of the ulnar nerve.[96]

A combination of sustained flexion and a restriction in joint play decreases the overall volume within the cubital tunnel, which can further increase the potential of ulnar nerve compression.[96,97]

CLINICAL PEARL

The pronated forearm position, combined with elbow flexion, wrist extension, and cyclic finger flexion and extension, creates shearing and compressive forces at several soft-tissue interfaces in the forearm.[98,99] The pronators and EDC adaptively shorten over time because of prolonged contractions in their most shortened positions.[94,98]

Palpation

Since they are superficial, most of the elbow structures are easily palpable (Figs. 17-11 and 17-12), making it easier for the clinician to pinpoint the specific area of pain. However, in cases in which the pain is more diffuse, the diagnosis becomes somewhat more difficult.

Palpation of the elbow complex is best performed with the patient seated or supine, so they are able to relax. A logical sequence based on surface anatomy is outlined below.

Bony Structures

Bony structures feel hard, whereas ligamentous structures feel firm. Bony palpation of the elbow should start with assessment for crepitus during flexion and extension of the elbow. The presence of pain, swelling, or temperature elevation should also be appreciated.

- ***Medial epicondyle (Fig 17-12).*** The medial epicondyle can be palpated on the medial aspect of the distal humerus. Just anterior and distal to the medial epicondyle one can palpate from proximal to distal the muscle origins of the pronator teres, FCR, palmaris longus, FDS, and FCU.[100] Just posterior to the medial epicondyle, the ulnar groove can be palpated, as can the ulnar nerve traveling within.
- ***Olecranon process.*** The olecranon (see Fig. 17-11) should be easy to locate on the posterior aspect of the elbow. The olecranon bursa will not be palpable unless inflamed or thickened. The olecranon ends distally in a point. Just distal to this point, the posterior border of the ulna can be palpated along its entire length (see Fig. 17-11). The clinician should assess for crepitus in the olecranon fossa as well as for any subtle extension blockage suggestive of synovitis, or the presence of intra-articular loose bodies.
- ***Lateral epicondyle (Fig. 17-11).*** Midway between the olecranon and the lateral epicondyle is the anconeus muscle. The lateral epicondyle is more difficult to palpate than the medial epicondyle as the former is covered by a large mass of extensor muscle, called the extensor bundle or wad.
- ***Supracondylar ridge (see Fig. 17-11).*** The supracondylar ridge is just superior to the lateral epicondyle. A number of tendons/muscles are located in the region between the lateral supracondylar ridge and the lateral epicondyle. The muscles from proximal to distal are the brachioradialis, ECRL, ECRB, and the EDC. By asking the patient to make a fist with the wrist in slight extension, the ECRL can be felt on the supracondylar ridge.[89]
- ***The joint line.*** The joint line is located at a point approximately 2 cm down from an imaginary line joining the two epicondyles, which passes medially and inferiorly. The joint lines are firm on palpation, and lie between two structures that are harder.[89]
- ***Head of the radius.*** The radial head is located in the skin depression immediately distal to the lateral epicondyle. To palpate the radial head (see Fig. 17-11) at the humeroradial joint, the clinician places the index finger on the lateral humeral epicondyle. From here, the index finger slides posteriorly and distally between the humerus and the radial head (see Fig. 17-11). Rotation of the radial head will be noted with pronation and supination.[89] A traumatically dislocated radius will appear out of position and tender to palpation.

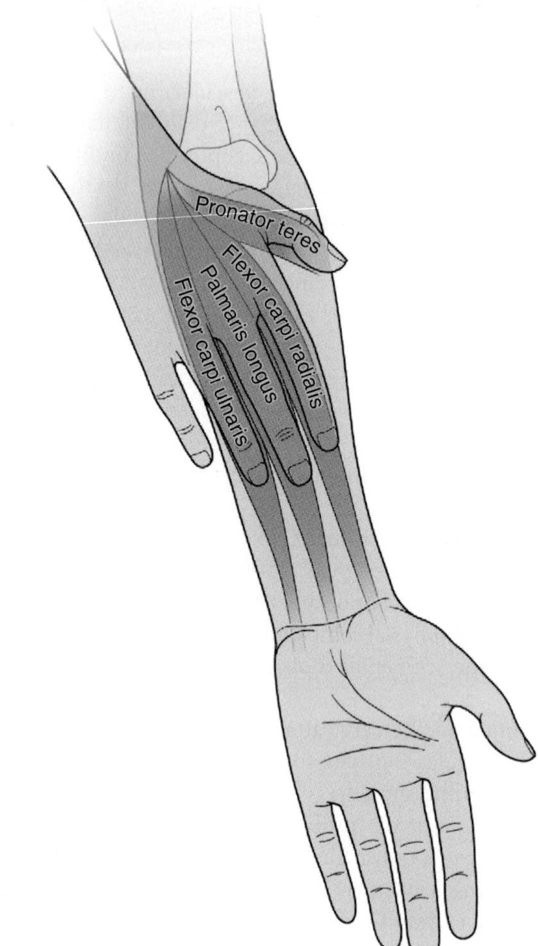

FIGURE 17-13 The wrist flexor–pronator muscle group

After examining the elbow's bony components, attention should be turned to the elbow's soft-tissue structures, which may be divided into four clinical zones: medial, posterior, lateral, and anterior.[89] The elbow's soft-tissue structures are best appreciated in 90 degrees of flexion. Swelling of the elbow can be localized as in a swollen olecranon bursa or diffuse as in a supracondylar fracture.

The medial aspect of the elbow contains the ulnar nerve, the wrist flexor–pronator muscle group (Fig. 17-13), and the MCL. The ulnar nerve can be felt as a soft tubule coursing through the groove between the medial epicondyle and the olecranon process. Secondary damage to the ulnar nerve can occur in supracondylar or epicondylar injuries.[89] The four muscles of the wrist flexor–pronator muscle group, pronator teres, FCR, palmaris longus, and FCU (see Fig. 17-13), originate from the medial epicondyle before diverging into separate paths down the forearm (see "Muscles," later). Overuse of the flexor mass results in pain and palpable tenderness at the medial epicondyle, extending approximately 1–3 cm distal to the epicondyle. Pain due to medial elbow tendinosis will be intensified with provocative testing, such as resistive wrist flexion and forearm pronation with the elbow extended and, in advanced cases, with the elbow flexed as well. The fan-shaped MCL connects the medial epicondyle to the medial margin of the ulna's trochlear notch. The anterior bundle of the MCL ligament is usually palpable with the elbow flexed from 30 to 60 degrees. Tenderness in this area can be due to MCL sprain. The valgus stress test is performed to assess MCL stability (see later).

Within the lateral aspect of the elbow are the wrist extensors, the LCL, and the AL. The three muscles of the wrist extensor group, brachioradialis, ECRL, and ECRB, are palpated as a unit, with the forearm in a neutral position and the wrist at rest (see "Muscles," later). These three muscles are commonly involved in lateral epicondylitis or "tennis elbow." Palpable tenderness over the ECRB is common in this condition. Pain due to lateral elbow tendinosis is intensified with resisted wrist and finger extension with the elbow extended and, in advanced cases, with the elbow flexed as well.[89] The LCL extends from the lateral epicondyle to the side of the AL, a ring-shaped band located deep to the extensor aponeurosis, cupping the radial head and neck. Although the LCL is difficult to directly palpate because of the overlying musculature, disruption of either the LCL or the AL can be assessed by palpation of the area and by the varus stress test (see later).

Muscles

- ***Biceps.*** The short head of the biceps is located at the coracoid process (together with the coracobrachialis muscle).[89] The long head of the biceps cannot be palpated at its origin, but it is palpable in the intertubercular groove of the proximal humerus. The muscle belly of the biceps is easily identifiable, especially with resisted elbow flexion and forearm supination.
- ***Brachialis.*** The origin of the brachialis can be palpated posterior to the deltoid tuberosity. Its insertion can be palpated at a point medial to the musculotendinous junction of the biceps, at the proximal border of the bicipital aponeurosis.[89]
- ***Brachioradialis.*** The brachioradialis can be palpated from the radial border of the cubital fossa distally to the radial styloid process.
- ***Common flexor origin at the medial epicondyle.***
- ***Common extensor origin at the lateral epicondyle.***
- ***Supinator.*** The borders of the supinator within the cubital fossa are formed by the brachioradialis (radially), pronator teres (ulnarly), and tendon of the biceps (proximally).[89]
- ***Triceps.*** Palpation of the triceps can be simplified by having the patient abduct the arm to 90 degrees. The lateral head of the triceps borders directly on the brachial muscle, whereas the medial head runs underneath both the long and lateral heads of the triceps. These two heads of the triceps can be palpated until their common insertion at the olecranon (Fig. 17-14).[89]
- ***Anconeus.*** This small muscular triangle can be palpated between the olecranon, the posterior border of the ulna, and the lateral epicondyle. If crepitus is felt at full elbow extension, the clinician can manually push the subanconeus bursa superiorly during elbow extension. If the crepitus decreases, a dysfunction of the anconeus should be

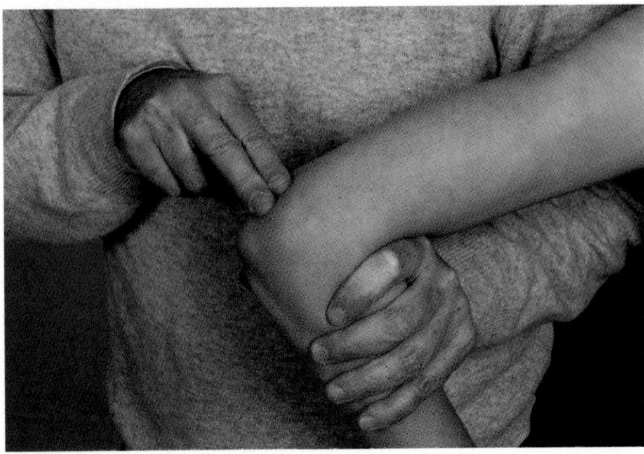

FIGURE 17-14 Palpation of the triceps at the elbow.

suspected, which can be treated with electrical stimulation and mobilization of the olecranon in a medial or lateral direction.

Active Range of Motion with Passive Overpressure

The patient with elbow pain should have a detailed assessment of his or her motion (Figs. 17-15 and 17-16). Range of motion can be assessed with the patient seated, although elbow extension is better evaluated with the patient standing. The patient is asked to perform active flexion and extension of the elbow, pronation and supination of the forearm, and wrist flexion and extension, with the ranges being recorded using a goniometer VIDEO:

- Flexion: active elbow flexion (Fig. 17-17) is 140–150 degrees.
- Extension: active elbow extension is 0 degree, although up to a 10-degree hyperextension is not uncommon, especially in women. This hyperextension is considered normal if it is equal on both sides and there is no history of trauma.
- Supination: active supination (Fig. 17-18) should be 90 degrees with no substitute motions (adduction) occurring at the shoulder.
- Pronation: active pronation is approximately 8–90 degrees with no substitute motions (abduction) occurring at shoulder.

Wrist flexion and extension, and forearm supination and pronation should be tested with the elbow flexed to 90 degrees and then fully extended.

In a study by Armstrong et al.,[101] the intratester, intertester, and interdevice (universal standard goniometers, a computerized goniometer, and a mechanical rotation measuring device) reliability of range-of-motion measurements of the elbow and forearm was assessed. Intratester reliability was high for all three measuring devices.[101] Intertester reliability was high for flexion and extension measurements with the computerized goniometer and moderate for flexion and extension measurements with the universal goniometer.[101] Intertester reliability was high for pronation and supination with all three devices.[101] The authors concluded that reliable measurements of elbow and forearm movement are obtainable,

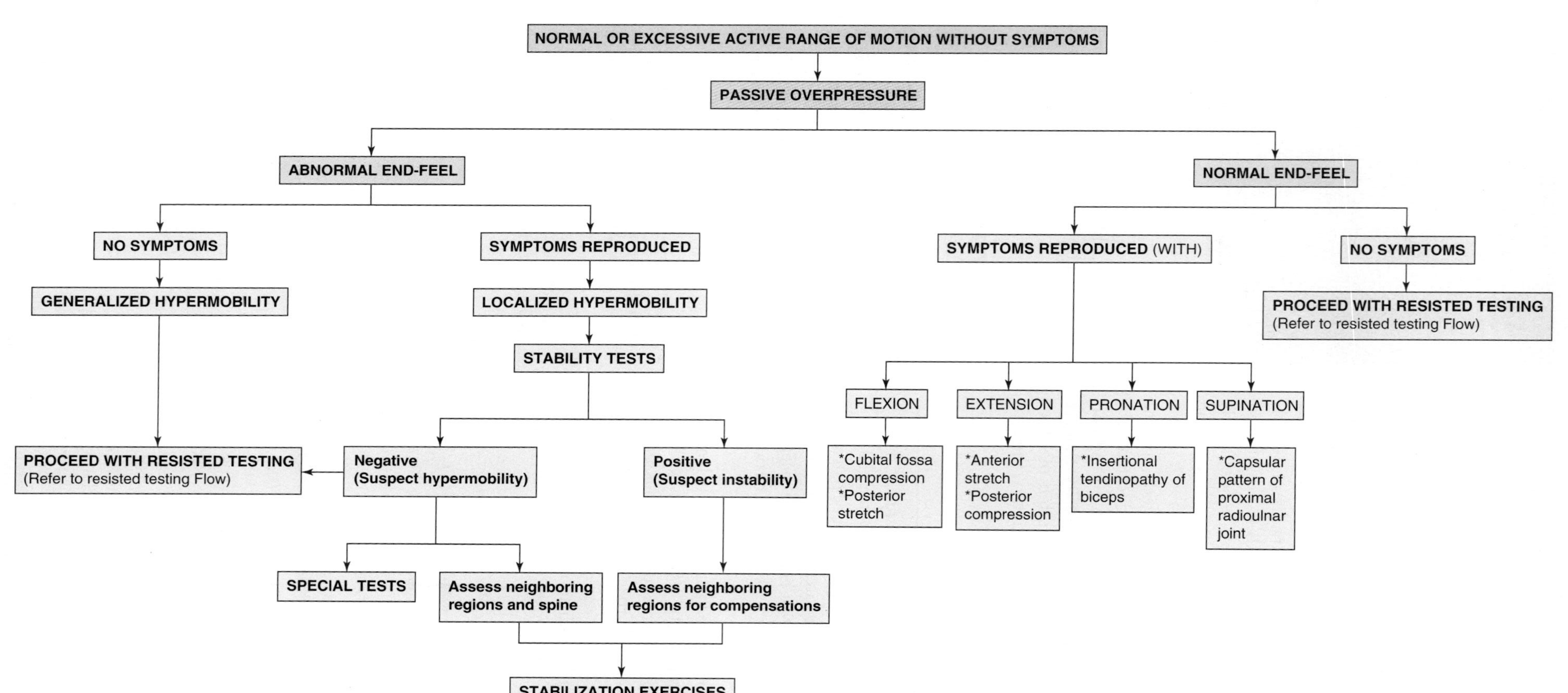

FIGURE 17-15 Examination sequence in the presence of symptoms with normal or excessive active range of motion in the elbow.

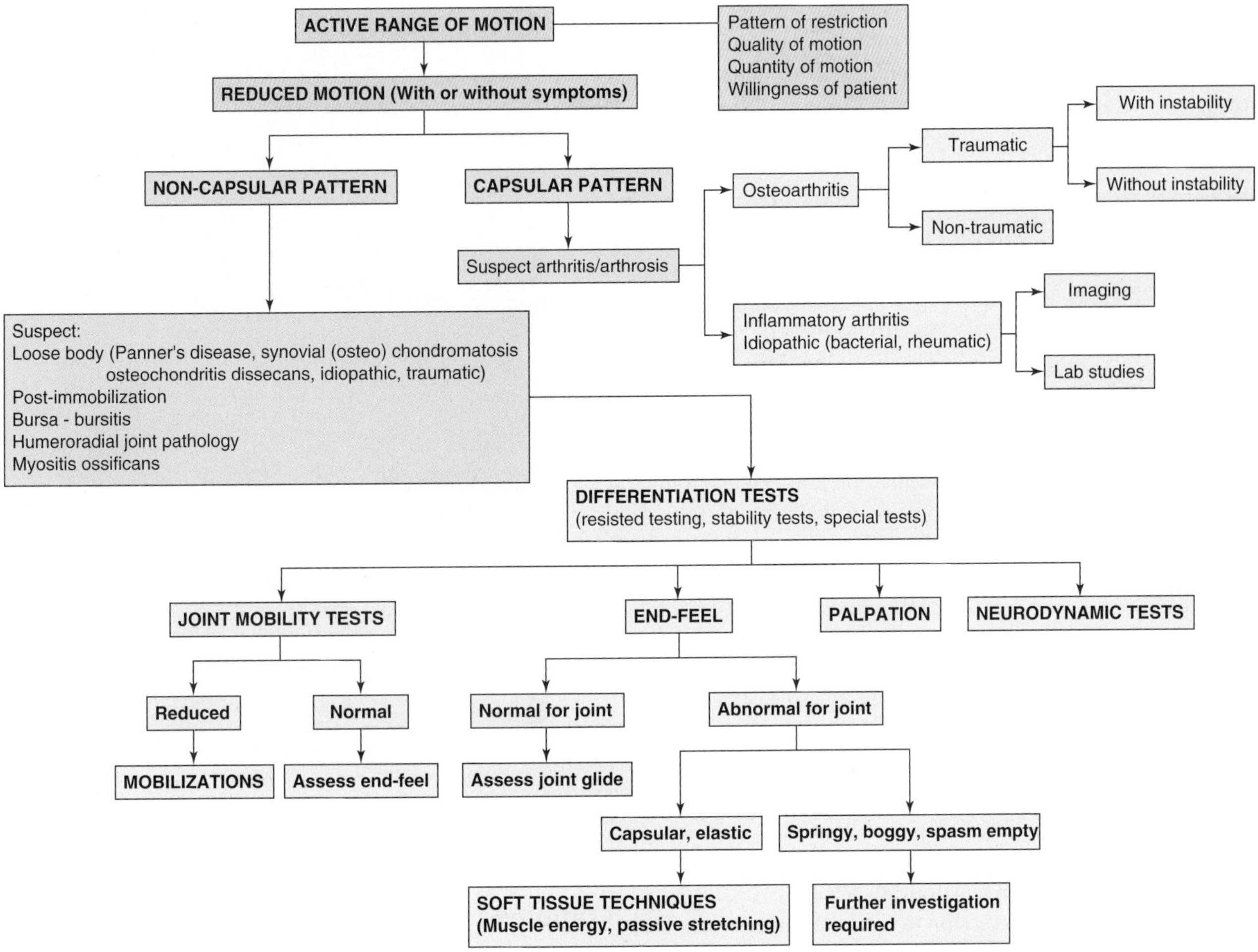

ACTIVE RANGE OF MOTION

Pattern of restriction
Quality of motion
Quantity of motion
Willingness of patient

REDUCED MOTION (With or without symptoms)

NON-CAPSULAR PATTERN

CAPSULAR PATTERN

Suspect arthritis/arthrosis

Osteoarthritis

Traumatic

With instability

Without instability

Non-traumatic

Inflammatory arthritis
Idiopathic (bacterial, rheumatic)

Imaging

Lab studies

Suspect:
Loose body (Panner's disease, synovial (osteo) chondromatosis osteochondritis dissecans, idiopathic, traumatic)
Post-immobilization
Bursa - bursitis
Humeroradial joint pathology
Myositis ossificans

DIFFERENTIATION TESTS
(resisted testing, stability tests, special tests)

JOINT MOBILITY TESTS

Reduced → MOBILIZATIONS

Normal → Assess end-feel

END-FEEL

Normal for joint → Assess joint glide

Abnormal for joint

Capsular, elastic → SOFT TISSUE TECHNIQUES (Muscle energy, passive stretching)

Springy, boggy, spasm empty → Further investigation required

PALPATION

NEURODYNAMIC TESTS

FIGURE 17-16 Examination sequence in the presence of painful flexion and/or extension at the elbow.

regardless of the level of experience, when standardized methods are used.[101]

Capsular or noncapsular patterns should be determined. The capsular pattern at the elbow is characterized by limitation of more flexion than extension. If motion restrictions are present, the nature and location of the motion barrier, and the relationship of pain to the motion barrier should be noted.[102]

The end-feels of elbow motion should be classified as either compliant, suggesting soft-tissue restriction, or rigid, suggesting a mechanical bony limit. Passive limitation warrants further investigation for the source of mechanical blockage. Pain that occurs at the limit(s) of motion suggests bony impingement. The clinician should also note the degree of ulnar adduction or abduction that occurs with the elbow motions.

Passive pronation and supination are applied by grasping the proximal aspect of the forearm. Passive overpressure is superimposed at the end of the available ranges of flexion and extension, using the appropriate conjunct rotations. Internal rotation of the forearm (pronation) is the conjunct rotation

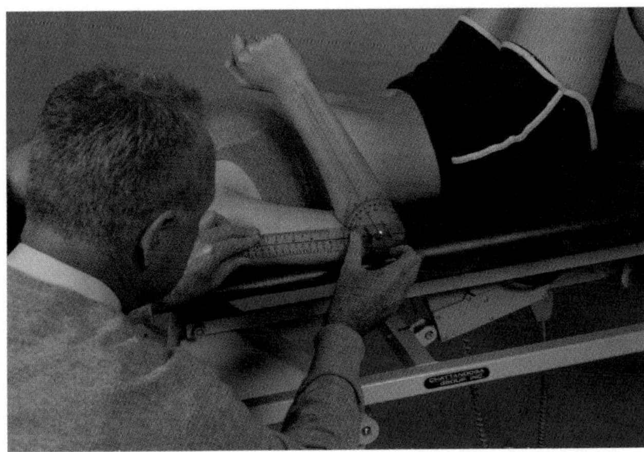

FIGURE 17-17 Elbow flexion.

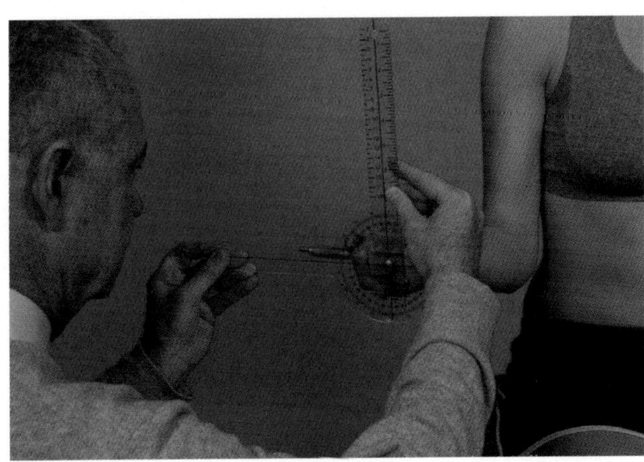

FIGURE 17-18 Forearm supination.

associated with elbow extension; external rotation of the forearm (supination) is the conjunct rotation associated with elbow flexion.[77,85] Normal values for elbow pronation and supination are approximately 75-degree pronation and 85-degree supination.[5]

CLINICAL PEARL

Decreased supination and pronation are frequent sequelae of a Colles' fracture, advanced degenerative changes, dislocations, and fractures of the forearm and elbow.

If there is a gross loss of pronation and supination post-trauma, a fractured radial head is a possibility. Of particular interest is the acute limitation of supination and extension in children, which likely results from a "pulled elbow" (also referred to as "nursemaid's elbow," see "Intervention Strategies" section).

Passive elbow flexion (Fig. 17-19) should have an end-feel of soft-tissue approximation. Elbow flexion combined with supination should have a capsular end-feel, whereas elbow flexion combined with pronation should have a bony end-feel. Passive flexion may aggravate an ulnar nerve neuropathy.[77] Loss of normal elbow flexion (~140 degrees) may be caused by osteophytic arthritis, intra-articular loose bodies, posterior capsule tightness, or possibly triceps tendinosis.

Passive elbow extension (Fig. 17-20) should have a bony end-feel. A springy end-feel may indicate a loose body. Elbow extension is usually the first motion to be limited and the last to be restored with intrinsic joint problems.[77,85] The clinician should be particularly careful of an elbow that has lost a gross amount of extension posttrauma, especially if accompanied by a painful weakness of elbow extension, as this may indicate an olecranon fracture. A significant loss of motion, with no accompanying weakness, could indicate myositis ossificans.

CLINICAL PEARL

Pain throughout the central arc of flexion and extension, or pronation and supination, implies degeneration of the humeroulnar or proximal radioulnar joints, respectively.

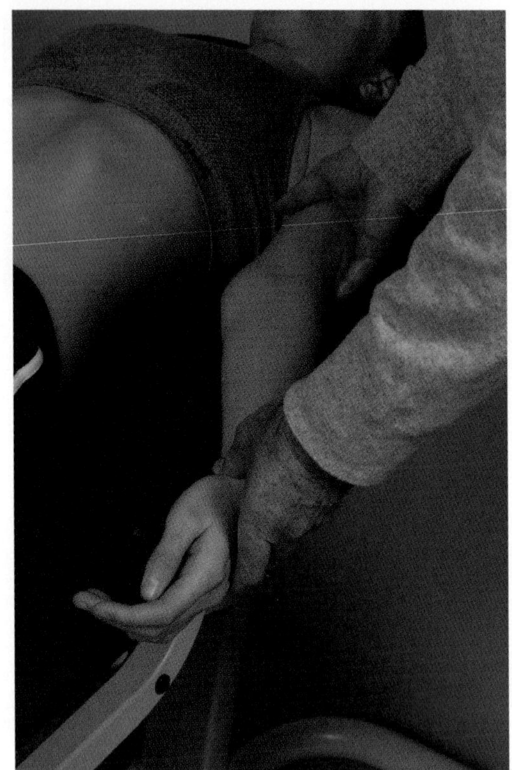

FIGURE 17-20 Passive elbow extension.

Combined Motions

Combined movement testing is used to assess the patient who has full range of motion but still has complaints of pain. The following combinations are assessed:

- Elbow flexion, adduction, and forearm pronation (Fig. 17-21)
- Elbow flexion, abduction, and forearm supination (see Fig. 17-22)
- Elbow extension, abduction, and forearm pronation (Fig. 17-23)
- Elbow extension, adduction, and forearm supination (see Fig. 17-24)

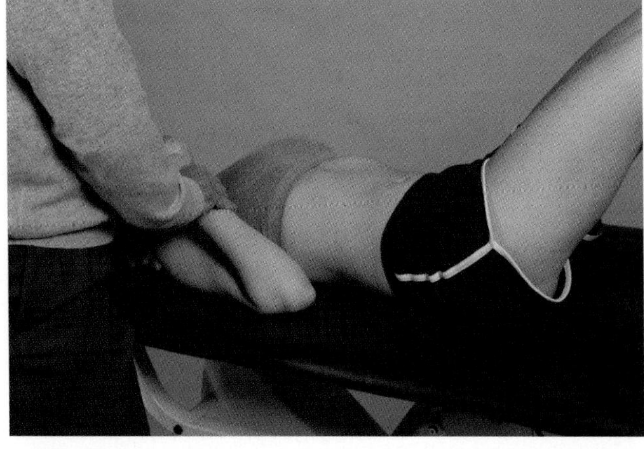

FIGURE 17-19 Passive elbow flexion.

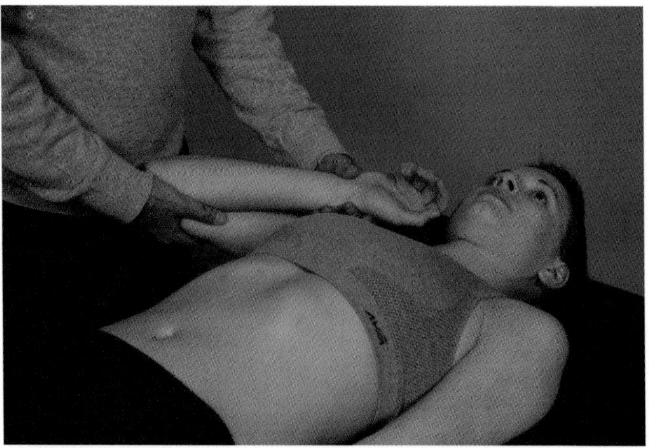

FIGURE 17-21 Combined motion of elbow flexion and pronation.

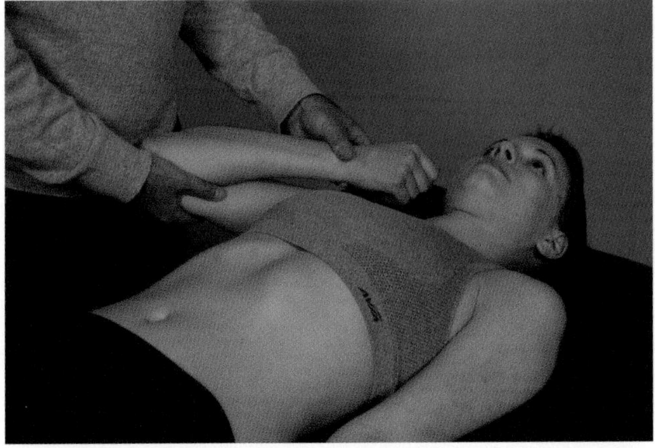

FIGURE 17-22 Combined motion of elbow flexion and pronation.

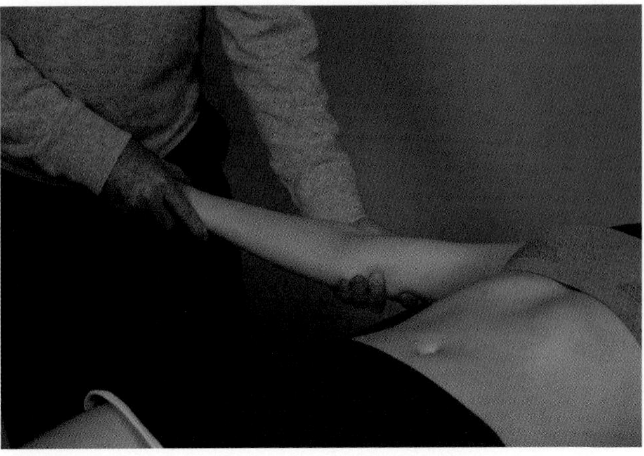

FIGURE 17-24 Combined motion of elbow extension and supination.

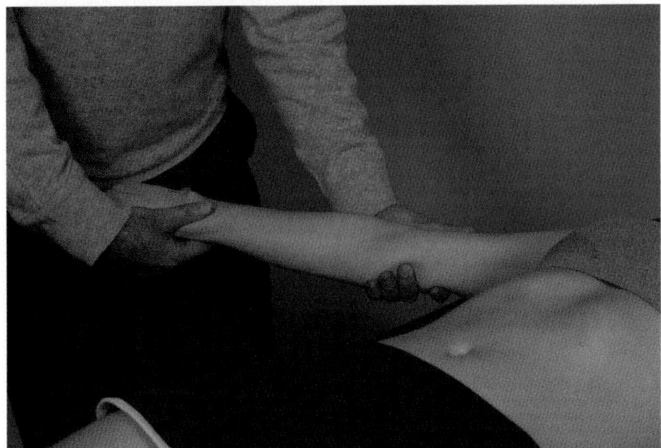

FIGURE 17-23 Combined motion of elbow extension and pronation.

Resistive Testing

In addition to all of the shoulder muscles that insert at or near the elbow (biceps, brachialis, and triceps), the clinician must also test the other muscles responsible for elbow flexion (Fig. 17-25) and extension and the muscles involved with forearm supination, pronation, and wrist flexion and extension. Elbow flexion strength is normally 70% greater than extension strength.[103] Muscle flexion power is greatest in the range of 90–110 degrees of flexion with the forearm supinated. In contrast, the flexion power is only 75% of maximum when the elbow is positioned in 45–135 degrees of flexion.[104] Supination strength is normally 15% greater than pronation strength.[103] The use of a dynamometer for testing upper extremity muscle groups has been found to be reliable.[105] Using make or break tests produce reliable results.[106] The most painful movement or movements should be tested last.

Elbow Flexion (C5–6)

Resisted elbow flexion is tested with the elbow flexed to 90 degrees, with the forearm in pronation VIDEO, then in supination VIDEO, and then in neutral rotation (Fig. 17-26) VIDEO. Pain with resisted elbow flexion most frequently implicates the biceps, especially if resisted supination is also painful. The brachialis is implicated if resisted elbow flexion with the forearm in full pronation is painful. The brachioradialis is rarely involved. Both sides are tested for comparison.

Elbow Extension (C7)

Resisted elbow extension is tested with forearm pronation, supination, and neutral. Both sides are tested for comparison. Pain with resisted elbow extension implicates the triceps muscle, although the anconeus muscle could also be involved.

Forearm Pronation/Supination (C5–7)

The clinician should test the strength of the forearm muscles by grasping the patient's hand in a handshake. The patient

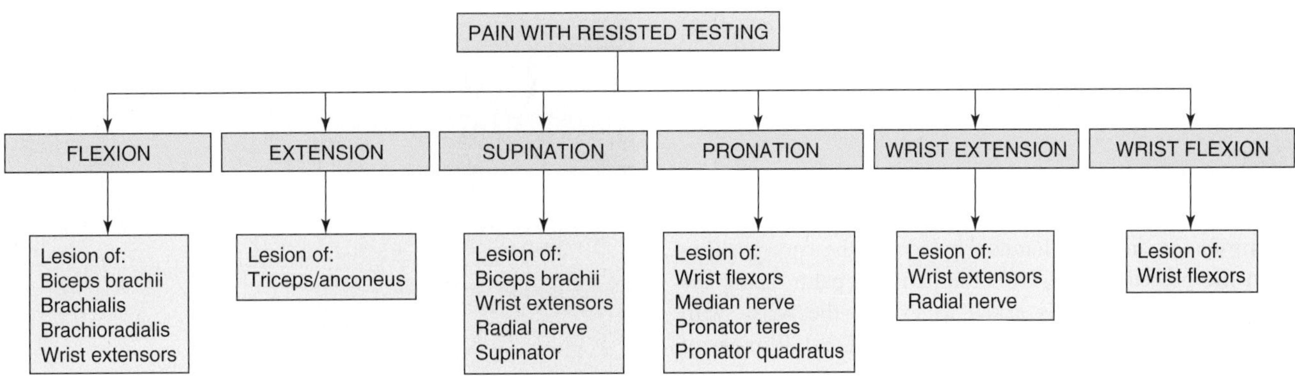

FIGURE 17-25 Symptoms reproduced with resisted testing at the elbow.

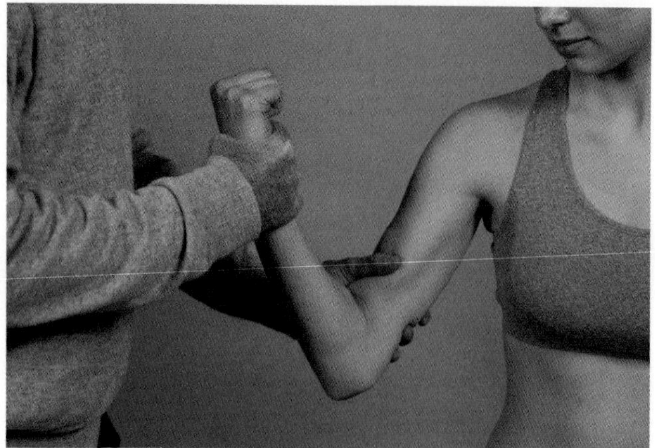

FIGURE 17-26 Resisted elbow flexion.

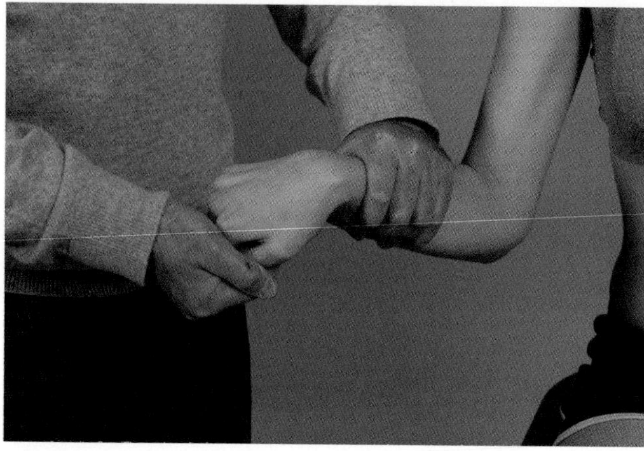

FIGURE 17-27 Resisted wrist flexion.

should be asked to exert maximum pressure to turn the palm first up (using supinators) and then down (using pronators). Supination is primarily the function of the supinator muscle, with augmentation from the biceps brachii for quickness or to overcome resistance. Supinator function can be effectively isolated during clinical assessment, by placing the elbow in extension VIDEO or near terminal elbow flexion VIDEO. Both these positions decrease the mechanical advantage of the biceps brachii. Weakness with supination may indicate a rupture, or a subluxation of the biceps tendon at the shoulder. It may also indicate a C5–6 nerve root lesion, radial nerve lesion (supinator), or musculocutaneous nerve lesion (biceps). The supinator muscle is rarely injured.

Pronator weakness is associated with rupture of the pronator teres from the medial epicondyle, fracture of the medial elbow, and lesions of the C6–7 or median nerve roots. Pronator quadratus weakness, which is tested with the elbow held in a flexed position VIDEO to neutralize the humeral head of the pronator teres muscle could indicate a lesion of the AIN. The pronator teres or quadratus muscles, which can be tested together VIDEO are rarely injured. Individuals with medial or lateral epicondylitis will also find the aforementioned maneuvers painful, and resisted wrist flexion and extension can be used to help differentiate the former and the latter, respectively.

Wrist Flexion

The FCU is the strongest wrist flexor. To test the flexors, the clinician stabilizes the patient's mid-forearm with one hand while placing the fingers of the other hand in the patient's palm, with the palm facing the patient (Fig. 17-27). The patient attempts to flex the wrist, with the elbow flexed and then extended. Weakness is evident in rupture of the muscle origin, lesions involving the ulnar (C8, T1) or median nerve (C6, C7), or tendinitis at the medial elbow if there is pain.

Wrist Extension

The most powerful wrist extensor is the ECU. To test the wrist extensors, the clinician's hands are placed in the same position as in the preceding test, with the patient's palm facing the clinician. The patient is asked to extend the wrist, with the elbow flexed and then extended (Fig. 17-28). Rupture of the extensor origin, lesions of the C6–8 nerve root, or lateral epicondylitis can cause weakness.

Radial Deviation

Resisted radial deviation is tested with the elbow at 90 degrees of elbow flexion, and at full elbow extension (see Chap. 18). Pain with resisted radial deviation is usually the result of lateral epicondylitis.

Ulnar Deviation

Resisted ulnar deviation, although rarely affected, is tested with the fingers in full flexion, and then in full extension (see Chap. 18).

Extension of Fingers 2–5

For resisted extension of fingers 2–5, the elbow is positioned in full extension, the wrist in neutral, and the metacarpophalangeal (MCP) joints at 90 degrees of flexion. Pain here is usually the result of extensor digitorum tendinitis, or lateral epicondylitis.

Extension of Fingers 2–3

For resisted extension of fingers 2–3, the patient is positioned as above. Pain with resistance implicates lateral epicondylitis.

If the above testing procedures are negative, or if the patient has complained that the combined movements cause the symptoms, resisted testing can be performed using combined movements. For example, testing elbow flexion in supination/pronation in varying degrees of elbow flexion.

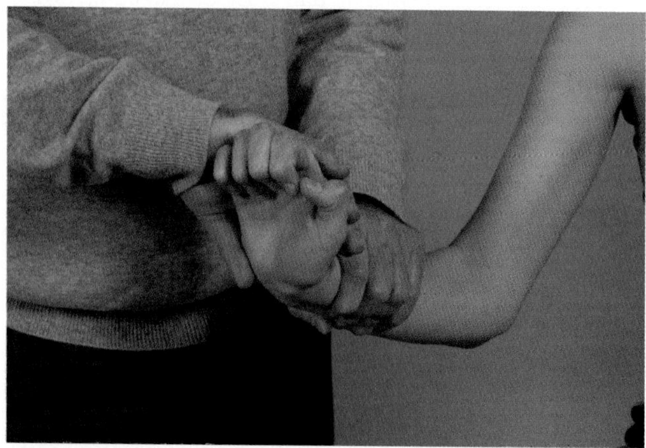

FIGURE 17-28 Resisted wrist extension.

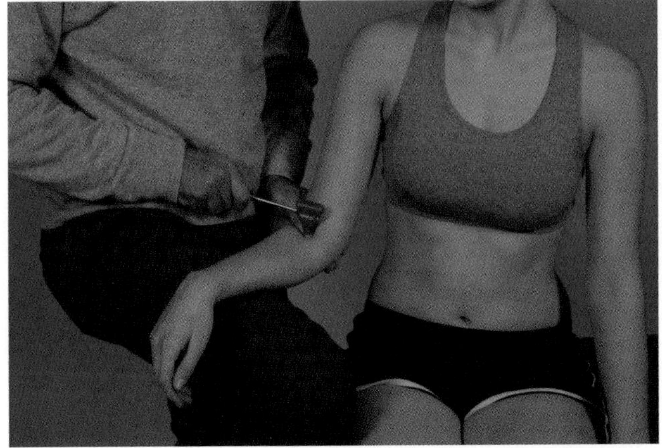

FIGURE 17-29 Biceps DTR.

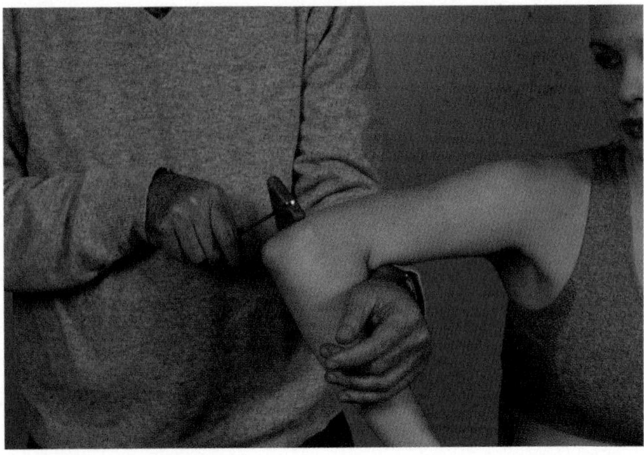

FIGURE 17-31 Triceps DTR.

Neurologic Examination

Sensation about the elbow is supplied by four different nerves and is evaluated as follows: lateral arm (axillary nerve, C5), lateral forearm (musculocutaneous nerve, C6), medial forearm (antebrachial cutaneous nerve, C8), and the medial arm (brachial cutaneous nerve, T1). Sensory testing may include Semmes–Weinstein sensibility and two-point discrimination (see Chaps. 3 and 18). An EMG evaluation can supplement the neuromuscular physical examination as needed. The three major muscle stretch reflexes of the elbow are the biceps (musculocutaneous nerve, C5), brachioradialis (radial nerve, C6), and the triceps (radial nerve, C7). The biceps reflex is elicited by placing a thumb over the biceps tendon in the cubital fossa and striking it with a reflex hammer while the patient's arm is relaxed and partially flexed (Fig. 17-29). The biceps muscle should be felt or seen to jerk slightly. The brachioradialis reflex is a radial jerk elicited by tapping the brachioradialis tendon at the distal end of the radius (Fig. 17-30). The triceps reflex can be elicited with the arm in the same position of partial, relaxed flexion (Fig. 17-31). The triceps muscle should jerk when the triceps tendon is tapped where it crosses the olecranon fossa. Depressed, exaggerated, or absent upper extremity reflexes are noted and compared with reflex testing at the other elbow.

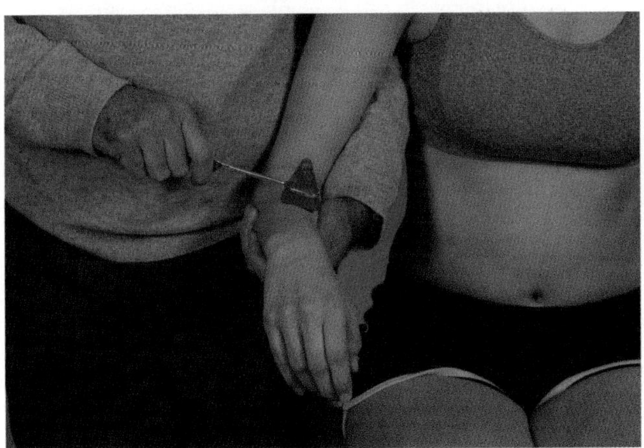

FIGURE 17-30 Brachioradialis DTR.

Functional Assessment

The functional strength of the elbow complex can be assessed using the tests outlined in Table 17-5. Like the shoulder, the elbow serves to position the hand for functional activities. A number of studies have reported the range-of-motion requirements for everyday activities. A total range of motion of 60–100 degrees of elbow flexion and 100 degrees of supination–pronation are required for tasks such as eating, dressing, and daily hygiene. The range of motion required for athletic activities, such as throwing a baseball, requires at least 10–20% greater range of motion.

Passive Articular Motion Testing

The passive articular mobility tests are used to examine the arthrokinematic motions of a joint or the accessory joint glides (see Chap. 4).

Ulnohumeral Joint

The patient is positioned in supine, with their head supported. The clinician sits or stands facing the patient.

Distraction/Compression. The clinician wraps the fingers around the proximal third of the forearm (Fig. 17-32). The clinician applies a longitudinal force through the proximal forearm, at an angle that is in 45 degrees less flexion than the position of the ulnar shaft, to either distract or compress the ulnohumeral joint. The quality and quantity of motion is noted. The test is repeated on the opposite extremity and the findings compared. An alternative method involves positioning the patient in prone, with the humerus being supported on the table and the arm hanging over the edge of the table (Fig. 17-33). Using one hand to stabilize the humerus, the clinician uses the other hand to apply a distraction force at the ulnohumeral joint. This position can also be used to assess the medial and lateral glides of this joint (Fig. 17-34).

Medial Glide. The clinician glides the ulna medially on the fixed humerus along the mediolateral plane of the joint line. The quality and quantity of motion is noted. The test is repeated on the opposite extremity and the findings compared.

Lateral Glide. The clinician glides the ulna laterally on the fixed humerus along the mediolateral plane of the joint line. The quality and quantity of motion is noted. The test

TABLE 17-5 Functional Testing of the Elbow

Starting Position	Action	Functional Test
Sitting, cuff weight attached to wrist	Elbow flexion	5-lb weight: functional 3–4-lb weight: functionally fair Active flexion (0 lb): functionally poor Cannot flex elbow: nonfunctional
Standing	Elbow extension with wall push-up	5 reps: functional 3–4 reps: functionally fair 1–2 reps: functionally poor 0 reps: nonfunctional
Standing facing door	Turning door knob into supination	5 reps: functional 3–4 reps: functionally fair 1–2 reps: functionally poor 0 reps: nonfunctional
Standing facing door	Turning door knob into pronation	5 reps: functional 3–4 reps: functionally fair 1–2 reps: functionally poor 0 reps: nonfunctional

Data from Palmer ML, Epler M: *Clinical Assessment Procedures in Physical Therapy*. Philadelphia, PA: JB Lippincott, 1990.

is repeated on the opposite extremity and the findings compared.

Radiohumeral Joint

The patient is positioned in sitting or supine, with their arm resting on the table. The following tests are performed[107,108]:

Anterior Glide. The clinician stabilizes the humerus and applies an anterior glide of the radius (Fig. 17-35), to assess the accessory glide that accompanies flexion.

Posterior Glide. The clinician stabilizes the humerus and applies a posterior glide of the radius (see Fig. 17-35) to assess the accessory glide that accompanies extension.

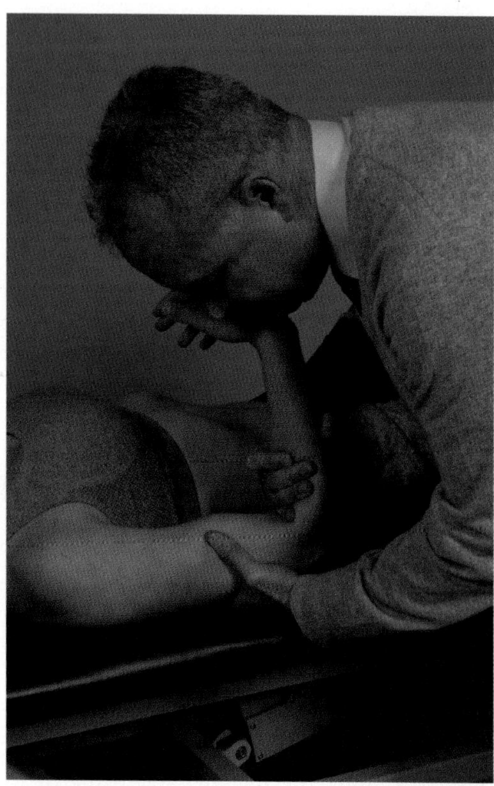

FIGURE 17-32 Ulnohumeral distraction/compression.

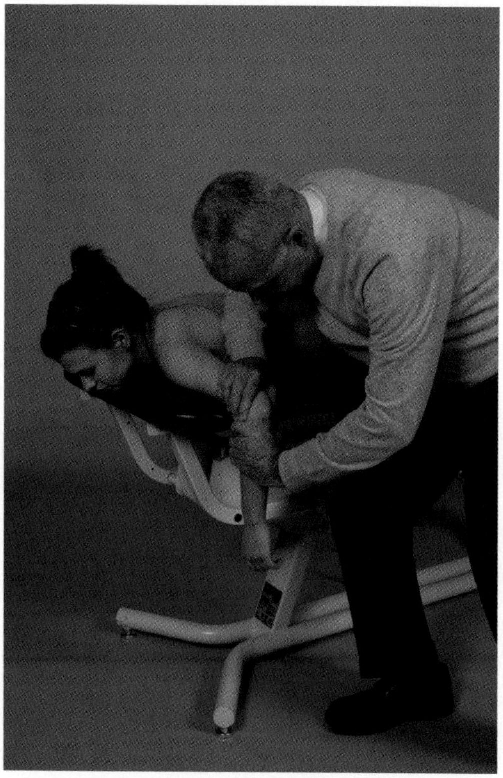

FIGURE 17-33 Ulnohumeral distraction.

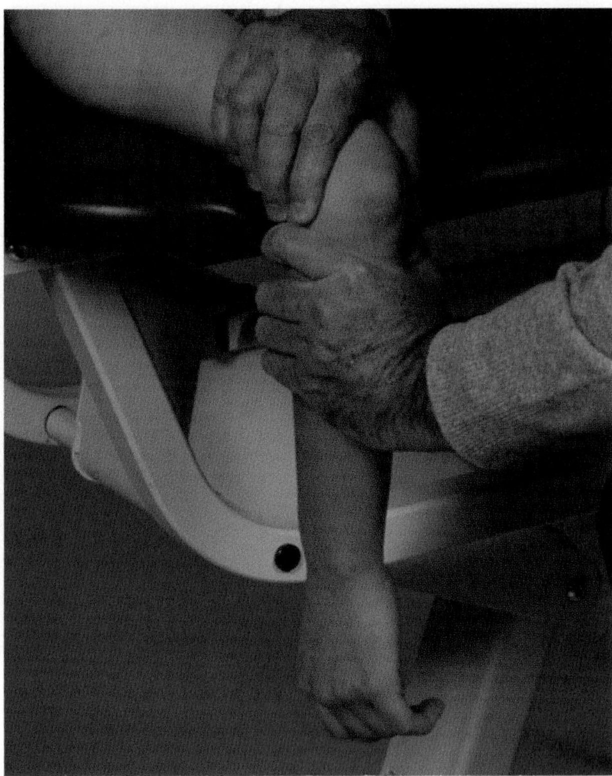

FIGURE 17-34 Medial and lateral glides of the ulnohumeral joint.

Distraction. The clinician stabilizes the radial head and the lateral epicondyle with one hand. With the other hand, the clinician grasps the radius and applies a longitudinal distraction force along the length of the radius (Fig. 17-36). A longitudinal compression force can be applied using the same patient–clinician position.

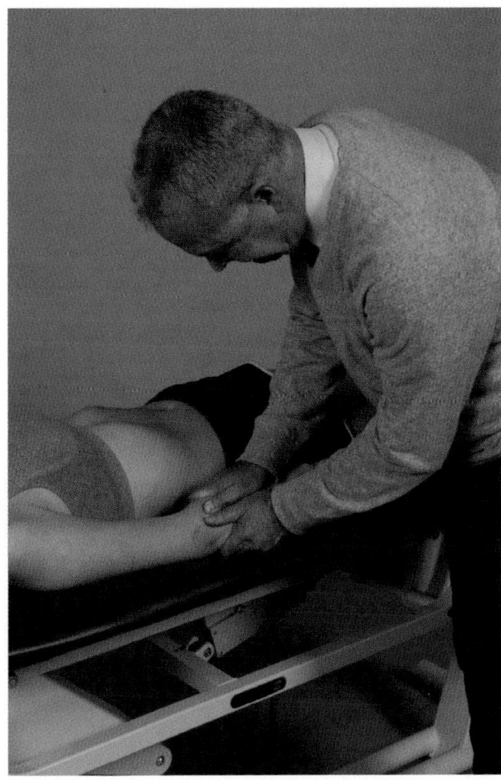

FIGURE 17-35 Radiohumeral joint glides.

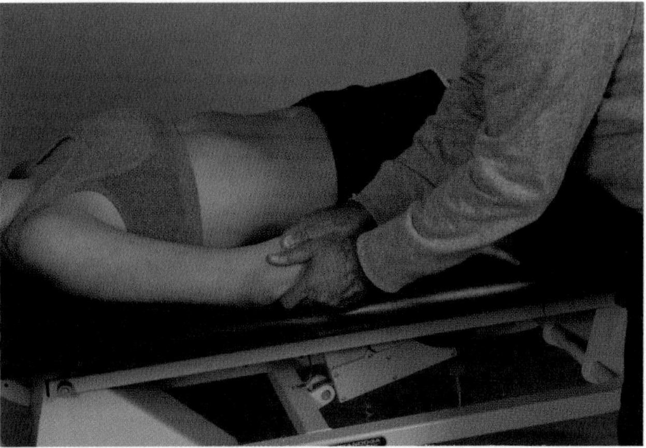

FIGURE 17-36 Distraction of radius.

Motion Testing of the Radial Head. The patient is positioned in sitting or supine, with the clinician facing the patient. The radial head is located by flexing and extending the elbow. Once located, the radial head is grasped by the clinician between the thumb and the index finger (see Fig. 17-36). The radial head is moved in an anterior and posterior direction, and any restriction of motion is noted. The posterior glide of the radius is coupled with pronation/extension, and anterior glide is coupled with supination/flexion. The most common dysfunction of the radial head is a posterior-radial head, which is accompanied by a loss of the anterior glide.

Stress Tests

Medial (Ulnar) Collateral Ligament (Valgus Test)

The patient is positioned in supine, with their head supported. The clinician stabilizes the distal humerus with one hand and palpates the distal forearm with the other. The anterior band of the MCL tightens in the range of 20–120 degrees of flexion, becoming lax in full extension, before tightening again in hyperextension. The posterior bundle is taut in flexion beyond 55 degrees.[3,14,23,85]

The anterior band is tested by flexing the elbow to between 20 and 30 degrees to unlock the olecranon from its fossa, as a valgus stress is applied continuously (Fig. 17-37).[25,60]

The posterior band is best tested using a "milking" maneuver. The patient is seated and the arm is positioned in shoulder flexion, elbow flexion beyond 55 degrees, and forearm supination. The clinician pulls downward on the patient's thumb (Fig. 17-38).[25] This maneuver generates a valgus stress on the flexed elbow. A positive sign is indicated by the reproduction of pain.

The tests are repeated on the opposite extremity and the findings compared. No diagnostic accuracy studies have been performed to determine the sensitivity or specificity of this test.

Lateral Pivot Shift Apprehension Test

The lateral pivot shift test is used in the diagnosis of posterolateral rotatory instability.[36] The patient is positioned in supine, with the involved extremity overhead. The clinician grasps the patient's wrist and elbow. The elbow is supinated with a mild force at the wrist, and a valgus moment and

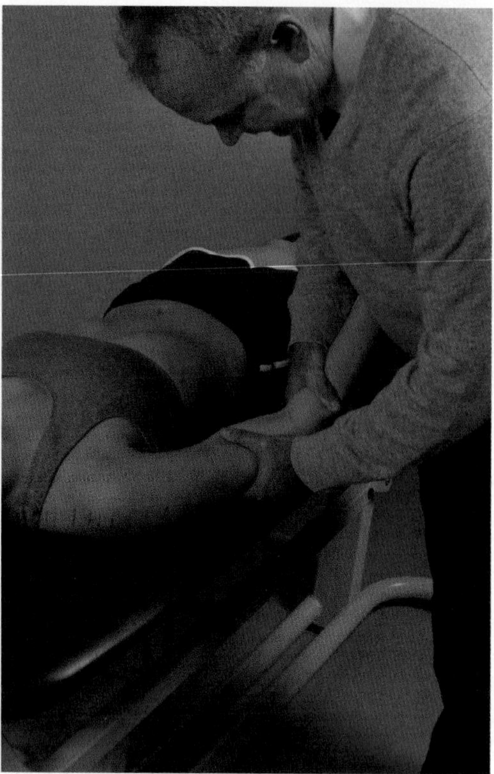

FIGURE 17-37 Ulnar collateral ligament stress test.

compressive force is applied to the elbow during flexion (Fig. 17-39).[109] This results in a typical apprehension response with reproduction of the patient's symptoms and a sense that the elbow is about to dislocate. Reproducing the actual subluxation, and the clunk that occurs with reduction, usually can only be accomplished with the patient under general anesthesia or occasionally after injecting local anesthetic into the elbow.

Lateral (Radial) Collateral Ligament (Varus Test)

The LCL is tested with the elbow positioned in 5–30 degrees short of full extension. The clinician stabilizes the humerus and adducts the ulna, producing a varus force at the elbow (Fig. 17-40). The end-feel is noted. No diagnostic accuracy studies have been performed to determine the sensitivity or specificity of this test.

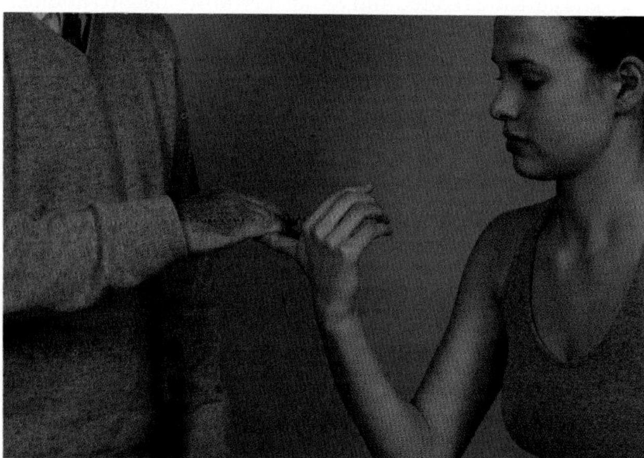

FIGURE 17-38 Milking maneuver.

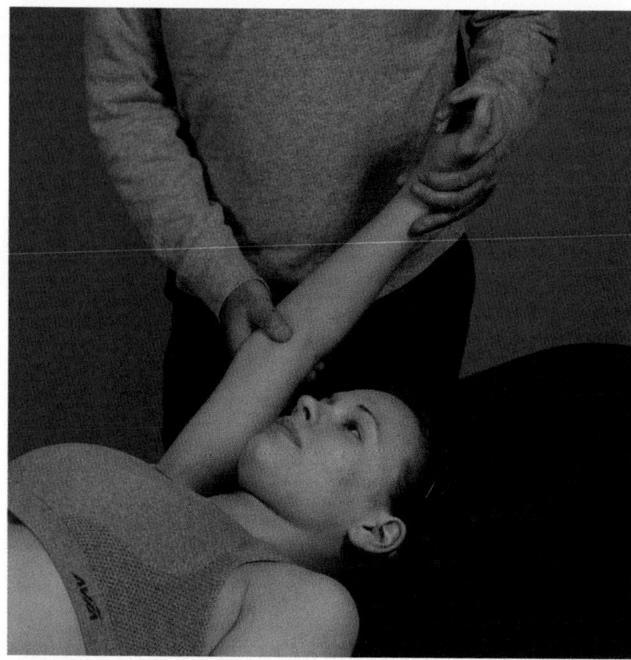

FIGURE 17-39 Lateral pivot shift apprehension test.

Special Tests

A number of special tests for the elbow exist. The diagnostic usefulness for some of these tests is outlined in Table 17-6.

Tennis Elbow

A number of tests exist for tennis elbow (lateral epicondylitis). Three are described here.

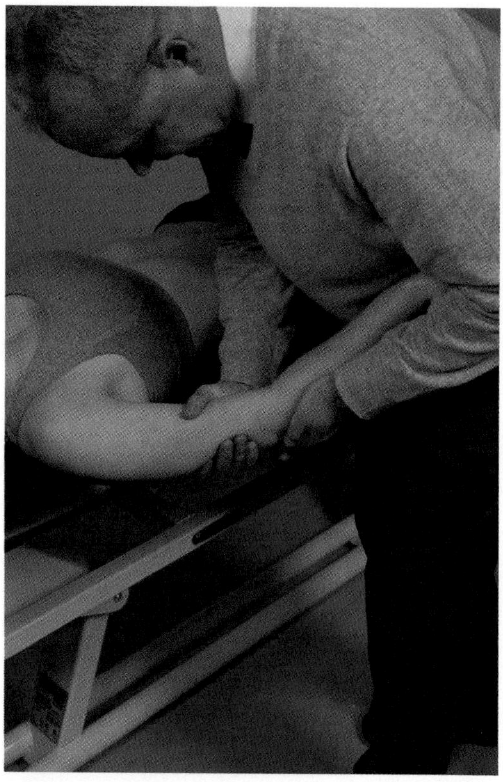

FIGURE 17-40 Radial collateral ligament stress test.

TABLE 17-6 Diagnostic Usefulness of Some Special Tests for the Elbow								
Test and Related Diagnosis	**Study Description**	**Reliability**	**Sensitivity**	**Specificity**	**LR+**	**LR−**	**DOR**	**QUADAS Score**
Elbow flexion (cubital tunnel syndrome)	Evaluated the clinical usefulness of provocative testing in 32 subjects with electrodiagnostically proven cubital tunnel syndrome using Tinel's sign, elbow flexion (without wrist extension and with forearm supination held for 60 seconds), pressure provocation, and combined elbow flexion and pressure provocation.[a]	NT	75	99	75	0.25	297	7
Pressure provocation (cubital tunnel syndrome)		NT	89	98	45	0.11	396	7
Percussion test/Tinel's sign (cubital tunnel syndrome		NT	70	98	35	0.31	114	7
Elbow extension (elbow fracture)	110 of 114 patients with acute elbow injury underwent radiographic evaluation. Inability to extend the elbow was found in 37 of 38 patients with bone injury.[b]	NT	97	69	3.1	0.04	72	10
Moving valgus stress (chronic medial collateral ligament tear of the elbow)	21 patients, who underwent surgical intervention for medial elbow pain due to medial collateral ligament insufficiency or other abnormality of chronic valgus overload, were assessed preoperatively with this test.[c]	NT	100	75	4	0	NA	10
Biceps squeeze test (distal biceps tendon rupture)	25 consecutive patients with presumptive distal biceps tendon ruptures were evaluated using this test. The test was positive in 24 patients. 21 of 22 patients had operative confirmation of a complete distal biceps tendon rupture.[d]	NT	96	100	N/A	0.04	N/A	9

[a]Novak CB, Lee GW, Mackinnon SE, et al: Provocative testing for cubital tunnel syndrome. *J Hand surg* 19:817–820, 1994.

[b]Docherty MA, Schwab RA, Ma OJ: Can elbow extension be used as a test of clinically significant injury? *South Med J* 95:539–541, 2002.

[c]O'Driscoll SW, Lawton RL, Smith AM: The "moving valgus stress test" for medial collateral ligament tears of the elbow. *Am J Sports Med* 33:231–239, 2005.

[d]Ruland RT, Dunbar RP, Bowen JD: The biceps squeeze test for diagnosis of distal biceps tendon ruptures. *Clin Orthop Relat Res* 128–131, 2005.

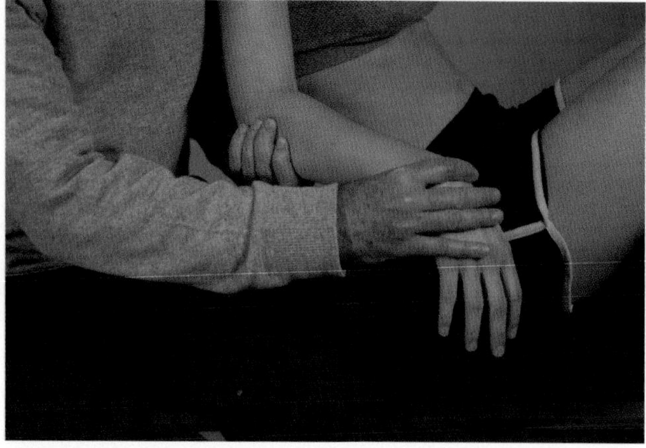

FIGURE 17-41 Cozen's test.

Cozen's Test. The clinician stabilizes the patient's elbow with one hand, and the patient is asked to pronate the forearm and extend and radially deviate the wrist against the manual resistance of the clinician (Fig. 17-41). A reproduction of pain in the area of the lateral epicondyle indicates a positive test. No diagnostic accuracy studies have been performed to determine the sensitivity or specificity of this test.

Mills' Test. The clinician palpates the patient's lateral epicondyle with one hand, while pronating the patient's forearm, fully flexing the wrist, and extending the elbow (Fig. 17-42). A reproduction of pain in the area of the lateral epicondyle indicates a positive test. No diagnostic accuracy studies have been performed to determine the sensitivity or specificity of this test.

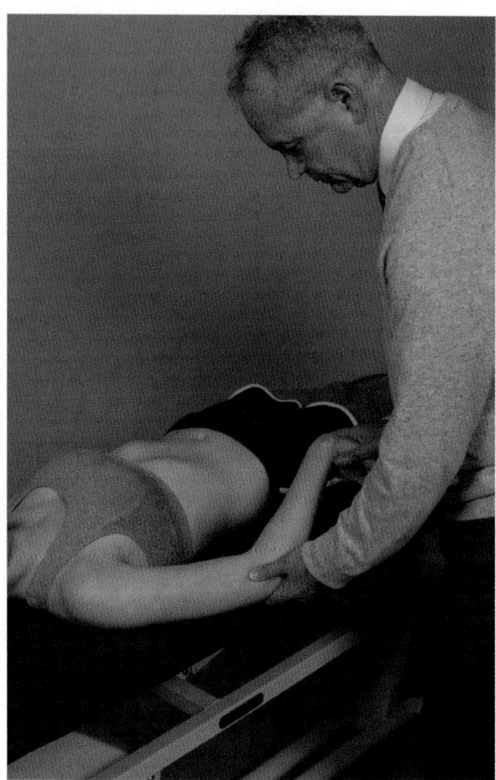

FIGURE 17-42 Mills' test.

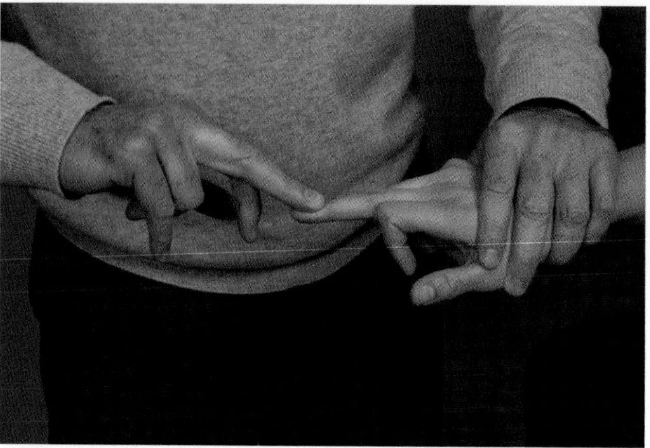

FIGURE 17-43 Maudsley test.

Maudsley Test. The patient is seated facing the clinician. Using one hand, the clinician grasps the patient's wrist, and using the other hand, resists third digit extension, stressing the extensor digitorum muscle (Fig. 17-43). A positive test is reproduction of pain along the lateral epicondyle. No diagnostic accuracy studies have been performed to determine the sensitivity or specificity of this test.

Golfer's Elbow (Medial Epicondylitis)

The clinician palpates the medial epicondyle with one hand, while supinating the forearm and extending the wrist and elbow with the other hand. A reproduction of pain in the area of the medial epicondyle indicates a positive test.

Elbow Flexion Test for Cubital Tunnel Syndrome

The patient is positioned in sitting or standing with both arms and shoulders in the anatomic position. The patient is asked to depress both shoulders, flex both elbows maximally, and supinate the forearms (Fig. 17-44). The patient is then asked to extend the wrists.[110] This position is maintained for 3–5 minutes and then the patient is asked to describe any symptoms. Tingling or paresthesia in the ulnar distribution of the forearm and hand indicates a positive test.

Pressure-Provocative Test for Cubital Tunnel Syndrome

Pressure is applied by the clinician, proximal to the cubital tunnel, with the elbow held in 20 degrees of flexion and the forearm in supination (Fig. 17-45).[111]

Percussion Test/Tinel's Sign (at the Elbow) for Cubital Tunnel Syndrome

The clinician locates the groove between the olecranon process and the medial epicondyle through which the ulnar nerve passes. This groove is tapped 4 to 6 times by the index finger of the clinician (Fig. 17-46). A positive sign is indicated by a tingling sensation in the ulnar distribution of the forearm and hand distal to the tapping point.

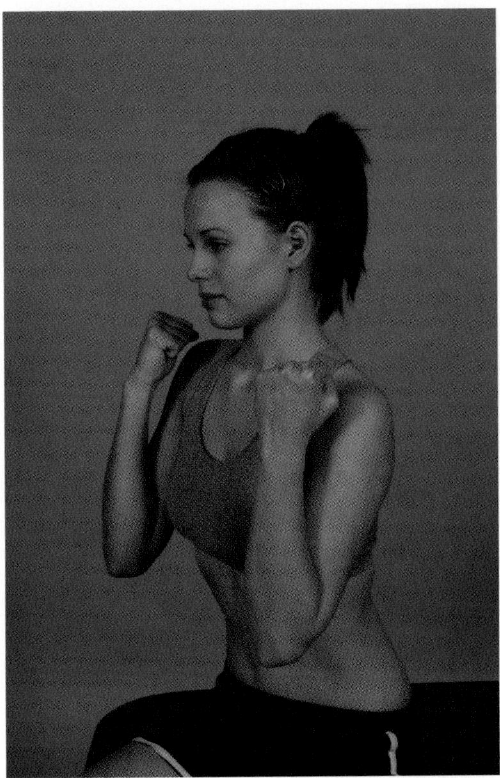

FIGURE 17-44 Elbow flexion test.

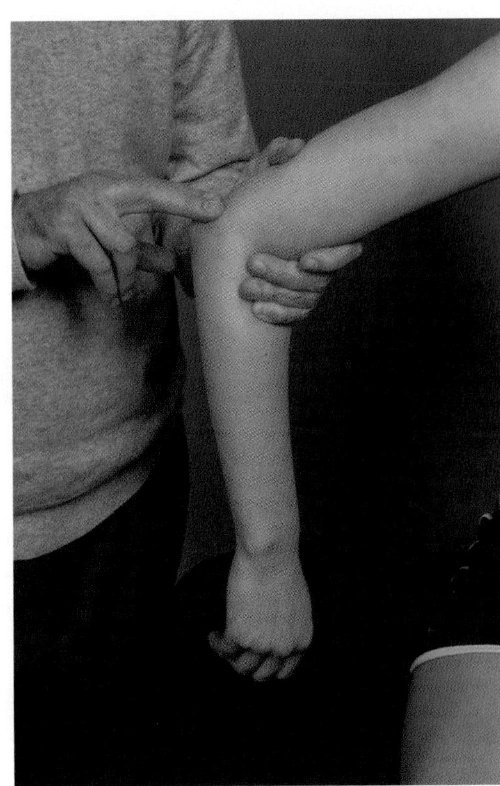

FIGURE 17-46 Percussion test/Tinel's sign (at the Elbow).

Elbow Extension Test

The patient is positioned in supine and is asked to fully extend the elbow. A positive test for elbow fracture is indicated by the patient's inability to fully extend the elbow.

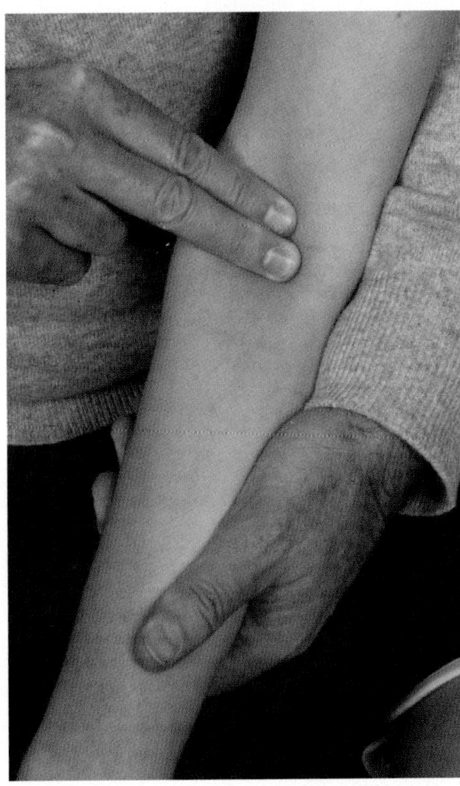

FIGURE 17-45 Pressure-provocative test for cubital tunnel syndrome.

Moving Valgus Stress Test

The patient is positioned in sitting and the clinician stands behind the patient. The clinician positions the patient's shoulder in 90 degrees of abduction and 120 degrees of elbow flexion. The clinician applies a modest valgus torque to the elbow until the shoulder reaches full external rotation. While applying a constant valgus torque, the elbow is quickly extended to 30 degrees (Fig. 17-47). A positive test for a chronic MCL tear of the elbow is the reproduction of medial elbow pain when forcibly extending the elbow from a flexed position between 120–70 degrees.

Biceps Squeeze Test

The patient is seated with the forearm resting comfortably in the patient's lap with the elbow flexed to approximately 60–80 degrees and the forearm in slight pronation. Standing on the

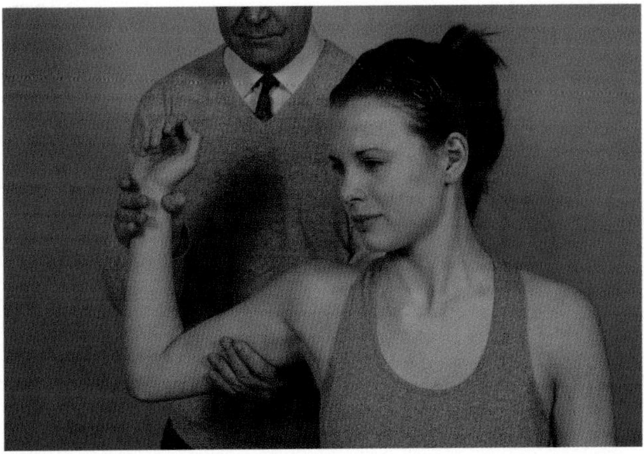

FIGURE 17-47 Moving valgus stress test.

involved side, the clinician squeezes the biceps firmly with one hand stablizing the upper extremity and the other hand around the belly of the biceps brachii (Fig. 17-48). A positive test for a distal biceps tendon rupture is a loss of forearm supination as the biceps brachii is squeezed.

Radiographic Evaluation

The standard X-ray series of the elbow includes anteroposterior (A-P) and lateral views (see Chap. 7).

THE EVALUATION

Following the examination, and once the clinical findings have been recorded, the clinician must determine a specific diagnosis or a working hypothesis, based on a summary of all of the findings. This diagnosis can be structure related (medical diagnosis) (Tables 17-7 and 17-8), or a diagnosis based on the preferred practice patterns as described in the Guide to Physical Therapist Practice.

INTERVENTION STRATEGIES

The intervention following elbow injury or elbow surgery follows a sequential and progressive multiphase approach. However, due to the unique orientation of the elbow complex,

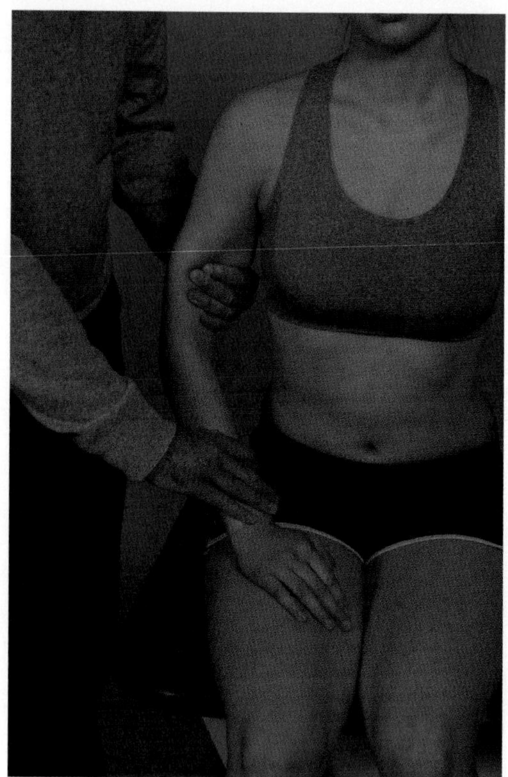

FIGURE 17-48 Biceps squeeze test.

TABLE 17-7 Differential Diagnosis for Common Causes of Elbow Pain

Condition	Patient Age (y)	Mechanism of Injury	Area of Symptoms	Symptoms Aggravated by	Observation
Bicipital tendinitis	20–50	Repetitive hyperextension of the elbow with pronation or repetitive stressful pronation–supination	Anterior aspect of the distal part of the arm	Elbow extension and shoulder extension	Unremarkable
Triceps tendinitis	20–50	Overuse of the upper arm and elbow, especially in activities like throwing and hammering	Posterior aspect of elbow	Activities involving elbow extension or full elbow flexion	Possible swelling near the point of the elbow
Lateral epicondylitis	35–55	Gradual overuse	Lateral aspect of elbow	Activities involving wrist extension/grasping	Possible swelling (over lateral elbow)
Medial epicondylitis	35–55	Gradual overuse	Anteromedial aspect of elbow	Activities involving wrist flexion	Possible swelling (over medial elbow)
Olecranon bursitis	20–50	Trauma	Posterior aspect of elbow	Contact with posterior elbow	Swelling over posterior elbow
Ulnar collateral ligament injury	20–45	Excessive valgus force to medial compartment of the elbow	Ulnar aspect of the elbow	Valgus stress of the elbow, throwing, and pitching	May have ecchymosis over ulnar aspect
Ulnar nerve entrapment	20–40	Gradual overuse Trauma	Medial elbow, forearm, and hand Medial 11/2 fingers	Activities involving elbow and wrist extension	Atrophy of hand muscles if chronic
Radial nerve entrapment	Varies	Can be overuse, direct trauma	Lateral elbow	Varies	Usually unremarkable
Median nerve entrapment	20–40	Gradual overuse	Anterior forearm Lateral 31/2 fingers	Activities involving full elbow extension or pronation of the forearm	Atrophy of anterior forearm and hand muscles if chronic

AROM, active range of motion; PROM, passive range of motion; ECRB, extensor carpi radialis brevis; ECRL, extensor carpi radialis longus.

AROM	PROM	End-Feel	Resisted	Special Tests	Tenderness with Palpation
Possible pain with elbow flexion	Pain with passive shoulder and elbow extension		Pain on elbow flexion and supination		Distal biceps belly The musculotendinous portion of the biceps Bicipital insertion of the radial tuberosity
Elbow extension Possible pain with extreme elbow flexion	Pain with passive shoulder and elbow flexion		Pain on elbow extension		Posterior aspect of elbow
Possible pain on wrist flexion with elbow extension	Pain on wrist flexion with the forearm pronated and the elbow extended		Pain on resisted wrist extension and radial deviation, with the elbow extended Pain on finger extension	Cozen Mills'	Lateral elbow (over the ECRB and ECRL)
Pain on wrist extension	Pain on combined wrist extension and forearm supination		Pain on pronation with wrist flexion	Passive supination of the forearm and extension of the wrist and elbow	Anteromedial elbow
Possible pain with extreme elbow flexion	Pain on full elbow flexion		Strong and pain free	Valgus stress with elbow flexed at ~25 degrees and humerus in external rotation	Posterior elbow
Pain with full extension possible	Passive extension of the elbow, valgus stress	Depends on severity	Usually unremarkable		Ulnar aspect of elbow
Inability to fully close hand	Full and pain free		Weakness of grip	Elbow flexion and pressure-provocative test Tinel's at elbow Wartenberg's sign Froment's sign	Anteromedial elbow
Usually unremarkable	Usually unremarkable		Pain with resisted forearm supination, resisted extension of middle finger		Maximal tenderness is usually elicited over the radial tunnel if radial tunnel syndrome
Pain on forearm pronation	Full and pain free		Weakness on pronation, wrist flexion, and thumb opposition	Benediction sign Inability to perform "OK" sign (anterior interosseous syndrome) Resisted supination (compression of the lacertus fibrosus)	Over the pronator teres 4 cm distal to the cubital crease, with concurrent resistance against pronation, elbow flexion, and wrist flexion—pronator syndrome

TABLE 17-8 **Findings in Common Conditions of the Elbow and Forearm**

Condition	Findings
Valgus extension overload syndrome	Tenderness around the tip of the olecranon Pain with forced passive elbow extension Increased valgus laxity (variable)
Cubital tunnel syndrome	Tenderness over the course of the ulnar nerve Abnormal Tinel's sign over the ulnar nerve, as it passes through the cubital tunnel (medial elbow) Ulnar nerve compression test abnormal Elbow flexion test abnormal (variable) Abnormal sensation (two-point discrimination or light touch), in the ulnar distribution: little finger; ulnar aspect of ring finger; ulnar aspect of hand Possible weakness and atrophy of the ulnar-innervated intrinsic muscles of the hand Possible weakness of flexor digitorum profundus to the little finger Possible signs of concomitant ulnar nerve instability, elbow instability, or elbow deformity
Radial tunnel syndrome	Tenderness in the extensor muscle mass of the forearm (distal to lateral epicondyle) at the arcade of Fröhse Long finger extension test reproduces pain Weakness of finger and thumb extensors and extensor carpi ulnaris
Pronator teres syndrome	Tenderness over the pronator teres in the proximal forearm Possible abnormal sensation (two-point discrimination or light touch) in the median nerve distribution: thumb, index finger, long finger, and radial side of ring finger On occasion, prolonged resisted pronation reproduces symptoms of weakness of median-innervated muscle Rare, but often incorrectly diagnosed as carpal tunnel Resisted elbow flexion and forearm supination reproduce symptoms due to compression at the lacertus fibrosus Resisted long finger proximal interphalangeal joint flexion reproduces symptoms due to compression by the flexor digitorum superficialis Possible weakness of median-innervated muscles
Anterior interosseous nerve syndrome	Weakness of flexor pollicis longus and flexor digitorum profundus to index finger Weakness of pronator quadratus
Distal biceps tendon rupture	Swelling Ecchymosis Palpable gap in the biceps tendon Weak or absent elbow flexion and supination
UCL strain or tear	Medial elbow joint pain in a thrower Complete tears open on valgus stress testing with the elbow flexed at 25 degrees compared to the uninvolved side, whereas incomplete tears are tender on palpation of the UCL but do not open on valgus stressing
Nursemaid's elbow (pulled elbow syndrome)	Mean age is 2–3 years History is critical to making diagnosis: reports of longitudinal traction on an extended elbow, resulting in a partial slippage of the annular ligament over the head of the radius and into the radiocapitellar joint Child typically holds the arm at the side, with the hand pronated (palm down) Closed reduction with manipulation is highly successful
Little league elbow	Covers a spectrum of pathologies about the elbow joint in young developing (pediatric) throwers Four distinct vulnerable areas to throwing stress: (1) medial elbow tension overload; (2) lateral articular surface compression overload; (3) posterior-medial shear forces; and (4) extension overload of the lateral restraints May present as Panner's disease (necrosis of the capitellum), OCD, medial epicondylar fracture, medial apophysitis, medial ligament rupture, and posterior osteophyte formation at the tip of the olecranon

UCL, ulnar collateral ligament.

Data from Birnie R, Reider B: Elbow and forearm. In: Reider B, ed. *Orthopaedic Physical Examination*. Philadelphia, PA: WB Saunders, 1999:67–98. With permission from WB Saunders.

the clinician is faced with multiple clinical challenges to successfully rehabilitate the injured elbow and should always consider the functional expectations of the individual patient when determining the most appropriate intervention.[7]

The techniques to increase joint mobility and the techniques to increase soft-tissue extensibility are described in the "Therapeutic Techniques" section.

ACUTE PHASE

The goals of the acute phase of elbow rehabilitation include:

- protection of the injury site;
- restoration of pain-free range of motion in the entire kinetic chain;
- improvement of patient comfort by decreasing pain and inflammation;
- retardation of muscle atrophy;
- minimization of the detrimental effects of immobilization and activity restriction;[112–117]
- maintenance of general cardiovascular fitness;
- ensuring that the patient is independent with a home exercise program.

During the early stages of the acute phase, the principles of PRICEMEM (protection, rest, ice, compression, elevation, manual therapy, early motion, and medication) are applied as appropriate. Icing for 20–30 minutes, three to four times a day, concurrent with nonsteroidal anti-inflammatory drugs (NSAIDs) or aspirin, can aid in reducing pain and swelling.

CLINICAL PEARL

Corticosteroid injections have been advocated for elbow injuries to promote and progress healing. Although the use of local injections increases the risks of disrupting tissue planes, fenestration of the area of tendinosis may be beneficial because of the bleeding that occurs in the new channels, which has the potential for transforming a failed intrinsic healing process into an extrinsic response.[118,119]

Early active-assisted and passive exercises are performed in all planes of the shoulder, elbow (Fig. 17-49) VIDEO, and wrist motions VIDEO, to nourish the articular cartilage and assist in collagen tissue synthesis and organization.[7,120–123] As the available range at the elbow occurs at the humeroulnar, humeroradial, and proximal and distal radioulnar joints, restrictions or laxities at any of these joints can affect the eventual outcome of the rehabilitative process.

The formation of an elbow flexion contracture must be avoided, as this contracture can place abnormal stresses on the elbow complex, especially during athletic activities.[124] One of the most common causes of joint contracture at the elbow is scarring of the anterior capsule, and at the insertion site of the brachialis.[7] This scarring can be minimized by performing joint mobilizations to the humeroulnar and humeroradial joints. A posterior glide of the ulna on the humerus is used to help restore elbow extension. The anterior capsule can be stretched using long-duration, low-intensity stretching to produce a plastic response from the collagen tissue.[7,125,126] Such a stretch can be accomplished by positioning the patient in supine, with a towel roll placed under the elbow joint, and the forearm hanging over the edge of the bed (Fig. 17-50). A

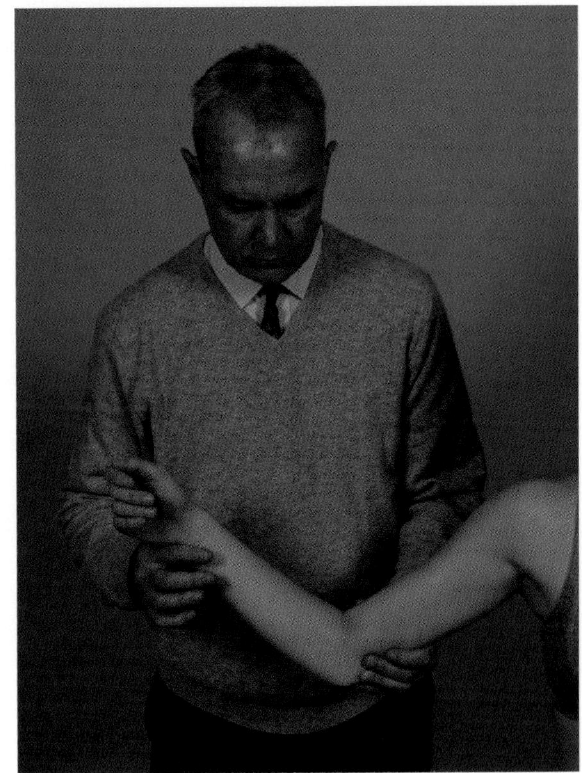

FIGURE 17-49 PROM/AAROM of elbow flexion.

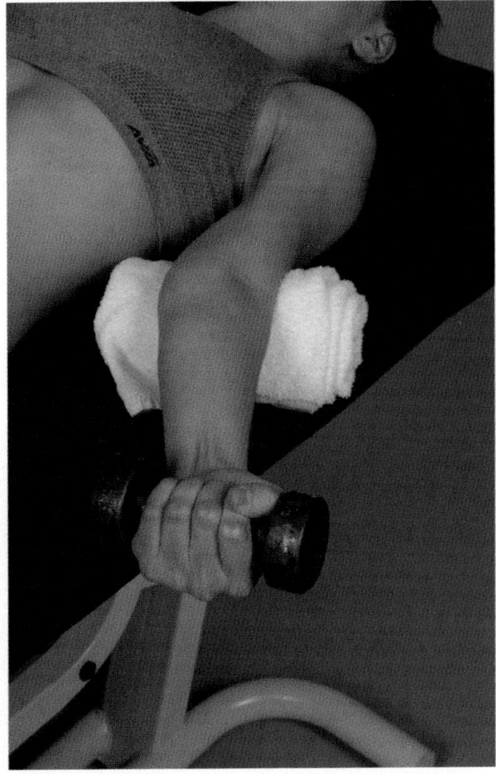

FIGURE 17-50 Passive elbow extension using weight in hand.

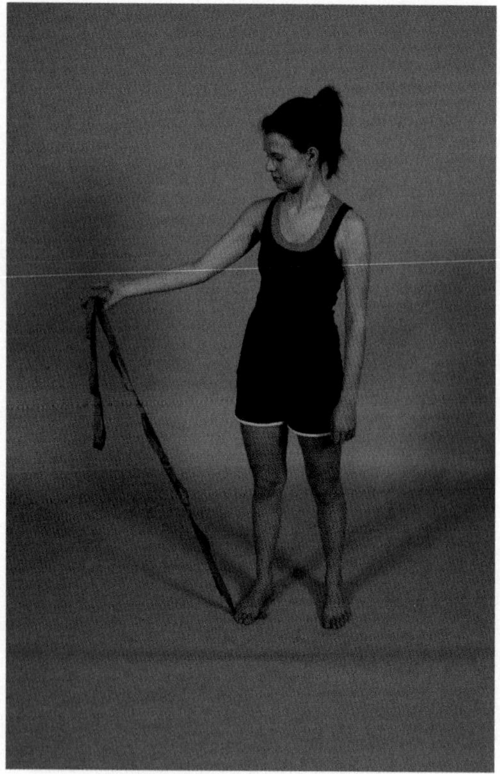

FIGURE 17-51 Elbow and wrist flexor stretch.

light weight (2–4 lb) is placed in the hand, and the elbow is extended as far as is comfortable. The passive stretch is maintained for 5–7 minutes, avoiding excessive pain manifested by a protective muscle response. This exercise becomes an important component of the patient's home exercise program. The elbow flexors (Fig. 17-51) and wrist flexors (Fig. 17-52) can also be stretched manually by the patient as part of the home exercise program.

Initially, the patient is advised to decrease the level of activity with the level of pain as the limiting factor, but without immobilizing the injured part completely.

Patients are initially instructed to perform submaximal isometric exercises at multiple angles for the elbow flexors and extensors, the forearm supinators and pronators, and the wrist flexors and extensors. Once full pain-free range

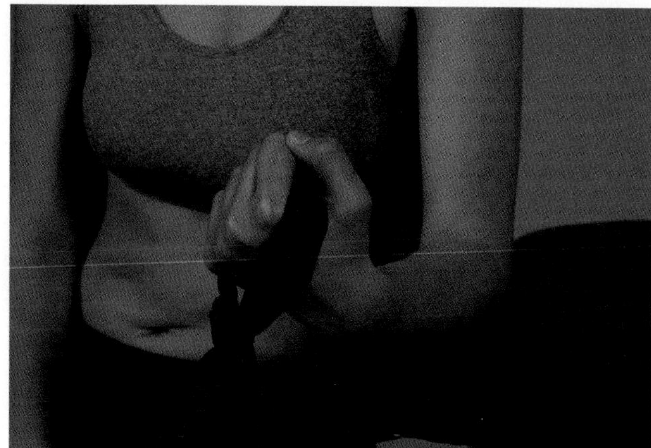

FIGURE 17-53 Wrist flexor PREs.

of motion has been achieved, the patient's strengthening program is progressed from the multiple angle isometrics to concentric progressive resistance exercises (PREs) using dumbbells or surgical tubing. Low resistance is used initially with one to two sets of 10 repetitions, progressing as tolerated to five sets of 10 repetitions. Once five sets of 10 repetitions can be performed without pain and in a slow and controlled manner, additional resistance is added in 1–3-lb increments.[7] The resistance-based exercise program is the mainstay of nonoperative intervention for the elbow and serves to retard muscle atrophy of the elbow and wrist musculature. Patients are advanced in concordance with their ability to participate in the program. Patients should be taught how to perform these exercises independently at the earliest opportunity.

Specific exercises to increase strength should include the following:

- Concentric exercises to the wrist flexors VIDEO and extensors VIDEO, elbow flexors VIDEO and extensors VIDEO, and radial VIDEO and ulnar deviators VIDEO, performed at varying speeds and resistance. These include wrist curls (Fig. 17-53), reverse wrist curls (Fig. 17-54) VIDEO, neutral wrist curls VIDEO, biceps curl (Fig. 17-55), and triceps strengthening (Fig. 17-56) resisted pronation (Fig. 17-57), resisted supination (Fig. 17-58) VIDEO. The exercises are initially performed using low speeds and resistance; the speed and the intensity of resistance are then gradually increased.

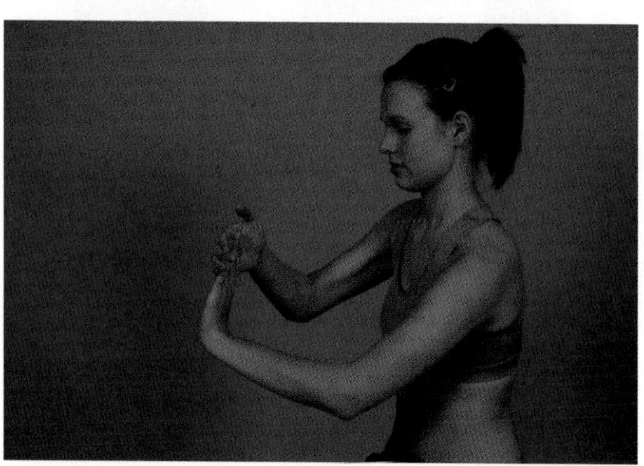

FIGURE 17-52 Wrist flexor and elbow flexor stretch.

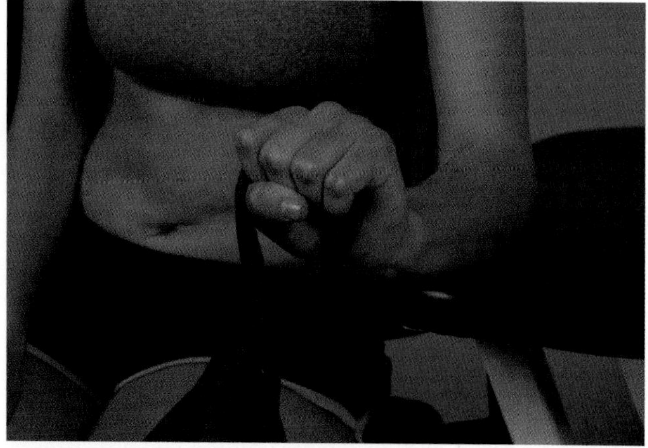

FIGURE 17-54 Wrist extensor PREs.

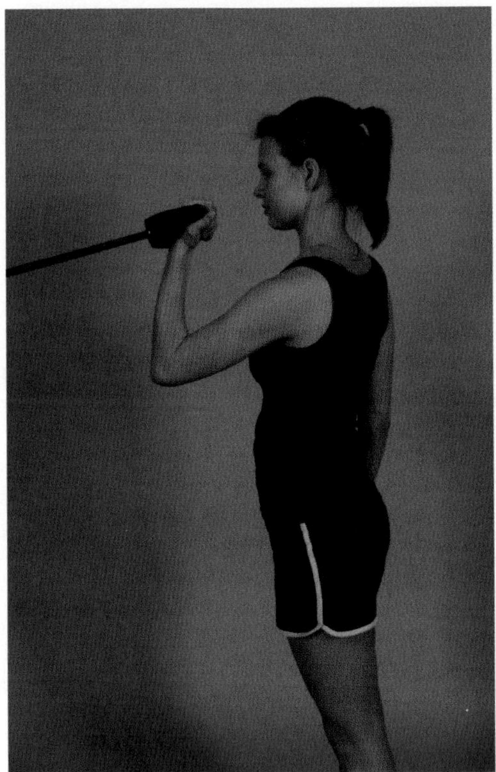

FIGURE 17-55 Elbow flexion PREs.

▸ The broom-handle exercise, which is a recommended exercise for the wrist flexors and extensors. A weight is tied to a rope or piece of string approximately 3 ft in length, which is then tied to a broom handle or dowel. The broom handle is held out in front of the patient with the palms down (for wrist extensors, see Fig. 17-59) or palms up

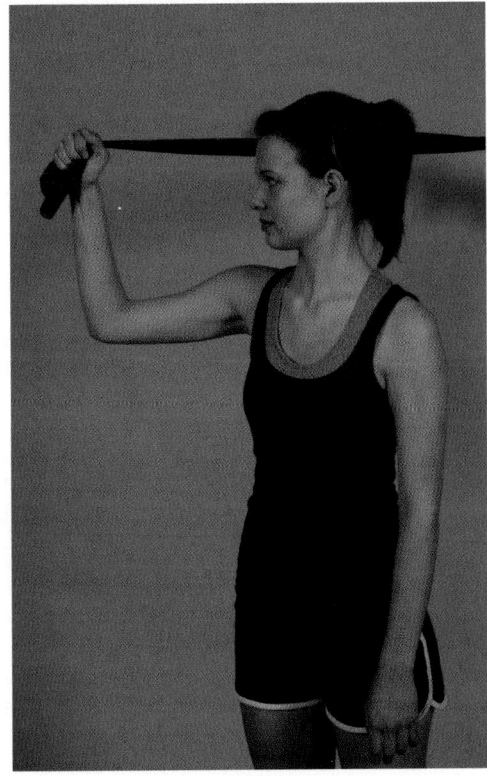

FIGURE 17-56 Triceps strengthening.

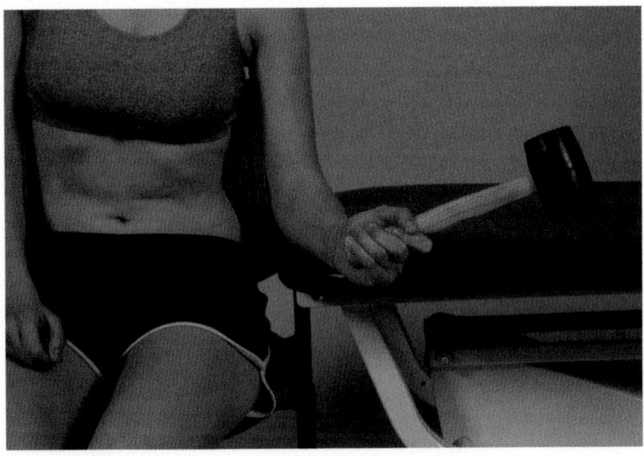

FIGURE 17-57 Strengthening exercise for pronators.

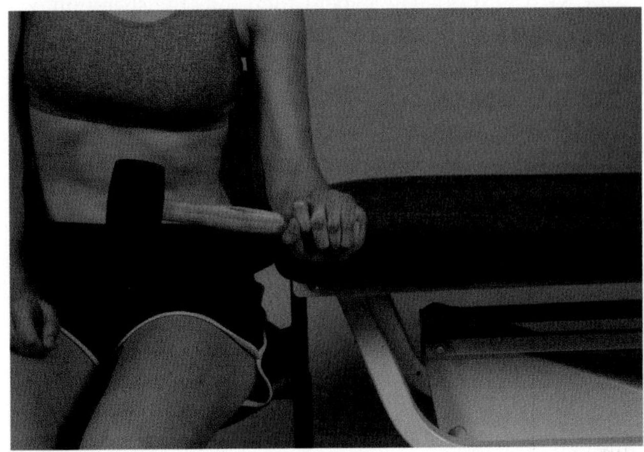

FIGURE 17-58 Strengthening exercise for supinators.

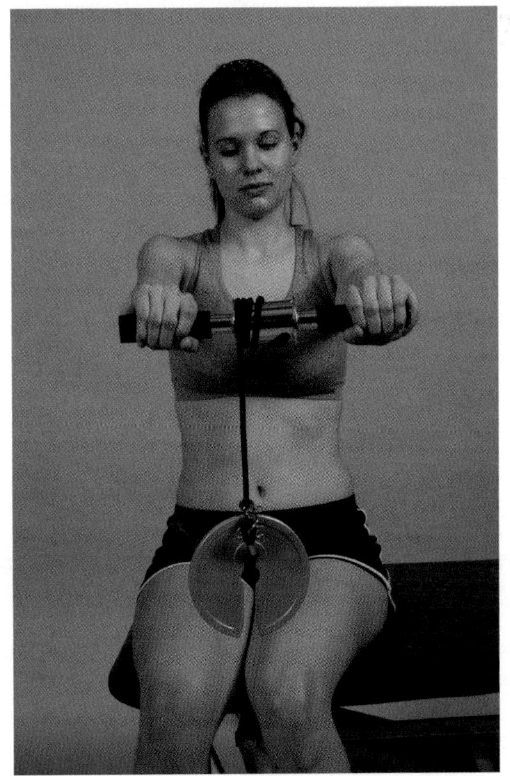

FIGURE 17-59 Broom-handle exercise.

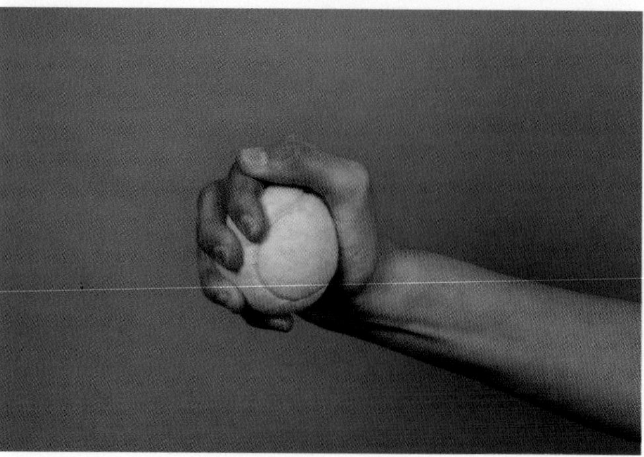

FIGURE 17-60 Tennis ball squeezes.

(for wrist flexors). The patient then rolls the string onto the handle/dowel to raise and then lower the weight.

- Tennis ball squeezes (Fig. 17-60) to improve grip strength (once symptoms have subsided).
- Exercises to increase the strength in opposing muscles, such as the flexors of the wrist and digits, in order to balance the force couple.

Shoulder exercises should also be introduced as early as possible, although caution should be used with shoulder external rotation exercises because of the potential for valgus stress to the elbow.[7,119,127,128] In the earlier phases of pain, modification of activity may involve alternating between low- and high-intensity workouts.[129,130] Endurance is developed over time, as the patient becomes able to tolerate more repetitions and sustained activities. If endurance is not developed and the muscle–tendon unit becomes fatigued, the muscular portion can no longer absorb the stresses and greater stresses are absorbed by the tendon.[131] Throughout all phases of rehabilitation and exercise, training should be within physiologic limits for cellular response and homeostasis.[132] Therefore, relative rest is sometimes advised during painful periods.

Stability at the shoulder and the elbow is extremely important for those patients returning to overhead sports and can be addressed using proprioceptive neuromuscular facilitation (PNF) patterns with increasing resistance.

In the presence of joint laxity that is not controllable with adequate exercise or ergonomic modifications, bracing can be effective.

Progression to the next phase occurs when the patient has full, pain-free range of motion, and strength at least 70% of the contralateral limb.

FUNCTIONAL PHASE

The functional phase addresses any tissue overload problems and functional biomechanical deficits. The goals of the functional phase include:

- restoring normal joint kinematics;
- improving muscle strength to within normal limits (WNL);
- improving neuromuscular control;
- restoring the normal strength and relationships of the muscle force couples.

If the feet and trunk are stabilized during an activity, the upper quarter kinetic chain involves the cervical spine, thoracic outlet, thoracic spine, shoulder, elbow, wrist, and hand. The upper quarter operates as a mechanical unit whose links are functionally interdependent on one another.

The clinician must be aware of any substitutions as individuals will instinctively modify their exercises to avoid motions involving painful, injured tissues, and to prevent further abuse of the overused tissues.[130,132] In such cases, the exercises must be corrected or discontinued.

Cocontraction of the muscles around the elbow can be produced with closed chain exercises such as the push-up, quadruped exercises, and dips, incorporating a wide range of equipment such as gymnastic balls, BAPS boards, mini-tramp, and slide board (see Chap. 16).

Training can also involve dynamic muscle cocontractions in an open kinetic chain by using ballistic movement patterns, with elastic tubing incorporating PNF diagonals. These ballistic movements, which can be increased in terms of speed based on tolerance, result in synchronous activation of agonists and antagonists.[133–135]

The function of the biceps is integral to the stability of the elbow complex and must be exercised, emphasizing slow and fast muscular contractions in both concentric and eccentric modes.[7] Wilk and colleagues[7] advocate the following drill to enhance the dynamic stability of the elbow:

- The patient flexes the elbow against resistance provided by elastic tubing.
- The patient holds a position isometrically, while the clinician employs rhythmic stabilization resistance anteriorly and posteriorly.
- The procedure is repeated for the wrist flexors–extensors and the forearm pronators–supinators.

Plyometric exercises are introduced as tolerated and as appropriate[136]:

- The patient grasps a length of elastic tubing and fully flexes the elbow, with the shoulder flexed to about 60 degrees (Fig. 17-61). This position is maintained briefly. The patient then releases the isometric hold, allowing the elbow to extend rapidly. As full extension is reached, the movement is quickly reversed back into full elbow flexion.[136] The forearm pronators–supinators can all be exercised in a similar fashion.
- For overhead athletes, ER exercises can be performed with elastic tubing at 90 degrees of shoulder abduction and 90 degrees of elbow flexion (Fig. 17-62).
- Plyometric weighted ball throws into IR at 0 degree of shoulder abduction (Fig. 17-63), and at 90 degrees of shoulder abduction (Fig. 17-64).
- Prone plyometric weighted ball throws with the patient's arm positioned at 90 degrees of shoulder abduction and 90 degrees of elbow flexion (Fig. 17-65).
- Plyometric wrist flips and snaps (Figs. 17-66 and 17-67)

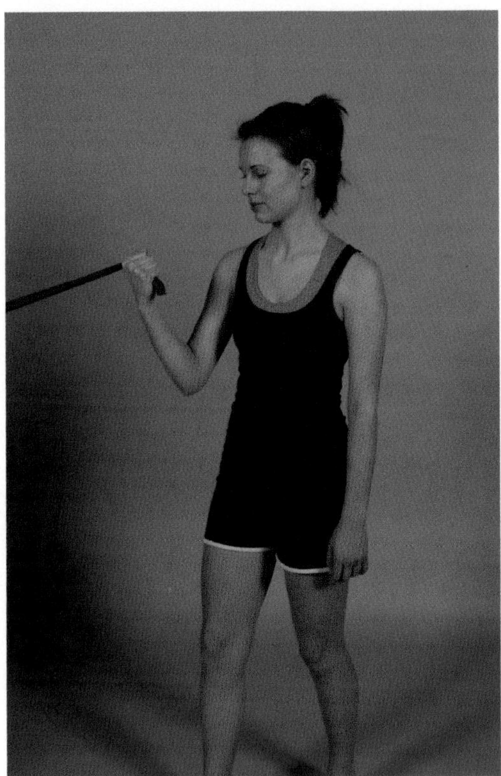

FIGURE 17-61 Plyometric exercise with elastic tubing.

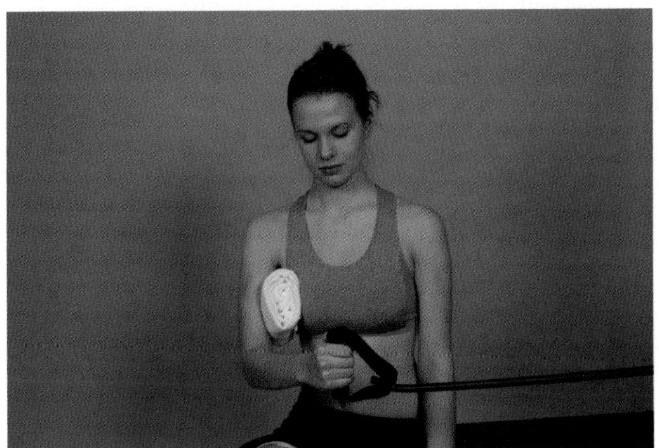

FIGURE 17-62 ER exercises performed at 90 degrees of shoulder abduction and 90 degrees of elbow flexion.

The shoulder stabilizers, triceps, and the wrist flexors–extensors can be trained as a unit using Swiss ball push-ups (Fig. 17-68), PNF patterns using T-band (Figs. 17-69 and Fig. 17-70), and medicine ball throws (Fig. 17-71).

Sport-specific training is essential before an athlete returns to play. There should be a gradual transition back to sports activities and other strenuous activities of daily living, depending on the recovery of the involved tissues and the restoration of the athletic skills required to perform the activity. Too often, patients return to full activity prematurely, with resulting reinjury. This is both frustrating and discouraging for the patient.

In order for the athlete to begin the return to sporting activities, the elbow must have full, pain-free range of motion; no pain or tenderness on physical examination; and adequate muscle strength, power, and endurance that is 90% of the uninvolved side.[7]

Those athletes who are returning to throwing can undergo a strength comparison through isokinetic testing. This can be

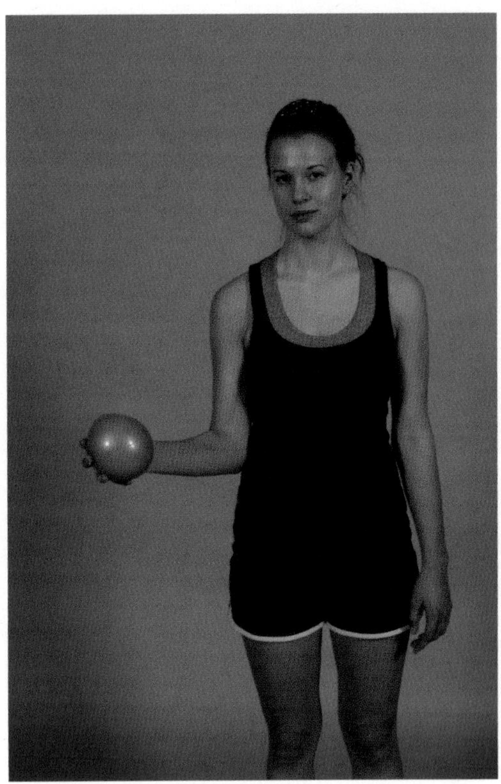

FIGURE 17-63 Plyometric medicine ball throws into IR at 0 degree of shoulder abduction.

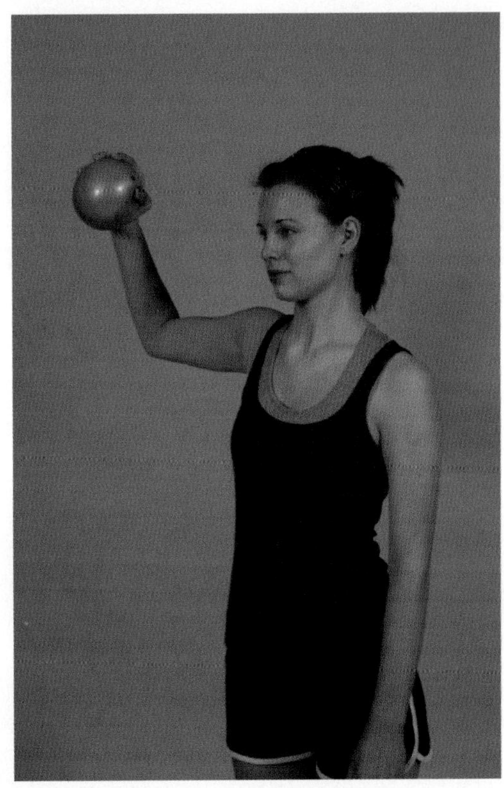

FIGURE 17-64 Plyometric medicine ball throws into IR at 90 degrees of shoulder abduction.

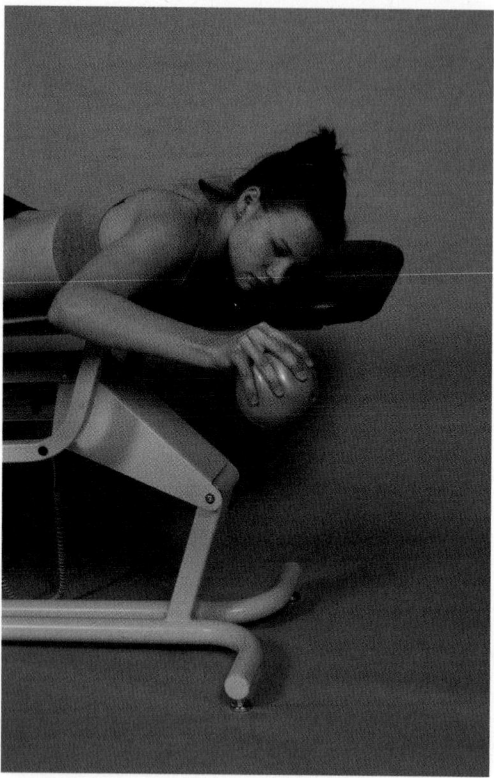
FIGURE 17-65 Prone weighted ball throws.

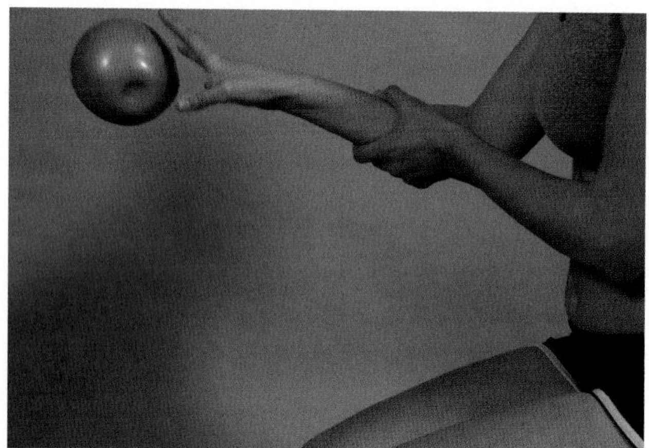
FIGURE 17-66 Plyometric wrist flips.

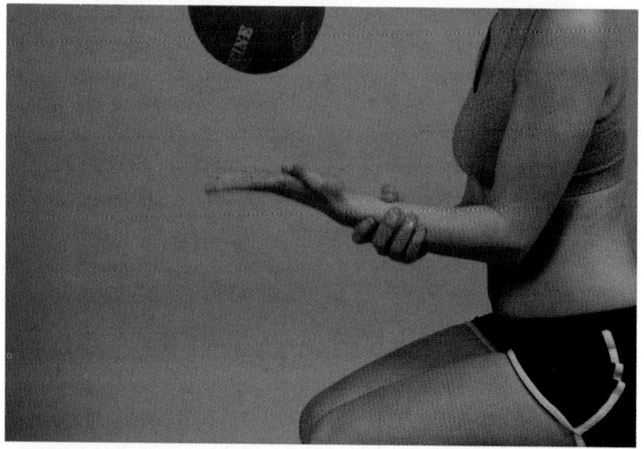
FIGURE 17-67 Plyometric wrist snaps.

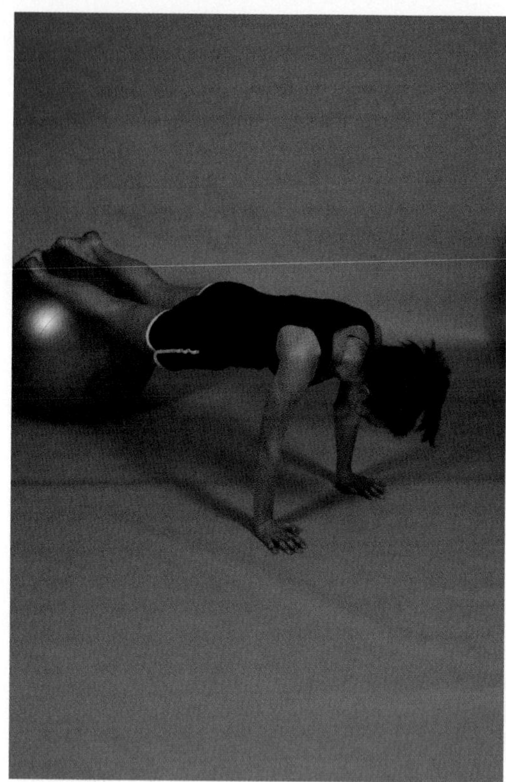
FIGURE 17-68 Swiss ball push-ups.

achieved with the patient in the seated position. Speeds of 180 degrees per second and 300 degrees per second are used. A bilateral comparison should indicate that the overhead athlete's elbow flexors are 10–20% stronger, the elbow extensors are 5–15% stronger when compared to the uninvolved

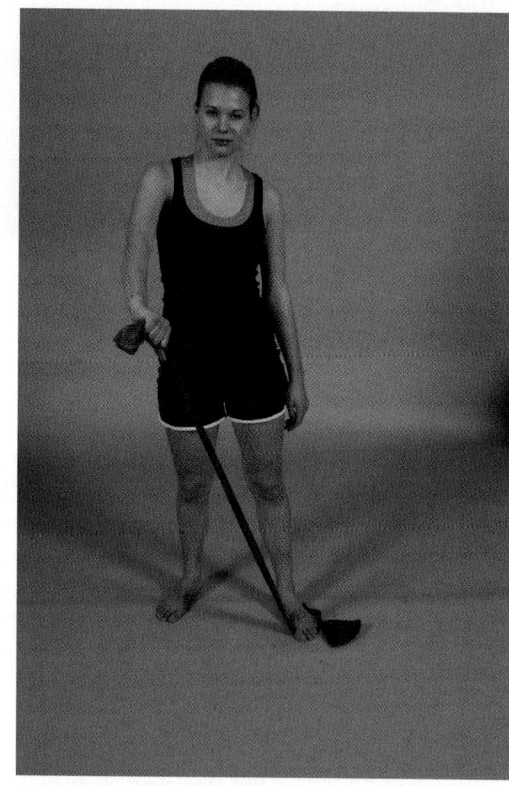
FIGURE 17-69 UE PNF using T-band.

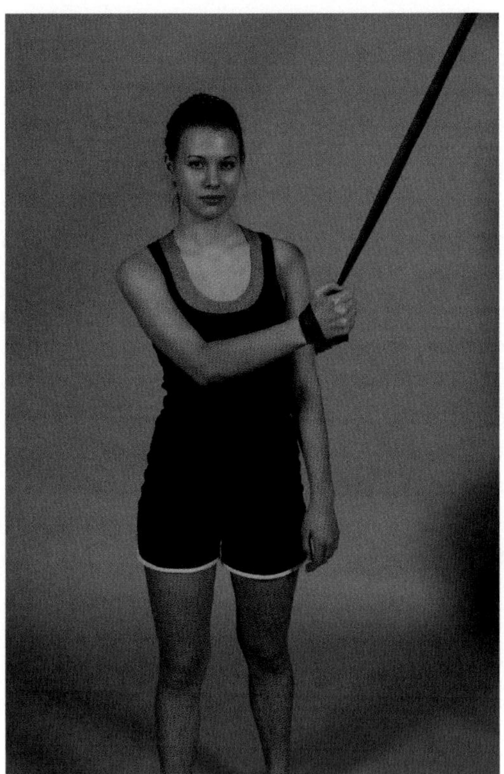

FIGURE 17-70 UE PNF using T-band.

side, and that the flexor–extensor ratio should be 70–80% at 180 degrees per second, and 63–69% at 300 degrees per second.[7]

Advanced strengthening exercises specific for the patient's activity/position are emphasized during the later part of this phase. These include high-speed/high-energy strengthening and eccentric muscular contractions performed in functional positions.[7]

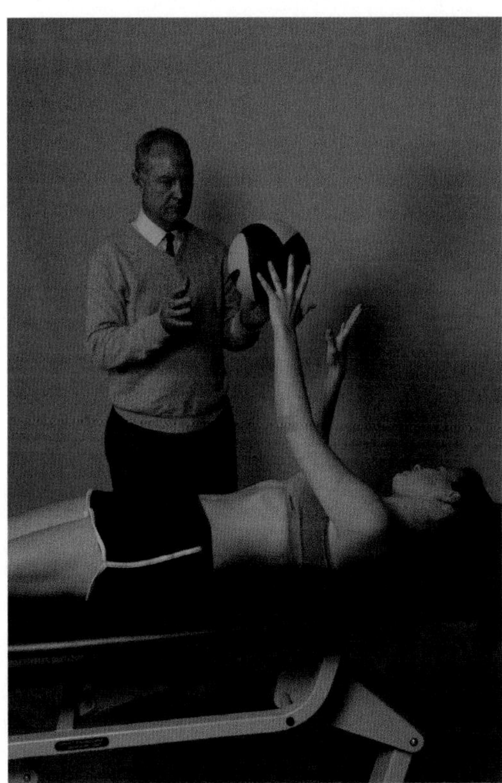

FIGURE 17-71 Medicine ball throws.

PRACTICE PATTERN 4D: IMPAIRED JOINT MOBILITY, MOTOR FUNCTION, MUSCLE PERFORMANCE, AND RANGE OF MOTION ASSOCIATED WITH CONNECTIVE TISSUE DYSFUNCTION

Impairments involving capsular restriction include every form of arthritis. It is important that the clinician establish the cause of the arthritis using the history, the tests and measures, results from any imaging studies, and findings from any laboratory tests before initiating treatment.

Traumatic Arthritis

Trauma at the elbow has the potential to produce a traumatic arthritis. The most common mechanism is the hyperextension injury, resulting in a sprain of the anterior capsule and the anterior band of the medial (ulnar) collateral ligament. The patient typically complains of diffuse elbow pain, especially on the medial aspect. Upon examination, a capsular pattern of passive flexion more limited than extension is present, whereas the motions of pronation and supination are unaffected. Traumatic arthritis at the elbow is usually treated with a corticosteroid injection in adults, whereas in children a brief period of immobilization in a sling, followed by gentle passive and active range of motion (AROM), is recommended.

Arthrosis

See Chapter 5.

Osteochondritis Dissecans Capitellum

Osteochondritis dissecans occurs in many areas of the adolescent skeleton, and patients usually present with an insidious onset of diffuse lateral elbow pain accompanied by a decrease in the range of motion, including locking.[137] The etiology of this condition is not completely understood, but its occurrence in the elbows of adolescents probably relates to a focal arterial injury and subsequent bone necrosis resulting from increased radiohumeral lateral compression forces.[138]

Pain is usually felt at the radiocapitellar joint and is increased with activities that involve pronation and supination. Physical examination usually demonstrates a loss of full active and passive elbow extension. Resistive testing can produce crepitus, in addition to pain at the humeroradial joint.[138] X-rays may reveal a flattening or focal distortion of the capitellum and perhaps even loose bodies.

Intervention for this condition depends on the findings from the radiographic, clinical, and, on occasion, arthroscopic examination but usually focuses on the control of pain.[138] Usually 3–4 months of nonabusive activity with exercises directed toward minimizing the strength loss during the rest period often proves effective. The exercises prescribed are similar to those for lateral epicondylitis with an emphasis on biceps and triceps strength and muscular balance to control elbow extension forces. A motion-limiting brace can be used to reduce stress.

Surgical intervention is reserved for patients who do not respond to conservative measures, or those with loose bodies or separation of the cartilage cap.[138]

Radiocapitellar Chondromalacia

Radiocapitellar chondromalacia of the elbow occurs because of repetitive valgus forces, such as those encountered in throwing sports. Such activities can result in lateral elbow joint compression of the radiocapitellar articulation, and sometimes subsequent damage to the radial head, the capitellum, or both. Frank osteochondral fracture and loose bodies may also occur (osteochondritis dissecans).

The typical presenting symptoms are crepitus, catching, locking, and lateral elbow pain with active flexion and extension and pronation–supination of the elbow. Swelling and localized tenderness are noted at the involved site.

An axial load applied with passive supination and pronation often provokes pain and can be helpful in differentiating this condition from lateral epicondylitis. Radiographs may show a loss of joint space, marginal osteophytes, and, possibly, loose bodies.

Mild cases of this condition respond to NSAIDs and those exercises prescribed for lateral epicondylitis. However, care must be taken to perform exercises within pain-free ranges only to ensure joint safety.

Posterior Elbow Impingement

Posterior elbow impingement results from mechanical abutment of bone and soft tissues in the posterior compartment of the elbow. Pathologic processes such as fibrous tissue deposits in the olecranon fossa, chondral injury, osteophytes, and loose bodies are sometimes responsible.[139] MCL insufficiency may also be present.

Radiography may show posterior or posteromedial osteophytes and loose bodies.

Surgical removal of the osteophytes and loose bodies is indicated if symptoms do not resolve with conservative treatment consisting of range-of-motion and strengthening exercises.

Malpositioning of the Elbow

Abducted Ulna Lesion

This lesion usually results from a FOOSH injury, forcing the ulna medially into full extension and abduction. Clinical findings include the following[140]:

- An increased carrying angle and apparent longer radius that is forced to glide distally. Initially, the hand is held in slight ulnar deviation due to a relative distal shift of the radius. However, this usually adapts, producing an ulnar carpal shift due to the pull of the radial deviators and wrist extensors.
- The elbow flexion may be decreased, but usually only an abnormal hard end-feel is detected.
- The forearm supination may be decreased, but usually only an abnormal hard end-feel is detected.
- The lateral glide at the elbow is decreased with an abnormally hard end-feel (the ulna is unable to adduct).
- decreased wrist extension.

There are potentially many and varied consequences of this lesion, including[140]

- the development of tennis-elbow symptoms as the radial deviators overwork to correct the ulnar deviation;
- an ulnar nerve traction injury, MCL sprain, and medial epicondylitis due to the increased carrying angle;
- carpal dysfunction due to the abnormal wrist biomechanics because of the distally displaced radius;
  - MCL laxity due to the adaptation occurring to correct the ulnar deviation;
  - hypertonicity and overuse of the radial deviators and extensors as the hand attempts to adopt a neutral position by attempting to radially deviate or extend.

The intervention for these conditions includes a correction of the malposition with either joint mobilizations or a high-velocity thrust.

Adducted Ulna Lesions

In the adducted ulna lesion, there is no involvement of the wrist. In fact, the head of the radius impacts the capitellum, resulting in decreased elbow extension and forearm pronation, and clinical findings that are exactly the opposite of those described above. The consequences of this lesion are less severe than with the abducted ulna, as the shift of the wrist is less due to the accommodation by the ulnar meniscus, but they include[140]:

- the development of tennis-elbow symptoms due to the prolonged stretch on the common extensor tendon;
- LCL laxity;
- minor carpal dysfunction;
- ulnar meniscus tearing due to continuous compression.

Posterior-Radial Head (External Rotation of the Ulna) Lesion

With this lesion, the radial head shifts posteriorly into extension on the humerus and the ulna. There is typically a history involving forced or excessive supination. Range-of-motion testing demonstrates decreased elbow extension and forearm pronation. Passive accessory motion testing reveals a decreased medial radial glide and decreased gapping space between the ulna and the radius.

Anterior-Radial Head (Internal Rotation of the Ulna) Lesion

With this lesion, the radial head shifts anteriorly into flexion on the humerus and the ulna. There is typically a history involving forced or excessive pronation. Range-of-motion testing demonstrates decreased elbow flexion and forearm supination. Passive accessory motion testing reveals a decreased lateral-radial glide.

Medial (Ulnar) Collateral Ligament Sprain

The most common mechanisms associated with MCL sprains are a chronic attenuation of valgus and external rotation forces,[22,31,60,141,142] as seen with a tennis serve or during a baseball throwing pitch,[143,144] and posttraumatic, usually following a FOOSH injury.[19] Related injuries after trauma may include fractures of the radial head, olecranon, or medial humeral epicondyle.[22,31] An MCL injury can also be iatrogenic, secondary to an excessive medial epicondylectomy for cubital tunnel syndrome,[145,146] or irritation of the ulnar nerve, secondary to inflammation of the ligamentous complex.[60,147,148]

The most common patient complaint is medial elbow pain at the site of the ligament's origin,[138] or at the insertion site in cases of an acute avulsion.[19] As the primary restraint to valgus stress is the anterior bundle of the MCL,[14,20–24,28] the physical examination of an individual with presumed medial joint insufficiency should focus on palpation of the course of the MCL.[19] Valgus stress testing of the elbow must also be performed.

An important secondary stabilizer of the elbow is the articular geometry of the joint complex.[3,21] Repetitive stress to the joint can lead to osteophyte formation and degenerative changes, which can produce medial elbow pain.

The intervention for an MCL injury includes rest and activity modification or restriction for about 2–4 weeks, range-of-motion exercises, modalities, and NSAIDs.[30] During the acute phase, the goals are as follows:

- To increase ROM
- To promote healing of MCL
- To retard muscular atrophy
- To decrease pain and inflammation (ice and compression)

Methods to increase range of motion during this period include:

- brace (optional) nonpainful ROM (20–90 degrees);
- active-assisted ROM, passive ROM elbow and wrist (nonpainful range).

Strengthening and stretching of the FCU, pronator teres, and FDS are initiated once the acute inflammatory stage has subsided. These exercises are performed in the pain-free mid-range of motion.[48,143,149,150] Emphasis is placed on isometric exercises of the forearm flexors, ulnar deviators, and pronators, in order to enhance their role as secondary stabilizers of the medial joint. In addition, strengthening of the shoulder and elbow muscles are incorporated to prevent or minimize injury and to facilitate rehabilitation of the upper extremity.[48,138] During the subacute phase, the goal is to gradually increase motion 0–135 degrees (increase 10 degrees/week). Concentric exercises are initiated, which should include:

- wrist curls;
- wrist extension PREs;
- pronation–supination PREs;
- biceps–triceps PREs.

Criteria to advance to the chronic phase include:

- full ROM;
- no pain or tenderness;
- no increase in laxity;
- strength $^4/_5$ of elbow flexors–extensors.

The goals during the chronic phase include:

- improve strength, power, and endurance;
- improve neuromuscular control.

These goals can be achieved using the following exercises:

- initiating exercise tubing and shoulder program;
- biceps–triceps program;
- supination–pronation PREs;
- wrist extension–flexion PREs;

As appropriate, a well-supervised throwing and conditioning program is initiated at approximately 3 months.[30] Criteria for progression to return to throwing include:

- full, nonpainful ROM;
- no increase in laxity;
- isokinetic testing fulfills criteria.

Operative repair of the MCL typically is required only in competitive throwing athletes or those involved in heavy manual labor,[19] as valgus laxity has been shown to cause minimal functional impairment with normal activities of daily living.[31] The surgical repair or reconstruction can be performed with or without ulnar nerve transposition.[151] The Tommy John technique is a surgical procedure in which the UCL is replaced with a tendon from elsewhere in the body. The palmaris longus tendon, which has been found to have a tensile strength of 357 N, is the most frequently used graft,[152] although the plantaris and toe extensor tendons can also be used.[141]

Lateral (Radial) Collateral Ligament (LCL) Sprain

Posterolateral rotatory instability results from insufficiency of the lateral soft-tissue support of the elbow, especially the LCL complex.[34,109,153] The mechanism of injury typically involves a combination of axial compression, external rotation, and valgus force applied to the elbow.[154,155] It may also have an iatrogenic origin and has been reported after overly aggressive debridement of the lateral soft tissues for patients with recalcitrant tennis elbow.[153,156]

Elbow Instability

Both the humeroulnar and the humeroradial articulation provide approximately 50% of the overall stability of the elbow.[21,24,25] Additional support is supplied by ligaments and muscles.

Although elbow instability has been documented for decades, the clinical tests for making the diagnosis of elbow instability are relatively recent.[109,154]

The following 5-item classification system for elbow instability is useful for correct diagnosing and treatment decision-making[157–159]:

1. *The timing* (acute, chronic, or recurrent).
2. *The articulation(s) involved.* Since the elbow is a complex joint, there are two categories of elbow instability, according to the articulation(s) involved, although the instability can involve both joints in a combined fashion[157]:
   a. *The ulnohumeral joint.* The instability of this hinge joint, which is most commonly predisposed to recurrent instability, can be congenital or acquired, although the former is rare.
   b. *The proximal radioulnar joint.* This involves a subluxation or dislocation of the radial head from the ulna, which can be congenital or acquired. Dislocation of the radial head from the ulna is usually traumatic and often part of a Monteggia fracture–subluxation.
3. *The direction of displacement (valgus, varus, anterior, or posterolateral rotatory).*
   a. *Valgus displacement.* The medial stabilizers of the elbow are the strongest. The mechanism of injury for a valgus displacement is usually a FOOSH injury and occurs in individuals who perform overhead movements such as sledgehammer users and baseball pitchers and javelin throwers.[142] The instability is characterized by pain in the anteromedial aspect of the arm, a moderate-to-severe flexion limitation (acute), and a positive valgus test at 20 degrees of flexion. Valgus instability is seen in one of two varieties: posttraumatic or chronic overload.[157]

Posttraumatic Valgus Instability. This type is often associated with disruption of the soft tissues on the medial side of the elbow, including the MCL, and the common flexor and pronator origin.[160] Valgus instability is usually found in patients with radial head fractures associated with tears of the MCL, or in patients with severe elbow instability following a dislocation that has disrupted the lateral ligament complex.

Chronic. This type typically occurs from repetitive microtrauma or overload, resulting in attenuation or rupture of the anterior band of the MCL.

   b. *Varus displacement.* Because of the anatomic design of the elbow, any force across the elbow principally distorts the elbow in a valgus direction, usually in combination with external rotation rotatory force as occurs from a FOOSH injury. Thus a pure varus mechanism of injury is uncommon.[139] Lateral instability can also occur acutely in patients with elbow dislocations and in many patients with recurrent or chronic instability when the LCL fails to heal.[157] Patients with a varus instability are unlikely to complain of symptoms except when using their arms as weight-bearing extremities (using crutches).[157]
   c. *Anterior displacements.* These injuries, which are rare, usually occur from a blow to the flexed elbow, which drives the olecranon anteriorly.[161] Associated injuries include fractures of the olecranon, with varying degrees of sprain to the collateral ligaments and damage to the vessels and nerves around the joint. On examination, the arm appears shorter, while paradoxically the forearm appears elongated and held in supination. The elbow is usually held in extension.
   d. *Posterior displacements.* Posterior elbow displacements, which are much more common than anterior or lateral displacements, involve a posteriorly displaced ulna in relation to the distal humerus. The patient's arm is held in 45 degrees of flexion. Posterior displacements can be further subdivided into three types: posterior, posterior-medial, and posterior-lateral.[153,159] The most common is usually posterior-lateral rather than direct posterior, so that the coronoid passes inferior to the trochlea, and the ulnar displacement on the humerus is three dimensional (the radius moves with the ulna), such that the ulna supinates (externally rotates) away from the trochlea.[157] The most common mechanism for a posterolateral instability involves proximal attenuation or avulsion of the ligamentous and muscular origins from the lateral epicondyle during a traumatic event.[33] The LCL is the primary static restraint against posterolateral rotatory instability.[15434,160,162–164] The lateral pivot shift test, also called the posterolateral rotatory instability test, is commonly used to assist in the diagnosis.[139] The surgical intervention for posterolateral rotatory instability involves a repair of the common tendon and ligament origins to the lateral epicondyle.[19]
4. *The degree of displacement (subluxation or dislocation).* Posterolateral rotatory instabilities typically consist of three stages, each of which has specific clinical, radiographic, and pathologic features that are predictable and have implications for treatment[157]:
   a. *Stage 1.* The elbow subluxates in a posterolateral rotatory direction, and the patient has an associated positive lateral pivot shift test.
   b. *Stage 2.* The elbow dislocates incompletely so that the coronoid is perched under the trochlea.
   c. *Stage 3.* The elbow dislocates fully so that the coronoid rests behind the humerus.
5. *The presence or absence of associated fractures.* Elbow subluxations and dislocations can be associated with elbow fractures. Fracture–dislocations most commonly involve the coronoid and/or radial head, an injury so difficult to treat and prone to unsatisfactory results that it has been termed the "terrible triad" of the elbow.[165]

The diagnosis for elbow instability is made by the history and a careful physical examination. Patients typically present with a history of recurrent painful clicking, snapping, clunking, or locking of the elbow, that occurs in the extension portion of the arc of motion with the forearm in supination.[157] An examination of the peripheral nerves and distal pulses is necessary to help determine the severity of the instability. Swelling may make the diagnosis of elbow instability difficult. However, if the clinician palpates the two epicondyles and the tip of the olecranon, the following findings help determine the diagnosis:

- If the three points are on the same plane, a supracondylar fracture is suspected.
- If the olecranon is displaced from the plane of the epicondyles, a posterior dislocation is suspected.

The diagnosis of a dislocation can be confirmed by a radiograph.

With patients presenting with a history of dislocation, the diagnosis of recurrent elbow instability is to be suspected. This diagnosis should also be considered when there has been trauma without dislocation. Recurrent instability may also be caused by surgeries such as tennis-elbow surgery or surgery on the radial head.[109,153,156,157]

Conservative intervention for elbow instability should focus on the entire kinetic chain, including the lower extremities and trunk. Posterior capsular tightness in the shoulder must be addressed.[166,167,168,169]

During the inflammatory phase, the intervention includes:

- immobilization of the elbow positioned at 90 degrees of flexion in a well-padded posterior splint for 3–4 days;
- initiation of light gripping exercises (putty or tennis ball);
- avoidance of any passive ROM (patient to perform active ROM when the posterior splint is removed and replaced with a hinged elbow brace or sling), and any valgus stresses to the elbow;
  - use of cryotherapy and high-voltage galvanic stimulation.
  - At days 4–14 the posterior splint is replaced with a hinged elbow brace initially set at 15–90 degrees. Exercises during this phase should include:
- wrist- and finger-active ROM in all planes;
- active elbow ROM (while *avoiding* valgus stress)—flexion–extension–supination–pronation;
- multiangle flexion isometrics;
- multiangle extension isometrics (while avoiding valgus stress);
- wrist curls/reverse wrist curls;
- light biceps curls;
- Shoulder exercises (avoidance of external rotation of shoulder, because this places valgus stress at the elbow). The elbow should be stabilized during shoulder exercises.

At around 2–6 weeks, the hinged brace is set from 0 degree to full flexion. Exercises include:

- PRE progression of elbow and wrist exercises;
- gentle low-load, long-duration stretching is initiated around 5–6 weeks to enhance extension;
- gradual progression of weight with curls, elbow extension, and so on;
- initiation of sports-specific exercises and drills;
- External rotation and internal rotation exercises of the shoulder may be incorporated at 6–8 weeks.

An interval throwing program can be initiated at around 8 weeks, however there should be no return to play until strength is 85–90% of the uninvolved limb. PNF, rhythmic stabilization, and plyometric exercises are used to improve functional stabilization of the joint, beginning with two-handed exercises in the nonprovocative ranges with the elbow close to the body, and progressing to one-handed activities with the involved arm in functional or sports-related positions.[37]

Surgical intervention is reserved for those patients in whom conservative measures fail.

PRACTICE PATTERN 4E: IMPAIRED JOINT MOBILITY, MOTOR FUNCTION, MUSCLE PERFORMANCE, AND RANGE OF MOTION ASSOCIATED WITH LOCALIZED INFLAMMATION

Overuse injuries at the elbow, which are relatively common, result from repetitive trauma that leads to inflammation and/or local tissue damage in the form of cellular and extracellular degeneration, which can be cumulative and result in tendinitis or tendinosis, stress fractures, ligament sprains, or muscle myositis. Both intrinsic and extrinsic factors contribute to overuse injuries. Intrinsic factors include biomechanical abnormalities; extrinsic factors are primarily training errors (incorrect technique, improper equipment, and changes in the duration or frequency of an activity).

Olecranon Bursitis

Because of its superficial location, the olecranon bursa is easily injured through direct trauma or can be irritated through repetitive grazing and weight bearing, resulting in bursitis. Olecranon bursitis is common in individuals who spend long periods weightbearing through the elbows, such as students, or where the potential for falling and striking an elbow on hard playing surfaces is high.[170]

Acute bursitis presents as a swelling over the olecranon process that can vary in size from a slight distension to a large mass several centimeters in diameter.[171] In chronic cases, the pain and swelling can be gradual, or sudden as in acute injury or an infection.[171] An inflamed bursa can occasionally become infected, requiring differentiation between septic and non-septic bursitis.[172]

Redness and heat suggest infection, whereas exquisite tenderness indicates trauma or infection as the underlying cause. Patients often note a decreased range of motion or an inability to don a long-sleeved shirt.[173] While the simple posttraumatic bursitis can be treated with the principles of PRICEMEM, the infected bursa needs prompt medical attention.[173]

Included in the differential diagnoses of olecranon bursitis are acute fractures, rheumatoid arthritis, gout, and synovial cysts.[171] If the patient is experiencing significant pain or discomfort with movement of the elbow, a sling helps to reduce these symptoms and calm the joint.[171] In those cases of marked swelling, or to distinguish between a septic and nonseptic bursitis, aspiration is the appropriate management. Aspiration also helps to reduce the level of discomfort and restriction of movement. The aspirated fluid is cultured and evaluated for crystals to rule out infection or gout. After aspiration, the elbow should be maintained in a splint and sling and reevaluated after 1 week. Bursitis that recurs despite three or more repeated aspirations, or an infection that does not respond to antibiotics, requires evaluation for surgical excision.[171,173]

Injection of corticosteroids is used to manage chronic bursitis once the diagnosis of infection has been excluded.[171]

Olecranon Impingement Syndrome

Repetitive impingement of the olecranon in the olecranon fossa may occur with valgus stresses in throwing sports. Stress to both articular surfaces of the joint may result in the formation of loose bodies, osteophytes, chondromalacia, and synovitis.[174]

The patient may report catching, clicking, and crepitus, which are worsened by elbow extension. Full elbow extension may be limited by a mechanical block. X-rays confirm loose bodies, olecranon osteophytes, and commonly associated anterior elbow changes.

Mild cases respond to a rehabilitation program focusing on restoration of normal motion, strength, and endurance. Continued pain, loose bodies, or mechanical blockage are indications for surgery.

Tendon Injuries of the Elbow

Tendon injuries of this region can be divided into several categories on the basis of the nature of their onset and the tissues involved. While acute tendon injuries are traumatic in nature, chronic overuse injuries are the result of multiple microtraumatic events that cause disruption of the internal structure of the tendon and produce tendinitis or tendinosis.

Bicipital Tendinosis

Bicipital tendinosis typically results from repetitive hyperextension of the elbow with pronation, or repetitive flexion combined with stressful pronation–supination.[85] Typically the patient complains of pain located at the anterior aspect of the distal part of the arm, with tenderness to palpation of the distal biceps belly, the musculotendinous portion of the biceps, or the bicipital insertion of the radial tuberosity.[77,85] Other findings include a reproduction of pain with resisted elbow flexion and supination, and with passive shoulder and elbow extension.

The conservative intervention focuses on regaining the strength, endurance, and flexibility of the flexor/supinator mechanism, and on strengthening the shoulder stabilizers. Other approaches involve electrotherapeutic and thermal modalities, transverse friction massage, trigger point assessment, and specific elbow joint mobilizations.

Biceps Tendon Rupture

The biceps tendon can be avulsed partially or completely either at the musculotendinous junction or at the radial tuberosity.[175] Avulsions of the biceps tendon at the elbow occur almost exclusively in males,[176] and the most common scenario is a rupture of the dominant elbow of a muscular male in his fifth decade of life.[139] Biceps ruptures typically involve a sudden contracture of the biceps against a significant load with the elbow in 90 degrees of flexion.[177]

Clinical findings vary depending on the extent of the rupture; whether it is partial or complete. The typical history includes a report of a sharp, tearing pain concurrent with an acute injury in the antecubital fossa.[139] The objective findings may include ecchymosis in the antecubital fossa, a palpable defect of the distal biceps, loss of strength of elbow flexion and grip, but especially a loss of forearm supination strength.[178]

In active individuals, the normal recommendation is primary repair of the acute tendon avulsion as if not repaired, a 30% loss of elbow flexion and a 40% loss of supination strength can be expected.[178] Postoperatively, the elbow is protected for 6–8 weeks, after which unrestricted range of motion and gentle strengthening exercises are initiated. Return to unrestricted activity is usually not allowed until nearly 6 months of healing has passed.[139]

Triceps Tendinosis

Triceps tendinosis results from repetitive extension, which can occur in such activities as competitive weightlifting, boxing, gymnastics, throwing, and racquet sports.

Subjectively, the patient reports localized tenderness of the triceps insertion at the olecranon that is aggravated with resisted elbow extension.

X-rays are indicated to rule out olecranon apophysitis in adolescence and an avulsion fracture in adults.

The initial stages of the intervention emphasize the principles of PRICEMEM. Therapeutic exercises emphasize strength of the elbow extensor mechanism, with a focus on closed chain exercises for the involved upper extremity.[174] In addition, shoulder strengthening and scapular stabilization exercises are introduced.

Triceps Tendon Rupture

These ruptures usually occur when a deceleration force occurs during elbow extension or with an uncoordinated contraction of the triceps muscle against the flexing elbow.[179] As with the biceps tendon rupture, the physical findings depend on whether the avulsion is partial or complete, but the most common findings include a loss of elbow extension strength, and an inability to extend overhead against gravity. A tendon defect may be present if the tear is complete.[139]

Primary repair is the treatment of choice in acute complete ruptures. Partial injury may be treated conservatively with immobilization for about 3 weeks, followed by a gradual progression of range of motion and strengthening.

Brachialis Strain

A brachialis strain is relatively rare, but the brachialis is prone to myositis ossificans, a pathologic bone formation, due to the fact that it is likely to hemorrhage when injured (see later).

Typically, the patient reports pain that is felt on the anterior aspect of the distal part of the arm, and there is palpable tenderness in the muscle belly of the brachialis. Resisted supination is not painful, although resisted elbow flexion combined with forearm pronation is.

The conservative intervention involves electrotherapeutic and thermal modalities, transverse friction massage, trigger point assessment, correction of muscle imbalances, and specific elbow joint mobilizations.

Epicondylitis

The term epicondylitis suggests an inflammation at one of the epicondyles. Epicondylitis are common in persons who frequently overuse the upper arm, particularly with activities that involve rotation of the arm with flexion and extension. Two types of epicondylitis are commonly described: lateral epicondylitis (tennis elbow) and medial epicondylitis (golfer's elbow). Lateral epicondylitis is four to seven times more common than medial epicondylitis.[180]

Lateral Epicondylitis (Tennis Elbow)

Lateral epicondylitis represents a pathologic condition of the common extensor muscles at their origin on the lateral humeral epicondyle. Specifically, the condition involves the tendons of the muscles that control wrist extension and radial deviation resulting in pain on the lateral side of the elbow with contraction of these muscles.[138]

The first description of tennis elbow is attributed to Runge,[181] but the name derives from lawn tennis arm described by Morris in the *Lancet* in 1882.[182] This was followed in 1883 by Dr H.P. Major describing his own affliction in 1883.[183] In Runge's original description, he called it writer's cramp (Schreibekrampf) and attributed it to a periostitis of the lateral humeral epicondyle.[181] Since then, it has been referred to by a number of names including epicondylalgia, epicondyle pain, musician's palsy (Musikerlähmung), [184] and tennis pain (Tennisschmerz), although most authors have used the terms epicondylitis or tennis elbow.

Tennis elbow affects between 1 and 3% of the population, occurs most commonly between 35 and 50 years of age with a mean age of 45,[185] is seldom seen in those under 20 years of age, and usually affects the dominant arm.[186–188] Cyriax[189] noted that the origin of the ECRB was the primary site of this injury, and pathologic changes have been consistently documented at this location,[190–193] although findings are also found in the ECRL, and the ECU.[131] One-third of patients also have involvement of the origin of the EDC.[189,192,193]

The proposed presence of macro- or microtears in the ECRB tendon was based on findings extrapolated from abnormal physical and intraoperative examinations showing gross alterations in the ECRB tendon.[189–191,194]

However, a recent study involving gross and microscopic dissections found that it was not possible to separate the origin of the ECRB from that of the common extensor tendon and that at times the two tendons appeared to interdigitate, indicating that any pathology believed to be isolated to the ECRB must be common to both.[195]

Over 25 conditions have been suggested as causes of tennis elbow,[189] including periostitis,[181,186,189,196] infection,[197,198] bursitis,[186,189,199–203] fibrillation of the radial head,[204] radioulnar joint disease,[205] AL lesion,[183,206,207] nipped synovial fringe,[208–213] calcific tendinitis,[214] neurogenic causes,[215,216] osteochondritis dissecans, and radial nerve entrapment.[70,72,215,217–219]

Capsular and ligamentous lesions have been mentioned by a number of authors. Landelius[220] regarded the pull of the radial head on the orbicular ligament and the capsule to be the cause. Bosworth[207,221,222] considered the impingement of the orbicular ligament on the head of the radius to be the sole problem.

Dysfunction of the cervical spine has also been speculated to cause tennis elbow. Theoretically, a frank radiculopathy may weaken the extensor muscles to the point at which normal use is traumatic and induces a grade I tear in the muscle belly or tendon. Less definite compression of the nerve root may compromise axoplasmic transportation, producing a trophic malnutrition of the muscle, resulting in damage. A facilitated segment at C5–6, with its resulting hypertonicity, might lead to a chronic overuse syndrome, or poor coordination. Wright and colleagues[223] found that neuronal changes within the spinal cord may be more important than peripheral nociceptor sensitization in the development of such disorders as tennis elbow. Gunn and Milbrandt[224] discussed a reflex localization of pain from radiculopathy at the cervical spine in patients with an intervention-resistant tennis elbow who had hypomobility of the lower cervical motion segments.[225] Maitland[226] has also reported improving the symptoms of lateral epicondylitis with a program of heat, mobilization, and traction of the cervical segments.[225]

The shoulder has also been speculated to be a cause of tennis elbow, due to the effect of an abnormal tension in the clavipectoral fascia on the brachial plexus. This fascia is attached to the clavicle around the subclavius muscle. From there it passes down to the upper border of the pectoralis minor and extends from the anterior intercostal membrane to the coracoid process. The fascia encloses the pectoralis minor and becomes the suspensory ligament of the axilla. It is speculated that if the fascia is distorted due to clavicular malposition, the traction exerted on the brachial plexus could lead to similar problems as those encountered with a cervical lesion. In these cases, altering the position of the shoulder girdle (protracting, retracting, elevating, and depressing it) would alter the symptoms produced during the isometric tests.

Whatever the cause, tennis elbow usually results from overuse although it can be traumatic in origin. The overuse injuries tend to involve abusive tissue trauma secondary to repetitive activity, which promotes microtraumatic tissue failure. Those tendons that wrap around a convex surface or the apex of a concavity, and those that cross two joints, are particularly vulnerable to overuse injuries, as are those with areas of scant vascular supply, or those subjected to repetitive tension.[227–232] One possible etiology for overuse at the elbow is the fact that the hand does not have a supportive function but functions predominantly to grasp some object. Repetitive grasping, with the wrist positioned in extension, places the elbow particularly at risk. Participants of tennis, baseball, javelin, golf, squash, racquetball, swimming, and weight lifting are all predisposed to this risk.[139]

While the terms *epicondylitis* and *tendinitis* are commonly used to describe tennis elbow, histopathologic studies have demonstrated that this condition is often not an inflammatory condition; rather, it is a degenerative condition, a tendinosis.[180,192]

Nirschl previously categorized the stages of repetitive microtrauma[233]:

- A stage 1 injury is probably inflammatory, is not associated with pathologic alterations, and is likely to resolve.
- A stage 2 injury is associated with pathologic alterations such as tendinosis or angiofibroblastic degeneration. It is this stage that is most commonly associated with sports-related tendon injuries such as tennis elbow, and with overuse injuries in general. Within the tendon, there is a fibroblastic and vascular response (tendinosis) rather than an immune blood-cell response (inflammation).
- A stage 3 injury is associated with pathologic changes (tendinosis) and complete structural failure (rupture).
- A stage 4 injury exhibits the features of a stage 2 or 3 injury and is associated with other changes such as fibrosis, soft

matrix calcification, and hard osseous calcification. The changes that are associated with a stage 4 injury may also be related to the use of cortisone.

Nirschl[234] postulates that some patients who have tennis elbow may have a genetic predisposition that makes them more susceptible to tendinosis at multiple sites. He terms this condition *mesenchymal syndrome* on the basis of the stem-cell line of fibroblasts and the presence of a potentially systemic abnormality of cross-linkage in the collagen produced by the fibroblasts. Patients may have mesenchymal syndrome if they have two or more of the following conditions[229,234]:

- Bilateral lateral tennis elbow
- Cubital tunnel syndrome
- CTS
- De Quervain tenosynovitis
- Trigger finger
- Rotator cuff tendinosis

Clinical Presentation. Three types of tennis elbow are recognized based on the mode of onset:

- The acute onset (indirect) type of tennis elbow is associated with a recognizable mechanism with acute pain, associated bruising on occasion,[235] and a feeling of something giving way within the elbow.[189]
- Rupture of the ECRL with tenderness in the muscles[236,237] is associated with direct trauma to the lateral side of the elbow, but with no tearing of the ligaments.[186,238]
- The chronic type is associated with a gradual onset and is occasionally termed occupational neuralgia (Beschaftigungensneuralgie).[239]

The pain of tennis elbow is often related to activities that involve wrist extension/grasp, as it is the wrist extensors that must contract during grasping activities to stabilize the wrist. Diffuse achiness and morning stiffness are also common complaints.[138] Occasionally the pain is experienced at night and the patient may report dropping objects frequently, especially if they are carried with the palm facing down.

Palpable tenderness is usually found over the ECRB and ECRL, especially at the lateral epicondyle, with the site of maximum tenderness most commonly being over the anterior aspect of the lateral epicondyle.[138] The next most common site is tenderness over the radial head, or where the lateral part of the common extensor tendon arises from the bone.[189] Tenderness can be found in other sites as well, in addition to swelling, but not consistently.[189] Differentiation between the various tendons is obviously important. Five types of tendon lesions of the elbow are recognized:

- a lesion of the muscle origin of the ECRL, which is usually located just proximal to the lateral epicondyle (type 1);
- An insertion tendinopathy of the ECRB (type 2). This is the most common site and is usually associated with type 5. As the ECRB also originates from the radial collateral ligament, involvement of the tendon can produce pain here, or at the radial head (type 3).
- an ECRB muscle belly strain (type 4);
- inflammation at the origin of the extensor digitorum (type 5).

The range-of-motion tests typically reveal the following:

- active motions are usually painless, although there may be pain with wrist flexion when combined with elbow extension.
- passive motion can produce pain, especially with passive wrist flexion with the forearm pronated and the elbow extended.

The resisted tests typically reproduce symptoms with resisted wrist extension and radial deviation with the elbow extended. Pain on resisted finger extension has also been reported. Cozen's or Mills' special tests are typically positive.

The cervical spine, shoulder, and wrist must also be examined. As a large number of tennis elbows appear to be secondary to a dysfunction of either the cervical spine or the shoulder, testing isometric wrist extension in varying positions of the cervical spine or shoulder will help differentiate the cause. If the primary cause is remote, the amount of discomfort on testing will vary with changes of the head or shoulder girdle position. If the pain disappears entirely during these maneuvers, there can be no symptomatic pathologic changes at the elbow, and no local treatment is required. However, usually the pain is reduced rather than being eliminated, indicating that the cause may be remote and local pathologic changes have since supervened.

Tennis elbow is normally a self-limiting complaint; without intervention, the symptoms will usually resolve within 8–12 months.

Intervention. There are numerous interventions cited for this condition, both medical and surgical.[240] In fact, more than 40 treatments have been suggested, indicating that the ideal remedy has yet to be found, although there is agreement that the initial management should be conservative. Many studies of the use of physical therapy in the management of tennis elbow are poorly designed and statistically weak.[241,242] The effectiveness of ultrasound for tennis elbow is undetermined. One study[243] found ultrasound to be effective in a placebo-controlled, double-blind trial,[244] but another study[245] found no difference. A recent randomized pilot study by Struijs et al.[246] of 31 patients diagnosed with tennis elbow found that the manipulation of wrist was more effective at a follow-up of 3–6 weeks than ultrasound, friction massage, and muscle stretching and strengthening exercises. The wrist manipulation used was an anterior (ventral) manipulation of the scaphoid (refer to Chap. 18), which was repeated 15 times, two times a week, with a maximum of nine intervention sessions. In a randomized study of 18 subjects,[247] joint mobilization to the radial head combined with neurodynamic techniques to the radial nerve was compared with a program consisting of ultrasound, transverse friction massage, and strengthening and stretching exercises. At 3-month follow-up, only the group receiving joint mobilizations and neurodynamic interventions had improved.

More recently, there has been a trend toward treatment of the cervical and thoracic spines with this disorder. Vicenzino and colleagues[248] demonstrated that cervical lateral glides resulted in immediate improvement in pain at the lateral elbow, in pain-free grip strength, and in increased range of motion during upper limb neurodynamic testing in patients with lateral epicondylalgia. A retrospective study by Cleland and colleagues[249] demonstrated that patients receiving manual therapy techniques directed at the cervical spine achieved similar success rates as a group who received treatment solely directed at the elbow, but that they achieved this success in significantly fewer visits ($p = 0.01$). Another clinical trial by Cleland et al.[250] which compared the outcomes of 10 patients with lateral epicondylalgia who were randomly assigned to receive localized treatment or localized treatment plus manual therapy to the cervicothoracic spine, found that the latter group demonstrated greater improvement in all outcome measures as compared to the treatment group receiving the localized management. Replication of these results is needed in a large-scale randomized clinical trial with a control group and a longer-term follow-up before any meaningful conclusions can be drawn.

In a randomized trial by Bisset and colleagues[251] investigated the efficacy of physical therapy for tennis elbow (combining mobilizations with movement (MWM) techniques and exercise) compared with a wait-and-see approach or corticosteroid injections over a 52-week period concluded that the physical therapy intervention had a superior benefit to wait and see in the first 6 weeks and to cortisone injections after 6 weeks.

Other forms of physical therapy including electrotherapy and thermotherapy have not been proven to be effective.[243]

The patient may be prescribed an orthotic device as a treatment strategy, and many different types of braces and other orthotic devices are available. The main type is a band or strap around the muscle belly of the wrist extensors. Theoretically, binding the muscle with a clasp, band, or brace should limit expansion and thereby decrease the contribution to force production by muscle fibers proximal to the band.[252] However, the benefits of tennis-elbow braces remain unproven. Snyder-Mackler and Epler reported on a comparison of a "standard" tennis-elbow brace and one with an air-filled bladder,[253] but it is not possible to extrapolate from their findings to the efficacy of tennis-elbow braces in the management of tennis elbow. Counterforce bracing[194] (such as the Count-R-Force brace from Medical Sports, Arlington, VA) has been shown to

- beneficially impact force couple imbalances and altered movements[127,254,255];
- decrease angular acceleration at the elbow[256];
- decrease EMG activity.[256]

However, tennis-elbow braces have been shown to have little effect in vibrational dampening.[257] As an alternative to bracing, Gellman[258] recommends a protective 20-degree wrist extension splint for tennis elbow to help offload the ECRB.[138] In a study by Struijs and colleagues[252] a total of 180 patients were randomized into three groups: brace-only treatment, physical therapy, and a combination of these. Main outcome measures were success rate, severity of complaints, pain, disability, and satisfaction. Physical therapy was superior to brace only at 6 weeks for pain, disability, and satisfaction. Contrarily, brace-only treatment was superior on ability of daily activities. Combination treatment was superior to brace on severity of complaints, disability, and satisfaction. At 26 and 52 weeks, no significant differences were identified.[252] The results from the study would tend to indicate that the brace treatment might be useful as an initial therapy.

The Mills' manipulation (see Intervention section), a thrust technique that is intended to maximally stretch the ECRB tendon in order to try to pull apart the two surfaces of the painful scar, has been recommended to treat true tennis elbow.[189] Manipulation of this kind has also been advocated in other studies.[259–261]

Nirschl and Sobel[119] have attempted to determine whether the presenting symptoms are helpful in both diagnosing and directing the intervention. This information was previously published in the form of a table.[119]

- ***Types 1 and 2.*** Benign (nonharmful) pain: Type 1 pain is characterized by stiffness or mild soreness after activity and resolves within 24 hours. Type 2 pain is marked by stiffness or mild soreness after exercise, lasts more than 48 hours, is relieved with warm-up exercises, is not present during activity, and resolves within 72 hours after the cessation of activity. The pain associated with types 1 and 2 may be due to peritendinous inflammation.
- ***Type 3.*** Semibenign (likely nonharmful) pain: Type 3 pain is characterized by stiffness or mild soreness before activity and is partially relieved with warm-up exercises. The pain does not prevent participation in activity and is only mild during activity. However, minor adjustments in the technique, intensity, and duration of activity are needed to control the pain. Type 3 pain may necessitate the use of nonsteroidal anti-inflammatory medications.
- ***Type 4.*** Semiharmful pain: Type 4 pain is more intense than type 3 pain and produces changes in the performance of a specific sport- or work-related activity. Mild pain accompanies the activities of daily living. Type 4 pain may reflect tendon damage.
- ***Types 5–7.*** Harmful pain: Type 5 pain, which is characterized as moderate or severe before, during, and after exercise, greatly alters or prevents performance of the activity. Pain accompanies but does not prevent the performance of activities of daily living. Complete rest controls the pain. Type 5 pain reflects permanent tendon damage. Type 6 pain, which is similar to type 5 pain, prevents the performance of activities of daily living and persists despite complete rest. Type 7 pain is a consistent, aching pain that intensifies with activity and that regularly interrupts sleep.

The pain of types 1 and 2 is usually self-limiting when proper precautions are taken. Types 3 and 4 usually respond to nonoperative medical therapy. The pain types of 5–7 are more likely to necessitate operative treatment.[119]

Johnson[262] recommends an exercise regimen consisting of PREs to the wrist extensors, with the elbow flexed to 90 degrees and also with the elbow straight is recommended. The exercises are performed as a 10-repetition maximum, morning and night. Gradually, the weight is increased so that the 10-repetition maximum is always maintained. The pain may increase for the first week or two or three, but by the fifth or sixth weeks, the elbow pain will be better. An ice pack or heating pad can be used during the painful period.[262]

The goals during the acute phase are to decrease inflammation/pain, promote tissue healing, increase flexibility, and retard muscle atrophy. Methods to accomplish this include[88]:

- cryotherapy;
- whirlpool;
- HVGS;
- phonophoresis;
- iontophoresis (with an anti-inflammatory such as dexamethasone);
- stretches for
  - wrist extension–flexion;
  - elbow extension–flexion;
  - forearm supination–pronation;
- avoidance of painful movements (such as gripping).

During the subacute phase, the goals should be to[88]

- improve flexibility;
- increase muscular strength and endurance;
- increase functional activities and return to function;
- emphasize concentric–eccentric strengthening with a focus on:
  - wrist extension–flexion;
  - forearm pronation–supination;
  - elbow flexion—extension;
- initiate shoulder strengthening (if deficiencies are noted);
- continue flexibility exercises;
- use counterforce brace;
- continue use of cryotherapy after exercise or function;
- initiate gradual return to stressful activities;
- gradually reinitiate previously painful movements.

During the chronic phase, the goal should be to:[88]

- improve muscular strength and endurance;
- maintain/enhance flexibility;
- gradually return to high-level sport activities;
- continue strengthening exercises (emphasize eccentric–concentric);
- continue to emphasize deficiencies in shoulder and elbow strength;
- continue flexibility exercises;
- gradually diminish use of the counterforce brace;
- continue to use cryotherapy as needed;
- initiate gradual return to sport activity;
- equipment modifications (grip size, string tension, and playing surface); and
- emphasize maintenance.

Incorrect technique, particularly with racquet sports, is the cause of many elbow problems. Emphasis should be placed on recruiting the whole of the shoulder and trunk when hitting the ball, so as to dissipate the forces as widely as possible. It is important to hit strokes with a firm wrist and not by means of wrist movements to return the ball. A late backhand in tennis should be corrected as this stroke is the most common cause of stress to the elbow if performed incorrectly.[130,180,233] Whereas the forehand demonstrates good weight transfer, the faulty backhand has no forward weight transfer, and the front shoulder is usually elevated.[173] The trunk leans away from the net at the time of impact, and the racquet head is down.[173] The elbow and wrist extend before impact, and the power source is forearm extension in the pronated position, resulting in a stroke that is nonrhythmic and jerky and with sharp pronation at follow-through.[173] Sometimes the use of a two-handed backhand may be helpful. One theory to support this is that the one-handed backhand links five body parts prior to impact (hips to trunk to shoulder to elbow to wrist), while the two-handed backhand only links two body parts (hips to trunk) prior to impact with the ball.[138]

The ball should be hit with the center point of the strings, or "sweet spot." When the ball is hit incorrectly, the forces are transmitted as an acute strain up and along the muscle mass to the extensor origin at the elbow.[233]

In addition to correcting poor technique, patient education should address racquet size, grip size, and string tension. A fiberglass, graphite, or wood racquet is more forgiving than a metal one. Tennis racquets with larger head sizes reduce arm vibration.[263] Tennis racquets should be strung with gut, as it is more resilient than nylon strings, to 52–55 pounds to allow the impact to be spread over slightly more time and decrease the forces transmitted to the forearm muscles.[264,265] Currently, the use of a mid-sized medium-flex, graphite tennis racquet with loosely strung nylon monofilament is recommended. The grip size should not be too large or too small,[266] and an increased racquet handle diameter is helpful for players with relatively weak wrist extensors.

If the symptoms are not controlled with the above measures, local injection of corticosteroid may be helpful. It was not until the 1950s that the injection of corticosteroids was first reported.[213,267,268] Freeland and Gribble found that hydrocortisone was neither more nor less effective than procaine and concluded that the short-term relief of pain was a nonspecific response that may be due to the volume of fluid injected or to the trauma of introducing the needle.[267] Subsequently a number of studies have shown steroids to be beneficial, and this has remained one of the mainstays of conservative treatment.[269–271]

Operative Intervention. Surgery is indicated if the symptoms do not resolve despite a properly performed conservative intervention lasting 6 months.[139] A simple handshake test can help to determine whether surgical intervention is required.[272] The patient is asked to perform a firm handshake with the elbow extended, and then supinate the forearm against resistance. The clinician notes whether the patient reports having pain at the origin of the extensors of the wrist. The elbow is then flexed to 90 degrees, and the same maneuver is performed. If pain is decreased in the flexed position, operative treatment is less likely to be needed. If the pain is equally severe with the elbow flexed and extended, then operative intervention is more likely to be needed.[272]

The goals of operative treatment of tendinosis of the elbow are to resect the pathologic material to stimulate neovascularization by producing focused local bleeding, and to create a healthy scar while doing the least possible structural damage to the surrounding tissues. Postoperatively, a carefully guided resistance-based rehabilitation program is recommended.

Medial Epicondylitis (Golfer's Elbow)

Medial epicondylitis is only one-third as common as lateral epicondylitis.[100] It primarily involves a tendinopathy of the common flexor origin, specifically the FCR and the humeral head of the pronator teres.[48,100,185] To a lesser extent, the palmaris longus, FCU, and FDS may also be involved.[233]

The mechanism for medial epicondylitis is not usually related to direct trauma, but rather to overuse. This commonly occurs for three reasons:

- Fatigue of the flexor–pronator tissues in response to repeated stress.
- A predisposition for medial ligamentous injury due to a sudden change in the levels of stress.[273]
- The MCL fails to sufficiently stabilize against the valgus forces.[274]

Medial epicondylitis usually begins as a microtear at the interface between the pronator teres and FCR origins with subsequent development of fibrotic and inflammatory granulation tissue.[30] An inflammation develops in an attempt to speed up tissue production to compensate for the increased rate of microdamage caused by increased use and decreased recovery time.[275] Chronic symptoms result from a loss of extensibility of the tissues, leaving the tendon unable to cope effectively against tensile loads.

Clinical Presentation. The typical clinical presentation for medial epicondylitis is pain and tenderness over the flexor–pronator origin, slightly distal and anterior to the medial epicondyle. The symptoms are typically reported to be exacerbated with either resisted wrist flexion and pronation or passive wrist extension and supination.[30,100]

Differential diagnosis for medial elbow symptoms includes[276]:

- MCL injury or insufficiency[22,277,278];
- ulnar nerve entrapment;
- medial elbow intra-articular pathology.[279]

Intervention. Conservative intervention for medial epicondylitis has been shown to have success rates as high as 90%.[100] The conservative intervention for this condition initially involves rest, activity modification, and local modalities. Complete immobilization is usually not recommended as it eliminates the stresses necessary for maturation of new collagen tissue. Once the acute phase has passed, the focus switches to restoring range of motion and correcting any imbalances of flexibility and strength. The strengthening program initially includes multi-angle isometrics, and then concentric and eccentric exercises of the flexor–pronator muscles.

Splinting or the use of a counterforce brace may be a useful adjunct.[30]

INTEGRATION OF PRACTICE PATTERNS 4F AND 5F: IMPAIRED JOINT MOBILITY, MOTOR FUNCTION, MUSCLE PERFORMANCE, AND RANGE OF MOTION, OR REFLEX INTEGRITY SECONDARY TO SPINAL DISORDERS, PERIPHERAL NERVE ENTRAPMENTS, COMPARTMENT SYNDROME, AND MYOFASCIAL PAIN DYSFUNCTION

Compressive Neuropathies

In the region of the elbow, there are a multitude of sites where the peripheral nerves can be entrapped or compressed (Table 17-9), with involvement of the ulnar and median and radial

TABLE 17-9 Nerve Injuries about the Elbow

Nerve	Motor Loss	Sensory Loss	Functional Loss
Median nerve (C6–8, T1)	Pronator teres Flexor carpi radialis Palmaris longus Palmaris longus Flexor digitorum superficialis Flexor pollicis longus Lateral half of flexor digitorum profundus Pronator quadratus Thenar eminence Lateral two lumbricals	Palmar aspect of hand with thumb, index, middle, and lateral half of ring finger Posterior (dorsal) aspect of distal third of index, middle, and lateral half of ring finger	Pronation weakness Wrist flexion and abduction weakness Loss of radial deviation at wrist Inability to oppose or flex thumb Thumb abduction weakness Weak grip Weak or no pinch (ape hand deformity)

(Continued)

TABLE 17-9 Nerve Injuries about the Elbow (Continued)			
Nerve	**Motor Loss**	**Sensory Loss**	**Functional Loss**
Anterior interosseous nerve (branch of median nerve)	Flexor pollicis longus Lateral half of flexor digitorum profundus Pronator quadratus Thenar eminence muscles Lateral two lumbricals	None	Pronation weakness, especially at 90-degree elbow flexion Weakness of opposition and thumb flexion Weak finger flexion Weak pinch (no tip to tip)
Ulnar nerve (C7–8, T1)	Flexor carpi ulnaris Medial half of flexor digitorum profundus Palmaris brevis Hypothenar eminence Adductor pollicis Medial two lumbricals All interossei	Posterior (dorsal) and palmar aspect of little and medial half of ring finger	Weak wrist flexion Loss of ulnar deviation at wrist Loss of distal flexion of little finger Loss of abduction and adduction of fingers Inability to extend second and third phalanges of little and ring fingers (benediction hand deformity) Loss of thumb adduction
Radial nerve (C5–8, T1)	Anconeus Brachioradialis Extensor carpi radialis longus and brevis Extensor digitorum Extensor pollicis longus and brevis Abductor pollicis longus Extensor carpi ulnaris Extensor indicis Extensor digiti minimi	Posterior aspect of hand (lateral two-thirds) Posterior aspect and lateral aspect of thumb Proximal two-thirds of posterior aspect of index, middle, and half of ring finger	Loss of supination Loss of wrist extension (wrist drop) Inability to grasp Inability to stabilize wrist Loss of finger extension Inability to abduct thumbs
Posterior interosseous nerve (branch of radial nerve)	Extensor carpi radialis and brevis Extensor digitorum Extensor pollicis longus and brevis Abductor pollicis longus Extensor carpi ulnaris Extensor indicis Extensor digiti minimi	None	Weak wrist extension Weak finger extension Difficulty stabilizing wrist Difficulty with grasping Inability to abduct thumb

Data from Magee DJ: *Orthopaedic Physical Assessment*, 2nd ed. Philadelphia, PA. WB Saunders, 2008.

nerves and their branches being by far the most common.[67] Table 17-10 outlines a summary of conservative management strategies for the various nerve entrapments.

Ulnar Nerve Entrapment (Cubital Tunnel Syndrome)

Although the ulnar nerve is well protected above the elbow, the nerve can be compressed or entrapped at a number of locations. Nirschl has divided the medial epicondylar groove into three zones[280,281]:

- zone I: proximal to the medial epicondyle;
- zone II: the level of the medial epicondyle (retrocondylar groove);
- zone III: distal to the medial epicondyle (cubital tunnel).

Repetitive overuse can result in compression of the ulnar nerve in zone III by a tight FCU muscle.[174] Entrapment can also be precipitated in zones II and III by a subluxating ulnar nerve, in zone II by elbow synovitis, in zone I or II by a cubitus valgus deformity, or in zone I by the medial intermuscular septum, which slopes from a thick wide base at the medial epicondyle, to a weak and thin edge more proximal on the humeral shaft.[59,65,174]

It has been suggested that because of the superficial location of the ulnar nerve, repetitive motion may initiate a cycle of inflammation and edema that inhibits the normal gliding of the nerve.[54,282] Additional injury occurs when traction forces caused by elbow flexion produce an additional compressive force on the internal architecture of the nerve.[57,283] The severity of nerve injury will be dependent on the magnitude, duration, and character of the applied forces.[54,282]

TABLE 17-10 Summary of Conservative Management for Nerve Entrapments

Nerve	Entrapment Site	Intervention
Median	Carpal tunnel Proximal forearm	Splint wrist in neutral position at night Stretching exercises for pronator teres Rest periods in supination
Ulnar	Guyon's canal Cubital tunnel	Splint wrist in neutral position at night Elbow pad Education: positioning in elbow extension and decreasing direct pressure on nerve Stretch the flexor carpi ulnaris
Radial (posterior interosseous) Radial (sensory)	Arcade of Fröhse Forearm	Positioning in supination and avoid repetitive pronation and supination activities Positioning in supination and avoid repetitive pronation and supination activities
Brachial plexus	Supraclavicular	Avoid provocative positions Stretch shortened muscles and strengthen weakened scapular muscles

The anconeus has also been reported as a cause of cubital tunnel syndrome and has been found to occur in 3–28% of human anatomic specimen elbows,[56,284] and in as many as 9% of patients undergoing surgical treatment for cubital tunnel syndrome.[285]

The clinical findings for an ulnar nerve entrapment depend on the location of the lesion and may include[286]:

- activity-related pain or paresthesias involving the fourth and fifth digits, accompanied by pain that may extend proximally or distally in the medial aspect of the elbow;
- pain or paresthesias worse at night;
- decreased sensation in the ulnar distribution of the hand;
- progressive inability to separate the fingers;
- loss of grip power and dexterity;
- atrophy or weakness of the ulnar intrinsic muscles of the hand (late sign);
- clawing contracture of the ring and little fingers (late sign)[287];
- positive elbow flexion and pressure-provocative test;
- positive Wartenberg's sign and Froment's sign (see Chap. 18);
- positive Tinel's sign at the elbow.

Conservative intervention is recommended for patients with intermittent symptoms and without changes in two-point discrimination or muscle atrophy. Activity modification with protection over the cubital tunnel with an elbow pad placed on the medial-posterior aspect,[286] limiting repetitive extreme elbow flexion, and night splinting at 40–60 degrees may be helpful.[57] In severe cases, the splint is worn during the day, or the elbow is cast at about 45 degrees. Exercises must not reproduce the distal nerve symptoms and may, therefore, initially need to be performed in limited arcs of motion.[174] For those patients who fail to respond to conservative management after 3–4 months, and who have muscle atrophy, persistent sensory changes, or persistent symptoms, surgical decompression, or an anterior transposition of the ulnar nerve is available.[65]

Median Nerve Entrapment (Humeral Supracondylar Process Syndrome)

Median nerve entrapment at the elbow is relatively rare, although it is often misdiagnosed as CTS.[97] The most proximal site at which the median nerve can be compressed is in the distal arm by the ligament of Struthers, an anatomic variant present in 0.7–2.7% of the population.[288] Very few cases of a ligament of Struthers neuropathy are described in the literature.[66,289,290] The patient may complain of pain in the wrist or medial forearm, which is exacerbated with full elbow extension or pronation of the forearm.[66,290] The patient may also report paresthesias in the index or long finger.[66]

In the antecubital area, there are three sites of potential median nerve entrapment.[97] One site is as the nerve passes under the lacertus fibrosus, or bicipital aponeurosis, a fascial band extending from the biceps tendon to the forearm fascia.[291] The second site is at the level of the pronator teres muscle, after the nerve crosses the elbow. The third potential site is as the median nerve travels under the FDS. Compression of the median nerve at any one of these three sites constitutes what is described in the literature as the pronator syndrome (PS).

Pronator Syndrome. The patient typically complains of an insidious onset of pain that is usually felt on the anterior aspect of the elbow, radial side of the palm, and the palmar side of the first, second, third, and half of the fourth digits. There is often associated "heaviness" of the forearm.[97] Unlike CTS, there is no Tinel's sign at the wrist, and there are no nocturnal symptoms.[292,293] Pain can be reproduced with[63]:

- pressure applied over the pronator teres 4 cm distal to the cubital crease with concurrent resistance against pronation, elbow flexion, and wrist flexion[294];
- resisted supination (due to compression of the lacertus fibrosus);

- resistance of the long finger flexors (due to compression by the FDS arch).

Diagnosis is confirmed electromyographically. PS typically responds well to activity modification (removing the causative activity), rest, NSAIDs, ice, and the restoration of proper flexibility and strength of the wrist flexors and forearm pronators. Rehabilitation will most benefit those cases in which compression is related to medial elbow tendinosis. In these cases, gentle massage along the fibers may aid in the breaking of adhesions. Surgical relief may be needed in recalcitrant cases.[292]

Anterior Interosseous Syndrome. Anterior interosseous syndrome was first described by Tinel in 1918, and was further delineated by Kiloh and Nevin in 1952.[292]

Potential sources of entrapment of the AIN include the Gantzer's muscle (an accessory head of the FPL), and the FCR muscle.[97,291,295]

Compression of the AIN results in forearm pain, and motor loss of the FPL, pronator quadratus, and the lateral half of the FDP, such that the patient is unable to perform the "OK" sign with the index finger and thumb. This must be differentiated from a rupture of the muscle or its tendon. No sensory changes occur, even though the AIN carries sensory information from the distal radioulnar joint, radiocarpal joint, and intercarpal joints.[296]

Pain and weakness are typically provoked with resisted flexion of the interphalangeal (IP) joint of the thumb and with the distal interphalangeal (DIP) joint of the index finger.

The differential diagnosis includes neuralgic amyotrophy, FPL tendon rupture, and index finger FDP rupture. Most cases of AIN syndrome typically resolve spontaneously.[297]

Although PS and AIN syndrome are relatively rare, it is important to be able to differentially diagnose the syndromes in cases of suspected CTS. Paresthesia is absent in AIN and present in both PS and CTS.[298] CTS involves paresthesia in the lateral $3^1/_2$ digits, whereas PS involves paresthesia in the lateral $3^1/_2$ digits and often in the distribution of the palmar cutaneous branch of the median nerve.[298] The paresthesia in CTS may be reproduced by compression over the wrist or Phalen's test, whereas PS requires compression at the pronator teres to reproduce paresthesia. Tinel's sign is present at the wrist in 80% of cases of CTS and is present at the pronator teres in PS in less than 50% of cases.[298] AIN syndrome is easily differentiated from CTS by the lack of paresthesia complaints.[298]

Radial Nerve Entrapment

The radial nerve is the most commonly injured peripheral nerve (see Chap. 3) and, because of its spiral course across the back of the mid-shaft of the humerus, and its relatively fixed position in the distal arm as it penetrates the lateral intermuscular septum, it is the most frequently injured nerve associated with fractures of the humerus.

A number of radial nerve entrapments are recognized and are named according to the location at which they occur. Four radial nerve entrapments are commonly cited: high radial nerve palsy, posterior interosseous nerve syndrome (PINS), radial tunnel syndrome (RTS), and superficial radial nerve palsy. The various symptoms of these entrapments can aid the clinician to determine the level of entrapment.

CLINICAL PEARL

There is motor and sensory involvement with the high radial nerve palsy, motor involvement with the PINS, pain with the RTS, and sensory disturbances with the superficial radial nerve palsy.[299] Symptoms of pain, cramping, and tenderness in the proximal posterior (dorsal) forearm, without muscle weakness, are associated with RTS, whereas PINS involves the loss of motor function of some or all of the muscles innervated by the PIN and is thus characterized by weakness.[299]

High Radial Nerve Compression. A spontaneous nerve compression may occur in the mid-arm at the level of the lateral head of the triceps due to strenuous muscular exercise.[300] A mid-shaft humerus fracture can result in a radial neuropathy at the spiral groove of the humerus in 14% of humeral fractures.[301] Regardless of the cause, a high radial nerve palsy will result in a loss of wrist extension, an inability to extend the fingers and thumb, and a decrease in sensibility of the first posterior (dorsal) web space.[299] Involvement of the triceps muscle is dependent on the level of compression. A cervical radiculopathy and thoracic outlet syndrome must be considered in the differential diagnosis.

Posterior Interosseous Nerve Syndrome (PINS). There are five potential sites of compression of the PIN as it traverses through the radial tunnel[67,70,216,299]:

- the fibrous bands that connect the brachialis to the brachioradialis[72,302];
- the vascular leash of Henry, a fan of blood vessels that cross the nerve at the level of the radial neck[70,72,303];
- medial proximal portion (leading edge) of the ECRB[70,72];
- Between fibrous bands at the proximal and distal edge of the supinator.[304] The proximal border of the supinator, through which the radial nerve passes, is referred to as the arcade of Fröhse.

Symptoms of PIN entrapment include lateral elbow pain that radiates into the distal forearm and is aggravated by repetitive pronation and supination, most specifically resisted supination. Tenderness is noted 3–4 cm distal to the lateral epicondyles where the radial nerve crosses the radial head and penetrates the supinator muscle. PIN palsy produces an inability to extend the MCP joints of the thumb, index, long, ring, or small fingers either individually or in combination.[305,306] Additionally, there is a loss of thumb IP extension and radial abduction of the thumb.[299] Since the PIN can innervate the ECRB prior to the nerve's entrance into the radial tunnel, this muscle may not be involved in the PIN palsy. Thus, when compression within the radial tunnel is sufficient to cause paralysis but there is no palsy, the condition is termed PINS.[292]

Initial conservative intervention includes rest, activity modification, and the use of a cock-up splint. Regular gentle stretching of the wrist extensor muscles, with the elbow held in full extension is begun after a spontaneous recovery.[292]

Radial Tunnel Syndrome. RTS involves compression of the deep branch of the radial nerve. Michele and Krueger[307] have been credited with recognizing RTS as a distinct entity and gave it the name radial PS. The term RTS was introduced by Roles and Maudsley,[72] who suggested that RTS was the cause of resistant tennis-elbow pain.

The same structures implicated in PIN compression syndrome can cause RTS, although RTS is often thought of as a dynamic compression syndrome.[218] This is because compression of the nerve occurs during elbow extension, forearm pronation, and wrist flexion, which causes the ECRB and the fibrous edge of the superficial part of the supinator to tighten around the nerve. The symptoms from this compression can mimic those of tennis elbow, namely tenderness over the lateral aspect of the elbow, pain on passive stretching of the extensor muscles, and pain on resisted extension of the wrist and fingers.[72,218] Men and women are equally affected, and the compression appears to be common in the fourth to sixth decades of life.[70]

Pain, which is poorly localized over the radial aspect of the proximal forearm, is the most common primary presenting symptom in RTS. In fact, it is the only nerve compression syndrome in which the signs and symptoms are not based on the nerve distribution.[308]

Upon palpation, maximal tenderness is usually elicited over the radial tunnel, some 5 cm distal to the lateral epicondyle, anterior to the radial neck. Resisted middle finger extension,[72] which tightens the fascial origin of the ECRB, and resisted supination of the forearm with the elbow fully extended[70] should reproduce the pain at the point of maximal tenderness. Positioning the arm in elbow extension, forearm pronation, and wrist flexion produces significant compression of the radial nerve.[292]

Conservative intervention should focus on education to avoid the provocative positioning of the arm into forceful extension and supination of the wrist and forearm and should include rest, stretching, and splinting.[72,309]

If a wrist immobilization splint is used, it is fitted in 45 degrees of extension for continual wear.

Surgical intervention is reserved for patients whose symptoms are not relieved by conservative intervention.

Radial Sensory Nerve Entrapment. The term *Wartenberg's syndrome*[310] or *cheiralgia paresthetica* is used to describe a mononeuritis of the superficial radial nerve, which can become entrapped where it pierces the fascia between the brachioradialis and ECRL tendons.[291,299] Symptoms include shooting or burning pain along the posterior-radial forearm, wrist, and thumb, associated with wrist flexion and ulnar deviation.[299] These symptoms can lead the clinician to believe that the first carpometacarpal joint and/or tendons of the anatomic snuffbox are involved and that de Quervain's disease is present.

Musculocutaneous Nerve Entrapment

The brachialis is a pure elbow flexor, whereas the biceps brachii is an elbow flexor and supinator of the forearm.[45,311] With complete loss of motor function of these two muscles due to a lesion of the musculocutaneous nerve, functional elbow flexion strength can still be obtained with contraction of the brachioradialis and pronator teres.[312] The ECRL, FCU, FCR, and palmaris longus may also assist with flexing the elbow.[313] The brachioradialis has a better mechanical advantage when the elbow is flexed to 90 degrees and is more active when the forearm is in the pronated or neutral position.[313] The pronator teres can produce full elbow flexion, but this is accompanied by forearm pronation.[312,314] Thus, with a complete musculocutaneous nerve palsy, full antigravity elbow flexion can still be obtained but is strongest with the elbow flexed at 90 degrees and the forearm pronated.

Acute Compartment Syndrome

See Chapter 5.

Myofascial Pain Dysfunction

Elbow pain, when not related to the joint or to microtearing of the common flexor or extensor tendons, is commonly referred into the elbow from a number of sources, including myofascial. Even if microtearing is present, trigger points can also be present in the relevant muscles, placing a chronic strain on that tendon.

Supinator

This muscle refers pain and tenderness primarily to the lateral epicondyle of the elbow, but also to the posterior (dorsal) web space between the thumb and index finger. According to Travell and Simons,[315] each of the common sites for tennis elbow can be accounted for by trigger points in the supinator, ECRL, and triceps muscles.

Supinator pain referral is activated by playing tennis with an extended elbow, which does not allow the biceps brachii to take part in the supination required to control the head of the tennis racquet.[316]

Triceps Brachii

A trigger point in the medial head of the triceps is a common cause of lateral elbow pain from the lateral side of this muscle or of medial elbow pain from the medial side of this muscle.[316]

INTEGRATION OF PRACTICE PATTERNS 4G AND 4I: IMPAIRED JOINT MOBILITY, MOTOR FUNCTION, MUSCLE PERFORMANCE, AND RANGE OF MOTION, ASSOCIATED WITH FRACTURES AND BONY OR SOFT-TISSUE SURGICAL PROCEDURES

Radial Head Fractures

Radial head fractures and dislocations are traumatic injuries (except for the occurrence of congenital radial head dislocations), usually from a FOOSH with the force of impact transmitted up the hand through the wrist and forearm to the radial head, which is forced into the capitellum. Both of these conditions require adequate treatment to prevent disability from stiffness, deformity, posttraumatic arthritis, nerve damage, or other serious complications.[317] These fractures and dislocations may be isolated just to the radial head (and neck) and the lateral elbow (and proximal forearm), or they may be part of a combined complex fracture pattern, involving other structures of the elbow, and even the distal humerus, or forearm and wrist. Blunt or penetrating trauma rarely causes radial head injury. The wrist, especially the distal radioulnar joint, may be damaged simultaneously, and the presence of wrist pain, grinding, or swelling should be determined. The presence of bleeding, even with small puncture wounds, should alert the clinician to the possibility of open injury. Neurovascular symptoms of numbness, tingling, or loss of sensation should be identified to rule out nerve or vascular injury. The presence of severe pain should alert the clinician to the possibility of compartment syndrome.

Patients with radial head fractures and dislocations present with localized swelling, tenderness, and decreased motion. The clinician should palpate the elbow, especially the radial head, feeling for deformity, and the wrist should be examined, especially feeling for stability of the distal radioulnar joint. All three major nerves of the forearm are at risk with elbow fractures and dislocations, so the clinician should also carefully assess neurovascular function for all of the nerves of the forearm and hand.

Radial head fractures present several challenges, as the radial head is a secondary stabilizer for valgus forces at the elbow as well as a restraint against longitudinal forces along the forearm.[318] Compromise of the MCL makes the radial head a more important stabilizer of the elbow.[5,318,319] A successful outcome correlates directly with the accuracy of anatomic reduction, restoration of mechanical stability that allows early motion, and consideration of the soft tissues. Surgical options for radial head fractures or dislocations include closed reduction with casting or early motion or open reduction with internal fixation (ORIF), replacement, or resection. Open management (including internal fixation, replacement, or excision depending on the fracture) is associated with better long-term function.

In the Mason classification, the fracture is type I if it is undisplaced and is generally treated nonoperatively with a splint or a sling for 3 days, and active elbow flexion exercises being initiated immediately. The fracture is type II if a single fragment is displaced, but may still be treated nonoperatively if the displacement is minimal. A type III fracture is comminuted and usually requires operative intervention but may occasionally be treated closed with early motion if the radial head is not reconstructible.

Following immobilization, as much early mobilization as the patient can tolerate is the key to a favorable outcome. Strengthening, initially involving isometric exercises, begins at 3 weeks and progresses to concentric exercises at 5–6 weeks. Heavy resistance is not performed until after 8 weeks, or when adequate healing is demonstrated on radiographs. What follows is a postfracture or postsurgical protocol for type I fracture, or a type II or III fracture that has been stabilized with ORIF.[82,88]

Acute Phase

During the acute phase, the goals are to decrease pain and inflammation, regain full wrist and elbow range of motion, and to retard muscular atrophy. Active-assisted and active range-of-motion exercises are initiated at the elbow with the goal to regain a minimum of 15–105 degrees after two weeks. Gripping exercises using putty can be initiated in addition to isometric strengthening exercises of the elbow and wrist. Finally, concentric strengthening exercises for the wrist can be initiated.

Subacute Phase

The goals during this phase are to maintain full elbow range of motion, progress to elbow strengthening, and to gradually increase functional demands. Shoulder strengthening exercises are initiated and progressed that focus on the rotator cuff, while the range-of-motion exercises for the elbow are continued. Active-assisted range of motion and passive range of motion exercises are initiated into supination–pronation to tolerance.

Chronic Phase

The goals during this phase are to maintain full elbow range of motion, increase strength, power, and endurance, and to gradually initiate sporting activities as appropriate. Eccentric elbow flexion–extension and plyometric exercises are initiated and continued until about 12 weeks.

Fractures with radial head surface involvement of more than 30%, fracture fragment displacement, and type III characteristics require management by an orthopaedic surgeon.[171]

Monteggia Fracture

Monteggia fracture–dislocations are a particular type of radial head injury, involving a combination of a dislocation of the proximal end of the radius and a fracture of the ulna. Instead of the radial head dislocation, the radial head or neck may be fractured. These lesions typically result from a direct blow to the forearm or a FOOSH injury with the arm positioned in either hyperextension or hyperpronation. The classification of Monteggia fracture–dislocations is outlined in Table 17-11.

Although relatively rare, these fractures can present with serious problems and poor functional outcomes without proper care.[222,320] Such complications include damage to the

TABLE 17-11 Classification of Monteggia Fracture Dislocations

Type	Description	Equivalent(s)	%
Type I	Anterior dislocation of the radial head and anterior angulation of the ulna fracture	Radial head or neck fracture instead of dislocation	60
Type II	Posterior dislocation of the radial head and posterior angulation of the ulna fracture	Posterior elbow dislocation. Radial head or neck fracture instead of dislocation	105
Type III	Lateral dislocation of the radial head with proximal ulna fracture	Radial head or neck fracture instead of dislocation	20
Type IV	Anterior dislocation of the radial head and proximal shafts of both bones fractured at same level	Radial head or neck fracture instead of dislocation	5

Data from Rabin SI: *Radial Head Fractures*. Available at: http://www.emedicine.com/orthoped/topic276.htm, 2005.

posterior branch of the radial nerve, AIN, and the ulnar nerve, as well as nonunion and poor AROM.[222]

For Monteggia fracture–dislocations, best treatment includes open reduction internal fixation of the ulna diaphyseal fracture. Following the surgery, the elbow is immobilized for about 4 weeks in 90–120 degrees of elbow flexion, after which AROM exercises for elbow flexion and forearm supination are initiated. AROM into extension beyond 90 degrees begins 4–6 weeks postoperatively.

Coronoid Fracture

The coronoid forms a significant portion of the articular surface of the proximal ulna. It serves as an important attachment site for muscles and ligaments about the elbow, and is essential for elbow stability.[1] Coronoid fractures, which are most commonly seen with high-energy injuries, are classified according to the size of the fragment type[1,321]:

- Type I: Tip avulsion. These fractures are generally stable and can be treated as simple dislocations with early motion.
- Type II: involves less than 50% of the height of the coronoid. Many of these are unstable and require ORIF.
- Type III: involve more than 50% of the height of the coronoid and frequently are accompanied by instability of the elbow. ORIF or a hinged external fixator may be required to maintain reduction.

Essex-Lopresti Fractures

This type of fracture is defined as a fracture of the radial head with proximal radius migration and disruption of the distal radioulnar joint and interosseous membrane,[322] which typically results from a FOOSH injury.[323]

Gentle AROM for forearm rotation is initiated about 6 weeks after surgery and immobilization in a Muenster cast.

Panner's Disease

Panner's disease (osteochondrosis deformans or osteochondritis) is an aseptic or osteonecrosis of the epiphysis.[324] Although related to direct trauma or to changes in the circulation, the actual etiology is unknown. Panner's disease is rarely seen before the age of 5 years and after the age of 16 years, and it almost exclusively (90%) affects boys. The main presenting symptoms are pain to the lateral aspect of the elbow, swelling, and a limitation of elbow movement in a noncapsular pattern. If a displaced fragment is present, there is often a painless limitation of elbow extension, with a soft end-feel, but a hard end-feel when flexion is limited.[12]

Conservative intervention involves rest from throwing or impact-loading stress, with a short period of splint immobilization sometimes being necessary. The exercise progression is based on clinical findings and patient tolerance.

Olecranon Fracture

An olecranon process fracture is fairly common due to its subcutaneous location and is usually caused by either a high- or a low-energy injury, such as a fall backward onto the elbow or a FOOSH injury, which produces passive elbow flexion combined with a sudden powerful contraction of the triceps muscle, resulting in an avulsion fracture of the olecranon.[325,326]

The classic signs of an avulsion fracture involving the triceps is a loss of active elbow extension; a palpable gap, pain, and swelling at the fracture site; and a large hematoma developing into diffuse ecchymosis.[327]

The focus on the intervention for the nondisplaced or minimally displaced fractures is to allow restoration of the articular surfaces and maintaining triceps function, while allowing early range of motion. The elbow is immobilized in a posterior splint or elbow immobilizer, with the elbow flexed at 90 degrees. Pronation and supination are started at 2–3 days, and pain-free flexion and extension motions begin at 2 weeks. The range of motion exercises avoid full flexion for up to 2 months, and resistance exercises are avoided for up to 3 months. Protected immobilization should continue until there is evidence of union (~ 6 weeks).

All other fractures require an ORIF or excision of the bone fragments with repair of the extensor mechanism.[222,325,326,328] Rehabilitation following the surgical procedure is dependent on the extent of the surgery and the length of the immobilization, although the emphasis on regaining early motion remains the same.

Pathologic Bone Formation

Pathologic bone formation about the elbow occurs in several distinct forms, which include heterotopic ossification, myositis ossificans, periarticular calcification, and ectopic ossification. [329]

Heterotopic ossification is defined as the formation of mature lamellar bone in nonosseous tissues.

Myositis ossificans refers to heterotopic ossification that forms in inflammatory muscle. Although heterotopic ossification and myositis ossificans are radiographically and histologically similar, these processes are distinguished by their anatomic locations.[330]

Periarticular calcification refers to collections of calcium pyrophosphates within soft tissues such as the collateral ligaments or joint capsule.

The term ectopic ossification includes heterotopic ossification and myositis ossificans. Since most cases of pathologic bone formation about the elbow consist of heterotopic ossification and myositis ossificans, ectopic ossification is the most appropriate descriptive term for this process.

Ectopic ossification about the elbow can result from direct injury, neural axis trauma, burns, and genetic disorders,[331] although direct elbow trauma is the most common cause.[332] Although elbow ectopic ossification may be asymptomatic, it frequently causes severe elbow stiffness or even ankylosis, and a resultant loss of function.[85,102]

Regan and Reilly[333] outlined following three factors that predispose the elbow to posttraumatic stiffness:

- The high degree of articular congruity
- The conformity of the elbow joint
- The covering of the anterior joint capsule by the brachialis, predisposing it to posttraumatic ectopic ossification. Posttraumatic elbow ectopic ossification typically begins to form 2 weeks after trauma, surgery, burn, or neurologic insult,[333–335] resulting in localized tissue swelling and tenderness, hyperemia, and pain.

Mobilization after elbow injury often is delayed, because it is difficult to achieve rigid internal fixation of comminuted elbow fractures. Furthermore, posttraumatic elbow stiffness may occur despite early aggressive motion and prophylactic measures.

Elbow stiffness may develop 1–4 months after an initial phase of motion recovery after injury.[336] The patient's chief complaint may be pain, stiffness, instability, sensory loss, weakness, or locking. If pain is present, it is located anteriorly, in the middle third of the arm.

Limited active and passive elbow flexion and extension are characteristics of ectopic ossification formation about the elbow. However, in some patients, active and passive elbow motion may remain normal, especially in the early phase. However, even with aggressive intervention, including static and dynamic splinting and frequent active and passive ROM exercises, elbow motion may diminish. Strength testing reveals weak and painful elbow flexion and extension, and the end-feels of elbow ROM become rigid or abrupt. Once the ectopic ossification matures, usually at 3–9 months after injury, elbow ROM remains stable as long as the active and passive ROM program is continued.

Ectopic ossification about the elbow may lead to delayed nerve palsy. The ulnar nerve is most commonly affected; however, tardy median and radial palsies have also been reported.[337–339] This complication may occur several months or many years after the formation of ectopic bone.

Plain radiographs establish the diagnosis of ectopic ossification, define its location, and show its maturity. Radiographs show ectopic ossification as early as 2 weeks after injury, and joint incongruity, osteophytes, and/or malunion will also be apparent.

Nearly all patients who present with elbow stiffness and ectopic ossification should be started on an aggressive active motion program to combat the progressive loss of motion that occurs during ectopic ossification maturation. In some patients, elbow motion may improve; however, in others, loss of motion occurs and ankylosis may result. Active exercises, passive exercises, continuous passive motion, dynamic splinting, and static splinting have all been advocated, although some authors suggest that passive elbow exercises enhance elbow ectopic ossification formation and exacerbate elbow stiffness,[340] even though there is little evidence to support this belief. Until there is a prospective study comparing patients with elbow injuries treated with passive stretching with patients treated without passive stretching, the relationship between passive elbow motion and ectopic ossification formation will remain unclear. However, the passive force should be applied slowly and progressively so as not to cause any further damage to the soft tissues and thereby provoke an exacerbation.

Unless there is a contraindication, all patients are started on an active and active-assisted ROM program.

Splinting is also commonly used to restore elbow ROM. Spring-loaded hinged dynamic splints may be used to counteract flexion and extension contractures. Patients are instructed to wear these splints for six 1-hour sessions daily and while they sleep. If flexion and extension are limited, the patient is issued a dynamic flexion splint and a dynamic extension splint and instructed to alternate use of them. Turnbuckle splints also are available and are typically used for rigid contractures. This splint allows the patient to impart a static constant stretch to the soft tissues by tightening the turnbuckle.[332]

Elbow ectopic ossification can be prevented in many cases with prophylactic measures. Patients who sustain an elbow injury and have a risk factor for ectopic ossification should be treated to prevent this complication. Two forms of prophylaxis are available:

- ***Chemotherapeutic agents.*** These include NSAIDs. NSAIDs have been shown to decrease the incidence and severity of ectopic ossification about the hip. No studies exist regarding its effect on elbow ectopic ossification.
- ***Low-dose external beam radiation.*** Clinical studies showed that this modality inhibits ectopic ossification formation after total hip arthroplasty.[341,342]

PEDIATRIC PATHOLOGY

Acquired and congenital pediatric conditions of the elbow are described in Chapter 30.

Supracondylar Fracture of Humerus

This type of fracture, which occurs most commonly in children, involves the flat and flared distal metaphysis of the humerus, as a result of hyperextension or a fall on a flexed elbow. The forces are transmitted through the elbow joint to the distal humerus. The distal humeral fragment is usually posteriorly displaced (extension type). Sometimes, a "follow-through" of fragments results in a proximal fragment piercing the anterior periosteum, brachialis muscle, and possibly the brachial artery and median nerve (flexion type). If the brachial artery is pierced, the injury is potentially limb threatening.

The child typically presents with marked swelling above the elbow with an obvious deformity and ecchymosis. Because of the nature of this condition, peripheral circulation and nerve function must be assessed.

The intervention is dependent on severity. Nondisplaced fractures are immobilized in a simple sling or shoulder immobilizer, with the elbow flexed for 3 weeks, whereas displaced fractures require closed reduction and immobilization in a cast that does not constrict circulation, for 3 weeks. During the period of immobilization, the patient is closely monitored for changes in peripheral circulation. Following the period of immobilization, if the postreduction evaluation is acceptable, AROM exercises are initiated in an effort to regain full extension. Strengthening of the biceps and triceps is also addressed.

THERAPEUTIC TECHNIQUES

TECHNIQUES TO INCREASE JOINT MOBILITY

A number of techniques exist to increase joint mobility and range of motion from general techniques to very specific techniques.

Passive Accessory Mobilizations

With some slight variations, the same techniques that are used to examine the passive accessory motions of the elbow complex can be used to mobilize the joints, with the clinician varying the amplitude and the velocity of the technique (i.e., grade) of the mobilizations based on the intent of the treatment, the patient response, the stage of tissue healing, and the irritability of the joint.

Ulnohumeral

Distraction/Compression

These are general techniques that can be used to improve overall elbow motion into flexion and extension.

Medial Glide. This technique is commonly used as part of the intervention for medial epicondylitis.

Lateral Glide. This technique is commonly used as part of the intervention for lateral epicondylitis.

Radiohumeral

Anterior Glide (Fig. 17-36). This technique can be used to improve elbow flexion.

Posterior Glide (see Fig. 17-36). This technique can be used to improve elbow extension.

Distraction (Fig. 17-37). This technique is commonly used as part of the intervention for a humeroradial joint compression positional fault.

Compression (Fig. 17-37). This technique is commonly used as part of the intervention for a humeroradial joint distraction positional fault.

Proximal Radioulnar Joint

Anteromedial/Posterolateral Glide (see Fig. 17-38)

The clinician glides the radial head anteromedially (to increase supination)/posterolaterally (to increase pronation) at the proximal radioulnar joint.

Mobilizations with Movements

To Increase Motion at the Elbow and for Tennis Elbow[343,344]

The patient is positioned in supine with the involved arm on the bed and the forearm supinated. A belt is wrapped around the posterior aspect of the clinician and around the patient's forearm so that the belt edge is level with the elbow joint (Fig. 17-72). Using one hand, the clinician stabilizes the patient's humerus, while the other hand supports the patient's forearm and wrist (see Fig. 17-72). From this position, the ulna is glided laterally as the clinician gently moves their hips backward. Adjustments in the direction of the mobilization glide are made with respect to the carrying angle of the elbow. If there is no pain, the patient actively flexes or extends their elbow while the mobilization force is maintained. The active motion can be progressed to resisted wrist extension or resisted gripping performed during the mobilization.

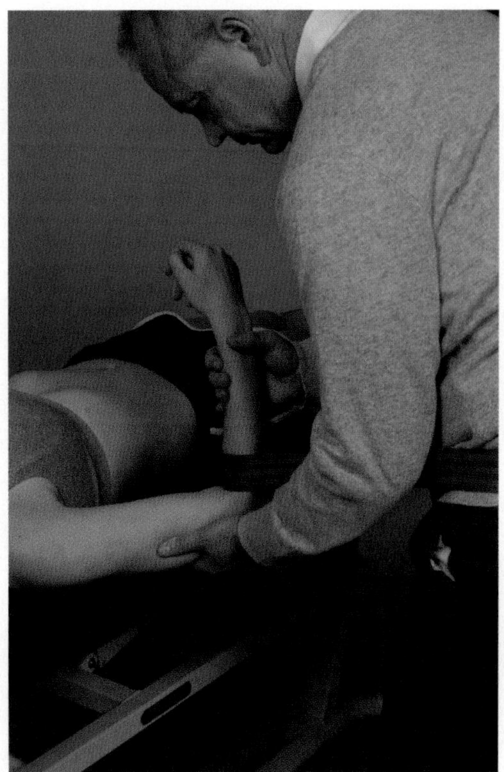

FIGURE 17-72 Mobilizations with movement to increase elbow motion.

Transverse Frictional Massage

TFM is used to treat a number of soft-tissue structures around the elbow.

Strain or Overuse of the Brachialis Muscle Belly. Although uncommon, lesions of the brachialis muscle belly are most often seen in long-distance cross-country skiers with inadequate training. In the following example, the right brachialis is treated.

The patient is positioned next to the short side of the treatment table, sitting, with the elbow in 90 degrees of flexion and the forearm resting on the table in maximal supination. The clinician sits next to the long side of the treatment table diagonally facing the patient. The clinician locates the site of the lesion by palpation. In most cases, the involved site is directly in the middle (between medial and lateral) of the muscle belly, at the level of the biceps musculotendinous junction. The clinician places the middle finger just lateral to the musculotendinous junction of the biceps (Fig. 17-73). The other hand holds the patient's forearm. The biceps musculotendinous junction is passively moved medially, as far as possible, with the thumb. After exerting pressure posteriorly, the clinician performs TFM in a lateral direction.

Strain or Overuse of the Muscle Belly—Musculotendinous Junction of the Biceps. Lesions of the biceps muscle belly or musculotendinous junction can occur as a result of carrying a heavy object or from forceful throwing activities. In the following example, the right biceps tendon is treated.

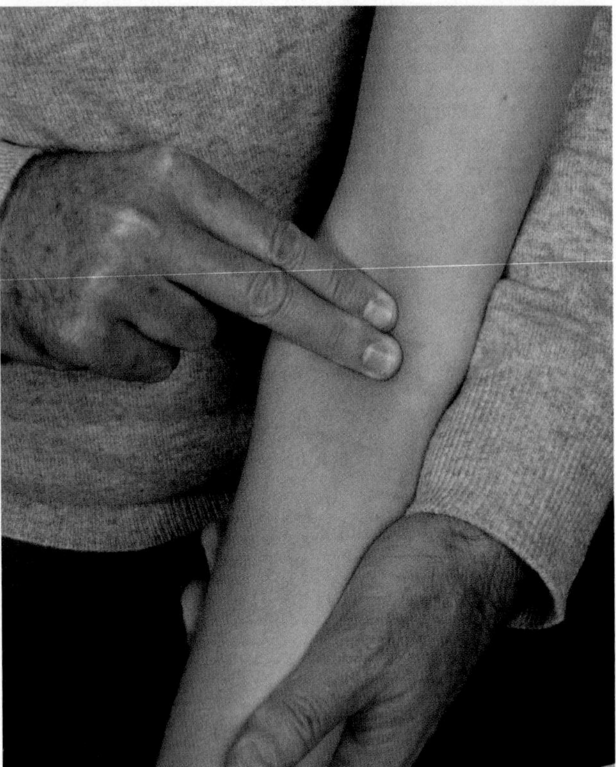

FIGURE 17-73 TFM to brachialis muscle belly.

The patient is positioned next to the short side of the treatment table, sitting, with the elbow in 90 degrees of flexion and the forearm resting on the table in supination. The clinician sits next to the long side of the treatment table diagonally facing the patient. The clinician locates the site of the lesion by palpation.

This is done by means of a pinch grip between the clinician's thumb and index finger of the right hand, which grasps the posterior aspect of the muscle belly, while the other hand fixes the patient's forearm. The transverse friction occurs through a "flat" pinching together of the thumb and index finger. Simultaneous extension of the wrist can be added to pull the muscle belly fibers transversely through the fingers.

The biceps musculotendinous junction is treated in much the same way.

Insertion Tendinopathy of the Triceps. Transverse friction is indicated for lesions in the musculotendinous junction (rare), the tendon, or the teno-osseous insertion of the triceps. Insertion tendinopathy of the triceps can occur as a result of chronic abuse or macrotrauma.

The patient is positioned prone on the treatment table, with the upper arm resting on the table and the forearm hanging over the edge of the table. The clinician sits next to the patient at the patient's involved side. The exact site of the lesion is confirmed by palpation. With one hand, the clinician holds the patient's elbow in slightly more than 90 degrees of flexion. The fingers of the other hand are placed at the site of the lesion (Fig. 17-74).

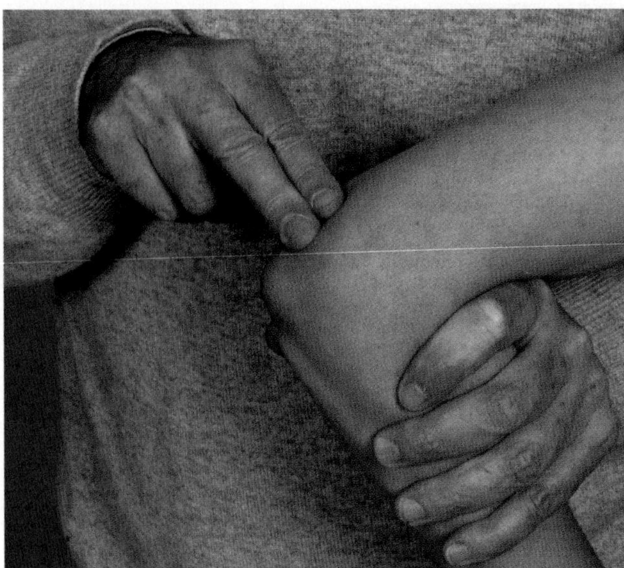

FIGURE 17-74 TFM to triceps.

Static stretching of the triceps is combined with the transverse friction.

Insertion Tendinopathy at the Medial Humeral Epicondyle (Golfer's elbow). The patient sits with the involved arm elevated sideways to just below the horizontal. The elbow is extended and the forearm, supinated. The clinician sits on a chair or stool next to the patient. If the right elbow is to be treated, the clinician stabilizes the patient's forearm and holds the elbow in slight flexion. To determine the most painful site of the lesion, the tip of the index finger carefully palpates the anterior plateau of the medial humeral epicondyle (Fig. 17-75). During the friction, the joint position of the finger does not change. The friction motion consists of minimal wrist extension and an even smaller amount of adduction of the arm.

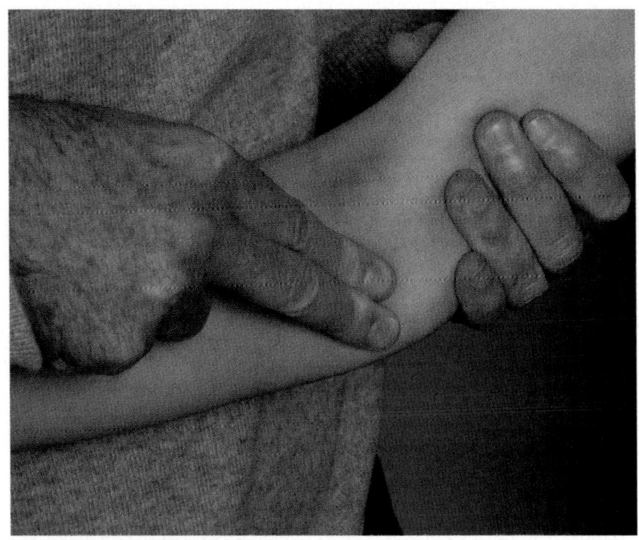

FIGURE 17-75 TFM of medial epicondyle.

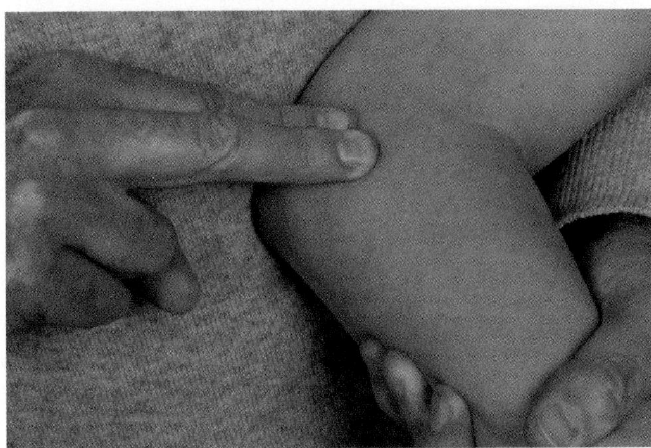

FIGURE 17-76 TFM at radial head for ECRB.

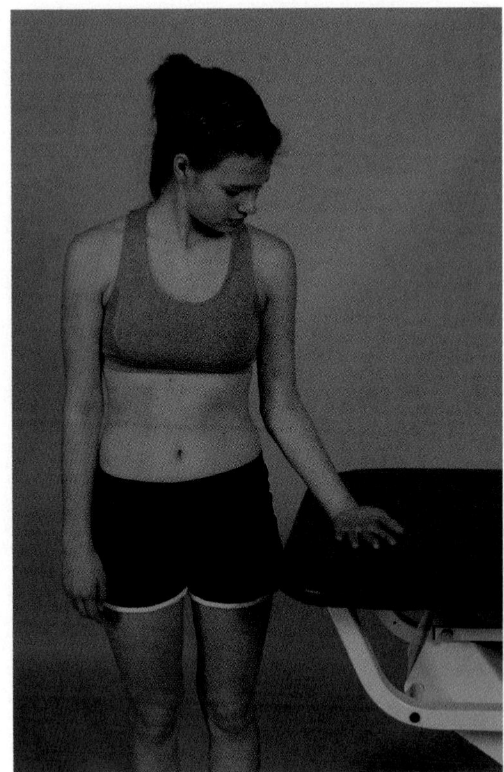

FIGURE 17-77 Biceps stretch.

Tendinitis of the Extensor Carpi Radialis Brevis. The patient is positioned, sitting, next to the short end of the treatment table. The upper arm is positioned in 45 degrees of abduction, with the elbow in approximately 80 degrees of flexion and the forearm in pronation. The clinician sits diagonally facing the patient. The tendon of the ECRB brevis is located. In the pronated forearm, the ECRB tendon runs over the radial head (Fig. 17-76). In most cases, the tendon felt is, in fact, the common tendon of the ECRB and the extensor digitorum. Sometimes, two tendons are palpated; the medial one is the ECRB. TFM is performed by moving the finger in a medial-to-lateral direction over the tendon.

Techniques to Increase Soft-Tissue Extensibility

An increase in flexibility is achieved through a routine stretching program that may be instituted early in the course of treatment, with emphasis on stretching the entire hand, forearm, and shoulder complex. Stretching should follow the application of local heat such as that afforded by a hot pack, ultrasound or transverse friction massage. Patients should be taught how to perform these techniques on themselves at the earliest opportunity.

In each of the following techniques, the stretch is maintained for approximately 30 seconds.

Biceps

The patient stands by a table and places the back of the hand on the tabletop with the forearm supinated. The elbow is gradually extended and the forearm is moved into further supination (Fig. 17-77).

Elbow and Wrist Flexors

The patient is positioned in standing. A stretching strap is secured to the patient's foot and grasped by the hand of the involved side. Maintaining the forearm in a supinated position and the elbow extended as far as possible, the patient raises their arm out to the side (Fig. 17-51) until a stretch it felt.

Wrist and Finger Extensors

Stretching of the ECRB is always combined with stretching of the ECRL and extensor digitorum and is indicated in all types of tennis and golfer's elbow.

The patient is positioned in sitting. The upper arm is held horizontally, with the elbow flexed 90 degrees, the forearm pronated, and the wrist flexed. The patient uses the left hand to grasp their right hand and positions the wrist in maximal flexion and ulnar deviation, with the forearm in maximal pronation (Fig. 17-78). The elbow is brought very slowly into extension.

Stretch for Golfer's Elbow

The function of the long wrist flexors is flexion of the elbow, pronation of the forearm, and flexion of the wrist. The patient sits on a chair, with the involved arm elevated approximately 60 degrees. The elbow is slightly flexed, the forearm supinated, and the wrist extended (Fig. 17-52). The patient brings the wrist and fingers into as much extension as possible using the uninvolved hand (see Fig. 17-52). While holding the wrist in maximal extension, the clinician very slowly extends the patient's elbow. As soon as pain or muscle guarding occurs, the motion is stopped and the elbow is brought slightly back into more flexion. If the pain disappears after a few seconds, the elbow can be brought further into extension.

Weight-Bearing Wrist Flexor Stretch

This stretch is performed by asking the patient to position the hand palm side down on a table and to position the elbow in slight flexion, the wrist into maximal ulnar

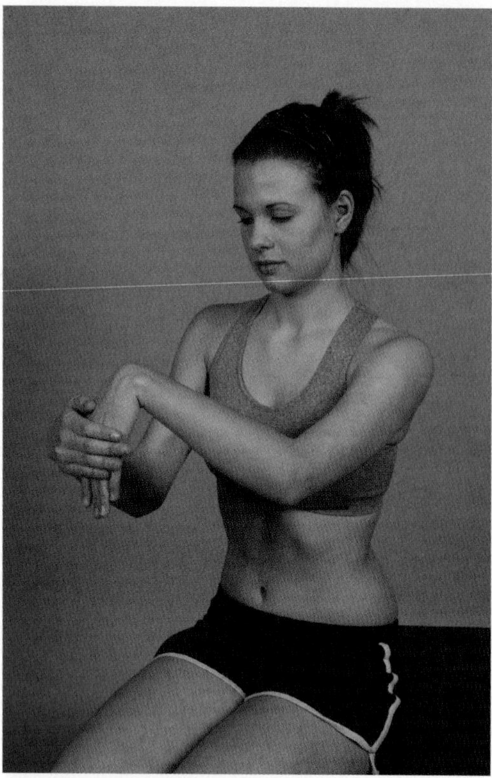

FIGURE 17-78 Wrist and finger extensor stretch.

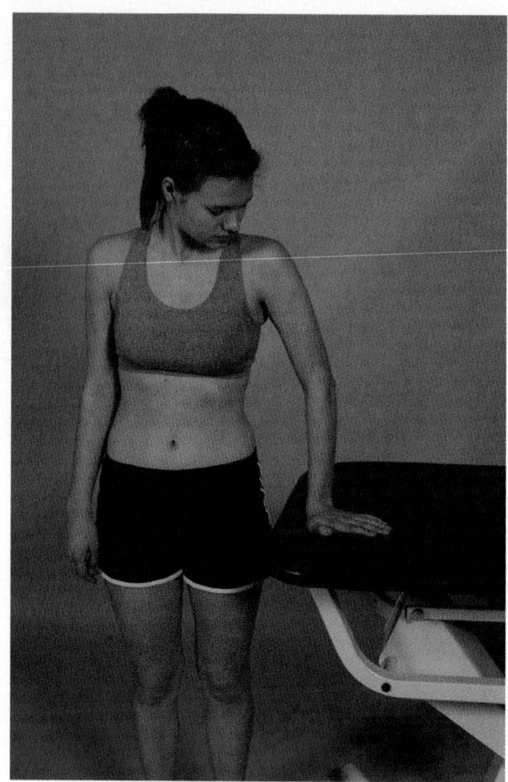

FIGURE 17-79 Weight-bearing wrist flexor stretch.

deviation and extension, and the forearm in maximal pronation (Fig. 17-79). Being careful to avoid pain and muscle splinting, the patient slowly straightens the elbow. The stretch should be held for approximately 40 seconds. At this point, the patient can gently pull the fingers up from the table to stretch the flexor muscles of the palm. Against very slight resistance (performed by the other hand), the arm is then brought back to the original position. This stretching procedure is repeated six times before repeating the entire procedure on the uninvolved side.

High-Velocity, Low-Amplitude Thrusting

Mills' Manipulation[12]

This technique is designed to break adhesions of the common extensor tendon and let the orbicular ligament slip back to its normal position. The Mills' manipulation is used instead of slowly stretching the tissues during the last few degrees of maximal elbow extension.

This manipulation is indicated only for certain patients, namely, those

- who demonstrate full active and passive elbow extension with a normal end-feel;
- whose elbow demonstrates only a slight limitation of motion with a myofascial end-feel.

Prior to the manipulation, transverse frictions should be applied to the site in order to soften the scar.

The patient is positioned in sitting, with the clinician standing behind the patient's shoulder (see Fig. 17-42). The patient's wrist is flexed. Maintaining the position of the patient's wrist, the clinician extends the elbow. The Mills' maneuver involves a forcible extension of the elbow, while simultaneous digital pressure is exerted over the point of maximum tenderness. If the wrist flexion is not maintained, the force will be through the elbow joint. Mills stressed the need to elicit an audible click during the procedure, although in practice many normal elbows can be made to click by the same maneuver,[345] indicating that the click is probably coincidental.

A modification to the patient position can be used for this manipulation. The patient is positioned in supine, with their arm off the edge of the table. The clinician adjusts the table height so that the patient's elbow joint can be rested on their thigh, while the clinician's foot is in contact with the floor. The patient's arm is then placed in slight shoulder extension and full internal rotation (palm down). In this position, the various tendons can be tested as to their level of involvement by having each one contract. The involved tendon is then softened up using transverse friction before the manipulation is applied using the aforementioned positions. The patient's elbow is then slightly raised off the clinician's thigh and then dropped quickly back onto the thigh.

Following the manipulation, exercises to stretch the scar should be carried out.

CASE STUDY

LATERAL ELBOW PAIN

HISTORY

History of Current Condition

A 43-year-old female patient presents with complaints of left elbow pain, which she reports having for about a year. The patient describes the onset of elbow pain as gradual and attributes it to her work as an electronics assembler, where she spends the day pulling out plugs. Over time, the pain has worsened to the point where it hurts all of the time. Although the patient has tried a course of anti-inflammatories, they were discontinued due to an adverse reaction. The patient has been placed on light duty at work, with a lifting restriction of 10 lb.

Past History of Current Condition

No past history of left elbow pain.

Past Medical and Surgical History

Unremarkable.

Medications

None.

Living Environment

Lives in a two-story house.

Occupational, Employment, and School

Assembly line worker. High school education.

Functional Status and Activity Level

The patient's goals were to decrease pain with activities of daily living and to be able to return to work without pain.

Health Status (Self-Report)

In general good health, but pain interferes with tasks at home and at work.

Questions

1. What is the most common diagnosis characterized by lateral elbow pain?
2. What can a history of gradual onset tell the clinician?
3. What can a history of repetitive activity tell the clinician?
4. What findings do you expect to note in the physical examination in terms of palpation, resistive tests, and special tests?
5. What additional questions would you ask to help rule out referral of pain from the cervical spine or shoulder?
6. List the various diagnoses that could present with these signs and symptoms, and the tests you would use to rule out each one.
7. Does this presentation and history warrant an upper quarter scanning examination? Why or why not?

CASE STUDY

MEDIAL ELBOW PAIN

HISTORY

History of Current Condition

A 23-year-old apprentice carpenter was seen in the clinic with complaints of right elbow pain, which he reported having for the last few months. The patient described the onset of elbow pain as gradual and attributed it to his work, where he spends most of the day using carpentry tools. Over time, the pain had worsened to the point where it hurt all of the time. The patient went to see his physician who prescribed a course of anti-inflammatory medications and physical therapy and placed the patient on light duty at work.

Past History of Current Condition

No past history of elbow pain.

Past Medical and Surgical History

Unremarkable.

Medications

Ibuprofen, 800 mg a day.

Functional Status and Activity Level

The patient's goals were to decrease pain with activities of daily living and recreational sports and to be able to return to work without pain.

Health Status (Self-Report)

In general good health, but pain interferes with tasks at home and at work.

Questions

1. What structure(s) do you suspect to be at fault with complaints of medial elbow pain?
2. What is the probable mechanism of injury for this patient?
3. What type of activities would you expect to exacerbate this condition?
4. What additional questions would you ask?
5. List the various diagnoses that could present with these signs and symptoms and the tests you would use to rule out each one.

REVIEW QUESTIONS*

1. True/False: The primary restraint to valgus stress at the elbow is bony congruity.
2. What is the maximal close-packed position of the humeroulnar joint?
3. Which muscles are involved with forearm pronation?
4. In which direction do most elbow dislocations occur?
5. Which muscle could flex the elbow if the three major elbow flexors were *not* available?
   A. The pronator teres
   B. The FPL
   C. The supinator
   D. The pronator quadratus

*Additional questions to test your understanding of this chapter can be found in the Online Learning Center for *Orthopaedic Assessment, Evaluation, and Intervention* at www.duttononline.net.

REFERENCES

1. Aviles SA, Wilk KE, Safran MR: Elbow. In: Magee DJ, Zachazewski JE, Quillen WS, eds. *Pathology and Intervention in Musculoskeletal Rehabilitation*. St. Louis, MI: Saunders, 2009:161–212.
2. Safran MR, Baillargeon D: Soft-tissue stabilizers of the elbow. *J Shoulder Elbow Surg* 14:179S–185S, 2005.
3. Morrey BF, An KN: Articular and ligamentous contributions to the stability of the elbow joint. *Am J Sports Med* 11:315–319, 1983.
4. Sobel J, Nirschl RP: Elbow injuries. In: Zachazewski JE, Magee DJ, Quillen WS, eds. *Athletic Injuries and Rehabilitation*. Philadelphia, PA: WB Saunders, 1996:543–583.
5. An KN, Morrey BF: Biomechanics of the Elbow. In: Morrey BF, ed. *The Elbow and Its Disorders*, 2nd ed. Philadelphia, PA: WB Saunders Co, 1993:53–73.
6. O'Driscoll SW, Morrey BF, An K-N: Intraarticular pressure and capacity of the elbow. *J Arthrosc Rel Surg* 6:100–103, 1990.
7. Wilk KE, Arrigo C, Andrews JR: Rehabilitation of the elbow in the throwing athlete. *J Orthop Sports Phys Ther* 17:305–317, 1993.
8. Neumann DA: Elbow and forearm complex. In: Neumann DA, ed. *Kinesiology of the Musculoskeletal System: Foundations for Physical Rehabilitation*. St. Louis, MO: Mosby, 2002:133–171.
9. Potter HP: The obliquity of the arm of the female in extension. The relation of the forearm with the upper arm in flexion. *J Anat Physiol* 29:488–491, 1895.
10. Atkinson WB, Elftman H: The carrying angle of the human arm as a secondary sex character. *Anat Rec* 91:42–49, 1945.
11. An K-N, Morrey BF, Chao EY: The carrying angle of the human elbow joint. *J Orthop Res* 1:369–378, 1984.
12. Cyriax J: *Textbook of Orthopaedic Medicine, Diagnosis of Soft Tissue Lesions*, 8th ed. London: Bailliere Tindall, 1982.
13. Pfaeffle HJ, Fischer KJ, Manson TT, et al: Role of the forearm interosseous ligament: is it more than just longitudinal load transfer? *J Hand Surg [Am]* 25:683–688, 2000.
14. Morrey BF, An KN: Functional anatomy of the ligaments of the elbow. *Clin Orthop* 201:84–90, 1985.
15. Ochi N, Ogura T, Hashizume H, et al: Anatomic relation between the medial collateral ligament of the elbow and the humero-ulnar joint axis. *J Shoulder Elbow Surg* 8:6–10, 1999.
16. O'Driscoll SW, Jaloszynski R, Morrey BF, et al: Origin of the medial ulnar collateral ligament. *J Hand Surg Am* 17A:164–168, 1992.
17. Floris S, Olsen BS, Dalstra M, et al: The medial collateral ligament of the elbow joint: Anatomy and kinematics. *J Shoulder Elbow Surg* 7:345–351, 1998.
18. Neill-Cage DJ, Abrams RA, Callahan JJ, et al: Soft tissue attachments of the ulnar coronoid process: An anatomic study with radiographic correlation. *Clin Orthop* 320:154–158, 1995.
19. Cohen MS, Bruno RJ: The Collateral Ligaments of the Elbow: Anatomy and. Clinical Correlation. *Clin Orthop Relat Res* 1:123–130, 2001.
20. Hotchkiss RN, Weiland AJ: Valgus stability of the elbow. *J Orthop Res* 5:372–377, 1987.
21. Morrey BF, Tanaka S, An KN: Valgus stability of the elbow: A definition of primary and secondary constraints. *Clin Orthop* 265:187–195, 1991.
22. Schwab GH, Bennett JB, Woods GW, et al: Biomechanics of elbow instability: The role of the medial collateral ligament. *Clin Orthop* 146:42–52, 1980.
23. Morrey BF: Applied anatomy and biomechanics of the elbow joint. *Inst Course Lect* 35:59–68, 1986.
24. Sojbjerg JO, Ovesen J, Nielsen S: Experimental elbow instability after transection of the medial collateral ligament. *Clin Orthop Relat Res* 218:186–190, 1987.
25. Jobe FW, Kvitne RS: Elbow instability in the athlete. *Inst Course Lect* 40:17–23, 1991.
26. Callaway GH, Field LD, Deng XH, et al: Biomechanical evaluation of the medial collateral ligament of the elbow. *J Bone Joint Surg* 79A:1223–1231, 1997.
27. Fuss FK: The ulnar collateral ligament of the human elbow joint. Anatomy, function and biomechanics. *J Anat* 175:203–212, 1991.
28. Regan WD, Korinek SL, Morrey BF, et al: Biomechanical study of ligaments around the elbow joint. *Clin Orthop* 271:170–179, 1991.
29. Guterieriez L: A contribution to the study of limiting factors of elbow extension. *Acta Anat* 56:145, 1964.
30. Chen FS, Rokito AS, Jobe FW: Medial elbow problems in the overhead-throwing athlete. *J Am Acad Orthop Surg* 9:99–113, 2001.
31. Kuroda S, Sakamaki K: Ulnar collateral ligament tears of the elbow joint. *Clin Orthop* 208:266–271, 1986.
32. Berg EE, DeHoll D: Radiography of the medial elbow ligaments. *J Shoulder Elbow Surg* 6:528–533, 1997.
33. Josefsson PO, Johnell O, Wendeberg B: Ligamentous injuries in dislocations of the elbow joint. *Clin Orthop* 221:221–225, 1987.
34. Cohen MS, Hastings H: Diagnosis and surgical management of the acute elbow dislocation. *J Am Acad Orthop Surg* 6:16–23, 1998.
35. Cohen MS, Hastings H: Rotatory instability of the elbow: The role of the lateral stabilizers. *J Bone Joint Surg* 79A:225–233, 1977.
36. O'Driscoll SW, Bell DF, Morrey BF: Posterolateral rotatory instability of the elbow. *J Bone Joint Surg Am* 73:440–446, 1991.
37. Ryan J: Elbow. In: Wadsworth C, ed. *Current Concepts of Orthopedic Physical Therapy - Home Study Course*. La Crosse, WI: Orthopaedic Section, APTA, 2001.
38. Jobe FW, Nuber G: Throwing injuries of the elbow. *Clin Sports Med* 5:621, 1986.
39. Schuind F, Garcia-Elias M, Cooney WP, et al: Flexor tendon forces: In vivo measurements. *J Hand Surg* 17A:291–298, 1992.
40. Schuind FA, Goldschmidt D, Bastin C, et al: A biomechanical study of the ulnar nerve at the elbow. *J Hand Surg [Br]* 20:623–627, 1995.

41. Jackson-Manfield P, Neumann DA: Structure and function of the elbow and forearm complex. In: Jackson-Manfield P, Neumann DA, eds. *Essentials of Kinesiology for the Physical Therapist Assistant*. St. Louis, MO: Mosby Elsevier, 2009:91–122.
42. Pauly JE, Rushing JL, Schering LE: An electromyographic study of some muscles crossing the elbow joint. *Anat Rec* 1:42, 1967.
43. Basmajian JV, Latif A: Integrated actions and functions of the chief flexors of the elbow: a detailed electromyographic analysis. *J Bone Joint Surg* 39A:1106–1118, 1957.
44. Funk DA, An KA, Morrey BF, et al: Electromyographic analysis of muscles across the elbow joint. *J Orthop Res* 5:529–538, 1987.
45. Basmajian JV, Deluca CJ: *Muscles Alive*, 5th ed. Baltimore, MD: Williams & Wilkins, 1985:268–269.
46. Thepaut-Mathieu C, Maton B: The flexor function of the muscle pronator teres in man: a quantitative electromyographic study. *Eur J Appl Physiol* 54:116–121, 1985.
47. An KN, Hui FC, Morrey BF, et al: Muscles across the elbow joint: a biomechanical analysis. *J Biomech* 14:659–669, 1981.
48. Davidson PA, Pink M, Perry J, et al: Functional anatomy of the flexor pronator muscle group in relation to the medial collateral ligament of the elbow. *Am J Sports Med* 23:245–250, 1995.
49. Basmajian JV, Deluca CJ: *Muscles Alive: Their Functions Revealed by Electromyography*. Baltimore, MD: Williams & Wilkins, 1985.
50. Reid DC: *Functional Anatomy and Joint Mobilization*, 2nd ed. Edmonton, AB: University of Alberta Press, 1975.
51. Hirasawa Y, Sawamura H, Sakakida K: Entrapment neuropathy due to bilateral epitrochlearis muscles: A case report. *J Hand Surg Am* 4:181–184, 1979.
52. Feindel W, Stratford J: The role of the cubital tunnel in tardy ulnar palsy. *Can J Surg* 1:287, 1958.
53. Apfelberg DB, Larson SJ: Dynamic anatomy of the ulnar nerve at the elbow. *Plast Reconstr Surg* 51:76–81, 1973.
54. Idler RS: General principles of patient evaluation and nonoperative management of cubital syndrome. *Hand Clin* 12:397–403, 1996.
55. Khoo D, Carmichael SW, Spinner RJ: Ulnar nerve anatomy and compression. *Orthop Clin North Am* 27:317–338, 1996.
56. O'Driscoll SW, Horii E, Carmichael SE, et al: The cubital tunnel and ulnar neuropathy. *J Bone Joint Surg* 73B:613–617, 1991.
57. Bozentka DJ: Cubital tunnel syndrome pathophysiology. *Clin Orthop Relat Res* 351:90–94, 1998.
58. Vanderpool DW, Chalmers J, Lamb DW, et al: Peripheral compression lesions of the ulnar nerve. *J Bone Joint Surg* 50B:792–803, 1968.
59. Folberg CR, Weiss APC, Akelman E: Cubital tunnel syndrome Part I: Presentation and diagnosis. *Orthop Rev* 23:136–144, 1994.
60. Conway JE, Jobe FW, Glousman RE, et al: Medial instability of the elbow in throwing athletes: Treatment by repair or reconstruction of the ulnar collateral ligament. *J Bone Joint Surg* 74A:67–83, 1992.
61. Gabel GT, Morrey BF: Operative treatment of medial epicondylitis: Influence of concomitant ulnar neuropathy at the elbow. *J Bone Joint Surg* 77:1065–1069, 1995.
62. Lee DG: "Tennis elbow": A manual therapist's perspective. *J Orthop Sports Phys Ther* 8:134–142, 1986.
63. Spinner M, Linscheid RL: Nerve entrapment syndromes. In: Morrey BF, ed. *The Elbow and Its Disorders*. Philadelphia, PA: Saunders, 1985:691–712.
64. Amadio PC, Beckenbaugh RD: Entrapment of the ulnar nerve by the deep flexor-pronator aponeurosis. *J Hand Surg Am* 11A:83–87, 1986.
65. Gabel GT, Amadio PC: Reoperation for failed decompression of the ulnar nerve in the region of the elbow. *J Bone Joint Surg* 72A:213–219, 1990.
66. Smith RV, Fisher RG: Struthers ligament: A source of median nerve compression above the elbow. *J Neurosurg* 38:778–779, 1973.
67. Barnum M, Mastey RD, Weiss APC, et al: Radial tunnel syndrome. *Hand Clin* 12:679–689, 1996.
68. Hrayama T, Takemitsu Y: Isolated paralysis of the descending branch of the posterior interosseous nerve. *J Bone Joint Surg* 70A:1402–1403, 1988.
69. Spinner M: *Injuries to the Major Branches of the Peripheral Nerves of the Forearm*. Philadelphia, PA: WB Saunders, 1978.
70. Lister GD, Belsoe RB, Kleinert HE: The radial tunnel syndrome. *J Hand Surg Am* 4:52–59, 1979.
71. Carr D, Davis P: Distal posterior interosseous nerve syndrome. *J Hand Surg Am* 10:873–878, 1985.
72. Roles NC, Maudsley RH: Radial tunnel syndrome: Resistant tennis elbow as a nerve entrapment. *J Bone Joint Surg Br* 54B:499–508, 1972.
73. Morrey BF, Chao EY: Passive motion of the elbow joint. *J Bone Joint Surg Am* 58:501–508, 1976.
74. Kibler BW: Clinical biomechanics of the elbow in tennis: implications for evaluation and diagnosis. *Med Sci Sports Exerc* 26:1203–1206, 1994.
75. Cummings GS: Comparison of muscle to other soft tissue in limiting elbow extension. *J Orthop Sports Phys Ther* 5:170, 1984.
76. Kapandji IA: *The Physiology of the Joints, Upper Limb*. New York, NY: Churchill Livingstone, 1991.
77. Hammer WI: *Functional Soft Tissue Examination and Treatment By Manual Methods*. Gaithersburg, MD: Aspen, 1991.
78. Kleinman WB, Graham TJ: The distal radioulnar joint capsule: clinical anatomy and role in posttraumatic limitation of forearm rotation. *J Hand Surg [Am]* 23:588–599., 1998.
79. Bert JM, Linscheid RL, McElfresh EC: Rotatory contracture of the forearm. *J Bone Joint Surg Am* 62:1163–1168, 1980.
80. Goel VK, Singh D, Bijlani V: Contact areas in human elbow joints. *J Biomech Eng* 104:169–175, 1982.
81. van Riet RP, Van Glabbeek F, Baumfeld JA, et al: The effect of the orientation of the radial head on the kinematics of the ulnohumeral joint and force transmission through the radiocapitellar joint. *Clin Biomech (Bristol, Avon)* 21:554–559. 2006.
82. Morrey BF, An KN, Stormont TJ: Force transmission through the radial head. *J Bone Joint Surg Am* 70:250–256, 1988.
83. Kibler BW, Press JM: Rehabilitation of the elbow. In: Kibler BW, Herring JA, Press JM, eds. *Functional Rehabilitation of Sports and Musculoskeletal Injuries*. Gaithersburg, MD: Aspen, 1998:171–182.
84. Watrous BG, Ho G Jr: Elbow pain. *Prim Care* 15:725–735, 1988.
85. Morrey BF, An KN, Chao EYS: Functional Evaluation of the Elbow. In: Morrey BF, ed. *The Elbow and Its Disorders*, 2nd ed. Philadelphia, PA: WB Saunders, 1993:86–97.
86. Polley HF, Hunder GG: *Physical Examination of the Joints*. Philadelphia, PA: WB Saunders, 1978:81–89.
87. Hochholzer T, Keinath C: Soweit die hande greifen (4). Wenn die arme knarren. *Rotpunkt* 2:62–65, 1991.
88. Wilk KE, Andrews JR: Elbow Injuries. In: Brotzman SB, Wilk KE, eds. *Clinical Orthopaedic Rehabilitation*. Philadelphia, PA: Mosby, 2003:85–123.
89. Winkel D, Matthijs O, Phelps V: *Examination of the Elbow, Diagnosis and Treatment of the Upper Extremities*. Gaithersburg , MD: Aspen, 1997:207–233.
90. Bollen SR: Soft tissue injury in extreme rock climbers. *Br J Sports Med* 22:145–147, 1988.
91. Hochholzer T, Keinath C: Soweit die hande greifen (3). Wenn die finger kribbeln. *Rotpunkt* 1:46–49, 1991.
92. Katz WA: *Rheumatic Diseases, Diagnosis and Management*. Philadelphia, PA: JB Lippincott, 1977.
93. American Academy of Orthopaedic Surgeons: *Orthopedic Knowledge Update 4: Home Study Syllabus*. Rosemont, IL: The Academy, 1992.
94. Kiser DM: Physiological and biomechanical factors for understanding repetitive motion injuries. *Semin Occup Med* 2:11–17, 1987.
95. Lewit K: *Manipulative Therapy in Rehabilitation of the Motor System*, 3rd ed. London: Butterworths, 1999.
96. Pecina M, Krmpotic-Nemanic J, Markiewitz A: *Tunnel Syndromes*. Boca Raton, FL: CRC, 1991.
97. Vennix MJ, Wertsch JJ: Entrapment neuropathies about the elbow. *J Back Musculoskel Rehabil* 4:31–43, 1994.
98. Keller K, Corbett J, Nichols D: Repetitive strain injury in computer keyboard users: pathomechanics and treatment principles in individual and group intervention. *J Hand Ther* 11:9–26, 1998.
99. Anderson M, Tichenor CJ: A patient with de Quervain's tenosynovitis: A case report using an Australian approach to manual therapy. *Phys Ther* 74:314–326, 1994.
100. Jobe FW, Ciccotti MG: Lateral and medial epicondylitis of the elbow. *J Am Acad Orthop Surg* 2:1–8, 1994.
101. Armstrong AD, MacDermid JC, Chinchalkar S, et al: Reliability of range-of-motion measurement in the elbow and forearm. *J Shoulder Elbow Surg* 7:573–580, 1998.
102. Morrey BF, Askew LJ, Chao EYS: A biomechanical study of normal functional elbow motion. *J Bone Joint Surg* 63A:872–877, 1981.
103. Bell S: Examination of the elbow. *Aust Fam Physician* 17:391–392, 1988.
104. Madsen OR: Torque, total work, power, torque acceleration energy and acceleration time assessed on a dynamometer: reliability of knee and elbow extensor and flexor strength measurements. *Eur J Appl Physiol Occup Physiol* 74:206–210, 1996.

105. Agre JC, Magness JL, Hull SZ, et al: Strength testing with a portable dynamometer: reliability for upper and lower extremities. *Arch Phys Med Rehabil.* 68:454–458, 1987.
106. Bohannon RW: Make tests and break tests of elbow flexor muscle strength. *Phys Ther* 68:193–194., 1988.
107. Kaltenborn FM: *Manual Mobilization of the Extremity Joints: Basic Examination and Treatment Techniques*, 4th ed. Oslo: Olaf Norlis Bokhandel, Universitetsgaten, 1989.
108. Maitland G: *Peripheral Manipulation*, 3rd ed. London: Butterworth, 1991.
109. O'Driscoll SW, Bell DF, Morrey BF: Posterolateral rotatory instability of the elbow. *J Bone Joint Surg* 73A:440–446, 1991.
110. Buehler MJ, Thayer DT: The elbow flexion test: A clinical test for cubital tunnel syndrome. *Clin Orthop* 233:213–216, 1988.
111. Novak CB, Lee GW, Mackinnon SE, et al: Provocative testing for cubital tunnel syndrome. *J Hand Surg Am* 19:817–820, 1994.
112. Booth FW: Physiologic and biochemical effects of immobilization on muscle. *Clin Orthop Relat Res* 219:15–21, 1987.
113. Eiff MP, Smith AT, Smith GE: Early mobilization versus immobilization in the treatment of lateral ankle sprains. *Am J Sports Med* 22:83–88, 1994.
114. Akeson WH, Amiel D, Mechanic GL, et al: Collagen cross-linking alterations in the joint contractures: changes in the reducible cross-links in periarticular connective tissue after 9 weeks immobilization. *Connect Tissue Res* 5:15, 1977.
115. Akeson WH, Amiel D, Abel MF, et al: Effects of immobilization on joints. *Clin Orthop* 219:28–37, 1987.
116. Akeson WH, Amiel D, Woo SL-Y: Immobility effects on synovial joints: The pathomechanics of joint contracture. *Biorheology* 17:95–110, 1980.
117. Woo SL-Y, Matthews J, Akeson WH, et al: Connective tissue response to immobility: A correlative study of biochemical and biomechanical measurements of normal and immobilized rabbit knee. *Arthritis Rheum* 18:257–264, 1975.
118. Kraushaar BS, Nirschl RP: Tendinosis of the elbow (tennis elbow). Clinical features and findings of histological, immunohistochemical, and electron microscopy studies. *J Bone Joint Surg (AM)* 81:259–278, 1999.
119. Nirschl RP, Sobel J: *Arm Care. A Complete Guide to Prevention and Treatment of Tennis Elbow.* Arlington, VA: Medical Sports, 1996.
120. Coutts RD: Continuous passive motion in the rehabilitation of the total knee patient. It's role and effect. *Orthop Rev* 15:27, 1986.
121. Dehne E, Tory R: Treatment of joint injuries by immediate mobilization based upon the spiral adaption concept. *Clin Orthop* 77:218–232, 1971.
122. Haggmark T, Eriksson E: Cylinder or mobile cast brace after knee ligament surgery. *Am J Sports Med* 7:48–56, 1979.
123. Noyes FR, Mangine RE, Barber S: Early knee motion after open and arthroscopic anterior cruciate ligament reconstruction. *Am J Sports Med* 15:149–160, 1987.
124. Andrews JR, Frank W: Valgus extension overload in the pitching elbow. In: Andrews JR, Zarins B, Carson WG, eds. *Injuries to the Throwing Arm.* Philadelphia, PA: WB Saunders, 1985:250–257.
125. Kottke FJ: Therapeutic exercise to maintain mobility. In: Kottke FJ, Stillwell GK, Lehman JF, eds. *Krusen's Handbook of Physical Medicine and Rehabilitation.* Baltimore, MD: WB Saunders, 1982:389–402.
126. Warren CG, Lehmann JF, Koblanski JN: Elongation of rat tail: Effect of load and temperature. *Arch Phys Med Rehabil* 52:465–474, 1971.
127. Kibler WB: Concepts in exercise rehabilitation of athletic injury. In: Leadbetter WB, Buckwalter JA, Gordon SL, eds. *Sports-Induced Inflammation: Clinical and Basic Science Concepts.* Park Ridge, IL: American Academy of Orthopaedic Surgeons, 1990:759–769.
128. Kibler WB, Chandler TJ, Pace BK: Principles of rehabilitation after chronic tendon injuries. *Clin Sports Med* 11:661–671, 1992.
129. Kibler WB: *Clinical Implications of Exercise: Injury and Performance, Instructional Course Lectures, American Academy of Orthopaedic Surgeons.* Rosemont, IL: American Academy of Orthopaedic Surgeons, 1994:17–24.
130. Leadbetter WB: Corticosteroid injection therapy in sports injuries. In: Leadbetter WB, Buckwalter JA, Gordon SL, eds. *Sports-Induced Inflammation: Clinical and Basic Science Concepts.* Park Ridge, IL: American Academy of Orthopaedic Surgeons, 1990:527–545.
131. Woo SL-Y, Tkach LV: The cellular and matrix response of ligaments and tendons to mechanical injury. In: Leadbetter WB, Buckwalter JA, Gordon SL, eds. *Sports-Induced Inflammation: Clinical and Basic Science Concepts.* Park Ridge, IL: American Academy of Orthopaedic Surgeons, 1990:189–202.
132. Novacheck TF: Running injuries: a biomechanical approach. *J Bone Joint Surg* 80-A:1220–1233, 1998.
133. Freund HJ, Budingen HJ: The relationship between speed and amplitude of the fastest voluntary contractions of human arm muscles. *Exp Brain Res* 35:407–418, 1978.
134. Marsden CD, Obeso JA, Rothwell JC: The function of the antagonist muscle during fast limb movements in man. *J Physiol* 335:1–13, 1983.
135. Wierzbicka MM, Wiegner AW, Shahani BT: Role of agonist and antagonist muscles in fast arm movements in man. *Exp Brain Res* 63:331–340, 1986.
136. Wilk KE, Voight ML, Keirns MA, et al: Stretch-shortening drills for the upper extremities: theory and clinical application. *J Orthop Sports Phys Ther* 17:225–239, 1993.
137. Woodward AH, Bianco AJ: Osteochondritis dissecans of the elbow. *Clin Orthop* 110:35–41, 1975.
138. Field LD, Savoie FH: Common elbow injuries in sport. *Sports Med* 26:193–205, 1998.
139. Kandemir U, Fu FH, McMahon PJ: Elbow injuries. *Curr Opin Rheumatol* 14:160–167, 2002.
140. Fryette HH: *Principles of Osteopathic Technique.* Colorado: Academy of Osteopathy, 1980.
141. Azar FM, Andrews JR, Wilk KE, et al: Operative treatment of ulnar collateral ligament injuries of the elbow in athletes. *Am J Sports Med* 28:16–23, 2000.
142. Jobe FW, Stark H, Lombardo SJ: Reconstruction of the ulnar collateral ligament in athletes. *J Bone Joint Surg* 68A:1158–1163, 1986.
143. Jobe FW, Tibone JE, Moynes DR, et al: An EMG analysis of the shoulder in pitching and throwing: A preliminary report. *Am J Sports Med* 11:3–5, 1983.
144. Jobe FW, Radovich M, Tibone JE, et al: An EMG analysis of pitching. A second report. *Am J Sports Med* 12:218–220, 1984.
145. Froimson AI, Anouchi YS, Seitz WH, et al: Ulnar nerve decompression with medial epicondylectomy for neuropathy at the elbow. *Clin Orthop* 265:200–206, 1991.
146. Heithoff SJ, Millender LH, Nalebuff EA, et al: Medial epicondylectomy for the treatment of ulnar nerve compression at the elbow. *J Hand Surg Am* 15A:22–29, 1990.
147. Glousman RE: Ulnar nerve problems in the athlete's elbow. *Clin Sports Med* 9:365–370, 1990.
148. Ciccotti MG, Jobe FW: Medial collateral ligament instability and ulnar neuritis in the athlete's elbow. *Instr Course Lect* 48:383–391, 1999.
149. Glousman R, Jobe FW, Tibone JE: Dynamic EMG analysis of the throwing shoulder with glenohumeral instability. *J Bone Joint Surg* 70:220–226, 1988.
150. Sisto DJ, Jobe FW, Moynes DR, et al: An electromyographic analysis of the elbow in pitching. *Am J Sports Med* 15:260–263, 1987.
151. Smith GR, Altchek DW, Pagnani MJ, et al: A muscle splitting approach to the ulnar collateral ligament of the elbow: Neuroanatomy and operative technique. *Am J Sports Med* 24:575–580, 1996.
152. Wright PE: Flexor and extensor tendon injuries. In: Crenshaw AH, ed. *Campbell's Operative Orthopaedics*, 8th ed. St Louis, MO: Mosby-Year Book, 1992:3003–3054.
153. Nestor BJ, O'Driscoll SW, Morrey BF: Ligamentous reconstruction for posterolateral rotatory instability of the elbow. *J Bone Joint Surg* 74A:1235–1241, 1992.
154. O'Driscoll SW, Morrey BF, Korinek S, et al: Elbow subluxation and dislocation: a spectrum of instability. *Clin Orthop* 280:186–197, 1992.
155. Sojbjerg JO, Helmig P, Kjaersgaard-Andersen P: Dislocation of the elbow: an experimental study of the ligamentous injuries. *Orthopedics* 12:461–463, 1989.
156. Morrey BF: Reoperation for failed surgical treatment of refractory lateral epicondylitis. *J Shoulder Elbow Surg* 1:47–49, 1992.
157. O'Driscoll SW: Classification and Evaluation of Recurrent Instability of the Elbow. *Clin Orthop Relat Res* 370:34–43, 2000.
158. O'Driscoll SW: Classification and spectrum of elbow instability: recurrent instability. In: Morrey BF, ed. *The Elbow and Its Disorders.* Philadelphia, PA: WB Saunders Company, 1993:453–463.
159. O'Driscoll SW: Elbow instability. *Hand Clin* 10:405–415, 1994.
160. Josefsson PO, Gentz CF, Johnell O, et al: Surgical vs. non-surgical treatment of ligamentous injuries following dislocation of the elbow. *J Bone Joint Surg* 69A:605–608, 1987.
161. Torchia M, DiGiovine N: Anterior dislocation of the elbow in an arm wrestler. *J Shoulder Elbow Surg* 7:539–541, 1998.

162. Doria A, Gil E, Delgado E, et al: Recurrent dislocation of the elbow. *Int Orthop* 14:41–55, 1990.
163. Durig M, Muller W, Ruedi TP, et al: The operative treatment of elbow dislocation in the adult. *J Bone Joint Surg* 61A:239–244, 1979.
164. Josefsson PO, Gentz CF, Johnell O, et al: Dislocations of the elbow and intraarticular fractures. *Clin Orthop* 246:126–130, 1989.
165. Hotchkiss RN: Fractures and Dislocations of the elbow. In: Rockwood CA, Green DP, Bucholz RW, et al, eds. *Fractures in Adults*. Philadelphia, PA: Lippincott Raven, 1996:980–981.
166. Wilson FD, Andrews JR, Blackburn TA, et al: Valgus extension overload in the pitching elbow. *Am J Sports Med* 11:83–88, 1983.
167. Azar FM, Wilk KE: Nonoperative treatment of the elbow in throwers. *Oper Tech Sports Med* 4:91–99, 1996.
168. Pappas AM, Zawacki RM, Sullivan TJ: Biomechanics of baseball pitching: a preliminary report. *Am J Sports Med* 13:216–222, 1985.
169. Burkhart SS, Morgan CD, Kibler WB: Shoulder injuries in overhead athletes: the "dead arm" revisited. *Clin Sports Med* 19:125–158, 2000.
170. Reilly J, Nicholas JA: The chronically inflamed bursa. *Clin Sports Med* 6:345–370, 1987.
171. Onieal M-E: Common wrist and elbow injuries in primary care. *Lippincotts Prim Care Pract* 3:441–450, 1999.
172. Shell D, Perkins R, Cosgarea A: Septic olecranon bursitis: recognition and treatment. *J Am Board Fam Pract* 8:217–220, 1995.
173. Reid DC, Kushner S: The elbow region. In: Donatelli RA, Wooden MJ, eds. *Orthopaedic Physical Therapy*, 2nd ed. New York, NY: Churchill Livingstone, 1994:203–232.
174. O'Connor FG, Wilder RP, Sobel JR: Overuse injuries of the elbow. *J Back Musculoskel Rehabil* 4:17–30, 1994.
175. Hempel K, Schwencke K: About avulsions of the distal insertion of the biceps brachii tendon. *Arch Orthop Unfallchir* 79:313–319, 1974.
176. McReynolds IS: Avulsion of the insertion of the biceps brachii tendon and its surgical treatment. *J Bone Joint Surg* 45A:1780–1781, 1963.
177. D'Alessandro DF, Shields CL Jr, Tibone JE, et al: Repair of distal biceps tendon ruptures in athletes. *Am J Sports Med* 21:114–119, 1993.
178. Morrey BF, Askew LJ, An KN, et al: Rupture of the distal tendon of the biceps brachii: a biomechanical study. *J Bone Joint Surg* 67A:418–421, 1985.
179. Farrrar EL, Lippert FG: Avulsion of triceps tendon. *Clin Orthop* 161:242–246, 1981.
180. Nirschl RP: Elbow tendinosis: tennis elbow. *Clin Sports Med* 11:851–870, 1992.
181. Runge F: Zur genese und behandlung des schreibekrampfs. *Berliner klinische Wochenschr* :245–246, 1873.
182. Morris H: The rider's sprain. *Lancet* 29:133–134, 1882.
183. Major HP: Lawn-tennis elbow. *BMJ* 15:557, 1883.
184. Brandesky W: Über den Epicondylusschmerz. *Dtsch Zeitschr Chir* 219:246–255, 1929.
185. Nirschl RP: Muscle and tendon trauma: tennis elbow. In: Morrey BF, ed. *The Elbow and Its Disorders*, 2nd ed. Philadelphia, PA: WB Saunders, 1993:681–703.
186. Fischer AW: Üeber die Epicondylus: und Styloidesneuralgie, ihre Pathogenese und zweckmäßige therapie. *Arch Klin Chir* 125:749–775, 1923.
187. Fischer E: Zur Röntgenbehandlung der Epikondylitis und verwandter Krankheitszustände. *Münch Med Wochenschr* 83:149, 1936.
188. Wiesner H: Die Epicondylitis humeri lateralis und ihre Behandlung unter besonderer Berücksichtigung der Hohmannschen Operation. *Zentralbl Chir* 77:787–791, 1952.
189. Cyriax JH: The pathology and treatment of tennis elbow. *J Bone Joint Surg* 18:921–940, 1936.
190. Coonrad RW, Hooper WR: Tennis elbow: its course, natural history, conservative and surgical management. *J Bone Joint Surg* 55-A:1177–1182, 1973.
191. Goldie I: Epicondylitis lateralis humeri (epicondylalgia or tennis elbow). *Acta Chir Scand Suppl* 6:339, 1964.
192. Nirschl RP: Tennis elbow tendinosis: pathoanatomy, nonsurgical and surgical management. In: Gordon SL, Blair SJ, Fine LJ, eds. *Repetitive Motion Disorders of the Upper Extremity*. Rosemont, IL: American Academy of Orthopaedic Surgeons, 1995:467–479.
193. Regan W, Wold LE, Coonrad R, et al: Microscopic histopathology of chronic refractory lateral epicondylitis. *Am J Sports Med* 20:746–749, 1992.
194. Nirschl RP, Pettrone FA: Tennis elbow. *J Bone Joint Surg [Am]* 61-A:832–839, 1979.
195. Greenbaum B, Itamura J, Vangsness CT, et al: Extensor carpi radialis brevis. An anatomical analysis of its origin. *J Bone Joint Surg [Br]* 81:926–929, 1999.
196. Vulliet H: Die Epicondylitis humeri. *Zentralbl Chir* 40:1311–1312, 1910.
197. Franke F: Ueber Epicondylitis humeri. *Dtsch Med Wochenschr* 36:13, 1910.
198. Elmslie RC: Tennis elbow. *Proc Royal Soc Med* 23(Part 1):328, 1929.
199. Osgood RB: Radiohumeral bursitis, epicondylitis, epicondylalgia(tennis elbow): a personal experience. *Arch Surg* 4:420–433, 1922.
200. Gruber W: *Monographie der Bursae Mucosae Cubitales*. St Petersburg: Mém. de l'Acad. Imp. d. Science de St Petersburg, 1866.
201. Schmitt J: Bursitis calcarea am Epicondylus externus humeri: ein beitrag zur Pathogenese der epicondylitis. *Arch Orthop UnfallChir* 19:215–221, 1921.
202. Crawford HD: Discussion to epicondylitis humeri (Hansson). *N.Y State J Med* 43:32–33, 1943.
203. Swensen L: Tennis elbow. *J Mich State Med Soc* 48:997, 1949.
204. Neuman JH, Goodfellow JW: Fibrillation of head of radius as one cause of tennis elbow. *BMJ* 2:328–330, 1975.
205. Preiser G: Ueber 'Epicondylitis humeri'. *Dtsch Med Wochenschr* 36:712, 1910.
206. Mills PG: The treatment of 'tennis elbow'. *BMJ* 1:12–13, 1928.
207. Bosworth DM: The role of the orbicular ligament in tennis elbow. *J Bone Joint Surg Am* 37A:527–533, 1955.
208. Trethowan WH: Tennis elbow. *BMJ* 2:1218, 1929.
209. Trethowan WH: Minor injuries of the elbow joint. *BMJ* 2:1109, 1929.
210. Ogilvie WH: Tennis elbow. *Proc Royal Soc Med* 14:319, 1929.
211. Bell Allen JC: Epicondylitis: traumatic radio-humeral synovitis. *Med J Aust* 1:273–274, 1944.
212. Moore M: Radiohumeral synovitis, a cause of persistent elbow pain. *Surg Clin North Am* 33:1363–1371, 1953.
213. Murley AHG: Tennis elbow: treated with hydrocortisone acetate. *Lancet* 2:223–225, 1954.
214. Paul NW: Radio-humeral bursitis—Is it traumatic? Analysis and report of 314 cases. *Ind Med Surg* 26:383–390, 1957.
215. Winkworth CE: Lawn-tennis elbow. *BMJ* 6:708, 1883.
216. Kaplan EB: Treatment of tennis elbow (epicondylitis) by denervation. *J Bone Joint Surg Am* 41A:147–151, 1959.
217. O'Sullivan S: Tennis-elbow. *BMJ* 8:1168, 1883.
218. Moss SH, Switzer HE: Radial tunnel syndrome: a spectrum of clinical speculations. *J Hand Surg* 8:414–418, 1983.
219. Morrison DL: Tennis elbow and radial tunnel syndrome: differential diagnosis and treatment. *J Am Osteopath Assoc* 80:823–826, 1981.
220. Landelius ESK: Tennisarmbåge eller epicondylalgi. *Nord Med* 10:1176–1177, 1941.
221. Bosworth DM: Surgical treatment of tennis elbow: a followup study. *J Bone Joint Surg* 47A:1533–1536, 1965.
222. Crenshaw AH: Shoulder and elbow injuries. In: Crenshaw AH, ed. *Campbell's Operative Orthopaedics*, 8th ed. St Louis: Mosby-Year Book Inc., 1992.
223. Wright A, Thurnwald P, O'Callaghan J, et al: Hyperalgesia in tennis elbow patients. *J Musculoske Pain* 2:83–96, 1994.
224. Gunn C, Milbrandt W: Tennis elbow and the cervical spine. *Can Med Assoc J* 114:803–809, 1976.
225. Rompe JD, Riedel C, Betz U, et al: Chronic lateral epicondylitis of the elbow: a prospective study of low-energy shockwave therapy and low-energy shockwave therapy plus manual therapy of the cervical spine. *Arch Phys Med Rehab* 82:578–582, 2001.
226. Maitland G: *Vertebral Manipulation*. Sydney: Butterworth, 1986.
227. Curwin S, Stanish WD: *Tendinitis, Its Etiology and Treatment*. Lexington, MA: Collamore Press, 1984.
228. Leadbetter WB: Cell-matrix response in tendon injury. *Clin Sports Med* 11:533–578, 1992.
229. Nirschl RP: Patterns of failed tendon healing in tendon injury. In: Leadbetter WB, Buckwalter JA, Gordon SL, eds. *Sports-Induced Inflammation: Clinical and Basic Science Concepts*. Park Ridge, IL: American Academy of Orthopaedic Surgeons, 1990:609–618.
230. Teitz CC, Garrett WE Jr, Miniaci A, et al: Tendon problems in athletic individuals. *J Bone Joint Surg* 79-A:138–152, 1997.
231. Woo SL-Y, Gomez MA, Woo YK, et al: Mechanical properties of tendons and ligaments. II. The relationships of immobilization and exercise on tissue remodeling. *Biorheology* 19:397–408, 1982.
232. Woo SL-Y, An K-N, Arnoczky SP, et al: Anatomy, biology, and biomechanics of tendon, ligament, and meniscus. In: Simon SR, ed.

Orthopaedic Basic Science. Rosemont, IL: American Academy of Orthopaedic Surgeons, 1994:45–87.
233. Nirschl RP: Prevention and treatment of elbow and shoulder injuries in the tennis player. *Clin Sports Med* 7:289–308, 1988.
234. Nirschl RP: Mesenchymal syndrome. *Virginia Med Monthly* 96:659–662, 1969.
235. Claud NL: Tennis-arm. *Le Progrès Médical* 16:273–277, 1902.
236. Rosenburg G: Tennisellenbogen und Muskelriß. *Med Klin* 21:771–773, 1925.
237. Heald CB: *Injuries and Sport: A General Guide for the Practitioner*. London: Humphrey Milford and Oxford University Press, 1931.
238. von Goeldel W: Beitrag zum Wesen und der Behandlung der Epikondylitis. *Münch Med Wochenschr* 67:1147–1148, 1920.
239. Bernhardt M: Ueber eine wenig bekannte Form der Beschäftigungsneuralgie. *Neurolog Centralbl* 15:13–17, 1896.
240. Friedlander HL, Reid RL, Cape RF: Tennis elbow. *Clin Orthop* 51:109–116, 1967.
241. Foley AE: Tennis elbow. *Am Fam Physician* 48:281–288, 1993.
242. Labelle H, Guibert R, Joncas J, et al: Lack of scientific evidence for the treatment of lateral epicondylitis of the elbow: an attempted meta-analysis. *J Bone Joint Surg* 74B:646–651, 1992.
243. Ernst E: Conservative therapy for tennis elbow. *Br J Clin Pract* 46:55–57, 1992.
244. Binder A, Hodge G, Greenwood AM, et al: Is therapeutic ultrasound effective in treating soft tissue lesions? *Br Med J (Clin Res Ed)* 290:512–514, 1985.
245. Lundeberg T, Abrahamsson P, Haker E: A comparative study of continuous ultrasound, placebo ultrasound and rest in epicondylalgia. *Scand J Rehabil* 20:99–101, 1988.
246. Struijs PA, Damen PJ, Bakker EW, et al: Manipulation of the wrist for management of lateral epicondylitis: a randomized pilot study. *Phys Ther Rev* 83:608–616, 2003.
247. Drechsler WI, Knarr JF, Snyder-Mackler L: A comparison of two treatment regimens for lateral epicondylitis: a randomized trial of clinical interventions. *J Sport Rehabil* 6:226–234, 1997.
248. Vicenzino B, Collins D, Wright A: The initial effects of a cervical spine manipulative physiotherapy treatment on the pain and dysfunction of lateral epicondylalgia. *Pain* 68:69–74, 1996.
249. Cleland J, Whitman JM, Fritz J: Effectiveness of manual physical therapy to the cervical spine in the management of lateral epicondylalgia: a retrospective analysis. *J Orthop Sports Phys Ther* 34:713–724, 2004.
250. Cleland JA, Flynn TW, Palmer JA: Incorporation of manual therapy directed at the cervicothoracic spine in patients with lateral epicondylalgia: a pilot clinical trial. *J Man Manip Ther* 13:143–151, 2005.
251. Bisset L, Beller E, Jull G, et al: Mobilisation with movement and exercise, corticosteroid injection, or wait and see for tennis elbow: randomised trial. *BMJ* 29:29, 2006.
252. Struijs PA, Kerkhoffs GM, Assendelft WJ, et al: Conservative treatment of lateral epicondylitis: brace versus physical therapy or a combination of both-a randomized clinical trial. *Am J Sports Med* 32:462–469, 2004.
253. Snyder-Mackler L, Epler M: Effect of standard and Aircast tennis elbow bands on integrated electromyography of forearm extensor musculature proximal to the bands. *Am J Sports Med* 17:278–281, 1989.
254. Froimson A: Treatment of tennis elbow with forearm support. *J Bone Joint Surg* 43:100–103, 1961.
255. Ilfeld FW, Field SM: Treatment of tennis elbow: use of special brace. *JAMA* 195:67–71, 1966.
256. Groppel J, Nirschl RP: A biomechanical and electromyographical analysis of the effects of counter force braces on the tennis player. *Am J Sports Med* 14:195–200, 1986.
257. Chiumento AB, Bauer JA, Fiolkowski P: A comparison of the dampening properties of tennis elbow braces. *Med Sci Sports Exerc* 29:123, 1997.
258. Gellman H: Tennis elbow (lateral epicondylitis). *Orthop Clin North Am* 23:75–79, 1992.
259. Marlin T: Treatment of 'tennis elbow': with some observations on joint manipulation. *Lancet* 1:509–511, 1930.
260. Bryce A: A case of 'tennis elbow' treated by luminous heat. *Br J Actinother Physiother* 5:55, 1930.
261. Kininmonth DA: (Discussion on manipulation.) Tennis elbow. *Ann Phys Med* 1:144, 1953.
262. Johnson EW: Tennis elbow. Misconceptions and widespread mythology. *Am J Phys Med Rehabil* 79:113, 2000.
263. Hennig EM, Rosenbaum D, Milani TL: Transfer of tennis racket vibrations onto the human forearm. *Med Sci Sports Exerc* 24:1134–1138, 1992.
264. Legwold G: Tennis elbow: joint resolution by conservative treatment and improved technique. *Phys Sportsmed* 12:168, 1984.
265. Liu YK: Mechanical analysis of racquet and ball during impact. *Med Sci Sports Exerc* 15:388, 1983.
266. Hatze H: The effectiveness of grip bands in reducing racquet vibration transfer and slipping. *Med Sci Sports Exerc* 24:226–229, 1992.
267. Freeland DE, de Gribble MG: Hydrocortisone in tennis-elbow. *Lancet* 2:225, 1954.
268. Quin CE, Binks FA: Tennis elbow (Epicondylalgia externa): Treatment with hydrocortisone. *Lancet* 2:221–222, 1954.
269. Clarke AK, Woodland J: Comparison of two steroid preparations to treat tennis elbow using the hypospray. *Rheumatol Rehabil* 14:47–49, 1975.
270. Day BH, Govindasamy N, Patnaik R: Corticosteroid injections in the treatment of tennis elbow. *Practitioner* 220:459–462, 1978.
271. Hughes GR, Currey HL: Hypospray treatment of tennis elbow. *Ann Rheum Dis* 28:58–62, 1969.
272. Kraushaar BS, Nirschl RP: Pearls: handshake lends epicondylitis cues. *Phys Sportsmed* 24:15, 1996.
273. Krischek O, Hopf C, Nafe B, et al: Shock-wave therapy for tennis and golfer's elbow–1 year follow-up. *Arch Orthop Trauma Surg* 119:62–66, 1999.
274. Glousman RE, Barron J, Jobe FW, et al: An electromyographic analysis of the elbow in normal and injured pitchers with medial collateral ligament insufficiency. *Am J Sports Med* 20:311–317, 1992.
275. Bauer M, Jonsson K, Jesefsson PO, et al: Osteochondritis dissecans of the elbow: a long-term follow-up study. *Clin Orthop* 284:156–162, 1992.
276. Balasubramaniam P, Prathap K: The effect of injection of hydrocortisone into rabbit calcaneal tendons. *J Bone Joint Surg* 54:729–736, 1972.
277. Baumgard SH, Schwartz DR: Percutaneous release of the epicondylar muscles for humeral epicondylitis. *Am J Sports Med* 10:233–238, 1982.
278. Barry NN, McGuire JL: Overuse syndromes in adult athletes. *Rheum Dis Clin North Am* 22:515–530, 1996.
279. Bennett JB: Articular injuries in the athlete. In: Morrey BF, ed. *The Elbow and its Disorders*, 2nd ed. Philadelphia, PA: WB Saunders, 1993:803–831.
280. Nirschl RP: Tennis injuries. In: Nicholas JA, Herschman EB, eds. *The Upper Extremity in Sports Medicine*. St. Louis, MO: Mosby, 1990:827–842.
281. Nirschl RP: Soft tissue injuries about the elbow. *Clin Sports Med*. 5:637–652, 1986.
282. Lundborg G: Surgical treatment for ulnar nerve entrapment at the elbow. *J Hand Surg Am* 17B:245–247, 1992.
283. Wilgis EF, Murphy R: The significance of longitudinal excursion in peripheral nerves. *Hand Clin* 2:761–766, 1986.
284. Dellon AL: Musculotendinous variations about the medial humeral epicondyle. *J Hand Surg Am* 11B:175–181, 1986.
285. Macnicol MF: The results of operation for ulnar neuritis. *J Bone Joint Surg* 61B:159–164, 1979.
286. Piligian G, Herbert R, Hearns M, et al: Evaluation and management of chronic work-related musculoskeletal disorders of the distal upper extremity. *Am J Ind Med* 37:75–93, 2000.
287. Preston D, Shapiro B: *Electromyography and Neuromuscular Disorders. Clinical Electrophysiologic Correlations*. Boston, MA: Butterworth-Heinemann, 1998.
288. Terry RJ: A study of the supracondyloid process in the living. *Am J Phys Anthropol* 4:129–139, 1921.
289. Gross PT, Jones HR: Proximal median neuropathies: Electromyographic and clinical correlation. *Muscle Nerve* 15:390–395, 1992.
290. Symeonides PP: The humerus supracondylar process syndrome. *Clin Orthop* 82:141–143, 1972.
291. Anto C, Aradhya P: Clinical diagnosis of peripheral nerve compression in the upper extremities. *Orthop Clin North Am* 27:227–245, 1996.
292. Lubahn JD, Cermak MB: Uncommon nerve compression syndromes of the upper extremity. *J Am Acad Orthop Surg* 6:378–386, 1998.
293. Werner CO, Rosen I, Thorngren KG: Clinical and neurophysiological characteristics of the pronator syndrome. *Clin Orthop* 197:231–236, 1985.
294. Gainor BJ: The pronator compression test revisited. A forgotten physical sign. *Orthop Rev* 19:888–892, 1990.
295. Mangini V: Flexor pollicis longus: Its morphology and clinical significance. *J Bone Joint Surg* 42A:467–470, 1960.
296. Spinner M: The anterior interosseous nerve syndrome with special attention to its variations. *J Bone Joint Surg* 52A:84–94, 1970.

297. Nakano KK, Lundergran C, Okihiro MM: Anterior interosseous nerve syndromes: Diagnostic methods and alternative treatments. *Arch Neurol* 34:477–480, 1977.
298. Lee MJ, LaStayo PC: Pronator syndrome and other nerve compressions that mimic carpal tunnel syndrome. *J Orthop Sports Phys Ther*. 34:601–609, 2004.
299. Plate A-M, Green SM: Compressive radial neuropathies. *AAOS Instr Course Lect* 49:295–304, 2000.
300. Manske PR: Compression of the radial nerve by the triceps muscle. *J Bone Joint Surg* 59A:835–836, 1977.
301. Wright PE II, Jobe MT: Peripheral nerve injuries. In: Canale ST, Daugherty K, Jones L, eds. *Campbell's Operative Orthopaedics*, 9th ed. St Louis, MO: Mosby Year Book, 1998:3827–3894.
302. Sharrard WJW: Posterior interosseous neuritis. *J Bone Joint Surg* 48B:777–780, 1966.
303. Thompson WAL, Kopell HP: Peripheral entrapment neuropathies of the upper extremity. *N Engl J Med* 260:1261–1265, 1959.
304. Derkash RS, Niebauer JJ: Entrapment of the posterior interosseous nerve by a fibrous band in the dorsal edge of the supinator muscle and erosion of a groove in the proximal radius. *J Hand Surg Am* 6:524–526, 1981.
305. Steichen JB, Christensen AW: Posterior interosseous nerve compression syndrome. In: Gelberman RH, ed. *Operative Nerve Repair and Reconstruction*. Philadelphia, PA: JB Lippincott, 1991:1005–1022.
306. Hirayama T, Takemitsu Y: Isolated paralysis of the posterior interosseous nerve: Report of a case. *J Bone Joint Surg* 70A:1402–1403, 1988.
307. Michele AA, Krueger FJ: Lateral epicondylitis of the elbow treated by fasciotomy. *Surgery* 39:277–284, 1956.
308. Verhaar J, Spaans F: Radial tunnel syndrome: An investigation of compression neuropathy as a possible cause. *J Bone Joint Surg* 73: 539–544, 1991.
309. Eaton CJ, Lister GD: Radial nerve compression. *Hand Clin* 8:345–357, 1992.
310. Wartenberg R: Cheiralgia paresthetica (isolierte neuritis des ramus superficialis nervi radialis). *Ztschr Ges Neurol Psychiatr* 141:145–155, 1932.
311. Sunderland S: The musculocutaneous nerve. In: Sunderland S, ed. *Nerves and Nerve Injuries*, 2nd ed. Edinburgh: Churchill Livingstone, 1978:796–801.
312. Sunderland S: Voluntary movements and the deceptive action of muscles in peripheral nerve lesions. *Aust N Z J Surg* 13:160–183, 1944.
313. Kendall FP, McCreary EK, Provance PG: *Muscles: Testing and Function*. Baltimore, MD: Williams & Wilkins, 1993.
314. Bartosh RA, Dugdale TW, Nielen R: Isolated musculocutaneous nerve injury complicating closed fracture of the clavicle: A case report. *Am J Sports Med* 20:356–359, 1992.
315. Travell JG, Simons DG: *Myofascial Pain and Dysfunction - The Trigger Point Manual*. Baltimore, MD: Williams & Wilkins, 1983.
316. Smolders JJ: Myofascial pain and dysfunction syndromes. In: Hammer WI, ed. *Functional Soft Tissue Examination and Treatment by Manual Methods - The Extremities*. Gaithersburg, MD: Aspen, 1991:215–234.
317. Rabin SI: *Radial Head Fractures*. Available at: http://www.emedicine.com/orthoped/topic276.htm, 2005.
318. Hotchkiss RN: Displaced fractures of the radial head: internal fixation or excision. *J Am Acad Orthop Surg* 5:1–10, 1997.
319. King GJW, Morrey BF, An K-N: Stabilizers of the elbow. *J Shoulder Elbow Surg* 2:165–170, 1993.
320. Bado JL: The Monteggia lesion. *Clin Orthop* 50:71, 1967.
321. Regan W, Morrey B: Fractures of the coronoid process of the ulna. *J Bone Joint Surg Am* 71:1348–1354, 1989.
322. Bowers WH: The distal radioulnar joint. In: Green DP, Hotchkiss RN, eds. *Operative Hand Surgery*, 3rd ed. New York, NY: Churchill Livingstone, 1993:995.
323. Morgan WJ, Breen TF: Complex fractures of the forearm. *Hand Clin* 10:375, 1994.
324. Panner HJ: A peculiar affection of the capitellum humeri resembling Calve-Perthes' disease of the hip. *Acta Radiol* 10:234, 1929.
325. Rettig AC, Waugh TR, Evanski PM: Fracture of the olecranon: a problem of management. *J Trauma* 19:23–28, 1979.
326. Horne JG, Tanzer TL: Olecranon fractures: a review of 100 cases. *J Trauma* 21:469–472, 1981.
327. Bach BR, Warren RF, Wickiewicz TL: Triceps rupture. A case report and literature review. *Am J Sports Med* 15:285–289, 1987.
328. O'Driscoll SW: Technique for unstable olecranon fracture-subluxations. *Oper Tech Orthop* 4:49–53, 1994.
329. Viola RW, Hastings H II: Treatment of ectopic ossification about the elbow. *Clin Orthop Relat Res* 370:65–86, 2000.
330. Ackerman LV: Extra-osseous localized non-neoplastic bone and cartilage formation (so-called myositis ossificans). *J Bone Joint Surg* 40A:279–298, 1958.
331. Connor JM, Evans DA: Fibrodysplasia ossificans progressiva: The clinical features and natural history of 34 patients. *J Bone Joint Surg* 64B:76–83, 1982.
332. Green DP, McCoy H: Turnbuckle orthotic correction of elbow-flexion contractures after acute injuries. *J Bone Joint Surg* 61A:1092–1095, 1979.
333. Regan WD, Reilly CD: Distraction arthroplasty of the elbow. *Hand Clin* 9:719–728, 1993.
334. Hastings H: Elbow Contractures and Ossification. In: Peimer CA, ed. *Surgery of the Hand and Upper Extremity*. New York, NY: McGraw-Hill, 1996:507–534.
335. Hastings H, Graham TJ: The classification and treatment of heterotopic ossification about the elbow and forearm. *Hand Clin* 10:417–437, 1994.
336. Thompson HC, Garcia A: Myositis ossificans: Aftermath of elbow injuries. *Clin Orthop* 50:129–134, 1967.
337. Garland DE, O'Hollaren RM: Fractures and dislocations about the elbow in the head-injured adult. *Clin Orthop* 168:38–41, 1982.
338. Keenan MA, Kauffman DL, Garland DE, et al: Late ulnar neuropathy in the brain-injured adult. *J Hand Surg Am* 13A:120–124, 1988.
339. Wainapel SF, Rao PU, Schepsis AA: Ulnar nerve compression by heterotopic ossification in a head-injured patient. *Arch Phys Med Rehabil* 66:512–514, 1985.
340. Stover SL, Hataway CJ, Zeiger HE: Heterotopic ossification in spinal cord-injured patients. *Arch Phys Med Rehabil* 56:199–204, 1975.
341. Ritter MA, Seiber JM: Prophylactic indomethacin for the prevention of heterotopic bone following total hip arthroplasty. *Clin Orthop* 196:217–225, 1985.
342. Schmidt SA, Kjaersgaard-Andersen P, Pedersen NW, et al: The use of indomethacin to prevent the formation of heterotopic bone after total hip replacement: a randomized, double-blind clinical trial. *J Bone Joint Surg* 70A:834–838, 1988.
343. Mulligan BR: *Manual Therapy: "NAGS", "SNAGS", "PRP'S" etc.* Wellington: Plane View Series, 1992.
344. Mulligan BR: Manual Therapy Rounds: Mobilisations with movement (MWM's). *J Man Manip Ther* 1:154–156, 1993.
345. Lahz JRS: Concerning the pathology and treatment of tennis elbow. *Med J Aust* 2:737–742, 1947.

The Forearm, Wrist, and Hand

CHAPTER 18

CHAPTER OBJECTIVES

At the completion of this chapter, the reader will be able to:

1. Describe the anatomy of the joints, ligaments, muscles, blood and nerve supply that comprise the forearm, wrist, and hand.
2. Describe the biomechanics of the forearm, wrist, and hand, including open- and close-packed positions, normal and abnormal joint barriers, and stabilizers.
3. Describe the purpose and components of the tests and measures for the forearm, wrist, and hand.
4. Describe the relationship between muscle imbalance and functional performance of the forearm, wrist, and hand.
5. Perform a comprehensive examination of the forearm, wrist, and hand, including palpation of the articular and soft-tissue structures, specific passive mobility and passive articular mobility tests, and stability tests.
6. Outline the significance of the key findings from the tests and measures and establish a diagnosis.
7. Summarize the various causes of forearm, wrist, and hand dysfunction.
8. Develop self-reliant intervention strategies based on clinical findings and established goals.
9. Evaluate the intervention effectiveness in order to progress or modify an intervention.
10. Plan an effective home program and instruct the patient in same.

OVERVIEW

A hand is a very personal thing. It is the interface between the patient and his or her world. It is an emblem of strength, beauty, skill, sexuality and sensibility. When it is damaged it becomes a symbol of vulnerability of the whole patient.

—*Paul W. Brand (1914–2003)*

In a sense, the shoulder, elbow, and wrist joints (Fig. 18-1) are merely mechanical devices that contribute to the usefulness of the hand.[1] The correct synchronization of these biological devices, coupled with patient motivation, produce a remarkable level of dexterity and precision.

The carpus, or wrist, represents a highly complex anatomic structure, comprising a core structure of 8 bones; more than 20 radiocarpal, intercarpal, and carpometacarpal (CMC) joints; 26 named intercarpal ligaments; and 6 or more parts of the triangular fibrocartilage complex (TFCC).[2] While these structures can be differentiated anatomically, they are functionally interrelated with movement in one joint having an effect on the motion of neighboring joints. This relationship extends as far as the elbow.

The hand accounts for about 90% of upper limb function.[3] The thumb, which is involved in 40–50% of hand function, is the more functionally important of the digits.[3] The index and middle fingers are each involved in about 20% of hand function, and are the second most important, with the ring finger being the least important. The middle finger is the strongest finger and is important for both precision and power functions.[3]

The following sections describe the respective bones, joints, soft tissues, and nerves, detailing both their individual and collective functions. For simplicity's sake, the forearm, wrist, and hand are separated into their various compartments.

ANATOMY

Distal Radioulnar Joint

The distal radioulnar joint (DRUJ) plays an important role in wrist and forearm function. The DRUJ is a uniaxial pivot joint that joins the distal radius and ulna and an articular disk (Fig. 18-1). The articular disk, known as the TFCC, assists in binding the distal radius and is the main stabilizer of the DRUJ (see next section).[4]

At its distal end, the radius widens to form a broad concave articular surface. The articular surface has an ulnar inclination in the frontal plane, which averages 23 degrees, and a anterior (palmar) inclination in the sagittal plane, which averages 11 degrees.[5] The distal end of the ulna expands slightly laterally into a rounded head and medially into an ulnar styloid process

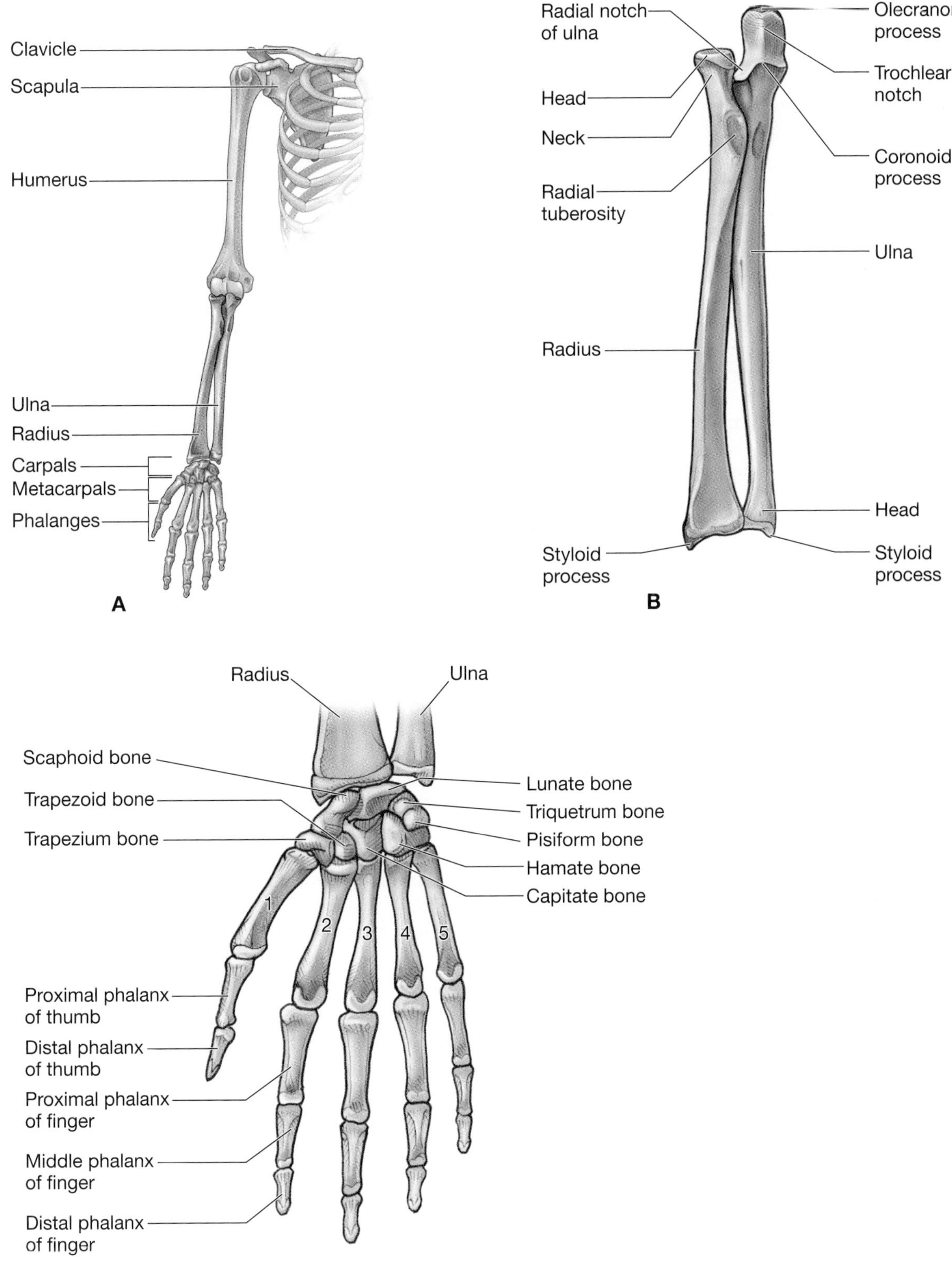

FIGURE 18-1 Arm, wrist, and hand joint structures. (Reproduced with permission from Morton DA, Foreman KB, Albertine KH: *The Big Picture: Gross Anatomy,* McGraw-Hill, 2011.)

(Fig. 18-1). The rounded head of the ulnar head contacts both the ulnar notch of the radius laterally and the TFCC distally.[6] The ulnar styloid process is approximately one-half inch shorter than the radial styloid process, resulting in more ulnar deviation than radial deviation being available.[6] The articular capsule, which attaches to the articular margins of the radius and ulna and to the disk enclosing the inferior radioulnar joint, is lax. Anterior (palmar) and posterior (dorsal) radioulnar ligaments strengthen the capsule anteriorly and posteriorly. Forearm supination tightens the anterior capsule and pronation tightens the posterior part, adding to the overall stability of the wrist.[7]

The DRUJ functions to transmit the loads from the hand to the forearm.

CLINICAL PEARL

The resting or open-packed position for the DRUJ is 10 degrees of supination.

The close-packed position for the DRUJ is 5 degrees of supination.

The capsular pattern for the DRUJ is pain at extremes of pronation/supination.

Triangular Fibrocartilage Complex

The TFCC essentially comprises a fibrocartilage disk interposed between the medial proximal row and the distal ulna within the medial aspect of the wrist.[8] The primary function of the TFCC is to enhance joint congruity and to cushion against compressive forces. Indeed the TFCC transmits about 20 percent of the axial load from the hand to the forearm.[7] The broad base of the disk is attached to the medial edge of the ulnar notch of the radius, and its apex is attached to the lateral aspect of the base of the ulnar styloid process. The disk's anterior and posterior borders are thickened.

A number of ligaments originate from the TFCC and provide support to it. These include the ulnolunate and ulnotriquetral ligaments, the ulnar collateral and the radio-ulnar ligaments. Other structures that lend support to the TFCC include the following:

- The ulnocarpal ligaments.
- The sheath of the extensor carpi ulnaris (ECU) tendon, which is the only wrist tendon that broadly connects to the TFCC.

Both the superior and the inferior articular surfaces of the TFCC are smooth and concave.[8] The disk separates the distal ulna from direct contact with the carpals but allows gliding between the carpals, disk, and ulna during forearm pronation and supination.[8,9]

The TFCC is innervated by branches of the posterior interosseous, ulnar, and posterior (dorsal) sensory ulnar nerves.[9]

The Wrist

The wrist comprises the distal radius and ulna, eight carpal bones, and the bases of five metacarpals (Fig. 18-1). The carpal bones lie in two transverse rows. The proximal row contains (lateral to medial) the scaphoid (navicular), lunate, triquetrum, and pisiform. The distal row holds the trapezium, trapezoid, capitate, and hamate.

Radiocarpal Joint

The radiocarpal joint, a biaxial ellipsoid joint, is formed by the large articular concave surface of the distal end of the radius, the proximal carpal row, and the TFCC. The lunate and triquetrum articulate with the TFCC. A radial styloid process projects distally from the lateral side of the radius. A cartilage-covered ulnar notch occupies the distal medial side of the radius.[10] Posteriorly, a posterior (dorsal) (Lister's) tubercle arises near the center of the radius, forming a pulley around which the extensor pollicis longus (EPL) tendon passes.[9] Lister's tubercle is a common site of attritional changes and potential tendon rupture.[11]

CLINICAL PEARL

The resting or open-packed position for the radiocarpal joint is neutral with slight ulnar deviation.

The close-packed position for the radiocarpal joint is extension with radial deviation.

The capsular pattern for the radiocarpal joint is flexion and extension equally limited.

The Carpals

Scaphoid. The scaphoid (Fig. 18-1) is the largest of the proximal carpal row bones, and its shape resembles that of a boat or canoe (thus the old term *navicular*).[9] The scaphoid bone links the proximal and distal carpal rows and helps provide stability to the wrist joint.

The scaphoid is tethered to the proximal carpal row by a number of strong ligamentous attachments, and two-thirds of its surface area is articular. The proximal surface of the scaphoid is convex and articulates with the radius. The medial surface is concave and articulates with the capitate.[10] The articulating surface for the lunate is flat. The distal surface consists of two convex facets for articulation with the trapezium and trapezoid (the scaphotrapeziotrapezoid joint).[9] The round tubercle on the inferolateral part of its anterior (palmar) surface serves as the attachment of the flexor retinaculum and the abductor pollicis brevis (APB).[10] The blood vessels to this bone enter the scaphoid at or distal to the wrist. This configuration predisposes a fracture on the proximal aspect to aseptic necrosis.[12] In addition, as the scaphoid plays a critical role in coordinating and stabilizing movements between the proximal and the distal rows of the carpals, damage to the intrinsic and extrinsic ligaments that support the scaphoid can result in persistent pain and dysfunction with loading activities.[13–15]

Lunate. The lunate (Fig. 18-1) articulates between the scaphoid and the triquetrum in the proximal carpal row. Its smooth convex proximal surface articulates with the radius and the TFCC at the lunate fossa.[10] Its lateral surface contains a flat semilunar facet for the scaphoid. The medial surface articulates with the triquetrum. The distal surface is deeply concave and articulates with the edge of the hamate in adduction and the medial aspect of the capitate.[10]

Triquetrum. The triquetrum (Fig. 18-1) is a pyramid-shaped bone. It articulates with the pisiform on its distal anterior (palmar) surface at the pisiform–triquetral joint.[10] The almost square distal–medial surface of the triquetrum articulates with the concavo–convex surface of the hamate. The ulnar collateral ligament (UCL) attaches to the medial and posterior (dorsal) surfaces of the triquetrum.[10] The proximal surface of the triquetrum articulates with the TFCC in full adduction.[9] The lateral surface of the triquetrum articulates with the lunate.

Pisiform. The pisiform (Fig. 18-1), as its name implies, is shaped like a "P" with a posterior (dorsal) flat articular facet for the triquetrum.[10] The pisiform, formed within the tendon of the flexor carpi ulnaris (FCU), is a sesamoid bone and serves as an attachment for the flexor retinaculum, abductor digiti minimi (ADM), UCL, pisohamate ligament, and pisometacarpal ligament. The pisiform also functions to increase the flexion moment of the FCU.[9]

As mentioned, the pisiform articulates with the anterior (palmar) surface of the triquetral and is thus separated from the other carpal bones, all of which articulate with their neighbors. The pisiform is closely related to the ulnar artery and nerve on its radial border, the nerve being the closer.[16]

Trapezium. The trapezium (Fig. 18-1) has a groove on its medial anterior (palmar) surface which contains the tendon of the flexor carpi radialis (FCR).[10] To its margins are attached two layers of the flexor retinaculum. The opponens pollicis (OP) is between the flexor pollicis brevis (FPB) distally and the APB proximally.[10] The lateral surface serves as an attachment site for the radial collateral ligament and capsular ligament of the first CMC joint. The distal articulating surface of the trapezium is saddle shaped. Medially, its concave surface articulates with the trapezoid, whereas more distally its convex surface articulates with the second metacarpal base.[10] Proximally, its concave surface articulates with the scaphoid.

Trapezoid. The trapezoid (Fig. 18-1) is small and irregular. The distal surface articulates with the grooved second metacarpal base. The medial surface articulates via a concave facet with the distal part of the capitate. The lateral surface of the trapezoid articulates with the trapezium, and its proximal surface articulates with the scaphoid bone.[10]

Capitate. The capitate (Fig. 18-1) is the most central and the largest of the carpal bones. Its distal aspect articulates with the third metacarpal base. Its lateral border articulates with the medial side of the second metacarpal base.[10] The convex proximal head of the capitate articulates with the lunate and scaphoid. The medial surface of the head articulates with the lunate, and the lateral aspect of the head articulates with the scaphoid.[10] Medially, the capitate articulates with the hamate.

With its central location, the capitate serves as the keystone of the proximal transverse arch. This arch is important to the prehensile activity of the hand.[9,17,18]

Hamate. The hamate (Fig. 18-1) is a cuneiform bone and contributes to the medial wall of the carpal tunnel. To the hook (hamulus) of the hamate is attached the flexor retinaculum. The hamate articulates with three carpal bones and two metacarpals.[9] The medial surface articulates with the triquetrum and by association with the pisohamate ligament, the pisiform. The lateral surface articulates with the capitate.[10] On its distal aspect the hamate articulates with the fourth and fifth metacarpal heads.

CLINICAL PEARL

The resting or open-packed position for the intercarpal joint is neutral or slight flexion.

The close-packed position for the intercarpal joint is extension.

There is no recognized capsular pattern of the intercarpal joints.

Midcarpal Joints

The midcarpal joint lies between the two rows of carpals. It is referred to as a "compound" articulation because each row has both a concave and a convex segment. Wrist flexion, extension, and radial deviation are mainly midcarpal joint motions. Approximately 50 percent of the total arc of wrist flexion and extension occur at the midcarpal level with more flexion (66 percent) occurring than extension (34 percent).[19]

The proximal row of the carpals is convex laterally and concave medially. The scaphoid, lunate, trapezium trapezoid, and triquetrum present with a concave surface to the distal row of carpals. The scaphoid, capitate, and hamate present a convex surface to a reciprocally arranged distal row.

CLINICAL PEARL

The resting or open-packed position for the midcarpal joint is neutral or slight flexion with ulnar deviation.

The close-packed position for the midcarpal joint is extension with ulnar deviation.

The capsular pattern for the midcarpal joint is equal limitation of flexion and extension.

First CMC Joint

The thumb is the most important digit of the hand and greatly magnifies the complexity of human prehension.[20,21] Functionally, the sellar (saddle-shaped) CMC joint is the most important joint of the thumb and consists of the articulation between the base of the first metacarpal and the distal aspect of the trapezium.

The articular surfaces of the trapezium and the proximal end of the first metacarpal are reciprocally shaped. Three other adjacent articulations are functionally related to this joint, which include the joints between the trapezium and the scaphoid, the trapezium and the trapezoid, and the base of the first metacarpal and the radial side of the base of the second metacarpal.[20,21]

Motions that can occur at this joint include flexion/extension, adduction/abduction, and opposition, the latter of which includes varying amounts of flexion, internal rotation, and anterior (palmar) adduction (see "Biomechanics"). Although the joint capsule of the first CMC joint is large and relatively loose, motions at the joint are controlled and supported by muscle actions and by at least five ligaments: anterior oblique, ulnar collateral, intermetacarpal, posterior oblique, and radial collateral. In general, most of the thumb ligaments are placed on tension with abduction, extension, and opposition.[20,21]

CLINICAL PEARL

The resting or open-packed position of the first CMC joint is midway between abduction and adduction, and flexion and extension.

The close-packed position of the first CMC joint is full opposition.

The capsular pattern of the first metacarpal joint is thumb abduction, then extension.

Other CMC Joints

The distal borders of the distal carpal row bones articulate with the bases of the metacarpals, thereby forming the CMC joints. The CMC articulations of the fingers permit only gliding movements. The CMC joints progress in mobility from the second to the fifth, with the second and third metacarpal joints being relatively immobile, and thus the primary stabilizing joints of the hand. The fourth and fifth CMC joints are more mobile to permit the hand to adapt to objects of different shapes during grasping.

Stability for the CMC joints is provided by the anterior (palmar) and posterior (dorsal) CMC and intermetacarpal ligaments. While the trapezoid articulates with only one metacarpal, all of the other members of the distal carpal row combine one carpal bone with two or more metacarpals.

CLINICAL PEARL

The resting or open-packed position of the CMC joints of the fingers is midway between flexion and extension.

The close-packed position of the CMC joints of the fingers is full flexion.

The capsular pattern of the CMC joints of the fingers is equal limitation in all directions.

Metacarpophalangeal Joints

The five metacarpals resemble miniature versions of the long bones of the body, with elongated shafts and expanded ends. The metacarpophalangeal (MCP) joint of the thumb is a hinge joint. Its bony configuration, which resembles the interphalangeal (IP) joints, provides it with some inherent stability. In addition, support for the joint is provided by anterior (palmar) and collateral ligaments. The MCP joint of the thumb consists of a convex surface on the head of the metacarpal and a concave surface on the base of the phalanx. The area of the articulating surface is increased by the presence of a volar plate, which allows greater range of motion than would be available otherwise. Approximately 75–80 degrees of flexion is available at this joint. The extension movements as well as the abduction and adduction motions are negligible. Traction, gliding, and rotatory accessory movements are also present.

The second through fifth metacarpals articulate with the respective proximal phalanges within biaxial joints. Their widened, proximal bases articulate with the carpals and with one another in plane joints.[10] Their biconvex distal heads are broader anteriorly than posteriorly, the significance of which is discussed later.

The MCP joints allow flexion–extension and medial–lateral deviation associated with a slight degree of axial rotation. The design of the MCP joint allows for great amplitude of movement, at the expense of stability.

Approximately 90 degrees of flexion is available at the second MCP, with the amount of available flexion progressively increasing toward the fifth MCP. Active extension at these joints is 25–30 degrees, while 90 degrees can be obtained passively. A loss of flexion and extension at the CMC joint of the little finger reduces the amount of opposition available, resulting in dysfunction of the prehensile pattern and difficulty in making a fist.[6] Approximately 20 degrees of abduction/adduction can occur in either direction at the MCP, with more being available in extension than in flexion. Abduction–adduction movements of the MCP joints are restricted in flexion and free in extension.

CLINICAL PEARL

The resting or open-packed position of the MCP joints is slight flexion.

The close-packed position of the MCP joints is full opposition (thumb)/full flexion (fingers).

The capsular pattern of the MCP joints is flexion, then extension.

The joint capsules are attached to the articular margins of the metacarpals and phalanges and surround the MCP joints. The joint capsule of these joints is relatively lax and redundant, but is endowed with collateral ligaments that pass posterior to the joint axis for flexion/extension of the MCP joints (Fig. 18-11). Although, these collateral ligaments are lax in extension, they become taut in approximately 70–90 degrees of flexion of the MCP joint.[22]

CLINICAL PEARL

Contracture of the collateral ligaments is a major cause of loss of MCP flexion. The MCP joints should never, under any circumstances, be immobilized in extension or hyperextension by a retraction of the collateral ligaments, which would result in their locking.[23] Instead the fingers should be splinted with the MCP joints flexed to 70–90 degrees.

The posterior (dorsal) hood apparatus reinforces (or replaces) the posterior (dorsal) joint capsules. The fibrocartilaginous volar plates reinforce the anterior (palmar) aspects of the joints (Fig. 18-12). The volar plates attach firmly to the phalangeal bases but connect only loosely to the metacarpal heads by membranous fibers. Their posterior (dorsal) surface contributes to the joint area, whereas their anterior (palmar) surface channels the finger flexor tendons.[23]

The asymmetry of the metacarpal heads as well as the difference in length and direction of the collateral ligaments also explains the rotational movement of the proximal phalanx during flexion–extension and why the ulnar deviation of the digits normally is greater than the radial deviation.[23] The rotary movements that occur are called conjunct rotations. The index finger has a conjunct rotation of internal rotation with abduction and flexion, whereas the ring and little finger each have a conjunct rotation of external rotation with abduction and flexion. The middle finger is not thought to have a conjunct rotation.

CLINICAL PEARL

In contrast to the IP articulations, which are stable throughout most of their range of movements, the MCP joints are stable only in flexion.[23]

IP Joints

Adjacent phalanges articulate in hinge joints that allow motion in only one plane: sagittal. The congruency of the IP joint surfaces contributes greatly to IP joint stability. In addition, the IP joints are surrounded by joint capsules that are attached to the articular margins of the phalanges.

Proximal Interphalangeal Joint

The proximal interphalangeal (PIP) joint is a hinged joint capable of flexion and extension. The supporting ligaments and tendons provide the bulk of the static and dynamic stability of this joint as it travels through a normal range of 110 degrees.[22,24–27] The capsule surrounding the articular surface of the joint is composed of the volar plate, lateral and accessory collateral ligaments, and extensor expansion.

The proximal IP joint is stable in all positions. The configuration of the volar plate allows it to function as a static restraint to hyperextension and to influence the mechanical advantage of the flexor tendons at the initiation of PIP joint flexion.[22] The volar plate also increases the surface area. This allows for a greater range of motion than would be available otherwise.

The thick collateral ligaments (true and accessory) of the PIP joint combine with the volar plate to provide lateral stability: the collateral ligaments of the PIP joints are maximally taut at 25 degrees of finger flexion.[22] For this reason, the IP joints are usually splinted in 25 degrees of flexion following surgery to prevent joint contractures. The splinting position is changed as the patient resumes function.

The flexor tendon system at the level of the PIP joint is less complex than the extensor mechanism and contributes very little to injuries about the PIP joint.[22]

The phalangeal bases effectively form a sellar surface, with bone projections allowing for a wide range of accessory movements to accommodate the gripping of a large array of irregular surfaces.

The motions available at these joints consist of approximately 110 degrees of flexion at the PIP joints and 90 degrees at the thumb IP joint. Extension reaches 0 degrees at the PIP joints and 25 degrees at the thumb IP joint. Traction, gliding, and accessory movements also occur at the IP joints.

Distal Interphalangeal Joints

The distal interphalangeal (DIP) joint has similar structures as the PIP joint but less stability and allows some hyperextension. The motions available at these joints consist of approximately 90 degrees of flexion and 25 degrees of extension. Traction, gliding, and accessory movements also occur at the DIP joints.

CLINICAL PEARL

The resting or open-packed position for the IP joints is slight flexion.

The close-packed position for the IP joints is full extension.

The capsular pattern of the IP joints is flexion, and then extension.

TABLE 18-1 Ligaments of the Wrist

Interosseous	Intrinsic Midcarpal	Extrinsic Radiocarpal/ Ulnocarpal
Distal row	*Posterior (dorsal)*	*Posterior (dorsal)*
Trapezium-trapezoid	Scaphotriquetral	Posterior (dorsal) radiocarpal
Trapezoid-capitate	Posterior (dorsal) intercarpal	
Capitohamate		
Proximal row	*Anterior (palmar)*	*Anterior (palmar)*
Scapholunate	Scaphotrapeziotrapezoid	Radioscaphocapitate
Lunotriquetral	Scaphocapitate	Long radiolunate
Triquetrocapitate	Short radiolunate	
Triquetrohamate	Radioscapholunate	
		Ulnolunate Ulnotriquetral Ulnocapitate

Carpal Ligaments

Excessive migration of the carpal bones is prevented by strong ligaments (Table 18-1) and by the ulnar support provided by the TFCC. The major ligaments of the wrist are depicted in Fig. 18-2.

The ligaments of the wrist provide support for the region. These ligaments can be divided into two types: extrinsic and intrinsic (Table 18-1). The extrinsic anterior (palmar) ligaments provide the majority of wrist stability. The intrinsic ligaments serve as rotational restraints, binding the proximal row into a unit of rotational stability.[28] The proximal row of carpals has no muscle insertions. Its stability depends entirely on the capsular and interosseous ligaments between the scaphoid, lunate, and triquetrum.[29] The ligaments between the proximal and the distal carpal rows provide support, centering especially on the capitate.[10] The midcarpal ligaments, which are longer than the interosseous ligaments, cross the midcarpal joint and connect bones of the distal and proximal rows on both the posterior (dorsal) and the anterior (palmar) surfaces.[9] No midcarpal ligaments directly attach to the lunate.

Antebrachial Fascia

The antebrachial fascia is a dense connective tissue that encases the forearm and maintains the relationships of the tendons that cross the wrist. The fascia is firmly attached to the subcutaneous border of the ulna, from which it sends a septum to the radius. This septum divides the forearm into an anterior compartment and a posterior compartment (see Muscles of the Wrist and Forearm).

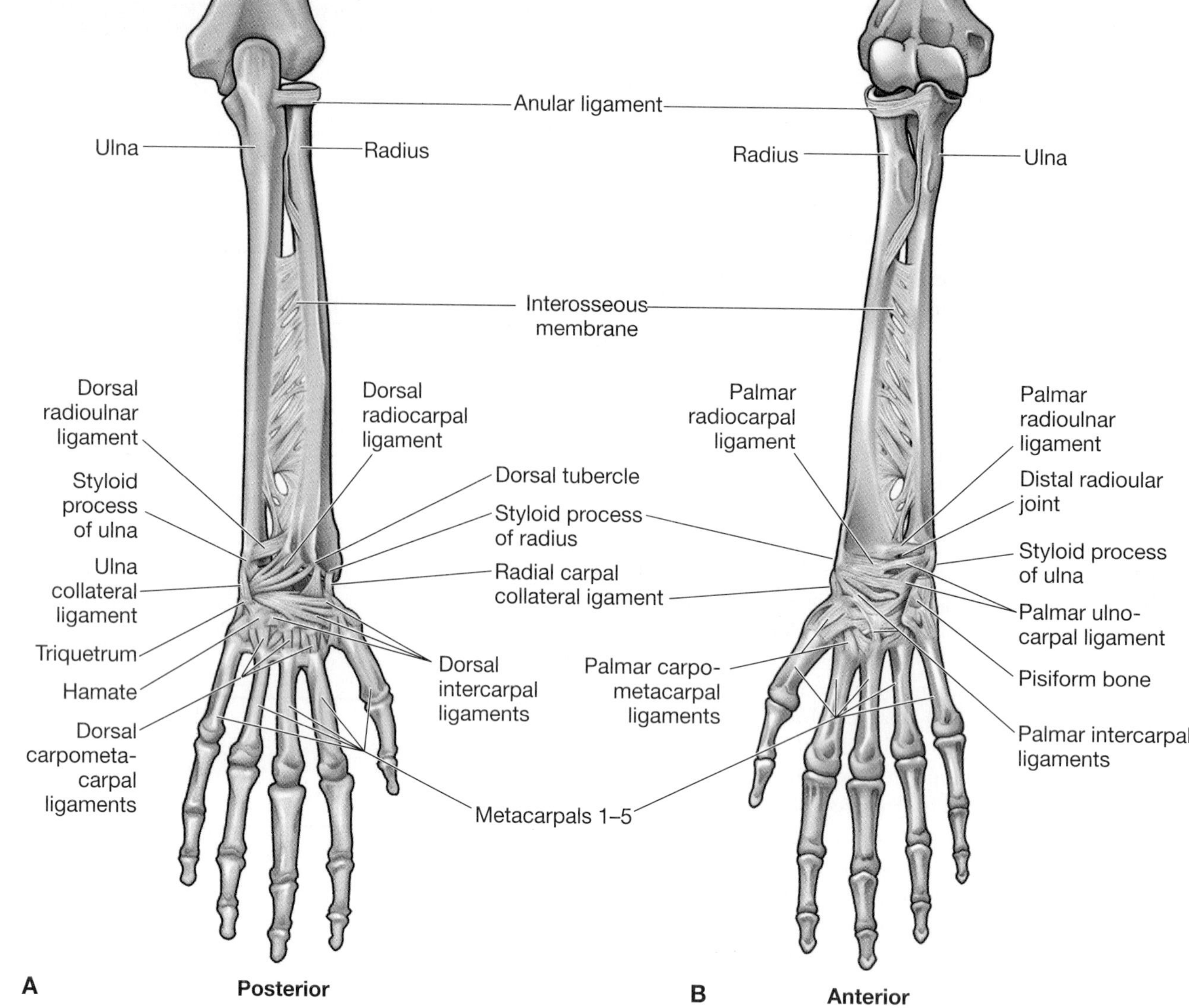

FIGURE 18-2 The major ligaments of the wrist. (Reproduced with permission from Morton DA, Foreman KB, Albertine KH: *The Big Picture: Gross Anatomy,* McGraw-Hill, 2011.)

The Extensor Retinaculum

At the point where the tendons cross the wrist, there is a ligamentous structure called a retinaculum that appears to lay over the tendons and their sheaths (Fig. 18-3). This retinaculum serves to prevent the tendons from "bowstringing" when the tendons turn a corner at the wrist.[30] The extensor retinaculum extends from the lateral border of the distal radius across the posterior (dorsal) surface of the distal forearm onto the posterior surface of the distal ulna and ulnar styloid process. It then wraps part way around the ulna to attach to the triquetrum and pisiform bones. The retinaculum and the underlying bones form six tunnel-like structures called fibro-osseous compartmentson the dorsum of the wrist (Fig. 18-3). The compartments, from lateral to medial, contain the tendons of

1. abductor pollicis longus (APL) and extensor pollicis brevis (EPB)
2. extensor carpi radialis longus (ECRL) and brevis (ECRB)
3. extensor pollicis longus (EPL)
4. extensor digitorum (ED) (four tendons) and extensor indicis (EI) (not shown)
5. extensor digiti minimi (EDM)
6. ECU.

CLINICAL PEARL

The mnemonic 2 2 1 2 1 1 can be used to remember the number of tendons in each compartment.[9]

As these tendons pass through the compartments, they are invested with synovial sheaths.

The posterior (dorsal) compartments serve to enhance the efficiency and effectiveness of the wrist and finger extensors (see "Extensor Hood") (Fig. 18-4). Proximal to the metacarpal heads, juncturae tendineae connect the four tendons of the ED muscles, limiting their independent motion.[6] For example, flexion of the middle and little fingers restricts extension of the ring finger MCP joint because the juncturae tendineae pulls the ring finger extensor tendon distally. Conversely, extension

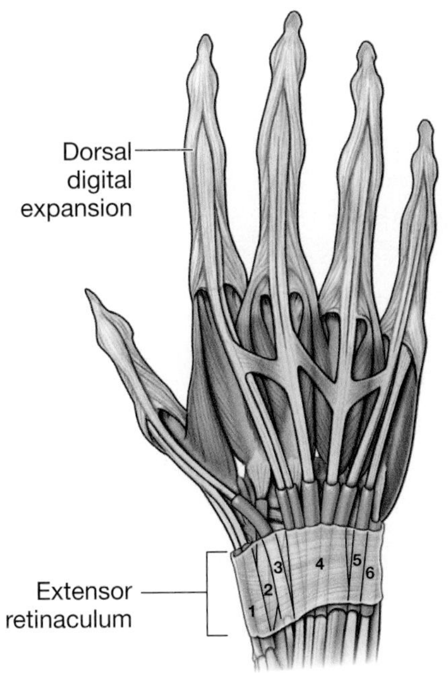

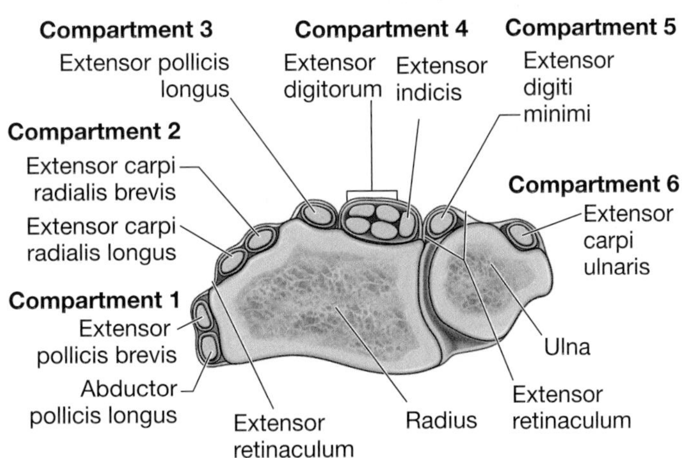

FIGURE 18-3 Extensor retinaculum and extensor tendons. (Reproduced with permission from Morton DA, Foreman KB, Albertine KH: *The Big Picture: Gross Anatomy,* McGraw-Hill, 2011.)

of the ring finger exerts an extensor force upon its neighbors, such that they can be actively extended even if the middle and little finger extensor tendons are severed proximal to the juncturae.[6]

The Flexor Retinaculum

The flexor retinaculum (transverse carpal ligament) spans the region between the pisiform, hamate, scaphoid, and trapezium, transforming the carpal arch into a tunnel, through which the median nerve and some of the tendons of the hand pass. (Fig. 18-5) The proximal attachment of the retinaculum is at the tubercle of the scaphoid and the pisiform. The hook of the hamate and the tubercle of the trapezium serve as its distal attachment. The retinaculum also[6]

- serves as an attachment site for the thenar and hypothenar muscles;
- helps maintain the transverse carpal arch;
- acts as a restraint against bowstringing of the extrinsic flexor tendons,
- protects the median nerve.

In the condition known as carpal tunnel syndrome (CTS), the median nerve is compressed in this relatively unyielding space (see "Intervention Strategies"). The structures that pass *deep* to the flexor retinaculum (Fig. 18-5) include

- flexor digitorum superficialis (FDS),
- flexor digitorum profundus (FDP),
- flexor pollicis longus (FPL),
- flexor carpi radialis (FCR).

The structures that pass *superficial* to the flexor retinaculum include

- the ulnar nerve and artery,
- the tendon of the palmaris longus,

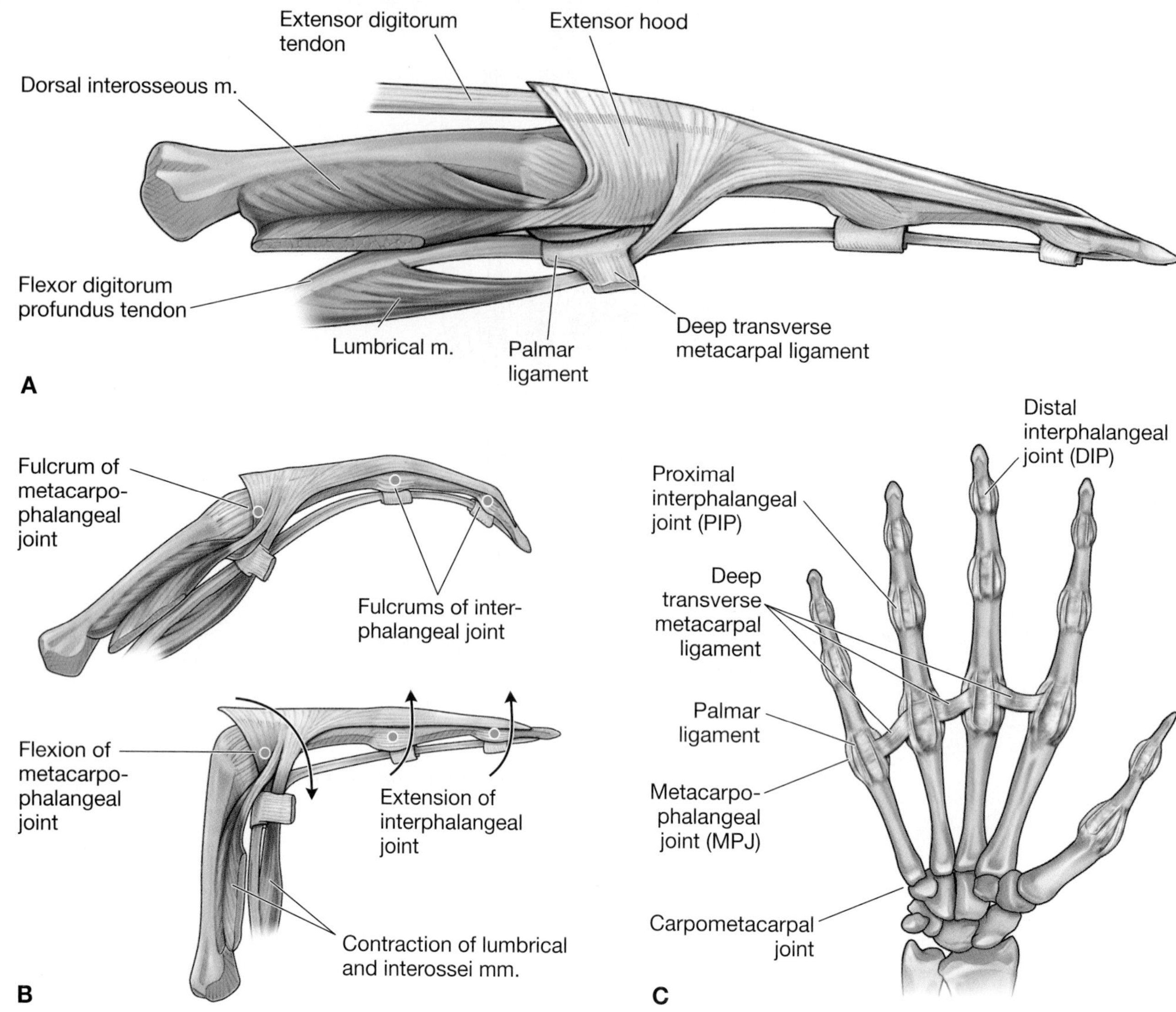

FIGURE 18-4 Extensor hood and smaller ligaments of the hand. (Reproduced with permission from Morton DA, Foreman KB, Albertine KH: *The Big Picture: Gross Anatomy,* McGraw-Hill, 2011.)

- the sensory branch (anterior (palmar) branch) of the median nerve.

Fibrous sheaths between the distal anterior (palmar) crease and the PIP joints bind the flexor tendons to the fingers. Some surgeons refer to the area where the sheaths contain two tendons as "no man's land."[6]

Carpal Tunnel

The carpal tunnel serves as a channel for the median nerve and nine flexor tendons (Fig. 18-5). The floor of the tunnel is formed by the anterior (palmar) radiocarpal ligament and the anterior (palmar) ligament complex. As mentioned previously, the roof of the tunnel is formed by the flexor retinaculum. The radial and ulnar are formed by carpal bones (hook of hamate and trapezium , respectively). The median nerve divides into a motor branch and distal sensory branches within the tunnel.

Tunnel of Guyon

The tunnel of Guyon is located superficial to the flexor retinaculum, between the hook of the hamate and the pisiform bones. The anterior (palmar) carpal ligament, palmaris brevis muscle, and the anterior (palmar) aponeurosis form its roof. Its floor is formed by the flexor retinaculum (transverse carpal ligament), pisohamate ligament, and pisometacarpal ligament.[6] The tunnel functions as a passageway for the ulnar nerve and artery into the hand.

Phalanges

The 14 phalanges each consist of a base, shaft, and head (Fig. 18-1). Two shallow depressions, which correspond to the pulley-shaped heads of the adjacent phalanges, mark the concave proximal bases. Two distinct convex condyles produce the pulley-shaped configuration of the phalangeal heads.[6]

Anterior (palmar) Aponeurosis

The anterior (palmar) aponeurosis, which consists of a dense fibrous structure continuous with the palmaris longus tendon and fascia covering the thenar and hypothenar muscles, is located just deep to the subcutaneous tissue

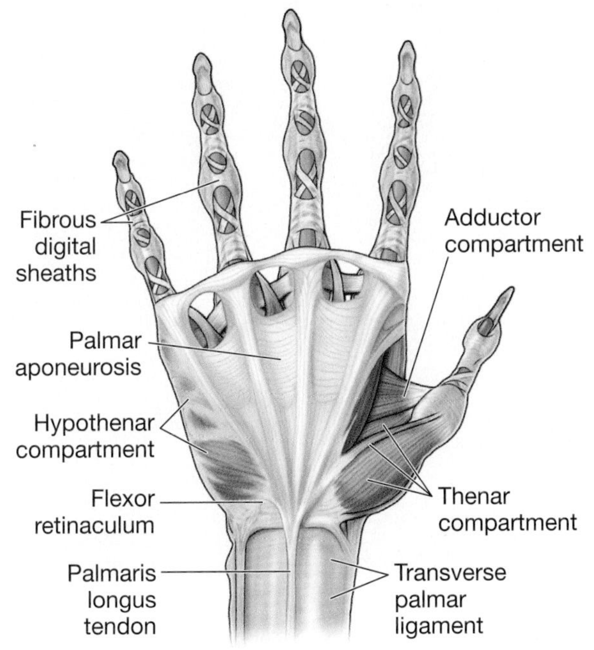

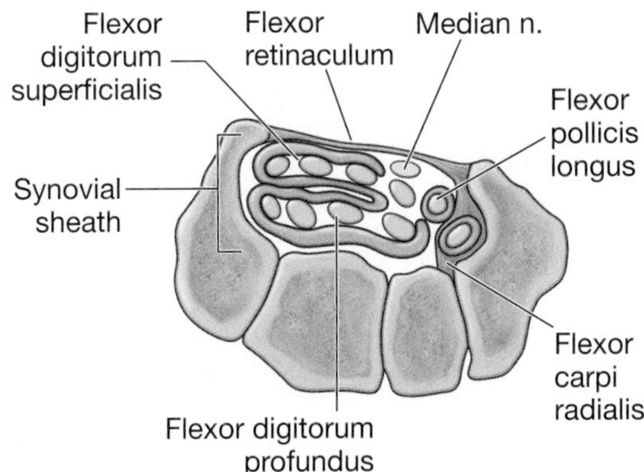

FIGURE 18-5 Flexor retinaculum and flexor tendons. (Reproduced with permission from Morton DA, Foreman KB, Albertine KH: *The Big Picture: Gross Anatomy,* McGraw-Hill, 2011.)

(Fig. 18-5). The aponeurosis travels distally to attach to the transverse metacarpal ligaments and flexor tendon sheaths. The aponeurosis offers some protection for the ulnar artery and nerve, and digital vessels and nerves. From the central region of the palm, the aponeurosis continues toward the fingers and splits into four slips. As these slips approach the MCP joints, they split and wrap around the tendons of their respective digit. Dupuytren contracture is a fibrotic condition of the anterior (palmar) aponeurosis that results in nodule formation or scarring of the aponeurosis and which may ultimately cause finger flexion contractures (see "Intervention Strategies").

Extensor Hood

At the level of the MCP joint, the tendon of the ED fans out to cover the posterior (dorsal) aspect of the joint in a hood-like structure (Fig. 18-4). A complex tendon that covers the posterior (dorsal) aspect of the digits is formed from a combination of the tendons of insertion from the ED, EI, and

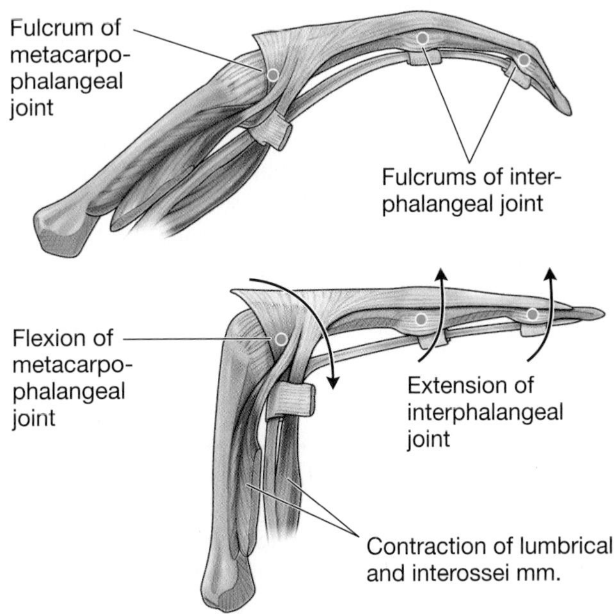

FIGURE 18-6 The tendons of the intrinsic muscles in relation to the joints. (Reproduced with permission from Morton DA, Foreman KB, Albertine KH: *The Big Picture: Gross Anatomy,* McGraw-Hill, 2011.)

EDM. The distal portion of the hood receives the tendons of the lumbricals and interossei over the proximal phalanx. The tendons of the intrinsic muscles pass anterior (palmar) to the MCP joint axes but posterior (dorsal) to the PIP and DIP joint axes (Fig. 18-6). Between the MCP and the PIP joints, the complete, complex ED tendon (after all contributions have been received) splits into three parts: a central slip and two lateral bands[6]:

- ***A central band.*** This band inserts into the proximal posterior (dorsal) edge of the middle phalanx.
- ***The lateral bands.*** These bands rejoin over the middle phalanx into a terminal tendon, which inserts into the proximal posterior (dorsal) edge of the distal phalanx. Rupture of the tendon insertion into the distal phalanx produces a "mallet" finger (see "Intervention Strategies"). The lateral bands, comprise fibers from both extrinsic and intrinsic tendons, are prevented from dislocating posteriorly (dorsally) by the transverse retinacular ligaments, which link them to the volar plates of the PIP joints.[6]

The arrangement of the muscles and tendons in this expansion hood creates a cable-like system that provides a mechanism for extending the MCP and IP joints and allows the lumbrical and possibly interosseous muscles to assist in the flexion of the MCP joints.

Stretching or laxity of these supporting structures allows "bowstringing" of the lateral bands, which transmit excessive extension force to the PIP joint.[6]

The oblique retinacular ligament (Landsmeer ligament) assists in the extensor hood mechanism. The ligament attaches between the PIP volar plate, where it is anterior (palmar) to the PIP joint axis, and the terminal tendon, where it is posterior (dorsal) to the DIP joint axis. This relationship to the PIP and DIP joints is essentially the same as that of the intrinsic muscles (lumbricals and interosseous) to the MCP and PIP joints—when the PIP joint extends, the oblique retinacular ligament exerts a passive extensor force on the DIP joint, and when the PIP joint flexes, it allows the DIP joint to flex.[31]

PIP joint position also may influence DIP joint position through lateral band action. The lateral bands normally slip palmarly upon PIP joint flexion, decreasing the excursion required for full DIP joint flexion. If scar tissue tethers the lateral bands so that they do not move palmarly, then simultaneous full flexion at both the PIP and the DIP joints is not possible.[6]

Synovial Sheaths

Synovial sheaths can be thought of as long narrow balloons filled with synovial fluid, which wrap around a tendon so that one part of the balloon wall (visceral layer) is directly on the tendon, while the other part of the balloon wall (parietal layer) is separate.[30] During wrist motions, the sheaths move longitudinally, reducing friction.

At the wrist, the tendons of both the FDS and the FDP are essentially covered by a synovial sheath and pass posterior (dorsal) (deep) to the flexor retinaculum. The FDP tendons are posterior (dorsal) to those of the FDS.

In the palm, the FDS and FDP tendons are covered for a variable distance by a synovial sheath.

At the base of the digits, both sets of tendons enter a "fibro-osseous tunnel" formed by the bones of the digit (head of the metatarsals and phalanges) and a fibrous digital tendon sheath on the anterior (palmar) surface of the digits.

Flexor Pulleys

Annular (A) and cruciate (C) pulleys restrain the flexor tendons to the metacarpals and phalanges and contribute to fibro-osseous tunnels through which the tendons travel.[11] The A1 pulley arises from the MCP joint and volar plate; A2 from the proximal phalanx; A3 from the PIP joint volar plate; A4 from the middle phalanx; and A5 from the DIP joint volar plate.[11] The C1 pulley originates near the head of the proximal phalanx; C2 near the base of the middle phalanx; and C3 near the head of the middle phalanx.[11]

The pulley system of the thumb includes the A1 arising from the MCP joint anterior (palmar) plate, A2 from the IP joint anterior (palmar) plate, and the oblique pulley from the proximal phalanx.[11]

Anatomic Snuffbox

The anatomic snuffbox (Fig. 18-7) is a depression on the posterior (dorsal) surface of the hand at the base of the thumb, just distal to the radius. This structure can be observed during active radial abduction of the thumb. The radial border of the snuffbox is formed by the tendons of the APL and EPB, while the ulnar border is formed by the tendon of the EPL. Along the floor of the snuffbox are the deep branch of the radial artery and the tendinous insertion of the ECRL. Underneath these structures, the scaphoid and trapezium bones are found.

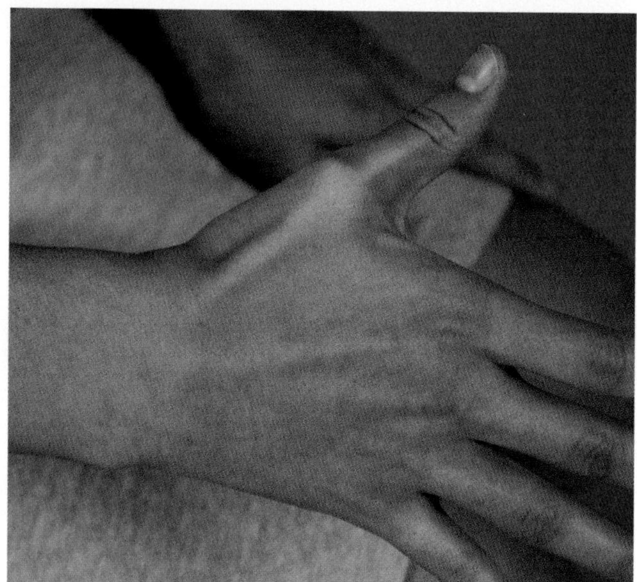

FIGURE 18-7 Anatomic snuffbox. (Reproduced with permission from Morton DA, Foreman KB, Albertine KH: *The Big Picture: Gross Anatomy*, McGraw-Hill, 2011.)

CLINICAL PEARL

Tenderness with palpation in the anatomic snuffbox suggests a scaphoid fracture but also can be present in minor wrist injuries or other conditions.[4]

MOBILE ARCH SYSTEMS

The bones and soft tissues of the hand form a number of functional arches of the hand that provide a perfect balance of force distribution in an equiangular spiral. The arches of the hand, which are all concave palmarly, serve to enhance prehensile function. This prehensile function is best illustrated by the ability of the human hand to grasp an egg. A number of arches are commonly recognized:

- ***The transverse arch.*** The proximal, relatively immobile transverse arch is formed within the anterior (palmar) concavity of the carpal bones.[6] This carpal arch, deepened by the anterior (palmar) projections of the scaphoid and trapezium laterally and the pisiform and hamate medially, should correspond to the concavity of the wrist. The distal transverse arch is more mobile and is defined by the alignment of the metacarpals. This arch allows the hand to adapt to objects held in the palm.[11]
- ***The metacarpal arch.*** This arch, formed by the metacarpal heads, is a relatively mobile transverse arch.
- ***The longitudinal arch.*** This is specifically the arch of the middle finger and the arch of the index finger. The longitudinal arch, which contributes to powerful gripping, spans the hand lengthwise, with its keystone at the MCP joints.[6]
- ***The oblique arches.*** These arches are formed by the thumb in opposition to the other fingers.

TABLE 18-2 Muscles of the Wrist and Hand: Their Actions and Nerve Supply

Action	Muscles	Nerve Supply
Wrist extension	Extensor carpi radialis longus	Radial
	Extensor carpi radialis brevis	Posterior interosseous
	Extensor carpi ulnaris	Posterior interosseous
Wrist flexion	Flexor carpi radialis	Median
	Flexor carpi ulnaris	Ulnar
Ulnar deviation of wrist	Flexor carpi ulnaris	Ulnar
	Extensor carpi ulnaris	Posterior interosseous
Radial deviation of wrist	Flexor carpi radialis	Median
	Extensor carpi radialis longus	Radial
	Abductor pollicis longus	Posterior interosseous
	Extensor pollicis brevis	Posterior interosseous
Finger extension	Extensor digitorum communis	Posterior interosseous
	Extensor indicis	Posterior interosseous
	Extensor digiti minimi	Posterior interosseous
Finger flexion	Flexor digitorum profundus	Anterior interosseous, lateral two digits
		Ulnar, medial two digits
	Flexor digitorum superficialis	Median
	First and second: median	
	Lumbricals	Third and fourth: ulnar
	Interossei	Ulnar
	Flexor digiti minimi	Ulnar
Abduction of fingers	Posterior (dorsal) interossei	Ulnar
	Abductor digiti minimi	Ulnar
Adduction of fingers	Anterior (palmar) interossei	Ulnar
Thumb extension	Extensor pollicis longus	Posterior interosseous
	Extensor pollicis brevis	Posterior interosseous
	Abductor pollicis longus	Posterior interosseous
Thumb flexion	Flexor pollicis brevis	Superficial head: median
		Deep head: ulnar
	Flexor pollicis longus	Anterior interosseous
	Opponens pollicis	Median
Abduction of thumb	Abductor pollicis longus	Posterior interosseous
	Abductor pollicis brevis	Median
Adduction of thumb	Adductor pollicis	Ulnar
Opposition of thumb and little finger	Opponens pollicis	Median
	Flexor pollicis brevis	Superficial head: median
	Abductor pollicis brevis	Median
	Opponens digiti minimi	Ulnar

Muscles of the Wrist and Forearm

The muscles of the forearm, wrist, and hand (Table 18-2) (Figs. 18-8 through 18-10) can be subdivided into 19 intrinsic muscles and 24 extrinsic muscles.[4] The intrinsic muscles are located entirely within the hand; they arise and insert within the hand. The extrinsic muscles, whose muscle bellies lie proximal to the wrist, originate in the forearm and insert within the hand. The flexors, which are located in the anterior compartment, flex the wrist and digits while the extensors, located in the posterior compartment, extend the wrist and the digits.

The design of the extrinsic and intrinsic muscle groups provides for a large number of muscles to act on the hand without excessive bulkiness. The extrinsic tendons enhance wrist stability by balancing flexor and extensor forces and compressing the carpals.

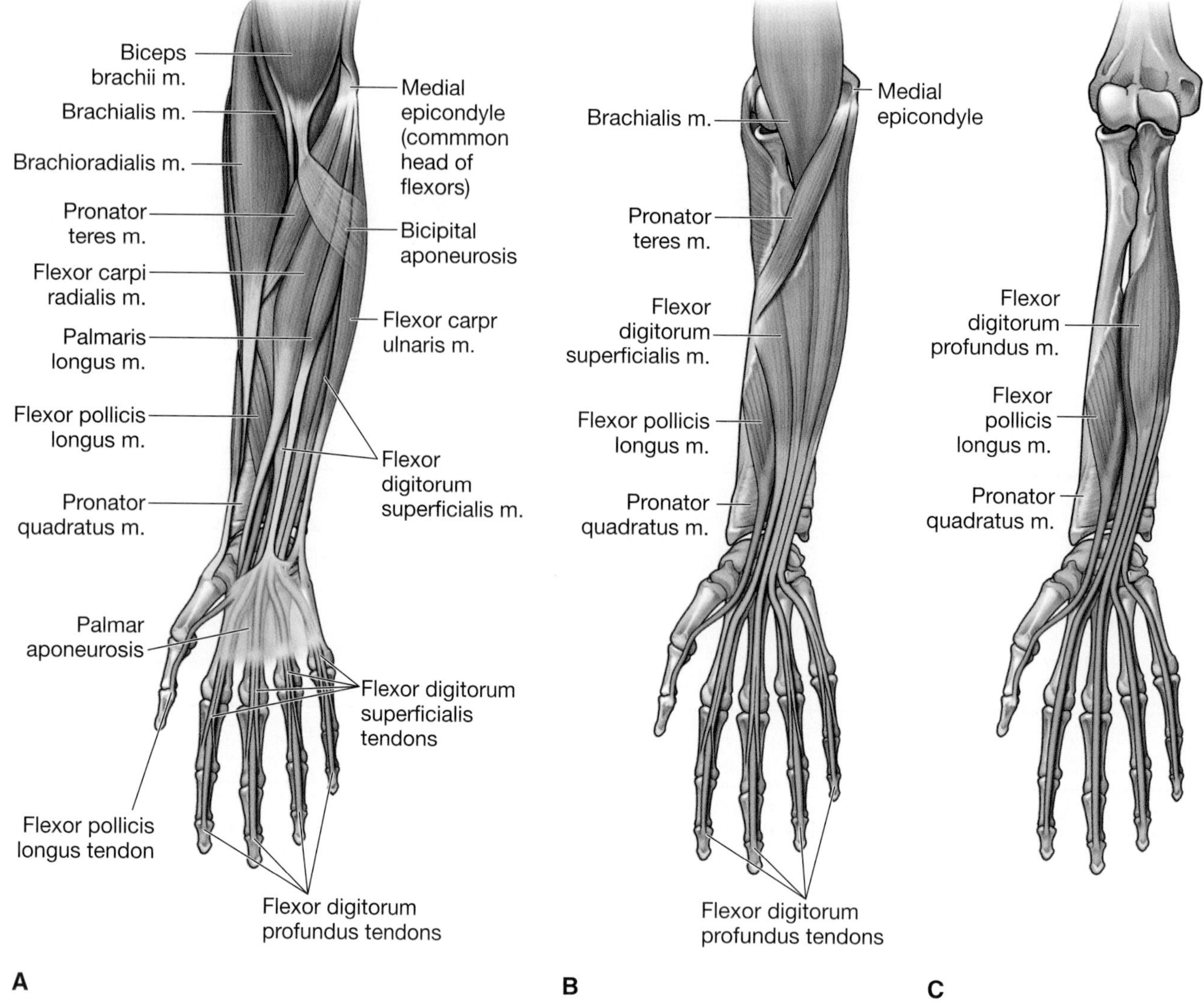

FIGURE 18-8 Muscles of the forearm, wrist, and hand. (Reproduced with permission from Morton DA, Foreman KB, Albertine KH: *The Big Picture: Gross Anatomy*, McGraw-Hill, 2011.)

The amount of tendon excursion determines the available range of motion at a joint. To calculate the amount of tendon excursion needed to produce a certain number of degrees of joint motion involves an appreciation of geometry. A circle's radius equals approximately 1 radian (57.29 degrees). The mathematical radius, which is equivalent to the moment arm, represents the amount of tendon excursion required to move the joint through 1 radian.[32] For example, if a joint's moment arm is 10 mm, the tendon must glide 10 mm to move the joint 60 degrees (approximately 1 radian) or 5 mm to move the joint 30 degrees (1/2 radian).[11]

Anterior Compartment of the Forearm

Superficial Muscles

Pronator Teres. The pronator teres is described in Chapter 17.

Flexor Carpi Radialis. The FCR originates from the medial humeral epicondyle as part of the common flexor tendon. It inserts on the anterior surface and base of the second metacarpal, possibly providing a slip to the third metacarpal. The FCR is innervated by the median nerve and functions to flex and radially deviate the wrist.

Palmaris Longus. The inconsistent palmaris longus arises from the medial humeral epicondyle as part of the common flexor tendon and inserts on the transverse carpal ligament and anterior (palmar) aponeurosis. It receives its innervation from the median nerve. The function of the palmaris longus is to flex the wrist, and it may play a role in thumb abduction in some people.[18]

Flexor Carpi Ulnaris. The FCU arises from two heads. The humeral head arises from the medial humeral epicondyle as part of the common flexor tendon, while the ulnar head arises from the proximal portion of the subcutaneous border of the ulna. The FCU inserts directly onto the pisiform, the hamate via the pisohamate ligament, and onto the anterior surface of the base of the fifth metacarpal, via the pisometacarpal

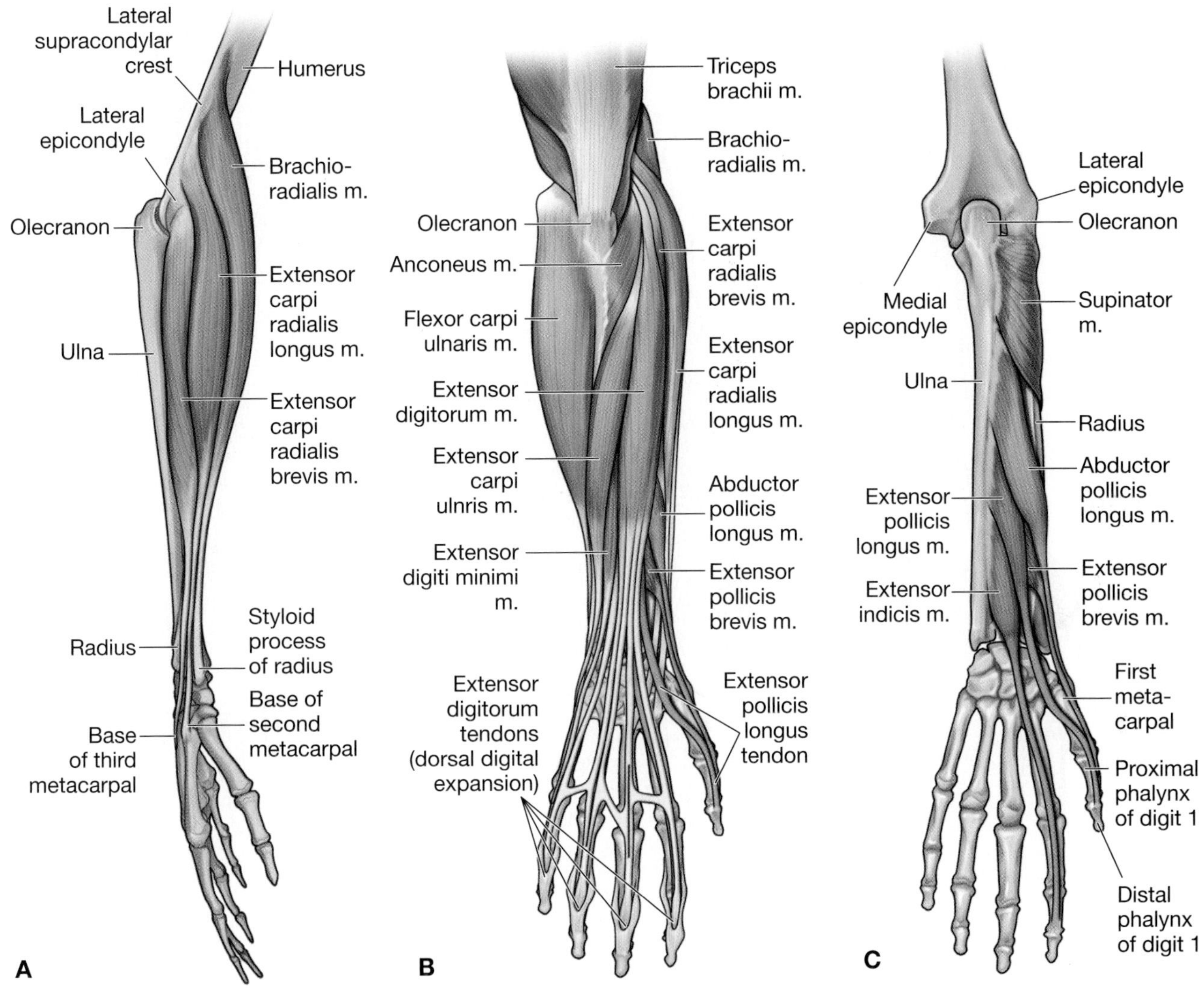

FIGURE 18-9 Muscles of the forearm, wrist, and hand. (Reproduced with permission from Morton DA, Foreman KB, Albertine KH: *The Big Picture: Gross Anatomy*, McGraw-Hill, 2011.)

ligament. The FCU is innervated by the ulnar nerve and functions to flex and ulnarly deviate the wrist.

Intermediate Muscle

Flexor Digitorum Superficialis. The FDS has a three-headed origin. The humeral head arises from the medial humeral epicondyle as part of the common flexor tendon. The ulnar head arises from the coronoid process of the ulna. The radial head arises from the oblique line of the radius. The FDS inserts on the middle phalanx of the medial four digits via a split, "sling" tendon. This muscle is innervated by the median nerve and serves to flex the proximal and middle IP joints of the medial four digits and assist with elbow flexion and wrist flexion. The FDS possesses tendons that are capable of relatively independent action at each finger.

Deep Muscles

Flexor Pollicis Longus. The FPL has its origin on the ventral surface of the radius, medial border of the coronoid process of the ulna, and the adjacent interosseous membrane. It inserts on the distal phalanx of the thumb. The FPL is innervated by the anterior interosseous branch of the median nerve, and it functions to flex the thumb.

Flexor Digitorum Profundus. The FDP arises from the medial and anterior (ventral) surfaces of the proximal ulna, the adjacent interosseous membrane, and the deep fascia of the forearm. The FDP inserts on the base of the distal phalanges of the medial four digits. The FDP has a dual nerve supply: the medial two heads are supplied by the ulnar nerve, while the lateral two heads are supplied by the anterior interosseous branch of the median nerve. The FDP functions to flex the DIP joints, after the FDS flexes the second phalanges, and assists with flexion of the wrist. The tendons of the FDS and FDP are held against the phalanges by a fibrous sheath. At strategic locations along the sheath, the previously mentioned five dense annular pulleys (designated A1, A2, A3, A4, and A5) and three thinner cruciform pulleys (designated C1, C2, and C3) prevent tendon bowstringing.[33]

Unlike the FDS tendons, the FDP tendons cannot act independently. To isolate the PIP joint flexor function of these two muscles, a clinician holds the adjoining finger(s) in extension while the patient attempts to flex the finger being tested. This anchors the profundus muscle of the finger being tested distally and allows the superficialis muscle to act alone at the PIP joint.

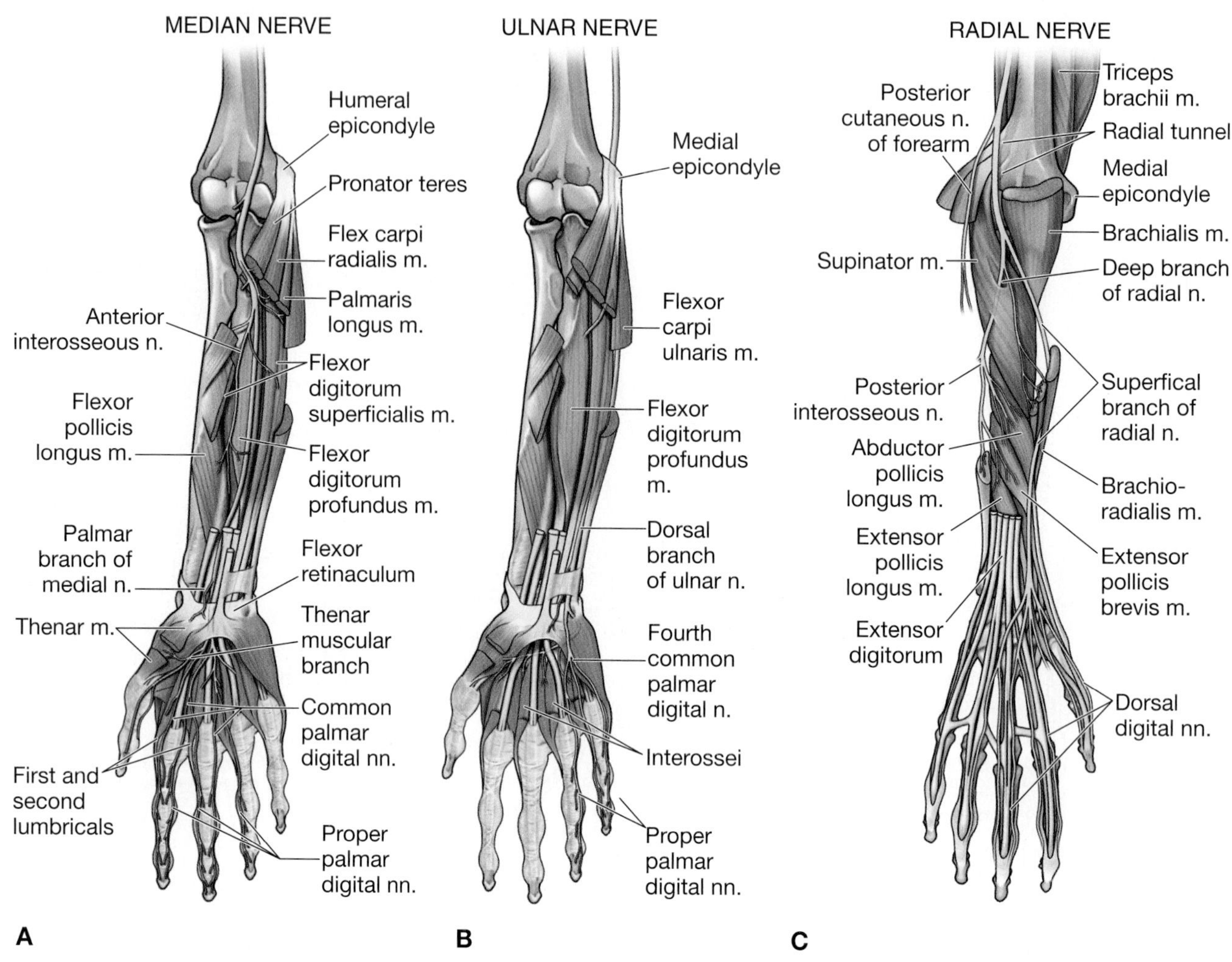

FIGURE 18-10 Muscles and nerve supply of the forearm, wrist, and hand. (Reproduced with permission from Morton DA, Foreman KB, Albertine KH: *The Big Picture: Gross Anatomy,* McGraw-Hill, 2011.)

Tendinous connections between the FDP and the FPL are a common anatomic anomaly, which have been linked to a condition causing chronic forearm pain, called Linburg syndrome,[34] although the association is by no means conclusive.[35]

Pronator Quadratus. The pronator quadratus arises from the anterior (ventral) surface and distal quarter of the ulna and inserts on the anterior (ventral) surface and distal quarter of the radius. The muscle functions to pronate the forearm, and it is innervated by the anterior interosseous branch of the median nerve. The pronator quadratus is well-designed biomechanically as an effective torque producer and a stabilizer of the DRUJ—its line of force is oriented almost perpendicular to the forearm's axis of rotation.[36]

Posterior Compartment of the Forearm

Superficial Muscles

Extensor Carpi Radialis Longus. The ECRL takes its origin at the supracondylar ridge of the humerus about 4–5 cm proximal to the epicondyle, and the thickest part of the muscle is proximal to the elbow joint. The ECRL inserts on the base of the second metacarpal and functions to extend and radially deviate the wrist. It also plays a role in elbow flexion, losing a part of its wrist action when the elbow is flexed.[23]

Extensor Carpi Radialis Brevis. The ECRB arises from the common extensor tendon on the lateral epicondyle of the humerus (see Chap. 17) and from the radial collateral ligament. It inserts on the posterior surface of the base of the third metacarpal bone and receives its nerve supply from the posterior interosseous branch of the radial nerve. The muscle stretches across the radial head during forearm pronation, resulting in increased tensile stress when the forearm is pronated, the wrist is flexed, and the elbow is extended. The more medial location of the ECRB compared to the ECRL makes it the primary wrist extensor, but it has also a slight action of radial deviation.

ED and EDM. The ED arises from the lateral humeral epicondyle, part of the common extensor tendon, while the EDM arises from a muscular slip from the ulnar aspect of the ED muscle. The ED inserts on the lateral and posterior (dorsal) aspect of the medial four digits, while the EDM inserts on the proximal phalanx of the fifth digit. Both muscles are innervated by the posterior interosseous branch of the radial nerve. While the ED functions to extend the medial four digits, the EDM extends the fifth digit.

Extensor Carpi Ulnaris. The ECU arises from the common extensor tendon on the lateral epicondyle of the humerus and the posterior border of the ulna. It inserts on the medial side of the base of the fifth metacarpal bone. It is innervated by the posterior interosseous branch of the radial nerve. The ECU is an extensor of the wrist in supination and primarily causes ulnar deviation of the wrist in pronation, working in synergy with the FCU to prevent radial deviation during pronation.[23]

Extension of the wrist is dependent on three muscles:

- ECRL
- ECRB
- ECU

The ECRB and ECRL are commonly considered to be similar muscles, but in fact they differ in many respects and have very different moment arms of extension.[37] The ECRB, because of its origin on the epicondyle, is not affected by the position of the elbow, so that all of its action is on the wrist, making it the most effective extensor of the wrist (because it has the greatest tension and the most favorable moment arm).[23] Taken together, both ECR tendons comprise about 10 percent of the muscle mass of the forearm and 76 percent of the muscle mass of the extensors of the wrist.[38] The ECRL has longer muscular fibers, mostly at the level of the elbow. The ECRL only becomes a wrist extensor after radial deviation is balanced against the ulnar forces of the ECU.

The ECU, the antagonist of EPL, has the weakest moment of extension, which becomes zero when the wrist is in complete pronation.

Deep Muscles

Abductor Pollicis Longus. The APL arises from the posterior (dorsal) surface of the proximal portion of the radius, ulna, and interosseous membrane and inserts on the ventral surface of the base of the first metacarpal. The APL is innervated by the posterior interosseous branch of the radial nerve and functions in abduction, extension, and external rotation of the first metacarpal.

Extensor Pollicis Brevis. The EPB arises from the posterior (dorsal) surface of the radius and interosseous membrane, just distal to the origin of the APL. It inserts on the posterior (dorsal) surface of the proximal phalanx of the thumb via the extensor expansion. The EPB is innervated by the posterior interosseous branch of the radial nerve and functions to extend the proximal phalanx of the thumb.

Extensor Pollicis Longus. The EPL arises from the posterior (dorsal) surface of the midportion of the ulna and interosseous membrane. It inserts on the posterior (dorsal) surface of the distal phalanx of the thumb via the extensor expansion. The EPL is innervated by the posterior interosseous branch of the radial nerve. It functions in extension of the distal phalanx of the thumb and is thus involved in extension of the middle phalanx and the MCP joint of the thumb.

Extensor Indicis. The EI arises from the posterior (dorsal) surface of the ulna, distal to the other deep muscles, and inserts on the extensor expansion of the index finger. It is innervated by the posterior interosseous branch of the radial nerve and is involved in extension of the proximal phalanx of the index finger.

Muscles of the Hand

The muscles of the hand (Fig. 18-11) are those that originate and insert within the hand and are responsible for fine finger movements.

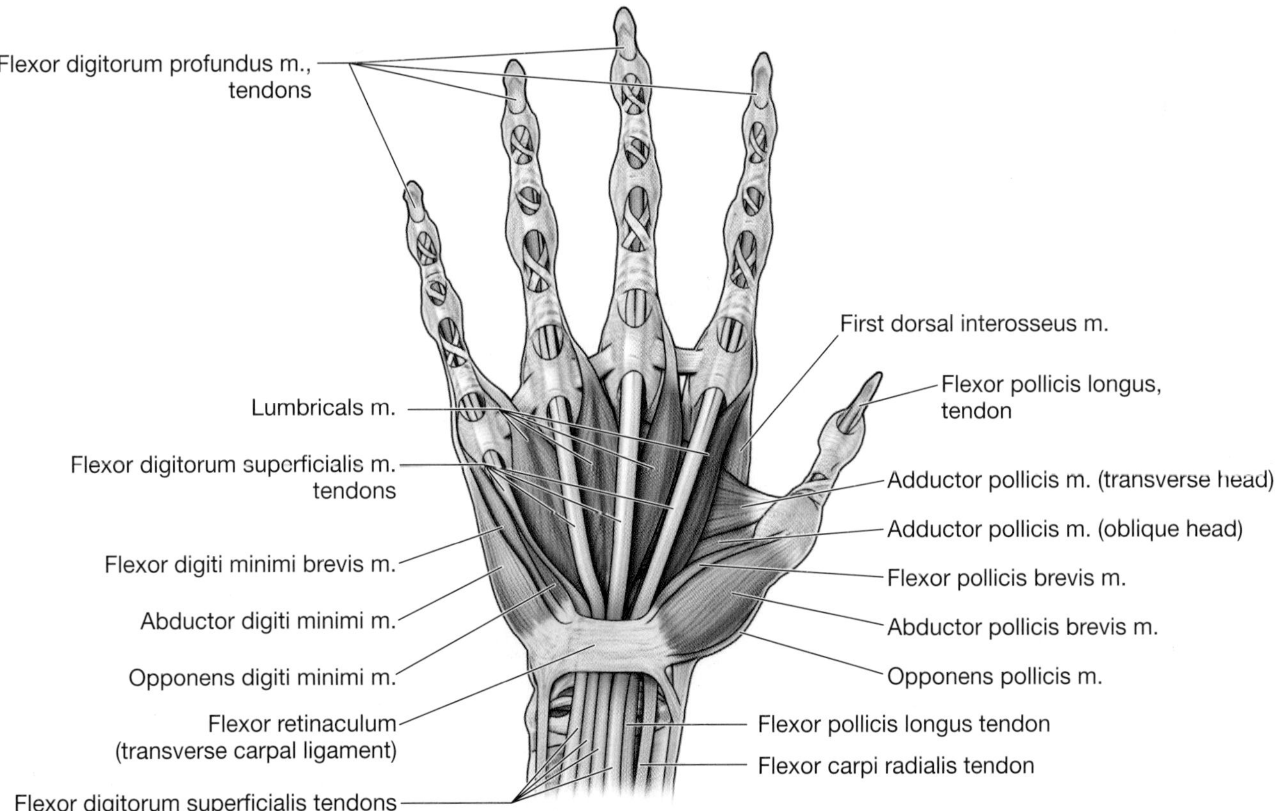

FIGURE 18-11 Muscles of the hand. (Reproduced with permission from Morton DA, Foreman KB, Albertine KH: *The Big Picture: Gross Anatomy*, McGraw-Hill, 2011.)

Short Muscles of the Thumb

Abductor Pollicis Brevis. The APB arises from the flexor retinaculum and the trapezium bone and inserts on the radial aspect of the proximal phalanx of the thumb. It is innervated by the median nerve and functions to abduct the first metacarpal and proximal phalanx of the thumb.

Flexor Pollicis Brevis. The FPB arises from two heads. The superficial head arises from the flexor retinaculum and the trapezium bone, while the deep head arises from the floor of the carpal canal. The FPB inserts on the base of the proximal phalanx of the thumb. The superficial head receives its innervation from the median nerve, while the deep head is innervated by the ulnar nerve. The FPB functions to flex the proximal phalanx of the thumb.

Opponens Pollicis. The OP arises from the flexor retinaculum and the trapezium bone and inserts along the radial surface of the first metacarpal. The OP is innervated by the median nerve and functions to flex, rotate, and slightly abduct the first metacarpal across the palm to allow for opposition with each of the other digits.

Adductor Pollicis (AP). The AP arises from two heads. The transverse head originates from the ventral surface of the shaft of the third metacarpal, while the oblique head originates from the trapezium, trapezoid, and capitate bones, and the base of the second and third metacarpal bone. The AP inserts on the ulnar side of the base of the proximal phalanx of the thumb and is innervated by the deep branch of the ulnar nerve. The AP functions to adduct the thumb and aids in thumb opposition.

Short Muscles of the Fifth Digit

Abductor Digiti Minimi. The ADM arises from the pisiform bone and the tendon of the FCU. It inserts on the ulnar aspect of the base of the proximal phalanx of the fifth digit, together with the flexor digiti minimi (FDM) brevis. It is innervated by the deep branch of the ulnar nerve and functions to abduct the fifth digit.

Flexor Digiti Minimi. The FDM originates from the flexor retinaculum and the hook of the hamate bone. It inserts on the ulnar aspect of the base of the proximal phalanx of the fifth digit, together with the ADM. It is innervated by the deep branch of the ulnar nerve and functions to flex the proximal phalanx of the fifth digit.

Deep branches of the ulnar artery and nerve enter the thenar mass and course into the deep region of the hand by passing between the ADM and the FDM.

Opponens Digiti Minimi (ODM). The ODM arises from the flexor retinaculum and the hook of the hamate bone and inserts on the ulnar border of the shaft of the fifth metacarpal bone. It is innervated by the deep branch of the ulnar nerve and functions to provide a small amount of flexion and external rotation of the fifth digit.

Interosseous Muscles of the Hand

The interossei muscles of the hand are divided by anatomy and function into anterior (palmar) and posterior (dorsal) interossei.

Anterior (palmar) Interossei. The three anterior (palmar) interossei have a variety of origins and insertions. The first interosseus originates from the ulnar surface of the second metacarpal bone and inserts on the ulnar side of the proximal phalanx of the second digit. The second anterior (palmar) interosseus arises from the radial side of the fourth metacarpal bone and inserts into the radial side of the proximal phalanx of the fourth digit. The third anterior (palmar) interosseus originates from the radial side of the fifth metacarpal bone and inserts into the radial side of the proximal phalanx of the fifth digit. The anterior (palmar) interossei are innervated by the deep branch of the ulnar nerve, and each muscle functions to adduct the digit to which it is attached toward the middle digit. The anterior (palmar) interossei also function to extend the distal and then the middle phalanges.

Posterior (dorsal) Interossei. The four posterior (dorsal) interossei have a similar varied origin and insertion as their anterior (palmar) counterparts. The posterior (dorsal) interossei originate via two heads from adjacent sides of the metacarpal bones. The first posterior (dorsal) interosseus muscle inserts into the radial side of the proximal phalanx of the second digit. The second inserts into the radial side of the proximal phalanx of the third digit. The third inserts into the ulnar side of the proximal phalanx of the third digit and the fourth inserts into the ulnar side of the proximal phalanx of the fourth digit. The posterior (dorsal) interossei receive their innervation from the deep branch of the ulnar nerve. The posterior (dorsal) interossei abduct the index, middle, and ring fingers from the midline of the hand.

Lumbricals

The lumbrical muscles are usually four small intrinsic muscles of the hand that originate from the FDP tendons and insert into the posterior (dorsal) hood apparatus. Occasionally, more than four lumbricals are found in one hand.[39]

During contraction, they pull the FDP tendons distally, thus possessing the unique ability to relax their own antagonist.[6] They function to perform the motion of IP joint extension with the MCP joint held in extension and can assist in MCP flexion.[23]

The lumbrical muscles also serve an important role in the proprioception of the hand, providing feedback about the position and movement of the hand and finger joints.[6]

In instances of lumbrical spasm or contracture, attempts to flex the fingers via the profundus result in transmission of force through the lumbricals into the extensor apparatus, producing extension rather than flexion.[6] A "lumbrical plus" deformity occurs if there is excessive lumbrical force or if there is imbalance of opposing forces, which produces exaggerated lumbrical action (i.e., MCP joint flexion and IP joint extension).[6]

The lumbricals have dual innervation. Lumbricals I and II are innervated typically by the median nerve, while the third and fourth lumbricals are innervated by the ulnar nerve.

Neurology

The three peripheral nerves that supply the skin and muscles of the wrist and hand include the median, ulnar, and radial nerves (Fig. 18-12).

Median Nerve

The median nerve enters the forearm by coursing anteriorly through the medial aspect of the cubital fossa and passing deep

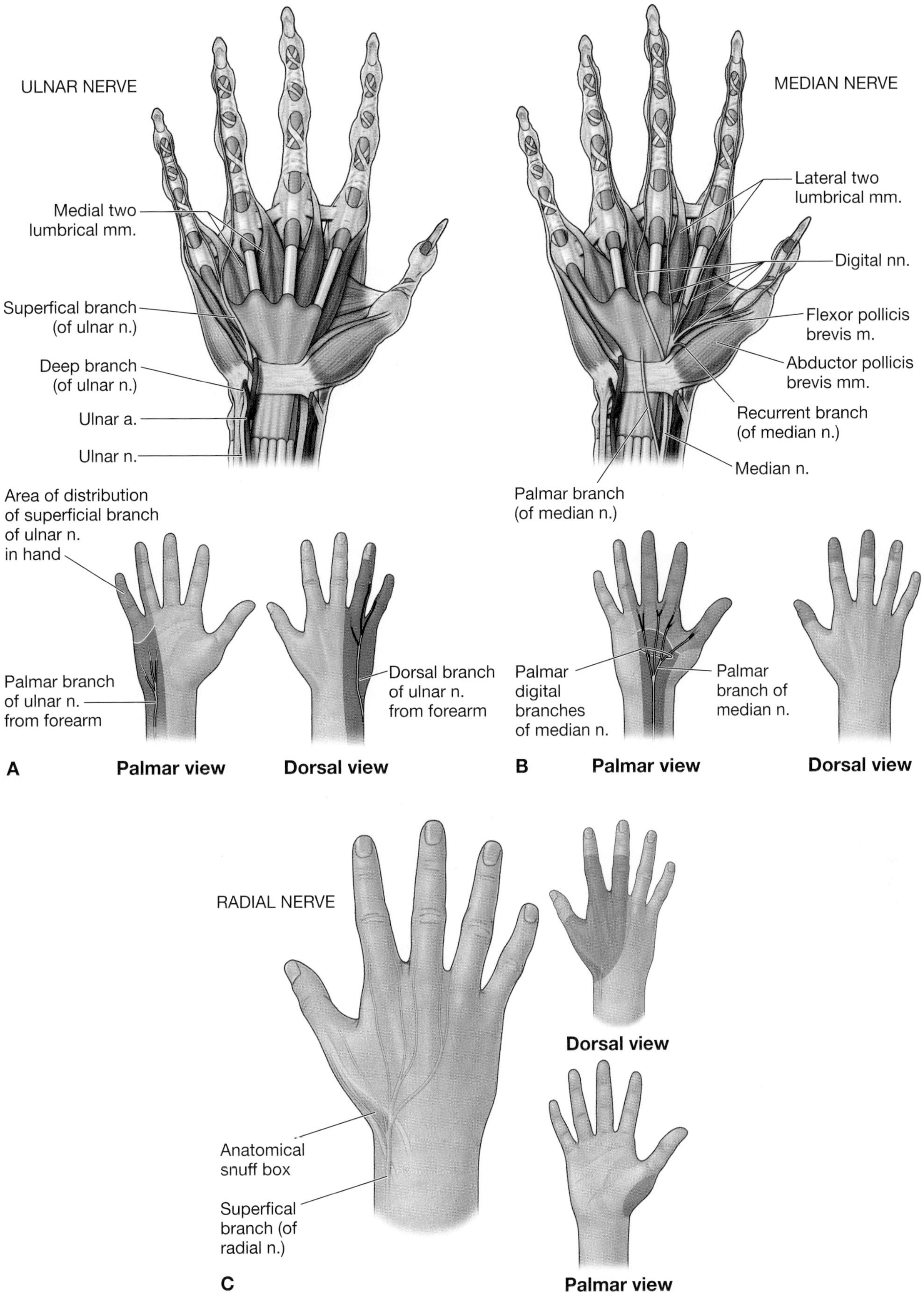

ULNAR NERVE
Medial two lumbrical mm.
Superfical branch (of ulnar n.)
Deep branch (of ulnar n.)
Ulnar a.
Ulnar n.
Area of distribution of superficial branch of ulnar n. in hand
Palmar branch of ulnar n. from forearm
Dorsal branch of ulnar n. from forearm
A
Palmar view
Dorsal view
MEDIAN NERVE
Lateral two lumbrical mm.
Digital nn.
Flexor pollicis brevis m.
Abductor pollicis brevis mm.
Recurrent branch (of median n.)
Median n.
Palmar branch (of median n.)
Palmar digital branches of median n.
Palmar branch of median n.
B
Palmar view
Dorsal view
RADIAL NERVE
Anatomical snuff box
Superfical branch (of radial n.)
C
Dorsal view
Palmar view

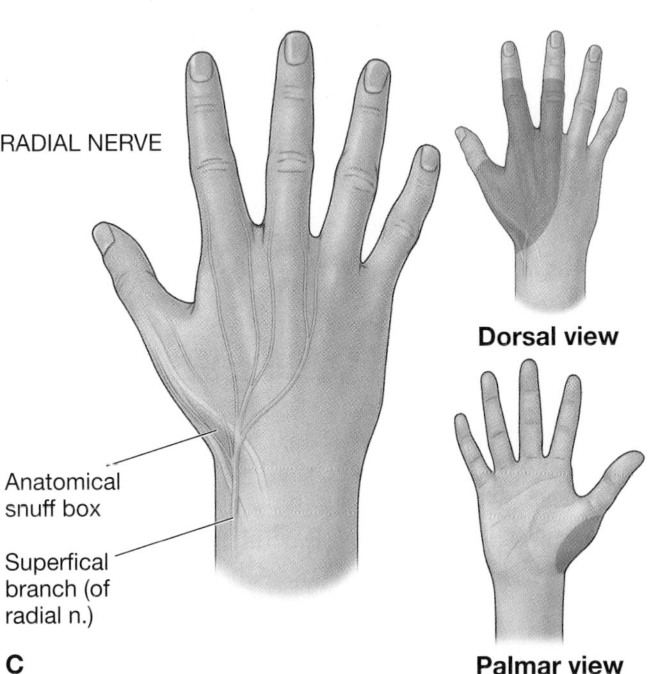

FIGURE 18-12 Nerves of the hand. (Reproduced with permission from Morton DA, Foreman KB, Albertine KH: *The Big Picture: Gross Anatomy*, McGraw-Hill, 2011.)

to the lacertus fibrosis, between the heads of the pronator teres muscle. Below the elbow, muscular branches leave the nerve and innervate the FCR, palmaris longus, and pronator teres muscles. The anterior interosseous branch innervates the pronator quadratus, FPL, and the FDP to the index finger and middle fingers and sometimes the ring finger.

Approximately 8 cm proximal to the wrist, the median nerve gives off a sensory branch, the anterior (palmar) cutaneous nerve that passes superficial to the flexor retinaculum and remains outside the carpal tunnel. This nerve innervates the skin in the central aspect of the palm, over the thenar eminence. The rest of the median nerve passes distally to the wrist, where it enters the carpal tunnel, which passes deep to the flexor retinaculum.

The nerve enters the hand through the carpal tunnel, deep to the tendon of the palmaris longus and in between the tendons of the FPL and FDS (the more radial of the two). From this point, the nerve divides into two branches: a motor branch which passes posterior (dorsal) to the flexor retinaculum and a sensory branch.

Motor Branch. This short branch enters the thenar eminence, where it usually supplies the APB and OP muscles, the FPB (occasionally), and the first and second lumbrical muscles.

Sensory Branch. The sensory anterior (palmar) digital branch innervates the anterior (palmar) surface and posterior (dorsal) aspect of the distal phalanges of the thumb, second and third fingers, and the radial half of the forefinger.

A number of median nerve entrapment syndromes exist (refer to "Peripheral Nerve Entrapment"), each with their own clinical features and functional implications. For example, entrapment of the median nerve in the carpal tunnel may result in numbness, pain, or paresthesia of the fingers and thumb and may severely hinder a patient's ability to perform precision maneuvers due to loss of critical sensory and motor function in the thumb, index, and middle fingers.

Ulnar Nerve

The ulnar nerve has been referred to as the nerve of fine movements of the hand. The ulnar nerve originates from the inferior roots of the brachial plexus (C 8–T 1). Two branches of the ulnar nerve arise in the midforearm:

1. ***The anterior (palmar) cutaneous branch.*** The anterior (palmar) cutaneous branch supplies a portion of the skin over the hypothenar eminence.
2. ***The posterior (dorsal) cutaneous branch.*** About 8–10 cm proximal to the ulnar styloid process, the posterior (dorsal) cutaneous branch of the ulnar nerve splits from the main trunk. The posterior (dorsal) cutaneous branch terminates into two posterior (dorsal) digital branches that supply sensation to the posterior (dorsal) and ulnar aspect of the middle phalanx of the ring and little fingers.[40]

Before reaching the wrist, the ulnar nerve branches to innervate the FDP and the FCU.

At the wrist, the ulnar nerve emerges just lateral to the tendon of the FCU as it passes superficial to the flexor retinaculum. The ulnar nerve passes into the hand via the tunnel of Guyon, where it divides into its superficial and deep terminal branches. The deep (motor) branch supplies the FDM, ADM, ODM, AP, palmaris brevis, third and fourth lumbricals, deep head of the FPB, and the interossei. The superficial branch, which is primarily sensory with the exception of its innervation to the palmaris brevis, divides into three branches.[40] The first of these three branches is a sensory branch to the ulnar aspect of the little finger, and the second is a sensory branch to the central ulnar anterior (palmar) area. The third branch, often referred to as the common digital nerve, innervates the fourth intermetacarpal space. The common digital nerve further divides into two proper digital nerves supplying the ulnar portion of the ring finger and the radial portion of the little finger.[40]

A number of ulnar nerve entrapment syndromes exist (refer to "Peripheral Nerve Entrapment"), each with their own clinical features and functional implications.

Radial Nerve

As the radial nerve enters the cubital fossa, it typically splits into a superficial and deep branch. The superficial branch typically courses distally along the lateral border of the forearm under cover of the brachioradialis muscle and tendon. At the wrist this branch divides into four to five digital branches, which provide cutaneous and articular innervation. The cutaneous innervation includes the lateral two-thirds of the dorsum of the hand and the posterior (dorsal) lateral 21/2 fingers to the proximal phalanx.

All of the motor branches of the radial nerve are located in the forearm. The deep branch (posterior interosseous nerve) typically penetrates the anterior (ventral) surface of, and passes through, the supinator muscle. It reaches the deep region of the posterior forearm by passing through the arcade of Fröhse. The nerve courses subcutaneously from the midportion of the forearm to an area adjacent to the styloid process of the radius and terminates on the posterior aspect of the wrist.

CLINICAL PEARL

Radial nerve entrapment (refer to "Peripheral Nerve Entrapment") may result in a loss of extension at the wrist and MCP joints of the fingers, and thumb extension and abduction. Since the wrist extensor muscles are synergists and stabilizers for the finger flexor muscles during gripping, this loss can significantly hamper hand function.

Vasculature of the Wrist and Hand

The brachial artery bifurcates at the elbow into radial and ulnar branches, which are the main arterial branches to the hand (Fig. 18-13).

Radial Artery

The radial artery is formed from the lateral branch of the bifurcation of the brachial artery. The artery gives off branches in the proximal portion of the forearm that form an anastomosis around the elbow joint. It runs distally under the cover of the brachioradialis muscle. Just proximal to the wrist, it is located between the brachioradialis and the FCR tendons. A small branch called the superficial anterior (palmar) artery leaves the radial artery 5–8 mm proximal to the tip of the radial

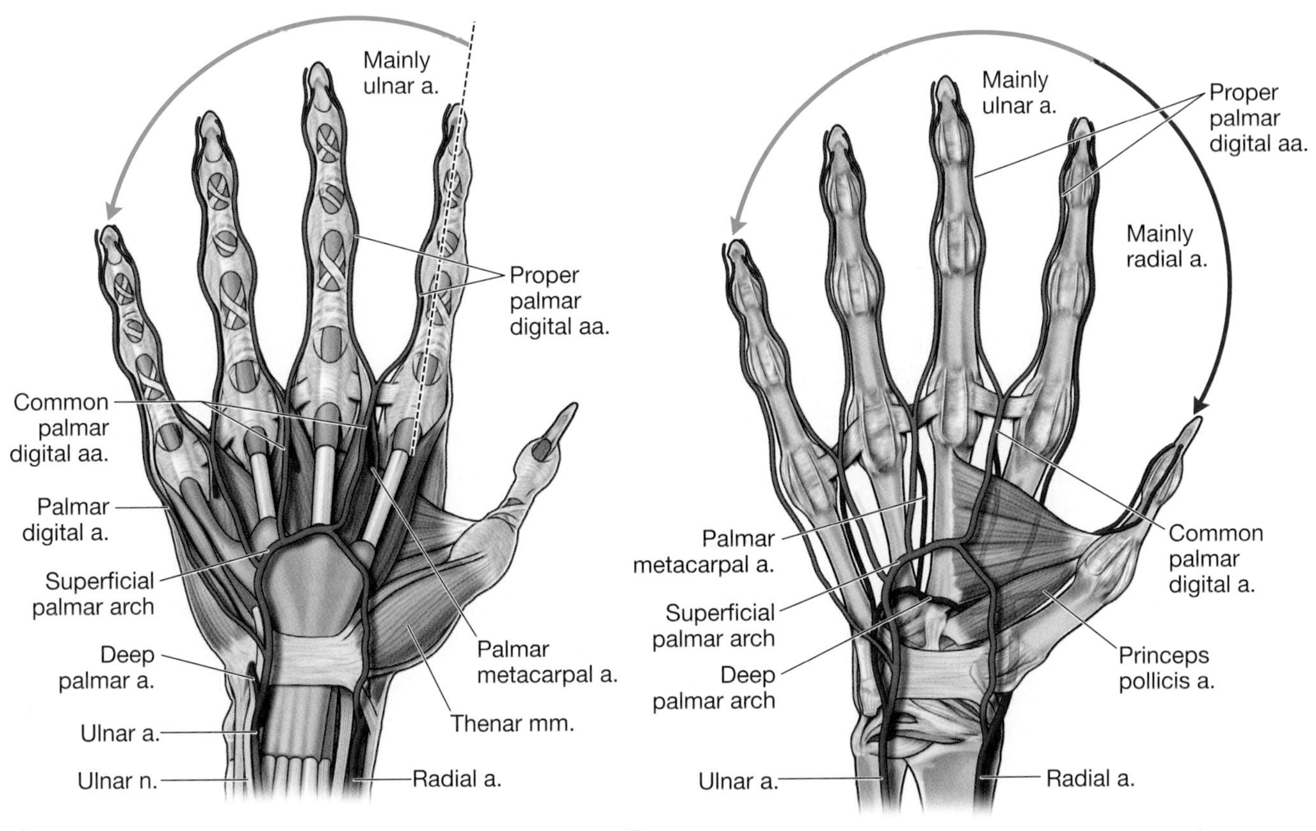

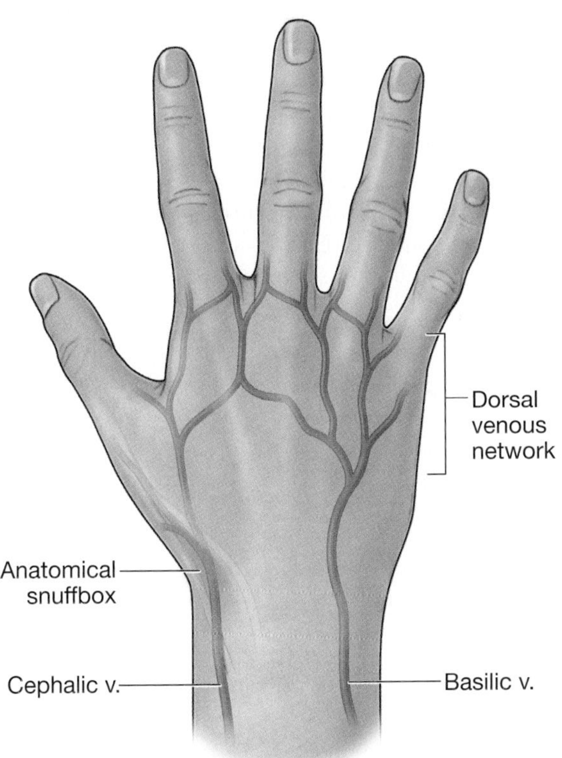

FIGURE 18-13 Vascular supply to the hand. (Reproduced with permission from Morton DA, Foreman KB, Albertine KH: *The Big Picture: Gross Anatomy*, McGraw-Hill, 2011.)

styloid, passes between the FCR and the brachioradialis, and continues distally to contribute to the superficial anterior (palmar) arch, which supplies the thenar mass. The radial artery has seven major carpal branches: three posterior (dorsal), three anterior (palmar), and a final branch that continues distally (see below).

Ulnar Artery

The ulnar artery originates as the medial branch from the bifurcation of the brachial artery. It too gives off branches in the proximal portion of the forearm that form an anastomosis around the elbow joint. The artery passes posterior (dorsal) to the ulnar head of the pronator teres and courses distally deep to the FDS, at which point it passes in the groove between the FCU and FDP, in the company of the ulnar nerve. In the proximal portion of the forearm, the artery gives off a common interosseous branch. The artery bifurcates, giving rise to the anterior and posterior interosseous arteries, which provide blood to structures in the deep anterior and posterior compartments of the forearm. The artery emerges at the wrist, just lateral to the tendon of the FCU. It then passes through the tunnel of Guyon and enters the superficial compartment of the hand. At the level of the carpus, the ulnar artery gives off a latticework of fine vessels that span the posterior (dorsal) and anterior (palmar) aspects of the medial carpals. Proximal to the end of the ulna, there are three branches: a branch to the posterior (dorsal) radiocarpal arch, one to the anterior (palmar) radiocarpal arch, and one to the proximal pole of the pisiform and to the anterior (palmar) aspect of the triquetrum.[41]

Vascular Arches of the Hand

Posterior (dorsal) Arches. The posterior (dorsal) arches are connected longitudinally at their medial and lateral aspects by the ulnar and radial arteries. They are connected centrally by the posterior (dorsal) branch of the anterior interosseous artery. There are three posterior (dorsal) transverse arches: the radiocarpal, the intercarpal, and the basal metacarpal[41]:

- ***Posterior (dorsal) radiocarpal.*** The radiocarpal arch is supplied by branches of the radial and ulnar arteries and the posterior (dorsal) branch of the anterior interosseous artery.
- ***Posterior (dorsal) intercarpal.*** The posterior (dorsal) intercarpal arch has a variable supply, which can include the radial, ulnar, and anterior interosseous arteries.
- ***Basal metacarpal.*** The basal metacarpal arch is supplied by perforating arteries from the second, third, and fourth interosseous spaces. It contributes to the vascularity of the distal carpal row through anastomoses with the intercarpal arch.

Anterior (palmar) Arches. Similar to the posterior (dorsal) vascularity, the anterior (palmar) vascularity is composed of three transverse arches: the anterior (palmar) radiocarpal, the anterior (palmar) intercarpal, and the deep anterior (palmar) arch[41]:

- ***Anterior (palmar) radiocarpal.*** This arch supplies the anterior (palmar) surface of the lunate and triquetrum.
- ***Anterior (palmar) intercarpal.*** This arch is small and is not a major contributor of nutrient vessels to the carpals.
- ***Deep anterior (palmar).*** This arch contributes to the radial and ulnar recurrent arteries and sends perforating branches to the posterior (dorsal) basal metacarpal arch and to the anterior (palmar) metacarpal arteries.

BIOMECHANICS

The wrist is the key joint of the hand and contains several segments whose combined movements create a total range of motion that is greater than the sum of its individual parts.[23] The osteokinematics of the wrist are limited to two degrees of freedom: flexion–extension and ulnar–radial deviation (Fig. 18-14). Wrist circumduction—a full circular motion made by the wrist—is a combination of these movements.[42] The apparent axial rotation of the palm—called pronation and supination—occurs at the proximal and DRUJs, with the hand moving with the radius, not separately from it.[42]

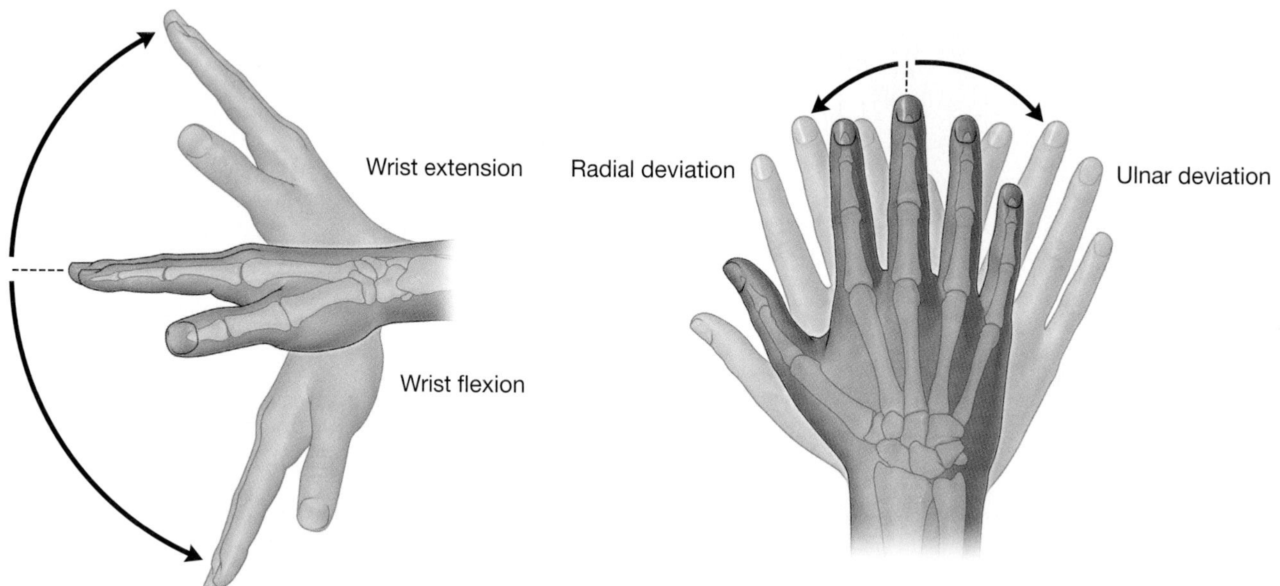

FIGURE 18-14 Movements of the wrist. (Reproduced with permission from Morton DA, Foreman KB, Albertine KH: *The Big Picture: Gross Anatomy*, McGraw-Hill, 2011.)

Pronation and Supination

The true axis for pronation–supination at the wrist may be situated anywhere between the radial and ulnar styloid, resulting in not one, but many pronation–supination axes.[43,44]

- Approximately 75–90 degrees of forearm pronation is available. During pronation, the concave ulnar notch of the radius glides around the peripheral surface of the relatively fixed convex ulnar head. Pronation is limited by the bony impaction between the radius and the ulna.
- Approximately 85–90 degrees of forearm supination is available. Supination is limited by the interosseous membrane and the bony impaction between the ulnar notch of the radius and the ulnar styloid process.

Congruency of the DRUJ surfaces is maximal at midrange of motion, although the joint is not considered to be truly locked in this position.[6] At this position, the TFCC is maximally stretched and the interosseous membrane is relatively lax.

The proximal and DRUJs are intimately related biomechanically, with the function and stability of both joints dependent on the configuration of, and distance between, the two bones. This configuration and distance maintains ligament and muscle tension.[45] A change in the length of the ulna of as little as 2 mm results in a change in the transmission of forces of 5–40 percent.[46]

Movement of the Hand on the Forearm

Due to the morphology of the wrist, movement at this joint complex involves a coordinated interaction between a number of articulations. These include the radiocarpal joint, the proximal row of carpals, and the distal row of carpals. All of these joints permit motion to occur around two axes: anterior–posterior in flexion–extension, and transverse in radial and ulnar deviation. Wrist extension is accompanied by a slight radial deviation and pronation of the forearm. Wrist flexion is accompanied by a slight ulnar deviation and supination of the forearm.

A number of concepts have been proposed over the years to explain the biomechanics of wrist motion.[47–60] The essential kinematics of the sagittal plane involve the mechanism of the carpal bone motions related to the central column of the wrist formed by the series of articulations among the radius, lunate, capitate, and third metacarpal bone.[42] Within this concept

- the radiocarpal joint is represented by the articulation between the radius and lunate composed of the radius, scaphoid, trapezoid, trapezium, and the column of the thumb;
- the CMC joint is assumed to be a rigid articulation between the capitate and the base of the third metacarpal;
- The ulnar or medial compartment of the midcarpal joint is represented by the articulation between the lunate and capitate. This column strongly supports the movements in the central column, while simultaneously anchoring the wrist to the radius.[48]

Under the column concept, the radial and ulnar columns are proposed to move with the central column due to mutual displacements between the proximal facets of the scaphoid and lunate. In addition, the proximal carpals are considered to move at the radiocarpal and midcarpal levels.[23,49]

Flexion and Extension Movements of the Wrist

The movements of flexion and extension of the wrist are shared between the radiocarpal articulation and the intercarpal articulation in varying proportions.[19] The arthrokinematics are based on synchronous convex-on-concave rotations at the radiocarpal and midcarpal joints.[42]

- During wrist extension, most of the motion occurs at the radiocarpal joint (66.5 percent or 40 degrees versus 33.5 percent or 20 degrees at the midcarpal joint) and is accompanied with slight radial deviation and pronation of the forearm.[19]
- During wrist flexion, most of the motion occurs in the midcarpal joint (60 percent or 40 degrees, versus 40 percent or 30 degrees at the radiocarpal joint) and is accompanied with slight ulnar deviation and supination of the forearm.[19]

Extension

At the radiocarpal joint, extension occurs as the convex surface of the lunate rolls posteriorly (dorsally) on the radius and simultaneously slides anteriorly (palmarly).[42] Rotation directs the lunate's distal surface in an extended, posterior (dorsal) direction. At the midcarpal joint, the head of the capitate rolls posteriorly (dorsally) on the lunate and simultaneously slides in an anterior (palmar) direction.[42] When the wrist is extended, the radiolunotriquetral and radiocapitate ligaments are stretched and tension develops within the wrist and finger flexor muscles. Tension within the structures stabilizes the wrist in its close-packed position of extension.[42,61,62]

Loss of active extension in the wrist constitutes a considerable functional impairment, including the following[23]:

- A reduction in grip strength.
- Changes in muscle length-tension relationships, which has serious implications when considering the action of the extrinsic muscles of the hand. For example, the strength of the thumb and finger flexors requires normal motion and function of wrist extension.

Flexion

The arthrokinematics of wrist flexion are similar to those described in extension, but occurs in a reverse fashion.

Frontal Lateral Movements of the Wrist

Like flexion and extension, the movements of ulna and radial deviation of the wrist are shared between the radiocarpal articulation and the intercarpal articulation in varying proportions (Fig. 18-15).[19] The amount of deviation is approximately 40 degrees of ulnar deviation and 15 degrees of radial deviation. There is a physiological ulnar deviation at rest, which is easily demonstrated clinically and radiographically.

Ulnar Deviation

Ulnar deviation occurs primarily at the radiocarpal joint.[62] When the hand is observed at rest, there is a physiological ulnar deviation. During ulnar deviation, the radiocarpal and midcarpal joints contribute fairly equally to the overall

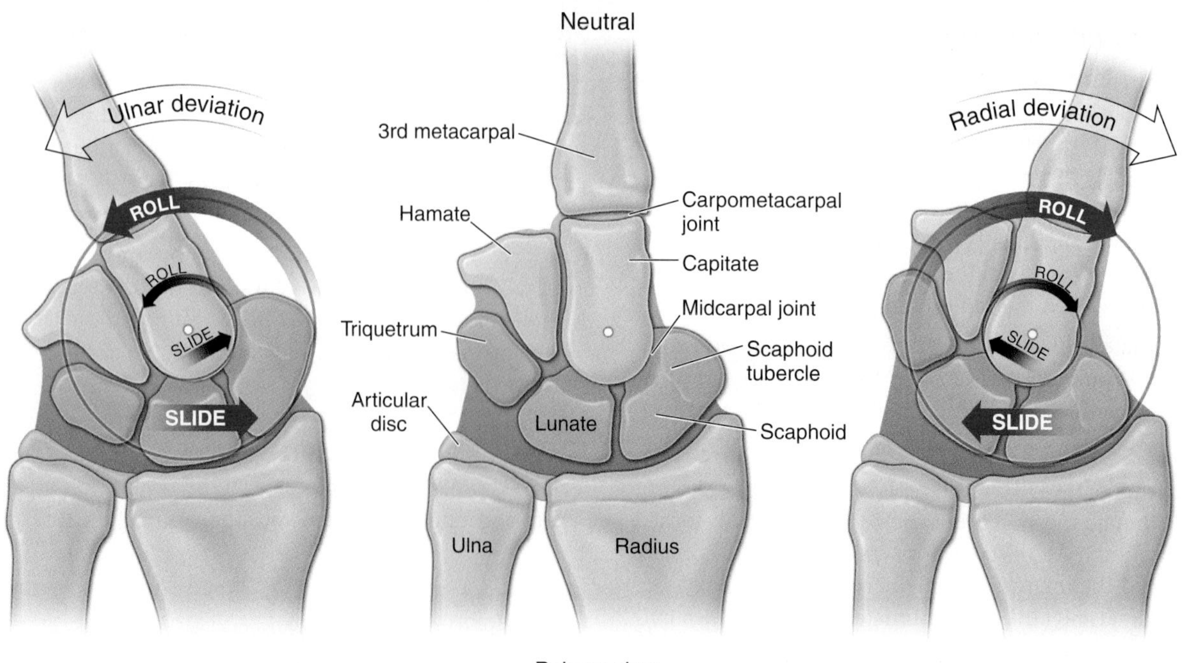

FIGURE 18-15 A model of the central column of the right wrist showing ulnar and radial deviation.

motion (Fig. 18-15).[42] At the radiocarpal joint, the scaphoid, lunate, and triquetrum roll ulnarly and slide a significant distance radially.[42] Ulnar deviation of the midcarpal joint occurs primarily from the capitate rolling ulnarly and sliding slightly radially.[42] Ulnar deviation is limited by the radial collateral ligament.[62] Although ulnar deviation brings the triquetrum into contact with the TFCC, the lack of direct ulnar-triquetral articulation permits a greater range of ulnar deviation. The muscle with the best biomechanical advantage to produce ulnar deviation of the wrist in pronation is the ECU.[23]

Radial Deviation

Radial deviation at the wrist occurs through similar arthrokinematics as described for ulnar deviation (Fig. 18-15).[42] Radial deviation occurs primarily between the proximal and the distal rows of the carpal bones. The motion of radial deviation is limited by impact of the scaphoid onto the radial styloid and the UCL. The APL and EPB are best suited to produce radial deviation of the wrist.[23]

CLINICAL PEARL

Extension of the wrist is accompanied by radial deviation, and flexion of the wrist is accompanied by ulnar deviation. The wrist also allows relatively extensive traction and gliding accessory movements.

A number of studies have examined the necessary range of motion at the wrist to perform functional activities. These studies report that at least 5 degrees of wrist flexion, 35 degrees of wrist extension, 10 degrees of radial deviation, and 15 degrees of ulnar deviation are needed to perform common personal care activities comfortably.[63,64] Less motion is required for 90 percent of personal care activities: 5 degrees of flexion, 6 degrees of extension, 7 degrees of radial deviation, and 6 degrees of ulnar deviation.[65]

Wrist Movements and the Digits

The position of the wrist in flexion or extension influences the tension of the long or "extrinsic" muscles of the digits. The position of the wrist also has important repercussions on the position of the thumb and fingers. Neither the flexors nor the extensors of the fingers are long enough to allow maximal range of motion at the wrist and the fingers simultaneously.[23] In fact, due to the restraining action of the long antagonistic muscles, complete flexion of the fingers is possible only if the wrist is in approximately 20 degrees of extension, which corresponds to the optimal position for hand function.[23] Thus the movements of the wrist reinforce the action of the extrinsic muscles of the fingers, and are synergistic with the more powerful digital flexors. As the wrist position changes, the functional lengths of the digital flexor tendons change and the resultant forces in finger flexion vary. In order for grip to be effective and have maximal force, the wrist must be stable and positioned in slight extension and ulnar deviation.[23]

CLINICAL PEARL

Studies have evaluated the effect of wrist position on the force generated at the middle and distal phalanges and found that the greatest force is exerted in ulnar deviation and then extension, with the least force being generated in flexion.[66]

Articulations of the Fingers

There are notable differences between the IP and MCP articulations of the digits and even between the articulations at the same level for each digit.[23] These differences are produced by

- the shape of the articulations;
- the orientation of the articular surface;
- the synovial insertion;
- the disposition of the collateral ligaments;
- the degree of play in the volar plate.

These elements determine the degree of mobility and stability of these articulations and the orientation of the distal segments. As the thumb pulp pronates in opposition, the pulps of the fingers supinate in external rotation when the MCP joints flex, or when the index finger moves radially. These variations in orientation allow for optimal use of the finger pulps for functional tasks of the hand (see Functional Position of the Hand).[23]

CLINICAL PEARL

The goal of functional restoration for the MCP joint flexion is 75 degrees for the index finger and middle finger, 80 degrees for the ring finger, and 85 degrees for the little finger.[23]

Thumb Movements

The first CMC joint is a saddle joint. The characteristic feature of a saddle joint is that each articular surface is concave in one diameter and convex in the other. Within the first CMC joint, the longitudinal diameter of the articular surface of the trapezium is generally concave from an anterior (palmar) to posterior (dorsal) direction, while the transverse diameter is generally convex along a medial to lateral direction. The proximal articular surface of the first metacarpal is reciprocally shaped to that of the trapezium. This articular relationship produces the following (Fig. 18-16):

- Thumb flexion and extension occur around an anterior–posterior axis in the frontal plane that is perpendicular to the sagittal plane of finger flexion and extension. In this plane, the metacarpal surface is concave, and the trapezium surface is convex. Flexion is accompanied by a conjunct rotation of internal rotation of the metacarpal. Extension is accompanied bya conjunct rotation of external rotation of the metacarpal. A total range of 50–70 degrees is available.
- Thumb abduction and adduction occur around a medial–lateral axis in the sagittal plane that is perpendicular to the frontal plane of finger abduction and adduction. During thumb abduction and adduction, the convex metacarpal surface moves on the concave trapezium. Abduction is accompanied by a conjunct rotation of internal rotation. Adduction is accompanied bya conjunct rotation of external rotation. A total range of 40–60 degrees is available.
- Opposition of the thumb involves a wide arc motion comprising sequential anterior (palmar) abduction and flexion from the anatomic position, accompanied by internal rotation of the thumb. Retroposition of the thumb returns the thumb to its anatomic position, a motion that incorporates the elements of adduction with extension and external rotation of the metacarpal.

Normal Ulnar Inclination of the Fingers

A normal ulnar inclination of the fingers occurs at the MCP joints due to a number of factors[23]:

- Asymmetry of the metacarpal heads and the collateral ligaments.
- Tendon factors: the extrinsic tendons, extensors, and flexors cross into the hand on the ulnar side of the longitudinal axis of the MCP joint.
- Muscle factors: the intrinsic muscles have a predominantly ulnar inclination and predominate over those with a radial inclination.
- The physiologic action of the thumb, which in lateral grip pushes the fingers in an ulnar direction.

The inclination is most marked in the index finger, less in the middle and little fingers, and almost nonexistent in the ring finger. The ulnar inclination is normally limited by the capsuloligamentous resistance at the MCP joints and by the action of the interosseous muscles, which act in a radial direction.[23] The weakness of these stabilizing elements, particularly in rheumatoid arthritis (RA), allows the ulnar inclination to be accentuated, resulting in pathologic ulnar deviation.

Functional Position of the Hand

Grips

The grip is typically divided into following stages[67,68]:

- Opening of the hand.
- Positioning and closing of the fingers to grasp an object and adapt to the object's shape.

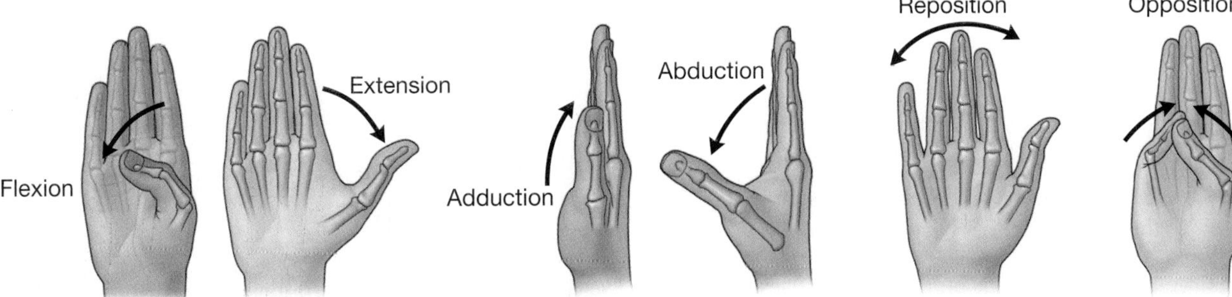

FIGURE 18-16 Thumb motions.

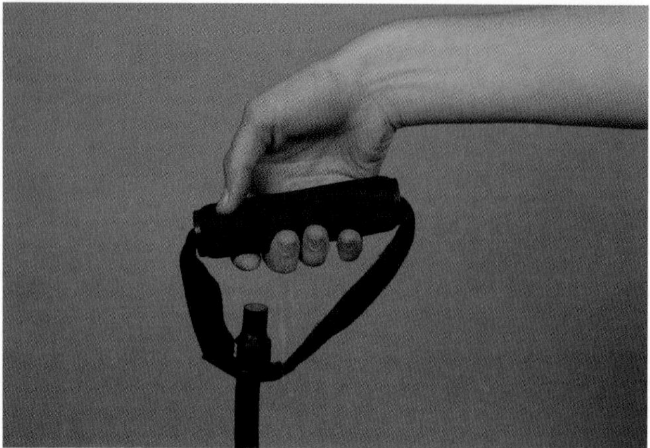

FIGURE 18-17 Hook grasp.

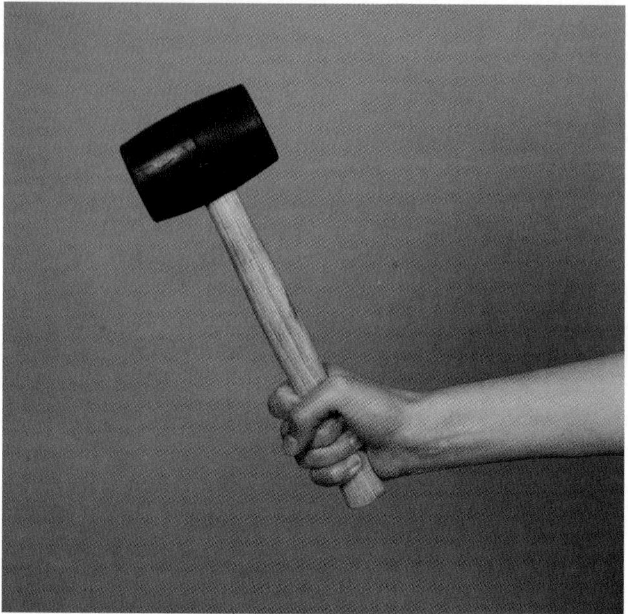

FIGURE 18-18 Fist grasp.

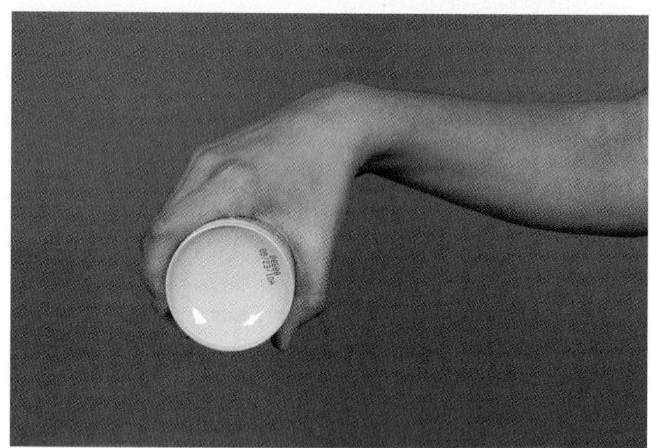

FIGURE 18-19 Cylindrical grasp.

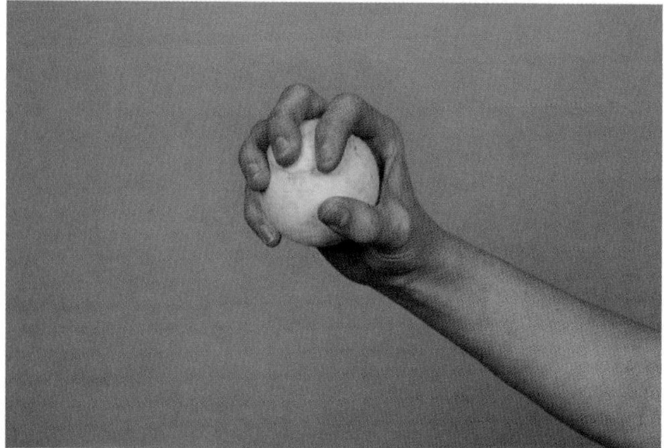

FIGURE 18-20 Spherical grasp.

- Controlled approach and purposeful closing of the fingers and/or palm. The amount of force exerted is determined by the weight, surface characteristics, and fragility of the object.[69]
- Maintenance and stabilization of the grip. This phase is not used in precision tasks.
- The release of the object.

Two major types of grips have been recognized: power grip and the precision or prehension grip.

Power Grip. The power grip involves the use of force to stabilize an object in the hand. The strength and power of a grip comes from a combination of

- thumb adduction,
- isometric flexion,
- an approximation of the thenar and hypothenar eminences,
- intact function of the ulnar side of the hand.

The power grips include the following:

- ***Hook grasp.*** This grasp involves all or the second and third fingers (the IP joint only for the IP and MCP joints of the fingers) and is controlled by the forearm flexors and extensors (Fig. 18-17).
- ***Fist grasp.*** In this grasp the hand moves around a narrow object (Fig. 18-18)
- ***Cylindrical grasp.*** In this grasp, the thumb is used and the entire hand wraps around an object (Fig. 18-19)
- ***Spherical grasp.*** This grasp involves the hand moving around a spherical object as it moves into position (Fig. 18-20)

Participation of the intrinsic muscles follows specific patterns in the various power grips. For example,

- the hook grip involves the fourth posterior (dorsal) interosseus, fourth lumbrical, and the ADM;
- the spherical grip involves all of the interossei (except the second), the ADM, and the fourth lumbrical.[70,71]

Precision Grip. In the precision grip, the muscles primarily function to provide exact control of finger and thumb position, so the position of the handled object can be changed either in space or about its own axis.[67,71] Due to the higher levels of sensory input required during these tasks, the areas with the most sensory receptors are used. A number of precision grips are recognized[23,62]:

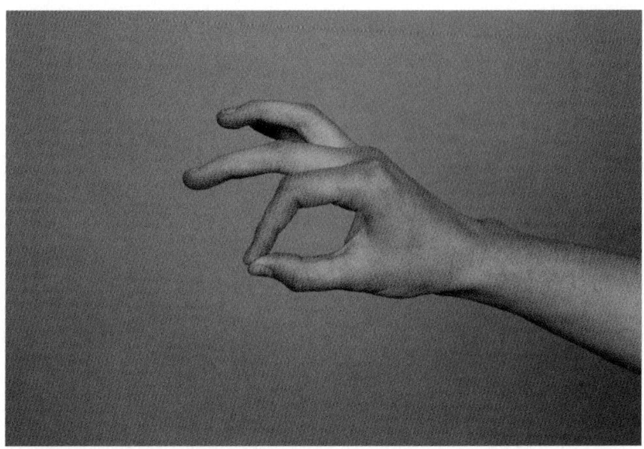

FIGURE 18-21 Pulp-to-pulp pinch prehension.

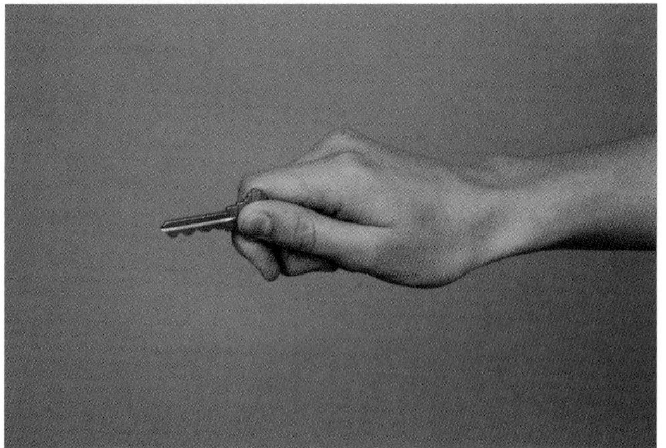

FIGURE 18-22 Lateral prehension.

- *Pulp-to-pulp pinch,* in which the pad of the thumb is opposed to the pad of one or more fingers (Fig. 18-21).
- *Lateral prehension,* where the anterior (palmar) aspect of the thumb presses against the radial aspect of the first phalanx of the index finger (Fig. 18-22).
- *Tip prehension,* in which the extreme tip of the thumb pad is opposed to the tip of the index or middle finger.
- *Three-fingered pinch* (thumb, index finger, and middle finger), as in sprinkling herbs, and multi-fingered pinch (Fig. 18-23).

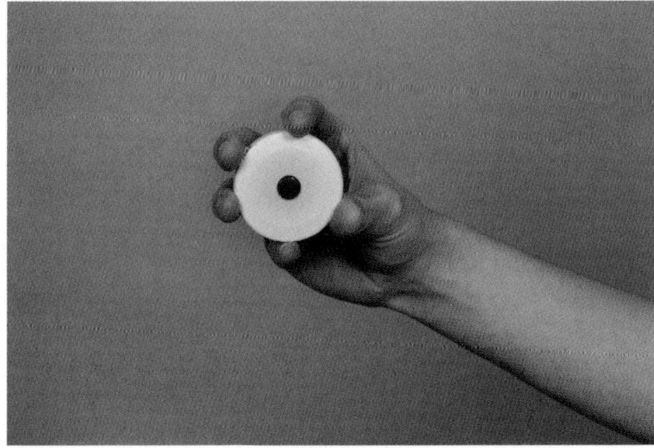

FIGURE 18-23 Multi-fingered pinch.

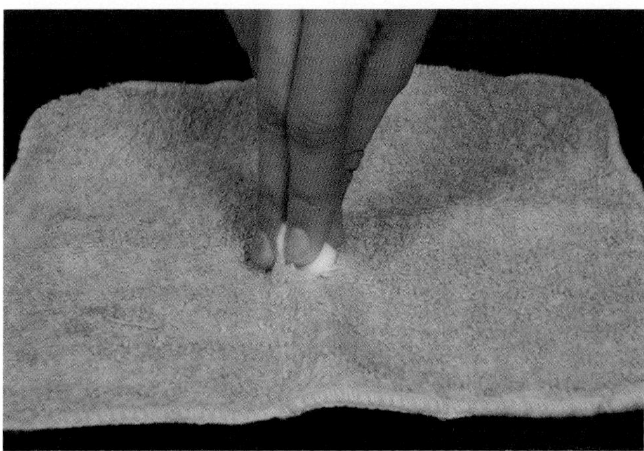

FIGURE 18-24 Five-fingered pinch.

- *Five-fingered pinch,* as in picking up a face towel (Fig. 18-24).

The radial side of the hand and the MCP joints are involved more in the precision or prehensile types of grips.[23,62]

Different grip patterns are used regularly during daily functional activities (Table 18-3).[1,72]

EXAMINATION

Elucidating the cause of forearm, wrist, and hand pain can be challenging. The examination must include all regions that may contribute to the symptoms of forearm, wrist, and hand pain or numbness. This requires a sound knowledge of differential diagnosis and often incorporates an examination of the entire upper kinetic chain, including the cervical and thoracic spine.

The common pathologies for the forearm, wrist, and hand and their interventions are detailed after the "Examination" section. An understanding of both is obviously necessary. As mention of the various pathologies occurs with reference to the tests and measures and vice versa, the reader is encouraged to switch between the two.

History

The assessment of the forearm, wrist, and hand begins by recording a detailed history to help focus the examination. All

TABLE 18-3 Estimated Use of Grips for Activities of Daily Living

Type of Grip	Estimated Use (%)
Pulp-to-pulp pinch	20
Lateral pinch	20
Five-fingered pinch	15
Fist grip	15
Cylinder grip	14
Three-fingered pinch	10
Spherical grip	4
Hook grip	2

Data from McPhee SD: Functional hand evaluations: a review. *Am J Occup Ther* 41:158–163, 1987.

relevant information must be gathered about the site, nature, behavior, and onset of the current symptoms. This should include information about the patient's age, hand dominance, avocational activities, and occupation.

CLINICAL PEARL

The non-neutral position of the hand is extension, flexion, or ulnar deviation.[73,74] Sustained non-neutral positions of the hand and wrist subject nerves to prolonged stretch and periods of high pressure.[75] In addition, these positions place muscles in inefficient length–tension relationships,[74] resulting in decreased transmission of contractile forces to the fingers.[74,76]

In addition to those questions covered in Chapter 4, the following questions should be asked:

- ***When did the symptoms occur?*** The date of injury is particularly important, especially as simple traumatic arthritis of the wrist does not last more than a few days if the wrist is rested.
- ***Was there a mechanism of injury?*** If the problem is trauma related, the clinician should ascertain the following:
  - The forces applied. For example, a rotational force applied to the wrist region may lead to a fracture of the radius and dislocation of the distal end of the ulna (Galeazzi fracture).
  - Where and when the injury occurred.
  - The position of the wrist and hand at the time of the trauma. For example, a fall on the outstretched hand (FOOSH) injury can lead to a lunate dislocation, Colles fracture, or scaphoid fracture.
  - Whether the environmental conditions were clean or dirty (if a wound is present).
  - Whether there was an accompanying "pop" or "click."
  - Whether swelling occurred.

If the problem is nontrauma related, the onset of pain or sensory change, swelling, or contracture should be ascertained.

- ***Are there any local areas of tenderness?*** Localized tenderness may indicate a carpal fracture, particularly of the scaphoid. Scaphoid fractures are associated with a load applied to the radial side of the palm when the wrist is in extreme extension,[77] and can be ongoing sources of pain and dysfunction (refer to "Intervention Strategies"). Pain along the radial aspect of the wrist and forearm is a common symptom for several pathoanatomical diagnoses, including de Quervain disease, intersection syndrome, intercarpal instabilities, scaphoid fracture, superficial radial neuritis, C6 cervical radiculitis/radiculopathy, and arthrosis of the first CMC, intercarpal, or radiocarpal joints.[78]
- ***How does the patient rate his or her pain?*** The patient's perception of their pain can be measured using a visual analog scale.
- ***What is the behavior of the symptoms?*** The clinician should note the sequence of symptoms, the level of functional impairment, the progression of symptoms, the time of day the symptoms are worse, and whether the symptoms appear to be posture related or work related. Knowledge of the past behavior of previous wrist, hand, and finger disorders and their interventions can help in assessing the nature and prognosis of the patient's current problem.
- ***Which hand is the dominant hand (DH) of the patient?*** Dysfunction of the DH can be very disabling, so inquiries concerning the functional demands of the patient must be made.

Systems Review

A complete review of the medical history and general health of the patient should be included along with a review of systems, and the presence of other orthopaedic, neurologic, or cardiopulmonary conditions. An upper quarter scanning examination is performed to provide an overview of the upper extremity, the direction for a more detailed examination, and to rule out referral from the cervical, thoracic, shoulder girdle, and elbow joints.

The clinician should be able to determine the suitability of the patient for physical therapy. All inflammatory conditions, whether infectious or not, are accompanied by diffuse pain or tenderness with movement. RA often affects this region with more severity and frequency than elsewhere. Therefore questions concerning other joint involvement and general debility must be asked. The presence of CTS, which is usually felt more at night, may also indicate RA.

If the clinician is concerned with any signs or symptoms of a visceral, vascular, neurogenic, psychogenic, spondylogenic, or systemic disorder that is out of the scope of physical therapy (see Chapter 5), the patient should be referred back to their physician.

Tests and Measures

Observation

The physical examination should begin with a general observation of the patient's posture—especially the cervical spine, the thoracic spine, and the position of the hand in relation to the body. For example, is the arm held against the chest in a protective manner, does the arm swing during the gait pattern, or does it just hang loosely? The patient's hands can be highly informative (Table 18-4). Although very subtle, the DH tends to be larger than the nondominant hand. The posture and alignment of the involved wrist and hand are examined. Wrist angulation into ulnar deviation increases shearing in the first posterior (dorsal) compartment. This angulation can predispose the patient to de Quervain syndrome (see "Intervention Strategies").[79] A prominence of the distal ulna may indicate DRUJ instability.[80] The posture of the hand should be analyzed. The clinician should observe how the patient appears to relate to the involved hand and if or how the patient attempts to use the hand.[11] The contour of the anterior (palmar) surface, including the arches, should be examined. If a finger

TABLE 18-4 Outline of Physical Findings of the Hand

Variations in size and shape of hand

- A. Large, blunt fingers (spade hand)
  - 1. Acromegaly
  - 2. Hurler disease (gargoylism)
- B. Gross irregularity of shape and size
  - 1. Paget disease of bone
  - 2. Maffucci syndrome
  - 3. Neurofibromatosis
- C. Spider fingers, slender palm (arachnodactyly)
  - 1. Hypopituitarism
  - 2. Eunuchism
  - 3. Ehlers–Danlos syndrome, pseudoxanthoma elasticum
  - 4. Tuberculosis
  - 5. Asthenic habitus
  - 6. Osteogenesis imperfecta
- D. Sausage-shaped phalanges
  - 1. Rickets (beading of joints)
  - 2. Granulomatous dactylitis (tuberculosis, syphilis)
- E. Spindliform joints (fingers)
  - 1. Early rheumatoid arthritis
  - 2. Systemic lupus erythematosus
  - 3. Psoriasis
  - 4. Rubella
  - 5. Boeck sarcoidosis
  - 6. Osteoarthritis
- F. Cone-shaped fingers
  - 1. Pituitary obesity
  - 2. Frohlich dystrophy
- G. Unilateral enlargement of hand
  - 1. Arteriovenous aneurysm
  - 2. Maffucci syndrome
- H. Square, dry hands
  - 1. Cretinism
  - 2. Myxedema
- I. Single, widened, flattened distal phalanx
  - 1. Sarcoidosis
- J. Shortened fourth and fifth metacarpals (bradymetacarpalism)
- K. Shortened, incurved fifth finger (symptom of DuBois)
  - 1. Mongolism
  - 2. Behavioral problem
  - 3. Gargoylism (broad, short, thick-skinned hand)
- L. Malposition and abduction, fifth finger
  - 1. Turner syndrome (gonadal dysgenesis, webbed neck, etc.)
- M. Syndactylism
  - 1. Congenital malformations of the heart, great vessels
  - 2. Multiple congenital deformities
  - 3. Laurence-Moon-Biedl syndrome
  - 4. In normal individuals as an inherited trait
- N. Clubbed fingers
  - 1. Subacute bacterial endocarditis
  - 2. Pulmonary causes
    - a. Tuberculosis
    - b. Pulmonary arteriovenous fistula
    - c. Pulmonic abscess
    - d. Pulmonic cysts
    - e. Bullous emphysema
    - f. Pulmonary hypertrophic osteoarthropathy
    - g. Bronchogenic carcinoma
  - 3. Alveolocapillary block
    - a. Interstitial pulmonary fibrosis
    - b. Sarcoidosis
    - c. Beryllium poisoning
    - d. Sclerodermatous lung
    - e. Asbestosis
    - f. Miliary tuberculosis
    - g. Alveolar cell carcinoma
  - 4. Cardiovascular causes
    - a. Patent ductus arteriosus
    - b. Tetralogy of Fallot
    - c. Taussig-Bing complex
    - d. Pulmonic stenosis
    - e. Ventricular septal defect
  - 5. Diarrheal states
    - a. Ulcerative colitis
    - b. Tuberculous enteritis
    - c. Sprue
    - d. Amebic dysentery
    - e. Bacillary dysentery
    - f. Parasitic infestation (gastrointestinal tract)
  - 6. Hepatic cirrhosis
  - 7. Myxedema
  - 8. Polycythemia
  - 9. Chronic urinary tract infections (upper and lower)
    - a. Chronic nephritis
  - 10. Hyperparathyroidism (telescopy of distal phalanx)
  - 11. Pachydermoperiostosis (syndrome of Touraine, Solente, and Gole)
- O. Joint disturbances
  - 1. Arthritides
    - a. Osteoarthritis
    - b. Rheumatoid arthritis
    - c. Systemic lupus erythematosus
    - d. Gout
    - e. Psoriasis
    - f. Sarcoidosis
    - g. Endocrinopathy (acromegaly)
    - h. Rheumatic fever
    - i. Reiter syndrome
    - j. Dermatomyositis
  - 2. Anaphylactic reaction-serum sickness
  - 3. Scleroderma

II. Edema of the hand

- A. Cardiac disease (congestive heart failure)
- B. Hepatic disease
- C. Renal disease
  - 1. Nephritis
  - 2. Nephrosis
- A. Hemiplegic hand
- B. Syringomyelia
- C. Superior vena caval syndrome
  - 1. Superior thoracic outlet tumor
  - 2. Mediastinal tumor or inflammation
  - 3. Pulmonary apex tumor
  - 4. Aneurysm
- A. Generalized anasarca, hypoproteinemia
- B. Postoperative lymphedema (radical breast amputation)
- C. Ischemic paralysis (cold, blue, swollen, numb)
- D. Lymphatic obstruction
  - 1. Lymphomatous masses in axilla
- A. Axillary mass
  - 1. Metastatic tumor, abscess, leukemia, Hodgkin disease
- A. Aneurysm of ascending or transverse aorta or of axillary artery
- B. Pressure on innominate or subclavian vessels
- C. Raynaud disease
- D. Myositis
- E. Cervical rib
- F. Trichiniasis
- G. Scalenus anticus syndrome

III. Neuromuscular effects

- A. Atrophy
  - 1. Painless
    - a. Amyotrophic lateral sclerosis
    - b. Charcot–Marie–Tooth peroneal atrophy
    - c. Syringomyelia (loss of heat, cold, and pain sensation)
    - d. Neural leprosy
  - 2. Painful
    - a. Peripheral nerve disease
  - 3. Radial nerve (wrist drop)
    - a. Lead poisoning, alcoholism, polyneuritis, trauma

(Continued)

TABLE 18-4 Outline of Physical Findings of the Hand *(Continued)*

b. Diphtheria, polyarteritis, neurosyphilis, anterior poliomyelitis
4. Ulnar nerve (benediction palsy)
 a. Polyneuritis, trauma
5. Median nerve (claw hand)
 a. Carpal tunnel syndrome
6. Rheumatoid arthritis
7. Tenosynovitis at wrist
8. Amyloidosis
9. Gout
10. Plasmacytoma
11. Anaphylactic reaction
12. Menopause syndrome
13. Myxedema

B. Extrinsic pressure on the nerve (cervical, axillary, supraclavicular, or brachial)
 1. Pancoast tumor (pulmonary apex)
 2. Aneurysms of subclavian arteries, axillary vessels, or thoracic aorta
 3. Costoclavicular syndrome
 4. Superior thoracic outlet syndrome
 5. Cervical rib
 6. Degenerative arthritis of cervical spine
 7. Herniation of cervical intervertebral disk

C. Shoulder–hand syndrome
 1. Myocardial infarction
 2. Pancoast tumor
 3. Brain tumor
 4. Intrathoracic neoplasms
 5. Discogenic disease
 6. Cervical spondylosis
 7. Febrile panniculitis
 8. Senility
 9. Vascular occlusion
 10. Hemiplegia
 11. Osteoarthritis
 12. Herpes zoster

D. Ischemic contractures (sensory loss in fingers)
 1. Tight plaster cast applications

E. Polyarteritis nodosa

F. Polyneuritis
 1. Carcinoma of lung
 2. Hodgkin disease
 3. Pregnancy
 4. Gastric carcinoma
 5. Reticuloses
 6. Diabetes mellitus
 7. Chemical neuritis
  a. Antimony, benzene, bismuth, carbon tetrachloride, heavy metals, alcohol, arsenic lead, gold, emetine
 8. Ischemic neuropathy
 9. Vitamin B deficiency
 10. Atheromata
 11. Arteriosclerosis
 12. Embolic

G. Carpodigital (carpopedal spasm) tetany
 1. Hypoparathyroidism
 2. Hyperventilation
 3. Uremia
 4. Nephritis
 5. Nephrosis
 6. Rickets
 7. Sprue
 8. Malabsorption syndrome
 9. Pregnancy
 10. Lactation
 11. Osteomalacia
 12. Protracted vomiting
 13. Pyloric obstruction
 14. Alkali poisoning
 15. Chemical toxicity
  a. Morphine, lead, alcohol

H. Tremor
 1. Parkinsonism
 2. Familial disorder
 3. Hypoglycemia
 4. Hyperthyroidism
 5. Wilson disease (hepatolenticular degeneration)
 6. Anxiety
 7. Ataxia
 8. Athetosis
 9. Alcoholism, narcotic addiction
 10. Multiple sclerosis
 11. Chorea (Sydenham, Huntington)

Data from Berry TJ: *The Hand as a Mirror of Systemic Disease*. Philadelphia: FA Davis Co, 1963; Juddge RD, Zuidema GD, Fitzgerald FT: General appearance. In: Judge RD, Zuidema GD, Fitzgerald FT, eds. *Clinical Diagnosis*, 4th ed. Boston, Little, Brown and Company, 1982:29–47.

is involved, its attitude should be observed. Digital deformities are the hallmark of RA.[81]

A visual inspection of the involved wrist and hand is made and is compared with the uninvolved side. The clinician inspects for lacerations, surgical scars, masses, swelling, or erythema.

- Scars should be examined for degree of adherence, degree of maturation, hypertrophy (excess collagen within the boundary of the wound), and keloid (excess collagen that no longer conforms to wound boundaries).
- The location and type of edema should be noted. Edema, the accumulation of fluid in the intercellular spaces, is a common consequence of surgery or injury to the hand. A determination is made as to whether the swelling is generalized or localized, hard or soft. Anterior effusion over the flexor tendons at the wrist may indicate rheumatoid tenovaginitis. Swelling that persists more than a few days following trauma probably suggests a carpal fracture. Localized swelling accompanied by redness and tenderness may indicate an infection. Measuring edema is an important part of the physical examination of individuals with conditions affecting the wrist and hand. Volumetry, a clinical application of Archimedes principle of water displacement as a measure of volume, is considered the gold standard for measuring hand size.[82] This method involves lowering the limb into a water-filled Plexiglass or metal tank (the volumeter) and measuring the amount of water displaced.[83] The reliability and validity of volumetric measurements is well established.[82] However, this method is time consuming and requires specialized equipment. An alternative method of measuring is the figure-of-eight method. Compared to volumetric method, the figure-of-eight method is more practical for clinical use as the procedure takes less time to perform and requires equipment that is less expensive and is readily available in most clinical settings.[82] The correct application of the tape is described in Table 18-5. Leard and colleagues[82] reported the figure-of-eight method to be a reliable and valid measure of hand size in individuals with conditions affecting the hand.

TABLE 18-5	Figure-of-Eight Taping Method
Step	**Description**
1	The starting point for the tape measure is the outermost aspect (medial surface using anatomical position as a reference) of the most distal aspect of the ulna styloid process.
2	The tape measure is drawn across the ventral surface of the wrist to the most distal aspect of the radial styloid process.
3	The tape measure is placed diagonally across the posterior (dorsal) aspect of the hand with the proximal surface of the tape measure placed over the fifth metacarpophalangeal (MCP) joint line.
4	The tape measure is then brought across the ventral surface of the MCP joints and the proximal surface of the tape measure is positioned over the second MCP joint line.
5	The tape measure is wrapped diagonally across the dorsum of the hand back to the starting point.

Data from Leard JS, Breglio L, Fraga L, et al: Reliability and concurrent validity of the Figure-of-Eight method of measuring hand size in patients with hand pathology. *J Orthop Sports Phys Ther* 34:335–340, 2004.

CLINICAL PEARL

The normal physiologic angles for relaxed hand posture are 14–15 degrees of ulnar deviation for the index finger, 13 degrees for the middle finger, 4 degrees for the ring finger, and 7–8 degrees for the little finger.

The swan-neck deformity is one of the most frequently encountered deformities of the fingers (see "Intervention Strategies").[81] When it occurs at the thumb it is referred to as a zigzag deformity. Any other finger deformities such as mallet finger and boutonniere (see "Rheumatoid Arthritis") are noted (Table 18-6). Other hand deformities include the following:

- ***Ulnar drift.*** The classic deformity of ulnar shift and ulnar deviation is associated with RA (although it can occur in other conditions) and the MCP joints. The deformity occurs due to the cumulative effects of various factors. Initially, the MCP joint capsule and ligamentous structures are stretched by the proliferation of the synovium, which loosens the collateral ligaments and decreases joint stability (see "Rheumatoid Arthritis").
- ***Extensor plus.*** This deformity results from either shortening of the extensor communis tendon or adherence of the tendon to the first part of the proximal phalanx at the extensor hood. It results in the inability to flex the PIP and MCP joints simultaneously, although each joint can be flexed normally individually.
- ***Myelopathy hand.*** This deformity, which is characterized by a loss of power in abduction and extension of the ulnar fingers, is caused by cervical spinal cord pathology in conjunction with cervical spondylosis.[86] Confirmation of this finding is made when lower motor neuron findings are seen at the level of the lesion while upper motor neuron findings are seen below the level of the lesion.

The nails should be inspected to see if they are healthy and pink (Table 18-7). Local trauma to the nails seldom involves more than one or two digits. The nails should be checked for hangnail infection or whether they appear ridged, which could indicate a RA dysfunction. Clubbed nails are an indication of hypertrophy of underlying structures. The presence of a paronychia or a pale paronychia should prompt the clinician to probe the axilla and neck lymph nodes for tenderness and swelling. Beau lines are transverse furrows that begin at the lunula and progress distally as the nail grows. They result from a temporary arrest of growth of the nail matrix occasioned by trauma or systemic stress.[87] With the knowledge that nails grow about 0.1 mm/day, by measuring the distance between the Beau lines and the cuticle, one may be able to approximately determine the date of the stress. For example, if the distance is 5 mm, the stress event occurred approximately 50 days before. Spoon nails (koilonychias) may occur in a form of iron deficiency anemia (Plummer–Vinson syndrome), coronary disease, and with the use of strong detergents.[87] Clubbing of the nails, characterized by a bulbous enlargement of the distal portion of the digits, may occur in association with cardiovascular disease, subacute endocarditis, advanced cor pulmonale, and pulmonary disease.[87]

Finger color should be observed. Fingers that are white in appearance might indicate Raynaud disease. Blotchy or red fingers might indicate liver disease. Blue fingers may indicate a circulatory problem.

Intrinsic muscle fibrosis is characterized by stiffness at the IP joints. On flexion of the MCP joint, extension of the fingers becomes tight and flexion is restricted. On extension of the MCP joint, flexion of the IP joints is possible.

- Adhesions proximal to the MCP joint allow lumbrical action (i.e., MCP flexion and PIP and DIP joint extension).
- Adhesions distal to the MCP joints result in the ability to extend the MCP and flex the PIP and DIP joints, but there is no extension possible in the fingers.

Palpation. Palpation of the wrist and hand is an integral component of the physical examination. Palpation may be performed separately or with the range-of-motion tests. Fortunately, most of the structures are superficial (Fig. 18-25), so a sound knowledge of surface anatomy is essential. The findings from palpation can often be confirmed using a specific special test (see "Special Tests"). Palpation of the following muscles, tendon, insertions, ligaments, capsules, and bones should occur as indicated and be compared with the uninvolved side for tenderness and/or swelling.

Trapezium. The trapezium is located immediately proximal to the base of the first metacarpal bone, just distal to the scaphoid. The tubercle of the trapezium lies anteriorly at the base of the thenar eminence. It can be made more prominent by opposing the thumb to the little finger and ulnarly deviating the wrist. Tenderness over this carpal may

TABLE 18-6 Hand and Finger Deformities and Their Possible Causes	
Deformity	**Possible Cause**
MCP joint flexion	Rupture of the extensor tendon just proximal to the MCP joint
Hyperextension of the MCP joint	Paralysis of the interossei
Deepening of the anterior (palmar) gutter and an inability to fully stretch out the palm	Tightness of the anterior (palmar) aponeurosis
Wasting of the hypothenar eminence and a clawed hand with flexion of the fourth and fifth digits (hand of benediction)	Ulnar nerve palsy
Wrist drop with increased flexion of the wrist, flexion of the MCP joint, and extension of the DIP joints	Radial nerve lesion
Isolated thenar atrophy	Arthritis of the carpometacarpal joint Median nerve lesion C8 or T1 nerve root lesion
Ape-hand deformity with a wasting of the thenar eminence and an inability to oppose or flex the thumb or abduct it in its own plane[84]	Median nerve palsy
Z-deformity of the wrist	Pattern of deformity in the rheumatoid hand[85]
Atrophy of the hand intrinsics	Pancoast tumor
Claw-hand deformity	Loss of ulnar nerve motor innervation to the hand, with resultant paralysis of the interosseous muscles, and muscle atrophy of the hypothenar eminence; this deformity is more severe in lesions distal to innervation of the FDP muscle, as this muscle adds to the flexion force upon the IP joints[6]
PIP hyperextension and slight flexion of the DIP	Rupture or paralysis of the flexor digitorum superficialis (FDS)
A fixed flexion deformity of the MCP and PIP joints, especially in the ring or little finger	Dupuytren contracture
A hook-like contracture of the flexor muscles, which is worse with wrist extension as compared to flexion	Volkmann ischemic contracture

DIP, distal interphalangeal; FDP, flexor digitorum profundus; MCP, metacarpophalangeal; PIP, proximal interphalangeal.

indicate scaphotrapezial arthritis secondary to scaphoid instability.[13]

Thumb CMC Joint. To examine the thumb CMC joint, the clinician palpates carefully along the shaft of the thumb metacarpal down to its proximal flare. Just proximal to this flare is a small depression where the CMC joint is located. By applying direct radial and ulnar stresses to the joint, the clinician can determine the overall stability of the joint as compared to the other thumb. Tenderness here is usually indicative of degenerative arthritis.

EPB, APL, and FCR Tendons. The EPB and APL tendons make up the first extensor compartment on the dorsum of the wrist and together form the radial border of the anatomic snuffbox. The APL is the first prominent tendon medially. Prominence of these tendons can be enhanced by extending and radially abducting the thumb. Tenderness over these tendons may indicate de Quervain tenosynovitis. Just medial to the APL is the radial artery with the FCR tendon, which inserts on the second metacarpal, situated medially.

Flexor Retinaculum. The flexor retinaculum, which can be palpated just medial to the FCR, transforms the carpal arch into the carpal tunnel. It is attached medially to the pisiform and hook of the hamate and laterally to the tubercle of the scaphoid and tubercle of the trapezium. Its proximal edge is at the distal crease of the wrist. The retinaculum can be the location for a retinacular cyst which, because of its firmness, is frequently mistaken for a bony spur.

Hamate. The hook of the hamate is palpated just distal and radial (in the direction of the thumb web space) to the pisiform on the anterior (palmar) aspect. Locating the hamate can be made easier if the clinician places the middle of the distal phalanx of the thumb on the pisiform, with the thumb pointing between the web space between the index and long finger. The clinician flexes the IP joint of the thumb and presses into the hypothenar eminence to feel the firm hook. The hook of the hamate is concave laterally, and the ulnar nerve's superficial division, which is just lateral and proximal to the hook, can be rolled on it. Tenderness over this carpal is common, and so the clinician should compare

TABLE 18-7 Glossary of Nail Pathology

Condition	Description	Occurrence
Beau lines	Transverse lines or ridges marking repeated disturbances of nail growth	Systemic diseases, toxic or nutritional deficiency states of many types, trauma (from manicuring)
Defluvium unguium (onychomadesis)	Complete loss of nails	Certain systemic diseases such as scarlet fever, syphilis, leprosy, alopecia areata, and exfoliative dermatitis; dermatoses such as nail infection, psoriasis, eczema; arsenic poisoning.
Diffusion of lunula unguis	Spreading of lunula	Dystrophies of the extremities
Eggshell nails	Nail plate thin, semitransparent bluish-white, with a tendency to curve upward at the distal edge	Syphilis
Fragilitas unguium	Friable or brittle nails	Dietary deficiency, local trauma
Hapalonychia	Nails very soft, split easily	Following contact with strong alkalis; endocrine disturbances, malnutrition, syphilis, chronic arthritis
Hippocratic nails	Watch-glass nails associated with drumstick fingers	Chronic respiratory and circulatory diseases, especially pulmonary tuberculosis; hepatic cirrhosis
Koilonychia	"Spoon nails"; nails are concave on the outer surface	Dysendocrinisms (acromegaly), trauma, dermatoses, syphilis, nutritional deficiencies, hypothyroidism
Leukonychia	White spots or striations or rarely the whole nail may turn white (congenital type)	Local trauma, hepatic cirrhosis, nutritional deficiencies, and many systemic diseases
Mees lines	Transverse white bands	Hodgkin granuloma, arsenic and thallium toxicity, high fevers, local nutritional derangement
Moniliasis of nails	Infections (usually paronychial) caused by yeast forms (*Candida albicans*)	Occupational (common in food handlers, dentists, dishwashers, and gardeners)
Onychatrophia	Atrophy or failure of development of nails	Trauma, infection, dysendocrinism, gonadal aplasia, and many systemic disorders.
Onychauxis	Nail plate is greatly thickened	Mild persistent trauma, systemic diseases such as peripheral stasis, peripheral neuritis, syphilis, leprosy, hemiplegia, or at times may be congenital
Onychia	Inflammation of the nail matrix causing deformity of the nail plate	Trauma, infection, many systemic diseases
Onychodystrophy	Any deformity of the nail plate, nail bed, or nail matrix	Many diseases, trauma, or chemical agents (poisoning, allergy)
Onychogryposis	"Claw nails"; extreme degree of hypertrophy, sometimes with horny projections arising from the nail surface	May be congenital or related to many chronic systemic diseases (see "Onychauxis")
Onycholysis	Loosening of the nail plate beginning at the distal or free edge	Trauma, injury by chemical agents, many systemic diseases
Onychomadesis	See defluvium unguium.	
Onychophagia	Nail biting	Neurosis
Onychorrhexis	Longitudinal ridging and splitting of the nails	Dermatoses, nail infections, many systemic diseases, senility, injury by chemical agents, hyperthyroidism
Onychoschizia	Lamination and scaling away of nails in thin layers	Dermatoses, syphilis, injury by chemical agents

(Continued)

TABLE 18-7 Glossary of Nail Pathology *(Continued)*

Condition	Description	Occurrence
Onychotillomania	Alteration of the nail structures caused by persistent neurotic picking of the nails	Neurosis
Pachyonychia	Extreme thickening of all the nails; the nails are more solid and more regular than in onychogryposis	Usually congenital and associated with hyperkeratosis of the palms and soles
Pterygium unguis	Thinning of the nail fold and spreading of the cuticle over the nail plate	Associated with vasopastic conditions such as Raynaud phenomenon and occasionally with hypothyroidism

Data from Berry TJ: *The Hand as a Mirror of Systemic Disease*. Philadelphia, PA: FA Davis Co, 1963; Judge RD, Zuidema GD, Fitzgerald FT: General appearance. In: Judge RD, Zuidema GD, Fitzgerald FT, eds. *Clinical Diagnosis*, 4th ed. Boston, MA: Little, Brown and Company, 1982:29–47.

findings with the other side. Severe tenderness could indicate a fracture of the hamate, especially if associated with a FOOSH injury or a missed hit swing of a racket or bat.[88] The FCU tendon surrounds the hamate as it inserts on the pisiform.

Pisiform. The pisiform is located on the flexor aspect of the palm, on top of the triquetrum, at the distal crease. Tenderness of this structure may indicate pisotriquetral arthritis or inflammation of the FCU tendon.[4] The pisiform may be fractured from a direct fall or blow to the hypothenar aspect of the hand.

Triangular Fibrocartilage Complex. The TFCC is located distal to the ulnar styloid and proximal to the pisiform. Tenderness over this structure indicates an injury to the TFCC.[4]

Ulnar Head and Styloid Process. The ulnar head forms a rounded prominence on the ulnar side of the wrist, which is easily palpated on the posterior aspect of the hand with the forearm in pronation.[80] The ulnar styloid process is ulnar and distal to the head of the ulna. It is best located with the forearm in supination.

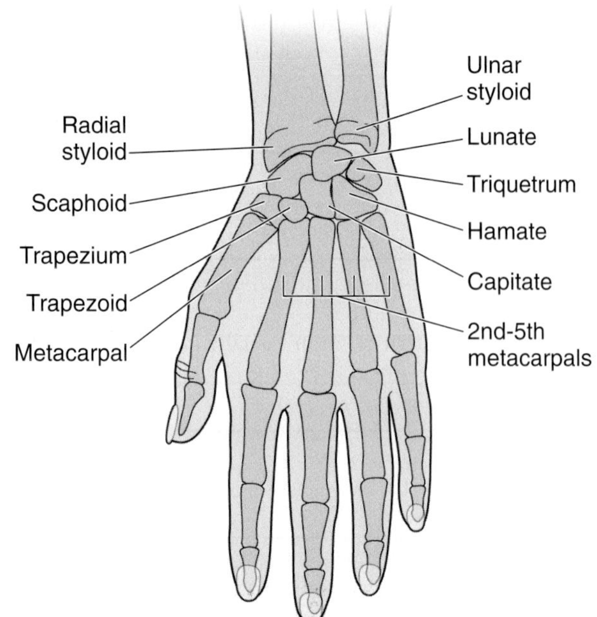

FIGURE 18-25 Bony structures of the hand.

Radial Styloid Process. The radial styloid process is larger and rounder than the ulnar styloid process. It is best palpated at the most proximal point of the anatomic snuffbox (see below), during radial abduction of the thumb. With simultaneous radial deviation of the wrist, this prominence becomes visible. Tenderness over the styloid, especially with radial deviation, may indicate contusion, fracture, or radioscaphoid arthritis.[89]

Lister's Tubercle. This is a small bony prominence on the posterior (dorsal) and distal end of radius. It is found by sliding a finger proximally from a point between the index and the middle fingers. Just distal to Lister's tubercle is the joint line of the scaphoid and radius. The ECRL and ECRB tendons travel radial to Lister's tubercle and insert on the base of the second and third metacarpals. The extensor digitorum communis (EDC) tendon travels ulnarly to Lister's tubercle. Radial to Lister's tubercle and proceeding further radially are the tendons of the ECRB, ECRL, EPB, and APL.

Scaphoid. The scaphoid is palpated just distal to the radial styloid in the anatomic snuffbox. The neck of the scaphoid is located on the floor of the anatomic snuffbox. Palpation can be made easier by positioning the wrist in ulnar deviation. The scaphoid may be grasped and moved passively by firm pressure between an opposed index finger and thumb applied to the anterior (palmar) surface and anatomic snuffbox simultaneously. In most individuals, the scaphoid is mildly tender to palpation, but those with a scaphoid fracture, nonunion, or scaphoid instability have severe discomfort (see "Special Tests").[2,90]

Lunate. The lunate is located just distal and ulnar to Lister's tubercle with the wrist flexed and is immediately proximal to, and in line with, the capitate. The mobile lunate can be felt to glide posteriorly (dorsally) with extension. It is the most commonly dislocated carpal and the scapholunate articulation is the most common area for carpal instability. Scapholunate synovitis (posterior (dorsal) wrist syndrome) or a scapholunate ligament injury presents with tenderness or fullness in this region.[2] Tenderness specific to the lunate can indicate Kienböck disease or osteonecrosis of the lunate.[91,92]

Capitate. The capitate is localized by palpating proximally over the posterior (dorsal) aspect of the third metacarpal until a small depression is felt. While palpating in this depression, as the wrist is flexed, the clinician should feel the capitate, the central bone of the carpals, move posteriorly (dorsally). Tenderness in this depression may indicate scapholunate or lunotriquetral instability, or capitolunate degenerative joint disease.

Second and Third Metacarpals. The base of the second and third metacarpals and the CMC joints are localized by palpating proximally along the posterior (dorsal) surfaces of the index and long metacarpals to their respective bases.[80] A bony prominence found at the base of the second or third metacarpal may be a carpal boss, a variation found in some individuals due to hypertrophic changes of traumatic origin.[80]

Triquetrum. The triquetrum is located by radially deviating the wrist while palpating just distal to the ulnar styloid. With ulnar deviation, the triquetrum articulates with the TFCC, which functions as a buffer between the styloid and the triquetrum. Tenderness and swelling in the triquetral hamate region are often present with midcarpal instability, which occurs when the anterior (palmar) triquetral–hamate–capitate ligament is ruptured or sprained.[93]

Tunnel of Guyon. The tunnel of Guyon is located in the space between the hamate and the pisiform.[6]

Carpal Tunnel. The distal wrist crease marks the proximal edge of the carpal tunnel. The boundaries of the carpal tunnel are as follows:

- ***Radial:*** scaphoid tubercle and trapezium.
- ***Ulnar:*** pisiform and hamate.
- ***Posterior (dorsal):*** the carpal bones.
- ***Anterior (palmar):*** transverse carpal ligament.
- ***Proximal:*** antebrachial fascia.
- ***Distal:*** distal edge of the retinaculum at the CMC level, FCR, and scaphoid tubercle.

PIP Joints. Palpation of the PIP joint offers important information. Palpation of the joint over four planes (posterior (dorsal), anterior (palmar), medial, and lateral) allows assessment of point tenderness over ligamentous origins and insertions that is highly suggestive of underlying soft-tissue disruption.[22] In cases in which the joint is grossly swollen and tender, this part of the examination may provide more accurate information several days after the injury.[22]

Active Range of Motion (AROM), then Passive Range or Motion with Overpressure. The gross motions of wrist, hand, finger, and thumb flexion, extension, and radial and ulnar deviations are tested (Fig. 18-14), first actively and then passively (Table 18-8). Horger[94] conducted a reliability study to determine (a) the intrarater and interrater reliability of goniometric measurement of active and passive wrist motions under clinical conditions and (b) the effect of a therapist's specialization on the reliability of measurement. The results indicated that measurement of wrist motion by individual therapists is highly reliable and that intrarater reliability is higher than interrater reliability for all active and passive motions.[94] Interrater reliability was generally higher among specialized therapists for reasons not immediately apparent from this study.[94] With the exception of pain, identified sources of error were found to have surprisingly little effect on the reliability of measurement.[94]

TABLE 18-8 Active Range-of-Motion Norms for the Forearm, Wrist, and Hand

Motion	Degrees
Forearm pronation	85–90
Forearm supination	85–90
Radial deviation	15
Ulnar deviation	30–45
Wrist flexion	80–90
Wrist extension	70–90
Finger flexion	MCP: 85–90; PIP: 100–115; DIP: 80–90
Finger extension	MCP: 30–45; PIP: 0; DIP: 20
Finger abduction	20–30
Finger adduction	0
Thumb flexion	CMC: 45–50; MCP: 50–55; IP: 85–90
Thumb extension	MCP: 0; IP: 0–5
Thumb adduction	30
Thumb abduction	60–70

CMC, carpometacarpal; DIP, distal interphalangeal; IP, interphalangeal; MCP, metacarpophalangeal; PIP, proximal interphalangeal.

Any loss of motion compared with the contralateral, asymptomatic wrist and hand should be noted.

During measurement of motion, one must be aware that finger joint positions may affect wrist joint ranges (and vice versa) due to the constant length of the extrinsic tendons that cross multiple joints. Forearm pronation and supination can have a similar impact on joint ranges. For example,

- greater wrist flexion occurs with finger extension than with finger flexion because the ED tendons are not stretched maximally;
- less deviation range of motion is available when the wrist is fully extended or flexed.

Thus during the examination, the clinician should maintain all joints in a consistent position (usually neutral), except the one being measured. In addition, the clinician should identify wrist and finger joint position when measuring the strength of related muscles.

Somatic dysfunction of the wrist permits motion toward the dysfunction; motion away from the dysfunction will be restricted.

Fanning and folding of the hand is performed by palpating the anterior (palmar) surface of the pisiform, scaphoid, hamate, and trapezium with the index and middle fingers and the posterior (dorsal) surface of the capitate with the thumbs as the hand is alternately fanned and folded. During these motions, the clinician should note the quantity and quality of the conjunct rotations. An absence of the conjunct rotations may indicate an intercarpal dysfunction.

The uninvolved joint should always be examined first. This allows for a determination of the normal function, allays the patient's anxiety, and allows for a true comparison of function.[4] During palpation, the clinician should be on the alert for any thickening over tendons, tenderness, or areas of fluctuation.[4] During active and passive testing, the presence of crepitus must be determined. The presence of crepitus with motion may indicate a tendon sheath synovitis or vaginitis.

CLINICAL PEARL

Crepitus usually accompanies a particularly acute tendonitis.

Pronation and supination. Pronation and supination of the wrist on the forearm will provisionally test the TFCC and the proximal and DRUJs. Full forced pronation–supination without evoking pain eliminates the DRUJ and the TFCC as potential sources of the patient's complaints.[2] Normal ranges for pronation and supination are approximately 85–90 degrees with approximately 75 degrees occurring in the forearm articulations and the remaining 15 degrees the result of wrist action. The normal end feel for these motions is tissue stretch, although in cachexic patients, the end feel of pronation may be bone to bone.

Radial and ulnar deviation. Normal radial deviation is approximately 15 degrees, while normal ulnar deviation is between 30 and 45 degrees. The normal end feel for these motions is bone to bone.

Wrist flexion. The normal range of motion of wrist flexion is 80 to 90 degrees with an end feel of tissue stretch. According to Watson,[2] any loss of passive wrist flexion is a sign of underlying organic carpal pathology. To determine whether painful wrist flexion is due to a problem between the scaphoid and radius, or the scaphoid and the trapezium and trapezoid, the wrist is placed in full flexion, with the posterior (dorsal) surface of the hand resting on the treatment table. The clinician pushes on the scaphoid and second metacarpal in a posterior (dorsal) direction. An increase in pain with this maneuver may indicate a problem at the scaphoid–radius articulation.

If there is no increase in pain with this maneuver, the wrist is placed in a neutral position with regard to flexion and extension. The clinician stabilizes the trapezium and trapezoid and pushes the scaphoid posteriorly (dorsally). An increase in pain with this maneuver may indicate a problem at the trapezium/trapezoid–scaphoid articulation.

To determine whether the painful wrist flexion is due to a problem between the capitate and the lunate or the lunate and the radius, the wrist is placed in full flexion. The clinician pushes the lunate in an anterior (palmar) direction. An increase in pain with this maneuver may indicate a problem at the capitate–lunate articulation. If the pain is not increased with this maneuver, the wrist is placed in full flexion and the clinician pushes the lunate in a posterior (dorsal) direction. An increase in pain with this maneuver may indicate a problem at the lunate–radius articulation. A decrease in pain with this maneuver may indicate a problem at the capitate–lunate articulation.

Wrist extension. The normal range of motion for wrist extension is 70–90 degrees with an end feel of the tissue stretch. According to Watson,[2] any loss of passive wrist extension is a sign of underlying organic carpal pathology. To determine whether the pain with wrist extension is due to a problem between the scaphoid and the radius or the scaphoid and the trapezium/trapezoid, the wrist is positioned in full extension with the palm positioned on the table. The clinician pushes on the radius in an anterior (palmar) direction, thus increasing the amount of wrist extension. An increase in pain with this maneuver may indicate a problem at the scaphoid–radius articulation. If this maneuver does not increase pain, the wrist is positioned as before. The clinician now pushes on the radius in a posterior (dorsal) direction. A decrease in pain with this maneuver may indicate a problem at the scaphoid–radius articulation. An increase in pain with this maneuver may indicate a problem at the scaphoid and trapezium/trapezoid articulation.

This is confirmed by placing the wrist as before in full extension and pushing on the scaphoid in a posterior (dorsal) direction. A decrease in pain with this maneuver indicates a problem between the scaphoid and the radius, whereas an increase in pain with this maneuver indicates the problem is between the scaphoid and the trapezium/trapezoid.

The clinician fixes the scaphoid and pushes the trapezium/trapezoid in an anterior (palmar) direction. A decrease in pain with this maneuver may indicate a problem at the scaphoid–trapezium/trapezoid articulation. If the pain remains unchanged with this maneuver, the problem is likely to be at the scaphoid–radius articulation. To confirm this hypothesis, the scaphoid can be pushed in an anterior (palmar) direction while the wrist is maintained in the position of full extension. This should increase the pain if the hypothesis is correct.

To determine whether pain is due to a problem between the capitate and lunate or the lunate and radius, the wrist is positioned in full extension, with the palm of the hand on the table. The clinician pushes on the radius in an anterior (palmar) direction. An increase in pain with this maneuver indicates a problem at the capitate–lunate articulation.

If the pain is increased by pushing the lunate and capitate in an anterior (palmar) direction, this may indicate a problem at the lunate–radius articulation.

If fixing the lunate and pushing the capitate in an anterior (palmar) direction (a relative motion of the lunate posteriorly [dorsally] in relation to the capitate) increases the pain, the problem is likely at the capitate–lunate articulation.

Thumb. The following motions are tested in varying degrees of wrist flexion and extension:

- CMC abduction, adduction, flexion, extension, and opposition (Fig. 18-16). During opposition, the clinician should observe for the conjunct rotation component of the motion.

- MCP and IP flexion and extension.

Fingers. It should never be assumed that lack of full active flexion or extension of the PIP is merely secondary to joint pain or fusion, because closed rupture of the middle slip of the extensor hood is easily missed until the appearance of a boutonniere deformity.[22] During flexion of the fingers, the overall area of the fingers should converge to a point on the wrist corresponding to the radial pulse. This can only occur if the index finger flexes in a sagittal plane and all the others in an increasingly oblique plane. A skyline view of the knuckles is made. In full flexion, a posteriorly (dorsally) subluxed capitate may be seen as a local swelling on the back and middle of the flexed wrist.

Total active motion of the fingers is the sum of all angles formed by the MCP, PIP, and DIP joints in simultaneous maximum active flexion, minus the total extension deficit at the MCP, PIP, and DIP joints (including hyperextension at the IP joints) in maximum active extension.

A normal value for total AROM in the absence of a normal contralateral digit for comparison is 260 degrees, based on 85 degrees of MCP flexion, 110 degrees of PIP motion, and 65 degrees of DIP motion.[95]

A comparison of active and passive motion indicates the efficiency of flexor and extensor excursion and/or degree of muscle strength within the available passive range of motion (PROM).[95] Instances of greater passive than active motion may indicate a limited tendon glide due to adherence of the tendon to surrounding structures or relative lengthening of the tendon due to injury or surgery, weakness, or pain.[95]

Due to the multitude of joints and multiarticular muscles found in the hand, the clinician may need to differentiate between various structures in order to determine the cause of a motion restriction (see "Special Tests").[95] For example, adherence of the extrinsic flexors is tested by passively maintaining the fingers and thumb in full extension while passively extending the wrist. In the presence of flexor tightness, the increasing flexor tension that develops as the wrist is passively extended will pull the fingers into flexion. Adherence of the extensor tendons is simply a reverse process. The digits are passively maintained in full flexion while the wrist is passively flexed. If tension pulling the fingers into extension is detected by the clinician's hand as the wrist is brought into flexion, extrinsic extensor tightness exists.

Strength Testing

Isometric tests are carried out in the extreme range, and if positive, in the neutral range. These isometric tests must include the interossei and lumbricals. The straight plane motions of wrist flexion, extension, and ulnar and radial deviation are tested initially. Pain with any of these tests requires a more thorough examination of the individual muscles. The clinician should be able to extrapolate hand placements for these tests by noting the anatomy of these muscles from the figures. The muscles controlling wrist extension (see Chapter 17), wrist flexion (see Chapter 17), radial deviation, and ulnar deviation are tested first.

Wrist

FCR/FCU. During the testing of these muscles, substitution by the finger flexors should be avoided by not allowing the patient to make a fist. The clinician applies the resistive force into extension and radial deviation for the FCU, and extension and ulnar deviation for the FCR.

ECRL/ECRB. Any action of the EDC should be ruled out by having the patient make a fist while extending the wrist. The clinician applies the resistive force on the dorsum of the second and third metacarpals, with the force directed into flexion and ulnar deviation.

Extensor Carpi Ulnaris. The ECU is tested by having the patient make a fist in wrist extension, while the clinician applies resistance on the ulnar dorsum of hand, with the force directed into flexion and radial deviation.

Thumb

APL/APB. The forearm is positioned midway between pronation and supination, or in maximal supination. The MCP and IP joints are positioned in flexion. The muscles are tested with anterior (palmar) abduction of the thumb in the frontal plane for the longus and in the sagittal plane for the brevis.

Opponens Pollicis. The forearm is positioned in supination and the posterior (dorsal) aspect of the hand rests on the table. The patient is asked to touch the finger pads of the thumb and little finger together. Using one hand, the clinician stabilizes the first and fifth metacarpals and the palm of the hand. With the other hand, the clinician applies a force to the distal end of the first metacarpal in the opposite direction of opposition (retroposition).

FPL/FPB. The forearm is positioned in supination and supported by the table, and the hand is positioned so that the posterior (dorsal) aspect rests on the table. The thumb is adducted. The longus is tested by resistance applied to the distal phalanx, whereas both heads of the brevis are tested by resistance applied to the proximal phalanx.

Adductor Pollicis. This muscle is tested by having the patient hold a piece of paper between the thumb and radial aspect of the index finger's proximal phalanx while the clinician attempts to remove it. If weak or nonfunctioning, the IP joint of the thumb flexes during this maneuver due to substitution by the FDP (Froment sign).

Extensor Pollicis Longus/EPB. Both of these muscles can be tested with the patient's hand flat on the table, palm down, and asking the patient to lift only the thumb off the table. To test each individually, resistance is applied to the posterior (dorsal) aspect of the distal phalanx for the EPL while stabilizing the proximal phalanx and metacarpal and to the posterior (dorsal) aspect of the proximal phalanx for the EPB while stabilizing the first metacarpal.

Intrinsics

Lumbricals. The four lumbricals are tested by applying resistance to the posterior (dorsal) surface of the middle and distal phalanges, while stabilizing under the proximal phalanx of the finger being tested. The anterior (palmar) and posterior (dorsal) interossei act with the lumbricals to achieve MCP flexion coupled with PIP and DIP extension.

Anterior (palmar) Interossei. The three anterior (palmar) interossei adduct the second, fourth, and fifth fingers to midline.Resistance is applied by the clinician to the radial aspect of the distal end of the proximal phalanx of the second, fourth, and fifth fingers, after first stabilizing the hand and fingers not being tested.

Posterior (dorsal) Interossei/ADM. The four posterior (dorsal) interossei abduct the second, third, and fourth fingers from midline. The ADM abducts the fifth finger from midline.

The intrinsic muscles are tested in the frontal plane to avoid substitution by the extrinsic flexors and extensors. Resistance is applied by the clinician to the ulnar aspect of the distal end of the proximal phalanx of each of the four fingers, after first stabilizing the hand and fingers not being tested.

Fingers

Flexor Digitorum Profundus. This muscle is tested with DIP flexion of each digit, while the MCP and PIP are stabilized in extension and wrist neutral. Due to the variability of nerve innervation for this muscle group, each of the fingers can be tested to determine whether a peripheral nerve lesion is present. The index finger is served by the anterior interosseous nerve, the middle finger by the main branch of the median nerve, and the ring and little finger by the ulnar nerve.

Flexor Digitorum Superficialis. There is normally one muscle tendon unit for each finger; however, an absent flexor digitorum superficialis to the little finger is common. The clinician should only allow the finger to be tested to flex by firmly blocking all joints of the nontested fingers, with the wrist in neutral.

ED/Extensor Indicis Proprius. There is only one muscle belly for this four-tendon unit. These three muscles are the sole MCP joint extensors. With the wrist in neutral, the strength is tested with the metacarpals in extension and the PIP/DIP flexed. The extensor indicis proprius can be isolated by positioning the index finger and hand in the "number one" position—the index finger in extension with other fingers clenched in a fist. The EDM muscle is tested with resistance of little finger extension with the other fingers maintained in a fist.

To isolate intrinsic muscle function, the patient is asked to actively extend the MCP joint and then to attempt to actively extend the PIP joint. Because the ED, EI, and EDM tendons are "anchored" at the MCP joint by active extension, only the intrinsic muscles can now extend the PIP joint.[17] To test the terminal extensor tendon function, the clinician stabilizes the middle phalanx and asks the patient to extend the DIP joint.[11]

Flexor Digiti Minimi. The forearm is positioned in supination and the posterior (dorsal) aspect of the hand rests on the table. The clinician stabilizes the fifth metacarpal and the palm with one hand, and then applies resistance to the anterior (palmar) surface of the proximal phalanx of the fifth digit with the other hand.

Opponens Digiti Minimi. The forearm is positioned in supination and the posterior (dorsal) aspect of the hand rests on the table. The patient is asked to touch the finger pads of the thumb and little finger together. Using one hand, the clinician stabilizes the first and fifth metacarpals and palm of the hand. With the other hand, the clinician applies a force to the distal end of the fifth metacarpal in the opposite direction of opposition (retroposition).

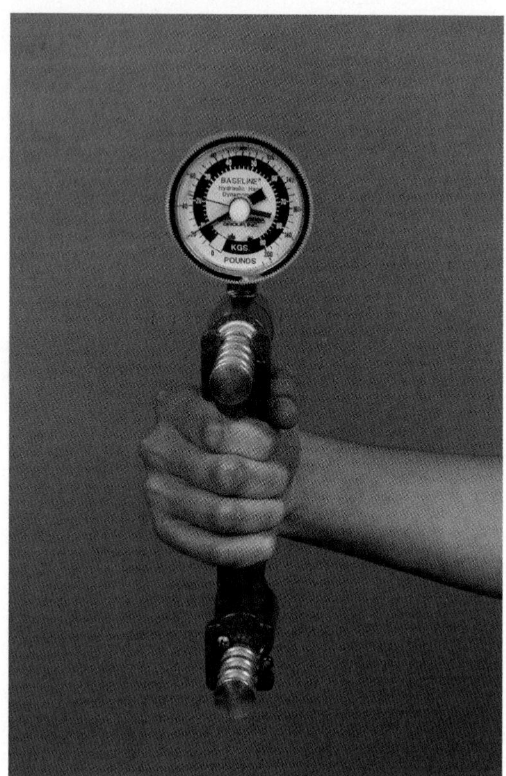

FIGURE 18-26 Grip strength.

Grip Strength. A loss of grip or pinch is a measurable factor used in the determination of permanent disability by compensation boards in some states.[96]

The assessment of grip strength (Fig. 18-26) and pinch strength (Fig. 18-27) is used to assess function of the hand, using a dynamometer. The average values for grip strength are given in Table 18-9. Normal grip strength, which provides statistical analysis of males versus females.[97] The mean value for the nondominant hand can be calculated from the values of the DH and the ratio.

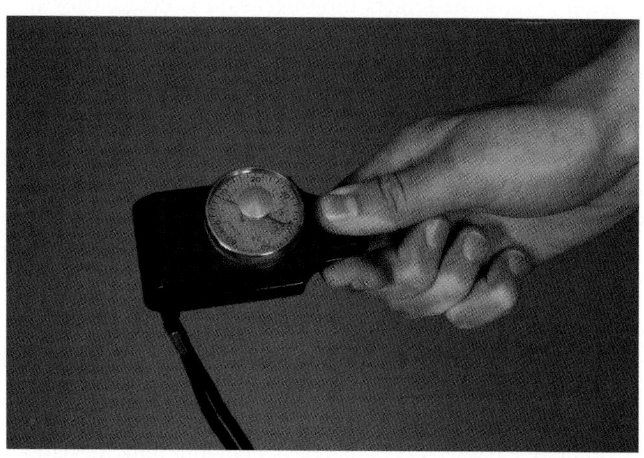

FIGURE 18-27 Pinch meter.

TABLE 18-9 Grip Strength in Normal Men and Women of Various Ages for the Dominant Hand (DH) in Kilopound per Square Centimeter (kp/cm²) and the Ratio dominant Hand/Nondominant Hand (DH/NDH), Based on 25 Determinations

	Men		Women	
Age	DH	DH/NDH	DH	DH/NDH
21–25	1.13 ± 0.18	1.07 ± 0.08	1.03 ± 0.16[a]	1.10 ± 0.12 NS
26–30	1.16 ± 0.23	1.05 ± 0.08	0.96 ± 0.16[b]	1.10 ± 0.08[a]
31–35	1.12 ± 0.17	1.06 ± 0.08	0.95 ± 0.17[b]	1.07 ± 0.14 NS
36–40	1.10 ± 0.18	1.07 ± 0.10	0.95 ± 0.19[c]	1.06 ± 0.15 NS
41–45	1.06 ± 0.14	1.05 ± 0.10	0.90 ± 0.19[b]	1.09 ± 0.1Z NS
46–50	0.97 ± 0.19	1.03 ± 0.08	0.82 ± 0.22[c]	1.06 ± 0.17 NS
51–55	0.97 ± 0.17	1.05 ± 0.10	0.79 ± 0.18[b]	1.12 ± 0.11[a]
56—60	0.81 ± 0.16	1.09 ± 0.13	0.74 ± 0.17 NS	1.05 ± 0.14 NS
61–65	0.79 ± 0.16	1.06 ± 0.16	0.66 ± 0.18[c]	1.09 ± 0.13 NS

Values = means ± standard deviations
[a]$0.01 < P < 0.05$
[b]$P < 0.001$
[c]$0.001 < P < 0.01$
NS $P > 0.05$
Data from Thorngren KG, Werner CO: Normal grip strength. *Acta Orthop Scand* 50:255–259, 1979.

A number of protocols using a sealed hydraulic dynamometer, such as the Jamar dynamometer (Fig. 18-26) (Asimow Engineering Co., Santa Monica, CA), have been shown to be accurate, reliable, and valid in measuring grip strength.[98,99] These dynamometers register force in pounds per square inch, or kilopound per square centimeter, and have adjustable handles to accommodate any sized hand, or any hand that may have a limitation of finger joint motion.[100]

Studies have demonstrated that the second handle setting of the Jamar dynamometer allows for the maximum grip strength from the patient.[100,101] The widest grip uses mostly the profundus muscles. At the narrowest grip, the profundus and superficialis muscle excursion are fully used, preventing much in the way of their contribution to the overall grip strength.[96,100]

Unfortunately, these tests are not purely objective, as they rely on the sincerity of effort from the patient.[102] Thus a number of tests have been introduced in an attempt to aid in the detection of insincerity of effort:

- ***The five-position grip strength test.***[96] This test uses the Jamar dynamometer and uses the five handle settings to measure grip strength at the five different grip widths. In normal and motivated patients, maximum grip strength occurs at the second or third grip width. The maximum grip strength, recorded at the first or fifth width setting, is supposed to be indicative of an insincerity of effort, although the reliability of the five-position grip strength test has been questioned.[101,103]
- ***The rapid exchange grip test, rapid simultaneous grip strength tests.*** The first test was developed by Lister.[104] Both of these tests use the Jamar dynamometer and compare the maximum grip strength during a five-position static grip strength test, with the maximum grip strength recorded when gripping the dynamometer repeatedly at a fast rate (80 times per minute).[105,106] In normal and motivated patients the static measure of grip strength of grip strength should be approximately 15 percent greater than the dynamic measure, while in patients demonstrating insincerity of effort, the dynamic measure is equal to or greater than the initial static measure.[106] The rapid exchange and the rapid simultaneous grip strength tests are time consuming and frequently performed erroneously in the clinical setting.[102]
- ***The rapid repeat test.*** The patient is seated with their arm by their side, the elbow in 90 degrees of flexion, and the forearm and wrist in neutral. The dynamometer, set at the second handle setting, is supported by the clinician and the patient alternately grips with both right and left hands on ten occasions, or until the patient has to stop due to fatigue or discomfort. This test has been found to be an unreliable discriminator of true and faked hand weakness.[102]

It is probably wise to combine the results of different grip strength tests before making any decisions.[107]

Functional Assessment. The hand serves many important functions that allow us to interact with others and the environment. In addition to providing a wealth of sensory information, the hand functions to grasp objects.

Hand functions have been further categorized by adding the terms *grasp* and *prehension*. These terms are used to describe functions of power or precision.[20,21]

The *functional position* of the wrist is the position in which optimal function is likely to occur.[62,108] This position involves wrist extension of between 20 and 35 degrees, ulnar deviation of 10 to 15 degrees, slight flexion of all of the finger joints, midrange thumb opposition, and slight flexion of the thumb

MCP and IP joints.[62] In this position, which minimizes the restraining action of the long extensor tendons, the pulps of the index finger and thumb are in contact.

A number of motions can be used to quickly assess hand function, including the following:

1. Opposition of the thumb and little finger.
2. Pad to pad mobility of the thumb and other fingers. The majority of the functional activities of the hand require at least 5 cm of opening of the fingers and thumb.[109]
3. The ability to make three different fists:
   a. The hook fist (placing fingertips onto MCP joints).
   b. Standard fist.
   c. Straight fist (placing fingertips on the thenar and hypothenar eminences). The ability to flex the fingers to within 1–2 cm of the distal anterior (palmar) crease is an indication of functional range of motion for many hand activities.[109]

The *functional range of motion* for the hand is the range in which the hand can perform most of its grip and other functional activities (Table 18-10).

The percentage losses of digital function are as follows: thumb, 40–50%; index finger, 20%; long finger, 20%; ring finger, 10%; little finger, 5%. Loss of the hand is 90% of the upper extremity and 54% of the whole person.

Function of the digits is related to nerve distribution. Flexion and sensation of the radial digits, important in precision grips, are controlled mainly by the median nerve, whereas flexion and sensation of the ulnar digits, important to the power grip, are controlled by the ulnar nerve. The muscles of the thumb, used in all forms of gripping, are controlled by both the median and the ulnar nerves. The release of a grip or opening of the hand is controlled by the radial nerve. A loss of the relationship between the thumb and the index finger results in an inability to perform fine motor skills that involve pulp-to-pulp pinch, as well as functions that require power.

TABLE 18-10 Functional Range of Motion of the Hand and Wrist

Joint Motion	Functional Range of Motion (Degrees)
Wrist flexion	5–40
Wrist extension	30–40
Radial deviation	10–20
Ulnar deviation	15–20
MCP flexion	60
PIP flexion	60
DIP flexion	40
Thumb MCP flexion	20

DIP, distal interphalangeal; MCP, metacarpophalangeal; PIP, proximal interphalangeal.

Data from Tubiana R, Thomine J-M, Mackin E: *Examination of the Hand and Wrist*. London: Mosby, 1996; Palmer AK, Werner FW, Murphy D, et al: Functional wrist motion: A biomechanical study. *J Hand Surg Am* 10A:39–46, 1985; Ryu J, Cooney WP, Askew LJ, et al: Functional ranges of motion of the wrist joint. *J Hand Surg Am* 16A:409–420, 1991.

Hand Disability Index.[84] The patient is asked to rate the following seven questions on a scale of zero to three, with three being the most difficult.

Unable to perform task = 0

Able to complete task partially = 1

Able to complete task but with difficulty = 2

Able to perform task normally = 3

Are you able to do the following:

1. Dress yourself, including tying shoelaces and doing buttons?
2. Cut your meat?
3. Lift a full cup or glass to your mouth?
4. Prepare your own meal?
5. Open car doors?
6. Open jars that have previously been opened?
7. Turn taps on and off?

A variety of evaluation tools have been devised for the hand, and they can be categorized into assessments of the neurovascular system, range of motion, sensibility, and function (Table 18-11).[109]

Dexterity tests include the following:

Minnesota Rate of Manipulation Test. This test, which primarily measures gross coordination and dexterity, consists of following five functions:

1. Placing
2. Turning
3. Displacing
4. One-hand turning and placing
5. Two-hand turning and placing

The activities are timed and compared with the time taken by the other hand and then compared with normal values.[109,110]

Jebsen–Taylor Hand-Function Test.[111] This test, which requires the least amount of extremity coordination, measures prehension and manipulative skills and consists of following seven subtests:

1. Writing
2. Card turning
3. Picking up small objects
4. Simulated feeding
5. Stacking
6. Picking up large, light objects
7. Picking up large, heavy objects

The subtests are timed and compared with the time taken by the other hand. The results are also compared with normal values.[109,110]

Nine-Hole Peg Test. This test was designed to assess finger dexterity of each hand.[112] The patient is asked to use one hand to place nine 3.2-cm (1.3-inch) pegs in a 12.7 by 12.7 cm (5 by 5 in.) board and is then asked to remove them. The task is timed and compared with the time taken by the other hand. The results are compared with normal values.[109,110]

TABLE 18-11 Functional Testing of the Wrist and Hand

Starting Position	Action	Functional Test
1. Forearm supinated, resting on table	Wrist flexion	Lift 0 lb: Nonfunctional Lift 1–2 lb: functionally poor Lift 3–4 lb: functionally fair Lift 5+ lb: functional
2. Forearm pronated, resting on table	Wrist extension lifting 1–2 lb	0 repetitions: nonfunctional 1–2 repetitions: functionally poor 3–4 repetitions: functionally fair 5+ repetitions: functional
3. Forearm between supination and pronation, resting on table	Radial deviation lifting 1–2 lb	0 repetitions: nonfunctional 1–2 repetitions: functionally poor 3–4 repetitions: functionally fair 5+ repetitions: functional
4. Forearm between supination and pronation, resting on table.	Thumb flexion with resistance from rubber band around thumb	0 repetitions: nonfunctional 1–2 repetitions: functionally poor 3–4 repetitions: functionally fair 5+ repetitions: functional
5. Forearm resting on table, rubber band around thumb and index finger	Thumb extension against resistance of rubber band	0 repetitions: nonfunctional 1–2 repetitions: functionally poor 3–4 repetitions: functionally fair 5+ repetitions: functional
6. Forearm resting on table, rubber band around thumb and index finger	Thumb abduction against resistance of rubber band	0 repetitions: nonfunctional 1–2 repetitions: functionally poor 3–4 repetitions: functionally fair 5+ repetitions: functional
7. Forearm resting on table	Thumb adduction, lateral pinch of piece of paper	Hold 0 s: nonfunctional Hold 1–2 s: functionally poor Hold 3–4 s: functionally fair Hold 5+ s: functional
8. Forearm resting on table	Thumb opposition, pulp-to-pulp pinch of piece of paper	Hold 0 s: nonfunctional Hold 1–2 s: functionally poor Hold 3–4 s: functionally fair Hold 5+ s: functional
9. Forearm resting on table	Finger flexion, patient grasps mug or glass using cylindrical grasp and lifts off table	0 repetitions: nonfunctional 1–2 repetitions: functionally poor 3–4 repetitions: functionally fair 5+ repetitions: functional
10. Forearm resting on table	Patient attempts to put on rubber glove keeping fingers straight	21+ s: nonfunctional 10–20 s: functionally poor 4–8 s: functionally fair 2–4 s: functional
11. Forearm resting on table	Patient attempts to pull fingers apart (finger abduction) against resistance of rubber band and holds	Hold 0 s: Nonfunctional Hold 1–2 s: functionally poor Hold 3–4 s: functionally fair Hold 5+ s: functional
12. Forearm resting on table	Patient holds piece of paper between fingers while clinician pulls on paper	Hold 0 s: nonfunctional Hold 1–2 s: functionally poor Hold 3–4 s: functionally fair Hold 5+ s: functional

Data from Palmer ML, Epler M: *Clinical Assessment Procedures in Physical Therapy.* Philadelphia, PA: JB Lippincott, 1990.

Purdue Pegboard Test.[113,114] This test evaluates finer coordination, requiring prehension of small objects, with measurement categories divided into

1. right hand
2. left hand
3. both hands
4. right, left, and both hands
5. assembly.

The subtests are timed and compared with normal values based on gender and occupation.[109,110]

Crawford Small Parts Dexterity Test.[115] This test involves the use of tweezers and a screwdriver and requires patients to control not only their hands but also small tools. This test correlates positively with vocational activities that demand fine coordination skills.[109]

The problem with most of these tests and others is that the critical measure of function used is time, even though time is not an accurate measure of function.

Although not standardized, a few other simple tests can be used to assess hand dexterity. These include writing in a straight line, buttoning and unbuttoning different-sized buttons, and zipping and unzipping using a variety of zipper sizes. The following scale can be used to grade these activities:

Unable to perform task = 0.

Able to complete task partially = 1.

Able to complete task but with difficulty = 2.

Able to perform task normally = 3.

Passive Accessory Joint Mobility Tests

In the following tests, the patient is positioned in sitting or supine, with the arm resting comfortably. In each of the tests, the clinician notes the quantity of joint motion as well as the joint reaction. The tests are always repeated on, and compared to, the same joint in the opposite extremity.

Distal Radioulnar Joint

Anterior–Posterior Glide. The patient is positioned in sitting with the forearm resting on the table. Using a pinch grip with both hands, the clinician places both thumbs on the posterior (dorsal) aspects of the ulnar and radial styloid processes (Fig. 18-28). The distal radius is stabilized and the distal ulna is moved posteriorly (dorsally) or anteriorly (palmarly) relative to the distal radius (Fig. 18-28). Alternatively, the distal ulna may be stabilized and the distal radius moved. This technique is used to assess joint plane motions necessary for pronation (posterior glide) and supination (anterior glide), or in the case of joint mobilizations to increase the joint play necessary for these motions.

Radiocarpal Joint. The patient's hand rests on the table with the wrist supported with a towel. The radiocarpal and ulnocarpal joints are placed in the resting position.

Distraction. Using one hand, the clinician grasps the distal radius and ulna. Using the other hand, the clinician grips the proximal row of carpals. A perpendicular distraction force is applied to separate the proximal level of carpals from the distal radius and ulna (Fig. 18-29).

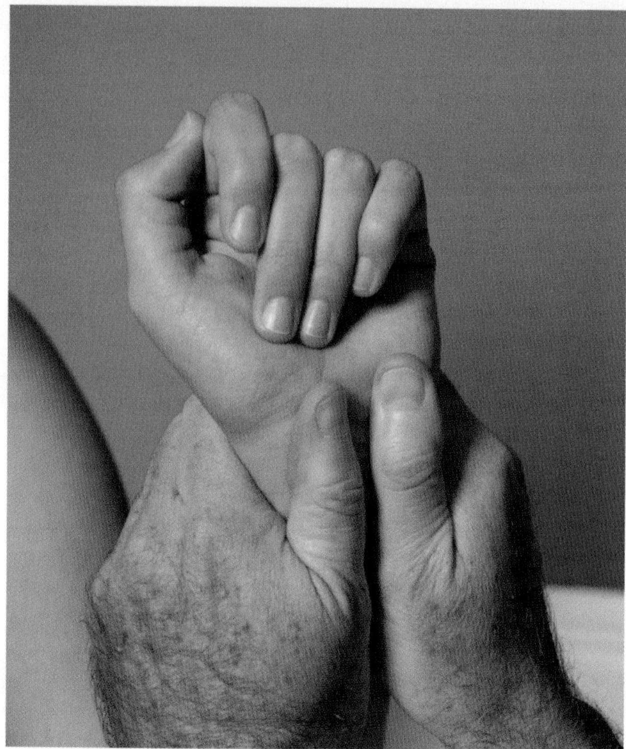

FIGURE 18-28 Mobility testing of the distal radioulnar joint.

Posterior–anterior glide. Using one hand to stabilize the patient's distal forearm, the clinician grasps the patient's hand with the other hand using the styloid processes and pisiform for landmarks. The proximal row of carpals is then moved posteriorly (dorsally) and anteriorly (palmarly) (Fig. 18-30). The posterior glide tests the joint's ability to flex, whereas the anterior glide assesses the ability of the joint to extend.

Ulnar and radial glide. The patient's hand rests on the table with the wrist supported with a towel (Fig. 18-31). Using one hand to stabilize the patient's distal forearm, the clinician grasps the patient's hand with the other hand using the styloid processes and pisiform for landmarks. The proximal row of carpals is then moved posteriorly (dorsally) and anteriorly (palmarly). The ulnar (medial) glide tests the joint's ability to radially deviate, whereas the radial (lateral) glide assesses the ability of the joint to ulnarly deviate.

Intercarpal Joints

Distal row. The patient's hand rests on the table or is held forward by the clinician. The clinician grasps the patient's hand with both hands, with the index fingers and thumbs of each

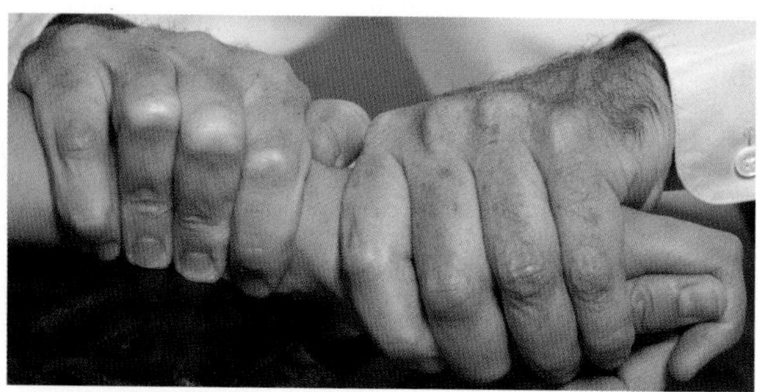

FIGURE 18-29 Radiocarpal distraction.

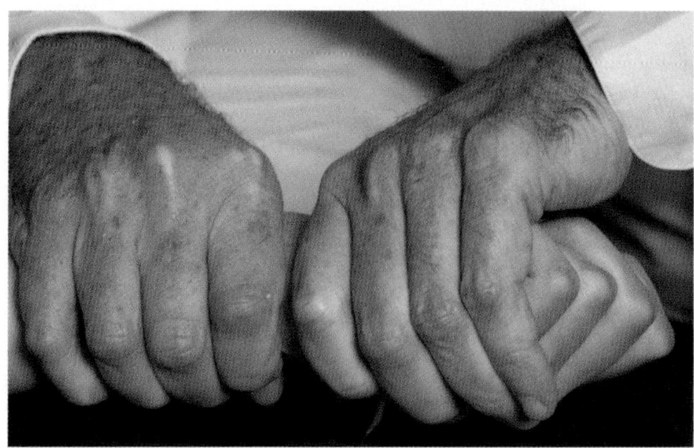

FIGURE 18-30 Anterior glide of the radiocarpal joint.

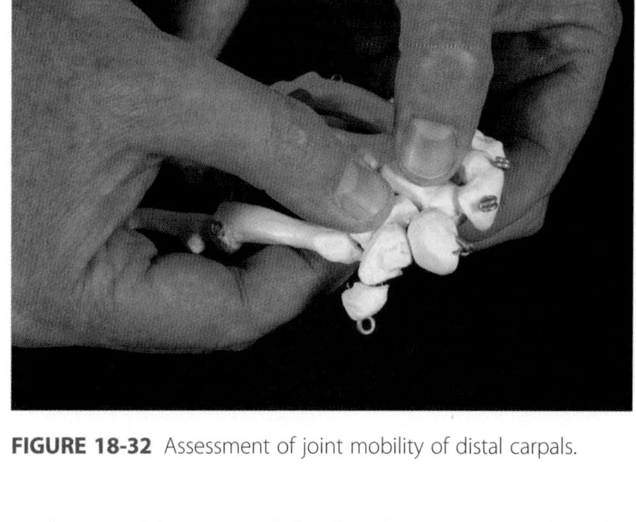

FIGURE 18-32 Assessment of joint mobility of distal carpals.

hand used to pinch an individual carpal and the adjacent carpal (Fig. 18-32). One carpal is moved anteriorly relative to the other and the clinician assesses the motion of the carpal in relation to the other. For example, the clinician assesses the motion of the capitate in relation to the hamate. An anterior glide of one carpal on another is a relative posterior glide of the other. For example, an anterior glide of the capitate on the hamate is a relative posterior glide of the hamate on the capitate.

Proximal row. The same technique is used to assess the proximal row of carpals.

Midcarpal Joints. The articulation between the proximal row of carpals and the distal row of carpals can be assessed using distraction, anterior glide, posterior glide, radial glide, and ulnar glide (Fig. 18-33). While assessing the distraction and anterior and posterior glides provides little information, the assessment of the radial glide can provide information about the ability of the wrist joint to ulnarly deviate, and the assessment of the ulnar glide can provide information about the ability of the wrist joint to radially deviate.

CMC Joints. Using one hand, the clinician uses a pinch grip of the index finger and thumb to palpate and stabilize the carpal bone that articulates with the metacarpal bone being tested (Fig. 18-34). With a pinch grip of the index finger and thumb of the other hand, the clinician palpates the metacarpal (Fig. 18-34).

The carpal bone is stabilized and the metacarpal is distracted (Fig. 18-35) and then glided posterior anteriorly along the plane of the CMC joint.

First CMC (trapeziometacarpal) Joint. The patient is positioned in sitting or supine.

Ulnar (medial) glide. The clinician applies a glide in an ulnar direction through the thenar eminence toward the radial

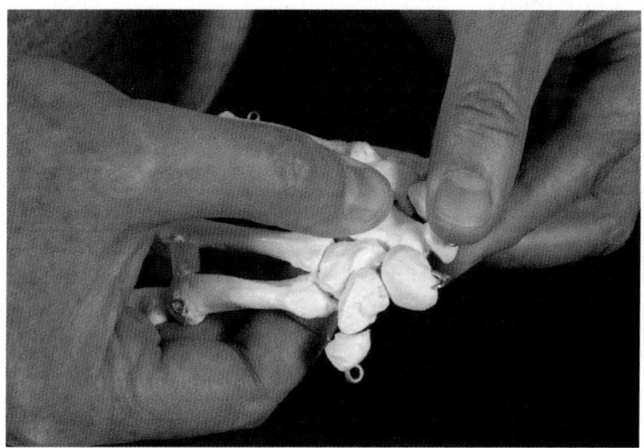

FIGURE 18-33 Assessment of joint mobility of intercarpals between distal and proximal rows.

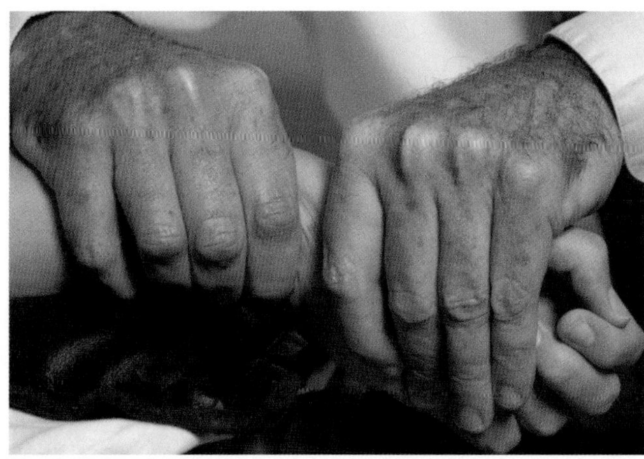

FIGURE 18-31 Ulnar glide of the radioulnar joint.

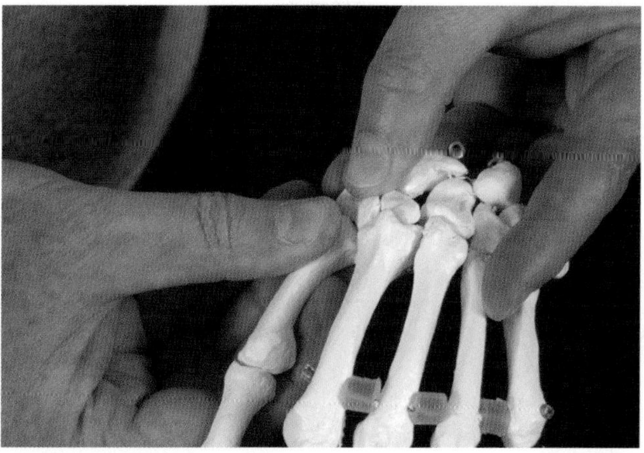

FIGURE 18-34 Carpometacarpal joint testing.

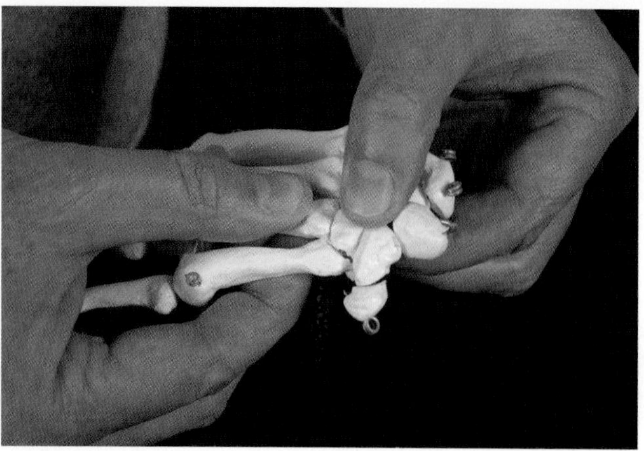

FIGURE 18-35 Distraction of the carpometacarpal joint.

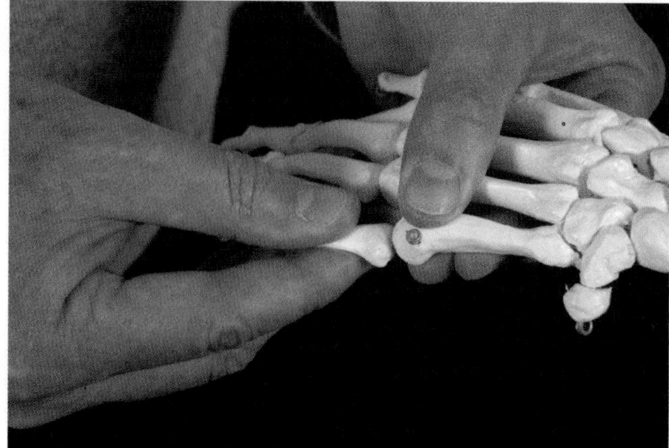

FIGURE 18-37 Long axis distraction of the MCP or IP joints.

aspect of the patient's metacarpal (Fig. 18-36). The ulnar glide is used to assess trapeziometacarpal joint flexion.

Radial (lateral) glide. The clinician applies a glide in a radial direction through the thenar eminence toward the ulnar aspect of the patient's metacarpal. The radial glide is used to assess trapeziometacarpal joint extension.

Distraction. The distraction technique may be used to decrease pain and to stretch the joint capsule.

MCP/IP Joints. Using a pinch grip of the index finger and thumb of one hand, the clinician palpates and stabilizes the metacarpal/phalanx. With a pinch grip of the index finger and thumb of the other hand, the clinician palpates the adjacent phalanx.

Distraction. The clinician stabilizes the proximal bone, and then applies a long axis distraction (Fig. 18-37).

Posterior–Anterior Glide. The clinician stabilizes the proximal bone, and then glides the phalanx posteroanteriorly along the plane of the joint (Fig. 18-37).

Ulnar (Medial)–Radial (Lateral) Glide. The clinician stabilizes the proximal bone, and then glides the phalanx mediolaterally along the plane of the joint (Fig. 18-37).

First MCP Joint. Using a pinch grip of the index finger and thumb of one hand, the clinician stabilizes the trapezium on the radial and ulnar surfaces. With a pinch grip of the index finger and thumb of the other hand, the clinician grips the proximal metacarpal on the radial and ulnar surfaces. A radial–ulnar glide is then performed by the mobilizing hand. A radial glide is necessary for trapeziometacarpal extension, whereas the ulnar glide is necessary for trapeziometacarpal flexion.

Distal and PIP Joints. Using a pinch grip of the index finger and thumb of one hand, the clinician stabilizes the distal end of the more proximal phalanx. Using the other hand the clinician grips the proximal end of the more distal phalanx. The PIP joint (Fig. 18-38) and DIP joint (Fig. 18-39) can then be distracted, or glided anteriorly or posteriorly. The anterior glide assesses the ability of the joint to move into flexion, whereas posterior glide assesses the ability of the joint to move into extension.

Special Tests

The special tests for the wrist and hand can be subdivided based on intent:

- Motion restriction
- Pain provocation
- Tendinous integrity
- Ligamentous stability
- Neurovascular status
- Sensibility testing
- Adverse neural tension.

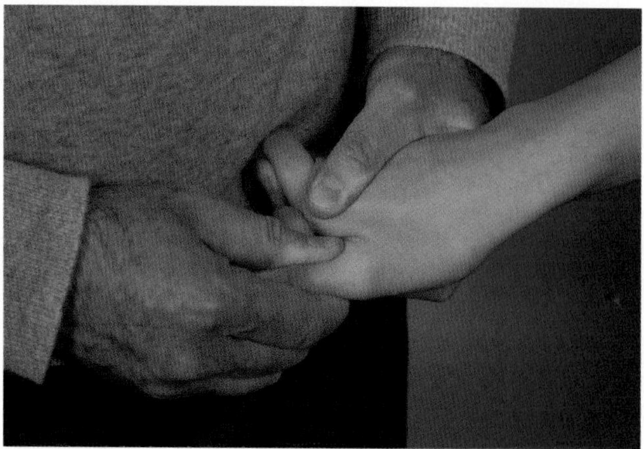

FIGURE 18-36 Ulnar glide of the first carpometacarpal joint.

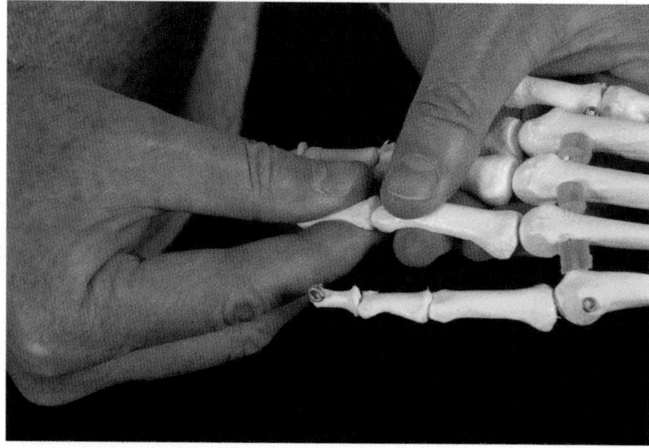

FIGURE 18-38 Assessment of proximal interphalangeal joint.

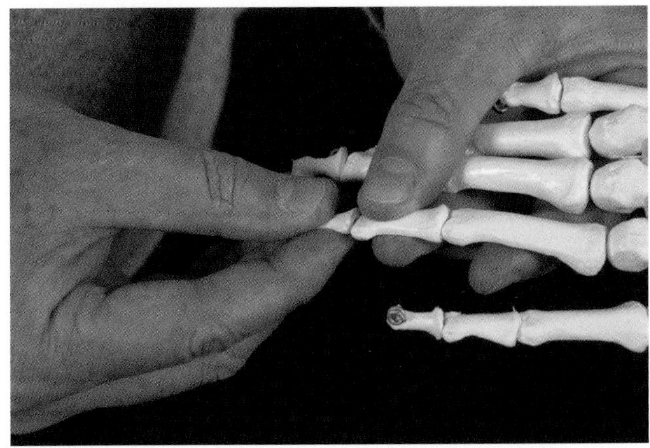

FIGURE 18-39 Assessment of distal interphalangeal joint.

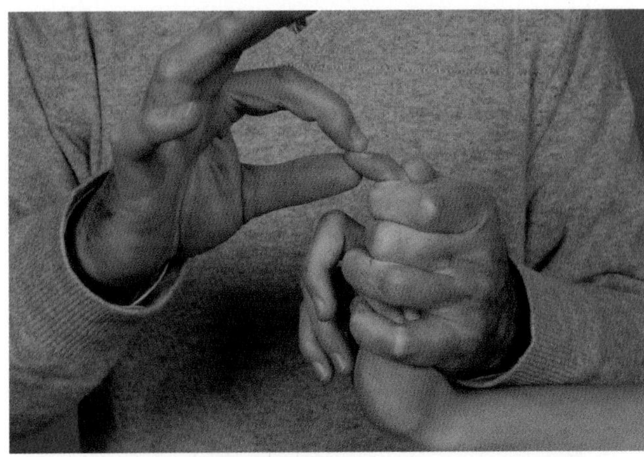

FIGURE 18-41 Haines–Zancolli test.

Motion Restriction

- The Bunnell–Littler test is used to determine whether flexion restriction of the PIP is due to tightness of the intrinsic muscles or due to a restriction of the MCP joint capsule. The MCP joint is held by the clinician in a few degrees of extension with one hand, while the other hand attempts to flex the PIP joint. If the joint cannot flex, tightness of the intrinsics or a joint capsular contraction should be suspected.[116] From this position, the clinician now slightly flexes the MCP joint, thereby relaxing the intrinsics, and attempts to flex the PIP joint (Fig. 18-40). If the joint can now flex, the intrinsics are tight. If the joint still cannot flex, the restriction is probably due to a capsular contraction of the joint. This test is also called the intrinsic-plus test.[23]
- The Haines–Zancolli test is used to determine whether restricted flexion in the DIP joints is due to a restriction of the PIP joint capsule or tightness of the oblique retinacular ligament. The test for a contracture of this ligament is the same as the Bunnell–Littler test, only at the PIP and DIP joints. The clinician positions and holds the PIP joint in a neutral position with one hand and attempts to flex the DIP joint with the other hand (Fig. 18-41). If no flexion is possible, it can be due to either a tight retinacular ligament or capsular contraction. The PIP joint is then slightly flexed to relax the retinacular ligament. If the DIP can now flex, the restriction is due to tightness in the retinacular ligament. If the DIP cannot flex, then the restriction is due to a capsular contraction.

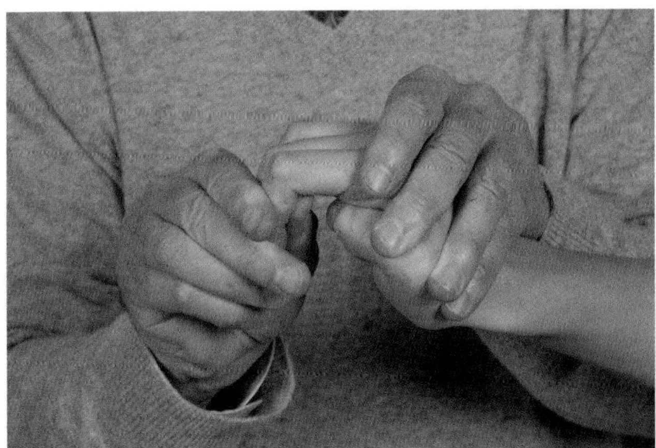

FIGURE 18-40 Bunnell–Littler test.

Pain Provocation Tests

Thumb CMC Grind Test. The grind test is used to assess the integrity of the thumb CMC joint by axially loading the thumb metacarpal into the trapezium.[9,117] The clinician grasps the thumb metacarpal using the thumb and index finger of one hand and the proximal aspect of the thumb CMC joint with the other hand (Fig. 18-42). An axial compressive force, combined with rotation, is applied to the thumb CMC joint. Reproduction of the patient's pain and crepitus is a positive test for arthrosis and synovitis.

Lichtman Test. The Lichtman test is a provocative test for midcarpal instability.[9] The patient's forearm is positioned in

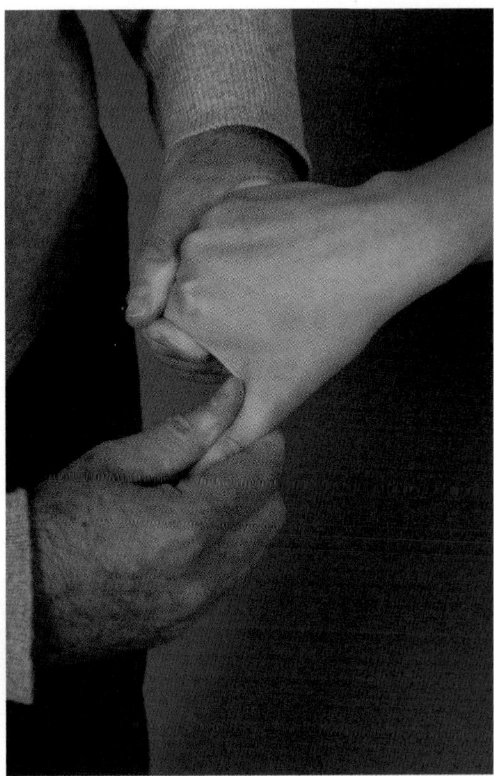

FIGURE 18-42 CMC grind test.

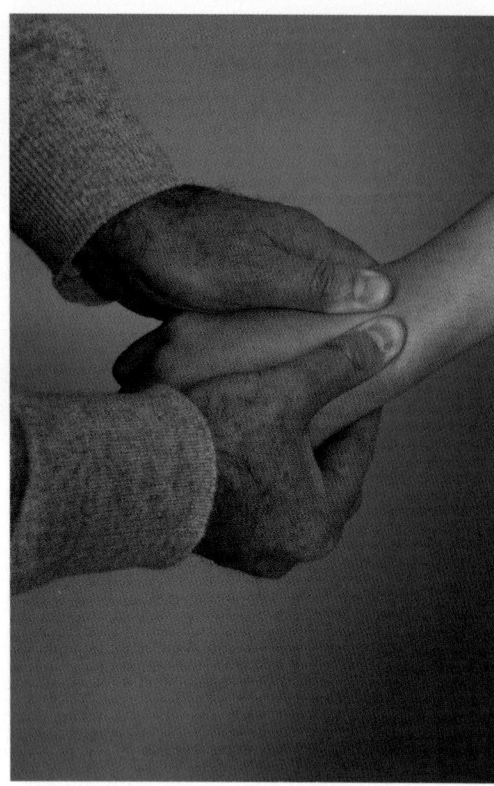

FIGURE 18-43 Lichtman test.

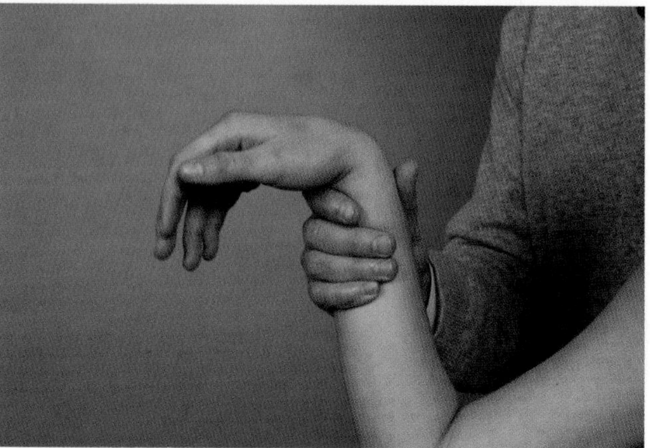

FIGURE 18-45 Carpal shake test.

pronation and the hand is held relaxed and supported by the clinician. The clinician gently moves the patient's hand from radial to ulnar deviation while compressing the carpus into the radius (Fig. 18-43). A positive test is when the midcarpal row appears to jump or snap from an anteriorly (palmarly) subluxed position to the height of the proximal row.[9]

Linscheid Test. The Linscheid test is used to detect ligamentous injury and instability of the second and third CMC joints. The test is performed by supporting the metacarpal shafts and pressing distally over the metacarpal heads in anterior (palmar) (Fig. 18-44) and posterior (dorsal) directions.[80] A positive test produces pain localized to the CMC joints.[118]

Carpal Shake Test. This test is used if intercarpal synovitis is suspected.[9] The clinician grasps the patient's distal forearm (Fig. 18-45). The patient is asked to relax and the clinician shakes the wrist (Fig. 18-45). Pain or resistance to this test indicates a positive test.

Wrist flexion and finger extension test. The patient is positioned in sitting with the elbow placed on the table. The clinician holds the patient's wrist in flexion and asks the patient to extend the fingers against manual resistance (Fig. 18-46). A positive test for scapholunate pathology is identified by pain over the scaphoid. No diagnostic accuracy studies have been performed to determine the sensitivity and specificity of this test.

Press (Sit to Stand) Test. This test is used if a tear of the TFCC is suspected.[9] The patient is instructed to place both hands on the armrests of a chair and attempt to lift their body slightly off the chair (Fig. 18-47). Pain or resistance to this test indicates a positive test. Lester and colleagues[119] reported a sensitivity of 100% compared with arthroscopic surgery and a sensitivity of 79% when compared with magnetic resonance imaging (MRI) arthrogram. Specificity could not be determined based on the methodology of this test design.

Supination lift test.[120] The patient is positioned in sitting with the elbows flexed to 90 degrees and the forearms supinated. The patient is asked to place the palms flat on the underside of the heavy table or against the clinician's hands. The patient is asked to lift the table or push up against the resisting clinician's hands (Fig. 18-48). A positive test for a TFCC tear is pain

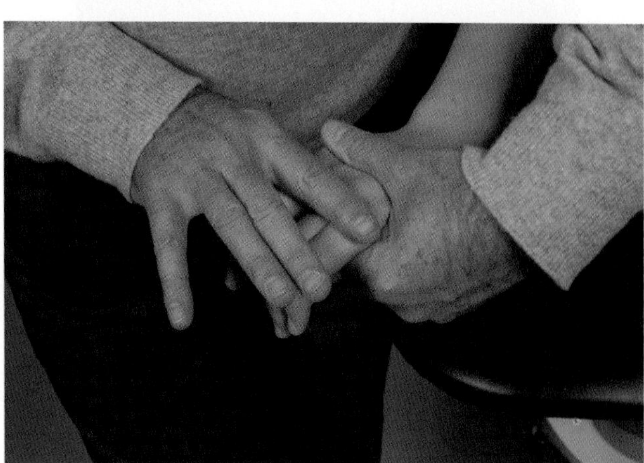

FIGURE 18-44 Linscheid test.

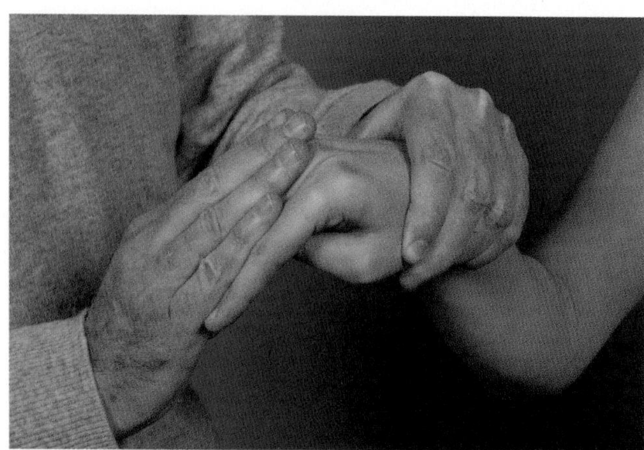

FIGURE 18-46 Wrist flexion and finger extension test.

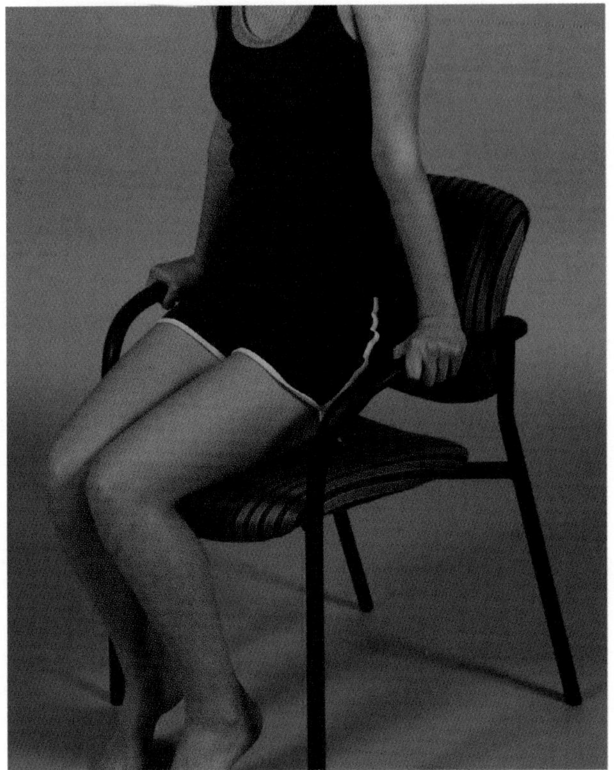

FIGURE 18-47 Press (sit to stand) test.

localized to the ulnar side of the wrist with difficulty applying force.

Ulnar Impaction Test. This test is used to assess the articulation between the ulnar carpus and the TFCC.[9] The patient is positioned in sitting, with the elbow flexed to about 90 degrees and the wrist positioned in ulnar deviation, and the fingers positioned in a slight fist. The clinician loads the wrist by applying a compressive force through the ring and small metacarpals (Fig. 18-49). Pain with this test indicates a possible tear of the TFCC or ulnar impaction syndrome (see "Intervention Strategies").

Finkelstein Test.[121] This test is used to detect stenosing tenosynovitis of the APL and EPB. The clinician grasps the patient's thumb, stabilizes the forearm with one hand, and then deviates the wrist to the ulnar side with the other hand

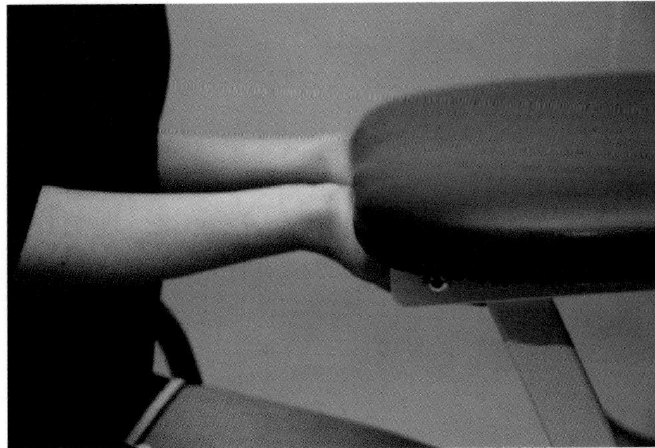

FIGURE 18-48 Supination lift test.

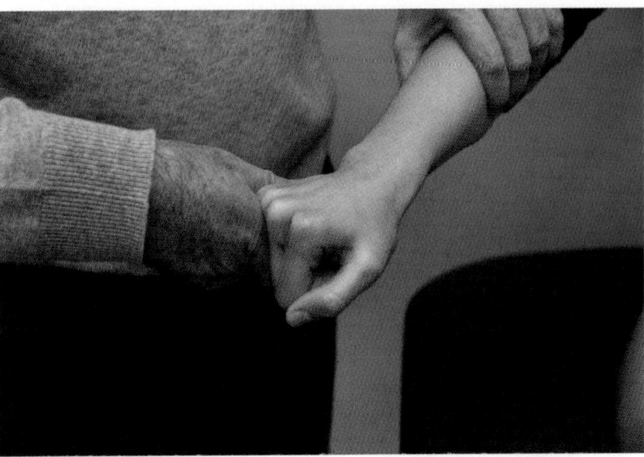

FIGURE 18-49 Ulnar impaction test.

(Fig. 18-50). No diagnostic accuracy studies have been performed to determine the sensitivity and specificity of this test, so the results of this test must be interpreted with caution,[122] as it may also be positive in Wartenberg syndrome (entrapment of the superficial radial sensory nerve),[123–125] basilar thumb arthrosis, EPB entrapment, or intersection syndrome (see "Intervention Strategies").[125] Deviating the wrist using pressure over the index metacarpal avoids confusion with thumb conditions.[126] A variation of Finkelstein test can be used to rule out an incomplete release of previous de Quervain disease.[127] If the usual Finkelstein test is positive, full abduction of the APL followed by flexion of the thumb's MCP joint will isolate the action of the EPB. Pain with this test will occur if the EPB lies in a separate sheath and was not released (EPB

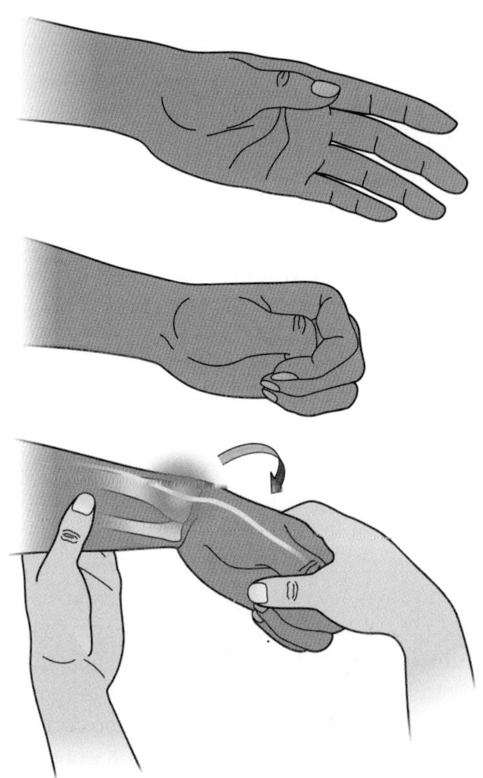

FIGURE 18-50 Finkelstein test.

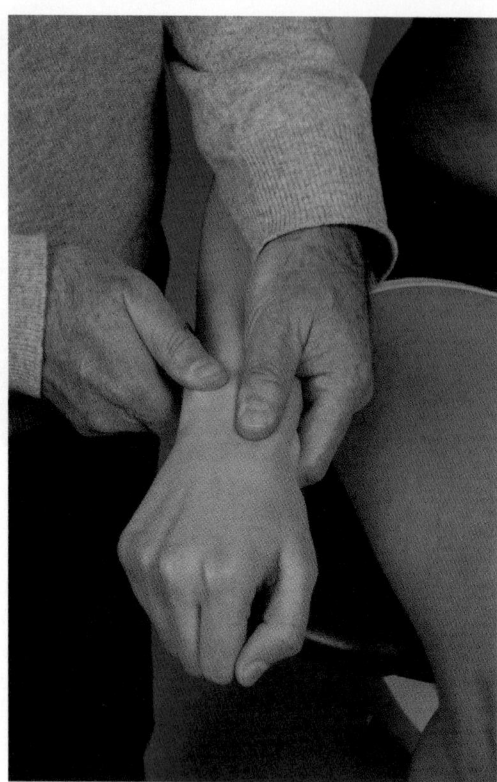

FIGURE 18-51 Radioulnar ballottement test.

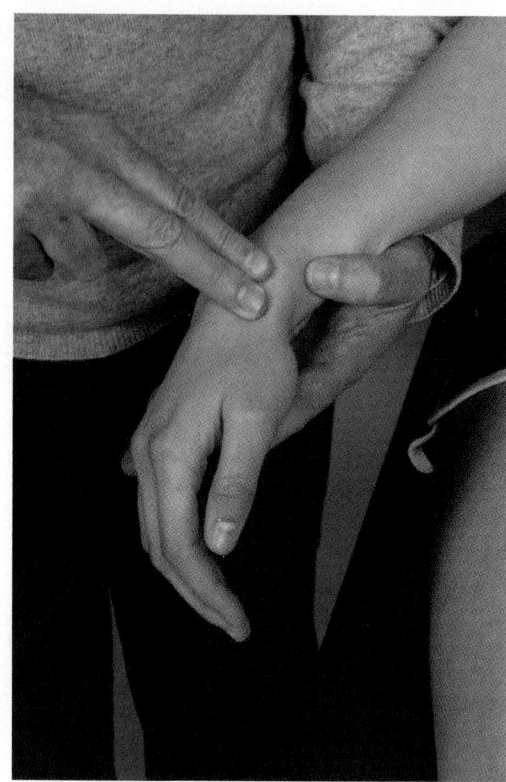

FIGURE 18-52 Wartenberg Test.

entrapment syndrome).[127] This test has been found to have a sensitivity of 81% and a specificity of 50%.[128]

Radioulnar Ballottement Test. The radioulnar ballottement test is used to assess DRUJ instability. The patient's elbow is flexed and the clinician uses their thumb and index finger to stabilize the radius radially and the ulnar head ulnarly (Fig. 18-51). Stress is applied in an anterior–posterior direction. Normally there is no movement in the anterior or posterior direction in maximum supination or pronation. Pain or mobility with this test is suggestive of radioulnar instability.

Wartenberg Test. The Wartenberg test is used with patients who complain of pain over the distal radial forearm associated with paresthesias over the posterior (dorsal) radial hand (Wartenberg syndrome). These patients frequently report symptom magnification with wrist movement or when tightly pinching the thumb and index digit together. The Wartenberg test involves tapping the index finger over the superficial radial nerve (similar to the Tinel test for CTS) on the posterior and radial side of the wrist (Fig. 18-52). A positive test is indicated by local tenderness and paresthesia with this maneuver. Hyper-pronation of the forearm can also cause a positive Tinel sign.

Finger Extension Test. This test is used to demonstrate posterior (dorsal) wrist syndrome, a localized scapholunate synovitis.[13] The clinician instructs the patient to fully flex the wrist and then actively extend the digits at both the IP and MCP joints. The clinician then applies pressure on the fingers into flexion at the MCP joints while the patient continues to actively extend (Fig. 18-53). A positive test occurs when there is production of central posterior (dorsal) wrist pain and indicates the possibility of Kienböck disease, carpal instability, joint degeneration, or synovitis (see "Intervention Strategies").[9]

Scapholunate Shear Test. The patient is positioned in sitting with their forearm pronated. With one hand, the clinician grasps the scaphoid. With the other hand, the clinician grasps the lunate between the thumb and the index finger (Fig. 18-54). The lunate and scaphoid are then sheared in an anterior (palmar) and then posterior (dorsal) direction.[2] Laxity and reproduction of the patient's pain are positive signs for this test.[9]

Tendinous Integrity

FDS Test. This test is used to test the integrity of the FDS tendon. The clinician holds the patient's fingers in extension

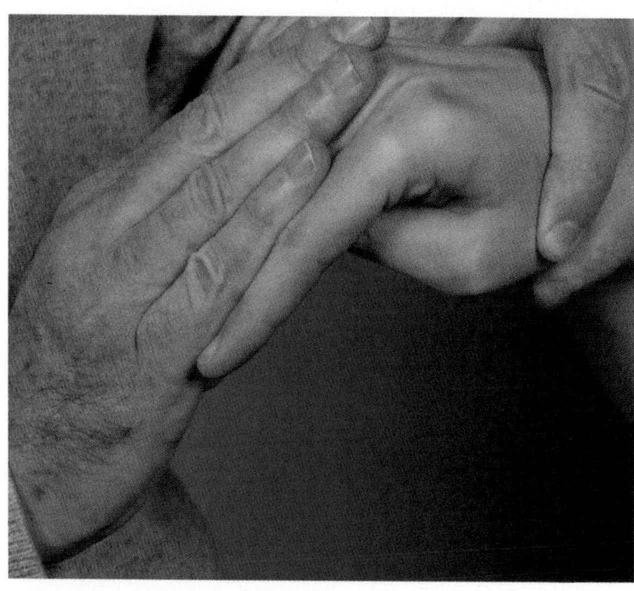

FIGURE 18-53 Finger extension test.

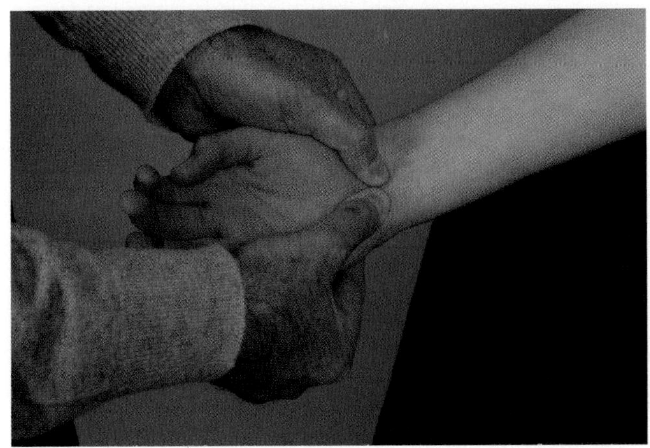

FIGURE 18-54 Scapholunate shear test.

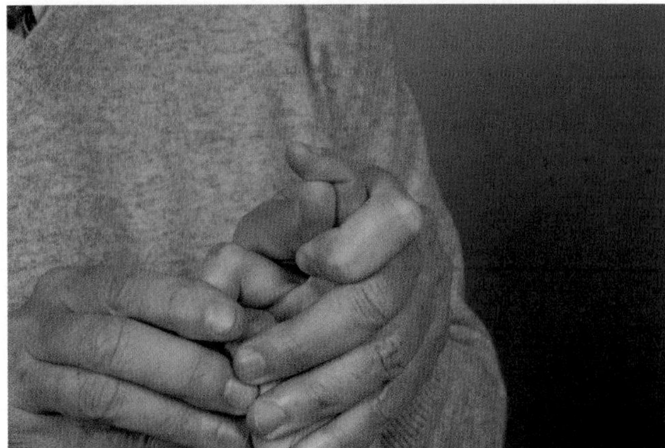

FIGURE 18-56 Flexor digitorum profundus test.

except for the finger being tested (this isolates the FDS tendon). The patient is instructed to flex the finger at the PIP joint (Fig. 18-55). If this is possible, the FDS tendon is intact. Since this tendon can act independently because of the position of the finger, it is the only functioning tendon at the PIP joint. The DIP joint, motored by the FDP, has no power of flexion when the other fingers are held in extension.

FDP Test. These tendons work only in unison. To test the FDP, the PIP joint and the MCP joints are stabilized in extension (Fig. 18-56). The patient is asked to flex this finger at the DIP joint. If flexion occurs, the FDP is intact. If no flexion is possible, the tendon is severed or the muscle denervated.

Integrity of the Central Slip (Extensor Hood Rupture).[129] The patient flexes the finger to 90 degrees at the PIP joint over the edge of the table. The patient is then asked to extend the PIP joint while the clinician palpates the middle phalanx (Fig. 18-57). The absence of extension force at the PIP joint, and fixed extension at the distal joint, indicates complete rupture of the central slip.[22] No diagnostic accuracy studies have been performed to determine the sensitivity and the specificity of the clinical test.

Ligamentous Stability. A number of tests are available to evaluate the ligamentous stability of the forearm, wrist, hand, and finger joints. In the following tests, the patient is positioned in sitting, and the clinician is standing or sitting, facing the patient. The clinician must remember to perform these tests on the uninvolved side to provide a basis for comparison.

Piano Key Test. The piano key test evaluates the stability of the ulnomeniscotriquetral joint.[4] The clinician firmly stabilizes the distal radius with one hand and grasps the head of the ulna between the thumb and the index finger of the other hand. The ulnar head is depressed in an anterior direction (as in depressing a key on a piano) (Fig. 18-58).[9] The test is positive for a TFCC tear or triquetral instability if there is excessive movement in an anterior (palmar) direction or if upon release of the ulna, the bone springs back into its high posterior (dorsal) position. There may also be discomfort reported during the test.[80] LaStayo and Howell[130] found this test to have a sensitivity of 66% and a specificity of 64%.

Lunotriquetral Shear (Reagan) Test. This test is designed to assess the integrity of the lunotriquetral ligament.[4] The clinician grasps the triquetrum between the thumb and the second finger of one hand and the lunate with the thumb and second finger of the other hand. The lunate is moved posteriorly (dorsally) with the thumb of one hand, while the triquetrum is pushed palmarly in the anteroposterior (AP) plane by the index finger of the other hand (Fig. 18-44). Crepitation, clicks, or discomfort in this area suggests injury to the ligament.[9,131] LaStayo and Howell[130] found this test to have a sensitivity of 64% and a specificity of 44% (LR+ 1.14; LR− 0.82).

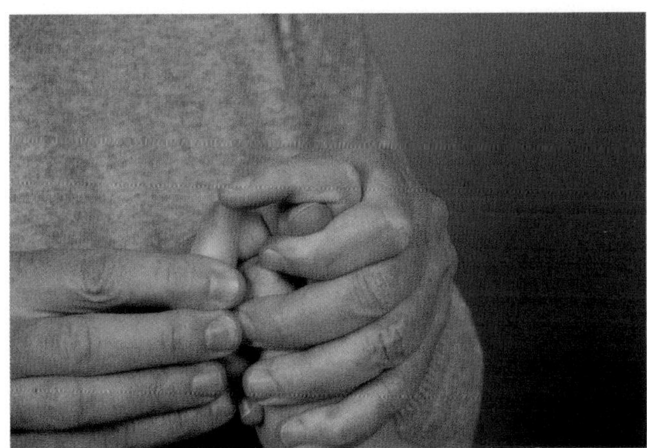

FIGURE 18-55 Flexor digitorum superficialis (FDS) test.

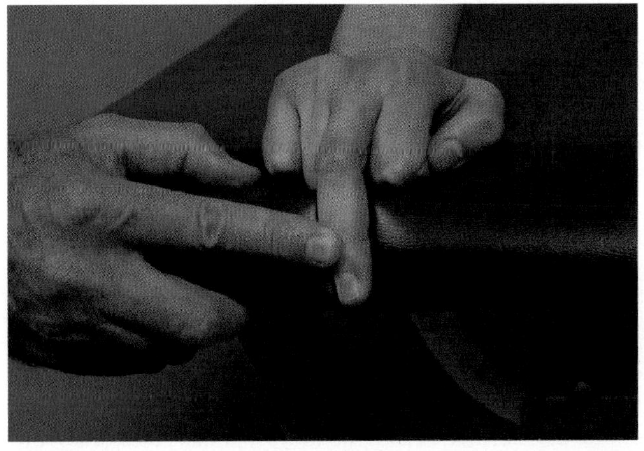

FIGURE 18-57 Integrity of the central slip (extensor hood rupture).

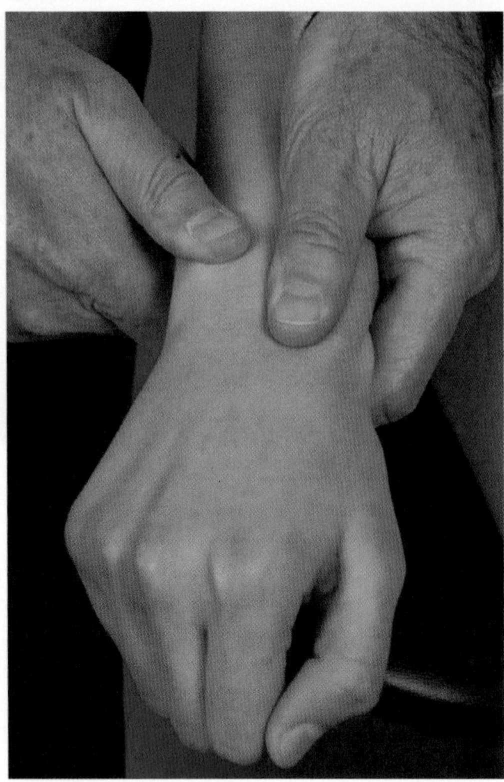

FIGURE 18-58 Piano key test.

The Pisotriquetral Shear Test. The pisotriquetral shear test assesses the integrity of the pisotriquetral articulation.[9] The clinician stabilizes the wrist with the fingers posterior (dorsal) to the triquetrum and the thumb over the pisiform. The pisiform is rocked back and forth in a medial and lateral direction. A positive test is manifested with pain during this maneuver. No diagnostic accuracy studies have been performed to determine the sensitivity and specificity of this test.

Pivot Shift Test of the Midcarpal Joint. The patient is positioned in sitting with the elbow flexed to 90 degrees and the forearm supinated. The clinician uses one hand to stabilize the forearm, while using the other hand to take the patient's hand into full radial deviation (Fig. 18-59). The patient's hand is then taken into full ulnar deviation. A positive test results if the capitate is felt to shift away from the lunate and indicates an injury to the anterior capsule and interosseous ligaments.[23] No diagnostic accuracy studies have been performed to determine the sensitivity and the specificity of this test.

Watson Test for Carpal Instability. The scaphoid shift maneuver examines the dynamic stability of the wrist, in particular the integrity of the scapholunate ligament.[13] The patient is positioned in sitting with their elbow in approximately 90 degrees of flexion, the forearm slightly pronated, and the wrist ulnarly deviated. The clinician grasps the wrist from the radial side and stabilizes the scaphoid tubercle with the thumb and the posterior (dorsal) aspect of the scaphoid with the index finger. The clinician uses the other hand to grasp the metacarpals. Starting in ulnar deviation in slight extension, the wrist is moved into radial deviation and slight flexion. As the wrist is brought passively into radial deviation, the normal flexion of the proximal row forces the scaphoid tubercle into an anterior (palmar) direction (into

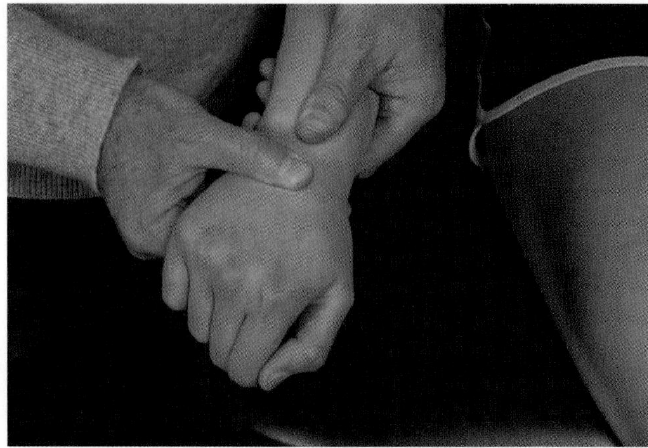

FIGURE 18-59 Pivot shift test of the midcarpal joint.

the clinician's thumb). The clinician attempts to prevent the anterior (palmar) motion of the scaphoid. When the scaphoid is unstable, its proximal pole is forced to sublux posteriorly (dorsally).[9] Pain at the posterior (dorsal) wrist or a clunk suggests instability.[26,29] The results are compared with the other hand. The results from the scaphoid shift test, which has been found to have a sensitivity of 69 percent and a specificity of between 64 and 68 percent,[91,92,130,132] should be used with caution, as the test can be positive in up to one-third of uninjured individuals.[14]

Scaphoid shift test. This is a slight modification to the Watson test. The patient positioning is similar to the Watson test except that the wrist is positioned in neutral to slight (0–10 degrees) radial deviation and neutral wrist flexion/extension. The clinician then quickly pushes the tubercle of the scaphoid in a posterior (dorsal) direction, noting a clunk, crepitus, or pain in comparison to the opposite wrist.[133] No diagnostic accuracy studies have been performed to determine the sensitivity and the specificity of this test.

Gamekeeper's or skier's thumb. The patient is positioned in sitting. The clinician stabilizes the patient's hand with one hand and takes the patient's thumb into extension with the other hand. While maintaining the thumb into extension, the clinician applies a valgus stress to the MCP joint of the thumb to stress the UCL (Fig. 18-60). A positive test is present

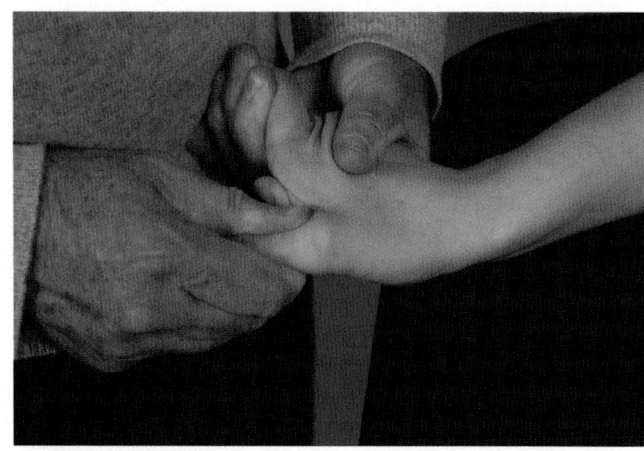

FIGURE 18-60 Gamekeeper's or skier's thumb.

if the valgus movement is greater than 30–35 degrees, indicating a complete tear of the UCL and the accessory collateral ligaments. Heymen and colleagues[134] reported a high sensitivity with this test (94%) and a 100% sensitivity and 46% specificity for detection of a palpable mass proximal to the MCP joint to indicate a complete tear of the UCL of the thumb.

Murphy Sign. The patient is asked to make a fist. If the head of the third metacarpal is level with the second and fourth metacarpals, the sign is positive for the presence of a lunate dislocation.[135]

Neurovascular Status. The assessment of sensibility and vasculature of the hand is an important component of every hand examination. Sensation is essential for precision movements and object manipulation. A number of tests can be used to document the neurovascular status of the wrist and hand.

Allen Test. The Allen test is used to determine the patency of the vessels supplying the hand. The clinician compresses both the radial and ulnar arteries at the wrist (Fig. 18-61), and then asks the patient to open and clench the fist three to four times to drain the venous blood from the hand. The patient is then asked to hold the hand open while the clinician releases the pressure on the ulnar artery and then the radial artery. The fingers and palm should be seen to regain their normal pink color. This procedure is repeated with the radial artery released and compression on the ulnar artery maintained. Normal filling time is usually less than 5 seconds. A distinct difference in the filling time suggests the dominance of one artery filling the hand.[131]

Tinel (Percussion) Test for CTS. The Tinel test is used to assist in the diagnosis of CTS. The area over the median nerve is tapped gently at the anterior (palmar) surface of the wrist (Fig. 18-62). If this produces tingling in the median nerve distribution, then the test is positive.[136] Variations exist between studies on the location and number of taps necessary to elicit a positive response, and in some studies the test is performed by tapping the median nerve in 20 degrees of wrist extension, while others tap along the path of the median nerve up to where the median nerve enters the carpal tunnel. The Tinel test has demonstrated a sensitivity of 60 percent and a specificity of 67 percent,[137] indicating that it is moderately acceptable for use in clinical practice.[138–141]

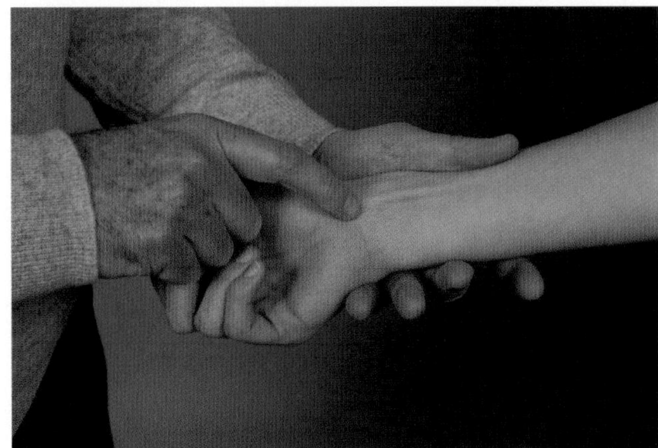

FIGURE 18-62 Tinel test at the wrist.

APB Weakness for CTS. The patient is positioned in sitting with their hand resting on the table. The clinician asked the patient to touch the pads of the thumb and small finger together. After asking the patient to keep the pads of the thumb and small finger together, the clinician applies a strong force in order to resist thumb abduction (Fig. 18-63). A positive test is weakness in some abduction with resisted testing as compared to the other hand. Studies performed to determine weakness in the APB are relatively consistent, demonstrating moderate diagnostic accuracy. For example, in a study by Gerr and Letz[142] the test was found to have a sensitivity of 63% and a specificity of 62%, compared to a Kuhlman and Hennessy study[143] that found the sensitivity to be 66% and the specificity to be 66%.

Phalen Test for CTS.[144,145] For the Phalen test, the patient sits comfortably with the wrists and elbows flexed (Fig. 18-64). The test is positive if the patient experiences numbness or tingling throughout the median nerve distribution of the hand within 45 seconds. For some patients, performance of this test recreates their wrist, thumb, or forearm ache.[146] Some studies have varied this test to be performed by the patient with wrist in complete flexion and elbow extended, bilateral wrist flexion with the posterior aspect of the hand pressing against one another, or passive wrist flexion by the clinician. The original Phalen test has demonstrated a sensitivity of 75 percent and a

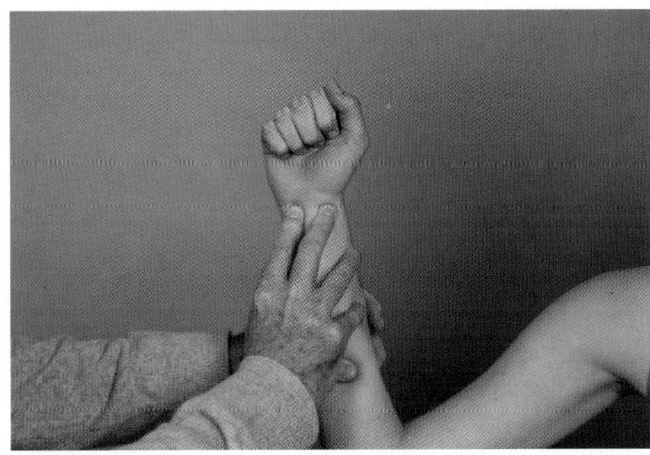

FIGURE 18-61 Allen test.

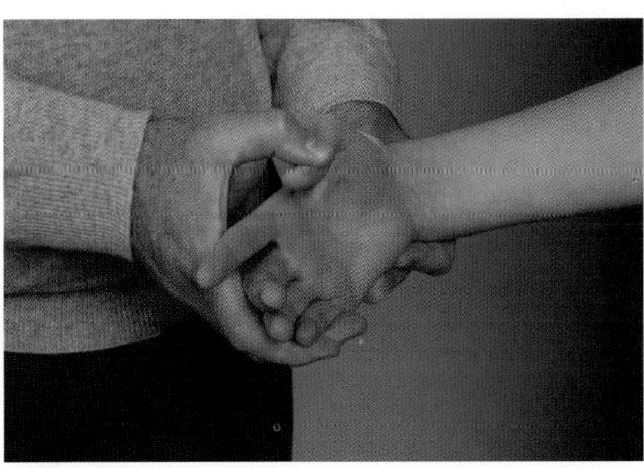

FIGURE 18-63 Abductor pollicis brevis weakness.

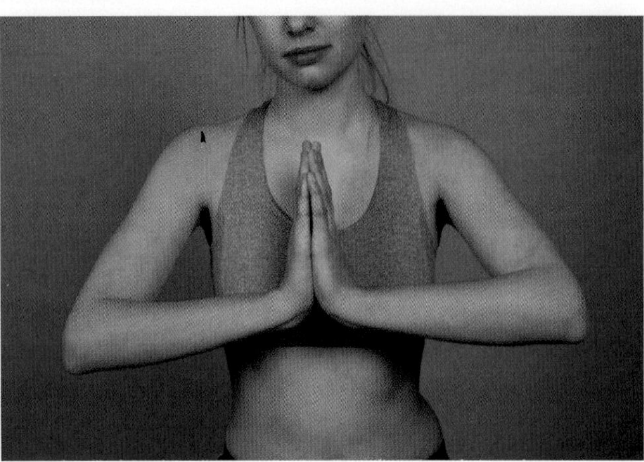

FIGURE 18-64 Phalen test.

specificity of 47 percent,[147] making it moderately acceptable for use in clinical practice.

Reverse Phalen Test for CTS. A reverse Phalen position is the same as the Phalen except the palms are placed together (Fig. 18-65). The patient is asked to keep both hands with the wrists in complete extension for 60 seconds (wrist and finger extension). A study by de Krom and colleagues[148] found the test to have a sensitivity of 41 percent and a specificity of 55 percent (LR+ 0.9; LR– 1.1). In another study, Werner and colleagues[149] showed that this maneuver results in a significantly higher intracarpal canal hydrostatic pressure as compared to a traditional Phalen or a modified Phalen maneuver and may add to the sensitivity of conventional screening methods.[136,150]

Hand Elevation Test for CTS. The patient is seated or standing and is asked to elevate both arms above the head (Fig. 18-66) and maintain them in this position until the patient feels paresthesia or numbness.[151] A positive test is the reproduction of symptoms such as paresthesia and numbness along the median nerve distribution after raising the arms for no greater than 2 minutes. A study by Ahn[152] found this test to have a sensitivity of 76 percent and a specificity of 99 percent (LR+ 76; LR– .24). In another study[151], this test was found to be more specific than the Phalen and Tinel tests. Although this clinical test has high diagnostic values there are numerous procedural biases in both study designs. In addition the test may be positive in patients with thoracic outlet syndrome.

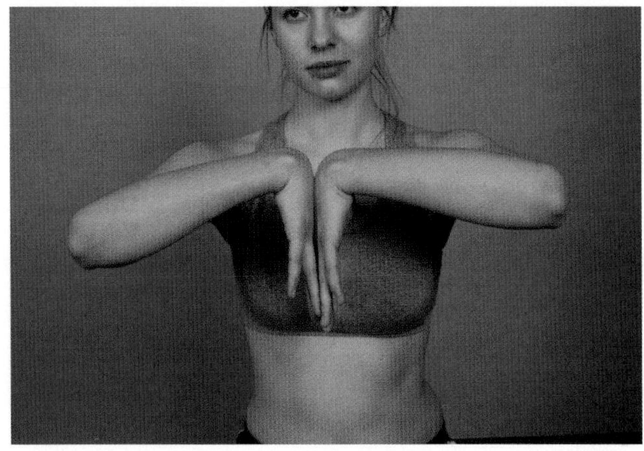

FIGURE 18-65 Reverse Phalen test.

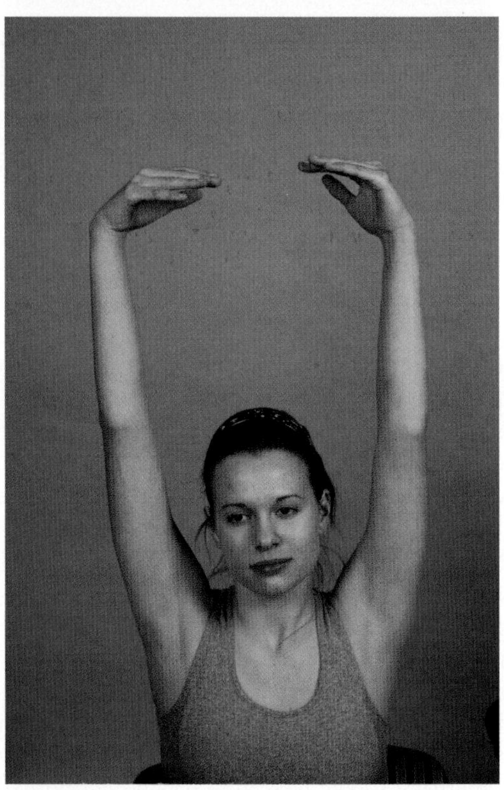

FIGURE 18-66 Hand elevation test.

Wrist flexion and median nerve compression. The patient is positioned in sitting with the elbow fully extended, the forearm in supination, and the wrist flexed to 60 degrees. The clinician applies an even constant pressure over the median nerve at the carpal tunnel using the thumb. A positive test for CTS is the reproduction of symptoms along the median nerve distribution within 30 seconds. Tetro and colleagues found this test to have a sensitivity of 86 percent and a specificity of 95 percent (LR+ 17; LR– 0.1).[153]

Median nerve compression test/pressure provocation test. The clinician sits opposite to the patient and holds the patient's hand with the clinician's thumbs directly over the course of the median nerve as it passes under the flexor retinaculum between the FCR and the palmaris longus. The clinician places gentle sustained pressure with the thumbs for 15 seconds to 2 minutes. The clinician then removes the pressure and questions the patient on the relief of symptoms, which may take a few minutes. A positive test is the reproduction of pain, paresthesia, or numbness distal to the site of compression during the compression in the distribution of the median nerve. Williams and colleagues[154] found this test to have a sensitivity of 100 percent and a specificity of 97 percent (LR+ 33; LR– 0).

Flick maneuver. The patient is positioned in sitting and is asked to vigorously shake his or her hands (Fig. 18-67). A positive test, indicating CTS, is the resolution of the paresthesia symptoms during or following administration of flicking the wrist. There appears to be some confusion as to what constitutes a flick. Some studies define a flick as a rapid, alternating movement up and down of the wrist, whereas

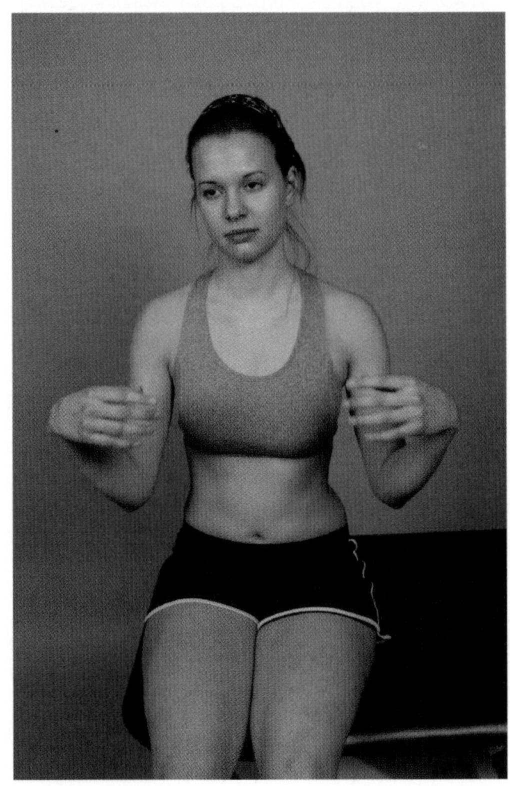

FIGURE 18-67 Flick maneuver.

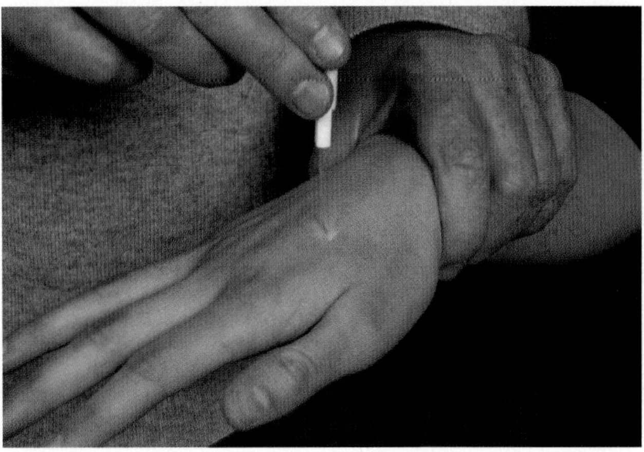

FIGURE 18-68 Semmes–Weinstein monofilament testing.

others describe the positive flick with as little movement as elbow extension. The diagnostic usefulness of this test is outlined in Table 18-12.

Semmes–Weinstein Monofilament Testing. The palm of the hand is divided into several areas, and only one point (usually in the center) is tested in each area.

- Between the fingertip and DIP joint.
- Between the DIP joint and PIP joint.
- Between the PIP joint and finger web.
- Between the finger web and the distal anterior (palmar) crease.
- Between the distal anterior (palmar) crease and the central palm.
- Base of palm and wrist.
- Superficial radial nerve distribution (Fig. 18-68)

The clinician applies a monofilament perpendicular to the surface, and the pressure is increased until the monofilament begins to bend (Fig. 18-69). Filament 2.83 MN is considered the "Normal" filament and indicates normal light touch perception. A positive test for CTS is when the patient with eyes closed cannot report which digit is receiving pressure at 2.83 mg. Normal values are depicted in Table 18-13. The diagnostic usefulness of this test based on some of the studies is outlined in Table 18-14.

Weber (Moberg) Two-Point Discrimination Test. The two-point discrimination tests were first introduced by Weber in

TABLE 18-12 The Diagnostic Usefulness of the Flick Maneuver

Study Description	Reliability	Sensitivity	Specificity	LR+	LR−	DOR	QUADAS Score
Hundred persons referred with suspected carpal tunnel syndrome underwent clinical and neurophysiological examinations blinded from each other. The gold standard for the CTS diagnosis was based on the results of these examinations but relief of CTS symptoms after surgery was also required[a]	NT	90	30	1.3	0.3	3.9	13
One hundred forty-two subjects referred for electrodiagnostic evaluation of possible CTS were first clinically evaluated with the flick, Phalen, and Tinel maneuvers before undergoing nerve conduction studies[b]	NT	37	74	1.4	0.9	1.7	11
The validity of 12 provocative tests for CTS in a random sample of 504 people from the general population was assessed[c]	NT	50	61	1.3	0.8	1.6	10

[a]Gunnarsson LG, Amilon A, Hellstrand P, et al: The diagnosis of carpal tunnel syndrome. Sensitivity and specificity of some clinical and electrophysiological tests. *J Hand Surg Br* 22:34–37, 1997.
[b]Hansen PA, Micklesen P, Robinson LR: Clinical utility of the flick maneuver in diagnosing carpal tunnel syndrome. *Am J Phys Med Rehabil* 83:363–367, 2004.
[c]de Krom MC, Knipschild PG, Kester AD, et al: Efficacy of provocative tests for diagnosis of carpal tunnel syndrome. *Lancet* 335:393–395, 1990.

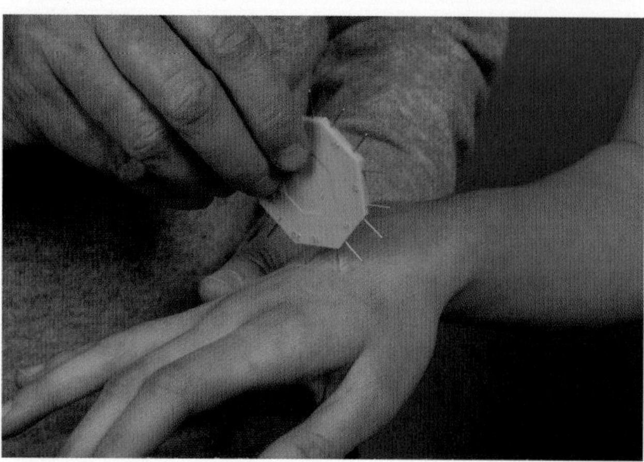

FIGURE 18-69 Disk-criminator.

TABLE 18-13	Light Touch Testing Scale and Filament Forces Using Semmes–Weinstein Monofilaments	
Color	**Pressure (mg)**	**Monofilament (MN)**
Green	50	2.83
Blue	200	3.61
Purple	2	4.31
Red	4	4.56
Red/orange	300	6.65
Diagonal redline	No response	0

1953 using calipers and by Moberg in 1958[155] using a paper clip.

Today it is recommended that a two-point aesthesiometer tool such as a Disk-Criminator (Fig. 18-69) be used. The instrument is explained and demonstrated to the patient until an appreciation can be made between one and two points in an area of normal sensibility. The instrument is applied, in a perpendicular fashion, to all of the fingertips in a mixed series of two and one points for five consecutive applications. The patient should be able to recognize at least four out of the five or seven out of ten.[23] The clinician repeats the tests in an attempt to find the minimal distance at which the patient can distinguish between the two stimuli, decreasing or increasing the distance between the points depending on the response by the patient.[23] This distance is called the threshold for discrimination. Normal discrimination distance is less than 6 mm, although this can vary between individuals, and in the area of the hand, with normal fingertip scores between 2 and 5 mm and finger surface scores between 3 and 7 mm.[156] Studies investigating the sensitivity and the specificity of this test indicate that the test has a high specificity but low sensitivity. For example, Buch-Jaeger and Foucher[157] found the test to have a sensitivity of 6 percent and a specificity of 99 percent. Another study by Gellman and colleagues[138] found the sensitivity to be 33 percent and the specificity to be 100 percent. These findings suggest that the test is useful for ruling in CTS.

Froment Sign. This is more of a sign than a test and may present as a complaint from the patient who reports an inability to pinch between the index finger and the thumb without flexion occurring at the DIP joint (Fig. 18-70).[158] A positive Froment sign, which results from a weakness in the AP and short head of the FPB muscles, indicates an ulnar nerve entrapment at the elbow or at the wrist.

Wrist ratio index. Sliding calipers are used to measure the mediolateral wrist width and then the AP height in centimeters. The caliper jaws are aligned with the distal wrist crease for both measurements. The wrist ratio index is calculated by dividing the AP measurement by the mediolateral measurement. A positive test for CTS is a wrist ratio of greater than 0.67. When used in isolation, the wrist ratio index does not appear to have strong diagnostic accuracy (Table 18-15).

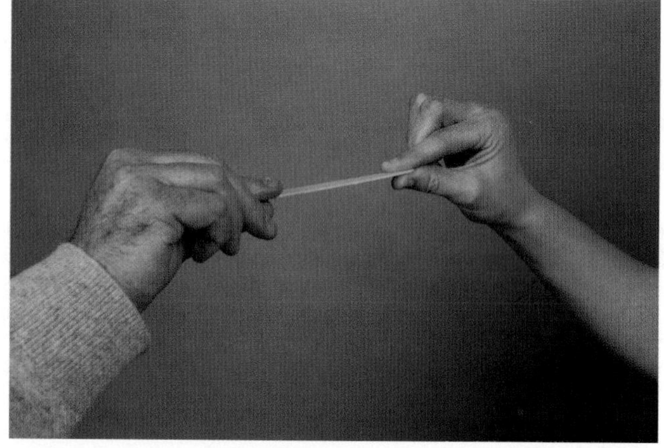

FIGURE 18-70 Froment sign.

TABLE 18-14 Diagnostic Usefulness of the Semmes–Weinstein Monofilament Test

Study	Reliability	Sensitivity	Specificity	LR+	LR−	DOR	QUADAS Score
Koris et al.[a]	NT	82	86	5.9	0.2	28	11
Pagel et al.[b]	NT	98	15	1.2	0.1	8.6	10
Buch-Jaeger and Foucher[c]	NT	59	59	1.4	0.7	2.1	9
Szabo et al.[d]	NT	83	NT	N/A	N/A	N/A	NT

[a]Koris M, Gelberman RH, Duncan K, et al: Carpal tunnel syndrome. Evaluation of a quantitative provocational diagnostic test. *Clin Orthop Relat Res* 157–161, 1990.
[b]Pagel KJ, Kaul MP, Dryden JD: Lack of utility of Semmes–Weinstein monofilament testing in suspected carpal tunnel syndrome. *Am J Phys Med Rehabil* 81:597–600, 2002.
[c]Buch-Jaeger N, Foucher G: Correlation of clinical signs with nerve conduction tests in the diagnosis of carpal tunnel syndrome. *J Hand Surg Br* 19:720–724, 1994.
[d]Szabo RM, Slater RR Jr, Farver TB, et al: The value of diagnostic testing in carpal tunnel syndrome. *J Hand Surg Am* 24:704–714, 1999.

TABLE 18-15 The Diagnostic Usefulness of the Wrist Ratio Index

Study Description	Reliability	Sensitivity	Specificity	LR+	LR−	DOR	QUADAS Score
The sensitivity and specificity of six CTS signs were determined by evaluating 143 subjects (228 hands) with symptoms of CTS. Immediately after performing the tests, standard nerve conduction studies were performed on all 228 hands to determine the presence or absence of CTS.[a]	NT	69	73	2.6	0.4	6.0	10
The average wrist ratio and median nerve latencies were determined in 665 patients with symptoms involving at least one hand or forearm.[b]	NT	47	83	2.8	0.6	4.3	10
Attempt to develop a CPR using a prospective diagnostic test study with blind comparison to a reference criterion of a compatible clinical presentation and abnormal electrophysiologic findings with 82 patients.[c]	ICC 0.77 (AP) 0.86 (ML)	93	26	1.3	0.3	4.7	12

[a]Kuhlman KA, Hennessey WJ: Sensitivity and specificity of carpal tunnel syndrome signs. *Am J Phys Med Rehabil* 76:451–457, 1997.
[b]Radecki P: A gender specific wrist ratio and the likelihood of a median nerve abnormality at the carpal tunnel. *Am J Phys Med Rehabil* 73:157–162, 1994.
[c]Wainner RS, Fritz JM, Irrgang JJ, et al: Development of a clinical prediction rule for the diagnosis of carpal tunnel syndrome. *Arch Phys Med Rehabil* 86:609–618, 2005.

The Katz Hand Diagram. Katz and colleagues[159] developed a hand symptom diagram rating system, which categorizes the distribution of current neuropathic hand symptoms using a key of numbness, tingling, pain, and decreased sensation. The diagram is designed to help diagnose those patients who have classic, probable, possible, and unlikely categories for CTS based on completion of the diagram. A number of studies have examined the diagnostic usefulness of the Katz Hand Diagram (Table 18-16).

The Wazir sign.[160] The patient, wrist is rested in extension, supination, and a relaxed position supported by the clinician. Using a reflex hammer or finger tip, the clinician gently taps on the extended wrist around the palmaris longus tendon (Fig. 18-71). A positive sign, indicating cervical myelopathy, exaggerates response of finger flexion, thumb flexion, and wrist flexion. The basis of this sign can be explained on the basis of disinhibition of tendon stretch reflex of the long flexor tendons of the fingers (C7 and C8), wrist flexors (C6 and C7), and/or with the involvement of pyramidal tracts.

Adverse Neural Tension

The Median Nerve. The patient is positioned in supine lying or sitting. The cervical spine is side bent and rotated to the

TABLE 18-16 The Diagnostic Usefulness of the Katz Hand Diagram

Study Description	Reliability	Sensitivity	Specificity	LR+	LR−	DOR	QUADAS Score
Comparison of diagnostic tests including hand pain diagram with neurophysiologic testing in 110 patients.[a]	NT	61	71	2.1	0.5	3.8	13
Diagram ratings of 63 patients (85 hands) evaluated in a hand clinic were compared with diagnoses established independent of diagram results by objective clinical criteria.[b]	NT	80	90	3.6	0.1	65	11
A study to determine the validity of tests or a combination of tests for the diagnosis of carpal tunnel syndrome in three groups of 50 subjects.[c]	NT	76	98	38	0.2	155	9
One hundred fifty-six consecutive new patients presenting with pain, numbness, or tingling of the upper extremity completed the carpal tunnel outcome instrument and the self-administered hand diagram developed by Katz[d]	NT	80	90	8.0	0.2	36	8

[a]Katz JN, Larson MG, Sabra A, et al: The carpal tunnel syndrome: diagnostic utility of the history and physical examination findings. *Ann Intern Med* 112:321–327, 1990.
[b]Katz JN, Stirrat CR: A self-administered hand diagram for the diagnosis of carpal tunnel syndrome. *J Hand Surg Am* 15:360–363, 1990.
[c]Szabo RM, Slater RR Jr, Farver TB, et al: The value of diagnostic testing in carpal tunnel syndrome. *J Hand Surg Am* 24:704–714, 1999.
[d]Atroshi I, Breidenbach WC, McCabe SJ: Assessment of the carpal tunnel outcome instrument in patients with nerve-compression symptoms. *J Hand Surg Am* 22:222–227, 1997.

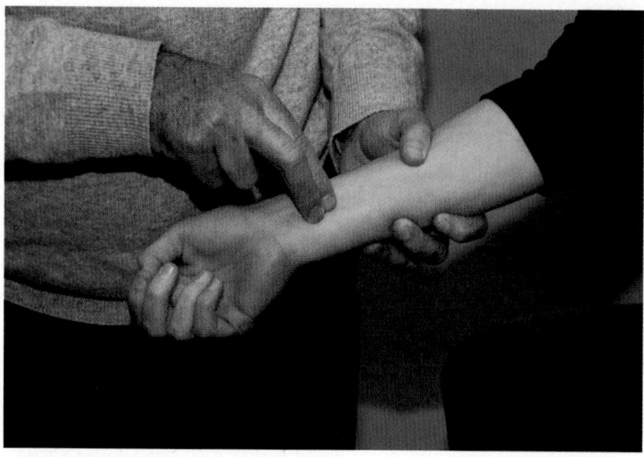

FIGURE 18-71 The Wazir sign.

opposite side. The shoulder girdle is positioned in retraction, depression, extension, and external rotation. The elbow is positioned in extension, the forearm in supination, and the wrist in extension (Chapter 11). The fingers are positioned in extension. Nerve irritation is suspected if

- with the cervical spine in the resting position, the upper extremity position described above results in symptoms in the anterior (palmar)/radial side of the hand;
- if the symptoms increase with cervical side bending and rotation away from the tested extremity;
- if the symptoms decrease with side bending and rotation toward the tested extremity.

If adherence of the nerve is suspected at the wrist, the cervical spine is positioned in the resting position and the extremity is positioned as before. Neural involvement should be suspected if

- with wrist flexion the symptoms decrease, but increase when the cervical spine is side bent and rotated away from the tested extremity;
- with wrist extension and the cervical spine side bent and rotated to the tested extremity, the symptoms decrease.

Radial Nerve. The patient is positioned in a supine or sitting position and the shoulder is positioned in retraction, depression, extension, and internal rotation. The elbow is positioned in extension, the forearm in pronation, the wrist in flexion and ulnar deviation, and the fingers in flexion (Chapter 11). If a nerve adhesion is suspected at the wrist, the procedure is as for the median nerve, except that the wrist is placed in extension and then taken back into flexion.

The posterior (dorsal) sensory nerve, which can become implicated (Wartenberg syndrome; see "Intervention Strategies") in a variety of radial-sided injuries because of its superficial location, can be stretched with a combination of wrist flexion and ulnar deviation.

Ulnar Nerve. The shoulder girdle positioning used to describe the test for the median nerve is used. The elbow is flexed and supinated, the wrist is extended and radially deviated, and the fingers extended (Chapter 11). If a nerve adhesion at the wrist is suspected, the procedure is as for the median nerve.

Diagnostic Imaging

Diagnostic testing of the forearm, wrist, and hand is limited to plain radiographs for most patients (see chapter 7). Bony tenderness with a history of trauma or a suspicion of bone or joint disruption indicates a need for radiographs. Standard projections for the wrist are the posteroanterior, lateral, and oblique. For the patient with a suspicion of a scaphoid injury, a scaphoid view should be added.[4] Wrist conditions rarely require computed tomography scans and MRI scans.[131]

The Evaluation

Following the examination, and once the clinical findings have been recorded, the clinician must determine a specific diagnosis or a working hypothesis, based on a summary of all of the findings. This diagnosis can be structure related (medical diagnosis) (Tables 18-17 and 18-18) or a diagnosis based on the preferred practice patterns as described in the Guide to Physical Therapist Practice.

INTERVENTION STRATEGIES

To restore the balance and beauty and power to a disabled hand is an adventure. The stakes are high. The rewards are exciting. The penalties of failure are grievous.

—Paul W. Brand (1914–2003)

Functional rehabilitation of the upper extremity emphasizes the restoration of functional use of the hand.[109] Hand functions can range from activities that require a strong gripping action to those that require fine precision and gentle touch. Stability of the wrist and hand is provided by a combination of muscular effort and ligamentous support. Motion of the hand and wrist is provided by a vast array of muscles and tendons and several articulated linkages. The hand and wrist can be involved in both open- and closed-kinetic chain activities.

Pain is perhaps the most common complaint with wrist and hand injuries, with stiffness following closely behind. Some conditions, such as peripheral nerve injury (as a result of fracture, dislocation, disease, etc.), diabetes mellitus, Raynaud, and complex regional pain syndrome (CRPS), are characterized by a loss of sensibility to varying degrees. Sensory recovery progresses in time and space according to the following successive stages:[161]

- Perception of pain and temperature—establishment of protective sensation
- Perception of low-frequency vibratory stimuli (30 Hz) as well as moving sense
- Per static tactile sense, at the same time as perception of high-frequency vibratory stimuli (256 Hz)
- Two-point discrimination—the last form of sensation to develop

Motor recovery is always slower than sensory recovery with the first sign of motor recovery being the regression of the atrophy in the territory normally supplied by the injured nerve.[161] Later, a weak contraction can be detected in the first muscle supplied by the nerve distal to the lesion, although this contraction is not powerful enough to produce joint movement or to overcome gravity.[161]

TABLE 18-17 Differential Diagnosis for Common Causes of Wrist and Hand Pain

Condition	Patient Age	Mechanism of Injury	Symptoms Aggravated by	Observation	AROM	PROM	End Feel	Resisted	Special Tests	Tenderness with Palpation
Carpal tunnel syndrome	35–55	Gradual overuse Wide-variety of factors	Repetitive activities of wrist Sustained positioning of wrist in flexion	Thenar muscle atrophy (later stages)	Full and pain-free			Weakness of grip on radial side (chronic) Strong and pain free (acute)	Tinel Phalen	Reproduction of symptoms with compression applied on anterior aspect of wrist
Wrist extensor tendonitis	20–50	Repetitive or prolonged activities, forceful exertion, awkward and static postures, vibration, and localized mechanical stress		Unremarkable		Wrist pain with finger flexion combined with radial/ulnar deviation		Pain with wrist extension		Anterior carpus
Wrist flexor tendonitis	20–50	Forceful gripping, rapid wrist movements, moving the wrist and fingers to the extremes of range	Activities involving wrist extension	Unremarkable	Wrist extension	Pain with combined wrist extension and elbow extension		Pain with wrist flexion		Pisiform In palm over base of second metacarpal
OA of first CMC Joint	40–60	Repetitive trauma Degeneration	Repetitive use of thumb Strong gripping	Soft-tissue thickening at base of thumb	Midlimitation of all thumb movements	Pain with thumb rotation Pain on thumb extension and abduction		Weakness of grip on radial side (chronic)		Anatomic snuff box

(Continued)

TABLE 18-17 Differential Diagnosis for Common Causes of Wrist and Hand Pain *(Continued)*

Condition	Patient Age	Mechanism of Injury	Symptoms Aggravated by	Observation	AROM	PROM	End Feel	Resisted	Special Tests	Tenderness with Palpation
Trigger finger	50+	Disproportion between the flexor tendon and its tendon sheath		Thickening/ puckering of skin in palm	Decreased finger extension Clicing or jerking with movements	Full and pain-free	Soft-tissue resistance to finger extension	Strong and pain free		No pain, but snapping of flexor tendon felt with finger extension
De Quervains tenosynovitis	50+	Repetitive finger-thumb gripping combined with radial deviation	Overuse, repetitive tasks which involve overexertion of the thumb	Swelling over lateral wrist/ thumb	Decreased ulnar deviation Decreased thumb flexion	Pain on thumb flexion combined with ulnar deviation of wrist		Pain with abduction and extension of thumb	Finkelstein	Lateral wrist and thumb
Duputryens contracture	40+	Multifactorial (alcohol, diabetes, epilepsy, smoking, trauma)		Thickening/ puckering of skin in palm	Decreased finger extension		Soft-tissue resistance to finger extension	Strong and pain free	Inability to place the palm of your hand completely flat on a hard surface	No tenderness, but thickening of soft tissues evident
Thumb ulnar collateral ligament injury	Varies	Forced hyperabduction and/or hyperextension stress of the thumb MCP joint	Extension of the thumb	Swelling at the ulnar side of the MCP joint	Usually unremarkable	Pain with passive hyperextension/ yperabduction		Usually unremarkable	Stress testing of the UCL	Ulnar side of the MCP joint of the thumb
Wrist sprain	20–40	Trauma (FOOSH injury)	Taking weight through the hand	Possible swelling around wrist joint	Extremes of all ranges	Wrist pain with ulnar or radial deviation		Pain with strong resistance in any direction		Medial or lateral joint line

TABLE 18-18 Findings in Common Conditions of the Hand and Wrist

Condition	Findings
de Quervain stenosing tenosynovitis	Tenderness and swelling over the first posterior (dorsal) compartment at the radial styloid Finkelstein test aggravates pain
Dupuytren disease	Palpable nodules and pretendinous cords in anterior (palmar) aponeurosis, most commonly affecting the ring or the little finger Secondary flexion contracture of the MCP and, occasionally, PIP joints
Flexor tendon sheath infection	Cardinal signs of Kanavel present Finger held in flexed position at rest Swelling along the volar surface of the finger Tenderness on the volar surface of the finger along the course of the flexor tendon sheath Pain exacerbated by passive extension of the involved finger
Injury to the ulnar collateral ligament of the MCP joint of the thumb (skier's or gamekeeper's thumb)	Swelling and tenderness over the ulnar aspect of the thumb MCP joint Pain exacerbated by stress of the UCL Increased laxity of the thumb UCL (more severe injuries)
Scapholunate instability	Swelling over the radial wrist. X-rays show increased scapholunate gap on clenched fist view (>1 mm) Tenderness over the posterior (dorsal) wrist over the scapholunate ligament Scaphoid shift test produces abnormal popping and reproduces the patient's pain
Mallet finger	Flexed or dropped posture of the finger at the DIP joint History of jamming injury (impact of a thrown ball) Inability to actively extend or straighten the DIP joint
Jersey finger (FDP avulsion)	Mechanism is hyperextension stress applied to a flexed finger (e.g., grabbing a player's jersey) Patient lacks active flexion at the DIP joint (FDP function lost) Swollen finger often assumes a position of relative extension compared to the other more flexed fingers
Degenerative arthritis of the fingers	Heberden nodes (most common) Bouchard nodes (common) Mucous cysts (occasional) Decreased motion at involved IP joints Instability of involved joints (occasional)

Data from Mass DP, Reider B: Hand and wrist. In: Reider B, ed. *The Orthopaedic Physical Examination*. Philadelphia, PA: WB Saunders, 1999:99–158.

Physical therapy techniques that can be used to help with motor and sensory recovery include the following:

- Activities and techniques to increase tactile input including electrical stimulation, high-frequency vibration, and tapping
- Contrast baths (for vasomotor disturbances)
- Protection through splinting
- Dexterity activities
- Weight-bearing activities through the affected extremity
- Neurodynamic mobilizations (Chapter 11)

The techniques to increase joint mobility and the techniques to increase soft-tissue extensibility are described in "Therapeutic Techniques".

Acute Phase

The goals of the acute phase include the following:

- Protection of the injury site to allow healing.
- Control pain and inflammation.
- Control and then eliminate edema.
- Restoration of pain-free range of motion in the entire kinetic chain.
- Improve patient comfort by decreasing pain and inflammation.
- Retard muscle atrophy.
- Minimize detrimental effects of immobilization and activity restriction.[162–167]
- Scar management if appropriate.
- Maintain general fitness.
- Patient to be independent with home exercise program.

Pain and inflammation control is the major focus of the intervention program in the acute phase. This may be accomplished using the principles of PRICEMEM (protection, rest, ice, compression, elevation, manual therapy, early motion, and medication). Icing for 20–30 minutes, three to four times a day, concurrent with nonsteroidal anti-inflammatory drugs (NSAIDs), or aspirin can aid in reducing pain and swelling.

One of the most significant problems a clinician faces with a hand-injured patient is the control and the elimination of edema. Edema can increase the risk of infection, decrease motion, and inhibit arterial, venous, and lymphatic flow.[168] Methods to control edema include elevation of the upper extremity and hand above the level of the heart, cryotherapy, active exercise, retrograde massage, intermittent compression, continuous compression wrapping, and contrast baths.

Therapeutic exercises are performed with the goal of regaining adequate soft-tissue rebalancing of the wrist by restoring the alignment of the extensor and the flexor tendons as near to normal as possible, and to prevent scarring or soft-tissue contractures by influencing the physiologic process of collagen formation. Movement is necessary to maintain joint mobility and gliding tendon function. Range-of-motion exercises are introduced as early as tolerated. These may be passive, active assisted, or active, as appropriate. If protected motion is necessary, it can be provided with taping, bracing, or in extreme cases, casting.

PROM exercises are performed through the available range of motion to maintain joint and soft-tissue mobility, or a passive stretch can be applied at the end range of motion to lengthen pathologically shortened soft-tissue structures, thereby increasing motion. Depending on the focus of the intervention, the PROM exercises may include

- MCP flexion and extension (Fig. 18-72).
- PIP and DIP flexion and extension (Fig. 18-73) and combined flexion and extension (Fig. 18-74).

AROM exercises should include specific and composite exercises. Composite exercises, which include fisting and thumb opposition to each digit in addition to exercises involving the wrist, elbow, and shoulder are designed to reproduce normal functional activities. Fast ballistic movements are discouraged if the goal is to restore mobility in the presence of increasing tissue resistance.[169] Examples of AROM exercises include the following:

- Active wrist and finger flexion and extension, wrist ulnar and radial deviation, finger adduction and abduction, and thumb opposition (Fig. 18-75), flexion, extension, abduction, and adduction. The wrist and hand muscles are usually exercised as a group if their strength is similar.

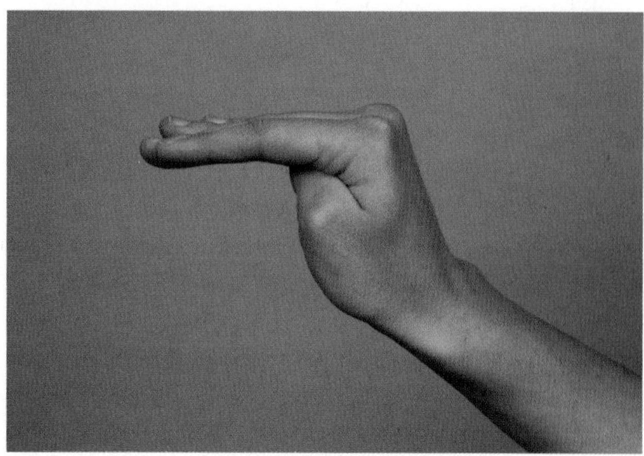

FIGURE 18-72 Isolated MCP flexion.

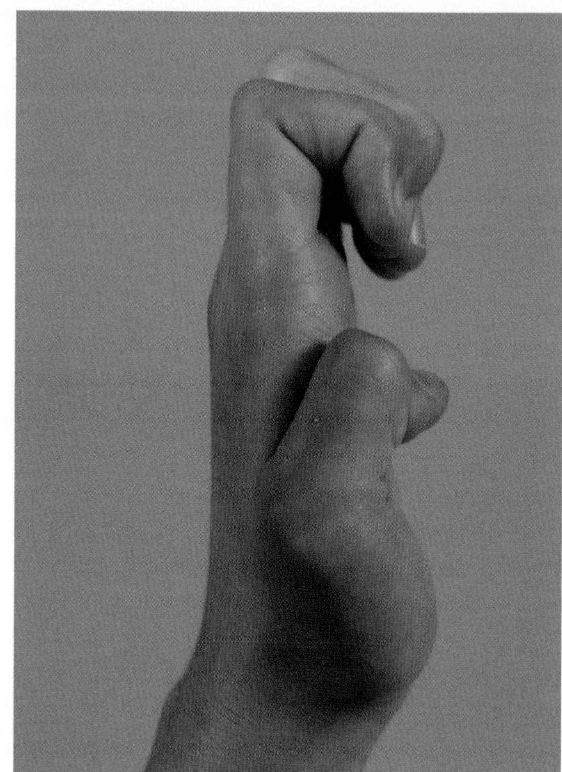

FIGURE 18-73 Isolated PIP and DIP flexion and extension.

Weaker muscles should be isolated in a similar fashion as that used when isolating the muscle for manual muscle testing. Protected range-of-motion exercises are performed to selectively mobilize joints and tendons while minimizing stress on repairing structures. As their name suggests, protected range-of-motion exercises are accomplished by placing the repaired structure in a protected position while adjacent tissues are carefully mobilized. An example of protective exercise can be seen following a radial nerve injury, where tendon transfers of the pronator teres, FCU,

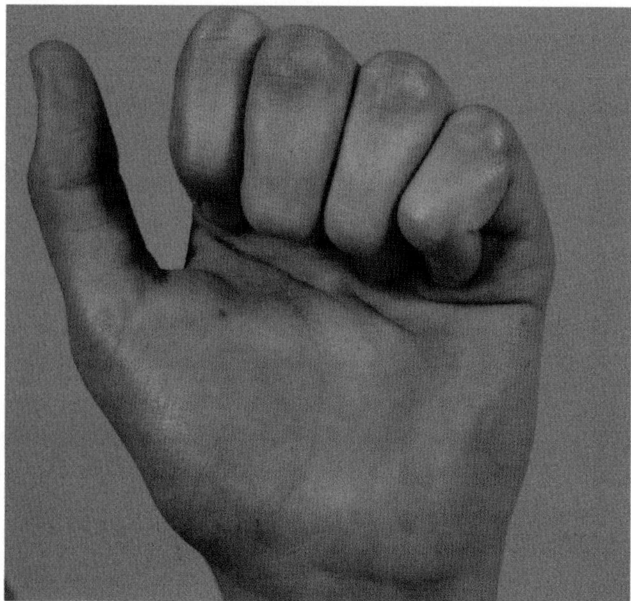

FIGURE 18-74 MCP, PIP and DIP flexion and extension.

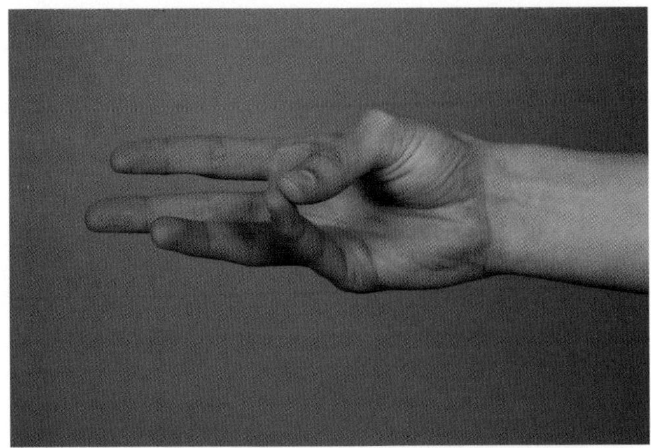

FIGURE 18-75 Thumb opposition.

and FDS may be performed.[169] Following the surgery the hand is immobilized with the wrist, MCP joints, and thumb in extension. At approximately 4 weeks, protective active motion exercises are introduced. These include MCP joint flexion and then PIP and DIP joint flexion with the MCP joint maintained in extension.[169]

- Active exercises of forearm pronation and supination.
- Active exercises of elbow flexion and extension

The AROM exercises are progressed to submaximal isometrics and muscle co-contractions. These early strengthening exercises are performed initially in the available pain-free ranges and, as pain subsides, are gradually progressed so that they are performed throughout the entire range.

Scar tissue management focuses on the control of stresses placed on healing tissues. Early active and passive motion provides controlled stress, encouraging optimal remodeling of scar tissue.[168] Methods to control scarring include the use of thermal agents, transverse friction massage (TFM) (see Chapter 11), mechanical vibration, compressive techniques, and splinting.

Splinting of the wrist and hand may be necessary. It is not within the scope of this text to provide comprehensive detail with regard to splinting. Entire texts are devoted to the subject.[170–173] However, splinting can often be an integral part of the rehabilitation program, and creative splinting can provide a useful adjunct to exercise. The general purposes of a splint are as follows[174,175]:

- ***Prevent or correct deformity or dysfunction.*** Maintain or re-establish normal tissue length, balance, and excursion.
- ***Immobilize/stabilize.*** To stabilize a mobile joint so the corrective exercise force can be directed to the stiff joint or adherent tendon.[169]
- ***Protect.*** Static splints have no moveable parts and maintain joints in one position to promote healing and minimize stress.
- ***Control/modify scar formation.***
- ***Substitute for dysfunctional tissue.***
- ***Provide exercise.*** *Dynamic splints* are used to provide active resistance in the direction opposite their line of pull to increase muscle strength, as well as to apply a corrective passive stretch to tendon adhesions and joint contractures.[169] *Drop-out* splints, which are commonly used with elbow flexion contractures, block joint motion in one direction but allow motion in another. Articulated splints contain at least two static components and are designed in such a way as to allow motion in one plane at a joint. *Static-progressive* splints involve the use of inelastic components to allow progressive changes in joint position as PROM changes without changing the structure of the splint. *Serial static* splints differ from static progressive splints in that they require the clinician to remold the splint to accommodate changes in range of motion.

Functional Phase

The functional phase of rehabilitation is usually initiated when normal wrist positions and co-contractions of the wrist flexors and extensors can be performed. The goals of the functional phase include the following:

- Attain full range of pain-free motion.
- Restore normal joint kinematics.
- Improve muscle strength to within normal limits.
- Improve neuromuscular control.
- Restore normal muscle force couple relationships.

The AROM exercises, initiated during the acute phase, are progressed until the patient demonstrates they have achieved the maximum range anticipated.

Normal joint kinematics are restored using joint mobilization techniques. Joint mobilization techniques refer to passive traction and/or gliding movements to joint surfaces that maintain or restore the joint play normally allowed by the capsule. The joint mobilization techniques for the forearm, wrist, and hand are described in "Therapeutic Techniques" at the end of this chapter.

Resistive exercises not only increase muscle strength and endurance, but also improve the ability of the patient to actively mobilize stiff joints.[169] Resistance exercises for the hand and wrist can be classified as either static (isometric) or dynamic (concentric, eccentric, or isokinetic). Strengthening of the muscles of the wrist and hand begins with specific exercises and progresses to exercises that involve the entire upper kinetic chain, including the trunk. Isometric exercises may be continued from the acute phase when the available range of motion remains restricted. Wherever possible, resistance exercises that strengthen functional muscle groups rather than individual muscles should be selected.[169] Specific exercises for the wrist and hand include the following:

- Resisted exercises into pronation (Fig. 18-76) and supination (Fig. 18-77).
- Hand and finger dexterity exercises including the nine-peg board (Fig. 18-78) or stroking exercises.
- Manually resisted exercises (Fig. 18-79). These are performed by the clinician initially, before becoming part of the patient's home exercise routine (Fig. 18-80).
- Resisted exercises can be performed using gripping with light resistive putty (Fig. 18-81) or a hand exerciser

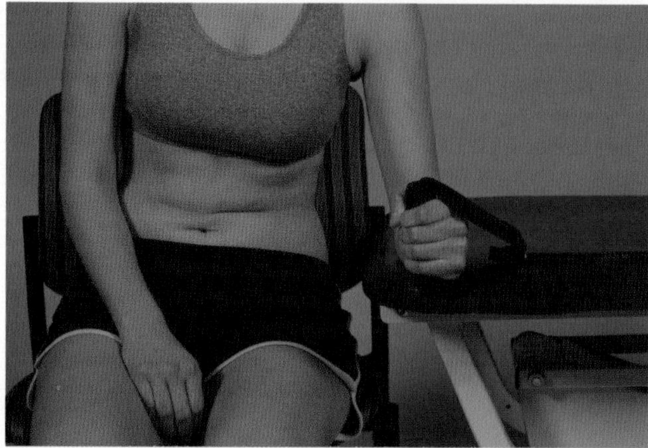

FIGURE 18-76 Resisted pronation.

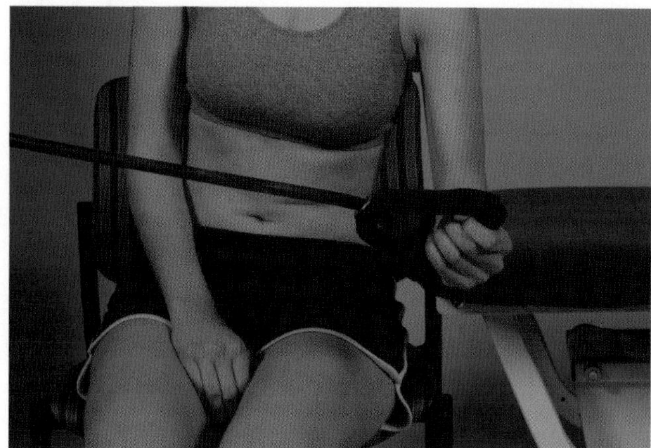

FIGURE 18-77 Resisted supination.

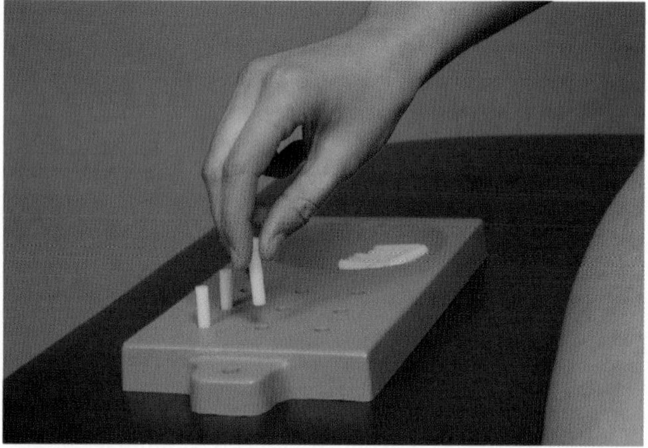

FIGURE 18-78 Nine-peg board.

(Fig. 18-82). Care must be taken with gripping or squeezing exercises because they typically restrict the use of the full range of motion.

- Resisted exercises can also be performed using elastic resistance (Fig. 18-83) or dumbbells (Fig. 18-84).
- Wrist extension should be done in pronation to work against gravity or in neutral forearm rotation to eliminate gravity. This exercise encourages the involvement of the ECRL, ECRB, and ECU. MCP flexion can be employed to eliminate any contribution from the ECU, thereby isolating the wrist musculature.

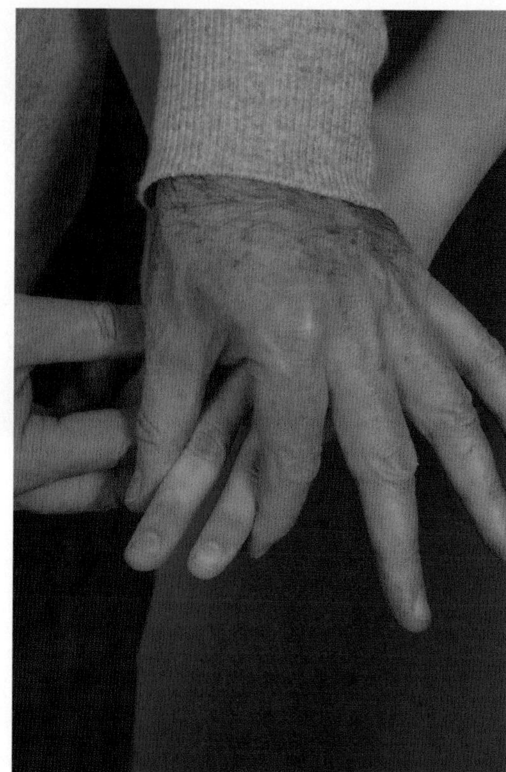

FIGURE 18-79 Manually resisted exercises.

- Wrist flexion should be done in supination to work against gravity or in neutral forearm rotation to eliminate gravity. Wrist flexion works the FCU and FCR.

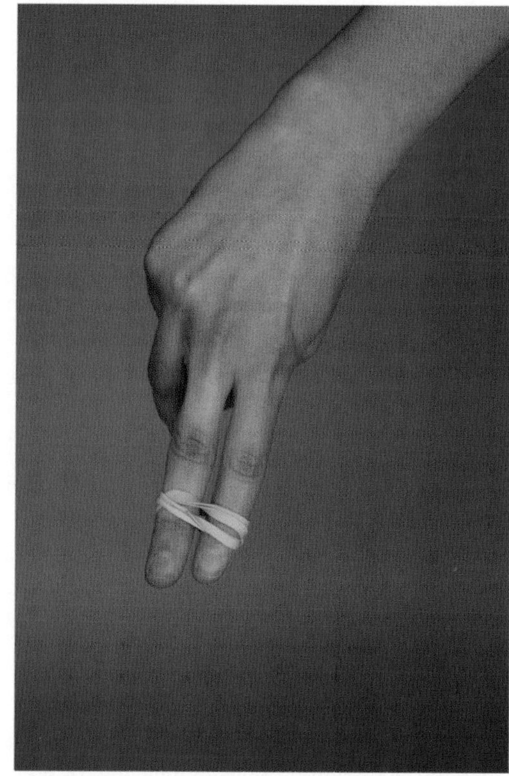

FIGURE 18-80 Resistance using elastic bands.

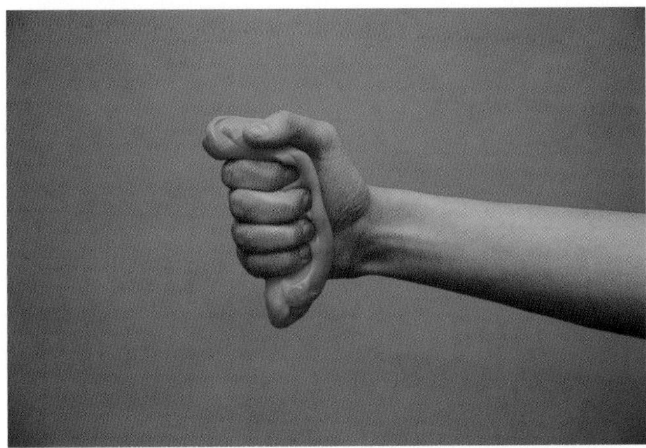
FIGURE 18-81 Putty exercises.

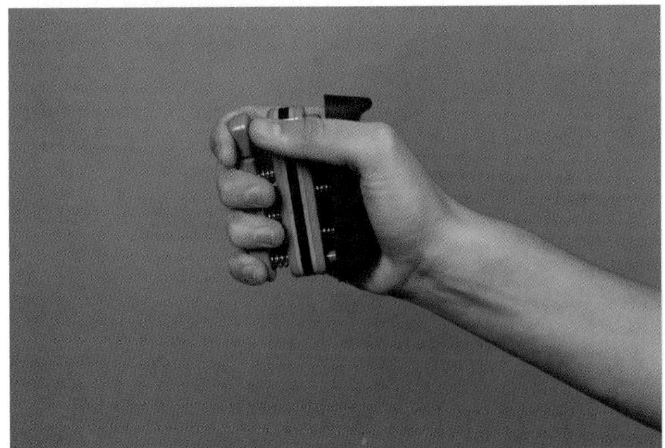
FIGURE 18-82 Hand exerciser.

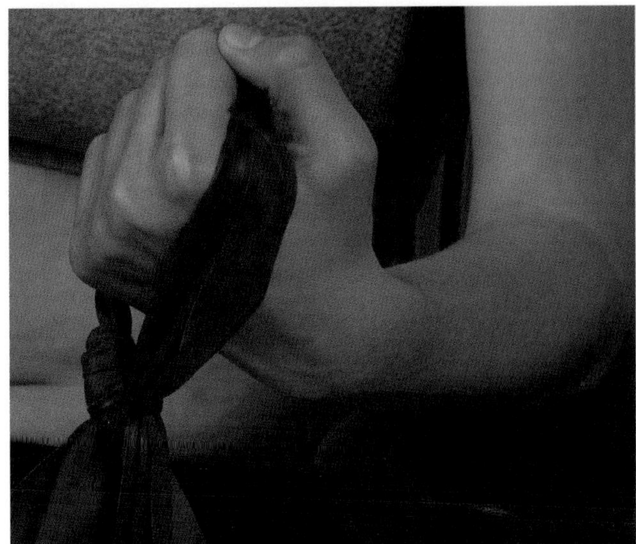
FIGURE 18-83 Resisted wrist flexion with elastic resistance.

- Proprioceptive neuromuscular facilitation patterns of the upper extremity are performed actively and then with resistance. These patterns incorporate the conjunct rotations involved with finger, hand, and wrist motions.

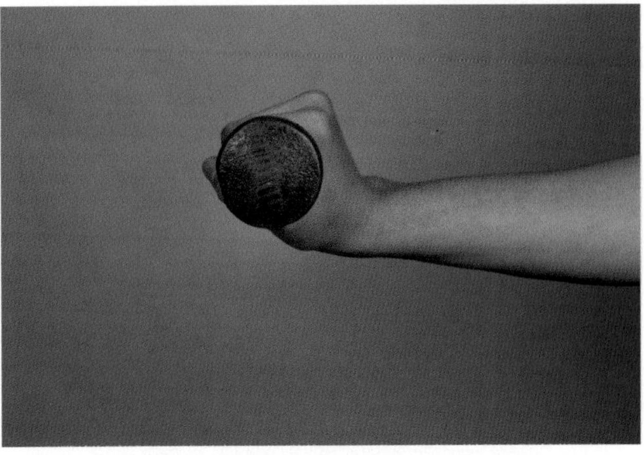
FIGURE 18-84 Resisted wrist extension with dumbbell.

- Wall push-ups encourage full wrist extension, while full push-ups require full, or close to full, wrist extension.
- ***Wrist flexion ball flips.*** Holding a small weighted ball, the patient leans forward over a treatment table so that the forearm is resting on the table but the hand and wrist is over the end, palm facing upward. The patient is asked to toss the ball in the air and then to catch it while keeping the elbow on the table.

The exercises for the other joints of the upper extremity are outlined in Chapters 16 and 17.

PRACTICE PATTERN 4D: IMPAIRED JOINT MOBILITY, MOTOR FUNCTION, MUSCLE PERFORMANCE, RANGE OF MOTION ASSOCIATED WITH CONNECTIVE TISSUE DYSFUNCTION

Rheumatoid Arthritis[176]

RA is a disease that affects the entire body and the whole person (see Chap. 5). It is a lifelong disease, which in the majority of people is only modified somewhat by intervention.[177] The cycle of stretching, healing, and scarring that occurs as a result of the inflammatory process seen in patients with RA causes significant damage to the soft tissues and periarticular structures.[178] As a consequence, these events may lead to pain, stiffness, joint damage, instability, and ultimately deformity. Many common hand and wrist deformities can be seen,[179] such as ulnar deviation of the MCP joints,[180] boutonnière deformity,[181] and swan-neck deformities of the digits.[182]

Ulnar Drift. The deformity of the ulnar drift and anterior (palmar) subluxation (Fig. 18-85A) is a result of a complex interaction of forces and damage to collateral ligaments and extensor mechanisms. Clinically, ulnar drift of the MCP articulations often precedes the wrist deformities.[23] The ulnar drift results in an imbalance that has the resultant effect of pulling the fingers into ulnar deviation, pronation, and

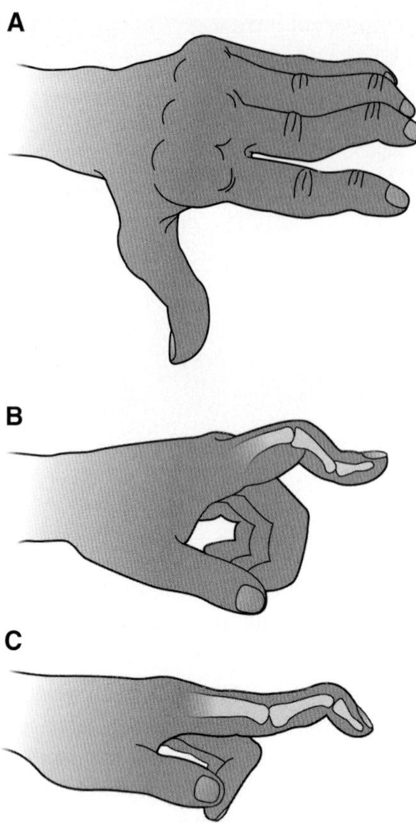

FIGURE 18-85 Finger deformities.

anterior (palmar) subluxation. The list of causes includes the following[179,183]:

- Subcollateral synovitis and weakening of the radial collateral ligament
- Distortion and attenuation of the sagittal fibers of the extensor hood
- A natural displacement of the extensor tendons to the ulnar side
- Radial deviation of the wrist
- Secondary contracture of the ulnar side intrinsic muscles
- Dysfunction of the radial side intrinsics
- Displacement of the flexor tendons to the ulnar side
- Appositional pinch (i.e., key pinch)
- Gravity
- The natural anatomic shape of the metacarpal head

Normally, in the flexed position, minimal lateral movement occurs at the MCP joint, but with increased laxity of the collateral ligaments, up to 45 degrees of lateral deviation occurs in this position.

Boutonnière Deformity. The boutonnière or buttonhole deformity (Fig. 18-85B) occurs when the common extensor tendon that inserts on the base of the middle phalanx is damaged. Damage to the central slip insertion requires extra effort to extend the joint, causing hyperextension at the DIP joint. The failure of the lateral bands to be connected to the central slip allows these bands to drift forward. Eventually they pass the axis of rotation of the PIP joint, and instead of extending this joint, they act as flexors while still hyperextending the distal joint. Such destruction also results in the loss of the influence of the interosseous muscles, ED longus, and lumbrical muscles on the PIP joints. Simultaneous with the loss of this muscle influence, the lateral bands of the extensor mechanism slide anteriorly. The realignment of the extensor mechanism, coupled with the loss of certain muscle influence, produces a deformity of extension of the MCP and DIP joints and flexion of the PIP joint. This is the classic boutonnière deformity.[182] The causes, namely synovitis, central slip rupture, and displaced lateral bands, are treatable by synovectomy,[184] repair, or reconstruction of the central slip and relocation of the lateral bands.

Other causes of boutonnière deformity include injuries caused by division, rupture, avulsion, or closed trauma to the common extensor tendon. The boutonnière deformity is the second most common closed tendon injury in sports.[26] In sports, the mechanism of injury is either a severe flexing force to the PIP joint or a direct blow to the posterior (dorsal) aspect of the PIP joint, which results in damage to the common extensor tendon. If traumatic in origin, this condition can be difficult to diagnose due to the degree of swelling, but if more than a 30-degree extension lag is present at the PIP joint, a boutonnière lesion should be suspected.[26]

The presence of a mobile correctable deformity requires little more than immobilizing the PIP in full extension for 6–8 weeks, with the DIP and MCP joints held free. Gentle AROM exercises can begin for flexion and extension of the PIP joint at 4–8 weeks, with the splint being reapplied between exercises. General strengthening usually begins at 10–12 weeks. For a return to competition an additional 2 months is required.[26]

Swan-Neck (Recurvatum) Deformity. The swan-neck deformity is characterized by a flexion deformity at the DIP and hyperextension of the PIP joint. This deformity is the least functional of all of the deformities that exist within the hand. Destruction of the oblique retinacular ligament of the extensor mechanism leads to posterior (dorsal) displacement of the lateral bands of the extensor mechanism. This rearrangement leads to an increased extensor force across the PIP joint with a resulting hyperextension of the PIP joint. The extended position of the PIP joint stretches the FDS and FDP tendons. The pull on the FDP tendon causes a passive flexion of the DIP joint. The resultant loss of function includes an inability to bring the tips of the fingers into grasp. The hypertrophy of rheumatoid synovitis displaces the tendon of the ECU forward. An alteration in posture at one joint leads to the reverse posture of the adjacent joint.[81] In addition to rheumatologic diseases, other etiologies include extensor terminal tendon injuries, spastic conditions, fractures to the middle phalanx that heal in hyperextension, and generalized ligamentous laxity.[182]

Clinical findings include a hyperextended PIP joint with a flexed DIP joint of the same digit (Fig. 18-85A).

The intervention for swan-neck deformity depends on the etiological status of the PIP joint and its related anatomic structures. The intervention for a swan-neck deformity with no loss of PIP joint flexion is usually conservative, with a Silver Ring splint used for the correction of the PIP hyperextension.[81]

Other deformities produced by RA

Radial Deviation of the CMC Block. This deformity is the result of the predominant action of the radial tendons (i.e., the FCR and the extensors carpi radialis longus and brevis), which radially deviate the CMC block. This deviation increases the angle between the radial border of the second metacarpal and the lower border for the distal radius, resulting in an important loss of muscular power in the flexors.[23,66]

The deviation of the wrist can involve an opposite deviation of the MCP joint, when the stabilizing elements of these joints (lateral ligament and volar plate) are weakened. The radial deviation of the CMC block may produce ulnar deviation of the MCP joints because of the interdependence of various articulations in the longitudinal chains.[23,185,186]

Effects of RA

The end result of the above-mentioned deformities is a reduction in the function of the hand and upper limb. Although humans are capable of significant compromise and adaptation, the loss of function that occurs with RA progressively accumulates to a point at which simple tasks become more difficult. The decreased excursion of tendons, weakness of muscles, and reduction of range of motion in joints multiplies the overall effects. Even when the muscle power is available, it may not be applied in the most effective direction. Joint laxity, which has been precipitated by synovitis and recurrent effusion, is progressively aggravated. Eventually the individual cannot cope with the resulting difficulties with doing activities of daily living. This is the characteristic end point of this progressive disease.

Interventions for RA of the Hand and Wrist

Because pain and instability of the wrist prevent much of the power from the forearm muscles from being transmitted from the wrist to the hand, some stabilization at the wrist level is necessary. The assessment of the thumb and finger problems involves careful evaluation of grasp and pinch. Based on the pathomechanics of the rheumatoid process, the following concepts form the foundation of any intervention to manage RA of the hand[187]:

1. Control the inflammation.
2. Focus on joint systems rather than isolated joints.
3. Consider the status of all tissues in the hand.
4. Consider the type of rheumatoid disease. The intervention is related to the type of rheumatoid disease:
    a. The type in which scarring outweighs the articular damage. Patients with stiff joints because of scarring do poorly after soft-tissue surgery. Patients in this group require aggressive and sustained therapy, often for 3–4 months.
    b. The type in which joint laxity and tissue laxity become difficult to stabilize after soft-tissue procedures. The patients in this group require careful intervention and control of the ROM and the direction of motion by the use of splints for many months after surgery.

The components of the intervention for patients with RA of the hand include the following:

1. ***Exercises.*** A combination of active exercises and isometric exercises are recommended to maintain muscle strength and improve range of motion. Range-of-motion exercises that encourage excursion of the long flexors are emphasized. The hand intrinsics are stretched by placing the MCP joints in extension and radial deviation while simultaneously flexing the PIP and DIP joints. Resistive exercises need to be introduced carefully due to the inflammatory nature of RA. Gentle squeezing exercises using a sponge in a tub of warm water are recommended. Bony and soft-tissue surgery will be less than successful in restoring function if there is residual severe imbalance in the forces acting across the joint.
2. ***Joint protection/energy conservation.*** Joint protection is the process of reducing internal and external stresses on the joints during functional activity and to help prevent poor use and abuse of the hand and wrist. Joint protection techniques include the following:
    a. Patient education to increase awareness of those activities that are stressful to the joints. In particular, tight and prolonged grasping should be avoided.
    b. The reduction of forces through the use of adaptive equipment and the avoidance of repetitive activities, positions of deformity, and the lifting of heavy weights. Many excellent self-help devices are available. Unless there is a reasonable use of the hand, any remaining imbalance will cause failure as shown in the secondary cycle of rheumatoid disease.
    c. The use of the larger/stronger and more proximal joints and muscles when available.
    d. The balance of rest and activity by planning ahead and using paced rests. Stress, rest, and sleep can have a significant effect on symptoms.
    e. The use of energy conservation techniques and labor-saving devices. Energy conservation involves sitting when able, organizing workspace and storage for accessibility, resting during activities when able, and using time savers such as prepared foods. Many different merchants offer adaptive equipments such as zipper pulls, kitchen utensils with enlarged handles, jar openers, and pens with a large grip.
    f. Elimination of some activities.
    g. Work simplification.
3. ***Splinting.*** Static splinting can be used to immobilize painful joints and prevent further deformity through positioning.
4. ***Pain management.*** The clinician should encourage the patient to investigate alternatives to pain medication, such as relaxation techniques, yoga, adopting a positive outlook, and the use of thermo- or cryotherapy.

TFCC Lesions

Injuries to the TFCC typically occur following a fall on the supinated outstretched wrist or as the result of chronic repetitive rotational loading.

Patients with lesions of the TFCC complain of medial wrist pain just distal to the ulna, which is increased with end-range forearm pronation/supination and with forceful gripping. Often there is a painful click during wrist motions. Tenderness is clearly localized to the posterior (dorsal) anatomic depression, which is immediately distal to the ulnar head.[188] Passive mobilization of the carpal condyle against the head of the ulna, with the wrist in passive or active ulnar deviation, will frequently elicit a painful crepitus or roughness, or more rarely an actual snap (McMurray test for the wrist). Passive supination combined with ulnar deviation can also reproduce the pain.

Initial radiographs are usually negative but can provide information as to whether an ulna-plus variance coexists with the triangular fibrocartilage tear (ulnocarpal impingement syndrome).[188] This condition is diagnosed on radiographs showing cystic or erosive changes in the ulnar head and along the proximal contour of the lunate.[189]

Injuries to the central, avascular portion of the disk are not amenable to spontaneous repair, whereas injuries to the vascularized periphery are.[188]

The conservative invention for a TFCC injury typically includes a long arm cast or splint fitted with the elbow in 90 degrees of flexion, and the forearm and wrist in ulnar deviation and extension for 6 weeks, if the TFCC is unstable.

While the wrist is in a cast or splint, the intervention should include proximal range-of-motion and strengthening exercises.

Active and active assisted exercises are initiated to the wrist and forearm after cast removal, with emphasis on flexion and extension initially, followed by pronation/supination, and radial/ulnar deviation. Two weeks after cast removal, assuming the patient is asymptomatic, progressive strengthening is initiated to the hand and wrist, taking care to prevent torsional loads to the wrist.

Osteoarthritis

Osteoarthritis (OA) is the most common joint disease (see Chap. 2). This condition can be primary or secondary, depending on the presence of a preexisting condition. While primary OA commonly involves the first CMC joint or sometimes the scaphotrapeziotrapezoid joint, it is uncommon in other parts of the joint.[188]

Secondary OA of the wrist attributable to an old trauma or infection is very common. In the case of malalignment of the scaphoid, degenerative arthritis will progress according to a very specific pattern that leads to an SLAC (scapholunate advanced collapse) wrist.[188] Degeneration occurs between the radius and the scaphoid and then between the lunate and the capitate. The radiolunate joint is almost never involved. Finally, a scapholunate diastasis develops and the capitate slides in between the lunate and the scaphoid.[190]

Patients with first CMC joint arthritis typically present with joint pain at the base of the thumb which is increased with use, restricted ROM in a capsular pattern, and joint crepitus.[188] First CMC arthritis is more common in women than men and is typically found in those 45 years and older.

Conservative intervention includes splinting, thermal modalities (moist heat or paraffin), and patient education.

Splinting. The splint should position the CMC joint in anterior (palmar) abduction to maximize the stability and anatomic alignment of the joint, with the IP joint free.[188]

Patient Education. The patient should be advised to

- minimize or avoid mechanical stresses including sustained pinching;
- avoid sleeping on the hands as this forces the thumb into adduction;
- use self-help devices such as jar lid openers and ergonomic scissors.

Gout

See Chapter 5.

Dupuytren Contracture (Palmar Fasciitis)

Population studies have shown that Dupuytren disease nearly always affects Caucasian races, particularly those of northern European descent.[191,192] The incidence increases with advancing age and it is exceedingly rare in children.[193] Men are 7–15 times more likely to have a clinical presentation requiring surgery than women, who tend to develop a more benign form of the disease that appears later in life.[194,195]

The etiology of Dupuytren disease is thought to be multifactorial. There is a higher incidence in the alcoholic population, the diabetic population, and the epileptic population.[195–197] Because of the association between smoking and microvascular changes in the hand, some believe that tobacco may also play a role in this disease.[195] Although not usually related to hand trauma, Dupuytren disease occasionally develops after significant hand injuries, including surgery.[198]

Dupuytren disease is an active cellular process in the fascia of the hand, which is characterized by the development of nodules in the palmar and digital fascia, which occur in specific locations along longitudinal tension lines.[191,195] The pathologic changes in the normal fascia result in the formation of tendon-like cords.[199–201] The characteritic contracture, which behaves similarly to the contracture and maturation of wound healing is caused by a thickening and shortening of the fascia.[195] The contractures form mainly at the MCP and PIP joint, and occasionally at the DIP joint.[202] The most commonly involved digit is the little finger, which is involved in approximately 70 percent of patients.

The diagnosis of Dupuytren disease in its early stages may be difficult and is based on the palpable nodule, characteristic skin changes, changes in the fascia, and progressive joint contracture. The skin changes are caused by a retraction of the overlying skin, resulting in dimples or pits.

Dupuytren disease can be classified into three biologic stages[200]:

- ***First stage.*** This proliferative stage is characterized by an intense production of myofibroblasts and the formation of nodules.
- ***Second stage.*** This involutional stage is represented by the alignment of the myofibroblasts along lines of tension.

- *Third stage.* During this residual stage, the tissue becomes mostly acellular and devoid of myofibroblasts, and only thick bands of collagen remain.[203]

The disease, which is usually bilateral, tends to be more severe in one hand, although there appears to be no association with hand dominance. Up to three rays may be involved in the more severely affected hand.

To date, conservative interventions have not yet proven to be clinically useful in the treatment of established contractures.[204] Some surgeons feel that any amount of PIP joint contracture warrants surgery, whereas others feel that 15 degrees or greater is an indication.[191,205] Surgery is the intervention of choice when the MCP joint contracts to 30 degrees and the deformity becomes a functional problem.[205]

Studies have shown that 50 percent of operative results depend on the postoperative management of effective splinting and exercise.[195,206] The intervention should be directed toward promoting wound healing, which in turn minimizes scarring and maximizes scar mobility so that hand function can be restored.[195]

Scar management and splinting are an important part of the postoperative management. The initial splint is positioned to provide slight MCP joint flexion of 10–20 degrees with PIP joint extension to allow maximal elongation of the wound.[195] Active, active assisted, and passive exercises are usually initiated immediately.

Wrist Sprains

The most common wrist sprain results from a downward force to the wrist exceeding its normal range of motion.[207] This forced movement of the joint is followed immediately by intense pain that subsides and then returns.[4]

Swelling typically occurs within 1–2 hours of the injury, with the degree of joint swelling indicating the severity of injury. With severe injuries, ecchymosis develops in 6–12 hours. Differential diagnosis includes a carpal fracture, particularly the scaphoid and lunate, traumatic instability, or a ligament tear.[208]

Conservative intervention depends on the severity of the sprain but likely includes some form of immobilization of the wristto avoid exacerbating the injury. Custom splints, which cover the palm and extend to about midforearm, are designed to allow for proper hand and wrist contouring while and to allow the fingers to move freely.[4] Cocking the wrist up about 10 degrees places the wrist in a position of rest.

Slight sprains typically remain splinted for 3–5 days. The splint is worn at all times except for removal for hygiene and exercise. More severe sprains take longer to recover, but should still be removed from the splint in 3–5 days to avoid stiffness.[4] Icing for 20–30 minutes, three to four times a day, concurrent with NSAIDs or aspirin can aid in reducing pain and swelling.

After splint removal, a rehabilitation program of AROM (wrist curls) should be started. Until the pain and swelling subside, wrist curls can be done in water to reduce muscle effort.[207] The clinician should consider taping the wrist to provide support and help decrease pain. The exercises are progressed to include a strengthening regime based on the hierarchy of strengthening exercises (see Chap. 12).

Perilunate Dislocation

A perilunate dislocation results from disruption of the scapholunate ligament, then extension of the injury to the capitolunate articulation and the lunotriquetral ligament.[209] Most carpal dislocations are of the perilunate variety with the lunate dislocating in an anterior (palmar) direction. This is accompanied by damage to both of the interosseous ligaments of the proximal row and possible injury to the median nerve.[9]

The usual mechanism of injury is hyperextension of the wrist. Physical examination is often limited, revealing swelling and a deformity, and the injury may be confused for a distal radius fracture. If the median nerve is involved, paresthesias or numbness in the median nerve distribution may be present. The dislocation is easily reduced if the intervention occurs soon after the injury. The reduction involves placing the wrist in extension and putting pressure on the lunate, after which the wrist is moved into flexion and immobilized.

Kienböck Disease

Kienböck disease is an aseptic necrosis, or osteonecrosis of the lunate. When the disease becomes advanced, carpal collapse, joint incongruity, and OA develop. The choice of treatment for patients with symptomatic Kienböck disease depends largely on the severity of the disease. Surgical intervention can include excision arthroplasty, limited intercarpal arthrodesis, revascularization, arthrodesis between the radius and the lunate, and vascular bundle implantation.[210] Conservative management of Kienböck disease involves immobilization in a short arm cast. Upon cast removal at 6–10 weeks, AROM exercises are initiated for the wrist, forearm, and thumb. Within 1–2 weeks following cast removal, PROM exercises are initiated. A wrist and thumb static splint is fitted with the wrist in neutral and the thumb midway between radial and anterior (palmar) abduction and is worn between exercise sessions and at night.

Intercarpal Instabilities

The integrity of the carpal relationship depends on the stability provided by both the interosseous ligaments and the midcarpal ligaments.[9] This relationship ensures that the carpal bones move as a unit. Conversely, disruption of this relationship allows abnormal independent motion of one or two carpal bones. Instability patterns are divided into those that are static and those that are dynamic. Static instability is the more severe of the two and usually involves a complete tear of one of the supporting ligaments or a fracture.[9] Dynamic instability patterns typically occur when the wrist is stressed. Carpal instability patterns that occur within the same row are classified as dissociative while those that occur across different rows are classified as nondissociative.

Dissociative. Two types of dissociative instability have been recognized[56]:

1. ***DISI (dorsal(posterior) intercalated segment instability).*** The most common dissociated instability is the scapholunate dissociation, in which the scapholunate angle is greater than 70 degrees when viewed on radiograph. Scapholunate instability usually follows a FOOSH injury where the primary forces are transferred through the wrist

in extension and ulnar deviation. As the scaphoid and lunate become disassociated, the lunate no longer follows the scaphoid into flexion, instead migrating with the triquetrum into a dorsal (posterior) angulation.[9] The patient with this type presents with difficulties and weakness with grasping and complains of chronic, vague wrist pain. The examination reveals tenderness over the scaphoid and/or lunate, laxity between the scaphoid and lunate, and a positive scaphoid-shift test.

2. ***VISI (ventral intercalated segment instability).*** The second most common dissociative instability is the lunatotriquetrum dissociation. Ventral refers to the ventral (anterior) tilt of the distal end of the lunate. The signs and symptoms for this instability are similar to those of the scapholunate instability, except for the location. In this type, the lunate remains tethered to the scaphoid by the interosseous ligament but not necessarily to the triquetrum.[9] During wrist motions, the lunate follows the scaphoid into a flexed posture, but the triquetrum does not. A scapholunate angle of less than 30 degrees indicates a VISI lesion.

Nondissociative. This is the most common dynamic instability of the wrist and usually results from an insufficiency of the posterior (dorsal) intercarpal ligaments. The nondissociative instability may not be symptomatic, and the patient may be able to sublux and reduce the joint at will.[9] A clunk can be felt to occur as the distal row jumps back into place at the extreme of ulnar deviation.[211]

Conservative intervention for carpal instabilities usually involves a trial period of cast immobilization. Surgery is reserved for chronic cases.

UCL Sprain of the Thumb

UCL injuries, also known as *gamekeeper's thumb*, and *skier's thumb*,[212] involve injury to the MCP joint of the thumb and are the most common ligament injury of the hand.[213]

The patient typically complains of pain or tenderness on the ulnar aspect of the MCP joint.

For the purposes of planning the intervention, these injuries can be divided into two categories:

- Grade I and II sprains, in which the majority of the ligament remains intact. The stability of the joint is tested in full extension and at 30 degrees of flexion, which stress the accessory collateral ligament and the UCL, respectively. An angulation of greater than 35 or 15 degrees greater than the uninvolved side indicates instability and the need for surgical intervention. Grade I and II tears are treated with immobilization in a thumb spica cast (a forearm-based splint fabricated from an anterior (palmar) or radial approach) for 3 weeks, with additional protective splinting for 2 weeks. Thumb spica splints are designed to immobilize the wrist, CMC, and MCP joints of the thumb, thereby permitting the radial wrist extensors and the proximal thumb to rest. Thumb spicas can be used for the intervention of a number of conditions including de Quervain disease and CMC arthritis.

When applying these splints, it is very important to ensure that the superficial radial nerve and the ulnar digital nerve of the thumb are not compromised. The splint is worn at all times except for removal for hygiene and exercise. AROM of flexion and extension begins at 3 weeks and progresses to strengthening exercises by 8 weeks, taking care not to apply any abduction stress to the MCP joint during the first 2–6 weeks.

- Grade III tears and displaced bony avulsions are treated with surgery and subsequent immobilization. If the ligament is completely torn, there is concern for a Stener lesion, in which the torn UCL protrudes beneath the adductor aponeurosis.[214] Postsurgical rehabilitation involves wearing a thumb spica splint for 3 weeks with an additional 2 weeks of splinting, except during the active flexion and extension exercises. Otherwise the exercise progression is the same as for the grade I and II sprains.
- Radial collateral sprains are classified and treated in a similar manner.

Ulnar Impaction Syndrome

The ulnar impaction syndrome can be defined as excessive impaction of the ulnar head against the TFCC and ulnar carpal bones. This results in a progressive degeneration of those structures.[215]

The patient with this syndrome typically presents with ulnar wrist pain and a limitation of motion. Upon physical examination, a combined motion of ulnar deviation and compression reproduces the pain (see "Special Tests").

The differential diagnosis includes ulnar impingement syndrome and arthrosis or incongruity of the DRUJ.[215]

It is important to remember that in the absence of obvious structural abnormalities, the ulnar impaction syndrome may result from daily activities that result in excessive intermittent loading of the ulnar carpal bones.

Conservative intervention includes the use of an ulnar gutter splint if there is evidence of wrist overloading.

Ganglia

Ganglia are thin-walled cysts containing mucoid hyaluronic acid that develop spontaneously over a joint capsule or tendon sheath. They are the most common soft-tissue tumor in the hand.[131,146] Common sites for ganglia are the anterior (volar) or posterior (dorsal) surfaces of the wrist and fingers.[4] Ganglia may not cause pain.[9] Frequently, as the ganglion begins to grow, the patient reports aching that is irritated by flexion and extension of the joint.[4]

At times, ganglia occur at other parts of the wrist, causing compression of the ulnar or median nerve.[4] When compression occurs, associated sensory symptoms in the digits or intrinsic muscle weakness may develop.[146] Upon examination, a ganglion is smooth, round, or multilobulated and tender with applied pressure.

For symptom relief, immobilization of the wrist through splinting is effective. This may cause the ganglion to shrink temporarily, although it is uncommon for the immobilization to be effective in resolving the ganglion.[146] Needle aspiration can resolve the ganglion. Occasionally, surgical excision is indicated for the patient with significant pain or cosmetic irritation (Table 18-19).

TABLE 18-19	Rehabilitation Protocol After Excision of Wrist Ganglion
Time Frame	**Intervention**
2 Wks	Remove the short arm splint and sutures Initiate active and active-assisted wrist extension and flexion Continue interval splint wear during the day between exercises and at night
2–4 Wks	Advance ROM exercises to resistive and gradual strengthening exercises Discontinue the splint at 4 wks
4–6 Wks	Allow normal activities to patient's tolerance
6 Wks	Allow full activity

Data from Brotzman SB, Calandruccio JH, Jupiter JB: Hand and wrist injuries. In: Brotzman SB, Wilk KE, eds. *Clinical Orthopaedic Rehabilitation*. Philadelphia, PA: Mosby, 2003:1–83.

Chondromalacia

Chondromalacia of the ulnar head is usually seen in young patients after a fall on the dorsiflexed wrist with the impact predominantly hypothenar, or repeated episodes of stressful pronation and supination (work or leisure activity).[188] The pain is localized to the posterior (dorsal) distal radioulnar area and manipulation of the ulnar head can elicit crepitation or a painful snap.[189]

Racquet Player's Pisiform

Racquet player's pisiform is a condition involving a minor subluxation of the pisiform, with occasional chondromalacia of the articular cartilage of the pisotriquetral joint.[16] The probable mechanism is a torsional stress upon the capsule of the pisotriquetral joint by the powerful and rapid pronation and supination movements at the wrist seen when wielding a racquet, particularly in badminton, racquetball, and squash players.

The typical clinical presentation is one of pain, disability, and swelling on the ulnar aspect of the wrist or proximal palm. The pain is reproduced with passive movement of the pisiform upon the triquetrum with the relaxed wrist flexed and ulnarly deviated.[16]

The typical intervention for this condition is surgical excision of the pisiform.[16]

PRACTICE PATTERN 4E: IMPAIRED JOINT MOBILITY, MOTOR FUNCTION, MUSCLE PERFORMANCE, RANGE OF MOTION ASSOCIATED WITH LOCALIZED INFLAMMATION

Tendonitis and Tenosynovitis

Tendonitis is a term that clearly indicates an inflammation of the tendon or tendon–muscle attachment, whereas tenosynovitis involves an inflammation of the tendon sheath.

Overuse syndromes are a common cause of tendonitis, particularly in the "weekend warrior." As a rule, the tendons of the APL and EPB are involved. There are, however, some uncommon locations and types of tendonitis. There has been a marked increase in reports of the so-called repetitive strain injury of the upper extremity.[188] One of the difficulties in evaluating this disorder is the establishment of a diagnosis in the absence of objective physical findings or confirmatory diagnostic images or laboratory data. These issues become more complicated when insurers and attorneys ask clinicians to establish a causal relation between the job and the complaints.[216,217]

Tenosynovitis is frequently seen in inflammatory rheumatic diseases, diabetes mellitus, or hypothyroid conditions (Table 18-20).

Conservative intervention includes nonsteroidal medications, splinting, patient education on the neutral rest position for the wrist, activity modification, and the avoidance of exacerbating activities (e.g., forceful gripping and heavy lifting). A stretching and icing regimen is recommended for the wrist flexors or extensors depending on the diagnosis. Occasionally, a series of steroid injections may be warranted. Patients are typically considered for surgery when a tenosynovitis has persisted for a period of 3 months of conservative treatment.

DeQuervain Disease. De Quervain disease[218] is a progressive tenosynovitis or tenovaginitis, which involves the tendon sheaths of the first posterior (dorsal) compartment of the wrist, resulting in a thickening of the extensor retinaculum, a stenosing of the fibro-osseus canal, and an eventual entrapment and compression of the tendons.[219] Although originally thought of as an active inflammatory condition, recent histological studies have found the disorder to be characterized by degeneration and thickening of the tendon sheath.[220]

In most instances, the first posterior (dorsal) compartment is a single compartment, which contains the APL and the EPB tendons and their associated synovial sheaths. The APL and EPB tendons allow the thumb to flex, extend, and grip objects. Overuse, repetitive tasks which involve overexertion of the thumb, or radial and ulnar deviation of the wrist, and arthritis are the most common predisposing factors, as they cause the greatest stresses on the structures of the first posterior (dorsal) compartment.[79,121] Such activities include scraping wallpaper, painting, , hammering, fly fishing, knitting, and cutting with scissors[79,221–224]

Typically, patients report a gradual and insidious onset[79,121,225] of a dull ache over the radial aspect of the wrist made worse by such activities as turning doorknobs or keys.[4] Patients also may note a "creak" in the wrist as the tendon moves.

Examination of the wrist may reveal the following:

- A localized swelling and tenderness in the region of the radial styloid process[121,225] and wrist pain radiating proximally into the forearm and distally into the thumb.[121,225–227]
- Severe pain[121,225] with wrist ulnar deviation and thumb flexion and adduction.[123] A reproduction of the pain can also be reported with thumb extension and abduction.[228]

TABLE 18-20 Clinical Findings in Common Forms of Tenosynovitis		
Tenosynovitis	**Findings**	**Differential Diagnosis**
Intersection syndrome	Edema, swelling, and crepitation in the intersection area; pain over the dorsum of the wrist that is exacerbated by wrist flexion and extension, unlike the pain of de Quervain tenosynovitis, which is exacerbated by radial and ulnar deviation; pain extends less radially than it does in de Quervain tenosynovitis	Wartenberg syndrome, de Quervain tenosynovitis
De Quervain	Pain along the radial aspect of the wrist that worsens with radial and ulnar wrist deviation; pain on performing Finkelstein maneuver is pathognomonic	Arthritis of the first carpometacarpal joint, scaphoid fracture and nonunion, radiocarpal arthritis, Wartenberg syndrome, intersection syndrome
Sixth posterior (dorsal) compartment	Pain over the ulnar dorsum of the wrist that is worsened by ulnar deviation and wrist extension; other planes of motion may also be painful; tenderness over the sixth posterior (dorsal) compartment; instability of the extensor carpi ulnaris is shown by having the patient circumduct the wrist while rotating the forearm from pronation to supination	Extensor carpi ulnaris instability, triangular fibrocartilage complex tears, lunotriquetral ligament tears, ulnocarpal abutment syndrome, distal radioulnar joint arthritis, traumatic rupture of the subsheath that normally stabilizes this tendon to the distal ulna
Flexor carpi radialis tunnel syndrome	Pain, swelling, and erythema around the anterior (palmar) radial aspect of the wrist at the flexor carpi radialis tunnel; pain exacerbated by resisted wrist flexion	Retinacular ganglion, scaphotrapezial arthritis, first carpometacarpal arthritis, scaphoid fracture/ nonunion, radial carpal arthritis, injury to the anterior (palmar) cutaneous branch of the median nerve, Lindberg syndrome (tendon adhesions between the flexor pollicis longus and the flexor digitorum profundus)
Trigger finger	Pain on digital motion, with or without associated triggering or locking at the interphalangeal joint of the thumb or proximal interphalangeal joint of other fingers; may be crepitus or a nodular mass near the first annular pulley that moves with finger excursion	Connective tissue disease, partial tendon laceration, retained foreign body, retinacular ganglion, infection, extensor tendon subluxation

Data from Brotzman SB, Calandruccio JH, Jupiter JB: Hand and wrist injuries. In: Brotzman SB, Wilk KE, eds. *Clinical Orthopaedic Rehabilitation*. Philadelphia, PA: Mosby, 2003:1–83; Idler RS: Helping the patient who has wrist or hand tenosynovitis. *J Musculoskel Med* 14:62, 1997.

- Crepitus of the tendons moving through the extensor sheath.[123,229]
- Palpable thickening of the extensor sheath and of the tendons distal to the extensor tunnel.[230]
- A loss of abduction of the CMC joint of the thumb.
- A positive Finkelstein test (Fig. 18-54) (see "Special Tests").[121]

Although the diagnosis is mostly clinical, posteroanterior and lateral radiographs of the wrist can be obtained to rule out any bony pathology, such as a scaphoid fracture, radioscaphoid, or triscaphoid arthritis; and Kienböck disease.[4]

CLINICAL PEARL

Isolation of the EPB tendon in a separate compartment has been reported to contribute to the pathogenesis of de Quervain disease.[128]

The intervention can be conservative or surgical. Conservative intervention usually includes rest, modification of activities, splinting, and anti-inflammatory medication. In a study by Lane and colleagues[231] wrist splints and NSAIDs were found to be effective only in patients with minimal symptoms and no restrictions in daily activities. No added benefit has been found in using a combined injection and splinting approach.[232] If splinting is appropriate, a thumb spica splint is fabricated with the wrist in 15 degrees of extension, the thumb midway between anterior (palmar) and radial abduction, and the thumb MCP joint in 10 degrees of flexion. As the splint is supposed be worn all day, when fitting the splint it is important that the thumb is able to oppose the index and long finger to aid with hand function. Following the removal of the splint after approximately 3–6 weeks, ROM exercises are prescribed, with a gradual progression to strengthening.

Three case reports have been published that describe manual physical therapy treatment for de Quervain disease. In the first report, Backstrom[233] reported the complete resolution of symptoms in a patient with a 2-month history of de Quervain tenosynovitis by incorporating Mulligan mobilization with movement techniques (radial gliding of the proximal carpal row and ulnar gliding of the trapezium), capitate manipulation, CMC joint mobilizations, and TFM over the first posterior (dorsal) tunnel, into an overall treatment plan. The second case report, by Anderson and Tichenor,[230] used an Australian (Maitland) approach consisting of central and unilateral cervical mobilizations, carpal bone mobilizations, cervical and upper extremity stretches, TFM to the APL and EPB tendon, and neural mobilizations. In this case report, the patient reported no wrist or hand pain following a 6-month treatment program. The third case report by Walker[78] used an impairment-based treatment approach for eight visits based on the examination findings of isolated radiocarpal, intercarpal, and CMC joint dysfunction. The treatments consisted of manual techniques and self-mobilizations applied to the radiocarpal, intercarpal, and CMC joints. At treatment completion, the patient achieved a pain-free state and nearly full function. These results were maintained at a long-term follow-up performed 10 months after treatment.[78]

The more invasive intervention begins with cortisone injections. If two to three injections do not give relief, surgical tendon sheath release is an option.[4]

Intersection Syndrome. Intersection syndrome is a tenosynovitis of the ECRL and ECRB (radial wrist extensors), where they cross under the APL and EPB.[217] Although similar to de Quervain, differentiation is made with the pain distribution. With the intersection syndrome, the pain is located over the distal forearm, 4–8 cm proximal to Lister's tubercle, approximately a hand's breadth proximal to the wrist joint..[217] posterior Symptoms are exacerbated by wrist flexion and extension and by resisted wrist extension.[234] The condition is common in rowers, weightlifters, and canoeists due to repetitive wrist flexion and extension.[126]

Intervention, in addition to NSAIDs, involves[217,235]

- splint immobilization of the wrist and thumb with the wrist in 15–20 degrees of extension;
- electrotherapeutic modalities including iontophoresis/phonophoresis;
- manual techniques including deep TFM followed by exercises for stretching and strengthening;
- patient education to emphasize the avoidance of any repetitive wrist flexion and extension in combination with a power grip.

EPL Tendonitis. This condition is rare except in RA, but it occurs when the EPL muscle extends into a tight third compartment.[236] Overuse (drummer boy palsy), direct trauma, forced wrist extension, and distal radius fractures may cause EPL tendonitis, which presents with the clinical signs and symptoms of decreased thumb flexion, pain, swelling, and crepitus at Lister's tubercle.[217]

EIP Syndrome. An increase in muscle size of the extensor indicis, caused by swelling or hypertrophy from repetitive exercise, may cause stenosis of the fourth posterior (dorsal) compartment and resultant tenosynovitis.[217]

A simple test of a resistance applied to active index finger extension while holding the wrist in a flexed position is a reliable provocative test.[237]

ECU Tendonitis. ECU tendonitis, a tenosynovitis of the sixth posterior (dorsal) compartment, usually presents as chronic dorsoulnar wrist pain, which is aggravated with forearm supination and ulnar deviation, which causes the tendon to sublux palmarly.[217,238]

FCU Tendonitis. The FCU is the most common wrist flexor tendon to become inflamed and is often associated with repetitive trauma and racquet sports.[16] The clinical signs and symptoms include pain and swelling localized just proximal to the pisiform, which is aggravated with wrist flexion and ulnar deviation.[217]

FCR Tendonitis. FCR tendonitis usually develops due to stenosis and tenosynovitis in the FCR fibro-osseous tunnel within the transverse metacarpal ligament. FCR tendonitis usually produces localized pain and swelling and painful deviation of the wrist.[217] FCR tendonitis frequently coexists with other conditions including fracture or arthritis around the CMC joint of the thumb.[217]

Digital Flexor Tendonitis and Trigger Digits. This condition is typically characterized by painful snapping or triggering of the fingers and thumb due to a disproportion between the flexor tendon and its tendon sheath. The condition invariably occurs at the metacarpal head level and at the A1 pulley (MCP joint pulley), with the result that the tendon is pulled through too narrow a canal.[217,239–241] The condition is more common in the fibrous flexor sheath of the thumb, ring, or middle finger.[242,243]

The etiology for this condition is unknown, although it is more common in patients with diabetes, young children, and menopausal women.[242,243] Trigger finger also commonly coexists with rheumatic changes of the hand and may be the earliest sign of RA.[244]

The base of the affected finger is often tender and is usually accompanied by the trigger phenomenon—pain on digital motion, with or without associated triggering or locking. As the condition progresses, it becomes very painful, and may result in limited or absent digital motion, especially in the PIP joint.[240] During excursion of the flexor tendon, the clinician may palpate crepitus or a moving nodular mass in the vicinity of, or slightly proximal to, the A1 pulley. The presence of swelling is most consistent with tenosynovitis that occurs secondary to connective tissue disease.

Conservative intervention involves the fitting of a hand-based MCP flexion block splint for the involved digit only, with the MCP joint only immobilized in full extension, for up to 6 weeks.[245] The purpose of this immobilization is to attempt to alter the mechanical forces on the proximal pulley system while encouraging maximal differential tendon gliding. Patient education plays an important role; the patient should be advised to eliminate any provocative movements such as repetitive grasping or the use of tools that apply pressure over the area.

Medical intervention usually involves one or a series of steroid injections,[246] with surgical release of the trigger finger reserved for those cases that do not respond to conservative measures.[217]

Tendon Ruptures

One of the main purposes of the hand is to grasp; therefore, the loss of flexor tendons imposes a catastrophic functional loss.[247] The purpose of a flexor tendon repair is to restore maximum active flexor tendon gliding to ensure effective finger joint motion.

Most flexor tendon ruptures occur silently after prolonged inflammatory tenosynovitis, although the causes can also be traumatic. When all nine flexor tendons to the digits have ruptured, little can be done. Single tendon ruptures are more common, and the FPL tendon is the most vulnerable to attrition rupture where it crosses the scaphotrapezial joint and where local synovitis can create a sharp spike of bone that abrades against this spur and ruptures during use. The FDP tendon to the index finger is also at risk from this bony spur.[248]

Tendon injuries are classified into five zones according to the level of injury. The zone within which the tendon is repaired dictates to some extent the intervention.

- *Zone 1.* This zone extends from the insertion of the FDP in the middle phalanx to that of the FDS in the base of the distal phalanx. Injuries at this level involve isolated lacerations of the FDS.
- *Zone 2.* This is the region in which both flexor tendons travel within the fibro-osseous tunnel from the A1 pulley to the FDP insertion. Usually, both flexor tendons are injured at this level.
- *Zone 3.* The area in the palm between the distal border of the carpal tunnel and the proximal border of the A1 pulley comprises zone 3. Common digital nerves and vessels, lumbrical muscles, and one or both flexor tendons may be injured in this region.
- *Zone 4.* This zone consists of that segment of the flexor tendons covered by the transverse carpal ligament. Injuries at this level involve median or ulnar nerves and tendons.
- *Zone 5.* The forearm from the musculotendinous junction of the extrinsic flexors to the proximal border of the transverse carpal ligament comprises zone 5. Interference with tendon gliding is less of a problem in this region.

There are a number of different procedures and rehabilitation protocols for flexor tendon repairs. In brief, the retracted ends of the tendon are retrieved either by hand and wrist positioning or with a surgical instrument. Although it is not within the scope of this text to discuss suturing techniques, it is important to mention that several suturing methods have been found to withstand an early active mobilization (EAM) protocol such as the one presented here. They include the Savage, Silfverskiold (modified Kirchmayer or modified Kessler),[249,250] Tang,[251] Robertson,[252] and cruciate[253] methods. In all of these methods, the anatomic relationship between the FDS and the FDP is maintained.

The rate of tendon healing following surgery depends on adequate nutrition (through vascular and synovial fluid perfusion), the part of the tendon affected, and the presence of the vinculum.

Early postoperative protected mobilization of repaired tendons has been popularly adopted as the postoperative treatment protocol after tendon repair.[254–260] Researchers have shown that early mobilization can prevent the formation of scar tissue without jeopardizing tendon healing. Several post-surgical protocols and modifications exist based on individual characteristics, the zone involved, the suture strength, and surgeon preferences. While it is not within the scope of this text to discuss all of the various types of protocols, it is important for the clinician to have an understanding of the concepts behind the two major types:[261]

- Early passive mobilization consists of passive flexion with active extension within the confines of a protective splint.[262] One of the original controlled motion protocols was developed by Kleinert and colleagues, who used a posterior ((dorsal) block splint with a rubber-band traction device and early active extension of the digit against the tension of the passive rubber-band flexion.[263] The block splint positioned the wrist in 40 degrees of flexion and the MCP joints in 40–60 degrees of flexion. In the 1970s, Duran and Houser[264] presented a controlled passive motion method that has become the basis for many of the early passive mobilization protocols used today. Various modified Duran protocols have since been developed.
- EAM consists of active flexion and extension of the involved finger within certain parameters of a protective splint.[262] In recent years, based on an improved understanding of connective tissue physiology and the success achieved with other types of surgical repairs, various active mobilization protocols have been attempted to obtain better function of repaired tendons.[257,258,265] It has been demonstrated that active mobilizations of the tendons are a more effective way to increase excursion and decrease adhesions of repaired tendons.[265–270] In addition, the tension added to the repaired tendon by active mobilization seems to help initiate proliferation of the teknocytes (tendon forming cells) and increase the rate of collagen synthesis of the repaired tendon, thereby enhancing the tendon healing process.[271,272] Considering the resistance of the sheath during tendon gliding and a decrease in suture strength during the initial weeks after repair, most investigators believe that sufficient suture strength is vital to the performance of gentle or moderate active finger motion.[249,252,253] The typical EAM protocol allows active flexion and extension of the involved fingers within the first 3–5 days by incorporating a concept known as *place and hold*, in which the involved finger is passively flexed to a certain position and the patient is then asked to hold it there through active contraction of that muscle.[262]

CLINICAL PEARL

Surgical repairs and treatment protocols can vary greatly, necessitating a high level of communication between the surgeon and the clinician.

Mallet Finger Deformity. Mallet finger deformity, one of the most common hand injuries sustained by the athletic population, is a traumatic disruption of the terminal tendon. This condition is especially common in the baseball catcher and the football receiver and results in a loss of active extension of the DIP joint.. The initial injury usually results from the delivery of a longitudinal force to the tip of the finger, which produces a sudden acute flexion force and a subsequent rupture of the extensor tendon just proximal to its insertion into the third phalanx or a fracture at the base of the distal phalanx.[26]

The physical examination reveals a flexion deformity of the DIP joint, which can be extended passively but not actively. This lack of active extension at the DIP joint is due to the zero tension being provided by the EDC, in addition to the resulting increased tone in the FDP.

The primary goal of treatment is to maximize function and range of motion of the involved DIP joint. Mallet deformities with an associated large fracture fragment are typically treated with 6 weeks of immobilization following open reduction and internal fixation (ORIF), usually with K-wires.[26] Closed reduction is used for other types, followed by 6 weeks of continuous posterior (dorsal) splinting of the DIP in 0 degrees of extension to 15 degrees of hyperextension.[26] The PIP joint should be free to move. If splinted, the splint is removed once a day while simultaneously holding the DIP joint in extension to allow air to reach the anterior (palmar) aspect of the middle and distal phalanx. Following the period of immobilization, the splint or fixators are removed and the terminal tendon is evaluated. If the tendon is unable to maintain extension of the DIP joint, a splint is reapplied and the tendon is retested periodically. Once the tendon has healed sufficiently to perform active extension of the DIP, AROM exercises to 20–35 degrees are initiated to the DIP joint. The clinician should continue to monitor for an extensor lag, and it is recommended that the patient continues to wear the splint between exercise sessions, at night, and when competing (as appropriate). Gentle progressive resistive exercises (PREs) using putty or a hand exerciser are initiated at week 8. Usually the splint is discontinued at 9 weeks if the DIP extension remains at 0–5 degrees and there is no extensor lag. Unrestricted use usually occurs after 12 weeks.

Rupture of the Terminal Phalangeal Flexor (Jersey Finger). A jersey finger rupture involves a rupture of the FDP tendon from its insertion in the distal phalanx. As there is no characteristic deformity associated with this type of rupture, this condition is often misdiagnosed as a sprained or " jammed" finger[26]

The injury commonly occurs in football when the flexed finger is caught in a jersey while the athlete is attempting to make a tackle, hence the term jersey finger. However, any forceful passive extension that is applied while the FDP muscle is contracting can cause this type of rupture. Although this condition can occur in any finger, the most commonly injured is the ring finger.[273]

Three types are recognized:

- In Type I, the tendon retracts into the palm with or without a bony fragment.
- Type II is the most common. The tendon retracts to the PIP joint and the long vinculum remains intact. As in type I, type II injuries may have a small bony avulsion.
- Type III injuries involve a large bony fragment.

To test the integrity of the tendon, the clinician isolates the FDP by holding the MCP and PIP joints of the affected finger in full extension and then asks the patient to attempt to flex the DIP. If the patient is able to flex the DIP, it is intact. If not, it is ruptured.

The intervention depends on the severity of the injury. If function is not seriously affected the condition is just monitored. However, if function is impacted, one option is surgical reattachment of the tendon, which requires a 12-week course of rehabilitation.

INTEGRATION OF PRACTICE PATTERNS 4F AND 5F

This includes conditions involving impaired joint mobility, motor function, muscle performance, and range of motion, or reflex integrity secondary to referred pain, spinal disorders, peripheral nerve entrapment, myofascial pain syndrome (MPS), and complex regional pain syndrome (CRPS).

Referred Pain

A number of structures can refer pain to the wrist and hand, and these include visceral structures, neurologic structures, and the more proximal joints (Chapter 5). The most common joints, which refer pain to the wrist and hand, include the cervical, thoracic, shoulder, and elbow joints.

Tumors

See Chapter 5.

Peripheral Nerve Entrapment

Peripheral nerve entrapments are common in this region and are typically associated with a history of pain or vague sensory disturbances.[274] Due to the vagueness of the signs and symptoms, nerve injuries are frequently overlooked as a source of acute, or more commonly chronic, symptomatology.[188] An early indicator of peripheral compression neuropathy may be the loss of vibration sensibility.[150] Nerve conduction studies may be performed, focusing on the sites of interest. Diabetes, with its associated neuropathies or cheiroarthropathy, may be an underlying cause of chronic wrist pain.[188]

Radial Nerve. The posterior interosseous nerve can be compressed as it enters the posterior (dorsal) wrist capsule by repetitive wrist extension maneuvers, inciting symptomatic inflammation.[275]

The major disability associated with radial nerve injury is weak wrist and finger extension, with the wrist and fingers adopting a position termed "wrist drop." The hand grip is weakened as a result of poor stabilization of the wrist and finger joints, and the patient typically demonstrates an inability to extend the thumb, proximal phalanges, wrist, and elbow, depending on the level. Supination of the forearm and adduction of the thumb are also affected. There is also decreased or impaired sensation on the posterior (dorsal) surface of the first interosseous space.

Wartenberg Syndrome. Wartenberg syndrome is a compression of the superficial sensory radial nerve. Inflammation of the tendons of the first posterior (dorsal) compartment can result in superficial radial neuritis. This results in pain, paresthesias, and numbness of the radial aspects of the hand and wrist.[276] In addition, the tendons of the brachioradialis and ECRL muscles can press on the nerve in a scissor-like fashion when the forearm is pronated, causing a proximal tethering on the distal segment of the nerve at the wrist.[277]

Wartenberg sign is described wherein the patient is asked to extend the fingers and abduction or clawing of the little finger occurs.[158]

Median Nerve Compression at the Wrist. CTS is a cause of chronic wrist pain and functional impairment of the hand. It results from an ischemic compression of the median nerve at the wrist as it passes through the carpal tunnel. Compression of the nerve in the carpal tunnel is compounded by an increase in synovial fluid pressure and tendon tension, which decreases the available volume.

Moersch[278] provided the first description of spontaneous median nerve compression and is credited with coining the term *carpal tunnel syndrome.*[279] The compression of the median nerve may result from a wide variety of factors that compromise the tunnel space such as fluid retention, which occurs during pregnancy,[280] infection,[281,282] and conditions such as renal dysfunction. In addition, several disease conditions, such as gout or pseudogout,[283] acromegaly, or amyotrophy[284] can also decrease the tunnel size. However, about half of the cases of CTS are related to repetitive and cumulative trauma in the workplace.[285,286] Forceful and repetitive contraction of the finger flexors can also provoke CTS.[287] Acute wrist trauma has also been associated with CTS. A FOOSH injury or other trauma can cause an anterior (palmar) subluxation of the lunate[288] or a distal radius fracture.[289,290] The degree of compression can be so great that profound neurologic deficit can rapidly follow, and if not treated appropriately, it can become permanent due to the decrease in capillary blood flow producing ischemia of the nerve.[291] A manipulative reduction should be carried out. If manipulation fails, the patient should be referred to a surgeon for immediate decompression.

Other causes include collagen disorders,[292,293] flexor tenosynovitis,[294] RA,[295] diabetes, hypothyroidism, and hemodialysis.[296] Less common causes include instances where the lumbrical muscles encroach within the tunnel during finger movements[297,298] or become hypertrophied.[299]

Although it occurs in all age groups, CTS more commonly occurs between the fourth and sixth decades. CTS is the most common compression neuropathy, with a prevalence of 9.2 percent in women and 0.6 percent in men.[300,301]

Carpal tunnel pressure appears to be an important factor in the pathophysiology of CTS, as increased pressure on the median nerve can produce short-term sensory and motor nerve conduction deficits and elicit symptoms of median nerve neuropathy.[291] Extreme wrist and finger postures can increase the tunnel pressure.[302] In addition, the angle of the MCP joint has been found to have a significant effect on carpal tunnel pressure during active wrist flexion and extension and radioulnar maneuvers. Motions performed in 0 degrees MCP flexion exhibit the highest pressures, followed by an MCP angle of 90 degrees.[303] This information should be considered in the design of splints for CTS patients. Fingertip loading has also been found to increase pressure in the carpal tunnel.[304]

The diagnosis of CTS is typically made after a review of the patient's history and physical examination.[147] The initial characteristic features of CTS include intermittent pain and paresthesias in the median nerve distribution of the hand (although the symptoms may radiate proximally into the forearm and arm), which progressively become more persistent as the condition progresses.[292,305–307] If the condition is allowed to progress, muscle weakness and paralysis can occur. The symptoms of CTS are typically worse at night due to the position of wrist flexion typically adopted during sleep and can be associated with morning stiffness.

Differential diagnosis for this condition includes cervical radiculitis,[308] thoracic outlet syndrome, pronator syndrome,[309] coronary artery ischemia, tendonitis, fibrositis, and wrist joint arthritis.[310,311] Cervical radiculopathy may be identified by the occurrence of proximal radiation of pain above the shoulder, paresthesias with coughing or sneezing, or a pattern of motor or sensory disturbances outside of the territory of the median nerve.[305] Ulnar neuropathy must be considered since no more than half of patients with CTS can reliably report the location of their paresthesias.[312] Thoracic outlet syndrome is occasionally a concern. Transient cerebral ischemia, not a rare occurrence, can be recognized by the absence of pain during an episode of numbness. Finally, when the symptoms persist following conservative or surgical intervention aimed to the site of the carpal tunnel, median nerve neuropathies proximal to the carpal tunnel should be suspected. Median nerve neuropathies can be due to diabetes, human immunodeficiency virus, nutritional deficiencies, and entrapment/compression of the nerve.[313] Median nerve compression proximal to the carpal tunnel may be divided into two major categories: pronator syndrome and anterior interosseus nerve syndrome (Chapter 17).[313]

The physical assessment focuses on an examination of the motor and sensory functions of the hand as compared to the uninvolved hand and includes Phalen test and Tinel sign.[141,305,314] A study[315] that examined the effect of upper extremity position on median nerve tension found the upper limb tension test for the median nerve to be specific.

Another study[316] described a maneuver that abolishes paresthesias in the carpal tunnel. The authors of this study suggest that this maneuver could be useful in the diagnosis of the syndrome, as well as providing a means of relieving symptoms and providing the basis for the design of a splint. With the involved hand positioned palm up, the clinician gently squeezes the distal metacarpal heads together.[316] If the basic maneuver does not relieve the symptoms, it may also be necessary to pronate the forearm while simultaneously stretching digits three and four.[316]

A number of medical tests can be used to help diagnose CTS. These include the median nerve conduction study (NCS) and EMG study. Median nerve conduction studies have been found to be normal in 5 percent of patients with symptoms.[146] The EMG study was found in one study[157] to confirm a diagnosis of CTS in only 61 percent of cases. However, radiculopathy due to disease of the cervical spine, diffuse peripheral neuropathy, or proximal median neuropathy can pose clinical questions that electrodiagnostic testing can settle.[305]

A carpal tunnel view radiograph may be the only view that shows abnormalities within the carpal tunnel.[29]

The conservative intervention for mild cases typically includes the use of splints, activity modification, diuretics, and NSAIDs.[317] The rationale for splints is based on observations that CTS symptoms improve with rest and worsen with activity.[318] However, prescription parameters for the type of splint are not standardized,[319] with some advocating neutral positioning,[320] and some recommending 0–15 degrees of wrist extension. The length of time for wearing the splint is also undetermined, with some recommending day and night use,[321] while others instruct patients to wear the brace at night and during activities stressful to the wrist.[322] Still others recommend only night use.[320] Rigid splints have been found to be superior to flexible ones in controlling carpal tunnel pressure,[323] although the softer flexible ones enhance compliance in RA patients.[324]

Night splints appear to allow the wrist to rest fully, although one study found that night splints did not significantly reduce intracarpal pressure when compared to controls who did not wear them.[85] Splints during the day are helpful only if they do not interfere with normal activity. The positioning of the splint may be significant.

Yoga that focuses on upper body postures was found to be of benefit in one study,[325] although the sample size was small and the results were not conclusive.

Ergonomic modifications can help reduce the incidence of CTS and alleviate symptoms in the already symptomatic patient. Patient education is also important to avoid sustained pinching or gripping, repetitive wrist motions, and sustained positions of full wrist flexion.

Isolated tendon excursion exercises for the finger flexor tendons and nerve gliding of the median nerve exercises are performed. These include isolated tendon gliding of the FDS and FDP of each digit. The exercises are thought to have a positive effect by facilitating venous return or edema dispersion in the median nerve.[320]

Contrast baths can be used in 10-minute sessions to assist in the reduction of inflammation and edema.

Evaluation for surgical management is necessary for patients with atrophy of the thenar muscles, decreased sensation, and persistent symptoms that are intolerable despite conservative therapy.[296]

Ulnar Nerve. Entrapment of the ulnar nerve can occur at the elbow in the cubital tunnel (Chapter 17). Entrapment of the ulnar nerve at the wrist can occur at Guyon canal. The clinical features of an ulnar nerve entrapment at the wrist are described in chapter 3.

If ulnar neuropathy at Guyon canal is suspected, it is often helpful to evaluate the pisotriquetral joint and the hook of the hamate. Abnormalities may be present at either site, resulting in secondary ulnar neuropathy.[326] In addition, the clinician must ask the patient whether they have any medical history involving diabetes and peripheral neuropathies.

The intervention for ulnar nerve compression can be surgical or conservative depending on the severity. Indications for surgical intervention include preventing deformity and increasing functional use of the hand. Conservative intervention for mild compression involves the application of a protective splint and patient education to avoid positions and postures that could compromise the nerve.

Hand-Arm Vibration Syndrome

Vibration is a physical stressor to which many people are exposed at work, in the home, or in their social activities. Humans respond characteristically to certain critical vibration frequencies at which there is maximum energy transfer from source to receiver.[327]

Hand-arm vibration syndrome (HAVS) is frequently underdiagnosed and misdiagnosed as CTS since the two entities typically coexist.[328] HAVS is associated with occupations involving exposure to sources of vibration including air-compressed drilling, grinding, and electric drills and saws.[329]

The pathophysiology of HAVS is poorly understood, but chronic exposure to vibration may produce circulatory, neurologic–sensory–motor, and musculoskeletal disturbances. Khilberg[330] has studied the acute effects and symptoms of work with vibrating hand-held power tools. He found that workers using nonimpact tools (grinders) had a lower prevalence of elbow and shoulder symptoms than those using low-frequency impact tools (chipping hammers), but it did not differ in this respect from workers using high-frequency impact tools. Work with impact tools in general was associated with a higher prevalence of pain in the wrist than work with nonimpact tools.[327]

The diagnosis of HAVS is based on a history of HAV exposure and sensorineural or vascular signs and symptoms, which include the following[228]:

- Blanching white fingers (Raynaud phenomenon). This is the most common symptom, and it occurs on exposure to cold. Its extent and frequency of occurrence determines the severity of the vascular grading.[327]
- Episodic tingling and numbness. The numbness or tingling can be graded.
- Mild to severe sensory deficits.
- Swelling of the digits and forearm tissue.
- Trophic skin changes.

The intervention for HAVS includes maintaining central body temperature, avoiding exposure to cold and vibrating tools, job modification, and splinting at night.[228]

Myofascial Pain Syndrome

The most frequent cause of wrist, hand, and finger pain is myofascial referral from the forearm flexors and especially from the forearm extensors. Trigger points in these muscles increase tendon tension and therefore relative compression of the carpal joints, which causes cracking and crepitus at the wrist due to abnormal joint glide.[331] The patient often reports a sense of stiffness in the wrist and hand, and pain exacerbated with wrist and finger flexion, which stretches these muscles, and on full wrist extension, which shortens these muscles.[331]

Complex Regional Pain Syndrome

The term CRPS refers to a classification of disorders, which can occur even after minor injury to a limb and which is a major cause of disability.[332]

CRPS, originally termed *causalgia*, has since been referred to by a number of names including posttraumatic osteoporosis, Sudeck atrophy, transient osteoporosis, algoneurodystrophy, shoulder–hand syndrome, gardenalic rheumatism, neurotrophic rheumatism, reflex neurovascular dystrophy, and reflex sympathetic dystrophy (RSD).[333]

Two types of CRPS are recognized by the International Association for the Study of Pain:

- *CRPS 1.* This type refers to the pain syndrome, previously termed RSD, which involves a pain syndrome triggered by a noxious event that is not limited to a single peripheral nerve.
- *CRPS 2.* This type refers to the pain syndrome, previously termed causalgia, which involves a pain syndrome that involves direct partial or complete injury to a nerve or one of its major branches.

The signs and symptoms for both types include pain, edema, stiffness, skin temperature changes, and sweating.[334] More recently, it has been suggested that a third type may exist. This type is characterized by irreversible changes in the skin and bones, marked muscle atrophy, unyielding pain, and severely limited mobility of the affected area.

Type I CRPS. The pain of type I CRPS is classified as sympathetically maintained pain or sympathetically independent pain, where sympathetically maintained pain is characterized by an abnormal reaction of the sympathetic nervous system.[334]

The edema, which can be pitting or nonpitting, is often present throughout all stages of CRPS and may be the result of vasomotor instability coupled with a lack of motion.[333]

The stiffness is one of the components of CRPS 1 that increases with time and is due to increased fibrosis in the ligamentous structures and adhesion formation around the tendons.[333]

The reported incidence of CRPS 1 is 1–2 percent after various fractures,[335] 2–5 percent after peripheral nerve injury,[336] and 7–35 percent in prospective studies of Colles fracture.[337,281] In 10–26 percent of cases no precipitating factor can be found.[338,282] A number of psychological components have been proposed, including the following:

1. A significant period of stress, anxiety, or depression
2. Childhood experiences.
   a. Sexual abuse
   b. Physical abuse
   c. Emotional abuse
   d. Abandonment
   e. Family history of drug or alcohol abuse
3. Adult experiences
   a. Care provider for aging or ill parent(s) or other relative
   b. Problem children, parents, or siblings
   c. Unhappy marriage
   d. Alcoholism
   e. Grief
   f. Abuse of any type
4. A low self-esteem
5. A negative outlook on life

However, there has been no evidence to support such notions. Instead, it is thought that the emotional and behavioral changes noted are a result, rather than a cause, of the prolonged pain and disability.[339]

The diagnosis of CRPS is made from the physical examination and the patient's medical history, which may include past events of trauma, persistent pain, hyperalgesia, allodynia (perception of a nonpainful stimulus as painful), edema, and diminished function of the area.

The type of pain and its duration are perhaps the most important diagnostic signs. The pain is typically burning in nature and is of a much longer duration than would be expected from the injury.[339]

A number of other conditions need to be ruled out before establishing a diagnosis of CRPS 1, and these include, but are not limited to the following:

- Rheumatoid and septic arthritis
- Gout
- Disk herniation
- Peripheral neuropathy
- Peripheral nerve entrapment
- Peripheral vascular disease

Classically, CRPS 1 has been subdivided into three clinical phases[340,341]:

- An acute inflammatory phase that can last from 10 days to 2–3 months. The acute stage of CRPS lasts from 1 to 3 months. This stage is reversible if the patient is treated. The affected limb becomes flushed, warm, and dry because regional blood vessels are relaxed, and stimulation of the sweat glands is reduced.[334] The pain is diffuse, severe, and constant with a burning, throbbing, or aching quality. Edema and increased hair and nail growth can also occur. By the end of this stage, the limb turns cold, sweaty, and cyanotic from vasoconstriction caused by paradoxical sympathetic stimulation.[334]
- A phase of vasomotor instability that can last for several months. This is the dystrophic stage, which lasts another 3–6 months. Constricted blood vessels can cool limb temperature by nearly 10 degrees.[334] The area will be pale, mottled, edematous, and sweaty. Pain remains continuous, burning, or throbbing but is more severe.[334] Nails may crack or become brittle and heavily grooved. Limb movement is limited by muscle wasting and joint stiffness. Osteoporosis and contractures can develop.[334]
- A cold end phase. The atrophic stage is characterized by irreversible damage to muscles and joints. Over the next 2–3 months the bones atrophy and the joints become weak, stiff, or even ankylosed.[334] The pain lessens and may become spasmodic or breakthrough but is no longer mediated by the sympathetic nervous system.[334] The skin is cool and looks glossy and pale or cyanotic.

No prospective studies are available in which this staging is confirmed. However, a prospective study of 829 patients[333] indicated that the following:

- In its early phase, CRPS is characterized by regional inflammation and not of a disturbance of the sympathetic nervous system. The regional inflammation increases after muscular exercise.

- Tremor was found in 49 percent and muscular incoordination in 54 percent of patients.
- Sympathetic signs such as hyperhidrosis are infrequent.

These data support the concept of an exaggerated regional inflammatory response to injury or operation in CRPS.[333,342]

The most effective intervention for CRPS 1 is disputed. However, most agree that the intervention requires a team approach, in which the physical therapist plays a pivotal role and that the earlier the intervention is instituted, the better the prognosis. Immobilization and overprotecting the affected limb may produce or exacerbate demineralization, vasomotor changes, edema, and trophic changes.[343]

Physical therapy is the first line of intervention, whether it be the sole intervention or performed immediately following a nerve block.[339,344]

The most important rule is to minimize pain while employing physical therapy. When excessive pain is created, sympathetically mediated pain may worsen.[339] It is vital to not reinjure the region or aggravate the problem with aggressive physical rehabilitation.[345]

The patient's involved limb must be elevated as often as possible to counteract the vascular stasis and actively mobilized several times per day.[339,346]

Recovery from muscle dysfunction, swelling, and joint stiffness requires appropriate physical activity and exercise, and pressure and motion are necessary to maintain joint movement and prevent stiffening.[339] The progression should occur slowly and gently with strengthening, active assisted range-of-motion, and AROM exercises.

Weight-bearing exercises and active stress loading exercises should also be incorporated. Active stress loading exercises include scrubbing and carrying. Scrubbing is a form of closed kinetic chain exercise for the upper or lower extremity in which the patient in a variety of positions performs a scrubbing action on a firm surface. As its name suggests, carrying exercises for the upper extremity involve having the patient carry small objects in the hand on the affected side and gradually increasing the weight of the object. For the lower extremity stress loading can be achieved through weight bearing.

Sensory threshold techniques can be used. These include fluidotherapy, vibration desensitization, transcutaneous electrical nerve stimulation, contrast baths, and desensitization using light and heavy pressure of various textures over the sensitive area.

Topical capsaicin is helpful, as are NSAIDs.

INTEGRATION OF PRACTICE PATTERNS 4G AND 4I

This includes conditions that result in impaired joint mobility, motor function, muscle performance, and range of motion that are associated with fractures and bony or soft tissue surgical procedures.

Distal Radius Fractures

Fracture of the distal radius is the most common wrist injury for any age group. While the older patient usually sustains an extra-articular metaphyseal fracture, the younger patient tends to sustain the more complicated intra-articular fracture.[208] Physical examination reveals swelling of the wrist, possible gross deformity, limited range of motion, and point tenderness over the distal radius. Successful management of a distal radius fracture must take into account the integrity and function of the soft tissues, while restoring anatomic alignment of the bones. The clinician should avoid distracting or placing the wrist in a flexed position, so that the mechanical advantage of the extrinsic tendons is maintained, pressure in the carpal canal is not increased, any carpal ligament injury is not exacerbated, and stiffness is not encouraged. The rehabilitation after fracture of the distal radius is nearly uniform among the various fracture types outlined below. The more specific guidelines are listed after each fracture description.

Colles Fracture.[4] Colles fracture is a complete fracture of the distal radius with posterior (dorsal) displacement of the distal fragment. The typical mechanism of injury is a FOOSH. The fracture displacement and angulation are evident on the lateral film—the Colles fracture has the characteristic dorsiflexion or "silver fork" deformity. Radiographs of the AP view show the usual comminuted fracture.

Management of this fracture requires a precise reduction of the fracture in order to maintain the normal length of the radius. Although the method of reduction, as well as the position of immobilization, is quite variable, in most cases closed reduction and a cast are chosen. However, the more complicated cases may require open reduction and external fixations.[347] A common sequelae of this fracture is a loss of full rotation of the forearm.

Smith Fracture. A Smith fracture, sometimes called a reverse Colles fracture, is defined as a complete fracture of the distal radius with anterior (palmar) displacement of the distal fragment.[348] The usual mechanism for this type of fracture is a fall on the back of a flexed hand. Smith fractures are classified into three types[349]:

- *Type I.* This is described as a transverse fracture through the distal radial shaft.
- *Type II.* This is an oblique fracture through the distal shaft starting at the posterior (dorsal) articulating lip.
- *Type III.* This type (also referred to as a reverse Barton fracture) is an oblique fracture beginning more distally on the articular surface of the radius.

The typical management for a Smith fracture is with closed reduction and long arm casting in supination for 3 weeks, followed by 2–3 weeks in a short-arm cast.[348] However, because Types II and III are frequently unstable, they may require an ORIF.

Barton Fracture. A Barton fracture involves a posterior (dorsal) or anterior (volar) articular fracture of the distal radius resulting in a subluxation of the wrist.[348] This type of fracture usually results from some form of direct and aggressive injury to the wrist or from a sudden pronation of the distal forearm on a fixed wrist. A technique to reduce these dislocations under anesthesia has been described in the literature.[350] The technique involves applying traction to the wrist and then placing the patient's wrist in full supination, mid-extension, and ulnar deviation, which closes the diastasis by reducing the scaphoid to its correct anatomic plane. An above-elbow cast is then applied for 4 weeks, followed by a forearm cast for a further 3 weeks with the wrist positioned in ulnar deviation. More complicated fractures may require an ORIF with 16 weeks being the average healing time.

Buckle Fracture. A buckle fracture is an incomplete, undisplaced fracture of the distal radius, which is commonly seen in children. Immobilization for 3–4 weeks in a short-arm cast or anterior (palmar) splint is adequate.[146] The possibility of abuse should be considered in the child with a fracture. Consultation with an orthopedist is advisable for fractures in the pediatric population.

The fracture is treated with a cast, external fixation, or ORIF. The fracture site is immobilized for 6 weeks if casted, 8 weeks with an external fixator, or 2 weeks if an ORIF with plate and screws is performed. If the fracture is nondisplaced, 2–6 weeks of rehabilitation is recommended, whereas displaced fractures typically require 8–12 weeks.

Conservative intervention usually begins while the fracture is immobilized and involves AROM of the shoulder in all planes, AROM of elbow flexion and extension, and finger flexion and extension. The finger exercises must include isolated MCP flexion, composite flexion (full fist), and intrinsic minus fisting (MCP extension with IP flexion). If a fixator or pins are present, pin site care should be performed.

Following the period of immobilization, extension and supination are commonly limited and need to be mobilized. AROM exercises of wrist flexion and extension and ulnar and radial deviation are initiated at this time. Wrist extension exercises are performed with the fingers flexed (especially at the MCP joints). The initiation of PROM occurs according to physician preference, either immediately or after 1–2 weeks.

Strengthening exercises are introduced as tolerated, using light weights and tubing. Putty can be used to increase grip strength if necessary.

Plyometrics and neuromuscular re-education exercises are next, followed by return to function or sports activities as appropriate.

Fractured Scaphoid

The scaphoid is the most commonly fractured carpal bone due to its location and is the only bone fractured in approximately 70 percent of all carpal fracture cases.[131,146,207,280] Most commonly, the injury results from a FOOSH with the wrist pronated. Although a fracture can occur in any part of the scaphoid, the common areas are at the waist and at the proximal pole.

Patients typically complain of posterior (dorsal) radial-sided wrist pain and have tenderness over the anatomic snuffbox. On physical examination, little swelling may be noted, although loss of the concavity of the anatomic snuffbox is frequently seen.[351] It may be good practice to treat all cases of wrist sprain that are accompanied with pain and swelling in the anatomic snuffbox as a scaphoid fracture until proven otherwise. Many investigators feel a reliable test for scaphoid injury is axial compression of the thumb along its longitudinal axis.[352,353] Described by Chen,[352] this test translates force directly across the scaphoid and should elicit pain if there is a fracture. Even with appropriate radiographs, fractures of the scaphoid can be difficult to visualize.[351] In cases in which there is a high clinical suspicion, a scaphoid view of the wrist is usually obtained. This is a clenched fist view with the wrist held in ulnar deviation. This view reduces the foreshortening of the scaphoid that occurs on a normal PA view and clearly displays the entire length of the scaphoid.[351] If plain radiographs are normal and clinical suspicion is high, MRI is warranted.

Accurate early diagnosis of scaphoid fracture is critical as the morbidity associated with a missed or delayed diagnosis is significant and can result in long-term pain, loss of mobility, and decreased function.[12] This degree of morbidity is related to the scant blood supply to the scaphoid, which results in a high incidence of delayed healing or nonunion, and the fact that scaphoid fractures are inherently unstable.

Conservative management of a scaphoid fracture remains controversial. For example, there is no agreement on the optimum position for immobilization. Current management is immobilization in a long-arm or short-arm thumb spica cast, with the wrist position and length of immobilization dependent on the location of the fracture:

- ***Proximal pole.*** Immobilization for 16–20 weeks in a long-arm or short-arm thumb spica, with the wrist positioned in slight extension and radial deviation.
- ***Central third.*** Immobilization for 6 weeks in a long-arm thumb spica, followed by a further 6 weeks in a short-arm thumb spica.
- ***Distal third.*** Immobilization for 6–8 weeks in a short-arm thumb spica.
- ***Tuberosity.*** Immobilization for 5–6 weeks in a long-arm or short-arm thumb spica.

For the patient with pain over the anatomic snuffbox but normal initial radiographs, application of a thumb spica cast for 3 weeks followed by repeat radiographs is indicated. If the radiographs remain normal but pain persists, a bone scan is the next step. If the bone scan is positive, management is continued as for an acute fracture. Chronic pain, loss of motion, and decreased strength from prolonged immobilization or early arthritis is common following a scaphoid fracture.

Following the removal of the splint, a capsular pattern of the wrist is usually evident. In addition, there will be a painful weakness of the thumb and/or wrist extension/radial deviation. AROM exercises for wrist flexion and extension, and radial and ulnar deviation are initiated as early as possible, with PROM to the same motions beginning after 2 weeks. A wrist and thumb immobilization splint is typically worn between exercises and at night for comfort and protection.

At about the same time as the PROM exercises are initiated, gentle strengthening exercises are introduced using 1- to 2-lb weights or putty. Over a period of several weeks, the exercise program is progressed to include weight-bearing activities, plyometrics, open- and closed-chain exercises, and neuromuscular reeducation, before finally progressing to functional and sport-specific exercises and activities as appropriate.

Because of the precarious nature of the blood supply and potential for movement at the fracture line, nonunion can occur in 8–10 percent of cases,[354,355] with the rate of nonunion varying with the actual fracture site (up to 20–30 percent of proximal third fractures and 10–20 percent of middle third fractures, with distal third fractures being relatively rare).[351354,355]

SLAC wrist is a late complication of scaphoid fracture, scapholunate dissociation, Kienböck disease, fracture of the distal radius, Preiser disease, and deposition of crystals of calcium pyrophosphate dehydrate.[356] The SLAC wrist is thought to result from a loss of the stabilizing effect of the scaphoid, with the development of an arthrosis at the radioscaphoid articulation. When the injury has progressed to this state, proximal row carpectomy or wrist fusion is the only option for the hand surgeon.[357]

Carpal Boss

A carpal boss is a rounded bony prominence that presents between the base of second and third metacarpal and the trapezoid and capitate, resulting from repetitive forced extension of the wrist and subsequent irritation of soft tissues. The ECRL and ECRB are commonly involved. This prominence resembles a ganglion and is not necessarily pathologic, although it can cause pain and irritation of the local soft tissues.[358] Confirmation is through radiographs.

Conservative intervention includes a wrist immobilization splint with the wrist positioned in slight extension (10–15 degrees) to reduce tension on the radial wrist extensors.

Metacarpal Fractures

Injuries to the metacarpals are the result of either direct or indirect trauma, with nature and direction of the applied force determining the exact type of fracture or dislocation. Most metacarpal fractures occur in the active and working population, particularly adolescents and young adults.[359,360] Specific injury patterns that occur from commonly seen trauma are as follows:

- ***CMC injuries.*** Metacarpal base fractures and dislocations of the CMC joint commonly result from an axial load or other stress on the hand with the wrist flexed.[359,360] CMC joints, especially the central joints, are quite stable. The metacarpal bases are held in position by posterior (dorsal) and anterior (palmar) CMC ligaments, as well as by interosseous ligaments. CMC dislocations may occur with or without fracture. Fracture-dislocation of the fifth metacarpal base is a common intra-articular injury and has been dubbed the reverse Bennett fracture. A direct blow to the ulnar border of the hand tends to cause an extra-articular fifth metacarpal base fracture.
- ***Metacarpal shaft injuries.*** Metacarpal shaft fractures are typically produced by either axial loading,direct trauma, or torsional forces on the digits. Usually, the fractures are classified anatomically as transverse, oblique, or spiral.[359,360] The fracture pattern often denotes the mechanism of injury, with direct or axial injury leading to transverse or oblique fractures and torsion leading to spiral fracture.
- ***Metacarpal neck fractures.*** The most common metacarpal fractures usually result from striking a solid object with a clenched fist and thus are dubbed boxer fractures, although this injury almost never occurs during boxing. Fractures of the fifth metacarpal neck are among the most common fractures in the hand.[359,360]
- ***Metacarpal head injuries.*** Metacarpal head fractures, which are rare injuries, result from axial loading or direct trauma. Fractures of the metacarpal head are intra-articular and periarticular.[359,360] If displaced, metacarpal head fractures usually require ORIF.
- ***Avulsion fracture at the origin of the collateral ligaments.*** This type of fracture is caused by forced deviation of the flexed MCP joint.[359,360]
- ***MCP dislocations.*** Almost all MCP dislocations occur with the proximal phalanx displaced posterior (dorsal)ly on the metacarpal head, as there is no specific posterior (dorsal) restraint to the MCP joint other than the joint capsule and extensor mechanism.[359,360]

The management of a patient with a metacarpal fracture depends on a variety of factors including the location, degree of displacement, angulation, and rotation. In addition, the patient's age, occupation, general health, and concomitant injuries must also be considered. Most metacarpal injuries are managed by closed reduction and immobilization or sometimes controlled mobilization utilizing a posterior (dorsal) block splint. Specific indications are further described below.

- Impaction fractures of the metacarpal bases that are not significantly displaced can be treated with splinting, followed by early mobilization.
- CMC dislocations and fracture dislocations, especially when multiple, are unstable injuries. In the past, these fractures were managed by closed reduction and external immobilization, which frequently led to grip weakness and residual pain. The current literature supports closed reduction, if joint congruity can be obtained, but with the addition of internal fixation.
- Displaced fracture dislocations of the fourth and fifth metacarpals, which are accompanied by fracture of the posterior (dorsal) hamate, require ORIF. Reverse Bennett fractures frequently need K-wire stabilization to counteract the deforming forces. If little articular incongruity is present, this may be a closed procedure.

As the major complication of these fractures is adherence of soft tissues, the primary goals of rehabilitation, once bony healing has occurred, are to restore an optimized soft-tissue balance and glide to allow pain-free motion and strength while simultaneously protecting the healing tissues.

Finger Fractures

Fractures of the finger (phalangeal), which are more common than metacarpal or carpal fractures, represent approximately 45 percent of fractures of the hand and wrist.[361] Phalangeal fractures can be divided into base, shaft, and neck and head fractures. Conservative intervention for the more stable fractures involves closed reduction in as near normal alignment as possible with an appropriate cast or splint[362]:

Distal Phalanx Fractures

Tuft Fracture. This is the most common fracture of the fingers, frequently resulting from a crush injury. These fractures are often associated with injuries to the nail matrix.

Shaft Fracture. This type of fracture is either longitudinal or more commonly transverse in orientation. If displaced, this type of fracture is usually associated with an injury to the nail matrix.

Intra-articular Fracture. This fracture in adults usually involves either the volar or posterior (dorsal) lip at the end of the bone, whereas in children an epiphyseal separation also may occur.

Volar Lip Fracture. This type of fracture, also referred to as Jersey finger or sweater finger, is also a tendon avulsion injury where the FDP remains attached to the small fracture fragment.

Unstable displaced articular fractures require surgical intervention. Generally speaking, following a fracture of the distal phalanx, a protective splint is worn for 2–4 weeks until the fracture site is nontender. AROM begins at 2–4 weeks or earlier if the fracture is stable enough. PROM begins at 5–6 weeks. PREs normally begin at 7–8 weeks.

Fractures of the Proximal and Middle Phalanges

Shaft Fracture. The type of shaft fracture depends largely on the mechanism of injury. A direct blow frequently causes transverse fractures, whereas twisting injuries often cause spiral or oblique fractures.

The intervention for this type of fracture depends on the location and the severity:

Proximal Phalanx Fractures. Nondisplaced extra-articular fractures are splinted with buddy tape. AROM is initiated immediately, with PROM being initiated at 6–8 weeks. Nondisplaced intra-articular fractures are splinted in the intrinsic plus position for 2–3 weeks. AROM begins at 2–3 weeks, with PROM being initiated at 4–8 weeks. PREs normally begin at clinical union (8–12 weeks).

Middle Phalanx Fractures. If nondisplaced, these fractures are splinted in the intrinsic plus position for approximately 3 weeks. Buddy splinting, the taping of a neighboring finger to the involved finger, may also be an option. AROM is initiated when pain and edema subsides. PROM begins at 4–6 weeks, with PREs normally beginning at 6–8 weeks.

THERAPEUTIC TECHNIQUES

Myofascial Release

Carpal Tunnel Release. A number of myofascial techniques can be used to treat CTS

Opening the Canal. The patient is positioned in sitting or supine lying with their palms facing upward. The clinician applies pressure centrally from the posterior (dorsal) surface of the carpal bones simultaneously with pressure applied from the ventral edges of the carpal bones, using a three-point-opposing-pressure technique.[363]

Abductor Brevis Release. The patient is positioned in sitting or supine lying with their palm facing upward. The clinician grasps the thumb with one hand and pulls it back into hyperextension with abduction, while simultaneously performing the opening canal technique described above.[363]

Carpal Tunnel Stretch. The patient is positioned in sitting or supine lying with their palm facing upward. The clinician stabilizes the patient's wrist with one hand and simultaneously hyperextends the digits and wrist of the patient with the other hand.[363]

Techniques to Increase Joint Mobility

The majority of the joint mobility tests described in the tests and measures section can also be utilized as mobilization techniques. For each of the techniques, the patient is positioned in sitting with their forearm and wrist in a neutral position, with the clinician positioned to the side of the patient. The amplitude and the velocity of each of the techniques (i.e., grade) is varied according to the stage of healing and the irritability of the joint.

The clinician must be cognizant of the joints that are responsible for the individual motions that occur at the wrist and hand and which ones present with convex or concave joint surfaces in order to deliver the most specific technique.

- Supination–pronation occurs primarily at the ulnomeniscotriquetral joint and the proximal and inferior radioulnar joints.
- Wrist flexion occurs primarily at the radiocarpal joint (distal radius and the articulating surfaces of the navicular and lunate).
- Wrist extension occurs primarily at the midcarpal joints (articulating surface of the scaphoid, lunate, and triquetral bones proximally, and the trapezium, trapezoid, capitate, and hamate bones distally).

Passive Accessory Mobilizations

Distal Radioulnar Joint

Anterior–posterior Glide. The clinician glides the radius in an anterior direction to improve forearm pronation and in a posterior direction to improve forearm supination. The intensity of the technique (i.e., grade) is varied according to the irritability of the joint.

Radiocarpal

Posterior–anterior glide (Fig. 18-30). The posterior glide is used to improve the joint's ability to flex, whereas the anterior glide is used to improve the ability of the joint to extend.

Ulnar and radial glide (Fig. 18-31). The ulnar (medial) glide is used to improve the joint's ability to radially deviate, whereas the radial (lateral) glide is used to improve the ability of the joint to ulnarly deviate.

Ulnocarpal, Midcarpal, CMC, MCP, and IP Joints

Distraction. Using a pinch grip of the index finger and thumb of one hand, the clinician palpates and stabilizes the proximal bone of the joint being distracted. With a pinch grip of the index finger and thumb of the other hand, the clinician palpates and mobilizes the distal bone longitudinally (Fig. 18-36).

Posterior–Anterior Glide (Flexion/Extension). Using a pinch grip of the index finger and thumb of one hand, the clinician palpates and stabilizes the proximal bone of the joint being mobilized in a posterior (dorsal)–anterior (palmar) plane. With a pinch grip, the clinician glides the distal bone along the posterior (dorsal)–anterior (palmar) plane of the corresponding joint. The appropriate conjunct rotation of the bone may be added. For example, to restore flexion at the radioscaphoid joint, the clinician rotates the scaphoid toward the center of the palm, while simultaneously gliding the scaphoid in a posterior (dorsal) direction.

The clinician can make the technique patient-assisted by flexing/extending the distal bone about the appropriate intra-articular axis to the limit of the physiologic range of motion. From this position, the patient is instructed to perform an isometric contraction against the clinician's equal resistance. The contraction is held for 3–5 seconds, following which the patient is instructed to completely relax. The new barrier of flexion/extension is localized and the mobilization repeated.

First CMC (Trapeziometacarpal) Joint

Posterior glide. This technique is used to improve range of motion into trapeziometacarpal joint abduction.

Anterior glide. This technique is used to improve range of motion into trapeziometacarpal joint adduction.

Medial–Lateral Glide (Abduction/Adduction). The medial glide technique is used to improve range of motion into trapeziometacarpal joint flexion. The lateral glide technique is used to improve range of motion into trapeziometacarpal joint extension.

The clinician can make the technique patient assisted by abducting/adducting the distal bone about the appropriate intra-articular axis to the limit of the physiologic range of motion. From this position, the patient is instructed to perform an isometric contraction against the clinician's equal resistance. The contraction is held for 3–5 seconds, following which the patient is instructed to completely relax. The new barrier of motion is localized and the mobilization repeated.

Intermetacarpal Loints. Using a pinch grip of the index finger and thumb of one hand, the clinician palpates and stabilizes one metacarpal. With the thumb and index finger of the other hand, the clinician mobilizes the neighboring metacarpal into an anterior or posterior glide, with the appropriate conjunct rotation

MCP Joints.

Posterior–Anterior Glide. A posterior glide is used to improve range of motion into extension for digits two through five, whereas an anterior glide is used to improve range of motion into flexion for digits two through five.

Ulnar (Medial)–Radial (Lateral) Glide. An ulnar glide is used to improve range of motion into ulnar deviation for digits two through five, whereas a radial glide is used to improve range of motion into radial deviation for digits two through five.

First MCP/IP Joint. A radial glide is used to improve trapeziometacarpal extension, while the ulnar glide is used to improve trapeziometacarpal flexion.

IP joints. The anterior glide can be used to improve the ability of the joint to move into flexion, whereas posterior glide can be used to improve the ability of the joint to move into extension.

High-Velocity, Low-Amplitude Thrusting

High-velocity thrust techniques can be used with any of the carpals. The following example describes the technique for a posteriorly (dorsally) displaced scaphoid:

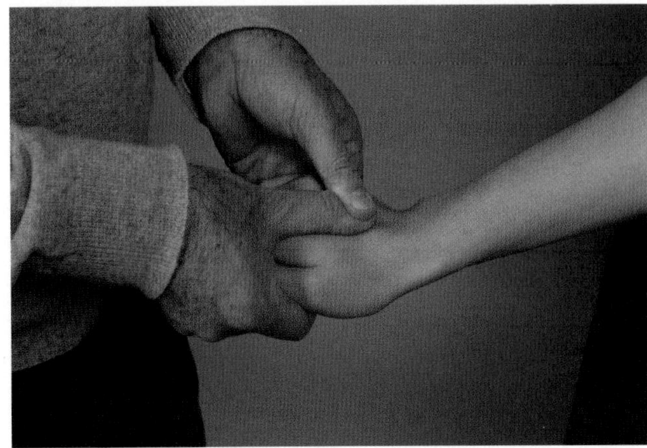

FIGURE 18-86 High-velocity thrust technique to the scaphoid.

The patient is positioned in sitting with the forearm of their affected side resting on a table with the anterior (palmar) side facing down. The clinician sits or stands at right angles to the patient's affected side. The clinician grips the patient's scaphoid bone between their thumb and index finger (Fig. 18-86). The clinician reinforces this grip by placing the thumb and the index of the other hand on top of them. The patient's wrist is then passively extended to the end range. At the end of the available range, the scaphoid is thrusted anteriorly (ventrally) while passively extending the wrist slightly.

Transverse Friction Massage

Common Sheath of APL and EPB. Transverse friction can be applied to the common shared sheath of the APL and EPB (Fig. 18-87) or at the point where the tendons pass over the wrist extensors.

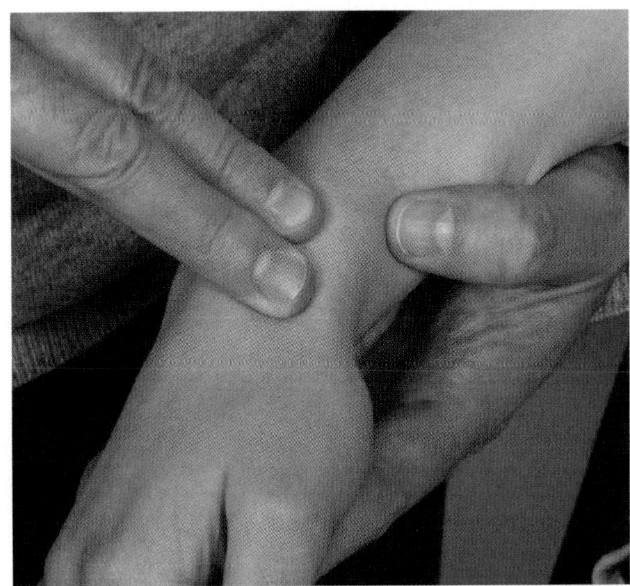

FIGURE 18-87 TFM to common shared sheath of the abductor pollicis longus and extensor pollicis.

Techniques to Increase Soft Tissue Extensibility

A number of techniques can be used to increase the extensibility of the soft tissues of the wrist, hand, and forearm. These include passive or AROM exercises that can be performed by the patient:

- Wrist flexion and extension
- Wrist ulnar and radial deviation
- Finger flexion and extension
- Finger adduction and abduction
- Thumb opposition, flexion, extension, abduction, and adduction

CASE STUDY

PAINFUL LEFT THUMB

HISTORY

History of Current Condition

A 23-year-old female patient complained of left thumb pain following a home do-it-yourself project that involved a lot of hammering of nails. The patient described a gradual onset of pain about 2 months ago and described the pain as burning located at the base of the left thumb. The patient also reported some swelling at the wrist. The patient attributed the pain to the hammering of nails as subsequent attempts to use the hammer reproduced the pain. Over time, the pain had worsened to the point where it hurt all of the time, even at night. The NSAIDs prescribed by the physician 2 weeks ago appeared to be helping.

Past History of Current Condition

No past history of left elbow, wrist, or hand pain.

Past Medical/Surgical History

Unremarkable except for removal of ganglion cysts from her right wrist/hand about 1 year ago.

Growth and Development

Right-hand dominant.

Medications

None, except for the prescribed NSAIDs.

Occupational/Employment/School

Office worker. College education.

Functional Status/Activity Level

The patient reported experiencing pain with vacuuming and lifting heavy pots and pans. The patient's goals were to decrease pain with activities of daily living.

Health Status (Self-Report)

In general good health, but pain interferes with gripping tasks at home and at work.

Questions

1. What are some of the more common diagnoses characterized by thumb pain?
2. What does the history of the gradual onset and of repetitive activity tell the clinician?
3. What findings do you expect to note in the physical examination in terms of palpation, resistive tests, and special tests?
4. What additional questions would you ask to help rule out referral of pain from the cervical spine or shoulder?
5. List the tests you would use to rule out the various diagnoses that you listed in question 1.
6. Does this presentation/history warrant an upper quarter scanning examination? Why or why not?

CASE STUDY

PAIN, WEAKNESS, AND NUMBNESS OF THE HAND

HISTORY

History of Current Condition

A 49-year-old female secretary complains of insidious onset of right hand numbness and pain, which began about 5 weeks previously. The symptoms are felt mainly in the right index finger, especially when working at her computer at work but also in her right thumb and middle finger after a day at work and at night. The symptoms are also reported to be worse during the night and early morning. The patient has also noted a slight decrease in her grip strength, which prompted her to see a MD, who prescribed PT, ibuprofen, vitamin B6, and a short course of diuretics. The patient denies any neck pain.

Past Medical/Surgical History

Unremarkable, including no history of previous symptoms or of diabetes mellitus reported by the patient.

Medications

800 mg of ibuprofen daily.

Other Tests and Measures

None. X-rays 1 year ago were unremarkable (per patient). Physician mentioned that further testing may be warranted (nerve conduction velocity, EMG).

Social Habits (Past and Present)

Smoker (1/2 pack per day).

Growth and Development

Right-hand dominant.

Occupational/Employment/School

Full-time secretary at local community hospital for last 6 years. Recently promoted which has meant an increase in computer work.

Functional Status/Activity Level

Symptoms interfering with work and at home with her needle craft. Symptoms also interfering with sleep approximately two times per night.

Questions

1. What are some of the more common diagnoses characterized by symptoms in this distribution?
2. What does the history of the gradual onset and of repetitive activity tell the clinician?
3. What findings do you expect to note in the physical examination in terms of palpation, resistive tests, and special tests?
4. What additional questions would you ask to help rule out referral of pain from the cervical and thoracic spine?
5. What additional questions would you ask to help rule out referral of pain from the shoulder or elbow?
6. List the tests you would use to rule out the various diagnoses that you listed in question 1.
7. Does this presentation/history warrant a scan? Why or why not?

REVIEW QUESTIONS*

1. Which two carpal bones does the radius articulate with?
2. Name the carpal bones in the distal row.
3. Which structures run through Guyon canal?
4. Which combination of symptoms indicates injury to the median nerve?
   a. The middle and index fingers lose the ability to flex and the thumb cannot adduct or extend.
   b. The ring and little fingers lose the ability to flex, and the little finger cannot abduct or oppose.
   c. The inability of the wrist and fingers to extend interferes with grasp.
   d. The middle and index fingers lose their ability to flex, and the thumb cannot oppose.
5. Finkelstein test is designed to assess involvement of which of the following contractile structures?
   a. EPL and APB muscles.
   b. EPB and APL muscles.
   c. Extensor pollicis longus and abductor pollicis longus muscles.
   d. EPB and APB muscles.

*Additional questions to test your understanding of this chapter can be found in the Online Learning Center for *Orthopaedic Assessment, Evaluation, and Intervention* at www.duttononline.net.

REFERENCES

1. McPhee SD: Functional hand evaluations: A review. *Am J Occup Ther* 41:158–163, 1987.
2. Watson HK, Weinzweig J: Physical examination of the wrist. *Hand Clin* 13:17–34, 1997.
3. Hume MC, Gellman H, McKellop H, et al: Functional range of motion of the joints of the hand. *J Hand Surg Am* 15A:240–243, 1990.
4. Onieal M-E: Common wrist and elbow injuries in primary care. *Lippincotts Prim Care Pract* 3:441–450, 1999.
5. Frykman GK, Kropp WE: Fractures and traumatic conditions of the wrist. In: Hunter JM, Mackin EJ, Callahan AD, eds. *Rehabilitation of the Hand: Surgery and Therapy*. St Louis, MO: Mosby-Year Book, Inc., 1995:315–336.
6. Wadsworth CT: *Anatomy of the Hand and Wrist, Manual Examination and Treatment of the Spine and Extremities*. Baltimore, MD: Williams & Wilkins Co, 1988:128–138.
7. Ward LD, Ambrose CG, Masson MV, et al: The role of the distal radioulnar ligaments, interosseous membrane, and joint capsule, in distal radioulnar joint stability. *J Hand Surg Am* 25:341–351, 2000.
8. Palmer AK, Werner FW: The triangular fibrocartilage complex of the wrist – anatomy and function. *J Hand Surg Am* 6:153–162, 1981.
9. Waggy C: Disorders of the wrist. In: Wadsworth C, ed. *Orthopaedic Physical Therapy Home Study Course – The Elbow, Forearm, and Wrist*. La Crosse, WI: Orthopaedic Section, APTA, Inc., 1997.
10. Gray H: *Gray's Anatomy*. Philadelphia, PA: Lea & Febiger, 1995.
11. Wadsworth C: Wrist and hand. In: Wadsworth C, ed. *Current Concepts of Orthopedic Physical Therapy – Home Study Course*. La Crosse, WI: Orthopaedic Section, APTA, 2001.
12. Wackerle JF: A prospective study identifying the sensitivity of radiographic findings and the efficacy of clinical findings in carpal navicular fractures. *Ann Emerg Med* 16:733–737, 1987.
13. Watson HK, Ashmead D, Makhlouf MV: Examination of the scaphoid. *J Hand Surg Am* 13A:657–660, 1988.
14. Wolfe SW, Gupta A, Crisco JJ III: Kinematics of the scaphoid shift test. *J Hand Surg Am* 22A:801–806, 1997.
15. Taleisnik J: Scapholunate dissociation. In: Taleisnik J, ed. *The Wrist*. New York: Churchill Livingstone, 1985:239–278.
16. Helal B: Racquet player's pisiform. *Hand* 10:87, 1978.
17. Chase RA: Anatomy and kinesiology of the hand. In: Hunter DM, Mackin E, Callaghan M, eds. *Rehabilitation of the Hand*. St Louis, MO: Mosby, 1995.
18. Kaplan EB: Anatomy and kinesiology of the hand. In: Flynn JE, ed. *Hand Surgery*, 2nd ed. Baltimore, MD: Williams and Wilkins, 1975.
19. Sarrafian SK, Melamed JL, Goshgarian GM: Study of wrist motion in flexion and extension. *Clin Orthop Relat Res* 126:153–159, 1977.
20. Tylor C, Schwartz R: The anatomy and mechanics of the human hand. *Artif limbs* 2:49–62, 1955.
21. Napler JR: The prehensile movements of the human hand. *J Bone Joint Surg Br* 38B:902–913, 1956.
22. Freiberg A, Pollard BA, Macdonald MR, et al: Management of proximal interphalangeal joint injuries. *J Trauma* 46:523–528, 1999.
23. Tubiana R, Thomine J-M, Mackin E: *Examination of the Hand and Wrist*. London: Mosby, 1996.
24. Kuczymski K: The proximal interphalangeal joint: anatomy and causes of stiffness in the fingers. *J Bone Joint Surg Br* 50:656–663, 1968.
25. Eaton RG: *Joint Injuries in the Hand*. Springfield, IL: Charles C Thomas, 1971:15–32.
26. Burton RI, Eaton RG: Common hand injuries in the athlete. *Orthop Clin North Am* 4:809–838, 1973.
27. Bowers WH, Wolf JW Jr, Nehil JL, et al: The proximal interphalangeal joint volar plate. I. An anatomical and biochemical study. *J Hand Surg Am* 5:79–88, 1980.
28. Culver JE: Instabilities of the wrist. *Clin Sports Med* 5:725–740, 1986.
29. Taleisnik J: Classification of carpal instability. In: Taleisnik J, ed. *The Wrist*. New York: Churchill Livingstone, 1985:229–238.
30. Moore JS: De Quervain's tenosynovitis: Stenosing tenosynovits of the first posterior (dorsal) compartment. *J Occup Environ Med* 39:990–1002, 1997.
31. Zancolli E: *Structural and Dynamic Basis of Hand Surgery*, 3rd ed. Philadelphia, PA: JB Lippincott, 1979.
32. Brand PW, Hollister AM, Agee JM: Transmission. In: Brand PW, Hollister AM, eds. *Clinical Mechanics of the Hand*. St Louis, MO: Mosby Inc, 1999:61–99.
33. Holtzhausen L-M, Noakes TD: Elbow, forearm, wrist, and hand injuries among sport rock climbers. *Clin J Sports Med* 6:196–203, 1996.
34. Linburg RM, Conmstock BE: Anomalous tendon slips from the pollicis longus to the flexor digitorum profundus. *J Hand Surg Am* 4:79–83, 1979.
35. Rennie WRJ, Muller H: Linburg syndrome. *Can J Surg* 41:306–308, 1998.
36. Stuart PR: Pronator quadratus revisited. *J Hand Surg Br* 21:714–722, 1996.
37. Brand PW: *Clinical Mechanics of the Hand*. St. Louis: CV Mosby, 1985.
38. Ketchum LD, Thompson DE: An experimental investigation into the forces internal to the human hand. In: Brand PW, ed. *Clinical Mechanics of the Hand*. St. Louis, MO: CV Mosby, 1985.
39. Hollinshead WH: *Anatomy for Surgeons*, 2nd ed. New York: Harper & Row, 1969.
40. Bowers WH, Tribuzi SM: Functional Anatomy. In: Stanley BG, Tribuzi SM, eds. *Concepts in Hand Rehabilitation*. Philadelphia, PA: FA Davis, 1992:3–34.
41. Freedman DM, Botte MJ, Gelberman RH: Vascularity of the carpus. *Clin Orthop* 383:47–59, 2001.
42. Neumann DA: Wrist. In: Neumann DA, ed. *Kinesiology of the Musculoskeletal System: Foundations for Physical Rehabilitation*. St. Louis, MO: Mosby, 2002:172–193.
43. Carpener N: The hand in surgery. *J Bone Joint Surg Br* 38B:128, 1956.
44. Kapandji AI: *Physiologie Articulaire*. Paris: Librairie Maloine, 1963.
45. Bonnel F, Allieu Y: Les articulations radio cubito carpienne et medio carpienne: Organisation anatomique et bases biomechaniques. *Ann Chir Main* 3:287–296, 1984.
46. Palmer AK: The distal radioulnar joint. *Hand Clin* 3:31, 1987.
47. Kauer JMG: The interdependence of carpal articulation chains. *Acta Anat (Basel)* 88:481–501, 1974.
48. Kauer JMG: The mechanism of the carpal joint. *Clin Orthop Relat Res* 202:16–26, 1986.
49. de Lange A, Kauer JM, Huiskes R: Kinematic behavior of the human wrist joint: a roentgen-stereophotogrammetric analysis. *J Orthop Res* 3:56–64, 1985.
50. Patterson RM, Nicodemus CL, Viegas SF, et al: High-speed, three-dimensional kinematic analysis of the normal wrist. *J Hand Surg Am* 23:446–453, 1998.
51. Patterson RM, Nicodemus CL, Viegas SF, et al: Normal wrist kinematics and the analysis of the effect of various dynamic external fixators for treatment of distal radius fractures. *Hand Clin* 13:129–141, 1997.
52. Patterson R, Viegas SF: Biomechanics of the wrist. *J Hand Ther* 8:97–105, 1995.
53. Ritt MJ, Stuart PR, Berglund LJ, et al: Rotational stability of the carpus relative to the forearm. *J Hand Surg Am* 20:305–311, 1995.
54. Ruby LK, Cooney WP 3rd, An KN, et al: Relative motion of selected carpal bones: A kinematic analysis of the normal wrist. *J Hand Surg Am* 13:1–10, 1988.
55. Gilford WW, Bolton RH, Lambrinudi C: The mechanism of the wrist joint with special reference to fractures of the scaphoid. *Guys Hosp Rep* 92:52–59, 1943.
56. Linscheid RL, Dobyns JH, Beabout J: Traumatic instability of the wrist; Diagnosis, classification and pathomechanics. *J Bone Joint Surg Am* 54A:1612–1632, 1972.
57. Navarro A: Anatomia y fisiologie del carpo. *Ann Inst Clin Quir Chir Exp* 1:162–250, 1937.
58. Landsmeer JMF: Les coherences spatiales et l'equilibre spatial dans la region carpienne. *Acta Anat Suppl (Basel)* 70:1–84, 1968.
59. Landsmeer JMF: *Atlas of Anatomy of the Hand*. Edinburgh: Churchill Livingstone, 1976.
60. Kauer JMG: *Een analyse van de carpale flexie*, Thesis Leiden, 1964.
61. MacConnail MA, Basmajian JV: *Muscles and Movements: A Basis for Human Kinesiology*. New York: Robert Krieger Pub Co, 1977.
62. Kapandji IA: *The Physiology of the Joints, Upper Limb*. New York: Churchill Livingstone, 1991.
63. Brumfield RH, Champoux JA: A biomechanical study of normal functional wrist motion. *Clin Orthop Relat Res* 187:23–25, 1984.
64. Palmer AK, Werner FW, Murphy D, et al: Functional wrist motion: A biomechanical study. *J Hand Surg Am* 10A:39–46, 1985.
65. Nelson DL: Functional wrist motion. *Hand Clin* 13:83–92, 1997.
66. Hazelton FT, Smidt GL, Flatt AE, et al: The influence of wrist position on the force produced by the finger flexors. *J Biomech* 8:301–306, 1975.
67. Landsmeer JMF: The anatomy of the posterior (dorsal) aponeurosis of the human finger and its functional significance. *Anat Rec* 104:31–45, 1949.

68. Bendz P: Systematization of the grip of the hand in relation to finger motion systems. *Scand J Rehabil Med* 6:158–165, 1974.
69. Magee DJ: *Orthopedic Physical Assessment*, 2nd ed. Philadelphia, PA: W. B. Saunders Company, 1992.
70. Landsmeer JMF: Power grip and precision handling. *Ann Rheum Dis* 21:164–170, 1962.
71. Long C, Conrad DW, Hall EA: Intrinsic-extrinsic muscle control of the hand in power grip and precision handling. *J Bone Joint Surg Am* 52A:853–867, 1970.
72. Sollerman C, Sperling L: Evaluation of activities of daily living function – especially hand function. *Scand J Rehabil Med* 10:139–145, 1978.
73. Armstrong TJ: Ergonomics and cumulative trauma disorders. *Hand Clin* 2:553–565, 1986.
74. Kiser DM: Physiological and biomechanical factors for understanding repetitive motion injuries. *Semin Occup Med* 2:11–17, 1987.
75. Butler DS: *Mobilization of the Nervous Sysytem*. New York: Churchill Livingstone, 1992.
76. Keller K, Corbett J, Nichols D: Repetitive strain injury in computer keyboard users: pathomechanics and treatment principles in individual and group intervention. *J Hand Ther* 11:9–26, 1998.
77. Weber ER, Chao EY: An experimental approach to the mechanism of scaphoid waist fractures. *J Hand Surg Am* 3:142–153, 1978.
78. Walker MJ: Manual physical therapy examination and intervention of a patient with radial wrist pain: A case report. *J Orthop Sports Phys Ther* 34:761–769, 2004.
79. Muckart RD: Stenosing tendovaginitis of abductor pollicis brevis at the radial styloid (de Quervain's disease). *Clin Orthop* 33:201–208, 1964.
80. Skirven T: Clinical examination of the wrist. *J Hand Ther* 9:96–107, 1996.
81. Nalebuff EA: The rheumatoid swan-neck deformity. *Hand Clin* 5:215–214, 1989.
82. Leard JS, Breglio L, Fraga L, et al: Reliability and concurrent validity of the figure-of-eight method of measuring hand size in patients with hand pathology. *J Orthop Sports Phys Ther* 34:335–340, 2004.
83. Beach RB: Measurement of extremity volume by water displacement. *Phys Ther* 57:286–287, 1977.
84. Eberhardt K, Malcus Johnson P, Rydgren L: The occurrence and significance of hand deformities in early rheumatoid arthritis. *Br J Rheumatol* 30:211–213, 1991.
85. Luchetti R, Schoenhuber R, Alfarano M, et al: Serial overnight recordings of intracarpal canal pressure in carpal tunnel syndrome patients with and without wrist splinting. *J Hand Surg Br* 19:35–37, 1994.
86. Ono K, Ebara S, Fuji T, et al: Myelopathy hand. New clinical signs of cervical cord damage. *J Bone Joint Surg Br* 69:215–219, 1987.
87. Judge RD, Zuidema GD, Fitzgerald FT: General Appearance. In: Judge RD, Zuidema GD, Fitzgerald FT, eds. *Clinical Diagnosis*, 4th ed. Boston, MA: Little, Brown and Company, 1982:29–47.
88. Polivy KD, Millender LH, Newberg A, et al: Fractures of the hook of the hamate – a failure of clinical diagnosis. *J Hand Surg Am* 10A:101–104, 1985.
89. Whipple TL: Preoperative evaluation and imaging. In: Whipple TL, ed. *Athroscopic Surgery: The Wrist*. Philadelphia, PA: JB Lippincott, 1992:11–36.
90. Osterman AL, Mikulics M: Scaphoid nonunion. *Hand Clin* 14:437–455, 1988.
91. Alexander AH, Lichtman DM: Kienbock's disease. In: Lichtman DM, ed. *The Wrist and its Disorders*. Philadelphia, PA: WB Saunders, 1988.
92. Kienböck R: Concerning traumatic malacia of the lunate and its consequences: degeneration and compression fractures. *Clin Orthop Relat Res* 149:4–5, 1980.
93. Rao SB, Culver JE: Triquetralhamate arthrodesis for midcarpal instability. *J Hand Surg Am* 20A:583–589, 1995.
94. Horger MM: The reliability of goniometric measurements of active and passive wrist motions. *Am J Occup Ther* 44:342–348, 1990.
95. Nicholson B: Clinical Evaluation. In: Stanley BG, Tribuzi SM, eds. *Concepts in Hand Rehabilitation*. Philadelphia, PA: FA Davis, 1992:59–91.
96. Stokes HM: The seriously uninjured hand – weakness of grip. *J Occup Med* 25:683–684, 1983.
97. Thorngren KG, Werner CO: Normal grip strength. *Acta Orthop Scand* 50:255–259, 1979.
98. Mathiowetz V, Weber K, Volland G, et al: Reliability and validity of grip and pinch strength evaluations. *J Hand Surg Am* 9A:222–226, 1984.
99. Schreuders TA, Roebroeck ME, Goumans J, et al: Measurement error in grip and pinch force measurements in patients with hand injuries. *Phys Ther* 83:806–815, 2003.
100. Bechtol CO: Grip test: The use of a dynamometer with adjustable hand spacings. *J Bone Joint Surg Am* 36A:820–824, 1954.
101. Tredgett MW, Pimble LJ, Davis TRC: The detection of feigned hand weakness using the five position grip strength test. *J Hand Surg Br* 24B:426–428, 1999.
102. Tredgett MW, Davis TRC: Rapid repeat testing of grip strength for detection of faked hand weakness. *J Hand Surg Br* 25B:372–375, 2000.
103. Niebuhr BR, Marion R: Voluntary control of submaximal grip strength. *Am J Phys Med Rehabil* 69:96–101, 1990.
104. Lister G: *The hand: Diagnosis and Indications*, 2nd ed. New York: Churchill Livingstone, 1984.
105. Joughin K, Gulati P, Mackinnon SE, et al: An evaluation of rapid exchange and simultaneous grip tests. *J Hand Surg Am* 18A:245–252, 1993.
106. Hildreth DH, Breidenbach WC, Lister GD, et al: Detection of submaximal effort by use of the rapid exchange grip. *J Hand Surg Am* 14A:742–745, 1989.
107. Stokes HM, Landrieu KW, Domangue B, et al: Identification of low effort patients through dynamometry. *J Hand Surg Am* 20A:1047–1056, 1995.
108. Norkin C, Levangie P: *Joint Structure and Function: A Comprehensive Analysis*. Philadelphia, PA: F.A. Davis Company, 1992.
109. Blair SJ, McCormick E, Bear-Lehman J, et al: Evaluation of impairment of the upper extremity. *Clin Orthop* 221:42–58, 1987.
110. Fess EE: The need for reliability and validity in hand assessment instruments. *J Hand Surg Am* 11A:621–623, 1986.
111. Jebsen RH, Taylor N, Triegchmann R, et al: An objective and standardized test for hand function. *Arch Phys Med Rehabil* 50:311, 1969.
112. Beckenbaugh RD, Shives TC, Dobyns JH, et al: Kienböck's disease : The natural history of Kienböck's disease and consideration of lunate fractures. *Clin Orthop* 149:98–106, 1980.
113. *Purdue Pegboard Test of Manipulative Dexterity*. Chicago, IL: Service Research Associates, 1968.
114. Tiffin J, Asker E: The Purdue pegboard: Norms and studies of reliability and validity. *J Appl Psychol* 32:324, 1948.
115. Crawford J: *Crawford Small Parts Dexterity Test (CSPDT), Psychological Corp (catalog): Tests, Products and Services for Business, Industry, and Government*. Cleveland, OH: Harcourt Brace Jovanovich, 1985:32.
116. Hoppenfeld S: *Physical Examination of the Spine and Extremities*. East Norwalk, CT: Appleton-Century-Crofts, 1976.
117. Swanson A: Disabling arthritis at the base of the thumb: Treatment by resection of the trapezium and flexible implant arthroplasty. *J Bone Joint Surg Am* 54A:456, 1972.
118. Beckenbaugh RD: Accurate evaluation and management of the painful wrist following injury. *Orthop Clin North Am* 15:289–306, 1984.
119. Lester B, Halbrecht J, Levy IM, et al: "Press test" for office diagnosis of triangular fibrocartilage complex tears of the wrist. *Ann Plast Surg* 35:41–45, 1995.
120. Buterbaugh GA, Brown TR, Horn PC: Ulnar-sided wrist pain in athletes. *Clin Sports Med* 17:567–583, 1998.
121. Finkelstein H: Stenosing tenovaginitis at the radial styloid process. *J Bone Joint Surg Am* 12A:509, 1930.
122. Elliot BG: Finkelstein's test; a descriptive error that can produce a false positive. *J Hand Surg Am* 17B:481–482, 1992.
123. Arons MS: De Quervain's release in working women: report of failures, complications, and associated diagnoses. *J Hand Surg Am* 12:540–544, 1987.
124. Belsole J: De Quervain's tenosynovitis diagnostic and operative complications. *Orthopedics* 12A:899, 1981.
125. Saplys R, Mackinnon SE, Dellon LA: The relationship between nerve entrapment versus neuroma complications and the misdiagnosis of de Quervain's disease. *Contemp Orthop* 15:51, 1987.
126. Williams JG: Surgical management of traumatic noninfective tenosynovitis of the wrist extensors. *J Bone Joint Surg Br* 59B:408, 1977.
127. Louis DS: Incomplete release of the forst posterior (dorsal) compartment – a diagnostic test. *J Hand Surg Am* 12A:87, 1987.
128. Alexander RD, Catalano LW, Barron OA, et al: The extensor pollicis brevis entrapment test in the treatment of de Quervain's disease. *J Hand Surg Am* 27:813–816, 2002.
129. Elson RA: Rupture of the central slip of the extensor hood of the finger: a test for early diagnosis. *J Bone Joint Surg Br* 68:229–231, 1986.
130. LaStayo P, Howell J: Clinical provocative tests used in evaluating wrist pain: A descriptive study. *J Hand Ther* 8:10–17, 1995.
131. Onieal M-E: *The hand: Examination and diagnosis, American Society for Surgery of the Hand*, 3rd ed. New York: Churchill Livingstone, 1990.

132. Easterling KJ, Wolfe SW: Scaphoid shift in the uninjured wrist. *J Hand Surg Am* 19A:604–606, 1994.
133. Lane LB: The scaphoid shift test. *J Hand Surg Am* 18:366–368, 1993.
134. Heyman P, Gelberman RH, Duncan K, et al: Injuries of the ulnar collateral ligament of the thumb metacarpophalangeal joint. Biomechanical and prospective clinical studies on the usefulness of valgus stress testing. *Clin Orthop Relat Res* 292: 165–171, 1993.
135. Booher JM, Thibodeau GA: *Athletic Injury Assessment*. St Louis, MO: CV Mosby, 1989.
136. Werner CO, Elmqvist D, Ohlin P: Pressure and nerve lesion in the carpal tunnel. *Acta Orthop Scand* 54:312–316, 1983.
137. Stewart JD, Eisen A: Tinel's sign and the carpal tunnel syndrome. *BMJ* 2:1125–1126, 1978.
138. Gellman H, Gelberman RH, Tan AM, et al: Carpal tunnel syndrome. An evaluation of the provocative diagnostic tests. *J Bone Joint Surg Am* 68A:735–737, 1986.
139. Marx RG, Hudak PL, Bombardier C, et al: The reliability of physical examination for carpal tunnel syndrome. *J hand Surg Br* 23B:499–502, 1998.
140. Golding DN, Rose DM, Selvarajah K: Clinical tests for carpal tunnel syndrome: an evaluation. *Br J Rheum* 25:388–390, 1986.
141. Heller L, Ring H, Costeff H, et al: Evaluation of Tinel's and Phalen's signs in diagnosis of the carpal tunnel syndrome. *Eur Neurol* 25:40–42, 1986.
142. Gerr F, Letz R: The sensitivity and specificity of tests for carpal tunnel syndrome vary with the comparison subjects. *J Hand Surg Br* 23:151–155, 1998.
143. Kuhlman KA, Hennessey WJ: Sensitivity and specificity of carpal tunnel syndrome signs. *Am J Phys Med Rehabil* 76:451–457, 1997.
144. Phalen GS: The carpal tunnel syndrome: Clinical evaluation of 598 hands. *Clin Orthop* 83:29–40, 1972.
145. Phalen GS: Spontaneous compression of the median nerve at the wrist. *JAMA* 145:1128–1133, 1951.
146. Onieal M-E: *Essentials of Musculoskeletal care*, 1st ed. Rosemont, IL: American Academy of Orthopaedic Surgeons, 1997.
147. Katz JN, Larson MG, Sabra A, et al: The carpal tunnel syndrome: diagnostic utility of the history and physical examination findings. *Ann Intern Med* 112:321–327, 1990.
148. de Krom MC, Knipschild PG, Kester AD, et al: Efficacy of provocative tests for diagnosis of carpal tunnel syndrome. *Lancet* 335:393–395, 1990.
149. Werner RA, Bir C, Armstrong TJ: Reverse Phalen's maneuver as an aid in diagnosing carpal tunnel syndrome. *Arch Phys Med Rehabil* 75:783–786, 1994.
150. Brain WR, Wright AD, Wilkinson M: Spontaneous compression of both median nerves in the carpal tunnel: Six cases treated surgically. *Lancet* 1:277–282, 1947.
151. Duck-Sun A: Hand elevation: A new test for carpal tunnel syndrome. *Ann Plast Surg* 46:120–124, 2001.
152. Ahn DS: Hand elevation: A new test for carpal tunnel syndrome. *Ann Plast Surg* 46:120–124, 2001.
153. Tetro AM, Evanoff BA, Hollstien SB, et al: A new provocative test for carpal tunnel syndrome. Assessment of wrist flexion and nerve compression. *J Bone Joint Surg Br* 80:493–498, 1998.
154. Williams TM, Mackinnon SE, Novak CB, et al: Verification of the pressure provocative test in carpal tunnel syndrome. *Ann Plast Surg* 29:8–11, 1992.
155. Moberg E: Objective methods for determining the functional value of sensibility in the hand. *J Bone Joint Surg Br* 40A:454–476, 1958.
156. Omer GE: Report of committee for evaluation of the clinical result in peripheral nerve injury. *J Hand Surg* 8:754–759, 1983.
157. Buch-Jaeger N, Foucher G: Correlation of clinical signs with nerve conduction tests in the diagnosis of carpal tunnel syndrome. *J Hand Surg Br* 19:720–724, 1994.
158. Preston D, Shapiro B: *Electromyography and Neuromuscular Disorders. Clinical Electrophysiologic Correlations*. Boston, MA: Butterworth-Heinemann, 1998.
159. Katz JN, Stirrat CR: A self-administered hand diagram for the diagnosis of carpal tunnel syndrome. *J Hand Surg Am* 15:360–363, 1990.
160. Wazir NN, Kareem BA: New clinical sign of cervical myelopathy: Wazir hand myelopathy sign. *Singapore Med J* 52:47–49, 2011.
161. Tubiana R, Thomine J-M, Mackin E: Examination of the peripheral nerve function in the upper limb. In: Tubiana R, Thomine J-M, Mackin E, eds. *Examination of the Hand and Wrist*. London: Mosby, 1996:261–369.
162. Booth FW: Physiologic and biochemical effects of immobilization on muscle. *Clin Orthop Relat Res* 219:15–21, 1987.
163. Eiff MP, Smith AT, Smith GE: Early mobilization versus immobilization in the treatment of lateral ankle sprains. *Am J Sports Med* 22:83–88, 1994.
164. Akeson WH, Amiel D, Mechanic GL, et al: Collagen cross-linking alterations in the joint contractures: changes in the reducible cross-links in periarticular connective tissue after 9 weeks immobilization. *Connect Tissue Res* 5:15, 1977.
165. Akeson WH, Amiel D, Abel MF, et al: Effects of immobilization on joints. *Clin Orthop* 219:28–37, 1987.
166. Akeson WH, Amiel D, Woo SL-Y: Immobility effects on synovial joints: The pathomechanics of joint contracture. *Biorheology* 17:95–110, 1980.
167. Woo SL-Y, Matthews J, Akeson WH, et al: Connective tissue response to immobility: A correlative study of biochemical and biomechanical measurements of normal and immobilized rabbit knee. *Arthritis Rheum* 18:257–264, 1975.
168. Walsh M, Muntzer E: Wound Management. In: Stanley BG, Tribuzi SM, eds. *Concepts in Hand Rehabilitation*. Philadelphia, PA: FA Davis, 1992:153–177.
169. Stanley BG: Therapeutic exercise: maintaining and restoring mobility in the hand. In: Stanley BG, Tribuzi SM, eds. *Concepts in Hand Rehabilitation*. Philadelphia, PA: FA Davis, 1992:178–215.
170. Fess EE, Phillips CA: *Hand Splinting: Principles and Methods*, 2nd ed. St Louis, MO: CV Mosby, 1987.
171. Malick MH: *Manual on static hand splinting*. Pittsburgh: Harmarville Rehabilitation Center, 1972.
172. Lohman H, Schultz-Johnson K, Coppard BM: *Introduction to Splinting: A Clinical-Reasoning & Problem-Solving Approach*. St Louis, MO: Mosby, Inc, 2001.
173. Cannon NM: *Manual of Hand Splinting*. New York: Churchill Livingstone, 1985.
174. Gribben MG: Splinting principles for hand injuries. In: Moran CA, ed. *Hand Rehabilitation: Clinics in Physical Therapy*. New York: Churchill Livingstone, 1986:166.
175. Schultz-Johnson K: Splinting – A problem-solving approach. In: Stanley BG, Tribuzi SM, eds. *Concepts in Hand Rehabilitation*. Philadelphia, PA: FA Davis, 1992:238–271.
176. Stanley JK: Soft tissue surgery in rheumatoid arthritis of the hand. *Clin Orthop Relat Res* 366:78–90, 1999.
177. Brewerton DA: The rheumatoid hand. *Proc R Soc Med* 59:225–228, 1966.
178. Wynn-Parry CB, Stanley JK: Synovectomy of the hand. *Br J Rheumatol* 32:1089–1095, 1993.
179. Flatt AE: Some pathomechanics of ulnar drift. *Plast Reconstr Surg* 37:295–303, 1966.
180. Shapiro JS: The etiology of ulnar drift: A new factor. *J Bone Joint Surg* 50A:634, 1968.
181. Ferlic DC: Boutonniere deformities in rheumatoid arthritis. *Hand Clin* 5:215–222, 1989.
182. Kiefhaber TR, Strickland JW: Soft tissue reconstruction for rheumatoid swan-neck and boutonniere deformities: Long-term results. *J Hand Surg Am* 18A:984–989, 1993.
183. Hastings DE, Evans JA: Rheumatoid wrist deformities and their relation to ulnar drift. *J Bone Joint Surg Am* 57A:930–934, 1975.
184. Pahle J: Die Synovektomie der Proximalen Interphalangealgelenke. *Orthopaede* 2:13–17, 1973.
185. Pahle JA, Raunio P: The influence of wrist position on finger deviation in the rheumatoid hand. *J Bone Joint Surg Br* 51B:664, 1969.
186. Stack GH, Vaughan-Jackson OJ: The zig-zag deformity in the rheumatoid hand. *Hand* 3:62–67, 1971.
187. Marx H: Rheumatoid arthritis. In: Stanley BG, Tribuzi SM, eds. *Concepts in Hand Rehabilitation*. Philadelphia, PA: FA Davis, 1992:395–418.
188. van Vugt RM, Bijlsma JWJ, van Vugt AC: Chronic wrist pain: diagnosis and management. Development and use of a new algorithm. *Ann Rheum Dis* 58:665–674, 1999.
189. Taleisnik J: Pain on the ulnar side of the wrist. *Hand Clin* 3:51–68, 1987.
190. Watson HK, Brenner LH: Degenerative disorders of the wrist. *J Hand Surg Am* 10A:1002–1006, 1985.
191. McFarlane RM, Albion U: Dupuytren's disease. In: Hunter JM, Schneider LH, Mackin EJ, et al, eds. *Rehabilitation of the Hand*, 3rd ed. St. Louis, MO: CV Mosby, 1990:867.
192. Sladicka MS, Benfanti P, Raab M, et al: Dupuytren's contracture in the black population: A case report and review of the literature. *J Hand Surg Br* 21:898, 1996.
193. Urban M, Feldberg L, Janssen A, et al: Dupuytren's disease in children. *J Hand Surg Br* 21:112, 1996.
194. Ross DC: Epidemiology of Dupuytren's disease. *Hand Clin* 15:53, 1999.

195. Saar JD, Grothaus PC: Dupuytren's Disease: An Overview. *Plast Reconstr Surg* 106:125–136, 2000.
196. Noble J, Arafa M, Royle SG, et al: The association between alcohol, hepatic pathology and Dupuytren's disease. *J Hand Surg Br* 17:71, 1992.
197. Yi IS, Johnson G, Moneim MS: Etiology of Dupuytren's disease. *Hand Clin* 15, 1999.
198. Lanzetta M, Morrison WA: Dupuytren's disease occurring after a surgical injury to the hand. *J Hand Surg Br* 21:481, 1996.
199. Hill NA, Hurst LC: Dupuytren's contracture. In: Doyle JR, ed. *Landmark Advances in Hand Surgery. Hand Clinics*. Philadelphia, PA: WB Saunders, 1989:349.
200. Luck JV: Dupuytren's contracture: A new concept of the pathogenesis correlated with surgical management. *J Bone Joint Surg Am* 41:635, 1959.
201. Rayan GM: Clinical presentation and types of Dupuytren's disease. *Hand Clin* 15:87, 1999.
202. Strickland JW, Leibovic SJ: Anatomy and pathogenesis of the digital cords and nodules. *Hand Clin* 7:645, 1991.
203. Tomasek JJ, Vaughan MB, Haaksma CJ: Cellular structure and biology of Dupuytren's disease. *Hand Clin* 15:21, 1999.
204. Hurst LC, Badalamente MA: Nonoperative treatment of Dupuytren's disease. *Hand Clin* 15:97, 1999.
205. Eckhaus D: Dupuytren's disease. In: Clark GL, Aiello B, Eckhaus D, et al, eds. *Hand Rehabilitation*. Edinburgh: Churchill Livingstone, 1993:37–42.
206. Gosset J: Dupuytren's disease and the anatomy of the palmodigital aponeuroses. In: Hueston JT, Tubiana R, eds. *Dupuytren's Disease*. Edinburgh: Churchill Livingstone, 1985.
207. Onieal M-E: Common wrist and ankle injuries. *Adv Nurse Pract* 4:31–36, 1996.
208. Chin HW, Visotsky J: Wrist fractures in the hand in emergency medicine. *Emerg Med Clin North Am* 11:703–735, 1993.
209. Mayfield JK, Johnson RP, Kilcoyne RK: Carpal dislocations: Pathomechanics and progressive perilunar instability. *J Hand Surg Am* 5:226–241, 1980.
210. Takase K, Imakiire A: Lunate excision, capitate osteotomy, and intercarpal arthrodesis for advanced Kienbock disease. Long-term follow-up. *J Bone Joint Surg Am* 83-A:177–183, 2001.
211. Ambrose L, Posner MA: Lunate-triquetral and midcarpal joint instability. *Hand Clin* 8:653–668, 1992.
212. Husband JB, McPherson SA: Bony skier's thumb injuries. *Clin Orthop Rel Res* 327:79–84, 1996.
213. Rettig AC: Current concepts in management of football injuries of the hand and wrist. *J Hand Ther* 4:42–50, 1991.
214. Stener B: Displacement of the ruptured ulnar collateral ligament of the metacarpophalangeal joint of the thumb. *J Bone Joint Surg Br* 44B:869–879, 1962.
215. Friedman SL, Palmer AK: The ulnar impaction syndrome. *Hand Clin* 7:295–310, 1991.
216. Kasdan ML, Millender LH: Occupational soft-tissue and tendon disorders. *Orthop Clinic North Am* 27:795–803, 1996.
217. Thorson E, Szabo RM: Common tendinitis problems in the hand and forearm. *Orthop Clin North Am* 23:65–74, 1992.
218. de Quervain F: Uber eine Form von chronischer Tendovaginitis. *Cor-Bl f schweiz Aertze* 25:389–394, 1895.
219. Lapidus PW, Fenton R: Stenosing tenovaginitis at the wrist and fingers: Report of 423 cases in 269 patients. *Arch Surg* 64:475–487, 1952.
220. Clarke MT, Lyall HA, Grant JW, et al: The histopathology of de Quervain's disease. *J Hand Surg Br* 23:732–734, 1998.
221. Patterson DC: DeQuervain's disease: stenosing tendovaginitis at the radial styloid. *N Engl J Med* 214:101–102, 1936.
222. Cotton FJ, Morrison GM, Bradford CH: DeQuervain's disease: Radial styloid tendovaginitis. *N Engl J Med* 219:120–123, 1938.
223. Diack AW, Trommald JP: DeQuervain's disease: A frequently missed diagnosis. *West J Surg* 47:629–633, 1939.
224. Wood CF: Stenosing tendovaginitis at the radial styloid. *South Surg* 10:105–110, 1941.
225. Lamphier TA, Crooker C, Crooker JL: DeQuervain's disease. *Ind Med Surg* 34:847–856, 1965.
226. Lamb DW, Hooper G, Kuczynski K: *Practice of Hand Surgery*. London: Blackwell Scientific Publications Ltd., 1989.
227. Reid DAC, McGrouther DA: *Surgery of the Thumb*. London: Butterworth & Co. Ltd, 1986.
228. Piligian G, Herbert R, Hearns M, et al: Evaluation and management of chronic work-related musculoskeltal disorders of the distal upper extremity. *Am J Ind Med* 37:75–93, 2000.
229. Harrington JM, Carter JT, Birrell L, et al: Surveillance case definitions for work related upper limb pain syndrome. *Occup Environ Med* 55:264–271, 1998.
230. Anderson M, Tichenor CJ: A patient with de Quervain's tenosynovitis: A case report using an Australian approach to manual therapy. *Phys Ther* 74:314–326, 1994.
231. Lane LB, Boretz RS, Stuchin SA: Treatment of de Quervain's disease: Role of conservative management. *J Hand Surg Br* 26:258–260, 2001.
232. Weiss AP, Akelman E, Tabatabai M: Treatment of de Quervain's disease. *J Hand Surg Am* 19:595–598, 1994.
233. Backstrom KM: Mobilization with movement as an adjunct intervention in a patient with complicated de Quervain's tenosynovitis: A case report. *J Orthop Sports Phys Ther* 32:86–94; discussion 94–97, 2002.
234. Grundberg AB, Reagan DS: Pathologic anatomy of the forearm: Intersection syndrome. *J Hand Surg Am* 10A:299, 1985.
235. Hunter SC, Poole RM: The chronically inflamed tendon. *Clin Sports Med* 6:371, 1987.
236. Mogensen BA, Mattson HS: Stenosing tenovaginitis of the third compartment of the hand. *Scand J Plast Reconstr Surg* 14:127, 1980.
237. Spinner M, Olshansky K: The extensor indicis proprius syndrome. *Plast Reconstr Surg* 51:134, 1973.
238. Hajj AA, Wood MB: Stenosing tenosynovitis of the extensor carpi ulnaris. *J Hand Surg Am* 11A:519, 1986.
239. Hueston JT, Wilson WF: The aetiology of trigger finger. *Hand* 4:257, 1972.
240. Kolind-Sorensen V: Treatment of trigger fingers. *Acta Orthop Scand* 41:428–432, 1970.
241. Lipscomb PR: Tenosynovitis of the hand and wrist: Carpal tunnel syndrome, de Quervain's disease, trigger digit. *Ann Surg* 134:110, 1951.
242. Nasca RJ: "Trigger finger." A common hand problem. *J Ark Med Soc* 76:388–390, 1980.
243. Medl WT: Tendonitis, tenosynovitis, "Trigger finger," and Quervain's disease. *Orthop Clin North Am* 1:375–382, 1970.
244. Pulvertaft RG: *Clinical Surgery of the Hand*. London: Butterworths, 1966.
245. Evans BE, Hunter JM, Burkhalter WE: Conservative management of the trigger finger: A new approach. *J Hand Ther* 1:59–68, 1988.
246. Newport ML, Lane LB, Stuchin SA: Treatment of the trigger finger by steroid injection. *J Hand Surg Am* 15A:748, 1990.
247. Ertel AN, Millender LH, Nalebuff E: Flexor tendon ruptures in patients with rheumatoid arthritis. *J Hand Surg Am* 13A:860–866, 1988.
248. Mannerfelt L, Norman O: Attrition rupture of flexor tendons in rheumatoid arthritis caused by bony spurs in the carpal tunnel. A clinical and radiological study. *J Bone Joint Surg Br* 51B:270–277, 1969.
249. Silfverskiold KL, May EJ, Tornvall AH: Gap formation during controlled motion after flexor tendon repair in zone II: A prospective clinical study. *J Hand Surg Am* 17:539, 1992.
250. Silfverskiold KL, May EJ: Flexor tendon repair in zone II with a new suture technique and early program combining passive and active flexion. *J Hand Surg Am* 19:53, 1994.
251. Tang JB, Shi D, Gu YQ, et al: Double and multiple looped suture tendon repair. *J Hand Surg Br* 19:699, 1994.
252. Robertson GA, Al-Qattan MM: A biomechanical analysis of a new interlock suture technique for flexor tendon repair. *J Hand Surg Br* 17:92, 1992.
253. McLarney E, Hoffman H, Wolfe SW: Biomechanical analysis of the cruciate four-strand flexor tendon repair. *J Hand Surg Am* 24:295, 1999.
254. Ejeskar A: Flexor tendon repair in no-man's-land: Results of primary repair with controlled mobilization. *J Hand Surg Am* 9:171, 1984.
255. Strickland JW, Glogovac SV: Digital function following flexor tendon repair in zone II: A comparison of immobilization and controlled passive motion techniques. *J Hand Surg Am* 5:537, 1980.
256. Chow JA, Thomes LJ, Dovelle S, et al: A combined regimen of controlled motion following flexor tendon repair in "no man's land.". *Plast Reconstr Surg* 9:447–455, 1987.
257. Cullen KW, Tohurst P, Lang D, et al: Flexor tendon repair in zone 2 followed by controlled active mobilisation. *J Hand Surg Br* 14B:392–395, 1989.
258. Elliot D, Moiemen NS, Flemming AFS, et al: The rupture rate of acute flexor tendon repairs mobilized by the controlled active motion regimen. *J Hand Surg Br* 19B:607–612, 1994.
259. Lister GD, Kleinert HE, Kutz JE, et al: Primary flexor tendon repair followed by immediate controlled mobilization. *J Hand Surg Am* 2:441–451, 1977.

260. Tang JB, Shi D: Subdivision of flexor tendon "no man's land" and different treatment methods in each subzone. *Clin Med J* 105:60–69, 1992.
261. Stewart KM: Review and comparison of current trends in the postoperative management of tendon repair. *Hand Clin* 7:447–460, 1991.
262. Green JB, Ranger HE, Draghetti JG, et al: Hand, wrist, and digit injuries. In: Magee DJ, Zachazewski JE, Quillen WS, eds. *Pathology and Intervention in Musculoskeletal Rehabilitation.* St. Louis, MI: Saunders, 2009:213–305.
263. Kleinert HE, Kutz JE, Atasoy E, et al: Primary repair of flexor tendons. *Orthop Clin North Am* 4:865–876, 1973.
264. Duran RJ, Houser RG: *Controlled Passive Motion Following Flexor Tendon Repair in Zones 2 and 3, American Academy of Orthopaedic Surgeons: Symposium on Flexor Tendon Surgery in the Hand.* St Louis: CV Mosby, 1975.
265. Taras JS, Skahen JR, James R, et al: The double-grasping and cross-stitch for acute flexor tendon repair: Applications with active motion. *Atlas Hand Clin* 1:13–28, 1996.
266. Aoki M, Kubota H, Pruitt DL, et al: Biomechancial and histological characteristics of canine flexor tendon repair using early postoperative mobilization. *J Hand Surg Am* 22A:107–114, 1997.
267. Panchal J, Mehdi S, Donoghue JO: The range of excursion of flexor tendons in zone V: A comparison of active vs passive flexor mobilization regimes. *Br J Plast Surg* 50:517–522, 1997.
268. Small JO, Bernnen MD, Colville J: Early active mobilisation following flexor tendon repair in zone 2. *J Hand Surg Br* 14:383–391, 1989.
269. Ingari JV, Pederson WC: Update on tendon repair. *Clin Plast Surg* 24:161, 1997.
270. Gelberman RH, Siedel DB, Woo SL-Y: Healing of digital flexor tendons: Importance of the interval from injury to repair. A biomechanical, biochemical, and morphological study in dogs. *J Bone Joint Surg Am* 73A:66–75, 1991.
271. Hitchcock TF, Light TR, Bunch WH, et al: The effect of immediate constrained digital motion on the strength of flexor tendon repairs in chickens. *J Hand Surg Am* 12A:590–595, 1987.
272. Kubota H, Manske PR, Aoki M, et al: Effect of motion and tension on injured flexor tendons in chickens. *J Hand Surg Am* 21A:456–463, 1996.
273. Lubahn JD, Hood JM: Fractures of the distal interphalangeal joint. *Clin Orthop Relat Res* 327:12–20, 1996.
274. Weinstein SM: Nerve problems and compartment syndromes in the hand. *Clin Sports Med* 11:161–188, 1992.
275. Carr D, Davis P: Distal posterior interosseous nerve syndrome. *J Hand Surg Am* 10:873–878, 1985.
276. Rask MR: Superficial radial neuritis and de Quervain's disease. *Clin Orthop* 131:176–178, 1979.
277. MacKinnon EJ, Dellon AL: *Surgery of the peripheral nerve.* New York: Thieme Medical Publishers Inc, 1988.
278. Moersch FP: Median thenar neuritis. *Proc Surg Meet Mayo Clin* 13:220–222, 1938.
279. Slater RR Jr, Bynum DK: Diagnosis and treatment of carpal tunnel syndrome. *Orthop Rev* 22:1095–1105, 1993.
280. Gates SJ, Mooar PA: *Orthopaedics and Sports Medicine for Nurses: Common Problems in Management.* Baltimore, MD: Williams & Wilkins, 1999.
281. Flynn JM, Bischoff R, Gelberman RH: Median nerve compression at the wrist due to intracarpal canal sepsis. *J Hand Surg Am* 20A:864–867, 1995.
282. Gerardi JA, Mack GR, Lutz RB: Acute carpal tunnel syndrome secondary to septic arthritis of the wrist. *J Am Osteopath Assoc* 89:933–934, 1989.
283. Ogilvie C, Kay NRM: Fulminating carpal tunnel syndrome due to gout. *J Hand Surg Br* 13:42–43, 1988.
284. Rosenbaum R: Disputed radial tunnel syndrome. *Muscle Nerve* 22:960–967, 1999.
285. Center for Disease Control: Occupational diseases surveillance: Carpal tunnel syndrome. *JAMA* 77:889, 1989.
286. Rempel DM, Harrison RJ, Barnhart S: Work-related cumulative trauma disorders of the upper extremity. *JAMA* 267:838–842, 1992.
287. Rowe L: The diagnosis of tendon and tendon sheath injuries. *Semin Occup Med* 1:1–6, 1987.
288. Robbins H: Anatomical study of the median nerve in the carpal canal and etiologies of the carpal tunnel syndrome. *J Bone Joint Surg Am* 45:953–956, 1963.
289. Bauman TD, Gelberman RH, Mubarak SJ, et al: The acute carpal tunnel syndrome. *Clin Orthop* 156:151–156, 1981.
290. Paley D, McMurtry RY: Median nerve compression by volarly displaced fragments of the distal radius. *Clin Orthop* 215:139–147, 1987.
291. Gelberman R, Szabo RM, Williamson RV, et al: Tissue pressure threshold for peripheral nerve viability. *Clin Orthop* 178:285–291, 1983.
292. Barnes CG, Curry HLE: Carpal tunnel syndrome in rheumatoid arthritis: A clinical and electrodiagnostic survey. *Ann Rheum Dis* 26:226–233, 1970.
293. Stanley JK: Conservative surgery in the management of rheumatoid disease of the hand and wrist. *J Hand Surg Am* 17B:339–342, 1992.
294. Vainio K: Carpal canal syndrome caused by tenosynovitis. *Acta Rheumatol Scand* 4:22–27, 1957.
295. Gelberman RH: Carpal tunnel syndrome. In: Gelberman RH, ed. *Operative Nerve Repair.* Philadelphia, PA: JB Lippincott, 1991:939–948.
296. Von Schroeder HP, Botte MJ: Carpal tunnel syndrome. *Hand Clin* 12:643–655, 1996.
297. Cobb TK, An K, Cooney WP, et al: Lumbrical muscle incursion into the carpal tunnel during finger flexion. *J Hand Surg Br* 19B:434–438, 1994.
298. Yii NW, Elliot D: A study of the dynamic relationship of the lumbrical muscles and the carpal tunnel. *J Hand Surg Br* 19B:439–443, 1994.
299. Robinson D, Aghasi M, Halperin N: The treatment of carpal tunnel syndrome caused by hypertrophied lumbrical muscles. *Scand J Plast Reconstr Surg* 23:149–151, 1989.
300. DeKrom MC, Knipschild PG, Kester AD, et al: Carpal tunnel syndrome: prevalence in the general population. *J Clin Epidemiol* 45:373–376, 1992.
301. Stevens JC, Sun S, Beard CM, et al: Carpal tunnel syndrome in Rochester, Minnesota, 1961–1980. *Neurology* 38:134–138, 1988.
302. Szabo RM, Chidgey LK: Stress carpal tunnel pressures in patients with carpal tunnel syndrome and normal patients. *J Hand Surg Am* 14A:624–627, 1989.
303. Keir PJ, Bach JM, Rempel DM: Effects of finger posture on carpal tunnel pressure during wrist motion. *J Hand Surg Am* 23A:1004–1009, 1998.
304. Rempel D, Keir PJ, Smutz WP, et al: Effects of static fingertip loading on carpal tunnel pressure. *J Orthop Res* 15:422–426, 1997.
305. D'Arcy CA, McGee S: Does this patient have carpal tunnel syndrome? *JAMA* 283:3110–3117, 2000.
306. Feuerstein M, Burrell LM, Miller VI, et al: Clinical management of carpal tunnel syndrome: A 12 year review of outcomes. *Am J Ind Med* 35:232–245, 1999.
307. Szabo RM: Carpal tunnel syndrome-general. In: Gelberman RH, ed. *Operative Nerve Repair and Reconstruction.* Philadelphia, PA: J. B. Lippincott, 1991:882–883.
308. Bowles AP Jr, Asher SW, Pickett JB: Use of Tinel's sign in carpal tunnel syndrome [letter]. *Ann Neurol* 13:689–690, 1983.
309. Hartz CR, Linscheid RL, Gramse RR, et al: The pronator teres syndrome: Compressive neuropathy of the median nerve. *J Bone Joint Surg Am* 63:885–890, 1981.
310. Anto C, Aradhya P: Clinical diagnosis of peripheral nerve compression in the upper extremities. *Orthop Clin North Am* 27:227–245, 1996.
311. Cambell WW: diagnosis and management of common compression and entrapment neuropathies. *Neurol Clin* 15:549–567, 1997.
312. Loong SC: The carpal tunnel syndrome: a clinical and electrophysiological study of 250 patients. *Proc Aust Assoc Neurol* 14:51–65, 1977.
313. Lee MJ, LaStayo PC: Pronator syndrome and other nerve compressions that mimic carpal tunnel syndrome. *J Orthop Sports Phys Ther* 34:601–609, 2004.
314. Kenneally M, Rubenach H, Elvey R: The upper limb tension test: the SLR of the arm. In: Grant R, ed. *Physical Therapy of the Cervical and Thoracic Spine.* New York: Churchill Livingstone, 1988.
315. Kleinrensink GJ, Stoeckart R, Vleeming A, et al: Mechanical tension in the median nerve. The effects of joint positions. *Clin Biomech* 10:240–244, 1995.
316. Manente G, Torrieri F, Pineto F, et al: A relief maneuver in carpal tunnel syndrome. *Muscle Nerve* 22:1587–1589, 1999.
317. Chang MH, Chiang HT, Lee SSJ, et al: Oral drug of choice in carpal tunnel syndrome. *Neurology* 51:390–393, 1998.
318. Roaf R: Compression of median nerve in carpal tunnel [letter to the editor]. *Lancet* 1:387, 1947.
319. Sailer SM: The role of splinting and rehabilitation in the treatment of carpal and cubital tunnel syndromes. *Hand Clin* 12:223–241, 1996.
320. Burke DT, Burke MM, Stewart GW, et al: Splinting for carpal tunnel syndrome: In search of the optimal angle. *Arch Phys Med Rehabil* 75:1241–1244, 1994.
321. Kruger VL, Kraft GH, Deitz JC, et al: Carpal tunnel syndrome: Objective measures and splint use. *Arch Phys Med Rehabil* 72:517–520, 1991.
322. Dolhanty D: Effectiveness of splinting for carpal tunnel syndrome. *Can J Occup Ther* 53:275–280, 1986.

323. Rempel D, Manojlovik R, Levinsohn DG, et al: The effect of wearing a flexible wrist splint on carpal tunnel pressure during repetitive hand activity. *J Hand Surg Am* 19:106–110, 1994.
324. Callinan NJ, Mathiowetz V: Soft versus hard resting hand splints in rheumatoid arthritis: pain relief, preference and compliance. *Am J Occup Ther* 50:347–353, 1995.
325. Garfinkel MS, Singhal A, Katz WA, et al: Yoga-based intervention for carpal tunnel syndrome: a randomized trial. *JAMA* 280:1601–1603, 1998.
326. Chidgey LK: Chronic wrist pain. *Orthop Clin North Am* 23:49–64, 1992.
327. Pelmear P, Wills M: Impact vibration and hand-arm vibration syndrome. *J Occup Environ Med* 39:1092–1096, 1997.
328. Miller RF, Lohman WH, Maldonado G, et al: An epidemiologic study of carpal tunnel syndrome and hard-arm vibration in relation to vibration syndrome. *J Hand Surg Am* 19A:99–105, 1994.
329. Pelmear P: Vibration-related occupational injuries. In: Herrington TN, Morse LH, eds. *Occupational Injuries – Evaluation, Management, Prevention*. St Louis, MO: Mosby, 1995:411–421.
330. Khilberg S: Acute effects and symptoms of work with vibrating handheld powered tools exposing the operator to impact and reaction forces [Thesis]. *Arbete och Hälsa* 10:1–50, 1995.
331. Smolders JJ: Myofascial pain and dysfunction syndromes. In: Hammer WI, ed. *Functional Soft Tissue Examination and Treatment by Manual Methods – The Extremities*. Gaithersburg, MD: Aspen, 1991:215–234.
332. Subarrao J, Stillwell GK: Reflex sympathetic dystrophy syndrome of the upper extremity: Analysis of total outcome of management of 125 cases. *Arch Phys Med Rehabil* 62:549–554, 1981.
333. Veldman PHJM, Reynen HM, Arntz IE, et al: Signs and symptoms of reflex sympathetic dystrophy: Prospective study of 829 patients. *Lancet* 342:1012–1016, 1993.
334. Metules TJ: When a simple fall turns into years of pain. *RN* 63:65–66, 2000.
335. Bohm E: Das Sudecksche Syndrom. *Hefte Unfallheilkd* 174:241–250, 1985.
336. Omer GC, Thomas MS: Treatment of causalgia. *Tex Med* 67:93–96, 1971.
337. Atkins RM, Duckworth T, Kanis JA: Features of algodsytrophy after Colles' fracture. *J Bone Joint Surg Br* 72:105–110, 1990.
338. Acquaviva P, Schiano A, Harnden P, et al: Les algodystrophies: terrain et facteurs pathogeniques. Resultats d'une enquete multicentrique portant sur 765 observations (Rapport). *Rev Rhum Mal Osteoartic* 49:761–766, 1982.
339. Dunn D: Chronic Regional Pain Syndrome, Type 1: Part I. *AORN J* 72:421–424,426,428–432,435,437–442,444–449,452–458, 2000.
340. Maurer G: Umbau, Dystrophie und Atrophie an den Gliedmassen (Sogenannte Sudecksche Knochenatrophie). *Erg Chir* 33:476–531, 1940.
341. Steinbrocker O: The shoulder-hand syndrome. Associated painful homolateral disability of the shoulder and hand with swelling and atrophy of the hand. *Am J Med* 3:402–407, 1947.
342. Sudeck P: Ueber die acute entzundliche Knochenatrophie. *Arch Klin Chir* 62:147–156, 1900.
343. Walker SM, Cousins MJ: Complex regional pain syndromes: Including ' reflex sympathetic dystrophy' and 'causalgia'. *Anaesth Intensive Care* 25:113–125, 1997.
344. Kingery WS: A critical review of controlled clinical trials for peripheral neuropathic pain and complex regional pain syndromes. *Pain* 73:123–139, 1997.
345. Wilson PR: Post-traumatic upper extremity reflex sympathetic dystrophy: Clinical course, staging, and classification of clinical forms. *Hand Clin* 13:367–372, 1997.
346. Gordon N: Review article: Reflex sympathetic dystrophy. *Brain Dev* 18:257–262, 1996.
347. McLatchie GR: *Essentials of Sports Medicine*, 2nd ed. Edinburgh: Churchill Livingstone, 1993.
348. Wilson RL, Carter MS: Management of hand fractures. In: Hunter J, Schneider LH, Mackin EJ, et al, eds. *Rehabilitation of the Hand*. St Louis, MO: CV Mosby, 1990:284.
349. Sorenson MK: Fractures of the wrist and hand. In: Moran CA, ed. *Hand Rehabilitation: Clinics in Physical Therapy*. New York: Churchill Livingstone, 1986:191–225.
350. King RJ: Scapholunate diastasis associated with a Barton fracture treated by manipulation or Terry-Thomas and the wine waiter. *J R Soc Med* 76:421–423, 1983.
351. Perron AD, Brady WJ, Keats TE, et al: Orthopedic pitfalls in the ED: scaphoid fracture. *Am J Emerg Med* 19:310–316, 2001.
352. Chen SC: The scaphoid compression test. *J Hand Surg Br* 14:323–325, 1989.
353. Waizenegger M, Barton NJ, Davis TR, et al: Clinical signs in scaphoid fractures. *J Hand Surg Br* 19B:743–747, 1994.
354. Ritchie JV, Munter DW: Emergency department evaluation and treatment of wrist injuries. *Emerg Med Clin North Am* 17:823–842, 1999.
355. Ring D, Jupiter JB, Herndon JH: Acute fractures of the scaphoid. *J Am Acad Orthop Surg* 8:225–231, 2000.
356. Watson HK, Kao SD: Degenerative disorders of the carpus. In: Lichtman DM, Alexander AH, eds. *The Wrist and its Disorders*, 2nd ed. Philadelphia, PA: W. B. Saunders, 1997:583–591.
357. Watson HK, Weinzweig J, Zeppieri J: The natural progression of scaphoid instability. *Hand Clin* 13:39–49, 1997.
358. Joseph RB, Linscheid R, Dobyns JH, et al: Chronic sprains of the carpometacarpal joints. *J Hand Surg Am* 6:172–180, 1981.
359. Al-Qattan MM: The triad of multiple metacarpal fractures and/or dislocations of the fingers, severe hand swelling and clinical evidence of acute median nerve dysfunction. *J Hand Surg Eur Vol* 33:298–304, 2008.
360. Ashkenaze DM, Ruby LK: Metacarpal fractures and dislocations. *Orthop Clin North Am* 23:19–33, 1992.
361. Hove LM: Fractures of the hand. Distribution and relative incidence. *Scand J Plast Reconstr Surg Hand Surg* 27:317–319, 1993.
362. Hritcko G: Finger fracture rehabilitation. In: Clark GL, Aiello B, Eckhaus D, et al, eds. *Hand Rehabilitation: A Practical Guide*, 2nd ed. Philadelphia, PA: Churchill Livingstone, 1998:319–327.
363. Sucher BM: Myofascial release of carpal tunnel syndrome. *J Am Osteopath Assoc* 93:92–101, 1993.

Hip CHAPTER 19

CHAPTER OBJECTIVES

At the completion of this chapter, the reader will be able to:

1. Describe the anatomy of the joint, ligaments, muscles, and blood and nerve supply that comprise the hip joint complex.
2. Describe the biomechanics of the hip joint, including the open- and close-packed positions, normal and abnormal joint barriers, force couples, and the static and dynamic stabilizers of the joint.
3. Describe the purpose and components of the examination of the hip joint.
4. Perform a comprehensive examination of the hip joint, including palpation of the articular and soft tissue structures, specific passive mobility, passive articular mobility tests, and stability stress tests.
5. Evaluate the total examination data to establish a diagnosis.
6. Describe the relationship between muscle imbalance and functional performance of the hip.
7. Summarize the various causes of hip dysfunction.
8. Develop self-reliant intervention strategies based on clinical findings and established goals.
9. Develop a working hypothesis.
10. Describe and demonstrate intervention strategies and techniques based on clinical findings and established goals.
11. Evaluate the intervention effectiveness in order to progress or modify an intervention.
12. Plan an effective home program and instruct the patient in same.

OVERVIEW

The hip articulation is a ball-and-socket joint formed between the head of the femur and the acetabulum of the pelvic bone (Fig. 19-1). Structurally, the hip is suited for stability first, then mobility.[1] The primary function of the hip is to support the weight of the head, arms, and trunk during the static erect posture and during dynamic activities such as ambulation, running, and stair climbing.[2] In addition, the hip joint provides a pathway for the transmission of forces between the pelvis and the lower extremities. The hip joint is a marvel of physics, transmitting truly impressive loads, both tensile and compressive. For example, during walking, the hip supports 1.3–5.8 times the body weight, and 4.5–8 times the body weight while running.[3] Finally, the hip joint functions to provide a wide range of lower limb movement.

The hip joint is well designed to provide such an important service, provided that it is permitted to grow and develop normally.

Normal hip joint growth and development occur because of a genetically determined balance of growth of the acetabulum and the presence of a strategically located spherical femoral head.[4–8]

- Absence of a normal femoral head during growth, such as in developmental dysplasia of the hip (DDH), causes the acetabulum to have a flat shape.
- A deformed head stimulates the formation of a correspondingly deformed acetabulum if the deformation occurs at a young enough age.[4]

ANATOMY

Bony Anatomy

The os coxa (hip bone) initially begins life as three individual bones: the ilium, the ischium, and the pubis.

Ilium

The ilium (see Fig. 19-1) is the largest of these three bones. It is composed of a large fan-like wing (ala) and an inferiorly

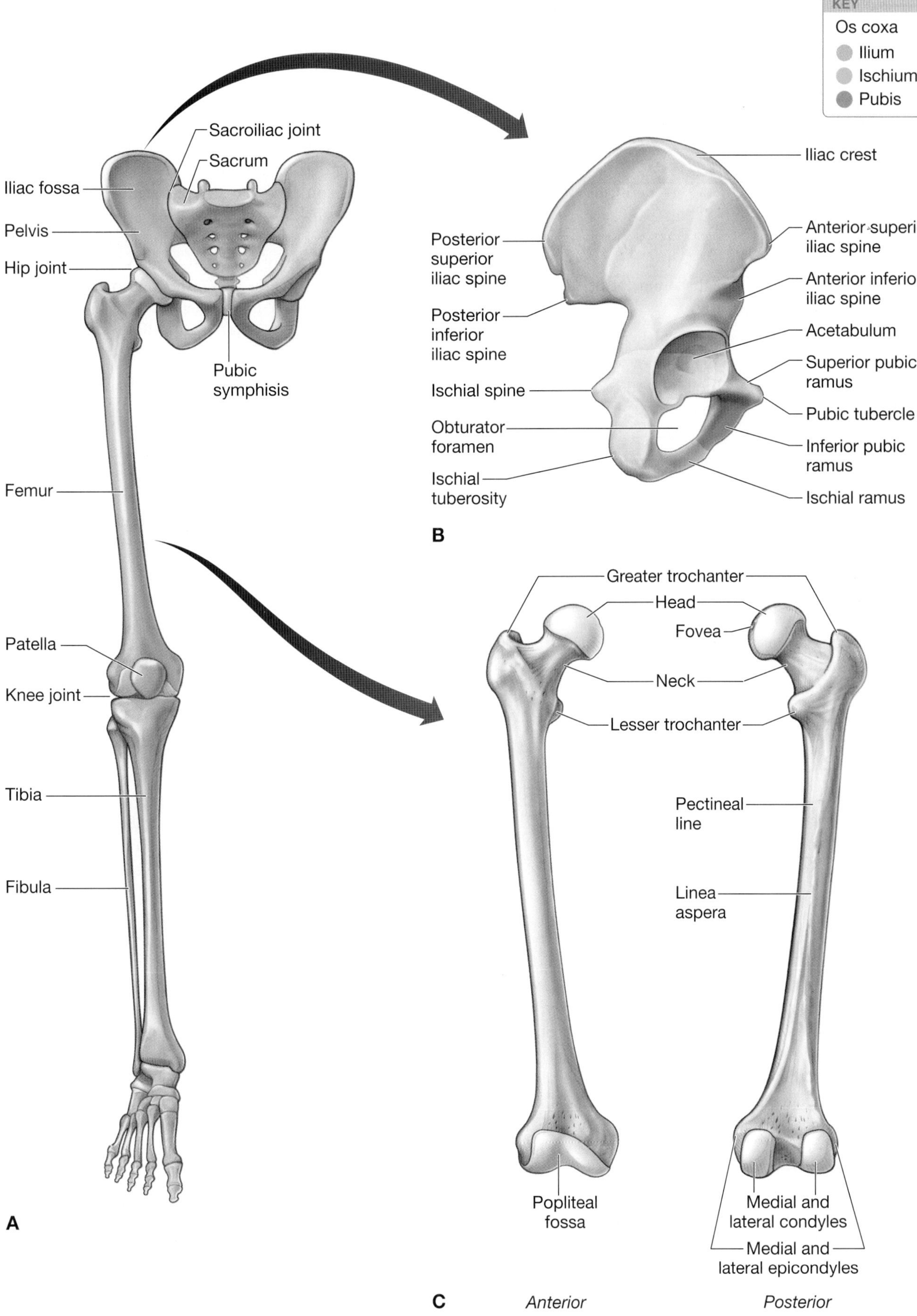

FIGURE 19-1 Bones of the lower extremity. (Reproduced, with permission, from Morton DA, Foreman KB, Albertine KH: *The Big Picture: Gross Anatomy,* McGraw-Hill, 2011.)

TABLE 19-1 Muscles that Attach to the Ischial Tuberosity
Semimembranosus
Semitendinosus
Long head of the biceps femoris
Adductor magnus
Quadratus femoris
Gemellus inferior

positioned body. The body of the ilium forms the superior two-fifths of the acetabulum.

- The wing of the ilium spans superiorly from the posterior superior iliac spine (PSIS) to the anterior superior iliac spine (ASIS). The wing serves as the insertion for the gluteus minimus, medius, and maximus.
- The anterior surface of the ilium forms a fossa and serves as the proximal attachment of the iliacus muscle.

Ischium

The ischium (see Fig. 19-1) is composed of a body, which contributes to the acetabulum, and a ramus. The ischium forms the posterior two-fifths of the acetabulum. Together, the ischium and the ramus form the ischial tuberosity. The ischial tuberosity is an important landmark for palpation, as it serves as the attachment for several muscles (Table 19-1) and the sacrotuberous ligament. The ischial spine, located on the body of the ischium, serves as the attachment for the sacrospinous ligament.

Pubis

The pubis (see Fig. 19-1) is the smallest of the three bones and consists of a body and inferior and superior rami. The pubis forms the anterior fifth of the acetabulum.

Acetabulum

The ilium, ischium, and pubis fuse together within the acetabulum and form a deep-seated depression in the lateral pelvis, which allows for the proximal transmission of weight from the axial skeleton to the lower extremity.[9] The surface of the acetabulum faces laterally, inferiorly, and anteriorly (see Fig. 19-1). The superior and posterior margins of the acetabulum are reinforced with a compact cortical bone, which extends the peripheral brim of the fossa, enhancing the stability of the joint during weight-bearing from both flexed and extended positions.[9] While the majority of acetabular development is determined by the age of eight,[10–12] the depth of the acetabulum increases additionally at puberty, because of the development of three secondary centers of ossification.[4,5,13] Around the periphery of the acetabulum is a thickened collar of fibrocartilage known as the acetabular rim, or labrum (see "The Acetabular Labrum" section), that further deepens the concavity and grasps the head of the femur.[9] The transverse acetabular ligament is a fibrous tissue link spanning the inferior acetabular notch that connects the anteroinferior and posteroinferior horns of the semilunar surface of the acetabulum. The posterior aspect of the ligament attaches to the bone beneath the lunate surface, and the anterior aspect attaches to the labrum.[14] The transverse acetabular ligament contains no cartilage cells.[15] The function of this ligament in the hip is currently unknown.

The articular surface of the acetabulum is limited to an inverted horseshoe-shaped area covering the anterior, superior, and posterior margins.[9] This relatively small contact area, may contribute to the prevalence of hip degenerative joint disease in humans.[16] The articular surface is covered by a thickened layer of hyaline cartilage, which thins near the center of the joint, and is absent over the acetabular notch (see Fig. 19-1), the area occupied by the ligamentum teres and obturator artery. The diameter of the acetabulum is slightly less than that of the femoral head and results in an incongruous fit of the joint surfaces. This incongruity unloads the joint during partial weight-bearing (PWB), by allowing the femoral head to sublux laterally out of the cup, while in full weight-bearing, the femoral head is forced into the acetabulum.[9] In addition, elastic deformation of the acetabulum increases joint congruency of the two-joint surfaces in weight-bearing.[17] Finally, a strong vacuum contributes to the joint coaptation.[1] The position of maximum articular congruence corresponds to a quadriped position: 90 degrees flexed, slightly abducted, and externally rotated.

Femur

The femur is the strongest and the longest bone in the body. The proximal end of the femur consists of a head, a neck, and a greater and lesser trochanter (see Fig. 19-1). Approximately two-thirds of the femoral head is covered with a smooth layer of cartilage except for a depression, the fovea capitis, which serves as the attachment of the ligamentum teres.

The femoral head is composed of a trabecular bone core encased in a thin cortical bone shell. Both the trabecular framework of the head and its pliable hyaline cartilage covering contribute toward the shaping of the femoral head within the acetabulum during full weight-bearing.[9] The trabecular bone in the femoral neck and head is specially designed to withstand high loads because of the incorporation of both primary and secondary compressive and tensile patterns. However, within this trabecular system, there is a point of weakness called the Ward triangle, which is a common site of osteoporotic fracture.[18]

The neck of the femur is located between the shaft of the femur and its head. On the anterior surface of the femoral neck is the rough intertrochanteric line. The femoral neck serves to extend the weight-bearing forces lateral and inferior to the joint fulcrum. The intertrochanteric crest marks the posterior junction between the neck and the shaft of the femur. The greater trochanter serves as the insertion site for several muscles that act on the hip joint (Table 19-2). The lesser trochanter, located on the posteromedial junction of the neck and the shaft of the femur, is created from the pull of the iliopsoas muscle.

The head of the femur is angled anteriorly, superiorly, and medially. The femoral neck is externally rotated with respect to the shaft. The angle that the femoral neck makes with the

TABLE 19-2	Muscles that Attach to the Greater Trochanter
Piriformis	
Gluteus medius	
Gluteus minimus	
Obturator internus	
Gemellus superior	
Gemellus inferior	

acetabulum is called the angle of anteversion/declination (see "Biomechanics" section).

Joint Capsule

The joint capsule of the hip (Fig. 19-2), a substantial fibrous sleeve, attaches proximally to the pelvis just lateral to the acetabular labrum and extends laterally over the femoral head and neck to attach to the intertrochanteric line anteriorly. Posteriorly, the capsule attaches to the lateral one-third of the femoral neck allowing for the attachment of the obturator externus tendon in the posterior intertrochanteric fossa.[9] Both the articular cartilage and the joint capsule are thicker anterosuperiorly, where maximal stress and weight-bearing occurs, and thinnest posteroinferiorly. The joint capsule has three thickened regions that constitute the capsular ligaments. These anterior capsular thickenings include the iliofemoral ligament and the pubofemoral ligament.

- The iliofemoral ligament (Y ligament of Bigelow) (Fig. 19-2) consists of two parts: an inferior (medial) portion and a superior (lateral) portion. The iliofemoral ligament is the strongest ligament in the body. The ligament is oriented superior laterally and blends with the iliopsoas muscle. By limiting the range of hip extension, this ligament, with the assistance of the pubofemoral ligament, allows maintenance of the upright posture and reduces the need for contraction of the hip extensors in a balanced stance. Hip adduction tightens the superior portion of the iliofemoral ligament.
- The pubofemoral ligament (Fig. 19-2) blends with the inferior band of the iliofemoral, and with the pectineus muscle. The orientation of the pubofemoral ligament is more inferior-medial. Its fibers tighten in extension and abduction and reinforce the joint capsule along the medial surface.

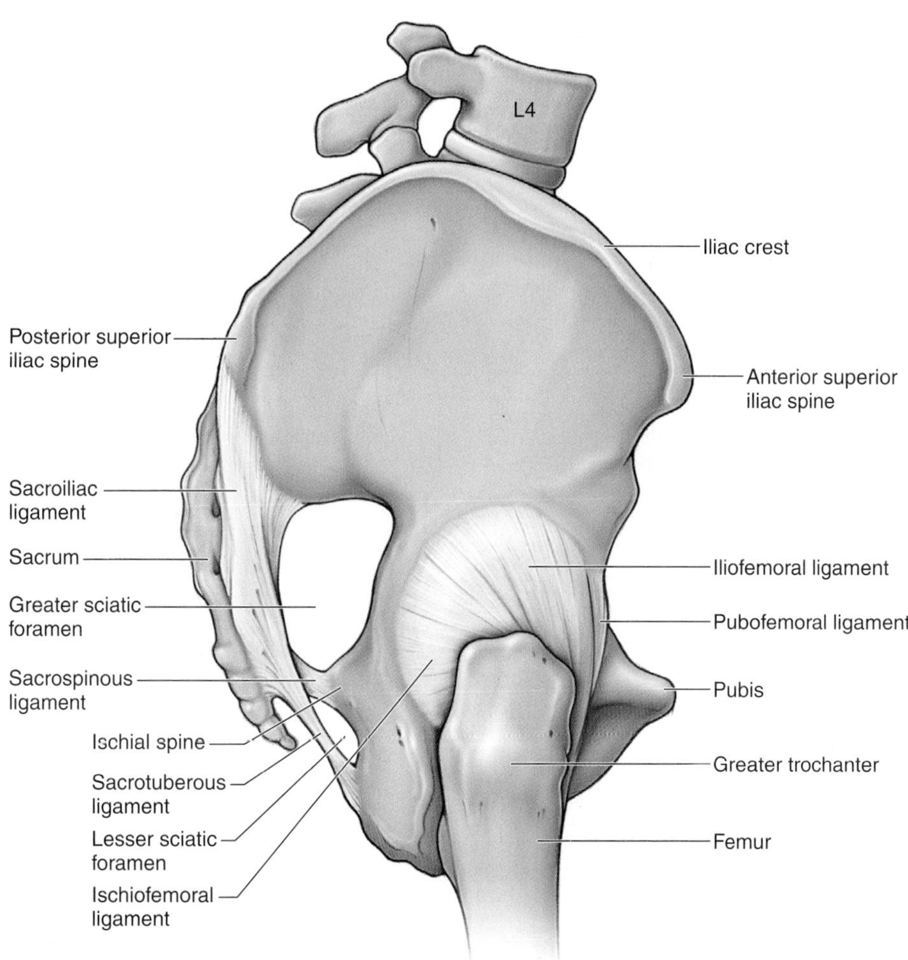

FIGURE 19-2 The hip joint capsule. (Reproduced, with permission, from Morton DA, Foreman KB, Albertine KH: *The Big Picture: Gross Anatomy*, McGraw-Hill, 2011.)

The posterior thickening of the capsule accounts for the ischiofemoral ligament (Fig. 19-2), which winds posteriorly around the femur and attaches anteriorly, strengthening the capsule. This ligament, which tightens with internal rotation of the hip, is more commonly injured than the other hip ligaments.

All these capsular thickenings/ligaments are taut in hip extension, especially the inferior portion of the iliofemoral ligament. Conversely, all the ligaments are relaxed in hip flexion. In external rotation of the hip, the superior portion of the iliofemoral ligament and the pubofemoral ligament are both taut. Because of their inherent strength, the hip ligaments are only usually compromised with severe macrotrauma involving a fracture/dislocation of the hip.

The ligamentum teres, or capitis femoris ligament (Fig. 19-3), is a structure seen only in the hip joint.[9] This ligament spans the hip joint running from the acetabular notch to the fovis capitis of the femur, attaching the femoral head to the inferior acetabular rim. The ligament is entirely enclosed by synovial membrane, which forms a sheath around the ligament. Within this sheath, vessels and nerves pass to the femoral head, providing an important source of arterial blood from a tiny posterior branch of the internal iliac artery. This arterial supply is a significant source of blood to the femoral head in infants and children[19] but becomes less significant in adulthood, because of collateral circulation from the circumflex arteries (see "Vascular Supply" section) surrounding the femoral neck, although chronic interruption the blood supply of the femoral head has been associated with avascular necrosis and degenerative arthritis.[20]

The ligamentum teres tightens during adduction, flexion, and external rotation and, although it provides very little to stability, it can contribute to symptoms when injured.

The Acetabular Labrum

The acetabular labrum (Fig. 19-3) is a ring consisting of fibrocartilage and dense connective tissue[21] that encases the femoral head and is attached to the acetabular margin. The acetabular labrum of the hip, to a large extent, is analogous to the meniscus of the knee (see Chap. 20) and the labrum of the glenohumeral joint (see Chap. 16) in that it enhances joint stability, decreases the forces transmitted to the articular cartilage,[22,23] and provides proprioceptive feedback.[22,23] The majority of the acetabular labrum is thought to be avascular. However, cadaver studies have shown blood vessels entering primarily the peripheral part of the labrum, with penetration only into the outer one-third of the substance of the labrum.[21] Nerve-endings and sensory end organs in the superficial layers of the labrum participate in nociceptive and proprioceptive mechanisms.[17,24] The osseous acetabulum in the hip provides substantial static stability to the hip joint.[24] Deepening of the socket that is provided by the labrum would, therefore, appear to be less important at the hip. Some research does indicate,

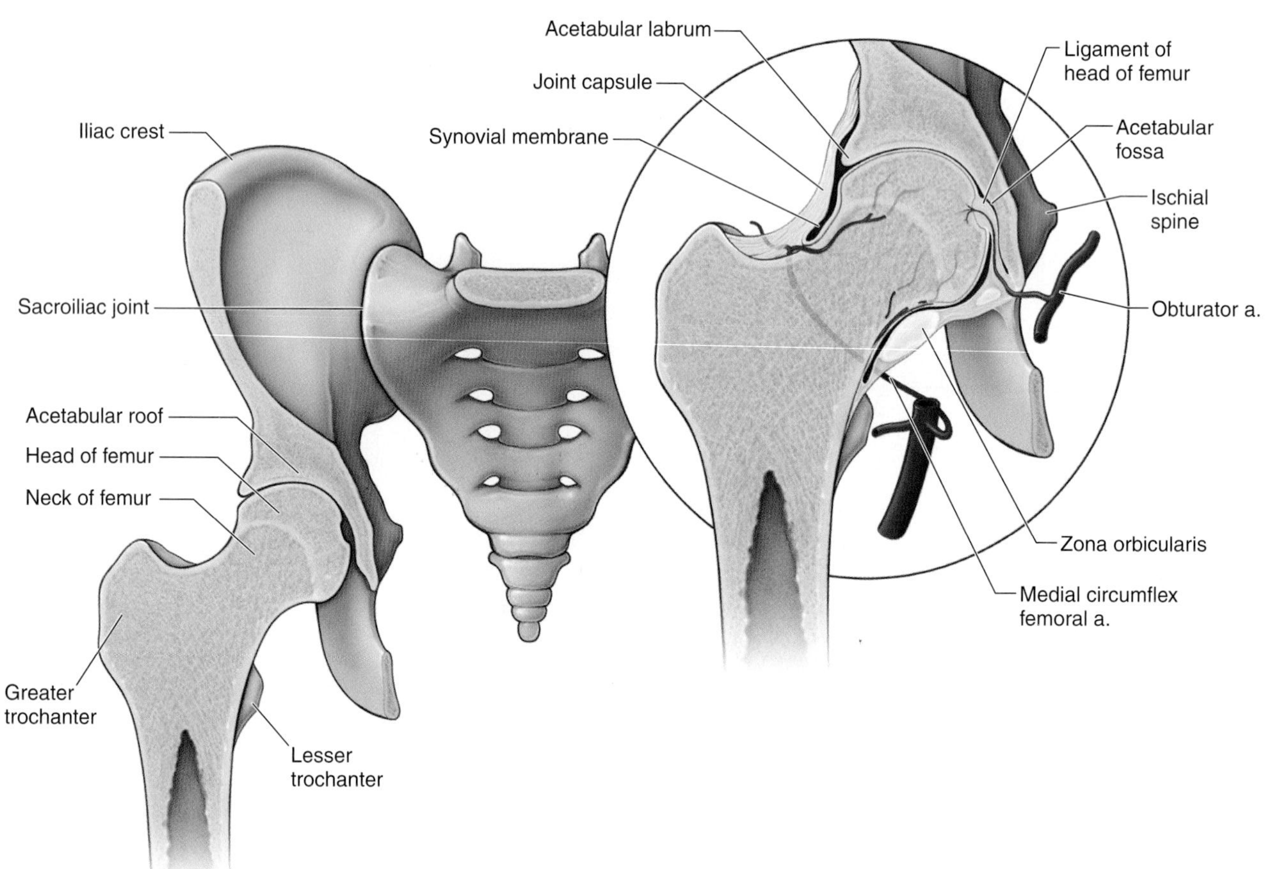

FIGURE 19-3 The hip joint. (Reproduced, with permission, from Morton DA, Foreman KB, Albertine KH: *The Big Picture: Gross Anatomy*, McGraw-Hill, 2011.)

however, that the labrum may enhance stability by providing negative intra-articular pressure in the hip joint.[25] Another study, by Konrath et al.,[17] examined the role of the acetabular labrum in load transmission in a biomechanical study. The distribution of contact area and pressure between the acetabulum and the femoral head was measured in cadaver hips before and after removal of the acetabular labrum. No appreciable changes with regard to contact area, load, and mean pressure were noted after removal of the labrum.[17]

Another proposed function of the labrum is to improve the mobility of the hip by providing an elastic alternative to the bony rim.[17] The labrum, which varies greatly in form and thickness, has a triangular cross section: an internal articular surface, an external surface contacting the joint capsule, and a basal surface attached to the acetabular bone and transverse ligaments.[15] Most of the labrum is composed of thick, type I collagen fiber bundles principally arranged parallel to the acetabular rim, with some fibers scattered throughout this layer running obliquely to the predominant fiber orientation.[26] The normal microvasculature of the acetabular labrum consists of a group of small vessels located in the substance of the labrum traveling circumferentially around the labrum at its attachment site on the outer surface of the bony acetabular extension.[27] In addition, the labrum is surrounded by highly vascularized synovium that is present in the capsular recess.[27]

Muscles

The hip joint is surrounded by a wide variety of muscles that accelerate, decelerate, and stabilize the hip joint. Indeed 21 muscles cross the hip, providing both tri-planar movement and stability between the femur and the acetabulum.[28] Consequently, abnormal performance of the muscles of the hip may alter the distribution of forces across the joint articular surfaces, potentially causing, or at least predisposing, degenerative changes in the articular cartilage, bone, and surrounding connective tissues.[28] The origin, insertion, and innervation of these muscles are outlined in Table 19-3. Since the hip joint is able to move through a wide range of motion (ROM), a muscle's line of pull may be altered with changing hip position, which makes describing a muscle's action difficult. For example, the orientation of the gluteus medius allows it to work as an internal rotator in hip flexion yet as a weak external rotator in hip extension.[29] Similarly, the tensor fascia latae (TFL) is a hip abductor and flexor, depending upon the hip position, while being a weak internal rotator in all positions.[30] The hip muscles and their respective actions are outlined in Table 19-3 and Table 19-4.

Iliopsoas

The iliopsoas muscle, formed by the iliacus and psoas major muscles (see Fig. 19-4), is the most powerful hip flexor, while also functioning as a weak adductor and external rotator of the hip. The iliopsoas attaches to the hip joint capsule, thereby giving it some support. Since the muscle spans both the axial and appendicular components of the skeleton, it also functions as a trunk flexor, and affords an important element to the vertical stability of the lumbar spine, especially when the hip is in full extension and passive tension is greatest in the muscle.[28,31] Theoretically, a sufficiently strong and isolated bilateral contraction of any hip flexor muscle will either rotate the femur toward the pelvis, the pelvis (and possibly the trunk) toward the femur, or both actions simultaneously.[28]

Gluteus Maximus

The gluteus maximus (Fig. 19-5) is the largest and most important hip extensor. It is also an important external rotator of the hip. The larger, superficial portion of this muscle inserts at the proximal part of the ITB, while the deep portion inserts into the gluteal tuberosity of the femur. The inferior gluteal nerve, which innervates the muscle, is located on the deep portion.

The gluteus maximus is normally active only when the hip is in flexion, as during stair climbing or cycling, or when extension of the hip is resisted.[32]

Gluteus Medius

The gluteus medius (Fig. 19-5) is critical for balancing the pelvis in the frontal plane during one leg stance,[33] which accounts for approximately 60% of the gait cycle (see Chap. 6).[34] During one leg stance, approximately 3 times the body weight is transmitted to the hip joint with two-thirds of that being generated by the hip-abductor mechanism.[34] In addition to its role as a stabilizer, the gluteus medius also functions as a decelerator of hip adduction.

Because of its shape, the gluteus medius is known as the deltoid of the hip. The muscle can be divided into two functional parts: an anterior portion and a posterior portion. The anterior portion works to flex, abduct, and internally rotate the hip. The posterior portion extends and externally rotates the hip. On the deep surface of this muscle is located the superior gluteal nerve and the superior and inferior gluteal vessels.

Gluteus Minimus

The gluteus minimus (Fig. 19-6), the major internal rotator of the femur, is a relatively thin muscle situated between the gluteus medius muscle and the external surface of the ilium. It receives support from the TFL, semitendinosus, semimembranosus, and gluteus medius.[32] The gluteus minimus also abducts the thigh, as well as helping the gluteus medius with pelvic support.

Piriformis

The piriformis (Fig. 19-6) is an external rotator of the hip at less than 60 degrees of hip flexion. At 90 degrees of hip flexion, the piriformis reverses its muscle action, becoming an internal rotator and abductor of the hip.[35] Because of its close association with the sciatic nerve, the piriformis can be a common source of buttock and leg pain.[36–39]

Rectus Femoris

The rectus femoris muscle (Fig. 19-7), one of the four quadriceps muscles (see Chap. 20), is a two-joint muscle that arises from two tendons: one, the anterior or straight, from the anterior inferior iliac spine (AIIS); the other, the posterior or reflected, from a groove above the brim of the

TABLE 19-3 Origin, Insertion, and Innervation of Muscles Acting Across the Hip Joint			
Muscle	**Origin**	**Insertion**	**Innervation**
Adductor brevis	External aspect of the body and inferior ramus of the pubis	The line from the greater trochanter of the linea aspera of the femur	Obturator nerve
Adductor longus	In angle between pubic crest and symphysis	The middle third of the linea aspera of the femur	Obturator nerve
Adductor magnus	Inferior ramus of pubis, ramus of ischium, and the inferolateral aspect of the ischial tuberosity	To the linea aspera and adductor tubercle of the femur	Obturator nerve and tibial portion of the sciatic nerve
Biceps femoris	Long head arises from the sacrotuberous ligament and posterior aspect of the ischial tuberosity. Short head does not act across the hip	On the lateral aspect of the head of the fibula, the lateral condyle of the tibial tuberosity, the lateral collateral ligament, and the deep fascia of the leg	Tibial portion of the sciatic nerve, S1
Gemelli (superior and inferior)	Superior–posterior (dorsal) surface of the spine of the ischium and inferior-upper part of the tuberosity of the ischium	Superior- and inferior-medial surface of the greater trochanter	Sacral plexus
Gluteus maximus	Posterior gluteal line of the ilium, iliac crest, aponeurosis of the erector spinae, posterior (dorsal) surface of the lower part of the sacrum, side of the coccyx, sacrotuberous ligament, and intermuscular fascia	Iliotibial tract of the fascia latae and gluteal tuberosity of the femur	Inferior gluteal nerve
Gluteus medius	Outer surface of the ilium between the iliac crest and the posterior gluteal line, anterior gluteal line, and fascia	Lateral surface of the greater trochanter	Superior gluteal nerve
Gluteus minimus	Outer surface of the ilium between the anterior and inferior gluteal lines, and the margin of the greater sciatic notch	On the anterior surface of the greater trochanter	Superior gluteal nerve
Gracilis	The body and inferior ramus of the pubis	The superior medial surface of the proximal tibia, just proximal to the tendon of the semitendinosus	Obturator nerve
Iliacus	Superior two-thirds of the iliac fossa and upper surface of the lateral part of the sacrum	Fibers converge with tendon of the psoas major to lesser trochanter	Femoral nerve
Obturator externus	Rami of the pubis, ramus of the ischium, and medial two-thirds of the outer surface of the obturator membrane	Trochanteric fossa of the femur	Obturator nerve
Obturator internus	Internal surface of the anterolateral wall of the pelvis and obturator membrane	Medial surface of the greater trochanter	Sacral plexus
Pectineus	Pectineal line	Along a line extending from the lesser trochanter to the linea aspera	Femoral or obturator or accessory obturator nerves
Piriformis	Pelvic surface of the sacrum, gluteal surface of the ilium, capsule of the sacroiliac joint, and sacrotuberous ligament	Upper border of the greater trochanter of femur	Sacral plexus
Psoas major	Transverse processes of all the lumbar vertebrae bodies and intervertebral disks of the lumbar vertebrae	Lesser trochanter of the femur	Lumbar plexus
Quadratus femoris	Ischial body next to the ischial tuberosity	Quadrate tubercle on femur	Nerve to quadratus femoris
Rectus femoris	By two heads, from the anterior–inferior iliac spine, and a reflected head from the groove above the acetabulum	Upper border of the patella	Femoral nerve
Sartorius	Anterior–superior iliac spine and notch below it	Upper part of the medial surface of the tibia in front of the gracilis	Femoral nerve
Semimembranosus	Ischial tuberosity	The posterior-medial aspect of the medial condyle of the tibia	Tibial nerve
Semitendinosus	Ischial tuberosity	Upper part of the medial surface of the tibia behind the attachment of the sartonus and below that of the gracilis	Tibial nerve
Tensor fascia latae	Anterior part of outer lip of the iliac crest and the lateral surface of the anterior–superior iliac spine	Iliotibial tract	Superior gluteal nerve

TABLE 19-4 Hip Actions and Muscles if in Anatomic Position

Hip Action	Prime Movers	Assistant Movers
Flexors	Iliopsoas Sartorius Tensor fascia latae Rectus femoris Pectineus Adductor longus	Adductor brevis Gracilis Gluteus minimus (anterior fibers)
Extensors	Gluteus maximus Semitendinosus Semimembranosus Biceps femoris (long head) Adductor Magnus (posterior head)	Gluteus medius (middle and posterior fibers) Adductor magnus (anterior head)
Abductors	Gluteus medius (all fibers) Gluteus minimus (all fibers) Tensor fascia latae	Sartorius Rectus femoris Piriformis
Adductors	Adductor magnus (anterior and posterior heads) Adductor longus Adductor brevis Gracilis Pectineus	Biceps femoris (long head) Gluteus maximus (posterior fibers) Quadratus lumborum Obturator externus
External rotators	Gluteus maximus Gemellus inferior Gemellus superior Obturator internus Quadratus femoris Piriformis (at less than 60 degrees hip flexion)	Gluteus medius (posterior fibers) Gluteus minimus (posterior fibers Biceps femoris (long head) Sartorius Obturator externus
Internal rotators	Not applicable	Semitendinosus Semimembranosus Gracilis Piriformis (at 90 degrees hip flexion) Gluteus medius (anterior fibers) Adductor longus Adductor brevis Pectineus Adductor Magnus (posterior head) Gluteus minimus (anterior fibers) Tensor fascia latae

Data from Anderson LC: The anatomy and biomechanics of the hip joint. *J Back Musculoskeletal Rehabil* 4:145–153, 1994; and Neumann DA: Kinesiology of the hip: a focus on muscular actions. *J Orthop Sports Phys Ther* 40:82–94, 2010.

acetabulum. The rectus femoris combines movements of flexion at the hip and extension at the knee. It functions more effectively as a hip flexor when the knee is flexed, as when a person kicks a ball.[32]

Obturator Internus

The obturator internus (Fig. 19-6) is normally an external rotator of the hip and an internal rotator of the ilium but becomes an abductor of the hip at 90 degrees of hip flexion.[40]

Obturator Externus

The obturator externus (Fig. 19-6), named for its location external to the pelvis, is an adductor and external rotator of the hip.[15]

Gemelli

The superior and inferior gemelli muscles (Fig. 19-6) are considered extensions of the obturator internus tendon. The superior gemellus is the smaller of the two. Both the gemelli function as minor external rotators of the hip.[15]

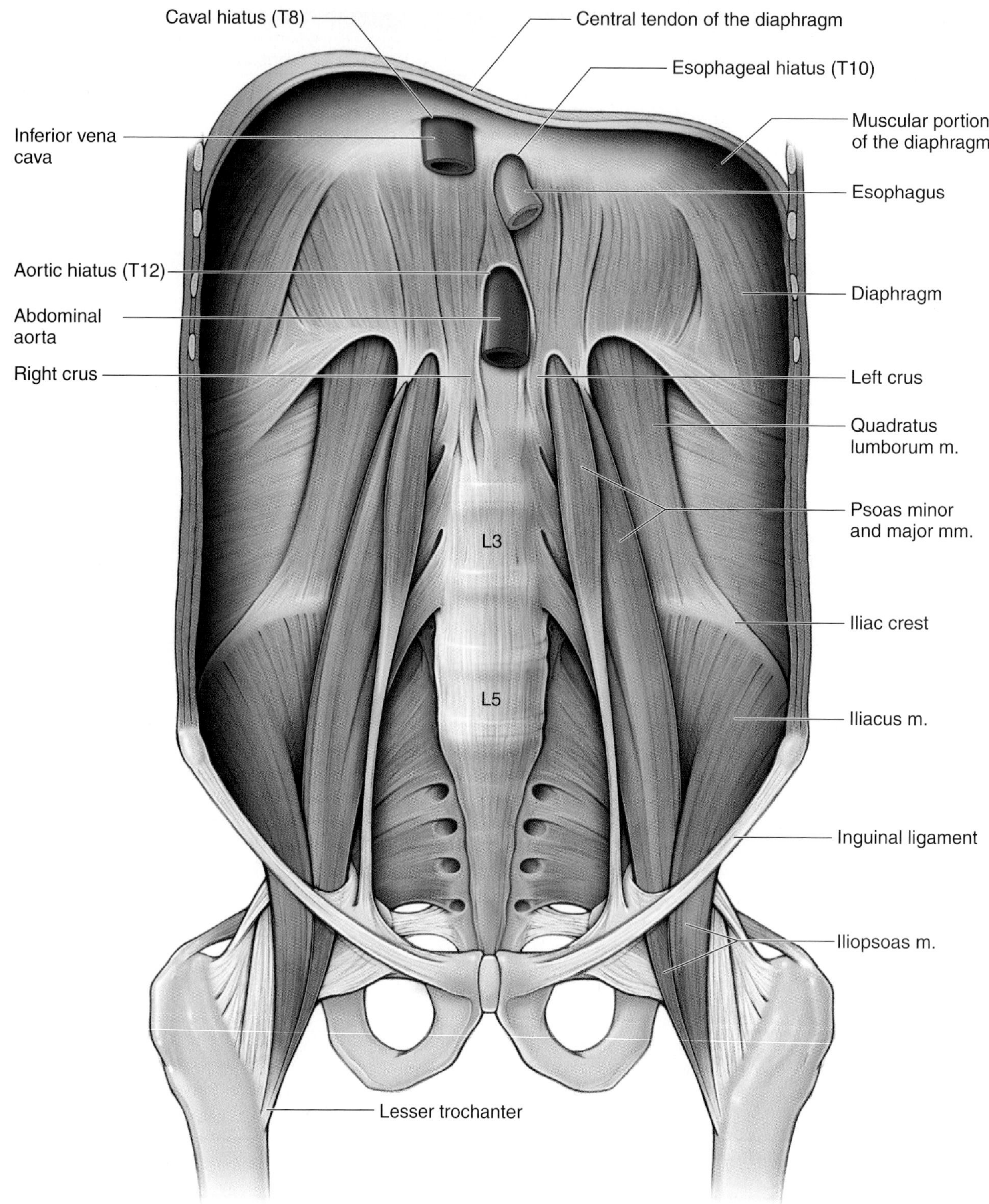

FIGURE 19-4 Muscles of the anterior hip. (Reproduced, with permission, from Morton DA, Foreman KB, Albertine KH: *The Big Picture: Gross Anatomy*, McGraw-Hill, 2011.)

Quadratus Femoris

The quadratus femoris muscle (Fig. 19-6), another external rotator of the hip, is a flat, quadrilateral muscle, located between the inferior gemellus and the superior aspect of the adductor magnus. The quadratus femoris and the inferior gemellus share the same innervation (L4–L5).[15] The obturator internus and superior gemellus also share the same innervation (L5–S1).[15]

CLINICAL PEARL

In a manner, generally, similar to the infraspinatus and teres minor at the glenohumeral joint, the short external rotators of the hip provide an important element of mechanical stability to the hip articulation[34] Interestingly, the popular posterior surgical approach to a total hip arthroplasty (THA), used by some surgeons, necessarily cuts through at least

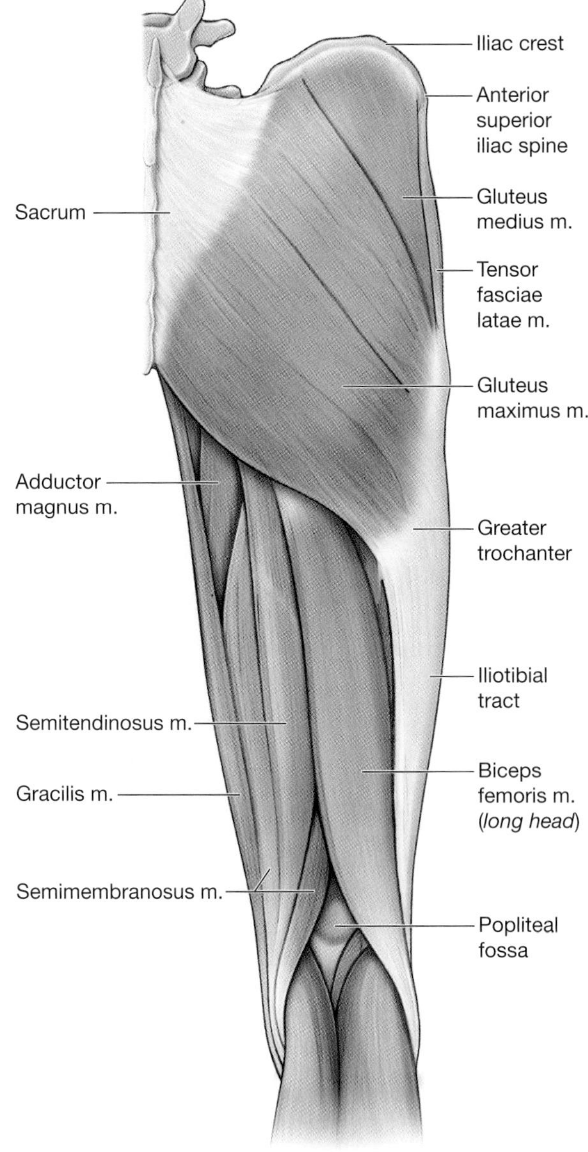

FIGURE 19-5 Superficial muscles of the posterior hip. (Reproduced, with permission, from Morton DA, Foreman KB, Albertine KH: *The Big Picture: Gross Anatomy,* McGraw-Hill, 2011.)

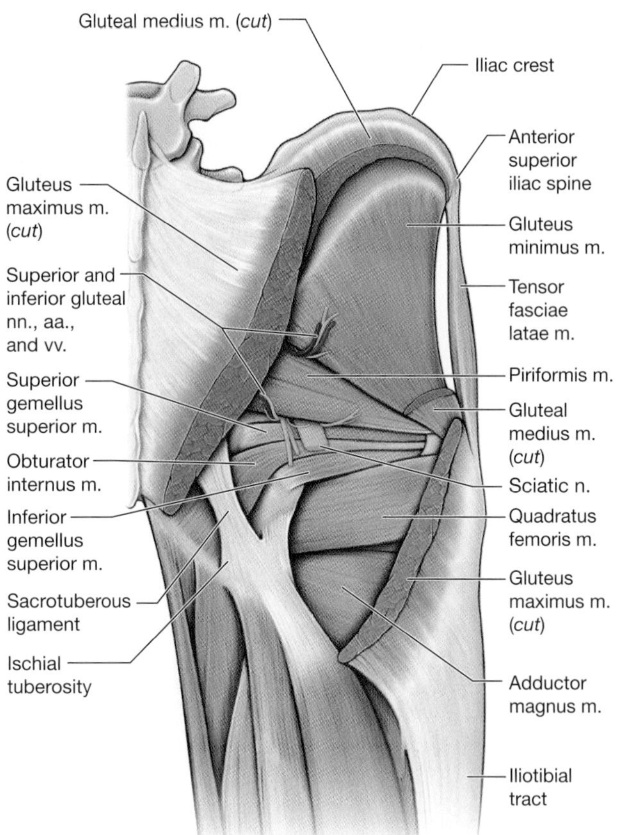

FIGURE 19-6 Deeper muscles of the posterior hip. (Reproduced, with permission, from Morton DA, Foreman KB, Albertine KH: *The Big Picture: Gross Anatomy,* McGraw-Hill, 2011.)

part of the hip's posterior capsule, potentially disrupting several of the short external rotators tendons.[28] Studies have reported a significant reduction in the incidence of posterior hip dislocation when the surgeon carefully repairs the posterior capsule and external rotator tendons.[28,41,42]

Pectineus

The pectineus (see Fig. 19-7) is an adductor, flexor, and internal rotator of the hip. Like the iliopsoas, the pectineus attaches to and supports the joint capsule of the hip.

Tensor Fascia Latae

The TFL (see Fig. 19-5) envelops the muscles of the thigh. The TFL counteracts the backward pull of the gluteus maximus on the iliotibial band (ITB). The TFL also flexes, abducts, and externally rotates the hip. The trochanteric bursa is found deep to this muscle, as it passes over the greater trochanter (see later).[43] The attachment of the TFL via the ITB to the anterolateral tibia provides a flexion moment in knee flexion and an extension moment in knee extension.[2]

Sartorius

The sartorius muscle (see Fig. 19-7) is the longest muscle in the body. The sartorius is responsible for flexion, abduction, and external rotation of the hip, and some degree of knee flexion.[44]

Hamstrings

The hamstrings muscle group consists of the biceps femoris, the semimembranosus, and the semitendinosus.

Biceps Femoris. The biceps femoris (see Fig. 19-8) arises by way of a long and short head. Only the long head acts on the hip. The long head is active during conditions that require lower amounts of force, such as decelerating the limb at the end of the swing phase and during forceful hip extension.[45] The biceps femoris extends the hip, flexes the knee, and externally rotates the tibia. The biceps femoris (53%) is the most commonly strained muscle of the hamstring complex. The anatomy of the biceps femoris may help to explain its higher rate of injury. Firstly, it has a long and a short head, both with separate nerve supplies. This dual innervation may lead to asynchronous stimulation of the two heads. Mistimed contraction of the different parts of the muscle group may mean a reduced capacity to generate effective tension to control the imposed loads of the muscle. There may also be

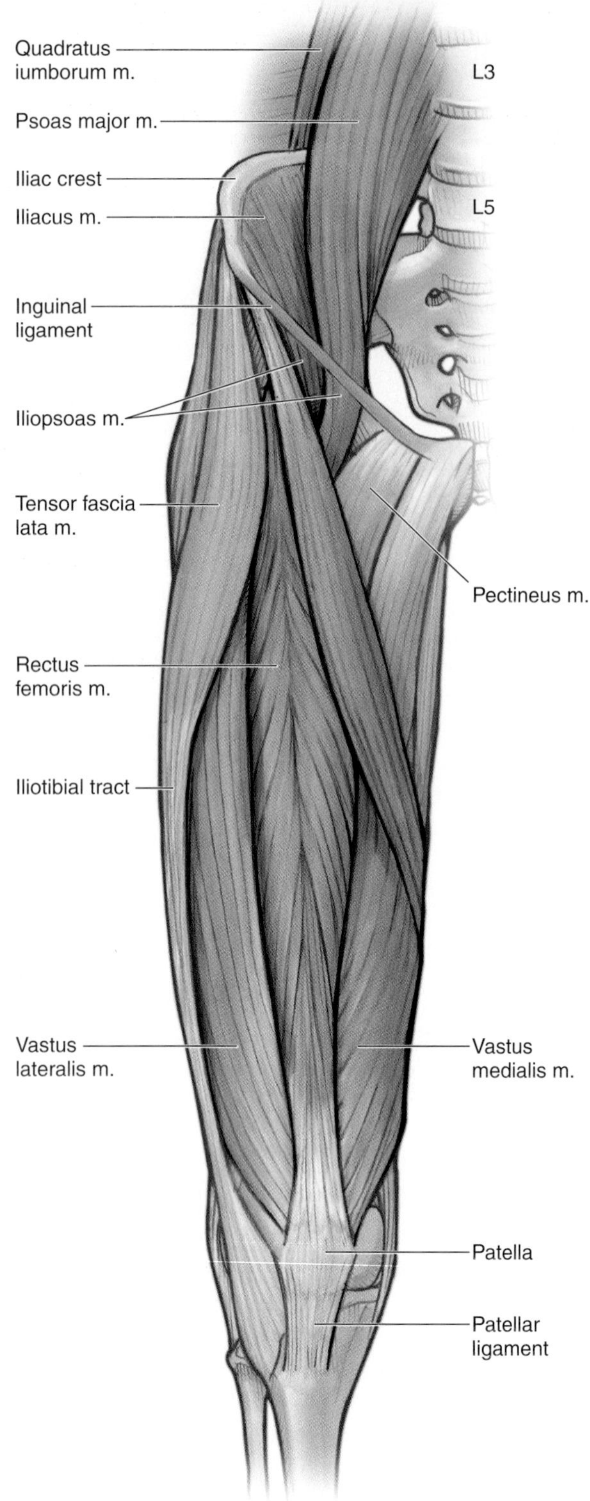

FIGURE 19-7 Muscles of the anterior hip and thigh. (Reproduced, with permission, from Morton DA, Foreman KB, Albertine KH: *The Big Picture: Gross Anatomy,* McGraw-Hill, 2011.)

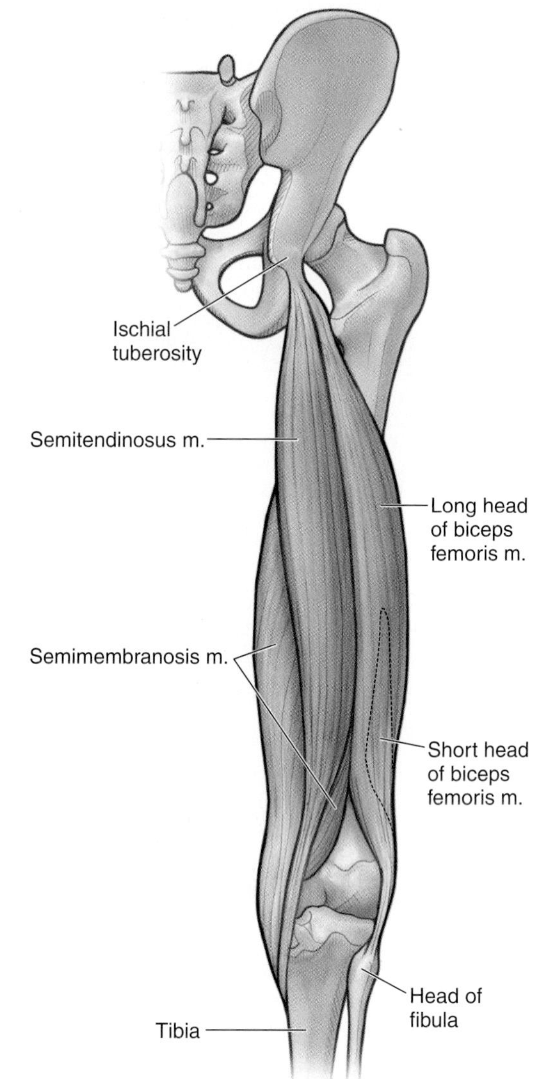

FIGURE 19-8 The hamstrings. (Reproduced, with permission, from Morton DA, Foreman KB, Albertine KH: *The Big Picture: Gross Anatomy,* McGraw-Hill, 2011.)

anatomical variations in the attachments of biceps femoris, which may predispose certain people to injury. Burkett suggested that an extensive femoral attachment of the short head of the biceps femoris with an overlying strength deficit predisposes to hamstring strain. The long head of the biceps femoris originates from the lower part of the sacrotuberous ligament; therefore, it could be argued that the biceps femoris has a triarticular function and is, therefore, more predisposed to injury than the other hamstring muscles. The insertion of the biceps femoris into the head of the fibula may also be a predisposing factor to injury. A previous knee or ankle injury resulting in alteration in the movement of the superior tibiofibular joint may affect the biomechanics of the biceps femoris, although this notion is speculative. However, incomplete knee excursion caused by meniscal damage may lead to excessive loading of the biceps femoris.[46] The biceps femoris acts as an external rotator of the semiflexed knee and the extended hip. Given the rotational demands of many sports, this function may also predispose the biceps femoris to injury.

Semimembranosus. The semimembranosus (see Fig. 19-8) gains its name from its membranous origin at the ischial tuberosity.

Semitendinosus. The semitendinosus (see Fig. 19-8) arises from the ischial tuberosity and inserts as part of the pes anserinus on the superior and medial aspect of the tibia, and deep fascia of the leg.

All three muscles of the hamstring complex (except for the short head of the biceps) work with the posterior adductor magnus and the gluteus maximus to extend the hip. The hamstrings also flex the knee and weakly adduct the hip. The long head of the biceps femoris helps with external rotation of the thigh and leg; the more medial semimembranosus and semitendinosus muscles assist with internal rotation of the thigh and leg. When the hamstrings contract, their forces are exerted at both the hip and knee joints simultaneously; functionally, however, they can actively mobilize only one of the two joints at any one time. Compared to walking and jogging, running is a stressful activity for the hamstrings and increases the high demands on their tendon attachments, especially during eccentric contractions. During running, the hamstrings have three main functions:

1. They decelerate knee extension at the end of the forward swing phase of the gait cycle. Through an eccentric contraction, the hamstrings decelerate the forward momentum (i.e., leg swing) at approximately 30 degrees short of full knee extension. This action helps provide dynamic stabilization to the weight-bearing knee.
2. At foot strike, the hamstrings elongate to facilitate hip extension through an eccentric contraction, thus further stabilizing the leg for weight-bearing.
3. The hamstrings assist the gastrocnemius in paradoxically extending the knee during the takeoff phase of the running cycle.

Hip Adductors

The adductors of the hip (Fig. 19-9) are found on the medial aspect of the joint.

Adductor Magnus. The adductor magnus is the most powerful adductor, and it is active to varying degrees in all hip motions except abduction. The posterior portion of the adductor magnus is sometimes considered functionally as a hamstring because of its anatomic alignment. Because of its size, the adductor magnus is less likely to be injured than the other hip adductors.[47]

Adductor Longus. The adductor longus is the most prominent muscle of the adductors during resisted adduction, and forms the medial border of the femoral triangle. The adductor

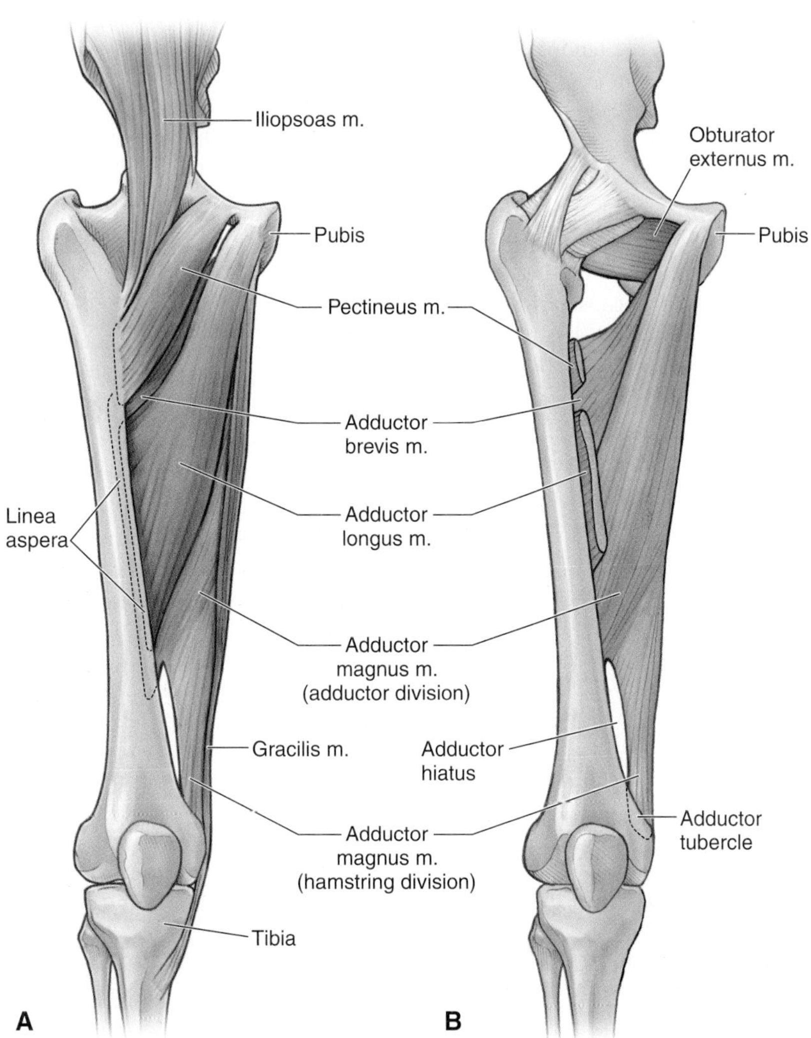

FIGURE 19-9 The hip adductors. (Reproduced, with permission, from Morton DA, Foreman KB, Albertine KH: *The Big Picture: Gross Anatomy*, McGraw-Hill, 2011.)

longus also assists with external rotation, in extension, and internal rotation in other positions. The adductor longus is the most commonly strained adductor muscle.[48]

Gracilis. The gracilis (see Fig. 19-9), the longest of the hip adductors, is also the most superficial and medial of the hip adductor muscles. The gracilis functions to adduct and flex the thigh and flex and internally rotate the leg.

The other adductors of the hip include the adductor brevis, obturator externus, and the pectineus muscles. The main action of this muscle group is to adduct the thigh in the open kinetic chain and stabilize the lower extremity to perturbation in the closed kinetic chain. Each individual muscle can also provide assistance in femoral flexion and rotation.[49]

Bursa

There are more than a dozen bursae in this region.[50] The more clinically significant ones are described below.

Iliopsoas Bursa

Many names have been used to describe the iliopsoas bursa (IPB), including the iliopsoas, iliopectineal, iliac, iliofemoral, and subpsoas bursa.[51] The IPB is the largest and most constant bursa about the hip, present in 98% of normal adult individuals, usually bilaterally.[52] The IPB is situated deep to the iliopsoas tendon and serves to cushion the tendon from the structures on the anterior aspect of the hip joint capsule. Its dimensions may be up to 7 cm in length and 4 cm in width.[52] Anatomic boundaries of the bursa include the iliopsoas muscle anteriorly, the pectineal eminence and the hip joint capsule posteriorly, the iliofemoral ligament laterally, and the acetabular labrum medially.[53]

In 15% of patients, the IPB communicates with the hip joint via a 1-mm-to-3-cm point of relative capsular thinning between the iliofemoral and pubofemoral ligaments.[18,51] While this connection may occur on a congenital basis,[51] this number rises to 30–40% in patients with hip joint pathology.[54]

As with other bursae, the IPB can become inflamed and distended. Inflammation and distension of this bursa are most commonly associated with rheumatoid arthritis, but it is also seen in association with athletic activity, overuse and impingement syndromes, osteoarthrosis, pigmented villonodular synovitis, synovial chondromatosis, infection, pseudogout, metastatic bone disease, and, in rare cases, after THA (see "Interventions" section).[55]

Trochanteric Bursa

Three bursae are consistently present at the greater trochanter, two major bursae and one minor bursa. The two clinically significant trochanteric bursae are the subgluteus medius bursa, and the more superficial subgluteus maximus bursa:

- Subgluteus medius bursa: located at the superoposterior tip of the greater trochanter and functions to prevent friction between the gluteus medius muscle and the greater trochanter and also between the gluteus medius and gluteus minimus muscles.
- Subgluteus maximus bursa: located between the greater trochanter and the fibers of the gluteus maximus and tensor fascia lata muscles as they blend into the ITB

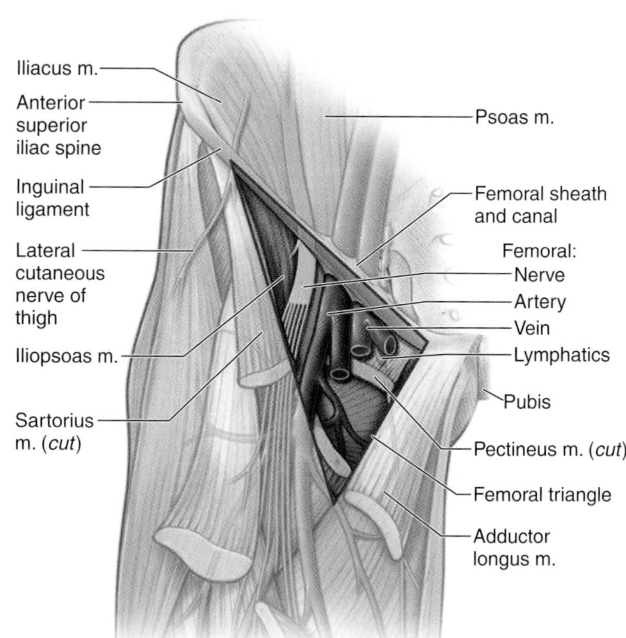

FIGURE 19-10 The femoral triangle. (Reproduced, with permission, from Morton, DA, Foreman KB, Albertine KH: *The Big Picture: Gross Anatomy*, McGraw-Hill, 2011.)

Ischiogluteal Bursa

The ischiogluteal bursa is located between the ischium and the gluteus maximus muscle. It can be painfully squeezed between the ischial tuberosity and the hard surface of a chair during sitting, producing an ischial bursitis. This condition is often referred to as *weaver's bottom*.

Femoral Triangle

For topographic reasons, it is important to have an understanding of the anatomy of the femoral triangle. The femoral triangle is defined superiorly by the inguinal ligament, medially by the adductor longus, and laterally by the sartorius (Fig. 19-10). The floor of the triangle is formed by portions of the iliopsoas on the lateral side and by the pectineus on the medial side (Fig. 19-10). A number of neurovascular structures pass through this triangle. These include (from medial to lateral) the femoral vein, artery, and nerve (Fig. 19-10). Thus, the clinician should use caution when palpating in this area or applying soft tissue techniques.

Neurology

The posterior gluteal region receives cutaneous innervation by way of the subcostal nerve; the iliohypogastric nerve; the posterior (dorsal) rami of L1, L2, and L3; and the posterior (dorsal) primary rami (cluneal nerves) of S1, S2, and S3 (Figs. 19-11, and 19-12A).[56]

The anterior region of the hip has its cutaneous supply divided around the inguinal ligament. The area superior to the ligament is supplied by the iliohypogastric nerve. The area inferior to the ligament is supplied by the subcostal nerve, the femoral branch of the genitofemoral nerve, and the ilioinguinal nerve (see Chap. 3).[56]

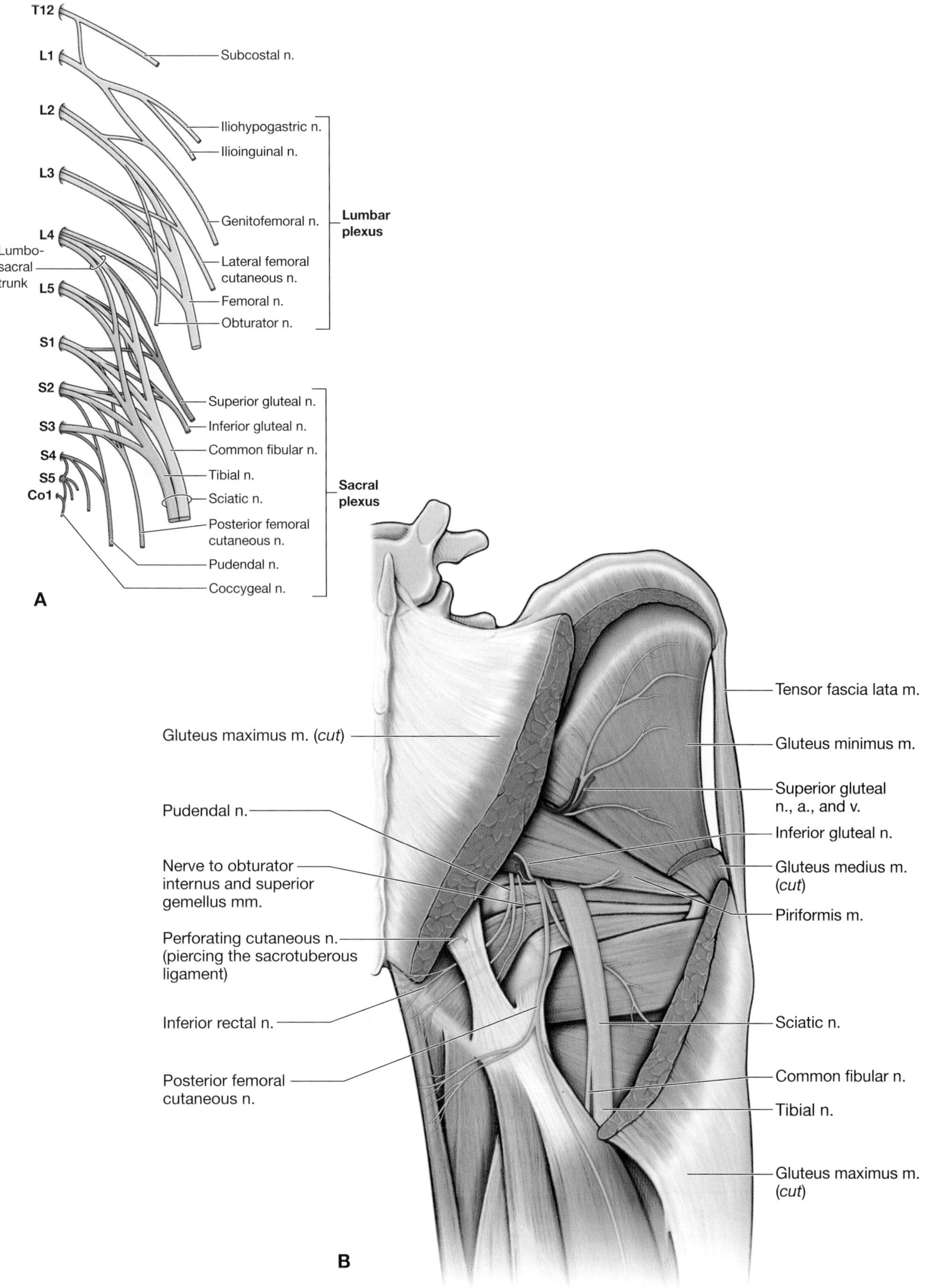

FIGURE 19-11 Neurology and vasculature of the posterior hip. (Reproduced, with permission, from Morton DA, Foreman KB, Albertine KH: *The Big Picture: Gross Anatomy*, McGraw-Hill, 2011.)

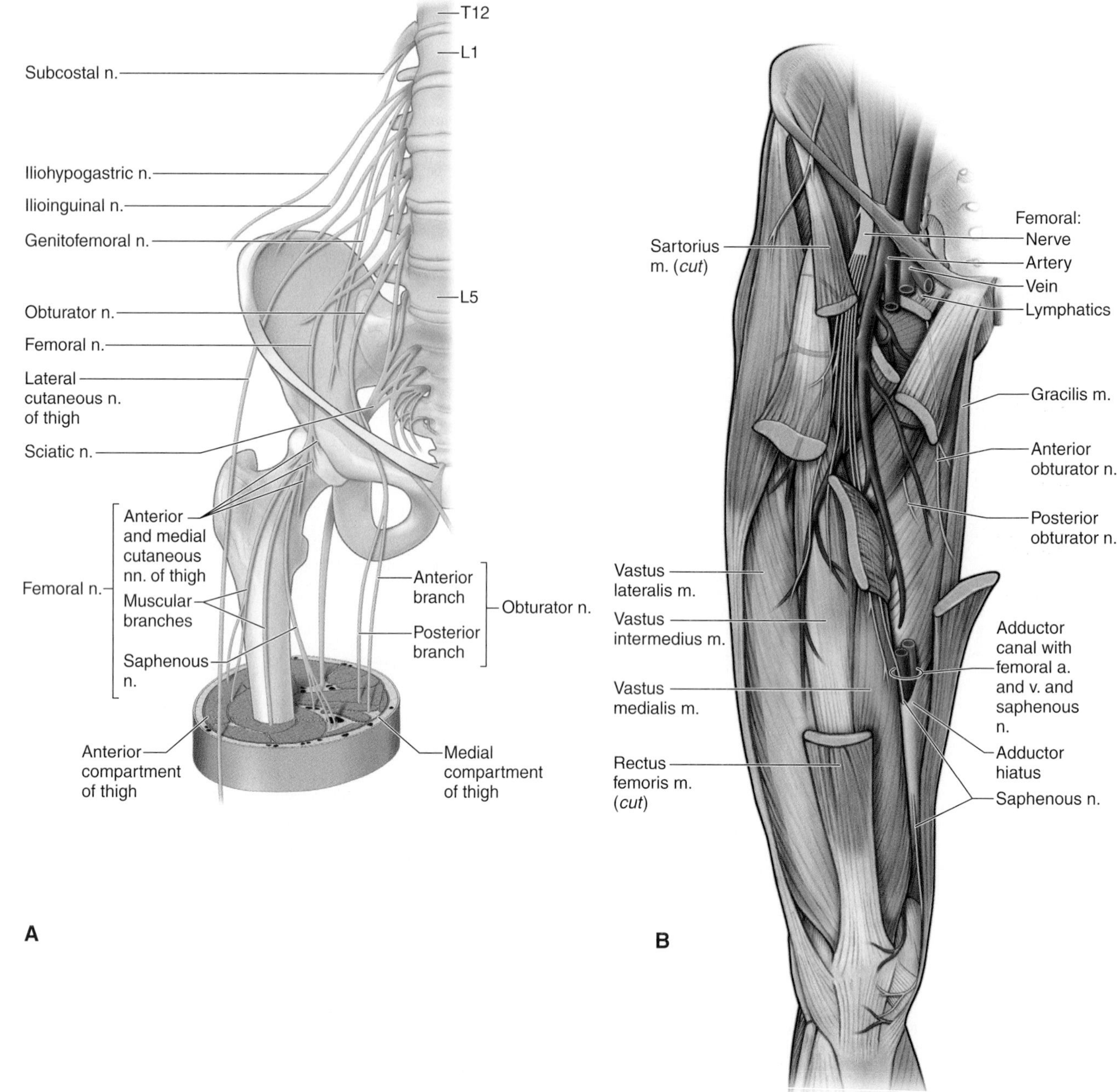

FIGURE 19-12 Neurology and vasculature of the anterior hip. (Reproduced, with permission, from Morton DA, Foreman KB, Albertine KH: *The Big Picture: Gross Anatomy*, McGraw-Hill, 2011.)

The nerves of the muscles that cross the hip joint (femoral, obturator, superior gluteal, and the nerve to the quadratus femoris) also supply the joint capsule and the joint. Therefore, pain referred from the hip joint may be felt anywhere in the thigh, leg, or foot.

Vascular Supply

The internal iliac artery becomes the femoral artery (Figs. 19-12B and 19-13), as it passes underneath the inguinal ligament. The femoral artery forms two branches. The anterior portion of the femoral neck and the anterior portion of the capsule of the hip joint are supplied by the lateral femoral circumflex artery. The medial femoral circumflex artery (MFCA) perforates and supplies the posterior hip joint capsule and the synovium.[56] The deep branch of the MFCA gives rise to two to four superior retinacular vessels and, occasionally, to inferior retinacular vessels.[57,58]

Most of the femoral head, comprising its upper one-half or upper two-thirds, is supplied by the obturator artery and a terminal branch of the MFCA (Fig 19-3).[20] The inferior epiphyseal artery, a branch of the lateral circumflex artery, contributes to the vascularization of the lower area of the femoral head. The supply to the femoral head from the ligamentum teres artery is extremely variable.[59] The blood supply to the weight-bearing portion of the head of the femur is derived from the MFCA.[60]

Two other branches are formed from the internal iliac artery: the inferior and superior gluteal arteries. These arteries supply the superior portion of the capsule and the gluteus maximus muscle.

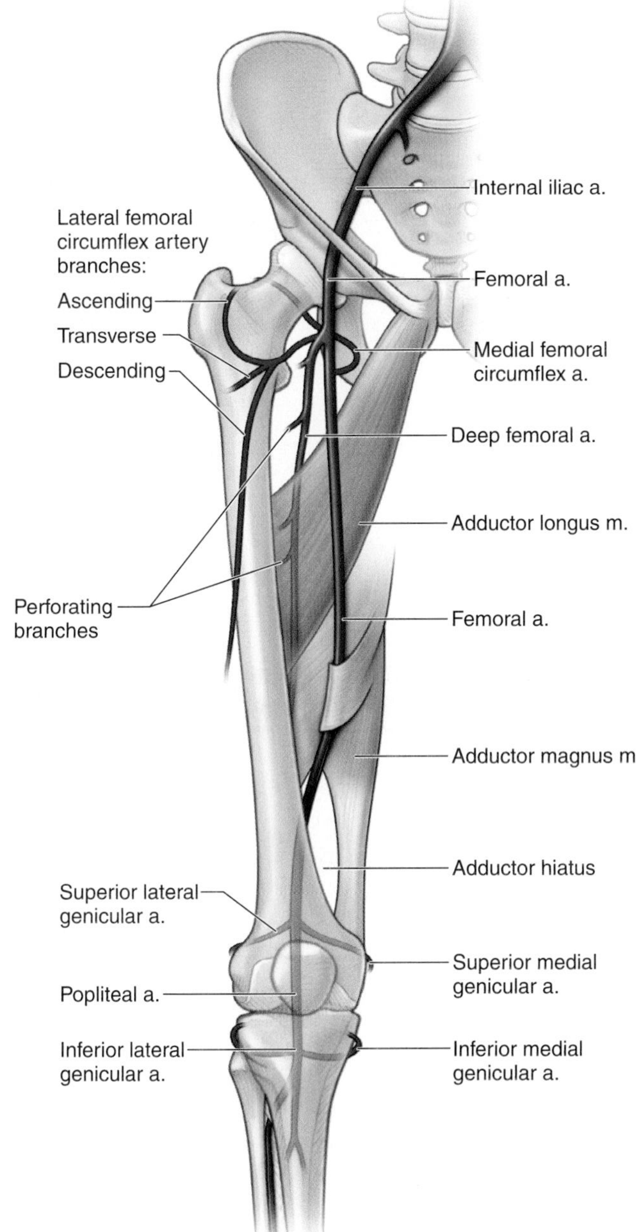

FIGURE 19-13 Vasculature of the hip and thigh. (Reproduced, with permission, from Morton DA, Foreman KB, Albertine KH: *The Big Picture: Gross Anatomy*, McGraw-Hill, 2011.)

BIOMECHANICS

The hip joint, classified as an unmodified ovoid joint, has three degrees of freedom, which permits motion in three planes: sagittal (flexion and extension around a transverse axis), frontal (abduction and adduction around an antero-posterior axis), and transverse (internal and external rotation around a vertical axis) (Fig. 19-14). All three of these axes pass through the center of the femoral head.

Active range of motion (AROM) of the hip is variable. Hip flexion averages 110–120 degrees, extension 10–15 degrees, abduction 30–50 degrees, and adduction 25–30 degrees. Hip external rotation averages 40–60 degrees and internal rotation averages 30–40 degrees (Table 19-5). Motions about the hip joint can occur independently; however, the extremes of motion require motion at the pelvis.[61]

CLINICAL PEARL

End-range hip flexion is associated with a posterior rotation of the ilium bone. The end range of hip extension is associated with an anterior rotation of the ilium. Hip abduction/adduction are associated with an upward/downward tilting of the pelvis (see Table 19-6).

The structure and design of the hip allows for both mobility and stability. The stability is particularly important for weight-bearing and ambulation. In the human body, the center of gravity is located at the second sacral vertebral level, several segments above and medial to the femoral head. Control of the body mass from such a distant fulcrum requires the generation of significant counterbalance forces as well as the ability of the joint to sustain both high compression and tensile strains.[62]

Quantitative and qualitative analysis of the generation of compressive forces at the hip and the muscular mechanisms during weight-bearing have been thoroughly documented.[63–70] During walking, the hip extensors have a vital, stabilizing role at the onset of each stride. As body weight is dropped onto the forward limb, the extensor muscles contract sharply to preserve upright stance by resisting the forward fall of the pelvis and the trunk.[71] The hip's flexed position, before attaining the passive stability provided by full extension in midstance, creates the demand (see Chap. 6). In a standing position, weakness of the hip extensors causes the pelvis to fall forward.[71]

The relationship between the proximal femur, the greater trochanter, and the overall femoral neck width is affected by muscle pull and the forces transmitted across the hip joint. In addition, normal joint nutrition, circulation, and muscle tone during development play an important role.[4,72–74]

In the anatomic position, the orientation of the femoral head causes the contact force between the femur and the acetabulum to be high in the anterosuperior region of the joint.[75] Since the anterior aspect of the femoral head is somewhat exposed in this position, the joint has more flexibility in flexion than extension.[76]

The femoral neck is subjected to shearing and torsional strains because of its oblique orientation to the shaft of the femur.[9] Downward forces act to displace the femoral head inferiorly and to bend the femoral neck downward. To counter these forces, the femoral neck has developed a unique system of obliquely oriented trabeculae that traverse the head and the neck.[9] The angle between the femoral shaft and the neck is called the collum/inclination angle (Fig. 19-15). This angle is approximately 125–130 degrees (Fig. 19-15)[35] but can vary with body types. In a tall person, the collum *angle* is larger. The opposite is true with a shorter individual. The collum angle has an important influence on the hips. An increase in the collum angle causes the femoral head to be directed more superiorly in the acetabulum and is known as coxa valga (Fig. 19-15). Coxa valga has the following effects at the hip joint:

- It alters the orientation of the joint reaction force (JRF) from the normal vertical direction to one that is almost parallel to the femoral shaft.[77,78] This lateral shift of the JRF reduces the

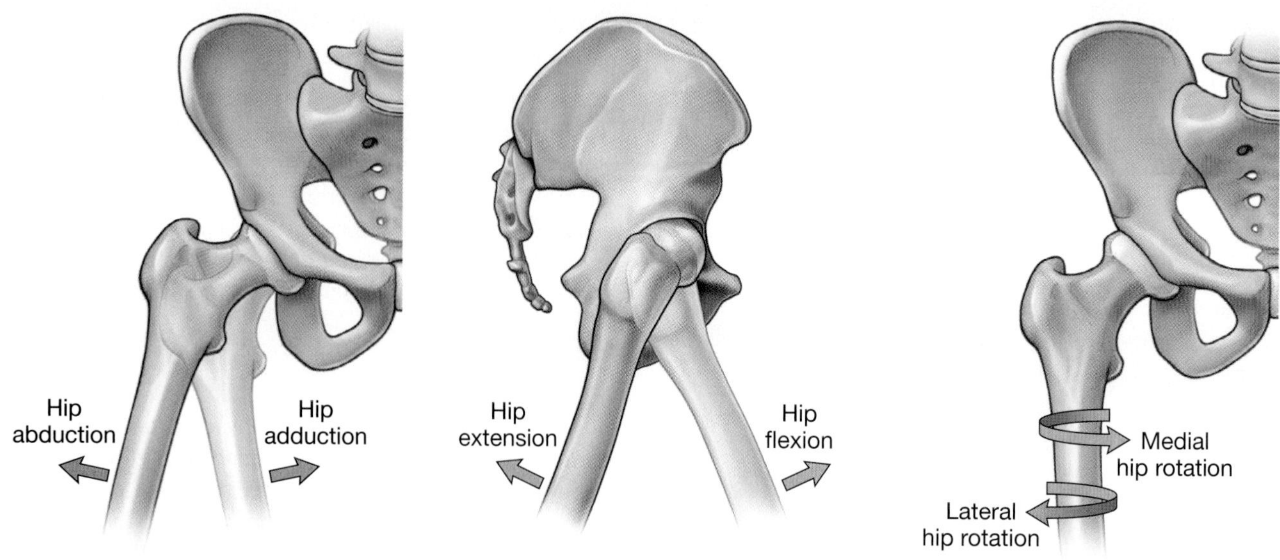

FIGURE 19-14 Movements of the hip. (Reproduced, with permission, from Morton DA, Foreman KB, Albertine KH: *The Big Picture: Gross Anatomy*, McGraw-Hill, 2011.)

TABLE 19-5 Normal Ranges and End-Feels at the Hip

Motion	Range of Motion (Degrees)	End-Feel
Flexion	110–120	Tissue approximation or tissue stretch
Extension	10–15	Tissue stretch
Abduction	30–50	Tissue stretch
Adduction	25–30	Tissue approximation or tissue stretch
External rotation	40–60	Tissue stretch
Internal rotation	30–40	Tissue stretch

Data from Beattie P: The hip. In: Malone TR, McPoil T, Nitz A, eds. *Orthopaedic and Sports Physical Therapy*, 3rd edn. St. Louis, MO: CV Mosby, 1996:506.

TABLE 19-6 Hip Motion and Associated Innominate Motions

Flexion (posterior rotation)
Extension (anterior rotation)
Abduction (upward)
Adduction (downward)
Internal rotation
External rotation

available weight-bearing surface, resulting in an increase in stress applied across joint surfaces not specialized to sustain such loads.

- The moment arm of the hip abductors is shortened, placing these muscles in a position of mechanical disadvantage.[78]

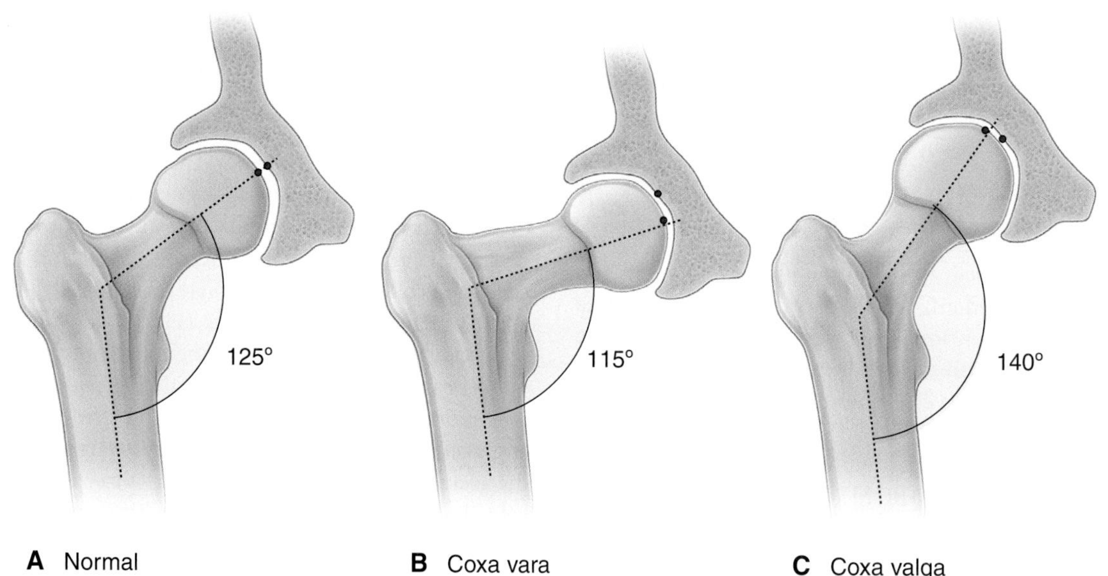

FIGURE 19-15 Angle of inclination and coxa vara/valga.

This causes the abductors to contract more vigorously to stabilize the pelvis, producing an increase in the JRF.[76]

- It increases the overall length of the lower extremity, impacting other components in the kinetic chain. For example, coxa valga decreases the normal physiologic angle at the knee, which places an increased mechanical stress on the medial aspect of the knee joint and more tensile stress on the lateral aspect of the joint.

If the collum angle is reduced, resulting in a more horizontal orientation of the femoral neck, it is known as coxa vara (Fig. 19-15). This position increases the downward shear forces on the femoral head and the tensile stretching forces through the superior trabecular bone along the lateral portion of the neck.[9] In coxa vara, the joint compression forces are significantly reduced as the greater trochanter is displaced lateral and superior, which increases the effective angle of pull and the lever arm of the hip abductors.[79] While the reduced compressive forces generated across the joint surfaces serve to decrease the incidence of articular cartilage damage, the increase in shearing and torsional forces at the femoral head/neck junction significantly increases the incidence of damage to the epiphyseal plate.[9]

Femoral alignment in the transverse plane also influences the mechanics of the hip joint. The *torsion angle* of the femur describes the relative rotation that exists between the shaft and the neck of the femur. Normally, as viewed from above, the femoral neck projects on average 5–15 degrees anterior to a mediolateral axis to the femoral condyles. An anterior orientation of the femoral neck to the transverse axis of the femoral condyles, is known as anteversion (Fig. 19-16), or a reverse orientation known as retroversion.[76,80,81] The normal range for femoral alignment in the transverse plane in adults is 5 degrees of anteversion (Fig. 19-16).[81,82] Typically, an infant is born with about 30 degrees of femoral anteversion.[83,84] This angle usually decreases to 15 degrees by 6 years of age because of bone growth and increased muscle activity. Subjects with excessive anteversion usually have more hip internal rotation ROM than external rotation, and gravitate to the typical "frog-sitting" posture as a position of comfort. There is also associated in-toeing while weight-bearing.[76]

Excessive anteversion directs the femoral head toward the anterior aspect of the acetabulum when the femoral condyles are aligned in their normal orientation. Some studies have supported the hypothesis that a persistent increase in femoral anteversion predisposes to osteoarthritis (OA) of the hip,[79,85–88] and knee,[89–91] although other studies have refuted this.[92–94]

The most stable position of the hip is the normal standing position: hip extension, slight abduction, and slight internal rotation.[15,70,95] The commonly cited open-packed (resting) positions of the hip are between 10 and 30 degrees of flexion, 10–30 degrees of abduction, and 0–5 degrees of external rotation.

When body weight is evenly distributed across both legs during upright standing, the forces acting on the hip joint are equivalent to half the partial weight made up of the trunk, head, and upper extremities.[96] Were this partial body weight to represent 60% of total body mass, then each hip would be compressed by a force equal to 30% of the total body weight. In a

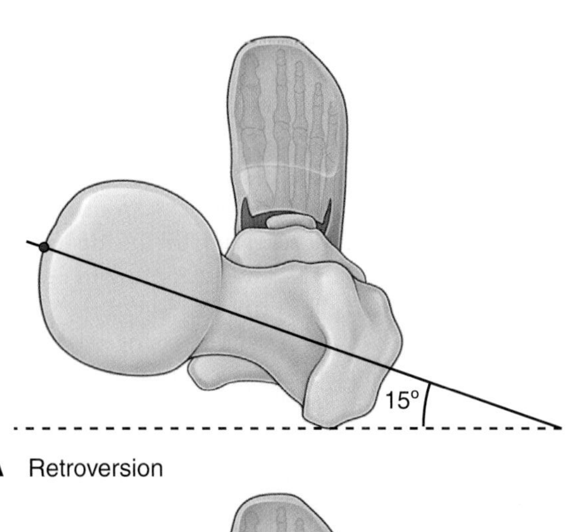

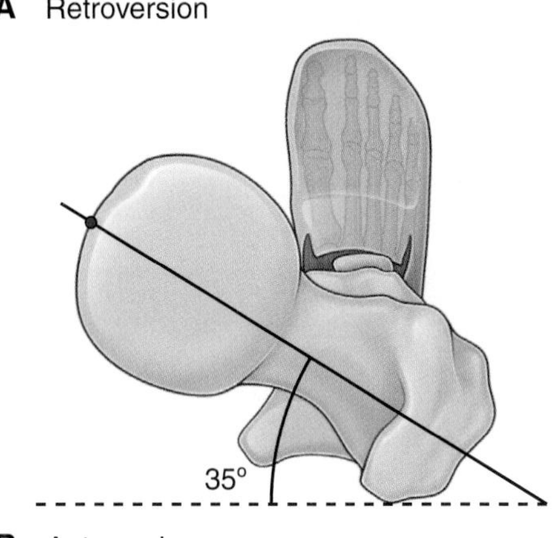

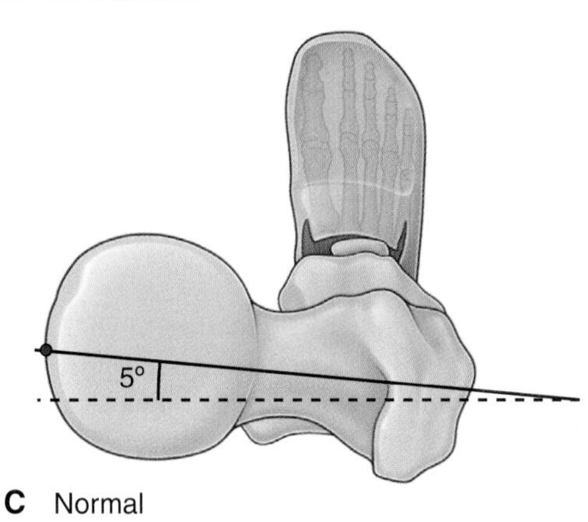

FIGURE 19-16 Angle of torsion: Anteversion and retroversion.

single-limb support, however, shifts in the center of gravity away from the supporting limb dramatically change the equilibrium forces necessary to maintain balance and create a state of disequilibrium. This state of disequilibrium requires the generation of compensatory forces by the hip musculature, in order to maintain balance. The hip joint is the fulcrum for all of the forces. Depending on the length of the moment arm created by the abductor muscles, the added force of the hip abductors acting on the hip joint can increase the pressures translated across the joint to levels exceeding three times body weight.[96]

During ambulation, these compressive joint forces are further multiplied by ground reaction forces and inertial forces related to acceleration and deceleration of the lower limb. Because of muscle tension, compression on the hip is approximately the same as body weight during the swing phase.[97]

However, during the support phase, peak joint forces can range from 300 to 400% of body weight at normal walking speed, to 550% of body weight during fast walking and jogging, and as high as 870% of body weight during stumbling.[32,98] Stair climbing and descending increase the loads on the hip by approximately 10% and 20%, respectively.[32,99] When pain accompanies degeneration of the hip joint articulation, the body compensates by attempting to reduce the forces generated across the articular surfaces. Since the contribution of body mass cannot be changed, the patient attempts to reduce joint pressures by shifting the upper trunk over the supporting limb during the stance phase. While this maneuver decreases the joint compression forces, the energy expended by laterally bending the trunk during stance significantly increases the energy cost of gait. For a patient with a painful hip, the use of a cane or crutch in the hand contralateral to the involved hip can be used to substantially reduce the excessive trunk motion and to decrease pressure on the hip joint.[2]

CLINICAL PEARL

Rapid flexion of the hip is generally associated with abdominal muscle activation that slightly precedes the activation of the hip flexor muscles.[100] This anticipatory activation may reflect a feedforward mechanism intended to stabilize the lumbopelvic region by increasing intra-abdominal pressure and increasing the tension in the thoracolumbar fascia.[101,102] Without sufficient stabilization of the pelvis by the abdominal muscles, a strong contraction of the hip flexor muscles may inadvertently tilt the pelvis anteriorly, thereby accentuating the lumbar lordosis, which may contribute to low back (LB) pain in some individuals.[28]

Bending forward at the waist requires a coordinated sequence of movements between the lumbar spine, pelvis, and hips. As the head and the upper trunk initiate flexion, the pelvis shifts posteriorly to maintain the center of gravity over the base of support. The trunk continues to forward bend, being eccentrically controlled by the extensor muscles of the spine, until approximately 45 degrees at which point the posterior ligaments of the spine become taut, and the facets of the zygapophyseal joints approximate. Once all of the vertebral segments are at the end of the range and stabilized by the posterior ligaments and facets, the pelvis begins to rotate forward (anterior pelvic tilt), being controlled eccentrically by the gluteus maximus and hamstring muscles. The pelvis continues to rotate forward until the full length of the muscles is reached. The return to the upright position begins with the hip extensor muscles rotating the pelvis posteriorly through reverse muscle action, then the back extensor muscles extending the spine from the lumbar region upward.

The hip extensor muscles, as a group, produce the greatest torque across the hip of any of the muscle groups.[103] This extensor torque is often used to rapidly accelerate the body upward and forward from a position of hip flexion, such as when pushing off into a sprint, arising from a deep squat, or climbing a very steep hill.[28] Furthermore, with the hip markedly flexed, many of the adductor muscles produce an extensor torque, thereby assisting the primary hip extensors.[104] With the trunk held relatively stationary, contraction of the hip extensors and abdominal muscles (with the exception of the transversus abdominis) functions as a force couple to posteriorly tilt the pelvis (Fig. 19-17).[28] Assuming the trunk remains upright during this action, the lumbar spine must flex slightly, thereby reducing its natural lordotic posture.[28]

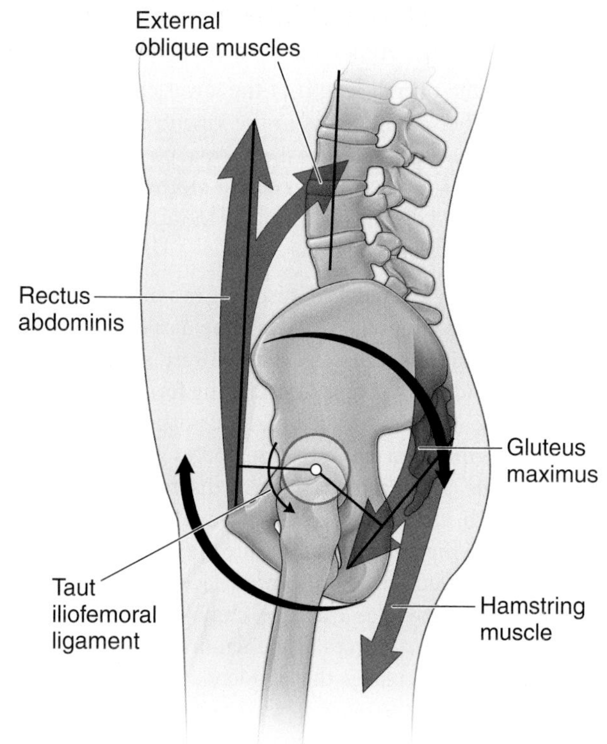

FIGURE 19-17 Force couples at the hip.

The functional potential of the entire external rotator muscle group at the hip is most fully recognized while performing pelvic and trunk rotation activities while bearing weight over one limb. With the right femur held relatively fixed, contraction of the external rotators would rotate the pelvis and the attached trunk to the left. This action of planting the limb and cutting to the opposite side is a natural way to abruptly change direction while running.[28] The gluteus maximus appears uniquely designed to perform this action as, with the right limb securely planted, a strong contraction of the gluteus maximus would, in theory, generate a very effective extension and external rotation torque about the right hip, helping to provide the necessary thrust to the combined-cutting and propulsion action.[28]

In sharp contrast to the external rotators, no muscle with any potential to internally rotate the hip lies even close to the horizontal plane in the anatomic position, making it difficult to assign any muscle as a primary internal rotator of the hip.[28,105] Since the overall orientation of the internal rotator muscles is positioned closer to the vertical and horizontal position, these muscles possess a far greater biomechanical potential to generate torque in the sagittal and frontal planes than in the horizontal plane.[28]

The adductors of the hip are found on the medial aspect of the joint. The primary function of this muscle group is to create an adduction torque bringing the lower extremity toward the midline.[106] This adduction torque can also bring the pubis symphysis region of the pelvis closer to the femur.[106] From the anatomic position, the adductors are also considered hip flexor muscles.

The most frequent demands placed on the hip abductors occur while walking during the single-limb support phase of walking.[28] The external (gravitational) abduction torque about the hip dramatically increases within the frontal plane as soon as the contralateral limb leaves the ground.[107] The hip abductors respond by generating an abduction torque about the stance hip that stabilizes the pelvis relative to the femur.[107] In addition, the hip abductors can hike the hip when working concentrically, and can lower the pelvis when working eccentrically.

According to Cyriax,[108,109] the capsular pattern of the hip is a marked limitation of flexion, abduction, and internal rotation. Kaltenborn[95] considers the capsular pattern of the hip to be extension more limited than flexion, internal rotation more limited than external rotation, and abduction more limited than adduction. Klassbo and colleagues[110] performed a theory-testing, observational, cross-sectional, and descriptive study involving 168 patients (mean age 61.7 years, range 36–90 years), of whom 50 had no hip OA, 77 had unilateral hip OA, and 41 had bilateral OA, based on radiological reports. The purpose of the study was to arrange and describe passive range of motion (PROM) patterns and to count the number of hips presenting with Cyriax's or Kaltenborn's capsular patterns. One examiner tested PROM bilaterally, using a goniometer and a standardized protocol. PROM limitations were calculated by comparing norms from the symptom-free hips ($n = 100$) in the study, from Kaltenborn, and, in patients with unilateral hip OA ($n = 77$), from the non-OA hip. The limitations were arranged by size in PROM patterns. The patterns and the numbers of hips with patterns corresponding to Cyriax's and Kaltenborn's capsular patterns were counted. Between 68 and 138 PROM patterns were identified by the use of different PROM norms for defining limitations. The results from this study showed that few OA hips showed Cyriax's capsular pattern and none demonstrated Kaltenborn's capsular pattern. In addition, it was concluded that it is impossible to anticipate radiological evidence of hip OA from the multitude of PROM patterns. A more useful determination can be made by assessing hip ROM in all planes and, if three planes of motion or more are restricted, OA is likely present.[111]

EXAMINATION

Although injuries of the hip are not as common as injuries to the knee or shoulder, they can create diagnostic and therapeutic challenges, and diseases of the hip can be very disabling. The common pathologies and the interventions for the hip joint are detailed after the examination. Table 19-7 outlines the clinical findings, differential diagnosis, and intervention strategies of some hip conditions, and Table 19-8 describes some of the physical findings for some of the more common causes of hip and thigh pain. An understanding of the pathology and the clinical findings is obviously necessary. Identifying the primary source of the pain is essential if one hopes to provide long-lasting relief of the symptoms. Acute presentations usually have a clear and identifiable cause, whereas in chronic conditions the true etiology may not be as obvious. For example, a protracted hip joint disorder can result in compensations that can develop secondary dysfunctions, which in turn may lead to symptoms such as trochanteric bursitis or chronic gluteal discomfort. As mention of the various pathologies occurs with reference to the examination and vice versa, the reader is encouraged to switch between the two.

CLINICAL PEARL

One study demonstrated that the clinical assessment of the hip can be 98% reliable at detecting the presence of the hip joint problem; although the exam may be poor at defining the exact nature of the intra-articular disorder.[112] However, as many structures can refer pain to the hip and groin region, the symptoms are often both confusing to the patient and challenging to the clinician. For example, hip joint disease may coexist with lumbar spine disease.

History

The importance of history taking cannot be overemphasized as the potential causes of hip pain are numerous (Table 19-9). The history should determine the onset of the symptoms, the mechanism of injury, if any, and the patient's chief complaint. A medical screening questionnaire for the pelvis, hip, and thigh is provided in Table 19-10. It is important for the clinician to determine:

Patient Age. The patient's age may help in the diagnosis. OA of the hip is diagnosed most often in patients over 60 years of age, although it can occur earlier.

Pain Location. The location of the pain can provide the clinician with some useful information (Table 19-12). Complaints of hip or groin pain, morning stiffness, stiffness after sitting, and hip pain with weight-bearing are suggestive of joint involvement, such as OA. It is important to identify patients with symptomatic OA correctly and to exclude conditions that may be mistaken for or coexist with OA.[113,114] Periarticular pain that is not reproduced by passive motion and direct joint palpation suggests an alternate etiology such as bursitis, tendinitis, or periostitis. Groin pain can result from local and referred sources. One of the more common causes of groin pain in the older patient is OA of the hip. However, OA of the hip may also cause pain behind the greater trochanter, anterior thigh, and knee because of the various nerves that cross the hip.[115]

Lateral and posterior hip (buttock) and thigh pain may be referred from the lumbar spine.

Distribution of Symptoms. The distribution of painful joints is helpful to distinguish OA from other types of arthritis because MCP, wrist, elbow, ankle, and shoulder arthritis are unlikely locations for OA except after trauma.

Symptom Fluctuations. The time of day that appears to change the pain for better or worse can provide some clues.

TABLE 19-7 History, Clinical Findings, Differential Diagnosis, and Intervention Strategies of Some Hip Conditions

Diagnosis	Medical Findings	Intervention	Whether to Refer
Legg–Calvé–Perthes disease	Insidious onset (1–3 months) of limp with hip or knee pain	Limited hip abduction, flexion, and internal rotation	Juvenile arthritis and other inflammatory conditions of the hip
Slipped capital femoral epiphysis	Acute (<1 month) or chronic (up to 6 months) presentation; pain may be referred to knee or anterior thigh	Pain and limited internal rotation, leg more comfortable in external rotation; chronic presentation may have leg length discrepancy	Muscle strain and avulsion fracture
Avulsion fracture	Sudden, violent muscle contraction; may hear or feel a "pop"	Pain on passive stretch and active contraction of involved muscle; pain on palpation of involved apophysis	Muscle strain and slipped capital femoral epiphysis
Hip pointer	Direct trauma to iliac crest	Tenderness over iliac crest; may have pain on ambulation and active abduction of hip	Contusion and fracture
Contusion	Direct trauma to soft tissue	Pain on palpation and motion and ecchymosis	Hip pointer, fracture, and myositis ossificans
Myositis ossificans	Contusion with hematoma approximately 2–4 wks earlier	Pain on palpation; firm mass may be palpable	Contusion, soft tissue tumors, and callus formation from prior fracture
Femoral neck stress fracture	Persistent groin discomfort increasing with activity, history of endurance exercise, and female athlete triad (eating disorder, amenorrhea, and osteoporosis)	ROM may be painful, pain on palpation of greater trochanter	Trochanteric bursitis, osteoid osteoma, and muscle strain
Osteoid osteoma	Vague hip pain present at night and increased with activities	Restricted motion and quadriceps atrophy	Femoral neck stress fracture and trochanteric bursitis
Iliotibial band syndrome	Lateral hip, thigh, or knee pain; snapping as iliotibial band passes over the greater trochanter	Positive Ober test	Trochanteric bursitis
Trochanteric bursitis	Pain over greater trochanter on palpation; pain during transitions from standing to lying down to standing	Pain on palpation of greater trochanter	Iliotibial band syndrome and femoral neck stress fracture
Avascular necrosis of the femoral head	Dull ache or throbbing pain in groin, lateral hip, or buttock; history of prolonged steroid use; prior fracture; and slipped femoral capital epiphysis	Pain on ambulation, abduction, and internal and external rotation	Early degenerative joint disease
Piriformis syndrome	Dull posterior pain, may radiate down the leg mimicking radicular symptoms, and history of track competition or prolonged sitting	Pain on active external rotation, passive internal rotation of hip, and palpation of sciatic notch	Nerve root compression and stress fractures
Iliopsoas bursitis	Pain and snapping in medial groin or thigh	Reproduce symptoms with active and passive flexion/extension of hip	Avulsion fracture
Meralgia paresthetica	Pain or paresthesia of anterior or lateral groin and thigh	Abnormal distribution of lateral cutaneous nerve of the thigh on sensory examination	Other causes of peripheral neuropathy
Degenerative arthritis	Progressive pain and stiffness	Reduction in internal rotation early, in all motion later, and pain on ambulation	Inflammatory arthritis

(Continued)

TABLE 19-7 History, Clinical Findings, Differential Diagnosis, and Intervention Strategies of Some Hip Conditions *(Continued)*

Diagnosis	Medical Findings	Intervention	Whether to Refer
Legg–Calvé–Perthes disease	Normal CBC and ESR; plain films positive (early with changes in the epiphysis, later with flattening of the femoral head)	Maintain ROM, and follow position of femoral head in relation to acetabulum radiographically	Orthopaedic surgery if unresolved
Slipped capital femoral epiphysis	Plain films show widening of epiphysis early, later slippage of femur under epiphysis	Non–weight-bearing, and surgical pinning	Urgent orthopaedic surgery with acute, large slips
Avulsion fracture	Plain films; if these are negative, CT or MRI	Rehabilitation program of progressive increase in ROM and strengthening	Orthopaedic surgery of >2-cm displacement
Hip pointer	Plain films if suspect fracture	Rest, ice, NSAIDs, local steroid, and anesthetic injection for severe pain; gradual return to activities with protection of site	PT appropriate
Contusion	Plain films negative	Rest, ice, compression, static stretch, and NSAIDs	PT appropriate
Myositis ossificans	Radiograph or ultrasound examination reveals typical calcified, intramuscular hematoma	Ice, stretching of involved structure, NSAIDs; surgical resection after 1 year if conservative treatment fails	PT appropriate; orthopaedic surgery if resection needed
Femoral neck stress fracture	Plain films may show cortical defects in femoral neck (superior or inferior surface); bone scan, MRI, and CT may also be used if plain films are negative and diagnosis is suspected	Inferior surface fracture; no weight-bearing until evidence of healing (usually 2–4 wks) with gradual return to activities; superior surface fracture: ORIF	Orthopaedic surgery for ORIF
Osteoid osteoma	Plain films; if these are negative and symptoms persist, MRI or CT	Surgical roemoval if unresponsive to medical therapy with aspirin or NSAIDs	Orthopaedic surgery
Iliotibial band syndrome		Modification of activity, footwear; stretching program, ice massage, and NSAIDs	PT appropriate
Trochanteric bursitis	Plain films, bone scan, and MRI negative for bony involvement	Ice, NSAIDs, stretching of iliotibial band, protection from direct trauma, and steroid injection	PT appropriate
Avascular necrosis of the femoral head	Plain films and MRI	Protected weight-bearing, exercises to maximize soft tissue function (strength and support), and total hip replacement	PT trial appropriate; orthopaedic surgery
Piriformis syndrome	EMG studies may be helpful; MRI of lumbar spine, if nerve root compression is suspected	Stretching, NSAIDs, relative rest, and correction of offending activity	PT appropriate
Iliopsoas bursitis	Plain films are negative	Iliopsoas stretching and steroid injection	PT appropriate
Meralgia paresthetica	Nerve conduction velocity testing may be helpful	Avoid external compression of nerve (clothing, equipment, and pannus)	—
Degenerative arthritis	Plain films help with diagnosis and prognosis	Maximizing support and strength of soft tissues, ice, NSAIDs, modification of activities, cane, and total hip replacement	PT trial appropriate; orthopaedic surgery

CBC, complete blood count; CT, computed tomography; EMG, electromyelography; ESR, erythrocyte sedimentation rate; MRI, magnetic resonance imaging; NSAIDs, nonsteroidal anti-inflammatory drugs; ORIF, open reduction with internal fixation; PT, physical therapy; ROM, range of motion.
Data from Adkins SB, Figler RA: Hip pain in athletes. *Am Fam Phys* 61:2109–2118, 2000.

TABLE 19-8 Physical Findings in Some of the More Common Causes of Hip and Thigh Pain

Condition	Description of Findings
Osteoarthritis of the hip	Tenderness over the anterior hip capsule Pain reproduced by passive rotation of the hip Restricted range of motion (rotation is usually first affected) Pain reproduced by Stinchfield's test (see "Special Tests" section) Abductor limp (more severe cases) Functional leg length discrepancy (if abduction contracture has developed)
Meralgia paresthetica	Altered sensation over the anterolateral thigh Symptoms reproduced by pressure or percussion just medial to the anterior–superior iliac spine
Piriformis tendinitis	Tenderness to deep palpation near the hook of the greater trochanter. Pain reproduced by piriformis stretch
Gluteus medius tendinitis	Tenderness just proximal to the greater trochanter Pain reproduced by resisted abduction of the hip
Trochanteric bursitis	Tenderness over the lateral aspect of the greater trochanter Popping or crepitation felt with flexion–extension of the hip (occasionally) Tight iliotibial tract revealed by Ober test (variable)—see "Special Tests" section
Quadriceps strain or contusion	Tenderness and swelling of the involved area of the quadriceps Weakness of quadriceps contraction Restriction of knee flexion, especially when the hip is extended Palpable divot in the quadriceps (more severe strains) Warmth and firmness in quadriceps (impending myositis ossificans)
Hamstring strain	Localized tenderness and swelling at the site of injury Ecchymosis (frequently) Restricted knee extension and straight-leg raising Palpable divot in the injured hamstring (more severe injuries) Abnormal tripod sign

Data from: Martell JM, Reider B: Pelvis, hip and thigh. In: Reider B, ed. *The Orthopaedic Physical Examination.* Philadelphia, PA: WB Saunders, 1999:159–199.

Hip joint pathology is usually associated with stiffness of the hip in the morning on arising. Such pathologies include

- OA of the hip joint;
- rheumatoid arthritis of the hip joint; prolonged morning stiffness (greater than 1 hour) should raise suspicion for this type of inflammatory arthritis;
- avascular necrosis of the femoral head.

Motion Restrictions. The first two motions that are diminished in hip OA are usually hip internal rotation and hip flexion, although as previously discussed, this can vary significantly.[116] A significant decrease or loss of motor function will always necessitate imaging studies to rule out an avulsion fracture, and/or nerve injury (see Chap. 7).

Mechanism of Injury. Patients who present with acute macrotrauma (e.g., falls and motor vehicle accidents) and who report having difficulty moving the hip or bearing weight require radiographs to rule out a fracture and/or dislocation. Falls on the outside of the hip are a common cause of trochanteric bursitis or contusion of the iliac crest (hip pointer). Such an injury may also involve the abdominal and/or gluteal muscles at their attachment sites. When the abdominal muscles are involved, patients may complain of pain with deep inspiration or have difficulty with trunk rotation.[117] Macrotraumatic forces applied along the femur such as those that occur with dashboard injuries and falls on the knee can result in damage to the articular cartilage, an acetabular labrum tear, a pelvic fracture, or a hip subluxation. An immediate loss of movement following direct trauma to this area usually indicates the presence of a hip or pelvic fracture, or a dislocation. Posterior contusions to the gluteus maximus and sciatic nerve can occur from a direct blow to the buttock.[117] In such cases, the patient may complain of pain in the buttocks and of pain, numbness, and/or tingling radiating down the course of the sciatic nerve. Both the athlete and nutritionally compromised individual are at risk of pelvic rami or femoral neck stress fractures. Anterior blows to the thigh can produce quadriceps contusions. These contusions can also result in myositis ossificans. The femoral nerve is fairly well protected and not usually injured. Acute muscle strains in the hip and thigh region, especially of the hamstrings, are usually seen in the athletic individual, most often occurring following a

TABLE 19-9 Potential Causes of Hip Pain	
Type of Pain/Structure Involved	**Cause**
Articular cartilage	Chondral lesion Osteoarthritis
Childhood disorders	Congenital dysplasia Legg–Calvé–Perthes disease Slipped capital femoral epiphysis
Inflammation	Trochanteric bursitis Psoas bursitis Tendinitis Toxic synovitis
Infection	Septic arthritis Osteomyelitis
Labral tear	
Neoplasm	
Neurologic	Local nerve entrapment
Overuse	Stress fractures of the femur Muscle strains Inguinal hernia Femoral hernia
Referred	Lumbar disk pathology Lumbar spine-degenerative joint disease Athletic pubalgia Radiculopathy Piriformis syndrome Sacroiliac joint pathology Genitourinary tract pathology Abdominal wall pathology
Systemic	Rheumatoid arthritis Crohn's disease Psoriasis Reiter's syndrome Systemic lupus erythematosus
Trauma	Soft tissue contusion Fractures of the femoral head Dislocation of the femoral head Avulsion injury Myositis ossificans
Vascular	Avascular necrosis Osteonecrosis

Data from Martin RL, Enseki KR, Draovitch P, et al.: Acetabular labral tears of the hip: Examination and diagnostic challenges. *J Orthop Sports Phys Ther* 36:503–515, 2006.

short sprint, jump kick, fall, or collision.[117] Quadriceps strains, usually involving the rectus femoris, occur in sprinters and kickers. The most frequently strained adductors are the longus and magnus, while hamstring injuries usually involve the biceps femoris.[118–120]

CLINICAL PEARL

Ironically, in general, a history of a significant traumatic event is a good prognostic indicator of a potentially correctable problem,[121] whereas arthritis is an indicator of poor long-term outcomes.[122]

If the patient is unable to recall a specific mechanism, the clinician should suspect a systemic (see "Systems Review" section and Chap. 5) or biomechanical cause. The hip is a region that is prone to overuse injuries. Walking or running can aggravate trochanteric bursitis, ITB friction syndrome, hamstring and adductor strains, or a femoral neck stress fracture. Pain with bursitis is frequently referred along the course of the muscle it underlies and nearby neurologic structures.[117] Obturator internus bursitis can refer pain to the back and buttock or along the course of the sciatic nerve. Subtrochanteric bursitis commonly refers pain to the LB, lateral thigh, knee, and hip.[117] Iliopectineal bursitis can refer pain along the course of the femoral nerve and anterior thigh. Ischiogluteal bursitis can refer pain along the posterior femoral cutaneous or sciatic nerve.[117]

Behavior of Symptoms. Reports of twinges of pain with weight-bearing activities may indicate the presence of a loose body within the joint. Noises in and around the joint can result from many causes so are not particularly diagnostic. One of the more common causes for clicking is a "snapping" hip, especially if the snapping consistently occurs at approximately 45 degrees of hip flexion. This type of snapping hip is thought to be because of the iliopsoas tendon riding over the greater trochanter or anterior acetabulum. The other types of snapping hip are described in the "Interventions" section. If pain is associated with the clicking, it requires further investigation.

CLINICAL PEARL

Mechanical symptoms such as locking, catching, popping, or ones that are sharp stabbing in nature are better prognostic indicators of a correctable problem.[123]

Aggravating or Relieving Factors. Information must be gathered with regard to the activities or positions that appear to aggravate or lessen the symptoms. For example, prolonged sitting on a hard surface may aggravate the ischial bursa, whereas buttock pain with prolonged sitting on a soft surface is more likely to be the result of a lumbar disk lesion. Rising from a seated position can be especially painful and the patient may experience an accompanying catching or sharp stabbing sensation. Entering and exiting an automobile is often difficult, because the hip is in a flexed position along with twisting maneuvers. As the hip is a weight-bearing joint and weight-bearing tends to aggravate articular pathologies, it is very important to gather information concerning the role of weight-bearing in painful activities, particularly whether the patient has pain at rest as well as during weight-bearing, or whether specific weight-bearing activities (e.g., stair climbing and walking) are the cause of increased pain.

TABLE 19-10 Medical Screening Questionnaire for the Pelvis, Hip, and Thigh Region

	Yes	No
Have you recently had a trauma, such as a fall?		
Have you ever had a medical practitioner tell you that you have osteoporosis?		
Have you ever had a medical practitioner tell you that you have a problem with the blood circulation in your hips?		
Are you currently taking steroids or have you been on prolonged steroid therapy?		
Do you have a history of cancer or has a member of your immediate family (i.e., parents or siblings) ever been diagnosed with cancer?		
Have you recently lost weight even though you have not been attempting to eat less or exercise more?		
Have you had a recent change in your bowel functioning such as black stools or blood in your rectum?		
Have you had diarrhea or constipation that has lasted for more than a few days?		
Do you have groin, hip, or thigh aching pain that increases with physical activity, such as walking or running?		

Data from DuVall RE, Godges J: Introduction to physical therapy differential diagnosis: The clinical utility of subjective examination. In: Wilmarth MA, ed. *Medical Screening for the Physical Therapist. Orthopaedic Section Independent Study Course 14.1.1*. La Crosse, WI: Orthopaedic Section, APTA, Inc, 2003:1–44.

Questions about work environment, athletic participation, and other daily and recreational activities help the clinician identify risk factors for cumulative trauma that might not be apparent to the patient.[117] Activities and positions that aggravate and alleviate symptoms should be identified (Table 19-11).

The hip and pelvic areas are also common sites for pain referral (Table 19-12). The differential diagnosis of hip pain is described in Chapter 5. To help determine the symptom distribution, a pain diagram should be completed by the patient (see Chap. 4). Following its completion, the patient should be encouraged to describe the type of symptoms experienced for each of the areas highlighted on the diagram, as well as the motions or positions that increase or decrease the symptoms. Since the lumbar spine can refer symptoms to the hip region, the clinician should always rule out involvement of the lumbar spine before a hip problem is suspected. The most common source of referred pain from the LB includes both neurogenic (nerve root compression) and spondylogenic (facet or sacroiliac joint) causes. Brown and colleagues[124] identified a limp, groin pain, and limited hip internal rotation as signs that significantly predicted a hip problem rather than a lumbar problem.

Finally, the clinician should determine the impact that the patients' condition has on their activities of daily living (ADL).

Systems Review

Referred pain to the hip is common and should be considered in the absence of acute trauma or when symptoms do not clearly originate from the hip. Pain may be referred to the hip region from a number of neuromusculoskeletal sources (see Chap. 5). In addition to those already mentioned, these can include

- pubic symphysis dysfunction;
- sacroiliac joint dysfunction;

TABLE 19-11 Subjective Reports and Possible Diagnoses

Subjective Report	Possible Diagnosis
Pain that is usually worse with sitting on hard surfaces, cycling, and prolonged standing	Ischiogluteal bursitis
Pain with squatting, lying on the involved side, climbing stairs, and walking	Subtrochanteric bursitis
A clicking or popping sound that occurs during running and dancing activities	Snapping hip syndrome
Pain with prolonged sitting, trunk flexion, and coughing/sneezing	Lumbar disk herniation
Pain with activities that involve lumbar extension	Spinal stenosis, spondylolisthesis, or facet syndrome
Pain at night unrelated to movement	Malignancy
Pain with walking, which is relieved with cessation of the activity	Vascular claudication
Pain that appears to be affected by the weather	Arthritic condition or fibromyalgia syndrome
Progressive loss of or change in motor, bowel, bladder, or sexual function	Myelopathy, conus medullaris syndrome, or cauda equinus syndrome

Data from Feinberg JH: Hip pain: Differential diagnosis. *J Back Musculoskeletal Rehabil* 4:154–173, 1994.

TABLE 19-12 Differential Diagnosis for Pain in the Hip or Buttock Area

Pain Distribution	Potential Cause	Pain Distribution	Potential Cause
Groin area	Stress fractures of the pelvis and femur	Groin and inner thigh region	Transient synovitis
	Crystal-induced synovitis (gout)		Infection
	An inguinal/femoral hernia		Loosened prosthesis
	Muscle calcification		Inflamed lymph nodes
	Hip adductor strain		Lower abdominal muscle strain
	Iliopectineal bursitis		Referred pain from viscera or spinal nerve
	Iliopsoas strain or avulsion fracture of the lesser	Pubic area	Sprain of pubic symphysis
		Lateral buttock area	Osteitis pubis
	Trochanter	Anterior and lateral thigh	Abdominal muscle strain
	Arthritis of the hip	Medial thigh	Bladder infection
	Hip arthrosis	Anterior–superior iliac spine	Trochanteric bursitis
	Femoral neck fracture	Iliac crest	Tendinitis of abductors or external rotators
	Osteonecrosis of the femoral head		
	Pubic symphysis dysfunction:		Apophysitis of greater trochanter
	▸ Osteitis pubis		Referred pain from mid or lower lumbar spine
	▸ Osteomyelitis pubis		Thrombosis of gluteal arteries
	▸ Pyogenic arthritis		Strain of quadriceps
	▸ Pubic fracture		Meralgia paresthetica
	▸ Pubic osteolysis		Entrapment of femoral nerve
	▸ Postpartum symphyseal pain		Thrombosis of femoral artery or great saphenous vein
	Sacroiliac joint lesion		
	Tumor		Stress fracture of femur
	Ureteral stone		Referred pain from hip or mid-lumbar spine
	Hernia		
	Inflammatory synovitis (e.g., rheumatoid arthritis, ankylosing spondylitis, and systemic lupus erythematosus)		Strain of adductor muscles
			Entrapment of obturator nerve
			Referred pain from hip or knee
	Subluxation		Apophysitis or sartorius or rectus femoris
	Dislocation		Strain of gluteal, oblique abdominals, tensor fascia, latae, and quadratus lumborum
			Entrapment of iliohypogastric nerve
			Referred pain from upper lumbar spine

Data from Beattie P: The hip. In: Malone TR, McPoil T, Nitz A, eds. *Orthopaedic and Sports Physical Therapy*, 3rd ed. St. Louis, MO: CV Mosby 1996:506.

- lumbar and low thoracic disk degenerative disease,
- lumbar stenosis with neurogenic claudication;
- peripheral nerve entrapments (lateral cutaneous nerve of the thigh);
- myofascial pain syndrome;
- spondyloarthropathy.

Complaints associated with referred pain include

- thigh pain, knee pain, and leg pain with or without hip pain, which may be indicative of lumbar radiculopathy;
- pain that is decreased with walking up stairs, which may indicate the presence of lumbar spine stenosis.

Referred pain is often related to posture and positioning. Other conditions that can refer symptoms to the pelvis, hip, and thigh region in an adult include cancer, pathological fractures of the femoral neck, and osteonecrosis of the femoral head (avascular necrosis). In the child, pain and loss of range at the hip joint should always alert the clinician to the possibility of transient synovitis, Legg–Calvé–Perthes disease, or a slipped femoral capital epiphysis (Table 19-13).

The Cyriax lower quarter scanning examination can be used to screen for the presence of upper or lower motor neuron lesions or the referral of symptoms from the spine (see Chap. 4). Key muscle testing is used to test for neurologic weakness. (see also "Active, Passive, and Resistive Tests" section).

TABLE 19-13 Red Flags for the Pelvis, Hip, and Thigh Region	
Condition	**Red Flags**
Colon cancer	Age over 50 yr Bowel disturbances (e.g., rectal bleeding or black stools) Unexplained weight loss History of colon cancer in immediate family Pain unchanged by positions or movement
Pathological fractures of the femoral neck	Older women (>70 yr) with hip, groin, or thigh pain History of a fall from a standing position Severe, constant pain that is worse with movement A shortened and externally rotated lower extremity
Osteonecrosis of the femoral head (avascular necrosis)	History of long-term corticosteroid use (e.g., in patients with rheumatoid arthritis, systemic lupus erythematosus, or asthma) History of avascular necrosis of the contralateral hip Trauma

Data from: DuVall RE, Godges J: Introduction to physical therapy differential diagnosis: The clinical utility of subjective examination. In: Wilmarth MA, ed. *Medical Screening for the Physical Therapist. Orthopaedic Section Independent Study Course 14.1.1*. La Crosse, WI: Orthopaedic Section, APTA, Inc., 2003:1–44.

Trigger points in patients with myofascial pain syndrome can cause both localized and referred symptoms that often closely resemble the referral patterns of a radiculopathy.[117]

Evidence of intense inflammation on examination suggests infectious or microcrystalline processes such as gout or pseudogout. Weight loss, fatigue, fever, and loss of appetite should be sought out, because these are clues to a systemic illness such as polymyalgia rheumatica, rheumatoid arthritis, lupus, or sepsis.

Examples of viscerogenic referred pain (see Chap. 5) include renal calculi (pain radiates into the groin), ovarian cysts or an ectopic pregnancy (pain radiating into the back or hip, or along the course of the sciatic nerve when there is direct compression), and diverticulitis or inguinal hernias (pain radiating across the abdomen or back or into the groin).[117]

Referred pain to the buttock can be a form of vasculogenic pain (see Chap. 5) and occurs in patients who have vascular claudication from stenosis of the distal aorta or common iliac vessels.[117]

If, following the history and systems review, the clinician is concerned with any signs or symptoms of a visceral, vascular, or systemic disorder, the patient should be referred to the appropriate health-care professional.

Tests and Measures

The hip can be one of the more challenging joints to examine. Unlike the knee or ankle, the joint is not readily palpable, and one must rely on a number of provocative tests and maneuvers to identify intra-articular or bony abnormalities.[117] Even many of the soft tissue structures are difficult to manually identify but can usually be isolated with proper clinical skills.

Observation

The most important aspect of inspection is stance (standing and sitting) and gait. The patient is observed from the front, back, and sides for general alignment of the hip, pelvis, spine, and lower extremities (see Chap. 6). While standing, a slightly flexed position of the involved hip and the ipsilateral knee is a common finding associated with hip pathology. In the seated position, slouching or listing to the uninvolved side avoids extremes of flexion. An antalgic gait may or may not be present depending on the severity of the symptoms.

The clinician observes the hip region, noting any scars, anatomical abnormalities, muscle atrophy, bruising, swelling, etc.

- A localized soft tissue mass or swelling may indicate a bursitis, an acute muscle contusion or tear with a hematoma, an avulsion fracture, myositis ossificans, a tumor, infection, or deep vein thrombosis.[117]
- Asymmetric muscle atrophy is usually an indication of a radiculopathy or peripheral neuropathy, but can also be seen with a tendon rupture.
- An ecchymosis may be seen with contusions, muscle tear, fracture, and patients with a bleeding diathesis.[117]
- Vesicular skin lesions that have a dermatomal distribution may be found in cases of herpes zoster. Café au lait spots greater than 3 cm and greater than six in number are characteristic of neurofibromatosis.
- Skin rashes may be because of secondary psoariatic arthritis, drug reactions, or one of the collagen vascular diseases.
- Obvious joint or bony deformity should raise suspicion of a fracture or dislocation.

Both pain and musculotendinous dysfunction can produce movement and postural dysfunctions at the hip joint.[125] According to Kendall,[126] the ideal alignment of the pelvis is indicated when the ASIS is on the same vertical plane as the symphysis pubis. The degree of pelvic tilt, which is measured as the angle between the horizontal plane and a line connecting the ASIS with the PSIS, varies from 5 to 12 degrees in normal individuals.[127] Both a low ASIS in women and a structurally flat back in men can cause structural variations in pelvic alignment, which can be misinterpreted as acquired postural impairments.[125] According to Sahrmann, all of the following are necessary to indicate the presence of a postural impairment of the hip[125]:

- An increase or decrease in the depth of the normal lumbar curve.
- A marked deviation from the horizontal line between the ASIS and PSIS.
- An increase or decrease in the hip joint angle in the anterior–posterior plane, with neutral knee joint alignment.

The following should be examined[125]:

- The glutei should be symmetrical and well rounded, not hanging loosely. The pelvic crossed syndrome (see Chap. 6) demonstrates weakness and inhibition of the glutei muscles.[128] This syndrome can be easily identified by having the patient perform a partial bridge with single leg support. This maneuver results in cramping of the hamstrings within a few seconds if the pelvic crossed syndrome is present. Atrophy of one buttock cheek compared with the other side may also indicate a superior or inferior gluteal nerve palsy. A balling-up of the gluteal muscle typically indicates a grade III tear of the gluteal muscles. Buttock swelling occurs with the "sign of the buttock."[108]

CLINICAL PEARL

The pelvic crossed syndrome is exhibited by adaptively shortened hip flexors and hamstrings, and inhibited glutei muscles and lumbar erector spinae.

- Swelling over the greater trochanter could indicate trochanteric bursitis.
- Adaptive shortening of the short hip adductors is indicated by a distinct bulk in the muscles of the upper third of the thigh.[128]
- The bulk of the TFL should not be distinct. A visible groove passing down the lateral aspect of the thigh may indicate that the TFL is overused, and both it and the ITB are adaptively shortened.[128]

The architecture and position of the hip joint and lower extremity is observed.

- In acute arthritis and gross osteoarthrosis, the hip joint is usually held in flexion and external rotation. This may be compensated for by an anterior tilt of the pelvis, together with an increased lordosis of the lumbar spine.
- Excessive external rotation of the leg, accompanied with toeing-out, occurs in extreme femoral neck retroversion, or a slipped femoral epiphysis.
- Increased hip flexion in standing can result from weakness or excessive lengthening of the external oblique or rectus abdominis muscles. Increased hip flexion may also be because of a hip flexion contracture.
- Increased hip extension in relaxed standing is indicative of a swayback posture. This is characterized by a posterior pelvic tilt and hyperextension of the knees, and results in a stretch on the anterior joint capsule of the hip and stress on the iliopsoas muscle and tendon.
- Lateral asymmetry in relaxed standing is characterized by a high iliac crest on one side. The difference in height between the two crests must be greater than one-half inch to have clinical significance. Lateral asymmetry may indicate a positive Trendelenburg sign (see "Special Tests" section), which indicates hip-abductor weakness.

Observation of the lower components of the kinetic chain includes

- the degree of genu varum/valgus (see Chap. 20);
- the degree of tibial torsion (see Chap. 20);
- the amount of calcaneal inversion/eversion (see Chap. 21).

Gait. Analysis of both the stance and swing phases of gait is essential (see Chap. 6). Determinants of the stance-phase of gait involve interaction between the pelvis and hip and distal limb joints (knee and ankle)[129,130] The clinician should note whether[70]

- the patient is using an assistive device. If they are, is it fitted at the correct height and do they use it correctly?
- there is a lack of hip motion, particularly extension. A lack of hip extension can have an impact on gait (see Chap. 6).
- there is a lateral horizontal shift of the pelvis and trunk over the stance leg during the swing phase. This may indicate a positive Trendelenburg sign (see "Special Tests" section). Activation of the abductor mechanism on weight-bearing is necessary to stabilize the hip and pelvis and prevent excessive lateral tilting of the pelvis to the contralateral side during the swing phase.
- the ankle alignment is neutral. Increased ankle pronation increases the degree of hip internal rotation which can place greater stress on hip rotators. This can be especially traumatic to those hip rotators that cross bony prominences, increasing the risk of bursitis; conversely, supination causes greater external rotation.

Strong activation of the hip extensors (with the abductors) is necessary at initial contact into early stance, from 30 degrees initial flexion to approximately 10 degrees of extension at terminal stance.[129] If the hip flexors are short or stiff in relation to the abdominal muscles, there may be an exaggeration in the anterior pelvic tilt and increased lumbar extension during this phase.[125]

Joint Loading Tests. Pain on weight-bearing is a common complaint in some patients with hip joint pathology, including rheumatoid arthritis and OA.[70] Depending on the capability of the patient, the following weight-bearing tests may produce pain:

- ***High step.*** The patient places one foot on a chair and then leans onto it (Fig. 19-18). This maneuver flexes the raised hip and extends the other. The test is repeated on the other side. This test gives the clinician an indication as to the range of flexion and extension at the hip.
- ***Unilateral standing.*** The patient stands on one leg (Fig. 19-19). An inability to maintain the pelvis in a horizontal position during unilateral standing is called a positive Trendelenburg (see "Special Tests" section).

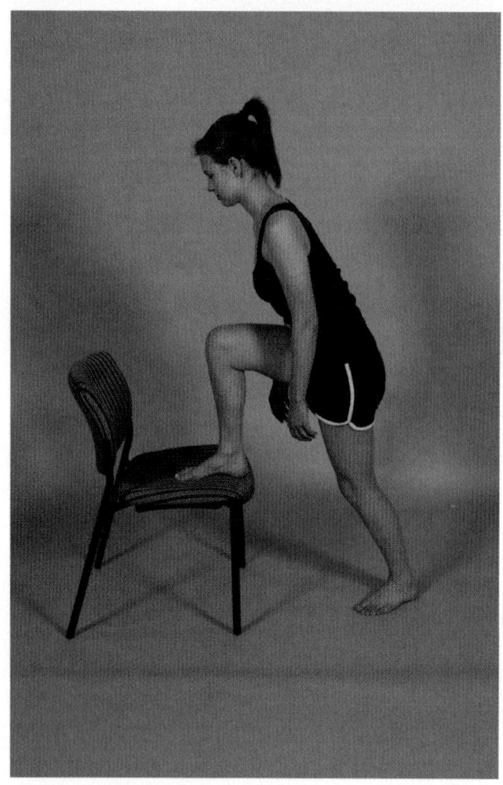

FIGURE 19-18 High step.

Palpation

The palpatory exam is done to identify both anatomic abnormalities and potential sources of symptoms other than from the hip joint itself. Given the location of the hip joint, palpation is usually unrevealing as far as any specific areas of discomfort related to an intra-articular source of hip symptoms. A palpable mass following acute trauma that is not well defined usually indicates a muscle tear, a muscle spasm, or hematoma.[117] A mass that developed 2–3 weeks after the initial injury and is warm and erythematous may be the first indication of myositis ossificans. A bursitis usually presents with some localized swelling, warmth, and erythema, and no history of acute trauma. Trigger points are usually identified as discrete nodules or bands within muscle tissue. There is no associated swelling and no warmth or erythema. Postural or bony malalignment can increase the risk of both acute traumatic and overuse injuries. The anatomic relationships of the joints of the lower extremity should be compared, looking for valgus and varus deformities, pes cavus or planus, spine mobility, hip anteversion, pelvic asymmetry, and leg length discrepancies (see Chap. 29).[117]

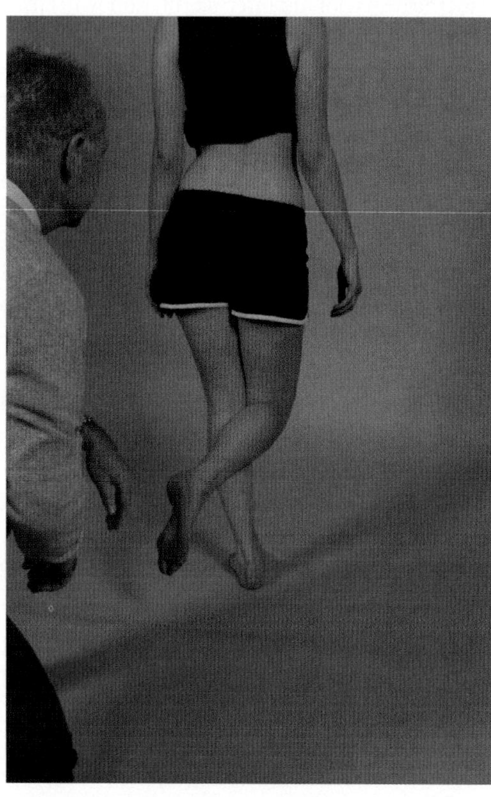

FIGURE 19-19 Trendelenburg sign indicating weakness of the left hip abductors.

Hoppenfeld[131] advocates an approach to palpation that is organized by region. Under this system, the palpation of bony structures occurs separately from the palpation of the soft tissues. While this may be helpful to the clinician, time constraints often dictate that the two are examined concurrently.

CLINICAL PEARL

The following are useful landmarks to use when locating the hip joint center of rotation[18]:

- The midpoint between the ASIS and pubic symphysis, lies over the femoral pulse.
- The superior tip of the greater trochanter is in line with the center of rotation.

Anterior Aspect of Hip and Groin

Anterior–Superior Iliac Spine. The anterior iliac spine serves as the origin for the sartorius muscle and the TFL. Both can be located by flexing and abducting the patient's hip, which produces a groove that resembles an inverted **V** close to the ASIS. The lateral side of the inverted **V** is formed by the TFL, while the medial side is formed by the tendon of the sartorius.

Anterior–Inferior Iliac Spine. The anterior–inferior iliac spine can be palpated in the space formed by the sartorius and the TFL, during passive flexion of the hip in the space known as the *lateral femoral triangle*. The lateral cutaneous nerve of the thigh passes through this triangle. Compression of this nerve produces a condition called *meralgia paresthetica* (see Chap. 5). The AIIS serves as the origin for the rectus femoris tendon.

Pubic Tubercle. The pubic tubercle is located by finding the groin crease and then traveling in an inferomedial direction, or by following the tendon of the adductor longus proximally. In males, the spermatic cord runs directly over the tubercle and can be tender to palpation in normal individuals. Inguinal hernias are usually found superior and medial to the tubercle, while femoral hernias are located lateral to the tubercle.

Adductor Magnus. The adductor magnus is palpable in a small triangle in the distal thigh, posterior to the gracilis muscle and anterior to the semimembranosus.

Rectus Femoris. The rectus femoris has its origin at the AIIS, which is located just distal to the ASIS, between the TFL and sartorius.

Iliopsoas Bursa. At the iliopectineal eminence, the iliopsoas muscle makes an angle of about 30 degrees in a posterolateral direction. To palpate this bursa, the patient is positioned in supine, with the hip being positioned in approximately 40 degrees of flexion and external rotation, and resting on a pillow. At the proximal end of the femur, the clinician palpates the adductor tubercle and then moves to the ASIS. From there, the clinician proceeds to the inguinal ligament, under the fold of the external oblique, and into the femoral triangle. The psoas bursa is located under the floor of the triangle, close to the pubic ramus.

Femoral Triangle. The femoral artery lies superficial and medial to the iliopsoas muscle and is easily located by palpation of the pulse. The femoral nerve is the most lateral structure in the femoral triangle. To examine the femoral triangle, the patient is positioned in supine and, if it is possible for the patient to do this, the heel of the leg is placed upon the opposite knee. This places the patient in a position of flexion–abduction and external rotation.

Inguinal Ligament. The inguinal ligament is located in the fold of the groin, running from the ASIS to the pubic tubercle. It can be located by using transverse palpation.

Adductor Longus. Together with the gracilis, the adductor longus forms the medial border of the femoral triangle. The gracilis is located medial and posterior to the adductor longus. The adductor longus is best viewed during resisted adduction, when it forms a cord-like structure just distal to the pubic tubercle, before crossing under the sartorius. It is often tender in dancers, cheerleaders, and others who perform strenuous activities requiring abduction at the hip.

Lateral Aspect of the Hip. The patient is positioned in side lying.

Iliac Crest. The iliac crest is easy to locate. The cluneal nerves are superficial structures and can be located just superior to the crest.

Greater Trochanter. The superior border of the greater trochanter represents the transverse axis of hip, and when the leg is abducted, an obvious depression appears above the greater trochanter. The gluteus medius inserts into the upper portion of the trochanter and can be palpated on the lateral aspect.[132]

Palpation of the greater trochanter is also used to assess the angle of anteversion and retroversion using the Craig test (see "Special Tests" section).

Lesser Trochanter. The lesser trochanter, covered as it is with the iliopsoas and adductor magnus, is very difficult to palpate directly, but it can be located on the posterior aspect if the hip is placed in extension and internal rotation, and the palpation is performed deeply lateral to the ischial tuberosity.

Piriformis Attachment. The origin of the piriformis can be found on the medial aspect of the superior point of the greater trochanter. Moving inferiorly from this point and the quadratus femoris located on the quadrate tubercle, the following tendon insertions can be palpated: superior gemellus, obturator internus, and inferior gemellus.

Psoas. The insertion for the psoas is located on the inferior aspect of the greater trochanter and can be found by placing the patient's hip in maximum internal rotation. Once the superior aspect of the greater trochanter is located, the clinician moves in a posterior/medial/inferior direction to locate the inferior aspect of the greater trochanter.

Subtrochanteric Bursa. The subtrochanteric bursa cannot be palpated directly. However, it can be tested by positioning the patient's leg in hyperadduction. At this point, the patient is asked to abduct the hip isometrically against the clinician's resistance. The contraction of the hip abductors compresses the bursa and may cause pain if the bursa is inflamed.

Posterior Aspect of the Hip. The patient is positioned in side lying or prone.

Quadratus Lumborum. Palpation of the quadratus lumborum is best accomplished with the patient in side lying, with the arm abducted overhead to open the space between the iliac crest and the 12th rib.

Ischial Tuberosity. A number of structures have their attachments on the ischial tuberosity. These include the ischial bursa, the semimembranosus tendon, the sacrotuberous ligament, the biceps femoris and semitendinosus tendons, and the tendons of the quadratus femoris, adductor magnus, and inferior gemellus. The ischial tuberosity is best palpated in the side lying position with the hip flexed to 90 degrees (see Chap. 29). This position moves the gluteus maximus upward, permitting direct palpation at the tuberosity. The *ischial bursa* is located on the inferior and medial aspect of the ischial tuberosity. A diagnosis of ischial bursitis is usually based on a history of pain with sitting on a hard surface and finding tenderness with palpation of the ischial tuberosity.

Sciatic Nerve. One of the most important structures to palpate in this area is the sciatic nerve. It can be located for palpation at a point halfway between the greater trochanter and ischial tuberosity. Tenderness of this nerve can be produced by a piriformis muscle spasm or by direct trauma.

Active, Passive, and Resistive Tests

The clinical procedures for performing ROM measurements vary, and disagreement exists about the accuracy of visual estimates compared to goniometer measurements. A study by Holm and colleagues[133] comprising 25 patients (6 M, 19 F; mean age 68.5 years, range 46–76 years) with osteoarthrosis of the hip, verified both clinically and radiologically, examined the reliability of goniometric measurements and visual estimates of hip ROM. Hip ROM measurements (abduction VIDEO, adduction VIDEO, extension VIDEO, flexion VIDEO, and internal VIDEO/external rotation VIDEO) were recorded by four different teams on the same day and were repeated 1 week later. Teams 1, 2, and 3 consisted of physiotherapists using standardized goniometric measurements. Team 4 involved an experienced orthopaedic surgeon making the assessments from visual estimates only. With the exception of abduction ($p = 0.03$), there were no significant differences between the measurements recorded on the first and second occasions for the same teams. The coefficient of variance was 5.5% for flexion (lowest) and 26.1% for extension (highest). Reproducibility was best for flexion. There was also high reliability when all the arcs of motion were summed up (abduction + adduction + extension + flexion + internal/external rotation). With the exception of internal rotation, there were highly significant differences between the teams when two people performed the measurements compared to the values measured by a single individual.

Concordance, expressed as the standardized agreement index, between visual estimates made by one individual (the orthopaedic surgeon) and goniometric measurements made by two experienced physiotherapists, was 0.77–0.83, which indicates good agreement.

Bierma-Zeinstra and colleagues[134] performed a study to compare the reliability of measurements of hip motions obtained with two instruments, an electronic inclinometer and a two-arm goniometer, and to investigate whether the two instruments, and different body positions, produce the same measurement data. Maximal active and passive hip movements were measured simultaneously with both instruments, in nine subjects during 10 consecutive measurements at short intervals. The results from the study demonstrated the following[134]:

- The intraobserver variability was lower with the inclinometer in measurements of passive hip rotations.
- The two instruments showed equal intraobserver variability for hip movements in general.
- The inclinometer showed lower interobserver variability in the measurements of active internal rotation.
- More rotational movement was measured with the two-arm goniometer and more extension and flexion with the inclinometer. Also, more rotational movement was found in the prone position compared to the sitting and supine positions.

The study concluded that the inclinometer is more reliable in measurements of hip rotation; for hip movements, in general, the two-arm goniometer is just as accurate when used by only one observer; and the two instruments, and some positions, are not interchangeable during consecutive measurements.[134]

During the examination of the ROM, the clinician should note which portions of the ROM are pain free and which portion causes the patient to feel pain. An assessment of the lumbopelvic rhythm can alert the clinician to the primary area of a particular limitation. During normal forward bending, the patient should be able to touch their toes without bending the knees and with a flattening of the lordosis (Fig. 19-20). However, if the hamstrings are adaptively shortened, toe touching, cannot be accomplished even with a flattening of the lordosis. If the tightness is located in the LB, as the patient bends forward, no flattening of the lordosis occurs, and the patient is unable to touch the toes even with good hamstring flexibility.

The capsular pattern of the hip appears variable and is an unreliable method for determining the presence of OA when used alone,[110] Twinges of pain with active motions may indicate the presence of a loose body within the joint. At the end of available AROM, passive overpressure is applied to determine the end-feel. The normal ranges and end-feels for the various hip motions are outlined in Table 19-5. Abnormal end-feels common in the hip include a firm capsular end-feel before expected end range; empty end-feel from severe pain, as in the sign of the buttock; and bony block in cases of advanced OA.[18] Horizontal abduction and adduction of the femur occur when the hip is in 90 degrees of flexion. Since these actions require the simultaneous, coordinated actions of several muscles, they can be used to assess the overall strength of the hip muscles.

Resisted testing of the muscles that cross the hip joint (Table 19-4) is performed to provide the clinician with information

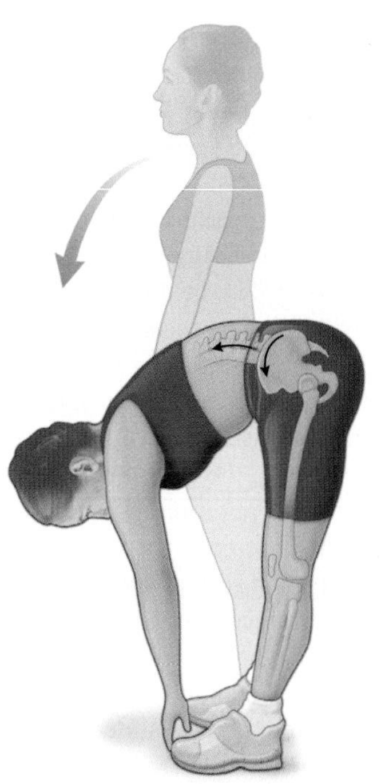

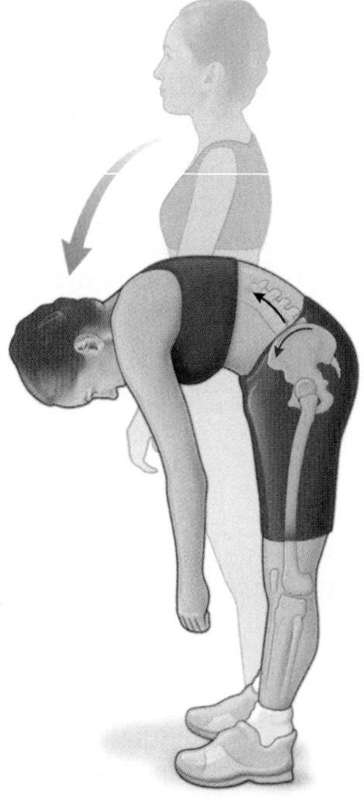

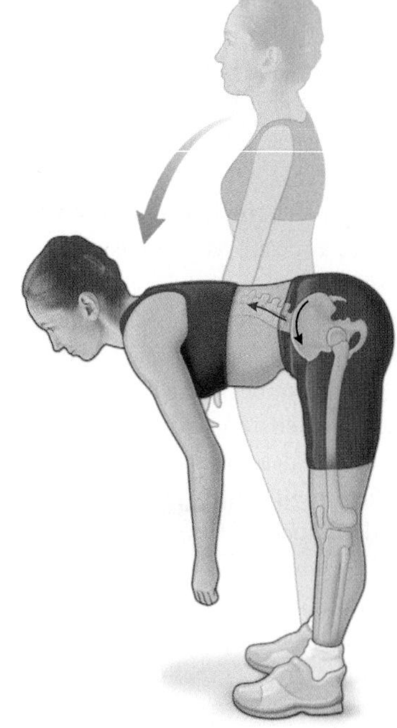

FIGURE 19-20 Lumbopelvic rhythm.

about the integrity of the neuromuscular unit, and to highlight the presence of muscle strains (see "Systems Review" section).[131]

If the history indicates that repetitive motions or sustained positions cause the symptoms, the clinician should have the patient reproduce these motions or positions.[135]

CLINICAL PEARL

In the child, pain and loss of range at the hip joint should always alert the clinician to the possibility of transient synovitis, Legg–Calvé–Perthes disease, or a slipped femoral capital epiphysis (see Chap. 30).

In addition to reports of pain and overall ROM, the clinician also notes information about weakness, joint end-feel, palpation of the moving joint, and muscle tightness.

Flexion. The six muscles primarily responsible for hip flexion are the iliacus, psoas major, pectineus, rectus femoris, sartorius, and TFL (Table 19-4). The primary hip flexor is the iliopsoas muscle.

Hip flexion motion can be tested in sitting or supine, first with the knee flexed (Fig. 19-21) and then with the knee extended. With the hip flexed, the ROM should be approximately 110–120 degrees. More hip flexion should be available with the knee flexed.

Resisted tests are then performed.

- To test the strength of the iliopsoas, the patient is seated with the thigh raised off the bed and resistance is applied by the clinician VIDEO.
- The action of the sartorius muscle, which flexes, abducts, and externally rotates the hip, is tested by asking the patient to bring the plantar aspect of the foot toward the opposite knee VIDEO. The clinician applies resistance at the medial malleolus and at the lateral aspect of the thigh to resist flexion, abduction, and external rotation.

A painless weakness of hip flexion is rarely a good sign. Although it may indicate a disk protrusion at the L1 or L2 level, these protrusions are not common. A more likely scenario is compression of the nerves by a neurofibroma or a metastatic invasion. Pain with the active motion or resisted tests should prompt the clinician to examine the contractile tissues individually. Passive stretching can also produce pain in a contractile structure.

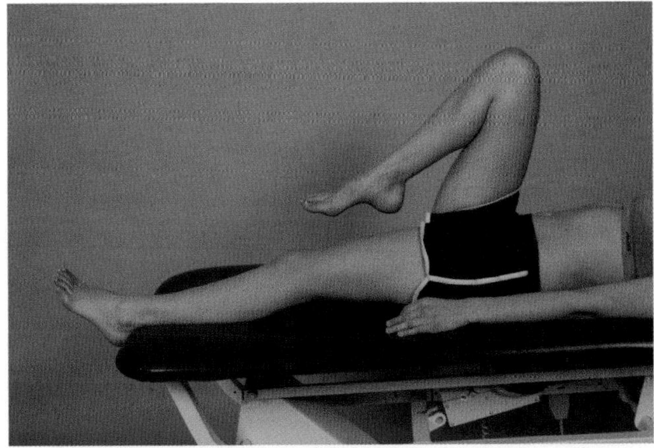

FIGURE 19-21 Hip flexion with knee flexed.

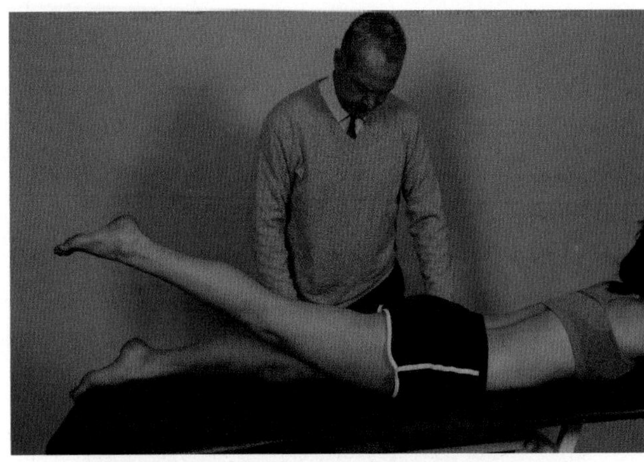

FIGURE 19-22 Hip extension.

Extension. The primary hip extensor is the gluteus maximus (Table 19-4). The hamstrings also serve as hip extensors. Hip extension also involves assistance from the adductor magnus, gluteus medius and minimus, and indirect assistance from the abdominals and the erector spinae.[136]

The patient is positioned in prone or over the end of a table. As the clinician monitors motion at the pelvis to ensure the lumbar spine does not extend, the patient is asked to lift the thigh toward the ceiling (Fig. 19-22). With a normal recruitment pattern, the order of firing should be gluteus maximus, opposite erector spinae, and then the ipsilateral erector spinae and hamstrings.[128] Poor recruitment patterns are demonstrated as follows:

1. An initial activation of the hamstrings and erector spinae with a delayed contraction of the gluteus maximus. The biceps femoris has a tendency to become shortened and overactive, resulting in delayed activation of the gluteus maximus.[137]
2. The erector spinae initiate the movement with a delayed activity of the gluteus maximus. This would lead to little, if any, extension of the hip joint, as the leg lift would be achieved by an anterior pelvic tilt and a hyperextension of the lumbar spine. This is a very poor movement pattern.

The normal ROM for hip extension is approximately 10–15 degrees. Reduced hip extension with the knee flexed can be the result of a number of reasons, including

- adaptive shortening of the iliopsoas, characterized by an increased lumbar lordosis, an externally rotated lower extremity, and a noticeable groove in the ITB in standing[138];
- a hip flexion contracture.

As before, the pelvis is monitored, and the patient is asked to raise the thigh off the table. The strength of the gluteus maximus is tested with the knee flexed (Fig. 19-23) VIDEO. The role of the hamstrings at the hip can be tested with the knee extended. By observing the patient's shoulder during this test, the recruitment pattern can be analyzed.

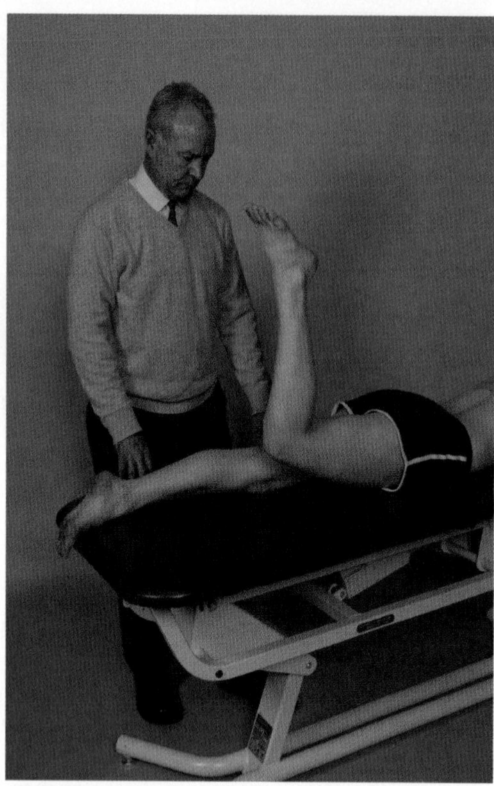

FIGURE 19-23 Hip extension with knee flexed.

The opposite shoulder should be seen to rise off the bed. With the abnormal pattern, the same shoulder rises off the bed. Patients who use this abnormal recruitment pattern will often have well-developed thoracic musculature on the posterior aspect and, as a result, develop problems at the thoracolumbar junction.[128]

Resistance is then applied by the clinician. A strong and painful finding with resisted hip extension may indicate a grade I muscle strain of the gluteus maximus or hamstrings. It may also indicate a gluteal bursitis or a lumbosacral strain. The strength of the medial and lateral hamstrings is also tested using resisted knee flexion, with the patient positioned in prone (see Chap. 20).

CLINICAL PEARL

Although hip extensor strength in the elderly has been identified as the primary predictor of walking ability, physical performance and balance, assessment of hip extensor strength in this population is commonly overlooked, as the presence of pain, contractures, and reduced mobility often limits the ability of the elderly patient with hip or spine impairment to adopt the prone position.[71] In these situations, the clinician should modify the testing position to accommodate the patient (e.g., have the patient lean over a table).

Abduction/Adduction. Hip adduction (Fig. 19-24) and abduction (Fig. 19-25) ROM can be tested in supine or side-lying making sure that both ASIS are level, and the legs are perpendicular to a line joining the ASIS.

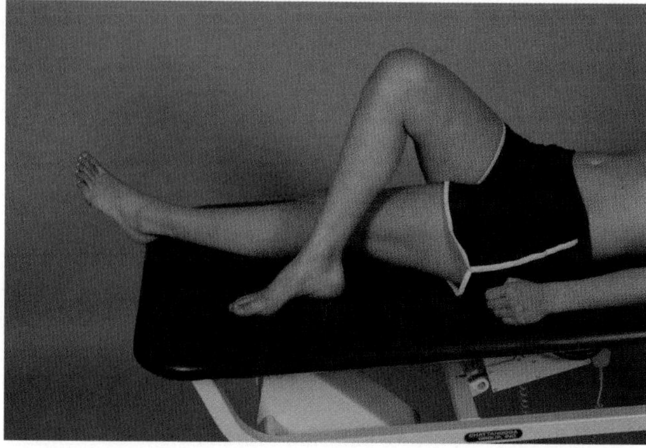

FIGURE 19-24 Hip adduction ROM using anti-gravity position.

Abduction. The clinician monitors the ipsilateral ASIS, and the patient is asked to abduct the leg. The abduction motion is stopped when the ASIS is felt to move. The prime movers for this movement are the gluteus medius/minimus and the TFL. The quadratus lumborum functions as the stabilizer of the pelvis. The strength of the gluteus medius and minimus can be tested against gravity in the sidelying position VIDEO. The patient is asked to perform hip abduction of the uppermost leg without any flexion or external rotation occurring (Fig. 19-25). The clinician applies resistance to the distal thigh.

The correct sequence of firing for hip abduction in side lying should be gluteus medius, followed by the quadratus lumborum and TFL after approximately 15 degrees of hip abduction. Altered patterning demonstrates the following:

1. External rotation of the leg during the upward movement, indicating an initiation and dominance of the movement by the TFL, accompanied by a weakness of the gluteus medius/minimus. The TFL has a tendency to become shortened and overactive.[137]
2. Full external rotation of the leg occurs during the leg lift, indicating a substitution of hip flexion and iliopsoas activity for the true abduction movement. If the piriformis is shortened and overactive, the external rotation of the leg is reinforced.[137]

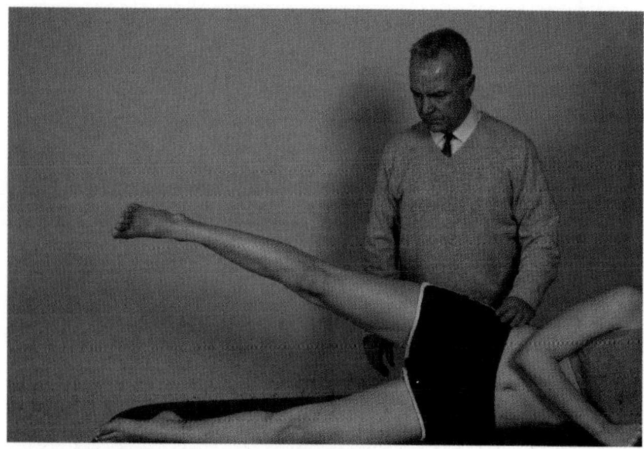

FIGURE 19-25 Hip abduction ROM.

3. A lateral pelvic tilt at the initiation of movement, indicating that the quadratus lumborum, which has a tendency to become shortened and overactive, is both stabilizing the pelvis and initiating the movement.[137] This is indicative of a very poor movement pattern.

Adduction. Hip adduction is tested with the patient supine and with the uninvolved leg adducted over the other leg or held in flexion (Fig. 19-24). As before, the ASIS is monitored for motion, indicating the end of range for adduction. The primary hip adductor is the adductor longus. Adaptive shortening of the hip adductors can theoretically result in inhibition of the gluteus medius, a decrease in frontal stability, ITB tendinitis, and anterior knee pain. Pain can be referred from the hip adductors into the anterolateral hip, groin, medial thigh, the anterior knee, and medial tibia. Pain in these regions with passive abduction, or active adduction, may indicate a strain of one of the adductors. The cause of the pain can be differentiated between the two-joint gracilis and the other hip adductors (longus, brevis, and pectineus) in the following manner. The patient is positioned in supine, with the tested leg over the edge of the table, monitored by the clinician. The clinician places the involved hip into the fully abducted position and the knee is flexed (Fig. 19-26). If no pain is reproduced with this maneuver, the patient is asked to extend the knee (Fig. 19-27), thereby bringing in the gracilis and implicating it if the pain is now reproduced. This can be confirmed with resisted hip adduction and knee flexion. If the other adductors are implicated, this can be confirmed with resisted adduction (longus and brevis) or resisted hip adduction and hip flexion (pectineus).

The strength of the hip-adductor muscle group can also be tested in side lying VIDEO, by flexing the uninvolved leg over the tested leg or by supporting the upper leg and then applying resistance. This position also stretches the hip abductors and can be a source of pain in the case of an ITB syndrome.

A strong and painful finding with resisted adduction is usually the result of an adductor longus lesion, whereas a painless weakness with resisted abduction is often found in a palsy of the fifth lumbar root because of a disk herniation of the same level.

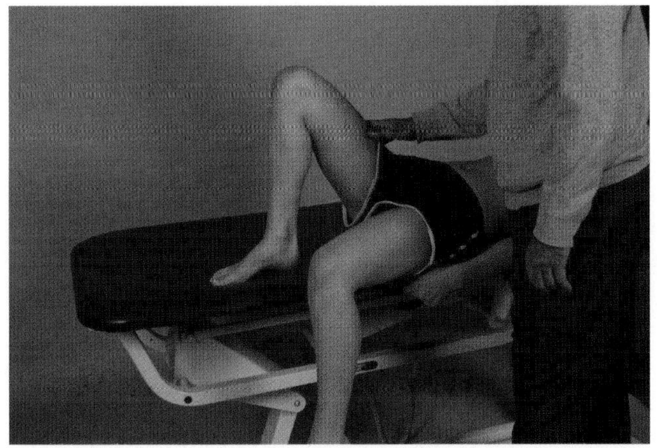

FIGURE 19-26 Differentiating hip-adductor muscles—knee flexed.

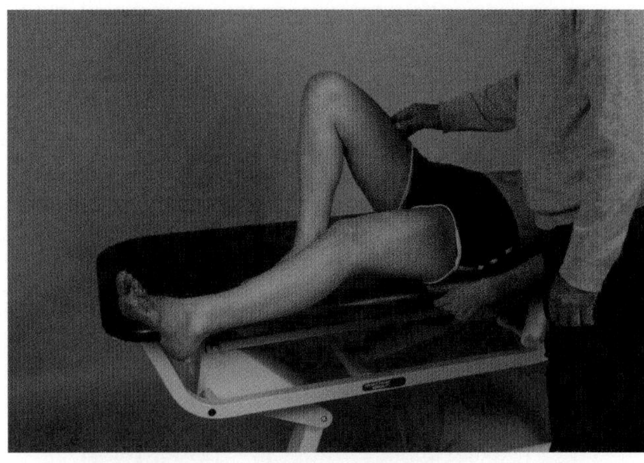

FIGURE 19-27 Differentiating hip-adductor muscles—knee extended.

Internal and External Rotation. Although a number of muscles contribute to external rotation of the femur (see Table 19-4), six muscles function solely as external rotators.[32] These are the piriformis, gemellus superior, gemellus inferior, obturator internus, obturator externus, and quadratus femoris. Normal ROM for hip external rotation is approximately 40–60 degrees. Excessive external rotation of the hip may indicate hip retroversion.

The major internal rotator of the femur is the gluteus minimus, assisted by the gluteus medius, TFL, semitendinosus, and semimembranosus. The internal rotators of the femur are estimated to be only approximately one-third the strength of the external rotators.[96] Normal ROM for hip internal rotation is approximately 30–40 degrees. Excessive internal rotation of the hip may indicate hip anteversion.

If an asymmetry exists between the two positions such that more ROM is available in the prone position compared with supine, a muscle restriction is likely present.[139] When the asymmetry of internal rotation ROM is much greater than the external rotation range in both the hip flexed and hip extended positions, structural anteversion may be present.[139] If retroversion is present, the range of external rotation is greater than the range of internal rotation in both the flexed and extended positions of the hip.[139]

To assess the ROM of the hip rotators, the patient is positioned in supine, with the leg in 90 degrees of hip flexion and 90 degrees of knee flexion. Hip IR (Fig. 19-28) and ER (Fig. 19-29) is then assessed. Alternatively, the patient can be positioned in prone, with the knee flexed to 90 degrees and the hip in neutral. Once the ROM measurements have been established, the strength of the internal rotators VIDEO and external rotators VIDEO is then assessed.

Functional Assessment

In addition to gait analysis, the function of the hip can be assessed through observation during functional activities such as sit to stand, or through use of a self-report measure, which allow a patient to rate his or her capacity to perform ADL. Table 19-14 outlines a functional assessment tool for the hip.

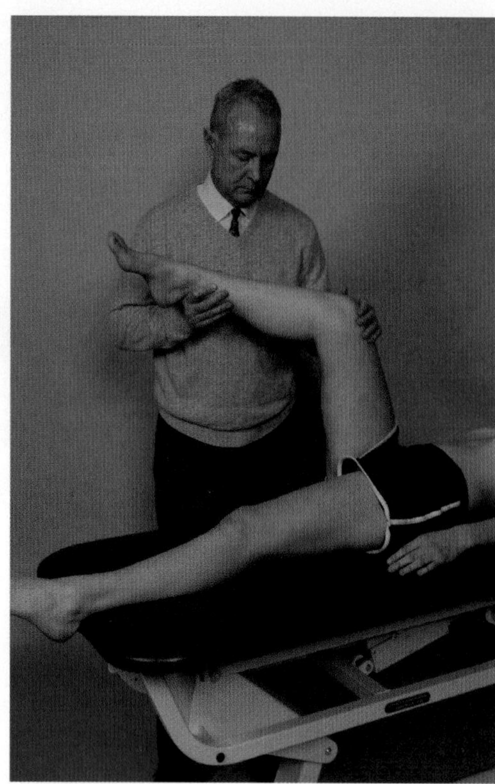

FIGURE 19-28 Supine hip IR.

The Harris Hip Rating Scale (Table 19-15) is the most commonly used functional outcome assessment for the hip and can be used to assess patient status following the onset of traumatic arthritis, and a variety of hip disorders.

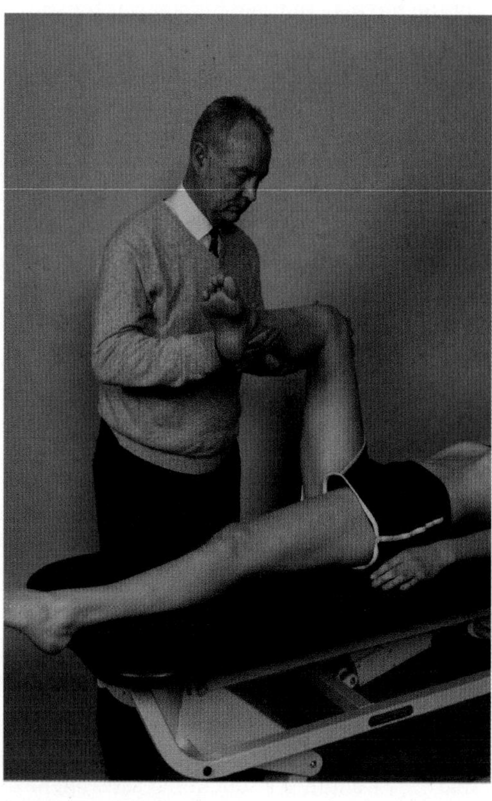

FIGURE 19-29 Supine hip ER.

Examination of Movement Patterns

Some of the movement patterns were assessed in the "Active, Passive, and Resistive Tests" section. One further test is described here.

Trunk Curl Up. This test assesses the patient's ability to sit up from a supine position and the relationship between the abdominal and iliopsoas muscles. The patient is positioned

TABLE 19-14 Functional Tests of the Hip

Starting Position	Action	Functional Test
Standing	Hip flexion: lift foot onto an 8-inch/20-cm step and return	5–6 repetitions: functional 3–4 repetitions: functionally fair 1–2 repetitions: functionally poor Zero repetitions: nonfunctional
Standing	Hip extension: sit in a chair and return to standing	5–6 repetitions: functional 3–4 repetitions: functionally fair 1–2 repetitions: functionally poor Zero repetitions: nonfunctional
Standing	Hip abductors: lift leg to the articular surfaces balance on one leg while keeping pelvis level	Hold 1–1.5 min: functional Hold 30–59 s: functionally fair Hold 1–29 s: functionally poor Cannot hold: nonfunctional
Standing	Hip adductors: walk sideways 6 m	6–8 m one way: functional 3–6 m one way: functionally fair 1–3 m one way: functionally poor 0 m: nonfunctional
Standing	Hip internal rotation: test leg off floor (holding onto object for balance if necessary), internally rotate non–weight-bearing hip	10–12 repetitions: functional 5–9 repetitions: functionally fair 1–4 repetitions: functionally poor Zero repetitions: nonfunctional
Standing, facing closed door	Hip external rotation: test leg off floor (holding onto object for balance if necessary), externally rotate non–weight-bearing hip	10–12 repetitions: functional 5–9 repetitions: functionally fair 1–4 repetitions: functionally poor Zero repetitions: nonfunctional

Data from Palmer ML, Epler M: *Clinical Assessment Procedures in Physical Therapy*. Philadelphia: JB Lippincott, 1990.

TABLE 19-15	Harris Hip Rating Scale

Harris Hip Function Scale

(Circle one in each group)

Pain (44 points maximum)

None/ignores	44
Slight, occasional, no compromise in activity	40
Mild, no effect on ordinary activity, pain after unusual activity, uses aspirin	30
Moderate, tolerable, makes concessions, occasional codeine	20
Marked, serious limitations	10
Totally disabled	0

Function (47 points maximum)

Gait (walking maximum distance) (33 points maximum)

1. Limp:	
None	11
Slight	8
Moderate	5
Unable to walk	0
2. Support:	
None	11
Cane, long walks	7
Cane, full time	5
Crutch	4
Two canes	2
Two crutches	0
Unable to walk	0
3. Distance walked:	
Unlimited	11
Six blocks	8
Two to three blocks	5
Indoors only	2
Bed and chair	0

Functional activities (14 points maximum)

1. Stairs:	
Normally	4
Normally with banister	2
Any method	1
Not able	0
2. Socks and tie shoes:	
With ease	4
With difficulty	2
Unable	0
3. Sitting:	
Any chair, 1 h	5
High chair, $\frac{1}{2}$ h	3
Unable to sit $\frac{1}{2}$ h any chair	0
4. Enter public transport:	
Able to use public transportation	1
Not able to use public transportation	0

Absence of deformity (requires all four) (four points maximum)

1. Fixed adduction <10 degrees	4
2. Fixed internal rotation in extension <10 degrees	0
3. Leg length discrepancy less than $1\frac{1}{4}$"	
4. Pelvic flexion contracture <30 degrees	

Range of motion (five points maximum)

Instructions

Record 10 degrees of fixed adduction as "–10 degrees abduction, adduction to 10 degrees"

Similarly, 10 degrees of fixed external rotation as "–10 degrees internal rotation, external rotation to 10 degrees"

Similarly, 10 degrees of fixed external rotation with 10 degrees further external rotation as "–10 degrees internal rotation, external rotation to 20 degrees"

Permanent flexion (1)_____	Range	Index Factor	Index Value*
A. Flexion to	_____ degrees		
(0–45 degrees)		1.0	
(45–90 degrees)		0.6	
(90–120 degrees)		0.3	
(120–140 degrees)		0.0	
B. Abduction to	_____ degrees		
(0–15 degrees)		0.8	
(15–30 degrees)		0.3	
(30–60 degrees)		0.0	
C. Adduction to	_____ degrees		
(0–15 degrees)		0.2	
(15–60 degrees)		0.0	
D. External rotation in extension to	degrees		
(0–30 degrees)		0.4	
(30–60 degrees)		0.0	
E. Internal rotation in extension to	_____ degrees		
(0–60 degrees)		0.0	

*Index Value = Range × Index Factor

Total index value (A + B + C + D + E)__

Total range of motion points___

(multiply total index value × 0.05)

Pain points: ___

Function points: ___

Absence of deformity points: ____

Range-of-motion points: ___

Total points: ____

(100 points maximum)

Comments:

Data from Harris WH: Traumatic arthritis of the hip after dislocation and acetabular fractures. Treatment by mold arthroplasty: An end-result study using a new method of result evaluation. *J Bone Joint Surg* 51:737–755, 1969.

in supine with the hips and knees flexed, both feet flat on the bed.

The patient is then asked to perform a sit-up while actively plantar flexing their ankles, thus removing the effect of the iliopsoas.[136] The patient progressively flexes the spine, starting at the cervical region, until the lumbar region is flexed. As soon as the iliopsoas becomes involved in the motion, the patient's feet will lift from the bed. Normally, the patient should be able to curl up so that the thoracic and lumbar spines are clear of the bed before the feet lift. A patient in excellent condition can complete a full sit-up without the feet lifting from the bed.

Passive Accessory Movements

Because of the extreme congruency of the joint partners at the hip joint, this is a difficult area to assess with any degree of accuracy, especially as the glides that occur are very slight. Unless otherwise indicated, the patient is positioned supine with the hip in its resting position. The clinician can wrap a belt around the patient's pelvis and the treatment table to help stabilize the pelvis.

Distraction. A joint distraction can be used to assess for pain and any hypomobility at the hip joint. The patient's thigh is grasped by the clinician as proximal as possible, and a distraction force is applied along the line of the femoral neck (see Fig. 19-30).

Leg Traction. The clinician grasps the patient's ankle and applies a longitudinal force along the length of the leg (Fig. 19-31).

Posterior Glide. The clinician stands on the medial side of the patient's thigh. A belt can be placed around the clinician's shoulder and under the patient's thigh, to help hold the weight of the lower extremity. The clinician places one hand on the distal thigh of the patient and the other hand on the anterior surface of the patient's proximal thigh (Fig. 19-32). Keeping the elbows extended and flexing the knees, the clinician applies a force through the patient's hip in a posterior direction (Fig. 19-32).

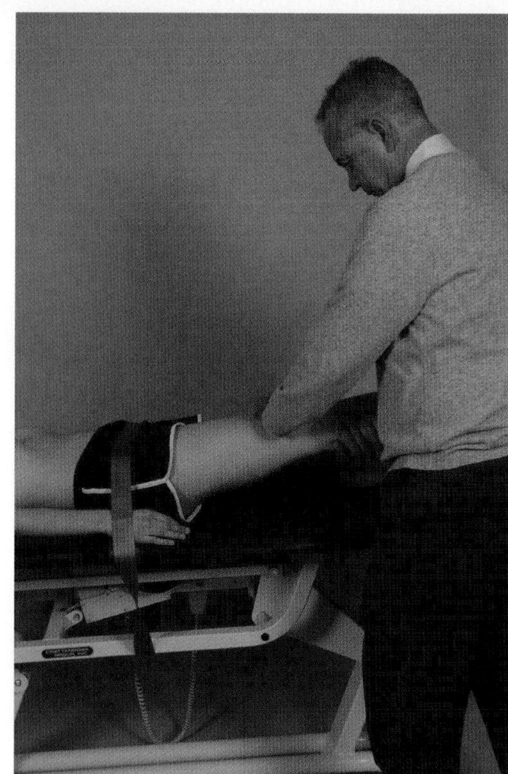

FIGURE 19-31 Leg traction for hip.

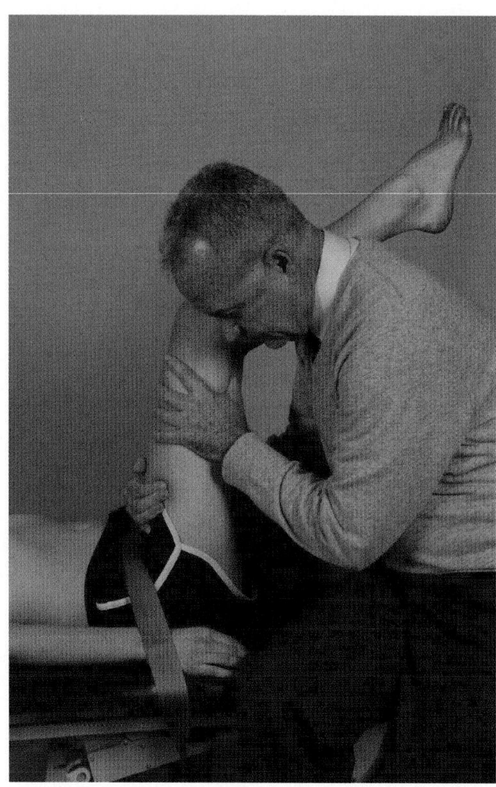

FIGURE 19-30 Hip joint distraction.

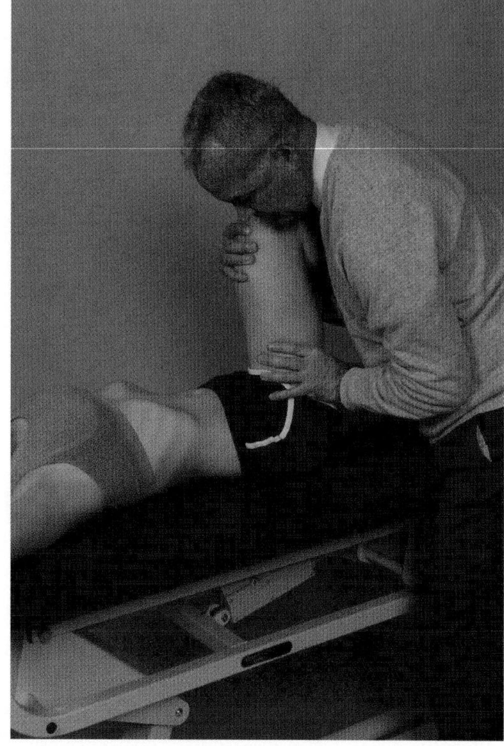

FIGURE 19-32 Posterior glide of the hip.

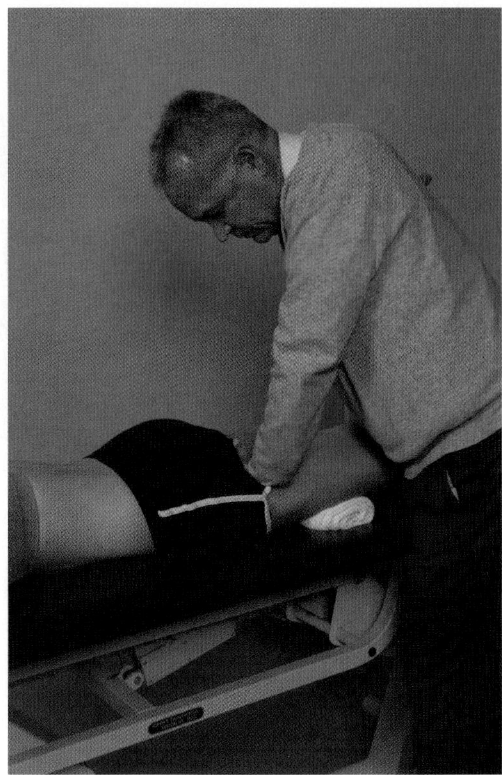

FIGURE 19-33 Anterior glide of the hip.

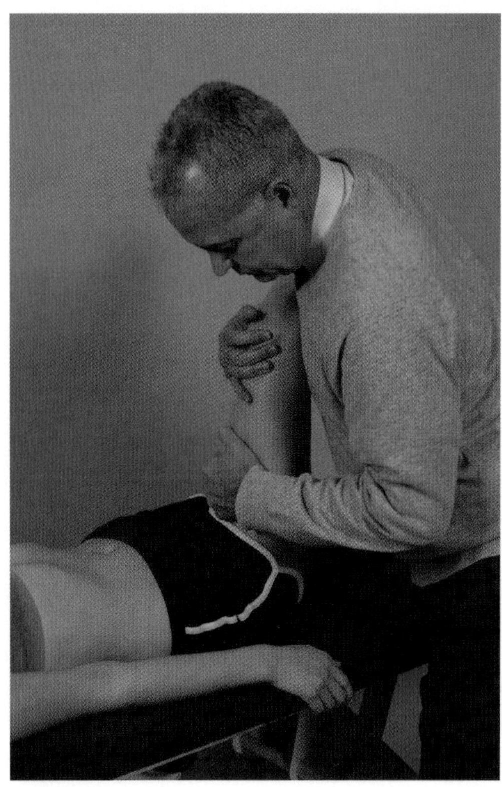

FIGURE 19-34 Inferior glide of the hip.

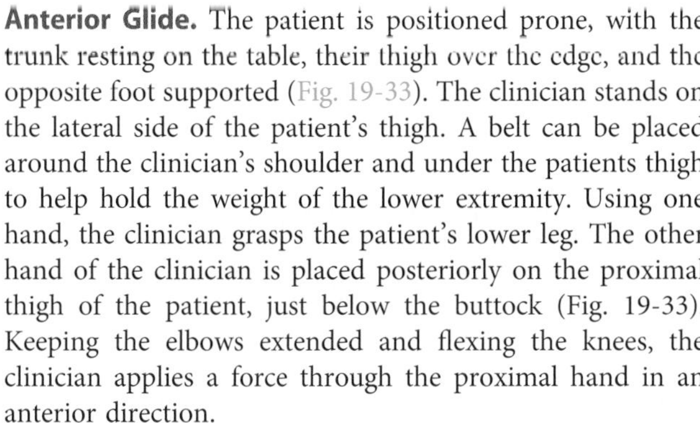

Anterior Glide. The patient is positioned prone, with the trunk resting on the table, their thigh over the edge, and the opposite foot supported (Fig. 19-33). The clinician stands on the lateral side of the patient's thigh. A belt can be placed around the clinician's shoulder and under the patients thigh to help hold the weight of the lower extremity. Using one hand, the clinician grasps the patient's lower leg. The other hand of the clinician is placed posteriorly on the proximal thigh of the patient, just below the buttock (Fig. 19-33). Keeping the elbows extended and flexing the knees, the clinician applies a force through the proximal hand in an anterior direction.

Inferior Glide. The patient is positioned with the hip and knee each flexed to 90 degrees and the lower leg placed against the clinician's shoulder. The clinician grasps the anterior aspect of the proximal femur as far proximally as possible with one hand. An inferior glide is imparted using the hands, while simultaneously rocking the patient's thigh into flexion (Fig. 19-34).

Neurological Tests

For sensation testing, the clinician should be aware of the dermatomal pattern as well as the areas supplied by the peripheral nerves (inferior femoral cutaneous nerve, lateral cutaneous nerve of the thigh, and posterior femoral cutaneous nerve).

Paresthesia or anesthesia is not commonly found in the buttock, hip, or groin region because of the degree of dermatome overlap. However, paresthesia in the "saddle" region should be considered indicative of a sign of cauda equina compression.

Special Tests

Special tests are merely confirmatory tests and should not be used alone to form a diagnosis. The results from these tests are used in conjunction with the other clinical findings to help guide the clinician. To assure accuracy with these tests, both sides should be tested for comparison.

Quadrant (Scour) Test. The quadrant or scour test is a dynamic test of the inner and outer quadrants of the hip joint surface.[140]

The patient is positioned in supine, close to the edge of the bed, with their hip flexed and foot resting on the bed. The clinician places one hand over the top of the patient's knee. The patient's hip is placed in 90 degrees of flexion, with the knee being allowed to flex comfortably. From this point, the clinician adducts the hip to the point at which the patient's pelvis begins to lift off the bed, to assess the inner quadrant (Fig. 19-35). At the end range of flexion and adduction, a compression force is applied through the knee along the longitudinal axis of the femur. From this point, the clinician moves the hip into a position of flexion and abduction to examine the outer quadrant. Throughout the entire movement, the femur is held midway between internal and external rotation, and the movement at the hip joint should follow the smooth arc of a circle. An abnormal finding is resistance, apprehension, or pain felt anywhere during the arc. The pain can result from compression of, or stress to, a number of structures including[140]

- the articular surfaces of the hip joint;
- the labrum;
- the hip joint capsule;
- the insertion of the TFL and the sartorius;

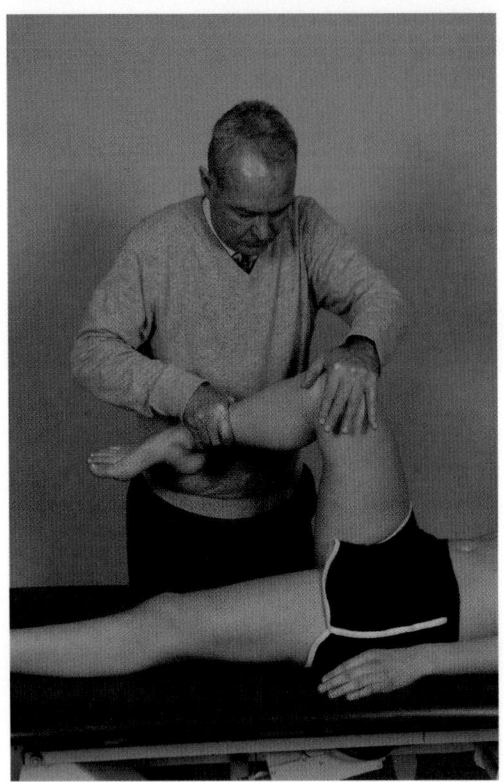

FIGURE 19-35 Scour test.

- the iliopsoas muscle;
- the IPB and neurovascular bundle;
- the insertion of the pectineus;
- the insertion of the adductor longus;
- the femoral neck.

The resistance may be caused by capsular tightness, an adhesion, a myofascial restriction, or a loss of joint congruity. Given all of the possible diagnoses, extreme care must be taken when interpreting the results from this test. Of the various studies that have looked at the Scour test, most have had poor study designs. Given the wide range of possible diagnoses with a positive finding, and the variety of patients this test is used with, bias is likely to result.

FABER or Patrick's Test. The FABER (flexion, abduction, external rotation) test (Fig. 19-36) is a screening test for hip, lumbar, or sacroiliac joint dysfunction, or an iliopsoas spasm (see Chap. 29).

SI Provocation Tests. A number of tests can be used to examine the sacroiliac joint (see Chap. 29).

In addition to the provocative tests, the passive motions of the hip can be examined with the innominate stabilized. The hip motions and their respective innominate motions in parenthesis are outlined in Table 19-6.

Craig Test. The Craig test is used to assess femoral anteversion/retroversion. The patient is positioned in prone with the knee flexed to 90 degrees. The clinician rotates the hip through the full ranges of hip internal and external rotation, while palpating the greater trochanter and determining the point in the range at which the greater trochanter is the most prominent laterally. If at this point the angle is greater than 8–15 degrees in the direction of internal rotation, when measured from the vertical and long axis of the tibia, the femur is considered to be in anteversion.[80,87,139,141]

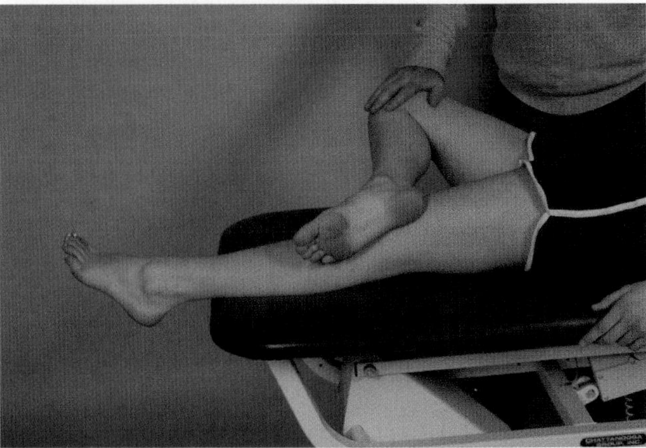

FIGURE 19-36 FABER test.

One study[141] showed this test to be accurate to within 4 degrees of intraoperative measurements, for the assessment of femoral anteversion/retroversion, and was more accurate than radiographic measurement techniques.

Flexion–Adduction Test. This test is used as a screening test for early hip dysplasia.[142] The patient is positioned in supine, and the hip is passively flexed to 90 degrees and in neutral rotation while maintaining the contact of the patient's pelvis to the bed. From this position, the clinician monitors the pelvis and the hip is passively adducted (Fig. 19-37). The resultant end-feel, restriction, discomfort, or pain is noted and

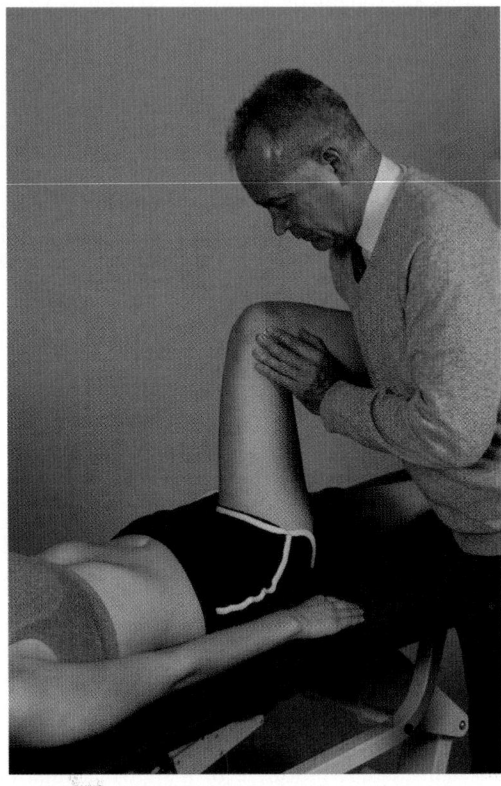

FIGURE 19-37 Flexion–Adduction test.

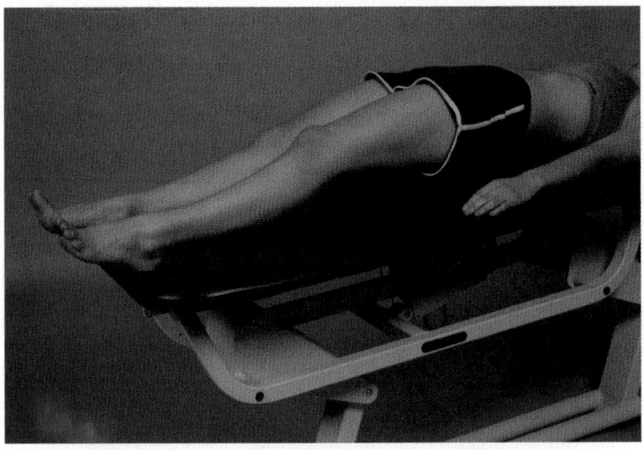

FIGURE 19-38 Supine Plank test.

compared with the normal side. A positive test for an early sign of hip dysplasia is the inability to adduct the flexed hip past midline toward the opposite hip. Although Woods and Macnicol[142] found the sensitivity to be 100% with this test, the test was performed on adolescents and demonstrated many design flaws.

Supine Plank Test. This test is used to detect hamstring weakness or injury. The patient is positioned in supine, resting on his or her arms and heels. The patient is asked to elevate the pelvis while maintaining their body weight on the arms and heels (Fig. 19-38). The patient is then asked to alternately lift one leg at a time. The test is positive for weakness if pelvic collapse or rotation occurs, or for injury if pain occurs at the ischial origin or in the hamstring musculature.

Trendelenburg Sign. The Trendelenburg sign indicates weakness of the gluteus medius muscle during unilateral weight-bearing. This position produces a strong contraction of the gluteus medius, which is powerfully assisted by the gluteus minimus and TFL, in order to keep the pelvis horizontal. For example, when the body weight is supported by the left foot (Fig. 19-19), the left hip abductors contract both isometrically and eccentrically to prevent the right side of the pelvis from being pulled downward by gravity.

The clinician crouches or kneels behind the patient so that the eyes are level with the patient's pelvis, and ensures that the patient does not lean to one side during the testing. The patient is asked to stand on one limb for approximately 30 seconds, and the clinician notes whether the pelvis remains level. If the hip remains level, the test is considered negative. A positive Trendelenburg sign is indicated if during unilateral weight-bearing the pelvis drops toward the the side of the unsupported limb (Fig. 19-19). A number of dysfunctions can produce the Trendelenburg sign. These include superior gluteal nerve palsy, lumbar disk herniation, weakness or tear of the gluteus medius, and advanced degeneration of the hip. Thus, if used in isolation, this test has little diagnostic value.

Pelvic Drop Test.[92] The patient is asked to place one foot on a 20-cm (8-inch) stool or step and to stand up straight. The patient then lowers the non–weight-bearing leg to the floor (Fig. 19-39). On lowering the leg, there should be no arm abduction, anterior or pelvic motion, trunk flexion, or any hip

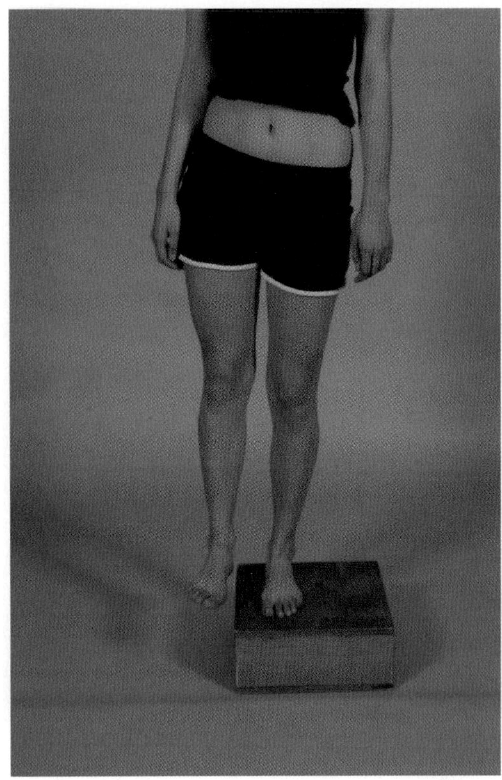

FIGURE 19-39 Pelvic Drop test.

adduction or internal rotation occuring at the weight-bearing hip. These compensations are indications of weak external rotators or an unstable hip.

Piriformis Compression of the Sciatic Nerve.[117] Piriformis compression of the sciatic nerve can be reproduced by maximally stretching the piriformis muscle. The patient lies supine with both legs flat on the exam table. The clinician raises one leg, and positions it in maximum flexion of the hip and knee. The hip is then internally rotated and fully adducted (Fig. 19-40). Pain radiating down the leg constitutes a positive test for piriformis syndrome.

Stinchfield's Test. Stinchfield's test is designed to help determine the source of a patient's back, buttock, groin, and/or leg pain. The patient is positioned in supine and asked to lift their leg, without bending the knee, to about 30 degrees. If this maneuver does not reproduce any pain, the clinician applies pressure downward on the patient's raised leg, in an attempt to extend the flexed hip, while the patient resists the force (Fig. 19-41). Pain produced either with or without resistance is assessed for location. If the pain is felt in the groin or anterior thigh, it is considered to arise from the hip; if from the buttock or lumbar spine, the sacroiliac joint or lumbar spine is the likely source. Stinchfield's test should not be confused with the straight-leg raise test used to detect neuromeningeal problems (see Chap. 11). Stinchfield's test is not dependent on the range obtained but rather on the location of symptoms. The only manner in which the two diagnoses could be confused is if a lumbar lesion was producing a restriction of the SLR at or below 30 degrees, but other signs and symptoms would help differentiate between the two. Unfortunately, Stinchfield's test has not been subjected to

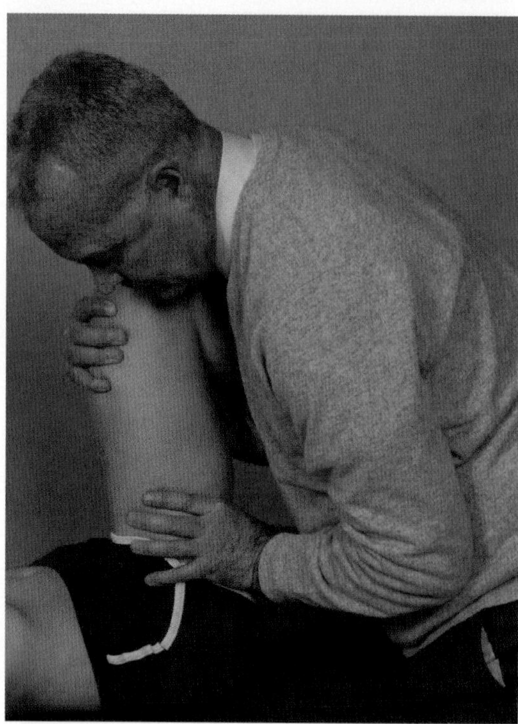

FIGURE 19-40 Piriformis Stretch.

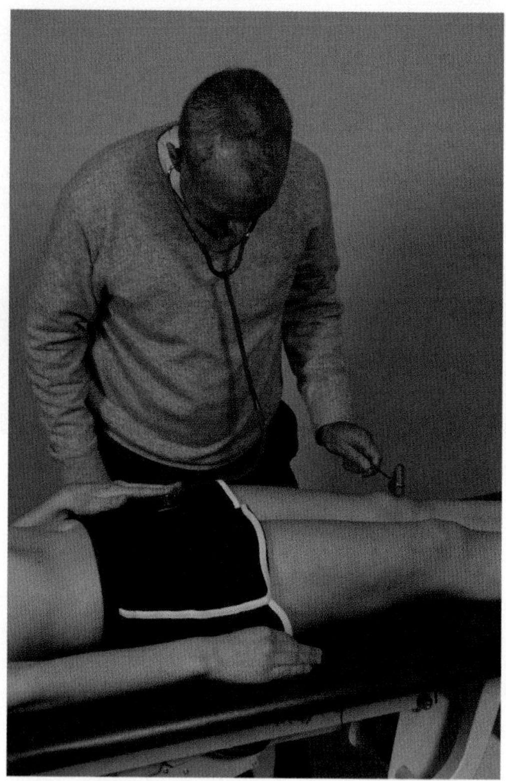

FIGURE 19-42 Auscultatory Patellar-Pubic Percussion test.

criteria validity research, so no sensitivity or specificity numbers are available.

Auscultatory Patellar-Pubic Percussion Test.[143–145] The ausculatory patellar-pubic percussion test is used when there is a suspicion of occult hip fracture. The patient is positioned in supine, and the clinician places the head of a stethoscope over the pubic symphysis. With the lower extremities extended and positioned symmetrically, the clinician taps (percusses) each patella with a finger or reflex hammer and compares the generated sound (Fig. 19-42). The percussion note should have symmetrical quality and intensity of sound. Any bony disruption along the conduction path (femur) will result in a diminished or muffled sound intensity of a duller quality. Reliability and validity of the technique has been demonstrated.[143] Tiru and colleagues[146] noted a positive predictive value of 0.98, sensitivity of 0.96, and specificity of 0.76. Although the study design was not without fault, the test does appear to have diagnostic value as a screening tool and as a diagnostic tool. Thus, a positive patellar-pubic percussion test should prompt a referral for diagnostic imaging.[143]

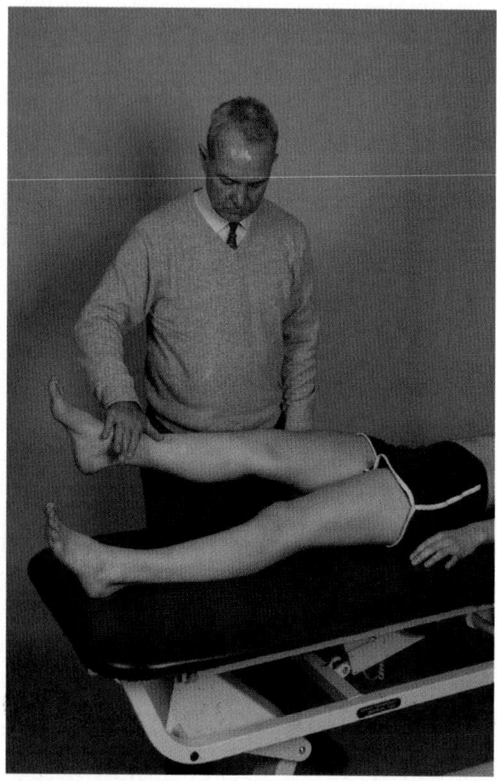

FIGURE 19-41 Stinchfield's test.

Muscle Length Tests

Restrictions in motion limit functional capacity, decrease muscle strength (by adversely affecting the muscle length–tension relationship), and can have an adverse effect on muscle and joint biomechanics.

Thomas Test and Modified Thomas Test. The original Thomas test was designed to test the flexibility of the iliopsoas complex but has since been modified and expanded to assess a number of other soft tissue structures. Neither the original test nor the suggested variations have ever been substantiated for reliability, sensitivity, or specificity.

The original test involves positioning the patient in supine, with one knee being held to the chest at the point where the lumbar spine is felt to flex (Fig. 19-43). The clinician assesses whether the thigh of the extended leg maintains full contact with the surface of the bed. If the thigh is raised off the surface

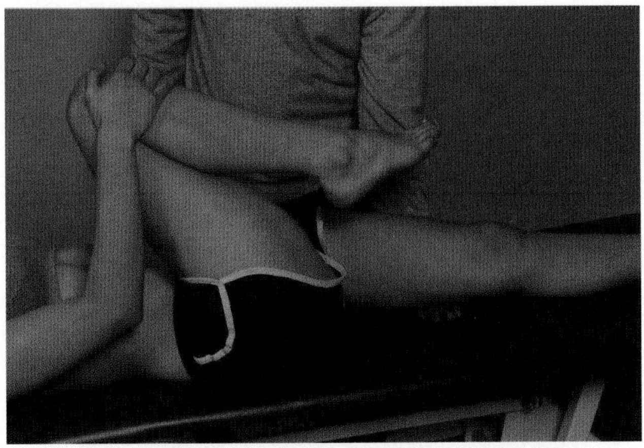

FIGURE 19-43 Thomas test demonstrating adaptive shortening.

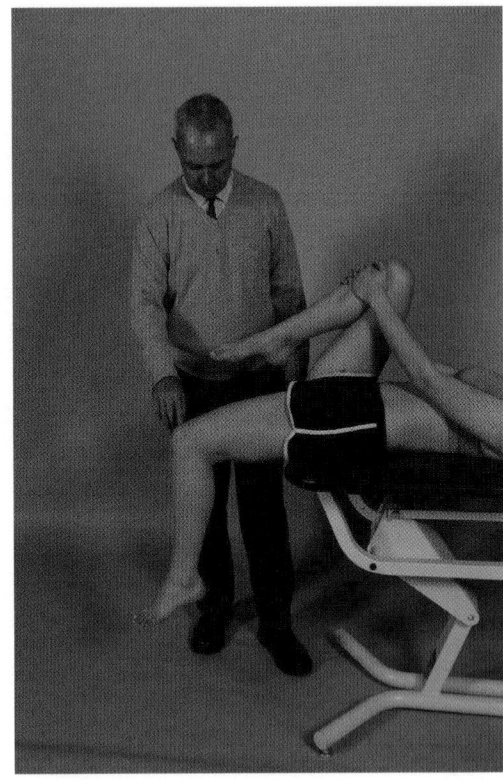

FIGURE 19-44 Modified Thomas test.

of the table, the test is positive. A positive test indicates a decrease in flexibility in the rectus femoris or iliopsoas muscles or both. One of the limitations of this test is that it merely determines the amount of hip extension possible at any given degree of pelvic flexion.[147] Another problem is that there are better methods of measuring the flexibility of the iliopsoas complex. For example, positioning the patient in prone, stabilizing the pelvis, and then extending the thigh. The precise point at which the pelvis begins to rise marks the end of the hip motion and the beginning of pelvic and spine motion.

A modified version of this test is commonly used to help eliminate the effect of the lumbar curve. For the modified version, the patient is positioned in sitting at the end of the bed. From this position, the patient is asked to lie back, while bringing both knees against the chest. Once in this position, the patient is asked to perform a posterior pelvic tilt. While the contralateral hip is held in maximum hip flexion by the patient's hands, the tested limb is lowered over the end of the bed toward the floor (Fig. 19-44). If normal, the thigh should be parallel with the bed, in neutral rotation, and neither abducted nor adducted, with the lower leg being perpendicular to the thigh and in neutral rotation. There should be 100–110 degrees of knee flexion present with the thigh in line with the table.

If the thigh is raised compared to the table, a decrease in the flexibility of the iliopsoas muscle complex should be suspected. If the rectus femoris is adaptively shortened, the amount of knee extension should increase with the application of overpressure into hip extension.[136] If the decrease in flexibility lies with the iliopsoas, attempts to correct the hip position should result in an increase in the external rotation of the thigh.[136]

The application of overpressure into knee flexion can also be used. If the increase in knee flexion produces an increase in hip flexion (the thigh rises higher off the bed), the rectus femoris is implicated, whereas if the overpressure produces no change in the degree of hip flexion, the iliopsoas is implicated.

This test can also be used to assess the flexibility of the TFL, if the hip of the tested leg is maximally adducted while monitoring the ipsilateral ASIS for motion. There should be 20 degrees of hip adduction available.

Two things must be remembered when interpreting the results of this test:

- The criteria are arbitrary and have been shown to vary between genders and limb dominance and to depend on the types and the levels of activity undertaken by the individual.[148]
- The apparent tightness might simply be normal tissue tension, producing a deviation of the leg because of an increased flexibility of the antagonists.

As always, the cause of the asymmetry must be found (or at least looked for) and addressed.

Ely's Test. This is a test designed to assess the flexibility of the rectus femoris. The patient is positioned in prone and the knee is passively flexed by the clinician (Fig. 19-45). If the rectus is tight, the hip flexes on the same side and the pelvis is observed to anteriorly rotate early in the range of knee flexion. The other side is tested for comparison. No diagnostic accuracy studies have been performed to determine the sensitivity and specificity of this test.

Ober Test. The Ober test is used extensively to evaluate the flexibility of the ITB and TFL (see Thomas test).[149] The patient is placed in the side lying position, and with the hip extended and abducted and the knee flexed to 90 degrees, the proximal part of the tested leg is released and allowed to drop passively (Fig. 19-46). The test is considered positive when the leg fails to lower. However, there have been some doubts expressed as to the reliability of the Ober test as a measure for ITB tightness and to date, no diagnostic accuracy studies have been performed to determine the sensitivity and specificity of this test.[150]

Modified Ober Test. The modified Ober test is performed in the same fashion as the Ober test except that the knee of the

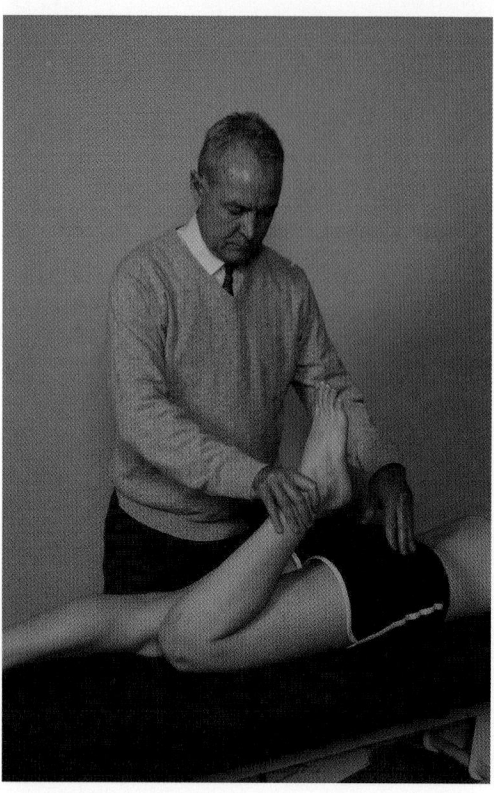
FIGURE 19-45 Ely's test.

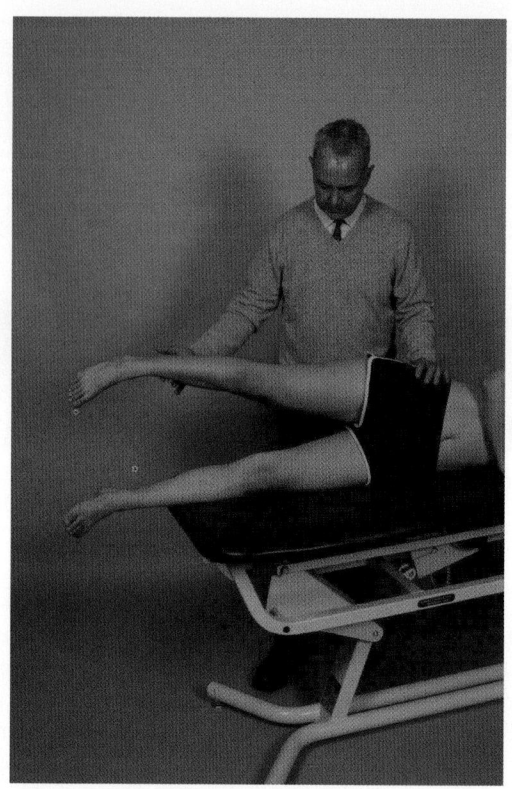
FIGURE 19-47 Modified Ober test.

tested leg is extended (Fig. 19-47).[151] A study by Reese and Bandy[151] was performed to determine the intrarater reliability of the Ober test and the modified Ober test for the assessment of IT band flexibility using an inclinometer to measure the hip adduction angle and to determine if a difference existed

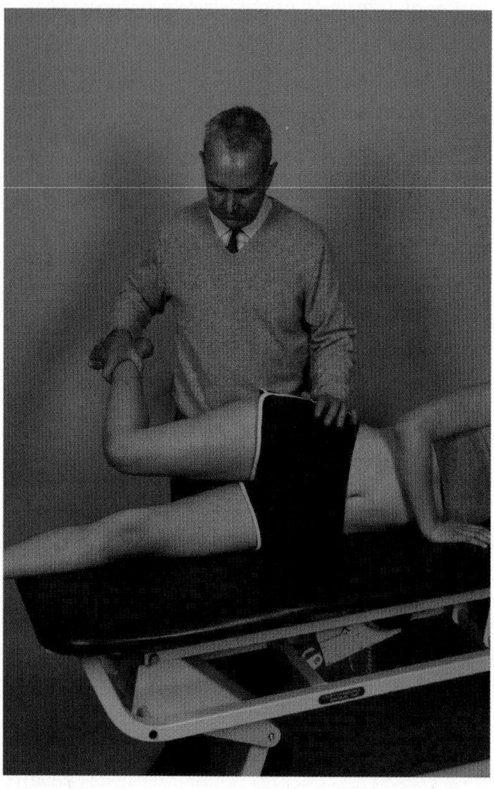
FIGURE 19-46 Ober test.

between the measurements of IT band flexibility between the Ober and the modified Ober test. Sixty-one subjects, with a mean age of 24.2 (SD = 4.3) years, were measured during two measurement sessions over 2 consecutive days.[151] During each measurement session, subjects were positioned on their left side and, with an inclinometer at the lateral epicondyle of the femur, hip adduction was measured during the Ober test (knee at 90 degrees of flexion) and the modified Ober test (knee extended).[151] If the limb was horizontal, it was considered to be at 0 degrees, if below horizontal (adducted), it was recorded as a positive number, and if above horizontal (abducted), it was recorded as a negative number. The ICC values calculated for the intrarater reliability of the repeated measurement were 0.90 for the Ober test and 0.91 for the modified Ober test.[151] Results of the dependent *t* test indicated a significantly greater ROM of the hip in adduction using the modified Ober test as compared to the Ober test.[151] The study concluded that the use of an inclinometer to measure hip adduction using both the Ober test and the modified Ober test appears to be a reliable method for the measurement of IT band flexibility, and the technique is quite easy to use.[151] However, given that the modified Ober test allows significantly greater hip adduction ROM than the Ober test, the two examination procedures should not be used interchangeably as a measurement of IT band flexibility.[151]

Straight-Leg Raise Test for Hamstring Length. The patient is positioned in supine with the legs staright and together resting on the table. The clinician stands on the side of the leg to be tested and grasps the patient's ankle with one hand, while visually monitoring, or palpating the patient's opposite ASIS. With the patient's knee extended, the clinician lifts the

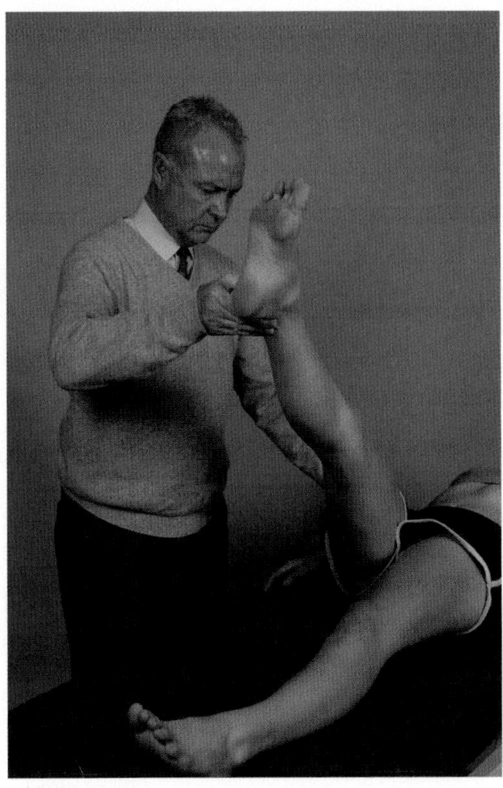

FIGURE 19-48 Straight-Leg Raise test for Hamstring Length.

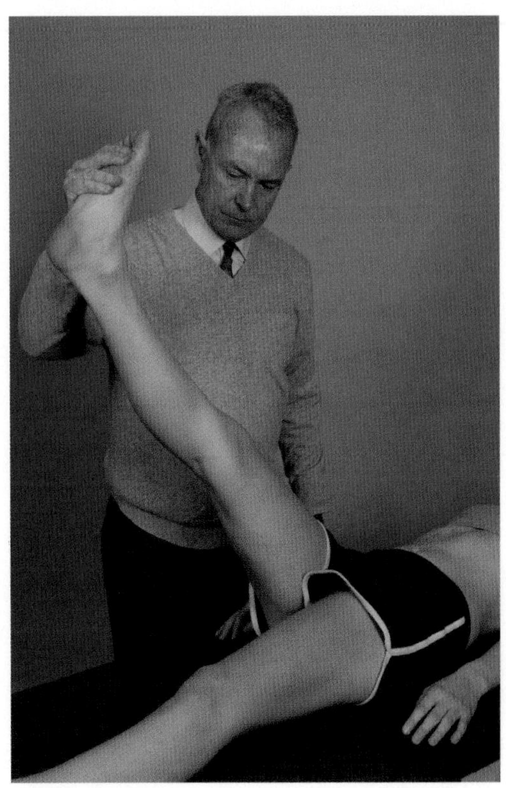

FIGURE 19-49 Straight-Leg Raise test with ankle dorsiflexion.

patient's leg, flexing it at the hip until motion is detected at the opposite ASIS (Fig. 19-48). The angle of hip flexion from the table is measured. The clinician returns the leg to the table and repeats the maneuver from the other side of the table with the other leg. The hamstrings are considered shortened if a straight leg cannot be raised to an angle of 80 degrees from the horizontal, while maintaining the other leg straight.[128] Any limitation of flexion is interpreted as being caused by adaptively shortened hamstring muscles.

This straight-leg raise test may also be used as a screen for adverse neural tension, particularly of the sciatic nerve (see Chap. 11), and to differentiate between a hamstring lesion and a sciatic nerve lesion by adding ankle dorsiflexion (Fig. 19-49)—adding dorsiflexion places tension through the sciatic nerve but does not alter hamstring length.

90–90 Straight-Leg Raise. Hamstring length can also be assessed with the patient positioned in supine and the tested leg flexed at the hip and knee to 90 degrees. From this position, the patient is asked to extend the knee of the involved side without extending the hip (Fig. 19-50). A measurement of knee motion is taken at the first resistance barrier.

Piriformis. The FAIR (flexion, adduction, and internal rotation) test is designed to detect compression of the sciatic nerve by the piriformis. The patient is positioned in side lying or supine with the involved extremity by the clinician. Holding the patient's knee, the clinician brings the involved extremity into a position of hip flexion, adduction, and internal rotation (Fig. 19-51). If pain is elicited at a point corresponding to the intersection of the sciatic nerve and the piriformis during this test, the result is considered positive.[152,153] The FAIR test has been demonstrated to have a

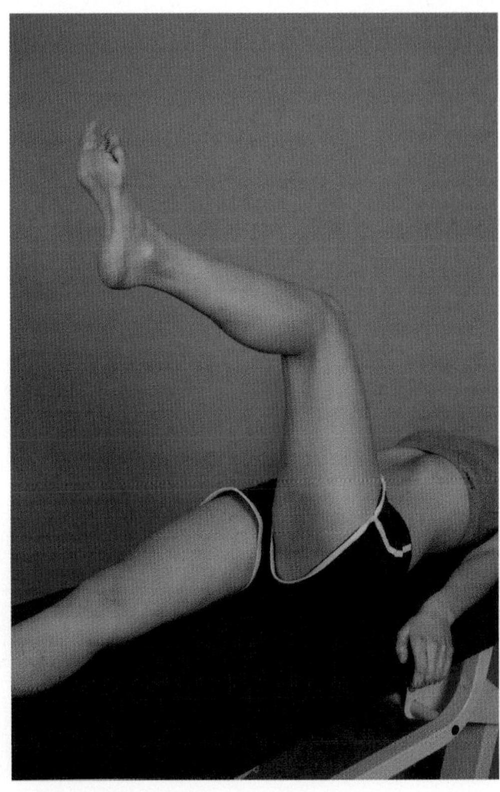

FIGURE 19-50 90–90 Straight-Leg Raise.

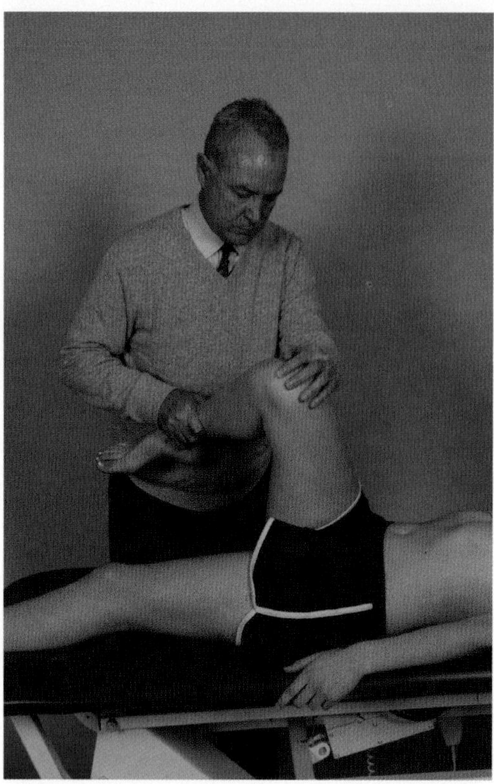

FIGURE 19-51 FAIR test.

sensitivity of 0.88, a specificity of 0.83, a + LR of 5.2, and a –LR of 0.14.[152,154]

Leg Length Discrepancy. The tests used to detect the presence of a leg length discrepancy are described in Chapter 29.

Fulcrum Test. The fulcrum test[155] is used to test for the presence of a stress fracture of the femoral shaft. The patient is positioned in sitting, with their knees bent over the edge of the bed and feet dangling. The clinician positions his or her arm under the thigh to be tested and moves it proximal to distal, as gentle pressure is applied on the thigh with the clinician's hand (Fig. 19-52). A positive test is when the patient reports sharp pain or expresses apprehension when the fulcrum arm is placed under the fracture site. The fulcrum test has not been subjected to criteria validity research, so no sensitivity or specificity numbers are available.

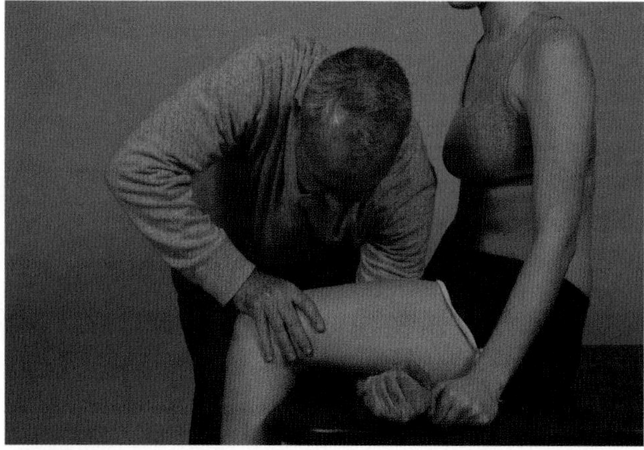

FIGURE 19-52 Fulcrum test.

Diagnostic Imaging

The standard radiographic views of the hip include anteroposterior views and axial or frog leg views (see Chap. 7).

INTERVENTION STRATEGIES

The hip joint and surrounding tissues are prone to a number of common conditions, including joint dysfunction, soft tissue injuries, impingement syndromes, and muscle imbalances of strength and flexibility. Also, because of the high potential of symptom referral from other regions to this area, any intervention for the hip joint must take the entire lower kinetic chain (lumbar spine, pelvis, and lower extremities) into consideration.

The techniques to increase joint mobility and soft tissue extensibility are described in the "Therapeutic Techniques" section.

Acute Phase

During the acute phase, the principles of PRICEMEM (protection, rest, ice, compression, elevation, manual therapy, early motion, and medication) are applied as appropriate. Elevation of the hip joint is usually not applicable or possible. The goals of the acute phase include

- protection of the injury site;
- restoration of pain-free ROM in the entire kinetic chain;
- improvement of patient comfort by decreasing pain and inflammation;
- retardation of muscle atrophy;
- minimization of the detrimental effects of immobilization and activity restriction[156–161];
- maintenance of general fitness;
- independence with home exercise program.

The promotion and progression of healing ususally involves a decrease in weight-bearing with rest and/or modification of activities, or through use of an assistive device. Assistive devices are often used to offset the load through the hip joint and to promote a symmetric gait pattern.[70,162] The use of a walker for maximum functional ambulation and safety may be required for some patients, particularly those with poor balance.[70]

The use of shoes with specially made cushion heels may further aid in diminishing the pain associated with weight-bearing.

According to patient tolerance, the clinician should also attempt to remove any other stresses to the hip joint such as joint restrictions in the lumbar spine or sacroiliac joint, and any muscle imbalances.

The approach during this phase may depend on the specific tissue involved:

- Contractile tissue lesions are treated with rest, gentle friction massage, submaximal isometric exercises (glut sets, quad sets, ham sets), pain-free range-of-motion exercises (heel slides, supine hip abduction/adduction), and with appropriate modalities. Whenever possible, active exercises are performed within a functional context.

- Articular lesions are best treated by placing the joint in the open-packed position (flexion, abduction, and external rotation) and with grade I and II joint mobilizations.

A progressive stretching program is initiated for those muscles that are prone to adaptive shortening (the hip flexors, short hip adductors, sartorius, piriformis, rectus femoris, hamstrings, TFL, and ITB), and those that are prone to be weak or inhibited (glutei muscles and the lumbar erector spina. Initially, the stretches can be performed using the milder techniques of postisometric relaxation techniques and myofascial release before progressing to other techniques (see "Techniques" section) as symptoms subside. The stretch positions used are those that are used for testing muscle length. Self-stretching is taught to the patient at the earliest opportunity.

Balance and coordination retraining activities are usually performed in some form of weight-bearing (sitting then standing), provided that there are no contraindications (pain or instability) to weight-bearing.[70] Simultaneous contraction of hip extensors and abductors in weight-bearing is the normal co-activation pattern used in early stance-phase of gait.[70,129] Once the patient is able to weight bear, these exercises are initially performed with double limb support (Fig. 19-53) and then progressed to single leg support as the patient progresses (Fig. 19-54). Once the static weight-bearing exercises can be performed, sit–stand transfers and gait activities are introduced. Functional exercises such as sit–stand–sit require simultaneous activation of hip muscles coordinated with other trunk and limb patterns normally used to accomplish the activity.[70] Gait-training procedures[163,164] during this phase involve the use of manual contacts at the pelvis to guide and stretch, and to apply joint approximation or resistance to help promote the development of appropriate patterns of neuromuscular control.

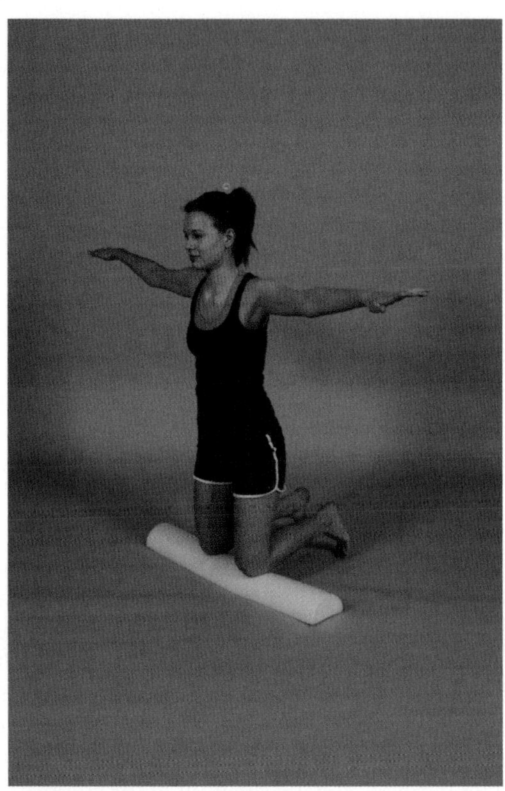

FIGURE 19-53 Weight shifting on fitter.

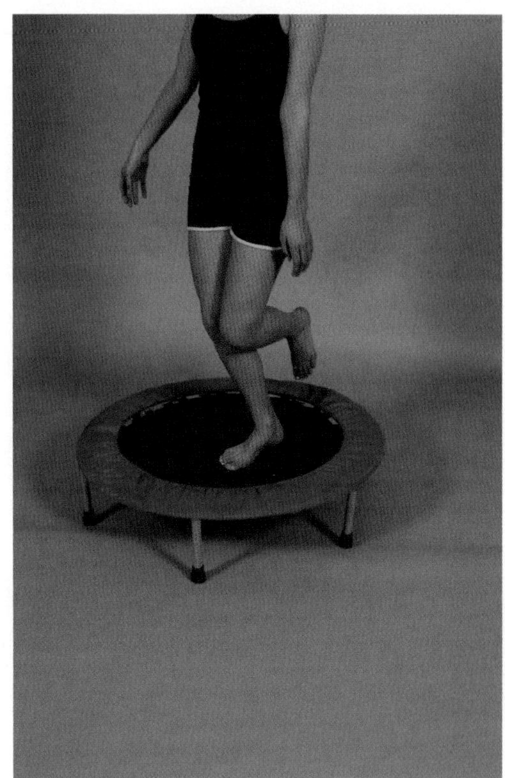

FIGURE 19-54 Unilateral balancing.

The essential components of normal swing-phase gait[129,164] to develop are

- posterior rotation of the pelvis during swing-phase flexion of the hip;
- a pelvic dip (drop) of no more than approximately 5 degrees on the side of swing limb;
- flexion of the hip to a maximum of 30 degrees (activation of hip flexors) with simultaneous knee flexion and dorsiflexion.

While standing, active hip flexion with adduction, combined with knee flexion, and dorsiflexion simulates the normal swing phase of gait, and promotes balance control in weight-bearing on the contralateral stance leg.[70] A multi-hip machine can be introduced as the hip muscles become stronger.

Cardiovascular fitness can be maintained during this phase using an upper body ergometer. If tolerated, a stationary bicycle can be used.

Functional Phase

Once there is no pain, and when the ROM is equal to that of the uninvolved limb, the patient progresses to the functional stage. The patient should also be able to perform normal walking and

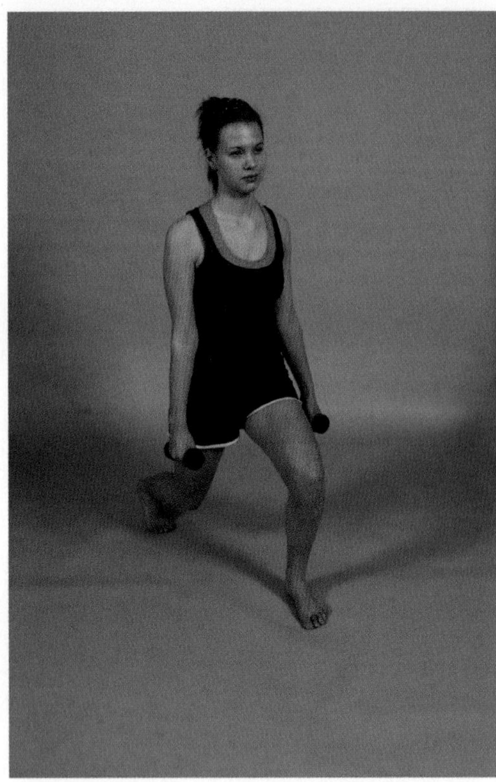

FIGURE 19-55 Lunge.

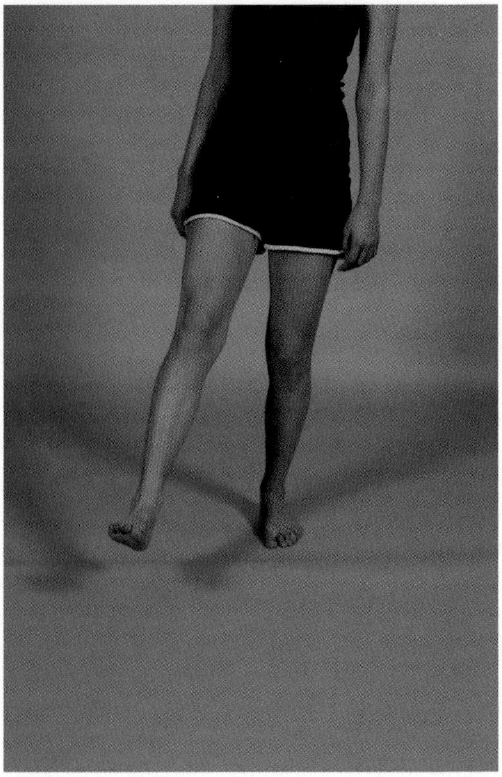

daily activities without pain. The goals of the functional phase include

- restoring normal joint kinematics;
- improving muscle strength to within normal limits;

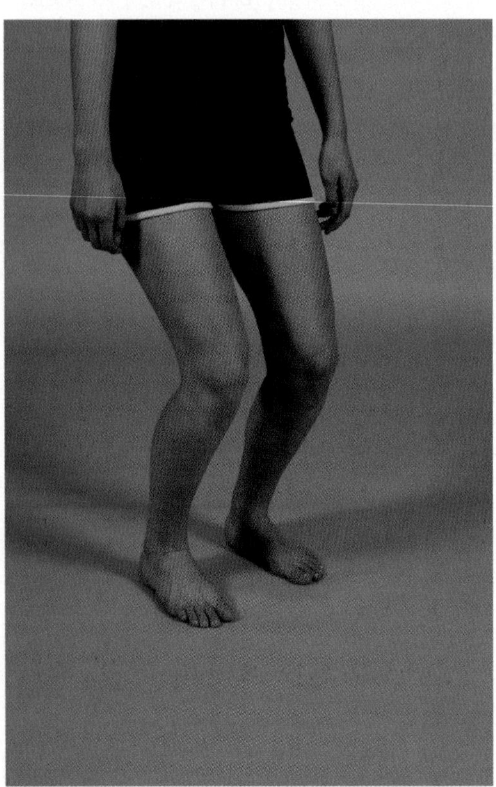

FIGURE 19-56 Squat.

FIGURE 19-57 Hip circumduction.

- improving neuromuscular control;
- restoring normal muscle force couple relationships.
- Return to normal function or athletic performance as appropriate

The following exercises are recommended during this phase:

- Quadruped exercises incorporating rocking forward and backward. These exercises help to stretch the joint capsule and apply joint compression.
- Lunging (Fig. 19-55) **VIDEO**, squatting (Fig. 19-56) **VIDEO**, and hip circumduction (Fig. 19-57). These exercises increase functional ROM and strength while simultaneously stretching the capsule.
- Open-chain exercises using cuff weights or tubing may be used to develop strength and endurance of all of the hip musculature **VIDEO** (Fig. 19-58). The exercises are initially performed using concentric contractions and then advanced to eccentric contractions using a variety of speeds and resistance.
- Bridging. Bridging utilizes body weight as a resistance force to the hip extensors and abductors.[70] A variety of bridging exercises exist, from the traditional, where the patient lies supine with the hips and knees flexed and the feet resting on the table and then raises the trunk until it is parallel with the thighs, (Fig. 19-59), **VIDEO** to the more difficult unilateral bridging exercises (Fig. 19-60) **VIDEO**. Manually applied resistance can be superimposed on the pelvis or thighs to generate maximal muscular tension in the contracting muscles.

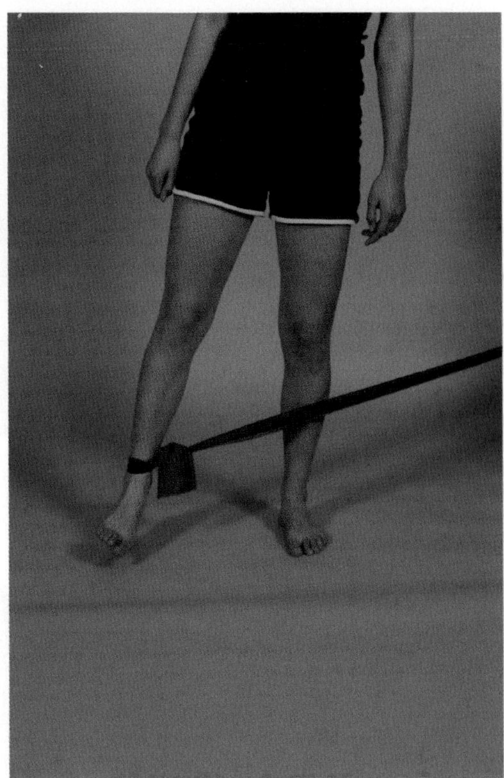

FIGURE 19-58 Hip abduction with T-band.

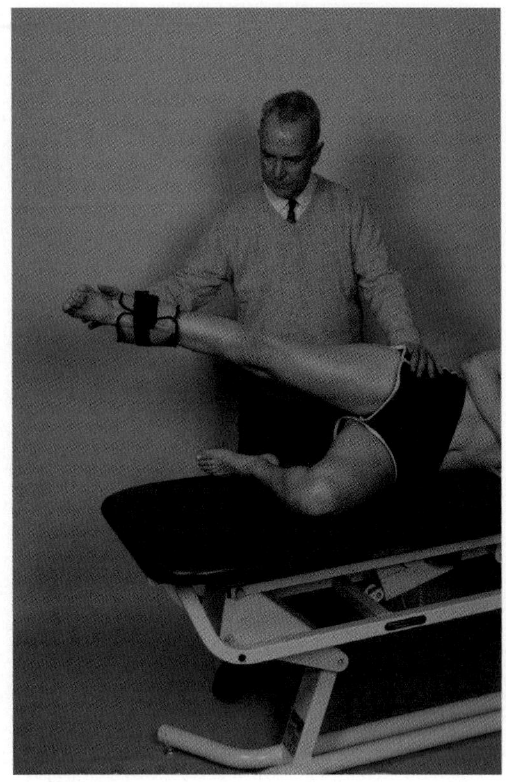

FIGURE 19-61 Gluteus medius strengthening.

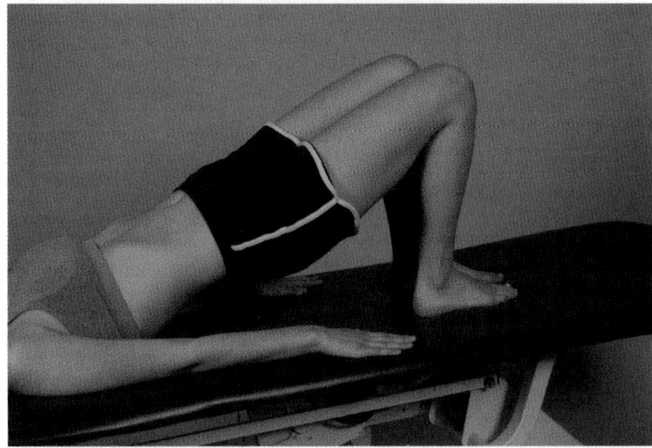

FIGURE 19-59 Bridging.

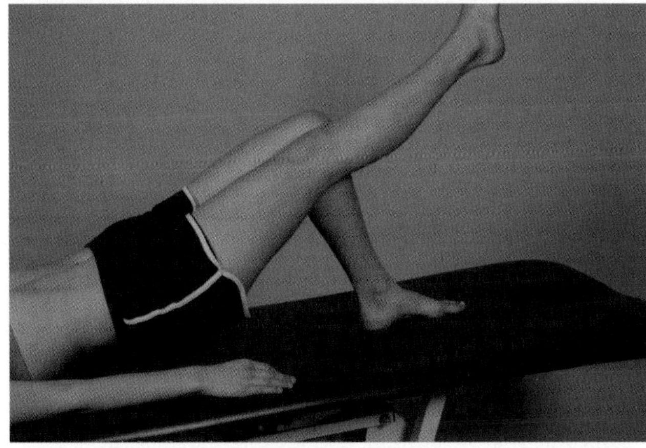

FIGURE 19-60 Unilateral bridging.

- Strengthening of the gluteus medius muscle is often an important component of the hip rehabilitation program. The gluteus medius can be strengthened in side lying, with the upper leg in slight hip extension and external rotation VIDEO (Fig. 19-61), the pelvic rise and drop exercise (Fig. 19-62), which also strengthens the quadratus lumborum, stool rotations (Fig. 19-63) and the clam shell exercise progression (Figs. 19-64 through 19-67).
- Strengthening of the hamstrings, including supine bent knee bridge walk-outs (Fig. 19-68 and Fig. 19-69), the supine single-leg chair bridge (Fig. 19-70 and Fig. 19-71), unilateral good mornings with rotations (Fig. 19-72 and Fig. 19-73), lunges with torso rotations (Fig. 19-74), hamstring lowers (Fig. 19-75), and grapevine stepping (Fig. 19-76). The grapevine stepping exercise, using the right leg as an example, is performed by asking the patient to stand with the feet together. The patient is then asked to take one step to the right, and then using the left leg to step behind and slightly to the right of the right foot, thereby crossing the left leg behind the right leg. The left foot should be pointed toward the right heel, but not directly behind it (Fig 19-76). The patient is then asked to take a step to the right with the right foot, and then to move the left foot so that the feet are together again. The routine is then repeated. The exercise is then performed moving to the left.
- The stationary bicycle can be used to increase lower extremity strength, endurance, and range during repetitive reciprocal movements of the lower extremities.[70] Electromyographic (EMG) analysis of lower limb muscles during pedaling has shown that the highest peak of activity

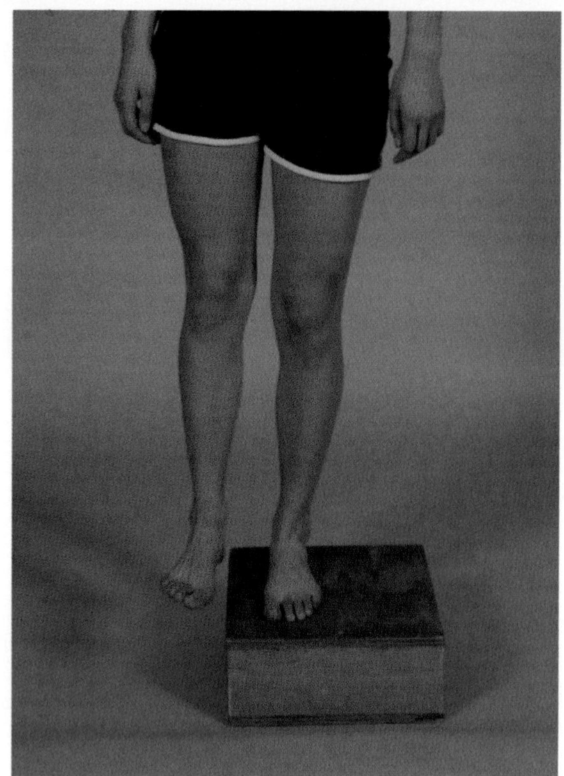

FIGURE 19-62 Pelvic rise and drop exercise.

for the gluteus maximus and biceps femoris muscles (as hip extensors) occurs during the pedal downstroke.[165] Stationary bicycling has also been found to be as effective for increasing ROM at the hip joint as static stretching.[166] The stationary bicycle is a convenient mode of exercise for home

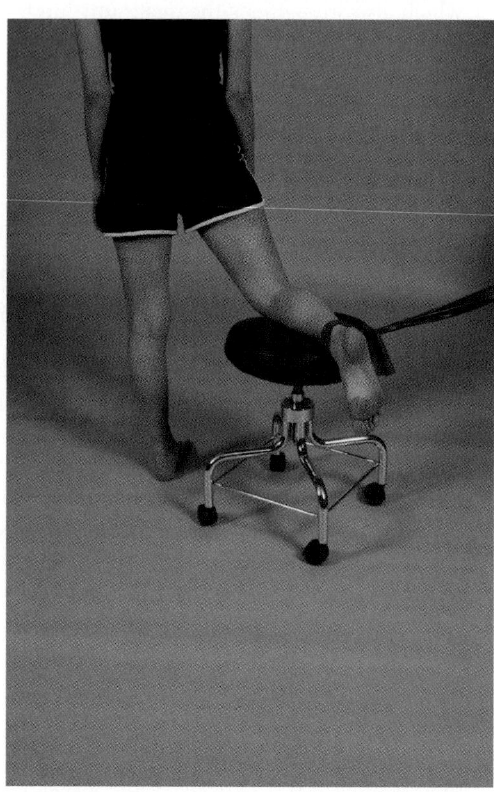

FIGURE 19-63 Stool rotations.

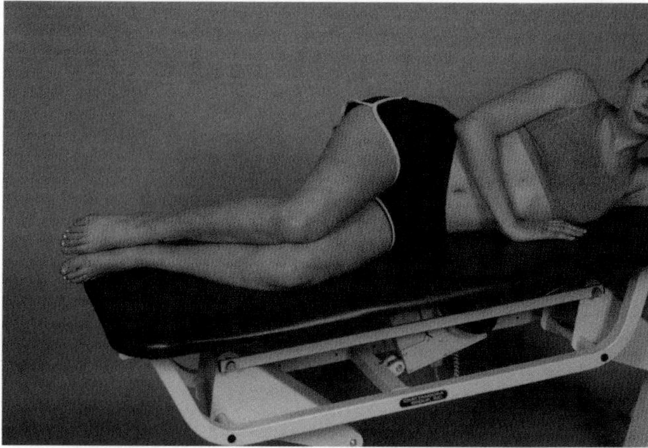

FIGURE 19-64 Clam shell progression.

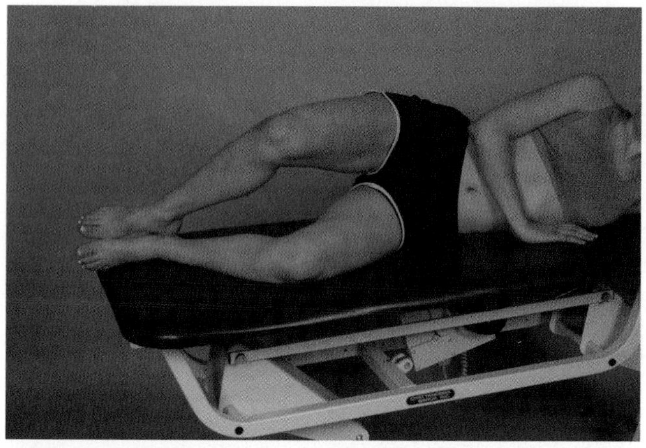

FIGURE 19-65 Clam shell progression.

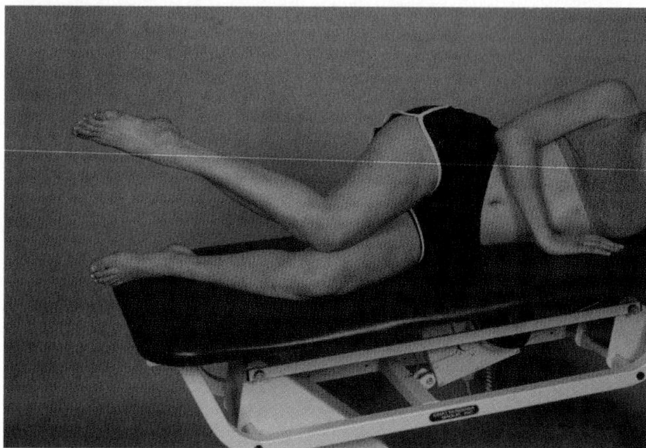

FIGURE 19-66 Clam shell progression.

use; however, the use of vigorous protocols should be carefully monitored for cardiac effects, especially in light of the fact that both blood pressure and heart rates have been found to increase markedly during this type of exercise.[70,167]

- Pool walking, swimming, and kicking may also be incorporated if available.

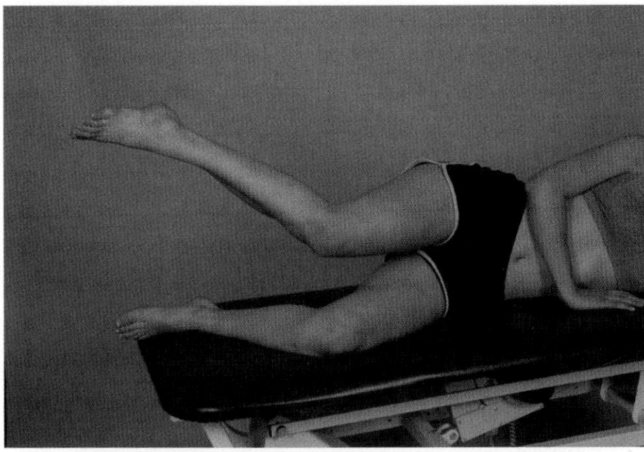

FIGURE 19-67 Clam shell progression.

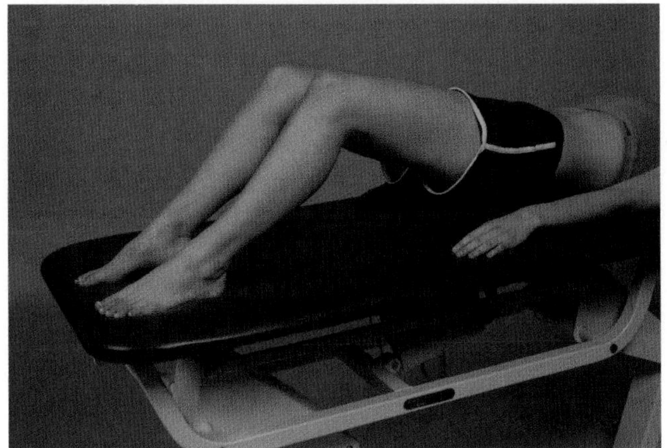

FIGURE 19-68 Supine bent knee bridge walk-outs—start position.

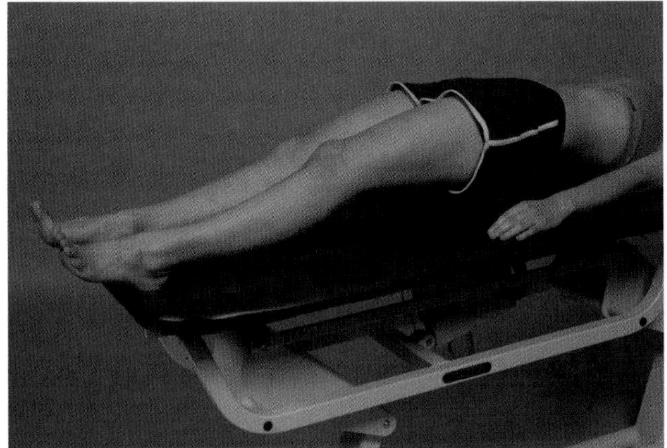

FIGURE 19-69 Supine bent knee bridge walk-outs—end position.

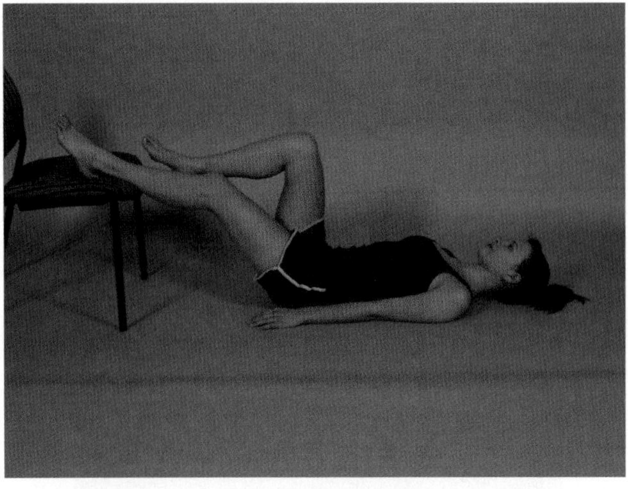

FIGURE 19-70 Supine single-leg chair bridge—start position.

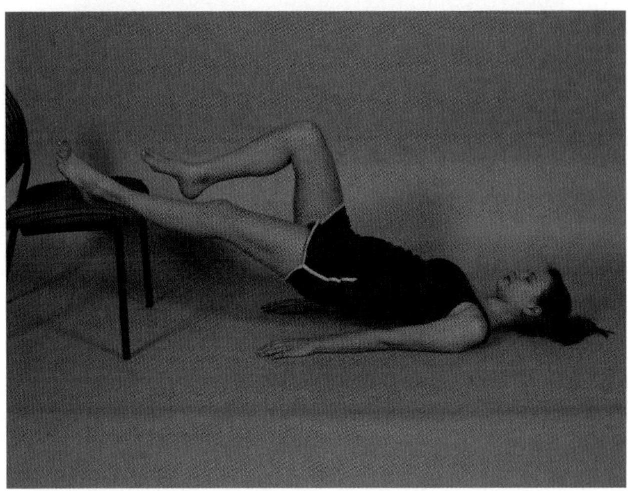

FIGURE 19-71 Supine single-leg chair bridge—end position.

Neuromuscular reeducation exercises for the hip are prescribed to emphasize specific movement patterns and sequencing of muscle contractions. These exercises demand a high level of control and coordination.[168–171] Ambulation activities can be used initially, progressing to more difficult unilateral extremity exercises.

Task-oriented exercise programs (work hardening) should be instituted for the patient who intends to resume a type of employment that requires a predetermined level of work performance. A more aggressive protocol needs to be adopted for the returning athlete. These exercise programs attempt to incorporate activities that simulate the actual circumstances and patterns of contraction used in the sport.[70,172] Examples of two such protocols are outlined in Tables 19-16 and 19-17.

Practice Pattern 4A: Primary Prevention/Risk Factor Reduction for Skeletal Demineralization

Idiopathic transient osteoporosis of the hip

Osteoporosis is the most prevalent bone disease among the aging population, and osteoporotic hip fractures account for substantial morbidity, mortality, and health-care costs.[173] Two types of osteoporosis are distinguished on the basis of age of presentation[174] and differing rates of loss of cortical or trabecular bone.[175] Type I is characterized by vertebral fractures in postmenopausal women at about the age of 65 years; type II may occur in both sexes at about 75 years of age and produces mainly osteoporotic hip fractures.[175]

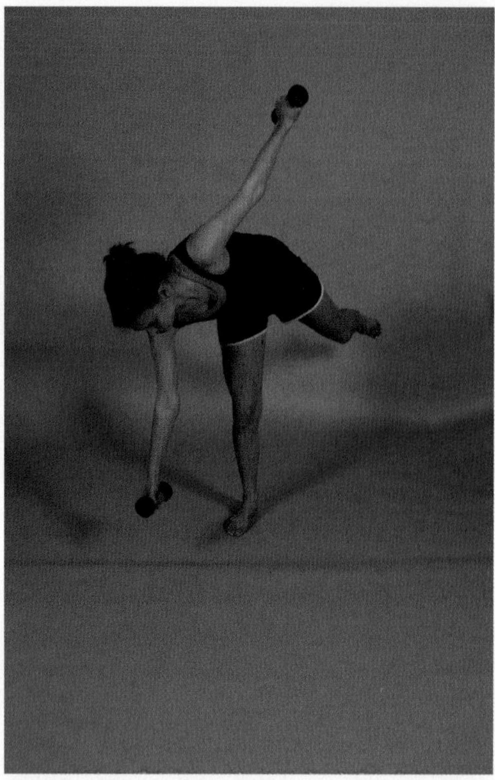

FIGURE 19-72 Unilateral good mornings with rotations.

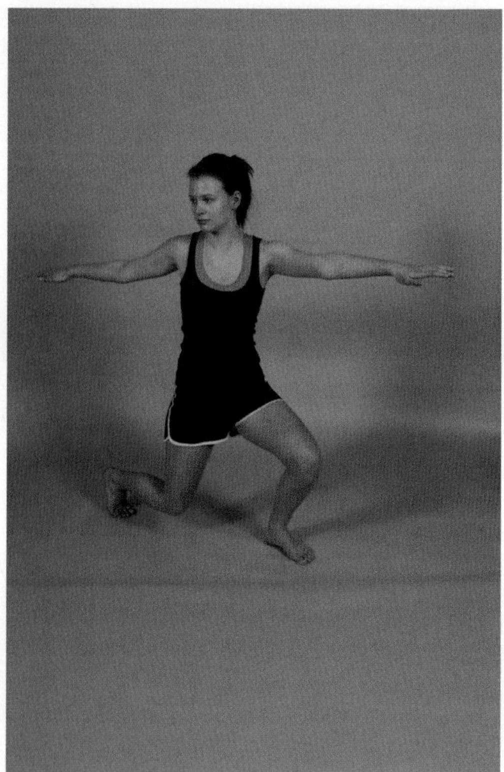

FIGURE 19-74 Lunge with torso rotations.

Men with osteoporosis of the hip are likely to have an underlying metabolic abnormality contributing to bone loss. The most common etiologies in men are hypogonadism, alcohol and corticosteroid use, anticonvulsant use, malabsorption syndromes, hyperthyroidism, and neoplasias.[176] Many factors have been cited for women, including decreased bone mass with an accelerated loss after menopause, parity, smoking, alcohol consumption, various medications, and diet. Although the reasons are unclear, in male patients either hip may be involved, whereas in women, the left hip is involved much more frequently.[177]

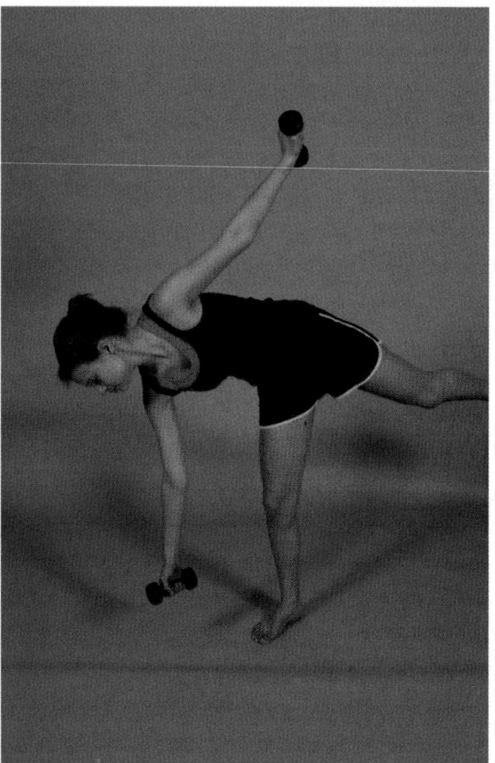

FIGURE 19-73 Unilateral good mornings with rotations.

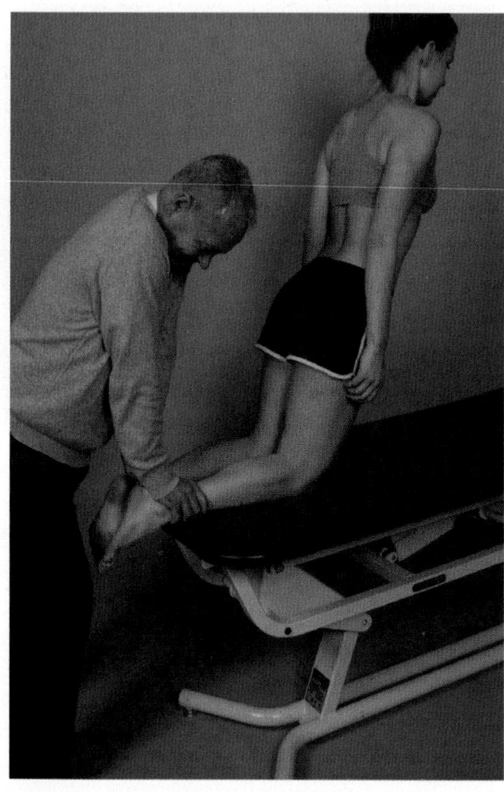

FIGURE 19-75 Hamstring lowers.

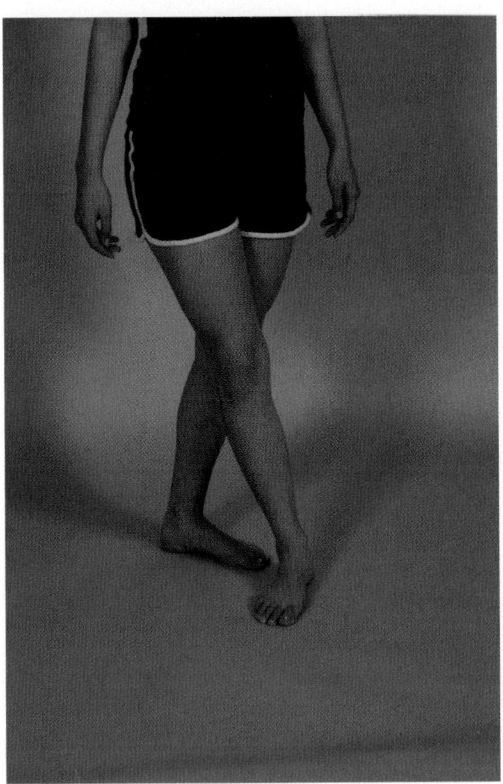

FIGURE 19-76 Grapevine stepping.

Hip pain begins spontaneously, without an antecedent history of trauma. The condition is aggravated by weight-bearing. The symptoms may become severe enough to result in a limp. The clinical findings are self-limiting and resolve in 2–6 months without permanent sequelae.[177] Biopsy of the synovium reveals normal findings or slight (mild, minimal, or equivocal) chronic inflammation.[178]

Radiographic findings are characteristic and become apparent within weeks or months of the onset of clinical findings. Osteoporosis is not usually found in the acetabulum but may be seen in the femoral neck. Progressive and marked osteoporosis of the femoral head is identified on plain radiographs.[178] The joint space is normal and the femoral subchondral bone is usually intact.

The differential diagnosis includes avascular necrosis, OA, septic arthritis, and rheumatoid arthritis.[178] The intervention for osteoporosis is discussed in Chapter 5.

Practice Pattern 4D: Impaired Joint Mobility, Motor Function, Muscle Performance, and ROM Associated with Connective Tissue Dysfunction

Osteoarthritis

OA involves a focal loss of articular cartilage with variable reaction of the subchondral bone. The prevalence of hip OA ranges from 7 to 25% in adults aged 55 years and older in the

TABLE 19-16 Return to Sport for Runners Following Soft Tissue Injury

Aerobic capacity and endurance

Cycling

- Incorporating appropriate warm-up and cool-down intervals, cardiovascular conditioning may be performed on stationary bicycle as symptoms permit or regular
- Attention to proper bike fit is important, as hip and back pain may result from improper biking biomechanics.
- If biking has not been used as a cross-training method in the past, an appropriate base building period is necessary:
- 3–5 min warm-up at 70–90 rpm, at 55–65% of age-estimated maximum heart rate.
- 10–15 min at 80–90 rpm, at 70–75% of age-estimated maximum heart rate, building this phase at no more than 3–5 min per session, as symptoms and cardiovascular condition permit.
- 3–5 min cool-down at 70 rpm, at 55–65% of age-estimated maximum heart rate.

Aqua jogging

- Deep-water jogging has been shown to be an effective mode of cross-training for runners, with good specificity of carryover.
- Use of a flotation device (Wet Vest) will enhance the comfort of beginners.
- Appropriate warm-up and cool-down intervals should be incorporated, as well as a base building period if this is an unfamiliar activity.

Running

As soon as symptoms permit, a return to running should be initiated. This should consist of level-ground or treadmill running at first, at a speed that brings the heart rate no higher than 60% of age-estimated maximum (warm-up pace), for durations that do not exacerbate symptoms (generally less than 15 min). As symptoms permit, duration (mileage) should be increased by no more than 10% per week. Once a substantial base of mileage has been built with no return of symptoms, the addition of speed-specific training may be incorporated. This may consist of "fartlek" (short bursts of acceleration within a longer run) or "tempo" (runs of longer duration at or near race pace), or it may be more regimented intervals using a track and stopwatch.

- For marathoners, the distance covered on any interval may range from 400 m at 10K race pace to 3–5 miles at marathon race pace.
- For shorter-distance runners, the intervals would be relatively shorter. For example, a 10K racer may do intervals of 100–400 m at 5K-race pace and 400 m up to 2 miles at 10K-race pace.

Speed-specific intervals should be performed no more than once per week initially and should be pursued cautiously. Total speedwork distance should make up no more than 10% of total weekly mileage.

Additional strengthening may be obtained with the incorporation of hill repeats.

(Continued)

TABLE 19-16 Return to Sport for Runners Following Soft Tissue Injury *(Contiinued)*

Specific hill training should be performed no more than twice per week and pursued cautiously.

- Monitoring of heart rate will assist in avoiding excessive speed on the uphill.
- Maintaining proper form on the downhill will reduce risk of impact injuries.
- To avoid overuse injury, periodization of mileage, terrain, interval training, proper footwear, etc., is crucial. For example, the following beginning marathon training schedule demonstrates good periodization of intensity, duration, and terrain:
    - Sun: 10 miles at 70% of age-estimated maximum heart rate on rolling trails.
    - Mon: 3 miles at 70% of age-estimated maximum heart rate on rolling hills.
    - Tues: 6 miles at 70% of age-estimated maximum heart rate on rolling hills.
    - Wed: Off or alternate form of training (e.g., swimming and biking)
    - Thurs: 5 miles, consisting of 1-mile warm-up, 2–3 miles of interval work at 80–85% of age-estimated maximum heart rate, and 1-mile cool-down (track).
    - Fri: 3 miles at 70% of age-estimated maximum heart rate on flat pavement.
    - Sat: Off or alternate form of training.

Balance/proprioceptive re-education

Balance/reach drills

The following exercises are performed at three to five sets of 10–15 reaches:

- Unilateral stance balancing, reaching one or both arms in various directions to maximum distance, avoiding use of other leg for counterbalance. Additional challenges can be added by holding a light weight or medicine ball or by using resistive tubing.
- Anterior reach: the anterior reach stimulates hamstrings, soleus, gastrocnemius, and hip/back extensors (depending on height of reach).
- Posterior overhead reach: the posterior overhead reach stimulates the gluteals, quadriceps, and hip/back extensors.
- Rotational reach to side: this reaching exercise stimulates the gluteals, quadriceps, trunk stabilizers, hip abductors, and abdominals.

Strengthening

Open-kinetic chain exercises

The following exercises are performed using weight machines, cuff weights, or resistive tubing, at three to five sets of 15–18 repetitions:

- Hip flexion
- Hip extension
- Hip abduction
- Hip adduction

Closed-kinetic chain functional exercises

The following exercises are performed: three to five sets of 15–18 repetitions, observing for deterioration of proper form because of fatigue.

Squats. Progression is made from mini-squats to deeper squats as symptoms permit, with additional challenges from additional weight.

Lunges. Progression is made from straight anterior/posterior and lateral lunges to rotational lunges as appropriate, increasing distance lunged or using additional weight as appropriate.

Step-ups/step-downs. Variations are made with step height and direction of step (lateral, anterior, posterior, or rotational) as appropriate, with additional challenges of increasing distance from step or use of additional weight as appropriate.

Flexibility

Flexibility exercises

These exercises are performed once the athlete has warmed up, for example after walking at least 3–5 min, or after a warm shower or bath. Emphasis should be on proper technique and form. The stretch should be held for at least 15–30 s.

The patient performs three to five repetitions of each stretch on both sides on a regular basis.

- Gastrocnemius/soleus
- Hamstrings
- Quadriceps
- Gluteals
- Psoas

Data from Schunk C, Reed K: *Clinical Practice Guidelines*. Gaithersburg, MD: Aspen, 2000.

TABLE 19-17	**Return to Sport Following Osteitis Pubis**

Phase I

1. Static adduction against soccer ball placed between feet when lying supine; each adduction is held for 30 s and is repeated 10 times.
2. Abdominal sit-ups performed both in straight direction and in oblique direction. The patient performs five sets to fatigue.
3. Combined abdominal sit-up and hip flexion (crunch). The patient starts from supine position and with a soccer/ basketball placed between knees. The patient performs five sets to fatigue.
4. Balance training on wobble board for 5 min.
5. One-foot exercises on sliding board, with parallel feet as well as with a 90-degree angle between feet. Five sets of 1-min continuous work are performed with each leg, and in both positions.

Phase II (from third week)

1. Leg abduction and adduction exercises in side lying. The patient performs five series of 10 repetitions of each exercise.
2. Low-back extension exercises while in prone over the end of treatment table. The patient performs five series of 10 repetitions.
3. One-leg weight-pulling abduction/adduction standing. The patient performs five series of 10 repetitions of the exercise for each leg.
4. Abdominal sit-ups both in straightforward direction and in oblique direction. The patient performs five sets to fatigue.
5. One-leg coordination exercise, flexing and extending knee and swinging arms in same rhythm (cross-country skiing on one leg). The patient performs five sets of 10 repetitions for each leg.
6. Skating movements on sliding board. This is performed five times for 1-min continuous work.

Data from Holmich P, Uhrskou P, Ulnits L, et al: Effectiveness of active physical training as treatment for long-standing adductor-related groin pain in athletes: Randomised trial. *Lancet* 353:439–443, 1999.

white European population.[179] Studies of the natural history of hip OA clearly demonstrate heterogeneity of disease progression, and the lack of a universal agreement as to the definition of progression of hip OA. Most define progression by radiological features such as loss of joint space, osteophytes, and sclerosis.[180,181] However, the demonstration of a correlation between radiographic features and clinical symptoms is not easy in OA: factors differentiating symptomatic OA from asymptomatic disease are unknown.[182] The two clinical sequelae of OA are joint pain and functional impairment.

Hip OA usually begins insidiously, although in a few cases it may start abruptly. The development of OA at any joint site depends on a generalized predisposition to the condition and abnormalities of biomechanical loading, which act at specific joints.[183] Individual risk factors, which may be associated with a generalized vulnerability to the disorder, include family history, obesity, and hypermobility of the joint.[182] Those that reflect local biomechanical insults include minor trauma to an already diseased joint, abnormalities of joint shape, and physical activity.[182]

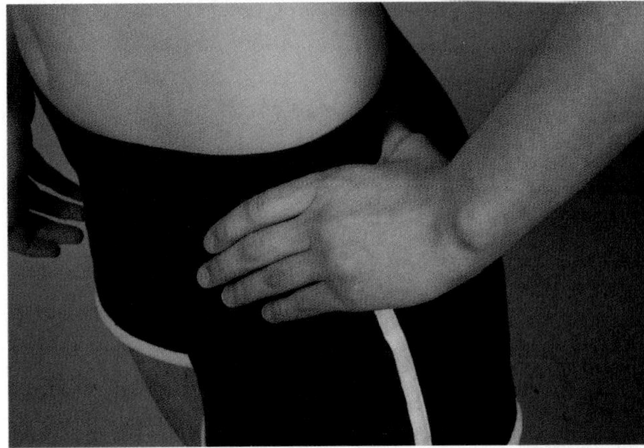

FIGURE 19-77 The C sign.

The pain of hip OA can vary greatly in both its site and its nature, sometimes making early diagnosis difficult.[184] The pain may be felt in the buttock, groin, thigh, or knee and varies in character from a dull ache to sharp and stabbing. The C sign (Fig. 19-77) may be encountered when asking the patient describe the location of the pain—the patient will cup the hand above the greater trochanter with the thumb posterior and the fingers gripping deep into the anterior groin when describing deep interior hip pain.[185] The discomfort associated with hip OA is generally related to activity and the bouts of pain can last for several hours.[184] Stiffness of the hip is usual, particularly after inactivity, and can be the presenting feature. As the disease progresses, the patient experiences difficulty in climbing stairs with the involved leg and may have difficulty in donning socks or stockings.[186] In advanced cases of the disease, the patient may complain of severe pain that is present at night or during rest, and there is a marked decline in the participation of recreational activities.

Early physical signs include restriction of internal rotation and abduction or flexion of the affected hip, with pain at the end of the range.[184] Birrell et al.[111] notes that as the number of restricted planes of hip motion increases, the specificity, or ruling in of the diagnosis of hip OA, increases. As specificity increases, sensitivity, or the ruling out of a diagnosis of hip OA, decreases in those patients with mild-to-moderate and severe OA of the hip.[111,116] This trade-off, where sensitivity decreases while specificity increases, is common with sensitivity and specificity.[116] The diagnostic value of decreased ROM in the hip is best when present in two or three planes of motion (positive likelihood ratio of 2.5–5), as compared to just one plane of motion (positive likelihood ratio of 1.9).[111,116]

A diagnosis of hip OA can usually be confirmed by radiography; joint space width of 2.5 mm or less indicates substantial loss of cartilage in the hip joint, and osteophytes, subchondral bone sclerosis, or cysts are usually present.[184] As mentioned, though, radiographs can be misleading because of the relative insensitivity of the their findings with clinical signs and symptoms. Two separate studies by Bierma-Zeinstra et al.[187] and Altman et al.[188] examined the relationship between patients with clinical signs and symptoms of hip OA and radiographic findings. The clinical diagnosis of early hip

OA according to Bierma-Zeinstra et al.[187] includes such variables as decreased external rotation, no pain aggravation with sitting, and over 60 years of age. The criteria from the Altman et al. study included hip internal rotation less than 15 degrees and an age of over 50 years. Diagnostic measurement properties, like sensitivity, specificity, and likelihood ratios, are probabilistic statistics; consequently, false-positive and false-negative results will always be potentially possible.[116]

The narrowing of the joint space associated with OA could potentially slacken the supporting ligaments, rendering them less effective and producing changes in proprioceptive input. Indeed, OA of the hip has been associated with deficits in a patient's proprioception and balance.[189,190] The joint space narrowing may also result in a relative decrease in the length of the muscles that cross the hip joint, which could feasibly result in a mechanical disadvantage of the muscles that act on the hip joint. In addition, OA of the hip can have many manifestations in neighboring joints, particularly the lumbar spine and the foot. This is likely because the joint stiffness associated with the disease diminishes the amount of rotation available at the hip, forcing the lumbar spine and foot to compensate for this loss.

Systematic reviews have concluded that exercise reduces the pain and disability associated with hip OA. Weigl et al.[191] demonstrated that strengthening exercises, flexibility, relaxation, and endurance training decreased pain and improved physical function in patients with OA.[116] van Baar and colleagues[192] showed that exercise improved function and reduced pain in patients with hip OA, but later found that the beneficial effect of exercise declined over time.[116,193] Research on the use of manual physical therapy in the treatment of hip OA is limited. Hoeksma and colleagues,[194] in a randomized clinical trial comparing the effectiveness of two different therapy programs in a group of patients with hip OA, demonstrated the superiority of manual physical therapy plus exercise over exercise alone for improving pain and ROM. MacDonald and colleagues,[195] in a case series describing the outcomes of individual patients with hip OA treated with manual physical therapy and exercise reported that all patients exhibited reductions in pain and increases in PROM, as well as a clinically meaningful improvement in function. The inherent limitations of the case series, however, do not allow for the identification of a cause-and-effect relationship. Further research, including randomized clinical trials, is necessary to uncover the exact effect of manual physical therapy and exercise in the treatment of hip OA.[195]

Based on the above research, the intervention goals for hip OA include relieving symptoms, minimizing disability, and reducing the risk of disease progression.[184] Intervention in the earlier stages includes:

- Patient education and empowerment through advice about what patients can do for themselves. Patients are often frightened that use of the hip will "wear out" an already damaged joint and feel they need "permission" to use it.[184] Evidence suggests that the involved joint will benefit from regular loading to help maintain its integrity.
- Modalities for muscle relaxation, pain relief, and anti-inflammation.
- Modification of ADL and self-care. Patients need to learn an appropriate balance and intersperse periods of activity with rest, as prolonged or heavy activity involving the diseased hip may cause further damage.[196]
- It is important to maintain a full range of hip movement, if possible. In addition to specific exercises for hip ROM, recreations such as swimming or cycling may help. Contact sports and activities such as jogging, which can cause repetitive high impact loading of the hip, are probably best avoided.[196]
- Diet and weight. There is no evidence for the involvement of any dietary factor in the etiopathogenesis of hip OA.[184] However, it is possible that obesity may accelerate progression or cause more pain. A reduction in weight can significantly improve a patient's symptoms, increase mobility, and improve health status.[197]
- Many people with arthritis of the spine or legs are more comfortable wearing trainers or other shoes with good shock-absorbing properties than they are in regular footwear. Sorbithane and other shock-absorbing insoles, which are available in sports and shoe shops, may be helpful.[184]
- A simple walking stick can make a big difference, reducing loading on a hip by 20–30%, but attention must be given to its length, characteristics, and use. In most cases, it will be most beneficial if it is held on the uninvolved side of the body and that it comes to the top of the pelvis and has a good ferrule and comfortable handle.[184]

The patient should be advised

- to engage in adequate warm-ups before exercising;
- to pay attention and respect the limitations of their body and not exercise if in discomfort;
- not to use medication to cover up pain from exercising.

Other measures include:

- manual techniques to mobilize the joint and passive stretches of the capsule, particularly distractive techniques.[195] Following these techniques, a fairly vigorous stretching program into flexion, abduction, and external rotation should be initiated. The FABER position, or cross-legged sitting, is ideal for this. Stretching the hip joint capsule involves maintaining the stretch for as long as an hour.
- strengthening exercises for the trunk stabilizers and the major muscle groups of the hip region, especially the gluteus medius.

The surgical intervention for advanced OA of the hip is addressed later in the chapter.

Rheumatoid arthritis

Rheumatoid arthritis is a systemic, inflammatory, and chronic disorder of unknown etiology, which is characterized with periods of exacerbation and remission, and which eventually result in destruction of the joint surfaces and progressive disability.[186]

In the early phases of the disease, systemic manifestations such as malaise, weight loss, and ability fatigue are seen.[186] The patient typically experiences vague pain and stiffness in the hip, especially when arising from bed in the morning. With time, the stiffness and pain becomes more severe and persistent and is accompanied by protective muscle spasms. Eventually, a hip flexion contracture develops.

Conservative intervention involves pharmacologic management and active exercises of the hip within the limits of pain to preserve joint motion and maintain good muscle tone.[186] The activity modifications outlined for OA of the hip are also advocated during periods of remission. The patient is instructed on joint protection skills and to take frequent breaks.

Ankylosing spondylitis

Ankylosing spondylitis (AS), also known as Marie–Strümpell disease or rheumatoid spondylitis, is a form of inflammatory arthritis, usually characterized by initial involvement of the sacroiliac joints, later involvement of the spinal joints, and occasional involvement of the hip joints and other joints of the body (refer to Chap. 5).[186] The patient is usually between 15 and 40 years, and AS affects one to three per 1000 people. Although males and females are affected evenly, mild courses of AS are more common in the latter.[198] Clinical findings in the hip may include an early capsular pattern of motion restriction.

An exercise program is particularly important for these patients to maintain functional outcomes (see Chap. 5).[199] The goal of exercise therapy is to maintain the mobility of the involved joints for as long as possible and to prevent stiffening. A strict regime of daily exercises, which include positioning and spinal extension exercises, breathing exercises, and exercises for the peripheral joints must be followed. Several times a day, the patient should lie prone for 5 minutes to help maintain hip and spinal extension, and they should be encouraged to sleep on a hard mattress and avoid side lying. Swimming is the best routine sport.

Avascular necrosis of the femoral head

Avascular necrosis of the femoral head is a condition in which there is progressive ischemia and secondary death of osteocytes or bone cells of the femoral head, resulting in the collapsing of bone of the femoral head and the later development of degenerative arthritis.[186] Avascular necrosis of the femoral head is described in more detail in Chapter 5.

Acetabular labral tear

Labral tears of the hip are more common than previously thought.[18] In the last 15 years, there have been numerous studies on the location and anatomical features of acetabular labral tears, including cadaver, arthroscopic, and MRI studies.[200] In studies of people with a tear of the labrum, researchers have attributed the injury to a variety of causes.[201] Direct trauma, sporting activities, and certain movements of the hip including torsional or twisting movements have been cited to cause labral tears.[201] However, a large percentage of labral tears are not associated with any known specific event or cause. Two common types of mechanisms have been recognized:

1. A young person with a twisting injury to the hip, usually an external rotation force in a hyperextended position.
2. An older person with a history of hip and/or acetabular dysplasia, or the result of repeated pivoting and twisting.

Acetabular labral tears represent the most common cause for mechanical hip symptoms—in a recent study, they were found to be the cause of groin pain in more than 20% of athletes presenting with groin pain.[202]

Labral tears can be classified according to location, etiology, and type[203]:

- ***Location.*** With respect to location, tears can be anterior, posterior, or superior (lateral), although anterior and anterosuperior tears appear to be the most common.[203] Anterior labral tears are also common in patients with degenerative hip disease or acetabular dysplasia. The most likely reason for the prevalence of anterior labral tears is that this region is subjected to higher forces or greater stresses than other regions of the labrum.[201] Because of the anterior orientation of both the acetabulum and the femoral head, the femoral head has the least bony constraint anteriorly and relies instead on the labrum, joint capsule, and ligaments for stability.[201]
- ***Etiology.*** With respect to etiology, tears can be degenerative, dysplastic, traumatic, or idiopathic. Degenerative tears can also be seen in association with inflammatory arthropathies.
- ***Type.*** Labral tears have been classified into four types: radial flap (the most common type), radial fibrillated, longitudinal peripheral, and abnormally mobile.[204] Seldes et al.[27] classified acetabular labral tears into type 1 and type 2 on the basis of their anatomical and histological features.
  - Type 1 tears consist of detachment of the labrum from the articular cartilage surface. These tears tend to occur at the transition zone between the fibrocartilaginous labrum and the articular hyaline cartilage.[27] They are perpendicular to the articular surface and, in some cases, extend to the subchondral bone.
  - Type 2 tears consist of one or more cleavage planes of variable depth within the substance of the labrum.[27]

Both types of tears are associated with chondrocyte proliferation and hyalinization of the labral fibrocartilage along the edges of the defect. All labral tears are associated with increased microvascularity within the substance of the labrum at the base of the tear adjacent to the labrum's attachment to bone.[26] Osteophyte formation is also sometimes seen within the labral tears.

Diagnosis can be made on the basis of the history and physical examination. However, it must be remembered that labral tears can have a variety of clinical presentations associated with a wide degree of clinical findings.[26]

- ***History.*** Since a labral lesion produces a decrease of pressure within the joint and causes an increase in the laxity of that joint, symptoms of a labral tear are usually mechanical: buckling, twinges, locking, instability, and painful clicking. There may or may not be a history of trauma. In the presence of a recalled incident, the trauma can vary from severe to very mild.[26] The injury is usually caused by the hip joint being stressed while in rotation. The pain is mainly in the anterior groin (most commonly) but can be in the thigh and/or medial knee, trochanteric, or buttock region.[26] It can have an acute onset or be gradual, and it is common for it to be sharp with a clicking, snapping, catching, or locking sensation.[26] Activities that involve forced adduction of the hip joint in association with rotation in either direction tend to aggravate the pain.[26]

- ***Physical examination.*** On examination, ROM of the hip may not be limited, but there may be pain at the extremes.[26] There is little information regarding the sensitivity, specificity, or likelihood ratios associated with a single clinical test or a cluster of tests in diagnosing a labral tear.[204] Generally speaking, the combined movement of flexion and rotation causes pain in the groin. More precisely, the specific maneuvers that may cause pain in the groin include:[205]
  - flexion, adduction, and internal rotation of the hip joint (impingement test/scour test) while it is held in at least 90 degrees of flexion and at least 15 degrees of abduction—positive with anterior—superior tears, anterior labral tears, and iliopsoas tendinitis;
  - passive hyperextension, abduction, and external rotation (with posterior tears), with the patient lying supine at the edge of the table; a positive finding with this test is apprehension or exquisite pain and suggests anterior hip instability, an anterior labral tear, or posteroinferior impingement;
  - resisted straight-leg raise test;
  - flexion of the hip with external rotation and full abduction, followed by extension, abduction, and internal rotation (anterior tears)[206];
  - extension, abduction, and external rotation brought to a flexed, adducted, and internally rotated position (posterior tears).[206]

In general, the clinician should suspect an acetabular labral tear when a patient has the following combination of signs and symptoms:

- no restrictions in ROM
- normal radiographs
- complaints of a long duration involving anterior hip or groin pain and clicking
- pain with passive hip flexion combined with adduction and internal rotation
- pain with an active straight-leg raise[201]

The diagnosis is typically confirmed with arthrography, MRI with intravenous or intra-articular administration of contrast medium, or arthroscopy.[17]

The appropriate physical therapy intervention for a patient with an acetabular labral tear has yet to be established.[201] Conservative intervention has traditionally included bed rest with or without traction, followed by a period of protected weight-bearing and use of nonsteroidal anti-inflammatory medication. Lewis and Sahrmann[201] recommend the use of key elements of the examination to develop a plan of intervention (Table 19-18). Operative treatment consists of arthrotomy or arthroscopy with resection of the entire labrum or the portion of the labrum that is torn. Postoperatively, the protocol can be divided into three phases[202,206,207]:

Phase 1 (days 1–7):

- Weight-bearing to tolerance with crutches.
- Isometric quadriceps, gluteal sets.
- AROM in all planes of motion.
- Closed-chain bridging, weight shifts, and balancing exercise.
- Open-chain standing abduction, adduction, flexion, and extension with no resistance.
- Avoidance of straight-leg raise exercises.

Phase 2 (weeks 2–3):

- Progress off crutches and normalize gait.
- Progress ROM exercises to gradual end-range stretch within tolerance.
- Stationary bike, if tolerated.
- Open-chain above the knee-resistive theraband or light pulley exercises.

Phase 3 (weeks 4–6):

- Continue flexibility exercises.
- Progress resisted strengthening and closed-chain exercises.
- Functional activities introduced as tolerated.

Femoral acetabular impingement

Femoral acetabular impingement (FAI) occurs when there is decreased joint clearance between the femur and the acetabulum.[204] Two types of FAI have been described: cam and pincer.

- Cam. Cam impingement occurs when the femoral head has an abnormally large radius, with a loss of the normal spherical junction between the femoral head and the neck. This deformity causes abnormal contact between the femur and the acetabulum, particularly when hip flexion is combined with adduction, and internal rotation. The cam impingement has been implicated in the etiology of anteriosuperior labral and chondral lesions.
- Pincer. The pincer type of impingement is caused by an abnormal acetabulum with increased overcoverage. This overcoverage can be general (coxa profunda) or local anterior (acetabular retroversion).

Pincer impingements are thought to be more common in middle-aged women participating in athletics, while cam impingements are more common in young athletic males.

Loose bodies

In advanced cases of OA, the hip joint becomes susceptible to loose bodies of cartilage or bone within the joint. If the loose body is large enough, it will cause a distraction in the joint, which will produce muscle inhibition and problems with gait and weight-bearing.

The patient typically reports sudden leg pain twinges with weight-bearing and periodic giving way of the leg. Clinical findings include a springy end-feel in the hip during passive hip extension (the close-packed position of the joint), which is often painless.

Confirmation and intervention usually involves arthroscopic techniques to identify and then remove the loose body.

The limping child

Examination and evaulation of the pediatric hip is very difficult because of the many changes the joint undergoes

TABLE 19-18 Conservative Intervention for Acetabular Labral Tears Based on Examination Findings	
Examination	**Intervention**
Positions and movement tests	Standing alignment, particularly noting the presence of hip hyperextension, as evident in the hyperextension or pelvic posterior tilt, or both In a sitting position, femoral motions accompanying the extension Precision of both active and passive hip flexions In the prone position, the pattern of hip extension as an indication of the relative participation of the hamstring and gluteus maximus muscles Effect of passive knee flexion on femoral motion in the prone position Pattern and range of hip rotation in prone and sitting positions; this assessment includes asymmetric ranges, suggesting the presence of femoral anteversion or retroversion In the quadruped position, the alignment of the hip joint and the presence of symptoms both while in the position and when rocking backward toward the heels
Muscle strength (force-generating capacity of muscle) and pattern of control	Hip abductor, gluteus maximus, iliopsoas, and deep external rotator muscles when not painful; the deep external rotator muscles are best tested with the hip flexed
Muscle length and stiffness	Medial and lateral hamstring muscles
Gait assessment	Particularly noting a lack of appropriate knee flexion at heel strike and early stance phase, prolonged foot flat during stance, and knee hyperextension that causes hip hyperextension Walking with the hip in external rotation as an improper correction of femoral anteversion
Modification of functional activities	Avoid sitting ▸ with knees lower than hips; ▸ with legs crossed or sitting on legs so that the hip is rotated; ▸ on the edge of deceit and contracting hip flexor muscles; ▸ with pressure on the femur, which can cause forces into the hip joint; instead, the pressure should be on the ischial tuberosity. When getting up from a chair that is behind a desk or out of the car, patients should avoid pushing or rotating the pelvis on a loaded femur. When walking on a treadmill, patients must be careful not to let the moving tread contribute to excessive hip hyperextension. Patients should avoid weight training of quadriceps femoris and hamstring muscles and avoid any exercises causing hip hyperextension

Data from Lewis CL, Sahrmann SA: Acetabular labral tears. *Phys Ther* 86:110–121, 2006.

throughout development. With infants, myelomeningocele (spina bifida), arthrogryposis, and development dysplasia of the hip (DDH) are the major concerns. Hip conditions to consider in children include the potentially serious diseases: bone or joint sepsis, primary or metastatic tumors of the bone, Legg–Calvé–Perthes disease, and slipped femoral capital epiphysis (see Chap. 30). A more benign cause for the limp is "irritable hip"/transient synovitis. A proportion of limping children will have a preceding history of injury, but often this is absent. The main concerns are not to miss serious pathology and to begin appropriate management for the underlying condition.

The watershed age for prognosis of pediatric hip conditions is 8 years old. This is the age when most acetabular development is complete.[4] In children younger than 8 years of age, deformities in the femoral head as a result of a disease process such as Perthes disease or osteonecrosis secondary to the intervention of DDH may be accommodated for by secondary changes in acetabular development.[4] After 8 years of age, accommodation of acetabular shape to a deformed femoral head may not be possible.

The flexion–adduction test (see "Special Tests") can provide an early indication of underlying hip disease, often before any noticeable or measurable change in abduction, internal rotation, or total flexion arc.[142]

It is often the first quadrantric movement to be restricted.[208,209]

Transient Synovitis. This is the most common cause of hip pain and of limp in preschool and early grade school-age children. Transient synovitis is also known as toxic synovitis, irritable hip, and observation hip. The child usually presents with a limp of acute onset, with no history of an inciting episode. There is usually unilateral pain at the hip, knee, or thigh and the child may refuse to move the involved leg in any direction because of pain. If ROM can be examined, it is usually limited in abduction and internal rotation, although with gentle, slow ROM it is possible to obtain full passive range of the hip. The intervention for transient synovitis is decreased weight-bearing for 1–2 weeks, along with nonsteroidal anti-inflammatory drugs (NSAIDs). The condition should be self-limiting unless there is a more serious condition such as septic arthritis or juvenile rheumatoid arthritis present.[210]

Integration of Practice Patterns 4C and 4D: Impaired Joint Mobility, Motor Function, Muscle Performance, and ROM Associated with Muscle Performance Because of Impaired Muscle Performance and Connective Tissue Dysfunction

Snapping hip (Coxa saltans)

Multiple etiologies for snapping hip (coxa saltans) exist. The etiologies are categorized as internal, external, or intraarticular.[211,212]

1. The internal type has been attributed to
   a. the iliopsoas snapping over structures just deep to it, namely the femoral head, proximal lesser trochanter, pectineus fascia, and iliopectineal eminence, which produces a snapping in the anterior groin region[213–216];
   b. stenosing tenosynovitis of the iliopsoas insertion.[217]
2. The external causes include snapping of the ITB or gluteus maximus over the greater trochanter.[213,215,216,218–220] This condition is more common in females with a wide pelvis and prominent trochanters and is exacerbated with running on banked surfaces.[221]
3. The intra-articular causes have included synovial chondromatosis, loose bodies, fracture fragments, and labral tears.[222–224] Snapping of the iliofemoral ligament over the anterior femoral head has also been described,[214,225,226] as has snapping of the long head of biceps origin over the ischium.[227]

When no cause can be identified, as in most patients, the condition is classified as a myopathy of idiopathic origin.

Particular areas of attention during the examination include observation of genu recurvatum, leg length, knee flexion contracture, overpronation of the foot, hip flexion contracture, and the amount of internal or external rotation of the lower extremity during static standing.

The intervention is based on etiology. If an imbalance of the TFL or iliopsoas is producing the symptoms, the intervention is focused on reconditioning and prevention. This includes increasing the flexibility of the soft tissues, and the correction of any strength imbalances. For example, if the flexibilty of the ITB is decreased, the emphasis is on stretching the ITB.

Flexion contracture

A flexion contracture at the hip is a common occurrence. Hip flexion contractures can result from

- adaptive shortening of the iliopsoas muscle or rectus femoris muscles;
- contracture of the anterior hip capsuloligamentous complex.

These changes to the soft tissue and connective tissues around the hip can result from OA, injury, or sustained postures involving hip flexion.

The resulting anterior rotation of the pelvis shifts the weight-bearing of the hip to a thinner region of hyaline cartilage, in both the femur and the acetabulum, and places the hip extensors in a state of low-level tension.[18]

Flexion contractures can be diagnosed using the Thomas test (see "Special Tests").

The intervention for the contracture is based on the cause. Adaptive shortening of the contractile tissues may be addressed using muscle energy, passive stretching, and myofascial techniques. Stretching of the capsuloligamentous complex is accomplished by grade III distraction mobilizations and by prolonged stretching.

Movement impairment syndromes of the hip

Three of the movement impairment syndromes detailed by Sahrmann in her excellent book, *Movement Impairment Syndromes*,[125] are described. The intervention for these syndromes focuses on the correction of muscle imbalances. The adaptively shortened structures are stretched and the weak muscles are strengthened.

Femoral Anterior Glide Syndrome. The characteristic findings for this condition result from an insufficient posterior glide of the femoral head during hip flexion. Typically, the patient complains of groin pain, particularly during hip flexion, gait, and running. The consequences of this syndrome are

- stretching of the anterior joint capsule and tightening of the posterior structures resulting in excessive hip extension ROM;
- an increase or decrease in the length of the hip external rotators;
- a decreased posterior glide of the femoral head;
- a decrease in length of the TFL on the involved side;
- weakness and lengthening of the iliopsoas on the involved side;
- dominance of hamstring activity over gluteus maximus activity, both of which are shortened.

Hip Extension with Knee Extension Syndrome. The characteristic findings for this condition result from an insufficient participation of the gluteus maximus during hip extension or the quadriceps during knee extension. Typically, the patient complains of pain at the hamstring insertion site on the ischial tuberosity and along the muscle belly, particularly during resisted hip extension, knee flexion, or both. The consequences of this syndrome are

- a decrease in hip flexion because of the hypertrophy of the hamstrings;
- dominance of hamstring activity over gluteus maximus activity;
- weakness of the gluteus maximus and hip external rotators;
- a decrease in the length of the hamstrings;
- an increase in the frequency of hamstring strains.

Femoral Accessory Motion Hypermobility. The characteristic findings for this condition result from early degenerative changes and increased compression at the hip joint because of stretching forces on the rectus femoris and hamstrings. Typically, the patient complains of pain deep in the hip joint and anterior groin that may extend along the medial and the anterior thigh, particularly during gait. The consequences of this syndrome are

- a slight antalgic gait;
- internal rotation of the hip during single-leg stance;
- external rotation of the hip with passive knee flexion in prone;
- medial rotation of the femur with knee extension in sitting;
- stiffer rectus femoris and hamstrings as compared to the iliopsoas and intrinsic hip internal rotators;
- anterior hip joint pain with FABER test.

Practice Pattern 4E: Impaired Joint Mobility, Motor Function, Muscle Performance, and ROM Associated with Localized Inflammation

In addition to those conditions producing impaired ROM, motor function, and muscle performance attributed to inflammation, practice pattern E includes conditions that cause pain and muscle guarding without the presence of structural changes. Such conditions include

- sprains of the hip ligaments;
- strains of the hip muscles;
- internal derangements of the hip joint;
- periarticular syndromes: tendinitis, bursitis, capsulitis, and tenosynovitis;
- pubalgia.

Overuse injuries of the hip result from repetitive microtrauma that leads to inflammation and local tissue damage in the form of cellular and extracellular degeneration. This tissue damage can be cumulative, resulting in myositis, bursitis, joint synovitis, cartilaginous degeneration, stress fractures, and neuropraxic or axonal nerve injury. Successful intervention requires a correct identification of the injury.

Hip joint sprains

The classic history of a hip joint sprain is a vigorous twisting of the lower extremity or trunk.[228] Clinical findings include an inability to circumduct the leg because of pain.[229]

Conservative intervention includes an ACE wrap hip spica. Crutches are used for partial weight-bearing ambulation. The crutch walking continues until the patient is able to ambulate without pain.[230] The patient is progressed to strengthening and flexibility exercises, and the functional tests of hopping, sprinting, running backward, cutting, and pivoting in the athlete must be satisfactorily passed prior to return of play.[228]

Muscle strains

First- and second-degree muscle strains are frequent injuries in sports activities.[70] The adductors, iliopsoas, rectus abdominis, gluteus medius, and hamstrings muscles are commonly involved.

Gluteus Medius/Gluteus Minimus. Tendinosis and tears of the gluteus medius and gluteus minimus were a common finding in an MRI study of patients presenting with buttock, lateral hip, or groin pain.[231] Gluteus medius syndrome is manifested by tenderness to palpation of the gluteus medius muscle, which can be triggered by sudden falls, prolonged weight-bearing on one extremity for long periods, activity overuse, or sporting injuries. Most commonly, this condition is observed in middle-aged women who have embarked upon a vigorous walking program, or who have started working out at a health club. Patients may present with pain that is transient and worsening over a time period, a Trendelenburg gait, a leg-length discrepancy and weakness. These symptoms also affect runners, as there is tilting of the pelvis with running. Hip-abduction strengthening should be avoided in the initial stages of gluteus medius syndrome because it only provokes tendinitis. As the acute stage resolves, hip-abductor strengthening is important and is best achieved in the aquatic environment.

Adductor. The hip-adductor muscles, especially the adductor longus and magnus are the most frequent cause of muscle-induced groin region pain.[48,232] Adductor strains have been known to cause long-standing problems.[233]

There are a number of causative factors for an adductor strain, including fatigue or an abduction overload.[234] Laboratory studies have shown that strengthening exercises can protect these muscles from injury.[235]

Adductor strains are associated with running, jumping, and twisting activities, particularly when external rotation of the affected leg is an added part of the activity.[229] Soccer players with a history of forceful kicking are particularly vulnerable to an adductor strain. In fact, the incidence of groin pain among male soccer players is 10–18% per year.[236–238] Adductor muscle strains are also commonly encountered in ice hockey.[239–241] These sports require a strong eccentric contraction of the adductor musculature during competition.[242,243] Risk factors associated with adductor strains include an imbalance between strength and flexibility,[244] and an imbalance between adductor and abductor strength.[243]

The signs and symptoms that are easily recognizable[245]:

- Pain on palpation of the adductor tendons or their insertion on the pubic bone, or both
- Twinging or stabbing pain in the groin area associated with quick starts and stops
- Edema or ecchymosis several days postinjury
- Pain with passive abduction or manual resistance to hip adduction when tested in different degrees of hip flexion (0 degrees [gracilis], 45 degrees [adductor longus and brevis], and 90 degrees [if combined with adduction, pectineus])
- A possible palpable defect in severe ruptures accompanied by muscle guarding

Groin strains are graded as a first-degree strain if there is pain, a minimal loss of strength and minimal restriction of motion; second degree if there is compromise to the strength of the muscle, but not including complete loss of strength and function; and third degree if there is complete disruption of the muscle tendon units, including complete loss of function of the muscle.[246] The differential diagnosis includes abdominal muscle strains, inguinal hernia, osteitis pubis, piriformis syndrome, and referred pain from the hip joint (osteoarthrosis), rectum, or lumbar spine.

Conservative intervention involves the principles of PRICEMEM in the acute stage (see Chap. 8). This is followed by heat applications, hip-adductor isometrics, and gentle stretching during the subacute phase, progressing to a graded resistive program for the adductors, including concentric and eccentric exercises, PNF diagonal motions to promote balance strength and flexibility around the joint, and then a gradual return to full activity. As part of the rehabilitation program, any imbalance between the adductors, abductors, and the abdominals needs to be addressed. In addition, the clinician should examine the patient's technique in their required activity, as poor technique can overload and fatigue the adductors.

Sports Hernia. A sports hernia occurs when weakening of the muscles or tendons of the lower abdominal wall occur but there is no palpable hernia. The symptoms of a sports hernia are characterized by pain during sports movements, particularly twisting and turning during single-limb stance. The pain usually radiates to the adductor muscle region, although it is often difficult for patients to pinpoint. Any exertion that increases intra-abdominal pressure, such as coughing or sneezing can cause pain. Currently, no clinical special test exists with a high degree of specificity to diagnosis this condition so the diagnosis is based on the patient's history and clinical signs when all other causes are ruled out. Conservative treatment usually involves a short period of rest followed by an exercise program focusing on abdominal strengthening. If the conservative approach fails, surgical repair is required.

Iliotibial Band Friction Syndrome. An iliotibial band friction syndrome (ITBFS) can manifest itself at the hip and at the knee (see Chap. 20). At the hip, an ITB contracture can lead to trochanteric bursitis by increasing compression and friction of the sub gluteus maximus bursa between the ITB and the greater trochanter.[34] The classic test for ITB contracture is the Ober test. A comprehensive approach of soft tissue mobilization and hold/relax stretching of the ITB, rectus femoris, and iliopsoas is necessary to decrease the stresses on the bursa.

Iliopsoas. With the exception of the adductors and hamstrings, the iliopsoas is one of the most frequently strained muscles of this region.[247] The mechanism of injury is forced extension of the hip while it is being actively flexed. Clinical findings include

- complaints of pain with attempts at acceleration and high-stepping activities;
- increased pain with resisted hip flexion, adduction, and external rotation.[228]

Conservative intervention involves rest, ice, and compression during the acute phase, progressing to prone lying, heat, a graded resistive exercise program, and specific instructions on proper warm-up and cool-down. Recovery from this condition can be lengthy, and recurrences are frequent.

Quadriceps. Strains of the quadriceps most commonly occur during sports involving sprinting, jumping, or kicking. The rectus femoris is the most commonly involved. Typically, the patient complains of local pain and tenderness in the anterior thigh, which may be gradual in onset or sudden during an explosive muscle contraction. Grade I strains result in pain with resisted testing and with passive stretching. Grade II strains cause significant pain with resisted testing and with passive and unopposed active stretching. Complete tears of the rectus feminists are rare and are usually associated with a palpable defect. During the initial period following injury, the principles of PRICEMEM are applied. Pain-free stretching and soft-tissue mobilization are instituted early to preserve ROM. Straight-leg raises are initiated in the supine position and are progressed to long sitting. Short arc quad sets in pain-free ranges are progressed to full range as tolerated. Closed-kinetic-chain exercises at sub-maximal weight are initiated using short arcs before being progressed to full range. Both concentric and eccentric exercises are performed. Attention must be given to hip flexor and hamstring strength and flexibility to ensure correct muscular balance.

Rectus Abdominis. Rectus abdominis strains usually occur when the muscle is strongly contracting, as it is being moved into a stretched and lengthened position. These strains are common in such sports as tennis, wrestling, pole vaulting, weight lifting, and soccer. Abdominal strains are primarily the result of inadequate abdominal strength and/or incorrect technique.[228] As it may be difficult to differentiate this condition from an inflammation of one of the internal abdominal organs, a physician should be consulted whenever there is any doubt.[247]

These are difficult injuries to heal. Although mild strains may only take 2–3 weeks to heal, premature return to play can create large muscle ruptures, leading to hernia formation in the abdominal wall.[228]

Conservative intervention is the same as for other muscle strains and involves rest, ice, and compression during the acute phase, progressing to heat and gentle stretching, a graded resistive exercise program, and specific instructions on proper warm-up and cool-down. Training and retraining of the rectus abdominis should include half sit-ups, done slowly with the knees bent, to eliminate compensation by the iliopsoas.[228,247]

Hamstrings. The hamstrings are the most commonly strained muscles of the hip,[229] with the biceps femoris being the most commonly injured hamstring. Hamstring tears are typically partial rather than complete, and usually occur during the eccentric phase of muscle usage, when the muscle develops tension as it lengthens. These running related hamstring injuries typically occur along and intramuscular tendon, or aponeurosis, and the adjacent muscle fibers.[248] Another type of hamstring injury, which involves the semimembranosus and its proximal free tendon, can occur during activities such as kicks that involve simultaneous hip flexion and knee extension.[249] This type of injury tends to require a prolonged recovery before an individual is able to return to his or her preinjury level of performance.[250]

A hamstring strain has a varied list of contributing factors including[230]:

- ***Previous hamstring injury.*** There is a strong correlation between a history of prior hamstring injury and recurrence. This is likely because of the fact that the initial injury results in a loss of extensibility and a loss of eccentric strength.

- ► ***Degenerative joint disease of the lumbar spine.*** LB pain and injury result in restricted ROM and decreased hamstring extensibility. In addition, research has demonstrated that LB pain decreases proprioception and neuromuscular control of the lower extremities.
- ► ***Advancing age.*** It is not clear why injuries to soft tissues served by the L5 and S1 nerves, which supply the hamstring and calf muscles, have such a strong correlation with advancing age, whereas there is little or no correlation between age and the soft tissue injuries with an L2–4 nerve supply. One could summize that the lumbar nerve roots of L5 and S1 are more likely to be affected by age-related spinal degeneration than the nerve supply of the quadriceps muscles (L2, L3, and L4).[251]
- ► ***Anterior pelvic tilt.*** A common finding is anterior tilt of the innominate bones on the injured side that increases tension in the hamstrings and causes a relative lengthened position of their origin and insertion. This altered pelvic position can also contribute to decreased hamstring strength. Cibulka et al.[252] researched manipulative treatment to correct an anterior innominate position in patients who had hamstring injuries. After only one treatment, isokinetic hamstring peak torque increased by 21.5% when compared with controls.[252] However, functional improvement from this torque increase was not addressed. One of the reasons cited for the significantly increased incidence in hamstring injuries in athletes of black origin is because they tend to have an increased anteriorly tilted pelvis.
- ► ***Leg length inequality.*** The shorter leg can develop overly tight hamstrings.
- ► ***Anatomical arrangement.*** Being a biarticular muscle group means that the hamstrings are more susceptible to adaptive shortening[253] and can also be subjected to large length changes. Everyday movements, such as walking, squatting, and sitting, flexion of the hip and knee occur together, with opposing effects on hamstring length. In contrast, the knee is extended and the hip is flexed in running and kicking, which places the hamstrings at longer lengths thereby increasing the risk of muscle tears. Antagonists to prime movers, muscles that are used to control or resist motion, are also at a greater risk of injury than the prime movers themselves. While decelerating the body, these muscles contract while rapidly lengthening. Therefore, they are performing "eccentric contractions."
- ► ***Poor posture.*** For example, Janda's lower crossed syndrome, which is associated with adaptive shortening of the hip flexors and the erector spinae, weak/inhibited gluteal and abdominal muscles, an increased anterior pelvic tilt and a hyperlordosis of the spine.
- ► ***Muscle imbalance.*** Muscle balance is a term used to describe the relationship between either:
  - Agonist to antagonist muscle groups. The hamstrings are directly antagonistic to the quadriceps during the first 160–165 degrees of leg extension but assume a paradoxical extensor action concurrent with initial contact.
  - The relationship of agonist muscle groups between limbs (inhibited gluteus maximus).
  - Eccentric to concentric muscle ratios.
  - The strength ratios between the hamstrings and trunk stabilizers.
- ► ***Decreased flexibility.*** Although there is little to no evidence to support this theory, decreased flexibility of the hamstrings has long been cited as the primary cause of hamstring injuries. In fact, the evidence has demonstrated that there is no correlation between passive hip flexion measurements and hamstring injuries provided that the minimum range is between 85 and 90 degrees. However, a differentiation must be made between active flexibility (the absolute range of movement in a joint or series of joints that is attainable in a momentary effort) and passive flexibility (the ability to assume and maintain extended positions) as research has shown that active flexibility is more closely related to sports achievement than is passive flexibility.

CLINICAL PEARL

Jonhagen and colleagues[254] found decreased flexibility and lower eccentric hamstring torques in runners who sustained a hamstring strain when compared with uninjured subjects matched for age and speed.

- ► ***Hamstring strength.*** The relationship between strength and the potential for a hamstring injury is not made clear in the studies available. Many authors have commented on the limitations of isokinetic testing and the specificity of the types of training. Few studies have reported on the relationship between concentric and eccentric strengths and the frequency of hamstring injury, but those that have suggested that poor eccentric strength in the hamstring muscle group might be a causative factor in hamstring strains. Kibler[255] stated that sports- or activity-specific testing is more appropriate for evaluating an athlete. Zachazewski[256] commented that for a test to have a predictive value it must incorporate some of the dynamic characteristics specific to that sport. Lephart et al.[257] states that low peak torque values are not necessarily related to functional capacity.
- ► ***Precipitating activity.*** Most hamstring injuries occur during running at the end of the swing phase or at foot strike when the hamstrings are working to decelerate the limb, while also controlling extension of the knee. At this point the greatest muscle–tendon stretch is incurred by the biceps femoris, which may contribute to its tendency to be more often injured than the other two hamstring muscles during high-speed running.[248] With the forceful flexion of the hip and extension of the knee during the swing phase of sprinting, the hamstring muscle groups are put under extremely high loads in a lengthened position where they must change from functioning eccentrically, to decelerate knee extension in the late swing, to concentrically, becoming an active extensor of

the hip joint. It has been proposed that this rapid changeover from eccentric to concentric function of the hamstring is when the muscle is most vulnerable to injury. Kujala et al.[46] also suggested that, during this swing phase, the hamstrings are placed under extremely high loads in an elongated position.

- ***Inadequate warm-up.*** Although most clinicians prescribe warm-up and stretching to help reduce the incidence of muscle strains, the evidence supporting this idea is weak and largely based on retrospective studies.[258]
- ***Fatigue.*** In a study of professional soccer players, nearly half (47%) of the hamstring injuries sustained during matches occurred during the last third of the first and second halves of the match. Kyrolainen et al.[259] looked at the recruitment pattern of leg muscles during different running speeds. The greatest changes in muscle activity pattern were observed in the biceps femoris muscles as the speed increased from a slow jog to maximum speed. Pinniger et al[260] found that, when footballers became fatigued during sprinting, there was earlier activation of the biceps femoris and semitendinosus muscles. Asynchrony may be because of local muscle fatigue and/or neural fatigue as a result of "irritation or damage along the path of the nerve supplying the muscle." General fatigue secondary to poor sleep patterns, stress, or suboptimal nutrition could result in central nervous system fatigue.
- ***Poor coordination.*** Many hamstring strains occur during the last part of the swing phase or at heel strike, during which time the hamstrings work maximally eccentrically to decelerate the leg.

Other unsubstantiated predisposing factors include cleat design, playing surface, level of hydration, adverse neural tension, experience of the coach, and hormonal levels (abnormally low resting levels of testosterone and unfavorable testosterone/cortisol ratio during recuperation after exercise).[46,119,261–263]

It is likely that a combination of the aforementioned factors play a role in hamstring injuries. Some of these factors are modifiable, others are not. The modifiable factors include muscle imbalances between flexibility and strength, overall conditioning, and playing surface.

Clinical findings associated with hamstring injury include:

- patient reports of a distinctive mechanism of injury with immediate pain during sprinting or while decelerating quickly.[228] In acute cases, the patient may report a "pop" or tearing sensation.
- tenderness elicited with passive stretching of the hamstrings.
- posterior thigh pain, often near the buttock, which is worsened with resisted knee flexion.
- tenderness to palpation, which is generally located at the muscle origin at the ischial tuberosity but may also be present in the muscle belly and distal insertions.

Hamstring strains can be graded according to findings:[228]

- Grade I: gait appears normal but there is pain with extreme range of a straight-leg raise.
- Grade II: antalgic gait or gait with a flexed knee. Resisted knee flexion and hip extension are both painful and weak.
- Grade III: usually requires the use of crutches for ambulation. In severe cases, ecchymosis, hemorrhage, and a muscle defect may be visible several days postinjury.

The differential diagnosis for posterior thigh pain includes neoplasms, overt lumbar disk protrusions with definite signs of nerve root impingement, ischial tuberosity apophysitis, or an avulsion fracture. Examination of the lumbar spine is important, because muscle injury may be related to referred pain with subsequent muscle inhibition and weakness.[264]

No consensus exists for rehabilitation of the hamstring muscles after strain. Despite differences in injury mechanisms and recovery time, current examination and rehabilitation approaches generally do not consider injury location (i.e., proximal free tendon injuries versus intramuscular tendon and adjacent muscle fibers) as part of the clinical decision making process. [249] Since in noninjured subjects, the performance of controlled eccentric strength training exercises has been shown to facilitate a shift in peak force development to longer muscle–tendon lengths,[265] eccentric exercises have been advocated in the rehabilitation of hamstring injuries.[266] A recent prospective investigation determined through isokinetic testing that a strength imbalance (≥20% bilateral deficit) between the eccentric hamstrings (30 degrees per second) and concentric quadriceps (240 degrees per second) resulted in a four-fold increase in risk ratio of hamstring injury (risk ratio, 4.66; 95% confidence interval: 2.01–10.8) compared to a normal strength profile.[267]

A number of eccentric strengthening protocols have been proposed that include such exercises as hamstring lowers, and the use of Yo-Yo™ flywheel ergometry. Although these protocols appear to decrease the severity of an initial injury, they tend to have an increased participant dropout rate because of the occurrence of muscle soreness and delayed onset muscle soreness (DOMS).[261,268,269]

As with all strains, the rehabilitation protocol is based on the stage of healing. Patients with a grade I strain can usually continue activities as much as possible. A grade II strain typically requires 5–21 days for rehabilitation, whereas a patient with a grade III strain may require 3–12 weeks of rehabilitation.

The protocol outlined in Table 19-19 is recommended. Muscle imbalances of strength and flexibility are addressed with proper techniques to stretch and strengthen the hamstrings. Exercises to enhance eccentric loading include the supine bent knee bridge walk out (Fig. 19-68), the supine single-limb chair bridge (Fig. 19-70), unilateral good mornings with rotations (Fig. 19-72), and increasing intensities of grapevine stepping (Fig. 19-76).

Finally, when appropriate, the biomechanical factors, including excessive anterior tilt of the pelvis, lumbar spine and sacroiliac joint dysfunction (trunk stabilization exercises) and leg length discrepancies, should be addressed and corrected.

TABLE 19-19 Rehabilitation Protocol for Hamstring Injury

Phase	Protocol
I (acute): 1–7 days	Rest, ice, compression, and elevation to control hemorrhaging and minimize inflammation and pain. Nonsteroidal anti-inflammatory drugs are an almost universally accepted treatment, and the only controversial aspect to their use is the appropriate timing of administration. The most common recommendation in the literature is short-term use (3–7 d), starting immediately after the injury. However, theoretically it would be beneficial to delay the treatment until 2–4 d after the injury, because they interfere with chemotaxis of cells, which is necessary for the repair and remodeling of regenerating muscle. Early motion exercise is theoretically important to prevent or decrease adhesion within the connective tissue. Active knee flexion and extension exercises could be performed during the treatment with ice. It is important that the exercises are pain free to prevent further injury during the rehabilitation.
II (subacute): day 3 to 3 wks	Begins when the signs of inflammation (swelling, heat, redness, and pain) begin to resolve. In this phase, it is important to continue muscle action to prevent atrophy and promote healing. Regular concentric strength exercises can begin in this phase when the athlete has achieved full range of motion without pain. The common recommendation in this stage is multiple joint angle, submaximal isometric contraction. If the athlete experiences pain, the intensity should be decreased. In this phase, other activities can be initiated to maintain cardiovascular fitness. This could be stationary bike riding, swimming, or other controlled resistance activities.
III (remodeling); 1–6 wks	To avoid the hamstring muscle becoming less flexible after the injury, hamstring stretching can begin in the third phase. Eccentric strengthening can begin (see text).
IV (functional): 2 wks to 6 months	The goal in this phase is return to sport without reinjury. This is achieved by increasing hamstring strength and flexibility to the normal values for the individual athlete. Simultaneously, pain-free running activities are increased from jogging at low intensity to running and finally sprinting. Pain-free participation in sports-specific activities is the best indicator of readiness to return to play.
V (return to competition): 3 wks to 6 months	When the athlete has returned to competition, the goal is to avoid reinjury. The focus should, therefore, be on maintaining stretching and strengthening.

Data from Clanton TO, Coupe KJ: Hamstring strains in athletes: Diagnosis and treatment. *J Am Acad Orthop Surg* 6:237–248, 1998.

CLINICAL PEARL

Rehabilitation of hamstring strains using progressive agility and trunk stabilizing exercises has been found to be more effective than a program emphasizing isolated hamstring stretching and strengthening.[270] An athlete should not be permitted to return to full participation in sports until flexibility and strength ratios have been restored, and before plyometric and functional exercises are able to be performed pain free.[228,230]

Tendinitis

Rectus Femoris. Rectus femoris tendinitis is typically sports-related, resulting from acute or chronic overuse. The pain is usually located at the origin (ASIS), or just distal to it. The patient often complains of groin pain during sprinting or lifting the knee. In most cases, the cause is adaptive shortening of the rectus. Intervention involves stretching and transverse friction massage (TFM).

Iliopsoas. Tendinitis of the iliopsoas complex almost always involves an overstretching of the muscle belly. The patient complains of groin pain, which can radiate into the anterior thigh. Resisted hip flexion and external rotation are often painful. In addition, passive hip flexion or passive hip extension/internal rotation are painful. The involved site is almost always just distal to the inguinal ligament, and just medial to the sartorius muscle. Conservative intervention involves TFM and stretching.

Quadriceps contusion

The term *charley horse* is synonymous with a contusion of the quadriceps muscle. These contusions are quite common and can vary in their degree of discomfort. They are usually because of a direct blow to the anterior thigh, with the vastus lateralis and intermedius being the most frequently involved.

The patient usually describes a specific mechanism and complains of a dull aching pain over the thigh. Clinical findings include

- palpable tenderness over the anterior lateral aspect of the thigh;
- variable swelling; extreme swelling should alert the clinician to the possibility of an injury to major vessels;

- pain increased with knee flexion, which is sometimes accompanied by spasm;
- a palpable hematoma on occasion.

Quadriceps contusions can be graded according to functional loss[271]:

- ***Grade I.*** In a mild contusion, the patient has localized tenderness with no alteration of gait. Knee motion can be performed without pain up to at least 90 degrees of flexion.
- ***Grade II.*** In a moderate contusion, the patient displays swelling and a tender muscle mass. Knee flexion motion is restricted to less than 90 degrees and an antalgic gait is present. The patient is unable to climb stairs or arise from a chair without considerable discomfort.
- ***Grade III.*** In a severe contusion, the patient cannot bend their knee beyond approximately 45 degrees. The patient is unable to walk unaided. Marked tenderness and swelling are present.

Conservative intervention involves a gradual progression of ROM and strengthening exercises.

Hip pointer

A hip pointer is a subcutaneous contusion of the iliac crest resulting from a direct blow, usually at or near the ASIS. The contusion is graded from I to III, depending on the extent of damage. Grade I hip pointers functionally limit the patient for about 5–14 days, while grade II and III hip pointers can functionally limit the patient for 14–21 days.

Usually, the patient reports point tenderness over the ASIS. The pain is increased with passive hip extension, resisted hip flexion, external rotation and abduction, active trunk motions, and with such activities as laughing, coughing, or sneezing.[228]

Early intervention within 2–4 hours is critical to avoid severe pain and limited trunk motion. The early intervention includes ice, compression, rest, and anti-inflammatory measures. Early motion exercises, which emphasize trunk side flexion to the side opposite the injury, should be initiated as tolerated and can be accompanied with transcutaneous electrical nerve stimulation (TENS). As the symptoms subside, gentle-graded stretching exercises are added in addition to trunk-strengthening exercises. Especially effective exercises include long sitting, straight-leg raises with the hip externally rotated, as well as the PNF diagonal flexion adduction, external rotation to extension, abduction, and internal rotation.

Prophylactic prevention of the injury with adequate padding of the iliac crest using materials such as high-density foam and orthoplast is recommended.

Pubalgia

Pubalgia is a collective term for all disorders that cause chronic pain in the region of the pubic tubercle and the structures attached to the pubic bone (inguinal region), including osteitis pubis, a chronic inflammatory and overuse condition of the pubic symphysis and adjacent ischial rami. A number of abnormalities in joints and muscles around the groin may increase the mechanical stress placed on the pubic region:

- limited hip ROM;
- increased adductor muscle tone;
- increased rectus abdominis tone;
- iliopsoas muscle shortening, often associated with hypomobility of the upper lumbar spine;
- lumbar spine/SIJ dysfunction;
- decreased lumbopelvic stability.

Pubalgia typically results from a sports injury. It usually results from a single-leg movement, where the weight-bearing leg is rotated as the other leg performs a movement such as kicking, or during activities such as sprinting and pivoting. During this kind of motion, small shearing movements occur in the pubic symphysis. The condition is rarely found in women—this may be because of variations in pelvic anatomy between men and women and strength differences or participation levels between genders.

Pubalgia typically presents as lower abdominal pain with exertion, minimal to no pain at rest, and increased pain with activities that involve resisted hip adduction. After the initial pain, the pain disappears when the patient is warmed up, only to return, often more intensely, after the activity. Eventually, the pain will increase with exertion and only slightly diminish with rest.

In most cases, the pain is unilateral at onset, with progression to bilateral pain in about 40% of cases.[272] Examination findings include the following:

- Pain may be elicited with passive hip flexion, when combined with hip adduction, or with passive abduction with a straight or bent knee. However, in some cases, ROM may appear normal.
- Point tenderness at the pubic tubercles, rectus abdominis insertion, adductor origin, and inferior pubic rami.
- Pain is intensified with sit-ups and resisted hip adduction.

Groin pain is a common complaint and can be ascribed to various disorders (see Table 19-20 and Table 19-21), necessitating a thorough knowledge of differential diagnosis. Palpation of the relevant structures should help in locating the cause, as will resistive testing of the various muscles.

Once the diagnosis has been established, the conservative intervention should be causal:

- A period of relative rest and anti-inflammatory medications.
- TFM can be applied locally.
- Ultrasound, electrical stimulation, thermotherapy, and cryotherapy as appropriate.
- Stretching as tolerated to the muscles surrounding the injured area:
  - The short and long adductors.
  - Hip flexors (iliopsoas and rectus femoris).
  - Hip internal rotators.
  - Abdominals.
  - Gluteal muscles.
- Strengthening of the same muscle groups. The strengthening exercises are performed isometrically initially, and then concentrically and eccentrically, and finally isokinetically as appropriate.
- Core stability training. A particularly effective form of core strengthening for athletic pubalgia, developed by Alex

TABLE 19-20 Differentiation of Hip Pathologies

Factor	Congenital Hip Dislocation	Septic Arthritis	Legg–Calvé–Perthes Disease	Transient Synovitis	Slipped Femoral Capital Epiphysis	Avascular Necrosis	Degenerative Joint Disease	Fracture
Age	Birth	Less than 2 yr; rare in adults	2–13 yr	2–12 yr	Males 10–17 yr; females 8–15 yr	30–50 yr	40 yr	Older adults
Incidence	Female > male; left > right; blacks < whites		Male > female; rare in blacks; 15% bilateral	Male > female; unilateral	Male > female; blacks > whites	Male > female	Female > male	Female > male
Observation	Short limb, associated with torticollis	Irritable child; motionless hip; prominent greater trochanter; mild illness	Short limb; high greater trochanter; quad atrophy; adductor spasm	Decreased flexion, abduction, and external rotation; thigh atrophy; and muscle spasm	Short limb, obese, quadriceps atrophy, and adductor spasm		Frequently obese, joint crepitus, and atrophy of gluteal muscles	Ecchymosis; may be swelling; short limb
Position	Flexed and abducted	Flexed, abducted, and externally rotated			Flexed, abducted, and externally rotated			External rotation
Pain		Mild pain with palpation and passive motion; often referred to knee	Gradual onset; aching in hip, thigh, and knee	Acute: severe pain in knee; moderate: pain in thigh and knee; tenderness over hip	Vague pain in knee, suprapatellar area, thigh, and hip; pain in extreme motion	50% sharp pain and 50% insidious and intermittent pain in extreme ends of range	Insidious onset and pain with fall in barometric pressure	Severe pain in groin area
History	May be breech birth	Steroid therapy; fever	20–25% familial, low birth weight, and growth delay	Low-grade fever	May be trauma		May be prolonged trauma and faulty body mechanics	May be trauma and fall
Range of motion	Limited abduction	Decreased (capsular pattern)	Limited abduction and extension	Decreased flexion, limited extension, and internal rotation	Limited internal rotation, abduction, and flexion; increased external adductor spasm	Decreased range of motion	Decreased motion, external and internal rotation, and extreme flexion	Limited
Special tests	Galeazzi's sign, Ortolani's sign, and Barlow's sign;	Joint aspiration						
Gait		Refuses to walk	Antalgic gait after activity	Refuses to walk and antalgic limp	Acute: antalgic; chronic: Trendelenberg external rotation	Coxalgic limp	Limp	
Radiologic findings	Upward and lateral displacement and delayed development of acetabulum	CT scan: localized abscess; increased separation of ossification	In stages: increased density, fragmentation, and flattening of epiphysis center	Normal at first, widened medial joint space	Displacement of upper femoral epiphysis, especially in frog position	Flattening followed by collapse of femoral head	Increased bone density, osteophytes, and subarticular cysts; degenerated articular cartilage	Fracture line and possible displacement; short femoral neck

Data from Richardson JK, Iglarsh ZA: *The Hip, Clinical Orthopaedic Physical Therapy*. Philadelphia, PA: WB Saunders, 1994:367–368.

TABLE 19-21 Differential Diagnosis for Common Causes of Hip Pain

Condition	Patient Age (yr)	Mechanism of Injury/Onset	Area of Symptoms	Symptoms Aggravated by	Observation
Trochanteric bursitis	15–45	Direct trauma Microtrauma	Lateral aspect of hip/thigh	Lying on involved side	Unremarkable
Groin strain	20–40	Sudden overload	Anteromedial thigh Medial thigh	Running	Possible bruising around medial thigh
Hamstring muscle tear	15–45	Sudden overload	Buttock and posterior thigh	Running	Possible bruising around posterior thigh
Piriformis syndrome	25–55	Gradual	Buttock and posterior thigh Back of leg	Prolonged sitting	Unremarkable
Hip OA	50+	Gradual	Anterior thigh Anteromedial thigh	Weight-bearing	Possible atrophy of thigh muscles Altered gait
Iliotibial band syndrome	25–55	Overuse	Lateral aspect of thigh Lateral aspect of knee		Unremarkable
Psoas bursitis	20–40	Overuse	Anteromedial thigh		Unremarkable
Lumbar/thoracic disk pathology	20–50	Gradual Sudden overload	Varies according to spinal nerve root involved but occurs in dermatomal distribution	Lumbar/thoracic flexion (bending/sitting) Activities that increase intrathecal pressure	May have associated deviation of trunk

OA, osteoarthritis; AROM, active range of motion; ER, external rotation; SLR, straight-leg raise; IR, internal rotation; PROM, passive range of motion.

AROM	PROM	Resisted	Tenderness with Palpation
Painful hip abduction with rotation	Pain at end-range hip ER Pain with hip ER with abduction	Pain with resisted hip abduction Pain with resisted hip IR	Lateral thigh over greater trochanter
Hip extension only limited movement	Pain at end-range hip extension Pain at end-range hip abduction	Pain with resisted hip adduction	Proximal medial thigh
Hip ER limited and painful	Pain at end-range hip flexion		
SLR limited and painful	Pain at end-range hip extension Pain with passive SLR	Pain with resisted hip extension Pain with resisted knee flexion	Posterior thigh
SLR limited and painful	Pain at end-range hip ER Pain with passive SLR	Pain with resisted hip ER	Buttock
Limited hip IR and extension	Pain at end-range hip IR	Weak hip abduction	Anterior hip
Painful hip IR	All movements feel stiff	General weakness of hip muscles	
Painful hip extension			
Pain on moving from knee extension to flexion	Pain at end-range hip ER with abduction	All resistive tests negative	Lateral epicondyle of femur Lateral aspect of knee
Hip extension with only limited movement	Pain at end-range hip extension	Pain with resisted hip flexion	Anterior hip
Increased symptoms with trunk flexion	Symptoms invariably increased with passive SLR	Fatigable weakness of associated myotome	Possible tenderness over involved spinal segment
Increased symptoms with hip flexion with knee extended (SLR)			

McKechnie, uses diagonal elastic tubing resistance between the upper and lower extremities. These exercises combine a contraction of the pelvic floor and transversus abdominis muscles while performing activities such as squats (Fig. 19-56), lunges (Fig. 19-55), and sport-specific movements.

- Proprioception training.

Effective warm-ups and preparation before the sporting activity can play an important preventative role.

In cases of failed conservative intervention, which is common, surgical intervention (pelvic floor repair) or cessation from the offending activity becomes the patient's only choice.[272] Post-surgical rehabilitation uses many of the same exercises and modalities as in the traditional rehabilitation program outlined above.

Bursitis

Trochanteric/Subtrochanteric. Trochanteric bursitis is the shared name given to inflammation of any one of the three trochanteric bursae. It has been suggested that trochanteric bursitis should be considered as a clinical diagnosis rather than an anatomical diagnosis, because it cannot be distinguished from gluteal tendinitis by signs and symptoms alone.[34] Trochanteric bursitis is the second most frequent cause of lateral hip pain, with a peak incidence occurring between 40 and 60 years of age,[50] and is more common in arthritic conditions and fibromyalgia and leg length discrepancy.[34,273] It is also more common in females than males (2–4:1 ratio).[34]

The bursae can become inflamed through either friction or direct trauma, such as a fall on the side of the hip.

The history may reveal complaints of aching lateral thigh, groin, and gluteal pain, especially when lying on the involved side.[274] Although the pain is typically local to the hip region, it can radiate distally to the knee and the lower leg.

Objectively, the clinical findings include

- the reproduction of pain with palpation or with stretching of the ITB across the trochanter with hip adduction or the extremes of internal or external hip rotation[275];
- that resisted abduction, extension, or external rotation of the hip are also painful;
- that there is often associated tightness of the hip adductors, which cause the patient's feet to cross the midline, resulting in increased stress on the trochanteric bursa.

Differential diagnosis should include[43,276]

- tendopathy of the gluteus medius or maximus muscles, with or without calcification;
- inguinal and femoral hernia;
- an irritation of the L4–5 nerve root;
- meralgia paresthetica;
- a "snapping" hip;
- lower spinal neoplasm;
- pelvic tumor;
- hip infection;
- avascular necrosis;
- stress fracture of the femur;
- bone or soft tissue tumor.

There is very little research on physical therapy interventions for trochanteric bursitis.[277] The intervention typically consists of the removal of the causative factors by stretching the lateral thigh tissues, especially the TFL and ITB, and emphasizing flexibility of the external rotators, quadriceps, and hip flexors. Strengthening of the hip abductors and correction of any muscle imbalances between the adductors and abductors is also important. Other interventions include heat and ultrasound. TFM has also been advocated.[278] Orthotics may be prescribed if there is a biomechanical fault in the kinetic chain. A steroid injection at the area of tenderness over the greater trochanter may be useful in particularly intense or recalcitrant cases.

Iliopsoas/Iliopectineal. The IPB is located between the anterior aspect of the hip joint capsule and the musculotendinous junction of the iliopsoas. Iliopsoas bursitis seems to be under-recognized by the medical community despite reports that continue to be published. This may be because the entity often exists for years without being identified. The usual complaint is one of anterior hip or groin pain, which is aggravated by lumbar or hip hyperextension or power walking. In the older populations, psoas bursitis can mimic such conditions as hip joint pathology, an L2–3 nerve root pathology, and meralgia paresthetica.

Objective findings are few, and they include

- pain with passive hip flexion and adduction at the end range;
- pain with passive hip extension and external rotation, which is increased if the hip flexors are resisted in this position;
- palpable tenderness of the involved bursa.

Conservative intervention consists of a stretching and strengthening program of the hip rotators and hip flexors. Johnston and colleagues[279] have published a conservative approach to iliopsoas bursitis, based on a retrospective study of nine patients with the condition. The recommended protocol consists of the following exercises:

- seated hip internal and external elastic resistance exercises;
- side-lying abduction/external rotation elastic resistance exercises;
- mini-squats, weight-bearing on the affected leg;
- stretching of the hip flexor, quadriceps, and lateral hip/piriformis, and hamstring muscles.

Ischial. An ischial bursitis, also referred to as Weaver's bottom, involves two different bursae, one between the ischial tuberosity and the inferior part of the gluteus maximus belly, and the other between the tendons of the biceps femoris and semimembranosus. Inflammation of these bursae usually results from chronic compression or direct trauma.

Subjectively, the patient typically reports pain with sitting in a firm chair, almost as soon as the buttocks touch the chair. Ischial bursitis tends to affect thinner people more than obese individuals and women more than men. It is also common in cyclists.

Differential diagnosis should include lumbar nerve root impingement, hamstring syndrome, piriformis syndrome, and hamstring insertion tendopathy. These can be differentiated between using the history, palpation, and resistive testing, as patients with ischial bursitis generally will not complain of pain in the posterior thigh or demonstrate hamstring flexibility and strength inadequacies.

Conservative intervention is based on the cause, and typically involves relative rest, the use of a padded seat cushion, soft tissue massage, correction of hamstring strength and flexibility deficits, anti-inflammatory measures such as ice massage, and ultrasound.

Gluteal. Inflammation of the gluteal bursa, which is located above and behind the greater trochanter, and underneath the gluteus maximus and medius, is one of the most frequent causes of pseudoradicular pain in the lower extremity. The patient, who is usually in their fourth or fifth decade, typically complains of pain in the gluteal or trochanteric area, which may spread to the outer or posterior thigh, and down to the calf muscles and the malleolus. Unlike the pain caused by a lumbar disk lesion, the symptoms are not related to sitting, but only to walking and going up stairs. A typical pattern is pain on passive internal rotation and abduction, and resisted external rotation or abduction.

Conservative intervention is based on the cause, and usually involves the use of a padded seat cushion, anti-inflammatory measures such as ice massage, and ultrasound.

Integration of Practice Patterns 4C, 4F, and 5F: Impaired Joint Mobility, Motor Function, Muscle Performance, ROM Associated with Spinal Disorders, Sign of the Buttock, Myofascial Pain Dysfunction (Referred Pain Patterns), and Peripheral Nerve Entrapments

If the tests and measures of the hip are negative for a hip disorder or a dysfunction of the lower kinetic chain, the clinician should examine the lumbar spine and sacroiliac joint, both of which can refer pain to this region.

Many internal disorders such as femoral and inguinal hernias, pelvic inflammatory disease, prostatitis, and nephrolithiasis can produce pain in the lower abdomen and groin region (see Chap. 5). These are all out of the scope of practice for the physical therapist, and a proper referral to an internist, urologist, or gynecologist should be sought.

Sign of the buttock

The sign of the buttock is a collection of signs that indicate the presence of serious pathology posterior to the axis of flexion and extension in the hip. Among the causes of the syndrome are osteomyelitis, fracture of the sacrum/pelvis, infections, sacroilitiis, gluteal hematoma, septic bursitis, ischiorectal abscess, tumor, and rheumatic bursitis. Typical findings include gross hip weakness with empty end-feel. The involved buttock looks larger. The seven signs of the buttock are

- a limited straight-leg raise;
- limited hip flexion;
- limited trunk flexion;
- a noncapsular pattern of hip restriction;
- painful and weak hip extension;
- gluteal swelling;
- an empty end-feel on hip flexion.

If the sign of the buttock is present, a medical referral is necessary.

Meralgia paresthetica

Patients with meralgia paresthetica typically describe burning, coldness, lightning-type pain, deep muscle achiness, and tingling or frank anesthesia in the anterolateral thigh (see Chap. 5). There may also be local hair loss in the anterolateral thigh.[280] The symptoms may be exacerbated when the hip is extended, as in prone lying, or when standing erect. Sitting may relieve the symptoms in some patients but exacerbate them in others. Eventually, there may be no position that provides relief.[280]

The initial intervention of meralgia paresthetica is conservative, and patients may benefit from analgesics, NSAIDs, looser clothing, and weight loss.

Piriformis syndrome

Piriformis syndrome is the result of entrapment of the sciatic nerve by the piriformis muscle, as it passes through the sciatic notch (see Chap. 5). Clinical findings include[281]

- restriction in ROM of hip adduction and internal rotation;
- positive FABER test;
- weak gluteus maximus, gluteus medius, and biceps femoris;
- neurologic symptoms in the posterior lower limb if the fibularis (peroneal) nerve is involved;
- ipsilateral short leg.

Conservative intervention for this condition includes gentle, pain-free static stretching of the piriformis muscle, strain–counterstrain techniques, soft tissue therapies (longitudinal gliding combined with passive internal hip rotation, as well as transverse gliding and sustained longitudinal release, with the patient lying on one side), ice massage to the gluteal region, and spray and stretch techniques.[228,282] Local corticosteroid or botox injections may be useful in more acute cases.[283]

Entrapment of the obturator nerve

Compression of the anterior division of the obturator nerve in the thigh has been described recently as one possible cause for adductor region pain, and entrapment of this nerve has been documented by nerve conduction studies.[284] The fascia over the nerve is thought to contribute to compression of the nerve, or perhaps allow for the development of a compartment syndrome.[284]

Myofascial pain dysfunction

Myofascial pain is referred into the hip from the following muscles: quadratus lumborum, piriformis, gluteus minimus, and adductor longus.

Quadratus Lumborum. This muscle is perhaps one of the most overlooked sources of hip pain. The more superficial trigger points of this muscle refer pain to the lateral ilium and greater trochanter and may also refer pain into the groin in the region of the inguinal ligament. The tenderness in the trochanteric region can be misdiagnosed as trochanteric bursitis.

Clinical findings can include

- restriction of hip joint movements by lumbar spasm;
- trochanteric and buttock tenderness;
- a contralateral short leg;
- an ipsilateral flexed innominate.

Conservative intervention includes gentle, pain-free static stretching of the muscle, soft tissue techniques, and progressive strengthening.

Gluteus Minimus. Trigger points may be located in the posterior and anterior portions of this muscle. The posterior trigger point refers pain to the medial lower buttock and into the posterior thigh and calf. These trigger points have the potential to increase the tone in the hamstring and calf muscles. Stretching the gluteus minimus before hamstring and calf stretching allows these two muscles to lengthen much more readily. The anterior trigger point refers symptoms to the lower buttock, and down the lateral thigh and leg as far as the lateral malleolus, on occasion.

Conservative intervention includes gentle, pain-free static stretching of the muscle, soft tissue techniques, and progressive strengthening.

Adductor Longus. Trigger points in this muscle strongly refer to the anterior hip and anterior knee. Clinical findings include

- pain with resisted strength testing;
- positive FABER test for pain;
- marked restriction of hip abduction.

Conservative intervention includes gentle, pain-free static stretching of the muscle, soft tissue techniques, and progressive strengthening.

Practice Pattern 4G: Impaired Joint Mobility, Motor Function, Muscle Performance, and ROM Associated with Fractures

Avulsions

Apophyseal avulsions of the pelvis and proximal femur occur most commonly to male athletes 10–20 years old, usually as the direct result of vigorous or uncoordinated activities such as kicking, jumping, hurdling, sprinting, and punting, involving the sartorius or TFL.[228,285] The anterior iliac spine is a common site for the injury, especially during the middle-to-late teenage years when the iliac crest unites with the ilium. Clinical findings can include[286]

- point tenderness;
- crepitus;
- hematoma;
- limited hip motion;
- pain with resisted hip flexion and passive hip extension that increase pain at the site.

Conservative intervention includes ice and hip spica compression, followed by bed rest, progressing to crutch ambulation and activity modification. Return to normal activity follows a period of strength, flexibility, and functional training.[228]

Stress fractures of the femoral neck/head

Stress fractures result from accelerated bone remodeling in response to repeated stress. Although stress fractures are a relatively uncommon etiology of hip pain, if not diagnosed in a timely fashion, progression to serious complications can occur.[287] It is estimated that up to 5% of all stress fractures involve the femoral neck, with another 5% involving the femoral head.[288] The fracture typically occurs on the superior side (tension-side fractures) or the inferior side (compression-side fractures) of the femoral neck.[289] These fractures may develop into a complete and displaced fracture if left untreated.

The most frequent symptom is the onset of sudden hip pain, usually associated with a recent change in training (particularly an increase in distance or intensity) or a change in training surface. The earliest and most frequent symptom is pain in the deep thigh, inguinal, or anterior groin area.[289] Pain can also occur in the lateral aspect or anteromedial aspect of the thigh. The pain usually occurs with weight-bearing or at the extremes of hip motion and can radiate into the knee. Less severe cases may only have pain following a long run. Night pain may occur if the fracture progresses. Stress fractures are generally classified as fatigue or insufficiency fractures[145]:

- Fatigue stress fractures are caused by repetitive and abnormally high forces from muscle action and/or weight-bearing torques and are often found in persons with normal bone densities. This type of stress fracture at the hip is most common in athletes involved in intense training, including military personnel.
- Insufficiency stress fractures are associated with individuals who have compromised bone densities. Since insufficiency stress fractures are associated with decreased bone mineral density, they tend to be most common in the elderly, especially postmenopausal women. Other predisposing factors for poor bone density include radiation treatments, rheumatoid arthritis due at least in part to the associated disuse and either corticosteroid or methotrexate treatment, renal failure, coxa vara, metabolic disorders, and Paget's disease.

The physical examination is often negative, although there may be a noncapsular pattern of the hip,[145] an empty end-feel, or pain at the extremes of hip internal or external rotation or pain with resisted hip external rotation.[290] In addition, the auscultatory patellar-pubic percussion test may be positive (see "Special Tests" section).

Differential diagnosis includes OA of the hip, referred symptoms from the spine, trochanteric bursitis, or septic arthritis.

Radiographs taken soon after the symptoms begin have been reported to be positive in only 20% of cases.[289] Diagnosis is best confirmed with bone scintigraphy (scan), although these have been shown to be prone to false negatives.[291] The intervention varies according to the bone scintigraphy findings.[289]

- If there is a positive scan only, or sclerosis and no fracture line on the radiographs, the intervention ranges from modified bed rest to non–weight-bearing with crutches until symptoms subside. Once pain free, weight-bearing is progressed. When significant PWB is pain free, cycling and swimming may be permitted. Weekly radiographs are obtained until the athlete is full weight-bearing without pain. Water running and water walking are progressed. If these remain pain free, running on land is commenced, with the initial run being no further than one-quarter mile.
- If there is an overt fracture line on the radiographs with no displacement, and provided that only the cortex is involved, an initial period of either bed rest or complete non–weight-bearing is necessary. The patient is progressed to partial and then full weight-bearing on crutches as symptoms permit. Roentgenograms every 2–3 days during the first week are necessary to detect any widening of the fracture line. If healing does not occur, internal fixation with some form of hip pin is indicated.

An overt fracture with radiographic evidence of opening or displacement is significant and requires surgical intervention, usually in the form of a hip screw and plate. Displaced fractures must be treated as an orthopaedic emergency.

HIP FRACTURE

Hip fracture, defined as a fracture of the proximal third of the femur, is the orthopaedic problem with the highest incidence, cost, and risk.[292] The morbidity rates after fracture is 32% to 80%.[293] Hip fractures are associated with substantial morbidity and mortality in the elderly. Approximately 90% of hip fractures result from a simple low energy fall.[294] The most common risk factors for falls (and thus hip fractures) are age, gender, race, institutionalization/hospitalization, medical comorbidities (cardiac disease, stroke, dementia, poor hip fracture, osteoporosis), hip geometry, medication, bone density, diet, smoking, alcohol consumption, fluorinated water, urban versus rural residents, and climate.[295] A number of hip fractures exist:

- Intertrochanteric: occur on the proximal, upper part of the femur or thigh bone between the greater trochanter, where the gluteus medius and minimus muscles attach, and the lesser trochanter, where the iliopsoas muscle attaches.
- Femoral neck: Fractures of the femoral neck are proximal to intertrochanteric fractures, whereas subtrochanteric fractures are distal or below to the trochanters.

Intertrochanteric

The intertrochanteric area of the femur, the area of the lesser and the greater trochanters and where the femur changes from an essentially vertical bone to a bone angling at a 45-degree angle from the near-vertical to the acetabulum or pelvis, is proximal to the femoral shaft and distal to the femoral neck. The etiology of intertrochanteric fractures is typically a combination of increased bone fragility of the intertrochanteric area of the femur associated with decreased muscle tone of the muscles in the area secondary to the aging process.

The current approach for intertrochanteric fractures is surgical intervention. With few exceptions, open reduction and internal fixation (ORIF) is used to treat essentially all intertrochanteric fractures. Following the procedure, a preventive protocol of antiembolism stockings and anticoagulants is followed. Physical therapy involves functional and gait training according to the weight-bearing status, and a progressive exercise program of ROM and strengthening.

CLINICAL PEARL

Hip fractures are associated with a high risk of deep vein thrombosis (DVT). Early mobilization, may reduce the risk of venous thromboembolism.

Subtrochanteric

The subtrochanteric region of the femur is exposed to high stresses during ADL; during normal ADL, up to six times the body weight is transmitted across the subtrochanteric region of the femur.[98] These fractures are most frequently seen in two patient populations; older osteopenic patients after a low-energy fall and younger patients involved in high-energy trauma. This region of the femur consists primarily of cortical bone, so healing in this region is predominantly through a primary cortical healing, which makes fracture consolidation quite slow to occur. Surgical treatment can be divided into three main techniques:

- External fixation: rarely used but is indicated in severe open fractures. External fixation is usually temporary, and conversion to internal fixation can be made if and when the soft tissues have healed sufficiently.
- Open reduction with plates and screws. Following ORIF and plate fixation, minimal protected weight-bearing can begin immediately but is advanced slowly beginning approximately 4 weeks after surgery, with full weight-bearing anticipated at 8–12 weeks.
- Intramedullary fixation. Following intramedullary nailing, if the bone quality and cortical contact is adequate, 50% partial weight-bearing can be allowed immediately. With less stability, patients can perform touchdown weight-bearing.

As most elderly patients may have difficulty complying with the weight-bearing restrictions, they are often permitted to progress to full postoperative weight-bearing status.

Femoral Neck Fracture

Femoral neck fractures are often associated with multiple injuries and high rates of avascular necrosis and nonunion. Hip fractures are common and are often devastating in the geriatric population. A number of factors predispose the elderly population to fractures, including decreased physical activity, osteoporosis, impaired vision, neurologic disease, and poor balance. The decision for operative or nonoperative treatment of femoral neck fractures and the type of surgical intervention are based on many factors. Compression fractures are more stable than tension-type fractures, and they can be treated nonoperatively. Treatment for nondisplaced fractures is bed rest and/or the use of crutches until passive hip movement is pain free and X-ray films show evidence of callus formation. Tension fractures may require operative stabilization as they are potentially unstable. Nondisplaced femoral neck fractures may need to be stabilized with multiple screws or pins. In the elderly population, premorbid cognitive function, walking ability, and independence in ADL are considered when determining the optimal method of surgical repair.

The prognosis for femoral neck fractures depends on the extent of injury (i.e., amount of displacement, amount of comminution, whether circulation has been disturbed), the adequacy of the reduction, and the adequacy of fixation. Maintaining aerobic conditioning throughout the rehabilitation process is important.

The weight-bearing status following the surgical procedure depends on the stability of reduction, bone, and method of fixation. The exercises performed initially include quadriceps sets, gluteal sets, heel slides, active-assisted hip abduction and adduction, and supine internal and external hip rotation. Once partial weight-bearing ambulation is allowed, aquatic training such as swimming or deep-water running may be used if available. Once full weight-bearing is achieved, exercises begin to address functional strengthening of the gluteus medius, the iliopsoas, gluteus maximus, adductors (magnus, longus, and brevis), quadriceps, and hamstrings.

If protected or non–weight-bearing ambulation is necessary, then upper body exercise, such as an upper body ergometer, can be used.

TOTAL HIP ARTHROPLASTY

The THA is a common procedure performed in cases of severe joint damage resulting from OA, rheumatoid arthritis, displaced femoral neck fractures, and avascular necrosis.[296] Arthroplasty of the hip may be categorized as a THA or a hemiarthroplasty. In a THA, the articular surfaces of both the acetabulum and femur are replaced. This involves either replacement of the femoral head and neck (conventional THA) or replacement of the surface of the femoral head (resurfacing THA); both procedures also replace the acetabulum. In contrast to a THA, a hemiarthroplasty involves replacement of the articular surface of the femoral head without any surgical alteration to the acetabular articular surface. Two main types of hemiarthroplasty exist:

- Unipolar. This involves replacement of the femoral head and the neck and tends to be used with less active and older patients who are unlikely to outlive the hip implant.
- Bipolar. This involves replacement of the femoral head and the neck with an additional acetabular cup that is not attached to the pelvis (bipolar hemiarthroplasty), or replacement of the surface of the femoral head (resurfacing hemiarthroplasty).

More recently, the minimally invasive anterior approach, using one or two small incisions, has become more popular. The rationale for minimally invasive procedures is that the use of small incisions potentially lessens soft tissue trauma during surgery and, therefore, should improve and accelerate a patient's postoperative recovery. Other benefits include reduced blood loss, reduce postoperative pain, shorter length of hospital stay and lower cost of hospitalization, a more rapid recovery of functional mobility and a better cosmetic appearance of the surgical scar.

A review of the literature reveals inconsistent practice patterns in the physical therapy management of THA patients. Most surgeons have designed their own post-surgical protocols, which should be strictly adhered to. Standard precautions are observed with patients who underwent a lateral or posterolateral approach to prevent posterior hip dislocation. These include the following:

- Avoidance of hip adduction. Typically an abduction wedge or pillow is prescribed. A pillow is placed between the legs if the patient wants to lie on the side.
- Avoidance of hip internal rotation. Combinations of hip flexion, internal rotation, and adduction must be avoided for up to 4 months after surgery or until physician clearance.
- Avoidance of hip flexion greater than 90 degrees (bending forward at the hip, reaching for objects or tying shoes). Elevated chairs or toilet seats can be used to increase compliance, as can an assistive device or reacher

Precautions for a patient who underwent an anterior/anterior lateral or direct lateral approach, with or without trochanteric osteotomy include:

- Avoidance of hip flexion greater than 90 degrees
- Avoidance of hip extension, adduction, and external rotation past neutral
- Avoidance of the combined motions of flexion, abduction, and external rotation

If a trochanteric osteotomy was performed, or the gluteus medius was incised and repaired, the patient should not perform active, anti-gravity hip abduction for at least 6–8 weeks or until approved by the surgeon.

THERAPEUTIC TECHNIQUES

Techniques to Increase Joint Mobility

Passive Articular Mobilization Techniques

In a single-blind randomized study[194] investigating interventions for hip OA, 109 subjects were randomly assigned to receive mobilization and manipulation to the hip joint or active exercises designed to improve strength and ROM for nine visits over a period of 5 weeks. Success rates after 5 weeks were 81% in the manual therapy group and 50% in the exercise group. Furthermore, patients in the manual therapy group had significantly better outcomes on pain, stiffness, hip function, and ROM. The effects of manual therapy on the improvement of pain, hip function, and ROM remained after 29 weeks.

Mobilizations of this joint are typically performed using a sustained stretch to decrease a hip joint capsular restriction, with the stretch being governed by the direction of the restriction, rather than by the concave–convex rule. For example, if hip joint extension is restricted, the distal femur is moved into the direction of hip extension.[209]

The joint is initially positioned in its neutral position and is progressively moved closer to the end of range. A belt can also be used for this technique. Rotations can be combined with any sustained stretch performed in a cardinal plane. Distraction or compression techniques can be used alone or combined with rotations.

Distraction. Joint distraction mobilizations are indicated for pain and any hypomobility at the hip joint, as in the case when pain is reported by the patient before tissue resistance is felt by the clinician. The lateral distraction technique (see Fig. 19-30) can be used to increase hip joint ROM into adduction and internal rotation.

Leg Traction (Inferior Glide). An inferior distraction (Fig. 19-31) can be used for temporary relief of joint pain, to increase ROM into hip joint abduction and for stretching capsular adhesion that is pronounced in the inferior portion of the joint capsule.[63,70]

Quadrant (Scouring) Mobilizations. Quadrant mobilizations involve flexion and adduction of the hip, combined with simultaneous joint compression through the femur.[70,209,297,298] The flexed and adducted thigh is swept through a 90–140-degree arc of flexion, while maintaining joint compression. This arc of motion should feel smooth and should be pain free. In an abnormal joint, pain or an obstruction to the arc occurs during the movement. In selected nonacute cases, the procedure may be used as an effective mobilizing procedure, where grade II to III mobilizations are applied perpendicular to the arc throughout.[70,297]

Posterior Glide. The posterior glide mobilization (Fig. 19-32) is used to increase flexion and to increase internal rotation of the hip.

Anterior Glide. The anterior glide (Fig. 19-33) is used to increase extension and to increase external rotation of the hip.

Inferior Glide. The inferior glide is used to increase abduction of the hip.

Mobilizations with Movement. *To Restore Internal Rotation of the Hip.*[299–301] This technique is employed when the patient presents with early signs of hip joint degeneration, as indicated by minor capsular signs and slight degenerative changes on radiographs. A belt that can be altered in length is required for the technique.

The patient is positioned in supine with the involved hip and knee flexed and the foot just off the edge of the bed, with the clinician standing on the involved side, facing the patient's head. A belt is placed around the back of the clinician, just below the hip joints, and around the patient's thigh as proximal as possible, so that the belt is approximately horizontal. Using the hand closest to the patient's head, the clinician grasps the lateral iliac crest of the involved side, with the elbow in the crease of the clinician's groin to stabilize the pelvis during the maneuver. The clinician wraps the other hand around the patient's midthigh. From this position, the clinician slowly extends their own hips to apply a distraction force to the patient's hip joint, while maintaining the fixation of the ilium.

If the maneuver produces any pain, it should be discontinued. This should be differentiated from discomfort, which might be caused by inappropriate placement of the belt.

To Restore Flexion of the Hip. The technique to restore flexion of the hip is identical to the one described above, except that during the distraction, the clinician passively flexes the patient's hip into flexion by side bending at the waist.[301]

Techniques to Increase Soft Tissue Extensibility

The efficacy of manual techniques for improving hip ROM has been reported in the literature. Crosman and colleagues[302] studied the effects of hamstring massage (effleurage, petrissage, and friction) on hip flexion range in normal individuals and noted significant range improvements after the soft tissue massage.[70] Godges and colleagues[303] reported improved hip flexion and hip extension ranges in normal individuals after the application of manual stretches to muscle groups opposing each respective motion, combined with exercise of agonistic muscles.

Iliopsoas. The patient is positioned in side lying (Fig. 19-78). The patient is instructed to flex the uninvolved hip and maintain its position by using their arms to help stabilize the lumbopelvic region. While monitoring the lumbopelvic motion with one hand, the clinician passively extends the thigh with the other arm/hand. The advantage of this technique is that varying degrees of hip adduction/abduction and knee flexion/extension can be controlled. The disadvantage is that the technique is more physically demanding for the clinician.

Iliopsoas and Rectus Femoris. Although a number of exercises have been advocated to stretch these muscle groups, because of their potential to increase the anterior shear of the

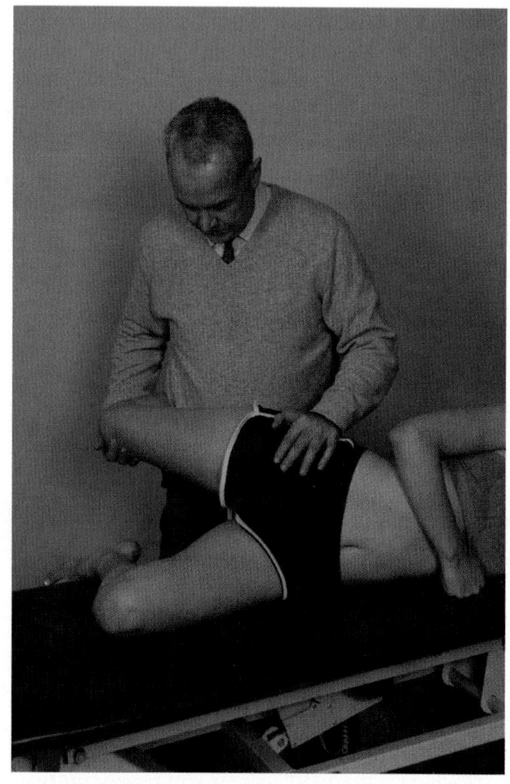

FIGURE 19-78 Sidelying hip flexor stretch.

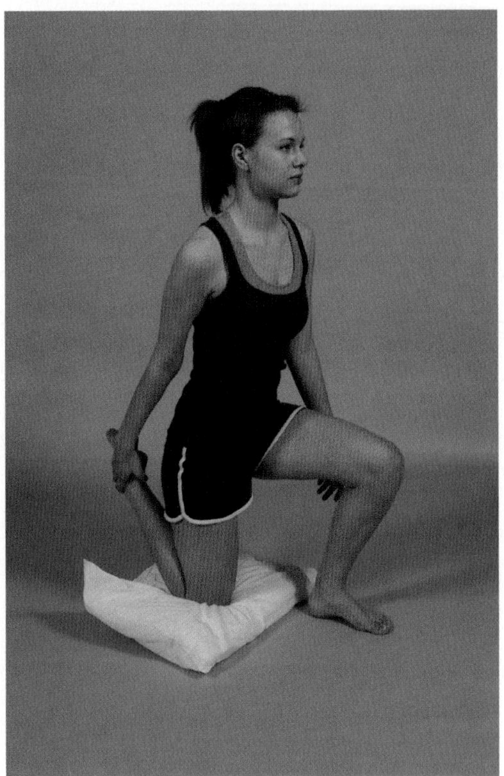

FIGURE 19-79 Iliopsoas and rectus femoris stretch.

lumbar vertebrae either directly or indirectly, the standing/kneeling position is preferred.

A pillow is placed on the floor, and the patient kneels down on the pillow with the other leg placed out in front in the typical lunge position (Fig. 19-79). The patient is asked to

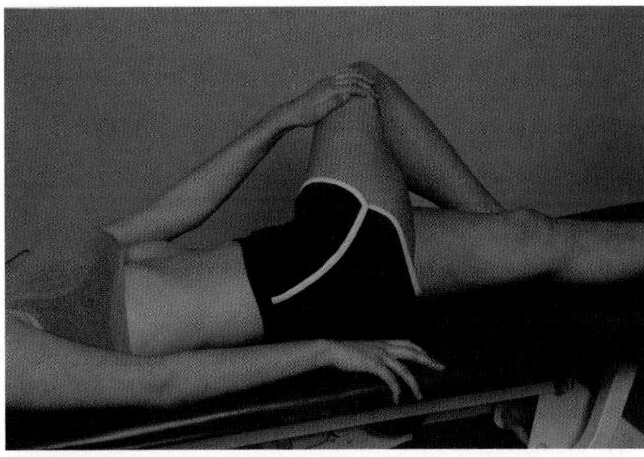

FIGURE 19-80 Tensor fascia latae stretch.

perform a posterior pelvic tilt and to maintain an erect position with respect to the trunk. From this starting position, the patient glides the trunk anteriorly, maintaining the trunk in a near vertical position. A stretch on the upper aspect of the anterior thigh of the kneeling leg should be felt. The rectus femoris can be stretched further from this position by grasping the ankle of the kneeling leg and raising the foot toward the buttock (Fig. 19-79).

Tensor Fascia Latae. The patient is positioned supine with the legs straight. The foot of the leg to be stretched is placed on the table on the outside of the uninvolved straight leg. The patient reaches and grasps the knee of the involved leg and pulls the knee across and over the straight leg (Fig. 19-80). Both shoulders should be kept flat against the table. At the point the stretch is felt, the position is maintained for approximately 30 seconds. The stretch is repeated 10 times.

CASE STUDY

Right Groin Pain

History

General Demographics

A 62-year-old male

History of Current Condition

A patient presents with complaints of aching pain in the right groin that varies in severity and extends down the anterior thigh to the knee. The pain began gradually about 3 months before. Initially, the patient felt stiffness whenever he sat for prolonged periods of time or after a night's sleep. The patient reports that he can no longer walk as far as he once did and that negotiating stairs was especially painful.

Past History of Current Condition

A long history of OA of the spine and occasional twinges of pain in the right groin. The patient also has a history of right-sided sciatica.

Past Medical/Surgical History

The patient had a total joint replacement of the right knee approximately 4 months ago.

Medications

Celecoxib.

Other Tests and Measures

Radiographs of right hip are negative for loose bodies, tumors, and fracture. Advanced OA of right hip was noted.

Social Habits (past and present)

Nonsmoker. Drinks occasionally. Active life style.

Social History

Married. Two children, both live close by.

Family History

No relevant history of hip problems in family.

Growth and Development

Normal development; left-handed.

Living Environment

Lives in an apartment. One flight of stairs to negotiate.

Occupational/Employment/School

Retired railroad laborer. High school education.

Functional Status/Activity Level

The patient demonstrates difficulty rising from a chair and transferring from bed to chair.

Health Status (self-report)

In general good health, but pain interferes with tasks at home and with helping his sick wife.

Systems Seview

Unremarkable.

Questions

1. List the possible structure(s) that can produce groin pain.
2. What might the history of pain with early morning stiffness and pain with stair negotiation tell the clinician?
3. What other activities might increase the patient's symptoms? Why?
4. To help rule out the various causes of groin pain, what other questions can you ask?
5. What is your working hypothesis at this stage? List the various diagnoses that could present with these signs and symptoms and the tests you would use to rule out each one.
6. Does this presentation/history warrant a Cyriax lower quarter scanning examination? Why or why not?

CASE-STUDY

Thigh Pain

History

History of Current Condition

A 22-year-old male sustained a kick to the right thigh approximately 2 weeks ago while playing college soccer. He complains of a dull ache on the anterior aspect of his thigh. The pain is worse with activities that involve attempting to squat or kick. The patient also reports feeling a lump on the front of his thigh. The patient saw his physician who diagnosed the condition as a deep quadriceps contusion and prescribed 8 weeks of physical therapy.

Past History of Current Condition

No previous history of thigh pain.

Past Medical/Surgical History

- No history of previous knee or hip injury.
- No back pain/surgery reported.
- No knee surgeries reported.
- History of chronic ankle sprains.

Medications

None.

Other Tests and Measures

Radiograph results pending.

Occupational/Employment/school

Full-time student at local college for the past 2 years.

Functional Status/Activity Level

Very active. In addition to soccer, the patient also plays tennis and racquetball.

Health Status (self-report)

In general, good health.

Questions

1. Given the specific mechanism of injury, list all of the structures you suspect could be injured and will require a specific examination.
2. What condition could be present with the history of pain in a muscle belly following a contusion?
3. What other activities do you suspect would increase the patient's symptoms? Why?
4. In a patient with an insidious onset of pain, what questions would you ask to help rule out the various causes of anterior thigh pain?
5. What is your working hypothesis at this stage?
6. Does this presentation/history warrant a lower quarter scan? Why or why not?

REVIEW QUESTIONS*

1. What is the close-packed position of the hip?
2. In which direction is the acetabulum angled?
3. Which ligament contains the blood supply to the femoral head?
4. The pubofemoral ligament is taut in which three directions?
5. Which muscle is known as the deltoid of the hip?

---

*Additional questions to test your understanding of this chapter can be found in the Online Learning Center for *Orthopaedic Assessment, Evaluation, and Intervention.*

REFERENCES

1. Rose J: Dynamic lower extremity stability. In: Hughes C, ed. *Movement Disorders and Neuromuscular Interventions for the Trunk and Extremities – Independent Study Course 18.2.5.* La Crosse, WI: Orthopaedic Section, APTA, Inc, 2008:1–34.
2. Norkin C, Levangie P: *Joint Structure and Function: A Comprehensive Analysis.* Philadelphia, PA: F.A. Davis Company, 1992.
3. van Mechelen W: Running injuries. A review of the epidemiological literature. *Sports Med* 14:320–335, 1992.
4. Weinstein SL: Natural history and treatment outcomes of childhood hip disorders. *Clin Orthop Relat Res* 344:227–242, 1997.
5. Ponseti IV: Growth and development of the acetabulum in the normal child. Anatomical, histological, and roentgenographic studies. *J Bone Joint Surg* 60A:575–585, 1978.
6. Skirving AP, Scadden WJ: The African neonatal hip and its immunity from congenital dislocation. *J Bone Joint Surg Br* 61-B: 339–341, 1979.
7. Coleman CR, Slager RF, Smith WS: The effect of environmental influence on acetabular development. *Surg Forum* 9:775–780, 1958.
8. Harrison TJ: The influence of the femoral head on pelvic growth and acetabular form in the rat. *J Anat* 95:127–132, 1961.
9. Anderson LC: The anatomy and biomechanics of the hip joint. *J Back Musculoskel Rehabil* 4:145–153, 1994.
10. Harris NH: Acetabular growth potential in congenital dislocation of the hip and some factors upon which it may depend. *Clin Orthop* 119:99–106, 1976.
11. Harris NH, Lloyd-Roberts GC, Gallien R: Acetabular development in congenital dislocation of the hip with special reference to the indications of acetabuloplasty and pelvic or femoral realignment osteotomy. *J Bone Joint Surg* 57B:46–52, 1975.
12. Lindstrom JR, Ponseti IV, Wenger DR: Acetabular development after reduction in congenital dislocation of the hip. *J Bone Joint Surg* 61A:112–118, 1979.
13. Harrison TJ: The growth of the pelvis in the rat-A mensural and morphological study. *J Anat* 92:236–260, 1958.
14. Maquet PG, Van de Berg AJ, Simonet JC: Femorotibial weight – bearing areas. Experimental determination. *J Bone and Joint Surg* 57-A:766–771, 1975.
15. Williams PL, Warwick R, Dyson M, et al: *Gray's Anatomy.* 37th ed. London: Churchill Livingstone, 1989.
16. Kessler RM, Hertling D: *Management of Common Musculoskeletal Disorders.* Philadelphia, PA: Harper and Row, 1983:379–443.
17. Konrath GA, Hamel AJ, Olson SA, et al: The role of the acetabular labrum and the transverse acetabular ligament in load transmission in the hip. *J Bone Joint Surg* 80A:1781–1788, 1998.
18. Fagerson TL: Hip. In: Wadsworth C, ed. *Current Concepts of Orthopedic Physical Therapy – Home Study Course.* La Crosse, WI: Orthopaedic Section, APTA, 2001.
19. Agus H, Omeroglu H, Ucar H, et al: Evaluation of the risk factors of avascular necrosis of the femoral head in developmental dysplasia of the hip in infants younger than 18 months of age. *J Pediatr Orthop B* 11:41–46, 2002.
20. Trueta I, Harrison MHM: The normal vascular anatomy of the femoral head in adult man. *J Bone Joint Surg* 35B:442–461, 1953.
21. Petersen W, Petersen F, Tillmann B: Structure and vascularization of the acetabular labrum with regard to the pathogenesis and healing of labral lesions. *Arch Orthop Trauma Surg* 123:283–288. Epub 2003 Jun 7, 2003.
22. Adeeb SM, Sayed Ahmed EY, Matyas J, et al: Congruency effects on load bearing in diarthrodial joints. *Comput Methods Biomech Biomed Engin* 7:147–157, 2004.
23. Narvani AA, Tsiridis E, Kendall S, et al: A preliminary report on prevalence of acetabular labrum tears in sports patients with groin pain. *Knee Surg Sports Traumatol Arthrosc* 11:403–408, 2003.
24. Kim YT, Azuma H: The nerve endings of the acetabular labrum. *Clin Orthop* 320:176–181, 1995.
25. Takechi H, Nagashima H, Ito S: Intra-articular pressure of the hip joint outside and inside the limbus. *Nihon Seikeigeka Gakkai Zasshi* 56:529–536, 1982.
26. Narvani AA, Tsiridis E, Tai CC, et al: Acetabular labrum and its tears. *Br J Sports Med* 37:207–211, 2003.
27. Seldes R, Tan V, Hunt J, et al: Anatomy, histologic features, and vascularity of the adult acetabular labrum. *Clin Orthop Relat Res* 382:232–240, 2001.
28. Neumann DA: Kinesiology of the hip: a focus on muscular actions. *J Orthop Sports Phys Ther* 40:82–94, 2010.
29. Delp SL, Hess WE, Hungerford DS, et al: Variation of rotation moment arms with hip flexion. *J Biomech* 32:493–501, 1999.
30. Basmajian JV, Deluca CJ: *Muscles Alive: Their Functions Revealed by Electromyography.* Baltimore, MD: Williams & Wilkins, 1985.
31. Yoshio M, Murakami G, Sato T, et al: The function of the psoas major muscle: passive kinetics and morphological studies using donated cadavers. *J Orthop Sci* 7:199–207, 2002.
32. Hall SJ: *The Biomechanics of the Human Lower Extremity, Basic Biomechanics.* 3rd ed. New York, NY: McGraw-Hill, 1999:234–281.
33. Janda V: On the concept of postural muscles and posture in man. *Aust J Physiother* 29:83–84, 1983.
34. Fagerson TL: Hip pathologies: diagnosis and intervention. In: Magee DJ, Zachazewski JE, Quillen WS, eds. *Pathology and Intervention in Musculoskeletal Rehabilitation.* St. Louis, MO: Saunders, 2009:497–527.
35. Kapandji IA: *The Physiology of the Joints, Lower Limb.* New York, NY: Churchill Livingstone, 1991.
36. Durrani Z, Winnie AP: Piriformis muscle syndrome: an underdiagnosed cause of sciatica. *J Pain Symptom Manage* 6:374–379, 1991.
37. Julsrud ME: Piriformis syndrome. *J Am Podiat Med Assn* 79:128–131, 1989.
38. Pace JB, Nagle D: Piriformis syndrome. *Western J Med* 124:435–439, 1976.
39. Steiner C, Staubs C, Ganon M, et al: Piriformis syndrome: pathogenesis, diagnosis, and treatment. *J Am Osteopath Assn* 87:318–323, 1987.
40. Harvey G, Bell S: Obturator neuropathy. An anatomic perspective. *Clin Orthop Relat Res* 363:203–211, 1999.
41. Dixon MC, Scott RD, Schai PA, et al: A simple capsulorrhaphy in a posterior approach for total hip arthroplasty. *J Arthroplasty* 19:373–376, 2004.
42. Mihalko WM, Whiteside LA: Hip mechanics after posterior structure repair in total hip arthroplasty. *Clin Orthop Relat Res* 420:194–198, 2004.
43. Gordon EJ: Trochanteric bursitis and tendinitis. *Clin Orthop* 20:193–202, 1961.
44. Johnson CE, Basmajian JV, Dasher W: Electromyography of the sartorius muscle. *Anat Rec* 173:127–130, 1972.
45. Anderson MA, Gieck JH, Perrin D, et al: The relationship among isokinetic, isotonic, and isokinetic concentric and eccentric quadriceps and hamstrings force and three components of athletic performance. *J Orthop Sports Phys Ther* 14:114–120, 1991.
46. Kujala UM, Orava S, Jarvinen M: Hamstring injuries. Current trends in treatment and prevention. *Sports Med* 23:397–404, 1997.
47. Holmich P: Adductor related groin pain in athletes. *Sports Med Arth Rev* 5:285–291, 1998.
48. Hasselman CT, Best TM, Garrett WE: When groin pain signals an adductor strain. *Physician Sports Med* 23:53–60, 1995.
49. Lynch SA, Renstrom PA: Groin injuries in sport: treatment strategies. *Sports Med* 28:137–144, 1999.
50. Shbeeb MI, Matteson EL: Trochanteric bursitis (greater trochanter pain syndrome). *Mayo Clin Proc* 71:565–569, 1996.
51. Melamed A, Bauer C, Johnson H: Iliopsoas bursal extension of arthritic disease of the hip. *Radiology* 89:54–58, 1967.
52. Armstrong P, Saxton H: Ilio-psoas bursa. *Br J Radiol* 45:493–495, 1972.
53. Chandler SB: The iliopsoas bursa in man. *Anat Rec* 58:235–240, 1934.
54. Sartoris DJ, Danzig L, Gilula L, et al: Synovial cysts of the hip joint and iliopsoas bursitis: a spectrum of imaging abnormalities. *Skeletal Radiol* 14:85–94, 1985.

55. Yamamoto T, Marui T, Akisue T, et al: Dumbbell-shaped iliopsoas bursitis penetrating the pelvic wall: a rare complication of hip arthrodesis. A case report. *J Bone Joint Surg Am* 85-A:343–345, 2003.
56. Croley TE: Anatomy of the hip. In: Echternach JL, ed. *Physical Therapy of the Hip*. New York, NY: Churchill Livingstone, 1990:1–16.
57. Bruce J, Walmsley R, Ross JA: *Manual of Surgical Anatomy*. Edinburgh: Churchill Livingstone, 1964.
58. Sevitt S, Thompson RG: The distribution and anastomoses of arteries supplying the head and neck of the femur. *J Bone Joint Surg Br* 47-B:560–573, 1965.
59. Bachiller FG, Caballer AP, Portal LF: Avascular necrosis of the femoral head after femoral neck fracture. *Clin Orthop Relat Res* 399:87–109, 2002.
60. Gautier E, Ganz K, Krugel N, et al: Anatomy of the medial femoral circumflex artery and its surgical implications. *J Bone Joint Surg Br* 82:679–683, 2000.
61. Cibulka MT, Sinacore DR, Cromer GS, et al: Unilateral hip rotation range of motion asymmetry in patients with sacroiliac joint regional pain. *Spine* 23:1009–1015, 1998.
62. Inman VT: Functional aspects of the abductor muscles of the hip. *J Bone Joint Surg Am* 29:607–619, 1947.
63. Turek SL: *Orthopaedics – Principles and Their Application*. 4th ed. Philadelphia, PA: JB Lippincott, 1984.
64. Cailliet R: *Soft Tissue Pain and Disability*. Philadelphia, PA: FA Davis, 1980.
65. Yamomoto S, Suto Y, Kawamura H, et al: Quantitative gait evaluation of hip diseases using principal component analysis. *J Biomech* 16:717, 1983.
66. Neumann DA, Cook TM: Effects of load and carry position on the electromyographic activity of the gluteus medius muscles during walking. *Phys Ther* 65:305–311, 1985.
67. Clark JM, Haynor DR: Anatomy of the abductor muscles of the hip as studied by computed tomography. *J Bone Joint Surg* 69A:1021, 1987.
68. Isacson J, Brostrom LA: Gait in rheumatoid arthritis: an electromyographic investigation. *J Biomech* 21:451, 1988.
69. Neumann DA, Soderberg GL, Cook TM: Electromyographic analysis of the hip abductor musculature in healthy right-handed persons. *Phys Ther* 69:431–440, 1989.
70. Yoder E: Physical therapy management of nonsurgical hip problems in adults. In: Echternach JL, ed. *Physical Therapy of the Hip*. New York, NY: Churchill Livingstone, 1990:103–137.
71. Perry J, Weiss WB, Burnfield JM, et al: The supine hip extensor manual muscle test: a reliability and validity study. *Arch Phys Med Rehabil* 85:1345–1350, 2004.
72. Gage JR, Camy JM: The effects of trochanteric epiphysiodesis on growth of the proximal end of the femur following necrosis of the capital femoral epiphysis. *J Bone Joint Surg* 62A:785–794, 1980.
73. Osborne D, Effmann E, Broda K, et al: The development of the upper end of the femur with special reference to its internal architecture. *Radiology* 137:71–76, 1980.
74. Schofield CB, Smibert JG: Trochanteric growth disturbance after upper femoral osteotomy for congenital dislocation of the hip. *J Bone Joint Surg* 72B:32–36, 1990.
75. Afoke NYP, Byers PD, Hutton WC: Contact pressures in the human hip joint. *J Bone Joint Surg Am* 69B:536, 1987.
76. Oatis CA: Biomechanics of the hip. In: Echternach J, ed. *Clinics in Physical Therapy: Physical Therapy of the Hip*. New York, NY: Churchill Livingstone, 1990:37–50.
77. Pauwels F: *Biomechanics of the Normal and Diseased Hip*. Berlin: Springer-Verlag, 1976.
78. Maquet PGJ: *Biomechanics of the Hip as Applied to Osteoarthritis and Related Conditions*. Berlin: Springer-Verlag, 1985.
79. Menke W, Schmitz B, Schild H, et al: Transversale skelettachsen der unteren extremitat bei coxarthrose. *Zeitschr Orthop* 129:255–259, 1991.
80. Pizzutillo PT, MacEwen GD, Shands AR: Anteversion of the femur. In: Tonzo RG, ed. *Surgery of the Hip Joint*. New York, NY: Springer-Verlag, 1984.
81. Lausten GS, Jorgensen F, Boesen J: Measurement of anteversion of the femoral neck, ultrasound and CT compared. *J Bone Joint Surg Am* 71B:237, 1989.
82. Gross MT: Lower quarter screening for skeletal malalignment – suggestions for orthotics and shoewear. *J Orthop Sports Phys Ther* 21:389–405, 1995.
83. Fabry G: Torsion of the femur. *Acta Orthop Belg* 43:454–59, 1977.
84. Fabry G, MacEwen GD, Shands AR Jr: Torsion of the femur. A follow-up study in normal and abnormal conditions. *J Bone Joint Surg Am* 55:1726–1738, 1973.
85. Giunti A, Moroni A, Olmi R, et al: The importance of the angle of anteversion in the development of arthritis of the hip. *Ital J Orthop Traumatol* 11:23–27, 1985.
86. Reikeras O, Hoiseth A: Femoral neck angles in osteoarthritis of the hip. *Acta Orthop Scand* 53:781–784, 1982.
87. Reikeras O, Bjerkreim I, Kolbenstvedt A: Anteversion of the acetabulum and femoral neck in normals and in patients with osteoarthritis of the hip. *Acta Orthop Scand* 54:18–23, 1983.
88. Terjesen T, Benum P, Anda S, et al: Increased femoral anteversion and osteoarthritis of the hip. *Acta Orthop Scand* 53:571–575, 1982.
89. Eckhoff DG: Femoral anteversion in arthritis of the knee [letter]. *J Pediat Orthop* 15:700, 1995.
90. Eckhoff DG, Montgomery WK, Kilcoyne RF, et al: Femoral morphometry and anterior knee pain. *Clin Orthop* 302:64–68, 1994.
91. Aranow S, Zippel H: Untersuchung zur femoro-tibialen Torsion bei Patellainstabilitaten. Ein Beitrag zur Pathogenese rezidivierender und habitueller Patellaluxationen. *Beitr Orthop Traumat* 37:311–326, 1990.
92. Swanson AB, Greene PW Jr, Allis HD: Rotational deformities of the lower extremity in children and their clinical significance. *Clin Orthop* 27:157–175, 1963.
93. Hubbard DD, Staheli LT, Chew DE, et al: Medial femoral torsion and osteoarthritis. *J Pediat Orthop* 8:540–542, 1988.
94. Kitaoka HB, Weiner DS, Cook AJ, et al: Relationship between femoral anteversion and osteoarthritis of the hip. *J Pediat Orthop* 9:396–404, 1989.
95. Kaltenborn FM: *Manual Mobilization of the Extremity Joints: Basic Examination and Treatment Techniques*. 4th ed. Oslo, Norway: Olaf Norlis Bokhandel, Universitetsgaten, 1989.
96. Johnston RC: Mechanical considerations of the hip joint. *Arch Surg* 107:411, 1973.
97. Paul JP, McGrouther DA: Forces transmitted at the hip and knee joint of normal and disabled persons during a range of activities. *Acta Orthop Belg* 41:78, 1975.
98. Bergmann G, Graichen F, Rohlmann A: Hip joint loading during walking and running, measured in two patients. *J Biomech* 26:969, 1993.
99. Bergmann G, Graichen F, Rohlmann A: Is staircase walking a risk for the fixation of hip implants. *J Biomech* 28:535, 1995.
100. Hodges PW, Richardson CA: Contraction of the abdominal muscles associated with movement of the lower limb. *Phys Ther* 77:132–142; discussion 142–144, 1997.
101. Hodges PW, Eriksson AE, Shirley D, et al: Intra-abdominal pressure increases stiffness of the lumbar spine. *J Biomech* 38:1873–1880, 2005.
102. Urquhart DM, Hodges PW, Story IH: Postural activity of the abdominal muscles varies between regions of these muscles and between body positions. *Gait Posture* 22:295–301, 2005.
103. Cahalan TD, Johnson ME, Liu S, et al: Quantitative measurements of hip strength in different age groups. *Clin Orthop Relat Res* 246:136–145, 1989.
104. Hoy MG, Zajac FE, Gordon ME: A musculoskeletal model of the human lower extremity: the effect of muscle, tendon, and moment arm on the moment-angle relationship of musculotendon actuators at the hip, knee, and ankle. *J Biomech* 23:157–169, 1990.
105. Dostal WF, Soderberg GL, Andrews JG: Actions of hip muscles. *Phys Ther* 66:351–361, 1986.
106. Jackson-Manfield P, Neumann DA: Structure and function of the hip. In: Jackson-Manfield P, Neumann DA, eds. *Essentials of Kinesiology for the Physical Therapist Assistant*. St. Louis, MO: Mosby Elsevier, 2009:227–271.
107. Hurwitz DE, Foucher KC, Andriacchi TP: A new parametric approach for modeling hip forces during gait. *J Biomech* 36:113–119, 2003.
108. Cyriax J: *Textbook of Orthopaedic Medicine, Diagnosis of Soft Tissue Lesions*. 8th ed. London: Bailliere Tindall, 1982.
109. Cyriax JH, Cyriax PJ: *Illustrated Manual of Orthopaedic Medicine*. London: Butterworth, 1983.
110. Klassbo M, Harms-Ringdahl K, Larsson G: Examination of passive ROM and capsular patterns in the hip. *Physiother Res Int* 8:1–12, 2003.
111. Birrell F, Croft P, Cooper C, et al: Predicting radiographic hip osteoarthritis from range of movement. *Rheumatology (Oxford)* 40:506–512, 2001.
112. Byrd JW, Jones KS: Diagnostic accuracy of clinical assessment, magnetic resonance imaging, magnetic resonance arthrography, and intra-articular injection in hip arthroscopy patients. *Am J Sports Med* 32:1668–1674, 2004.
113. Spiera H: Osteoarthritis as a misdiagnosis in elderly patients. *Geriatrics* 42:37–42, 1987.

114. Schon L, Zuckerman JD: Hip pain the elderly: Evaluation and diagnosis. *Geriatrics* 43:48–62, 1988.
115. Wroblewski BM: Pain in osteoarthrosis of the hip. *Practitioner* 1315:140–141, 1978.
116. Cibulka MT, Threlkeld J: The early clinical diagnosis of osteoarthritis of the hip. *J Orthop Sports Phys Ther* 34:461–467, 2004.
117. Feinberg JH: Hip pain: differential diagnosis. *J Back Musculoskel Rehabil* 4:154–173, 1994.
118. Hoskins W, Pollard H: The management of hamstring injury–Part 1: Issues in diagnosis. *Man Ther* 10:96–107, 2005.
119. Brockett CL, Morgan DL, Proske U: Predicting hamstring strain injury in elite athletes. *Med Sci Sports Exerc* 36:379–387, 2004.
120. Verrall GM, Slavotinek JP, Barnes PG, et al: Clinical risk factors for hamstring muscle strain injury: a prospective study with correlation of injury by magnetic resonance imaging. *Br J Sports Med* 35:435–439; discussion 440, 2001.
121. Byrd JW, Jones KS: Prospective analysis of hip arthroscopy with 2-year follow-up. *Arthroscopy* : the journal of arthroscopic & related surgery : official publication of the Arthroscopy Association of North America and the International Arthroscopy Association 16:578–587, 2000.
122. Byrd JW, Jones KS: Prospective analysis of hip arthroscopy with 10-year followup. *Clin Orthop Relat Res* 468:741–746, 2010.
123. O'Leary JA, Berend K, Vail TP: The relationship between diagnosis and outcome in arthroscopy of the hip. *Arthroscopy* : the journal of arthroscopic & related surgery : official publication of the Arthroscopy Association of North America and the International Arthroscopy Association 17:181–188, 2001.
124. Brown MD, Gomez-Marin O, Brookfield KF, et al: Differential diagnosis of hip disease versus spine disease. *Clin Orthop Relat Res* 280–284, 2004.
125. Sahrmann SA: Movement impairment syndromes of the hip. In: Sahrmann SA, ed. *Movement Impairment Syndromes.* St Louis, MO: Mosby, 2001:121–191.
126. Kendall FP, McCreary EK, Provance PG: *Muscles: Testing and Function.* Baltimore, MD: Williams & Wilkins, 1993.
127. Deusinger R: Validity of pelvic tilt measurements in anatomical neutral position. *J Biomech* 25:764, 1992.
128. Jull GA, Janda V: Muscle and motor control in low back pain. In: Twomey LT, Taylor JR, eds. *Physical Therapy of the Low Back: Clinics in Physical Therapy.* New York, NY: Churchill Livingstone, 1987:258–278.
129. Inman VT, Ralston HJ, Todd F: *Human Walking.* Baltimore, MD: Williams & Wilkins, 1981.
130. Lehmkuhl LD, Smith LK: *Brunnstrom's Clinical Kinesiology.* Philadelphia, PA: F.A. Davis, 1983.
131. Hoppenfeld S: *Physical Examination of the Hip and Pelvis, Physical Examination of the Spine and Extremities.* East Norwalk, CT: Appleton-Century-Crofts, 1976:143.
132. Echternach JL: Evaluation of the hip. In: Echternach JL, ed. *Physical Therapy of the Hip.* New York, NY, Churchill Livingstone, 1990:17–32.
133. Holm I, Bolstad B, Lutken T, et al: Reliability of goniometric measurements and visual estimates of hip ROM in patients with osteoarthrosis. *Physiother Res Int* 5:241–248, 2000.
134. Bierma-Zeinstra SM, Bohnen AM, Ramlal R, et al: Comparison between two devices for measuring hip joint motions. *Clin Rehabil* 12:497–505, 1998.
135. McKenzie R, May S: History. In: McKenzie R, May S, eds. *The Human Extremities: Mechanical Diagnosis and Therapy.* Waikanae: Spinal Publications New Zealand Ltd, 2000:89–103.
136. Janda V: *Muscle Function Testing.* London: Butterworths, 1983.
137. Vasilyeva LF, Lewit K: Diagnosis of muscular dysfunction by inspection. In: Liebenson C, ed. *Rehabilitation of the Spine: A Practitioner's Manual.* Baltimore, MD: Lippincott Williams & Wilkins, 1996:113–142.
138. Clark MA: *Integrated Training for the New Millenium.* Thousand Oaks, CA: National Academy of Sports Medicine, 2001.
139. Gelberman RH, Cohen MS, Hekhar S, et al: Femoral anteversion. *J Bone Joint Surg* 69B:75, 1987.
140. Maitland GD: *The Peripheral Joints: Examination and Recording Guide.* Adelaide: Virgo Press, 1973.
141. Ruwe PA, Gage JR, Ozonoff MB, et al: Clinical determination of femoral anteversion: a comparison with established techniques. *J Bone and Joint Surg* 74:820, 1992.
142. Woods D, Macnicol M: The flexion-adduction test: an early sign of hip disease. *J Pediatr Orthop* 10:180–185, 2001.
143. Adams SL, Yarnold PR: Clinical use of the patellar-pubic percussion sign in hip trauma. *Am J Emerg Med* 15:173–175, 1997.
144. Peltier LF: The diagnosis of fractures of the hip and femur by auscultatory percussion. *Clin Orthop Relat Res* 123:9–11, 1977.
145. Gurney B, Boissonnault WG, Andrews R: Differential diagnosis of a femoral neck/head stress fracture. *J Orthop Sports Phys Ther* 36:80–88, 2006.
146. Tiru M, Goh SH, Low BY: Use of percussion as a screening tool in the diagnosis of occult hip fractures. *Singapore Med J* 43:467–469, 2002.
147. Milch H: The acromio-femoral angle. *Bull Hosp Joint Dis* 8:150–154, 1947.
148. Harvey D: Assessment of the flexibility of elite athletes using the modified Thomas test. *Br J Sports Med* 32:68–70, 1998.
149. Grelsamer RP, McConnell J: *The Patella: A Team Approach.* Gaithersburg, MD: Aspen, 1998.
150. Melchione WE, Sullivan MS: Reliability of measurements obtained by the use of an instrument designed to indirectly measure ilio-tibial band length. *J Orthop Sports Phys Ther* 18:511–515, 1993.
151. Reese NB, Bandy WD: Use of an inclinometer to measure flexibility of the iliotibial band using the Ober test and the modified Ober test: differences in magnitude and reliability of measurements. *J Orthop Sports Phys Ther* 33:326–330, 2003.
152. Fishman LM, Dombi GW, Michaelsen C, et al: Piriformis syndrome: diagnosis, treatment, and outcome – a 10-year study. *Arch Phys Med Rehabil* 83:295–301, 2002.
153. Fishman LM, Schaefer MP: The piriformis syndrome is underdiagnosed. *Muscle Nerve* 28:646–649, 2003.
154. Fishman LM, Zybert PA: Electrophysiologic evidence of piriformis syndrome. *Arch Phys Med Rehabil* 73:359–364, 1992.
155. Johnson AW, Weiss CB, Wheeler DL: Stress fractures of the femoral shaft in athletes – more common than expected: A new clinical test. *Am J Sports Med* 22:248–256, 1994.
156. Booth FW: Physiologic and biochemical effects of immobilization on muscle. *Clin Orthop Relat Res* 219:15–21, 1987.
157. Eiff MP, Smith AT, Smith GE: Early mobilization versus immobilization in the treatment of lateral ankle sprains. *Am J Sports Med* 22:83–88, 1994.
158. Akeson WH, Amiel D, Mechanic GL, et al: Collagen cross-linking alterations in the joint contractures: changes in the reducible cross-links in periarticular connective tissue after 9 weeks immobilization. *Connect Tissue Res* 5:15, 1977.
159. Akeson WH, Amiel D, Abel MF, et al: Effects of immobilization on joints. *Clin Orthop* 219:28–37, 1987.
160. Akeson WH, Amiel D, Woo SL-Y: Immobility effects on synovial joints: The pathomechanics of joint contracture. *Biorheology* 17:95–110, 1980.
161. Woo SL-Y, Matthews J, Akeson WH, et al: Connective tissue response to immobility: A correlative study of biochemical and biomechanical measurements of normal and immobilized rabbit knee. *Arthritis Rheum* 18:257–264, 1975.
162. Mennet P, Egger B: *Hüftdisziplin.* Rheinfelden: Solbadklink Rheinfelden, 1986.
163. Rothstein JM: Muscle biology: clinical considerations. *Phys Ther* 62:1823, 1982.
164. Carr JH: *A Motor Relearning Programme for Stroke.* Rockville, MD: Aspen, 1987.
165. Mohr TM, Allison JD, Patterson R: Electromyographic analysis of the lower extremity during pedalling. *J Orthop Sports Phys Ther* 2:163, 1981.
166. Hubley CL, Kozey JW, Stanish WD: The effects of static stretching exercises and stationary cycling on range of motion at the hip joint. *J Orthop Sports Phys Ther* 6:104, 1984.
167. Negus RA, Rippe JM, Freedson P, et al: Heart rate, blood pressure, and oxygen consumption during orthopaedic rehabilitation exercise. *J Orthop Sports Phys Ther* 8:346, 1987.
168. Knott M, Voss DE: *Proprioceptive Neuromuscular Facilitation.* 2nd ed. New York, NY: Harper & Row Pub Inc, 1968.
169. Malone T, Nitz AJ, Kuperstein J, et al: Neuromuscular concepts. In: Ellenbecker TS, ed. *Knee Ligament Rehabilitation.* Philadelphia, PA: Churchill Livingstone, 2000:399–411.
170. Risberg MA, Mork M, Krogstad-Jenssen H, et al: Design and implementation of a neuromuscular training program following anterior cruciate ligament reconstruction. *J Orthop Sports Phys Ther* 31:620–631, 2001.
171. Saliba V, Johnson G, Wardlaw C: Proprioceptive neuromuscular facilitation. In: Basmajian JV, Nyberg R, eds. *Rational Manual Therapies.* Baltimore, MD: Williams & Wilkins, 1993.

172. Stanton PE: Hamstring injuries in sprinting – the role of eccentric exercise. *J Orthop Sports Phys Ther* 10:343, 1989.
173. Bukata SV, Rosier RN: Diagnosis and treatment of osteoporosis. *Curr Opin Orthop* 11:336–340, 2000.
174. Gallagher JC: The pathogenesis of osteoporosis. *Bone Miner* 9:215–217, 1990.
175. Riggs BL, Wahner HW, Duun WL, et al: Differential changes in bone mineral density of the appendicular and axial skeleton with aging: relationship to spinal osteoporosis. *J Clin Invest* 67:328–335, 1981.
176. Kelepouris N, Harper KD, Gannon F, et al: Severe osteoporosis in men. *Ann Intern Med* 123:452–460, 1995.
177. Wilson A, Murphy W, Hardy D, et al: Transient osteoporosis: transient bone marrow edema? *Radiology* 167:757–760, 1988.
178. Major NM, Helms CA: Idiopathic transient osteoporosis of the hip. *Arthritis Rheum* 40:1178–1179, 1997.
179. Tepper S, Hochberg MC: Factors associated with hip osteoarthritis: data from the first National Health and Nutrition Examination Survey (NHANES-I). *Am J Epidemiol* 137:1081–1088, 1993.
180. Danielsson L: Incidence and prognosis of coxarthrosis. *Acta Orthop Scand* 66(suppl):9–87, 1964.
181. Seifert MH, Whiteside CG, Savage O: A 5-year follow-up of fifty cases of idiopathic osteoarthritis of the hip. *Ann Rheum Dis* 28:325–326, 1969.
182. Cooper C, Campbell L, Byng P, et al: Occupational activity and the risk of hip osteoarthritis. *Ann Rheum Dis* 55:680–682, 1996.
183. Felson DT: Epidemiology of hip and knee osteoarthritis. *Epidemiol Rev* 10:1–28, 1988.
184. Dieppe P: Management of hip osteoarthritis. *BMJ* 311:853–857, 1995.
185. Byrd JW: *Physical Examination, Operative Hip Arthroscopy*. New York, NY, Springer, 2005:36–50.
186. Spear CV: Common pathological problems of the hip. In: Echternach JL, ed. *Physical Therapy of the Hip*. New York, NY: Churchill Livingstone, 1990:51–69.
187. Bierma-Zeinstra SM, Oster JD, Bernsen RM, et al: Joint space narrowing and relationship with symptoms and signs in adults consulting for hip pain in primary care. *J Rheumatol* 29:1713–1718, 2002.
188. Altman R, Alarcon G, Appelrouth D, et al: The American College of Rheumatology criteria for the classification and reporting of osteoarthritis of the hand. *Arthritis Rheum* 33:1601–1610, 1990.
189. Guralnik J, Ferrucci L, Simonsick EM, et al: Lower-extremity function in persons over the age of 70 years as a predictor of subsequent disability. *N Engl J Med* 332:556–560, 1995.
190. Fried LP, Guralnik JM: Disability in older adults: Evidence regarding significance, etiology, and risk. *J Am Geriatr Soc* 45:92–100, 1997.
191. Weigl M, Angst F, Stucki G, et al: Inpatient rehabilitation for hip or knee osteoarthritis: 2 year follow up study. *Ann Rheum Dis* 63:360–368, 2004.
192. van Baar ME, Dekker J, Oostendorp RA, et al: The effectiveness of exercise therapy in patients with osteoarthritis of the hip or knee: a randomized clinical trial. *J Rheumatol* 25:2432–2439, 1998.
193. van Baar ME, Dekker J, Oostendorp RA, et al: Effectiveness of exercise in patients with osteoarthritis of hip or knee: nine months' follow up. *Ann Rheum Dis* 60:1123–1130, 2001.
194. Hoeksma HL, Dekker J, Ronday HK, et al: Comparison of manual therapy and exercise therapy in osteoarthritis of the hip: a randomized clinical trial. *Arthritis Rheum* 51:722–729, 2004.
195. MacDonald CW, Whitman JM, Cleland JA, et al: Clinical outcomes following manual physical therapy and exercise for hip osteoarthritis: a case series. *J Orthop Sports Phys Ther* 36:588–599, 2006.
196. Minor MA, Hewett JE, Webel RR, et al: Efficacy of physical conditioning exercise in patients with rheumatoid arthritis and osteoarthritis. *Arthritis Rheum* 32:1396–405, 1989.
197. Felson DT: The epidemiology of osteoarthritis: Prevalence and risk factors. In: Keuttner KE, Goldberg VM, eds. *Osteoarthritic Disorders*. Rosemont, IL: American Academy of Orthopaedic Surgeons, 1995:13–24.
198. Haslock I: Ankylosing spondylitis. *Baillieres Clin Rheumatol* 7:99, 1993.
199. Kraag G, Stokes B, Groh J, et al: The effects of comprehensive home physiotherapy and supervision on patients with ankylosing spondylitis: an 8-month follow-up. *J Rheumatol* 21:261–263, 1994.
200. Byrd JW: Labral lesions: an elusive source of hip pain case reports and literature review. *Arthroscopy* 12:603–612, 1996.
201. Lewis CL, Sahrmann SA: Acetabular labral tears. *Phys Ther* 86:110–121, 2006.
202. Narvani AA, Tsiridis E, Kendall S, et al: A preliminary report on prevalence of acetabular labrum tears in sports patients with groin pain. *Knee Surg Sports Traumatol Arthrosc* 11:403–408, 2003.
203. McCarthy J, Noble P, Aluisio F, et al: Anatomy, pathologic features, and treatment of acetabular labral tears. *Clin Orthop Relat Res* 406:38–47, 2003.
204. Martin RL, Enseki KR, Draovitch P, et al: Acetabular labral tears of the hip: examination and diagnostic challenges. *J Orthop Sports Phys Ther* 36:503–515, 2006.
205. Leunig M, Werlen S, Ungersbock A, et al: Evaluation of the acetabulum labrum by MR arthrography. *J Bone Joint Surg* 79B:230–234, 1997.
206. Fitzgerald RH: Acetabular labrum tears. Diagnosis and treatment. *Clin Orthop* 311:60–68, 1995.
207. Burnett RS, Rocca GJ, Prather H, et al: Clinical presentation of patients with tears of the acetabular labrum. *J Bone Joint Surg Am* 88:1448–1457, 2006.
208. Lesquesne M: Diseases of the hip in adult life. *Folia Rheumatol* 17A:5–24, 1967.
209. Maitland G: *Peripheral Manipulation*. 3rd ed. London: Butterworth, 1991.
210. Adkins SB, Figler RA: Hip pain in athletes. *Am Fam Phys* 61:2109–2118, 2000.
211. Allen WC, Cope R: Coxa saltans: the snapping hip revisited. *J Am Acad Orthop Surgeons* 3:303–308, 1995.
212. Teitz CC, Garrett WE Jr, Miniaci A, et al: Tendon problems in athletic individuals. *J Bone and Joint Surg* 79-A:138–152, 1997.
213. Jacobson T, Allen WC: Surgical correction of the snapping ilipsoas tendon. *Am J Sports Med* 18:470–474, 1990.
214. Lyons JC, Peterson LFA: The snapping iliopsoas tendon. *Mayo Clin Proc* 59:327–329, 1984.
215. Sammarco GJ: The dancer's hip. *Clin Sports Med* 2:485–498, 1983.
216. Schaberg JE, Harper MC, Allen WC: The snapping hip syndrome. *Am J Sports Med* 12:361–365, 1984.
217. Micheli LJ: Overuse injuries in children's sports. *Orthop Clin North Am* 14:337–360, 1983.
218. Binnie JF: The snapping hip. *Ann Surg* 58:59–66, 1913.
219. Mayer L: Snapping hip. *Surg Gynecol Obstet* 29:425–428, 1919.
220. Brignall CG, Brown RM, Stainsby GD: Fibrosis of the gluteus maximus as a cause of snapping hip. A case report. *J Bone Joint Surg Am* 75:909–910, 1993.
221. Faraj AA, Moulton A, Sirivastava VM: Snapping iliotibial band: report of ten cases and review of the literature. *Acta Orthop Belg* 67:19–23, 2001.
222. Altenberg AR: Acetabular labrum tears: a cause of hip pain and degenerative arthritis. *South Med J* 70:174–175, 1977.
223. Dorrell JH, Catterall A: The torn acetabular labrum. *J Bone Joint Surg* 68B:400–403, 1986.
224. Ikeda T, Awaya G, Suzuki S: Torn acetabular labrum in young patients: Arthroscopic diagnosis and management. *J Bone Joint Surg* 70B:13–16, 1988.
225. Howse AJG: Orthopaedists aid ballet. *Clin Orthop* 89:52–63, 1972.
226. Quirk R: Ballet injuries: the Australian experience. *Clin Sports Med* 2:507–514, 1983.
227. Rask MR: "Snapping bottom": Subluxation of the tendon of the long head of the biceps femoris muscle. *Muscle Nerve* 3:250–251, 1980.
228. Lambert SD: Athletic injuries to the hip. In: Echternach J, ed. *Physical Therapy of the Hip*. New York, NY: Churchill Livingstone, 1990:143–164.
229. Klaffs CE, Arnheim DD: *Modern Principles of Athletic Training*. St Louis, MO: CV Mosby, 1989.
230. Ellison AE, Boland AL Jr, DeHaven KE, et al: *Athletic Training and Sports Medicine*. Chicago, IL: American Academy of Orthopaedic Surgery, 1984.
231. Kingzett-Taylor A, Tirman PF, Feller J, et al: Tendinosis and tears of gluteus medius and minimus muscles as a cause of hip pain: MR imaging findings. *AJR Am J Roentgenol* 173:1123–1126, 1999.
232. Lovell G: The diagnosis of chronic groin pain in athletes: a review of 189 cases. *Aust J Sci Med Sport* 27:76–79, 1995.
233. Renstrom P, Peterson L: Groin injuries in athletes. *Br J Sports Med* 14: 30–36, 1980.
234. Holmich P, Uhrskou P, Ulnits L, et al: Effectiveness of active physical training as treatment for long-standing adductor-related groin pain in athletes: randomised trial. *Lancet* 353:439–443, 1999.
235. Garrett WEJ, Safran MR, Seaber AV, et al: Biomechanical comparison of stimulated and nonstimulated skeletal muscle pulled to failure. *Am J Sports Med* 15:448–454, 1987.

236. Ekstrand J, Gillquist J: Soccer injuries and their mechanisms: a prospective study. *Med Sci Sports Exerc* 15:267–270, 1983.
237. Nielsen AB, Yde J: Epidemiology and traumatology of injuries in soccer. *Am J Sports Med* 17:803–807, 1989.
238. Engstrom B, Forssblad M, Johansson C, et al: Does a major knee injury definitely sideline an elite soccer player? *Am J Sports Med* 18:101–105, 1990.
239. Tegner Y, Lorentzon R: Ice hockey injuries: incidence, nature and causes. *Br J Sports Med* 25:87–89, 1991.
240. Merrifield HH, Cowan RF: Groin strain injuries in ice hockey. *J Sports Med* 1:41–42, 1973.
241. Benson BW, Meeuwisse WH: Ice hockey injuries. *Med Sport Sci* 49:86–119, 2005.
242. Malliaras P, Hogan A, Nawrocki A, et al: Hip flexibility and strength measures: reliability and association with athletic groin pain. *Br J Sports Med* 43:739–744, 2009.
243. Tyler TF, Nicholas SJ, Campbell RJ, et al: The association of hip strength and flexibility with the incidence of adductor muscle strains in professional ice hockey players. *Am J Sports Med* 29:124–128, 2001.
244. Ekstrand J, Gillquist J: The avoidability of soccer injuries. *Int J Sports Med* 4:124–128, 1983.
245. Casperson PC, Kauerman D: Groin and hamstring injuries. *Athletic Training* 17:43, 1982.
246. Taylor DC, Meyers WC, Moylan JA, et al: Abdominal musculature abnormalities as a cause of groin pain in athletes. Inguinal hernias and pubalgia. *Am J Sports Med* 19:239–242, 1991.
247. Peterson L, Renstrom P: *Sports Injuries – Their Prevention and Treatment.* Chicago, IL: Year Book Medical Publishers, 1986.
248. Askling CM, Tengvar M, Saartok T, et al: Acute first-time hamstring strains during high-speed running: a longitudinal study including clinical and magnetic resonance imaging findings. *Am J Sports Med* 35:197–206, 2007.
249. Askling C, Saartok T, Thorstensson A: Type of acute hamstring strain affects flexibility, strength, and time to return to pre-injury level. *Br J Sports Med* 40:40–4, 2006.
250. Askling CM, Tengvar M, Saartok T, et al: Acute first-time hamstring strains during slow-speed stretching: clinical, magnetic resonance imaging, and recovery characteristics. *Am J Sports Med* 35:1716–1724, 2007.
251. Orchard JW, Farhart P, Leopold C: Lumbar spine region pathology and hamstring and calf injuries in athletes: is there a connection? *Br J Sports Med* 38:502–504; discussion 502–504, 2004.
252. Cibulka MT, Delitto A, Koldehoff RM: Changes in innominate tilt after manipulation of sacro-iliac joint in patients with low back pain. An experimental study. *Phys Ther* 68:1359–1363, 1988.
253. Janda V: Muscle strength in relation to muscle length, pain and muscle imbalance. In: Harms-Ringdahl K, ed. *Muscle Strength.* New York, NY: Churchill Livingstone, 1993:83–91.
254. Jonhagen S, Nemeth G, Eriksson E: Hamstring injuries in sprinters: the role of concentric and eccentric hamstring strength and flexibility. *Am J Sports Med* 22:262–266, 1994.
255. Kibler WB: Concepts in exercise rehabilitation of athletic injury. In: Leadbetter WB, Buckwalter JA, Gordon SL, eds. *Sports-Induced Inflammation: Clinical and Basic Science Concepts.* Park Ridge, IL: American Academy of Orthopaedic Surgeons, 1990:759–769.
256. Zachazewski JE: Flexibility for sports. In: Sanders B, ed. *Sports Physical Therapy.* Norwalk, CT: Appleton and Lange, 1990:201–238.
257. Lephart SM, Perrin DH, Fu FH, et al: Relationship between selective physical characteristics and functional capacity in the anterior cruciate ligament-deficient athlete. *J Orthop Sports Phys Ther* 16:174–181, 1992.
258. Dadebo B, White J, George KP: A survey of flexibility training protocols and hamstring strains in professional football clubs in England. *Br J Sports Med* 38:388–394, 2004.
259. Kyrolainen H, Avela J, Komi PV: Changes in muscle activity with increasing running speed. *J Sports Sci* 23:1101–1109, 2005.
260. Pinniger GJ, Steele JR, Groeller H: Does fatigue induced by repeated dynamic efforts affect hamstring muscle function? *Med Sci Sports Exerc* 32:647–653, 2000.
261. Askling C, Karlsson J, Thorstensson A: Hamstring injury occurrence in elite soccer players after preseason strength training with eccentric overload. *Scand J Med Sci Sports* 13:244–250, 2003.
262. Croisier JL, Forthomme B, Namurois MH, et al: Hamstring muscle strain recurrence and strength performance disorders. *Am J Sports Med* 30: 199–203, 2002.
263. Proske U, Morgan DL, Brockett CL, et al: Identifying athletes at risk of hamstring strains and how to protect them. *Clin Exp Pharmacol Physiol* 31:546–550, 2004.
264. Tafazzoli F, Lamontagne M: Mechanical behaviour of hamstring muscles in low-back pain patients and control subjects. *Clin Biomech (Bristol, Avon)* 11:16–24, 1996.
265. Brockett CL, Morgan DL, Proske U: Human hamstring muscles adapt to eccentric exercise by changing optimum length. *Med Sci Sports Exerc* 33:783–790, 2001.
266. Heiderscheit BC, Sherry MA, Silder A, et al: Hamstring strain injuries: recommendations for diagnosis, rehabilitation, and injury prevention. *J Orthop Sports Phys Ther* 40:67–81, 2010.
267. Croisier JL, Ganteaume S, Binet J, et al: Strength imbalances and prevention of hamstring injury in professional soccer players: a prospective study. *Am J Sports Med* 36:1469–1475, 2008.
268. Arnason A, Andersen TE, Holme I, et al: Prevention of hamstring strains in elite soccer: an intervention study. *Scand J Med Sci Sports* 18:40–48, 2008.
269. Gabbe BJ, Branson R, Bennell KL: A pilot randomised controlled trial of eccentric exercise to prevent hamstring injuries in community-level Australian Football. *J Sci Med Sport* 9:103–109, 2006.
270. Sherry MA, Best TM: A comparison of 2 rehabilitation programs in the treatment of acute hamstring strains. *J Orthop Sports Phys Ther* 34:116–125, 2004.
271. Jackson DW: Quadriceps contusions in the young athlete. *J Bone and Joint Surg* 55:95, 1973.
272. Meyers WC, Foley DP, Garrett WE, et al: Management of severe lower abdominal or inguinal pain in high-performance athletes. *Am J Sports Med* 28:2–8, 2000.
273. Roberts WN, Williams RB: Hip pain. *Primary Care* 15:783–793, 1988.
274. Traycoff RB: Pseudotrochanteric bursitis: the differential diagnosis of lateral hip pain. *J Rheumatol* 18:1810–1812, 1991.
275. Hammer WI: The use of transverse friction massage in the management of chronic bursitis of the hip or shoulder. *J Man Physiol Ther* 16:107–111, 1993.
276. Buckingham RB: Bursitis and tendinitis. *Compr Ther* 7:52–57, 1981.
277. Cibulka MT, Delitto A: A comparison of two different methods to treat hip pain in runners. *J Orthop Sports Phys Ther* 17:172–176, 1993.
278. Hammer WI: Friction massage. In: Hammer WI, ed. *Functional Soft Tissue Examination and Treatment by Manual Methods.* Gaithersburg, MD: Aspen, 1991:235–249.
279. Johnston CAM, Kindsay DM, Wiley JP: Treatment of iliopsoas syndrome with a hip rotation strengthening program: a retrospective case series. *J Orthop Sports Phys Ther* 29:218–224, 1999.
280. Ivins GK: Meralgia paresthetica, the elusive diagnosis: clinical experience with 14 adult patients. *Annals of Surgery* 232:281–286, 2000.
281. Smolders JJ: Myofascial pain and dysfunction syndromes. In: Hammer WI, ed. *Functional Soft Tissue Examination and Treatment by Manual Methods – The Extremities.* Gaithersburg, MD: Aspen, 1991:215–234.
282. Roy S, Irvin R: *Sports Medicine – Prevention, Evaluation, Management, and Rehabilitation.* Englewood Cliffs, NJ: Prentice-Hall, 1983.
283. Fishman LM, Anderson C, Rosner B: BOTOX and physical therapy in the treatment of piriformis syndrome. *Am J Phys Med Rehabil* 81:936–942, 2002.
284. Bradshaw C, McCrory P, Bell S, et al: Obturator neuropathy a cause of chronic groin pain in athletes. *Am J Sports Med* 25:402–408, 1997.
285. Miller ML: Avulsion fractures of the anterior superior iliac spine in high school track. *Athletic Training* 17:57, 1982.
286. Andersen JL, George F, Krakauer LJ, et al: *Year Book of Sports Medicine.* Chicago, IL: Year Book Medical Publishers, 1982.
287. Boden BP, Osbahr DC: High-risk stress fractures: evaluation and treatment. *J Am Acad Orthop Surg* 8:344–353, 2000.
288. Clough TM: Femoral neck stress fracture: the importance of clinical suspicion and early review. *Br J Sports Med* 36:308–309, 2002.
289. Fullerton LR Jr, Snowdy HA: Femoral neck stress fractures. *Am J Sports Med* 16:365–367, 1988.
290. Jones DL, Erhard RE: Diagnosis of trochanteric bursitis versus femoral neck stress fracture. *Phys Ther* 77:58–67, 1997.
291. Keene JS, Lash EG: Negative bone scan in a femoral neck stress fracture. *Am J Sports Med* 20:234–236, 1992.
292. Guccione AA, Fagerson TL, Anderson JJ: Regaining functional independence in the acute care setting following hip fracture. *Phys Ther* 76:818–826, 1996.

293. Braithwaite RS, Col NF, Wong JB: Estimating hip fracture morbidity, mortality and costs. *J Am Geriatr Soc* 51:364–370, 2003.
294. Liporace FA, Egol KA, Tejwani N, et al: What's new in hip fractures? Current concepts. *Am J Orthop* 34:66–74, 2005.
295. Cummings SR, Nevitt MC: A hypothesis: the causes of hip fractures. *J Gerontol* 44:M107–M111, 1989.
296. Harris WH: Traumatic arthritis of the hip after dislocation and acetabular fractures. Treatment by mold arthroplasty: an end-result study using a new method of result evaluation. *J Bone Joint Surg* 51:737–755, 1969.
297. Grieve GP: The hip. *Physiotherapy* 69:196, 1983.
298. Maitland GD: The hypothesis of adding compression when examining and treating synovial joints. *J Orthop Sports Phys Ther* 2:7, 1980.
299. Mulligan BR: *Manual Therapy: "NAGS", "SNAGS", "PRP'S" etc.* Wellington: Plane View Series, 1992.
300. Mulligan BR: Manual Therapy Rounds: Mobilisations with movement (MWM's). *J Man Manip Ther* 1:154–156, 1993.
301. Mulligan BR: Mobilisations with Movement (MWMS) for the hip joint to restore internal rotation and flexion. *J Man Manip Ther* 4:35–36, 1996.
302. Crosman LJ, Chateauvert SR, Weisberg J: The effects of massage to the hamstring muscle group on range of motion. *J Orthop Sports Phys Ther* 6:168, 1984.
303. Godges JJ, MacRae H, Longdon C, et al: The effects of two stretching procedures on hip range of motion and gait economy. *J Orthop Sports Phys Ther* 10:350, 1989.

CHAPTER 20 The Knee

CHAPTER OBJECTIVES

At the completion of this chapter, the reader will be able to:

1. Describe the anatomy of the joint, ligaments, muscles, and blood and nerve supply that comprise the knee joint complex.
2. Describe the biomechanics of the tibiofemoral and patellofemoral joints, including the forces involved with closed-chain and open-chain activities, the open- and close-packed positions, normal and abnormal joint barriers, force couples, and joint stabilizers.
3. Describe the purpose and components of an examination for the knee joint complex.
4. Perform a detailed examination of the knee joint complex, including palpation of the articular and soft tissue structures, specific passive and active mobility tests, stability tests, and special tests.
5. Understand the purpose of muscle function testing and extrapolate information from the findings.
6. Describe the significance of muscle imbalance in terms of functional muscle performance.
7. Outline the significance of the key findings from the history, the tests and measures of the knee complex, and establish a diagnosis.
8. Describe the common pathologies of the knee joint complex and their relationship to impairment.
9. Develop self-reliant intervention strategies based on clinical findings and established goals.
10. Apply active and passive techniques to the knee joint complex and its surrounding structures, using the correct intensity and duration.
11. Evaluate intervention effectiveness to progress or modify the intervention.
12. Plan an effective home program, and instruct the patient in this program.
13. Help the patient to develop self-reliant intervention strategies.

OVERVIEW

The knee joint complex is extremely elaborate and includes three articulating surfaces, which form two distinct joints contained within a single-joint capsule: the patellofemoral and tibiofemoral joints. Anatomically and biomechanically the tibiofemoral joint and the patellofemoral joint can be considered as separate entities, in much the same way as the craniovertebral joints are when compared with the rest of the cervical spine. In 15–20% of the population, an accessory sesamoid bone occurring in the gastrocnemius, the fabella, is present as part of the knee joint complex.[1,2] The fabella, when present, articulates with the lateral femoral condyle and is hence an articular sesamoid.

The knee is one of the most commonly injured joints in the body. The types of knee injuries seen clinically can be generalized into the following categories:

- Unspecified sprains or strains, and other minor injuries, including overuse injuries
- Contusions
- Meniscal or ligamentous injuries

It is important that the clinician be familiar with the diagnostic and therapeutic procedures appropriate for all of the categories of injury. It is also important that the clinician have a good understanding of differential diagnosis as thigh, knee, and calf pain can result from a broad spectrum of conditions.

ANATOMY

TIBIOFEMORAL JOINT

The tibiofemoral joint consists of the distal end of the femur and the proximal end of the tibia (Fig. 20-1). The tibiofemoral joint has great demands placed on it in terms of both stability and mobility. The femur is the largest bone in the body and represents approximately 25% of a person's height.[3] Its distal

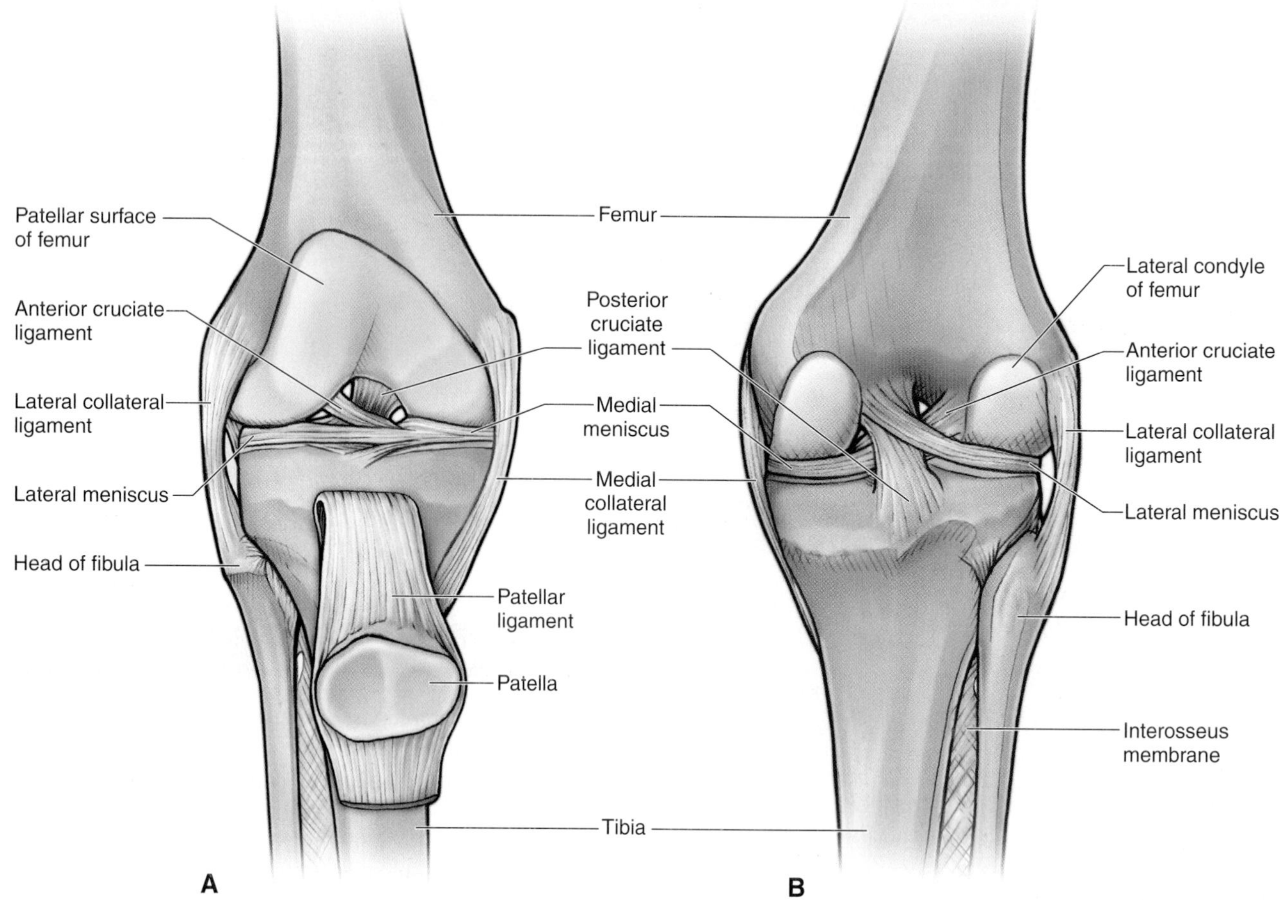

FIGURE 20-1 Anterior and posterior views of the bones of the tibiofemoral joint. (Reproduced with permission from Morton DA, Foreman KB, Albertine KH: *The Big Picture: Gross Anatomy*, McGraw-Hill, 2011.)

aspect (Fig. 20-1) is composed of two femoral condyles that are separated by an intercondylar notch or fossa. The intercondylar notch serves to accept the anterior cruciate ligament (ACL) and the posterior cruciate ligament (PCL).

CLINICAL PEARL

A narrow intercondylar notch has been associated with an increase in injuries to the ACL.[4]

The femoral condyles (see Fig. 20-1) project posteriorly from the femoral shaft. The smaller lateral femoral condyle is ball-shaped and faces outward, whereas the elliptical-shaped medial femoral condyle faces inward. The lateral condyle serves as the origin of the popliteus, whereas the lateral epicondyle serves as the origin for the lateral head of the gastrocnemius and the lateral collateral ligament (LCL). The medial epicondyle (see Fig. 20-1) serves as the insertion site for the adductor magnus, the medial head of the gastrocnemius, and the medial collateral ligament (MCL).

The anteroposterior length of the adult medial femoral condyle is on average 1.7 cm greater than that of its lateral counterpart, resulting in an increased length of the articular surface on the medial femoral condyle as compared with that of the lateral femoral condyle.[5] Thus, the articulating surfaces are asymmetric, yet work in unison.[2] The distal and the posterior portion of the femoral condyles articulate with the tibia.

The proximal tibia (see Fig. 20-2) is composed of two plateaus separated by the intercondylar eminence, including the medial and lateral tibial spines.[6] The tibial plateaus are concave in a mediolateral direction. In the anteroposterior direction, the medial tibial plateau is also concave, whereas the lateral is convex, producing more asymmetry and an increase in lateral mobility. The medial plateau has a surface area that is approximately 50% greater than that of the lateral plateau, and its articular surface is three times thicker.[7] The concavity of the tibial plateaus is accentuated by the presence of the menisci (see later).

PATELLOFEMORAL JOINT

The patellofemoral joint is a complex articulation, dependent on both dynamic and static restraints for its function and stability.

The patella (Fig. 20-1), a ubiquitous sesamoid bone found in birds and mammals, plays an important role in the biomechanics of the knee. Its articular anatomy is uncomplicated: it

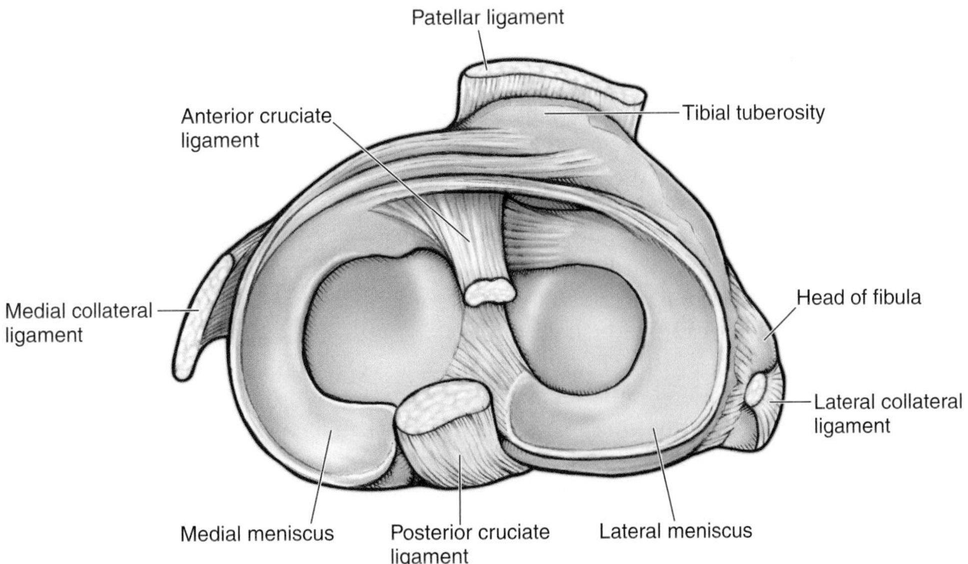

FIGURE 20-2 Articulating surfaces of the tibia. (Reproduced with permission from Morton DA, Foreman KB, Albertine KH: *The Big Picture: Gross Anatomy*, McGraw-Hill, 2011.)

is a very hard, triangular-shaped bone, situated in the intercondylar notch and embedded in the tendon of the quadriceps femoris muscle above and the patellar tendon below. The thickness of the patella varies considerably, attaining a maximum height of 2–2.5 cm (0.77–1 inch) at its central portion.[8] The posterior surface of the patella can include up to seven facets. A smaller facet, known as the odd facet, exists medially and is delineated by a second vertical ridge.[9] These concave medial and lateral facets are separated by a vertical ridge and are covered with aneural hyaline cartilage, the thickest cartilage in the body (up to 7-mm thick).[8] The articular cartilage of the patella is unique because it lacks conformity with the underlying bone.[10] The hyaline cartilage, here as elsewhere, functions to minimize the friction that occurs at the functional contact areas of the joint surfaces.

Radiographic and cadaver studies have classified the patella into four types based on the size and shape of these lateral and medial facets.[11]

The patellar surface of the femur is divided into medial and lateral facets that closely correspond to those on the posterior surface of the patella.[12] The patellofemoral joint functions to[13]

- provide the articulation with low friction;
- protect the distal aspect of the femur from trauma and the quadriceps from attritional wear;
- improve the cosmetic appearance of the knee;
- improve the moment arm (distance between the center of gravity and the center of rotation) of the quadriceps. This is achieved by elevating the quadriceps femoris muscle from the center of knee rotation. This increases the efficiency of the quadriceps muscle and provides it with leverage for extending the leg. The patellar contribution to the knee extensor moment arm increases with increasing amounts of knee extension;
- decrease the amount of anteroposterior tibiofemoral shear stress placed on the joint.

JOINT CAPSULE AND SYNOVIUM

The capsule of the knee joint complex is composed of a thin, strong fibrous membrane and is the largest synovial capsule in the body. The capsule ascends anteriorly approximately 2 finger breadths above the patella to form the suprapatellar pouch. Posteriorly, it ascends to the origins of the gastrocnemius. Inferiorly, the capsule attaches along the edges of the articulating surfaces of the tibial plateaus, with the exception of the intercondylar eminence, and a small portion of the anterior intercondylar region.[14] A synovial membrane lines the inner portion of the knee joint capsule. By lining the joint capsule, the synovial membrane excludes the cruciate ligaments from the interior portion of the knee joint, making them extrasynovial yet intra-articular.

The articularis genu, located superior to the patella, is thought to function to retract the knee capsule during knee extension. Thus, it serves a similar function as the anconeus in the elbow.

PROXIMAL TIBIOFIBULAR JOINT

The proximal, or superior, tibiofibular joint (see Fig. 20-1) is an almost plane joint with a slight convexity on the oval tibial facet and a slight concavity of the fibular head. The joint is located below the tibial plateau on the lateral condyle of the tibia. The tibial articulating facet faces laterally, posteriorly, and inferiorly. Although the joint is often described as a simple, synovial, modified ovoid, it functions as a modified sellar when combined with the distal, or inferior, tibiofibular joint (see Chap. 21).

The joint capsule of the proximal tibiofibular joint complex is thicker anteriorly than posteriorly and, in 10% of the population, the synovium is continuous with that of the knee joint.[15] The joint receives support from anterior and posterior ligaments, and an interosseous membrane. The interosseous membrane attaches between the medial border of the fibula and the lateral border of the tibia, providing attachment to the deep anterior and posterior muscles of the leg. The majority of its fibers pass obliquely in an inferior and lateral direction.

The proximal tibiofibular joint has more motion than its distal partner. The motion occurring at the proximal joint consists of two glides, one in a superoinferior direction and the other in an anteroposterior direction.[7] These motions are possible because of the orientation of the joint line, which also facilitates an osteokinematic spin of the fibula. The motion at this joint can be decreased by articular fibrosis or by soft tissue restraints; the biceps femoris can pull or hold it posteriorly, whereas the tibialis anterior can pull or hold it anteriorly.

Although the capsular pattern of restriction for this joint is unclear, it is probably indicated by pain during an isometric contraction of the biceps femoris with the knee at 90 degrees of flexion. The close-packed position for this joint, equally debatable, is probably weight-bearing ankle dorsiflexion.

Both the tibia and fibula are vulnerable to fracture at the lower third of their shaft. Anterior joint subluxations occur at this joint as a result of medial knee joint strain or an inversion sprain of the ankle. Posterior joint subluxation can occur as a result of a lateral knee joint strain, but is often missed because of the more serious ligament damage to the knee.

The nerve supply for this joint is provided by the common fibular (peroneal) and recurrent articular nerves. The joint receives its blood supply from a perforating branch of the fibular (peroneal) artery, and the anterior tibial artery.

LIGAMENTS

The static stability of the knee joint complex depends on four major knee ligaments, which provide a primary restraint to abnormal knee motion:

- Anterior cruciate (Fig. 20-1). Provides the primary restraint for anterior translation and medial rotation of the tibia on the femur and is a secondary restraint to valgus and varus rotation of the tibia.
- Posterior cruciate (see Fig. 20-1). Provides the primary restraint for posterior translation and medial rotation of the tibia on the femur and is a secondary restraint to valgus and varus rotation of the tibia.
- Medial (tibial) collateral (see Fig. 20-1). Provides the primary restraint for valgus and lateral rotation of the tibia, and is a secondary restraint to anterior and posterior translation of the tibia on the femur.
- Lateral (fibular) collateral (see Fig. 20-1). Provides the primary restraint for varus and lateral rotation of the tibia, and is a secondary restraint to anterior and posterior translation of the tibia on the femur.

Cruciate Ligaments

The two central intra-articular cruciate ligaments derive their name from the Latin word *crucere* (cross) because they cross each other (Fig. 20-1). Both the ACL and PCL lie in the center of the joint, and each are named according to their attachment sites on the tibia.[15] The cruciate ligaments, which differ from those of other joints in that they restrict normal, rather than abnormal, motion, are the main stabilizing ligaments of the knee and restrain against anterior (ACL) and posterior (PCL) translations of the tibia on the femur. They also restrain against excessive internal and external rotation and varus movement of the tibia.[16]

CLINICAL PEARL

One study[17] analyzed the coupled internal–external rotation of the tibia, finding that when an anterior force was applied to the tibia of a knee with intact ligaments, internal rotation occurred, whereas a posterior force produced external rotation of the tibia. These movements, rotations with coupled anterior and posterior translation, were found to be greater in flexion than near extension.[18] Another study[19] found this increase to be more marked at an angle of 20 degrees of flexion than at full extension or at 90 degrees of flexion.

The blood supply to the cruciate ligaments is largely provided from the middle and inferior geniculate branches of the popliteal artery. The cruciate ligaments are innervated by the posterior articular nerve, a branch of the posterior tibial nerve.[20] The function of this nerve supply is questionable although it may serve as proprioceptive in nature.[21] In addition, the cruciate ligaments contain mechanoreceptors, suggesting that disruption of the ligament structure can produce partial deafferentation of the joint.[22] Evidence of a proprioceptive function of the ACL comes from extensive histologic observations demonstrating that the ACL appears to contain proprioceptive nerve endings.[23,24] Indeed, Krauspe et al.,[20] in single-fiber studies, identified a total of 26 mechanoreceptors of the cruciate ligament among 13 animals.

Although these cruciate ligaments function together, they are described separately.

Anterior Cruciate Ligament

The ACL is a unique structure and one of the most important ligaments to knee stability, serving as a primary restraint to anterior translation of the tibia relative to the femur, and a secondary restraint to both internal and external rotation in the non–weight-bearing knee.[25–28] An injury to this ligament has terminated many a promising sports career.[29,30]

The ACL (see Fig. 20-1) is composed of a vast array of individual fascicles. These, in turn, are composed of numerous interlacing networks of collagen fibrils. The fascicles originate on the inner aspect of the lateral femoral condyle in the intercondylar notch and travel obliquely and distally through the knee joint.[16] They enter the anterior intercondylar surface of the tibial plateau, where they partially blend with the lateral meniscus. As the fascicles of the ACL course through the knee joint and attach to their insertion sites, they fan out and give a slight spiral appearance to the ligament, a phenomenon that is more pronounced during knee flexion.[31,32]

The synovial tissue that enfolds the ACL consists of an intimal layer, facing the joint cavity, and a subsynovial layer.[16] The subsynovial layer is in direct contact with the ACL and contains neurovascular structures. The ACL is considered

TABLE 20-1 Rank Comparison of Peak ACL Strain Values During Commonly Prescribed Rehabilitation Activities		
Rehabilitation Activity	**Peak Strain (Mean ± ISD)**	**No. of Subjects**
Isometric quads contraction at 15 degrees (30 Newton meters [Nm] of extension torque)	4.4 (0.6)%	8
Squatting with sport cord	4.0 (1.7)%	8
Active flexion–extension of the knee with 45-N weight boot	3.8 (0.5)%	9
Lachman test (150 N of anterior shear load: 30 degrees of flexion)	3.7 (0.8)%	10
Squatting	3.6 (1.3)%	8
Active flexion–extension (no weight boot) of the knee	2.8 (0.8)%	18
Simultaneous quadriceps and hamstring contraction at 15 degrees	2.8 (0.9)%	8
Isometric quadriceps contraction at 30 degrees (30 Nm of extension torque)	2.7 (0.5)%	18
Stair climbing	2.7 (2.9)%	5
Anterior drawer (150 N of anterior shear load: 90 degrees of flexion)	1.8 (0.9)%	10
Stationary bicycling	1.7 (1.9)%	8
Isometric hamstring contraction at 15 degrees (10 Nm of flexion torque)	0.6 (0.9)%	8
Simultaneous quadriceps and hamstring contraction at 30 degrees	0.4 (0.5)%	8
Passive flexion–extension of the knee	0.1 (0.9)%	10
Isometric quads contraction at 60 degrees (30 Nm of extension torque)	0.0%	8
Isometric quadriceps contraction at 90 degrees (30 Nm of extension torque)	0.0%	18
Simultaneous quadriceps and hamstring contraction at 60 degrees	0.0%	8
Simultaneous quadriceps and hamstring contraction at 90 degrees	0.0%	8
Isometric hamstring contraction at 30 degrees, 60 degrees, and 90 degrees to −10 Nm of flexion torque	0.0%	8

ACL, anterior cruciate ligament; ISD, implied standard deviation.
Data from Beynnon BD, Fleming BC: Anterior cruciate ligament strain in-vivo: A review of previous work. *J Biomech* 31:519–525, 1998.

intra-articular yet extrasynovial because of the posterior invagination of the synovial membrane.

Although the posterior articular nerve is the major nerve for the ACL, afferent fibers have also been demonstrated in the medial and lateral articular nerves.[33]

Like all ligaments, the ACL behaves as a viscoelastic structure, allowing it to dissipate energy and to adjust its length and internal load distribution as a function of load history.[34,35] This means that the normal ACL is capable of microscopic adjustments to internal stresses over time, thus influencing the laxity, stresses, and kinematics of the joint in subtle but potentially important ways.[36] One anatomic factor that contributes to selective fiber recruitment during tensile loading is the specific location of the insertions of the ACL on the femur and the tibia. These differing insertion sites allow different fibers of the ACL to be recruited with every subtle three-dimensional change in the position of the joint.[31,36–38]

Butler et al.[39] have shown that whatever the angle of knee flexion, the ACL absorbs nearly 90% of the force causing anterior translation. The anteromedial bundle of the ACL is taut in flexion, whereas in extension, the posterolateral fibers are stretched. These unique properties not only make the ACL the "crucial" ligament of the knee joint, but also increase its potential for injury.[28,40,41]

The tensile strength of the ACL is equal to that of the knee collaterals, but is half that of the PCL.[42] Since its fibers are unyielding, forcing the ACL more than 5% beyond its resting length may result in rupture.[28] Several factors can influence the amount of tension on the ACL.

- Compressive loading of the tibiofemoral joint, such as that occurs during weight-bearing, has been shown to reduce anteroposterior laxity and stiffen the joint when compared with the non–weight-bearing position.[43] These changes appear to reflect the increased strain borne by the ACL during the transition from non–weight-bearing to weight-bearing.[44] Thus, the popular belief in the beneficial effects of early weight-bearing and closed-kinetic chain exercises (CKCEs) following anterior cruciate reconstruction may be open to question (Table 20-1).[44]
- Stair-climbing exercises using exercise equipment such as the Stairmaster 4000PT (Randall Sports Medicine, Kirkland, WA) have been shown to produce moderate strain on the ACL compared with other rehabilitation activities.[45]
- The circumstances that cause the highest loads and strains on the ACL during daily function are[36] quadriceps-powered extension of the knee, moving it from approximately 40 degrees of flexion to full extension; hyperextension of the knee; excessive internal tibial rotation; or excessive varus or valgus stress on the tibia if a collateral ligament is torn.

Both estimates[46,47] and measurements[25,26] have shown that the maximum measured strain differential in the ACL is approximately 5% during any rehabilitation exercise.[36,48] This strain represents only approximately one-quarter of the failure strain of the normal ACL, suggesting that these exercises load the normal ACL to only a small fraction of its failure capacity.[34,36,38]

Posterior Cruciate Ligament

The PCL attaches posteriorly to the insertion of the posterior horns of the lateral and medial menisci on the posterior part of the posterior intercondylar fossa of the tibia.[49] From here, the PCL extends obliquely medially, anteriorly, and superiorly to attach to the lateral surface of the medial femoral condyle (see Fig. 20-1). Overall, the ligament is wider at its femoral origin and narrowest near the tibial insertion.[50] The PCL is covered by synovial lining and is therefore considered to be extra-synovial yet intra-articular.

Information regarding the biomechanical function of the PCL is scant compared with that of the ACL. It is known that the PCL is 50% thicker and has twice the tensile strength of the ACL.[51] The PCL is more vertical in extension and horizontal in flexion.[52] Like the ACL, the PCL consists of two bundles: anterior lateral and posterior medial. Overall, the ligament is most taut with further flexion of the knee.[53] Specifically, the anterior lateral bundle is taut in flexion, while the posterior medial bundle is taut in extension. According to Butler et al.,[39] the PCL provides 90–95% of the total restraint to posterior translation of the tibia on the femur, with the remainder being provided by the collateral ligaments, posterior portion of the medial and lateral capsules, and the popliteus tendon. The contribution percentage resisting posterior translation decreases as the knee extends. The PCL is significantly loaded if a posteriorly directed force is applied to the tibia when the knee is flexed to 90 degrees or greater while in neutral rotation.[54] If the same force is applied to the tibia when the knee is in terminal extension, the load on the PCL is not increased.[54] This is contrary to the popular belief that hyper-extension of the knee is the mechanism of injury of the PCL. The PCL also restrains internal rotation of the tibia on the femur and helps prevent posterior-medial instability at the knee.[55]

Other functions of the PCL include acting as a secondary restraint to external rotation of the tibia on the femur at 90 degrees of flexion,[56] assisting with a rolling/gliding mechanism of the tibiofemoral joint, and resisting varus/valgus forces at the knee after the collateral ligaments have failed.

A significant force is needed to tear the PCL. Thus, tears of the PCL are usually the result of severe contact injuries that often occur in traumatic situations, such as a dashboard injury during a motor vehicle accident.

In concert with the PCL are the anterior and posterior meniscofemoral ligaments, which comprise approximately 22–50% of the cross-sectional area of the PCL.[50,57] Although these ligaments arise from the common PCL origin they are distinct structures having different insertion sites.[58] Both are named with respect to the orientation to the PCL (see "Lateral Meniscus" section). Since the insertion site of the meniscofemoral ligaments are different from that of the PCL, if a midsubstance tear of the PCL occurs, it is possible that one or both of the meniscofemoral ligaments may remain intact.[59]

Medial Collateral Ligament

Both the MCL and the LCL are considered to be extra-articular ligaments.

The MCL, or tibial collateral ligament (see Fig. 20-1), develops as a thickening of the medial joint capsule.[60] It can be subdivided into a superficial band and a deep band.

- The superficial band is a thick, flat band, and has a fan-like attachment proximally on the medial femoral condyle, just distal to the adductor tubercle, from which it extends to the medial surface of the tibia approximately 6 cm below the joint line, covering the medial inferior genicular artery and nerve.[61] The superficial band blends with the posteromedial corner of the capsule and, when combined, is referred to as the posterior oblique ligament.[62] The superficial band is separated from the deep layer of the ligament by a bursa. Since the superficial band is farther from the center of the knee, it is the first ligament injured when a valgus stress is applied.[63]
- The deep band (medial capsular ligament) is a continuation of the capsule. It blends with the medial meniscus and consists of an upper meniscofemoral portion and a lower meniscotibial portion.

The anterior fibers of the MCL are taut in flexion and can be palpated easily in this position. The posterior fibers, which are taut in extension, blend intimately with the capsule and with the medial border of the medial meniscus, making them difficult to palpate.

Information regarding the biomechanical function of the collateral ligaments is quite scarce compared with that of the ACL. It would appear that the MCL is the primary stabilizer of the medial side of the knee against valgus forces, and external rotation of the tibia, especially when the knee is flexed.[64] Grood et al.[65] determined that the MCL was the primary restraint, providing 57% and 78% of the total restraining moment against valgus force at 5 and 25 degrees of flexion.[66]

Lateral Collateral Ligament

The LCL, or fibular collateral ligament (see Fig. 20-1), arises from the lateral femoral condyle and runs distally and posteriorly to insert into the head of the fibula. The LCL forms part of the so-called arcuate-ligamentous complex. This complex also comprises the biceps femoris tendon, iliotibial tract, and the popliteus.

The cord-like LCL develops independently, and remains completely free from the joint capsule and the lateral meniscus. It is separated from these structures by the popliteus tendon, and straddled by the split tendon of the biceps femoris. The LCL can be divided into three parts:

1. ***Anterior.*** This part consists of the joint capsule.
2. ***Middle.*** This part is considered to be part of the iliotibial band (ITB) and covers the capsular ligament.
3. ***Posterior.*** This Y-shaped portion of the ligament is part of the arcuate-ligamentous complex, which supports the posterior capsule.[67,68]

The main function of the LCL is to resist varus forces. It offers the majority of the varus restraint at 25 degrees of knee flexion,[69,70] and in full extension.

OTHER RESTRAINTS

Some structures in the knee clearly augment the functions of the ACL and the PCL. These structures are known as secondary restraints.[36] The secondary restraints include the structures in the posterolateral and posteromedial corners of the knee, which serve to control anterior tibial translation relative to the femur.[36,54,71,72]

Dynamic stability synergistic to the PCL is provided by unopposed contraction of the quadriceps complex, which increases anterior tibial translation. Conversely, an isolated contraction of the hamstrings results in a posterior translation of the tibia, which is synergistic to the ACL. Cocontraction of the hamstrings and the quadriceps has been theorized to minimize tibial translation in either direction.[36] The popliteus muscle–tendon complex (PMTC) contributes to both static and dynamic posterolateral knee joint stabilization.[73] During concentric activation, the popliteus internally rotates the tibia on the femur. During eccentric activation, it serves as a secondary restraint to tibial external rotation on the femur (see "Popliteus" section).[74]

The knee joint is also strengthened externally by the patellar ligament, oblique popliteal ligaments, and the fabella.

- The patellar ligament, or patellar tendon, lies in the thickened portion of the quadriceps femoris tendon between the top of the patella and the tibia (Fig. 20-1). The patellar ligament strengthens the anterior portion of the knee joint and prevents the lower leg from being flexed excessively.
- The oblique popliteal ligament, located on the posterior surface of the knee joint, is a dense thickening in the posterior capsule made up of a continuation of the popliteal tendon and part of the insertion of the semimembranosus.[65] It arises posterior to the medial condyle of the tibia and extends superomedially to attach to the posterior fibrous capsule. The oblique popliteal ligament provides reinforcement to the lateral capsule, limits anteromedial rotation of the tibia, and prevents hyperextension of the knee.[16]
- The fabella is located in the posterolateral corner of the knee and may be osseous or cartilaginous in makeup. When the fabella is present, there is a fabellofibular ligament, which courses superiorly and obliquely from the lateral head of the gastrocnemius to the fibular styloid.[68] The fabellofibular ligament helps prevent excessive internal rotation of the tibia and adds further ligamentous support on the lateral and posterolateral aspects of the knee.[75] Seebacher et al. found through dissection that the arcuate ligament was quite large in the absence of a fabella.[1]

CLINICAL PEARL

Purists classify the patellar tendon as a ligament, because it serves as the connection between two bones (tibia and patella). However, because this structure attaches the quadriceps unit to the tibia, it functions as a tendon.

MENISCI

The crescent-shaped lateral and medial menisci (Fig. 20-2), attached on top of the tibial plateaus, lie between the articular cartilage of the femur and the tibia. The knee menisci, once described as "the functionless remains of leg muscles,"[76] are now recognized as being integral to normal knee function. The blood supply of the meniscus, which is key to successful meniscal repair, comes from the perimeniscal capsular arteries, which are branches of the lateral, medial, and middle genicular arteries.[16] The outer 25% of the lateral meniscus (with the exception of the posterolateral corner of the lateral meniscus adjacent to the popliteus tendon) and the outer 30% of the medial menisci are vascularized, giving these areas the potential for healing.[77] The remaining inner portions of the menisci are considered avascular. Despite the lack of vascularity to the inner portions, tears involving the avascular zone may heal. This healing capacity may be improved with the addition of a fibrin clot or with such techniques as trephination.[78,79]

Medial Meniscus

The semilunar or U-shaped medial meniscus (see Fig. 20-2), with the wider separation of its anterior and posterior horns, is larger and thicker than its lateral counterpart and sits in the concave medial tibial plateau.[80] The medial meniscus is wider posteriorly than anteriorly. It is attached to the anterior and posterior tibial plateau by coronary ligaments. These ligaments connect the outer meniscal borders with the tibial edge and restrict movement of the meniscus. The medial meniscus also has an attachment to the deeper portion of the MCL and the knee joint capsule. The horns of the medial meniscus are further apart than those of the lateral, which makes the former nearly semilunar and the latter almost circular (see Fig. 20-2). The posterior horn of the medial meniscus receives a piece of the semimembranosus tendon.

The transverse genicular ligament serves as a link between the lateral and medial menisci.

Lateral Meniscus

The lateral meniscus, which forms a C-shaped incomplete circle,[80] sits atop the convex lateral tibial plateau (see Fig. 20-2). It is smaller, thinner, and more mobile than its medial counterpart.

The lateral meniscus has an interesting relationship with the popliteus tendon, which supports it during knee extension and separates it from the joint (see later discussion).[73]

The periphery of the lateral meniscus attaches to the tibia, the capsule, and the coronary ligament, but not to the LCL. Two meniscofemoral ligaments, the ligaments of Humphrey and Wrisberg attach to the lateral meniscus.[5]

- The ligament of Humphrey, also known as the anterior meniscofemoral ligament, runs anteriorly to the PCL and inserts on the posterior aspect of the lateral meniscus.[58]
- The ligament of Wrisberg, also known as the posterior meniscofemoral ligament, runs posteriorly to the PCL to insert either into the superior/lateral aspect of the tibia, the

posterior aspect of the lateral meniscus, or the posterior capsule.[81]

The meniscofemoral ligaments become taut with internal rotation of the tibia and help with stabilization of the meniscus.[61]

The lateral meniscus often is associated with the appearance of synovial-filled cysts, which may occur following a minor injury to the meniscus and produce a small internal tear. As fluid begins to congregate within this tear, it is pushed deeper and deeper into the meniscus. The swelling eventually produces a small bulge on the lateral aspect of the meniscus.

Menisci Function

The menisci assist in a number of functions, including load transmission, shock absorption, joint lubrication and nutrition, secondary mechanical stability (particularly the posterior horn of the medial meniscus that blocks anterior translation of the tibia on the femur),[80] and the guiding of movements.[82]

Load Transmission

The meniscus is viscoelastic, with greater stiffness at higher deformation rates. Many studies have confirmed the role of the menisci in load transmission by showing decreased contact area and increased peak articular stresses following partial or total meniscectomy.[83–85] The lateral meniscus carries 70% of the compressive load in the lateral compartment, compared with just 40% by the medial meniscus in its respective compartment.[80,86–88] By converting joint loading forces to radial-directed hoop stresses on their circumferential collagen fibers, and taking advantage of their viscoelastic nature, the menisci transmit 50–60% of the joint load when the knee is in extension, and 85–90% when the knee is in flexion.[86–95]

Shock Absorption

Because of their viscoelastic nature, the menisci are able to assist in shock absorption. During the normal gait pattern, the articular surface of the knee bears up to six times the body weight, with over 70% of that load borne by the medial tibial plateau.[80,96] The medial tibial plateau bears most of this load during stance when the knee is extended, with the lateral tibial plateau bearing more of the much smaller loads imposed during the swing phase.[96] This is compensated for by the fact that the medial tibial plateau has a surface area roughly 50% larger than the lateral plateau, and articular cartilage that is approximately three times thicker than the lateral articular cartilage.[97]

CLINICAL PEARL

A meniscectomy can reduce the shock-absorbing capacity of the knee by 20%.[98] Loss of just 20% of a meniscus can lead to a 350% increase in contact forces.[99]

Joint Lubrication

The menisci assist in joint lubrication by helping to compress synovial fluid into the articular cartilage, which reduces frictional forces during weight-bearing. A meniscectomy increases the coefficient of friction within the knee, thereby increasing the stresses on the articular surfaces.[100]

Joint Stability

The menisci deepen the articulating surfaces of tibial plateaus. This increases the stability of the knee, especially during axial rotation and valgus–varus stresses.[100–104]

If the ACL is intact, the menisci do not significantly contribute to anteroposterior stability.[43,105,106,107] However, in an ACL-deficient knee, the posterior horn of the medial meniscus functions as a secondary restraint to anteroposterior translation by wedging between the femur and the tibia.[106,108] In contrast, the increased mobility of the lateral meniscus prevents it from contributing to anteroposterior stability.[105] This difference helps to explain the higher incidence of medial meniscus tears seen in ACL-deficient knees.[109]

Guiding Movement

During flexion and extension of the knee, the menisci move posteriorly and anteriorly, respectively. The lateral meniscus has greater mobility because it does not attach to the LCL, and, as mentioned previously, its capsular attachment is interrupted by the passage of the popliteus tendon.[73,110] During knee motion, the menisci move on the tibial plateau with the femoral condyles to maintain joint congruence.[110] The femur, accompanied by the menisci, rolls anteriorly on the tibia during extension, and posteriorly during flexion (Fig. 20-3).[100,110,111] Thompson et al.[112] demonstrated that the mean anteroposterior excursion of the menisci during a 120-degree arc of motion was 5.1 mm at the medial meniscus, and 11.2 mm at the lateral. The inner sides of the menisci, which are attached by their horns to the tibial plateau, move with the tibia. As the body of each meniscus is fixed around the femoral condyle, they move with the femur. Therefore, during movements between tibia and femur, distortion of the menisci is inevitable.

- During flexion of the knee, the menisci move posteriorly. The medial meniscus is moved about 5 mm by the pull of the semimembranosus tendon, and the lateral meniscus is pulled about 11 mm by the popliteus, resulting in an external rotation of the tibia.
- During extension, the menisci move anteriorly.
- During external rotation of the tibia, the menisci will follow the displacement of the femoral condyles, which means that the medial meniscus is pushed posteriorly and the lateral meniscus is pulled anteriorly. During internal rotation, the opposite occurs. These rotations are conjunct, integral with flexion and extension, but can also be adjunct and independent, best demonstrated with the knee semiflexed. Conjunct external rotation of the tibia on the femur during the last stages of knee extension is part of a locking mechanism called the "screw home" mechanism, described later.
- The medial coronary ligament is stretched during external rotation of the tibia, whereas the lateral coronary ligament is stretched during internal rotation of the tibia.

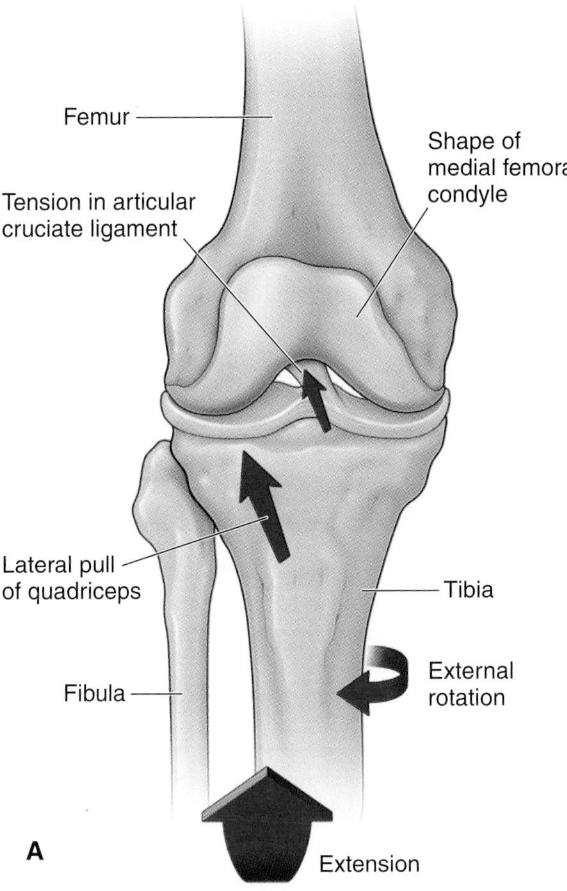

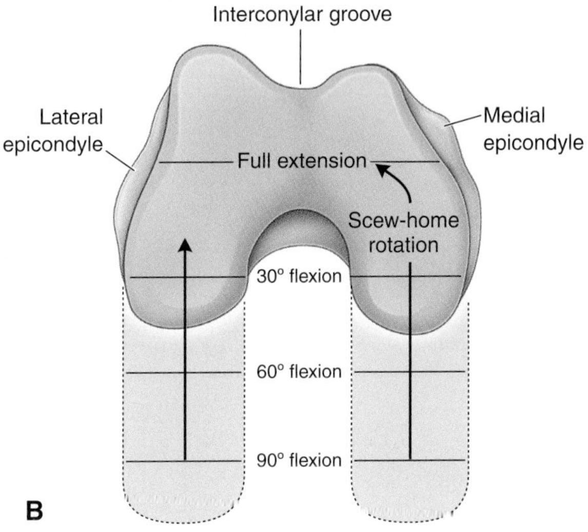

FIGURE 20-3 Tibiofemoral motions.

BURSAE

There are a number of bursae situated in the soft tissues around the knee joint. The bursae serve to reduce friction and to cushion the movement of one body part over another.

Superficial and Deep Infrapatellar Bursae

The superficial infrapatellar bursa is located between the patellar tendon and the skin, whereas the deep infrapatellar bursa is located between the patellar tendon and the tibia.

Prepatellar Bursa

The prepatellar bursa is located between the skin and the anterior aspect of the patella.

Tibiofemoral Bursa

The tibiofemoral bursae consist of a bursa between the head of the gastrocnemius muscle and the joint capsule on both sides, a bursa between the LCL and both the biceps femoris and popliteus, and a bursa between the MCL and the femoral condyle. There are also a number of bursae between the various tendons of the pes anserinus and between the MCL and the superficial pes anserinus.

The bursae around the knee can have contact with each other and with the knee joint capsule.

CLINICAL PEARL

A "Baker's cyst" may occur with fluid accumulation when there is a natural connection between the semimembranosus bursa and the knee joint.

Fat Pads

There are three fat pads located at the anterior knee: the quadriceps fat pad, the prefemoral fat pad, and the infrapatellar (Hoffa's) fat pad. The fat pads of the knee house neurovascular projections. The functions of the fat pads include the following:

- Synovial fluid secretion
- Joint stability
- Neurovascular supply
- Occupiers of dead space

PLICA

Synovial plicae of the knee were first described in the beginning of the last century.[113,114] Postmortem studies have shown plica to be present in 20–50% of knees,[10,115,116] with the highest prevalence in individuals of Japanese descent.[114,117–120]

Synovial plica represents a remnant of the three separate cavities in the synovial mesenchyme of the developing knee. These cavities are supposed to coalesce into one cavity at the 12-week stage of fetal growth.[121,122] The size and extent of this remnant depends on the degree of reabsorption.[123]

The three joints involved in the developing knee from which the remnants evolve are[112]

1. the joint between the fibular and the femur;
2. the joint between the tibia and the femur;
3. the joint between the patella and the femur.

The most common plica in the knee is called the anterior or inferior plica, or mucous ligament.[121,124] This plica is represented by tape-like fold running from the fat pad to the intercondylar notch of the femur and overlying the ACL. The plicae to the medial and lateral sides of the patella, which run in a horizontal plane from the fat pad to the side of the patellar retinaculum, are referred to as the superomedial or superolateral plicae or the suprapatellar membrane, or the medial or lateral synovial shelf. [121]

It has been suggested that symptomatic synovial plicae are one of the causes of anterior pain in the knee in children and adolescents.[125–127]

RETINACULA

The wing-like retinacula of the knee are formed from structures in the first and second layers of the knee joint. The retinacula can be subdivided into the medial and the lateral retinacula for clinical examination and intervention purposes.[128,129] The retinacula serve to connect the patella to a number of structures, including the femur, menisci, and tibia, both medially and laterally.[9]

The lateral retinaculum is the stronger and thicker of the two. It consists of two distinct layers of fibrous connective tissue: the superficial and deep retinacula. These structures are oriented longitudinally with the knee extended.[129]

- The superficial retinaculum consists of fibers from the vastus lateralis (VL) and the ITB.[130]
- The deep retinaculum consists of the lateral patellofemoral ligament, the deep fibers of the ITB, and the lateral patellotibial ligament.[130] These structures connect the patella to the ITB and help prevent medial patellar excursion.[131]

Although partially located deep to the ITB, the lateral retinaculum is blended with the biceps femoris to form a so-called conjoint tendon.[1,129] This relationship may explain why adaptively shortened hamstrings can lead to patellofemoral symptoms.[9] It is also well established that adaptive shortening of the lateral retinaculum is a common finding in patellofemoral dysfunction.[132–136]

Given the fact that the medial retinaculum is thinner than the lateral retinaculum, it is not thought to be as significant to patella position and tracking as its lateral counterpart.

MUSCLES

The major muscles that act on the knee joint complex are the quadriceps, the hamstrings (semimembranosus, semitendinosus, and biceps femoris), the gastrocnemius, the popliteus, and the hip adductors (Table 20-2).

Quadriceps

The four muscles that make up the quadriceps are the rectus femoris, the vastus intermedius, the VL, and the vastus medialis (Fig. 19-7). The quadriceps tendon represents the convergence of all four muscles tendon units, and it inserts

TABLE 20-2 Muscles of the Knee: Actions, Nerve Supply, and Nerve Root Derivation

Action	Primary Muscles	Peripheral Nerve Supply	Nerve Root Derivation
Flexion of knee	Biceps femoris	Sciatic	L5, S1–2
	Semimembranosus	Sciatic	L5, S2–2
	Semitendinosus	Sciatic	L5, S1–2
	Gracilis	Obturator	L2–3
	Sartorius	Femoral	L2–3
	Popliteus	Tibial	L4–5, S1
	Gastrocnemius	Tibial	S1–2
	Tensor fascia latae	Superior gluteal	L4–5
Extension of knee	Rectus femoris	Femoral	L2–4
	Vastus medialis	Femoral	L2–4
	Vastus intermedius	Femoral	L2–4
	Vastus lateralis	Femoral	L2–4
	Tensor fascia latae	Superior gluteal	L4–5
Internal rotation of flexed leg (non–weight-bearing)	Popliteus	Tibial	L4–5
	Semimembranosus	Sciatic	L5, S1–2
	Semitendinosus	Sciatic	L5, S1–2
	Sartorius	Femoral	L2–3
	Gracilis	Obturator	L2–3
External rotation of flexed leg (non–weight-bearing)	Biceps femoris	Sciatic	L5, S1–2

Data from Magee DJ: *Orthopaedic Physical Assessment*, 2nd ed. Philadelphia, PA: WB Saunders, 1992.

into the anterior aspect of the superior pole of the patella. The quadriceps muscle group is innervated by the femoral nerve. The quadriceps muscles can act to extend the knee when the foot is off the ground, although more commonly, they work as decelerators, preventing the knee from buckling when the foot strikes the ground.[137,138]

Rectus Femoris

The rectus femoris (see Fig. 19-7), which originates at the anterior inferior iliac spine (AIIS) is the only quadriceps muscle that crosses the hip joint. The other quadriceps muscles originate on the femoral shaft. This gives the hip joint substantial significance with respect to the knee extensor mechanism in the examination and intervention.[138] The line of pull of the rectus femoris, with respect to the patella, is at an angle of about 5 degrees with the femoral shaft[138] (see Fig. 20-12).

Vastus Intermedius

The vastus intermedius (see Fig. 19-7) has its origin on the proximal part of the femur, and its line of action is directly in line with the femur.

Vastus Lateralis

The VL (Fig. 19-7) is composed of two functional parts: the VL and the vastus lateralis oblique (VLO).[137] The VL has a line of pull of about 12–15 degrees to the long axis of the femur in the frontal plane, whereas the VLO has a pull of 38–48 degrees.[138]

Vastus Medialis

The vastus medialis (Fig. 19-7) is composed of two parts that are anatomically distinct[137]: the vastus medialis obliquus (VMO) and the vastus medialis proper, or longus (VML).[139] The VML appears to have little biomechanical significance unlike its counterpart, the VMO.

Vastus Medialis Obliquus. The VMO arises from the adductor magnus tendon.[140] The insertion site of the normal VMO is the medial border of the patella, approximately one-third to one-half of the way down from the proximal pole. If the VMO remains proximal to the proximal pole of the patella and does not reach the patella, there is an increased potential for malalignment.[11]

The vector of the VMO is medially directed, and it forms an angle of 50–55 degrees with the mechanical axis of the leg.[137,140–142] The VMO is least active in the fully extended position[143–145] and plays little role in extending the knee, acting instead to realign the patella medially during the extension maneuver. It is active in this function throughout the whole range of extension.

According to Fox,[146] the vastus medialis is the weakest of the quadriceps group and appears to be the first muscle of the quadriceps group to atrophy and the last to rehabilitate.[147] The normal VMO/VL ratio of electromyographic (EMG) activity in standing knee extension from 30 to 0 degrees is 1:1,[148] but in patients who have patellofemoral pain, the activity in the VMO decreases significantly; instead of being tonically active, it becomes phasic in action.[149] The presence of swelling also inhibits the VMO, and it requires almost half of the volume of effusion to inhibit the VMO as it does to inhibit the rectus femoris and VL muscles.[150]

The VMO is frequently innervated independently from the rest of the quadriceps by a separate branch from the femoral nerve.[137]

Vastus Medialis Longus. The VML originates from the medial aspect of the upper femur and inserts anteriorly into the quadriceps tendon, giving it a line of action of approximately 15–17 degrees off the long axis of the femur in the frontal plane.[138]

Since the quadriceps group is aligned anatomically with the shaft of the femur and not with the mechanical axis of the lower extremity, any quadriceps muscle contraction (regardless of knee flexion angle) results in compressive forces acting on the patellofemoral joint.[151]

Hamstrings

As a group, the hamstrings primarily function to extend the hip and to flex the knee. The hamstrings are innervated by branches of the sciatic nerve.

Semimembranosus Muscle

The semimembranosus muscle (Fig. 19-8) arises from the lateral facet of the ischial tuberosity and the ischial ramus. This muscle inserts into the posteromedial aspect of the medial tibial condyle and has an key expansion that reinforces the posteromedial corner of the knee capsule. The semimembranosus pulls the meniscus posteriorly, and internally rotates the tibia on the femur, during knee flexion, although its primary function is to extend the hip and flex the knee.

Semitendinosus Muscle

The semitendinosus muscle (see Fig. 19-8) arises from the upper portion of the ischial tuberosity via a shared tendon with the long head of the biceps femoris. From there, it travels distally, becoming cord-like about two-thirds of the way down the posteromedial thigh. Passing over the MCL, it inserts into the medial surface of the tibia and deep fascia of the lower leg, distal to the gracilis attachment, and posterior to the sartorius attachment. These three structures are collectively called the *pes anserinus* ("goose foot") at this point. Like the semimembranosus, the semitendinosus functions to extend the hip, flex the knee, and internally rotate the tibia.

Biceps Femoris

The biceps femoris (see Fig. 19-8) muscle is a two-headed muscle. The longer of the two heads arises from the inferomedial facet of the ischial tuberosity, whereas the shorter head originates from the lateral lip of the linea aspera of the femur. The muscle inserts on the lateral tibial condyle and the fibular head. The biceps femoris functions to extend the hip, flex the knee, and externally rotate the tibia. The superficial layer of the common tendon has been identified as the main force creating external tibial rotation and controlling internal rotation of the femur.[152] The pull of the biceps on the tibia retracts the joint capsule and pulls the iliotibial tract posteriorly, keeping it tight throughout flexion.

Gastrocnemius

The gastrocnemius originates from above the knee by two heads, each head connected to a femoral condyle and to the

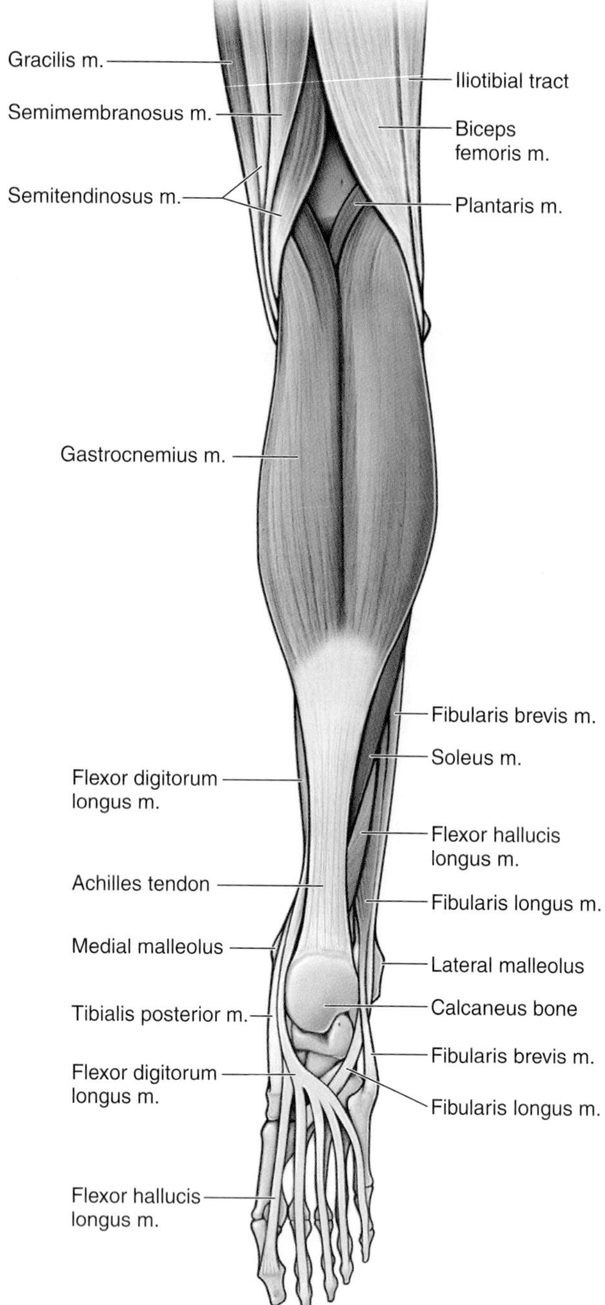

FIGURE 20-4 Gastrocnemius muscle.

joint capsule (Fig. 20-4). Approximately halfway down the leg, the gastrocnemius muscles merge to form an aponeurosis. As the aponeurosis gradually contracts, it accepts the tendon of the soleus, a flat broad muscle deep to the gastrocnemius. The aponeurosis and the soleus tendon end in a flat tendon, called the *Achilles tendon,* which attaches to the posterior aspect of the calcaneus. The two heads of the gastrocnemius and the soleus are collectively known as the *triceps surae* (see Chap. 21).

Although the primary function of the gastrocnemius–soleus complex is to plantar flex the ankle and to supinate the subtalar joint, the gastrocnemius also functions to flex or extend the knee, depending on whether the lower extremity is weight-bearing or not. It has been proposed that weakness of the gastrocnemius may cause knee hyperextension.[153]

In addition, it has been theorized that the gastrocnemius acts as an antagonist to the ACL, exerting an anteriorly directed pull on the tibia throughout the range of knee flexion–extension motion, particularly when the knee is near extension.[154,155]

Popliteus

The popliteus originates from the lateral femoral condyle near the LCL. The muscle has several attachments, including the lateral aspect of the lateral femoral condyle, the posterior-medial aspect of the head of the fibula and the posterior horn of the lateral meniscus.[156] The larger base of this triangular muscle inserts obliquely into the posterosuperior part of the tibia above the soleal line. The muscle has several important functions, including the reinforcement of the posterior third of the lateral capsular ligament[67] and the unlocking of the knee during flexion from terminal knee extension. It performs this latter task by internally rotating the tibia on the femur (a good example of an arcuvial muscle), preventing impingement of the posterior horn of the lateral meniscus by drawing it posteriorly, and, with the PCL, preventing a posterior glide of the tibia.[67,157–159] Since knee joint injury frequently involves some component of transverse-plane rotation and the popliteus muscle has been described as an important, primary, dynamic, transverse-plane, rotatory knee joint stabilizer, an understanding of its function in relation to other posterolateral knee joint structures is important.[160] Attached to the popliteus tendon is the popliteofibular ligament, which forms a strong attachment between the popliteal tendon and the fibula. This ligament adds to posterolateral stability.[161–164] A medial portion of the popliteus penetrates the joint, becoming intracapsular with the lateral meniscus. This part of the popliteus tendon is pain sensitive, and an injury here can often mimic a meniscal injury on the lateral aspect of the joint line.[73] Differentiation between these two lesions can be elucidated with the reproduction of pain with resisted flexion in an extended and externally rotated position of the tibia if the popliteus is involved.

Hip Adductors

The hip adductors, which play an indirect role in the medial stability of the knee (Table 20-3), are described in Chapter 19. The exception to this is the two-joint gracilis muscle, the third member of the pes anserinus group, which in addition to adducting and flexing the hip, assists in flexion of the knee and internal rotation of the lower leg.

Tensor Fascia Latae

The tensor fascia latae (TFL) arises from the outer lip of the iliac crest and the lateral surface of the anterior superior iliac spine (ASIS) (Fig. 19-5). Over the flattened lateral surface of the thigh, the fascia latae thickens to form a strong band, the iliotibial tract.[16] When the hip is flexed, the TFL is anterior to the greater trochanter and helps maintain the hip in flexion. As the hip extends, the TFL moves posteriorly over the greater trochanter to assist with hip extension. The TFL is also a weak extensor of the knee, but only when the knee is already

TABLE 20-3 Hip Adductors Involved in Knee Stability			
Muscle	**Proximal Attachment**	**Distal Attachment**	**Innervation**
Adductor longus	Pubic crest and symphysis	By an aponeurosis to middle third of linea aspera of femur	Obturator nerve, L3
Adductor magnus	Inferior ramus of pubis, ramus of ischium, and inferolateral aspect of ischial tuberosity	By an aponeurosis to linea aspera and adductor tubercle of femur	Obturator nerve and tibial portion of sciatic nerve, L2–4
Gracilis	Thin aponeurosis from medial margins of lower half of body of pubis, whole of inferior ramus, and joining part of ramus of ischium	Upper part of medial surface of tibia, below tibial condyle and just proximal to tendon of semitendinosus	Obturator nerve, L2

extended. The muscle is innervated by the superior gluteal nerve, L4–L5.

Iliotibial Band (Tract)

The ITB or tract begins as a wide covering of the superior and lateral aspects of the pelvis and thigh in continuity with the fascia latae (Fig. 20-4 and Fig. 19-5). It inserts distal and lateral to the patella at the tubercle of Gerdy on the lateral condyle of the tibia. Anteriorly, it attaches to the lateral border of the patellar. Posteriorly, it is attached to the tendon of the biceps femoris. Laterally, it blends with an aponeurotic expansion from the VL[165] (see Chap. 19).

Like the patella tendon, the ITB can be viewed as a ligament or a tendon. Its location adjacent to the center of rotation of the knee allows it to function as an anterolateral stabilizer of the knee in the frontal plane[166] and to both flex and extend the knee.[138,167] During stationary standing, the primary function of the ITB is to maintain knee and hip extension, providing the thigh muscles an opportunity to rest. While walking or running, the ITB helps maintain flexion of the hip and is a major support of the knee in squatting from full extension until 30 degrees of flexion. In knee flexion greater than 30 degrees, the iliotibial tract becomes a weak knee flexor, as well as an external rotator of the tibia.

MAJOR NERVES AND BLOOD VESSELS

The posterior structure of the knee joint is a complex of nerves and blood vessels. The major blood supply to this area comes from the femoral, popliteal, and genicular arteries.[16]

Femoral Nerve

The course and distribution of the femoral nerve is described in Chapter 3.

Saphenous Nerve

The saphenous nerve is the largest cutaneous branch of the femoral nerve (L2–L4). It leaves the subsartorial canal approximately 8–10 cm above the medial condyle of the knee and gives off branches to the medial aspect of the knee. Entrapment of the saphenous nerve during its course here can occur because of direct trauma, genu valgus, or knee instability, resulting in saphenous neuritis.

Sciatic Nerve

The sciatic nerve (see Chap. 3) provides motor branches to the hamstrings and all muscles below the knee.[168] It also provides the sensory innervation to the posterior thigh and entire leg and foot below the knee (except the medial aspect, which is innervated by the saphenous nerve).[168] The tibial and fibular (peroneal) divisions of the sciatic nerve serve the posterior aspect of the knee. The common fibular (peroneal) nerve is formed by the upper four posterior divisions (L4, L5, and S1, S2) of the sacral plexus, and the tibial nerve, is formed from all five anterior divisions (L4, L5, and S1–S3).

Common Fibular (Peroneal) Nerve

The common fibular (peroneal) nerve is a component of the sciatic nerve as far as the upper part of the popliteal space. At the apex of the popliteal fossa, the common fibular (peroneal) nerve begins its independent course, descending along the posterior border of the biceps femoris, before traveling diagonally across the posterior aspect of the knee joint to the upper external portion of the leg near the head of the fibula.[16] Sensory branches are given off in the popliteal space. These include the superior and inferior articular branches to the knee joint, and the lateral sural cutaneous nerve.[16] The latter nerve joins the medial calcaneal nerve (from the tibial nerve) to form the sural nerve, supplying the skin of the lower posterior aspect of the leg, the external malleolus, and the lateral side of the foot and fifth toe.[16]

The common fibular (peroneal) nerve curves around the lateral aspect of the fibula toward the anterior aspect of the bone, before passing deep to the two heads of the fibularis (peroneus) longus muscle, where it divides into three terminal branches: the recurrent articular, and the superficial and deep fibular (peroneal) nerves. The recurrent articular nerve accompanies the anterior tibial recurrent artery, supplying branches to the proximal tibiofibular and knee joints, and a twig to the tibialis anterior muscle.

Tibial Nerve

The tibial nerve, the larger of the two branches of the sciatic nerve, begins its own course in the upper part of the popliteal space. It descends vertically through this space, passing between the heads of the gastrocnemius muscle to the posterior aspect of the leg, and to the posteromedial aspect of the ankle, where its terminal branches serve the foot and ankle (see Chap. 21).

The tibial nerve supplies the gastrocnemius, plantaris, soleus, popliteus, tibialis posterior, flexor digitorum longus pedis, and flexor hallucis longus muscles. Articular branches pass to the knee and ankle joints.

BIOMECHANICS

Tibiofemoral Joint

The tibiofemoral joint, or knee joint, is a ginglymoid, or modified hinge joint, which has six degrees of freedom. The bony configuration of the knee joint complex is geometrically inappropriate and lends little inherent stability to the joint. Joint stability is therefore reliant on the static restraints of the joint capsule, ligaments, and menisci, and the dynamic restraints of the quadriceps, hamstrings, and gastrocnemius.[36,169] Since the ligaments share tensile load-carrying functions with the musculotendinous units, these structures can be considered to complement each other's functions directly.[36] The PCL is located very near the long axis of tibial rotation and has been described as the main stabilizer of the knee.[170]

The motions that occur about the knee consist of flexion and extension, coupled with other motions such as varus and valgus motions, and external and internal rotation. This is because the longitudinal axis of the knee is not perpendicular to the sagittal plane, but lies along a line that connects the origins of the collateral ligaments on the medial and lateral femoral epicondyles.[12,171]

All the motions about the tibiofemoral joint consist of a rolling, gliding, and rotation between the femoral condyles and the tibial plateaus (Fig. 20-5). This rolling, gliding, and rotation occurs almost simultaneously, albeit in different directions, and serves to maintain joint congruency.[5,172]

- Flexion and extension occur with a mediolateral translation around a mediolateral axis. In the relaxed standing position, with the knee straight or slightly flexed, the vector force is behind the knee; therefore there is a tendency for further knee flexion unless the quadriceps contracts.[110]
- A varus–valgus angulation occurs with anteroposterior translation around an anteroposterior axis.
- External and internal rotation of the joint occurs with superior–inferior translation around a superoinferior axis and transverse plane. The available range of motion (ROM) in rotation is dependent on the flexion–extension position of the knee.[173] The amount of rotation progressively increases from no rotation at terminal extension to 70 degrees of rotation (40 degrees of external rotation and 30 degrees of internal rotation) available at 90 degrees of flexion. The amount of available rotation decreases as further flexion occurs.[5,111]

During the initial 30 degrees of knee flexion, the LCL provides a greater contribution to resisting tibial varus and the PMTC provides a greater contribution to resisting tibial external rotation and posterior translation.[160,174] For flexion to be initiated from a position of full extension, the knee joint must first be "unlocked." As mentioned previously, the service of locksmith is provided by the popliteus muscle, which acts to internally rotate the tibia with respect to the femur, enabling flexion to occur.[97]

During flexion of the knee, the femur rolls posteriorly and glides anteriorly, with the opposite motion occurring during extension of the knee. This arrangement resembles a twin wheel, rolling on a central rail. Available knee flexion can vary between 120 and 160 degrees, depending on the position of the

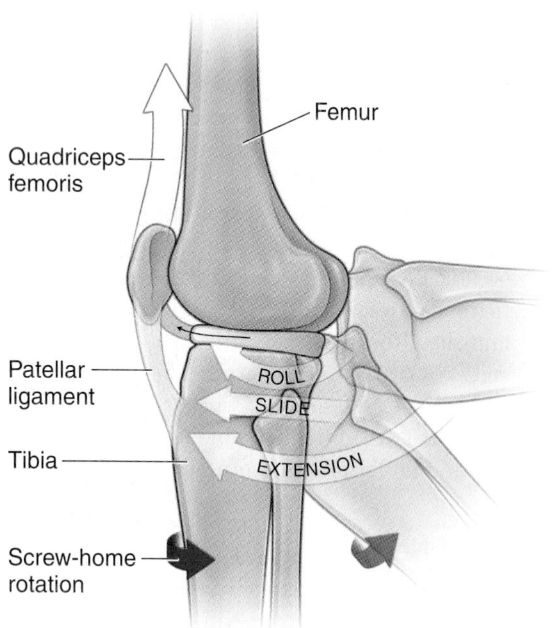

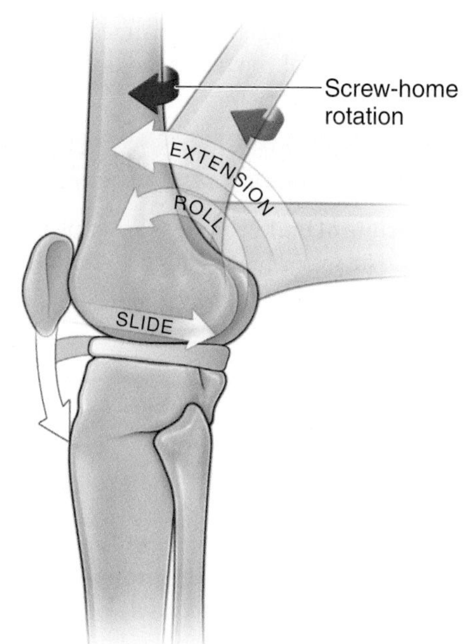

FIGURE 20-5 The arthrokinematics of knee motions.

hip and the girth of the soft tissues around the leg and the thigh.

From 30–5 degrees of weight-bearing knee extension (moving toward full knee extension), the lateral condyle of the femur, together with the lateral meniscus, become congruent, moving the axis of movement more laterally. The tibial glide now becomes much greater on the medial side, which produces internal rotation of the femur, and the ligaments, both extrinsic and intrinsic, start to tighten near terminal extension. At this point, the cruciates become crossed and are tightened.

In the last 5 degrees of extension, rotation is the only movement accompanying extension. This rotation is referred to as the "screw home" mechanism and is a characteristic motion in the normal knee, in which the tibia externally rotates and the femur internally rotates as the knee approaches extension (Fig. 20-3). This motion is known to be a complex function of surface geometry, tension in the ligamentous structures, and the action of muscles,[175,176] and has been described both in vivo[177–180] and in vitro.[181,182]

Knee hyperextension is usually available from 0 to 15 degrees.[183] During knee hyperextension, the femur does not continue to roll anteriorly but instead tilts forward. This creates anterior compression between the femur and the tibia.[153] In the normal knee, bony contact does not limit hyperextension as it does at the elbow. Rather, hyperextension is checked by the soft tissue structures. When the knee hyperextends, the axis of the thigh runs obliquely inferiorly and posteriorly, which tends to place the ground reaction force anterior to the knee. In this position, the posterior structures are placed under tension, which helps to stabilize the knee joint, negating the need for quadriceps muscle activity.[157]

CLINICAL PEARL

The transition from non–weight-bearing to weight-bearing has been found to produce a threefold increase of anterior translation of the tibia relative to the femur in the ACL-deficient knee compared with the contralateral normal knees.[184]

The normal capsular pattern of the knee joint is gross limitation of flexion and slight limitation of extension. The ratio of flexion to extension is roughly 1:10; thus, 5 degrees of limited extension corresponds to a 45–60-degree limitation of flexion. The causes of a capsular pattern in the knee are the same as for any other joint. These include traumatic arthritis, rheumatoid and reactive arthritis, osteoarthrosis, monarticular and steroid-sensitive arthritis, crystal synovitis or gout, hemarthrosis, and septic arthritis.

Open-kinetic chain (OKC) and closed-kinetic chain (CKC) exercises have different effects on tibial translation and ligamentous strain and load:

- During active OKC knee extension, the shear component produced by unopposed contraction of the quadriceps depends on the angle of knee flexion, increasing as the knee flexion angle increases.
- During CKC exercises for the lower extremity, the flexion moment arms of the knee and hip increase as a squat is performed.

Patellofemoral Joint

The patella is an inactive component of the knee extensor mechanism, in which the static and dynamic interactions of the underlying tibia and femur determine the patellar-tracking pattern. As the knee flexes, the compression forces between the patella and the femur increase (see "Patellofemoral Joint Reaction Force" section) as the contact surface area increases, in an attempt to normalize the contact stress unit load. Even though the surface area increases with knee flexion, it cannot keep up with these increased joint reaction forces. To assist in the control of the forces around the patellofemoral joint, there are a number of static and dynamic restraints. The static restraints include the following:

- ***Medial retinaculum.*** Although not as robust as its lateral counterpart, the medial retinaculum is the primary static restraint to lateral patellar displacement at 20 degrees of knee flexion, contributing 60% of the total restraining force.[185]
- ***Bony configuration of the trochlea.*** The patellofemoral joint is intrinsically unstable because the tibial tubercle lies lateral to the long axis of the femur and the quadriceps muscle and the patella is therefore subject to a laterally directed force.[186] If the patella fails to engage securely in the patellar groove at the start of flexion, it slips laterally, and as flexion continues, it can dislocate completely or slip back medially to its correct position.[186] The causes of insufficient engagement include
  - an abnormally high patella,
  - patellar dysplasia,
  - a poorly developed patellar groove (trochlea).
- ***Medial patellomeniscal ligament and lateral retinaculum.*** These structures contribute 13% and 10% of the restraint to translation of the patella, respectively.
- ***Passive restraints.*** The passive restraints to translation of the patella are provided by the structures that form the superficial and deep lateral retinaculum.

The primary dynamic restraints to patellar motion are the quadriceps muscles, particularly the VMO. The activity of the VMO increases as the torque around the knee increases, and it provides the only dynamic medial stability for the patella.[145,150] However, the muscle vector of the VMO is more vertical than normal when a patellar malalignment is present, making it less effective as a dynamic stabilizer.[187,188] The timing of the VMO contractions relative to those of other muscles, especially the VL, also appears to be critical and has been found to be abnormal with patellar malalignment.[137,189–192]

Deficits in the timing of muscle activity have been identified in other musculoskeletal conditions such as lower back pain, in which the EMG activity of transversus abdominus has been shown to be delayed compared with a control group[191,193] (see Chap. 28).

A study by Cowan et al.,[191] which found that on average the onset of EMG activity of the VL occurred before that of VMO in subjects with patellofemoral pain syndrome, appears to lend support to this theory. Thus, specific retraining of the VMO is believed to improve patellar tracking.[191]

QUADRICEPS ANGLE

The quadriceps (Q) angle can be described as the angle formed by the bisection of two lines, one line drawn from the ASIS to the center of the patella, and the other line drawn from the center of the patella to the tibial tubercle[194] (Fig. 20-6). The angle is a measure of the tendency of the patella to move laterally when the quadriceps muscles are contracted.[195,196]

The Q-angle was originally described by Brattström,[197] although many authors had previously described the importance of genu valgus and its relationship to patellofemoral instability. Brattström described the Q-angle as the angle formed by the resultant vector of the quadriceps force and the patellar tendon with the knee in an "extended, end-rotated" position.

Various normal values for the Q-angle have been reported.[126,194,198–201] The most frequent ranges cited are 8–14 degrees for males and 15–17 degrees for females. The discrepancy between males and females allegedly results from the wider pelvis of the female, although this has yet to be proven. Indeed, it is not even clear that, on average, women have a significantly greater Q-angle.[199,202] Angles of greater than 20 degrees are considered abnormal and may be indicative of potential displacement of the patella.[203–205]

The Q-angle can vary significantly with the degree of foot pronation and supination, and when compared with measurements made in the supine position.[201,206] Confusing this issue is that the Q-angle is increased in patients with a lateralized tibial tuberosity, but it can be falsely normal when the patella is laterally displaced.[11]

The significance of a normal Q-angle was highlighted in a study by Huberti and Hayes[207] who concluded that, with a normal physiologic Q-angle, the pressure distributions on the patella were remarkably uniform at each of the angles of knee flexion tested (20, 30, 60, 90, and 120 degrees) between the medial and lateral facets. In contrast, when the physiologic Q-angle was decreased by 10 degrees, the patellar contact pressure increased by 53% at 20 degrees of knee flexion. However, when the knee flexion angle increased beyond 20 degrees, the contact pressure actually decreased, with the lowest value at 90 degrees.[207]

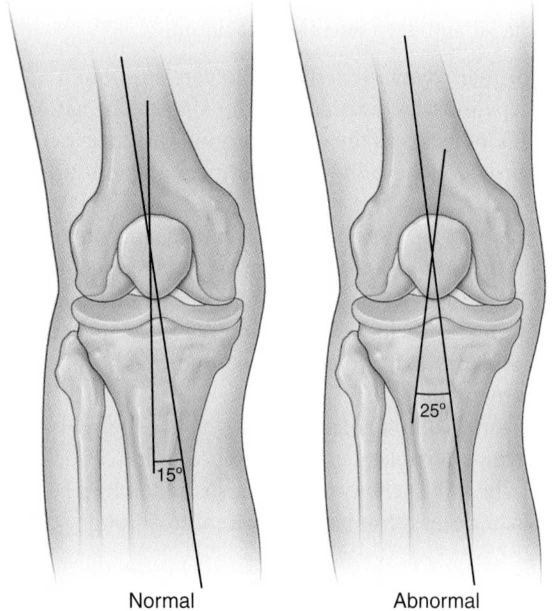

FIGURE 20-6 The Q-angle.

Although this measurement has been used to evaluate and treat patellofemoral joint pathology, few studies have examined its reliability. Greene et al.[208] evaluated the interobserver and intraobserver reliability of the Q-angle measurement comparing clinically derived Q-angle measurements with radiographically derived measurements. A reliability analysis was performed using intraclass correlation coefficients (ICCs). For interobserver measurements, the ICCs ranged from 0.17 to 0.29 for the four variables evaluated (right and left, extension and flexion). For intraobserver measurements, the ICCs ranged from 0.14 to 0.37. The average ICC between the clinically and radiographically derived measurements ranged from 0.13 to 0.32, which demonstrates poor interobserver and intraobserver reliability of Q-angle measurement and poor correlation between clinically and radiographically derived Q-angles.

CLINICAL PEARL

Although an increased Q-angle is traditionally associated with valgus knees, some of the highest Q-angles are found in patients with a combination of genu varus and proximal tibial torsion.[196,209]

The A angle is another measurement that has been used to evaluate and treat patellofemoral joint pathology and as a quantitative measurement of patellar realignment. The A angle is defined as the relationship between the longitudinal axis of the patellar and the patella tendon, or the patella's orientation to the tibial tubercle. The angle is created by drawing imaginary lines through the patella longitudinally and from the tibial tuberosity to the apex of the inferior pole of the patella. An A angle greater than 35 degrees is often cited as a cause of patellar pathomechanics. Ehrat et al.[210] performed a study to determine intrarater and interrater reliability for the A angle. The results of the study indicated that the A angle was not reproducible and further study is needed before the A angle can be used as a reliable assessment tool for patellar position.

Patella–Femur Contact and Loading

In view of the frequent problems associated with the patellofemoral joint, it is remarkable that, for much of the time, the articulating surfaces of this joint are not even in contact.[211] Indeed, there is no bone-to-bone contact with the femur in full knee extension, or during standing or walking on level ground[11,212,213] (Table 20-4).

The amount of contact between the patella and the femur appears to vary according to a number of factors, including (1) the angle of knee flexion, (2) the location of contact, (3) the

TABLE 20-4 Patella–Femur Contact During Range of Knee Flexion	
Knee Range of Flexion (Degrees)	**Facet Contact**
0	No contact
15–20	Inferior pole
45	Middle pole
90	All facets
Full flexion (135 degrees)	Odd facet and lateral aspect

Data from Goodfellow JW, Hungerford DS, Woods C: Patellofemoral joint mechanics and pathology: I and II. *J Bone Joint Surg* 58B:287–299, 1976; Aglietti P, Insall JN, Walker PS, et al.: A new patella prosthesis. *Clin Orthop* 107:175–187, 1975.

surface area of contact, and (4) the patellofemoral joint reaction force (PJRF).[211] Each of these factors is discussed separately.

Angle of Knee Flexion

As knee flexion proceeds, the quadriceps vector becomes more perpendicular, and the force on the patella gradually increases (Fig. 20-7).[214] This increasing force is somewhat dissipated by the increased patellofemoral contact with increasing flexion (see later discussion).[147] However, because the force increases more rapidly than the surface area, the stress on the patella increases significantly with flexion.[212] Any muscle imbalance between the lateral and medial quadriceps muscles can affect the patellar alignment and distribution of pressure in the lower flexion angles of less than 60 degrees.[211] This can produce a rotation of the patella in the coronal plane.[215] At higher flexion angles, imbalances are likely to produce a tilt of the patella in the sagittal plane.[215]

Location of Contact

In the normal knee, as the knee flexes from 10 to 90 degrees, the contact area shifts gradually from the distal to the proximal pole of the patella.[207,213,216,217] At full extension, the patella is not in contact with the femur, but rests on the supratrochlear fat pad.[215] From full extension to 10 degrees of flexion, the tibia internally rotates, allowing the patella to move into the trochlea.[211] This brings the distal third of the patellar into contact with the femur. From 10 to 20 degrees of flexion, the patella contacts the lateral surface of the femur on the inferior patellar surface.[213,218] The middle surfaces of the inferior aspect of the patellar come into contact with the femur at around 30–60 degrees of flexion, at which point the patella is well seated in the groove.[213,218] As the knee continues to flex to 90 degrees, the patella moves laterally, and the area of patella contact moves proximally.[211] At 90 degrees of knee flexion, the entire articular surface of the patella (except the odd facet) is in contact with the femur.[213,218] Beyond 90 degrees, the patella rides down into the intercondylar notch. At this point, the medial and lateral surfaces of the patella are in contact with the femur, and the quadriceps tendon articulates with the patellar groove of the femur.[211] At approximately 120 degrees of knee flexion, there is no contact between the patella and the medial femoral condyle.[188,219] At 135 degrees of knee flexion, the odd facet of

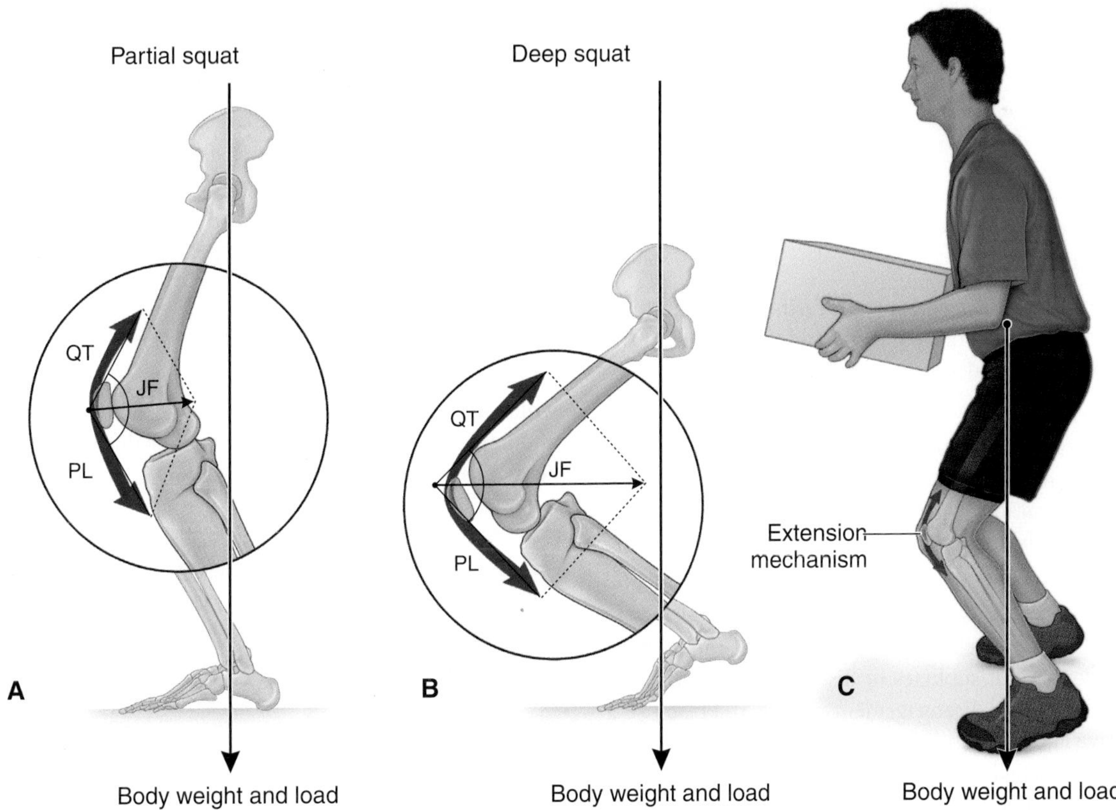

FIGURE 20-7 The relationship between the depth of the squat position and the compression force within the patellofemoral joint.

the patella makes contact with the medial femoral condyle.[213,218]

Surface Area of Contact

Knowledge of the patellofemoral contact pattern is useful for determining the limits of motion when patients with patellofemoral symptoms perform OKC and CKC exercises.[216] Some authors have proposed that the contact area quadruples as the knee flexes from 20 to 90 degrees.[86,192]

Patellofemoral Joint Reaction Force

The PJRF is a function of quadriceps and patellar tendon tension and of the angle formed between the quadriceps and patellar tendon. These forces are caused by the increase in patellar and quadriceps tendon tension and the increase in the acuity of the Q-angle that occurs during knee flexion.[192,217,220,221]

OKC and CKC exercises produce different effects on PJRF and contact stress per unit area:

- During OKC extension, the flexion moment arm for the knee increases as the knee extends from 90 degrees of flexion to full extension (0 degree), resulting in increased quadriceps and patellar tendon tension and increasing PJRFs. Clinicians most often allow OKC exercises at 90–40 degrees of knee flexion as this range provides the lowest PJRF while producing the greatest amount of patellofemoral contact area.
- During CKC exercises, the flexion moment arm of the knee increases as the angle of knee flexion increases (Fig. 20-7). Maximum force in the quadriceps muscle and patellar tendon is generated at 60 degrees of flexion with values approaching 3000 N.[217] CKC, such as the leg press and wall squat, are typically prescribed initially at 0–16 degrees and then progressed to 0–30 degrees where the PJRFs are lower.

Patellar Stability

Once engaged, the patella is held in place as flexion proceeds by two mechanisms:

1. ***Static restraints.*** The primary static restraints for this joint are the medial and lateral retinacula and the contact of the patella with the lateral edge of the patellar groove.
   a. Appropriate tension within the retinacula assures patellar tracking through the groove. Inappropriate tensioning may result in excessive pressure on the lateral patellofemoral joint surfaces (lateral patellofemoral pressure syndrome) or medial subluxation of the patella from the groove.
   b. The trochlea acts as a lateral buffer to the patella. Sometimes the patella engages correctly at the start of the flexion but subluxes or dislocates as flexion proceeds.[186] This disengagement may be the result of a defective lateral trochlear margin, an unusually shallow groove, or malalignment (if excessive genu valgus is present, the laterally directed force applied to the patella is greater).
2. ***Dynamic restraints.*** The dynamic restraints of the patellofemoral joint are the quadriceps muscle and the extensor mechanism in general. The tension provided by these soft tissues can prevent the patella from slipping laterally. However, excessively tight lateral structures or deficient medial structures may increase the laterally directed force. This may result in maltracking of the patella or possible subluxation.[146] The lateral structures (VL, lateral retinaculum, and iliotibial band) may be tight from fibrosis of the VL[222] or adaptively shortened for no obvious reason.[186] The medial structures (medial retinaculum) may be loose after injury to the medial retinaculum, from stretching after repeated dislocations, or from severe wasting of the vastus medialis.[186]

Patellar Tracking

Patellar tracking, specifically patella maltracking, continues to be the subject of much study.[188,192,223–225] In the normal knee, the patella glides in a sinuous path inferiorly and superiorly during flexion and extension, respectively, covering a distance of 5–7 cm with respect to the femur.[226] A concave, lateral, C-shaped curve is produced by the patella as it moves from approximately 120 degrees of knee flexion toward approximately 30 degrees of knee extension. The lateral curve produces a gradual medial glide of the patella from 45 to 15 degrees of knee flexion in the frontal plane and a medial tilt (from 45 to 0 degrees of knee extension) in the sagittal plane.[192,224] Further extension of the knee (between 15 and 0 degrees) produces a lateral glide of the patella in the frontal plane and a lateral tilt in the sagittal plane.[192,224]

One proposed mechanism for abnormal patellar tracking is an imbalance in the activity or tension of the medial and lateral restraints.[190,191,227]

The cause of the imbalance tends to be hypertonus of the VL, or an excessively tight TFL or ITB.[211] Other joints within the lower kinetic chain can also influence the tracking of the patella.

CLINICAL SIGNIFICANCE OF OKC AND CKC ACTIVITIES

As previously discussed, in relation to the lower kinetic chain, which includes the lumbar spine, pelvic joints, hip, knee, foot, and ankle joints, the motions that occur during activities can be described as CKC or OKC motions.

CLINICAL PEARL

A CKC motion at the knee joint complex occurs when the knee bends or straightens while the lower extremity is weight-bearing, or when the foot is in contact with any firm surface. An OKC motion occurs when the knee bends or straightens when the foot is not in contact with any surface.

Since the knee joint complex is an integral part of the lower kinetic chain, movement at any portion of the kinetic chain will influence knee joint mechanics, necessitating an examination of the entire chain as part of a comprehensive assessment. Kinetic chain exercises need to be monitored carefully to detect the influence of any abnormal motion that occurs in one portion of the segment on the remaining portions of the kinetic chain.[228] For example, normal biomechanics dictate that the tibiofemoral joint extends during midstance as the body traverses the fixed foot. Excessive pronation in either magnitude or duration prevents the knee joint from acquiring the necessary external rotation of the tibia for this extension, which in turn may affect patella tracking.[150,229]

Another example occurs during the descending phase of a squat, which requires simultaneous flexion at the hip and knee, and dorsiflexion at the ankle. If ankle dorsiflexion motion is limited, subtalar joint pronation will increase to compensate for the lack of dorsiflexion.[228,229] This increased pronation, which is coupled with internal rotation of the lower extremity, results in an increase in the functional Q angle and may contribute to persistent patellofemoral pain.[228]

Whether the motion occurring at the knee joint complex occurs as a CKC or OKC has implications on the biomechanics and the joint compressive forces induced. A significant number of studies[42,230–242] have examined the biomechanics of the knee during OKC and CKC activities and have attempted to quantify and compare cruciate ligament tensile forces, tibiofemoral compressive forces, and muscle activity about the knee during these activities.

Closed-Kinetic Chain Motion

Tibiofemoral Joint

During CKC knee flexion, the femoral condyles roll backward and glide forward on the tibia. During CKC knee extension, the femoral condyles roll forward and slide backward. During CKC knee flexion, as the femur rolls posteriorly, the distance between the tibial and femoral insertions of the ACL increases. Since the ACL cannot lengthen, it guides the femoral condyles anteriorly.[183] In contrast, during CKC extension of the knee, the distance between the femoral and tibial insertions of the PCL increases. Since the PCL cannot lengthen, the ligament pulls the femoral condyles posteriorly as the knee extends.[183]

It has been suggested by some studies that the CKCE, with its axial loading of the joint, and resultant joint compressive forces and minimization of shear forces exerted across the knee, may protect the anterior cruciate-graft during quadriceps exercises through use of the contours of the joint, thereby providing greater stabilization to the knee.[243,244] Other studies have shown that CKCEs such as squatting do not necessarily protect the ACL any more than OKC flexion and extension exercises[245] (see Table 20-4). However, increasing the resistance during the CKCEs does not produce a significant increase in ACL strain values, unlike increasing the resistance during OKC flexion–extension exercises.[245]

It would appear that CKCEs are only beneficial if performed in a restricted range, with some studies demonstrating that CKCEs at greater than 30 degrees of knee flexion can exacerbate patellofemoral problems.[232,234]

Thus, a "paradox of exercise"[233] is encountered for the patient recovering after an ACL reconstruction, whereby the patient risks excessive ACL strain if these exercises are performed at less than 30 degrees of knee flexion, but patellofemoral joint complications if the exercises are performed at greater than 30 degrees of knee flexion.[235] Consequently, patients undergoing ACL rehabilitation who are susceptible to patellofemoral pain should be forewarned about potential patellofemoral joint complications when performing these exercises. These patients should also be advised to inform the clinician of any anterior knee pain that develops during their rehabilitative process.

Patellofemoral Joint

During CKCEs, the flexion moment of the arm increases as the angle of knee flexion increases. In addition, the joint-reaction force increases proportionately more during knee flexion than the magnitude of the contact area.[188] Thus, the articular pressure gradually increases as the knee flexes from 0 to 90 degrees,[188] with maximum values occurring at 90 degrees of flexion.[207] However, because this increasing force is distributed over a larger patellofemoral contact area, the contact stress per unit area is minimized. Changes in the Q-angle of 10 degrees can increase patellofemoral contact pressures by 45% at 20 degrees of flexion.[207] As the Q-angle increases, the patella tends to track more laterally.[147] A 50% decrease in tension in the VMO can displace the patella laterally by up to 5 mm.[215]

From 90 to 120 degrees of flexion, the articular pressure remains essentially unchanged because the quadriceps tendon is in contact with the trochlea, which effectively increases the contact area.[246]

Thus, for the patellofemoral joint, CKCEs are performed in the 0–45-degree range of flexion, with caution used when exercising between 90 and 50 degrees of knee flexion, where the PJRFs can be significantly greater.[246]

Open-Chain Motion

Tibiofemoral Joint

During OKC flexion, the tibia rolls and glides posteriorly on the femur, while during extension the opposite occurs. OKC knee extension involves a conjunct external rotation of the tibia, while OKC knee flexion involves a conjunct internal rotation of the tibia.

OKC activities produce shear forces at the tibiofemoral joint in the direction of tibial movement. For example, OKC knee extension produces anterior shear stresses.[247] As the ACL provides 85% of the restraining force to this tibial shear,[39] OKC knee extension may compromise a repaired or reconstructed ACL,[248] especially in the last 45 degrees of knee extension,[247,249,250] although at full extension, the ACL is under no tension.[26,231,248,251–253] However, if resistance is applied to the lower leg during OKCEs, an increase in strain on the ACL is demonstrated,[26] particularly in the last few degrees of extension.[36] OKCE is preferred over CKCE if minimal PCL tensile force is desired. Since PCL tension generally increases with knee flexion, knee ROMs that are less than 60 degrees will minimize PCL tensile force.[235] The higher compressive forces that occur during the beginning and end ranges of knee flexion in OKCE may serve to unload some of the tensile force in these respective cruciate ligaments.[235]

Both OKCEs and CKCEs appear equally effective in minimizing ACL tensile force, except during the final 25 degrees of knee extension in OKCEs.

OKC flexion, resulting from an isolated contraction of the hamstrings, reduces ACL strain throughout the ROM,[26] but increases the strain on the PCL as flexion increases from 30 to 90 degrees.[251]

CLINICAL PEARL

It may be prudent to exclude the final 25 degrees of knee extension range for the patient using OKCE for rehabilitation immediately following an ACL injury.[235]

Patellofemoral Joint

In an OKC activity, the forces across the patella are their lowest at 90 degrees of flexion. As the knee extends from this position, the flexion moment arm (contact stress/unit) for the knee increases, peaking between 35 and 40 degrees of flexion, while the patella contact area decreases.[232,254] This produces an increase in the PJRF at a point when the contact area is very small. At 0 degrees of flexion (full knee extension), the quadriceps force is high, but the contact stress/unit is low.

Thus OKCEs for the patellofemoral joint should be performed from 25 to 90 degrees of flexion (60–90 degrees if there are distal patellar lesions), or at 0 degree of extension (or hyperextension) from a point of view of cartilage stress.[246] OKCEs are not recommended for the patellofemoral joint between 0 and 45 degrees of knee flexion, especially if there are proximal patellar lesions, as the PJRFs are significantly greater.[246]

CLINICAL PEARL

Increased tension in the PCL occurs at greater than 65 degrees of knee flexion in CKCE and at greater than 30 degrees with OKCE.[235] Therefore, it may be prudent to limit knee flexion during both OKCE and CKCE to knee angles of less than 30 degrees following a PCL injury.[235]

EXAMINATION

The common pathologies for the knee joint complex are detailed after this section. An understanding of both is obviously necessary. Since mention of the various pathologies occurs with reference to the examination, and vice versa, the reader is encouraged to switch between the two discussions.

History

With the vast number of specific tests available for the knee joint complex, it is tempting to overlook the important role of the history, which can detail both the chronology and mechanism of events. The diagnosis of most tibiofemoral and patellofemoral joint disorders often can be made on the basis of a thorough history and physical examination alone. The patient's family history, medical history, and history of the present knee problem are necessary for a complete diagnosis. A medical screening questionnaire for the knee, leg, ankle, and foot region is provided in Table 20-5. In addition to those questions outlined in "History" section in Chapter 4, the clinician should determine the following:

Chief Complaint

It is important to elucidate the exact nature and location of the patient's chief complaint. Does the complaint relate to pain or instability, or both? If the chief complaint is pain, is there a history of recent trauma?

Onset of Symptoms

Questions about the onset of symptoms (traumatic versus insidious) are, as with any joint, important. Acute injuries are often traumatic and can be associated with both pain and instability. Reports of immediate pain associated with an inability to weight bear can indicate a muscle, ligament, or fracture injury and should be related to the patient's current complaints to identify the likely cause. As always, an insidious onset of pain should alert the clinician to the possibility of a serious condition. Pain in the knee can be referred from the

TABLE 20-5 Medical-Screening Questionnaire for the Knee, Leg, Ankle, and Foot Region

	Yes	No
Have you recently had a fever?		
Have you recently taken antibiotics or other medicines for an infection?		
Have you had a recent surgery?		
Have you had a recent injection to one or more of your joints?		
Have you recently had a cut, scrape, or open wound?		
Have you been diagnosed as having an immunosuppressive disorder?		
Do you have a history of heart trouble?		
Do you have a history of cancer?		
Have you recently taken a long car ride, bus trip, or plane flight or been bedridden for any reason?		
Have you recently begun a vigorous physical training program?		
Do you have growing, hip, thigh, or calf aching or pain that increases with physical activity, such as walking or running?		
Have you recently sustained a blow to your shins or any other trauma to either of your legs?		

Data from DuVall RE, Godges J: Introduction to physical therapy differential diagnosis: The clinical utility of subjective examination. In: Wilmarth MA, ed. *Medical Screening for the Physical Therapist. Orthopaedic Section Independent Study Course* 14.1.1 La Crosse, WI: Orthopaedic Section, APTA, 2003:1–44.

hip, the back, and the sacroiliac joint. Complaints of shooting pain, burning pain, and pain that travels down the thigh should be carefully investigated using a lumbar screen to rule out radicular symptom production. A gradual, nontraumatic onset of knee pain could also indicate patellofemoral joint dysfunction or symptomatic degenerative joint disease of the knee joint complex. The characteristic clinical features in an uncomplicated osteoarthritis (OA) of the knee joint are a dull and aching pain that occurs at the end of the day or after prolonged periods of standing or walking.[255] As the disease progresses, there is pain and stiffness on rising in the morning, which eases with activity or rest, and a limitation of movement in the capsular pattern.

Mechanism of Injury

The clinician should determine how exactly the injury happened—was it a traumatic blow, a contact injury, a noncontact injury, or did the patient fall? The position of the joint at the time of the traumatic force dictates which anatomic structures are at risk for injury; hence, an important aspect of obtaining the patient's history for acute injuries is to allow him or her to describe the position of the knee and direction of forces at the time it was injured.[256] The direction the patient was turning to and the direction of the blow help to determine the structures likely affected.[257] Twisting injuries can result in injuries to the ligaments or meniscus. Contact injuries can result in deep bone bruising, muscle contusions, and ligamentous or meniscal injury when combined with twisting or hyperextension.

The primary mechanisms of injury in the knee are direct trauma, a varus or valgus force (with or without rotation), hyperextension, flexion with posterior translation, a twisting force, and overuse.[258]

- ***Direct trauma.*** A direct blow to the anterior aspect of the knee may cause a patellar injury. Repetitive microtrauma to the patella may also be a factor. For example, Bloom[259] describes a condition called *airplane knee,* in which the frequent flyer in coach class gets repetitive knee bumps from the passenger in front when the seat is dropped back suddenly.
- ***Valgus force.*** A history of a valgus force to the knee without rotation could indicate damage to the medial meniscus, collateral ligament, epiphyseal plate, or patellar dislocation–subluxation.[256] A history of a valgus force with rotation could indicate damage to the ACL, or the posteromedial capsule (the so-called unholy triad).
- ***Varus force.*** A history of a varus force with rotation can involve the LCL, the posterolateral capsule, and the PCL.[256]
- ***Hyperextension.*** A hyperextension force can result in ACL injuries and associated medial meniscal tears. Complaints of buckling or giving way after the injury can reinforce a suspicion of ligamentous involvement.
- ***Flexion.*** During flexion, as the tibia internally rotates, the posterior horn of the medial meniscus is pulled toward the center of the joint. If excessive, this movement can produce a traction injury of the medial meniscus, tearing it from its peripheral attachment and producing a longitudinal tear of the substance of the meniscus.[257]
- ***Flexion with a posterior translation.*** This mechanism can result in a PCL injury.
- ***Twisting force.*** Meniscal injuries are usually associated with a torsional force that combines compression and rotation, often in activities that require cutting maneuvers.[259] In addition, the ACL often is injured during traumatic twisting injuries in which the tibia moves forward with respect to the femur, often accompanied by valgus stress.[257] No direct blow to the knee or leg is required, but the foot is usually planted and the patient may remember a "popping" sensation at the time of the injury. Similar to the ACL, PCL injuries often occur during twisting with a planted foot in which the force of the injury is directed posteriorly against the tibia with the knee flexed.[257]
- ***Overuse.*** Patellar injury is most often a result of overuse.[259] Typically, there is an associated 4–6-week training program change. These changes can include (1) increasing a training load more than 10% per week; (2) not allowing a 15% decrease for a week off; (3) not using an alternate-day or hard-easy pattern; (4) changing quickly from flat to hill training; (5) running in one direction on a canted road; (6) running in worn-out shoes; or (7) biking in cleated shoes that fix the tibial rotation relative to the pedal.[259]

Location of Symptoms

The location of the symptoms may afford the clinician clues as to the cause. Initially, the clinician should consider the anatomical structures underlying the area of pain to ascertain the cause. Medial knee pain can be caused by a spectrum of possibilities ranging from localized musculoskeletal to nonmusculoskeletal pathology (Table 20-6).[260] For example, medial meniscal lesions frequently result in posterior medial joint line pain and mild medial joint line pain.[256] Medial knee pain also may suggest an MCL injury. MCL injury can produce pain at the medial femoral condyle, medial joint line, or proximal tibia.[256] Lateral joint line pain may be caused by an LCL injury. Localized swelling over specific knee structures, such as the MCL or LCL, also may accompany the pain. Midlateral joint line pain often is caused by a lateral meniscal lesion. Patellofemoral joint pain usually is anterior, radiating medially and laterally, but primarily in, around, or under the patella.[259] Posterior knee pain may be secondary to joint effusion producing distention of the posterior capsule, a mild strain of one of the gastrocnemius muscles or a PCL tear.[256] Posterior knee pain accompanied by snapping could indicate a Baker's cyst.

Behavior of Symptoms

Symptoms that are not alleviated with rest could indicate a nonmechanical source, or a chemically induced source, such as an inflammatory reaction. A hot and swollen joint without a history of trauma should provoke suspicions about hemophilia, rheumatoid arthritis, an infection, or gout.

Quality of the Symptoms

Deep knee pain may indicate damage to one of the cruciate ligaments. Generalized pain in the knee region is characteristic of referred pain, or pain from a contusion or partial tear of a muscle or ligament.[261] Often a patient with a chronic

TABLE 20-6 Differential Diagnosis of Medial Knee Pain

Cause	Condition
Local musculoskeletal	Patellofemoral syndrome Medial meniscus tear Patellar tendinitis Lateral patellar subluxation Pes anserine tendinitis Pes anserine bursitis Vastus medialis strain Saphenous neuropathy Medial collateral ligament sprain Medial tibial plateau fracture Medial tibial plateau stress fracture Proximal tibia stress fracture
Tumors	Osteochondroma Chondroblastoma Giant cell tumor Osteoid osteoma Osteosarcoma Ewing sarcoma Chondrosarcoma Fibrosarcoma Pigmented villonodular synovitis (PVNS) Localized nodular synovitis (LNS)
Systemic disease	Thyroid disorder (Grave's disease) Lymphoma Leukemia Myeloma
Vascular/inflammatory	Rheumatoid arthritis Reiter's syndrome Saphenous thrombophlebitis Deep vein thrombosis
Remote neuromusculoskeletal	Hip dysplasia Lumbosacral pathology Obturator neuropathy

Data from Rosenthal MD, Moore JH, DeBerardino TM: Diagnosis of medial knee pain: Atypical stress fracture about the knee joint. *J Orthop Sports Phys Ther* 36:526–534, 2006.

condition has several complaints, and a historical investigation can help identify the original cause. Patients do not always recognize the significance that an old injury may play in their current condition, but these options must be considered if the clinician is unable to make a diagnosis with the information available.

Reports of Swelling

In the presence of trauma, the main thrust of the history should be to establish whether the patient experienced an effusion or hemarthrosis (the assessment of swelling is described in "Observation" section.) An effusion is the method by which the joint reacts to stress and usually takes several hours to accumulate. The effusion can result from blood filling the joint or from an increased production of synovial fluid. The time frame of onset provides the clinician with clues as to the nature of the effusion. Synovial effusion usually takes 6–12 hours to develop and produces a dull, aching pain as the joint capsule is distended. By contrast, an acute hemarthrosis is usually well formed after 1–2 hours, leaving a very tense and inflamed knee. The two diagnoses that represent over 80% of the causes of an acute tense hemarthrosis are an ACL tear and patellar dislocation.[262] Other causes of an intra-articular effusion include MCL rupture and intra-articular fracture. Patients with a meniscal lesion often report repetitive episodes of effusion.[259]

Reports of Joint Noise

Reports of grinding, popping, and clicking in the knee with a particular maneuver are common but may not be related to a pathologic process.[167] However, reports of a "pop" involving sudden rotation of the femur or tibia may indicate damage to the ACL, MCL, coronary ligament, or meniscus, or an osteochondral fracture.[167] Sprains to the ligaments of the knee are often more painful than complete ruptures, because the latter have no intact fibers from which pain of a mechanical origin can occur. Instability of the knee often is described as a sensation of "giving way," sliding, or buckling. Sharp, catching pain usually indicates a mechanical problem.

Aggravating Positions or Activities

Questions should be asked to determine whether certain kinds of activities bring on the symptoms. For example, the pain may be noticed after resting or after certain activities. Morning pain and stiffness that lessens with activity or movement may indicate a degenerative joint complaint. Complaints of locking or pseudolocking during active or passive flexion and extension can highlight a dysfunctional structure. True locking of the knee is rare; however, loose bodies can cause recurrent locking or the sensation of something catching or getting in the way of movement. "Locking" that occurs with extension could indicate a lesion of the meniscus, a hamstring muscle spasm or an entrapment of the cruciate ligament. "Locking" that occurs with flexion could indicate a lesion to the posterior horn of the medial meniscus. With patellar irritability, there is no true mechanical blocking, although there may be stiffness, grating, or rapid movement inhibition.[259]

Impact on Function

The clinician should determine which functional activities reproduce the pain or exacerbate the symptoms. The following statements should be viewed as generalizations, as there are always exceptions.

- Weight-bearing activities involving a twisting weight-bearing load (e.g., getting in and out of a car with low seats) tend to aggravate a meniscal lesion.
- Patellofemoral joint pain often develops as a result of extended activity, such as in the middle of a long run or bike ride, continues into the evening or night, and can disturb sleep.[259]

- Walking upstairs or downstairs is usually difficult for patients with knee pathology. Usually, patients with a meniscal lesion complain of increased pain with stair climbing, whereas patients with a patellofemoral joint lesion complain of increased pain when descending stairs.
- Patients with a meniscal lesion or patellofemoral pain rarely can do a full squat without pain.
- Complaints of pain with kneeling activities are more likely to indicate a patellofemoral lesion than a meniscal lesion.
- Sitting tends to provoke more symptoms in patients with patellofemoral dysfunction than it does in those with meniscal or ligamentous lesions.

Anterior Knee Pain

Due to the prevalence of patellofemoral related disorders, there is a significant temptation to cut corners with a patient who presents with anterior knee pain, and to proceed directly to the diagnosis of patellofemoral pain.[147] However, this should be avoided, especially in light of the fact that the literature is replete with descriptions of physical examination techniques for the evaluation of the patellofemoral joint.[133,226,263–268]

CLINICAL PEARL

The differential diagnosis of anterior knee pain (see Chap. 5) should include tears of the menisci, medial synovial plica syndrome, inflammatory or degenerative arthritis, tumors of the joint, ligament injuries that mimic patellar instability, osteochondritis dissecans of the medial femoral condyle, prepatellar bursitis, patellar tendinitis, inflammation of the patellar fat pad, and Sindig–Larsen–Johansson syndrome.[8,147,269–271]

Classically, the pain from patellofemoral joint dysfunction is anterior, but it also can be medial,[196,272] lateral,[196,272] or popliteal (posterior).[194] Particular activities can help with differential diagnosis. Pain from rotational malalignment of the patella is typically exacerbated by activity and relieved by rest. Complaints of pain that occur when a patient arises from a seated position, negotiates stairs, or squats are associated with patellofemoral dysfunction. The so-called movie-theater sign[196]—pain with prolonged sitting—traditionally has been associated with patellar pain from any source. Venous congestion and stretching of painful tissues are potential explanations for this symptom.[246] Activities that involve eccentric loading of the knee, and increased hill work with running, tend to provoke patellar tendinitis, whereas inferior patellar pain following vigorous kicking, flip turns in swimming, or delivery of a fast ball in cricket would tend to implicate the fat pad.[273] The fat pad also may be irritated with the straight leg raise exercise.[266]

If a patellofemoral disorder is suspected, the clinician should look for evidence of an anatomical variant and/or a biomechanical dysfunction involving the lower quadrant. These anatomical variants can occur in any of the following joints: hip, patellofemoral, tibiofemoral, subtalar, intertarsal, or any combination of these joints. Examples of biomechanical dysfunctions that can cause patellofemoral disorders include excessive femoral anteversion, excessive genu valgum, excessive tibial external rotation, excessive pronation, and VMO dysplasia.

Edema rarely is reported with insidious onset overuse injuries, except in the case of plical irritation, ITB friction syndrome (ITBFS), irritation of the pes anserine or Osgood–Schlatter's disease.[167] Following the history, a hypothesis is made and this hypothesis is then tested with the physical examination. Ideally, the clinician is able to process and identify responsible structures for the patient's complaints and the history of injury to aid in the differential diagnosis.

Systems Review

Knee pain and dysfunction can arise from multiple sources. Knee pain that has gradually worsened over time should lead to an evaluation of systemic illness and overuse complications such as tendinitis. A subjective complaint of stiffness may imply swelling, and the joint mobility and effusion should be assessed. Complaints of weakness should be followed by an examination of the patient's strength and gait pattern.

The clinician needs to consider the likelihood of a specific diagnosis based on age. For example, a slipped capital femoral epiphysis (SCFE) is less likely to be the cause of a recent onset of pain in a 40-year-old fully developed man that it would be in an adolescent. Knee pain can be referred to the knee from the lumbosacral region (L3–S2 segments) or from the hip. For example, anteromedial pain can be referred from the L2 and L3 spinal levels, whereas posterolateral knee pain can be referred from the L4, L5, and S1 to S2 levels. The peripheral nerves are also capable of referring pain to this area. Medial knee pain having a burning quality could indicate saphenous nerve neuritis. A family history of knee problems, rheumatoid arthritis, or OA may need further investigation with a laboratory work-up or X-ray films. Pain that is constant and burning in nature should alert the clinician to the possibility of complex regional pain syndrome (CRPS), gout, or radicular pain. Intermittent pain usually indicates a mechanical problem (meniscus). The health intake questionnaire should be designed to provide evidence of undiagnosed systemic problems that relate to the knee dysfunction (e.g., Lyme disease). Chapter 5 describes some of the more common causes of referred knee pain, and causes of a more serious nature.

TESTS AND MEASURES

Observation

The observation component of the examination begins as the clinician meets the patient and ends as the patient is leaving. This informal observation should occur at every visit.

Swelling or Effusion

The amount of swelling present may provide the clinician with valuable information regarding the internal damage that may have resulted. Diffuse swelling indicates fluid in the joint or synovial swelling, or both. An effusion can be detected by noticing the loss of the peripatellar groove and by palpation of

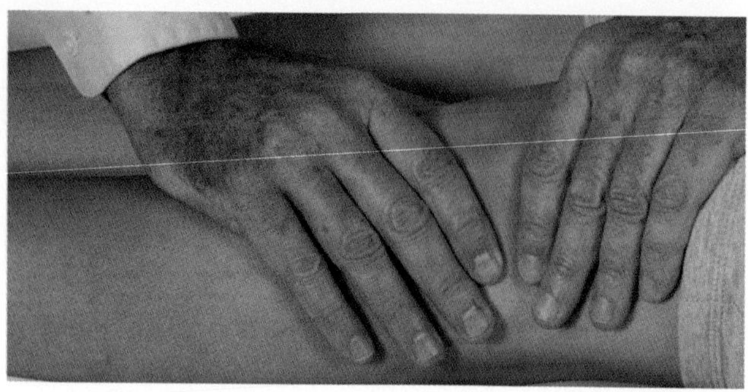

FIGURE 20-8 Patellar ballottement test.

the fluid. A perceptible bulge on the medial aspect suggests a small effusion; this sign may not be present with larger effusions. The swelling is examined with the patient positioned in supine, in the following manner[274]:

- ***Patellar ballottement (maximal effusion).*** Ballottement of the patella is a useful technique for detecting an effusion. Using one hand, the clinician grasps the patient's thigh at the anterior aspect about 10 cm above the patella, placing the fingers medial and the thumb lateral. The patient's knee is extended. With the other hand, the clinician grasps the patient's lower leg about 5 cm distal to the patella, placing the fingers medial and the thumb lateral. The proximal hand exerts compression against the anterior, lateral, and medial aspects of the thigh and, while maintaining this pressure, slides distally. The distal hand exerts compression in a similar way and slides proximally (Fig. 20-8). Using the index finger of the distal hand, the clinician now taps the patella against the femur. In the normal knee joint with minimal free fluid, the patella moves directly into the femoral condyle and there is no tapping sensation underneath the clinician's fingertips. However, in the knee with excess fluid, the patella is "floating"; thus, ballottement causes the patella to tap directly against the femoral condyle. This sensation is transmitted to the clinician's fingertips. A positive test is indicative of a significant synovial effusion or hemarthrosis in the knee joint. However, sometimes, this test can produce false-positive results. When this is the case, the uninvolved side usually tests positive as well.

If there is no swelling but there is evidence of bruising or bleeding into the tibial area, disruption of the joint capsule may be present, or a SCFE, if the patient is an adolescent. Popliteal swelling, which can compress the tibial or common fibular (peroneal) nerves, or both, can produce complaints of paresthesia and anesthesia.

The formal observation of the patient is divided into three sections: standing and walking, seated, and lying examinations.

Patient Standing

The patient is asked to stand with the feet slightly apart and aligned straight ahead. This position can be used to assess overall limb alignment as well as to identify possible foot abnormalities. A careful physical examination of the hip, knee, and ankle is performed, observing for both static restraints, and, to a great degree, dynamic restraints.[127] Following this position, the patient is asked to stand with the feet shoulder-width apart. The entire trunk and lower extremities are observed. Areas of atrophy should be noted and correlated with other findings. Common areas include the medial aspect of the quadriceps following trauma, nerve injury, or knee surgery.

Degree of Femoral Retroversion or Anteversion

Femoral retroversion–anteversion is indicated by whether the feet are rotated outward or inward, respectively, in the relaxed standing position. The position of the patella is examined to see whether it looks inward (the so-called squinting patella), which could indicate femoral anteversion. Femoral anteversion results in internal rotation of the femoral sulcus, and an increase in the Q-angle. Femoral anteversion has been associated with abnormal patellofemoral mechanics.[147,275] Even if the patella looks straight in the presence of femoral anteversion, it may be held there by tight lateral structures.[266]

Leg-Length Discrepancy

Compensations for leg-length discrepancies include excessive foot pronation, toeing-out (forefoot abduction), and a flexed knee gait or stance.[276,277]

Degree of Genu Varum/Genu Valgum

Genu varus ("bow legs") can be the result of bowing of the tibia or varus at the knee joint. An increased varus moment can contribute to early degeneration of the knee and, when exaggerated, is most often an indication of advanced degenerative joint disease (DJD).[278] On the basis of the relationship between the proximal and distal aspects of the femur, a change in the orientation between the shaft and the neck will change the orientation of the tibiofemoral joint, thereby altering the weight-bearing forces through the knee joint. For example, an increase in the normal angle of inclination at the hip (coxa valga) will redirect the femoral shaft more laterally than normal, resulting in a decrease in the normal physiologic valgus angle of the knee (genu varus). This results in a shifting of the mechanical axis to the medial compartment of the knee, increasing the compression forces medially.[66]

Genu valgus ("knock knees") can result from a change of angulation of the femur caused by femoral anteversion, tibial torsion, or excessive foot pronation. A valgus knee increases the Q-angle by displacing the tibial tuberosity laterally and can be associated with patellofemoral pain.[279]

To observe genu varum and genu valgum, the patient is positioned in standing so that the patellae face anteriorly and the medial aspect of the knees and the medial malleoli of both lower extremities are as close together as possible. A distance of 9–10 cm (3.5–4 inches) between the malleoli of the ankles with the knees touching is considered excessive and indicates genu valgum, whereas a distance of 4 cm (1.6 inches) measured between the knees when the ankles are together, indicates genu varum.[280–282]

Degree of Knee Flexion

A flexed knee in the relaxed standing position is often indicative of arthritic changes of the knee.

Degree of Genu Recurvatum or Hyperextension

Knee recurvatum may be an expression of a generalized ligamentous laxity or may be associated with patella alta.[205] Hyperextension of knee produces stress on the posterior capsule, slackening of the ACL, and alterations in the compressive forces acting on the anterior articulating surface of the tibia.[278] The anterior compressive forces can cause the inferior pole of the patella to be driven posteriorly into the fat pad, producing an irritation.

Q-Angle Assessment

A properly measured Q-angle can contribute significantly to the evaluation of patellofemoral malalignment. However, relying solely on the Q-angle measurement to determine patellofemoral alignment is an oversimplification. As with other clinical signs, an abnormal value does not necessarily identify the source of pain. The Q-angle itself is not pathologic and is increased in only a small percentage of patients with patellar pain.[283]

The Q-angle should be assessed dynamically and statically. It is important that this angle be measured in a consistent fashion. The preferred position for this test is the one-legged standing position without shoes. Hyperpronation of the feet can be masked unless the foot and ankle are placed in a subtalar neutral position[284] (see Chap. 21). A measurement is then taken using an imaginary line drawn from the ASIS to the center of the patella, and a second line from the tibial tuberosity to the center of the patella (Fig. 20-6). The weight-bearing position can be simulated in a supine patient by dorsiflexing the ankles, extending the knees, and pointing the toes to the ceiling. With the knee flexed to 90 degrees, the tibial tubercle should lie less than 20 mm lateral to the midline of the femur at the upper edge of the femoral condyles; a distance of more than 20 mm indicates an abnormally lateral tubercle.[11] Both tight hamstrings and a decrease in ankle dorsiflexion can result in an increase in the dynamic Q angle.[188]

Degree of Tibial Torsion[285]

External tibial torsion increases the Q-angle, whereas internal torsion decreases it.[147] The vast majority of the studies focusing on anterior knee pain have examined the coronal relationships at the knee (Q-angle, patellar tilt, patellar subluxation). Few studies have addressed the rotational relationships, specifically the rotational orientation of the tibia to the femur.[286] This rotational relationship of the tibia to the femur in the transverse plane is referred to as *knee version*. Knee version often is recognized as a factor in the context of the osteoarthritic knee.[287–289] The significance of this rotational characteristic of the knee with anterior pain is that the patella is tethered to the tibia by the infrapatellar tendon and retinaculum, and if the tibia is rotated externally with respect to the femur, the patella will be pulled laterally by virtue of this attachment.[286] If the patella is not free to translate laterally, because of its soft tissue attachments and its conformity with the patellar groove, increased pressure may be placed on the lateral facet. This pressure may produce a condition called a *lateral patellar compression syndrome*.[286,290]

Tibia-to-Floor Angle

If the tibia-to-floor angle is 10 degrees or greater, the extremity requires an excessive amount of subtalar joint pronation to produce a plantigrade foot.[205]

Patella Tendon-to-Patella Height Ratio

This measurement is best performed radiographically. The patella tendon length should be equal, or slightly longer than the height of the patella.[291] If a ratio of greater than 15–20% exists, patella alta should be suspected. If the ratio is less than 15–20%, patella baja should be suspected.

Foot Alignment

An often-neglected feature, which directly impacts the patellofemoral joint, is that of foot alignment. The normal weight-bearing foot exhibits a mild amount of pronation. If the foot pronates excessively, a compensatory internal rotation of the tibia may occur. This produces an increased amount of rotatory stress and dynamic abduction movement at the knee that has to be absorbed through the peripatellar soft tissues at the knee joint.[205,226,275,292] These stresses can force the patella to displace laterally.[293,294] In addition, a change in the position of the talus can affect the functional leg length. Subtalar supination may cause the leg to lengthen, whereas subtalar pronation shortens the leg.

Gait

Abnormal foot mechanics are manifested during ambulation, and abnormal gait patterns may suggest an underlying condition (see Chap. 6). The gait assessment relative to the knee allows the clinician to identify deviations of the foot, ankle, knee, or hip joint, such as excessive subtalar and midtarsal joint pronation, limited ankle dorsiflexion, tibial or femoral torsion abnormalities, and excessive varus or valgus at the knee, all of which could place the knee structures at risk for further microtrauma.[167]

During normal gait, the knee should be observed to flex to approximately 15 degrees at initial contact before extending to the neutral position at terminal stance.[278] An increase in 5 degrees of pronation at midstance, a period where the foot should be in supination, holds more potential for producing pain than if the 5 degrees occurs during the contact phase.[229]

Since the joint reaction forces are reported to increase with the magnitude of quadriceps contraction and the knee-flexion angle,[295] patients with patellofemoral pain often adopt compensatory gait strategies to reduce the muscular demands at the knee. Evidence in support of this premise was reported by Dillon et al.,[296] who found that subjects with patellofemoral pain limited the amount of stance phase knee flexion during level and ramp walking.

An injury to the ACL produces distinct changes in lower extremity biomechanics during gait.[297] Although healthy individuals demonstrate an extensor torque at the knee for 10–45% of the stance phase,[298–300] gait analysis of individuals with recent ACL deficiency shows functional adaptations in a high proportion of patients, with an extensor torque that lasts for nearly the entire stance phase.[298] Other analysis has also shown a decrease in the flexion moment of the knee in the range of 0–40 degrees of flexion in patients who have a chronic tear of the ACL.[301,302]

When the normal limb moves into the midstance phase, gravity and inertia generate a moment that tends to flex the knee. Since the quadriceps muscles balance this moment, a decrease in the flexion moment suggests a decrease in the quadriceps muscle moment.[303] Such a decrease has been noted in both limbs of patients who had only one knee with a torn ACL.[302]

Andriacchi[303] termed this finding the *quadriceps-avoidance gait,* although not all patients who have a torn ACL have such a gait, and its prevalence appears to be partly related to the time since the injury.[304] In activities that involve knee-flexion angles of less than 30 degrees (i.e., those involving normal gait), the quadriceps-avoidance gait is most effective in preventing anterior tibial translation.[303,305,306] In activities that involve knee-flexion angles of 40 degrees or more (e.g., jumping or sharp changes in running direction), increased contraction of the hamstrings is effective in preventing anterior tibial translation.[154,306–308]

Gait adaptations in individuals with ACL injury who have reconstruction surgery are less clear for two reasons[297]:

1. Very few comprehensive gait analyses have been conducted on this population.
2. The large variations in surgical and rehabilitation procedures and patient characteristics, and in patient compliance with rehabilitation, limit the generalization of these potential results.

Gait can also be affected by genu recurvatum, because during the loading response in gait, an individual with genu recurvatum transfers body weight directly from the femur to the tibia without the usual muscle energy absorption and cushioning of a flexed knee provided. This may lead to pain in the medial tibiofemoral joint (compression) and posterolateral ligamentous structures (tensile). In individuals with quadriceps weakness, compensation may occur by hyperextending the knee to provide greater knee stability.

Patient Sitting

Active Knee Extension

Although formally assessed as part of the active range of motion (AROM) with passive overpressure tests (see later), active knee extension may also be used during the observation phase of the examination. The patient should fully extend the knee from a flexed position. Normally, the patella follows a straight line, or a slight and smooth, gradual, lateral concave "C" curve as the knee extends. The presence of a "J sign," in which the patella slips off laterally as the knee approaches extension, or apprehension with motion involving lateral or medial stress, is necessary to confirm patellar instability.[11]

The patella may be compressed with the palm of the hand through the full ROM, as ulcerated lesions can be tender with this provocative test.[11] However, care should be taken with this maneuver, because it can provoke pain in otherwise asymptomatic patients.

Distal patellar lesions are often tender with this test in the early degrees of knee flexion, whereas proximal lesions are tender at approximately 90 degrees.[11] This information can help guide the clinician with the intervention. Crepitus at the knee is a nonspecific finding and can be associated with both cartilaginous and synovial lesions.[11] Although often a concern to patients because they believe it to be indicative of arthritis, crepitus is often a result of tight, deep, lateral retinacular structures and can be improved with retinacular stretching techniques.[266]

In addition to observing the patella during active knee extension, the clinician should also note any evidence of a quadriceps lag manifested by an inability to fully extend the knee. This lag can result from muscle atrophy, pain, effusion, reflex inhibition, or a loss of mechanical advantage. Quadriceps reflex inhibition has been well documented throughout the literature and is thought to result from pain or effusion, or both, although the exact etiology has yet to be determined.[262,309–314]

Some of the proposed causes for this reflex inhibition include

- the result of capsular stretching;[313]
- the result of increased intra-articular pressure.[310]

In the presence of various pain syndromes, such as CRPS,[309] additional muscle inhibition can occur. In most patients, limitations of motion resolve as the pain and effusion dissipate. However, this quadriceps inhibition may allow scar tissue to form while the knee is held in a flexed position. Atrophy of the quadriceps muscle and flexion contracture usually results, and activities of daily living become more difficult to perform. Joint immobilization can complicate all of these factors. Disuse may induce abnormal cross-links between collagen fibers at abnormal locations,[315,316] decreasing their extensibility[317] and promoting intra-articular and extra-articular scarring.

Patient Lying Supine

Malalignment can be observed on certain the supine, resting patients, whereas in other subjects a dynamic evaluation (walking, jumping, squatting, etc.) is required to detect an abnormal alignment. The lateral pull test can be performed to assess patellar tracking.[318] The patient lies supine with the knee extended and the clinician asks the patient to perform an isometric quadriceps contraction. The clinician observes patellar tracking during the contraction. The test is considered positive if the patella tracks more laterally than superiorly, and negative if superior displacement is equal to lateral displacement.[318] However, since the lateral pull test has been found to have only fair intrarater, and poor interrater reliability, care must be taken in placing too much emphasis on this test when making clinical decisions.

Hip Screening

With the patient supine and then prone, the hip is flexed and rotated as the clinician checks for a source of referred pain.[196]

Since patellar malalignment can be associated with adaptive shortening, the following structures (in decreasing order of frequency) are assessed[187,196]:

- ***Lateral retinaculum (see "Special Tests" section).*** A tight lateral retinaculum may pull the patella laterally.
- ***Hamstrings (see "Special Tests" section).*** When an individual with tight hamstrings runs, there is a decrease in

stride length and a potential for the quadriceps to fatigue in an effort to overcome the passive resistance of the hamstrings.[319] Tightness of the hamstrings also produces an increase in knee flexion at heel strike. Since the knee cannot straighten, an increased dorsiflexion is required to position the body over the planted foot.[266] If the range of full dorsiflexion has already occurred at the talocrural joint, further range is achieved by subtalar pronation. This has the effect of increasing the valgus vector force and the dynamic Q-angle.[266,320]

- ***Iliotibial band (see "Special Tests" section).*** The ITB is maximally taut at 20–30 degrees of flexion. Adaptive shortening of this band can cause a lateral tracking and tilting of the patella, and often a stretching of the medial retinaculum.[229]
- ***Tensor fascia latae and rectus femoris (see Chap. 19).*** Adaptive shortening of these structures can increase the amount of compression of the patella on the femur.[229]
- ***Hip rotators.*** The hip rotators can accentuate anteversion or retroversion (see Chap. 19).[229]
- ***Achilles–Soleus Length.*** A decrease in talocrural joint dorsiflexion ROM may result in a compensatory subtalar pronation during ambulation and weight-bearing.[321] Soft tissue tightness is particularly prevalent during the adolescent growth spurt, in which the long bones are growing faster than the surrounding soft tissues.[322]

Active Range of Motion

ROM testing for the tibiofemoral joint should include assessment of knee flexion and extension, tibial internal and external rotation. Normal knee motion (Table 20-7) has been described as 0 degrees of extension to 140 degrees of flexion, although hyperextension is frequently present to varying degrees.[323] In general, however, the best way to ascertain normal motion is to examine the contralateral knee, provided that it has no abnormal conditions.

The ROM testing can often be diagnostic and provides the clinician with some clues as to the cause of the problem. Examining the uninvolved knee first allays a patient's fears and helps to determine what the normal ROM is. In addition, observation of the uninvolved knee can afford the clinician information about the patellofemoral joint and the tracking of the patella.[324]

TABLE 20-7 Normal Ranges and End-Feels at the Knee

Motion	Range of Motion (degrees)	End-Feel
Flexion	0–140	Tissue approximation or tissue stretch
Extension	0–15	Tissue stretch
External rotation of tibia on femur	30–40	Tissue stretch
Internal rotation of tibia on femur	20–30	Tissue stretch

CLINICAL PEARL

Full active range of knee motion requires the following:

- Congruent articular surfaces
- Adequate muscle function
- An articular capsule with suitable capacity and flexibility
- Effective space in the medial and lateral articular recesses, intercondylar notch, and suprapatellar pouch
- Sufficient meniscal motion[325]

A number of studies have demonstrated that goniometric measurements of knee ROM performed in a clinical setting can be highly reliable.[326–330] Rothstein et al. showed that intratester and intratester reliability for flexion of the knee VIDEO was high ($r = 0.91$–0.99 and $r = 0.88$–0.97, respectively).[326] Watkins et al. showed that the intertester reliability for measurements of knee ROM obtained by visual estimation was 0.83 for flexion and 0.82 for extension.[330]

Flexion

The amount of knee flexion should be assessed to see if the motion is restricted by tight structures. If no restriction is suspected, tests are required for generalized ligament laxity and for abnormally loose patellar retinacula (see later discussion).

The primary flexors of the knee are the three hamstring muscles, assisted by the gracilis, sartorius, popliteus, and gastrocnemius muscles, and the TFL (in 45–145 degrees of flexion; see Table 20-2). The patient lies in the supine position. Using one hand, the clinician grasps the anterior aspect of the patient's lower leg, just proximal to the malleoli, while the other hand grasps the anterior aspect of the patient's thigh, just above the patella. The patient's hip is flexed to about 90 degrees and stabilized with one hand, while the clinician flexes the knee with the other hand (Fig. 20-9). At the end of the ROM, the clinician exerts slight overpressure. The normal end-feel is usually one of soft tissue approximation. A flexion limitation other than soft tissue approximation is usually the result of an articular lesion, such as arthritis or arthrosis (capsular pattern), a lesion of one of the menisci, or a loose body.[274]

Rotation of the tibia relative to the femur is possible when the knee is flexed and non–weight-bearing, with

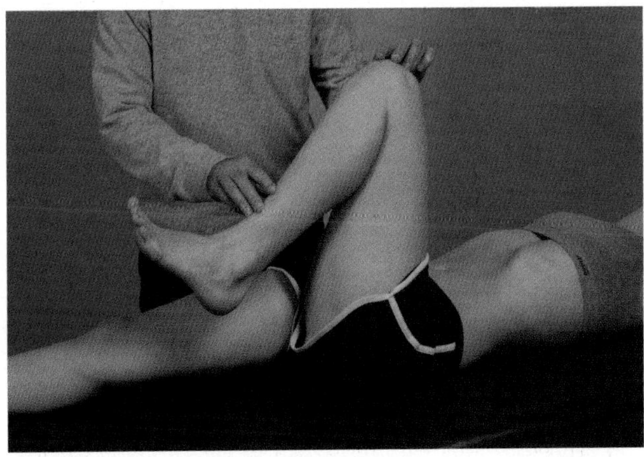

FIGURE 20-9 Knee flexion.

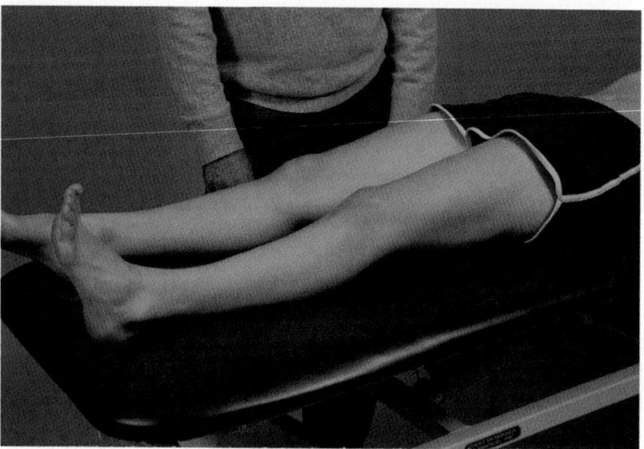

FIGURE 20-10 Knee extension

rotational capability greatest at approximately 90 degrees of flexion.[97]

Extension

The primary extensors of the knee are the quadriceps muscles, consisting of the rectus femoris, VL, vastus medialis, and vastus intermedius (see Table 20-2). Also assisting with knee extension in the 0–30-degree flexion range is the ITB and TFL.

The patient extends the knee (see Fig. 20-10), and the clinician applies overpressure by stabilizing the thigh and pulling the ankle up to the ceiling, while allowing the conjunct external rotation of the tibia. Under normal conditions, the end-feel is usually hard.

A limitation of active knee motion can have a number of causes. The patient may have a neurologic deficit from a lumbar intervertebral disk (IVD) herniation, with loss of knee motion as the primary symptom. Any acute injury causing pain may limit active knee motion as a result of muscle inhibition.[310]

Passive Range of Motion

Passive movements, as elsewhere, can determine the amount of available motion, the presence or absence of a capsular pattern, and the end-feel. At the tibiofemoral joint, the end-feel of flexion should be tissue approximation, whereas the end-feel of extension and medial and lateral rotation of the tibia on the femur is tissue stretch. Passive hyperextension of the knee with overpressure is performed to assess (from the end-feel) whether the knee extension is limited as a result of an articular disorder. Such articular disorders include arthritis or arthrosis, a lesion of one of the menisci, or a loose-body involvement. Hayes et al.[331] found the intrarater reliability of end-feel and pain/resistance judgments at the knee to be generally good, especially after accounting for subject change and unbalanced distributions. Interrater reliability, however, was generally not acceptable, even after accounting for these factors.[331] In a separate study, Hayes et al.[332] explored the construct validity and test–retest reliability of the passive motion component of the Cyriax soft tissue diagnosis system and compared the hypothesized and actual patterns of restriction, end-feel, and pain/resistance sequence (P/RS) of 79 subjects with OA of the knee and examined associations among these indicators of dysfunction and related constructs of joint motion, pain intensity, and chronicity. The results of the study are discussed next.

Consistent with the hypotheses based on Cyriax's assertions about patients with OA, most subjects had capsular end-feels for extension; subjects with tissue approximation end-feels for flexion had more flexion ROM than did subjects with capsular end-feels, and the P/RS was significantly correlated with pain intensity ($\rho = 0.35$, extension; $\rho = 0.30$, flexion).[332]

Contrary to the hypotheses based on Cyriax's assertions, most subjects had noncapsular patterns, tissue approximation end-feels for flexion, and what Cyriax called pain synchronous with resistance for both motions.[332]

Pain intensity did not differ depending on end-feel. The P/RS was not correlated with chronicity ($\rho = 0.03$, extension; $\rho = 0.01$, flexion).[332]

Reliability, as analyzed by ICCs (ICC[3,1]) and Cohen's κ coefficients, was acceptable (≥ 0.80) or nearly acceptable for ROM (ICC = 0.71–0.86, extension; ICC = 0.95–0.99, flexion) but not for end-feel ($\kappa = 0.17$, extension; $\kappa = 0.48$, flexion) and P/RS ($\kappa = 0.36$, extension; $\kappa = 0.34$, flexion).[332]

The study concluded that the use of a quantitative definition of the capsular pattern, end-feels, and P/RS as indicators of knee OA should be reexamined and the validity of the P/RS as representing chronicity and the reliability of end-feel and the P/RS are questionable.[332]

Others have found that a ratio of loss of extension to loss of flexion during passive range of motion (PROM) of between 0.03 and 0.50 was more likely than a noncapsular pattern in patients with an inflamed knee or osteoarthrosis (likelihood ratio = 3.2).[333]

According to the osteopathic theories of somatic dysfunction,[334] the following guidelines are used:

- If the restriction to movement is opposite to the direction that the bone seems to have traveled (e.g., the tibia has a reduced joint glide), a mobilization or a manipulation is the intervention of choice.
- If the restriction to movement is in the same direction that the bone seems to have moved and the opposite movement seems to be excessive (a change has occurred in the overall starting position), a muscle imbalance should be suspected, and a muscle energy technique used.
- If the patient demonstrates normal range but pain with movement, the joint cannot be at fault.
- If a muscle is very hypertonic, a spinal dysfunction may be present (unless trauma is involved), producing a hypermobility.

Even minor losses of knee motion may have adverse effects. It is common to lose both flexion and extension; however, loss of extension is usually more debilitating.[335] A loss of extension of more than 5 degrees may cause patellofemoral pain and a limp during walking,[336] whereas restricted flexion does not severely affect gait as long as the knee can be flexed to at least 60 degrees. [337] Diminished running speed is associated with loss of flexion of 10 degrees or more,[338] whereas an extension deficit of more than 10 degrees is poorly tolerated by active people.[339] A loss of more than 20 degrees of extension may cause a significant functional limb-length discrepancy.[338]

Patellar Motion Tests

Probably the most important part of the patellofemoral examination is the observation of the dynamics of patellar tracking in weight-bearing and non–weight-bearing.

A unilateral squat (Waldron test) can be used to assess patellofemoral function.[340] The patient stands on the involved leg, and the clinician sits or squats next to the patient. Using the entire surface of the palm, the clinician exerts slight pressure in an anteroposterior direction against the patient' s patella (Fig. 20-11). From this position, the patient is asked to bend the knee slowly, if possible, to about 90 degrees, while the clinician palpates for crepitus and locking of the patella and assesses the course of movement of the patella. Crepitus or locking can indicate the presence of patellofemoral chondropathy or patellofemoral arthrosis. However, Nijs et al.[341] reported unimpressive positive and negative likelihood ratios for this test.

In patellar malalignment or pathologies of the corresponding femoral joint surface, movement of the patella can be disturbed. The patella is observed while the patient initiates flexion of the knee to see if it engages smoothly at the proximal end of the trochlea or more distally than normal. Lateralization of the patella can occur during flexion, particularly when the Q-angle is excessive.

The passive mobility tests for the patella are outlined in "Patellar Stability Tests" section.

Kinetic Chain Assessment

Ankle Motions

Ankle motions are tested because, as has been discussed, a number of structures share a common relationship with the foot, ankle, and knee joint complex (see Chap. 21) and can therefore have an impact on knee function. For example, adaptive shortening of the gastrocnemius, particularly in the presence of adaptively shortened hamstring muscles, may produce increased knee flexion at initial contact and during the stance phase of gait.[215]

Hip Motions

Several muscles cross both the hip and the knee. These include the rectus femoris, gracilis, sartorius, and hamstrings muscles. Adaptive shortening of any of these structures may cause alterations in postural mechanics and gait. The hip rotators can also influence other aspects of the lower kinetic chain. Sahrmann advocates the testing of length–strength relationship of the hip external rotators because of their CKC function of decelerating lower extremity internal rotation.[167,342]

Passive Accessory Motion Testing

The passive accessory motion tests, or joint glides, are performed at the end of the patient's available range to determine if the joint itself is responsible for the loss of motion.

Tibiofemoral Distraction

The patient lies in the prone position. The clinician is beside the patient. Using one hand to stabilize the thigh, the clinician uses the other hand to grip the distal tibia from the medial and lateral sides. The clinician then applies a force perpendicular to the tibial joint surface (Fig. 20-12).

Posterior Glide of the Tibia on the Femur

The patient lies in the supine position with the thigh supported by a towel. Standing to the side of the patient,

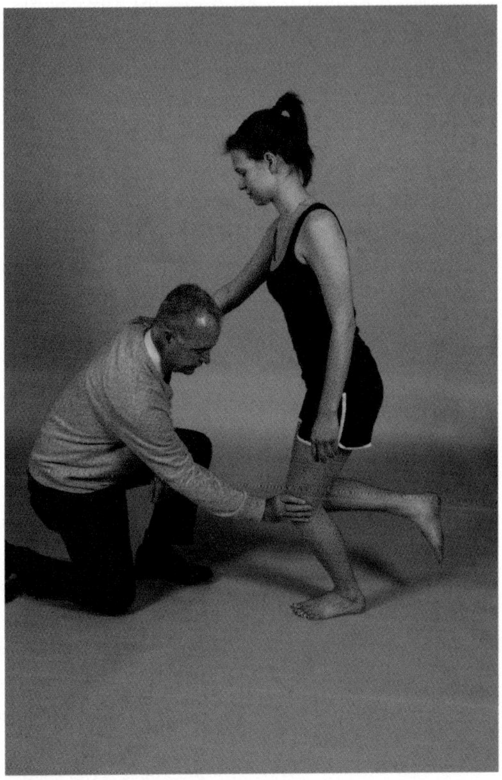

FIGURE 20-11 Waldron test.

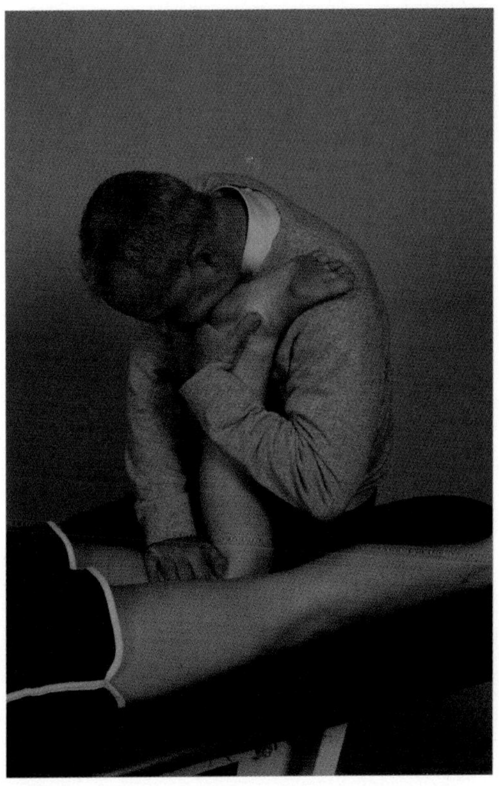

FIGURE 20-12 Tibiofemoral distraction.

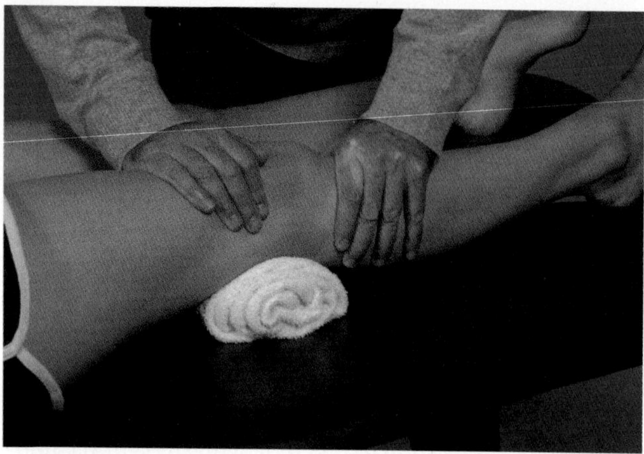

FIGURE 20-13 Posterior glide of the tibia on the femur.

the clinician applies a posterior glide through the tibia (Fig. 20-13).

Anterior Glide of the Tibia on the Femur

The patient lies in the supine position with the knee flexed and the foot placed on the table. The clinician stands to the side of the patient. Using both hands, the clinician applies an anterior glide of the tibia (Fig. 20-14).

Proximal Tibiofibular Joint

The proximal tibiofibular joint can be assessed with the patient in the supine position and the knee flexed to approximately 90 degrees. The clinician stabilizes the tibia using one hand and uses the other hand to grasp the fibular head and to assess the anterolateral and posteromedial glides (Fig. 20-15).

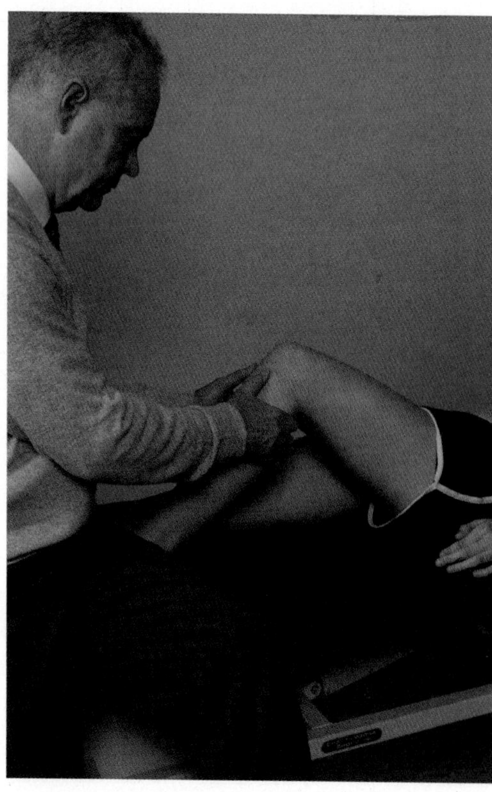

FIGURE 20-14 Anterior glide of the tibia on the femur.

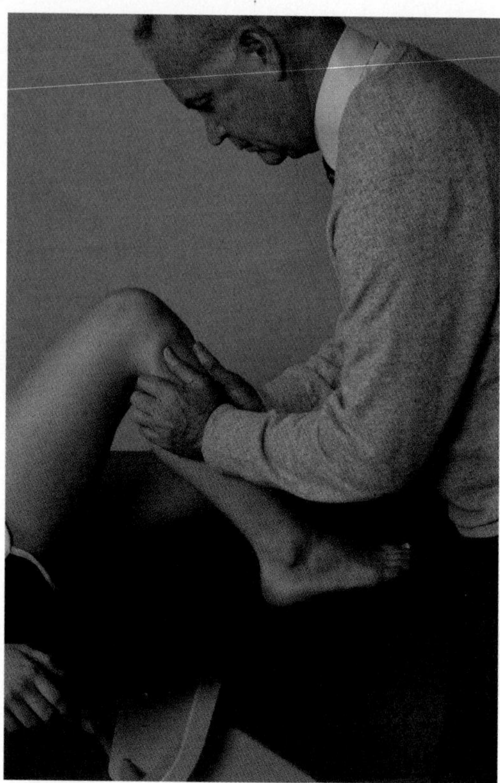

FIGURE 20-15 Mobility testing of the proximal tibiofibular joint.

Passive Tibial External Rotation

The patient lies in the supine position. Using one hand, the clinician grasps the patient's foot and brings the ankle into maximal plantar flexion. The other hand is positioned to monitor the joint space.[274] The patient's knee is flexed to 90 degrees and the hip to approximately 45 degrees. The distal hand performs an external rotation of the tibia while maintaining the ankle in maximum plantar flexion (see Fig. 20-16). At the end of the ROM, the clinician exerts slight overpressure. Under normal conditions, the end-feel is firm. The clinician notes whether the pain is provoked or whether there is a hypermobility or hypomobility[274]:

- Pain with passive external rotation of the tibia can be the result of a lesion of the medial meniscotibial ligament, medial meniscus, MCL, or the posteromedial capsuloligamentous complex.
- Hypermobility with this maneuver can be the result of a lesion of the posteromedial capsuloligamentous complex, often in combination with lesions of the MCL and the ACL. Hypermobility may also be seen in ballet dancers.
- Hypomobility of passive tibial external rotation is seen only in severe articular disorders with significant capsular limitations of motion.

Passive Tibial Internal Rotation

The patient lies in the supine position. Using one hand, the clinician grasps the patient's foot and brings the ankle into maximal plantar flexion. The other hand is positioned to monitor the joint space. The patient's knee is flexed to 90 degrees and the hip to about 45 degrees. The distal hand performs an internal rotation of the tibia while maintaining

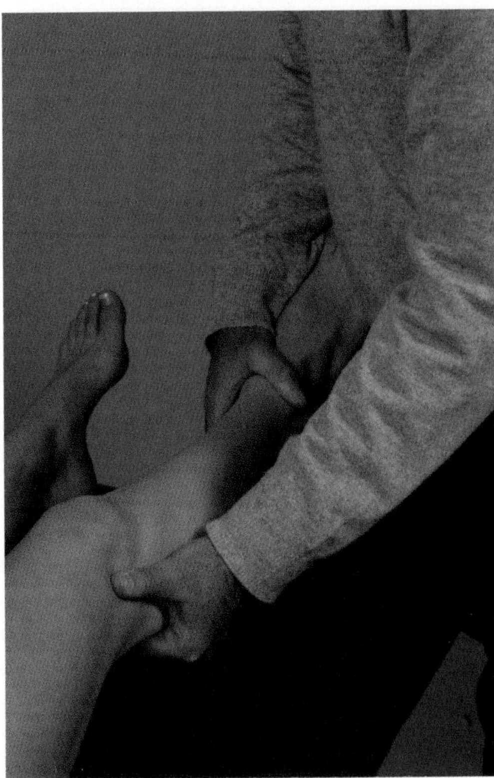

FIGURE 20-16 Passive external rotation of tibia.

the ankle in maximum plantar flexion (see Fig. 20-17). At the end of the ROM, the clinician exerts slight overpressure. Under normal conditions, the end-feel is firm. The clinician notes whether pain is provoked or whether there is hypermobility or hypomobility[274]:

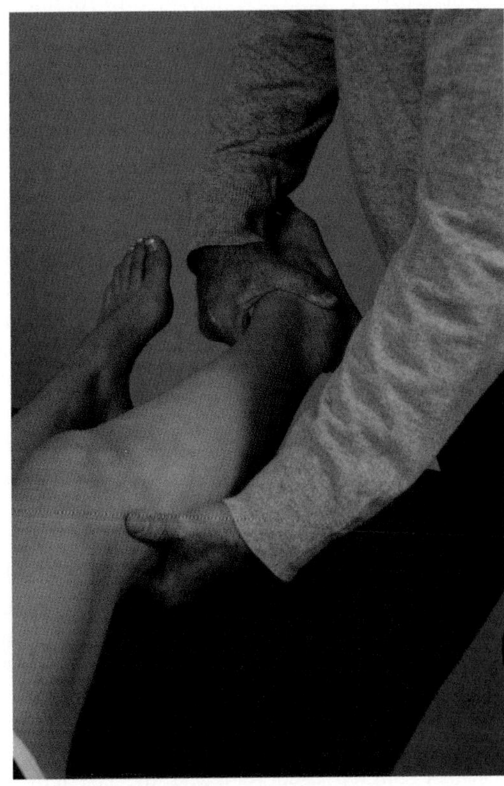

FIGURE 20-17 Passive tibial internal rotation.

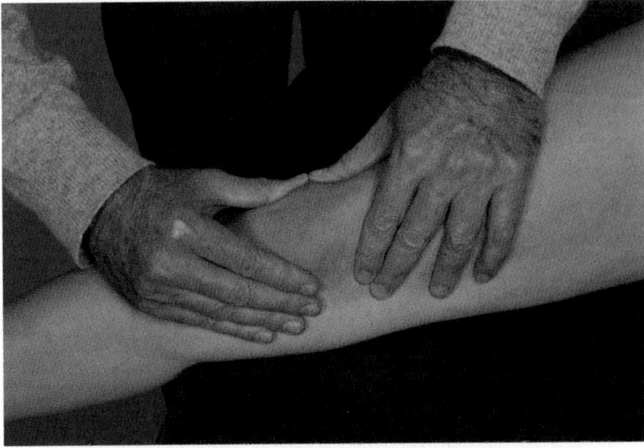

FIGURE 20-18 Patellar mobility testing.

- Pain can be the result of a lesion of the lateral meniscotibial ligament, lateral meniscus or posterolateral capsuloligamentous complex.
- Hypermobility can be the result of a lesion of the posterolateral capsuloligamentous complex.
- Hypomobility is seen only in severe articular disorders with significant capsular limitations of motion.

Patellofemoral Joint Mobility Tests

The patient lies in the supine position with the involved knee supported in slight flexion. The clinician moves the patella superiorly, inferiorly, medially, and laterally (Fig. 20-18). Caution must be used with the lateral glide in case the joint is hypermobile, as this is the most common direction for patella dislocations. To assess the various tilts of the patella, both hands are wrapped around the patella and the thumbs are used to tilt the patella medially and laterally (Fig. 20-19). The findings are compared with the contralateral side.

Strength Testing

Gross muscle testing is useful in checking for deficits in the lower extremities. Strength testing involves the performance of resisted isometric tests. The joint is placed in its resting position to minimize any joint compression forces.

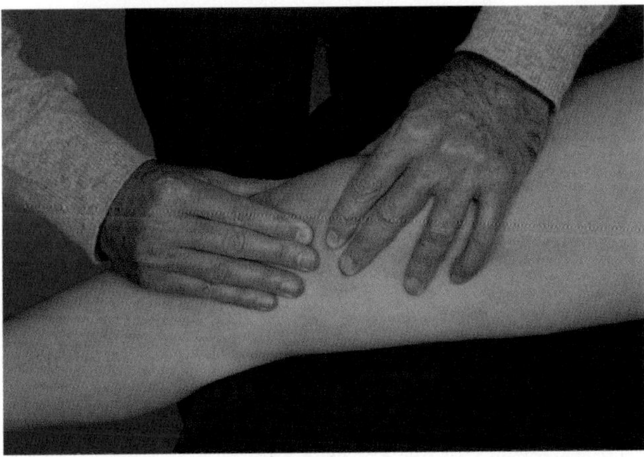

FIGURE 20-19 Patellar tilting test.

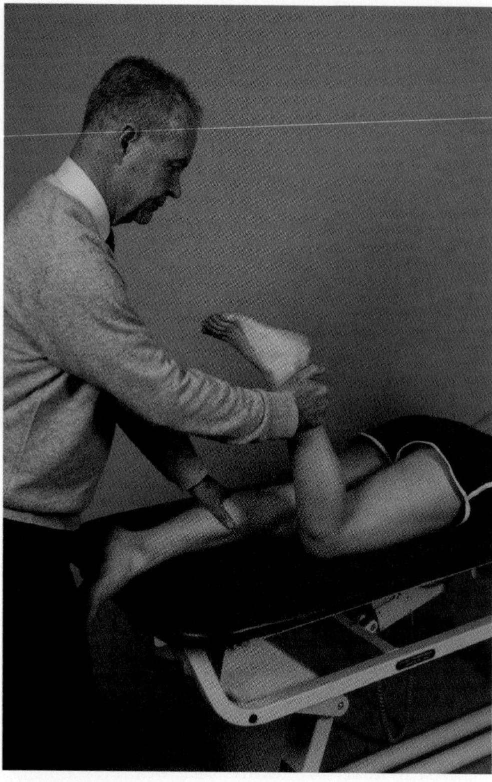

FIGURE 20-20 Strength testing the medial hamstrings.

Knee Flexion

The strength of the knee flexors (the hamstrings) can be assessed by positioning the patient prone with the knee flexed to approximately 80–90 degrees. By internally rotating the tibia (Fig. 20-20) and resisting knee flexion, the clinician can theoretically assess the integrity of the medial hamstrings (semimembranosus and semitendinosus). The biceps femoris is assessed similarly by externally rotating the tibia and resisting knee flexion (Fig. 20-21) VIDEO.

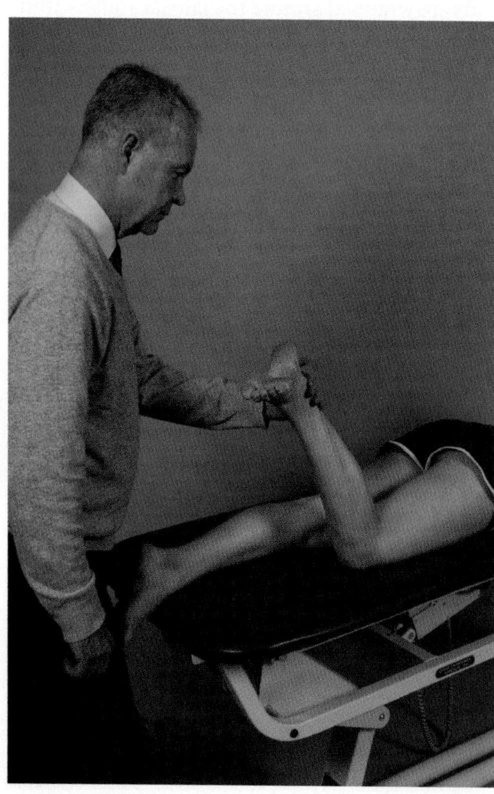

FIGURE 20-21 Strength testing the biceps femoris.

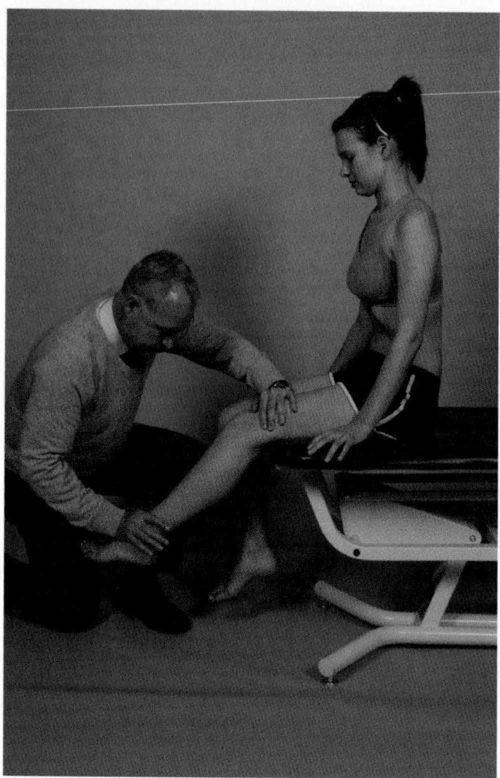

FIGURE 20-22 Strength testing of knee extensors at 60 degrees.

Knee Extension

Pain may be reproduced, and localized, with multiple angle isometric testing of the quadriceps, as described by McConnell.[189] Thus, the strength of the knee extensors (the quadriceps) is tested in 0, 30, 60 (Fig. 20-22), 90, and 120 degrees of knee flexion and held for 1 second with the femur externally rotated, to see if the pain can be reproduced or localized. The reproduction of pain with these tests suggests excessive pain from patellar compression. Any abnormal tibial movement with these tests may suggest ligamentous instability.[343] If pain is noted during this testing, McConnell suggests returning the knee to full extension, producing and maintaining a medial glide of the patella, and then returning the knee to the painful position to retest. This action should reduce the pain if it is of a patellofemoral origin.[189]

The final 15 degrees of knee extension require a 60% increase in muscle firing.[137] An extension lag (passive knee extension that is greater than active knee extension) indicates a slight loss of quadriceps muscle function.[167,266,344]

Siegel and Jacob[343] suggest testing the quadriceps muscle at 0, 30, 60, and 90 degrees while observing for any abnormal tibial movement. Any abnormal tibial movement would suggest ligament instability or excessive pain from patellar compression.

Plantar Flexion

The heel raise can be used to assess the strength of the gastrocnemius. The strength of the gastrocnemius muscle

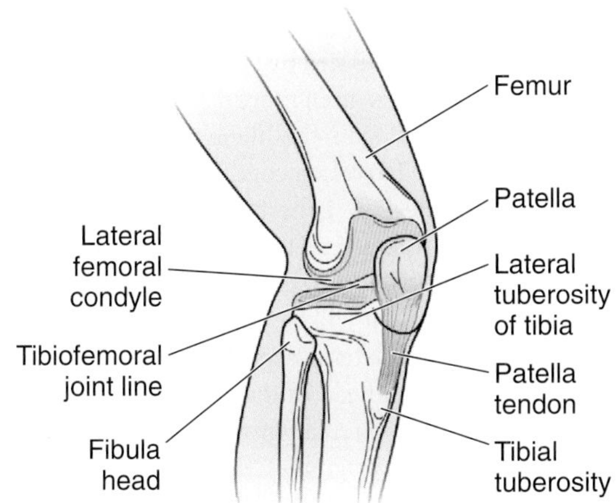

FIGURE 20-23 Palpable structures on the anterolateral surface of the knee.

is tested because of its intimate relationship to the knee and its importance in lower extremity function. The patient is positioned in standing, leaning against a wall, or supported by the clinician with the knees extended. One foot is tested at a time as the patient rises up on the toes for 10–20 repetitions (depending on age and physical ability) while standing.

- The patient everts the foot and raises up on the toes to test the lateral head.
- The patient inverts the foot and raises up on the toes to test the medial head.

The soleus muscle can be tested similarly by having the patient perform a unilateral heel raise while keeping the knee flexed.

Palpation

Palpation of the soft tissues about the knee is critical and often reveals more important information than any imaging tool. For palpation to be reliable, the clinician must have a sound knowledge of surface anatomy (Figs. 20-23 and 20-24), and the results from the palpation examination should be correlated with other findings. A logical sequence should be employed by the clinician. The skin, retinacula, quadriceps tendon, and patellar tendon are palpated to rule out any soft tissue sources of pain. Differences in temperature between the knees suggest inflammation in the warmer of the two. The following structures should be identified and palpated.

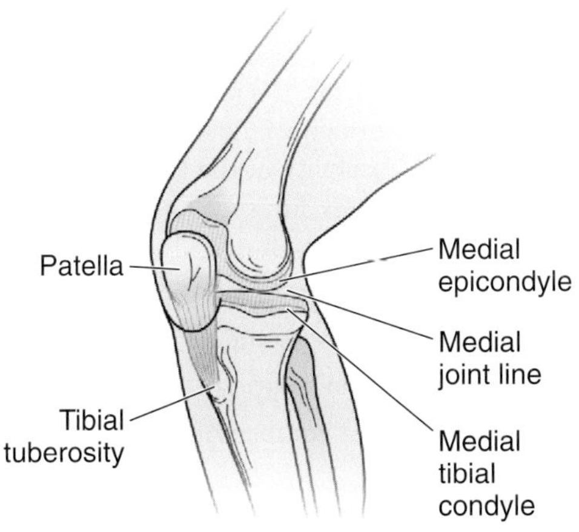

FIGURE 20-24 Palpable structures on the anteromedial surface of the knee.

Posterior Aspect

The patient lies in the prone position. The clinician locates the popliteal fossa. The semimembranosus and semitendinosus form the proximal medial border of the fossa. Deep inside this fossa, a Baker's cyst can be palpated if it is present. With the knee in a slightly flexed position, the thin round tendon of the semitendinosus should be easy to palpate. Medial and lateral to this tendon are the deeper parts of the semimembranosus. The popliteal pulse can be located just below the crease of the knee, more to the lateral side than to the medial side, and posterior to the tibial plateau. Medial to the pulse is the tendon of semimembranosus. At this point, if the thumb is pushed deeper, the attachment of the PCL can be located as it arises from the back of the tibia. Even under normal circumstances, this attachment will be tender. A little lateral to this is the attachment of the meniscofemoral ligament. The PCL and meniscofemoral ligament curve inward, to attach on the inner aspect of the medial condyle of the femur.

At the proximal lateral part the fossa, the biceps femoris tendon is found. This tendon is palpable together with the common fibular (peroneal) nerve. The tendon of the gracilis is medial and anterior to the medial part of the semimembranosus. Palpation performed medially and anteriorly to this point leads to the sartorius muscle. The tendons of the sartorius, gracilis, and semitendinosus form the pes anserinus. The sartorius and gracilis muscles can be differentiated as follows: the gracilis contracts during hip adduction, while the sartorius contracts during hip abduction. Palpation more anteriorly leads to the medial femoral condyle and the adductor tubercle. Tenderness at the anterior aspect of the medial femoral condyle, associated with a snapping sensation as the knee is flexed, can indicate a symptomatic plica.[345] The adductor tubercle serves as the attachment site for the patellar retinaculum and the medial patellofemoral ligament, and is a hallmark site of tenderness with lateral patellar dislocation.[274] The adductor tubercle is also the attachment site of the adductor magnus, and the origin of the MCL. The distal borders of the popliteal fossa are palpated by positioning the patient's knee in slight flexion. The medial head of the gastrocnemius can be palpated deep within and medial to the fossa, while the lateral head can be found deep within and medial to the tendon of the biceps femoris muscle.

Anterior Aspect

The patient lies supine with the hip and thigh positioned in extension. The clinician palpates the medial and lateral edges of the patella. The VMO normally inserts into the upper third or half of the medial patella and is readily palpable. In patients with patella malalignment, the VMO may be dysplastic and virtually invisible inserting proximal to the superior pole of the patella.[346] Palpation of the rectus femoris insertion on the superior aspect of the patella is only possible with the patella tipped slightly forward.[274] Complaints of pain distal to the patella during extension of the knee may indicate a patella tendon–ligament lesion at the inferior pole. In some individuals, the continuation of the tendon of the VL muscle, the lateral patellar retinaculum, can be palpated at the lateral side of the patella.[274]

Palpation of the joint space is made easier when the tibia is rotated internally and externally while in the flexed position. The anterior part of the medial meniscus is palpable in the medial joint space with the tibia externally rotated, between the patellar tendon–ligament and the anterior edge of the MCL. Under normal circumstances, the medial meniscus is not palpable beyond 30 degrees of flexion.[274] The medial meniscotibial or coronary ligament, which attaches the medial meniscus to the tibia, is palpable anteriorly with the knee positioned at 90 degrees of flexion and the tibia maximally externally rotated, proximal to the tibia (passive external rotation of the knee will provoke the patient's pain, if the ligament is damaged).[274]

CLINICAL PEARL

Joint line tenderness usually is associated with a tibiofemoral injury, such as a meniscal or collateral ligament tear, but it can also be associated with patellar pathology, although the reasons are probably multifactorial.[205,269,272] Numerous studies have shown that joint line tenderness, when used in isolation, is of little value in specifically diagnosing a meniscus tear.

Other structures to palpate for tenderness on the anterior aspect of the knee include the following:

- ***Base (inferior pole) of patella.*** Tenderness at the inferior tip of the patella indicates patellar tendinitis.
- ***Infrapatellar fat pad (Hoffa's fat pad).*** This structure is located between the patella ligament (anteriorly) and the anterior joint capsule (posteriorly).
- ***Lateral retinaculum.***
- ***Apex of patella.***
- ***Accessory retinaculum from the ITB.***
- ***Medial retinaculum.***
- ***Medial and lateral patellar facets.*** These facets, which are readily palpated using the thumb and index finger, can be tested for tenderness and alignment, as can the overhang of the lateral facet over the patellar groove, by pushing the patella to one side and then the other (glide test), and then curling the fingers around and under the borders of the patella. Palpation of the facets should not elicit pain. The clinician should be able to palpate under one-third of the patella. A tilt of the patella (lateral side down) reflects a tight retinaculum, especially if the tilt cannot be passively corrected by the clinician.[346] When the patella is laterally displaced by the clinician and the patient reports sudden and considerable discomfort as the knee approaches extension, this is termed the apprehension sign (see "Special Tests" section).[346] The combination of tilt and lateral facet tenderness in the absence of any other positive findings on physical examination suggests clinically significant patella malalignment.[346]
- ***Dynamic restraints.*** The patient is asked to contract the quadriceps. In patients with malalignment, the VMO typically cannot be identified by sight or palpation; it inserts no farther distally than the proximal pole of the patella and it remains soft, even with maximal quadriceps contraction.[196] In the normal knee, the VMO should be felt to contract simultaneously with the VL.

Lateral Aspect

The fibular head can be palpated by following the tendon of the biceps femoris distally. It is often more distal and posterior than imagined. On the lateral side, the highest point on the lateral femoral condyle is the lateral epicondyle, which serves as the origin of the LCL. The LCL is best palpated when the hip is maximally externally rotated and the knee is flexed to 90 degrees in the "figure-four" cross-legged stance.[274] If the LCL is followed down to the fibular head, it will be felt to blend with the biceps femoris. On the posterolateral aspect of the condyle is the attachment for the lateral head of the gastrocnemius. Anterior to this, there is a small circular groove, which is where the tendon of the popliteus originates from the lateral condyle. Tenderness in this location, just behind the LCL, either anterior or posterior to it, would suggest damage to the popliteus muscle.[274] On the anterolateral aspect of the knee is Gerdy's tubercle, the largest bony prominence medial to the apex of the fibular head, which serves as the attachment site for the ITB.

The lateral joint space is palpated starting at a point just lateral to the patellar tendon–ligament. The anterior part of the lateral meniscus is best palpated with the knee in an extended position.

Medial Aspect

The highest point of the medial aspect of the femur is the medial epicondyle, which serves as the origin for the MCL. Superior to this point is the adductor tubercle, and superior to that is the supracondylar ridge, which is the attachment for the VMO. Very localized tenderness at the medial aspect of the knee, away from the joint line, may indicate a neuroma.[344]

Special Tests

Numerous special tests exist for the knee joint complex based on the intent and diagnostic purpose.

Stress Tests

The stress tests are used to determine the integrity of the joint, ligaments, and the menisci. A complete history and physical examination can diagnose approximately 90% of ligamentous injuries. The goal of the stress tests is to identify the degree of separation and the quality or end-feel of the separation when a stress is applied in a specific direction. Intact ligaments have an abrupt and firm end-feel, whereas sprained ligaments have a soft or indistinct end-feel depending on the degree of injury. A comparison should always be made with the uninvolved knee before a determination is made. It is important to remember that both pain and swelling can hamper the sensitivity of these tests.[347]

Serious functional instability of the knee appears to occur unpredictably. The reasons for such discrepancies are unknown, but they may be a result of[36]

- varying definitions of instability;
- varying degrees of damage to the ACL;[348,349]
- different combinations of injuries;[71]
- different mechanisms of compensation for the loss of the ACL;
- differences in rehabilitation;
- the diverse physical demands and expectations of different populations.

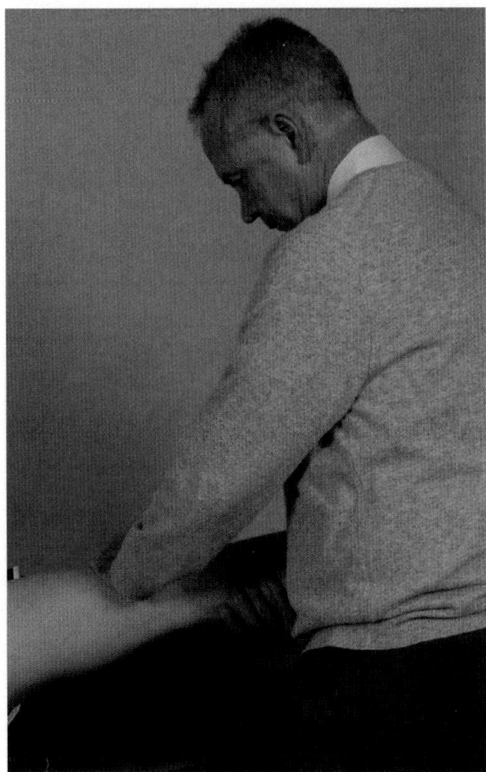

FIGURE 20-25 Valgus test.

Valgus Stress

The patient lies in the supine position, with the involved knee extended. The clinician applies a strong valgus force, with a counterforce applied at the lateral femoral condyle (Fig. 20-25). Normally, there is little or no valgus movement in the knee, and, if present, it should be less than the amount of varus motion. Under normal conditions, the end-feel is firm. With degeneration of the medial or lateral compartments, varus and valgus motions may be increased, while the end-feels will be normal.

With the knee tested in full extension, any demonstrable instability is usually very significant. Pain with this maneuver is caused by an increase in tension of the medial collateral structures or the connection of these structures with the medial meniscus. If pain or an excessive amount of motion is detected compared with the other extremity, a hypermobility or instability should be suspected. The following structures may be implicated:

- Superficial and deep fibers of the MCL
- Posterior oblique ligament
- Posteromedial capsule
- Medial capsular ligament
- ACL
- PCL

CLINICAL PEARL

A study by Garvin et al.[350] looked at 23 patients with a surgically proven tear of the MCL, where findings from magnetic resonance imaging (MRI) of the knee were evaluated retrospectively. MRI revealed the tear in all cases, although when the injury was severe, distinguishing high-grade partial tears from complete tears was difficult.[350] Physical examination had indicated a tear in 22 (96%) of the cases.[350] A high prevalence of associated cruciate and meniscal injuries was seen (in 23 [100%] and 12 [52%] of the cases, respectively). Tears of the LCL occurred in 13 (57%) of the patients and at least one bony infarction in 22 (96%); most of the infarctions were in the lateral compartment. Infarctions of the lateral femoral condyle were frequently geographic (in 14 [70%] of the 20 cases) or impacted (in 5 [25%]).[350]

To further assess the MCL, posterior oblique ligament, and PCL, the test is then repeated at 20–30 degrees of flexion. Hughston[55] concluded that a valgus stress test positive at 30 degrees and negative at 0 degree indicates a tear limited to the medial compartment ligaments (posterior oblique ligament) and posterior medial capsule, whereas a valgus stress test positive at 0 degree indicates a tear of both the PCL and the medial compartment ligaments.

The posterior fibers of the MCL can be isolated, by placing the knee in 90 degrees of flexion with full external rotation of the tibia.[274] The femur is prevented from rotating by the clinician's shoulder. The clinician places one hand on the posterior aspect of the foot and the other on the heel, and an external rotation force is applied using the foot as a lever.

These tests can be graded by the following:[63]

- Grade I: The joint space opening is within 2 mm of the contralateral side.
- Grade II: The joint space opens 3–5 mm more than the contralateral side in 20 degrees of knee flexion and less than 2 mm more than the normal knee in full extension.
- Grade III: The joint space opens 5–10 mm more than that of the normal knee in 20 degrees of flexion and full extension.

More research is needed to evaluate the diagnostic accuracy and reliability of this test.

Varus Stress

The patient lies in the supine position, with the involved knee in full extension. The clinician applies a strong varus force, thereby gapping the lateral aspect of the knee (see Fig. 20-26). To be able to assess the amount of varus movement, the clinician should repeat the maneuver several times, applying slight overpressure at the end of the ROM. Under normal conditions, the end-feel is firm, after slight movement. Unlike the valgus stress test, the varus test has been shown to be highly unreliable with many false-negative findings.[351]

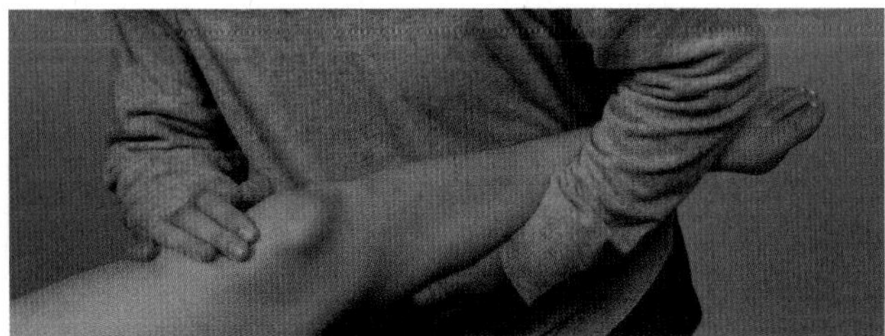

FIGURE 20-26 Varus test.

Theoretically, if this test is positive for pain or excessive motion compared with the other extremity, the following structures may be implicated:

- LCL
- Lateral capsular ligament
- Arcuate-popliteus complex
- ACL
- PCL

If the instability is gross, one or both cruciate ligaments as well as, occasionally, the biceps femoris tendon and the ITB may be involved, leading to a rotary instability if not in the short term, certainly over a period of time.[159]

The test is then repeated at 10–30 degrees of flexion with the tibia in full external rotation to further assess the LCL, posterolateral capsule, and arcuate–popliteus complex.

Grading of these injuries is the same as for MCL injuries and is based on the degree of opening of the lateral joint line.[63]

More research is needed to evaluate the diagnostic accuracy and reliability of this test.

One-Plane Anterior Instability

Ensuring the integrity of the ACL is crucial for maintaining the normal biomechanical properties of the knee joint, protecting its periarticular structures, and preventing premature OA. Knee joints with ACL deficiencies have rotary instabilities that expose supporting ligaments and menisci adjacent to the ACL to further damage and degenerative joint disease.[28] Signs and symptoms of chronic rotary knee instabilities from ACL deficiencies include swelling, pain, a "giving way" of patients' knee joints, arthritis, and possible subsequent meniscal injuries.

Several tests have been advocated for testing the integrity of the ACL. Three of the more commonly used ones are the Lachman test, the anterior drawer test, and the pivot shift (see "Anterolateral Rotary Instability" section).

Lachman Test. Torg et al.[352] were the first to publish a description of the Lachman test, whereby the knee is held in 30 degrees of flexion while the tibia is anteriorly translated with respect to the femur (Fig. 20-27).

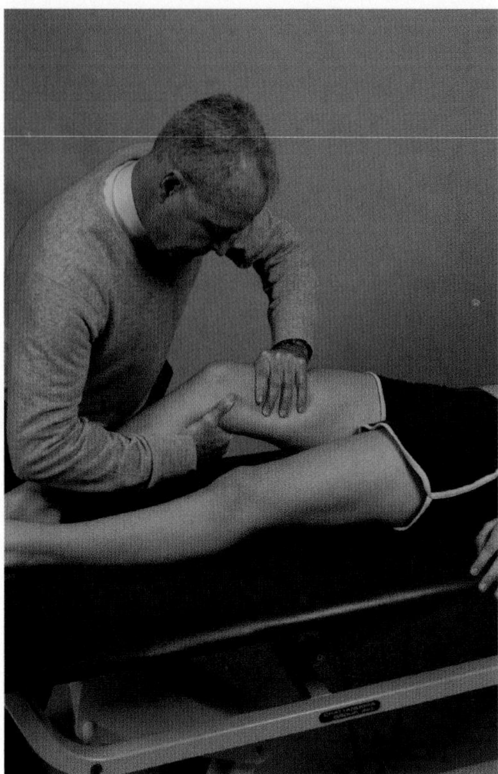

FIGURE 20-27 Lachman test.

The accuracy and reliability of the Lachman appears to vary. Katz et al. found that in the hands of an experienced clinician, accuracy of this test was 81.8% sensitive and 96.8% specific,[353] increasing to 100% if the patient was anesthetized.[354,355] In contrast, Cooperman et al.[356] reported that the predictive value of a positive test was 47% for all examiners, whereas the predictive value of a negative test was 70%, results that would indicate that Lachman test judgments have limited reliability and may be more useful for predicting that a patient does not have an ACL injury than for predicting that the ACL is injured.[357]

These discrepancies likely occur as there are a number of factors that can influence the results. These include

- an inability of the patient to relax;
- the degree of knee flexion;
- the size of the clinician's hand;
- the stabilization (and thus relaxation) of the patient's thigh.

According to Weiss et al.,[358] these factors can be minimized by the use of the modified Lachman test. In this modification, the patient lies in the supine position, with the feet resting firmly on the end of the table and the knees flexed 10–15 degrees. The clinician stabilizes the distal end of patient's femur using the thigh rather than the hand, as in the Lachman test, and then attempts to displace patient's tibia anteriorly. If the tibia moves forward, and the concavity of the patellar tendon–ligament becomes convex, the test is considered positive.

The grading of knee instability is as follows[55,359,360]:

1 + (mild): 5 mm or less

2 + (moderate): 5–10 mm

3 + (serious): more than 10 mm

With this test, false-negatives can occur. False-negatives may be caused by a significant hemarthrosis, protective hamstring spasm, or tear of the posterior horn of the medial meniscus.[352]

Active Lachman Test. The patient lies in the supine position with a bolster under the distal femur so that the knee is flexed to 30–40 degrees. The patient is asked to actively extend the involved knee and then to relax back to the starting position. A positive test for a torn ACL is indicated by an anterior glide of the proximal tibia during the knee extension. The one study[361] that examined this test did not report reliability or diagnostic accuracy.

Anterior Drawer Test. The aforementioned Lachman test is a modification of the anterior drawer test.[274] The patient lies in the supine position with the clinician standing to the side of

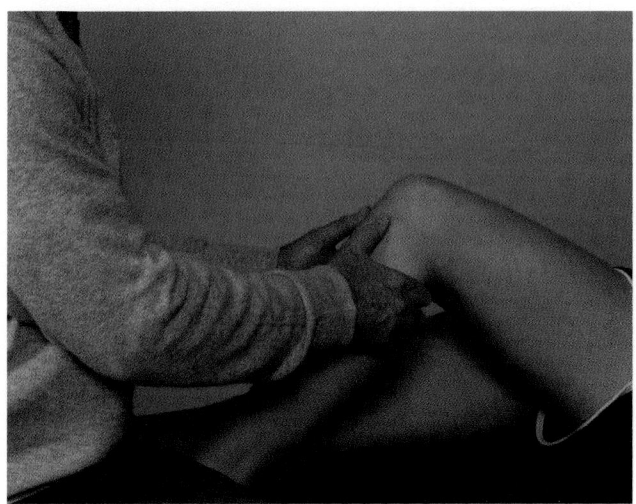

FIGURE 20-28 The anterior drawer test.

the patient's involved knee. The clinician grasps the lower leg of the patient just distal to the joint space of the knee and the patient's knee is flexed to 90 degrees so that the foot is flat and the lower leg is not rotated. The clinician fixates the patient's leg by sitting on the foot. The clinician can place the thumbs either in the joint space or just distal to it to assess mobility. The clinician tests the tension in the musculature. It is important that all muscles around the knee be relaxed to allow any translatory movement to occur. With both hands, the clinician now abruptly pulls the lower leg forward (Fig. 20-28). This test is positive for an ACL tear when an abnormal anterior movement of the tibia occurs compared with the other extremity. Overall, there is wide variation in the reported sensitivities of the anterior drawer test. The anterior drawer test in 80 degrees of flexion without rotation has been found to be 40.9% sensitive and 96.8% specific.[353] This test appears to be a specific test helpful at ruling in a torn ACL when the test is positive.[352,362,363] False-negatives may occur with this test for the same reasons as those in the Lachman test. Given the low sensitivity of this test, the clinician should not rule out an acute ACL injury solely on the basis of a negative anterior drawer.

There are a number of variations to the anterior drawer test, all of which involve positioning the patient supine[274]:

- ***Anterior drawer test and maximal external rotation.***[274] The initial positions of the patient and clinician are the same as in the anterior drawer test in 80 degrees of flexion without rotation, except that the lower leg is positioned in maximum external rotation. For the performance, refer to the preceding description. The ACL and the medial and posteromedial capsuloligamentous structures are tested in this position. If this test is positive, there is likely to be an anteromedial rotatory instability. The specific medial and posteromedial structures that are affected can be further differentiated by the abduction (valgus) stress tests previously described. No diagnostic accuracy studies have been performed to determine the sensitivity and specificity of this test.
- ***Anterior drawer test and maximal internal rotation.***[274] The initial positions of the patient and clinician are the same as in the anterior drawer test in 80 degrees of flexion without rotation, except that the lower leg is now maximally internally rotated. Performance of the test is the same as described earlier for that test. When in maximal internal rotation, the PCL can completely restrict anterior translation of the tibia. Thus, for this test to demonstrate excessive anterior translation, the PCL, ACL, and lateral or posterolateral capsuloligamentous structures have to be affected. No diagnostic accuracy studies have been performed to determine the sensitivity and specificity of this test.

Comparison of the Lachman and Anterior Drawer Tests. The Lachman test has two advantages over the anterior drawer test in 90 degrees of knee flexion. First, all parts of the ACL are more or less equally taut. Second, in acute lesions it is often impossible to position the knee in 90 degrees of flexion because of a hemarthrosis. In a study of patients with an ACL rupture, the Lachman test was positive in 80% of nonanesthetized patients and 100% of anesthetized patients. In comparison, the anterior drawer sign was positive in 9% of nonanesthetized patients and 52% of anesthetized patients.[364]

Jonsson et al.[365] compared both the Lachman and anterior drawer tests in 45 patients with an acute ACL injury and 62 patients with a chronic knee injury. Patients were tested while nonanesthetized and anesthetized, and the diagnosis was verified by arthroscopy. The Lachman test results for the acute injury group was 87% (conscious) and 100% (anesthetized). The anterior drawer test results were 33% and 98%, respectively. The chronic injury group scored a positive Lachman test in 97% (conscious) and 99% (anesthetized). The anterior drawer test was positive in 92% and 100%, respectively.

According to Larson,[366] the Lachman test proved to be the most sensitive test for an ACL rupture. However, this article lacked statistical data to verify this assertion. Another study[355] that compared the two tests reported a sensitivity of 99% for the Lachman test and a sensitivity of 70% for the anterior drawer sign.

One-Plane Posterior Instability

The PCL is very strong and is rarely completely torn. It is typically injured in a dashboard injury or in knee flexion activities (falling on the patella). Several tests have been advocated to test the integrity of the PCL.[274]

Posterior Sag (Godfrey) Sign. The patient lies in the supine position with the knees flexed to approximately 90 degrees and the legs supported under the lower calf/heel by the clinician's arm. The clinician assesses the contour of the tibial tuberosities (Fig. 20-29). If there is a rupture (partial) of the PCL, the tibial tuberosity on the involved side will be less visible than that on the noninvolved side.[367] This discrepancy is caused by an abnormal posterior translation, resulting from a rupture of the PCL. In cases of doubt, the patient can be asked to contract the hamstrings slightly by pushing the heels into the clinician's arm. This maneuver usually results in an increase in the posterior translation of the tibia and is often performed as a quick test of the integrity of the PCL. This test may have

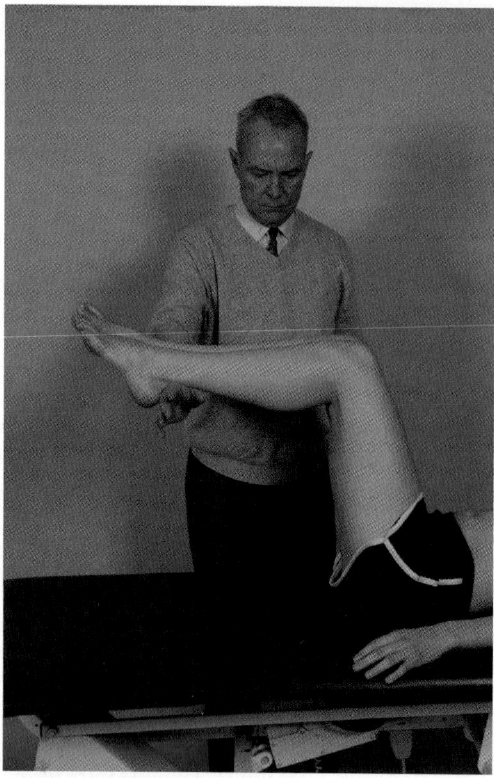

FIGURE 20-29 Godfrey sign.

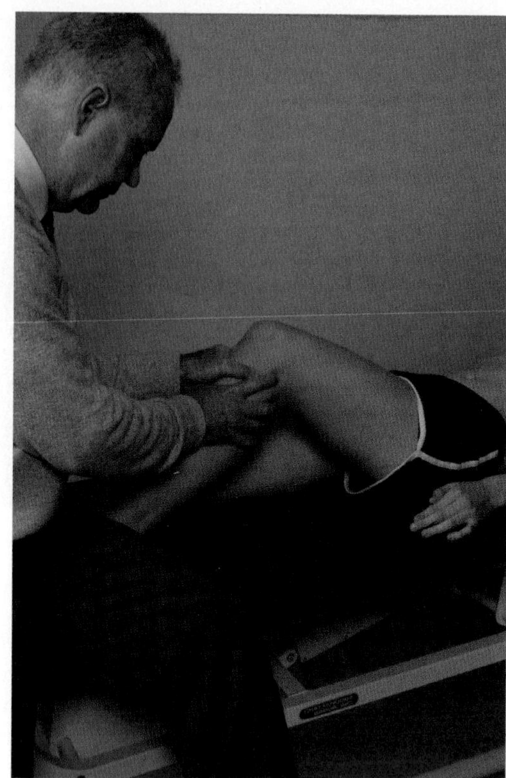

FIGURE 20-30 Posterior drawer.

some value as a screening test when negative due to its high sensitivity.[368,369]

Posterior Drawer Test. The patient lies in the supine position, with the involved knee flexed to 90 degrees. The clinician attempts a posterior displacement of the tibia on the femur (Fig. 20-30). In a blinded, randomized, and controlled study involving 39 patients to assess the clinical examination skills of orthopaedic surgeons with fellowship training in sports medicine, Rubinstein et al.[370] reported that the accuracy for detecting a PCL tear was 96%, with a 90% sensitivity and a 99% specificity. The examination accuracy was higher for grades II and III posterior laxity than for grade I laxity.[370] Eighty-one percent of the time, the examiners agreed on the grade of the PCL tear for any given patient.[370]

Functional Posterior Drawer Test.[371] The patient lies in the prone position with the foot in neutral rotation and the knee flexed to 80–90 degrees. The patient is asked to isometrically contract the hamstrings while the clinician stabilizes the foot (Fig. 20-31). A positive result for a PCL tear is a posterior subluxation of the lateral tibial plateau.

Quadriceps Active Test. The patient lies in the supine position and the relaxed limb is supported with the knee flexed to 90 degrees in the drawer-test position. The patient is asked to execute a gentle quadriceps contraction to shift the tibia without extending the knee. If the PCL is ruptured, the tibia sags into posterior subluxation (~2 mm or more), and the patellar ligament is then directed anteriorly. Studies have shown significantly different sensitivities for this test. Rubinstein et al.[370] reported a sensitivity of 54% and a specificity of 97% whereas Daniel[372] reported a sensitivity of 98%.

Rotary Instabilities

Rotary or complex instabilities occur when the abnormal or pathologic movement is present in two or more planes. The ligamentous laxities present at the knee joint in these situations allow motion to take place around the sagittal, coronal, and horizontal axes.

Posterolateral Instability. This type of instability is relatively rare, because it requires complete posterior cruciate

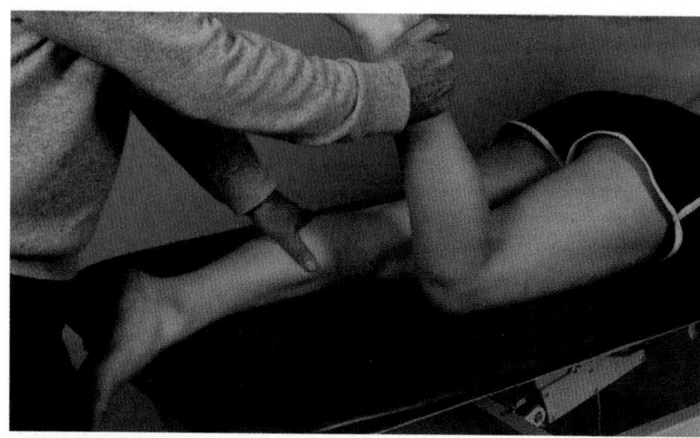

FIGURE 20-31 Functional posterior drawer test.

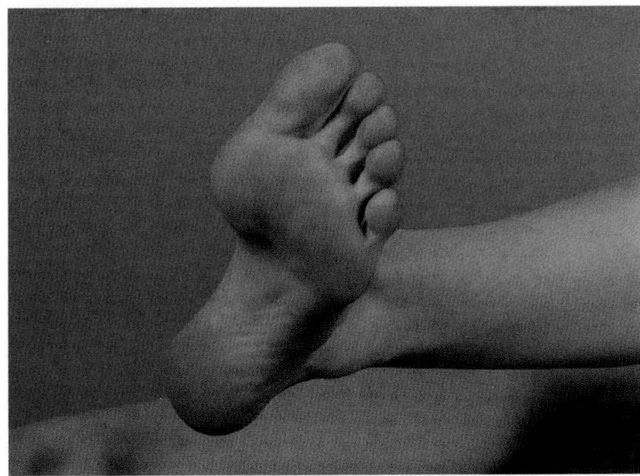

FIGURE 20-32 Modified posterolateral drawer.

laxity. It occurs when the lateral tibial plateau subluxes posteriorly on the femur, with the axis shifting posteriorly and medially to the medial joint area. With a hyperextension test, this posterior displacement is obvious and has been labeled as the *external rotation recurvatum sign.*

Modified Posterolateral Drawer (Loomer's) Test.[55,360] The patient lies in the supine position with the hip and knee flexed to 90 degrees, and the lower leg in external rotation (Fig. 20-32).[373] If the tibia rotates posteriorly during the test, the test is positive for posterolateral instability, indicating that the following structures may have been injured:

- PCL
- Arcuate–popliteus complex
- LCL
- Posterolateral capsule

The one-plane medial and lateral stability tests, described earlier, can be used to further differentiate which lateral and posterolateral structures are affected.

Dial Test. This test is used to assess abnormal external tibial rotation to help differentiate between an isolated posterolateral corner injury and combined ACL/PCL injuries. The patient lies in the supine position with the knee flexed to 30 degrees over the edge of the table.[374] The clinician applies an external rotation force to the patient foot by placing the fingers and thumb alongside the talocalcaneal bone contours (Fig. 20-33). The foot–thigh angle is measured and compared with the uninjured knee. The test is then performed with 90 degrees of knee flexion and the foot–thigh angle is remeasured. When comparing the two angles, a difference of 10 degrees or more is significant. As the knee is flexed to 90 degrees, a reduction in increased rotation may occur although the amount of motion remains greater than the uninjured side if the PCL is still intact. This increased rotation occurs because the PCL is a secondary stabilizer to external rotation and gains mechanical advantage when the knee is flexed.[375]

Posteromedial Displacement with Valgus Stress Test. The patient lies in the supine position, with the involved leg slightly flexed.[373] The clinician pushes the lower leg posteriorly into hyperextension while applying a valgus stress (Fig. 20-34). If the tibia sags posteriorly during the test, the test is positive for posteromedial instability, indicating that the following structures may have been injured:

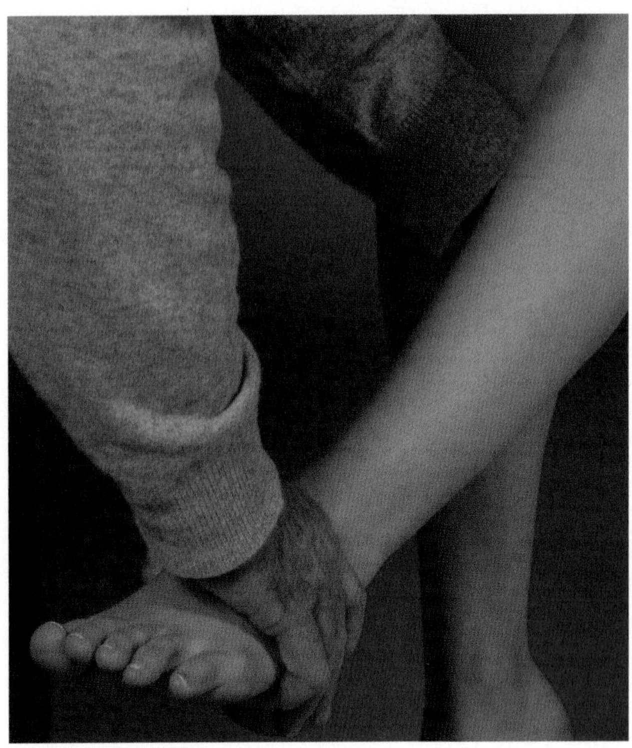

FIGURE 20-33 Dial test.

- PCL
- Posterior oblique ligament

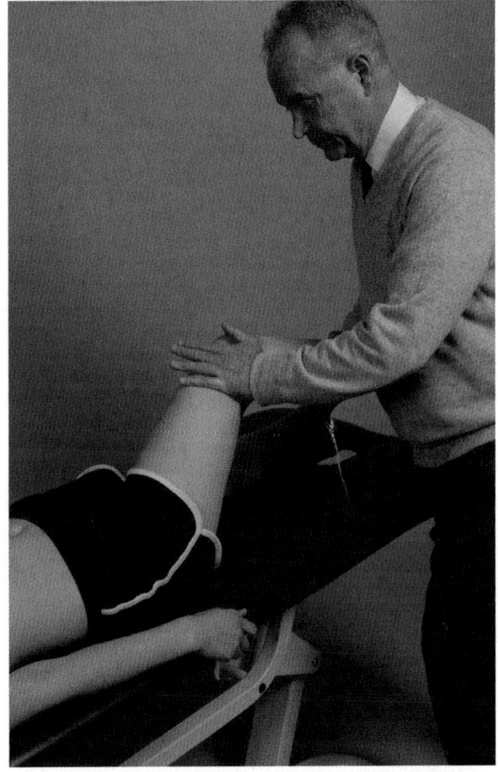

FIGURE 20-34 Posteromedial displacement with valgus stress test.

- MCL
- Posteromedial capsule
- ACL

The one-plane medial and lateral stability tests, described earlier, can be used to further differentiate which medial and posteromedial structures are affected.

Anterolateral Rotary Instability. The pathology for this condition almost certainly involves the ACL and, clinically, the instability allows the medial tibial condyle to sublux posteriorly, because the axis of motion has moved to the lateral joint compartment.[159]

The diagnosis of anterolateral instability is based on the demonstration of a forward subluxation of the lateral tibial plateau as the knee approaches extension and the spontaneous reduction of the subluxation during flexion, in the lateral pivot-shift test.[159] This form of instability usually occurs when the individual is either decelerating or changing direction, and the sudden shift of the lateral compartment is experienced as a "giving way" phenomenon, often associated with pain.[159]

Pivot-Shift Test

This test was first described by Galway et al.[376] in 1972 and has been described since by a number of authors.[377–380]

The pivot shift is the anterior subluxation of the lateral tibial plateau that occurs when the lower leg is stabilized in (almost) full extension, whereby further flexion produces a palpable spring-like reduction.[381] The pivot shift is the most widely recognized dynamic instability of the knee, and it has been shown to correlate with reduced sports activity,[382] degeneration of the cartilage,[383,384] reinjury, meniscal damage,[385] joint arthritis,[385] and a history of instability symptoms.[357,386]

Since the majority of patients with an ACL rupture complain of a "giving way" sensation, the pivot-shift test is regarded in current literature as capable of identifying rotational instability.[377,378,380]

The patient lies in the supine position with the clinician standing to the side of the patient's involved knee. There are two main types of clinical tests to determine the presence of the pivot shift: the reduction test and the subluxation test.

- ***Reduction test.*** The clinician stabilizes the patient's lower leg and flexes the knee to 90 degrees with one hand while using the palm of the other hand to medially rotate the tibia, effectively subluxing the lateral tibial plateau (Fig. 20-35).[386] A sudden reduction of the anteriorly subluxed lateral tibial plateau is seen as the pivot shift.[376]
- ***Subluxation test.*** This test is effectively the reverse of the reduction test.[55] The test begins with patient's knees flexed. The clinician internally rotates the patient's tibias with one hand and applies a valgus stress to the knee joint with the other hand (Fig. 20-36). The clinician slowly extends the knee, maintaining rotation of the tibia. As the patient's knee reaches full extension, the tibial plateau will be felt to relocate. However, only 35–75% of patients whose knees pivot while the patient is under anesthesia will experience such a pivot when awake.[355,387–389]

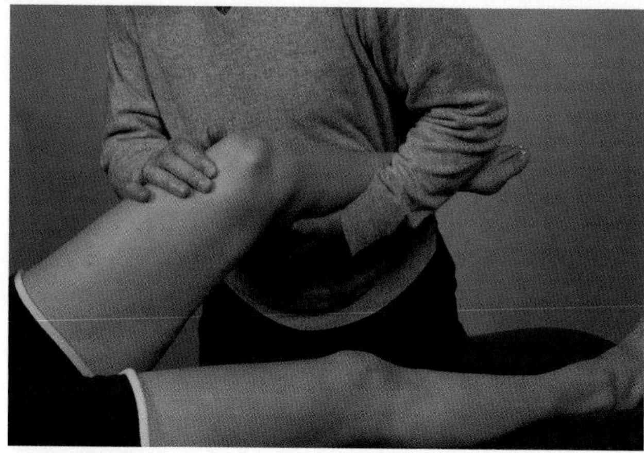

FIGURE 20-35 Pivot-shift test—reduction.

Although the specificity of the pivot shift test is very high, namely 98% (95% CI, 25–38), there is little agreement in the literature with regard to the sensitivity of the test, which varies between 0% and 98%.[355,364,390] However, in a meta-analysis that looked at 28 studies to assess the accuracy of clinical tests for diagnosing ACL ruptures, Benjaminse et al.[391] found the pivot shift test to be very specific both in acute as well as in chronic conditions, and recommended that both the Lachman and pivot-shift tests be performed in all cases of suspected ACL injury.

It is worth noting that the pivot-shift test can be positive with an isolated ACL injury[355,392] or a tear or stretching of the lateral capsule,[379,393] although an injury to the MCL reduces the likelihood of a pivot shift even with ACL injury.[355,394]

Patellar Stability Tests

Patellar stability is assessed by gently pushing the patella medially and laterally while the knee is in a position of 90 degrees of flexion. This position is used because it places all of the retinacula on stretch. If this test is positive for laxity, further testing is performed by applying medial and lateral patellar glides, tilts, and rotations, with the knee in relaxed extension, and noting any limitations of motion or excessive excursion (Table 20-8).[266]

- ***Glide.*** The glide component determines the amount of lateral deviation of the patella in the frontal plane. A 5-mm

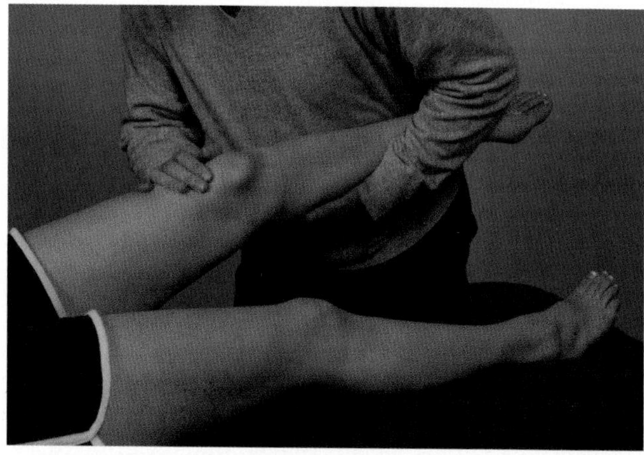

FIGURE 20-36 Pivot-shift test—subluxation.

TABLE 20-8	Assessing the Tilt, Orientation, and Glide of the Patella		
Test and Measure	**Procedure and Determination of Positive Finding**	**Population**	**Reliability Kappa Values**
Superoinferior tilt[a]	Clinician visually estimates patellar alignment while palpating superior and inferior patellar poles Patellar orientation graded according to an ordinal scale extending from −2 to +2, with −2 representing inferior patellar pole below superior pole, and +2 representing inferior patellar pole above superior pole	27 asymptomatic subjects	Intraexaminer κ = 0.50 Interexaminer κ = 0 30
Anterior tilt[b]	Clinician palpates inferior patellar pole If the clinician can palpate inferior pole, no anterior tilt exists; if downward pressure on superior pole is required to palpate inferior pole, it is considered to have an anterior tilt	66 patients referred to physical therapy who would normally undergo evaluation of patellofemoral alignment	Interexaminer κ = 0.24
Anterior/posterior tilt component[c]	Clinician palpates inferior and superior patellar poles Scored 0, 1, or 2: 0 if inferior patellar pole is as easily palpable as superior pole; 1 if inferior patellar pole is not as easily palpable and superior pole; 2 if inferior pole is not clearly palpable compared with superior pole	56 subjects, 25 had symptomatic knees	Intraexaminer κ = 0.03–0.23 Interexaminer κ = 0.04
Rotation[a]	Clinician positions index fingers along longitudinal axes of patellar and estimates acute angle formed Graded according to ordinal scale extending from −2 to +2: −2 indicates that longitudinal axis of patella is more lateral than axis of femur; +2 indicates that patella is more medial than axis of femur	27 asymptomatic subjects	Intraexaminer κ = 0.41 Interexaminer κ = −0.03
Patellar rotation[b]	Clinician determines relationship between longitudinal axis of patella and femur Longitudinal axis of patellar should be in line with ASIS; if distal end of patella is medial, it is considered to be medially rotated; if distal end is lateral, it is considered to be laterally rotated	66 patients referred to physical therapy who would normally undergo evaluation of patellofemoral alignment	Interexaminer κ = 0.36
Patellar rotation component[c]	Clinician determines relationship between longitudinal axis of patella and femur Scored as −1, 0, or + 1: 0 when patellar long axis is parallel to long axis of femur; 1 when inferior patellar pole is lateral to axis of femur and classified as lateral patellar rotation; −1 when inferior pole is medial to axis of femur and classified as medial patellar rotation		Intraexaminer κ = −0.06 to 0.00 Interexaminer κ = −0.03
Mediolateral tilt[a]	Clinician estimates patellar alignment while palpating medial and lateral aspects of patella Patellar orientation graded according to an ordinal scale extending from −2 to +2 with −2 representing a lateral tilt, 0 no appreciable tilt, and +2 a medial tilt	27 asymptomatic subjects	Intraexaminer κ = 0.57 Interexaminer κ = 0.18
Medial/lateral tilt[b]	Clinician palpates medial and lateral borders of patella with thumb and index finger If digit palpating the medial border is higher than that palpating the lateral border, then the patella is considered laterally tilted; if digit palpating the lateral border is higher than that palpating the medial patella, then the patella is medially tilted	66 patients referred to physical therapy who would normally undergo an evaluation of patellofemoral alignment	Intraexaminer κ = 0.28–0.33 Interexaminer κ = 0.21

(Continued)

TABLE 20-8 Assessing the Tilt, Orientation, and Glide of the Patella *(Continued)*			
Test and Measure	**Procedure and Determination of Positive Finding**	**Population**	**Reliability Kappa Values**
Medial/lateral tilt[c]	Clinician attempts to palpate posterior surface of medial and lateral patella borders Scored 0, 1, or 2: 0 if clinician palpates posterior border on both medial and lateral sides; 1 if >50% of lateral border can be palpated but posterior surface cannot; 2 if <50% of lateral border can be palpated	56 subjects, 25 had symptomatic knees	Intraexaminer κ = 0.44–0.50 Interexaminer κ = 0.19
Patellar tilt test[c]	Clinician lifts lateral edge of patella from lateral femoral epicondyle Graded as having positive, neutral, or negative angle with respect to horizontal plane	99 knees, of which 26 were symptomatic	Interexaminer κ = 0.20–0.35
Mediolateral position[a]	Clinician visually estimates patellar alignment while palpating sides of lateral epicondyles with index fingers, and patella midline with thumbs Patellar orientation graded according to an ordinal scale extending from −2 to +2 with −2 representing a lateral displacement, 0 no appreciable displacement, and +2 a medial displacement	27 asymptomatic subjects	Intraexaminer κ = 0.40 Interexaminer κ = 0.03
Mediolateral orientation[d]	With knee supported in 20 degrees of flexion, the clinician identifies medial and lateral epicondyles of femur and midline of patella. Clinician then marks medial and lateral epicondyles and patellar midline with tape Distances between patella midline and medial and lateral condyles are measured	20 healthy physiotherapy students	Interexaminer Medial distance: ICC = 0.91 Lateral distance: ICC = 0.94
Medial/lateral displacement[b]	Clinician palpates medial and lateral epicondyles with index fingers while simultaneously palpating midline of patella with thumbs Distance between index fingers and thumbs should be the same; when distance to index finger palpating lateral epicondyles is less, patella is laterally displaced; when distance to index finger palpating medial epicondyles is less, patella is medially displaced	66 patients referred to physical therapy who would normally undergo evaluation of patellofemoral alignment	Interexaminer κ = 0.10
Medial/lateral glide[c]	Clinician uses a tape measure to record distance from medial and lateral femoral condyles to mid-patella Scored 0 or 1: 0 if distance from medial epicondyle to mid-patella equals distance from lateral epicondyle to mid-patella; 1 if distance from medial epicondyle to mid-patella is 0.5 cm greater than that from lateral condyle to mid-patella	56 subjects, 25 had symptomatic knees	Intraexaminer κ = 0.11–0.35 Interexaminer κ = 0.02

Data from Cleland J: Knee. *Orthopaedic Clinical Examination: An Evidence-Based Approach for Physical Therapists*. Carlstadt, NJ: Icon Learning Systems, LLC, 2005:271–320.

[a]Data from Tomsich DA, Nitz AJ, Threlkeld AJ, et al.: Patellofemoral alignment: Reliability. *J Orthop Sports Phys Ther* 23:200–208, 1996.

[b]Data from Fitzgerald GK, McClure PW: Reliability of measurements obtained with four tests for patellofemoral alignment. *Phys Ther* 75:84–92, 1995.

[c]Data from Watson CJ, Propps M, Galt W, et al.: Reliability of McConnell's classification of patellar orientation in symptomatic and asymptomatic subjects. *J Orthop Sports Phys Ther* 29:378–385; 1999; discussion 386–393.

[d]Data from Herrington LC: The Inter-tester reliability of a clinical measurement used to determine the medial-lateral orientation of the patella. *Man Ther* 7:163–167, 2002.

lateral displacement of the patella causes a 50% decrease in VMO tension.[395] In the normal knee when fully extended and relaxed, the patella can be passively displaced medially and laterally approximately 1 cm in each direction, or approximately one-third of the width of the patella.[187] Displacement of more than half the patella over the medial or lateral aspect is considered abnormal.[9] If the patient is apprehensive as the glide maneuver is being performed, the problem is likely to be one of poor patellar engagement. A decreased medial glide of the patella has been found to be related to ITB and/or lateral retinaculum tightness.[131]

- ***Tilt.*** The degree of patellar tilt is assessed by comparing the height of the medial patellar border with the height of the lateral border, which helps to determine the degree of tightness in the deep retinacular fibers. A slight lateral tilt of the patella is normal. An increased medial tilt results from a tight lateral retinaculum. If the passive lateral structures are too tight, the patella will tilt so that the medial border is higher than the lateral border (lateral tilt), making the posterior edge of the lateral border difficult to palpate.[266] A posterior tilt results in fat pad irritation.
- ***Rotation.*** The rotation component determines whether there is any deviation of the long axis of the patella from the long axis of the femur. If the inferior pole is sitting lateral to the long axis of the femur, the patient has an externally rotated patella, whereas if the inferior pole is sitting medial to the long axis, the patient has an internally rotated patella.

If the patient has one or more of these components present, the clinician needs to determine which of them, if any, is abnormal.

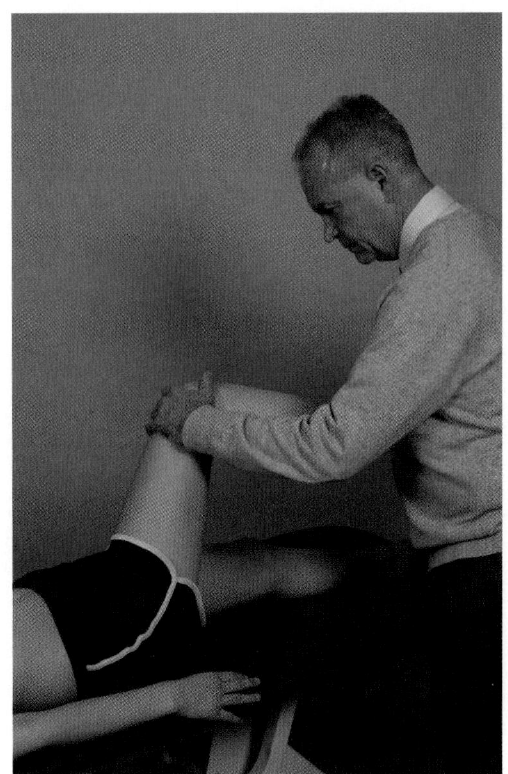

FIGURE 20-37 McMurray test.

Meniscal Lesion Tests

McMurray's Test

The McMurray test was originally developed to diagnose posterior horn lesions of the medial meniscus. The patient lies in the supine position, and the clinician, standing on the same side as the involved knee, maximally flexes the hip and knee. This is accomplished by grasping the patient's foot in such a way that the thumb is lateral, the index and middle fingers are medial, and the ring and little fingers hold the medial edge of the foot (Fig. 20-37). The thumb of one hand is placed against the lateral aspect of the patient's knee (see Fig. 20-37). To test the medial meniscus, the clinician rotates the tibia into external rotation, then slowly extends the knee. To test the lateral meniscus, the clinician flexes the knee again but now internally rotates the patient's tibia and then slowly extends the knee. A positive test traditionally is indicated by an audible or palpable *thud* or *click*. In a study by Dervin et al.[396] to determine clinicians' accuracy and reliability for the clinical diagnosis of unstable meniscus tears in patients with symptomatic OA of the knee, a positive McMurray test was the only positive predictor of an unstable meniscal tear.[396]

Numerous variations exist for the McMurray test, including the addition of varus/valgus stresses. An examination of the variation seemed to indicate that the McMurray test has some value as a specific test where a positive test would rule in the disease.

Apley's Test[397]

The patient is placed in the prone position, with the knee flexed to 90 degrees. The patient's thigh is stabilized by the clinician's knee. The clinician grasps the patient's foot with one hand, distracts the tibia, and rotates the tibia internally and externally, noting whether or not pain is reproduced. A positive test is indicated by worse pain with rotation and is indicative of a *rotation sprain* of soft tissue. The clinician then applies internal and external rotation with compression to the lower leg, noting any pain and the quality of motion (Fig. 20-38). A positive test for a meniscus tear is indicated by more pain in compression than distraction. It would appear from a number of studies that the Apley test can be used as a specific test to rule in a meniscus tear when positive.

Steinmann's Sign[274]

Steinmann's test can be used to diagnose meniscal lesions. The patient is placed in the supine position, while the clinician stands to the side. Using one hand, the clinician grasps the patient's lower leg just proximal to the malleolus. The other hand grasps the lateral side of the patient's lower leg as proximal to the knee as possible while also palpating the medial joint space with the fingers (Fig. 20-39). The knee is extended, and the joint line between the patellar tendon and the MCL is palpated. After the painful site is located with the fingers, pressure against this site is maintained while the knee is flexed. After several degrees of motion, the pain disappears, and the painful site can sometimes again be palpated more posteriorly in the joint space. If the most painful site is found in the joint space at the level of the MCL, the test is less reliable, because both the medial meniscus and the ligament move posteriorly during flexion.

Anderson Mediolateral Grind Test

The Anderson mediolateral grind test[398] can be used to detect meniscal lesions. The patient is placed in the supine position, and the clinician grasps the involved leg between the trunk and arm. The clinician places the index finger and thumb of the

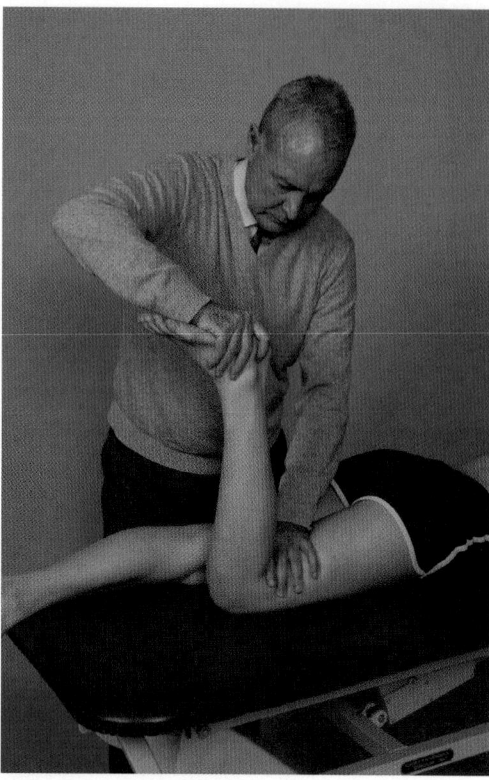

FIGURE 20-38 Apley's grind test.

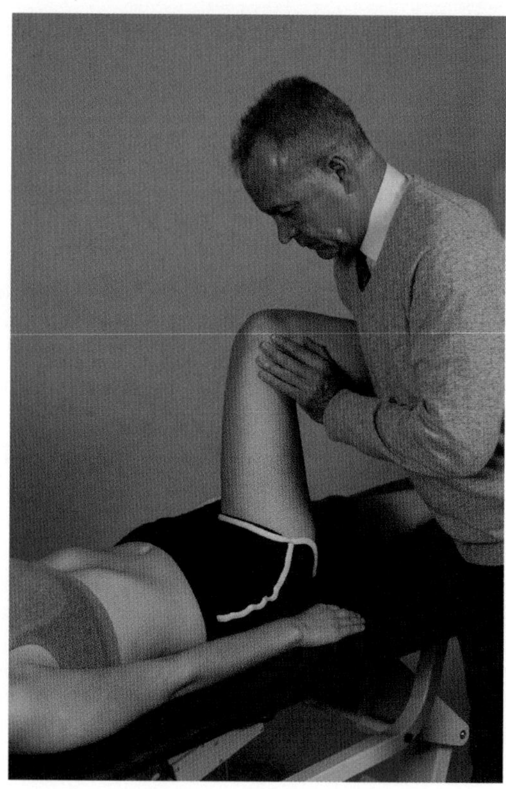

FIGURE 20-40 Anderson mediolateral grind test.

other hand over the anterior knee joint line. With the patient's knee flexed at 45 degrees, a valgus stress is applied as the knee is simultaneously slightly flexed (Fig. 20-40), followed by a varus component while the knee is extended, producing a circular motion of the knee. The maneuver is repeated, increasing the valgus and varus stresses with each rotation.

In one study[398] that examined 100 knees with the Anderson mediolateral grind test, as well as arthroscopy, the test was found to have a sensitivity of 70% and a specificity of 67%. However further research needs to be performed to corroborate the statistics reported in this study.

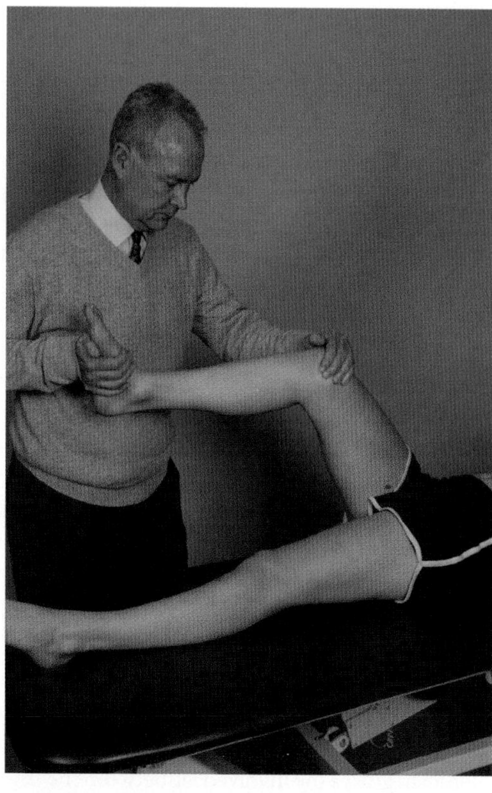

FIGURE 20-39 Steinmann's I sign.

Bounce Home Test

The patient is placed in the supine position and the clinician extends the involved knee to end range (Fig. 20-41). A positive test for meniscus tear is indicated by a block preventing full extension, or pain at end-range extension. A number of studies seem to indicate that neither pain at full extension nor an extension block seem to indicate a torn meniscus.[399–401]

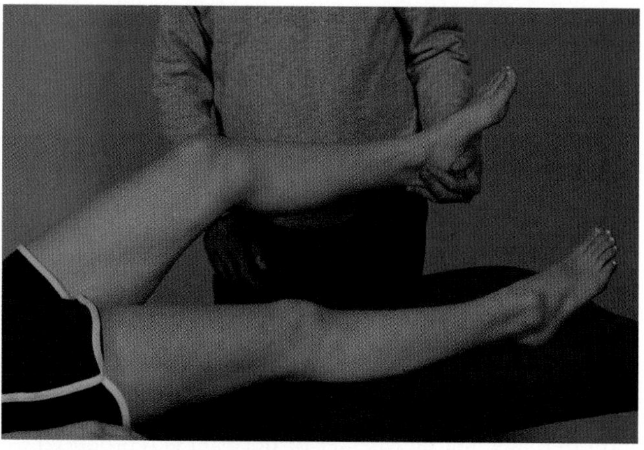

FIGURE 20-41 Bounce home test.

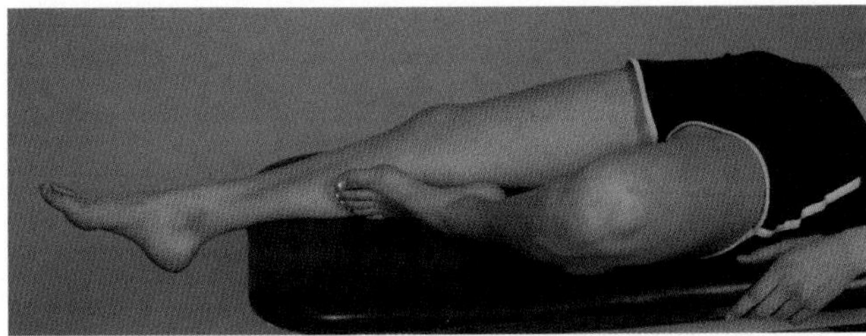

FIGURE 20-42 Figure-4 test.

Figure-4 Test

This test was developed to detect popliteomeniscal fascicle tears, which create instability of the lateral meniscus. The patient lies in the supine position and is asked to place the foot of the involved knee by the contralateral knee, forming a figure 4 (Fig. 20-42). The clinician pushes the involved knee toward the bed. A positive test is indicated by pain over the lateral joint line at the popliteal hiatus. In a very small study[402] involving only six patients the test demonstrated a sensitivity of 100%. Further research is necessary before diagnostic conclusions can be made from this test.

Payr Sign

The patient is placed in the supine position or sits and places the foot of the involved knee on the medial aspect of the contralateral knee, forming a figure 4. The clinician pushes the involved knee toward the floor (Fig. 20-43). A positive test for a posterior horn lesion of the medial meniscus is indicated by reproduction of the patient's pain over the medial joint line. In a study by Jerosch and Riemer[403] this test was found to have a sensitivity of 54% and a specificity of 44%, demonstrating a diagnostic value similar to that of a coin toss.

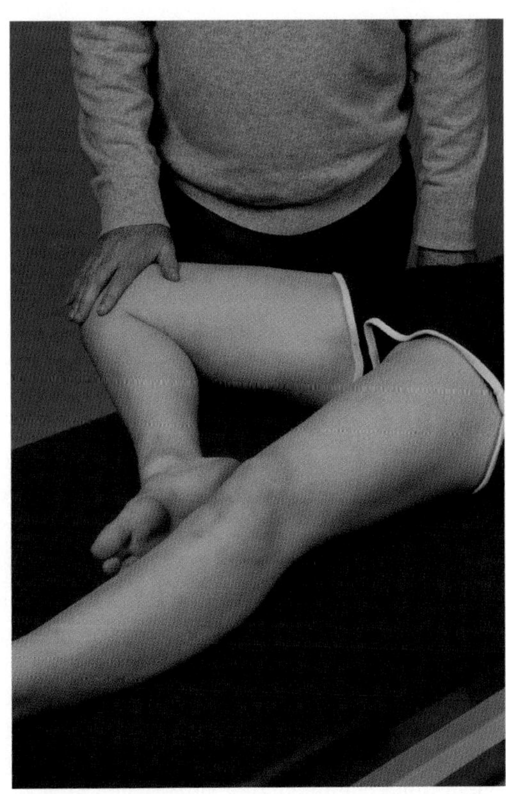

FIGURE 20-43 Payr sign.

Other Special Tests

The remaining special tests for the knee joint complex are dependent on the clinician's needs, the structure of each joint, and the subjective complaints (Table 20-9). These tests are only performed if there is some indication that they would by helpful in arriving at a diagnosis. The special tests help confirm or implicate a particular structure and may also provide information as to the degree of tissue damage.

Plical Irritation

Plical irritation has a characteristic pattern of presentation. The anterior pain in the knee is episodic and associated with painful clicking, "giving way," and the feeling of something catching in the knee. Careful palpation of the patellar retinaculum and fat pad, with the knee extended and then flexed, can be used to detect tender plicae and to differentiate tenderness within the fat pad from tenderness over the anterior horn of the menisci.

- ***Medial plica test.*** This test can also be used to detect plical irritation. Using the heel of the cranial hand, the clinician pushes the patella medially and maintains it there (Fig. 20-44). While the patella is maintained in this position, the clinician flexes the patient's knee and internally rotates the tibia with the other hand. The knee is then extended from the flexed position while the clinician palpates for any clunks.
- ***Medial plica shelf test.*** The patient lies in the supine position on the bed, with the knee supported in about 30 degrees of flexion by either a bolster or the clinician's thigh. The clinician places both thumbs together at the lateral aspect of the patella and pushes the patella medially (Fig. 20-45). If a painful click is elicited during this test, there is likely to be a symptomatic mediopatellar synovial plica.

Suprapatellar or Infrapatellar Tendinitis

The patient is placed in the supine position, with the lower extremity extended.

- ***Infrapatellar test.*** The clinician pushes down on the suprapatellar aspect, palpates under the inferior pole of the patella, and checks for tenderness, which may indicate infrapatellar tendinitis.
- ***Suprapatellar test.*** The clinician pushes on the infrapatellar aspect of the patella, palpates under the superior pole of the patella, and checks for tenderness, which may indicate suprapatellar tendinitis.

Integrity of Patellofemoral Articulating Surfaces

These tests involve the application of manual compression to the patella in an attempt to elicit pain.

TABLE 20-9 Subjective Complaint, Potential Diagnosis, and Confirmatory Test

Subjective Complaint	Potential Diagnosis	Confirmatory Test(s)
My knee hurts when I get up from a chair or go up steps	Patellofemoral dysfunction	Patellofemoral grind test
My knee gives out when I step down from the curb	Subluxation/dislocation of the patella	Patella apprehension test
My knee locks	1. Torn medial meniscus 2. Loose body within the knee joint	McMurray test and Apley grinding and distraction tests
My knee feels swollen and tight	Fluid within the knee	Patellar effusion tests
My knee buckles; it gives out	1. Unstable knee joint (torn collateral or cruciate ligament) 2. Torn medial meniscus	Valgus and varus stress tests, anterior drawer, Lachman, Posterior sag, strength testing (neuro screen), meniscus tests
I cannot straighten my knee out	1. Fluid in the knee 2. Torn meniscus	Meniscus tests, patellar ballottement test, bounce home test
I have pain on the inside of my leg	1. Torn medial collateral ligament 2. Bursitis, pes anserinus bursa	Valgus stress test Palpation of the pes anserinus bursa
I made a quick turn while playing sports while my foot was planted, and my leg suddenly collapsed and the knee became swollen	Torn medial meniscus	Apley test and McMurray test
I have bow legs and they hurt	1. Osteoarthritis 2. Ligamentous instability	Range of motion (capsular) Patellofemoral grinding test Ligament stability tests
I have swelling in the back of my knee	Popliteal cyst	Palpation of popliteal fossa
I landed heavily on the front of my knee and it hurts	1. Patellar fracture 2. Chondromalacia 3. Fat pad syndrome 4. Prepatellar bursitis 5. Infrapatellar bursitis	Radiograph Palpation
I cannot move my knee in any direction without pain	Infected knee joint	Joint aspiration

Data from Hoppenfeld S: Physical examination of the knee joint by complaint. *Orthop Clin North Am* 10:3–20, 1979.

Zohler's Sign

The patient is placed in the supine position, with the knee extended and resting on the table. The clinician pulls the patient's patella in a distal direction. While continuing to exert pressure in a distal direction, the clinician instructs the patient to contract the quadriceps muscle (Fig. 20-46). If this test is painful, there is likely to be a symptomatic patellar chondromalacia, although this test may be positive in a large proportion of asymptomatic individuals. One study[367] to examine this test did not record reliability or diagnostic accuracy.

Clarke's Test

This test is similar to Zohler's test, except that the clinician applies an increasing compressive force to the base of the patella while the patient actively contracts the quadriceps. Like Zohler's test, this test may be positive in a large proportion of asymptomatic individuals.

Waldron Test

See "Patella Motion Tests" Section.

Patellar Mobility and Retinaculum Tests

Patellar glides can be used to examine retinacular mobility. The patella should be able to translate at least 33% of its width both medially and laterally. Inability to do this indicates tightness of the retinacula. Hypermobility of the patella is demonstrated if the patella can be translated 100% of its width medially or laterally.

The lateral retinaculum is assessed by way of a patellar tilt and a mediolateral displacement (glide).[189,404–406] A number of patient positions can be used to assess the flexibility of the retinacular tissue.

- ***Medial shift.***[274] The patient is supine, with the knee extended. The clinician places both thumbs together at the lateral aspect of the patella and pushes the patella medially. The amount of motion and the end-feel are assessed. Often the patella is found to have less ROM medially than laterally. Whether this condition is pathologic is best determined by comparison to the noninvolved side. This patellar movement often is limited after surgery and after immobilization.

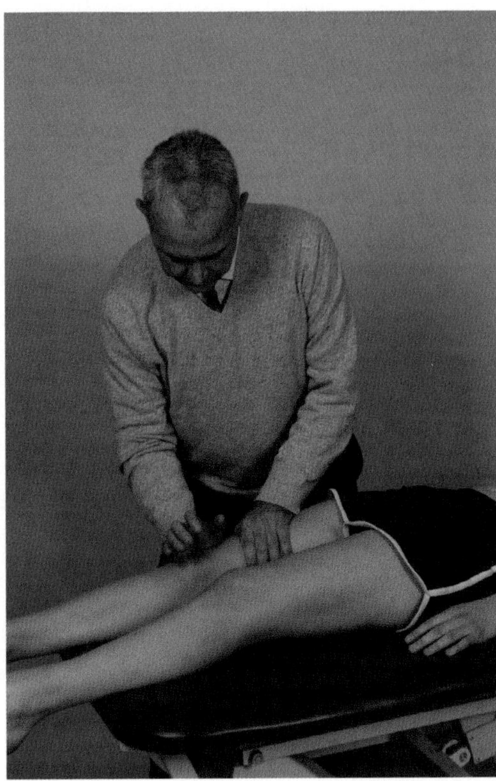

FIGURE 20-44 Medial plica test.

- ***Lateral shift.*** The patient is supine, with the knee extended. The clinician places the fingertips of both hands against the medial aspect of the patella and pushes the patella laterally. The amount of motion and the end-feel are assessed. Usually the patella has more ROM laterally than medially. When there are instabilities of the patella, the lateral mobility is usually abnormally increased. This patellar movement often is limited after surgery and after immobilization.
- ***Distal shift.*** The patient is supine, with the knee extended. With the thenar and hypothenar eminences placed against the base of the patient's patella, the clinician pushes the patella in a distal direction. As with the previous two shift tests, the amount of motion and end-feel are assessed. The motion usually is limited in instances of patella alta (a high position of the patella), after surgery, and after immobilization.

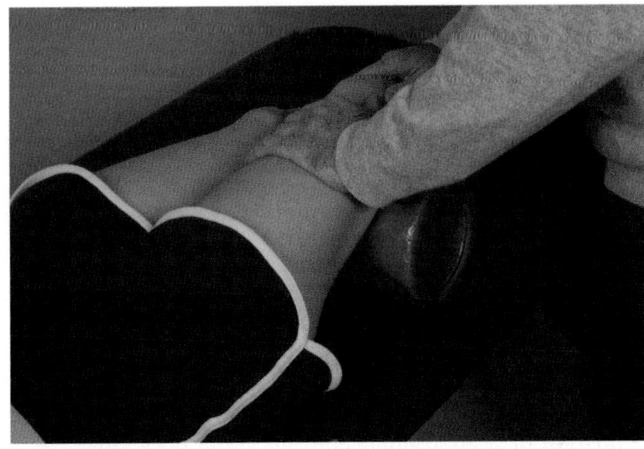

FIGURE 20-45 Medial plica shelf test.

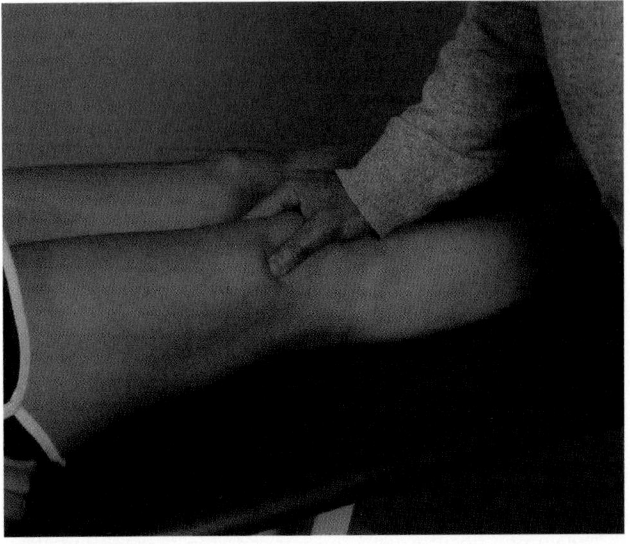

FIGURE 20-46 Zohler's sign.

- ***Prone technique.*** The clinician passively flexes the patient' s knee to 90 degrees and internally rotates the tibia. The lower extremity is then moved into hip adduction. The test is positive for tightness of the lateral structures if the hip cannot be fully adducted. This test also can be performed in the side-lying position, with the involved side uppermost.
- ***Lateral tilt of the patella.*** The patient lies in the supine position, with the knee extended and relaxed. The clinician attempts to lift the lateral border of the patella. An inability to lift the lateral border of the patella above the horizontal plane is an indication of tightness of the lateral retinaculum.
- ***Side-Lying technique.***[266] With the knee of the uppermost leg flexed to 20 degrees, the patella is moved in a medial direction toward the treatment table. The clinician should be able to expose the lateral femoral condyle, unless the tissues of the superficial lateral retinacula are tight. To test the deep fibers, the clinician places a hand on the middle of the patella, takes up the slack of the glide, and applies an anteroposterior pressure on the medial border of the patella. The lateral femoral condyle should move freely away from the femur. This test also can be used as an intervention technique.[266]

Fairbank's Apprehension Test for Patellar Instability

The Fairbank test[407] is best performed with the patient in the supine position and the patient's leg supported at approximately 30 degrees of knee flexion. The clinician places both thumbs on the medial aspect of the patella and applies a laterally directed force to the medial aspect of the patella, attempting to sublux it laterally while applying a small amount of passive flexion to the knee.[205] This test appears to be more specific than sensitive, meaning a positive test would help rule in patellofemoral instability.[341,408]

Wilson Test for Osteochondritis Dissecans

The following accessory test can be performed when osteochondritis dissecans of the knee is suspected. The patient is supine. The clinician flexes the patient's hip and knee to 90 degrees. Axial compression is exerted at the knee by pushing proximally, in line with the tibia, with the distal hand. The lower leg is held in internal rotation as the knee is slowly extended, maintaining the axial compression. In many cases of osteochondritis dissecans, the patient experiences pain because the pressure on the medial cartilaginous surfaces is increased significantly with this maneuver.

Hamstring Flexibility

The popliteal angle is the most popular method reported in the literature for assessing hamstring tightness, especially in the presence of a knee flexion contracture.[409] The patient is placed in the supine position and the opposite hip is extended. The popliteal angle is determined by measuring the angle that the tibia subtends with the extended line of the femur when the ipsilateral hip is flexed to 90 degrees and the knee of the limb under examination is maximally passively extended to initial tissue resistance.[410] The popliteal angle is at the maximum of 180 degrees from birth to age 2 years.[409] This angle then decreases to an average of 155 degrees by age 6 years and remains steady thereafter.[409] An angle less than 125 degrees suggests significant hamstring tightness.[409]

Hamstring flexibility can also be assessed with a passive straight leg raise, while ensuring that the lumbar spine is flattened on the treatment table and the pelvis is stabilized. However, this method may be used only if there is full extension at the knee of the leg being examined. Normal hamstring length should allow 80–85 degrees of hip flexion when the knee is extended and the lumbar spine is flattened.[266]

ITB Flexibility

The cardinal sign of iliotibial contracture is the presence in a supine patient of an abduction contracture when the hip and knee are extended, which is eliminated when the hip and knee are flexed.[411] Other tests include the following:

Retinacula Test. The patient is placed in the side-lying position and the knee is fully flexed. This position tightens the ITB. The clinician applies a medial and oblique force to the patella with the thumbs. Approximately 0.5–1 cm of patella motion should be available.

Ober's Test. The Ober test for ITB length is described in Chapter 19.

Quadriceps Flexibility. Quadriceps flexibility is examined by placing the patient in prone position and passively flexing the knee, bringing the heel toward the buttocks. The lumbar spine is monitored and stabilized if necessary to prevent motion. The heel should touch the buttocks. An adaptively shortened rectus femoris is usually the structure that prevents this motion (see later discussion).

Functional Tests

Functional outcome following knee injury must consider the patient's perspective and not just objective measurements of instability. Functional motion requirements of the knee vary according to the specific task. In normal level ground walking, 60–70 degrees of knee flexion is required. This requirement increases to 80–85 degrees for stair climbing and to 120–140 degrees for running.[3] Approximately 120 degrees of knee flexion are necessary for activities such as squatting to tie a shoelace or to don a sock.[412] Table 20-10 outlines the amounts of knee ROM that must be available for common activities of daily living.

TABLE 20-10 Approximate Range of Motion Required for Common Activities of Daily Living

Activity	Required Flexion Range of Motion (Degrees)
Running	120–140
Squatting	120
Tying shoelace	120
Donning a sock	120
Climbing downstairs	110
Sitting and rising	85
Climbing upstairs	80
Swing phase of gait	70
Stance phase of gait	20

Data from Laubenthal KN, Smidt GL, Kettelkamp DB: A quantitative analysis of knee motion for activities of daily living. *Phys Ther* 52:34–42, 1972.

Subjective Tests

Clinical research studies are placing an increased emphasis on the perspective of the patient with use of health-related quality-of-life instruments. Many patient-based knee-rating scales have been developed (Table 20-11). These include the following.

WOMAC Index. The Western Ontario and McMaster Universities Osteoarthritis Index (WOMAC) (Table 20-12) is a widely used measure of symptoms and physical disability, originally developed for people with OA of the hip or knee.[413] The measure was developed to evaluate clinically important, patient-relevant changes in health status as a result of intervention.[414] Evidence of the reliability (test–retest), validity, and responsiveness of the WOMAC has been provided in OA patients undergoing total knee or hip arthroplasty[413] and in OA patients receiving nonsteroidal anti-inflammatory drugs (NSAIDs).[415] The WOMAC evaluates three dimensions: pain, stiffness, and physical function with 5, 2, and 17 questions, respectively[416] (see Table 20-12). Each subscale is summated to a maximum score of 20, 8, and 68, respectively. There is also an index score or global score, which is most commonly calculated by summating the scores for the three subscales.[416]

International Knee Documentation Committee Questionnaire. The International Knee Documentation Committee (IKDC) questionnaire was formed to set standards for the evaluation of knee ligament injury.[417] The IKDC form uses four domains for the final rating: patient's self-reported

TABLE 20-11 Knee Questionnaire Indices

Indices	Indication	Reliability	Validity	Comment
Western Ontario and McMaster Universities Osteoarthritis Index Bellamy[a]	Osteoarthritis	Strong for osteoarthritis	Strong for osteoarthritis	Strong for pain, stiffness, and physical function in osteoarthritis
International Knee Documentation Committee Questionnaire[b]	Knee ligament injury	Good	Strong	Not sensitive for sports related function Not as responsive to changes over time
Lysholm Knee Score[c]	Ligament and meniscal injuries	Good	Unclear	Not useful for high functioning individuals Score is heavily weighted on pain and instability ratings Acceptable psychometric performances as outcome measures for patients with a meniscal injury of the knee
Cincinnati Knee Rating System[d]	Nonspecific knee injury	Unknown	Unclear	Allows assessment of outcome based on the patient's usual activities
Knee Outcome Survey[e]	Nonspecific knee injury	Strong for functional limitations	Strong for functional limitations	Responsive for functional limits for a variety of impairments
Lower extremity function scale[f]	All lower extremity conditions	Strong for hip and knee total arthroplasty	Strong for hip and knee total arthroplasty	Useful with patients following arthroplasty

Data from Manal TJ, Dickerson-Schnatz A: Disorders of the tibiofemoral joint. In: Wilmarth MA, ed. *Evidence-Based Practice for the Upper and Lower Quarter. Orthopaedic Physical Therapy Home Study Course* 13.2.2. La Crosse, WI: Orthopaedic Section, APTA, 2003:1–44.

[a]Data from Bellamy N, Buchanan WW, Goldsmith CH, et al.: Validation study of WOMAC: a health status instrument for measuring clinically important patient-relevant outcomes following total hip or knee arthroplasty in osteoarthritis. *J Orthop Rheumatol* 1:95–108, 1988.

[b]Data from Hefti F, Muller W, Jakob RP, et al.: Evaluation of knee ligament injuries with the IKDC form. *Knee Surg Sports Traumatol Arthrosc* 1:226–234, 1993; Irrgang JJ, Anderson AF, Boland AL, et al.: Responsiveness of the international knee documentation committee subjective knee form. *Am J Sports Med* 34:1567–1573, 2006. Epub Jul 26, 2006; Anderson AF, Irrgang JJ, Kocher MS, et al.: The international knee documentation committee subjective knee evaluation form: Normative data. *Am J Sports Med* 34:128–135, 2006. Epub Oct 11, 2005; Irrgang JJ, Anderson AF, Boland AL, et al.: Development and validation of the international knee documentation committee subjective knee form. *Am J Sports Med* 29:600–613, 2001; Irrgang JJ, Ho H, Harner CD, et al.: Use of the International Knee Documentation Committee guidelines to assess outcome following anterior cruciate ligament reconstruction. *Knee Surg Sports Traumatol Arthrosc* 6:107–114, 1998.

[c]Data from Tegner Y, Lysholm J: Rating systems in the evaluation of knee ligament injuries. *Clin Orthop* 198:43–49, 1985; Briggs KK, Kocher MS, Rodkey WG, et al.: Reliability, validity, and responsiveness of the Lysholm knee score and Tegner activity scale for patients with meniscal injury of the knee. *J Bone Joint Surg Am* 88:698–705, 2006.

[d]Data from Tegner Y, Lysholm J: Rating systems in the evaluation of knee ligament injuries. *Clin Orthop* 198:43–49, 1985; Phillips N, Benjamin M, Everett T, et al.: Outcome and progression measures in rehabilitation following anterior cruciate ligament injury. *Phys Ther Sports* 1:106–118, 2000; Noyes FR, McGinniss GH, Mooar LA: Functional disability in the anterior cruciate insufficient knee syndrome. Review of knee rating systems and projected risk factors in determining treatment. *Sports Med* 1:278–302, 1984.

[e]Data from Irrgang JJ, Snyder-Mackler L, Wainner RS, et al.: Development of a patient-reported measure of function of the knee. *J Bone Joint Surg* 80A: 1132–1145, 1998.

[f]Data from Binkley JM, Stratford PW, Lott SA, et al.: The Lower Extremity Functional Scale (LEFS): scale development, measurement properties, and clinical application. North American Orthopaedic Rehabilitation Research Network. *Phys Ther* 79:371–383, 1999.

function, self-reported symptoms, ROM, and ligament examination. The worst rating in any one of the four domains (normal, nearly normal, abnormal, or severely abnormal) determines the final rating of the knee.

Lysholm Knee Scoring Scale. The Lysholm Knee Scale[418] is commonly used as a subjective report scoring system designed to evaluate the intervention outcome and postsurgical result of knee patients. The scale consists of eight items related to limping; the need for an assistive device; ability to squat or climb stairs; and the presence of pain, swelling, locking, or "giving way," and leg atrophy.[419] Points are given for each level of ability or disability reported, with the perfect score being 100 (Table 20-13). The designers of this scale found that patients suffering from knee instability scored significantly lower than patients with minimal or no instability (average = 75.6 and 93.6, respectively).

Cincinnati Knee Rating System. The Cincinnati knee rating system self-report version uses a combination of functional level and symptom reporting to arrive at an overall disability rating for the knee.[420] The scale provides a point scoring system

TABLE 20-12 Western Ontario and McMaster Universities Osteoarthritis Index (WOMAC)

Name: ____________________

Primary Care Physician: ____________________

This survey asks for your views about the amount of pain, stiffness, and disability you are experiencing. Please answer every question by filling in the appropriate response. If you are unsure about how to answer a question, please give the best answer you can. (Please mark your answers with an "X")

SECTION A: PAIN

The following questions concern the amount of pain you are currently experiencing due to arthritis in your hips and/or knees. For each situation, please enter the amount of pain recently experienced.

***Question:* How much pain do you have?**

	None	Mild	Moderate	Severe	Extreme
1. Walking on a flat surface.	☐	☐	☐	☐	☐
2. Going up or down stairs.	☐	☐	☐	☐	☐
3. At night while in bed.	☐	☐	☐	☐	☐
4. Sitting or lying.	☐	☐	☐	☐	☐
5. Standing upright.	☐	☐	☐	☐	☐

SECTION B: JOINT STIFFNESS

The following questions concern the amount of joint stiffness (not pain) you are currently experiencing in your hips and/or knees. Stiffness is a sensation of restriction or slowness in the ease with which you move your joints.

	None	Mild	Moderate	Severe	Extreme
1. How severe is your stiffness after first wakening in the morning?	☐	☐	☐	☐	☐
2. How severe is your stiffness after sitting, lying, or resting later in the day?	☐	☐	☐	☐	☐

SECTION C: PHYSICAL FUNCTION

The following questions concern your physical function. By this we mean your ability to move around and to look after yourself. For each of the following activities, please indicate the degree of difficulty you are currently experiencing due to arthritis in your hips and/or knees. (Please mark your answers with an "X")

***Question:* What degree of difficulty do you have with:**

	None	Mild	Moderate	Severe	Extreme
1. Descending stairs.	☐	☐	☐	☐	☐
2. Ascending stairs.	☐	☐	☐	☐	☐
3. Rising from sitting.	☐	☐	☐	☐	☐
4. Standing.	☐	☐	☐	☐	☐
5. Bending to floor.	☐	☐	☐	☐	☐
6. Walking on flat.	☐	☐	☐	☐	☐
7. Getting in/out of car.	☐	☐	☐	☐	☐
8. Going shopping.	☐	☐	☐	☐	☐
9. Putting on socks/stockings.	☐	☐	☐	☐	☐
10. Rising from bed.	☐	☐	☐	☐	☐
11. Taking off socks/stockings.	☐	☐	☐	☐	☐
12. Lying in bed.	☐	☐	☐	☐	☐
13. Getting in/out of bath.	☐	☐	☐	☐	☐
14. Sitting.	☐	☐	☐	☐	☐
15. Getting on/off toilet.	☐	☐	☐	☐	☐
16. Heavy domestic duties.	☐	☐	☐	☐	☐
17. Light domestic duties.	☐	☐	☐	☐	☐

for the type of sports-related activity and frequency of participation, which allows an assessment outcome that is based on the patient's usual activities.

Knee Outcome Survey. The Knee Outcome Survey (KOS) consists of two separate scales: the activities of daily living scale (ADLS) and the sports activity scale (SAS). The ADLS (Table 20-14)[421] assesses the full spectrum of symptoms and functional limitations that may occur due to knee disorders.[419] The test–retest reliability of this scale is 0.97.[422] The SAS scale includes factors commonly experienced during sports activities.

Lower Extremity Function Scale. The lower extremity function scale was designed to be applicable to all lower extremity conditions of musculoskeletal origin.[423]

TABLE 20-13 Lysholm Knee Scoring Scale	
Category	**Score**
LIMP	
None	5
Slight or periodic	3
Serve and constant	0
SUPPORT	
None	5
Stick or crutch	3
Weight-bearing impossible	0
LOCKING	
No locking and no catching sensations	5
Catching, but no locking sensation	4
Locking	
Occasionally	2
Frequently	3
Locked joint on examination	0
INSTABILITY	
Never giving way	30
Rarely during athletics or other severe exertion	25
Frequently during athletics or other severe exertion (incapable of participation)	20
Occasionally in daily activities	10
Often in daily activities	5
With every step	0
PAIN	
None	30
Inconstant and slight during severe exertion	25
Marked on giving way	20
Marked during severe exertion	15
Marked on or after walking more than 2 km	10
Marked on or after walking less than 2 km	5
Constant	0
SWELLING	
None	10
With giving way	7
On severe exertion	5
On ordinary exertion	2
Constant	0
STAIR CLIMBING	
No problems	10
Slightly impaired	6
One step at a time	2
Impossible	0
SQUATTING	
No problems	5
Slightly impaired	4
Not beyond 90 degrees	2
Impossible	0

Data from Tegner Y, Lysholm J: Rating systems in the evaluation of knee ligament injuries. *Clin Orthop* 198:43–49, 1985.

Although these instruments have been commonly used to evaluate patients following knee surgery or trauma, relatively little work has been done to compare these knee instruments for the evaluation of athletic patients, and those that have been cross-sectional in design and therefore have not assessed reliability or how the instruments performed over time. Marx et al. performed a study to determine the reliability, validity, and responsiveness of the Lysholm scale, the American Academy of Orthopaedic Surgeons (AAOS) sports knee-rating scale (see "Advanced Functional Tests" section), the ADLS of the KOS, and the Cincinnati knee-rating system in athletic patients with a wide variety of disorders of the knee. According to the study, the reliability was high for all scales, with the ICC ranging from 0.88 to 0.95. As for construct validity, the correlations among the knee scales ranged from 0.70 to 0.85 and those between the knee scales and the physical component scale of the Short Form-36 (SF-36) and the patient and clinician severity ratings ranged from 0.59 to 0.77. Responsiveness, measured with the standardized response mean, ranged from 0.8 for the Cincinnati knee-rating system to 1.1 for the ADLS.

Patellar Joint Evaluation Scale. This scale assesses seven components of patellofemoral joint function (Table 20-15).

Objective Functional Tests

The functional tests for the knee are introduced once the patient is able to perform active and resisted motions without pain.

Aggregated Locomotor Function Score. The aggregated locomotor function (ALF) score was formed by summating the mean timed scores (seconds) from three locomotor functions (walking time, stair ascent, and stair descent) and time taken to transfer from sitting to standing.[424]

- ***Eight meter walk time.*** The patient is asked to walk 8 m at their own naturally preferred comfortable pace with or without walking aids as appropriate. Three repetitions of the walk are undertaken and the mean time is recorded.
- ***Stair ascent and descent time.*** The patient is asked to ascend and then descend seven steps (4 of 15 cm and 3 of 20 cm) at their naturally preferred comfortable pace. The method that the patient employs to negotiate the stairs is recorded, that is, whether they use alternate legs, use the banisters, or always lead with one leg. The patient is timed (in seconds) and asked to repeat the test four times. The mean time of the four repetitions is calculated.
- ***Transferring time.*** The patient is asked to walk, at their own natural pace, a distance of 2 m to a chair (with a seat height of 0.46 m, typical of a toilet seat) and sit down, then immediately stand up and walk back to the start. The patient is timed (in seconds) as they approach and retreat from the chair. The patient is asked to perform the test three times and the mean time is calculated.

The ALF score has demonstrated excellent intratester reliability with a high ICC statistic, narrow confidence

TABLE 20-14 Patient Reported Measure of Knee Function

ACTIVITIES OF DAILY LIVING SCALE

Instructions: The following questionnaire is designed to determine the symptoms and limitations that you experience because of your knee while you perform your usual daily activities. Please answer each question by checking the statement that best describes you over the last 1–2 days. For a given question, more than one of the statements may describe you, but please mark ONLY the statement that best describes you during your usual daily activities.

SYMPTOMS

1. To what degree does pain in your knee affect your daily activity level?
   5 I never have pain in my knee.
   4 I have pain in my knee, but it does not affect my daily activity.
   3 Pain affects my activity slightly.
   2 Pain affects my activity moderately.
   1 Pain affects my activity severely.
   0 Pain in my knee prevents me from performing all daily activities.
2. To what degree does grinding or grating of your knee affect your daily activity level?
   5 I never have grinding or grating in my knee.
   4 I have grinding or grating in my knee, but it does not affect my daily activity.
   3 Grinding or grating affects my activity slightly.
   2 Grinding or grating affects my activity moderately.
   1 Grinding or grating affects my knee slightly.
   0 Grinding or grating in my knee prevents me from performing daily activities.
3. To what degree does stiffness in your knee affect your daily activity level?
   5 I never have stiffness in my knee.
   4 I have stiffness in my knee, but it does not affect my daily activity.
   3 Stiffness affects my activity slightly.
   2 Stiffness affects my activity moderately.
   1 Stiffness affects my activity severely.
   0 Stiffness in my knee prevents me from performing all daily activities.
4. To what degree does swelling in your knee affect your daily activity level?
   5 I never have swelling in my knee.
   4 I have swelling in my knee, but it does not affect my daily activity.
   3 Swelling affects my activity slightly.
   2 Swelling affects my activity moderately.
   1 Swelling affects my activity severely.
   0 Swelling in my knee prevents me from performing all daily activities.
5. To what degree does slipping of your knee affect your daily activity level?
   5 I never have slipping of my knee.
   4 I have slipping of my knee, but it does not affect my daily activity.
   3 Slipping affects my activity slightly.
   2 Slipping affects my activity moderately.
   1 Slipping affects my activity severely.
   0 Slipping of my knee prevents me from performing all daily activities.
6. To what degree does buckling of your knee affect your daily activity level?
   5 I never have buckling of my knee.
   4 I have buckling of my knee, but it does not affect my daily activity level.
   3 Buckling affects my activity slightly.
   2 Buckling affects my activity moderately.
   1 Buckling affects my activity severely.
   0 Buckling of my knee prevents me from performing all daily activities.

(Continued)

TABLE 20-14 Patient Reported Measure of Knee Function *(Continued)*

SYMPTOMS

7. To what degree does weakness or lack of strength of your leg affect your daily activity level?
   5 My leg never feels weak.
   4 My leg feels weak, but it does not affect my daily activity.
   3 Weakness affects my activity slightly.
   2 Weakness affects my activity moderately.
   1 Weakness affects my activity severely.
   0 Weakness of my leg prevents me from performing all daily activities.

FUNCTIONAL DISABILITY WITH ACTIVITIES OF DAILY LIVING

8. How does your knee affect your ability to walk?
   5 My knee does not affect my ability to walk.
   4 I have pain in my knee when walking, but it does not affect my ability to walk.
   3 My knee prevents me from walking more than 1 mile.
   2 My knee prevents me from walking more than $^1/_2$ mile.
   1 My knee prevents me from walking more than 1 block.
   0 My knee prevents me from walking.
9. Because of your knee, do you walk with crutches or a cane?
   3 I can walk without crutches or a cane.
   2 My knee causes me to walk with 1 crutch or a cane.
   1 My knee causes me to walk with 2 crutches.
   0 Because of my knee, I cannot walk even with crutches.
10. Does your knee cause you to limp when you walk?
   2 I can walk without a limp.
   1 Sometimes my knee causes me to walk with a limp.
   0 Because of my knee, I cannot walk without a limp.
11. How does your knee affect your ability to go upstairs?
   5 My knee does not affect my ability to go upstairs.
   4 I have pain in my knee when going upstairs, but it does not limit my ability to go upstairs.
   3 I am able to go upstairs normally, but I need to rely on use of a railing.
   2 I am able to go upstairs one step at a time with use of a railing.
   1 I have to use crutches or a cane to go upstairs.
   0 I cannot go upstairs.
12. How does your knee affect your ability to go downstairs?
   5 My knee does not affect my ability to go downstairs.
   4 I have pain in my knee when going downstairs, but it does not limit my ability to go downstairs.
   3 I am able to go downstairs normally, but I need to rely on use of a railing.
   2 I am able to go downstairs one step at a time with use of railing.
   1 I have to use crutches or a cane to go downstairs.
   0 I cannot go downstairs.
13. How does your knee affect your ability to stand?
   5 My knee does not affect my ability to stand. I can stand for unlimited amounts of time.
   4 I have pain in my knee when standing, but it does not limit my ability to stand.
   3 Because of my knee, I cannot stand for more than 1 hour.
   2 Because of my knee, I cannot stand for more than half an hour.
   1 Because of my knee, I cannot stand for more than 10 minutes.
   0 I cannot stand because of my knee.

(Continued)

TABLE 20-14 Patient Reported Measure of Knee Function *(Continued)*

14. How does your knee affect your ability to kneel on the front of your knee?
   5 My knee does not affect my ability to kneel on the front of my knee. I can kneel for unlimited amounts of time.
   4 I have pain when kneeling on the front of my knee, but it does not limit my ability to kneel.
   3 I cannot kneel on the front of my knee for more than 1 hour.
   2 I cannot kneel on the front of my knee for more than half an hour.
   1 I cannot kneel on the front of my knee for more than 10 minutes.
   0 I cannot kneel on the front of my knee.
15. How does your knee affect your ability to squat?
   5 My knee does not affect my ability to squat. I can squat all the way down.
   4 I have pain when squatting, but I can still squat all the way down.
   3 I cannot squat more than $^3/_4$ of the way down.
   2 I cannot squat more than $^1/_2$ of the way down.
   1 I cannot squat more than $^1/_4$ of the way down.
   0 I cannot squat at all.
16. How does your knee affect your ability to sit with your knee bent?
   5 My knee does not affect my ability to sit with my knee bent. I can sit for unlimited amounts of time.
   4 I have pain when sitting with my knee bent, but it does not limit my ability to sit.
   3 I cannot sit with my knee bent for more than 1 hour.
   2 I cannot sit with my knee bent for more than half an hour.
   1 I cannot sit with my knee bent for more than 10 minutes.
   0 I cannot sit with my knee bent.
17. How does your knee affect your ability to rise from a chair?
   5 My knee does not affect my ability to rise from a chair.
   4 I have pain when rising from the seated position, but it does not affect my ability to rise from the seated position.
   3 Because of my knee, I can only rise from a chair if I use my hands and arms to assist.
   0 Because of my knee, I cannot rise from a chair.

intervals, low standard error of measurement (SEM), and low smallest detectable difference (SDD).[424] Importantly, the measure demonstrates moderately sized correlation with two validated self-report questionnaires of physical function (SF-36 and WOMAC) and appears to be more responsive to change induced by exercise intervention, than either.[424]

Simple Functional Weight-Bearing Tests

The simplest functional weight-bearing test for the knee is the squat position. The patient should be able to perform this maneuver without pain.

Duck Walk/Childress Sign. The patient squats with the toes pointing outward and walks forward. This maneuver is similar to the McMurray test for meniscal lesion (although more stressful). Pain, or crepitus, with this test supposedly indicates a lesion of the posterior horn of the meniscus or the MCL.[367] A positive test for meniscus tear is indicated by a block preventing full flexion or pain at end range flexion. However, studies have shown that pain neither with squatting nor with a duck walk seem to indicate a torn meniscus.[401,425]

Incidentally, a patient with a patellofemoral lesion can duck walk without difficulty, but experiences difficulty coming up out of the squat.[259]

Advanced Functional Tests

More advanced functional tests for the knee include the following AAOS sports knee-rating scale, vertical jump, functional hop, single-leg squat, and running tests.[419]

American Academy of Orthopaedic Surgeons Sports Knee-Rating Scale. The AAOS sports knee-rating scale was included in the Musculoskeletal Outcomes Data Evaluation and Management System (MODEMS) for athletic patients with disorders of the knee. This instrument has five parts with a total of 23 questions: a core section (seven questions) on stiffness, swelling, pain, and function, and four sections (four questions each) on locking or catching on activity, giving-way on activity, current activity limitations due to the knee, and pain on activity due to the knee.

Vertical Jump. Vertical jumping is an explosive movement, in which the vertical velocity of the trunk is of decisive importance for jump height. The vertical jump test is commonly used in sports medicine, and investigators have found it to be significantly related to athletic performance.[426–432] The vertical jump is performed in the following manner. A baseline measurement is made of the highest point that the patient can reach while remaining flat footed. The patient's fingertips are covered with chalk and he or she is then asked to jump as high

TABLE 20-15 Patellofemoral Joint Evaluation Scale	
Function	**Points**
Limp	
None	5
Slight or episodic	3
Severe	0
Assistive devices	
None	5
Cane or brace	3
Unable to bear weight	0
Stair climbing	
No problem	20
Slight impairment	15
Very slowly	10
One step at a time, always same leg first	5
Unable	0
Crepitation	
None	5
Annoying	3
Limits activities	2
Severe	0
Instability (giving way)	
Never	20
Occasionally with vigorous activities	10
Frequently with vigorous activities	8
Occasionally with daily activities	5
Frequently with daily activities	2
Every day	0
Swelling	
None	10
After vigorous activities only	5
After walking or mild activities	2
Constant	0
Pain	
None	35
Occasionally with vigorous activities	30
Marked with vigorous activities	20
Marked after walking 1 mile or mild or moderate rest pain	15
Marked with walking <1 mile	10
Constant and severe	0

Scoring: 90–100 points, excellent; 80–90 points, good; 60–79 points, fair: <60 points, poor.
Data from Karlson J, Thomee R, Sward L: Eleven year follow-up of patellofemoral pain syndromes. *Clin J Sports Med* 6:23, 1996.

as possible, marking the wall with the chalk on the fingertips. The patient is allowed three jumps, after which the clinician subtracts the baseline reach from the maximum vertical jump to obtain the vertical jump distance.

Functional Hop Tests

- ***Hop for distance.*** This test has good test–retest reliability (0.79–0.99),[429,430,432–437] although its correlation with power and isokinetic strength testing is unclear.[336,428,430,437–440] The patient stands on the involved leg, with the toes as close to the starting position as possible. The hands are placed behind the back or on the hips. The patient then tries to hop as far as possible, landing on the same extremity. Three attempts are permitted. The distance is measured from the take-off toe to the landing heel and is compared with the hop distance of the uninvolved leg, and scored as a percentage. The distances hopped are influenced by age and sex.[436] Norms for this test in high school athletes are an average of 155 cm for boys and an average of 121 cm for girls.[441] The sensitivity of this test has been found to be 52% and the specificity to be 97%.[442] Barber et al.[430] found a significant relationship between the one-legged hop and the subjective limitations of sprinting, jumping, and landing.
- ***Triple hop.***[429,443] The triple-hop test is similar to the hop-for-distance test, except that the patient hops for three consecutive hops, and the score is the distance measured from the take-off toe to the landing heel of the third jump. One study reported a high correlation between concentric isokinetic strength of the quadriceps muscle and the triple hop for distance.[440]
- ***Timed 6-m hop.***[430,432,434] This test is reliable, with an ICC ranging from 0.66 to 0.77,[429,433] and is considered to be one of the best indicators of function.[438] The clinician marks off a distance of 6 m and the patient performs single-leg hops over the distance. The time taken is measured to the nearest 0.01 second and compared with the uninvolved leg. This functional test evaluates the strength, endurance, proprioception, balance, and power of the various knee structures. The test is recommended for use with athletes returning to sport. The sensitivity of this test has been found to be 49%, and the specificity to be 94%.[442]
- ***Crossover hop.*** The crossover hop has an ICC of 0.96 for test–retest reliability.[429] The results of this test have a relationship with the isokinetic parameter of acceleration range and are considered to be the best indicator of knee function.[438] The test is performed as follows: the patient places his or her feet behind the start line and a tape measure is laid perpendicular to that line. The patient is asked to stand on one leg to the right of the tape measure. The patient is then asked to jump, on one leg, to the left side of the tape, back to the right, and then back to the left, attempting to propel himself or herself forward as far as possible with each hop. The score is the distance measured from the take-off toe to the landing heel of the third jump. Three attempts are permitted, and two sides are compared as a percentage of each other.
- ***Stairs hop.*** The patient is timed as he or she hops up and down several steps (20–25 steps are recommended), first on the uninvolved leg and then on the involved leg.[443]
- ***Side-to-side hop.*** Steadman[444] advocates the use of the side-to-side Heiden hop. The Heiden hop involves the patient jumping from side to side, to a line placed approximately 5–6 feet (1.5–1.8 m) apart. The landing is

controlled with a soft flexion of the knee, balancing the body on the foot closest to the line. The patient then leaps sideways to the other line, landing on the opposite foot in a controlled fashion, gently assuming a semisquat position on the single leg.[445] This exercise is performed side to side for 5–10 minutes. Evidence of an ungraceful landing, loss of balance, or shaking muscles on the involved side indicates weakness of the quadriceps.[445]

Single-Leg Squat Test. The patient is asked to balance on one leg and then to squat down on that leg while keeping the trunk erect. The amount of flexion at the knee is measured with a goniometer and is compared with a similar measure of the uninvolved leg. If a hand or the opposite extremity touches the ground, the measurement is retaken. Although seemingly a static test, this is a test of the dynamic ability of the quadriceps, hamstring, gluteal, and gastrocnemius muscles to maintain eccentric control, and for the patient to maintain balance.

Running Tests

- *Figure-of-eight running.* Two cones are positioned 10 m apart. The patient is asked to run around the cones in a figure-of-eight pattern, for a certain number of rotations, rounding the turns rather than planting and cutting, while the clinician times the run. The time ratio of figure-of-eight running to straight running is one of the most definitive ways to compare patients with an ACL-deficient knee to those with normal knees.[446]
- *Carioca test.* The carioca test involves the patient running laterally with a crossover of the legs and a weaving of the feet, beginning with the trailing leg in front, then trailing the leg in back of the leading leg, for a distance of either 8 feet[447] or 24.4 m.[448]
- *Shuttle run.*[439,449] The shuttle run involves having the patient run between cones or varying distances.

Imaging Studies

Radiographic imaging of the knee is described in Chapter 7. Arthrograms of the knee are used primarily to diagnose tears in the menisci and plica, although their use is gradually being replaced by arthroscopy, which allows the surgeon to diagnose and repair lesions simultaneously.

THE EVALUATION

Following the examination, and once the clinical findings have been recorded, the clinician must determine a specific diagnosis or a working hypothesis, based on a summary of all of the findings. This diagnosis can be structure related (medical diagnosis) (Table 20-16), or a diagnosis based on the preferred practice patterns as described in the *Guide to Physical Therapist Practice.*

Intervention Strategies

Acute knee injuries are a common occurrence. One study[450] demonstrated, perhaps not surprisingly, that the most common type of acute knee injuries were sports related, occurred in men younger than 35 years of age, and were of moderate severity. Studies[450–452] that compare the two sexes report higher rates of sports injuries in men. This finding could be a result of the greater numbers of men participating in sports activities or the greater frequency of injuries in men who do participate in sports.

Of particular interest are non–sports-related falls, which are experienced two to three times more frequently in women than in men, except in the group older than 55 years, for whom the incidence of falls is equal in both sexes.[450]

Most knee pain of nontraumatic origin improves with conservative intervention.[453] Different approaches have been emphasized over the years, including patient education,[454–456] activity modification ,[147,455,457,458] progressive muscle stretching and strengthening,[136,147,454,456–461] functional lower extremity training,[462] external patellar supports and braces,[147,454,456,463,464] foot orthotics (Table 20-17),[464,465] and taping to improve patella tracking.[454,457,460,466,467]

This wide range of interventions raises the question of whether any of them are efficacious, or whether a combination of some is to be recommended. What is clear is that the impairments and functional limitations found during the examination must guide the intervention. The successful intervention requires detailing the factors that influence these impairments and functional limitations, and determining the stage of healing.

Whatever the knee injury, the goal of the rehabilitation program is to return the patient to an optimum level of function. The emphasis during knee rehabilitation must focus on achieving a balance between allowing the damaged structures to heal, improving muscle control, and increasing the competence of the static restraints. Consideration must also be given to the various forces placed on the knee during CKC and OKC exercises. The techniques to increase joint mobility and soft tissue extensibility are described in "Therapeutic Techniques" section.

Acute Phase

Every attempt is made to protect the joint to promote and progress the healing. The goals during the acute phase are to

- reduce pain and swelling;
- control inflammation;
- regain ROM;
- minimize muscle atrophy and weakness;
- attain early neuromuscular control;
- maintain or improve the patient's general cardiovascular fitness.

The reduction of pain and the control of swelling are extremely important as both can inhibit normal muscle function and control. The principles of PRICEMEM (protection, rest, ice, compression, elevation, manual therapy, early motion, and medication) are used to minimize pain, swelling, and inflammation.

TABLE 20-16 Differential Diagnosis of Common Causes of Knee Pain

Condition	Patient Age (years)	Mechanism of injury	Area of Symptoms	Aggravated by Symptoms	Observation
Patellofemoral syndrome	20–50	Gradual Macrotrauma Microtrauma	Anterior knee	Prolonged sitting Stairs Kneeling	Possible soft tissue thickening/swelling at anterior knee
Patellar tendinitis	15–50	Gradual (repeated eccentric overloading during deceleration activities)	Anterior knee	Squatting, jumping	Usually unremarkable
Quadriceps muscle tear	20–40	Sudden overload	Anterior thigh	Squatting	Possible bruising over anterior thigh/knee Possible swelling over anterior thigh/knee
Knee osteoarthritis	50+	Gradual due to microtrauma Macrotrauma	Generalized knee	Weight-bearing	Possible soft tissue thickening/swelling around knee
Anterior cruciate ligament sprain/tear	15–45	Trauma to knee (sudden deceleration, an abrupt change of direction, valgus force, rotary force) while foot is fixed	Varies according to number of associated structures involved Typically associated with immediate swelling of knee (acute hemarthrosis)	Weight-bearing	Knee swelling
Collateral ligament injury	Varies	Trauma to contralateral aspect of knee (valgus or varus)	Distal femur on medial or lateral aspect depending on whether MCL or LCL is involved	Varus stress (LCL) Valgus stress (MCL)	Swelling may be present depending on extent of trauma
Prepatellar bursitis	15–50	Direct trauma to anterior aspect of knee	Anterior knee	Kneeling	Local swelling, fluctuation
Patellar subluxation/dislocation	Varies	Twisting injury with the femur internally rotating on a fixed foot, although there may be no history of trauma	Varies according to tissues involved	Weight-bearing	Dependent on the degree of trauma
Lumbar disk pathology	20–50	Gradual Sudden overload of lumbar spine	L3 dermatome	Trunk flexion Bearing down	May have associated trunk deviation

(Continued)

TABLE 20-16 Differential Diagnosis of Common Causes of Knee Pain *(Continued)*

AROM	PROM	End-Feel	Resisted	Tenderness with Palpation
Usually no limited ranges	Pain at end range knee flexion	Usually unremarkable	Usually no pain with resisted tests	Anterior knee especially with patella compression
Usually unremarkable	Pain at end range knee flexion	Usually unremarkable	May have pain with resisted knee extension	Over the patellar tendon, inferior or superior to the patellar
Limited knee flexion	Pain with combined hip extension and knee flexion	Spasm/empty depending on extent of injury	Pain with resisted hip flexion;;; Pain with resisted knee extension	Anterior thigh
Loss of motion in a capsular pattern	Pain at end range knee flexion and extension	Unremarkable	Generalized weakness	Typically posterior knee if present at all
Loss of some knee flexion and extension (depending on extent of swelling)	Pain at end ranges	Loss of firm end-feel with Lachman/anterior drawer	Pain with resisted knee rotation	Depends on associated injuries
Depends on extent of trauma	Possible pain at end range of tibial rotation	Depends on extent of injury	Usually negative	Distal medial femur to medial joint line (MCL) Distal lateral femur to lateral joint line (LCL)
Unremarkable	Sometimes passive flexion is painful	Usually unremarkable	Usually unremarkable	Anterior aspect of knee
Dependent on extent of trauma	Dependent on extent of trauma, usually apprehension present	Spasm/empty	Usually unable to perform secondary to pain	Lateral femoral condyle, retinacular, patellar facet
Usually pain with trunk flexion	Unremarkable	May have painful SLR	Fatiguable weakness in associated myotome	May have tenderness over involved spinal segment

TABLE 20-17 Randomized Clinical Trials and Other Experimental Studies Related to Foot Orthotics and Patellofemoral Pain Syndrome

Investigators	Independent Variables	Dependent Variables	N	Statistical Significance	Clinical Importance	Study Design
Eng JJ and Pierrynowski MR[a]	Exercise group (isometric quadriceps set, straight leg raise, stretching) and soft orthotic group	Maximum pain (visual analog scale) with activities (walking, running, stair ascent, stairs descent, sitting one hour, squatting)	20 women with patellofemoral pain (comparison group, $n = 10$; experimental group, $n = 10$)	Statistically significant ($P < 0.05$) at weeks 4, 6, and 8.	Clinically important as compared with the compassion group	Randomized clinical trial
Eng JJ and Pierrynowski MR[b]	Walking and running with and without orthotics	Knee, talocrural, and subtalar joints range of motion for each plane of motion	10 women with patellofemoral pain syndrome and forefoot varus and calcaneal valgus >6 degrees	No significant difference at the knee except transverse and frontal plane range of motion	Could not determine	Repeated measures analysis
Hung Y and Gross MT[c]	Three foot positions (supinated, pronated, and neutral)	Vastus medialis obliquus–vastus lateralis EMG ratio (isometric quadriceps set; one leg squat, 0–50 degrees)	16 nonimpaired subjects (20 subjects started the study)	No significant difference	Not clinically important	Repeated measures analysis
Tomaro J and Burdett RG[d]	Walking with and without orthotics	EMG: tibialis anterior, fibularis (peroneus) longus, gastrocnemius	10 subjects with a history of like pathology (three men and seven women)	Average muscle electromyogram, no significant difference; duration and tibialis anterior/stance × 100% $P < 0.05$	Not clinically important	Repeated measures with randomization
Nawoczenski DA et al.[e]	Running with orthotics	Tibial internal rotation	20 recreational runners with lower limb pain	A decrease of 2.1 degrees in tibial rotation	Clinically important	Repeated measures analysis

Data from Lohman EB, Harp T: Patellofemoral pain: A critical appraisal of the literature. In: Wilmarth MA, ed.: *Evidence-Based Practice for the Upper and Lower Quarter. Orthopaedic Physical Therapy Home Study Course* 13.2.1 La Crosse, WI: Orthopaedic Section, APTA, 2003:1–44. With permission from Orthopaedic Section, APTA.

[a]Data from Eng JJ, Pierrynowski MR: The effect of soft foot orthotics on three-dimensional lower-limb kinematics during walking and running. *Phys Ther* 74:836–844, 1994.

[b]Data from Eng JJ, Pierrynowski MR: Evaluation of soft foot orthotics in the treatment of patellofemoral pain syndrome. *Phys Ther* 73:62–68; discussion 68–70, 1993.

[c]Data from Hung YJ, Gross MT: Effect of foot position on electromyographic activity of the vastus medialis oblique and vastus lateralis during lower-extremity weight-bearing activities. *J Orthop Sports Phys Ther* 29:93–102, 1999; discussion 103–105.

[d]Data from Tomaro J, Burdett RG: The effects of foot orthotics on the EMG activity of selected leg muscles during gait. *J Orthop Sports Phys Ther* 18:532–536, 1993.

[e]Data from Nawoczenski DA, Cook TM, Saltzman CL: The effect of foot orthotics on three-dimensional kinematics of the leg and rearfoot during running. *J Orthop Sports Phys Ther* 21:317–327, 1995.

Therapeutic Exercises

Numerous clinical trials have used therapeutic exercise as part of a comprehensive intervention program for both the tibiofemoral and patellofemoral joints.[235,243,250,468–470,471]

Once the pain, swelling, and inflammation are under control, early controlled ROM exercises are initiated. In the acute phase of healing, the interventions focus on decreased loading of the joint complex, which might include postural correction, activity modification, or the use of an assistive device. Bracing may be needed to provide adequate protection (see the discussion in "Functional Phase" section). Exercises prescribed for the knee joint complex must include those that promote neuromuscular control, timing, balance, and proprioception.

Exercises recommended for this phase include isometric muscle setting (quadriceps sets VIDEO, hamstring sets, gluteal sets), active knee flexion (heel slides VIDEO), straight leg raises (if appropriate) (Fig. 20-47), hip swings VIDEO and patellar mobilizations. Proprioceptive neuromuscular facilitation (PNF) activities may be initiated with slow-speed, low-force, controlled exercises. Electrical stimulation can be used to facilitate muscle activity and to promote muscle reeducation.[472] The training of the VMO should be regarded as a motor skill acquisition rather than a strengthening procedure,[150,473] with the goal of the training to produce a modification of the length–tension relationship between the VMO and its antagonist, the VL. This may result in a change of the equilibrium point, which will enable the appropriate alignment of the patella.[474] If the muscle control of the VMO is poor, biofeedback can be used to augment the hip adductor training.[475] Taping can be used as an adjunct (see later discussion).

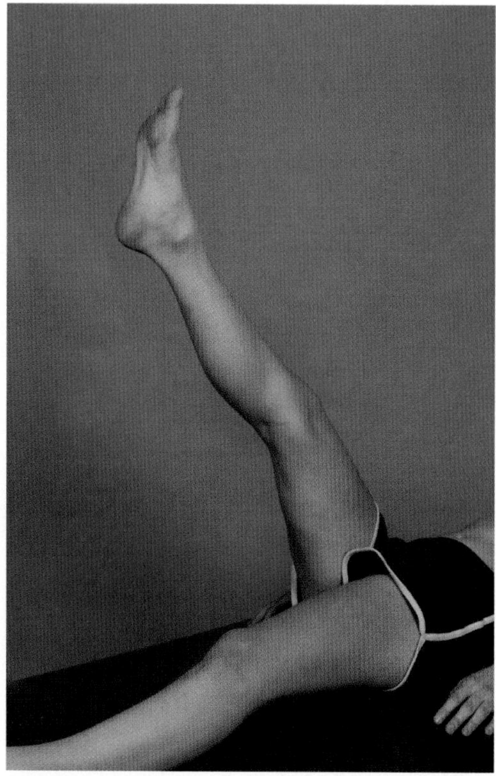

FIGURE 20-47 Straight leg raise.

Once the muscle control is achieved, gentle CKC exercises are initiated. CKC exercises initially include small-range wall slides and heel raises. Contractions of the quadriceps should be encouraged in the functional knee positions that provoke pain, such as sitting, and stair negotiation. The benefit of CKCEs is that they decrease shear forces and emphasize cocontractions.[476,477] General recommendations for CKC exercise at the knee are from 0 to 20 degrees,[471] or 0–40 degrees of flexion.[234] All the exercises performed in the clinic should be performed by the patient at home whenever possible.

Tibiofemoral Joint

The CKC exercises previously mentioned are progressed to include the supine leg press, the hip sled with minimal resistance.[478231] These exercises are performed bilaterally initially and then unilaterally once there is evidence of good dynamic stability.

Cocontraction exercises for the hamstrings and quadriceps, which further reduce tibiofemoral shear forces,[243,244,308,479,480] can be achieved by having the patient perform single-leg bridges by leaning back on a Swiss ball (Fig. 20-48) and raising the uninvolved leg off the floor, while the involved leg is used to maintain balance. Cocontraction also can be accomplished by "single-leg" wall slides using the Swiss ball (Fig. 20-49), with the uninvolved leg supporting most of the body weight.

Stationary bicycling has long been recognized as a useful therapeutic exercise for knee rehabilitation to control the ROM and impact forces at the knee.

- The ROM at the knee can be controlled by adjusting the seat height.
- The impact forces can be adjusted on most exercise bicycles by varying the resistance at the pedal–foot interface.

The amount of strain on the ACL during stationary bicycling is relatively low compared with other rehabilitation activities[481] (see Table 20-1).

Patellofemoral Joint

Rehabilitation that includes a combination of painless muscle strengthening, stretching, and patellofemoral taping often is beneficial in creating an internal biomechanical environment that encourages maximal tissue healing.[482] A number of

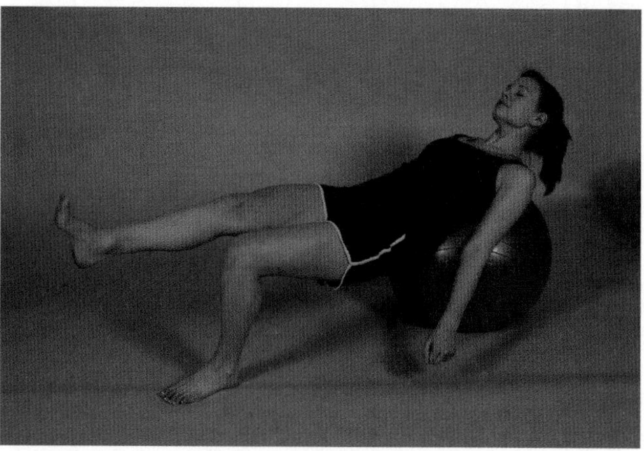

FIGURE 20-48 Single-leg bridges on Swissball.

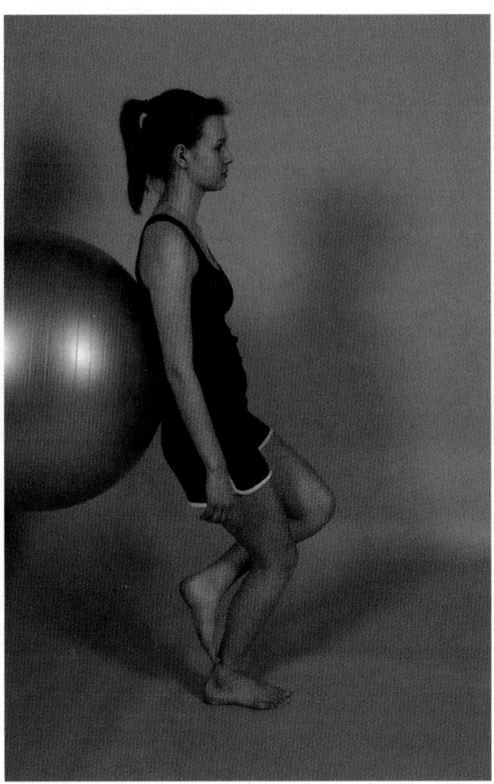

FIGURE 20-49 Wall slide with Swissball.

classification systems have been used to categorize individuals with patellofemoral disorders (Table 20-18). As with any disorder, although the use of a classification system may help, the clinician must formulate effective treatment interventions based on the findings from the history, subjective examination, physical examination, functional assessment, and the patient's response to the prescribed exercises.

A number of activities have been identified that increase patellofemoral compression. These include jumping, stair climbing, squatting, prolonged sitting with the knee flexed beyond 40 degrees, prolonged kneeling, arising from chairs, prone lying, or standing in genu recurvatum.[9,147] During the early stages of healing, the patient must try to avoid these activities or at least minimize exposure. In the presence of biomechanical dysfunctions of the foot, including pronation, correct footwear must be worn. If the malalignment of the lower extremity is severe, a foot orthosis can be prescribed.[463,474] The type of orthosis used is dependent on the diagnosis. Most commonly, an orthosis is used to correct a flat foot so that the patella no longer squints. Foot pronation imparts internal torsion to the tibia and a valgus moment at the knee. Klingman et al.[483] have shown that medial rearfoot-posted orthoses result in a more medial position of the patella during static weight-bearing radiographs. In the presence of genu recurvatum, a heel raise can be issued for use during

TABLE 20-18 Classification Systems for Nonoperative Patellofemoral Syndrome

Lohman[a]	Wilk et al.[b]	Holmes et al.[c]
1. Overconstrained—tight lateral or inferior structures (tilt, glide, anteroposterior tilt) 2. Combination—tight lateral structures and loose medial structures 3. Underconstrained—loose lateral and medial structures (excessive joint play) resulting in instability (subluxation or dislocation) 4. Normal—normal alignment but painful (e.g., tendinitis, apophysitis, or bursitis) 5. Unable or not specified—the underlying cause of patellofemoral pain syndrome cannot be determined 6. Other causation—osteochondrosis dissecans, chondromalacia patellae, sympathetically maintained pain, fractures, synovial plicae	1. Patellar compression syndrome—excessive lateral pressure syndrome; global pressure syndrome 2. Patellar instability—chronic patellar subluxation; recurrent patellar dislocation 3. Biomechanical dysfunction 4. Direct patella trauma—articular cartilage lesion (isolated); fracture and dislocation; articular cartilage lesion with associated malalignment 5. Soft tissue lesions—suprapatellar plica, fat pad syndrome; medial patellofemoral ligament pain; iliotibial band friction syndrome 6. Overuse syndromes—tendinitis; apophysitis 7. Osteochondritis dissecans 8. Neurologic disorders—complex regional pain syndrome; sympathetically maintained pain	1. Patellofemoral instability—subluxation or dislocation, single episode; lateral or medial subluxation or dislocation, recurrent; chronic dislocation of patella, congenital or acquired; associated fractures, osteochondral or avulsion 2. Patellofemoral pain with malalignment—increased functional quadriceps angle (femoral anteversion, external tibial torsion, genu valgum, foot hyperpronation); tight lateral retinaculum; grossly inadequate medial stabilizers; electrical dissociation; patella alta; patella baja; dysplastic femoral trochlea 3. Patellofemoral pain without malalignment—tight medial and lateral retinaculum; plica (medial, lateral, suprapatellar); osteochondritis dissecans; traumatic patellar chondromalacia; fat pad syndrome; patellofemoral osteoarthritis; patella tendinitis; quadriceps tendinitis; prepatellar bursitis; apophysitis; symptomatic bipartite patella; other trauma (quadriceps tendon rupture, patella tendon rupture, patella fracture, proximal tibial epiphysis fracture, contusion, turf knee or wrestler's knee, cruciate ligament instability)

Data from: Lohman EB, Harp T: Patellofemoral pain: A critical appraisal of the literature. In: Wilmarth MA, ed. *Evidence-Based Practice for the Upper and Lower Quarter. Orthopaedic Physical Therapy Home Study Course* 13.2.1 La Crosse, WI: Orthopaedic Section, APTA, 2003:1–44.

[a]Data from Lohman EB: Diagnosis and management of patellofemoral pain. In: Godges J, Deyle G, eds. *Lower Quadrant: Evidence-Based Description of Clinical Practice. Orthop Phys Ther Clin North Am*, 1998:367–396.

[b]Data from Wilk KE, Davies GJ, Mangine RE, et al.: Patellofemoral disorders: a classification system and clinical guidelines for nonoperative rehabilitation. *J Orthop Sports Phys Ther* 28:307–322, 1998.

[c]Data from Holmes SWJ, Clancy WGJ: Clinical classification of patellofemoral pain and dysfunction. *J Orthop Sports Phys Ther* 28:299–306, 1998.

exercise. It is therefore reasonable, for selected patients, to prescribe an orthotic device for the shoe.[188,484]

It remains unclear to what extent there are specific exercises to strengthen the VMO.[11,146,485] A study by Mirzabeigi et al.[486] attempted to isolate the VMO from the VL, vastus intermedius, and VML, using nine sets of strengthening exercises. These exercises included isometric knee extension with the hip in neutral, 30 degrees of external rotation, and 30 degrees of internal rotation; isokinetic knee extension through full range; isokinetic knee extension in the terminal 30-degree arc; side-lying ipsilateral and contralateral full knee extension; and stand and jump from a full squat. Although the study concluded that isometric exercises in neutral and external rotation of the hip challenged both the VMO and VL, none of the exercises demonstrated isolation of the VMO.[486] Indeed, a thorough review of the existing literature shows that isolated contraction of the VMO, independent of the VL has never been documented.[487] The VMO does not extend the knee and is not, therefore, activated by the traditional straight leg raise,[488] even with the addition of adduction.[489] However, because of the relationship of the VMO to the adductor magnus, and its separate nerve supply in most cases,[137] the clinician should still emphasize adduction of the thigh, while minimizing internal rotation of the hip, to facilitate a VMO contraction.[475] According to Hodges and Richardson,[490] activation of the adductor magnus significantly improves the VMO contraction in weight-bearing, but maximum contraction of the adductor magnus in non–weight-bearing is required before facilitating VMO activity.

The hip external rotators and abductors affect lower limb control, and a strengthening program that addresses these muscle groups should be integrated into the overall progression. For example, weakness of the hip external rotators may allow uncontrolled and excessive pronation of the foot to occur along with excessive femoral internal rotation, both contributing to an increase in the valgus alignment of the knee, thereby increasing the Q-angle.[167] Strengthening of the hip rotators may need to be initiated in the OKC, but should be advanced to strengthening in the CKC as soon as functional muscular control is present.[167]

Exercises during this phase include the following:

- Isometric quadriceps sets at 20 degrees of flexion, progressing to multiple angle isometrics.
- Heel slides with the tibia positioned in internal and then external rotation.
- Straight leg raises performed with the thigh externally rotated and the knee flexed to 20 degrees. Performing the exercise in this fashion is reported to allow the least amount of patellofemoral contact force while maximally stressing the vastus medialis component of the quadriceps muscle.[207,232,491] The resistance is progressed from 0 to 5 lb.
- Straight leg raises performed into abduction with the thigh externally rotated to enhance strengthening of the gluteus medius.
- Low-resistance knee extension (short-arc quadriceps) exercises, performed with the leg externally rotated, from 50 to 20 degrees (avoiding terminal knee extension) (Fig. 20-50). During non–weight-bearing knee extension, the amount of quadriceps muscle force required to extend the knee steadily increases as in the moves from 90 degrees to full knee extension. The resistance is progressed from 0 to 5 lb.
- Hip adduction exercises performed in the side-lying position on the involved side (Fig. 20-51). The exercise can also be performed with the hip internally rotated and the knee flexed to 20 degrees.[140,492] This position of knee flexion places the patella midway between the two femoral condyles.

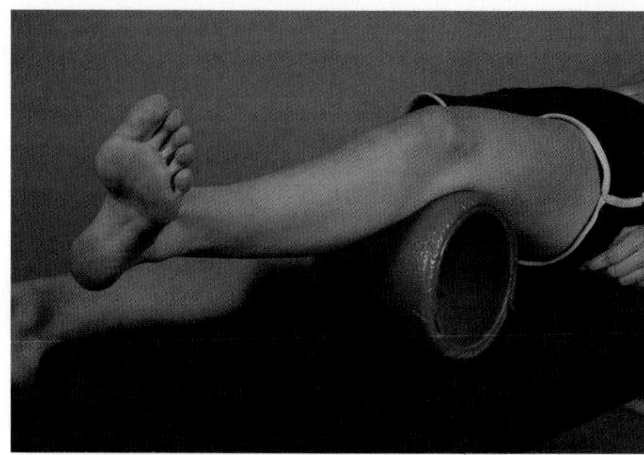

FIGURE 20-50 Short arc quad in external rotation.

Functional exercises that incorporate the entire lower kinetic chain are implemented as soon as tolerated. Kibler[493] advocates the following protocol:

- Active hip extension and quadriceps activation with the foot flat on the floor or stepping on or off a flat step (Fig. 20-52). This reactivates the normal sequencing pattern for the entire leg.
- Isolation and maximal activation of the quadriceps in a CKC position by working with the foot on a slant board (Fig. 20-53), effectively removing the hip and ankle from full activation, but placing maximal load on the slightly flexed knee. Care must be taken not to exercise through pain as this may indicate that muscle control is insufficient.[150] During weight-bearing exercises, the quadriceps muscle force is relatively minimal when the knee is extended and steadily increases as the knee flexes.
- Unilateral stance with hip extension, slight knee flexion, and hip and trunk rotation.

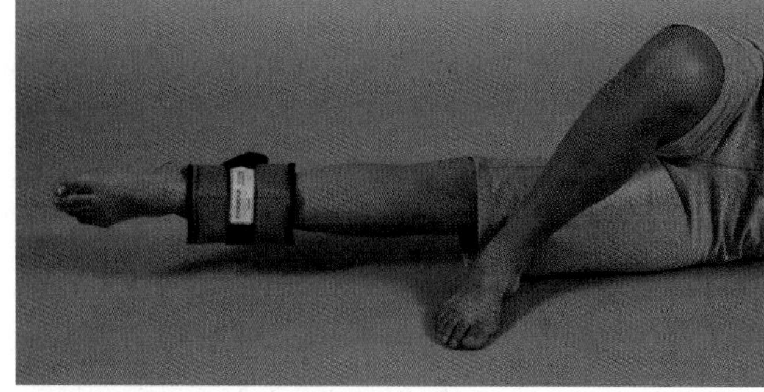

FIGURE 20-51 SLR into adduction.

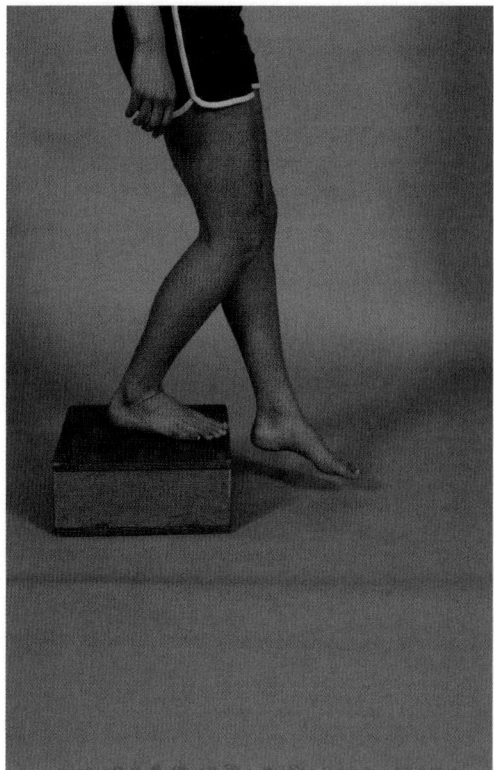

FIGURE 20-52 Step downs.

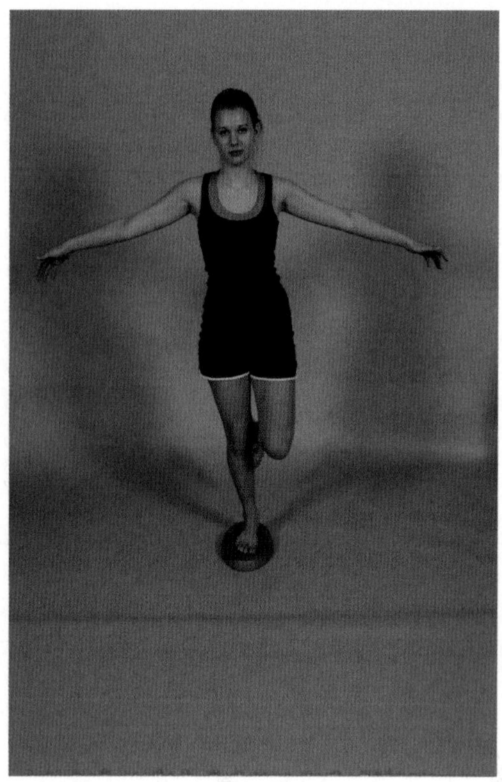

FIGURE 20-54 Unilateral stance on soft surface.

The correction of muscle inflexibilities is very important in the rehabilitative process. This activity can be made more challenging using softer surfaces (Fig. 20-54).

Stretching of the quadriceps VIDEO hip flexors, ITB, lateral retinaculum, hamstrings, and gastrocnemius are usually initiated during this phase. The rationale for stretching the ITB and lateral retinaculum is well recognized.[129,454,494] Adaptive shortening in the hamstrings and gastrocnemii has been associated with a compensatory pronation.[320] In addition, adaptively shortened hamstrings may cause increased flexion of the knee and increased patellofemoral compression forces, especially during the stance phase of gait.[300] Correction of muscle imbalances is based on a full analysis as to the effect that these interventions will have on the pathologic process, or on other structures within the kinetic chain. For example, stretching the hamstrings of an elderly patient to relieve the stresses at the knee may exacerbate the symptoms of lateral recess stenosis, because the adaptively shortened hamstrings may be helping to maintain the pelvis in a posterior pelvic tilt.[495]

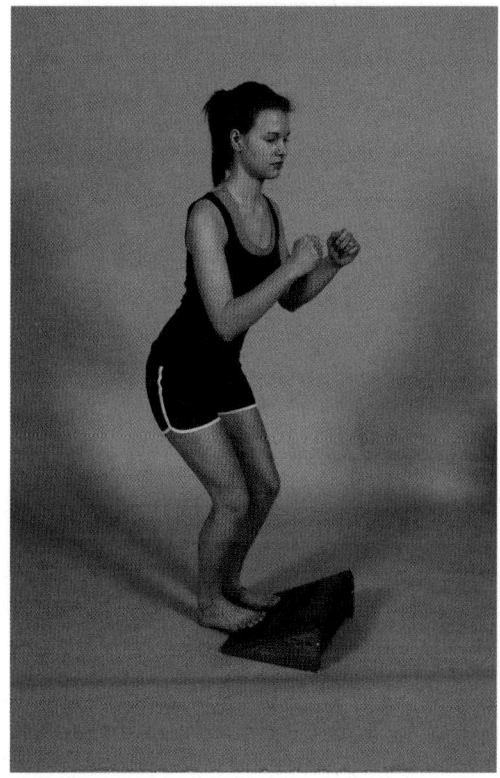

FIGURE 20-53 Squat on slant board.

Functional Phase

The functional phase of the knee rehabilitation program should be designed to addresses any tissue overload problems and functional biomechanical deficits once the painful symptoms have improved. During this phase, the patient gradually and incrementally increases joint-loading activities. As an approximation, patients typically progress to this phase when terminal knee extension exercises can be done with 25–30-lb weights.[9] Among the goals for this phase are to

- attain full range of pain-free motion;
- restore normal joint kinematics;
- improve muscle strength;
- improve neuromuscular control;
- restore normal muscle force–couple relationships.

ROM exercises during this phase include flexion and extension exercises; stationary cycling progressing to moderate resistance; and standing wall slides VIDEO. The stationary bike exercises are initially performed with a high seat (providing about 15 degrees of knee flexion in the extended leg).

There is controversy about whether knee exercises should be performed in an OKC or CKC manner.[234] CKCEs, such as the squat, leg press, dead lift, and power clean, have long been used as core exercises by athletes to enhance performance in sport.[496,497] These multijoint exercises have biomechanical and neuromuscular similarities to many athletic movements.[235] OKCEs appear to be less functional in terms of many athletic movements and primarily serve a supportive role in strength and conditioning programs. However, it is advised that a combination of the OKC and CKC exercises be used.

Closed-Chain Exercises

CKCEs during this phase include a continued progression of those exercises introduced during the acute phase. Other exercises are introduced including sideways step-ups (Fig. 20-55) and step-downs VIDEO, single knee toe raises VIDEO (Fig. 20-56) and dips, partial (Fig. 20-57) to full squats with added resistance,[454] the seated leg press, front and side lunges VIDEO (Fig. 20-58), jumping and landing exercises VIDEO (Fig. 20-59 and Fig. 20-60), Fitter-board exercises (Fig. 20-61), resisted walking in all four planes VIDEO (flexion, extension, abduction, and adduction) using elastic tubing (Fig. 20-62), balance activities VIDEO and obstacle jumping[498] VIDEO (Fig. 20-63).

In the presence of knee version, an adjunct to the usual exercise regimen may be strengthening of the internal tibial rotators (semimembranosus, gracilis, semitendinosus, sartorius), with greater emphasis placed on hamstring stretching, particularly the biceps femoris, while adding stretching of the ITB.[286] CKCEs to strengthen the hamstrings, gastrocnemii, and quadriceps in a functional manner include a variety of exercises on a stair climber. The patient stands on the machine backward for the quadriceps and forward for the hamstrings.

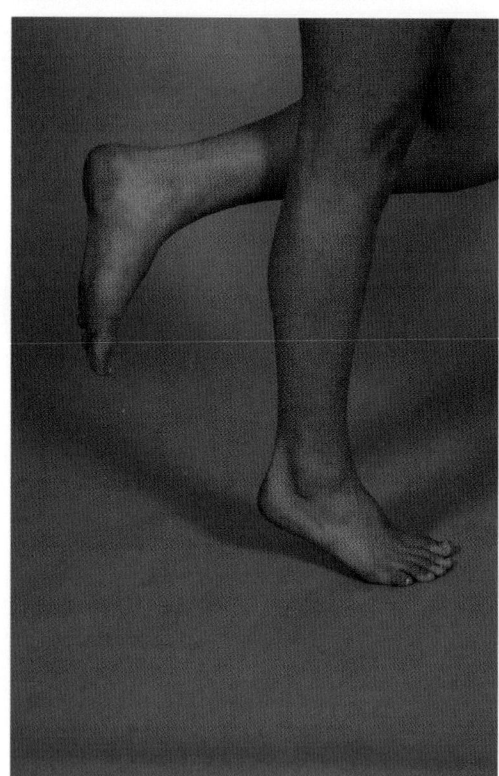

FIGURE 20-56 Single leg heel raises.

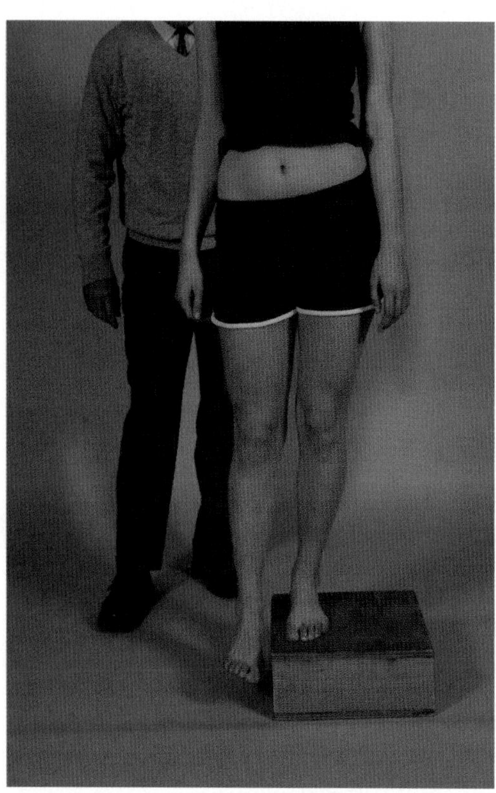

FIGURE 20-55 One quarter step up to the side.

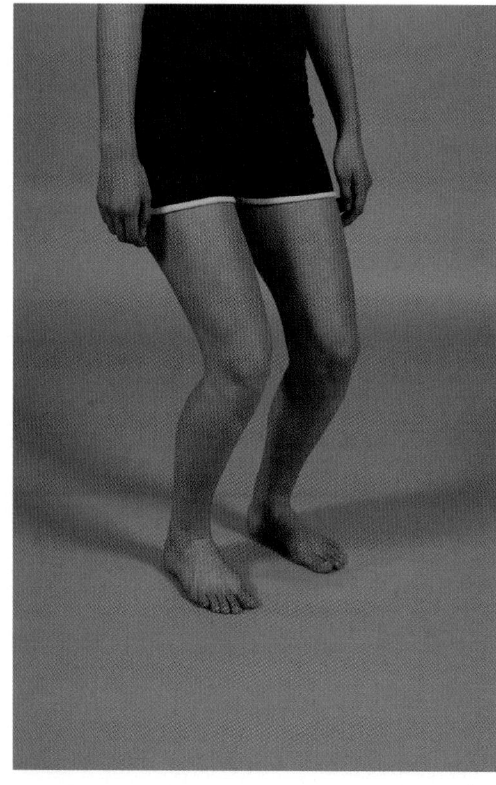

FIGURE 20-57 Partial squat.

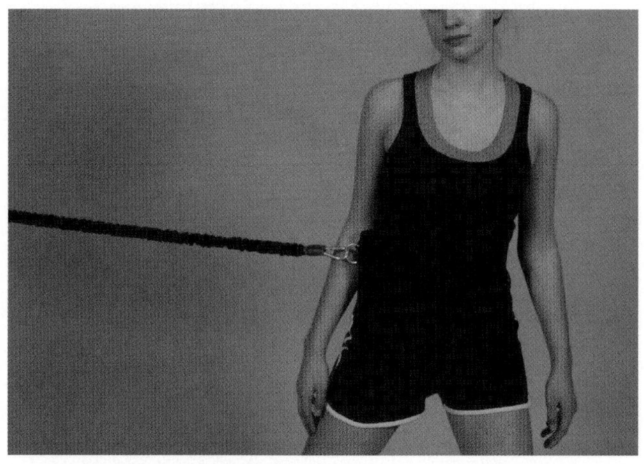

FIGURE 20-58 Resisted side lunges.

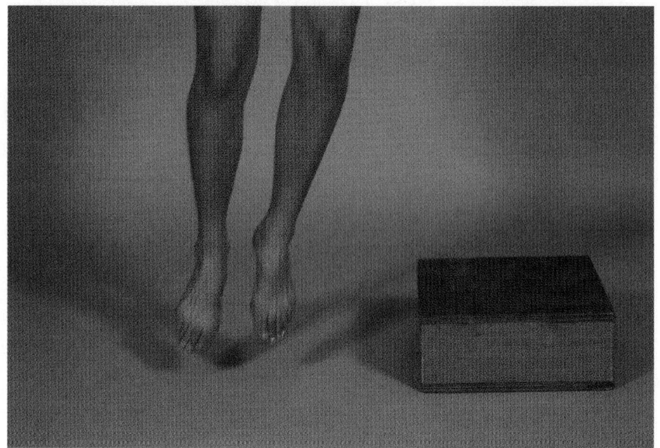

FIGURE 20-59 Jumping and landing.

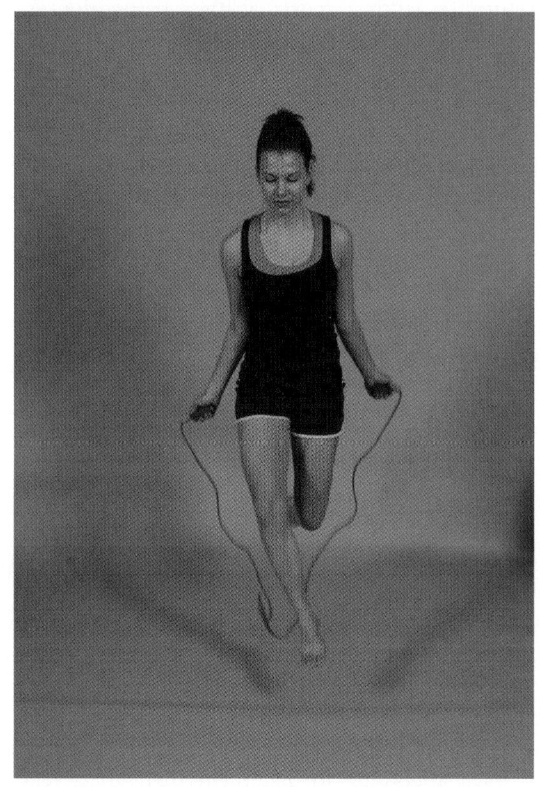

FIGURE 20-60 Jump roping as a plyometric exercise.

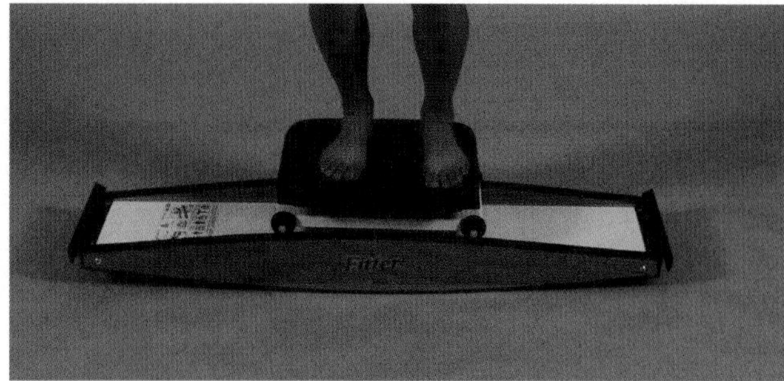

FIGURE 20-61 Fitter board exercises.

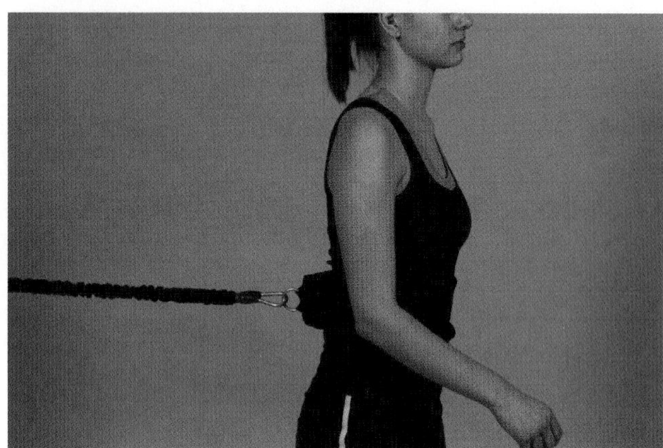

FIGURE 20-62 Resisted walking exercise.

The use of an inclined treadmill can also be used to selectively exercise the hamstrings, gastrocnemii, and quadriceps as follows:

- Walking or running downhill works the quadriceps eccentrically.
- Walking or running uphill works the gastrocnemii and hamstrings concentrically.
- Walking or running downhill backward works the gastrocnemii and hamstrings eccentrically.
- Walking backward uphill uses the quadriceps concentrically.

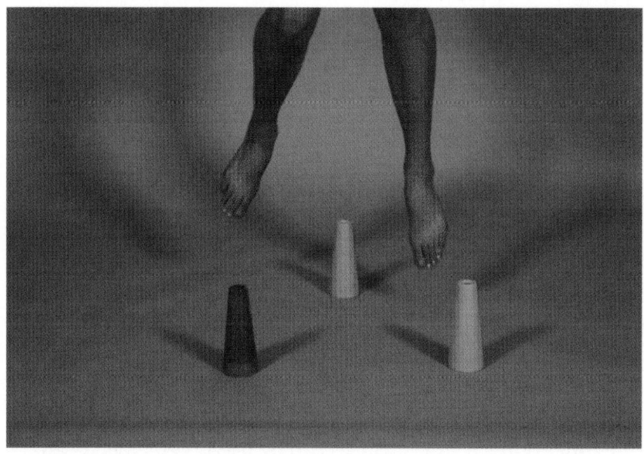

FIGURE 20-63 Obstacle jumping.

Uphill and retrotreadmill walking have been found to produce less patellofemoral joint restrictive forces than forward walking.[499]

For those patients with patellofemoral pain, or weak hip abductors, hip abductor action can be facilitated during a lunge task by creating an adduction force using elastic tubing that the patient is instructed to counteract.

Open-Chain Exercises

OKCEs during this phase can include a wide variety of exercises including seated knee extension and knee flexion exercises that are viewed as single-joint, single-muscle-group exercises.[235] Using the knowledge of the compressive forces at the joint, OKCEs (e.g., short-arc quadriceps VIDEO, multiple-angle isometrics) should be performed in the 50–90-degree or 90–50-degree range of knee flexion.[234,488] Other exercises include

- straight leg raises in all four planes (flexion, extension, abduction, and adduction), progressing to about 10% of body weight in resistance;
- supine leg lowering;
- seated leg lowering;
- short-arc quadriceps progression to about 10% of body weight in resistance;
- Side-lying (clam) exercise to strengthen the gluteus medius (see Chap. 19). The patient is positioned in side lying with the hips and knees flexed to about 45 degrees. A piece of Theraband is wrapped around both sides and the patient is asked to abduct and externally rotate the uppermost leg against the resistance of the Theraband.

Swenson et al.[500] recommend the use of the 4-minute OKC exercise for patellofemoral pain. The exercise protocol was developed by Glen Porter, ATC, a basketball trainer at Michigan State University, MI, and Alan Glock, MD, an orthopaedic surgeon in Richmond, IN. The exercise is performed as follows.

The patient sits on the edge of a chair, with the upper leg supported. The patient is asked to contract the quadriceps muscle with the knee in full extension. The contraction is held for 1 minute, after which the leg is flexed to 45 degrees for 30 seconds. Four cycles of extension and flexion constitute the 4-minute VMO program. Initially, the exercise is performed four to six times a day. Ankle weights are added after 1–2 weeks and the number of sets is decreased.[500]

The functional rehabilitation strategy should be to progressively improve three-dimensional dynamic lower extremity postural stability. This can be achieved using a multiplanar task progression integrating both non–weight-bearing and weight-bearing lower extremity function.[160] An example of a non–weight-bearing exercise is standing in unilateral knee flexion in conjunction with tibial internal rotation and hip external rotation, performed either actively or with a resistive band.[160] To make efficient use of elastic resistance, quick concentric activation should be followed by a slower eccentric activation.[160] For weight-bearing exercises, both forward and side lunges on varying surfaces can be used. Task speed can be progressively increased and spontaneous responses can be achieved by having the patient respond to random cues to provide the direction of movement. Simultaneous use of different size and weight balls for catching and tossing may increase specificity and serve as a distractor to better assess the patient's true ability to maintain appropriate, well-controlled, three-dimensional, dynamic, lower extremity postural stability.[160]

For some patients, a return to sports may be a goal. Since strenuous activities may exert five times more force than is imparted with the various ligament stress tests,[501] the clinician cannot rely on the results from the ligament stress tests as a means to assess a patient's readiness to return to sport. Once strength and endurance have reached at least 70% of the uninvolved extremity with isokinetic testing, the more advanced (PNF) exercises involving high-speed, high-force, uncontrolled movements are initiated, stopping short of cutting, jumping, and twisting maneuvers if symptoms of instability develop.[502,503] Running, jumping, and twisting activities must be included in the clinical examinations of such patients to enable true assessment.[443] Criteria for progression into the return to sport phase include the following:

- Full AROM and PROM compared with the uninvolved knee. It has been suggested that the patient should have 8–118 degrees of knee motion, demonstrate a normal gait pattern, ascend and descend stairs, and demonstrate no gait deviation when running, before participating in athletic activity.[445,504]
- A quadriceps-to-hamstring ratio of 2:3 and equal to or greater than 75% of the uninvolved leg.
- Ability to perform a one-leg squat for 15–20 repetitions.
- Normal joint kinematics.

A return to cutting sports at the competition level is permitted when the quadriceps strength index is 85–90% of the uninvolved leg at 60 degrees per second with isokinetic testing. Sport-specific drills are added late in the functional phase as the athlete approaches return to play. Activity-specific progressions must be completed to test all of the working parts involved in the activity before full return to function is advised.

Bracing

Patellofemoral Bracing

External patellar supports are commonly employed in the management of patellofemoral pain as an adjunct to other intervention methods. Although they relieve symptoms in many patients, their mode of action remains theoretical and their usefulness is unpredictable.[267]

Theoretically, the brace is designed to centralize the patella within the patellar groove, thereby reducing symptoms and improving function.[463,505] The various commercially available patellofemoral braces use a number of methods to improve patellar tracking, including patellar cut-outs, lateral buttresses, air bladders, and positioning straps.

Despite the wide use of patellofemoral bracing, only a few studies have attempted to document their effectiveness in correcting patellar alignment. Using MRI, Koskinen and

Kujala[506] reported a quantitative decrease in lateral patellar displacement using the safety brace (Axini, Boliden, Sweden), while Worrell et al.[507] found that the Palumbo brace (Dynorthotics LP, Vienna, VA) reduced lateral patellar displacement and increased patellofemoral congruence at 10 degrees of flexion. These studies, however, used static imaging techniques and, therefore, actual patellar tracking was not assessed. This is an important limitation because patellar tracking is considered to be a dynamic entity. Studies comparing active and passive procedures have shown that patellar motion is significantly influenced by the degree of quadriceps contraction.[217,267,508,509] Finestone et al.[510] found that some braces were less effective and more harmful to the skin than conservative therapy (i.e., maintaining activity and avoiding pain-causing activity, or no therapy, or simple muscle stretching and strengthening).[511]

Although it is debatable whether bracing can influence patellar tracking, it appears that external supports must, in some way, interact mechanically with the patellofemoral joint because many patients report significant clinical improvements.

Tibiofemoral Bracing

Functional knee braces are commonly prescribed following an ACL injury or reconstruction to promote healing, by reducing anterior translation of the tibia with respect to the femur and thereby restoring normal joint kinematics.[22,512,513]

The efficacy of knee bracing with regard to providing adequate protection is controversial, because the compliance of the soft tissues around the thigh decreases the ability of the brace to function correctly, particularly at high loads.[513,514]

A study by Fleming et al.[513] using the Legend brace (dj Orthopaedics LLC, Vista, CA) indicated that a functional knee brace can protect the ACL during anteroposterior shear loading in the non–weight-bearing and weight-bearing knee and during internal torques in the non–weight-bearing knee. However, this study used only one brace and one knee flexion angle (20 degrees).

Risberg et al.,[515] who used randomized, prospective clinical trials of bracing after ACL injury or reconstruction, found no difference in joint laxity, pain, muscle strength, and functional knee tests between patients who wore a functional knee brace and those who did not wear a functional brace during post-surgical rehabilitation.

Several studies have indicated that subjects with chronic ACL-deficient knees have impaired proprioception.[516–518] Whether functional knee braces enhance proprioception in ACL-deficient knees remains unclear. Although a few studies have addressed the relationship between proprioception and functional outcome measures,[516,517] the studies that have compared the effect of functional braces on proprioception between ACL-reconstructed knees and the contralateral uninvolved knee have as yet demonstrated no improvement in proprioception with the wearing of such braces,[519] and no effect on long-term outcome.[22]

Interestingly, bandaging of the knee, or the use of a neoprene brace, has been shown to improve proprioception in both normal individuals and those with different types of knee disorders, including knee OA and an ACL tear.[22,520]

Taping

The primary goal of taping[189,521] is to pull the patella away from a painful area, thereby unloading it and reducing pain, rather than as a adjustment for patellofemoral malalignment.[454,522,523] The extent to which this is possible and the amount of displacement required to provide pain relief varies from patient to patient and from study to study (Table 20-19).[11] Indeed, the displacement does not need to be perceptible to effect improvement. Bockrath et al.[522] found that taping did affect perceived pain but was not associated with patellar position changes. A recent computed tomography (CT) study,[524] involving 16 female patients (aged 16–25 years) who had anterior knee pain related to patellofemoral incongruence, evaluated the effect of patellar taping on patellofemoral incongruence. The subjects underwent CT examination with their quadriceps muscles relaxed and contracted, both before and after patellar taping. The study found that patellar taping did not significantly affect patellofemoral lateralization, or tilt, and concluded that although patellar taping may well be effective in controlling anterior knee pain, it does not do so by medializing the patella.[524] Another study found that McConnell taping was effective in moving the patella medially but ineffective in maintaining this difference after exercise.[525]

A secondary function of taping is to increase the beneficial proprioceptive characteristics of the patellofemoral joint.[526,527] Grabiner et al.[528] have postulated that the VMO needs time to develop force, relative to the VL, to optimally track the patella. This lag time can cause the patella to track laterally. By applying tape across an overly powerful VL, the clinician may be able to change the relative excitation of the VMO and VL, diminishing the pull of the VL,[11,189,521] although the mechanisms by which this works are unknown.

One other function of taping for malalignment of the patella is to position the patella optimally so that the area of contact between the patella and femur is maximized.[266] This position places the patella parallel to the femur in the frontal and sagittal planes, and the patella is midway between the two condyles when the knee is flexed to 20 degrees.[266]

Once the tape is applied, the clinician assesses the following:

- The overall limb alignment. This includes an assessment when walking normally, on the heels, and with the feet in the inverted and everted positions; stair climbing; and squatting.
- The effect on functional painful and pain-free ranges.

From this information, the patellar position is adjusted by taping. The most obvious deviation is always corrected first. The glide component can be corrected by firmly gliding the patella medially and taping the lateral patellar border (Fig. 20-64). The tilt component can be corrected by firm taping from the middle of the patella medially, which lifts the lateral border and provides a passive stretch to the lateral structures (Fig. 20-65). To correct external rotation of the patella, firm taping from the middle inferior pole upward and medially is required. For correction of internal rotation, firm taping from the middle superior pole downward and medially is needed.

In addition to the taping, biofeedback, stretching of the lateral structures, and a home exercise program are recommended. For a more detailed description of the application of

TABLE 20-19 The Effects of Patellofemoral Taping on Patellofemoral Pain

Investigators	Study Design	Number of Interventions	Percentage Improvement and Clinical Importance
Eburne and Bannister[a]	Single-blind randomized control trial	3 months or until pain-free	Both groups 50%—no clinical importance
McConnell[b]	Experimental	Eight sessions	92%, no control—could not determine
Gerrard[c]	Experimental	Five sessions	96%, no control—could not determine
Powers et al.[d]	Experimental	One session	78%, no control—clinical importance
Salsich et al.[e]	Experimental	One session	92.6%, no control—clinical importance
Bockrath et al.[f]	Experimental	One session	54%, no control—clinical importance
Kowall et al.[g]	Randomized control trial	Eight sessions over 1 month	44%, no control—no statistical difference between groups but clinical importance
Clark et al.[h]	Single-blind randomized control trial	Six sessions (five taping sessions)	No statistical difference between groups or clinical importance

Data from Lohman EB, Harp T: Patellofemoral pain: A critical appraisal of the literature. In: Wilmarth MA, ed.: *Evidence-Based Practice for the Upper and Lower Quarter. Orthopaedic Physical Therapy Home Study Course* 13.2.1 La Crosse, WI: Orthopaedic Section, APTA, 2003:1–44. With permission from Orthopaedic Section, APTA.

[a]Data from Eburne J, Bannister G: The McConnell regime versus isometric quadriceps exercises in the management of anterior knee pain. A randomized prospective controlled trial. *The Knee* 3:151–153, 1996.

[b]Data from McConnell JS: Patella alignment and quadriceps strength. *Proceedings of the MTAA Conference. Adelaide*, 1987.

[c]Data from Gerrard B: The patello-femoral pain syndrome: a clinical trial of the McConnell programme. *Aust J Physiother* 35:71–80, 1989.

[d]Data from Powers CM, Landel R, Perry J: Timing and intensity of vastus muscle activity during functional activities in subjects with and without patellofemoral pain. *Phys Ther* 76:946–955, 1996; discussion 956–967.

[e]Data from Salsich GB, Brechter JH, Farwell D, et al.: The effects of patellar taping on knee kinetics, kinematics, and vastus lateralis muscle activity during stair ambulation in individuals with patellofemoral pain. *J Orthop Sports Phys Ther* 32:3–10, 2002.

[f]Data from Bockrath K, Wooden C, Worrell T, et al.: Effects of patella taping on patella position and perceived pain. *Med Sci Sports Exerc* 25:989–992, 1993.

[g]Data from Kowall MG, Kolk G, Nuber GW, et al.: Patellar taping in the treatment of patellofemoral pain. A prospective randomized study. *Am J Sports Med* 24:61–66, 1996.

[h]Data from Clark HD, Wells GA, Huet C, et al.: Assessing the quality of randomized trials: reliability of the Jadad scale. *Control Clin Trials* 20:448–452, 1999.

the tape, the reader is referred to an excellent book, *The Patella: A Team Approach*.[188]

Lesher et al.[529] attempted to determine the predictive validity and interrater reliability of selected clinical examination items and to develop a clinical prediction rule (CPR) to determine which patients would respond successfully to a medial glide patellar taping technique. A CPR is, by definition, an optimum number of clinical examination items use for predicting a diagnosis or prognosis. Two examination items (positive patella tilt test or tibial varum >5 degrees, +LR = 4.4 [95% CI = 1.3–12.3] and a −LR of 0.53 [0.38–0.86]) comprised the CPR. Application of the CPR improved the probability of a successful outcome from 52% to 83%. As the CPR in this study represented a level IV CPR, it requires validation in a separate sample before it can be implemented on a broad basis.[530]

Taping can also be used with patients who have patellar OA. A controlled clinical trial[531] found that patients achieved significant reduction in pain after medial knee taping to realign the patella.

Walking Poles

Results from a number of studies[532–534] have demonstrated that walking poles reduce the forces on the lower extremity

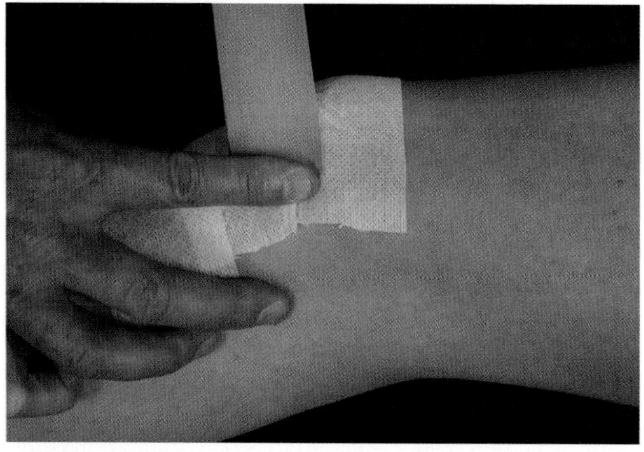

FIGURE 20-64 Patellar taping for correction of tilt.

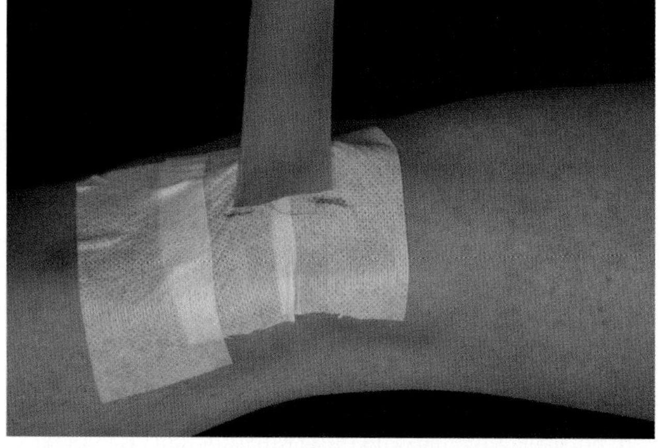

FIGURE 20-65 Patellar taping for correction of glide.

during level walking when walking velocity is controlled. Schwameder et al.[535] reported 12–25% reduction in peak and average ground reaction force, knee joint moments, and tibiofemoral compressive and shear forces walking down a 25-degree gradient.

A study by Willson et al.[532] found that the use of the poles tended to reduce the vertical joint reaction forces at the knee over the no-poles condition. Differences of 4.4% were found in vertical joint reaction forces at the knee between the no-poles, pole-back, and pole-front conditions.[532] However, knee extensor angular impulse was greater with all pole conditions compared with no-poles. Thus, walking with poles caused a more flexed knee position through stance, reducing the vertical bone-on-bone forces and increasing the internal (muscular) knee extensor kinetics.[532] This reduction of lower extremity stress during a faster walking velocity may symbolize a less harmful mode of exercise for healthy and pathologic populations alike. Thus, the use of walking poles may lead to an increased training stimulus as a result of the greater walking velocity and reduced lower extremity loading conditions compared with a self-selected walking velocity.[532]

PREFERRED PRACTICE PATTERN 4C: IMPAIRED MUSCLE PERFORMANCE

Patellofemoral Pain

Patellofemoral-related problems are characterized by pain in the vicinity of the patella that is worsened by sitting and climbing stairs,[147,536] inclined walking and squatting.[491] It is a common reason for referral to physical therapy.[457] A British sports injury clinic study showed that 5.4% of the total injuries seen and 25% of all knee problems treated for a 5-year period were attributed to patellofemoral pain.[537]

Although patellofemoral pain can occur in anyone, particularly athletes, women who are not athletic appear to be more prone to this problem (2:1 ratio) than men who are not athletic.[538] However, among athletes, the incidence is higher in males (4:1).[461]

Numerous authors have proposed classification systems for patellofemoral pain using various clinical, radiographic, etiologic, and pathologic criteria to categorize patients.[134,285,538–543] The purpose of a physical therapy classification system is to aid in proper diagnosis and intervention based on impairment. To help in the determination of the classification, the clinician must answer the following questions:

- Is the problem truly related to the patellofemoral joint or its related structures?
- Is a muscle imbalance present?
- Is inflammation present?
- Is instability present?

Determining the classification gives significant guidance to intervention options. Patellofemoral instability, especially recurrent, usually requires surgical intervention, whereas patellofemoral pain resulting from inflammation or a muscle imbalance usually responds well to conservative intervention.[284]

The term *malalignment* implies that the static or dynamic restraints of the patellofemoral joint are insufficient to allow normal patellar tracking. Malalignment appears to be a necessary but not sufficient condition for the onset of patellofemoral pain. Symptoms seem to be set off by a trigger, or combination of structural and dynamic factors, the nature of which varies from patient to patient.[284]

Anatomic Variance

A number of anatomic features can have an impact on the function of the patellofemoral joint and subsequent dysfunction:

- Femoral trochlear dysplasia.[182]
- Patellar morphology and the amount of congruence of the patellofemoral joint
- The natural positioning of the patella (alta or baja)[194,291,544–546]

Gender[216]

A commonly cited reason as to why women have more anterior knee pain than men is the difference in the orientation and alignment of the lower extremity. The broader pelvis of the female moves the hip joints farther lateral relative to the mid-line. This produces an increased valgus angle from the hip to the knee and then to the ground. Females also have a higher prevalence of increased femoral anteversion, which also increases the valgus angle.[547] Although the increased valgus thrust on the patella is not necessarily a problem, it increases the tendency for excessive lateral pressure on the patella, which then can lead to retinacular stress around the patella and, in some people, concavity of the lateral facet and anterior knee pain.

Tibial Rotation

The Q angle can be influenced distally through motions of the tibia. For example, external rotation of the tibia moves the tibial tuberosity laterally, thereby increasing the Q angle, whereas tibial internal rotation decreases the Q angle by moving the tibial tuberosity medially.

Subtalar Joint Position

Tibial rotation is influenced by subtalar joint motion. For example, subtalar joint pronation causes internal rotation of the tibia, whereas subtalar joint supination causes the tibia to rotate laterally.

Femoral Rotation

As with tibial rotation, the Q angle can be influenced through motions of the femur. For example increased femoral internal rotation results in a larger Q angle, whereas femoral external rotation minimizes the Q angle.

The impairments resulting from patellofemoral dysfunction have been related to problems that cannot be improved by physical therapy and those that can. EMG evidence of poorly coordinated muscle activation has been documented in other joints, such as the shoulder and low back.[548] At the knee, the VMO may be proximally positioned and abnormally oriented, and the timing of its contractions may be poorly synchronized with those of the surrounding muscles.[146,196,454,489,492,549] Since coordinated firing of the dynamic stabilizing muscles is important for the normal functioning of the patellofemoral joint it would be reasonable to assume that physical therapy would be of benefit to enhance the dynamic stabilizers. Thus, the intervention for a maltracking patella must seek to restore the balance of force production of the medial and lateral stabilizers of the patellofemoral joint and to attempt the reestablishment of functional control of the VMO (see "Intervention Strategies" section).[188,189,284,454,457,466,467,521]

Patellar Compression Syndromes

Patellar compression syndromes result from an overconstrained patella whose motion is severely restricted by surrounding soft tissues.

Lateral Patellar Compression Syndrome[131,146,187,550]

A tight lateral retinaculum may be responsible for patellar tilt and excessive pressure on the lateral patellar facet, producing the excessive lateral pressure syndrome as described by Ficat and Hungerford.[265] The patient typically complains of pain over the lateral retinaculum.[187,551,552] The diagnosis is confirmed clinically by a decreased medial patellar glide and evidence of a lateral patellar tilt.

The medial stabilizers play a role in the lateral pressure syndrome, and the VMO frequently becomes atrophied, probably as a result of the new patellar position, the associated pain, and the resultant inflammation.[319] The presence of nerve-fiber changes in the lateral retinaculum[129,187] raises the possibility that these changes might be a catalyst for pain, although it is not clear whether the malalignment precedes the nerve changes or vice versa. The major long-term problem with excessive lateral pressure syndrome is a chronic imbalance of facet loading and the subsequent effect on the articular cartilage and surrounding soft tissue.

Fortunately, this condition seems to respond well to a conservative approach consisting of[319]

- stretching of the lateral retinacular structures;
- patellar taping to correct the excessive lateral tilt and to apply a long duration, low-load stretch of the lateral retinaculum;
- stretching of the hamstrings, quadriceps, and ITB;
- strengthening of the VMO;
- anti-inflammatory measures;
- activity modification through minimization of stair ambulation and deep knee squats.

Infrapatellar Contracture Syndrome[553]

The term *infrapatellar contracture syndrome* (IPCS) was first coined by Paulos et al. in 1987.[339] This condition is characterized by a restriction of patellar movement because both the medial and lateral retinaculum are excessively tight. This restriction may result in a decrease in knee flexion and extension. Another term for this condition, *global patellar pressure syndrome,* was proposed by Wilk et al.[319]

The development of this condition appears to be related to direct trauma and subsequent pathologic fibrous hyperplasia in the peripatellar tissues or secondary to prolonged immobilization after surgery.[339]

IPCS has been described as having three progressive stages: a prodromal stage, an active stage, and a residual stage.[554]

Prodromal Stage. The prodromal stage begins between 2 and 8 weeks after trauma to the knee. Knee ROM is painful, there is a decrease in patellar mobility, and an extensor lag is present. This scenario is usually noted with patients who fail routine postoperative rehabilitation. Without recognition, patients can progress to the second stage within 6–20 weeks. Early detection of IPCS is important because only the prodromal stage is amenable to nonsurgical intervention. Rehabilitation should be initiated with early patellar mobilization, stretching of the hamstrings, hip flexors, quadriceps, gastrocnemius, and ITB, with the emphasis on restoring full knee extension. Other components in the prodromal stage should include active ROM, multiangle isometric strengthening of the quadriceps, neuromuscular stimulation, transcutaneous electrical nerve stimulation (TENS), and NSAIDs. When performing the patella mobilizations, the glides should be held for a long duration (1–12 minutes) to enhance the remodeling of the soft tissue.[319,555] Activities such as bicycling, resisted knee extensions, deep knee bends, or deep squats (beyond 60 degrees) should not be initiated until patellar mobility is restored to prevent excessive patellar compression and patellofemoral joint contact pressures.[319]

Active Stage. In the second stage, there is loss of the extensor lag because of the restriction of passive and active knee ROM. There are also tissue texture changes in the patella tendon. This creates a positive shelf sign: an abrupt step-off or "shelf" from the patellar tendon to the tibial tubercle.[339] Patients who progress to this stage require surgery, with open intra-articular and extra-articular debridement. Immediate daily rehabilitation with continuous passive motion (CPM), full AROM, and extension splints at night also can be used.

Residual Stage. The third stage is notable for significant patellofemoral arthrosis and a residual low-riding patella at 8 months or even years after the onset of IPCS. Additional classifications distinguish whether the patellar entrapment is primary, caused by infrapatellar contracture (see separate section), or secondary, as a result of surgical intervention or postoperative immobilization. The patient history typically includes complaints of knee pain and stiffness, swelling, and crepitus, and "giving way" may also be reported. On physical examination, the diagnosis may be made by a 10-degree or greater loss of extension, a 25-degree or greater loss of flexion, and significantly reduced patellar mobility as demonstrated by decreased patellar glide. Additional findings include atrophy of the quadriceps femoris, palpable patellofemoral crepitus, diffuse synovitis, and an antalgic or flexed knee gait.

PREFERRED PRACTICE PATTERN 4D: IMPAIRED JOINT MOBILITY, MOTOR FUNCTION, MUSCLE PERFORMANCE, RANGE OF MOTION ASSOCIATED WITH CONNECTIVE TISSUE DYSFUNCTION

Articular Cartilage Defects

Articular cartilage defects of the knee are a common cause of pain and functional disability. Since nonoperative rehabilitation and palliative care for this condition are frequently unsuccessful, many patients opt for surgical procedures designed to facilitate the repair or transplantation of autogenous cartilage tissue.[556] Reparative techniques include the following:

- ***Arthroscopic lavage and debridement.*** This procedure is performed to reduce the inflammation and mechanical irritation within a given joint. Debridement can include smoothing of the fibrillated articular or meniscal surfaces, shaving of motion-limiting osteophytes, and removal of inflamed synovium.[557]
- ***Microfracture.*** The surgical objective of microfracture is the controlled perforation of the subchondral bone plate to permit an efflux of pluripotent marrow elements into a chondral defect.[557]
- ***Autologous osteochondral mosaicplasty grafting.*** This is a method to transplant bone and hyaline cartilage, using small osteochondral plugs, to a region of chondral or osteochondral defect.
- ***Autologous chondrocyte implantation (ACI).*** This is a cartilage restorative procedure in which a concentrated solution of autologous chondrocytes is implanted into a defect with the goal of restoring hyaline cartilage to the injured area.[557]
- ***Osteochondral autograft transfer (OAT).*** Osteochondral autograft is most clearly indicated for a symptomatic, unipolar lesion of the distal femoral condyle in a nondegenerative joint that has proper limb alignment, as well as ligamentous stability and meniscal competence.[557]
- ***Osteochondral allograft transplantation.*** In contrast to OAT, osteochondral allograft transplantation relies upon tissue taken from cadaveric donors rather than from the patient's own knee. The benefits of allografting include elimination of donor site morbidity and the ability to provide fully formed articular cartilage without specific limitation with respect to defect size. The drawbacks to the procedure are graft availability, cell viability, immunogenicity, and risk of disease transmission.[557]

The postsurgical rehabilitation progression is designed based on the four biologic phases of cartilage maturation: proliferation, transitional, remodeling, and maturation. The duration of each phase that follows varies depending on the lesion, patient, and the specifics of the surgery.[556]

- ***Proliferation phase.*** This phase generally lasts 4–6 weeks following surgery. The goals during this phase are to protect the repair, decrease swelling, gradually restore PROM and weight-bearing and to enhance volitional control of the quadriceps.
- ***Transition phase.*** This phase typically consists of weeks 4 through 12 postsurgery. During this phase, the patient progresses from partial to full weight-bearing while full ROM and soft tissue flexibility is achieved.[556] It is during this phase in which patients typically resume most normal activities of daily living.
- ***Remodeling phase.*** This phase generally takes place from 3 to 6 months postoperatively. At this point, the patient typically notes improvement of symptoms and has normal ROM. During this phase, low-to-moderate impact activities, such as bicycle riding, golfing, and recreational walking, are gradually incorporated.
- ***Maturation phase.*** This phase begins in a range of 4–6 months and can last up to 15–18 months postsurgery. The duration of this phase varies based on lesion size and location, and the specific surgical procedure performed.

Tibiofemoral Osteoarthritis

OA has been acknowledged as the most common cause of disability in the United States.[558,559] Thirty-three percent of persons aged 63–94 years are affected by OA of the knee, which often limits the ability to rise from a chair, stand comfortably, walk, and use stairs.[560,561]

OA may affect one or more of the three compartments of the knee: medial tibiofemoral, lateral tibiofemoral, and patellofemoral.

OA has long been regarded as a "wear-and-tear" or "degenerative" condition, a view supported by epidemiologic surveys that demonstrated associations with certain occupations and life choices and its increased prevalence with advancing age.[562] Recognized risk factors include physically demanding occupations, particularly jobs that involve kneeling or squatting,[335,563–566] certain sports,[567,568] older age, female sex, evidence of OA in other joints, obesity,[569] and previous injury or surgery of the knee.[570]

The clinical findings of OA at the knee include swelling, which can vary from minimal to severe, depending on the clinical stage and severity. The joint can also be warm to touch, although that again depends on the stage and severity. Usually, the patient reports pain with weight-bearing activities and, at times, pain at rest. The loss of motion, if present, is typically in a capsular pattern. Muscle weakness is probably the longest documented and best established correlate of functional limitation in individuals with OA, particularly with knee OA.[563,571–573]

Regular partaking in physical activity has been recognized for several years as being of benefit in the management of knee OA,[574–580] and exercises to strengthen the quadriceps are becoming established as a useful adjunct in the treatment for OA of the knee.[581] Although there is agreement that strengthening exercises can be helpful, the effect of exercise therapy on pain, quadriceps strength, and physical function appears to be small to moderate in most clinical trials.

Puett and Griffin[574] reviewed 15 controlled trials of conservative intervention for hip and knee OA from 1966 through 1993 and concluded that exercise reduces pain and improves function in patients with OA of the knee, but that the optimal exercise regimen has yet to be determined.[574] In addition to strengthening exercises, fitness walking and aerobic exercise have both been reported to result in functional improvement in patients with OA of the knee.[574–580] However, unweighted treadmill walking has not been shown to decrease pain associated with OA of the knee.[582]

Deyle et al.[469] conducted a randomized trial comparing the use of manual therapy techniques to the knee, hip, foot and ankle, and lumbar spine combined with exercises for lower extremity strengthening, ROM and endurance to a group of patients with knee OA that received a placebo ultrasound treatment. The study concluded that patients with OA of the knee who were treated with manual physical therapy and exercise experienced clinically and statistically significant improvements in self-perceptions of pain, stiffness, and functional ability, and the distance walked in 6 minutes. The beneficial effects of intervention, which were achieved in eight clinic visits, persisted at 4 weeks and 1 year after the conclusion of clinical treatment.[469] An important aspect of the treatment described by Deyle et al. was that the impairments that were present at other joints in addition to the knee were addressed. This emphasizes the need to evaluate and address a variety of problems that a patient with knee OA may have to optimize the response to treatment.[583]

In addition to the exercises that recover lower extremity strength, ROM, and cardiovascular endurance, it is now being recommended that therapy programs also include techniques to improve balance and coordination and provide patients with an opportunity to practice various skills that they will likely encounter during normal day activities.[584]

Other conservative interventions for OA of the knee include NSAIDs, cortisone injections, patient education, weight loss, and thermal modalities.[469,581] The use of shoes with a well-cushioned sole is recommended, as are frequent rest periods during the day. Wedged insoles with an angle of 5–10 degrees on a frontal section have been shown to be helpful for OA of the medial compartment knee OA.[585,586] The patient is instructed in principles of joint protection, and advised to seek alternatives to prolonged standing, kneeling, and squatting.[581]

CLINICAL PEARL

Isokinetic and concentric/eccentric exercises must be prescribed carefully to avoid excessive compressive forces or shear forces at the knee.

Total Knee Arthroplasty

Total knee arthroplasty (TKA) has been shown to be an effective long-term intervention for the elderly population to relieve knee pain, improve function, increase social mobility and interaction, and contribute to psychologic well-being.[587–589]

Although pain and loss of function are the primary reasons for a TKA, the procedure can also be used to correct knee instability and lower extremity alignment and for the treatment of isolated but severe patellofemoral disease.[66,590] Since TKA is generally contraindicated in younger and more active patients, those with unicompartmental osteoarthritis of the knee may be considered candidates for a high tibial osteotomy or a distal femoral osteotomy. The high tibial osteotomy is used with isolated medial compartment arthritis. The distal femoral osteotomy is used in lateral compartment arthritis. The short-term results for these procedures have been very successful,[591,592] even to the point where the need for TKA is eliminated.[593] However, permanent pain relief with high tibial osteotomy is as yet unlikely.

Absolute and relative contraindications for a TKA include, but are not limited to

- active infection of the knee;
- significant genu recurvatum;
- severe obesity;
- return to high-impact sports or occupations;
- arterial insufficiency;
- neuropathic joint;
- mental illness.

Several techniques are at the surgeon's disposal. The choice of approach is determined by surgeon's familiarity and comfort. Three approaches are commonly described: anterior, subvastus, and lateral.[594]

- ***Anterior approach.*** The anterior approach is generally through an anterior midline longitudinal skin incision and median parapatellar arthrotomy. The advantages of this approach include its extensile potential and its wide exposure medially and laterally. The disadvantages include its violation of the quadriceps mechanism, and the potential for patellar devascularization.[594]
- ***Subvastus approach.*** The subvastus approach uses the same midline anterior skin incision as the anterior approach. The advantages of this approach include maintenance of the quadriceps mechanism with decreased postoperative pain and earlier functional recovery.[594] The disadvantage is its somewhat limited exposure.
- ***Lateral approach.*** The lateral approach occurs lateral to the patella and through the medial edge of Gerdy's tubercle. Proponents of this technique feel that it is a superior method in the correction of valgus deformity.[594]

Most primary arthroplasties rely upon the patient's anatomy to confer stability to the articulation. Anatomic structures that can confer stability include the PCL and a balancing of the soft tissues around the knee. The fate of the PCL in primary TKA remains controversial. If the PCL is sacrificed, a posterior stabilizer (see later) is used. However, the long-term results of PCL-retaining and posterior-stabilized TKAs are similar.[595,596] PCL substitution may be indicated in patients requiring TKA who present with end-stage DJD with varus or valgus malalignment and an associated flexion contracture, with a combined deformity greater than 15 degrees.[597,598]

Many of the earlier designs of TKA replaced only the tibiofemoral joint and did not address the patellofemoral articulation. The posterior stabilizer was developed to increase the arc of motion of these earlier models and thereby improve the functional results of TKA. Although the ROM improved substantially with these components, patellofemoral complications emerged as a key problem after knee replacement. Errors in sizing, alignment, and rotation of the tibial and femoral components were eventually highlighted as contributing factors to many of these patellofemoral problems. In addition, many of these complications appear to be secondary to patellar resurfacing which may be a part of the procedure. Whether to resurface the patella remains among the most controversial topics in TKA.

Following a knee replacement, there is a decrease in the contact area and consequent increase in the contract stress at the patellofemoral joint.[599] A study by Matsuda et al.[599] showed that resurfacing the patella reduced the contact area to a larger degree compared with not resurfacing the patella. In addition, kinematic studies of motion of the patellofemoral joint after knee replacement have consistently shown some degree of altered kinematics.[600]

Preoperative instruction is believed to be invaluable in the early postoperative setting. Preoperative instruction should include education regarding the ice–compression–elevation program, ROM exercises, isometric quadriceps strengthening, patellofemoral mobilization, and gait training with the appropriate postoperative assistive devices.[601]

Complications associated with TKA include the following[602]:

- Thromboembolic disease
- Fat embolism
- Poor wound healing
- Infection
- Periprosthetic fractures
- Neurologic problems, including fibular nerve palsy
- Vascular injuries
- Arthrofibrosis
- Disruption of the extensor mechanism

Postoperative rehabilitation for the TKA continues to be studied in an effort to decrease the cost while still providing the quality of clinical results expected by the surgeon and the patient.[603]

A review of the literature divulges conflicting practice patterns in the physical therapy management of TKA patients.[604–607]

The success of the rehabilitation program for this patient population is dependent on knowledge of the surgical procedure, communication with the surgeon and the patient, and above all, the ability of the rehabilitation team to educate the patient to participate actively in the treatment program.[601]

Patellofemoral Osteoarthritis

Patellofemoral OA is diagnosed by correlating patellofemoral pain with radiographic changes consistent with joint degeneration. Differentiation of idiopathic and posttraumatic subtypes is based on the history. Intervention for patellofemoral OA is usually conservative unless it coexists with severe tibiofemoral degenerative joint disease, in which case a total knee replacement may be warranted.

The term *chondromalacia patella* has long been a catch-all category of anterior and, specifically, retropatellar knee pain. The term *chondromalacia* was first used by Aleman in 1928.[608] He used the term "chondromalacia posttraumatica patellae" to describe lesions of the patella found at surgery and thought to be caused by prior trauma. With time, "chondromalacia" became an all-inclusive term with no agreed-on classification system or definitions of terms.[284]

True chondromalacia refers to a softening of the cartilage on the posterior aspect of the patella and is estimated to occur in fewer than 20% of persons who present with anterior knee pain.[204] The syndrome is most common in the 12–35-year-old age group, and most studies show a predominance in females.[125,203,204,461,500,609]

Two types of chondromalacia have been described. One type involves surface degeneration of the patella that is age dependent and most often asymptomatic. The other type involves basal degeneration. This type results from trauma and abnormal tracking of the patella and is symptomatic.[213]

Chondromalacia is classified into four grades, according to the degree of degeneration noted arthroscopically[610]:

- ***Grade 1.*** Closed disease. This grade is characterized by an intact joint surface that is spongy. The softening is reversible. A blister or raised portion of the articular surface is seen.
- ***Grade 2.*** Open disease. This grade is characterized by fissures that may or may not be obvious initially.
- ***Grade 3.*** Severe exuberant fibrillation or "crabmeat" appearance.
- ***Grade 4.*** The fibrillation is full-thickness and the erosive changes extend down to bone, which may be exposed. This is, in effect, OA and its extent depends on the size of the lesion.

Since cartilage has no nerve supply, chondral lesions themselves are usually asymptomatic,[611] although cartilage that is worn down to bone remains a potential source of pain due to irritation of, or abnormal pressure on, the richly innervated subchondral bone.[500]

The conservative intervention for patellofemoral OA includes the removal of any muscle imbalances of flexibility or strength. Occasionally, surgical realignment may prove beneficial when the articular degeneration is isolated to the lateral patellofemoral joint.

Arthrofibrosis

The term *arthrofibrosis* has been used to describe a spectrum of knee conditions in which loss of motion is the major finding.[497,612–616] It is perhaps best defined as a condition of restricted knee motion characterized by dense proliferative scar formation, in which intra-articular and extra-articular adhesions can progressively spread to limit joint motion.[617] This dense scar tissue can obliterate the parapatellar recesses, suprapatellar pouch, intercondylar notch, and eventually the articular surfaces.[338] Patella infera and chronic patellar entrapment also may develop as a consequence of this process.[338]

Arthrofibrosis may occur as the result of the inflammatory cascade after injury or operative treatment. Although inflammation is undoubtedly present in a large number of individuals, it is not clear why an aggressive form of this condition may develop in some patients.

To diagnose arthrofibrosis accurately, other causes of restricted active and passive motion of the knee must first be eliminated. Mechanical causes include loss of articular congruency (e.g., as a result of fracture, meniscal tear, or loose body), interruption of the extensor or flexor mechanism, substantial effusion,[618,619] or nonisometric placement of a graft during reconstruction of the ACL.[315,339,614] Some investigators believe that an ACL reconstruction performed within 3 weeks after an injury may increase the likelihood of arthrofibrosis[620,621] although others disagree.[622] Poor or unsupervised rehabilitation[315] preoperatively or postoperatively, with delayed motion protocols, may further increase the risk.[623]

Symptoms vary and often do not correlate with the severity of the condition. Since arthrofibrosis usually occurs after trauma or an operative procedure, pain and stiffness may be the initial symptoms.

- The presence of pain may complicate preexisting knee stiffness.[338,624] Although pain can be present early, it often becomes more prominent when joint degeneration and arthritis occur because of long-standing arthrofibrosis. Pain may also be constant, especially when it is associated with CRPS.[338,624]
- Stiffness is usually the primary symptom and is often worse in the morning hours.[617] Patients may complain of a warm, swollen knee that is painful with attempted motion.

Global arthrofibrosis of the knee manifests as marked limitation of flexion, extension, and patellar glide associated with widespread joint inflammation as well as intra-articular formation of fibrous tissue. This can progress to chondrification and ossification of soft tissues.[617]

Quadriceps function can be decreased or absent because of pain.[624] As function of the quadriceps muscle decreases, the ability of the muscle to act as a shock absorber is lessened, which may lead to additional articular degeneration. Often, the knee is held in a flexed position, which encourages tightening of the posterior part of the capsule and the hamstrings.

Crepitus and weakness are frequently present with swelling following prolonged standing or walking. Even when the patient does not have pain, loss of motion and quadriceps weakness can be substantial impediments to the performance of activities of daily living. An antalgic, flexed-knee gait is often seen.[339] Although effusion may be present, swelling is more often a result of inflamed, thickened capsular and pericapsular tissues.

Active and passive knee flexion and extension often are restricted in a capsular pattern, and the mediolateral and superoinferior patellar glides are reduced. This restriction of passive motion often has a spring-like end-feel, reflecting the density and stiffness of the thickened, inflamed, or scarred peripatellar tissue.

Intervention includes ROM exercises and the stretching of specific structures. When a plateau has been reached during rehabilitative efforts to restore motion or when there is progressive loss of motion, additional intervention of a gentle manipulation of the knee under anesthesia may result in improvement. Closed manipulation or vigorous attempts to gain passive motion may cause indiscriminate tearing of intra-articular tissue,[613] excessive tibiofemoral and patellofemoral compression with the risk of chondral damage or fracture,[325,613,625] rupture of the patellar ligament,[613,625] and even femoral fracture.[613] Manipulation has also been noted to initiate CRPS.[625]

Anteroposterior Slide Dysfunction: Tibia on Femur

In this condition, the tibia demonstrates a restricted anterior or posterior joint glide. This motion is coupled to knee flexion–extension.[334] Movement of the tibia on the femur into extension is coupled with an anterior glide. Movement of the tibia on the femur into flexion is coupled with a posterior glide. The initial complaints or findings are restrictions of flexion or extension movements.

The technique used to treat this dysfunction is a modification of the anterior drawer test. The patient is placed in the supine position, with the involved knee flexed and the foot flat on table, while the clinician sits on the patient's foot, anchoring it to the table. The clinician wraps both hands around the proximal tibia, placing the thumbs in front of the medial and lateral condyles and pressing on them. The clinician's hand encircles the leg and grasps it firmly below the popliteal space. The clinician creates a direct anteroposterior translatory glide of the tibia on the femur by first pulling the tibia forward with both hands, before pushing it backward with both thumbs.

Tibiofemoral Instability

Both intrinsic and extrinsic trauma to the knee occurs frequently. Several factors can predispose an individual to knee joint laxity:

- Repetitive microtrauma
- Severe macrotrauma
- Genetics[626]
- Gender[626]
- Ethnic factors[626]

Knee laxity may contribute to the development and progression of knee OA. It may also be a consequence of moderate to severe OA, although some knees become more stable with time because of the formation of osteophytes. Laxity is associated with more abrupt joint motion, large displacements, and suboptimal distribution of larger forces over the articular cartilage.[627,628] Since significant instability or damage to the internal structures of the knee joint can damage the articular surfaces and lead to degenerative changes, it is imperative that these injuries be treated as soon as possible.

There is no typical clinical presentation for knee instability in terms of the history. However, a history of "giving way" should always be taken seriously, as well as any evidence of locking or "catching" within the joint.[159]

The examination may reveal laxity. The direction of the laxity will determine the intervention. The intervention usually consists of muscle strengthening, correcting muscle imbalances, and the use of passive restraints, such as orthotics.

Anterior Cruciate Ligament Tear

More than 250,000 athletes are diagnosed with ACL injuries each year, making the management of sports-related ACL injuries the most widely discussed subject in the field of sports medicine.[629] This emphasis could be a result of the increasing frequency of the problem and the controversy surrounding its management. ACL injury factors have been divided into intrinsic and extrinsic factors.[630] Intrinsic factors include a narrow intercondylar notch, weak ACL, generalized overall joint laxity, and lower extremity malalignment; extrinsic factors include quadriceps and hamstring imbalances, altered neuromuscular control, shoe-to-surface interface, playing surface, and athlete's playing style.

Gender has also been implicated, with women being two to eight times more likely to sustain an ACL injury than men participating in the same sports.[630,631] Theories about the higher rates of ACL injury in women have centered on:[632]

- ***Anatomic alignment and structural differences.*** These include the differences in pelvic width and tibiofemoral angle between males and females, which can affect the entire lower extremity.[633] The magnitude of the quadriceps femoris angle (Q-angle) and the width of the femoral notch are thought to be anatomic factors that have contributed to the disparity of ACL injury rates between males and females.[632] Hypothetically, a larger Q-angle increases the lateral pull of the quadriceps femoris muscle on the patella placing medial stress on the knee,[633] and decreasing the effectiveness of the quadriceps as a knee extensor and diminishing the hamstrings' ability to exert its protective influence on the ACL.
- ***Femoral notch.*** A narrow intercondylar notch appears to increase the potential for ACL ruptures.[634] In a cadaver study, Norwood and Cross[635] showed that the ACL impinges on the anterior intercondylar notch with the knee in full extension.[632] The shape of the femoral notch varies with gender and may contribute to the incidence of ACL injury.[636] A small, A-shaped notch may be a sign of a congenitally smaller ACL.[636]
- ***Joint laxity.*** Joint laxity tends to be greater in women than in men,[637–639] although the correlation between ligamentous laxity and injury is not clear.
- ***Hormonal influence.*** Hormones, especially estrogen, estradiol, and relaxin, may be involved indirectly in increased ACL injury in females.[640,641]
- ***ACL size.*** Females typically have a smaller ACL than males, which would tend to enhance the risk of tissue failure.[642]
- ***Muscular strength and muscular activation patterns.*** Several studies have demonstrated that women have significantly less muscle strength in the quadriceps and hamstrings compared with men, even when muscle strength is normalized for body weight.[639,643–646] Approximately 30% of all ACL injuries are classified as contact injuries and the remaining 70% are not related to direct contact and are therefore classified as noncontact.[647,648] The most common noncontact of ACL injury in females are as follows[647,648]:
  - Planting and cutting
  - Straight knee landings
  - One-step stop with the knee hyperextended
  - Sudden deceleration

While landing injuries to the ACL are common in both males and females, male athletes appear to employ different mechanisms to compensate for high landing forces than females, resulting in a decrease in both varus and valgus laxity of the knee during the landing.[649–652]

The observation about the varying orientation and tensions of the ACL has clinical importance in a number of ways, and can help to define the following[36]:

- ***Mechanism of injury.*** Since the posterolateral portion of the ligament is taut when the knee is in extension, it is the most commonly injured portion.[36]
- ***How diagnostic tests are performed.*** When the ACL is tested for torn fibers, the knee joint should be assessed for stability in various positions, especially in slight flexion.
- ***Operative reconstruction.*** Reconstruction should be aimed at replacing the damaged portions of the ACL at the relevant angles of the joint.

All ACL tears (i.e., sprains) are categorized as grade I, II, or III injuries. Ligament tears are classified according to the degree of injury, which ranges from overstretched ligament fibers (i.e., partial or moderate tears) to ligament ruptures (i.e., complete tears or disruptions). The term *midsubstance tear* refers to the site of the ACL injury and indicates a central ligament tear as opposed to a tear at one of the ligament's bony attachment sites. Almost all ACL tears are complete midsubstance tears.[40,41] Young athletes may sustain growth plate injuries (e.g., avulsion fractures) rather than midsubstance tears because the epiphyseal cartilage in their growth plates is structurally weaker than their ligaments, collagen, or bones. In the past, research has shown that tears in ACL complexes of young athletes usually resulted in avulsion fractures not midsubstance tears. Recent studies, however, now suggest that young athletes may sustain midsubstance tears similar to those in adult athletes.[2,653]

Symptomatic ACL deficiencies in young athletes' knee joints are subject to the same long-term detrimental effects that occur in adult athletes.[654] Young athletes also may be more predisposed to more long-term degenerative knee conditions as the result of more years of chronic rotary knee instabilities from ACL deficiencies.[655]

Associated Knee Injuries

ACL injuries rarely occur in isolation, because the ACL functions in conjunction with other structures of the knee. For example, when the outer aspect of the knee sustains a direct blow that produces a valgus stress, the MCL is often torn first, followed by the ACL.[28] Debate continues regarding clinical intervention for the patient with combined ACL and MCL injury. For example, the following protocol is used at the University of Cincinnati Sports Medicine:[656]

- Grade 1 MCL: injury with or without meniscus damage. ACL surgery performed within 1 week; no presurgery motion restriction.
- Grade 2 MCL: injury with or without meniscus damage. ACL surgery performed within 2 weeks; a 7-day period of

motion limitation (brace locked at 30 degrees of full motion performed in rehabilitation on a daily basis, and after 7 days the brace is unlocked to full motion).

- Grade 3 MCL: injury with or without meniscus damage. ACL surgery performed after 3 weeks with a 10-day motion restriction (brace locked at 30 degrees and full motion is performed in rehabilitation starting day 7 after injury, and brace unlocked after 14 days).

Meniscal injuries can also occur, with the medial meniscus being more commonly involved. Approximately 49% of patients with sports-related ACL injuries have meniscal tears.[657]

Transection of the ACL leads to slight degenerative changes in the cartilage, but additional deafferentation of the knee joint produces severe degenerative changes.[658,659] This suggests that sensory input from the joint may play a role in adapting movement strategies so that potentially harmful positions and loads are prevented.

Mechanism of Injury

Most published studies of the ACL are directed toward the basic mechanics of the ligament, method of surgical repair, and rehabilitation.[247,603,660–662] Unfortunately, little is known about the actual mechanism of injury during sport activity, although one sport that has been studied in some detail is alpine (downhill) skiing,[663,664] in which three common causes of ACL injury have been discussed:

- The first is referred to as the "phantomfoot" mechanism.[664] This mechanism occurs when a skier falls backward with the knee flexed and the tibia internally rotated. The combination of a strong quadriceps contraction (to maintain balance) with a rigid boot that fails to release may lead to an ACL disruption.[665] As a result, the ligament disruption occurs during a hard landing when the skier is off balance.
- In the second mechanism, when the skier lands on the ski's tail, the stiff posterior shell of the boot combined with a strong quadriceps contraction to maintain balance slides the tibia anteriorly, leading to an anterior drawer maneuver.
- The third mechanism, valgus rotation, seems to be more common in men who participate in downhill or cross-country skiing. It occurs when the inside (medial) edge of the front of the ski becomes caught in the snow. The leg is abducted and externally rotated while the skier is driven forward by momentum. High-speed skiing and poorly groomed ski slopes also are factors that contribute to this type of injury.

Regrettably, little attention has been directed to the mechanism of ACL injuries in other sports, although sudden deceleration, an abrupt change of direction, and a fixed foot have all been cited as key elements of an ACL injury.[665] For example, a common mechanism of injury to the ACL occurs when excessive lateral force (i.e., valgus stress) is applied to the outer aspect of the knee joint. This type of injury often is seen in contact sports activities (e.g., football, soccer, and rugby), resulting from tackles or blows to the lateral side of the knee. A twisting injury to the ACL occurs when the knee is in full extension and the femur is rotated externally on a fixed tibia. This mechanism of injury usually occurs because of abrupt changes in speed, direction, or velocity that torque the knee. Maneuvers often seen in sports activities, such as football, basketball, and soccer, can cause twisting injuries to the ACL. Snowboarders also may experience the same mechanism of injury when their feet and ankles are locked in ski boots and their knees are torqued. A less common mechanism of injury to the ACL occurs with extreme hyperflexion or hyperextension of the knee joint.[28]

Examination

Diagnoses of sports-related ACL injuries can be difficult, and clinicians must consider many factors when determining the best treatment options for patients with ACL injuries. A thorough patient history and physical examination are essential for accurate diagnoses of ACL injuries. Patients commonly describe the sensation of their knee "popping" or "giving out" as the tibia subluxes anteriorly. Other signs and symptoms of ACL injuries include pain, immediate dysfunction, instability in the involved knee, and the inability to walk without assistance. In rare instances, when patients have isolated ACL injuries that do not involve related collateral or meniscal tears, local tenderness around the knee joint may be absent.[655]

The classic sign of ACL injuries is acute hemarthrosis (i.e., extravasation of blood into a joint or synovial cavity).[666] The signs and symptoms of hemarthrosis (i.e., pain, edema, and joint stiffness) make clinical examinations more difficult for clinicians and very uncomfortable for patients.

Atrophy of the quadriceps is a regular finding with patients who have a torn ACL.[667–671] Several authors found a decrease in extensor torque that was larger than would be expected on the basis of the decrease in the volume of the quadriceps as measured with CT,[668,669,672–674] whereas the hamstring muscles do not have a comparable force deficit. It would appear that even specific conservative intervention can only partially correct the deficit.[675] The difference in torque has been reported to persist after reconstruction of the ACL with use of autogenous grafts or allografts from the patellar ligament[675,676] or with use of semitendinosus grafts.[677,678]

During the examination, it is important for the clinician to examine the patient's contralateral knee for baseline comparisons. This especially is true in children who have inherent or congenital laxities, such as knock-knee (genu valgum) or saber legs (genu recurvatum). It is also important to remember that the pain the patient experiences during the examination may affect the accuracy of the test results. Common manual tests to assess the ACL include the anterior drawer and the Lachman test (see "Stress Testing" section).

Arthrometer

An arthrometer, such as a KT1000, is a noninvasive mechanical testing device for measuring anteroposterior knee motion. This device assesses the amount of displacement between the femur and the tibia at a given force in millimeters. Intratester reliability and intertester reliability for the KT1000 have been reported to be high, both within and between days.[359] In addition, based on a number of studies, the KT1000 appears to be a clinically applicable instrument that can be used to assess anterior laxity in patients with an ACL deficient knee.[63] Before using the KT1000 to assess anteroposterior laxity of the knee, the clinician must screen for PCL injury.

Although most patients who have a complete tear of the ACL have increased tibial translation on instrumented testing,[679] it is not known exactly how many of these patients will have "giving way" of the knee or how many knees will have overt or latent damage of the cartilage within a few years.[36,680,681]

Imaging Studies

Radiographs can identify arthritic changes that may be associated with chronic rotary instability from ACL deficiencies. They can also demonstrate avulsion fractures of the tibial spine, or hypoplastic intracondylar notches with diminished tibial spines, which indicate a congenital absence of the cruciate ligaments.[27]

MRI scans are useful for diagnosing ACL injuries, although their use in discriminating between complete and partial ACL tears is limited. Diagnostic MRI scans, however, can detect associated meniscal tears that routine radiographs cannot show.[2] Both MRI scans and radiographs are necessary to assess whether young athletes' growth plates are closed or open, a factor that may affect treatment decisions.

The primary healing potential of the ACL has been reported to be extremely poor in both clinical and experimental studies.[385,682–685] This is probably due to its minimal blood supply and the presence of joint fluid, both of which contribute to a reduced healing potential.[685–687] One study[687] did report two rare cases of spontaneous healing of an acute tear of the ACL, although the injuries were either near the origin or near the insertion of the ACL.

Patients with either partial (grades I and II) ACL tears (negative pivot shifts) or "isolated" ACL tears, who lead a less active lifestyle and participate in linear, nondeceleration activities are considered to be candidates for conservative intervention.[502] However, to return to normal preinjury activity levels, patients must be thoroughly rehabilitated and protective measures (e.g., knee bracing and activity restrictions) must be taken to prevent further knee injuries. Conservative intervention for these patients does not mean "nonintervention," because these patients require aggressive treatment to decrease pain and swelling, protect the joint from further injury, regain motion, increase strength and endurance, and return to function.[502] Numerous lower extremity rehabilitation protocols following injury or surgery have been reported in the literature.[233,268,444,623,688–698] For the middle-aged and older athlete, physical therapy often is the treatment of choice, unless the patient plans to participate in sports activities that expose the knees to vigorous twisting forces. Certain sports activities, however, must be avoided, especially those involving jumping, quick starts and stops, and abrupt lateral movements (e.g., soccer, basketball).

ROM exercises, which are initiated as early as possible, must be performed carefully so as not to further aggravate soft tissue injury and prolong pain and effusion. Failure of the pain and effusion to resolve, and ROM to improve, should arouse suspicion of a displaced torn meniscus.[502]

Most authors stress the importance of strengthening the quadriceps, gastrocnemius-soleus, and hamstrings muscles to prevent, or minimize, atrophy and maintain or improve strength.[233,268,623,688–692,694,696,697,699] The strengthening exercises should be performed through a limited ROM, determined by patient tolerance and response to the exercises.[231,233,444,689,690,696,697] Others recommend CKC exercises[243,623,689,696] to promote cocontraction of the thigh musculature and limit anterior tibial translation. A comprehensive knee rehabilitation protocol should include all of these factors.

Surgical treatment of the torn ACL includes direct repair, repair with augmentation, and reconstruction with autographs or allografts. Currently, arthroscopic reconstruction remains the treatment of choice. Numerous surgical approaches and postsurgical rehabilitation protocols exist that are beyond the scope of this text. Generally speaking, the rehabilitation progression following ACL reconstruction can either be accelerated, when used for young, athletic patients, or slower when used for older patients whose needs are more recreational. Normal return to sports activities occur at about 6 months for the accelerated patient and 6–9 months for the general orthopaedic patient.

Genu Recurvatum ("Saber Legs")

Genu recurvatum is a position of the knee joint complex in which the ROM occurs beyond neutral or 0 degrees of extension.[157] Genu recurvatum appears to be more common in females than in males and may exist due to postural habit, increased joint laxity, or knee injury.[700]

Traditionally, rehabilitation has only been used to address this condition when poor muscle control of the knee exists, such as occurs following trauma or a neurologic insult such as a cerebral vascular accident (CVA). However, one might question whether genu recurvatum predisposes an individual to knee injury. Certainly, the posterior structures of the knee (the capsular and noncapsular soft tissue structures, including the arcuate complex, posterior capsule, lateral meniscus, fabellofibular ligament, and biceps femoris muscle) are likely to be stressed with genu recurvatum. The posterior capsule forms two pouches that extend over the articular surface of the femoral condyle and tibial plateaus.[156] The capsule is thin over the posterior aspect of the femoral condyles but is supported by the two heads of the gastrocnemius and reinforced by the oblique popliteal ligament. The arcuate ligament also reinforces the capsule laterally. Stability is further enhanced internally by the lateral meniscus, which forms a concave articular surface for articulation with the convex lateral femoral condyle.[5]

A thorough history will guide the clinician to suspect genu recurvatum as a contributing factor in knee or another lower-leg injury. Individuals with genu recurvatum may present with one of a variety of lower extremity diagnoses as it is doubtful that their primary diagnosis will be genu recurvatum. Patients may have a history of an injury that forced them into hyperextension. Examples include landing from a jump on an extended knee; a blow to the anteromedial aspect of the proximal tibia, forcing the knee into hyperextension; and a noncontact external rotation hyperextension injury. From the anatomic and biomechanical review, it appears that the possible consequence of genu recurvatum in the active individual may be an increase in stress placed on the ACL, the anterior joint, or the posterolateral corner of the knee. Symptoms attributable to genu recurvatum include the following:

- ***Anteromedial joint pain.*** This pain results from the compressive forces at the medial tibiofemoral compartment. This pain may be accentuated if a varus alignment is present.
- ***Posterolateral knee pain.*** This pain results from the tension placed on the posterior structures and is aggravated by stepping or forceful knee extension in weight-bearing.[101]

The patient may also complain of knee instability during activities of daily living. Noyes et al. have described the posterolateral syndrome as an injury to the posterolateral structures in conjunction with a torn ACL.[701] This syndrome is usually characterized by no history of injury and a gradual onset of knee pain. Loudon et al.[702] found a positive correlation between genu recurvatum and ACL injury in female athletes. Hutchison and Ireland[638] attributed the recurvatum posture and laxity in the posterior capsule to habitual posture.

Patients with genu recurvatum are easily identified during static standing, with the sagittal view best demonstrating this posture. Individuals also may present with excessive femoral internal rotation, genu varum or valgum, tibial varum, or excessive subtalar joint pronation, which is more noticeable in the frontal plane.

When performing activities such as step-ups, patients will use momentum to straighten the lower extremity, and they will be unable to control weight-bearing terminal knee extension. Kendall et al.[153] report that the hyperextension posture of the knee is caused from weakness in the gastrocnemius.

Proprioception in individuals with genu recurvatum may be deficient, especially near the end range of extension. One study[702] demonstrated that individuals who stood in hyperextension and without knee injury were unable to reproduce knee joint angles in the last 15 degrees of extension compared with other knee angles of 45 and 60 degrees on a leg-press machine. Individuals may perceive the hyperextended knee position as "normal" and, when they are introduced to a more vigorous activity, they may have a tendency to stay in hyperextension, putting the knee at risk for injury.[702,638]

If genu recurvatum is suspected as contributing to the patient's symptoms, special attention is needed to identify posterolateral instability. This can be achieved using the posterolateral drawer test and the varus stress test at 30 degrees. If the recurvatum is unilateral, the clinician should assess the lumbar spine and pelvis for obliquity or muscle imbalance. In addition, the hip should be evaluated for excessive internal rotation, which contributes to genu recurvatum, and the subtalar and midfoot joints should be checked for excessive pronation, which allows excessive internal rotation of the tibia (see Chap. 19).

Patients with genu recurvatum need to learn that 0 degree of knee extension is the normal knee position, and hyperextension is to be avoided.[703] The patient is taught to keep the knee in the same plane as the foot. Verbal cueing is helpful, but other strategies, such as the temporary use of posterior knee taping, can give the patient direct sensory feedback. This neutral position should then be carried over to dynamic strengthening exercises.

Muscle sequencing is the key, with the hamstrings and gastrocnemius firing in conjunction with the quadriceps to guide the knee into extension rather than using the passive force of gravity.[639] Patients should progress through weight-bearing exercises that require sequential use of eccentric and concentric control of the lower extremity, such as resistive terminal extension, single leg balance, mini-dips, squats, forward and backward step-ups, lunges, and jump landings.

Knee control during gait can be taught in conjunction with the previously mentioned exercises. Noyes et al. recommend that the patient maintain knee flexion of 5 degrees throughout the stance phase of gait. A 1–2-inch elevated heel may be used in the initial training to create a flexion moment at the knee, and the trunk should be maintained in an upright position versus a forward lean or flexed hip during midstance to avoid an anterior shift of body weight.[701] Excessive internal femoral rotation also should be controlled during this phase of gait.[701]

Continued training of the patient with genu recurvatum should focus on functional tasks. These include stair climbing and sit-to-stand transfers, such as stair climbing. During the pull-up phase of stair climbing, patients should be trained to refrain from thrusting into knee extension. Individuals may have a tendency to hyperextend their knees with other daily activities, such as bending forward to brush their teeth or prolonged standing.

The final phase of rehabilitation focuses on more complex activities and sports-specific skills. It is important that athletes involved in jumping and cutting sports master a flexed knee position. Henning et al.[231] have suggested that extreme loads are placed on the ACL when the knee is straight or near-straight during planting and cutting, landing from jumps, and sudden stops while running. Emphasis should thus be placed on flexing the knee during these sports activities to prevent injuries to the ACL. Hamstrings that are adaptively shortened offer protection to these joints and should not be stretched.

Meniscal Tears

Because of the interrelationship of the menisci with other structures of the knee, a torn meniscus is the most common cause of mechanical symptoms in the knee. Knee injuries may result in isolated or combined meniscal lesions. Collagen and proteoglycan damage can be caused by mechanical factors (tears or surgical resection), enzymatic degradation, or synthesis of new, poorly functioning molecules.[80] Meniscal lesions usually occur when the patient attempts to turn, twist, or change direction when weight-bearing, but they can also occur from contact to the lateral or medial aspect of the knee while the lower extremity is planted.[66] Collagen damage leads to abnormal hydration and an irreversible cascade of tissue alteration.[80] When proteoglycans are damaged (and the collagen remains intact), these tissue changes are reversible. For example, immobilization leads to proteoglycan loss, which is reversed after return of motion stimulates fibrochondrocytes to synthesize new proteoglycan molecules.[80] With aging, the meniscal tissue degenerates and can delaminate, thus making it more susceptible to splitting from shear stress, resulting in horizontal cleavage tears.[704] Without the menisci, the loads on the articular surfaces are increased significantly, leading to a greater potential for articular cartilage injuries and degenerative arthritis. Since the menisci are without pain fibers, it is the tearing and bleeding into the peripheral attachments as well as traction on the capsule that most likely produce a patient's symptoms.[257] In fact, 16% of asymptomatic patients have meniscal tears demonstrated on MRI, with the incidence increasing to 36% for patients older than 45 years.[705]

Patients with meniscal injuries typically present with a history of swelling, popping, or clicking, and pain along the joint line. With posterior horn tears, the meniscus may return to its anatomic position with extension. If the tear extends anteriorly beyond the MCL, creating a bucket-handle tear, then the unstable meniscus fragment cannot always move back into an anatomic position.[257] Such a meniscal tear can result in locking of the knee in a flexed position. The lateral meniscus, being more mobile, is less likely to be associated with locking when torn. The patient may also note a "clicking" sensation while walking as a result of traction against a torn medial or lateral meniscus.[705] Locking of the knee is more common in younger patients with meniscal tears, because older patients are more likely to have degenerative meniscal tears with less mechanical symptoms and an insidious onset.[257]

The joint line pain is thought to result from capsular irritation. Meniscal tears are symptomatic as they render a portion of the meniscus abnormally mobile.[706] The shape and location of the meniscal tear determines the symptoms and clinical findings.

At the time of writing, four conservative approaches exist for the intervention of meniscal injuries: rehabilitation, meniscectomy, meniscus repair, and allograft transplantation.[66] The choice of intervention depends on several factors, including age, activity demands, size and location of the tear, and collateral tissue damage.[707]

Meniscal lesions that can be treated conservatively (~one-third) include the diffusely degenerative meniscus. Unless a tear is acute, peripheral, and stable, the relative avascularity of the middle third and the inner third of both menisci indicates a poor healing potential in these areas.

The conservative intervention for meniscal tears focuses on the resolution of impairments such as swelling, restricted ROM, and strength by using exercises, bracing, and oral medications.[708]

If the knee is locked or cannot be fully extended, the torn meniscal fragment is displaced and must be treated surgically. Although most peripheral tears are successfully repaired because of the healing capabilities of the meniscus, tears of the inner third of the meniscus are usually treated by meniscectomies.[66]

A number of surgical techniques exist for meniscal repair:

- Open repair. Open meniscal repair currently is most useful with multiple-ligament injuries in which the collateral ligament injuries may require open repair or tibial plateau fractures require open reduction and internal fixation.
- Arthroscopic. This technique allows evaluation and treatment of meniscal tears that are not possible with open techniques.

Rehabilitation after meniscal repair depends on whether ACL reconstruction was performed at the same time. For example, if ACL reconstruction is performed concurrently with the meniscal repair, more aggressive ROM exercises should be performed although flexion should be limited to 90 degrees for the first 4–6 weeks. Although many protocols exist, the principles of rehabilitation include an initial period of non–weight-bearing and limitation of flexion. Arnoczky et al.[78] have demonstrated that the meniscus is subject only to small amounts of motion and stress between 15 and 60 degrees of knee flexion.

An example of a rehabilitation protocol for a postsurgical lateral meniscal repair is outlined in Box 20-1.

Allograft Meniscal Transplantation[239]

Studies demonstrating the ability of meniscal tissue to heal if attached to a well-vascularized periphery led to the hypothesis that transplanted allographic meniscal tissue would have the potential to revascularize and function within the recipient's knee.[240–244]

Meniscal transplantation was first performed in humans in 1984 by Milachowski et al..[245] Since that time, preliminary reports and case studies have appeared in the literature. These reports have shown good or satisfactory results in 85–95% of patients.[241,245–248]

The topic of postoperative rehabilitation for the meniscal transplant is not fully developed within the current literature. Most reports advocate the use of a brace on the involved knee, 5–6 weeks of partial or non–weight-bearing status on the involved extremity and immediate ROM of the knee joint.[241,246,248,249] Restoring full extension immediately after surgery is emphasized, particularly in medial transplants, because this often involves removal and reattachment of the posterior oblique ligament and deep portion of the MCL. Loss of motion after ACL reconstruction has been correlated with repairs of these structures.[250] As rehabilitation progresses, CKC activities are limited from 0 to 60 degrees of flexion, because the load borne by the menisci increases as the knee approaches 90 degrees.[216] Proprioceptive training is emphasized, because the menisci contain mechanoreceptors and likely have a proprioceptive role.[251] On the basis of the findings from a variety of studies,[241–245,247] the initiation of functional activities can occur at approximately 9 months, with a full return to functional activities at approximately 1 year after surgery. The functional progression initially includes jogging, and progresses to running straight ahead. Cutting activities, which are added slowly, are monitored carefully. Returning to hard cutting and pivoting activities following meniscal transplant surgery is not recommended because of the high stresses these activities place on the menisci and the increased risk of reinjury they present.

Posterior Cruciate Ligament Tear

Injury to the PCL is thought to account for 3–20% of all knee injuries depending on the source, which suggests that many go undiagnosed.[709,710] Because of its inherent strength, damage to the PCL usually only occurs with significant trauma such as a dashboard injury associated with a motor vehicle accident,[711] or by a fall on a hyperflexed knee with the foot positioned in plantarflexion.[712] Isolated injuries of the PCL are less frequent as compared with combined injuries. For example, Fanelli[713,714] reported that 96.5% of traumatic knee injuries that involved the PCL were combined injuries. High energy mechanisms are

Box 20-1 Rehabilitation Protocol for Postsurgical Lateral Meniscus Repair

Week 1

- Continuous passive motion (CPM): PROM 10–70 degrees (knee extension/flexion), 3 × 60 min/d
- No AROM exercises
- Partial weight-bearing with crutches (20% of body weight)
- Knee brace locked in extension (for 4 weeks); wear brace day and night; remove brace for exercising and CPM
- Modalities to decrease swelling and pain: ice 6 × 10 min/d, transcutaneous electrical nerve stimulation (TENS) 2 × 20 min/d
- Patella mobilizations, low grade, 5 min/d
- Soft tissue massage (posterolateral, suprapatellar), 15 min/d
- Isometric quadriceps contractions (in 20 degrees of flexion), 10 × 30 s/d
- Electrical muscle stimulation (EMS) for quadriceps (in 20 degrees of flexion): 30 contractions per day (4-s duration [85 Hz], 20-s rest time per day)
- Upper body ergometer aerobic program, 10 min/d
- Upper extremity and trunk strengthening program, 30 min/d

Week 2

- Continue with the above program
- Partial weight-bearing with crutches (20% of body weight)
- PROM goal: 0–90 degrees
- AROM exercises for extension (in available range)
- No AROM for flexion
- Seated concentric quadriceps contractions, 60–0 degrees of flexion (against manual resistance, Theraband), 6 × 20 reps/d
- EMS for quadriceps (60 degrees of flexion), 30 contractions per day (4-s duration [85 Hz], 20-s rest time)
- Pool exercises (gait, balance, coordination), 20 min/d

Week 3

- Continue with the above program
- Partial weight-bearing with crutches (50% of body weight)
- ROM goal: 0 degree, 120 degrees, discontinue CPM when goal reached
- Flexibility exercises for quadriceps (Thomas position), 6 × 30 s/d
- Bilateral proprioceptive exercises (knee flexion, 10–20 degrees), on different unstable surfaces, 6 × 1 min/d
- Bilateral balance exercises (Biodex Stability System), 6 × 30 s/d
- Isokinetics (speeds 30 degrees/s and 60 degrees/s) in limited ROM (40–90 degrees of flexion) for quadriceps, 3 × 20 reps/d
- Stationary bike for gentle ROM exercise (low resistance), 3 × 15 min/d

Week 4

- Continue with the above program
- Partial weight-bearing with crutches (70% of body weight)
- ROM goal: 0–130 degrees
- Begin gentle AROM exercises for flexion
- Bilateral mini-squats (0–40 degrees), 6 × 20 reps/d
- Unilateral proprioceptive and balance training (knee flexion, 10–20 degrees), 6 × 20 s/d
- Isometric hamstring exercises (in 0, 20, 40, 60, and 80 degrees of flexion), 6 × 30 reps/d
- Simulated leg press on the CKC attachment (Biodex Systems), range 0–60 degrees, speed 90 degrees/s, 3 × 30 reps/d
- Deep-water running program (with wet vest), 20 min/d

Week 5

- Continue with the above program
- Full weight-bearing for *level* gait (avoid stairs), discontinue the use of crutches
- ROM goal: ensure 0–130 degrees with active and passive exercises
- Discontinue knee brace, use of knee neoprene sleeve

Box 20-1 Rehabilitation Protocol for Postsurgical Lateral Meniscus Repair *(Continued)*

- Flexibility exercises: add stretching for hamstrings, gastrocnemius/soleus, iliotibial hand, hip flexors, adductors, 3 × 30 s for each muscle group
- Unilateral proprioceptive and balance training (knee flexion, 10–20 degrees), 6 × 30 s/d
- Isokinetics quadriceps (speeds, 30, 60, 90, 120, 150, and 180 degrees/s; range, 110–0 degrees), 6 × 10 reps (each speed)/d
- Hamstring exercises (0–90 degrees of flexion) with Theraband, 5 × 20 reps/d
- Stationary bike (increase resistance), 3 × 20 min/d

Week 6

- Continue with the above program
- Exercise passive flexion end of ROM (unloaded flexion), 6 × 10 min/d
- Bilateral semi-squats (0–60 degrees), 6 × 20 reps/d
- Bilateral reactive/quickness training, 10 × 30 s/d
- Agility training (lateral movements with Sport Cord), 3 × 15 min/d

Week 7

- Continue with the above program
- "Sit back on heels" exercise (loaded flexion), 12 × 1 min/d
- Stairs allowed
- Unilateral mini-squats (0–40 degrees), 6 × 20 reps/d
- Isokinetics quadriceps AND hamstring (speeds 180, 210, 240, 270, and 300 degrees/s; range, 110–0 degrees), 6 × 10 reps (each speed)/d
- Strengthening program on weight machines (leg press, leg curls), 1 × 30 min/d
- Endurance program on bike, 1 × 45 min/d

Week 8

- Continue with the above program
- PROM goal: symmetrical
- Progress unilateral mini-squats to semisquats
- Lunges program (front, lateral, diagonal), 3 × 25 each
- Stairmaster, 1 × 30 min/d

Week 9

- Continue with the above program
- Intensify strengthening (2 × 45 min/d) and endurance program (1 × 60 min/d)

Week 10

- Continue with the above program
- "Sit back on heels" goal: symmetrical
- Plyometrics program (bilateral vertical and horizontal jumping), 1 × 20 min/d
- Controlled return to sports

Week 11 to 14

- Continue with the above program
- If no problems, discontinue rehabilitation by end of week 12
- Intensify sport-specific ice training until complete integration in the team training

Data from Bizzini M, Gorelick M, Drobny T: Lateral meniscus repair in a professional ice hockey goaltender: A case report with a 5-year follow-up. *J Orthop Sports Phys Ther* 36:89–100, 2006.

thought to result in a higher portion of combined injuries, whereas lower energy mechanisms are thought to result in a high proportion of isolated injuries.[715]

Clinical findings for a PCL tear include the following:

- Reports of hearing a "pop."
- Pain in the posterior aspect of the knee joint that may be aggravated with kneeling. Minimal pain typically occurs with extension, but is typically increased past 90 degrees of flexion and the patient may lack 10–20 degrees of flexion.[716]
- Minimal swelling.

- Possible abrasion or contusion on the superior, anterior aspect of the tibia, suggesting the occurrence of a posteriorly directed force of the tibia on the femur.
- Instability may or may not be present, depending on the severity of the tear. If present, the patient may complain of "giving way."
- Positive special tests, such as the posterior drawer, posterior sag, and quadriceps active test (see "Special Tests" section).
- Variable neurovascular findings based on severity. Structures to be assessed include the posterior tibial artery and vein (palpation of the distal posterior tibialis and dorsal pedis pulses and the fibular (peroneal) nerve (motor and sensory distributions of the nerve).

It is important for the clinician to delineate between isolated and combined lesions as intervention recommendations between these groups is different.[716] Specifically, isolated injuries (grades I and II, where the posterior translation is <10 mm) are generally treated conservatively, whereas combined injuries frequently necessitate a more aggressive intervention.[368]

Diagnostic studies may include radiographs, MRI, instrumented testing and stress radiographs. In acute cases, routine radiographs are essential to determine the absence or presence of associated fracture or an avulsion.

CLINICAL PEARL

MRI has been heralded as the gold standard for assessing PCL injuries.[717] Sensitivity and specificity for detection of PCL tears with MRI has been reported at 99%.[718]

Although it is not possible to predict which patients will obtain a favorable clinical results from conservative intervention and which will worsen over time, it would appear that the prognosis for an injury that occurs at high velocities and force levels is less favorable when compared with injury that occurred at low velocities and lower force levels.[719,720]

The focus of conservative intervention for isolated PCL injuries is to restore ROM and to strengthen the quadriceps and gastrocnemius, while delaying hamstring strengthening (for approximately 6–8 weeks) and protecting the articular surfaces.

- Quadriceps strengthening is performed to help reduce posterior tibial translation.[721] Theoretically, with the distal end fixed, a concentric contraction of the gastrocnemius can glide the femoral condyles posteriorly thereby reducing posterior subluxation of the tibia on the femur.
- Hamstring strengthening is delayed following the injury to decrease the potential for PCL stress. Resisted OKC knee flexion exercises should be avoided. Instead the hamstrings should be strengthened in a CKC environment to minimize any posterior shear stresses due to joint compression as well as substantially decreasing the angle of pull of the hamstrings on the posterior tibia.

A combination of OKCEs and CKCEs are initiated to promote dynamic stability of the knee.

CLINICAL PEARL

Many isolated PCL injuries heal with conservative intervention, especially in light of the fact that many PCL-deficient patients do not experience functional instability.[716] However, the long-term follow-up studies of PCL injuries reveal a progressive development of pain and degeneration of the medial compartment of the tibiofemoral joint.[722]

Important exercises include squats, lunges, and CKC knee extensions. Heavy resistance OKC knee extension exercises through a range of 45–20 degrees of flexion are avoided to protect the patellofemoral joint.[232,254] Balance and proprioceptive exercises also are performed. For the symptomatic patient, the use of a PCL brace may be advantageous. In addition, for patients with medial compartment pain, a trial of a lateral heel wedge may be beneficial.

Plyometrics are introduced for appropriate patients such as athletes. Return to sport may occur in as little as 6–8 weeks, but on average takes 12–16 weeks, providing that there are no complicating factors. These complicating factors include significant varus or valgus alignment, or damage to additional tissues.

Surgical intervention of isolated PCL injuries is an area of continued controversy and there is yet no clear consensus as to which techniques or graft designs are best. Complicating matters is that outcomes between the various surgical treatments are difficult to compare due to the wide range of injury patterns, differences in surgical and rehabilitation protocols. As the outcomes of conservative management are good or excellent in 50–80% of patients with isolated grade I or grade II PCL injuries, a trial period of rehabilitation as described above is typically recommended initially.[719,723]

The surgical management of patients who have PCL injuries combined with other ligament or capsular injuries is somewhat clearer and is recommended in the presence of pain and/or significant instability. As with postsurgical ACL protocols, a wide variety exists, a summary of which follows:

- Day 1–1 month: the goals during this phase are to control inflammation and promote healing, achieve full knee extension, knee flexion range of motion to 90 degrees, and quadriceps strength $\geq$3/5. Exercises during this phase include quad sets, ankle pumps, supine straight leg raise, and hip abduction/adduction. Any added resistance is applied proximal to the knee.
- 1–3 months: the goals during this phase are to achieve knee flexion ROM equal to 125 degrees, and quadriceps strength $\geq$4/5. At approximately 8 weeks postoperatively, exercises can include stationary bike without toe clips, leg press from 0 to 90 degrees, CKC terminal knee extension, and balance and proprioceptive exercises.
- 3–9 months: the goals during this phase are to have no limitation with activities of daily living and a limited resumption of low impact recreational activities. The CKCEs are progressed.
- 9–12 months: During this phase steps should be taken to return to previous levels of physical function and athletic pursuits.

Patellofemoral Instability

Patella instability can be produced by the following:

- ***A small patella.*** A smaller patella decreases the stability of the patella during its tracking.[11,724,725]
- ***A shallow patellar groove.*** The term *dysplastic femoral trochlea* implies a shallow intercondylar sulcus, especially at the lateral ridge, which often contributes to instability.[11,724,725]

There is strong evidence that implicates the depth of the trochlear groove of the femur for abnormal patella malalignment relative to the femur.[726] Powers[726] compared the trochlear groove or sulcus angle, using pneumatic MRI, of 23 women with patellofemoral disorders, 12 of whom had no history of patellofemoral disorders, at various degrees of knee flexion (45, 56, 27, 18, 9, and 0 degrees). The study indicated that the trochlear groove depth correlated with patella kinetics. Trochlear groove shallowness was found to be predictive of lateral tilt at the angles studied between 27 and 0 degrees and lateral patella displacement at 9 and 0 degrees.[726] These findings suggest that the depth of the trochlear sulcus affects the orientation of the patella in the first 30 degrees of knee flexion for lateral tilt and the first 10 degrees for lateral glide.[727]

- ***An abnormal patellar position.*** The patella may lie too far proximally or distally relative to the trochlea, conditions called *patella alta* and *patella baja* (or patella infera), respectively.[227,728,729] Patella alta, as a separate entity, does not necessarily contribute to knee pain, but it can certainly contribute to lateral maltracking by causing the patella to enter into the patellar groove late in knee flexion. Patella baja occurs rarely in otherwise normal individuals. It is seen in achondroplastic dwarfs, who seldom have anterior knee pain, and as a postoperative complication of knee surgery.[339,730,554] Several radiographic methods for diagnosis of patella alta and baja have been reported in the literature.[729,731–733]
- ***A muscle imbalance between the VMO and VL.***[133,146,460] These imbalances are discussed in the "Biomechanics" Section.
- ***Generalized ligamentous laxity or complex malalignments of the entire extremity (genu recurvatum).***[187,285,734]

Instability is usually identified through the history, with the patient reporting either dislocation or subluxation episodes. A subluxation needs to be differentiated from "giving way," as this can be simply a reflex inhibition of the quadriceps secondary to pain. The direction of instability is usually lateral, with medial instability almost always secondary to iatrogenic causes.[284] On palpation, medial retinacular and distal patellar pole tenderness or distal quadriceps tenderness may be elicited.[319]

The number of episodes is important because patients who are first-time dislocators and infrequent subluxators should have a trial of conservative intervention or limited arthroscopic evaluation for documented osteochondral lesions,[187] whereas, recurrent instability is an indication for surgical intervention.[284] Once the instability and its direction have been established, the anatomic cause of the instability is determined.

Cruciate ligament instabilities can lead to secondary patellofemoral pain through increased patellofemoral contact pressures and abnormal joint loading patterns.

Symptomatic Plica

The plica syndrome has been associated with anterior pain as well as clicking, catching, locking, or pseudolocking of the knee, and it may even mimic acute internal derangement of the knee.[119,345,735–740]

There is some controversy regarding the prevalence of the plica syndrome, with some reports suggesting that it does not exist.[741–743] Jackson et al.,[119,743] Dandy,[742] and others[115,116,227,345,744–747] have stated that although plicae may indeed cause symptoms, the syndrome is overdiagnosed and many normal synovial plicae are removed. Conversely, other authors consider the plica syndrome to be a common cause of anterior pain in the knee that is often misdiagnosed, and believe that a suprapatellar membrane is virtually never asymptomatic.[124,748,749]

Sherman and Jackson[750] have proposed a set of criteria for the diagnosis of symptomatic synovial plica:

- History of the appropriate clinical symptoms.
- Failure of nonoperative intervention.
- Arthroscopic finding of a plica with an avascular fibrotic edge that impinges on the medial femoral condyle during flexion of the knee. This is often a diagnosis of exclusion and can only be confirmed at arthroscopy.
- No other abnormality in the knee that would explain the symptoms. It has also been suggested that a localized area of chondromalacia at the site of impingement by a plica on the femoral condyle is evidence that a plica is the cause of the symptoms.

Clinical Findings

The mediopatellar plica (also termed *Lino's shelf*), although the least common, this variety is often the cause of problems if it becomes thickened, resulting in pain with palpation over the medial parapatellar area. The severity of symptoms is not proportional to the size or breadth of the synovial plica.[119] There also appears to be no correlation between the duration of symptoms and the presence of pathologic changes in the plica.[751]

A palpable band or snapping, especially over the medial femoral condyle, should be sought. In one study of plicae in the knee, clicking was reported in 64%, "giving way" in 59%, and pseudolocking in 45% of the patients.[345] A number of special tests exists for the detection of plical irritation (see "Special Tests" section).

Plicae are not visualized well on plain radiographs, but a double-contrast arthrogram may demonstrate a suprapatellar plica or an anterior plica.[746,752–756] A skyline radiograph may demonstrate a synovial shelf.[736,757,758]

The conservative intervention for plica syndrome involves stretching of the quadriceps, hamstrings, and gastrocnemius as well as isometric strengthening, cryotherapy, ultrasound, patellar bracing, anti-inflammatory medication, and an altered sports-training schedule.[116,735,759–762] In an uncontrolled study,[763] this type of intervention resulted in an improvement in 40% of patients over a 1-year period.

Injection of the synovial plicae with corticosteroids and a local anesthetic in another uncontrolled study[764] was reported to have an excellent result in 73% of patients.

When patients are truly symptomatic, or when conservative measures have failed, surgical excision is usually curative.

PREFERRED PRACTICE PATTERN 4E: IMPAIRED JOINT MOBILITY, MOTOR FUNCTION, MUSCLE PERFORMANCE, RANGE OF MOTION ASSOCIATED WITH LOCALIZED INFLAMMATION

Tendinitis

Patellar tendinitis (jumper's knee) and quadriceps tendinitis are overuse conditions that are frequently associated with eccentric overloading during deceleration activities (e.g., repeated jumping and landing, downhill running). The association of patellar tendinitis with jumping was first described by Maurizio,[765] but the term *jumper's knee* originated from Blazina et al.. [766] Some authors feel that the term *patellar tendinitis* is a misnomer because the patellar "tendon," which connects two bones, is in fact a ligament.[767,768]

The high stresses placed on these areas during CKC functioning place them at high risk for overuse injuries. Overuse is simply a mismatch between stress on a given structure and the ability of that structure to dissipate the forces, resulting in inflammatory changes.[769]

The diagnosis of tendinitis is based on a detailed history and careful palpation of the tendon in both flexion and extension. Pain on palpation near the patellar insertion is present in both patellar and quadriceps tendinitis. These are usually self-limiting conditions that respond to rest, stretching, eccentric strengthening,[470,770,771] bracing, and other conservative techniques. When treating overuse injuries, it is essential that the clinician limit both the chronic inflammation and degeneration by working on both sides of the problem: tissue strength should be maximized through proper training, and adequate healing time must be allowed before returning to full participation.[769]

Several protocols have been advocated for the conservative intervention of patellar tendinitis. Stanish et al.[771] proposed the following strengthening program of eccentric exercise for chronic patellar tendinitis.

A 5-minute warm-up period consisting of a series of three to five static stretches held for 15–30 seconds each is performed. Next, the patient, from a standing position, flexes the knees, abruptly drops to a squatting position, and then recoils to the standing position. The velocity of the drop is increased until the patient is able to perform it as quickly as possible without pain. At this point, sandbags are added to the patient's shoulders to increase the load on the tendon. Apart from some minor discomfort during the exercises and some post-exercise muscle soreness, the procedures should be performed without pain.[771]

Reid[772] proposes a protocol based on the severity of the lesion. Grade I lesions, which are characterized by no undue functional impairment and pain only after the activity, are addressed with adequate warm-up before training and ice massage after training. With grade II to III strains, activity modification, localized heating of the area, a detailed flexibility assessment, and an evaluation of athletic techniques are recommended. In addition, a concentric–eccentric program for the anterior tibialis muscle group is prescribed, which progresses into a purely eccentric program as the pain decreases.[773]

The patient is positioned in supine with the foot in full plantar flexion. The clinician applies overpressure on the posterior aspect of the foot, placing the foot into further plantar flexion and stretching the anterior tibialis. The patient is asked to perform a concentric contraction into full dorsiflexion, which is resisted by the clinician. An eccentric contraction is then performed by the patient by returning the foot into its plantar flexed position as the clinician resists the motion from full dorsiflexion to full plantar flexion. This maneuver is repeated to the point of fatigue of the anterior tibialis.[773] As soon as possible, the eccentric loading program is added.

It is not clear why a program initially directed at the anterior tibialis muscle group should be therapeutic for the infrapatellar tendon and ligament, but it is theorized that the program may stretch the infrapatellar ligament, change the quadriceps-to-foreleg strength ratio or alter the biomechanics of take-off and landing.[772]

Surgical intervention is usually required only if significant tendonosis develops and is successful in the majority of patients.[774]

Iliotibial Band Friction Syndrome

As its name suggests, ITBFS is a repetitive stress injury that results from friction of the ITB as it slides over the prominent lateral femoral condyle at approximately 30 degrees of knee flexion.[775] The friction has been found to occur at the posterior edge of the band, which is felt to be tighter against the lateral femoral condyle than the anterior fibers.[775,776] The friction causes a gradual development of a reddish-brown bursal thickening at the lateral femoral condyle.

ITBFS is the most common overuse syndrome of the knee, being particularly common in long-distance runners (20–40 miles/week). In addition, long-distance runners who train on hilly terrain, graded slopes, or road cambers are also at risk, especially if their runs include downhill running,[776,777] which positions the knee in significantly less flexion than normal at initial contact. Finally, running on canted surfaces can result in a leg-length inequality and a change in the Q-angle, which can increase the stress on the ITB.

Although most cases of ITBFS have been reported in distance runners, anyone engaging in activity that requires repetitive knee flexion and extension, such as downhill skiing, circuit training, weight lifting, and jumping sports, is prone to developing this pathology.[494] ITBFS is also common in cyclists.[778–780] This is thought to be due to the pedaling stroke, which causes the ITB to be pulled anteriorly on the downstroke and posteriorly on the upstroke. Extrinsic factors include excessive bike seat height or cleat position on the pedal. If the cleats are excessively internally rotated on the pedal, the tibia also internally rotates, resulting in a valgus force on the knee and increased tension of the ITB.

A study of six cadavers by Muhle et al.[781] found that in four of six individuals, some fibers of the ITB remained in contact with the lateral femoral condyle during extension. With further flexion, the ITB moves posteriorly and contacts the lateral femoral epicondyle and LCL, indicating a phase during knee flexion during which an impingement of the band occurs. In runners, this impingement phase occurs predominantly during the early stance phase, very soon after initial contact.[494] In general, the faster the speed of running, the less the time spent in the impingement zone, because the knee flexion angle at initial contact increases with speed of running.[782–784]

Subjectively, the patient reports pain with the repetitive motions of the knee. There is rarely a history of trauma. Although walking on level surfaces does not generally reproduce symptoms, especially if a stiff-legged gait is used,[165,776] climbing or descending stairs often aggravates the pain.[785] Patients do not usually complain of pain during sprinting, squatting, or during such stop-and-go activities as tennis, racquetball, or squash.[776] The progression of symptoms is often associated with changes in training surfaces, increased mileage, or training on crowned roads. The lateral knee pain is described as diffuse and hard to localize.

Objectively, there is localized tenderness to palpation at the lateral femoral condyle or Gerdy's tubercle on the anterolateral portion of the proximal tibia. The resisted tests are likely to be negative for pain. The special tests for the ITB (Ober's test, Noble compression test, and creak test) should be positive for pain, or crepitus, or both, especially at 30 degrees of weight-bearing knee flexion. There may also be associated biomechanical changes. In addition to an adaptively shortened ITB, the following findings have all been associated with ITB friction problems, although they have yet to be substantiated: cavus foot (calcaneal varus) structure,[786] leg-length difference (with the syndrome developing on the shorter side),[787,788] fatigue,[789] internal tibial torsion (increased lateral retinaculum tension), anatomically prominent lateral femoral epicondyle, and genu varum.[790]

A study by Fredericson et al.[791] found that long-distance runners with ITBFS have weaker hip abduction strength in the involved leg compared with the uninvolved leg and symptoms improved with a successful return of hip abductor strength. To control coronal plane movement during stance phase, the gluteus medius and TFL must exert a continuous hip abductor movement. Fatigued runners or those with weak gluteus medius muscles are prone to increased thigh adduction and internal rotation at midstance. This, in turn, leads to an increased valgus vector at the knee and increased tension on the ITB, making it more prone to impingement.[791]

Conservative intervention for ITBFS consists of activity modification to reduce the irritating stress (decreasing mileage, changing the bike seat position, and changing the training surfaces), using new running shoes,[792] heat or ice applications, strengthening of the hip abductors, and stretching of the ITB.[203] Surgical intervention, consisting of a resection of the posterior half of the ITB at the level that passes over the lateral femoral condyle, is reserved for the more recalcitrant cases.[780]

Bursitis

Several types of bursitis are differentiated:

- ***Superficial and deep infrapatellar bursitis.*** Inflammation of these bursae usually results from a mechanical irritation during such activities as kneeling ("nun's knee") or direct trauma.
- ***Prepatellar bursitis ("housemaid's knee").*** Inflammation of this bursa is seen in patients who experience recurrent minor trauma of the anterior knee. Those whose occupations require long periods of kneeling are particularly at risk. Diagnosis is straightforward, with pain and possibly swelling present on palpation of the prepatellar bursa.
- ***Superficial pes anserinus bursitis.*** This condition can involve any of the bursae lying between the various tendons of the superficial pes anserinus or a bursa between the MCL and the superficial pes anserinus. Inflammation of these bursae is common in novice swimmers and long-distance runners. Clinical findings may include medial knee pain just distal to the joint line, and an externally rotated tibia, compared with the uninvolved side.
- ***MCL bursitis.***[553] MCL bursitis was first described by Brantigan and Voshell[793] as inflammation of the bursae deep to the MCL.[793–795] Because of the proximity of this bursa to the medial meniscus or medial meniscotibial ligament, this condition is often misdiagnosed. Patients describe pain along the medial joint line, confirmed on physical examination by a tender palpable mass that can be exacerbated by placing the knee under a valgus load. Because of the proximity of the semimembranosus tendon to the bursa, internal and external rotation can also impinge on the bursa and cause pain.[793] Imaging is not essential, but an MRI scan may show the inflamed bursa.[261]

The intervention for bursitis includes the removal of the irritation. This may involve the stretching of adaptively shortened structures or joint mobilizations to help correct alignment.

Sindig–Larson–Johansson Syndrome and Osgood–Schlatter Disease

This condition is an apophysitis of the tibial tubercle (Osgood–Schlatter disease) and inferior pole of the patella (Sinding–Larsen–Johanssen syndrome) that occurs in skeletally immature individuals, especially those involved in sports requiring repetitive-loaded knee flexion.

Osgood–Schlatter disease presents between the ages of 8 and 13 years in females and 10 and 15 years in males, who are affected about three times as often.[772] In 25–33% of the cases, there is bilateral involvement.[796] The condition is the result of a retrograde ossification of the tibial tubercle, which produces an apophysitis. Although usually self-limiting, it can progress to an osteonecrosis.

Sinding–Larsen–Johanssen syndrome usually occurs prior to the growth spurt. Fragmentation of the tibial tubercle or irregular calcification of the inferior patellar pole may be seen on radiographs. Pain is usually reported with use of the knee in activities such as athletics, cycling, or resisted knee extension. The involved area is tender and usually prominent on physical examination.

The intervention for these conditions is usually symptomatic, including short courses of anti-inflammatory medications, a focus on hamstring flexibility, and moderate-intensity quadriceps strengthening. The traditional approach of activity limitations is no longer considered necessary. Rarely, individuals will require excision of symptomatic ossicles or degenerated tendons for persistent symptoms at skeletal maturity. More persistent cases may require immobilization for 6–8 weeks.[772]

Quadriceps Contusion

Quadriceps contusions, resulting from a direct blow, can be very disabling.[797] Contusions of the anterior portion of the muscle are usually more serious than those involving the lateral portion of the muscle because of the differences in muscle mass present in the two areas.

As elsewhere in the body, contusions are graded according to severity. A grade I contusion produces only mild discomfort, with no swelling and no detrimental effect on gait. The patient with a grade II contusion may or may not have a normal gait cycle. Grade III contusions in this muscle are very rare due to the lack of muscle belly tissue.

These are frustrating injuries for the clinician and the patient, because there are often few clinical and radiographic findings to establish the diagnosis, resulting in a diagnosis made by way of exclusion. MRI may be helpful in the acute phase, but this remains a diagnosis that is largely based on the history.

If the intervention for these contusions occurs too early, or is too aggressive, myositis ossificans can develop. Myositis ossificans is a pathologic bone formation resulting from muscle tissue damage, bleeding, and damage to the periosteum of the femur, and producing ectopic bone formation.[798,799]

The intervention includes ice and 24-hour compression applied immediately, which should be continued until all of the signs and symptoms are absent. Gentle pain-free quadriceps-stretching exercises are begun on the first day, progressing to resistive exercises as tolerated, usually on the second day. If an abnormal gait is present, the patient may be issued crutches until the normal gait returns.

Patients with a grade I contusion can continue with normal activities as tolerated. A patient with a grade II contusion may require 3–21 days for rehabilitation. Grade III contusions may require 3 weeks to 3 months to fully heal.

Turf Knee or Wrestler's Knee

Turf knee, or wrestler's knee, is an injury to the soft tissue overlying the knee. It is caused by a shearing mechanism within the subcutaneous tissues. Swelling and tenderness are present, but the swelling is present in the extra-articular tissues and should be differentiated from a true joint effusion. A joint effusion is characterized by a ballotable patella, and the intra-articular fluid is mobile and can be pushed to and from the suprapatellar pouch. With turf knee, these signs are absent, but there is boggy swelling in the soft tissue and a sense of subcutaneous fluid is present on palpation. This injury usually responds well to rest and avoidance of the aggravating trauma.

Hoffa's (Fat Pad) Syndrome

The infrapatellar fat pad may be a cause of anterior knee pain. This syndrome was first described by Hoffa[800] in 1904. It is thought to represent hypertrophy and inflammation of the infra-patellar fat pad secondary to impingement between the femoral condyles and tibial plateau during knee extension. Direct trauma and overuse have also been attributed as causes. Irritation also can be produced by a posterior tilt of the inferior pole of patella.

Symptoms include anterior knee pain that is inferior to the pole of the patella. Pain is exacerbated by knee extension, particularly hyperextension, but not by knee flexion.[319] Inspection may reveal inferior patellar edema and associated tenderness of the fat pad when palpated through the tendon. Direct palpation of the fat pad on either side of the patellar tendon as the knee is brought from flexion into full extension is painful if the fat pad is inflamed. A diagnostic test, termed the *bounce test* (eliciting pain with passive knee hyperextension), is sometimes useful.[261] One must be careful to look for other causes of inflammation, such as OA, before concluding that the fat pad is the primary source of pain.[284] Plain radiographs are invariably negative, but abnormalities of the fat pad can be noted on MRI.[801]

Conservative intervention includes rest, ice, anti-inflammatory medications, and iontophoresis or phonophoresis. Local corticosteroid injections into the fat pad are preferred by some physicians because they can be both diagnostic and therapeutic.

Biomechanical interventions include addressing the causes of hyperextension through orthotic interventions, such as heel lifts or taping the superior pole posteriorly and holding the patella in a superior glide with tape.

In recalcitrant cases, surgical resection of portions of the fat pad is indicated.

Medial Retinaculitis

Medial retinaculitis is a rare condition seen almost exclusively in runners. It probably represents a fatigue tear in the medial capsular insertion into the patella. A positive bone scan in the medial edge of the patella confirms this diagnosis.

Baker's Cyst

Usually a Baker's cyst is asymptomatic, but in the presence of a synovial effusion, the cyst can swell up with fluid and become painful. On occasion, the cyst can become so large that it protrudes through the soft tissues, just proximal to the popliteal fossa, between the heads of the gastrocnemius. Ruptures of the cyst can occur, and these can mimic the symptoms of a tear of the gastrocnemius.

Clinical findings with the larger cysts include pain with active and passive knee flexion and extension, with weight-bearing, and pain and an increased prominence of the swelling with resisted knee flexion.

The conservative intervention for this condition normally involves treating the articular disorder that caused the cyst to swell. The medical management includes aspiration or surgical resection.

Popliteus Tendinitis

Popliteus tendinitis is common in runners who used canted surfaces, which produce oblique lateral rotary stresses to the knee, or who run downhill frequently. The condition typically manifests as point tenderness in the lateral aspect of the knee corresponding to the popliteus insertion site, which is exacerbated with eccentric loading.

Popliteus tendinitis can be diagnosed by having the patient sit so that the leg is in the figure-4 position, with the lateral aspect of the ankle resting on the contralateral knee.

Intervention involves a modification in the training regimen, ultrasound, and transverse friction massage.

Breaststroker's Knee

This condition of pain and tenderness localized on the medial aspect of the knee is often associated with performance of the whip-kick, the kick used with breaststroke.[97] The forceful whipping together of the lower legs often forces the lower leg into slight abduction at the knee, with subsequent irritation and inflammation to the MCL of the knee.

In a study of breaststroke kinematics,[802] it was found that angles of hip abduction of less than 37 degrees, or greater than 42 degrees at the initiation of the kick, resulted in a dramatic increase in the incidence of knee pain.[97]

PREFERRED PRACTICE PATTERN 4G: IMPAIRED JOINT MOBILITY, MUSCLE PERFORMANCE, RANGE OF MOTION ASSOCIATED WITH FRACTURE

Tendon Ruptures or Fractures

Quadriceps and patellar tendon ruptures, and patellar fractures, usually result from eccentric overload of the extensor mechanism or direct trauma. These are usually easy to diagnose, because the patient is unable to actively extend the knee, and there is a palpable defect at the site of injury. Radiographs will confirm fractures or avulsions. In skeletally immature individuals, fractures involving the proximal tibial epiphysis can occur. These are usually evident on radiographs and often require surgical intervention.

INTEGRATION OF PREFERRED PATTERNS 4 F AND 5 F: IMPAIRED JOINT MOBILITY, MOTOR FUNCTION, MUSCLE PERFORMANCE, AND RANGE OF MOTION SECONDARY TO COMPLEX REGIONAL PAIN SYNDROME (REFLEX SYMPATHETIC DYSTROPHY), MYOFASCIAL PAIN SYNDROMES (REFERRED PAIN SYNDROMES), PERIPHERAL NERVE ENTRAPMENT

Peripheral Nerve Entrapment

Compression Neuropathy of the Saphenous Nerve[553]

Saphenous nerve palsy is an impingement of the large cutaneous branch of the femoral nerve by the fascia of its three bordering muscles (anterolaterally by the vastus medialis, posterolaterally by the adductor longus, and medially by the sartorius) as it exits the adductor canal.[794,803–805] Occasionally, branches of the femoral vessels also may impinge on the nerve. The onset can be insidious or secondary to trauma or surgery about the knee.

Entrapment of the saphenous nerve often results in marked pain at the medial aspect of the knee. Patients describe a burning sensation in the nerve's sensory distribution, which typically worsens at night and is exacerbated by lower limb activity. The pain can be confused with an internal derangement of the knee or an anserine bursitis.

Physical examination reveals a Tinel's sign at the adductor canal. Often there is associated local tenderness. Sensory changes may be seen within the sensory distribution of the nerve. There is no motor weakness. Confirmation of a saphenous lesion can be made using resisted flexion of the knee or resisted adduction of the thigh, which should increase the pain, or pressure over the saphenous opening, in the subsartorial fascia, producing a radiation of the pain. Active flexion of the knee beyond 60 degrees can also reproduce the pain.

EMG and nerve conduction studies can help eliminate L-3 and L-4 radiculopathies and aid in the diagnosis.[803] Diagnostic peripheral nerve blocks with lidocaine also may be performed. Mild-to-moderate cases can be treated with rest, anti-inflammatory medications, ice, ultrasound, and TENS.[794,805,806] Second-line interventions include therapeutic nerve blocks with phenol.[804] Cases refractory to these interventions can be managed with surgical release of fascial bands and neurectomy.[805]

Compression Neuropathy of Superficial Fibular (Peroneal) Nerve

This nerve can be entrapped as a result of fibrosis following a direct blow,[807,808] or surgery. Symptoms typically include pain over the lateral distal aspect of the leg and ankle, mimicking symptoms of a disk herniation, with irritation of the L5 nerve root. However, differentiation can be made with percussion or pressure over the nerve at its point of exit, which will cause reproduction of the symptoms in this syndrome.[809]

Myofascial Pain Dysfunction: Vastus Medialis

This muscle refers pain deep to the patella, and patients typically complain of knee joint stiffness and loud cracking noises as the patella suddenly releases during knee flexion.[810] Dysfunction of the vastus medialis, which counters the lateral pull of the other three quadriceps muscles and ensures proper patellar tracking, can lead to patellofemoral dysfunction and pain. Structural deformities, such as valgus deviation of the knee or overpronation of the foot, put additional strain on this muscle and perpetuate trigger point activity.[810]

Complex Regional Pain Syndrome (Reflex Sympathetic Dystrophy)

This condition is characterized by intractable knee pain of considerable duration. The patient may appear severely disabled, often using crutches, and may appear anxious and depressed. The presence of cyanosis or mottling indicates autonomic dysfunction. There also may be a noticeable difference in temperature between the involved area and the contralateral limb. In late cases, trophic changes of the skin occur. In addition, wasting of the quadriceps and stiffness of the joint may be evident.

Early diagnosis is the key to a successful intervention. The intervention should include a comprehensive team approach involving the physician and physical therapist. The most important rule is to avoid excessive pain.[811] Complete rest to the involved region, particularly immobilization in a cast, is harmful.[812,813]

It is important to not reinjure the region or aggravate the problem with aggressive physical rehabilitation.[813] Thus, the progression should occur slowly and gently.

- Exercises are prescribed for strengthening, active assistive ROM, and AROM. Weight-bearing exercises and active stress loading exercises also should be incorporated.
- Sensory threshold techniques, including fluidotherapy, vibration desensitization, TENS, contrast baths, and desensitization using light and heavy pressure of various textures over the sensitive area, should be used.
- Affected joints should be rested and elevated to counteract the vascular stasis, but the joint also should be mobilized gently several times per day.[812]

THERAPEUTIC TECHNIQUES

Techniques to Increase Joint Mobility

A number of techniques can be used to increase joint mobility.

Joint Mobilizations

The mobilizations described in this section should always be complimented with exercises or automobilization techniques performed at home by the patient.

Patellofemoral Mobilizations

Numerous studies in the literature recommend using patellar mobilizations as one of the components of a physical therapy intervention for patellofemoral disorders.[191,814] These mobilizations are advocated to be performed in a variety of directions to increase the mobility of the patella, presumably to improve tracking. These include superior mobilizations, inferior mobilizations, and medial and lateral glides. However, from an evidence-based perspective, there is not one randomized study supporting the efficacy of patellofemoral mobilizations in the treatment of patellofemoral disorders at present.

The mobilizations for the tibiofemoral joint are identical to the techniques used to assess the joint, which are described in the passive physiologic articular mobility tests of the examination.

Distraction of the Tibiofemoral Joint

A variety of techniques can be used to apply a long-axis traction force to the tibiofemoral joint. Joint distraction is used for pain control and general mobility. Distraction at this joint tends to occur when moving into flexion. Using the resting position of the joint as a starting point, and the tibia rotated into either neutral, external rotation, or internal rotation, different ranges of flexion can be used.

Posterior Glide of the Tibia on the Femur

This technique is used to increase the joint glide associated with flexion of the tibiofemoral joint, with the emphasis of the mobilization technique varying according to the ROM being treated. For example, in the midranges of flexion, the posterior glide of the tibia is applied along the plane of the joint, whereas in the last few degrees of flexion, the posterior glide is applied with the congruent rotation of internal rotation of the tibia. Active mobilization can also be employed by positioning the patient's foot and leg into internal rotation, and asking the patient to pull isometrically with the hamstrings.

Anterior Glide of the Tibia on the Femur

This technique is used to increase the joint glide associated with extension of the tibiofemoral joint. If the clinician is attempting to regain the last 10–30 degrees of extension, the emphasis is placed on positioning the tibia in external rotation.

Proximal Tibiofibular Joint

The mobilizations for this joint are identical to the techniques used to assess the joint, which are described in the passive physiologic articular mobility tests of the examination. Myofascial restrictions of this joint present with the fibular head in an anterior or posterior position, and in the absence of adaptive shortening, the passive mobility tests will be normal. The intervention should be aimed at the cause of the muscle imbalance, but if direct treatment is attempted, active mobilization (muscle energy) techniques are used.

- To increase the posterior movement, the patient is asked to contract the hamstrings. The biceps femoris is attached to the fibular head and will help draw the fibular posteriorly.

- To increase the anterior glide, the patient is asked to contract the anterior tibialis, whose attachment will pull the fibula anteriorly.

Pericapsular hypomobility restrictions also present with the fibular head positioned anteriorly or posteriorly. The passive mobility test demonstrates reduced motion with a capsular end-feel. Treatment is by anterolateral (foot in plantar flexion) or posteromedial (foot in dorsiflexion) capsular stretches.

High-Velocity Correction for a Posterior Fibular Head

The patient is placed in the supine position, with the clinician standing beside the table, opposite the dysfunction. The clinician grasps the patient's foot and ankle on the side of the dysfunction with the nonthrusting hand and flexes the patient's hip and knee to 90 degrees. The clinician first places the index finger of his or her thrusting hand into the patient's popliteal crease, monitoring the dysfunctional fibular head. Next, the clinician locks the patient's foot on the side of the dysfunction in his or her armpit. The clinician then exerts a rapid downward thrust on the distal tibia and fibula while simultaneously pulling the fibular head anteriorly with his or her index finger.

AUTOMOBILIZATIONS

To Increase Extension

- Towel hyperextensions. A towel of sufficient height to elevate the calf and thigh off the table is placed under the heel (Fig. 20-66). A weight can be added to the tibia or femur to assist in regaining hyperextension at the knee (Fig. 20-67).
- Prone hangs (Fig. 20-68) **VIDEO**.
- Quadriceps setting. These exercises are done repeatedly during the day and can also be performed during the towel extension exercise.
- Standing extension (Fig. 20-69) with foot placed on a stool or chair.

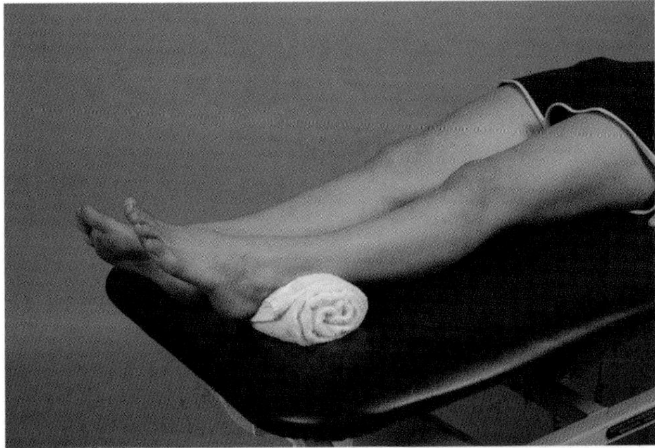

FIGURE 20-66 Towel hyperextensions.

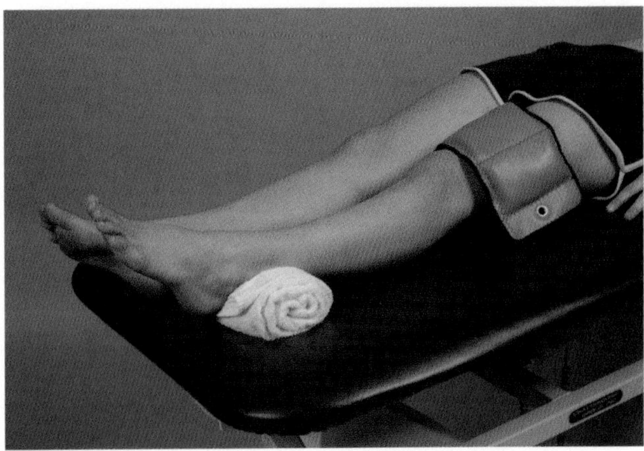

FIGURE 20-67 Towel hyperextensions with weight.

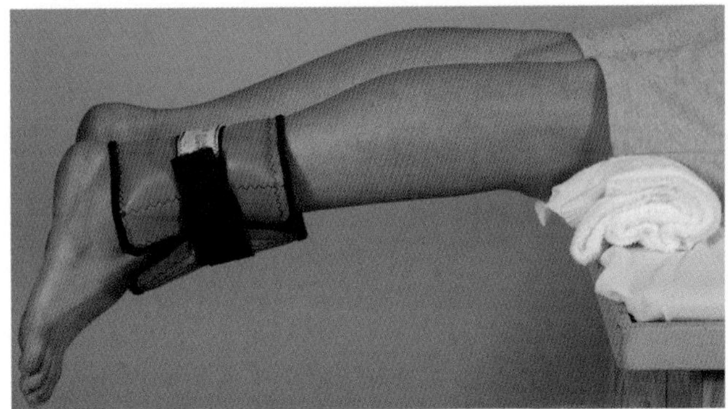

FIGURE 20-68 Prone hangs.

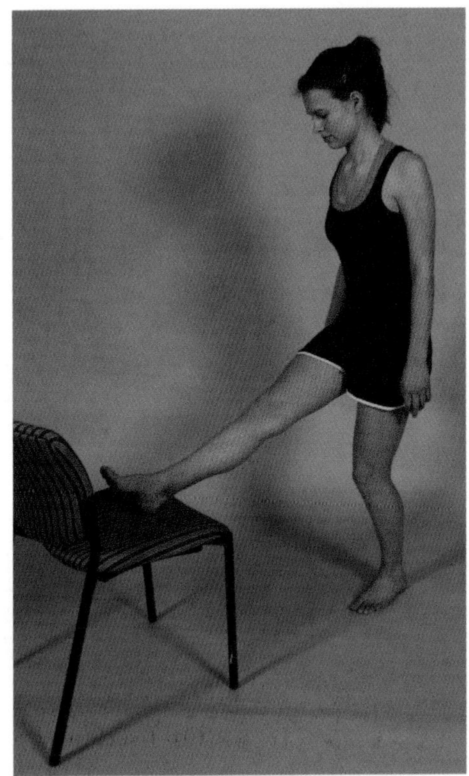

FIGURE 20-69 Standing extension.

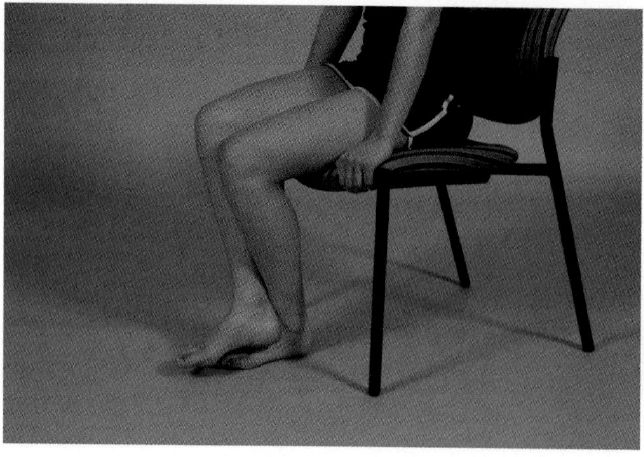

FIGURE 20-70 Seated heel slides with passive overpressure.

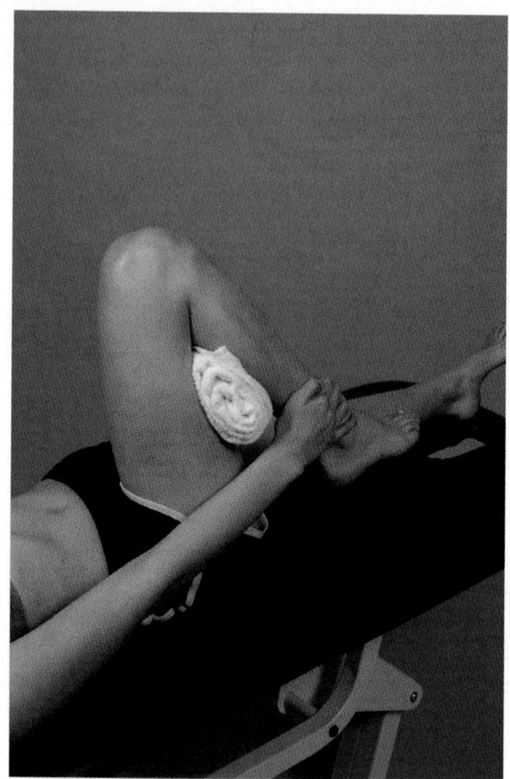

FIGURE 20-71 Passive knee flexion with towel roll behind knee.

To Increase Flexion

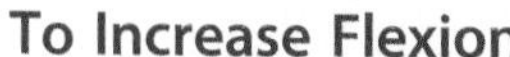

- Wall slides in supine with the sole of the foot on the wall are performed until 90 degrees of flexion is obtained, and then seated heel slides with passive overpressure are initiated (Fig. 20-70).
- The patient is placed in the supine or sitting position. A rolled-up towel/pillow of sufficient size is placed behind the knee so that with the knee actively flexed, the towel/pillow can be held in place and act as a fulcrum. Using one or both hands, the patient grasps the anterior aspect of the lower leg (Fig. 20-71). By gently pushing the lower leg posteriorly, flexion of the knee can be increased.

Techniques to Increase Soft Tissue Extensibility

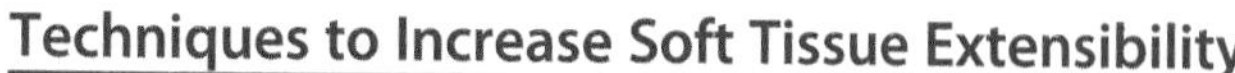

Increasing soft tissue extensibility is the hallmark of the functional knee rehabilitation protocol and includes stretching of the ITB, hamstring muscles, quadriceps, hip flexors, and Achilles tendon[189,319] (Table 20-20). The stretching techniques for the ITB, hamstring muscles, quadriceps, and hip flexors are described in Chapter 19. The technique for the Achilles tendon is described in Chapter 21.

Patients with marked internal rotation of the hip may require stretching of the anterior hip structures to increase the available external rotation and to help the gluteal muscles work in the inner range.[475]

TABLE 20-20 Muscle Stretching: Positions of Maximal Elongation and Stretch

Muscle	Maximal Elongation	Stretch
Gastrocnemius	Subtalar joint neutral, knee extension	Ankle dorsiflexion
Soleus	Subtalar joint neutral, knee flexion	Ankle dorsiflexion
Medial hamstrings	Hip external rotation, abduction, and flexion	Knee extension
Lateral hamstrings	Hip internal rotation and flexion	Knee extension
Rectus femoris	Hip extension	Knee flexion
Tensor fascia lata	Knee flexion, hip extension and external rotation	Hip adduction
Iliotibial band	Hip extension, neutral hip rotation, slight knee flexion	Hip adduction

CASE-STUDY

LEFT ANTERIOR KNEE PAIN

HISTORY

History of Current Condition

A 30-year-old woman presented with a 2-month history of progressive anterior left-knee pain.[553] The pain had started insidiously 3 months after she began playing field hockey. She denied any traumatic inciting mechanism. The pain was increased with hyperflexion and weight-bearing activities, abated with rest, but seemed aggravated with prolonged sitting. The patient also noted difficulty achieving full knee extension and had intermittent swelling and stiffness. Previous trials of oral anti-inflammatories had only mildly improved her pain.

History of Current Condition

No previous history of knee surgery or injury.

Past Medical/Surgical History

Unremarkable.

Medications

None.

Other Tests and Measures

Radiographs were negative for loose bodies, tumors, and fracture.

Social Habits (Past and Present)

Nonsmoker and drinker; active lifestyle.

Social History

Single; living alone.

Family History

No relevant history of knee problems in family.

Growth and Development

Normal development; right-handed.

Living Environment

Two-storey house.

Occupational/Employment/School

Full-time laborer; high-school education.

Functional Status/Activity Level

The patient denied any locking of her left knee, although there had been occasions when she felt the knee gave way because of pain. Pain increases with stair negotiation, particularly ascending stairs, and with prolonged sitting.

Health Status (Self-report)

The patient reported being in generally good health, but pain interferes with tasks at home and at work.

Questions

1. What structure(s) do you suspect to be at fault in this patient and require a specific examination?
2. What might the history of pain with prolonged sitting and stair negotiation tell the clinician?
3. What other activities do you suspect would increase the patient's symptoms? Why?
4. To help rule out the various causes of anterior knee pain, what other questions can you ask?
5. What is your working hypothesis at this stage? List the various diagnoses that could present with these signs and symptoms, and the tests you would use to rule out each one.
6. Does this presentation/history warrant a scan? Why or why not?

CASE-STUDY

LATERAL KNEE PAIN WITH RUNNING

HISTORY

History of Current Condition

A 22-year-old male runner complained of lateral right-knee pain that radiated from the lateral aspect of the knee, up the lateral thigh, and down to the proximal aspect of the lateral tibia. The pain was aggravated with running, especially on hills, and had begun about 6 weeks ago when he began training for a triathlon. The patient reported no pain with walking. The patient saw his physician, who prescribed a course of NSAIDs and recommended physical therapy.

History of Current Condition

No previous history of lower extremity pain.

Medical/Surgical History

Unremarkable.

Medications

Ibuprofen, 800 mg daily.

Functional Status/Activity Level

Pain was interfering with training for a triathlon. The patient also experienced pain with stair climbing.

Health Status (Self-report)

The patient reported being in generally good health.

Questions

1. What structure(s) could be at fault with complaints of lateral knee pain aggravated with running?
2. What might the history of a gradual onset of pain related to a change in training tell the clinician?
3. Why do you think the patient's symptoms are worsened with running on hills but not affected with walking?
4. What additional questions would you ask to help rule out referred pain from the lumbar spine?
5. What is your working hypothesis at this stage? List the various diagnoses that could present with these signs and symptoms, and the tests you would use to rule out each one.
6. Does this presentation/history warrant a scan? Why or why not?

REVIEW QUESTIONS*

1. Name a structure of the knee joint that is extra-articular and extrasynovial.
2. List three functions of the menisci.
3. Which peripheral nerve is primarily responsible for knee extension?
4. Anteversion of the hip may result in which knee deformity?
5. Which facet of the patella is likely to be involved if pain is reproduced at 20–30 degrees of knee flexion?

*Additional questions to test your understanding of this chapter can be found in the Online Learning Center for *Orthopaedic Assessment, Evaluation, and Intervention* at www.duttononline.net.

REFERENCES

1. Seebacher JR, Inglis AE, Marshall JL, et al: The structure of the posterolateral aspect of the knee. *J Bone Joint Surg* 64A:536–541, 1982.
2. Clasby L, Young MA: Management of sports-related anterior cruciate ligament injuries. *AORN J* 66:609–625, 628, 630; quiz 632–636, 1997.
3. Reinking MF: Knee anatomy and biomechanics, In: Wadsworth C, ed. *Disorders of the Knee—Home Study Course.* La Crosse, WI: Orthopaedic Section, APTA, Inc., 2001:1-8.
4. Kirkendall DT, Garrett WEJ: The anterior cruciate ligament enigma. Injury mechanisms and prevention. *Clin Orthop Relat Res* 372:64–68, 2000.
5. Kapandji IA: *The Physiology of the Joints, Lower Limb.* New York, NY: Churchill Livingstone, 1991.
6. Tortora GJ, Anagnostakos NP: *Principles of Anatomy and Physiology,* 5th ed. New York, NY: Harper Row Publishers, Inc, 1987.
7. Nordin M, Frankel VH: *Basic Biomechanics of the Musculoskeletal System.* 2nd ed. Philadelphia, PA: Lea & Febiger, 1989.
8. Reider B, Marshall JL, Koslin B, et al: The anterior aspect of the knee joint: An anatomical study. *J Bone and Joint Surg [Am]* 63A:351–356, 1981.
9. Bourne MH, Hazel WA, Scott SG, et al: Anterior knee pain. *Mayo Clinic Proc* 63:482–491, 1988.
10. Grelsamer RP: Patellar malalignment. *J Bone Joint Surg Am* 82-A:1639–1650, 2000.
11. Wiberg G: Roentgenographic and anatomic studies on the femoropatellar joint. *Acta Orthop Scandinavica* 12:319–410, 1941.
12. Yoshioka Y, Siu D, Cooke TDV: The anatomy and functional axes of the femur. *J Bone Joint Surg Am* 69-A: 873–879, 1987.
13. Brick GW, Scott RD: The patellofemoral component of total knee arthroplasty. *Clin Orthop* 231:163–178, 1988.
14. Jouanin T, Dupont JY, Lassau FP: The synovial folds of the knee joint: Anatomical study. *Anat Clin* 4:47, 1983.
15. Gray H: The joints: Articulation of the lower limb, In: Clemente CD, ed. *Anatomy of the Human Body,* 13th ed. Philadelphia, PA: Lea & Febiger, 1985:309–310, 397, 401.
16. Pick TP, Howden R: *Gray's Anatomy,* 15th ed. New York, NY: Barnes & Noble Books, 1995.
17. Gollehon DL, Torzilli PA, Warren RF: The role of the posterolateral and cruciate ligaments in the stability of the human knee. *J Bone Joint Surg Am* 69-A:233–242, 1987.
18. Lerat JL, Moyen BL, Cladiere F,et al: Knee instability after injury to the anterior cruciate ligament. Quantification of the Lachman test. *J Bone Joint Surg Br* 82:42–47, 2000.
19. Markolf KL, Kochan A, Amstutz HC: Measurement of knee stiffness and laxity in patients with documented absence of the anterior cruciate ligament. *J Bone Joint Surg Am* 66-A:242–253, 1984.
20. Krauspe R, Schmidt M, Schaible H-G: Sensory innervation of the anterior cruciate ligament. An electrophysiological study of the response properties of single identified mechanoreceptors in the cat. *J Bone Joint Surg Am* 74-A:390–397, 1992.
21. Schultz RA, Miller DC, Kerr CS, et al: Mechanoreceptors in human cruciate ligaments. A histological study. *J Bone Joint Surg Am* 66:1072–1076, 1984.
22. Beynnon BD, Good L, Risberg MA: The effect of bracing on proprioception of knees with anterior cruciate ligament injury. *J Orthop Sports Phys Ther* 32:11–15, 2002.
23. Biedert RM, Stauffer E, Friederich NF: Occurrence of free nerve endings in the soft tissue of the knee joint. A histologic investigation. *Am J Sports Med* 2:430–433, 1992.
24. Haus J, Halata Z, Refior HJ: Proprioception in the human anterior cruciate ligament. Basic morphology. A light microscopic, scanning and transmission electron microscopic study. *Zeitschr Orthop* 130:484–494, 1992.
25. Beynnon B, Howe JG, Pope MH, et al: The measurement of anterior cruciate ligament strain in vivo. *Int Orthop* 16:1–12, 1992.
26. Beynnon BD, Fleming BC, Johnson RJ, et al: Anterior cruciate ligament strain behavior during rehabilitation exercises in vivo. *Am J Sports Med* 23:24–34, 1995.
27. Canale ST, Tolo VT: Fractures of the femur in children. *Instr Course Lect* 44:255–273, 1995.
28. Stanish WD, Lai A: New concepts of rehabilitation following anterior cruciate reconstruction. *Clin Sports Med* 12:25–58, 1993.
29. Erikson E: Acute sports injuries: An introduction and brief overview. In: Harries M, Williams C, Stanish WD, et al., eds: *Oxford Textbook of Sports Medicine.* New York, NY: Oxford University Press, 1994:341.

30. Johnson RJ: Acute knee injuries: An introduction. In: Harries M, Williams C, Stanish WD, et al., eds. *Oxford Textbook of Sports Medicine*. New York, NY: Oxford University Press, 1994:342–344.
31. Arnoczky SP, Matyas JR, Buckwalter JA, et al: Anatomy of the anterior cruciate ligament. In: Jackson DW, Arnoczky SP, Woo SL-Y, et al, eds. *The Anterior Cruciate Ligament. Current and Future Concepts*. New York, NY: Raven Press, 1993:5–22.
32. Samuelson TS, Drez D, Maletis GB: Anterior cruciate ligament graft rotation: Reproduction of normal graft rotation. *Am J Sports Med* 24:67–71, 1996.
33. Gomez-Barrena E, Munuera L, Martinez-Moreno E: Neural pathways of anterior cruciate ligament traced to the spinal ganglia. *Trans Orthop Res Soc* 17:503, 1992.
34. Haut RC: The mechanical and viscoelastic properties of the anterior cruciate ligament and of ACL fascicles. In: Jackson DW, Arnoczky SP, Woo SL-Y, et al, eds. *The Anterior Cruciate Ligament. Current and Future Concepts*. New York, NY: Raven Press, 1993:63–73.
35. Kwan MK, Lin TH, Woo SL-Y: On the viscoelastic properties of the anteromedial bundle of the anterior cruciate ligament. *J Biomech* 26:447–452, 1993.
36. Frank CB, Jackson DW: The science of reconstruction of the anterior cruciate ligament. *J Bone Joint Surg* 79:1556–1576, 1997.
37. Takai S, Woo SL-Y, Livesay GA, et al: Determination of the in situ loads on the human anterior cruciate ligament. *J Orthop Res* 11:686–695, 1993.
38. Butler DL, Guan Y, Kay MD, et al: Location-dependent variations in the material properties of the anterior cruciate ligament. *J Biomech* 25:511–518, 1992.
39. Butler DL, Noyes FR, Grood ES: Ligamentous restraints to anterior posterior drawer in the human knee: A biomechanical study. *J Bone Joint Surg Am* 62-A:259–270, 1980.
40. Arnoczky SP: Anatomy of the anterior cruciate ligament. In: Urist MR, ed. *Clinical Orthopedics and Related Research*. Philadelphia, PA: J.B. Lippincott, 1983:19–20.
41. Cabaud HE: Biomechanics of the anterior cruciate ligament. In: Urist MR, ed. *Clinical Orthopedics and Related Research*. Philadelphia, PA: J.B. Lippincott, 1983:26–30.
42. Kennedy JC, Hawkins RJ, Willis RB: Strain gauge analysis of knee ligaments. *Clin Orthop* 129:225–229, 1977.
43. Bargar WL, Moreland JR, Markolf KL, et al: In vivo stability testing of post meniscectomy knees. *Clin Orthop* 150:247–252, 1980.
44. Fleming BC, Renstrom PA, Beynnon BD, et al: The effect of weightbearing and external loading on anterior cruciate ligament strain. *J Biomech* 34:163–170, 1999.
45. Fleming BC, Beynnon BD, Renstrom PA, et al: The strain behavior of the anterior cruciate ligament during stair climbing: An in vivo study. *J Arthrosc Rel Surg* 15:185–191, 1999.
46. O'Connor JJ, Zavatsky A: Anterior cruciate ligament function in the normal knee. In: Jackson DW, Arnoczky SP, Woo SL-Y, et al, eds. *The Anterior Cruciate Ligament, Current and Future Concepts*. New York, NY: Raven Press, 1993:39–52.
47. O'Connor JJ, Zavatsky A: Anterior cruciate ligament forces in activity. In: Jackson DW, Arnoczky SP, Woo SL-Y, et al, eds. *The Anterior Cruciate Ligament, Current and Future Concepts*. New York, NY: Raven Press, 1993:131–140.
48. Beynnon BD, Johnson RJ, Fleming BC: The mechanics of anterior cruciate ligament reconstruction. In: Jackson DW, Arnoczky SP, Woo SL-Y, et al, eds. *The Anterior Cruciate Ligament Current and Future Concepts*. New York, NY: Raven Press, 1993:259–272.
49. Noyes FR, Grood ES, Butler DL, et al: Clinical biomechanics of the knee: Ligamentous restraints and functional stability. In: Funk FJJ, ed. *American Academy of Orthopedic Surgeon's Symposium on the Athlete's Knee*. St. Louis, MI: C.V. Mosby, 1980:1–35.
50. Harner CD, Xerogeanes JW, Livesay GA, et al: The human posterior cruciate ligament complex: An interdisciplinary study. Ligament morphology and biomechanical evaluation. *Am J Sports Med* 23:736–745, 1995.
51. Kennedy JC, Hawkins RJ, Willis RB, et al: Tension studies of human knee ligaments, yield point, ultimate failure, and disruption of the cruciate and tibial collateral ligaments. *J Bone Joint Surg* 58-A:350, 1976.
52. Van Dommelen BA, Fowler PJ: Anatomy of the posterior cruciate ligament. A review. *Am J Sports Med* 17:24–29, 1989.
53. Grover JS, Bassett LW, Gross ML, et al: Posterior cruciate ligament: MR imaging. *Radiology* 174:527–530, 1990.
54. Markolf KL, Wascher DC, Finerman GAM: Direct in vitro measurement of forces in the cruciate ligaments. Part II: The effect of section of the posterolateral structures. *J Bone Joint Surg* 75-A:387–394, 1993.
55. Hughston JC, Andrews JR, Cross MJ, et al: Classification of knee ligament instabilities. Part 1. *J Bone Joint Surg* 58A:159–172, 1976.
56. Grood ES, Stowers SF, Noyes FR: Limits of movement in the human knee. Effect of sectioning the posterior cruciate ligament and posterolateral structures. *J Bone Joint Surg Am* 70:88–97, 1988.
57. Heller L, Langman J: The Menisco-Femoral Ligaments of the Human Knee. *J Bone Joint Surg Br* 46:307–313, 1964.
58. Amis AA, Gupte CM, Bull AM, et al: Anatomy of the posterior cruciate ligament and the meniscofemoral ligaments. *Knee Surg Sports Traumatol Arthrosc* 14:257–63, 2006.
59. Clancy WG, Jr., Shelbourne KD, Zoellner GB, et al: Treatment of knee joint instability secondary to rupture of the posterior cruciate ligament. Report of a new procedure. *J Bone Joint Surg Am* 65:310–322, 1983.
60. Merida-Velasco JA, Sanchez-Montesionos I, Espin-Ferra J, et al: Development of the human knee joint ligaments. *Anat Rec* 248:259–268, 1997.
61. Gray H: *Gray's Anatomy*. Philadelphia, PA: Lea & Febiger, 1995.
62. Hughston JC, Jacobson KE: Chronic posterolateral rotatory instability of the knee. *J Bone Joint Surg* 67A:351–359, 1985.
63. Reinold MM, Berkson EM, Asnis P, et al: Knee: Ligamentous and patella tendon injuries. In: Magee DJ, Zachazewski JE, Quillen WS, eds. *Pathology and intervention in musculoskeletal rehabilitation*. St. Louis, MI: Saunders, 2009:528–578.
64. Tria AJ: Ligaments of the knee. New York, NY: Churchill Livingstone, 1995.
65. Grood ES, Noyes FR, Butler DL, et al: Ligamentous and capsular restraints preventing medial and lateral laxity in intact human cadaver knees. *J Bone Joint Surg* 63A:1257–1269, 1981.
66. Greenfield B, Tovin BJ, Bennett JG: Knee. In: Wadsworth C, ed. *Current Concepts of Orthopedic Physical Therapy*. La Crosse, WI: Orthopaedic Section, APTA, 2001.
67. Sudasna S, Harnsiriwattanagit K: The ligamentous structures of the posterolateral aspect of the knee. *Bull Hosp Joint Dis Orthop Inst* 50:35–40, 1990.
68. Kaplan EB: The fabellofibular and short lateral ligaments of the knee joint. *J Bone Joint Surg* 43A:169–179, 1961.
69. DeLee JC, Riley MD: Acute straight lateral instability of the knee. *Am J Sports Med* 11:404–411, 1983.
70. Nicholas JA: Lateral instability of the knee. *Orthop Rev* 6:33–44, 1977.
71. Terry GC, Norwood LA, Hughston JC, et al: How iliotibial tract injuries of the knee combine with acute anterior cruciate ligament tears to influence abnormal anterior tibial displacement. *Am J Sports Med* 21:55–60, 1993.
72. Wroble RR, Grood ES, Cummings JS, et al: The role of the lateral extraarticular restraints in the anterior cruciate ligament-deficient knee. *Am J Sports Med* 21:257–262, 1993.
73. Last RJ: The popliteus muscle and the lateral meniscus. *J Bone Joint Surg* 32B:93–99, 1950.
74. Pasque C, Noyes FR, Gibbons M, et al: The role of the popliteofibular ligament and the tendon of popliteus in providing stability in the human knee. *J Bone Joint Surg Br* 85:292–298, 2003.
75. Watanabe Y, Moriya H, Takahashi K, et al: Functional anatomy of the posterolateral structures of the knee. *J Arthroscopy Rel Surg* 9:57–62, 1993.
76. Sutton JB: *Ligaments: Their Nature and Morphology*. London: M.K. Lewis, 1897.
77. Arnoczky SP, Warren RF: Microvasculature of the human meniscus. *Am J Sports Med* 10:90–95, 1982.
78. Arnoczky SP, Warren RF, Spivak JM: Meniscal repair using an exogenous fibrin clot: An experimental study in dogs. *J Bone Joint Surg* 70A:1209–1217, 1988.
79. Barber FA, Click SD: Meniscus repair rehabilitation with concurrent anterior cruciate reconstruction. *Arthroscopy* 13:433, 1997.
80. Alford W, Cole BJ: The indications and technique for meniscal transplant. *Orthop Clin North Am* 36:469–84, 2005.
81. Wallace LA, Mangine RE, Malone T: The knee. In: Gould JA, Davies GJ, eds. *Orthopaedic and Sports Physical Therapy*. St. Louis, MI: C.V. Mosby, 1985:342–363.
82. Fritz JM, Irrgang JJ, Harner CD: Rehabilitation following allograft meniscal transplantation: A review of the literature and case study. *J Orthop Sports Phys Ther* 24:98–106, 1996.

83. Jackson DW, McDevitt CA, Simon TM, et al: Meniscal transplantation using fresh and cryopreserved allografts. *Am J Sports Med* 20:644–656, 1992.
84. Baratz ME, Fu FH, Mengato R: Meniscal tears: The effect of meniscectomy and of repair on intraarticular contact areas and stress in the human knee. A preliminary report. *Am J Sports Med* 14:270–275, 1986.
85. Radin EL, Delamotte F, Maquet P: The role of the menisci in the distribution of stress in the knee. *Clin Orthop* 185:290–294, 1984.
86. Ahmed AM, Burke DL: In vitro measurement of static pressure distribution in synovial joints: I. Tibial surface of the knee. *J Biomed Eng* 105:216–225, 1983.
87. Seedholm BB, Hargreaves DJ: Transmission of the load in the knee joint with special reference to the role of the menisci—Part II. *Med Eng* 8:220–228, 1979.
88. Walker PS, Erkman MJ: The role of the menisci in force transmission across the knee. *Clin Orthop* 109:184–192, 1975.
89. Fukubayashi T, Kurosawa H: The contact area and pressure distribution pattern of the knee: A study of normal and osteoarthritic knee joints. *Acta Orthop Scand* 51:871–879, 1980.
90. Kettlekamp DB, Jacobs AW: Tibiofemoral contact area: Determination and implications. *J Bone Joint Surg* 54A:349–356, 1972.
91. Shrive NG, O'Connor JJ, Goodfellow JW: Load bearing in the knee joint. *Clin Orthop* 131:279–287, 1978.
92. Anderson DR, Woo SL-Y, Kwan MK, et al: Viscoelastic shear properties of the equine medial meniscus. *J Orthop Res* 9:550–558, 1991.
93. Arnoczky SP, Adams M, DeHaven K, et al: Meniscus. In: Woo SL, Buckwalter JA, eds. *Injury and Repair of the Musculoskeletal Soft Tissues.* Chicago, IL: American Academy of Orthopaedic Surgeons, 1987:487–537.
94. Bullough PG, Vosburgh F, Arnoczky SP: The menisci of the knee. In: Insall JN, ed. *Surgery of the Knee.* New York, NY: Churchill Livingstone Inc, 1984:135–146.
95. Rosenberg LC, Buckwalter JA, Coutts R, et al: Articular cartilage. In: Woo SL-Y, Buckwalter JA, eds. *Injury and Repair of the Musculoskeletal Soft Tissues.* Chicago, IL: American Academy of Orthopaedic Surgeons, 1988:401–482.
96. Morrison JB: The mechanics of the knee joint in relation to normal walking. *J Biomech* 3:51, 1970.
97. Hall SJ: *The Biomechanics of the Human Lower Extremity, Basic Biomechanics*, 3rd ed. New York, NY: McGraw-Hill, 1999:234–281.
98. Voloshin AS, Wosk J: Shock absorption of meniscectomized and painful knees. A comparative in vivo study. *J Biomed Eng* 5:157–193, 1983.
99. Fukuda Y, Takai S, Yoshino N, et al: Impact load transmission of the knee joint-influence of leg alignment and the role of meniscus and articular cartilage. *Clin Biomech (Bristol, Avon).* 15:516–521, 2000.
100. Renstrom P, Johnson RJ: Anatomy and biomechanics of the menisci. *Clin Sports Med* 9:523–538, 1990.
101. Markloff KL, Bargar WL, Shoemaker SC, et al: The role of joint load in knee stability. *J Bone Joint Surg* 63A:570–585, 1981.
102. Smillie IS: *Injuries of the Knee Joint.* London: Churchill Livingstone Inc., 1971.
103. Shields CL, Silva I, Yee L, et al: Evaluation of residual instability after arthroscopic meniscectomy in anterior cruciate deficient knees. *Am J Sports Med* 15:129–131, 1987.
104. Wang CJ, Walker PS: Rotational laxity of the human knee. *J Bone Joint Surg* 56A:161–170, 1974.
105. Levy M, Torzelli PA, Gould JD, et al: The effect of lateral meniscectomy on the motion of the knee. *J Bone Joint Surg* 71A:401–406, 1989.
106. Levy M, Torzelli PA, Warren RF: The effect of medial meniscectomy on anterior-posterior motion of the knee. *J Bone Joint Surg* 64A:883–888, 1982.
107. Hsieh HH, Walker PS: Stabilizing mechanisms of the loaded and unloaded knee joint. *J Bone Joint Surg* 58A:87–93, 1976.
108. Sullivan D, Levy IM, Sheskier S, et al: Medial restraints to anterior-posterior motion of the knee. *J Bone Joint Surg* 66A:930–936, 1984.
109. Thompson WO, Fu FH: The meniscus in the cruciate-deficient knee. *Clin Sports Med* 12:771–796, 1993.
110. Kapandji IA: *The Physiology of Joints, Lower Limb*, 2nd ed. New York, NY: Churchill Livingstone, Inc., 1970.
111. Norkin C, Levangie P: *Joint Structure and Function: A Comprehensive Analysis.* Philadelphia, PA: F.A. Davis Company, 1992.
112. Thompson WO, Thaete FL, Fu FH, et al: Tibial meniscal dynamics using three-dimensional reconstruction of magnetic resonance imaging. *Am J Sports Med* 19:210–215, 1991.
113. Fullerton A: The surgical anatomy of the synovial membrane of the knee-joint. *British J Surg* 4:191–200, 1916.
114. Mayeda P: Ueber das Strangartige Gebilde in der Knigel–Enkhoehle (Chordi Cavi Artioularis Genu). *Mitt Med Fak Kaisert Univ Tokyo* 21:507–553, 1918.
115. Hardaker WT, Whipple TL, Bassett FH, III: Diagnosis and treatment of the plica syndrome of the knee. *J Bone and Joint Surg* 62-A:221–225, 1980.
116. Zanoli S, Piazzai E: The synovial plica syndrome of the knee. Pathology, differential diagnosis and treatment. *Ital J Orthop Traumatol* 9:241–250, 1983.
117. Aoki T: The "ledge" lesion in the knee. Proceedings of the Twelfth Congress of Orthopaedic Surgery and Traumatology. Excerpta Medica International Congress Series. *Amsterdam, Excerpta Medica* 1972:462.
118. Iino S: Normal arthroscopic findings in the knee joint in adult cadavers. *J Jpn Orthop Assoc* 14:467–523, 1939.
119. Jackson RW, Marshall DJ, Fujisawa Y: The pathologic medial shelf. *Orthop Clin North Am* 13:307–312, 1982.
120. Sakakibara J: Arthroscopic study on Iino's band (plica synovialis mediopatellaris). *J Jpn Orthop Assoc* 50:513–522, 1976.
121. Johnson DP, Eastwood DM, Witherow PJ: Symptomatic Synovial Plicae of the Knee. *J Bone Joint Surg Am* 75-A:1485–1496, 1993.
122. Gray DJ, Gardner E: Prenatal development of the human knee and superior tibiofibular joints. *Am J Anat* 86:235–287, 1950.
123. Ogata S, Uhthoff HK: The development of synovial plica in human knee joints: An embryologic study. *Arthroscopy* 6:315–321, 1990.
124. Johnson LL: *Diagnostic and Surgical Arthroscopy: The Knee and Other Joints.* St. Louis, MI: C.V. Mosby, 1981.
125. Dugdale TW, Barnett PR: Historical background: Patello-femoral pain in young people. *Orthop Clin North Am* 17:211–219, 1986.
126. Fairbank JCT, Pynsent PB, van Poortvliet JA, et al: Mechanical factors in the incidence of knee pain in adolescents and young adults. *J Bone Joint Surg* 66B:685–693, 1984.
127. Cox JS, Cooper PS: Patellofemoral Instability. In: Fu FH, Harner CD, Vince KG, eds. *Knee Surgery.* Baltimore, MD: Williams & Wilkins, 1994:959–962.
128. Warren LF, Marshall JL: The supporting structures and layers on the medial side of the knee. *J Bone Joint Surg Am* 61:56–62, 1979.
129. Fulkerson JP, Gossling HR: Anatomy of the knee joint lateral retinaculum. *Clin Orthop* 153:183–188, 1980.
130. Terry GC, Hughston JC, Norwood LA: The anatomy of the iliopatellar band and iliotibial tract. *Am J Sports Med* 14:39–44, 1986.
131. Puniello MS: Iliotibial band tightness and medial patellar glide in patients with patellofemoral dysfunction. *J Orthop Sports Phys Ther* 17:144–148, 1993.
132. Fulkerson JP: The etiology of patellofemoral pain in young, active patients: A prospective study. *Clin Orthop* 179:129–133, 1983.
133. Fulkerson JP: *Disorders of the Patellofemoral Joint: Evaluation and Treatment, Evaluation and Treatment of Injured Athletes Course.* Cap Cod, MA: Boston University, 1993.
134. Insall JN: Chondromalacia patellae: Patellar malalignment syndrome. *Orthop Clin North Am* 10:117–127, 1979.
135. Kramer P: Patellar malalignment syndrome: Rationale to reduce excessive lateral pressure. *J Orthop Sports Phys Ther* 8:301–309, 1986.
136. Paulos L, Rusche K, Johnson C, et al: Patellar malalignment: A treatment rationale. *Phys Ther* 60:1624–1632, 1980.
137. Lieb F, Perry J: Quadriceps function. *J Bone Joint Surg Am* 50:1535, 1968.
138. Grelsamer RP, McConnell J: Normal and abnormal anatomy of the extensor mechanism. In Grelsamer RP, McConnell J, eds: *The Patella: A Team Approach.* Gaithersburg, MD: Aspen, 1998:11–24.
139. Hallisey MJ, Doherty N, Bennett WF, et al: Anatomy of the junction of the vastus lateralis tendon and the patella. *J Bone Joint Surg Am* 69: 545–549, 1987.
140. Bose K, Kanagasuntheram R, Osman MBH: Vastus medialis oblique: An anatomic and physiologic study. *Orthopedics* 3:880–883, 1980.
141. Koskinen SK, Kujala UM: Patellofemoral relationships and distal insertion of the vastus medialis muscle: A magnetic resonance imaging study in nonsymptomatic subjects and in patients with patellar dislocation. *Arthroscopy* 8:465–468, 1992.
142. Raimondo RA, Ahmad CS, Blankevoort L, et al: Patellar stabilization: A quantitative evaluation of the vastus medialis obliquus muscle. *Orthopedics* 21:791–795, 1998.

143. Nakamura Y, Ohmichi H, Miyashita M: EMG relationship during maximum voluntary contraction of the quadriceps. *IX Congress of the International Society of Biomechanics*, Waterloo,Ontario, 1983.
144. Knight KL, Martin JA, Londerdee BR: EMG comparison of quadriceps femoris activity during knee extensions and straight leg raises. *Am J Phys Med* 58:57–69, 1979.
145. Brownstein BA, Lamb RL, Mangine RE: Quadriceps torque and integrated electromyography. *J Orthop Sports Phys Ther* 6:309–314, 1985.
146. Fox TA: Dysplasia of the quadriceps mechanism: Hypoplasia of the vastus medialis muscle as related to the hypermobile patella syndrome. *Surg Clin North Am* 55:199–226, 1975.
147. Tria AJ, Palumbo RC, Alicia JA: Conservative care for patellofemoral pain. *Orthop Clin North Am* 23:545–554, 1992.
148. Reynolds L, Levin TA, Medeiros JM, et al: EMG activity of the vastus medialis oblique and the vastus lateralis in the their role in patellar alignment. *Am J Sports Med* 62:62–70, 1983.
149. Moller BN, Krebs B, Tideman-Dal C,et al: Isometric contractions in the patellofemoral pain syndrome. *Arch Orthop Trauma Surg* 105:24, 1986.
150. Reid DC: *Anterior Knee Pain and the Patellofemoral Pain Syndrome, Sports Injury Assessment and Rehabilitation.* New York, NY: Churchill Livingstone, 1992:345–398.
151. Larson RL, Jones DC: Dislocations and ligamentous injuries of the knee. In: Rockwood CA, Green DP, eds. *Fractures in Adults*, 2nd ed. Philadelphia, PA: J.B. Lippincott, 1984:1480–1591.
152. Gill DM, Corbacio EJ, Lauchle LE: Anatomy of the knee. In: Engle RP, ed. *Knee Ligament Rehabilitation.* New York, NY: Churchill Livingstone, 1991:1–15.
153. Kendall FP, McCreary EK, Provance PG: *Muscles: Testing and Function.* Baltimore, MD: Williams & Wilkins, 1993.
154. O'Connor JJ: Can muscle co-contraction protect knee ligaments after injury or repair? *J Bone Joint Surg* 75-B:41–48, 1993.
155. Fleming BC, Renstrom PA, Goran O, et al: The gastrocnemius muscle is an antagonist of the anterior cruciate ligament. *J Orthop Res* 19:1178–1184, 2001.
156. Timm KE: Knee. In: Richardson JK, Iglarsh ZA, eds. *Clinical Orthopaedic Physical Therapy.* Philadelphia, PA: W.B. Saunders, 1994:399–482.
157. Brownstein B, Noyes FR, Mangine RE, et al: Anatomy and biomechanics. In: Mangine RE, ed. *Physical Therapy of the Knee.* New York, NY: Churchill Livingstone, 1988:1–30.
158. Magee DJ: *Orthopedic Physical Assessment*, 2nd ed. Philadelphia, PA: W. B. Saunders, 1992.
159. Reid DC: Knee ligament injuries, anatomy, classification, and examination. In: Reid DC, ed. *Sports Injury Assessment and Rehabilitation.* New York, NY: Churchill Livingstone, 1992:437–493.
160. Nyland J, Lachman N, Kocabey Y, et al: Anatomy, function, and rehabilitation of the popliteus musculotendinous complex. *J Orthop Sports Phys Ther* 35:165–179, 2005.
161. Veltri DM, Deng XH, Torzilli PA, et al: The role of the cruciate and posterolateral ligaments in stability of the knee. A biomechanical study. *Am J Sports Med* 23:436–443, 1995.
162. Veltri DM, Deng XH, Torzilli PA, et al: The role of the popliteofibular ligament in stability of the human knee. A biomechanical study. *Am J Sports Med* 24:19–27, 1996.
163. Maynard MJ, Deng XH, Wickiewicz TL, et al: The popliteofibular ligament. Rediscovery of a key element in posterolateral stability. *Am J Sports Med* 24:311–316, 1996.
164. Veltri DM, Warren RF, Wickiewicz TL, et al: Current status of allographic meniscal transplantation. *Clin Orthop* 306:155–162, 1994.
165. Renne JW: The iliotibial band friction syndrome. *J Bone and Joint Surg* 57.1110–1111, 1975.
166. Evans P: The postural function of the iliotibial tract. *Ann R Coll Surg Engl* 61:271–280, 1979.
167. Pease BJ, Cortese M: *Anterior Knee Pain: Differential Diagnosis and Physical Therapy Management, Orthopaedic Physical Therapy Home Study Course 92-1.* La Crosse, WI: Orthopaedic Section, APTA, Inc, 1992.
168. Vloka JD, Hadzic A, E. A, et al. The division of the sciatic nerve in the popliteal fossa: Anatomical implications for popliteal nerve blockade. *Anesth Analg* 92:215–7, 2001.
169. Wojtys EM, Huston LJ: Neuromuscular performance in normal and anterior cruciate ligament-deficient lower extremities. *Am J Sports Med* 22:89–104, 1994.
170. Hughston JC, Bowden JA, Andrews JR, et al: Acute tears of the posterior cruciate ligament. Results of operative treatment. *J Bone Joint Surg Am* 62:438–450, 1980.
171. Hollister AM, Jatana S, Singh AK, et al: The axes of rotation of the knee. *Clin Orthop* 290:259–268, 1993.
172. Goodfellow J, O'Connor J: The mechanics of the knee and prosthesis design. *J Bone and Joint Surg* 60B:358, 1978.
173. Boeckmann RR, Ellenbecker TS: Biomechanics. In: Ellenbecker TS, ed. *Knee Ligament Rehabilitation.* Philadelphia, PA: Churchill Livingstone, 2000:16–23.
174. Nielsen S, Helmig P: The static stabilizing function of the popliteal tendon in the knee. An experimental study. *Arch Orthop Trauma Surg* 104:357–362, 1986.
175. Blankevoort L, Huiskes R, De Lange A: The envelope of passive knee joint motion. *J Biomech* 21:705–720, 1988.
176. Ishii Y, Terajima K, Koga Y, et al: Screw home motion after total knee replacement. *Clin Orthop Relat Res* 358:181–187, 1999.
177. Asai O: [The combination method for diagnosis of meniscus lesion in the knee (Translation by O Asai)]. *Nippon Seikeigeka Gakkai Zasshi* 7:625–633, 1981.
178. Kuriwaka Y: [A biomechanical study of osteoarthritis of the knee with special reference to the rotatory movement of the knee joint. (Translation by Y. Kunuaka)]. *Nippon Seikeigeka Gakkai Zasshi* 56:713–726, 1982.
179. Lafortune MA, Cavanagh PR, Sommer HJ, III, et al: Three-dimensional kinematics of the human knee during walking. *J Biomech* 25:347–357, 1992.
180. Tasker T, Waugh W: Articular changes associated with internal derangement of the knee. *J Bone Joint Surg* 64B:486–488, 1982.
181. Eckhoff DG, Smith D, Schecter R, et al: Automatic rotation (screw-home) in the cruciate deficient and prosthetic knee. *Trans Orthop Res Soc* 21:216, 1996.
182. Schlepckow P: [Experimental studies of the kinematics of the stable and unstable human knee joint.] Experimentelle Untersuchungen zur Kinematik des stabilen and instabilen menschlichen Kniegelenkes. *Z Orthop Ihre Grenzgeb* 127:711–715, 1989.
183. McGinty G, Irrgang JJ, Pezzullo D: Biomechanical considerations for rehabilitation of the knee. *Clin Biomech* 15:160–166, 2000.
184. Beynnon BD, Fleming BC, Labovitch R, et al: Chronic anterior cruciate ligament deficiency is associated with increased translation of the tibia during the transition from non-weightbearing to weightbearing. *J Orthop Res* 20:332–337, 2002.
185. Desio SM, Burks RT, Bachus KN: Soft tissue restraints to lateral patellar translation in the human knee. *Am J Sports Med* 26:59–65, 1998.
186. Dandy DJ: Chronic patellofemoral instability. *J Bone Joint Surg Br* 78:328–335, 1996.
187. Fulkerson JP: *Disorders of the Patellofemoral Joint.* Baltimore, MD: Williams & Wilkins, 1997.
188. Grelsamer RP, McConnell J: *The Patella: A Team Approach.* Gaithersburg, MD: Aspen, 1998.
189. McConnell J: *Conservative management of patellofemoral problems, The Patella. A Team Approach.* Gaithersburg, MD: Aspen, 1998:119–136.
190. Voight M, Weider D: Comparative reflex response times of the vastus medialis and the vastus lateralis in normal subjects and subjects with extensor mechanism dysfunction. *Am J Sports Med* 10:131–137, 1991.
191. Cowan SM, Bennell KL, Hodges PW, et al: Delayed onset of electromyographic activity of vastus medialis obliquus relative to vastus lateralis in subjects with patellofemoral pain syndrome. *Arch Phys Med Rehab* 82:183–189, 2001.
192. Ahmed AM, Burke DL, Hyder A: Force analysis of the patellar mechanism. *J Orthop. Res* 5:69–85, 1987.
193. Hodges P, Richardson C: Inefficient muscular stabilisation of the lumbar spine associated with low back pain: A motor control evaluation of transversus abdominis. *Spine* 21:2540–2650, 1996.
194. Insall JN, Falvo KA, Wise DW: Chondromalacia patellae. A prospective study. *J Bone Joint Surg* 58A:1–8, 1976.
195. Grana WA, Kriegshauser LA: Scientific basis of extensor mechanism disorders. *Clin Sports Med* 4:247–257, 1985.
196. Hughston JC, Walsh WM, Puddu G: *Patellar Subluxation and Dislocation, Saunders Monographs in Clinical Orthopaedics.* Philadelphia, PA: W.B. Saunders, 1984.
197. Brattström H: Shape of the intercondylar groove normally and in recurrent dislocation of the patella. *Acta Orthop Scand* 68:1–48, 1964.
198. Aglietti P, Insall JN, Cerulli G: Patellar pain and incongruence. *Clin Orthop* 176:217–224, 1983.
199. Horton MG, Hall TL: Quadriceps femoris muscle angle: Normal values and relationships with gender and selected skeletal measures. *Phys Ther* 69:897–901, 1989.

200. Hsu RWW, Himeno S, Coventry MB, et al: Normal axial alignment of the lower extremity and load-bearing distribution at the knee. *Clin Orthop* 255:215–227, 1990.
201. Woodland LH, Francis RS: Parameters and comparisons of the quadriceps angle of college aged men and women in the supine and standing positions. *Am J Sports Med* 20:208–211, 1992.
202. Kernozek TW, Greer NL: Quadriceps angle and rearfoot motion: Relationships in walking. *Arch Phys Med Rehab* 74:407–410, 1993.
203. Cox JS: Patellofemoral problems in runners. *Clin J Sports Med* 4:699–715, 1985.
204. Percy EC, Strother RT: Patellalgia. *Phys Sportsmed* 13:43–59, 1985.
205. Carson WG: Diagnosis of extensor mechanism disorders. *Clin Sports Med* 4:231–246, 1985.
206. Olerud C, Berg P: The variation of the quadriceps angle with different positions of the foot. *Clin Orthop* 191:162–165, 1984.
207. Huberti HH, Hayes WC: Patellofemoral contact pressures. The influence of Q-angle and tendofemoral contact. *J Bone and Joint Surg* 66-A:715–724, 1984.
208. Greene CC, Edwards TB, Wade MR, et al: Reliability of the quadriceps angle measurement. *Am J Knee Surg* 14:97–103, 2001.
209. Harrison MM, Cooke TDV, Fisher SB, et al: Patterns of knee arthrosis and patellar subluxation. *Clin Orthop* 309:56–63, 1994.
210. Ehrat M, Edwards J, Hastings D, et al: Reliability of assessing patellar alignment: The A angle. *J Orthop Sports Phys Ther* 19:22–27, 1994.
211. Rand JA: The patellofemoral joint in total knee arthroplasty. *J Bone Joint Surg Am* 76:612–620, 1994.
212. Aglietti P, Insall JN, Walker PS, et al: A new patella prosthesis. *Clin Orthop* 107:175–187, 1975.
213. Goodfellow JW, Hungerford DS, Woods C: Patellofemoral joint mechanics and pathology: I and II. *J Bone Joint Surg* 58B:287–299, 1976.
214. Kaufer H: Patellar biomechanics. *Clin Orthop* 144:51–54, 1979.
215. McConnell J, Fulkerson JP: The Knee: Patellofemoral and Soft Tissue Injuries. In: Zachazewski JE, Magee DJ, Quillen WS, eds. *Athletic Injuries and Rehabilitation*. Philadelphia, PA: W.B. Saunders, 1996:693–728.
216. Hehne H-J: Biomechanics of the patellofemoral joint and its clinical relevance. *Clin Orthop* 258:73–85, 1990.
217. Huberti HH, Hayes WC, Stone JL, et al: Force ratios in the quadriceps tendon and ligamentum patellae. *J Orthop Res* 21:49–54, 1984.
218. Fujikawa K, Seedholm BB, Wright V: Biomechanics of the patellofemoral joint. Parts 1 and 2. Study of the patellofemoral compartment and movement of the patella. *Eng Med* 12:3–21, 1983.
219. Kwak SD, Colman WW, Ateshian GA, et al: Anatomy of the human patellofemoral joint articular cartilage: surface curvature analysis. *J Orthop. Res* 15:468–472, 1997.
220. Bishop RED, Denham RA: A note on the ratio between tensions in the quadriceps tendon and infrapatellar ligament. *Eng Med* 6:53–54, 1977.
221. Buff HU, Jones JC, Hungerford DS: Experimental determination of forces transmitted through the patello-femoral joint. *J Biomech* 21:17–23, 1988.
222. Lloyd-Robert GC, Thomas TG: The etiology of quadriceps contracture in children. *British J Bone Joint Surg* 46-B:498–502, 1964.
223. Heegaard J, Leyvraz P-F, Van Kampen A, et al: Influence of soft structures on patellar three-dimensional tracking. *Clin Orthop* 299:235–243, 1994.
224. van Kampen A, Huiskes R: The three-dimensional tracking pattern of the human patella. *J Orthop Res* 8:372–382, 1990.
225. Ateshian GA, Kwak SD, Soslowsky LJ, et al: A stereophotogrammetric method for determining in situ contact areas in diarthrodial joints, and a comparison with other methods. *J Biomech* 27:111–124, 1994.
226. Carson WG, James SL, Larson RL, et al: Patellofemoral disorders—Physical and radiographic examination. Part I. Physical examination. *Clin Orthop* 185:178–186, 1984.
227. Insall JN: Patellar pain: Current concepts review. *J Bone Joint Surg* 64A:147–152, 1982.
228. Irrgang JJ, Rivera J: Closed kinetic chain exercises for the lower extremity: Theory and application. *Sports Physical Therapy Section Home Study Course: Current Concepts in Rehabilitation of the Knee. Home Study Course.* La Crosse, WI: Orthopaedic Section, APTA, Inc., 2001.
229. Tiberio D: The effect of excessive subtalar joint pronation on patellofemoral mechanics: A theoretical model. *J Orthop Sports Phys Ther* 9:160–165, 1987.
230. Arms SW, Pope MH, Johnson RJ, et al: The biomechanics of anterior cruciate ligament rehabilitation and reconstruction. *Am J Sports Med* 12:8–18, 1984.
231. Henning CE, Lynch MA, Glick C: An in vivo strain gauge study of elongation of the anterior cruciate ligament. *Am J Sports Med* 13:22–26, 1985.
232. Hungerford DS, Barry M: Biomechanics of the patellofemoral joint. *Clin Orthop* 144:9–15, 1979.
233. Paulos LE, Noyes FR, Grood ES: Knee rehabilitation after anterior cruciate ligament reconstruction and repair. *Am J Sports Med* 9:140–149, 1981.
234. Steinkamp LA, Dilligham MF, Markel MD,et al: Biomechanical considerations in patellofemoral joint rehabilitation. *Am J Sports Med* 21:438–444, 1993.
235. Escamilla RF, Fleisig GS, Zheng N, et al: Biomechanics of the knee during closed kinetic chain and open kinetic chain exercises. *Med Sci Sports Exerc* 30:556–569, 1998.
236. Ariel BG: Biomechanical analysis of the knee joint during deep knee bends with heavy loads. In: Nelson R, Morehouse C, eds. *Biomechanics IV*. Baltimore, MD: University Park Press, 1974:44–52.
237. Dahlkvist NJ, Mayo P, Seedhom BB: Forces during squatting and rising from a deep squat. *Eng. Med* 11:69–76, 1982.
238. Nisell R, Nemeth G, Ohlsen H: Joint forces in extension of the knee. Analysis of a mechanical model. *Acta Orthop Scand* 57:41–46, 1986.
239. Meglan D, Lutz G, Stuart M: Effects of closed chain exercises for ACL rehabilitation upon the load in the capsule and ligamentous structures of the knee. *Orthop Trans* 17:719–720, 1993.
240. Andrews JG, Nay JG, Vaughan CL: Knee shear forces during a squat exercise using a barbell and a weight machine. In: Matsui H, Kobayashi K, eds. *Biomechanics VIII-B*. Champaign, IL: Human Kinetics, 1983: 923–927.
241. Harttin HC, Pierrynowski MR, Ball KA: Effect of load, cadence, and fatigue on tibio-femoral joint force during a half squat. *Med Sci Sports Exerc* 21:613–618, 1989.
242. Stuart MJ, Meglan DA, Lutz GE, et al: Comparison of intersegmental tibiofemoral joint forces and muscle activity during various closed kinetic chain exercises. *Am J Sports Med* 24:792–799, 1996.
243. Palmitier RA, An KN, Scott SG, et al: Kinetic chain exercises in knee rehabilitation. *Sports Med* 11:402–413, 1991.
244. Ohkoshi Y, Yasuda K, Kaneda K, et al: Biomechanical analysis of rehabilitation in the standing position. *Am J Sports Med* 19:605–611, 1991.
245. Beynnon BD, Johnson RJ, Fleming BC, et al: The strain behavior of the anterior cruciate ligament during squatting and active flexion and extension: A comparison of an open and a closed kinetic chain exercise. *Am J Sports Med* 25:823–829, 1997.
246. Grelsamer RP, McConnell J: *Applied Mechanics of the Patellofemoral Joint, The Patella: A Team Approach*. Gaithersburg, MD: Aspen, 1998:25–41.
247. Grood ES, Suntay WJ, Noyes FR, et al: Biomechanics of the knee extension exercise. *J Bone Joint Surg* 66A:725–734, 1984.
248. Yasuda K, Sadaki T: Exercise after anterior cruciate ligament reconstruction: the force exerted on the tibia by the separate isometric contractions of the quadriceps of the hamstrings. *Clin Orthop* 220:275–283, 1987.
249. Kaufman KR, An KN, Litchy WJ, et al: Dynamic joint forces during knee isokinetic exercise. *Am J Sports Med* 19:305–316, 1991.
250. Yack HJ, Collins CE, Whieldon TJ: Comparison of closed and open kinetic chain exercise in the anterior cruciate ligament-deficient knee. *Am J Sports Med* 21:49–54, 1993.
251. Lutz GE, Palmitier RA, An KN, et al: Comparison of tibiofemoral joint forces during open-kinetic-chain and closed-kinetic-chain exercises. *Am J Bone Joint Surg* 75:732–739, 1993.
252. Nisell R, Ekholm J: Joint load during the parellel squat in powerlifting and force analysis of in vivo bilateral quadriceps tendon rupture. *Scand J. Sports Sci* 8:63–70, 1986.
253. Sawhney R, Dearwater S, Irrgang JJ,et al: Quadriceps exercise following anterior cruciate ligament reconstruction without anterior tibial translation. *American Conference of the American Physical Therapy Association,*. Anaheim, CA, 1990.
254. Reilly DT, Martens M: Experimental analysis of the quadriceps muscle force and patello-femoral joint reaction force for various activities. *Acta Orthop Scand* 43:126–137, 1972.
255. Dieppe P: The classification and diagnosis of osteoarthritis. In: Kuettner KE, Goldberg WM, eds. *Osteoarthritic Disorders*. Rosemont, IL: American Academy of Orthopaedic Surgeons, 1995: 5–12.

256. Clancy WG: Evaluation of acute knee injuries. In: Finerman G, ed. *American Association of Orthopaedic Surgeons, Symposium on Sports medicine: The Knee.* St Louis, MI: CV Mosby, 1985:185–193.
257. Solomon DH, Simel DL, Bates DW, et al: The rational clinical examination. Does this patient have a torn meniscus or ligament of the knee? Value of the physical examination. *JAMA* 286:1610–1620, 2001.
258. Tria AJ: *Ligaments of the knee.* New York, NY: Churchill Livingston, 1995:xi, 324.
259. Bloom MH: Differentiating between meniscal and patellar pain. *Phys Sports Med* 17:95–108, 1989.
260. Rosenthal MD, Moore JH, DeBerardino TM: Diagnosis of medial knee pain: Atypical stress fracture about the knee joint. *J Orthop Sports Phys Ther* 36:526–534, 2006.
261. Safran MR, Fu FH: Uncommon causes of knee pain in the athlete. *Orthop Clin North Am* 26:547–559, 1995.
262. Fahrer H, Rentsch HU, Gerber NJ, et al: Knee effusion and reflex inhibition of the quadriceps. *J Bone Joint Surg* 70B:635–638, 1988.
263. Boden BP, Pearsall AW, Garrett WE, Jr, et al: Patellofemoral instability: Evaluation and management. *J Am Acad Orthop Surg* 5:47–57, 1997.
264. Brody LT, Thein JM: Nonoperative treatment for patellofemoral pain. *J Orthop Sports Phys Ther* 28:336–344, 1998.
265. Ficat P, Hungerford DS: *Disorders of the Patellofemoral Joint.* Baltimore, MD: Williams & Wilkins, 1977.
266. Grelsamer RP, McConnell J: *Examination of the patellofemoral joint, The Patella: A Team Approach.* Gaithersburg, MD: Aspen, 1998:109–118.
267. Shellock FG, Mink JH, Deutsch AL, et al: Patellofemoral joint: Identification of abnormalities using active movement, "unloaded" vs "loaded" kinematic MR imaging techniques. *Radiology* 188:575–578, 1993.
268. Zappala FG, Taffel CB, Scuderi GR: Rehabilitation of patellofemoral joint disorders. *Orthop Clin North Am* 23:555–565, 1992.
269. Bentley G, Dowd G: Current concepts of etiology and treatment of chondromalacia patella. *Clin Orthop* 189:209, 1984.
270. Insall JN: Patella pain syndromes and chondromalacia patellae. *Inst Course Lect* 30:342–356, 1981.
271. Kummel B: The treatment of patellofemoral problems. *Primary Care* 7:217–229, 1980.
272. Karlson S: Chondromalacia patellae. *Acta Chir Scand* 83:347–381, 1940.
273. McConnell J: Fat pad irritation—A mistaken patellar tendinitis. *Sports Health* 9:7–9, 1991
274. Winkel D, Matthijs O, Phelps V: *Examination of the Knee.* Gaithersburg, MD: Aspen, 1997
275. James SL: Chondromalacia patella. In: Kennedy JC, ed. *The Injured Adolescent Knee.* Baltimore, MD: Williams & Wilkins, 1979.
276. Wallace L: *Lower Quarter Pain: Mechanical Evaluation and Treatment.* Cleveland, OH: Western Reserve Publishers, 1984.
277. Wallace L: Rehabilitation following patellofemoral surgery. In: Davies GJ, ed. *Rehabilitation of the Surgical Knee.* Ronkonkoma, NY: Cypress, 1984:60–62.
278. Sahrmann SA: Movement impairment syndromes of the hip. In: Sahrmann SA, ed. *Movement Impairment Syndromes.* St Louis, MI: CV Mosby, 2001:121–191.
279. Larson RL: Subluxation-dislocation of the patella. In: Kennedy JC, ed. *The Injured Adolescent Knee.* Baltimore, MD: Williams & Wilkins, 1979.
280. Schiedel F, Probst A, Buller TC, et al: The postoperative patella height: A comparison of additive and subtractive high tibial osteotomy in correcting the genu varum. *Arch Orthop Trauma surg* 129:1271–1277, 2009.
281. Hinterwimmer S, von Eisenhart-Rothe R, Siebert M, et al: Patella kinematics and patello-femoral contact areas in patients with genu varum and mild osteoarthritis. *Clin Biomech(Bristol, Avon)* 19:704–710, 2004.
282. Greene WB: Genu varum and genu valgum in children: Differential diagnosis and guidelines for evaluation. *Compr Ther* 22:22–29, 1996.
283. Post WR: Clinical evaluation of patients with patellofemoral disorders. *Arthroscopy* 15:841–851, 1999.
284. Holmes SWJ, Clancy WGJ: Clinical classification of patellofemoral pain and dysfunction. *J Orthop Sports Phys Ther* 28:299–306, 1998.
285. Merchant AC: Classification of patellofemoral disorders. *Arthroscopy* 4:235–240, 1988.
286. Eckhoff DG, Brown AW, Kilcoyne RF, et al: Knee version associated with anterior knee pain. *Clin Orthop Relat Res* 339:152–155, 1997.
287. Eckhoff DG, Johnston RJ, Stamm ER, et al: Version of the osteoarthritic knee. *J Arthroplasty* 9:73–80, 1994.
288. Takai S, Sakakida K, Yamashita F, et al: Rotational alignment of the lower limb in osteoarthritis of the knee. *Int Orthop (SICOT)* 9:209–216, 1985.
289. Yagi T, Sasaki T: Tibial torsion in patients with medial-type osteoarthritic knee. *Clin Orthop* 213:177–182, 1986.
290. Ficat P, Ficat C, Bailleux A: Syndrome d'hyperpression externe de la rotule (S.H.P.E.). *Rev Chir Orthop* 61:39–59, 1975.
291. Insall JN, Goldberg V, Salvati E: Recurrent dislocation and the high-riding patella. *Clin Orthop* 88:67–69, 1972.
292. James SL, Bates BT, Osternig LR: Injuries to runners. *Am J Sports Med* 6:40–49, 1978.
293. Sammarco GJ, Hockenbury RT: Biomechanics of the foot and ankle. In: Frankel VH, Nordin M, eds. *Basic Biomechanics of the Musculoskeletal System.* Baltimore, MD: Williams and Wilkins, 2000.
294. Wright DG, Desai SM, Henderson WH: Action of the subtalar and ankle joint complex during stance phase of walking. *J Bone and Joint Surg* 46A:361–382, 1964.
295. Maquet PG: *Biomechanics of the Knee.* New York, NY: Springer-Verlag, 1984.
296. Dillon P, Updyke W, Allen W: Gait analysis with reference to chondromalacia patellae. *J Orthop Sports Phys Ther* 5:127–131, 1983.
297. DeVita P, Hortobagyi T, Barrier J: Gait biomechanics are not normal after anterior cruciate ligament reconstruction and accelerated rehabilitation. *Med Sci Sports Exerc* 30:1481–1488, 1998.
298. Devita P, Hortobagyi T, Barrier J, et al: Gait adaptations before and after anterior cruciate ligament reconstruction surgery. *Med Sci Sports Exerc* 29:853–859, 1997.
299. Devita P, Torry M, Glover K, et al: A functional knee brace alters joint torque and power patterns during walking and running. *J Biomech* 29:583–588, 1996.
300. Winter DA: Biomechanical motor patterns in normal walking. *J Motor Behav* 15:302–329, 1983.
301. Andriacchi TP, Birac D: Functional testing in the anterior cruciate ligament-deficient knee. *Clin Orthop* 288:40–47, 1993.
302. Berchuck M, Andriacchi TP, Bach BR, et al: Gait adaptations by patients who have a deficient anterior cruciate ligament. *J Bone Joint Surg* 72-A:871–877, 1990.
303. Andriacchi TP: Dynamics of pathological motion: Applied to the anterior cruciate deficient knee. *J Biomech* 23:99–105, 1990.
304. Birac D, Andriacchi TP, Bach BR, Jr: Time related changes following ACL rupture. *Trans Orthop Res Soc* 16:231, 1991.
305. Mikosz RP, Andriacchi TP, Andersson GBJ: Model analysis of factors influencing the prediction of muscle forces at the knee. *J Orthop Res* 6:205–214, 1988.
306. Mikosz RP, Wu CD, Andriacchi TP: Model interpretation of functional adaptations in the ACL-deficient patient. *Proc North Am Congress Biomech* 2:441, 1992.
307. More RC, Karras BT, Neiman R, et al: Hamstrings—An anterior cruciate ligament protagonist. An in vitro study. *Am J Sports Med* 21:231–237, 1993.
308. Renstrom P, Arms SW, Stanwyck TS, et al: Strain within the anterior cruciate ligament during hamstring and quadriceps activity. *Am J Sports Med* 14:83–87, 1986.
309. Stanton-Hicks M, Janig W, Hassenbusch S, et al: Reflex sympathetic dystrophy: Changing concepts and taxonomy. *Pain* 63:127–133, 1995.
310. DeAndrade JR, Grant C, Dixon ASJ: Joint distension and reflex muscle inhibition in the knee. *J Bone Joint Surg* 47A:313–322, 1965.
311. Jensen K, Graf BK: The effects of knee effusion on quadriceps strength and knee intraarticular pressure. *Arthroscopy* 9:52–56, 1993.
312. Jones DW, Jones DA, Newham DJ: Chronic knee effusion and aspiration: The effect on quadriceps inhibition. *Br J Rheumatol* 26: 370–374, 1987.
313. Snyder-Mackler L, De Luca PF, Williams PR, et al: Reflex inhibition of the quadriceps femoris muscle after injury or reconstruction of the anterior cruciate ligament. *J Bone Joint Surg Am* 76:555–560, 1994.
314. Stratford P: Electromyography of the quadriceps femoris muscles in subjects with normal knees and acutely effused knees. *Phys Ther* 62: 279–283, 1981.
315. Sprague NF, III.: Motion-limiting arthrofibrosis of the knee: the role of arthroscopic management. *Clin Sports Med* 6:537–549, 1987.
316. Steadman JR, Burns TP, Peloza J, et al: Surgical treatment of arthrofibrosis of the knee. *J Orthop Tech* 1:119–127, 1993.
317. Akeson WH, Woo SL, Amiel D, et al: The connective tissue response to immobility: Biochemical changes in periarticular connective tissue of the immobilized rabbit knee. *Clin Orthop* 93:356–362, 1973.

318. Watson CJ, Leddy HM, Dynjan TD, et al: Reliability of the lateral pull test and tilt test to assess patellar alignment in subjects with symptomatic knees: Student raters. *J Orthop Sports Phys Ther* 31:368–74, 2001.
319. Wilk KE, Davies GJ, Mangine RE, et al: Patellofemoral disorders: A classification system and clinical guidelines for nonoperative rehabilitation. *J Orthop Sports Phys Ther* 28:307–322, 1998.
320. Root M, Orien W, Weed J: *Clinical Biomechanics*. Los Angeles: Clinical Biomechanics Corp, 1977.
321. Powers CM, Maffucci R, Hampton S: Rearfoot posture in subjects with patellofemoral pain. *J Orthop Sports Phys Ther* 22:155–160, 1995.
322. Subotnick SI: The foot and sports medicine. *J Orthop Sports Phys Ther* 2:53–54, 1980.
323. Barber-Westin SD, Noyes FR, Andrews M: A rigorous comparison between the sexes of results and complications after anterior cruciate ligament reconstruction. *Am J Sports Med* 25:514–526, 1997.
324. Mendelsohn CL, Paiement GD: Physical examination of the knee. *Primary Care* 23:321–8, 1996.
325. Enneking WF, Horowitz M: The intra-articular effects of immobilization on the human knee. *J Bone Joint Surg* 54-A:973–985, 1972.
326. Rothstein JM, Miller PJ, Roettger RF: Goniometric reliability in a clinical setting. Elbow and knee measurements. *Phys Ther* 63:1611–1615, 1983.
327. Clapper MP, Wolf SL: Comparison of the reliability of the Orthoranger and the standard goniometer for assessing active lower extremity range of motion. *Phys Ther* 68:214–218, 1988.
328. Brosseau L, Tousignant M, Budd J, et al: Intratester and intertester reliability and criterion validity of the parallelogram and universal goniometers for active knee flexion in healthy subjects. *Physiother Res Int* 2:150–66, 1997.
329. Gogia PP, Braatz JH, Rose SJ, et al: Reliability and validity of goniometric measurements at the knee. *Phys Ther* 67:192–5., 1987.
330. Watkins MA, Riddle DL, Lamb RL, et al: Reliability of goniometric measurements and visual estimates of knee range of motion obtained in a clinical setting. *Phys Ther* 71:90–96; discussion 96–97., 1991.
331. Hayes KW, Petersen CM: Reliability of assessing end-feel and pain and resistance sequence in subjects with painful shoulders and knees. *J Orthop Sports Phys Ther* 31:432–445, 2001.
332. Hayes KW, Petersen C, Falconer J: An examination of Cyriax's passive motion tests with patients having osteoarthritis of the knee. *Phys Ther* 74:697–707; discussion 707–709, 1994
333. Fritz JM, Delitto A, Erhard RE, et al: An examination of the selective tissue tension scheme, with evidence for the concept of a capsular pattern of the knee. *Phys Ther* 78:1046–1056; discussion 1057–61, 1998.
334. Schiowitz S: Diagnosis and Treatment of the Lower Extremity—The Knee. In: DiGiovanna EL, Schiowitz S, eds. *An Osteopathic Approach to Diagnosis and Treatment*. Philadelphia, PA: J.B. Lippincott, 1991:330–346.
335. Cooper C, McAlindon T, Coggon D, et al: Occupational activity and osteoarthritis of the knee. *Ann Rheum Dis* 53:90–93, 1994.
336. Sachs RA, Daniel DM, Stone ML, et al: Patellofemoral problems after anterior cruciate ligament reconstruction. *Am J Sports Med* 17:760–765, 1989.
337. Benum P: Operative mobilization of stiff knees after surgical treatment of knee injuries and posttraumatic conditions. *Acta Orthop Scand* 53:625–631, 1982.
338. Cosgarea AJ, DeHaven KE, Lovelock JE: The surgical treatment of arthrofibrosis of the knee. *Am J Sports Med* 22:184–191, 1994.
339. Paulos LE, Rosenberg TD, Drawbert J, et al: Infrapatellar contracture syndrome. An unrecognized cause of knee stiffness with patella entrapment and patella infera. *Am J Sports Med* 15:331–341, 1987.
340. Waldron VD: A test for chondromalacia patella. *Orthop Rev* 12:103, 1983.
341. Nijs J, Van Geel C, Van der auwera C, et al: Diagnostic value of five clinical tests in patellofemoral pain syndrome. *Man Ther* 11:69–77, 2006.
342. Sahrmann SA: *Diagnosis and Treatment of Muscle Imbalances Associated with Regional Pain Syndromes*. Lecture Outline. St. Louis, MO: Washington University, 1992.
343. Segal P, Jacob M: *The Knee*. Chicago: Year Book Medical Publishers, 1983.
344. Grelsamer RP, McConnell J: *The History and Physical Examination, The Patella: A Team Approach*. Gaithersburg, MD: Aspen, 1998:43–55.
345. Broom HJ, Fulkerson JP: The plica syndrome: A new perspective. *Orthop Clin North Am* 17:279–281, 1986.
346. Grelsamer RP, Stein DA: Rotational malalignment of the patella. In: Fulkerson JP, ed. *Common Patellofemoral Problems*. Rosemont, IL: American Academy of Orthopaedic Surgeons, 2005:19–28.
347. Austermuehle PD: Common knee injuries in primary care. *Nurse Practitioner* 26:32–45; quiz 46–47, 2001.
348. Rauch G, Wirth T, Dorner P, et al: Is conservative treatment of partial or complete anterior cruciate ligament rupture still justified? An analysis of the recent literature and a recommendation for arriving at a decision. *Zeitschr Orthop* 129: 438–446, 1991.
349. Sommerlath K, Odensten M, Lysholm J: The late course of acute partial anterior cruciate ligament tears. A nine to 15-year follow-up evaluation. *Clin Orthop Related Res* 281:152–158, 1992.
350. Garvin GJ, Munk PL, Vellet AD: Tears of the medial collateral ligament: Magnetic resonance imaging findings and associated injuries. *Can Assoc Radiol J* 44:199–204., 1993
351. Harilainen A: Evaluation of knee instability in acute ligamentous injuries. *Ann Chir Gynaecol* 76:269–273, 1987.
352. Torg JS, Conrad W, Kalen V: Clinical diagnosis of anterior cruciate ligament instability in the athlete. *Am J Sports Med* 4:84–93, 1976.
353. Katz JW, Fingeroth RJ: The diagnostic accuracy of ruptures of the anterior cruciate ligament comparing the Lachman's test, the anterior drawer sign, and the pivot-shift test in acute and chronic knee injuries. *Am J Sports Med* 14:88–91, 1986.
354. DeHaven K: Arthroscopy in the diagnosis and management of the anterior cruciate deficient knee. *Clin Orthop* 172:52–56, 1983.
355. Donaldson WF, Warren RF, Wickiewicz TL: A comparison of acute anterior cruciate ligament examinations. *Am J Sports Med* 13:5–10, 1985.
356. Cooperman JM, Riddle DL, Rothstein JM: Reliability and validity of judgments of the integrity of the anterior cruciate ligament of the knee using the Lachman's test. *Phys Ther* 70:225–233, 1990.
357. Kujala UM, Nelimarkka O, Koskinen SK: Relationship between the pivot shift and the configuration of the lateral tibial plateau. *Arch Orthop Trauma Surg* 111:228–229, 1992.
358. Weiss JR, Irrgang JJ, Sawhney R, et al: A functional assessment of anterior cruciate ligament deficiency in an acute and clinical setting. *J Orthop Sports Phys Ther* 11:372–373, 1990.
359. Hanten WP, Pace MB: Reliability of measuring anterior laxity of the knee joint using a knee ligament arthrometer. *Phys Ther* 67:357–359, 1987.
360. Hughston JC, Andrews JR, Cross MJ, et al: Classification of knee ligament instabilities. Part 2. *J Bone Joint Surg* 58A:173–179, 1976.
361. Cross MJ, Schmidt DR, Mackie IG: A no-touch test for the anterior cruciate ligament. *J Bone Joint Surg Br* 69:300, 1987.
362. Bomberg BC, McGinty JB: Acute hemarthrosis of the knee: Indications for diagnostic arthroscopy. *Arthroscopy* 6:221–225, 1990.
363. Lee JK, Yao L, Phelps CT, et al: Anterior cruciate ligament tears: MR imaging compared with arthroscopy and clinical tests. *Radiology* 166:861–864, 1988.
364. DeHaven KE: Diagnosis of acute knee injuries with hemarthrosis. *Am J Sports Med* 8:9–14, 1980.
365. Jonsson T, Althoff B, Peterson L, et al: Clinical diagnosis of ruptures of the anterior cruciate ligament. *Am J Sports Med* 10:100–102, 1982.
366. Larson RL: Physical examination in the diagnosis of rotatory instability. *Clin Orthop* 172:38–44, 1983.
367. Strobel M, Stedtfeld HW: *Diagnostic Evaluation of the Knee*. Berlin: Springer-Verlag, 1990.
368. Fowler PJ, Messieh SS: Isolated posterior cruciate ligament injuries in athletes. *Am J Sports Med* 15:553–557, 1987.
369. Clendenin MB, DeLee JC, Heckman JD: Interstitial tears of the posterior cruciate ligament of the knee *Orthopedics* 3:764–772, 1980.
370. Rubinstein RA, Jr., Shelbourne KD, McCarroll JR, et al: The accuracy of the clinical examination in the setting of posterior cruciate ligament injuries. *Am J Sports Med* 22:550–557, 1994.
371. Shino K, Horibe S, Ono K: The voluntary evoked posterolateral drawer sign in the knee with posterolateral instability. *Clin Orthop* 215:179–186, 1987.
372. Daniel DM, Stone ML, Barnett P, et al: Use of the quadriceps active test to diagnose posterior cruciate-ligament disruption and measure posterior laxity of the knee. *J Bone Joint Surg Am* 70:386–391, 1988.
373. Hughston JC, Norwood LA: The posterolateral drawer test and external rotation recurvatum test for posterolateral rotary instability of the knee. *Clin Orthop* 147:82–87, 1980.
374. Gollehon DL, Torzilli PA, Warren RF: The role of the posterolateral and cruciate ligaments in the stability of the human knee. A biomechanical study. *J Bone Joint Surg Am* 69:233–242, 1987.

375. Romeyn RL, Davies GJ, Jennings J: The multiple ligament-injured knee: Evaluation, treatment and rehabilitation. In: Manske RC, ed. *Postsurgical Orthopedic Sports Rehabilitation: Knee and Shoulder*. St. Louis, MI: CV Mosby, 2006:279–317.
376. Galway HR, Beaupre A, MacIntosh DL: Pivot shift: A clinical sign of symptomatic anterior cruciate deficiency. *J Bone Joint Surg* 54B:763–764, 1972.
377. Jensen K: Manual laxity tests for anterior cruciate ligament injuries. *J Orthop Sports Phys Ther* 11:474–481, 1990.
378. Jakob RP, Stäubli HU, Deland JT: Grading the pivot shift. *J Bone Joint Surg* 69B:294–299, 1987.
379. Losee RE: Concepts of the pivot shift. *Clin Orthop* 172:45–51, 1983.
380. Noyes FR, Grood ES, Cummings JF, et al: An analysis of the pivot shift phenomenon. *Am J Sports Med* 19:148–155, 1991.
381. Neeb TB, Aufdemkampe G, Wagener JH, et al: Assessing anterior cruciate ligament injuries: The association and differential value of questionnaires, clinical tests, and functional tests. *J Orthop Sports Phys Ther* 26:324–331, 1997.
382. Kaplan N, Wickiewicz TL, Warren RF: Primary surgical treatment of anterior cruciate ligament ruptures. A long-term follow-up study. *Am J Sports Med* 18:354–358, 1990.
383. Conteduca F, Ferretti A, Mariani PP, et al: Chondromalacia and chronic anterior instabilities of the knee. *Am J Sports Med* 19:119–123, 1991.
384. Tamea CD, Henning CE: Pathomechanics of the pivot shift maneuver. *Am J Sports Med* 9:31–37, 1981.
385. Noyes FR, Mooar PA, Matthews DS, et al: The symptomatic anterior cruciate-deficient knee. Part I. The long-term functional disability in athletically active individuals. *J. Bone and Joint Surg* 65-A:154–162, 1983.
386. Bull AM, Andersen HN, Basso O, et al: Incidence and mechanism of the pivot shift. An in vitro study. *ClinOrthop Relat Res* 363:219–231, 1999.
387. Bach BR, Jr., Jones GT, Sweet FA, et al: Arthroscopy-assisted anterior cruciate ligament reconstruction using patellar tendon substitution. Two- to four-year follow-up results. *Am J Sports Med* 22:758–767, 1994.
388. Daniel DM, Stone ML, Riehl B: Ligament Surgery: The Evaluation of Results. In: Daniel DM, Akeson WH, O'Connor JJ, eds. *Knee Ligaments, Structure, Function and Repair*. New York, NY: Raven Press, 1990:521–534.
389. Norwood LA, Andrews JR, Meisterling RC, et al: Acute anterolateral rotatory instability of the knee. *J Bone Joint Surg* 61A:704–709, 1979.
390. Otter C, Aufdemkampe G, Lezeman H: Diagnostiek van knieletsel en relatie tussen de aanwezigheid van knieklachten en de resultaten van functionele testen en Biodex-test, Jaarboek 1994 Fysiotherapie Kinesitherapie. Houten, Bohn, Stafleu, van Loghum, 1994:195–228.
391. Benjaminse A, Gokeler A, van der Schans CP: Clinical diagnosis of an anterior cruciate ligament rupture: a meta-analysis. *J Orthop Sports Phys Ther* 36:267–288, 2006.
392. Harilainen A, Sandelin J, Osterman K, et al: Prospective preoperative evaluation of anterior cruciate ligament instability of the knee joint and results of reconstruction with patellar ligament. *Clin Orthop* 297:17–22, 1993.
393. Losee RE, Johnson TR, Southwick WO: Anterior subluxation of the lateral tibial plateau. A diagnostic test and operative repair. *J Bone Joint Surg* 60A:1015–1030, 1978.
394. Gerber C, Matter P: Biomechanical analysis of the knee after rupture of the anterior cruciate ligament and its primary repair. An instant-centre analysis of function. *J Bone Joint Surg* 65B:391–399, 1983.
395. Ahmed AM, Shi S, Hyder A, et al: The effect of quadriceps tension characteristics on the patellar tracking pattern. Transactions of the 34th Orthopaedic Research Society. Atlanta, GA: 1988.
396. Dervin GF, Stiell IG, Wells GA, et al: Physicians' accuracy and interrator reliability for the diagnosis of unstable meniscal tears in patients having osteoarthritis of the knee. *Can J Surg* 44:267–274, 2001.
397. Apley AG: The diagnosis of meniscus injuries: Some new clinical methods. *J Bone and Joint Surg* 29B:78–84, 1947.
398. Anderson AF: Clinical diagnosis of meniscal tears: Description of a new manipulation test. *Am J Sports Med* 14:291–296, 1982.
399. Kurosaka M, Yagi M, Yoshiya S, et al: Efficacy of the axially loaded pivot shift test for the diagnosis of a meniscal tear. *Int Orthop* 23:271–274, 1999.
400. Dervin GF, Stiell IG, Wells GA, et al: Physicians' accuracy and interrator reliability for the diagnosis of unstable meniscal tears in patients having osteoarthritis of the knee. *Can J Surg* 44:267–274, 2001.
401. Noble J, Erat K: In defence of the meniscus. A prospective study of 200 meniscectomy patients. *J Bone Joint Surg Br* 62-B:7–11, 1980.
402. LaPrade RF, Konowalchuk BK: Popliteomeniscal fascicle tears causing symptomatic lateral compartment knee pain: Diagnosis by the figure-4 test and treatment by open repair. *Am J sports med* 33:1231–1236, 2005.
403. Jerosch J, Riemer S: [How good are clinical investigative procedures for diagnosing meniscus lesions?]. *Sportverletz Sportschaden*, 18:59–67, 2004.
404. Fithian DC, Mishra DK, Balen PF, et al: Instrumented measurement of patellar mobility. *Am J Sports Med* 23:607–615, 1995.
405. Kolowich PA, Paulos LE, Rosenberg TD, et al: Lateral release of the patella: Indications and contraindications. *Am J Sports Med* 18:359–365, 1990.
406. Teitge RA, Faerber W, Des Madryl P, et al: Stress radiographs of the patellofemoral joint. *J Bone Joint Surg* 78-A:193–203, 1996.
407. Fairbank HA: Internal derangement of the knee in children. *Proc R Soc Med* 3:11, 1937.
408. Niskanen RO, Paavilainen PJ, Jaakkola M, et al: Poor correlation of clinical signs with patellar cartilaginous changes. *Arthroscopy* 17:307–310, 2001.
409. Kuo L, Chung W, Bates E,et al: The hamstring index. *J Pediatr Orthop* 17:78–88, 1997.
410. Thompson NS, Baker RJ, Cosgrove AP, et al: Musculoskeletal modelling in determining the effect of botulinum toxin on the hamstrings of patients with crouch gait. *Dev Med Child Neurol* 40:622–625, 1998.
411. Gautam VK, Anand S: A new test for estimating iliotibial band contracture. *J Bone Joint Surg* 80B:474–475, 1998.
412. Laubenthal KN, Smidt GL, Kettelkamp DB: A quantitative analysis of knee motion for activities of daily living. *Phys Ther* 52:34–42, 1972.
413. Bellamy N, Buchanan WW, Goldsmith CH, et al: Validation study of WOMAC: A health status instrument for measuring clinically important patient-relevant outcomes following total hip or knee arthroplasty in osteoarthritis. *J Orthop Rheumatol* 1:95–108, 1988.
414. Bellamy N: Outcome measurement in osteoarthritis clinical trials. *J Rheumatol* 43 (Suppl):49–51, 1995.
415. Bellamy N, Buchanan WW, Goldsmith CH, et al: Validation study of WOMAC: A health status instrument for measuring clinically important patient relevant outcomes to antirheumatic drug therapy in patients with osteoarthritis of the hip or knee. *J Rheumatol* 15:1833–1840, 1988.
416. McConnell S, Kolopack P, Davis AM: The Western Ontario and McMaster Universities Osteoarthritis Index (WOMAC): A review of its utility and measurement properties. *Arthritis Rheum* 45:453–461, 2001.
417. Hefti F, Muller W, Jakob RP, et al: Evaluation of knee ligament injuries with the IKDC form. *Knee Surg Sports Traumatol Arthrosc* 1:226–234, 1993.
418. Lysholm J, Gilquist J: Evaluation of knee ligament surgery results with special emphasis on the use of a scoring scale. *Am J Sports Med* 10:150–154, 1982.
419. Manske R, Vequist SW: Examination of the knee with special and functional testing. In: Wadsworth C, ed. *Disorders of the Knee—Home Study Course*. La Crosse, WI: Orthopaedic Section, APTA, Inc., 2001.
420. Noyes FR, McGinniss GH, Mooar LA: Functional disability in the anterior cruciate insufficient knee syndrome. Review of knee rating systems and projected risk factors in determining treatment. *Sports Med* 1:278–302, 1984.
421. Irrgang JJ, Safran MC, Fu FH: The knee: ligamentous and meniscal injuries. In: Zachazewski JE, Magee DJ, Quillen WS, eds. *Athletic Injuries and Rehabilitation*. Philadelphia, PA: W.B. Saunders, 1996:623–692.
422. Irrgang JJ, Snyder-Mackler L, Wainner RS, et al: Development of a patient-reported measure of function of the knee. *J Bone Joint Surg* 80A:1132–1145, 1998.
423. Binkley JM, Stratford PW, Lott SA, et al: The Lower Extremity Functional Scale (LEFS): Scale development, measurement properties, and clinical application. North American Orthopaedic Rehabilitation Research Network. *Phys Ther* 79:371–383, 1999.
424. McCarthy CJ, Oldham JA: The reliability, validity and responsiveness of an aggregated locomotor function (ALF) score in patients with osteoarthritis of the knee. *Rheumatology (Oxford)*. 43:514–517.
425. Pookarnjanamorakot C, Korsantirat T, Woratanarat P: Meniscal lesions in the anterior cruciate insufficient knee: The accuracy of clinical evaluation. *J Med Assoc Thai* 87:618–623, 2004.
426. Wilson G, Murphy A: The efficacy of isokinetic, isometric and vertical jump tests in exercise science. *Aust J Sci Med Sport* 27:20–24, 1995.
427. Curl WW, Markey KL, Mitchell WA: Agility training following anterior cruciate ligament reconstruction. *Clin Orthop* 172:133–136, 1983.

428. Delitto A, Irrgang JJ, Harner CD, et al: Relationship of isokinetic quadriceps peak torque and work to one-legged hop and vertical jump in ACL reconstructed subjects. *Phys Ther* 73:S85, 1993.
429. Bolga LA, Keskula DR: Reliability of lower extremity functional performance tests. *J Orthop Sports Phys Ther* 26:138, 1997.
430. Barber SD, Noyes FR, Mangine RE, et al: Quantitative assessment of functional limitations in normal and anterior cruciate ligament-deficient knees. *Clin Orthop* 255:204–214, 1990.
431. Blackburn JR, Morrissey MC: The relationship between open and closed kinetic chain strength of the lower limb and jumping performance. *J Orthop Sports Phys Ther* 27:430–435, 1998.
432. Fitzgerald GK, Lephart SM, Hwang JH, et al: Hop tests as predictors of dynamic knee stability. *J Orthop Sports Phys Ther* 31:588–597, 2001.
433. Booher LD, Hench KM, Worrell TW, et al: Reliability of three single hop tests. *J Sports Rehabil* 2:165–170, 1993.
434. Daniel D, Malcolm L, Stone ML, et al: Quantification of knee instability and function. *Contemp Orthop* 5:83–91, 1982.
435. Hu HS, Whitney SL, Irrgang JJ, et al: Test-retest reliability of the one-legged vertical jump test and the one-legged standing hop test. *J Orthop Sports Phys Ther* 15:51, 1992.
436. Ageberg E, Zatterstrom R, Moritz U: Stabilometry and one-leg hop test have high test-retest reliability. *Scand J Med Sci Sports* 8:198–202, 1998.
437. Sekiya I, Muneta T, Ogiuchi T, et al: Significance of the single-legged hop test to the anterior cruciate ligament-reconstructed knee in relation to muscle strength and anterior laxity. *Am J Sports Med* 26:384–388, 1998.
438. Wilk KE, Romaniello WT, Soscia SM, et al: The relationship between subjective knee scores, isokinetic testing, and functional testing in the ACL-reconstructed knee. *J Orthop Sports Phys Ther* 20:60–73, 1994.
439. Tegner Y, Lysholm J, Lysholm M, et al: A performance test to monitor rehabilitation and evaluate anterior cruciate ligament injuries. *Am J Sports Med* 14:156–159, 1986.
440. Shaffer SW, Payne ED, Gabbard LR, et al: Relationship between isokinetic and functional tests of the quadriceps. *J Orthop Sports Phys Ther* 19:55, 1994.
441. DeCarlo MA, Snell KE: Normative data for range of motion and single-leg hop in high school athletes. *J Sport Rehabil* 6:246–255, 1997.
442. Noyes FR, Barber SD, Mangine RE: Abnormal lower limb asymmetry determined by function hop tests after anterior cruciate ligament rupture. *Am J Sports Med* 19:513–518, 1991.
443. Risberg MA, Ekeland A: Assessment of functional tests after anterior cruciate ligament surgery. *J Orthop Sports Phys Ther* 19:212, 1994.
444. Steadman JR: Rehabilitation of acute injuries of the anterior cruciate ligament. *Clin Orthop* 172, 1983.
445. Markey KL: Functional rehabilitation of the anterior cruciate deficient knee. *Sports Med* 12:407–417, 1991.
446. Fonseca ST, Magee KF, Wessel J, et al: Validation of a performance test for outcome evaluation of knee function. *Clin J Sports Med* 2:251–256, 1992.
447. Lephart SM, Perrin DH, Fu FH, et al: Functional performance tests for the anterior cruciate ligament insufficient athlete. *Athletic Trainer* 26:44–50, 1991.
448. Lephart SM, Perrin DH, Fu FH, et al: Relationship between selective physical characteristics and functional capacity in the anterior cruciate ligament-deficient athlete. *J Orthop Sports Phys Ther* 16:174–181, 1992.
449. Barber SD, Noyes FR, Mangine RE, et al: Rehabilitation after ACL reconstruction: Function testing. *Sports Med Rehabil Series* 8:969–974, 1992.
450. Yawn BP, Amadio P, Harmsen WS, et al: Isolated acute knee injuries in the general population. *J Trauma-Injury Infect Crit Care* 48:716–23, 2000.
451. Kannus P, Jarvinen M: Incidence of knee injuries and the need for further care: A one-year prospective follow-up study. *J Sports Med Phys Fitness* 29:321–325, 1989.
452. Nielsen AB, Yde J: Epidemiology of acute knee injuries: A prospective hospital investigation. *J Trauma* 31:1644–1648, 1991.
453. Henry JH, Crosland JW: Conservative treatment of patellofemoral subluxation. *Am J Sports Med* 7:12–14, 1979.
454. McConnell J: The management of chondromalacia patellae: A long-term solution. *Australian J Physiother* 32:215–223, 1986.
455. Reid DC: The myth, mystic and frustration of anterior knee pain [editorial]. *Clin J Sports Med* 3:139–143, 1993.
456. Shelton GL: Conservative management of patellofemoral dysfunction. *Prim Care* 19:331–350, 1992.
457. Hilyard A: Recent advances in the management of patellofemoral pain: The McConnell programme. *Physiotherapy* 76:559–565, 1990.
458. Kujala UM: Patellofemoral problems in sports medicine. *Ann Chir Gynaecol* 80:219–223, 1991.
459. Garrick JG: Anterior knee pain (chondromalacia patella). *Physician Sportsmed* 17:75–84, 1989.
460. Fulkerson JP, Shea KP: Current concepts review: disorders of patellofemoral alignment. *J Bone Joint Surg Am* 72:1424–1429, 1990.
461. Levine J: Chondromalacia patellae. *Physician Sportsmed* 7:41–49, 1979.
462. O'Neill DB: Arthroscopically assisted reconstruction of the anterior cruciate ligament. *J Bone Joint Surg* 78A:803–813, 1996.
463. Palumbo PM: Dynamic patellar brace: A new orthosis in the management of patellofemoral pain. *Am J Sports Med* 9:45–49, 1981.
464. Walsh WM, Helzer-Julin M: Patellar tracking problems in athletes. *Prim Care* 19:303–330, 1992.
465. Whitelaw GP, Rullo DJ, Markowitz HD, et al: A conservative approach to anterior knee pain. *Clin Orthop* 246:234–237, 1989.
466. Gerrard B: The patello-femoral pain syndrome: A clinical trial of the McConnell programme. *Aus J Physiother* 35:71–80, 1989.
467. Gilleard W, McConnell J, Parsons D: The effect of patella taping on the onset of vastus medialis obliquus and vastus lateralis muscle activity in persons with patellofemoral pain. *Phys Ther* 78:25–32, 1998.
468. Andriacchi TP: Functional analysis of pre- and post-knee surgery: Total knee arthroplasty and ACL reconstruction. *J Biomech Eng* 115:575–581, 1993.
469. Deyle GD, Henderson NE, Matekel RL, et al: Effectiveness of manual physical therapy and exercise in osteoarthritis of the knee. A randomized, controlled trial. *Ann Intern Med* 132:173–81, 2000.
470. Bennett JG, Stauber WT: Evaluation and treatment of anterior knee pain using eccentric exercise. *Med Sci Sports Exerc* 18:526–530, 1986.
471. Doucette SA, Child DP: The effect of open and closed chain exercise and knee joint position on patellar tracking in lateral patellar compression syndrome. *J Orthop Sports Phys Ther* 23:104–110, 1996.
472. Bohannon RW: The effect of electrical stimulation to the vastus medialis muscle in a patient with chronically dislocating patella. *Phys Ther* 63:1445–1447, 1983.
473. Mariani P, Caruso I: An electromyographic investigation of subluxation of the patella. *J Bone and Joint Surg Br* 61:169, 1979.
474. Villar RN: Patellofemoral pain and the infrapatellar brace: A military view. *Am J Sports Med* 13:313, 1985.
475. Grelsamer RP, McConnell J: Conservative management of patellofemoral problems. In: Grelsamer RP, McConnell J, eds. *The Patella: A Team Approach.* Gaithersburg, MD: Aspen, 1998:109–118.
476. Chu DA: Rehabilitation of the lower extremity. *Clin Sports Med* 14:205–222, 1995.
477. Lehman RC, Host JV, Craig R: Patellofemoral dysfunction in tennis players. A dynamic problem. *Clin J Sports Med* 14:177–205, 1995.
478. Griffin LY: Ligamentous injuries. In: Griffin LY, ed. *Rehabilitation of the Injured Knee* 2nd ed. St Louis, MI: CV Mosby, 1995:149–164.
479. Baratta R, Solomonow M, Zhou BH, et al: Muscular coactivation: The role of the antagonist musculature in maintaining knee stability. *Am J Sports Med* 16:113–122, 1988.
480. Hawkins RJ, Misamore GW, Merritt TR: Follow-up of the acute non-operated isolated anterior cruciate ligament tear. *Am J Sports Med* 14:205–210, 1986.
481. Fleming BC, Beynnon BD, Renstrom PA: The strain behavior of the anterior cruciate ligament during bicycling: An in vivo study. *Am J Sports Med* 26:109–118, 1998.
482. Dye S: Patellofemoral pain without malalignment: A tissue homeostasis perspective. In: Fulkerson JP, ed. *Common patellofemoral problems.* Rosemont, IL: American Academy of Orthopaedic Surgeons, 2005:1–9.
483. Klingman RE, Liaos SM, Hardin KM: The effect of subtalar joint posting on patellar glide position in subjects with excessive rearfoot pronation. *J Orthop Sports Phys Ther* 25:185–191, 1997.
484. Pedowitz WJ, Kovatis P: Flatfoot in the adult. *J Am Acad Orthop Surgeons* 3:293–302, 1995.
485. LeVeau BF, Rogers C: Selective training of the vastus medialis muscle using EMG biofeedback. *Phys Ther* 60:1410–1415, 1980.
486. Mirzabeigi E, Jordan C, Gronley JK, et al: Isolation of the vastus medialis oblique muscle during exercise. *Am J Sports Med* 27:50–53, 1999.
487. Powers CM: Rehabilitation of patellofemoral joint disorders: A critical review. *J Orthop Sports Phys ther* 28:345–354, 1998.
488. Soderberg G, Cook T: An electromyographic analysis of quadriceps femoris muscle settings and straight leg raising. *Phys Ther* 63:1434, 1983.
489. Karst GM, Jewett PD: Electromyographic analysis of exercises proposed for differential activation of medial and lateral quadriceps femoris muscle components. *Phys Ther* 73:286–295, 1993.

490. Hodges P, Richardson C: An investigation into the effectiveness of hip adduction in the optimization of the vastus medialis oblique contraction. *Scand J Rehabil Med* 25:57–62, 1993.
491. Doucette SA, Goble EM: The effect of exercise on patellar tracking in lateral patellar compression syndrome. *Am J Sports Med* 20:434–440, 1992.
492. Hanten WP, Schulthies SS: Exercise effect on electromyographic activity of the vastus medialis oblique and the vastus lateralis muscles. *Phys Ther* 70:561–565, 1990.
493. Kibler BW: Closed kinetic chain rehabilitation for sports injuries. *Phys Med Rehabil North Am* 11:369–384, 2000.
494. McNicol K, Taunton JE, Clement DB: Iliotibial band friction syndrome in athletes. *Can J Appl Sport Sci* 6:76–80, 1981.
495. Laus M, Tigani D, Alfonso C, et al: Degenerative spondylolisthesis: Lumbar stenosis and instability. *Chir Organi Mov* 77:39–49, 1992.
496. Cahill BR, Griffith EH: Effect of preseason conditioning on the incidence and severity of high school football knee injuries. *Am J Sports Med* 6:180–184, 1978.
497. Klein W, Shah N, Gassen A: Arthroscopic management of postoperative arthrofibrosis of the knee joint: Indication, technique, and results. *Arthroscopy* 10:591–597, 1994.
498. Thomeé R: A comprehensive treatment approach for patellofemoral pain syndrome in young women. *Phys Ther* 77:1690–1703, 1997.
499. Flynn TW, Soutas-Little RW: Patellofemoral joint compressive forces in forward and backward running. *J Orthop Sports Phys Ther* 21:277–282, 1995.
500. Swenson EJ, Jr., Hough DO, McKeag DB: Patellofemoral dysfunction: How to treat, when to refer patients with problematic knees. *Postgrad Med* 82:125–141, 1987.
501. Noyes FR, Grood ES, Butler DL, et al: Knee ligament tests: What do they really mean? *Phys Ther* 60:1578–1581, 1980.
502. Williams JS, Bernard RB: Operative and nonoperative rehabilitation of the ACL-injured knee. *Sports Med Arth Rev* 4:69–82, 1996.
503. Engle RP, Canner GC: Proprioceptive neuromuscular facilitation (PNF) and modified procedures for anterior cruciate ligament (ACL) instability. *J Orthop Sports Phys Ther* 11:230, 1989.
504. Lephart SM, Borsa PA: Functional rehabilitation of knee injuries. In: Fu FH, Harner C, eds. *Knee Surgery*. Baltimore, MD: Williams & Wilkins, 1993. 88–121
505. Hunter LY: Braces and taping. *Clin Sports Med* 4:439–454, 1985.
506. Koskinen SK, Kujala UM: Effect of patellar bracing on patellofemoral relationships. *Scand J Med Sci Sports* 1:119–122, 1991.
507. Worrell T, Ingersoll CD, Bockrath-Puliese K, et al: Effect of patellar taping and bracing on patellar position as determined by MRI in patients with patellofemoral pain. *Athl Train* 33:16–20, 1998.
508. Brossmann J, Muhle C, Schroder C, et al: Patellar tracking patterns during active and passive knee extension: Evaluation with motion-triggered cine MR imaging. *Radiology* 187:205–212, 1993.
509. Sasaki T, Yagi T: Subluxation of the patella. *Int Orthop* 10:115–120, 1986.
510. Finestone A, Radin EL, Lev B, et al: Treatment of overuse patellofemoral pain: Prospective randomized controlled clinical trial in a military setting. *Clin Orthop* 293:208–210, 1993.
511. Arroll B, Ellis-Pegler E, Edwards A, et al: Patellofemoral pain syndrome: A critical review of the clinical trials on nonoperative therapy. *Am J Sports Med* 25:207–212, 1997.
512. Branch TP, Hunter R, Donath M: Dynamic EMG analysis of anterior cruciate deficient legs with and without bracing during cutting. *Am J Sports Med* 17:35–41, 1989.
513. Fleming BC, Renstrom PA, Beynnon BD, et al: The influence of functional knee bracing on the anterior cruciate ligament strain biomechanics in weightbearing and nonweightbearing knees. *Am J Sports Med* 28:815–824, 2000.
514. Liu SH, Daluiski A, Kabo JM: The effects of thigh soft tissue stiffness on the control of anterior tibial displacement by functional knee orthoses. *J Rehabil Res Dev* 32:135–140, 1995.
515. Risberg MA, Holm I, Steen H, et al: The effect of knee bracing after anterior cruciate ligament reconstruction: A prospective, randomized study with two years' follow-up. *Am J Sports Med* 27:76–83, 1999.
516. Borsa PA, Lephart SM, Irrgang JJ, et al: The effects of joint position and direction of joint motion on proprioceptive sensibility in anterior cruciate ligament-deficient athletes. *Am J Sports Med* 25:336–340, 1997.
517. Barrett DS: Proprioception and function after anterior cruciate ligament reconstruction. *J Bone Joint Surg* 73B:833–837, 1991.
518. Corrigan JP, Cashman WF, Brady MP: Proprioception in the cruciate deficient knee. *J Bone Joint Surg* 74-B:247–250, 1992.
519. Risberg MA, Beynnon BD, Peura GD, et al: Proprioception after anterior cruciate ligament reconstruction with and without bracing. *Knee Surg Sports Traumatol Arthrosc* 7:303–309, 1999.
520. Barrett DS, Cobb AG, Bentley G: Joint proprioception in normal, osteoarthritic and replaced knees. *J Bone Joint Surg* 73-B:53–56, 1991.
521. McConnell J: Promoting effective segmental alignment. In: Crosbie J, McConnell J, eds. *Key Issues in Musculoskeletal Physiotherapy*. Boston, MA: Butterworth Heinemann, 1993:172–194.
522. Bockrath K, Wooden C, Worrell T, et al: Effects of patella taping on patella position and perceived pain. *Med Sci Sports Exerc* 25:989–992, 1993.
523. Gerrard B: The patello-femoral pain syndrome in young, active patients: A prospective study. *Clin Orthop* 179:129–133, 1989.
524. Gigante A, Pasquinelli FM, Paladini P,et al: The effects of patellar taping on patellofemoral incongruence. A computed tomography study. *Am J Sports Med* 29:88–92, 2001.
525. Larsen B, Andreassen E, Urfer A, et al: Patellar taping: A radiographic examination of the medial glide technique. *Am J Sports Med* 23:465–471, 1995.
526. Marumoto JM, Jordan C, Akins R: A biomechanical comparison of lateral retinacular releases. *Am J Sports Med* 23:151–155, 1995.
527. Masse Y: "La trochléoplastie." Restauration de la gouttière trochléene dans les subluxations et luxations de la rotule. *Rev Chir Orthop* 64:3–17, 1978.
528. Grabiner M, Koh T, Draganich L: Neuromechanics of the patellofemoral joint. *Med Sci Sports Exerc* 26:10–21, 1994.
529. Lesher JD, Sutlive TG, Miller GA, et al: Development of a clinical prediction rule for classifying patients with patellofemoral pain syndrome who respond to patella taping. *J Orthop Sports Phys Ther* 36:854–866, 2006.
530. McGinn TG, Guyatt GH, Wyer PC, et al: Users' guides to the medical literature: XXII: How to use articles about clinical decision rules. Evidence-Based Medicine Working Group. *JAMA*. 284:79–84, 2000.
531. Cushnaghan J, McCarthy C, Dieppe P: Taping the patella medially: A new treatment for osteoarthritis of the knee joint? *BMJ* 308:753–755, 1994.
532. Willson J, Torry MR, Decker MJ, et al: Effects of walking poles on lower extremity gait mechanics. *Med Sci Sports Exerc* 33:142–147, 2001.
533. Brunelle EA, Miller MK: The effects of walking poles on ground reaction forces. *Res Q Exerc Sport* 69, 1998.
534. Neureuther G: Ski poles in the summer. Landesarszt der Bayerischen Bergwacht Munich Med. *Wacherts* 13:123, 1981.
535. Schwameder H, Roithner R, Muller E, et al: Knee joint forces during downhill walking with hiking poles. *J Sport Sci* 17:969–978, 1999.
536. Heng RC, Haw CS: Patello-femoral pain syndrome. *Curr Orthop* 10:256–266, 1996.
537. Devereaux MD, Lachman SM: Patello-femoral arthralgia in athletes attending a sports injury clinic. *Br J Sports Med* 18:8–21, 1984.
538. Hughston JC: Subluxation of the patella. *J Bone Joint Surg* 50A:1003–1026, 1968.
539. Ficat P, Bizou H: Luxations récidivantes de la routle. *Rev Orthop* 53:721, 1967.
540. Fulkerson JP, Kalenak A, Rosenberg TD, et al: Patellofemoral pain. *Am Acad Orthop Surg Instruct Course Lect*, 1992:57–71.
541. Martinez S, Korobkin M, Fondren FB, et al: Diagnosis of patellofemoral malalignment by computed tomography. *J Comput Assist Tomogr* 7:1050–1053, 1983.
542. Merchant AC, Mercer RL, Jacobsen RH, et al: Roentgenographic analysis of patellofemoral congruence. *J Bone Joint Surg* 56A:1391–1396, 1974.
543. Minkoff J, Fein L: The role of radiography in the evaluation and treatment of common anarthrotic disorders of the patellofemoral joint. *Clin Sports Med* 8:203–260, 1989.
544. Geenen E, Molenaers G, Martens M: Patella alta in patellofemoral instability. *Acta Orthop Belg* 55:387–393, 1989.
545. Hvid I, Andersen L, Schmidt H: Chondromalacia patellae: the relation to abnormal patellofemoral joint mechanics. *Acta Orthop Scand* 52:661–666, 1981.
546. Moller BN, Krebs B, Jurik AG: Patellar height and patellofemoral congruence. *Arch Orthop Trauma Surg* 104:380–381, 1986.
547. Hvid I, Andersen LI: The quadriceps angle and its relation to femoral torsion. *Acta Orthop Scand* 53:577–579, 1982.
548. Rowe CR, Pierce DS, Clark JG: Voluntary dislocation of the shoulder: A preliminary report on a clinical, electromyographic, and psychiatric study of 26 patients. *J Bone Joint Surg* 55A:445–460, 1973.

549. Wise HH, Fiebert IM, Kates JL: EMG biofeedback as treatment for patellofemoral pain syndrome. *J Orthop Sports Phys Ther* 6:95–103, 1984.
550. Jeffreys TE: Recurrent dislocation of the patella due to abnormal attachment of the ilio-tibial tract. *J Bone Joint Surg* 45-B:740–743, 1963.
551. Fulkerson JP, Schutzer SF: After failure of conservative treatment of painful patellofemoral malalignment: Lateral release or realignment? *Orthop Clin North Am* 17:283–288, 1996.
552. Fulkerson JP, Tennant R, Jaivin J, et al: Histologic evidence of retinacular nerve injury associated with patellofemoral malalignment. *Clin Orthop* 197:196–205, 1985.
553. Ellen MI, Jackson HB, DiBiase SJ: Uncommon causes of anterior knee pain: A case report of infrapatellar contracture syndrome. *Am J Phys Med Rehabil* 78:376–380, 1999.
554. Paulos LE, Wnorowski DC, Greenwald AE: Infrapatellar contracture syndrome: Diagnosis, treatment, and long-term followup. *Am J Sports Med* 22:440–449, 1994.
555. Woo SL-Y, Buckwalter JA: *Injury and Repair of the Musculoskeletal Tissue.* Park Ridge, IL: American Academy of Orthopaedic Surgeons, 1988.
556. Reinold MM, Wilk KE, Macrina LC, et al: Current concepts in the rehabilitation following articular cartilage repair procedures in the knee. *J Orthop Sports Phys Ther* 36:774–94, 2006.
557. Lewis PB, McCarty LP, III, Kang RW, et al: Basic science and treatment options for articular cartilage injuries. *J Orthop Sports Phys Ther* 36:717–727., 2006.
558. Prevention FtCfDCa: Prevalence of disabilities and associated health conditions-United States, 1991–1992. *JAMA* 272:1735–1736, 1994.
559. Panush RS, Lane NE: Exercise and the musculoskeletal system. *Baillieres Clin Rheumatol* 8:79–102, 1994.
560. Felson DT, Naimark A, Anderson JJ, et al: The prevalence of knee osteoarthritis in the elderly. The Framingham Osteoarthritis Study. *Arthritis Rheum* 30:914–918, 1987.
561. Felson DT: The epidemiology of knee osteoarthritis: Results from the Framingham Osteoarthritis Study. *Sem Arthritis Rheum* 20:42–50, 1990.
562. Peyron JG, Altman RD: The epidemiology of osteoarthritis. In: Moskowitz RW, Howell DS, Goldberg VM, et al, eds. *Osteoarthritis: Diagnosis and Medical/Surgical Management.* Philadelphia, PA: W.B. Saunders, 1992:15–37.
563. Anderson JJ, Felson DT: Factors associated with osteoarthritis of the knee in the first National Health and Nutrition Examination Survey. *Am J Epidemiol* 128:179–189, 1988.
564. Felson DT, Hannan MT, Naimark A: Occupational physical demands, knee bending and knee osteoarthritis: Results from the Framingham study. *J Rheumatol* 18:1587–1592, 1991.
565. Jensen LK, Eenberg W: Occupation as a risk factor for knee disorders. *Scand J Work Environ Health* 22:165–175, 1996.
566. Maetzel A, Makela M, Hawker G, et al: Osteoarthritis of the hip and knee and mechanical occupational exposure: A systematic overview of the evidence. *J Rheum* 24:1599–1607, 1997.
567. Kujala UM, Kaprio J, Sarna S: Osteoarthritis of weight bearing joints of lower limbs in former elite male athletes. *BMJ* 308:231–234, 1994.
568. Kujala UM, Kettunen J, Paananen H, et al: Knee osteoarthritis in former runners, soccer players, weight lifters, and shooters. *Arthr Rheum* 38:539–546, 1995.
569. Felson DT, Zhang Y, Hannan MT, et al: Risk factors for incident radiographic knee osteoarthritis in the elderly: The Framingham Study. *Arthr Rheum* 40:728–733, 1997.
570. Felson DT: Epidemiology of hip and knee osteoarthritis. *Epidemiol Rev* 10:1–28, 1988.
571. Baker K, McAlindon T: Exercise for knee osteoarthritis. *Curr Opin Rheumatol* 12:456–463, 2000.
572. Wessel J: Isometric strength measurements of knee extensors in women with osteoarthritis of the knee. *J Rheumatol* 23:328–331, 1996.
573. Slemenda C, Heilman DK, Brandt KD, et al: Quadriceps weakness and osteoarthritis of the knee. *Ann Intern Med* 127:97–104, 1998.
574. Puett DW, Griffin MR: Published trials of nonmedicinal and noninvasive therapies for hip and knee osteoarthritis. *Ann Intern Med* 121:133–140, 1994.
575. Fisher NM, Pendergast DR, Gresham GE, et al: Muscle rehabilitation: Its effect on muscular and functional performance of patients with knee osteoarthritis. *Arch Phys Med Rehabil* 72:367–374, 1991.
576. Fisher NM, Gresham GE, Pendergast DR: Effects of a quantitative progressive rehabilitation program applied unilaterally to the osteoarthritic knee. *Arch Phys Med Rehabil* 74:1319–1326, 1993.
577. Fisher NM, Gresham GE, Abrams M, et al: Quantitative effects of physical therapy on muscular and functional performance in subjects with osteoarthritis of the knees. *Arch Phys Med Rehabil* 74:840–847, 1993.
578. Kovar PA, Allegrante JP, MacKenzie CR, et al: Supervised fitness walking in patients with osteoarthritis of the knee. A randomized, controlled trial. *Ann Intern Med* 116:529–534, 1992.
579. Ettinger WH, Jr, Burns R, Messier SP, et al: A randomized trial comparing aerobic exercise and resistance exercise with a health education program in older adults with knee osteoarthritis. The Fitness Arthritis and Seniors Trial. *JAMA* 277:25–31, 1997.
580. Lane NE, Buckwalter JA: Exercise: A cause of osteoarthritis? *Rheum Dis Clin North Am* 19:617–633, 1993.
581. Brandt KD: Nonsurgical management of osteoarthritis, with an emphasis on nonpharmacologic measures. *Arch Fam Med* 4:1057–1064, 1995.
582. Mangione KK, Axen K, Haas F: Mechanical unweighting effects on treadmill exercise and pain in elderly people with osteoarthritis of the knee. *Phys Ther* 76:387–394, 1996.
583. Fitzgerald GK, Oatis C: Role of physical therapy in management of knee osteoarthritis. *Curr Opin Rheumatol* 16:143–147, 2004.
584. Fitzgerald GK, Childs JD, Ridge TM, et al: Agility and perturbation training for a physically active individual with knee osteoarthritis. *Phys Ther* 82:372–382, 2002.
585. Yasuda K, Sasaki T: The mechanics of treatment of the osteoarthritic knee with a wedged insole. *Clin Orthop* 215:162–172, 1985.
586. Yasuda K, Sasaki T: Clinical evaluation of the treatment of osteoarthritic knees using a newly designed wedged insole. *Clin Orthop* 221:181–187, 1985.
587. Rorabeck CH, Murray P: The benefit of total knee arthroplasty. *Orthopedics* 19:777–779, 1996.
588. Diduch DR, Insall JN, Scott WN,et al: Total knee replacement in young, active patients. Long-term follow-up and functional outcome. *J Bone Joint Surg* 79A:575–582, 1997.
589. Ritter MA, Herbst SA, Keating EM, et al: Long-term survival analysis of a posterior cruciate-retaining total condylar total knee arthroplasty. *Clin Orthop* 309:136–145, 1994.
590. Kolettis GT, Stern SH: Patellar resurfacing for patellofemoral arthritis. *Orthop Clin North Am* 23:665–673, 1992.
591. Aglietti P, Rinonapoli E, Stringa G, et al: Tibial osteotomy for the varus osteoarthritic knee. *Clin Orthop* 176:239–251, 1983.
592. Insall JN, Shoji H, Mayer V: High tibial osteotomy: A five year evaluation. *J Bone Joint Surg* 56A:1397–1405, 1974.
593. Windsor RE, Insall JN, Vince KG: Technical considerations of total knee arthroplasty after proximal tibial osteotomy. *J Bone Joint Surg* 70A:547–555, 1988.
594. Larcom P, Lotke PA: Treatment of inflammatory and degenerative conditions of the knee. In: Dee R, Hurst LC, Gruber MA, et al, eds. *Principles of Orthopaedic Practice*, 2nd ed. New York, NY: McGraw-Hill, 1997:945–983.
595. Aglietti P, Buzzi R, De Felice R, et al: The Insall-Burstein total knee replacement in osteoarthritis: A 10-year minimum follow-up. *J Arthroplasty* 14:560–565, 1999.
596. Banks SA, Markovich GD, Hodge WA: In vivo kinematics of cruciate-retaining and substituting knee arthroplasties. *J Arthroplasty* 12:297–304, 1997.
597. Laskin RS: Total knee replacement with posterior cruciate ligament retention in patients with a fixed varus deformity. *Clin Orthop* 331:29–34, 1996.
598. Laskin RS, Rieger M, Schob C, et al: The posterior-stabilized total knee prosthesis in the knee with a severe fixed deformity. *Am J Knee Surg* 1:199–203, 1988.
599. Matsuda S, Ishinishi T, White SE, et al: Patellofemoral joint after total knee arthroplasty: Effect on contact area and contact stress. *J Arthroplasty* 12:790–797, 1997.
600. Chew JTH, Stewart NJ, Hanssen AD, et al: Differences in patellar tracking and knee kinematics among three different total knee designs. *Clin Orthop* 345:87–98, 1997.
601. Auberger SS, Mangine RE: *Innovative Approaches to Surgery and Rehabilitation, Physical Therapy of the Knee.* New York, NY: Churchill Livingstone, 1988:233–262.
602. Ecker ML, Lotke PA: Postoperative care of the total knee patient. *Orthop Clin North Am* 20:55–62, 1989.
603. Kumar PJ, McPherson EJ, Dorr LD, et al: Rehabilitation after total knee arthroplasty: A comparison of 2 rehabilitation techniques. *Clin Orthop Relat Res* 331:93–101, 1996.

604. Enloe LJ, Shields RK, Smith K, et al.: Total hip and knee replacement treatment programs: a report using consensus. *J Orthop Sports Phys Ther* 23:3–11, 1996.
605. Manske PR, Gleeson P: Rehabilitation program following polycentric total knee arthroplasty. *Phys Ther* 57:915–918, 1987.
606. Waters EA: Physical therapy management of patients with total knee replacement. *Phys Ther* 54:936–942, 1974.
607. Schunk C, Reed K: *Clinical Practice Guidelines.* Gaithersburg, MD: Aspen, 2000.
608. Aleman O: Chondromalacia post-traumatica patellae. *Acta Chir Scand* 63:149–190, 1928.
609. Beck JL, Wildermuth BP: The female athlete's knee. *Clin J Sports Med* 4:345–66, 1985.
610. Outerbridge RE: The aetiology of chondromalacia patellae. *J Bone Joint Surg* 43B:752–757, 1961.
611. Dye SF, Vaupel GL: The pathophysiology of patellofemoral pain. *Sports Med Arthrosc Rev* 2:203–210, 1994.
612. Gillespie MJ, Friedland J, DeHaven K: Arthrofibrosis: Etiology, classification, histopathology, and treatment. *Op Tech Sports Med* 6:102–110, 1998.
613. Parisien JS: The role of arthroscopy in the treatment of postoperative fibroarthrosis of the knee joint. *Clin Orthop* 229:185–192, 1988.
614. Richmond JC, Assal M: Arthroscopic management of arthrofibrosis of the knee, including infrapatellar contraction syndrome. *Arthroscopy* 7:144–147, 1991.
615. Sebastianelli WJ, Gillespie MJ, Hicks DG, et al: The histopathology of arthrofibrosis. *Arthroscopy* 9:359–360, 1993.
616. Shelbourne KD, Johnson GE: Outpatient surgical management of arthrofibrosis after anterior cruciate ligament surgery. *Am J Sports Med* 22:192–197, 1994.
617. Lindenfeld TN, Wojtys EM, Husain A: Operative Treatment of Arthrofibrosis of the Knee. *J Bone Joint Surg Am* 81-A:1772–1784, 1999.
618. Delcogliano A, Franzese S, Branca A, et al: Light and scan electron microscopic analysis of cyclops syndrome: Etiopathogenic hypothesis and technical solutions. *Knee Surg Sports Traumatol Arthrosc* 4:194–199, 1996.
619. Jackson DW, Schaefer RK: Cyclops syndrome: Loss of extension following intra-articular anterior cruciate ligament reconstruction. *Arthroscopy* 6:171–178, 1990.
620. Shelbourne KD, Wilckens JH, Mollabashy A, et al: Arthrofibrosis in acute anterior cruciate ligament reconstruction. The effect of timing of reconstruction and rehabilitation. *Am J Sports Med* 19:332–336, 1991.
621. Wasilewski SA, Covall DJ, Cohen S: Effect of surgical timing on recovery and associated injuries after anterior cruciate ligament reconstruction. *Am J Sports Med* 21:338–342, 1993.
622. Hunter RE, Mastrangelo J, Freeman JR, et al: The impact of surgical timing on postoperative motion and stability following anterior cruciate ligament reconstruction. *Arthroscopy* 12:667–674, 1996.
623. Shelbourne KD, Nitz P: Accelerated rehabilitation after anterior cruciate ligament reconstruction. *Am J Sports Med* 18:292–299, 1990.
624. Lindenfeld TN, Bach BR, Jr. Wojtys EM: Reflex sympathetic dystrophy and pain dysfunction in the lower extremity. *J Bone and Joint Surg* 78-A:1936–1944, 1996.
625. Christel P, Herman S, Benoit S, et al: A comparison of arthroscopic arthrolysis and manipulation of the knee under anaesthesia in the treatment of post-operative stiffness of the knee. *French J Orthop Surg* 2:348–355, 1988.
626. Silman AJ, Day SJ, Haskard DO: Factors associated with joint mobility in an adolescent population. *Ann Rheum Dis* 46:209–212, 1987.
627. Woo SL Y, Lewis JL, Suh J-K, et al: Acute injury to ligament and meniscus as inducers of osteoarthritis. In: Kuettner KE, Goldberg VM, eds. *Osteoarthritic Disorders.* Rosemont, IL: American Academy of Orthopaedic Surgeons, 1995:185–196.
628. Buckwalter JA, Lane NE, Gordon SL: Exercise as a cause for osteoarthritis. In: Kuettner KE, Goldberg BA, eds. *Osteoarthritic Disorders.* Rosemont, IL: American Academy of Orthopaedic Surgeons, 1995:405–417.
629. Johnson DL: Acute knee injuries: An introduction. *Clin Sports Med* 12:344, 1993.
630. Arendt E, Dick R: Knee injury patterns among men and women in collegiate basketball and soccer. NCAA data and review of literature. *Am J Sports Med* 23:694–701, 1995.
631. Bjordal JM, Arnly F, Hannestad B, et al: Epidemiology of anterior cruciate ligament injuries in soccer. *Am J Sports Med* 25:341–345, 1997.
632. Huston LJ, Greenfield ML, Wojtys EM: Anterior cruciate ligament injuries in the female athlete. Potential risk factors. *Clin Orthop Relat Res* 372:50–63, 2000.
633. Shambaugh JP, Klein A, Herbert JH: Structural measures as predictors of injury in basketball players. *Med Sci Sports Exerc* 23:522–527, 1991.
634. Muneta T, Takakuda K, Yamomoto H: Intercondylar notch width and its relation to the configuration of cross-sectional area of the anterior cruciate ligament. *Am J Sports Med* 25:69–72, 1997.
635. Norwood LA, Cross MJ: The intercondylar shelf in the anterior cruciate ligament. *Am J Sports Med* 5:171–176, 1977.
636. Ireland ML: Special Concerns of the Female Athlete. In: Fu FH, Stone DA, eds. *Sports Injuries: Mechanism, Prevention, and Treatment*, 2nd ed. Baltimore, MD: Williams & Wilkins, 1994:153–162.
637. Grana WA, Moretz JA: Ligamentous laxity in secondary school athletes. *JAMA* 240, 1978.
638. Hutchinson MR, Ireland ML: Knee injuries in female athletes. *Sports Med* 19:288–302, 1995.
639. Huston LJ, Wojtys EM: Neuromuscular performance characteristics in elite female athletes. *Am J Sports Med* 24:427–436, 1996.
640. Liu SH, Al-Shaikh RA, Panossian V, et al: Estrogen affects the cellular metabolism of the anterior cruciate ligament. A potential explanation for female athletic injury. *Am J Sports Med* 25:704–709, 1997.
641. Slauterbeck JR, Narayan RS, Clevenger C, et al: Effects of estrogen level on the tensile properties of the rabbit anterior cruciate ligament. *J Orthop Res* 17:405–408, 1999.
642. Ireland ML: The female ACL: Why is it more prone to injury? *Orthop Clin North Am* 33:637–651, 2002.
643. Griffin JW, Tooms RE, Zwaag RV, et al: Eccentric muscle performance of elbow and knee muscle groups in untrained men and women. *Med Sci Sports Exerc* 25:936–944, 1993.
644. Hakkinen K, Kraemer WJ, Newton RU: Muscle activation and force production during bilateral and unilateral concentric and isometric contractions of the knee extensors in men and women at different ages. *Electromyogr Clin Neurophysiol* 37:131–142, 1997.
645. Kanehisa H, Okuyama H, Ikegawa S, et al: Sex difference in force generation capacity during repeated maximal knee extensions. *Eur J Appl Physiol* 73:557–562, 1996.
646. Miller AEJ, MacDougall JD, Tarnopolsky MA, et al: Gender differences in strength and muscle fiber characteristics. *Eur J Appl Physiol* 66:254–262, 1993.
647. Griffin LY, Albohm MJ, Arendt EA, et al: Understanding and preventing noncontact anterior cruciate ligament injuries: A review of the Hunt Valley II meeting, January 2005. *Am J Sports Med* 34:1512–1532, 2006.
648. Griffin LY, Agel J, Albohm MJ, et al: Noncontact anterior cruciate ligament injuries: Risk factors and prevention strategies. *J Am Acad Orthop Surg* 8:141–150, 2000.
649. Hewett TE, Zazulak BT, Myer GD, et al: A review of electromyographic activation levels, timing differences, and increased anterior cruciate ligament injury incidence in female athletes. *Br J Sports Med* 39:347–350, 2005.
650. Hewett TE, Torg JS, Boden BP: Video analysis of trunk and knee motion during non-contact anterior cruciate ligament injury in female athletes: Lateral trunk and knee abduction motion are combined components of the injury mechanism. *Br J Sports Med* 43:417–22, 2009.
651. Hewett TE, Myer GD, Ford KR, et al: Dynamic neuromuscular analysis training for preventing anterior cruciate ligament injury in female athletes. *Instr Course Lect* 56:397–406, 2007.
652. Hewett TE, Myer GD, Ford KR, et al: Biomechanical measures of neuromuscular control and valgus loading of the knee predict anterior cruciate ligament injury risk in female athletes: A prospective study. *Am J Sports Med* 33:492–501, 2005.
653. Mizuta H, et al: The conservative treatment of complete tears of the anterior cruciate ligament in skeletally immature patients. *J Bone Joint Surg* 77:890, 1995.
654. Parker AW, Drez D, Cooper JL: Anterior cruciate injuries in patients with open physes. *Am J Sports Med* 22:47, 1994.
655. Micheli LJ, Jenkins M: Knee injuries. In: Micheli LJ, ed. *The Sports Medicine Bible.* Scranton, PA: Harper & Row, 1995:118–151.
656. Mangine RE, Minning SJ, Eifert-Mangine M, et al: Management of the patient with an ACL/MCL injured knee. *NAJSPT* 3:204–211, 2008.
657. Daniel DM, et al: Fate of the ACL-injured patient. *Am J Sports Med* 22:642, 1994.
658. O'Connor BL, Visco DM, Brandt KD, et al: Neurogenic acceleration of osteoarthrosis. The effects of previous neurectomy of the articular nerves

on the development of osteoarthrosis after transection of the anterior cruciate ligament in dogs. *J. Bone and Joint Surg* 74-A:367–376, 1992.
659. Vilensky JA, O'Connor BL, Brandt KD, et al: Serial kinematic analysis of the canine hindlimb joints after deafferentation and anterior cruciate ligament transection. *Osteoarth Cartilage* 5:173–182, 1997.
660. Gillquist J, Messner K: Anterior cruciate ligament reconstruction and the long-term incidence of gonarthrosis. *Sports Med* 27:143–156, 1999.
661. Hoher J, Moller HD, Fu FH: Bone tunnel enlargement after anterior cruciate ligament reconstruction: Fact or fiction? *Knee Surg Sports Traumatol Arthrosc* 6:231–240, 1998.
662. Howell SM: Principles for placing the tibial tunnel and avoiding roof impingement during reconstruction of a torn anterior cruciate ligament. *Knee Surg Sports Traumatol Arthrosc* 6:S49–S55, 1998.
663. Elmqvist L-G, Johnson RJ: Prevention of Cruciate Ligament Injuries. In: Feagin JA, ed. *The Crucial Ligaments: Diagnosis and Treatment of Ligamentous Injuries About the Knee*, 2nd ed. New York, NY: Churchill Livingstone, 1994:495–505.
664. Ettlinger CF, Johnson RJ, Shealy JE: A method to help reduce the risk of serious knee sprains incurred in alpine skiing. *Am J Sports Med* 23:531–537, 1995.
665. Feagin J, J.A., Lambert KL: Mechanism of injury and pathology of anterior cruciate ligament injuries. *Orthop Clin North Am* 16:41–45, 1985.
666. Liu SH, et al: The diagnosis of acute complete tears of the anterior cruciate ligament. *J Bone Joint Surg* 77:586, 1995.
667. Gerber C, Hoppeler H, Claassen H, et al: The lower-extremity musculature in chronic symptomatic instability of the anterior cruciate ligament. *J Bone Joint Surg* 67-A:1034–1043, 1985.
668. Kariya Y, Itoh M, Nakamura T, et al: Magnetic resonance imaging and spectroscopy of thigh muscles in cruciate ligament insufficiency. *Acta Orthop Scand* 60:322–325, 1989.
669. Lorentzon R, Elmqvist LG, Sjostrom M, et al: Thigh musculature in relation to chronic anterior cruciate ligament tear: Muscle size, morphology, and mechanical output before reconstruction. *Am J Sports Med* 17:423–429, 1989.
670. Noyes FR, Mangine RE, Barber S: Early knee motion after open and arthroscopic anterior cruciate ligament reconstruction. *Am J Sports Med* 15:149–160, 1987.
671. Yasuda K, Ohkoshi Y, Tanabe Y, et al: Quantitative evaluation of knee instability and muscle strength after anterior cruciate ligament reconstruction using patellar and quadriceps tendon. *Am J Sports Med* 20:471–475, 1992.
672. Elmqvist LG, Lorentzon R, Johansson C, et al: Knee extensor muscle function before and after reconstruction of anterior cruciate ligament tear. *Scand J Rehabil Med* 21:131–139, 1989.
673. Fink C, Hoser C, Benedetto KP, et al: (Neuro)Muskulare Veranderungen der kniegelenksstabilisierenden Muskulatur nach Ruptur des vorderen Kreuzbandes. *Sportverletz Sportsch* 8:25–30, 1994.
674. Lopresti C, Kirkendall DT, Streete GM: Quadriceps insufficiency following repair of anterior cruciate ligament. *J Orthop Sports Phys Ther* 9:245–249, 1988.
675. Snyder-Mackler L, Delitto A, Bailey SL, et al: Strength of the quadriceps femoris muscle and functional recovery after reconstruction of the anterior cruciate ligament. A prospective, randomized clinical trial of electrical stimulation. *J Bone Joint Surg Am* 77:1166–1173, 1995.
676. Yahia LH, Newman N, Rivard CH: Neurohistology of lumbar spine ligaments. *Acta Orthop Scand* 59:508–512, 1988.
677. Rosenberg TD, Pazik TJ, Deffner KT: *Primary Quadrupled Semitendinosus ACL Reconstruction: A Comprehensive 2-Year Evaluation, Proceedings of the Twentieth SICOT Congres.* Amsterdam: SICOT, 1996:177–178.
678. Kramer J, Nusca D, Fowler P, et al: Knee flexor and extensor strength during concentric and eccentric muscle actions after anterior cruciate ligament reconstruction using the semitendinosus tendon and ligament augmentation device. *Am J Sports Med* 21:285–291, 1993.
679. Daniel DM, Malcom LL, Losse G, et al: Instrumented measurement of anterior laxity of the knee. *J Bone Joint Surg* 67-A:720–725, 1985.
680. Indelicato PA, Bittar ES: A perspective of lesions associated with ACL insufficiency of the knee. A review of 100 cases. *Clin Orthop* 198:77–80, 1985.
681. Irvine GB, Glasgow MMS: The natural history of the meniscus in anterior cruciate insufficiency. Arthroscopic analysis. *J Bone Joint Surg* 74-B:403–405, 1992.
682. Andersson C, Odensten M, Good L, et al: Surgical or non-surgical treatment of acute rupture of the anterior cruciate ligament. A randomized study with long-term follow-up. *J Bone Joint Surg* 71-A:965–974, 1989.
683. Hefti FL, Kress A, Fasel J, et al: Healing of the transected anterior cruciate ligament in the rabbit. *J Bone Joint Surg* 73-A:373–383, 1991.
684. Kleiner JB, Roux RD, Amiel D, et al: Primary healing of the anterior cruciate ligament (ACL). *Trans Orthop Res Soc* 11:131, 1986.
685. Nagineni CN, Amiel D, Green MH, et al: Characterization of the intrinsic properties of the anterior cruciate and medial collateral ligament cells: An in vitro cell culture study. *J Orthop Res* 10:465–475, 1992.
686. Andrish J, Holmes R: Effects of synovial fluid on fibroblasts in tissue culture. *Clin Orthop* 138:279–283, 1979.
687. Kurosaka M, Yoshiya S, Mizuno T, et al: Spontaneous healing of a tear of the anterior cruciate ligament. A report of two cases. *J Bone Joint Surg Am* 80:1200–1203, 1998.
688. Antich TJ, Brewster CE: Rehabilitation of the nonreconstructed anterior cruciate ligament-deficient knee. *Clin Sports Med* 7:813–826, 1988.
689. Bynum EB, Barrack RL, Alexander AH: Open versus closed kinetic chain exercises in rehabilitation after anterior cruciate ligament reconstruction: A prospective randomized study. *Annual conference of the American Academy of Orthopaedic Surgeons*, New Orleans, LA, 1994.
690. Frndak PA, Berasi CC: Rehabilitation concerns following anterior cruciate ligament reconstruction. *Sports Med* 12:338–346, 1991.
691. Mangine RE, Noyes FR, DeMaio M: Minimal protection program: Advanced weight bearing and range of motion after ACL reconstruction-Weeks 1 to 5. *Orthopedics* 15:504–515, 1992.
692. Pevsner DN, Johnson JRG, Blazina ME: The patellofemoral joint and its implications in the rehabilitation of the knee. *Phys Ther* 59:869–874, 1979.
693. Seto JL, Brewster CE, Lombardo SJ: Rehabilitation of the knee after anterior cruciate ligament reconstruction. *J Orthop Sports Phys Ther* 11:8–18, 1989.
694. Shelbourne KD, Wilckens JH: Current concepts in anterior cruciate ligament rehabilitation. *Orthop Rev* 19:957–964, 1990.
695. Silfverskold JP, Steadman JR, Higgins RW: Rehabilitation of the anterior cruciate ligament in the athlete. *Sports Med* 6:308–319, 1988.
696. Steadman JR, Forster RS, Silfverskold JP: Rehabilitation of the knee. *Clin Sports Med* 8:605–627, 1989.
697. Steadman JR, Sterett WI: The surgical treatment of knee injuries in skiers. *Med Sci Sports Exerc* 27:328–333, 1995.
698. Timm KE: Postsurgical knee rehabilitation. A five-year study of four methods and 5,381 patients. *Am J Sports Med* 16:463–468, 1988.
699. Gryzlo SM, Patek RM, Pink M: Electromyographic analysis of knee rehabilitation exercises. *J Orthop Sports Phys Ther* 20:36–43, 1994.
700. Loudon JK, Goist HL, Loudon KL: Genu recurvatum syndrome. *J Orthop Sports Phys Ther* 27:361–367, 1998.
701. Noyes FR, Dunworth LA, Andriacchi TP, et al: Knee hyperextension gait abnormalities in unstable knees. *Am J Sports Med* 24:35–45, 1996.
702. Loudon JK, Jenkins WJ, Loudon KL: The relationship between static posture and ACL injury in female athletes. *J Orthop Sports Phys Ther* 24:91–97, 1996.
703. Rubinstein RA, Shelbourne KD, VanMeter CD, et al: Effect on knee stability if hyperextension is restored immediately after autogenous bone-patellar tendon-bone anterior cruciate ligament reconstruction. *Am J Sports Med* 23:365–368, 1995.
704. Egner E: Knee joint meniscal degneration as it relates to tissue fiber structure and mechanical resistance. *Pathol Res Pract* 173:310–324, 1982.
705. Boden SD, Davis DO, Dina TS, et al: A prospective and blinded investigation of magnetic resonance imaging of the knee: Abnormal findings in asymptomatic subjects. *Clin Orthop* 282:177–185, 1992.
706. O'Connor RL: *Arthroscopy.* Philadelphia, PA: J.B. Lippincott, 1977.
707. Diment MT, DeHaven KE, Sebastianelli WJ: Current concepts in meniscal repair. *Orthopedics* 16:973–977, 1993.
708. Tria AJ, Klein KS: *An Illustrated Guide to the Knee.* New York, NY: Churchill Livingstone, 1992.
709. Miyasaka KC, Daniel DM, Stone ML, et al: The incidence of knee ligament injuries in the general population. *Am J Knee Surg* 4:3–8, 1991.
710. Cooper DE, Warren RF, Warner JJP: The PCL and posterolateral structures of the knee: Anatomy, function and patterns of injury. *Inst Course Lect* 40:249–270, 1991.
711. Trickey EL: Injuries to the PCL: Diagnosis and treatment of early injuries and reconstruction of late instability. *Clin Orthop* 147:76–81, 1980.

712. Insall JN, Hood RW: Bone block transfer of the medial head of the gastrocnemius for posterior cruciate insufficiency. *J Bone and Joint Surg* 65A:691–699, 1982.
713. Fanelli GC, Edson CJ: Posterior cruciate ligament injuries in trauma patients: Part II. *Arthroscopy* 11:526–529, 1995.
714. Fanelli GC: Posterior cruciate ligament injuries in trauma patients. *Arthroscopy* 9:291–294, 1993.
715. Petrigliano FA, McAllister DR: Isolated posterior cruciate ligament injuries of the knee. *Sports Med Arthrosc Rev* 14:206–212, 2006.
716. Harner CD, Hoher J: Evaluation and treatment of posterior cruciate ligament injuries. *Am J Sports Med* 26:471–482, 1998.
717. Feltham GT, Albright JP: The diagnosis of PCL injury: Literature review and introduction of two novel tests. *Iowa Orthop J* 21:36–42, 2001.
718. Fischer SP, Fox JM, Del Pizzo W, et al: Accuracy of diagnoses from magnetic resonance imaging of the knee. A multi-center analysis of one thousand and fourteen patients. *J Bone Joint Surg Am* 73:2–10, 1991.
719. Shelbourne KD, Muthukaruppan Y: Subjective results of nonoperatively treated, acute, isolated posterior cruciate ligament injuries. *Arthroscopy* 21:457–461, 2005
720. Cross MJ, Powell JF: Long-term followup of posterior cruciate ligament rupture: A study of 116 cases. *American J Sports Med* 12:292–297, 1984.
721. Tibone JE, Antich TJ, Perry J, et al: Functional analysis of untreated and reconstructed posterior cruciate ligament injuries. *Am J Sports Med* 16:217–223, 1988.
722. Dejour H, Walch G, Peyrot J, et al: The natural history of rupture of the PCL. *French J Orthop Surg* 2:112–120, 1988.
723. Parolie JM, Bergfeld JA: Long-term results of nonoperative treatment of isolated posterior cruciate ligament injuries in the athlete. *Am J Sports Med* 14:35–38, 1986.
724. Picard F, Saragaglia D, Montabaron E, et al: Étude morphométrique de l' articulation fémoro-patellaire à partir de l'incidence radiologique de profil. *Rev Chir Orthop* 83:104–111, 1997.
725. Dejour H, Walch G, Neyret P, et al: La dysplasie de la trochlée fémorale. *Rev Chir Orthop* 76:45–54, 1990.
726. Powers CM: Patellar kinematics. Part II. The influence of the depth of the trochlear groove in subjects with and without patellofemoral pain. *Phys Ther* 80:965–973, 2000.
727. Lohman EB, Harp T: Patellofemoral Pain: A Critical Appraisal of the Literature. In: Wilmarth MA, ed. *Evidence-Based Practice for the Upper and Lower Quarter. Orthopaedic Physical Therapy Home Study Course 13.2.1.* La Crosse, WI: Orthopaedic Section, APTA, Inc, 2003:1–44.
728. Brattström H: Patella alta in non-dislocating knee joints. *Acta Orthop Scand* 41:578–588, 1970.
729. Blackburn J, Peel T: A new method of measuring patellar height. *J Bone Joint Surg* 58B:241–245, 1977.
730. Noyes FR, Wojtys EM, Marshall MT: The early diagnosis and treatment of developmental patella infera syndrome. *Clin Orthop* 265:241–252, 1991.
731. Blumensaat C: Die lageabweichungen und verrunkungen der kniescheibe. *Ergeb Chir Orthop* 31:149–223, 1938.
732. Fulkerson JP, Schutzer SF, Ramsby GR, et al: Computerized tomography of the patellofemoral joint before and after release or realignment. *Arthroscopy* 3:19–24, 1987.
733. Grelsamer RP, Meadows S: The modified Insall-Salvati ratio for assessment of patellar height. *Clin Orthop* 282:170–176, 1992.
734. Turner MS: The association between tibial torsion and knee joint pathology. *Clin Orthop* 302:47–51, 1994.
735. Amatuzzi MM, Fazzi A, Varella MH: Pathologic synovial plica of the knee. Results of conservative treatment. *Am J Sports Med* 18:466–469, 1990.
736. De la Caffinière JY, Mignot M, Bruch JM: Pli synovial interne et chondropathie rotulienne. *Rev Chir Orthop* 67:479–484, 1981.
737. Hughston JC, Whatley GS, Dodelin RA, et al: The role of the suprapatellar plica in internal derangement of the knee. *Am J Orthop* 5:25–27, 1963.
738. Patel D: Arthroscopy of the plicae–synovial folds and their significance. *Am J Sports Med* 6:217–225, 1978.
739. Pipkin G: Knee injuries: the role of suprapatellar plica and suprapatellar bursa in simulating internal derangements. *Clin. Orthop* 74:161–176, 1971.
740. Vaughan-Lane T, Dandy DJ: The synovial shelf syndrome. *J Bone Joint Surg* 64-B:475–476, 1982.
741. Dandy DJ: *Arthroscopic Surgery of the Knee.* New York, NY: Churchill Livingstone, 1981.
742. Dandy DJ: Arthroscopy in the treatment of young patients with anterior knee pain. *Orthop Clin North Am* 17:221–229, 1986.
743. Jackson RW: The sneaky plicae (editorial). *J. Rheumat* 7:437, 1980.
744. Apple JS: Infrapatellar plica on lateral knee arthrograms. *AJR Am J Roentgenol* 141:843, 1983.
745. Dupont JY: La place des replis synoviaux dans la patholgie du genou. *Rev Chir Orthop* 71:401–403, 1985.
746. Lupi L, Bighi S, Cervi PM, et al: Arthrography of the plica syndrome and its significance. *Eur J Radiol* 11:15–18, 1990.
747. Patel D: Plica as a cause of anterior knee pain. *Orthop Clin North Am* 17:273–277, 1986.
748. Fujisawa Y, Jackson R, Marshall DM: Problems caused by the medial and lateral synovial folds of the patella. *Kansetsukyo* 1:40–44, 1976.
749. Reid GD, Glasgow M, Gordon DA, et al: Pathologic plicae of the knee mistaken for arthritis. *J Rheumat* 7:573–576, 1980.
750. Sherman RMP, Jackson RW: The pathological medial plica: Criteria for diagnosis and prognosis. *J Bone Joint Surg* 71-B:351, 1989.
751. Richmond JC, McGinty JB: Segmental arthroscopic resection of the hypertrophic retropatellar plica. *Clin Orthop* 178:185–189, 1983.
752. Apple JS, Martinez S, Hardaker WT, et al: Synovial plicae of the knee. *Skel Radiol* 7:251–254, 1982.
753. Aprin H, Shapiro J, Gershwind M: Arthrography (plica views). A noninvasive method for diagnosis and prognosis of plica syndrome. *Clin Orthop* 183:90–95, 1984.
754. Brody GA, Pavlov H, Warren RF, et al: Plica synovialis infrapatellaris: Arthrographic sign of anterior cruciate ligament disruption. *AJR Am J Roentgenol* 140:767–769, 1983.
755. Pipkin G: Lesions of the suprapatellar plica. *J Bone and Joint Surg* 32-A:363–369, 1950.
756. SanDretto MA, Wartinbee DR, Carrera GF, et al: Suprapatellar plica synovialis: A common arthrographic finding. *J Canadian Assn. Radiol* 33:163–166, 1982.
757. Deutsch AL, Resnick D, Dalinka MK, et al: Synovial plicae of the knee. *Radiology* 141:627–634, 1981.
758. Thijn CJP, Hillen B: Arthrography and the medial compartment of the patello-femoral joint. *Skel Radiol* 11:183–190, 1984.
759. Fisher RL: Conservative treatment of patellofemoral pain. *Orthop Clin North Am* 17:269–272, 1986.
760. Morrison RJ: Synovial plicae syndrome. *J Manip Physiol Ther* 11:296–299, 1988.
761. Newell SG, Bramwell ST: Overuse injuries to the knee in runners. *Phys Sports Med* 12:80–92, 1984.
762. Subotnick SI, Sisney P: The plica syndrome: A cause of knee pain in the athlete. *J Am Podiatr Med Assoc* 76:292–293, 1986.
763. Rovere GD, Nichols AW: Frequency, associated factors, and treatment of breaststroker's knee in competitive swimmers. *Am J Sports Med* 13:99–104, 1985.
764. Rovere GD, Adair DM: The medial synovial shelf plica syndrome. Treatment by intraplical steroid injection. *Am J Sports Med* 13:382–386, 1985.
765. Maurizio E: La tendinite rotulea del giocatore di pallavolo. *Arch Soc Tosco Umbra Chir* 24:443–445, 1963.
766. Blazina ME, Kerlan RK, Jobe F, et al: Jumper's Knee. *Orthop Clin North Am* 4:665–678, 1973.
767. Anderson JE: *Grant's Atlas of Anatomy*, 7th ed. Baltimore, MD: Williams & Wilkins, 1980.
768. Hollinshead WH, Rosse C: *Textbook of Anatomy.* Philadelphia, PA: Harper & Row, 1985.
769. Fredberg U, Bolvig L: Jumper's knee. *Scand J Med Sci Sports* 9:66–73, 1999.
770. Fyfe I, Stanish WD: The use of eccentric training and stetching in the treatment and prevention of tendon injuries. *Clin J Sports Med* 11:601–624, 1992.
771. Stanish WD, Rubinovich RM, Curwin S: Eccentric exercise in chronic tendinitis. *Clin Orthop Relat Res* 208:65–68, 1986.
772. Reid DC: Bursitis and knee extensor mechanism pain syndromes. In: Reid DC, ed. *Sports Injury Assessment and Rehabilitation.* New York, NY: Churchill Livingstone, 1992:399–437.
773. Black JE, Alten SR: How I manage infrapatellar tendinitis. *Phys Sports Med* 12:86–90, 1984.
774. Popp JE, Yu SS, Kaeding CC: Recalcitrant patellar tendinitis, magnetic resonance imaging, histologic evaluation, and surgical treatment. *Am J Sports Med* 25:218–222, 1997.
775. Noble CA: The treatment of iliotibial band friction syndrome. *Br J Sports Med* 13:51–54, 1979.

776. Noble CA: Iliotibial band friction syndrome in runners. *Am J Sports Med* 8:232–234, 1980.
777. Lindenberg G, Pinshaw R, Noakes TD: Iliotibial band friction syndrome in runners. *Phys Sportsmed* 12:118–130, 1984.
778. Sutker AN, Jackson DW, Pagliano JW: Iliotibial band syndrome in distance runners. *Phys Sportsmed* 9:69–73, 1981.
779. Holmes JC, Pruitt AL, Whalen NJ: Iliotibial band syndrome in cyclists. *Am J Sports Med* 21:419–424, 1993.
780. Biundo JJ, Jr., Irwin RW, Umpierre E: Sports and other soft tissue injuries, tendinitis, bursitis, and occupation-related syndromes. *Curr Opin Rheumatol* 13:146–149, 2001.
781. Muhle C, Ahn JM, Yeh L: Iliotibial band friction syndrome: MR imaging findings in 16 patients and MR arthrographic study of six cadaveric knees. *Radiology* 212:103–110, 1999.
782. Mann RA, Hagy J: Biomechanics of walking, running, and sprinting. *Am J Sports Med* 8:345–350, 1980.
783. Mann RA: *Biomechanics of running, AAOS Symposium on the Foot and Leg in Running Sports.* St. Louis, MI: CV Mosby, 30–44, 1982.
784. Orchard JW, Fricker PA, Abud AT, et al: Biomechanics of the iliotibial band friction syndrome in runners. *Am J Sports Med* 24: 375–379, 1996.
785. Barber FA, Sutker AN: Iliotibial band syndrome. *Sports Med* 14:144–148, 1992.
786. Lineger JM, Christensen CP: Is iliotibial band syndrome often overlooked? *Phys Sportsmed* 20:98–108, 1984.
787. Krissoff WB, Ferris WF: Runners' injuries. *Physician Sportsmed* 7:55–63, 1979.
788. Krivickas LS: Anatomical factors associated with overuse sports injuries. *Sports Med* 24:132–146, 1997.
789. Messier SP, Pittala KA: Etiologic factors associated with selected running injuries. *Med Sci Sports Exerc* 20:501–505, 1988.
790. Schwellnus MP: Lower limb biomechanics in runners with the iliotibial band friction syndrome. *Med Sci Sports Exerc* 25:S68, 1993.
791. Fredericson M, Cookingham CL, Chaudhari AM, et al: Hip Abductor Weakness in Distance Runners with Iliotibial Band Syndrome. *Clin J Sport Med* 10:169–175, 2000.
792. Pinshaw R, Atlas V, Noakes TD: The nature and response to therapy of 196 consecutive injuries seen at a runners' clinic. *S Afr Med J* 65:291–298, 1984.
793. Brantigan OC, Voshell AF: The tibial collateral ligament: Its function, its bursae and its relation to the medial meniscus. *J Bone Joint Surg Am* 25:121–131, 1943.
794. Worth RM, Kettlekamp DB, Defalque RJ, et al: Saphenous nerve entrapment: A cause of medial knee pain. *Am J Sports Med* 12:80–81, 1984.
795. Voshell AF, Brantigan OC: Bursitis in the region of the tibial collateral ligament. *J Bone Joint Surg Am* 26:793–798, 1944.
796. Mital MA, Matza RA: Osgood-Schlatter's disease: the painful puzzler. *Physician Sports Med* 5:60, 1977.
797. Ryan J, Wheeler J, Hopkinson W: Quadriceps contusion: West Point update. *Am J Sports Med* 19:299–303, 1991.
798. Beauchesne RP, Schutzer SF: Myositis ossificans of the piriformis muscle: An unusual cause of piriformis syndrome. A case report. *J Bone Joint Surg Am* 79:906–910, 1997.
799. Thompson HC, Garcia A: Myositis ossificans: Aftermath of elbow injuries. *Clin Orthop* 50:129–134, 1967.
800. Hoffa A: The influence of the adipose tissue with regard to the pathology of the knee joint. *J Am Med Assoc* 43:795–796, 1904.
801. Jacobson JA, Lenchik L, Ruhoy MK, et al: MR imaging of the infrapatellar fat pad of Hoffa. *Radiographics* 17:675–691, 1997.
802. Vizsolyi P, et al. Breaststroker's knee. *Am J Sports Med* 15:63, 1987.
803. Kimura J: Diseases of the root and plexus in electrodiagnosis. In: Kimura J, ed. *Diseases of Nerve and Muscle: Principles and Practice*, 2nd ed. Philadelphia, PA: F.A. Davis, 1989:507.
804. Lippitt AB: Neuropathy of the saphenous nerve as a cause of knee pain. *Bull Hosp Joint Dis Orthop Institute* 52:31–33, 1993.
805. Romanoff ME, Cory PC, Kalenak A, et al: Saphenous nerve entrapment in the adductor canal. *Am J Sports Med* 17:478–481, 1989.
806. Magora F, Aladjemoff L, Tannenbaum J, et al: Treatment of pain by transcutaneous electrical stimulation. *Acta Anaesthesiol Scand* 22:589–592, 1978.
807. Sunderland S: Traumatized nerves, roots and ganglia: Musculoskeletal factors and neuropathological consequences. In: Knorr IM, Huntwork EH, eds. *The Neurobiologic Mechanisms in Manipulative Therapy*. New York, NY: Plenum Press, 1978:137–166.
808. Tibrewall SB, Goodfellow JW: Peroneal nerve palsy at the level of the lower third of the leg. *J R Soc Med* 77:72–73, 1984.
809. Sridhara CA, Izzo KL: Terminal sensory branches of the superficial peroneal nerve: An entrapment syndrome. *Arch Phys Med Rehab* 66:789–791, 1985.
810. Smolders JJ: Myofascial pain and dysfunction syndromes. In: Hammer WI, ed. *Functional Soft Tissue Examination and Treatment by Manual Methods – The Extremities*. Gaithersburg, MD: Aspen, 1991: 215–234.
811. Dunn D: Chronic Regional Pain Syndrome, Type 1: Part I. *AORN Journal* 72:421–424, 426, 428–432, 435, 437–442, 444–449, 452–458, 2000.
812. Gordon N: Review article: Reflex sympathetic dystrophy. *Brain Dev* 18:257–262, 1996.
813. Wilson PR: Post-traumatic upper extremity reflex sympathetic dystrophy: Clinical course, staging, and classification of clinical forms. *Hand Clinics* 13:367–372, 1997.
814. Cowan SM, Bennell KL, Crossley KM, et al: Physical therapy alters recruitment of the vasti in patellofemoral pain syndrome. *Med Sci Sports Exerc.* 34:1879–1885, 2002.

CHAPTER 21 The Ankle and Foot

CHAPTER OBJECTIVES

At the completion of this chapter, the reader will be able to:

1. Describe the anatomy of the joints, ligaments, muscles, and blood and nerve supply that comprise the ankle and foot complex.
2. Describe the biomechanics of the ankle and foot complex, including the open- and close-packed positions, normal and abnormal joint end-feels, kinesiology, and the effects of open- and closed-chain activities.
3. Outline the purpose and components of the tests and measures of the ankle and foot complex.
4. Perform a detailed examination of the ankle and foot complex, including palpation of the articular and soft tissue structures, range-of-motion (ROM) testing, passive articular mobility tests, and stability tests for the ankle and foot complex.
5. Discuss the significance of the key findings from the tests and measures.
6. Evaluate the total examination data to establish a physical therapy diagnosis.
7. Describe the significance of muscle imbalance in terms of functional muscle performance and the deleterious effects on the lower kinetic chain.
8. Develop self-reliant examination and intervention strategies.
9. Describe the intervention strategies based on clinical findings and established goals.
10. Apply manual techniques to the ankle and foot complex, using the correct grade, direction, and duration.
11. Incorporate appropriate therapeutic exercises into the intervention progression.
12. Evaluate intervention effectiveness in order to progress or modify the intervention.
13. Plan an effective home program and instruct the patient in same.

OVERVIEW

The ankle and foot is a complex structure of 28 bones (including two sesamoid bones) and 55 articulations (including 30 synovial joints), interconnected by ligaments and muscles.

The foot has undergone a number of evolutionary adaptations, which make it very effective for bipedal locomotion.[1] First, the foot has become plantigrade, which allows most of the sole to be a weight-bearing surface. Second, the great toe has come to lie in a position with the other toes and, because of the relative immobility of the first metatarsal at the metatarsophalangeal (MTP) joint, is now relatively nonprehensile. Third, the metatarsals and phalanges have progressively shrunk and become small in comparison to the hypertrophied tarsus. Last, the medial side of the foot has become larger and stronger than that of any other primate.

The ankle joint sustains the greatest load per surface area of any joint of the body.[2] Peak vertical forces reach 120% of body weight during walking and they approach 275% during running.[3] The joints and ligaments of the ankle and foot complex act as stabilizers against these forces and constantly adapt during weight-bearing activities, especially on uneven surfaces. It is estimated that an average 180-lb man absorbs 76.2 tons on each foot while walking 1 mile and that the same man absorbs 121.5 tons per foot while running 1 mile.[4] Approximately 60% of this weight-bearing load is carried out by the rearfoot, and 28% by the metatarsal heads.[5,6] Although the ankle and foot complex normally adapts well to the stresses of everyday life, sudden or unanticipated stresses to this region have the potential to produce dysfunction.

ANATOMY

The ankle and foot complex is a sophisticated musculoskeletal arrangement designed to facilitate numerous and various weight-bearing and non–weight-bearing functions.[7] Anatomically and biomechanically, the foot can be subdivided into the

TABLE 21-1 The Joints of the Foot and Ankle: Their Open- and Close-Packed Positions and Capsular Patterns

Joints of the Hind Foot	Open-Packed Position	Close-Packed Position	Capsular Pattern
Tibiofibular joint	Plantar flexion	Maximum dorsiflexion	Pain on stress
Talocrural joint	10 degrees of plantar flexion and midway between inversion and eversion	Maximum dorsiflexion	Plantar flexion and dorsiflexion
Subtalar joint	Midway between the extremes of ROM	Supination	Varus and valgus
Joints of the Midfoot			
Midtarsal joints	Midway between the extremes of ROM	Supination	Dorsiflexion, plantar flexion, adduction, and internal rotation
Joints of the Forefoot			
Tarsometatarsal joints	Midway between the extremes of ROM	Supination	None
Metatarsophalangeal joints	10 degrees of extension	Full extension	Great toe: extension and flexion of second to fifth toes: variable
Interphalangeal joints	Slight flexion	Full extension	Flexion and extension

rearfoot or hindfoot (tibia, fibula, talus and calcaneus), the midfoot (the navicular, cuboid, and the three cuneiforms), and the forefoot (the 14 bones of the toes, the five metatarsals, and the medial and lateral sesamoids) (Table 21-1 and Fig. 21-1). The seven tarsal bones occupy the proximal half of the foot (see Fig. 21-1). Although described separately, the joints of the lower leg, ankle, and foot act as functional units and not in isolation. The joints of the foot and ankle, their open- and close-packed positions, and capsular patterns are outlined in Table 21-1. The shapes of the articulating surfaces of the leg and foot are outlined in Table 21-2. An appreciation of the shapes of the articulating surfaces is important when examining the joint glides and when performing joint mobilizations. Most of the stability of the foot and ankle is provided by a vast array of ligaments (Table 21-3).

REARFOOT

The joints of the rearfoot are the tibiofibular joint, talocrural (ankle) joint, and the subtalar (talocalcaneal) joint. The proximal row of tarsals comprises the talus (astragalus) (see Fig. 21-1), and calcaneus (or calcis). The function of the rearfoot is as follows:

- to influence the function and movement of the midfoot and forefoot;
- to convert the transverse rotations of the lower extremity into sagittal, transverse, and frontal plane movements.[8]

MIDFOOT

The joints of the midfoot include the talocalcaneonavicular joint, cuneonavicular joint, cuboideonavicular joint, intercuneiform joints, cuneocuboid joint, and the calcaneocuboid joint. The distal tarsal row contains, medial to lateral, the medial, intermediate, and lateral cuneiforms and the cuboid, which is roughly in parallel with the proximal row and which forms a transverse arch, posteriorly (dorsally) convex. Medially, the navicular is positioned between the talus and the cuneiforms (see Fig. 21-1). Laterally, the cuboid is positioned between the calcaneus and the lateral cuneiform and the fourth and fifth metatarsals (see Fig. 21-1). The function of the midfoot is to transmit motions from the rearfoot to the forefoot and to promote stability.[8]

CLINICAL PEARL

The midtarsal, or Chopart's joint, consists of the calcaneocuboid joint and talonavicular joint and connects the rearfoot to the midfoot. The midtarsal joint facilitates adduction and abduction of the forefoot.[7] The tarsometatarsal, or Lisfranc's joint, connects the midfoot and the forefoot.[7]

FOREFOOT

The joints of the forefoot include the tarsometatarsal joints, the intermetatarsal joints, the MTP joints, and the interphalangeal (IP) joints. The function of the forefoot is to adapt to the terrain, adjusting to uneven surfaces. The first metatarsal is the shortest and the strongest (see Fig. 21-1), whereas the second is the longest and the least mobile, serving as the anatomic touchstone for abduction and adduction of the foot.[9] The phalanges of the foot, although similar in number and distribution to those in the hand, are shorter and broader than their counterparts.

DISTAL TIBIOFIBULAR JOINT

The distal tibiofibular joint (Fig. 21-1) is classified as a syndesmosis, except for approximately 1 mm of the inferior portion, which is covered in hyaline cartilage. The joint consists of a concave tibial surface and a convex or plane surface on the medial distal end of the fibula. There is an

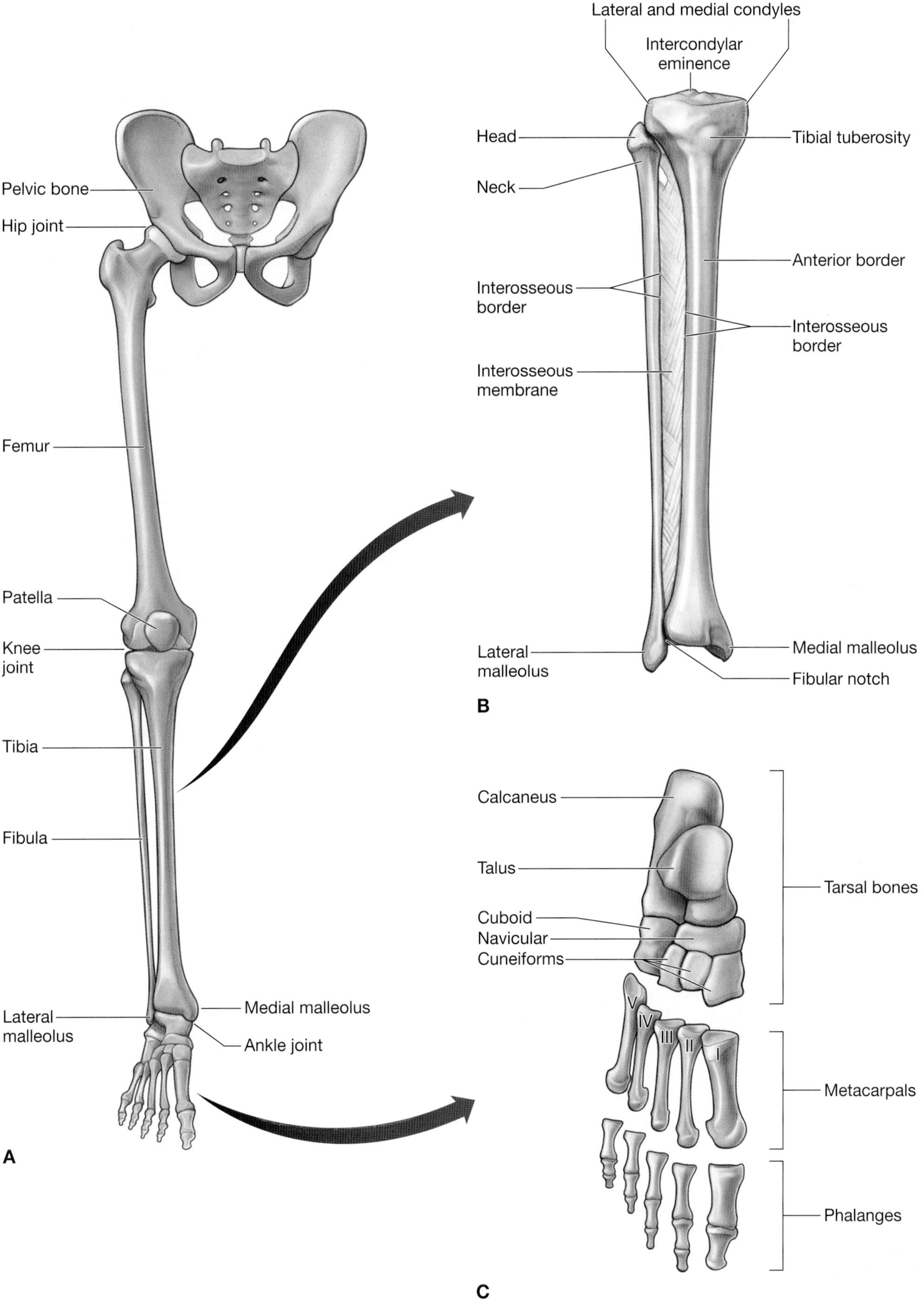

FIGURE 21-1 Bones of the lower extremity and foot. (Reproduced with permission from Morton DA, Foreman KB, Albertine KH: *The Big Picture: Gross Anatomy,* McGraw-Hill, 2011.)

TABLE 21-2 Shapes of the Articulating Surfaces of the Leg and Foot		
Joint	**Proximal Bone and Shape of Its Joint Surface**	**Distal Bone and Shape of Its Joint Surface**
Inferior tibiofibular	Tibia—concave	Fibula—convex
Talocrural	Tibia—concave in anterior–posterior direction and concave–convex–concave in mediolateral direction	Fibula—convex in anterior–posterior direction and convex–concave–convex in mediolateral direction
Talocalcaneal	Talus—posterior facet biconcave, middle facet biconvex, and anterior facet convex	Calcaneus—posterior facet biconvex, middle facet biconcave, and anterior facet concave
Talonavicular	Talus—biconvex	Navicular—biconcave
Calcaneocuboid	Calcaneus—convex in mediolateral direction and concave in superior–inferior direction (saddle shaped)	Cuboid—concave in mediolateral direction and convex in superior–inferior direction (saddle shaped)
Cuboideonavicular	Navicular—planar	Cuboid—planar
Cuneonavicular	Navicular—slightly convex	Cuneiforms—slight concave
Intercuneiform	Cuneiforms (medial and middle)—planar	Cuneiforms (middle and lateral)—planar
Cuneocuboid	Lateral cuneiform—planar	Cuboid—planar
Tarsometatarsal	Cuneiforms and cuboid—planar to slightly convex	Bases of metatarsals—planar to slightly concave
Metatarsophalangeal	Metatarsals—biconvex	Proximal phalanges—biconcave
Interphalangeal	Proximal phalanges—convex in superior–inferior and concave in medial–lateral direction	Middle phalanges—concave in superior–inferior and convex in medial–lateral direction

elongation into the joint by the synovium of the talocrural joint, the fibers of which are oriented inferiorly and laterally. The fibula serves as a site for muscular and ligamentous attachment, providing stability for the talus at the talocrural joint. The tibia is the second longest bone of the skeleton and is a major weight-bearing bone.

As at the proximal tibiofibular joint (see Chap. 20), support for this joint is provided primarily by ligaments. The joint is stabilized by four ligaments, collectively known as the syndesmotic ligaments. These include the inferior interosseous ligament, the anterior inferior tibiofibular ligament, the posterior inferior tibiofibular ligament, and the inferior transverse ligament. Of these ligaments, the inferior interosseous ligament is the primary stabilizer.

THE TALOCRURAL (ANKLE) JOINT

The talocrural (tibiotalar) joint is the articulation between the talus and the distal tibia. The talus serves as the link between the foot and the leg through the ankle joint and functions to distribute the body weight posteriorly toward the heel and anteriorly to the midfoot. The talus is divided into an anterior head and a posterior neck and body:

- ***Body.*** The superior dome-shaped surface of the body articulates with the tibia. The body is convex in the anteroposterior (A-P) direction and slightly concave in the mediolateral (M-L) and superior directions. The shape of this articulating surface can be compared with that of a cone, with the base of the cone facing laterally and the apex medially. Since the superior aspect of the body of the talus is wedge shaped with the wider portion anterior, no varus/valgus movement is possible when the ankle is positioned in maximum dorsiflexion, unless the mortise or the tibiofibular ligaments are compromised.
- ***Neck.*** The neck of the talus is a narrow region between the head and the body of the talus, and it is medially inclined. Its rough surfaces serve as attachments for ligaments. Inferior to the neck of the talus is the sulcus tali, which, when the talus and the calcaneus are articulated, roofs the sinus tarsi and is occupied by the talocalcaneal interosseous and cervical ligaments.
- ***Head.*** The plantar surface of the head has three articular areas separated by smooth ridges. The most posterior and largest of the articular areas is oval, slightly convex, and rests on a shelf-like medial calcanean projection called the *sustentaculum tali*. The other two articulating facets connect the talus with the navicular and the plantarcalcaneonavicular ligament.

The medial malleolus extends distally to approximately one-third of the height of the talus, whereas the lateral malleolus extends distally to approximately two-thirds the height of the talus.

The fibrous capsule of the ankle joint is relatively thin on its anterior and posterior aspects. It is lined with synovial membrane and reinforced by the collateral ligaments (see later).

CLINICAL PEARL

No tendons, with the exception of a small slip from the posterior tibialis, attach to the talus. However, the talus serves as the attachment for many ligaments.

TABLE 21-3	Ankle and Foot Joints and Associated Ligaments		
Joint	**Associated Ligament**	**Fiber Direction**	**Motions Limited**
Distal tibiofibular	Anterior tibiofibular	Distolateral	Distal and posterior glide of fibula
	Posterior tibiofibular	Distolateral	Distal and anterior glide of fibula
	Interosseous	Distolateral	Separation of tibia and fibula
Ankle	Deltoid (medial collateral)		
	Superficial		
	Tibionavicular	Plantar–anterior	Lateral translation and external rotation of the talus
	Calcaneotibial	Plantar, plantar–posterior	Eversion (abduction of talus, calcaneus and navicular)
	Posterior talotibial	Plantar–posterior	Dorsiflexion, lateral translation and external rotation of the talus
	Deep		
	Anterior talotibial	Anterior	Abduction of the talus when in plantar flexion or eversion
	Lateral or fibular collateral		
	Anterior talofibular	Anterior–medial	Inversion and plantar flexion Anterior displacement of the talus Internal rotation of the talus
	Calcaneofibular	Posterior distal and medial	Inversion and dorsiflexion
	Posterior talofibular	Horizontal	Dorsiflexion Posterior displacement of foot Inversion
Subtalar	Lateral (anterior) talocalcaneal	Distal anterolateral	Joint separation during inversion and dorsiflexion
	Medial (posterior) talocalcaneal	Distal	Anterior translation of talus and inversion
	Cervical ligament	Distal–posterior–lateral	Inversion
	Interosseous	Distal and lateral	Joint separation
Main ligamentous support of longitudinal arches	Long plantar	Anterior, slightly medial	Eversion
	Short plantar	Anterior	Eversion
	Plantar calcaneonavicular	Dorsal–anterior–medial	Eversion
	Plantar aponeurosis	Anterior	Eversion
Midtarsal or transverse	Bifurcated		Joint separation
	Medial band	Longitudinal	Plantar flexion
	Lateral band	Horizontal	Inversion
	Dorsal talonavicular	Longitudinal	Plantar flexion of talus on navicular
	Dorsal calcaneocuboid	Longitudinal	Inversion, plantar flexion
Intertarsal	Dorsal and plantar ligaments		Joint motion in direction causing ligament tautness
	Interosseous ligaments connecting cuneiforms, cuboid, and navicular		Flattening of the transverse or longitudinal arch
Tarsometatarsal	Dorsal, plantar, and interosseous		Joint separation
Intermetatarsal	Dorsal, plantar, and interosseous		Joint separation Joint separation
	Deep transverse metatarsal		Flattening of the transverse arch
Metatarsophalangeal	Fibrous capsule		
	Dorsal, thin—separated from extensor tendons by bursae		Flexion
	Plantar— inseparable from deep surface of plantar and collateral ligaments		Extension
	Collateral		Flexion, abduction, or adduction in flexion
Interphalangeal	Collateral		Flexion, abduction, or adduction in flexion
	Plantar		Extension

The talus receives its blood supply from the branches of the anterior and posterior tibial arteries and is very susceptible to aseptic necrosis, particularly with proximal fractures.[10]

Talocrural Ligaments

The most important ligaments of the talocrural joint can be divided into two main groups: lateral collaterals and medial (deltoid) collaterals.

Lateral Collaterals

The lateral collateral ligament complex consists of three separate bands, which function together as the static stabilizers of the lateral ankle. Each of the lateral ligaments has a role in stabilizing the ankle and/or subtalar joint, depending on the position of the foot. As such, these ligaments are commonly involved in ankle sprains.[11–15]

Anterior Talofibular Ligament. This thickening of the anterior capsule extends from the anterior surface of the fibular malleolus, just lateral to the articular cartilage of the lateral malleolus, to just anterior to the lateral facet of the talus and to the lateral surface of the talar neck (Fig. 21-2).

The anterior talofibular ligament (ATFL) is an intracapsular structure and is approximately 2–5-mm thick and 10–12-mm long.[16] The ATFL functions to resist ankle inversion in plantarflexion. Regardless of ankle position, the ATFL is usually the first ankle ligament to be torn in an inversion injury.[16] The accessory functions of the ATFL include providing resistance against anterior talar displacement from the mortise and resistance against internal rotation of the talus within the mortise.[17]

CLINICAL PEARL

The ATFL requires the lowest maximal load to produce failure of the lateral ligaments, although it has the highest strain of failure in that group.

Calcaneofibular Ligament. The calcaneofibular ligament (CFL) (see Fig. 21-2), an extra-articular structure covered by the fibular (peroneal) tendons, is larger and stronger than the ATFL. It fans out at 10–40 degrees from the tip of the fibular malleolus to the lateral side of the calcaneus, paralleling the horizontal axis of the subtalar joint. This ligament effectively spans the ankle and subtalar joints, which have markedly different axes of rotation.[18–21] Thus, its attachment is designed so that it does not restrict motion in either joint, whether they move independently or simultaneously.[20,22,23] As the ankle joint passes from dorsiflexion to plantarflexion, the CFL is less able to resist talar tilt to inversion, although the ATFL is more able to resist this tilt.[22]

Posterior Talofibular Ligament. The posterior talofibular ligament (PTFL) (see Fig. 21-2) is the strongest of the lateral ligament complex,[16] and serves to indirectly aid talofibular stability during dorsiflexion due to its anatomic location, where it can act as a true collateral ligament and prevent talar tilt into inversion.[22,24] The PTFL is rarely injured except in severe ankle sprains. The ligament is coalescent with the joint capsule, and its orientation is relatively horizontal. Its attachment on the talus involves nearly the entire nonarticular portion of the posterior talus to the groove for the flexor hallucis longus (FHL)

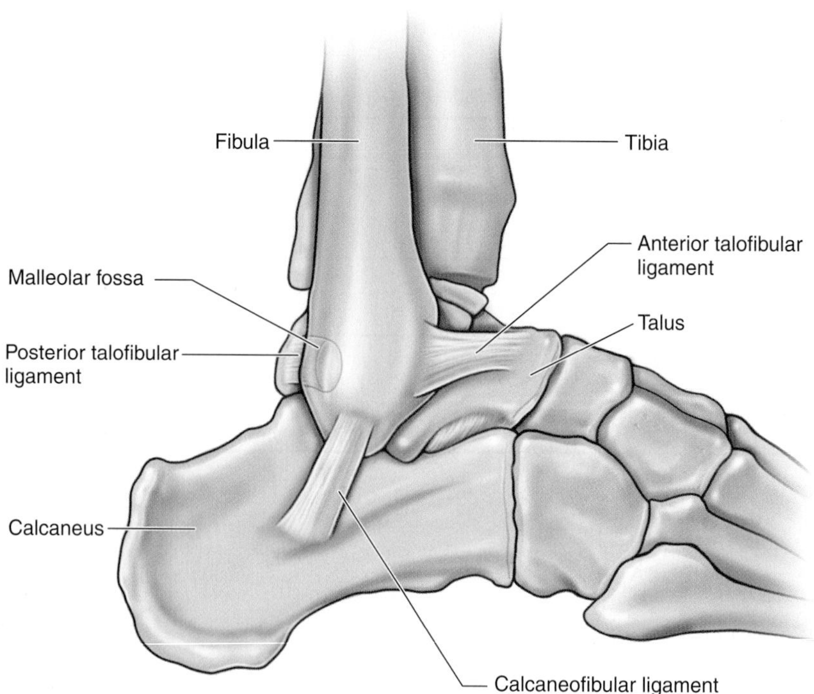

FIGURE 21-2 Lateral ligaments. (Reproduced with permission from Morton DA, Foreman KB, Albertine KH: *The Big Picture: Gross Anatomy*, McGraw-Hill, 2011.)

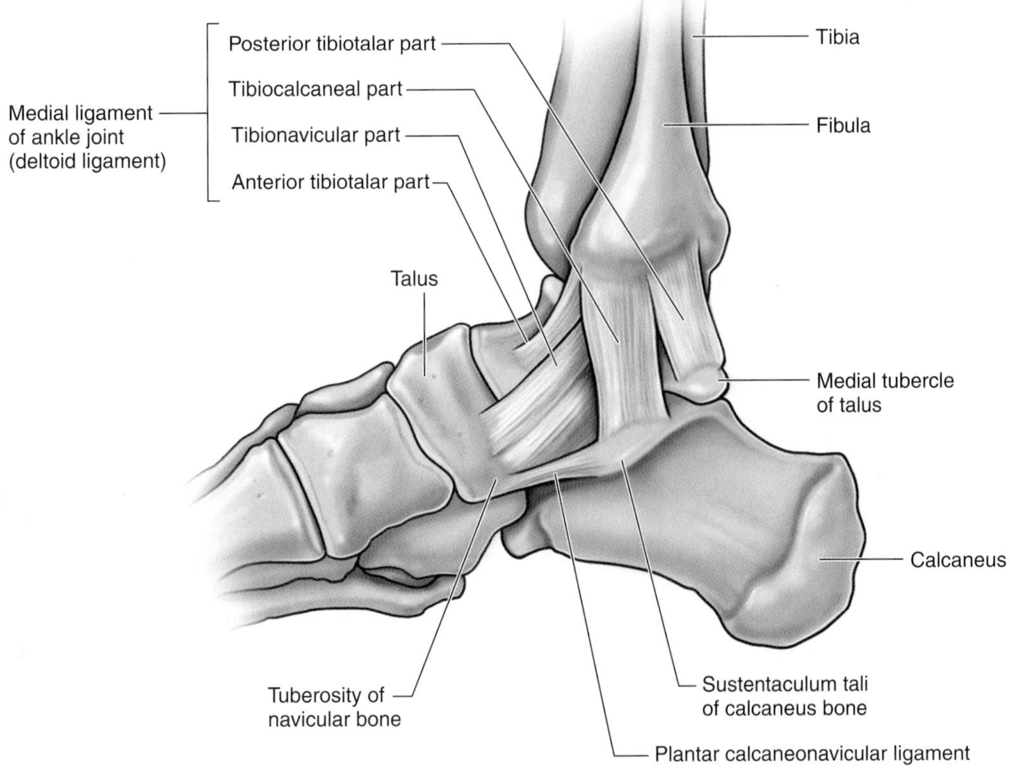

FIGURE 21-3 Medial ligaments. (Reproduced with permission from Morton DA, Foreman KB, Albertine KH: *The Big Picture: Gross Anatomy,* McGraw-Hill, 2011.)

tendon, and anteriorly to the digital fossa of the fibula, which transmits the vessels that supply the talus and the fibula.[25,26]

Lateral Talocalcaneal Interosseous. The lateral talocalcaneal interosseous (LTCIL) ligament is sometimes included in this group as it does play a role in lateral ankle and subtalar stability (see Talocalcaneal Ligaments).[16,27]

CLINICAL PEARL

In dorsiflexion, the PTFL is maximally stressed, and the CFL is taut, whereas the ATFL is loose. Conversely, in plantarflexion, the ATFL is taut, and the CFL and PTFL become loose.[26,28–30]

Besides maintaining lateral ankle stability, the lateral ankle ligaments play a significant role in maintaining rotational ankle stability.[22] Significant compromise to the ATFL and/or CFL leads to a measurable increase in inversion without any tilting of the talus or subtalar gapping.[22] A loss of ATFL function permits an increase in external rotation of the leg and unlocks the subtalar joint, allowing further inversion, which may lead to symptomatic instability.[22]

Medial Collaterals. Collectively, the medial collateral ligaments form a triangular-shaped ligamentous structure known as the deltoid ligament of the ankle (Fig. 21-3). Wide variations have been noted in the anatomic description of the deltoid ligament of the ankle but is generally agreed that it consists of both superficial and deep fibers. The superficial fibers consist of the following:

- ***Tibionavicular fibers (see Fig. 21-3).*** These fibers extend from the medial malleolus to the tuberosity of the navicular and serve to resist lateral translation and external rotation of the talus.
- ***Posterior talotibial fibers (see Fig. 21-3).*** These fibers travel in a posterolateral direction from the medial malleolus to the medial side of the talus and medial tuberosity of the talus. These fibers resist ankle dorsiflexion and lateral translation and external rotation of the talus.
- ***Calcaneotibial fibers (see Fig. 21-3).*** These thin fibers extend from the medial malleolus to the sustentaculum tali. The fibers are oriented in such a way that they resist abduction of the talus, calcaneus, and navicular, when the foot and ankle are positioned in plantar flexion and eversion.[19]

The deep fibers consist of the following:

- ***Anterior talotibial fibers (see Fig. 21-3).*** The fibers of this strong ligament extend from the tip of the medial malleolus to the anterior aspect of the medial surface of the talus. These fibers are oriented in such a way that they resist abduction of the talus, when it is in plantar flexion and eversion. Such is the strength of these fibers that an injury to this ligament is often associated with an avulsion fracture.

Although the calcaneotibial ligament is very thin and supports only negligible forces before failing, the talotibial ligaments are very strong.[31,32] Rasmussen et al.[33,34] found that the superficial fibers of the deltoid ligament of the ankle specifically limited talar abduction or negative talar tilt and that the deep layers of the deltoid ligament of the ankle ruptured with external rotation of the leg, without the superficial portion being involved.

CLINICAL PEARL

The strength of the ankle ligaments from weakest to strongest is the ATFL, PTFL, CFL, and deltoid complex.[35]

SUBTALAR (TALOCALCANEAL) JOINT

The subtalar joint consists of two separate, modified ovoid surfaces with their own joint cavities. The two anterior and posterior articulations are connected by an interosseous membrane.

- The anterior joint consists of a concave facet on the calcaneus and a convex facet on the talus. The anterior component is situated more medial than the posterior, giving the plane of the joint an average 42 degrees (±9 degrees) superior from the transverse foot plane and 23 degrees (±11 degrees) medial from the sagittal foot plane.[36]
- The posterior joint consists of a convex facet on the calcaneus and a concave facet on the talus.

This relationship ensures that the anterior and posterior aspects can move in opposite directions to each other during functional movements (while the anterior aspect is moving medially, the posterior aspect is moving laterally).

The calcaneus, the largest tarsal bone and the most frequently fractured, projects further posteriorly than the tibia and fibula. It serves as a weight-bearing bone and as a short lever for muscles of the calf, which are attached to its posterior surface. The skin and fat over the distal-inferior area of the calcaneus are specialized for friction and shock absorption.[37]

CLINICAL PEARL

The skin on the sole of the foot is thicker than anywhere else in the body. Located beneath the skin in the heel area is a fat pad, which is designed to handle compressive loads beyond what other fat pads in the body will tolerate. This fat pad comprises a honeycombed pattern of subcutaneous fat globules in fibroelastic septae 13–21 mm thick, which abuts the calcaneus.[38] The septae closest to the calcaneus are aligned concentrically, in a pattern that opposes a concentrically aligned reversed pattern closest to the skin. These opposing patterns create a torsion effect that resists compression, thereby providing a cushion for initial contact by the heel and allowing the skin to resist forces up to five times the body weight during running.[38] However, after the age of 40, the thickness of the subcutaneous fat decreases, with a resultant loss of shock absorbency.[3940] This can be counteracted by using a heel cup/counter, which confines the overall volume of the fat pad around the calcaneus.

The retrocalcaneal bursa lies anterior to the posterosuperior calcaneal tuberosity of the calcaneus. It lubricates the Achilles tendon anteriorly, as well as the superior aspect of the calcaneus.[39] The superior or proximal surface of the calcaneus is divisible into thirds.

- ***The posterior third.*** This is a roughened surface that is concavoconvex in extension, the convexity transverse. It supports fibroadipose tissue between the calcaneal tendon and the ankle joint. Distal to the posterior articular facet is a rough depression that narrows into a groove on the medial side—the sulcus calcanei—which completes the sinus tarsi with the talus.
- ***The middle third.*** This surface carries the posterior talar facet and is oval and convex anteroposteriorly.
- ***The anterior third.*** This surface is only partly articular.

Talocalcaneal Ligaments

A number of ligaments provide support to this joint, although some confusion exists in the descriptions and nomenclature of these ligaments. In relation to the sinus tarsi, the most medial ligament is the talocalcaneal interosseous ligament, which branches superiorly into medial and lateral bands.[22] The cervical ligament and portions of the retinaculum are located more laterally. The talocalcaneal interosseous and cervical ligaments are often collectively referred to as the interosseous ligaments.[41]

Medial (Posterior) Talocalcaneal Interosseous

The medial talocalcaneal interosseous ligament extends from the medial tubercle of the talus to the posterior aspect of the sustentaculum tali and the area of the calcaneus just posterior to the sustentaculum tali. It functions to stabilize against anterior translation of the talus (especially at the initial contact phase of the gait cycle) by producing passive eversion of the talus. This results in a close packing of the lateral foot and fibula. Damage to this ligament, which typically occurs with inversion sprains and rotational compression fractures of the calcaneus, can permit excessive anterior motion of the talus. This excessive motion may result in posterior tibialis tendinitis[42] and on occasion, Achilles' tendinitis.[43]

Lateral (Anterior) Talocalcaneal Interosseous

The lateral (anterior) talocalcaneal interosseous ligament (LTCIL) originates from the roof of the sinus tarsi and extends in a posteroinferior direction from the lateral process of the talus to the lateral surface of the calcaneus, just anterior to the CFL. This ligament functions to prevent the talus and the calcaneus from separating during inversion movements. This highly innervated structure is typically injured with a dorsiflexion and inversion mechanism.[44]

MIDTARSAL (TRANSVERSE TARSAL) JOINT COMPLEX

The midtarsal joint complex consists of the talonavicular and calcaneocuboid articulations.

Talonavicular

The talonavicular joint is classified as a synovial, compound, modified ovoid joint.

The joint is actually formed by components of the talus, navicular, calcaneus, and plantar calcaneonavicular (spring) ligament. The rounded convex anterior head of the talus fits into the concavity of the posterior navicular and the anterior component of the subtalar joint and rests on the posterior (dorsal) surface of the spring ligament. The joint capsule is only well developed posteriorly, where it forms the anterior part of the interosseus ligament.

Calcaneocuboid

The calcaneocuboid joint is classified as a simple, synovial, modified sellar joint.

The anterior surface of the calcaneus, which articulates with the reciprocally shaped posterior surface of the cuboid, is relatively convex in an oblique horizontal direction and relatively concave in an oblique vertical direction.[45] The cuboid, most lateral in the distal tarsal row, is located between the calcaneus proximally and the fourth and fifth metatarsals distally. To the posterior (dorsal) surface are attached posterior (dorsal) calcaneocuboid, cubonavicular, cuneocuboid, and cubometatarsal ligaments, and to the proximal edge of the plantar ridge, deep fibers of the long plantar ligament. To the projecting proximal–medial part of the plantar surface are attached a slip of the tendon of tibialis posterior and flexor hallucis brevis (FHB). To the rough part of the medial cuboidal surface are attached the interosseous, cuneocuboid, and cubonavicular ligaments, and proximally the medial calcaneocuboid ligament, which is the lateral limb of the bifurcated ligament.[46] The capsule is thickened posteriorly (dorsally) to form the posterior (dorsal) calcaneocuboid ligament. The joint has a large plantar phalanx to provide additional support during weight-bearing.

A number of ligaments help provide support to this region. The spring ligament (plantar calcaneonavicular Fig. 21-3) connects the navicular bone to the sustentaculum tali on the calcaneus. The ligaments of the calcaneocuboid joint include the long plantar ligament and a portion of the bifurcate ligament posterior (dorsally).

- The long and strong plantar ligament attaches to the plantar surface of the calcaneus, the tuberosity on the plantar surface of the cuboid bone, and to the bases of the second, third, and fourth (and possibly fifth) metatarsals.[46] The plantar ligament functions to provide indirect plantar support to the joint, by limiting the amount of flattening of the lateral longitudinal arch of the foot.[47] Together with the groove in the cuboid bone, it forms a tunnel for the passage of the fibularis (peroneus) longus tendon across the plantar surface of the foot.[46]
- The bifurcate ligament functions to support the medial and lateral aspects of the foot when weight-bearing in a plantar flexed position (twisted).

The plantar calcaneocuboid ligament, sometimes referred to as the short plantar ligament, is a relatively broad and strong strap-like structure that extends from the area of the anterior tubercle of the calcaneus to the adjacent plantar surface of the cuboid bone. It provides plantar support to the joint and possibly helps to limit flattening of the lateral longitudinal arch.

CUNEONAVICULAR

The cuneonavicular joint is classified as a compound, synovial, modified ovoid joint. The navicular presents a convex surface to the concave surface of the combined cuneiforms. The wedge-like cuneiform bones articulate with the navicular proximally and with the bases of the first to third metatarsals distally (see Fig. 21-1). The medial cuneiform is the largest and the intermediate, the smallest. In the intermediate and lateral cuneiforms, the posterior (dorsal) surface is the base of the wedge, but in the medial, the wedge is reversed, a prime factor in shaping the transverse arch. The wedge shape of these bones also provides a cavity for the neurovascular and musculotendinous structures of the foot.

The cuneiforms, together with articulations with the metatarsal bones, form Lisfranc's joint.[9] The proximal surface of all three cuneiforms form a concavity for the convex surface of the navicular. In the intermediate and lateral cuneiforms, the posterior (dorsal) surface is the base of the wedge, but in the medial, the wedge is reversed, which assists in the formation of the transverse arch. The medial cuneiform is the largest, the intermediate the smallest. The ligament of Lisfranc runs between the medial cuneiform and second metatarsal base. Disruption of this ligament can lead to a dislocation of the medial aspect of the foot, as the first metatarsal and medial cuneiform separate from the second metatarsal and intermediate cuneiform.

The joint cavity and capsule of the cuneonavicular joint is continuous with that of the intercuneiform and cuneocuboid joints, and the synovium is continuous with that of these joints, the second and third cuneometatarsal joints, and the intermetatarsal joints of each base except the fifth.

INTERCUNEIFORM AND CUNEOCUBOID JOINTS

These joints (see Fig. 21-1) are classified as compound, synovial, modified ovoid joints. The joint capsule and synovium is contiguous between all of these joints and with that of the cuneonavicular joint.

Dysfunctions in the cuneocuboid joint result from a collapse of the plantar supporting structures or from direct trauma. Such dysfunctions may result in the cuboid subluxing in a plantar direction (medial border of cuboid moves inferiorly). At the intercuneiform joints, the third cuneiform may sublux on the second cuneiform.

CUBOMETATARSAL

Laterally, the cuboid bone articulates with the fourth and fifth metatarsals distally, and with the calcaneus proximally. When considered alone, the cubometatarsal joint is classified as a compound, modified ovoid, synovial joint. When the cubometatarsal joints are considered together, they form a modified sellar joint. The joint capsule and synovium of the fourth and fifth cubometatarsal joints are separated from the other tarsometatarsal joints by an interosseous ligament.

CUBONAVICULAR

The cubonavicular joint (see Fig. 21-1) is classified as a syndesmosis or a plane surfaced joint. If the joint is synovial, the capsule and synovium is continuous with the cuneonavicular joint.

INTERMETATARSAL

The first intermetatarsal joint (see Fig. 21-1) is classified as a simple, synovial, modified ovoid joint, whereas the second, third, and fourth are classified as compound joints. If the joint is synovial, the capsule and synovium is continuous with the cuneonavicular joint. Motion at these joints is confined to posterior (dorsal)/anterior (plantar) gliding, producing a fanning and folding motion of the foot. Proximally, the five metatarsals articulate with the tarsals and with themselves through broad concavities.[9]

METATARSOPHALANGEAL

The MTP joints (see Fig. 21-1) are classified as simple, synovial, modified ovoid joints. The capsule and synovium in each of these joints is confined to its own joint and posteriorly (dorsally) is thin, whereas plantarly (anteriorly), it is blended with the plantar and collateral ligaments. Rotation occurring in the early stages of development of the limbs results in the thumb being the most lateral digit in the hand, whereas the hallux (great toe) is the most medial digit in the foot.[48]The concave bases of the proximal phalanges (see Fig. 21-1) articulate with the convex heads of the metatarsals. The first MTP joint, with its more extensive articular surface on the anterior (plantar) aspect of the metatarsal than on the posterior (dorsal), allows for a greater freedom of motion,[48] and its anterior (plantar) surface forms two grooves for articulation with the hallucal sesamoids (see next section). The fifth metatarsal has a lateral styloid process at its base, which serves as the insertion site for the tendon of the fibularis (peroneus) brevis. The styloid area is often avulsed during acute inversion injuries of the foot.[9] Three types of forefoot are recognized based on the length of the metatarsal bones, although it is unclear whether these various types affect foot function in any way[48]:

- ***Index plus.*** This type is characterized by the first metatarsal being longer than the second, with the other three of progressively decreasing lengths, so that $1 > 2 > 3 > 4 > 5$.
- ***Index plus–minus.*** In this type, the first metatarsal is of the same length as the second, with the others progressively diminishing in length, so that $1 = 2 > 3 > 4 > 5$.
- ***Index minus.*** With this type, the second metatarsal is longer than the first and third metatarsals. The fourth and fifth metatarsals are progressively shorter than the third, so that $1 < 2 > 3 > 4 > 5$.

Stability of the MTP joints is primarily provided by a musculocapsular ligamentous complex anteriorly (plantarly), and medially and laterally by the medial and lateral collateral ligaments, respectively.

First MTP Joint

The first MTP joint is the articulation between the head of the first metatarsal and the proximal phalanx. Although there is some anatomic variation from patient to patient, the first MTP joint is typically a cam-shaped, condylar-hinged joint.[49] The MCP joint has little inherent stability because the proximal phalanx has a fairly shallow cavity in which the metatarsal head articulates. The joint is stabilized posteriorly (dorsally) by the capsule and expansion of the extensor hallucis tendon. Fan-shaped medial and lateral collateral ligaments provide valgus and varus stability, respectively. The plantar surface of the capsule is reinforced by a fibrocartilaginous plate, called the plantar accessory ligament. In addition, the MTP joints are dynamically stabilized by the short flexor complex (FHB and the two sesamoids embedded in the FHB tendons), the adductor hallucis, and the abductor hallucis tendons.

> **CLINICAL PEARL**
>
> The sesamoids are contained within the tendon of the FHB and serve to increase the lever arm for flexion of the MTP joint, analogous to the function of the patella at the knee.[50]

The sesamoids are connected distally to the base of the proximal phalanx by extensions of the FHB called the plantar plate. Typically, the sesamoids are anterior (plantar) to the medial and lateral condyles of the metatarsal pad. The sesamoids are separated on the anterior (plantar) aspect of the first metatarsal head by a cresta, which helps to stabilize the sesamoids, and are connected to one another by the intersesamoidal ligament. The abductor hallucis inserts into the medial sesamoid, and the adductor hallucis inserts into the lateral sesamoid. The FHL (Fig. 21-4) pierces the two heads of the FHB muscle to run just anterior (plantar) to the intersesamoidal ligament. In normal gait, the capsuloligamentous complex of the first MTP joint must withstand 40–60% of body weight, but in athletic activity, this can reach as much as eight times body weight.[47,51–56]

INTERPHALANGEAL

The hallux has two phalanges, whereas each of the remaining toes have three (see Fig. 21-1). The IP joints are classified as simple, synovial, modified sellar joints. The saddle-shaped articular fossa of the head of the proximal phalanx articulates with the base of the intermediate phalanx. This in turn receives the smaller and flatter distal phalanx.

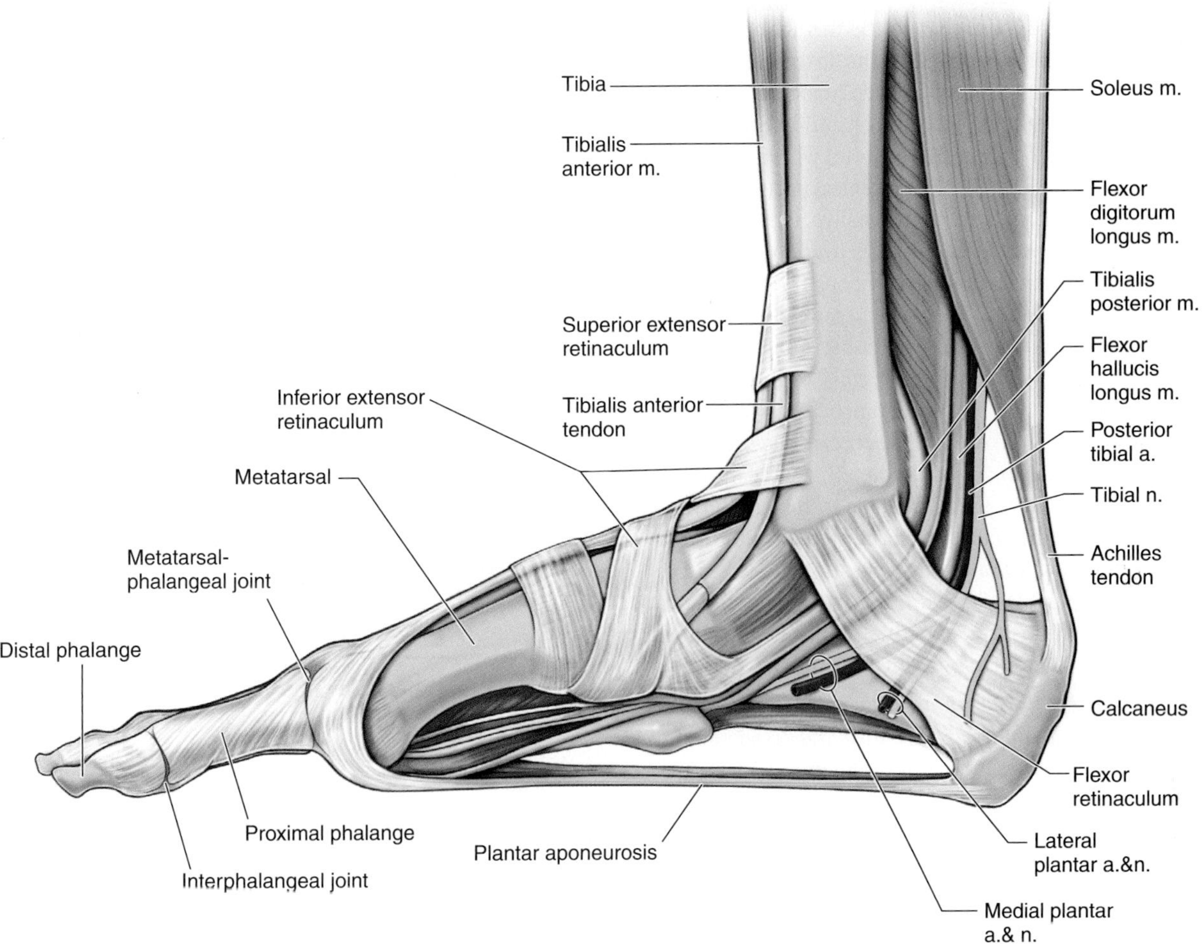

FIGURE 21-4 Medial aspect of the ankle and foot. (Reproduced with permission from Morton DA, Foreman KB, Albertine KH: *The Big Picture: Gross Anatomy*, McGraw-Hill, 2011.)

ACCESSORY OSSICLE

An accessory ossicle (accessory bone) is an anomalous bone that fails to unite during developmental ossification. Common locations include the fibular malleolus, tibiar malleolus, navicular, and talus.

The accessory navicular is the most common accessory bone in the foot.[57] It occurs on the medial, anterior (plantar) border of the navicular, at the site of the tibialis posterior tendon insertion.[58] The incidence in the general population has been reported to be 4–14%[58,59] The posterior aspect of the talus often exhibits a separate ossification center, appearing at 8–10 years of age in girls and 11–13 years of age in boys. Fusion usually occurs 1 year after its appearance.[60,61] When fusion does not occur, an *os trigonum* is formed (see "Pathologies" section).

CLINICAL PEARL

An accessory bone can be differentiated from a fracture radiographically, because an accessory bone will have rounded edges, where a fracture will have sharp edges.[62]

PLANTAR FASCIA/PLANTAR APONEUROSIS

The terms *plantar fascia* and *plantar aponeurosis* (Fig. 21-4) are often used interchangeably, although strictly speaking only the central part of the plantar fascia is extensively aponeurotic.[63] The plantar fascia is the investing fascial layer of the anterior (plantar) aspect of the foot that originates from the os calcis and inserts through a complex network to the anterior (plantar) forefoot. It is a tough, fibrous layer, composed histologically of both collagen and elastic fibers. The plantar fascia is often regarded as being analogous to the palmar fascia of the hand. However, unlike the fascial layer of the palm, which is generally thin, the plantar fascia is a thick structure, and not only serves a supportive and protective role, but is also intricately involved with the weight-bearing function of the foot.[63] The plantar fascia is divided into three major areas: a central portion and medial and lateral sections, each oriented longitudinally on the anterior (plantar) surface of the foot.[26]

- ***Central portion.*** The central portion is the major portion of the plantar fascia both anatomically and functionally.[63] This portion is the thickest and the strongest and is narrowest proximally where it attaches to the medial process of the calcaneal tuberosity, proximal to the flexor digitorum brevis (FDB). This attachment site is often involved in a condition called plantar heel pain (see "Intervention Strategies" section); however, pain can occur anywhere along the structure. From its insertion, the central portion of the fascia fans out and becomes thinner distally. Its fibers are longitudinally oriented and adhere to the underlying FDB muscle.[63] The central portion envelops the FDB muscle on both sides, forming the medial and lateral intermuscular septums, which anchor the plantar fascia to the deep plantar pedis.[63] At the midshaft of the second to fifth MTP joints, the body of the central portion branches into five superficial longitudinal tracts.[63] All five superficial longitudinal tracts terminate by inserting into, and blending with, the overlying subcutaneous tissues and skin. Due to the anatomical connections of the central portion, dorsiflexion of the toe slides the plantar pads distally, placing tension on the plantar aponeurosis. The central portion of the fascia primarily functions as a dynamic stabilizer of the medial longitudinal arch during weight-bearing activities.

- ***Lateral and medial portions.*** The smaller and thinner lateral and medial portions are thin and cover the under surface of the abductor digiti minimi and abductor hallucis muscles, respectively.

With standing and weight-bearing, the plantar fascia plays a major role in the support of the weight of the body, by virtue of its attachments across the longitudinal arch. During the different phases of gait, the plantar fascia assumes different biomechanical functions. For example, during the toe-off portion of the gait cycle, the windlass effect on the plantar fascia helps to reconstitute the arch and generates a more rigid foot for propulsion.[*62] During heel strike, and during the first half of the stance phase of the gait cycle with the toes in neutral, the plantar fascia relaxes, flattening the arch. This allows the foot to accommodate to irregularities in the walking surface and to absorb shock.[62] As the foot proceeds from midstance to terminal stance, the toes dorsiflex and, through its attachments to the toes via the plantar plate, the plantar fascia tightens. The plantar fascia is pulled over the metatarsal heads, causing the metatarsal heads to be depressed and the longitudinal arch to rise.[63] During the swing phase of gait, the plantar fascia is under little tension and appears to serve no important functional role.

RETINACULA

There are four important ankle retinacula, which function to tether the leg tendons as they cross the ankle to enter the foot (Fig. 21-4).[64]

- ***Extensor retinaculum.*** The extensor retinaculum consists of two parts: superior and inferior. The superior part functions to contain the tendons of the extensor digitorum longus, extensor hallucis longus, tibialis anterior, and fibularis (peroneus) tertius. The Y-shaped inferior part consists of an upper and a lower band, which prevent "bow-stringing" of the posterior (dorsal) tendons.
- ***Superiofibular (peroneal) retinacula.*** This firmly tethers the fibularis (peroneus) longus and brevis tendons behind the fibular malleolus.
- ***Flexor retinaculum.*** The flexor retinaculum provides a firm support structure for the flexor digitorum longus, FHL, tibialis posterior, and the neurovascular bundle.

EXTRINSIC MUSCLES OF THE LEG AND FOOT

The extrinsic muscles of the foot (Table 21-4) can be divided into anterior, posterior superficial, posterior deep, and lateral compartments.

Anterior Compartment

This compartment contains the dorsiflexors (extensors) of the foot. These include the tibialis anterior, extensor digitorum longus, and extensor hallucis longus (see Fig. 21-5).

Posterior Superficial Compartment

This compartment, located posterior to the interosseous membrane, contains the calf muscles that plantar flex the foot. These include the gastrocnemius, soleus (see Fig. 21-5), and the plantaris muscle (Fig. 21-6).

Triceps Surae

The triceps surae comprises the two heads of the gastrocnemius, which arise from the posterior aspects of the distal femur, and the soleus, which arises from the tibia and fibula, which combine to form the Achilles tendon.[65] The medial head of the gastrocnemius is by far the largest component and, according to electromyographic (EMG) studies, is the most active of the two during running.[66,67] The soleus (Fig. 21-5), because it does not cross the knee joint, is subject to early disuse atrophy with undertraining and/or immobilization.[66] The Achilles tendon is formed from the conjoint tendons of the gastrocnemius and soleus muscles. The fibers from the gastrocnemius and soleus interweave and twist as they descend, producing an area of high stress 2–6 cm above the distal tendon insertion.[68] A region of relative avascularity exists in the same area,[69] which correlates well with the site of some Achilles tendon injuries, including complete spontaneous rupture.[66,70,71] The plantaris muscle has its own tendon and contributes no fibers to the Achilles tendon.[72]

Achilles Tendon. The Achilles tendon is the thickest, strongest tendon in the body.[65] As the Achilles tendon comes off the posterior calf muscles, it courses distally to attach approximately three-quarters of an inch below the superior portion of the os calcis, on the medial aspect of the calcaneus. Two bursae occur at the point of insertion of the Achilles tendon into the calcaneus. The retrocalcaneal bursa lies deep into the tendon, adjacent to the calcaneus. The superficial bursa of the tendo

*The orientation of the aponeurosis promotes inversion of the calcaneus and supination of the subtalar joint when it is under tension, which raises the longitudinal arch and provides a rigid lever for propulsion.

TABLE 21-4 Extrinsic Muscle Attachments and Innervation

Muscle	Proximal	Distal	Innervation
Gastrocnemius	Medial and lateral condyle of femur	Posterior surface of calcaneus through Achilles tendon	Tibial S2 (S1)
Plantaris	Lateral supracondylar line of femur	Posterior surface of calcaneus through Achilles tendon	Tibial S2 (S1)
Soleus	Head of fibula, proximal third of shaft, soleal line and midshaft of posterior tibia	Posterior surface of calcaneus through Achilles tendon	Tibial S2 (S1)
Tibialis anterior	Distal to lateral tibial condyle, proximal half of lateral tibial shaft, and interosseous membrane	First cuneiform bone, medial and plantar surfaces, and base of first metatarsal	Deep fibular (peroneal) L4 (L5)
Tibialis posterior	Posterior surface of tibia, proximal two-thirds posterior of fibula, and interosseous membrane	Tuberosity of navicular bone and tendinous expansion to other tarsals and metatarsals	Tibial L4 and L5
Fibularis (peroneus) longus	Lateral condyle of tibia, head, and proximal two-thirds of fibula	Base of first metatarsal and first cuneiform, lateral side	Superficial fibular (peroneal) L5 and S1 (S2)
Fibularis (peroneus) brevis	Distal two-thirds of lateral fibular shaft	Tuberosity of fifth metatarsal	Superficial fibular (peroneal) L5 and S1 (S2)
Fibularis (peroneus) tertius	Lateral slip from extensor digitorum longus	Tuberosity of fifth metatarsal	Deep fibular (peroneal) L5 and S1
Flexor hallucis longus	Posterior distal two-thirds fibula	Base of distal phalanx of great toe	Tibial S2 (S3)
Flexor digitorum longus	Middle three-fifths of posterior tibia	Base of distal phalanx of lateral four toes	Tibial S2 (S3)
Extensor hallucis longus	Middle half of anterior shaft of fibula	Base of distal phalanx of great toe	Deep fibular (peroneal) L5 and S1
Extensor digitorum longus	Lateral condyle of tibia proximal anterior surface of shaft of fibula	One tendon to each lateral four toes, to middle phalanx, and extending to distal phalanges	Deep fibular (peroneal) L5 and S1

achillis lies superficial to the distal portion of the tendon, between the tendon itself and the subcutaneous tissues, but is not visible unless it is pathologically inflamed. Deeper to the Achilles tendon is the pre-Achilles fat pad, a triangular area of adipose tissue, also known as Kager's triangle. Further anterior to this fat pad are the deep flexor tendons of the calf, predominantly the FHL, which overlies the posterior tibia and the talus.

There is no synovial sheath surrounding the Achilles tendon. The peritendon covers the endotendon and is composed of a thin sheath, called the epitenon, and another fine outer sheath, the peritenon, composed of fatty areola tissue, which fills the interstices of the fascial compartment in which the tendon is situated.[73] The peritenon is able to stretch 2–3 cm with tendon movement, which allows the Achilles tendon to glide smoothly.[74]

Posterior Deep Compartment

This compartment contains the flexors of the foot. These muscles course behind the medial malleolus. They include the posterior tibialis, flexor digitorum longus, and FHL (see Fig. 21-7).

The primary function of the tibialis posterior muscle is to invert and plantar flex the foot. It also provides support to the medial longitudinal arch.[75] The flexor digitorum longus functions to flex the phalanges of the lateral four toes and assists with plantar flexion of the foot.

The FHL flexes the great toe and also assists with plantar flexion of the foot.

Lateral Compartment

This compartment contains the fibularis (peroneus) longus and brevis (see Fig. 21-5). The fibular (peroneal) tendons lie behind the lateral malleolus in a fibro-osseous tunnel formed by a groove in the fibula and the superficial fibular (peroneal) retinaculum. The fibular (peroneal) retinaculum and the posterior CFL form the posterior wall of this tunnel.

CLINICAL PEARL

The fibularis (peroneal) muscles serve as both plantar flexors and evertors of the foot.[76,77] The fibularis (peroneus) longus also abducts the forefoot in the transverse plane, thereby serving as a support for the medial longitudinal arch.[78]

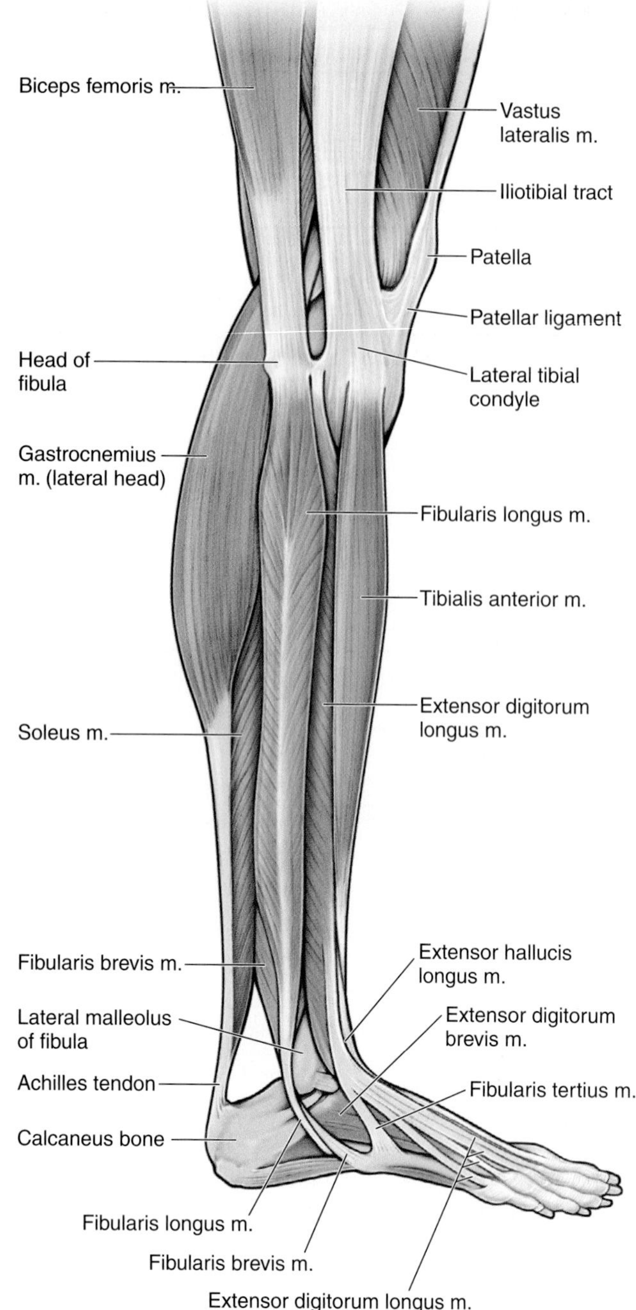

FIGURE 21-5 Lateral aspect of foot and ankle. (Reproduced with permission from Morton DA, Foreman KB, Albertine KH: *The Big Picture: Gross Anatomy,* McGraw-Hill, 2011.)

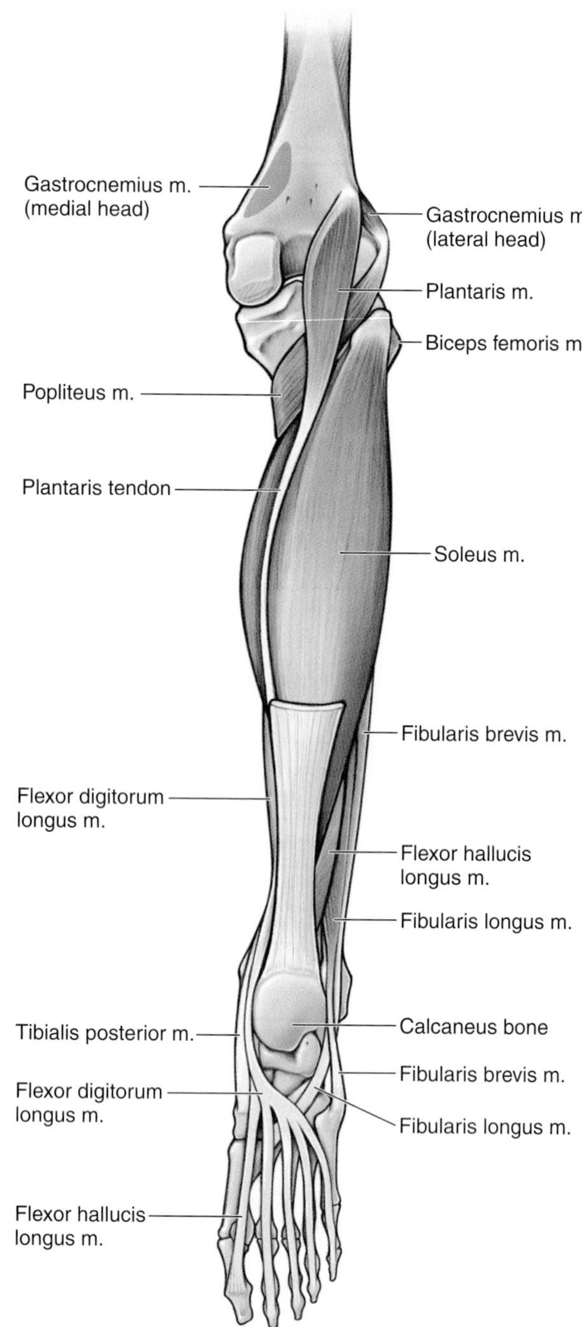

FIGURE 21-6 Posterior superficial muscles. (Reproduced with permission from Morton DA, Foreman KB, Albertine KH: *The Big Picture: Gross Anatomy,* McGraw-Hill, 2011.)

INTRINSIC MUSCLES OF THE FOOT

Beneath the plantar aponeurosis–plantar fascia are the four muscular layers of the intrinsic muscles of the anterior (plantar) foot (Table 21-5), as well as the plantar ligaments of the rear- and midfoot. The intrinsic muscles provide support to the foot during propulsion.[79]

First Layer

The first layer is the most anterior (plantar) and consists of the following:

- ***Abductor hallucis*** (Fig. 21-8). This muscle arises from the medial process of the calcaneal tuberosity and inserts into the medial side of the base of the proximal phalanx of the great toe.
- ***Abductor digiti minimi (see Fig. 21-8).*** This muscle arises from the lateral process of the calcaneal tuberosity as well as the plantar aponeurosis and inserts into the lateral side of the base of the proximal phalanx of the little toe.
- ***Flexor digitorum brevis (see Fig. 21-8).*** This muscle arises from the medial process of the calcaneal tuberosity, lateral to the abductor hallucis and deep into the central portion of the

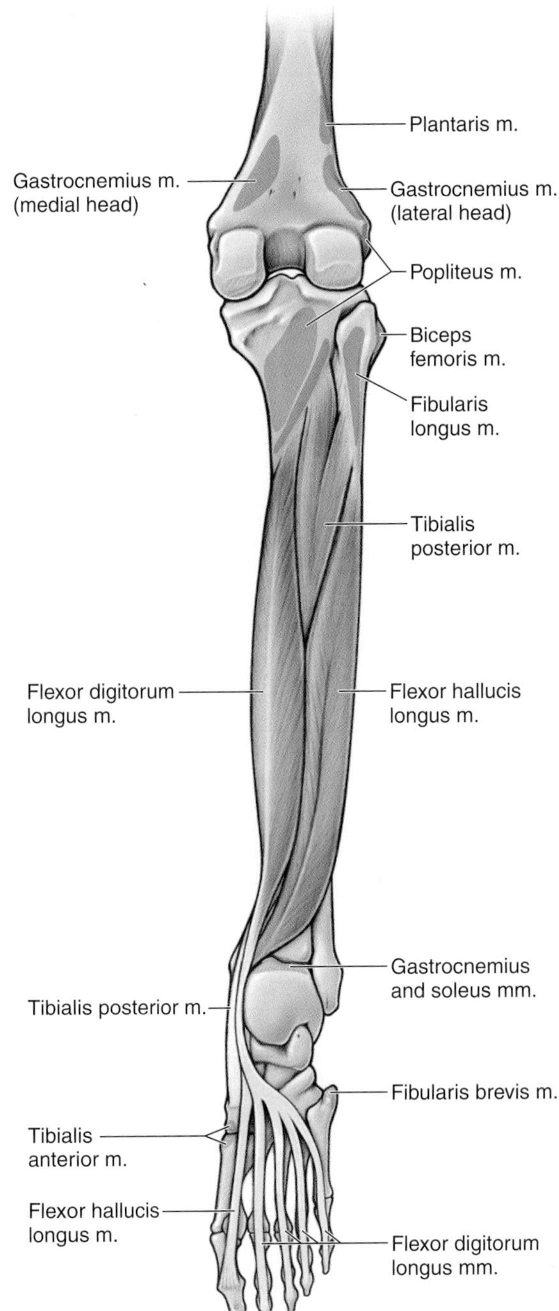

FIGURE 21-7 Posterior Deep Muscle Compartment. (Reproduced with permission from Morton DA, Foreman KB, Albertine KH: *The Big Picture: Gross Anatomy*, McGraw-Hill, 2011.)

plantar fascia, and inserts into the middle phalanx of the lateral four toes.

Second Layer

- ***Flexor digitorum accessorius (quadratus plantae; Fig. 21-8).*** This muscle arises from the calcaneal tuberosity via two heads. The medial head arises from the medial surface of the calcaneus and the medial border of the long plantar ligament, whereas the lateral head arises from the lateral border of the anterior (plantar) surface of the calcaneus and the lateral border of the long plantar ligament. The muscle terminates in tendinous slips, joining the long flexor tendons to the second, third, fourth, and occasionally fifth toes.
- ***Lumbricales.*** There are four lumbricales (see Fig. 21-8), all of which arise from the tendon of the flexor digitorum longus. The first arises from the medial side of the tendon of the second toe, the second from adjacent sides of the tendons for the second and third toes, the third from adjacent sides of the tendons for the third and fourth toes, and the fourth from adjacent sides of tendons for the fourth and fifth toes. They insert with the tendons of the extensor digitorum longus and interossei into the bases of the terminal phalanges of the four lateral toes. The function of the lumbricales is to flex the MTP joint and extend the proximal IP (PIP) joint.

Third Layer

- ***Flexor hallucis brevis (Fig. 21-8).*** This muscle arises from the medial part of the anterior (plantar) surface of the cuboid bone, the adjacent portion of the lateral cuneiform, and the posterior tibialis tendon and inserts on the medial and lateral side of the proximal phalanx of the great toe.
- ***Flexor digiti minimi (see Fig. 21-8).*** This muscle arises from the sheath of the fibularis (peroneus) longus, the base of the fifth metatarsal bone, and inserts into the lateral side of the base of the proximal phalanx of the little toe.
- ***Adductor hallucis (see Fig. 21-8).*** This muscle arises via two heads: an oblique and a transverse head. The oblique head arises from the bases of the second, third, and fourth metatarsal bones and the sheath of the fibularis (peroneus) longus. The transverse head arises from the joint capsules of the second, third, fourth, and fifth MTP heads and the deep transverse metatarsal ligament. The adductor hallucis inserts on the lateral side of the base of the proximal phalanx of the great toe.

Fourth Layer

- ***Posterior (dorsal) interossei.*** The four posterior (dorsal) interossei are bipennate, and they arise from adjacent sides of the metatarsal bones. The first inserts into the medial side of the proximal phalanx of the second toe. The second inserts into the lateral side of the proximal phalanx of the second toe. The third inserts into the lateral side of the proximal phalanx of the third toe, and the fourth inserts into the lateral side of the proximal phalanx of the fourth toe. The posterior (dorsal) interossei function to abduct the second, third, and fourth toes from an axis through the second metatarsal ray.
- ***Anterior (plantar) interossei (Fig. 21-8).*** The three anterior (plantar) interossei are unipennate and arise from the bases and medial sides of the third, fourth, and fifth metatarsal bones. They insert into the medial sides of the bases of the proximal phalanges of the third, fourth, and fifth toes. The anterior (plantar) interossei function to adduct the lateral three toes.

TABLE 21-5 Intrinsic Muscles of the Foot

Muscle	Proximal	Distal	Innervation
Extensor digitorum brevis	Distal superior surface of calcaneus	Posterior (dorsal) surface of second through fourth toes and base of proximal phalanx	Deep fibular (peroneal) S1 and S2
Flexor hallucis brevis	Plantar surface of cuboid and third cuneiform bones	Base of proximal phalanx of great toe	Medial plantar S3 (S2)
Flexor digitorum brevis	Tuberosity of calcaneus	One tendon slip into base of middle phalanx of each of the lateral four toes	Medial and lateral plantar S3 (S2)
Extensor hallucis brevis	Distal superior and lateral surfaces of calcaneus	Posterior (dorsal) surface of proximal phalanx	Deep fibular (peroneal) S1 and S2
Abductor hallucis	Tuberosity of calcaneus and plantar aponeurosis	Base of proximal phalanx and medial side	Medial plantar L5 and
Adductor hallucis	Base of second, third, and fourth metatarsals and deep plantar ligaments	Proximal phalanx of first digit lateral side	Medial and lateral plantar S1 and S2
Lumbricals	Medial and adjacent sides of flexor digitorum longus tendon to each lateral digit	Medial side of proximal phalanx and extensor hood	Medial and lateral plantar L5, S1, and S2 (L4)
Plantar interossei			
First	Base and medial side of third metatarsal	Base of proximal phalanx and extensor hood of third digit	
Second	Base and medial side of fourth metatarsal	Base of proximal phalanx and extensor hood of fourth digit	Medial and lateral plantar S1 and S2
Third	Base and medial side of fifth metatarsal	Base of proximal phalanx and extensor hood of fifth digit	
Posterior (dorsal) interossei			
First	First and second metatarsal bones	Proximal phalanx and extensor hood of second digit medially	
Second	Second and third metatarsal bones	Proximal phalanx and extensor hood of second digit laterally	Medial and lateral plantar S1 and S2
Third	Third and fourth metatarsal bones	Proximal phalanx and extensor hood of third digit laterally	
Fourth	Fourth and fifth metatarsal bones	Proximal phalanx and extensor hood of fourth digit laterally	
Abductor digiti minimi	Lateral side of fifth metatarsal bone	Proximal phalanx of fifth digit	Lateral plantar S1 and S2

POSTERIOR (DORSAL) INTRINSIC MUSCLES

The posterior (dorsal) intrinsic muscles of the foot are the extensor hallucis brevis (EHB) and extensor digitorum brevis (EDB). The EHB inserts into the base of the proximal phalanx of the great toe, whereas the EDB inserts into the base of the second, third, and fourth proximal phalanges. Both of these muscles are innervated by the lateral terminal branch of the deep fibular (peroneal) nerve.

ARCHES OF THE FOOT

The arches of the foot support the foot by three mechanisms[80]

- The osseous relationship of the tarsal and metatarsal bones.
- Ligamentous support from the plantar aponeurosis and anterior (plantar) ligaments.
- Muscle support.[81] There are three main arches: the medial longitudinal, the lateral longitudinal, and the transverse arches.

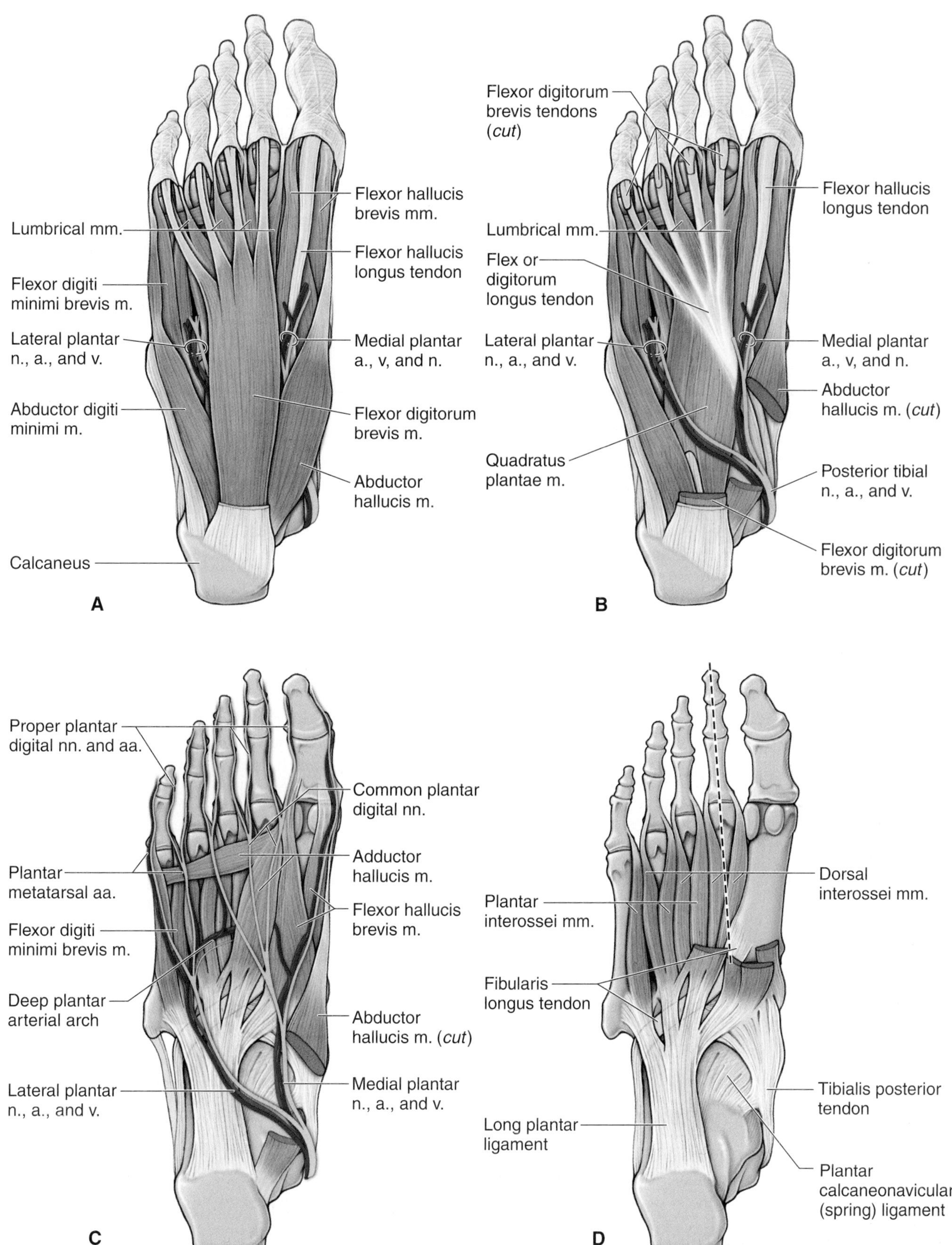

FIGURE 21-8 Intrinsic Muscles of the Foot. (Reproduced with permission from Morton DA, Foreman KB, Albertine KH: *The Big Picture: Gross Anatomy*, McGraw-Hill, 2011.)

- The *medial longitudinal arch* plays an important role in foot function during weight-bearing activities. The arch comprises the calcaneus, talus, navicular, three cuneiforms, and the three medial metatarsals (including the two sesamoids). Although some of the integrity of the arch depends on the bony architecture, support is also provided by the ligaments and muscles, including the anterior (plantar) calcaneonavicular (spring) ligament, the plantar fascia, the tibialis posterior, fibularis (peroneus) longus, flexor digitorum longus, FHL, and fibularis (peroneus) longus.[78,82,83] The soleus and gastrocnemius muscle group has also been noted to have an effect on the arch and can flatten it with adaptive shortening.[78] Not only is the arch a major source of frontal plane motion of the foot, but it also is a major load-bearing structure.[84] Analysis of the medial longitudinal arch has long been used by clinicians to make determinations about foot abnormalities, with a high arch indicating a supinated foot and a low or collapsed arch being associated with a pronated or flatfoot, respectively.[85] Studies have found a higher incidence of stress fractures, plantar heel pain, metatarsalgia, and lower extremity injuries, including knee strains and iliotibial band syndrome, in individuals with high arches, compared with those who have low arches.[86–88] This difference has always been attributed to the decreased shock-absorbing ability of the higher-arched foot,[89] although one study reported that arch height does not affect shock absorption.[90]
- The *lateral longitudinal arch*, which is more stable and less mobile than the medial longitudinal arch, consists of the calcaneus, cuboid, and fourth and fifth metatarsals. The superior and deep longitudinal plantar ligament supports the calcaneocuboid and cubometatarsal joints, together with the fibularis (peroneus) brevis, longus, and tertius, and the abductor digiti minimi and FDB muscles.[91]
- The *transverse arch* forms the convexity of the posterior aspect of the foot and consists of metatarsal heads one through five, including the sesamoids (arch I); cuneiforms one through three and the cuboid (arch II); and the navicular and cuboid (arch III). The adductor hallucis, fibularis (peroneus) longus, posterior tibialis, and anterior tibialis all add dynamic support to this arch.

NAIL PLATE

The nail plate is composed of keratinized squamous cells, bordered by proximal and lateral nail folds.[92] The hyponychium lies between the distal portion of the nail bed and the distal nail fold and marks the transition to normal toe epidermis.[92] Fingernail plates grow on average at a rate of 3 mm per month, and toenail plates grow at one-half to one-third that rate.[92]

NEUROLOGY

The saphenous nerve, the largest cutaneous branch of the femoral nerve, provides cutaneous distribution to the medial aspect of the foot. Branches of the sciatic nerve provide the sensory and motor innervation for the foot and leg (see Chap. 3). The branches are the common fibular (peroneal) and tibial nerves. The common fibular (peroneal) nerve, in turn, divides into the superficial fibular (peroneal) and deep fibular (peroneal) nerves (Fig. 21-9). The tibial nerve divides into the sural, medial calcaneal, medial anterior (plantar), and lateral anterior (plantar) nerves.[92]

VASCULAR SUPPLY

Two branches of the popliteal artery, the anterior tibial artery and the posterior tibial artery, form the main blood supply to the foot (Fig. 21-9).

Anterior Tibial Artery

The anterior tibial artery supplies the anterior compartment of the leg and enters the posterior aspect of the foot under the superior and inferior retinacula as the posterior (dorsal) pedis artery. The posterior (dorsal) pedis artery gives rise to the arcuate artery and the first posterior (dorsal) and anterior (plantar) metatarsal artery, which serve the posterior aspect of the foot and the digits.

Posterior Tibial Artery

The posterior tibial artery, which supplies the posterior and lateral compartments and 75% of the blood to the foot, enters the foot after traveling around the medial malleoli. At this point, the artery divides into the medial and lateral anterior (plantar) arteries, which serve the anterior (plantar) aspect of the foot. A main branch of the posterior tibial artery, the fibular (peroneal) artery, supplies the lateral compartment as well as many hindfoot structures.

BIOMECHANICS

Terminology

Motions of the leg, foot, and ankle consist of single- and multiplane movements. The single-plane motions include the following:

- ***The frontal plane motions of inversion and eversion.*** Eversion is a frontal plane motion of the foot about an anteroposterior axis, in which the medial aspect of the sole of the foot moves in an anterior (plantar) direction (Fig. 21-10). Inversion is a frontal plane motion of the foot about an anteroposterior axis, in which the lateral aspect of the sole of the foot moves in an anterior (plantar) direction (Fig. 21-10).
- ***The sagittal plane motions of dorsiflexion and plantar flexion.*** These movements at the ankle and at the midtarsal jointoccur in the sagittal plane about a M-L axis.[93] Plantar flexion is a movement of the foot downward toward the ground, and dorsiflexion is a movement of the foot upward toward the tibia.

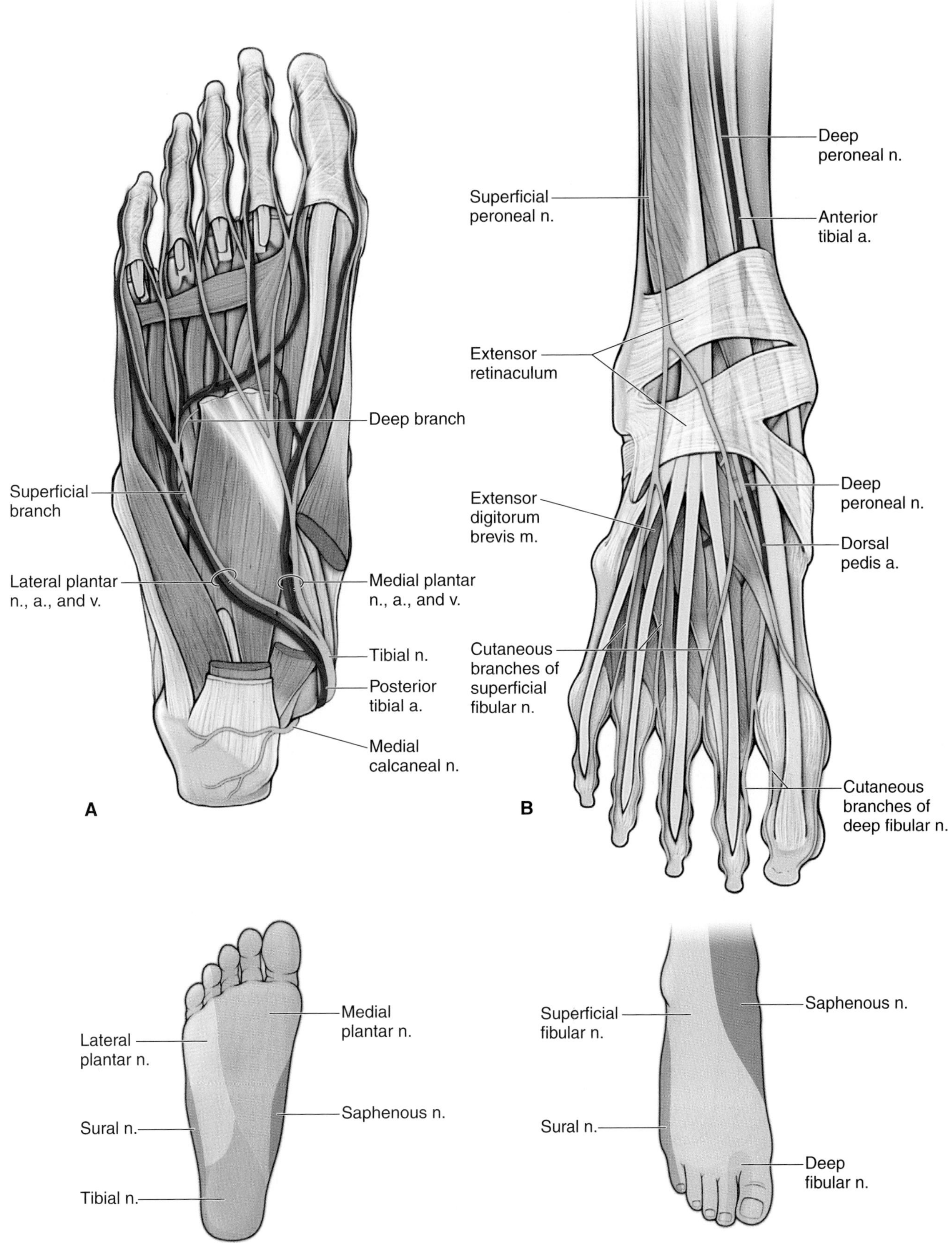

FIGURE 21-9 Neurovascular supply of the ankle and foot. (Reproduced with permission from Morton DA, Foreman KB, Albertine KH: *The Big Picture: Gross Anatomy*, McGraw-Hill, 2011.)

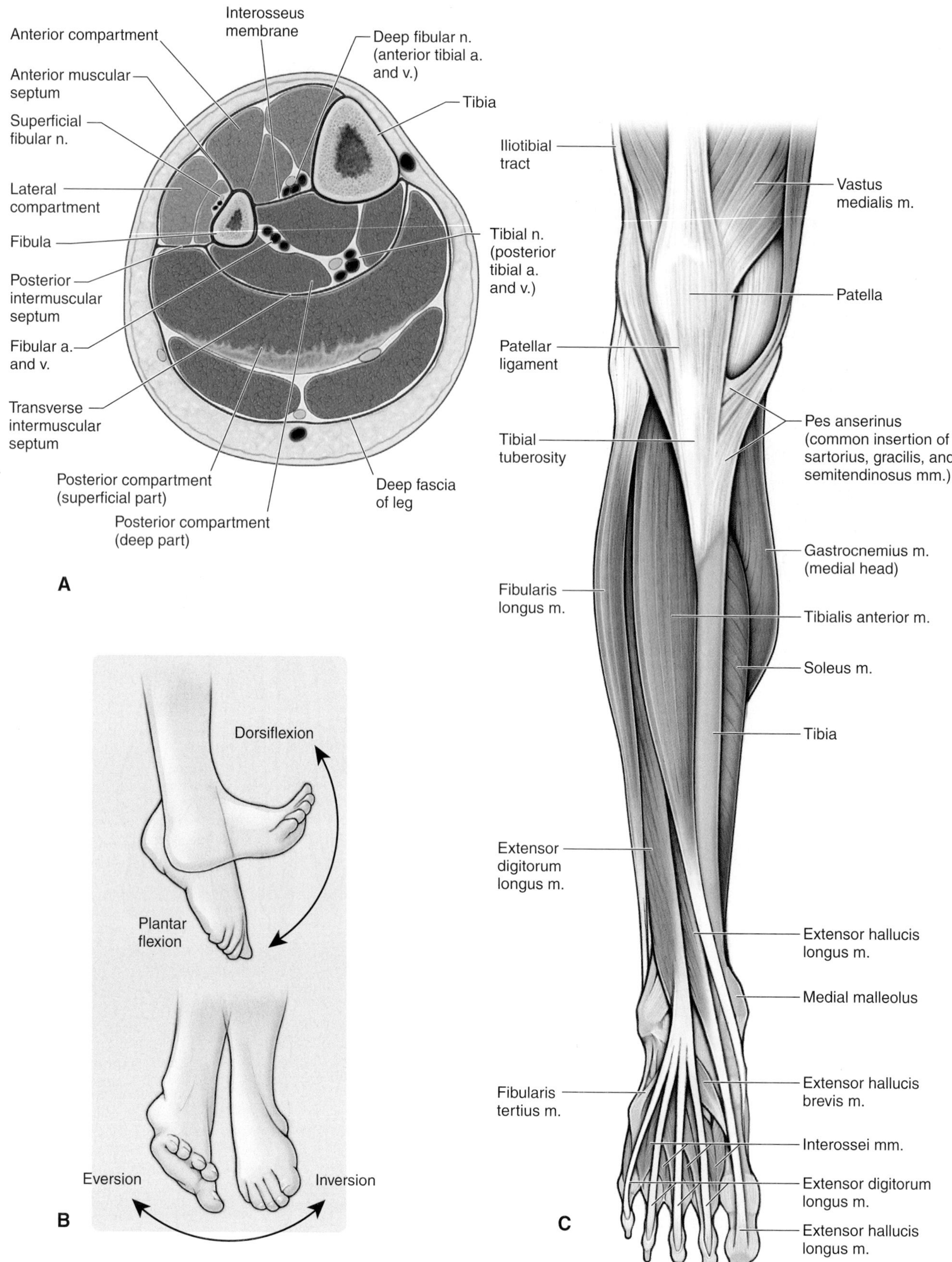

FIGURE 21-10 Ankle motions and related musculature. (Reproduced with permission from Morton DA, Foreman KB, Albertine KH: *The Big Picture: Gross Anatomy,* McGraw-Hill, 2011.)

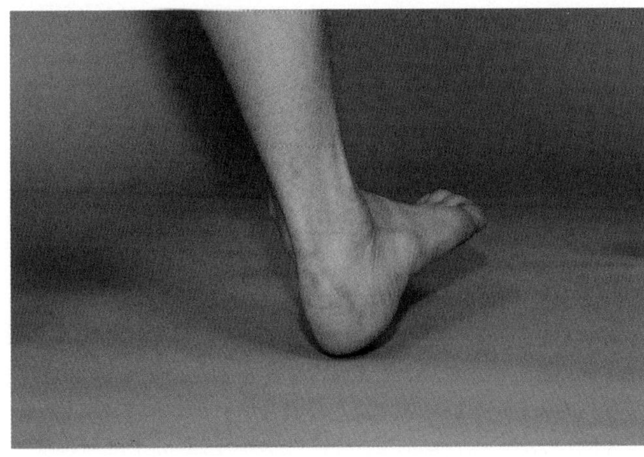

FIGURE 21-11 Pronation in non–weight-bearing.

- ***The horizontal plane motions of adduction and abduction.*** These motions of the forefoot occur in the horizontal plane about a superoinferior axis.[93] Abduction moves the forefoot laterally, whereas adduction moves the forefoot medially.

A triplane motion describes a movement about an obliquely oriented axis through all three body planes. Triplanar motions occur at the talocrural, subtalar, and midtarsal joints and at the first and fifth rays.[94] Pronation and supination are examples of triplanar motions. The three body plane motions in pronation are abduction in the transverse plane, dorsiflexion in the sagittal plane, and eversion in the frontal plane (Fig. 21-11).[94] The three body plane motions in supination are adduction, plantar flexion, and inversion (Fig. 21-12).[94] In pronation, the forefoot is rotated in such a manner so that the big toe moves downward and little toe moves upward, whereas in supination, the reverse occurs.

Distal Tibiofibular Joint

Although the two tibiofibular joints (proximal and distal) are described as individual articulations, they function as a pair. The movements that occur at these joints are primarily a result of the ankle's influence.

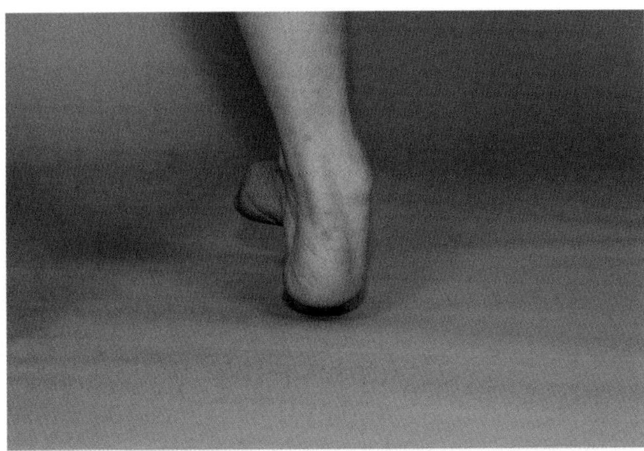

FIGURE 21-12 Supination in non–weight-bearing.

- Supination of the foot produces a distal and posterior glide of the head of the fibula.
- Pronation produces a proximal and anterior glide with an external rotation of the fibula.
- Plantar flexion of the foot produces a distal glide with a slight medial rotation of the fibula.
- Dorsiflexion of the ankle yields a proximal glide. The fibula rotates externally around its longitudinal axis.

During these movements, however, it is the tibia that performs the greatest amount of movement, as it rotates around the fibula. This is probably a consequence of more body weight falling through the larger bone. During ipsilateral rotation, both the tibia and the fibula rotate laterally, but in relative terms, the tibia moves more laterally than the fibula, causing a relative anterior and superior glide of the fibular head on the tibia at the superior joint. During contralateral rotation, the tibia rotates more medially, producing a relative posterior and inferior fibular glide at the joint.

The ligaments of the distal tibiofibular joint are more commonly injured than the ATFL.[95] Injuries to the ankle syndesmosis most often occur as a result of forced external rotation of the foot or during internal rotation of the tibia on a planted foot.[17] Hyperdorsiflexion may also be a contributing mechanism.[96]

The capsular pattern of this joint is probably pain with weight-bearing dorsiflexion of the ankle, as this produces the greatest ligamentous tension (Table 21-1). For the same reason, the close-packed position is considered as weight-bearing dorsiflexion of the ankle.

CLINICAL PEARL

Because of the interaction between the proximal and distal tibiofibular joints with the knee and the ankle function, the clinician should always assess the functional mobility of both these complexes when treating one or the other.

Talocrural Joint

The talocrural joint is classified as a synovial hinge or modified sellar joint. There is general agreement that motion between the tibia and the foot is a complex combination of talocrural and subtalar joint motion, which is limited by the shape of the articulations and soft tissue interaction.[22] Stability for this joint in weight-bearing is provided by the articular surfaces, while in non–weight-bearing, the ligaments appear to provide the majority of stability.[24]

The primary motions at this joint are dorsiflexion and plantar flexion (Fig. 21-10), with a total range of 70–80 degrees. The maximum amount of dorsiflexion necessary at the talocrural joint during human gait is approximately 10 degrees of the normally available 20 degrees,[94,97,98] and occurs during the stance phase, just prior to heel rise.[99] The orientation of the talocrural joint axis, which is oriented on average 20–30 degrees posterior to the frontal plane as it passes posteriorly from the medial malleolus to the lateral malleolus,[23,83,100] can be estimated clinically as a line that passes inferiorly from the medial malleolus to the lateral malleolus (with a mean orientation of 10 degrees to the horizontal plane), with the adult distal leg being oriented vertically.[83,100,101] Although the majority of talocrural motion occurs in the sagittal plane, an significant amount of horizontal motion occurs in the horizontal plane, especially during internal rotation of the tibia or pronation of the foot.[83,100]

Because of the fit of the saddle-shaped talus within the mortise, the talus is able to produce a slight separation of the tibial and fibula malleoli during the extremes of dorsiflexion and plantar flexion.[102] In addition, because of this fit, the tibia follows the talus during weight-bearing so that the talocrural joint externally rotates with supination and internally rotates with pronation.[103] Conversely, the tibia internally rotates during pronation and externally rotates during supination.[104]

Theoretically, the capsular pattern of the ankle joint is more restriction of plantar flexion than dorsiflexion, although clinically this appears to be reversed (Table 21-1). The close-packed position is weight-bearing dorsiflexion, whereas the open-packed position is midway between supination and pronation.

Subtalar Joint

The subtalar (talocalcaneal) joint functions to provide inversion and eversion of the hindfoot—approximately 50% of apparent ankle inversion observed actually comes from the subtalar joint.[105] The axis of motion for the subtalar joint, which is approximately 45 degrees from horizontal and 20 degrees medial to the midsagittal plane,[21,36,83] moves during subtalar joint motion,[106–108] which allows the subtalar joint to produce a triplanar motions of pronation/supination. This motion has been compared with a ship on the sea or an oblique mitered hinge.[109] The various components of the triplanar motion at this joint vary according to whether the joint is weight-bearing or non–weight-bearing.[110]

- During weight-bearing (close chain) activities, pronation involves a combination of calcaneal eversion, adduction, and plantar flexion of the talus and internal rotation of the tibia, whereas supination involves a combination of calcaneal inversion, abduction and dorsiflexion of the talus and external rotation of the tibia.[111]
- During non–weight-bearing (open chain) activities, pronation involves a combination of calcaneal eversion and abduction and dorsiflexion of the talus (see Fig. 21-11), whereas supination involves a combination of calcaneal inversion and adduction and plantar flexion of the talus (see Fig. 21-12).[111]

The subtalar joint controls supination and pronation in close conjunction with the transverse tarsal joints of the midfoot. Subtalar joint supination and pronation are measured clinically by the amount of calcaneal or hindfoot inversion and eversion. In normal individuals, there is an inversion to eversion ratio of 2:3 to 1:3, which amounts to an average of approximately 20 degrees of inversion and 10 degrees of eversion.[20,83,94,109] For normal gait, a minimum of 4–6 degrees of eversion and 8–12 degrees of inversion are required.[108]

During normal gait, the foot needs to pronate and supinate 6–8 degrees from the neutral position.[112] If the foot pronates excessively, a compensatory internal rotation of the tibia may occur. This produces an increased amount of rotatory stress and dynamic abduction moment at the knee, which has to be absorbed through the peripatellar soft tissues at the knee joint.[113–116] These stresses can force the patella to displace laterally and may result in patellofemoral dysfunction.[3,117] In addition, a change in the position of the talus can affect the functional leg length. Subtalar supination may cause the leg to lengthen, while subtalar pronation shortens the leg. Thus, the mid-position of the subtalar joint, subtalar joint neutral, is considered the range at which the subtalar joint should act to prevent dysfunction. The subtalar joint neutral position is actually a measurement of the angle between a line that bisects the distal third of the lower leg and a line that bisects the calcaneus.[118] The bisection of the calcaneus represents the position of the anterior (plantar) condyles, because the calcaneus is almost perpendicular to the condyles. The angle between the bisections should be 0 degree in the normal foot but is actually 2–3 degrees of varus (inverted in most subjects).[119]

CLINICAL PEARL

Mathematically, the subtalar joint neutral position is that angle at which the ratio of calcaneal inversion to eversion is approximately 2:1.[94]

Stability for the subtalar joint is provided by the CFL, the cervical ligament, the interosseous ligament, the lateral talocalcaneal ligament, the fibulotalocalcaneal ligament (ligament of Rouviere), and the extensor retinaculum.[120]

The capsular pattern of this joint varies. In chronic arthritic conditions, there is an increasing limitation of inversion, but with traumatic arthritis, eversion appears most limited clinically. The close-packed position for this joint is full inversion, whereas the open-packed position is inversion/plantar flexion (Table 21-1).

Midtarsal (Transverse Tarsal) Joint Complex

The function of the midtarsal joint complex is to provide the foot with an additional mechanism for raising and lowering the arch and to absorb some of the horizontal plane tibial motion that is transmitted to the foot during stance.[103,121] Motions around the two axes at the midtarsal joint involve[80]

- a rotational motion about a longitudinal axis into inversion and eversion, which can be observed in the elevation and depression of the medial arch of the foot during the stance phase of gait,[20,21]
- an oblique axis, producing the near sagittal motions of forefoot dorsiflexion and abduction, and forefoot plantar flexion and adduction.[20]

Both axes are dependent on the position of the subtalar joint.[20,108,121] When the subtalar joint is pronated, the two sets of axes are parallel to one another, allowing for the maximum amount of motion at the midtarsal joint. When the subtalar joint is supinated, the two sets of axes are in opposition, allowing little motion to occur, thereby enhancing stability.

During gait, the midtarsal joint has following two functions[80]:

- To permit adaptation of the foot to uneven terrain in the early stance
- To provide a stable foot during terminal stance

Theoretically, as a modified ovoid, the joint complex can sublux into dorsiflexion/plantar flexion, abduction/adduction, with or without rotation. In practice, the most commonly found subluxations may be considered as inversion/dorsiflexion or eversion/plantar flexion lesions.[46] The capsular pattern of the midtarsal joint complex is a limitation of dorsiflexion, plantar flexion, adduction, and internal rotation (Table 21-1). The close-packed position for the midtarsal joint is supination (Table 21-1). The open-packed position is midway between the extremes of ROM.

Cuneonavicular Joint

The cuneonavicular joint has one to two degrees of freedom: plantar/dorsiflexion, inversion/eversion. The capsular pattern of this joint is a limitation of dorsiflexion, plantar flexion, adduction, and internal rotation. The close-packed position is supination. The open-packed position is considered to be midway between the extremes of ROM (Table 21-1).

Intercuneiform and Cuneocuboid Joints

Due to their very plane curvature, these joints have only one degree of freedom: inversion/eversion. The close-packed position for these joints is supination. The open-packed position is considered to be midway between extremes of ROM (Table 21-1).

Cubometatarsal Joint

The capsular pattern of this joint is a limitation of dorsiflexion, plantar flexion, adduction, and internal rotation. The close-packed position is pronation. The open-packed position is considered to be midway between extremes of ROM (Table 21-1).

Cubonavicular Joint

The close-packed position for this joint is supination. The open-packed position is midway between extremes of ROM (Table 21-1).

Intermetatarsal Joints

The close-packed position for these joints is supination. The open-packed position is midway between extremes of ROM (Table 21-1).

MTP Joints

The MTP joints have two degrees of freedom: flexion/extension and abduction/adduction. ROM of these joints is variable, ranging from 40 to 100 degrees dorsiflexion (with a mean of 84 degrees), 3–43 degrees (mean, 23 degrees) plantar flexion, and 5–20 degrees varus and valgus.[122] The closed-packed position for the MTP joints is full extension. The capsular pattern for these joints is variable, with more limitation of extension than flexion. The open-packed position is 10 degrees of extension.

First MTP Joint

The function of the great toe is to provide for normal propulsion during gait and to provide stability to the medial aspect of the foot. Normal alignment of the first MTP joint varies between 5 degrees varus and 15 degrees valgus.[123] The most important motion at the first MTP is dorsiflexion. During normal gait, the first MTP joint dorsiflexes approximately 60 degrees. During sprinting (running sports), squatting (football and baseball), and relevé (in dance), greater than 90 degrees of dorsiflexion is necessary.

The first MTP is characterized by having a remarkable discrepancy between active and passive motion.The first ray of the foot consists of the first metatarsal and the first (medial) cuneiform bone. These two bones act as a functional unit, playing an important role in providing structural integrity to the foot during weight-bearing activities.[83] Three extrinsic muscles of the foot insert at the base of the first ray: the anterior tibialis, posterior tibialis, and fibularis (peroneus) longus. The need for clinical assessment of the posterior (dorsal) mobility of the first ray is based on its functional role during weight-bearing activities. Any disruption to its normal motion (hypo- or hypermobility) reduces the ability of the first ray to adequately stabilize the medial column of the foot and the longitudinal arch, increasing the potential for injury to the head of the first metacarpal.[124]

IP Joints

Each of the IP joints has one degree of freedom: flexion/extension. The capsular pattern is more limitation of flexion than of extension. The close-packed position is full extension (Table 21-1). The open-packed position is slight flexion.

EXAMINATION

The examination is used to identify static and dynamic, and structural or mechanical foot abnormalities. The clinical diagnosis is based on an assessment of the changes in joint mobility and tissue changes at the foot and ankle and the effect these have on the function of the foot and ankle and the remainder of the lower kinetic chain.

The exact form of the examination is very much dependent on the acuteness of the condition. For example, weight-bearing tests cannot be done if the patient cannot bear weight, and most stress tests will prove impossible if the joints cannot be taken to their full range. In these cases, the clinician must rely heavily on the history.

CLINICAL PEARL

With an acute lesion, the purpose of the examination is to try to determine if a serious injury might have occurred, and whether there is a need to refer the patient back for further medical examination or treatment. Due to the acute pain and inflammatory state of the tissues in the acute stage, the physical examination may need to be modified and sometimes curtailed.

HISTORY

The primary purposes of the history are to do the following:

- Determine the patient's chief complaint.
- Determine the mechanism of injury, if any. Information about the mechanism of injury should include when, where, how, and if an injury occurred. Details about the mechanism of injury allow the clinician to infer the pathologic status and structures involved, although it must be remembered that the patient's recollection of the mechanism involved frequently does not necessarily correspond to the structures damaged.[16,125] Most ankle sprains occur when the foot is plantar flexed, inverted, and adducted (Table 21-6). This same mechanism can also lead to a malleolar or talar dome fracture. A history involving sudden changes in training patterns may indicate an overuse injury. A dorsiflexion injury with associated snapping and pain on the lateral aspect of the ankle that rapidly diminishes may indicate a tear of the fibular (peroneal) retinaculum.[126] If there is no traumatic event, the clinician must determine if there has been a change in exercise or activity intensity (e.g., increased mileage with runners), training surface, or changes in body weight or shoe wear (causal agents).[16,125] In addition, the clinician must determine whether the symptoms vary with activity, type of terrain, or changes in position. Complaints of cramping may accompany muscular fatigue or intermittent claudication from arterial insufficiency. Plantar heel pain associated with plantar fasciitis is typically associated with an insidious onset. Achilles tendinitis is an overuse injury associated with an insidious onset of posterior calcaneal pain. Increased symptoms when walking or running on uneven terrain as compared with an even terrain may suggest ankle instability. Increased symptoms when walking or running on hard surfaces as compared with a softer surface may suggest a lack of shock absorbency of the foot or shoe. Pain that is related to a certain time of day may indicate an activity-related problem or a condition such as plantar heel pain if the pain is felt when first bearing weight in the morning.
- Determine the patient's occupation, if any. The impact of the injury on the patient's personal life, work, and athletic demands will largely direct the early intervention.[16,125]
  - If painless ambulation is essential, then rigid immobilization (i.e., a cast) may be appropriate.
  - If rapid return to sports competition is of paramount importance, functional immobilization is preferred.

TABLE 21-6 Examination Sequence in the Presence of a History of Inversion Trauma of the Foot and Ankle

History of Inversion Trauma
Possible pathology/structure involved
Ligamentous
Lesion of the anterior talofibular/calcaneofibular ligament
Lesion of the bifurcate ligament
Lesion of the cuboid-fifth metatarsal ligament
Lesion of the anterior tibiotalar and tibionavicular ligaments
Lesion of the tibiofibular interosseous ligament
Articular
Traumatic arthritis of the talocrural joint (TCJ)
Traumatic arthritis of the subtalar joint (STJ)
Traumatic arthritis of the transverse tarsal joints (TTJ)
Posterior tibiotalar compression syndrome
Sinus tarsi syndrome
Tibio fibular syndesmosis instability
Muscular
Tenosynovitis of the fibularis muscles
Tendinitis of the fibularis muscles
Rupture of the superior extensor retinaculum
Achillodynia
Tenosynovitis or tendinitis of the EHL
Tenosynovitis or tendinitis of the EDL
Neurologic
Overstretching of common fibular nerve/superficial fibular/deep fibular nerve
Osseous
Avulsion fracture of the base of the fifth metatarsal
Fracture of the shaft of the fifth metatarsal
Avulsion fracture at the lateral calcaneus
Avulsion fracture at the cuboid
Fracture of the anterior calcaneal process
Osteochondral fracture of the talus
Fracture of the lateral tubercle of the talus
Navicular fracture
Talar neck fracture
Talar head fracture

Data from Winkel D, Matthijs O, Phelps V: Appendix F. In: Winkel D, Matthijs O, Phelps V, eds. *Diagnosis and Treatment of the Lower Extremities.* 1997, Gaithersburg, MD: Aspen, 1997:645–646.

- Determine the location and severity of the condition. Most often, the patient can point to the location of the pain. The site and severity of the pain can be measured using a body diagram and visual analog scale, respectively. The distribution of pain is important, and the clinician should determine whether the pattern is referred, associated with a structure, related to a dermatome or peripheral nerve, or systemic in nature.[127] A stress fracture or tendinitis typically has a localized site of pain, whereas diffuse pain is associated with compartment syndromes.

- Determine which activities and positions aggravate the symptoms. Information should be gleaned about whether activities aggravate the symptoms and if so, which. For example, pain with forced dorsiflexion and eversion and with squatting activities may suggest ankle instability. Pain after activity suggests an overuse or chronic injury. Pain during an activity suggests stress on the injured structure.
- Ascertain the area, nature, and behavior of the symptoms.[128] Information about the time of injury, the time of the onset of swelling, and its location are important. The patient may report hearing a "snap," "crack," or "pop" at the time of injury, which could indicate a ligamentous injury or a fracture. The patient may report that their ankle felt weak and/or unstable at the time of the initial trauma or sometime thereafter. An inability to bear weight or the presence of severe pain and rapid swelling indicates a serious injury such as a capsular tear, fracture, or grade III ligament sprain.[129–132]
- Help determine the specific structure at fault.[133]
- Detect systemic conditions (e.g., collagen disease, neuropathy, radiculopathy, and vascular problems) or the presence of serious pathology.

In addition, questions regarding previous ankle injury, goals of the patient regarding functional goals, level and intensity of sports involvement, and past medical history are important to help the clinician individualize the intervention to the patient.

SYSTEMS REVIEW

As symptoms can be referred distally to the leg, foot, and ankle from a host of other joints and conditions, the clinician must be able to differentially diagnose from the presenting signs and symptoms (see Chap. 5). The cause of the referred symptoms may be neurologic or systemic in origin. If a disorder involving a specific nerve root (L4, L5, S1, or S2) is suspected, the necessary sensory, motor, and reflex testing should be performed. Peripheral nerve injuries may also occur in this region and often go unrecognized. These include Morton's neuroma and entrapment of the tibial nerve or its branches, the deep fibular (peroneal) nerve, superficial fibular (peroneal) nerve, and sural and saphenous nerves.[134]

Systemic problems that may involve the leg, foot, and ankle include diabetes mellitus (peripheral neuropathy), osteomyelitis, gout and pseudogout, sickle cell disease, complex regional pain syndrome, peripheral vascular disease, and rheumatoid arthritis (refer to Chap. 5). A systemic problem such as rheumatoid arthritis may be associated with other signs and symptoms, including other joint pain, although the other joint pain may also be the result of overcompensation in the rest of the kinetic chain.

Warning signs at the ankle and foot that should alert the clinician to a more insidious condition include:

- immediate and continuous inability to bear weight, which may indicate a fracture;
- nocturnal pain, which may indicate a malignancy, hemarthrosis, fracture, or infection;
- gross pain during ankle valgus and tenderness with pressure on the distal fibula, which may indicate a fractured fibula;
- pain and weakness during resisted eversion, which may indicate fracture of the fifth metatarsal bases;
- calf pain and/or tenderness, swelling with pitting edema, increased skin temperature, superficial venous dilatation, or cyanosis, which may indicate the presence of a deep vein thrombosis (DVT), requiring immediate medical attention (see Chap. 5);
- feelings of warmth or coldness in the foot. An abnormally warm foot can indicate local inflammation but can also originate from a tumor in the pelvic or lumbar region.[135] An abnormally cold foot usually indicates a vascular problem.[135]

TESTS AND MEASURES

Observation

Observation of the lower extremity is extensive. It is extremely important to observe the entire kinetic chain when assessing the leg, foot, and ankle. Weight-bearing and non–weight-bearing postures of the foot are compared.

Observing the patient while they move from sitting to standing and walk to the treatment area gives the clinician a sense of the patient's functional ability in weight-bearing and provides the first opportunity for gait analysis.[101] An important part of the examination of the foot and ankle is the gait assessment (see Chap. 6). During gait, the transverse and longitudinal arches can be grossly assessed—the lateral longitudinal arch bears the body weight in the early stance, whereas the medial longitudinal arch provides support in the mid- and late-stance phase of gait.[136] The foot should touch the ground, the heel first and the heel should begin to rise at approximately 35% of the gait cycle.[136] Early heel rise may occur due to tightness of the gastrocnemius–soleus complex, whereas late heel rise may be secondary to weakness of the calf musculature.[136] Normally, the foot pronates during the early stance phase, but the foot should not remain pronated during heel rise and toe off.[136]

CLINICAL PEARL

Patients with an ankle injury usually avoid the normal heel-to-toe progression to decrease weight-bearing and painful ankle dorsiflexion.[137] Instead, the patient is likely to adopt a toe-to-heel progression, with varying amounts of hip circumduction and external rotation of the lower leg, or steppage gait, to further unload the ankle.[138]

The following are assessed with the patient standing:

- ***Shoulder and pelvic heights (see Chaps. 16 and 29).***
- ***Spinal curvature (see Chap. 27).***
- ***Pelvic rotation (see Chap. 29).***

- ***The degree of hip rotation.*** In the femur, anteversion and retroversion angles should be noted (refer to Chap. 19). Excessive internal rotation of the hip toward the opposite hip (anteversion) may result in a flattening of the medial longitudinal arch and toeing-in/internal torsion of the tibia (pigeon toes). Excessive external rotation of the hip away from the opposite hip (retroversion) may result in an elevation of the medial longitudinal arch.
- ***The degree of knee flexion or hyperextension.*** A genu recurvatum (hyperextension) places the talocrural joint in more plantar flexion than normal and can often be a compensatory mechanism in the longer limb of individuals who have a leg-length inequality; see Chap. 29.[139] An increase in knee flexion accomplishes the same compensation for a leg-length inequality.[139]
- ***The degree of varus and valgus of the knee and tibia.*** Excessive tibia varum, genu varus, or forefoot varus can increase the frontal angle of the talocrural joint, which promotes excessive weight-bearing on the lateral aspect of the foot unless compensatory pronation is available within the foot to bring the medial aspect of the foot to the support surface.[139] Tibia varum refers to the frontal plane position of the distal one-third of the leg, as it relates to the supporting surface.[107]
- ***Rotational components of the tibia.*** Tibial torsion is assessed with the patient in sitting, with their feet hanging over the end of the bed so that their knees are in approximately 90 degrees of flexion.[101] The thumb of one hand is placed over the apex of one malleolus, and the index finger of the same hand is placed over the apex of the other malleolus. A qualitative estimate of the direction and magnitude of tibial torsion can be made by envisioning a line that passes through the malleoli and estimating its orientation to the frontal plane of the proximal tibia.[139] Alternatively, tibial torsion can be measured with the patient in prone with the knee flexed to 90 degrees and the subtalar joint positioned and stabilized in subtalar neutral.*

CLINICAL PEARL

The neutral subtalar position is calculated based on a normal 2:1 ratio of inversion to eversion. To locate subtalar neutral, the patient is positioned in prone with the opposite hip flexed, abducted, and externally rotated. If evaluating the right ankle, the clinician uses the thumb and forefinger of the left hand to palpate the hollows over the neck of the talus on either side of the anterior portion of the ankle. Using the thumb and forefinger of the other hand, the clinician grasps the head of the fourth and fifth metatarsals and rocks the foot back and forth. As the foot is inverted, a bulge can be felt on the lateral aspect of the foot. With eversion, the bulge can be felt to bulge medially. The point at which the talar head is felt to bulge equally on the medial and lateral sides is the subtalar neutral position.

Once the subtalar neutral position has been established, a line is drawn on the sole of the foot parallel to the length of the femur. A second line is drawn in line with the foot. The angle between these lines is the tibial torsion angle.[64] There is normally an angle of 12–18 degrees to the frontal plane.[140] Tibial torsion is generally less in children. A position of relative internal rotation of the tibia produces an increase in rigidity to the subtalar joint prior to midstance, due to premature stabilization of the longitudinal arch of the foot.[141] Excessive external rotation of the tibia places an increased strain along the longitudinal arch, as well as the first MTP joint.[141]

- ***Rearfoot to leg orientation.*** This can be an indicator of weight-bearing subtalar position. It is assessed by measuring the acute angle formed between a line representing the posterior aspect of the distal third of the leg, and a line approximately 1-cm distal to the first mark, representing the midline of the posterior aspect of the calcaneus (see Fig. 21-13).[139] The angle is assessed as the patient shifts weight on the lower extremity to simulate single-limb support. If the lines are parallel or in slight varus (2–8 degrees), the leg–rearfoot orientation is considered normal.[142] Movement of the rearfoot into eversion (rearfoot valgus) during this maneuver is indicative of subtalar pronation.[94] Pronation of the foot is manifested by eversion of the heel, abduction of the forefoot, a decrease in the medial longitudinal arch, internal rotation of the leg in relation to the foot, and dorsiflexion of the subtalar and midtarsal joints. If the heel is in too much valgus, the forefoot is excessively abducted, or there is excessive external rotation of the tibia, more toes can be seen on the affected side than the normal side when viewing the leg from behind ("too-many-toes sign").[42] If the patient is asked to raise up on the toes, the calcaneus should be observed to move into a position of inversion. An inability of the calcaneus to invert with this maneuver could

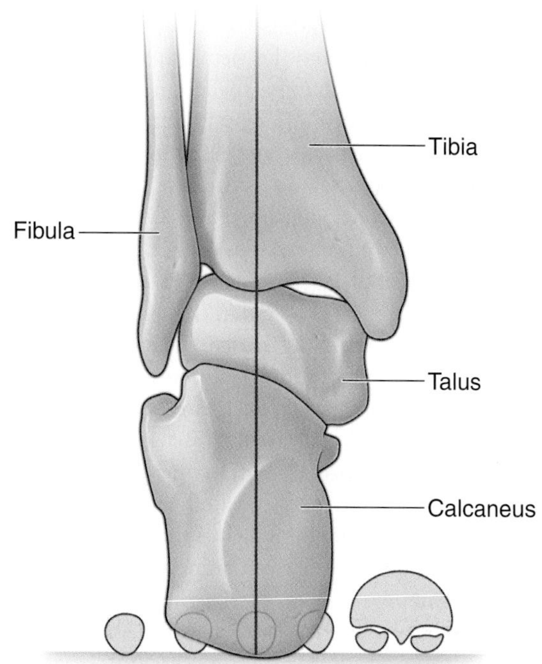

FIGURE 21-13 Rearfoot to leg orientation.

*The subtalar neutral position refers to the position in which all bones of the subtalar joints and the talocrural joints line up optimally in their open-packed positions—a position of neither pronation nor supination.

indicate the presence of an abnormality within the subtalar joint mechanism or a weakness of the posterior tibialis.[42,141]

- ***The weight-bearing foot.*** The following are major components of the normal weight-bearing foot:[119,143]
  - Both planar condyles of the calcaneus are on the floor surface. An imaginary plane representing the ground surface is applied to the anterior (plantar) surface of the calcaneus. The metatarsal heads should rest upon this plane. If the plane of the metatarsal heads is perpendicular to the bisection of the calcaneus, the forefoot-to-rearfoot relationship is normal, or neutral.
  - The "normal" foot should demonstrate 6–8 degrees of calcaneal eversion during gait. The foot should pronate initially, just after initial contact (see Chap. 6).
  - All of the metatarsal heads lie in one plane, which is in the same plane as the anterior (plantar) condyles of the calcaneus[94]
  - The ball of the foot is level with the plantar surface of the heel.
  - A normal forefoot-to-rearfoot relationship (see later).
  - The orientation of the distal third of the lower leg should be vertical, to position the foot properly for the stance phase.
  - The midtarsal joint is maximally pronated, while the subtalar joint, MTP, and IP joints are in neutral.
  - The presence of a well-formed static medial arch should be noted, as well as its dynamic formation with heel raising.
- ***Forefoot-to-rearfoot relationship.*** Goniometric measurement of forefoot position relative to the rearfoot is a routine procedure used by rehabilitation specialists. This measurement is also frequently made by visual estimation. Neutral alignment of the forefoot relative to the rearfoot is present when a line representing the anterior (plantar) aspect of the metatarsal heads is perpendicular to the line bisecting the rearfoot. The forefoot-to-rearfoot angle is approximately 10–12 degrees.[119,143] Forefoot varus is the term used to describe inversion of the forefoot away from this neutral position, while forefoot valgus describes an everted forefoot position.[139] The relationship can be assessed with the patient positioned in prone with their knee extended and their feet over the end of the table. The subtalar neutral position is located using the method described previously. Slight pressure is applied to the metatarsal heads while maintaining subtalar neutral. This will determine the relationship of the forefoot to rearfoot, and both of these to the bisection of the lower leg. A varus or valgus tilt of the forefoot in relation to the hindfoot becomes significant when the first metatarsal is in a plantar flexed position, as this positions the hindfoot into an inverted position during weight-bearing.[141] Somers et al. examined the reliability of goniometric and visual estimation of forefoot position measurements when experienced and inexperienced testers performed the evaluation. Two clinicians ($\geq$ 10 years' experience) and two physical therapy students were recruited as testers. Ten subjects (20–31 years old), free from pathology, were measured. Each foot was evaluated twice with the goniometer and twice with visual estimation by each tester. Intraclass correlation coefficient (ICC) and coefficients of variation method error were used as estimates of reliability. There was no dramatic difference in the intratester or intertester reliability between experienced and inexperienced testers, regardless of the evaluation used. Estimates of intratester reliability (ICC 2,1), when using the goniometer, ranged from 0.08 to 0.78 for the experienced clinicians and from 0.16 to 0.65 for the inexperienced clinicians. When using visual estimation, ICC (2,1) values ranged from 0.51 to 0.76 for the experienced clinicians and 0.53 to 0.57 for the inexperienced clinicians. The estimate of intertester reliability [ICC (2,2)] for the goniometer was 0.38 for the experienced clinicians and 0.42 for the inexperienced clinicians. When using visual estimation, ICC (2,2) values were 0.81 for the experienced clinicians and 0.72 for the inexperienced clinicians. Although experience does not appear to influence forefoot position measurements, of the two evaluation techniques, visual estimation may be the more reliable.
- ***Foot deviations in weight-bearing.*** These include pes planus (low inclined subtalar joint axis), pes cavus (high inclined subtalar joint axis), talipes equinus (plantar flexed foot), talipes equinovarus (supinated foot), and hallux valgus.[101]
- ***Degree of foot pronation or supination in non-weight-bearing.*** The patient lies in the prone position, with the foot over the edge of the table. The clinician holds the foot over the fourth and fifth metatarsal heads with one hand. Both sides of the talus are palpated on the posterior aspect of the foot using the thumb and index finger of the other hand. The clinician then passively dorsiflexes the foot until a resistance is felt. At this point, and while maintaining the dorsiflexed position, the clinician moves the foot back and forth through the arc of supination and pronation. During supination, the talus should be felt to bulge laterally, while during pronation, the talus should be felt to bulge medially. Supination at the subtalar joint occurs in association with 20 degrees of calcaneal inversion, while pronation occurs in association with 10 degrees of calcaneal inversion.
- ***Degree of toe-out.*** The normal foot in relaxed standing adopts a slight toe-out position of approximately 12–18 degrees from the sagittal axis of the body (Fick angle).[134]
- ***Forefoot equinus.*** To assess for forefoot equinus, the clinician stabilizes the rearfoot with one hand and applies pressure on the entire forefoot via pressure across the metatarsal heads, into dorsiflexion. If the plantar declination of the lateral structures cannot be reduced so that the plantar flexed attitude is no longer visible, a positive identification of forefoot equinus can be made.[143]
- ***Presence of a talar bulge.*** The patient is positioned in standing, and the clinician observes to see whether the talar head bulges excessively on the medial side of the midfoot, indicating excessive subtalar joint pronation in weight-bearing. Adaptive shortening of the gastrocnemius/soleus group is indicated with a prominence of the soleus, particularly on the medial side of the teno-calcaneum.

Other areas that should be examined include the following:

- ***Condition of the nails.*** When examining the nails a systematic approach is used, involving an inspection of the shape, contour, and color of the nails. The clinician should observe for the presence of subungual hematomas, subungual exostosis, onychocryptosis, onychia, onychauxis, onychomycosis, paronychia, tinea pedis, or blisters.
- ***Toe deformities.*** Contractions of the capsule of the IP or MTP joints of the toes in association with tendon shortening may produce a series of deformities, ranging from hammer toe to mallet toe to claw toe. *Hammer toe* usually involves a flexion contracture of the anterior (plantar) surface of the PIP, with a mild associated extension contracture of the MTP joint. *Mallet toe* results from a flexion deformity of the distal interphalangeal joint (DIP) with plantar contracture. Often a corn or callus is present on the posterior aspect of the affected joint. Corns are similar to calluses but have a central nidus. *Claw toe* deformity is a more advanced contracture of capsules and intrinsic musculature, which may also be associated with pes cavus and neurologic or primary muscle pathology to the lumbrical and interosseous muscles. The claw toe results in hyperextension of the MTP joints and flexion of the PIP and DIP joints.
- ***Functional hallux limitus.*** Clinically, the presence of functional hallux limitus, an inability of the first MTP joint to extend, can be determined by assessing the ROM available at the first MTP joint, while the first ray is prevented from plantar flexing. The patient is positioned in standing, the feet shoulder-width apart. The patient is asked to actively raise the great toe off the floor, while keeping the remaining toes and foot on the ground. The amount of hallux extension is measured; less than 10 degrees is considered limited.[144] This test has been found to have a sensitivity of 0.72 and a specificity of 0.66.[144]
- ***The leg, foot, and ankle are examined for the presence of bruising, swelling, or unusual angulation.*** Ecchymosis may be present, but the blood usually settles along the medial or lateral aspects of the heel.[16,125] The appearance of bluish-black plaques on the posterior and posterolateral aspect of one or both heels in a young distance runner is found in a condition called *black-dot heel*, which results from a shearing stress or a pinching of the heel between the counter and the sole of the shoe at initial contact during running.

Extracellular fluid pools on the posterior aspect of the foot and around the malleoli after injury or surgery.[101] Shortly after a lateral ligament sprain, the swelling is limited to the lateral ankle. Subsequently, the swelling is diffuse, and the localization of tenderness may be difficult. An objective measure of the amount of swelling present can be made using the figure-of-eight method (see "Special Tests" section).

- ***Callus formation.*** Calluses provide the clinician with an index as to the degree of shear stresses applied to the foot and clearly outline abnormal weight-bearing areas.[145] In adequate amounts calluses provide protection, but in excess they may cause pain. Callus formation under the second and third metatarsal heads could indicate excessive pronation in a flexible foot, or Morton's (interdigital) neuroma (see Chap. 5) if under the second through fourth. A callus under the fifth and sometimes the fourth metatarsal head may indicate an abnormally rigid foot.
- ***Any evidence of circulatory impairment or vasomotor changes.*** Brick-red coloring or cyanosis when the leg is dependent is an indication of vascular impairment, especially if the color changes when the leg is elevated. Vasomotor changes include toenail changes, changes in skin texture, abnormal skin moisture or dryness, and loss of hair on the foot. Vasomotor changes may be associated with complex regional pain syndrome (see Chap. 5).
- ***The type of shoes.*** High-heeled shoes have been associated with adaptive shortening of the gastrocnemius soleus complex, knee pain, and low-back pain.[50,146] They have also been associated with an increased potential for ankle sprains, hallux valgus, bunions, metatarsalgia, interdigital neuromas, peripheral nerve compression, and stress fractures.[50,146] Shoes with a negative heel may result in hyperextension of the knees.
- ***The weight-bearing and wear patterns of the shoe.*** The greatest amount of wear on the sole of the shoe should occur beneath the ball of the foot, in the area corresponding to the first, second, and third MTP joints and slight wear to the lateral side of the heel. Old running shoes belonging to patients who excessively pronate tend to display overcompression of the medial arch of the midsole and extensive wear of the lateral regions of the heel counter and medial forefoot. The upper portion of the shoe should demonstrate a transverse crease at the level of the MTP joints. A stiff first MTP joint can produce a crease line that runs obliquely, from forward and medial to backward and lateral.[147] The cup at the rear of the shoe, which is formed by the heel counter (Fig. 21-34), should be vertical and symmetrical with respect to the shoe and should be of a durable enough material to hold the heel in place.[148] A medial inclination of the cup, with bulging of the lateral lip of the counter, indicates a pronated foot.[147] A lateral bulge of the heel counter indicates a supinated foot. Scuffing of the shoe might indicate tibialis anterior weakness.[80] The shape of the last influences the amount of motion that the shoe permits.[149] As the degree of curvature in the last increases, more foot mobility is available.

The non–weight-bearing component of the examination is initiated by having the patient seated on the edge of the bed, feet dangling. The feet should adopt an inverted and plantar flexed position. A mobile or nonstructural flatfoot will take on a more normal configuration in non–weight-bearing, whereas a fixed or structural flatfoot will maintain its planus state. By placing one hand on the patella and the other hand on the tips of the malleoli, the clinician should note approximately 20–30 degrees of external rotation of the ankle in relation to the knee.[141]

Palpation

Careful palpation should be performed around the leg, foot, and ankle to differentiate tenderness of specific ligaments and other structures. Areas of localized swelling and ecchymosis over the ligaments on the medial or lateral aspects of the foot and ankle should be noted.

Posterior Aspect of Foot and Ankle

Achilles Tendon

The Achilles tendon is inspected for contour changes such as swelling, erythema, and thickening. Any gaps or nodules in the tendon and specific sites of pain should be carefully examined. Palpable gaps in the tendon accompanied by an inability to rise up on the toes could indicate a rupture of the tendon.

Calcaneus

At the distal end of the Achilles tendon is the calcaneal tuberosity. The posterior aspect of the calcaneus and surrounding soft tissue is palpated for evidence of exostosis ("pump bump" or Haglund's deformity) and associated swelling (retrocalcaneal bursitis). The inferior medial process of the calcaneus, just distal to the weight-bearing portion of the calcaneus, serves as the attachment of the plantar fascia and is often tender with plantar heel pain.

Anterior and Anteromedial Aspects of the Foot and Ankle

While reading the next section, the reader may find it helpful to remove a shoe and sock and self-palpate.

Great Toe and the Phalanges

Beginning medially, the clinician locates and palpates the great toe and its two phalanges. The first metatarsal bone is more proximal, the head of which should be palpated for tenderness on the lateral aspect (bunion) and inferior aspect (sesamoiditis).

Moving laterally from the phalanges of the great toe, the clinician palpates the phalanges and metatarsal heads of the other four toes.

Tenderness of the second metatarsal head could indicate the presence of Freiberg's disease, an osteochondritis of the second metatarsal head (see Chap. 5). A callus under the second and the third metatarsal head may indicate a fallen metatarsal arch. Palpable tenderness in the region of the third and fourth metatarsal heads could indicate a Morton's neuroma, especially if the characteristic sharp pain between the toes of this condition is relieved by walking barefoot. Tenderness on the lateral aspect of the fifth metatarsal head could indicate the presence of a tailor's bunion.

Cuneiform

The first cuneiform is located at the proximal end of the first metatarsal (see Fig. 21-1) and is palpated for tenderness.

Navicular

The navicular is the most prominent bone on the medial aspect of the foot. The navicular tuberosity can be located by moving proximally from the medial aspect of the first cuneiform (see Fig. 21-1). The talonavicular joint line lies directly proximal to the navicular tuberosity. In addition, the posterior tibialis, which can be made more prominent with resisted plantar flexion, adduction, and supination, can be used as a reference as it inserts on the plantar surface of the navicular (see later). Tenderness of the navicular could indicate the presence of a fracture or osteochondritis of the navicular (Köhler's disease).

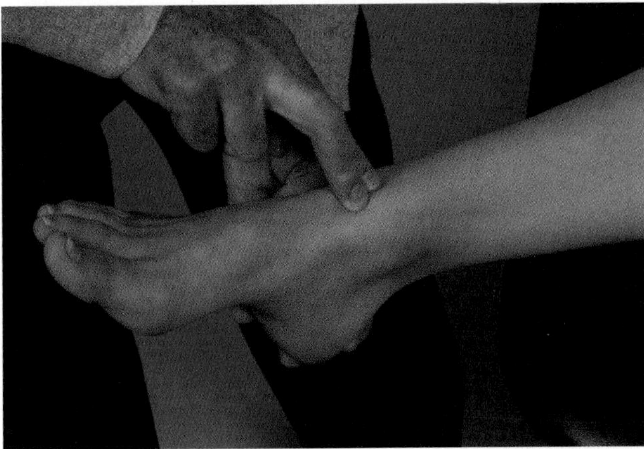

FIGURE 21-14 Dorsal pedis pulse.

Second and Third Cuneiforms

These two bones can be palpated by moving laterally from the first cuneiform (see Fig. 21-1). Tenderness of these bones may indicate a cuneiform fracture.

Posterior (Dorsal) Pedis Pulse

The pulse of the posterior (dorsal) pedis artery, a branch of the anterior tibial artery, can be palpated over the talus, cuneiform bones (Fig. 21-14), between the first and second cuneiforms, or between the first and second metatarsal bones.

Medial Malleolus

The medial malleolus is palpated for swelling or tenderness. Moving proximally from the anterior aspect of the medial malleolus, the distal aspect of the tibia is palpated. Distal to that is the talus bone. Moving distal from the tibia, the clinician palpates the long extensor tendons, the tibialis anterior, and the superior and inferior extensor retinaculum. The tendon of the tibialis anterior is visible at the level of the medial cuneiform and the base of the first metatarsal bone, especially if the foot is positioned in dorsiflexion and supination.

Talus

The talus can be located by moving from the distal aspect of the medial malleolus along a line joining the navicular tuberosity. It can be more easily located by everting and inverting the foot. Eversion causes the talar head to become more prominent, while inversion causes the head to be less visible.

Sustentaculum Tali

Distal and inferior to the medial malleolus, a shelf-like bony prominence of the calcaneus, the sustentaculum tali, can be palpated. At the posterior aspect of the sustentaculum tali, the talocalcaneal joint line can be palpated.

Posterior Tibialis Tendon

This tendon is palpable at the level of the medial malleolus, especially with the foot held in plantar flexion and supination. Distal and medial to this tendon, the crossing of the flexor digitorum longus and flexor hallucis tendons can be felt.

Posterior Tibial Artery

The posterior tibial artery (Fig. 21-9) can be located posterior to the medial malleolus and anterior to the Achilles tendon.

Medial (Deltoid) Ligament of the Ankle

The medial (deltoid) ligament of the ankles is very difficult to differentiate, so they are usually palpated as a group on the medial aspect of the ankle (see Fig. 21-4).

Anterior and Anterolateral Aspects of the Foot and Ankle

Tibial Crest

The tibial crest is palpated for tenderness, which may indicate the presence of shin splints. Swelling in this area may indicate the presence of anterior compartment syndrome. The muscles of the lateral (peronei) and anterior compartments (tibialis anterior and the long extensors) are palpated here for swelling or tenderness. Swelling or tenderness of these structures usually indicates inflammation.

Lateral Malleolus

The lateral malleolus is located at the distal aspect of the fibula. Distal to the lateral malleolus is the calcaneus.

Fibularis (Peroneus) Longus

The tendon of the fibularis (peroneus) longus runs superficially behind the lateral malleolus. Resisted pronation and plantar flexion of the foot make the tendon more prominent.

Fibularis (Peroneus) Brevis

The origin for the fibularis (peroneus) brevis is more distal to the fibularis (peroneus) longus and lies deeper. It becomes superficial on the lateral aspect of the foot, at its insertion at the tuberosity of the fifth metatarsal.

Anterior Talofibular Ligament

The ATFL can be palpated two to three finger-breadths anteroinferior to the lateral malleolus (see Fig. 21-5).[129] This is usually the area of most extreme tenderness following an inversion sprain. The anterior aspect of the distal tibiofibular syndesmosis may also be tender following this type of sprain.

Calcaneofibular Ligament

The CFL can be palpated one to two finger-breadths inferior to the lateral malleolus (see Fig. 21-5).[129]

Posterior Talofibular Ligament

The PTFL can be palpated posteroinferior to the posterior edge of the lateral malleolus (see Fig. 21-5).[129]

Sinus Tarsi

The sinus tarsi is visible as a concave space between the lateral tendon of the extensor digitorum longus muscle and the anterior aspect of the lateral malleolus. The origin of the EDB is at the level of this tunnel.

Cuboid

The cuboid bone can be palpated by moving distally approximately one finger-breadth from the sinus tarsi.

Active and Passive Range of Motion

ROM testing is divided into active range of motion (AROM) and passive range of motion (PROM), with overpressure being superimposed at the end of available range to assess the end-feel. AROM tests are used to assess the patient's willingness to move and the presence of movement restriction patterns such as a capsular or noncapsular pattern. The end-feel may provide the clinician with information as to the cause of a motion restriction. The normal ranges of motion and end-feels for the lower leg, ankle, and foot are outlined in Table 21-7. The open- and close-packed positions and capsular patterns for the ankle and foot are outlined in Table 21-1.

General AROM of the foot and ankle in the non–weight-bearing position is assessed first, with painful movements being performed last. The hip and knee joints may also be examined as appropriate. Weight-bearing tests are usually performed after the non–weight-bearing tests.

If the symptoms are experienced during the general tests, then passive, active, and resisted tests of specific structures must be performed. If the general tests are negative, there is probably no immediate need to proceed with a more detailed examination, although this may have to be done if no other region appears to be the cause of the problem.

Although specific motions at the distal tibiofibular joint cannot be produced voluntarily, the function of this joint can be assessed indirectly by asking the patient to twist around both feet in each direction while bearing weight.

TABLE 21-7 Normal Ranges of Motion and End-Feels for the Lower Leg, Ankle, and Foot

Motion	Normal Range (Degrees)	End-Feel
Plantar flexion	50	Tissue stretch
Dorsiflexion	20	Tissue stretch
Supination	45–60	
Pronation	15–30	
Hindfoot inversion	20	Tissue stretch
Hindfoot eversion	10	Tissue stretch
Toe flexion	Great toe: MTP, 45; IP, 90 Lateral four toes: MTP, 40; PIP, 35; DIP, 60	Tissue stretch
Toe extension	Great toe: MTP, 70; IP, 0 Lateral four toes: MTP, 40; PIP, 0; DIP, 30	Tissue stretch

Data from Rasmussen O: Stability of the ankle joint. *Acta Orthop Scand Suppl* 211:56–78, 1985; Seto JL, Brewster CE: Treatment approaches following foot and ankle injury. *Clin Sports Med* 13:295, 1985.

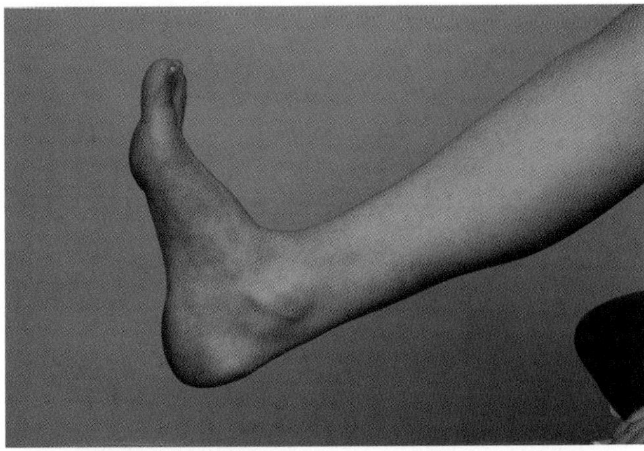

FIGURE 21-15 Ankle dorsiflexion.

Dorsiflexion

The patient lies in the supine position, with the knee slightly flexed and supported by a pillow, while the clinician stands at the foot at the table, facing the patient VIDEO.

Active dorsiflexion is initially performed with the knee flexed (Fig. 21-15). Care must be taken to prevent pronation at the subtalar and oblique midtarsal joint during dorsiflexion. The foot is slightly inverted to lock the longitudinal arch.[141] Passive overpressure is applied. With the knee flexed to approximately 90 degrees, the length of the soleus muscle is examined. Passive overpressure into dorsiflexion when the knee is flexed assesses the joint motion, as well as the soleus length. The soleus is implicated if pain is produced in this test, especially if resisted plantar flexion is painful or more painful with the knee flexed than with the knee extended. With the knee flexed, 20 degrees of dorsiflexion past the anatomic position (the foot at 90 degrees to the bones of the leg) is found in the normally flexible person.[150] The flexibility of the soleus muscle may also be assessed in standing in able-bodied individuals by asking the patient to perform a deep squat or a lunge.

- *Squat.* If the muscle length is normal, the patient should be able to place the whole foot on the floor, including the heel, while in the full squat position (Fig. 21-16). If the soleus is short, the heel will not touch the floor.
- *Lunge.* A standard goniometer is aligned along the lateral aspect of the leg and the floor. The subject steadies themselves and then performs a weight-bearing lunge maneuver (Fig. 21-17). The angle recorded on the goniometer indicates the range of dorsiflexion under load. If the goniometer is set so that vertical is zero, the arm of the goniometer always aligns to the vertical and the scale rotates to indicate the inclination from the vertical. This angle is then recorded as the ankle dorsiflexion range. This method is considered the most appropriate method of measuring ankle dorsiflexion range, as it reflects the functionally available range for the individual. Bennell et al.[151] evaluated the interrater and intrarater reliability of a weight-bearing dorsiflexion lunge using a gravity goniometer in 13 healthy subjects. Two methods were used to assess the dorsiflexion lunge: (1) the distance from the great toe to the wall and (2) the angle between the tibial shaft and the vertical using an inclinometer. The average of three trials was used in data analysis. Intrarater ICCs ranged from 0.97 to 0.98. Interrater ICC values were 0.97 (angle) and 0.99 (distance), indicating excellent reliability for both methods of assessing a DF lunge.[151]

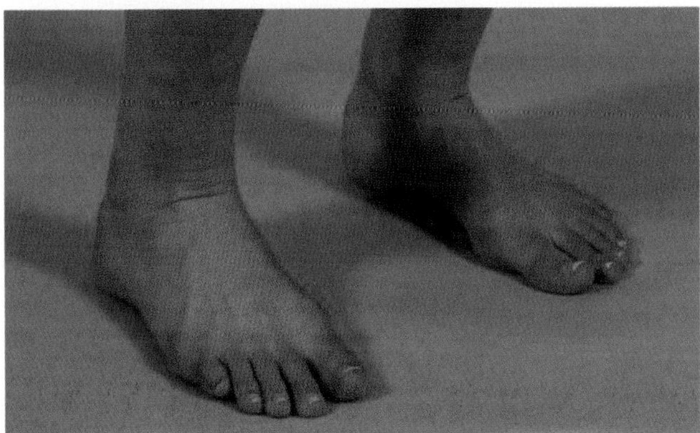

FIGURE 21-16 Ankle dorsiflexion during squat.

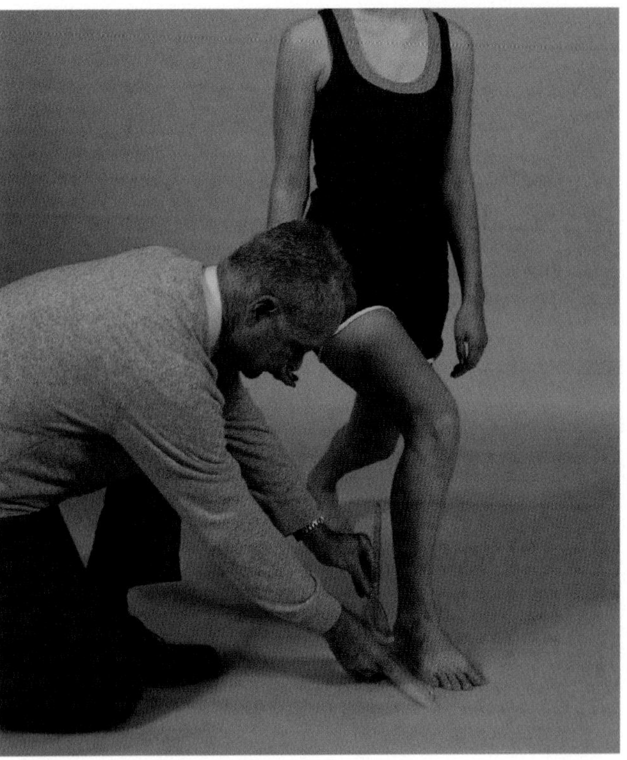

FIGURE 21-17 Ankle dorsiflexion during lunge with goniometer.

CLINICAL PEARL

Chronic adaptive shortening of the soleus muscle can be caused by excessive running, a weak posterior tibialis, or a weak quadriceps. Adaptive shortening of the soleus can result in forefoot pronation and a valgus stress at the knee.

To assess the length of the gastrocnemius, the patient is placed in the supine position with the knee extended, and the ankle positioned in subtalar neutral. The patient is then asked to dorsiflex the ankle (Fig. 21-18). Passive overpressure into

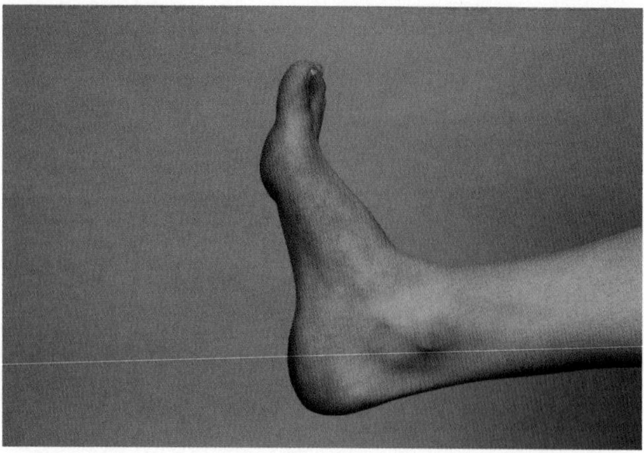

FIGURE 21-18 Active ankle dorsiflexion (knee extended).

dorsiflexion is applied. The normal range is 20 degrees. If the gastrocnemius is shortened, dorsiflexion of the ankle will be reduced as the knee is extended, and increased as the knee is flexed. A muscular end-feel should be felt with the knee extended, and a capsular end-feel should be felt with the knee flexed.

CLINICAL PEARL

A decrease in the flexibility of the gastrocnemius can result from a number of dysfunctions, including dysfunction of the subtalar joint or transtarsal joint, an ankle sprain, high-heeled footwear, or poor gait/running mechanics.

Plantar Flexion

The patient is placed in the supine position, while the clinician stands at the foot of the table, facing the patient VIDEO. The patient is asked to plantar flex the ankle (Fig. 21-19). Plantar flexion of the ankle is approximately 30–50 degrees.[94] When tested in weight-bearing with the unilateral heel raise, heel inversion should be seen to occur. Failure of the foot to invert may indicate instability of the foot/ankle, posterior tibialis dysfunction, or adaptive shortening.[152]

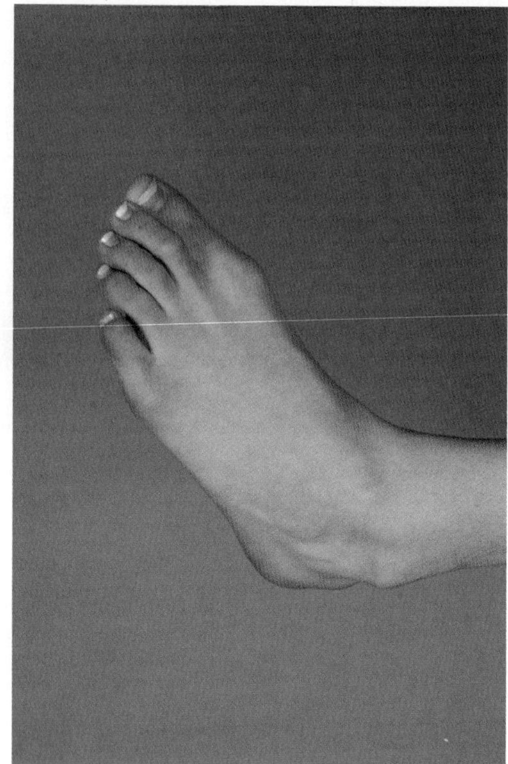

FIGURE 21-20 Ankle inversion.

Hindfoot Inversion (Supination) and Hindfoot Eversion (Pronation)

Both hindfoot inversion (Fig. 21-20) and hindfoot eversion (Fig. 21-21) are tested by lining up the longitudinal axis of the leg and vertical axis of the calcaneus. Passive motion of hindfoot inversion (supination) is normally 20 degrees.[94] The amount of hindfoot eversion (pronation) is normally 10 degrees.[94]

Great Toe Motion

The patient is positioned in supine, with the leg being supported by a pillow, while the clinician stands at the foot at the table, facing the patient. Active extension of the great toe is performed and assisted passively without dorsiflexing the first

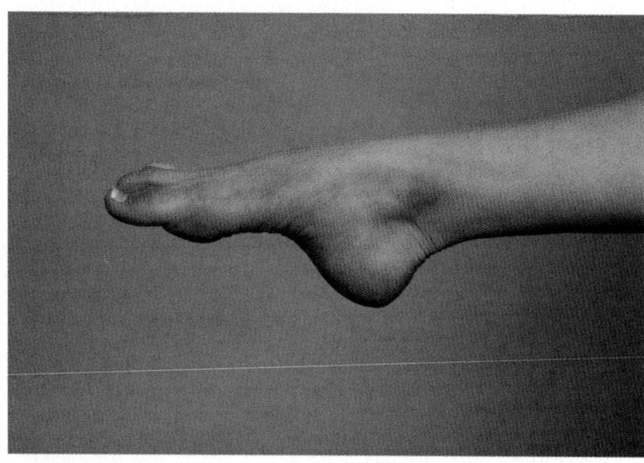

FIGURE 21-19 Ankle plantar flexion.

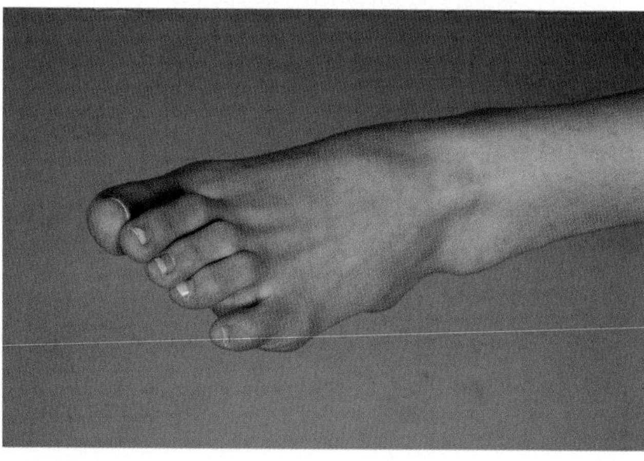

FIGURE 21-21 Ankle eversion.

ray. The amount of posterior (dorsal) mobility is usually classified as normal, hypomobile, or hypermobile. Although this method of assessment is common, its reliability and validity have been shown to be poor.[122] Extension of the great toe occurs primarily at the MTP joint. Passive extension of the great toe at the MTP joint should demonstrate elevation of the medial longitudinal arch (windlass effect), and external rotation of the tibia.[153] Passive MTP joint extension of between 55 and 90 degrees is necessary at terminal stance,[154] depending on length of stride, shoe flexibility, and toe-in/toe-out foot placement angle.[139] Forty-five degrees of first MTP flexion and 90 degrees of IP joint flexion are considered normal.[141]

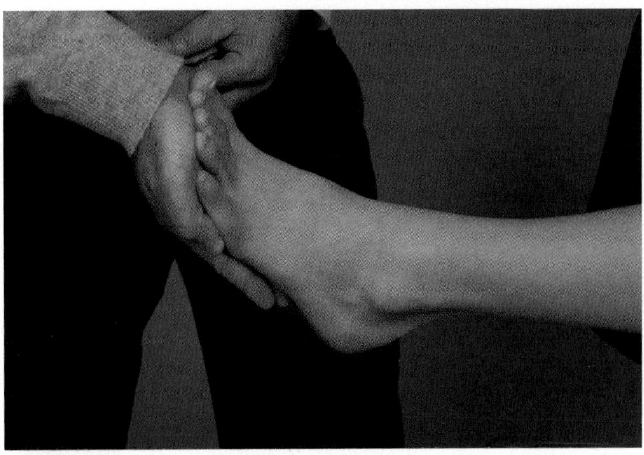

FIGURE 21-22 Manual muscle testing of the plantar flexors.

Strength Testing

Ankle

Gastrocnemius and Plantaris Muscles. Plantar flexion strength can be tested initially in non–weight-bearing (Fig. 21-22). If no plantar flexion weakness is apparent in non–weight-bearing, a heel raise test is performed in the functional position, standing with the knee extended and the opposite foot off the floor VIDEO. Technically, one heel raise through full ROM, while standing with support on one leg, scores a 3/5 (fair) with manual muscle testing, with five single-limb heel raises scoring a 4/5 (good) and 10 single-limb heel raises scoring a 5/5 (normal). From a functional viewpoint, a wider range of scoring can sometimes prove more useful. Table 21-8 outlines an alternative scoring method.

TABLE 21-8 Functional Testing of the Foot and Ankle

Starting Position	Action	Functional Test
Standing on one leg	Lift toes and forefeet off ground (dorsiflexion)	10–15 repetitions: functional 5–9 repetitions: functionally fair 1–4 repetitions: functionally poor 0 repetition: nonfunctional
Standing on one leg	Lift heels off ground (plantar flexion)	10–15 repetitions: functional 5–9 repetitions: functionally fair 1–4 repetitions: functionally poor 0 repetition: nonfunctional
Standing on one leg	Lift lateral aspect of foot off ground (ankle eversion)	5–6 repetitions: functional 3–4 repetitions: functionally fair 1–2 repetitions: functionally poor 0 repetition: nonfunctional
Standing on one leg	Lift medial aspect of foot off ground (ankle inversion)	5–6 repetitions: functional 3–4 repetitions: functionally fair 1–2 repetitions: functionally poor 0 repetitions: nonfunctional
Seated	Pull small towel up under the toes or pick up and release small object (i.e., pencil, marble, cotton ball) (toe flexion)	10–15 repetitions: functional 5–9 repetitions: functionally fair 1–4 repetitions: functionally poor 0 repetitions: nonfunctional
Seated	Lift toes off ground (toe extension)	10–15 repetitions: functional 5–9 repetitions: functionally fair 1–4 repetitions: functionally poor 0 repetitions: nonfunctional

Data from Palmer ML, Epler M: *Clinical Assessment Procedures in Physical Therapy*. Philadelphia, PA: JB Lippincott, 1990.

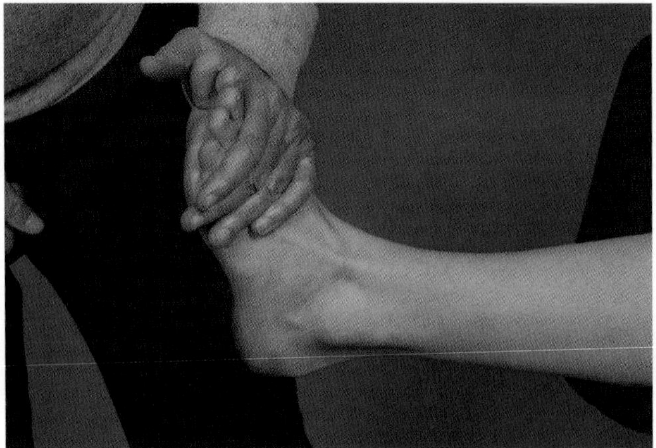

FIGURE 21-23 Manual muscle testing of the tibialis anterior.

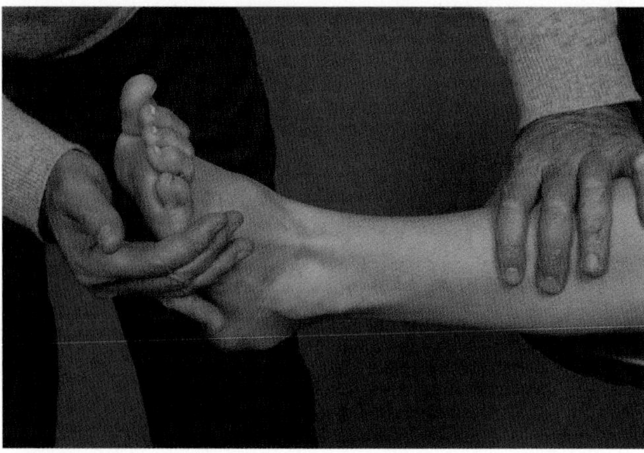

FIGURE 21-25 Manual muscle testing of the fibularis (peroneus) muscle group.

Soleus Muscle. The soleus muscle produces plantar flexion of the ankle joint, regardless of the position of the knee. To determine the individual functioning of the soleus as a plantar flexor, the knee is flexed to minimize the effect of the gastrocnemius muscle. The soleus is tested in a similar manner to that of the gastrocnemius, except that the patient performs the unilateral heel raise with some degree of knee flexion. Ability to perform 10–15 raises in this fashion is considered normal, five to nine raises graded as fair, one to four raises graded as poor, and zero repetitions graded as nonfunctional. Alternatively, the strength of the soleus can be tested with the patient in prone VIDEO.

Tibialis Anterior Muscle. The tibialis anterior muscle produces the motion of dorsiflexion and inversion. The knee must remain flexed during the test to allow complete dorsiflexion. The patient's foot is positioned in dorsiflexion and inversion. The leg is stabilized, and resistance is applied to the medial posterior aspect of the forefoot into plantar flexion and eversion (Fig. 21-23) VIDEO.

Tibialis Posterior Muscle. The tibialis posterior muscle produces the motion of inversion in a plantar flexed position. The leg is stabilized in the anatomic position, with the ankle in slight plantar flexion. Resistance is applied to the medial border of the forefoot into eversion and dorsiflexion (Fig. 21-24) VIDEO.

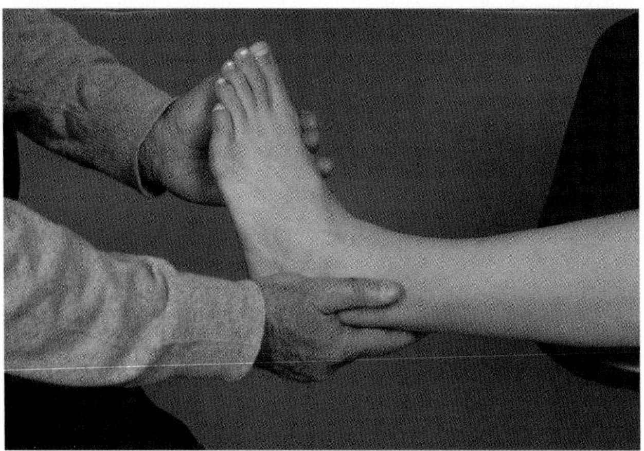

FIGURE 21-24 Manual muscle testing of the tibialis posterior.

Fibularis (Peroneus) Longus, Fibularis (Peroneus) Brevis, and Fibularis (Peroneus) Tertius Muscles. VIDEO The lateral compartment muscles and the fibularis (peroneus) tertius muscle VIDEO produce the motion of eversion. The patient is positioned in supine, with the foot over the edge of the table and the ankle in the anatomic position. Resistance is applied to the lateral border of the forefoot (Fig. 21-25).

Digits. Grades for the toes differ from the standard format because gravity is not considered a factor.

0: No contraction.

Trace or 1: Muscle contraction is palpated, but no movement occurs.

Poor or 2: Subject can partially complete the ROM.

Fair or 3: Subject can complete the test range.

Good or 4: Subject can complete the test range but is able to take less resistance on the test side than on the opposite side.

N or 5: Subject can complete the test range and take maximal resistance on the test side as compared with the normal side.

Flexor Hallucis Brevis and Longus Muscles. The flexor hallucis brevis VIDEO and FHL muscles VIDEO produce MTP joint flexion and IP joint flexion. The foot is maintained in midposition. The first metatarsal is stabilized, and resistance is applied beneath the proximal and distal phalanx of the great toe into toe extension.

Flexor Digitorum Brevis and Longus Muscles. The flexor digitorum longus and brevis muscles produce IP joint flexion. The motion is tested with the foot in the anatomic position. If the gastrocnemius muscle is shortened, preventing the ankle from assuming the anatomic position, the knee is flexed. The toes may be tested simultaneously.

The foot is held in the midposition and the metatarsals are stabilized. Resistance is applied beneath the distal and proximal phalanges VIDEO.

Extensor Hallucis Longus and Brevis Muscles. VIDEO The extensor hallucis longus and the EHB muscles produce the motion of extension of the IP and MTP joints. The foot is maintained in midposition. Resistance is applied to the posterior aspect of both phalanges of the first digit into toe flexion.

Extensor Digitorum Longus and Brevis Muscles. The extensor digitorum longus and the EDB muscles produce the motion of extension at the MTP and IP joints of the lateral four digits from a flexed position VIDEO. Resistance is applied to the posterior (dorsal) surface of the proximal and distal phalanges into toe flexion.

Intrinsic Muscles of the Foot. The intrinsic muscles of the foot are tested with the patient in either the supine or the sitting position. Most subjects are unable to voluntarily contract the intrinsic muscles of the foot individually.

Abductor Hallucis Muscle. The metatarsals are stabilized, and resistance is applied medially to the distal end of the first phalanx VIDEO.

Adductor Hallucis Muscle. The metatarsals are stabilized, and resistance is applied to the lateral side of the proximal phalanx of the first digit VIDEO.

Lumbrical Muscles. The lateral four metatarsals are stabilized, and resistance is applied to the middle and distal phalanges of the lateral four digits.

Plantar Interossei Muscles. The lateral three metatarsals are stabilized, and resistance is applied to the middle and distal phalanges.

Posterior (Dorsal) Interossei and Abductor Digiti Minimi Muscles. The metatarsals are stabilized and resistance is applied:

- ***Posterior (Dorsal) interossei.*** Applied to the middle and distal phalanges.
- ***Abductor digiti minimi.*** Applied to the lateral side of the proximal phalanx of the fifth digit.

Functional Tests

Subjective Tests

The Ankle Joint Functional Assessment Tool. The Ankle Joint Functional Assessment Tool (AJFAT)[155] is composed of 12 questions rating the ankle's functional ability (Table 21-9). The AJFAT questions are based on assessment tools previously used for evaluating the functional level of the knee.[156–158]

The Foot Function Index. The Foot Function Index (FFI)[159] is a functional outcome measure that consists of three subsections: pain, disability (Table 21-9), and activity. A study by Budiman-Mak et al.[159] examined test–retest reliability (intraclass correlation coefficient, ICC = 0.87), internal consistency (0.96), and construct and criterion validity of the questionnaire.

Objective Tests

Weight-Bearing Tests

In weight-bearing, with the feet fixed, the patient should be asked to perform the following while the clinician notes any reproduction of pain or abnormal motion:

TABLE 21-9 Ankle Joint Functional Assessment Tool (AJFAT)

1. How would you describe the level of pain you experience in your ankle?
   - ________(0) Much more than the other ankle
   - ________(1) Slightly more than the other ankle
   - ________(2) Equal in amount to the other ankle
   - ________(3) Slightly less than the other ankle
   - ________(4) Much less than the other ankle
2. How would you describe any swelling of your ankle?
   - ________(0) Much more than the other ankle
   - ________(1) Slightly more than the other ankle
   - ________(2) Equal in amount to the other ankle
   - ________(3) Slightly less than the other ankle
   - ________(4) Much less than the other ankle
3. How would you describe the ability of your ankle when walking on uneven surfaces?
   - ________(0) Much less than the other ankle
   - ________(1) Slightly less than the other ankle
   - ________(2) Equal in ability to the other ankle
   - ________(3) Slightly more than the other ankle
   - ________(4) Much more than the other ankle
4. How would you describe the overall feeling of stability of your ankle?
   - ________(0) Much less stable than the other ankle
   - ________(1) Slightly less stable than the other ankle
   - ________(2) Equal in stability to the other ankle
   - ________(3) Slightly more stable than the other ankle
   - ________(4) Much more stable than the other ankle

(Continued)

TABLE 21-9 Ankle Joint Functional Assessment Tool (AJFAT) *(Continued)*
5. How would you describe the overall feeling of strength of your ankle? ________(0) Much less strong than the other ankle ________(1) Slightly less strong than the other ankle ________(2) Equal in strength to the other ankle ________(3) Slightly stronger than the other ankle ________(4) Much stronger than the other ankle
6. How would you describe your ankle's ability when you descend stairs? ________(0) Much less than the other ankle ________(1) Slightly less than the other ankle ________(2) Equal in amount to the other ankle ________(3) Slightly more than the other ankle ________(4) Much more than the other ankle
7. How would you describe your ankle's ability when you jog? ________(0) Much less than the other ankle ________(1) Slightly less than the other ankle ________(2) Equal in amount to the other ankle ________(3) Slightly more than the other ankle ________(4) Much more than the other ankle
8. How would you describe your ankle's ability to "cut," or change direction, when running? ________(0) Much less than the other ankle ________(1) Slightly less than the other ankle ________(2) Equal in amount to the other ankle ________(3) Slightly more than the other ankle ________(4) Much more than the other ankle
9. How would you describe the overall activity level of your ankle? ________(0) Much less than the other ankle ________(1) Slightly less than the other ankle ________(2) Equal in amount to the other ankle ________(3) Slightly more than the other ankle ________(4) Much more than the other ankle
10. Which statement best describes your ability to sense your ankle beginning to "roll over"? ________(0) Much later than the other ankle ________(1) Slightly later than the other ankle ________(2) At the same time as the other ankle ________(3) Slightly sooner than the other ankle ________(4) Much sooner than the other ankle
11. Compared with the other ankle, which statement best describes your ability to respond to your ankle beginning to "roll over"? ________(0) Much later than the other ankle ________(1) Slightly later than the other ankle ________(2) At the same time as the other ankle ________(3) Slightly sooner than the other ankle ________(4) Much sooner than the other ankle
12. Following a typical incident of your ankle "rolling," which statement best describes the time required to return to activity? ________(0) More than 2 days ________(1) 1 to 2 days ________(2) More than 1 hour and less than 1 day ________(3) 15 minutes to 1 hour ________(4) Almost immediately

Data from Rozzi SL, Lephart SM, Sterner R, et al: Balance Training for Persons with Functionally Unstable Ankles. *J Orthop Sports Phys Ther* 29:478–486, 1999.

- *Weight-bearing on the foot borders.* The patient is asked to bear weight on the medial borders of the feet while keeping the knees extended. The patient is then asked to bear weight on the lateral borders of the feet while maintaining the knee extension.
- *Heel raising.* In addition to being a general screening test, heel raising also assesses the ability of the medial arch to increase and produce a supinated/inverted arch. Under normal conditions, the tibialis posterior tendon inverts the hind foot as the patient raises their heel. With poor or absent tibialis posterior function, the patient just rolls on the outside of the foot and demonstrates a decreased ability to unilaterally raise the heel.
- *Twisting of the lower leg.* Twisting tests the ability of the foot to supinate on the ipsilateral side, and its ability to pronate on the contralateral side.

The results of these tests may not be helpful in forming an actionable diagnosis, but they may be the only way to reproduce the patient's symptoms and will therefore be of use in the formation of a diagnosis.

Single-leg Stance Test

Chronic ankle instability is a frequent consequence after lateral ankle sprain. The inability to maintain quiet stance during single standing has consistently been shown to be associated with ankle instability.[160]

Star Excursion Balance Test

The star excursion balance test (SEBT) is a clinical test purported to detect functional performance deficits associated with lower extremity pathology in otherwise healthy individuals.[160] The SEBT consists of a series of lower extremity reaching tasks in directions that challenge subjects' postural control, strength, ROM, and proprioceptive abilities. The farther a subject can reach with one leg while balancing on the opposite leg, the better the functional performance they are deemed to have. The subject stands barefoot at the center of the grid with eight lines extending in a star pattern at 45-degree increments from the center of the grid.[161] Subjects are asked to maintain a single-leg stance while reaching with the contralateral leg to touch as far as possible along the chosen line, and then to return to a bilateral stance while maintaining their equilibrium.[161] The test is then repeated using the other leg.

Functional Examination

See Table 21-8.

Passive Articular Mobility

Passive articular mobility tests assess the accessory motions available between the joint surfaces. These same techniques can be used to increase joint play using the varying grades of mobilization (see "Joint Mobilizations" in Techniques to Increase Joint Mobility). As with any other joint complex, the quality and quantity of joint motion must be assessed to determine the level of joint involvement. The joint play movement tests must be performed on both sides so that comparisons can be made. The patient is positioned in lying.

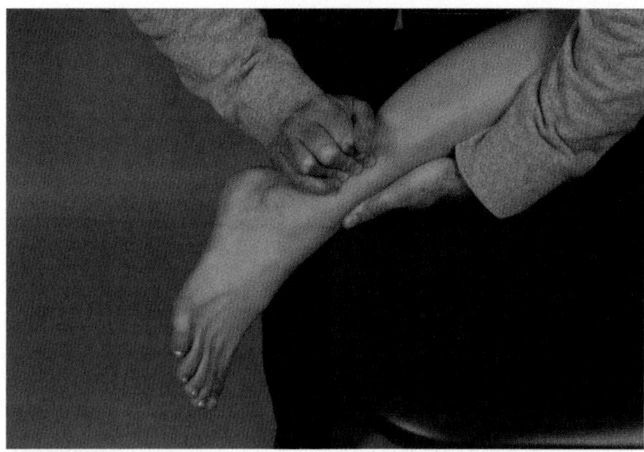

FIGURE 21-26 Mobility testing of the distal tibiofibular joint.

Distal Tibiofibular Joint

Although the glide at this joint would appear to be negligible, Mulligan has proposed that some ankle inversion injuries may be the result of a distal fibular positional fault. One study[162] examined the distal tibiofibular posterior glide of the ankles of 25 subjects for joint excursion. Of the 50 ankles, six had been diagnosed with an acute ankle sprain. Two ankles exhibited an increase in excursion, both of which of had been sprained suggesting that in approximately one-third of diagnosed ankle sprains, the true cause might be an anterior positional fault of the distal fibular on the tibia.

To perform the mobility tests of this joint, the patient is placed in supine and the clinician grips the tibia and fibula using one hand for each (Fig. 21-26). While one hand prevents downward motion of the medial malleolus, the other hand glides the fibula anteriorly and posteriorly in relation to the tibia. To assess the motion of the tibial component, one hand stabilizes the fibula and lateral malleolus, while the other hand glides the tibia anteriorly and posteriorly in relation to the fibula. Theoretically, a superior and inferior glide can be assessed at this joint, but it is unclear whether information provided by such testing would help the clinician in making a diagnosis or designing a plan of care.

Long-Axis Distraction of Ankle and Foot

The clinician stabilizes the proximal segment and applies traction to the distal segment. This test is performed at the talocrural joint (Fig. 21-27), the subtalar joint (Fig. 21-28), the MTP joints (Fig 21-29), and the IP joints (Fig 21-30).

Anterior–Posterior Glide

To test the anterior glide of the talocrural joint, the clinician stabilizes the tibia and fibula and draws the talus and foot forward together (Fig. 21-31). Pushing the talus and foot together in a posterior direction on the tibia and fibula (Fig. 21-32) tests the posterior movement. The anterior glide of the talus assesses the joint's ability to move into plantar flexion,

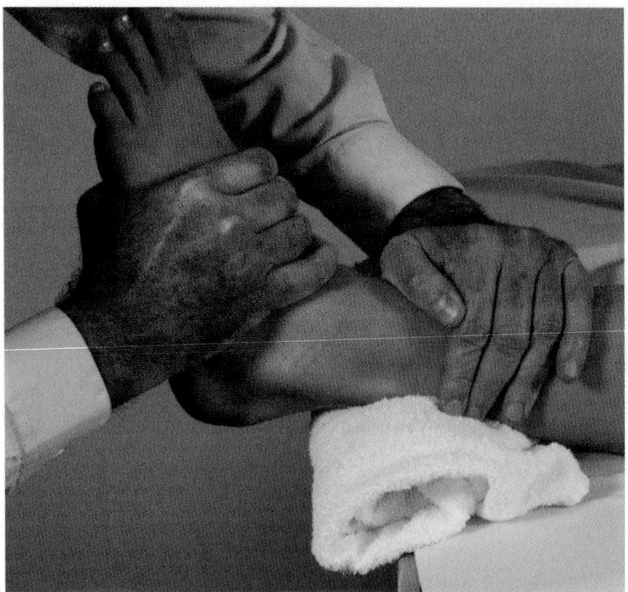
FIGURE 21-27 Long-axis distraction of talocrural joint.

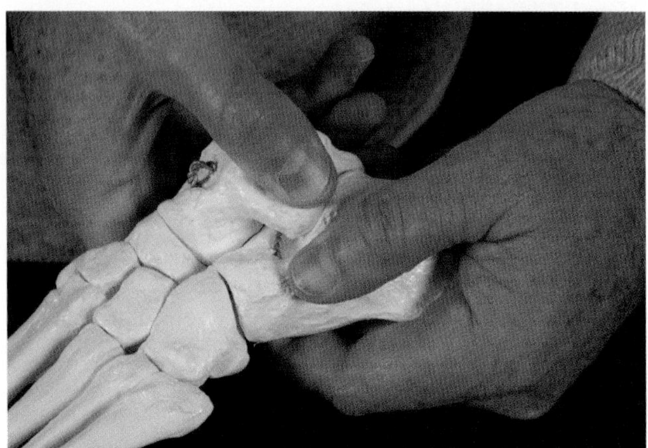
FIGURE 21-28 Long-axis distraction of subtalar joint.

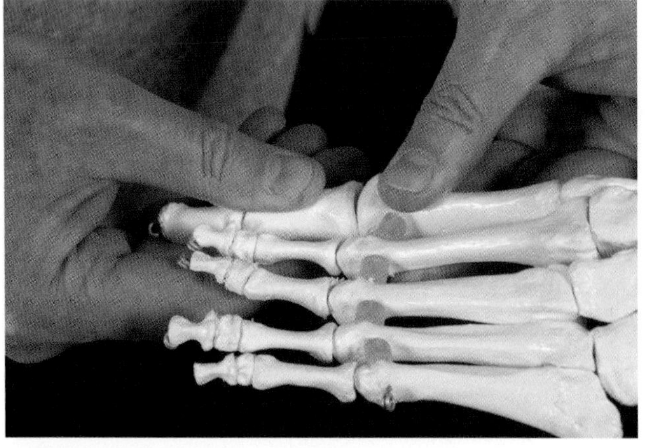
FIGURE 21-29 Long-axis distraction of the IP joint.

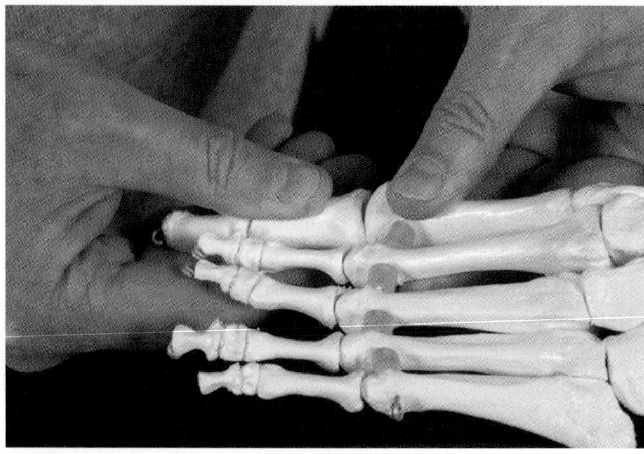
FIGURE 21-30 Long-axis distraction of the MTP joint.

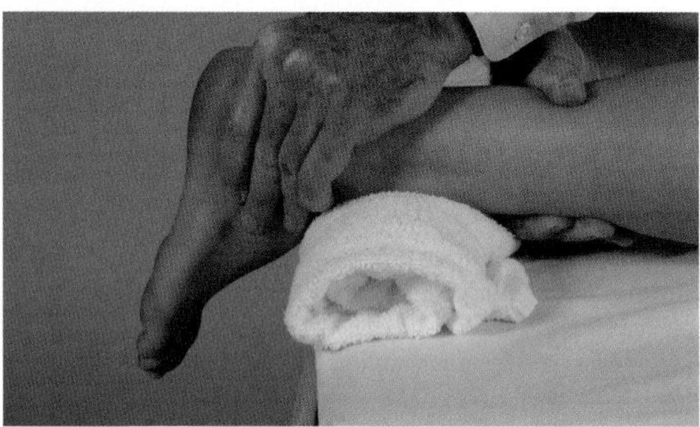
FIGURE 21-31 Anterior glide of the talocrural joint.

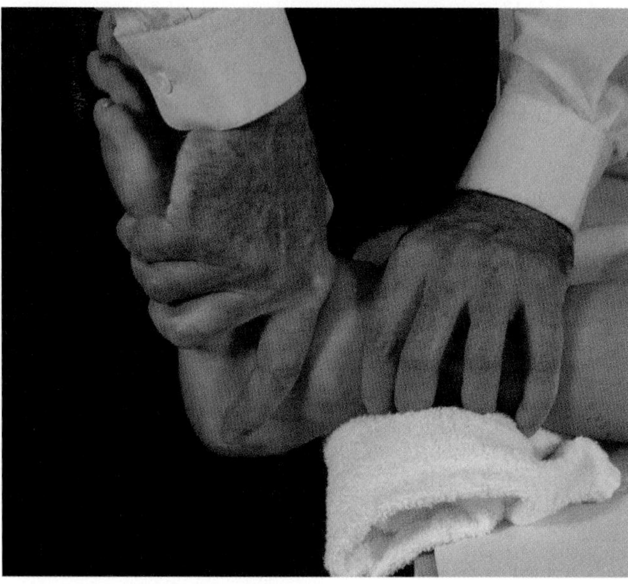
FIGURE 21-32 Posterior glide of the talocrural joint.

whereas the posterior glide of the talus assesses the joint's ability to move into dorsiflexion.

The anterior–posterior glides can also be applied to the midtarsal (Fig. 21-33), intertarsal (Figs. 21-34 and 21-35), MTP (Fig. 21-36), and IP (Fig. 21-37) joints.

Calcaneal Inversion–Eversion (Subtalar)

Subtalar joint motion is extremely important to normal foot function. A loss of eversion causes weight-bearing to occur along the lateral side of the ankle joint. The patient lies in the prone position with the knee slightly flexed and supported by a

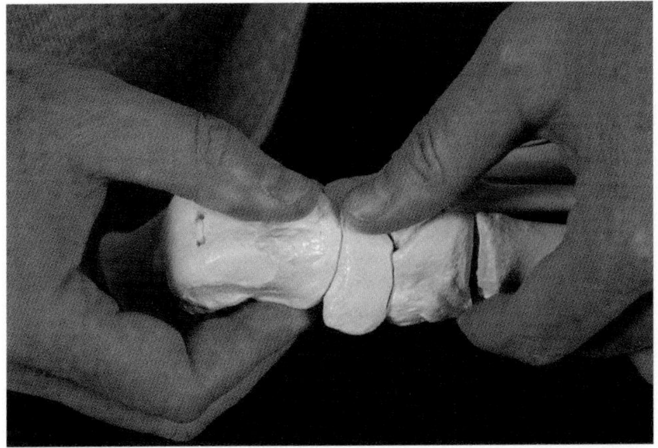

FIGURE 21-33 A-P glide of mid-tarsal joints.

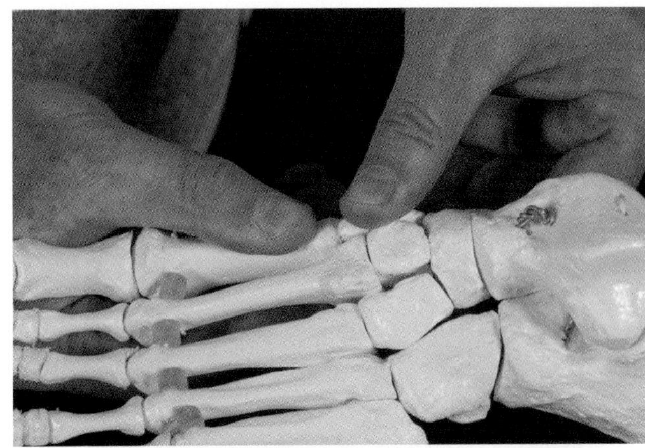

FIGURE 21-36 A-P glide of MTP.

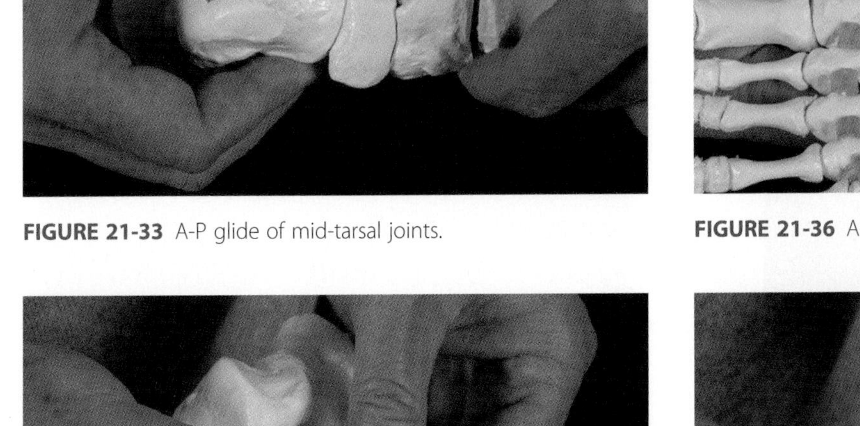

FIGURE 21-34 A-P glide of intertarsals.

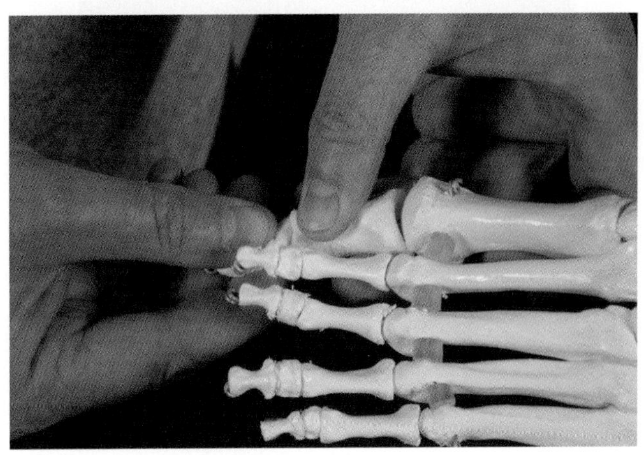

FIGURE 21-37 A-P glide of IP joints.

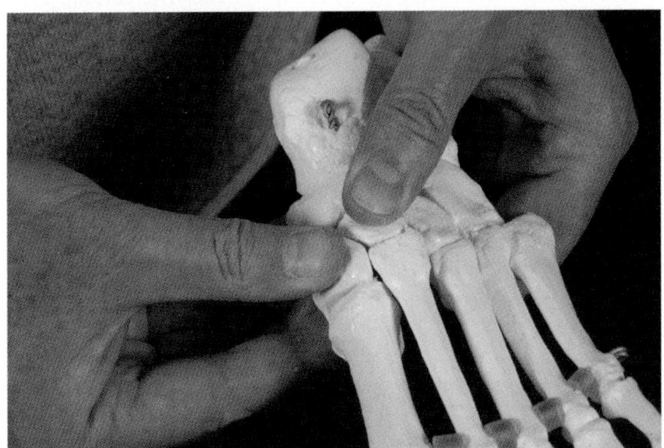

FIGURE 21-35 A-P glide of intertarsals.

pillow, while the clinician stands at the foot of the table, facing the patient. The clinician grasps the calcaneus in one hand, while the other hand locks the talus. The calcaneus is passively inverted (varus) and everted (valgus) on the talus (Fig. 21-38). The amount and quality of the motions as compared with the other foot are noted. Although some differences exist, generally calcaneal eversion will measure 5–10 degrees, while calcaneal inversion will measure approximately 20–30 degrees.[20,94,141] A similar technique can be used to assess

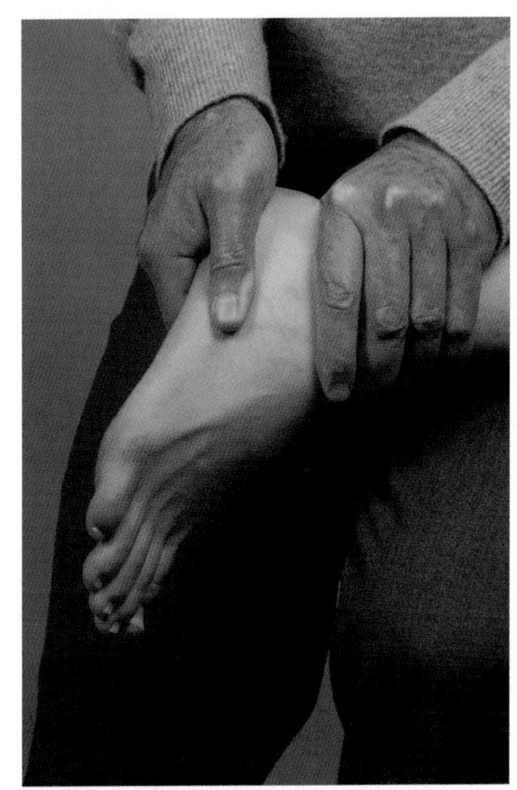

FIGURE 21-38 Calcaneal inversion and eversion.

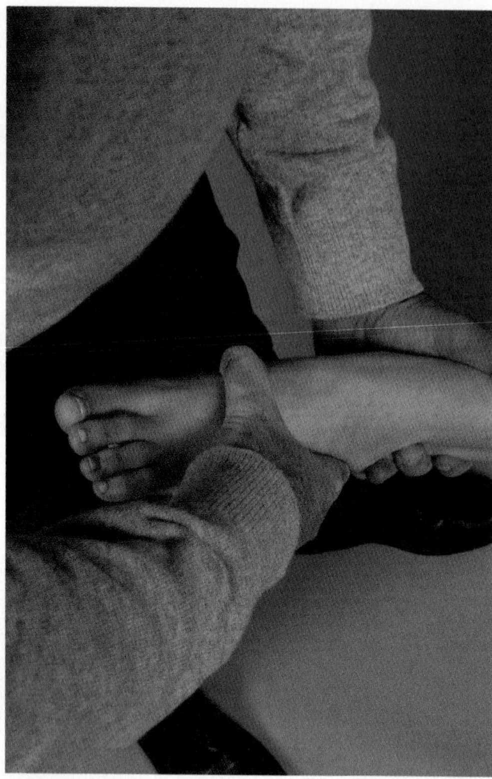

FIGURE 21-39 Mobility testing midtarsal inversion/eversion.

medial and lateral gapping at this joint. Medial gapping is associated with subtalar joint eversion, whereas lateral gapping is associated with subtalar joint inversion.

Midtarsal Joint Motion

The rotational movements of the midtarsal joint, which allow the forefoot to twist on the rearfoot, can be observed in the non–weight-bearing position. The clinician stabilizes the calcaneus with one hand, while inverting and everting the foot at the midtarsal joint with the other hand (Fig. 21-39).[85]

First MTP Joint (First Ray) Motion

The patient lies in supine position, with the clinician at the foot of the table facing away from the patient. The clinician grasps and locks the first MTP joint, before grasping the great toe and moving it into extension and flexion (posteriorly (dorsally) and anteriorly (ventrally), respectively) (Fig. 21-40). Long-axis distraction and compression can also be applied (Fig. 21-41) to assess capsular and articular integrity, respectively.

Limited range may result from a combination of biomechanical factors such as excessive pronation or joint glide restriction.[163] To examine the conjunct rotation of the metatarsals, the clinician locks the second metatarsal to evaluate the first and locks the third to evaluate the second. The quantity and quality of motion is noted and compared with the other side.

Special Tests

Special tests are merely confirmatory tests and should not be used alone to form a diagnosis. Selection for their use is at the

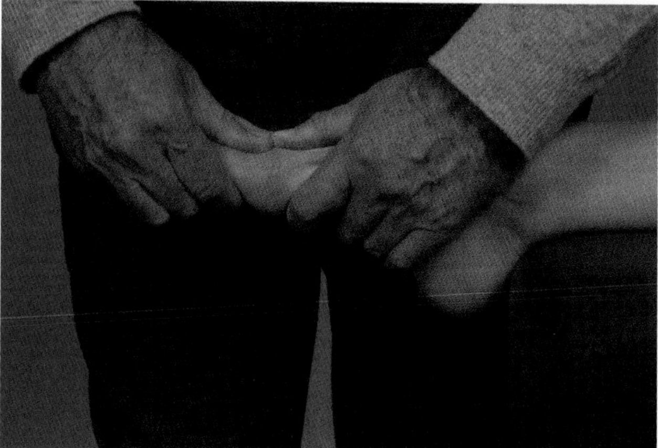

FIGURE 21-40 First MTP motion.

discretion of the clinician and is based on a complete patient history. The results from these tests are used in conjunction with the other clinical findings. To assure accuracy with these tests, both sides should be tested for comparison.

Assessing Ankle Girth

Physical therapists need a reliable method by which to measure ankle girth following injury so that there can be clinical quantification of the volume of edema. Two methods are described:

- ***Figure-of-eight tape method.*** The patient lies in the supine position or seated. The clinician places a tape measure midway between the tibialis anterior tendon and lateral malleolus. The tape is then drawn medially and is placed just distal to the navicular tuberosity. The tape is then pulled across the arch and just proximal to the fifth metatarsal. The tape is then pulled across the tibialis anterior tendon and around the ankle to a point just distal to the medial malleolus, before being finally pulled across the Achilles tendon and placed just distal to the lateral malleolus and across the start of the tape. Tatro-Adams et al.[164] reported the ankle figure-of-eight method to be a reliable tool for measuring ankle girth. (Fig. 21-42)
- ***Volumetry method.*** A volumeter is filled with water, and the patient's foot is placed into the volumeter with toe tips

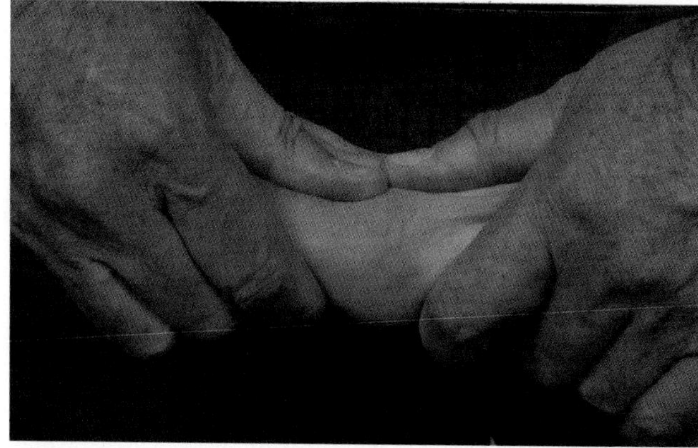

FIGURE 21-41 Long-axis distraction and compression at the 1st MTP joint.

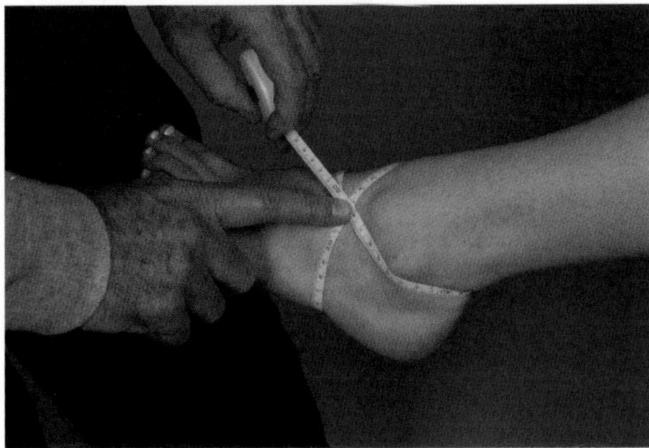

FIGURE 21-42 Figure-of eight tape method.

touching the front wall. The amount of water displaced is measured.

Petersen et al. performed a study to determine the interrater and intrarater reliability of water volumetry and the figure-of-eight method on subjects with ankle joint swelling and found high interrater reliability for both the water volumetry (ICC = 0.99) and the figure-of-eight methods (ICC = 0.98). In addition, intrarater reliability was high for both (ICCs = 0.98–0.99). The authors concluded that both methods are reliable measures of ankle swelling, although they recommended the figure-of-eight method because of its ease of use, time efficiency, and cost effectiveness. However, water volumetry may be more appropriate when measuring diffuse lower extremity swelling.

Ligamentous Stress Tests

The examination of the ligamentous structures in the ankle and foot is essential, not only because of their vast array but also because of the amount of stability that they provide. Positive results for the ligamentous stability tests include excessive movement, as compared with the same test on the uninvolved extremity, pain (depending on the severity), or apprehension.

Mortise/Syndesmosis

Cotton (Clunk) Test

The patient lies in supine position with their foot over the end of the bed. One hand is used to stabilize the distal leg on the bed, while the clinician uses the other hand to grasp the heel and move the calcaneus laterally (see Fig. 21-43).[165] A clunk can be felt as the talus hits the tibia and fibula, if there has been significant mortise widening.[129] Beumer et al.[166] found this test to have a sensitivity of 46%.

Kleiger (External Rotation) Test

The Kleiger (external rotation) test[17,137,167] is a general test to implicate the syndesmosis if pain is produced over the anterior or posterior tibiofibular ligaments and the interosseous membrane, but can also be used to assess the integrity of the medial (deltoid) ligament of the ankle complex.[168,169] If this test is positive, further testing is necessary to determine the source of the symptoms.

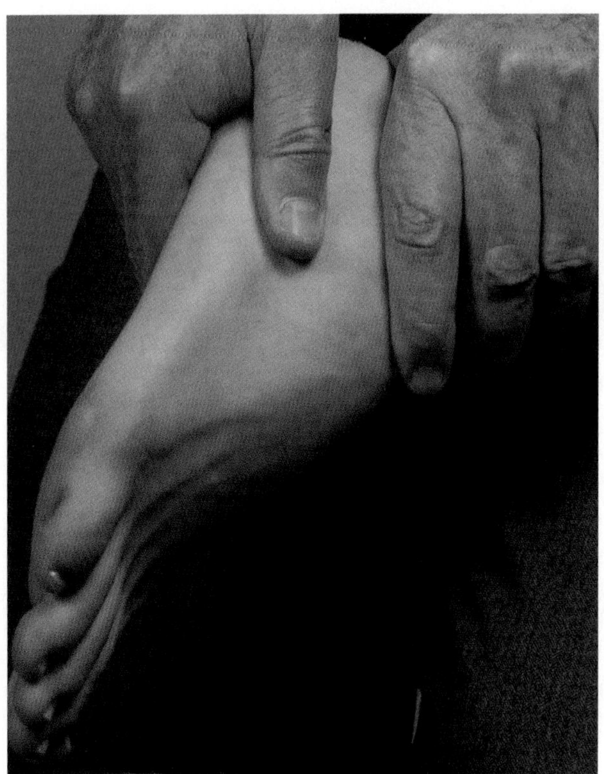

FIGURE 21-43 Cotton (Clunk) Test.

The patient sits with their legs dangling over the end of the bed, the knee flexed to approximately 90 degrees, and the foot relaxed. The clinician stabilizes the lower leg with one hand and, using the other hand, grasps the foot and externally rotates it (Fig. 21-44). Pain experienced at the anterolateral aspect of the distal tibiofibular syndesmosis is a positive sign for syndesmosis injury,[170] whereas pain on the medial aspect of the ankle and/or displacement of the talus from the medial malleolus (depending on severity) with the ankle positioned in plantar flexion may indicate a tear of the medial (deltoid) ligament of the ankle. Alonso et al.[170] reported data that indicate that the external rotation stress test is more reliable than the squeeze test and the dorsiflexion–compression test for diagnosing syndesmosis injuries.

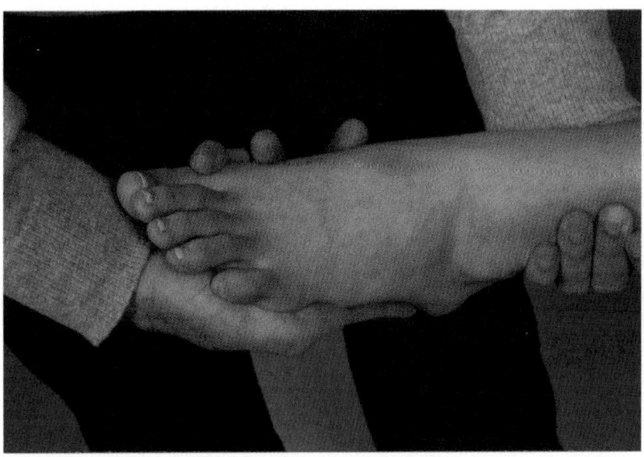

FIGURE 21-44 Kleiger (external rotation) test.

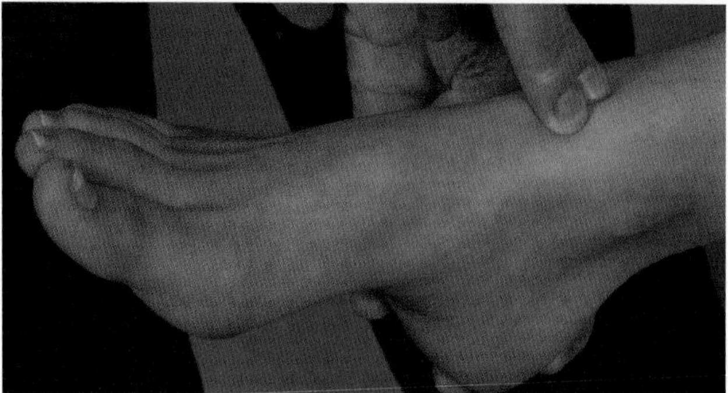

FIGURE 21-45 The point test.

The Point Test[170,171]

The point test, also referred to as the palpation test, is used to impose pressure on the anterior distal tibiofibular syndesmosis. The patient can be positioned in supine or sitting. The clinician applies pressure directly over the anterior aspect of the distal tibiofibular syndesmosis (Fig. 21-45). Pressure is applied gradually, and a positive test involves a report of pain by the patient.

The Dorsiflexion Maneuver[171,172]

The dorsiflexion maneuver is performed to force the wider anterior portion of the talar dome into the ankle mortise, thereby inducing separation of the distal fibula and tibia. The patient sits at the edge of the examination table, and the clinician stabilizes the patient's leg with one hand, while the clinician's other hand passively moves the foot into dorsiflexion (Fig. 21-46). Pain experienced at the distal tibiofibular syndesmosis is a positive test result. A variation of the dorsiflexion maneuver exists, known as the dorsiflexion compression test,[170] which involves patients moving their ankle joints into extreme dorsiflexion in bilateral weight-bearing. Patients are asked to note the pain they experience in this position and the position of the tibia is noted with an inclinometer. The patient then assumes an upright position, and the clinician applies medial–lateral compression with two hands on the malleoli of the injured leg. The clinician maintains the medial–lateral compression, as the patient is asked to move the ankles into dorsiflexion again and to report if the end-range pain has changed compared with the previous movement. A positive test result is either a reported reduction in the end-range pain or an increase in dorsiflexion ROM.

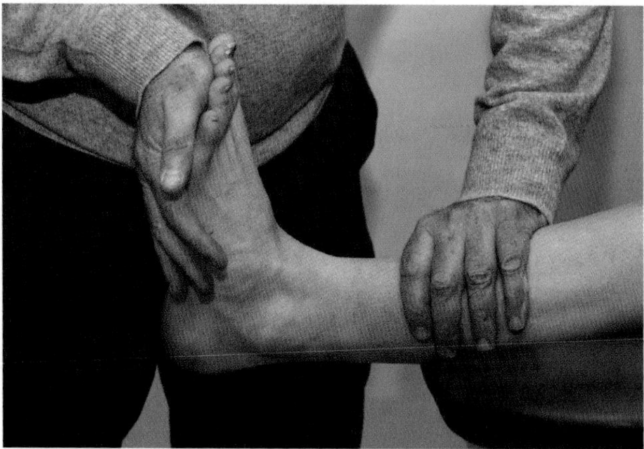

FIGURE 21-46 The dorsiflexion maneuver.

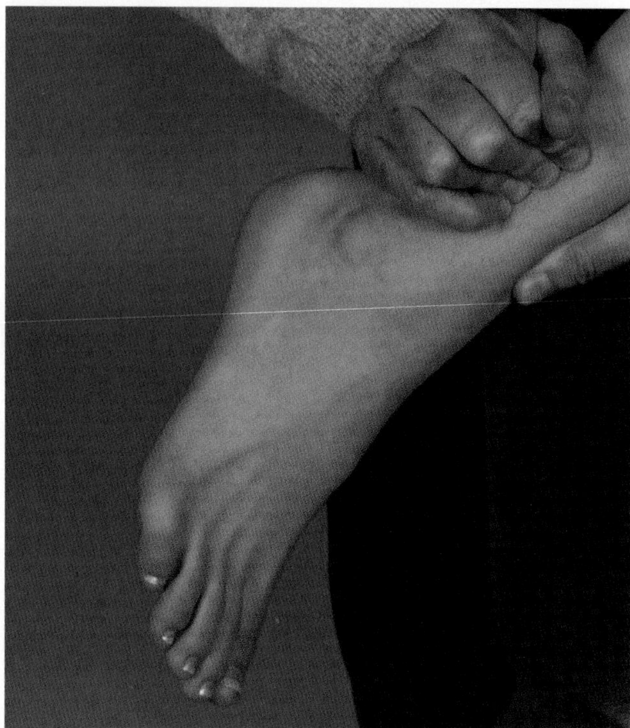

FIGURE 21-47 Fibula translation test.

Fibula Translation Test

The patient is placed in the side-lying position with the tested leg uppermost. The clinician applies an anterior and posterior force on the fibula at the level of the syndesmosis (Fig. 21-47). A positive test is pain during translation and more displacement of the fibula than the compared side. Although a cadaver study by Beumer et al.[166] found this test to have a sensitivity of 82% and specificity of 88% (LR+ 6.8; LR− 0.2), the study only found increased translation when all ligaments were removed in the cadavers.

The One-legged Hop Test[171,173]

The one-legged hop test is performed by having the patient stand on the injured leg and hop continuously. Nussbaum et al.[173] reported that patients with syndesmosis injuries could not complete 10 repetitions of unilateral hopping without significant pain. However, the one-legged hop test should be used with caution, and perhaps only if the other special tests are negative, because performing this test may impose further separation of the distal tibiofibular syndesmosis.[171]

The Crossed-Leg Test[171,174]

The crossed-leg test mimics the squeeze test (see later) and attempts to induce separation of the distal syndesmosis. The patient sits in a chair, with the injured leg resting across the knee of the uninjured leg. The resting point should be at approximately mid-calf. The clinician then applies a gentle

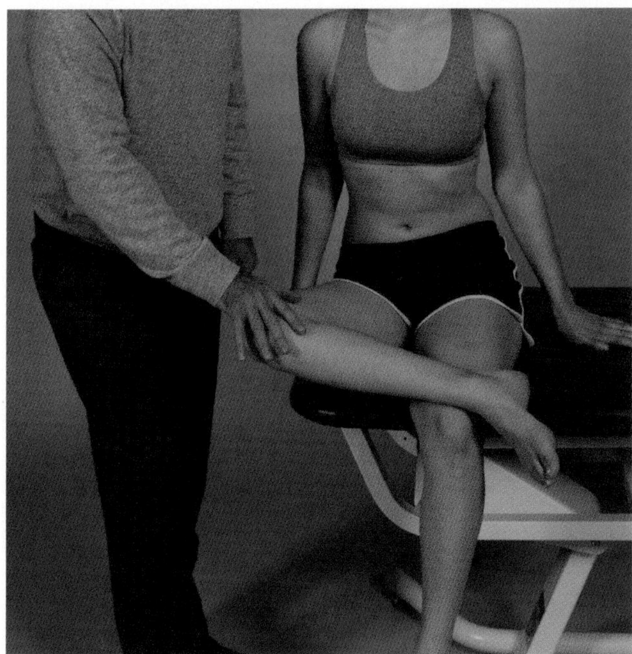

FIGURE 21-48 The crossed-leg test.

force on the medial aspect of the knee of the test leg (Fig. 21-48). Pain experienced in the area of the distal syndesmosis suggests the presence of injury. This test may not be useful for patients with knee or hip pathology because it may be difficult for them to assume the test position. Reliability and validity data for this test are not yet available.

The Heel-Thump Test[171,175]

The heel-thump test is performed to force the talus into the mortise, in an attempt to impose separation of the distal syndesmosis. The patient lies at the edge of the examination table, with the ankle resting in plantar flexion. The clinician holds the patient's leg with one hand and with the other hand applies a gentle but firm thump on the heel with their fist (Fig. 21-49). This force is applied at the center of the heel and in line with the long axis of the tibia. Pain experienced at the distal tibiofibular syndesmosis suggests the presence of injury. Although the heel thump test has been recommended to help differentiate between a syndesmotic sprain and a lateral ankle sprain, this test may not be specific for a syndesmotic sprain as the test has also been recommended to assess the possible presence of tibial stress fractures.[176] Reliability and validity data for this test are not yet available.

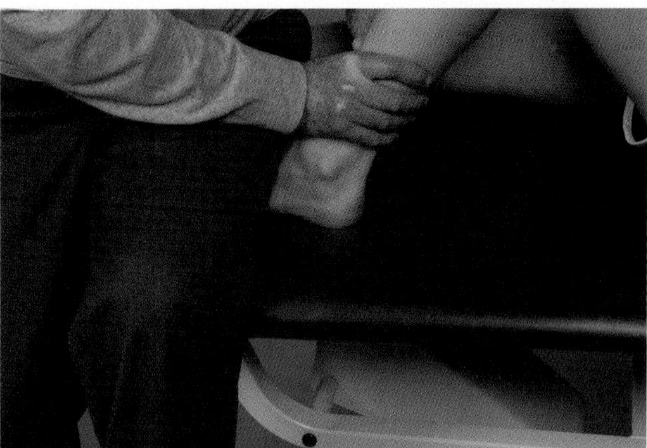

FIGURE 21-50 Posterior drawer test.

Posterior Drawer Test

The posterior drawer test can also be used to test for the presence of instability at the distal tibiofibular joint. The patient is supine. The hip and knee are flexed to provide as much dorsiflexion of the ankle as possible. This drives the wide anterior part of the talus back into the mortise. An anterior stabilizing force is then applied to the cruris, and the foot and talus are translated posteriorly (Fig. 21-50). If the distal tibiofibular joint is stable, there will be no drawer available, but if there is instability, there will be a drawer.

Squeeze (Distal Tibiofibular Compression) Test

In the squeeze test, the patient lies in supine or side-lying position and the clinician squeezes the upper to middle third of the leg at a point approximately 6–8 inches below the knee (Fig. 21-51).[137] Pain felt in the distal third of the leg may indicate a compromised syndesmosis, if the presence of a tibia and/or fibula fracture, calf contusion, or compartment syndrome has been ruled out.[126,168]

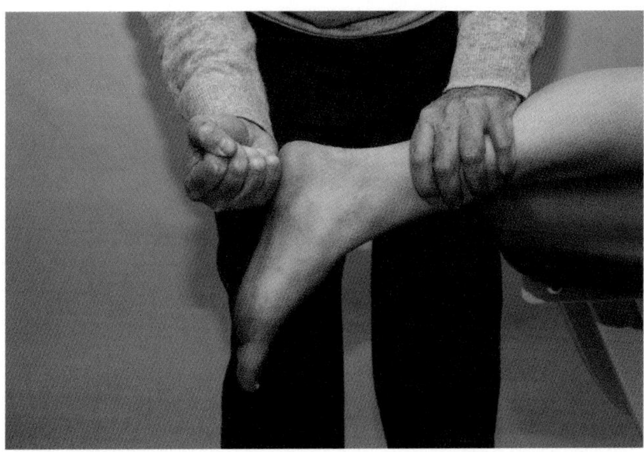

FIGURE 21-49 The heel-thump test.

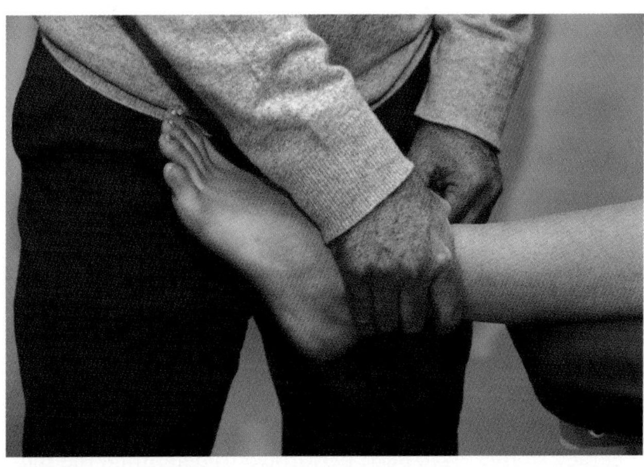

FIGURE 21-51 Squeeze test.

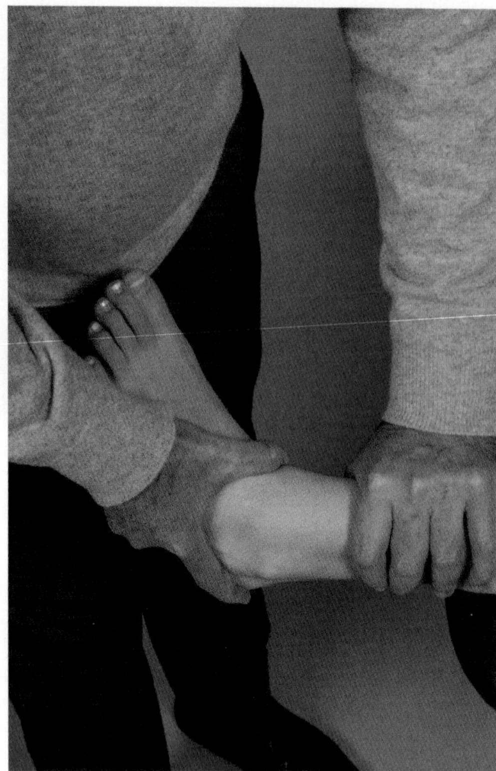

FIGURE 21-52 Calcaneus tilt.

Lateral Collaterals

The lateral collateral ligaments of the ankle resist inversion. An additional function is to prevent excessive varus movement, especially during plantar flexion. In extreme plantar flexion, the mortise no longer stabilizes the broader anterior part of the talus, and varus movement of the ankle is then possible.

Calcaneus Tilt

The patient lies in the supine position. The lower leg is stabilized using a lumbrical grip, while the other hand grasps the foot and calcaneus. The clinician applies a medially directed force in an attempt to adduct the calcaneus, thereby gapping the lateral side of the ankle (Fig. 21-52). Pain on the lateral aspect of the ankle with this test, and/or displacement (depending on severity), may indicate a sprain of the ligament. Hertel et al.[177] found this test to have a sensitivity of 78% and a specificity of 75% (LR+ 3.1; LR− 0.29).

Talar Tilt

This test is used to determine whether the CFL is torn. The patient lies in a supine or side-lying position with the foot relaxed and the knee flexed. The clinician places the foot in the anatomical (90 degrees) position to bring the CFL perpendicular to the long axis of the talar. The talus is then tilted from side to side into adduction and abduction (Fig. 21-53). Adduction tests the CFL and, to some degree, the ATFL, whereas abduction stresses the deltoid ligament. No diagnostic accuracy studies have been performed to determine the sensitivity and specificity of this test.

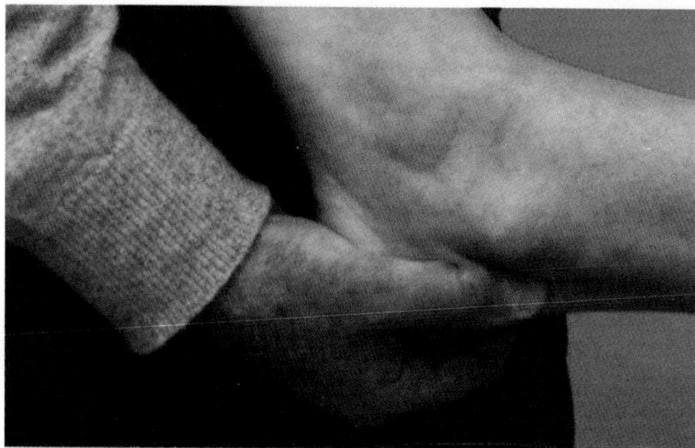

FIGURE 21-53 Talar tilt.

Anterior Drawer Test

The anterior drawer stress test is performed to estimate the stability of the ATFL.[28,178,179] The test is performed with the patient seated at the end of the bed or lying supine with their knee flexed, to relax the gastrocnemius–soleus muscles, and the foot supported perpendicular to the leg.[180,178] The clinician uses one hand to stabilize the distal aspect of the leg, while the other hand grasps the patient's heel and positions the ankle in 10–15 degrees of plantar flexion (Fig. 21-54). The heel is very gently pulled forward, and if the test is positive, the talus, and with it the foot, rotates anteriorly out of the ankle mortise around the intact medial (deltoid) ligament of the ankle, which serves as the center of rotation. Tohyama et al.[179] reported that a relatively low anterior load (30 N) during this test was more sensitive than a higher load (60 N) in distinguishing a significant distance between injured to normal anterior displacement. This seemingly occurs because a greater load would tend to elicit a protective muscle contraction that could mask the anterior talar displacement.

This test has limited reliability, particularly if it is negative or if it is performed without anesthesia in the presence of muscle guarding.[181] It has been reported that 4 mm of laxity in the ATFL, resulting from posttraumatic attenuation or fibrosis, will give a clinically apparent anterior drawer (2 mm is normal)—false-positive findings may be seen in up to 19%

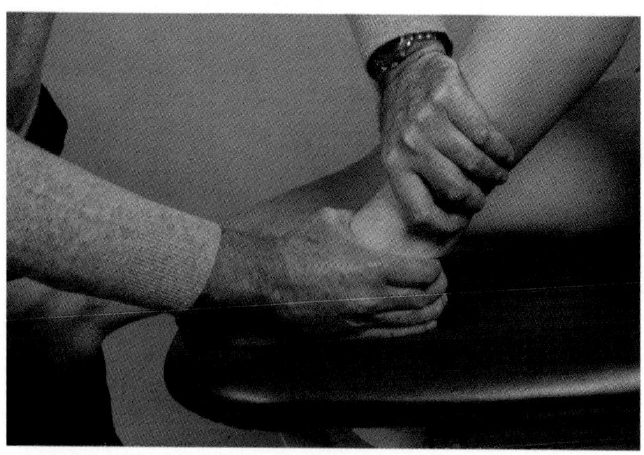

FIGURE 21-54 Anterior drawer test.

of uninjured ankles in those with ligamentous laxity.[182–184] As is often the case, when combining the results from several tests, diagnostic accuracy can be enhanced. For example, van Dijk et al.[185] reported that when the combination of pain on lateral ligament palpation, hematoma formation of the lateral ankle, and a positive anterior drawer test were used a lateral ligament lesion was correctly diagnosed in 95% of cases.

The Dimple Sign

Another positive sign for a rupture of the ATFL, if pain and spasm are minimal, is the presence of a dimple located just in front of the tip of the lateral malleolus during the anterior drawer test.[186] This results from a negative pressure created by the forward movement of the talus, which draws the skin inwards at the site of the ligament rupture.[187] This dimple is also seen with a combined rupture of the ATFL and CFLs.[186] However, the dimple is only present within the first 48 hours after injury, due to organized hematoma and repair tissue blocking the communication between the joint and the subcutaneous tissues.[186]

Medial Collaterals (Deltoid Complex)

The medial collaterals function to resist eversion. Given their strength, these ligaments are usually only injured as the result of a major trauma.

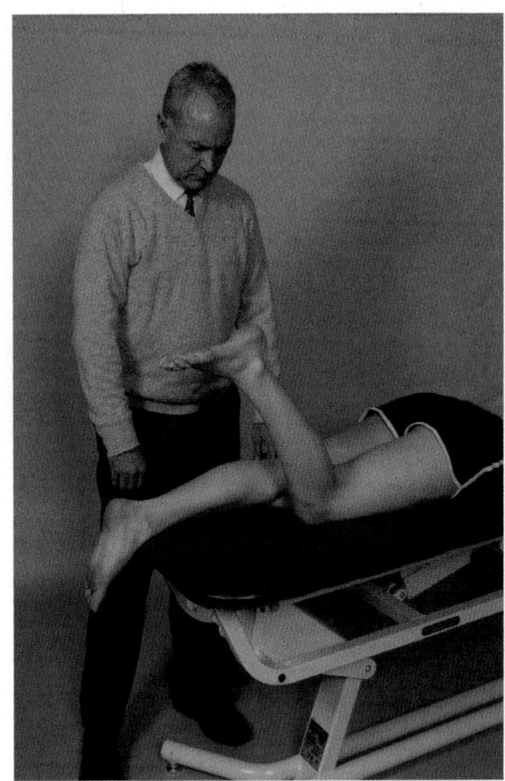

FIGURE 21-56 Matles test for Achilles tendon rupture.

Tendon Tests

Thompson Test for Achilles Tendon Rupture

In this test, the patient lies in the prone position or in kneeling with the feet over the edge of the bed (Fig. 21-55). With the patient relaxed, the clinician gently squeezes the calf muscle and observes for the production of plantar flexion. An absence of plantar flexion indicates a complete rupture of the Achilles tendon.[188] This test has been found to have surprisingly low sensitivity (40%).[188]

Matles Test for Achilles Tendon Rupture

The patient lies in the prone position with the foot over the end of the table and the clinician stands at the end of the table. The patient is asked to actively flex the knee to 90 degrees while the position of the foot is observed throughout the motion (Fig. 21-56). If the foot falls into neutral or slight dorsiflexion, the test is positive for Achilles tendon rupture (in normal patients, the foot remains in plantar flexion). Maffulli[189] found this test to have a sensitivity of 0.88, a specificity of 0.85, and a positive predictive value of 0.92.

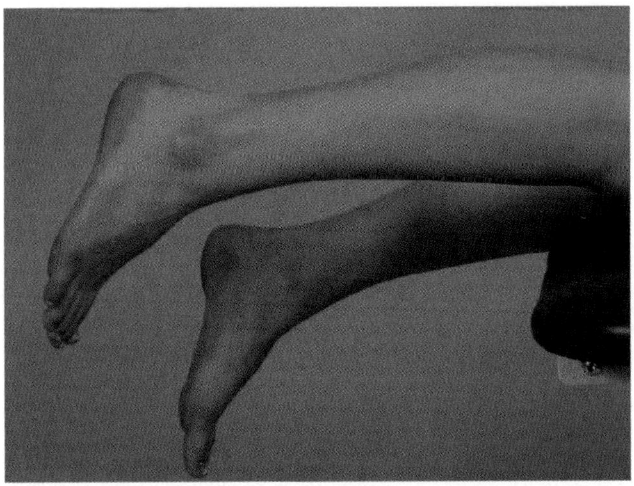

FIGURE 21-55 Patient position for the Thompson test.

Articular Stability Tests

Navicular Drop Test

The navicular drop test is a method to assess the degree to which the talus plantar flexes in space on a calcaneus that has been stabilized by the ground, during subtalar joint pronation.[190,191]

The clinician palpates the position of the navicular tubercle as the patient's foot is non–weight-bearing but resting on the floor surface, with the subtalar joint maintained in neutral. The clinician then attempts to quantify the amount of inferior displacement of the navicular tubercle, as the patient assumes 50% weight-bearing on the tested foot (relaxed standing).[139] A navicular drop that is greater than 10 mm from the neutral position to the relaxed standing position suggests excessive medial longitudinal arch collapse of abnormal pronation.[191,192]

This test has been found to have an intratester reliability that ranged from ICC = 0.61 to 0.79 and intertester reliability of ICC = 0.57.[139] However, it is questionable whether a significant drop is also indicative of dysfunction.

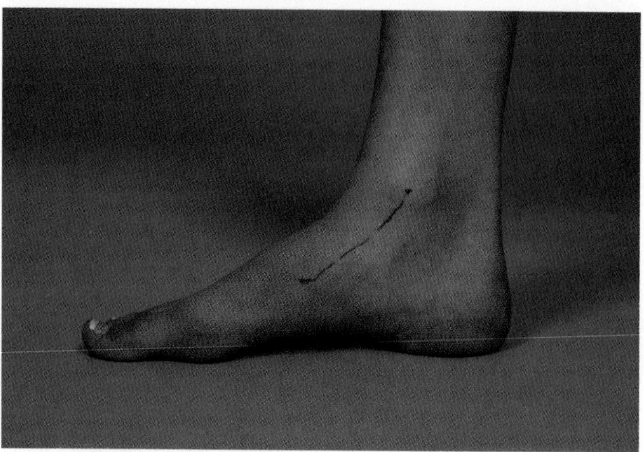

FIGURE 21-57 Feiss line.

Feiss Line[193]

The Feiss line test is used to assess the height of the medial arch, using the navicular position. With the patient non-weight-bearing, the clinician marks the apex of the medial malleolus and the plantar aspect of the first MTP joint, and a line is drawn between the two points (Fig. 21-57). The navicular is palpated on the medial aspect of the foot, and an assessment is made of the position of the navicular relative to the imaginary line. The patient is then asked to stand with their feet approximately 3–6 inches apart. In weight-bearing, the navicular normally lies on or very close to the line. If the navicular falls one-third of the distance to the floor, it represents a first-degree flatfoot; if it falls two-thirds of the distance, it represents a second-degree flatfoot; and if it rests on the floor, it represents a third-degree flatfoot. No diagnostic accuracy studies have been performed to determine the sensitivity and specificity of this test.

Vascular Status

Homans' Sign

This was the traditional test used to detect a deep vein thrombophlebitis (DVT). The patient lies in the supine position with their knee extended. The clinician stabilizes the thigh with one hand and passively dorsiflexes the patient's ankle with the other. Pain in the calf with this maneuver was considered a positive sign for DVT. However, a positive Homan's sign has been found to be insensitive, nonspecific, is present in fewer than 30% of documented cases of DVT,[194,195] and the performance of the test may increase the risk of producing a pulmonary embolism (PE).

Buerger's Test

The patient is placed in the supine position with the knee extended. The clinician elevates the patient's leg to approximately 45 degrees and maintains it there for at least 3 minutes. Blanching of the foot is positive for poor arterial circulation, especially if, when the patient sits with the legs over the end of the bed, it takes 1–2 minutes for the limb color to be restored.

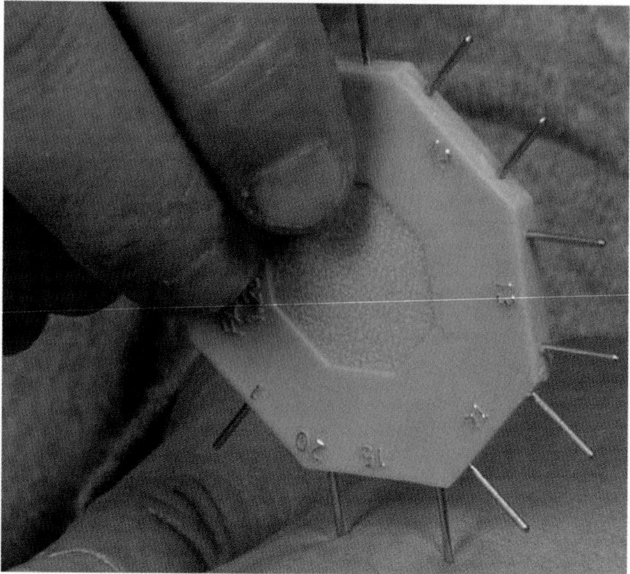

FIGURE 21-58 Sensory testing using pinprick.

Posterior (Dorsal) Pedis Pulse

The posterior (dorsal) pedis pulse can be palpated just lateral to the tendon of the extensor hallucis longus over the posterior aspect of the foot (see Fig. 21-14).

Neurologic Tests

The applicable sensory, motor, and reflex tests should be performed if a disorder related to a spinal nerve root (L4–S2) or peripheral nerve is suspected. A neurogenic cause of foot pain must be considered in a patient, especially if the pain is refractory. The patient usually complains of pain that is poorly localized, which is aggravated by activity but may also occur at rest. Any difference in sensation between extremities should be noted and can be mapped out in more detail by testing pinprick sensation (Fig. 21-58). The segmental and peripheral nerve innervations are listed in Chapter 3. Common muscle stretch reflexes tested in this area are the Achilles reflex (S1–2) and the posterior tibialis reflex (L4–5). Specific pathologies associated with peripheral nerve entrapment are described in the intervention strategies section.

The pathologic reflexes (Babinski and Oppenheim), tested when an upper motor neuron lesion is suspected, are described in Chapter 3.

Morton's Test.[196]

The patient is positioned in supine. The clinician grasps the foot around the metatarsal heads and squeezes the heads together. The reproduction of pain with this maneuver indicates the presence of a neuroma or a stress fracture. No diagnostic accuracy studies have been performed to determine the sensitivity and specificity of this test.

Tinel's Sign

The posterior tibial nerve may be tapped behind the medial malleolus (Fig. 21-59). Tingling or paresthesia with this test is considered a positive finding. As with all Tinel's test

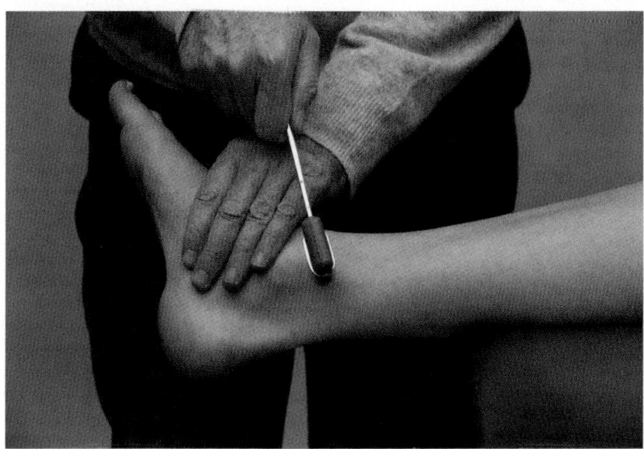

FIGURE 21-59 Tinel's sign.

throughout the body, this test provides only marginal sensitivity (58%).[197]

Imaging Studies

Radiography

According to the Ottawa rules for ankle X-rays (with Buffalo modifications),[198,199] X-rays are indicated to rule out fracture of the ankle when there is bone tenderness in the posterior half of the lower 6 cm of the fibula or tibia and an inability to bear weight immediately after injury.[198–200] Similarly, if there is bone tenderness over the navicular and/or fifth metatarsal, and an inability to bear weight immediately after injury, then radiographs of the foot are indicated (see Chap. 7).[198,200]

Other imaging techniques include arthrography, fibular (peroneal) tenography, and magnetic resonance imaging (MRI).

THE EVALUATION

Following the examination, and once the clinical findings have been recorded, the clinician must determine a specific diagnosis or a working hypothesis, based on a summary of all of the findings. This diagnosis can be structure related (medical diagnosis) (Table 21-10) or a diagnosis based on the preferred practice patterns as described in the *Guide to Physical Therapist Practice*.

INTERVENTION STRATEGIES

Due to the incorporated nature of the foot and ankle structures in functional activities, the rehabilitation for this region is best organized around a common framework for most foot and ankle pathologies.[201]

The techniques to increase joint mobility and the techniques to increase soft tissue extensibility are described in the "Therapeutic Techniques" section.

Acute Phase

The goals during the acute phase include:

- decreasing pain, inflammation, and swelling;
- protecting the healing area from reinjury;
- re-establishing pain-free ROM;
- preventing muscle atrophy;
- increasing weight-bearing tolerance;
- increasing neuromuscular control;
- maintaining fitness levels;
- attaining patient independence with a home-exercise program.

The control of pain, inflammation, and swelling is accomplished by applying the principles of PRICEMEM (protection, rest, ice, compression, elevation, manual therapy, early motion, and medication). Icing for 20–30 minutes several times a day, concurrent with nonsteroidal anti-inflammatory drugs (NSAIDs) can aid in reducing pain and swelling.

The injured ankle should be positioned and supported in the maximum amount of dorsiflexion allowed by pain and effusion. Maximal dorsiflexion places the joint in its close-packed position or position of greatest congruency.[202] This allows for the least capsular distention and resultant joint effusion. With ankle sprains, this position produces an approximation of the torn ligament ends in grade III injuries to reduce the amount of gap scarring and reduces the tension in the grades I and II injured ligaments.[16,125]

The means by which to support or protect the joint during this phase will vary depending on the severity of the injury and the anticipated compliance of the patient to any restrictions placed on them by the physician.[16,125] For example, mild-to-moderate ankle sprains (grade I and II sprains) can be readily supported by the use of an elastic bandage, open Gibney strapping (with or without felt-pad incorporation), taping,[203–208] or the use of some type of thermoplastic stirrup such as an Air Cast (see next section).[209,210] One of the main advantages of this type of immobilization is that pain-free protected plantar flexion and dorsiflexion are possible, whereas inversion and eversion are minimized.

To increase ROM, the clinician can perform gentle capsular stretches and grades I–II joint mobilizations. Exercises in this phase include towel stretches VIDEO (Fig. 21-60), ankle circles VIDEO and pumps, VIDEO low-level biomechanical ankle platform system (BAPS) exercises (Fig. 21-61), and active and active assist exercises in straight planes (plantar flexion, dorsiflexion, inversion, and eversion) and proprioceptive neuromuscular facilitation (PNF) planes. Exercises for the foot intrinsics may include toe curl exercises with a towel VIDEO (Fig. 21-62) or having the patient pick up marbles from the floor with their toes and place the marbles in a small container or bowl VIDEO.

Isometric exercises within the patient's pain tolerance and pain-free ROM are initiated for all motions. These exercises are initially performed submaximally at multi-angles, progressing to maximal isometric contractions as tolerated. Mild manual resistive isometrics in all planes may also be started throughout the pain-free range. Active motion and exercise

TABLE 21-10 Differential Diagnosis of Common Causes of Leg, Foot, and Ankle Pain

Condition	Patient Age	Mechaism of Injury	Area of Symptoms	Symptoms Aggravated by	Observation	AROM	PROM	Resisted	Special Tests	Tenderness with Palpation
Gastrocnemius strain	20–40	Sudden overload	Upper calf	Heel raise	Antalgic gait	Painful and limited DF	Pain with overpressure into DF Restricted range of DF with knee extended	Pain on PF		Mid to upper calf
Plantar fascitis	20–60	Gradual with no known cause	Sole of foot (under heel)	Weight-bearing especially first thing in the morning	Unremark able Flattened arches Pronated foot	Full and pain free	Pain with overpressure into great toe extension	Weak foot intrinsics	Pressure applied over plantar fascial insertion site on the calcaneus	Plantar aspect of heel
Achilles tendinitis	20–40	Overuse	Posterior ankle	Jumping, running	Minor swelling of posterior ankle	Painful and limited DF	Pain with overpressure into DF Restricted range of DF with knee extended	Pain on PF		Posterior ankle
Posterior tibialis tendinitis	20–40	Overuse with a flat pronated foot	Medial ankle, along the course of the tendon	Activities involving weight-bearing plantar flexion	Possible peritendinous swelling over medial ankle	Pain on eversion Pain on PF	Pain with overpressure into eversion Pain with overpressure into PF	Pain on resited inversion with the foot plantar flexed	Rule out tear with heel raise symmetry	Medial ankle
Morton's neuroma	40–60	Gradual with no known cause	Sole of foot	Weight-bearing	Pronated foot Flattened arches	Full and pain free	Pain with overpressure into toe extension	Strong and painless		Web spaces of toes

Retrocalcaneal bursitis	Varies	Direct irritation of bursa. usually from shoe	Hindfoot	Friction	Possible swelling, erythema of hindfoot	Usually unremarkable	Usually unremarkable	Usually unremarkable	Palpation	Just above the insertion site of the Achilles tendon on the calcaneus
Anterior tibialis tendinitis	15–45	Overuse	Anterior lower leg	Activities involving repetitive dorsiflexion	Unremarkable	Pain with combined PF and inversion	Pain with overpressure into PF	Pain on DF		Anterolateral lower leg
Tarsal tunnel syndrome	25–50	Posttraumatic, neoplastic, inflammatory, rapid weight gain, fluid retention, abnormal foot/ankle mechanics or a valgus foot deformity	Medial malleolus, distribution of posterior tibial nerve up the leg, or down into the medial arch, plantar surface of the foot and toes	Excessive dynamic pronation in walking or running	Pronated foot, pes planus, possible swelling	Full and pain free	Pain with extreme plantar flexion and eversion	Weak toe flexion (late)	Positive Tinel's over tarsal tunnel	No tenderness usually
Midfoot Sprain	15–40	High impact landing sports Foot twisted when in fixed position	Midfoot	Walking on toes	Usually unremarkable	Usually unremarkable	Usually unremarkable	Usually unremarkable	Weight-bearing lateral and anterior–posterior radiographs	Generalized tenderness of midfoot
Medial tibial stress syndrome	15–30	Overuse	Anterior lower leg Posterior-medial lower leg	Exercise involving involved lower extremity		Pain with combined PF and inversion	Full and pain free	Pain on PF Pain on eversion		Posteromedial calf

(Continued)

TABLE 21-10 Differential Diagnosis of Common Causes of Leg, Foot, and Ankle Pain *(Continued)*

Condition	Patient Age	Mechaism of Injury	Area of Symptoms	Symptoms Aggravated by	Observation	AROM	PROM	Resisted	Special Tests	Tenderness with Palpation
Metatarsal stress fracture	15–45	Overuse	Forefoot	Weight-bearing activities	Possible edema over fracture site	Usually unremarkable	Usually unremarkable	Usually unremarkable	Palpation, ultrasound, tuning fork, bone scan, MRI, CT scan	Maximal point tenderness over the bone at the fracture site
Referred	Varies	Symptoms can be referred from the lumbar spine, hip, knee, or from systemic diseases such as diabetes mellitus (DM), spondyloarthropathy (Reiter's syndrome)	May be dermatomal if spinal nerve involved; stocking-like if DM, bilateral heels if Reiter's	Activities unrelated to foot and ankle; unrelated to activity	Varies, but may be unremarkable	Usually unremarkable	Usually unremarkable	Usually unremarkable, but weakness may be present if spinal nerve root involved	Sensation, DTR, lab tests	Tenderness of joint if spondyloarthropathy

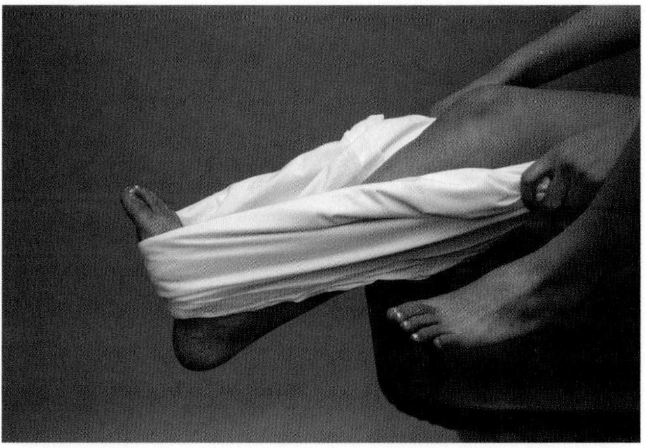

FIGURE 21-60 Towel stretch.

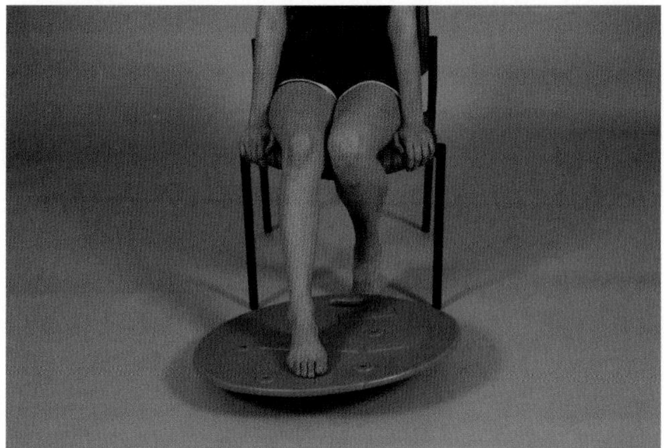

FIGURE 21-61 BAPS exercise.

may also be used to effectively increase local circulation and further promote the resorption of any persistent edema.[211,212] Exercises are progressed to include concentric exercises, once the isometric exercises are pain free. Seated lower extremity closed kinetic-chain exercises (Fig. 21-63) may also be performed during this phase.

Each muscle or muscle group should be strengthened with a specific exercise that isolates the muscle or group. Resistance

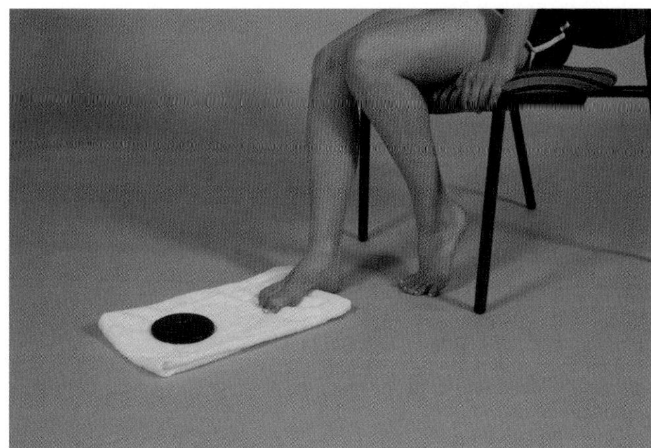

FIGURE 21-62 Towel toe curls.

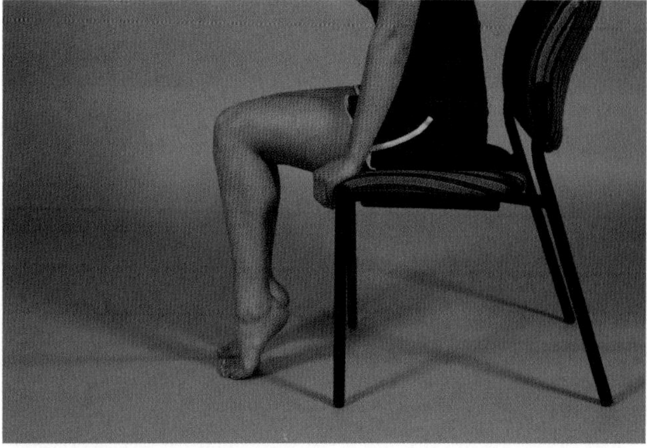

FIGURE 21-63 Seated heel raises.

(rubber tubing/bands, weights, isokinetic devices, body weight exercises, etc.) is increased as tolerated. Emphasis should initially be at low resistance and endurance in all pain-free positions. As the program progresses, the joint range is increased from a stress-free position to a more stressful position. As with all exercises, the patient should become an active participant at the earliest opportunity. The exercises learned in the clinic need to be integrated appropriately into a home-exercise regimen.

Pain-free weight-bearing as tolerated is encouraged with the use of any appropriate support or assistive device, such as taping, a brace, a cane or crutches VIDEO.[213,214] The use of an assistive device is usually continued until the patient has a pain-free uncompensated gait. Even when using an assistive device, pain-free ankle motion during the normal gait cycle and as normal a gait as possible continues to be encouraged VIDEO.

Specific joint mobilization techniques[215] and muscle stretching are initiated to begin to increase ROM.

Bracing

Braces can play an important role in both the initial intervention and prevention of ankle injuries. Acutely, their role is to compress, protect, and support the ankle. They also function to limit ROM of the injured ankle, most importantly plantar flexion and inversion, which is a precarious position for the sprained ankle.[129]

Functional braces that provide medial–lateral stabilization such as the Air Cast (Air Cast, Inc., Summit, NJ) also provide compressive force that assists in decreasing effusion.[16,125] Patients who suffer a grade III ligament injury may require more protection and support than can be afforded by a thermoplastic device. In cases such as this, consideration should be given to using a functional walking orthosis, either with a fixed ankle or a hinged ankle (which can be motion restricted) that allows only plantar flexion and dorsiflexion.[16,125] The advantage of the orthosis is that it is removable to allow the patient to continue to ice to minimize inflammation.

Overall, braces have been demonstrated to be biomechanically effective in preventing, decreasing, or slowing motions that cause injury to the lateral ankle ligaments.[216]

Although, one study[217] reported that braces were not as effective as freshly applied tape (see taping), clinically, braces appear to be as effective, if not more effective, than tape in the prevention of lateral ankle sprains.[218–222] The injury rate in one study by Sitler et al.[220] reported that the ankle injury rate was more than triple in the nonbraced players compared with braced players during intramural basketball at West Point.

In the presence of instability, the ankle joint is best supported by a commercial brace, with or without taping, depending on the stress of the sport.[16,125]

Night Splinting

Night splinting of the ankle in dorsiflexion has been postulated to prevent nocturnal contracture of the gastrocnemius–soleus complex, which is thought to be detrimental to plantar fascia healing.[223–225] The splint holds the ankle fixed in 5 degrees of dorsiflexion and the toes slightly stretched into dorsiflexion (i.e., at a functional length).[38] For most patients, this orthosis reduces morning pain considerably.[225] Powell et al.[224] performed a crossover study using splinting with the ankle in dorsiflexion as the sole method of treatment in 47 patients. This study also showed improvement in 80% of involved feet.

Functional Phase

For the patient to progress to the functional phase of the rehabilitation program, pain-free weight-bearing, and an uncompensated gait pattern must be present. However, pain may still be felt with activities more vigorous than walking. In addition, there should be minimal pain and tenderness, full PROM and strength rated at 4/5 to 5/5 with manual muscle testing as compared with the uninvolved side.[201] A recurrence of symptoms should not be provoked. The goals of this phase are as follows:

- to restore normal joint kinematics;
- to attain full range of pain-free motion;
- to improve neuromuscular control of the lower extremity in a full-weight-bearing posture on both level and uneven surfaces;
- to improve or regain lower extremity strength and endurance through integration of local and kinetic chain exercises;
- to return to previous level of function or recreation.

Exercises during this phase include manually resisted exercises, concentric exercises with tubing into dorsiflexion (Fig. 21-64), VIDEO plantar flexion VIDEO, inversion VIDEO, and eversion (Fig. 21-65) VIDEO. Exercise tubing can also be used for toe flexion VIDEO and extension VIDEO. Closed-chain exercises include, but are not limited to, seated marching on the floor VIDEO or pillow VIDEO, unilateral stance on the floor VIDEO, weight shifting VIDEO, standing bilateral or unilateral heel raises VIDEO, standing gastrocnemius stretch VIDEO, wall slide VIDEO, toe walking VIDEO, heel walking VIDEO, and supine leg press VIDEO. Emphasis should be placed on regaining any dorsiflexion that was lost. Regaining dorsiflexion can also be assisted by the use of a tilt board or heel cord stretching box. The

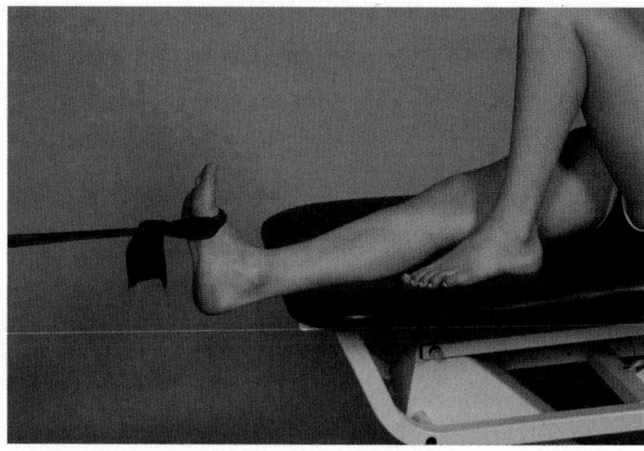

FIGURE 21-64 Dorsiflexion PRE with resistive tubing.

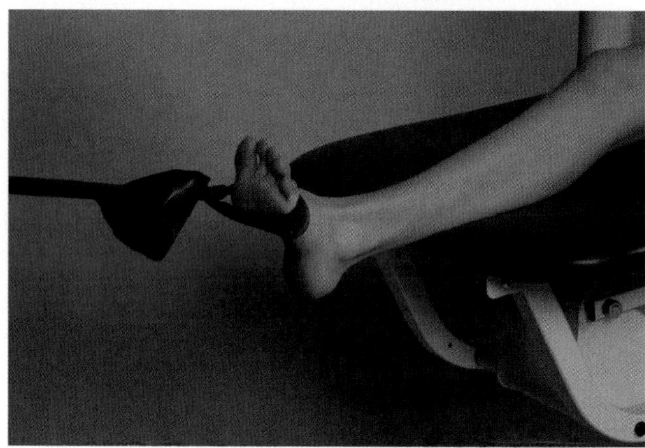

FIGURE 21-65 Eversion PRE with resistive tubing.

gastrocnemius is stretched by keeping the knee straight (Fig. 21-66) and the soleus is stretched by flexing the knee (Fig. 21-67).[205,214]

Proprioceptive exercises are especially important for full functional return and injury prevention.[16,125] Three factors are thought to cause functional instability of the ankle joint:[226]

- Anatomic or mechanical instability.
- Muscle weakness.
- Deficits in joint proprioception.

One of the all-to-common consequences of an ankle injury is an alteration of the motor conduction velocity of the fibular (peroneal) nerve and the protective function of the fibularis (peroneal) muscles on the ankle joint.[209,227,228] A decrease in fibular (peroneal) reaction time has been demonstrated to continue for up to 12 weeks after injury[209,227] despite a nearly full return of strength (96%) in comparison with the contralateral side.[227] An increase in the latency response of the fibularis (peroneal) muscles has also been demonstrated in normal subjects with an increase in plantar flexion, indicating a loss of protective reflexes when in this position.[229] The patient must train and be rehabilitated in all potential positions of injury.[16,125]

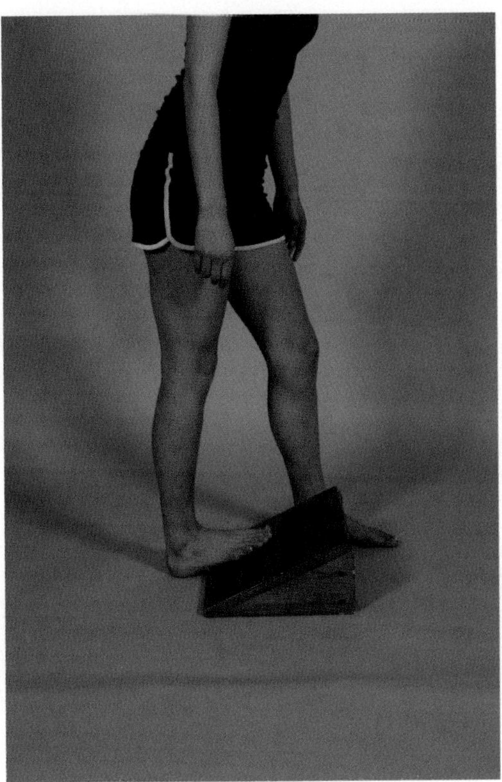

FIGURE 21-66 Gastrocnemius stetch.

A study by Rozzi et al.[155] demonstrated that a 4-week course of single-leg balance training showed an improvement in balance ability in both the trained and the untrained limbs. Examples of exercises to perform to enhance proprioception include unilateral stance on a pillow VIDEO, side (lateral) step up VIDEO, standing unilateral heel raise VIDEO, lunges onto VIDEO, or over VIDEO a pillow, backward step ups VIDEO, and cross-over walking VIDEO.

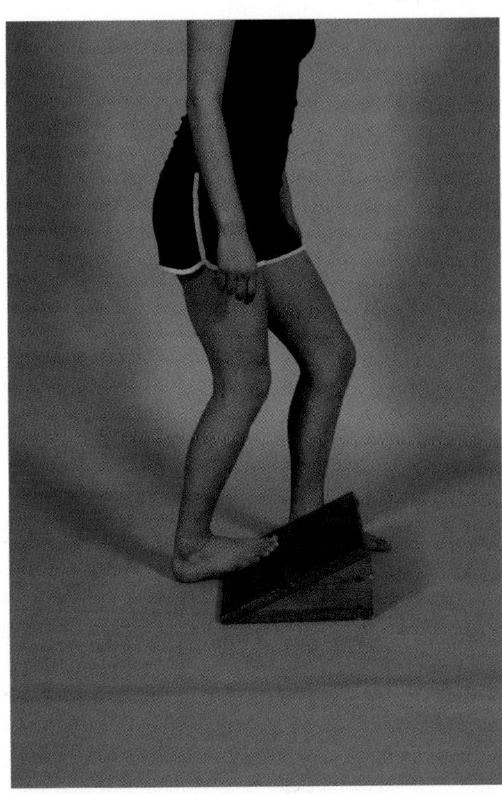

FIGURE 21-67 Soleus stretch.

After isolated strength exercises are initiated in the early portion of this phase, multidirectional, multijoint exercises should begin. Ankle PNF exercises are started based on the patient's tolerance.[230]

Multidirectional balance activities should progress from the non–weight-bearing, open-chained exercises until the ROM is full and painless, at which time closed-chain exercises are introduced with a progression to full-weight-bearing.[16,125] The greater the severity of injury, the more significant the need for multidirectional balance and weight-bearing rehabilitation activities.[231–238] These activities are effective in progressing the patient toward a progressive return to function. This progression involves beginning with a phase of walking or jogging on flat surfaces, ascending and descending stairs both forwards and backwards, with a progression to turning, changing directions and lateral movements while running, and eccentric loading with stair running.[127]

Further work is needed to fully determine the effect of training the responsiveness to ankle musculature to counteract potentially injurious stimuli. Until then, multidirectional balance activities and proprioceptive training should continue to be stressed as part of a clinical rehabilitation program.

Tests found to correlate well with good recovery are descending stairs, walking on heels and toes, and balancing on a square beam.[127,239] For some patients, the goal may be to return to sport. Progression to this level occurs when there is[201]:

- full pain-free active and passive ROM;
- no complaints of pain or tenderness;
- 75–80% strength of the plantar flexors, dorsiflexors, invertors, and evertors compared to the uninvolved side;
- adequate unilateral stance balance (30 seconds with eyes closed).

Before being allowed to return to full competition, the patient should be put through a functional test that simulates all requirements of his or her sport.[16,125] Observational analysis should be made of the patient's quality of movement and whether or not they are favoring the injured extremity in any way.[16,125] Activities during this phase involve cutting drills, shuttle runs, carioca crossover drills, and sports-specific activities such as lay-ups and dribbling.[129]

Full-strength, fibular (peroneal) latency response time and proprioceptive sense about the ankle may not return for many weeks even though the patient has returned to activity.[209,227,240]

Taping

Historically, ankle taping has been the athletic trainer's method of choice to attempt to prevent ankle sprains. Ankle taping is effective in restricting the motion of the ankle and has also been proved to decrease the incidence of ankle sprains.[241–246]

However, although taping initially restricts motion, the tape loses 50% of its net support after as little as 10 minutes of exercise.[217,246–254] Because of this deterioration of support, and the cost of tape, removable and reusable ankle braces were designed as an alternative to taping.[16,125]

The use of tape for increased proprioception remains controversial. It is hypothesized that the tape can either provide additional cutaneous cues or provide a general facilitation at spinal or higher levels, thereby enhancing the perception of movement signals from other proprioceptive sources,[255–258] although this has yet to be proved conclusively.[256,259,260]

The more common instabilities treated with taping include splaying of the mortise, inversion instability of the ankle, plantar instability of the talonavicular joint, and inversion or eversion instability of the talocalcaneal joint.[16,125]

- The mortise is taped circumferentially around the lateral and medial malleolus.
- Talocalcaneal instabilities are taped around the neck of the talus and the heel. With the exception of the inferior tibiofibular joint (which is a syndesmosis), the taping can effect a temporary improvement in symptoms and function.

The decision whether or not to use some type of protective taping or bracing upon return to activity to prevent reinjury is a decision based on the individual athlete and his or her case. No type of taping or bracing will prevent all injuries.[16,125]

CLINICAL PEARL

Often a player may argue that their performance will be adversely affected by the use of taping or bracing.[16,125] A review of the literature demonstrates that for normal athletic movement and function there does not appear to be an adverse impact on function or performance.[218,253,261–265] Indeed, one study involving soccer players, demonstrated a fivefold decrease in the incidence of recurrent ankle sprains when using semirigid orthoses, without significantly affecting sports performance.[222]

Footwear

The type of sneaker worn during basketball, high top versus low top, has been studied and shown to have no relationship to the incidence of injury.[242] However, it does appear that increased shoe height can enhance the passive resistance to inversion when the foot is in plantar flexion and can also increase the passive resistance afforded by tape and orthoses.[217]

One of the many contributing factors to running injuries is improper or worn out footwear. On average, running shoes wear out between 300 to 500 miles, although these figures are merely estimates and the actual distance at which a shoe breaks down may vary according to running style, training techniques and environmental conditions, including terrain and weather. Running in a shoe that no longer provides the correct protection in terms of cushioning, traction, and support may lead to heel pain, shin splints, tendinitis, and stress fractures.

CLINICAL PEARL

In general, a runner with a high medial longitudinal arch and a C-shaped foot, often characterized as a "supinator," tends to underpronate during midstance and should therefore be using a shoe with a softer midfoot and one that is more cushioned, especially on the lateral edge of the shoe.

Similarly, a runner with a low medial longitudinal arch, often characterized as a "pronator," tends to produce an excessive medial roll of the foot during the stance phase and should therefore be using a shoe designed for motion control of the rearfoot and with hard or rigid midsoles made from plastic or high-density foam that permit only minimal pronation.[266]

Orthotics

An orthosis can be defined as any device used to support, align, or protect joints or body segments, thus improving function.[267] If significant biomechanical variations from normal are noted during the examination, an orthosis may be indicated.

The principal purpose of a foot or ankle orthosis is as follows[267]:

- evenly distribute the weight-bearing forces on the plantar aspect of the foot;
- reduce stress on anatomic structures local or proximal to the foot and ankle by either force attenuation or control of joint motion;
- prevent, correct, or compensate for the presence of foot or ankle deformities.

A wide variety of materials are available for the fabrication of custom-made orthotics, which vary in elasticity, plasticity, compliance, and rigidity. A rigid orthosis is usually constructed from a hard thermoplastic, graphite, or fiberglass material. Semirigid devices can be composed of materials including leather, rubber, cork, polypropylene, and copolymers.

Biomechanical foot orthoses incorporate the concept of posting. The posts may be an addition of an extrinsic (relatively noncompressible) material to the shell of the orthoses, or an intrinsic post (using relatively rigid material) built into the design of the shell, which functions to balance the malalignment of the foot. Extrinsic posts offer the advantage of being easy to adjust, whereas intrinsic posts are much more difficult to adjust. Despite the widespread use of orthoses, questions are arising as to the theoretical basis for their use for the following reasons:[267]

- Any definition of "normal" foot alignment assumes that anything that falls outside the criteria for "normal" must be abnormal and associated with pathology; yet, studies have shown that the criteria we use to describe "normal" apply to very few individuals and that many asymptomatic individuals display foot abnormalities but meet those criteria.[268–270] Before correcting a malalignment using an orthotic, the clinician needs to determine more definitively the causal relationship between the malalignment and the patient's symptoms.

- The determination of subtalar neutral, the measurement that is the cornerstone for the prescription of orthotics, is relatively unreliable. While the intrarater reliability in determining subtalar neutral has been found to be acceptable,[271] the interrater reliability scores have demonstrated that therapists are frequently unable to agree with other therapists in determining subtalar neutral.[268,271]

Heel Lifts

The use of heel lifts is advocated in the literature for a variety of conditions, including Achilles tendinitis, plantar fasciitis, and calcaneal apophysitis.[43]

The material used to make the heel lift can be modified to increase shock absorption in cases of calcaneal bruising and heel spurs.[272]

Heel Cups

Heel cups are used for similar conditions as heel lifts, with the added benefit that the heel cup is able to help redistribute the forces through the heel better, and because the medial and lateral walls help contain the fat pads of the calcaneus, thus improving the natural shock-absorptive ability.[39,267,273]

Wedges

Prefabricated or custom-made wedges are referred to as a "post" when used in functional foot orthoses. Wedges are typically used to slant the entire foot or part of the foot either medially or laterally to prevent motion or change the weight-bearing aspect of the foot.

PREFERRED PRACTICE PATTERN 4B: IMPAIRED JOINT MOBILITY, MOTOR FUNCTION, MUSCLE PERFORMANCE, AND ROM ASSOCIATED WITH IMPAIRED POSTURE

Clinical findings with this pattern can include pain with sustained positions, structural deformities and deviations, limited ROM in a noncapsular pattern of restriction, and altered kinematics.

The Pronated Foot

In the normal foot, the angle of the rearfoot and forefoot intersect at 90 degrees, with a downward projection of the center of mass at 135 degrees, such that all of the forces counteract one another, resulting in zero net force and zero rotational velocity.[274] Any changes in this anatomical relationship can affect the static equilibrium. Pronation of the foot creates an angle greater than 90 degrees between the rearfoot and the forefoot. Static equilibrium can only now be maintained through a counteracting force such as the passive stretch of the passive plantar mechanism. Pronation of the ankle and foot during the stance phase of gait is in essence a temporary collapse of the ankle, rearfoot, and midfoot, which serves to provide a more adaptable structure. This adaptability allows for shock absorption and ground terrain changes and helps to prevent excessive strain on the joints or ligaments.[85] Although some pronation of the foot is necessary during functional activities, excessive pronation has been linked to lower limb overuse injuries, because maintenance of the equilibrium becomes the function of the muscles, specifically the fibularis (peroneus) brevis and the posterior tibialis.[43,275–278] Excessive pronation can occur as a result of a number of different factors, including the following:[143]

- Congenital, including tarsal coalitions, metatarsus varus, and convex pes valgus.[4,48,279]
- Developmental, including talipes calcaneovalgus, talipes calcaneovarus, ligament laxity, and/or a tight Achilles tendon and forefoot varus.[4,48,279,280]
- Equinus at the ankle, resulting in increased dorsiflexion of the forefoot at the rearfoot around the oblique midtarsal joint axis;
- Subtalar varus;
- A plantar flexed lateral column, which results in pronation due to the fact that the fourth and fifth metatarsals are lower than the adjacent third metatarsal, which produces a pronatory force with weight-bearing;
- Rearfoot varus associated with excessive forefoot pronation and delayed resupination.

The patient with a symptomatic pronated foot typically complains of pain along the medial longitudinal arch. Occasionally, there is pain laterally beneath the tip of the fibula secondary to impingement of the calcaneus against the fibula. The pain is usually aggravated with prolonged standing and walking and relieved with rest.[281] Often these patients become symptomatic when they suddenly increase their level of activity.

The examination often reveals a flattening of the longitudinal arch associated with a valgus deformity of the heel, a medial bulge at the talonavicular joint, a low medial longitudinal arch, and abduction of the forefoot on the rearfoot at the transverse tarsal joint.[281,282]

Two terms can be used to describe the pronated foot: weak and hypermobile. Both the weak and the hypermobile flatfoot can cause symptoms in everyday weight-bearing activities due to postural fatigue.

The Weak Foot

The weak foot produces moderate pronation. Severe pronation with flattening of the foot is associated with congenital or ligamentous laxity and is deemed to be occurring if the foot is pronating beyond 25% of the stance phase.[4,112,143,283] Acquired flatfoot deformity is a symptomatic and progressive flatfoot deformity, resulting from the loss of function of the tibialis posterior muscle/tendon and/or the loss of integrity of the ligamentous structures supporting the joints of the arch and the rearfoot. The weak foot is characterized by a general increase in the ROM at the subtalar and midtarsal joints, with the heel positioned in valgus, and the medial arch is dropped. In addition, the forefoot is externally positioned on the rearfoot, and the foot is usually toed out.[143]

The Hypermobile Foot

Occasionally, a foot that appears normal in non–weight-bearing (static examination) can excessively pronate during running (dynamic examination). Consequently, it is usual for this type of foot to only give symptoms with running, which emphasizes the importance of performing both a static and a dynamic examination of the foot.

Hypermobility at the foot and ankle can lead to increased stress on the bone and soft tissues, especially the ligaments, and an overreliance on muscular support.[80]

The intervention for an abnormally and symptomatic pronated foot depends on the type, but typically involves the following:

- Removal or alleviation of the abnormal tissue stress.
- Stretching of the gastrocnemius–soleus complex.
- Activity and shoe modification.[80,284] A straighter last is more desirable for a person with excessive pronation.
- Taping or arch strapping: can be used to limit excessive pronation.[285,286]
- Orthotics.

THE FLATFOOT

A flatfoot or pes planus is manifested by little or no longitudinal arch with full-weight-bearing, which is present beyond the the age of 6 years.[287]

In most cases, a pes planus is flexible demonstrated by the fact that the arch can be recreated with the patient standing up on their toes. Flexible pes planus has been reported to occur in 15% of the general population,[288] with the majority being asymptomatic.[289] If a flatfoot is painful, other causes must be sought out, such as tarsal coalition, vertical talus, or accessory navicular.[58]

A rigid flatfoot, a relatively rare condition, positions the calcaneus in a valgus position and the midtarsal region in pronation, resulting in a displaced navicular (posteriorly (dorsally)) and a talus that faces medially and inferiorly.

Extrinsic congenital deformities can cause abnormal pronation. These include hip dysplasia, femoral anteversion, tibial torsions, and genu varum or valgus. These deformities produce a rotation of the lower limb, which can have the following consequences:

- ***Excessive external rotation of the lower limb.*** This may shift the center of gravity in weight-bearing to the medial aspect of the foot. Ideally, the center of gravity during weight-bearing should pass through the center of the foot. This increase in medial stress causes the talus to plantar flex and adduct, while the calcaneus tilts laterally (into valgus).
- ***Excessive internal rotation of the lower limb.*** This produces excessive weight-bearing on the lateral aspect of the foot. In an attempt to shift the center of gravity more medially, the forefoot abducts on the rearfoot, or the foot abducts on the leg. These compensations produce excessive pronation of the subtalar joint.

THE STIFF FOOT

Pes cavus is an abnormally supinated and stiff foot. While normal supination is designed to allow the foot to function as a rigid lever during push-off, torque conversion, and a lengthening mechanism of the leg,[85] the stiff foot prevents normal pronation from occurring during the stance phase of gait. Without the normal amount of pronation needed to allow the dissipation of stresses, the foot loses its ability to absorb shock. The stiff foot is characterized by a high arch, increased external rotation of the tibia, and increased forefoot varus.

There are three classifications of abnormal supination:[4,143]

- ***Pes cavus.*** This classic type is characterized by a fixed plantar flexed forefoot, or an equinus forefoot, which places the rearfoot in neutral during weight-bearing.[280] The high longitudinal arch of the cavus foot results in limited weight-bearing on the plantar aspect of the foot. This produces increased pressure on the heel and on the metatarsal heads.[281] The physical examination reveals a varus configuration of the heel, a marked elevation of the longitudinal arch, no medial bulge at the talonavicular joint, an adducted forefoot relative to the rearfoot, and external rotation of the leg.[281,282]
- ***Pes cavovarus.*** This type is characterized by a fixed plantar flexed medial column or first ray. This places the calcaneus in varus or inversion during weight-bearing, so that the foot lands on its lateral border.[280]
- ***Pes equinovarus.*** This foot type demonstrates a fixed plantar flexed forefoot and rearfoot, with no compensation occurring with weight-bearing.

The intervention for a symptomatic case of cavus foot is supportive and involves having the patient wear a soft shoe with adequate padding to increase the weight-bearing surface of the foot and provide more midsole cushion for the plantar aspect of the foot.[281290]

SPECIFIC JOINT DEFORMITIES AND DEVIATIONS

Talocrural Joint

Talipes Equinus

The lack of a minimum of 10 degrees of dorsiflexion at the talocrural joint is termed as talipes equinus.[94] A common cause for a lack of dorsiflexion at the ankle is adaptive shortening of the gastrocnemius and soleus muscle groups. Other causes include trauma, spasticity, structural bone deformities, and inflammatory disease. This dysfunction often results in excessive forces being transferred to the forefoot and increased pronation at the subtalar joint.[140]

Common problems associated with this foot type include medial arch pain, posterior leg pain, plantar heel pain, metatarsalgia, lateral ankle sprain, and talonavicular pain.[80]

Subtalar Joint

Rearfoot Varus

This is the most common structural foot deformity and is the most common abnormality of the subtalar joint. The most important component of a rearfoot varus is a calcaneal varus (subtalar varus). A calcaneus varus is characterized by an inverted position of the calcaneus when in the subtalar joint neutral position. This may result in limited eversion and pronation of the subtalar joint when the foot is in contact with the ground. The combination of calcaneal varus and any medial inclination of the tibia produce a total rearfoot varus. A 2–3-degree rearfoot varus is common and generally presents no problems.[291]

The practical significance of a rearfoot varus is that at heel strike, the calcaneus is inverted more than normal and the medial condyle of the calcaneus is farther from the ground, resulting in an increase in lateral heel contact. To bring the medial side of the foot to the ground, the calcaneus must evert. Eversion of the calcaneus is produced by the subtalar joint pronating.

Thus, a rearfoot varus forces the subtalar joint to go through an excessive amount of pronation. In addition, the pronation occurs too rapidly. Rapid pronation from this varus contact position can result in retrocalcaneal exostosis.

Partial compensation occurs if the subtalar joint pronates abnormally but does not have enough available pronation ROM to bring the medial condyle of the calcaneus to the ground.[119] In response to a rearfoot varus, a callus will often form under the second metatarsal head and, to a lesser degree, under the third and fourth metatarsal heads.[119] The callus does not occur under the first metatarsal head, because the stability of the latter depends on the fibularis (peroneus) longus muscle.

If no compensation occurs at the subtalar joint, the midtarsal may compensate with increased mobility and medial longitudinal arch collapse.[85]

When the rearfoot varus is large, the metatarsal joint and the forefoot may be excessively mobile, when the heel rises from the ground during propulsion. In addition, the foot may not become rigid until after the heel rises, instead of just before heel rise.

Other tissue disorders that can result from rearfoot varus include plantar heel pain, metatarsalgia, or stress factors of the second ray and hallux valgus. The proximal effects of subtalar joint compensation for a rearfoot varus are substantial. The excessive and rapid pronation that occurs during the contact phase of gait puts a tremendous stress on the primary muscle that decelerates subtalar joint pronation, the tibialis posterior muscle, producing symptoms of overuse in this muscle.[119]

In addition to the extreme stress placed upon the tibialis posterior muscle, abnormal subtalar joint pronation may produce an excessive internal rotation of the lower leg.[119] Normally, the tibia rotates an average of 19 degrees during ambulation.[20] At the beginning of the stance phase, the tibia internally rotates as the talus plantar flexes and adducts. At the end of the stance phase, the tibia must externally rotate, pushing the talus into dorsiflexion and abduction. Any extra rotation must be absorbed in the knee, hip, or sacroiliac joint, or between the lumbar vertebral segments. For example, abnormal subtalar joint pronation increases the valgus stress on the knee, and symptoms of a mild strain of the medial collateral ligament can arise.[119]

Rearfoot varus commonly occurs with tibia vara or pes cavus.[80]

Rearfoot Valgus

Rearfoot valgus involves eversion of the calcaneus when the subtalar joint is in its neutral position. The midtarsal and subtalar joints supinate to compensate. This structural deformity is often associated with genu valgum, or with tibia valgus, and can lead to excessive pronation and limited supination.

Midtarsal Joint

Forefoot Varus

Forefoot varus is defined as inversion of the forefoot on the rearfoot, when the subtalar joint is held in neutral.[94] Some forefoot varus is normal, and in asymptomatic individuals, there is usually approximately 7 degrees of forefoot varus.[292]

This sagittal plane osseous deformity of the forefoot/first ray,[293] with increased stress applied to the medial plantar aspect of the foot, is considered to be the single most common intrinsic cause of mechanical pain and dysfunction within the foot, lower one-third of the leg, and knee (Table 21-11).[280]

TABLE 21-11 Effects of a Forefoot Varus
Talus adducts/plantar flexes
↓
Foot muscles fire out of sync
↓
Lower extremity internally rotates
↓
Midtarsal joint hypermobile
↓
Cuboid pulley is less efficient
↓
Fibularis tendon less functional
↓
First ray hypermobile
↓
Second and third metatarsals bear too much weight
↓
Metatarsals splay apart
↓
Bunions, fractures, and calluses

Data from Hunter S, Prentice WE: Rehabilitation of the ankle and foot. In: Prentice WE, Voight MI, eds. *Techniques in Musculoskeletal Rehabilitation*. New York: McGraw-Hill, 2001:605. With permission from McGraw-Hill.

Since the medial side of the foot is higher than the lateral side, the forefoot assumes an inverted or varus position. To assist the medial side of the forefoot in reaching the ground, the subtalar joint may excessively pronate as the midstance phase begins. This compensation places the midtarsal joint in its maximally mobile position, at the time when it should be in a stable supinated position (just before and during propulsion). The compensation can create the following:

- extreme stresses on the fibularis (peroneus) longus and the forefoot;
- dorsiflexion and subsequent hypermobility of the first ray.[94,119]
- plantar heel pain;[119]
- hallux valgus, bunion deformity, and a subluxation of the first MTP joint.[280]

Since the first-ray complex cannot effectively contribute to propulsion, the second metatarsal head will experience excessive loading, with the potential for callus formation under the second metatarsal head, or metatarsalgia or stress fracture of the second metatarsal.[119,294]

In addition, the forefoot-to-rearfoot alignment in the frontal plane is abnormal, which predisposes the fifth toe to receive pressure from the shoe, which can result in a fifth-digit hammer toe.[143] Terminal knee extension during the midstance phase requires the tibia to externally rotate on the femur. If the knee joint compensates by having the femur rotate medially with the tibia, the problem is transferred to a more proximal structure, mainly the hip joint, or the sacroiliac joint, increasing stress to both contractile and noncontractile tissues.[119]

Forefoot Valgus

This dysfunction occurs when the plane of the metatarsal head is in an everted, or valgus, position. Two structural types of forefoot valgus deformities exist.

- All of the metatarsal heads may be everted.
- The first metatarsal head may be plantar flexed, while the second to fifth metatarsal heads lie in the appropriate plane (pes cavovarus).

If the first ray is plantar flexed, compensation may occur at the subtalar joint in the form of rapid supination of the subtalar joint. This shifts the weight laterally to the fifth metatarsal head.[94,280] If no subtalar joint compensation occurs in response to a forefoot valgus, the body weight is borne on the medial side of the forefoot.[119] To bring the lateral side of the foot to the ground, compensatory supination must occur at the subtalar joint.[119] This supination occurs at a rate that is much sooner than in a normal foot.[143] One of the distal effects of the abnormally supinated foot is that the midtarsal joint is unable to adapt to uneven surfaces, which leads to an increased susceptibility to lateral inversion sprains (Table 21-12).[119]

In addition, the shock-absorbing ability of the knee is also compromised, as the necessary internal rotation of the lower leg required for flexion is delayed. This may play a role in the development of problems around the lateral aspect of the knee or patellofemoral joint.[94,118] The increased forces may also travel up the lower extremity and contribute to the development of sacral and low-back dysfunction.

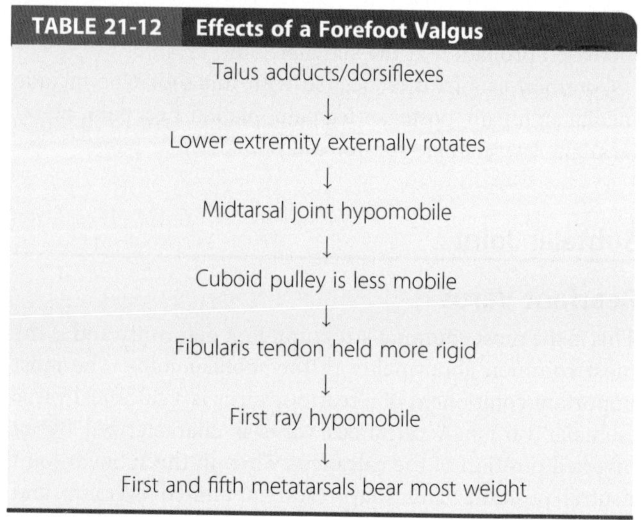
TABLE 21-12 Effects of a Forefoot Valgus

Talus adducts/dorsiflexes
↓
Lower extremity externally rotates
↓
Midtarsal joint hypomobile
↓
Cuboid pulley is less mobile
↓
Fibularis tendon held more rigid
↓
First ray hypomobile
↓
First and fifth metatarsals bear most weight

Data from Hunter S, Prentice WE: Rehabilitation of the ankle and foot. In: Prentice WE, Voight MI, eds. *Techniques in Musculoskeletal Rehabilitation*. New York, NY: McGraw-Hill, 2001:605. With permission from McGraw-Hill.

Forefoot Equinus

This is also a forefoot deformity, but it occurs in the sagittal plane. The metatarsal heads, although possibly perpendicular to the calcaneal bisection, are not level with the plantar condyles of the calcaneus. This results in a relative plantar flexion of the forefoot structures when compared with the rearfoot. The functional effect of this deformity is that the ankle joint must move through a greater excursion of dorsiflexion to allow the body to move forward over the foot during the midstance phase.[119]

The subtalar joint itself is unable to compensate directly for a forefoot equinus because it has very little dorsiflexion. Thus, the midtarsal joint usually becomes the source of the dorsiflexion. If the midtarsal joint is to provide the necessary dorsiflexion, the subtalar joint must be pronated. However, the time when maximum subtalar pronation is needed by the midtarsal joint (at terminal stance) coincides with the time when the subtalar joint should be in a supinated position for propulsion.

More proximally, if the foot and ankle are not able to provide the necessary dorsiflexion, the motion in the sagittal plane may be achieved at the knee joint. This may result in a hyperextension force at the knee, as the body progresses forward over the foot and the tibia.

Combined Rearfoot and Forefoot Deformities

Combinations of deformities frequently occur together.

- A rearfoot varus can occur with either a forefoot varus or a forefoot valgus.[119] In a foot that exhibits a rearfoot and a forefoot varus, the compensatory subtalar joint pronation is accentuated throughout the initial contact, midstance, and terminal stance phases of the gait cycle.[119]

- A rearfoot varus may be combined with a flexible forefoot valgus.[119] Clinically, this foot type demonstrates a significant amount of pronation during stance. As the subtalar joint begins to pronate, the midtarsal joint mobility increases and the forefoot valgus becomes flexible.[119] The foot is abnormally pronated, but the abnormal pronation occurs at the midtarsal joint as well as at the subtalar joint.
- A rigid forefoot valgus can occur with a rearfoot varus.[119] This combination creates extreme bone stress in the middle of the foot, particularly the tarsal bones. Degenerative joint changes and tarsal stress fractures are potential problems, as are lateral ankle sprains and the more proximal problems that occur with a forefoot valgus.[119]

Congenital Variations of the Foot

Clubfoot

The term *clubfoot* encompasses a wide range of deformities, most of which involve the heel to some degree. The most common clubfoot deformity is talipes equinovarus. Two categories exist: a flexible form and a resistant form. The former is amenable to conservative intervention with orthotics and footwear modification. The latter type is invariably associated with stiffness and requires surgical intervention.

Convex Pes Valgus

This deformity is also known as "rocker bottom" foot. It is characterized by a primary posterior (dorsal) and lateral dislocation of the talocalcaneonavicular joint. This results in the navicular articulating with the posterior aspect of the talus, locking it in the vertical position and preventing normal dorsiflexion of the rearfoot.[280,295] The compensation for this loss of rearfoot dorsiflexion is dorsiflexion at the midfoot.[85]

Metatarsal Deformities

Four metatarsal deformities are commonly recognized[293]:

- ***Metatarsus adductus.*** This is a transverse plane deformity with adduction of all of the five metatarsals, which occurs at the tarsometatarsal joint.
- ***Metatarsus varus.*** This deformity is characterized by a medial subluxation of the tarsometatarsal joints with an adduction and inversion deformity of the metatarsals. This results in an inability of the forefoot to be passively abducted to the neutral position.[280]
- ***Metatarsus adductovarus.*** This is a combined transverse and frontal plane deformity of forefoot adduction and inversion that occurs at the tarsometatarsal joint.
- ***Forefoot adductus.*** This is a combined transverse and frontal plane deformity of forefoot adduction and inversion that occurs at the midtarsal joint.

PREFERRED PRACTICE PATTERN 4D: IMPAIRED JOINT MOBILITY, MOTOR FUNCTION, MUSCLE PERFORMANCE, AND ROM ASSOCIATED WITH CONNECTIVE TISSUE DYSFUNCTION

Seronegative Spondyloarthropathies

Ankylosing spondylitis (AS), psoriatic arthritis, and Reiter's syndrome are all capable of producing foot and ankle pain. Although AS predominantly affects the axial skeleton, it can also affect the MTP joints.[281]

Psoriatic arthritis usually occurs with accompanying skin lesions. However, in 10–15% of cases, no dermatologic problems exist.[281] The condition is characterized by symmetrical involvement of the hands and feet, most often at the level of the DIP joints.[281]

Reiter's syndrome consists of a triad of conjunctivitis, urethritis, and asymmetric arthritis. This condition usually affects the knees, feet, and ankles.[281]

Posttraumatic Arthritis

Posttraumatic arthritis, which is associated with repeated inversion sprains, is more common than osteoarthritis at the ankle. The trauma may result from direct injuries to the cartilage and/or altered biomechanics (malalignment, altered weight-bearing forces, and incongruent joint loading). Individuals with posttraumatic arthritis of the ankle generally report isolated ankle pain and stiffness and complaints of catching, locking, clicking, and painful giving-way episodes.[296] The objective examination typically reveals swelling and limited and painful ankle dorsiflexion and plantar flexion ROM. Because of unique set of challenges presented, posttraumatic arthritis in this region is difficult to treat conservatively. The conservative treatment approach can include medication (NSAIDs, corticosteroid), patient education (weight loss, activity modification or avoidance, the use of a cane), shoe modification (heel lift to reduce dorsiflexion) bracing (AFO), stretching, mobilization, strengthening, and symptom management (heat, ice, and/or electrical stimulation), as appropriate. Surgical options include ankle arthrodesis and arthroplasty.

Osteochondrosis

Osteochondrosis is an injury to an ossification center, resulting in inflammation, degeneration, recalcification, necrosis, and/or fragmentation. It can occur at an epiphyseal center of a long bone or apophyseal area where a tendon inserts. Osteochondrosis at an apophyseal area is typically referred to as an apophysitis. An adolescent may develop apophysitis due to an overuse injury, while an adult typically develops tendinitis.[297] Common examples of osteochondrosis include Sever disease (see later) and Freiberg disease.

- Freiberg disease. Osteochondrosis of the epiphyseal center of the metatarsal (the second metatarsal is most commonly involved) due to abnormal stress on the metatarsal, resulting in localized pain and swelling. Freiberg disease can result from abnormal pronation or an excessively long second metatarsal. The intervention for Freiberg disease includes the restoration of normal biomechanics, including the use of a metatarsal pad or bar to reduce the weight-bearing forces on the metatarsal.

Osteochondritis Dissecans

Osteochondritis dissecans[297] and osteochondral lesions represent the same entity and relate to an injury of the articular cartilage and/or the underlying bone. The anterolateral and posteromedial locations on the talus are susceptible to injury when the talocrural joint undergoes torsional stress, through either impact or cyclical loading.[298] When the subchondral bone is involved, avascular necrosis with resulting bone infarction can occur. If the overlying articular cartilage remains intact, a space is created between the living bone and articular cartilage. An in-growth of fibrous tissue may result, and, if this tissue is not displaced, healing takes place. The associated symptoms are related to the stability of the fragment and can be similar to those commonly reported after an ankle sprain. If the fragment is maintained by the cartilage, symptoms may be mild. The symptoms will be more severe if a fragment breaks off into the joint, with sensations of giving way secondary to sharp pain, catching, and/or locking. The intervention and prognosis depend on the size and location of the lesion as well as the stability of the fragment. Activities that may disrupt the healing fragment must be avoided. This would include weight-bearing activities where twisting may occur, such as challenging balance and proprioceptive exercises. Surgical treatment can involve debridement and stabilization of the fragment. In cases when significant bone necrosis has occurred, bone grafting may be required.

Hallux Rigidus

Hallux rigidus is characterized by decreased dorsiflexion of the first MTP joint, and pain and swelling in the posterior (dorsal) aspect of the joint.[50] Two types of hallux rigidus have been described: adolescent and adult.

- ***Adolescent.*** The adolescent type is consistent with an osteochondritis dissecans or localized articular disorder.
- ***Adult.*** The adult type is a more generalized degenerative arthritis.[49] The cause of this degenerative process is unknown. Possible etiologies include crystal-induced arthropathy (gout and pseudogout), rheumatoid arthritis, the seronegative spondyloarthropathies, posttraumatic degeneration, an intra-articular fracture, or an osteochondrotic lesion of the first metatarsal head.[49,299] Repetitive dorsiflexion of the first MTP joint could also potentially lead to the development of hallux rigidus, although no studies have linked levels of physical activity to the development of hallux rigidus.[299]

The characteristics of both types include stiffness and pain in the MTP joint. This is associated with difficulty during the gait cycle, especially when walking or running up hills, climbing stairs or during the terminal stance phase of gait.[49] Since approximately 75 degrees of hallux dorsiflexion is needed for normal gait, limited extension of the great toe gives the feeling of vaulting over the toe. This may necessitate external rotation of the foot to allow for toe clearance. Thus, patients may present with lateral stress transfer as they attempt to unload the hallux MTP joint. This may produce synovitis of the lesser MTP joints or even stress fractures of the lesser metatarsals.[49]

A posterior (dorsal) metatarsal head osteophyte, or posterior (dorsal) bunion, may rub against footwear, causing an abrasion or ulceration. The patient may also experience tingling and numbness on the posterior aspect of the toe due to compression of the cutaneous nerves.

Tenderness is usually present on palpation of the posterior (dorsal), and especially lateral, aspects of the joint. Radiographs demonstrate loss of the first MTP joint space, the formation of posterior (dorsal) and lateral osteophytes on the metatarsal head, and occasionally loose fragments about the joint.[163]

The initial intervention involves shoe modifications, rest, and NSAIDs. A shoe with an extra-deep toe box can be helpful to decrease posterior (dorsal) pressure on the first MTP joint, while a stiff-soled shoe or a rigid custom orthotic with a Morton's extension can be helpful in limiting toe dorsiflexion. A rocker-bottom sole can also help to decrease the extension of the hallux during normal gait. An intra-articular corticosteroid injection may be considered as a temporizing measure. If symptoms increase, or when conservative measures fail, surgical intervention may provide the solution.

The most common surgical procedure is the cheilectomy, which is an excision of the posterior (dorsal) 25–33% of the metatarsal head. This removes the offending osteophytes, improves toe dorsiflexion, and preserves the good articular cartilage on the middle and plantar aspects of the metatarsal head.[300] A dorsiflexion osteotomy of the proximal phalanx (Moberg procedure) may be used concurrently with a cheilectomy in selected patients to increase functional toe dorsiflexion.[301]

Tarsal Coalition

Tarsal coalition is a fibrous, cartilaginous, or bony connection of two or more bones in the midfoot or hindfoot.[58,302] It usually presents during adolescence, at an average age of 13 years,[303] when the coalition is ossifying and subtalar motion becomes more limited. Most tarsal coalitions are bilateral,[302,304] and have been reported to occur in less than 1% of the general population.[302] Calcaneonavicular and talocalcaneal are the most common coalitions seen.[58,302,303,305,306]

A partial or complete talocalcaneal coalition significantly alters the mechanics of the ankle joint complex, as compensatory motions occur at the ankle joint level.

The patient with a tarsal coalition typically presents with pain that is vague and has an insidious onset. They may present with a history of frequent "ankle sprains" or generalized hindfoot or midfoot pain.[303] Symptoms often begin or are exacerbated by athletic training.

The physical examination will show limited or no subtalar motion compared with the other foot and occasional tight fibularis (peroneal) muscles.[307] Spastic fibularis (peroneal) muscles have been reported to occur in less than 1% of these patients.[306]

The diagnosis of such malformations is often very difficult. Plain radiographs should include AP, lateral, and oblique views of the foot.[58,302]

The goal of conservative treatment of tarsal coalition is to reduce stress in the foot, relax the fibularis (peroneal) muscles, and support the foot. This can usually be accomplished with orthotics and exercise, although temporary casting may be necessary.[58,302] If conservative treatment fails, however, a resection may be necessaryto restore mobility and decrease pain.[302,303]

Os Trigonum

An os trigonum has been reported to be present in approximately 10% of the general population and is often unilateral.[60,134,308,309] The origin of this ossicle may be congenital or acquired. Congenitally, it can be a persistent separation of the secondary center of the lateral tubercle from the remainder of the posterior talus secondary to repeated microtrauma during development.[60,309] The acquired form may be secondary to an actual fracture that has not united.[60,309,310]

Symptoms associated with os trigonum include pain with maximum plantar flexion as the posterior talus impinges on the posterior tibia.[297] The intervention involves symptom reduction with restoration of normal strength, ROM, and biomechanics as needed. If symptoms persist, surgical removal of the bone may be required but is delayed until skeletal maturity is achieved.[297]

Hallux Valgus

Hallux valgus describes a deformity of the first MTP joint, in which the proximal phalanx is deviated laterally with respect to the first metatarsal. It may also be used to describe varying degrees of metatarsus primus varus/valgus deviation of the proximal phalanx, medial deviation of the first metatarsal head, and bunion formation.

Hallux valgus occurs almost exclusively in populations that wear shoes, although there are also some predisposing anatomic factors. Women are more likely than men to have hallux valgus (a ratio of 9:1),[311] and the condition has been reported to affect 22–36% of adolescents.[312–317]

The deformity results from a lateral subluxation of the FHL muscle, which transforms the FHL and brevis from flexors to adductors, which then pull the PIP medially and the DIP laterally.[163] In addition, the abductor hallucis muscle slides underneath the metatarsal head and brings about pronation of the great toe, approaching 70–90% of pronation in severe cases.[318]

With increasing lateral deviation of the hallux, the MTP joint becomes incongruent, the sesamoids subluxate laterally, the hallux pronates, the medial aspect of the first metatarsal head becomes more prominent, and weight-bearing shifts from the first metatarsal head to the second metatarsal, and possibly the third.[50,141] This weight transfer may result in the formation of a painful plantar keratosis, or a hammer toe or a crossover toe deformity of the second toe.[50]

The cause of hallux valgus is unclear, but various factors are cited such as tight shoes, metatarsus primus varus, pes planus, forefoot pronation, joint hyperlaxity, and heredity.[312,313] Hallux valgus is often associated with medial deviation of the first metatarsal, known as metatarsus primus varus.[50]

A compensated bunion is a mild deformity without MTP joint subluxation and without marked lateral sesamoid subluxation.[319] A decompensated bunion is a moderate-to-severe deformity characterized by hallux valgus angle greater than 25 degrees, intermetatarsal angle greater than 15 degrees, lateral sesamoid subluxation, and great toe pronation.

The intervention for hallux valgus begins conservatively and the intervention for the bunion includes advice on wearing wider shoes, or an orthotic prescription.[312,313,315] A silicone bunion pad placed over the bunion may be helpful in alleviating direct pressure on the prominence.[50] Other interventions are based on the causative factors:

- Achilles stretching is used in cases of Achilles contracture.
- A simple toe spacer can be used between the first and second toes if they require separating.
- In cases of pes planus associated with hallux valgus, a medial longitudinal arch support with Morton's extension under the first MTP joint can be used to help alleviate symptoms.[50]

If pain persists, however, structural realignment of the first metatarsal varus is usually necessary, as the bunion deformity becomes more severe and decompensated.

Turf Toe

The term "turf toe" is used to describe a sprain of the first MTP joint.[50] Turf toe is more common in football, baseball, and soccer players. Football players are at higher risk of this injury, if they are tackled while landing from a jump or if another player lands on the back of their heel, forcing the first MTP joint into hyperdorsiflexion.[7,320] Soccer players tend to develop the sprain in the great toe of the nonkicking foot due to the forced dorsiflexion on the stance leg as the other leg kicks the ball. It was originally thought that the artificial grass surface on football fields caused athletes to stop more quickly during planting and cutting, thus, slamming the toe into the front of the shoe. However, it is more likely that the lighter flexible turf shoes that are designed for the surface are more responsible. This increase in shoe flexibility causes a repetitive hyperextension injury of the great toe. The tendency of artificial turf to become hard and stiff over time may be a contributing factor.[321] Hypermobility of the first ray reportedly leads to biomechanical problems. It has been theorized that during gait, the medial longitudinal arch collapses because of excess posterior (dorsal) motion of the first ray. This collapse decreases the ability of the foot to effectively propel the body forward during walking. The increased posterior (dorsal) excursion of the first ray causes the foot to roll inward (pronation), and the second metatarsal must support an excessive proportion of the body weight.[125] The resulting increased magnitude and duration of pronation significantly diminishes the ability of the fibularis (peroneus) longus muscle to stabilize the first metatarsal.[124] As a result, ligamentous tissues that usually limit the end-range dorsiflexion movement of the first metatarsal undergo increased stress, and joint laxity occurs.[124] Because of these mechanical consequences, hypermobility of the first ray has been implicated in numerous conditions frequently accompanied by excessive or prolonged for pronation, including lesser metatarsalgia, acquired flatfoot, posterior tibialis tendinitis, plantar fasciitis, and shin splints.[124,322]

The mechanism of injury for turf toe can also involve hyperflexion and varus and valgus stresses of the first MTP joint.[7,320] With forced hyperflexion of the hallux, tearing of the plantar plate and collateral ligaments can occur. In the more severe injury, the capsule can actually tear off from the metatarsal head.[57] A fracture of the sesamoids can also occur, and posterior (dorsal) dislocation of the first MTP joint is possible.[53]

Clinically, patients with turf toe present with a swollen, stiff, and red, first MTP joint. They may have a history of a single dorsiflexion injury or multiple injuries to the great toe. The joint may be tender, both plantarly and posteriorly (dorsally). Players may have a limp and be unable to run or jump because of pain.

Turf toe typically develops into a chronic injury and long-term results include decreased first MTP joint motion, impaired push-off, and hallux rigidus.[320] Fifty percent of athletes will have persistent symptoms 5 years later.[323]

Clanton and Ford[323] have classified the severity of turf toe injuries from grades I to III:

- Grade I: a minor stretch injury to the soft tissue restraints with little pain, swelling, or disability.
- Grade II: a partial tear of the capsuloligamentous structures with moderate pain, swelling, ecchymosis, and disability.
- Grade III: a complete tear of the plantar plate with severe swelling, pain, ecchymosis, and inability to bear weight normally.

The intervention for turf toe in the acute phase is rest, ice, a compressive dressing, and elevation. NSAIDs are often prescribed, and the toe is taped with multiple loops of tape placed over the posterior (dorsal) aspect of the hallucal proximal phalanx and criss-crossed under the ball of the foot plantarly to limit dorsiflexion.[53] Occasionally, a forefoot steel plate is used.[57] Passive ROM and progressive resistance exercises are begun as soon as patient tolerance allows.[53,163] return to normal activities is based on the initial severity:

- Patients with grade I sprains are usually allowed to return to sports as soon as symptoms allow, sometimes immediately.
- Patients with grade II sprains usually require 3–14 days' rest from athletic training.
- Grade III sprains usually require crutches for a few days and up to 6 weeks' rest from sports participation.

A return to sports training too early after injury could result in prolonged disability. Return to play is indicated when the toe can be dorsiflexed 90 degrees.[323]

Sprains

Ankle sprains are the most common injuries in sports and recreational activities,[324] and they remain a difficult diagnostic and therapeutic challenge. If left untreated, ankle sprains can lead to chronic instability and impairment.[129]

Ankle ligament injuries constitute 4.7–24.4% of all injuries incurred in an individual sport,[325] and 10–28% of all injuries that occur in running and jumping sports.[326,327] Most acute ankle injuries occur in people 21–30 years old, although injuries in the younger and older age groups tend to be more serious.[328] More than 40% of ankle sprains can potentially progress to chronic problems.[184,329–338]

Dynamic stability is provided to the lateral ankle by the strength of the fibularis (peroneus) longus and brevis tendons. Stormont et al.[24] recently showed that ankle instability, and thus sprains, could only occur during systematic loading and unloading, but not while the ankle is fully loaded, due to the articular restraints. In the neutral position or dorsiflexion, the ankle is stable because the widest part of the talus is in the mortise. However, in plantar flexion, ankle stability is decreased, as the narrow posterior portion of the talus is in the mortise.[129] Thus, the most common mechanism of an ankle sprain is one of inversion and plantar flexion.[16,57] With eversion and external rotation, the deltoid and/or ligaments of the distal tibiofibular joint can be injured, producing the so-called medial and central sprains, respectively. Eversion injuries to the medial (deltoid) ligament of the ankles account for 5% of ankle sprains.[11,131,339]

The prognosis for ankle sprains is inversely proportional to the severity and grade of the initial injury (Table 21-13),[340] the age of the patient (younger patients do not fair as well), and the rate of recurrence (the prognosis is worse when the ankle has been previously sprained).[16,125,332]

Lateral Ankle (Inversion) Sprain

Sprains of the lateral ligamentous complex represent 85% of ankle ligament sprains.[206,324] In the younger population, serious ankle sprains are unusual in the skeletally immature, because the ligaments are usually stronger than the bone,[304,341,342] necessitating a physeal fracture to be ruled out.[16,57]

The ATFL, which is the least elastic of the lateral ligaments,[145] is involved in 60–70% of all ankle sprains, while 20% involve both the ATFL and the CFL.[11,131,339] The sequence of lateral ligament tears is first the ATFL, then the anterolateral capsule, then the distal tibiofibular ligament, then the CFL, and finally the PTFL, the strongest of the lateral ligaments.[13,206] This rupture may be associated with ankle dislocation, distal lateral malleolar avulsion or spiral fracture, medial malleolar fracture, or talar neck or medial compression fractures.[206] Most (86%) ankle ligament tears are midsubstance; thus, only 14% are avulsion injuries.[131]

The high-ankle sprain, or syndesmotic sprain, which involves disruption of the ligamentous structures between the distal fibula and tibia, just proximal to the ankle joint, is a less-understood form of ankle sprain injury in comparison with the lateral ankle sprain. The mechanisms of injury for syndesmotic ankle sprains include[171,174,343]:

- forceful external rotation of the foot, resulting in widening of the ankle mortise, as the talus is driven into external rotation within the ankle mortise;
- forceful eversion of the talus, which widens the mortise;
- forceful dorsiflexion, which widens the mortise, as the wider anterior aspect of the talar dome enters the joint space.

TABLE 21-13 The West Point Ankle Sprain Grading System			
Criterion	**Grade I**	**Grade II**	**Grade III**
Location of tenderness	ATFL	ATFL and CFL	ATFL, CFL, and PTFL
Edema and ecchymosis	Slight and local	Moderate and local	Significant and diffuse
Weight-bearing ability	Full or partial	Difficult without crutches	Impossible without significant pain
Ligament damage	Stretched	Partial tear	Complete tear
Instability	None	None or slight	Definite

ATFL, anterior talofibular ligament; CFL, calcaneofibular ligament; PTFL, posterior talofibular ligament.
Data from Gerber JP, Williams GN, Scoville CR, et al.: Persistent disability associated with ankle sprains: A prospective examination of an athletic population. *Foot Ankle Int* 19:653–660, 1998.

With all of the above mechanisms, the distal fibula is pushed laterally away from its articulation with the distal tibia. Chronic instability of the syndesmosis may then result in increased shear stress and altered contact pressure patterns that might predispose the individual to degenerative articular cartilage changes in the ankle joint.[171,174,343]

Although a physical examination is reliable for the diagnosis of an ankle fracture,[198] the reliability for detecting lateral ankle sprains may not be as definitive, especially if the examination is performed immediately after the injury.[187] The place of a physical examination in diagnosis has been reviewed in a series of 160 patients,[187] comparing the accuracy within 48 hours of injury with that at 4–7 days. The specificity and sensitivity of delayed physical examination for the presence or absence of a lateral ligament injury were 84% and 96%, respectively, indicating that a reasonably precise clinical diagnosis is possible if the examination is delayed for approximately 4 days post-injury.[344] Injuries to the foot and ankle may quickly be dismissed as ankle sprains, particularly in the adolescent population (Table 21-14). A clinician examining the foot and ankle needs to be aware of other potential pathologies to consider when an adolescent patient is referred to physical therapy with the diagnosis of ankle sprain. These pathologies include osteochondrosis, osteochondritis dissecans, accessory ossicle, anterior impingement syndrome, sinus tarsi syndrome, tarsal coalition, and epiphyseal fractures.[297]

The mechanism of injury can afford some clues. As mentioned, a history of a forced dorsiflexion can result in a sprain

TABLE 21-14 Potential Pathologies Associated with Adolescent Ankle Injuries		
Pathology	**Definition**	**Signs and Symptoms**
Sever ostoechondrosis	Calcaneal apophysitis	Localized pain and tenderness at the Achilles attachment
Talocrural osteochondritis dissecans	Injury to articular cartilage and/or underlying bone	Catching, locking, and/or sudden sharp stabbing pains
Accessory ossicles at the distal tiba or fibula	Ossification centers that have not fused	Localized pain and tenderness Accessory bone with rounded edges on radiographs
Accessory os trigonum	Accessory ossicle on the posterior-lateral process of the talus	Pain posteriorly with maximum plantar flexion Accessory bone with rounded edges on radiographs
Anterior ankle impingement	Thickening of joint capsule with or without bone spurs at the anterior talocrural joint	Pain anteriorly with sudden dorsiflexion Decreased dorsiflexion ROM—a hard end-feel if bone spurs are present
Sinus tarsus syndrome	Injury to the structures contained within the sinus tarsus	Hindfoot instability Tenderness inferior and anterior to the anterior talofibular ligament
Tarsal coalition	Congenital union between two tarsal bones: usually calcaneonavicular or talocalcaneal coalition	Localized tenderness over the involved joint Rigid flatfoot and peroneal muscle spasm with inversion
Distal tibal epiphyseal fractures	Growth plate injury	Tenderness at the distal tibia Inability to weight bear

Data from Martin R: Considerations for differential diagnosis of an ankle sprain in the adolescent. *Orthop Pract* 16:21–22, 2004.

of the distal tibiofibular syndesmosis. Distal tibiofibular syndesmosis sprains are usually accompanied by complaints of pain that greatly exceed the amount of swelling and that increase with external rotation of the foot.[129] Forced plantar flexion can result in anterior capsular sprains. These are characterized by pain that worsens with passive plantar flexion and resisted dorsiflexion.[129]

No single symptom or test can provide a completely accurate diagnosis of a lateral ankle ligament rupture, but the collection of findings can be strongly indicative[187]:

- The absence of swelling at the time of the delayed (after 4 days) physical examination suggests that there is no ligament rupture, whereas extensive swelling at this time is indicative of ligament rupture.[345]
- Pain on palpation of the involved ligament suggests involvement.
- Presence of a hematoma suggests a rupture.
- Positive anterior drawer test suggests a rupture.
- Impairment of walking ability after injury suggests involvement.

One study[187] demonstrated that a combination of tenderness at the level of the ATFL, a lateral hematoma, discoloration, and a positive drawer test indicated a ligament rupture in 95% of cases, whereas the absence of these findings always indicated an intact ligament.

Lateral ankle sprains can be categorized as follows:

- Grade I: characterized by minimal to no swelling and localized tenderness over the ATFL. These sprains require on the average 11.7 days before the full resumption of athletic activities.[346]
- Grade II: characterized by localized swelling and more diffuse lateral tenderness. These sprains require approximately 2–6 weeks for return to full athletic function.[347,348]
- Grade III: characterized by significant swelling, pain, and ecchymosis and should be referred to a specialist.[349] Grade III injuries may require greater than 6 weeks to return to full function. For acute grade III ankle sprains, the average duration of disability has been reported to be anywhere from 4.5 to 26 weeks, and only 25–60% of patients are symptom free 1–4 years after injury.[350] In a summary of all prospective and controlled studies on grade III sprains, it was concluded that the long-term prognosis is good to excellent in 80–90% of patients with this injury, regardless of the type of intervention chosen.[351]

Intervention

Conservative intervention has been found to be consistently effective in treating grades I and II ankle sprains,[352] and high-ankle sprains (Table 21-15).

TABLE 21-15 Summary of Conservative Treatment for Ankle Sprains

Phase/Criteria	Description of Intervention
Phase I	
	Pain and edema control: rest, ice, compression, elevation, electrical stimulation, toe curls, ankle pump, and cryotherapy
	Temporary immobilization/stabilization (i.e., short leg cast, splint, brace, and heel lift)
	Non–weight-bearing with crutches
Phase II	
Pain and swelling subside	Patient can ambulate using partial weight-bearing without pain.
Partial weight-bearing with assistive device	Lower-level balance training: bilateral standing activity or standing on a balance pad or several layers of towels
	Lower-level strengthening using theraband
Phase III	
Patient can ambulate full-weight-bearing without pain, possibly still needing protection from heel lift or ankle brace.	Unilateral balance training
	Progress from double-heel raises to single-heel raises
	Treadmill walking or over ground walking
	Progress to fast walking
Phase IV	
Able to perform heel raises in unilateral stance	Fast pain-free walking without heel lift
	Jog to run progression
	Shuttle runs and cutting maneuvers
	Sport-specific training

The timeline for progression of an individual patient is dependent on the severity of the injury and the ability of the patient and the criteria listed in the table for progression to each phase.

Data from Lin CF, Gross ML, Weinhold P: Ankle syndesmosis injuries: Anatomy, biomechanics, mechanism of injury, and clinical guidelines for diagnosis and intervention. *J Orthop Sports Phys Ther* 36:372–384, 2006.

Intervention in the acute stage centers around aggressive attempts as follows:

- minimize effusion so as to speed healing;
- promote early protected motion;
- foster early supported/protected weight-bearing as tolerated;
- foster protected return to activity;
- prevent reinjury.

Early intervention incorporates cryotherapy, compression, and elevation to assist in the reduction of pain, swelling, and secondary hypoxic effects.[353] Although early motion and mobility rather than immobilization have demonstrated the stimulation of collagen bundle orientation and the promotion of healing,[354] it must be remembered that full ligamentous strength is not regained for several months or longer.[355–358]

Active ROM exercises, such as ankle pumping and toe curls (30 reps, four times/day each), are encouraged during this phase, but within pain-free limits.[137]

Protected weight-bearing with an orthosis is permitted, with weight-bearing to tolerance as soon as possible following injury.[17] As the healing progresses and the patient is able to bear more weight on his or her ankle, there is a corresponding increase in the use of weight-bearing (closed-chain) exercises. A recommended activity during this phase is the "cross drill." The patient stands independently or with minimal assistance on the involved limb, with the other leg flexed. The patient then moves the uninvolved limb into hip flexion, hip extension, hip abduction, and hip adduction. The exercise is performed initially on a firm surface with the eyes open, and then, as the patient improves, the exercise is performed on a foam surface or balance board, first with the eyes open and then with the eyes closed.

In the subacute stages of the rehabilitation process (4–14 days), the patient begins dynamic balance and proprioceptive exercises. The external support may still be required during this phase. Using a balance board, the patient balances on the involved limb, while playing "catch" with the clinician. The intensity of this exercise can be varied by using balls of different sizes and different weights. The clinician may also make the exercises more challenging by throwing the ball to a variety of locations. This will require a shift in the center of gravity and an instantaneous adjustment of balance from the patient.

Long-sitting gastrocnemius stretching with a strap or sheet can be introduced in this phase (six reps of 20 seconds each) to promote ankle dorsiflexion past the neutral position, enabling a closer to normal walking pattern.[137] Open-chain (non-weight-bearing) progressive resistive exercises with elastic resistance are performed (two sets of 30 reps each) for isolated plantar flexion, dorsiflexion, inversion, and eversion. Stationary cycling can also be performed (at a comfortable intensity for up to 30 minutes), to provide cardiovascular endurance training and controlled ankle ROM.[142]

In the advanced healing stage (2–4 weeks postinjury), the goals are as follows:

- the restoration of normal AROM;
- normal gait without an assistive device;
- pain-free performance of full-weight-bearing functional activities;
- enhancement of proprioception.

Activities to help achieve these goals include heel-to-toe anterior–posterior walking (10 m for 20 reps), carioca drills, and mini-trampoline balancing exercises (unilateral stance with eyes open and then closed, and catching and passing activities with a medicine ball).

Plyometric activities are introduced during the functional challenge/return to activity phase. These can include two-foot ankle hopping, single-ankle hops, and then multidirection single-ankle hops. If appropriate, barrier jumps or hops may be introduced.

Recurrent Ankle Sprains

Recurrent ankle sprains may be due to the following[16,125]:

- healing of the ligaments in a lengthened position;
- weakness of the healed ligaments due to inherent weakness of the scar;
- fibular (peroneal) muscle weakness (the incompletely rehabilitated ankle sprain);
- distal tibiofibular instability;
- hereditary hypermobility;
- loss of ankle proprioception;
- impingement by the distal fascicle of the anterior tibiofibular ligament, and/or impingement of capsular scar tissue (meniscoid tissue) in the talofibular joint;
- undiagnosed associated problems such as cuboid subluxation or subtalar instability.

The associated complication of ankle sprains include early degenerative changes.[179,334] Talar displacement of greater than 1 mm reduces the ankle's weight-bearing surface by 42.3%,[359–361] resulting in asymmetric load-bearing of the articular surface.

Chronic lateral instability is manifested by recurrent injuries with pain, tenderness, and sometimes bruising over the lateral ligaments.[184,332,362–365] Many, approximately 30%,[332] may be asymptomatic between the events. Others may manifest with chronic lateral pain, tenderness, swelling, or induration with great difficulties in sports and daily activities.[184,332,363] A history of insecurity, instability, and giving way[27,364,366] is far more important in diagnosis than the physical examination in acute and recurrent sprains.[332,367]

In general, subjective complaints include

- frequent sprains[330,336];
- difficulty in running on uneven surfaces;[330]
- difficulty in cutting and jumping in athletic events.[184,330,337]
- feelings of "giving way."[330,333,336]
- Recurrent pain[184,331,333,335,336] and swelling.[330,333,335–337]
- Tenderness.[330,331,333]
- Inability to run.[329]
- Weakness.[184,329]

Recurrent ankle sprains are typically treated conservatively for 2–3 months,[329,330,338,368,369] using a combination of some or all of the following: a lateral heel wedge, fibular (peroneal) muscle strengthening, proprioceptive/coordination exercises, taping, elastic or thermoplastic ankle supports, and/or a short leg brace.

If the conservative trial fails late repair or reconstruction of the lateral ligaments is recommended.[332,370–375]

According to Hinterman et al.,[22] a number of conditions can mimic ankle instability:

- Fibularis (peroneal) tendon subluxation.
- Instability of the Chopart joint. Inversion and plantar flexion trauma of the foot may result in avulsion by the bifurcate ligament and, sometimes, additionally by the talonavicular ligament. Injuries at the Chopart joint level are, however, frequently missed acutely and misdiagnosed as lateral ankle sprain, if the clinical examination is not carefully carried out.[376]
- Talocalcaneal and talonavicular coalition.
- Posterior tibial dysfunction.

MIDFOOT SPRAIN

A sprain of the tarsometatarsal joint usually occurs from an indirect axial load on a plantar flexed and rotated foot, with or without abduction.[377] On examination, the patient will have tenderness to palpation directly over this area, and pain with passive midfoot pronation and supination while the rearfoot is stabilized.[377]

Radiographs of the foot should include weight-bearing AP and lateral and oblique views to rule out dislocation. The metatarsals should be lined up with their respective cuneiforms.[57]

Conservative intervention can proceed if displacement of the metatarsals on a radiograph is less than 2 mm and includes an orthotic or a fracture boot if the patient is unable to bear weight comfortably.[57] A stiff shoe and orthotics to support the medial longitudinal arch are recommended for return to athletics.[378]

Sinus Tarsi Syndrome

The sinus tarsi is located between the inferior neck of the talus and the superior aspect of the calcaneus. It is inferior and slightly anterior to the ATFL. Sinus tarsi syndrome is a sprain of the subtalar joint, with injury to the talocalcaneal interosseous ligament. The mechanism of injury involves an inversion sprain in a plantar flexed position that injures both the talocrural and subtalar joint and is sometimes difficult to distinguish from a routine ankle sprain.[57]

Symptoms can include a feeling of hindfoot instability when walking on uneven ground. Observation usually reveals swelling in the sinus tarsi. There is usually pain with palpation and pronation,[342] usually due to scarring in the soft tissue elements of the sinus tarsi.[378]

The intervention may include joint-specific mobilization and manipulation, followed by strengthening and proprioceptive exercises. An orthotic can be used to limit pronation and maintain the foot in a functional neutral position.

Selective cortisone injection into the subtalar joint can also be diagnostic and therapeutic.[342]

Cuboid Syndrome

Cuboid syndrome (locked cuboid, calcaneal cuboid fault syndrome, and subluxed cuboid) is common but poorly recognized.[379] The calcaneocuboid joint is usually very mobile but can be repetitively subluxed laterally and posteriorly (dorsally) with strong forces. The subluxation is usually a temporary occurrence. The etiology has been proposed to be secondary to overuse, increasing body weight, training on uneven surfaces, or a lateral ankle or lateral foot sprain.[379,380]

Cuboid syndrome usually presents with a gradual onset of lateral midfoot pain. The pain is usually localized near the fourth and fifth metatarsals at the posterior (dorsal) aspect of the cuboid or the calcaneocuboid joint.[379] Often, the patient feels as if he or she is walking with a small stone in their shoe. Maximum discomfort is elicited by pressure directed over the fibular (peroneal) groove on the plantar surface of the calcaneus.[57] On occasion, the hook of the bone under the cuboid breaks or the short plantar ligament tears, producing heel pain.

Common findings in the physical examination are a subtle forefoot valgus and a pronated foot, as well as a tight fibularis (peroneus) longus tendon.[379,381,382] The pronated foot produces an unstable midtarsal joint. Careful gait analysis will often reveal that the pain is reproduced in terminal stance, at the onset of heel rise. Other findings include asymmetrical weakness of the fibularis (peroneus) longus muscle and decreased ROM of the lateral foot.

The intervention for this condition includes a manipulation of the midfoot (see "Cuboid Whip" section), stretching the fibularis (peroneal) tendons and strapping/plantar padding.[379,381]

Talocrural Joint Subluxation

There are essentially two types of subluxations at this joint, anterior and posterior, which result in a loss of plantar flexion and dorsiflexion, respectively.

- The anterior subluxation is commonly caused by an inversion, plantar flexion force. The clinical findings include a limitation of dorsiflexion, a decreased posterior talar glide, and/or conjunct external rotation of the talus.
- The posterior subluxation may be from a compensatory or other type of flatfoot or from a dorsiflexion injury. The clinical findings include a loss of the plantar flexion talar swing, anterior glide, and/or medial conjunct talar rotation.

The intervention for this type of injury is usually a high-velocity thrust technique applied to the joint.

PREFERRED PRACTICE PATTERN 4E: IMPAIRED JOINT MOBILITY, MOTOR FUNCTION, MUSCLE PERFORMANCE, AND ROM ASSOCIATED WITH LOCALIZED INFLAMMATION

The list of potential pathology for soft tissue injuries to the foot, accompanied with localized inflammation, is extensive.

Inflammation or Infection of the Nails and Skin

Subungual Hematoma

A subungual hematoma is also called "black toenails" or "runner's toe" and results from bleeding under the toenails due to chronic friction or bumping of the toe against ill-fitting shoes, or from overt trauma to the posterior (dorsal) aspect of the toe.[383] Due to the extreme sensitivity of the nail bed, significant pulsating pain is often associated with this problem, with or without palpation.

In the case of poorly fitting shoes, prophylactic treatment is recommended. Athletic shoes should be one size longer than street shoes in most cases.[145]

For an existing hematoma, the treatment of choice involves decompression of the hematoma using a red-hot paper clip or 18-gauge needle, heated in an alcohol burner, which is used to burn a hole through the nail.[384]

Subungual Exostosis

A subungual exostosis is a hypertrophic bone, usually affecting the medial border of the hallux, as the result of excessive pressure, that produces pain on ambulation.[385] An accurate diagnosis of this condition requires a radiograph.[384]

Conservative intervention involves using a deep toe box and decreasing the width of hypertrophic nails.

Onychocryptosis

Onychocryptosis is more commonly referred to as ingrown toenails. It is commonly associated with a secondary pyogenic infection or paronychia. Onychocryptosis without paronychia is treated conservatively by removing the offending portion of the nail and then smoothing the nail border with a curette.[384]

Onychia

Onychia is an infection of one or both sides of the nail and nail plate, which can result from a number of factors including chronic pressure on the nail plate, allergies, nail polish, improperly cutting the nails, or certain soaps.[384]

Onychauxis

Onychauxis is an overgrowth of the nail that can be the result of microtrauma or macrotrauma, peripheral neuritis, old age, nutritional disturbances, or decreased circulation, producing future nail growth distortion.[383,384,386] The diagnosis is made by the hallmark characteristics of a hypertrophic, dystrophic, and discolored nail plate.[387]

The conservative intervention for this condition involves the mechanical or chemical debridement of the nail plate.[387]

Onychomycosis

Onychomycosis is a chronic fungal condition of the nails, which is often responsible for causing onychauxis.[388]

Tinea Pedis

Tinea pedis is more commonly known as athlete's foot. It usually presents with redness or itchiness but can also appear as dry and flaky skin.[384]

Treatment is simple and involves soaking the foot in one-half cup of vinegar in a pan of water once a day and applying a topical antifungal agent.[384]

Blisters

Blisters occur secondary to friction and shearing and can give the clinician valuable information as to where the stresses of the foot are occurring. Besides the obvious fact that tight shoes cause blisters, other causes include excessive motion such as pronation and supination.

Tendinitis

Overuse of the ankle and foot tendons occurs as the result of training errors, abrupt changes in training patterns, muscle–tendon imbalances, anatomic malalignment, or improper footwear.[342] This overuse causes the tendons to break down, resulting in tendinitis. Although more common in the adult population, tendinitis can also be seen in the adolescent due to a sudden growth spurt or the resumption of play after a period of decreased training.[389] The intervention for tendinitis/tenosynovitis includes identifying and removing the causative factor, an initial period of PRICEMEM followed by a program of stretching and strengthening of the tendon. On occasion, the intervention may require casting, orthotics, and/or prophylactic bracing.

Fibularis (Peroneal) Tendinitis

This form of tendinitis is particularly common in young ice skaters and dancers, but can also be seen in any running athlete. A number of conditions are associated with fibularis tendinitis including repeated inversion strains, which stretch and inflame the sheaths of the fibularis (peroneus) longus and brevis tendons (runner's foot), or with instability between the fourth and fifth metatarsals.

The patient usually presents with pain behind and distal to the lateral malleolus.[389] There may be associated swelling in the acute phase. There will also be pain with resisted foot eversion.

Fibularis (Peroneal) Tendon Subluxation

Subluxation of the fibularis (peroneal) tendons is an infrequent but potentially disabling condition that mainly affects young athletes.[390] In its early and later phases, the condition is often difficult to distinguish from a lateral ankle sprain, as the acute symptoms include pain at the posterior distal fibula, swelling, ecchymosis, and apprehension, or inability to evert the foot against resistance.[57,391] The chronic symptoms include lateral ankle pain, popping or snapping, and instability.[57] Confusing the issue is the fact that a chronic fibularis tendon subluxation can both mimic and coexist with chronic ankle instability.

One of the causes of this condition is that, in some individuals, there may be a number of anatomic anomalies that predispose the fibularis tendon to sublux including, an absent or shallow fibula groove,[76,342,392,393] probably combined with pes planus, hindfoot valgus, or lax/absent fibular retinaculum.[76,77,389,392,394] A subluxation can also occur from a traumatic rupture of the retinaculum as the result of a violent forced dorsiflexion of the ankle with reflex contraction of the fibularis muscles and subsequent dislocation.[76,77,308,342,394–396]

As with many tendon conditions, fibularis tendon subluxation can be an acute episode that turns into a chronic problem due to misdiagnosis.[57] Many of these subluxations are incorrectly diagnosed at the acute stage as simple ankle sprains.[397] The young patient may present acutely after a supposed ankle sprain, with pain and swelling over the posterolateral aspect of the ankle. More commonly though, the initial presentation may occur weeks to months after the injury.[307] The adolescent may complain of recurrent inversion ankle sprains and lateral ankle instability, with a painful snapping across the ankle.[398] Chronic ankle instability can also contribute to chronic fibularis tendon subluxation, with the development of an incompetent superficial fibular retinaculum.[76,398] This can also be confused with the rare isolated injury to the PTFL.[76,77,393,394]

On physical examination, subluxation may be provoked with forceful ankle dorsiflexion and eversion. There may be pain posterior to the lateral malleolus in an acute situation, as well as a negative anterior drawer test.[57]

A number of surgical procedures have been described for a chronic fibularis tendon subluxation, including tendon transfer, repair of the fibular retinaculum, groove deepening procedures, and tendon rerouting.[76,390,394,396,397]

Tibialis Posterior Tenosynovitis

The tibialis posterior tendon is lined with a tenosynovial sheath that can become inflamed, resulting in a tenosynovitis. If the tenosynovitis is left untreated, it can progress to an eventual rupture of the tibialis posterior tendon.[399]

Posterior tibial dysfunction is a complex disorder of the hindfoot. Controversy exists as to whether a persisting rotational instability after ankle sprain may cause posterior tibial dysfunction or vice versa. Posterior tibial dysfunction may cause ankle instability by overloading the ankle ligaments, especially the medial (deltoid) ligament of the ankle.[42]

The symptoms associated with this condition are usually felt in one of three locations:

- Distal to the medial malleoli in the area of the navicular.
- Proximal to the medial malleoli.
- At the musculotendinous origin, or insertion.

Posterior tibialis tenosynovitis is seen relatively frequently in participants of dance and ice-skating who have a pronated foot and flattened longitudinal arch.[150] The condition is also seen in running sports that require rapid changes in direction (basketball, tennis, and soccer) as abrupt changes in direction place increased stress across the tendon.[75] Other contributing factors include an adaptive shortening of the gastrocnemius–soleus complex and weakness of the posterior tibialis.

On physical examination, the patient will present with pain on resisted ankle plantar flexion and inversion,[75] with tenderness to palpation along the tendon's course posterior to the medial malleolus through to its insertion into the navicular. Swelling may sometimes be seen. Sometimes pain may be secondary to an accessory navicular.[75] With a complete rupture, the navicular subluxes inferiorly, and the patient ambulates in a flat-footed position, as they are unable to produce any toe-off at terminal stance.

Plain radiographs are rarely helpful, although MRI or bone scan[400] may aid in the diagnosis.

Patla and Haxby[152] describe a condition called tibialis posterior myofascial tightness (TPMT) as a factor in heel pain. In contrast to tibialis posterior tenosynovitis, TPMT is not characterized by inflammation of the tendon sheath. The patient with TPMT complains of immediate heel pain on weight-bearing in the morning. The pain is increased with increased load from activities but typically decreases during the day. There is no specific injury or activity identified as the cause. Physical findings include[152]

- depression of the medial arch with standing;
- neutral or inverted calcaneus in standing;
- flatfoot appearance and diminished push-off with gait;
- decreased full ROM of plantar flexion and calcaneal inversion with weight-bearing heel raising;
- full PROM of dorsiflexion and plantar flexion, with possible end-range discomfort;
- that posterior tibialis length test (see "Special Tests" section) shows decreased extensibility and often produces pain.

The intervention for this condition is geared toward correcting the impairments of the tibialis posterior muscle. The same technique and contacts used in the test are used for treatment, except that the manual stretch is maintained for approximately 2 minutes and is repeated approximately four times, with slightly stronger pressure being used each time.

Tibialis Anterior Tendinitis

Tibialis anterior tendinitis is most commonly seen in runners, especially in those who participate in up or down hill training. The examination will show point tenderness over the tendon, as it crosses the ankle.

FHL Tenosynovitis

As with the posterior tibialis, the FHL is lined by a tenosynovial sheath, which can become inflamed. FHL tendinitis is characterized by pain posterior to the medial malleolus, which is most often confused with posterior tibialis tenosynovitis.[401]

FHL tendinitis will usually present itself as pain with resisted great toe flexion in the young patient, as well as pain posterior and inferior to the medial malleolus. Dancers who assume the repeated plantar flexed posture of demipointe or pointe are particularly susceptible to this condition.[381,402,403] Runners and gymnasts are also susceptible.

The tendon sheath becomes inflamed due to forceful push-offs with the forefoot, where the FHL is stretched between the posterior talar tubercle and the sustentaculum tali. The tendon sheath can also be irritated with plantar flexion, where it is compressed over the posterior talar tubercle.[401,404]

Achilles Tendinitis

It is probably no accident that Homer decided that the heels of his Greek hero, Achilles, would be the one vulnerable area of the body.[405] This vulnerability of the heel continues to this day, with Achilles tendinitis being the most common overuse syndrome of the lower leg,[71] accounting for 5–18% of the total number of running injuries.

The Achilles tendon is placed under extreme and rapid eccentric loading forces during such activities as running, standing up while cycling, ballet, gymnastics, soccer, and basketball.[404,406]

The underlying mechanism of Achilles tendinitis is not well understood, but a number of mechanisms have been proposed of which the biomechanical hypothesis is the most popular. Immediately after the foot makes contact with the ground in a supinated position, it pronates and then supinates again as the propulsion phase approaches.[43,115] The pronated foot imparts an internal rotation force through the tibia, whereas knee extension imparts an external rotation force through the tibia.[406] The overpronated foot places the medial aspect of the tendon under tension, generating an obligatory internal tibial rotation, which tends to draw the Achilles tendon medially.[407] The rapid and repeated transitions from pronation to supination cause the Achilles tendon to undergo a "whipping" or "bow-string" action.[408] Moreover, if the foot remains in a pronated position after knee extension has begun, the external tibial rotation at the knee and the internal tibial rotation at the foot result in a "wringing" or twisting action of the tendon.[43]

Another proposed mechanism involves the eccentric contraction of the triceps surae during support. Maximal triceps sural contraction is associated with adduction and supination of the foot. At heel strike, the calf muscles undergo a rapid shortening before lengthening, as the tibia rotates forward over the foot. The calf muscles then shorten again during the forward propulsion phase.[409] These abrupt alternations in muscle action may cause microtears in the tendon.

In addition to those causes already described, a number of other factors appear to have some influence on the development of Achilles tendinitis:

- ***Stretching.*** McCrory et al.[408] determined that injured runners were less likely to incorporate stretching into their regular training routines. However, whether stretching habits can be related to the incidence of overuse injuries remains uncertain.[410–413]
- ***Training variables.*** Overuse injuries of the tendons have been strongly associated with a number of training variables including training at a faster pace,[66,410,414] and hill training.[68,409,415]
- ***Fatigue.*** Overtraining has been found to correlate with muscle fatigue and microtears of a tendon.[43,115]
- ***Exercise variables.*** Muscular insufficiency has been proposed as a significant factor in the inability to eccentrically control dorsiflexion during the beginning of the initial contact phase of running.[408,414–416]
- ***Anthropometric variables.*** One study determined that 20% of the injured runners with Achilles tendinitis had cavus feet.[115] Clement et al.,[415] suggested that a potential cause was compensatory overpronation resulting from the inflexibility of the cavus foot. A high-arched foot has also been found to be related to the incidence of various overuse syndromes by a number of other studies.[66,277,417,418]
- Age. Some studies have found a correlation between age and the pathogenesis of running injuries,[408,419] whereas others[412,418,420–422] have found no associations.
- ***Shoe type.*** Spiked running shoes, which provide minimal shock absorption and which lock the feet on the surface during the single support phase during running have been correlated with Achilles tendinitis. Theoretically, this type of shoe transfers the lateral and vertical torque shear forces directly to the foot and ankle and through the Achilles tendon, thereby increasing the overloading of the tendon, and causing microtrauma and inflammation of the tendon.[407,423]
- Sacroiliac joint dysfunction.[407] The primary function of the pelvis appears to be as a shock absorber, transmitting the weight of the trunk and upper extremities to the lower limbs and distributing the ground reaction forces.[93,424] The ground forces, which tend to rotate the innominate posteriorly, and the trunk forces combine to provide a mechanism of stability.[93,424] Posterior dysfunction is reported to be the most common lesion of the sacroiliac articulation by several authors.[425–427] This results in a functional shortening and external rotation of the involved leg,[428–430] both of which may influence the kinematic chain of the lower extremity in the following manner:[407]
- The ankle and foot position will be in external rotation, instead of neutral, at heel strike.
- Due to the transfer of body weight over the involved leg during the rest of the stance phase, the loading of the lateral aspect of the heel will be short, the following pronation prolonged, and the inversion delayed. This may decrease the amount of dorsiflexion in the ankle, thus minimizing the tension in the plantar soft tissues. This, in turn, decreases the leverage of the Achilles tendon and the truss mechanism[423] may not be activated due to insufficient hyperextension of the big toe.
- Because of the relative ineffectiveness of the foot's truss mechanism at terminal stance, together with the decrease in leverage of the Achilles tendon, the triceps surae will have to activate more motor units to ensure continued performance, thus putting additional loading on the Achilles tendon.

Achilles tendinitis typically occurs as one of two types of tendinitis: insertional and noninsertional, with the former involving the tendon–bone interface and the latter occurring just proximal to the tendon insertion on the calcaneus in or around the tendon substance.[406]

Noninsertional tendinitis can be referred to as peritendinitis, peritendinitis with tendinosis, or tendinosis.[406,431]

- ***Peritendinitis.*** The inflammation in peritendinitis is limited to the peritendon, and thickening can result.
- ***Peritendinitis with tendinosis.*** This condition describes a second stage of inflammation, in which a portion of the Achilles tendon itself is involved in the disease process.

- *Pure tendinosis.* This condition, which typically affects the *weekend warrior*, is characterized by microscopic and macroscopic mucoid degeneration of the tendon.

Clinical symptoms associated with Achilles tendinitis consist of a gradual onset of pain and swelling in the tendon 2–3 cm proximal to its insertion, which is exacerbated by activity. Some patients will present with pain and stiffness along the Achilles tendon when rising in the morning or complain of pain at the start of activity, which improves as the activity progresses. In fact, in the early stages of the condition, morning stiffness may be the only symptom, whereas pain is felt even at rest in the advanced stages.[65]

The vast majority of symptomatic patients are runners who complain of pain in the posterior aspect of the heel, approximately 2 cm proximal to the superior margin of the calcaneus, which increases during running activities.[73] The pain typically worsens over time, until it inhibits the individual from running, at which point they usually seek medical attention.

The differential diagnosis for posterior heel pain includes retrocalcaneal bursitis,[73] metabolic diseases, arthritis and chondropathic diseases of the ankle joint, tibia vara, os trigonum, a calcaneal contusion, plantar heel pain, calcaneal stress fracture impingement syndrome and stress fractures of the fibula or tibia (see Chap. 5).[407,432]

The Achilles tendon and heel may be examined with the patient in sitting or prone. Upon observation, the patient will often be found to have pronated feet, and the presence of swelling around the tendon is common.

Systematic palpation is performed along the tendon, over the heel, along the posterior border of the calcaneus, and down to the heel pad. Localization of the tenderness is extremely important. Tenderness located 2–6 cm proximal to the insertion is indicative of noninsertional tendinitis, whereas pain at the bone–tendon junction is more indicative of insertional tendinitis.[406] If there is an area in the tendon itself, which is discrete and painful with side-to-side pressure of the fingers, this often indicates an area of mucoid degeneration or a small partial rupture of the tendon.[73] If the tenderness is in the area of the retrocalcaneal bursa, which is noted by side-to-side pressure in that area, this is the primary area of involvement.[73]

A lack of 20 degrees of dorsiflexion in knee extension signifies adaptive shortening of the gastrocnemius, and an inability to dorsiflex 30 degrees in knee flexion implicates the soleus as well.[73]

Analysis of gait may reveal an antalgic gait, with the involved leg held in external rotation during both the stance and swing phases. There is often pain with resisted testing of the gastrocnemius/soleus complex.

The intervention for Achilles tendinitis in relation to exercise intensity varies according to the severity of the symptoms[72]:

- *Type I.* Characterized by pain that is only experienced after activity. These patients should reduce their exercise by 25%.
- *Type II.* Characterized by pain that occurs both during and after activity but does not affect performance. These patients should reduce their training by 50%.
- *Type III.* Characterized by pain during and after activity that does affect performance. These patients should temporarily discontinue running.

The conservative intervention, which almost always involves modification of extrinsic factors (training errors including a sudden increase in mileage, excessive hill running, and improper shoes), includes Achilles stretching, eccentric strengthening of the calf muscles, the correction of any lower chain asymmetries (low-back, pelvic, and hip flexor asymmetries; knee flexion contracture; femoral anteversion; and foot pronation),[433,434] electrotherapeutic modalities as appropriate, correct shoe wear, and orthotics—appropriately designed orthoses made from a mold of the foot held in subtalar neutral, and non–weight-bearing can be of significant benefit.[65]

A literature review[435] that investigated the best intervention for a patient with recurrent Achilles tendinitis, based on its validity and strength, recommended the 12-week eccentric program as outlined by Alfredson et al.[436] The program consists of two types of eccentric exercises—eccentrically loading the calf muscles with the knee bent and the knee straight and three sets of 15 repetitions using just body weight to start, with the patient instructed to continue unless the pain becomes disabling. The exercises are performed two times per day, each day of the week, for 12 weeks. If only minor pain or discomfort is experienced, the patient is instructed to increase the load by using a backpack loaded with weight. The 37-year-old patient in this study was compliant with the program and was able to successfully progress to marathon training within 3 weeks of beginning the program.[435]

Rupture of the Achilles Tendon

Rupture of the Achilles tendon was first described in 1575, and first reported in the literature in 1633.[437] Although the etiology of a spontaneous rupture remains incompletely understood, a number of theories have been proposed, including microtrauma,[438] inhibitor mechanism malfunction,[439] hypoxic and mucoid tendon degeneration,[440] decreased perfusion,[441] and systemic or locally injected steroids.[442] However, the fact that the peak incidence of Achilles' tendon rupture occurs in the middle age group rather than in the older population tends to lend credence to a mechanical etiology.[443] Three specific activities have been implicated in rupturing the Achilles tendon:[444]

- Pushing off on the forefoot while extending the knee.
- Sudden dorsiflexion with full-weight-bearing as might occur with a slip or fall.
- Aggressive dorsiflexion such as that occurs when jumping or falling from a height and landing on a plantar flexed foot.

The diagnosis of an Achilles tendon rupture is based almost solely on the history and physical findings. The classic history includes reports of sudden pain in the calf area, often associated with an audible snap, followed by difficulty in stepping off on the foot.[443] Physical examination reveals swelling of the calf as well as a palpable defect in the tendon (hatchet strike), as well as ecchymosis around the malleoli.[445] Perhaps, the most reliable sign of a complete rupture is a positive result on the Thompson squeeze test (see Fig. 21-51).[188,446]

Treatment options for an Achilles tendon rupture include surgical and non-surgical approaches, although opinions are divided as to what is the best course of action. The conservative intervention of Achilles tendon rupture traditionally consisted of short- or long-leg cast immobilization in the gravity equinus position (10–20 degrees of plantar flexion). However, this approach was found to result in a high incidence of re-rupture (10–30%)[447–450] and a decrease in maximal function.[439,451,452] This may be because it is impossible to restore the correct length of the Achilles' tendon with nonoperative treatment.[443] Recent studies have produced superior results with a much quicker rehabilitation using fixed or hinged boots.[453–456]

The results from the surgical approaches have varied with the recent studies reporting small, but statistically significant benefits from surgery.[457,458]

Sever Disease (Calcaneal Apophysitis)

Sever disease is a traction apophysitis at the insertion of the Achilles tendon and is a common cause of heel pain in the athletically active child, with 61% of cases occurring bilaterally.[459]

The calcaneal apophysis serves as the attachment for the Achilles tendon superiorly and for the plantar fascia and the short muscles of the sole of the foot inferiorly.[460] This os calcis secondary center of ossification appears at 9 years of age and usually fuses at 16 years of age.[57] The average age of onset for this condition is 8–13 years.[461]

Factors involved in the etiology of Sever disease include beginning a new sport or season, foot pronation, and a tight gastrocnemius–soleus complex.[462] Young gymnasts and dancers are particularly susceptible to this condition because of their repetitive jumping or landing from a height.[462] The tight Achilles' tendon is usually associated with a recent growth spurt and is not related to a specific injury.[57]

Although radiographs are often normal, sclerosis or fragmentation of the apophysis may be seen on plain radiographs.[57]

The location of the pain differs from that of plantar heel pain in that its focal point is more posterior than it is plantar.

The intervention for Sever disease begins with stretching the heel cord, using heel cups or heel wedges, and avoiding barefoot walking until becoming asymptomatic.[342]

Iselin's Disease

Iselin's disease is a traction apophysitis of the tuberosity of the fifth metatarsal. It is more commonly seen in athletically active older children and adolescents. The secondary center of ossification appears as a small, shell-shaped fleck of bone oriented slightly oblique to the metatarsal shaft and is located on the lateral plantar aspect of the tuberosity of the fifth metatarsal. This apophysis is located within the insertion site of the fibularis (peroneus) brevis tendon. The center appears in girls at an average of 9 years and in boys at 12 years and usually fuses to the shaft by 11 and 14 years, respectively.

The patient is usually involved in sports with running, cutting, and jumping. These activities may result in an inversion stress to this area. There is usually pain over the area, but no specific history of trauma. Resisted eversion typically reproduces the pain. A bone scan will usually be positive. Iselin's disease can be differentiated from an avulsion fracture of the base of the fifth metatarsal because the apophysis is located parallel to the long axis of the shaft and an avulsion fracture is usually transverse in nature.

The intervention for Iselin's disease includes immobilization for acute pain and physical therapy for strengthening of the fibularis (peroneal) tendons.[463]

Plantar Heel Pain

Plantar heel pain, which is the term used to describe pain arising from the insertion of the plantar fascia, with or without heel spur, has been experienced by 10% of the population.[464–466] The condition, often referred to as plantar fasciitis, is an inflammatory process. Waugh[467] has recently proposed that previously accepted inflammatory conditions, such as epicondylitis and plantar fasciitis, may be more accurately referred to as chronic pain syndromes.[468]

A number of factors have been proposed for the etiology of this condition:

- ***Obesity.***[469] Obesity has been shown to occur in 40% of men and 90% of women with plantar heel pain.[470,471] A body mass index greater than 30 kg/m^2 increases the risk of developing plantar heel pain.[472]
- ***Occupational.*** There is an association between plantar heel pain and prolonged standing or walking ("policeman's heel"),[62] or a sudden change in the stresses placed upon the feet likening this condition to other repetitive stress disorders such as carpal tunnel syndrome and tennis elbow.
- ***Acute injury.*** Although less common, plantar heel pain may be associated with an acute injury to the heel. Some people recall stepping on a pebble, or other hard object, before the pain began ("stone bruise").[62]
- ***Anatomical.*** The heel pad is specially constructed as an efficient shock absorber to attenuate peaks in dynamic forces and to dampen vibrations.[473] Part of the impact energy involved in displacement of the heel pad during ambulation is dissipated, and part of the energy is recovered in the subsequent elastic recoil. Two studies that examined the mechanical properties of the heel pad[474,475] found that thickness and compressibility index (CI; ratio of thickness of the loaded heel pad to that of the unloaded one) were greater in patients with plantar heel pain. This finding implies that loss of elasticity of the heel pad may be a factor in plantar heel pain syndrome.
- ***Biomechanical causes.*** People with high arches (pes cavus) or low arches (pes planus) are at increased risk because of the increased repetitive stress being placed on the fascia.[62] Likewise, adaptive shortening of the calf muscles and Achilles tendon, excessive rearfoot motion (especially overpronation), or a rigid varus hindfoot may also put the patient at risk, by placing excess stress on the plantar fascia.[277,476–478] Amis et al.[477] found that 78% of patients with painful heels had ankle dorsiflexion limitations of at least 5 degrees. Kibler et al.[478] noted that 90% of running athletes with plantar fasciitis had either a lack of 5 degrees dorsiflexion beyond neutral on the affected side or a lack of 10 degrees or more dorsiflexion compared with the noninvolved side. Weakness of the intrinsic foot muscles has also been cited as a cause. These factors may increase the moment of maximum tension in the fascia, which, even under normal circumstances, endures tension that is approximately two times body weight during walking at the

moment when the heel of the trailing leg begins to lift off the ground. Thus, an accurate history of footwear should be obtained: Often patients wear shoes with poor cushioning or inadequate arch support or they walk barefoot on hard floors.

Although more common in active individuals, plantar heel pain can also affect the sedentary, although the reasons for this remain elusive. Despite the fact that modern shoes are designed with every conceivable type of heel cushioning, plantar heel pain continues to be a pervasive entity. Although more common in middle-aged individuals, plantar heel pain can occur in the younger individual, although it rarely exists alone in this age group and usually coincides with calcaneal apophysitis.[57] As the plantar fascia assists in the development of the push-off power during running and jumping, it is not surprising that plantar heel pain is particularly prevalent in joggers and tennis players, as well as in athletes participating in racquet sports, soccer, gymnastics, and basketball.[62]

The role of the heel spur in plantar heel pain is controversial.[62] Half of patients with plantar heel pain have heel spurs,[470] whereas 16–27% of the population have heel spurs without symptoms.[148,479] The greater pull of the plantar fascia was thought to lead to periosteal hemorrhage and inflammatory reaction and to laying down of new bone and heel spur formation,[480] but the heel spur is more often associated with the FDB muscle than the plantar fascia.[150,404,477,481–484]

Since chronic subcalcaneal heel pain is a common manifestation of many conditions, the following diagnoses must be excluded:

- ***Inflammatory spondyloarthropathies.*** These disorders should be considered when multiple joints or areas are involved. Up to 16% of patients presenting with subcalcaneal pain will later be diagnosed with a systemic arthritic disorder.[38,62]
- ***Calcaneal stress fracture.***[485] The history for calcaneal stress fractures usually involves a sudden increase in a running activity, such as that seen in a military recruit at boot camp or a reservist.
- ***Nerve entrapment.***[485–487] Heel pain was recently reported to involve the nerve to abductor digiti quinti, the first branch of the lateral plantar nerve.[488] In a fifth of cases of inferior heel pain, the pain may be caused by this nerve being trapped between the abductor digiti quinti muscle and the quadratus plantae muscle or affected by inflammation of the plantar fascia.[488] Positive percussion (Tinel's sign) on the medial aspect of the heel should lead to a suspicion of entrapment of the nerve to abductor digiti quinti or a tarsal tunnel syndrome (TTS).[38]
- ***Tumors.*** Tumors in this area are quite rare, presenting as palpable masses or bony erosions of the calcaneus.
- ***Infections.***[489] As with infections in other parts of the body, there will usually be some swelling and/or erythema and a history of malaise or fever.
- ***Neuropathy (diabetic, alcoholic).***[485] A history of burning pain, numbness, or paresthesias can often be elicited in patients with neuropathic pain. A thorough neurologic exam will confirm the diagnosis.
- ***The fat-pad syndrome.***[37,490] Pain while hopping on the toes may help distinguish this entity from the fat-pad syndrome.

The diagnosis of plantar heel pain is typically made on the basis of clinical findings. Common findings include a history of pain and tenderness on the plantar medial aspect of the heel, especially during initial weight-bearing in the morning. This is thought to be due to the fact that in the morning, the plantar fascia is cold, contracted, or stiff.[491] The patient may also report pain that radiates up the calf and toward the toes. In severe cases, the pain may have a throbbing or burning quality. Interference with daily activities is common.[492] Plantar heel pain is usually unilateral, although in 15–30% of people, both feet are affected.[62,493] The heel pain often decreases during the day but worsens with increased activity (such as jogging, climbing stairs, or going up on the toes) or after a period of sitting.

On physical examination, there will be localized pain on palpation along the medial edge of the fascia or at its origin on the anterior edge of the calcaneus, although firm finger pressure is often necessary to localize the point of maximum tenderness.[38] The main area of tenderness is typically just over and distal to the medial calcaneal tubercle, and usually there is one small extremely painful area. Tenderness in the center of the posterior part of the heel may be due to bruising or atrophy of the heel pad or to subcalcaneal bursitis.[470] Slight swelling in the area is common.[477] Tightness of the Achilles tendon is found in 78% of patients.[470,477]

To test for plantar heel pain, the fascia needs to be put on stretch with a bowstring-type test. The patient's heel is manually fixed in eversion. The clinician takes hold of the first metatarsal and places it in dorsiflexion before extending the great toe as far as possible. Pain should be elicited at the medial tubercle.

It has been reported that almost 90% of patients with plantar heel pain who undergo a conservative intervention improve significantly within 12 months, although approximately 10% can develop persistent and often disabling symptoms.[494] This time frame for resolution of symptoms suggests that present interventions are ineffective and that time alone heals the patient. A recent review of the literature at the plantar heel pain interventions concluded that there was no quality information regarding the effectiveness of treatments of the heel pain.[465] The interventions thus far attempted include the following:

- ***Night splinting.*** There is limited evidence for night splints to treat chronic symptoms.[495]
- ***Orthotics.*** Most of the orthotics are designed to correct biomechanical faults, especially over pronation.
- ***Heel cups/taping.*** Lynch et al.[496] performed an unblinded prospective trial of 103 subjects with plantar heel pain randomized into one of three groups of treatment: anti-inflammatory (NSAIDS and steroid injections), accommodative (viscoelastic heel cup), or mechanical (taping for 4 weeks followed by custom orthoses). At the end of 3 months, there was no significant difference in activity level and first step pain between the groups. However, the mechanical treatment group (taping) had significantly better visual analog scales (VAS) scores than the accommodative group (heel cup) and had a significantly better rate of fair or

excellent outcomes. A randomized controlled trial by Hyland et al.[468] found calcaneal taping to invert the heel and raise the medial longitudinal arch to be a more effective tool for the relief of plantar heel pain than stretching, sham taping, or no treatment after 1 week. Taping can be considered as a means of reinforcing either the calcaneal fat pad and/or the medial longitudinal arch. The tape of choice is a low-die 1-inch tape.[73] Prior to applying the tape, the patient should be relaxed and the heel and foot placed in neutral. Excessive tension through the strips will lead to complaints during activity. The patient should be in weight bearing throughout the foot before applying the final closing strips. Care must be taken when applying the tape on the medial, lateral, or posterior (dorsal) aspect of the foot. Tension in the tape flow is critical, if skin breakdown is to be avoided with repeated taping.[73]

- ***Stretching and strengthening.*** Some evidences exist for plantar fascia stretching to address chronic plantar fasciitis.[497]
- ***Deep frictional massage.*** This can be applied manually VIDEO or through the use of a tennis ball VIDEO, or golf ball VIDEO.
- ***Corticosteroid injection.*** There is limited evidence for topical corticosteroids administered via iontophoresis for pain relief.[495]
- ***Dexamethasone iontophoresis.***
- ***Shoe modifications.***
- ***NSAIDs.***
- ***Casting.*** Recalcitrant or long-standing cases of plantar heel pain may require casting. This can take the form of a short-leg walking cast positioned in neutral (plantigrade) for 4–6 weeks. Patients with severe pain and marked limitation of activity are best treated with a molded, below-knee, walking cast for 3–4 weeks.[39] It provides relative rest, reduces pressure on the heel at heel strike, provides an arch support, and prevents tightening of the Achilles tendon. A night splint positioned in 5 degrees of dorsiflexion is worn for an additional 6 weeks once the cast is removed, and the patient can resume the stretching and strengthening program for an additional 6 weeks once the cast is removed.[62]
- ***Extracorporeal shock wave lithotripsy***[498]
- ***Radiofrequency lesioning.***
- ***Open and endoscopic plantar fasciotomy and surgical neurolysis (in extremely recalcitrant cases).*** It has been reported that approximately 5% of patients who are diagnosed with plantar heel pain undergo surgery for the condition.[496,499]

A number of clinical trials have attempted to examine the efficacy of intervention combinations for plantar heel pain. The University of Pittsburgh Medical Center Foot and Ankle Clinic has advocated nonsurgical treatment of insertional plantar heel pain using a standardized regimen since 1992.[500] The regimen is as follows:

- Take NSAIDs as directed for 4 weeks.
- Attend the University of Pittsburgh Sports Medicine Clinic for a one-time instructional home-exercise program of Achilles stretching (four exercises) and plantar fascia stretching (two exercises). The subject is instructed to continue the exercises for six sets, holding each for 30 seconds × 3/day.
- Wear a night splint every night to bed.
- Use an orthosis or heel cup at all times when wearing shoes.

The reported outcomes in this study were not as good as the average outcome reported in other published studies, with only 51% being asymptomatic after 4 months.[500] The authors cited that the reasons for this were that other studies may have included subjects with causes of subcalcaneal heel pain other than true plantar heel pain, making direct comparison difficult.

The lack of a universal intervention for plantar heel pain, and the poor level of long-term success, likely stems from its many causes. A poor response to an intervention may be due, in part, to inappropriate and nonspecific techniques or an inaccurate diagnosis. The etiological trauma for plantar heel pain occurs after the peak loads of initial contact are reached and as the center of mass advances beyond the ankle. This would tend to indicate that the forces associated with initial contact are not directly linked with the stresses that are applied to the plantar fascia. Indeed, the highest force loads on the foot during gait occur at the forefoot. These forces have been found to be 15–25% higher than those occurring during initial contact. Fortunately, the foot has a built-in mechanism to deal with these loads—the Windlass mechanism. As the heel rises about the rotating MTP joints, the plantar fascia, through its insertion into the bases of the digits, "winds" itself around the drum-like metatarsal heads. This creates a winch-like effect that pulls the proximal aspect of the heel closer to the ball of the foot and elevates the medial longitudinal arch, which, in turn, provides a stable platform upon which propulsion can occur. Critical to the efficiency of the Windlass mechanism is the ability of the first MTP joint to dorsiflex during the heel-raise phase of gait. An inability to dorsiflex the first MTP is called functional hallux limitus (see "Examination" section).

Given that plantar heel pain appears to be impairment based, an impairment-based physical therapy examination and intervention approach would appear to be logical.[495] Such an approach has been investigated in several randomized controlled trials. Pollard and So[501] reported full recovery in a 35-year-old male with a 3-month history of right inferior heel pain, using a combination of talocrural and talocalcaneal joint mobilization, stretching, strengthening, custom orthosis, and pain modalities. Patla and Abbott[152] reported restoration of pain-free functional activities with the use of manual posterior tibialis stretching in two patients with primary complaints of heel pain. Young et al.,[495] in a case series, treated four patients with plantar heel pain, using an impairment-based physical therapy approach, which emphasized manual therapy. All four patients demonstrated complete pain relief and full return to activities.[495]

On the basis of the above-mentioned studies, the intervention for plantar heel pain should include the following:

- Rest or at least aviodance of any activity that continually provides axial loading of the heel and tensile stresses on the fascia.
- A recommendation of shoes that provide good shock absorption at the heel and support to the medial longitudinal arch and plantar fascia.
- The identification of the cause of any tissue overloading that is occurring, as well as any functional biomechanical deficits (plantar flexor inflexibility and weakness) and functional adaptations (running on toes, shortened stride length, and foot inversion).
- Strengthening exercises. A number of strengthening exercises have been devised for plantar heel pain:
  - ***Towel curls.*** A towel is placed on a smooth surface, with the foot placed on the towel. The patient is instructed to pull the towel toward the body by curling up the toes, and then attempt to move the towel in the reverse direction VIDEO.
  - ***Marble pick-ups.*** A few marbles are placed on the floor near a cup. While keeping the heel on the floor, the patient uses the toes to pick up the marbles and drop them in the cup.
  - ***Toe taps.*** The patient is instructed to keep the heel on the floor and lift all of the toes off the floor. The patient is asked to tap the big toe to the floor, while keeping the outside four toes in the air. Next, the patient keeps the big toe in the air, while tapping the other four toes to the floor.
- A regimen of stretching of the gastrocnemius and the medial fascial band, especially before arising in the morning and after sedentary periods during the day, as well as before and after exercise.[502]
  - ***Gastrocnemius and soleus.*** Patients are taught how to stretch the gastrocnemius and soleus VIDEO components of the triceps surae independently while minimizing stress on the plantar fascia. After a warm-up, the patient stands against a wall, with his or her hands placed against the wall. With one foot forward and one behind, the patient leans his or her trunk toward the wall, shifting their weight over the front foot, while straightening the knee of the back leg. The heel of the back foot should remain on the floor while the front of the foot is internally rotated and supinated, to stabilize the medial longitudinal arch, putting the foot in the close-packed position and allowing for the stretch to be isolated to the Achilles tendon.[62] The stretch is then repeated on the other leg. A similar stretch can be done by standing on a stair step, with only the toes on the stairs and the back two-thirds of the feet hang off the step. By leaning forward to balance, the heel, Achilles tendon, and calf will be stretched. The stretch can also be performed when standing, where the heel is on the floor and the front part of the foot is on a wooden 2 × 4.
  - ***Plantar fascia stretch.*** The plantar fascia stretch is performed with the patient sitting with their legs crossed, with the involved leg over the contralateral leg. Then, while using the hand on the affected side, the patient places his or her fingers across the base of the toes on the bottom of the foot (distal to the MTP joints) and pulls the toes back toward the shin until a stretch is felt in the arch of the foot. The correct stretch is confirmed by palpating the tension in the plantar fascia with the contralateral hand, while performing the stretching. In a prospective randomized trial from DiGiovanni et al.,[497] 101 patients who had chronic proximal plantar heel pain for at least 10 months were randomized into one of two treatment groups. The mean age was 46 years. All patients received prefabricated soft insoles and a 3-week course of celecoxib, and they also viewed an educational video on plantar heel pain. The patients received instructions for either a plantar fascia tissue-stretching program (Group A) or an Achilles-tendon-stretching program (Group B). All patients completed the pain subscale of the FFI and a subject-relevant outcome survey that incorporated generic and condition-specific outcome measures related to pain, function, and satisfaction with treatment outcome. The patients were reevaluated after 8 weeks. Eighty-two patients returned for follow-up evaluation. With the exception of the duration of symptoms ($P < 0.01$), covariates for baseline measures revealed no significant differences between the groups. The pain subscale scores of the FFI showed significantly better results for the patients managed with the plantar fascia-stretching program with respect to item 1 (worst pain; $P = 0.02$) and item 2 (first steps in the morning; $P = 0.006$).[497] Analysis of the response rates to the outcome measures also revealed significant differences with respect to pain, activity limitations, and patient satisfaction, with greater improvement seen in the group managed with the plantar fascia-stretching program.

The stretches are performed twice daily, beginning with a sustained stretch for 1 minute and progressing to 3 minutes based on tolerance.[488] The rest period should involve gentle active dorsiflexion and plantar flexion exercises, while resting the Achilles tendon and calf on a hot pack to enhance the stretch.[62] Massage to the foot in the area of the arch and heel or rolling the foot over a tennis ball or a 15-ounce can may also be helpful.

- Orthotics may be prescribed, but only after careful examination of the footwear to ensure a firm, well-fitting heel counter, good heel cushioning, and an adequate longitudinal arch support.[503] A wide variety of rigid, semirigid, and soft shoe inserts are commercially available, although rigid plastic orthoses rarely alleviate the symptoms and often aggravate the heel pain.[472] Orthoses made of softer materials provide cushioning by reducing the shock of walking by up to 42%.[38] Since the plantar fascia is stretched during flattening of the foot, orthoses should be designed to maintain the medial longitudinal arch during ambulation, and should be prescribed in full length or three-quarters length-accommodative inlays of medium-density plastazote.[38]

The type of orthotic prescribed depends on the findings:[62]

- ***Normal foot.*** Off-the-shelf heel cups should be used to cushion the heel. Cyriax recommended heel lifts to relieve the strain on the plantar fascia during early treatment,[133] and bilateral heel lifts of ¼ to ⅜ inch are sometimes successful, but their use should be discontinued at the earliest possible time.[73]

- *Pes planus (flatfoot).* For this foot type, the orthotic is used to stabilize the arch and thereby decrease the strain on the plantar fascia. A University of California-Biomechanics Laboratory (UC-BL) type of orthotic is indicated.
- *Pes cavus (high arch).* An excessively high arch or cavus foot can cause an inability to evert the foot to dissipate stress. In this situation, the orthotic of choice would be one that focuses on cushioning to increase the total contact area of the foot.

Bursitis

Retrocalcaneal Bursitis

Retrocalcaneal bursitis is a distinct entity denoted by pain that is anterior to the Achilles tendon, just superior to its insertion on the os calcis. This type of bursitis appears to be more common in older individuals and low-level recreational athletes.[73,504]

The bursa becomes inflamed, hypertrophied, and adherent to the underlying tendon, resulting in deep pain and visible swelling.[39,74] Characteristic findings include pain with a two-finger squeeze just superior and anterior to the Achilles insertion and pain with passive dorsiflexion.[57]

Retrocalcaneal bursitis is treated conservatively with shoe modifications (open backed if necessary) and a heel lift.[57] In rare cases, a bursectomy with associated resection of the posterior superior margin of the os calcis is necessary.

A small percentage of the population has an adventitious subcalcaneal bursa, which may become inflamed and cause heel pain.[478]

Anterior Ankle Bursitis

Anterior ankle bursitis is commonly seen in young figure skaters and ice hockey players.[57] This condition can present with swelling over the anterior ankle or over either malleoli. A doughnut pad inside the skate over the irritable area will usually decrease the pressure at this point.[57]

Haglund's Deformity

Haglund's deformity[505] refers to an abnormal prominence of the posterior superior lateral border of the calcaneus. Because of its association with various shoe types, it is often referred to as a "pump bump,"[506] "high heel,"[507] and "winter heel."[508,509]

The prominence is frequently a bony spur or osteophyte acquired as the result of poorly fitting of shoes in adolescent females, ice skaters, soccer players, and runners,[150] but is also thought to be a congenital variation.

Whatever the etiology of these various prominences, they frequently aggravate the retrocalcaneal bursa on the deep surface of the Achilles tendon, producing an associated retrocalcaneal bursitis or Achilles tendinitis.[57]

On physical examination, a bump, which is 2–3 cm in diameter, is usually located more to the lateral side of the heel, and there is often an accompanying thickening of the overlying skin. Pain is often noted on palpation just proximal and slightly lateral to the insertion of the Achilles tendon.[502] Sometimes a varus hindfoot is found. A cavus or high-arched foot is believed to change the calcaneal position and increase the prominence of this ridge.[502]

Before intervention is initiated, the differential diagnosis must be considered, including systemic disease, Achilles tendinitis, or intrinsic conditions of the calcaneus, such as infection and tumor.[57]

Intervention involves relieving the friction imposed by the shoe counter by using a softer heel counter, increasing shoe size by one-half, padding the prominence, or using a heel lift to actually raise the heel out of the shoe.[74,509,510] Achilles stretching and strengthening and the use of local modalities, such as ultrasound, are also recommended.[57]

Surgical excision of the deformity is reserved for persistent symptoms in the young athlete.[506,509,511]

Metatarsalgia

During the normal gait cycle, the center of pressure progresses along the plantar aspect of the foot from the heel at initial contact to the toes at terminal stance. The center of pressure is initially located in the central heel and then accelerates rapidly across the midfoot to reach the forefoot, where it is located under the second and the third metatarsal head, rather than under the first and the fifth metatarsal head and the calcaneus, as was once thought.[50,85,89] This weight-bearing force is approximately equal to the body weight, which is more than twice the load carried by the other toes combined.

Any biomechanical intrinsic or extrinsic condition that increases stress on the metatarsal heads may result in metatarsal head pain and the development of painful plantar keratoses or calluses.[149] Plantar keratoses may be diffuse and large or small and discrete.

- A Morton's foot with a short first metatarsal and a relatively long second metatarsal may result in increased loading of the second metatarsal head and the development of a painful callus.[512]
- Patients with abnormally lax first metatarsal–cuneiform joints, resulting in a hypermobile first ray, can experience increased weight-bearing under the second and third metatarsals, which often results in painful diffuse calluses.[50]
- A prominent lateral condyle of a lesser metatarsal can result in a smaller discrete plantar keratosis, which can be exquisitely tender to palpation.
- A tight Achilles tendon can increase the forefoot load in late stance phase and may result in metatarsalgia.[50]
- The use of high-heeled shoes extrinsically increases forefoot load and may lead to diffuse metatarsalgia.

The intervention for metatarsalgia involves the use of a metatarsal pad that is placed proximal to the painful metatarsal heads. Adhesive-backed metatarsal pads of different shapes and sizes are available to unload one or several metatarsal heads. Custom orthotics may also be molded specifically for the cavus foot to decrease load on the plantar flexed first and second rays, to distribute weight evenly across the forefoot. A patient with a hypermobile first ray will benefit from a custom longitudinal arch support with medial forefoot post. A trial of Achilles stretching is helpful in the initial treatment of metatarsalgia. The wearing of high heels should be discouraged in patients with metatarsalgia.

If unresponsive to conservative intervention, surgical plantar condylectomy may be required for resolution of a discrete plantar keratosis. More generalized diffuse painful calluses such as those seen under the first and second metatarsal heads in the cavus foot may require posterior (dorsal) closing wedge osteotomies of the metatarsal bases to achieve pain relief.[149]

Idiopathic Synovitis

Idiopathic synovitis of the second or third MTP joint is another cause of metatarsalgia. This condition results in painful distension of the joint, swelling of the second toe, warmth, and limited MTP joint motion.[513] Second MTP joint synovitis probably occurs as a result of attrition of the plantar plate due to a long second metatarsal.[514] Posterior (dorsal) instability of the MTP joint may develop with joint subluxation or dislocation. A hammer toe or claw toe deformity is common.

Initially, the patient develops pain on palpation in the plantar and posterior (dorsal) aspects of the MTP joint. Joint instability can be diagnosed with passive articular mobility testing.

Conservative intervention includes NSAID, a metatarsal pad, taping the toe in a plantar flexed position, and an accommodative shoe. An intra-articular corticosteroid injection in combination with a rocker-sole modification has been shown to result in improvement in 93% of 15 cases.[515] Persistent pain in the second MTP joint despite conservative measures may necessitate operative synovectomy to avert toe dislocation or deformity.

Metatarsalgia of the Fifth Toe

This is usually due to overwork of the fibularis (peroneus) longus/brevis secondary to an unstable ankle. The overwork of the brevis leads to an instability of the fifth metatarsal at the intermetatarsal or cubometatarsal joints. The patient will point to the tubercle of the fifth metatarsal and complain of pain along the proximal part of the fibularis (peroneus) muscle. Conservative intervention involves taping a strip of tape over the posterior aspect of the foot and then one strip on the medial aspect, going proximal to distal. These two strips are then connected with strips of tape under the foot, across the sole.

Anterior Ankle Impingement

Anterior ankle impingement can be bony or soft tissue related. Patients with this problem usually present with anterior ankle pain exacerbated by extreme dorsiflexion.[16,57]

A bony impingement can be seen in young ballet dancers who exercise in extreme ankle dorsiflexion, irritating the periosteum on the talar neck, and leading to an exostosis and discomfort with pliés.[462]

A form of soft tissue impingement can be secondary to generalized synovitis or capsulitis. This can develop after acute or recurrent episodes of an inversion ankle sprain or in adolescent gymnasts who sustain repeated forced dorsiflexion in landing and dismount.

Chronic anterolateral ankle impingement due to a thickened and scarred joint capsule is a frequent sequela of recurrent ankle sprains. Wolin et al.[516] reported in 1950 that recurrent pain and swelling after injury to the lateral ligaments without instability in patients with a history of previous ankle sprains was due to hyalinized connective tissue arising from the anteroinferior portion of the talofibular joint capsule. They believed that the symptoms resulted from this connective tissue becoming pinched in the talofibular joint with motion. As this mass of tissue and synovium increases in size, impingement of the tissue mass between the talus, tibia, and fibula causes further irritation and pain. This has since been confirmed arthroscopically and by MRI.[517–524]

Bassett et al.[525] reported a cause of chronic pain in the ankle after inversion sprain in seven patients as being due to talar impingement by a distal fascicle of the anterior–inferior tibiofibular ligament.

On physical examination, there is usually pain to palpation anteriorly, with no palpable swelling.[304] Plain ankle radiographs can be helpful in determining a bony problem, but a bone scan is usually necessary for a definitive diagnosis. MRI may also be diagnostic.

The intervention for the soft tissue impingement variety includes discontinuing landing temporarily, icing,[404] anti-inflammatories, and exercises to stretch the Achilles tendon and strengthen the dorsiflexors. Occasionally, a pad taped over the anterior ankle may provide temporary relief.[304] Arthroscopy may be indicated if conservative treatment fails. A partial synovectomy[526] or excision of osteophytes is successful but must be followed by exercises to prevent recurrence.

Posterior Ankle Impingement

Posterior ankle impingement or talar compression syndrome[60] is seen most often in young female dancers, ice skaters, or gymnasts.[57] These sports require excessive plantar flexion of the ankle, compressing the posterior structures of the ankle.[60,401]

On physical examination, the patient will have pain on palpation of the posterior ankle, dramatically increased with forced plantar flexion.[57]

Plain radiographs of the ankle can be taken to rule out a bony etiology (i.e., os trigonum).[60] Soft tissue etiology includes FHL irritation, a thickened or invaginated posterior capsule, synovitis, and calcific debris.[401,527,528]

Sesamoiditis

This condition has been defined as inflammation and swelling of the peritendinous structures of the sesamoids. The tibial (medial) and fibular (lateral) sesamoids are situated under the first metatarsal head. These sesamoids are prone to injury in repetitive high-impact and contact sports.[50] Since the tibial sesamoid bears most of the force under the first metatarsal head, it is most commonly injured.[50]

Although direct trauma or forced dorsiflexion of the great toe can acutely fracture the sesamoids, most sesamoid injuries are overuse injuries. Twelve percent of injuries to the great toe complex are sesamoid injuries.[51]

The etiologies of sesamoid injuries include stress fracture (40%), acute fractures (10%), chondromalacia, synovitis, sesamoiditis (30%), osteochondritis (10%), arthritis (5%), and bursitis (5%).[51] Bipartite or multipartite sesamoids occur in 5–33% of the population and are bilateral in 25%.[54,529]

The diagnosis of sesamoiditis is one of exclusion.[530] Sesamoiditis is associated with local trauma, pain on weight-bearing, and plantar soft tissue swelling.[531] Passive dorsiflexion of the MTP joint while palpating the sesamoids exacerbates the pain. Sesamoidal bursitis presents with swelling, erythema, and tenderness with a side-to-side pinch. A plantar fullness or fluid-filled bursal cyst may be palpated under the sesamoids.

Conservative intervention involves rest from the offending activity, NSAIDs, and low-heeled shoes with a soft metatarsal support proximal to the metatarsal head, to decrease the load on the involved sesamoid.[532] One or two injections of corticosteroids into the region of the sesamoids may be helpful.[50] Failure of several months of conservative care may result in the need for surgical excision of the offending sesamoid to alleviate symptoms.[532]

MEDIAL TIBIAL STRESS SYNDROME

Exercise-induced anterior and medial leg pain has been reported to account for 60% of all injuries causing leg pain in athletes.[533] A number of generic terms such as "medial tibial syndrome," "tibial stress syndrome," "shin splints," "posterior tibial syndrome," "soleus syndrome," and "periostitis" have evolved over the years to describe exercise-related leg pain. Of all these terms, medial tibial stress syndrome (MTSS) is the most appropriate.

MTSS appears to involve periosteal irritation indicated by a diffuse linear uptake on a bone scan along the length of the tibia.[534] The anatomic site of the abnormality has been fairly well localized to the fascial insertion of the medial soleus.

The characteristic complaint in these patients is a dull aching pain along the middle or distal posteromedial tibia. Early in this process, the pain usually occurs at the beginning of a run, resolves with continued exertion, only to recur toward the end or after a workout.[535] At this stage, the pain typically subsides quickly with rest.[535] With continued training the pain usually becomes more severe, and persistent, and with increasing chronicity, the pain may be present with ambulation or at rest.[535]

Overuse or weakness of the tibialis anterior, EDL, or EDB may be the causative factors in anterior shin splints, as are excessive or abnormal pronation, restricted ankle joint dorsiflexion, training errors, and inadequate footwear.[80]

With the exception of pain and point tenderness at the anteromedial aspect of the tibia, which is increased with active dorsiflexion and passive stretching into plantar flexion, there are few objective findings. However, the pain is usually provoked with activity and relieved with rest.

As with most overuse injuries, the intervention for shin splints involves activity modification, followed by a gradual return to sports, making sure to identify and correct any training errors or abnormal foot biomechanics.

PREFERRED PRACTICE PATTERN 5F: IMPAIRED JOINT MOBILITY, MOTOR FUNCTION, MUSCLE PERFORMANCE, AND ROM, OR REFLEX INTEGRITY SECONDARY TO PERIPHERAL NERVE INJURY

An entrapment neuropathy is characterized by an entrapment of a peripheral nerve by fascia, a ligament, a bony groove, or a tendinous arch of a muscle origin. Sural nerve neuropraxias and fibular (peroneal) nerve palsies are an infrequent complication of lateral ligamentous injuries of the ankle but are quite problematic.[16,125] EMG evaluation of patients with ankle sprains reveals that up to 80% of patients with severe ankle sprains have some evidence of fibular (peroneal) nerve injury.[16,125]

Interdigital Neuroma

The name of the condition is a misnomer, as a true neuroma does not exist. Rather, there is a thickening of the tissues around the nerve due to perineural fibrosis, fibrinoid degeneration, demyelination, and endoneural fibrosis.[50,536] In a study of 91 patients with interdigital neuromas, the male: female ratio was 1:9.[537]

Although a common cause of this condition is chronic compression of the interdigital nerve, it can also occur due to an acute dorsiflexion injury to the toes, with an associated injury to the collateral ligaments of the MTP joint.[50,146]

Symptoms are usually aggravated with weight-bearing and somewhat relieved by rest and forefoot massage.[50,146] Incorrect shoe selection, such as wearing a cross-training or racket shoe for long-distance running, may increase the impact forces on the forefoot and contribute to the symptoms.[50] Narrow shoes and high-heeled shoes have also been implicated.

Physical examination reveals tenderness in the web space plantarly between the metatarsal heads.[50] Squeezing the forefoot with one hand, while carefully palpating the involved interspace with the thumb and index fingers of the other hand, will usually elicit marked discomfort,[50] or produce a painful audible click, known as Mulder's sign.[538] Careful palpation of the MTP joint, metatarsal head, and proximal phalanx should be performed to rule out localized joint or bone pathology such as MTP joint synovitis, stress fracture, or Freiberg's disease, which can also cause symptoms of forefoot pain.[50] A positive Tinel's sign over the tarsal tunnel or multiple symptomatic web spaces should alert the clinician to the possibility of a more proximal nerve compression or underlying peripheral neuropathy.[50] EMG studies and nerve conduction velocity testing should be performed in these cases.[146]

The intervention initially involves an avoidance of the offending activity, cross-training using lower-impact sports, and a modification of footwear—a switch to wider, more accommodating shoes with soft soles and better shock absorption.[50] In addition, a metatarsal pad, placed proximal to the symptomatic interspace, may prove helpful.[50] The metatarsal pad can also be incorporated into a custom-made full-length semirigid orthotic.[50] A trial of NSAIDs is indicated in an attempt to decrease inflammation around the interdigital nerve.[50] A trial of vitamin B6 has been used successfully in the treatment of carpal tunnel syndrome and may also be useful in the treatment of interdigital neuritis.[539]

Recalcitrant cases that fail to respond after 2–3 months of the above conservative measures may benefit from an injection of corticosteroids.[50] One to two injections can be tried, but multiple injections should be avoided, as corticosteroids may cause atrophy of the plantar fat pad.[50] Surgery is the intervention of last resort.

Deep Fibular (Peroneal) Nerve Entrapment/Anterior TTS

Entrapment of the deep fibular (peroneal) nerve was first reported in 1963[540] and was given the name anterior TTS in 1968.[541]

At the ankle level, both motor and sensory branches of the deep fibular (peroneal) nerve are present.

Anterior tarsal syndrome[542] occurs when there is a contusion to the terminal branch of the deep fibular (peroneal) nerve, as it travels beneath the posterior tibialis and EHB tendons, and above the first and second cuneiforms, where it is relatively unprotected.[543] The compression usually results from tight boots or from the shoe straps of high heels, a ganglion, pes cavus, or from direct trauma.[542,544] A partial anterior TTS[545] occurs when either the motor branch to the EDB or only the sensory branch of the deep fibular (peroneal) nerve is compressed beneath the inferior extensor retinaculum.[543]

Patients with anterior TTS complain of a deep aching pain in the medial and posterior (dorsal) aspect of the foot, burning around the nail of the great toe, and pins and needles at the adjacent borders of the great and second toes that are exacerbated with plantar flexion and improved with rest.[543,544,546,547]

The examination reveals weakness or atrophy of the EDB muscle and diminished movement with toe extension.[543]

Conservative intervention for these patients involves an alteration of daily and sports activities, alteration in footwear, orthotics, and if necessary NSAIDs.[543]

Surgical intervention, reserved for those who do not respond to conservative measures within 3 months, involves decompression of the nerve.[543]

Superficial Fibular (Peroneal) Nerve

Although injuries to the superficial nerve at the level of the ankle are relatively rare, the nerve can be stretched with lateral (inversion) ankle sprains or can become entrapped as it pierces the deep fascia to become subcutaneous approximately 4–5 inches above the lateral malleolus.[146,548–552]

Patients complain of diminished sensation on the posterior aspect of the foot, which is exacerbated with activity.

Tarsal Tunnel Syndrome

TTS is an entrapment neuropathy of the tibial nerve, as it passes through the anatomic tunnel between the flexor retinaculum and the medial malleolus (also see Chap. 5). In addition, the terminal branches of the tibial nerve, the medial, and lateral plantar nerves, may be involved. These latter nerves are often collectively called the posterior tibial nerve. The onset of TTS may be acute or insidious. Differential diagnosis includes plantar heel pain, chronic heel pain syndrome, and FHL tenosynovitis. The clinical findings for TTS are outlined in Chapter 5. Etiologic factors for TTS can be classified as internal or external. Internal factors include anatomical variations such as an accessory flexor digitorum longus muscle. External factors include excessive pronation, which can tighten the flexor retinaculum and the calcaneonavicular ligament. Conservative intervention for TTS includes the use of orthotics to correct biomechanical gait abnormalities. Specifically, a foot orthosis with a rearfoot varus post can limit excessive pronation. In cases of early excessive rearfoot pronation and subtalar joint pronation at heel strike, an orthosis with a deepened heel cup can help to control rearfoot motion. In cases of severe hyperpronation, a rearfoot wedge may be helpful.

Peripheral Neuropathy

Peripheral neuropathy is characterized by a progressive loss of nerve fibers that predisposes the patient to painful or insensitive extremities, vascular compromise, and neuropathic ulceration.[553,554] In more severe cases, uncontrolled peripheral neuropathy can result in amputation. Affected nerve functions associated with peripheral neuropathy include reduced nerve conduction velocity, decreased temperature sensation, decreased tendon reflex response, alterations in autonomic function, and a decreased ability to detect vibration and touch. Peripheral neuropathy is a complication of both insulin-dependent (type 1) and noninsulin-dependent (type 2) diabetes mellitus.[543,554]

A loss of sensation in the legs and feet prevents the patient from detecting minor cuts or trauma, which can become infected, placing these patients at high risk of developing a neuropathic ulcer. Motor neuropathy may cause muscle atrophy and imbalances, which can lead to foot deformity and increased pressure on the plantar aspect of the foot. This is particularly true with the diabetic patient who participates in sports, where the forces acting on the sole of the foot can be significant. Autonomic dysfunction may lead to decreased perspiration and sebaceous oil production, which can cause dryness, cracking, and, eventually, fissures in the skin. Good foot care is thus essential for these patients. It is recommended that the clinician regularly assess the general skin condition of the patient's foot and leg (dryness, cracks, and fissures) and the skin temperature. Red and warm skin may indicate the presence of infection, cellulitis, or an undetected bone infection or fracture. Cold skin and pallor may indicate decreased blood flow. Other signs of vascular compromise can include diminished pulses and toe pressures, dry and shiny skin with no hair growth, and thickened flaky nails. Skin rashes and foul odor may be indicative of a fungal infection. Callus and corn formation, blisters, and bunions may highlight the presence of an ill-fitting shoe or a deformity (equinus contracture, claw toes, and charcot arthropathy). Charcot (rocker-bottom) foot occurs when the bones at the plantar aspect are prominent, resulting in a diminished longitudinal arch and an increased potential for fracture. Other conditions to observe for include plantar warts and ingrown toenails.

Sensation of the foot can be tested using Semmes–Weinstein filaments, which are calibrated nylon monofilaments with increasing stiffness indicated by increasing numbers (see Chap. 3).[553,554] Protective sensation of the foot has been defined as the ability to sense a 5.07 monofilament, whereas absent sensation is defined as the inability to sense a 6.10 monofilament.[553]

The primary focus of intervention with this patient population is patient education regarding proper foot and nail inspection and care.

The following advice should be given:

- The feet should be washed everyday in warm, not hot, water. Hot water dries the skin and can easily burn the foot. The water temperature can be tested using a thermometer. The feet should not be soaked to avoid skin maceration.
- The skin should be inspected at least once a day for cuts, bruises, blisters, swelling, and calluses. A mirror can be used where necessary. If the skin is dry, lotion can be applied on the tops, bottoms, and sides of the feet, but not between the toes, which can create a moist environment for fungal and bacterial infections.
- Toenails should be trimmed straight across with a nail clipper once a week. Rounding off the corners of the nails increases the potential of ingrown toenails and increases the potential for cutting the skin. If the patient has retinal neuropathy and poor eyesight, the nails are best trimmed by a family member or by a professional.
- The patient should avoid walking barefoot or wearing sandals.
- The feet should be protected from hot or cold temperatures.
- The patient should exercise a little every day. Appropriate nonimpact exercises include cycling or swimming. Gait training may be appropriate to maintain mobility and alter gait patterns to decrease abnormal plantar pressures.[553]
- If possible, the patient should stop smoking. Smoking causes the blood vessels to constrict.

Appropriate footwear and orthotics should be prescribed where appropriate to reduce plantar pressures and increase the weight-bearing area of the foot.[80] The total contact cast is considered the gold standard for ambulating patients, due to its ability to reduce pressure on the midfoot and forefoot by distributing pressure over the total foot surface.[80] Alternatively, the patient may be prescribed a prefabricated walker boot, or a bivalved ankle foot orthosis.

In the presence of a diabetic wound, frequent sharp debridement of nonviable tissue has been shown to be an effective method to speed wound healing.[555] This can be performed with a scalpel and tweezers. Enzymatic and autolytic debridements can be used as adjuncts to sharp debridement.[555] Enzymatic debridement uses ointments that contain papain-urea or other enzymes that help break the bonds between necrotic tissue and wound bed. Autolytic debridement uses moisture-retentive secondary dressings (hydrogels and hydrocolloids) to provide a moist environment, which helps to keep the wound fluids in contact with the wound bed.

Complex Regional Pain Syndrome

The more classic patient with complex regional pain syndrome will present with severe regional pain, swelling, dysesthesia to light touch (allodynia) and vasomotor instability, and the subjective report will be one of pain out of proportion to the degree of injury (see Chap. 5).[556]

Myofascial Pain Syndrome

Ankle or foot pain can arise, and trigger points in the tibialis anterior, extensor digitorum, or fibularis (peroneus) longus muscle are the most likely causes.[557]

Tibialis Anterior

Trigger points of this muscle can refer pain, tenderness, and stiffness deep into the anterior ankle and the great toe. These trigger points can be activated due to excessive pronation of the foot and excessive dorsiflexion.[557]

Extensor Digitorum

Trigger points of this muscle can refer pain and tenderness over the posterior aspect of the foot and into the middle three toes.

Fibularis (Peroneus) Longus

Trigger points of this muscle can refer to just posterior to the lateral malleolus. This muscle is usually strained on inversion sprain injuries of the ankle and can therefore be the source of residual pain at the lateral ankle.[557]

PREFERRED PRACTICE PATTERN 4G: IMPAIRED JOINT MOBILITY, MOTOR FUNCTION, MUSCLE PERFORMANCE, AND ROM ASSOCIATED WITH FRACTURES

Stress Fractures

A stress or fatigue fracture involves a break that develops in bone after cyclical, submaximal loading. A number of extrinsic factors are associated with stress fractures of the leg and foot including running on hard surfaces, improper running shoes, or sudden increases in jogging or running distance. Biomechanical factors, including malalignment of the lower extremity, particularly excessive pronation, should also be considered when evaluating stress fractures. In the foot, the two most common locations for stress fractures are the metatarsal shaft and the calcaneus.[558]

Metatarsal Stress Fracture

The second and third metatarsals are the most frequently injured.[559] A number of studies have found stress fractures to be more common in women, older individuals, and Caucasians.[560,561] Amenorrhea is present in up to 20% of robustly exercising women and may be as high as 50% in elite runners and dancers.[562] Patients with amenorrhea for more than 6 months experience the same bone loss as postmenopausal women, predisposing them to stress fracture.[563] Muscular fatigue of the foot may also play a role in the etiology.[564]

Although numerous studies have attempted to correlate foot shape, footwear, and orthotics to the incidence of stress fractures, none have conclusively shown a direct relationship,[272,565–567] although one study showed a decrease in the incidence of metatarsal fractures in low-arched feet by using a semirigid orthotic.[86]

The typical clinical findings with this type of fracture include reports of mild forefoot discomfort, which may initially be relieved by rest, but which occurs while walking and even at rest as the fracture worsens.[50] Occasionally, there is point tenderness over the involved metatarsal, swelling, and a palpable mass.[559,568]

Anteroposterior, lateral, and oblique radiographs of the foot may not show a fracture for 3–6 weeks, although a technetium bone scan is positive as early as 48–72 hours after onset of symptoms.[50]

The intervention for metatarsal stress fractures includes rest from the offending activity and cross-training in a low-impact sport.[50] Weight-bearing to tolerance may be allowed in comfortable shoes of choice or a wooden shoe. If weight-bearing is painful, or the fracture is diagnosed late, a short leg cast or hard-soled shoe is worn for 4–6 weeks until healing callus is seen radiographically.[559,568]

Proximal Second Metatarsal

This type of metatarsal stress fracture differs from other metatarsal stress fractures since it can be difficult to heal and may result in chronic nonunion. The anatomy in this area tends to encourage an abnormal amount of stress, particularly in young ballet dancers.[569–572]

Other predisposing factors can include amenorrhea, anorexia nervosa, cavus foot, and anterior ankle impingement with resulting hyperpronation.[569]

On physical examination, there will be pain in the first web space, usually accompanied by proximal second metatarsal pain.[573]

Initial foot radiographs will most often be negative; hence, a bone scan is usually necessary. The bone scan may be nonspecific, with synovitis, stress reaction, and stress fracture as differential.[573]

The intervention for second metatarsal stress fracture usually consists of 6–8 weeks of rest in a hard shoe or cast,[569,573] with gradual return to activities when the tenderness resolves.

Navicular Stress Fracture

Although navicular stress fractures occur infrequently, they are the most common midfoot fracture. A navicular fracture typically presents with an insidious onset or with a history of acute flexion and inversion.[7] The patient complains of chronic pain that is vague in nature but tender to palpation on the posterior aspect of the foot and/or medial aspect of the midfoot.[559]

This condition is most commonly seen in basketball players, hurdlers, and runners, in whom repeated cyclic loading results in fatigue failure through the relatively avascular central portion of the tarsal navicular.[57,308,574] The cyclic loading across the navicular may be exacerbated due to a short first metatarsal, metatarsus adductus, or limited dorsiflexion or subtalar motion.[57]

To confirm the diagnosis, bone scan or CT scan may be necessary, as plain films are rarely diagnostic.[574]

The intervention varies according to the type of fracture. Nondisplaced fractures are treated with a short-leg non-weight-bearing cast for 6–8 weeks.[342,574]

If the fracture fails to heal or is displaced, operative intervention of fixation with compression screw, and additional bone grafting where necessary, is used.[342,574]

Return to sport may take as long as 16–20 weeks.[559]

Sesamoid Stress Fracture

The young patient with a sesamoid stress fracture will present with the insidious onset of pain and swelling over the plantar aspect of the first MTP joint.[308,575] Pain is usually aggravated by activity and relieved with rest. Differential diagnosis includes metatarsalgia, bursitis, sesamoiditis, and bipartite sesamoid.[575]

The intervention for a sesamoid fracture is initially rest from the offending high-impact activity and a wooden-soled shoe or a short-leg cast for 6–8 weeks. If cast, a CT scan is performed at 8 weeks to detect signs of avascular necrosis. If avascular necrosis is present and the young patient has persistent symptoms, re-section may be necessary.[52] Surgical choices include excision of the involved sesamoid or bone grafting, in an attempt to achieve union and preserve the sesamoid.

An alternative treatment is the use of a "C" or "J" pad, which unloads the injured sesamoid. Pads with adhesive backing may be fixed to the insole of the shoe or may be incorporated into a custom-molded orthotic to unload the sesamoid.

Fractures

Pilon Fractures

These fractures result from an axial compression force, where the tibia is driven inferiorly into the talus, splitting and shattering the distal end of the tibia and completely disrupting the ankle joint, resulting in long-term morbidity in the majority of cases.[576]

Talar Dome Fractures

These are the most common chondral fractures and are also known as osteochondritis dissecans, transchondral fractures, or flake fractures.[7]

These injuries, which present with persistent swelling, pain with walking, locking of the ankle, and crepitus, tend to present as a "sprained ankle that did not heal."[7]

Intervention varies from none, to casting, to arthroscopy for larger fragments.[7]

Talar Fractures

Major fractures of the talar head, neck, and body are associated with high-energy mechanisms, with one-half of major talar injuries involving fractures of the talar neck, 15–20% involving talar body fractures, and the remainder involving talar head fractures.[7] The mechanism of injury usually involves an axial load with the foot positioned in plantar flexion or excessive dorsiflexion, resulting in compression of the talar head against the anterior aspect of the tibia.[577]

The intervention varies according to location and severity, with nondisplaced fractures treated with a short-leg non-weight-bearing cast for 6–8 weeks and displaced fractures involving immediate reduction.[7]

Unimalleolar Fractures

Unimalleolar fractures are the most common fractures of the ankle.[7] The degree of stability of these fractures is dependent on their location, with those located below the tibiotalar joint tending to be stable.[7] Approximately 85% of lateral malleolar fractures occur without damage to the medial aspect of the ankle joint and do not cause abnormal displacement of the talus.[578,579]

Medial malleolar fractures are often seen in conjunction with other fractures.

Bimalleollar and Trimalleolar Fractures

These fractures, as their name implies, involve two or three malleoli. The bimalleolar fracture usually results from a severe pronation/abduction/external rotation force, which shears the lateral malleoli and avulses the medial malleolus. The trimalleolar fracture involves a fracture of the medial, lateral, and "posterior" malleolus, which typically results from an abduction and severe external rotation force so strong that the talus moves sufficiently posteriorly to shear off the posterior margin of the tibia.

The intervention for bimalleolar fractures remains controversial, whereas it is generally agreed that trimalleolar fractures require open reduction and internal fixation.[580]

Calcaneus

The calcaneus is the most frequently fractured tarsal, accounting for over 60% of foot fractures,[581] and one that can be a frequent and often misdiagnosed cause of heel pain.[582] With the increasing number of middle-aged and elderly people involved in active recreational pursuits, sports medicine has had to incorporate the way these conditions are related to these different age groups.[57] Jumping activities or unaccustomed activities may precipitate crushing of the fragile architecture of an osteoporotic calcaneus, leading to fractures.[57]

Tenderness on M-P compression of the heel (squeeze test) should lead to a suspicion of a stress fracture of the calcaneus.[38]

Conservative intervention of calcaneal fractures has shown poor long-term clinical results with significant loss of ankle function.[583,584]

Fifth Metatarsal Fractures

All fractures of the proximal fifth metatarsal have been arbitrarily labeled a "Jones fracture." The most common fifth metatarsal base fracture is an avulsion fracture of the tuberosity caused by traction of the fibularis (peroneus) brevis and lateral band of the plantar fascia during hindfoot inversion.[585]

The proximal fifth metatarsal has a poor blood supply and is at significant risk for delayed union or nonunion. These fractures should be treated with non–weight-bearing short-leg cast immobilization for 6–8 weeks or until healing is seen radiographically. If an established nonunion develops, screw fixation and/or bone grafting may be required.[586]

THERAPEUTIC TECHNIQUES

Techniques to Increase Joint Mobility

Joint Mobilizations

With some slight variations, the same techniques that are used to examine the joint glides described in the test and measures section can be used to mobilize the joints, with the clinician varying the intensity of the mobilizations based on the intent of the technique, the patient's response, and the stage of tissue healing. The purposes for the various mobilizations include the following:

- Posterior glide of the talocrural joint can be used to increase ankle joint dorsiflexion, whereas an anterior glide of the talocrural joint can be used to increase ankle joint plantar flexion.
- Medial gapping of the subtalar joint can be used for increasing ROM into subtalar joint eversion, whereas lateral gapping of the subtalar joint can be used for increasing ROM into subtalar joint inversion.
- A posterior glide of the intermetatarsal joints can be used to assist flattening of the transverse arch of the foot, whereas an anterior glide can be used to help increase the transverse arch of the foot.
- A posterior glide of the MTP joint can be used to increase ROM into MTP joint extension, whereas an anterior glide of the MTP joint can be used to increase ROM into MTP joint flexion.
- A posterior glide of the interphalangeal joint can be used to increase ROM into interphalangeal joint extension, whereas an anterior glide of the interphalangeal joint can be used to increase ROM into interphalangeal joint flexion.

Intervention following successful manual treatment should consist of strengthening of the plantar flexors, particularly the fibularis (peroneal) muscles. If the patient has a history of recurrent ankle sprains, then appropriate proprioceptive retraining should be instituted. Pain relief and improved function should be immediate and long lasting; however, if the condition reoccurs, follow-up care could include foot taping (for example using the Low-dye technique), use of arch supports or foot orthoses (over the counter or custom made), stretching and/or soft tissue mobilization of the fibularis (peroneus) muscles, and adjustment to any asymmetrical training or daily habitual usage patterns.

CASE STUDY

BILATERAL HEEL PAIN

HISTORY

History of Current Condition

A 54-year-old female presents with insidious onset of a constant dull ache in both heels, which is worse in the morning, especially when first putting her feet on the ground and at the end of the day. The patient denies numbness or tingling in either foot or ankle area or any history of trauma. Pain has increased this past week, prompting her to see an MD who prescribed physical therapy and an anti-inflammatory medication.

Past History of Current Condition

Bilateral heel pain of approximately 2 months duration a few years ago, which resolved spontaneously.

Past Medical/Surgical History

Unremarkable.

Medications

NSAIDs are prescribed for pain relief and decreasing the inflammation.[470]

Other Tests and Measures

Radiographs showed the presence of a heel spur in both heels.

Social Habits (Past and Present)

Sedentary lifestyle.

Growth and Development

Overweight as a child.

Living Environment

Lives in a ranch-type home with carpeting throughout, except for a tiled bathroom.

Occupational/Employment/School

Works in a warehouse stacking boxes of tissues and has been working there for 6 years.

Functional Status/Activity Level

Soreness occurs first hour in morning, especially when she initially bears weight, and again at the end of the day after working. Walking on the concrete floor at work is reported to aggravate the condition.

Health Status

General good health, but feels her pain interferes with tasks at home and at work.

Questions

1. List all of the structures that could be at fault with complaints of bilateral heel pain of an insidious onset.
2. Does the history of heel pain with initial weight-bearing in the morning give the clinician any clues as to the diagnosis?
3. Why do you think the patient's symptoms are worsened with weight-bearing?
4. What additional questions would you ask to help rule out referral from the hip, knee, or lumbar spine?
5. Do you have a working hypothesis at this stage? List the various tests you would use to rule out each of the possible causes.
6. Does this presentation/history warrant a scan? Why or why not?

CASE STUDY

HEEL PAIN

HISTORY

History of Current Condition

A 34-year-old female complains of insidious onset of pain in the posterior aspect of the right ankle, which began approximately 3 months ago when she began a jogging program but which had not worsened significantly until last week. The pain is worse in the morning and after prolonged positions. The patient denies numbness or tingling in the foot or ankle area. The increase in pain this past week had prompted the patient to visit her MD, who prescribed physical therapy and gave her a heel lift to wear in each of her shoes.

Past History of Current Condition

Similar right posterior heel pain of approximately 1-month duration a few years ago, which resolved spontaneously.

Past Medical/Surgical History

Unremarkable.

Medications

Naproxen (daily).

Functional Status/Activity Level

Soreness occurs first hour in the morning.

Health Status

In good health but feels the pain interferes with tasks at home and at work.

Questions

1. List the structure(s) and differential diagnoses that may be involved with complaints of unilateral heel pain related to running.
2. What does the history of no significant worsening of the pain tell the clinician?
3. Why do you think the patient's symptoms are worse after rest?
4. What additional questions would you ask?
5. What is your working hypothesis at this stage? If you have a number of hypotheses, which tests would you use to rule out each one?
6. Does this presentation/history warrant a lower quarter scanning examination? Why or why not?

REVIEW QUESTIONS*

1. Name the three ligaments associated with the distal tibiofibular joint.
2. Which nerve is involved with TTS?
3. What structures maintain the longitudinal arch?
4. Supination of the foot in weight-bearing is a combination of which movements of the calcaneus and talus?
5. Morton's neuroma most commonly involves which nerve?

*Additional questions to test your understanding of this chapter can be found in the Online Learning Center for *Orthopaedic Assessment, Evaluation, and Intervention* at www.duttononline.net.

REFERENCES

1. Schiowitz S: Diagnosis and treatment of the lower extremity—The Knee. In: DiGiovanna EL, Schiowitz S, eds. *An Osteopathic Approach to Diagnosis and Treatment.* Philadelphia, PA: JB Lippincott, 1991:330–346.
2. Sartoris DJ: Diagnosis of ankle injuries: The essentials. *J Foot Ankle Surg* 33:101–107, 1994.
3. Sammarco GJ, Hockenbury RT: Biomechanics of the foot and ankle. In: Frankel VH, Nordin M, eds. *Basic Biomechanics of the Musculoskeletal System.* Baltimore, MD: Williams and Wilkins, 2000.
4. Mann RA: *Biomechanics of running, AAOS Symposium on the Foot and Leg in Running Sports.* St. Louis, MO: Mosby, 1982:30–44.
5. Cavanagh PR, Rodgers MM, Iiboshi A: Pressure distribution under symptom-free feet during barefoot standing. *Foot Ankle Int* 7:262–276, 1987.
6. Gieve DW, Rashi T: Pressures under normal feet in standing and walking as measured by foil pedobarography. *Ann Rheum Dis* 43:816, 1984.
7. Wedmore IS, Charette J: Emergency department evaluation and treatment of ankle and foot injuries. *Emerg Med Clin North Am* 18:86–114, 2000.
8. Donatelli RA: Normal anatomy and biomechanics. In: Donatelli RA, ed. *Biomechanics of the Foot and Ankle.* Philadelphia, PA: WB Saunders, 1990:3–31.
9. Subotnick SI: Normal anatomy. In: Subotnick SI, ed. *Sports Medicine of the Lower Extremity*, 2nd ed. Philadelphia, PA: Churchill Livingstone, 1999:75–111.
10. Mulfinger G, Trueta J: The blood supply to the talus. *J Bone Joint Surg* 52B:160, 1970.
11. Brostrom L: Sprained ankles: I. Anatomic lesions on recent sprains. *Acta Chir Scand* 128:483–495, 1964.
12. Cailliet R: *Foot and Ankle Pain*, 2nd ed. Philadelphia, PA: F. A. Davis, 1983:148–158.
13. Cox JS: Surgical and nonsurgical treatment of acute ankle sprains. *Clin Orthop* 198:118–126, 1985.
14. Hamilton WG: Surgical anatomy of the foot and ankle. *Clin Symp* 37:1–32, 1985.
15. Moseley HF: Traumatic disorders of the ankle and foot. *Clin Symp* 17:1–30, 1965.
16. Safran MR, Benedetti RS, Bartolozzi AR, III, et al: Lateral ankle sprains: A comprehensive review: part 1: etiology, pathoanatomy, histopathogenesis, and diagnosis. *Med Sci Sports Exerc* 31:S429–S437, 1999.
17. Hockenbury RT, Sammarco GJ: Evaluation and treatment of ankle sprains—clinical recommendations for a positive outcome. *Phys Sports Med* 24:57–64, 2001.
18. Close JR: Some applications of the functional anatomy of the ankle joint. *J. Bone Joint Surg* 38-A:761–781, 1956.
19. Hintermann B, Nigg BM, Sommer C, et al: Transfer of movement between calcaneus and tibia in vitro. *Clin Biomech* 9:349–355, 1994.
20. Inman VT: *The Joints of the Ankle.* Baltimore, MD: Williams & Wilkins, 1991.
21. Manter JT: Movements of the subtalar and transverse tarsal joints. *Anat. Rec* 80:397–400, 1941.
22. Hintermann B, et al: Biomechanics of the unstable ankle joint and clinical implications. *Med Sci Sports Exerc* 31:S459–S469, 1999.
23. Mann RA: Functional anatomy of the ankle joint ligaments. In: Bateman JE, Trott AW, eds. *The Foot and Ankle.* New York, NY: BC Decker Inc, 1980:161–170.
24. Stormont DM, Morrey BF, An K-N, et al: Stability of the loaded ankle. *Am J Sports Med* 13:295–300, 1985.
25. Burks RT, Morgan J: Anatomy of the lateral ankle ligaments. *Am J Sports Med* 22:72–77, 1994.
26. Sarrafian SK: *Anatomy of Foot and Ankle.* Philadelphia, PA: Lippincott, 1994:239–240.
27. Anderson KJ, Lecocq JF: Operative treatment of injury to the fibular collateral ligaments of the ankle. *J. Bone Joint Surg* 36A:825–832, 1954.
28. Colville MR, Marder RA, Boyle JJ, et al: Strain measurement in lateral ankle ligaments. *Am J Sports Med* 18:196–200, 1990.
29. Rasmussen O: Stability of the ankle joint. *Acta Orthop Scand* 211 (Suppl):56–78, 1985.
30. Renstrom PA, Wertz M, Incavo S, et al: Strain in the lateral ligaments of the ankle. *Foot Ankle* 9:59–63, 1988.
31. Harper MC: Deltoid ligament: An anatomical evaluation of function. *Foot Ankle* 8:19–22, 1987.

32. Siegler S, Block J, Schneck CD: The mechanical characteristics of the collateral ligaments of the human ankle joint. *Foot Ankle* 8:234–242, 1988.
33. Rasmussen O, Kroman-Andersen C, Boe S: Deltoid ligament: Functional analysis of the medial collateral ligamentous apparatus of the ankle joint. *Acta Orthop Scand* 54:36–44, 1983.
34. Rasmussen O, Tovberg-Jensen I: Mobility of the ankle joint: Recording of rotatory movements in the talocrural joint in vitro with and without the lateral collateral ligaments of the ankle. *Acta Orthop Scand* 53:155–160, 1982.
35. Attarian DE, McCracken HJ, Devito DP, et al: Biomechanical characteristics of human ankle ligaments. *Foot Ankle* 6:54–58, 1985.
36. Isman RE, Inman VT: Anthropometric studies of the human foot and ankle. *Bull Prosthetic Res* 4:97–129, 1969.
37. Jahss MH, Kummer F, Michelson JD: Investigations into the fat pads of the sole of the foot: Heel pressure studies. *Foot Ankle* 13:227–232, 1992.
38. Singh D, Angel J, Bentley G, et al: Fortnightly review. Plantar fasciitis. *BMJ* 315:172–175, 1997.
39. Frey CC, Rosenburg Z, Shereff M, et al: The retrocalcaneal bursa: Anatomy and bursography. *Foot Ankle* 13:203–207, 1982.
40. Jorgensen U, Bojsen-Möller F: Shock absorbency factors in the shoe/heel interaction—with special focus on role of the heel pad. *Foot Ankle* 9:294–299, 1989.
41. Williams PL, Warwick R, Dyson M, et al: *Gray's Anatomy*, 37th ed. London: Churchill Livingstone, 1989.
42. Hintermann B: Tibialis posterior dysfunction: A review of the problems and personal experience. *Foot Ankle Surg* 3:61–70, 1997.
43. Clement DB, Taunton JE, Smart GW: Achilles tendinitis and peritendinitis: Etiology and treatment. *Am J Sports Med* 12:179–183, 1984.
44. Gagey O, Hue E: Mechanics of the deltoid muscle. A new approach. *Clin Orthop Relat Res* 375:250–257, 2000.
45. Bojsen-Möller F: Calcaneocuboid joint and stability of the longitudinal arch of the foot at high and low gear push off. *J Anat* 129:165–176, 1979.
46. Pick TP, Howden R: *Gray's Anatomy*, 15th ed. New York, NY: Barnes & Noble, 1995.
47. Jahss MH: The sesamoids of the hallux. *Clin Orthop* 157:88–97, 1981.
48. Jahss MH: *Disorders of the Foot*. Philadelphia, PA: WB Saunders, 1982.
49. Weinfeld SB, Schon LC: Hallux Metatarsophalangeal arthritis. *Clin Orthop Relat Res* 349:9–19, 1998.
50. Hockenbury RT: Forefoot problems in athletes. *Med Sci Sports Exerc* 31: S448–S458, 1999.
51. McBryde AM, Jr, Anderson RB: Sesamoid problems in the athlete. *Clin Sports Med* 7:51–60, 1988.
52. Richardson EG: Injuries to the hallucal sesamoids in the athlete. *Foot Ankle* 7:229–244, 1987.
53. Sammarco GJ: Turf toe. *Instr Course Lect* 42:207–212, 1993.
54. Scranton PE, Rutkowski R: Anatomic variations in the first ray. Part B. Disorders of the sesamoids. *Clin Orthop* 151:256–264, 1980.
55. Van Hal ME, Keeve JS, Lange TA, et al: Stress fractures of the sesamoids. *Am J Sports Med* 10:122–128, 1982.
56. Whittle AP: Fractures of the foot in athletes. *Op Tech Sports Med* 2:43–57, 1994.
57. Omey ML, Micheli LJ: Foot and ankle problems in the young athlete. *Med Sci Sports Exerc* 31:S470–S486, 1999.
58. Sullivan JA: The child's foot. In: Morrissy RT, ed. *Lovell and Winter's Pediatric Orthopaedics*, 4th ed. Philadelphia, PA: Lippincott, 1996:1077–1135.
59. Chen YJ, Shih HN, Huang TJ, et al: Posterior tibial tendon tear combined with a fracture of the accessory navicular: A new subclassification? *J Trauma-Injury Inf Crit Care* 39:993–996, 1995.
60. Brodsky AE, Khalil MA: Talar compression syndrome. *Am J Sports Med* 14:472–476, 1986.
61. McDougall A: The os trigonum. *J Bone Joint Surg* 37B:257–265, 1955.
62. Charles LM: Why does my foot hurt? Plantar fasciitis. *Lippincott's Primary Care Pract* 3:408–409, 1999.
63. Hedrick MR: The plantar aponeurosis. *Foot Ankle Int* 17:646–649, 1996.
64. Scioli MW: Achilles tendinitis. *Orthop Clin North Am* 25:177–182, 1994.
65. Soma CA, Mandelbaum BR: Achilles tendon disorders. *Clinics Sports Med* 13:811–823, 1994.
66. Gerdes MH, Brown TW, Bell A, et al: A flap augmentation technique for Achilles tendon repair. Postoperative strength and functional outcome. *Clin Orthop* 280:241–246, 1992.
67. Reynolds NL, Worrell TW: Chronic Achilles peritendinitis: Etiology, pathophysiology, and treatment. *J Orthop Sports Phys Ther* 13:171–176, 1991.
68. Carr AJ, Norris SH: The blood supply of the calcaneal tendon. *J Bone Joint Surg* 71B:100–101, 1989.
69. Lagergren C, Lindholm A: Vascular distribution in the Achilles tendon: An angiographic and microangiographic study. *Acta Chir Scand* 116:491–495, 1958.
70. Nelen G, Martens M, Bursens A: Surgical treatment of chronic Achilles tendinitis. *Am J Sports Med* 17:754–759, 1989.
71. Nichols AW: Achilles tendinitis in running athletes. *J Am Bd Fam Pract* 2:196–203, 1989.
72. Reid DC: Heel pain and Problems of the Hindfoot. In: Reid DC, ed. *"Sports Injury Assessment and Rehabilitation."* New York, NY: Churchill Livingstone, 1992:437–493.
73. Myerson MS, McGarvey W: Disorders of the Achilles tendon insertion and Achilles tendinitis. *AAOS Instr Course Lect* 48:211–218, 1999.
74. Conti SF: Posterior tibial tendon problems in athletes. *Orthop Clin North Am* 25:109–121, 1994.
75. Clarke HD, Kitaoka HB, Ehman RL: Peroneal tendon injuries. *Foot Ankle* 19:280–288, 1998.
76. Brage ME, Hansen ST: Traumatic subluxation/dislocation of the peroneal tendons. *Foot Ankle* 13:423–431, 1992.
77. Thordarson DB, Schotzer H, Chon J, et al: Dynamic support of the human longitudinal arch. *Clin Orthop* 316:165–172, 1995.
78. Mann R, Inman V: Phasic activity of intrinsic muscles of the foot. *J Bone Joint Surg* 46A:469–480, 1964.
79. Appling SA, Kasser RJ: Foot and Ankle. In: Wadsworth C, ed. *Current Concepts of Orthopedic Physical Therapy—Home Study Course*. La Crosse, WI: Orthopaedic Section, APTA, 2001.
80. Reeser LA, Susman RL, Stern JT: Electromyographic studies of the human foot: Experimental approaches to hominid evolution. *Foot Ankle* 3:391–406, 1983.
81. Huang C, Kitaoka HB, An K, et al: Biomechanical evaluation of longitudinal arch stability. *Foot Ankle* 14:352–357, 1993.
82. Hicks JH: Mechanics of the foot. *J Anat* 87:345–357, 1953.
83. Saltzman CL, Nawoczenski DA: Complexities of foot architecture as a base of support. *J Orthop Sports Phys Ther* 21:354–360, 1995.
84. Donatelli R: Normal anatomy and pathophysiology of the foot and ankle. In: Wadsworth C, ed. *Contemporary Topics on the Foot and Ankle*. La Crosse, WI: Orthopedic Section, APTA, Inc., 2000.
85. Simkin A, Leichter I, Giladi M, et al: Combined effect of foot structure and an orthotic device on stress fractures. *Foot Ankle* 10:25–29, 1989.
86. Giladi M, Milgrom C, Stein M, et al: The low arch, a protective factor in stress fractures: A prospective study of 295 military recruits. *Orthop Review* 14:709–712, 1985.
87. Cowan DN, Jones BH, Robinson JR: Foot morphological characteristics and risk of exercise-related injury. *Arch Fam Med* 2:773–777, 1993.
88. Roy KJ: Force, pressure, and motion measurements in the foot. *Clin Podiatr Med Surg* 5:491–508, 1988.
89. Nachbauer W, Nigg B: Effects of arch height of the foot on ground reaction forces in running. *Med Sci Sports Exerc* 23:1264–1269, 1992.
90. MacConnail MA, Basmajian JV: *Muscles and Movements: A Basis for Human Kinesiology*. New York, NY: Robert Krieger, 1977.
91. Mayeaux EJ, Jr.: Nail disorders. *Dermatology* 27:333–351, 2000.
92. Williams PL, Warwick R: *Gray's Anatomy*, 36th ed. Philadelphia, PA: WB Saunders, 1980.
93. Root M, Orien W, Weed J: *Clinical Biomechanics: Normal and Abnormal Function of the Foot*. Los Angeles, CA: Clinical Biomechanics, 1977.
94. Vaes PH, Duquet W, Casteleyn PP, et al: Static and dynamic roentgenographic analysis of ankle stability in braced and non-braced stable and functionally unstable ankles. *Am J Sports Med* 26:692–702, 1998.
95. Edwards GS, DeLee JC: Ankle diastasis without fracture. *Foot Ankle* 4:305–312, 1984.
96. Murray MP: Gait as a total pattern of movement. *Am J Phys Med* 46:290, 1967.
97. Perry J: The mechanics of walking: A clinical interpretation. In: Perry J, Hislop HJ, eds. *Principles of Lower Extremity Bracing*. New York, NY: American Physical Therapy Association, 1967:9–32.
98. Scott SH, Winter DA: Talocrural and talocalcaneal joint kinematics and kinetics during the stance phase of gait. *J Biomech* 24:743–752, 1991.
99. Barnett CH, Napier JR: The axis of rotation at the ankle joint in man: Its influence upon the form of the talus and mobility of the fibula. *J Anat* 86:1–9, 1952.
100. Giallonardo LM: Clinical evaluation of foot and ankle dysfunction. *Phys Ther* 68:1850–1856, 1988.
101. Close JR, Inman VT: The action of the ankle joint. *Prosthetic Devices Research Project*. Institute of Engineering Research 11:5, 1952.

102. Lundberg A, Goldie I, Kalin B, et al: Kinematics of the ankle/foot complex: Plantar flexion and dorsiflexion. *Foot Ankle* 9:194–200, 1989.
103. Levens AS, Inman VT, Blosser JA: Transverse rotations of the lower extremity in locomotion. *J Bone Joint Surg* 30A:859–872, 1948.
104. Stephens MM, Sammarco GJ: The stabilizing role of the lateral ligament complex around the ankle and subtalar joints. *Foot Ankle* 13:130–136, 1992.
105. O'Connor JJ, Leardini A, Catani F: The one degree of freedom nature of the human ankle/subtalar complex. *J Bone Joint Surg [Br]* 79-B:364–365, 1997.
106. Hunt GC: *Functional Biomechanics of the Subtalar Joint, Orthopaedic Physical Therapy Home Study Course 92-1: Lower Extremity*. La Crosse, WI: Orthopaedic Section, APTA, Inc., 1992.
107. Subotnick SI: Biomechanics of the subtalar and midtarsal joints. *J Am Podiatry Assoc* 65:756–764, 1975.
108. Close JR, Inman VT, Poor PM, et al: The function of the subtalar joint. *Clin Orthop* 50:159–179, 1967.
109. Oatis CA: Biomechanics of the foot and ankle under static conditions. *Phys Ther* 68:1815–1821, 1988.
110. Green DR, Whitney AK, Walters P: Subtalar joint motion. *J Am Podiat Med Assn* 69:83–91, 1979.
111. Mann RA, Hagy J: Biomechanics of walking, running, and sprinting. *Am J Sports Med* 8:345–350, 1980.
112. Carson WG: Diagnosis of extensor mechanism disorders. *Clin Sports Med* 4:231–246, 1985.
113. Carson WG, James SL, Larson RL, et al: Patellofemoral disorders—Physical and radiographic examination. Part I. Physical examination. *Clin Orthop* 185:178–186, 1984.
114. James SL, Bates BT, Osternig LR: Injuries to runners. *Am J Sports Med* 6:40–49, 1978.
115. James SL: Chondromalacia patella. In: Kennedy JC, ed. *The Injured Adolescent Knee*. Baltimore, MD: Williams & Wilkins, 1979.
116. Wright DG, Desai SM, Henderson WH: Action of the subtalar and ankle joint complex during stance phase of walking. *J Bone Joint Surg* 46A:361–382, 1964.
117. McPoil TG, Jr, Brocato RS: The foot and ankle: Biomechanical evaluation and treatment. In: Gould JA, Davies GJ, eds. *Orthopaedic and Sports Physical Therapy*. St Louis, MO: Mosby, 1985:313–341.
118. Tiberio D: Pathomechanics of structural foot deformities. *Phys Ther* 68:1840–1849, 1988.
119. Harper MC: The lateral ligamentous support of the subtalar joint. *Foot Ankle* 11:354–358, 1991.
120. Elftman H: The transverse tarsal joint and its control. *Clin Orth Rel Res* 16:41–45, 1960.
121. Joseph J: Range of movement of the great toe in men. *J Bone Joint Surg* 36B:450–457, 1954.
122. Hardy RH, Clapham JCR: Observations on hallux valgus: Based on a controlled series. *J Bone Joint Surg* 33B:376–391, 1951.
123. Cornwall MW, Fishco WD, McPoil TG, et al: Reliability and validity of clinically assessing first-ray mobility of the foot. *J Am Podiatr Med Assoc* 94:470–476, 2004.
124. Safran MR, Zachazewski JE, Benedetti RS, et al: Lateral ankle sprains: A comprehensive review part 2: treatment and rehabilitation with an emphasis on the athlete. *Med Sci Sports Exerc* 31:S438–S447, 1999.
125. Marder RA: Current methods for the evaluation of ankle ligament injuries. *J Bone Joint Surg* 76A:1103–1111, 1994.
126. Magee DJ: Lower Leg, Ankle, and Foot. In: Magee DJ, ed. *Orthopedic Physical Assessment*. Philadelphia, PA: WB Saunders, 2002:765–845.
127. Maitland G: *Peripheral Manipulation*, 3rd ed. London: Butterworth, 1991.
128. Adamson C, Cymet T: Ankle sprains: Evaluation, treatment, rehabilitation. *Maryland Med J* 46:530–537, 1997.
129. Bordelon RL: Clinical assessment of the foot. In: Donatelli RA, ed. *Biomechanics of the Foot and Ankle*. Philadelphia, PA: WB Saunders, 1990:85–98.
130. Brostrom L: Sprained ankles: III. Clinical observations in recent ligament ruptures. *Acta Chir Scand* 130:560–569, 1965.
131. Cox JS: The diagnosis and management of ankle ligament injuries in the athlete. *Athl Training* 18:192–196, 1982.
132. Cyriax J: *Textbook of Orthopaedic Medicine, Diagnosis of Soft Tissue Lesions*, 8th ed. London: Bailliere Tindall, 1982.
133. Kelikian H, Kelikian AS: *Disorders of the Ankle*. Philadelphia, PA: WB. Saunders, 1985.
134. Winkel D, Matthijs O, Phelps V: Examination of the Ankle and Foot. In: Winkel D, Matthijs O, Phelps V, eds. *Diagnosis and Treatment of the Lower Extremities*. Maryland, MD: Aspen, 1997:375–401.
135. Hyman GS, Soloman J, Dahm D: Physical examination of the foot and ankle. In: Malanga GA, Nadler SF, eds. *Musculoskeletal Physical Examination—An Evidence-Based Approach*. Philadelphia, PA: Elsevier-Mosby, 2006:315–343.
136. Brosky T, Nyland A, Nitz A, et al: The ankle ligaments: Consideration of syndesmotic injury and implications for rehabilitation. *J Orthop Sports Phys Ther* 21:197–205, 1995.
137. Turco VJ: Injuries to the foot and ankle in athletes. *Orthop Clin North Am* 8:669–682, 1977.
138. Gross MT: Lower quarter screening for skeletal malalignment—suggestions for orthotics and shoewear. *J Orthop Sports Phys Ther* 21:389–405, 1995.
139. Staheli LT: Rotational problems of the lower extremity. *Orthop Clin North Am* 18:503–512, 1987.
140. Hunt GC, Brocato RS: Gait and foot pathomechanics. In: Hunt GC, ed. *Physical Therapy of the Foot and Ankle*. Edinburgh: Churchill Livingstone, 1988:39–57.
141. Mann RA: Biomechanical approach to the treatment of foot problems. *Foot Ankle* 2:205–212, 1982.
142. Roy S, Irvin R: *Sports Medicine—Prevention, Evaluation, Management, and Rehabilitation*. Englewood Cliffs, NJ: Prentice-Hall, 1983.
143. Subotnick SI: Clinical Biomechanics. In: Subotnick SI, ed. *Sports Medicine of the Lower Extremity*. Philadelphia, PA: Churchill Livingstone, 1999:127–156.
144. Payne C, Chuter V, Miller K: Sensitivity and specificity of the functional hallux limitus test to predict foot function. *J Am Podiatr Med Assoc* 92:269–271, 2002.
145. Reid DC: *Sports Injury Assessment and Rehabilitation*. New York, NY: Churchill Livingstone, 1992.
146. Schon LC: Nerve entrapment, neuropathy, and nerve dysfunction in athletes. *Orthop Clin North Am* 25:47–59, 1994.
147. Hertling D, Kessler RM: *Management of Common Musculoskeletal Disorders: Physical Therapy Principles and Methods*, 3rd ed. Philadelphia, PA: Lippincott Williams & Wilkins, 1996.
148. Baxter DE: The heel in sport. *Clin Sports Med* 13:683–693, 1994.
149. Baxter DE, Zingas C: The foot in running. *J Am Acad Orthop Surg* 3: 136–145, 1995.
150. Leach RE, Dizorio E, Harvey RA: Pathologic hindfoot conditions in the athlete. *Clin Orthop* 177:116–121, 1983.
151. Bennell KL, Talbot RC, Wajswelner H, et al: Intra-rater and inter-rater reliability of a weight-bearing lunge measure of ankle dorsiflexion. *Aust J Physiother* 44:175–180, 1998.
152. Patla CE, Abbott JH: Tibialis posterior myofascial tightness as a source of heel pain: Diagnosis and treatment. *J Orthop Sports Phys Ther* 30:624–632, 2000.
153. Rose GK, Welton GA, Marshall T: The diagnosis of flat foot in the child. *J Bone Joint Surg* 67B:71–78, 1985.
154. Bojsen-Möller F, Lamoreux L: Significance of dorsiflexion of the toes in walking. *Acta Orthop Scand* 50:471–479, 1979.
155. Rozzi SL, Lephart SM, Sterner R, et al: Balance training for persons with functionally unstable ankles. *J Orthop Sports Phys Ther* 29:478–486, 1999.
156. Lysholm J, Gilquist J: Evaluation of knee ligament surgery results with special emphasis on the use of a scoring scale. *Am J Sports Med* 10:150–154, 1982.
157. Tegner Y, Lysholm J, Lysholm M, et al: A performance test to monitor rehabilitation and evaluate anterior cruciate ligament injuries. *Am J Sports Med* 14:156–159, 1986.
158. Noyes FR, Barber SD, Mooar LA: A rationale for assessing sports activity levels and limitations in knee disorders. *Clin Orthop* 246:238–249, 1989.
159. Budiman-Mak E, Conrad KJ, Roach KE: The foot function index: A measure of foot pain and disability. *J Clin Epidemiol* 44:561–570, 1991.
160. Forkin DM, Koczur C, Battle R, et al: Evaluation of kinesthetic deficits indicative of balance control in gymnasts with unilateral chronic ankle sprains. *J Orthop Sports Phys Ther* 23:245–250, 1996.
161. Hertel J, Braham RA, Hale SA, et al: Simplifying the star excursion balance test: Analyses of subjects with and without chronic ankle instability. *J Orthop Sports Phys Ther* 36:131–137, 2006.
162. Kavanagh J: Is there a positional fault at the inferior tibiofibular joint in patients with acute or chronic ankle sprains compared to normals? *Man Ther* 4:19–24, 1999.

163. Katcherian DA: Pathology of the first ray. In: Mizel MS, Miller RA, Scioli MW, eds. *Orthopaedic Knowledge Update, Foot and Ankle*. Rosemont, IL: American Academy of Orthopaedic Surgeons, 1998:157–159.
164. Tatro-Adams D, McGann SF, Carbone W: Reliability of the figure-of-eight method of ankle measurement. *J Orthop Sports Phys Ther* 22:161–163, 1995.
165. Peng JR: Solving the dilemna of the high ankle sprain in the athlete. *Sports Med Arthrosc Rev* 8:316–325, 2000.
166. Beumer A, Swierstra BA, Mulder PG: Clinical diagnosis of syndesmotic ankle instability: Evaluation of stress tests behind the curtains. *Acta Orthop Scand* 73:667–669, 2002.
167. Kleiger B: Mechanisms of ankle injury. *Orthop Clin North Am* 5:127–146, 1974.
168. Hopkinson WJ, et al: Syndesmosis sprains of the ankle. *Foot Ankle Int* 10:325, 1990.
169. Katznel A, Lin M: Ruptures of the ligaments about the tibiofibular syndesmosis. *Injury* 25:170–172, 1984.
170. Alonso A, Khoury L, Adams R: Clinical tests for ankle syndesmosis injury: Reliability and prediction of return to function. *J Orthop Sports Phys Ther* 27:276–284, 1998.
171. Lin CF, Gross ML, Weinhold P: Ankle syndesmosis injuries: Anatomy, biomechanics, mechanism of injury, and clinical guidelines for diagnosis and intervention. *J Orthop Sports Phys Ther* 36:372–384, 2006.
172. Taylor DC, Englehardt DL, Bassett FH: Syndesmosis sprains of the ankle. The influence of heterotopic ossification. *Am J Sports Med* 20:146–150, 1992.
173. Nussbaum ED, Hosea TM, Sieler SD, et al: Prospective evaluation of syndesmotic ankle sprains without diastasis. *Am J Sports Med* 29:31–35, 2001.
174. Kiter E, Bozkurt M: The crossed-leg test for examination of ankle syndesmosis injuries. *Foot Ankle Int* 26:187–188, 2005.
175. Lindenfeld T, Parikh S: Clinical tip: Heel-thump test for syndesmotic ankle sprain. *Foot Ankle Int* 26:406–408, 2005.
176. Starkey C, Ryan JL: *Evaluation of Orthopedic and Athletic Injuries*. Philadelphia, PA: F.A. Davis, 2002.
177. Hertel J, Denegar CR, Monroe MM, et al: Talocrural and subtalar joint instability after lateral ankle sprain. *Med Sci Sports Exerc* 31:1501–1508, 1999.
178. Landeros O, Frost HM, Higgins CC: Anteriorly unstable ankle due to trauma: A report of 29 cases. *J Bone Joint Surg* 48A:1028, 1966.
179. Landeros O, Frost HM, Higgins CC: Post traumatic anterior ankle instability. *Clin Orthop* 56:169–178, 1968.
180. Tohyama H, Beynnon BD, Renstrom PA, et al: Biomechanical analysis of the ankle anterior drawer test for anterior talofibular ligament injuries. *J Orthop Res Official Publ Orthop Res Soc* 13:609–614, 1995.
181. Frost HM, Hanson CA: Technique for testing the drawer sign in the ankle. *Clin Orthop* 123:49–51, 1977.
182. Kaikkonen A, Hyppanen E, Kannus P, et al: Long-term functional outcome after primary repair of the lateral ligaments of the ankle. *Am J Sports Med* 25:150–155, 1997.
183. Gould N, Selingson D, Gassman J: Early and late repair of lateral ligaments of the ankle. *Foot Ankle* 1:84–89, 1980.
184. Staples OS: Rupture of the fibular collateral ligaments of the ankle. *J Bone Joint Surg* 57A:101–107, 1975.
185. van Dijk CN, Lim LS, Bossuyt PM, et al: Physical examination is sufficient for the diagnosis of sprained ankles. *J Bone Joint Surg Br* 78:958–962, 1996.
186. Aradi AJ, Wong J, Walsh M: The dimple sign of a ruptured lateral ligament of the ankle: Brief report. *J Bone Joint Surg [Br]* 70-B:327–328, 1988.
187. Thompson TC, Doherty JH: Spontaneous rupture of tendon of Achilles: A new clinical diagnostic test. *J Trauma* 2:126, 1962.
188. Maffulli N: The clinical diagnosis of subcutaneous tear of the Achilles tendon. A prospective study in 174 patients. *Am J Sports Med* 26:266–270, 1998.
189. Picciano AM, Rowlands MS, Worrell T: Reliability of open and closed kinetic chain subtalar joint neutral positions and navicular drop test. *J Orthop Sports Phys Ther* 18:553–558, 1993.
190. Mueller MJ, Host JV, Norton BJ: Navicular drop as a composite measure of excessive pronation. *J Am Podiat Med Assn* 83:198–202, 1993.
191. Brody DM: Techniques in the evaluation and treatment of the injured runner. *Orthop Clin North Am* 13:541–558, 1982.
192. Palmer ML, Epler M: *Clinical Assessment Procedures in Physical Therapy*. Philadelphia, PA: JB Lippincott, 1990.
193. McRae SJ, Ginsberg JS: Update in the diagnosis of deep-vein thrombosis and pulmonary embolism. *Curr Opin Anaesthesiol* 19:44–51, 2006.
194. Aschwanden M, Labs KH, Engel H, et al: Acute deep vein thrombosis: Early mobilization does not increase the frequency of pulmonary embolism. *Thromb Haemost* 85:42–46, 2001.
195. Evans RC: *Illustrated Essentials in Orthopedic Physical Assessment*. St. Louis, MO: Mosby-Year Book, 1994.
196. Oloff LM, Schulhofer SD: Flexor hallucis longus dysfunction. *J Foot Ankle Surg* 37:101–109, 1998.
197. Stiell IG, McKnight RD, Greenberg GH, et al: Implementation of the Ottawa Ankle Rules. *JAMA* 271:827–832, 1994.
198. Leddy JJ, Smolinski RJ, Lawrence J, et al: Prospective evaluation of the Ottawa Ankle Rules in a University Sports Medicine Center. With a modification to increase specificity for identifying malleolar fractures. *Am J Sports Med* 26:158–165, 1998.
199. Stiell IG, Greenberg GH, McKnight RD, et al: Decision rules for the use of radiography in acute ankle injuries: Refinement and prospective validation. *JAMA* 269:1127–1132, 1994.
200. Kibler BW: Rehabilitation of the ankle and foot. In: Kibler BW, Herring JA, Press JM, eds. *Functional Rehabilitation of Sports and Musculoskeletal Injuries*. Gaithersburg, MD: Aspen, 1998:273–283.
201. Kessler RM, Hertling D: *Management of Common Musculoskeletal Disorders*. Philadelphia, PA: Harper and Row, 1983:379–443.
202. Hettinga DL: Inflammatory response of synovial joint structures. In: Gould JA, Davies GJ, eds. *Orthopaedic and Sports Physical Therapy*. St. Louis, MO: CV Mosby, 1985:87–117.
203. Maadalo A, Waller JF: Rehabilitation of the foot and ankle linkage system. In: Nicholas JA, Hershman EB, eds. *The Lower Extremity and Spine in Sports Medicine*. St. Louis, MO: Mosby, 1986:560–583.
204. McClusky GM, Blackburn TA, Lewis TA: A treatment for ankle sprains. *Am J Sports Med* 4:158–161, 1976.
205. O'Donoghue DH: Treatment of ankle injuries. *Northwest Med* 57: 1277–1286, 1958.
206. Vegso JJ, Harmon LE: Non-operative management of athletic ankle injuries. *Clin Sports Med* 1:85–98, 1982.
207. Wilkerson GB: Treatment of ankle sprains with external compression and early mobilization. *Phys Sports Med* 13:83–90, 1985.
208. Konradsen L, Olesen S, Hansen HM: Ankle sensorimotor control and eversion strength after acute ankle inversion injuries. *Am J Sports Med* 26:72–78, 1998.
209. Korkala O, Rusanen M, Jokipii P, et al: A prospective study of the treatment of severe tears of the lateral ligament of the ankle. *Int Orthop* 11:13–17, 1987.
210. Knight KL, Aquino J, Johannes SM, et al: A re-examination of Lewis' cold induced vasodilation in the finger and ankle. *Athl Training* 15:248–250, 1980.
211. Knight KL, Londeree BR: Comparison of blood flow in the ankle of uninjured subjects during therapeutic applications of heat, cold, and exercise. *Med Sci Sports Exerc* 12:76–80, 1980.
212. Knue J, Hitchings C: The use of a rigid stirrup for prophylactic ankle support. *Athl Training* 18:121, 1982.
213. Quillen WS: An alternative management protocol for lateral ankle sprains. *J Orthop Sports Phys Ther* 2:187–190, 1981.
214. Kaltenborn FM: *Manual Mobilization of the Extremity Joints: Basic Examination and Treatment Techniques*, 4th ed. Oslo: Olaf Norlis Bokhandel, Universitetsgaten, 1989.
215. Löfvenberg R, Karrholm J: The influence of an ankle orthosis on the talar calcaneal motions in chronic lateral instability of the ankle: A stereophotogrammetric analysis. *Am J Sports Med* 21:224–230, 1993.
216. Shapiro MS, Kabo JM, Mitchell PW, et al: Ankle sprain prophylaxis: An analysis of the stabilizing effects of braces and tapes. *Am J Sports Med* 22:78–82, 1994.
217. Gross MT, Clemence LM, Cox BD, et al: Effect of ankle orthosis on functional performance for individuals with recurrent ankle sprains. *J Orthop Sports Phys Ther* 25:245–252, 1997.
218. Sharpe SS, Knapik J, Jones B: Ankle braces effectively reduce recurrence of ankle sprains in female soccer players. *J Athl Training* 32:21–24, 1997.
219. Sitler M, Ryan J, Wheeler B, et al: The efficacy of a semirigid ankle stabilizer to reduce acute ankle injuries in basketball: A randomized clinical study at West Point. *Am J Sports Med* 22:454–461, 1994.
220. Stover CN: Air stirrup management of ankle injuries in the athlete. *Am J Sports Med* 8:360–365, 1980.
221. Surve I, Schwellnus MP, Noakes T, et al: A fivefold reduction in the incidence of recurrent ankle sprains in soccer players using the sport-stirrup orthosis. *Am J Sports Med* 22:601–606, 1994.

222. Mizel MD, Marymont JV, Trapman E: Treatment of plantar fasciitis with a night splint and shoe modification consisting of a steel shank and anterior rocker bottom. *Foot Ankle Int* 17:732–735, 1997.
223. Powell MW, Post WR, Keener JK: Effective treatment of chronic plantar fasciitis with dorsiflexion night splints: A cross-over prospective randomized study. *Foot Ankle Int* 19:10–18, 1998.
224. Wapner KL, Sharkey PF: The use of night splints for treatment of recalcitrant plantar fasciitis. *Foot Ankle* 1:135–137, 1991.
225. Lentell GL, Katzman LL, Walters MR: The relationship between muscle function and ankle stability. *J Orthop Sports Phys Ther* 11:605–611, 1990.
226. Kleinrensink GJ, Stoeckart R, Meulstee J, et al: Lowered motor conduction velocity of the peroneal nerve after inversion moments. *Am J Sports Med* 24:362–369, 1996.
227. Nawoczenski DA, Owen MG, Ecker ML, et al: Objective evaluation of peroneal response to sudden inversion stress. *J Orthop Sports Phys Ther* 7:107–109, 1985.
228. Lynch SA, Edlund U, Gottlieb D, et al: Electromyographic latency changes in the ankle musculature during inversion moments. *Am J Sports Med* 24:362–369, 1996.
229. Voss DE, Ionta MK, Myers DJ: *Proprioceptive Neuromuscular Facilitation: Patterns and Techniques*, 3rd ed. Philadelphia, PA: Harper and Row, 1985:1–342.
230. Docherty CL, Moore JH, Arnold BL: Effects of strength training on strength development and joint position sense in functionally unstable ankles. *J Athl Training* 33:310–314, 1998.
231. Fiore RD, Leard JS: A functional approach in the rehabilitation of the ankle and rear foot. *Athl Training* 16:231–235, 1980.
232. Hoffman M, Payne VG: The effects of proprioceptive ankle disk training on healthy subjects. *J Orthop Sports Phys Ther* 21:90–93, 1995.
233. Keggereis S: The construction and implementation of functional progressions as a component of athletic rehabilitation. *J Orthop Sports Phys Ther* 5:14–19, 1985.
234. Mattacola CG, Lloyd JW: Effects of a 6 week strength and proprioception training program on measures of dynamic balance: A single case design. *J Athl Training* 32:127–135, 1997.
235. Sheth P, Yu B, Laskowski ER, et al: Ankle disk training influences reaction times of selected muscles in a simulated sprain. *Am J Sports Med* 25:538–543, 1997.
236. Tropp H, Askling C, Gillquist J: Prevention of ankle sprains. *Am J Sports Med* 13:259–262, 1985.
237. Wester JU, Jespersen SM, Nielsen DK, et al: Wobble board training after partial sprains of the lateral ligaments of the ankle: A prospective randomized study. *J Orthop Sports Phys Ther* 23:332–336, 1996.
238. Kaikkonen A, Kannus P, Järvinen M.: A performance test protocol and scoring scale for evaluation of ankle injuries. *Am J Sports Med* 22:462–469, 1994.
239. Leanderson J, Eriksson E, Nilsson C, et al: Proprioception in classical ballet dancers: A prospective study on the influence of an ankle sprain proprioception in the ankle joint. *Am J Sports Med* 24:370–374, 1996.
240. Abdenour TE, Saville WA, White RC, et al: The effect of ankle taping upon torque and range of motion. *Athl Training* 14:227–228, 1979.
241. Barnett JR, Tanji JL, Drake C, et al: High versus low top shoes for the prevention of ankle sprains in basketball players: A prospective randomized study. *Am J Sports Med* 21:582–596, 1993.
242. Delacerde FG: Effect of underwrap conditions on the supportive effectiveness of ankle strapping with tape. *J Sports Med Phys Fitness* 18:77–81, 1978.
243. Garrick JG, Requa RK: Role of external support in the prevention of ankle sprains. *Med Sci Sports Exerc* 5:200–203, 1973.
244. Metcalfe RC, Schlabach GE, Looney MA, et al: A comparison of moleskin tape, linen tape and lace up brace on joint restriction and movement performance. *J Athl Training* 32:136–140, 1997.
245. Pederson TS, Richard MD, Merrill G, et al: The effects of spatting and ankle taping on inversion before and after exercise. *J Athl Training* 32:29–33, 1997.
246. Bunch RP, Dednarski K, Holland D, et al: Ankle joint support: A comparison of reusable lace on braces with taping and wrapping. *Physician Sportsmed* 13:59–62, 1985.
247. Fumich RM, Ellison AE, Guerin GJ, et al: The measured effect of taping on combined foot and ankle motion before and after exercise. *Am J Sports Med* 9:165–170, 1981.
248. Glick JM, Gordon RB, Nishimoto D: The prevention and treatment of ankle injuries. *Am J Sports Med* 4:136–141, 1976.
249. Laughman RK, Carr TA, Chao EY, et al: Three-dimensional kinematics of the taped ankle before and after exercise. *Am J Sports Med* 8:425–431, 1980.
250. Malina RM, Plagenz LB, Rarick GL: Effect of exercise upon measurable supporting strength of cloth and tape on ankle wraps. *Res Q* 34:158–165, 1963.
251. Manfroy PP, Ashton-Miller JA, Wojtys EM: The effect of exercise, prewrap and athletic tape on the maximal active and passive ankle resistance to ankle inversion. *Am J Sports Med* 25:156–163, 1997.
252. Paris DL, Vardaxis V, Kokkaliaris J: Ankle ranges of motion during extended activity periods while taped and braced. *J Athl Training* 30: 223–228, 1995.
253. Rarick GL, Bigley G, Karst R, et al: The measurable support of the ankle joint by conventional methods of taping. *J Bone Joint Surg* 44A:1183–1190, 1962.
254. Karlsson J, Andreasson GO: The effect of external ankle support in chronic lateral ankle joint instability. *Am J Sports Med* 20:257–261, 1992.
255. Refshauge KM, Kilbreath SL, Raymond J: The effect of recurrent ankle inversion sprain and taping on proprioception at the ankle. *Med Sci Sports Exerc* 32:10–15, 2000.
256. Gandevia SC, McCloskey DI: Joint sense, muscle sense, and their combination as position sense, measured at the distal interphalangeal joint of the middle finger. *J Physiol* 260:387–407, 1976.
257. Provins KA: The effect of peripheral nerve block on the appreciation and execution of finger movements. *J Physiol* 143:55–67, 1958.
258. Jerosch J, Hoffstetter I, Bork H, et al: The influence of orthoses on the proprioception of the ankle joint. *Knee Surg Sports Traumatol Arthrosc* 3:39–46, 1995.
259. Robbins S, Waked E, Rappel R: Ankle taping improves proprioception before and after exercise in young men. *Br J Sports Med* 29:242–247, 1995.
260. Lindley TR, Kernozed TW: Taping and semirigid bracing may not affect ankle functional range of motion. *J Athl Training* 30:109–112, 1995.
261. MacKean LC, Bell G, Burnham RS: Prophylactic ankle bracing versus taping: Effects of functional performance in female basketball players. *J Orthop Sports Phys Ther* 22:77–82, 1995.
262. MacPherson K, Sitler M, Kimura I, et al: Effects of a semirigid and soft shell prophylactic ankle stabilizer on selected performance tests among high school football players. *J Orthop Sports Phys Ther* 21:147–152, 1995.
263. Verbrugge JD: The effects of semirigid air stirrup bracing versus adhesive ankle taping on motor performance. *J Sports Orthop Phys Ther* 23:320–325, 1996.
264. Wiley JP, Nigg BM: The effect of an ankle orthosis on ankle range of motion and performance. *J Orthop Sports Phys Ther* 23:362–369, 1996.
265. Wilk BR, Gutierrez W: Shoes and athletic injuries: Analyzing shoe design, wear pattern and manufacturers' defects. *AMAA Q* 2000.
266. Cornwall MW: Foot and Ankle Orthosis. In: Wadsworth C, ed. *Contemporary Topics in the Foot and Ankle.* La Crosse, WI: Orthopaedic section, APTA, Inc., 2000.
267. Smith-Oricchio K, Harris BA: Interrater reliability of subtalar neutral, calcaneal inversion and eversion. *J Orthop Sports Phys Ther* 12:10–15, 1990.
268. McPoil TG, Knecht HG, Schuit D: A survey of foot types in normal females between the ages of 18 and 30 years. *J Orthop Sports Phys Ther* 9:406–409, 1988.
269. Garbalosa JC, McClure MH, Catlin PA, et al: The frontal plane relationship of the forefoot to the rearfoot in an asymptomatic population. *J Orthop Sports Phys Ther* 20:200–206, 1994.
270. Elveru RA, Rothstein JM, Lamb RL: Goniometric reliability in a clinical setting: Subtalar and ankle measurements. *Phys Ther* 68:672–677, 1988.
271. Milgrom C, Giladi M, Kashton H, et al: A prospective study of the effect of a shock-absorbing orthotic device on the incidence of stress fractures in military recruits. *Foot Ankle* 6:101–104, 1985.
272. Nawoczenski DA: Orthoses for the foot. In: Nawoczenski DA, Epler ME, eds. *Orthotics in Functional Rehabilitation of the Lower Limb.* Philadelphia, PA: WB Saunders, 1997:116–155.
273. Hamill J, Knutzen KM: *Biomechanical Basis of Human Movement.* Media, PA: Williams & Wilkins, 1995.
274. Lutter L: Injuries in the runner and jogger. *Minn Med* 63:45–52, 1980.
275. Viitasalo JT, Kvist M: Some biomechanical aspects of the foot and ankle in athletes with and without shin splints. *Am J Sports Med* 11:125–130, 1983.
276. Messier SP, Pittala KA: Etiologic factors associated with selected running injuries. *Med Sci Sports Exerc* 20:501–505, 1988.
277. DeLacerda FG: A study of anatomical factors involved in shin splints. *J Orthop Sports Phys Ther* 2:55–59, 1980.

278. Mann RA: Biomechanics of the foot. *Instructional Course Lectures, AAOS,* 31:167–180, 1982.
279. Donatelli RA: Abnormal biomechanics of the foot and ankle. *J Orthop Sports Phys Ther* 9:11–16, 1987.
280. Mann RA: Pain in the foot. *Postgrad Med* 82:154–162, 1987.
281. Dahle LK, Mueller MJ, Delitto A, et al: Visual assessment of foot type and relationship of foot type to lower extremity injury. *J Orthop Sports Phys Ther* 4:70–74, 1991.
282. Buchbinder MR, Napora NJ, Biggs EW: The relationship of abnormal pronation to chondromalacia of the patella in distance runners. *J Am Podiatr Med Assoc* 69:159, 1979.
283. Johanson MA, Donatelli R, Wooden MJ, et al: Effects of three different posting methods on controlling abnormal subtalar pronation. *Phys Ther* 74:149–161, 1994.
284. Hadley A, Griffiths S, Griffiths L, et al: Antipronation taping and temporary orthoses: Effects on tibial rotation position after exercise. *J Am Podiatr Med Assoc* 89:118–123, 1999.
285. Keenan AM, Tanner CM: The effect of high-dye and low-dye taping on rearfoot motion. *J Am Podiat Med Assoc* 91:255–261, 2001.
286. Staheli LT: Evaluation of planovalgus foot deformities with special reference to the natural history. *J Am Podiatr Med Assoc* 77:2–6, 1987.
287. Barry RJ, Scranton J, P.E: Flatfeet in children. *Clin Orthop* 181:68–75, 1983.
288. Griffin LY: Common sports injuries of the foot and ankle seen in children and adolescents. *Orthop Clin North Am* 25:83–93, 1994.
289. McPoil TG: The foot and ankle. In: Malone TR, McPoil TG, Nitz AJ, eds. *Orthopaedic and Sports Physical Therapy*, 3rd ed. St Louis, MO: Mosby-Year Book, 1997:261–293.
290. Subotnick SI: The foot and sports medicine. *J Orthop Sports Phys Ther* 2:53–54, 1980.
291. McCrea JD: *Pediatric Orthopaedics of the Lower Extremity.* Mt Kisco, NY: Futura, 1985.
292. Hutton WC, Dhanedran M: The mechanics of normal and hallux valgus feet—a quantitative study. *Clin Orthop* 157:7–13, 1981.
293. Herdon CH, Heyman CH: Problems in the recognition and treatment of congenital convex pes valgus. *J Bone Joint Surg* 45A:413–418, 1963.
294. Martin RL, Stewart GW, Conti SF: Posttraumatic ankle arthritis: An update on conservative and surgical management. *J Orthop Sports Phys Ther* 37:253–259, 2007.
295. Martin R: Considerations for differential diagnosis of an ankle sprain in the adolescent. *Orthop Pract* 16:21–22, 2004.
296. Thein LA: The child and adolescent athlete. In: Zachazewski JE, Magee DJ, Quillen WS, eds. *Athletic Injuries and Rehabilitation.* Philadelphia, PA: WB Saunders, 1996:933–956.
297. Mann RA: Hallux rigidus. *Instr Course Lect* 39:15–21, 1990.
298. Mann RA: Hallux rigidus: Treatment by cheilectomy. *J Bone Joint Surg* 70A:400–406, 1988.
299. Moberg E: A simple operation for hallux rigidus. *Clin Orthop* 142:55–56, 1979.
300. Elkus RA: Tarsal coalition in the young athlete. *Am J Sports Med* 14:477–480, 1986.
301. O'Neill DB, Micheli LJ: Tarsal coalition: A follow-up of adolescent athletes. *Am J Sports Med* 17:544–549, 1989.
302. Hunter-Griffin LY: Injuries to the leg, ankle, and foot. In: Sullivan JA, Grana WA, eds. *The Pediatric Athlete.* Park Ridge, IL: American Academy of Orthopaedic Surgeons, 1990:187–198.
303. Mitchell GP, Gibson JMC: Excision of calcaneonavicular bar for painful spasmodic flatfoot. *J Bone Joint Surg* 49B:281–287, 1967.
304. Stormont DM, Peterson HA: The relative incidence of tarsal coalition. *Clin Orthop* 181:28–36, 1983.
305. Harris RI, Beath T: Etiology of peroneal spastic flatfoot. *J Bone Joint Surg* 30B:624–634, 1948.
306. Keene JS, Lange RH: Diagnostic dilemmas in foot and ankle injuries. *JAMA* 256:247–251, 1986.
307. Marotta JJ, Micheli LJ: Os trigonum impingement in dancers. *Am J Sports Med* 20:533–536, 1992.
308. Ihle CL, Cochran RM: Fracture of the fused os trigonum. *Am J Sports Med* 10:47–50, 1982.
309. Frey C: Foot health and shoewear for women. *Clin Orthop Relat Res* 372:32–44, 2000.
310. Geissele AE, Stanton RP: Surgical treatment of adolescent hallux valgus. *J Pediatr Orthop* 10:642–648, 1990.
311. McDonald MD, Stevens. DB: Modified Mitchell bunionectomy for management of adolescent hallux valgus. *Clin Orthop* 332:163–169, 1996.
312. Cole S: Foot inspection of the school child. *J Am Podiatr Assoc* 49:446–454, 1959.
313. Coughlin MJ: Juvenile bunions. In: Mann RA, Coughlin MJ, eds. *Surgery of the Foot and Ankle*, 6th ed. St. Louis, MO: Mosby-Year Book, 1993:297–339.
314. Craigmile DA: Incidence, origin, and prevention of certain foot defects. *Br Med J* 2:749–752, 1953.
315. Scranton PE, Jr, Zuckerman JD: Bunion surgery in adolescents: Results of surgical treatment. *J Pediatr Orthop* 4:39–43, 1984.
316. Mann RA: The great toe. *Orthop Clin North Am* 20:519–533, 1989.
317. Baxter DE: Treatment of the bunion deformity in athletes. *Orthop Clin North Am* 25:33–39, 1994.
318. Rodeo SA, O'Brien S, Warren RF, et al: Turf-toe: An analysis of metatarsophalangeal joint sprains in professional football players. *Am J Sports Med* 18:280–285, 1990.
319. Bowers KD, Jr, Martin RB: Impact absorption: New and old Astroturf at West Virginia University. *Med Sci Sports Exerc* 6:217–221, 1974.
320. Glasoe WM, Yack HJ, Saltzman CL: Anatomy and biomechanics of the first ray. *Phys Ther* 79:854–859, 1999.
321. Clanton TO, Ford JJ: Turf toe injury. *Clin Sports Med* 13:731–741, 1984.
322. Garrick JG: The frequency of injury, mechanism of injury, and epidemiology of ankle sprains. *Am J Sports Med* 5:241–242, 1977.
323. Garrick JG: Characterization of the patient population in a sports medicine facility. *Physician Sportsmed* 13:73–76, 1985.
324. Barker HB, Beynnon BD, Renstrom. P: Ankle injury risk factors in sports. *Sports Med* 23:69–74, 1997.
325. Kaeding CC, Whitehead R: Musculoskeletal injuries in adolescents. *Primary Care Clin Office Pract* 25:211–223, 1998.
326. Vargish T, et al: The abnkle injury-indications for the selective use of X-rays. *Injury* 14:507, 1983.
327. Anderson KJ, Lecocq JF, Lecocq. EA: Recurrent anterior subluxation of the ankle joint: A report of two cases and an experimental study. *J Bone Joint Surg* 34A:853–860, 1952.
328. Brand RL, Black HM, Cox JS: The natural history of inadequately treated ankle sprains. *Am J Sports Med* 5:248–249, 1977.
329. Brostrom L, Sundelin P: Sprained ankles: IV. Histologic changes in recent and "chronic" ligament ruptures. *Acta Chir Scand* 132:248–253, 1966.
330. Brostrom L: Sprained ankles: V. Treatment and prognosis in recent ligament ruptures. *Acta Chir Scand* 132:537–550, 1966.
331. Brostrom L: Sprained ankles: VI. Surgical treatment of "chronic" ligament ruptures. *Acta Chir Scand* 132:551–565, 1966.
332. Harrington KD: Degenerative arthritis of the ankle secondary to long standing lateral ligament instability. *J Bone Joint Surg* 61A:354–361, 1979.
333. Javors JR, Violet JT: Correction of chronic lateral ligament instability of the ankle by use of the Brostrom procedure. *Clin Orthop* 198:201–207, 1985.
334. Lauttamus L, Korkala O, Tanskanen P: Lateral ligament injuries of the ankle: Surgical treatment of the late cases. *Ann Chir Gynaecol* 71:164–167, 1982.
335. Riegler HF: Reconstruction for lateral instability of the ankle. *J Bone Joint Surg* 66A:336–339, 1984.
336. Stewart MJ, Hutchings WC: Repair of the lateral ligament of the ankle. *Am J Sports Med* 6:272–275, 1978.
337. Brostrom L, Liljedahl S-O, Lindvall N: Sprained ankles: II. Arthrographic diagnosis of recent ligament ruptures. *Acta Chir Scand* 129:485–499, 1965.
338. Gerber JP, Williams GN, Scoville CR, et al: Persistent disability associated with ankle sprains: A prospective examination of an athletic population. *Foot Ankle Int* 19:653–660, 1998.
339. Dias LS: Fractures of the distal tibial and fibular physes. In: C.A. Rockwood J, Wilkins KE, King RE, eds. *Fractures in Children*, 3rd ed. Philadelphia, PA: Lippincott, 1991:1314–1381.
340. McManama GB, Jr.: Ankle injuries in the young athlete. *Clin Sports Med* 7:547, 1988.
341. Pena FA, Coetzee JC: Ankle syndesmosis injuries. *Foot Ankle Clin* 11: 35–50, viii, 2006.
342. Klenerman L: The management of sprained ankle. *J Bone Joint Surg Br* 80:11–20, 1998.
343. Prins JG: Diagnosis and treatment of injury to the lateral ligament lesion of the ankle: A comparative clinical study. *Acta Chir Scand* 486(Suppl): 3–149, 1978.
344. Thorndike A: *Athletic Injuries: Prevention, Diagnosis and Treatment.* Philadelphia, PA: Lea and Febiger, 1962.

345. Inman VT: Sprains of the ankle. In: Chapman MW, ed. *AAOS Instructional Course Lectures*, 1975:294–308.
346. O'Donoghue DH: *Treatment of Injuries to Athletes.* Philadelphia, PA: WB Saunders, 1976:698–746.
347. Gronmark T, Johnson O, Kogstad O: Rupture of the lateral ligaments of the ankle. *Foot Ankle* 1:84–89, 1980.
348. Iversen LD, Clawson DK: *Manual of Acute Orthopaedics.* Boston, MA: Little, Brown, and Company, 1982.
349. Kannus P, Renstrom P: Current concepts review: Treatment of acute tears of the lateral ligaments of the ankle. *J Bone Joint Surg* 73A:305–312, 1991.
350. Balduini FC, Tetzelaff J: Historical perspectives on injuries of the ligaments of the ankle. *Clin Sports Med* 1:3–12, 1982.
351. Prentice WE: Using therapeutic modalities in rehabilitation. In: Prentice WE, Voight ML, eds. *Techniques in Musculoskeletal Rehabilitation.* New York, NY: McGraw-Hill, 2001:289–303.
352. Eiff MP, Smith AT, Smith GE: Early mobilization versus immobilization in the treatment of lateral ankle sprains. *Am J Sports Med* 22:83–88, 1994.
353. Noyes FR, Torvik PJ, Hyde WB, et al: Biomechanics of ligament failure: II. An analysis of immobilization, exercise, and reconditioning effects in primates. *J Bone Joint Surg* 56A:1406–1418, 1974.
354. Tipton CM, James SL, Mergner W, et al: Influence of exercise in strength of medial collateral knee ligaments of dogs. *Am J Physiol* 218:894–902, 1970.
355. Tipton CM, Matthes RD, Maynard JA, et al: The influence of physical activity on ligaments and tendons. *Med Sci Sports Exerc* 7:165–175, 1975.
356. Vailas AC, Tipton CM, Mathes RD, et al: Physical activity and its influence on the repair process of medial collateral ligaments. *Connect Tissue Res* 9:25–31, 1981.
357. Dias LS: The lateral ankle sprain: An experimental study. *J Trauma* 19:266–269, 1977.
358. Johnson EE, Markolf K: The contribution of the anterior talofibular ligament to ankle laxity. *J Bone Joint Surg* 65A:81–88, 1983.
359. Ramsey PL, Hamilton WC: Lateral talar subluxation: The effect of tibiotalar contact surfaces. *J Bone Joint Surg* 57A:567–568, 1975.
360. Brand RL, Collins MDF, Templeton T: Surgical repair of ruptured lateral ankle ligaments. *Am J Sports Med* 9:40–44, 1981.
361. Freeman MAR, Dean MRE, Hanham IWF: The etiology and prevention of functional instability of the foot. *J Bone Joint Surg* 47B:678–685, 1965.
362. Karlsson J, Bergstern T, Peterson L: Reconstruction of the lateral ligaments of the ankle for chronic lateral instability. *J Bone Joint Surg* 70-A:581–588, 1988.
363. Ruth CJ: The surgical treatment of injuries of the fibular collateral ligaments of the ankle. *J Bone Joint Surg* 43A:229–239, 1961.
364. Hintermann B: Biomechanik der Sprunggelenke: Unfallmechanismen. [Biomechanics of the ankle joint: Injury mechanisms.]. *Swiss Surg* 4:63–69, 1998.
365. Orava S, Jaroma H, Suvela M: Radiological instability of the ankle after Evan's repair. *Acta Orthop Scand* 54:734–738, 1983.
366. Nicholas JA: Ankle injuries in athletes. *Orthop Clin North Am* 15:153–175, 1974.
367. Tropp H: *Functional Instability of the Ankle Joint.* Linkoping: Linkoping University, 1985.
368. Elmslie RC: Recurrent subluxation of the ankle joint. *Ann Surg* 100:364–367, 1934.
369. Hintermann B: Die anatomische Rekonstruktion des Aussenbandapparates mit der Plantarissehne. [Anatomical reconstruction of the lateral ligament complex of the ankle.]. *Operat Orthop Traumatol* 10:210–218, 1998.
370. Karlsson J, Bergsten T, Lansinger O, et al: Surgical treatment of chronic lateral instability of the ankle joint: A new procedure. *Am J Sports Med* 17:268–274, 1989.
371. Karlsson J, Eriksson BI, Bergsten T, et al: Comparison of two anatomic reconstructions for chronic lateral instability of the ankle joint. *Am J Sports Med* 25:48–53, 1997.
372. Rudert M, Wülker N, Wirth CJ: Reconstruction of the lateral ligaments of the ankle using a regional periosteal flap. *J Bone Joint Surg* 79-B:446–451, 1997.
373. Sammarco GJ, Diraimondo CV: Surgical treatment of lateral ankle instability syndrome. *Am J Sports Med* 16:501–511, 1988.
374. Rosenbaum D, Becker HP, Sterk J, et al: Functional evaluation of the 10-year outcome after modified Evans repair for chronic ankle instability. *Foot Ankle Int* 18:765–771, 1997.
375. Curtis MJ, Myerson M, Szura B: Tarsometatarsal joint injuries in the athlete. *Am J Sports Med* 21:497–502, 1993.
376. Clanton TO, Porter DA: Primary care of foot and ankle injuries in the athlete. *Clin Sports Med* 16:435–466, 1997.
377. Marshall P, Hamilton WG: Cuboid subluxation in ballet dancers. *Am J Sports Med* 20:169–175, 1992.
378. Blakeslee TJ, Morris JL: Cuboid syndrome and the significance of midtarsal joint stability. *J Am Podiat Med Assn* 77:638–642, 1987.
379. Khan K, Brown J, Way S, et al: Overuse injuries in classical ballet. *Sports Med* 19:341–357, 1995.
380. Newell SG, Woodie A: Cuboid syndrome. *Physician Sportsmed* 9:71–76, 1981.
381. Hefland AE: Nail and hyperkeratotic problems in the elderly foot. *Am Fam Phys* 39:101–110, 1989.
382. Subotnick SI: Foot Injuries. In: Subotnick SI, ed. *Sports Medicine of the Lower Extremity.* Philadelphia, PA: Churchill Livingstone, 1999:207–260.
383. Bendl BJ: Subungual exostosis. *Cutis* 26:260, 1980.
384. Zook EG: The perionychium: Anatomy, physiology, and care of injuries. *Clin Plast Surg* 8:27, 1981.
385. Bartolomei FJ: Onychauxis. *Clin Podiatr Med Surg* 12:215–220, 1995.
386. Krausz CE: Nail survey of 12,500 patients. *Br J Chiropody* 48:239, 1983.
387. Sammarco GJ: Peroneal tendon injuries. *Orthop Clin North Am* 25:135–145, 1994.
388. Micheli LJ, Waters PM, Sanders DP: Sliding fibular graft repair for chronic dislocation of the peroneal tendons. *Am J Sports Med* 17:68–71, 1989.
389. Clanton TO, Schon LC: Athletic injuries to the soft tissues of the foot and ankle. In: Mann RA, Coughlin MJ, eds. *Surgery of the Foot and Ankle*, 6th ed. St. Louis, MO: Mosby-Year Book, 1993:1167–1177.
390. Frey CC, Shereff MJ: Tendon injuries about the ankle in athletes. *Clin Sports Med* 7:103–118, 1988.
391. Niemi WJ, Savidakis J, Dejesus JM: Peroneal subluxation: A comprehensive review of the literature with case presentations. *J Foot Ankle Surg* 36:141–145, 1997.
392. Stover CN, Bryan DR: Traumatic dislocation of the peroneal tendons. *Am J Surg* 103:180–186, 1962.
393. Arrowsmith SR, Fleming LL, Allman FL: Traumatic dislocations of the peroneal tendons. *Am J Sports Med* 11:142–146, 1983.
394. Eckert WR, Davis FA: Acute rupture of the peroneal retinaculum. *J Bone Joint Surg* 58A:670–673, 1976.
395. Slatis P, Santavirta S, Sandelin J: Surgical treatment of chronic dislocation of the peroneal tendons. *Br J Sports Med* 22:16–18, 1988.
396. Sobel M, Geppert MJ, Warren RF: Chronic ankle instability as a cause of peroneal tendon injury. *Clin Orthop Relat Res* 296:187–191, 1993.
397. Kettlecamp D, Alexander H: Spontaneous rupture of the posterior tibilialis tendon. *J Bone Joint Surg* 51A:759, 1969.
398. Groshar D, Liberson A, Alperson M, et al: Scintigraphy of posterior tibial tendinitis. *J Nucl Med* 38:247–249, 1997.
399. Hamilton WG, Geppert MJ, Thompson FM: Pain in the posterior aspect of the ankle in dancers. *J Bone Joint Surg* 78A:1491–1500, 1996.
400. Garth WP: Flexor hallucis tendinitis in a ballet dancer. *J Bone Joint Surg* 63A:1489, 1981.
401. Koleitis GJ, Micheli LJ, Klein JD: Release of the flexor hallucis longus tendon in ballet dancers. *J Bone Joint Surg* 78A:1386–1390, 1996.
402. Teitz CC: Sports medicine concerns in dance and gymnastics. *Pediatr Clin North Am* 29:1399–1421, 1982.
403. Morford M, Lenardon RJ: *Classical Mythology.* New York, NY: Longman, 1985:3329–3335.
404. Clain MR, Baxter DE: Achilles tendinitis. *Foot Ankle* 13:482–487, 1992.
405. Voorn R: Case report: Can sacroiliac joint dysfunction cause chronic Achilles tendinitis? *J Orthop Sports Phys Ther* 27:436–443, 1998.
406. McCrory JL, Martin DF, Lowery RB, et al: Etiologic factors associated with Achilles tendinitis in runners. *Med Sci Sports Exerc* 31:1374–1381, 1999.
407. Smart GW, Taunton JE, Clement DB: Achilles tendon disorders in runners: A review. *Med Sci Sport Exerc* 12:231–243, 1980.
408. Jacobs SJ, Berson BJ: Injuries to runners: A study of entrants to a 10,000 meter race. *Am J Sports Med* 14:151–155, 1986.
409. Pinshaw R, Atlas V, Noakes TD: The nature and response to therapy of 196 consecutive injuries seen at a runners' clinic. *S Afr Med J* 65:291–298, 1984.
410. Brunet ME, Cook SD, Brinker MR, et al: A survey of running injuries in 1505 competitive and recreational runners. *J Sports Med Phys Fitness* 30:307–315, 1990.

411. van Mechelen W, Hlobil H, Kemper HCG, et al: Prevention of running injuries by warm-up, cool-down and stretching exercises. *Am J Sports Med* 21:711–719, 1993.
412. Hess GP, Cappiello WL, Poole RM, et al: Prevention and treatment of overuse tendon injuries. *Sports Med* 8:371–384, 1989.
413. Clement DB, Taunton JE, Smart GW, et al: A survey of overuse running injuries. *Physician Sportsmed* 9:47–58, 1981.
414. Renstrom P, Johnson RJ: Overuse injuries in sports: A review. *Sports Med* 2:316–333, 1985.
415. Lyshold J, Wiklander J: Injuries in runners. *Am J Sports Med* 15:168–171, 1987.
416. Sheehan GA: An overview of overuse syndromes in distance runners. *Ann N Y Acad Sci* 301:877–880, 1977.
417. Barry NN, McGuire JL: Overuse syndromes in adult athletes. *Rheum Dis Clin North Am* 22:515–530, 1996.
418. Gudas CJ: Patterns of lower extremity injury in 224 runners. *Exerc Sports Med* 12:50–59, 1980.
419. Hogan DG, Cape RD: Marathoners over sixty years of age: Results of a survey. *J. Am. Geriatr. Soc* 32:121–123, 1984.
420. Janis LR: Results of the Ohio runners sports medicine survey. *J Am Podiatr Med Assoc* 10:586–589, 1986.
421. Sarrafian SK: *Functional Anatomy, Anatomy of the Ankle and Foot.* Philadelphia, PA: J.B. Lippincott Company, 1992:559–590.
422. Kapandji IA: *The Physiology of Joints.* New York, NY: Churchill Livingstone, 1974.
423. Grieve GP: *Common Vertebral Joint Problems.* New York, NY: Churchill Livingstone, 1981.
424. Menell JB: *The Science and Art of Joint Manipulation, Spinal Column.* London: J & A Churchill, 1952.
425. Mennell JM: *Back Pain. Diagnosis and Treatment Using Manipulative Techniques.* Boston, MA: Little, Brown & Company, 1960.
426. Hartman SL: *Handbook of Osteopathic Technique*, 2nd ed. London: Unwin Hyman, 1990.
427. Magee DJ: *Lumbar Spine, Pelvic Joints, Orthopedic Physical Assessment.* Philadelphia, PA: WB Saunders, 1987:182–238.
428. Ombreght L, Bisshop P, Veer TJ, et al: *Applied Anatomy of the Sacroiliac Joint, A System of Orthopaedic Medicine.* Philadelphia, PA: WB Saunders, 1991:690–708.
429. Puddu G, Ippolito E, Postacchini F: A classification of Achilles tendon disease. *Am J Sports Med* 4:145–150, 1976.
430. Lohrer H: Seltene ursachen und differentialdiagnosen der achillodynie. *Sportverl Sportschad* 5:182–185, 1991.
431. Bates BT, Osternig LR, Mason B, et al: Foot orthotic devices to modify selected aspects of lower extremity mechanics. *Am J Sports Med* 7:338–342, 1979.
432. Leach RE, Schepsis AA: *Achilles Tendinitis.* Bulgaria: Forum Medicus, 1986.
433. Goodnite EA: The practical use of evidence-based practice in determining the best treatment for a patient with recurrent Achilles tendinitis. *Orthop Pract* 17:12–14, 2005.
434. Alfredson H, Pietila T, Jonsson P, et al: Heavy-load eccentric calf muscle training for the treatment of chronic Achilles tendinosis. *Am J Sports Med* 26:360–366, 1998.
435. Pare A: *Les Oeuvres*, 9th ed. Lyon: Claude Rigaud et Claude Obert, 1633.
436. Fox JM, Blazina ME, Jobe FW, et al: Degeneration and rupture of the Achilles tendon. *Clin Orthop* 107:221–224, 1975.
437. Inglis AE, Scott WN, Sculco TP, et al: Surgical repair of ruptures of the tendo Achillis. *J Bone Joint Surg* 58A:990–993, 1976.
438. Kager H: Zur Klinik und Diagnostik des Achillesshnenrisses. *Chirurgie* 11:691–695, 1939.
439. Langergren C, Lindholm A: Vascular distribution in the Achilles tendon. *Acta Chir Scand* 116:491–495, 1958.
440. Maffulli N, Dymond NP, Regine R: Surgical repair of ruptured Achilles tendon in sportsmen and sedentary patients: A longitudinal ultrasound assessment. *Int J Sports Med* 11:78–84, 1990.
441. Popovic N, Lemaire R: Diagnosis and treatment of acute ruptures of the Achilles tendon: Current concepts review. *Acta Orthop Belg* 65:458–471, 1999.
442. Arner O, Lindholm A, Orell SR: Histologic changes in subcutaneous rupture of the Achilles tendon. *Acta Chir Scand* 116:484, 1958/1959.
443. Wills CA, Washburn S, Caiozzo V, et al: Achilles tendon rupture: A review of the literature comparing surgical versus nonsurgical treatment. *Clin Orthop* 207:156–163, 1986.
444. Fierro NL, Sallis RE: Achilles tendon rupture: Is casting enough. *Postgrad Med* 98:145–151, 1995.
445. Cetti A, Christensen SE, Ejsted R, et al: Operative versus non-operative treatment of Achilles tendon rupture. *Am J Sports Med* 21:791–799, 1993.
446. Jacobs D, Martens M, Van Audekercke R, et al: Comparison of conservative and operative treatment of Achilles tendon rupture. *Am J Sports Med* 6:107–111, 1978.
447. Lea RB, Smith L: Non-surgical treatment of tendo Achilles rupture. *J Bone Joint Surg* 54A:1398–1407, 1972.
448. Leppilahti J, Orava S: Total Achilles tendon rupture. *Sports Med* 25:79–100, 1998.
449. Soma CA, Mandelbaum BR: Repair of acute Achilles tendon ruptures. *Orthop Clin North Am* 26:241–246, 1995.
450. Nistor L: Surgical and non-surgical treatment of Achilles tendon rupture. *J Bone Joint Surg* 63A:394–399, 1981.
451. Micheli LJ, Ireland ML: Prevention and management of calcaneal apophysitis in children: An overuse syndrome. *J Pediatr Orthop* 7:34–38, 1987.
452. Mafulli N: Intensive training in young athletes. *Sports Med* 9:229–243, 1990.
453. Gwynne-Jones DP, Sims M, Handcock D: Epidemiology and outcomes of acute Achilles tendon rupture with operative or nonoperative treatment using an identical functional bracing protocol. *Foot Ankle Int* 32:337–343, 2011.
454. Nilsson-Helander K, Silbernagel KG, Thomee R, et al: Acute achilles tendon rupture: a randomized, controlled study comparing surgical and nonsurgical treatments using validated outcome measures. *Am J Sports Med* 38:2186–2193, 2010.
455. Karkhanis S, Mumtaz H, Kurdy N: Functional management of Achilles tendon rupture: A viable option for non-operative management. *Foot and ankle surgery : official journal of the European Society of Foot and Ankle Surgeons* 16:81–86, 2010.
456. Chiodo CP, Glazebrook M, Bluman EM, et al: American Academy of Orthopaedic Surgeons clinical practice guideline on treatment of Achilles tendon rupture. *J Bone Joint Surg Am* 92:2466–2468, 2010.
457. Metz R, van der Heijden GJ, Verleisdonk EJ, et al: Recovery of calf muscle strength following acute achilles tendon rupture treatment: a comparison between minimally invasive surgery and conservative treatment. *Foot Ankle Spec* 2:219–226, 2009.
458. Willits K, Amendola A, Bryant D, et al: Operative versus nonoperative treatment of acute Achilles tendon ruptures: a multicenter randomized trial using accelerated functional rehabilitation. *J Bone Joint Surg Am* 92:2767–2775, 2010.
459. Stanitski C: Management of sports injuries in children and adolescents. *Orthop Clin North Am* 19:689–698, 1988.
460. Meeusen R, Borms J: Gymnastic injuries. *Sports Med* 13:337–356, 1992.
461. Canale ST, Williams KD: Iselin's disease. *J Pediatr Orthop* 12:90–93, 1992.
462. Crawford F: Plantar heel pain and fasciitis. *Clin Evid* 1589–1602, 2004.
463. Crawford F, Thomson C: Interventions for treating plantar heel pain. *Cochrane Database Syst Rev* 3, 2003.
464. Crawford F, Atkins D, Edwards J: Interventions for treating plantar heel pain. *Cochrane Database Syst Rev* 3, 2000.
465. Waugh EJ: Lateral epicondylalgia or epicondylitis: What's in a name? *J Orthop Sports Phys Ther* 35:200–202, 2005.
466. Hyland MR, Webber-Gaffney A, Cohen L, et al: Randomized controlled trial of calcaneal taping, sham taping, and plantar fascia stretching for the short-term management of plantar heel pain. *J Orthop Sports Phys Ther* 36:364–371, 2006.
467. Warren BL, Jones CJ: Predicting plantar fasciitis in runners. *Med Sci Sports Exerc* 19:71–73, 1987.
468. DeMaio M, Paine R, Mangine RE, et al: Plantar fasciitis. *Orthopedics* 16:1153–1163, 1993.
469. Williams PL, Smibert JG, Cox R, et al: Imaging study of the painful heel syndrome. *Foot Ankle* 7:345–349, 1987.
470. Riddle DL, Pulisic M, Pidcoe P, et al: Risk factors for Plantar fasciitis: A matched case-control study. *J Bone Joint Surg Am* 85-A:872–877, 2003.
471. Sarrafian SK: Functional anatomy of the foot and ankle. In: Sarrafian SK, ed. *Anatomy of the Foot and Ankle: Descriptive, Topographic, Functional*, 2nd ed. Philadelphia, PA: J.B. Lippincott, 1993:474–602.
472. Prichasuk S: The heel-pad in plantar heel pain. *J Bone Joint Surg* 76-B:140–142, 1994.
473. Tsai WC, Wang CL, Hsu TC, et al: The mechanical properties of the heel pad in unilateral plantar heel pain syndrome. *Foot Ankle Int* 20:663–668, 1999.

474. Schepsis AA, Leach RE, Gorzyca J: Plantar fasciitis: Etiology, treatment, surgical results, and review of the literature. *Clin Orthop* 266:185–196, 1991.
475. Amis J, Jennings L, Graham D, et al: Painful heel syndrome: Radiographic and treatment assessment. *Foot Ankle* 9:91–95, 1988.
476. Kibler WB, Goldberg C, Chandler TJ: Functional biomechanical deficits in running athletes with plantar fasciitis. *Am J Sports Med* 19:66–71, 1991.
477. Barrett SL, Day SV, Pugnetti TT, et al: Endoscopic heel anatomy: Analysis of 200 fresh frozen specimens. *J Foot Ankle Surg* 34:51–56, 1995.
478. DuVries HL: Heel spur (calcaneal spur). *Arch Surg* 74:536–542, 1957.
479. Tanz SS: Heel pain. *Clin Orthop* 28:169–178, 1963.
480. Wolgin M, Cook C, Graham C, et al: Conservative treatment of plantar heel pain: Long-term follow-up. *Foot Ankle* 15:97–102, 1994.
481. Kier R: Magnetic resonance imaging of plantar fasciitis and other causes of heel pain. *MRI Clin N Am* 2:97–107, 1994.
482. Rubin G, Witten M: Plantar calcaneal spurs. *Am J Orthop* 5:38–55, 1963.
483. Karr SD: Subcalcaneal heel pain. *Orthop Clin North Am* 25:161–175, 1994.
484. Hendrix CL, Jolly JP, Garbalosa JC, et al: Entrapment neuropathy: The etiology of intractable chronic heel pain syndrome. *J Foot Ankle Surg* 37:273–279, 1998.
485. Meyer J, Kulig K, Landel R: Differential diagnosis and treatment of subcalcaneal heel pain: A case report. *J Orthop Sports Phys Ther* 32:114–124, 2002.
486. Pfeffer GB: Planter heel pain. In: Baxter DE, ed. *The Foot and Ankle in Sport*. St Louis, MO: Mosby, 1995:195–206.
487. Kosinski M, Lilja E: Infectious causes of heel pain. *J Am Podiat Med Assn* 89:20–23, 1999.
488. Jahss MH, Michelson JD, Desai P, et al: Investigations into the fat pads of the sole of the foot: Anatomy and histology. *Foot Ankle* 13:233–242, 1992.
489. Chandler TJ, Kibler BW: A biomechanical approach to the prevention, treatment and rehabilitation of plantar fasciitis. *Sports Med* 15:344–352, 1993.
490. Kwong PK, Kay D, Voner RT, et al: Plantar fasciitis: Mechanics and pathomechanics of treatment. *Clin Sports Med* 7:119–126, 1988.
491. Furey JG: Plantar fasciitis: The painful heel syndrome. *J Bone Joint Surg* 57(A):672, 1975.
492. Davis PF, Severud E, Baxter DE: Painful heel syndrome: Results of nonoperative treatment. *Foot Ankle Int* 15:531–535, 1994.
493. Young B, Walker MJ, Strunce J, et al: A combined treatment approach emphasizing impairment-based manual physical therapy for plantar heel pain: A case series. *J Orthop Sports Phys Ther* 34:725–733, 2004.
494. Lynch DM, Goforth WP, Martin JE, et al: Conservative treatment of plantar fasciitis: A prospective study. *J Am Podiatr Med Assoc* 88: 375–380, 1998.
495. DiGiovanni BF, Nawoczenski DA, Lintal ME, et al: Tissue-specific plantar fascia-stretching exercise enhances outcomes in patients with chronic heel pain. A prospective, randomized study. *J Bone Joint Surg* 85-A:1270–1277, 2003.
496. Rompe JD, Schoellner C, Nafe B: Evaluation of low-energy extracorporeal shock-wave application for treatment of chronic plantar fasciitis. *Journal of Bone & Joint Surgery* 84-A:335–341, 2002.
497. Scherer PR: Heel spur syndrome. Pathomechanics and nonsurgical treatment. Biomechanics Graduate Research Group for 1988. *J Am Pod Med Assn* 81:68–72, 1991.
498. Martin RL, Irrgang JJ, Conti SF: Outcome study of subjects with insertional plantar fasciitis. *Foot Ankle Int* 19:803–811, 1998.
499. Pollard H, So V: Management of plantar fasciitis: A case report. *J Sports Chiropr Rehabil* 13:136–137, 2004.
500. Van Wyngarden TM: The painful foot, part II: Common rearfoot deformities. *Am Fam Phys* 55:2207–2212, 1997.
501. Tanner SM, Harvey JS: How we manage plantar fasciitis. *Physician Sports Med* 16:39, 1988.
502. Jones D, James S: Partial calcaneal osteotomy for retrocalcaneal bursitis. *Am J Sports Med* 12:72, 1984.
503. Haglund P: Beitrag zur Klinik der Achillessehne. *Z Orthop Chir* 49:49–58, 1927.
504. Dickinson PH, Coutts MB, Woodward EP, et al: Tendo achillis bursitis: A report of twenty-one cases. *J Bone Joint Surg* 48:77–81, 1966.
505. Fowler A, Philip JF: Abnormality of the calcaneus as a cause of painful heel: Its diagnosis and operative treatment. *Br J Surg* 32:494–498, 1945.
506. Nisbet NW: Tendo Achilles bursitis ("winter heel"). *Br J Surg* 2:1394–1395, 1954.
507. Stephens MM: Haglund's deformity and retrocalcaneal bursitis. *Orthop Clin North Am* 25:41–46, 1994.
508. Taylor GJ: Prominence of the calcaneus: Is operation justified? *J Bone Joint Surg* 68(B):467–470, 1986.
509. Keck S, Kelley P: Bursitis of the posterior part of the heel. *J Bone Joint Surg* 47(A):267–273, 1965.
510. Morton DJ: *The Human Foot: Its Evolution, Physiology, and Functional Disorders*. New York, NY: Columbia Press, 1935.
511. Mann RA, Mizel MS: Monarticular nontraumatic synovitis of the metatarsophalangeal joint: A new diagnosis? *Foot Ankle* 6:18–21, 1985.
512. Fortin PT, Myerson MS: Second metatarsophalangeal joint instability. *Foot Ankle Int* 16:306–313, 1995.
513. Trepman E, Yeo SJ: Nonoperative treatment of metatarsophalngeal synovitis. *Foot Ankle Int* 16:771–777, 1995.
514. Wolin I, Glassman F, Sideman S, et al: Internal derangement of the talofibular component of the ankle. *Surg Gynecol* 91:193–200, 1950.
515. Ferkel RD, Karzel RP, Pizzo WD, et al: Arthroscopic treatment of anterolateral impingement of the ankle. *Am J Sports Med* 19:440–446, 1991.
516. Ferkel RD, Fischer SP: Progress in ankle arthroscopy. *Clin Orthop* 240:210–220, 1989.
517. Guhl JF: *Soft tissue (synovial) pathology, Ankle Arthroscopy: Pathology and Surgical Technique*, 2nd ed. Thorofare, NJ: Slack, 1993:93–135.
518. Martin DF, Baker CL, Curl WW, et al: Operative ankle arthroscopy: Long-term follow-up. *Am J Sports Med* 17:16–23, 1989.
519. Martin DF, Curl WW, Baker CL: Arthroscopic treatment of chronic synovitis of the ankle. *Arthroscopy* 5:110–114, 1989.
520. McCarroll J, Schrader JW, Shelbourne KD, et al: Meniscoid lesions of the ankle in soccer players. *Am J Sports Med* 15:255–257, 1987.
521. Reynaert P, Gelen G, Geens G: Arthroscopic treatment of anterior impingement of the ankle. *Acta Orthop Belg* 60:384–388, 1994.
522. Schonholtz GJ: *Arthroscopic Surgery of the Shoulder, Elbow, and Ankle*. Springfield, IL: Charles C Thomas, 1989.
523. Bassett FH, Gates HS, III, Billys JB, et al: Talar impingement by the anteroinferior tibiofibular ligament. *J Bone Joint Surg* 72A:55–59, 1990.
524. Thein R, Eichenblat M: Arthroscopic treatment of sports-related synovitis of the ankle. *Am J Sports Med* 20:496–498, 1992.
525. Howse AJG: Posterior block of the ankle joint in dancers. *Foot Ankle* 3:81–84, 1982.
526. Johnson RP, Collier BD, Carrera GF: The os trigonum syndrome, use of bone scan in the diagnosis. *J Trauma* 24:761, 1984.
527. Scranton PE: Pathologic and anatomic variations of the sesamoids. *Foot Ankle* 1:321–326, 1981.
528. Dobas DC, Silvers MD: The frequency of partite sesamoids of the metatarsophalangeal joint. *J Am Podiatry Assoc* 67:880–882, 1977.
529. Coughlin MJ: Sesamoid pain: Causes and surgical treatment. *Instr Course Lect* 39:23–35, 1990.
530. Mann RA: Metatarsalgia: Common causes and conservative treatment. *Postgrad Med* 75:150–167, 1984.
531. Orava S, Puranen J: Athletes' leg pain. *Br J Sports Med* 13:92–97, 1979.
532. Blue JM, Mathews LS: Leg injuries. *Clin Sports Med* 16:467–478, 1997.
533. Andrish JT: Leg pain. In: DeLee JC, Drez D, eds. *Orthopedic Sports Medicine*. Philadelphia, PA: WB Saunders, 1994:1603–1607.
534. Graham CE, Graham DM: Morton's neuroma: A microscopic evaluation. *Foot Ankle* 5:150, 1984.
535. Wu KK: Morton's interdigital neuroma: A clinical review of its etiology, treatment, and results. *J Foot Ankle Surg* 35:112–119, 1996.
536. Mulder JD: The causative mechanism in Morton's metatarsalgia. *J Bone Joint Surg* 33B:94–95, 1951.
537. Szabo RM: Carpal tunnel syndrome-general. In: Gelberman RH, ed. *Operative Nerve Repair and Reconstruction*. Philadelphia, PA: JB Lippincott, 1991:882–883.
538. Koppell HP, Thompson WAL: *Peripheral Entrapment Neuropathies*. Baltimore, MD: Williams & Wilkins, 1963.
539. Marinacci AA: *Applied Electromyography*. Philadelphia, PA: Lea & Febriger, 1968.
540. Borges LF, Hullett M, Selker DJ, et al: The anterior tarsal tunnel syndrome. *J Neurosurg* 54:89–92, 1981.
541. Dellon AL: Deep peroneal nerve entrapment on the dorsum of the foot. *Foot Ankle* 11:73–80, 1990.
542. Zengzhao L, Jiansheng Z, Li Z: Anterior tarsal syndrome. *J Bone Joint Surg* 73B:470–473, 1991.
543. Krause KH, Witt T, Ross A: The anterior tarsal syndrome. *J Neurol* 217:67–74, 1977.
544. Gessini L, Jandolo B, Pietrangeli A: The anterior tarsal syndrome: Report of four cases. *J Bone Joint Surg* 66A:786–787, 1984.

545. Ombregt L, Bisschop P, ter Veer HJ, et al: Nerve Lesions and Entrapment Neuropathies of the Lower Limb. In: Ombregt L, ed. *A System of Orthopaedic Medicine*. London: WB Saunders, 1995:932–937.
546. Hyslop GH: Injuries to the deep and superficial peroneal nerves complicating ankle sprain. *Am J Surg* 51:436–439, 1941.
547. Pecina M, Krmpotic-Nemanic J, Markiewitz A: *Tunnel Syndromes*. Boca Raton, FL: CRC, 1991.
548. Acus RW, Flanagan JP: Perineural fibrosis of superficial peroneal nerve complicating ankle sprain: A case report. *Foot Ankle Int* 11:233–235, 1991.
549. Meals RA: Peroneal-nerve palsy complicating ankle sprain: Report of two cases and review of the literature. *J Bone Joint Surg* 59-A:966–968, 1977.
550. Nitz AJ, Dobner JJ, Kersey D: Nerve injury and grades II and III ankle sprains. *Am J Sports Med* 13:177–182, 1985.
551. Mueller MJ, Diamond JE, Delitto A, et al: Insensitivity, limited joint mobility, and plantar ulcers in patients with diabetes mellitus. *Phys Ther* 69:453–462, 1989.
552. Mueller MJ: Etiology, evaluation, and treatment of the neuropathic foot. *Crit Rev Phys Rehabil Med* 3:289–309, 1992.
553. Reddy M, Kohr R, Queen D, et al: Practical treatment of wound pain and trauma: A patient-centered approach. An overview. *Ostomy Wound Management* 49(4 Suppl):2–15, 2003.
554. Dietz FR, Matthews KD, Montogomery WJ: Reflex sympathetic dystrophy in children. *Clin Orthop* 258:225–231, 1990.
555. Smolders JJ: Myofascial pain and dysfunction syndromes. In: Hammer WI, ed. *Functional Soft Tissue Examination and Treatment by Manual Methods—The Extremities*. Gaithersburg, MD: Aspen, 1991:215–234.
556. McBryde AM, Jr.: Stress fractures in athletes. *J Sports Med* 3:212–217, 1975.
557. Monteleone GP: Stress fractures in the athlete. *Orthop Clin North Am* 26:423, 1995.
558. Brudvig TJ, Gudger TD, Obermeyer L: Stress fractures in 295 trainees: A one-year study of incidence as related to age, sex, and race. *Mil Med* 148:666–667, 1983.
559. Protzman PR: Physiologic performance of women compared to men at the U.S. Military Academy. *Am J Sports Med* 7:191–196, 1979.
560. Marshall LA: Clinical evaluation of amenorrhea. In: Agostini R, Titus S, eds. *Medical and Orthopedic Issues of Active and Athletic Women*. Philadelphia, PA: Hanley and Belfus, 1994:152–163.
561. Myburgh KH, Bachrach LK, Lewis B, et al: Low bone mineral density at axial and appendicular sites in amenorrheic athletes. *Med Sci Sports Exerc* 25:1197–1202, 1993.
562. Sharkey NA, Ferris L, Smith TS, et al: Strain and loading of the second metatarsal during heel life. *J Bone Joint Surg* 77A:1050–1057, 1995.
563. Pester S, Smith PC: Stress fractures in the lower extremities of soldiers in basic training. *Orthop Rev* 21:297–303, 1992.
564. Gardner LI, Dziados JE, Jones BH, et al: Prevention of lower extremity stress fractures: A controlled trial of a shock absorbent insole. *Am J Public Health* 78:1563, 1988.
565. Schwellnus MP, Jordaan G, Noakes TD: Prevention of common overuse injuries by the use of shock absorbing insoles: A prospective study. *Am J Sports Med* 18:636–641, 1990.
566. Gross RH: Fractures and dislocations of the foot. In: C.A. Rockwood J, Wilkins KE, King RE, eds. *Fractures in Children*, 3rd ed. Philadelphia, PA: Lippincott, 1991:1383–1453.
567. Harrington T, Crichton KJ, Anderson IF: Overuse ballet injury of the base of the second metatarsal: A diagnostic problem. *Am J Sports Med* 21:591–598, 1993.
568. Hamilton WG: Foot and ankle injuries in dancers. In: Mann RA, Coughlin MJ, eds. *Surgery of the Foot and Ankle*, 6th ed. St. Louis, MO: Mosby-Year Book, 1993:1241–1276.
569. Micheli LJ, Sohn RS, Solomon R: Stress fractures of the second metatarsal involving Lisfranc's joint in ballet dancers. *J Bone Joint Surg* 67A:1372–1375, 1985.
570. O'Malley MJ, Hamilton WG, Munyak J: Fractures of the distal shaft of the fifth metatarsal: "Dancer's fracture". *Am J Sports Med* 24:240–243, 1996.
571. O'Malley MJ, Hamilton WG, Munyak J, et al: Stress fractures at the base of the second metatarsal in ballet dancers. *Foot Ankle* 17:89–94, 1996.
572. Torg JS, Pavlov H, Cooley LH, et al: Stress fractures of the tarsal navicular: A retrospective review of twenty-one cases. *J Bone Joint Surg* 64A:700–712, 1982.
573. Biedert R: Which investigations are required in stress fracture of the great toe sesamoids? *Arch Orthop Trauma Surg* 112:94–95, 1993.
574. Bourne RB, Rorabeck CH, MacNab J: Intra-articular fractures of the distal tibia: The pilon fracture. *J Trauma* 23:591–595, 1983.
575. Tomaro JE: Injuries of the leg, foot, and ankle. In: Wadsworth C, ed. *Contemporary Topics on the Foot and Ankle—Home Study Course*. La Crosse, WI: Orthopaedic Section, APTA, Inc., 2000.
576. Clarke HJ, Michelson JD, Cox QGK, et al: Tibio-talar stability in bimalleolar ankle fractures: A dynamic in vitro contact area study. *Foot Ankle Int* 11:222–227, 1991.
577. Michelson JD, Clarke HJ, Jinnah RH: The effect of loading on tibiotalar alignment in cadaver ankles. *Foot Ankle Int* 10:280–284, 1990.
578. Ho R, Abu-Laban RB: Ankle and foot. In: Rosen P, Barker FJ, II, Braen G, et al, eds. *Emergency Medicine: Concepts and Clinical Practice*, 3rd ed. St Louis, MO: Mosby, 1998:821.
579. Starosta D, Sacceti A, Sharkey P, et al: Calcaneal fracture with compartment syndrome of the foot. *Ann Em Med* 17:144, 1988.
580. Leabhart JW: Stress fractures of the calcaneus. *J Bone Joint Surg* 41 (A):1285–1290, 1959.
581. Kitaoka HB, Schaap EJ, Chao EYS, et al: Displaced intra-articular fractures of the calcaneus treated non-operatively. *J Bone Joint Surg* 76A:1531–1540, 1994.
582. Thoradson DB, Kreiger LE: Operative vs. non-operative treatment of intra-articular fractures of the calcaneus: A prospective randomized trial. *Foot Ankle Int* 17:2–9, 1996.
583. Lawrence SJ, Botte MJ: Jones' fractures and related fractures of the proximal fifth metatarsal. *Foot Ankle* 14:358–365, 1993.
584. Torg JS, Balduini FC, Zelko RR, et al: Fractures of the fifth metatarsal distal to the tuberosity. *J Bone Joint Surg* 66A:209–214, 1984.
585. Landel R: Treatment of cuboid syndrome: Manual reduction via grade 5 mobilization. *Orthopaedic Practice* 17:37–38, 2005.
586. Mulligan BR: Manual Therapy: "NAGS", "SNAGS", "PRP'S" etc. Wellington: Plane View Series, 1992.

SECTION V THE SPINE AND TMJ

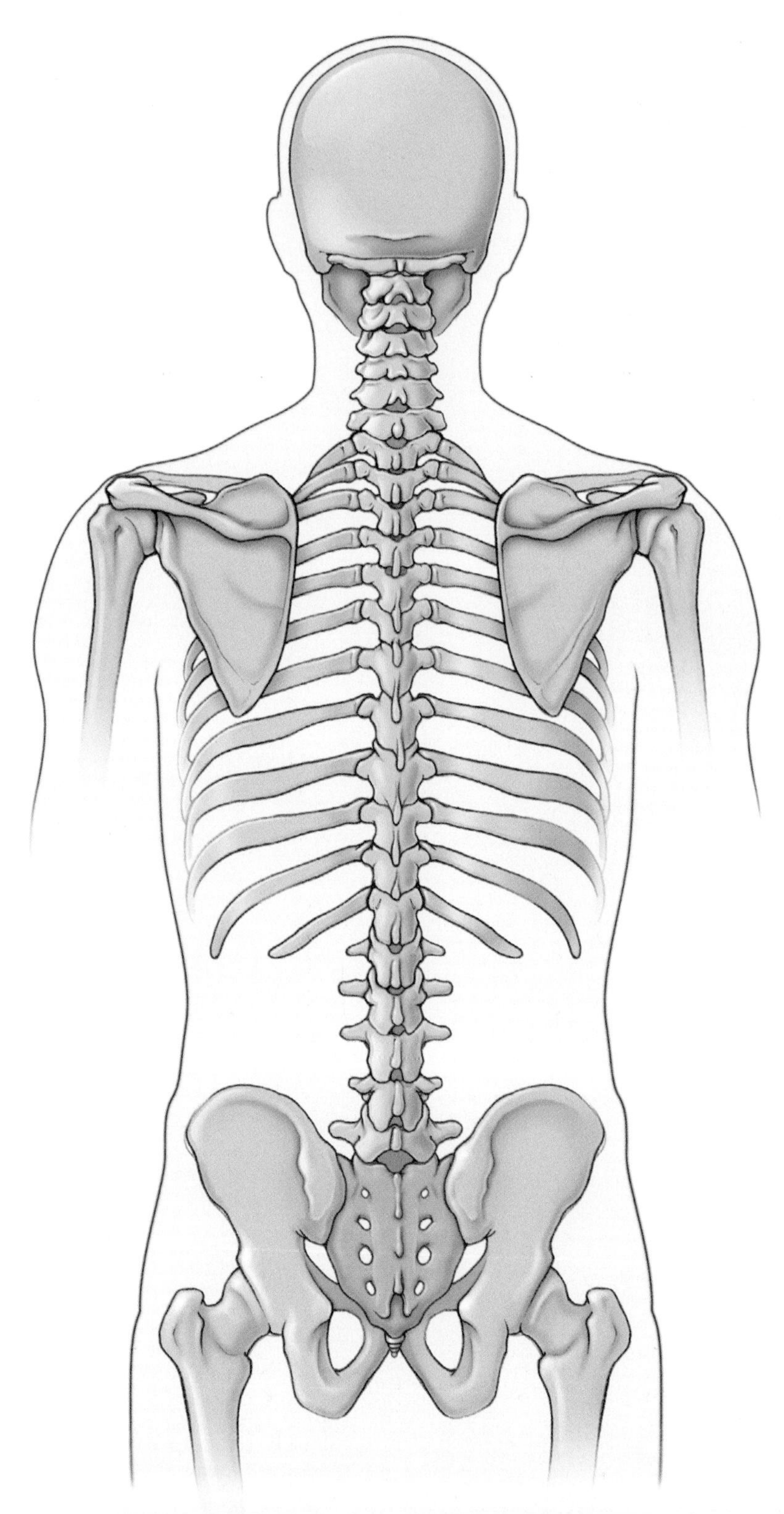

CHAPTER 22 Vertebral Column

STRUCTURE

The design specification for the human vertebral column is the provision of structural stability affording full mobility as well as protection of the spinal cord and axial neural tissues.[1] While achieving these seemingly disparate objectives, the spine also contributes to the functional requirements of gait and to the maintenance of static weight-bearing postures (see Chap. 6).[1]

At the component level, the basic building block of the spine is the vertebra. The vertebra serves as the weight-bearing unit of the vertebral column, and it is well designed for this purpose. Although a solid structure would provide the vertebral body with sufficient strength, especially for static loads, it would prove too heavy and would not have the necessary flexibility for dynamic load bearing.[2] Instead, the vertebral body is constructed with a strong outer layer of cortical bone and a hollow cavity, the latter of which is reinforced by vertical and horizontal struts called *trabeculae.*

The term *vertebral column* describes the entire set of vertebrae excluding the ribs, sternum, and pelvis (Fig. 22-1). The normal vertebral column is made up of 29 vertebrae (7 cervical, 12 thoracic, 5 lumbar, and 5 sacral) and four coccygeal segments. The adage that "function follows form" is very much applicable when studying the vertebral column. Although all vertebrae have similar characteristics, each has specific details that reflect its unique function (Table 22-1). The overall contour of the normal vertebral column in the coronal plane is straight. In contrast, the contour of the sagittal plane changes with development. At birth, a series of primary curves give a kyphotic posture to the whole spine. With development of the erect posture, secondary curves develop in the cervical and lumbar spines, producing a lordosis in these regions. The curves in the spinal column provide it with increased flexibility and shock-absorbing capabilities.[2]

A motion segment in the vertebral column is defined as two adjacent vertebrae and consists of three joints. One joint is formed between the two vertebral bodies and the intervertebral disk (IVD). The other two joints are formed by the articulation of the superior articular processes of the inferior vertebra and the inferior articular processes of the superior vertebra(Fig. 22-2). These latter joints are known as the facets or zygapophyseal joints.

The vertebral column contains 24 pairs of zygapophyseal joints, which are located posteriorly, and project from the neural arch of the vertebrae. The regional characteristics of the zygapophyseal joints are described in the relevant chapters. Mechanically, zygapophyseal joints are classified as plane joints as the articular surfaces are essentially flat.[3] The articular surfaces are covered in hyaline cartilage and like most synovial joints, have small fatty or fibrous synovial meniscoid-like fringes that project between the joint surfaces from the margins.[4] These intra-articular synovial folds act as space fillers during joint displacement and actively assist in the dispersal of synovial fluid within the joint cavity.[1] The articular processes act as a mechanical barricade, particularly against excessive torsion and shear, permitting certain movements while blocking others[3]:

- Horizontal articular surfaces favor axial rotation.
- Vertical articular surfaces (in either sagittal or frontal planes) act to block axial rotation.

Most zygapophyseal joint surfaces are oriented somewhere between the horizontal and vertical planes. In the cervical spine, the zygapophyseal joints are relatively horizontal while progressively increasing toward 45 degrees to the horizontal from the upper to the lower segments.[5–8] In the thoracic region, the joints assume an almost vertical direction while remaining essentially in a coronal orientation, which facilitates axial rotation and resists anterior displacement.[9] In the lumbar spine, the zygapophyseal joints are vertical with a curved, J-shaped surface predominantly in the sagittal plane, which restricts rotation and also resists anterior shear.[1] Understanding the variable structure and function of the human zygapophyseal joints and their relationship with the other components of the vertebral column is an important requirement in the examination and intervention of individuals with mechanical spinal pain disorders.[1]

The IVDs of the vertebral column lie between the adjacent superior and inferior surfaces of the vertebral bodies from C2 to S1 and are similar in shape to the bodies (Fig. 22-3). The IVD forms a symphysis or amphiarthrosis between two adjacent vertebrae and represents the largest avascular structure in the body.[10] Each disk is composed of an inner *nucleus pulposus* (NP), an outer *annulus fibrosus* (AF), and limiting cartilage end plates. The annulus and end plates anchor the IVD to the vertebral body. The IVDs contribute 20–25% of

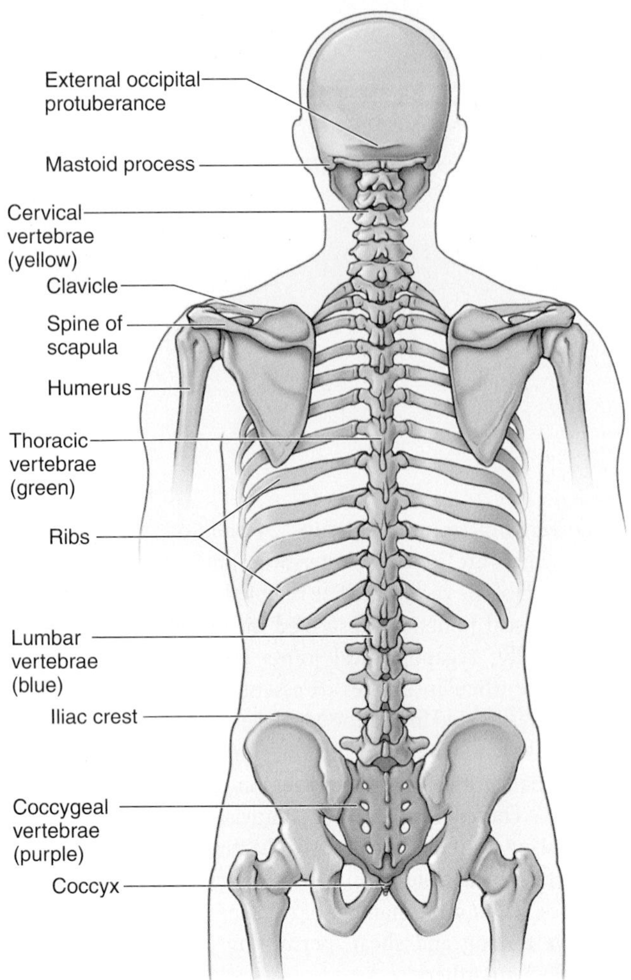

FIGURE 22-1 The vertebral column. (Reproduced, with permission, from Morton DA, Foreman KB, Albertine KH: *The Big Picture: Gross Anatomy,* McGraw-Hill, 2011.)

the length of the vertebral column. In cervical and lumbar regions, the IVDs are thicker anteriorly and this contributes to the normal lordosis. In the thoracic region, each of the IVDs is of uniform thickness. Phylogenically, the IVD is a relatively new structure. In the human spinal column, the combined

TABLE 22-1 Coupling in the Lumbar Spine

Author	Neutral	Flexion	Extension
Farfan[1]	—	Contralateral	Contralateral
Kaltenborn[2]	—	Ipsilateral	Ipsilateral
Grieve[3]	—	Ipsilateral	Contralateral
Fryette[4]	Contralateral	Ipsilateral	Ipsilateral
Evjenth[5]	—	Ipsilateral	Contralateral

Data from Farfan HF: *Mechanical Disorders of the Low Back.* Philadelphia, PA: Lea & Febiger, 1973; Kaltenborn FM: *The Spine: Basic Evaluation and Mobilization Techniques.* Wellington, New Zealand: University Press, 1993; Grieve GP: *Common Vertebral Joint Problems.* New York, NY: Churchill Livingstone, 1981; Fryette HH: *Principles of Osteopathic Technique.* Colorado Springs, CO: American Academy of Osteopathy, 1980; Evjenth O, Hamberg J: *Muscle Stretching in Manual Therapy, a Clinical Manual.* Alfta, Sweden: Alfta Rehab Forlag, 1984.

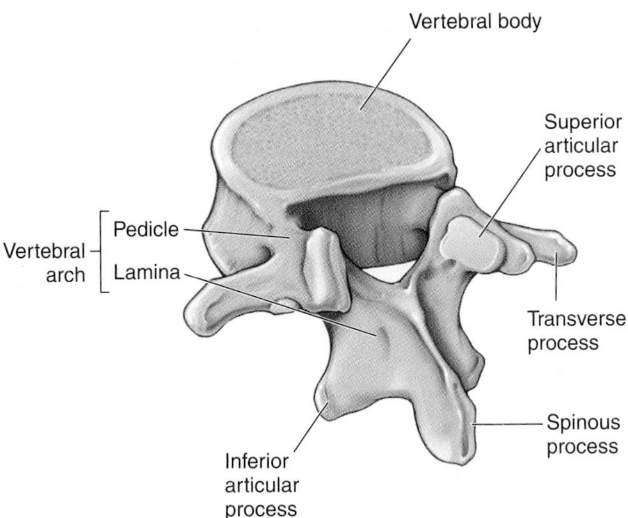

FIGURE 22-2 The vertebral body. (Reproduced, with permission, from Morton DA, Foreman KB, Albertine KH: *The Big Picture: Gross Anatomy,* McGraw-Hill, 2011.)

heights of the IVDs account for approximately 20–33% of the total length of the spinal column.[11] The presence of an IVD not only permits motion of the segment in any direction up to the point that the disk itself is stretched, but also allows for a significant increase in the weight-bearing capabilities of the spine.[12] A normally functioning disk is extremely important to permit the normal biomechanics of the spine to occur and to reduce the possibility of mechanical interference among any of the neural structures. Although the disk is incapable of independent motion, movement of the disk does occur during the clinically defined motions of flexion–extension, side bending, and axial rotation.[13] The major stresses that must be withstood

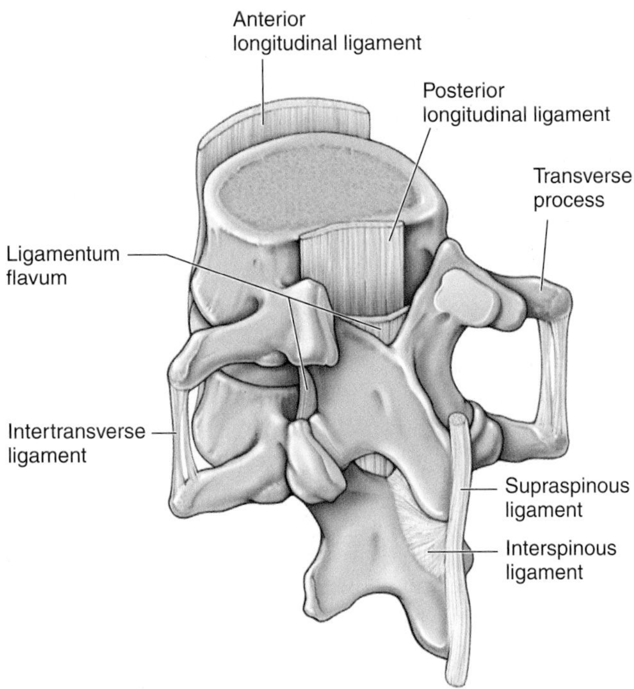

FIGURE 22-3 The intervertebral disk and intervertebral motion. (Reproduced, with permission, from Morton DA, Foreman KB, Albertine KH: *The Big Picture: Gross Anatomy,* McGraw-Hill, 2011.)

by the IVD are axial compression, shearing, bending, and twisting, either singly or in combination with each other.

The role of the IVD is unique because it operates as an osmotic system, holding neighboring vertebral bodies together, while simultaneously pushing them apart. As such, the IVD is a dynamic structure that responds to stresses applied from vertebral movement or from static loading.

There are regional differences within the spine, each with its own specific demands and function. As discussed, all vertebral disks have traditionally been described as being composed of three parts: the AF, the vertebral end plate, and a central gelatinous mass, called the NP (Fig. 22-1). However, this description is based on the anatomy of a lumbar disk, the region where most research has occurred and for which many authors have extrapolated the anatomy to all IVDs.[14] An appreciation of the differing anatomy of the IVDs throughout the spine is important when developing clinical examination and intervention models.[14]

SPINAL JUNCTIONS

The spine contains four junctions, each of which is different in posterior element orientation and spinal curvature. Transitional vertebrae can occur at any of the junctions. The transition can be "complete" but is more commonly partial. These junctions, described by Schmorl and Junghanns[15] as *ontogenically restless*, are often rich in anomalies[16]:

- The craniovertebral junction is located between the cervical spine and the atlas, axis, and head. This region is covered in Chapter 23.
- The cervicothoracic junction represents the region where the mobile cervical spine and the relatively stiffer superior segments of thoracic spine meet, and where the powerful muscles of the upper extremities and shoulder girdle insert. The cervicothoracic junction is described in Chapters 25 and 27.
- The thoracolumbar junction is located between the thoracic spine, with its large capacity for rotation, and the lumbar spine, with its limited rotation. This region is described in Chapter 27.
- The lumbosacral junction is located between the lumbar spine, with its ability to flex and extend, and the relative stiffness of the sacroiliac joints. This region is described in Chapters 28 and 29.

Although highly variable, the line of gravity acting on a standing person with ideal posture passes through the mastoid process of the temporal bone anterior to the second sacral vertebra, posterior to the hip, and anterior to the knee and ankle (see Chap. 6).[3] In the vertebral column, the line of gravity is on the concave side of the apex of each region's curvature. As a consequence, ideal posture allows gravity to produce a torque that helps maintain the optimal shape of each spinal curvature.[3]

SPINAL STABILITY

Spinal stability is characterized by the behavior of the spinal column and the coordination of muscles that surround the spine. There are two types of stability:

- Static. This type of stability refers to a state of equilibrium where the velocity of the object or body is zero. When a person is standing perfectly still with no swing back and forth, the person said to be in static equilibrium.
- Dynamic. This type of stability implies a change over time but the velocity is constant. Theoretically, if a perturbation is applied to the spine and the spine behaves as it did in its undisturbed state, it is said to be stable, whereas if the spine's kinematic behavior changes as a result of the disturbance, it is unstable.[17] States requiring dynamic stability are far more common than those requiring static stability.

From the mechanical point of view, the spinal system is inherently unstable. Panjabi[18,19] indicates that there are three subsystems that contribute to spinal stability:

- Passive system. The spinal column, which includes the vertebrae, IVDs, zygapophyseal joints, joint capsules, and ligaments (Fig. 22-4) are the load-bearing units and the source of passive stiffness for stabilizing the spine. Passive stiffness of the ligaments and joint capsules is mainly a factor at the extremes of range of motion (ROM). The effectiveness

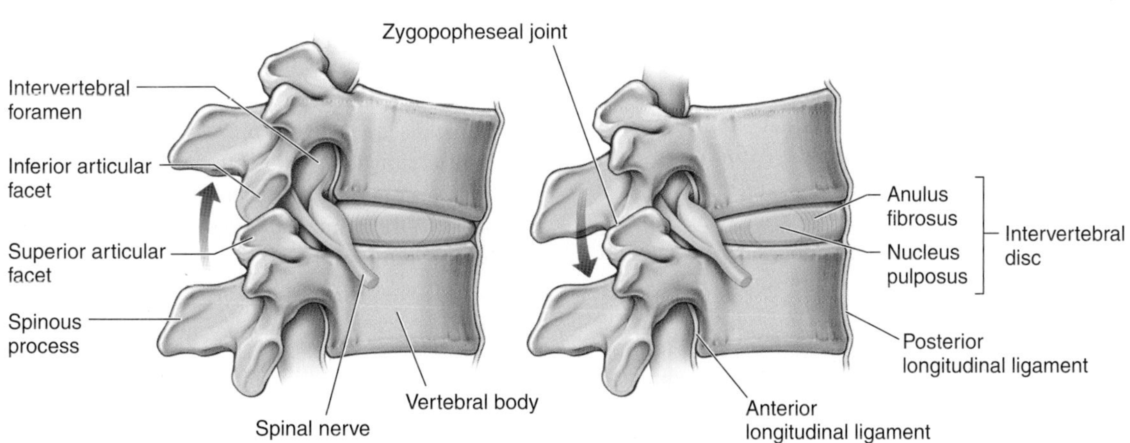

FIGURE 22-4 Ligaments of the spine. (Reproduced, with permission, from Morton DA, Foreman KB, Albertine KH: *The Big Picture: Gross Anatomy*, McGraw-Hill, 2011.)

of the passive support system is a factor of the ability of its structures to resist the forces of translation, compression, and torsion.

- Active system. Muscles, which serve to reduce or prevent movement and are the source of active stiffness (i.e., muscles act like stiff springs) by using stored elastic energy and the level of activation or force.[18,20] Because the passive stiffness is mainly engaged at the extremes of range, the primary source of stiffness for stability during movements in healthy individuals is from the active stiffness of the trunk muscles and not the passive stiffness from ligaments. A large number of muscles have a mechanical effect on the spine and pelvis and all muscles are required to maintain optimal control.[20] Muscle activity must be coordinated to maintain control of the spine within a hierarchy of interdependent levels: control of intervertebral translation and rotation, control of spinal posture/orientation, and control of body with respect to the environment, in addition to maintaining a number of homeostatic functions such as respiration and continence.[20–22] The concept of different trunk muscles playing differing roles in the provision of dynamic stability to the spine was proposed by Bergmark[23] and later refined by others.[24–29] The specific muscles that provide stability and their interactions are described in the relevant chapters.
- Central nervous system (CNS), which utilizes feedforward (anticipatory) control to generate active muscle stiffness and uses feedback (reflex) control to augment the stiffness.[30] The CNS must continually interpret the status of stability, plan mechanisms to overcome predictable challenges, and rapidly initiate activity in response to unexpected challenges.[20]

CLINICAL PEARL

Although trunk muscles must have sufficient strength and endurance to satisfy the demands of spinal control, the efficacy of the muscle system is dependent on its controller, the CNS.[18,20]

The *neutral zone* is a term used by Panjabi[18] to define a region of laxity around the neutral resting position of a spinal segment. The neutral zone is the position of the segment in which minimal loading is occurring in the passive structures (IVD, zygapophyseal joints, and ligaments) and the active structures (the muscles and tendons that control spinal motion), and within which spinal motion is produced with minimal internal resistance.[2] Panjabi and colleagues[31] have studied the effect of intersegmental muscle forces on the neutral zone and ROM of a lumbar functional spinal unit subjected to pure moments in flexion–extension, side bending, and rotation. Simulated muscle forces were applied to the spinous process of the mobile vertebra of a single motion segment using two equal and symmetric force vectors directed laterally, anteriorly, and inferiorly. The simulated muscle force maintained or decreased the motions of the lumbar segment for intact and injured specimens with the exception of the flexion ROM which increased.[31]

CLINICAL PEARL

Mechanoreceptors throughout the spine play an important role in spinal stability and provide excitatory or positive feedback control during rapid elongation of the ligaments.[32] For example, when large unexpected perturbations cause the spine to rapidly flex, the subsequent quick stretch to the posterior ligaments of the spine leads to a rapid activation of the trunk extensor muscles.[33] In addition, the mechanoreceptors can become desensitized when exposed to tissue creep, leading to impaired muscle responses.[34]

The interaction between the passive and active systems of the spine changes when there has been prolonged tension or cyclic loading of the passive system resulting in a change to the muscle responses in the form of a delayed response. Furthermore, it is hypothesized that these changes in muscle activation may lead to increased spinal compression forces, which have been recognized as a risk factor for vertebral end-plate fracture, especially if applied repetitively.[35,36] An alternate consequence is that muscle insufficiency resulting from fatigue may shift the loading to the passive tissues,[37,38] which may put the spine at increased risk of injury.

CLINICAL PEARL

Activities such as acute repetitive loading have been shown to have a significant effect on reducing the stiffness of the passive tissues of the spine, because of the viscoelastic nature of the muscles, tendons, ligaments, and IVDs.[39,40]

Under normal circumstances, when large perturbations are expected, preparatory coactivation of the spinal muscles enhances active stiffness, and reflexes augment the stiffness at the appropriate time.[41] These anticipatory postural adjustments and corrective responses are part of a motor control strategy executed by the CNS that was learned from previous experience when performing similar movements or activities.[42–45]

The emphasis on spinal stability exercises should be to:

- Strengthen the trunk muscles so that they are able to produce sufficiently large forces and active stiffness. The timing and sequencing of muscle activity, coupled with the appropriate magnitude of muscle activation, produces smooth, accurate, and efficient movement behavior that is adjusted to the immediate demands and consequences within the environment.[30]
- Increase the endurance of the trunk muscles so that the force output of the muscles does not deteriorate.
- Incorporate sound motor learning principles to address impaired motor control strategies.

The various strategies to incorporate with the intervention for spinal instability are addressed in the appropriate chapters.

SPINAL MOTION

The movements of the vertebral column occur in diagonal patterns as a combination of flexion or extension with a coupled motion of side bending and rotation. Movements of the spine, like those elsewhere, are produced by the coordinated action of nerves and muscles. Agonistic and synergistic muscles initiate and perform the movements, whereas the antagonistic muscles control and modify the movements. The amount of motion available at each region of the spine is a factor of a number of variables. These include

- disk-vertebral height ratio
- compliance of the fibrocartilage
- dimensions and shape of the adjacent vertebral end plates
- age
- disease
- gender

The type of motion available is governed by

- the shape and orientation of the articulations
- the ligaments and muscles of the segment, and the size and location of its articulating processes

Including translations and rotations around three different axes, the spine is considered to possess 6 degrees of freedom.[46] Although the ROM at each vertebral segment varies, the relative amounts of motion that occur at each region is well documented[11,47]:

- In the upper craniovertebral region (occiput to C2), there is comparatively little flexion–extension, whereas the mid to lower cervical spine permits increasing flexion–extension movements from approximately 10 degrees at the C2–3 level to about 20 degrees at C5–6 and C6–7. Axial rotation in the upper cervical spine is 30–40 degrees in each direction, whereas it is 5–6 degrees in the lower cervical spine.
- Flexion–extension movements (see Fig. 22-3) are about 4 degrees in the upper thoracic spine, 6 degrees in the midthoracic spine, and 12 degrees in the lower thoracic spine. Side bending in the upper thoracic spine is approximately 6 degrees. Axial rotation in the upper thoracic spine is 5–6 degrees.
- In the lumbar spine, there is a gradual increase of flexion–extension movements from about 12 degrees at L1–L2 to 20 degrees at the L5–S1 level. Side bending in the lumbar spine is greatest at L3–L4 where it is approximately 8–9 degrees. Axial rotation in the lumbar spine is minimal.
- Although various motion patterns have been proposed for the sacroiliac joint,[48–51] the precise model for sacroiliac motion has remained fairly elusive (see Chap. 29).[52–54] Postmortem analysis has shown that until an advanced age, small movements are measurable under different load conditions.[55,56]

In general, the human zygapophyseal joints of the spine are capable of only two major motions: gliding upward and gliding downward. If these movements occur in the same direction, flexion or extension occurs. If the movements occur in opposite directions, side bending occurs. Although rotation does occur as a motion component within intervertebral segments, it is always coupled and never an isolated motion.[57] Indeed during functional rotation of the spine, the actual motion occurring at any given zygapophyseal joint is a linear glide. Because the orientation of the articular facets of the zygapophyseal joints do not correspond exactly to pure planes of motion, pure motions of the spine occur very infrequently.[46] In fact, most motions of the spine occur three-dimensionally because of the phenomenon of coupling. Coupling involves two or more individual motions occurring simultaneously at the segment and has been found to occur throughout the lumbar,[58] thoracic,[59] and cervical regions.[60] Descriptions about the types of coupling that occurs in these regions are provided in the respective chapters. All normal motion in the cervical, thoracic, and lumbar regions involves both sides of the segment moving simultaneously around the same axis. That is to say, a motion of the right side of a segment produces an equal motion on the left side of that same segment. If both sides of a vertebral segment are equally impaired (equally hypomobile or hypermobile), there is no change in the axis of motion except in the case where it ceases to exist, as in a bony ankylosis. Where a symmetric motion impairment exists, there is no noticeable deviation from the path of flexion or extension (impaired side bending and rotation), but rather, the path is shortened with a hypomobility (producing decreased motion) or lengthened with a hypermobility (producing increased motion).

An alteration to the structures of the motion segment can result in a loss of motion, a loss of segment integrity (instability), or a loss of function. These changes result mainly from injury, developmental changes, fusion, fracture healing, healed infection, or surgical arthrodesis.[47] The loss of motion segment integrity, which can be measured with flexion–extension roentgenograms, is defined as an anteroposterior motion of one vertebra over another that is greater than 3.5 mm in the cervical spine, greater than 2.5 mm in the thoracic spine, and greater than 4.5 mm in the lumbar spine.[61] Loss of motion segment integrity also may be defined as a difference in the angular motion of two adjacent motion segments greater than

- 11 degrees in the cervical spine
- 15 degrees at L1–L2, L2–L3, and L3–L4
- 20 degrees at L4–L5
- 25 degrees between L5 and S1

Fryette's Laws of Physiologic Spinal Motion[62]

Although listed as laws, Fryette's descriptions of spinal motion are better viewed as concepts because they have undergone review and modifications over time. These concepts serve as useful guidelines in the evaluation and intervention of spinal dysfunction and are cited throughout many texts describing spinal biomechanics.

Fryette's First Law

"When any part of the lumbar or thoracic spine is in neutral position, side bending of a vertebra will be opposite to the side of the rotation of that vertebra."

The term *neutral*, according to Fryette, is interpreted as any position in which the zygapophyseal joints are not engaged in any surface contact, and the position where the ligaments and capsules of the segment are not under tension. This law describes the coupling for the thoracic and lumbar spines. The cervical spine is not included in this law because the zygapophyseal joints of this region are always engaged. When a lumbar or thoracic vertebra is side bent from its neutral position, the vertebral body will turn toward the convexity that is being formed, with the maximum rotation occurring near the apex of the curve formed.

Dysfunctions that occur in the neutral range are termed by osteopaths as *type I dysfunctions*.

Fryette's Second Law

"When any part of the spine is in a position of hyperextension or hyperflexion, the side bending of the vertebra will be to the same side as the rotation of that vertebra."

Put simply, when the segment is under load, the coupling of side bending and rotation occurs to the same side. The term *non-neutral*, according to Fryette, is interpreted as any position in which the zygapophyseal joints are engaged in surface contact, the position where the ligaments and capsules of the segment are under tension, or in positions of flexion or extension. This law describes the coupling that occurs in the C2–T3 areas of the spine.

Dysfunctions occurring in the flexion or extension ranges are termed by osteopaths as *type II dysfunctions*.

Fryette's Third Law

Fryette's third law tells us that if motion in one plane is introduced to the spine, any motion occurring in another direction is thereby restricted.

CLINICAL PEARL

Whereas it is commonly believed that coupled motions in the lower cervical spine occur toward the same side (a side bend to the right is accompanied with rotation to the right), it is important to remember that results from numerous studies are inconsistent regarding the specific spinal motions that are coupled with one another in the upper cervical, lumbar, and thoracic spines.[63]

Combined Motions

It would appear that, irrespective of the coupling that occurs, there is a great deal of similarity between a motion involving flexion followed by left side bending, and a motion involving left side bending followed by flexion. However, although both motions have the same end result, they use different methods to arrive there. The same could be said of the following combined motions:

- Flexion and right side bending followed by right side bending and flexion.
- Extension and right side bending followed by right side bending and extension.
- Extension and left side bending followed by left side bending and extension.

By using combined motions, the clinician can often reproduce a patient's symptom that was not reproduced using the planar motions of flexion, extension, side bending, and rotation.[64–66] However, care should be taken when utilizing combined motions, especially with the acute and subacute patient, when a reduction of symptoms through modalities and gentle exercise might be preferable to exacerbating the patient's condition through a comprehensive movement examination.

Using a biomechanical model, a restriction of extension, side bending, and rotation to the same side of the pain is termed a *closing* restriction, whereas a restriction of the opposite motions (flexion, side bending, and rotation to the opposite side of the pain) is termed an *opening* restriction. Motions that involve flexion and side bending away from the symptoms tend to invoke a stretch to the structures on the side of the symptoms, whereas motions that involve extension and side bending toward the side of the symptoms produce a compression of the structures on the side of the symptoms.[64–66] An example of a stretching pattern would be pain on the right side of the spine that is increased with either flexion followed by a left side-bending movement or a left side-bending motion followed by a flexion movement. A compression pattern would involve pain on the right side of the spine that is increased with a movement involving either extension followed by right side bending or right side bending followed by extension.

The symptom reproduction that occurs with combined motions usually follows a logical and predictable pattern. However, there are situations in which illogical patterns are found. Because the vertebral column consists of many articulating segments, movements are complex and usually involve several segments resulting in restrictions that may be complex and apparently illogical. An example of such a pattern would be pain on the right side of the spine that is increased with a flexion and right side bending combination but decreased with an extension and right side bending combination. The movements just described involve a combination of stretching and compression movements. These illogical patterns typically indicate that more than one structure is involved.[64–66] Of course, they could also indicate to the clinician that the patient does not have a musculoskeletal impairment.

EXAMINATION OF THE VERTEBRAL COLUMN AND PELVIS

The examination of the spine is complicated by the number of conditions that can cause pain in this region of the body. In addition, there is little scientific evidence for the establishment of many of the diagnostic labels attributed to spinal pain, such as instability, degenerative disc disease, and subluxation.[67]

The purpose of the examination is to correctly identify those patients who will benefit from a physical therapy intervention. The correct identification of a diagnosis requires the use of evidence-based measuring tools that are valid, specific, and sensitive. There are numerous methods for examining and evaluating the spine, and each results in a conclusion that determines the course of the intervention.[68,69] Unfortunately, many of the procedures that are used today to examine the spine demonstrate methodologic shortcomings.[67–69] The interventions for spinal conditions fair no better. Despite the ever-increasing numbers of randomized controlled trials evaluating interventions for low back pain (LBP),[70] treatment outcomes remain less than optimal.[71] One reason for this may be the fact that many trials test interventions in a heterogeneous population of patients with LBP and such a diverse group of patients may not correspond to the one treatment approach.[72] This hypothesis has led to the design of classification systems to identify subgroups of patients who may respond preferentially to certain treatments.[73]

Use of Traditional Classification Systems

In recent years, attempts have been made to use a variety of methods to classify spinal pain, particularly LBP, into syndromes. The term *syndrome* implies that the specific diagnosis is unknown. A syndrome is a collection of signs and symptoms that, collectively, characterizes a particular condition. In the spine, where determining a specific diagnosis has historically been proven to be extremely difficult, syndromes have become popular By classifying syndromes, it is proposed that a patient is more likely to respond to a type of intervention unique to that syndrome. The criteria that have thus been used to categorize a syndrome include the following:

- Pathoanatomy.[74,75] This strategy involves using correlations to produce categories. The disadvantage of using pathoanatomy is the difficulty in identifying a relevant pathoanatomic cause for most patients.[76]
- Presence or absence of radiculopathy.[77,78]
- Location and type of pain.[79]
- Duration of the symptoms (acute, subacute, or chronic).[80]
- Activity and work status.[78,81]
- Impairments identified during the physical examination.
- Direction of motion that reproduces, peripheralizes, or centralizes the symptoms.[82,83]

The more common classifications are outlined next. The use of such classification systems may have some prognostic value and can direct clinicians to specific interventions.[84]

Osteopathic System

Osteopaths rely on the results from the active motion tests and position tests to determine their intervention approach. *Note:* Osteopaths use the term side flexion instead of side bending.

Position Testing

Position testing involves palpation of the soft tissues over paired transverse processes of the spine, to detect palpable positional irregularity and altered tissue tension at a segmental level when the spine is positioned in flexion or extension compared with neutral. To locate the transverse process in the lumbar spine, the clinician first locates the spinous process to determine the level and then moves slightly laterally and superiorly by placing the thumbs on either side of the spinous process. Thus, the clinician must be very familiar with so-called *layer palpation* to be sure that the palpating fingers are monitoring the positions of the transverse processes at a particular segmental level. Vertebral dysfunctions occur as a combination of movements in the three planes. The key movement is rotation. Theoretically, the rotational dysfunction, which is a result of the altered axis of rotation produced by the stiffer of the two sides of the segment, will be palpated as a much firmer end-feel to the palpation on that side. The direction of the rotation is named after the more posterior of the two transverse processes, and the positional name is an osteokinematic one having no established relationship with any joint.

Position Testing in Extension. If a marked segmental rotation is evident at the limit of extension, this would indicate that one of the facets is unable to complete its inferior motion (i.e., it is being held in a relatively flexed or superior position). The direction of the resulting rotation (denoted in terms of the anterior part of the vertebral body) informs the clinician as to which of the facets is not moving. For example, if the segment is rotated to the *left* when palpated in extension, the *right* zygapophyseal joint is not moving normally. This impairment can be described in one of the three ways as follows:

1. The right zygapophyseal joint cannot extend or "close."
2. The right zygapophyseal joint is flexed (F), rotated (R), and side-flexed (S) left (L) around the axis of the right zygapophyseal joint.
3. The right zygapophyseal joint is unable to perform any motions that require an inferior glide, such as extension, right side bending, and right rotation.

FRS or extension impairments are more evident in the positional tests than ERS impairments (described next) because there is less overall motion available into extension.

Position Testing in Flexion. If a marked segmental rotation is evident in full flexion, this indicates that one of the facets cannot complete its superior motion. For example, if the segment is found to be left-rotated when palpated in flexion, the left zygapophyseal joint is not moving normally.

This impairment can be described in one of the three ways as follows:

1. The left zygapophyseal joint cannot flex or "open."
2. The left zygapophyseal joint is extended (E), rotated (R), and side-flexed (S) left (L).
3. The left zygapophyseal joint is unable to perform any motion that requires a superior glide such as flexion, right rotation, and right side bending.

Position Testing in Neutral. Positional testing is performed in the neutral spine position for three reasons as follows:

1. If a rotational impairment of a segment exists only in neutral and is not evident in either full flexion or full extension, the cause of the impairment is probably not mechanical in origin but rather neuromuscular. These neuromuscular impairments are usually found at the spinal junctions, particularly the thoracolumbar and cervicothoracic junctions.

2. If a marked rotation is evident at a segment and this rotation is consistent throughout flexion, extension, and neutral, then the cause is probably an anatomic anomaly (e.g., scoliosis) rather than an articular problem.
3. If the cause of the rotational impairment is articular (zygapophyseal joint), the positional testing in neutral gives the clinician an idea as to the starting position of the corrective technique.

The terminology used to describe the rotational disruption of the pure spinal motions (ERS or FRS) describes the positional and kinetic impairments only. It does not indicate what the pathology might be. Reasons for these impairments, other than movement dysfunctions, may include bony anomalies such as a deformed transverse process, compensatory adaptation, structural scoliosis, or a hemivertebra.

The analysis of the change in the rotational impairment between full flexion and full extension theoretically gives clues as to the pathology. Thus, in conjunction with other tests, such as active motion testing, this analysis can assist in ascertaining a biomechanical diagnosis.

Position testing has been found to be very reliable when used by experienced clinicians to identify segmental levels based on the relative position of spinous processes.[85] The results for inter-rater reliability have been mixed when clinicians are asked to determine lumbar segmental abnormality using position testing,[86,87] and poor when attempting to determine the segmental level of a marked spinous process.[88]

CLINICAL PEARL

The clinician should be aware that position testing is insensitive to symmetric impairments and thus can give false negatives.

McKenzie System[82,83]

The McKenzie mechanical diagnostic and classification approach is a noninvasive and an inexpensive method of assessing patients with cervical and LBP that uses physical signs, symptom behavior, and their relation to end range test movements to determine appropriate classification and intervention.

The McKenzie approach focuses on the following three components.

- Providing a mechanical diagnosis.
- Providing a mechanical treatment, based on the mechanical diagnosis.
- Prevention of recurrence which is achieved by
  - emphasizing the patient's responsibility for their own recovery
  - fully exploring the patient's self generated forces before progression to externally applied forces.

According to McKenzie, symptoms of lumbar and/or cervical pathology can demonstrate a phenomenon of centralization and peripheralization.[82,89,90]

- Centralization of symptoms is the immediate or eventual abolition of the most distal extent of referred or radicular pain toward the midline of the spine in response to therapeutic loading strategies. Centralization occurs more commonly with extension, especially with end range repeated movements. Although centralization of the symptoms can be associated with an increase in spinal pain, it normally indicates improvement in the patient's condition and provides the clinician with a directional preference.
- Peripheralization of symptoms indicates movement in the opposite direction and is usually associated with a poorer prognosis.

The history taking is an integral component of the McKenzie approach. The purpose of the history is to provide the clinician with information regarding

- an overall impression of the clinical presentation
- the site of pain
- the stage of the disorder
- the status of the presenting condition. The severity of problem is used to guide the vigor of the examination
- the identification of red flags
- the baseline of symptomatic/mechanical presentation against which improvements can be judged
- any aggravating/relieving factors (especially the role of posture). This helps the clinician to develop a hypothetical diagnosis by syndrome
- functional limits on the patient's quality of life

During the initial observation, the patient's sitting and standing postures are noted to reveal how the spine is habitually subjected to static loading by the patient. In addition, the patient is asked to perform a single movement of each movement plane direction (see below) while the clinician notes the quantity and quality of movement—the ability of the patient to achieve end range with spinal curve reversal and without deviating from the intended movement plane.[91] The accurate assessment of the effect of repeated movements/sustained positions on the patient's pain patterns is a key component of the McKenzie examination (Table 22-2). The movement plane directions evaluated for both the cervical and lumbar spines are those within which the clinically presenting antalgic postures occur.[91]

- ***Cervical spine.*** The movements observed include protrusion, flexion, retraction, extension, side bending right, side bending left, rotation right, and rotation left.
- ***Lumbar spine.*** The movements observed include flexion, extension, side gliding right, side gliding left.

After the quantity and quality of movement is assessed by the performance of single movements in each movement plane direction, dynamic and static tests are performed.[91] The effects of loading in a certain movement plane direction are highlighted best by repetition (dynamic) or sustained (static) loading. Static loading tests are generally used when dynamic tests do not provide a clear preferred loading strategy. With both the static and dynamic tests, loading in a sagittal movement plane direction is typically explored first, unless the patient has significant antalgia in a coronal movement plane direction, in which case, the coronal movement plane is

TABLE 22-2	Various Effects of Test Movements
Term	**Definition**
Produce	No symptoms at rest but are created with movement
Increased	Symptoms present are increased
Decreased	Symptoms present are decreased
Abolished	Movement eliminates those symptoms that occur with rest
Worse	Symptoms increase or remain worse
No worse	Symptoms increase with movement (don't remain worse)
No better	Symptoms reduced/abolished with movement (do not remain)
Better	Presenting symptoms decreased/abolished/ remain better
Pain during movements	Pain during movements
End range pain	Pain occurs at end ranges
No effect	Movement has no effect on symptoms

explored first.[91] Should loading in the coronal plane not provide satisfactory answers, the transverse movement plane is explored.

- ***Dynamic tests.*** These tests involve performing a single motion within the movement plane direction being studied, followed by repetitive motion in the same movement plane direction while the clinician closely monitors how mechanics and symptoms respond during motion, at end range, and after the dynamic loading. The testing progression applied includes the following[91]:
  - Cervical spine: flexion in sitting, retraction in sitting, retraction-then-extension in sitting, retraction in lying, and retraction extension in lying. If required, the following tests are also performed: protrusion in sitting, retracted side bending right in sitting, retracted side bending left in sitting, retracted rotation right in sitting, and retracted rotation left in sitting.
  - Lumbar spine: flexion in standing, extension in standing, flexion in lying, and extension in lying. If required, the following tests are also performed: side gliding right in standing or prone extension with right lateral shift and side gliding left in standing or prone extension with left lateral shift.
- ***Static tests.*** These tests are often used as ancillary tests to confirm dynamic testing or to further explore the effects of loading when dynamic testing yields no definitive conclusion.[91]
  - Cervical spine: protrusion, flexion, retraction (sitting or supine), retraction and extension (sitting, prone, or supine), retracted side bending right or left, and retracted rotation right or left.
  - Lumbar spine: sitting slouched, sitting erect, standing slouched, standing erect, lying prone in extension, long sitting, lateral shift right or left, and rotation in flexion.

The clinical reasoning intrinsic to the McKenzie method classifies mechanical and symptomatic responses to loading into three main syndromes: postural, dysfunction, and derangement (Table 22-3) and (Fig. 22-4).

The *posture syndrome* is proposed to result from sustained loading of the tissues during end range positions/postures. The pain associated with the postural syndrome is of a gradual onset, dull, local, midline, symmetric, and never referred. Prolonged postures worsen the pain, whereas movement abolishes it. On examination, the patient demonstrates no spinal deformity or loss of range and repeated movements do not produce the symptoms. The onset of symptoms, which is time-dependent (usually occurring after more than 15 minutes), is provoked with sustained end-of-range positions.

The *dysfunction syndrome* is proposed to result from an adaptive shortening of some soft tissues and an overstretching of others. The intermittent pain associated with this syndrome is local, adjacent to the midline of the spine, and not referred. The exception occurs in the case of an adherent nerve root (ANR) where the pain may be felt in the buttock, thigh, or calf (Table 22-4). The ANR represents the only time when distal pain is experienced in the dysfunction syndrome, and the only time when distal symptoms are repeatedly reproduced as part of its management. Activities and positions at the end of range worsen the pain of the dysfunction syndrome, whereas activities that avoid end ranges lessen the symptoms. On examination, the patient demonstrates a loss of motion or function that distinguishes this syndrome from the posture syndrome. Repeated movements do not alter the symptoms and the loss of motion, or function, may be symmetric or asymmetric.

The *derangement syndrome* is thought to result from a displacement or an alteration in the position of joint structures. The joint structure most commonly involved is the IVD, and McKenzie divides these disturbances into posterior disk and anterior disk derangements. The posterior derangements are further subdivided into seven derangement categories. Derangements 1 through 6 describe posterior derangements, whereas derangement 7 describes the anterior derangement (Table 22-5).

The pain of a derangement syndrome, which is usually of a sudden onset and associated with paresthesia or numbness, is dull or sharp and can be central, unilateral, symmetric, or asymmetric. Although the pain may be referred into the buttock, thigh, leg, or foot, it varies in both intensity and distribution. Bending, sitting, or sustaining positions worsen a posterior derangement, whereas walking and standing worsen an anterior derangement. Patients with a posterior derangement often feel better when walking and lying, whereas patients with an anterior derangement usually feel better in sitting and other flexed positions. On examination, a lateral shift may be noted. There is always a loss of motion and function. Certain motions produce, increase, or cause the symptoms to peripheralize (move away from the spine),

TABLE 22-3 Summary of the Three McKenzie Syndromes

	Mechanical or Symptomatic Responses	Frequency of Complaints (Responses)	Point of Response Elicitation	Rate of Response Elicitation	Response Persistence After Loading Cessation	Rate of Syndrome Resolution	Responses During Motion	Responses at Mechanically Unimpeded End Range	Responses at Mechanically Impeded End Range	Movement Plane Specific Responses	Preferred Loading Strategies	Reasons for Patient Failure
Postural	Symptomatic only	Intermittent	Sustained end range	Delayed onset after sustained end range positioning	None	Weeks	None	Symptomatic	None exist	Movement plane direction specific	Avoid symptoms	Ignorant, fatigue, self-conscious
Dysfunction	Symptomatic and mechanical	Intermittent	Restricted end range	Immediate at restricted end range	None	Months	None	None	Mechanical and symptomatic	Movement plane direction specific	Pursue symptoms	Avoiding symptoms
Derangement	Symptomatic and mechanical	Intermittent or constant	During motion, obstructed or unobstructed end range	Immediate or delayed, during motion, at obstructed or unobstructed end range	Often persists	Days	Yes	Mechanical and symptomatic	Mechanical and symptomatic	Loading in one movement plane direction may affect another	Pursue centralization, avoid peripheralization	Avoiding symptoms of centralization

Data from Jacob G, McKenzie R: Spinal therapeutics based on responses to loading. In: Liebenson C, ed. *Rehabilitation of the Spine: A Practitioner's Manual.* Baltimore, MD: Lippincott Williams & Wilkins, 1996:225–252.

TABLE 22-4	Characteristics of the Adherent Nerve Root

The ANR syndrome usually presents following the resolution of a derangement syndrome or postsurgically (6–12 wks).

History

- Sciatic or surgery in the few months that has improved but is now unchanging
- Intermittent leg symptoms, thigh/calf (tightness)
- Consistent activity produces symptoms: touching toes, long sitting, walking
- Pain in leg does not *persist* upon ceasing movement or when changing position

Exam

- Flexion in standing clearly restricted—consistently produces concordant pain/tightness at end range
- No rapid reduction/abolition of symptoms produced; no lasting distal symptoms
- Moderate/major loss of flexion (may demonstrate deviation)
- Flexion movement will improve if knee is flexed
- FIL has no effect
- No rapid change in mechanical presentation with repeated movement testing.

Intervention

- Flexion in sit with increasing knee extension
- Flexion in stand
- Flexion step stand (opposite leg on chair)
- End the session with EIL/EIS
- Monitor mechanical response to extension. Should remain unchanged following repeated flexion

FIL = flexion in lying; EIL = extension in lying; EIS = extension in standing.

whereas other motions decrease, abolish, or centralize the symptoms. McKenzie advocates a variety of loading principles for the reduction of the derangement.

- Extension
- Flexion
- Lateral movement
- Force progression
  - Start position: loaded versus unloaded
  - Positioning to mid range
  - Positioning at end range
- Dynamic patient-generated forces
  - Patient motion to mid range
  - Patient motion to end range
  - Patient motion to extreme ranges using patient overpressure (sag).
- Clinical generated forces
  - Patient motion to mid range with clinician's overpressure
  - Patient motion to end range with clinician's overpressure
  - Clinician mobilization
  - Clinician high-velocity thrust technique

TABLE 22-5 Comparison of the Lumbar and Cervical McKenzie Derangement Syndromes

Lumbar Derangements	Cervical Derangements
Derangement 1 Central or symmetrical pain across low back; rarely buttock and/or thigh pain; no deformity	**Derangement 1** Central or symmetrical pain about C5–7; rarely scapular and/or shoulder pain; no deformity
Derangement 2 Central or symmetrical pain across low back with or without buttock and/or thigh pain; deformity of lumbar kyphosis	**Derangement 2** Central or symmetrical pain about C5–7 with or without scapular, shoulder, or upper arm pain; deformity of cervical kyphosis
Derangement 3 Unilateral or asymmetrical pain across low back with or without buttock and/or thigh pain; no deformity	**Derangement 3** Unilateral or symmetrical pain about C3–7 with or without scapular, shoulder, or upper arm pain; no deformity
Derangement 4 Unilateral or asymmetrical pain across low back with or without buttock and/or thigh pain; deformity of lumbar scoliosis	**Derangement 4** Unilateral or symmetrical pain about C5–7 with or without scapular, shoulder, or upper arm pain; with deformity or acute wry neck or torticollis
Derangement 5 Unilateral or asymmetrical pain across low back with or without buttock and/or thigh pain with sciatica extending below knee; no deformity	**Derangement 5** Unilateral or symmetrical pain about C5–7 with or without scapular or shoulder pain and with arm symptoms distal to elbow; no deformity
Derangement 6 Unilateral or asymmetrical pain across low back with or without buttock and/or thigh pain with sciatica extending below knee; deformity of lumbar scoliosis	**Derangement 6** Unilateral or symmetrical pain about C5–7 with arm symptoms distal to the elbow with deformity of cervical kyphosis, acute wry neck or torticollis
Derangement 7 Symmetrical or asymmetrical pain across low back with or without buttock and/or thigh pain with deformity of accentuated lumbar lordosis	**Derangement 7** Symmetrical or asymmetrical pain about C4–6 with or without anterior/anterior-lateral pain; no deformity

Data from McKenzie RA: *The Cervical and Thoracic Spine: Mechanical Diagnosis and Therapy*. Waikanae, NZ: Spinal Publications, 1990; McKenzie RA. *The Lumbar Spine: Mechanical Diagnosis and Therapy*. Waikanae, NZ: Spinal Publication, 1981; Moss JM. Cervical and lumbar pain syndromes. In: Boyling JD, Palastanga N, eds. *Grieve's Modern Manual Therapy: The Vertebral Column*, 2nd ed. Edinburgh: Churchill Livingstone, 1994:291–400.

- Force alternatives
  - Static patient-generated forces
  - Strategy: sagittal/frontal/or combination
  - Time factor: sustained/repeated
  - Frontal plane angle during combined procedures

Once the subjective history and mechanical evaluation has been performed on the initial visit, the clinician should have an idea regarding which mechanical category the patient may belong. Depending upon the syndrome, a specific self-treatment program is prescribed for home use, and patients are encouraged to accept responsibility for their intervention and recovery. The specific programs relative to the cervical and lumbar spine are described in the respective chapters.

The inter-rater reliability of the McKenzie method in performing clinical tests and classifying patients with LBP into syndromes has been investigated in a number of studies.[68,89,92–99]

Repeated movements have been found to be a reliable part of the examination of the spine in a number of studies.[98,100]

In one study,[98] intertester reliability between two therapists trained in the McKenzie method seemed to be high for classifying patients with LBP into McKenzie syndromes, and excellent for judging pain status change, including the centralization phenomenon, during examination of the lumbar spine.[96,98] The results from a study by Kilpikoski also suggested that intertester reliability in performing clinical tests and classifying patients with LBP into the main McKenzie syndromes is high when the clinicians have been trained in the McKenzie method.[99]

Donahue and colleagues[92] suggested that the McKenzie method was unreliable for detecting the presence of a lateral shift, but that a relevant lateral component could be reliably detected using symptom response to repeated movements. In contrast, Tenhula and associates[95] noted a significant relation between positive results on a contralateral side-bending movement test and a lumbar lateral shift, indicating that the former is a useful clinical test for confirming the presence of a lateral shift in patients with LBP.

Kilby and colleagues[97] found the "McKenzie algorithm" (Fig. 22-5) to be reliable in the examination of pain behavior and pain response with repeated movements but unreliable in the detection of end range pain and lateral shift.

Riddle and Rothstein[68] found that the McKenzie approach was unreliable when physical therapists classified patients into McKenzie syndromes. They suggested that a potential source of unreliability was in determining whether the patient had a lateral shift and, if so, in which direction and whether the patient's pain centralized or peripheralized during test movements.[68]

Treatment-Based Classification System

This system, originally proposed by Delitto and colleagues,[101] uses information gathered from the physical examination and from the patient's self-reports of pain (pain scale and pain diagram) and disability (modified Oswestry questionnaire) to classify the patient with LBP.[101,102] The classification determines whether the patient's condition is amenable to physical therapy or whether care from another practitioner is required. The treatment-based classification (TBC) system is designed for patients judged to be in the acute stage, with the determination of acuity based on the alignment of various body structures, the effect of movements on symptoms, the nature of the patient's symptoms, the degree of disability, and the goals for management, instead of strictly on the elapsed time from injury.[102]

Patients in the acute stage are those with higher levels of disability (modified Oswestry scores generally greater than 30), who report substantial difficulty with basic daily activities such as sitting, standing, and walking. Intervention goals are to improve the ability to perform basic daily activities, reduce disability, and permit the patient to advance in his or her rehabilitation.[102] Patients judged to be in the acute stage are assigned to a classification that guides the initial intervention. Seven classifications are described for patients in the acute stage[101]:

1. Immobilization.
2. Lumbar mobilization.

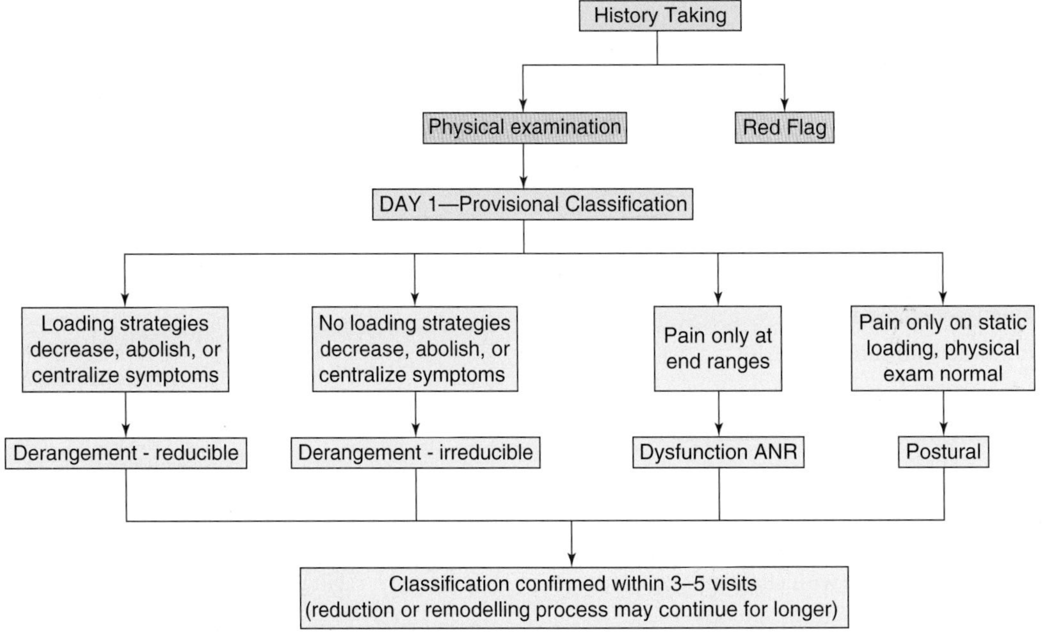

FIGURE 22-5 McKenzie classification algorithm.

3. Sacroiliac mobilization.
4. Extension syndrome.
5. Flexion syndrome.
6. Lateral shift.
7. Traction.

Each of the classifications has key examination findings and recommended interventions. To facilitate comparisons among classifications, these seven classifications may be collapsed further into four classifications based on similarities in the prescribed interventions.

1. Mobilization/manipulation.
2. Stabilization (either sacroiliac or lumbar).
3. Specific exercise (flexion, extension, or lateral shift correction).
4. Traction.

Mobilization/Manipulation

The mobilization classification includes patients believed to have indications for either sacroiliac or lumbar region mobilization or manipulation. Mobilization of the sacroiliac region is indicated by asymmetries of the pelvic landmarks (anterior superior iliac spines, posterior superior iliac spines, and iliac crests) with the patient in the standing position and by positive results in three of four tests as follows:

1. Asymmetry of posterior superior iliac spine heights with the patient sitting.
2. The standing flexion test.
3. The prone-knee flexion test.
4. The supine to long-sitting test.

Acute-stage intervention for this category involves a manipulation technique proposed to affect the sacroiliac joint region, muscle energy techniques, and ROM exercises for the lumbosacral spine.[96]

Lumbar mobilization is believed to be indicated by the presence of the following:

- Unilateral paraspinal pain in the lumbar region.
- Asymmetric amounts of lumbar side-bending ROM with the patient standing in either an "opening" pattern (limited and painful flexion and side-bending ROM to the side opposite the pain) or a "closing" pattern (limited and painful extension and side-bending ROM to the same side as the pain).

The intervention for this category consists of lumbar mobilization or manipulation techniques and ROM exercises for the lumbosacral spine.

Stabilization

The stabilization classification is purported to identify patients with lumbar segmental instability. Key examination findings are typically gleaned from the history and include a history of frequent episodes of symptoms precipitated by minimal perturbations, frequent use of manipulation with short-term relief of symptoms, trauma, or reduced symptoms with the prior use of a corset.[101]

The intervention for this category focuses on strengthening exercises for the back extensor and abdominal exercises as well as stabilization exercises designed to improve dynamic control of the lumbar spine.[102]

Specific Exercise

The key examination finding that places patients into a specific exercise classification is the presence of centralization with movement of the lumbar spine based on the McKenzie method.[82] When either lumbar flexion or extension is found to produce centralization, the patient is treated with specific exercises in the direction producing the centralization. Patients are also educated to avoid positions found to peripheralize symptoms during examination.

The primary examination findings that lead to a classification of a lateral shift, in which the shoulders are offset from the pelvis in the frontal plane, are a visible frontal plane deformity and asymmetric side-bending ROM in standing. If correction of the deformity produces centralization, the patient is taught specific exercises designed to correct the lateral shift (i.e., pelvic translocation).[82]

Traction

The traction classification is reserved for patients with signs and symptoms of nerve root compression who are unable to centralize with any lumbar movements. The acute stage intervention involves the use of mechanical traction or autotraction[103] in an attempt to produce centralization.

Under the TBC, patients judged to be in a more chronic stage are treated with a conditioning program designed to improve strength, flexibility, and conditioning, or with a work-reconditioning program.[101]

A recent cross-sectional study[73] to evaluate the TBC algorithm found that approximately one-half of patients with acute or subacute LBP met the criteria for only one treatment subgroup. In addition, although approximately 25% of the patients met the criteria for more than one subgroup, 25% of the patient's did not meet the criteria for any of the treatment subgroups. This latter finding suggests that further research is needed to refine the algorithm.

Canadian Biomechanical Model[104]

The Canadian model is an eclectic approach founded upon an amalgam of doctrines and techniques that incorporate the biomechanical concepts of the Norwegians,[105–108] the selective tissue tension principles of Cyriax,[79,109] the muscle energy concepts of the American osteopaths,[110–112] the combined movement testing of Edwards,[68] the manipulative techniques of Stoddard,[113] the various approaches to stabilization therapy,[25,114–116] the exercise protocols of McKenzie,[82,83] the muscle balancing concepts of Janda, Jull, and Sahrmann,[117–119] and the movement reeducation principles of the neurodevelopment and sensory integrationist clinicians.[120,121]

The basic tenet of the Canadian approach is that, given an understanding of the anatomy and biomechanics of a joint, segment or region, the pathologic mechanisms can be extrapolated using a series of testing procedures. These tests include the Cyriax upper and lower quarter scanning examinations for differential diagnosis (see Chap. 4), uncombined (plane) and combined movement testing, passive physiological intervertebral motion (PPIVM) tests, passive accessory intervertebral motion (PAIVM) tests, and segmental stability tests.

Following the active motion tests, the clinician should be able to determine the planar motions (flexion, extension, and side bending and rotation to both sides) that provoke symptoms. However, the clinician cannot yet determine whether a joint or soft tissue is responsible for the pain. Two tests are used to help determine the presence of articular involvement: the PPIVM tests and the PAIVM tests.

Passive Physiologic Intervertebral Mobility Testing

The PPIVM tests are used to determine the amount of segmental mobility available in the spine. The PPIVM tests assess the ability of each segment to move through its normal ROM. The adjacent spinous processes of the segment are palpated simultaneously and movement between them is assessed as the segment is passively taken through its physiologic range. If both spinous processes move simultaneously, there is no movement occurring at the segment and a hypomobility exists. If the movement between adjacent spinous processes appears excessive when compared with the level above or below, a hypermobility or instability may be suspected.

Thus, once the physiologic range has been assessed, it can be categorized as either normal, excessive, or reduced compared with the neighboring segment. Other positive findings for a hypomobility would be a reduced range in a capsular or noncapsular pattern in the active motion tests, a reduced joint glide, and a change in the end-feel from the expected norm for that joint. The end-feel and joint glide are both tested in the PAIVM tests (discussed next).

Therefore, one of three conclusions may be drawn from the PPIVM tests:

1. The joint motion is determined to be normal. If the PPIVM test of a spinal joint has a normal range and end-feel, the joint can usually be considered normal because in the spine, instability will invariably produce a hypermobility. However, in a peripheral joint, it is possible to have a normal range in the presence of articular instability. Thus, if a peripheral joint demonstrates a normal physiologic range, the stability of the joint needs to be tested using the segmental stability tests (see later discussion) before the clinician can deem the joint to be normal.
2. The joint motion is determined to be reduced (hypomobile). A hypomobility can be painful, suggesting an acute sprain of a structure, or painless, suggesting a contracture or an adhesion of the tested structure. If the motion is determined as being reduced (hypomobile), PAIVM testing is performed to determine, using the joint glides, whether the reduced motion is a result of an articular or extra-articular restriction.
3. The motion is determined to be excessive (hypermobile). If the motion is determined to be excessive, segmental stability tests are performed to determine whether a hypermobility or an instability is present (see later discussion).

It is worth noting that the judgments of joint stiffness made by experienced physical therapists examining patients in their own clinics have been found to have poor reliability in a number of studies. In two separate studies, [100,122] manual therapy tests that provoke patient's symptoms were found to be more reliable than judging stiffness in the spine. Smedmark and colleagues[123] investigated the interexaminer reliability of passive intervertebral motion testing. In their study, passive intervertebral motion of the cervical spine was assessed independently by two physical therapists whose backgrounds (education and clinical experience) were equal. Sixty-one patients seeking care for cervical problems at a private clinic were included in the study, in which three segments of the cervical spine and the mobility of the first rib were graded as stiff or not stiff. Data analyzed by percentage agreement and κ coefficient indicated an interexaminer reliability that was greater than expected by chance. Results demonstrated interexaminer reliability of between 70 and 87% and κ coefficients ranging between 0.28 and 0.43, considered to be only fair to moderate.

However, in a study by Gonnella and colleagues[124] the performance of five physical therapists in evaluating passive mobility of the vertebral column of five asymptomatic endomorphic subjects was assessed for the reliability within and between therapists, the criteria for grading, and the subjects themselves. Intratester reliability was found to be reasonable to good; there was no intertester reliability. Reliability was highest at L1–L3 and lowest at L5–S1. Problems identified were idiosyncratic behaviors that may develop with experience, subject characteristics, and the instrument itself.

Passive Accessory Intervertebral Mobility Testing

In the PAIVM tests, the clinician assesses the joint glides or accessory motions of each joint and determines the type of end-feel encountered.

Accessory motions are involuntary motions. With few exceptions, muscles cannot restrict the glides of a joint, especially if the glides are tested in the loose-pack position of a peripheral joint and at the end of available range in the spinal joints.[125] Thus, if the joint glide is restricted, the cause is an articular restriction such as the joint surface or capsule. If the glide is normal, then the restriction must be from an extra-articular source such as a periarticular structure or muscle.

Determining the type of end-feel is very important, particularly in joints that only have very small amounts of normal range such as those of the spine. To execute the end-feel, the point at which resistance is encountered is evaluated for quality and tenderness. Additional forces are needed as the end range of a joint is reached and the elastic limits are challenged. This space, termed as the *end-play zone*, requires a force of over-pressure to be reached and when that force is released, the joint springs back from its elastic limits. Because pain generally does not limit movement in specific and deliberate passive tests, the PAIVM tests are better for gauging the reliability of the limitation based on tissue resistance, rather than patient willingness, and are better at determining the pattern of restriction than the active tests. If pain is reproduced with end-feel testing, it is useful to associate the pain with the onset of tissue resistance to gain an appreciation of the acuteness of the problem. A normal end-feel indicates normal range, whereas an abnormal end-feel suggests abnormal range, either hypomobile or hypermobile. If the articular restraints are irritable, the range will be about normal but will be accompanied by a spasm end-feel because a reflex muscle contraction can prevent the motion into an abnormal and painful range.[125,126] If nonirritable, the physiologic range will be increased and the end-feel will be softer than the expected capsular one, suggesting a compromise of the structure under examination. A hard, capsular end-feel indicates a pericapsular hypomobility, whereas a jammed end-feel indicates a pathomechanical hypomobility.

The PAIVM tests can be performed symmetrically or asymmetrically. These tests are described in the relevant chapters of this text. Generally speaking, the symmetric tests are used when planar motions have produced pain in the active motion tests, whereas the asymmetric techniques are used when the combined motions have produced pain in the active motion tests.

Caution must be taken when basing clinical judgments on the results of accessory motion testing alone because few studies have examined the validity and reliability of accessory motion testing of the spine or extremities and little is known about the validity of these tests for most inferences.[127]

Hayes and Peterson[128] examined two physical therapists who used standardized positions to evaluate two knee motions and five shoulder motions. Evaluators did not interview subjects and were blinded to previous test results. Evaluators applied overpressure and noted the end-feel while subjects identified the moment their pain was reproduced. Following testing, subjects rated their pain intensity. Analyses included percentage of agreement κ, weighted κ, and maximum κ coefficients and confidence intervals. Analyses were repeated for subjects whose pain intensity during testing did not change between examinations. Intrarater κ coefficients varied from 0.65 to 1.00 for end-feel, and intrarater weighted κ coefficients varied from 0.59 to 0.87 for pain-resistance sequence. Most coefficients remained stable or improved for the unchanged subjects. Inter-rater κ coefficients for end-feel and weighted κ coefficients for pain resistance sequence varied from −0.01 to 0.70. The authors concluded that the reliability of end-feel and pain-resistance judgments at the knee and shoulder was generally good, especially after accounting for subject change and unbalanced distributions. Inter-rater reliability, however, was generally not acceptable, even after accounting for these factors.[128]

In a separate study by the same authors,[129] the relationship between pain and normal and abnormal (pathologic) end-feels during passive physiologic motion assessment at the knee and shoulder were examined. Physical therapists examined subjects with unilateral knee or shoulder pain, and each subject was examined twice. Passive physiologic motions, two at the knee and five at the shoulder, were tested by applying an overpressure at the end of ROM, using standardized positions. Subjects reported the amount of pain (0–10) immediately after the evaluator recorded the end-feel. The authors concluded that abnormal (pathologic) end-feels are associated with more pain than normal end-feels during passive physiologic motion testing at the knee or shoulder. Dysfunction should be suspected when abnormal (pathologic) end-feels are present.[129]

Based on review of the literature of the MEDLINE and CINAHL databases for the period of 1980 through 2000, using the keywords *motion palpation, accessory motion,* and *intervertebral motion,* Huijbregts[130] performed a review of 28 reliability studies. The following conclusions were made from this study:

- Intra-rater agreement varied from less than chance to generally moderate or substantial agreement.
- Inter-rater agreement only rarely exceeded poor to fair agreement.
- Rating scales measuring absence versus presence or magnitude of pain response yielded higher agreement values than mobility rating scales.

Segmental Stability Tests

These are tests for movements that should not exist to an appreciable degree. The tests include maneuvers that induce non-physiologic rotational, anterior, posterior, and transverse shears to the segment. The limitation in the clinical diagnosis of segmental instability lies in the difficulty of accurately detecting excessive intersegmental motion, because even conventional radiologic testing is often insensitive and unreliable.[131,132] Instability should be suspected in the presence of a positive stability test in conjunction with other clinical findings and symptoms of instability. A positive stability test in the absence of other clinical findings is probably irrelevant. Hypermobility is clinically manifested by the presence of increased physiologic range in one or more directions, or normal range with pain and spasm at the end of that range.

Research indicates that skilled clinicians can distinguish subjects with symptomatic spondylolysis from LBP based on the finding of increased intersegmental motion at the level above the pars defect.[133,134]

The various stability tests are described in the specific chapters of this text.

REFERENCES

1. Singer KP, Boyle JJW, Fazey P: Comparative anatomy of the zygapophyseal joints. In: Boyling JD, Jull GA, eds. *Grieve's Modern Manual Therapy: The Vertebral Column.* Philadelphia, PA: Churchill Livingstone, 2004:17–29.
2. Bogduk N, Twomey LT: Anatomy and biomechanics of the lumbar spine. In: Bogduk N, Twomey LT, eds. *Clinical Anatomy of the Lumbar Spine and Sacrum,* 3rd ed. Edinburgh: Churchill Livingstone, 1997:2–53; 81–152;171–176.
3. Neumann DA: Axial skeleton: osteology and arthrology. In: Neumann DA, ed. *Kinesiology of the Musculoskeletal System: Foundations for Physical Rehabilitation.* St. Louis, MO: Mosby, 2002:251–310.
4. Singer KP, Giles LGF: Manual therapy considerations at the thoracolumbar junction: an anatomical and functional perspective. *J Man Physiol Ther* 13:83–88, 1990.
5. Pal GP, Sherk HH: The vertical stability of the cervical spine. *Spine* 13:447, 1988.
6. Pal GP, Routal RV, Saggu SK: The orientation of the articular facets of the zygapophyseal joints at the cervical and upper thoracic region. *J Anat* 198:431–441, 2001.
7. Pal GP, Routal RV: The role of the vertebral laminae in the stability of the cervical spine. *J Anat* 188:485–489, 1996.

8. Pal GP, Routal RV: A study of weight transmission through the cervical and upper thoracic regions of the vertebral column in man. *J Anat* 148:245–261, 1986.
9. Gregersen GG, Lucas DB: An in vivo study of the axial rotation of the human thoracolumbar spine. *J Bone Joint Surg Am* 49:247–262, 1967.
10. Lundon K, Bolton K: Structure and function of the lumbar intervertebral disk in health, aging, and pathological conditions. *J Orthop Sports Phys Ther* 31:291–306, 2001.
11. White AA, Punjabi MM: *Clinical Biomechanics of the Spine*, 2nd ed. Philadelphia, PA: J.B. Lippincott Company, 1990.
12. Buckwalter JA: Spine update: aging and degeneration of the human intervertebral disc. *Spine* 20:1307–1314, 1995.
13. Huijbregts PA: Lumbopelvic region: anatomy and biomechanics. In: Wadsworth C, ed. *Current Concepts of Orthopaedic Physical Therapy – Home Study Course.* La Crosse, WI: Orthopaedic Section, APTA, 2001.
14. Mercer S: Comparative anatomy of the spinal disc. In: Boyling JD, Jull GA, eds. *Grieve's Modern Manual Therapy: The Vertebral Column.* Philadelphia, PA: Churchill Livingstone, 2004:9–16.
15. Schmorl G, Junghanns H: *The Human Spine in Health and Disease*, 2nd ed. New York, NY: Grune & Stratton, 1971.
16. Wigh R: The thoracolumbar and lumbosacral transitional junctions. *Spine* 5:215–222, 1980.
17. Reeves NP, Cholewicki J, Narendra KS: Converging on a stable definition of spine stability. *Clin Biomech* 22:487–488, 2007.
18. Panjabi MM: The stabilizing system of the spine. Part 1. Function, dysfunction adaption and enhancement. *J Spinal Disord* 5:383–389, 1992.
19. Panjabi MM: Clinical spinal instability and low back pain. *J Electromyogr Kinesiol* 13:371–379, 2003.
20. Hodges PW: Motor control of the trunk. In: Boyling JD, Jull GA, eds. *Grieve's Modern Manual Therapy: The Vertebral Column.* Philadelphia, PA: Churchill Livingstone, 2004:119–139.
21. Tencer AF, Ahmed AM: The role of secondary variables in the measurement of the mechanical properties of the lumbar intervertebral joint. *J Biomech Eng* 103:129–137, 1981.
22. Wilder DG, Pope MH, Seroussi RE, et al.: The balance point of the intervertebral motion segment: an experimental study. *Bull Hosp Jt Dis Orthop Inst* 49:155–169, 1989.
23. Bergmark A: Stability of the lumbar spine. A study in mechanical engineering. *Acta Orthop Scand* 230:20–24, 1989.
24. Hodges P, Richardson C: Inefficient muscular stabilisation of the lumbar spine associated with low back pain: a motor control evaluation of transversus abdominis. *Spine* 21:2540–2650, 1996.
25. Richardson CA, Jull GA, Hodges P, et al.: *Therapeutic Exercise for Spinal Segmental Stabilization in Low Back Pain.* London: Churchill Livingstone, 1999.
26. Cholewicki J, McGill S: Mechanical stability of the in vivo lumbar spine: implications for injury and chronic low back pain. *Clin Biomech* 11:1–15, 1996.
27. Stokes IAF, Gardner-Morse M: Lumbar spine maximum efforts and muscle recruitment patterns predicted by a model with multijoint muscles and joints with stiffness. *J Biomech* 27:1101–1104, 1994.
28. Comerford MJ, Mottram SL: Functional stability re-training: principles and strategies for managing mechanical dysfunction. *Man Ther* 6:3–14, 2001.
29. Comerford MJ, Mottram SL: Movement and stability dysfunction-contemporary developments. *Man Ther* 6:15–26, 2001.
30. Givens-Heiss D: Dynamic lumbar stability. In: Hughes C, ed. *Movement Disorders and Neuromuscular Interventions for the Trunk and Extremities – Independent Study Course 18.2.4.* La Crosse, WI: Orthopaedic Section, APTA, Inc., 2008:1–23.
31. Panjabi M, Abumi K, Duranceau J, et al.: Spinal stability and intersegmental muscle forces. A biomechanical model. *Spine* 14:194–199, 1989.
32. Solomonow M, Zhou BH, Harris M, et al.: The ligamento-muscular stabilizing system of the spine. *Spine* 23:2552–2562, 1998.
33. Stubbs M, Harris M, Solomonow M, et al.: Ligamento-muscular protective reflex in the lumbar spine of the feline. *J Electromyogr Kinesiol* 8:197–204, 1998.
34. Solomonow M, Zhou BH, Baratta RV, et al.: Biomechanics and electromyography of a cumulative lumbar disorder: response to static flexion. *Clin Biomech (Bristol, Avon)* 18:890–898, 2003.
35. Bowman SM, Keaveny TM, Gibson LJ, et al.: Compressive creep behavior of bovine trabecular bone. *J Biomech* 27:301–310, 1994.
36. Brinckmann P, Biggemann M, Hilweg D: Fatigue fracture of human lumbar vertebrae. *Clin Biomech* 3:(Suppl):S1–S23, 1988.
37. Mannion AF, Connolly B, Wood K, et al.: The use of surface EMG power spectral analysis in the evaluation of back muscle function. *J Rehabil Res Dev* 34:427–439, 1997.
38. Roy SH, De Luca CJ, Casavant DA: Lumbar muscle fatigue and chronic lower back pain. *Spine* 14:992–1001, 1989.
39. Best TM, McElhaney J, Garrett WE, Jr., et al.: Characterization of the passive responses of live skeletal muscle using the quasi-linear theory of viscoelasticity. *J Biomech* 27:413–419, 1994.
40. Keller TS, Spengler DM, Hansson TH: Mechanical behavior of the human lumbar spine, I: creep analysis during static compressive loading. *J Orthop Res* 5:467–478, 1987.
41. Heiss DG, Shields RK, Yack HJ: Anticipatory control of vertical lifting force and momentum during the squat lift with expected and unexpected loads. *J Orthop Sports Phys Ther* 31:708–723; discussion 724–729, 2001.
42. Bertucco M, Cesari P: Does movement planning follow Fitts' law? Scaling anticipatory postural adjustments with movement speed and accuracy. *Neuroscience* 171:205–213, 2010.
43. Toussaint HM, Michies YM, Faber MN, et al.: Scaling anticipatory postural adjustments dependent on confidence of load estimation in a bi-manual whole-body lifting task. *Exp Brain Res* 120:85–94, 1998.
44. Toussaint HM, Commissaris DA, Beek PJ: Anticipatory postural adjustments in the back and leg lift. *Med Sci Sports Exerc* 29:1216–1224, 1997.
45. Toussaint HM, Commissaris DA, Hoozemans MJ, et al.: Anticipatory postural adjustments before load pickup in a bi-manual whole body lifting task. *Med Sci Sports Exerc* 29:1208–1215, 1997.
46. Grieve GP: *Common Vertebral Joint Problems.* New York, NY: Churchill Livingstone Inc, 1981.
47. American Medical Association: *Guides to the Evaluation of Permanent Impairment.* 5th ed. Chicago, IL: American Medical Association, 2001.
48. Aiderink GJ: The sacroiliac joint: review of anatomy, mechanics and function. *J Orthop Sports Phys Ther* 13:71, 1991.
49. Lee DG: The pelvic girdle: an approach to the examination and treatment of the lumbo-pelvic-hip region. 2nd ed. Edinburgh: Churchill Livingstone, 1999.
50. Grieve GP: The sacroiliac joint. *Physiotherapy* 62:384–400, 1976.
51. Kirkaldy-Willis WH, Hill RJ: A more precise diagnosis for low back pain. *Spine* 4:102–109, 1979.
52. Wang M, Bryant JT, Dumas GA: A new in vitro measurement technique for small three-dimensional joint motion and its application to the sacroiliac joint. *Med Eng Phys* 18:495–501, 1996.
53. Van der Wurff P, Meyne W, Hagmeijer RHM: Clinical tests of the sacroiliac joint, a systematic methodological review. part 2: validity. *Man Ther* 5:89–96, 2000.
54. Ross J: Is the sacroiliac joint mobile and how should it be treated? *Br J Sports Med* 34:226, 2000.
55. Miller JAA, Schultz AB, Andersson GBJ: Load-displacement behaviour of sacroiliac joints. *J Orthop Res* 5:92–101, 1987.
56. Vleeming A, Van Wingerden JP, Dijkstra PF: Mobility in the sacroiliac joints in the elderly: a kinematic and radiological study. *Clin Biomech* 7:170–176, 1992.
57. Pettman E: Principles and practices. In: Pettman E, ed. *Manipulative Thrust Techniques – An Evidence-Based Approach.* Abbotsford, BC: Aphema Publishing, 2006:12–26.
58. Krag MH: *Three-Dimensional Flexibility Measurements of Preload Human Vertebral Motion Segments.* New Haven, CT: Yale University School of Medicine, 1975.
59. Seifert MH, Whiteside CG, Savage O: A 5-year follow-up of fifty cases of idiopathic osteoarthritis of the hip. *Ann Rheum Dis* 28:325–326, 1969.
60. Farfan HF: The scientific basis of manipulative procedures. *Clin Rheum Dis* 6:159–177, 1980.
61. White AA, Panjabi MM: *Clinical Biomechanics of the Spine.* In: White AA, Panjabi MM, eds. 2nd ed. Philadelphia, PA: Lippincott-Raven, 1990:106–108.
62. Fryette HH: *Principles of Osteopathic Technique.* Colorado, CO: Academy of Osteopathy, 1980.
63. Harrison DE, Harrison DD, Troyanovich SJ: Three-dimensional spinal coupling mechanics: part I. A review of the literature. *J Manipulative Physiol Ther* 21:101–113, 1998.
64. Brown L: An introduction to the treatment and examination of the spine by combined movements. *Physiotherapy* 74:347–353, 1988.
65. Edwards BC: Combined movements of the lumbar spine: examination and clinical significance. *Aust J Physiother* 25, 1979.
66. Edwards BC: Combined movements of the lumbar spine: examination and treatment. In: Palastanga N, Boyling JD, eds. *Grieve's Modern*

Manual Therapy of the Vertebral Column. Edinburgh: Churchill Livingstone, 1994:561–566.
67. Nachemson A, Vingard E: Assessment of patients with neck and back pain: a best evidence synthesis. In: Nachemson AL, Jonsson E, eds. *Neck and Back Pain: The Scientific Evidence of Causes, Diagnosis, and Treatment*. Philadelphia, PA: Lippincott Williams and Wilkins, 2000:189–235.
68. Riddle DL, Rothstein JM: Intertester reliability of McKenzie's classifications of the syndrome types present in patients with low back pain. *Spine* 18:1333–1344, 1993.
69. Riddle DL: Classification and low back pain; a review of the literature and critical analysis of selected systems. *Phys Ther* 78:708–737, 1998.
70. Maher CG, Moseley AM, Sherrington C, et al.: A description of the trials, reviews, and practice guidelines indexed in the PEDro database. *Physical Therapy* 88:1068–1077, 2008.
71. Machado LA, Kamper SJ, Herbert RD, et al.: Analgesic effects of treatments for non-specific low back pain: a meta-analysis of placebo-controlled randomized trials. *Rheumatology* 48:520–527, 2009.
72. Kent P, Keating J: Do primary-care clinicians think that nonspecific low back pain is one condition? *Spine* 29:1022–1031, 2004.
73. Stanton TR, Fritz JM, Hancock MJ, et al.: Evaluation of a treatment-based classification algorithm for low back pain: a cross-sectional study. *Phys Ther* 91: 496–509 2011.
74. Bernard TN, Kirkaldy-Willis WH: Recognizing specific characteristics of nonspecific low back pain. *Clin Orthop* 217:266–280, 1987.
75. Mooney V: The syndromes of low back disease. *Orthop Clin North Am* 14:505–515, 1983.
76. Abenhaim L, Rossignol M, Gobeille D, et al.: The prognostic consequences in the making of the initial medical diagnosis of work-related back injuries. *Spine* 20:791–795, 1995.
77. Bigos S, Bowyer O, Braen G, et al.: *Acute Low Back Problems in Adults*. Rockville, MD: Agency for Health Care Policy and Research, Public Health Service, U.S. Department of Health and Human Services, AHCPR Publication 95-0642; 1994.
78. Spitzer WO: Approach to the problem. In: Scientific Approach to the Assessment and Management of Activity-Related Spinal Disorders: A Monograph for Clinicians. *Spine* 12:9–11, 1987.
79. Cyriax J: *Textbook of Orthopaedic Medicine, Diagnosis of Soft Tissue Lesions*, 8th ed. London: Bailliere Tindall, 1982.
80. Von Korff M: Studying the natural history of back pain. *Spine* 19:2041–2046, 1994.
81. Quebec Task Force on Spinal Disorders: Scientific approach to the assessment and management of activity-related spinal disorders: a monograph for clinicians. Report of the Quebec Task Force on Spinal Disorders. *Spine* 12(Suppl):1–59, 1987.
82. McKenzie RA: *The Lumbar Spine: Mechanical Diagnosis and Therapy*. Waikanae, NZ: Spinal Publication, 1981.
83. McKenzie RA: *The Cervical and Thoracic Spine: Mechanical Diagnosis and Therapy*. Waikanae, NZ: Spinal Publications, 1990.
84. Bouter LM, van Tulder MW, Koes BW: Methodologic issues in low back pain research in primary care. *Spine* 23:2014–2020, 1998.
85. Downey BJ, Taylor NF, Niere KR: Manipulative physiotherapists can reliably palpate nominated lumbar spinal levels. *Man Ther* 4:151–156, 1999.
86. Keating JC, Bergmann TF, Jacobs GE, et al.: Interexaminer reliability of eight evaluative dimensions of lumbar segmental abnormality. *J Manipulative Physiol Ther* 13:463–470, 1990.
87. Deepak S, Covvath R: Reliability of palpation assessment in non-neutral dysfunctions of the lumbar spine. *Orthopaedic practice* 16: 23–26, 2004.
88. Binkley J, Stratford PW, Gill C: Interrater reliability of lumbar accessory motion mobility testing. *Phys Ther Rev* 75:786–792; discussion 793–795, 1995.
89. Donelson R, Silva G, Murphy K: Centralization phenomenon: its usefulness in evaluating and treating referred pain. *Spine* 15:211–213, 1990.
90. Donelson R, Aprill C, Medcalf R, et al.: A prospective study of centralization in lumbar referred pain. A predictor of symptomatic discs and anular competence. *Spine* 22:1115–1122, 1997.
91. Jacob G, McKenzie R: Spinal therapeutics based on responses to loading. In: Liebenson C, ed. *Rehabilitation of the Spine: A Practitioner's Manual*. Baltimore, MD: Lippincott Williams & Wilkins, 1996:225–252.
92. Donahue MS, Riddle DL, Sullivan MS: Intertester reliability of a modified version of McKenzie's lateral shift assessment obtained on patients with low back pain. *Phys Ther* 76:706–726, 1996.
93. Donelson R: Reliability of the McKenzie assessment. *J Orthop Sports Phys Ther* 30:770–773, 2000.
94. Donelson R, Grant W, Kamps C, et al.: Pain response to sagittal end-range spinal motion. A prospective, randomized, multicentered trial. *Spine* 16:S206–S212, 1991.
95. Tenhula JA, Rose SJ, Delitto A: Association between direction of lateral lumbar shift, movement tests, and side of symptoms in patients with low back pain syndromes. *Phys Ther* 70:480–486, 1990.
96. Fritz JM, Delitto A, Vignovic M, et al.: Interrater reliability of judgements of the centralisation phenomenon and status change during movement testing in patients with low back pain. *Arch Phys Med Rehabil* 81:57–60, 2000.
97. Kilby J, Stigant M, Roberts A: The reliability of back pain assessment by physiotherapists using a "Mckenzie algorithm." *Physiotherapy* 76:579–583, 1990.
98. Razmjou H, Kramer JF, Yamada R: Intertester reliability of the McKenzie evaluation in assessing patients with mechanical low back pain. *J Orthop Sports Phys Ther* 30:368–383, 2000.
99. Kilpikoski S, Airaksinen O, Kankaanpaa M, et al.: Interexaminer reliability of low back pain assessment using the McKenzie method. *Spine* 27:E207–E214, 2002.
100. Maher C, Adams R: Reliability of pain and stiffness assessments in clinical manual lumbar spine examination. *Phys Ther* 74:801–807, 1994.
101. Delitto A, Erhard RE, Bowling RW: A treatment-based classification approach to low back syndrome: identifying and staging patients for conservative management. *Phys Ther* 75:470–489, 1995.
102. Fritz JM, George S: The use of a classification approach to identify subgroups of patients with acute low back pain. Interrater reliability and short-term treatment outcomes. *Spine* 25:106–114, 2000.
103. Natchev E: *A Manual on Autotraction*. Stockholm, Sweden: Folksam Scientific Council, 1984.
104. Meadows JTS: *The Principles of the Canadian Approach to the Lumbar Dysfunction Patient, Management of Lumbar Spine Dysfunction – Independent Home Study Course*. La Crosse, WI: APTA, Orthopaedic Section, 1999.
105. Kaltenborn FM: *The Spine : Basic Evaluation and Mobilization Techniques*. Wellington, New Zealand: University Press, 1993.
106. Kaltenborn FM: *Manual Mobilization of the Extremity Joints: Basic Examination and Treatment Techniques*, 4th ed. Oslo, Norway: Olaf Norlis Bokhandel, Universitetsgaten, 1989.
107. Evjenth O, Gloeck C: *Symptom Localization in the Spine and Extremity Joints*. Minneapolis, MN: OPTP, 2000.
108. Evjenth O, Hamberg J: *Muscle Stretching in Manual Therapy, A Clinical Manual*. Alfta, Sweden: Alfta Rehab Forlag, 1984.
109. Cyriax JH, Cyriax PJ: *Illustrated Manual of Orthopaedic Medicine*. London: Butterworth, 1983.
110. Mennell JB: *The Science and Art of Joint Manipulation*. London: J & A Churchill, 1949.
111. Mennell JM: *Back Pain. Diagnosis and Treatment Using Manipulative Techniques*. Boston, MA: Little, Brown & Company, 1960.
112. Mitchell FL, Moran PS, Pruzzo NA: *An Evaluation and Treatment Manual of Osteopathic Muscle Energy Procedures*. Manchester, MO: Mitchell, Moran and Pruzzo Associates, 1979.
113. Stoddard A: *Manual of Osteopathic Practice*. New York, NY: Harper & Row, 1969.
114. McGill SM, Childs A, Liebenson C: Endurance times for low back stabilization exercises: clinical targets for testing and training from a normal database. *Arch Phys Med Rehab* 80:941–944, 1999.
115. Sweeney TB, Prentice C, Saal JA, et al.: Cervicothoracic muscular stabilization techniques. In: Saal JA, ed. *Physical Medicine and Rehabilitation, State of the Art Reviews: Neck and Back Pain*. Philadelphia, PA: Hanley & Belfus, 1990:335–359.
116. Hyman J, Liebenson C: Spinal stabilization exercise program. In: Liebenson C, ed. *Rehabilitation of the Spine: A Practitioner's Manual*. Baltimore, MD: Lippincott Williams & Wilkins, 1996:293–317.
117. Jull GA, Janda V: Muscle and Motor control in low back pain. In: Twomey LT, Taylor JR, eds. *Physical Therapy of the Low Back: Clinics in Physical Therapy*. New York, NY: Churchill Livingstone, 1987:258–278.
118. Janda V: Muscles and motor control in cervicogenic disorders: assessment and management. In: Grant R, ed. *Physical Therapy of the Cervical and Thoracic Spine*. New York, NY: Churchill Livingstone, 1994:195–216.

119. Sahrmann SA: *Diagnosis and Treatment of Movement Impairment Syndromes.* St Louis, MO: Mosby, 2001.
120. Knott M, Voss DE: *Proprioceptive Neuromuscular Facilitation.* 2nd ed. New York, NY: Harper & Row Pub Inc., 1968.
121. Feldenkrais M: *The Elusive Obvious.* Cupertino, CA: Meta Publications, 1981.
122. Maher C, Latimer J, Adams R: An investigation of the reliability and validity of posteroanterior spinal stiffness judgments made using a reference-based protocol. *Phys Ther* 78:829–837, 1998.
123. Smedmark V, Wallin M, Arvidsson I: Inter-examiner reliability in assessing passive intervertebral motion of the cervical spine. *Man Ther* 5:97–101, 2000.
124. Gonnella C, Paris SV, Kutner M: Reliability in evaluating passive intervertebral motion. *Phys Ther Rev* 62:436–444, 1982.
125. Exelby L: The locked lumbar facet joint: intervention using mobilizations with movement. *Man Ther* 6:116–121, 2001.
126. Janda V: Muscles, motor regulation and back problems. In: Korr IM, ed. *The Neurological Mechanisms in Manipulative Therapy*. New York, NY: Plenum, 1978:27–41.
127. Riddle DL: Measurement of accessory motion: critical issues and related concepts. *Phys Ther* 72:865–874, 1992.
128. Hayes KW, Petersen CM: Reliability of assessing end-feel and pain and resistance sequence in subjects with painful shoulders and knees. *J Orthop Sports Phys Ther* 31:432–445, 2001.
129. Petersen CM, Hayes KW: Construct validity of Cyriax's selective tension examination: association of end-feels with pain at the knee and shoulder. *J Orthop Sports Phys Ther* 30:512–527, 2000.
130. Huijbregts PA: Spinal motion palpation: a review of reliability studies. *J Man & Manip Ther* 10:24–39, 2002.
131. Dvorak J, Panjabi M, Novotny J, et al.: Clinical validation of functional flexion-extension roentgenograms of the lumbar spine. *Spine* 16:943–950, 1991.
132. Pope M, Frymoyer J, Krag M: Diagnosing instability. *Clin Orthop* 296:60–67, 1992.
133. Phillips DR, Twomey LT: Comparison of manual diagnosis with a diagnosis established by a uni-level spinal block procedure. In: Singer KP, ed. *Proceedings of the Eighth Biennial Conference, Manipulative Therapist Association of Australia*. Perth, Australia: 1993:55–61.
134. Avery A: *The Reliability of Manual Physiotherapy Palpation Techniques in the Diagnosis of Bilateral Pars Defects in Subjects with Chronic Low Back Pain.* Western Australia: Curtin University of Technology, 1996.

CHAPTER 23 The Craniovertebral Region

CHAPTER OBJECTIVES

At the completion of this chapter, the reader will be able to:

1. Describe the anatomy of the vertebrae, ligaments, muscles, and blood and nerve supply that comprise the craniovertebral segments.
2. Describe the biomechanics of the craniovertebral joints, including coupled movements, normal and abnormal joint barriers, and kinesiology.
3. Perform a comprehensive history and systems review for the craniovertebral region.
4. Perform a detailed examination of the craniovertebral musculoskeletal system, including palpation of the articular and soft tissue structures, specific passive mobility tests, passive articular mobility tests, and stability tests.
5. Evaluate the total examination data to establish a diagnosis.
6. Apply appropriate manual techniques to the craniovertebral joints, using the correct grade, direction, and duration.
7. Describe intervention strategies based on clinical findings and established goals.
8. Evaluate intervention effectiveness in order to progress or modify intervention.
9. Plan an effective home program and instruct the patient in this program.
10. Help the patient to develop self-reliant intervention strategies.

OVERVIEW

The craniovertebral region is a collective term that refers to the occiput, atlas, axis, and supporting ligaments, which accounts for approximately 25% of the vertical height of the entire cervical spine. Injuries to this region have the potential to involve the brain, brain stem and spinal cord, resulting in a myriad of symptoms ranging from headache and vertigo to cognitive and sympathetic system dysfunction.[1] Craniovertebral injuries that involve cognitive and sympathetic system dysfunction demonstrate a poorer prognosis and a lengthy recovery.

ANATOMY

The craniovertebral region is considered as a separate entity from the rest of the cervical spine because of its distinct embryology and anatomical structure. Kapandji[2] notes that the occiput, atlas, and axis actually form a primary kyphotic curve and that this curve serves as a delineation between the craniovertebral region and the cervical spine proper.

Foramen Magnum

The general shape of the foramen magnum is oval, with the longer axis oriented in the sagittal plane (Fig. 23-1).[3] The margin of the foramen is relatively smooth and serves as the most superior attachment for a variety of the ligaments of the vertebral column. The smaller anterior region of the foramen magnum is characterized by a pair of tubercles to which the alar ligaments attach. The posterior portion of the foramen magnum houses the brain stem–spinal cord junction.

On either side of the anterolateral aspect of the foramen magnum are two ovoid projections, called occipital condyles (Fig. 23-1). The long axis of these paired occipital condyles is situated in a posterolateral to anteromedial orientation. The occipital condyles articulate with the first cervical vertebra.

Atlas

The atlas is a ring-like structure that is formed by two lateral masses, which are interconnected by anterior and posterior arches (Fig. 23-1). The demarcation of the two regions is marked by a pair of tubercles to which the transverse ligament of the atlas attaches. Although the atlas has a smaller vertical dimension than any other cervical vertebrae, it is considerably wider. Because this vertebra does not have a spinous process, there is no bone posteriorly between the occipital bone and the spinous process of C2. This results in an increase in the potential for craniovertebral extension.

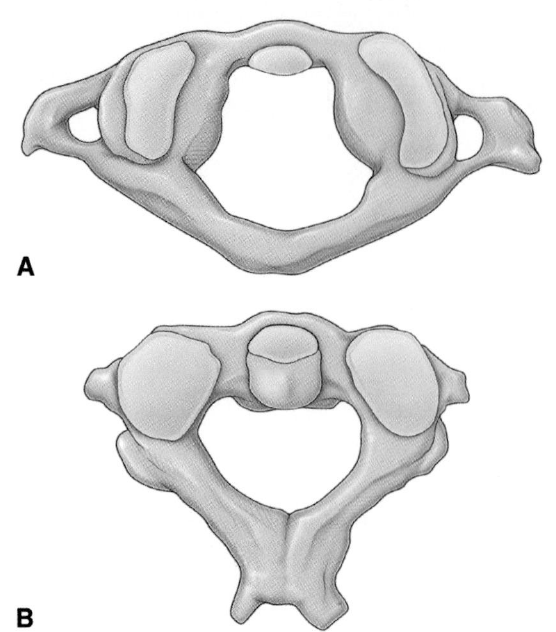

FIGURE 23-1 Bony structures of the craniovertebral joints. **A.** The atlas (C 1). **B.** The axis.

The superolateral aspect of each of the posterior arches has a transverse foramen to accommodate the vertebral artery (see Chap. 24). The articular surface of the inferior facet is circular and relatively flat and slopes inferiorly from medial to lateral. The upper articular facets of C1 are elongated from anterior to posterior, with the anterior ends closer together and more upwardly curved than their posterior counterparts.[3] This arrangement results in much more extension than flexion being available at the articulation between the occipital condyles and the atlas—the occipitoatlantal (O-A) joint.[4]

O-A Joint

The O-A joint represents the most superior zygapophyseal joint of the vertebral column and the only vertebral level that has an articulation characterized by a convex surface (occipital condyle) moving on a concave joint partner (articulating facet of the atlas).[5]

Axis

The axis serves as a transitional vertebra (Fig. 23-1), because it is the link between the cervical spine proper and the craniovertebral region.

The dimensions of the axis are significantly different from those of the atlas. The atlas is considerably wider than the axis, but because of the long spinous process, the axis extends much farther posteriorly and is the first palpable midline structure below the occiput.[6] Like the atlas, the transverse process of the axis has a transverse foramen to allow passage of the vertebral artery (not shown).

A unique feature of the axis is the odontoid process, or dens (Fig. 23-2). The dens, which develops with age, extends superiorly from the body to just above the C1 vertebra, before tapering to a blunt point. Very dense, thick trabecular bone is present in the center of the tip of the dens, and the cortical bone at the anterior base of the body of C2 (where the anterior longitudinal ligament attaches) is uniformly thick.[7] Hypodense bone, however, is present consistently beneath the odontoid process at the upper portion of the body of C2.[8] This area of hypodense bone is susceptible to fracture. The anterior aspect of the dens has a hyaline cartilage-covered mid-line facet for articulation with the anterior tubercle of the atlas (the median atlantoaxial (A-A) joint). The posterior aspect of the dens usually is marked with a groove where the transverse ligament passes. The dens functions as a pivot for the upper cervical joints and as the center of rotation for the A-A joint. The most variable dimension of the axis is the dens angle in the sagittal plane, which can range from –2 degrees (leaning slightly anterior) to 42 degrees (leaning posterior).[9] This extremely variable angle can make assessment of fracture reduction challenging.[7]

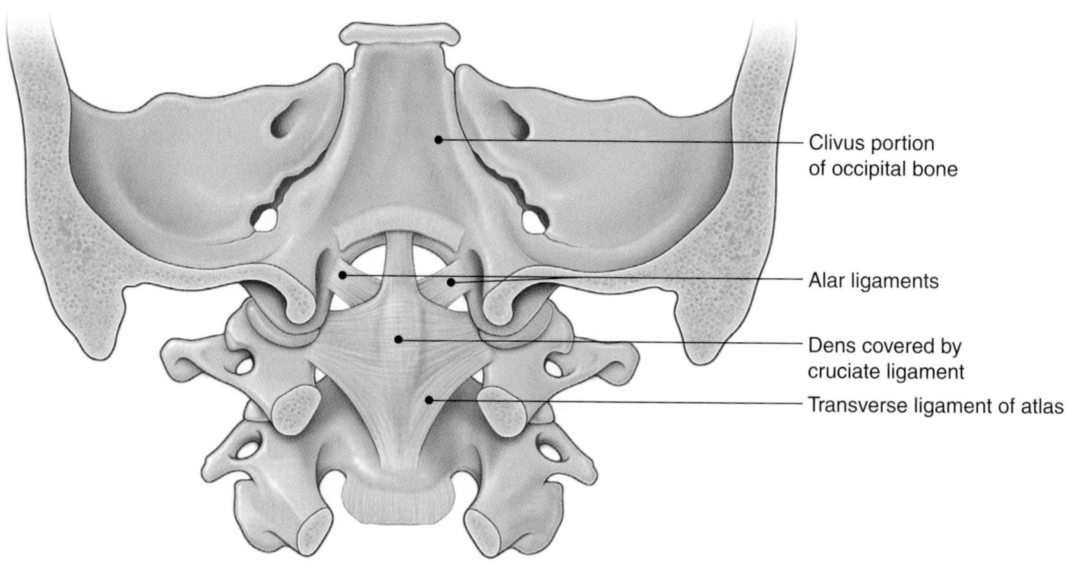

FIGURE 23-2 Ligamentous structures of the craniovertebral joints.

A-A Joint

This is a relatively complex articulation, which consists of

- two lateral zygapophyseal joints between the articular surfaces of the inferior articular processes of the atlas and the superior processes of the axis;
- two medial joints: one between the anterior surface of the dens of the axis and the anterior surface of the atlas, and the other between the posterior surface of the dens and the anterior hyalinated surface of the transverse ligament[6] (Fig. 23-2).

The relatively large superior articular facets of the axis (Fig. 23-2) lie lateral and anterior to the dens. These facets slope considerably downward from medial to lateral in line with the zygapophyseal facets of the mid-low cervical spine.[10] As the lateral A-A joints function to convey the entire weight of the atlas and the head to lower structures, the lamina and pedicles of the axis are quite robust.[11] The stout, moderately long spinous process serves as the uppermost attachment for muscles that are essentially lower cervical in nature and for muscles that act specifically on the craniovertebral joints.

One of the functions of the intervertebral disk (IVD) in the spine is to facilitate motion and provide stability. Thus, in the absence of an IVD in this region, the supporting soft tissues of the joints of the upper cervical spine must be lax to permit motion, while simultaneously being able to withstand great mechanical stresses.

Craniovertebral Ligaments

The craniovertebral region is noted for a variety of ligaments, some of which have been the focus of a number of clinical tests to determine their efficiency in preventing unwanted and potentially dangerous movements. The controlling structures for these segments, which must be considered together, are the

- ***Capsule and accessory capsular ligaments.*** The lateral capsular ligaments (anterolateral O-A ligament) of the O-A joints are typical of synovial joint capsules. These ligaments run obliquely from the basiocciput to the transverse process of the atlas. By necessity, they are quite lax, to permit maximal motion, so they provide only moderate support to the joints during contralateral head rotation.
- ***Apical ligament.*** The apical ligament of the dens extends from the apex of the dens to the anterior rim of the foramen magnum. The ligament is short and thick. It runs from the top of the dens to the basi-occiput and is thought to be a remnant of the notochord. The apical ligament appears to be only a moderate stabilizer against posterior translation of the dens relative to both the atlas and the occipital bone.[11]
- ***Vertical and transverse bands of the cruciform ligament.*** (See Fig. 23-2 and later discussion.)
- ***Alar and accessory alar ligaments.*** (See Fig. 23-2 and later discussion.)
- ***Anterior O-A membrane.*** The anterior O-A membrane is thought to be the superior continuation of the anterior longitudinal ligament. It connects the anterior arch of vertebra C1 to the anterior aspect of the foramen magnum.
- ***Posterior O-A membrane.*** The posterior O-A membrane is a continuation of the ligamentum flavum. This ligament interconnects the posterior arch of the atlas and the posterior aspect of the foramen magnum and forms part of the posterior boundary of the vertebral canal.[11]
- ***Tectorial membrane.*** The tectorial membrane is the most superficial of the three membranes and interconnects the occipital bone and the axis. This ligament is the superior continuation of the posterior longitudinal ligament and connects the body of vertebra C2 to the anterior rim of the foramen magnum. This bridging ligament is an important limiter of upper cervical flexion and holds the occiput off the atlas.[12]

A-A Ligaments

The anterior A-A ligament is continuous with the anterior O-A membrane above. [13] The posterior A-A ligament interconnects the posterior arch of the atlas and the laminae of the axis.

Occipitoaxial Ligaments

The O-A ligaments are very important to the stability of the upper cervical spine.

Alar Ligament[5]

The alar ligaments (see Fig. 23-2) connect the superior part of the dens to fossae on the medial aspect of the occipital condyles, although they can also attach to the lateral masses of the atlas.[14,15] A study of 44 cadavers[16] found the orientation of the ligament to be superior, posterior, and lateral. In another study, [14] 19 upper cervical spine specimens were dissected to examine the macroscopic and functional anatomy of alar ligaments. The study found that the most common orientation (10/19) was cauda-cranial, followed by transverse (5/19). In two of the specimens, a previously undescribed ligamentous connection was found between the dens and the anterior arch of the atlas, the anterior atlantodental ligament. In 12 specimens, the ligament also attached via caudal fibers to the lateral mass of the atlas. The posteroanterior orientation of the ligaments in 17 of the 19 subjects was directly lateral from the dens to the occipital attachment or slightly posterior.

The function of the ligament is to resist flexion, contralateral side bending, and contralateral O-A rotation.[17] In addition, the alar ligaments restrict anteroposterior translation of the occiput on C1 to some degree.[18] Because of the connections of the ligament, side bending of the head produces a contralateral or ipsilateral rotation of C2, depending on the source.[19]

CLINICAL PEARL

Insufficiency of the alar ligaments increases the potential for occipitoaxial instability. The degree of instability can be determined in conjunction with other clinical findings, such as neurologic or vascular compromise, pain, and deformity.

The Cruciform Ligament

The cruciform (cross-shaped) ligament has superior, inferior, and transverse portions (Fig. 23-2). The superior and inferior portions of this ligament attach to the posterior aspect of the body of the dens and the anterior rim of the foramen magnum. The transverse portion, which stretches between tubercles on the medial aspects of the lateral masses of the atlas, connects the atlas with the dens of the axis. The transverse portion of the ligament is so distinct and important that it is often considered a separate ligament (Fig. 23-2). The major responsibility of the transverse ligament is to counteract anterior translation of the atlas relative to the axis, thereby maintaining the position of the dens relative to the anterior arch of the atlas.[12]

The transverse ligament also limits the amount of flexion between the atlas and axis.[20] These limiting functions are of extreme importance because excessive movement of either type could result in the dens compressing the spinal cord, epipharynx, vertebral artery, or superior cervical ganglion. The integrity of the transverse ligament is also essential to the stability of atlas fractures; degenerative, inflammatory, and congenital disorders; and other abnormalities that affect the craniovertebral region.

The importance of the ligament is reflected in its physical properties. Spontaneous or isolated traumatic tears of this ligament are extremely rare events. The ligament is comprised almost entirely of collagen, with a parallel orientation close to the atlas and the dens, but with an approximately 30-degree obliquity at other points in the ligament. Dvorak and colleagues[21] found the transverse ligament to be almost twice as strong as the alar ligaments and to have a tensile strength of 330 Newtons (N) (33 kg/73 lb).

Craniovertebral Muscles

Anterior Suboccipital Muscles

Rectus Capitis Anterior. The rectus capitis anterior (RCA) runs vertically. It travels deep to the longus capitis from the anterior aspect of the lateral mass of the atlas to the inferior surface of the base of the occiput, anterior to the occipital condyle. The RCA flexes and minimally rotates the head. Thus, an adaptively shortened RCA on the right could feasibly produce a decreased left translation in extension during mobility testing of the O-A joint. The muscle is supplied by the anterior (ventral) rami of C1 and C2.

Rectus Capitis Lateralis. This muscle arises from the superior surface of the C1 transverse process and inserts into the inferior surface of the jugular process of the occiput. It is homologous to the posterior intertransverse muscle of the spine. The rectus capitis lateralis side bends the head ipsilaterally. It is supplied by the anterior (ventral) rami of C1 and C2.

Posterior Suboccipital Muscles. The posterior suboccipitals lie beneath the splenius capitis and trapezius muscles. These muscles function in the control of segmental sliding between C1 and C2[22] and may have an important role in proprioception, having more muscle spindles than any other muscle for their size.[22] All of the posterior suboccipital muscles are innervated by the posterior ramus of C1 and also are strongly linked with the trigeminal nerve.[23,24] The suboccipitals receive their blood supply from the vertebral artery.

Rectus Capitis Posterior Major. The rectus capitis posterior major is the largest of the posterior suboccipitals. It runs from the C2 spinous process, widening as it runs cranially to attach to the lateral part of inferior nuchal line (Fig. 23-3). Located inferior and lateral to the occipital

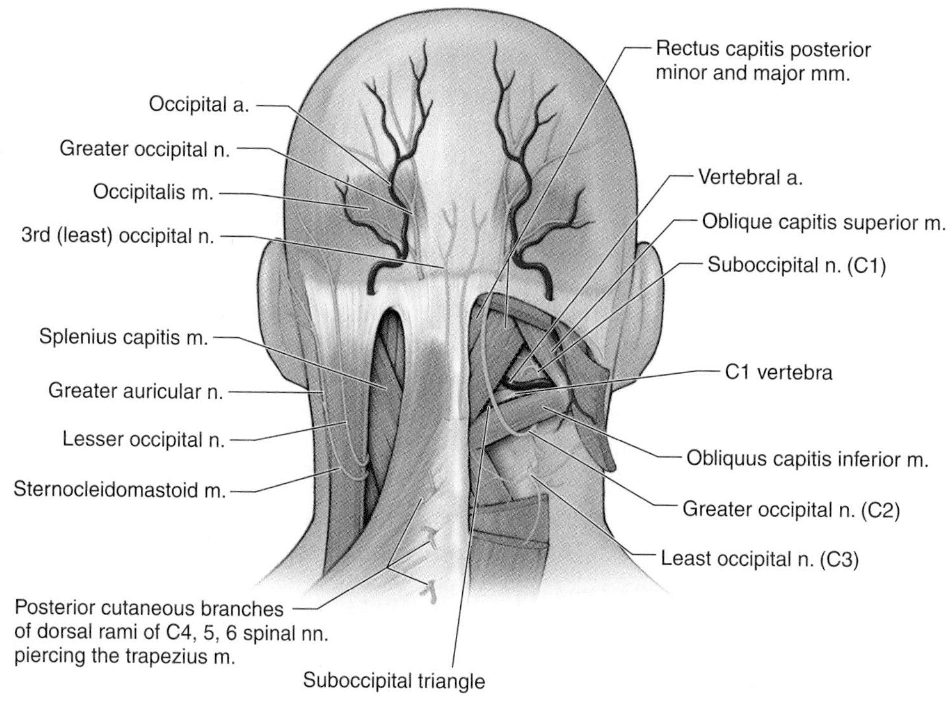

FIGURE 23-3 Muscles of the craniovertebral joints.

protuberances, the rectus capitis posterior major muscles, when working together, extend the head. When working individually, the muscles produce ipsilateral side bending and rotation of the head.

Rectus Capitis Posterior Minor. The rectus capitis posterior minor is a small unisegmental muscle that runs from the posterior arch tubercle of the atlas to the medial part of the inferior nuchal line (see Fig. 23-3). Because of the shortness of the atlantean tubercle, the muscle is very horizontal, running almost parallel with the occiput. The muscle functions to extend the head and provides minimal support during ipsilateral side bending of the head.

CLINICAL PEARL

Connective tissue attachments between the rectus capitis posterior minor and dura mater recently have been identified.[25] This finding has led to the use of cervical flexion with neurodynamic mobility tests (see Chap. 11). The differentiation between adverse neural tension and adaptive shortening of the muscle can be made by performing short neck flexion, with the neural system pretensioned and then relaxed.

Obliquus Capitis Inferior. This is the larger of the two oblique muscles and runs from the spinous process and lamina of the axis superolaterally to the transverse process of the atlas (see Fig. 23-3).

The inferior oblique muscle works to produce ipsilateral rotation of the atlas and skull and to control anterior translation and rotation of C1 (atlas). An adaptively shortened right inferior oblique may exert an inferior and posterior pull on the right transverse process of the atlas, producing a right rotated A-A joint.[26,27] This results in a gross limitation of left rotation of the head while in cervical flexion, but a minimal limitation of left rotation of the head in extension.

Obliquus Capitis Superior. The superior oblique arises from the transverse process of the atlas and runs superoposterior and medially to the bone between the superior and inferior nuchal lines, lateral to the attachment of rectus capitis posterior major (see Fig. 23-3). Because of its posteromedial orientation, the superior oblique functions to provide contralateral rotation and ipsilateral side bending of the O-A joint, when acting unilaterally. When working together, the two superior obliques can produce head extension. Dysfunction of this muscle has been implicated as a common cause of chronic headaches.[28–32]

The posterior sub-occipital muscles can work concentrically with the larger extensors and rotators of the cervical spine, or eccentrically, controlling the action of the flexors. Because two of these muscles parallel the occiput, their controlling influence may be more linear than angular, producing or guiding the arthrokinematic, rather than the osteokinematic, motion.[22]

Nerve Supply

The posterior (dorsal) ramus of spinal nerve C1 is larger than the anterior (ventral) ramus. It exits from the spinal canal by passing posteriorly between the posterior arch of the atlas and the rim of the foramen magnum, along with the vertebral artery. It then enters the suboccipital triangle and supplies most of the muscles that form that triangle. It usually has no cutaneous distribution.

The posterior (dorsal) ramus of spinal nerve C2 (see Fig. 23-3), also known as the greater occipital nerve, is larger than the anterior (ventral) ramus of C2. It exits from the vertebral canal by passing through the slit between the posterior arch of the atlas and the lamina of the axis. This nerve is the largest of the cervical posterior (dorsal) rami and is primarily a cutaneous nerve. It supplies most of the posterior aspect of the scalp, extending anteriorly to a line across the scalp that runs from one external auditory meatus to the other. Because this nerve has an extensive cutaneous distribution, it has a very large posterior (dorsal) root ganglion. This ganglion is commonly located in a vulnerable location, almost directly between the posterior arch of C1 and the lamina of C2 (see Fig. 23-3). The interval between these two bony structures is small, and it is reduced with extension of the upper cervical spine. Given the sensitivity of the posterior (dorsal) root ganglion to compression, the possible relationship between the forward head position and occipital headaches is apparent.[28–32] The O-A joints,[33] A-A joints,[34] and the C2 spinal nerve[35] have all been implicated as primary nociceptors in cervicogenic headaches (CHs). Among individuals with chronic neck pain, 58–88% describe associated headaches.[36,37] The prevalence of C2–3 zygapophyseal joint pain has been estimated at 50–53% in those patients with a chief complaint of headaches after whiplash injury.[36,37]

Blood Supply

The intradural vertebral artery supplies the most superior segments of the cervical spinal cord (see Chap. 24). The cervical cord is supplied by two arterial systems, central and peripheral, which overlap but are discrete. The first is dependent entirely on the single anterior spinal artery (ASA). The second, without clear-cut boundaries, receives supplies from the ASA and both posterior spinal arteries.[38] Because the ASA is medial and dominant, unilateral spinal cord infarctions are very rare. However, they may occur in the perfusion territory supplied by the ASA.[39,40] This is a result of obstruction of either a duplicated ASA[40] or one of the sulcal arteries, which arise from the ASA and turn alternatively left or right to supply one side of the central cord. [41] Peripheral hemicord infarction may result from ischemia, in the territory of the ASA[39] or posterior spinal artery.[42]

Biomechanics

The upper cervical spine is responsible for approximately 50% of the motion that occurs throughout the entire cervical spine. Motions at the O-A and A-A joints occur relatively independently, while below C2, normal motion is a combination of motion at other levels.

Articular facet asymmetry of the human upper cervical spine has been recognized for more than 30 years.[43,44] The implications of this anatomic observation in the human spine has been considered in relation to joint disease, specifically, facet tropism (the phenomenon observed in living tissue, of moving toward or away from a focus of stimulus), which is associated with subsequent degenerative joint disease.[45,46]

CLINICAL PEARL

Due to the proximity of vital structures, joint disease in this region can have severe consequences. These consequences can include

- vertebral artery compromise;
- compression of the spinal cord;
- brainstem lesions.

O-A Joint

The deep atlantal sockets of the atlas facilitate flexion–extension but impede other movements. In living individuals the average mean motion of flexion and extension at this joint is a combined range of 15–20 degrees.[47] However, the variability in range of motion in normal subject is large. Lind et al.[48] reported a mean of 14 degrees with a standard deviation of 15 degrees in normal subjects. Side bending motion occurs at an average of a little over 9 degrees to both sides,[49–51] with an axial rotation range of 0 degrees (8 degrees when the movement was forced).[50,51]

Although it is generally agreed that rotation and side bending at this joint occur to opposite sides when they are combined, particular rules for patterns of defined coupled motion are not supported by the current literature.[52]

CLINICAL PEARL

Clinical studies suggest that hypermobility of this joint should only be considered as a diagnosis if the range of axial rotation exceeds 8 degrees, making rotational mobility and stability testing necessary at this articulation.

A-A Joint

The design of the ligamentous and bony structures at the A-A joint allow for a large arc of rotation.

CLINICAL PEARL

Within the spine, only two articulations permit pure axial rotation:

- The A-A joint
- The thoracolumbar junction

The major motion that occurs at all three of the A-A articulations is axial rotation. Werne[49] reported 47 degrees to each side in cadavers. A more recent study using CT scanning observed 32 degrees (SD, 10) of axial rotation to either side.[51] This amount of rotation has the potential to cause compression of the vertebral artery (see Chap. 24).[53,54] To help prevent this compression, as the atlas rotates, the ipsilateral facet moves posteriorly while the contralateral facet moves anteriorly, so that each facet of the atlas slides inferiorly along the convex surface of the axial facet, telescoping the head downward.

The first 25 degrees of head rotation (approximately 60%) occur primarily at the A-A articulations.[55] However, the axial rotation of the atlas is not a pure motion, because it is coupled with a significant degree of extension (14 degrees) and, in some cases, flexion.[56]

In living individuals, the reported range of flexion–extension motion at this joint is highly variable, averaging 10 degrees.[57] Flexion at the A-A joint is limited by the tectorial membrane. Extension is limited by the anterior arch of C1, as it makes contact with the odontoid process. The flexion and extension motions are associated with small anteroposterior translational movements, which can create a small space between the back of the anterior arch of the atlas and the odontoid. This space is called the atlanto-odontoid interval (ADI). Because of the arthrokinematics of the joint, flexion increases the ADI, whereas extension decreases it. Excessive gapping of the ADI can have serious consequences, as it can lead to a compression of the spinal cord by the atlas.[58] An ADI of more than 3 mm in adults, and 4.5 mm in children younger than 12 years of age, detected on radiographs is indicative of gross instability and is strongly suggestive of a compromise of the transverse ligament.[58] An increased ADI can be associated with a history of trauma but also may be associated with severe ligamentous laxity in patients with rheumatoid arthritis (RA), neoplastic disease, Down's syndrome, and aplasia or dysplasia of the dens.[19]

Side bending at this joint is approximately 5 degrees. Although coupling at this joint is commonly cited as contralateral side bending during rotation, it is highly variable because of the passive nature of the kinematics of the atlas.[59] Whether the atlas flexes or extends during axial rotation depends on the geometry of the A-A joint and the precise direction of any forces acting through the atlas from the head.[59] The direction of the conjunct rotation appears to be dependent on the initiating movement.[60,61] If the initiating movement is side bending (latexion), the conjunct rotation of the joint is to the opposite side. If the initiating movement is rotation (rotexion), the conjunct motion (side bending) is to the same side.[60,61] If correct, this principle can be exploited in the assessment of the craniovertebral joints:

1. ***Rotexion.*** During rotation of the head to the right (rotexion):
   a. Left side bending and right rotation occur at the O-A joint, accompanied by a translation to the right.
   b. Right side bending and right rotation occur at the A-A joint and at C2–3.

   In other words, if the head motion is initiated with rotation, ipsilateral side bending of the A-A joint and C2–3 occurs, whereas at the O-A joint, contralateral side bending occurs.
2. ***Latexion.*** Side bending of the head to the right produces
   a. left rotation of the O-A joint, accompanied by a translation of the occiput to the left;
   b. left rotation of the A-A joint;
   c. right rotation of C2–3.

In other words, if head motion is initiated with side bending, contralateral rotation of both the O-A and the A-A joints occurs, but ipsilateral rotation occurs at C2–3.

EXAMINATION

The primary objective of the examination of this region is to rule out any serious injury, especially if the patient reports any recent trauma to the head or neck. The pain distribution from cervical structures is outlined in Table 23-1 and the differential diagnoses are described in Chapter 5. The initial examination should focus on the general appearance of the patient (including skin lesions such as rashes), vital signs (pulse, blood pressure, and temperature), and the presence of any upper motor neuron signs or symptoms.[62] Once serious injury has been ruled out, a biomechanical assessment of the craniovertebral joints can be performed. In addition, because of their close relationship with the craniovertebral joints, the cervical spine (see Chap. 25) and temporomandibular joint (see Chap. 26) should be assessed as part of a comprehensive examination of this region.

The biomechanical examination of the craniovertebral joints is best performed in a sequential manner (Fig. 23-4). In general, the O-A joint is examined and treated before the A-A joint to avoid confusion between findings from the combined testing of both joints. The examination and any intervention are terminated if any serious signs and/or symptoms are produced. In these instances, an appropriate referral is made.

History

The craniovertebral region, as with the rest of the neck, is a common area for myofascial pain syndromes. These syndromes are frequently associated with complaints of local muscle soreness, and muscle spasm.[63] Pain may also be referred to this region from trigger points in the upper trapezius muscle, splenius capitis, sternocleidomastoid (SCM) muscle, digastric muscle, cervicis muscles, posterior cervical muscles (semispinalis capitis, semispinalis cervicis, multifidus, and rotators), and sub-occipital muscles (rectus capitis posterior major and minor and inferior and superior obliques) (refer to "Intervention" section).[63]

TABLE 23-1 Pain Distribution from Cervical Structures

Structure	Pain Area
Occipital condyles	Frontal
Occipitocervical tissues	Frontal
C1 posterior (dorsal) ramus	Orbit, frontal, and vertex
C1—2	Temporal and suboccipital
C3 posterior (dorsal) ramus	Occiput, mastoid, and frontal

Data from Meadows J: *A Rationale and Complete Approach to the Sub-Acute Post-MVA Cervical Patient.* Calgary, AB: Swodeam Consulting, 1995.

Complaints of headaches are also common in patients with craniovertebral joint dysfunction.[33-35] Some of the more common types of headaches are described in Chapter 5. In all patients presenting with an unexplained or unusual headache, a full neurologic and general physical examination is required.[62] This examination should focus on the patient's mental status and speech, gait, balance and coordination, a cranial nerve and long tract examination, and an examination of visual fields, and acuity (see Chap. 3).[62]

Patients who complain of headaches should be asked to describe the headache. The clinician must always be alert to the potential coincidental occurrence of secondary headache syndromes. These include headache associated with trauma, vascular disease, nonvascular intracranial disorders, substance abuse or withdrawal, noncephalic infections, metabolic disorders, disorders of facial or cranial structures, and cranial neuralgia.[64] Several conditions may mimic episodic or chronic tension-type headache (see Chap. 5), including muscle tension. Chronic tension-type headaches are often erroneously attributed to chronic sinusitis, but clinical and radiologic evidence must be obtained before making this diagnosis. A causal relationship between tension-type headache and oromandibular dysfunction is controversial, but the two conditions often coexist.[65] The most important structures that register pain within the skull are the blood vessels, particularly the proximal part of the cerebral arteries, as well as the large veins and venous sinuses.[66] The chronic headache of intracranial hypotension is most often distinguished by an increase of pain on standing. Descriptions such as throbbing and pounding are suggestive of a vascular origin but can also inculpate migraine, fever, neuralgia, or hypertension. Chronic, recurrent headaches can be associated with eyestrain, excessive eating or drinking, or smoking.

Intrinsic to the understanding of the relationship of headache to the craniovertebral region are the intracranial pain pathways and their interconnections, especially the trigeminocervical pathway (see Chap. 3).

The location of the headache can provide the clinician with useful information as to the source.

- Forehead pain may be caused by sinusitis or a muscle spasm of the occipital or sub-occipital region.
- Occipital pain can be caused by eyestrain, herniated cervical disk, hypertension, neuralgia, or an ear or eye disorder.
- Parietal pain may be indicative of meningitis or a tumor.
- Facial pain can be caused by sinusitis, trigeminal neuralgia, dental problems, or a tumor.

Dizziness (vertigo) and nystagmus are nonspecific neurologic signs that require a careful diagnostic workup (see Chap. 3). A report of vertigo, although potentially problematic, is not a contraindication to the continuation of the examination.

CLINICAL PEARL

Dizziness associated with disorders of motor function, such as clumsiness, weakness, or paralysis, could suggest compromise of the vertebrobasilar system.

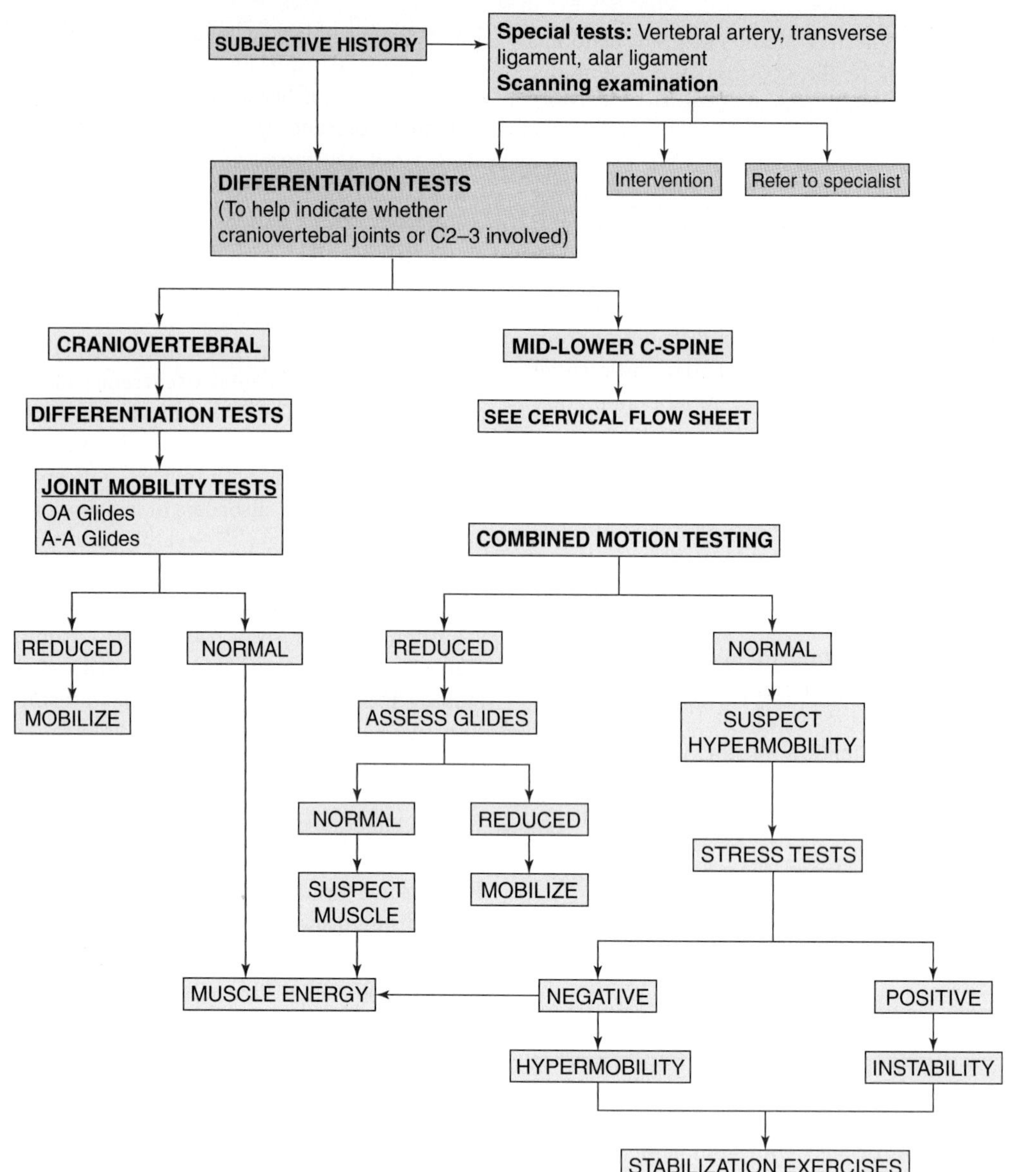

FIGURE 23-4 Craniovertebral examination algorithm.

Systems Review

The craniovertebral region houses many vital structures. These include the spinal cord, the vertebral artery, and the brain stem. It is extremely important for the clinician to approach this area with caution and to rule out the presence of serious pathology. Craniovertebral and cranial dysfunction can be responsible for a number of signs and symptoms that may be benign or may indicate the presence of serious pathology (Table 23-2).

Due to the proximity of the cranial structures, the clinician should develop the habit of quickly screening patients with neck and head pain for their ability to orient to time, place, and name; concentrate; reason and process information; make judgments; communicate effectively; and recall information. Obtaining this information needs to be done in a sensitive manner. Asking questions as to whether the patients know their own name and what day it is may be considered inappropriate by some patients. Most of the concerns about the patient's mental status can be addressed through general conversation, or as part of the history. Perhaps surprisingly, the incidence of neurologic involvement in upper cervical spine injury is relatively low (18–26%).[67] This may be because, significant cord damage in the upper cervical spine is usually fatal secondary to respiratory arrest.[7]

When compression of the spinal cord is suspected, a thorough neurologic examination should be performed. If confirmed, the appropriate medical services should be contacted. The cranial nerves should be assessed, particularly if there are complaints about vision or the patient appears to have problems with speech or swallowing. Patients with referred pain in the region of the trigeminal nerve commonly have an underlying disorder of the upper cervical spine, such as A-A instability caused by RA.[63,68] As described in Chapter 3, the various cranial nerve tests can be performed in approximately 5 minutes with practice.

Tests and Measures

The examination is terminated if any serious signs and symptoms are produced.

TABLE 23-2 Examination Findings and the Possible Conditions Causing Them

Findings	Possible Condition
Dizziness	Upper cervical impairment, vertebrobasilar ischemia, and craniovertebral ligament tear; also may be relatively benign
Quadrilateral paresthesia	Cord compression and vertebrobasilar ischemia
Bilateral upper limb paresthesia	Cord compression and vertebrobasilar ischemia
Hyperreflexia	Cord compression and vertebrobasilar ischemia
Babinski or clonus sign	Cord compression and vertebrobasilar ischemia
Consistent swallow on transverse ligament stress tests	Instability, retropharyngeal hematoma, and rheumatoid arthritis
Nontraumatic capsular pattern	Rheumatoid arthritis, ankylosing spondylitis, and neoplasm
Arm pain lasting >6–9 mo	Neoplasm
Persistent root pain <30 y	Neoplasm
Radicular pain with coughing	Neoplasm
Pain worsening after 1 mo	Neoplasm
>1 level involved	Neoplasm
Paralysis	Neoplasm or neurologic disease
Trunk and limb paresthesia	Neoplasm
Bilateral root signs and symptoms	Neoplasm
Nontraumatic strong spasm	Neoplasm
Nontraumatic strong pain in elderly patient	Neoplasm
Signs worse than symptoms	Neoplasm
Radial deviator weakness	Neoplasm
Thumb flexor weakness	Neoplasm
Hand intrinsic weakness or atrophy	Neoplasm, thoracic outlet syndrome, and carpal tunnel syndrome
Horner's syndrome	Superior sulcus tumor, breast cancer, cervical ganglion damage, and brain stem damage
Empty end-feel	Neoplasm
Severe post-traumatic capsular pattern	Fracture
Severe post-traumatic spasm	Fracture
Loss of ROM post-trauma	Fracture
Post-traumatic painful weakness	Fracture

Data from Meadows J. *Orthopaedic Differential Diagnosis in Physical Therapy.* New York: McGraw-Hill; 1999.
ROM, range of motion.

Observation

The patient is observed in the sagittal, coronal, and transverse planes.

Sagittal Plane. Observing the status of the cervical curve and the relative position of the patient's chin to the chest helps the clinician to assess postural alignment in the sagittal plane. A popular view among clinicians is that habitual adoption of extreme cervical posture may account for symptoms of pain and dysfunction arising from the head and neck area.[69] The argument is that alterations in spinal alignment may lead to changes in muscle activity and loading on the surrounding soft tissue and articular structures, which then predisposes patients to such complaints.[70,71] This argument has been supported in several studies, which have found a statistically significant correlation between the tendency to hold the head forward, relative to the true vertical in the so-called *forward head posture*, and symptoms of pain.[71,72] However, in other investigations, no such correlation has been confirmed.[73,74]

Tucking or elevation of the chin in the presence of a normal cervical curve may indicate craniovertebral dysfunction.[75]

The ears are observed for the presence of asymmetry in size, shape, or color. The top of the ear is normally in line with the eyebrow.

Coronal Plane. Alignment in the coronal plane is assessed by observing the orientation of the head relative to the trunk and shoulders, the leveling of the mastoid processes, and the symmetry of the cervical soft tissues. The face is observed for any asymmetry or indications of bruising, puffiness, prominence, swelling, perspiration, or abnormal skin color. Any asymmetry in the relative size of the pupils of the eyes and the distance between the upper and lower lids is noted. Pupillary size differences can occur in normal individuals but initially should arouse concern, because an abnormal unilateral change in size may be caused by an autonomic dysfunction or a central nervous system lesion.[76] The superior lid should cover a portion of the iris but not the pupil itself, unless ptosis or drooping of the eyelid is present[76] (see Chap. 3).

Missing teeth should be accounted for as a loss of teeth may be a result of trauma, avulsion, or loosening.

Transverse Plane. Alignment in the transverse plane is assessed by observing the patient from behind and noting the orientation of the head. The orientation of the head is best observed by noting any asymmetry in the position of the mastoids, which can indicate whether the head is more rotated or tilted to one side, both of which may indicate a positional fault of the craniovertebral joints. Bruising around the mastoids or around the crown of the head (Battle's sign), with a history of trauma, may indicate the presence of a cranial vault injury, such as a basilar fracture. A low hairline may indicate a condition such as Klippel–Feil syndrome,[77] defined as a short neck with decreased cervical movement and low posterior hairline. Radiologically, patients with Klippel–Feil syndrome show a failure of cervical segmentation. The etiology is unclear, but the syndrome is believed to be caused by faulty segmentation of the mesodermal somites.[78] The syndrome appears to be heterogeneous, with environmental factors possibly contributing.[79] Autosomal dominant and recessive patterns of inheritance also have been reported.[80]

Active Range of Motion, Passive Overpressure, and Resistance

Short Neck Flexion. The clinician instructs the patient to place his or her chin on the surface of the throat. This motion simulates flexion at the craniovertebral joints. If this maneuver produces tingling in the feet or electric shock sensations down the neck (Lhermitte's sign), it is highly indicative of serious pathology. Although Lhermitte's sign is not a specific symptom, it is commonly encountered in patients with meningitis (see Chap. 5) and cervical spinal cord demyelination caused by multiple sclerosis.[81] The sign also has been found in many other conditions that cause a traumatic or compressive cervical myelopathy, such as cervical spondylosis, cervical instability, and epidural or subdural tumors.[82,83]

If the patient reports a pulling sensation during short neck flexion, the cervicothoracic junction may be at fault. Active short neck flexion tests cranial nerve XI and the C1 and C2

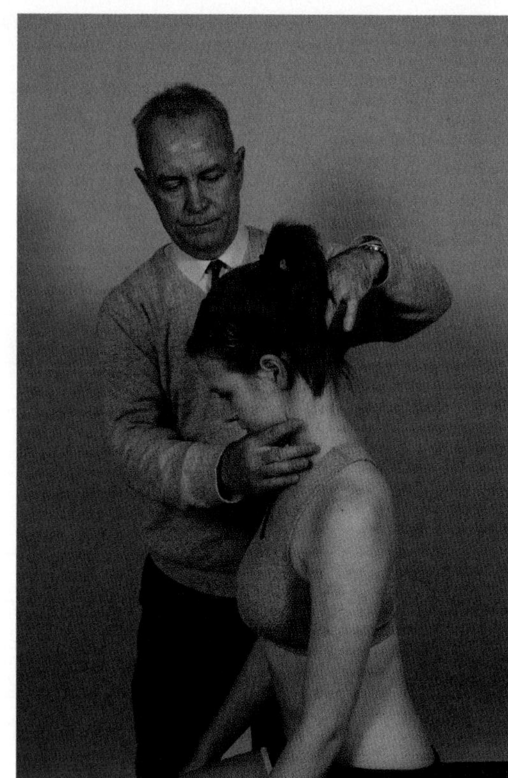

FIGURE 23-5 Short neck flexion with overpressure and resistance.

myotomes, as well as the patient's willingness to move. Placing the neck in short neck flexion places the short neck extensors (C1), which are innervated by the spinal accessory nerve, on stretch. The clinician applies overpressure and tests the short neck extensors by asking the patient to resist (Fig. 23-5). Positive findings with this test are severe pain, nausea, muscle spasm, or cord signs, the latter of which may indicate a dens fracture or a tumor and cause the examination to be terminated.[82] Thus, if a patient is able to perform short neck flexion, a cervical fracture or a transverse ligament compromise can be provisionally ruled out.

Short Neck Extension. The clinician instructs the patient to look upward by only lifting the chin. The patient extends the head on the neck and the clinician attempts to lift the occiput in the direction of the ceiling (Fig. 23-6). An inability to perform, or pain during, this motion (in the presence of normal motion in the other planes) may indicate significant tearing of the anterior cervical structures. If this test produces tingling in the feet, it is highly suggestive of compression to the spinal cord. This compression may occur because of "buckling" or ossification of the ligamentum flavum, with resultant loss of its elasticity.[84] A loss of balance or a drop attack with this maneuver would strongly suggest compromise of the vertebrobasilar system. A drop attack is defined as a loss of balance without a loss of consciousness (see Chap. 24). The short neck flexors (C1), which are innervated by the spinal accessory nerve, can be tested in this position by applying overpressure as though lifting the patient's chin toward the ceiling while the patient resists (see Fig. 23-6).

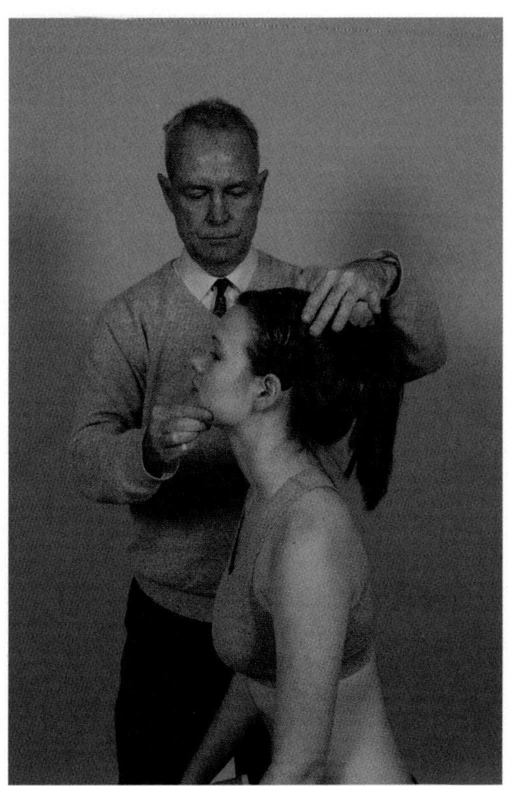

FIGURE 23-6 Short neck extension with overpressure and resistance.

CLINICAL PEARL

If the neck is unstable secondary to a dens fracture or a transverse ligament tear, the patient will be unable or unwilling to flex or extend the neck in the traditional manner, often because of severe muscle spasm.

Side Bending. The patient is asked to side bend their head around the appropriate axis (through the patient's nose). Side bending is included here for completeness. Much more a function of the lower cervical spine, side bending of the neck is nonetheless significantly decreased in cases of craniovertebral instability or articular fixation. It could be argued that, in the presence of serious ligamentous disruption due to a subluxation of the atlas under the occiput, this motion may provoke symptoms, but it is likely that such a significant incidence of instability would be detected earlier in the examination.[85] The side-bending motions that do occur in the craniovertebral joints are essentially conjunct motions, so the results from this test are unlikely to provide much in the way of additional information.

Rotation. Neck and head rotation could be considered as the functional motion of the craniovertebral joints. Thus, if the patient's symptoms and loss of motion are not reproduced with active rotation, it is doubtful that damage to tissues making up the craniovertebral joints is significant or even present. The patient is asked to perform active neck rotation. An inability to move any amount in either direction is potentially a very serious sign, as it could indicate the presence of a dens fracture or a C1–2 dislocation–fracture. Every measure must be taken to determine the cause of this inability to move. In cases of a suspected fracture or severe instability, the patient should be placed in a cervical collar and the physician immediately notified. In addition to the presence of a fracture, some of the other serious conditions that can be provoked by cervical rotation include vertebral artery compromise—cervical rotation is the most likely (single) motion to reproduce signs or symptoms of vertebral artery compromise (see Chap. 24).[82,86–88]

The findings from the cervical rotation tests may also afford the clinician some information with regard to a biomechanical lesion of the craniovertebral joints:

- A loss of rotation associated with pain and a history of recent trauma. This could indicate the presence of an acute/subacute, posttraumatic arthritis of the craniovertebral joints. Since it may also indicate a soft tissue injury, further testing would be required.
- A loss of rotation associated with pain and a history of chronic trauma. This finding could indicate a chronic painless hypomobility with an adaptive but painful ipsilateral hypermobility involving the craniovertebral joints (e.g., pain with right rotation could occur if the right O-A joint cannot flex and there is a hypermobility of the right A-A joint). It may also occur if the left O-A joint cannot extend. Again, further testing is needed to confirm this hypothesis.
- A loss of rotation range of motion associated with no pain, but with a history of chronic trauma. This finding, which could indicate a chronic, posttraumatic arthritis, is likely to be an incidental finding, since most patients seek help because of pain. However, depending on the extent of the loss of rotation, the patient may have become aware of a loss of function.
- Full rotation range of motion associated with pain and a history of chronic trauma. This could indicate a chronic fibrotic (painless) hypomobility with an adaptive but painful contralateral hypermobility (e.g., pain with right rotation could occur if the left O-A joint cannot flex and the right O-A joint develops a compensatory hypermobility).

Palpation

Objective palpation of this area is guided by a sound anatomic knowledge. Palpation usually proceeds layer by layer. It should be noted that asymmetric joint geometry is common in this region.[89] For spine palpation to be a valid indicator for manual techniques, the clinician applying it must first be able to differentiate between asymmetric motion caused by vertebral dysfunction and that caused by asymmetric joint anatomy.[89] However, examination of the skin overlying the spine has been found to be very helpful, because certain skin changes in a particular location may point in the direction of a dysfunctional spinal area.[90] The skin is assessed for its thickness, moisture, and ease of displacement in all directions. Abnormal autonomic skin reactions, such as erythematous changes, increased sweat production, and pain that can be induced with minimal palpatory pressure, may indicate a segmental dysfunction.[91]

Palpation may be started at that area indicated by the patient as painful. These painful sites must be correctly localized. The bony landmarks of this region that should be routinely palpated include the occiput, mastoid, atlas, and axis.

Occiput. The clinician locates the external occipital protuberance, which is the most prominent bony structure at the occiput in the midline. By following the external occipital protuberance laterally, the clinician can locate the superior nuchal line. The semispinalis capitis muscle is located about $1\frac{1}{2}$ fingerbreadths below the superior nuchal line.[91]

Mastoid. The mastoid processes are located behind each ear. Once this structure is located, the clinician moves the fingers inferiorly toward the tip of the mastoid process. Starting from the medial tip of the mastoid process, the palpating finger is moved superiorly to the upper pole of the mastoid sulcus, an important area in the examination of the irritation zones of the occiput and C1.[91]

Atlas. By placing the palpating fingers between the mastoid process and the descending ramus of the mandible, the clinician can locate the transverse process of the atlas. The inferior oblique and the superior oblique both have attachments to this site.

Axis. The spinous process of C2 is the first prominent bony landmark that is accessible to palpation below the external occipital protuberance of the occiput. The spinous process of C2 serves as the origin of the inferior oblique muscle and the rectus capitis posterior major muscle.

Passive Physiologic Mobility Testing of the Occiput, Atlas, and Axis

O-A Joint. When mobility testing this joint, the first point to remember is that the joint is capable of both flexion and extension, and that side bending and rotation also can occur, albeit slight. The second point to keep in mind is that the arthrokinematics of this joint are the reverse of those occurring in the other zygapophyseal joints and that they occur in a different plane (horizontal). The joint mobility of the O-A joint can be assessed in sitting VIDEO or in supine.

With the patient supine, the head is extended around the axis for the O-A joint VIDEO. The head is then side bent left and right. As the side bending is performed, a gradual translational force is applied in the direction opposite to the side bending. The range of movement of the side bending is assessed from side to side as is the end-feel of the translation. This procedure is then repeated for flexion.

During extension of the O-A joint (Fig. 23-7), the occipital condyles glide anteriorly to the limit of their symmetric extension range. During left side bending and right translation in extension, the coupled right rotation is produced. This rotation causes the right occipital condyle to return toward a neutral position, while the left condyle advances toward the extension barrier. If left side bending in extension is limited, then the limiting factor is on the left joint of the segment (ipsilateral to the side bending), which is preventing the advance of the condyle into its normal position. Thus, extension and right translation test the anterior glide of the left O-A joint, whereas extension and left translation stress the anterior glide of the right O-A joint (Table 23-3).

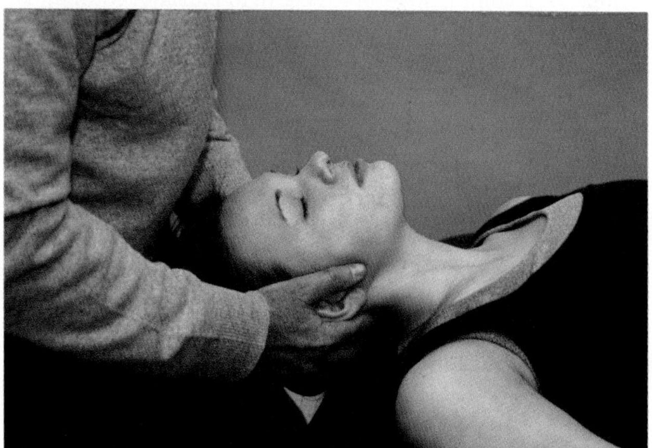

FIGURE 23-7 Passive mobility testing of O-A in extension.

TABLE 23-3 Movement Restrictions of the Craniovertebral Joints and Their Probable Causes

Movement Restriction	Probable Causes
Flexion and right side bending	Left flexion hypomobility Extensor muscle tightness Posterior capsular adhesions Left subluxation (into extension)
Extension and right side bending	Right extension hypomobility Left flexor muscle tightness Anterior capsular adhesions Right subluxation (into flexion)
Flexion and right side-bending motion greater than extension and left side bending	Left capsular pattern (arthritis and arthrosis)
Flexion and right side bending equal to extension and left side bending	Left arthrofibrosis (very hard capsular end-feel)
Right-side flexion in flexion and extension	Probably an anomaly

During flexion of the O-A joint, the occipital condyles glide posteriorly (Fig. 23-8). The right rotation associated with left side bending causes the left condyle to move away from the flexion barrier toward the neutral position, while the right condyle is moved posteriorly further into the flexion barrier. Thus, flexion and translation to the right tests the posterior glide of the right O-A joint, whereas flexion and left rotation tests the posterior glide of the left O-A joint (see Table 23-3).

It is apparent that during these tests, the arthrokinematic and osteokinematic movements are tested simultaneously; thus, the end-feel must be used to determine the cause of the restriction. The following patterns of impairment are more or less commonly seen, and the causes of the impairments can be deduced. However, it must be remembered that deductions are only of value if the resultant intervention is successful.[60]

- A patient who has a subluxation into flexion (loss of anterior glide) on the right O-A joint should demonstrate decreased extension, decreased right side bending and left rotation, and a jammed end-feel with translation to the left.
- A patient with a periarticular restriction of the left O-A joint into flexion (loss of posterior glide) should demonstrate decreased flexion, decreased right side bending and left rotation, and a capsular end-feel with translation to the left.

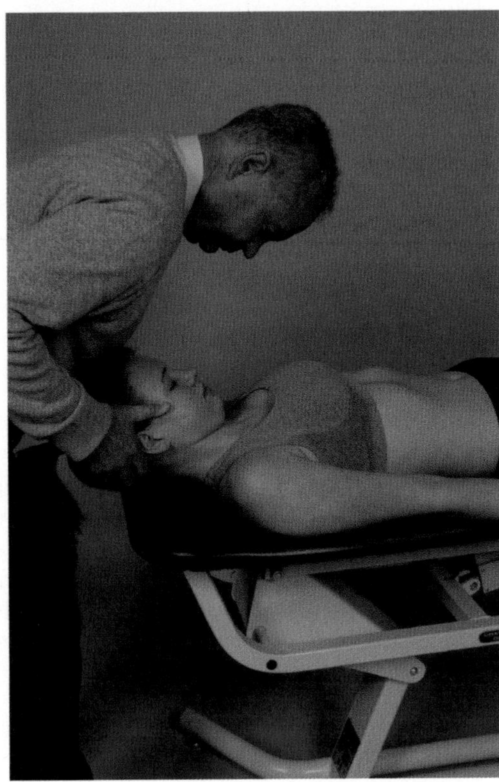

FIGURE 23-8 Passive mobility testing of O-A in flexion.

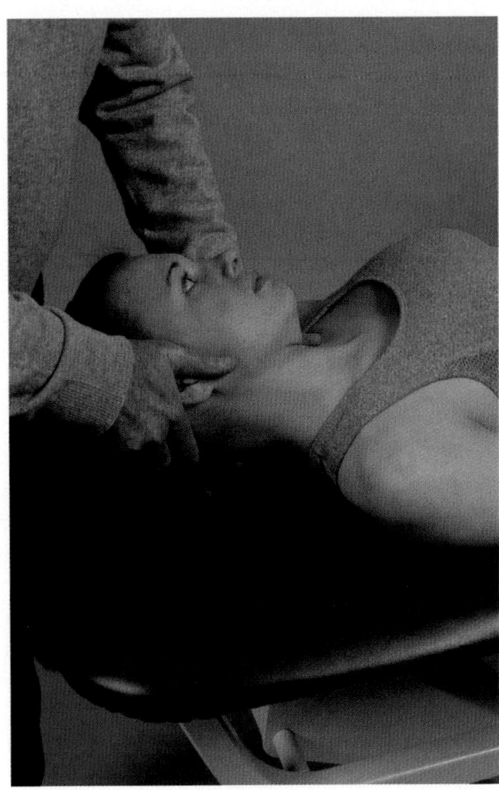

FIGURE 23-9 Passive mobility testing of A-A rotation in supine.

- A patient with a fibrous adhesion of the right O-A joint (loss of anterior and posterior guide) should demonstrate decreased extension and right side bending and decreased flexion and left side bending, with a hard capsular end-feel at both extremes.
- With motion testing, a decreased flexion and right side bending with a pathomechanic end-feel indicates a left O-A joint being subluxed into extension.
- With motion testing, a decreased extension and right side-bending limitation indicates a capsular pattern of the right O-A joint. A decreased extension and left side-bending limitation, with a spasmodic end-feel (flexion with greater range), indicates traumatic arthritis of the left O-A joint.
- A decreased right translation of the O-A in flexion may indicate a right posterior O-A joint dysfunction or an impaired or adaptively shortened right superior oblique muscle.

A-A Joint. There are a number of methods to assess the passive physiologic mobility of the A-A joint VIDEO. The most common method described in many texts involves the patient lying supine and the clinician passively applying full cervical flexion, and then introducing cervical rotation. The problem with this technique is that it relies on the fact that the mid-to-lower cervical spine will be locked with the flexion. Because the neck is often prevented from further flexion when the chin meets the sternum, the clinician has no way of knowing whether full cervical flexion has occurred. Thus, some of the subsequent rotation may be attributed to a combination of cervical spine and A-A motion. This assumption may not be important with asymmetric lesions but can result in false-negative findings with symmetric lesions.

A better method of assessment involves the use of cervical side bending. With the patient positioned in supine, the clinician side bends the head and neck around the craniovertebral axis and then rotates the head in the direction opposite to the side bending (Fig. 23-9). The clinician assesses the amount of range available and then assesses the other side.

CLINICAL PEARL

In a study by Smedmark and colleagues,[92] passive intervertebral motion of the cervical spine was assessed independently by two physical therapists. The therapists had equal backgrounds concerning education and clinical experience. Sixty-one patients seeking care for cervical problems at a private clinic were included in the study where three segments of the cervical spine and the mobility of the first rib were graded as stiff or not stiff. Data were analyzed by percentage agreement and kappa coefficient. Results demonstrated interexaminer reliability of between 70 and 87% and kappa coefficients ranging between 0.28 and 0.43 considered to be only "fair to moderate."

In a similar study by Pool and colleagues,[93] which assessed the interexaminer reproducibility of physical examination of the cervical spine, two physical therapists independently judged the general mobility and intersegmental mobility (segments C0–T2) of the neck and the pain that was provoked. Agreement for general mobility showed kappa between 0.05 and 0.61, and for the intersegmental mobility, it showed kappa values between −0.09 and 0.63. Agreement for provoked neck pain within one point of an 11-point numerical rating scale varied between 46.9 and 65.7% for general mobility and between 40.7 and 75.0% for intersegmental mobility. The ICCs varied between 0.36 and 0.71 for general mobility and between 0.22 and 0.80 for intersegmental mobility. The study concluded that despite the use of a standardized protocol to assess general mobility and intersegmental mobility of the cervical spine, it is difficult to achieve reasonable agreement and reliability between two examiners. Likewise, the patients were not able to score the same level of provoked pain in two assessments with an interval of 15 minutes.

Combined Motion Testing

Flexion and extension at the O-A joints involve a posterior and anterior gliding of the occipital condyles, respectively. The same gliding (although reciprocal in opposing facets) is utilized in rotation. At the A-A joint, flexion and extension primarily involve a "rolling" action of the condyles, with an insignificant amount of gliding. Therefore, craniovertebral flexion and extension will have a minimal effect on A-A rotation.[94] Thus, if a symptom or range of motion is drastically altered by craniovertebral flexion or extension, an assumption could be made that the dysfunction is at the O-A joint.[94] For example, if the right occipital condyle cannot glide posteriorly, the right joint will be unable to flex or to permit rotation to the right, as both of these motions involve a posterior glide at the right O-A joint. In the combined motion tests, the right rotation restriction will be more evident when combined with craniovertebral flexion but will be less evident when combined with craniovertebral extension.

The findings from the combined motion tests can be used to determine which joint glide is to be assessed. For example, if it was determined in the combined motion testing that the right O-A joint is restricted or painful with flexion (implicating the posterior glide), the O-A joint is positioned and assessed in its extreme of flexion and right rotation (the two motions associated with a posterior glide of the right O-A joint).

Linear Segmental Stress Testing

The craniovertebral region demonstrates a high degree of mobility, but little stability, with the ligaments affording little protection during a high-velocity injury. Instability of this region can result from a number of causes:

- Trauma (especially a hyperflexion injury to the neck).
- RA, psoriatic arthritis, or ankylosing spondylitis. Nontraumatic hypermobility or frank instability of the O-A joint has been reported in association with RA.[95]
- Corticosteroid use. Prolonged exposure to this class of drug can produce a softening of the dens and transverse ligament by deteriorating the Sharpey fibers, which attach the ligament to the bone. Steroid use also promotes osteoporosis, predisposing bones to fracture.
- Recurrent upper respiratory tract infections or chronic sore throats in children. Grisel's syndrome[96] is a spontaneous A-A dislocation, affecting children between the ages of 6 and 12 years. The outstanding symptom is a spontaneously arising torticollis. The most likely etiology seems to be an inflammation of the retropharyngeal space caused by upper respiratory tract infections or by adenotonsillectomy and producing pharyngeal hyperemia and bone absorption.
- Congenital malformation. Nontraumatic hypermobility or frank instability of the O-A joint has been reported in association with congenital bony malformations.[97]
- Down's syndrome. Nontraumatic hypermobility or frank instability of the O-A joint has been reported in children and adolescents with Down's syndrome.[98,99]
- Immature development. Patients younger than 12 years of age often have an immature or absent dens (see later).
- Osteoporosis.

It must be remembered that the A-A joint complex consists of three joints. The median joint, although it has no weight-bearing function, is extremely important in maintaining stability, while at the same time facilitating motion within this joint complex. Fielding and colleagues[100] found that the stability of the A-A joint depends greatly on the ligamentous structures and on a normal and intact dens. Occasionally, the integrity of the dens can be compromised because of:

1. Anomalies of the dens, including:
   a. Os odontoideum. This is a condition in which the IVD between the developing bodies of axis and atlas does not ossify.
   b. Congenital absence of the dens.
   c. An underdeveloped dens whose lack of height renders it unchecked by the transverse ligament. The body of the dens is not of sufficient size to be retained in the osseoligamentous ring of the atlas until a child is approximately 12 years old. Great care and justification are needed with any craniovertebral mobilization or manipulative technique with this age group.
2. Pathologies affecting the dens, including:
   a. Demineralization or resorption of the dens, such as occurs with Grisel's syndrome[96] or RA.
   b. An old, undisplaced fracture (especially of the dens), which originally escaped diagnosis and subsequently formed a pseudoarthrosis.

Indications for Stability Testing. The following findings are considered to be indications to perform stability or stress tests of the craniovertebral region[82]:

- History of neck trauma or any of the causes of instability listed previously.
- Patient report of neck instability usually described as the head feeling heavy.
- Presence of the following signs and symptoms:
  - A lump in the throat
  - Lip paresthesia
  - Nausea or vomiting
  - Severe headache and muscle spasm
  - Dizziness

The patient is positioned in supine to remove any muscular influences. If the patient is unable to lie down, the clinician may need to reconsider the appropriateness of performing these tests.

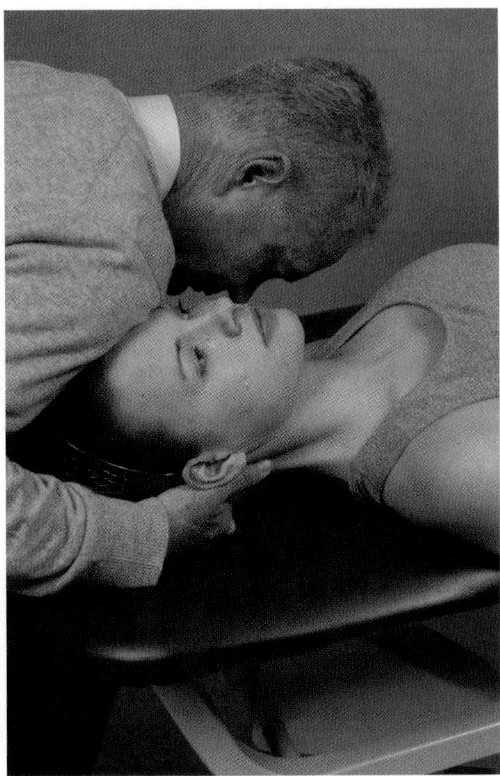

FIGURE 23-10 Longitudinal stability testing.

Longitudinal Stability. General traction is applied to the entire cervical region. If this maneuver does not reproduce the signs or symptoms, C2 is stabilized so that the traction force may be directed at the craniovertebral region (Fig. 23-10). The diagnostic value of this test is as yet unknown.

Anterior Shear: Transverse Ligament. The patient is positioned in supine, with his or her head cradled in the clinician's hands. The clinician locates the anterior arches of C2 by moving around the vertebra from the back to the front using the thumbs. Once the arches are located, the clinician pushes down on the anterior arches of C2 with the thumbs toward the table, while the patient's occiput and C1, cupped in the clinician's hands, is lifted, keeping the head parallel to the ceiling but in slight flexion[82] (Fig. 23-11) VIDEO. The patient is instructed to count backward aloud. The position is held for approximately 15 seconds or until an end-feel is perceived. The diagnostic value of this test is as yet unknown.

Sharp–Purser Test. This test was designed originally to test the sagittal stability of the A-A segment in patients with RA, because a number of pathologic conditions can affect the stability of the osseoligamentous ring of the median joints of this segment in this patient population. These changes result in degeneration and thinning of the articular cartilage between the odontoid process and the anterior arch of the atlas, or, occasionally, in a softening of the dens.

The aim of the test was to determine whether the instability was significant enough to provoke central nervous system's signs or symptoms. Uitvlugt and Indenbaum[101] assessed the validity of the Sharp–Purser test in 123 outpatients with RA. The study findings indicated a predictive value of 85% and a high specificity of 96%. The sensitivity was 88% when subluxation was greater than 4 mm.[101] The authors concluded that the Sharp–Purser test is a useful clinical examination to diagnose A-A instability in the RA population.[101]

However, the original test was poorly defined and only involved upper cervical flexion. Hence, a modified version was introduced which is described.

The patient is positioned in sitting. The patient is asked to segmentally flex the head around a craniovertebral axis (short neck flexion) and relate any signs or symptoms that this might evoke to the clinician. In addition, a positive test may be indicated by the patient hearing or feeling a clunk. Local symptoms, such as soreness, are ignored for the purposes of evaluating the test. If no serious signs or symptoms are provoked, the clinician stabilizes C2 posteriorly with one hand and applies a posteriorly oriented force to the forehead of the patient (Fig. 23-12) VIDEO.

In the presence of a positive test, a provisional assumption is made that the symptoms are caused by excessive translation of the atlas, compromising one or more of the sensitive structures listed previously, and the physical examination is terminated. No intervention should be attempted other than the issuing of a cervical collar to prevent craniovertebral flexion and an immediate referral to the patient's physician.

Coronal Stability: Alar Ligament. Rotation and side bending tighten the contralateral alar (e.g., rotation or side bending to the right tightens the left alar), whereas flexion typically tightens both alar ligaments.

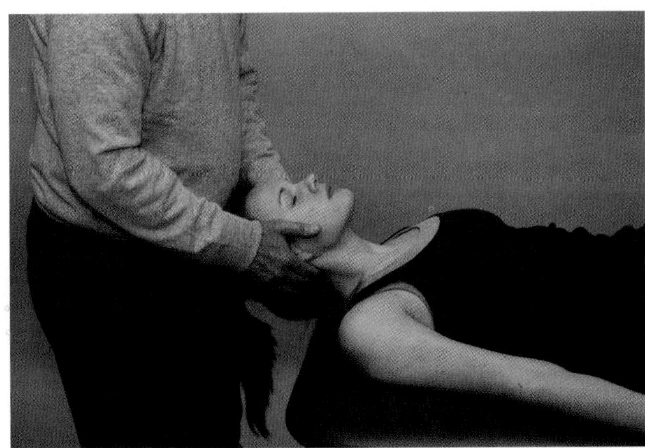

FIGURE 23-11 Transverse ligament test.

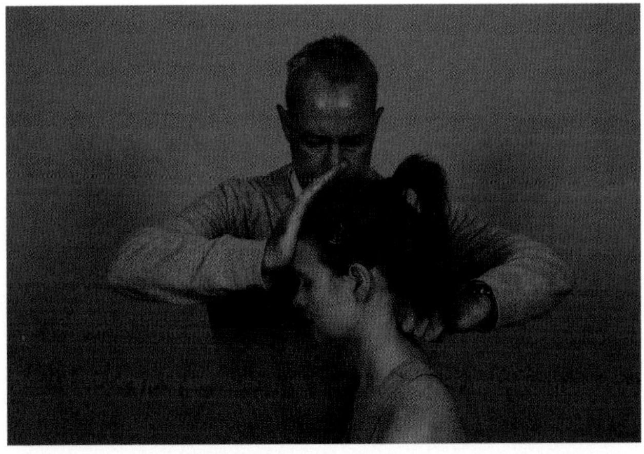

FIGURE 23-12 Modified Sharp–Purser test.

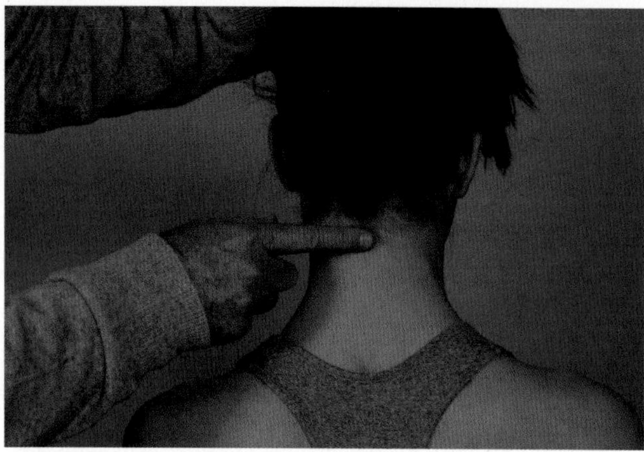

FIGURE 23-13 Alar ligament test in sitting.

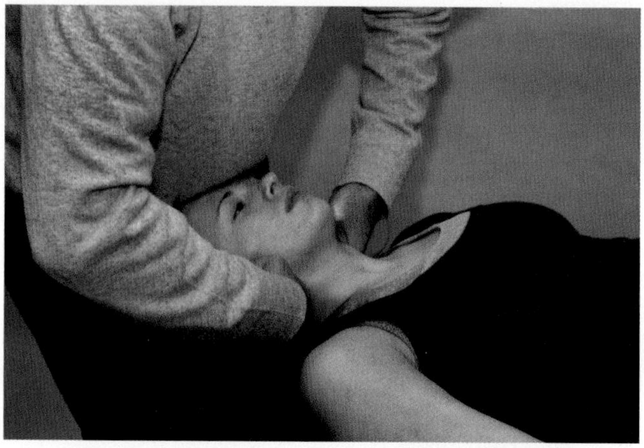

The posterior aspect of the transverse process of C2 is palpated with one hand, while the patient's head is side bent or rotated (Fig. 23-13). **VIDEO**. This is a test of immediacy. If the C2 transverse process does not move as soon as the head begins to rotate, laxity of the alar ligament should be suspected. To confirm the findings in this test, the point of rotation is maintained, as the patient's head is cradled by the clinician (Fig. 23-14), and while monitoring the motion at the C2 segment, the clinician introduces side bending through the craniovertebral joints to slacken the alar ligament. Further rotation should now be possible. The diagnostic value of this test is as yet unknown.

Transverse Shear.[82] Transverse shearing of the craniovertebral joints is performed with the patient supine. The clinician stabilizes the mastoid, and C1 is moved in a transverse direction, using the soft part of the metacarpophalangeal joint of the index finger (Fig. 23-15). The test is repeated by stabilizing C1 and translating the mastoid.

C1 and C2 can be tested similarly. The soft aspect of each second metacarpal head is placed on the opposite transverse processes and laminae of C1 and C2, with the palms facing each other. The clinician stabilizes C1 and then attempts to move C2 transversely using the soft part of metacarpals (Fig. 23-16). No movement should be felt. The diagnostic value of this test is as yet unknown.

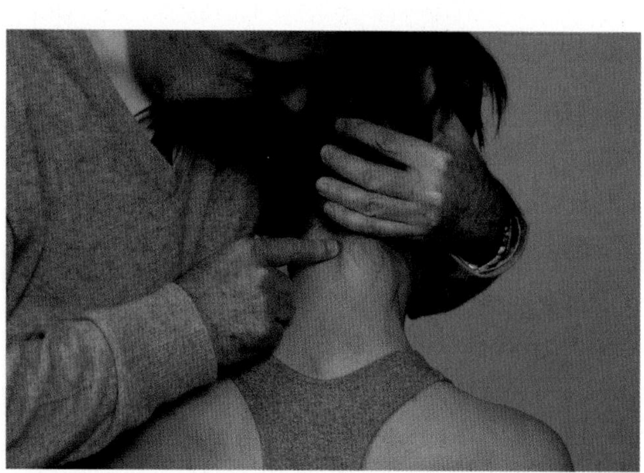

FIGURE 23-14 Confirmatory test for alar ligament in sitting.

FIGURE 23-15 Transverse shear of O-A joint.

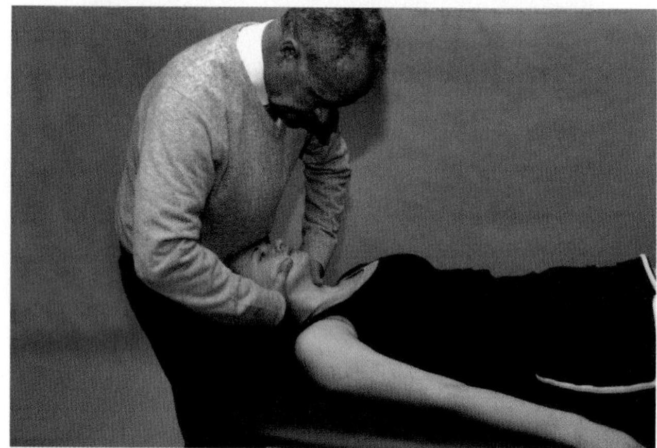

FIGURE 23-16 Transverse shear of A-A joint.

Neurologic Examination

The neurologic examination is performed to assess the normal conduction of the central and peripheral nervous systems. The presence of neurologic symptoms deserves special attention. Many of the symptoms that occur in the upper limb have their origins in the neck. The patient with neck trauma can report seemingly bizarre symptoms, but these need to be heeded until the clinician can rule out serious pathology. Cervical myelopathy, involving an injury to the spinal cord itself, is associated with multisegmental paresthesias, upper motor neuron (UMN) signs and symptoms such as spasticity, hyperreflexia, visual and balance disturbances, ataxia, and sudden changes in bowel and bladder function. The presence of any UMN sign or symptom requires an immediate medical referral.

In addition to the muscle stretch (deep tendon) reflexes and sensory tests outlined in Chapter 25, the clinician should perform the spinal cord reflexes of Babinski and Hoffman (see Chap. 3). Studies by Boden and colleagues[102] and Sung and Wang have demonstrated that the Hoffman test is the most sensitive reflex test in the detection of cervical myelopathy.[103]

Imaging Studies

The standard, initial cervical spine radiographic series in trauma patients includes a cross-table lateral view, an anteroposterior view, and an open-mouth view, the latter of which is used to help rule out a fracture of the dens (see Chap. 7).[7] The usefulness of the anteroposterior view has been questioned because it provides little additional information.[104] Although this three-view screening series can detect 65–95% of axis injuries,[105,106] the C2 vertebra often is obscured by overlying bony maxillary, mandibular, and dental structures; therefore, C2 fractures may be missed.[7] The clinician needs to be aware of the limitations of plain radiographs, as problems exist with both specificity and sensitivity. However, radiographs can provide a gross assessment of the severity of the degenerative changes of the spine.

Thin-section CT is the best study for evaluating C2 bony fractures.[107] Sagittal reconstruction of CT images is important because axial images may not detect a transverse odontoid fracture.[7] Although CT is excellent in evaluating bony injuries, it can miss soft tissue and significant ligamentous injuries.[7] Recently, therefore, dynamic flexion/extension lateral fluoroscopic evaluation has been advocated in polytrauma patients to identify occult ligamentous instabilities and confirm that the cervical spine is uninjured.[108] As with any diagnostic study, the findings must be correlated with the history and physical examination.

INTERVENTION STRATEGIES

The gamut of musculoskeletal injury to the craniovertebral region of the spine ranges from a simple strain (muscle) or sprain (ligament) to injuries of the bone and neurovascular injuries. The most common injuries seen clinically are muscle strains and postural dysfunctions.

Muscle strains are common in the cervical spine because most of the cervical muscles attach via myofascial tissue inserting into the periosteum rather than by the more resilient tendon.[109] The severity of the strain is dependent on the magnitude of forces involved. If the force is sufficient, both the muscle and the associated joint become involved. In an abnormal spine, the forces needed to cause injury are reduced. Repetitive microtrauma is a common cause of craniovertebral dysfunction.

Postural dysfunctions of this region, particularly the forward head posture (see Chap. 25), usually manifest themselves at the O-A joint, resulting in fixed capital extension and a loss of O-A flexion. Patients with postural dysfunctions may develop secondary myofascial trigger points (MTrPs) and myofascial pain syndromes. In postural dysfunctions and trauma-related injuries, other joints and regions may be involved and require further investigation.

Pain, tenderness, active range of motion restrictions, muscle imbalances, and segmental motion restrictions are common findings with craniovertebral dysfunction.

The structure at fault should determine the intervention[110]:

- If ligamentous tissue damage or an intra-articular lesion is suspected, the safest initial approach would be to help in unloading the joint and controlling the extremes of motion with a soft collar for a 7–10-day period.
- Within the patient's pain tolerance, contractile lesions should be treated aggressively once the acute phase has subsided, with the emphasis on regaining maximal muscle length.[110]

The techniques to increase joint mobility and soft tissue extensibility are described later, under "Therapeutic Techniques" section.

A correct diagnosis can usually be accomplished through detailed history and a comprehensive examination. Confirmation of the correct diagnosis can be made with an assessment of the response of the patient to the initial rehabilitation program. The intervention for the craniovertebral region may commence when the possibility of serious injury including fracture, dislocation, or injury to the spinal cord and vertebral artery have been ruled out.

Acute Phase

The goals of this phase include

- reducing pain, inflammation, and muscle spasm;
- reestablishing a nonpainful range of motion;
- improving neuromuscular postural control;
- retarding muscle atrophy;
- promotion of healing.

Various electrotherapeutic modalities and physical agents may be used during the acute phase to modulate pain and to decrease inflammation and muscle spasm (see Chap. 8). Therapeutic cold and electrical stimulation may be used for 48–72 hours. The cryotherapy is continued at home. A transcutaneous electrical nerve stimulation (TENS) unit may be prescribed to help control pain and encourage range of motion. Joint protection may be appropriate. In such cases, a soft or semirigid cervical collar may be prescribed for 7–10 days to reduce muscle guarding (see Chap. 25). Nonsteroidal anti-inflammatory drugs (NSAIDs) often are prescribed for 2–3 weeks to help decrease inflammation and to control pain, thereby increasing the potential for an early return to function. Bed rest, along with analgesics and muscle relaxants for no more than 2–3 days, is prescribed for patients with a severe injury. However, in less severe cases, bed rest has not been shown to improve recovery and, compared with mobilization or patient education, rest tends to prolong symptoms.[111,112]

The patient also is taught how to find the neutral position for the upper cervical spine. The neutral position is defined as the least painful position that minimizes mechanical stresses.

Range of motion exercises are initiated as early as possible, based on patient tolerance, to prevent hypomobility. Neck flexion and rotation exercises usually are performed first. Extension and side-bending exercises are introduced based on the response of the patient to the flexion and rotation exercises. The rotation and side-bending exercises are performed in the supine position and then progressed to weight bearing. All of the exercises should be performed in the pain-free range.

Upper extremity range of motion and strengthening exercises should also be introduced to promote early integration of the entire upper kinetic chain. Important muscles to include are the rhomboids, middle and lower trapezius, latissimus dorsi, serratus anterior, and deltoid. In addition, the muscles of the rotator cuff should be strengthened.

Gentle manual techniques (see "Therapeutic Techniques" section later), such as sustained or rhythmic specific traction (grade I or II) mobilizations and massage, may also be used. As the patient progresses, muscle stretching may be introduced. Manual techniques can have a mechanical effect on joint mobility and soft tissue extensibility. In addition, these techniques can have beneficial neurophysiologic effects, which can help alleviate pain and muscle spasm. Self-stretching and self-mobilization techniques are taught to the patient at the earliest and appropriate opportunity (see "Therapeutic Techniques" section later).

Active joint protection techniques may be part of the acute phase. Joint protection exercises work by supporting the joint and reducing the applied stresses. Joint protection exercises include cervical stabilization exercises. These exercises initially are performed in single planes and in the neutral position, using submaximal isometric contractions. As with the range of motion exercises, it is recommended that these exercises be performed initially in the supine position, and later, in sitting, as tolerance increases. As the pain-free ranges increase, the exercises are performed throughout the newly attained pain-free ranges.

Aerobic conditioning must also be included as part of the comprehensive rehabilitation program. A stationary bike, tread-mill, or a stair-stepping machine can be used.

The patient is advanced to the functional phase when

- the pain has significantly decreased so that there is minimal pain with activities of daily living;
- there is significant improvement in the pain-free ranges of motion.

Functional Phase

The duration of this phase can vary tremendously and depends on several factors:

- Severity of the injury.
- Healing capacity of the patient.
- How the condition was managed during the acute phase.
- Level of patient involvement in the rehabilitation program.

The goals of this phase are to

- significantly reduce or completely resolve the patient's pain;
- restore full and pain-free range of motion;
- fully integrate the entire upper kinetic chain;
- restore full cervical and upper quadrant strength and neuromuscular control.

During this phase, the range of motion exercises are continued until maximum range of motion is attained. The strengthening program is progressed from submaximal isometrics in single planes to maximal isometrics in single planes. Then the patient is progressed to isometrics in combined motions (flexion and side bending and extension and side bending). The strength training is then progressed to concentric and eccentric exercises in single planes, using elastic tubing, pulleys, or isolation exercises. Proprioceptive neuromuscular facilitation patterns are introduced when appropriate. Elastic tubing is issued to the patient to allow training at home.

For progression to return to play, the athlete should demonstrate

- normal and pain-free single-plane and multiplane range of motion;
- normal cervical, cervicothoracic, glenohumeral, and scapulothoracic strength;
- normal flexibility of cervical, cervicoscapular, and cervicothoracic musculature.

Return to sport activities should be designed to mimic the sport as closely as possible. The goal should be to improve the balance, power, and endurance of the cervical, cervicothoracic, glenohumeral, and scapulothoracic muscle groups and force couples.

Pattern 4D: Impaired Joint Mobility, Motor Function, Muscle Performance, and Range of Motion Associated with Connective Tissue Dysfunction

Transverse Ligament Injuries

Injuries to the transverse ligament are classified as follows[49,58]:

- *Type I injuries.* Disruptions of the substance of the transverse ligament, without an osseous component.
- *Type II injuries.* Fractures or avulsions involving the tubercle for insertion of the transverse ligament on the C1 lateral mass, without disruption of the ligament substance.

The medical literature supports the conclusion that a type I injury is incapable of healing without surgery for internal fixation but that most type II injuries heal when treated with an orthosis.[113]

Integration of Patterns 4B and 4D: Impaired Joint Mobility, Motor Function, Muscle Performance, and Range of Motion Secondary to Impaired Posture and Connective Tissue Dysfunction

Myofascial Pain Patterns

Myofascial pain syndromes are closely associated with tender areas that have come to be known as MTrPs (see Chap. 10). The term *myofascial trigger point* is a bit of a misnomer, because trigger points may also be cutaneous, ligamentous, periosteal, and fascial.[114] Dysfunctional joints also are associated with trigger points and tender attachment points.[115]

For a more detailed description of myofascial pain patterns in the upper quadrants, including their causes, signs and symptoms, and interventions, the reader is referred to the excellent book by Travell and Simons, *Myofascial Pain and Dysfunction: The Trigger Point Manual* (Volume 1, *The Upper Extremities*).[63]

The interventions for MTrPs are outlined in Chapter 10. These include stretch and spray, muscle stripping, massage therapy, myofascial release, ischemic compression, stretching, postural correction and education to eliminate any causative or perpetuating factors, electrotherapeutic and thermal modalities, cryotherapy, injections, and joint mobilizations.

Integration of Patterns 4D and 4E: Impaired Joint Mobility, Motor Function, Muscle Performance, and Range of Motion Secondary to Connective Tissue Dysfunction and Localized Inflammation

Osteoarthritis

Osteoarthrosis of the A-A joints, unrelated to trauma, is a rare cause of pain in the craniovertebral region and an even more uncommon cause of A-A instability. It could be argued that if osteoarthrosis of the lateral mass articulations progresses, the synovitis may gradually involve the ligamentous structures, thereby weakening them and rendering them prone to rupture.[116]

Inflammatory Arthritis

The greatest risk for complications with the spondyloarthropathies in the craniovertebral region occurs at the A-A joint, where there are two different synovial articulations: the two lateral facet joints and the articulation between the odontoid process of C2 and the anterior part of C1.[86] The transverse ligament is typically the weakest part of the complex in the presence of spondyloarthropathy.

Rheumatoid Arthritis. The most common inflammatory lesion found in the retro-odontoid space is RA, which induces abnormal proliferation of the synovial soft tissue (pannus) and frequently causes the destruction of the bony structure[117] (see Chap. 5).

Ankylosing Spondylitis. See Chapter 5.

Gout. See Chapter 5.

Craniovertebral Instability

There has been much controversy about defining and diagnosing spinal instability. Segmental spinal instability generally is defined as a greater displacement between vertebrae than that which occurs under physiologic load. Therefore, maximum flexion and extension radiographs usually are used to determine hypermobility between vertebrae. Craniovertebral instability frequently is encountered in inflammatory, neoplastic, degenerative, and traumatic disorders, in addition to congenital and developmental abnormalities. Clinically, instability appears as a subluxation or spinal deformity accompanied by severe pain or neurologic deficits. Several types of craniovertebral instability are recognized; among them are the following:

- ***Translational or rotary instability of C1.*** Translational anterior A-A instability is detected on lateral cervical radiographs as a widened, mobile atlantodental interval (ADI) of greater than 3 mm, caused by laxity or rupture of the transverse ligament or from an odontoid fracture.[118] Patients with congenital abnormalities of the odontoid process may develop chronic A-A subluxation. This leads to the formation of fibrous granulation tissue or a hypertrophic scar in the peri- or retro-odontoid epidural space, which is known as a "pseudotumor."[119] Chronic mechanical irritation associated with neck movement is speculated to be one of the causes of fibrous scar formation.[120] Posterior translation of C1 is also possible, but for this to occur, the dens or anterior arch of the atlas must be fractured or incompetent. Rotational A-A instability appears as asymmetric rotation of the C1 lateral masses on plain radiographs. Rotational subluxations that are irreducible, recurrent, or associated with transverse ligament disruption require surgery.[118] Patients with A-A subluxations exceeding 6 mm are at high risk for neurologic injury and sudden death and are, therefore, immediately considered for fusion.[121]
- ***O-A instability.*** O-A instability is demonstrated radiographically by movement between the dens and basion (the middle point on the anterior margin of the foramen magnum), by distraction or translation of the occipital condyles, or by vertical migration.[122]

Surgical stabilization is required to correct instability when conservative intervention has failed or when spontaneous healing with an orthosis, such as a halo brace, is unlikely.

Pattern 4F: Impaired Joint Mobility, Motor Function, Muscle Performance, and Range of Motion, or Reflex Integrity, Secondary to Spinal Disorders

Peripheral Vertigo

Dizziness is the third most common complaint among outpatients, after chest pain and fatigue.[123] There are several types of dizziness, some benign and some serious, and it is important that the clinician be able to make the distinction. Among the causes of dizziness that must be carefully considered by the clinician examining the cervical spine are the central and peripheral (Table 23-4) causes of vertigo or dizziness (see Chap. 3).[124]

TABLE 23-4 Peripheral Vestibular Disorders
Vestibular neuritis
Ramsay Hunt syndrome
Labyrinthitis
Benign proximal positional vertigo
Ménière's disease
Acute peripheral vestibulopathy
Otosclerosis
Head trauma
Cerebellopontine angle tumor
Toxic vestibulopathies
Acoustic neuropathy
Perilymphatic fistula
Autoimmune disease of the inner ear

Data from Huijbregts P, Vidal P: Dizziness in orthopaedic physical therapy practice: classification and pathophysiology. *J Man Manip Ther* 12:199–214, 2004.

Vestibular Neuritis. Vestibular neuritis is thought to represent a reactivated dormant herpes infection in Scarpa's ganglion, within the superior division of the vestibular nerve, which innervates the anterior and horizontal SCC.[125,126]

Ramsay Hunt Syndrome. Ramsay Hunt syndrome is caused by varicella zoster and is a variant of vestibular neuritis, with multiple cranial nerves involved. This involvement results in facial paresis, tinnitus, hearing loss, and a vestibular defect.[127,128] It may also involve cranial nerves V, IX, and X.

Labyrinthitis. Infection of the labyrinth can be viral or bacterial. Acute labyrinthitis usually presents with severe vertigo, sudden or progressive hearing loss, nausea, vomiting, and fever. The condition lasts for 1–5 days, with subsequent resolution of complaints over a 2–3-week period.

Benign Paroxysmal Positional Vertigo. Benign paroxysmal positional vertigo (BPPV) is the most common peripheral vestibular disorder and the most common cause of dizziness in the elderly, with the incidence increasing with age.[127] Causes of BPPV (see also Chap. 3) include head trauma, vestibular neuritis, insult to the labyrinth, surgical stapedectomy, degeneration of the inner ear, and vestibular artery compromise. Two pathophysiological theories have been proposed to explain the etiology of BPPV: cupulolithiasis, and canalithiasis[129]:

- *Cupulolithiasis.* Sedimentous material, possibly macular otoconia, is released into the endolymphatic fluid in the SCC. This release of sedimentous material is hypothesized to result from trauma or degenerative changes. When the head is upright, this material will settle on the SCC cupula. Fixed deposits on the cupula increased density at the structure making the cupula, which previously had the same density as the surrounding endolymphatic fluid now sensitive to gravity and, therefore, head position.
- *Canalithiasis.* An accumulation of utricle debris (otoconia), which can move within the posterior SCC and stimulate the vestibular sense organ (cupula), causing vertigo and nystagmus.[127]

The name BPPV implies that this type of vertigo is positional in nature. However, it may be more correct to call BPPV a positioning-type vertigo[129] Symptom duration is brief: 30–60 seconds; hence, it is a positioning-type vertigo rather than positional-type vertigo, as occurs in vertebrobasilar insufficiency.[129]

The diagnosis usually is made solely on the basis of the history, although it is possible to confuse BPPV with orthostatic hypotension, another common cause of dizziness in the elderly. Whereas orthostatic hypotension causes dizziness when the patient sits up or stands, BPPV can occur in all positions, especially with changes in head position.

The side of the lesion is diagnosed with a maneuver similar to the Dix–Hallpike test (see Fig. 3-26 in Chap. 3). The intervention for posterior canal BPPV involves performing a canalith-repositioning maneuver, which is designed to return the otoconia from the SCC back to the macule of the utricle, from whence it can be reabsorbed.

Canalith-Repositioning Procedure.[127] The patient is seated on the end of the bed with his or her feet dangling. The clinician stands to the side of the patient, supporting the patient's head. The patient is moved into the Dix–Hallpike position, toward the side of the involved ear and maintained there for 20 seconds. Then the head is slowly rotated through moderate extension of the cervical spine toward the uninvolved side and maintained in the new position for 20 seconds. The patient is then rolled to a side-lying position, with the head being turned 45 degrees down (toward the floor) and maintained there for 20 seconds. While keeping the head turned toward the uninvolved side and the head pitched down, the patient slowly sits up.

To maintain the otoconia in the utricle following the maneuver, the patient is fitted with a soft collar and is instructed not to bend over, lie back, move the head up or down, or tilt the head to either side for the remainder of the day.

Ménière's Disease. This condition is characterized by paroxysmal vertigo, lasting minutes to days, accompanied by tinnitus, fluctuating low-frequency hearing loss, and a sensation of fullness in the ear.[129,130] Attacks are often associated with nausea and vomiting. Age at onset is usually between the ages of 20 and 50 years, and men are more often affected than women.[130] The underlying cause is thought to be an increase in the volume of the endolymphatic fluid in the membranous labyrinth, which displaces the inner ear structures with resultant signs and symptoms of horizontal or rotary nystagmus.[130]

Acute Peripheral Vestibulopathy. This condition is characterized by a sudden onset of vertigo, nausea, and vomiting, which last for up to 2 weeks and is not associated with hearing loss. Differential diagnosis from central disorders characterized by acute vertigo is imperative.[130]

Otosclerosis. The pathophysiologic mechanism behind otosclerosis is immobility of the stapes and resultant conductive hearing loss. Associated signs and symptoms include vertigo and nystagmus.

Head Trauma. Head trauma may result in labyrinth damage and subsequent vertigo.

Cerebellopontine Angle Tumor. This is a benign acoustic neuroma that can produce insidious unilateral sensorineural hearing loss, vertigo, and tinnitus.[130]

Toxic Vestibulopathies. Ingested alcohol differentially distributes between the cupula and the endolymphatic fluid: It initially diffuses preferentially into the cupula, decreasing its density relative to that of the endolymphatic fluid, thus rendering the peripheral vestibular apparatus unusually sensitive to gravity.[129] The vertigo and nystagmus are evident in the lateral recumbent position and are accentuated when the eyes are closed.[129,130] Aminoglycosides (streptomycin, gentamicin, and tobramycin), salicylates (aspirin and derivatives) quinine and quinidine, and various chemotherapeutic drugs have all been associated with producing vertigo, nausea, and vomiting, and occasionally nystagmus.

Acoustic Neuropathy. Conditions such as basilar meningitis, hypothyroidism, diabetes mellitus, and Paget's disease can lead to compression of the vestibulocochlear nerve.[129,130]

Perilymphatic Fistula. A rare cause of vertigo, which can result from head injury, barotrauma due to diving or flying, or a very forceful Valsalva maneuver, which results in a rapid loss of perilymphatic fluid.[129,130]

Autoimmune Disease of the Inner Ear. Diseases such as RA, Crohn's disease, or polyarthritis are often concurrently present with fluctuating deafness and recurrent vertigo.[129,130]

Vestibular Rehabilitation. The use of a custom-designed physical therapy program in the rehabilitation of patients with unilateral peripheral vestibular hypofunction is aimed at promoting vestibular compensation, promoting central habituation, and readjusting the vestibulo-ocular and vestibulospinal reflexes (see Chap. 3).[131,132]

Repetition of movements and positions that provoke dizziness and vertigo form the basic premise of habituation training, even though many of the exercises may initially increase the patient's symptoms. Several progressions have been devised (Table 23-5 and Box 23-1). Brown and colleagues, in a retrospective case series of 48 patients with central vestibular dysfunction noted improvement in both subjective and objective measures of balance after physical therapy intervention.[134] The treatment consisted of one or more of the following: balance and gait training, general strengthening and flexibility exercises, vestibular adaptation exercises, education in the use of assistive devices and safety awareness techniques to avoid falls, and utilization of varied senses, particularly somatosensation and vision, to aid in maintaining balance.[134]

Cervical Vertigo

Cervical vertigo is a diagnosis and a disorder that seems to be poorly understood, and yet dizziness is a common clinical symptom in patients with cervical and upper quadrant syndromes.[124] Cervical or reflex vertigo is thought to originate from a disturbance of the tonic neck reflex input from the neck to the vestibular nucleus. This disturbance can be caused by a dysfunction in the cervical joints[135] or the SCM.[136] As early as 1926, Barré[137] described a syndrome involving sub-occipital pain and vertigo, which was usually precipitated by turning the head. Ryan and Cope[138] coined the term "cervical vertigo" in 1955 for this syndrome.

Cervical vertigo symptoms appear to result from an alteration to proprioceptive spinal afferents from the mechanoreceptors of the neck, usually, but not always, resulting from trauma.[139] Macnab[133] thought that the 575 patients he studied exhibited little evidence of overt neck damage, or of neurologic damage. He thought areas other than the neck itself, such as the brain, brain stem, cranial nerves, cervical nerve roots, or inner ear, might be responsible for the symptoms.

TABLE 23-5 Cawthorne–Cooksey Exercises for Patients with Vestibular Hypofunction

A. In bed
   1. Eye movements—at first slow, then quick
      a. Up and down
      b. From side to side
      c. Focusing on a finger moving from 3 to 1 ft away from face
   2. Head movements—at first slow, then quick; later with eyes closed
      a. Bending forward and backward
      b. Turning from side to side

B. Sitting
   1. Same as A1 and A2, above
   2. Shoulder shrugging and circling
   3. Bending forward and picking up objects from ground

C. Standing
   1. Same as A1 and A2 and B3, above
   2. Changing from sitting to standing position with eyes open and shut
   3. Throwing a small ball from hand to hand (above eye level).
   4. Throwing ball from hand to hand under knee
   5. Changing from sitting to standing and turning round in between

D. Moving about (in class)
   1. Circle around center person who will throw a large ball and to whom it will be returned
   2. Walk across room with eyes open and then closed
   3. Walk up and down slope with eyes open and then closed
   4. Walk up and down steps with eyes open and then closed
   5. Any game involving stooping and stretching and aiming, such as skittles, bowls, or basketball

   Diligence and perseverance are required, but the earlier and more regularly the exercise regimen is carried out, the faster and more complete will be the return to normal activity.

Data from Herdman SJ, Borello-France DF, Whitney SL: Treatment of vestibular hypofunction. In: Herdman SJ, ed. *Vestibular Rehabilitation*. Philadelphia, PA: FA Davis, 1994:287–315.

Data from Dix MR: The rationale and technique of head exercises in the treatment of vertigo. *Acta Oto-Rhino-Laryngol Belg* 33:370, 1979.

Box 23-1 Exercises to Improve Postural Stability[133]

These exercises are devised to incorporate head movement (vestibular stimulation) or to foster use of different sensory cues for balance.

1. The patient stands with his or her feet as close together as possible, with both or one hand helping maintain balance by touching a wall if needed. The patient then turns his or her head to the right and to the left horizontally, while looking straight ahead at the wall for 1 minute without stopping. The patient takes his or her hand or hands off the wall for longer and longer periods of the time while maintaining balance. The patient then tries moving his or her feet even closer together.
2. The patient walks, with someone for assistance if needed, as often as possible (acute disorders).
3. The patient begins to practice turning his or her head while walking. This will make the patient less stable, so the patient should stay near a wall as he or she walks.
4. The patient stands with his or her feet shoulder-width apart with eyes open, looking straight ahead at a target on the wall. He or she progressively narrows the base of support from feet apart to feet together to a semi-heel-to-toe position. The exercise is performed first with arms outstretched, then with arms close to the body, and then with arms folded across the chest. Each position is held for 15 seconds, before the patient does the next-most-difficult exercise. The patient practices for a total of 5–15 minutes.
5. The patent stands with his or her feet shoulder-width apart with eyes open, looking straight ahead at a target on the wall. The patient progressively narrows his or her base of support from feet apart to feet together to a semi-heel-to-toe position. The exercise is performed with eyes closed, at first intermittently and then for longer and longer periods of time. The exercise is performed first with arms outstretched, then with arms close to the body, and then with arms folded across the chest. Each position is held for 15 seconds, and then the patient tries the next position. The patient practices for a total of 5–15 minutes.
6. A headlamp can be attached to the patient's waist or shoulders, and the patient can practice shifting weight to place the light into targets marked on the wall. This home "biofeedback" exercise can be used, with the feet in different positions and the patient standing on surfaces of different densities.
7. The patient practices standing on a cushioned surface. Progressively more difficult tasks might be standing on hard floor (linoleum, wood), thin carpet, shag carpet, thin pillow, and sofa cushion. Graded-density foam can also be purchased.
8. The patient practices walking with a more narrow base of support. The patient can do this first, touching the wall for support or for tactile cues and then gradually touching only intermittently and then not at all.
9. The patient practices turning around while walking, at first making a large circle but gradually making smaller and smaller turns. The patient must be sure to practice turning in both directions.
10. The patient can practice standing and then walking on ramps, either with a firm surface or with more cushioned surface.
11. The patient can practice maintaining balance while sitting and bouncing on a Swiss ball or while bouncing on a trampoline. This exercise can be incorporated with attempting to maintain visual fixation of a stationary target, thus facilitating adaptation of the otolith-ocular reflexes.
12. Out in the community, the patient can practice walking in a mall before it is open and, therefore, while it is quiet; can practice walking in the mall while walking in the same direction as the flow of traffic; and can then walk against the flow of traffic.

Biesinger,[140] on the other hand, proposed two possible neurologic origins:

1. A contributor from the sympathetic plexus surrounding the vertebral arteries.
2. Functional disorders of proprioception in segments C1–2.

It would seem likely that direct damage to the vestibular apparatus, or severe damage to the vertebral artery, will produce immediate dizziness, whereas dizziness arising from the cervical joints or a less severely injured vertebral artery may not occur until the joints themselves became abnormal, or until the ischemia has had time to make itself felt (Table 23-6).[110] Because cervical pain also frequently is delayed, it is at least arguable that delayed dizziness commonly originates from injured cervical joints and less commonly from ischemia.[110]

The intervention for cervical vertigo generally begins with conservative physical therapy and anti-inflammatory medications, once testing rules out other causes. With time and therapy, most patients with abnormal electroneurograms end up having normal results at follow-up testing.[110]

Cervicogenic Headache

CHs, also known as cervical headaches, are loosely defined as "any headache beginning in the neck."[30] These types of headaches are difficult to define and classify because of their variable distribution and character of symptoms. Neck pain can arise from injuries of the cervical muscles, ligaments, disks, and joints. From lower cervical segments, the pain may be referred to the shoulder and upper limb (see Table 22-1). From upper segments, neck pain may be referred to the head and manifested as headache.[141] The World Cervicogenic Headache Society has defined CH as "referred pain perceived in any part of the head and caused by a primary nociceptive source in musculoskeletal tissues that are innervated by

TABLE 23-6 Differential Diagnostic Characteristics of Cervicogenic Dizziness, BPPV, and VBI			
	Vertigo Type	**Nystagmus Characteristics**	**Associated Signs and Symptoms**
Cervicogenic dizziness	Positioning type	No latency period	Nystagmus
		Brief duration Fatigable with repeated motion	Neck pain Suboccipital headaches Cervical motion abnormality
BPPV	Positioning type	Short latency: 1–5 s Brief duration: <30 s Fatigable with repeated motion	Nystagmus
VBI	Positional type	Long latency: 55 ± 18 s Increasing symptomatology with maintained head position Not fatigable with repeated motion	Dizziness Drop attacks Diplopia Dysarthria Dysphagia Ataxia of gait Nausea Numbness Nystagmus

BPPV, benign paroxysmal positional vertigo; VBI, vertebrobasilar insufficiency.
Data from Huijbregts P, Vidal P: Dizziness in orthopaedic physical therapy practice: classification and pathophysiology. *J Man Manip Ther* 12:199–214, 2004; Terrett AGJ: *Current Concepts in Vertebrobasilar Complications Following Spinal Manipulation*, 2nd edn. Norwalk, IA: Foundation for Chiropractic Education and Research, 2001.

cervical nerves." According to the International Headache Society (IHS),[142] a CH is defined as one that meets the following criteria: (1) pain localized to the neck and occipital region that may project to the forehead, orbital region, temples, vertex, or ears; (2) pain precipitated or aggravated by specific neck movements or sustained neck posture; and (3) resistance to or limitation of active or passive physiologic and accessory neck movements or abnormal tenderness of neck muscles, or both. In addition, the IHS guidelines require radiographic examination to diagnose CHs. According to the IHS, radiologic examination must reveal at least one of the following: (1) movement abnormalities during flexion–extension, (2) abnormal posture, or (3) fractures, bone tumors, RA, congenital abnormalities, or other distinct pathology other than spondylosis or osteochondrosis.[142] To help in the determination when examining a patient complaining of headache, the clinician is advised to follow the simple diagnostic clinical algorithm set out below:[62]

- Exclude possible intracranial causes on history and physical examination. If intracranial pathology is suspected, then an urgent workup is required, which may include neuroimaging studies and laboratory investigations.
- Exclude headaches associated with viral or other infective illness.
- Exclude a drug-induced headache or headache related to alcohol or substance abuse.
- Consider an exercise-related (or sex-related) headache syndrome (see Chap. 5).
- Differentiate between vascular, tension, cervicogenic, or other causes of headache.

With CHs, pain is precipitated or aggravated by specific neck movements or sustained neck posture.

CLINICAL PEARL

CHs tend to be unilateral and accompanied by tenderness of the C2–3 articular pillars on the affected side.[143] The patient with a CH usually reports a dull aching pain of moderate intensity, which begins in the neck or occipital region and then spreads to include a greater part of the cranium.[144]

CHs can emerge from a number of sources, including[145]

- irritation of the posterior (dorsal) root ganglia and nerve root components caused by compression of the C2 posterior (dorsal) root ganglia between the C1 posterior arch and the superior C2 articular process[146];
- compression of the C2 anterior (ventral) ramus at the articular process of C1–2[88];
- entrapment of the C2 posterior (dorsal) root ganglia by the C1–2 epistrophic ligament.[147]

Neck pain and headache are also the cardinal features of a whiplash mechanism.[37,148,149] According to the international classification, headache after whiplash is best classified as cervicogenic (group 11.2.1) and thus related to injured structures around the cervical spine.[142] The incidence of headache after whiplash injury is said to decrease during the first 6 months after trauma.[150] Headache after whiplash can be from cervical spine trauma as listed or from a possible coup–contracoup injury from the rapid acceleration–deceleration of the brain in a closed calverium. Particularly relevant is the relation between a history of headache and the development of a trauma-related headache after whiplash injury. In addition, psychological variables, which may be important in idiopathic headache,[151,152] should be evaluated in relation to the development and recovery from headache after whiplash.

Several interventions have been recommended for CHs, including posture training, manual therapy, exercise, rest, and minor analgesics.[64] Manual therapy studies have demonstrated positive effects at both the impairment (pain and muscle function) and the disability level, with most studies focusing on short-term outcomes.[153,154]

In a single case study, McDonnell and colleagues[153] described an intervention approach for CH, consisting of a specific active exercise program and modification of postural alignment, with good results after seven visits over a 3-month period. The intervention focused on

- increasing the strength and control of the abdominals;
- increasing the length of the anterior thorax muscles;
- increasing the length of the posterior cervical extensor muscles;
- improving the strength and decreasing the length of the posterior scapulothoracic muscles;
- increasing shoulder joint and cervical motion.

Schoensee et al.[155] found that a treatment regimen of joint mobilization to the upper cervical spine in 10 CH patients decreased headache frequency, duration, and intensity.[156] CH frequency remained lower 1 month after the study.[155]

McKenzie[157] recommends a home program of cervical retraction exercises to decrease CH symptoms and maintain correct cervical alignment VIDEO. These exercises, which are performed throughout the day, are progressed based on changes in symptom location and intensity. If an exercise fails to reduce CH pain, a new component is added and the prior exercise is discontinued.[156]

For the prevention of chronic tension-type headaches, behavioral approaches commonly involve regular sleep and meals, stress coping, meditation, or relaxation strategies, and avoidance of initiating or trigger factors, including work-related or family stress and emotional problems.[64]

Hammill and colleagues[158] conducted a study, in which 20 subjects with tension-type headaches were treated with posture training, massage, and stretches. The results showed a significant decrease in headache frequency and in sickness impact profile scores at the end of the 6-week treatment period and again 12 months after the treatment concluded.[156]

Bronfort and colleagues[159] performed a systematic review of randomized controlled trials to include nine trials of 683 subjects with chronic headaches. They found that spinal mobilization treatment had a better effect than massage for CH and that it had a comparable effect to commonly used prophylactic prescription medications for tension-type and migraine headaches.[156,159]

Chiari Malformations

Chiari malformations are a group of disorders that manifest varying degrees of inferior displacement of the cerebellum and brain stem through the foramen magnum. Four types are recognized[160]:

- ***Chiari type I malformation.*** This type consists of the inferior displacement of the cerebellar hemispheres (cerebellar tonsils) through the foramen magnum. This tongue-like projection of the medial inferior cerebellum envelops the medulla. The fourth ventricle is in a normal position. As the degree of descent increases, the outflow of cerebrospinal fluid decreases, and a tubular cavitation of the upper spinal cord, called syringomyelia, then occurs. Syringomyelia is distinct from hydromyelia, which is an enlargement of the central canal of the spinal cord.
- ***Chiari type II malformation.*** Chiari type II malformation is associated with inferior displacement of the brainstem and fourth ventricle through the foramen magnum into the vertebral canal, often with hydrocephalus and meningomyelocele.
- ***Chiari type III malformation.*** This type is associated with a herniation of the cerebellum into a high cervical meningocele.
- ***Chiari type IV malformation.*** In Chiari type IV malformation, the cerebellum is generally hypoplastic.

Chiari types II–IV typically present with florid symptoms and are usually diagnosed in infancy or childhood.[160] In contrast, in Chiari type I malformation, the signs of brainstem dysfunction evolve slowly over years and are, thus, more likely than the other types to be encountered in physical therapy.

The clinical manifestations of Chiari I malformation are among the most protean in clinical medicine, which can lead to a delay in diagnosis. The most common presenting symptoms are upper extremity weakness and various pain syndromes that often include neck and arm pain.[161] Occipital headaches, which are exacerbated by coughing, sneezing, stooping, or lifting, are also frequent.[161] Clumsiness, upper extremity sensory changes ataxia, vertigo, hearing loss, tinnitus, dysphagia, hiccups, dysarthria, and hoarseness of voice are some of the other reported symptoms.[161]

The diagnosis of Chiari malformation is most commonly made with MRI. If surgical intervention is necessary, it involves decompression of the Chiari malformation with or without drainage of the syringomyelia.[160]

Pattern 4G: Impaired Joint Mobility, Motor Function, Muscle Performance, and Range of Motion Associated with Fracture

Although the intervention for fractures is beyond the scope of practice for a physical therapist, being able to detect their presence, especially in this region, is critical. Clinical findings that could suggest the possibility of a craniovertebral fracture include[162,163]:

- painful neck muscle splinting;
- neck and occipital numbness;
- pain and stiffness in the neck, with a reluctance to move the head;
- presence or absence of neurological signs and symptoms.

Fractures of the Axis

There are three types of fractures of the C2 (axis) vertebra: odontoid fractures involving the dens, bilateral traumatic spondylolisthesis of the pars interarticularis ("hangman's" fracture), and nonodontoid/nonhangman's (miscellaneous) fractures.[164]

Odontoid Fractures

Odontoid fractures are a relatively common upper cervical spine injury, comprising nearly 60% of all fractures of the axis and 10–18% of all cervical spine fractures.[67,165–168] Although odontoid fractures occur in all age groups, the mean age is approximately 47 years with a bimodal distribution.[7] In younger patients, who comprise the first peak, these fractures are usually secondary to high-energy trauma; motor vehicle accidents are responsible for the majority of the odontoid injuries.[169] The second peak in the incidence of odontoid fractures is in the elderly.[106] In fact, odontoid fractures are the most common cervical spine fracture in patients older than age 70.[7] These fractures, unlike those in the younger patients, tend to result from low-energy injuries, such as falls from a standing height.[7] The mechanism of injury often is hyperextension resulting in posterior displacement of the odontoid.[7]

Described in 1974, the Anderson and D'Alonzo system divides fractures into three types based on anatomic location[166]:

- ***Type I.*** Type I is an oblique avulsion fracture from the tip of the odontoid above the transverse ligament, attached to the alar ligament. This fracture is clinically rare, accounting for 1–5% of odontoid fractures, and may be associated with O-A dislocation.[167]
- ***Type II.*** Type II fractures occur through the neck of the odontoid. They are the most common type of odontoid fracture (38–80%).
- ***Type III.*** Type III fractures extend into the body of C2. They account for 15–40% of all odontoid fractures.

Current management of odontoid fractures is based on three principles: timely diagnosis, reduction of the fracture, and sufficient immobilization to permit healing.[168] Numerous treatment methods have been developed to achieve anatomic alignment and optimal stability, including cervical orthoses, Minerva jackets, halo-thoracic vests, posterior cervical fusion, and direct anterior dens screw fixation.[170]

Jefferson Fracture. Jefferson fracture was defined as the association of a lateral mass fracture of C1 and the disruption of the C1 ring (either on the posterior or on the anterior arch).[171] Jefferson fractures now represent a spectrum of injuries from bilateral ring fractures, to lateral mass fracture, to the pathognomonic four-point fracture (both anterior and posterior arches) of the C1 ring that the fracture was originally named for.[172] Jefferson fracture classically results from axial loading on the atlas and is generally associated with minimal neurologic deficit and good prognosis for neurologic recovery.[173] Presently, three general types of Jefferson fractures are described[174]:

- ***Type I.*** Type I involves bilateral single-arch (anterior or posterior, but not both) fractures.
- ***Type II.*** Type II is the concurrent anterior and posterior arch fractures, which include the classic four-point break Jefferson fracture.
- ***Type III.*** Type III is the lateral mass fracture of C1, which may extend into the anterior or the posterior osseous arch.

No prognostic significance has been attached to the different types of Jefferson fracture.[174] Isolated Jefferson fracture can be treated effectively with external immobilization. The traditional mode of cervical immobilization is the halo vest.[172]

THERAPEUTIC TECHNIQUES

Techniques to Increase Soft Tissue Extensibility

Soft tissue techniques generally are applied before performing the local segmental examination and in preparation for a mobilization or manipulation intervention. Soft tissue techniques are capable of producing a strong analgesic, and relaxing, effect. With a reduction in cervical muscle tension, or spasm, it becomes much easier for the clinician to palpate and register movement.

General Kneading

General kneading techniques can be applied to the soft tissues of the craniovertebral region. These techniques are especially useful before performing a specific mobilization or manipulation VIDEO.

Suboccipital Massage

Soft tissue techniques can be performed at several sites in the cervical region. In principle, every tender site can be treated, even though it usually involves areas of referred pain or tenderness.[175]

The patient is positioned prone or sitting, and the head is positioned in slight flexion, without rotation. The clinician stands on the uninvolved side. The SCM may need to be displaced laterally, in order to palpate the muscles attaching to the transverse process of C1. The clinician locates the most tender area and places the thumb directly lateral to the tender spot (Fig. 23-17). During the massage, the thumb moves from laterally to medially and slightly cranially, while at the same

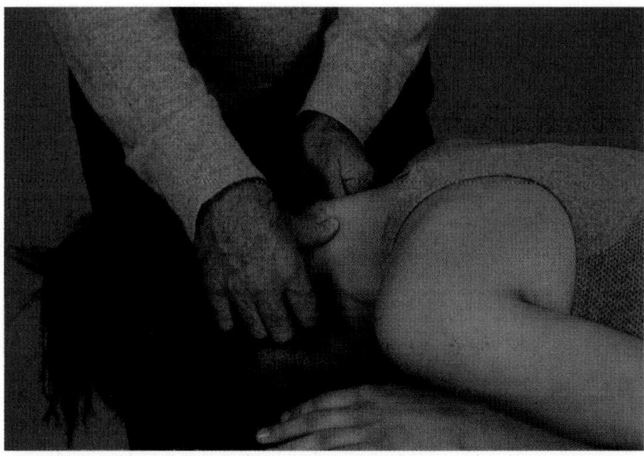

FIGURE 23-17 Suboccipital massage.

time, pressure is exerted in an anteromedial and superior direction.

A similar technique is used in a combination of upper cervical traction and soft tissue mobilization of the suboccipital muscles. This technique is best performed with the patient supine, because the neck is unloaded and the patient can relax more in the supine versus seated position. While one hand grasps the patient's head, the clinician uses the fingers of the other hand to press gently into the muscles between two vertebrae. While maintaining the pressure on the muscles, a slight traction force is applied and sustained for several seconds before being released. The procedure is repeated in a rhythmic manner.

The paravertebral muscles can be treated in a similar fashion. With one hand, the clinician stabilizes the patient's head at the forehead. With the index or middle finger of the left hand, or both fingers, the clinician pulls the musculature in a lateral and anterior direction. At the same time, the hand on the patient's forehead rotates the patient's head away from the side being treated. The end position is held for 2–3 seconds, before returning to the initial position. The clinician repeats this technique for several seconds or minutes in a rhythmic manner.

Muscle Stretching of the Suboccipital Muscles

Rectus Capitis Posterior Major and Minor. To stretch these muscles, the patient is positioned in supine or sitting. The clinician fixes C2 into craniovertebral flexion (see Fig. 23-18). To stretch the left muscle, a right side bending and right rotation motion is added, and the patient is instructed to not let the head drop back. Hold–relax or contract–relax techniques can be used.

Inferior Oblique. To stretch the left muscle, the patient's head and neck are positioned into flexion (see Fig. 23-19), left side bending, and right rotation. A massage to the muscle can be applied by stroking the muscle from the C1 transverse process to the C2 spinous process, applying a force in the direction of less pain.

Superior Oblique. The patient is positioned in sitting. The clinician places the index finger over the posterior aspect of the transverse process of C1, and the other hand wraps around the patient's head. To stretch the right superior oblique, the patient's head and neck must be placed in flexion, left side bending, and right rotation (see Fig. 23-20). Hold–relax or contract–relax techniques can be used.

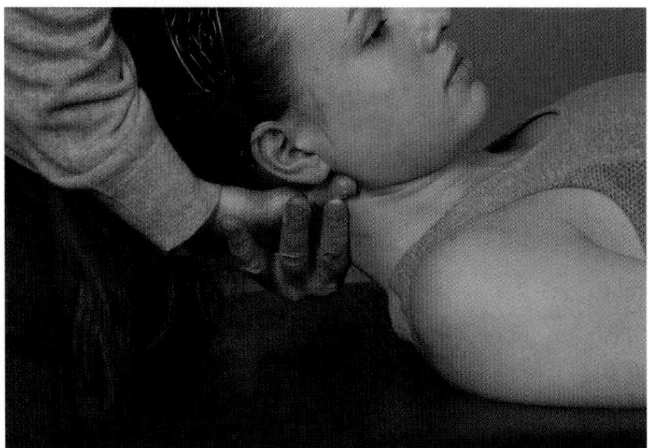

FIGURE 23-18 Stretch for rectus capitis posterior major and minor.

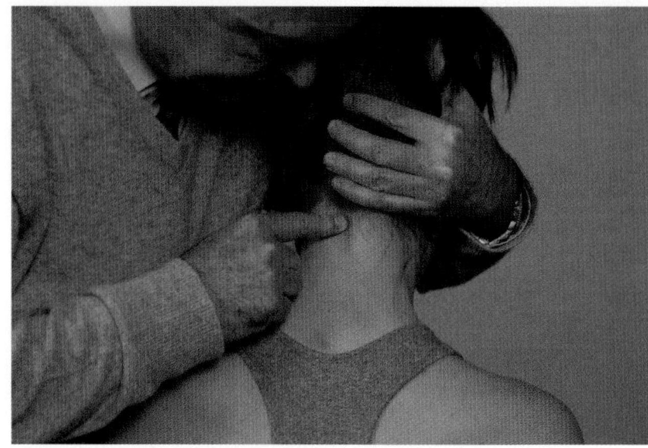

FIGURE 23-19 Stretch for inferior oblique.

Self-Stretching

The following exercises should be performed at an intensity level that achieves an improvement without a regression of status.

Chin Retraction. The patient is seated in the correct posture. The patient is instructed to attempt to move the head, as a unit, in a posterior direction, while maintaining eye level VIDEO. The clinician should limit the number of chin tucks the patient performs, to remove any potential for harm to the cervical structures from overuse.

C2–3 Side Bending and Rotation. The pattern of limitation for this area is usually one of a closing restriction. The patient is seated in the correct posture. The patient places both hands behind the neck, with the ulnar border of the little finger being just below the C2 spinous process and the rest of the hand covering as much of the midcervical region as possible. The

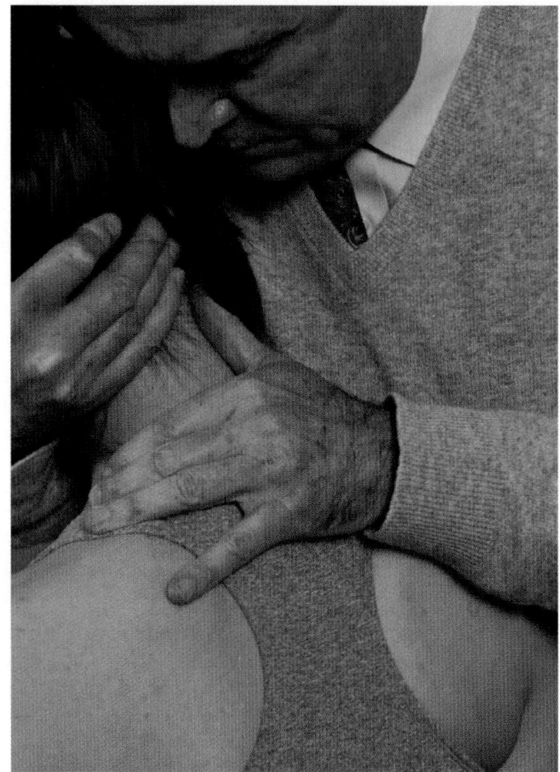

FIGURE 23-20 Stretch for superior oblique.

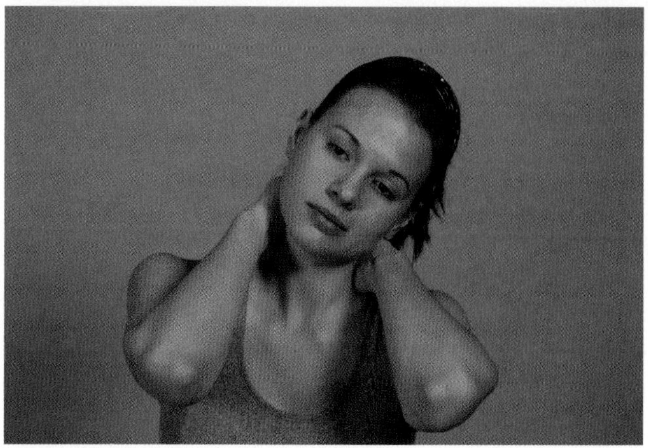

FIGURE 23-21 C2–3 side-bending and rotation exercise.

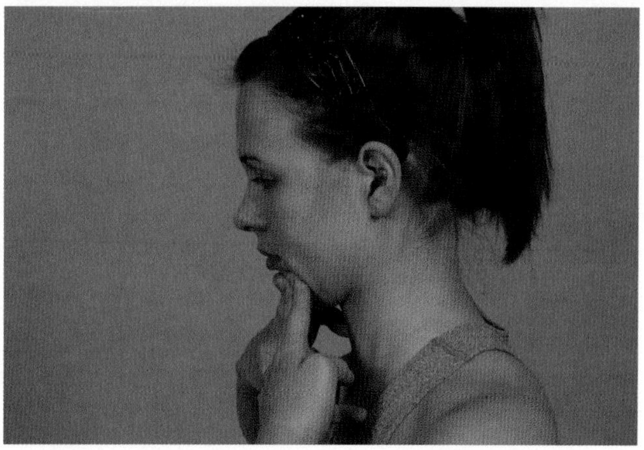

FIGURE 23-23 Home exercise for O-A flexion.

patient then simultaneously side flexes and rotates the neck and head in the direction of the restriction (Fig. 23-21), by attempting to look downward and backward (for a closing restriction).

A-A Rotation. The patient is seated in the correct posture. The patient places both hands behind the neck, with the ulnar border of the little finger being at the level of the C2 spinous process and the rest of the hand covering as much of the midcervical region as possible. The patient then gently turns the head in the direction of the restriction (Fig. 23-22) VIDEO. Coupled motions should be encouraged. For example, if the patient has a restriction with right rotation, right rotation and left side bending are emphasized.

O-A Flexion. The patient is seated in the correct posture. The patient performs a chin tuck. From the chin-tucked position, the patient is instructed to place the tips of the index and middle fingers of both hands over the anterior aspect of the chin (Fig. 23-23). The fingertips provide resistance for an attempted extension movement of the head on the neck. The patient then attempts to look upward, while resisting the motion with the fingertips. This is followed by relaxation and then another chin tuck. An alternative method involves asking the patient to clasp their figures behind the neck so that the little fingers are placed at the base of the skull VIDEO.

O-A Extension. The patient is seated in the correct posture. The patient places both hands behind the neck, with the ulnar border of the little finger being at the level of the C1 spinous process and the rest of the hand covering as much of the midcervical region as possible. The patient then gently lifts the chin around the appropriate axis (Fig. 23-24).

Techniques to Increase Joint Mobility

A series of studies that have investigated the efficacy of manual therapy in the treatment of upper cervical dysfunction and headache are outlined in Table 23-7.

Joint Mobilization Techniques

O-A Joint. ***Specific Traction.***[175] Specific traction is used here, as elsewhere in the spine, to apply a gentle degree of distraction and mechanical stimulation. It typically is used with acute conditions.

The patient is positioned in supine. The clinician stabilizes the C1 vertebra using a wide pinch grip, and the patient's forehead is stabilized against the clinician's shoulder (see Fig. 23-25). A traction force is then applied, a graded cranial force (I to II) by the occipital hand and the chest VIDEO.

Supine Technique for a Symmetrical Loss of O-A Extension. The patient is positioned in supine, head on a pillow, and knees flexed over a pillow. The clinician is positioned at the head of the table. The clinician cradles the patient's head in

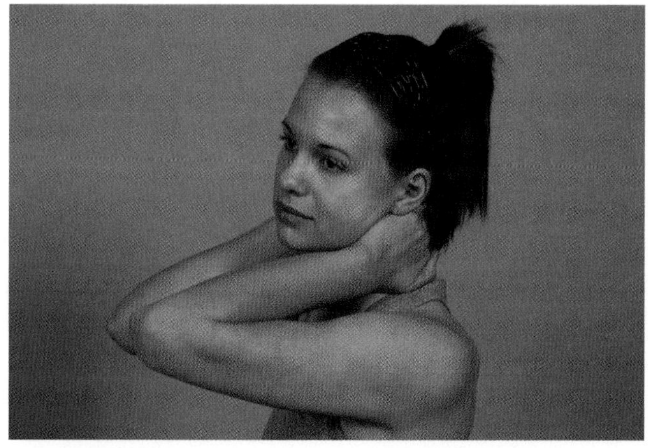

FIGURE 23-22 Exercise to increase right rotation at the A-A.

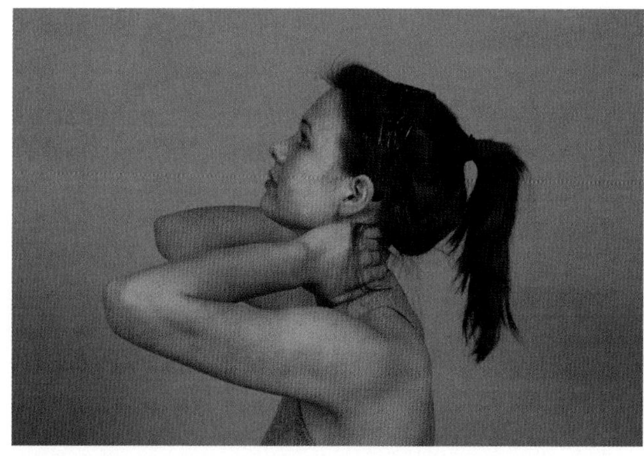

FIGURE 23-24 Home exercise for O-A extension.

TABLE 23-7 Summary of Published Studies Investigating Manual Therapy Treatment for Upper Cervical Dysfunction and Headache

Author	Sample Size	Intervention Group	Control Group	Outcome Measured	Number of Visits and Duration of Care
Boline et al.[a]	150	Manipulation	Medication	Headache frequency and intensity. Number of medications. SF-36 score	12 visits 6 wks
Howe et al.[b]	52	Manipulation ± Injection + Medication	Medication only	Cervical range of motion. Neck, scapular, arm, and hand pain. Neck stiffness. Headache intensity	1 visit only
Jensen et al.[c]	19	Mobilization Muscle energy	Cold packs	Frequency of medications. Pain intensity, dizziness, visual, and hearing	6 visits 12 wks
Nilsson[d]	39	Manipulation	Laser Friction massage	Headache duration and intensity. The number of nonsteroidal anti-inflammatory drugs	6 visits 3 wks
Nilsson et al.[e]	39	Manipulation	Laser Friction massage	Cervical passive range of motion	6 visits 3 wks
Osterbauer et al.[f]	20	Manipulation Electrical ± stimulation ± Medication	No treatment (10 nonimpaired)	Pain intensity. Cervical range of motion. Kinesthesia	2–3 visits per wk 6 wks
Parker et al.[g]	85	Manipulation by Chiropractor Manipulation by physical therapist	Mobilization by a physical therapist	Migraine frequency, intensity, and duration. Disability	Up to 16 visits 8 wks
Rogers[h]	20	Manipulation	Stretching	Pain. Kinesthesia	6 visits
Schoensee et al.[156,i]	10	Mobilization	None	Headache frequency, duration, and intensity	3–4 wks 9–12 visits 3–4 wks
Vernon[j]	33	Manipulation	None	Headache frequency, duration, and intensity	9 visits Unspecified
Whittingham et al.[k]	26	Manipulation at C1 and C2	None	Headache frequency, duration, and intensity	4 visits 2 wks
Yeomans[l]	58	Manipulation	None	Cervical intersegmental range of motion	3 visits per wk 2–6 wks

[a]Data from Boline PD, Kassak K, Bronfort G, et al.: Spinal manipulation vs. amitriptyline for the treatment of chronic tension-type headaches: a randomized clinical trial. *J Manip Physiol Ther* 18:148–154, 1995.

[b]Data from Howe DH, Newcombe RG, Wade MT: Manipulation of the cervical spine—a pilot study. *J R Coll Gen Pract* 33:574–579, 1983.

[c]Data from Jensen OK, Nielsen FF, Vosmar L: An open study comparing manual therapy with the use of cold packs in the treatment of post-traumatic headache. *Cephalalgia* 10:241–250, 1990.

[d]Data from Nilsson N: A randomized controlled trial of the effect of spinal manipulation in the treatment of cervicogenic headache. *J Manip Physiol Ther* 18:435–440, 1995.

[e]Data from Nilsson N, Christensen HW, Hartvigsen J: Lasting changes in passive range motion after spinal manipulation: a randomized, blind, controlled trial. *J Manip Physiol Ther* 19:165–168, 1996.

[f]Data from Osterbauer PJ, Derickson KL, Peles JD, et al.: Three-dimensional head kinematics and clinical outcome of patients with neck injury treated with spinal manipulative therapy: a pilot study. *J Manip Physiol Ther* 15:501–511, 1992.

[g]Data from Parker GB, Tupling H, Pryor DS: A controlled trial of cervical manipulation of migraine. *Aust N Z J Med* 8:589–593, 1978.

[h]Data from Rogers RG: The effects of spinal manipulation on cervical kinesthesia in patients with chronic neck pain: a pilot study. *J Manip Physiol Ther* 20:80–85, 1997.

[i]Data from Schoensee SK, Jensen G, Nicholson G, et al.: The effect of mobilization on cervical headaches. *J Orthop Sports Phys Ther* 21:184–196, 1995.

[j]Data from Vernon H: Chiropractic manipulative therapy in the treatment of headaches: a retrospective and prospective study. *J Manip Physiol Ther* 5: 109–112, 1982.

[k]Data from Whittingham W, Ellis WB, Molyneux TP: The effect of manipulation (toggle recoil technique) for headaches with upper cervical joint dysfunction: a pilot study. *J Manip Physiol Ther* 17:369–375, 1994.

[l]Data from Yeomans SG: The assessment of cervical intersegmental mobility before and after spinal manipulative therapy. *J Manip Physiol Ther* 15:106–114, 1992. With permission from Molina P: Upper cervical dysfunction and cervicogenic headache. In: Wilmarth MA, ed. *Evidence-Based Practice for the Upper and Lower Quarter. Orthopaedic Physical Therapy Home Study Course 13.2.1*. La Crosse, WI: Orthopaedic Section, APTA, Inc, 2003: 1–44.

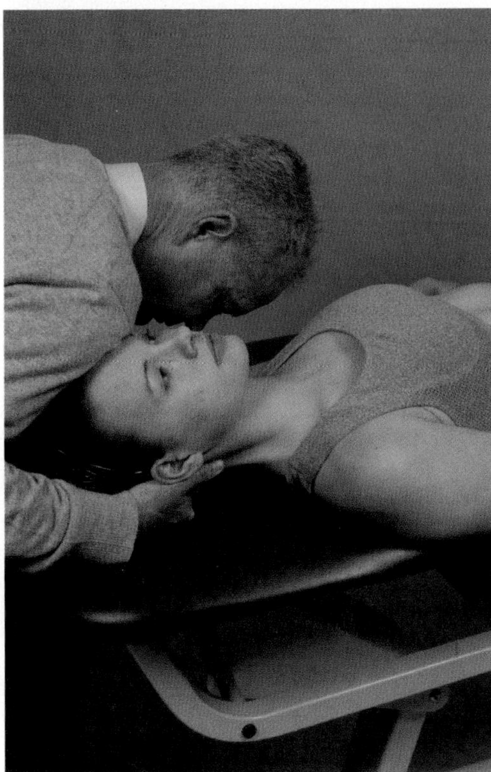

FIGURE 23-25 Specific traction to O-A joint in supine.

both hands with the finger pads under the occiput and places each thumb over the zygomatic arches of the patient. Using thumb pressure, the clinician tilts the patient's head into craniovertebral flexion, while the finger pads produce a posterior glide of the occipital condyles (see Fig. 23-26) VIDEO.

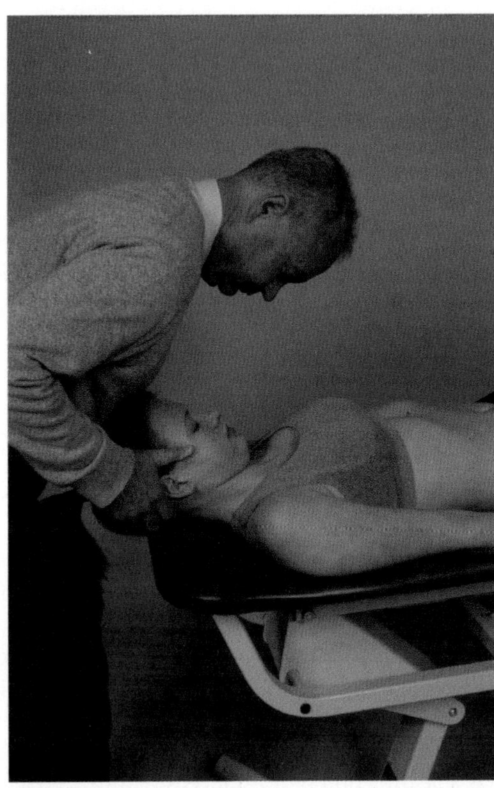

FIGURE 23-26 Supine technique for a symmetrical loss of O-A extension.

The joint slack is taken up. The patient is instructed to attempt to place the chin on their throat. After an isometric contraction of 3–5 seconds, the patient is instructed to relax, and the resultant joint slack is taken up by the clinician. When, following repeated muscle-assisted mobilizations, no further increased motion is apparent, it can be assumed that the inert barrier to motion has been reached. Passive soft tissue mobilization is then performed. This combination of muscle-assisted and passive mobilizations is continued until no further soft-tissue slack is appreciated.

Seated Technique for a Loss of Extension at the Left O-A Joint.[175] The following mobilization techniques can be used for a restriction of the anterior glide of the left O-A joint. The reader is expected to extrapolate the information to produce the necessary technique for a restriction of the anterior glide of the right joint.

The patient is seated with the clinician standing on the right side. C1 is stabilized anteriorly, using a wide pinch grip by the left hand and wrapping the pads of the index finger and thumbs around the front of the transverse process (Fig. 23-27). The right arm stabilizes the patient's head against the clinician's chest, and the right hand grasps the occiput. The patient's head is then extended and left side flexed around the appropriate axes, with right translation being produced by means of the side bending until the extension barrier is reached. The mobilization is then performed by applying a graded force against the translation barrier.

Active participation from the patient can be introduced. From the motion barrier, the patient is asked to gently meet the clinician's resistance. The direction of resistance is that which facilitates further extension, left side bending, and right rotation. The isometric contraction is held for up to 5 seconds and followed by a period of complete relaxation. The joint is then passively taken to the new motion barrier. The technique is repeated three times and followed by a reexamination.

Supine Technique for an Asymmetrical Loss of O-A Extension (e.g., Loss of Left O-A Joint Extension).[94] The patient is positioned in supine, head on a pillow, and knees flexed over a pillow. The clinician is positioned at the head of the table. The clinician cradles the patient's head in both hands. The left index and middle finger pads are placed just medial to the patient's left mastoid process, with the palm supporting

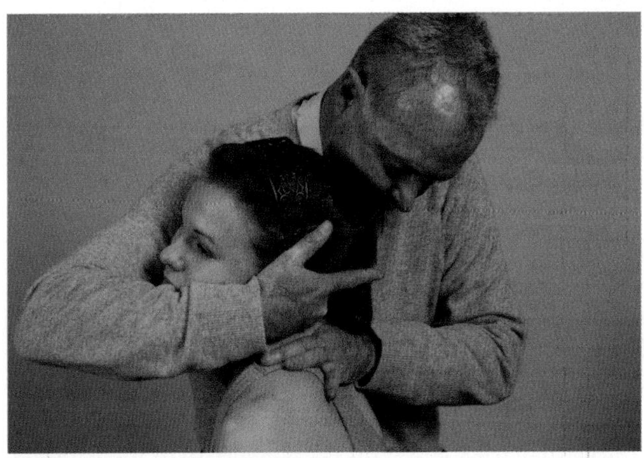

FIGURE 23-27 Seated technique for a loss of extension at the left O-A joint.

the occiput. The clinician's right hand is placed over the right side of the patient's head VIDEO.

Using both hands, the clinician passively moves the patient's head into craniovertebral extension and right translation, until the extension motion barrier of the left O-A joint is reached. The joint slack is taken up by the clinician using their left fingers to push upward toward the patient's lips and the clinician's right hand, thereby inducing side flexion of the patient's head to the left.

The patient is instructed to resist left side flexion of the O-A joint using the command "Don't let me pull your left ear upwards." The contraction is held for 3–5 seconds, and the patient is asked to relax. As the patient relaxes, the new joint slack is taken up by the clinician pushing further toward the patient's lips with the left finger pads and side flexing the patient's head to the left with clinician's right hand. To ensure that the extension is occurring around a craniovertebral axis, the clinician looks at the patient's face. As slack is taken up, flexion of the right O-A joint should simultaneously produce chin movement toward the ceiling, while the forehead moves toward the bed. To ensure that the left side flexion is occurring around the correct axis, the clinician should note the chin movement occurring to the right, while the forehead moves to the left. During the conjunct right rotation, the chin and forehead should both be seen to rotate to the right.

As with the technique to increase unilateral flexion, once the inert barrier is reached, the combined passive motion into the barrier is stressed with oscillatory passive stretch, and then muscle-assisted mobilizations are repeated. This is continued until there is no further "give" to the motion barrier.

Supine Technique for an Asymmetrical Loss of O-A Flexion (e.g., Loss of Left O-A Joint Flexion).[94] The patient is positioned in supine, head on a pillow, and knees flexed over a pillow. The clinician is positioned at the head of the table. The clinician cradles the patient's head in both hands, so that the right hand is placed over the right side of the patient's head and the clinician's left index and middle finger pads are placed just medial to the patient's left mastoid processes, with the palm supporting the patient's occiput VIDEO.

Using both hands, the clinician produces craniovertebral flexion to the barrier. At this point, the patient's head is translated to the left until a firm end-feel is encountered. This maneuver induces a right side bending and a left rotation at the O-A joints. The barrier to flexion of the left O-A joint is thus achieved.

Joint slack is taken up as the clinician uses a lumbrical action to pull on the patient's left mastoid process, in the direction toward the bed surface, with the left index and middle fingers. Simultaneously, the patient's head is side flexed to the right by the clinician's right hand. Using fingertip pressure through the right hand, the clinician instructs the patient: "Don't let me lift your right ear upwards." The clinician then attempts to draw the patient's right mastoid process superiorly. This produces an isometric resistance of right side flexion of the O-A joint (and, therefore, left rotation).

After an isometric contraction of 3–5 seconds, the patient is instructed to relax, and as the relaxation is felt by the clinician, the resultant joint slack is taken up by the clinician by simultaneously pulling the patient's left mastoid process toward the bed (with the left hand) and side bending the head to the right (with the right hand). When, following repeated muscle-assisted mobilizations, no further increased motion is apparent, it can be assumed that the inert barrier to motion has been reached. Passive soft tissue mobilization is then achieved by pushing further into the left O-A joint flexion barrier by simultaneously pulling the left mastoid process toward the bed (left hand) and right side bending of the head (right hand). This combination of muscle-assisted and passive mobilizations is continued until no further soft tissue slack is appreciated. To ensure that the flexion is occurring around a craniovertebral axis, the clinician looks at the patient's face. As slack is taken up, flexion of the left O-A joint should simultaneously produce

- a downward motion of the patient's chin and an upward motion of the patient's forehead (flexion);
- a left-sided motion of the patient's chin with a left-sided motion of the forehead (right side flexion);
- a rotation of chin and forehead to the left (left rotation).

If these facial movements are not seen, then the right hand is used to ensure that these motions are occurring, thus maintaining a craniovertebral axis.

A-A Joint. ***Loss of the Anterior-Inferior Glide of the Left A-A Joint (e.g., Loss of Right Rotation in A-A Joint—Loss of Left Anterior/Inferior Glide).***[94] The patient is positioned in supine, head on a pillow, and knees flexed over a pillow. The clinician is positioned at the head of the table. The clinician cradles the patient's head in both hands. The clinician's right index and middle finger pads are placed around the *left* side of the patient's C2 neural arch, making firm contact with the left side of the C2 spinous process VIDEO. The clinician's left hand supports the left side of the patient's head. The patient's head is side flexed by clinician's left hand. Using the fingers of the right hand, the clinician feels for the C2 spinous process to move to the right. At this point, the C2 spinous process is pulled by the index and middle fingers of the right hand until the motion barrier is detected. The patient is instructed to push their head into clinician's left hand, i.e., resisted left side flexion. The C2 spinous process should be felt to move to the right, and the clinician's right fingers move to fix it, as the patient is instructed to relax. As patient relaxes, the slack in left side bending of the head is taken up. This is repeated until no further motion of C2 spinous process is detected.

A similar technique can be performed with the patient in sitting (Fig. 23-28). Using one hand (left, in the photo), the clinician stabilizes the C2 segment and the inferior vertebral segments using a lumbrical grip. The fifth digit of the other hand wraps around the neural arch of C1 and supports the head. The patient's head is side flexed by clinician's shoulder and rotated by the clinician's right hand until the rotation barrier is reached. The mobilization is then performed by applying a graded force against the barrier. Active participation from the patient can be introduced. From the motion barrier, the patient is asked to gently meet the clinician's resistance. The direction of resistance is that which facilitates further rotation. The isometric contraction is held up to 5 seconds and followed by a period of complete relaxation.

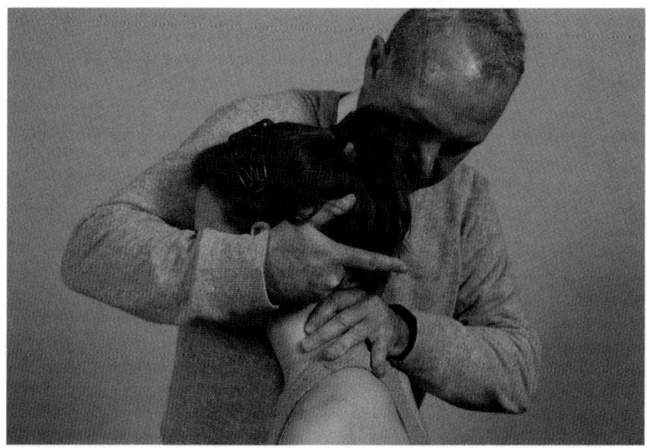

FIGURE 23-28 Seated technique for loss of right rotation in A-A joint—loss of left anterior/inferior glide.

The joint is then passively taken to the new motion barrier. The technique is repeated three times and followed by a reexamination.

Mobilizations with Movement[176]

Upper Cervical Traction. This is an excellent technique for the intervention of upper cervical headaches. The patient is positioned in sitting, with the clinician standing in front, facing the patient. The patient's head against the clinician's chest, and the fingers wrap around the patient's head to provide firm support (Fig. 23-29). The clinician's other hand is used to stabilize the inferior segment (see Fig. 23-29).

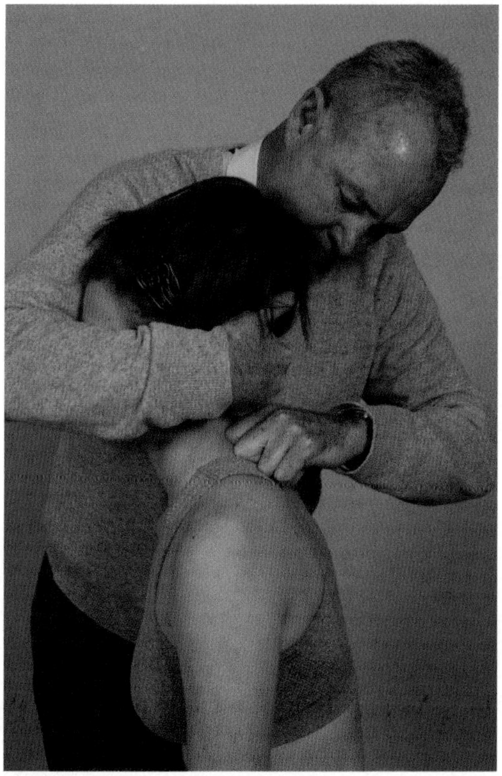

FIGURE 23-29 Upper cervical traction.

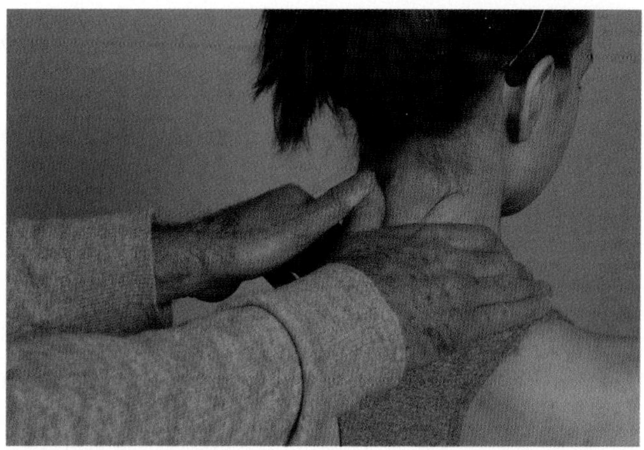

FIGURE 23-30 Mobilization to increase right rotation of the A-A.

The clinician applies pressure on the inferior segment while preventing motion of the head and applying a longitudinal force through the head. The end-feel is obtained and is maintained for 10–20 seconds.

To Improve Right Rotation of the A-A Joint. The patient is positioned in sitting, with the clinician sitting behind. The clinician places the thumb of one hand over the left aspect of the transverse process of C2, and the other thumb over the first thumb to help reinforce it. The remaining fingers of the hands are placed around the patient's neck and upper back, or to the side of the head (Fig. 23-30).

The patient is asked to rotate the head and neck slowly to the right, while the clinician simultaneously assists the movement using pressure from both thumbs, rotating C2 to the left.

This technique can be taught as part of the patient's home exercise program, using a to wel, belt, or a strap (Fig. 23-31). The same technique can be used to improve cervical rotation to the left by altering the position of the thumbs.

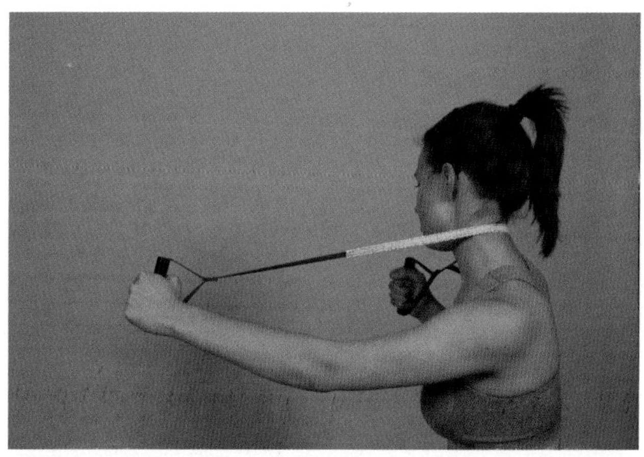

FIGURE 23-31 Home exercise to increase right rotation of the A-A.

CASE STUDY

HEADACHE AND NECK PAIN

HISTORY

A self-employed 42-year-old man presented to the clinic complaining of posterior upper neck pain and right suboccipital and occipital headache, which began 2 months earlier after a diving accident. He denied being knocked unconscious and could remember everything about the accident except for the period a few minutes after it. The posterior neck pain was felt immediately but was much worse the next morning upon waking. The occipital headaches started a few days later and became worse with fatigue or exertion. The patient also reported difficulty concentrating and sleeping and had occasional bouts of dizziness, especially when turning his head to the left, during which he would become unsteady, but denied vertigo. When the neck and occipital pain flared up, it spread from the occipital region over the head to the right eye. Previous interventions included physical therapy in the form of ultrasound, massage, spray and stretch, myofascial release, and cranial sacral therapy, which had provided no relief.

The patient had no history of back or neck pain, apart from the occasional ache, and his medical history was unremarkable.

Questions

1. List the concerns the clinician should have following this history.
2. Using a flow diagram describe how you would proceed with this patient following the history.
3. What special tests should be considered at this point?
4. Are additional questions needed with regard to the history?

REVIEW QUESTIONS*

1. Describe the anatomy of the craniovertebral region.
2. What structures provide stability in the craniovertebral region?
3. Which of the following is not a suboccipital muscle: rectus capitis lateralis, rectus capitis posterior major, rectus capitis posterior minor, obliquus capitis inferior, and obliquus capitis superior?
4. What is the extension of the posterior longitudinal ligament called?
5. Which muscle produces side bending of the O-A joint to the same side, as well as extension and contralateral rotation of the O-A?

*Additional questions to test your understanding of this chapter can be found in the Online Learning Center for *Orthopaedic Assessment, Evaluation, and Intervention* at www.duttononline.net.

REFERENCES

1. Radanov BP, Dvorak J, Valach L: Cognitive deficits in patients after soft tissue injury of the cervical spine. *Spine* 17:127–131, 1992.
2. Kapandji IA: *The Physiology of the Joints: Annotated Diagrams of the Mechanics of the Human Joints*, 2nd ed. Edinburgh: Churchill Livingstone, 1974.
3. Gray H: *Gray's Anatomy*. Philadelphia, PA: Lea & Febiger, 1995.
4. Panjabi M, Dvorak J, Duranceau J, et al.: Three-dimensional movement of the upper cervical spine. *Spine* 13:727, 1988.
5. Walsh R, Nitz AJ: Cervical spine. In: Wadsworth C, ed. *Current Concepts of Orthopedic Physical Therapy - Home Study Course*. La Crosse, WI: Orthopaedic Section, APTA, 2001.
6. Williams PL, Warwick R, Dyson M, et al.: *Gray's Anatomy*, 37th ed. London: Churchill Livingstone, 1989.
7. Sasso RC: C2 dens fractures: treatment options. *J Spinal Disord* 14:455–463, 2001.
8. Heggeness MH, Doherty BJ: The trabecular anatomy of the axis. *Spine* 18:1945–1949, 1993.
9. Doherty BJ, Heggeness MH: Quantitative anatomy of the second cervical vertebra. *Spine* 20:513–517, 1995.
10. Ellis JH, Martel W, Lillie JH, et al.: Magnetic resonance imaging of the normal craniovertebral junction. *Spine* 16:105, 1991.
11. Pick TP, Howden R: *Gray's Anatomy*, 15th ed. New York, NY: Barnes & Noble Books, 1995.
12. Pal GP, Sherk HH: The vertical stability of the cervical spine. *Spine* 13:447, 1988.
13. Yoganandan N, Pintar F, Butler J, et al.: Dynamic response of human cervical spine ligaments. *Spine* 14:1102, 1989.
14. Dvorak J, Panjabi MM: Functional anatomy of the alar ligaments. *Spine* 12:183, 1987.
15. Dvorak J, Panjabi MM, Gerber M, et al.: CT functional diagnostics of the rotary instability of the upper cervical spine and experimental study in cadavers. *Spine* 12:197–205, 1987.
16. Okazaki K: Anatomical study of the ligaments in the occipito-atlantoaxial complex (Japanese). *Nihon Seikeigeka Gakkai Zasshi* 69:1259–1267, 1995.
17. Panjabi M, Dvorak J, Crisco J, et al.: Flexion, extension, and lateral bending of the upper cervical spine in response to alar ligament transections. *J Spinal Disord* 4:157–167, 1991.
18. O'Brien MF, Lenke LG: Fractures and dislocations of the spine. In: Dee R, Hurst L, Gruber M, et al., eds. *Principles of Orthopaedic Practice*, 2nd ed. New York, NY: McGraw-Hill, 1997:1237–1293.
19. Vangilder JC, Menezes AH, Dolan KD: *The Craniovertebral Junction and its Abnormalities*. Mount Kisco, NY: Futura Publishing Co, 1987.
20. White AA, Johnson RM, Panjabi MM, et al.: Biomechanical analysis of clinical stability in the cervical spine. *Clin Orthop* 109:85–96, 1975.
21. Dvorak J, Schneider E, Saldinger P, et al.: Biomechanics of the craniocervical region; the alar and transverse ligaments. *J Orthop Res* 6:452–461, 1987.
22. Buckworth J: Anatomy of the suboccipital region. In: Vernon H, ed. *Upper Cervical Syndrome*. Baltimore, MD: Williams & Wilkins, 1988.
23. Bogduk N: Innervation and pain patterns of the cervical spine. In: Grant R, ed. *Physical Therapy of the Cervical and Thoracic Spine*. New York, NY: Churchill Livingstone, 1988.
24. Swash M, Fox K: Muscle spindle innervation in man. *J Anat* 112:61–80, 1972.

25. Hack GD, Koritzer RT, Robinson WL, et al.: Anatomic relation between the rectus capitis posterior minor muscle and the dura mater. *Spine* 20:2484–2486, 1995.
26. Fryette HH: *Principles of Osteopathic Technique*. Colorado, CO: Academy of Osteopathy, 1980.
27. DiGiovanna EL, Schiowitz S: *An Osteopathic Approach to Diagnosis and Treatment*. Philadelphia, PA: JB Lippincott, 1991.
28. Bellavance A, Belzile G, Bergeron Y, et al.: Cervical spine and headaches. *Neurology* 39:1269–1270, 1989.
29. Bogduk N: Cervical causes of headache and dizziness. In: Grieve GP, ed. *Modern Manual Therapy of the Vertebral Column*. New York, NY: Churchill Livingstone, 1986:289–302.
30. Bogduk N: The anatomical basis for cervicogenic headache. *J Manip Physiol Ther* 15:67–70, 1992.
31. Edmeads J: The cervical spine and headache. *Neurology* 38:1874–1878, 1988.
32. Fredriksen TA, Hovdal H, Sjaastad O: Cervicogenic headache: clinical manifestation. *Cephalalgia* 7:147–160, 1987.
33. Dreyfuss P, Michaelson M, Fletcher D: Atlanto-occipital and lateral atlanto-axial joint pain patterns. *Spine* 19:1125–1131, 1994.
34. Ehni GE, Benner B: Occipital neuralgia and the C1–2 arthrosis syndrome. *J Neurosurg* 61:961–965, 1984.
35. Bovim G, Berg R, Dale LG: Cervicogenic headache: anaesthetic blockade of cervical nerves (C2–5) and facet joint (C2/3). *Pain* 49:315–320, 1992.
36. Lord SM, Barnsley L, Wallis BJ, et al.: Third occipital nerve headache: a prevalence study. *J Neurol Neurosurg Psychiatry* 57:1187–1190, 1994.
37. Lord SM, Barnsley L, Wallis BJ, et al.: Chronic cervical zygapophyseal joint pain after whiplash: a placebo-controlled prevalence study. *Spine* 21:1737–1744, 1996.
38. Lazorthes G: Pathology, classification and clinical aspects of vascular diseases of the spinal cord. In: Vinken PJ, Bruyn GW, eds. *Handbook of Clinical Neurology*. Oxford: Elsevier, 1972:494–506.
39. Baumgartner RW, Waespe W: ASA syndrome of the cervical hemicord. *Eur Arch Psychiatry Clin Neurosci* 241:205–209, 1992.
40. Wells CEC: Clinical aspects of spinovascular disease. *Proc R Soc Med* 59:790–796, 1966.
41. Decroix JP, Ciaudo-Lacroix C, Lapresle J: Syndrome de Brown-Sequard du a un infarctus spinal. *Rev Neurol* 140:585–586, 1984.
42. Gutowski NJ, Murphy RP, Beale DJ: Unilateral upper cervical posterior spinal artery syndrome following sneezing. *J Neurol Neurosurg Psychiatry* 55:841–843, 1992.
43. Tulsi RS: Some specific anatomical features of the atlas and axis: dens, epitransverse process and articular facets. *Aust N Z J Surg* 48:570–574, 1978.
44. Singh S: Variations of the superior articular facets of atlas vertebrae. *J Anat* 99:565–571, 1965.
45. Noren R, Trafimow J, Andersson GBJ, et al.: The role of facet joint tropism and facet angle in disc degeneration. *Spine* 16:530–532, 1991.
46. Malmavaara A, Videman T, Kuosma E, et al.: Facet joint orientation, facet and costovertebral joint osteoarthritis, disc degeneration, vertebral body osteophytosis, and Schmorl's nodes in the thoracolumbar junctional region of cadaveric spines. *Spine* 12:458–463, 1987.
47. White AA, Panjabi MM: *Clinical Biomechanics of the Spine*. In: White AA, Panjabi MM, eds. 2nd ed. Philadelphia, PA: Lippincott-Raven, 1990: pp 106–108 [A1].
48. Lind B, Sihlbom H, Nordwall A, et al.: Normal range of motion of the cervical spine. *Arch Phys Med Rehabil* 70:692–695., 1989.
49. Werne S: The possibilities of movements in the cranio-vertebral joints. *Acta Orthop Scand* 28:165–173, 1959.
50. Penning L, Wilmink JT: Rotation of the cervical spine. A CT study in normal subjects. *Spine* 12:732–738, 1987.
51. Dvorak J, Hayek J, Zehender R: CT – functional diagnosis of the rotary instability of the upper cervical spine – 2. An evaluation on healthy adults and patients with suspected instability. *Spine* 12:726–731, 1987.
52. Mercer S: Kinematics of the spine. In: Boyling JD, Jull GA, eds. *Grieve's Modern Manual Therapy: The Vertebral Column*. Philadelphia, PA: Churchill Livingstone, 2004:31–37.
53. Selecki BR: The effects of rotation of the atlas on the axis: experimental work. *Med J Aust* 1:1012, 1969.
54. Fielding JW: Cineroentgenography of the normal cervical spine. *J Bone Joint Surg* 39A:1280, 1957.
55. White AA, Panjabi MM: The clinical biomechanics of the occipitoatlantoaxoid complex. *Orthop Clin North Am* 9:867–878, 1975.
56. Mimura M, Moriya H, Watanabe T, et al.: Three-dimensional motion analysis of the cervical spine with special reference to the axial rotation. *Spine* 14:1135, 1989.
57. Hohl M, Baker HR: The atlanto-axial joint. *J Bone Joint Surg* 46A:1739–1752, 1964.
58. Fielding JW, Cochran GV, Lawsing J.F. I, et al.: Tears of the transverse ligament of the atlas. A clinical and biomechanical study. *J Bone and Joint Surg* 56A:1683–1691, 1974.
59. Mercer SR, Bogduk N: Joints of the cervical vertebral column. *J Orthop Sports Phys Ther* 31:174–182; discussion 183. 2001.
60. Meadows JTS: *Manual Therapy: Biomechanical Assessment and Treatment, Advanced Technique*. Calgary, AB: Swodeam Consulting, Inc., 1995.
61. Meadows J, Pettman E: *Manual Therapy: NAIOMT Level II & III Course Notes*. Denver, CO: North American Institute of Manual Therapy, Inc., 1995.
62. McCrory P: Headaches and exercise. *Sports Med* 30:221–229, 2000.
63. Travell JG, Simons DG: *Myofascial Pain and Dysfunction – The Trigger Point Manual*. Baltimore, MD: Williams & Wilkins, 1983.
64. Welch KM: A 47-year-old woman with tension-type headaches. *JAMA* 286:960–966, 2001.
65. Jensen S, Graff-Radford S: Oromandibular function and tension-type headache. In: Olesen J, Tfelt-Hansen P, Welch KMA, eds. *The Headaches*. Philadelphia, PA: Lippincott Williams & Wilkins, 2000:593–597.
66. Wolff HG: *Headache and Other Head Pain*, 2nd ed. New York, NY: Oxford University Press, 1987:53–76.
67. Chutkan NB, King AG, Harris MB: Odontoid fractures: evaluation and management. *J Am Acad Ortho Surg* 5:199–204, 1997.
68. Viikara-Juntura E: *Examination of the Neck. Validity of Some Clinical, Radiological and Epidemiologic Methods*. Helsinki: University of Helsinki, Institute of Occupational Health, 1988.
69. Johnson GM: The correlation between surface measurement of head and neck posture and the anatomic position of the upper cervical vertebrae. *Spine* 23:921–927, 1998.
70. Braun BL, Amundson LR: Quantitative assessment of head and shoulder posture. *Arch Phys Med Rehabil* 70:322–329, 1989.
71. Braun BL: Postural differences between asymptomatic men and women and craniofacial pain patients. *Arch Phys Med Rehabil* 72:653–656, 1991.
72. Watson D, Trott P: Cervical headache: an investigation of natural head posture and upper cervical flexor muscle performance. *Cephalalgia* 13:272–284, 1993.
73. Grimmer K: The relationship between cervical resting posture and neck pain. *Physiotherapy* 82:45–51, 1996.
74. Griegel-Morris P, Larson K, Mueller-Klaus K, et al.: Incidence of common postural abnormalities in the cervical, shoulder, and thoracic regions and their association with pain in two age groups of healthy subjects. *Phys Ther* 72:426–430, 1992.
75. Bergmann TF, Peterson DH, Lawrence DJ: *Chiropractic Technique: Principles and Procedures*. New York, NY: Churchill Livingstone, 1993.
76. Kori AA, Leigh JL: The cranial nerve examination. In: Gilman S, ed. *Clinical Examination of the Nervous System*. New York, NY: McGraw-Hill, 2000:65–111.
77. Magee DJ: *Orthopedic Physical Assessment*. Philadelphia, PA: WB Saunders, 2002.
78. McGaughran JM, Kuna P, Das V: Audiological abnormalities in the Klippel-Feil syndrome. *Arch Dis Child* 79:352–355, 1998.
79. Bhandari S, Farr MJ: Case report: Klippel-Feil syndrome with coexistent hypoparathyroidism. *Am J Med Sci* 311:174–177, 1996.
80. Da-Silva EO: Autosomal recessive Klippel-Feil syndrome. *J Med Genet* 19:130–134, 1982.
81. Kanchandani R, Howe JG: Lhermitte's sign in multiple sclerosis: a clinical survey and review of the literature. *J Neurol Neurosurg Psychiatry* 45:308–312, 1982.
82. Pettman E: Stress tests of the craniovertebral joints. In: Boyling JD, Palastanga N, eds. *Grieve's Modern Manual Therapy: The Vertebral Column*, 2nd ed. Edinburgh: Churchill Livingstone, 1994:529–538.
83. Murphy DK, Gutrecht JA: Lhermitte's sign in cavernous angioma of the cervical spinal cord. *J Neurol Neurosurg Psychiatry* 65:954–955, 1998.
84. al-Orainy IA, Kolawole T: Ossification of the ligament flavum. *Eur J Radiol* 29:76–82, 1998.
85. Fuss FK: Sagittal kinematics of the cervical spine – how constant are the motor axes? *Acta Anatomica* 141:93–96, 1991.
86. Hardin J Jr.: Pain and the cervical spine. *Bull Rheum Dis* 50:1–4, 2001.

87. Bland JH: New anatomy and physiology with clinical and historical implications. In: Bland JH, ed. *Disorders of the Cervical Spine*, 2nd ed. Philadelphia, PA: WB Saunders, 1994:71–79.
88. Bogduk N: An anatomical basis for the neck-tongue syndrome. *J Neurol Neurosurg Psychiatry* 44:202–208, 1981.
89. Ross JK, Bereznick DE, McGill SM: Atlas-axis facet asymmetry. Implications in manual palpation. *Spine* 24:1203–1209, 1999.
90. Greenman PE: *Principles of Manual Medicine*, 2nd ed. Baltimore, MD: Williams & Wilkins, 1996.
91. Dvorak J, Dvorak V: General Principles of Palpation. In: Gilliar WG, Greenman PE, eds. *Manual Medicine: Diagnostics*, 2nd ed. New York, NY: Thieme Medical Publishers, 1990:71–75.
92. Smedmark V, Wallin M, Arvidsson I: Inter-examiner reliability in assessing passive intervertebral motion of the cervical spine. *Man Ther* 5:97–101, 2000.
93. Pool JJ, Hoving JL, de Vet HC, et al.: The interexaminer reproducibility of physical examination of the cervical spine. *J Manipulative Physiol Ther* 27:84–90, 2004.
94. Pettman E: *Level III course notes*. Berrien Springs, MI: North American Institute of Manual Therapy, Inc., 2003.
95. Martel W: The occipito-atlanto-axial joints in rheumatoid arthritis. *Am J Roentgenol* 86:223–240, 1961.
96. Parke WW, Rothman RH, Brown MD: The pharyngovertebral veins: an anatomical rationale for Grisel's syndrome. *J Bone Joint Surg* 66A:568, 1984.
97. Georgopoulos G, Pizzutillo PD, Lee MS: Occipito-atlantal instability in children. *J Bone Joint Surg* 69A:429–436, 1987.
98. El-Khoury GY, Clark CR, Dietz FR, et al.: Posterior atlantooccipital subluxation in Down syndrome. *Radiology* 159:507–509, 1986.
99. Brooke DC, Burkus JK, Benson DR: Asymptomatic occipito-atlantal instability in Down's syndrome. *J Bone Joint Surg* 69A:293–295, 1987.
100. Fielding JW, Hawkins RJ, Ratzan SA: Spine fusion for atlanto-axial instability. *J Bone and Joint Surg* 58A:400–407, 1976.
101. Uitvlugt G, Indenbaum S: Clinical assessment of atlantoaxial instability using the Sharp-Purser test. *Arthritis Rheum* 31:918–922, 1988.
102. Boden SD, McCowin PR, Davis DO, et al.: Abnormal magnetic resonance scans of the cervical spine in asymptomatic subjects: a prospective investigation. *J Bone Joint Surg* 72A:1178–1184, 1990.
103. Sung RD, Wang JC: Correlation between a positive Hoffman's reflex and cervical pathology in asymptomatic individuals. *Spine* 26:67–70, 2001.
104. Freemyer B, Knopp R, Piche J, et al.: Comparison of five-view and three-view cervical spine series in the evaluation of patients with cervical trauma. *Ann Emerg Med* 18:818–821, 1989.
105. Schaffer MA, Doris PE: Limitation of the cross table lateral view in detecting cervical spine injuries: a retrospective analysis. *Ann Emerg Med* 10:508–513, 1981.
106. Marchesi DG: Management of odontoid fractures. *Orthopaedics* 20:911–916, 1997.
107. Blacksin MF, Lee HJ: Frequency and significance of fractures of the upper cervical spine detected by CT in patients with severe neck trauma. *Am J Roentgenol* 165:1201–1204, 1995.
108. Harris MB, Waguespack AM, Kronlage S: "Clearing" cervical spine injuries in polytrauma patients: is it really safe to remove the collar? *Orthopedics* 20:903–907, 1997.
109. Press JM, Herring SA, Kibler WB: *Rehabilitation of Musculoskeletal Disorders. The Textbook of Military Medicine*. Washington, DC: Borden Institute, Office of the Surgeon General, 1996.
110. Meadows J: *A Rationale and Complete Approach to the Sub-Acute Post-MVA Cervical Patient*. Calgary, AB: Swodeam Consulting, 1995.
111. McKinney LA, Dornan JO, Ryan M: The role of physiotherapy in the management of acute neck sprains following road-traffic accidents. *Arch Emerg Med* 6:27–33, 1989.
112. McKinney LA: Early mobilisation and outcome in acute sprains of the neck. *BMJ* 299:1006–1008, 1989.
113. Lipson SJ: Fractures of the atlas associated with fractures of the odontoid process and transverse ligament ruptures. *J Bone Joint Surg* 59A:940–943, 1977.
114. Smolders JJ: Myofascial pain and dysfunction syndromes. In: Hammer WI, ed. *Functional Soft Tissue Examination and Treatment by Manual Methods – The Extremities*. Gaithersburg, MD: Aspen, 1991:215–234.
115. Liebenson C: Active muscular relaxation techniques (part 2). *J Manipulative Physiol Ther* 13:2–6, 1990.
116. Ghanayem AJ, Leventhal M, Bohlman HH: Osteoarthrosis of the atlanto-axial joints. Long-term follow-up after treatment with arthrodesis. *J Bone Joint Surg Am* 78A:1300–1307, 1996.
117. Semble EL, Elster AD, Loeser RF, et al.: Magnetic resonance imaging of the craniovertebral junction in rheumatoid arthritis. *J Rheumatol* 15:1367–1375, 1988.
118. Wilson BC, Jarvis BL, Haydon RC: Nontraumatic subluxation of the atlantoaxial joint: Grisel's syndrome. *Larynoscope* 96:705–708, 1987.
119. Lansen TA, Kasoff SS, Tenner MS: Occipitocervical fusion for reduction of traumatic periodontoid hypertrophic cicatrix. Case report. *J Neurosurg* 73:466–470, 1990.
120. Nishizawa S, Ryu H, Yokoyama T, et al.: Myelopathy caused by retro-odontoid disc hernia: case report. *Neurosurgery* 39:1256–1259, 1996.
121. Papadopoulos SM, Dickman CA, Sonntag VKH: Atlantoaxial stabilization in rheumatoid arthritis. *J Neurosurg* 74:1–7, 1991.
122. Dickman CA, Douglas RA, Sonntag VKH: Occipitocervical fusion: posterior stabilization of the craniovertebral junction and upper cervical spine. *BNI Q* 6:2–14, 1990.
123. Kroenke K, Mangelsdorff D: Common symptoms in ambulatory care: incidence, evaluation, therapy and outcome. *Am J Med* 86:262–266, 1989.
124. Aspinall W: Clinical testing for cervical mechanical disorders which produce ischemic vertigo. *J Orthop Sports Phys Ther* 11:176–182, 1989.
125. Furuta Y, Fukuda S, Chida E, et al.: Reactivation of herpes simplex virus type 1 in patients with Bell's palsy. *J Med Virol* 54:162–166, 1998.
126. Fetter M, Dichgans J: Vestibular neuritis spares the inferior division of the vestibular nerve. *Brain* 119:755–763, 1996.
127. Tusa RJ: Vertigo. *Neurol Clin* 19:23–55, 2001.
128. Adour KK: Otological complications of herpes zoster. *Ann Neurol* 35: S62-S64, 1994.
129. Huijbregts P, Vidal P: Dizziness in orthopedic physical therapy practice: classification and pathophysiology. *J Man Manip Ther* 12:199–214, 2004.
130. Simon RP, Aminoff MJ, Greenberg DA: *Clinical Neurology,* 4th ed. Stanford, CT: Appleton and Lange, 1999.
131. Courjon JH, Jeannerod M, Ossuzio I, et al.: The role of vision in compensation of vestibulo-ocular reflex after hemilabyrinthectomy in the cat. *Exp Brain Res* 5:67–107, 1977.
132. Fetter M, Zee DS: Recovery from unilateral labyrinthectomy in rhesus monkeys. *J Neurophysiol* 59:370–393, 1988.
133. Macnab I: Acceleration extension injuries of the cervical spine. In: Rothman RH, Simeoni FA, eds. *The Spine*. Philadelphia, PA: WB Saunders, 1982:515–527.
134. Brown KE, Whitney SL, Marchetti GF, et al.: Physical therapy for central vestibular dysfunction. *Arch Phys Med Rehabil* 87:76–81, 2006.
135. Wyke BD: Neurology of the cervical spinal joints. *Physiotherapy* 65:72–76, 1979.
136. Cohen LA: Role of eye and neck proprioceptive mechanisms in body orientation and motor coordination. *J Neurophysiol* 24:1–11, 1961.
137. Barré M: Sur un syndrome sympathetique cervical posterieur et sa cause frequente: l'arthrite cervicale. *Rev Neurol* 33:1246–1248, 1926.
138. Ryan GMS, Cope S: Cervical vertigo. *Lancet* 2:1355, 1955.
139. Wing LW, Hargrove-Wilson W: Cervical vertigo. *Aust N Z J Surg* 44:275, 1974.
140. Biesinger E: Vertigo caused by disorders of the cervical vertebral column. *Adv Otorhinolaryngol* 39:44, 1988.
141. Sjaastad O, Fredriksen TA, Pfaffenrath V: Cervicogenic headache: diagnostic criteria. The Cervicogenic Headache International Study Group Headache. *Headache* 38:442–445, 1998.
142. Headache Classification Committee of the International Headache Society: Classification and diagnostic criteria for headache disorders, cranial neuralgias and facial pain. *Cephalalgia suppl* 7:1–551, 1988.
143. Maigne R: La céphalée sus-orbitaire. Sa fréquente origine cervicale. Son traitement. *Ann Med Phys* 39:241–246, 1968.
144. Nicholson GG, Gaston J: Cervical headache. *J Orthop Sports Phys Ther* 31:184–193, 2001.
145. Sizer PS Jr. Phelps V, Brismee J-M: Diagnosis and management of cervicogenic headache and local cervical syndrome with multiple pain generators. *J Man & Manip Ther* 10:136–152, 2002.
146. Lu J, Ebraheim NA: Anatomical consideration of C2 nerve root ganglion. *Spine* 23:649–652, 1998.
147. Polletti CE, Sweet WH: Entrapment of the C2 root and ganglion by the atlanto-epitrophic ligament: clinical syndrome and surgical anatomy. *Neurosurg* 27:288–290, 1990.
148. Barnsley L, Lord SM, Wallis BJ, et al.: The prevalence of chronic cervical zygapophyseal joint pain after whiplash. *Spine* 20:20–26, 1995.
149. Barnsley L, Lord S, Bogduk N: The pathophysiology of whiplash. In: Malanga GA, ed. *Cervical Flexion-Extension/Whiplash Injuries. Spine: State of the Art Reviews*. Philadelphia, PA: Pa, Hanley & Belfus, 1998: 209–242.

150. Maimaris C, Barnes MR, Allen MJ: Whiplash injuries of the neck: a retrospective study. *Injury* 19:393–396, 1988.
151. Martin PR, Nathan PR, Milech D, et al.: The relationship between headaches and mood. *Behav Res Ther* 26:353–356, 1988.
152. Arena JG, Blanchard EB, Andrasik F: The role of affect in the etiology of chronic headache. *J Psychosom Res* 28:79–86, 1984.
153. McDonnell MK, Sahrmann SA, Van Dillen L: A specific exercise program and modification of postural alignment for treatment of cervicogenic headache: a case report. *J Orthop Sports Phys Ther* 35:3–15, 2005.
154. Hurwitz EL, Aker PD, Adams AH, et al.: Manipulation and mobilization of the cervical spine. A systematic review of the literature. *Spine* 21:1746–1759; discussion 1759–1760., 1996.
155. Schoensee SK, Jensen G, Nicholson G, et al.: The effect of mobilization on cervical headaches. *J Orthop Sports Phys Ther* 21:184–196., 1995.
156. Hanten WP, Olson SL, Weston AL, et al.: The effect of manual therapy and a home exercise program on cervicogenic headaches: a case report. *J Man Manip Ther* 13:35–43, 2005.
157. McKenzie RA: *The Cervical and Thoracic Spine: Mechanical Diagnosis and Therapy*. Waikanae, NZ: Spinal Publications, 1990.
158. Hammill JM, Cook TM, Rosecrance JC: Effectiveness of a physical therapy regimen in the treatment of tension-type headache. *Headache* 36:149–153., 1996.
159. Bronfort G, Assendelft WJJ, Evans R, et al.: Efficacy of spinal manipulation for chronic headache: a systematic review. *J Manip Physiol Ther* 24:457–466, 2001.
160. Aferzon M, Reams CL: Radiology quiz case 2. Chiari malformation (type I). *Arch Otolaryngol Head Neck Surg* 128:1104, 1106–1107, 2002.
161. Piper JG, Menezes AH: Chiari malformations in the adult. In: Menezes AH, Sonntag VKH, eds. *Principles of Spinal Surgery*. New York, NY: McGraw-Hill, 1996:379–394.
162. Lui TN, Lee ST, Wong CW, et al.: C1-C2 fracture-dislocations in children and adolescents. *J Trauma* 40:408–411, 1996.
163. Wong DA, Mack RP, Craigmile TK: Traumatic atlantoaxial dislocation without fracture of the odontoid. *Spine* 16:587–589, 1991.
164. Greene KA, Dickman CA, Marciano FF, et al.: Acute axis fractures: analysis of management and outcomes. *Spine* 22:1843–1852, 1997.
165. Pepin JW, Bourne RB, Hawkins RJ: Odontoid fractures, with special reference to the elderly patient. *Clin Orthop* 193:178–183, 1985.
166. Anderson LD, D'Alonzo RT: Fractures of the odontoid process of the axis. *J Bone Joint Surg* 56A:1663–1674, 1974.
167. Scott EW, Haid RW, Peace D: Type I fractures of the odontoid process: implications for atlantoaxial instability. *J Neurosurg* 72:488–492, 1990.
168. Heller J, Levy M, Barrow D: Odontoid fracture malunion with fixed atlantoaxial subluxation. *Spine* 18:311–314, 1993.
169. Appuzo ML, Heiden JS, Weiss MH, et al.: Acute fractures of the odontoid process: an analysis of 45 cases. *J Neurosurg* 48:85–91, 1978.
170. Seybold EA, Bayley JC: Functional outcome of surgically and conservatively managed dens fractures. *Spine* 23:1837–1846, 1998.
171. Jefferson G: Fracture of the atlas vertebra, report of four cases and a review of those previously recorded. *Br J Surg* 7:407–422, 1920.
172. Lee TT, Green BA, Petrin DR: Treatment of stable burst fracture of the atlas (Jefferson fracture) with rigid cervical collar. *Spine* 23:1963–1967, 1998.
173. Hadley MN, Dickman CA, Browner CM, et al.: Acute traumatic atlas fractures: management and long-term outcome. *Neurosurgery* 23:31–35, 1988.
174. Landells CD, Van Peteghem PK: Fractures of the atlas: classification, treatment, and morbidity. *Spine* 13:450–452, 1988.
175. Kaltenborn FM: *The Spine : Basic Evaluation and Mobilization Techniques*. Wellington: New Zealand University Press, 1993.
176. Mulligan BR: *Manual Therapy: "NAGS", "SNAGS", "PRP'S" etc.* Wellington: Plane View Series, 1992.

Vertebral Artery

CHAPTER 24

CHAPTER OBJECTIVES

At the completion of this chapter, the reader will be able to:

1. Describe the anatomy and distribution of the vertebral artery.
2. Describe the four commonly recognized portions of the vertebral artery.
3. Outline the causes of vertebral artery occlusion or compromise.
4. Recognize the characteristics of vertebral artery occlusion or insufficiency.
5. Describe various special tests used to assess the patency of the vertebrobasilar system and their diagnostic value.

OVERVIEW

The vertebral artery (VA), a component of the vertebrobasilar artery (VBA) system, supplies 20% of the blood to the brain (primarily the posterior cranial fossa), with the remaining 80% being supplied by the carotid system.[1] The first studies of the VA were recorded as far back as 1844.[2] Since that time, recognition of the importance of the VA has continued to grow, and it is now discussed in more detail than any other artery by physical therapists. For this reason, the VA is afforded its own chapter. To fully comprehend its significance, a review of its anatomy and function is in order.

ANATOMY

The VBA system consists of three key vessels: two VAs and one basilar artery. The basilar artery is formed by the two VAs joining each other at the midline (Fig. 24-1).

Along its course, the artery can be viewed as having four portions: proximal, transverse, suboccipital, and intracranial.[3,4]

Proximal Portion

This portion runs from the origin of the artery to its point of entry to the cervical spine. The VA usually originates from the posterior surface of the subclavian artery, but it can also originate from the aortic arch and common carotid artery.[5]

The VA runs vertically, slightly medial, and posteriorly lateral to the longus colli and medial to the anterior scalene muscles to reach the transverse foramen of the lower cervical spine, although its exact direction is dependent on its exact point of origin. Its anomalous origin in this region has been suggested as a potential factor increasing the chance of blood flow compromise due to compression by the longus colli or scalene muscles.

In approximately 88% of individuals, the artery enters the transverse foramen of C6, but it has been shown to enter as far superior as the transverse foramen of C4.[6]

CLINICAL PEARL

Tortuosity and compression of this portion of the artery are common. The reasons for this can be congenital or muscular (resulting from compression by the longus colli and medial aspect of the anterior scalene), or a consequence of advancing years.

Transverse Portion

The second portion of the VA runs from the point of entry at the spinal column to the transverse foramen of C2 (Fig. 24-2). As already described, the origin of this part of the artery is typically at the C6 level, but this may vary between individuals and even from side to side in the same individual.

Throughout this section of the spinal column, the artery travels vertically in a true canal called the transverse canal (TC). The TC is formed by the bony transverse foramina at each spinal level and the overlying anterior and posterior intertransverse muscles, the scaleni, and the longus colli muscle. The dimension of the TC is proportionate to the diameter of the artery which itself is variable. Within the TC, the artery is surrounded by a periosteal sheath that is adherent to the boundaries of the canal and affords protection for the artery. However, the artery is in close proximity to the uncinate processes of each vertebral body on its medial aspect

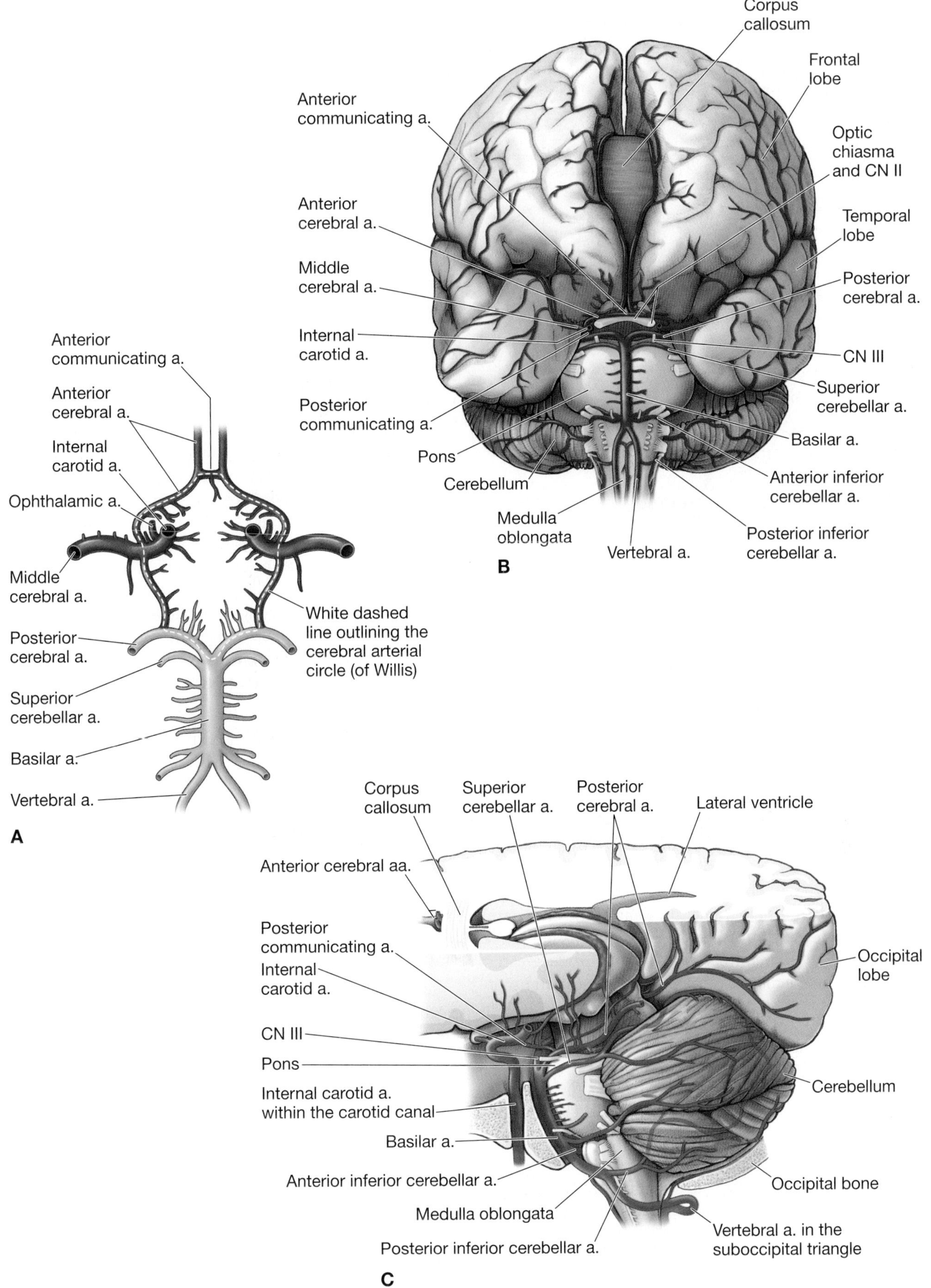

FIGURE 24-1 The vertebral artery and its relationship to the cranial arteries. (Reproduced with permission from Morton DA, Foreman KB, Albertine KH: *The Big Picture: Gross Anatomy*. New York: McGraw-Hill, 2011.)

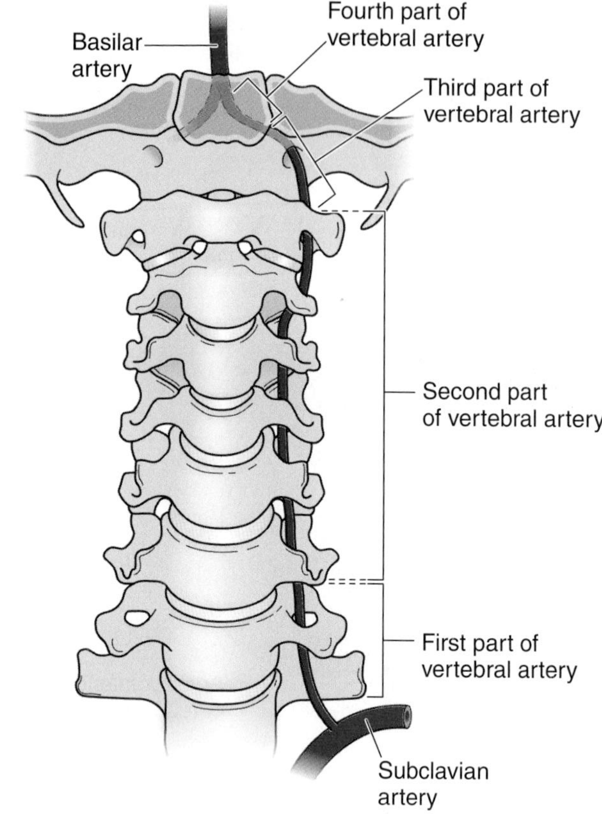

FIGURE 24-2 The left vertebral artery showing the four parts of its route.

and is prone to compression from osteophyte formation or subluxation from the zygapophyseal joint.[4,7] The VA in the transverse foramen is also adjacent to the anterior spinal roots. Arterial enlargement by an intramural hematoma or a dissecting aneurysm may cause radiculopathy by compressing or stretching the spinal root.[8]

Anomalies in this portion of the artery, which can include looping within the intervertebral foramina, can occur because of an abnormal origin of the artery from the aorta.[9]

The proximal and suboccipital portions of the artery are more elastic and less muscular than the transverse part.[10] This variation is believed to be an adaptation to the greater mobility required in the proximal and transverse portions of the artery.

Suboccipital Portion

This portion of the artery extends from its exit at the axis (C2) to its point of penetration into the spinal canal. This portion can be further subdivided into four parts:

1. Within the transverse foramen of C2 (see Fig. 24-2). This portion lies in a complete bony canal formed by the two curves of the transverse foramen of C2. The inferior curve is almost vertical, whereas the superior curve is more horizontal and orientated laterally.
2. Between C2 and C1 (see Fig. 24-2). The second part runs vertically upward to the transverse foramen of C2. Throughout its journey, it is covered by the intertransversarii, the levator scapulae muscle, and the inferior oblique capitis muscle. Compression of the VA may occur in conditions in which these muscles have increased tone or loss of flexibility.[11] It is also at this level that the VA is subjected to the most mechanical stress, as more than 50% of cervical spine rotation occurs here.
3. In the transverse foramen of C1 (see Fig. 24-2). In its third part, the suboccipital portion of the VA bends posteriorly and medially in the transverse foramen of C1 in which it is completely enclosed.
4. Between the posterior arch of the atlas and its entry into the foramen magnum (see Fig. 24-2). On exiting from the transverse foramen of C1, the artery and the nerve of C1 wind behind the mass of the superior articular process of the atlas (C1) to cross the posterior arch of the atlas in a groove in which the artery is held by a restraining ligament. Anomalies in this portion of the artery include ossification of the restraining ligament of the atlantal groove, turning this into a complete bony tunnel. From the medial end of this groove, the artery runs forward, inward, and upward to pierce the posterior atlantooccipital membrane. The artery penetrates the dura mater on the lateral aspect of the foramen magnum about 1.5 cm lateral to the midline of the neck. This upper portion of the extracranial VA is relatively superficial and covered only by the trapezius, semispinalis capitis, and rectus capitis muscles. Having unyielding bone beneath it, and only muscles above, the artery is vulnerable to direct blunt trauma at this part of its course, whereas in the remainder of its course, it is threatened more by penetrating trauma or disease processes such as osteophytosis or atherosclerosis.[12,13]

Although the artery is affected by cervical motion in the lower cervical region, it is affected even more between C2 and the occipital bone.[14]

CLINICAL PEARL

The VA is most vulnerable to compression and stretching at the level of C1–2 because of the amount of cervical rotation that can occur at the atlantoaxial joint.[15]

In addition, because the transverse foramen of C1 is more lateral than that of C2, the artery must incline laterally between the two vertebrae. At this point, the artery is vulnerable to impingement from the following:

- Cervical extension at the craniovertebral joints, such as that which occurs with a forward head posture.[11]
- Excursion of the transverse mass of C1 during rotation. Approximately 50% of the cervical axial rotation occurs between C1 and C2; hence, there is a large excursion of the transverse mass of C1 with rotation. The artery is stretched during this process and the size of the lumen can be reduced.[14,16] Any reduction in the size of the lumina is more profound in the presence of arterial disease.
- The atlantoaxial membrane. Ossification of this membrane can occur.

Intracranial Portion

This portion of the VA that runs from its penetration of the dura mater into the arachnoid space at the level of the foramen magnum to the formation of the basilar artery by the midline union of the two arteries at the lower border of the pons (Fig. 24-1).

> **CLINICAL PEARL**
>
> The VA that is most vulnerable to a stretch injury during neck rotation is usually the one that is contralateral to the side of the rotation.[17,18] For example, the left VA is more vulnerable with rotation to the right. During right rotation, the left transverse foramen of C1 moves anteriorly and slightly to the right. This movement imparts a marked stretch on the left VA, and it increases the acuteness of the angle formed between its ascending and posteromedial courses.

After its penetration of the cranium, the VA inclines medially toward the medulla oblongata. It courses up the front of the medulla to reach the lower border of the pons, where the artery from each side unites with its partner to form the basilar artery. A major change in the structure of the VA occurs as it becomes intracranial.[4] The tunica adventitia and tunica media become thinner, and there is a gross reduction in the number of elastic fibers in these coats.[10] This decrease in elasticity can result in the distortion of the VA during cervical extension and rotation.[14,16,19]

> **CLINICAL PEARL**
>
> The intracranial portion of the artery is prone to mechanical obstructions including atherosclerotic plaques and stenosis.[11]

Branches

Intracranially, the VA first generates small meningeal branches that supply the bone and dura mater of the cerebellar fossa. It is possible that ischemia of these tissues, which occurs with VA occlusion, could be responsible for the suboccipital pain that often accompanies damage to the artery.[15]

Spinal Branches[8]

Each of the vertebral arteries gives off single branches (Fig. 24-1), which fuse to form the anterior spinal artery (ASA) that descends in the median anterior fissure and is additionally supplied by anterior radicular arteries (typically two to four). While the ASA is bilaterally derived, the anterior radicular arteries may arise exclusively or predominately from one VA. This helps to explain how a unilateral insufficiency of the VA may cause bilateral spinal cord infarction.

The paired posterior spinal arteries (PSAs) originate superiorly from the vertebral arteries or posterior inferior cerebellar arteries (PICAs). The PSAs are also supplied by posterior radicular arteries (usually two or three), which themselves arise exclusively or predominately from one VA, again demonstrating how a unilateral VA dissection can lead to bilateral spinal cord infarction. The PSAs supply the posterior one-fifth to one-quarter of the spinal cord including the posterior columns, the posterior (dorsal) horns, and parts of the corticospinal and spinothalamic tracts. The ASA is the exclusive arterial supply to the gray matter of the cord. The watershed area between the PSA and ASA encompasses the anterior (ventral) horns and part of the corticospinal and spinothalamic tracts.

Muscular Branches

The muscular branches arise from the suboccipital part of the artery as it winds around the superior articular process of the atlas. They supply the deep suboccipital muscles and anastomose with the occipital and cervical arteries.

Posterior Inferior Cerebellar Artery

The PICA (see Fig. 24-1) is the largest branch of the VA, usually being formed opposite to the medulla oblongata about 1 cm below the formation of the basilar artery. It supplies, either directly or indirectly, the medulla and the cerebellum and, via the PSAs, the posterior (dorsal) portion of the spinal cord.

> **CLINICAL PEARL**
>
> The term cervical arterial dysfunction has been suggested for use when referring to arterial problems of the cervical spine, as the term embraces both the completeness of the arterial anatomy (i.e., the vertebrobasilar system, internal carotid arteries, and the Circle of Willis) and the range of pathologies that the clinician may encounter.[20]

Basilar Artery

The formation of the basilar artery at the lower border of the pons marks the termination of the VA. The basilar artery runs in a fissure on the anterior surface of the pons (see Fig. 24-1). Directly and indirectly, the basilar artery supplies the pons, the visual area of the occipital lobe, the membranous labyrinth, the medulla, the temporal lobe, the posterior thalamus, and the cerebellum.

Collateral Circulation

Fortunately, there is an inherent redundancy in the vascular supply to the brain. The posterior and anterior vessels, and the vessels stemming from the internal carotid arteries, form an anastomotic network via the circle of Willis. Thus, occlusion of the left VA may be compensated for by perfusion of the right VA, the occipital artery, the ascending and deep cervical arteries, and the internal carotid arteries.[21,22] In fact, there is evidence that suggests that blood flow velocity and blood flow volume can increase in the arteries to compensate for occlusion in another vessel.[23] It is worth considering that palpation of the carotid pulse would give the clinician information regarding the ability of the carotid to perform its normal function, and if the pulse appears excessively strong, this could be an indication that the carotid artery is compensating for loss of VA flow.[24,25]

VERTEBROBASILAR INSUFFICIENCY

Damage and occlusion of the vertebral arteries are felt to occur because of the close proximity of the VA and the bony and ligamentous structures of the cervical spine.[26] Trauma to this area may lead to thrombosis, dissection, transection, transmural hematoma, pseudoaneurysm, and spasm of the VA. VA insufficiency may also occur because of atherosclerotic involvement of the artery, sickle cell disease (see Chapter 5), rheumatoid arthritis, arterial fibroplasias, an arteriovenous fistula, and a number of congenital syndromes.

Whatever the cause of VA compromise, the diagnosis requires a high index of suspicion for prompt recognition and intervention. Vertebrobasilar insufficiency (VBI) is associated with signs and symptoms of focal neurologic compromise that are of sudden onset and brief duration and relate to the specific areas that are normally supplied by the vessels.

Occlusion

The VA is subject to occlusion from external and internal causes.

External Causes

Extracranial Compression

Extracranial compression of the VA may cause neurologic symptoms depending on the acuteness of the occlusion or the presence of underlying pathologic conditions such as atherosclerosis, sickle cell disease, fibromuscular dysplasia, rheumatoid arthritis, or osteogenesis imperfecta.

Many blood flow studies have demonstrated a change (reduction) in blood flow in the contralateral VA during cervical rotation.[27–30] Other studies, however, have found no change in blood flow.[31,32]

What is known is that the greatest mechanical stress affecting the contralateral artery occurs at a position of cervical rotation and extension. Furthermore, if this position is sustained, the arterial flow takes longer to return to normal.[32]

In addition to the C1–2 portion, the VA is vulnerable to compression in the portion that courses through the transverse foramen from C6 to C1. Because of its fixation to the spine in this segment, subluxations of one vertebral body on another may exert undue tension and traction on the artery. Positions of the cervical spine can cause compression of the VA.[19,33] Rotation–extension–traction appears to be the most stressful, followed by rotation–extension, rotation alone, side flexion alone, extension alone, and then flexion.[19,33,34]

If the main restraint to atlantoaxial rotation, the alar ligament, is ruptured, then the degree of C1–2 rotation has been shown to increase by 30%.[35] Insufficiency of the alar ligament has been shown to follow a rear-end collision in motor vehicle accidents, and it may also exist because of a congenital defect of the dens.[36] Other contributing factors to the preponderance of lesions occurring at the second cervical joint level are the fixation of the periosteal sheath of the artery to the dura mater, the superficiality of the artery in this region, and the hard neural arch beneath the artery.

Unilateral occlusion of the VA rarely results in a neurologic deficit because of the collateral supply through the contralateral vertebral and PICAs.[37]

CLINICAL PEARL

The most common mechanism for a nonpenetrating trauma injury to the VA is hyperextension of the neck, with or without rotation, or cervical side flexion.[38,39] These motions can result in stretching and tearing of the intima and media, especially at the points where the artery is tethered to a bone.[40,41]

After the primary tear of the intima, blood flows into the arterial wall between the intima and the media causing intramural hematoma and thickening of the vessel wall. Subintimal hemorrhage can produce various degrees of stenosis; subadventitial hemorrhage can cause a pseudoaneurysm. Tearing of the artery is not always related to remarkable trauma, and so this aspect may not appear in the history unless the symptoms appear immediately following the injury. The presence of a pseudoaneurysm has been a commonly noted angiographic feature following sudden head and neck movements. In this injury, the two internal coats of the VA are torn from the tunica adventitia, which under the influence of arterial pressure slowly balloons out and sometimes ruptures.

CLINICAL PEARL

Even in the absence of underlying trauma, cervical rotation (approximately 20 degrees) and extension (approximately 20 degrees) have been shown to reduce the lumen of the VA to the point where blood flow is compromised to the point of almost nonexistence.[42] An underlying pathology may therefore be quiescent, and the patient may not complain of vascular-like symptoms prior to an infarction except with specific movements.[43]

Extracranial Dissection

Extracranial VA dissection (vertebrobasilar infarction) is recognized with increasing frequency as a cause of stroke, and spontaneous dissections of the carotid and vertebral arteries are well-recognized causes of stroke in young and middle-aged adults.[44–47] Traumatic dissection can also occur in the extracranial part of the internal carotid arteries, often after only moderate blunt trauma.[48]

Postmortem studies have shown that neurologic deficits, or even death, have followed posterior neck injuries by up to 8 days after the accident.[49,50] The most common clinical findings are brain stem or cerebellar ischemic symptoms preceded by severe neck pain, occipital headache, or both. Occasionally, these patients report radicular symptoms.[45]

Spinal manipulation, in particular manipulation of the upper spine, has been associated with serious adverse occurrences, including dissection of the vertebral[51] and internal carotid artery,[52] resulting in strokes[53] and death.[54] However, the evidence implicating cervical manipulations with these serious consequences is conflicting, especially in light of the fact that even normal neck movements have been associated with spontaneous dissections. The reciprocal finding of increased blood flow through the carotid artery during VA occlusion was made by Stern,[55] who demonstrated that the flow rate in the contralateral carotid artery increased by one and a half to two times with experimental occlusion of the VA. These alterations in the flow rates following an occlusion of the parallel artery serve as an apparent safety mechanism and may explain why more patients are not injured during cervical manipulation.

CLINICAL PEARL

The potential risk of a VBA dissection after manipulation is reported to be somewhere between 1 in 1.3 million treatment sessions[56] and 1 in 400,000 manipulations.[57] The clinicians involved in such instances have stated that the patient's prognosis is greatly enhanced if they can be treated by anticoagulant therapy quickly enough.[24] This requires that the manipulative clinician is totally familiar with the signs and symptoms of VBA damage.

Frisoni and Anzola[58] concluded that VA dissection at the atlantoaxial joint with intimal tear, intramural bleeding, or pseudoaneurysm leading to thrombosis or embolism is the mechanism for VBI when associated with chiropractic manipulation. The same study found that possible risk factors for VBI after neck motion are VA size asymmetry, anomalous course of VA, atherosclerosis, osteoarthritis, and vertebral ligament laxity.[58] However, despite the reports of 115 cases of cerebrovascular accidents after manipulation in English language publications during the period of 1966–1998 (198 articles), there is virtually no detailed information on the magnitude of forces that were exerted or the type of procedure used. It has even been suggested that, in many cases, cervical manipulation may have been administered to patients who already had a spontaneous dissection in progress.[59]

CLINICAL PEARL

It is the responsibility of all health care providers who use cervical manipulation to be cognizant of the potential adverse consequences.

Internal Causes

Atherosclerosis and Thrombosis

Atherosclerosis of the extracranial part of the VA primarily affects the proximal and transverse portions, leaving the suboccipital part relatively free. Atherosclerosis in the transverse portion of the artery occurs at any level between C2 and C6 and tends to occur at levels of the artery opposite osteophytic spurs. Castaigne et al.[60] investigated 44 patients with VBA occlusions and found that the cause in almost 90% of cases was atherosclerosis, mostly affecting the proximal and intracranial portions of the artery. Approximately 40% of the patients in this study had concomitant carotid stenosis.

Atherosclerosis may, as with any other artery, produce signs and symptoms resulting from ischemia of the tissues supplied by the artery distal to the occlusion. However, if the contralateral artery is not occluded, and is of good caliber, the condition may be asymptomatic.

Thrombosis can occur at any level of the VA but is more common in the suboccipital and intracranial portions than in the transverse part.[61]

Arterial Fibrodysplasia

This condition is a nonatheromatous, noninflammatory segmental angiopathy of unknown etiology. It occurs in less than 1% of all patients receiving cerebral angiograms, but it is the third most frequent structural lesion affecting the VA following atherosclerosis and dissection.[62] Arterial fibrodysplasia is believed to be hereditary, affecting mainly young and middle-aged female patients.

Klippel–Trenaunay Syndrome

Klippel–Trenaunay syndrome consists of a constellation of anomalies including capillary malformation, varicose veins or venous malformations, and hypertrophy of both bony and soft tissues primarily involving limbs and to a much lesser degree, intra-abdominal, thoracic, or facial structures.[63,64] The vascular abnormalities commonly occur in the lower extremity but have been observed in other areas as well (head, neck, buttocks, abdomen, chest, and oral cavity). Klippel–Trenaunay syndrome is theorized to result from a mesodermal abnormality.[65] The syndrome is diagnosed on the basis of presence of any two of the three aforementioned features and any intervention is based on the severity of these features.

Arteriovenous Fistulas

An arteriovenous fistula is an abnormal communication between the extracranial VA, or one of its muscular or radicular branches, and an adjacent vein. It has variable causes, including traumatic dissections or dissecting aneurysms, and may occur spontaneously as a result of the existing disease, such as fibromuscular dysplasia, or as a congenital condition. Most spontaneous arteriovenous fistulas occur at the level of C2–3 and come directly from the VA through what is believed to be a tiny rupture in the wall of the artery.[66,67] Although rare, progressive myelopathy from an intracranial arteriovenous fistula can occur.[68] In these cases, endovascular embolization, either alone or followed by surgery, is the intervention of choice.

The Clinical Manifestations of Vertebrobasilar Insufficiency

The clinical manifestations of VBI are difficult to distinguish from other causes of brainstem ischemia (see later) and can include any or all of the following: dizziness, visual disturbance, drop attacks (a sudden loss of postural tone without loss of consciousness), ataxia, dysarthria, dysphagia, hemiplegia, hemianesthesia, nausea, and ringing in the ears. Indeed, no single consistent pattern of neurologic signs and symptoms is pathognomonic for VA insufficiency. The most common presenting symptoms are vertigo, nausea, and headache that can be subtle, intermittent, and even chronic in nature.[11,69–71]

CLINICAL PEARL

Terret[72] proposed the following pneumonic for the signs and symptoms associated with VBI: five D's and 3 N's:

- Dizziness
- Drop attacks
- Diplopia
- Dysarthria
- Dysphagia
- Nausea
- Numbness
- Nystagmus

Vertigo

Vertigo or dizziness is a commonly reported symptom in the physical therapy clinic.[11,70,71] Owing to the different areas of the brain that the VA and its branching arteries supply, dizziness, although the most common and usual symptom of VBI, is rarely an isolated symptom, especially in advanced stages of the condition. Tatlow and Bammer[16] proved that the cause of the vertigo in patients with VBI was cervical rather than vestibular. This was accomplished by placing symptomatic patients into a Stryker bed to determine whether the vertigo symptoms were being elicited by the movement of the entire body or by the movement of the head relative to the torso. Each patient who was secured within the Stryker bed had the entire body rotated up to a full 360 degrees en bloc (without movement of the head and neck relative to the torso), and the patients reported no symptoms. However, when the torso was fixed in a still position but the head and neck was moved relative to the torso, symptoms were reproduced.

Nausea

Nausea is the accompanying symptom for many different conditions including VBI.

Headache

The headache associated with VBI is typically a unilateral occipital headache with associated vertigo and nausea.[40] The pain is usually sharp and acute in its onset located on the same side as the insufficiency.

In addition to those signs and symptoms already mentioned, the following have also been linked, both directly and indirectly, to VBI[40,73,74]:

- Wallenberg, Horner, and similar syndromes
- Bilateral or quadrilateral paresthesia
- Hemiparesthesia
- Scotoma (a permanent or temporary area of depressed or absent vision)
- Periodic loss of consciousness
- Lip/perioral anesthesia
- Hemifacial paralysis/anesthesia
- Hyperreflexia
- Positive Babinski, Hoffman, or Oppenheim signs
- Clonus
- Gait ataxia
- Dysphasia

Clinicians need to be aware of these signs and symptoms and consider VA dissection early in the differential diagnosis because of the potential devastating neurological consequences and to decrease morbidity and mortality.[40]

Subclavian Steal Syndrome

The subclavian steal syndrome involves a proximal subclavian artery obstruction and reversed vertebral flow with resultant siphoning of blood from the brain and cerebrovascular symptoms.[75–77]

The subclavian steal syndrome can produce cerebral symptoms such as a "drop attack."[78] Headache, dizziness, and vertigo can occur while walking and turning the neck to look to the side or up.[79]

Imaging Studies

Conventional angiography has long been the gold standard in the diagnosis of arterial and venous pathology in the neck. Angiography can show the arterial lumen and allows extensive characterization of dissections of the carotid and vertebral arteries.[80] VA angiography is not, however, without risk. Magnetic resonance angiographic (MRA) techniques are less invasive and are replacing conventional angiography as the gold standard in the diagnosis of dissections of the carotid and vertebral arteries. MRA is highly sensitive and specific in identifying stenoses and occlusions and can show the intramural hematoma itself.[81]

Ultrasonographic techniques are useful in the initial assessment of patients who are thought to have a dissection of the carotid artery.[82] Doppler sonography allows a direct visualization of the vascular tree while assessing blood flow velocity and pressure waveforms. Although the site of dissection generally is not seen, an abnormal pattern of flow is identified in more than 90% of patients.[82]

Physical Therapy Examination of the Vertebral Artery

Screening procedures to identify patients at risk for VBI prior to manual therapy interventions have been widely advocated and routinely used by physical therapists for many years, being first described by Maitland in 1968.[83] It is widely recognized that passive therapeutic maneuvers applied to the cervical spine carry a small risk of developing iatrogenic stroke. This is especially pertinent with regard to cervical manipulations (high-velocity thrust or grade V techniques). It is therefore generally advised that all patients with neck pain receive a subjective screening examination for VBI and be evaluated for their ability to perform active neck movements.[84] The initial test consists of having the patient rotate the head to each side while in the sitting position. The longus colli and scalene muscles rotate the cervical spine and can squeeze the VA on the side contralateral to the rotation.[11]

The presence of muscular compression of the artery can be further tested by combining cervical flexion with rotation to place the inferior oblique capitis on stretch.[11] If dizziness is provoked with rotation, it is sometimes possible to implicate or exclude the vestibular apparatus of the inner ear as the source of dizziness.[85] In a standing position, the clinician holds the patient's head steady as the patient turns the trunk while keeping the feet fixed, thus producing sustained end-range cervical spine rotation.[86] Because the semicircular canal fluid is not disturbed by this test, a positive response theoretically excludes the labyrinth of the inner ear.[85]

CLINICAL PEARL

Following positive responses in the history or initial test, the patient must be handled very carefully and further intervention, particularly manipulation of the cervical spine, should not be delivered. The patient should not, under any circumstance, be allowed to leave the clinic until his or her physician has been contacted and until the necessary arrangements have been made for the safe transport of the patient to an appropriate facility.

Theoretically, patients with a negative subjective history and negative findings with the initial test should undergo additional passive physical examination procedures in the form of stress tests for the vertebrobasilar system to further assess the potential for VBI.[87] Traditionally, this has involved the use of manual premanipulative tests to determine the appropriateness of a grade V technique.

In those cases in which the clinician is to perform cervical mobilizations of grade I–IV rather than a grade V thrust technique, the Australian Physiotherapy Association's Protocol for Premanipulative Testing of the Cervical Spine continues to be recommended, although this cannot be viewed as a prescriptive guideline.[84] The protocol recommends that the clinician should maintain the immediate premobilization position for a minimum of 10 seconds to test the patency of the vertebrobasilar system. Others recommend assessing the patient's responses for a further 10 seconds to note any latent response.[17,37] Clinical testing of the VA should stop once positive signs or symptoms are noted. Throughout the tests, the clinician should observe the patient's eyes for possible nystagmus or changes in pupil size and should have the patient count backward to assess his or her quality of speech. The patient is asked to report any changes in symptoms however insignificant he or she may feel the changes to be.

Unfortunately, it is not clear how sensitive these premanipulative protocols are.[85,88] For example, studies by Haynes[89] and Cote et al.,[90] found these protocols to have poor predictiver value. Other studies have shown that the results of these tests are inconsistent[91] and inaccurate,[92] suggesting that the VA tests have very little, if any, diagnostic value. In addition, many of these premanipulative screening protocols involve the same combination of positions that have been suspected of causing spontaneous arterial dissections (cervical extension and rotation).

CLINICAL PEARL

A positive VA test is one in which signs or symptoms change, especially if the changes evoked include those previously mentioned. More subtle examination findings can include a significant delay in verbal responses to questions of orientation with some inconsistency of answers, changes in pupil size, and nystagmus.[15]

Although one could argue that if the VA was damaged or compromised, the patient would surely have signs and/or symptoms indicating this, the logical question still becomes, "How does one proceed in the absence of certainty?"[87] It would seem extremely prudent to avoid cervical thrust techniques on a patient with any degree of uncertainty. Even in the absence of any symptoms, it would be wise to either introduce the application of incrementally greater movements and loads or investigate VA flow using Doppler sonography or an MRA scan before performing a grade V technique in the cervical spine.[93] In addition to the specific tests of blood flow, the clinician should use a combination of the patient's description of the symptoms and medical history, and those considerations in Table 24-1, before reaching a conclusion.[94] Alternatively, the clinician should consider avoiding placing the patient's cervical spine in the extremes of rotation and side bending in both the examination and the subsequent intervention, which would obviate the need for these tests.

CLINICAL PEARL

Grade V techniques should never be performed when slow blood flow of the VA is displayed on neck Doppler sonography or MRA scan.[93]

The following case study[42] illustrates the problems associated when encountering a patient with a VBA insufficiency.

TABLE 24-1 Nine Factors to Consider with Vertebral Artery Testing

1. Inherent redundancy of blood supply—collateral circulation
2. Morphology of the vertebral artery at the atlantoaxial level
3. Biomechanics of upper cervical spine—concurrent contralateral side bending with cervical rotation
4. The nonvascular causes of dizziness (cervicogenic dizziness and benign paroxysmal positional vertigo)
5. The amount of cervical rotation to be used
6. Medical history (transient ischemic attack, cerebrovascular accident, cardiac risk factors, cervical spondylosis)
7. Psychometric properties of vertebral artery testing (0% sensitivity)
8. Force to be applied
9. Potential risk of injury with manipulation (thrust, rotational techniques vs nonthrust, nonrotational techniques)

Data from Vidal PG: Vertebral artery testing as a clinical screen for vertebrobasilar insufficiency: Is there any diagnostic value? *Orthop Pract* 16:7–12, 2004.

CASE STUDY

HISTORY

A 62-year-old woman with no history of vertigo or dizziness reported to the clinic for her scheduled physical therapy session for cervical degenerative joint disease. During the course of conversation, the patient reported experiencing dizziness after a shampoo treatment of her hair at a hairdressing salon. She had visited her hairdresser earlier that day and reported severe vertigo, occipital pain, difficulty in standing, and a periodic numbness of the right arm and leg. The patient also reported hypesthesia in a glove-and-stocking type of distribution.

Tests and Measures

Most of the findings of the physical therapy examination were negative. Although muscle stretch reflexes and muscle power were normal, disturbances of equilibrium were noted and nystagmus was present.[95] Given the presence of the nystagmus, the patient was referred back to her physician for further testing.

Following MRA, a diagnosis was made of VBA insufficiency with cerebellar infarction caused by neck hyperextension in the hairdressing salon. The patient was treated conservatively with rest and medication, and the vertigo improved 1 week after injury, enabling the patient to walk without assistance.

DISCUSSION

Beauty parlor stroke syndrome was first described by Weintraub[96] in 1993. Since then, various authors have reported similar cases.[97,98] Because this syndrome is not recognized widely, a careful history is necessary in the presence of symptoms such as those described. Such symptoms are often thought to be nonspecific and might be attributed to neurosis, psychogenic headache, or menopause, particularly when imaging studies do not show specific findings. Routine radiography, computed tomography, and magnetic resonance imaging studies usually do not help to identify lesions in this syndrome. Special care is therefore necessary to evaluate the clinical findings during examination of the nervous and auditory systems. The most likely pathophysiologic mechanism of the beauty parlor stroke syndrome is stenosis of the VA caused by compression at the atlantooccipital junction. This compression leads to damage of the intima, thrombus formation, stenosis of the artery by fibrosis, or embolism followed by infarction of the brain stem or cerebellum.

REVIEW QUESTIONS

1. From which artery does the VA normally arise?
2. What is the most common variation in the origin of the VA?
3. Describe the course of the third part of the artery (suboccipital).
4. List the branches generated directly by the basilar artery.
5. Which of the cranial nerves is (are) not vascularized by the VA?

REFERENCES

1. Hardesty WH, Whitacre WB, Toole JF, et al: Studies on vertebral artery blood flow in man. *Surg Gyn Obstet* 116:662, 1963.
2. Quain R: *The Anatomy of the Arteries of the Human Body and Its Application to Pathology and Operative Surgery, with a Series of Lithographic Drawings.* London, England: Taylor and Walton, 1844.
3. George B, Laurian C: *The Vertebral Artery: Pathology and Surgery.* New York, NY: Springer-Verlag Wien, 1987.
4. Thiel HW: Gross morphology and pathoanatomy of the vertebral arteries. *J Manipulative Phys Ther* 14:133–141, 1991
5. Gray H: *Gray's Anatomy.* Philadelphia, PA: Lea & Febiger, 1995.
6. Rieger P, Huber G: Fenestration and duplicate origin of the left vertebral artery in angiography. *Neuroradiology* 25:45–50, 1983.
7. Sheehan S, Bauer RB, Meyer JS: Vertebral artery compression in cervical spondylosis. *Neurology* 10:968–986, 1960.
8. Crum B, Mokri B, Fulgham J: Spinal manifestations of vertebral artery dissection. *Neurology* 55:304–306, 2000.
9. Anderson RE, Sheally CN: Cervical pedicle erosion and rootlet compression caused by a tortuous vertebral artery. *Radiology* 96:537–528, 1970.
10. Wilkinson IMS: The vertebral artery: extra and intra-cranial structure. *Arch Neurol* 27:393–396, 1972.
11. Aspinall W: Clinical testing for cervical mechanical disorders which produce ischemic vertigo. *J Orthop Sports Phys Ther* 11:176–182, 1989.
12. Hadley LA: Tortuosity and deflection of the vertebral artery. *Am J Roentgenol Radium Ther Nucl Med* 80:306–312, 1958.
13. Cooper DF: Bone erosion of the cervical vertebrae secondary to tortuosity of the vertebral artery. *J Neurosurg* 53:106–108, 1980.
14. DeKleyn A, Nieuwenhuyse P: Schwindelanfaalle und Nystagumus bei einer bestimmeten Lage des Kopfes. *Acta Otolaryngol* 11:155–157, 1927.
15. Feudale F, Liebelt E: Recognizing vertebral artery dissection in children: a case report. *Pediatr Emerg Care* 16:184–188, 2000.
16. Tatlow TWF, Bammer HG: Syndrome of vertebral artery compression. *Neurology* 7:331–340, 1957.
17. Fast A, Zincola DF, Marin EL: Vertebral artery damage complicating cervical manipulation. *Spine* 12:840, 1987.
18. Ouchi H, Ohara I: Extracranial abnormalities of the vertebral artery detected by selective arteriography. *J Cardio Surg* 18:250–261, 1973.
19. Toole J, Tucker S: Influence of head position upon cerebral circulation. *Arch Neurol* 2:616–623, 1960.
20. Kerry R, Taylor AJ, Mitchell J, et al: Manual therapy and cervical arterial dysfunction, directions for the future: a clinical perspective. *J Man Manipulative Ther* 16:39–48, 2008.
21. Bogduk N: Cervical causes of headache and dizziness. In: Grieve GP, ed. *Modern Manual Therapy of the Vertebral Column.* New York, NY: Churchill Livingstone, 1986:289–302.
22. Bogduk N: The anatomical basis for cervicogenic headache. *J Manipulative Physiol Ther* 15:67–70, 1992.
23. Kuether T, Nesbit G, Clark W, et al: Rotational vertebral artery occlusion: a mechanism of vertebrobasilar insufficiency. *Neurosurgery* 41:427–433, 1997.

24. Pettman E: Principles and practices. In: Pettman E, ed.: *Manipulative Thrust Techniques—an Evidence-Based Approach.* Abbotsford, British Columbia, Canada: Aphema Publishing, 2006:12–26.
25. Meadows J: *Orthopedic Differential Diagnosis in Physical Therapy.* New York, NY: McGraw-Hill, 1999.
26. Giacobetti FB, Vaccaro AR, Bos-Giacobetti MA, et al: Vertebral artery occlusion associated with cervical spine trauma. *Spine* 22:188–192, 1997.
27. Arnold C, Bourassa R, Langer T, et al: Doppler studies evaluating the effect of a physical therapy screening protocol on vertebral artery blood flow. *Man Ther* 9:13–21, 2004.
28. Mitchell JA: Changes in vertebral artery blood flow following normal rotation of the cervical spine. *J Manipulative Physiol Ther* 26:347–351, 2003.
29. Li YK, Zhang YK, Lu CM, et al: Changes and implications of blood flow velocity of the vertebral artery during rotation and extension of the head. *J Manipulative Physiol Ther* 22:91–95, 1999.
30. Mitchell J: Vertebral artery blood flow velocity changes associated with cervical spine rotation: a meta-analysis of the evidence with implications for Professional Practice. *J Man Manipulative Ther* 17:46–57, 2009.
31. Haynes M, Cala L, Melsom A, et al: Vertebral arteries and cervical rotation: modeling and magnetic resonance angiography studies. *J Manipulative Physiol Ther* 25:370–383, 2002.
32. Zaina C, Grant R, Johnson C, et al: The effect of cervical rotation on blood flow in the contralateral vertebral artery. *Man Ther* 8:103–109, 2003.
33. Brown BSJ, Tissington-Tatlow WF: Radiographic studies of the vertebral arteries in cadavers. *Radiology* 81:80–88, 1963.
34. Haynes MJ: Doppler studies comparing the effects of cervical rotation and lateral flexion on vertebral artery blood flow. *J Manipulative Physiol Ther* 19:378–384, 1996.
35. Panjabi M, Dvorak J, Crisco J, et al: Flexion, extension, and lateral bending of the upper cervical spine in response to alar ligament transections. *J Spinal Disord* 4:157–67, 1991.
36. Jónsson H, Jr., Cesarini K, Sahlstedt B, et al: Findings and outcome in whiplash-type neck distortions. *Spine* 19:2733–2743, 1994.
37. Golueke P, Sclafani S, Phillips T: Vertebral artery injury—diagnosis and management. *J Trauma* 27:856–865, 1987.
38. Hayes P, Gerlock AJ, Cobb CA: Cervical spine trauma: a cause of vertebral artery injury. *J Trauma* 20:904–905, 1980.
39. Schwarz N, Buchinger W, Gaudernak T, et al: Injuries of the cervical spine causing vertebral artery trauma: case reports. *J Trauma* 31:127–133, 1991.
40. Auer RN, Krcek J, Butt JC: Delayed symptoms and death after minor head trauma with occult vertebral artery injury. *J Neurol Neurosurg Psychiatry* 57:500–502, 1994.
41. Bose B, Northrup BE, Osterholm JL: Delayed vertebrobasilar insufficiency following cervical spine injury. *Spine* 10:108–110, 1985.
42. Endo K, Ichimaru K, Shimura H, et al: Cervical vertigo after hair shampoo treatment at a hairdressing salon: a case report. *Spine* 25:632, 2000.
43. Nagler W: Vertebral artery obstruction by hyperextension of the neck: report of three cases. *Arch Phys Med Rehabil* 54:237–240, 1973.
44. Hart RG, Easton JD: Dissections. *Stroke* 16:925–927, 1985.
45. Caplan LR, Zarins C, Hemmatti M: Spontaneous dissection of the extracranial vertebral artery. *Stroke* 16:1030–1038, 1985.
46. Biller J, Hingtgen WL, Adams HP, et al: Cervicocephalic arterial dissections. A ten-year experience. *Neurol Clin* 1:155–182, 1986.
47. Mas JL, Bousser MG, Hasboun D, et al: Extracranial vertebral artery dissections: a review of 13 cases. *Stroke* 18:1037–1047, 1987.
48. Mokri B: Traumatic and spontaneous extracranial internal carotid artery dissections. *J Neurol* 237:356–361, 1990.
49. Schmitt HP, Gladisch R: Multiple Frakturen des Atlas mit zweizeitiger todlicher Vertebralisthrombose nach Schleudertrauma der Halswirbelsaule. *Arch Orthop Unfachir* 87:235–244, 1977.
50. Schneider RC, Schemm GW: Vertebral artery insufficiency in acute and chronic spinal trauma. *J Neurosurg* 18:348–360, 1961.
51. Hillier CEM, Gross MLP: Sudden onset vomiting and vertigo following chiropractic neck manipulation. *J Postgrad Med* 74:567–568, 1998.
52. Peters M, Bohl J, Thömke F, et al: Dissection of the internal carotid artery after chiropractic manipulation of the neck. *Neurology* 45:2284–2286, 1995.
53. Jeret JS, Bluth MB: Stroke following chiropractic manipulation: report of 3 cases and review of the literature. *J Neuroimaging* 10:52, 2000.
54. Klougart N, Leboeuf-Yde C, Rasmussen LR: Safety in chiropractic practice, part 1: the occurrence of cerebrovascular accidents after manipulation to the neck in Denmark from 1978-1988. *J Manipulative Physiol Ther* 19:371–377, 1996.
55. Stern WE: Circulatory adequacy attendant upon carotid artery occlusion. *Arch Neurol* 21:455–465, 1969.
56. Assendelft WJ, Bouter SM, Knipschild PG: Complications of spinal manipulation: a comprehensive review of the literature. *J Fam Pract* 42:475–480, 1996.
57. Dvorak J, Orelli F: How dangerous is manipulation to the cervical spine? Case report and results of a survey. *Man Med* 2:1–4, 1985.
58. Frisoni G, Anzola G: Vertebrobasilar ischemia after neck motion. *Stroke* 22:1452–1460, 1991.
59. Haldeman S, Kohlbeck FJ, McGregor M: Risk factors and precipitating neck movements causing vertebrobasilar artery dissection after cervical trauma and spinal manipulation. *Spine* 24:785–794, 1999.
60. Castaigne P, Lhermitte F, Gautier JC, et al: Arterial occlusions in the vertebro-basilar system. A study of 44 patients with post-mortem data. *Brain* 96:133–154, 1973.
61. Viktrup L, Knudsen GM, Hansen SH: Delayed onset of fatal basilar thrombotic embolus after whiplash injury. *Stroke* 26:2194–2196, 1995.
62. Stanley JC, Fry WJ, Seeger JF, et al: Extracranial internal carotid and vertebral artery fibrodysplasia. *Arch Surg* 109:215–222, 1974.
63. Klippel M, Trenaunay P: Du naevus variqueux osteohypertrophique. *Arch Gen Med* 185:641, 1900.
64. Capraro PA, Fisher J, Hammond DC, et al: Klippel-Trenaunay syndrome. *Plast Reconstruct Surg* 109:2052–2060, 2002.
65. Baskerville PA, Ackroyd JS, Browse NL: The etiology of the Klippel-Trenaunay syndrome. *Ann Surg* 202:624, 1985.
66. van Dijk JM, terBrugge KG, Willinsky RA, et al: Clinical course of cranial dural arteriovenous fistulas with long-term persistent cortical venous reflux. *Stroke* 33:1233–1236, 2002.
67. Nair R, Chetty R, Woolgar J, et al: Spontaneous arteriovenous fistula resulting from HIV arteritis. *J Vasc Surg* 33:186–187, 2001.
68. Partington MD, Rufenacht DA, Marsh WR, et al: Cranial and sacral dural arteriovenous fistulas as a cause of myelopathy. *J Neurosurg* 76:615–622, 1992.
69. Ferbert A, Bruckmann H, Drummen R: Clinical features of proven basilar artery occlusion. *Stroke* 21:1135–1142, 1990.
70. Fisher CM: Vertigo in cerebrovascular disease. *Arch Otolaryngol* 85:529–534, 1967.
71. Troost BT: Dizziness and vertigo in vertebrobasilar disease. *Stroke* 11:413–415, 1980.
72. Terrett AGJ: *Current Concepts in Vertebrobasilar Complications Following Spinal Manipulation.* 2nd ed. Norwalk, IA: Foundation for Chiropractic Education and Research, 2001.
73. Woolsey RM, Hyung CG: Fatal basilar artery occlusion following cervical spine injury. *Paraplegia* 17:280–283, 1980.
74. Pettman E: Stress tests of the craniovertebral joints. In: Boyling JD, Palastanga N, eds. *Grieve's Modern Manual Therapy: The Vertebral Column.* 2nd ed. Edinburgh, Scotland: Churchill Livingstone, 1994: 529–538.
75. Contorni L: Il circolo collaterale vertebro-vertebrale nell' obliterazione dell'arteria succlavia alla sua origine. *Minerva Chir* 15:268–271, 1960.
76. Reivich M, Holling HE, Roberts B, et al: Reversal of blood flow through the vertebral artery and its effects on cerebral circulation. *N Engl J Med* 265:878–885, 1961.
77. Fisher CM: A new vascular syndrome: the subclavian steal syndrome. *N Engl J Med* 265:912–913, 1961.
78. Meissner I, Wiebers DO, Swanson JW, et al: The natural history of drop attacks. *Neurology* 36:1029–1034, 1986.
79. Dieter RA, Jr., Kuzycz GB: Iatrogenic steal syndromes. *Int Surg* 83: 355–357, 1998.
80. Schievink WI: Spontaneous dissection of the carotid and vertebral arteries. *N Engl J Med* 344:898–906, 2001.
81. Djouhri H, Guillon B, Brunereau L, et al: MR angiography for the long-term follow-up of dissecting aneurysms of the extracranial internal carotid artery. *AJR Am J Roentgenol* 174:1137–1140, 2000.
82. De Bray J-M, Lhoste P, Dubas F, et al: Ultrasonic features of extracranial carotid dissections: 47 cases studied by angiography. *J Ultrasound Med* 13:659–64, 1994.
83. Maitland G: *Vertebral Manipulation.* Sydney, New South Wales, Australia: Butterworth, 1986
84. Australian Physiotherapy Association: Protocol for pre-manipulative testing of the cervical spine. *Aust J Physiother* 34:97–100, 1988.
85. Grant ER: Clinical testing before cervical manipulation—can we recognise the patient at risk? *Proceedings of the Tenth International Congress of the World Confederation for Physical Therapy*, Sydney, New South Wales, Australia, 1987:192.

86. Rivett D: The vertebral artery and vertebrobasilar insufficiency. In: Boyling JD, Jull GA, eds. *Grieve's Modern Manual Therapy: The Vertebral Column.* Philadelphia, PA: Churchill Livingstone, 2004: 257–273.
87. Childs JD, Flynn TW, Fritz JM, et al: Screening for vertebrobasilar insufficiency in patients with neck pain: manual therapy decision-making in the presence of uncertainty. *J Orthop Sports Phys Ther* 35:300–306, 2005.
88. Rivett DA, Sharples KJ, Milburn PD: Effect of pre-manipulative tests on vertebral artery and internal carotid artery blood flow. A pilot study. *J Manipulative Physiol Ther* 22:368–375, 1999.
89. Haynes M: Vertebral arteries and cervical movement: Doppler ultrasound velocimetry for screening before manipulation. *J Manipulative Physiol Ther* 25:556–567, 2002.
90. Cote P, Kreitz B, Cassidy D, et al: The validity of the extension-rotation test as a clinical screening procedure before neck manipulation: a secondary analysis. *J Manipulative Physiol Ther* 19:159–164, 1996.
91. Bolton PS, Stick PE, Lord RS: Failure of clinical tests to predict cerebral ischemia before neck manipulation. *J Manipulative Physiol Ther* 12:304–307, 1989.
92. Westaway MD, Stratford P, Symons B: False-negative extension/rotation pre-manipulative screening test on a patient with an atretic and hypoplastic vertebral artery. *Man Ther* 8:120–127, 2003.
93. Young YH, Chen CH: Acute vertigo following cervical manipulation. *Laryngoscope* 113:659–662, 2003.
94. Vidal PG: Vertebral artery testing as a clinical screen for vertebrobasilar insufficiency: is there any diagnostic value? *Orthop Pract* 16:7–12, 2004.
95. Sakata E, Ohtsu K, Shimura H, et al: Transitory, counterolling and pure-rotatory positioning nystagmus caused by cerebellar vermis lesion [in Japanese with English abstract]. *Pract Otol* 78:2729–2736, 1985.
96. Weintraub MI: Beauty parlor strokes syndrome: report of five cases. *JAMA* 269:2085–2086, 1993.
97. Nakagawa T, Yamane H, Shigeta T, et al: Evaluation of vertebro-basilar hemodynamics by magnetic resonance angiography. *Equilib Res* 56:360–365, 1997.
98. Shimura H, Yuzawa K, Nozue M: Stroke after visit to the hairdresser. *Lancet* 350:1778, 1997.

CHAPTER 25 The Cervical Spine

CHAPTER OBJECTIVES

At the completion of this chapter, the reader will be able to:

1. Describe the anatomy of the vertebrae, ligaments, muscles, and blood and nerve supply that comprise the cervical intervertebral segment.
2. Describe the biomechanics of the cervical spine, including coupled movements, normal and abnormal joint barriers, kinesiology, and reactions to various stresses.
3. Perform a detailed objective examination of the cervical musculoskeletal system, including palpation of the articular and soft tissue structures, specific passive mobility tests, passive articular mobility tests, and stability tests.
4. Perform and interpret the results from combined motion testing.
5. Assess the static and dynamic postures of the cervical spine and implement the appropriate intervention.
6. Apply manual therapy techniques using the correct grade, intensity, direction, and duration.
7. Evaluate intervention effectiveness in order to progress or modify the intervention.
8. Plan an effective home program, including spinal care, and instruct the patient in this program.
9. Help the patient to develop self-reliant intervention strategies.

OVERVIEW

The cervical spine, (Fig. 25-1) which consists of 37 joints, permits more motion than any other region of the spine. The majority of the anatomy of the cervical spine can be explained in reference to the functions that the head and neck perform on a daily basis. To carry out these various tasks, the head has to be provided with the ability to perform extensive, detailed, and, at times, very quick motions. These motions allow for precise positioning of the eyes and the ability to respond to a host of postural changes that result from stimulation of the vestibular system (see Chap. 3).[1] In addition to providing this amount of mobility, the cervical spine has to afford some protection to several vital structures, including the spinal cord and the vertebral and carotid arteries. However, with stability being sacrificed for mobility, the cervical spine is rendered more vulnerable to both direct and indirect trauma.[2] Neck and upper extremity pain are common in the general population, with surveys finding the 1-year prevalence rate for neck and shoulder pain to be 16–18%.[2,3] This frequency is also reflected in the prevalence of neck pain in the outpatient physical therapy setting, which has been found to be between 15% and 34%.[3,4] In the younger population, cervical pathology is most commonly due to a ligament sprain or muscle strain, whereas in the older population cervical injuries are more commonly due to cervical spondylosis and/or spinal stenosis. Due to the complexity of this area, sufficient time must be allowed for a comprehensive examination to ensure that all causes of the signs and symptoms are determined.

ANATOMY

Bogduk and Mercer[5] divide the cervical spine into four anatomical units: the atlas, the axis, the C2–3 junction, and the remaining cervical vertebrae. For the sake of simplicity, these units are described in separate chapters. The atlas, axis, and C2–3 junction are described in Chapter 23. The remaining cervical vertebrae are described in this chapter.

Vertebrae

Compared with the rest of the spine, the vertebral bodies of the cervical spine are small and consist predominantly of trabecular (cancellous) bone.[1] The third to sixth cervical vertebrae can be considered typical, whereas the seventh is atypical. The third, fourth, and fifth vertebrae are almost identical, whereas the sixth has enough minor differences to distinguish it from the others.

The typical cervical vertebra has a larger transverse than anteroposterior dimension. The superior aspect of the centrum is concave transversely and convex anteroposteriorly, forming a sellar surface that reciprocates with the inferior surface of the centrum, superior to it.[1] The superior surface of

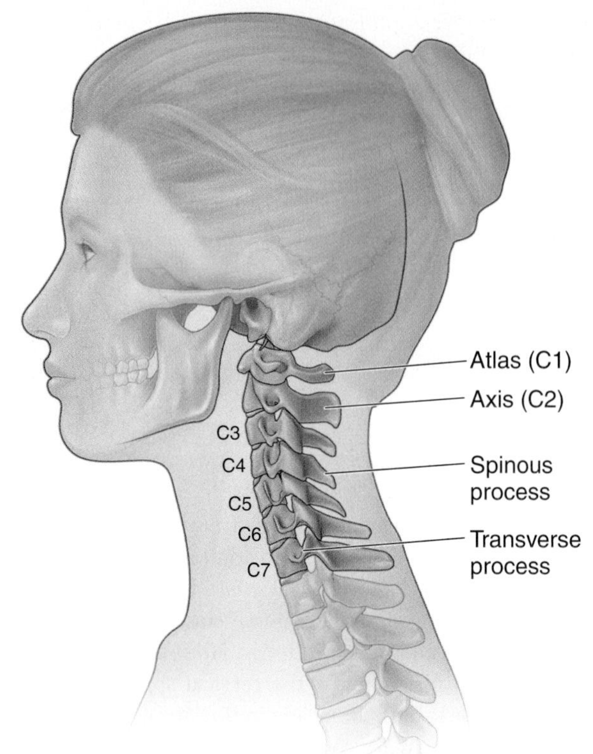

FIGURE 25-1 Cervical vertebra only.

the vertebral body is characterized by superiorly projecting processes on their superolateral aspects. Each of these hook-shaped processes is called an uncinate process and is composed of the raised lip of the superolateral aspect of the body, which articulates with a reciprocally curved surface at the synovial uncovertebral joint.

Variations in the lower cervical vertebrae are most commonly found in the spinous and transverse processes. The transverse processes are short and project anterolaterally and slightly inferiorly and are typified by a foramen in each. The transverse processes of vertebrae C3–6 are posterior and lateral to the transverse foramina, through which the vertebral artery, accessory vertebral vein, and the vertebral nerve all pass.

With the exception of the C2 vertebra (see Chap. 23), the superior aspect of the transverse process has a deep groove that mimics the orientation of the transverse process and the spinal nerve, both of which are parallel with the intervertebral foramen. The inferolateral orientation of the transverse process, and the fact that the spinal nerves are firmly anchored in the groove, makes the nerves vulnerable to a stretch injury around the distal end of the transverse process.[1]

The articular pillars and zygapophyseal (facet) joints of vertebrae C2–7 are located approximately 1 inch lateral to the spinous processes. The articular pillar is formed by the superior and inferior articular processes of the zygapophyseal joint, which bulge laterally at the pedicle–lamina junction. The articular facets on the superior articular process are concave and face superolaterally to articulate with the reciprocally curved and orientated facet on the inferior articular process of the vertebra above. The articular pillars bear a significant proportion of axial loading.[6]

As in the rest of the spine, the pedicles and laminae form the neural arch, which encloses the vertebral foramen. The pedicles project backward and laterally, whereas the long, narrow laminae run posteriorly and medially, to terminate in a short bifid spinous process, which projects slightly inferiorly.[1] The seventh cervical vertebra varies from the typical cervical vertebra. In addition to possessing a much longer and monoid spinous process to which the ligamentum nuchae attaches, the seventh vertebra has wider transverse processes, no inferior uncinate facet, and no transverse foramen.

Intervertebral Disk

In the cervical spine, there are five disks, with the first disk being located between C2 and C3. The cervical disks (Fig. 25-2) are named after the vertebra above (C4 disk lies between C4 and C5). The anatomy of the cervical disk is distinctly different from that of the lumbar intervertebral disk (IVD). The cervical nucleus pulposus (NP) at birth constitutes no more than 25% of the entire disk, not 50% as in lumbar disks.[7]

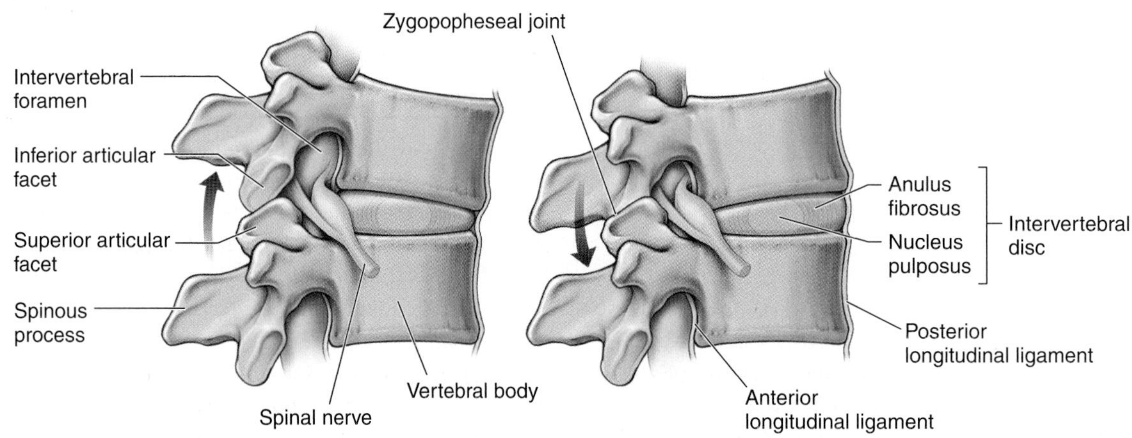

FIGURE 25-2 The intervertebral disk, articulations, ligaments, and neurologic structures. (Reproduced, with permission, from Morton, DA, Foreman KB, Albertine KH: *The Big Picture: Gross Anatomy*, McGraw-Hill, 2011.)

The IVD height-to-vertebral body height ratio (2:5) is the greatest in the cervical spine, and the IVDs make up approximately 25% of the superior-to-inferior height of the cervical spine.[8] This increase in height ratio allows for the greatest possible range of motion. The NP sits in, or near, the center of the disk, lying slightly more posteriorly than anteriorly. The inferior surface of the cervical IVD is concave, and the inferior–anterior surface of the centrum projects downward to partly cover the anterior aspect. The anterior margin of the IVD is attached to the anterior longitudinal ligament (ALL). This surface can be palpated by the clinician and is often tender in the presence of intervertebral instability. The diskal margins of the posterior surface of the vertebral body give rise to the posterior longitudinal ligament (PLL).

CLINICAL PEARL

The cervical IVD, and its development, is distinctly different from that of the lumbar disk.

A number of features distinguish the cervical disk from the lumbar disk[9]:

- Anteriorly, the cervical annulus fibrosis (AF) consists of interwoven alar fibers, whereas posteriorly, the AF lacks any oblique fibers and consists exclusively of vertically orientated fibers.
- Essentially, the cervical AF has the structure of a dense anterior interosseous ligament, with few fibers to contain the NP posteriorly.
- In no region of the cervical AF do successive lamellae exhibit alternating orientations. In fact, only in the anterior portion of the AF—where obliquely orientated fibers, upward and medially, interweave with one another—does a cruciate pattern occur.
- Posterolaterally, the NP is contained only by the alar fibers of the PLL, under or through which the nuclear material must pass if it is to herniate. Further protection against disk herniation is afforded by the uncovertebral joints, which reinforce the posterolateral aspect of the IVD.
- The absence of an AF over the uncovertebral region. In this region, collagen fibers are torn during the first 7–15 years of life, leaving clefts that progressively extend across the back of the disk. Rather than an incidental age change, this disruption has been interpreted either as enabling[10] or resulting from[11] rotatory movements of the cervical vertebrae (see next section).
- Axial rotation of a typical cervical vertebra occurs around an oblique axis perpendicular to the plane of its facets.[11]

As in the rest of the spine, the cervical IVD functions as a closed but dynamic system, distributing the changes in pressure equally to all components of the container (i.e., the end plates and the AF) and across the surface of the vertebral body. It has been observed that in the first and second decades of life, before complete ossification occurs, lateral tears occur in the AF, most probably induced by motion of the cervical spine in the bipedal posture.[12] The tears in the lateral part of the disk tend to enlarge toward the medial aspect of the IVD. The development of such tears through both sides may result in a complete transverse splitting of the disk. Such a process can be observed in the second and third decades of life in the lower cervical spine when the IVD is split in the middle into equal halves.[12] With this aging process, the NP rapidly undergoes fibrosis such that, by the third decade, it is fibrocartilaginous in nature.[13] Almost everyone older than 40 years of age has evidence of cervical disk degeneration.[14] According to Töndury and Theiler,[15] in the fourth and fifth decades of life, the NP usually dries out, and acute extrusion is not expected then. This development can be visualized on conventional radiographs as a flattening of the uncovertebral processes and a narrowing of the IVD space.[16] This may lead to a loss of elasticity and increased stresses on the vertebral end plates.

These age-related changes are evident chemically and morphologically and are much more evident in the NP than in the AF. Degenerative disk disease in this region results in diminished disk height, subjecting the bony elements to increased load.[8] The splitting of the IVD in the second and third decades of life may result in segmental instability.[12] Also, such splitting of the IVD can allow the NP to move toward the spinal canal, ultimately causing disk protrusion or extrusion and resulting in nerve root compression.[12]

In general, compression of the cervical nerve roots occurs at the entrance zone of the intervertebral foramina.[17] Anteriorly, compression of the nerve roots is likely caused by protruding disks and osteophytes of the uncovertebral region, whereas the superior articular process, the ligamentum flavum, and the periradicular fibrous tissues often affect the nerve posteriorly.[17–20] Osteophytes develop in response to this increased stress and from degenerative changes of the zygapophyseal and uncovertebral joints. The osteophytes effectively increase the available surface area and decrease the overall force on the end plates.[21] Radicular arteries within the dural root sleeves may become compressed by osteophytes, leading to spasm and decreased vascular perfusion.[21] In addition, venous obstruction may occur, resulting in edema and additional reduction in nerve root perfusion.[21]

The nerve root is divided into the anterior (ventral) and posterior (dorsal) roots (Fig. 25-2), which are responsible for motor and sensory functions, respectively. Ebraheim and colleagues[22] described the quantitative anatomy of the cervical nerve root groove and divided it into three zones: medial zone (pedicle), middle zone (vertebral artery foramen), and lateral zone. The medial zone of the cervical nerve root groove corresponds to the intervertebral foramen, and this zone is believed to play an important role in the etiology of cervical radiculopathy.[17] The intervertebral foramen, which can be further divided into an entrance zone (medial) and an exit zone (lateral), resembles a funnel in shape. The entrance zone corresponds to the narrow part of the funnel, and the shape of the radicular sheath is conical, with its takeoff points from the central dural sac being the largest part.[17] Consequently, nerve root compression occurs mostly in the entrance zone of the intervertebral foramina. Whether compression of the anterior (ventral) roots, posterior (dorsal) roots, or both occurs depends on various anatomic structures around the nerve roots. Anteriorly, compression of the nerve roots is likely caused by protruding disks and osteophytes of the uncovertebral region, whereas the superior articular process, the ligamentum flavum, and the periradicular fibrous tissues often affect the nerve posteriorly.[17–20] Osteophytes may develop in response to this increased stress and form degenerative changes of the zygapophyseal and uncovertebral joints. The osteophytes effectively increase the available surface area and decrease the overall force on the end plates.[21] Radicular arteries within the dural root sleeves may become compressed by osteophytes, leading to spasm and decreased vascular perfusion.[21] In addition, venous obstruction may occur, resulting in edema and additional reduction in nerve root perfusion.[21]

Articulations

The structure of the cervical vertebrae, combined with the orientation of the zygapophyseal facets, provides very little bony stability, and the lax soft tissue restraints permit large excursions of motion.[1] A narrow space exists between the spinal cord and the vertebral canal walls in this region. There also is a very small amount of extra space in the intervertebral foramina. Thus, a relatively small change to either the vertebral canal or the dimensions of the intervertebral foramen can result in significant compression of the spinal cord or the spinal nerve, respectively.[23]

Each pair of vertebrae in this region is connected by a number of articulations: a pair of zygapophyseal joints, two uncovertebral joints, and the IVD.

Zygapophyseal Joints

There are 14 zygapophyseal joints (Fig. 25-2) from the occiput to the first thoracic vertebra (C1–7). These joints are typical synovial joints and are covered with hyaline cartilage. The articular facets are teardrop shaped, with the superior facet facing up and posteriorly, while the inferior one faces down and anteriorly. In the middle to lower cervical regions, the dual requirements of stability and mobility are provisioned through zygapophyseal joints, with C5–6 contributing the greatest segmental mobility. The average horizontal angle of the joint planes of the middle segments is approximately 45 degrees between the frontal and transverse planes[24,25] with the upper cervical levels being closer to 35 degrees, and the lower levels at approximately 65 degrees.

CLINICAL PEARL

Clinically, the orientation of the zygapophyseal joint planes can be thought of as passing through a patient's nose.

The orientation of the zygapophyseal joint planes in the midcervical spine permits considerable flexibility in the motions of flexion and extension and encourages the coupling motions of rotation and side bending to the same side in the upper segments (see Chap. 22). However, the more caudal segments approaching the cervicothoracic junction show a tendency for a smaller range of motion—it is here that axial loading is higher and the segmental mobility becomes markedly diminished as the thoracic cage commences.[26]

The anterior joint capsule is strong, but it is lax in neutral and extension.[27] The posterior capsule is thin and weak. This laxity allows for translation between facets. The major constraints and supports of these joints are the ligaments of the vertebral column and the IVD.

Vascular, fat-filled, synovial intra-articular inclusions[5] have been observed in these joints. These structures have been described as fibroadipose meniscoids, synovial folds, and capsular rims. The meniscoids consist of connective and fatty tissue that is highly vascularized and innervated.[12] In the cervical spine, the meniscoids function as space fillers for the uneven articular surfaces, especially in regions where the elasticity of the relatively thin cartilage is not sufficient.[12] These inclusions, which are theorized to play some role in protecting the articular surfaces as they are sucked in or expelled during movements, are prone to entrapment and can play a potential role in intra-articular fibrosis and cervical spine pain.[28] Töndury and Theiler[15] have observed that the meniscoids atrophy and virtually disappear with increasing age.

The zygapophyseal joint receives its nerve supply from the medial branches of the cervical posterior rami from C2 to C8 and the recurrent meningeal (sinuvertebral) nerve. The recurrent meningeal (sinuvertebral) nerve also innervates the anterior dural sac, the posterior AF, and the PLL. The capsular pattern of the zygapophyseal joint is a limitation of extension and equal loss of rotation and side bending, with flexion being unaffected.

Uncovertebral Joints

From C3 to T1, there usually are a total of 10 saddle-shaped, diarthrodial articulations. These articulations, known as *joints of Luschka*, *uncinate processes*, or *uncovertebral joints*, are formed between the uncinate process found on the lateral aspect of the superior surface of the inferior vertebra and the beveled inferolateral aspect of the superior vertebra.[29] The uncovertebral joints develop within the first 12 years of life, as a result of loading from the head, and become fully developed by about 33 years of age.[30,31] Two of these uncovertebral joints are found between each pair of adjacent vertebrae in the cervical spine proper (C2–3 to C6–7). The uncovertebral joint maintains a synovial compartment and creates the posterior lateral border of the IVD.[32]

The biomechanical role of the uncovertebral joint is thought to be that of a sagittally oriented guiding rail during cervical flexion and extension that acts to transfer rotation forces into side bending and posterior translation motions.[29,33,34] This function is accomplished while simultaneously ensuring that the translation and, to some extent, the side bending (lateral flexion) between adjacent vertebral bodies are limited to the sagittal plane.[29,33,34] This stabilizing feature develops and changes with age and is based on alterations in the uncinate processes.[35]

CLINICAL PEARL

The uncovertebral joints serve to

- guide cervical flexion and extension;
- reduce side bending of the cervical spine;
- prevent posterior translation of neighboring vertebrae;
- reinforce the posterolateral aspect of the IVD.[36]

Penning and Wilmink[37] highlighted a possible correlation between uncovertebral joint configuration and the coupled cervical segmental motion of side bending and axial rotation. A more recent study of the C5–6 segment level by Clausen and colleagues[38] found that both the zygapophyseal joints and the uncovertebral joints are the major contributors to coupled motion in the lower cervical spine and that the uncinate processes effectively reduce motion coupling and primary cervical motion (motion in the same direction as load application), especially in response to axial rotation and side-bending loads.[38]

The onset of degenerative changes in the cervical spine has been shown to occur more commonly at the midcervical level than at the lower cervical level.[39] The reasons for the different degrees of involvement are not clear. The degenerative changes result in the substitution of a hinge-like motion, with the pivot point on the contralateral side, in place of the normal gliding motion at the uncovertebral joints.[1] This alteration effectively transforms the cervical segment into a sellar joint.[15,37,40]

CLINICAL PEARL

With a loss of disk height as a result of degeneration or degradation of the IVD, the potential for repeated contact between the bony surfaces of the uncovertebral joint increases. This repetitive contact may result in hypertrophic changes in the bone in the form of osteophytes.[1]

The nerve roots in the midcervical level are more predisposed to osteophytic compression because of a combination of

- higher uncinate process;
- smaller anteroposterior diameter of the intervertebral foramina;
- longer course of nerve roots in close proximity to the uncovertebral joints at C4–6 levels;
- greatest segmental mobility at C5 and C6.

The vertebral artery may also be compromised in the degenerative cervical spondylotic process. When involved, the vertebral artery (see Chap. 24) usually is compromised at the level of the inferior aspect of the superior vertebra, where the apical posterolateral uncovertebral osteophytes are present.

Intervertebral Foramina

The intervertebral foramina are found between all vertebrae of the spine, except in the upper cervical spine. Although there are seven cervical vertebrae, there are eight intervertebral foramina. This difference occurs because there is a nerve root existing between the occiput and the atlas (C1) that is designated to the C1 nerve root. The cervical intervertebral foramina are 4–5 mm long and 8–9 mm high. They extend obliquely anteriorly and inferiorly from the spinal canal at an angle of 45 degrees in the coronal plane.[41] The anterior boundary of the foramen is formed by the IVD and by portions of both vertebral bodies, with the zygapophyseal joints serving as the posterior boundaries. The pedicles form the superior and inferior boundaries. The medial to lateral depth of the posterior wall is formed by the lateral aspect of the ligamentum flavum.

The intervertebral foramina serve as the principal routes of entry and exit for the neurovascular systems to and from the vertebral canal. Within each foramen are

- a segmental mixed spinal nerve;
- from two to four recurrent meningeal nerves or sinuvertebral nerves;
- various spinal arteries;
- plexiform venous connections.

Because they contribute to the innervation of the upper limb, the lower cervical spinal nerves are quite large in diameter and nearly fill the foramina. This region is vulnerable to narrowing with certain motions, or with osteophyte growth. The dimensions of the intervertebral foramina decrease with full extension and ipsilateral side bending of the cervical spine such that uncovertebral osteophytes may compress the nerve root and cervical cord posteriorly.

The spinal nerves also are in close proximity to both the ligamentum flavum and the zygapophyseal joint. Thus, zygapophyseal joint arthritis or a hypertrophic ligamentum flavum can cause posterior impingement of these nerves.

Vertebral Canal

In the cervical region, the vertebral canal contains the entire cervical part of the spinal cord, as well as the upper part of the first thoracic spinal cord segment. There are eight cervical spinal cord segments, and thus eight cervical spinal nerves (see Chap. 3) on each side, but only seven cervical vertebrae.

Ligaments

Both the function and the location of the ligaments in this region are similar to that of the rest of the spine. For the purposes of these descriptions, the short ligaments that interconnect the adjacent vertebrae are classified as segmental, whereas those that attach to the peripheral aspects of all of the vertebrae are classified as continuous.

Continuous Ligaments

Anterior Longitudinal Ligament. The ALL (Fig. 25-1) is a strong band, extending along the anterior surfaces of the vertebral bodies and IVDs, from the front of the sacrum to the anterior aspect of C2. The ALL is narrower in the upper cervical spine but is wider in the lower cervical spine than it is in the thoracic region. It is firmly attached to the superior and inferior end plates of the cervical vertebrae, but not to the cervical disks. At the waist of the centrum, the ligament thickens to fill in the concavity of the body. The ALL functions to restrict spinal extension and is thus vulnerable to hyperextension trauma.

Posterior Longitudinal Ligament

Lying on the anterior aspect of the vertebral canal, the PLL extends from the sacrum to the body of the axis (C2), where it is continuous with the tectorial membrane (Fig. 25-1). The

PLL travels over the posterior aspect of the centrum, attaching to the superior and inferior margins of the body, but is separated from the waist of the body by a fat pad and the basivertebral veins. In addition, this ligament attaches firmly to the posterior aspect of the IVDs, laminae of hyaline cartilage, and adjacent margins of vertebral bodies. The PLL is broader and considerably thicker in the cervical region than in the thoracic and lumbar regions.[42] The PLL functions to prevent disk protrusions and also acts as a restraint to segmental flexion of the vertebral column.

The dura mater is strongly adherent to the PLL at the level of C3 and higher, but this attachment diminishes at lower levels.

Ligamentum Nuchae (Nuchal Ligament)

This bilaminar fibroelastic intermuscular septum spans the entire cervical spine, extending from the external occipital protuberance to the spinous process of the seventh cervical vertebra.[43] Some consider the ligament to be an extension or a replacement of the supraspinous and interspinous ligaments.[44,45] However, an observational study by Allia and Gorniak[46] suggest that it is a distinct ligamentous structure comprised of four portions formed by aponeurotic fibers from the trapezius, splenius capitis, rhomboid minor, and the serratus posterior superior.[45] The ligament is described as being a strong, thick band of elastic tissue that aids in the suspension of the head, neck.[45] However, the function of the nuchal ligament is controversial. While Mercer[47] suggests that the only contribution of the ligament to stability is at C7 and the occiput, others have proposed that the ligament may play a more important role in cervical stability,[46,48] while still others have proposed that it many play a role in posterior dural stretching and cervicogenic headaches. Studies[45–47] have shown that when the occipitoatlantal joint is flexed, the superficial fibers of the ligament tighten and pull on the deep laminae and muscular attachments, which, in turn, pull the vertebrae posteriorly, limiting the anterior translation of flexion and, therefore, flexion itself.

Segmental Ligaments

The interspinous ligaments are thin and almost membranous, interconnecting the spinous processes. The ligament is poorly developed in the upper cervical spine but well developed in the lower.[42]

The ligamentum flavum runs perpendicularly to the spine from C1 and C2, where it is referred to as the *posterior atlantoaxial ligament*, to L5 and S1. This ligament connects the laminae of successive vertebrae, from the zygapophyseal joint to the root of the spinous process. It is formed by collagen and yellow elastic tissue and, therefore, differs from all other ligaments of the cervical spine. The ligamentum flavum of the cervical spine is fairly long, allowing an appreciable amount of flexion to occur, while maintaining tension when the head and neck are in neutral. Scarring or fatty infiltration to the ligament in this region can compromise the degree of elasticity, making the ligament lax, particularly with cervical extension. This laxity increases the potential for the contents of the vertebral canal to be compressed by the buckling ligament.[49] Any enlargement of the ligament increases the likelihood that a spinal nerve or its posterior root will become impinged.[9] The ligament appears to function as a restrictor of flexion of the neck.

Muscles

The neck muscles are characteristically grouped in layers[50]:

- The superficial layer consists of muscles that connect the skull and shoulder girdle and include the trapezius (Fig. 25-3) and sternocleidomastoid (SCM) (Fig. 25-3). Other superficial muscles, which connect the scapula with the vertebral column, include the levator scapulae and the rhomboids. The scalene muscle group (Fig. 25-4) provides a relationship between the cervical spine and the first and second ribs.
- A deeper layer links the skull and vertebral column and includes long posterior (dorsal) (splenius capitis (Fig. 25-5), semispinalis capitis, and longissimus capitis).
- The deepest layers consist of muscles that link the cervical and thoracic vertebrae, splenius cervicis, semispinalis cervicis, and longissimus cervicis.

For the most part, the muscles of the neck function to support and move the head. Given the number of degrees of freedom available at the neck, it is likely that the muscles are organized as functional synergies. Muscle synergies are conceptualized as units of control, incorporating the muscles around the joint that will act together in a functional fashion.[50] Under this concept, the central nervous system (CNS) needs only trigger a synergic unit to produce a specific movement, instead of communicating with each individual muscle.[50] Synergistic movements incorporate both agonist and antagonist muscle groups, which results in a greater level of control.

Superficial Muscles

Trapezius

The trapezius muscle (Fig. 25-3) is the most superficial back muscle. It is a flat triangular muscle that runs from the superior nuchal line and external occipital protuberance of the occipital bone to the spinous process of T12 and is the largest muscle attachment in the body. Its insertion can be traced from the entire superior aspect of the spine of the scapula, the medial aspect of the acromion, and the posterior aspect of the lateral third of the clavicle.

This muscle traditionally is divided into middle, upper, and lower parts, according to anatomy and function.

- The middle part originates from C7 and forms the cervicothoracic part of the muscle.
- The lower part, attaching to the apex of the scapular spine, is relatively thin.
- The upper part (Table 25-1) is very thin, and yet it has the most mechanical and clinical importance to the cervical spine.[51]

The innervation for the trapezius comes from the accessory nerve (CN XI) and fibers from the anterior (ventral) rami of the third and fourth cervical spinal nerves, with the former being speculated to provide the motor innervation and the latter supplying the sensory information.[52–56] The greater

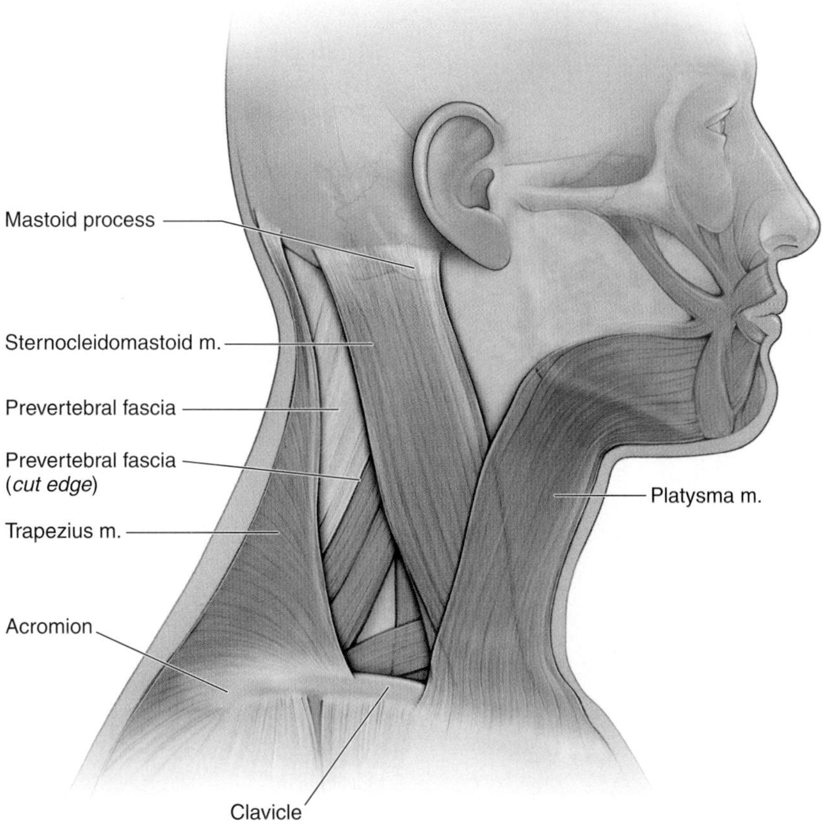

FIGURE 25-3 Muscles of the lateral and posterior cervical spine. (Reproduced, with permission, from Morton DA, Foreman KB, Albertine KH: *The Big Picture: Gross Anatomy*, McGraw-Hill, 2011.)

occipital nerve occasionally travels through the trapezius near its superior border to reach the scalp and can become entrapped by an adaptive shortening of the upper trapezius muscle or be traumatized by a blunt force.[56–58]

The different parts of this muscle provide a variety of actions on the shoulder girdle, including elevation and retraction of the scapula. When the shoulder girdle is fixed, the trapezius can produce ipsilateral side bending and contralateral rotation of the head and neck. Working together, the trapezius muscles can produce symmetric extension of the neck and head.[59] In addition, the trapezius muscle can produce scapular adduction (all three parts), and upward rotation of the scapula (primarily the superior and inferior parts). The importance of the trapezius to the shoulder joint is discussed in Chapter 16.

Sternocleidomastoid

The SCM (Fig. 25-3) is a fusiform muscle that descends obliquely across the side of the neck, forming a distinct landmark for palpatory purposes. It is the largest muscle in the anterior neck. It is attached inferiorly by two heads, arising from the posterior aspect of the medial third of the clavicle and the manubrium of the sternum. From here, it passes superiorly and posteriorly to attach on the mastoid process of the temporal bone. The motor supply for this muscle is from the accessory nerve (CN XI), whereas the sensory innervation is supplied from the anterior (ventral) rami of C2 and C3.[60] This muscle can provide the clinician with information regarding the severity of symptoms, and postural impairments, because of its tendency to become prominent when hypertonic. The SCM also is involved with a condition called torticollis, a postural deformity of the neck (see Chap. 5 and later).

In broad terms, the actions of this muscle are flexion, side bending, and contralateral rotation of the head and neck.[59] Acting together, the two muscles draw the head forward and can also raise the head when the body is supine. This head-raising action is a combination of upper cervical extension and lower cervical flexion. The muscle is also active on resisted neck flexion. With the head fixed, it is also an accessory muscle of forced inspiration.

Levator Scapulae

The levator scapulae (Fig. 16-5), is a slender muscle attached by tendinous slips to the posterior tubercles of the transverse processes of the upper cervical vertebrae (C1–4). The levator, located deep to both the upper and the middle parts of the trapezius, can be palpated just deep to the superior border of the trapezius. It descends posteriorly, inferiorly, and laterally to the superior angle and medial border of the scapula, between the superior angle and the base of the spine (Table

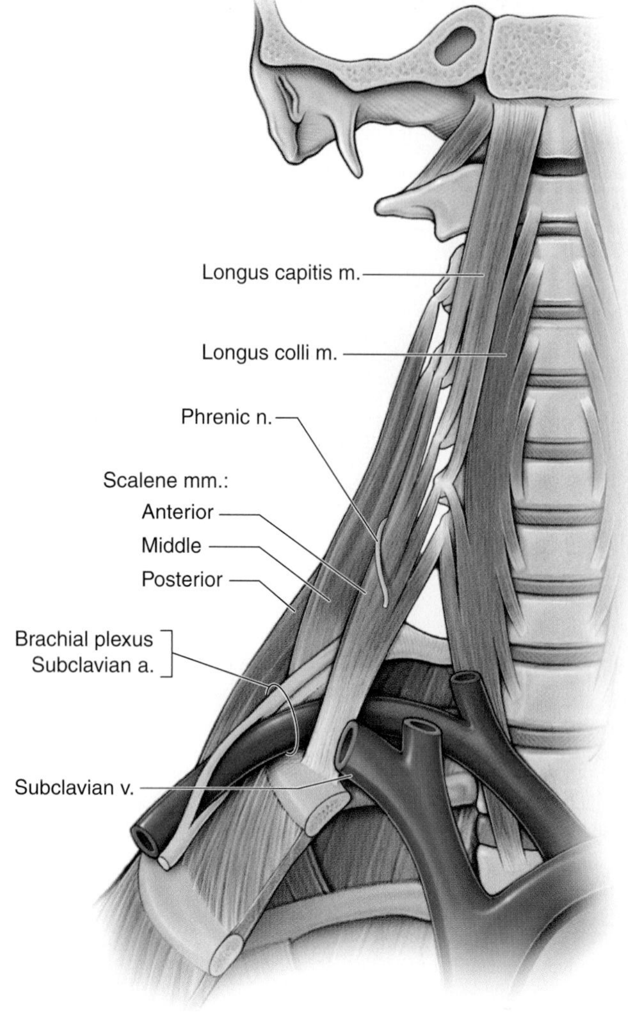

FIGURE 25-4 Muscles of the anterior cervical spine. (Reproduced, with permission, from Morton, DA, Foreman KB, Albertine KH: *The Big Picture: Gross Anatomy,* McGraw-Hill, 2011.)

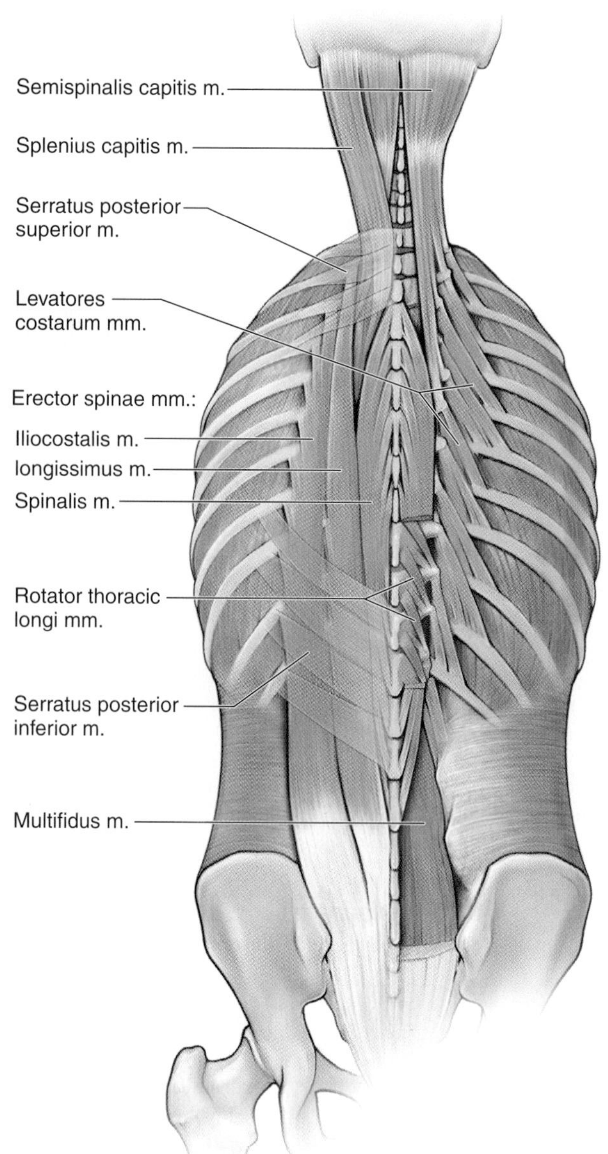

FIGURE 25-5 Deep cervical muscles. (Reproduced, with permission, from Morton, DA, Foreman KB, Albertine KH: *The Big Picture: Gross Anatomy,* McGraw-Hill, 2011.)

25-1). The levator is the major stabilizer and elevator of the superior angle of the scapula. With the scapula stabilized, the levator produces rotation and side bending of the neck to the same side; when acting bilaterally, cervical extension is produced. With a forward head posture, the potential for this extension moment increases.[1] This abnormal anterior translation is resisted by tension within the levator scapulae and the ligamentum nuchae.[61]

CLINICAL PEARL

If the levator scapulae is shorter on one side, it may provoke contralateral suboccipital muscle spasms and subsequent headaches.[1]

The levator is supplied by direct branches of the C3 and C4 cervical spinal nerves and from C5 through the posterior (dorsal) scapular nerve. It is heavily innervated with muscle spindles.

TABLE 25-1 Attachments of Upper Trapezius and Levator Scapulae Muscles

Muscle	Proximal	Distal	Innervation
Upper trapezius	Superior nuchal line Ligamentum nuchae	Lateral third of clavicle and the acromion process	Spinal accessory
Levator scapulae	Transverse processes of upper four cervical vertebrae	Medial border of scapula at level of scapular superior angle	Posterior (dorsal) scapular C5 (C3 and C4)

Rhomboids

The rhomboid major is a quadrilateral sheet of muscle, and the rhomboid minor muscle is small and cylindrical (see Chap. 16). Together they form a thin sheet of muscle that fills much of the interval between the medial border of the scapula and the midline. Although the rhomboid minor, with its attachment to the spinous processes of C7 and T1, has a slight association with the cervical spine, the rhomboid major, arising from the spinous processes of T1–5, is inactive during isolated head and neck movements. The two muscles descend from their points of origin, passing laterally to the posterior aspect of the vertebral border of the scapula, from the base of the spine to the inferior angle. Both of these muscles receive their nerve supply from the posterior (dorsal) scapular nerve (anterior (ventral) ramus of C4–5). The principal action of these muscles is to work with the levator scapulae to control the position and movement of the scapula. Both of the muscles are involved with concentric contractions during rowing exercises or other activities involving scapular retraction.

Scalenes

The scalenes (Fig. 25-4) extend obliquely like ladders (*scala* means ladder in Latin) and share a critical relationship with the subclavian artery. Tightness of these muscles will affect the mobility of the upper cervical spine. In addition, because of their distal attachments to the first and second ribs (Table 25-2), they can, if in spasm, elevate the ribs and be implicated in thoracic outlet syndrome (TOS).[62,63]

Scalenus Anterior. The scalenus anterior (see Fig. 25-4) runs vertically, behind the SCM on the lateral aspect of the neck. Arising from the anterior tubercles of the C3–6 transverse processes, it travels to the scalene tubercle on the inner border of the first rib. The osteal portion of the vertebral artery and the stellate ganglion are located lateral to the scalenus anterior. Acting from above, the scalenus anterior, like the rest of the scalenes, is an inspiratory muscle, even with quiet breathing.[64] Working bilaterally from below, it flexes the spine. Unilaterally, it side bends the spine ipsilaterally and rotates the spine contralaterally. It is supplied by the anterior (ventral) rami of C4, C5, and C6.

Scalenus Medius. The scalenus medius (see Fig. 25-4) is the largest and longest of the group, attaching to the transverse processes of all cervical vertebrae except the atlas (although it often attaches to this) and running to the upper border of the first rib. It is separated from the anterior scalene by the carotid artery, and cervical nerve, and is pierced by the nerve to the rhomboids (posterior (dorsal) scapular) and the upper two roots of the nerve to the serratus anterior (long thoracic). Working unilaterally on the cervical spine, the scalenus medius is an ipsilateral side bender of the neck. Working bilaterally, it is a cervical flexor.

Scalenus Posterior. The scalenus posterior (Fig. 25-4) is the smallest and deepest of the group, running from the posterior tubercles of the C4–6 transverse processes to attach to the outer aspect of the second rib. It functions to elevate or fix the second rib and side bends the neck ipsilaterally. It is innervated by the anterior (ventral) rami of C5, C6, and C7.

Scalenus Minimus (Pleuralis). The scalenus minimus is a small muscle slip, running from the transverse process of C7 to the inner aspect of the first rib and the dome of the pleura. It is a suprapleural membrane that is often considered to be the expansion of the tendon of this muscle. The muscle functions to elevate the dome of the pleura during inspiration, and is innervated by the anterior (ventral) ramus of C7.[65]

Platysma. The broad sheet of the platysma muscle is the most superficial muscle in the cervical region (Fig. 25-3). The platysma covers most of the anterolateral aspect of the neck, the upper parts of the pectoralis major, and deltoid, extending superiorly to the inferior margin of the body of the mandible. As a muscle of facial expression, it cannot affect bony motion, except perhaps as a passive restraint to head extension. It is supplied by the cervical branch of CN VII (facial).

Deeper Muscles of the Back

The deep or intrinsic muscles of the back are the primary movers of the vertebral column and head and are located deep

TABLE 25-2 Attachments of Scalene, Longus Colli, and Longus Capitis Muscles

Muscle	Proximal	Distal	Innervation
Scalenus			
Anterior	Anterior tubercles of C3–6	Superior crest of first rib	Anterior (ventral) primary rami of cervical spinal nerves
Middle	Posterior tubercles of C2–7	Superior crest of first rib	
Posterior	Posterior tubercles of C5–7	Outer surface of second rib	
Longus colli	Anterior tubercles of C3–5 Anterior surface of C5–7, T1–3	Tubercle of the atlas, anterior tubercles of C5 and C6, and anterior surface of C2–4	Anterior (ventral) primary rami of cervical spinal nerves
Longus capitis	Anterior tubercles of C3–6	Inferior occipital bone and basilar portion	Anterior (ventral) primary rami of cervical spine nerves

to the thoracolumbar fascia. The muscles in all of these groups are segmentally innervated by the lateral branches of the posterior (dorsal) rami of the spinal nerves.

Splenius Capitis

The splenius capitis (Fig. 25-5) extends upward and laterally, from the posterior (dorsal) edge of the nuchal ligament and the spinous processes of the lower cervical and upper thoracic vertebrae (T4–C7) to the mastoid process of the occipital bone just inferior to the superior nuchal line and deep to the SCM muscle.

Splenius Cervicis

The splenius cervicis is just inferior and appears continuous with the capitis, extending from the spines of the third to the sixth thoracic vertebrae to the posterior tubercles of the transverse processes of the upper cervical vertebrae.

The splenius capitis and splenius cervicis muscles are two important head and neck rotators. From their attachments (Table 25-3), it is clear that these two muscles are capable of producing ipsilateral rotation, side bending, and extension at the spinal joints they cross.

Cervical Erector Spinae

The erector spinae complex spans multiple segments, forming a large musculotendonous mass (Fig. 25-6) consisting of the iliocostalis, longissimus, and spinalis muscles (Tables 25-4 and 25-5).

- The iliocostalis cervicis appears to function as a stabilizer of the cervicothoracic junction and lower cervical spine.
- The semispinalis has thoracis, cervicis, and capitis divisions. The obliquus capitis superior (superior oblique) and inferior (inferior oblique) and the rectus capitis posterior major and minor (see Chap. 23) lie underneath the semispinalis capitis and splenius capitis muscles.[66] The semispinalis cervicis is a stout muscle that extends superiorly to the spinous process of vertebra C2, functioning as a strong extensor of the lower cervical spine.[1]

TABLE 25-3 Attachments of Splenius Capitis and Cervicis Muscles

Muscle	Proximal	Distal	Innervation
Splenius capitis	Inferior ligamentum nuchae, spinous process of C7 and T1–4 vertebrae	Mastoid process, occipital bone, and lateral third of superior nuchal line	Cervical spinal nerve and Anterior (ventral) primary rami of cervical spinal nerves
Splenius cervicis	Spinous processes of T3–6 vertebrae	Posterior tubercles of C1–3	

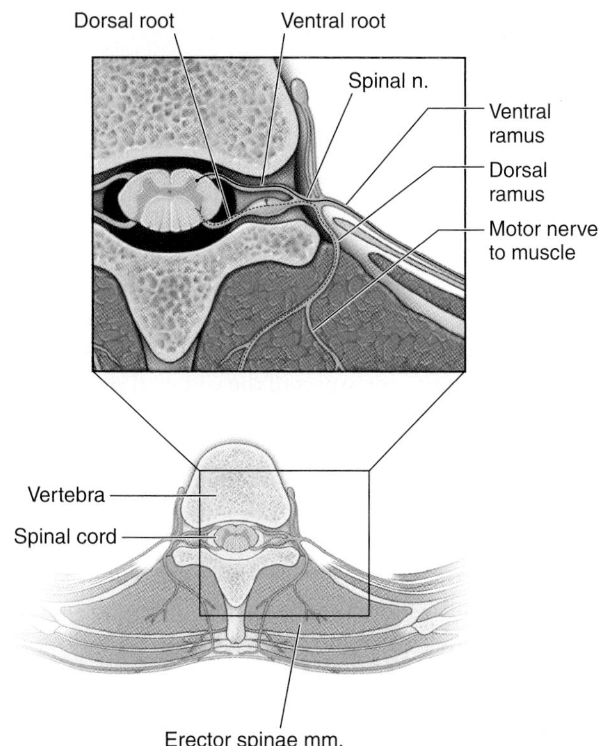

FIGURE 25-6 Erector spinae. (Reproduced, with permission, from Morton DA, Foreman KB, Albertine KH: *The Big Picture: Gross Anatomy*, McGraw-Hill, 2011.)

TABLE 25-4 Prime Movers of the Cervical Spine: Rotation and Side Bending

Muscles of Rotation and Side Bending	
Ipsilateral side bending	*Ipsilateral rotation*
Longissimus capitis	Splenius capitis
Intertransversarii posteriores cervices	Splenius cervices
Multifidus	Rotatores breves cervices
Rectus capitis lateralis	Rotatores longi cervices
Intertransversarii anteriores cervices	Rectus capitis posterior major
Scaleni	Obliquus capitis inferior
Iliocostalis cervicis	
Contralateral rotation	*Ipsilateral side bending and contralateral rotation*
Obliquus capitis superior	Sternocleidomastoid
	Scalenus anterior
	Multifidus
	Longus colli
Ipsilateral side bending and ipsilateral rotation	
Longus coli	
Scalenus posterior	

Data from Evjenth O, Hamberg J: *Muscle Stretching in Manual Therapy, a Clinical Manual.* Alfta, Sweden: Alfta Rehab Forlag, 1984.

TABLE 25-5 Prime Movers of the Cervical Spine: Extensors and Flexors		
Extensor Muscles		**Flexor Muscles**
Prime Movers	Accessory Muscles	Prime Movers
Trapezius	Multifidus	Sternocleidomastoid—anterior fibers
Sternocleidomastoid—posterior fibers	Suboccipitals	Accessory muscles
Iliocostalis cervices	Rectus capitis posterior major and minor	Prevertebral muscles
Longissimus cervices	Obliquus capitis superior	Longus colli
Splenius cervices	Obliquus capitis inferior	Longus capitis
Splenius capitis		Rectus capitis anterior
Interspinales cervices		Scalene group
Spinalis cervices		Scalenus anterior
Spinalis capitis		Infrahyoid group
Semispinalis cervices		Sternohyoid
Semispinalis capitis		Omohyoid
Levator scapulae		Sternothyroid Thyrohyoid

Data from Evjenth O, Hamberg J: *Muscle Stretching in Manual Therapy, a Clinical Manual.* Alfta, Sweden: Alfta Rehab Forlag, 1984.

- The interspinales and intertransversarii, which interconnect the processes for which they are named, produce only minimal motion because they can influence only one motion segment and are more likely to function as sensory organs for reflexes and proprioception.[67]

Deep Neck Flexors

The prevertebral muscles of the neck consist of:

- ***Longus colli.*** The longus colli (Fig. 25-4) consists of a vertical portion that originates from the bodies of the first three thoracic and last three cervical vertebrae, an inferior oblique portion that originates from the bodies of the first three thoracic vertebrae, and the superior oblique portion that originates from anterior tubercles of the transverse processes of C3–5. The various portions of the longus colli insert into the bodies of C2–4, the anterior tubercles of the transverse processes of C5–6, and the anterior tubercle of the atlas. The longus colli functions to flex (and assists in rotating) the cervical vertebrae and head. Acting singly, the longus colli side bends the vertebral column. The longus colli is innervated by branches of the anterior primary rami of C2–8.
- ***Longus capitis.*** The longus capitis (Fig. 25-4) originates from the anterior tubercles of the transverse processes of C3–6 and inserts onto the inferior surface of the basilar part of the occipital bone. The longus capitis functions to flex (and assists in rotating) the cervical vertebrae and head. It is innervated by the muscular branches of C1–4.
- ***Rectus capitis anterior.*** The rectus capitis anterior (RCA) originates from the lateral mass of the atlas and inserts onto the base of the occipital bone in front of the foramen magnum. The RCA flexes and rotates the head and is innervated by the muscular branches of C1–2.
- ***Rectus capitis lateralis.*** The rectus capitis lateralis (RCL) originates from the upper surface of the transverse process of the atlas and inserts onto the inferior surface of the jugular process of the occipital bone. The RCL side bends the head to the ipsilateral side and is innervated by branches of the anterior rami of C1–2.

CLINICAL PEARL

The longus colli and longus capitis play an important role in cervical stabilization (see "Muscle Control" section).

Neurology

The nerve supply to the cervical structures is rather unique because of the association that some of the muscles have with the cranial nerves. The cervical spine is the only region that has more nerve roots than vertebral levels.[8]

In general, structures supplied by the upper three cervical nerves can cause neck and head pain (see Table 23-1), whereas the mid to lower cervical nerves can refer symptoms to the shoulder, anterior chest, upper limb, and scapular area.[68]

Cervical proprioceptive input has considerable influence on posture through the tonic neck reflex and on eye movement and accommodation through the cervico-occular and vestibulo-ocular reflexes (see Chap. 3).[68–70] It is probably no accident that the two largest postural muscles of the head and neck, the trapezius and the SCM muscles, are partly innervated by the accessory nerve (CN XI).

Vascular Supply

The middle cervical segments are supplied by radicular branches off the extradural vertebral artery and are the most common segments to be affected in vertebral artery disease.[71] The vertebral artery is detailed in Chapter 24.

The common carotid artery bifurcates at the middle to upper cervical level into the internal and external carotid arteries. The carotid body, a specialized structure that senses oxygen and carbon dioxide levels in the blood, is located at this bifurcation.[8] The carotid sinus, which contains baroreceptors that monitor blood pressure, is located at a point before the bifurcation.[8]

Cervical Lordosis

The amount of cervical lordosis is a factor of the zygapophyseal joint planes and the cervical IVDs. Under normal conditions, the C4–5 interspace is considered the midpoint of the curve, and the center of gravity (COG) for the skull lies anterior to the foramen magnum. The longus colli has been shown to have an important supporting role on the cervical curve.[72]

A reduction in the cervical lordotic curve because of injury or abnormal posture results in more weight being borne by the vertebral bodies and IVDs, whereas an increase in the lordosis increases the compressive load on the zygapophyseal joints and posterior elements. Watson and Trout[73] have demonstrated a link between a lack of endurance capacity of the upper cervical and deep neck flexors and the forward head posture (see later).

Cervicothoracic Junction

The cervicothoracic junction comprises the C7–T1 segment, although functionally it includes the seventh cervical vertebra, the first two thoracic vertebrae, the first and second ribs, and the manubrium. In addition, the cervicothoracic junction forms the thoracic outlet, through which the neurovascular structures of the upper extremities pass. Lewit[74] considers the cervicothoracic junction to be the third major area of the spine for musculoskeletal problems, with the craniovertebral area and the lumbosacral junction being first and second, respectively.

BIOMECHANICS

The motions that occur at the cervical spine correspond to motions of the head, although the range of head movement bears little relation to the range of neck movement and that the total range is the sum of both the head and the neck motions.[75]

The cervical spine is a complex mechanical linkage composed of multiple degrees of freedom of movement about each of its joints and at least 20 pairs of muscles, many of which are capable of performing similar actions.[50] It is estimated that the osseoligamentous system contributes 20% to the mechanical stability of the cervical spine while 80% is provided by the surrounding neck musculature.[76] The role of the ligaments in stabilization occurs mainly at end of range postures,[77] while the muscles supply dynamic support in activities around neutral- and mid-range postures.[78]

At the zygapophyseal joints, there is a sagittal range of 50–80 degrees in each direction of flexion and extension.[79] The only significant arthrokinematic motions available to the zygapophyseal joint are an inferior, medial glide of the inferior articular process of the superior facet during extension and a superior, lateral glide during flexion. Segmental side bending is, therefore, extension of the ipsilateral joint and flexion of the contralateral joint. Rotation, coupled with ipsilateral side bending, also involves extension of the ipsilateral joint and flexion of the contralateral. Because of their multiple insertions, many of the neck muscles have multiple functions or can change their function depending on the initial position of each vertebral joint and the degree to which the joints are free to move in each of the planes of motion.[50] Thus, a voluntary motor task in the head and neck can be accomplished through a variety of combinations of kinematic and muscle actions. Considering that most functional daily tasks are performed in and around midrange postures, the muscles controlling the cervical spine are subject to constant external and internal forces.[78]

Flexion

Flexion may be divided into three sequential phases.[80,81] The initial phase begins in the lower cervical spine (C4–7) where C6–7 makes its maximum contribution followed by the C5–6 segment and then by C4–5. Motion in the second phase occurs initially at C0–2 followed by C2–3 and C3–4. The first phase of motion occurs again at the lower cervical spine (C4–7) initially, with the C4–5segment followed by C5–6 then the C6–7 segment.[80,81]

At the segmental level, flexion is described as an anterior osteokinematic rock tilt of the superior vertebra in the sagittal plane, a superoanterior glide of both superior facets of the zygapophyseal joints, and an anterior translation slide of the superior vertebra on the IVD (see Fig. 25-7). This produces an anterior (ventral) compression and a posterior (dorsal) distraction of the cervical disk. The uncovertebral joint lies on, or very near to, the axis of rotation for flexion and extension. Consequently, the main arthrokinematic motion that seems likely to be occurring here is an anterior spin (or very near spin).[82] This arthrokinematic spin appears especially probable, as impairments of the uncovertebral joint seem to be unaffected by flexion or extension. Thus, uncovertebral restrictions may be detected in all cervical positions, although flexion partly disengages the joint because of its posterior position on the vertebra.[82]

Although all of the following anatomic movement restrictors act to some degree on most of the components of flexion, they act particularly on the associated movement component.

- Anterior osteokinematic motion is restrained by the extensor muscles and the posterior ligaments (posterior longitudinal, interspinous, and ligamentum flavum).
- Superoanterior arthrokinematic is restrained by the joint capsule, whereas translation is restrained by the disk and the nuchal ligament.

Extension

Extension is described as a posterior osteokinematic sagittal rock, an inferoposterior glide and approximation of the superior facets of the zygapophyseal joints, and a posterior translation of the vertebra on the disk (see Fig. 25-8). The uncovertebral joint undergoes a posterior arthrokinematic spin. The osteokinematic motion of extension is restricted by the anterior prevertebral muscles and the ALL. The arthrokinematic motion is restricted by the zygapophyseal joint capsule.[82] The IVD restrains the posterior translation.

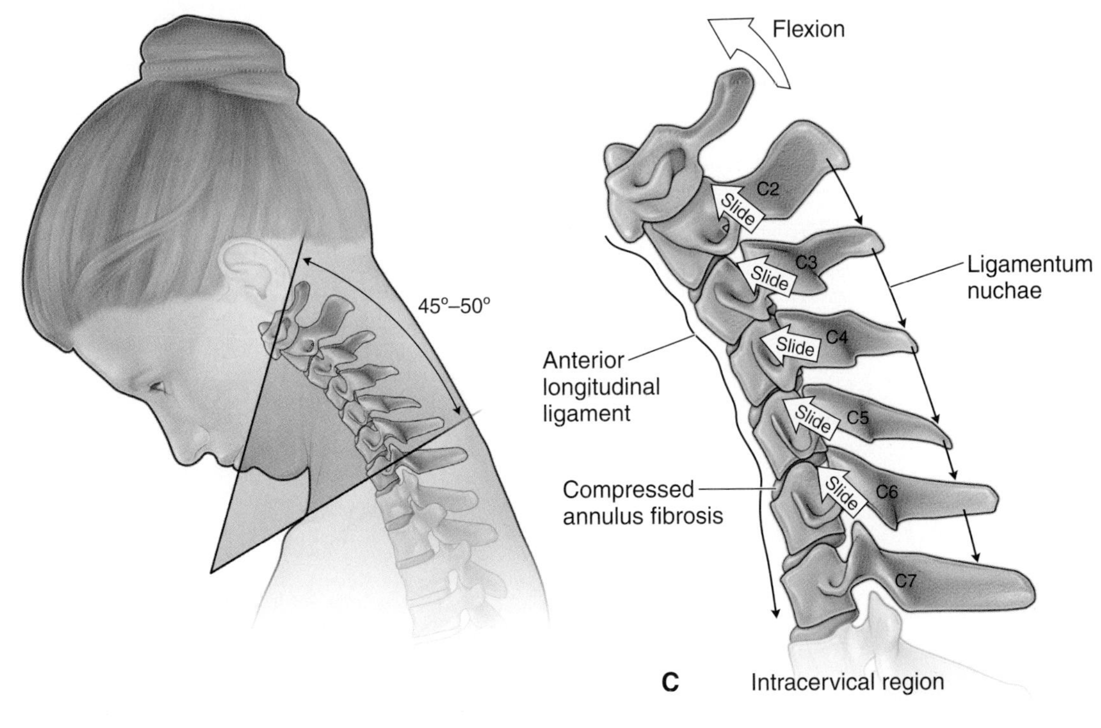

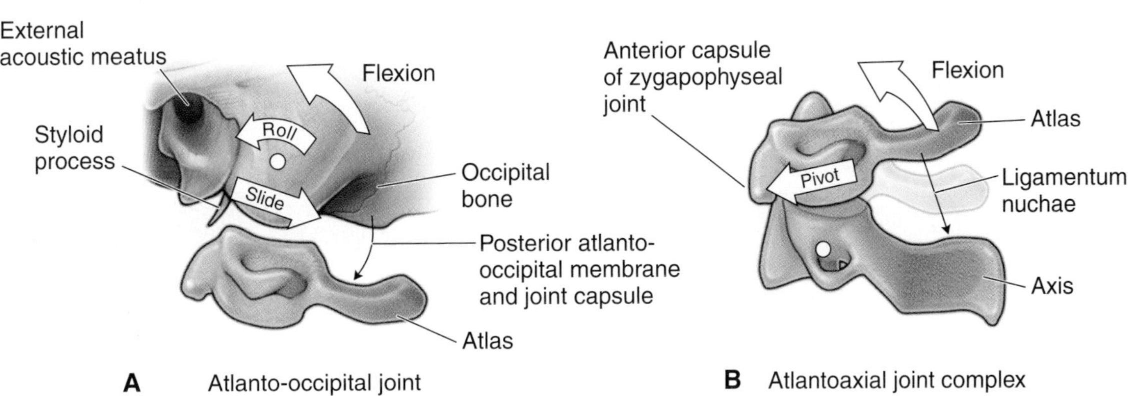

FIGURE 25-7 Kinematics of craniocervical flexion.

CLINICAL PEARL

Forward flexion occurs with rotation below the C5–6 level, and extension occurs with rotation above the C4–5 level. The net result is that whenever cervical spine rotation occurs, the greatest degree of weight bearing is on the anterior edge of the vertebral bodies below the C5 to C6 segments and on the posterior edge above C4 to C5 (this factor has been implicated in the cause of spondylosis in these areas).[1]

The greatest amount of cervical motion occurs at the C5 to C6 segment, with the C4 to C5 and C6 to C7 segments a close second.[79] Significant flexion occurs at C5 to C6, and extension around C6 to C7.[83] A coupled translation of between 2 and 3.5 mm occurs with flexion and extension. Side bending averages about 10 degrees to each side in the midcervical segments, decreasing in the caudal segments.[83]

Side Bending

Side bending (lateral flexion) is an ipsilateral osteokinematic rock, a superoanterior glide of the contralateral superior facet, and a posteroinferior glide of the ipsilateral facet (see Fig. 25-9). In addition, there is a contralateral translation of the vertebra on the disk, an inferomedial glide of the ipsilateral uncovertebral joint, and a superolateral glide of the contralateral uncovertebral joint. A composite curved translation results. This curve is formed by the superoinferior linear glides of the zygapophyseal joints, the oblique inferomedial and superomedial glides of the uncovertebral joints, and the linear translation across the disk.[82]

The osteokinematic rock can be limited by the contralateral scalenes and intertransverse ligaments. The uncovertebral and zygapophyseal arthrokinematic motions can be limited by the joint capsule, and the translation is limited by the IVD. If the side bending is limited but the translation is okay, it is unlikely

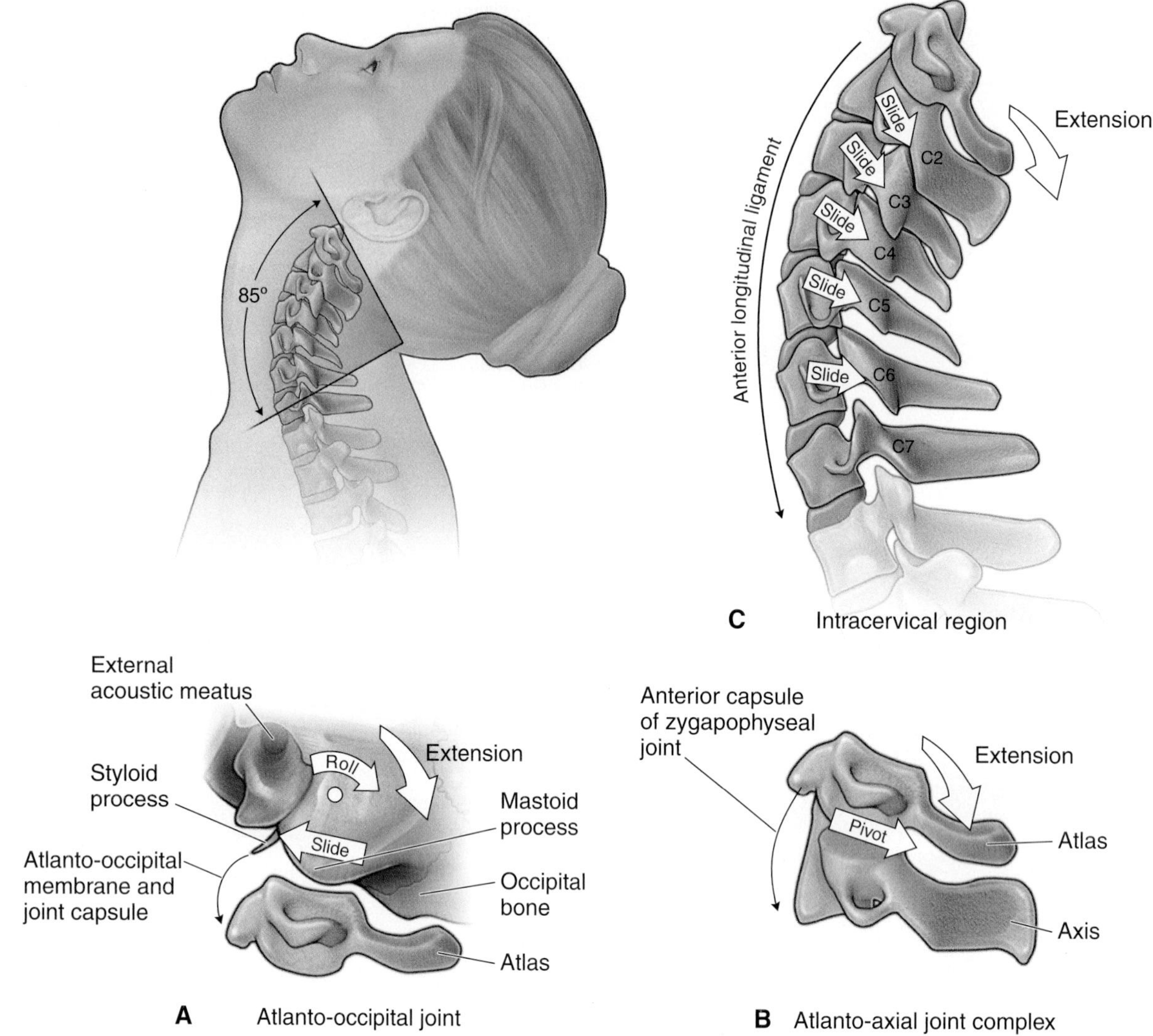

FIGURE 25-8 Kinematics of craniocervical extension.

that the joint complex (the zygapophyseal joint, disk, or uncovertebral joint) is impaired; instead, these findings may implicate adaptive shortening of the soft tissues.[82] However, if the translation is also limited, a problem with the joint complex also probably exists.

Rotation

Rotation is chiefly an osteokinematic motion of the vertebra about a vertical axis that is coupled with ipsilateral side bending (see Fig. 25-10). Presumably, the translation follows the side bending (i.e., contralateral), resulting in the same uncovertebral and zygapophyseal arthrokinematic motions as does side bending.[82]

Muscle Control

The control of head and neck postures and movements is a complex task, especially in the presence of pain or dysfunction. The muscle groups of the cervical region may be divided into those that sustain postures or stabilize the segments and those that produce movement.[84–86] Considerable biomechanical, physiological and clinical research in both the cervical and lumbar regions has been undertaken which supports Bergmark's[86,87] model for a functional division between the deep and more superficial muscles in their relative contributions to spinal support and control.[78] According to this model, the more superficial multisegmental (global) muscles have the responsibility for maintaining equilibrium of external forces (torque production and control of the head) so that the load transmitted to the spinal segments can be controlled efficiently by the deep intersegmental (local) muscle system.[68,78,86]

The SCM (anteriorly) and the semispinalis capitis and splenius capitis (posteriorly) are thought to be the global muscles of the neck, whereas the local system is thought to comprise the longus capitis and colli (Table 25-2),[72] semispinalis cervicis, and multifidus.[88] The longus colli and posterior (dorsal) neck muscles form a muscle sleeve that surrounds the cervical column to support the cervical spinal segments in functional movements.[72]

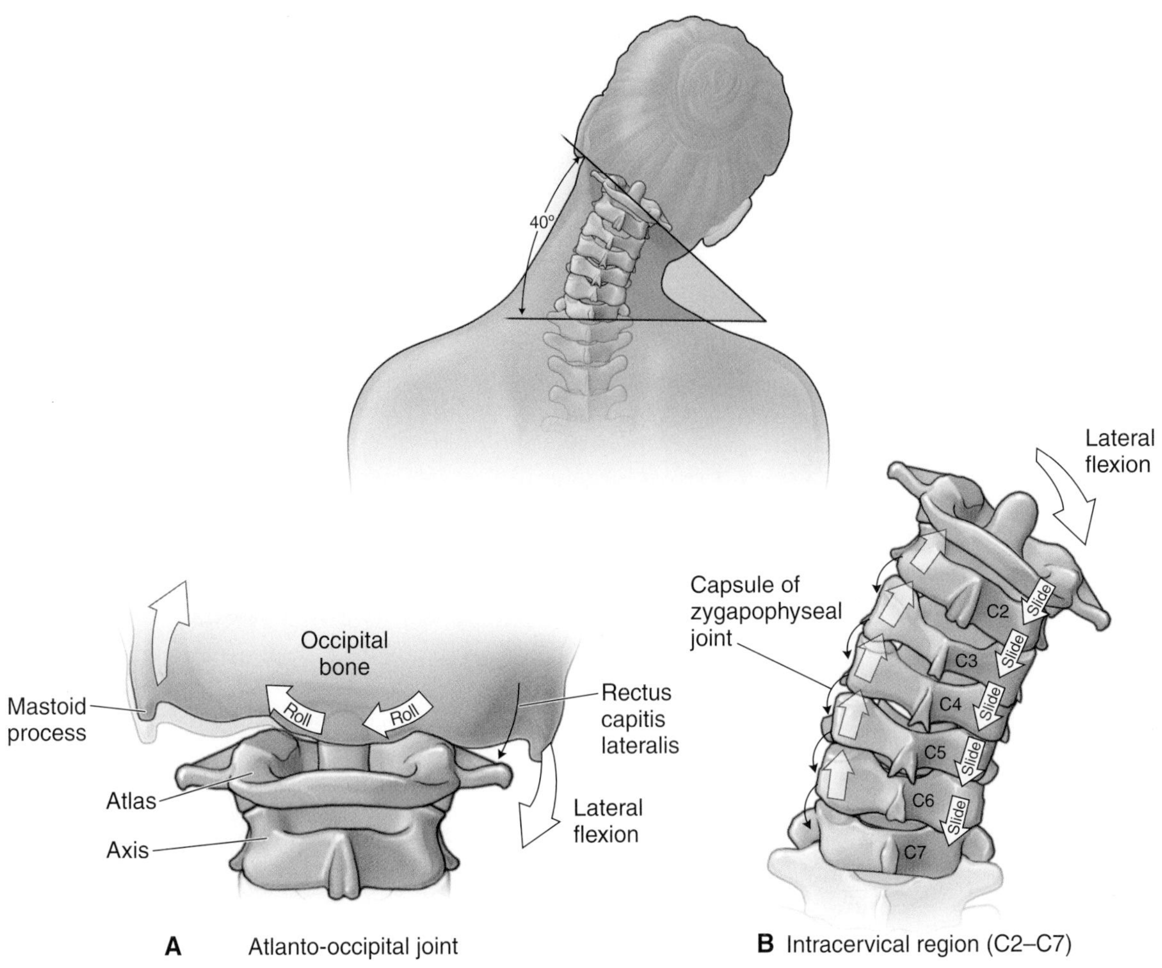

FIGURE 25-9 Kinematics of craniocervical side bending.

Patients with neck pain have been found to demonstrate generally less torque production (strength and endurance) in all planes, with a greater loss in the cervical flexors than extensors.[89] However, addressing strength alone in research and exercise programs may oversimplify the problems in the neuromuscular system associated with neck pain.[78] Recent research has recognized the vital role that activation of the deep neck flexor muscles plays in supporting the cervical segments and the cervical curve (see "Muscle Function Testing: Deep Neck Flexors" section later).[72,88,90] Indeed, impairment in the axioscapular-girdle muscles has been linked clinically to cervical pain syndromes.[84,91–95] The nature of the impairment in the cervical and cervicobrachial muscle systems indicates the need for careful and precise movement analysis and muscle testing to appreciate and accurately define the problem.[78]

EXAMINATION

The cervical spine is an area with a high potential for serious injury, which makes this a region of the body that needs to be examined with caution, especially when there is a history of acute and recent trauma of the neck, because of the potential for the examination itself to be harmful.[96] Although most conditions involving neck and upper limb symptoms can be diagnosed after a careful history and physical examination, in cases of significant trauma, imaging studies may be required to exclude a fracture or instability. Where possible, the patient should be examined for central and/or peripheral neurologic deficit, neurovascular compromise, and serious skeletal injury, such as fractures or craniovertebral ligamentous instability.

Winkel and colleagues[97] clinically categorize cervical disorders by the location of symptoms and the etiology of each condition:

- ***Local cervical syndrome (LCS).*** This syndrome manifests with local neck complaints, resulting from cervical muscle strain, ligament sprain, or a primary or secondary disk-related condition.
  - A primary disk-related LCS is characterized by symptoms that may result from a protrusion, prolapse, or extrusion of the disk.
  - A secondary disk-related LCS is characterized by symptoms resulting from gradual changes in the cervical spine that have been generated by previous degradation of

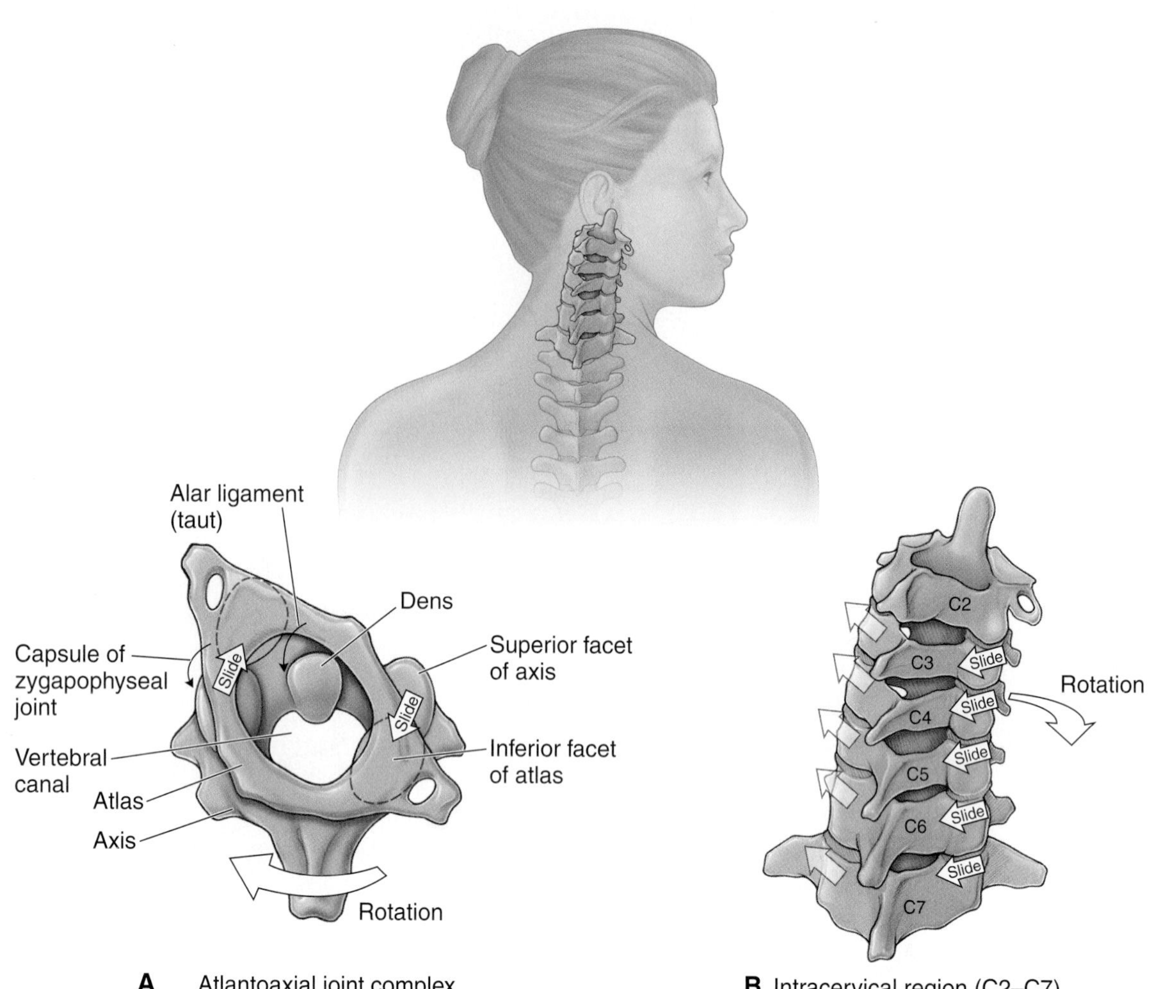

FIGURE 25-10 Kinematics of craniocervical rotation.

the IVD. These changes include internal disk disruption and synovitis or irritation of the zygapophyseal and uncovertebral joints. In the cervical spine, myofascial pain may be a secondary tissue response to an IVD or zygapophyseal joint injury.[98] The cervical zygapophyseal (facet) joints can be responsible for a significant portion of chronic neck pain. Established referral zones for the cervical zygapophyseal joint[99,100] overlap both myofascial and dermatomal pain patterns. Cervical zygapophyseal joint pain is typically unilateral and is described by the patient as a dull ache. Occasionally, the pain can be referred into the craniovertebral or interscapular regions.

- ***Cervicobrachial syndrome.*** This syndrome includes symptoms in the local cervical region, as well as in one or both upper extremities, as a result of nerve root irritation through compression or tension of the nerve root.
- ***Cervicocephalic syndrome.*** This syndrome is characterized by complaints in both the neck and the head and includes symptoms such as dizziness, tinnitus, and headache. These symptoms may result from articular, ligamentous, neurologic, organic, or vascular sources.
- ***Cervicomedullary syndrome.*** This syndrome is characterized by spinal cord symptoms associated with cord compression at the cervical spine (cervical myelopathy).

Clearing tests for the cervical spine include

- vertebral artery tests;
- Sharp–Purser test;
- articular stability tests;
- transverse ligament test;
- alar ligament test;
- temporomandibular joint (TMJ) assessment.

Once damage to the vertebral artery (see Chap. 24) and transverse ligament (see Chap. 23) has been ruled out, the most likely pain candidates are assessed first. These include the bone, muscles, ligaments, zygapophyseal joints, and IVD. In addition, because of its close proximity, a quick examination of the TMJ should be performed to rule out pain referral from this joint (see Chap. 26). The examination must be graduated and progressive so that the testing can be discontinued at the

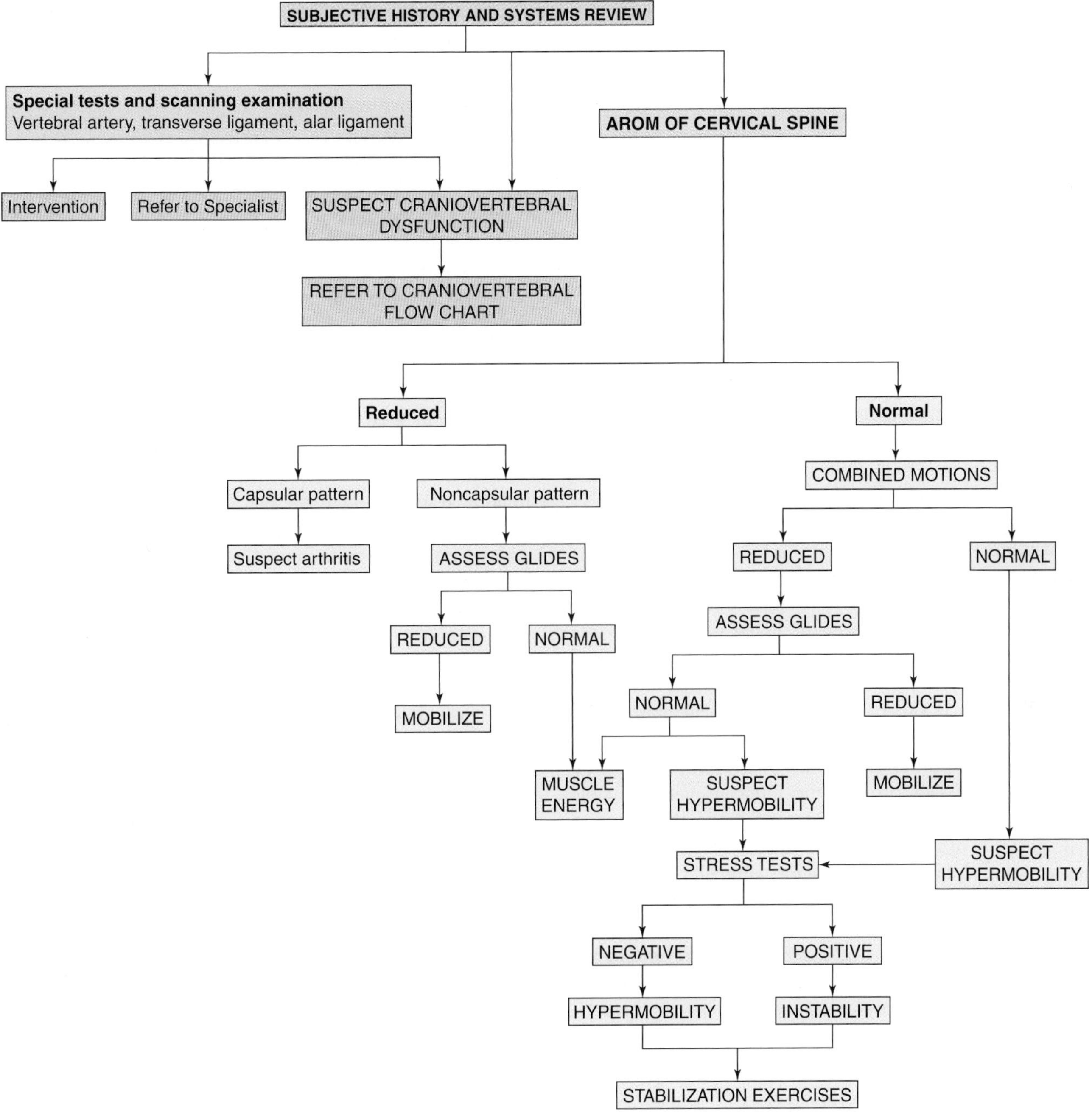

FIGURE 25-11 An examination and treatment algorithm for the mid-lower cervical spine.

first signs of serious pathology.[96] An examination and treatment algorithm for the mid-lower cervical spine is outlined in Figure 25-11.

History

The most common symptoms of cervical disorders are ongoing or motion-induced neck or arm pain, or both, and suboccipital headache.[12] In addition to the questions listed under History in Chapter 4, the clinician should obtain the following information.

The clinician must determine whether the trauma occurred and the exact mechanism. In acute sprains and strains, patients typically relate an activity that precipitated the onset of their symptoms. This may be lifting or pulling a heavy object, an awkward sleeping position, a hyperextension injury, or prolonged static postures. In whiplash-associated disorders (WADs), patients generally describe an accident in which they were unexpectedly struck from the rear, front, or side. Rotational injuries may also occur. If there were neurologic symptoms following the trauma (paresthesias, dizziness, tinnitus, visual disturbances, or loss of consciousness), more severe damage should be suspected.[101] If the patient reports electric shock-like symptoms down the spine with neck flexion (Lhermitte's sign), the clinician should consider the possibility of inflammation or irritation of the meninges.[102–104] A traumatic mechanism of injury with complaints of nonspecific cervical symptoms that are exacerbated in the vertical position, and relieved with the head supported in the supine position, is suggestive of cervical instability, especially if the patient reports that dysthesias of the face occur with neck movement.[105–107]

For the purposes of the examination, it is important to establish a baseline of symptoms so that the clinician is able to determine whether a particular movement aggravates or lessens the patient's symptoms. The history can provide the clinician with information as to the location of the patient's symptoms (head, neck, shoulder, arm, and hand), the nature of the symptoms (constant, intermittent, or variable), the type of symptoms (pain, paresthesia, numbness, weakness, and stiffness), the severity of the condition, and the activities or positions that appear to aggravate or improve the patient's condition. It is also important to determine the type of work the patient does and whether that work involves sustained postures, the potential for eye strain, repetitive motions of the head, neck and upper extremity, or heavy lifting. Symptoms associated with coughing and sneezing are often associated with disk pathology. Radicular pain may be accompanied by sensorimotor symptoms.[12]

The patient's chief complaint should be determined. The clinician should determine the location and boundaries of the symptoms. All symptoms present should be recorded on a body diagram, even those that may initially appear unrelated. If pain is the major symptom, the clinician should attempt to quantify the pain using a pain rating scale. It is also appropriate at this time to establish the patient's goals.

Asking the patient to describe his or her symptoms over a 24-hour period can provide the clinician with valuable information about the severity, the positions and activities that aggravate or relieve the symptoms, and the duration of the symptoms. Patients who report difficulty in sleeping because of pain may have an inflammatory condition, but the more insidious causes of night pain, such as malignancy, must be ruled out. The patient's sleeping position and habits should be investigated. Cervical symptoms often are increased when a foam or very firm pillow is used.[108] Sleeping in the prone position requires adequate cervical and upper thoracic rotation. Some degree of cervical extension also is required, depending on the number and type of pillow used. The onset of symptoms may also provide clues as to the type of tissue involved. Muscle or ligamentous pain may either occur immediately following trauma or be delayed for several hours or days. Bone pain usually occurs immediately.

The reports of headaches or facial pain, depending on frequency and severity warrant special attention (see Systems Review).

It is important for the clinician to determine whether the patient has had successive onsets of similar symptoms in the past, because recurrent injury tends to have a detrimental effect on the potential for recovery. If the patient has had a recurrent injury, the clinician should note how often, and how easily, the injury has recurred and the success or failure of previous interventions.

The clinician must determine whether there are musculoskeletal symptoms elsewhere. It is well established that the head, neck, upper thoracic regions, and upper extremities can be sites of referred pain. Thoracic interscapular pain, at a point level with T4–5, is a very common complaint, especially in women.[2] This pain is thought to be posture related.

CLINICAL PEARL

Referred symptoms that are cervical in origin can occur in the upper extremities, thoracic spine, scapula, and, occasionally, the upper chest. Pain may be referred to the tip of the acromion or scapular region via the cutaneous branches of the upper thoracic posterior (dorsal) rami.[109] The rib articulations of cervicothoracic region may produce local pain, or refer pain to the suprascapular fossa or shoulder.[110]

Neck pain accompanied by widespread musculoskeletal pain raises the strong possibility of fibromyalgia, whereas neck pain with synovitis of peripheral joints suggests an inflammatory arthropathy, such as rheumatoid arthritis.[111] Myofascial pain syndromes are characterized by generalized aching and the presence of trigger points (see Chap. 10). The basic pathologic impairment in myofascial pain has yet to be substantiated.[112,113] Pain that is constant in nature and unrelated to rest or activity may be inflammatory in origin, in which case physical therapy and, specifically, manual therapy may be inappropriate.[114]

A report of diffuse nonspecific neck pain that is exacerbated by neck movements is suggestive of mechanical neck pain, cervical facet syndrome,[115] or a cervical strain/sprain.[116] Conditions that have a mechanical origin usually are improved with rest, although they may worsen initially on retiring.[117] Pain caused by sustained positions and postures, such as the upper crossed postural syndrome,[84] may awaken the patient at night but usually is relieved with a change of position.

CLINICAL PEARL

An insidious onset of symptoms could suggest postural (e.g., TOS), degenerative, or myofascial origins; or a disease process, such as ankylosing spondylitis, cervical spondylosis, or facet syndrome. An insidious onset may also indicate the presence of a serious pathology such as a tumor.

Systems Review

General health questions provide information about the status of the cardiopulmonary system, the presence or absence of systemic disease, and medications the patient may be taking that might affect the examination or intervention. Warning signs in the cervical region include

- unexplained weight loss;
- evidence of compromise to two or three spinal nerve roots;
- gradual increase in pain;
- expansion of pain in terms of the regions involved;
- spasm with passive range of motion of the neck;
- visual disturbances;
- painful and weak resistive testing;

- hoarseness;
- limited scapular elevation;
- Horner's syndrome;
- T1 palsy (weakness and atrophy of the intrinsic muscles of the hand);
- arm pain in a patient who is younger than 35 years or in a patient for more than 6 months;
- side bending away from the painful side that causes pain (if this is the only motion that causes pain).

It must also be remembered that all cervical patients, especially the ones with a history of a hyperextension mechanism, are at potential risk of serious head and neck injuries, including vertebrobasilar injury (Chap. 24) and cervical myelopathy. Cervical myelopathy (Table 25-6), involving an injury to the spinal cord itself, is associated with multisegmental paresthesias and upper motor neuron (UMN) signs and symptoms such as spasticity, hyperreflexia, visual and balance disturbances, ataxia, and sudden changes in bowel and bladder function. Early indicators of this condition include reports of symptoms in multiple extremities and clumsiness when performing fine motor skills. Myelopathy may occur with compression of the spinal cord and is more likely to occur at the C5–6 level, because in this region the spinal cord is at its widest and the spinal canal, at its narrowest.[118] Usually, narrowing of the spinal canal occurs during the end stages of degenerative disease, although structural anomalies, such as a narrowed trefoil canal or shortened pedicles, can result in congenital stenosis.[8] Depending on the cause, the onset of myelopathy can be sudden or gradual.

TABLE 25-6 The Differential Diagnosis of Myelopathy

Compressive myelopathy
Cervical spondylosis with stenosis
Cervical disk herniation fracture
Spondylolisthesis
Tumor
▸ Vertebral column primary tumor
▸ Metastatic tumor infection
▸ Epidural abscess
▸ Discitis or osteomyelitis with epidural extension
Epidural hematoma syringomyelia
Medical myelopathy
Idiopathic acute or subacute transverse myelitis
Postinfectious and postvaccination myelitis
Multiple sclerosis
Amyotrophic lateral sclerosis
Infectious myelitis: viral, bacterial, fungal, and parasitic
Arachnoiditis
Vascular disease of the spinal cord
▸ Atherosclerosis
▸ Epidural arteriovenous malformation
Connective tissue disease
Paraneoplastic myelopathy
Metabolic and nutritional disease of the spinal cord
▸ Vitamin B_{12} deficiency
▸ Chronic liver disease
Toxins
Decompression illness (Caisson's disease)
Electrical injury
Radiation injury (postradiation therapy)
Necrotic myelopathy of unknown cause

Data from Spivak JM, et al.: *Orthopaedics: A Study Guide*. New York: McGraw-Hill, 1999:349.

The following signs and symptoms demand a cautious approach or an appropriate referral:

- recent trauma (occurring up to 6 weeks earlier);
- an acute capsular pattern;
- severe movement loss, whether capsular or noncapsular;
- strong spasm;
- paresthesia
- segmental paresis;
- segmental or multisegmental hyporeflexia or areflexia;
- UMN signs and symptoms (see Chap. 3). These can include reports of neck pain with bilateral upper extremity symptoms and occasional reports of loss of balance or lack of coordination of the lower extremities.
- Constant or continuous pain;
- moderate-to-severe radiating pain;
- moderate-to-severe headaches;
- tinnitus;
- history of loss of consciousness;
- memory loss or forgetfulness;
- difficulties with problem solving;
- reduced motivation;
- irritability;
- anxiety or depression;
- insomnia.

CLINICAL PEARL

Symptoms that respond to mechanical stimuli in a predictable manner are usually considered to have a mechanical source. Symptoms that show no predictable response to mechanical stimuli are unlikely to be mechanical in origin, and their presence should alert the clinician to the possibility of a more sinister disorder or one of central initiation, autonomic, or affective in nature.[114]

Neurologic Symptoms

The presence of neurologic symptoms, including sympathetic symptoms (e.g., blurred vision, sweating, tinnitus), deserves special attention. Many of the symptoms that occur in an upper limb have their origins in the neck. The patient with neck trauma can report seemingly bizarre symptoms, but these need to be heeded until the clinician can rule out serious pathology. Cervical radiculitis is most commonly associated with spinal nerve root irritation. Peripheral symptoms can also be caused by a host of other conditions, including TOS or an isolated peripheral nerve lesion.[119]

The systems review must include questions that will elicit any symptoms that might suggest a CNS condition or a vascular compromise to the brain. For example, lower limb symptoms associated with neck motions, difficulty walking, poor balance, or bowel or bladder dysfunction. One of the earlier indications of a balance disturbance can be elicited during the history or systems review with correct questioning. A simple question such as "Do you have difficulty with walking or with balance?" can provide the clinician with valuable information. Positive responses may indicate a cervical myelopathy or systemic neurologic impairment.[120] The neurologic examination, if appropriate, attempts to differentiate between nerve root and spinal cord compression. The presence of any UMN sign or symptom requires an immediate medical referral.

Vascular Compromise

A history of dizziness, falling, faintness, or seizures always warrants further investigation. It is not always an easy task for the clinician to determine whether the presenting dizziness is the result of a disturbed afferent input from the cervical spine, which can be extremely rewarding to treat, or has a more serious cause.[96] For example, dizziness provoked by head movements may indicate an inner ear or vertebral artery problem. A history of falling without loss of consciousness (drop attack) is strongly suggestive of vertebral artery compromise.[121] Testing of the vertebral artery (see Chap. 24) should be considered if the observation and history reveal any of the signs and symptoms that have been linked, directly or indirectly, to vertebral artery insufficiency. These include

- Wallenberg's, Horner's, and similar syndromes;
- bilateral or quadrilateral paresthesia;
- hemiparesthesia;
- ataxia;
- nystagmus;
- drop attacks;
- periodic loss of consciousness;
- lip anesthesia;
- hemifacial paresthesia or anesthesia;
- dysphasia;
- dysarthria.

Headache or Facial Pain

Does the patient have headaches and, if so, where? What is their frequency and intensity? Does a position alter the headache? If the patient reports relief of pain and referred symptoms with the placement of the hand or arm of the affected side on top of the head (Shoulder abduction/Bakody's sign), this usually is indicative of a disk lesion of the C4 or C5 level.[122]

A history of headaches may or may not be benign, depending on the frequency and severity. Differential diagnosis is important, especially in light of the fact that there is considerable overlap in symptoms among tension headaches; cervicogenic headaches (see Chap. 23); cervical, trigeminal, and glossopharyngeal neuralgia (see Chap. 5); the headache associated with Lyme disease (see Chap. 5); migraines without aura (see Chap. 5); and TMJ dysfunction (see Chap. 26).[123] Cervicogenic headaches, which can be mild, moderate, or severe, tend to be unilateral and located in the suboccipital region, with referral to the frontal, retro-orbital, and temporal areas.[69,124] The more serious causes of headache without a history of trauma include spontaneous subarachnoid hemorrhage, vertebral artery compromise, meningitis, pituitary tumor, brain tumor, and encephalitis (see Chap. 5).

Facial pain can be the consequence of temporomandibular dysfunction, temporal arteritis, acute sinusitis, orbital disease, glaucoma, trigeminal neuralgia, referred pain, and herpes zoster (see Chap. 5).

TESTS AND MEASURES

Observation

Static observation of general posture, as well as the relationship of the neck on the trunk, and the head on the neck, is carried out while the patient is standing and sitting, both in the waiting area and in the examination room (see Chap. 6). Once in the examination room, the patient is asked to assume an upright neutral postural position from a relaxed sitting position. This can help the clinician to gain an idea of which muscle strategy the patient is using to support the natural spinal curves.[78] A major contributor to cervicogenic pain is a lack of postural control resulting from poor neuromuscular function.[85,123,125,126] Sustained postures, or fatigue overloading of the deep spinal and postural muscles, can result in increased joint compressive forces and inefficient movement strategies.[112,113,127,128] A good pattern when assuming an upright neutral postural position would involve the pelvis being brought into an upright neutral position, with the formation of a low lumbar lordosis (lumbar multifidus) rather than with thoracolumbar extension (thoracopelvic extensors).[78] Postural misalignment of the head on the trunk is associated with complaints of pain in the neck and shoulder region and TMJ dysfunction, but is also observed in asymptomatic individuals.

The clinician should look for:

- Hair quality (i.e., brittle hair due to thyroid problems).
- The position of the patient's head. If it is shifted to one side, a disk protrusion may be present; if deviated, acute arthritis may be the cause. Severe or constant pain usually is manifested by the patient constantly changing his or her posture or remaining very still.
- Evidence of the patient being a mouth breather. Mouth breathing encourages forward head posture.
- Evidence of skin cancer, such as unusual looking moles.
- Torticollis.

- Sprengel's deformity, a congenital elevation and medial rotation of the scapula, which gives the patient the appearance of having no neck on one side, secondary to a high-riding scapula.
- Scars (long, transverse scars indicative of cervical surgery), lumps, rashes, thyroid enlargement (goiter), skin discoloration, or other lesions.
- Scoliosis in the thoracic spine.
- Soft tissue contours that can highlight swelling, muscle atrophy or hypertrophy.
- The position of the thoracic and cervical curves as well as the craniocervical posture.
- Scapular position in association with muscle bulk/tone of the axioscapular-girdle muscles both anteriorly and posteriorly.[78] Ideally, the resting scapulae should sit such that the superior angle lies level with the T2 or T3 spinous process, the root of the spine of the scapula level with the T3 or T4 spinous process, and the inferior angle level with the T7–9 spinous process.[129] Common "abnormal" postural positions of the scapula include a downwardly rotated and protracted scapula, which is often associated with a dominant action of the levator scapular and an increase resting length of the trapezius.[78,93,128] Conversely the scapula may appear slightly elevated, indicating an adaptively shortened upper trapezius, protective positioning, or neural tissue mechanosensitivity.[78]
- Bone deformities (i.e., endocrine disorders). Conditions include abnormal bony enlargement of the face, jaw, hands, and feet (acromegaly); a "moon-faced," buffalo hump (fatty deposits) at the neck, axial obesity, generalized atrophy of muscles, and kyphotic posture due to excess cortisol production (Cushing's syndrome) or bulging eyes due to excess thyroid hormone (Graves disease).[130]
- Autonomic skin changes (increased sweating, trophic changes, and texture changes).
- Birthmarks.
- Changes in the patient's facial expression suggesting pain with transitional movements.

SIDE VIEW

- The forehead should be vertical.
- The tip of the chin should be in line with the manubrium. If the chin is anterior to the manubrium, a forward head is present (see later discussion). The amount of forward head can be measured in two ways. The simplest method is to measure the distance between the tip of the chin and the manubrium. The more complex and expensive methods involve the use of computer-assisted digitizing systems.
- The clinician should observe the cervical lordosis. A flattened lordosis may be associated with stretched posterior cervical ligaments and extensor muscles, and adaptively shortened cervical flexors. An excessive lordosis is associated with a forward head and an adaptive shortening of the posterior ligaments and neck extensor muscles.
- The ears are inspected for signs of asymmetry, inflammation, rashes, lumps, scars, or other lesions. Discharge from within the external ear canal may indicate infection (i.e., otitis externa).[130]

POSTERIOR VIEW

- The clinician should assess muscular asymmetry, especially in the upper trapezius and SCM (see also Chap. 16).
- The spinous process of the axis should be in the midline.
- Usually the shoulder on the dominant side is slightly lower than that on the nondominant side.
- Is there any atrophy of the deltoid suggesting axillary nerve palsy?
- As the patient rotates the head to each side, the tips of the transverse processes of the atlas should be felt to rotate anteriorly and then posteriorly. Both sides are compared. The procedure is repeated for side bending. The transverse process should become less prominent and should approximate the mastoid process, on the side of the side bending.

ANTERIOR VIEW

- The clinician should assess whether the patient's head is shifted to one side. A cervical disk protrusion (C3–4 or C4–5) can produce a horizontal side shift of the head.[82] This side shift allows the patient to maintain eye level.
- A slight tilt of the head is normal but may indicate an upper cervical joint dysfunction.
- The eyes should be inspected for ptosis (droopy eyelid). The patient should be instructed to look up, while the clinician gently pulls down both lower eyelids to inspect the conjunctiva (for signs of anemia—bluish appearance and conjunctivitis—redness) and sclera (for jaundice—yellowish appearance).[130] The eyes should also be observed for other signs of discoloration, discharge, and any deformity of the iris. The clinician should also note any evidence of nystagmus (see Chap. 3), which may be positional and fatigable and which may be caused by a lesion anywhere from the eyes to the midbrain.[131] A Dix–Hallpike test (see Chap. 3) should be carried out in patients suspected of having a vestibular disorder.[131]
- Facial symmetry. The clinician visually splits the mass of the head into two vertical halves. Cerebral asymmetries in form and volume, associated with cranial asymmetries, are a common feature of the human race and are often associated with facial asymmetries.[132,133] This asymmetry is, in many cases, related to asymmetric cerebral growth, which is mostly accomplished in utero,[134,135] although it may also have a local origin, for instance, in the case of mandibular asymmetry. Facial asymmetry can also be due to facial nerve (CN VII) paralysis or partial weakness. The trigeminal nerve (CN V) may be involved if asymmetry (deviation) is observed in the mouth due to muscle weakness or atrophy on one side of the jaw.[130]

TABLE 25-7 Potential Consequences of the Forward Head

Deficit	Impairment	Effect
Cervical hyperlordosis	Overclosing of TMJ	Trigeminal facilitation
	Posterior compression	Suboccipital hypertonicity
	Capsular ligament injury	Scalene hypertonicity with first rib impairment
	Meniscal derangement	
	Craniovertebral hyperextension	Trigeminal facilitation
	O-A flexion hypomobility	Masticator hypertonicity
	A-A rotation hypomobility	TMJ impairment
	O-A extension hypermobility	
	Craniovertebral instability	
	Midcervical hyperextension	C4 facilitation
	Flexion hypomobility	Levator scapulae hypertonicity with adduction of scapula and overuse of supraspinatus
	Extension hypermobility	
	Anterior instabilities	C5 facilitation
		Rotator cuff hypertonicity
		Tennis elbow
Shoulder protraction	Glenohumeral instability	Supraspinatus tendonitis
	Acromioclavicular instability	Infraspinatus tendonitis
		Acromioclavicular sprain
Cervicothoracic hyperkyphosis	Extension hypomobilities	Shoulder girdle hypomobility
		Glenohumeral instability
		Acromioclavicular instability
		Supraspinatus tendonitis

A-A, atlantoaxial; O-A, occipitoatlantal; TMJ, temporomandibular joint.
Data from Troyanovich SJ, Harrison DE, Harrison DD: Structural rehabilitation of the spine and posture: Rationale for treatment beyond the resolution of symptoms. *J Manipulative Phys Ther* 21:37–50, 1998; Mannheimer JS: Prevention and restoration of abnormal upper quarter posture. In: Gelb H, Gelb M, eds. *Postural Considerations in the Diagnosis and Treatment of Cranio-Cervical-Mandibular and Related Chronic Pain Disorders.* St. Louis, MO: Ishiyaku EuroAmerica, 1991:93–161; Meadows JTS: *Manual Therapy: Biomechanical Assessment and Treatment, Advanced Technique.* Calgary: Swodeam Consulting, Inc., 1995.

Forward Head

The cervical and upper thoracic regions are highly prone to postural and degenerative dysfunctions. Poor posture and dysfunctional movement patterns may alter the normal segmental motion of the neighboring regions (Table 25-7). A forwardly inclined head increases the stresses at the cervicothoracic junction and increases the craniovertebral lordosis, producing compensatory occipitoatlantal extension.

In the forward head posture, the upper trapezius can be maintained in a constant state of contraction[33] (Table 25-7). This constant state of contraction can also occur as a result of a protective mechanism for the cervical joints, ligaments, or IVD.[136]

This hypertonicity of the upper trapezius produces a paravertebral area that is broader and more prominent than normal. Tightness or adaptive shortening of the levator scapulae results in the contour of the neckline appearing as a double line (wave) where the muscle inserts into the scapula.[84] This is described as Gothic shoulders, because it is reminiscent of the form of a Gothic church tower.

Movement patterns performed on a poor postural base contribute to repetitive microtrauma of cervical structures. These structures include the zygapophyseal facets, IVD, ligaments, joint capsules, and muscles, all of which are capable of propagating the cycle of pain and dysfunction.[137,138]

Active Range of Motion

The clinical examination of the mobility of the cervical spine should consist of a comparison between active and passive ranges and coupled movements of the cervical spine. Knowledge of cervical anatomy and kinematics should assist the clinician in determining the structure responsible, based on the pattern of movement restriction noted in the physical examination (Table 25-8). The range of motion assessment of the craniovertebral region is described in Chapter 23.

The range of motion available at the cervical spine is the result of such factors as the motion available at each segment, the shape and orientation of the zygapophyseal joint surfaces, the inherent flexibility of the restraining ligaments and joint capsules, the height and pliability of the IVD, and the range available in the craniovertebral and

TABLE 25-8 Movement Restriction and Possible Causes

Movement Restriction	Possible Causes
Extension and right side bending	Right extension hypomobility Left flexor muscle tightness Anterior capsular adhesions Right subluxation Right small disk protrusion
Flexion and right side bending	Left flexion hypomobility Left extensor muscle tightness Left posterior capsular adhesions Left subluxation
Extension and right side bending restriction greater than extension and left side bending	Left capsular pattern (arthritis and arthrosis)
Flexion and right side bending restriction equal to extension and left side flexion	Left arthrofibrosis (very hard capsular end-feel)
Side bending in neutral, flexion, and extension	Uncovertebral hypomobility or anomaly

upper thoracic joints. A movement restriction is a loss of movement in a specific direction, and one in which a movement toward or away from the restriction may alter the degree and location of those symptoms. When cervical range of motion (CROM) is painful or restricted, muscle pathology is suggested if the restricted motion exists in the direction opposite to the action of the involved muscles. The clinician can apply resistance to the indicated muscle group(s) to verify this hypothesis.

CLINICAL PEARL

A motion that is restricted but painless, or normal but painful, could indicate a hypomobility. Pain that is produced by the motion that is restricted indicates an acute or subacute injury, whereas pain that is produced by the motion that is not restricted, or excessive, could indicate a hypermobility.

Because of the close relationship of the shoulder to the cervical spine, active elevation of each upper extremity should be assessed to rule out symptom reproduction from the shoulder movements. If there is a loss of one of the cervical motions, the restricted motion should be examined more closely by separating the motion into its various components. For example, full cervical rotation requires motion at the craniovertebral joints, particularly the atlantoaxial joint, as well as segmental rotation at each of the cervical segments.

CLINICAL PEARL

Radiographic evaluation has long been considered the "gold standard" for studying CROM.[139–143] However, this method is invasive and is generally not feasible or practical. However, in situations in which an accurate and reliable cervical ROM evaluation is needed, radiographic evaluation is the method of choice because of its greater sensitivity.[143]

The major movements that are assessed clinically are rotations out of neutral position VIDEO flexion–extension, and side bending (Fig. 25-12A–D). The most painful movements are performed last so that no residual pain is carried over from the previous movement. The dual inclinometer method recommended in the American Medical Association's *Guides to the Evaluation of Permanent Impairment*[144] is often considered the clinical standard for assessing cervical ROM in the clinic.[145,146] This method requires accurate identification of anatomic landmarks (Table 25-9). Both inter- and intra-rater reliability studies have shown the inclinometry method to be reliable.[147–150] Others dispute this conclusion and contend that the inclinometer method is flawed and should not be used in clinical settings.[151,152] Using the inclinometer technique, the normal active ranges of motion for the cervical spine are as follows:

- forward flexion: 45–50 degrees;
- extension: 85 degrees;
- side bending: 40 degrees;
- rotation: 70–90 degrees.

The CROM instrument, introduced on the market by Performance Attainment Associates (Roseville, MN), measures the cervical range of motion for flexion, extension, side bending, and rotation using separate inclinometers. These inclinometers are attached to a frame similar to that for eyeglasses: one in the sagittal plane for flexion–extension, a second in the frontal plane for side bending, and a third in the horizontal plane for rotation.[141] Two of these inclinometers have a gravity-dependent needle (in the sagittal and frontal planes), and the other has a magnetic needle (in the horizontal plane).[141] A magnetic neck brace is worn by the patient. Several researchers have studied the instrument to investigate its intrarater and interrater reliability. Youdas and colleagues[151] reported and intraclass correlation coefficient (ICC) varying from 0.73 to 0.95 and an interrater reliability of 0.73 to 0.92 for six cervical movements assessed in 20 patients with orthopaedic disorders.[141] Capuano-Pucci and colleagues[147] obtain similar results with 20 healthy subjects.[141] In a study by Tousignant and colleagues,[141] which attempted to estimate the criterion validity of the CROM goniometer using a healthy population found the device to be valid for measurements of cervical flexion and extension. In a more recent study, which compared range of motion measurements using a CROM goniometer and an optoelectronic system (OPTOTRAK), Tousignant et al.[142] reported that the CROM device showed excellent criterion validity for measurements of cervical rotation. Wainner et al.[153] used an inclinometer and a goniometer in 50 patients with suspected cervical radiculopathy or carpal tunnel syndrome. The results of this study are summarized in Table 25-10.

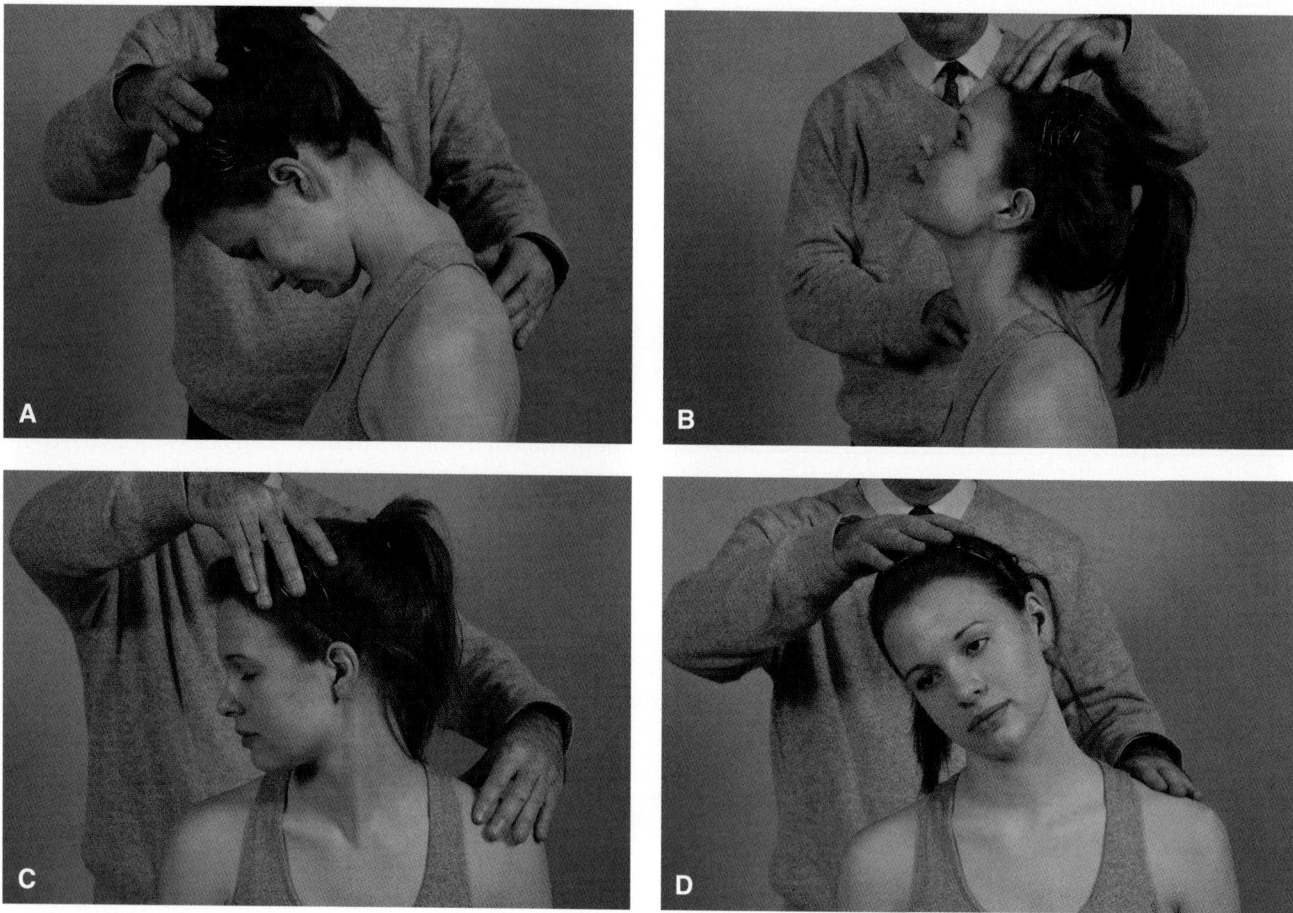

FIGURE 25-12 Cervical active range of motion with passive overpressure and resistance. **A** flexion. **B** extension. **C** rotation. **D** side bending.

Whichever method is chosen, it is important remember that, as with other joints in the body, the range of motion in the cervical spine may vary according to a number of factors including the structural ones already mentioned. The available range of motion may be reduced based on the individual's age, neck girth and length, body habitus, diurnal changes,[154] neurologic disease, or other factors unrelated to the disability for which the exam is being performed. Without taking body size into account, measurements may underestimate or overestimate range of motion.[155] The decrease due to age is probably because of the development of degenerative changes, the only exception being the rotation available at C1-2, which may increase.[156] Gender influences on cervical mobility are somewhat more controversial. Dvorak and colleagues[156] reported women having greater cervical range of motion compared with men, whereas other studies have shown men have greater available flexion,[157,158] women have a greater range in cervical extension only,[146] or that that gender is not a variable in cervical range of motion.[159]

Biomechanical studies have shown that during flexion of the cervical spine, the segments below the second vertebra are blocked.[12] Therefore, rotation out of maximum flexion of the cervical spine occurs in the atlantoaxial joint. However, rotation out of maximum extension occurs predominantly in the middle and lower cervical spine but includes the atlantoaxial joint, as well.[160]

Each of the active motions is tested with a gentle overpressure applied at the end of range if the active range appears to be full and pain free. With the exception of rotation, the weight of the head usually provides sufficient overpressure. It is necessary to apply overpressure even in the presence of pain, in order to achieve an end-feel. If the application of overpressure produces pain, the presence of an acute muscle spasm is possible. Caution must be taken when using overpressure in the direction of rotation, especially if the rotation is combined with ipsilateral side bending and extension, because this can compromise the vertebral artery.[161] Given the variability in CROM in the literature even with "normal" patients, recording absolute ranges of motion are perhaps not as important in the presence of pain and dysfunction as the assessment of:

- ***Quality and quantity of the motion.*** Quantity and quality of movement refers to the ability to achieve end range with curve reversal and without deviation from the intended movement plane.[162]
- ***Symptoms provoked.*** According to McKenzie, the use of repeated movements to provoke symptoms helps to differentiate between the postural, dysfunction, and derangement syndromes (see Chap. 22). For example, pain of postural origin does not occur with repeated movements and does not limit movement in any direction but is felt only when the patient is stationary or when static loading has been prolonged. In contrast, the pain experienced in the dysfunction syndrome is felt immediately when movement reaches the end of the limited range but stops immediately when the end range position is released. In addition, the pain

TABLE 25-9	The American Medical Association Inclinometer Technique for Measuring Cervical ROM
Range	**Method**
Flexion	Two inclinometers are used, which are aligned in the sagittal plane. The center of the first inclinometer is placed over the T1 spinous process. The center of the second one is placed on top of the head, parallel to a line drawn from the corner of the eye to the ear, where the temple of eyeglasses would sit. The patient is asked to flex the neck, and both inclinometer angles are recorded. The cervical flexion angle is calculated by subtracting the T1 from the calvarium inclinometer angle.
Extension	Two inclinometers can be used, which are aligned as for measuring cervical flexion. The patient is asked to extend the neck, and both inclinometer angles are recorded. The cervical extension angle is calculated by subtracting the T1 from the calvarium inclinometer angle.
Rotation	The patient is positioned supine. One inclinometer is used, and it is aligned in the transverse plane. The base of the inclinometer is placed over the forehead. The patient is asked to rotate the neck, and the inclinometer angle is recorded. The test is repeated on the other side.
Side bending	Two inclinometers are used, which are aligned in the coronal plane. The center of the first inclinometer is placed over the T1 spinous process. The center of the second one is placed on top of the head, over the calvarium. The patient is asked to side bend the neck, and both inclinometer angles are recorded. The cervical side-bending angle is calculated by subtracting the T1 from the calvarium inclinometer angle.

ROM, range of motion.
Data from American Medical Association: *Guides to the Evaluation of Permanent Impairment*, 5th ed. Chicago, IL: American Medical Association, 2001.

felt by the patient with a dysfunction syndrome is always intermittent and is the same each day, provided that their activity levels are consistent. In the derangement syndromes, the symptoms can be produced or abolished, increased or decreased, or centralized or peripheralized in response to repeated movements or sustained positions.

- ***Willingness of the patient to move.***
- ***Presence of specific patterns of restriction.*** According to Cyriax,[163] the capsular pattern of the cervical spine is full flexion in the presence of limited extension, and symmetric limitation of rotation and side bending.

When interpreting the motion findings, the position of the joint at the beginning of the test should be correlated with the subsequent mobility noted, because alterations in joint mobility may merely reflect an altered starting position.

TABLE 25-10	Reliability of Cervical ROM Testing Using a Goniometer and Inclinometer	
Motion	**Instrumentation**	**Interexaminer Reliability ICC (95% CI)**
Flexion	Inclinometer	0.79 (0.65, 0.88)
Extension	Inclinometer	0.84 (0.70, 0.95)
Left rotation	Goniometer	0.75 (0.59, 0.85)
Right rotation	Goniometer	0.63 (0.22, 0.82)
Left side bending	Inclinometer	0.63 (0.40, 0.78)
Right side bending	Inclinometer	0.68 (0.62, 0.87)

ROM, range of motion.
Data from Wainner RS, Fritz JM, Irrgang JJ, et al.: Reliability and diagnostic accuracy of the clinical examination and patient self-report measures for cervical radiculopathy. *Spine* 28:52–62, 2003; Cleland J: Cervical Spine, *Orthopaedic Clinical Examination: An Evidence-Based Approach for Physical Therapists.* Carlstadt, NJ: Icon Learning Systems, LLC, 2005:92–140.

Flexion

An assessment of gross range of motion of cervical flexion is performed (Fig. 25-12A), and the clinician makes note of any motion that reproduces or enhances the symptoms and the location of the symptoms. Considerable emphasis should be placed on the amount and quality of flexion available, and the symptoms it provokes, because flexion is the only motion normally tolerated well by the cervical spine. If the patient has poor concentric control of the deep neck flexors, the SCM will initiate the flexion movement, which will result in the jaw leading the movement instead of the nose (the SCM initially protrudes the chin before flexion occurs). The extreme of cervical flexion is normally found when the chin is able to reach the chest with the mouth closed, although a gap of up to two finger widths is also considered normal.

If end-range flexion is immediately painful, meningitis or acute radicular pain should be ruled out. If the pain is felt after a 15–20-second delay, ligament pain should be suspected. The most common restrictions to cervical flexion are an upper thoracic or cervicothoracic restriction or an occipitoatlantal joint restriction. If, during flexion, the patient pivots the head and neck over a hypomobile and fixed cervicothoracic region, excessive motion will be noted at the levels of C4–6.

Flexion may also be limited by acute or severe trauma (muscle spasms straighten the lordosis), fracture dislocations, or IVD dysfunction.

Extension

The patient is asked to extend the neck (Fig. 25-12B). Normal extension motion allows the face to be parallel with the ceiling. The deep cervical flexors with their extensive longitudinal intersegmental attachments from the upper thoracic spine to the skull are best suited to control extension.[78] If the patient has poor eccentric control of the deep neck flexors, two characteristic patterns of movement are evident[78]:

- There is minimal, if any, movement of the head posteriorly during extension.
- At some point during the extension, the head appears to drop or translate backward.

The return from a fully extended position to a neutral upright position requires a coordinated concentric contraction of the cranial cervical flexors.

Cervical flexion or cervical extension can provoke dizziness. This finding is thought to result from an osteophytic compression on the posterolateral aspect of the transverse foramen by the inferior articulating surface of the zygapophyseal joint.[164] Cervical distraction can be applied at the point of symptom provocation. If this maneuver increases the symptoms, manual or mechanical traction should not be part of the intervention plan.

Rotation

With rotation, the chin should be in line with the acromioclavicular joint at the end of rotation (see Fig. 25-12C).

Limitation of or pain on cervical rotation usually suggests pathology at the C1–2 (atlantoaxial) segment, because most rotation occurs at this joint.[111] However, if a patient is able to achieve 40–50 degrees of cervical rotation while maintaining eye level, atlantoaxial involvement is unlikely. If, on the other hand, the neck has to side bend early in the active rotation range in order to achieve full motion, the atlantoaxial joint is likely to be involved. If full rotation is limited and cannot be achieved even with the substitution of neck side bending, the problem is likely with the mid-to-low cervical spine segments.

Two screening tests can be used to highlight the level of a rotation restriction. Both of the tests utilize rotation of the neck, with the neck in various amounts of flexion.

1. Rotation with the neck in full side bending is reported to test the C1–2 level.
2. Rotation with the neck in a chin tuck tests the C2–3 level.

Side Bending

Side bending is performed to the left and right, while the ipsilateral and contralateral shoulder are monitored for movement by the clinician as stabilization of the ipsilateral shoulder merely tests the length of the upper trapezius, Fig. 25-12D.) The range of side bending is always greater in the supine than in the sitting position. Active side bending is typically the first motion to demonstrate problems of the cervical spine.[165] Restricted cervical side bending could be the result of joint restriction, muscle tightness, or lack of pain-free movement or extensibility of the neural tissues.[68]

Finally, if in the history, the patient has reported that repetitive movements or sustained postures have caused problems, these should be reproduced in an attempt to provoke the symptoms.

PASSIVE RANGE OF MOTION

In those situations where the patient does not have full active range of motion and even in those situations when overpressure has been applied at the end of active range of motion to determine the end-feel, passive range of motion must be assessed. This is best performed with the patient in supine to relax the muscles. Due to this muscle relaxation, passive range of motion in supine is greater than in sitting, particularly with side bending (approximately 45 degrees in sitting but 75 to 80 degrees in supine), so an assessment of the end-feel in sitting can often be misleading. With each of the cervical motions, the end-feel should be a solid tissue stretch. As with the active motions, the most painful movements are performed last. Further assessment of passive movements can include position testing, and passive physiological intervertebral motion testing (see Differing Philosophies).

Combined Motion Testing

Because normal cervical function involves complex and combined motions, and because symptoms may only occur with these combined motions, combined motion testing may need to be assessed. Combined motion testing typically occurs when the testing of single plane motions (flexion, extension, side bending, and rotation) and end-feels were found to be normal and pain-free.

Using a biomechanical model, a restriction of cervical extension, side bending, and rotation (Fig. 25-13) to the same side as the pain is termed a *closing* restriction. This restriction is the most common pattern producing distal symptoms. However, a limitation in cervical flexion accompanied by the production of distal symptoms can also occur.[165] Side bending toward or away from the side of the pain can also reproduce upper extremity symptoms, depending on the cause. Pain caused by intervertebral foraminal narrowing may be increased with ipsilateral side bending. Pain caused by an IVD protrusion may be increased with contralateral side bending.

A restriction of the opposite motions (cervical flexion, side bending, and rotation to the opposite side of the pain) is termed an *opening* restriction. Opening restrictions are slightly more difficult to identify in the cervical spine because, frequently, there is no actual restriction of cervical flexion, but rather a restriction of rotation and side bending, along with reproduction of pain on the contralateral side.[165]

McKenzie[117] advocates using neck retraction and protrusion, with other motions and positions being superimposed. Neck protrusion produces an extension of the upper cervical

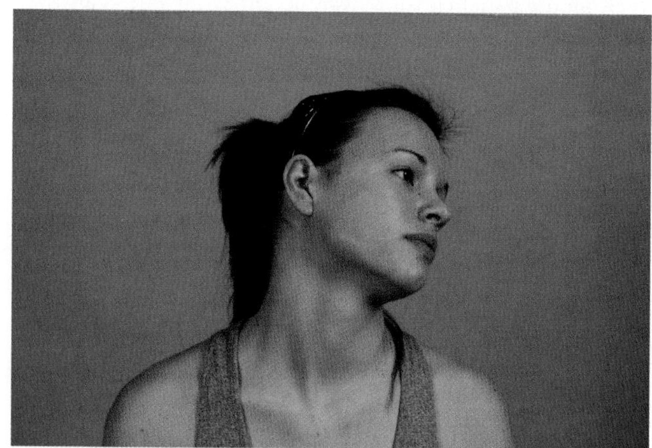

FIGURE 25-13 Cervical extension, side bending and rotation.

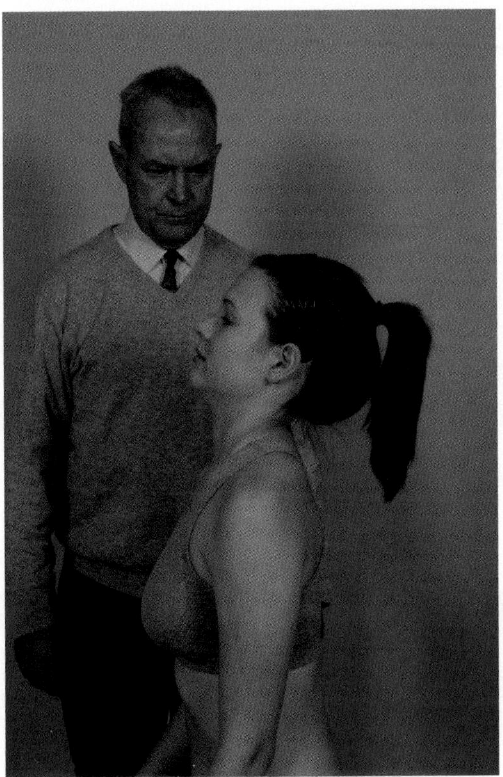

FIGURE 25-14 Neck retraction in extension.

spine and flexion of the mid and lower cervical spine, whereas neck retraction produces a flexion of the upper cervical spine and an extension of the mid and lower cervical spine. Neck retraction is performed with extension (Fig. 25-14), side bending (Fig. 25-15), and rotation to both sides in sitting

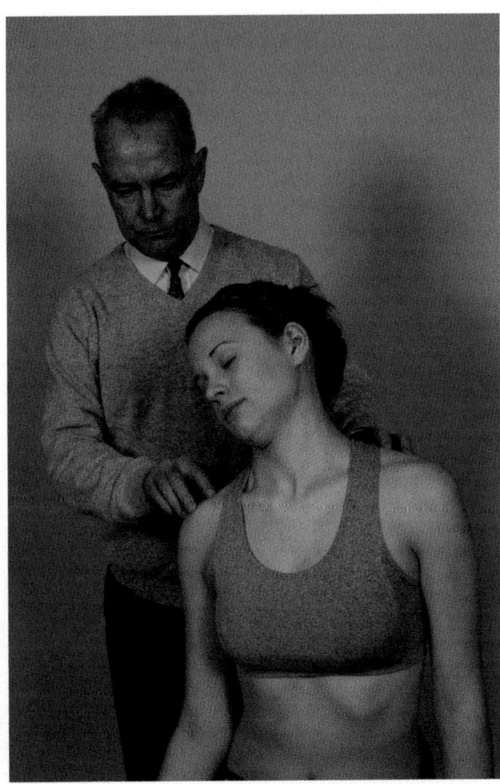

FIGURE 25-15 Neck retraction in side bending.

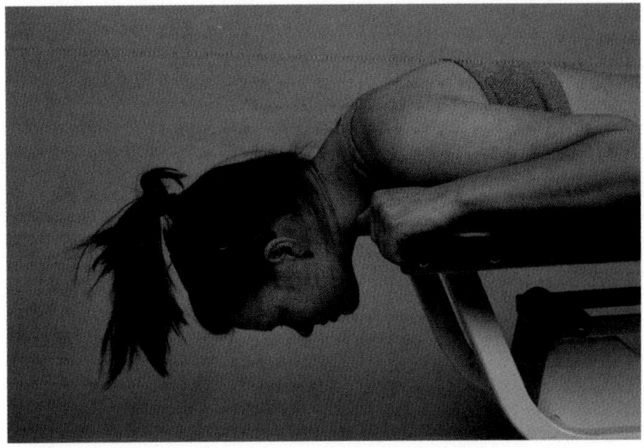

FIGURE 25-16 Neck retraction in prone—start position.

position and then prone, with the head off the end of the table (Figs. 25-16 and 25-17). The results from these motions are combined with the findings from the history and the single-plane motions to categorize the symptomatic responses into one of three syndromes: postural, dysfunction, or derangement. This information can guide the clinician as to which motions to use in the intervention.

Key Muscle Testing

The purpose of resisted testing is outlined in Chapters 3 and 4. There are numerous smaller muscles throughout this area, so resistance needs to be applied gradually. The same movements that were done actively are tested isometrically. Some of these muscles are also tested as part of the Cyriax upper quarter scanning examination (see Chap. 4) and are used as a peripheral joint scanning examination to determine muscle power and possible neurological weakness. Ideally, the clinician should place the joint in its resting position before testing each muscle and the contraction should be held for at least 5 seconds.

Resisted Cervical Flexion

Resisted cervical flexion tests the key muscle of C1–2, and cranial nerve XI (spinal accessory).

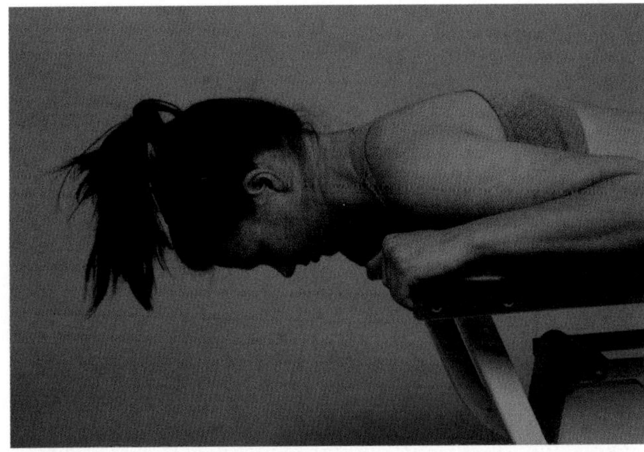

FIGURE 25-17 Neck retraction in prone—terminal position.

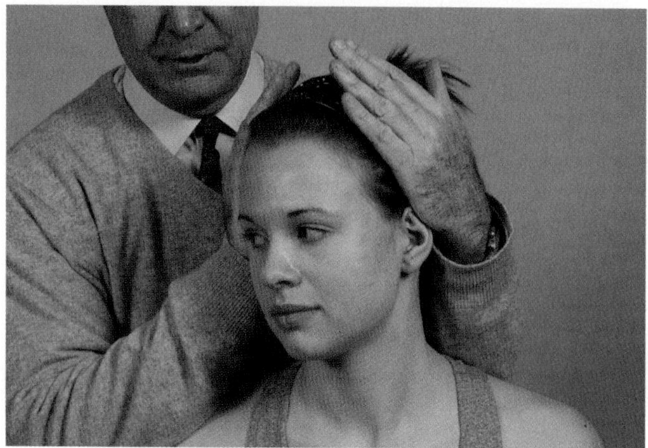

FIGURE 25-18 Resisted cervical rotation.

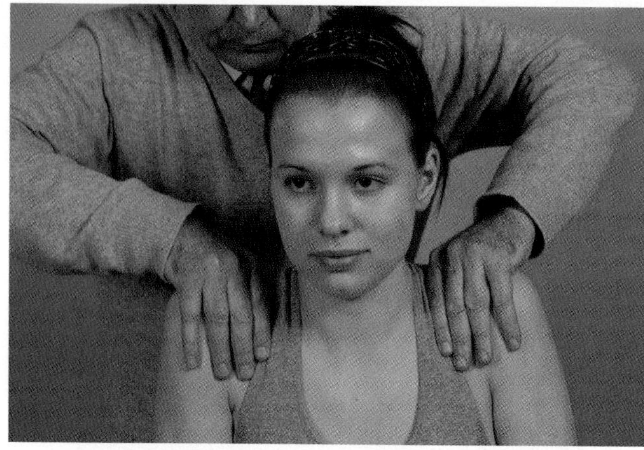

FIGURE 25-20 Resisted shoulder elevation.

Resisted Cervical Rotation

Resisted cervical rotation (Fig. 25-18) tests the key muscle of C2.

Resisted Cervical Side Bending

Resisted side bending tests the key muscle of C3, and cranial nerve XI (Fig. 25-19).

Scapular Elevators (C4 and cranial nerve XI)

The clinician asks the patient to elevate the shoulders about one-half of full elevation. The clinician applies a downward force on both shoulders, while the patient resists (Fig. 25-20).

Diaphragm (C4)

Using a tape measure, the clinician measures the amount of rib expansion that occurs with a deep breath (Fig. 25-21). A comparison is made to a similar measurement at rest. Four measurement positions are used:

1. fourth lateral intercostal space;
2. axilla;
3. nipple line;
4. tenth rib.

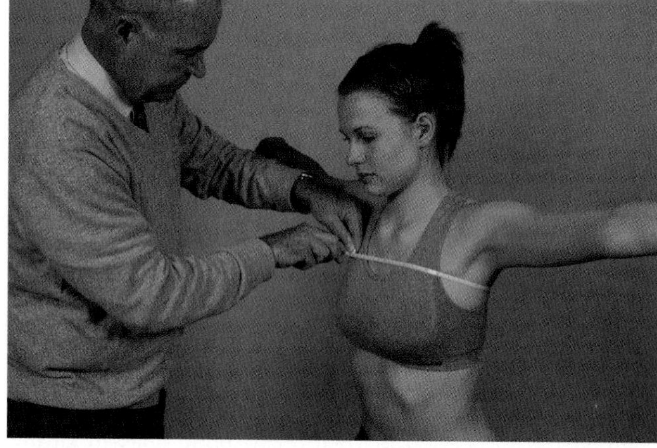

FIGURE 25-21 Chest expansion measurement.

Shoulder Abduction (C5)

The clinician asks the patient to abduct the arms to about 80–90 degrees, with the forearms in neutral. The clinician applies a downward force on the humerus, while the patient resists (Fig. 25-22).

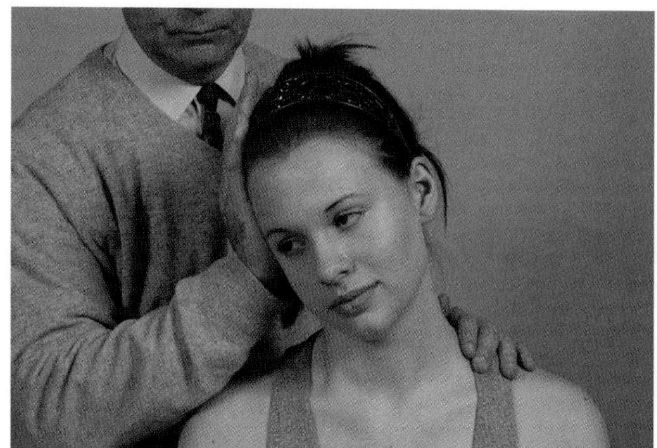

FIGURE 25-19 Resisted cervical side bending.

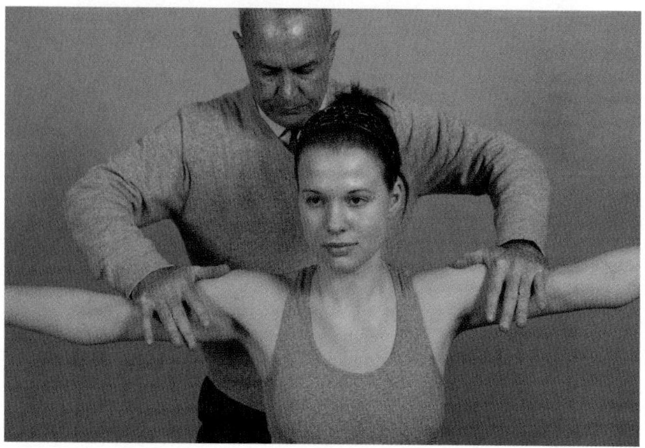

FIGURE 25-22 Resisted shoulder abduction.

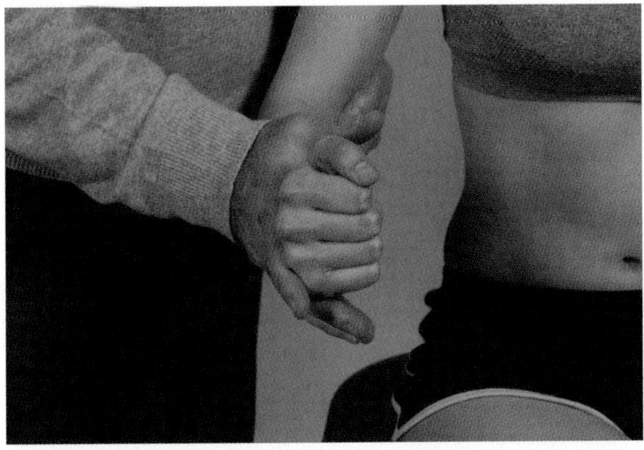

FIGURE 25-23 Resisted shoulder external rotation.

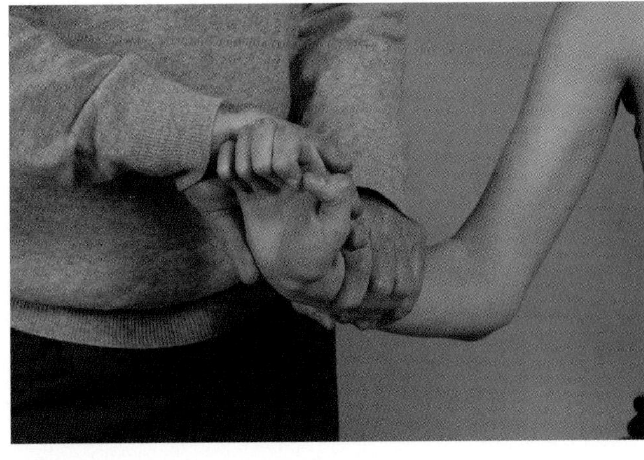

FIGURE 25-25 Resisted wrist extension.

Shoulder External Rotation (C5)

The clinician asks the patient to put the arms by the sides, with the elbows flexed to 90 degrees and the forearms in neutral. The clinician applies an inward force to the forearms (Fig. 25-23).

Elbow Flexion (C6)

The clinician asks the patient to position the arms, with the elbows flexed to 90 degrees and the forearms supinated. The clinician applies a downward force to the forearms (Fig. 25-24).

Wrist Extension (C6)

The clinician asks the patient to place the arms by the sides, with the elbows flexed to 90 degrees and the forearms, wrists, and fingers in neutral. The clinician applies a downward force to the back of the patient's hands (Fig. 25-25).

Shoulder Internal Rotation (C6)

The clinician asks the patient to put the arms by the sides, with the elbows flexed to 90 degrees and the forearms in neutral. The clinician applies an outward force to the forearms (Fig. 25-26).

Elbow Extension (C7)

The patient is seated with the arm above the head and the elbow flexed. The clinician stands beside the patient and tests

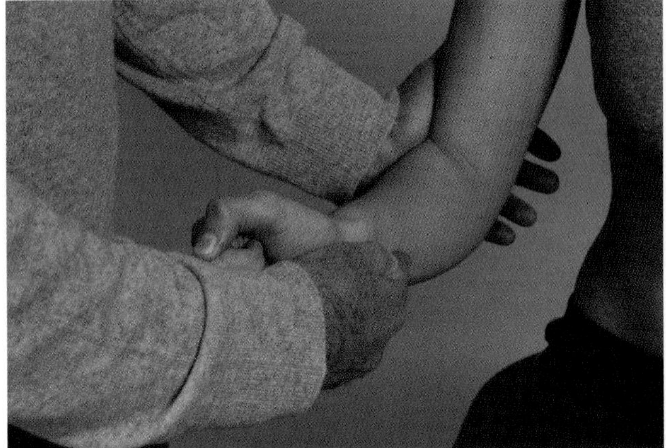

FIGURE 25-26 Resisted shoulder internal rotation.

the triceps by grasping the patient's forearm and attempting to flex the elbow (Fig. 25-27).

Wrist Flexion (C7)

The clinician asks the patient to place the arms out in front, with the elbows flexed slightly and the forearms, wrists, and fingers in neutral. The clinician applies an upward force to the palm of the patient's hands (Fig. 25-28).

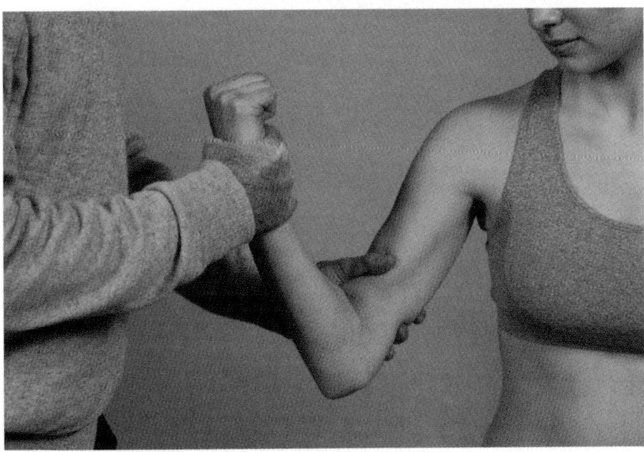

FIGURE 25-24 Resisted elbow flexion.

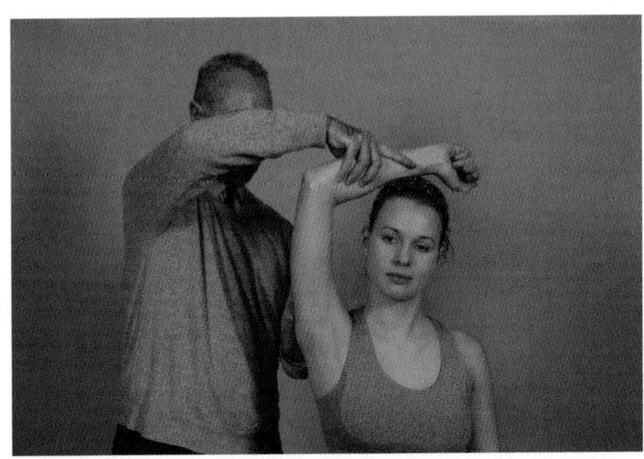

FIGURE 25-27 Resisted elbow extension.

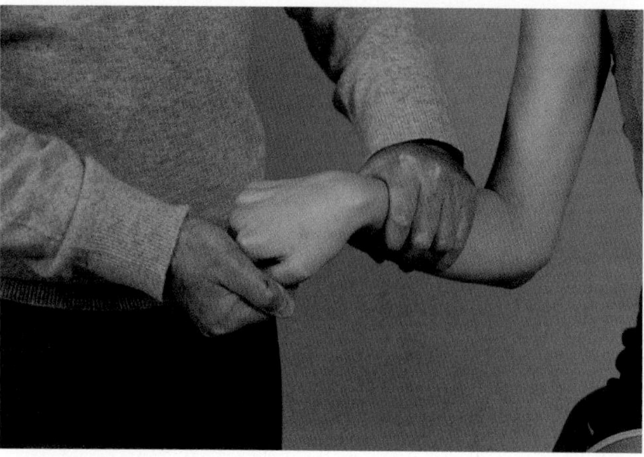

FIGURE 25-28 Resisted wrist flexion.

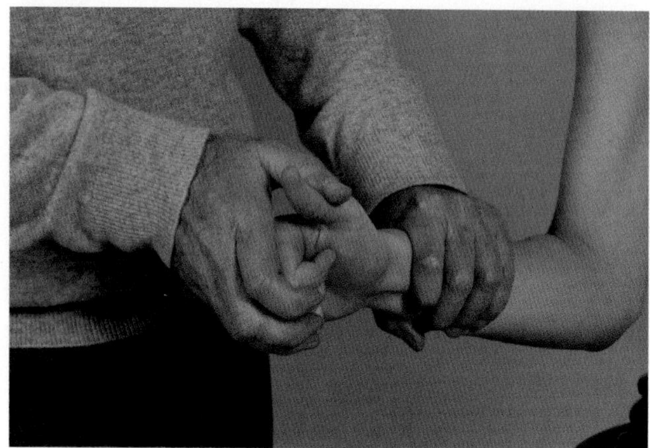

FIGURE 25-29 Resisted thumb extension.

Thumb Extension (C8)

The patient extends the thumb just short of full range of motion. The clinician stabilizes the patient's wrist with one hand and applies an isometric force into thumb flexion with the other (Fig. 25-29).

Hand Intrinsics (T1)

The patient is asked to squeeze the clinician's fingers between their fingers, while the clinician tries to pull their fingers away (Fig. 25-30).

Based on the findings from the history, systems review, and key muscle testing, a sensory examination may be necessary (see Chap. 3).

Strength Testing of the Deep Segmental and Postural Support Muscles

Deep Neck Flexors

The patient is positioned in supine, with the knees bent and the feet flat on the bed. The patient's head and neck are positioned in the desired midrange neutral position of the craniocervical region—where the line of the forehead and chin is in a horizontal plane and an imaginary line extending from the tragus and bisecting the neck longitudinally is parallel to the bed. If the patient does not adopt this position automatically, padding may be used. Once the correct position is obtained, an inflatable pressure sensor (Stabilizer, Chattanooga, South Pacific) is folded in three and positioned suboccipitally behind the neck (Fig. 25-31), such that it abuts the occiput. The bladder is inflated until the pressure is stabilized on the baseline of 20 mm Hg, a volume sufficient to just fill the space between the bed and the patient's neck, without exerting any pressure on the neck. The patient is instructed to gently nod the head slowly in an arc-like motion as if saying "yes," while

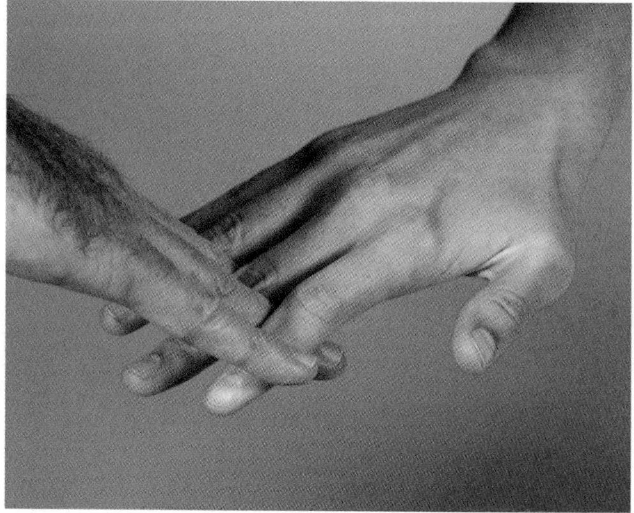

FIGURE 25-30 Strength test for finger adductors (hand intrinsics).

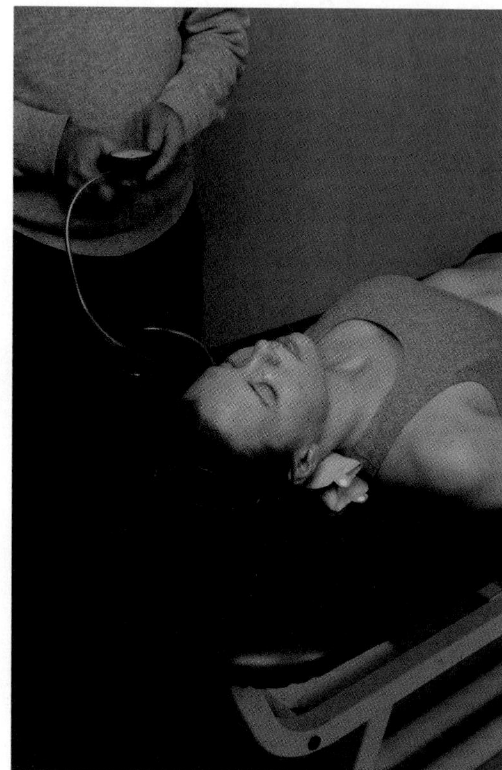

FIGURE 25-31 Muscle function testing of deep neck flexors.

TABLE 25-11	Common Faults in Performance of the Craniocervical Flexion Test and Suggestions for Correction
Common Faults	**Correction**
The patient performs a neck retraction movement rather than the rotation action of craniocervical flexion	Teach the patient to initiate the movement with their eyes. Look down with the eyes and follow with a slow and controlled chin nod. Look up to the ceiling with the eyes only and follow with the chin to resume the neutral position. Emphasize the sliding of the occiput on the bed to achieve the pure craniocervical flexion. The clinician may guide the movement with fingers placed on either side of the patient's head.
The pressure change is achieved using excessive superficial muscle activity	Palpate the sternocleidomastoid and scalene muscles during the test, to give the patient an awareness of the superficial muscle contraction. Limit the range of craniocervical flexion to the point just short of palpating the dominant superficial muscle activity. Teach the patient self-palpation and an awareness of the correct action. EMG biofeedback may also be beneficial, while the patient practices a slow and controlled craniocervical flexion.
The patient rests in a position of flexion, with associated tension in the scalene muscles	Re-educate the awareness of the neutral position by focusing the eyes on the ceiling above the head, lifting the chin, and palpating the relaxation in the scalenes. Relaxation training may be required in cases of anxiety. Diaphragmatic breathing training can help to relax the respiratory accessory muscles.
There is evident jaw clenching and use of the jaw muscles	Instruct the patient in the relaxed position of the mandible—the anterior one-third of the tongue on the roof of the mouth, lips together, teeth apart.
The patient is holding their breath	Instruct in relaxed nasal breathing while performing the exercise
The patient performs the action quickly and often overshoots the target pressure	Reteach the craniocervical flexion action and emphasize that the movement should be slow and controlled.

Data from Jull GA, Falla D, Treleaven J, et al.: A therapeutic exercise approach or cervical disorders. In: Boyling JD, Jull GA, eds. *Grieve's Modern Manual Therapy: The Vertebral Column*. Philadelphia, PA: Churchill Livingstone, 2004:451–470.

the clinician notes both the quality and the quantity of motion. Ideally, there should be a pattern of progressively increasing craniocervical flexion (Table 25-11). With weak deep neck flexors in the presence of a strong SCM, the jaw juts forward at the beginning of the movement, producing hyperextension of

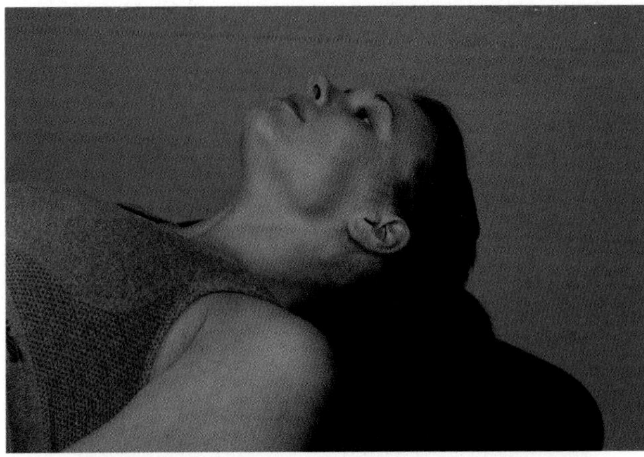

FIGURE 25-32 Patient demonstrating weak neck flexors in the presence of a strong SCM.

the craniovertebral junction[85] (Fig. 25-32). Confirmation is made by applying a very slight amount of resistance (2–4 g) against the patient's forehead.

Holding Capacity of Deep Segmental and Postural Support Muscles[68]

This test is designed to assess the ability of a muscle group to sustain a low-load isometric contraction and to replicate its function.

Deep Neck Flexors

The deep flexors of the craniovertebral and cervical regions are assessed by testing the patient's ability to sustain a precise inner range upper cervical flexion action.[68]

The patient is positioned in supine, with the head being supported on a folded towel, the knees flexed, and the feet flat on the bed. The inflatable pressure sensor is again positioned suboccipitally behind the neck (Fig. 25-31), and the bladder is inflated to 22 mm Hg to just fill the space between the bed and the patient's neck, without exerting any pressure on the neck.

The patient is asked to bring the chin toward the sternum in a gentle and slow manner. Ideally, the patient should attempt to target five incremental pressure targets (in increments of 2 mm Hg) from the baseline level of 22 mm Hg.[68]

Lower Scapular Stabilizers

The mid and lower trapezius, and serratus anterior muscles, can be assessed with the patient positioned in prone, the arm slightly abducted, and the arms placed by the side of the patient. The patient is asked to sustain the scapula against the chest wall in a position of retraction and depression (Fig. 25-33), while the clinician palpates over the muscles.[68] The end-range position is sustained for 10 seconds, and the test is repeated 10 times.

Retraining the postural support muscles initially involves postural education, an emphasis on the relaxation of unwanted muscle activity, and repeated repetitions of 10-second holds of the corrected scapula position.

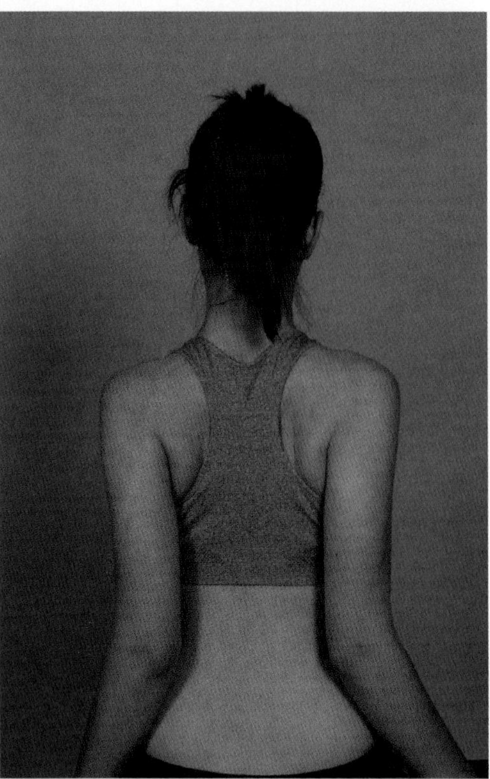

FIGURE 25-33 Testing the holding capacity of the lower scapular stabilizers (clinician not shown).

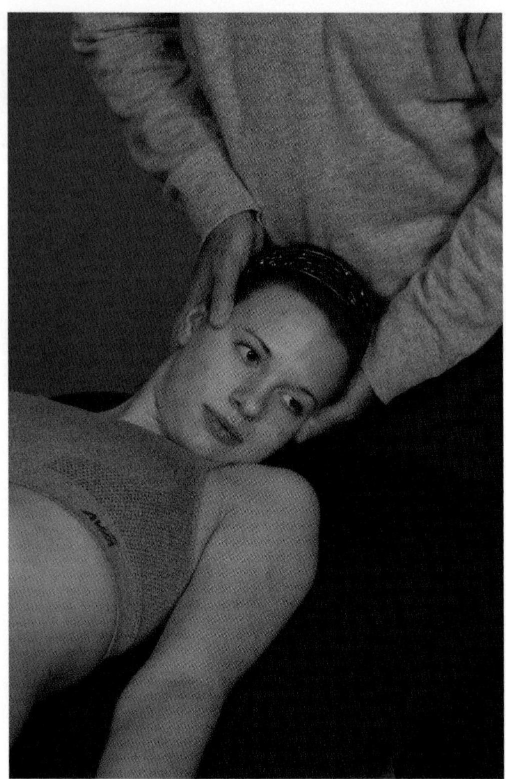

FIGURE 25-34 Cervical flexion, contralateral side flexion and ipsilateral rotation. The amount of available rotation is minimal.

Muscle Length Testing

Upper Trapezius

The upper trapezius has a tendency to become adaptively shortened and overactive, which can have the effect of pulling the head laterally, as well as increasing the craniovertebral and cervical lordosis.[166]

The patient is positioned in supine. The patient's head is maximally flexed, inclined to the contralateral side (Fig. 25-34), and ipsilaterally rotated. While stabilizing the head, the clinician depresses the shoulder distally. A normal finding is free movement of about 45 degrees of rotation, with a soft motion barrier. Tightness of this muscle results in a restriction in the range of motion and a hard barrier.

Levator Scapulae

A quick test to determine the extensibility of the levator involves positioning the patient sitting.[165] The patient is asked to place one hand above the head. For example, the right hand if the length of the right levator is to be tested, the patient's neck and head are positioned in left side flexion, and the patient is asked to abduct the left arm as far as possible. Normal extensibility of the levator and the rhomboids, and the absence of shoulder girdle pathology, should allow the patient to fully abduct the arm, while the head is side bent away (Fig. 25-35). The test is repeated on the other side for comparison.

The more specific test involves positioning the patient in supine. The clinician maximally flexes the patient's head, induces contralateral rotation, and inclines the head toward

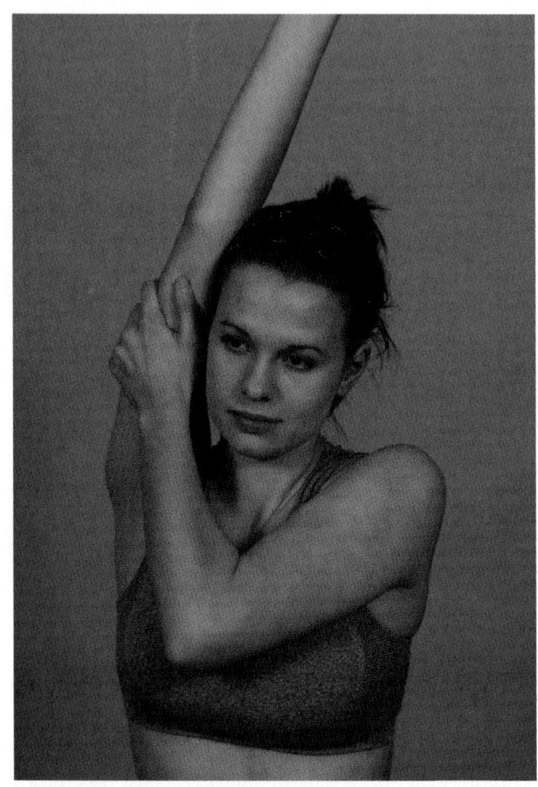

FIGURE 25-35 Muscle length test of levator scapulae.

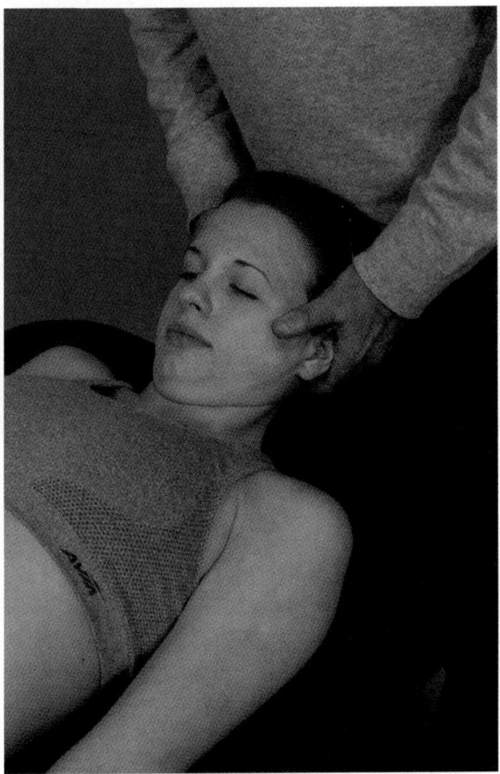

FIGURE 25-36 More specific test to assess the muscle length of the levator scapulae.

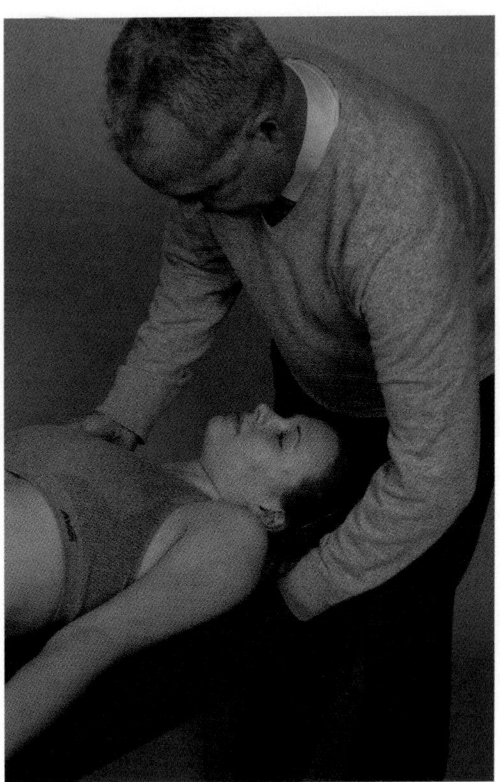

FIGURE 25-37 Muscle length test of the right sternocleidomastoid.

the contralateral side (Fig. 25-36). The clinician then depresses the patient's shoulder distally. If tightness is present, there will be tenderness at the levator insertion and a restriction of movement to less than 45 degrees.

Sternocleidomastoid

The SCM muscle has a tendency to become adaptively shortened and overactive, which can have the effect of altering the relationships between the head, neck, and shoulders and producing restrictions at the craniovertebral and cervicothoracic junctions.[166]

The patient is positioned in supine, with the head being supported. From this position, the clinician induces side bending of the neck to the contralateral side and extension of the neck (Fig. 25-37). The clinician stabilizes the scapula and rotates the patient's head and neck toward the ipsilateral side.

Scalenes

The patient is positioned in supine, with the clinician at the head of the bed. The clinician side flexes and extends the head to the contralateral side, while stabilizing the shoulder (Fig. 25-38). The normal range of motion should be 45 degrees.

Neurologic Examination

The neurologic examination is performed to assess the normal conduction of the central and peripheral nervous systems and to help rule out such conditions as brachial neuritis and TOS. The tests for the TOS are described under "Special Tests" section later. Depending on the results from the history, a cranial nerve examination may be warranted (see Chap. 3).

Sensory (Afferent System)

The clinician instructs the patient to say "yes" each time he or she feels something touching the skin. The clinician notes any hypoesthesia or hyperesthesia within the spinal and peripheral

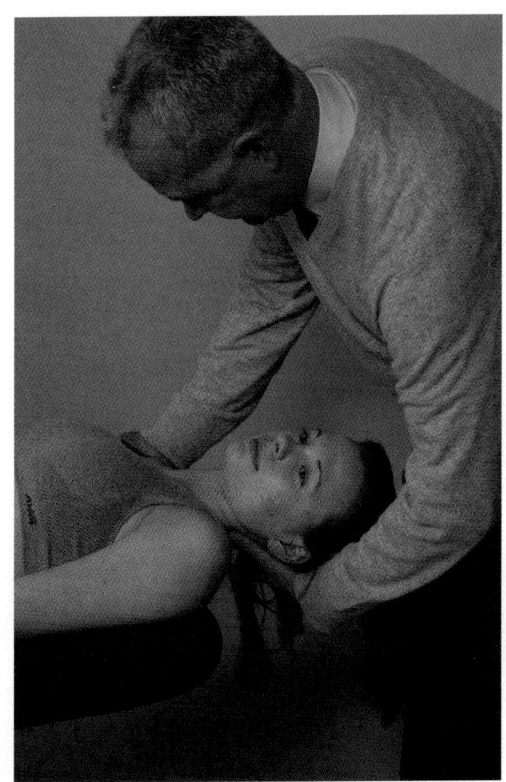

FIGURE 25-38 Muscle length test of scalenes.

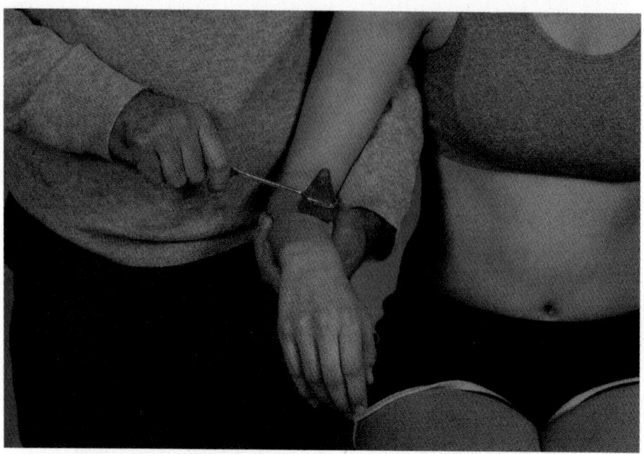

FIGURE 25-39 Brachioradialis reflex.

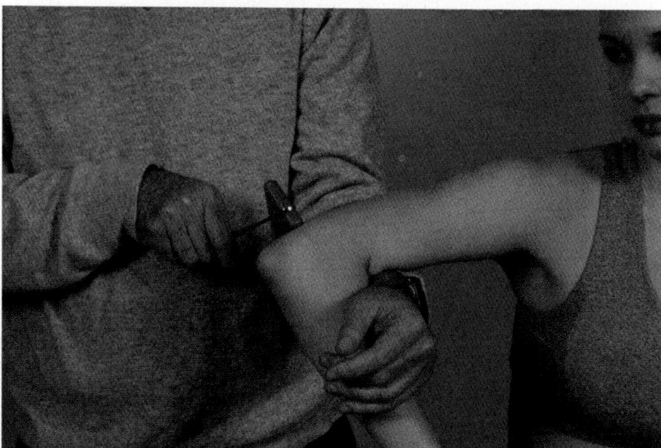

FIGURE 25-41 Triceps reflex.

nerve distributions. Light touch of hair follicles is used throughout the whole dermatome, followed by pinprick in the area of hypoesthesia. Remember that there is normally no C1 dermatome!

Muscle Stretch Reflexes

The following muscle stretch reflexes should be checked for differences between the two sides:

- C5–6: brachioradialis (Fig. 25-39)
- C6: biceps (Fig. 25-40)
- C7: triceps (Fig. 25-41)

Pathological Reflexes

The following reflexes are tested:

- Hoffmann's sign (Fig. 3-36)
- Babinski (Fig. 3-29)
- Lower limb deep tendon reflexes (Achilles and patellar) for hyperreflexia

Palpation

The results from palpation rely on the patient's subjective report; thus, changes in the patient's attention and pain tolerance affect reliability. It is important to place the patient in a position where the neck muscles can relax. Usually, this involves the patient lying supine with their head supported by a pillow and the clinician positioned at the patient's head.

In the neck, the major lymph nodes are located along the anterior and posterior aspects of the neck, which is divided by the SCM muscle.[131] Usually, the closer the lymph node is to the spinal cord, the greater the size of the lymph node.[131] The neck is the exception to the rule. Other lymph nodes are also located on the underside of the jaw and suboccipital areas.[131] The number and size of lymph nodes usually decrease with aging.

The anterior neck can be palpated for the thyroid gland by gently displacing the trachea laterally and palpating each side in turn. Asking the patient to swallow during the palpation can help locate the thyroid gland, as it should be felt to slide under the fingers while it moves upward.

Using the index fingers, the clinician slides the fingers under the SCM and begins to palpate the anterior aspect of the cervical vertebral bodies (from C7 to C3) for tenderness. The posterior aspects, including the facet joints, can be palpated with the other hand. If palpation reveals some tenderness, the clinician can further stress the segment by gently applying a posteroanterior pressure.[167] This is accomplished using the hand under the neck and applying an anterior shear at each segmental level. This pressure should result in a slight increase in the cervical lordosis. If it results in an excessive anterior glide at the segment compared with the segment above or below, the test can be considered positive and a stability test of that segment should be performed.

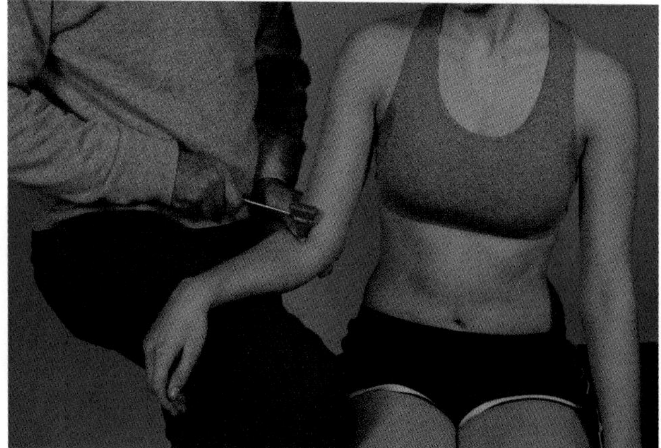

FIGURE 25-40 Biceps reflex.

CLINICAL PEARL

Sandmark and Nisell[168] reported that palpation over the facet joints was the most appropriate screening to corroborate self-reported neck dysfunction.

According to Hoppenfeld,[169] all of the spinous processes lower than C2 are usually palpable. The interval between the external occipital protuberance and the spine of C2 contains the posterior arch of vertebra C1, which is very deeply located and usually not palpable. The C2 spinous process can be palpated in the midline below the external occipital protuberance, the prominent midline elevation on the posteroinferior aspect of the occipital bone.[1] Occasionally, because of a bifid spine that is not symmetric, the spine may appear to be lateral to the midline, or two bony prominences may be felt at a single level between C3 and C6. C7 is usually the longest spinous process, being referred to as the *vertebra prominens,* although the spinous process of either C6 or T1 might be quite long, as well. The spinous process of C7 is located by either counting down to the correct level or using a motion test. The motion test involves the clinician feeling for the largest spinous process located at the base of the neck and then asking the patient to extend the neck. The C6 spinous process will be felt to move anteriorly with neck extension, whereas the spinous process of C7 does not.

CLINICAL PEARL

Palpation is a key component of the evaluation for cervical myofascial pain.[170]

The following muscles should be palpated for tenderness:

- trapezius;
- sternocleidomastoid;
- splenius;
- semispinalis;
- multifidus;
- suboccipitals (see Chap. 23).

The TMJ can be checked for clicking, limited range of motion, tenderness, or swelling by gently palpating the area immediately anterior of the tragus of each ear while the patient slowly opens and closes the mouth (see Chap. 26).[131]

Differing Philosophies

The next stage in the examination process depends on the clinician's background. Many manual techniques are used to examine the cervical spine, but the reproducibility of these techniques is questionable.[171–175] Clinicians who are heavily influenced by the muscle energy techniques of the osteopaths[176] use position testing to determine the segment on which to focus. Other clinicians omit the position tests and proceed to the combined motion and passive physiologic tests.

Position Testing

The position tests are screening tests that, like all screening tests, are valuable in focusing the attention of the clinician on one segment, but not appropriate for making a definitive statement concerning the movement status of the segment. However, when combined with the results of the active and passive movement testing, they help to form a working hypothesis.

The patient is positioned sitting, and the clinician stands behind the patient. Using the thumbs, the clinician palpates the articular pillars of the cranial vertebra of the segment to be tested (Fig. 25-42). The patient is asked to flex the neck, and the clinician assesses the position of the cranial vertebra relative to its caudal neighbor and notes which articular pillar of the cranial vertebra is the most posterior (dorsal). A posterior (dorsal) left articular pillar of the cranial vertebra relative to the caudal vertebra is indicative of a left-rotated position of the segment in flexion.[176]

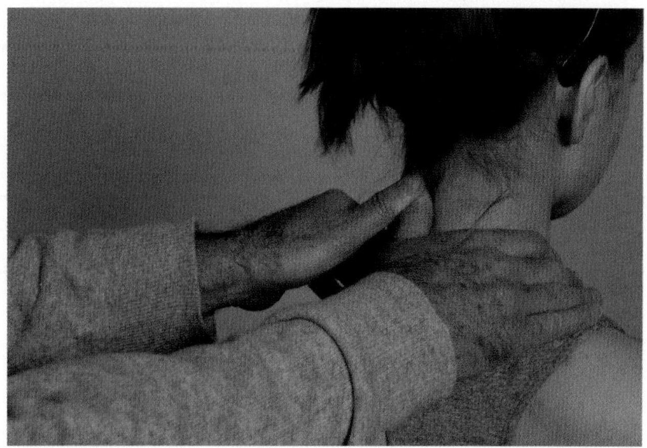

FIGURE 25-42 Palpating the articular pillar just lateral to the spinous process.

In the following example, the C4 and C5 segments are used. The patient is asked to extend the joint complex, while the clinician assesses the position of the C4 vertebra relative to C5 by noting which articular pillar is the most posterior (dorsal). A posterior (dorsal) left articular pillar of C4 relative to C5 is indicative of a left-rotated position of the C4–5 joint complex in extension.[176]

This test may also be performed with the patient supine. However, in the sitting position, one can better observe the effect of the weight of the head on the joint mechanics.

Passive Physiologic Intervertebral Mobility Testing

These screening tests examine intersegmental mobility. As with any other screening test, these tests quickly obviate the need for more exhaustive testing and focus the clinician's attention on a specific level or levels and specific movement(s). Manual examination of the cervical spine by experienced clinicians has shown good sensitivity and specificity to detect cervical zygapophyseal syndromes compared with other medical diagnostic tools, including radiographs, and are sensitive for identifying fused joint levels (Table 25-12).[98,177] However, the protocols used to assess general mobility and intersegmental mobility of the cervical spine have demonstrated difficulty achieving reasonable interexaminer agreement and reliability.[172,175]

To test the intersegmental mobility of the midcervical region, the patient is positioned in supine and the the patient's neck is placed in the neutral position of the head on the neck, and the neck on the trunk. Once in this position, lateral glides are performed, beginning at C2 and progressing inferiorly VIDEO. The lateral glides are usually tested in one direction before repeating the process on the other side. The lateral glides result in a relative side bending of the cervical spine in the direction opposite to the glide. Light pressure from the clinician's body can be applied against the top of the patient's skull to hold the head in position. This reinforces the

TABLE 25-12 Usefulness of Passive Physiological Testing in the Cervical Spine							
PPM Test Level	**Reliability (kappa)**	**Sensitivity**	**Specificity**	**LR+**	**LR−**	**DOR**	**QUADAS Score**
C2–3 block[a]	76	98	91	10.9	0.02	495.8	11
C5–6 block[a]	46	78	55	1.7	0.4	4.3	11

[a]Humphreys BK, Delahaye M, Peterson CK: An investigation into the validity of cervical spine motion palpation using subjects with congenital block vertebrae as a 'gold standard'. BMC Musculoskeletal Disorders 5:19, 2004.

stabilization caused by the weight of the patient's thorax against the table. Each spinal level is glided laterally to the left and right, while the clinician palpates for muscle guarding, range of motion, end-feel, and the provocation of symptoms VIDEO. Lateral glides are performed as far inferiorly as possible.

Following these procedures, the areas in which a restricted glide was found are targeted, and repetition of the lateral glides is performed in the flexed and then extended positions.

Flexion

The same considerations are pertinent for flexion hypomobilities. To test in flexion, the patient's head and neck are flexed without allowing a chin tuck, which would tighten the nuchal ligament (Fig. 25-43). For example, if left side bending is restricted in flexion, the right side of the segment is not flexing sufficiently (see Table 25-8). The opposite occurs if the restriction occurs with right-side bending (the left side is not flexing sufficiently).

Extension

With the patient supine, and the occiput cupped, the segment is extended by lifting the superior vertebra forward (obviating the need to extend the entire spinal region) and allowing the patient's head and neck to bend over the fulcrum, created by the clinician's fingers. While maintaining the extended position (by pushing the transverse processes of the segment anteriorly), the segment is side bent left and then right around its axis of motion and translated contralaterally (Fig. 25-44). During the translation, very slight head motion should occur. Rather, a slight tilting around each segmental axis occurs, using gentle pressure via the fingertips or the fleshy part of the second metacarpophalangeal joint. The slight side bending before the translation is to fix the axis at that segmental level. During left side bending, the left side of the segment is maximally extended, while the right side is moved toward its neutral position. The opposite occurs with right side bending.

The range of motion of the side bending and the end-feel of the translation is evaluated for normal, excessive, or reduced

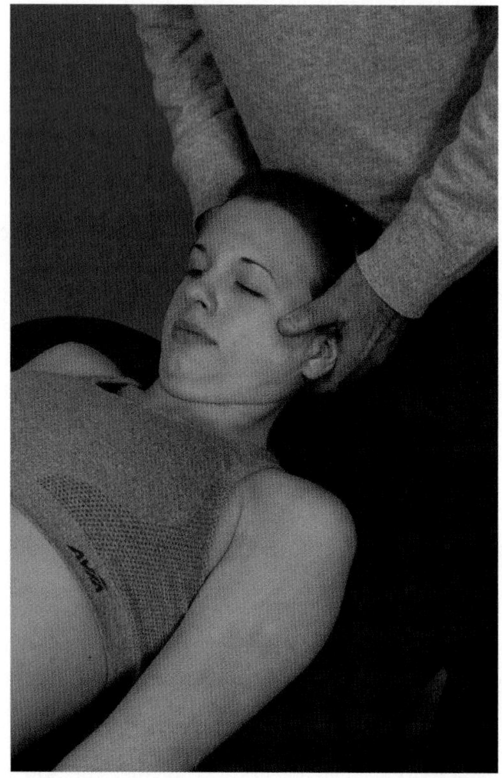

FIGURE 25-43 Translational glides of cervical spine in flexion.

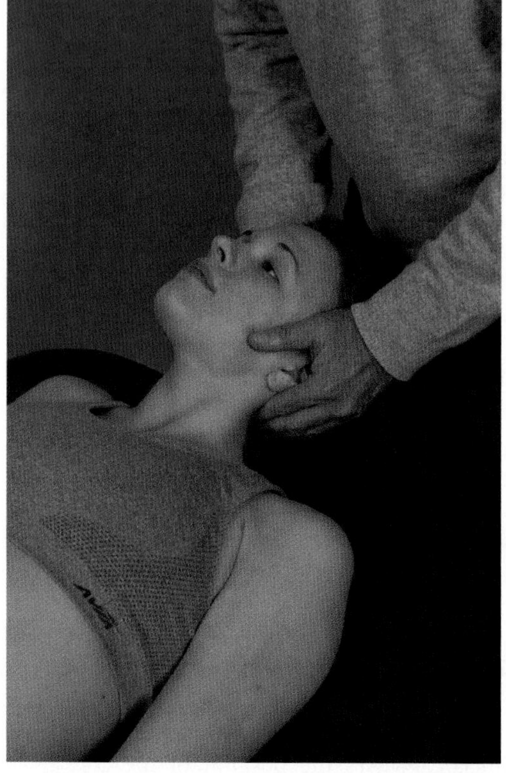

FIGURE 25-44 Translational glides of cervical spine in extension.

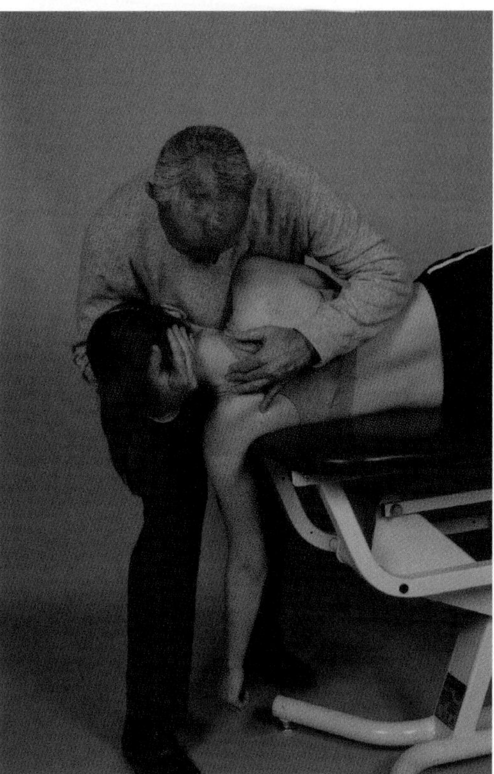

FIGURE 25-45 Segmental mobility testing of the cervicothoracic junction.

motion states. If the end-feel of the translation is normal, but the side bending is restricted, the hypomobility is extra-articular (myofascial) (see Table 25-8).

To test the intersegmental mobility of the lower cervical/upper thoracic region, the patient is positioned in side lying with their arm over the end of the table to stabilize the thorax and their head cradled by the clinician (Fig. 25-45). The patient's neck is placed in the neutral position of the head on the neck and the neck on the trunk. Once in this position, the clinician uses the index finger to monitor intersegment motion between the spinous processes, while passively moving the patient's head and neck into flexion, extension, side bending, and then rotation.

Because of the unreliability of mobility testing in extension, the information gleaned from motion testing is more likely to be more reliable in determining the side of the closing restriction.

Clinically, it would appear that the zygapophyseal joints are more involved with the rotational aspect of the coupling, functioning to prevent excessive rotation, whereas the uncovertebral joints appear to be more involved with pure side-bending motions. Although this concept may not hold up to scientific scrutiny, it tends to work well in the clinic. Thus, a glide restriction found in flexion, extension, and neutral would tend to implicate a problem with the uncovertebral joint.

While it is not necessary, or sometimes not possible, to make a diagnosis from these tests, some useful deductions can be made and these will direct the ensuing joint glide tests to the appropriate joint. Remember, that if the end-feel of the glide suggests that motion is still occurring at the end of available range, the joint is *not* the cause of restriction (think *muscle*).

Passive Physiologic Accessory Intervertebral Mobility Tests

The passive physiologic accessory intervertebral mobility (PPAIVM) tests investigate the degree of linear or accessory glide that a joint possesses and are used on segmental levels where there is a possible hypomobility, to help determine if the motion restriction is articular, periarticular, or myofascial in origin. In other words, they assess the amount of arthrokinematic motion, as well as the quality of the end-feel. The motion is assessed in relation to the patient's body type and age and the normal range for that segment, and the end-feel is assessed. A variety of techniques can be used to assess the joint glides in this region. Unless otherwise stated, the patient is positioned in supine with their head resting on the treatment table. The cervical spine is positioned in midrange in relation to flexion, extension, side bending, and rotation. The clinician is positioned at the patient's head. For each of the tests, the clinician assesses the quantity and quality of motion and makes comparisons to the contralateral side, or to the adjacent segment, as appropriate.

Distraction. Using both hands, the clinician wraps around the occiput of the patient using the web space of the hands. The clinician leans backward, and gently applies a force to the chin and occiput to distract the vertebral bodies from one another (Fig. 25-46). Most of the force should be directed to the occiput.

Segmental Translation. In the following example, a left side bending of C3–4 will be described. The patient is positioned in supine, with the clinician at the head of the bed. The clinician cradles the patient's head with both hands and places the pad of the index fingers of each hand across the neural arches of

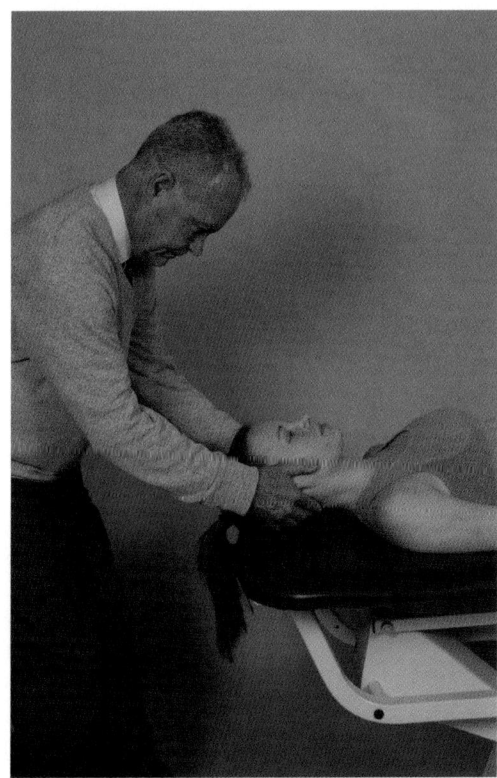

FIGURE 25-46 General distraction of cervical spine in supine.

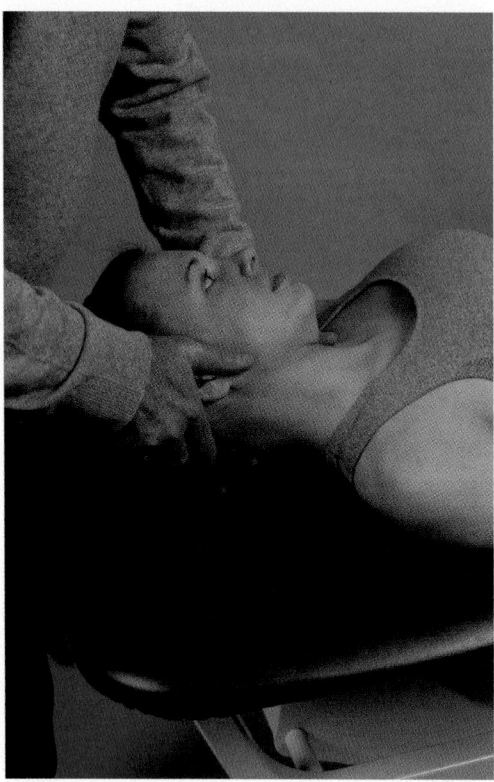

FIGURE 25-47 Left side bending/rotation with right translation at the C3–4 level.

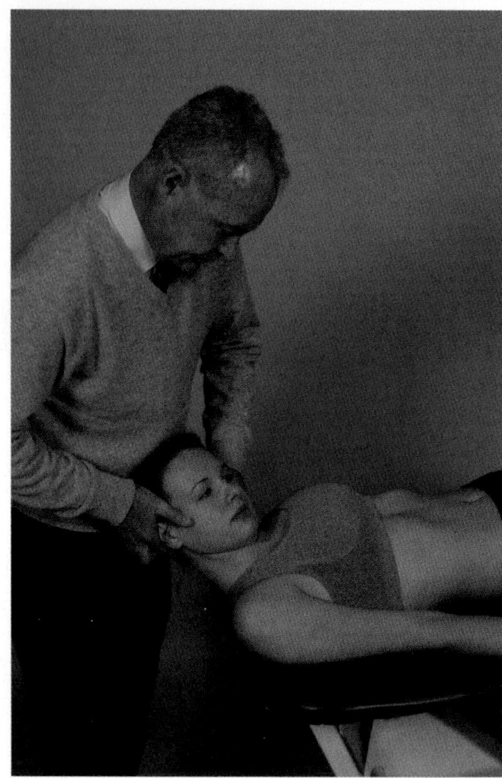

FIGURE 25-48 Rotation of superior segment in supine.

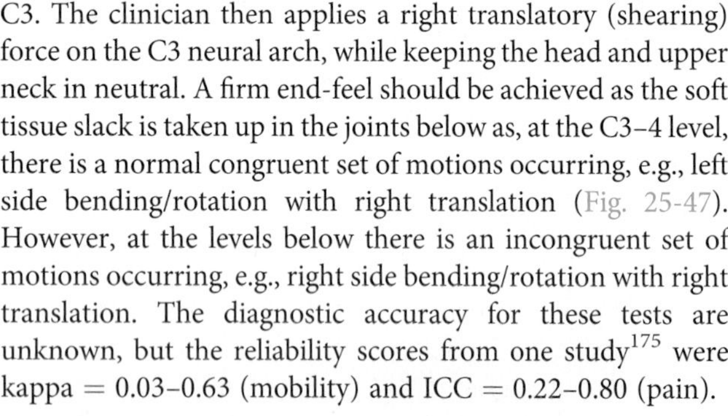

C3. The clinician then applies a right translatory (shearing) force on the C3 neural arch, while keeping the head and upper neck in neutral. A firm end-feel should be achieved as the soft tissue slack is taken up in the joints below as, at the C3–4 level, there is a normal congruent set of motions occurring, e.g., left side bending/rotation with right translation (Fig. 25-47). However, at the levels below there is an incongruent set of motions occurring, e.g., right side bending/rotation with right translation. The diagnostic accuracy for these tests are unknown, but the reliability scores from one study[175] were kappa = 0.03–0.63 (mobility) and ICC = 0.22–0.80 (pain).

Rotation. To test the motions involved with cervical rotation, the patient is positioned in supine and the cervical spine is placed in the range in relation to flexion, extension, side bending, and rotation. The clinician stands at the patient's head. Leaning forward, the clinician rests the abdomen against the top of the patient's head. Using one hand, the clinician grips the inferior segment posteriorly using the web space of the hand, and laterally with the index finger and thumb. Using a similar grip, the clinician uses the other hand to wrap around the superior segment. While stabilizing the inferior segment, the clinician glides the superior segment into rotation (Fig. 25-48).

Combined motions. Leaning forward, the clinician rests the abdomen against the top of the patient's head. Using one hand, the clinician grips the inferior segment posteriorly using the web space, and laterally with the index finger and thumb. Using a similar grip, the clinician uses the other hand to wrap around the superior segment. The patient's head is then guided into the four quadrants: flexion and rotation to the right (Fig. 25-49), flexion and rotation to the left, extension and rotation to the right, and extension and rotation to the left.

Cervical Stress Tests

Depending on the irritability of the segment, a variety of tests can be used to assess for instability. It is worthwhile to start gently with segmental palpation and gentle posteroanterior

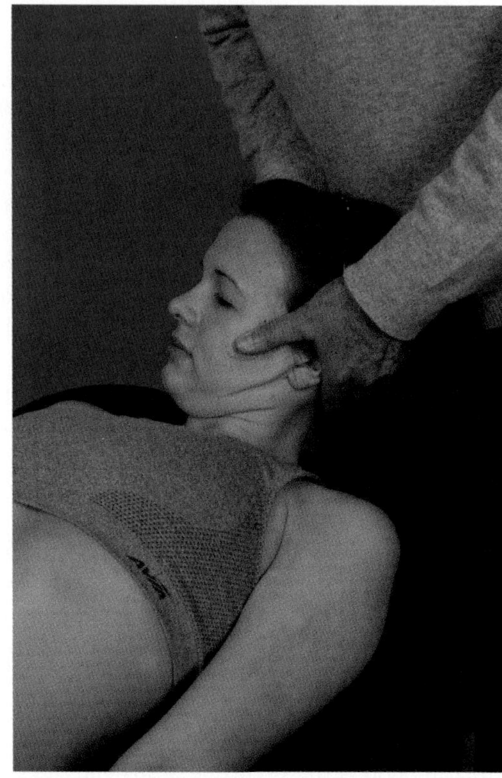

FIGURE 25-49 Flexion and rotation to the right in supine.

pressures before progressing to the other techniques. Unless indicated, the patient is positioned supine. The following tests are performed to examine segmental stability.

Posteroanterior Spring Test

The patient is positioned in prone for anterior stability testing; the clinician places his or her thumbs over the posterior aspects of the transverse processes of the inferior vertebra of the segment being tested. To ensure patient comfort during this test, the thumbs must be placed under (posterior to) the SCM, rather than over it, and must function merely to stabilize the maneuver, exerting no pushing force. The vertebra is then pushed anteriorly (Fig. 25-50), and the clinician feels for the quality and quantity of movement. A rotational component can be added to the test by applying force on only one of the transverse processes.

For posterior stability testing, the thumbs are placed on the anterior aspect of the superior vertebra, and the index fingers are on the posterior aspect (neural arch) of the inferior.[167] The inferior vertebra is then pushed anteriorly on the superior one, producing a relative posterior shear of the superior segment.

It is likely that this test is highly sensitive at implicating the dysfunctional level, but is not specific for the causative pathological process. However, the diagnostic value of this test is as yet unknown.

Transverse Shear

The transverse shear test should not be confused with the lateral glide tests previously mentioned. The lateral glide tests are used to assess joint motion, whereas the transverse shear test assesses the stability of the segment. Although motion is expected to occur in the lateral glide test, no motion should be felt to occur with the transverse shear test.[178]

The inferior segment is stabilized, and the clinician attempts to translate the superior segment transversely using the soft part of the metacarpophalangeal joint of the index finger[167] (Fig. 25-51). The end-feel should be a combination of capsular and slightly springy. The test is then reversed so that the superior segment is stabilized and the inferior segment is translated under it.

The test is repeated at each segmental level and for each side. The diagnostic value of this test is as yet unknown.

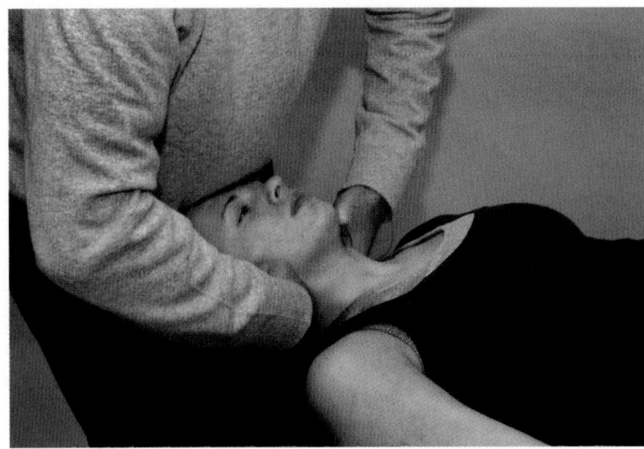

FIGURE 25-51 Transverse shear test.

Craniovertebral Ligament Stress Tests

The tests for these ligaments, which include the alar and transverse ligament, are described in Chapter 23.

Distraction and Compression

The patient is supine, and the clinician sits or stands at the patient's head. The clinician cups the patient's occiput in one hand and rests the anterior aspect of the ipsilateral shoulder on the patient's forehead. The other hand stabilizes at a level close to the base of the neck[167] (Fig. 25-46). A traction–compression–traction force is applied. This test can also be performed with the patient in sitting (Figs. 25-52 and 25-53). The clinician notes the quality and quantity of motion.

Pain reproduced with compression suggests the presence of

- disk herniation;
- vertebral end plate fracture;
- vertebral body fracture;
- acute arthritis or joint inflammation of a zygapophyseal joint;
- nerve root irritation, if radicular pain is produced.

Reproduction of pain with cervical distraction suggests the presence of

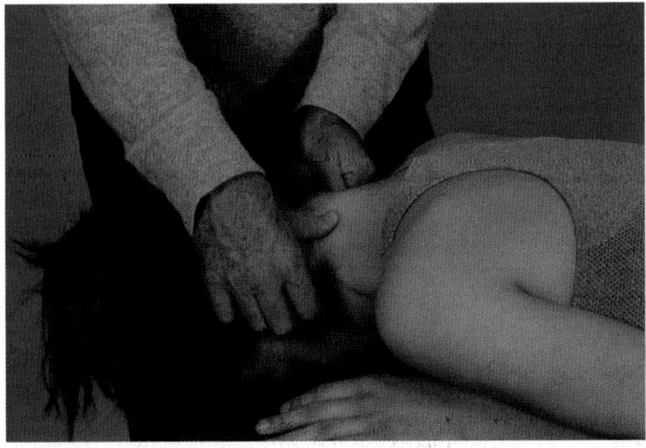

FIGURE 25-50 P-A pressures of cervical spine.

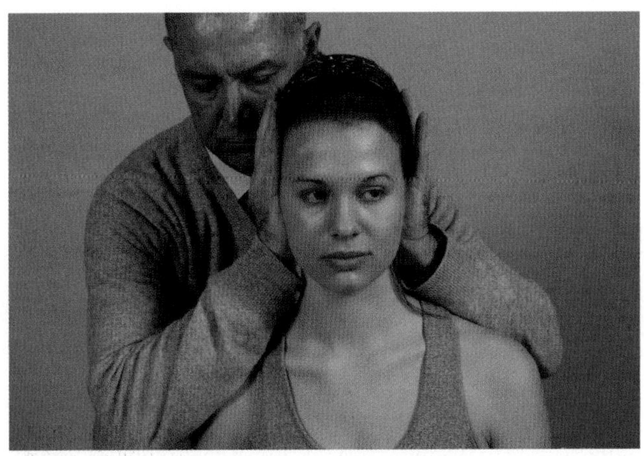

FIGURE 25-52 Cervical distraction in sitting.

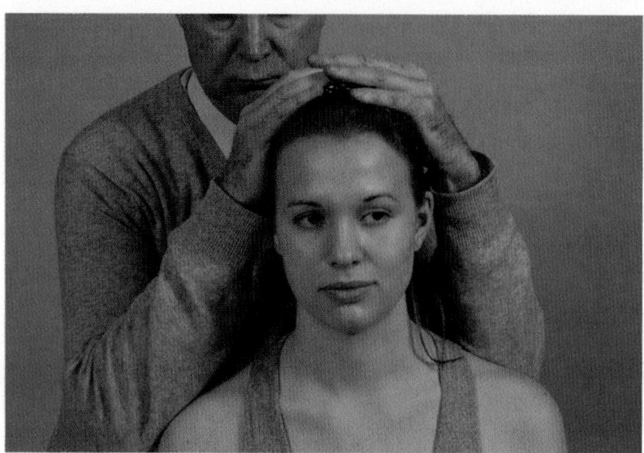

FIGURE 25-53 Cervical compression in sitting.

- spinal ligament tear;
- tear or inflammation of the AF;
- muscle spasm;
- large disk herniation;
- dural irritability (if nonradicular arm or leg pain is produced).

Functional Assessment

A number of formal ways of measuring neck function are available, and include the following:

- The neck disability index (NDI) is a patient survey instrument (see Table 5-3) that contains 10 items, seven related to activities of daily living, two related to pain, and one item related to concentration. The NDI is a revision of the Oswestry index and is designed to measure the level of reduction in activities of daily living in patients with neck pain. The NDI has been widely researched and validated,[179] and its test–retest reliability has been found to be 0.89.[179]
- The Northwick Park Neck Pain Questionnaire (Table 25-13)[180] contains nine sections that cover activities likely to affect neck pain. Each section contains five statements related to the patient's perceived level of difficulty performing the activity of the section. Scores on the questionnaire range from 0 to 100%, with 0% being associated with no disability and 100% with severe disability. The questionnaire has good short-term repeatability and internal consistency.[181]

Special Tests

In most cases, the special tests are only performed if there is some indication that they would be helpful in arriving at a diagnosis. However, in the cervical spine, in addition to the cervical stress tests, the vertebral artery should also be assessed (see Chap. 24), especially if the plan is to place the cervical spine in the extremes of extension, or extension and rotation as part of the examination or treatment.

Temporomandibular Joint Screen

Because the TMJ (see Chap. 26) can refer pain to this region, the clinician is well advised to rule out this joint as the cause for the patient's symptoms.

The patient is asked to open and close the mouth and to laterally deviate the jaw, as the clinician observes the quality and quantity of motion and notes any reproduction of symptoms.

Neurodynamic Mobility Tests

Upper limb tension testing (see Chap. 11) may serve a useful role in differentiating between the involvement of neural and nonneural structures.[8]

Lhermitte's Symptom or "Phenomenon"

This is not so much a test as it is a symptom, described as an electric shock-like sensation that radiates down the spinal column into the upper or lower limbs when flexing the neck (see Chap. 3).

Flexion Rotation Test

This test is used to determine the presence of a cervicogenic headache and is both a range of motion and provocation test. The patient is positioned in supine and resting symptoms are noted. The patient is asked to maximally flex his or her neck and to hold that position. Using both hands, the clinician applies a full rotational force to both sides and notes any changes in symptoms (Fig. 25-54). The test is considerd positive for a cervicogenic headache if a loss of 10 degrees or greater is noted when comparing both sides. Given the testing position, it is likely that C1–2 is the tested level. A single blind, age and gender matched, comparative measurement study by Hall and Robinson[182] found this test to have a sensitivity of 86% and a specificity of 100% (QUADAS score of 12).

Scalene Cramp and Relief Tests

For the scalene cramp test, the patient is positioned in sitting and is asked to turn the head toward the painful side and pull the chin down into the supraclavicular fossa (Fig. 25-55). This position causes contraction of the scalenes and should reproduce distal radiation of pain if the scalenes are involved. The scalene relief test is performed by asking the patient to actively place the forearm against the forehead on the involved side. This position increases the space between the clavicle and the scalenes and is positive for scalene dysfunction if it relieves the patient's pain. No diagnostic accuracy studies have been performed to determine the sensitivity and specificity of this test.

Spurling Test

Provocative tests for cervical radiculopathy include the foraminal compression test or Spurling test.[183] The patient is positioned in sitting. The test is performed by asking the patient to rotate the head to the uninvolved side and then the involved side (Fig. 25-56). The clinician then carefully applies a downward pressure on the head, with the head in neutral. The test is considered positive if pain radiates into the limb ipsilateral to the side at which the head is rotated.[184] Neck pain

TABLE 25-13 The Northwick Park Neck Pain Questionnaire		
Parameter	**Status**	**Points**
Neck pain intensity	I have no pain at the moment.	0
	The pain is mild at the moment.	1
	The pain is moderate at the moment.	2
	The pain is severe at the moment.	3
	The pain is the worst imaginable at the moment.	4
Neck pain and sleeping	My sleep is never disturbed by pain.	0
	My sleep is occasionally disturbed by pain.	1
	My sleep is regularly disturbed by pain.	2
	Because of pain I have less than 5 hours sleep in total.	3
	Because of pain I have less than 2 hours of sleep in total.	4
Pins and needles or numbness in the arms at night	I have no pins and needles or numbness at night.	0
	I have occasional pins and needles or numbness at night.	1
	My sleep is regularly disturbed by pins and needles or numbness.	2
	Because of pins and needles I have less than 5 hours sleep in total.	3
	Because of pins and needles or numbness I have less than 2 hours of sleep in total.	4
Duration of symptoms	My neck and arms feel normal all day.	0
	I have symptoms in my neck or arms on waking which last less than 1 hour.	1
	Symptoms are present on and off for a total period of 1–4 hours.	2
	Symptoms are present on and off for a total of more than 4 hours.	3
	Symptoms are present continuously all day.	4
Carrying	I can carry heavy objects without extra pain.	0
	I can carry heavy objects but they give me extra pain.	1
	Pain prevents me from carrying heavy objects but I can manage medium weight objects.	2
	I can lift only light-weight objects.	3
	I cannot lift anything at all.	4
Reading and watching TV	I can do this as long as I wish with no problems.	0
	I can do this as long as I wish if I'm in a suitable position.	1
	I can do this as long as I wish but it causes extra pain.	2
	Pain causes me to stop doing this sooner than I would like.	3
	Pain prevents me from doing this at all.	4
Working/housework	I can do my usual work without extra pain.	0
	I can do my usual work but it gives me extra pain.	1
	Pain prevents me from doing my usual work for more than half the usual time.	2
	Pain prevents me from doing my usual work for more than a quarter of the usual time.	3
	Pain prevents me from working at all.	4
Social activities	My social life is normal and causes me no extra pain.	0
	My social life is normal but increases the degree of pain.	1
	Pain has restricted my social life but I am still able to go out.	2
	Pain has restricted my social life to the home.	3
	I have no social life because of pain.	4
Driving[a]	I can drive whenever necessary without discomfort.	0
	I can drive whenever necessary but with discomfort	1
	Neck pain or stiffness limits my driving occasionally.	2
	Neck pain or stiffness limits my driving frequently.	3
	I cannot drive at all due to neck symptoms.	4
	TOTAL SCORE:	

Instructions: The questionnaire has been designed to give us information as to how your NECK PAIN has affected your ability to manage in everyday life. Please answer every question and mark in each section ONLY THE ONE BOX which applies to you. We realize you may consider that two of the statements in any one section relates to you but PLEASE JUST MARK THE BOX WHICH MOST CLOSELY DESCRIBES YOUR PROBLEM.

[a]The question on driving is omitted if the patient did not drive a car when in good health.

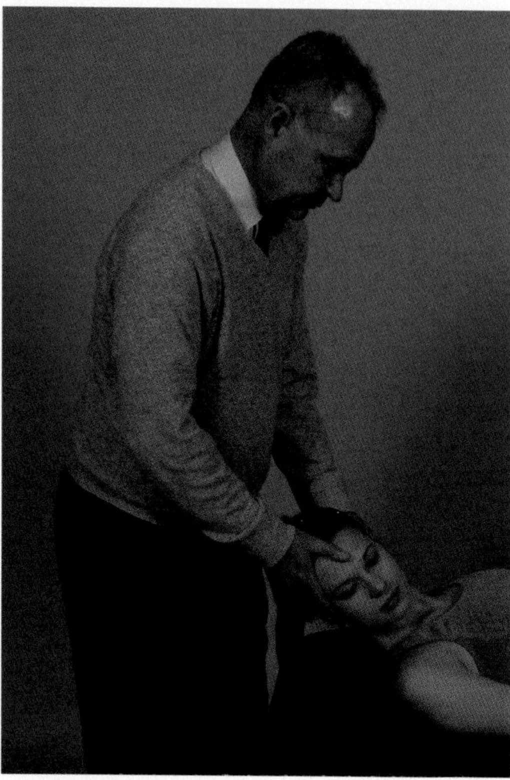

FIGURE 25-54 Flexion rotation test.

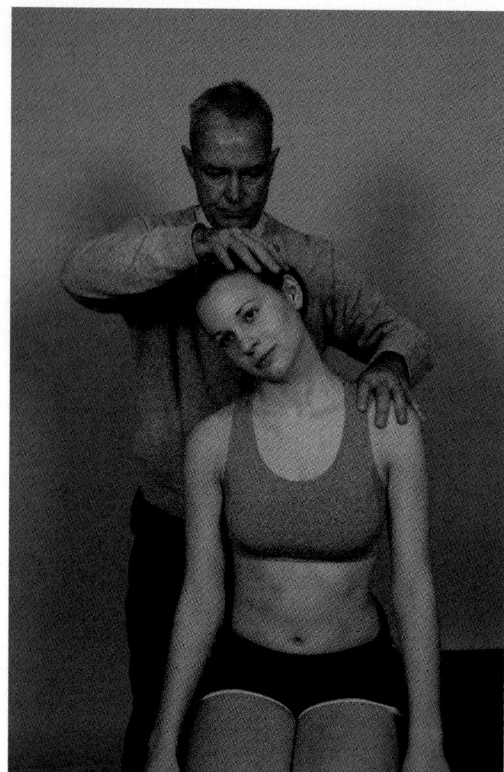

FIGURE 25-56 Spurling Test.

with no radiation into the shoulder or arm does not constitute a positive test. Conditions such as stenosis, cervical spondylosis, osteophytes, or disk herniation are implicated with a positive test. There are few methodologically sound studies that assess the interexaminer reliability, sensitivity, and specificity of this test. The literature appears to indicate high specificity and low sensitivity.[185] Therefore, the test is not useful as a screening test, but it is clinically useful in helping to confirm a cervical radiculopathy.

Modifications to this test have been advocated, which divide the test into three stages, each of which is more provocative.[120] If symptoms are reproduced, the clinician does not progress to the next stage. The first stage involves applying compression to the head in neutral. The second stage involves compression with the head in extension. The final stage involves compression with the head in extension and rotation to the uninvolved side, and then to the involved side. No diagnostic accuracy studies have been performed to determine the sensitivity and specificity of these variations.

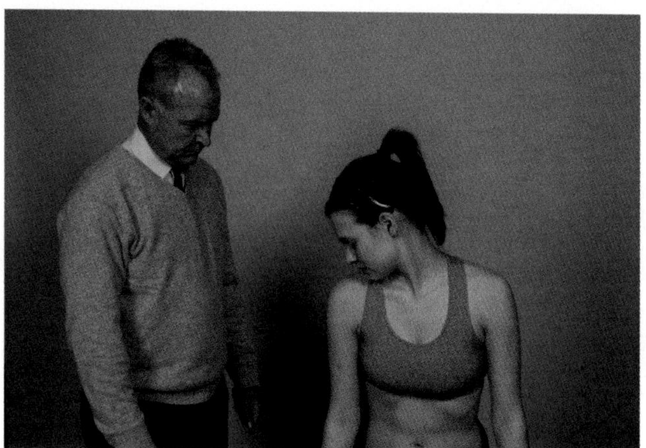

FIGURE 25-55 Scalene cramp and relief tests.

Valsalva

The patient is positioned in sitting and is instructed to hold his or her breath and then "bear down" as in performing a bowel movement. Reproduction of the consistent pain during bearing down is considered a positive response for a disk herniation (Table 25-14).

Shoulder Abduction Test

This test[186,187] is used to test for the presence of radicular symptoms. The patient is positioned sitting or supine and is asked to elevate the arm through abduction, so that the hand or forearm rests on top of the head (Fig. 25-57). If this position relieves or decreases the patient's symptoms, a cervical extradural compression problem, such as a herniated disk, or nerve root compression should be suspected. The literature seems to indicate high specificity with low sensitivity for this test (Table 25-14). The specific segmental level can be determined by the dermatome distribution of the symptoms. If the symptoms are increased with this maneuver, the implication is that pressure is increasing in the interscalene triangle.[187]

Brachial Plexus Compression Test

The patient is positioned in sitting and is asked to side bend the head to the uninvolved side. The clinician applies firm

TABLE 25-14 Evidence-based Tests for Cervical Radiculopathy							
Test	**Reliability**	**Sensitivity**	**Specificity**	**LR+**	**LR−**	**DOR**	**QUADAS Score**
Spurling[a]	NT	30	93	4.3	.75	5.69	9
Valsalva[b]	.69 kappa	22	94	3.67	0.82	4.41	10
Shoulder abduction[c]	NT	68	NT	N/A	N/A	N/A	8
Shoulder abduction[b]	.20 kappa	17	92	2.12	0.90	2.35	10
Brachial plexus compression test[d]	NT	69	83	4.1	0.37	10.8	8
Cervical hyperflexion[d]	NT	8	100	N/A	N/A	N/A	8
Cervical hyperflexion (limited <55°)[b]	.60 kappa	89	41	1.51	0.27	5.6	10
Cervical hyperextension[d]	NT	25	90	2.5	0.83	3	8
Cervical distraction[b]	.88 kappa	44	90	4.4	0.62	7.1	10

[a]Tong HC, Haig AJ, Yamakawa K: The Spurling test and cervical radiculopathy. *Spine* 27:156–159, 2002.
[b]Wainner RS, Fritz JM, Irrgang JJ, et al: Reliability and diagnostic accuracy of the clinical examination and patient self-report measures for cervical radiculopathy. *Spine* 28:52–62, 2003.
[c]Davidson RI, Dunn EJ, Metzmaker JN: The shoulder abduction test in the diagnosis of radicular pain in cervical extradural compressive monoradiculopathies. *Spine* 6:441–446, 1981.
[d]Uchihara T, Furukawa T, Tsukagoshi H: Compression of brachial plexus as a diagnostic test of cervical cord lesion. *Spine* 19:2170–2173, 1994.

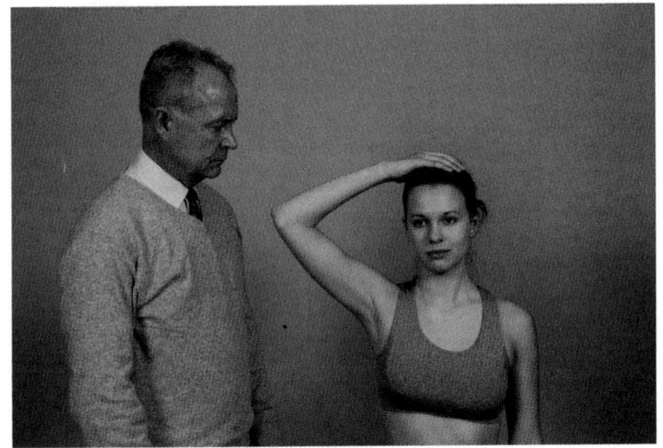

FIGURE 25-57 Shoulder abduction test.

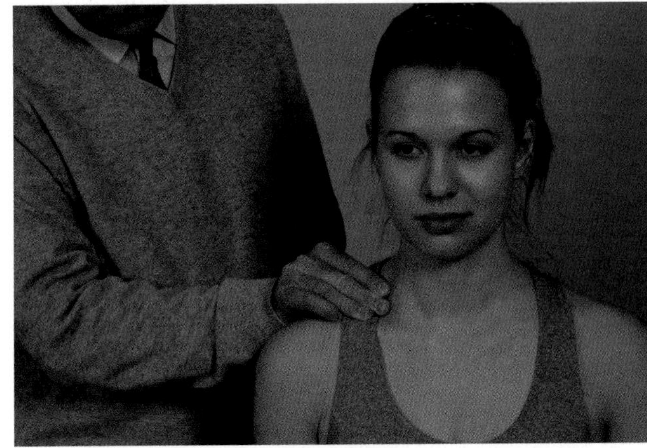

FIGURE 25-58 Brachial Plexus Compression Test without the sidebending.

pressure to the brachial plexus by squeezing the plexus lateral to the scalenus between the thumb and fingers (Fig. 25-58). Reproduction of shoulder or upper arm pain is positive for mechanical cervical lesions (Table 25-14), or a thoracic outlet dysfunction.[188]

Cervical Hyperflexion

The patient is positioned in sitting and is asked to flex his or her neck to the first point of pain or toward end range if no pain exists (Fig. 25-59). Reproduction of radicular symptoms during hyperflexion is considered a positive response (Table 25-14).

Cervical Hyperextension (Jackson's Test)

The patient is positioned in sitting and is asked to extend his or her neck to the first point of pain or toward the end range if no

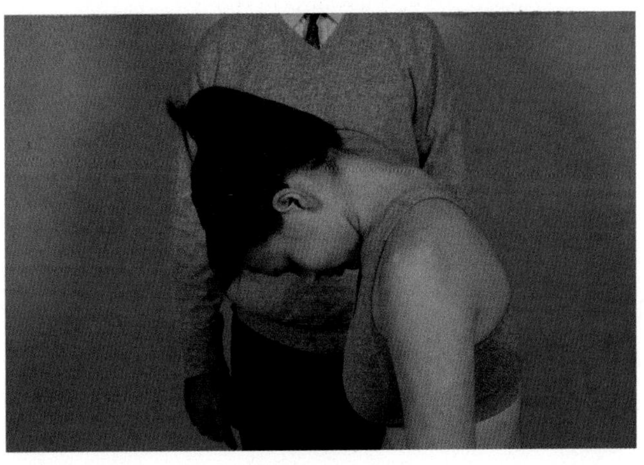

FIGURE 25-59 Cervical hyperflexion.

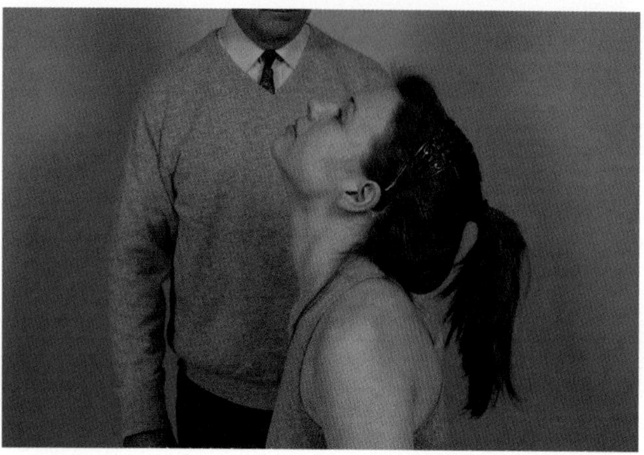

FIGURE 25-60 Cervical hyperextension (Jackson's test).

pain exists (Fig. 25-60). Reproduction of symptoms is considered a positive response (Table 25-14).

Cervical Distraction

The patient is positioned in supine. Using one hand the clinician uses a lumbrical grip around the occiput. Using the other hand the clinician wraps the hand gently around the patient's chin. A traction force is applied and the patient's symptoms are assessed (Fig. 25-61). A positive test is reduction of symptoms during traction and is indicative of some form of foraminal compression, or zygapophyseal joint irritation. This test appears to have high specificity but low sensitivity (Table 25-14).

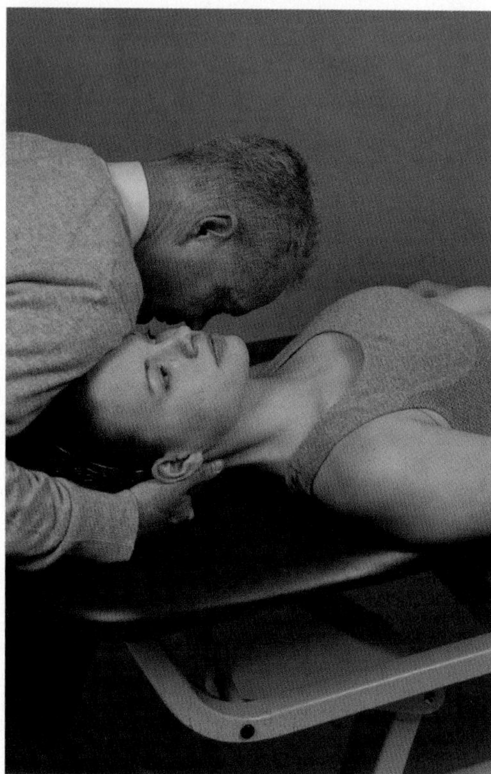

FIGURE 25-61 Cervical distraction.

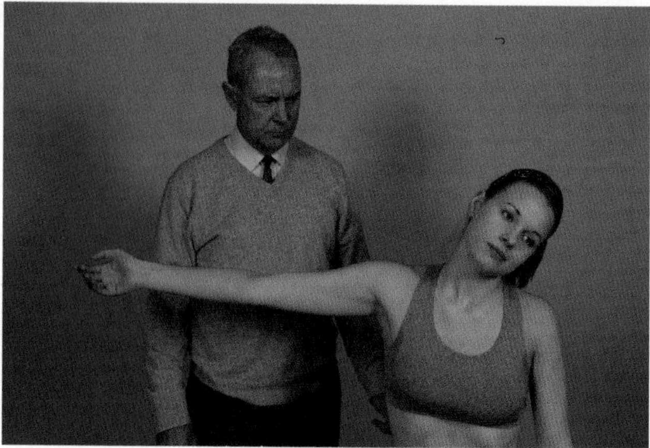

FIGURE 25-62 Stretch Test.

Brachial Plexus Tests

Stretch Test

The patient is positioned sitting or standing and is asked to raise the arm on the involved side (Fig. 25-62) and then to side bend the head to the uninvolved side. Pain and paresthesia along the involved arm are indicative of a brachial plexus irritation.

Cervical Rotation Lateral Flexion Test

This test is used as part of the examination of a patient presenting with brachialgia and thoracic outlet symptoms to assess first rib hypomobility. The motion of cervical rotation combined with lateral flexion (side bending) can be restricted in the presence of a subluxed first rib at the costotransverse joint.[189] The patient is seated and the cervical spine positioned in neutral with regard to flexion–extension. The clinician then passively rotates the cervical spine maximally, away from the side to be tested, and then flexes the neck forward as far as possible, moving the ear toward the chest (Fig. 25-63). The test is then repeated to the other side, and a comparison is made about the quantity and quality of motion. If the first rib is subluxed, the restriction to passive movement is felt abruptly. If restricted motion is found on

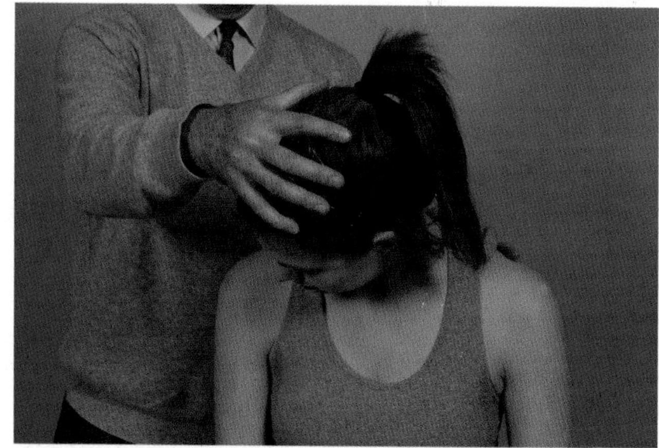

FIGURE 25-63 Cervical Rotation Lateral Flexion Test.

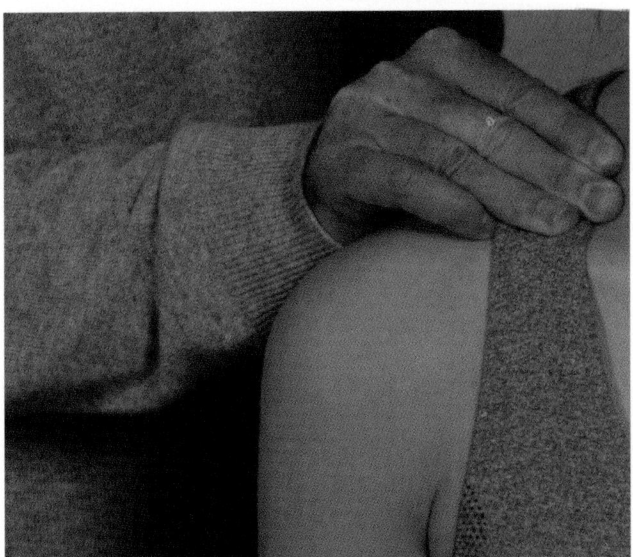

FIGURE 25-64 Tinel's Sign.

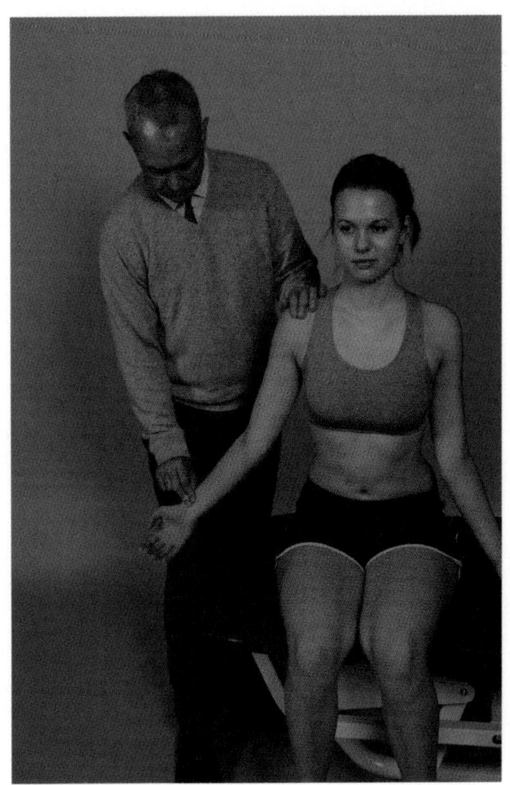

FIGURE 25-65 Adson's test.

one side, first-rib mobilizations are performed and then the patient is retested. Lindgren and colleagues found this test to have excellent interobserver repeatability and to have good agreement with a radiologic examination in the detection of a subluxed first rib.[190] However it is worth remembering that a number of additional factors may influence the finding, including TOS, cervical radiculopathy, and upper thoracic pain.

Tinel's Sign

The patient is positioned in sitting and is asked to side bend the head to the uninvolved side. The clinician taps or squeezes along the trunks of the brachial plexus using the fingers (Fig. 25-64). Local pain indicates a cervical plexus lesion. A tingling sensation in the distribution of one of the trunks may indicate a compression or neuroma of one or more trunks of the brachial plexus.[191]

Thoracic Outlet Tests

Despite their widespread use, no studies documenting the reliability of the common thoracic outlet maneuvers of Adson's, Allen's, or the costoclavicular maneuver have been performed.[192] Because TOS is a controversial diagnosis, most of the thoracic outlet tests examine specificity only.

When performing TOS tests, either the diminution or disappearance of pulse or reproduction of neurologic symptoms indicates a positive test. However, the aim of the tests should be to reproduce the patient's symptoms rather than to just obliterate the radial pulse.

Adson's Vascular Test

The patient is positioned in sitting with the arms placed at 15 degrees of abduction. The clinician palpates the radial pulse. The patient is asked to inhale deeply, and to hold his or her breath (Fig. 25-65). The patient is then asked to tilt the head back, and rotate the head, so that the chin is elevated and pointed towards the examined side **VIDEO**. The clinician records the radial pulse as diminished or occluded and asks the patient about the presence of paresthesia. The test position theoretically increases the scalenus angle and the tension of the anterior and middle scalenes thereby compromising the interscalene triangle.[193] However, biomechanically, the scalene angle actually increases, which should reduce the likelihood of compression. Moreover, to date, no studies have been performed to document the reliability of this test. Plewa and Delinger[194] found the specificity of this test to be 100% when assessing pain, 89% when assessing vascular changes, and 89% when assessing paresthesia.

Costoclavicular Test

The patient is positioned sitting straight in an exaggerated military posture and with both arms at the sides. The clinician assesses the radial pulse in this position. The patient is asked to retract and depress the shoulders while protruding the chest (Fig. 25-66) **VIDEO**. This position is held for 60 seconds. The clinician assesses changes in the radial pulse and asks the patient about the presence of paresthesia. It is likely that this test position reduces the volume of the costoclavicular space. Plewa and Delinger[194] found the specificity of this test to be 100% when assessing pain, 89% when assessing vascular changes, and 85% when assessing paresthesia.

Roos Test[195]

The patient is positioned sitting. The arm is positioned in 90 degrees of shoulder abduction, and 90 degrees of elbow flexion. The patient is asked to perform slow finger clenching for 3 minutes (Fig. 25-67). The radial pulse may be reduced or obliterated during this maneuver, and an infraclavicular bruit

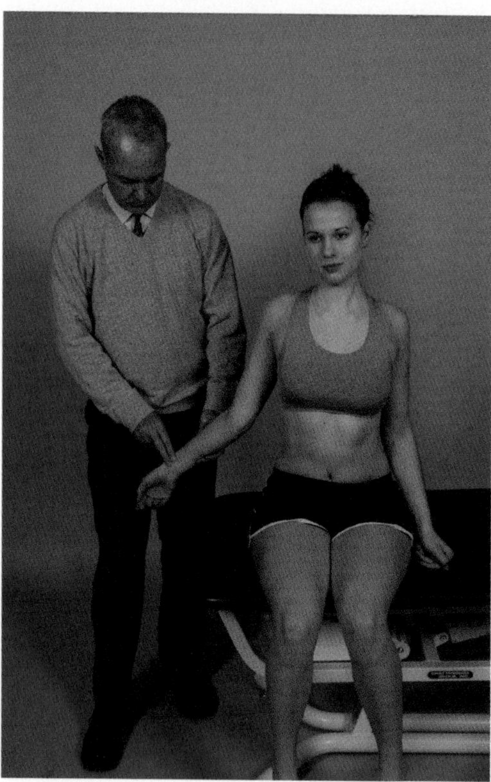

FIGURE 25-66 Costoclavicular test.

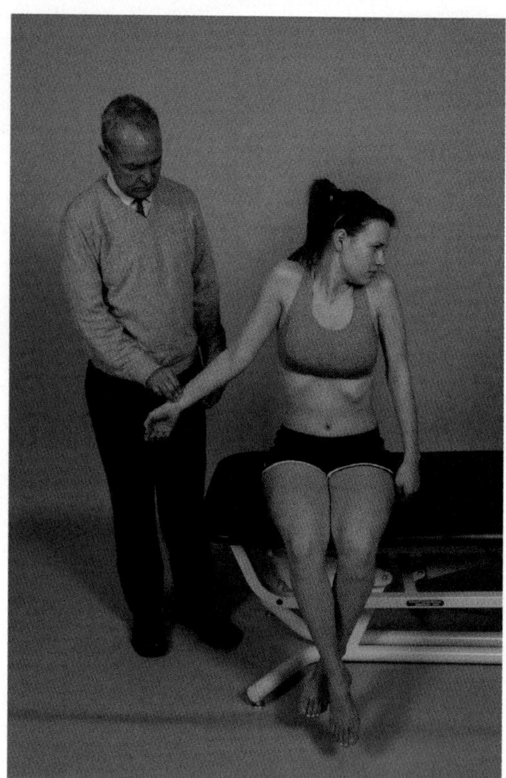

FIGURE 25-68 Hyperabduction Maneuver (Wright Test).

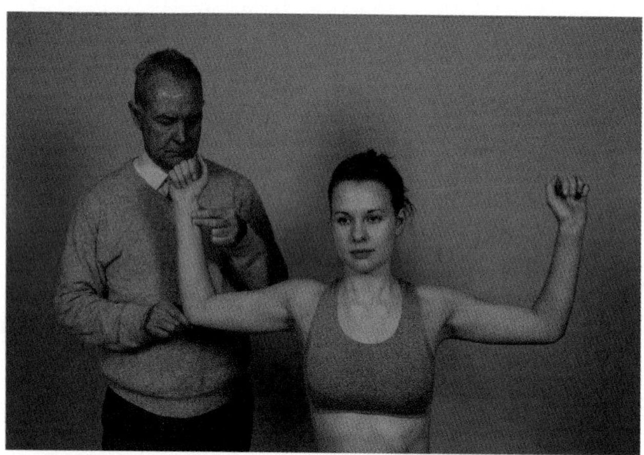

FIGURE 25-67 Roos test.

may be heard. If the patient is unable to maintain the arms in the start position for 3 minutes, or reports pain, heaviness, or numbness and tingling, the test is considered positive for TOS on the involved side. This test is also referred to as the hands-up test, or the elevated arm stress test. No diagnostic accuracy studies have been performed to determine the sensitivity and specificity of this test.

Hyperabduction Maneuver (Wright Test).[196]

The patient is positioned in relaxed sitting. The clinician palpates the radial pulse and then asks the patient to hyperabduct his or her shoulders and to turn the head away from the side being examined (Fig. 25-68). The position is held for 1–2 minutes. A positive test includes reproduction of paresthesia or a decrease in the radial pulse. No diagnostic accuracy studies have been performed to determine the sensitivity and specificity of this test. However, is important to note that a number of studies have found that arm elevation induces radial pulse obliteration in 60–69% of normal subjects.[197,198]

Passive Shoulder Shrug

This simple, but effective, test is used with patients who present with symptoms of TOS to help rule out this syndrome. The patient is seated with the arms folded, and the clinician stands behind. The clinician grasps the patient's elbows and passively elevates the shoulders up and forward (Fig. 25-69). This position is maintained for 30 seconds. Any changes in the patient's symptoms are noted. The maneuver has the effect of slackening the soft tissues and the brachial plexus. No diagnostic accuracy studies have been performed to determine the sensitivity and specificity of this test.

UPPER LIMB TENSION TESTS

The reader is encouraged to refer to Chapter 11 for the descriptions of these tests. The upper limb tension tests are equivalent to the straight leg raise test and others of the lower extremities and are designed to put stress on the neuromeningeal structures of the upper limb. A negative finding strongly suggests a lack of existence of radiculopathy (Table 25-15). Each test begins by testing the normal side first. Normal responses include

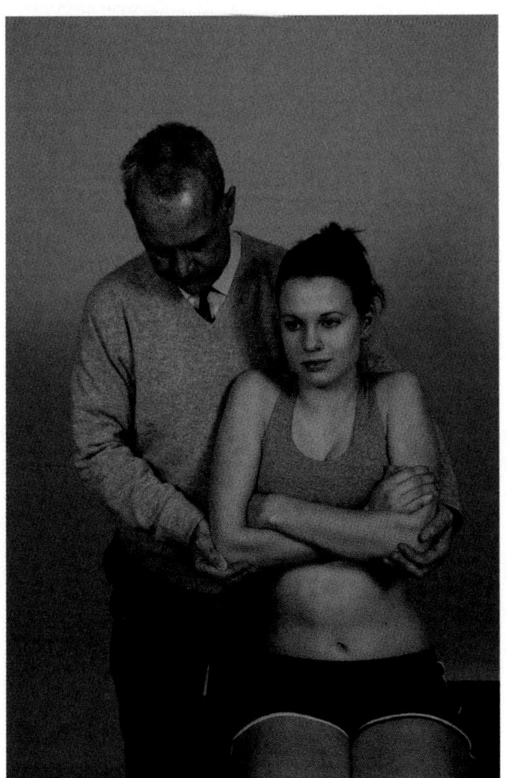

FIGURE 25-69 Passive Shoulder Shrug.

- deep stretch or ache in the cubital fossa;
- deep stretch or ache into the anterior or radial aspect of the forearm and radial aspect of hand;
- deep stretch in the anterior shoulder area;
- sensation felt down the radial aspect of the forearm;
- sensation felt in the median distribution of the hand.

Positive findings include

- reproduction of the patient's symptoms;
- a sensitizing test in the ipsilateral quadrant that alters the symptoms.

IMAGING STUDIES

It is recommended that the results of any imaging studies should be viewed after the clinical examination, so as to remove the potential for bias, especially in light of the fact that degenerative changes and anatomical variations are fairly common in the cervical spine, but that many of these changes have no relationship to the patient's complaints. A description of the various imaging studies and their relevance to a specific region are described in Chapter 7.

INTERVENTION STRATEGIES

Cervical impairments have the same causes as any other areas of the body, that is, a micro- or macrotraumatic impairment of the structures that compose the joint complex.

The clinician must discuss the diagnosis, prognosis, and the intervention with the patient. It is important that the clinician describe the basic anatomy and function of the cervical spine in a way that the patient will understand. Expectations of both the patient and the clinician must be clarified. Patients must realize at the outset that they are responsible for their own recovery and must participate actively in their treatment.

Based on a working hypothesis, the physical therapy intervention needs to be precise, and guided by the impairments, functional limitations, and disability found during the examination. The intervention should aim to reverse the dysfunction and to prevent the recurrence of future episodes. A study by Saturno and colleagues,[199] which assessed the reliability and validity of existing clinical guidelines on neck physiotherapy treatment and follow-up in Spain, determined the eight evidence-based recommendations listed in Table 25-16. Other studies have reported that physical therapy interventions that have included manual therapy, postural reeducation, neck-specific strengthening and stretching exercises, and ergonomic changes at work have been shown to be beneficial in reducing neck pain and improving mobility.[200–202] A pragmatic randomized clinical trial by Hoving et al.,[203] that compared the effectiveness of manual therapy (mainly spinal mobilizations), physical therapy (mainly exercise therapy), and continued care by the general practitioner (analgesics, counseling, and education) for cervical pain over a period of 1 year, found high improvement scores for the manual therapy group for all of the outcomes, followed by physical therapy and general practitioner care.

The joint mobilization techniques for the cervical spine and the manual techniques to increase soft tissue extensibility are described later, under "Therapeutic Techniques" section.

Systematic reviews of physical therapy modalities for neck pain report a lack of high-quality evidence of their efficacy and highlight poor methodologic quality in many studies.[204] Electrotherapy has a long history of use in physical therapy interventions and two high-quality trials reported that pulsed shortwave diathermy delivered by small portable units

TABLE 25-15 Clinical Usefulness of Upper Limb Tension Tests

Test	Reliability	Sensitivity	Specificity	LR+	LR−	DOR	QUADAS Score
Median nerve bias[a]	.76 kappa	97	22	1.24	.14	9.1	10
Radial nerve bias[a]	.83 kappa	72	33	1.07	0.84	1.26	10

[a]Wainner RS, Fritz JM, Irrgang JJ, et al: Reliability and diagnostic accuracy of the clinical examination and patient self-report measures for cervical radiculopathy. *Spine.* 28:52–62, 2003.

TABLE 25-16	Evidence-Based Recommendations for Cervical Intervention

Every patient with neck pain must receive ergonomic advice on the reduction of repetitive movements and/or postures. As a basic treatment for all patients, an active physical therapy program will be useful in neck and shoulder muscles. This will include

1. active stretching exercises;
2. dynamic muscular strengthening exercises;
3. exercises to do at home.

As a basic treatment for all patients with chronic neck pain (>3 months) a program of oculocervicokinetic reeducation (exercises to address eye–head coordination to improve cervicocephalic anesthesia—the ability to relocate accurately the head on the trunk after an active movement in the horizontal plane) will be used.

If trigger points are identified in some muscles, transcutaneous electrostimulation will be used.

If there is a dysfunction of the analytic joint passive mobility, joint mobilization/manipulative treatment will be used, which includes structural techniques of vertebral mobilization/manipulation, or contract–relax techniques, or both.

If there is pain radiating to the upper limb, mechanical intermittent cervical traction will be used.

Data from Saturno PJ, Medina F, Valera F, et al: Validity and reliability of guidelines for neck pain treatment in primary health care. A nationwide empirical analysis in Spain. *Int J Qual Health Care* 15:487–493, 2003; Levoska S, Keinanen-Kiukaanniemi S: Active or passive physiotherapy for occupational cervicobrachial disorders? A comparison of two treatment methods with a 1-year follow-up. *Arch Phys Med Rehabil* 74:425–430, 1993; Hsueh TC, Cheng PT, Kuan TS, et al: The immediate effectiveness of electrical nerve stimulation and electrical muscle stimulation on myofascial trigger points. *Am J Phys Med Rehabil* 76:471–476, 1997; Cassidy JD, Lopes A, Yong-Hing M: The immediate effect of manipulation versus mobilization on pain and range of motion in the cervical spine: A randomized controlled trial. *J Manip Physiol Ther* 15:570–575, 1992; Zylbergold RS, Piper MC: Cervical spine disorders. A comparison of three types of traction. *Spine* 10:867–871, 1985.

inserted into cervical collars significantly reduced pain in patients with mechanical neck pain.[205,206]

Acute Phase

During the acute phase, the patient should be encouraged to perform as many activities of daily living as possible. The return to activities should be encouraged and begin within 2–4 days after a cervical injury, depending on severity. Rest is usually advocated in the first 24–72 hours, depending on the severity of the injury, to give healing a chance. Indications for rest include pain reported with all neck and head motions, however, slight, and high irritability of the symptoms. Ignoring the need for rest in these situations increases the risk of delaying the recovery from the acute phase. In those situations where absolute rest is warranted, the patient is told that rest means just that. Pillows should be adjusted so that the head remains in neutral when sleeping in side-lying or supine position. The patient should be cautioned about prone lying.

Patients are encouraged to take up or resume a regular activity such as walking or, later in this phase, swimming and perhaps running, or anything else that will get them back to a normal mind set about their function, without reinjuring the area.

In general, two basic approaches are used to treat neck pain with exercises:

- General strengthening and endurance exercises for the neck flexor muscles.[207,208]
- Specific exercises designed to improve coordination and control of the muscles.[78]

Appropriate exercises must ensure proper motor control, performance, and endurance of a specific part of the body. When prescribing exercises to the patient, the clinician must decide on the type of muscle contraction, the patient's body position, the level of resistance or load, and the number of repetitions, and method of progression.[209,210] Gentle exercises are prescribed in the first part of the healing phase. The main reasons for these early exercises are

- to encourage patient involvement;
- to provide mechanoreceptor stimulation;
- to control pain and inflammation;
- to promote healing;
- to maintain the newly attained ranges;
- to provide neuromuscular feedback.

AAROM/AROM[211]

The patient is positioned in supine with the head supported on a pillow or a towel roll. Usually, the easiest and most comfortable exercise is rotation. The patient is asked to perform gentle, active, small-range, and amplitude rotational movements of the neck, initially in one direction, and then the other up to a maximum range of comfort. Care must be taken with these exercises to ensure that the normal movement pattern is performed and that the pattern is reinforced with repetition. The movements are repeated 10 times in each direction. According to Bird and colleagues,[212] to improve endurance, a repetition of 4–6 sets per exercise, with rest periods of 30–60 seconds between sets, is appropriate. To help relieve muscle tension, the exercises can be done in conjunction with breathing.[96] When the patient reaches the end of the comfortable range (at the point where some tissue resistance is first being felt), the patient takes a moderate breath in and then releases it. At the end of the release, a relaxation of the muscles allows a slight increase in range without stressing any tissues, and without causing pain. The focus of these exercises is on motor control rather the muscle strength.

Once these non–weight-bearing active assisted range of motion exercises can be performed without an exacerbation or recurrence of symptoms, active cervical range-of-motion exercises can be initiated in the sitting, and then standing positions.

Retraining of Craniovertebral Flexion

The patient is positioned in supine and is instructed by the clinician on how to perform correct craniovertebral flexion (CVF) using gentle nodding movements while eliminating any compensation strategies, such as neck retraction, excessive cervical flexion, and/or jaw clenching.[78]

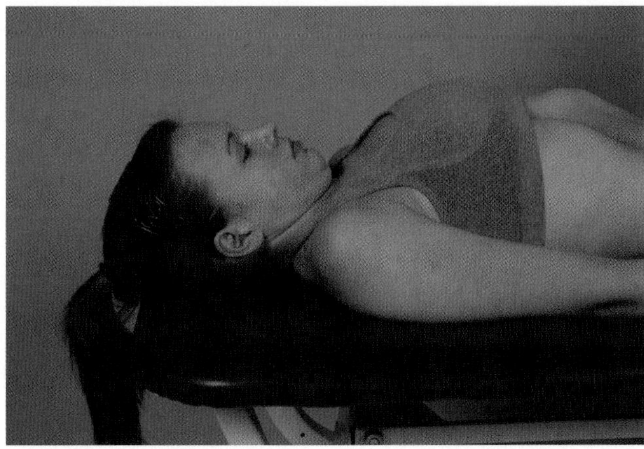

FIGURE 25-70 Head nod.

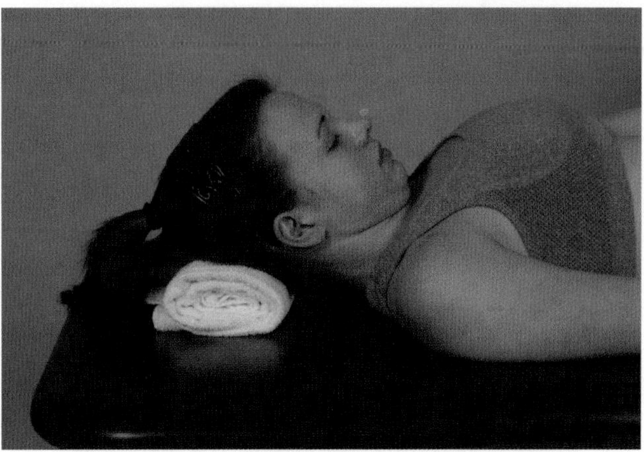

FIGURE 25-72 Head nod with towel roll in supine.

Head Nod.[211] The key exercise to recruit the deep cervical flexors, which are the most common muscles to become weak with neck dysfunction, is the head nod exercise (Fig. 25-70). Correct performance of the exercise ensures that the flexion only occurs at the junction between the head and neck (at the O-A joint) before continuing segmentally into midcervical flexion. The exercise is initially performed in sitting (gravity assisted) while ensuring that no forward movement of the head occurs (which would change the exercise into one of eccentric contraction of the cervical extensors), and to reduce the potential of using the SCM muscle. The patient can be taught to palpate the SCM and scalene muscles during the exercise for any unwanted contractions. As the patient gradually nods the chin down, the back of the head should be seen to move up toward the ceiling. The nod is stopped at the point in the range that can be achieved without superficial muscle activity, held for 10 seconds to promote the endurance function of the muscles, and is repeated 10 times. Once the patient is able to tolerate the exercise in the upright position, they are asked to perform the exercise in supine on an inclined board (Fig. 25-71). As the inclined board is tilted progressively backward toward horizontal the assistance from gravity is gradually reduced. Once in supine, the head is positioned in neutral, either resting on a pillow, or on a small folded towel placed under the occiput so that the normal cervical lordosis is supported (Fig. 25-72). In this position, the head nod exercise is performed with no lifting of the head off the surface, while the patient palpates anteriorly to ensure no superficial muscle activity. Once this is mastered, the exercise is progressed so that the head nod uses the towel roll as a fulcrum (making sure that the neck does not lose contact with the towel) and the back of the head may lift just off the bed during the motion, while preventing the chin from poking forward (this is a sign of excessive anterior translation caused by a relative dominance of the SCM and scalenes). At this time, it is no longer necessary to palpate the anterior structures as the superficial muscles must now be active to lift the head off the bed (Fig. 25-73). To highlight contraction of the flexors more unilaterally in cases of asymmetric weakness, a head nod into a flexion quadrant (e.g., flexion, side bending, rotation to the same side) can be used. The exercise can also be performed in prone over an exercise ball or in the quadruped position (Fig. 25-74). In the prone position, gravity draws the head forward into a position of upper cervical extension, which is opposed by the head nod motion into upper cervical flexion.

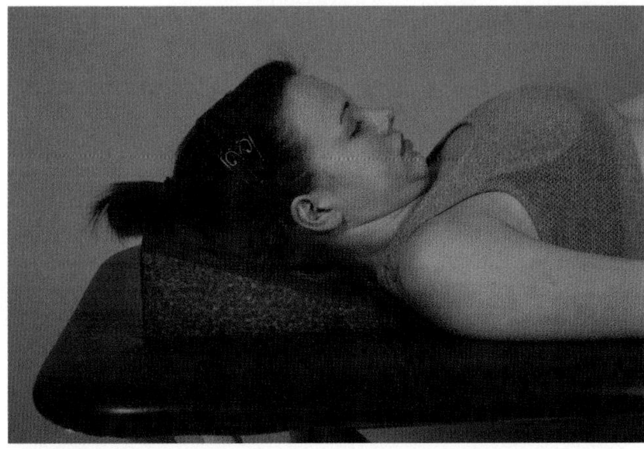

FIGURE 25-71 Head nod on incline.

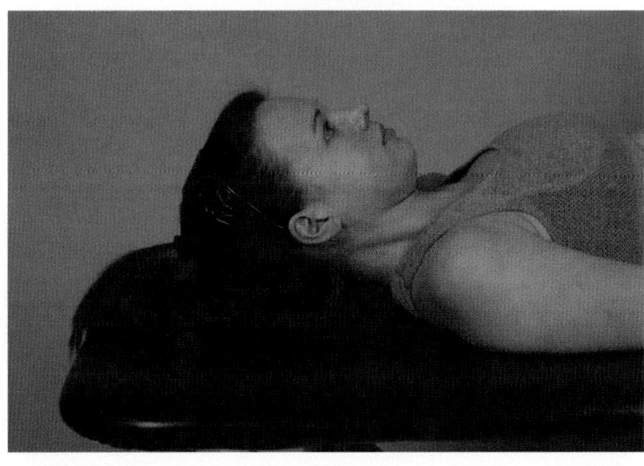

FIGURE 25-73 Head nod with head lift.

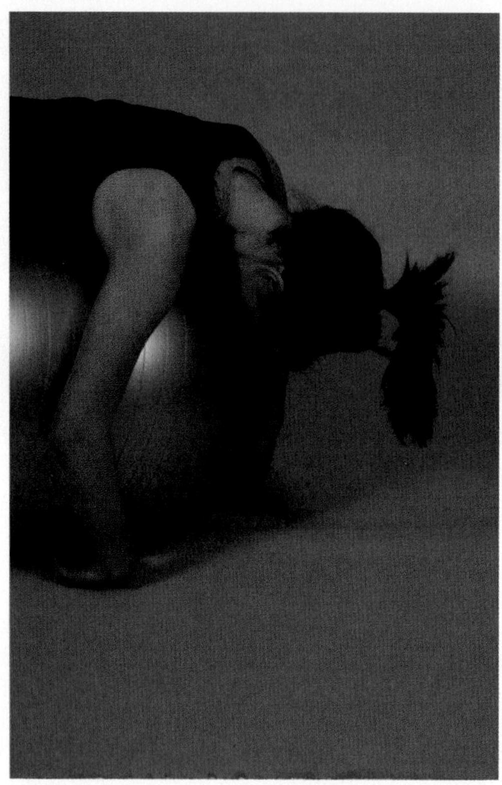

FIGURE 25-74 Head nod prone on Swissball.

Return to Neutral[211]

The return to neutral exercise is intended to recruit the deep cervical segmental extensors. The deep cervical extensor muscles include the semispinalis cervicalis and the multifidus. The craniovertebral extensor muscles include the rectus capitis and the suboccipital muscles. While in the sitting position, and starting from a position at the end of the head nod exercise, the patient is asked to gradually lift the chin and then look up toward the ceiling (eccentric contraction of the cervical flexor muscles), while preventing any chin retraction or cervical retraction, and to continue this movement, trying to look farther along the ceiling, until the end of the comfortable range is reached. At this point, the patient then returns to the start position (concentric contraction of the cervical flexor muscles). Once the patient is able to perform this exercise correctly, the start position is initiated from a position of CVF (Fig. 25-75). If the CV region can be sustained in flexion until the end of the motion, the capitis group of the erector spinae muscles will tend to be inhibited. The exercise is progressed by having the patient perform it on all fours (Fig. 25-76). Finally, isometric hold exercises in different parts of the range can be initiated and progressed based on patient tolerance. In cases of asymmetric weakness, the exercise can be made more specific by working into an extension quadrant (e.g., combined extension, side bending, and rotation to the same side).

Coupling Activation[211]

The primary side benders and rotators can be recruited by exercising into a quadrant position. For both of the following exercises, the patient is told to perform a preset nod to activate the deep stabilizing muscles before performing any motion of the head. These muscles can be trained more specifically and intensely in the sidelying position, with the head supported on a wedge (Fig. 25-77). As the head is lifted off the wedge, the muscles opposite to the side the patient is lying on contract

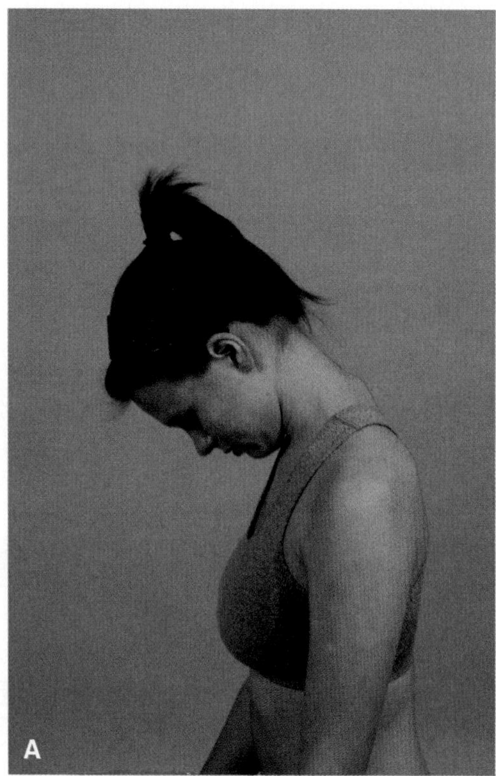

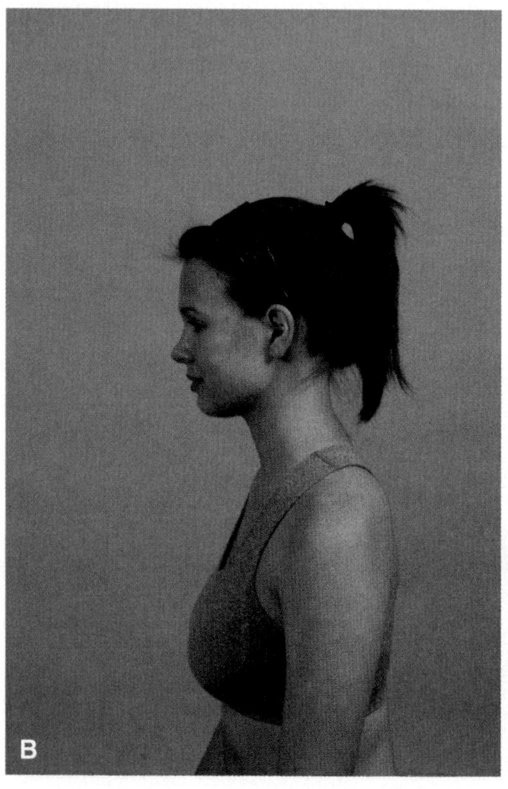

FIGURE 25-75 Seated head nod with return to neutral. A Start position. B End position

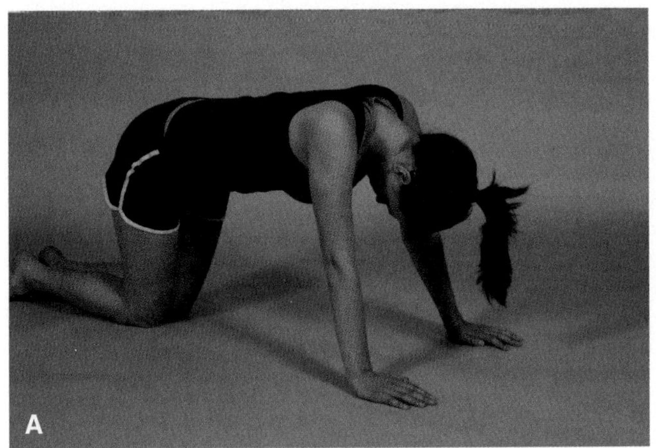

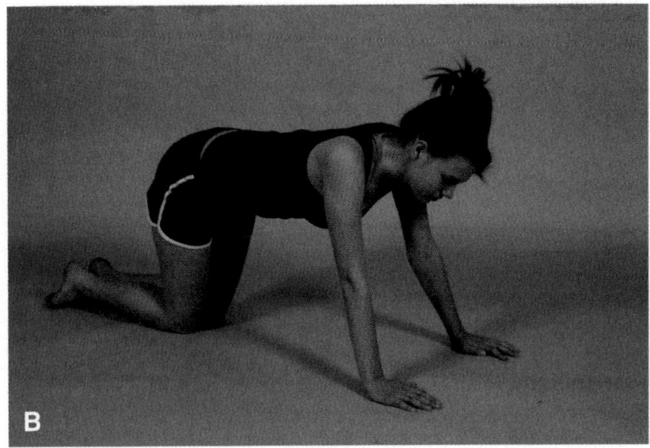

FIGURE 25-76 Return to neutral on all fours. **A** Start position. **B** End position.

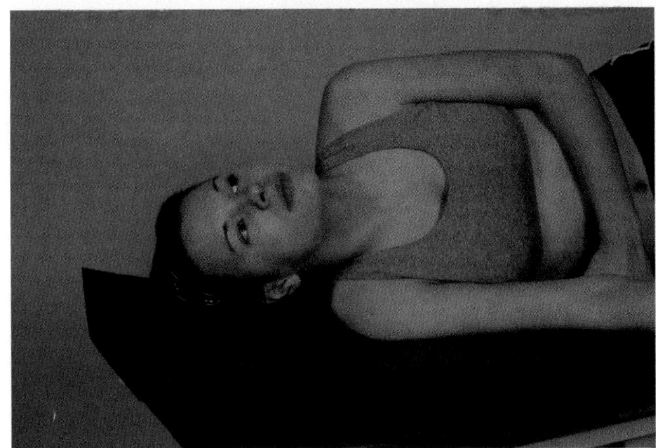

FIGURE 25-77 Combined flexion, side bending, and rotation on wedge in sidelying.

against gravity. The deeper muscles can be emphasized by ensuring that the neck remains in contact with the wedge, thereby decreasing the amount of translation.

Global Strengthening

The global strengthening exercises are initiated with submaximal isometric contractions throughout the single planes using multi-angle submaximal isometric contractions, including flexion VIDEO, extension VIDEO, side bending VIDEO, and rotation VIDEO (Fig. 25-78A–D). The manual resistance is initially applied by the clinician and then by the patient. Although these exercises should not cause sharp pain, they may produce mild delayed-onset muscle soreness. Minimal resistance is used in the neutral position to aid in venous return, stimulate the mechanoreceptors in the muscle, and allay any concerns regarding weakening of the neck from disuse or a cervical collar.[96]

The exercise progression proceeds using the following principles[213]:

- The hold time of the isometric contraction is increased.
- The number of repetitions of this holding activity is increased.
- Progression to the next level is based on the ability of the patient to stabilize and isolate the correct muscle action in the exercise positions.

Increasing the Holding Capacity of the Deep Neck Flexors

Once the patient is able to perform a correct CVF movement, the emphasis switches to increasing the endurance capacity of the involved muscles (deep neck flexors). It is recommended that a preinflated, air-filled pressure sensor is used to help guide and control the training of these muscles so as to provide visual feedback and motivation to the patient.[78] The starting point for the training is the pressure level the patient has reached and can hold without compensation for at least 10 seconds (typically at 22 or 24 mmHg). The patient is instructed on how to achieve the determined pressure level and then to hold it for a time without evidence of compensation or poor motor patterns. The aim is to the patient to hold the position for 10 seconds and then to repeat this 10 times. Practice should occur at least twice a day. The goal is for the patient to perform this exercise with a pressure level between 28 and 30 mmHg. Depending on the patient, achievement of this goal can take anywhere from 4 to 6 weeks to 12 weeks.[78]

Co-contraction of the Neck Flexors and Extensors

These exercises are initially performed with the patient positioned in sitting, and consist of a series of gentle, alternating self-resisted isometric rotation contractions, similar to those used with rhythmic stabilization protocols. A typical progression for training the cervical flexors and extensors to enhance dynamic stability is outlined in Table 25-17.

The other exercises prescribed early in the intervention include:

- exercises designed to regain correct scapular positioning. In patients with cervical problems, the scapula is typically protracted and downwardly rotated. Exercises are prescribed in an attempt to bring the coracoid upward and the acromion backward incorporating a slight retraction

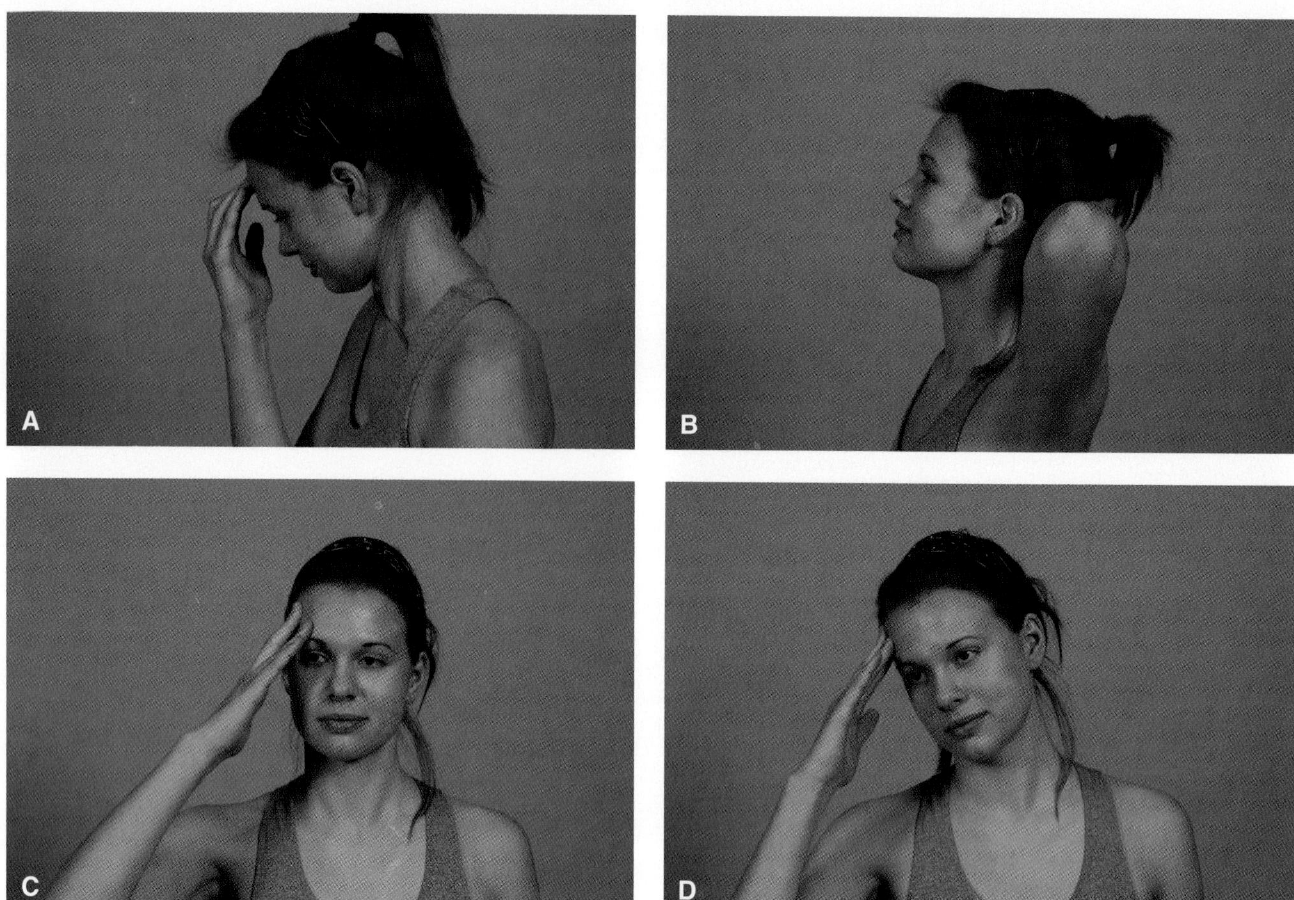

FIGURE 25-78 Cervical submaximal isometrics in four planes. **A** Flexion. **B** Extension. **C** Rotation **D** Side bending.

and lateral rotation of the scapula. Exercises include shoulder shrugging VIDEO, and shoulder square (retraction) exercises VIDEO. The scapula retraction exercises are initially performed supine, with the glenohumeral joint in internal and external rotation. The patient is asked to isometrically retract the shoulders against the bed.

- exercises designed to increase the endurance capacity of the scapular stabilizers, and scapular control with arm movements and loads (see Chap. 16).
- for nerve irritation hip and knee flexion–extension exercises and ankle dorsiflexion in non–weight-bearing position (to help move the dura).

TABLE 25-17 Retraining Progression for the Cervical Flexors and Extensors

Exercise	Patient Position	Description
Cervical bracing	Four-point kneeling	The patient is asked to protract the head and then to perform upper cervical flexion while maintaining the lower cervical spine in a neutral position. This position is held for at least 10 seconds.
Cervical bracing with extremity movements	Four-point kneeling	The patient is asked to combine cervical bracing with arm and leg movements. While maintaining the stability of the body and cervicothoracic region, the patient raises an arm. The patient then raises a leg. These movements are alternated (right arm, left leg; right leg, left arm) until the patient can maintain them and perform the correct movement pattern. To provide more challenge, the patient can be asked to balance a light book on the head.
Cervical bracing with extremity movements on unstable base	Push-up position with lower legs on a Swiss ball	The patient is asked to combine cervical bracing while balancing on a Swiss ball.

Data from Murphy DR: Conservative Management of Cervical Spine Syndromes. New York, NY: McGraw-Hill, 2000; O'Grady WH, Tollan MF: The role of exercise in treating cervical hypermobility or instability. *Orthop Phys Ther Clin North Am* 10:475–501, 2001.

- isometric, shoulder and abdominal exercises (using the Valsalva maneuver, not pelvic tilting or sit-ups).
- postural reeducation.

As with any exercise progression, these exercises are replaced with more challenging exercises, as the patient's healing progresses. Guidelines are provided for safe home exercising by teaching the patient to identify warning signs that could lead to exacerbation or recurrence of symptoms. In the event of an increase of symptoms, the techniques are adjusted by reducing either the amplitude of the movements or the number of movements, or both.

Other movements, such as cervical retraction VIDEO, and cervical protrusion can be added to the program, depending on which movements are found to be beneficial during the progression.

The efficacy of electrotherapeutic modalities has not been subjected to randomized clinical trials.[214] Although passive modalities have their uses in the acute phase, the clinician should remember that they must only be used as an adjunct to the more active program, and with a specific goal in mind, such as to help in the reduction of pain and inflammation. Thus, the patient should be weaned off the use of modalities as early as possible. Cervical traction (see Chap. 8) has been advocated for neck sprains, and for the pain of radiculopathy, but no clinical or statistically significant change in pain or overall range of motion has been identified.[215–218]

- ***Ultrasound.*** Pulsed ultrasound should be used precisely.[219] It can be applied to the posterior aspects of the zygapophyseal joints to control pain and reduce swelling or to a torn muscle.
- ***Non-thermal agents.*** Theoretically, ice is the preferred choice during this phase. However, ice can often increase pain that arises from trigger points. At the earliest opportunity the application of heat is introduced because of its ability to relax musculature, and stimulate vasodilation.[220]
- ***Electrical muscle stimulation.***[96] Providing that none of the muscles stimulated are torn, electrical muscle stimulation can be used in the early stages as an effective pain reliever and as a venous pump. The patient is positioned supine. A small electrode is placed on each of the left and right suboccipital muscles, and a large common electrode is placed along the upper thoracic spinous process. The channels are made to stimulate asynchronously with a long "on" ramp, and a contraction length of 2 or 3 seconds (certainly no longer than 5, because this becomes uncomfortable). The session can last anywhere from a few minutes to 30 minutes, once it is established that there are no adverse effects from the intervention.

Numerous manual therapy techniques are available to the clinician, each with its own uses. These techniques, described later under "Therapeutic Techniques" section, can be used with hypomobilities, and soft tissue injuries. The nature and location of the dysfunction, as well as the intention of its effect, guide the selection of a particular technique. Movement gained by a manual technique must be reinforced by both the mechanical and neurophysical benefits of active movement.[68]

No randomized controlled trials (RCTs) have been done on the efficacy of manipulations for patients with predominantly acute neck pain. A number of RCT studies have been done with subacute and chronic neck pain, most of which have shown that manipulation is probably slightly more effective than mobilization or other interventions.[221]

Cervical Collars

The use of cervical collars is controversial. Although several studies have concluded that the wearing of a cervical collar results in delayed recovery, these studies looked at the use of collars and other passive therapies versus other more active forms of intervention, such as early patient activation and exercise. A study by Mealy and colleagues[222] found that early active mobilization techniques following a WAD improved pain reduction and increased mobility, compared with a control group receiving 2 weeks' rest with a soft cervical collar and gradual mobilization thereafter. Another study[25] found physical therapy or exact instructions in a home program of self-mobilization to be better than 2 weeks' rest, with a soft collar at the 1- and 2-month follow-ups. A similar result was found at the 2-year follow-up.[224] Borchgrevink and colleagues[225] found that patients encouraged to continue with daily activities had a better outcome than patients prescribed sick leave and immobilization.

With those patients who have a severe capsular restriction of motion, however, a cervical collar should be issued. Soft cervical collars do not rigidly immobilize the cervical spine and if used judiciously can provide support for the head and neck in the very acute stages.[214,226]

The collar serves a number of functions, among them are

- providing support in maintaining the cervical spine erect;
- reminding the patient that the neck is injured and, thereby, preventing the patient from engaging in unexpected or excessive movements;
- allowing the patient to rest the chin during activities, thereby offsetting the weight of the head;
- allowing the patient to perform cervical rotations while the weight of the head is offset.

Prolonged reliance on the use of a collar may induce stiffness and weakness, but this can be avoided by recommending a time-limited use of the collar, which is based on specific factors such as the patient's condition and function. Certain situations warrant the use of a collar, such as long drives in a vehicle or prolonged postures of standing and sitting. However, patients should be weaned off the collar once there is significant improvement in the range of motion and pain levels.

Functional Phase

Although strengthening exercises have been advocated for the intervention of neck pain,[207,227] only a few controlled intervention studies have been conducted to examine their benefit. However, in one randomized study, investigators found that a multimodal intervention of postural, manual, psychological, relaxation, and visual training techniques was superior to traditional approaches involving ultrasound and electric stimulation.[228] Patients returned to work earlier, and they had better results in pain intensity, emotional response, and postural disturbances.[228]

The stabilization of this region must include postural stabilization retraining of the entire spine.

Cervicothoracic stabilization is a specific type of therapeutic exercise that can help the patient to (1) gain dynamic control of cervicothoracic spine forces, (2) eliminate repetitive injury to the motion segments, (3) encourage healing of the injured segment, and (4) possibly alter the degenerative process.[229]

Cervicothoracic stabilization exercises include the following:

Shoulder Shrugs and With Resistance

These exercises, initiated in the acute phase without resistance, are progressed so that the patient performs them with resistance added by asking the patient to hold a weight in each hand. The shrug strengthens the upper trapezius, levator scapulae, and rhomboids. The shoulder circles strengthen the upper trapezius, levator scapulae, and rhomboids.

Scapular Retraction

Once this exercise can be performed in supine without pain, the patient performs the exercise in the side-lying position and then prone or standing without resistance VIDEO. Resistance is added as tolerated. Scapular retraction in internal rotation of the glenohumeral joint strengthens the infraspinatus, teres minor, middle and posterior deltoids, and the rhomboids. Scapular retraction in external rotation of the glenohumeral joint strengthens the infraspinatus, teres minor, middle and posterior deltoids, and middle trapezius VIDEO.

Serratus Punch

This exercise is performed initially with the patient supine, one shoulder flexed to 90 degrees, and the elbow extended. From this position, the patient raises the extended arm toward the ceiling and protracts the shoulder girdle. This exercise can be progressed by adding a weight to the hand and performing it against a wall or a chair, before progressing to a push-up on the floor.

Tree Hug

The patient is asked to wrap a length of elastic tubing around the back and to hold the two ends, with the thumbs pointing forward and the arms in about 60 degrees of abduction (Fig. 25-79). From this position, the patient is asked to imagine hugging a tree and to reproduce that motion.

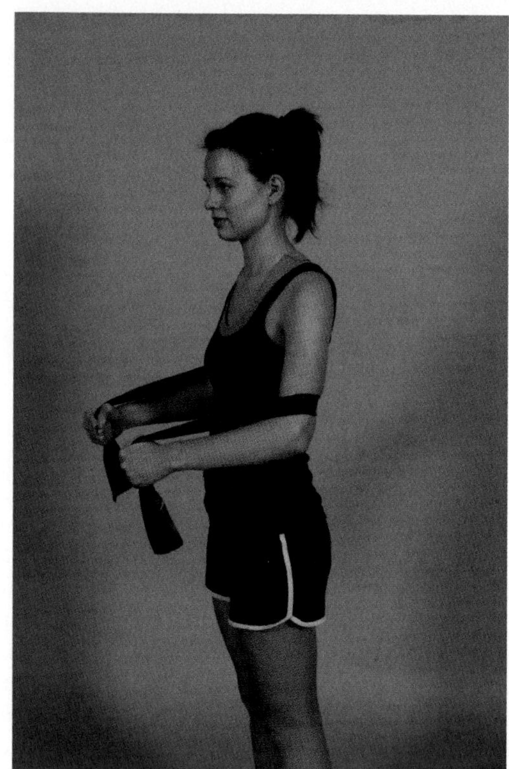

FIGURE 25-79 Tree hug.

Upright Rows Video

The muscles involved with this exercise (Fig. 25-80) include the deltoids, supraspinatus, clavicular portion of the pectoralis major, long head of the biceps, upper and lower portions of the trapezius, levator scapulae, and serratus anterior.

Elastic tubing is placed under the feet and the ends are held in each hand. Keeping the back straight, and the elbows out to the side, the patient raises their hands from about waist height to just below the chin (Fig. 25-80).

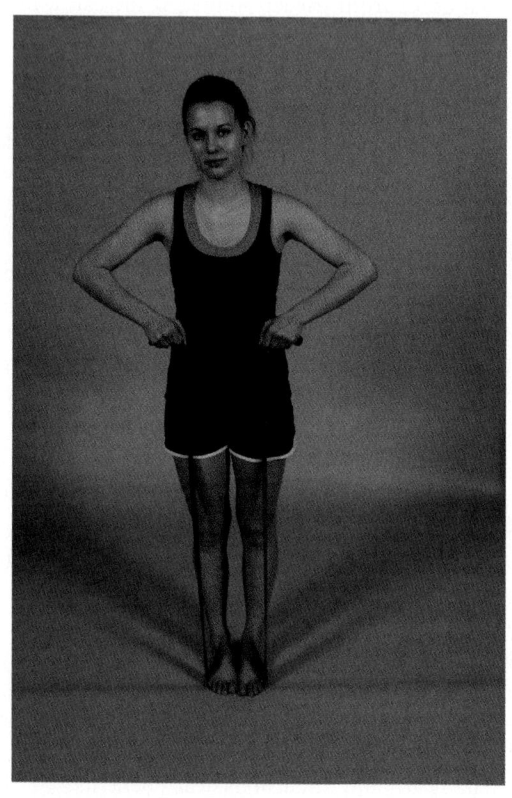

FIGURE 25-80 Upright rows.

Lateral Arm Raise

This exercise (Fig. 25-81) is initiated without resistance. Once it can be performed without pain, resistance in the form of

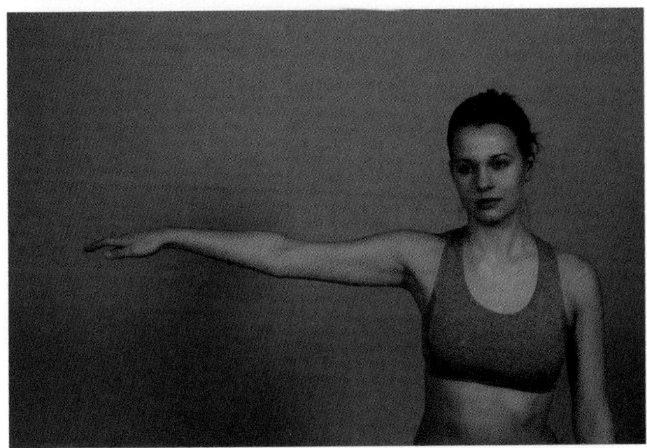

FIGURE 25-81 Lateral arm raise.

tubing or hand weights is added. Lateral arm raises involve the deltoid, supraspinatus, serratus anterior, and upper and lower trapezius.

Front Arm Raise

Again, this exercise (Fig. 25-82) is initiated without resistance. Once it can be performed without pain, resistance in the form of tubing or hand weights is added. Front arm raises involve the anterior deltoid, pectoralis major (upper portion), coracobrachialis, serratus anterior, and upper and lower trapezius.

Cervical Retraction Against Gravity

To strengthen the cervicothoracic stabilizers, the patient is positioned prone, with the head off the end of the bed and supported in a protracted position of the neck. The patient is asked to retract the chin from this position, raising the head toward the ceiling, while maintaining the face parallel to the floor (see Fig. 25-14).

Gravity Cervical Stabilization

These exercises can be performed into extension, rotation VIDEO, and side bending VIDEO. Cervical side translations also can be performed against gravity.

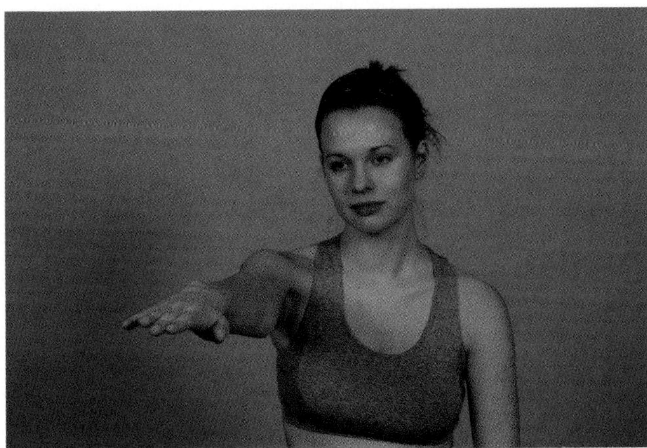

FIGURE 25-82 Front arm raise.

Closed kinetic chain activities can also be very helpful in rehabilitating weak shoulder girdle muscles and the cervical stabilizers (see Chap. 16).

It should be emphasized that all exercises should be performed correctly and without pain, although some degree of postexercise soreness can be expected. Isokinetic exercises of the neck are not functional and are not recommended as a strengthening tool.

Strength training can progress to manually resisted cervical stabilization exercises in various planes. Cervical proprioceptive neuromuscular facilitation patterns are ideal for this purpose (Chap. 10). Muscle cocontraction of agonist and antagonist can be used for joint stabilization, by increasing joint stiffness and supporting the independent torque-producing role of the muscles that surround the joint.[230–232]

Continued efforts must be made to progressively reduce the patient's pain and advance physical function through exercise.[137] However, the use of pain medication to help control pain and inflammation, probably helps patients to progress, while experiencing considerably less pain and enabling their return to work.

Ergonomics

The patient's workstation and lifestyle ergonomics should be addressed (Table 25-18). A chair that provides adequate support and encourages the patient to maintain lumbar lordosis provides a stable platform for the cervical spine.[233] The feet should easily touch the floor, and the thighs should be horizontal to the ground. Computer monitors should be positioned to allow a slight 20-degree downward slope of the eyes.

Postural Retraining

It is important to retrain the patient to assume a correct upright and neutral spine position and to be able to consciously activate and hold the supporting muscles in a variety of functional positions.[68] Few studies have investigated the association between posture and active range of motion. Hanten and colleagues[234] measured resting head posture and total range between full protraction and retraction in the horizontal plane, in subjects with and without neck pain, and found that the neck pain group had less range than the normal group. Lee and colleagues[235] investigated associations between subclinical neck pain/discomfort, and range of motion and physical dimensions of the cervicothoracic spine. Their data suggested that there are early range changes associated with the development of neck pain.

The retraining of the cervicothoracic postural muscles usually begins at the lumbopelvic region, ensuring that the patient does not adopt the chest-out, shoulders-back position, which results in an incorrect thoracolumbar or thoracic lordosis, rather than a correct balance between all of the spinal curves.[68]

Overall Strength and Fitness

Strengthening of the entire kinetic chain should always be a consideration but will depend on the physical requirements of the patient. Strengthening exercises for the kinetic chain can

TABLE 25-18 Workstation Setup and Keyboard Technique Checklist

Fault	Correction
Visual field	
Monitor positioned to side of keyboard	Monitor directly in front of chair and parallel to keyboard
Stationary monitor	Monitor mounted on adjustable support
Screen too high or too low	10–15-degree downward viewing angle to center of screen
Copy on desk surface	Copy secured along side of monitor
Glare from direct and reflected light	Clean antiglare screen (glare filter and angle screen away from window)
Overhead fluorescent lights	Task-appropriate lighting
Incorrect focal distance for visual acuity	Focal distance (eyeglasses) corrected for computer use (i.e., 20–24 in)
Posture	
Head forward	Ears aligned with shoulders; chin retracted
Shoulders elevated	Shoulder girdle muscle balance
Scapular winging	Scapulothoracic proximal stability
Hypertonic upper trapezii	Lower keyboard or desk height
Shoulder protraction/internal rotation	Neutral shoulder alignment
Elbow flexion >90 degrees	Keyboard parallel to or slightly below elbow level (i.e., 80–90 degrees of elbow flexion)
Elbow flexion <80 degrees	Keyboard moved closer to minimize reach
Wrist flexion or extension	Height of keyboard or chair adjusted to achieve wrist in position of function[a]
Elbows locked at sides	Arms stabilized from scapulothoracic region
Wrists against keyboard or desk edge	Hard keyboard or desk edge padded
Wrist extension	Keyboard positive incline eliminated; flat keyboard or negative incline
Wrist ulnar deviation	Reeducate neutral wrist positioning; split keyboard
Finger MCP joint hyperextension	Fingers in position of function
Flat of kyphotic back	Back supports in chair to match individual spinal contours
Stationary chair back and seat pan	Versatile chair allowing forward, upright, and reclined postures; seat pan inclined forward with "waterfall" edge
Hips lower than knees	Seat height raised; seat pan inclined to position hips slightly higher (5–10 degrees) than knees
Feet dangling	Feet flat on floor or foot rest
Keyboard technique	
Wrist extensor/flexor co-contraction	Light key touch; relaxation-biofeedback training
Wrist ulnar deviation	Wrist aligned with forearm
Intrinsic plus keystrike	Hand postures in position of function
Intrinsic minus keystrike (zig-zag)	
Digital extensor habitus	Thumb lightly resting on spacebar; spacebar use with thumb press versus lift and strike
Thumb held in horizontal abduction and extension	
Excessive force of keystrike	Keystrike with finger press versus lift and strike; keystrike with arm bounce
Ulnar deviation at wrist and fingers	Wrist aligned with forearm; use of external rotation–abduction at shoulder for lateral key reach with lateral keystrike
Excessive leaning on wrist rests	Wrist glide versus wrist rest technique
Fifth finger lateral reach and strike	Index finger use for lateral keystrike: slight supination with fifth finger keystrike
Hands play with combination keystrikes	Combination key command efficiency; macroprogram development
Typing too fast	Kinesthetic awareness training
Infrequent breaks and poor work–rest cycles	Periodic rest breaks and task rotation; computer programmed to signal rest breaks

MCP, metacarpophalangeal.

[a]Position of function: forearm, wrist, and hand aligned, 20–30-degree wrist extension, natural curve to digits with MCP joints at about 50 degrees of flexion, and thumb in line with radius.

Data from Rempel DM, Harrison RJ, Barnhart S: Work-related cumulative trauma disorders of the upper extremity. *JAMA* 267:838–842, 1992; Armstrong TJ: Ergonomics and cumulative trauma disorders. *Hand Clin* 2:553–565, 1986.

include lat pull-downs VIDEO, PREs for the middle trapezius and rhomboids VIDEO, and upper extremity PNF patterns VIDEO. It is important throughout the rehabilitation process for patients to maintain their level of cardiovascular fitness as much as possible. Aerobic exercise, which increases endurance and the general sense of well-being, should be a part of all exercise programs.[236,237] Cardiovascular conditioning should be started as soon as possible to prevent deconditioning. These exercises also serve as a great warm-up before a stretching program.

PRACTICE PATTERN 4B: IMPAIRED JOINT MOBILITY, MOTOR FUNCTION, MUSCLE PERFORMANCE, AND RANGE OF MOTION ASSOCIATED WITH IMPAIRED POSTURE

Fiber composition studies have demonstrated that the primary dysfunction in neck muscles is a loss in the tonic supporting capacity, with the dysfunction being greater within the neck flexors.[68,238] Several postural syndromes of the cervical have been identified over the years.

Upper (Proximal) Crossed Syndrome

This syndrome involves adaptive shortening of the levator scapulae, upper trapezius, pectoralis major and minor, SCM, and weakness of the deep neck flexors and lower scapular stabilizers. The syndrome is characterized by[84,85]

- elevation and protraction of the shoulder;
- rotation and abduction of the scapula;
- scapular winging;
- forward head (see discussion that follows);
- decreased stability of the glenohumeral joint;
- increased muscle activity of the levator scapula and trapezius.

The positional changes that occur with the proximal crossed syndrome may alter the structural relationships of the shoulder and the cervical spine. This alteration may result in changes in the length–tension relationships and the kinematics of the scapular and cervical muscles. The consequences of these changes may include posterior nerve root irritation, cervical radiculopathy, segmental hypermobility, and instability at C4–5.[117,239]

The intervention for this syndrome is based on the clinical findings. Any changes in the length–tension relationships should be addressed through stretching and strengthening.

Forward Head

Abnormal posture adaptations have long been considered by many to be the cause of numerous musculoskeletal and neurovascular impairments (see Chap. 6).[51,59,70,240–249] These adaptations are further perpetuated by the natural cycle of aging of the spine, which involves disk degeneration, vertebral wedging, ligamentous calcification, and reduction in the cervical and lumbar lordoses, producing a position of spinal flexion, or stooping.

Habitual movement patterns or positions may contribute to the development of these changes and produce muscular hyperactivity, ligamentous stress, and alteration of the anatomic and biomechanical relationship of the joints. It is theorized that if a muscle lengthens as part of this compensation, muscle spindle activity increases within that muscle, producing reciprocal inhibition of the muscle's functional antagonist, and resulting in an alteration in the normal force–couple and arthrokinematic relationship, thereby affecting the efficient and ideal operation of the movement system.[126,128,250–252]

Because the zygapophyseal joints in the midcervical region incur more weight bearing, as a result of the protruding head, marginal osteophytosis may occur. The common levels for this to occur are C5–6 and C6–7. These changes also alter the scapulothoracic rhythm because of alterations in the muscle tone of the rhomboids and serratus anterior. These altered relations increase the distance between the origin and insertion of the trapezius, of the rhomboid major and minor, and of the levator scapulae, which results in further stress.

The intervention for postural dysfunction focuses on the correction of any strength and flexibility imbalances. Once the mechanical source is identified, the focus is the simultaneous retraining of the muscles, by contracting the lengthened muscle when it is in a shortened position, and stretching the shortened muscle.[128] An exercise program for forward head posture should address underlying soft tissue imbalances by including deep cervical flexor and shoulder retractor strengthening and cervical extensor and pectoral muscle stretching. Therapeutic exercise programs initially should focus on the achievement of good movement patterns. Pearson and Walmsley[253] found that repeated upper cervical retractions changed resting neck posture. Roddey and colleagues[254] demonstrated improvements in resting scapular position following a stretching program of the pectoralis minor muscle. Wright and colleagues[255] in a randomized, controlled study of a postural correction program consisting of scapular strengthening and neck stretching exercises for clients with temporomandibular disorder and pain, reported a significant improvement in symptoms (jaw and neck pain) as compared to the control group.[256]

Recommended exercises include the following:

- The head nod exercise progression.
- The return to normal exercise progression.
- Resisted shoulder retraction exercises in standing using theraband. This is progressed to shoulder retraction in prone using weights.
- Unilateral and bilateral pectoralis minor stretches.
- Exercises to reposition the head into a natural head posture, as appropriate, using a mirror. Once the patient is able to reposition the head with the eyes open, the task is repeated with the eyes closed and the clinician providing feedback.[257]
- Exercises to retrain the oculomotor system. These exercises are initiated by asking the patient to keep the head stationary in the natural head posture and using the eyes to track objects.[257] Once this is mastered, the patient is asked to

combine eye movements and head movements. For example the patient is asked to rotate the head and eyes at the same time in the same direction, then to rotate the head and eyes in the opposite direction at the same time. Obviously, these exercises should not be performed if symptoms such as dizziness and unsteadiness appear. A study by Humphreys and Irgen found that these exercises reduced pain intensity and improved the accuracy of repositioning of the head after 4 weeks of treatment in patients with chronic neck pain, compared with patients who did not receive treatment. However, as the authors acknowledged, a link still has to be made to establish the connection between craniovertebral kinesthesia, head reposition accuracy, and neck pain.

PATTERN 4D: IMPAIRED JOINT MOBILITY, MOTOR FUNCTION, MUSCLE PERFORMANCE, AND FORMAT RANGE OF MOTION ASSOCIATED WITH CONNECTIVE TISSUE DYSFUNCTION

Cervical Disk Pathology

The cervical spine is vulnerable to the same impairments as those of the lumbar spine and any weakness in the surrounding structures results in either a disk bulge or a rupture. Cervical radiculopathy is, by definition, a disorder of the cervical spinal nerve root and, most commonly, is caused by a cervical disk herniation or other space-occupying lesion, resulting in nerve root inflammation, impingement, or both. Considering the structure of the cervical AF, the possibilities that emerge for mechanisms of diskogenic pain are strain or tears of the anterior AF, particularly after hyperextension trauma, and strain of the alar portions of the PLL when stretched by a bulging disk.[9]

Analysis of the anatomic proportions of the cervical spine indicates that cervical diskogenic disease can have an impact on neural structures in the bony spinal canal. The anterior–posterior diameter of the cervical spinal canal tends to be narrower in patients with herniation resulting in myelopathy.[75,258,259] That is, patients with wide canals might be nonmyelopathic even with the same degree of herniation. In the lumbar disk, a prolapse is common. In the cervical spine, a straightforward prolapse is uncommon, and a cervical disk herniation should not be considered as a miniature version of lumbar disk herniation. It is, unlike lumbar disk herniation, extremely rare under the age of 30 years, with the age range of peak incidence between 45 and 54 years, and only slightly less common in the 35–44-year-old group.[260] Acute disk herniations may result in compression of nerve roots. Cervical disks may become painful as part of the degenerative cascade, from repetitive microtrauma, or from macrotrauma. The indication that degeneration plays a greater role in cervical disk herniation may explain why cervical disk herniation is extremely rare in those less than 30 years of age and why the mean age is around 50 years.[261,262]

The most common level of cervical nerve root involvement has been reported at the seventh (C7, 60%) and sixth (C6, 25%),[20,263] followed by C4–5 disk (Table 20-4).[3,261,262] In a study of 18 cadavers by Tanaka et al.,[17] the C5 nerve roots were found to exit over the middle aspect of the IVD, whereas the C6 and C7 nerve roots were found to traverse the proximal part of the disk. The C8 nerve roots had little overlap with the C7–T1 disk in the intervertebral foramen. The C6 and C7 rootlets passed two disk levels in the dural sac. Also, a high incidence of the intradural connections between the dorsal rootlets of C5, C6, and C7 segments was found.[17] These intradural connections between dorsal nerve roots and the relation between the course of the nerve root and the IVD may explain the clinical variation of symptoms resulting from nerve root compression in the cervical spine.[17]

Cervical IVDs with herniation usually remain normal in height or change only slightly without abnormality in the uncovertebral joints.[261] Sclerosis and formation of osteophytes in the uncovertebral joints accompany narrowed disks in spondylosis. These facts indicate that the uncovertebral joints bear a part of the axial load to the IVD in the cervical spine. Accordingly, disk degeneration may play a more important role than trauma in the production of herniation in the cervical spine, and it is common for a patient to awake with a cervical disk herniation, misinterpreting it as a "crick" in the neck.

CLINICAL PEARL

Asymptomatic cervical disk herniation is often found in magnetic resonance images for other diseases.[20] Boden et al.[14] reported the incidence of cervical disk protrusions in the asymptomatic population to be 10–15%, depending on age.

Other factors associated with increased risk include heavy manual labor requiring lifting of more than 25 lb, smoking, and driving or operating vibrating equipment.[264]

Cervical disk degeneration occurs in a predictable fashion. The NP and AF form small cysts[265,266] and fissures as the first disruptive changes after the death of chondrocytes and the separation of fibers or fiber bundles. Subsequently, they extend and unite to form horizontal and vertical clefts.[261] Shearing stress to the disk by translational motion may lead to fibrillation of the matrix, as in osteoarthritic joint cartilage. Some of the vertical clefts extend to the cartilaginous end plate, and portions of the cartilaginous end plate may be torn off.

The cervical IVD is innervated by the sinuvertebral nerve, formed by branches from the anterior (ventral) nerve root and the sympathetic plexus.[267] Once formed, the nerve turns back into the intervertebral foramen along the posterior aspect of the disk, supplying portions of the AF, PLL, periosteum of the vertebral body and pedicle, and adjacent epidural veins. As in the lumbar spine, the pain associated with cervical disk lesions probably occurs from an inflammatory process initiated by nerve root compression, resulting in nerve root swelling.

Within the compressed nerve root, intrinsic blood vessels show increased permeability, which secondarily results in edema of the nerve root.[268] Chronic edema and fibrosis within the nerve root can alter the response threshold and increase the sensitivity of the nerve root to pain.[269] Neurogenic chemical mediators of pain released from the cell bodies of the sensory neurons and nonneurogenic mediators released from disk tissue may play a role in initiating and perpetuating this inflammatory response.[270] The posterior (dorsal) root ganglion has been implicated in the pathogenesis of radicular pain. Prolonged discharges originate from the cell bodies of the posterior (dorsal) root ganglion as a result of brief pressure.[268] In addition to the chemicals produced by the cell bodies of the posterior (dorsal) root ganglion, the membrane surrounding the posterior (dorsal) root ganglion is more permeable than that around the nerve root, allowing a more florid local inflammatory response.[268] The blood supply to the nerve root usually is not compromised by an acute herniation, unless the compression is severe.[21,271] A study involving patients under local anesthesia found that compression of the cervical nerve root produced limb pain, whereas pressure on the disk produced pain in the neck and the medial border of the scapula.[11,272] Intradiskal injection and electrical stimulation of the disk have also suggested that neck pain is referred by a damaged outer AF.[272,273] Muscle spasms of the neck have also been found after electrical stimulation of the disk.

The capacity of the disk to self-repair is restricted by the fact that only the peripheral aspects of the AF receive blood, and a small amount at that.

Numerous clinical examination findings are purported to be diagnostic of cervical radiculopathy including patient history, cervical range of motion limitations, neurologic examination, and specific maneuvers (e.g., Spurling). Most of these items have demonstrated a fair or better level of reliability.[153] However, because the clinical presentation of cervical radiculopathy is so variable, it is advisable to use a combination of test results before making a diagnosis.[153]

It is important to obtain a detailed history to establish a diagnosis of a cervical radiculopathy and to rule out other causes, such as TOS and brachial neuritis. The clinician should first determine the main complaint (i.e., head or neck pain, numbness, weakness, decreased neck function) and location of symptoms.[10,218] Anatomic pain drawings can be helpful by supplying the clinician with a quick review of the pain pattern.

CLINICAL PEARL

Patients with a cervical disk herniation are often younger, whereas patients with radicular symptoms due to cervical disk degeneration are often middle aged.

Henderson and colleagues reviewed the clinical presentations of cervical radiculopathy in 736 patients[274]: 99.4% had arm pain, 85.2% had sensory deficits, 79.7% had neck pain, 71.2% had reflex deficits, 68% had motor deficits, 52.5% had scapular pain, 17.8% had anterior chest pain, 9.7% had headaches, 5.9% had anterior chest and arm pain, and 1.3% had left-sided chest and arm pain (cervical angina). Neurologic deficits corresponded with the offending disk level in approximately 80% of patients.[268]

The patient usually reports a history of neck pain before the onset of arm pain. The onset of neck and arm discomfort with cervical disk herniation is usually insidious and can range from a dull ache to severe burning pain.[10,218] The symptoms may be referred to the medial scapula initially and then along the upper or lower arm and into the hand, depending on the nerve root that is involved.[10,218]

Patients with a cervical disk lesion typically have severe pain that prevents them from getting into a comfortable position.[268] The symptoms are usually aggravated by extension or rotation of the head to the side of the pain (the Spurling maneuver) (Fig. 25-56). Aggravation of the symptoms by neck extension often helps differentiate a radicular etiology from muscular neck pain or a pathologic condition of the shoulder with secondary muscle pain in the neck.[268]

The common radicular syndromes of the cervical spine are outlined in Table 25-19.

C2-3 disk herniations are rare,[275] in either traumatic or spontaneous etiology, and affected only 8 of 2786 patients (0.28%) of the surgical cervical spondylotic cases over 10 years in one study.[276] These herniations are difficult to identify on clinical examination, because these patients usually have no specific motor weakness or reflex abnormality. Radiculopathy of the third cervical nerve root results from pathologic changes

TABLE 25-19 Common Radicular Syndromes of the Cervical Spine

Disk Level	Nerve Root	Motor Deficit	Sensory Deficit	Reflex Compromise
C4–5	C5	Deltoid Biceps	Anterolateral shoulder and arm	Biceps
C5–6	C6	Wrist extensors Biceps	Lateral forearm and hand Thumb	Brachoradialis Pronator teres
C6–7	C7	Wrist flexors Triceps Finger extensors	Middle finger	Triceps
C7–T1	C8	Finger flexors Hand intrinsics	Medial forearm and hand and ring and little fingers	None
T1–2	T1	Hand intrinsics	Medial forearm	None

Data from American Medical Association: *Guides to the Evaluation of Permanent Impairment*, 5th ed. Chicago, IL: American Medical Association, 2001.

in the disk between the second and third cervical levels and is unusual. The posterior ramus of the third cervical nerve innervates the suboccipital region, and involvement of that nerve causes pain in this region, often extending to the back of the ear.

Radiculopathy of the fourth cervical nerve root may be an unexplained cause of neck and shoulder pain.[268] Numbness extending from the caudad aspect of the neck to the superior aspect of the shoulder may be present. Difficulty with breathing during exercise may be reported in diaphragmatic involvement (C3–5).

Radiculopathy of the fifth cervical nerve root can present with numbness in an "epaulet" distribution, beginning at the superior aspect of the shoulder and extending laterally to the midpart of the arm.[268] The absence of pain with a range of motion of the shoulder and the absence of impingement signs at the shoulder help to differentiate radiculopathy of the fifth cervical nerve root from a pathologic shoulder condition.[268]

Radiculopathy of the sixth cervical nerve root presents with pain radiating from the neck to the lateral aspect of the biceps, down the lateral aspect of the forearm, to the posterior (dorsal) aspect of the web space between the thumb and the index finger, and into the tips of those digits.[268] Numbness occurs in the same distribution.

The seventh cervical nerve root is considered to be the most frequently involved by cervical radiculopathy. The patient has pain radiating along the back of the shoulder, often extending into the scapular region, down along the triceps, and then along the posterior aspect of the forearm and into the posterior aspect of the long finger.[268] The patient usually pronates the forearm while trying to describe the location of the symptoms, and this is a useful observation in differentiating the hand symptoms from those of sixth cervical radiculopathy and carpal tunnel syndrome.[268]

Radiculopathy of the eighth cervical nerve root usually presents with symptoms extending down the medial aspect of the arm and forearm and into the medial border of the hand and the ulnar two digits.[268] Numbness usually involves the posterior and anterior aspects of the ulnar two digits and hand and may extend up the medial aspect of the forearm. The patient reports difficulty with using the hands for routine daily activities.[268]

Patients can also present with radicular symptoms that result from other pathologies. These can include schwannomas, meningiomas, and benign or malignant vertebral body tumors.[268] A Pancoast tumor of the apical lung can involve the more inferior cervical nerve roots and, additionally, the sympathetic chain.[268] Idiopathic brachial plexus neuritis is thought to be viral in nature and presents with severe arm pain that resolves and leaves behind polyradicular motor deficits. Polyradicular involvement may also be seen with epidural abscesses.[268]

In middle-aged and older patients, the symptoms are often the result of degenerative changes and compression of the neural structures by osteophytes rather than disk herniation. Prior episodes of similar symptoms or localized neck pain are important for the diagnosis and ultimate intervention. The older patient may have had previous episodes of neck pain or give a history of having arthritis of the cervical spine. Leg symptoms associated with neck dysfunction, especially in the elderly, should arouse the suspicion of cervical spondylotic myelopathy.[259]

The position of the head and neck at the time of injury should also be noted. Acute disk herniations and sudden narrowing of the neural foramen may occur from injuries involving cervical extension, side bending, or rotation and axial loading.[277,278]

The clinician should be aware that upper trunk brachial plexus disorders can be confused with a C5 or C6 radiculopathy. This condition, often referred to as a *burner*, or *stinger*, is thought to result from either traction or compressive forces to the brachial plexus or cervical nerve roots.[279,280] At times, electrodiagnostic studies and MRI are needed to establish the diagnosis.

Peripheral nerve entrapment within the upper limb, including entrapment or compression of the suprascapular, median, and ulnar nerves, may also be confused with a cervical radiculopathy[10,218]:

- A suprascapular neuropathy can be confused with a C5 or C6 radiculopathy but would spare the deltoid and biceps muscles.
- C6 and C7 radiculopathies are most likely to be confused with median neuropathies.
- A C8 radiculopathy must be differentiated from ulnar neuropathies and TOS.

It is important to differentiate an eighth cervical radiculopathy from ulnar nerve weakness. The function of the flexor digitorum profundus in the index and long fingers and of the flexor pollicis longus in the thumb can be affected by an eighth cervical radiculopathy, but they are not affected by ulnar nerve entrapment.[268] With the exception of the adductor pollicis, the short thenar muscles are spared with ulnar nerve involvement but are involved with an eighth cervical or first thoracic radiculopathy.[268] Entrapment of the anterior interosseus nerve may masquerade as an eighth cervical or first thoracic radiculopathy, but it does not cause the sensory changes or have thenar muscle involvement.[268]

The head and neck positions or motions that increase or decrease the symptoms can be used by the clinician both to help in the diagnosis and to plan the intervention. Typically, the patient with cervical radiculopathy has a head list away from the side of injury and holds the neck stiffly. These patients complain of increased posterior neck pain with neck positions that cause foraminal narrowing: extension, side bending, or rotation toward the symptomatic side.

Active range of motion is usually reduced in the direction of pain, which is usually extension, rotation, and side bending, either toward or away from the affected nerve root. Side bending away from the affected side can cause increased displacement of a disk herniation upon a nerve root, whereas same-side bending induces pain by an impingement of a nerve root at the site of the neural foramen.[277,278]

Anterior neck pain along the SCM muscle belly, which is aggravated by rotation to the contralateral side, is most often a result of muscular strain.[268] Pain in the posterior neck muscles, which is worsened by flexion of the head, suggests a myofascial etiology.[268] Patients who present with severe pain in the suboccipital region often have pathologic changes in the upper cervical spine.[268] The pain in these patients may radiate to the back of the ear or the lower neck. Rotation of the neck is often markedly restricted.

On palpation, a nonspecific finding is tenderness noted along the cervical paraspinals, along the ipsilateral side of the affected nerve root, and over the upper trapezius. There may also be muscle tenderness along muscles where the symptoms are referred (e.g., medical scapula, proximal arm, and lateral epicondyle), as well as associated hypertonicity or spasm in these painful muscles.

Manual muscle testing determines a nerve root level on physical examination and can detect subtle weakness in a myotomal, or key muscle, distribution. Weakness of shoulder abduction suggests C5 pathology, elbow flexion and wrist extension weakness suggests a C6 radiculopathy, weakness of elbow extension and wrist flexion can occur with a C7 radiculopathy, and weakness of thumb extension and ulnar deviation of the wrist is seen in C8 radiculopathies.[272]

On sensory examination, a dermatomal pattern of diminished, or loss of, sensation should be present. In addition, patients with radiculitis may have hyperesthesia to light touch and pinprick examination.[272] The sensory examination can be quite subjective, however, in as much as it requires patient response.

Muscle stretch reflexes are helpful (see Table 25-19). Any grade of reflex can be normal,[281] so the asymmetry of the reflexes is most helpful:

- The biceps brachii reflex occurs at the level of C5–6. The brachioradialis is another C5–6 reflex.
- The triceps reflex tests the C7–8 nerve roots.
- The pronator reflex can be helpful in differentiating C6 and C7 nerve root problems. If it is abnormal in conjunction with an abnormal triceps reflex, then the level of involvement is more likely to be C7. This reflex is performed by tapping the anterior aspect of the forearm, with the forearm in a neutral position and the elbow flexed.[281,282]

Little is known about the natural history of cervical radiculopathy, and there are few controlled randomized studies comparing operative with conservative intervention, although the outcome data support the concept that an extruded disk actually may have a more favorable prognosis than contained disk pathology.[217,283]

Conservative intervention consists of modified rest, a cervical collar, oral corticosteroid "dose-packs," and NSAIDs.[284,285] Oral corticosteroids have been used to reduce the associated inflammation from compression, although there is no controlled study to support their use in the intervention of cervical radiculopathy.[217,277] The beneficial effect of corticosteroids may occur as a result of the anti-inflammatory properties of these drugs. Cervical epidural corticosteroids have also been used in patients who have not responded to medications, traction, and a well-designed physical therapy program.

Exercise programs for patients with disk herniations are individualized.[218] Cervical and cervicothoracic stabilization exercises form the basis of the therapeutic exercise progression. Most patients obtain analgesia using the controlled use of cervical retraction or posterior gliding of the lower cervical spine, in combination with extension of the lower cervical spine and flexion of the upper cervical spine (chin tuck),[286] although repetitive use of this exercise has the potential to cause harm and should be used only as long as the patient is achieving benefit.

The majority of studies investigating the outcomes of patients with cervical radiculopathy have used generic self-report measures or measures of pain. Two condition-specific measures that have been shown to be reliable and valid in patients with cervical radiculopathy are the NDI (Chap. 5) and the Patient Specific Functional Scale.[287]

Surgical Intervention

Surgical intervention is reserved for patients with persistent radicular pain who do not respond to conservative measures (see later discussion).[288] In general, the decision to proceed with surgical intervention is made when a patient has significant extremity or myotomal weakness, progressive neurologic deficits, severe unremitting pain, or pain that persists beyond an arbitrary "conservative" intervention period of 8–12 weeks.[289] Based on this criteria, surgical treatment for cervical disk herniation is needed in only a very small percentage of individuals. Compressive pathologic lesions causing cervical radiculopathy (soft disk fragment herniation or spondylotic bone spurs) are most often located anterior to the nerve root.[290] Typically, lateral cervical disks are removed by the posterior approach, whereas the anterior approach is used with prolapsed midline disks that compromise the spinal cord, or some paramedian disks that compromise either the spinal cord or the nerve root but do not extend beyond the lateral margin of the cervical cord.[291]

The common surgical procedures for cervical disk injuries include (1) anterior cervical discectomy and fusion, (2) laminectomy and laminotomy–facetectomy, (3) laminectomy or laminoplasty (with or without fusion), and (4) anterior corpectomy and fusion.

Anterior Cervical Discectomy and Fusion

A herniated disk in the neck is commonly approached anteriorly. Both lateral and central disks can be removed through this anterior approach. The results from cervical diskectomy have shown an approximately 95% chance of good-to-excellent relief from the radiating arm pain.[285] Numbness in the upper extremity generally improves. Typically, the patient may resume full, unrestricted activities within 3–6 months following surgery. Complications from this surgery are very rare, with the most common being a transient sore throat, hoarseness, difficulty swallowing, failure of bony fusion, and pseudoarthrosis. Although fusions provide inherent stability to the motion segment and immobilize potentially painful degenerative disk and facet joints, the disadvantages, especially in a highly mobile cervical spine segment, include the increased possibility of further progression of degenerative changes at other disk levels, which eventually requires further surgery.[292]

Anterior Corpectomy and Fusion

The anterior approach for this technique is the same as for the anterior cervical discectomy and fusion. The appropriate disks are incised and removed back from the PLL. The cervical spine is stabilized after corpectomy with strut bone grafts. Internal fixation is often indicated to provide additional rigidity. Postoperatively a rigid cervical orthosis is typically used.

Laminectomy

This procedure, typically indicated for spinal stenosis, is designed to resect the lamina on one or both sides, to increase the axial space available for the spinal cord. The indication in the context of cervical disk disease is when more than three levels of disk degeneration with anterior spinal cord compression are present. Single-level cervical disk herniation is ideally managed from the anterior approach. The complications of the posterior approach include instability leading to kyphosis, recalcitrant myofascial pain, and occipital headaches. Post-laminectomy kyphosis requires revision surgery. If preexistent kyphosis is present, an anterior approach is favorable because in a patient with kyphosis, laminectomy may accelerate kyphosis. As an alternative to laminectomy, a foraminotomy can be used to remove a single-level unilateral lateral disk herniation. This involves removal of 50% of the zygapophyseal joint on one side. This procedure is effective when radicular arm pain is greater than axial neck pain. Foraminotomy can also be performed anteriorly and has a success rate of 91% in relieving radicular pain.[292]

Laminaplasty

Laminaplasty is commonly indicated for multilevel spondylotic myelopathy. Comparative studies with laminectomy have shown that patients with laminaplasty have superior functional recovery in spondylotic myelopathy.[293–296] The incidence of spinal cord injury with laminaplasty is approximately 10 times lower than that of laminectomy.[293–296] Nerve root injury is commonly seen in about 11% of the surgeries.[293–296] This complication is unique to laminaplasty, and the suggested etiology is traction on the nerve root with posterior migration of the spinal cord.[293–296]

In the best-case scenario, the surgeon chooses the technique that directly eliminates the nerve-compressing lesion, while preserving the motion segment of the spine. The anterior microforaminotomy procedure has shown promising results in preserving the remaining disk and the intervertebral space as much as possible, while directly eliminating the compressive pathologic lesion.[297,298] The advantages of this technique are many, including removal of only the offending mass, preservation of most of the disk and motion segment, a shorter operative procedure and hospital stay, avoidance of a fusion procedure and the attendant potential problems, and an earlier return to full activity. The disadvantages are the long-term issues related to disk degeneration and unilateral removal of an uncovertebral joint.[292]

Patients who undergo spinal surgery may receive physical therapy as part of their rehabilitation. Although there is a large amount of information from evidence-based clinical practice guidelines for the management of many musculoskeletal conditions, there is relatively little information available on the physical therapy management of patients who have undergone spinal surgery.

The RCTs comparing various physical activity programs[299–302] have demonstrated the benefits of these programs. These benefits have included less pain and disability, improved range of motion, and greater satisfaction with care.

Before the surgery, the patients may receive advice on spine care, postsurgical precautions, and instructions on basic exercises.

The postsurgical intervention following surgery is as varied as the number of types of surgery. The following are guidelines for postsurgical rehabilitation. The primary goals for the initial period following the surgery are

- reduction of pain and inflammation;
- prevention of postsurgical complications;
- protection of the surgical site;
- prevention of a recurrent herniation;
- maintenance of dural mobility;
- improvement of function;
- minimizing of the detrimental effects of immobilization.[303–308]
- Early return to appropriate functional activities. Patients usually are permitted to shower 1 week after the surgery.
- Safe return to occupational duties. Patients with a sedentary occupation may return to work within 7–10 days after the surgery. Prolonged positions and postures are to be avoided.
- Patient education on correct body mechanics and independent self-care.

The patient is given guidance on the gradual resumption of daily activities. Immobilization or prolonged rest should be avoided. Instead, the patient is encouraged to walk for short periods and distances several times a day.

Outpatient physical therapy, if appropriate, usually begins in the second or third week. The physical therapy examination includes

- a thorough history;
- inspection of the wound site;
- anthropometric data;
- postural examination;
- neural examination, including neurodynamic mobility, and strength testing.

The components of the physical therapy intervention include a graded exercise program, with gentle range of motion, submaximal isometrics, and arm and leg exercises as appropriate.

Additional interventions may include electrotherapeutic modalities, physical agents, and scar massage. Patient education is very important, particularly postural education and information on body mechanics.

Progressive strengthening exercises for the spinal stabilizers usually are initiated by the fourth postoperative week.

Cardiovascular conditioning exercises are introduced at the earliest opportunity based on patient tolerance. These include riding a stationary bicycle, using an upper body ergonometer and a stair-stepper, and swimming in a pool. The sessions for these exercises are initially brief (5–10 minutes) and are gradually increased up to 30–60 minutes.

Activities such as jogging are usually permitted at 6–8 weeks if there is minimal pain. When the patient does resume these activities, they should be done in the morning hours when the IVD is maximally hydrated.[309] High-impact sports such as basketball and soccer are usually permitted after the 12th week.

Cervical Spondylosis

Cervical spondylosis is a chronic degenerative condition affecting the contents of the spinal canal (nerve roots and/or spinal cord) and the cervical vertebral bodies and IVDs, is the most common cause of progressive spinal cord and nerve root compression. The characteristics of degenerative joint disease (DJD) and degenerative disk disease (DDD) relate to bony changes, and the two often occur concurrently.[8] Abnormalities in the osseous and the fibroelastic boundaries of the bony cervical spinal canal or in the lateral recess, and foramina affect the availability of space for spinal cord and nerve roots, resulting in a myelopathy or stenosis, respectively. Cyriax[163,106] reserved the term *spondylosis* for the end stage of spinal diseases, although the term is now used to describe varying levels of degenerative changes in the cervical spine.[8] Although this condition often remains asymptomatic for a long time, it can become a major influence in the production of radiculomyelopathic compressive disturbances, when other conditions such as spondylosis, diskal hernia, and trauma become superimposed. As the resulting space for neural structures becomes smaller, the risk of developing motor and/or sensory disturbances increases.

Progressive degenerative changes are expected to appear over time on radiographs as part of the natural history of the aging spine. Radiographic evidence of cervical degeneration is observed in some 30-year olds and is present in more than 90% of people older than 60 years of age.[310] The areas most commonly and most severely affected are C5–6 and C6–7.[33] Although aging of the cervical spine is ubiquitous, controversy remains about whether the process of spondylosis may be accelerated in patients with a history of soft tissue injuries to the neck and persistent pain. However, in the absence of pain, the finding of degenerative changes on radiographs should not be misconstrued as pathologic. One study reported evidence of cervical spondylosis in 35% of asymptomatic individuals.[311]

Kirkaldy-Willis[312] categorized spondylosis of the spine into three stages:

- Dysfunctional. During this stage, the patient complains of a gradual onset of neck or arm symptoms (radiculopathy), or both, that have increased frequency and severity.[8]
- Unstable. During this stage, the pain is often worse when the patient is in certain positions, and can interfere with sleep. Morning stiffness of the neck, which gradually improves throughout the day, is a common finding.
- Stabilization. During this stage, lateral nerve root entrapment becomes more common. In some cases the spinal cord or anterior spinal vessels may be compressed resulting in cervical myelopathy and/or vertebrobasilar insufficiency.[313] The blood supply of the spinal cord is an important anatomic factor in the pathophysiology. Radicular arteries in the dural sleeves tolerate compression and repetitive minor trauma poorly. The spinal cord and canal size are also factors.

CLINICAL PEARL

Osteoarthritis in the cervical spine is, in effect, the later stages of spondylosis, and is marked by progressive degeneration of the IVD and, especially, the zygapophyseal joint. Osteoarthritic changes can include osteophyte formation, hypertrophy of the synovial membrane and, in some cases, a chronic inflammatory response.

The physical examination findings depend on the degree of severity but can include reduced motion in the sagittal plane, with a decrease in side bending in the early stages. As the degeneration progresses, a capsular pattern develops.[163] Cervical spondylotic myelopathy is the most serious consequence of cervical IVD degeneration, especially when it is associated with a narrow cervical vertebral canal. Five categories of cervical spondylotic myelopathy are described in Table 25-20, based on the predominant neurologic findings.

TABLE 25-20 Characteristics of the Different Syndromes of Cervical Spondylotic Myelopathy

Syndrome	Pain	Gait Abnormality	Involvement of the Extremities	Laterality
Lateral (radicular)	Yes	Sometimes	Upper	Often unilateral
Medial (myelopathic)	No	Yes	Lower	Usually bilateral
Combined	Sometimes	Yes	Upper and lower	Unilateral in upper extremities and bilateral in lower extremities
Vascular	No	Yes	Upper and lower	Bilateral
Anterior (painless weakness of the upper extremity)	No	No	Upper	Often unilateral

Data from Spivak JM, DiCesare PE, Feldman DS: *Orthopaedics: A Study Guide*. New York: McGraw-Hill, 1999:349.

Myelography, with CT, is usually the imaging test of choice to assess spinal and foraminal stenosis.

The conservative intervention for cervical spondylosis without radiculopathy or myelopathy involves the use of electrotherapeutic modalities to control pain and increase the extensibility of the connective tissue. These modalities usually include moist heat, electrical stimulation, and ultrasound. Immobilization of the cervical spine may be considered for patients with nerve irritation to limit the motion of the neck and further irritation. In such instances, soft cervical collars are recommended initially. More rigid orthoses (e.g., Philadelphia collar and Minerva body jacket) can significantly immobilize the cervical spine. With the use of any of the braces, the patient's tolerance and compliance are under consideration. The use of the brace should be discontinued as soon as feasible. Molded cervical pillows can better align the spine during sleep and provide symptomatic relief for some patients. Manual techniques may be used to stretch the adaptively shortened tissues. Range-of-motion exercises are performed as tolerated. These exercises initially are performed in the pain-free direction and then in the direction of pain. As the patient regains motion, isometric exercises and cervical stabilization exercises are prescribed.

Zygapophyseal Joint Dysfunction

The patient with a zygapophyseal joint dysfunction typically reports an onset of unilateral neck pain, or "neck locking," following sudden backward bending, side bending, or rotation of the neck, or pain that followed a sustained head position. The condition is thought to result from entrapment of a small piece of synovial membrane by the zygapophyseal joint.[99,115,314]

Palpation just lateral to the midline often indicates regional soft tissue changes in response to the underlying zygapophyseal joint injury, and combined motion testing usually shows a closing pattern of restriction corresponding to the injured zygapophyseal joint.[98]

Because traditional images (plain radiographs, computed tomography, and MRI) are typically unremarkable in the presence of zygapophyseal joint pain,[314] clinical suspicions of these joint injuries can be confirmed if necessary by diagnostic intra-articular zygapophyseal joint injections, or a block of the joint's nerve supply.[315,316]

The conservative intervention involves the use of cryotherapy and electrotherapeutic modalities to control pain and inflammation. Joint mobilization techniques, involving combinations of flexion or extension and rotation, with traction superimposed, are applied initially in the pain-free direction and then in the direction of pain.

As the patient regains motion, range-of-motion and isometric exercises are prescribed until full range of motion is restored, at which time the strengthening exercises are progressed.

An interesting study by Cleland and colleagues[317] investigated the predictive validity [clinical prediction rule (CPR)] of variables from the initial examination to identify patients with neck pain who are likely to benefit from thoracic spine thrust manipulation. The study identified a CPR with six variables are as follows:

1. Symptoms of less than 30 days
2. No symptoms distal to the shoulder
3. Looking up does not aggravate symptoms
4. Fear avoidance-beliefs questionnaire (FABQ) (see Chap. 4) physical activity score less than 12.
5. Diminished upper thoracic spine kyphosis
6. Cervical extension range of motion less than 30 degrees

The study found that if three of these (positive likelihood ratio = 5.5) were present, the chance of experiencing a successful outcome from a thoracic spine thrust manipulation improved from 54 to 86%.

Acute Torticollis (Acute Wry Neck)

Torticollis is both a symptom and a disease. An acute form of torticollis, known as acute wryneck, typically develops overnight in young and middle-aged adults. The precise etiology is unclear, but as most patients appear to experience symptoms shortly after awakening, it may be the result of an injury to the muscles, joints, or ligaments through sleeping with the neck in an unusual position. This unusual position may place the involved joints in a position of extreme motion, stretching the structures and increasing the risk of impingement when the joint position is returned to normal.

The most common clinical presentation includes painful neck, which are both visible and palpable. There is a marked limitation in range of motion of the neck and the patient may hold the head in a position of comfort toward the side of the involved muscle. A common feature is the presence of limited to no radiographic correlation between the degree of pain presented by the patient in the neck and the degree of radiographic changes.

The hanging head method is a simple but successful method for treating acute painful wry neck of spontaneous onset.[318] The technique requires a table with the capacity to tilt the head down. The patient is positioned in supine at the end of the table and a head down tilt of about 20 degrees is provided. This position, which is maintained for 5–10 minutes, provides a gentle traction force allowing the SCM to relax. Alternatively, gentle traction can be applied manually. If this treatment is successful, no further intervention is necessary. In the cases where this technique is unsuccessful, the patient is reassured that they have a self limiting condition, and that the symptoms will usually resolve significantly within 7 days, with complete resolution within 2 weeks.[319]

Cervical Spine Instability

Punjabi defined clinical stability as "the ability of the spine, under physiological load, to limit patterns of displacement so as not to damage or irritate the spinal cord or nerve roots, and, in addition, to prevent incapacitating deformity or pain due to structural changes."[320] Cervical instability can occur secondary to trauma, surgery, systemic disease, or degenerative changes to the motion segment. Signs and symptoms associated with minor cervical instability include[107]

- history of major trauma;
- reports of catching/locking/giving way;
- unpredictability of symptoms;
- subjective reports of neck weakness (head feels heavy);
- altered range of motion;
- neck pain with or without muscle spasms;
- reports of headaches.

To date, there is no gold standard for diagnosing minor instability in the mid-cervical spine, only a high degree of suspicion based on signs and symptoms. In these cases, a cervicothoracic stabilization program is recommended to restore lost functional capacities, range of motion, muscular strength, and endurance.

PATTERN 4E: IMPAIRED JOINT MOBILITY, MOTOR FUNCTION, MUSCLE PERFORMANCE, AND RANGE OF MOTION ASSOCIATED WITH LOCALIZED INFLAMMATION

Whiplash-Associated Disorders

Over recent years, the role of the physical therapist in the intervention of the consequences of whiplash has increased dramatically. It is thus imperative that the clinician have a strong understanding of the mechanisms that produce the myriad of symptoms associated with this disorder.

The term *whiplash injury* was introduced in 1928 by the American orthopedist H. E. Crowe,[321] and it was defined as the effects of sudden acceleration–deceleration forces on the neck and upper trunk as a result of external forces exerting a "lash-like effect." Crowe emphasized that the term *whiplash* "describes only the manner in which a head was moved suddenly to produce a sprain in the neck."

Despite a great deal of attention, WADs remain an enigma as the subjective nature and high prevalence of the symptoms, in the absence of focal physical findings and positive imaging studies, have led to controversy over their cause.[322] In addition, the diagnosis has been associated with issues of financial compensation.[323–325]

Definition

There is little agreement as to the definition of WAD. Some authors of whiplash articles, such as Gay and Abbot,[326] do not define whiplash clearly. Neither Gotten,[327] nor Macnab[328,329] offered definitions, although Macnab noted that "a significant soft tissue injury can result from the application of an extension strain to the neck by sudden acceleration."[261] And Farbman[330] classified the whiplash injury as a musculoligamentous neck sprain, which did not involve nerve root damage, fractures, and other complications. Nordhoff[331] describes the whiplash injury in equally simplistic terms, as an injury that occurs because of occupant motions within a vehicle that is rapidly decelerating or accelerating, without reference to the body parts involved. Even the definition provided by the Quebec Task Force on WADs,[332] that, for whatever reason, did not include front-end collisions, offered the following vague definition:

Whiplash is an acceleration–deceleration mechanism of energy transfer to the neck. It may result from rear-end or side-impact motor vehicle collisions, but can also occur through diving and other mishaps. The impact may result in bony or soft tissue injuries (whiplash injury), which in turn may lead to a variety of clinical manifestations.

Mechanism

A number of mechanisms have been proposed that result in a WAD. These include

- motor vehicle accidents (MVAs);
- sporting injuries involving a blow to the head or neck, or a heavy landing;
- pulls and thrusts on the arms;
- falls, landing on the trunk or shoulder.

Perhaps the most common mechanism of WAD is the MVA. According to reports, more than 1 million whiplash injuries occur each year in the United States.[324] Eighteen percent of MVAs involving passenger cars in the United States in 1994 were rear-end impacts.[333]

The extent of injury from a WAD following an MVA depends, in part, on three factors: (1) the position of the head at the point of impact, (2) the amount of force involved, and (3) the direction of those forces.

Head Position

Pure extension injuries seem to be uncommon in a WAD, because most injuries involve forced combinations of motion. These include a flexion or extension force applied to a rotated head and neck, resulting from a turned position on impact.[334] As many as 57% of persons sustaining whiplash injury, with symptoms persisting 2 years after collisions, reported having their heads rotated out of the anatomic position at the time of impact.[335,336] In fact, head position has been reported as the only accident feature of a collision event that has a statistically significant correlation with symptom duration.[336]

Amount of Force

The amount of force applied to the neck is approximately equal to the weight of the head and the speed with which the head moves. Consequently, the heavier the head or the faster it moves, the greater the stress that is put through the neck. However, it is well recognized by clinicians with any experience with post-MVA patients that some patients who have survived high-velocity accidents do better than many who appear to have been involved in trivial impacts.

Force Direction

Force direction plays a significant role in the degree of damage sustained by the patient. The direction of the applied forces depends on[96]

1. where the car is hit, that is, front end, rear end, or side;
2. symmetry of the impact, that is, directly head on or rear end, or the forward or backward side;

3. whether the car is pushed ahead into another vehicle, the curb, or other stationary object;
4. the position of the victim in relation to the impact.

During the early phase of a rear-end collision, the occupant's trunk is forced upward toward the head, and the cervical spine undergoes a sigmoid deformation, resulting in the head being moved upward and backward.[337] During this motion, at about 100 milliseconds after impact, the lower cervical vertebrae undergo extension, but without translation.[337] This motion causes the vertebral bodies to separate anteriorly and the zygapophyseal joints to impact posteriorly.[337] These forces may lead to posterior dislocations.[328,338,339]

The reason for the greater severity of hyperextension injuries over the other force directions is believed to be related to several factors, including[331]

- whether the seat back breaks;
- whether the occupant hits the front of the occupant space;
- the differential motion between the seat back and occupant;
- hyperextension of the neck over the head restraint;
- rebound neck flexion as the head rebounds off the head rest.

Hyperflexion injuries are typically less severe because the amount of head excursion is limited by the chin striking the chest. The damage incurred by cervical side-bending traumas depends on whether the head hits an object or the shoulder.[96]

A number of other variables also determine the type and extent of the injury[331]

- seat position;
- occupant size, height, and posture;
- vehicle interior design;
- size of vehicle.
- Sex of driver. Women generally position their seats more forward than men, which places their bodies closer to the front car structures and, therefore, at higher risk of impacting the front interior.
- Seat belt. The subject of seat belts is controversial, because the seatbelt appears to be responsible for more injuries than any other contact source in the car, albeit minor ones.[340] This is, in part, because of their design, which restrains only one shoulder, and because the belt acts as a fulcrum for energy concentration on the occupant.[331] As of 1997, federal law has required all passenger vehicles to have air bags. Mortality reductions in frontal collisions associated with airbags have been estimated to be no greater than 25–30%[341] and perhaps substantially less[342] when compared with the approximately 50% reduction associated with proper use of seat belts.[343] Because airbags provide supplemental protection for occupants wearing a seat belt, it is necessary to compare the combined effect of airbags and seat belts either relative to device alone or completely unrestrained in order to adequately evaluate their effectiveness. A study by McGwin and colleagues[344] conducted a retrospective cohort study of front seat occupants involved in police-reported, tow-away, frontal motor vehicle collisions, using data from the 1995 to 2000 National Automotive Sampling System. Compared with completely unrestrained occupants, those using a seat belt alone or in combination with an airbag had a reduced overall risk of injury (relative risks, 0.42 and 0.71, respectively); no association was observed for those restrained with an airbag only (relative risk, 0.98). The study concluded that airbag deployment does not appear to significantly reduce the risk of injury either alone or in combination with seat belts.[344] Population-based studies of airbag effectiveness against less serious injuries, which have been rare, seem to suggest that airbags may merely be altering the distribution of injuries.[331,345]
- Headrest height. Headrest height appears to play a role, with the driver often setting the head rest too low, or sitting too far forward to obtain adequate support from the head rest.[346,347] However, the fatal accidents involving hyperextension appear to occur in the absence of a head restraint, where there is no structural limitation to the head movement except anatomic structures.

Clinical Findings

It should be obvious that a meticulous examination of the traumatized patient is of paramount importance.[348] Signs and symptoms to alert the clinician include

- UMN signs and symptoms;
- periodic loss of consciousness;
- that the patient does not move the neck, even slightly (fractured dens);
- painful weakness of the neck muscles (fracture);
- gentle traction and compression of the neck that are painful (fracture);
- severe muscle spasm (fracture);
- complaints of dizziness.

The symptoms following a WAD usually begin in the neck and interscapular area within a few hours of the injury. Headaches often accompany the neck and shoulder girdle symptoms.[111]

Sources of Symptoms

The causes for symptoms following a whiplash injury are numerous. The resulting damage from a WAD can include an injury to one or more of the following types of structures:

- ***Soft tissue structures.***[101] A cervical strain may be produced by an overload injury to the cervical muscle–tendon unit because of excessive forces. These forces can result in the elongation and tearing of muscles or ligaments, edema, hemorrhage, and inflammation. Many cervical muscles do not terminate in tendons but, instead, attach directly to bone by myofascial tissue that blends into the periosteum.[349] Muscles respond to injury in a variety of ways, including reflex contraction, which further increases the resistance to stretch and serves as a protection to the injured muscle.
- ***Joint capsule and ligaments.*** Both mechanoreceptors and nociceptors have been identified in the human cervical joint capsule[350] and ligaments,[314] indicating a neural input in

pain sensation and proprioception. Postmortem studies have found that after whiplash injuries, ligamentous injuries are extremely common in the cervical spine, but that herniation of the NP is a rare event.[351–354] The motion segment lesions found in the cervical spine included bruising and hemorrhage of the uncinate region, the so-called rim lesions or transections of the anterior annulus fibrosus, rupture of the alar ligaments, and avulsions of the vertebral end plate.[351–355] As in the lumbar spine, the outer layers of the cervical annulus are innervated,[356] and are, therefore, a reasonable source of pain.[357]

- ***Zygapophyseal joint.*** Fractures or contusions of the zygapophyseal joints can occur, although postmortem studies reveal that many of these injuries are undetectable by plain radiographs.[351,355,358,359] Zygapophyseal joint pain is the only basis for chronic neck pain after whiplash that has been subjected to scientific scrutiny.[115,360,361] However, it cannot be diagnosed clinically or by medical imaging. The diagnosis relies on fluoroscopically guided, controlled diagnostic blocks of the painful joint. Although there is uncertainty about the exact pathway that elicits neck pain, the cervical zygapophyseal joint has been identified as a source of pain in between 25 and 65% of people with neck pain.[115,314–316,362–364] Specifically, the prevalence of lower cervical facet joint pain has been reported to be 49%.[363] It is worth remembering that although the so-called neck sprains from MVAs usually involve the cervical spine, one of the upper eight thoracic spinal joints is sometimes found to be affected, so these structures should be assessed in the examination of a whiplash injury.[365]
- ***Central or peripheral neurologic systems.*** These systems may be injured secondary to traction, impingement, hemorrhage, avulsion, or concussion. Although neck pain and headache are the two most common symptoms of a whiplash injury,[4] other symptoms such as visual disturbances, balance disorders, and altered cerebral function are reported. In 1927, Klein and Nieuwenhuyse[366] first demonstrated that simple rotation of the patient's neck, while the head was maintained fixed, caused vertigo and nystagmus. In 1976, Toglia[367] reported objective electronystagmography (ENG) abnormalities in about 57% of 309 patients with whiplash injuries. Wing and Hargrove-Wilson[368] reported that all of their 80 patients showed nystagmus in ENG records with the head flexed, extended, or rotated to the right and left. Abnormal peripheral vestibular function was found using platform posturography in about 90% of the 48 patients examined by Chester.[369] Fractures and dislocations, many causing cord damage, have been demonstrated on human victims of hyperextension injuries, who had no radiographic evidence of the severity of these lesions.[96,370]
- ***Intervertebral disk.*** Experimental and clinical studies have consistently demonstrated how poorly and slowly disk lesions heal after a hyperextension trauma, with very small lesions taking as long as 18 months to heal.[359,371] A follow-up study, averaging a review time of nearly 11 years,[372] found that 40% of patients were still having intrusive or severe symptoms (12% severe and 28% intrusive). The same study also found that in general, the symptoms did not alter after 2 years postaccident.
- ***Posterior (dorsal) root ganglia.***[359]
- ***Vascular structures (vertebrobasilar arteries).*** Postmortem studies have shown that vertebral artery lesions are found in about one-third of fatally injured MVA victims with vertebral atlas injury.[373]
- ***Visceral structures (secondary to ruptures, or contusions).***

The physical examination usually reveals tenderness over the transverse and spinous processes, or over the anterior vertebral body, depending on the structures involved. Depending on the severity of the strain, motion can be markedly restricted as a result of muscle guarding.

Other than perhaps to screen for possible fractures, there is no valid indication for medical imaging after whiplash, unless the patient has neurologic signs.[322] Findings on plain films are typically normal, although there may be a loss of the cervical lordosis. MRI reveals nothing but age-related changes with the same prevalence as in asymptomatic individuals.[374–376] An enticing, but small, recent study suggests that, in patients with persisting acute neck pain, single photon emission computed tomography, at 4 weeks after injury revealed occult, small fractures of the vertebral rims or the synovial joints of the neck.[377]

Intervention

Once the physician has ruled out the possibility of fracture, dislocation, IVD injury, or neurovascular compromise, a conservative approach is recommended. Initially, brief use of a cervical collar may be prescribed to reduce muscle guarding. Bed rest, along with analgesics and muscle relaxants, for no more than 2–3 days is prescribed for patients with a severe injury. However, in less severe cases, bed rest has not been shown to improve recovery and, when compared with mobilization or patient education, rest tends to prolong symptoms.[25,224]

CLINICAL PEARL

A study by Scholten-Peeters[378] and colleagues reported that the physical prognostic factors associated with delayed recovery following a WAD included decreased mobility of the cervical spine immediately after injury, pre-existing neck trauma, older age, and female gender.

Ice and electrical stimulation are applied to the neck during the first 48–72 hours to help control pain and inflammation. Range-of-motion exercises in the pain-free ranges of flexion and rotation are initiated as early as possible to reduce the likelihood of hypomobility. Gentle cervical isometrics also are introduced. Aggressive strengthening of the cervical musculature should not begin until full range of motion is restored. Strengthening of the trapezius muscle and other scapular stabilizers can be performed using upper extremity exercises, taking care to avoid an increase in symptoms.

Many patients improve within 8 weeks, although complete resolution is less common.[286] If pain persists for more than

3 months, more severe ligamentous, disk, associated zygapophyseal joint injuries, or other factors (see later) should be suspected. If significant neck pain persists past 6–8 weeks, flexion and extension radiographs may be useful to exclude, or confirm, instability.

Outcomes

Studies addressing the natural history of WAD have yielded variable results. In one series, symptoms had resolved in 52% of patients at 8 weeks and in 87% of the patients at 5 months.[379] In another series, most patients rapidly recovered following an acute injury, with some 80% being asymptomatic by 12 months.[335] After 12 months, between 15 and 20% of patients remained symptomatic, and only about 5% were severely affected. In addition to the distress resulting from neck and upper extremity pain, costs to society associated with absenteeism from work also are incurred.

The majority of studies reveal that, although most patients with WAD have a spontaneous resolution of symptoms, a small subgroup of patients are symptomatic beyond 1 year.[322] This group of patients constitutes the major burden to insurance companies and to health care resources, because in spite of aggressive imaging and diagnostic testing, clinicians are routinely unable to identify the specific source of these symptoms or apply interventions that are successful. It is in this small subgroup of patients with persisting chronic symptoms that the need for a better understanding of the risk factors, pathophysiology, natural history, and effectiveness of intervention options is apparent.[322]

When symptoms persist beyond 6 months, evidence for preexisting degenerative disease is most often found.[380] Preexisting symptoms, such as headache, and radiologic degenerative changes appear to be important predictors for an unfavorable outcome.[124]

One study[335] examined a group of 117 consecutive patients, who were followed on a regular basis from shortly after the initial injury through 2 years, to determine whether preinjury status, mechanism of injury, physical examination, and somatic, radiographic, or neuropsychologic factors could be used to predict eventual outcome. At 2 years, the patients with persistent symptoms were found to have been older at the time of injury than the asymptomatic group and had a higher incidence of pretraumatic headache. There was a higher incidence of a rotated, or inclined, head position at the time of impact, as well as a higher intensity of initial neck pain and headache, a higher incidence of initial radicular symptoms, a greater number of initial overall symptoms, and a higher average score on a multiple symptom analysis.[335]

Financial compensation, which is determined by the continued presence of pain and suffering, appears to provide a barrier to recovery and may promote persistent illness and disability. The incidence of insurance claims for whiplash is about one per 1000 population per year,[360] yet not all persons involved in motor vehicle crashes develop symptoms, and not all symptomatic patients experience chronic injury. The differences in the rating of prolonged symptoms between systems with and without compensation raises questions about the real incidence of chronic WADs.[381]

INTEGRATION OF PATTERNS 4B, 4F, AND 5F: IMPAIRED JOINT MOBILITY, MOTOR FUNCTION, MUSCLE PERFORMANCE, RANGE OF MOTION SECONDARY TO IMPAIRED POSTURE, SYSTEMIC DYSFUNCTION (REFERRED PAIN SYNDROMES), SPINAL DISORDERS, MYOFASCIAL PAIN DYSFUNCTION, AND PERIPHERAL NERVE ENTRAPMENT

Thoracic Outlet Syndrome[193,382]

The thoracic outlet is the anatomic space bordered by the first thoracic rib, the clavicle, and the superior border of the scapula, through which the great vessels and nerves of the upper extremity pass (Fig. 25-4). TOS is a syndrome characterized by symptoms attributable to compression of the neural or vascular anatomic structures that pass through the thoracic outlet. The bony boundaries of the outlet include the clavicle, first rib, and scapula, and the outlet passage is further defined by the interscalene interval, a triangle with its apex directed superiorly. This triangle is bordered anteriorly by the anterior scalene muscle, posteriorly by the middle scalene muscle, and inferiorly by the first rib (see Fig. 25-4).

The other names used for TOS are based on descriptions of the potential sources for its compression. These names include cervical rib syndrome, scalenus anticus syndrome, hyperabduction syndrome, costoclavicular syndrome, pectoralis minor syndrome, and first thoracic rib syndrome.

TOS was first noted in 1743 when an association was made between the cervical rib and TOS, although it was not until 1818, that the medical management of TOS was discussed.[383] In the early twentieth century, Adson stressed the role of the scalene muscles in neurovascular compromise, and Wright showed that shoulder hyperabduction could produce thoracic outlet obstruction.[383] It was Peet[384] who coined the term "TOS" in 1956. Then, in the early 1960s, Roos[63] emphasized the importance of the first rib and its muscular and ligamentous attachments in causing thoracic outlet obstruction.

The lowest trunk of the brachial plexus, which is made up of rami from the C8 and T1 nerve roots, is the most commonly compressed neural structure in TOS. These nerve roots provide sensation to the fourth and fifth fingers of the hand and motor innervation to the hand intrinsic muscles.

The subclavian artery and the lower trunk of the plexus pass behind the clavicle, and into the costoclavicular space (see Fig. 25-4). From there they pass over the first rib, between the insertions of the anterior and middle scalene muscles and are joined by the subclavian vein.

Thus, the course of the neurovascular bundle can be subdivided into three different sections, based on the areas of potential entrapment:

1. As the brachial plexus and subclavian artery pass through the interscalene triangle (see Fig. 25-4), interscalene triangle compression can result from injury of the scalene or

scapular suspensory muscles. In some cases, fibromuscular bands can develop between the anterior and middle scalenes, or between the long transverse processes of the lower cervical vertebrae, producing entrapment. The subclavian vein is not involved, because it usually passes anterior to the anterior scalene muscle. Entrapment at this site may also result from cervical ribs, which are present in 0.2% of the population and occur bilaterally in 80% of those affected.[63] However, the presence of a cervical rib does not necessarily precipitate signs and symptoms, with fewer than 10% of individuals with cervical ribs ever experiencing TOS.[63]

2. As it passes the first rib, clavicle, and subclavius: the costoclavicular interval. Entrapment in this space between the ribcage and the posterior aspect of the clavicle may occur with clavicle depression, rib elevation caused by scalene hypertonicity, repetitive shoulder abduction, or a first rib-clavicular deformity. A postfracture callus formation of the first rib or clavicle can also increase the potential for entrapment.
3. As it passes the coracoid process, pectoralis minor, and clavipectoral fascia to enter the axillary fossa. At this point, the subclavian artery and vein become the axillary artery and vein. At this third site, the neurovascular bundle can be compromised with arm abduction or elevation, especially if external rotation is superimposed on the motion. Pectoralis minor tendon compression is associated with shoulder hyperabduction. During hyperabduction, the tendon insertion and the coracoid act as a fulcrum, about which the neurovascular structures are forced to change direction. Hypertrophy of the pectoralis minor tendon has also been noted as a cause of outlet compression.[383]

There may be multiple points of compression of the peripheral nerves between the cervical spine and hand, in addition to the thoracic outlet. When there are multiple compression sites, less pressure is required at each site to produce symptoms. Thus, a patient may have concomitant TOS, ulnar nerve compression at the elbow, and carpal tunnel syndrome. This phenomenon has been called the *multiple crush syndrome*.[385]

Symptoms vary from mild-to-limb threatening and often mimic common but difficult to treat conditions such as tension headache or fatigue syndromes. The chief complaint is usually one of diffuse arm and shoulder pain, especially when the arm is elevated beyond 90 degrees. Potential symptoms include pain localized in the neck, face, head, upper extremity, chest, shoulder, or axilla; and upper extremity paresthesias, numbness, weakness, heaviness, fatigability, swelling, discoloration, ulceration, or Raynaud phenomenon.[382] Neural compression symptoms occur more commonly than vascular symptoms.[63]

Karas[386] described five symptom patterns of TOS, characterized by the primary structures compressed.

1. The lower trunk pattern reflects lower plexus compression and manifests with pain in the supraclavicular and infraclavicular fossa, back of the neck, rhomboid area, axilla, and medial arm and may radiate into the hand and fourth and fifth fingers. The history includes reports of feelings of coldness, or electric shock sensations in the C8–T1 or ulnar nerve distributions.
2. The upper trunk pattern results from upper plexus compression and is distinguished by pain in the anterolateral neck, shoulder, mandible, and ear, and paresthesias that radiate into the upper chest and lateral arm in the C5–7 dermatomes.[386,387]
3. With venous involvement, the signs and symptoms can include swelling of the entire limb, nonpitting edema, bluish discoloration, and venous collateralization across the superior chest and shoulder.
4. Arterial involvement produces coolness, ischemic episodes, and exertional fatigue.[386]
5. The mixed pattern consists of a combination of vascular and neurologic symptoms.[386]

Mechanisms

Proposed mechanisms for TOS:

- ***Traumatic.*** Twenty-one percent to 75% of TOS patients have an association with trauma.[387] This may involve macro-trauma, as in the case of an MVA, or microtrauma, as in the case of a muscle strain of the scapular stabilizers, resulting from repetitive overhead activities.[388–390]
- ***Developmental.*** During the normal growth of children and adolescents, the scapulae gradually descend upon the posterior thorax, with the descent being slightly greater in women than in men. A strain injury to the scapular suspensory muscles, which lengthen in conjunction with scapular descent during normal development, is known to be associated with TOS. These facts help to explain the rarity of symptomatic TOS until after puberty, and the increased prevalence in women.[193,391]

Diagnosis

TOS is a clinical diagnosis, made almost entirely on the basis of the history and physical examination (see Special Tests). To help rule out other conditions that can mimic TOS, the physical examination should include the following:

- A careful inspection of the spine, thorax, shoulder girdles, and upper extremities for postural abnormalities, shoulder asymmetry, muscle atrophy, excessively large breasts, obesity, and drooping of the shoulder girdle.
- Palpation of the supraclavicular fossa for fibromuscular bands, percussion for brachial plexus irritability, and auscultation for vascular bruits that appear by placing the upper extremity in the position of vascular compression.
- Assessment of the neck and shoulder girdle for active and passive ranges of motion, areas of tenderness, or other signs of intrinsic disease.
- A thorough neurologic examination of the upper extremity, including a search for sensory and motor deficits and abnormalities of muscle stretch reflexes.
- Assessment of respiration to ensure patient is using correct abdominodiaphragmatic breathing.

- Assessment of the suspensory muscles: the middle and upper trapezius, levator scapulae, and SCM (thoracic outlet "openers"). These muscles typically are found to be weak.
- Assessment of the scapulothoracic muscles: the anterior and middle scalenes, subclavius, pectoralis minor and major (thoracic outlet "closers"). These muscles typically are found to be adaptively shortened.
- First rib position or presence of cervical rib.
- Clavicle position and history of prior fracture, producing abnormal callous formation or malalignment.
- Scapula position, acromioclavicular joint mobility, and sternoclavicular joint mobility.
- Neurophysiologic tests, which are useful to exclude coexistent pathologies such as peripheral nerve entrapment or cervical radiculopathy. An abnormal reflex F wave conduction and decreased sensory action potentials in the medial antebrachial cutaneous nerve may be diagnostic.[392]

Intervention

Conservative intervention should be attempted before surgery and should be directed toward muscle relaxation, relief of inflammation, and attention to posture. This intervention approach may require a change of occupation for the patient, because TOS is more common in those who stoop at work. Aggressive physical therapy, particularly traction, may worsen symptoms.[393]

The focus of the intervention is the correction of postural abnormalities of the neck and shoulder girdle, strengthening of the scapular suspensory muscles, stretching of the scapulothoracic muscles, and mobilization of the whole shoulder complex and the first and second ribs.

Kenny and colleagues[394] prospectively evaluated a group of eight patients, composed mainly of middle-aged women, whose TOS was treated with a supervised physical therapy program of graduated resisted shoulder elevation exercises.[193] All patients showed major symptomatic improvement.

If symptoms progress or fail to respond within 4 months, surgical intervention should be considered.[395] Lower plexus TOS is surgically treated by first rib and (if present) cervical rib excision.[396] Although it has been suggested that the insured patient is more likely to have an operation, results are independent of any associated litigation.[397]

THERAPEUTIC TECHNIQUES

TECHNIQUES TO INCREASE JOINT MOBILITY

Joint Mobilizations

Most joint mobilizations use the same technique as the assessment but, by using grades, convert it into a treatment method. The purpose of joint mobilization techniques is to

- reduce stresses through both the fixation and the leverage components of the spine;
- reduce stresses through hypermobile segments by mobilizing the hypomobile joints;
- reduce the overall force needed by the clinician, thus giving greater control.

The selection of a manual technique is dependent on several factors, including:

- The acuteness of the condition, the cause of the restriction, and the goal of the intervention. If the structure is acutely painful (pain is felt before resistance or pain is felt with resistance), pain relief, rather than a mechanical effect, is the major goal. Joint oscillations (grades I and II) that do not reach the end of range are used. The segment or joint is left in its neutral position, and the mobilization is carried out from that point.
- Whether the restriction is symmetric, involving both sides of the segment, or asymmetric, involving only one side of the segment.

A number of specific manual techniques can be employed. Spinal locking techniques can be used to augment the comfort and safety of a manual technique. Locking is simply a method of taking up any available soft tissue tension or slack, thereby making a manual technique more specific. Two types of locking techniques are commonly advocated: craniovertebral locking and locking through segmental translation. Because of the potential for vertebral artery compromise in the craniovertebral region, the craniovertebral joints are often "locked" first before continuing motion into the middle and/or lower cervical spine joints. In the following example, a left side-bending technique is used. Although this locking technique may be used with the patient positioned in sitting or supine, if it used in supine it is important to apply a small amount of compression to compensate for the loss of the spinal loading due to the weight of the head.

While palpating the C2 spinous process, the clinician slowly side-bends the patient's head to the left. If the side bending is performed around a sagittal craniovertebral axis, the C2 spinous process should be felt to move to the right, indicating left rotation of the C2 on the C3. Maintaining the left side-bent position, the head is now rotated to the right until the C2 spinous process regains a central position. The head is again side bent slightly to the left, and the C2 spinous process derotated back to midline. These motions are continued until a firm end-feel is reached. At this point, motion in the craniovertebral joints has now been exhausted, while the rest of the cervical joints remain in neutral. Being careful to maintain the position of the head, especially the right rotation, the side bending is continued left to the middle or lower cervical level required. As the cervical joints are prevented from rotating to the left, the middle cervical side bending motion is exhausted very quickly.

The vast majority of biomechanical dysfunctions of the cervical spine involve the posterior quadrant (a loss of extension and a loss of side bending and rotation to one side or both). The loss of cervical flexion is usually associated with a cervical disk protrusion, a cervicothoracic dysfunction, or a craniovertebral dysfunction. However, for completeness, the techniques described here will address a loss in both the anterior and the posterior quadrants.

The C4–5 level is used in the following examples. Midrange is considered the biomechanical neutral resting position of the joint, and is the ideal start point for techniques that are not intended to stress the barrier and that are intended to avoid causing pain or increasing inflammation. The various methods of grading manual therapy techniques are described in Chapter 10.

Basic Techniques to Restore Motion in the Posterior Quadrant

Seated Mobilization Technique to Restore Extension and Left Side Bending-Rotation VIDEO. If the clinician has large hands, mobilizing into extension can be a problem, because the stabilizing hand prevents the full glide into extension from occurring. To overcome this problem, the stabilization of the inferior segment is performed by pushing the thumb up against the side of its spinous process, thereby preventing the rotation induced by the mobilization of the superior segment. For example, if the left side of C4–5 is being mobilized into extension, left side bending, and left rotation by the upper hand, the thumb of the inferior hand is pushed against the right side of the C5 spinous process, preventing rotation of C5 to the left (Fig. 25-83).

Supine Mobilization Technique to Restore Extension and Left Side Bending-Rotation (Left Side Bending-Rotation shown on VIDEO*).*[167] The patient is positioned supine, with the head being supported. The clinician stands at the patient's head, facing the shoulders. With the radial aspect of the right index finger, the clinician palpates the spinous process and the right inferior articular process of the C4 vertebra. With the other hand, the clinician supports the head and neck superior to the level being treated (Fig. 25-84). A lock of the superior segment is accomplished by left side bending and right rotating the C3–4 joint complex, leaving the craniovertebral joints in a neutral position. The motion barrier for extension, left side bending, and left rotation of C4–5 is then localized by pushing the right inferior articular process of C4 in a posteroinferior and medial direction on C5.

- ***Passive.*** The clinician applies a grade I–V force to the C4 vertebra to produce a posteroinferor and medial glide of the left zygapophyseal joint at C4–5.

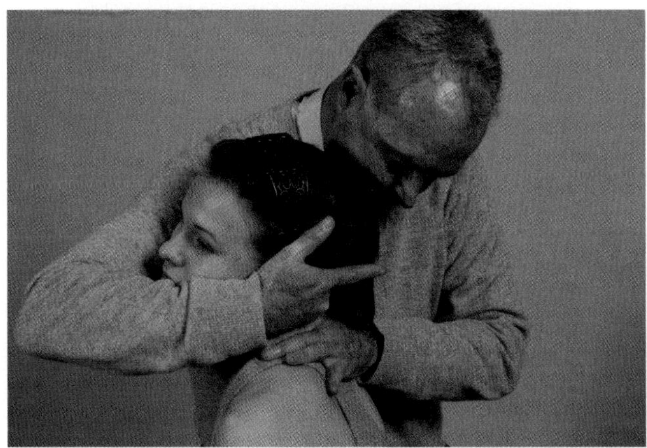

FIGURE 25-83 Seated mobilization to increase extension and left rotation.

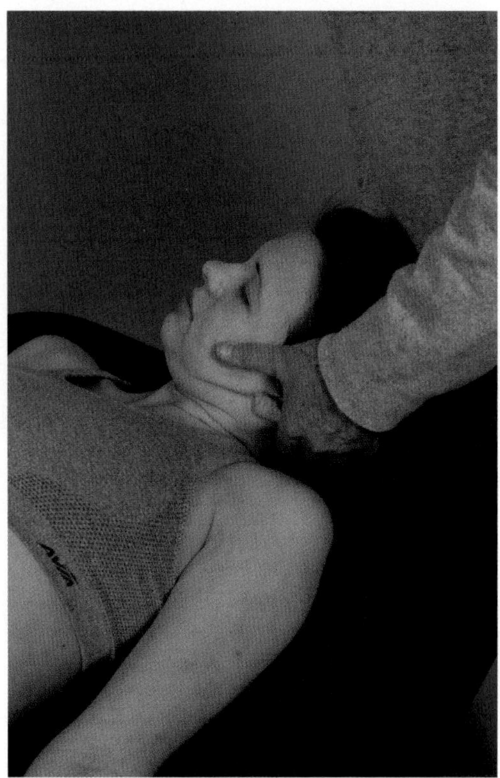

FIGURE 25-84 Supine Mobilization Technique to Restore Extension and Left Side Bending-rotation.

- ***Active.*** From the motion barrier, the patient is asked to turn the eyes in a direction that facilitates further extension, left side bending, and right rotation. The isometric contraction is held for up to 5 seconds and followed by a period of complete relaxation. The joint is then passively taken to the new motion barrier. The technique is repeated three times and followed by a reexamination of joint function.

Basic Techniques to Restore Motion in the Anterior Quadrant

Seated Mobilization Technique to Restore Flexion and Right rotation (Rotation Right Side Bending-Rotation shown on VIDEO). The patient is positioned sitting, and the clinician stands on the right side. Using one hand, the clinician stabilizes the C5 segment using a lumbrical grip (Fig. 25-85). The other hand reaches around the head of the patient, securing it to the clinician's chest, and the ulnar border of the fifth finger is applied to the left transverse process and neural arch of C4. The C4–5 segment is then flexed and rotated to the right to the barrier (see Fig. 25-85). The mobilization is carried out by the clinician applying pressure into flexion and right rotation.

- ***Passive.*** A grade I–IV mobilization force is applied to the C4 vertebra to produce a superoanterior glide at the zygapophyseal joints, thus flexing the C4–5 joint complex and feeling the spinous processes separate.
- ***Active.*** At the motion barrier, the patient is instructed to turn the eyes in a direction that facilitates further flexion at C4–5. The isometric contraction is held for up to 5 seconds

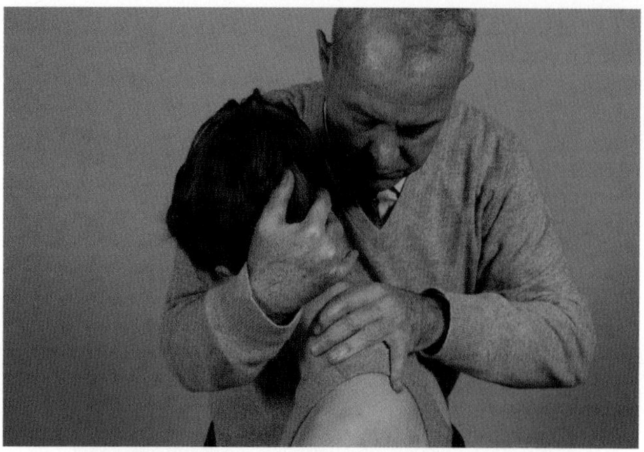

FIGURE 25-85 Seated mobilization into flexion and right rotation.

and followed by a period of complete relaxation. The joint is then passively taken to the new motion barrier. The technique is repeated three times and followed by a reexamination of joint function.

Supine Mobilization Technique to Restore Flexion and Right Side bending-Rotation (Left Side Bending-Rotation shown on VIDEO*).* The patient is positioned supine, with the head being supported. The clinician stands at the head of the table facing the patient. The C4–5 segment is flexed, right side bent, and left translated to bring the right joint to its flexion barrier. The clinician hooks a fingertip under the right articular process and lays a fingertip pad over the articular process on the right (see Fig. 25-86). The mobilization is achieved by pulling the left process cranially, as steady light pressure is applied to the back of the left process to maintain a normal axis of motion.

- ***Passive.*** A grade I–V mobilization force is applied to the C4 vertebra to produce a superoanterior and medial glide of the right zygapophyseal joint at C4–5.
- ***Active.*** At the motion barrier, the patient is instructed to turn the eyes in a direction that facilitates further flexion, right side bending, and rotation at C4–5. The isometric contraction is held for up to 5 seconds and followed by a period of complete relaxation. The joint is then passively taken to the new motion barrier. This technique is repeated three times and followed by a reexamination of function.

Techniques to Restore Motion in Bilateral Extension Hypomobility

Bilateral hypomobilities can be treated with unilateral techniques performed to each side when only the last part of the range of movement is absent.

Seated Technique for the Cervicothoracic Junction

The patient is seated with the arms behind the head. The clinician stands in front of the patient and threads the arms through the patient's arms, before resting both of the hands on the top, and back, of each of the patient's shoulders (Fig. 25-87). By gently leaning the patient forward, the cervical spine is extended until the stiff segment is located at the cervicothoracic junction. Gradually, the clinician increases

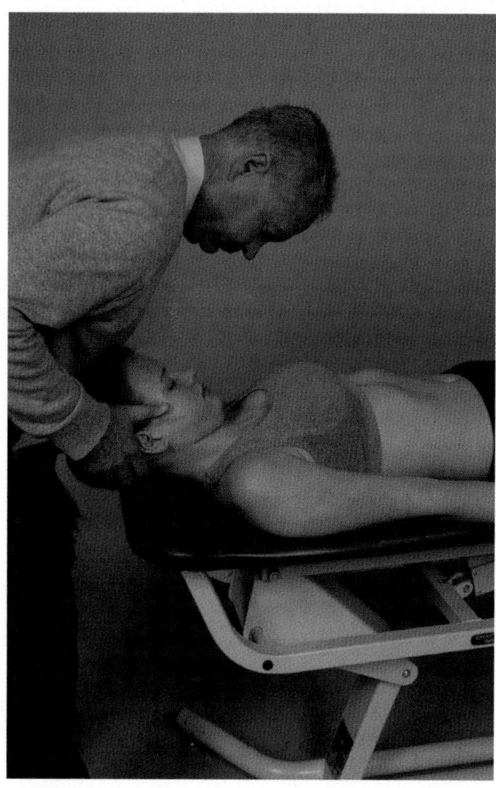

FIGURE 25-86 Supine Mobilization Technique to Restore Flexion and Left Side Bending-Rotation.

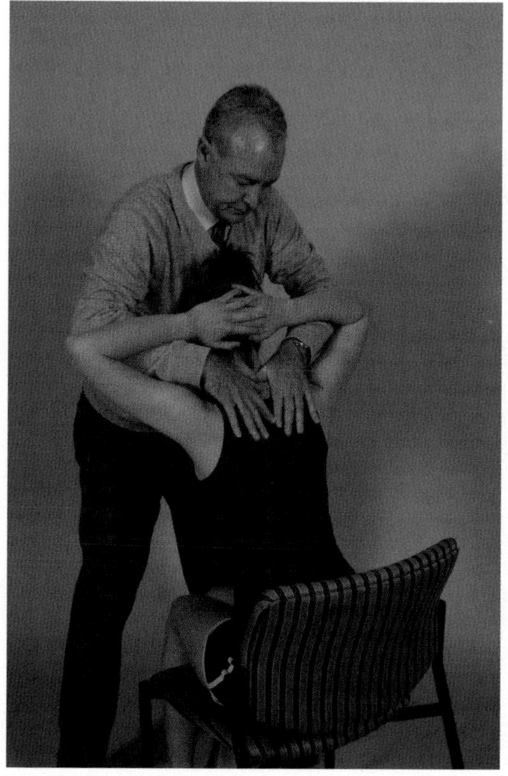

FIGURE 25-87 Seated Technique for the Cervicothoracic Junction.

the amount of cervicothoracic extension by gently kneading the mid-scapular area. Distraction, side flexion, or rotation motions can also be introduced. Care should be taken to avoid overextending the lumbar spine during this technique, by pulling the patient too far forward.

Mobilizations with Movement

To Improve Flexion. The patient is positioned sitting, with the clinician standing to the side, facing the patient.[398] The patient's head is held in neutral against the clinician's lower chest, and the distal phalanx of the little finger is hooked under the spinous process of the superior vertebra of the segment being treated. The rest of the fingers wrap around the patient's neck to provide firm support, and the wrist is extended, with the forearm placed in the plane of the facets. The lateral border of the thenar eminence of the other hand is placed below the little finger (see Fig. 25-88), and the palm of the hand rests on the upper back of the patient.

The patient is asked to flex the neck, and the glide of the superior segment is produced along the correct plane by a pull from the little finger in an anterior and superior direction, while the other hand stabilizes the lower segment.

This technique can be taught as part of the patient's home exercise program using a towel, belt, or strap.

To Improve Extension. The patient is positioned sitting, with the clinician standing to the side, facing the patient. The patient's head is held in neutral against the clinician's lower chest, and the distal phalanx of the little finger is hooked under the spinous process of the superior vertebra of the segment being treated. Using a key grip between the index finger and thumb, the clinician places the grip over the articular pillar on either side of the inferior spinous process of the segment (Fig. 25-89).

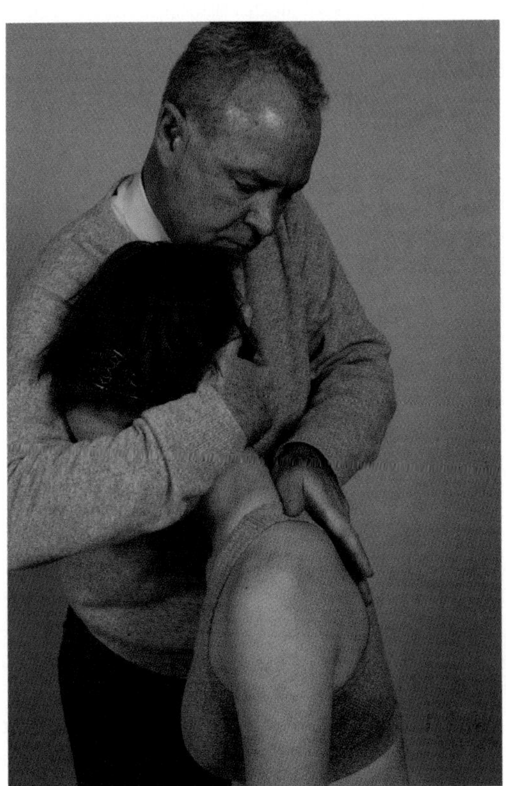

FIGURE 25-88 Mobilization with movement to improve cervical flexion.

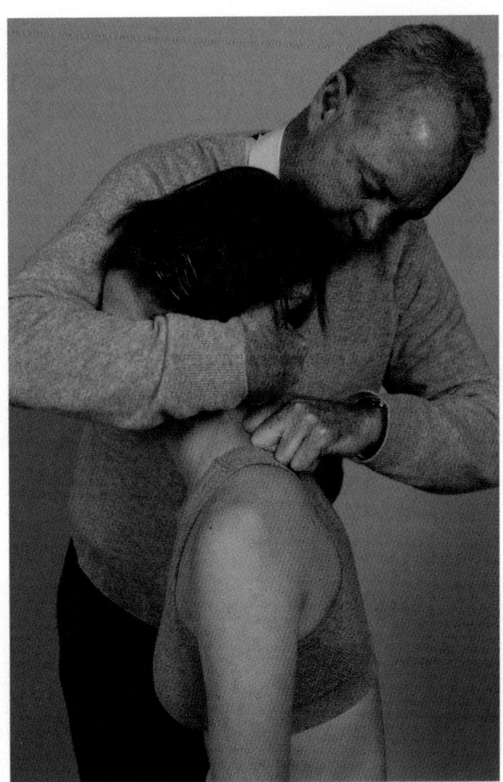

FIGURE 25-89 Mobilization with movement to improve cervical extension.

The patient is asked to extend the neck, while the clinician simultaneously applies a glide of the inferior vertebra by pushing with the key grip hand.

This technique can be taught as part of the patient's home exercise program using a towel, belt, or a strap.

To Improve Rotation to the Right. The patient is positioned sitting, with the clinician sitting behind. The clinician places the thumb of one hand over the articular pillar over the right aspect of the spinous process of the superior vertebra of the segment to be treated. The other thumb is placed over the first thumb to help reinforce. The remaining fingers of the two hands are placed around the neck and upper back.

The patient is asked to rotate the head and neck slowly to the right, while the clinician simultaneously applies the glide along the correct joint plane using pressure from both thumbs (see Fig. 25-90). The same technique can be used to improve cervical rotation to the right by altering the position of the thumbs.

This technique can be taught as part of the patient's home exercise program using a towel, belt, or a strap (Fig. 25-91).

Techniques to Increase Soft Tissue Extensibility

A variety of soft tissue techniques for the cervical region is available to the clinician. The choice of technique depends on the goals of the treatment and the dysfunction being treated.

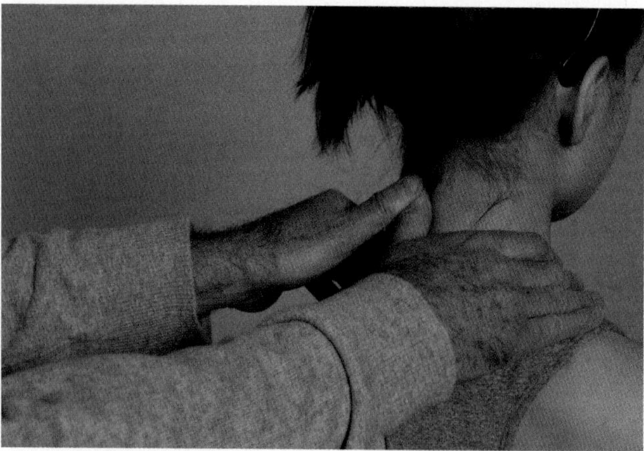

FIGURE 25-90 Mobilization with movement to improve cervical rotation to the left.

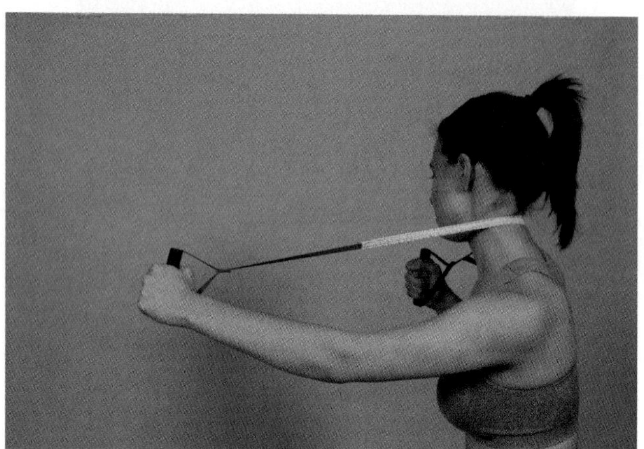

FIGURE 25-91 Home exercise to improve cervical rotation to the left.

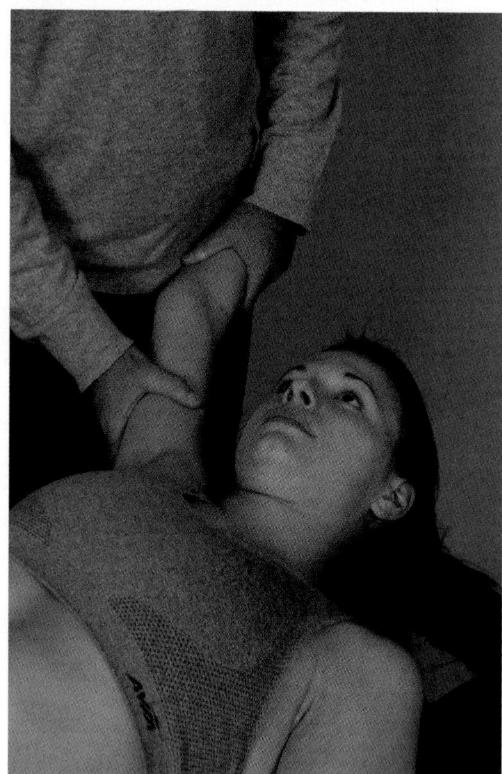

FIGURE 25-92 Pectoralis major stretch.

Myofascial Trigger Point Therapy

Ischemic compression is advocated for myofascial trigger points and is achieved by sustaining direct pressure over a trigger point, using the thumb to apply pressure.[286] The pressure is held for 5–7 seconds and then quickly withdrawn.[399] The procedure is repeated on each trigger point. After each trigger point has been treated, the clinician returns to the first trigger point. The procedure is repeated three times on each trigger point.[399]

To facilitate self-treatment for inaccessible regions such as the rhomboid muscles, lying on a tennis ball, or using the handle of a cane can be substituted for direct manual compression.[286]

Muscle Stretching

Pectoralis Minor. The pectoralis minor can be stretched effectively using a corner and placing the forearms on the walls. The patient needs to avoid adopting a forward head posture during the stretch. The patient attempts a contraction of horizontal aduction and internal rotation into the wall. The clinician is cautioned against using this exercise with any patient with shoulder pathology, especially an anterior instability.

Pectoralis Major. The pectoralis major can be specifically stretched if the orientation of its fibers is considered (clavicular and costosternal), by having the patient lie supine and extending the arm off the table in either approximately 140 degrees of shoulder abduction (costosternal fibers) or approximately 45–50 degrees of abduction (clavicular fibers) (see Fig. 25-92).

For the following muscles, the same technique that is used to assess the length of this muscle is used for the stretch:

Sternocleidomastoid. The SCM functions to flex and rotate the neck and extend the occipitoatlantal joint. The patient is positioned in sitting or supine (see Fig. 25-37). The patient is positioned supine, with the head supported. From this position, the clinician induces side bending of the neck to the contralateral side, and extension of the neck. The clinician stabilizes the scapula and rotates the patient's head and neck toward the ipsilateral side.

Anterior and Middle Scalenes. The patient is positioned in supine. After stabilizing the first two ribs with the heel of one hand, the clinician performs passive cervical extension, contralateral side bending, and ipsilateral rotation (see Fig. 25-38).

Levator Scapulae. The stretch can be passively applied by the clinician. The patient is positioned supine, with the head at the edge of the table. The elbow and hand of the side to be treated are placed above the head. The clinician stands at the head of the table and presses his or her thigh against the point of the patient's elbow, fixing it caudally. Using both hands, the clinician then flexes the neck and side flexes the patient's head to the opposite side, until resistance is felt. The patient is then asked to look toward the treated side, a motion that is resisted by the clinician. When the patient relaxes, the clinician moves the head into further side flexion and flexion.

Upper Trapezius. This procedure is similar to that of the levator scapulae except that the amount of neck flexion is reduced (see Fig. 25-34). The patient is positioned supine, with the head at the edge of the table. Using both hands, the clinician then flexes the neck and side bends the patient's head to the opposite side. Rotation to the ipsilateral side is then added until resistance is felt. The patient is then asked to look toward the treated side, a motion that is resisted by the clinician. When the patient relaxes, the clinician moves the head into further flexion, side bending, and rotation.

In addition to the muscles described here, the clinician should assess the following muscles for adaptive shortening:

- rectus capitis posterior major;
- rectus capitis posterior minor;
- obliquus capitis inferior;
- obliquus capitis superior.

The stretches for these muscles are described in Chapter 23.

Self-Stretching Techniques

Levator Scapulae

The patient is seated with good posture. The patient flexes the neck fully and then side bends the head, while maintaining the neck flexion (see Fig. 25-93). The side bending continues until a gentle stretch is felt. Gentle overpressure can be applied using one hand. The stretch is maintained for 8–10 seconds and then the patient relaxes. The stretch is repeated 10 times.

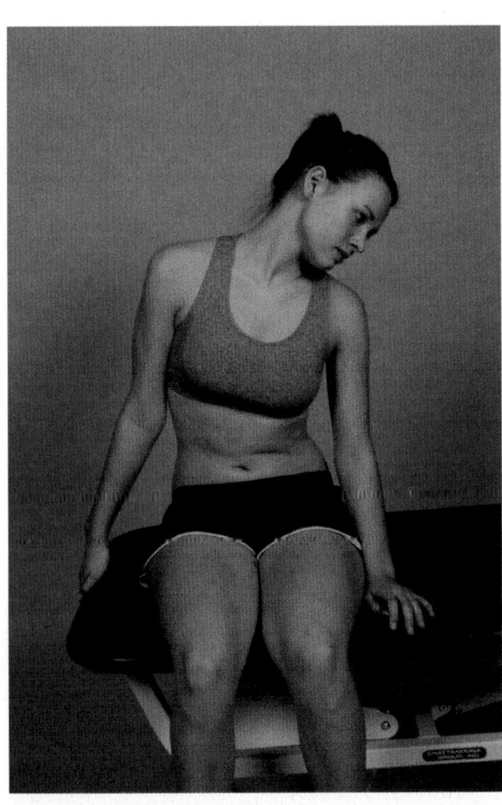

FIGURE 25-93 Self stretch of levator scapulae.

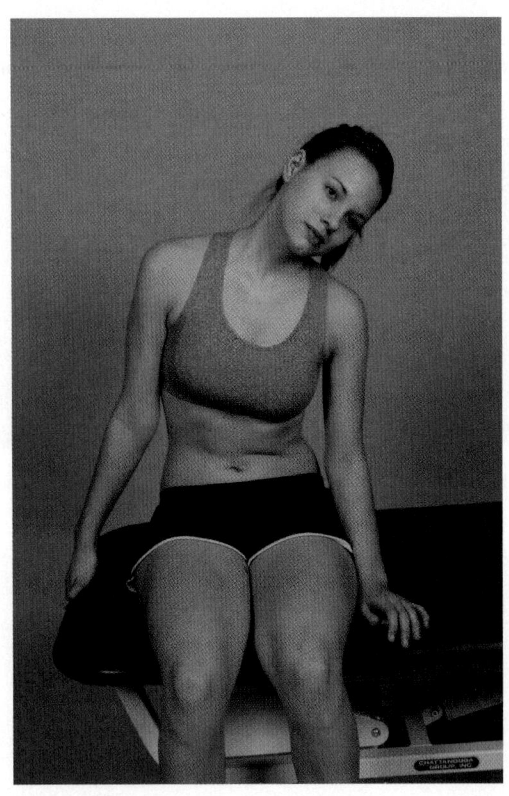

FIGURE 25-94 Self-stretch of upper trapezius.

Upper Trapezius

The self-stretch of the right upper trapezius depicted in Fig. 25-94, is described.[400] The stretch is maintained for 8–10 seconds, and then the patient relaxes. The stretch is repeated 10 times.

Three-Finger Exercise

Active range of motion in the cervical spine can be increased through patient participation, using the three-finger exercise.[401] The patient's mandible rests on digits two, three, and four. The motions of flexion (Fig. 25-95), side bending (Fig. 25-96), and rotation (Fig. 25-97) can all be performed.

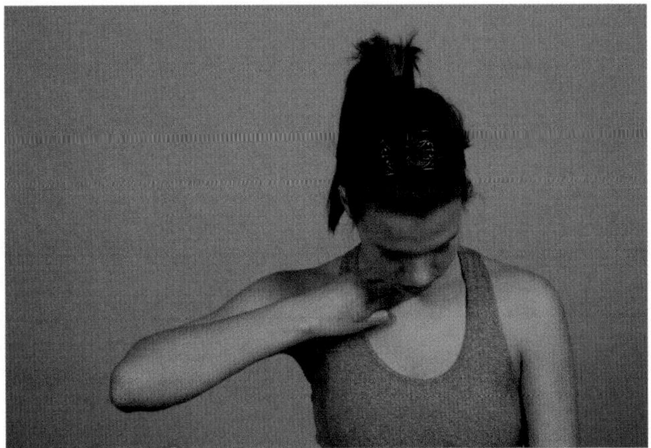

FIGURE 25-95 Three finger exercise into cervical flexion.

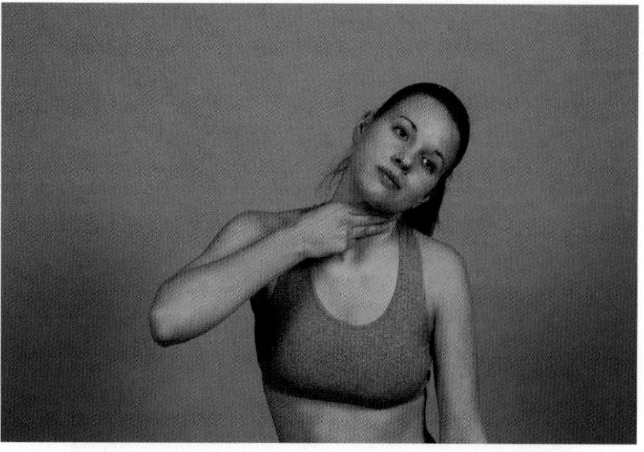
FIGURE 25-96 Three finger exercise into cervical side bending.

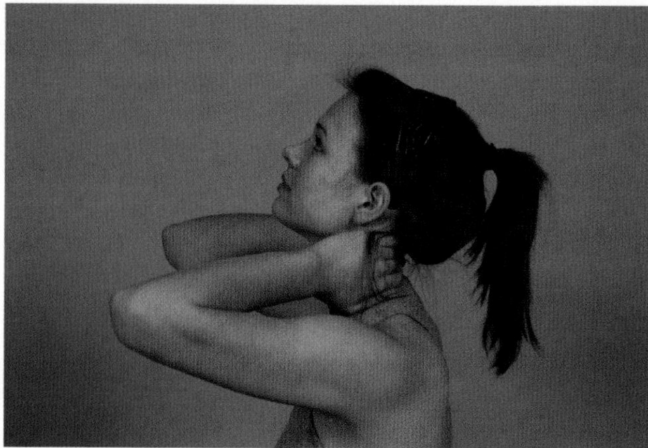
FIGURE 25-98 Active exercise into cervical extension.

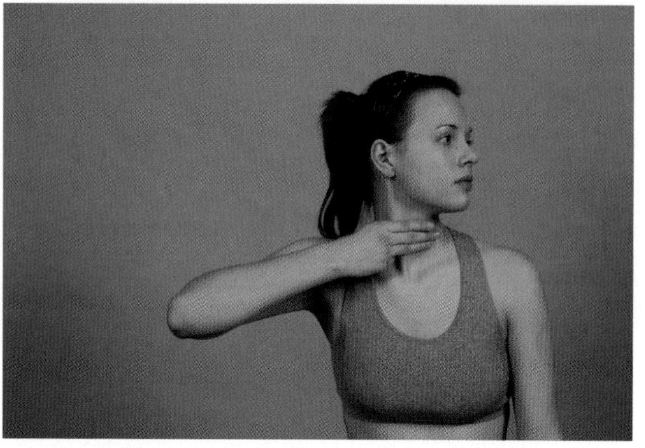
FIGURE 25-97 Three finger exercise into cervical rotation.

The patient is cautioned against reproducing sharp pain, while attempting to feel a stretch at the end of the available motion.

With a different hand position, cervical extension can be performed in a controlled and safe manner. The fingers are interlocked and placed behind the neck, with the little fingers at the lowest segmental level of the joint restriction (at C 5 for a C4-5 restriction). Using the little finger as a fulcrum, the patient extends the cervical spine to the point just shy of pain. This position is held for a few seconds and the neck is returned to the neutral position (Fig. 25-98).

CASE STUDY

NECK PAIN AND ARM PARESTHESIA

HISTORY

A 21-year-old woman presented to the clinic with complaints of right neck and shoulder pain, and paresthesias that often radiated into the medial arm, forearm, and fourth and fifth fingers of the right upper extremity. The patient also reported that her right upper extremity often felt tired and heavy and that her right hand occasionally would appear to have a weak grip. The patient reported that her symptoms began shortly after she was involved in an MVA about 2 months previously and have increased slightly since that time. The patient denied any history since the accident of dizziness, tinnitus, blurred vision, or headaches. No left-sided neck pain or left upper extremity symptoms were reported.

The patient described her overall health as good. Her past medical history was unremarkable, and there was no past history of any surgeries.

Questions

1. What are some of the potential causes for upper extremity paresthesias? Can you rule out any of these causes from the history given? What further questions would you ask to help rule out some of the causes?
2. Which conditions could be associated with a weak grip? Could you rule these in or out with the history?
3. Which conditions could be associated with a report of a tired and heavy upper extremity? How would you rule these in or out?
4. Would the results from any imaging studies be helpful in this case? If so, which ones and why?
5. Is an upper quarter scanning examination warranted in this case? Why or why not?
6. Is this an irritable condition? Why or why not?
7. What type of conditions were the questions about dizziness, tinnitus, blurred vision, and headaches designed to help rule out?

CASE STUDY

LOW NECK PAIN

HISTORY

A 33-year-old woman presented with a diagnosis of low neck and upper back pain that, over the past few weeks, had become constant. Initially, the pain had been minimal, but it had worsened progressively. The pain was localized to the midline at the base of the neck, and there was no report of arm pain or symptoms. The patient worked as a computer operator for a local bank. Sleeping had become difficult, and all motions of the neck were reported to reproduce the symptoms. The patient denied any dizziness or nausea, or history of neck trauma.

The patient described her overall health as excellent. The past medical history was unremarkable.

Questions

1. Make a list of all of the possible causes of midline neck pain.
2. What could the gradual onset of the pain tell the clinician?
3. What is your working hypothesis at this stage? List the tests you would use to rule out the various causes of midline neck pain.
4. Should the reports of night pain concern the clinician?
5. Does this presentation/history warrant a Cyriax upper quarter scanning examination? Why or why not?

CASE STUDY

BILATERAL ARM AND WRIST WEAKNESS

HISTORY

A 36-year-old man who sustained a left tibial plateau fracture presented at the clinic with complaints of bilateral arm and wrist weakness that had worsened progressively over the past month since his discharge from the hospital. The patient was ambulating with crutches and non–weight-bearing on the left side. There was no history of cervical trauma. The patient reported no pain in his upper extremities but had noticed a mild and vague numbness in his hands. There was no report or evidence of a preceding viral infection and no proximal migration of the weakness, nor did he have any other areas of weakness. The patient did complain of pain in his axillae, and commented that his crutches had been rubbing against his axillae.[402]

Questions

1. What structure(s) could be at fault when weakness is the major complaint?
2. Why was the history of no cervical trauma pertinent?
3. Why was the statement about preceding viral infection pertinent?
4. Why was the statement about the proximal migration of the weakness pertinent?
5. What is your working hypothesis at this stage? List the various diagnoses that could present with bilateral arm numbness and the tests you would use to rule out each one.
6. Does this presentation/history warrant a scanning examination? Why or why not?

CASE STUDY

RIGHT-SIDED NECK PAIN

HISTORY

A 45-year-old woman awoke with right-sided neck pain 10 days earlier. The pain was felt over the right neck on an intermittent basis. She related that the pain was worse with head turning to the right, and further aggravated with activities involving cervical extension. She described no neurologic pain or paresthesia. The pain sites and intensity were unchanged since the onset.

Further questioning revealed that the patient was otherwise in good health and had no reports of bowel or bladder impairment, night pain, dizziness, or radicular symptoms.

Questions

1. What structure(s) could be at fault with complaints of right-sided neck pain?
2. What should the motion pattern of restriction/pain tell you?
3. What is your working hypothesis at this stage? List the various diagnoses that could present with right-sided neck pain and the tests you would use to rule out each one.
4. What do the questions about night pain and dizziness pertain to?
5. Does this presentation/history warrant a scanning examination? Why or why not?

REVIEW QUESTIONS*

1. Contraction of one SCM muscle results in
   a. rotation of the face to the same side;
   b. side bending of the head and neck to the opposite side;
   c. flexion of the head and neck;
   d. rotation of the face to the opposite side.
2. Which of the following groups of muscles performs cervical rotation to the opposite side?
   a. longus capitis, RCP, and rectus capitis posterior;
   b. splenius cervicis and splenius capitis;
   c. SCM, scalenus anterior, and obliquus capitis;
   d. SCM and scalenus medius.
3. Which of the following muscles is thin and sheet-like and has fibers that extend from the chest upward over the neck?
   a. levator scapula;
   b. buccinator;
   c. orbicularis oris;
   d. platysma.
4. Which cervical structure is thought to help prevent cervical disk protrusions?
5. Which nerve trunk of the plexus is the most commonly compressed neural structure in TOS?

*Additional questions to test your understanding of this chapter can be found in the Online Learning Center for *Orthopaedic Assessment, Evaluation, and Intervention* at www.duttononline.net.

REFERENCES

1. Pratt N: *Anatomy of the Cervical Spine.* La Crosse, WI: Orthopaedic Section, APTA, 1996.
2. Maigne J-Y: Cervicothoracic and thoracolumbar spinal pain syndromes. In: Giles LGF, Singer KP, eds. *Clinical Anatomy and Management of the Thoracic Spine.* Oxford: Butterworth-Heinemann, 2000:157–168.
3. Kelsey JL: An epidemiological study of the relationship between occupations and acute herniated lumbar intervertebral discs. *Int J Epidemiol* 4:197–205, 1975.
4. Bovim G, Schrader H, Sand T: Neck pain in the general population. *Spine* 19:1307–1309, 1994.
5. Mercer S, Bogduk N: Intra-articular inclusions of the cervical synovial joints. *Br J Rheumat* 32:705–710, 1993.
6. Pal GP, Sherk HH: The vertical stability of the cervical spine. *Spine* 13:447, 1988.
7. Taylor JR: Regional variation in the development and position of the notochordal segments of the human nucleus pulposus. *J Anat* 110:131–132, 1971.
8. Walsh R, Nitz AJ: Cervical spine. In: Wadsworth C, ed. *Current Concepts of Orthopedic Physical Therapy - Home Study Course.* La Crosse, WI: Orthopaedic Section, APTA, 2001.
9. Mercer SB, Bogduk N: The ligaments and annulus fibrosus of human adult cervical intervertebral discs. *Spine* 24:619–626, 1999.
10. Kokubun S, Sakurai M, Tanaka Y: Cartilaginous endplate in cervical disc herniation. *Spine* 21:190–195, 1996.
11. Murphey F, Simmons JC: Ruptured cervical disc: experience with 250 cases. *Am J Surg* 32:83, 1966.
12. Dvorak J: Epidemiology, physical examination, and neurodiagnostics. *Spine* 23:2663–2673, 1998.
13. Oda J, Tanaka H, Tsuzuki N: Intervertebral disc changes with aging of human cervical vertebra: From neonate to the eighties. *Spine* 13:1205–1211, 1988.
14. Boden SD, McCowin PR, Davis DO, et al: Abnormal magnetic resonance scans of the cervical spine in asymptomatic subjects: A prospective investigation. *J Bone Joint Surg* 72A:1178–1184, 1990.
15. Tondury G, Theiler K: *Entwicklungsgeschichte und Fehlbildung der Wirbelsäule.* Stuttgart: Hyppokrates, 1958.
16. Garvey TA, Eismont FJ: Diagnosis and treatment of cervical radiculopathy and myelopathy. *Orthop Rev* 20:595–603, 1991.
17. Tanaka N, Fujimoto Y, An HS, et al: The anatomic relation among the nerve roots, intervertebral foramina, and intervertebral discs of the cervical spine. *Spine* 25:286–291, 2000.
18. Goodman BW: Neck pain. *Prim Care* 15:689–707, 1988.
19. Brooker AEW, Barter RW: Cervical spondylosis: A clinical study with comparative radiology. *Brain* 88:925–936, 1965.
20. Gore DR, Sepic SB, Gardner GM, et al: Roentgenographic findings in the cervical spine of asymptomatic people. *Spine* 6:521–526, 1987.
21. Manifold SG, McCann PD: Cervical radiculitis and shoulder disorders. *Clin Orth Rel Res* 368:105–113, 1999.
22. Ebraheim NA, An HS, Xu R, et al: The quantitative anatomy of the cervical nerve root groove and the intervertebral foramen. *Spine* 21:1619–1623, 1996.
23. Yoo JU, Zou D, Edwards T, et al: Effect of cervical motion on the neuroforaminal dimensions of the human cervical spine. *Spine* 17:1131–1136, 1992.
24. Williams PL, Warwick R, Dyson M, et al: *Gray's Anatomy*, 37th ed. London: Churchill Livingstone, 1989.
25. White AA, Panjabi MM: *Clinical Biomechanics of the Spine.* 2nd ed. Philadelphia, PA: Lippincott-Raven, 1990.
26. Singer KP, Boyle JJW, Fazey P: Comparative anatomy of the zygapophyseal joints. In: Boyling JD, Jull GA, eds. *Grieve's Modern Manual Therapy: The vertebral column.* Philadelphia, PA: Churchill Livingstone, 2004:17–29.
27. Lysell E: Motion in the cervical spine: an experimental study on autopsy specimens. *Acta Orthop Scand* 123S:1, 1969.
28. Giles LG, Taylor JR: Innervation of human lumbar zygapophyseal joint synovial folds. *Acta Orthop Scand* 58:43–46, 1987.
29. Kotani Y, McNulty PS, Abumi K, et al: The role of anteromedial foraminotomy and the uncovertebral joints in the stability of the cervical spine. A biomechanical study. *Spine* 23:1559–1565, 1998.
30. Tillman B, Tondury G, Ziles K: [*Human anatomy: Locomotor System*]. Stuttgart: Thieme, 1987.

31. Orofino C, Sherman MS, Schechter D: Luschka's joint—a degenerative phenomenon. *J Bone Joint Surg* 5A:853–858, 1960.
32. Panjabi MM, Duranceau J, Goel V, et al: Cervical human vertebrae. Quantitative three-dimensional anatomy of the middle and lower regions. *Spine* 16:861–869, 1991.
33. Porterfield J, De Rosa C: *Mechanical Neck Pain: Perspectives in Functional Anatomy*. Philadelphia, PA: WB Saunders, 1995.
34. Milne N: The role of zygapophyseal joint orientation and uncinate processes in controlling motion in the cervical spine. *J Anat* 178:189–201, 1991.
35. Yanagisawa E: Anatomy of the uncinate process. *Ear Nose Throat J* 79:228, 2000.
36. Norkin C, Levangie P: *Joint Structure and Function: A Comprehensive Analysis*. Philadelphia, PA: F.A. Davis Company, 1992.
37. Penning L, Wilmink JT: Rotation of the cervical spine. A CT study in normal subjects. *Spine* 12:732–738, 1987.
38. Clausen JD, Goel VK, Traynelis VC, et al: Uncinate processes and Luschka joints influence the biomechanics of the cervical spine: quantification using a finite element model of the C5-C6 segment. *J Orthop Res* 15:342–347, 1997.
39. Argenson C, Francke JP, Sylla S, et al: The vertebral arteries (segment V1 and V2). *Anat Clin* 2:29–41, 1980.
40. Penning L: Differences in anatomy, motion, development, and ageing of the upper and lower cervical disk segments. *Clin Biomech* 3:37–47, 1988.
41. Hadley LA: Intervertebral joint subluxation, bony impingement and foramen encroachment with nerve root changes. *Am J Roentgenol* 65:377–402, 1951.
42. Johnson RM, Crelin ES, White AA, et al: Some new observations on the functional anatomy of the lower cervical spine. *Clin Orth Rel Res* 111:192–200, 1975.
43. Buckworth J: Anatomy of the suboccipital region. In: Vernon H, ed. *Upper Cervical Syndrome*. Baltimore, MD: Williams & Wilkins, 1988.
44. Hollinshead WH: *Anatomy for Surgeons—The Back and Limbs*, 3rd ed. Philadelphia, PA: Harper and Row, 1982:300–308.
45. Johnson GM, Zhang M, Jones DG: The fine connective tissue architecture of the human ligamentum nuchae. *Spine* 25:5–9, 2000.
46. Allia P, Gorniak G: Human ligamentum nuchae in the elderly: Its function in the cervical spine. *J Man Manip Ther* 14:11–21, 2006.
47. Mercer SR, Bogduk N: Clinical anatomy of ligamentum nuchae. *Clin Anat* 16:484–493, 2003.
48. Fielding JW, Burstein AA, Frankel VH: The nuchal ligament. *Spine* 1:3–11, 1976.
49. Penning L: Normal movements of the cervical spine. *J Roentgenol* 130:317–326, 1978.
50. Keshner EA: Motor control of the cervical spine. In: Boyling JD, Jull GA, eds. *Grieve's Modern Manual Therapy: The Vertebral Column*. Philadelphia, PA: Churchill Livingstone, 2004:105–117.
51. Travell JG, Simons DG: *Myofascial Pain and Dysfunction—The Trigger Point Manual*. Baltimore, MA: Williams & Wilkins, 1983.
52. Karuman PM, Soo KC: Motor innervation of the trapezius muscle: A histochemical study. *Head Neck* 18:254–258, 1996.
53. Krause HR, Bremerich A, Herrmann M: The innervation of the trapezius muscle in connection with radical neck-dissection. An anatomical study. *J Craniomaxillofac Surg* 19:87–89, 1991.
54. Nori S, Soo KC, Green RF, et al: Utilization of intraoperative electroneurography to understand the innervation of the trapezius muscle. *Muscle Nerve* 20:279–285, 1997.
55. Soo KC, Guiloff RJ, Oh A, et al: Innervation of the trapezius muscle: A study in patients undergoing neck dissections. *Head Neck* 12:488–495, 1990.
56. Soo KC, Strong EW, Spiro RH, et al: Innervation of the trapezius muscle by the intra operative measurement of motor action potentials. *Head Neck* 15:216–221, 1993.
57. Fahrer H, Ludin HP, Mumenthaler M, et al: The innervation of the trapezius muscle. An electrophysiological study. *J Neurol* 207:183–188, 1974.
58. Krause HR: Shoulder-arm-syndrome after radical neck dissection: its relation with the innervation of the trapezius muscle. *Int J Oral Maxillofac Surg* 21:276–279, 1992.
59. Kendall FP, McCreary EK, Provance PG: *Muscles: Testing and Function*. Baltimore, MD: Williams & Wilkins, 1993.
60. Fitzgerald MJT, Comerford PT, Tuffery AR: Sources of innervation of the neuromuscular spindles in sternomastoid and trapezius. *J Anat* 134:471–490, 1982.
61. Eliot DJ: Electromyography of levator scapulae: New findings allow tests of a head stabilization model. *J Manipulative Phys Ther* 19:19–25, 1996.
62. Rayan GM, Jensen C: Thoracic outlet syndrome: provocative examination maneuvers in a typical population. *J Shoulder Elbow Surg* 4:113–117, 1995.
63. Roos DB: The place for scalenectomy and first-rib resection in thoracic outlet syndrome. *Surgery* 92:1077–1085, 1982.
64. Raper AJ, Thompson WT, Shapiro W, et al: Scalene and sternomastoid muscle function. *J Appl Physiol* 21:497–502, 1966.
65. Pick TP, Howden R: *Gray's Anatomy*, 15th ed. New York, NY: Barnes & Noble Books, 1995.
66. Hiatt JL, Gartner LP: *Textbook of Head and Neck Anatomy*. Baltimore, MD: Williams & Wilkins, 1987.
67. Murphy DR: *Conservative Management of Cervical Spine Syndromes*. New York, NY: McGraw-Hill, 2000.
68. Jull GA: Physiotherapy management of neck pain of mechanical origin. In: Giles LGF, Singer KP, eds. *Clinical Anatomy and Management of Cervical Spine Pain. The Clinical Anatomy of Back Pain*. London: Butterworth-Heinemann, 1998:168–191.
69. Bogduk N: Cervical causes of headache and dizziness. In: Grieve GP, ed. *Modern Manual Therapy of the Vertebral Column*. New York, NY: Churchill Livingstone, 1986:289–302.
70. Karlberg M, Persson L, Magnusson M: Reduced postural control in patients with chronic cervicobrachial pain syndrome. *Gait Posture* 3:241–249, 1995.
71. Crum B, Mokri B, Fulgham J: Spinal manifestations of vertebral artery dissection. *Neurology* 55:304–306, 2000.
72. Mayoux-Benhamou MA, Revel M, Valle C, et al: Longus colli has a postural function on cervical curvature. *Surg Radiol Anat* 16:367–371, 1994.
73. Watson D, Trott P: Cervical headache: an investigation of natural head posture and upper cervical flexor muscle performance. *Cephalalgia* 13:272–284, 1993.
74. Lewit K: *Manipulative Therapy in Rehabilitation of the Locomotor System*, 2nd ed. Oxford: Butterworth-Heinemann, 1996.
75. Adams CBT, Logue V: Studies in spondylotic myelopathy 2. The movement and contour of the spine in relation to the neural complications of cervical spondylosis. *Brain* 94:569–586, 1971.
76. Panjabi MM, Cholewicki J, Nibu K, et al: Critical load of the human cervical spine: An in vitro experimental study. *Clin Biomech (Bristol, Avon)* 13:11–17, 1998.
77. Harms-Ringdahl K, Ekholm J, Schuldt K, et al: Load moments and myoelectric activity when the cervical spine is held in full flexion and extension. *Ergonomics* 29:1539–1552, 1986.
78. Jull GA, Falla D, Treleaven J, et al: A therapeutic exercise approach or cervical disorders. In: Boyling JD, Jull GA, eds. *Grieve's Modern Manual Therapy: The vertebral column*. Philadelphia, PA: Churchill Livingstone, 2004:451–470.
79. Penning L: Functional Pathology of the Cervical Spine. Baltimore, MD: Williams & Wilkins, 1968.
80. Mercer S: Kinematics of the spine. In: Boyling JD, Jull GA, eds. *Grieve's Modern Manual Therapy: The Vertebral Column*. Philadelphia, PA: Churchill Livingstone, 2004:31–37.
81. Van Mameren H, Drukker J, Sanches H, et al: Cervical spine motions in the sagittal plane. I: Ranges of motion of actually performed movements, an x-ray cine study. *Eur J Morphol* 28:47–68, 1990.
82. Meadows J, Pettman E, Fowler C: *Manual Therapy, NAIOMT Level II & III Course Notes*. Denver, CO: North American Institute of Manual Therapy, 1995.
83. White AA, Panjabi MM: *Clinical Biomechanics of the Spine*, 2nd ed. Philadelphia, PA: J B Lippincott, 1990.
84. Janda V: Muscles and motor control in cervicogenic disorders: Assessment and management. In: Grant R, ed. *Physical Therapy of the Cervical and Thoracic Spine*. New York, NY: Churchill Livingstone, 1994:195–216.
85. Jull GA, Janda V: Muscle and Motor control in low back pain. In: Twomey LT, Taylor JR, eds. *Physical Therapy of the Low Back: Clinics in Physical Therapy*. New York, NY: Churchill Livingstone, 1987:258–278.
86. Bergmark A: Stability of the lumbar spine. *Acta Orthop Scand* 60:1–54, 1989.
87. Bergmark A: Stability of the lumbar spine. A study in mechanical engineering. *Acta Orthop Scand* 230:20–24, 1989.
88. Conley MS, Meyer RA, Bloomberg JJ, et al: Noninvasive analysis of human neck muscle function. *Spine* 20:2505–2512, 1995.

89. Vernon HT, Aker P, Aramenko M, et al: Evaluation of neck muscle strength with a modified sphygmomanometer dynamometer: reliability and validity. *J Man Physiol Ther* 15:343–349, 1992.
90. Mayoux-Benhamou MA, Revel M, Vallee C: Selective electromyography of dorsal neck muscles in humans. *Exp Brain Res* 113:353–360, 1997.
91. Behrsin JF, Maguire K: Levator scapulae action during shoulder movement: a possible mechanism for shoulder pain of cervical origin. *Aust J Physiother* 32:101–106, 1986.
92. Comerford MJ, Mottram SL: Functional stability re-training: principles and strategies for managing mechanical dysfunction. *Man Ther* 6:3–14, 2001.
93. Mottram SL: Dynamic stability of the scapula. *Man Ther* 2:123–131, 1997.
94. Bansevicius D, Salvesen R: [Cervicogenic headache]. *Tidsskr Nor Laegeforen* 123:2701–2704, 2003.
95. Bansevicius D, Sjaastad O: Cervicogenic headache: the influence of mental load on pain level and EMG of shoulder-neck and facial muscles. *Headache* 36:372–378, 1996.
96. Meadows J: *A Rationale and Complete Approach to the Sub-Acute Post-MVA Cervical Patient.* Calgary, AB: Swodeam Consulting, 1995.
97. Winkel D, Matthijs O, Phelps V: Cervical Spine. In: Winkel D, Matthijs O, Phelps V, eds. *Diagnosis and Treatment of the Spine.* Maryland, MD: Aspen, 1997:542–727.
98. Jull G, Bogduk N, Marsland A: The accuracy of manual diagnosis for cervical zygapophyseal joint pain syndromes. *Med J Aust* 148:233–236, 1988.
99. Dwyer A, Aprill C, Bogduk N: Cervical zygapophyseal joint pain patterns: a study from normal volunteers. *Spine* 15:453, 1990.
100. Aprill C, Dwyer A, Bogduk N: Cervical zygapophyseal joint pain patterns II: A clinical evaluation. *Spine* 15:458–61, 1990.
101. Hohl M: Soft-tissue injuries of the neck in automobile accidents. *J Bone Joint Surg* 56A:1675–1682, 1974.
102. Jamieson DRS, Ballantyne JP: Unique presentation of a prolapsed thoracic disk: Lhermitte's symptom in a golf player. *Neurology* 45:1219–1221, 1995.
103. Kanchandani R, Howe JG: Lhermitte's sign in multiple sclerosis: A clinical survey and review of the literature. *J Neurol Neurosurg Psychiatry* 45:308–312, 1982.
104. Ventafridda V, Caraceni A, Martini C, et al: On the significance of Lhermitte's sign in oncology. *J Neurooncol* 10:133–137, 1991.
105. Wang B, Liu H, Wang H, et al: Segmental instability in cervical spondylotic myelopathy with severe disc degeneration. *Spine* 31: 1327–1331, 2006.
106. Rabb CH: Cervical instability. *J Neurosurg Spine* 3:169; author reply 169, 2005.
107. Cook C, Brismee JM, Fleming R, et al: Identifiers suggestive of clinical cervical spine instability: a Delphi study of physical therapists. *Phys Ther* 85:895–906, 2005.
108. Grieve G: Common patterns of clinical presentation. In: Grieve GP, ed. *Common Vertebral Joint Problems*, 2nd ed. London: Churchill Livingstone, 1988:283–302.
109. Maigne J-Y, Maigne R, Guerin-Surville H: Upper thoracic dorsal rami: Anatomic study of their medial cutaneous branches. *Surg Radiol Anat* 13:109–112, 1991.
110. Bogduk N, Valencia F: Innervation and pain patterns of the thoracic spine. In: Grant R, ed. *Physical Therapy of the Cervical and Thoracic Spine*, 2nd ed. Melbourne: Churchill Livingstone, 1994:77–88.
111. Hardin J Jr: Pain and the cervical spine. *Bull Rheum Dis* 50:1–4, 2001.
112. White AA, Sahrmann SA: A movement system balance approach to management of musculoskeletal pain. In: Grant R, ed. *Physical Therapy for the Cervical and Thoracic Spine*. Edinburgh: Churchill Livingstone, 1994:339–358.
113. Gossman MR, Sahrmann SA, Rose SJ: Review of length-associated changes in muscle. *Phys Ther* 62:1799–1808, 1982.
114. Magarey ME: Examination of the cervical and thoracic spine. In: Grant R, ed. *Physical Therapy of the Cervical and Thoracic Spine*, 2nd ed. New York: Churchill Livingstone, 1994:109–144.
115. Bogduk N, Lord SM: Cervical zygapophyseal joint pain. *Neurosurg Q* 8:107–117, 1998.
116. Bogduk N: The rationale for patterns of neck and back pain. *Patient Manage* 8:13, 1984.
117. McKenzie RA: *The Cervical and Thoracic Spine: Mechanical Diagnosis and Therapy.* Waikanae, NZ: Spinal Publications, 1990.
118. Herkowitz HN: Syndromes related to spinal stenosis. In: Weinstein JN, Rydevik B, Sonntag VKH, eds. *Essentials of the Spine.* New York, NY: Raven Press, 1995:179–193.
119. Bush K, Hillier S: Outcome of cervical radiculopathy treated with periradicular/epidural corticosteroid injections: A prospective study with independent clinical review. *Eur Spine J* 5:319–325, 1996.
120. Bradley JP, Tibone JE, Watkins RG: History, physical examination, and diagnostic tests for neck and upper extremity problems. In: Watkins RG, ed. *The Spine in Sports.* St. Louis, MO: Mosby-Year-Book Inc., 1996.
121. Meadows J: *Orthopedic Differential Diagnosis in Physical Therapy.* New York, NY: McGraw-Hill, 1999.
122. Foreman SM, Croft AC: *Whiplash Injuries: The Cervical Acceleration/Deceleration Syndrome.* Baltimore, MD: Williams & Wilkins, 1988.
123. Jull GA, Treleaven J, Versace G: Manual examination: Is pain a major cue to spinal dysfunction. *Aust J Physiother* 40:159–165, 1994.
124. Radanov B, Sturzenegger M, Di Stefano G, et al: Factors influencing recovery from headache after common whiplash. *Br Med J* 307:652–655, 1993.
125. Richardson CA, Jull GA, Hodges P, et al: *Therapeutic Exercise for Spinal Segmental Stabilization in Low Back Pain.* London: Churchill Livingstone, 1999.
126. Janda V: Muscle strength in relation to muscle length, pain and muscle imbalance. In: Harms-Ringdahl K, ed. *Muscle Strength.* New York, NY: Churchill Livingstone, 1993:83–91.
127. Janda V: Muscles, motor regulation and back problems. In: Korr IM, ed. *The Neurological Mechanisms in Manipulative Therapy.* New York, NY: Plenum, 1978:27–41.
128. Sahrmann SA: *Diagnosis and Treatment of Movement Impairment Syndromes.* St Louis, MO: Mosby, 2001.
129. Sobush DC, Simoneau GG, Dietz KE, et al: The lennie test for measuring scapular position in healthy young adult females: a reliability and validity study. *J Orthop Sports Phys Ther.* 23:39–50, 1996.
130. Donato EB, DuVall RE, Godges JJ, et al: Practice analysis: Defining the clinical practice of primary contact physical therapy. *J Orthop Sports Phys Ther* 34:284–304, 2004.
131. Donato EB: Physical examination procedures to screen for serious disorders of the head, neck, chest, and upper quarter. In: Wilmarth MA, ed. *Medical Screening for the Physical Therapist. Orthopaedic Section Independent Study Course 14.1.1.* La Crosse, WI: Orthopaedic Section, APTA, Inc, 2003:1–43.
132. Geschwing N, Levitsky W: Human brain: Left-right asymmetries in temporal speech region. *Science* 161:186–187, 1968.
133. Galaburda AM, le May M: Right left asymmetries in the brain. *Science* 199:852–856, 1978.
134. Bledschmidt M: Principles of biodynamic differentiation in human. In: Bledschmidt M, ed. *Development of the Basicranium.* Bethesda, MD: Nat. Inst. Health, 1976:54–80.
135. Enlow DH: The prenatal and postnatal growth of the basicranium. In: Bledschmidt M, ed. *Development of the Basicranium.* Bethesda, MD: Nat. Inst. Health, 1976:192–204.
136. Cloward RB: Cervical discography: A contribution to the etiology and mechanism of neck, shoulder and arm pain. *Ann Surg* 150:1052–1064, 1959.
137. Sweeney TB, Prentice C, Saal JA, et al: Cervicothoracic muscular stabilization techniques. In: Saal JA, ed. *Physical Medicine and Rehabilitation, State of the Art Reviews: Neck and Back Pain.* Philadelphia, PA: Hanley & Belfus, 1990:335–359.
138. Saal JS: *Flexibility Training, Physical Medicine and Rehabilitation: State of the Art Reviews.* Philadelphia, PA: Hanley & Belfus, Inc., 1987:537–554.
139. Lantz CA, Chen J, Buch D: Clinical validity and stability of active and passive cervical range of motion with regard to total and unilateral uniplanar motion. *Spine* 24:1082–1089, 1999.
140. Lind B, Sihlbom H, Nordwall A, et al: Normal range of motion of the cervical spine. *Arch Phys Med Rehabil* 70:692–695, 1989.
141. Tousignant M, de Bellefeuille L, O'Donoughue S, et al: Criterion validity of the cervical range of motion (CROM) goniometer for cervical flexion and extension. *Spine* 25:324–330, 2000.
142. Tousignant M, Smeesters C, Breton AM, et al: Criterion validity study of the cervical range of motion (CROM) device for rotational range of motion on healthy adults. *J Orthop Sports Phys Ther* 36:242–248, 2006.
143. Wolfenberger VA, Bui Q, Batenchuk GB: A comparison of methods of evaluating cervical range of motion. *J Manipulative Physiol Ther* 25:154–160, 2002.

144. American Medical Association: *Guides to the Evaluation of Permanent Impairment*, 5th ed. Chicago, IL: American Medical Association, 2001.
145. Mayer TG, Kondraske G, Beals SB, et al: Spinal range of motion. Accuracy and sources of error with inclinometric measurement. *Spine.* 22:1976–1984, 1997.
146. Mayer T, Brady S, Bovasso E, et al: Noninvasive measurement of cervical tri-planar motion in normal subjects. *Spine* 18:2191–2195, 1993.
147. Capuano-Pucci D, Rheault W, Aukai J, et al: Intratester and intertester reliability of the cervical range of motion device. *Arch Phys Med Rehabil* 72:338–340, 1991.
148. Ordway NR, Seymour R, Donelson RG, et al: Cervical sagittal range-of-motion analysis using three methods. Cervical range-of-motion device, 3space, and radiography. *Spine* 22:501–508, 1997.
149. Nilsson N, Christensen HW, Hartvigsen J: The interexaminer reliability of measuring passive cervical range of motion, revisited. *J Manipulative Physiol Ther* 19:302–305, 1996.
150. Nilsson N: Measuring passive cervical motion: A study of reliability. *J Manipulative Physiol Ther* 18:293–297, 1995.
151. Youdas JW, Carey JR, Garrett TR: Reliability of measurements of cervical spine range of motion: Comparison of three methods. *Phys Ther* 71:98–104, 1991.
152. Chen SP, Samo DG, Chen EH, et al: Reliability of three lumbar sagittal motion measurement methods: Surface inclinometers. *J Occup Environ Med* 39:217–25, 1997.
153. Wainner RS, Fritz JM, Irrgang JJ, et al: Reliability and diagnostic accuracy of the clinical examination and patient self-report measures for cervical radiculopathy. *Spine* 28:52–62, 2003.
154. Wing P, Tsang I, Gagnon F: Diurnal changes in the profile shape and range of motion of the back. *Spine* 17:761–766, 1992.
155. Chibnall JT, Duckro PN, Baumer K: The influence of body size on linear measurements used to reflect cervical range of motion. *Phys Ther* 74:1134–1137, 1994.
156. Dvorak J, Antinnes JA, Panjabi M, et al: Age and gender related normal motion of the cervical spine. *Spine* 17:S393–S398, 1992.
157. Kuhlman KA: Cervical range of motion in the elderly. *Arch Phys Med Rehabil* 74:1071–1079, 1993.
158. Youdas JW, Garrett TR, Suman VJ, et al: Normal range of motion of the cervical spine: An initial goniometric study. *Phys Ther* 72:770–780, 1992.
159. Lowery WD Jr, Horn TJ, Boden SD, et al: Impairment evaluation based on spinal range of motion in normal subjects. *J Spinal Disord* 5:398–402, 1992.
160. Dvorak J, Herdmann J, Janssen B, et al: Motor-evoked potentials in patients with cervical spine disorders. *Spine* 15:1013–1016, 1990.
161. Toole J, Tucker S: Influence of head position upon cerebral circulation. *Arch Neurol* 2:616–623, 1960.
162. Jacob G, McKenzie R: Spinal therapeutics based on responses to loading. In: Liebenson C, ed. *Rehabilitation of the Spine: A Practitioner's Manual.* Baltimore, MD: Lippincott Williams & Wilkins, 1996:225–252.
163. Cyriax J: *Textbook of Orthopaedic Medicine, Diagnosis of Soft Tissue Lesions*, 8th ed. London: Bailliere Tindall, 1982.
164. Constantin P, Lucretia C: Relations between the cervical spine and the vertebral arteries. *ACTA Radiol* 6:91–96, 1971.
165. Ehrhardt R, Bowling RW: *Treatment of the Cervical Spine*, La Crosse, WI: APTA Orthopedic Section, Physical Therapy Home Study Course, 1996.
166. Vasilyeva LF, Lewit K: Diagnosis of muscular dysfunction by inspection. In: Liebenson C, ed. *Rehabilitation of the Spine: A Practitioner's Manual.* Baltimore, MD: Lippincott Williams & Wilkins, 1996:113–142.
167. Lee DG: *A Workbook of Manual Therapy Techniques for the Upper Extremity.* Delta, BC: Delta Orthopaedic Physiotherapy Clinics, 1989.
168. Sandmark H, Nisell R: Validity of five common manual neck pain provoking tests. *Scand J Rehabil Med* 27:131–136, 1995.
169. Hoppenfeld S: *Physical Examination of the Spine and Extremities.* East Norwalk, CT: Appleton-Century-Crofts, 1976.
170. Landes P, Malanga GA, Nadler SF, et al: Physical examination of the cervical spine. In: Malanga GA, Nadler SF, eds. *Musculoskeletal Physical Examination—An Evidence-Based Approach.* Philadelphia, PA: Elsevier-Mosby, 2006:33–57.
171. Fjellner A, Bexander C, Faleij R, et al: Interexaminer reliability in physical examination of the cervical spine. *J Manipulative Physiol Ther* 22:511–516, 1999.
172. Smedmark V, Wallin M, Arvidsson I: Inter-examiner reliability in assessing passive intervertebral motion of the cervical spine. *Man Ther* 5:97–101, 2000.
173. Strender LE, Lundin M, Nell K: Interexaminer reliability in physical examination of the neck. *J Manipulative Physiol Ther* 20:516–520, 1997.
174. Viikari-Juntura E: Interexaminer reliability of observations in physical examinations of the neck. *Phys Ther* 67:1526–1532, 1987.
175. Pool JJ, Hoving JL, de Vet HC, et al: The interexaminer reproducibility of physical examination of the cervical spine. *J Manipulative Physiol Ther* 27:84–90, 2004.
176. Mitchell FL, Moran PS, Pruzzo NA: *An Evaluation and Treatment Manual of Osteopathic Muscle Energy Procedures.* Manchester, MO: Mitchell, Moran and Pruzzo Associates, 1979.
177. Jensen OK, Justesen T, Nielsen EF, et al: Functional radiographic examination of the cervical spine in patients with post-traumatic headache. *Cephalalgia* 109:275–303, 1990.
178. Pettman E: Stress tests of the craniovertebral joints. In: Boyling JD, Palastanga N, eds. *Grieve's Modern Manual Therapy: The Vertebral Column*, 2nd ed. Edinburgh: Churchill Livingstone, 1994:529–538.
179. Vernon H, Mior S: The neck disability index: A study of reliability and validity. *J Manip Physiol Ther* 14:409–415, 1991.
180. Leak AM, Cooper J, Dyer S, et al: The Northwick Park Neck Pain Questionnaire, devised to measure neck pain and disability. *Br J Rheumatol* 33:469–474, 1994.
181. Hoving JL, O'Leary EF, Niere KR, et al: Validity of the neck disability index, Northwick Park neck pain questionnaire, and problem elicitation technique for measuring disability associated with whiplash-associated disorders. *Pain* 102:273–281, 2003.
182. Hall T, Robinson K: The flexion-rotation test and active cervical mobility—a comparative measurement study in cervicogenic headache. *Man Ther* 9:197–202, 2004.
183. Spurling RG, Scoville WB: Lateral rupture of the cervical intervetebral discs. A common cause of shoulder and arm pain. *Surg Gynecol Obstet* 78:350–358, 1944.
184. Jahnke RW, Hart BL: Cervical stenosis, spondylosis, and herniated disc disease. *Radiol Clin North Am* 29:777–791, 1991.
185. Tong HC, Haig AJ, Yamakawa K: The Spurling test and cervical radiculopathy. *Spine* 27:156–159, 2002.
186. Davidson RI, Dunn EJ, Metzmaker JN: The shoulder abduction test in the diagnosis of radicular pain in cervical extradural compressive monoradiculopathies. *Spine* 6:441–446, 1981.
187. Evans RC: *Illustrated Essentials in Orthopedic Physical Assessment.* St. Louis, MO: Mosby-Year book Inc, 1994.
188. Uchihara T, Furukawa T, Tsukagoshi H: Compression of brachial plexus as a diagnostic test of a cervical cord lesion. *Spine* 19:2170–2173, 1994.
189. Lindgren KA, Leino E, Hakola M, et al: Cervical spine rotation and lateral flexion combined motion in the examination of the thoracic outlet. *Arch Phys Med Rehabil* 71:343–344, 1990.
190. Lindgren KA, Leino E, Manninen H: Cervical rotation lateral flexion test in brachialgia. *Arch Phys Med Rehabil* 73:735–737, 1992.
191. Landi A, Copeland S: Value of the Tinel sign in brachial plexus lesions. *Ann R Coll Surg Engl* 61:470–471, 1979.
192. Marx RG, Bombardier C, Wright JG: What we know about the reliability and validity of physical examination tests used to examine the upper extremity. *J Hand Surg* 24A:185–193, 1999.
193. Nichols AW: The thoracic outlet syndrome in athletes. *J Am Board Fam Pract* 9:346–355, 1996.
194. Plewa MC, Delinger M: The false-positive rate of thoracic outlet syndrome shoulder maneuvers in healthy subjects. *Acad Emerg Med* 5:337–342, 1998.
195. Roos DB: Congenital anomalies associated with thoracic outlet syndrome. *J Surg* 132:771–778, 1976.
196. Wright IS: The neurovascular syndrome produced by hyperabduction of the arms. *Am Heart J* 29:1–19, 1945.
197. Gilroy J, Meyer JS: Compression of the subclavian artery as a cause of ischaemic brachial neuropathy. *Brain* 86:733–746, 1963.
198. Raaf J: Surgery for cervical rib and scalenus anticus syndrome. *J Am Med Assoc* 157:219–25, 1955.
199. Saturno PJ, Medina F, Valera F, et al: Validity and reliability of guidelines for neck pain treatment in primary health care. A nationwide empirical analysis in spain. *Int J Qual Health Care* 15:487–493, 2003.
200. Koes BW, Bouter LM, van Mameren H, et al: The effectiveness of manual therapy, physiotherapy and treatment by the general practitioner for nonspecific back and neck complaints: A randomized clinical trial. *Spine* 17:28–35, 1992.
201. Foley-Nolan D, Moore K, Codd M, et al: Low energy high frequency pulsed electromagnetic therapy for acute whiplash disorders. A double blind randomized controlled study. *Scand J Rehabil Med* 24:51–59, 1992.

202. Giebel GD, Edelmann M, Huser R: Sprain of the cervical spine: Early functional vs. immobilization treatment (in German). *Zentralbl Chir* 122:512–521, 1997.
203. Hoving JL, de Vet HC, Koes BW, et al: Manual therapy, physical therapy, or continued care by the general practitioner for patients with neck pain: Long-term results from a pragmatic randomized clinical trial. *Clin J Pain* 22:370–377, 2006.
204. Gross AR, Aker PD, Goldsmith CH, et al: Physical medicine modalities for mechanical neck disorders. *Cochrane Database Syst Rev* 2:CD000961, 2000.
205. Foley-Nolan D, Moore K, Codd M, et al: Low energy high frequency pulsed electromagnetic therapy for acute whiplash injuries. A double blind randomized controlled study. *Scand J Rehabil Med* 24:51–59, 1992.
206. Foley-Nolan D, Barry C, Coughlan RJ, et al: Pulsed high frequency (27 MHz) electromagnetic therapy for persistent neck pain. A double blind, placebo-controlled study of 20 patients. *Orthopedics* 13:445–451, 1990.
207. Berg HE, Berggren G, Tesch PA: Dynamic neck strength training effect on pain and function. *Arch Phys Med Rehabil* 75:661–665, 1994.
208. Jordan A, Ostergaard K: Rehabilitation of neck/shoulder patients in primary health care clinics. *J Manipulative Physiol Ther* 19:32–35, 1996.
209. Falla D: Unravelling the complexity of muscle impairment in chronic neck pain. *Man Ther* 9:125–133, 2004.
210. Falla DL, Jull GA, Hodges PW: Patients with neck pain demonstrate reduced electromyographic activity of the deep cervical flexor muscles during performance of the craniocervical flexion test. *Spine* 29:2108–2114, 2004.
211. Kennedy CN: The cervical spine. In: Hall C, Thein-Brody L, eds. *Therapeutic Exercise: Moving Toward Function*. Baltimore, MD: Lippincott Williams & Wilkins, 2005:582–609.
212. Bird SP, Tarpenning KM, Marino FE: Designing resistance training programmes to enhance muscular fitness: a review of the acute programme variables. *Sports Med* 35:841–851, 2005.
213. Richardson C, Jull G: Muscle control-pain control. What exercises would you prescribe? *Man Ther* 1:2–10, 1995.
214. Quebec Task Force on Spinal Disorders: Scientific approach to the assessment and management of activity-related spinal disorders: A monograph for clinicians. Report of the Quebec Task Force on Spinal Disorders. *Spine* 12(Suppl):1–59, 1987.
215. Zylbergold RS, Piper MC: Cervical spine disorders. A comparison of three types of traction. *Spine* 10:867–871, 1985.
216. Colachis SC, Strohm BR: Cervical traction: Relationship of traction time to varied tractive force with constant angle of pull. *Arch Phys Med Rehabil* 46:815–819, 1965.
217. Ellenberg MR, Honet JC, Treanor WJ: Cervical radiculopathy. *Arch Phys Med Rehabil* 75:342–352, 1994.
218. Saal JS, Saal JA, Yurth EF: Nonoperative management of herniated cervical intervertebral disc with radiculopathy. *Spine* 21:1877–83, 1996.
219. Ter Haar GR, Stratford IJ: Evidence for a non-thermal effect of ultrasound. *Br J Cancer* 45:172–175, 1982.
220. Michlovitz SL: The use of heat and cold in the management of rheumatic diseases. In: Michlovitz SL, ed. *Thermal Agents in Rehabilitation*. Philadelphia, PA: FA Davis, 1990:158–174.
221. Hurwitz E, Aker P, Adams A, et al: Manipulation and mobilization of the cervical spine. *Spine* 21:1746–1760, 1996.
222. Mealy K, Brennan H, Fenelon GC: Early mobilization of acute whiplash injuries. *BMJ* 292:656–657, 1986.
223. McKinney LA, Dornan JO, Ryan M: The role of physiotherapy in the management of acute neck sprains following road-traffic accidents. *Arch Emerg Med* 6:27–33, 1989.
224. McKinney LA: Early mobilisation and outcome in acute sprains of the neck. *BMJ* 299:1006–1008, 1989.
225. Borchgrevink GE, Kaasa A, McDonagh D, et al: Acute treatment of whiplash neck sprain injuries. *Spine* 23:25–31, 1998.
226. Gennis P, Miller L, Gallagher EJ, et al: The effect of soft cervical collars on persistent neck pain in patients with whiplash injury. *Acad Emerg Med* 3:568–573, 1998.
227. Dyrssen T, Svedenkrans M, Paasikivi J: Muskelträning vid besvär I nacke och skuldror effektiv behandling för att minska smärtan. *Läkartidningen* 86:2116–2120, 1989.
228. Provinciali L, Baroni M, Illuminati L, et al: Multimodal treatment of whiplash injury. *Scand J Rehabil Med* 28:105–111, 1996.
229. Cole AJ, Farrell JP, Stratton SA: Functional rehabilitation of cervical spine athletic injuries. In: Kibler BW, Herring JA, Press JM, eds. *Functional Rehabilitation of Sports and Musculoskeletal Injuries*. Gaithersburg, MD: Aspen, 1998:127–148.
230. Keshner EA, Campbell D, Katz RT: Neck muscle activation patterns in humans during isometric head stabilization. *Exp Brain Res* 75:335–344, 1989.
231. Andersson GBJ, Winters JM: Role of muscle in postural tasks: Spinal loading and postural stability. In: Winters JM, Woo SL-Y, eds. *Multiple Muscle Systems*. New York, NY: Springer-Verlag, 1990: 375–395.
232. O'Connor JJ: Can muscle co-contraction protect knee ligaments after injury or repair? *J Bone Joint Surg* 75-B:41–48, 1993.
233. Black KM, McClure P, Polansky M: The influence of different sitting positions on cervical and lumbar posture. *Spine* 21:65–70, 1996.
234. Hanten WP, Lucio RM, Russell JL, et al: Assessment of total head excursion and resting head posture. *Arch Phys Med Rehabil* 72:877–880, 1991.
235. Lee H, Nicholson LL, Adams RD: Cervical range of motion associations with subclinical neck pain. *Spine* 29:33–40, 2004.
236. Turk DC, Nash JM: Chronic pain: new ways to cope. In: Goleman D, Gurin J, eds. *Mind Body Medicine*. Yonkers, NY: Consumers Union of United States, 1993:111–131.
237. Jette DU, Jette AM: Physical therapy and health outcomes in patients with spinal impairments. *Phys Ther* 76:930–945, 1996.
238. Uhlig Y, Weber BR, Grob D, et al: Fiber composition and fiber transformations in the neck muscles of patients with dysfunction of the cervical spine. *J Orthop Res* 13:240–249, 1995.
239. Greenfield B: Upper quarter evaluation: Structural relationships and interindependence. In: Donatelli R, Wooden M, eds. *Orthopedic Physical Therapy*. New York, NY: Churchill Livingstone, 1989:43–58.
240. Cailliet R: *Neck and Arm Pain*, 3rd ed. Philadelphia, PA: FA Davis, 1990.
241. Darnell MW: A proposed chronology of events for forward head posture. *J Craniomandib Prac* 1:49–54, 1983.
242. Mannheimer JS: Prevention and restoration of abnormal upper quarter posture. In: Gelb H, Gelb M, eds. *Postural Considerations in the Diagnosis and Treatment of Cranio-Cervical-Mandibular and Related Chronic Pain Disorders*. St. Louis, MO: Ishiyaku EuroAmerica, 1991:93–161.
243. Kisner C, Colby LA: *Therapeutic Exercise. Foundations and Techniques*. Philadelphia, PA: FA Davis, 1997.
244. Kraus SL: Cervical spine influences on the craniomandibular region. In: Kraus SL, ed. *TMJ Disorders: Management of the Craniomandibular Complex*. New York, NY: Churchill Livingstone, 1988:367–396.
245. Kendall HO, Kendall FP, Boynton DA: *Posture and Pain*. Baltimore, MD: Williams and Wilkins, 1952.
246. Crawford HJ, Jull GA: The influence of thoracic posture and movement on range of arm elevation. *Physiother Theory Pract* 9:143–148, 1993.
247. Adams MA, McNally DM, Chinn H, et al: Posture and the compressive strength of the lumbar spine. International Society of Biomechanics Award Paper. *Clin Biomech* 9:5–14, 1994.
248. Ayub E: Posture and the Upper Quarter. In: Donatelli RA, ed. *Physical Therapy of the Shoulder*, 2nd ed. New York, NY: Churchill Livingstone, 1991:81–90.
249. Janda V: On the concept of postural muscles and posture in man. *Aust J Physiother* 29:83–84, 1983.
250. Janda V: *Muscle Function Testing*. London: Butterworths, 1983.
251. Lewit K: *Manipulative Therapy in Rehabilitation of the Motor System*, 3rd ed. London: Butterworths, 1999.
252. Lewit K, Simons DG: Myofascial pain: Relief by post-isometric relaxation. *Arch Phys Med Rehabil* 65:452–456, 1984.
253. Pearson N, Walmsley R: Trial into the effects of repeated neck retractions in normal subjects. *Spine* 20:1245–1251, 1995.
254. Roddey T, Olson S, Grant S: The effect of pectoralis muscle stretching on the resting position of the scapula in persons with varying degrees of forward head/rounded shoulder posture. *J Manual Manipulative Ther* 10:124–128, 2002.
255. Wright E, Domenech M, Fischer J: Usefulness of posture training for patients with temporomandibular disorders. *J Am Dent Assoc* 131:202–210, 2000.
256. Harman K, Hubley-Kozey CL, Butler H: Effectiveness of an exercise program to improve forward head posture in normal adults: A randomized, controlled 10-week trial. *J Manual Manipulative Ther* 13:163–176, 2005.
257. Humphreys BK, Irgens PM: The effect of a rehabilitation exercise program on head repositioning accuracy and reported levels of pain in chronic neck pain subjects. *J Whiplash Relat Disord* 1:99–112, 2002.
258. Ferguson RJ, Caplan LR: Cervical spondylitic myelopathy: History and physical findings. *Neurol Clin* 3: 373–82, 1985.

259. Young WF: Cervical spondylotic myelopathy: A common cause of spinal cord dysfunction in older persons. *Am Fam Phys* 62:1064–1070, 1073, 2000.
260. Kondo K, Molgaard C, Kurland L, et al: Protruded intervertebral cervical disc. *Minn Med* 64:751–753, 1981.
261. Kokubun S: Cervical disc herniation (In Japanese). *Rinsho Seikei Geka* 24:289–297, 1989.
262. O'Laoire SA, Thomas DGT: Spinal cord compression due to prolapse of cervical intervertebral disc (herniation of nucleus pulposus): Treatment in 26 cases by discectomy without interbody bone graft. *J Neurosurg* 59:847–853, 1983.
263. Ward R: Myofascial release concepts. In: Nyberg N, Basmajian JV, eds. *Rational Manual Therapies*. Baltimore, MD: Williams & Wilkins, 1993:25–241.
264. Leblhuber F, Reisecker F, Boehm-Jurkovic H, et al: Diagnostic value of different electrophysiologic tests in cervical disc prolapse. *Neurology* 38:1879–1881, 1988.
265. Motoe T: Studies on topographic architecture of the annulus fibrosus in the developmental and degenerative process of the lumbar intervertebral disc in man (In Japanese). *J Jpn Orthop Assoc* 60:495–509, 1986.
266. Yasuma T, Koh S, Okamura T, et al: Histological changes in aging lumbar intervertebral discs: Their role in protrusions and prolapses. *J Bone Joint Surg* 72A:220–229, 1990.
267. Bogduk N, Windsor M, Inglis A: The innervation of the cervical intervertebral discs. *Spine* 13:2–8, 1988.
268. Rao R: Neck pain, cervical radiculopathy, and cervical myelopathy: Pathophysiology, natural history, and clinical evaluation. *J Bone Joint Surg Am* 84-A:1872–1881, 2002.
269. Cooper RG, Freemont AJ, Hoyland JA, et al: Herniated intervertebral disc-associated periradicular fibrosis and vascular abnormalities occur without inflammatory cell infiltration. *Spine* 20:591–598, 1995.
270. Chabot MC, Montgomery DM: The pathophysiology of axial and radicular neck pain. *Semin Spine Surg* 7:2–8, 1995.
271. Farfan HF, Kirkaldy-Willis WH: The present status of spinal fusion in the treatment of lumbar intervertebral joint disorders. *Clin Orthop* 158:198, 1981.
272. Schutter H: *Intervertebral Disc Disorders, Clinical Neurology*. Philadelphia, PA: Lippincott-Raven, 1995:chap. 41.
273. Cloward RB: The clinical significance of the sinu-vertebral nerve of the cervical spine in relation to the cervical disk syndrome. *J Neurol Neurosurg Psychiatry* 23:321, 1960.
274. Henderson CM, Hennessy RG, Shuey HM Jr, et al: Posterior-lateral foraminotomy as an exclusive operative technique for cervical radiculopathy: A review of 846 consecutively operated cases. *Neruosurgery* 13:504–512, 1983.
275. Good DC, Couch JR, Wacaser L: Numb, clumsy hands and high cervical spondylosis. *Surg Neurol* 22:285–291, 1984.
276. Chen TY: The clinical presentation of uppermost cervical disc protrusion. *Spine* 25:439–442, 2000.
277. Cole AJ, Farrell JP, Stratton. SA: cervical spine athletic injuries. *Phys Med Rehabil Clin North Am* 5:37–68, 1994.
278. Marks MR: Cervical spine injuries and their neurologic implications. *Clin Sports Med* 9:263–278, 1990.
279. Barnes R: Traction injuries to the brachial plexus in adults. *J Bone Joint Surg* 31B:10–16, 1949.
280. Clancy WG: Brachial plexus and upper extremity peripheral nerve injuries. In: Torg JS, ed. *Athletic Injuries to the Head Neck and Face*. Philadelphia, PA: Lea & Febiger, 1982:215–222.
281. Braddom RL: Management of common cervical pain syndromes. In: Lisa JAD, ed. *Rehabilitation Medicine: Principles and Practice*, 2nd ed. Philadelphia, PA. J.B. Lippincott, 1993:1038.
282. Malanga GA, Campagnolo DI: Clarification of the pronator reflex. *Am J Phys Med Rehabil* 73:338–340, 1994.
283. Reiners K, Toyka KV: Management of cervical radiculopathy. *Eur Neurol* 35:313–316, 1995.
284. Grisoli F, Graziani N, Fabrizi AP, et al: Anterior discectomy without fusion for treatment of cervical lateral soft disc extrusion: A follow-up of 120 cases. *Neurosurgery* 24:853–859, 1989.
285. Gore DR, Sepic SB: Anterior cervical fusion for degenerated or protruded discs. A review of one hundred forty-six patients. *Spine* 9:667–671, 1984.
286. Dreyer SJ, Boden SD: Nonoperative treatment of neck and arm pain. *Spine* 23:2746–2754, 1998.
287. Cleland JA, Fritz JM, Whitman JM, et al: The reliability and construct validity of the Neck Disability Index and patient specific functional scale in patients with cervical radiculopathy. *Spine*. 31:598–602, 2006.
288. Dillin W, Booth R, Cuckeler J, et al: Cervical radiculopathy: A review. *Spine* 11:988–991, 1986.
289. Aldrich F: Posterolateral microdiscectomy for cervical monoradiculopathy caused by posterolateral soft cervical disc sequestration. *J Neurosurg* 72:370–377, 1990.
290. Jho HD, Kim WK, Kim MH: Anterior microforaminotomy for treatment of cervical radiculopathy: Part 1—disc-preserving "functional cervical disc surgery". *Neurosurgery* 51:46–53, 2002.
291. Houser OW, Onofrio BM, Miller GM, et al: Cervical disk prolapse. *Mayo Clin Proc* 70:939–945, 1995.
292. Johnson JP, Filler AG, McBride DQ, et al: Anterior cervical foraminotomy for unilateral radicular disease. *Spine* 25:905–909, 2000.
293. Aita I, Wadano Y, Yabuki T: Curvature and range of motion of the cervical spine after laminaplasty. *J Bone Joint Surg Am* 82-A:1743–1748, 2000.
294. Nowinski GP, Visarius H, Nolte LP, et al: A biomechanical comparison of cervical laminaplasty and cervical laminectomy with progressive facetectomy. *Spine*. 18:1995–2004, 1993.
295. Herkowitz HN: Cervical laminaplasty: Its role in the treatment of cervical radiculopathy. *J Spinal Disord* 1:179–188, 1988.
296. Kimura I, Oh-Hama M, Shingu H: Cervical myelopathy treated by canal-expansive laminaplasty. Computed tomographic and myelographic findings. *J Bone Joint Surg Am* 66:914–920, 1984.
297. Jho HD: Microsurgical anterior cervical foraminotomy: A new approach to cervical disc herniation. *J Neurosurg* 84:155–160, 1996.
298. Jho HD: Anterior microforaminotomy for cervical radiculopathy: Disc preservation technique. In: Rengachary SS, Wilkins RJ, eds. *Neurosurgical Operative Color Atlas*. Baltimore, MD: Williams & Wilkins, 1998:43–52.
299. Danielsen J, Johnsen R, Kibsgaard S, et al: Early aggressive exercise for postoperative rehabilitation after discectomy. *Spine* 25:1015–1020, 2000.
300. Johannsen F, Remvig L, Kryger P, et al: Supervised endurance training compared to home training after first lumbar diskectomy: A clinical trial. *Clin Exp Rheumatol* 12:609–614, 1994.
301. Kjellby-Wendt G, Styf J: Early active training after lumbar discectomy: A prospective, randomized and controlled trial. *Spine* 23:2345–2351, 1998.
302. Skall F, Manniche C, Nielsen C: Intensive back exercises 5 weeks after surgery of lumbar disk prolapse: A prospective randomized multicentre trial with historical control. *Ugeskr Laeger* 156:643–646, 1994.
303. Booth FW: Physiologic and biochemical effects of immobilization on muscle. *Clin Orthop Relat Res* 219:15–21, 1987.
304. Eiff MP, Smith AT, Smith GE: Early mobilization versus immobilization in the treatment of lateral ankle sprains. *Am J Sports Med* 22:83–88, 1994.
305. Akeson WH, Amiel D, Mechanic GL, et al: Collagen cross-linking alterations in the joint contractures: Changes in the reducible cross-links in periarticular connective tissue after 9 weeks immobilization. *Connect Tissue Res* 5:15, 1977.
306. Akeson WH, Amiel D, Abel MF, et al: Effects of immobilization on joints. *Clin Orthop* 219:28–37, 1987.
307. Akeson WH, Amiel D, Woo SL-Y: Immobility effects on synovial joints: The pathomechanics of joint contracture. *Biorheology* 17:95–110, 1980.
308. Woo SL-Y, Matthews J, Akeson WH, et al: Connective tissue response to immobility: A correlative study of biochemical and biomechanical measurements of normal and immobilized rabbit knee. *Arthritis Rheum* 18:257–264, 1975.
309. White T, Malone T: Effects of running on intervertebral disc height. *J Orthop Sports Phys Ther* 12:410, 1990.
310. Heine J: Uber die arthritis deformans. *Virchows Arch Pathol Anat* 260:521–663, 1926.
311. Friedenberg ZB, Miller WT: Degenerative disc disease of the cervical spine. *J Bone Joint Surg* 45:1171–1178, 1963.
312. Kirkaldy-Willis WH: *Managing Low Back Pain*, 2nd ed. New York, NY: Churchill Livingstone, 1988.
313. Jeffreys E: Cervical spondylosis. In: Jeffreys E, ed. *Disorders of the Cervical Spine*. Boston, MA: Butterworths, 1980:90–106.
314. Aprill C, Bogduk N: The prevalence of cervical zygapophyseal joint pain: A first approximation. *Spine* 17:744–747, 1992.
315. Barnsley L, Lord S, Bogduk N: Comparative local anaesthetic blocks in the diagnosis of cervical zygapophyseal joint pain. *Pain* 55:99–106, 1993.
316. Barnsley L, Lord SM, Wallis BJ, et al: The prevalence of chronic cervical zygapophyseal joint pain after whiplash. *Spine* 20:20–26, 1995.

317. Cleland JA, Childs JD, Fritz JM, et al: Development of a clinical prediction rule for guiding treatment of a subgroup of patients with neck pain: Use of thoracic spine manipulation, exercise, and patient education. *Phys Ther* 87:9–23, 2007.
318. Banerjee A: The hanging head method for the treatment of acute wry neck. *Arch Emerg Med* 7:125, 1990.
319. Bland J: *Disorders of the Cervical Spine: Diagnosis and Medical Management*. Philadelphia, PA: WB Saunders, 1994.
320. Panjabi M, Thibodeau L, Crisco JJ, et al: What constitutes spinal stability. *Clin Neurosurg* 34:313–319, 1988.
321. Crowe H: *Injuries to the cervical spine, Presentation to the annual meeting of the Western Orthopaedic Association*. San Francisco, CA, 1928.
322. Spitzer WO, Skovron ML, Salmi LR, et al: Scientific monograph of the Quebec Task Force on Whiplash-Associated Disorders: Redefining "whiplash" and its management. *Spine* 20:[Erratum, Spine 1995;20: 2372], 1995.
323. Reilly PA, Travers R, Littlejohn GO: Epidemiology of soft tissue rheumatism: The influence of the law. *J Rheumatol* 18:1448–1449, 1991.
324. Evans RW: Some observations on whiplash injuries. *Neurol Clin* 10:975–997, 1992.
325. Ferrari R, Russell AS: Epidemiology of whiplash: An international dilemma. *Ann Rheum Dis* 58:1–5, 1999.
326. Gay JR, Abbott KH: Common whiplash injuries of the neck. *JAMA* 152:1698–1704, 1953.
327. Gotten N: Survey of 100 cases of whiplash injury after settlement of litigation. *JAMA* 162:854–857, 1956.
328. MacNab I: Acceleration injuries of the cervical spine. *J Bone Joint Surg* 46A:1797–1799, 1964.
329. Macnab I: The whiplash syndrome. *Orthop Clin North Am* 2:389–403, 1971.
330. Farbman AA: Neck sprain. Associated factors. *JAMA* 25:1010–1015, 1973.
331. Nordhoff LS Jr: Cervical trauma following motor vehicle collisions. In: Murphy DR, ed. *Cervical Spine Syndromes*. New York, NY: McGraw-Hill, 2000:131–150.
332. Scientific monograph of the quebec task force on whiplash-associated disorders. *Spine* 20:33S, 38S–39S, 1995.
333. National Highway Traffic Safety Administration: *Traffic Safety Facts 1994: A Compilation of Motor Vehicle Crash Data from the Fatal Accident Reporting System and the General Estimates System*. Washington, DC: National Highway Traffic Safety Administration, 1995.
334. Pennie B, Agambar L: Patterns of injury and recovery in whiplash. *Injury* 22:57–60, 1991.
335. Radanov BP, Sturzenegger M, Di Stefano G: Long-term outcome after whiplash injury. A 2-year follow-up considering features of injury mechanism and somatic, radiologic, and psychosocial findings. *Med Sci Sports Exerc* 74:281–297, 1995.
336. Sturzenegger M, Radanov BP, DiStefano G: The effect of accident mechanisms and initial findings on the long-term course of whiplash injury. *J Neurol* 242:443–449, 1995.
337. Nikolai MD, Teasell R: Whiplash: The evidence for an organic etiology. *Arch Neurol* 57:590–591, 2000.
338. Forsyth HF: Extension injury of the cervical spine. *J Bone Joint Surg* 46A:1792–1797, 1964.
339. Barnes R: Paraplegia in cervical spine injuries. *J Bone Joint Surg* 30B:234, 1948.
340. Carrette S: Whiplash injury and chronic neck pain. *N Engl J Med* 330:1083–1084, 1994.
341. Zador PL, Ciccone MA: Automobile driver fatalities in frontal impacts: Air bags compared with manual belts. *Am J Public Health* 83:661–666, 1993.
342. Cummings P, McKnight B, Rivara FP, et al: Association of driver air bags with driver fatality: A matched cohort study. *BMJ* 324:1119–1122, 2002.
343. Evans L: The effectiveness of safety belts in preventing fatalities. *Accid Anal Prev* 18:229–241, 1986.
344. McGwin G Jr, Metzger J, Alonso JE, et al: The association between occupant restraint systems and risk of injury in frontal motor vehicle collisions. *J Trauma* 54:1182–1187, 2003.
345. Segui-Gomez M: Driver air bag effectiveness by severity of the crash. *Am J Public Health* 90:1575–1581, 2000.
346. Morris F: Do headrests protect the neck from whiplash injuries? *Arch Emerg Med* 6:17–21, 1989.
347. Maimaris C, Barnes MR, Allen MJ: Whiplash injuries of the neck: A retrospective study. *Injury* 19:393–396, 1988.
348. Grob D: Posterior surgery. In: Gunzburg R, Szpalski M, eds. *Whiplash Injuries: Current Concepts in Prevention, Diagnosis and Treatment of the Cervical Whiplash Syndrome*. Philadelphia: Lippincott-Raven Publishers, 1998:241–246.
349. Press JM, Herring SA, Kibler WB: *Rehabilitation of Musculoskeletal Disorders. The Textbook of Military Medicine*. Washington, DC: Borden Institute, Office of the Surgeon General, 1996.
350. McLain RF: Mechanoreceptor endings in human cervical facet joints. *Spine* 19:495–501, 1994.
351. Jonsson H, Cesarini K, Sahlstedt B, et al: Findings and outcomes in whiplash-type neck distortions. *Spine* 19:2733–2743, 1994.
352. Jonsson H, Bring G, Rauschning W, et al: Hidden cervical spine injuries in traffic accident victims with skull fractures. *J Spinal Disord* 4:251–263, 1991.
353. Rauschning W, McAfee PC, Jonsson H: Pathoanatomical and surgical findings in cervical spinal injuries. *J Spinal Disord* 2:213–222, 1989.
354. Twomey LT, Taylor JR: The whiplash syndrome: Pathology and physical treatment. *J Manual Manipulative Ther* 1:26–29, 1993.
355. Ommaya AR: The head: kinematics and brain injury mechanisms. In: Aldman B, Chapon A, eds. *The Biomechanics of Impact Trauma*. Amsterdam: Elsevier, 1984:117–138.
356. Mendel T, Wink CS: Neural elements in cervical intervertebral discs. *Anat Record* 78A:25, 1989.
357. Cloward RB: Cervical diskography. A contribution to the etiology and mechanism of neck pain. *Ann Surg* 150:1052, 1959.
358. Kaneoka K, Ono K, Inami S, et al: Motion analysis of cervical vertebrae during whiplash loading. *Spine* 24:763–769, 1999.
359. Taylor JR, Twomey LT: Acute injuries to cervical joints: An autopsy study of neck sprain. *Spine* 9:1115–1122, 1993.
360. Barnsley L, Lord S, Bogduk N: The pathophysiology of whiplash. In: Malanga GA, ed. *Cervical Flexion-Extension/Whiplash Injuries. Spine: State of the Art Reviews*. Philadelphia, PA: Hanley & Belfus, 1998:209–242.
361. Winkelstein B, Nightingale RW, Richardson WJ, et al: The cervical facet capsule and its role in whiplash injury: a biomechanical investigation. *Spine* 25:1238–1246, 2000.
362. Deans GT, Magalliard K, Rutherford WH: Neck sprain: A major cause of disability following car accidents. *Injury* 18:10–12, 1987.
363. Lord SM, Barnsley L, Wallis BJ, et al: Chronic cervical zygapophyseal joint pain after whiplash: A placebo-controlled prevalence study. *Spine* 21:1737–1744, 1996.
364. Bogduk N: Innervation and pain patterns of the cervical spine. In: Grant R, ed. *Physical Therapy of the Cervical and Thoracic Spine*. New York, NY: Churchill Livingstone, 1988.
365. Livingston M: *Common Whiplash Injury: A Modern Epidemic*. Springfield, IL: Charles C Thomas, 1999.
366. Klein de A, Nieuwenhuyse AC: Schwindelanfaalle und Nystagumus bei einer bestimmeten Lage des Kopfes. *Arch Otolaryngol* 11:155, 1927.
367. Toglia JU: Acute flexion-extension injury of the neck. *Neurology* 26:808, 1976.
368. Wing LW, Hargrove-Wilson W: Cervical vertigo. *Aust N Z J Surg* 44:275, 1974.
369. Chester JB Jr: Whiplash, postural control, and the inner ear. *Spine* 16:716, 1991.
370. Edeiken-Monroe B, Wagner LK, Harris JH Jr: Hyperextension dislocation of the cervical spine. *AJR* 146:803–808, 1986.
371. Osti OL, Vernon-Roberts B, Frazer RD: Annulus tears and intervertebral disc degeneration: A study using an animal model. *Spine* 15:762, 1990.
372. Gargan MF, Bannister GC: Long term prognosis of soft tissue injuries of the neck. *J Bone Joint Surg* 72B:901, 1990.
373. Viktrup L, Knudsen GM, Hansen SH: Delayed onset of fatal basilar thrombotic embolus after whiplash injury. *Stroke* 26:2194–2196, 1995.
374. Borchgrevink G, Smevik O, Nordby A, et al: MR Imaging and radiography of patients with cervical hyperextension-flexion injuries after car accidents. *Acta Radiol* 36:425–428, 1995.
375. Ronnen HR, de Korte PJ, Brink PRG, et al: Acute whiplash injury: Is there a role for MR imaging? A prospective study of 100 patients. *Radiology* 201:93–96, 1996.
376. Ellertsson AB, Sigurjonsson K, Thorsteinsson T: Clinical and radiographic study of 100 cases of whiplash injury. *Acta Neurol Scand* 57:269, 1978.

377. Seitz JP, Unguez CE, Corbus HF, et al: SPECT of the cervical spine in the evaluation of neck pain after trauma. *Clin Nucl Med* 20:667–673, 1995.
378. Scholten-Peeters GG, Verhagen AP, Bekkering GE, et al: Prognostic factors of whiplash-associated disorders: A systematic review of prospective cohort studies. *Pain* 104:303–322, 2003.
379. Pennie BH, Agambar LJ: Whiplash injuries. *J Bone Joint Surg* 72B:277–279, 1990.
380. Helliwell PS, Evans PF, Wright V: The straight cervical spine: Does it indicate muscle spasm? *J Bone Joint Surg* 76B:103–106, 1994.
381. Stovner LJ: The nosologic status of the whiplash syndrome: A critical review based on a methodological approach. *Spine* 21:2735–2746, 1996.
382. Thompson JF, Jannsen F: Thoracic outlet syndromes. *Br J Surg* 83:435–436, 1996.
383. Strukel RJ, Garrick JG: Thoracic outlet compression in athletes: A report of four cases. *Am J Sports Med* 6:35–39, 1978.
384. Peet RM, Hendriksen JD, Anderson TP, et al: Thoracic outlet syndrome: Evaluation of the therapeutic exercise program. *Proc Mayo Clin* 31:281–287, 1956.
385. MacKinnon EJ, Dellon AL: *Surgery of the Peripheral Nerve*. New York, NY: Thieme Medical Publishers Inc, 1988.
386. Karas SE: Thoracic outlet syndrome. *Clin Sports Med* 9:297–310, 1990.
387. Selke FW, Kelly TR: Thoracic outlet syndrome. *Am J Surg* 156:54–57, 1988.
388. Sanders RJ, Jackson CG, Banchero N, et al: Scalene muscle abnormalities in traumatic thoracic outlet syndrome. *Am J Surg* 159:231–236, 1990.
389. McCarthy WJ, Yao JST, Schafer MF, et al: Upper extremity arterial injury in athletes. *J Vasc Surg* 9:317–327, 1989.
390. Vogel CM, Jensen JE: "Effort" thrombosis of the subclavian vein in a competitive swimmer. *Am J Sports Med* 13:269–272, 1985.
391. Leffert RD: Thoracic outlet syndrome and the shoulder. *Clin Sports Med* 2:439–452, 1983.
392. Nishida T, Price SJ, Minieka MM: Medial antebrachial cutaneous nerve conduction in true neurogenic thoracic outlet syndrome. *Electromyogr Clin Neurophysiol* 33:285–288, 1993.
393. Cuetter AC, David MB: The thoracic outlet syndrome: Controversies, over diagnosis, over treatment, and recommendations for management. *Muscle Nerve* 12:410–419, 1989.
394. Kenny RA, Traynor GB, Withington D, et al: Thoracic outlet syndrome: A useful exercise treatment option. *Am J Surg* 165:282–284, 1993.
395. Silver D: Thoracic outlet syndrome. In: Sabiston DC, ed. *Textbook of Surgery: The Biological Basis of Modern Surgical Practice*, 13th ed. Philadelphia, PA: WB Saunders Company, 1986.
396. Crawford FA: Thoracic outlet syndrome. *Surg Clin North Am* 60:947–956, 1980.
397. Sanders RJ, Johnson RF: Medico-legal matters. In: Sanders RJ, Haug CE, eds. *Thoracic Outlet Syndrome: A Common Sequela of Neck Injuries*. Philadelphia, PA: JB Lippincott, 1991:271–277.
398. Mulligan BR: *Manual Therapy: "NAGS", "SNAGS", "PRP'S" etc.* Wellington: Plane View Series, 1992.
399. Cohen JH, Schneider MJ: Receptor-tonus technique. An overview. *Chiro Tech* 2:13–16, 1990.
400. Liebenson C: Manual resistance techniques and self stretches for improving flexibility and mobility. In: Liebenson C, ed. *Rehabilitation of the Spine: A Practitioner's Manual*. Baltimore, MD: Lippincott Williams & Wilkins, 1996:253–292.
401. Erhard RE: *Manual Therapy in the Cervical Spine, Orthopedic Physical Therapy Home Study Course*, La Crosse, WI: APTA, Orthopaedic Section, 1996.
402. Raikin S, Froimson MI: Bilateral brachial plexus compressive neuropathy (crutch palsy). *J Orthop Trauma* 11:136–138, 1997.

The Temporomandibular Joint

CHAPTER 26

CHAPTER OBJECTIVES

At the completion of this chapter, the reader will be able to:

1. Describe the anatomy of the temporomandibular joint (TMJ), including the bones, ligaments, muscles, and blood and nerve supply.
2. Describe the biomechanics of the TMJ, including the movements, normal and abnormal joint barriers, kinesiology, and reactions to various stresses.
3. Summarize the various causes of temporomandibular dysfunction (TMD).
4. Describe the close association between the TMJ, the middle ear, and the cervical spine.
5. Perform a comprehensive examination of the temporomandibular musculoskeletal system, including palpation of the articular and soft tissue structures, specific passive mobility and passive articular mobility tests, and stability tests.
6. Evaluate the total examination data to establish a diagnosis.
7. Recognize the manifestations of abnormal TMJ function and develop strategies to correct these abnormalities.
8. Apply active and passive mobilization techniques to the TMJ, using the correct grade, direction, and duration.
9. Describe and demonstrate intervention strategies and techniques based on clinical findings and established goals.
10. Evaluate the intervention effectiveness in order to progress or modify an intervention.
11. Plan an effective home program and instruct the patient in this program.

OVERVIEW

Housed within the skull are the components of the stomatognathic system, which includes the TMJ, the masticatory systems, and the related organs and tissues such as the inner ear and salivary glands.[1] An interrelationship exists between the stomatognathic system and the head and neck due to their proximity and shared embryological development. An understanding of this relationship is vital to understand the reasons for the myriad of symptoms that this region can exhibit.

The embryologic structures from which the head, the face, and the neck originate are segmentally organized during development with the appearance and modification of six paired branchial or pharyngeal arches.[1] These branchial arches contain the cranial nuclei of the trigeminal nerve (ophthalmic; maxillary and mandibular), the facial, the glossopharyngeal, and the laryngeal branch of the vagus nerve as well as the hypoglossal nerve.

The first of these arches, the mandibular arch, consists of a large anterior (ventral) part (mandibular process of Meckel's cartilage) and a small posterior (dorsal) (maxillary) process. As development progresses, both processes disappear except for two small portions at the posterior (dorsal) ends, which persist. The first brachial arch forms

- the mandible;
- the rudiments of the inner ear bones, the malleus, and incus;
- the anterior malleolar and sphenomandibular ligaments of the TMJ;
- the tensor tympani and the tensor veli palatini of the inner ear;
- the mylohyoid and the anterior belly of the digastric muscle;
- the trigeminal mandibular nerve.

The second pharyngeal arch (the hyoid arch) consists of Reichert's cartilage. This arch is involved in the formation of

- the superior component of the hyoid bone and the lesser cornu bone;
- the stapes muscle;
- the temporal styloid process;
- the stylohyoid ligament;
- the stapedius muscle;
- the stylohyoid muscle;
- the posterior belly of the digastric muscle;
- the muscles of facial expression and mastication;

- the platysma muscle;
- the glossopharyngeal nerve.

The third pharyngeal arch is involved in the formation of the greater cornu of the hyoid and its body, the stylopharyngeal muscle, and the sensory apparatus of the posterior one-third of the tongue.

The fourth pharyngeal arch combines with the sixth arch to form the thyroid, cricoid, and arytenoid cartilages of the larynx. The muscles derived from this arch are the pharyngeal constrictors (the cricothyroid) and the intrinsic muscles of the larynx. The pharyngeal constrictors are innervated by the superior laryngeal branch of the vagus nerve. The intrinsic muscles of the larynx are innervated by the recurrent laryngeal branch of the vagus nerve.

In primitive creatures, and the human fetus, vibrations through the jaw are used as a basis for hearing. At around $8^1/_2$ weeks, the small bones of the inner ear (the malleus, incus, and stapes) can be seen as distinct entities. The development of the malleus bone and the tensor tympani are intimately related to that of the lateral pterygoid muscle. Due to this embryological relationship, it is theorized that a spasm of the lateral pterygoid muscle can increase the tension within the tensor tympani (similar to that of a drum skin)[1] resulting in an increased sensitivity to pitch and vibration. Theoretically, this increased tension could produce sensorineural tinnitus, or ringing in the ears,[1] a common associated symptom of a temporomandibular disorder (TMD), and an injury to the craniovertebral region. TMD is a collective term used to describe a number of related disorders affecting the stomatognathic system and its related structures, all of which may have common symptoms. The term *TMJ dysfunction* as an overall descriptor of stomatognathic system dysfunction has been discontinued because it implies structural problems when none may exist, and does not include the many other factors that may be involved.[2]

The diagnosis of TMD, like that of whiplash syndrome, remains controversial.[3] This is due in part to a paucity of studies regarding the incidence, course, management, and prognosis of claimed TMDs.[4,5] However, reports of TMD appear to be quite common. About 60–70% of the general population has at least one sign of a TMD, yet only around one in four people with signs is actually aware of, or reports, any symptoms,[6,7] and only about 5% of people with one or more signs of a TMD will actually seek an intervention.[7–9] After a technology assessment conference in 1996 about managing TMD, the National Institutes of Health (NIH) concluded that the natural history and etiology of TMD are not well understood and that most TMD symptoms are self-limiting, can recur, and may fluctuate over time.[10] The most common TMD by far, comprising 90–95% of all TMD cases, is a condition with multiple musculoskeletal facial pain complaints and a variety of jaw impairments, without an identified structural cause.[11]

TMD is best approached as a biopsychosocial dysfunction. Although TMD originally was approached as one syndrome, current research supports the view that TMD is a cluster of related disorders in the stomatognathic system that have many common symptoms.[6,12] McNeill and colleagues[13] have described three etiologic factors of TMD: (1) predisposing factors, (2) precipitating or triggering factors, and (3) perpetuating or sustaining factors[14]:

- Predisposing factors include the structural, neurologic, hormonal, and metabolic features of an individual.
- Precipitating factors generally fall into the following four categories: (1) overt, extrinsic trauma to the head, the neck, or the jaw; (2) repeated low-grade extrinsic trauma, such as nail biting and chewing gum; (3) repeated low-grade intrinsic trauma such as teeth clenching or bruxism (grinding teeth); and (4) stress that passes a certain threshold, which is individual for each patient.
- Perpetuating or contributing factors are those that aid in the continuation of symptoms. These can include systemic disease and cervical pathology.

Thus, the clinical course of TMD does not reflect a progressive disease but rather a complex disorder that is molded by many interacting factors, such as stress, anxiety, and depression, which serve to maintain the disease.[12] Headaches, orofacial pain, earache, and neck pain are common complaints. Persistent or recurrent pain is considered the main reason that more than 90% of patients with TMD seek an intervention.[8,15] A diagnosis of TMD must, therefore, include an examination of all of the following:

- Jaw muscles
- Bone and cartilage joint structures
- Facial structures
- Soft tissue joint structures, including the articular disk and synovium
- Jaw and joint function
- Cervical and upper thoracic spine function
- Posture and dysfunction
- Systemic disease
- Psychosocial issues

Given the number of potential causes of jaw and face pain, a diagnosis of TMD can rarely be ascribed solely to the TMJ. Examples of appropriate diagnoses for TMD are more likely to include

- rheumatoid arthritis with synovitis, arthralgia, condylar degenerative disease, and open bite deformity;
- chronic pain with a behavioral disorder;
- myofascial pain and impairment;
- internal disk derangement, with displacement and reduction.

CLINICAL PEARL

Most of those who seek medical intervention for TMDs are female, outnumbering male patients by at least four to one.[8,9,16] The reason for the higher prevalence of TMD in women, and the overrepresentation of females at orofacial pain clinics, remains obscure. One explanation could be that women more readily seek treatment for illness than do men.[17]

Nonsurgical interventions such as counseling, physical therapy, pharmacotherapy, and occlusal splint therapy continue to be the most effective way of managing more than 80% of patients with TMD.[12] Although dentists are the primary professionals involved in the examination and intervention of TMD, physical therapists can play an important role in assisting the dentist in restoring function to the stomatognathic system. However, the procedures in physical therapy intervention are not well described in the literature in this area.

ANATOMY

The TMJ (Fig. 26-1) is a synovial, compound, modified ovoid bicondylar joint, which is formed between the articular eminence of the temporal bone, the intra-articular disk, and the head of the mandible.

The TMJ is unique in that, even though the joint is synovial, the articulating surfaces of the bones are covered not by hyaline cartilage but by fibrocartilage.[18,19] Fibrocartilage has the same general properties found in hyaline cartilage but tends to be less distensible, owing to a greater proportion of dense collagen fibers (see Chap. 1). The development of fibrocartilage over the load-bearing surface of the TMJ indicates that the joint is designed to withstand large and repeated stresses and that this area of the joint surface has a greater capacity to repair itself than would hyaline cartilage.[20]

The area of load bearing is affected by the congruity of the contacting tooth surfaces (occlusion), head position, and the coordination of muscle function. The fibrocartilage is at its thinnest at the roof of the fossa, but load bearing here occurs only in the presence of dysfunction.[21]

The mandible works like a class-three lever (see Chap. 1), with its joint as the fulcrum. Although there is no agreement among the experts concerning force transmission through the joint, there does appear to be agreement that postural impairments of the cervical and upper thoracic spine can produce both pain and impairment of the TMJ.[6]

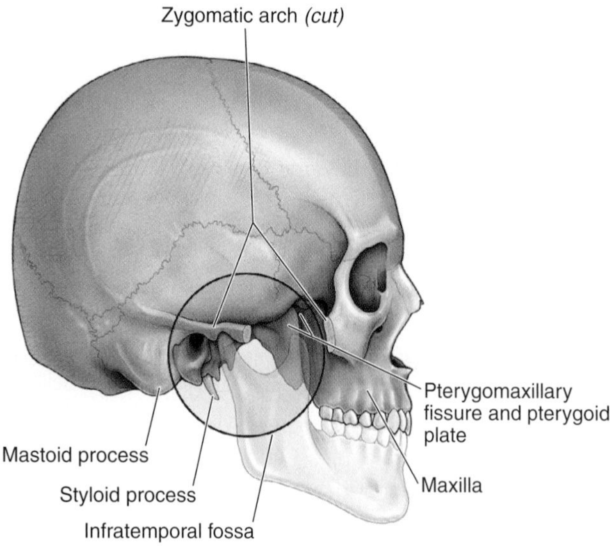

FIGURE 26-1 The temporomandibular joint. (Reproduced, with permission, from Morton DA, Foreman KB, Albertine KH: *The Big Picture: Gross Anatomy*, McGraw-Hill, 2011.)

Bony Anatomy

A number of bony components make up the masticatory system: the maxilla and the mandible, which support the teeth, and the temporal bone, which supports the mandible at its articulation with the skull. The sphenoid bone and the hyoid bone also could be included, because they provide important anatomic and functional links to the TMJ.

Maxilla

The borders of the maxillae extend superiorly to form the floor of the nasal cavity as well as the floor of each orbit (Fig. 26-1). Inferiorly, the maxillary bones form the palate and the alveolar ridges, which support the teeth. The maxillae and mandible each contain 16 permanent teeth. The structure of each tooth reflects its function in mastication.

Sphenoid Bone

The greater wings of the sphenoid bone form the boundaries of the anterior part of the middle cranial fossa. From these greater wings, the pterygoid laminae serve as the attachments for the medial and lateral pterygoid muscles.

Hyoid Bone

The U-shaped hyoid bone (Fig. 26-2), also known as the skeleton of the tongue, serves as the attachment for the infrahyoid muscles and for some of the extrinsic tongue muscles. The hyoid bone is involved with the mandible to provide reciprocal stabilization during swallowing and chewing. Theoretically, due to its muscle attachments, the position of the hyoid bone can be affected by cervical and shoulder positions, as occurs during forward head posture, which changes the length–tension relationships.

Mandible

The mandible, or jaw (Fig. 26-1), which supports the lower teeth, is the largest and the strongest bone in the face. It is suspended below the maxillae by muscles and ligaments that provide it with both mobility and stability. The medial surface of the mandible serves as the attachment for the medial pterygoid and the digastric muscles. The platysma, mentalis, and buccinator gain attachment on its lateral aspect.

Two broad, vertical rami extend upward from the mandible: the condyle and the coronoid process. The anterior of the two processes, the coronoid, serves as the attachment for the temporalis and masseter muscles.[22] The condyle process articulates with the temporal bone. The bony surfaces of the condyle and the articular portion of the temporal bone are made of dense cortical bone. The articulating surface of the condyle is flattened from front to back with its medial–lateral length twice as long as its anterior–posterior length. The condyles are generally convex, possessing short bony projections known as medial and lateral poles.[23]

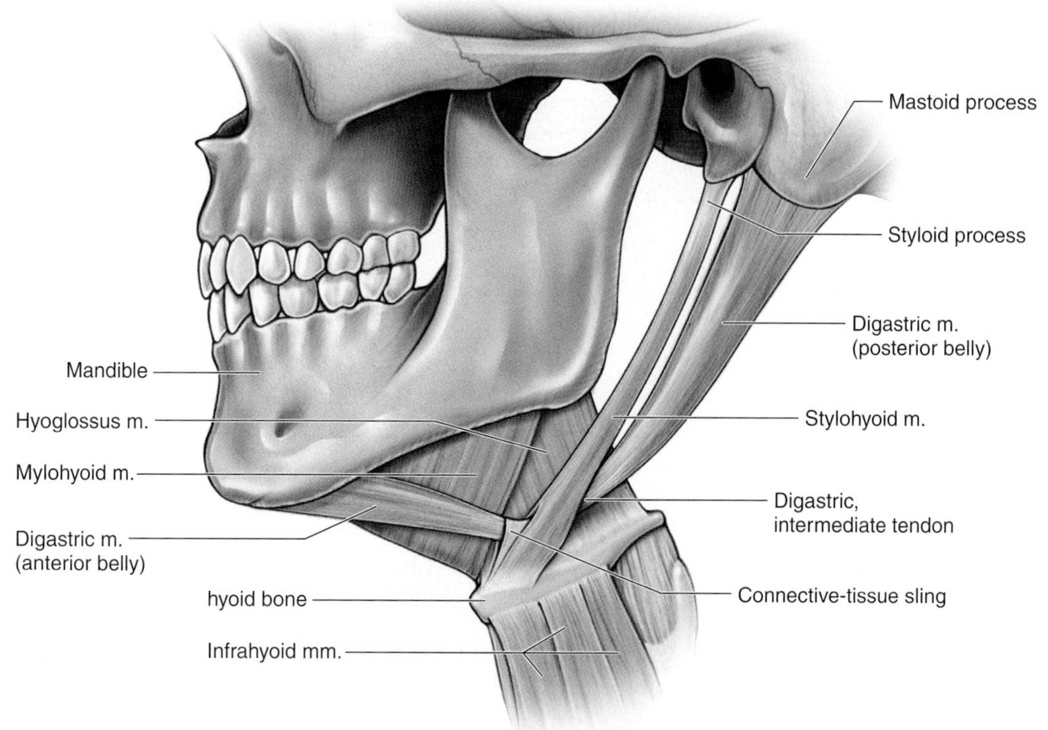

FIGURE 26-2 The hyoid bone and related muscles. (Reproduced, with permission, from Morton DA, Foreman KB, Albertine KH: *The Big Picture: Gross Anatomy,* McGraw-Hill, 2011.)

Temporal Bone

The mandibular fossa of the temporal bone is divided into two surfaces: articular and nonarticular.[23] The articulating surface of the temporal bone is made up of a concave mandibular, or glenoid, fossa and a convex bony prominence called the articular eminence.[24] The articular tubercle, situated anterior to the glenoid fossa, serves as an attachment for the temporomandibular (or lateral) ligament.[22] The nonarticular surface of the fossa consists of a very thin layer of bone and fibrocartilage that occupies much of the superior and posterior walls of the fossa.[23]

Fibrocartilaginous Disk

Located between the articulating surface of the temporal bone and the mandibular condyle is a fibrocartilaginous disk (sometimes inappropriately referred to as "meniscus") (Fig. 26-3). The biconcave shape of the disk is determined by the shape of the condyle and the articulating fossa.[25] Rees[19] has described the fibrocartilaginous disk as having three clearly defined transverse, ellipsoidal zones that are divided into three regions—posterior band, intermediate zone, and anterior band—of which the intermediate zone makes contact with the articular surface of the condyle.

Both the disk and the lateral pterygoid muscle develop from the first branchial arch, and there is very little differentiation among the muscle, the disk, and the joint capsule.[26,27] The fibrocartilaginous disk is tethered by a number of structures:

- Medial and lateral collateral diskal ligaments firmly attach the fibrocartilaginous disk to the medial and lateral poles of the condyle, permitting anterior and posterior rotation of the disk on the condyle during mouth opening and closing.[28,29]
- Posteriorly, the disk is attached by fibroelastic tissue to the posterior mandibular fossa and the back of the mandibular condyle.[28,29]
- Anteriorly, the disk is attached to the upper part of the tendon of the lateral pterygoid muscle[28,29] (Fig. 26-3).

The disk usually is located on top of the condyle in the 12 o' clock to 1 o'clock position on the mandibular head when the jaw is closed.[30] Since the only firm attachment of the disk to the condyle occurs medially and laterally, the disk can move somewhat independently of the condyle.[31]

The disk effectively divides the TMJ into a lower and an upper joint cavity (see Fig. 26-3):

- ***Lower compartment.*** This compartment, bordered by the mandibular condyle and the inferior surface of the articular disk, is where, under normal conditions, the osteokinematic spin (rotation) of the condyle occurs.[6]
- ***Upper compartment.*** This compartment, bordered by the mandibular fossa and the superior surface of the articular disk, primarily allows only translation of the disk and condyle along the fossa, and onto the articular eminence.[6]

Blood vessels and nerves are found only in the thickened periphery of this disk, especially its posterior attachment; its middle articular portion is avascular and aneural.[32]

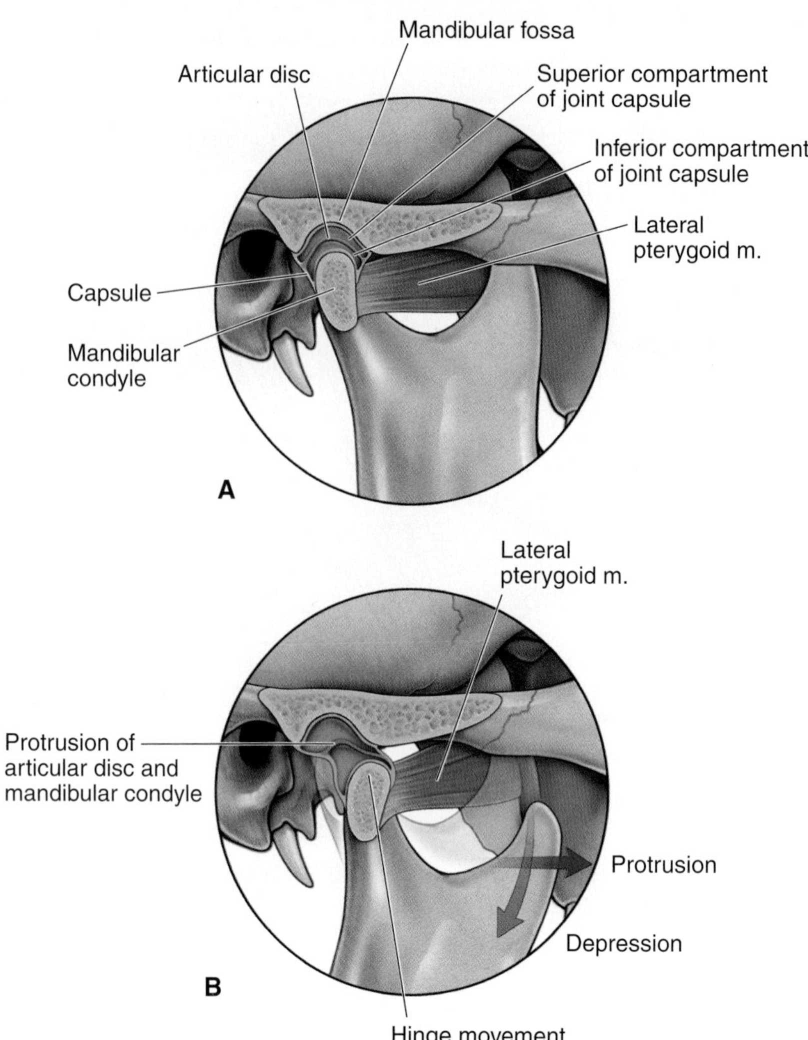

FIGURE 26-3 The TMJ disk and the pterygoid. (Reproduced, with permission, from Morton DA, Foreman KB, Albertine KH: *The Big Picture: Gross Anatomy*, McGraw-Hill, 2011.)

Supporting Structures

The supporting structures of the TMJ consist of periarticular connective tissue (ligament, tendon, capsule, and fascia). As its name implies, the periarticular connective tissue serves to keep the joints together and to limit the ranges of motion at the joint. For example, the ligaments of the TMJ protect and support the joint structures and act as passive restraints to joint movement. The synovial cavities are surrounded by loose connective tissue rather than by ligaments.

The intercapsular structures are located posteriorly to the condyle. Anterior to the joint are the muscles of the medial and lateral pterygoid (see next section). There are no well-defined anterior or posterior ligaments between the mandibular condyle and the temporal bone. However, two strong ligaments help to provide joint stability:

1. ***Joint capsule or capsular ligament.*** This structure, which surrounds the entire joint, is thought to provide proprioceptive feedback regarding joint position and movement.[33,34]
2. ***Temporomandibular (or lateral) ligament.*** The capsule of the TMJ is reinforced laterally by an outer oblique portion and an inner horizontal portion of the temporomandibular ligament, which function as a suspensory mechanism for the mandible during moderate opening movements. The ligament also functions to resist rotation and posterior displacement of the mandible.

Two other ligaments assist with joint stability:

- ***Stylomandibular ligament.*** The stylomandibular ligament is a specialized band that splits away from the superficial lamina of the deep cervical fascia to run deep to both pterygoid muscles.[24] This ligament becomes taut and acts as a guiding mechanism for the mandible, keeping the condyle, disk, and temporal bone firmly opposed.
- ***Sphenomandibular ligament.*** The sphenomandibular ligament is a thin band that runs from the spine of the sphenoid bone to a small bony prominence on the medial surface of the ramus of the mandible, called the lingula. This ligament acts to check the angle of the mandible from sliding

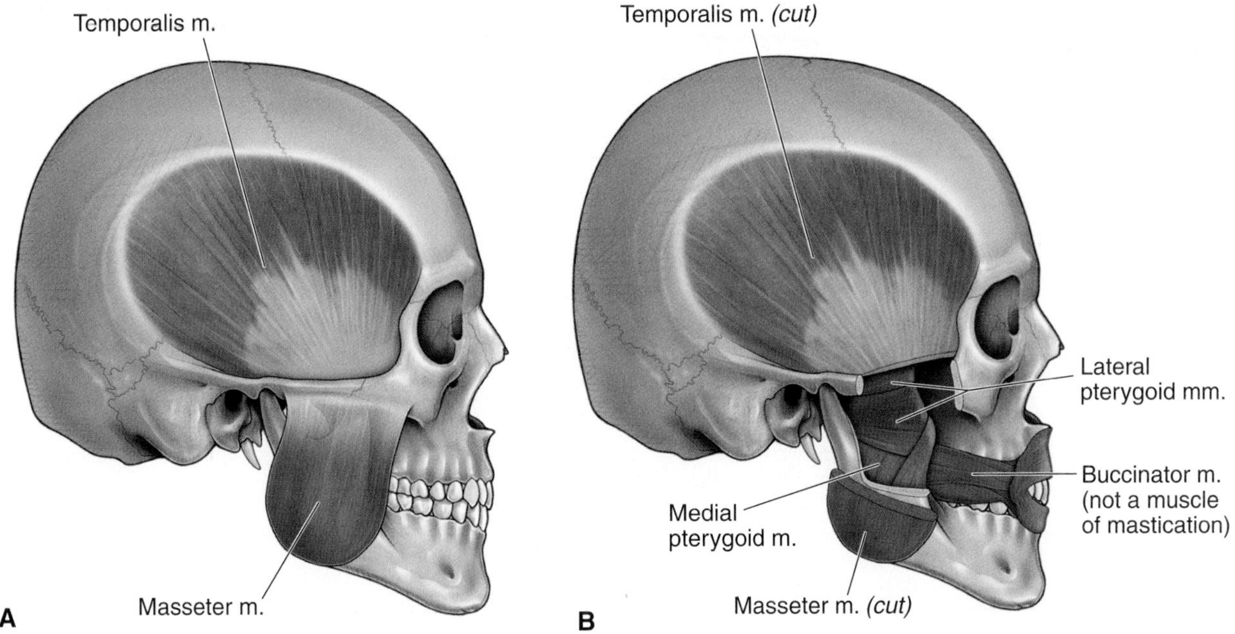

FIGURE 26-4 Lateral view of TMJ. (Reproduced, with permission, from Morton DA, Foreman KB, Albertine KH: *The Big Picture: Gross Anatomy*, McGraw-Hill, 2011.)

as far forward as the condyles during the translatory cycle and serves as a suspensory ligament of the mandible during wide opening.[24] It is this ligament that hurts with any prolonged jaw opening, such as that which occurs at the dentist.

CLINICAL PEARL

Pinto's ligament[35] is a vestige of Meckel's cartilage, an embryological tissue. It arises from the neck of the malleus of the inner ear and runs in a medial superior direction to insert into the posterior aspect of the TMJ capsule and the disk. While the role of this ligament in mandibular mechanics is thought to be negligible, its relationship to the middle ear and the TMJ could be a basis for the middle ear symptoms, which are often present with TMD. Stack[36] postulated that auditory symptoms of fullness and pressure in the middle ear may be present as a result of direct transmission of TMJ capsular tension to the ossicles of the middle ear through this ligament.

Muscles

The muscles of mastication are the key muscles when discussing TMD. Three of these muscles, the masseter, the medial pterygoid, and the temporalis (Fig. 26-4), function to raise the mandible during mouth closing. The lateral pterygoid and digastric muscles work together to depress the mandible during mouth opening.

Although these muscles work most efficiently in groups, an understanding of the specific anatomy and action(s) of the individual muscles is necessary for an appreciation of their coordinated function during masticatory activity (Tables 26-1 and 26-2).

Temporalis

The temporalis muscle (Fig. 26-4) has its origin from the floor of the temporal fossa and the temporal fascia. The muscle travels inferiorly and anteriorly to insert on the anterior border of the coronoid process and the anterior border of the ramus of the mandible. The temporalis muscle is innervated by a branch of the mandibular division of the trigeminal nerve. In addition to assisting with mouth closing and side-to-side grinding of the teeth, the temporalis muscle provides a good deal of stability to the joint.

The Masseter

The masseter (Fig. 26-4) is a two-layered quadrilateral-shaped muscle. The superficial portion arises from the anterior two-thirds of the lower border of the zygomatic arch. The deep portion arises from the medial surface of the zygomatic arch. Both sets of fibers blend anteriorly and form a raphe with the medial pterygoid.[24] The masseter inserts on the lateral surface of the coronoid process of the mandible, upper half of the ramus and angle of the mandible. The masseter muscle is innervated by a branch of the mandibular division of the trigeminal nerve. The major function of the masseter is to elevate the mandible, thereby occluding the teeth during mastication.

The Medial Pterygoid

The medial pterygoid muscle is a thick quadrilateral muscle, with a deep origin situated on the medial aspect of the mandibular ramus (Fig. 26-4). The muscle travels posteriorly to insert on the inferior and posterior aspects of the medial subsurface of the ramus and angle of the mandible. The medial pterygoid muscle is innervated by a branch of the mandibular division of the trigeminal nerve. Working bilaterally, and in

TABLE 26-1 Muscles of the Temporomandibular Joint

Muscle	Proximal	Distal	Innervation
Medial pterygoid	Medial surface of lateral pterygoid plate and tuberosity of maxilla	Medial surface of mandible close to angle	Mandibular division of trigeminal nerve
Lateral pterygoid	Greater wing of sphenoid and lateral pterygoid plate	Neck of mandible and articular cartilage	Mandibular division of trigeminal nerve
Temporalis	Temporal cranial fossa	By way of a tendon into medial surface, apex, and anterior and posterior borders of mandibular ramus	Anterior and posterior deep temporal nerves, which branch from anterior division of mandibular branch of trigeminal nerve
Masseter	Superficial portion: from anterior two-thirds of lower border of zygomatic arch; deep portion from medial surface of zygomatic arch	Lateral surfaces of coronoid process of mandible, upper half of ramus, and angle of mandible	Masseteric nerve from anterior trunk of mandibular division of trigeminal nerve
Mylohyoid	Medial surface of mandible	Body of hyoid bone	Mylohyoid branch of trigeminal nerve and mandibular division
Geniohyoid	Mental spine of mandible	Body of hyoid bone	Anterior (ventral) ramus of C1 via hypoglossal nerve
Stylohyoid	Styloid process of temporal bone	Body of hyoid bone	Facial nerve
Anterior and posterior digastric	Internal surface of mandible and mastoid process of temporal bone	By intermediate tendon to hyoid bone	Anterior: mandibular division of trigeminal nerve; posterior: facial nerve
Sternohyoid	Manubrium and medial end of clavicle	Body of hyoid bone	Ansa cervicalis
Omohyoid	Superior angle of scapula	Inferior body of hyoid bone	Ansa cervicalis
Sternothyroid	Posterior surface of manubrium	Thyroid cartilage	Ansa cervicalis
Thyrohyoid	Thyroid cartilage	Inferior body and greater horn of hyoid bone	C1 via hypoglossal nerve

association with the masseter and temporalis muscles, the medial pterygoids assist in mouth closing. Individually, the medial pterygoid muscle is capable of deviating the mandible toward the opposite side. The medial pterygoid muscle also acts as an assistance to the lateral pterygoid and anterior fibers of the temporalis muscle to produce protrusion of the mandible.

The Lateral Pterygoid

Two divisions of the lateral pterygoid muscles are recognized, each of which is functionally and anatomically separate (Fig. 26-3 and Fig. 26-4). The superior head arises from the infratemporal surface of the greater wing of the sphenoid. The inferior head arises from the lateral surface of the lateral pterygoid plate. Despite several investigations,[37–39] no consensus has been reached regarding the insertion of the lateral pterygoid muscle. However, the most commonly described insertion is at the anterior aspect of the neck of the mandibular condyle and capsule of the TMJ. The lateral pterygoid muscle is innervated by a branch of the mandibular division of the trigeminal nerve.

The superior head of the lateral pterygoid is involved mainly with chewing and functions to anteriorly rotate the disk on the condyle during the closing movement.[40,41] It has also been suggested that in normal function of the craniomandibular complex, the superior lateral pterygoid plays an important role in stabilizing and controlling the movements of the disk.[42]

The inferior head of the lateral pterygoid muscle exerts an anterior, lateral, and inferior pull on the mandible, thereby opening the jaw, protruding the mandible, and deviating the mandible to the opposite side.

Infrahyoid or "Strap" Muscles

The infrahyoid muscles comprise the sternohyoid, omohyoid, sternothyroid, and thyrohyoid muscles (Fig. 26-5).

Sternohyoid

The sternohyoid muscle is a strap-like muscle that functions to depress the hyoid and assist in speech and mastication.

Omohyoid

The omohyoid muscle, situated lateral to the sternohyoid, consists of two bellies and functions to depress the hyoid. In addition, the muscle has been speculated to tense the inferior aspect of the deep cervical fascia in prolonged inspiratory efforts, thereby releasing tension on the apices of the lungs and

TABLE 26-2 Actions of the Temporomandibular Joint Muscles

Action	Muscles Acting
Opening of mouth	Lateral pterygoid Mylohyoid Geniohyoid Digastric
Closing of mouth	Masseter Temporalis Medial pterygoid
Protrusion of mandible	Lateral pterygoid Medial pterygoid Masseter Mylohyoid Geniohyoid Digastric Stylohyoid Temporalis (anterior fibers)
Retraction of mandible	Temporalis (posterior fibers) Masseter Digastric Stylohyoid Mylohyoid Geniohyoid
Lateral deviation of mandible	Lateral pterygoid (ipsilateral muscle) Medial pterygoid (contralateral muscle) Temporalis Masseter

on the internal jugular vein, which are attached to this fascial layer.[24]

Sternothyroid and Thyrohyoid

The sternothyroid and thyrohyoid muscles (see Fig. 26-5) are located deep to the sternohyoid muscle. The sternothyroid muscle is involved in drawing the larynx downward, whereas the thyrohyoid depresses the hyoid and elevates the larynx.

These infrahyoid muscles are innervated by fibers from the upper cervical nerves. The nerves to the lower part of these muscles are given off from a loop, the ansa cervicalis (cervical loop) (see Chap. 3).

Suprahyoid Muscles

The suprahyoid muscles (Fig. 26-2), working with the infrahyoid muscles, play a major role in coordinating mandibular function, by providing a firm base on which the tongue and mandible can be moved.

Geniohyoid

The geniohyoid muscle is a narrow muscle situated under the mylohyoid muscle. The muscle functions to elevate the hyoid bone.

Digastric

As its name suggests, the digastric muscle consists of two bellies. The posterior belly arises from the mastoid notch of the temporal bone, while the anterior belly arises from the digastric fossa of the mandible. The posterior belly is innervated by a branch from the facial nerve. The anterior belly is innervated by the inferior alveolar branch of the trigeminal nerve. The two bellies of the digastric muscle are joined by a rounded tendon that attaches to the body and greater cornu of the hyoid bone through a fibrous loop or sling.[24]

Bilaterally, the two bellies of the digastric muscle assist in forced mouth opening by stabilizing the hyoid. The posterior bellies are especially active during coughing and swallowing.[24]

CLINICAL PEARL

Working in combinations, the muscles of the TMJ are involved as follows:

- Mouth opening—bilateral action of the lateral pterygoid and digastric muscles.
- Mouth closing—bilateral action of the temporalis, masseter, and medial pterygoid muscles.
- Lateral deviation—action of the ipsilateral masseter, and contralateral medial and lateral pterygoid muscles.
- Protrusion—bilateral action of the lateral pterygoid, medial pterygoid, and anterior fibers of the temporalis muscles.
- Retrusion—bilateral action of the posterior fibers of the temporalis muscle, the digastric, stylohyoid, geniohyoid, and mylohyoid muscles.

Mylohyoid

This flat, triangular muscle is functionally a muscle of the tongue, stabilizing or elevating the tongue during swallowing and elevating the floor of the mouth in the first stage of deglutition.[24]

Stylohyoid

The stylohyoid muscle elevates the hyoid and base of the tongue and has an undetermined role in speech, mastication, and swallowing.

Nerve Supply

The TMJ is primarily supplied from three nerves that are part of the mandibular division of the fifth cranial (trigeminal) nerve (Fig. 26-6) (Box 26 1). Portions of the middle ear ossicles, middle ear musculature, and muscles of mastication all originate from the first branchial arch and are innervated by this nerve. Therefore, in a patient with altered bite mechanics, spasm of the muscles of mastication caused by a displaced condyle may cause neuromuscular dysfunction of all the muscles innervated by the trigeminal nerve, including the tensor palatini.[43]

There is considerable clinical interest in the interactions between the cervical and craniofacial regions. This interest

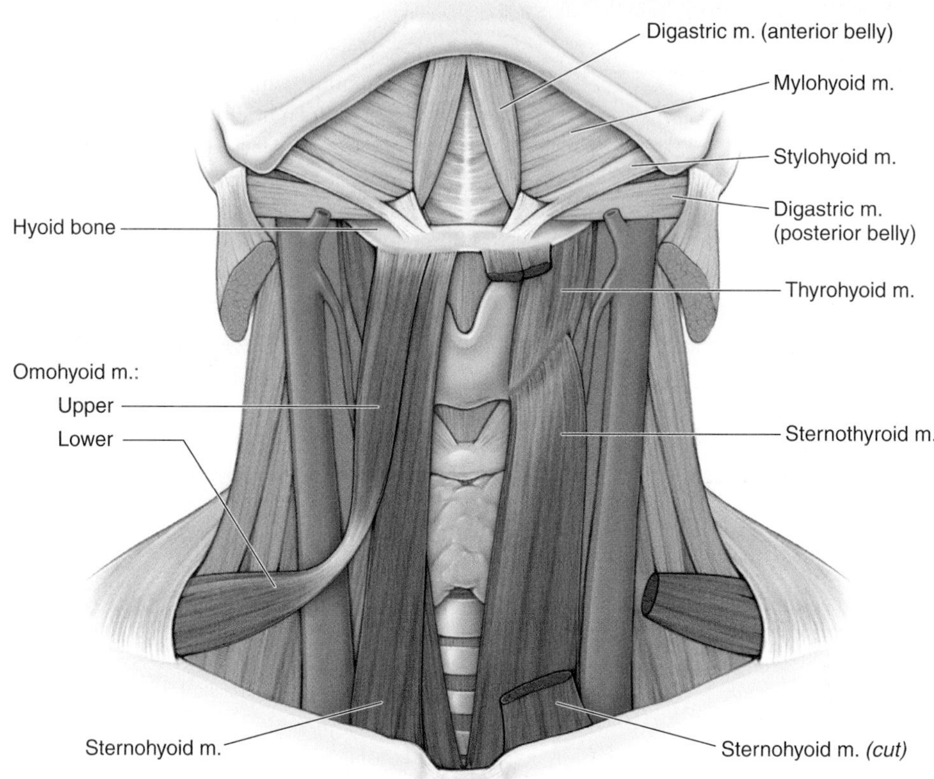

FIGURE 26-5 The infrahyoid muscles. (Reproduced, with permission, from Morton DA, Foreman KB, Albertine KH: *The Big Picture: Gross Anatomy,* McGraw-Hill, 2011.)

stems from a number of reports concerning patients who have pain in the cervical and craniofacial areas simultaneously.[31,44–47]

In the suboccipital region, a series of dense neural connections, called the *trigeminocervical complex,* exists among trigeminal, facial, glossopharyngeal, and vagus nerves, with those of the upper C1–4 cervical spinal nerves (Fig. 26-7).[14] Postural abnormalities resulting from various acute or chronic etiologies that produce suboccipital compression may, therefore, be responsible for craniofacial pain anywhere in the head, in addition to symptoms of dizziness or nystagmus.[5,14,48]

TMJ-related headaches usually include pain near the TMJ and ear, ear fullness, temporal headaches, and facial pain.[49] The dizziness associated with TMD tends to be of the nonvertiginous variety, with the patient complaining of unsteadiness, giddiness, or lightheadedness.[50] Although the exact mechanism is unclear, postural influences, alteration in the position of the jaw by the malocclusion, and the subsequent mismatching between the cervical muscles might be the cause.[50]

BIOMECHANICS

The movements that occur at the TMJ are extremely complex. The TMJ has three degrees of freedom, with each of the degrees of freedom being associated with a separate axis of rotation.[51] Two primary arthrokinematic movements (rotation and anterior translation) occur at this joint around three planes: sagittal, horizontal, and frontal.

Rotation occurs from the beginning to the midrange of movement. In addition to the rotational motions during mouth opening and closing and lateral deviations, movements at the TMJ involve arthrokinematic rolls and slides. Gliding, translation, or sliding movements occur in the upper cavity, whereas rotation or hinged movement occurs in the lower cavity. The motions of protrusion and retrusion are planar glides. Thus,

- mouth opening, contralateral deviation, and protrusion all involve an anterior osteokinematic rotation of the mandible and an anterior, inferior, and lateral glide of the mandibular head and disk;
- mouth closing, ipsilateral deviation, and retrusion all involve a posterior osteokinematic rotation of the mandible and an anterior, inferior, and lateral glide of the mandibular head and disk.

Occlusal Position

Occlusal positions are functional positions of the TMJ. The occlusal position is defined as the point at which contact between some or all of the teeth occurs. Under normal circumstances, the upper molars rest directly on the lower molars and the upper incisors slightly override the lower incisors. The ideal position provides mutual protection of the

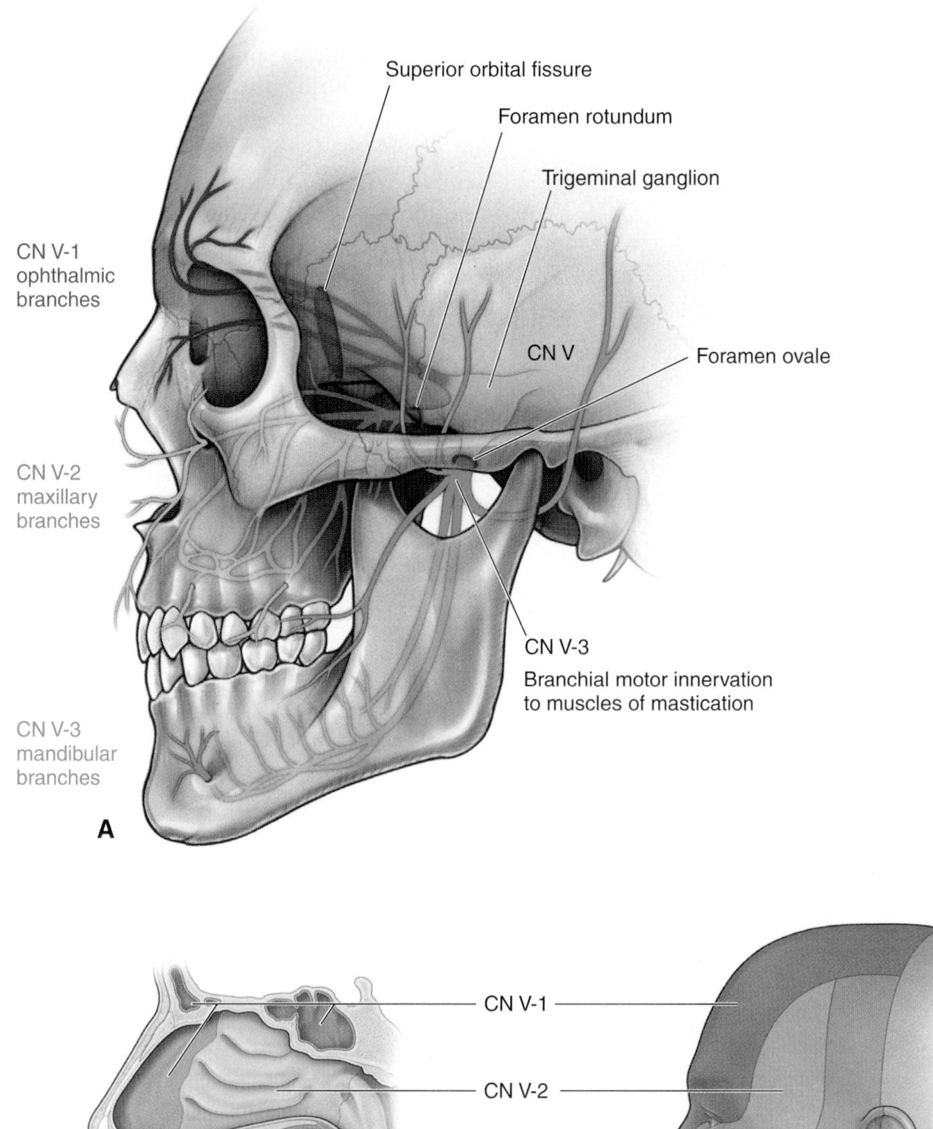

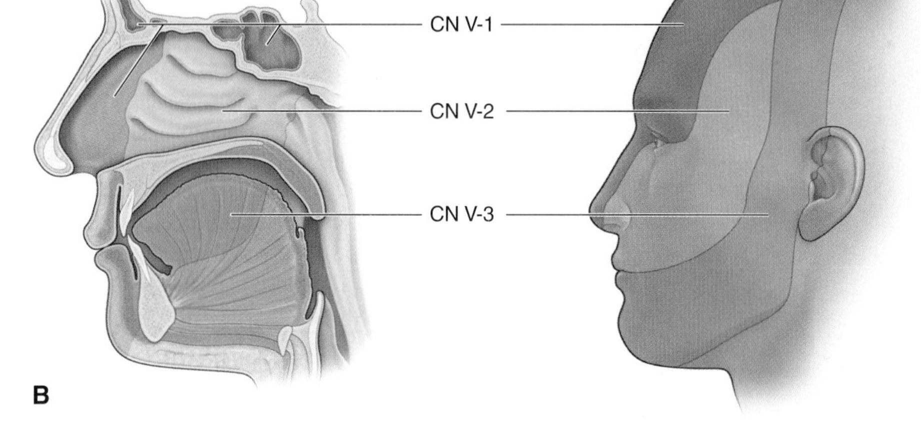

FIGURE 26-6 The trigeminal nerve. (Reproduced, with permission, from Morton DA, Foreman KB, Albertine KH: *The Big Picture: Gross Anatomy*, McGraw-Hill, 2011.)

anterior and posterior teeth, comfortable and painless mandibular function, and stability.[14]

- The median occlusal position corresponds to the position in which all of the teeth are fully interdigitated[18] and is considered the start position for all mandibular motions. The median occlusal position is dependent on the presence, shape, and position of the teeth. Protrusion of the upper or lower incisors, failure of the upper incisors to overlap with the lower incisors, absent or abnormally shaped teeth, and back teeth that do not meet are all causes of malocclusion.
- The centric position is considered to be the position that implies the most retruded, unstrained position of the mandible from which lateral movements are possible and the components of the oral apparatus are the most balanced.[52] Ideally, the centric position should coincide with the median occlusal position.[52] It is worth remembering that malocclusion is probably very common in the general nonsymptomatic patient and may or may not be relevant to the presenting symptoms.[53] Rather than being a primary etiologic factor in TMD, malocclusion is likely to have a secondary or contributory role.[14,54]

Box 26-1 Characteristics of the Trigeminal Nerve

Motor Nucleus

The anterolateral upper pons.

Sensory Nucleus

There are two nuclei: (1) the chief sensory nucleus in the posterior (dorsal)–lateral pons and (2) the mesencephalic nucleus, which extends from the chief sensory nucleus upward through the pons to the midbrain.

Spinal Nucleus

The spinal tract consists of small- and medium-sized myelinated nerve fibers and runs caudally to reach the upper cervical segments of the spinal cord. The lowest nerve fibers in the tract mix with the spinal fibers in the tract orf Lissauer.

Nerves

- Mandibular
- Ophthalmic
- Maxillary

Termination

- Muscles of mastication, both pterygoids, tensor veli palatini, tensor tympani, mylohyoid, and anterior belly of digastric.
- Skin of vertex, temporal area, forehead, and face; mucosa of sinuses, nose, pharynx, anterior two-thirds of tongue, and oral cavity.
- Lacrimal, parotid, and lingual glands; dura of anterior and middle cranial fossae.
- External aspect of tympanic membrane and external auditory meatus, TMJ, and teeth.
- Dilator pupillae and probably proprioceptors of extraocular muscles.
- Sensation from upper three or four cervical levels.

Mouth Opening

Mouth opening occurs in a series of steps (Table 26-3). In the erect position, the condyles begin to rotate anteriorly and translate inferiorly and laterally during the first 25 degrees of opening as the jaw opens. The upper head of the lateral pterygoid muscle and the anterior head of the digastric muscle draw the disk anteriorly and prepare for condylar rotation during movement.[31] This initial condylar rotation occurs as the mandibular elevators (masseter, temporalis, and medial pterygoid muscles) gradually relax and lengthen, allowing gravity to depress the mandible (see Fig. 26-8).[31] The directions of the fibers of the lateral and medial temporomandibular ligaments also keep the condyle from moving posteriorly. The fibrous capsule and parts of the temporomandibular ligament limit excessive lateral movement of the condyle. The rotation occurs through the two condylar heads between the articular disk and the condyle. As the mandible moves forward on opening, the disks move medially and posteriorly until the collateral ligaments and the lateral pterygoid stop their movement. During the last 15 degrees of opening, the rotation ceases due to tightening of the collateral ligaments, and is replaced by an anterior translation of the condyles (see Fig. 26-8).[55] During this translation, the condyle and disk move together. The anterior translation, which is produced mainly by muscle contraction, serves to prevent mandibular encroachment of the anterior neck structures. Opening is also assisted by the other suprahyoid muscles.[31] In extremely wide opening, such as that occurs with yawning, the functional joint contact is on the distal aspect of the condyle, and the anterior lateral aspect of the condyle contacts the posterior part of the masseter muscle. In this position, the soft tissue structures are in a position of stretch, making them more prone to dysfunction.[56]

Mouth Closing

Closing of the mouth involves a reversal of the movements described for mouth opening. The condyles translate posteriorly as a result of an interaction between the retracting portions of the masseter and temporalis muscle and the retracting portions of the mandibular depressors (see Fig. 26-8).[51] As the condyles translate posteriorly and glide medially, they hinge on the disks. The disks then glide posteriorly and superiorly on the temporal bone along with the condyles (as a result of the actions of the masseter, medial pterygoid, and temporalis muscles).[41] When the jaws are closed to maximal occlusal contact, the condyles contact the disks and the disks contact the posterior slopes of the articular tubercles and the glenoid fossae.

Protrusion

Protrusion is a forward movement of the mandible that occurs at the superior joint compartments, which consists of the disk and condyle moving downward, forward, and laterally. The muscles responsible for protrusion are the anterior fiber of the temporalis and the medial and lateral pterygoid muscles.

Retrusion

Retrusion is a backward movement of the mandible, produced by the posterior fiber of the temporalis and assisted by the suprahyoid muscles. The retrusive range is limited by the extensibility of the temporomandibular ligaments.[57]

Lateral Excursion

If a protrusion movement occurs unilaterally, it is called a *lateral excursion, or deviation.* For example, if only the left TMJ protrudes, the jaw deviates to the right.

Lateral movements of the mandible are the result of asymmetric muscle contractions (Fig. 26-9). During lateral excursion to the right, the condyle and the disk on the left side glide inferiorly, anteriorly, and laterally in the sagittal plane and medially in the horizontal plane along the articular eminence. The condyle and the disk on the right side rotate laterally on a sagittal plane and translate medially in the horizontal plane, while remaining in the fossa.

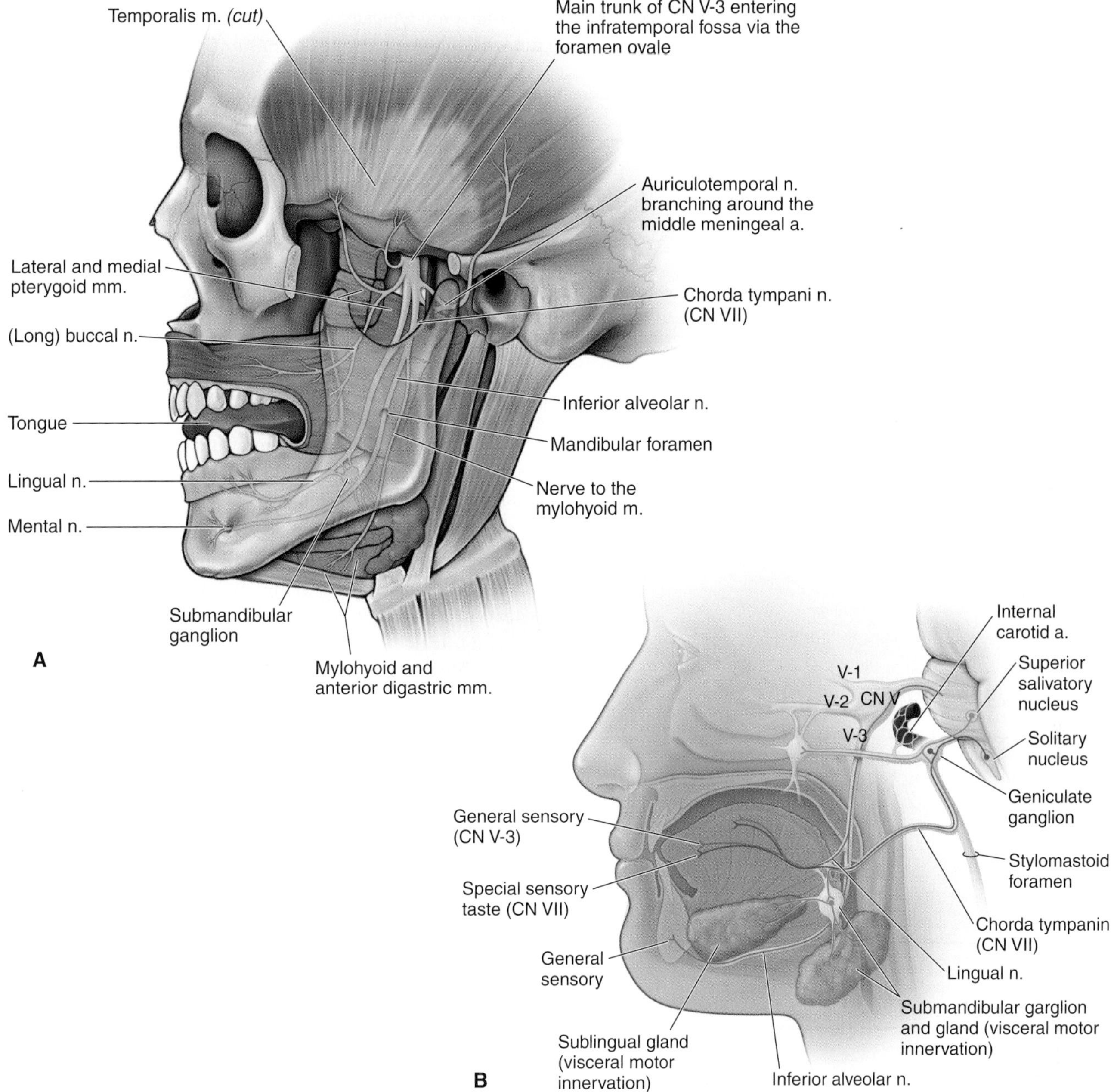

FIGURE 26-7 Neurology of the TMJ. (Reproduced, with permission, from Morton DA, Foreman KB, Albertine KH: *The Big Picture: Gross Anatomy*, McGraw-Hill, 2011.)

CLINICAL PEARL

The translation of the human condyle during jaw opening and lateral jaw movements is referred to as the *Bennett shift.*

The Close- and Open-Packed (Resting) Positions

The close-packed position of the TMJ is difficult to determine because the position of maximal muscle tightness is also the position of least joint surface congruity and vice versa. Rocabado[50] considers there to be two close-packed positions, named according to the end position of the mandibular head in the fossa:[55]

- ***Anterior close-packed position.*** This position is the position of maximum opening of the joint.
- ***Posterior close-packed position.*** This position is the maximum retruded position of the joint.

Under this premise, the open-packed, or "rest" position is any position away from the anterior or posterior close-packed positions of the joint.[55] The rest position, or "freeway space" corresponds to the position of the TMJ where the residual tension of the muscles is at rest and no contact occurs between maxillary and mandibular teeth. In this position, the tongue is against the palate of the mouth with its most anterior–superior tip in the area against the palate, just posterior to the rear of the upper central incisors.[58]

TABLE 26-3 Arthrokinematic Steps of the Temporomandibular Joint

Step	Movement
Rest position	Joint is in an open-packed position.
Rotation	There is a mid-opening. Condylar joint surfaces glide forward, inferior joint surface of disk has a relative posterior glide, upper lateral pterygoid relaxes, inferior pterygoid contracts, and posterior connective tissue is in a functional state of rest.
Functional opening	Disk and condyle experience a short anterior translatory glide; superior and inferior heads of lateral pterygoid contract to guide disk and condyle forward. Posterior connective tissue is in a functional tightening.
Translation	There is full opening. Disk and condyle glide anteriorly and caudally. Superior and inferior heads of lateral pterygoid contract to guide disk and condyle fully forward. Posterior connective tissues tighten.
Closure	Surface of condyle joint glides posteriorly, and disk glides relative to anterior surface. Superior head of lateral pterygoid contracts and inferior head relaxes. Posterior connective tissue returns to its functional length.

Data from Rocabado M: Arthrokinematics of the temporomandibular joint. In: Gelb H, ed. *Clinical Management of Head, Neck and TMJ Pain and Dysfunction.* Philadelphia, PA: WB Saunders, 1985.

Capsular Pattern

The capsular pattern of the TMJ is limitation of mouth opening. If one joint is more involved than the other, the jaw will laterally deviate to the same side during opening.

CLINICAL PEARL

The significance of the rest position is that it permits the tissues of the stomatognathic system to rest and undergo repair.[59]

EXAMINATION

Currently, clinical examination is the gold standard for diagnosing TMDs. Given the multifactorial causes of TMD, a comprehensive examination of the entire upper quadrant, including the cervical spine and shoulders, usually is warranted. In general, the TMJ and the upper three cervical joints all refer symptoms to the head, whereas the mid-to-low cervical spine typically refers symptoms to the shoulder and the arm.[60–62] An accurate diagnosis of TMD involves a careful evaluation of the information gleaned from the history, systems review, and tests and measures. In most chronic cases, a behavioral or psychological examination is required.[2,30,62–67] Since postural dysfunctions are closely related to TMJ symptoms, the clinician should always perform a postural examination as part of a comprehensive examination of this joint. An examination form for the TMJ examination is shown in Table 26-4.

History

During the history, the clinician should observe the patient's mouth to see whether the mouth moves comfortably while speaking, or whether mouth movements appear guarded.

The clinician should determine from the patient the main reason for the visit. There are three cardinal features of TMDs, which can be local or remote:

1. ***Restricted jaw function.*** Limited mouth opening, which may be reported as intermittent or progressive, is a key feature of TMD. Patients may describe a generalized tight feeling, which may indicate a muscular disorder, or capsulitis, or the sensation that the jaw suddenly "catches" or "locks," which usually is related to a mechanical interference within the joint (an internal derangement).[12] Associated signs of an internal derangement include pain and deviation of mandibular movements during opening and closing (refer to Practice Pattern 4D, under "Intervention Strategies" section later), and biting firm objects. Pain in the fully open position is probably caused by an extra-articular problem. Locking may imply that the mouth does not fully open or does not fully close and is often related to problems of the disk or joint degeneration.
2. ***Joint noises.*** Joint noises (crepitus) of the TMJ may or may not be significant, because joint sounds occur in approximately 50% of healthy populations.[68] Some joint sounds are not audible to the clinician, so a stethoscope may be required. "Hard" crepitus is a diffuse sustained noise that occurs during a significant portion of the opening or closing cycle, or both, and is an evidence of a change in osseous contour.[56] Clicking describes a brief noise that occurs at some point during opening, closing, or both (see the discussion of range of motion testing, later). Jaw clicking during mouth opening or closing may be suggestive of an internal derangement consisting of an anterior disk displacement with reduction.[69,70]

CLINICAL PEARL

TMJ sounds should be related to symptoms, as joint noise in of itself, is of little clinical importance in the absence of pain.[64,71]

3. ***Orofacial pain.*** Approximately 50% of all cases of TMD are masticatory myalgias.[72] TMJ pain should be evaluated carefully in terms of its onset, nature, intensity, site,

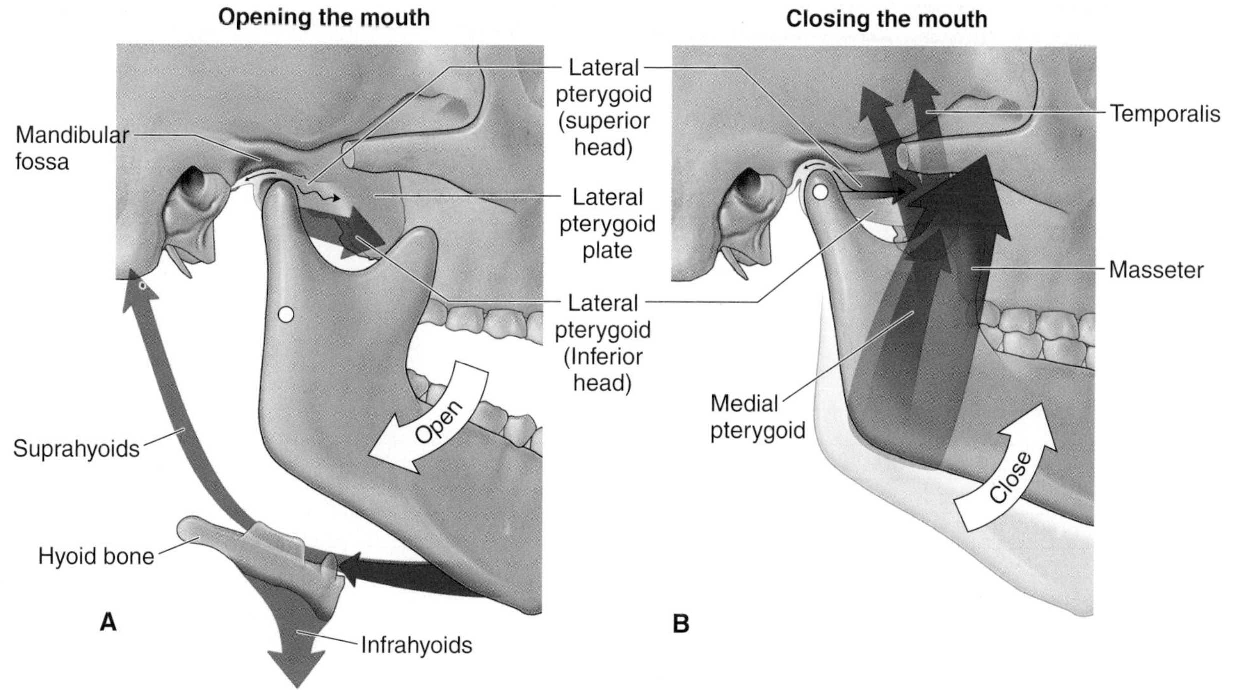

FIGURE 26-8 Mouth opening and closing.

duration, aggravating and relieving factors, and how it relates to joint noise and restricted mandibular movements.[12] Orofacial pain associated with mouth opening or closing, and jaw crepitus is suggestive of osteoarthrosis, capsulitis, or internal derangement consisting of an anterior disk displacement with reduction.[69,70,73–76] In a study by Magnusson and colleagues,[77] five different scales of self-assessment of pain were tested in patients with TMJ disorders. The precision and sensitivity and the capacity to register memory of pain and discomfort were compared for each of the five scales (Table 26-5). From these results, the behavior rating scale can be recommended when measuring pain and discomfort in patients with TMJ disorders.

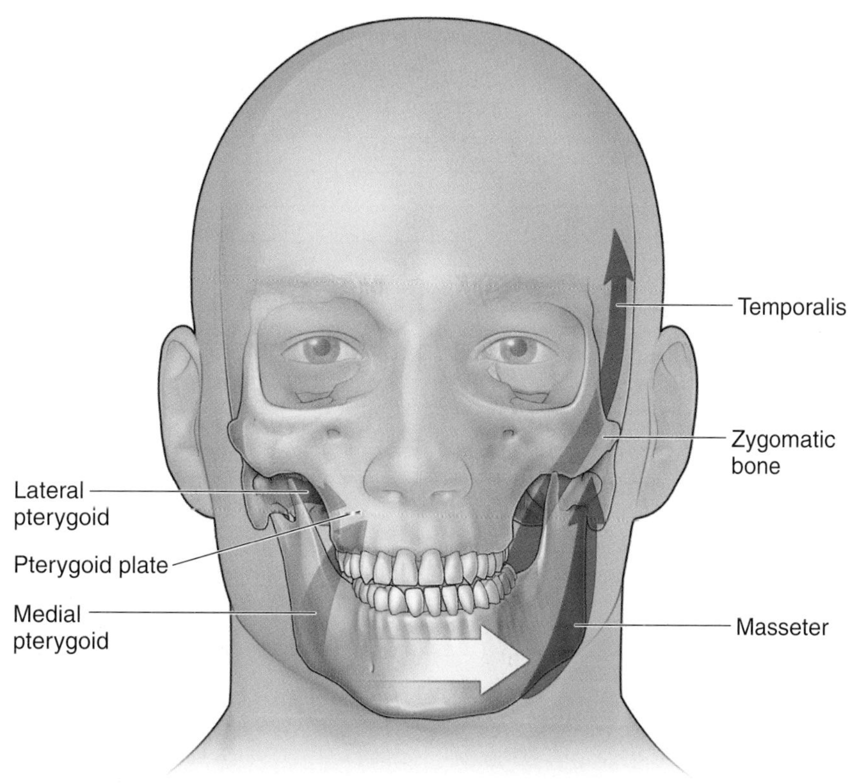

FIGURE 26-9 Lateral deviation to the left.

TABLE 26-4 Temporomandibular Examination Form

Name: ____________________ General Dentist: ____________________
Patient's Physician: ____________________ Phone (home): ____________________
Age: __________ Phone (bus): ____________________
Address: ____________________ Chief Complaint: ____________________
Occupation: ____________________
Phone: ____________________

Check all applicable

I. MEDICAL HISTORY

Arthritic Disease

1. Traumatic arthritis: ____________________
2. Osteoarthritis: ____________________
3. Rheumatoid arthritis: ____________________
4. Psoriatic arthritis: ____________________
5. Other: ____________________

ENT. Disorders

1. Salivary gland disorders: ____________________
2. Cysts: ____________________
3. Ear problems: ____________________
4. Polyps: ____________________
5. Nose/Throat problems: ____________________
6. Allergies: ____________________
7. Sinusitis: ____________________
8. Other: ____________________

Vascular Disease and Blood Dyscrasias ____________________

Head/Neck Trauma

Date: __________ Description ____________________

Headache/Neuralgia (location, character, frequency, duration)

Medication (current and past)

1. Type: ____________________
2. Allergy to medication: ____________________

Additional Medical Information (past and present)

1. Surgery: ____________________
2. Psychiatric: ____________________
3. ENT: ____________________
4. Orthopaedic: ____________________
5. Neurologic: ____________________
6. Internist: ____________________
7. Rheumatologic: ____________________
8. Chiropractic: ____________________
9. Physical therapy: ____________________
10. Endocrine: ____________________
    a. Do your nails break easily? ____________________
    b. Is your skin dry? ____________________
    c. Do you tire easily? ____________________
    d. Does the cold weather bother you? ____________________
11. Osteopathic: ____________________
12. Other: ____________________
13. Nutritional state: ____________________

(Continued)

TABLE 26-4 Temporomandibular Examination Form *(Continued)*

II. DENTAL HISTORY

A. Oral Conditions (describe general condition, presence of fixed or removable prosthesis, periodontal problems, and vertical dimension discrepancies)

____

____

____

B. Last Dental Examination and Films: ____________________

C. Recent Dental Treatment:

D. Previous Orthodontic Therapy Dates: ________ **Bicuspid Extraction?** ____________

E. Previous TMJ Treatment and Results (date/doctor): ________________

F. Pain Symptoms:

1. Date of onset: ____________________
2. Area of onset __________ Right __________ Left __________
3. Type: superficial, deep, sharp, dull
4. Quality: burning, aching
5. Frequency: ____________________
6. Duration: constant, intermittent
7. Period of greatest intensity: ____________________
8. Status of pain: increased, decreased, unchanged
9. Onset: abrupt, gradual
10. Disappearance: abrupt, gradual
11. Factors alleviating pain: ____________________
12. Triggering devices: eating, yawning, speaking, singing, shouting
13. Pain in specific teeth: ____________________
14. Additional pain information: ____________________

G. Oral Symptoms (other than pain)

1. Jaws clenched upon awakening
2. Clenching and grinding during sleep
3. Clenching and grinding during waking hours
4. Muscle fatigue ____________________

H. Vertigo, Syncope, Meniere's Disease (frequency, duration, circumstances): ________________

I. Ear Symptoms/Joint Noises

1. Tinnitus: (R) (L)
2. Popping, clicking, or grating noises on opening and closing: (R) (L)
3. Stuffiness of ears: (R) (L)

J. Skeletal–Facial Deformity: ____________________

K. Other Complaints: ____________________

III. CLINICAL EXAMINATION

Reported Pain

1. Temporomandibular joint	(R) (L)	6. Shoulder	(R) (L)
2. Upper back	(R) (L)	7. Arm	(R) (L)
3. Middle back	(R) (L)	8. Fingers	(R) (L)
4. Lower back	(R) (L)	9. Chest	(R) (L)
5. Scapula area	(R) (L)	10. Occipital area	(R) (L)

Tenderness and Pain on Palpation

1. Temporalis
   a. Anterior Fibers (R) (L)
   b. Middle Fibers (R) (L)
   c. Posterior Fibers (R) (L)

(Continued)

TABLE 26-4 Temporomandibular Examination Form *(Continued)*

III. CLINICAL EXAMINATION *(Continued)*	
2. Masseter	
a. Zygoma	(R) (L)
b. Body	(R) (L)
c. Lateral surface of angle of mandible	(R) (L)
3. Digastric	(R) (L)
4. Posterior cervicals	(R) (L)
5. Trapezius	(R) (L)
6. Sternocleidomastoid	(R) (L)
7. Lateral pterygoid: insertion	(R) (L)
8. Medial pterygoid: insertion	(R) (L)
9. Mylohyoid	(R) (L)
10. Coronoid process	(R) (L)
11. TMJ lateral aspect	(R) (L)
Lateral/Posterior aspect	(R) (L)
3a. Ear (anterior wall tenderness)	(R) (L)
TMJ Sounds	
(Stethoscopic and/or digital palpation)	
1. Crepitation	(R) (L)
2. Sagittal *opening* click:	
Immediate	(R) (L)
Intermediate	(R) (L)
Full Opening	(R) (L)
3. Sagittal *closing* click:	
Immediate	(R) (L)
Intermediate	(R) (L)
Terminal closure	(R) (L)
4. Nature of click (soft/loud)	(R) (L)
B. Occlusal Interferences	
Left nonworking side Right nonworking side	
Protrusive Centric Occlusion	
Occlusion: Angle's class ____	
Extruded labial or lingual version teeth ____	
Clinical Postural Observation	
1. Head posture (at rest): ____	
2. Range of motion: ____	
Summary of TMJ Imaging Findings: ____	
Mandibular Movement	
1. Widest interincisal opening ____	
2. Right lateral ____ Left lateral ____	
3. Pain present with movement? ____	
Diagnosis: ____	
Plan of Treatment: ____	
Prognosis: ____	
Remarks: ____	

ENT, ear, nose, and throat; TMJ, temporomandibular joint.
Data from McNeill C, Mohl ND, Rugh JD, et al.: Temporomandibular disorders: Diagnosis, management, education, and research. *J Am Dent Assoc* 120:253–257, 1990.

CLINICAL PEARL

Pain that is centered immediately in front of the tragus of the ear and that projects to the ear, temple, cheek, and along the mandible is highly diagnostic for TMD.[78]

A gradual onset of symptoms after minor or prolonged physical activity may be indicative of a mechanical derangement.[79] Symptoms of a mechanical nature generally are eased with rest. The irritability of a disorder is determined by the degree of activity necessary to provoke a symptom response.

TABLE 26-5 Patient Reports of Pain in TMJ Disorders

Test and Measure	Test Procedure	Population	Reliability Kappa Values
Visual analog scale	100 mm line with the end defined as no pain and worst pain imaginable	38 consecutive patients referred with TMJ disorders	κ = .38
Numeric scale	10-point scale with 0 indicating no paint and 10 representing worst pain		κ = .36
Behavior rating scale	Six-point scale ranging from minor discomfort to very strong discomfort		κ = .68
Verbal scale	Five-point scale ranging from no pain to very severe pain		κ = .44

Data from Magnusson T, List T, Helkimo M: Self-assessment of pain and discomfort in patients with temporomandibular disorders: A comparison of five different scales with respect to their precision and sensitivity as well as their capacity to register memory of pain and discomfort. *J Oral Rehabil* 22:549–556, 1995; Cleland J: *Temporomandibular Joint, Orthopaedic Clinical Examination: An Evidence-Based Approach for Physical Therapists.* Carlstadt, NJ: Icon Learning Systems, LLC, 2005:39–89. With permission from Icon Learning Systems.

The severity of the symptoms and the time before the symptoms subside provide the clinician with valuable information regarding possible pathology.[80] Specific questions about activities and postures of a sustained nature, such as sitting, sleeping, and driving, should be asked.[81] It is important to determine:

- If the presenting symptoms were caused by trauma or surgery, or if the onset of pain occurred gradually. Questions should focus on any history of trauma during birth or childhood, as well as more recently.
- If there are any emotional factors in the patient's background that may provoke habitual protrusion or muscular tension.
- If the patient is aware of any parafunctional habits (cheek biting, nail biting, pencil chewing, teeth clenching, or bruxism). For example, does the patient chew on one side more than the other? Chewing more on one side versus the other is typically the result of malocclusion (see later). In addition, favoring one side can lead to a loss of vertical dimension (the distance between any two arbitrary points on the face). A simple way to measure the aforementioned is to measure from the lateral edge of the eye to the corner of the mouth and from the base of the nose to the chin.
- The behavior of symptoms over a 24-hour period. This information assists the clinician in formulating causal relationships.
- Whether the symptoms are improving or worsening.
- The relationship of eating to the symptoms. Alcohol, chocolate, and other foods such as ice cream can cause head pain in some individuals, suggesting a vasomotor-related pain.
- The patient's past dental and orthodontic history.
- Whether the patient has experienced any locking, clicking, or catching of the jaw.[48]

Chronic head, neck, and back pain often are associated with psychogenic causes. Psychiatric disorders, usually, are manifested in patients whose afflictions seem to be excessive or persist beyond what would be normal for that condition. The checklist outlined in Table 26-6 can be used by the clinician to identify factors that may warrant an examination by a mental health professional.

Systems Review

Clinicians often see patients with a TMD who present with nonspecific symptoms such as neck pain, headaches, earaches, and tinnitus. However, because these symptoms are not considered specific for TMDs, other possible causes should be sought and ruled out during the systems review.[82–84] Pain or dysfunction in the orofacial region often results from non-musculoskeletal causes such as otolaryngologic, neurologic, vascular, neoplastic, psychogenic, and infectious diseases.

Unexplained weight loss, ataxia, weakness, fever with pain, nystagmus, and neurologic deficits are characteristic of intracranial disorders.[85] Neurovascular disorders are associated with migraine headache and its variants, carotidynia, and cluster headaches (see Chap. 5). Neuropathic disorders include trigeminal neuralgia, glossopharyngeal neuralgia, and occipital neuralgia.

TABLE 26-6 Checklist of Psychological and Behavioral Factors

Inconsistent, inappropriate, or vague reports of pain
Overdramatization of symptoms
Symptoms that vary with life events
Significant pain of >6 months' duration
Repeated failures with conventional therapies
Inconsistent response to medications
History of other stress-related disorders
Major life events (e.g., new job, marriage, divorce, and death)
Evidence of drug abuse
Clinically significant anxiety or depression
Evidence of secondary gain

Note: The significance of these factors depends on the particular patient. Data from McNeill C, Mohl ND, Rugh JD, et al.: Temporomandibular disorders: Diagnosis, management, education, and research. *J Am Dent Assoc* 120:253–260, 1990.

The seriousness of head, face, mouth, and neck disorders that are detectable by a careful history and physical examination runs the gamut from a trivial (though discomforting) viral upper respiratory tract infection to a malignant tumor.[86]

Once the possibility of cervical, systemic, psychogenic, or ear or sinus problems has been ruled out, the next step is to consider the possibility of TMJ pain and impairment, particularly if the pain is accompanied by jaw clicking and limited mouth opening.[87]

Tests and Measures

In a study by Lobbezoo-Scholte and colleagues,[88] the interexaminer reliability of six orthopaedic tests for the TMJ (palpation, active motions, joint compression and distraction, joint mobility testing, detection of joint sounds, and resistive tests) was determined in a group of 79 patients with signs and/or symptoms of craniomandibular disorders (CMD), subdivided into three subgroups of patients with a mainly arthrogenous, and a combination of myogenous and arthrogenous disorders. Multi-test scores were composed for each test and combinations of tests for the three main symptoms of CMD: pain, joint noises, and restriction of movement. Although the orthopaedic tests showed different reliability scores, overall reliability of the determination of these three main symptoms of CMD was satisfactory. In the subgroups, arthrogenous signs and symptoms could be determined reliably with the set of six tests, whereas the reliability of the tests in determining pain and joint noises in the myogenous group was rather low. It may be concluded that these tests are well suited to evaluate arthrogenous signs and symptoms, but that the clinician should be aware of erroneous results of the tests in evaluating pain of a myogenous origin.

In another study by Dworkin and colleagues,[89] the interexaminer reliability was found to be excellent for vertical range of motion measures and for summary indices measuring the overall presence of a clinical sign that could arise from several sources (for example, summary indices of muscle palpation and pain). However, many clinical signs important in the differential diagnosis of subtypes of TMD were not measured with high reliability. In particular, assessment of pain in response to muscle palpation and identification of specific TMJ sounds seemed to be possible only with modest, sometimes marginal, reliability.

Observation

The posture of the head and neck are assessed for asymmetry. The forward head posture (FHP–see Chaps. 6 and 25) frequently is associated with TMD.[33,90,91] This is likely because of the direct impact a FHP can have on oral symmetry during occlusion. Occlusion occurs when the teeth are in contact and the mouth is closed—when tapping the teeth together in the neutral position, all of the teeth appear to strike simultaneously. However, if the same task is attempted while placing the head forward, it is the anterior teeth that occlude first. A deviation from normal occlusion is defined as malocclusion—improper positioning of the teeth and jaws. Malocclusion is a variation of normal growth and development which can affect the bite, the ability to clean teeth properly, gum tissue health, jaw growth, speech development and appearance. The consequences of this repetitive functional malocclusion during food or gum chewing should be apparent. A chronic FHP may result in an adaptive shortening of the deep cervical fascia and muscles, which can exaggerate the functional malocclusion. Most people have some degree of malocclusion, although it is not usually serious enough to require treatment. Malocclusions can be divided mainly into three types, depending on the sagittal relations of teeth and jaws, by Angle's classification method, which is based on the relative position of the first maxillary molar:[92]

- Class I (Neutrocclusion): The molar relationship of the occlusion, but the other teeth have problems such as spacing, crowding, and over or under eruption.
- Class II (Distocclusion): The upper molars are placed anteriorly. There are two subtypes:
  - Class II Division 1 (large overjet): The molar relationships are like that of Class II and the anterior teeth are protruded.
  - Class II Division 2 (deep overbite): The molar relationships are like that of class II but there is lateral flaring of the lateral maxillary incisors.
- Class III (Mesiocclusions): The lower front teeth are more prominent than the upper front teeth. In this case the patient very often has a large mandible or a short maxillary bone.

The clinician should also note whether the teeth are normally aligned or whether there is any crossbite, underbite, or overbite.

- Crossbite: This occurs when the teeth of the mandible are lateral to the upper maxillary teeth on one side and medial on the opposite side. An anterior crossbite occurs when the lower incisors are anterior to the upper incisors, whereas a posterior crossbite occurs when there is a transverse abnormal relationship of the teeth.
- Underbite: This occurs when the mandibular teeth are anterior to the maxillary teeth either unilaterally, bilaterally, or in pairs.
- Overbite: This occurs when the anterior maxillary incisors extend below the anterior mandibular incisors when the jaw is in central occlusion.

CLINICAL PEARL

Overjet, not to be confused with overbite, is a measure of how far the top incisor teeth are ahead of the bottom incisors. Normally, the top and bottom front teeth should be touching upon closure leaving no or zero overjet. If the top teeth are ahead by some distance, this is referred to as positive overjet. If the top teeth are behind the bottom teeth, this is referred to as negative overjet, or underjet.

The face is also assessed for asymmetry, such as swelling or flattening of the cheek. Asymmetry is an important finding, because developmentally the facial structures evolve in a proportional relationship, some determined by genetics, others in response to the physical environment.[93]

Orthognathy relates to the amount of projection of the lower face in relation to an imaginary perpendicular line from the eyes when viewed from the side. Three types of facial profile are recognized:

- Orthognathic: A straight facial profile in which the upper and lower lips are in line with the tip of the chin.
- Retrognathic: Describes a facial profile in which the tip of the chin is posterior to the upper and lower lips.
- Prognathic: Describes a facial profile in which the tip of the chin is anterior to the upper and lower lips.

In addition, the clinician should note the presence of any abnormal jaw deviation, unusual dryness of the lips, changes in eye position, and signs of tissue stress such as overdeveloped masseter and mentalis muscles, or a hypertrophied lower lip.[31] A lateral deviation of the jaw, evidenced by a malalignment or malocclusion of the upper and lower teeth, or hypertonus of one of the masseter muscles, may cause an adaptive shortening of the mastication muscles on the ipsilateral side of the deviation, and a lengthening of the muscles on the contralateral side. Since the role that malocclusion plays in TMD remains unclear, the relevance of the malalignment to the patient's symptoms must be determined by passively attempting to correct the deformity.[53,57] An increase in pain with the correction suggests the presence of a protective deformity.

The teeth should be examined for symmetry. Cavities, wear patterns, and restored and missing teeth should be noted. Defects in dimensions can be measured radiographically.[94] The vertical dimension of dental occlusion (i.e., depth of bite) has been implicated as a possible craniomandibular component associated with TMD.[36] It has been proposed that a deep dental overbite may have pathologic effects on cranial nerve V, the tensor veli palatini, and the soft tissue surrounding the TMJ.[36,95] Seldin[96] and Sicher[97] proposed that a deep bite results in a displaced condyle, which causes inflammation and muscle spasm in the retrodiscal tissue and muscles surrounding the TMJ. Tooth wear and fracture are often destructive signs of parafunctional habits (abrasive diet, bruxism, and teeth clenching). Loss of teeth can cause disruption in the working and nonworking interfaces of the teeth, which may cause unilateral function and subsequent overloading of the remaining teeth and the TMJ.[14] The clinician should also ask the patient if there are any painful or sensitive teeth, which can lead to incorrect biting, and subsequent abnormal loading of the TMJs.

The tongue should be examined. The tongue should appear dull red, moist, and glistening. Its anterior portion should have a smooth yet roughened appearance.[86] The posterior portion should have a smooth, slightly uneven appearance.

- A hairy tongue with yellow–brown to black elongated papillae on the posterior surface sometimes follows antibiotic therapy.[86]
- A dry or white tongue may indicate a salivary gland dysfunction or an oral yeast or bacterial infection respectively.[86]

The tongue should be observed while the patient swallows to check for any deviations. The tongue is tested for frenulum length. A short frenulum may interfere with tongue function. The tongue should have no difficulty in touching the hard palate behind the upper incisors.[52] A large tongue can exert excessive pressure against the teeth and may interfere with occlusion, resulting in bite marks.

The rest position of the TMJ should be noted. The clinician can locate the rest position of the TMJ by gently placing the little finger with the palmar portion facing anteriorly into the external auditory meatus. From an open-mouth position, the patient is asked to slowly close the mouth. At the point of resting position, the patient's mandibular heads are felt to gently touch the finger. The space between the upper and lower incisors should be 2–4 mm. A greater distance may indicate hypermobility of both TMJs.

Range of Motion

The range of motion of the TMJ, the cervical spine, the craniovertebral joints, and the shoulders should be assessed with active range of motion (AROM), and then with passive overpressure, to assess the end-feel. During cervical flexion, the mandible moves superiorly and anteriorly, whereas during cervical extension, the mandible moves inferiorly and posteriorly. The patient should be able to open and close the mouth while keeping a fist in place under the chin. During side bending or rotation of the cervical spine, maximum occlusion occurs on the ipsilateral side. Although it is unclear how the individual components of the examination contribute to the final diagnosis, most clinicians would agree that substantially reduced mandibular motion is a strong indicator of the presence of a serious TMD and helps to distinguish TMD patients from non-TMD controls.[98,99] However, there is little evidence to suggest that mandibular motion measurements add critical information to the process of differential diagnosis among the common TMD subgroups.[98]

The clinician observes the opening and closing of the mouth, noting both the range and the quality of movement. All movements of the TMJ should be smooth and without noise or pain. Normally, the mandible should open and close in a straight line. To help detect crepitus, the clinician can palpate over the mandible heads during opening and closing (Fig. 26-10). If crepitus or clicking occurs on opening and/or closing, the clinician notes where they occur in the range. If pain occurs, a determination should be made as to where in the range the pain occurs, and the location of the pain. A Boley gauge, T-bar, or ruler, can be used to measure the range of the TMJ in millimeters.[93] Walker et al.[100] used a prospective descriptive study to determine the discriminant validity and intra- and interrater reliability of measurements of TMJ range of motion using a ruler. Two groups of subjects were tested: 15 subjects (two men, 13 women; mean age = 35.2 years) with a TMD and 15 subjects (three men, 12 women; mean age = 42.9 years) without a TMD. Six motions were measured (opening, left lateral deviation, right lateral deviation, protrusion, overbite, and overjet) by two physical therapists. The study concluded that mouth opening was the only TMJ ROM measurement to discriminate between subjects with and without a TMD (mean 36.2 ± 6.4 versus 43.5 ± 6.1 mm). The technical error of measurement of the measures varied from 0.2–2.5 mm. Intrarater reliability coefficients (ICC 3, 1) varied from 0.70 to 0.99. Interrater reliability coefficients (ICC 2, k) varied from 0.90 to 1.0.

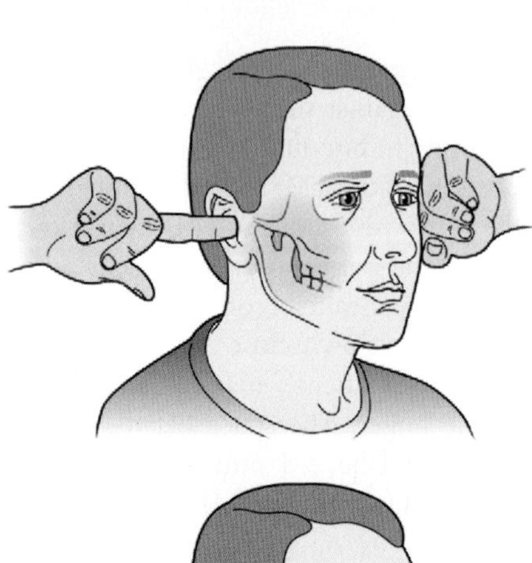

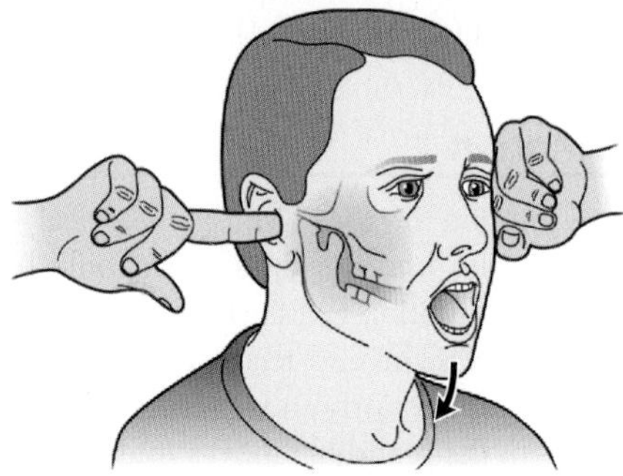

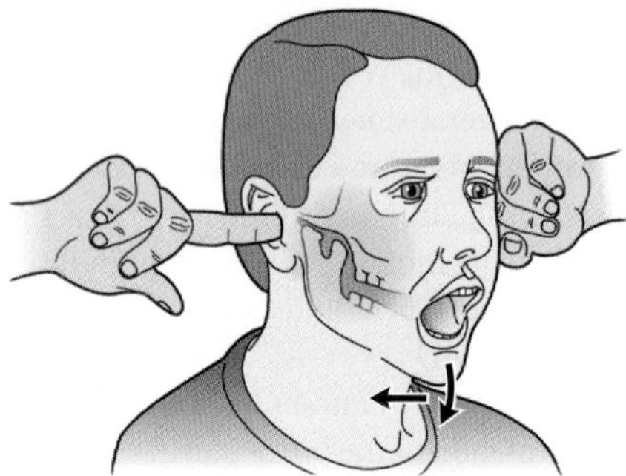

FIGURE 26-10 Palpation of TMJ during mouth opening and deviation.

CLINICAL PEARL

Joint clicking can be a normal occurrence or it may be caused by one of the types of internal derangement (refer to Practice Pattern 4D, later) including disk displacements, adhesive disk hypomobility, and deviation in form (articular surface damage). Clicking may also be a result of hypermobility or muscle incoordination.[101]

The type and temporal sequence of joint clicking can provide the clinician with the following information:

1. Reciprocal clicking is defined as clicking that occurs during opening and again during closing. The opening click occurs when the condyle moves under the posterior band of the disk until it snaps into its normal relationship on the concave surface of the disk, whereas the closing click reflects the reversal of this process.[102] Reciprocal clicks may be early, intermediate, or late, depending on the degree of opening at which they occur.[55]
   a. Early clicking usually indicates a small anterior displacement.
   b. Late clicking usually indicates that the disk has been further displaced.

Reciprocal clicking is a common finding in patients with a posterosuperior condylar positioning.[31]

2. Clicking that occurs at the end of opening often results from articular hypermobility and is accompanied by a deviation of the jaw toward the contralateral side.
3. The "soft" and "popping" opening and closing clicks associated with muscular incoordination are usually intermittent and inconsistent. They are thought to be caused by ligament movement or articular surface separation. Muscle tenderness to palpation is a frequently associated symptom.

Elevation of the Mandible (Mouth Closing)

The primary muscles involved with mouth closing are the masseter, the temporalis, and the medial pterygoid.[52] Since the maxillary teeth are fixed, the upper midline of the incisors can be used as a landmark to assess lower jaw deviation during mouth closing. Under normal conditions, the midline relationship between the upper and lower incisors should remain constant in the closed and open positions. Overpressure can be applied to the mouth closing by placing the fingers under the chin and pushing superiorly in a controlled fashion (Fig. 26-11). The normal end-feel for mouth closing should be bone on bone (teeth contact).

Depression of the Mandible (Mouth Opening)

The opening of the mouth is considered the most revealing and diagnostic movement for TMD.

While approximately only 25–35 mm of mouth opening measured between the maxillary and mandibular incisors is required for everyday activities, the maximum range of motion is approximately 50 mm.[78] At this extreme, the periarticular structures are stretched to 100% of their total length. The functional range of motion is considered to be closer to 40 mm, or approximately a two-to-three-knuckle width of the nondominant hand[12,55,103] (see Fig. 26-12). At this point in the range, the periarticular structures are stretched to 70–80% of their total length. Excessive opening is indicated when the patient is able to insert three or more knuckles between the incisors. Excessive opening is associated with large anterior translatory movements at the beginning of

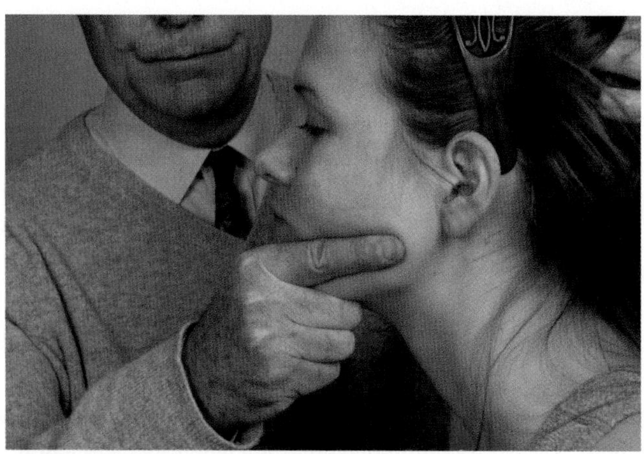

FIGURE 26-11 Mouth closing with overpressure.

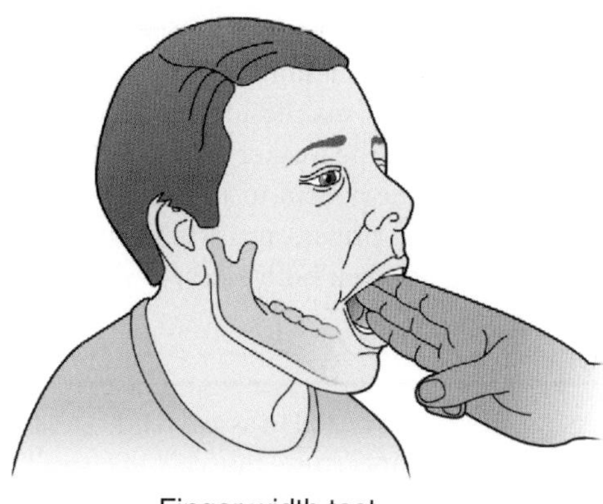

FIGURE 26-12 Three-knuckle width of mouth opening.

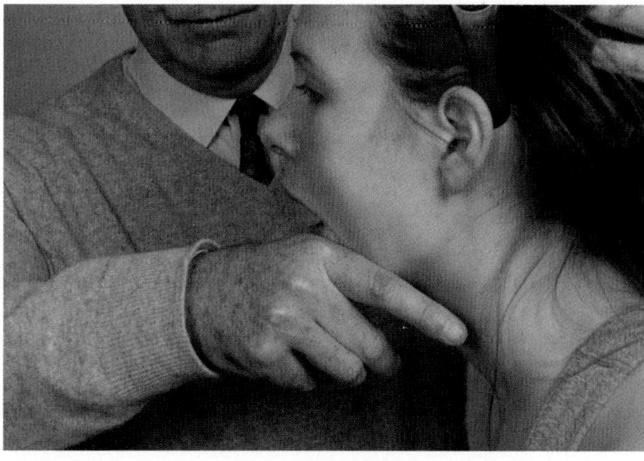

FIGURE 26-13 Mouth opening with overpressure.

mouth opening, accompanied by excessive protrusive movements of the mandible.[55]

If deviation occurs to the left on opening (a C-type curve) or to the right (a reverse C-type curve), hypomobility is evident toward the side of the deviation. If during mouth opening, an S-type or reverse S-type curve is noted, the problem is probably a muscular imbalance or medial displacement of the disk. Reduced mouth opening can result from a number of disorders including chronic muscle contraction, ankylosis, acute disk displacement without reduction, and severe trismus of the jaw muscles (the limitation of jaw opening caused by spasm of the masticatory muscles) and gross osteoarthritis.[82] Muscle contractures and ankylosis tend to develop after a substantial trauma or are developmental disorders occurring early in life and are not often misdiagnosed.[82] If contracture of the masticatory muscles is present, the mandibular opening can be as limited as 10–20 mm between the incisors.[104] Acute disk displacement without reduction and trismus are difficult to distinguish because both conditions present with recent onset, and painful limitation of jaw opening.[98] To be certain of the anatomic basis of acute disk displacement without reduction, most clinicians feel that joint imaging with magnetic resonance of the disk is required.[70,98,105] A limited opening of the jaw may also indicate joint hypomobility, muscle tightness, or the presence of trigger points within the elevator muscles: the temporalis, the masseter, and the medial pterygoid.

Translation of the lateral pole of the condyle should occur after 11 mm of mouth opening. If an opening deviation occurs, it is important to note where in the opening cycle it occurs. Opening and closing deviations are observed simply by taking a small ruler or tongue depressor and laying the edge down the midline of the face.[56] While the clinician "eyes" the straight edge, the patient opens and closes the mouth slowly[101]:

- Limited opening with deviation to one side should alert the clinician to an internal derangement without reduction, which limits the translation on the involved side and causes the jaw to deviate toward the less-mobile side, even if that is the normally mobile side and the other side is hypermobile. Early deviation suggests hypomobility, and late deviation indicates hypermobility.
- If hypomobility resulting from internal derangement with reduction of one TMJ is present, the mandible will deviate in a C pattern of motion to that side of the open mouth in the midrange of opening before returning to normal.
- The patient who demonstrates an S movement of the jaw while opening the mouth may have a muscle imbalance (often caused by trigeminal facilitation and masticatory hypertonicity), or it may be a momentary locking of a deranged disk. Lateral excursion of the mandible with mouth opening implicates contralateral structures such as the contralateral disk, the masseter, the medial and lateral pterygoid, or the lateral ligaments.

Overpressure can be applied to the opening movement using a lumbrical grip placed on the patient's chin, under the bottom lip (Fig. 26-13). The overpressure is applied to ensure that the jaw is maximally depressed. The normal end-feel should be tissue stretch. Locking of the jaw can be associated with three types of abnormal end-feel[56]:

- ***Hard.*** This type of end-feel is associated with osseous abnormalities.
- ***Springy.*** This type of end-feel is associated with a displacement of the disk.
- ***Capsular.*** This type of end-feel is associated with adaptive shortening of the periarticular tissues.

Excursion of the Mandible

The superior and inferior incisors are assessed for any deviation of the jaw laterally (cross-bite) or anteroposteriorly (overbite or underbite).

Protrusion of the Mandible. The patient opens the mouth slightly and protrudes the lower jaw. The normal movement of the lower teeth is greater than 7 mm, measured from the resting position to the protruded position.[93] The amount and direction of the protrusion are noted:

- An abnormal protrusive position may be associated with a residual pediatric tongue thrust (deviant swallowing) or an acquired adult tongue thrust secondary to a forward head posture or habitual protrusion.
- Any lateral excursion of the mandible during protrusion may indicate involvement of the contralateral structures, such as the contralateral disk, the masseter, the medial and lateral pterygoid, or the lateral ligaments.

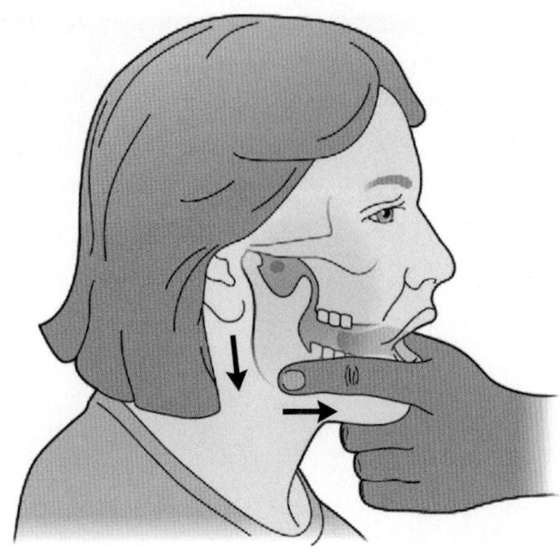

FIGURE 26-14 Manual jaw protrusion.

The clinician can apply overpressure by grasping the patient' s mandible with the index and the middle fingers behind the mandibular angles and the thumbs on the patient's cheeks, and then gently pulling the jaw anteriorly (Fig. 26-14).

Retrusion of the Mandible. The patient is asked to retrude the jaw as far back as possible. The normal movement is 3–4 mm.[57] Pain at the end range of retrusion may indicate an intracapsular injury.[6] Overpressure can be applied using a lumbrical grip positioned under the patient's bottom lip and pushing the mandible posteriorly (Fig. 26-15).

Lateral Deviation of the Mandible. The patient opens the mouth slightly and moves the lower jaw to the left and to the right. The right and left motions are compared. Normal range of motion for lateral deviation is approximately one-fourth of the opening range (10–15 mm).[34] Lateral deviation can be measured as the amount of lateral excursion between the center of the mandibular incisors and the center of the maxillary incisors. An appreciable difference between the two sides is more significant than a limited range occurring bilaterally.[31] Passive overpressure can be applied in a lateral direction. Pain reported on the side away from the direction of overpressure may indicate ligamentous or joint capsule damage.[31]

Tongue Movements. Tongue movements give valuable information about the function of the hypoglossal nerve (CN XII). Any deviation or atrophy of the tongue during tongue protrusion may indicate a lesion of this nerve. Unilateral weakness of the tongue is manifested by a deviation of the protruded tongue toward the weaker side. A test for weakness of the tongue is to ask the patient to stick the tongue into the cheek, while the clinician presses against the bulging cheek. A comparison is made between both sides.

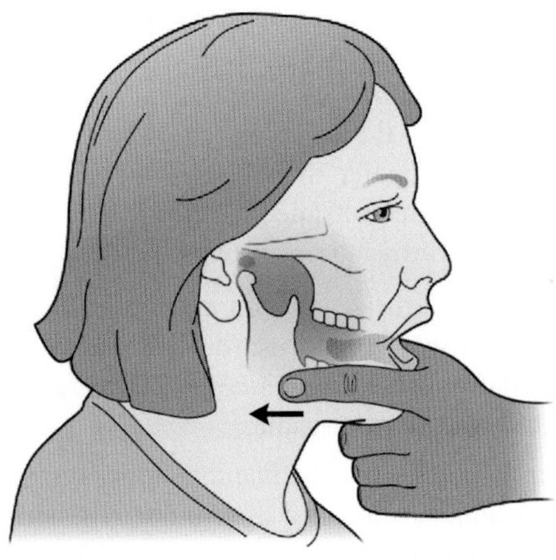

FIGURE 26-15 Manual jaw retrusion.

Palpation

Palpation of the TMJ can be used to assess tenderness, patterns of pain referral, skin temperature, muscle tone, swelling, skin moisture, and the location of trigger points. A study by de Wijer and colleagues[106] found the inter-examiner reliability of the multitest scores for muscle palpation and joint palpation in 79 patients referred to a TMD and orofacial pain department to be moderate (kappa = 0.51) and fair (kappa = 0.33), respectively. In a study by Manfredini and colleagues,[107] 61 patients with TMJ pain were assessed by means of a standardized clinical examination and magnetic resonance imaging (MRI). The aim of this work was to evaluate the predictive value of clinical symptoms for MRI findings of TMJ effusion. The study reported that a clinical examination based on the assessment of pain in the TMJ with lateral palpation, with posterior palpation, during motion, and during maximum-assisted opening, and the presence of click and crepitus sounds demonstrated an accuracy of 78.7% to predict TMJ effusion. Among the single clinical symptoms, the most reliable predictor of TMJ effusion was found to be the presence of pain with lateral palpation (accuracy 76.2%; *kappa* = 0.53).[107]

For comparison and expediency, palpation of the lateral and posterior aspects of the TMJs is performed bilaterally and simultaneously. The palpation begins with gentle touch and light pressure, because the muscles of mastication can be highly sensitive if they are in spasm.

Anterior Aspect

Zygomatic Arch. The zygomatic arch is located anterior to the condylar process of the mandible. The temporal muscle lies above and the masseter muscle lies below the zygomatic arch.

Hyoid Bone. The hyoid bone, located anterior to the C2 and C3 vertebrae, is palpated for normal, painless movement as the patient swallows.

Digastric Muscle (Anterior Belly). The anterior belly of the digastric muscle can be palpated from its origin on the lingual side of the mandible to its tendinous insertion on the hyoid bone.

Thyroid. The thyroid cartilage, located anterior to the C4 and C5 vertebrae, is palpated and moved. Crepitation of this structure may be felt during neck extension as the cartilage becomes taut.

Lateral Aspect

Temporomandibular Joint. The clinician palpates the lateral aspect of the TMJ by placing the tip of the forefinger just anterior to the tragus of the ear (see Fig. 26-10). As the individual opens the mouth wide, the clinician's finger will identify a depression posterior to the condylar head and overlying the joint that is created by the translating condyle. Tenderness in this depression may indicate inflammation.[31] Alternatively, the lateral aspect of the joint capsule can be palpated on the lateral pole of the condyle just anterior to the tragus. To facilitate identification of the lateral pole, the patient is asked to open and lightly hold a cotton roll in the premolar region.[98]

Mandible. The mandible should be palpated along its entire length. Any asymmetry from side to side should be noted. The mandibular angle serves as an important landmark for orientation. The mandibular ramus is covered by the masseter muscle. The condylar process of the mandible is located just in front of the ear. The parotid gland is located anterior to and below the auricle, and normally extends from the sternomastoid muscle anteriorly to the masseter muscle. Enlargement of the parotid gland causes the earlobe to move outward on the involved side. Enlargement of the parotid gland can have a number of causes, including infection, trauma, diabetes mellitus, lymphoma, or chronic alcoholism.[86] The submandibular gland is palpable in front of the mandibular angle and underneath the mandibular body, about halfway between the chin and the mandibular angle. Normally, the gland has a firm, irregular consistency.

Sternocleidomastoid Muscle. The sternocleidomastoid is palpated from its dual origin on the sternum and the clavicle along its course upward and posteriorly to its insertion on the mastoid process.

Trapezius Muscle. The trapezius muscle is palpated from its origin on the acromion process to its insertion along the midline of the spine to the base of the skull. The trapezius is perhaps the most common site for muscular trigger points and often refers pain to the base of the skull and the temporal region.[108]

Masseter Muscle. Both the superficial and deep portions of the masseter run from the zygomatic arch to the mandibular ramus. The clinician should place the palpating finger against the ramus and then ask the patient to gently clench the teeth.

Temporalis Muscle. The temporalis muscle can be palpated in front of, and above, the ear. The clinician places a finger against the temporal region and then asks the patient to gently clench the teeth.

Posterior Aspect. Posterior TMJ palpation is performed by placing the tip of the little finger in the patient's external auditory canal and exerting anterior pressure as the patient repeatedly opens and closes the mouth.[31] Alternatively, the palpation can be performed with the teeth in the intercuspal position.[98] If inflammation is present, pain is felt on jaw closing as the tissue is compressed between the clinician's finger and the condyle.[30] The examination also may reveal a posterosuperiorly positioned condyle and disk dysfunction. This posterosuperior position of the condyle can be a result of occlusal factors or trauma. The position results in an anteriorly displaced disk and an impingement by the condyle on the space normally occupied by the disk. This displacement may cause reciprocal clicking or locking.

The masseter, temporalis, and perihyoid muscles are palpated extraorally for hypertonicity and tenderness. In addition, the lateral aspect of the joint capsule and the lateral TMJ ligament are palpated for tenderness.

Medial Pterygoid. The patient is asked to move the tongue to the opposite side. The clinician slides a thumb onto the medial aspect of the lower gum and toward the back of the mouth and angle of the mandible. The thumb is maintained at the bottom of the mouth to prevent the gag reflex. The insertion site for the medial pterygoid is located on the medial aspect of the mandibular angle.

Lateral Pterygoid. It is questionable whether the lateral pterygoid can be palpated.[109] Nonetheless, descriptions detailing palpation of this muscle exist. The muscle is said to be palpated by sliding a thumb back to the medial aspect of the base of the upper molars. The patient is asked to open the mouth wider, and the clinician slides the thumb back and up at an angle of 45 degrees and inspects the muscle and area for tenderness.

Muscle Tests

It is important to be able to selectively stress the muscles of mastication and facial expression to determine whether they are implicated in the symptoms. All these tests cannot replace a thorough palpation of the muscles. All test positions, resisted motions, and attempted facial expressions may be used as exercises to rehabilitate any identified deficits. For each of the following, the patient is seated.

Temporalis

The clinician palpates the side of the head in the temporal fossa region. The patient is asked to elevate and retract the mandible. Resistance can be applied using a tongue depressor placed between the teeth. Both sides are tested.

Masseter

The clinician palpates the cheek, just above the angle of the mandible. The patient is asked to elevate the mandible, as in closing the jaw. Resistance can be applied using a tongue depressor placed between the teeth.

Lateral Pterygoid

The clinician palpates the pterygoid at the neck of the mandible and joint capsule. The patient is asked to protrude and depress the mandible against manual resistance.

Medial Pterygoid

The patient is asked to elevate and protrude the mandible. Resistance can be applied using a tongue depressor placed between the teeth.

Suprahyoid Muscles

The clinician palpates the floor of the mouth. The patient is asked to press the tip of the tongue against the front teeth. Resistance can be applied to the surface of the hyoid bone in an attempt to protrude the tongue.

Infrahyoid Muscles

The clinician palpates below the hyoid bone, immediately lateral to the midline. The patient is asked to swallow, while the clinician palpates for the movement of the hyoid and the larynx.

TABLE 26-7 Muscles of Facial Expression

Muscle	Action	Innervation
Occipitofrontalis	Wrinkles forehead by raising eyebrows	Facial nerve
Corrugator	Draws eyebrows together, as in frowning	Facial nerve
Procerus	Draws skin on lateral nose upward, forming transverse wrinkles over bridge of the nose	Facial nerve
Nasalis	Dilates and compresses aperture of the nostrils	Facial nerve
Orbicularis oculi	Closes eyes tightly	Facial nerve
Superior levator palpebrae	Lifts upper eyelid	Oculomotor nerve
Orbicularis oris	Closes and protrudes lips	Facial nerve
Major and minor zygomatic	Raises corners of mouth upward and laterally, as in smiling	Facial nerve
Levator anguli oris	Raises upper border of lip straight up, as in sneering	Facial nerve
Risorius	Draws corners of mouth laterally	Facial nerve
Buccinator	Presses cheeks firmly against teeth	Facial nerve
Levator labii superioris	Protrudes and elevates upper lip	Facial nerve
Depressor anguli oris and platysma	Draws corner of mouth downward and tenses skin over neck	Facial nerve
Depressor labii inferioris	Protrudes lower lip, as in pouting	Facial nerve
Mentalis	Raises skin on chin	Facial nerve

Muscles of Facial Expression

This group of muscles, most of which are innervated by the facial nerve, can be assessed by having the patient attempt to make the specific facial expression attributed to each muscle (Table 26-7). Facial strength can be evaluated with the House–Brackmann facial nerve grading system[110–113] (Table 26-8), which separates facial nerve paralysis into six grades, based on the severity of findings. In 1985, the American Academy of Otolaryngology, Head and Neck Surgery adopted the House–Brackmann six-point subjective grading scale as a universal standard. Parameters evaluated during the examination include:

- overall macroscopic and gross appearance;
- appearance at rest;
- forehead movement;
- eyelid closure;
- mouth appearance;
- synkinesis contracture or hemifacial spasm, or both.

Ligament Stress Tests

The ligament stress tests assess the integrity of the capsule and ligaments. Positive findings include excessive motion compared with the other side, or pain. The patient is seated.

Temporomandibular (Lateral) Ligament

This test is only performed if there is a painful loss of AROM of the TMJ. The purpose of the test is to determine if the painful restriction is caused by damage to one of the ligaments or the joint capsule.

The clinician cradles and stabilizes the patient's head with one hand. The index and middle fingers of this hand can be used to palpate the joint line. The patient is asked to open their mouth to the point of restriction; mandible is positioned slightly open. The clinician places the thumb of the mobilizing hand on the ipsilateral molars of the side to be tested. The clinician then applies a downward force on the molars creating a caudal shear (Fig. 26-14). There should be slight movement with this technique, and the end-feel should be capsular.

Joint Capsule

The clinician stands at the head of the patient. The patient's mandible is closed. The clinician places one hand on top of the patient's head, and the other hand on the ramus and angle of one side. The clinician then applies a contralateral protrusion and ipsilateral deviation force (Fig. 26-16).

Joint Loading Tests

Selective loading of the TMJ may be used to help determine the presence of an intracapsular pathology. A positive finding is pain with the test. These tests include dynamic loading and joint compression.[52]

Dynamic Loading

The patient is asked to bite forcefully on a cotton roll or tongue depressor on one side. This maneuver loads the contralateral TMJ.

Joint Compression

The patient is positioned supine, with the clinician standing at the head of the bed. The clinician places the fingers of each hand under each side of the mandible, with the thumbs resting on the ramus. The mandible is then tipped posteriorly and inferiorly to compress the joint surfaces.

TABLE 26-8 House–Brackmann Facial Nerve Grading System

Parameter	Grade I	Grade II	Grade III	Grade IV	Grade V	Grade VI
Overall appearance	Normal	Slight weakness on close inspection	Obvious but not disfiguring difference between both sides	Obvious weakness and/or disfiguring asymmetry	Only barely perceptible motion	No movement
At rest	Normal symmetry	Normal symmetry	Normal symmetry	Normal symmetry	Asymmetry	Asymmetry
Forehead movement	Normal with excellent function	Moderate-to-good function	Slight-to-Moderate Function	None	None	None
Eyelid closure	Normal closure	Complete with minimum effort	Complete with maximal effort	Incomplete closure with maximal effort	Incomplete closure with maximal effort	No movement
Mouth	Normal and symmetric	Slight asymmetry	Slight asymmetry with maximum effort	Asymmetry with maximum effort	Slight movement	No movement
Synkinesis contracture and/or hemifacial spasm	None	May have very slight synkinesis; no contracture or hemifacial spasm	Obvious but not disfiguring synkinesis contracture and/or hemifacial spasm	Synkinesis contracture and/or hemifacial spasm disfiguring or severe enough to interfere with function	Synkinesis contracture and/or hemifacial spasm usually absent	No movement

Data from House JW, Brackman DE: Facial nerve grading system. *Otolaryngol Head Neck Surg* 93:146–147, 1985.

Passive Articular Mobility Testing

The passive articular mobility tests assess the joint glides and the end-feels. The patient and clinician setup are identical to that described above for the temporomandibular (lateral) ligament stress test.

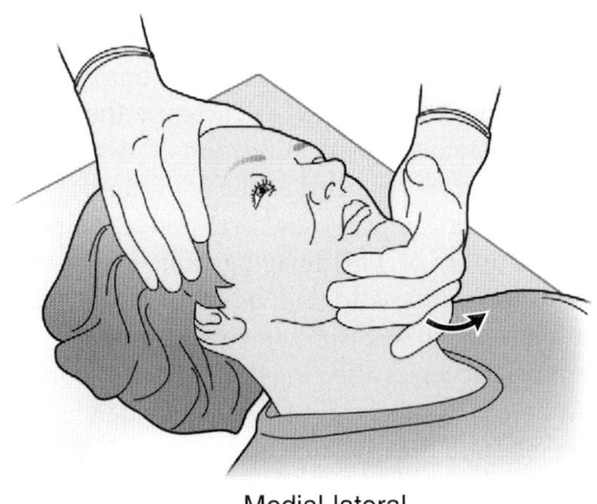

FIGURE 26-16 Contralateral protrusion and ipsilateral deviation force to TMJ.

From the end-range position (or as close as possible, given that the thumb is in the patient's mouth), the following maneuvers are performed assessing for range and end-feel. Findings are compared with each side. Pain, or a restricted glide, are positive findings and may indicate articular involvement or a capsular restriction. It is important to check the specific glides that are related to the loss of active motion. For example, if a patient demonstrated diminished mouth opening, the combined anterior, inferior, and lateral glide is assessed at each joint.

Limited opening can be caused by anterior disk displacement without reduction, elevator muscle spasm, or capsular restraint. By inducing a passive stretch to the joint after the patient has actively opened the mouth to the full extent, the "end-feel" can be used to differentiate between these causes. For example, if a displaced disk is responsible for limited opening, there will be a hard end-feel with little or no play. In contrast, a gummy end-feel is present when muscle spasm or capsular connective tissue is preventing full opening.[55] To help differentiate between elevator muscle spasm and a capsular restriction, passive motions can be used. With elevator muscle spasm, only vertical movement is restricted and protrusive and lateral excursions are normal. Anterior disk displacement without reduction, however, exhibits restrictions in both protrusive movements and contralateral excursions. Movement to the side of the involved

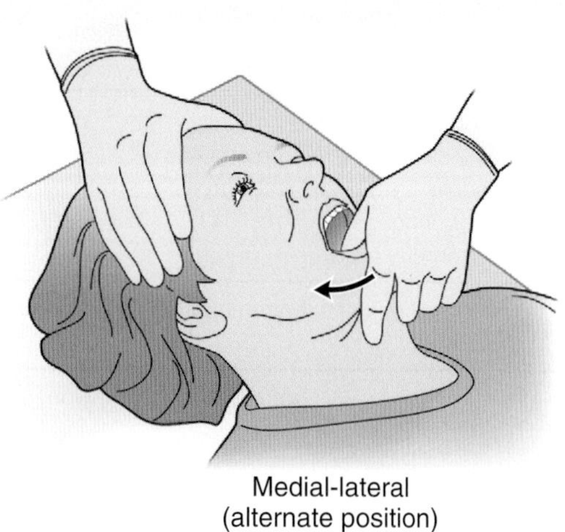

FIGURE 26-17 Medial glide.

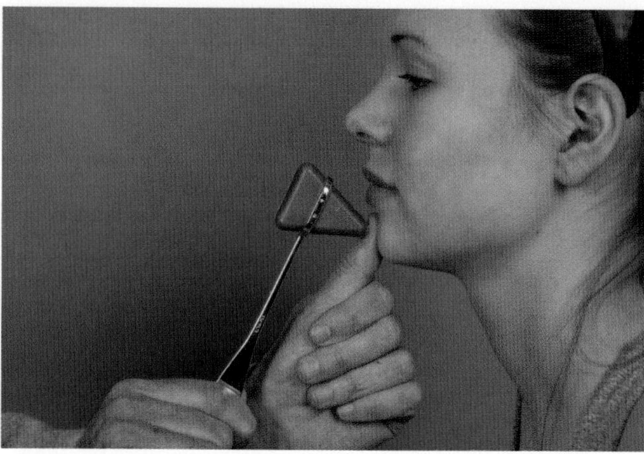

FIGURE 26-18 Jaw jerk test.

joint is usually not mechanically restricted because the main movement occurring in the joint is rotation. While hypomobility may be apparent with passive articular mobility testing, hypermobility is difficult to determine with these tests.

Most of the mobility tests can also be used for mobilizations by changing the grade and the intent. The clinician should remove the thumb from the patient's mouth every 10–15 seconds to allow the patient to swallow.

- Distraction (Fig. 26-14). The mandible is moved inferiorly in a direction perpendicular to the joint surface.
- Anterior glide (see Fig. 26-14). The mandible is moved anteriorly.
- Medial glide (see Fig. 26-17). The clinician stands to the side of the patient and stabilizes the patient's head. A medial force is applied by the other hand. This glide assesses the ability of the TMJ to side glide to the contralateral side from the side of the joint being tested.
- Posterior glide with lateral excursion for the posterior ligaments.

Neurologic Tests

Trigeminal Nerve (CN V)

Sensation. The skin near the midline (there is overlap from the anterior (ventral) rami of C2 and C3 if tested too laterally) of the forehead and face can be stroked with cotton wool or tissue paper or can be tested for pinprick sensation. It is best if the testing is carried out bilaterally and simultaneously.

Reflex. The jaw jerk can be used to test trigeminal function. A lesion superior to the pons would produce hyperreflexia, and a lesion below the pons would result in hyporeflexia or areflexia. The patient's mouth is relaxed and open in the resting position. The clinician places a thumb on the mandible and then lightly taps the thumb with the pointed end of a reflex hammer (Fig. 26-18). A normal response is one in which the mouth closes.

Facial Nerve (CN VII)

The facial nerve can be tested using the Chvostek (Weiss sign) test. The patient is positioned sitting. The clinician taps the parotid gland overlying the mass of the muscle. If the facial muscles twitch (typically a twitch of the nose or lips), the test is considered positive for hypocalcemia (i.e., from hypoparathyroidism, pseudohypoparathyroidism, hypovitaminosis D) with resultant hyperexcitability of the nerves.

Special Tests

At the time of writing, no routine special tests for the TMJ exist. Most, if not all, of the structures of the TMJ are isolated and tested during the standard examination previously described. Although cranial nerve testing (see Chap. 3) is not, strictly speaking, a special test, this testing should be performed if an injury to a cranial nerve is suspected. In addition, the special tests for thoracic outlet syndrome, brachial plexus stretching, and dural mobility should be performed to help rule out any referral of symptoms.

Imaging Studies

With the rapid progress made in TMJ imaging techniques, many studies have focused on the importance of internal derangement and osteoarthrosis as the underlying mechanisms in the etiology of TMJ-related pain and dysfunction. Despite the limitations, plain radiographs of the TMJ, such as high-level orthopantomograms and transcranial projections, are useful ways of visualizing any gross pathologic, degenerative, or traumatic changes in the bony component of the TMJ complex.[12,114] MRI is currently the most accurate imaging modality for identification of disk positions of the TMJ and may be regarded as the gold standard for disk position identification purposes.[115] However, many reports question the utility of TMJ imaging studies because of the number of asymptomatic individuals who demonstrate positive signs of disk displacements and joint arthrosis (degenerative processes affecting the TMJ).[1,116] Postmortem examinations of a total of 140 persons (dental histories unknown) showed that 40–80% had joint pathology or disk displacements.[116] The relevance of bony joint arthrosis was also disputed by evidence that patients with TMJ rheumatoid arthritic pathology actually had fewer symptoms than normal individuals.[117]

INTERVENTION STRATEGIES

The lack of a consistent method for identifying and diagnosing TMD in a research setting, varying durations of treatment, lack of control groups, lack of objective-dependent measures, and lack of specification of symptom duration have prevented significant research on the effectiveness of various treatment modalities for TMD.[118,119,120] Complicating matters is the fact that the majority of the symptoms associated with TMD are self-limiting and resolve without active intervention.[48] The chronic pain associated with TMD most likely occurs because of secondary factors. These factors include a fixed FHP, abnormal stress levels, depression, or oral parafunctional habits (such as bruxism). This prolonged pain is frequently due to adaptive shortening of the tissues, or from a secondary hypermobility. It is likely that the longer the duration of the symptoms, the smaller the likelihood that the patient will benefit from a conservative intervention.[78] A number of authors[121,122] have recommended that the intervention for TMD should be directed at the following factors[123]:

- Treatment of symptoms to reduce or eliminate pain or joint noises, or both.
- Treatment of the underlying cause or the predisposing factor (poor posture, stress, depression, and oral parafunctional habits).[68,124]
- The restoration of normal mandibular and cervical function.[101]

Recently, there has been an interest in the relative effectiveness of specific conservative interventions for TMD and, as a result, a number of systematic reviews have been performed in the area.[53,98,120,125–129] For example, Kulekcioglu and colleagues[127] reported that low-level laser therapy can be considered as an alternative physical modality in the management of TMD, and Tegelberg[130] and Au[131] have reported significant symptom reduction after exercise management of TMD. However, most of the studies have demonstrated the importance of a multifactorial approach in the conservative management of TMD. For example, the results of a systematic review by McNeely and colleagues[129] found manual therapy, and the use of active and passive oral exercises, and exercises to improve posture, as effective interventions to reduce symptoms associated with TMD. However, this review also found no evidence to support the use of electric physical modalities to reduce TMD pain.[129] A single case study by Cleland and Palmer[132] found manual physical therapy (anterior joint glides, distraction and contract–relax stretching to upper trapezius, levator scapulae, and posterior occipitals), therapeutic exercise (scapulothoracic muscles) and patient education with regards to posture, parafunctional habits, soft diet, tongue resting position, and activity modification to be an effective management strategy for a patient with bilateral disk displacement without reduction within 8 visits.[132] Gatchel and colleagues[120] conducted a randomized clinical trial with a 1 year follow-up to evaluate the efficacy of a biopsychosocial intervention for patients who were at high risk of progressing from acute to chronic TMD-related pain. The study reported that the group who received behavioral skills training and biofeedback demonstrated reduced pain levels, improved coping abilities, and reduced emotional distress at the 1 year point.[120]

It should be clear from the studies that TMD is complex and that there is a clear need for further well-designed RCTs examining physical therapy interventions for TMD, which include valid and reliable outcome measures.

Acute Phase

Acute injuries to the TMJ most frequently have a traumatic origin, such as a direct blow,[133–135] or from a sudden locking of the jaw caused by an internal derangement.[136,137]

The typical patient presentation for an acute injury demonstrates a capsular pattern of restriction (decreased ipsilateral opening and lateral deviation to the involved side), with pain and tenderness on the same side.

Physical Therapy

PRICEMEM (protection, rest, ice, compression, elevation, manual therapy, early motion, and medications) are recommended during the acute phase, with the exception of elevation, which is neither appropriate or feasible. Cold is applied to reduce edema, inflammation, and muscle spasm. Chapman[138] concluded that local application of cold provides short-term relief of pain, possibly because of its analgesic effects and ability to reduce inflammation. No single drug has been proved to be effective for all cases of TMD. Thus, a wide variety of drug classes have been described for chronic orofacial pain, ranging from short-term treatment with nonsteroidal anti-inflammatory drugs (NSAIDs), corticosteroids, and muscle relaxants for pain of muscular origin to chronic administration of antidepressants for less well-characterized pain. The analgesic effect of NSAIDs is specific only in cases of TMD, in which pain is the result of an inflammatory process such as synovitis or myositis. At the doses usually prescribed clinically, opiates are more effective in dampening the patient's emotional response to pain than eliminating the pain itself.[118]

The patient should receive instruction on how to obtain the rest position of the TMJ.[139]

Motion of the TMJ should be restricted to pain-free movements to allow the rest or immobilization of any painful muscular and articular structures. However, very gentle and pain-free active exercises should be performed frequently (every hour or so) to help stimulate the mechanoreceptors and modulate pain, as well as improve vascularization. Kropmans and colleagues[140] report at least 6 mm of change has to be seen to be a detectable difference when doing more than one measurement or to determine the effect of treatment.

Appropriate exercises during the acute stage include the so-called 6 × 6 exercise protocol of Rocabado,[141] which are thought to aid in strengthening, coordination, and the reduction of muscle spasm. The patient should be instructed to perform the following exercises six times each at a frequency of six times per day.

1. ***Tongue rest position and nasal breathing.*** The patient places the tip of the tongue on the roof of the mouth, just behind the front teeth. With the tongue in this position, the patient is asked to breathe through the nose and

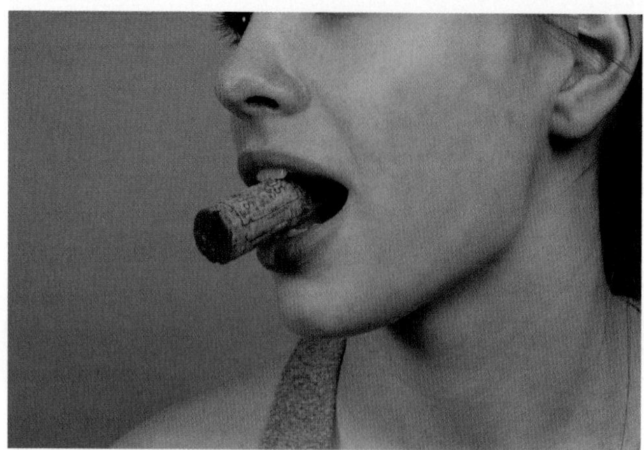

FIGURE 26-19 Cork exercise

to only use the diaphragm muscle for expiration (no accessory breathing muscles).

2. ***Controlled opening.*** The patient positions the tongue in the rest position and practices chewing and opening the mouth to the point where the tongue begins to leave the roof of the mouth. Another gentle exercise to help increase joint mobility and articulation is the 'cork' exercise. The size (height) of the cork depends on the available motion. The patient holds the cork between his or her teeth while talking for approximately 2 minutes (Fig. 26-19). The talking exercise is then repeated with the cork removed.
3. ***Rhythmic stabilization.*** The patient positions the tongue in the rest position and grasps the chin with one or both hands. The patient then applies a resistance sideways to right deviation and then left deviation. The patient then applies a resistance against mouth opening and closing. Throughout all of these exercises, the patient must maintain the resting jaw position.
4. ***Release of cervical flexion.*** The patient places both hands behind the neck and interlaces the fingers to stabilize the entire cervical region. The neck is kept upright while the patient performs craniovertebral flexion (see Chap. 23), which produces a distraction of the occiput from the atlas and helps to counteract the craniovertebral extension produced by the FHP.
5. ***Longitudinal neck extension.*** The patient is asked to glide the neck backward and stretch the head upward in one movement to improve the functional and mechanical relationship of the head to the cervical spine. This exercise needs to be monitored closely to prevent hypermobility of the cervical segments.
6. ***Shoulder retraction.*** The patient is asked to pull the shoulders back and downward in one motion while squeezing the shoulder blades together to help restore the shoulder girdle to an ideal postural position and to establish stability of the entire head–neck–shoulder complex.

Neuromuscular education techniques can be used to control premature or excessive translation. If premature translation has been found to be occurring, the patient is taught to maintain the tongue on the posterior portion of the palate and to monitor the lateral pole of the condyles during opening to ensure that only rotation occurs during the early phase of opening.[101]

One of the most commonly overlooked problems during TMJ intervention is altered swallowing sequence and tongue position.[101] Few other forces can match the ability of the tongue to cause occlusal and skeletal deformation.[142] The presence of a residual pediatric tongue thrust or an acquired adult tongue thrust secondary to a forward head posture can affect the response to all other interventions. Presence of a tongue thrust is manifested by the hyoid moving slowly up and down during swallowing, contraction of the suboccipitals during swallowing, or head rocking and excessive lip activity during swallowing.[101] Patients with these findings should be shown the normal resting position for the tongue, and swallowing should be practiced without movement of the head and with the correct sequencing of tongue movements.[142]

Patient Education

The clinician should explain the cause and nature of the disorder to the patient, and to reassure him or her of the benign nature of the condition.[124] A successful self-care program allows healing and prevents further injury and is often enough to control the problem.[143]

A typical self-care home program includes the following:[124]

- Limitation of mandibular function (rest). The patient is advised to eat soft foods and avoid those that need a lot of chewing and is discouraged from wide yawning, singing, chewing gum, and any other activities that would cause excessive jaw movement.
- An exercise program, including the 6×6 protocol.
- Habit awareness and modification.
- Stress avoidance. Patients should be advised to identify anysource(s) of stress and to try to change their lifestyle accordingly.
- The patient's sleeping position. If the intrinsic ligaments are injured, the patient should be advised to sleep on the back, with the neck supported by a cervical pillow.[68] The prone position should be avoided as it compresses the TMJ, and stresses the cervical spine by extending and rotating it.

Occlusal Appliance Therapy

The most common form of intervention provided by dentists for TMD is occlusal appliance therapy, alone or in combination with other interventions.[144] Occlusal appliances include bite-raising appliances, occlusal splints, or bite guards. These removable custom-made appliances are usually made of hard acrylic, which are custom made to fit over the occlusal surfaces of the teeth in one arch.[124] The function of the occlusal device is to provide a stable jaw posture by creating single contacts for all of the posterior teeth in centric relation and centric occlusion.[144]

Although occlusal appliance therapy has been shown clinically to alleviate symptoms of TMD, the experimental evidence has been lacking and thus the physiologic basis of the response to treatment has never been well understood.[145,146]

Malocclusion, in itself, is not established as an important factor in TMD,[54,147] because very few patients with malocclusion actually go on to develop TMD.[148] In an evidence-based assessment of occlusal adjustment as a treatment for TMDs, Tsukiyama and colleagues[53] concluded that the experimental evidence reviewed was neither convincing nor powerful enough to support the performance of occlusal therapy as a general method for treating a nonacute TMD, bruxism, or headache.[53]

Functional Phase

The interventions described for this phase are best used in combination and are dependent on the patient's needs.[1,78,149,150]

Postural Education

In a study of postural problems in 164 patients with head and neck pain, Fricton and colleagues[151] found poor sitting and standing posture in 96%, FHP in 84.7%, rounded shoulders in 82.3%, abnormal lordosis in 46.3%, and scoliosis in 15.9%. These findings indicate that there may be a correlation with TMJ dysfunction and poor posture, although comparisons would need to be made with a controlled group of normal individuals before final conclusions are drawn.

The focus of the postural intervention should be to educate the patient on correct posture of the head, neck, shoulder, and tongue, in order to help minimize symptoms. Oftentimes, the focus of the education is to teach the patient mental reminders to reduce the times spent in habitual positions during work and recreation. These positions, which cause an alteration in the tensile properties of the muscles and adaptive shortening of the joint capsule and ligaments, result in a variety of problems, including joint strain and improper weight-bearing through the joint.[152–154] The pathologic posture then becomes associated with, or the precursor of, other deformities. A balanced and relaxed position, on the other hand, affords the best mechanical advantage for the body.[144] Since these postural deviations do not always cause symptoms,[155] and the corrected positions require effort to maintain, patients need reassurance that the benefits in changing their posture may take time.[104,156]

Psychotherapy

Recent studies suggest that, on occasion, TMD may be the somatic expression of an underlying psychological or psychiatric disorder such as depression.[124,157–162] These studies have demonstrated increased psychometric scores denoting pain, chronic disability, and depression in TMD patients that far exceed the general population. A study by Gardea and colleagues[163] evaluated the relative long-term efficacy of electromyographic biofeedback, CBST, combined biofeedback and CBST, and no treatment in 108 patients suffering from chronic TMD. After an initial evaluation, patients were assigned to one of the four treatment groups. The three biobehavioral interventions consisted of 12 standardized sessions. Patients were reevaluated 1 year after completing treatment. Results demonstrated that patients who received the biobehavioral interventions reported significant improvement in subjective pain, pain-related disability, and mandibular functioning 1 year after receiving the treatment. The no-treatment comparison group did not demonstrate such improvements, whereas the combined biofeedback and CBST treatment produced the most comprehensive improvements across all outcome measures.

Where persistent habits exacerbate or maintain the TMD, a more structured program of behavioral therapy may be required. Such behavioral therapy may include counseling on lifestyle, relaxation therapy, sleep interruption devices, or hypnosis.[164] Medical hypnosis has been demonstrated to be an effective treatment modality for TMD, in terms of reducing both symptoms and medical use.[165,166]

Manual Therapy

The specific manual techniques for the TMJ are described under "Therapeutic Techniques" section later.

Trigger Point Therapy

The most common intervention for masticatory muscle disorders is trigger point therapy.[167] Chapter 11 reviews the basis for the various intervention procedures for trigger points, which include deep massage, soft tissue mobilizations, postural exercises, ultrasound, acupuncture, and trigger point injections. Spray and stretch techniques may also be used. These techniques involve the application of a vapocoolant spray during the stretching of soft tissues to reduce trigger points and eliminate referred pain.[108] Vapocoolants may also be applied to rapidly cool the skin and overlying musculature during stretching. When using vapocoolants in this region, care must be taken to cover the patient's eyes and to prevent any inhalation of the vapors.

Exercise

Some evidence suggests that exercise of the specific painful area during the functional phase is effective in strengthening the muscles, improving function, and reducing pain. Tegelberg and Kopp[168] ran parallel studies of jaw exercise versus a no-treatment control in subjects with rheumatoid arthritis and ankylosing spondylitis. Significant differences were detected for both conditions in mean maximal opening, but no between-group differences were detected for change in the subjective symptoms (pain and stiffness).

Because of the association of TMD and poor posture, the prescribed exercises for TMD include strengthening exercises for the cervicothoracic stabilizers (see Chap. 25) and the scapular stabilizers (see Chap. 16). Stretching exercises are prescribed for the scalenes, trapezius, pectoralis minor, and levator scapulae (see Chap. 25) and the suboccipital extensors (see Chap. 23).

A restriction of mouth opening is treated with range-of-motion exercises to elongate the soft tissues and with joint mobilizations. The patient should be encouraged to begin full active range-of-motion exercises as early as tolerated (see the discussion of automobilizations under "Therapeutic Techniques" section later). However, if jaw deviation is occurring, the exercises should be performed in a range in which the patient can control the deviation.

Excessive mandibular motion is treated by muscle reeducation, with isometrics performed at the desired opening range.

Thermal and Electrotherapeutic Modalities

A multitude of electrotherapeutic modalities, especially ultrasound and electrical stimulation, have been applied to patients with TMDs,[12,73,123] but there appears to be little evidence that passive modalities alone can cause long-lasting reductions, and very few studies have systematically evaluated the effect of these treatments.[123,149,150,169,170] The American Academy of Craniomandibular Disorders recommends the use of thermal and electrotherapeutic modalities and intraoral splints in conjunction with other interventions, including mobilization of the TMJ.[171]

Moist Heat Packs. Conventional hot packs or face packs may be used in the functional stage and are applied for approximately 15 minutes. Thermotherapy is used to help the soft tissues relax and to increase circulation.

High-Voltage Electric Stimulation. High-voltage stimulators deliver a monophasic, twin-peak waveform. Because of the short duration of this twin-peak wave, high voltages with high-peak current but low average current can be achieved. These electrical characteristics provide patient comfort and safety in application. In addition, in contrast to low-voltage direct-current devices, thermal and galvanic effects are minimized.[172]

High-voltage stimulators have been applied clinically to reduce or eliminate muscle spasm and soft tissue edema, as well as for muscle reeducation (non—CNS-produced muscle contraction), trigger point therapy, and increasing blood flow to tissues with decreased circulation.[62,63,172]

Ultrasound. The effects of ultrasound are partly thermal, because of the increase in blood flow and tissue temperature produced. Thus, ultrasound may be used to help the soft tissues relax and to increase circulation. Ultrasound is an ideal modality both before and during joint and soft tissue mobilization. There is also a mechanical effect associated with ultrasound, because the sound waves produce pressure changes in the tissues, which may result in a micromassage of the tissues.[123] A 3-MHz frequency is recommended, with an intensity of between 0.75 and 1.0 W/cm^2. Tongue depressors can be inserted in the patient's mouth to apply a gentle stretch during the ultrasound treatment.[101]

Iontophoresis. Iontophoresis may be used to introduce medications such as cortisol, dexamethasone, salicylates, and analgesics.[173,174] Kahn[175] found that following TMJ surgery, the use of iontophoresis in conjunction with ultrasound produced a decrease in pain, paresthesia, and trismus.

Surgical Intervention

Published reports show that about 5% of patients undergoing an intervention for TMD may eventually require surgery.[8,9] A range of surgical procedures is currently used to treat TMD, ranging from TMJ arthrocentesis and arthroscopy to the more complex open joint surgical procedures, referred to as *arthrotomy*.[9]

The proximity of the medial aspect of the TMJ to the structures of the infratemporal fossa raises the possibility of complications associated with TMJ surgery on the medial aspect of the joint.[176] These complications include involvement of the inferior alveolar, lingual, and auriculotemporal nerves.[177] A further study found that the location of such vital structures as the middle meningeal artery, the carotid artery, the internal jugular vein, and the trigeminal nerve varied, increasing the likelihood of significant intraoperative or postoperative complications.[178]

In terms of intervention, the postsurgical patient is treated as though in the acute phase of healing and is progressed gradually, as outlined under "Intervention Strategies" section earlier.

PRACTICE PATTERN 4D: IMPAIRED JOINT MOBILITY, MOTOR FUNCTION, MUSCLE PERFORMANCE, AND RANGE OF MOTION ASSOCIATED WITH CONNECTIVE TISSUE DYSFUNCTION

Internal Derangement: Intra-articular Disk Displacement

TMJ internal derangement is one of the most common forms of TMD and is associated with characteristic clinical findings such as pain, joint sounds, and irregular or deviating jaw function.[66,179] The term *internal derangement* when related to TMD denotes an abnormal positional relationship of the articular disk to the mandibular condyle and the articular eminence.[64] This abnormal positional relationship may result in mechanical interference and restriction of the normal range of mandibular activity. Theoretically, internal derangement of the TMJ involves the anterior (and medial) displacement of the disk, resulting from the action of the upper head of the lateral pterygoid muscle, a tear or thinning of the disk, osteoarthrosis, or malocclusion.[27,42,180]

The diagnosis of internal derangement of the TMJ requires the use of a classification system, such as the one devised by Pertes and Attanasio[181]:

1. Deviation in form
   a. frictional disk incoordination (FDI)
   b. articular surface defects
   c. disk thinning and perforation
2. Disk displacements
   a. partial anteromedial disk displacement
   b. anteromedial disk displacement with reduction
      -partial
      -complete
   c. anteromedial disk displacement with intermittent locking

d. anteromedial disk displacement without reduction
   -acute
   -chronic

3. Adhesive disk hypomobility
4. Displacement of disk–condyle complex
   a. subluxation
   b. dislocation

Deviation in Form

Frictional Disk Incoordination

FDI may occur when the intra-articular disk adheres to the eminence.[181] FDI usually occurs after a prolonged period of TMJ inactivity, such as that occurs with post surgical immobilization. Other causes of this condition include occlusion, bruxism, excessive biting force, and trauma. The adhesion can result in a loss of the translatory glide of the condyle, which in turn can result in excessive pressure between the disk and the eminence and a strain on the discal ligaments, predisposing the patient to a true disk displacement of the joint.

Clinical findings with this condition may include a discrete opening click with momentary discomfort, while the remainder of the translatory cycle is accomplished without difficulty.[182] The click associated with deviation in form usually occurs at the same point in the range of opening and closing.

The conservative intervention for this condition should focus on the elimination of any occlusal disharmony, the reduction of parafunctional habits, and methods to prevent the disk–condyle complex from returning to the closed position.[6] The latter goal can be accomplished by applying a permanent stabilization splint for a few months. When symptoms have been reduced, the patient should be weaned off the splint during the day and, eventually, night.

Articular Surface Defects

An articular surface defect located on the articulating surface of the eminence, the superior surface of the disk, or both, may cause an obstruction to the normal translatory movement of the disk.[183] The defect may be caused by trauma to the mandible when the teeth are apart, habitual abuse, or developmental and growth anomalies.[6]

Clinical findings for articular surface defects include a reciprocal click at the same point during both opening and closing movements. In addition, a lateral deviation frequently occurs on opening, as the patient attempts to circumvent the interference. Although the condition itself is painless, it can be worsened by any activities that increase intra-articular pressure.[6,184]

Conservative intervention for this condition includes habit training to develop a path of mandibular movement that avoids the interference. In addition, the patient is asked to make a conscious effort to reduce the force of chewing and eliminate parafunctional habits. Chewing on the affected side, by decreasing the intra-articular pressure, may also be helpful. A stabilization splint may serve to reduce pressure on the joint structures.[6,182]

Disk Thinning and Perforation

Disk thinning can result from the application of excessive pressure on the TMJ and can lead to a deformation of the joint structures. Continuous pressure eventually may cause perforation of the disk.

The symptoms of disk thinning and perforation depend on the extent of disk damage. Theoretically, thinning of the central part of the disk should be painless, because that part of the disk is not innervated. However, variable joint tenderness and muscle pain often is associated with any activity that deepens the central bearing area of the disk.

If the disk should perforate, grating sounds or crepitus during the translatory cycle are likely because of damage of the articular surfaces.[185,186] The diagnosis of disk perforation usually is made by imaging, arthrography, or arthroscopy. MRI, which is ideal for visualizing disk displacement, may not be so accurate for a perforation.[187]

Conservative intervention for disk thinning usually involves the application of a stabilization splint to prevent a perforation. If perforation has occurred and the patient can no longer tolerate the symptoms, surgical intervention is indicated.

Disk Displacements[181]

A pathologic click in a disk displacement may be caused by the condyle subluxing anteriorly or medially later than normal in the opening cycle. The click may also occur as the condyle relaxes onto the disk, or it may represent the sudden snapping back of the disk by the less than adequately elastic posterior ligament of the disk.

Partial Anteromedial Disk Displacement. In a healthy joint, the center of the posterior band of the disk is in the 12 o'clock position on the condyle when the teeth are occluded. With partial anterior disk displacement, the disk is permitted to slide anteriorly on the condyle and the terminal position of the posterior band of the disk occurs anteriorly to the normal position on the condyle in the closed-joint position. The anterior displacement is thought to occur because of two factors: some thinning of the posterior band and minimal elongation of the discal ligaments.[182]

The conservative intervention for partial displacements should focus on preventing any worsening of the disk displacement. This can be achieved using intraoral appliances in combination with psychological stress reduction.

Anteromedial Intra-articular Disk Displacement with Reduction. Disk displacement with reduction is both an anatomic and a functional disorder that is cyclic in nature.[187] Anteromedial disk displacement with reduction is described as an unexpected alteration or interference of the disk–condyle structural relation during mandibular translation with mouth opening and closing.[68] The misalignment of the disk is thought to be the result of articular surface irregularity, disk–articular surface adherence, synovial fluid degradation, or myofascial imbalances around the joint.[188]

The temporarily misaligned disk reduces or improves its structural relationship with the condyle when mandibular translation occurs with mouth opening. This change often is associated with an "opening click," and a reciprocal "closing click," which occurs just before the teeth occlude during mouth closing. Pain, if present, usually occurs at the time of the disk reduction.

Disk displacement with reduction may be characterized by five progressive stages.[93,189,190]

- *Stage I.* In stage I, the disk may be positioned slightly anteromedially on the mandibular head. Pain is usually mild or absent. As the disk becomes deformed from the repetitive microtrauma, it begins to interfere with the normal translation of the condyle.[68]
- *Stage II.* In this stage, the disk slips further anteromedially on the mandibular head. The reciprocal click may occur in the early phase of opening and late in the phase of closing.[68] Stage II is characterized by a loss of integrity of the ligamentous and intracapsular structures. This loss of integrity may result in increased mobility and a decrease in control of the disk, which increases the potential for impingement and deformation of the disk, resulting in severe pain, and increases the potential for intermittent *open locking* or subluxation of the joint.[102] An *open lock* is characterized by two opening clicks, and two clicks on closing. During opening, the first click occurs when the condyle moves over the posterior rim of the disk and the second click as the condyle moves over the anterior rim.[68] If, after the second click occurs on opening, the disk lies posterior to the condyle, the condyle may be prevented from sliding back.[191]
- *Stage III.* Stage III, often the most painful stage, is characterized by a reciprocal click that occurs later in the opening cycle and earlier in the closing cycle.[68] Occasionally, the intra-articular disk becomes adherent to the mandibular condyles in both the open and closed positions. This is known as a *closed-lock* position.[68] The sustained closed-lock condition produces a sudden limitation of opening, as the disk becomes permanently lodged anteriorly, thereby interfering with the normal condylar rotation and translation.[102] This closed-lock condition results in a hard end-feel in the joint when the clinician attempts to induce a passive stretch to the joint.[55] The impingement on the posterior attachment of the disk by the condylar head may result in a prolonged stretching of the tissue. The limitation of opening usually is restricted to 25–30 mm. Since condylar translatory mobility commonly is hindered only on the affected side, the mandible may deviate away from the midline toward the affected side with maximal jaw opening.[68] However, if this condition is chronic, there may be no deviation or limitation of jaw opening because of progressive tearing in the retrodiscal lamina. Tenderness of the masticatory muscles may also occur as a result of the protective splinting of the joint.
- *Stage IV.* In this stage, clicking is rare because the disk position is usually so incompatible. If clicking does occur, it is usually a single opening click because of the irregularities in translations.[68] Chronic locking with soft tissue remodeling can occur as a result of routine daily jaw function on the posteriorly or anteriorly positioned disk.[102] Known as *rotational displacement,* this condition is associated with pain and, commonly, with anterior displacement of the disk.[192]
- *Stage V.* This stage is characterized by radiographic degenerative changes on the condylar head and, occasionally, on the articular eminences, with evidence of remodeling and osteophytosis.[187] Marked deformity and thickening of the disk may occur, and the shape of the disk may change in configuration from biconcave to biconvex. The joint space typically is narrowed to the point where bone-on-bone contact is evident, resulting in coarse crepitus with jaw motions.

Stages I and II usually are amenable to physical therapy intervention. The focus for these stages is on reducing muscle dysfunction and improving the biomechanics of the joint.[102] The intervention usually involves using mandibular-repositioning appliances that stabilize a protrusive position to keep the disk in a more optimal relationship with the condyle.[193] The primary purpose of protrusive splint therapy may be to allow repair and regeneration to occur in the retrodiscal tissue and, possibly, in the discal ligaments.[194]

The intervention for stages III–V, and for those patients who are postsurgical, is directed at promoting and progressing the healing, restoring joint range of motion, and reducing the inflammation associated with capsulitis.[102]

Anteromedial Disk Displacement with Intermittent Locking. As mentioned in the previous section, if the disk remains displaced for longer periods of time, its shape becomes deformed and may slowly change from biconcave to biconvex. This change in shape makes the passage of the condyle under the disk more difficult. To return the disk, the patient must learn to move the mandible to the opposite side in order to activate the superior retrodiscal lamina.[102] Unfortunately, at this point, the retrodiscal tissue has thinned considerably and lost much of its elasticity, making disk reduction difficult to achieve.

The intermittent locking may occur at any time, but it most often occurs in the morning upon awakening, after a prolonged period of clenching, or after chewing on the involved side.[90] Conservative intervention usually involves a mandibular-repositioning appliance to keep the disk in correct alignment with the condyle.

Intra-articular Disk Displacement Without Reduction.[68] Although some patients may show progression through the various stages of disk displacement, it is unclear why some patients remain in the category of anterior disk displacement with reduction for years, whereas others proceed to intermittent locking and anterior disk displacement without reduction within a matter of months.

Disk displacement without reduction is described as an alteration or interference of the disk–condyle structural relation that is maintained during mandibular translation. As a result of continued disk deformation along with elongation of discal ligaments and a loss of tension in the posterior attachment, the disk may remain anteromedially displaced creating a "closed lock." Contact is lost among the condyle, disk, and articular eminence, and the articular disk space collapses, trapping the disk in front of the condyle and thereby preventing translation. Usually, the displacement of the disk becomes worse with jaw motions. Initially, there may be an associated locking with a sudden and marked limited jaw motion. In addition, there may be a deviation of the mandible toward the involved side during mouth opening, and a marked limitation of lateral deviation to the contralateral side.[68,102]

The limited opening resulting from anterior disk displacement without reduction may have a variety of causes. In addition to the more common causes, including muscle spasm and capsular tightness, limited mouth opening may occur when either the disk is lodged anteriorly to the condyle or the TMJ is dislocated or subluxed. Limited mouth opening as a result of elevator muscle spasm or capsular restraint can be differentiated by determining the end-feel. Elevator muscle spasm tends to limit only vertical movement; the protrusive and lateral excursions are usually normal. Anterior disk displacement without reduction, however, exhibits restrictions in both protrusive movements and contralateral excursions. Movement to the side of the involved joint is usually not mechanically restricted, because the main movement occurring in the joint is rotation. Pain restriction may be the result of impingement on inflamed retrodiscal tissues. Secondary muscle spasm of the elevator muscles may add to the restricted opening as well as capsular involvement.

In the acute phase, joint noise is usually absent. However, crepitus may be detected as the displacement becomes chronic and changes occur in the articular surfaces. As the condition becomes chronic, the pain often is markedly reduced and the range of motion may approach normal dimensions.

The intervention for the acute phase of this type of disk displacement should focus on a reduction of the displaced disk through mobilization of the joint. Since secondary elevator muscle spasm is usually present, as well as some inflammation of joint structures, it may be of benefit for the patient to take a skeletal muscle relaxant and an NSAID prior to physical therapy session. The reduction procedure involves the patient opening the mouth as wide as he/she is comfortable and then moving the mandible toward the opposite joint. If unsuccessful, the clinician may then attempt to reduce the disk manually through downward pressure on the last molar on the involved side.[184] Success in reducing the disk usually can be clinically determined by comparing the amount of vertical opening and contralateral movement after mobilization with the amount of movement before mobilization. This difference should be verified through imaging, because clinical criteria alone may not be accurate. Generally speaking, reductive mobilization is more successful in the more acute conditions. In cases in which changes in the connective tissue capsule may be contributing factors, manual stretching of the vertical fibers of the capsule may be indicated.

Adhesive Disk Hypomobility[181]

Although many cases of intracapsular restriction of mandibular movement or closed lock are caused by an anterior disk displacement without reduction, another frequent abnormality of the TMJ is the formation of intra-articular adhesions. The restriction may also be caused by an adhesion occurring in the superior joint cavity between the disk and the eminence, resulting in a loss of condylar translation. In addition, an adhesion may result in condylar displacement of the disk, with distortion of the disk itself on mandibular opening.[187]

Trauma frequently is implicated as a causative factor. If the trauma is slight, only mild surface damage to the disk may occur, resulting in FDI or an articulating surface defect. A more severe episode could cause intracapsular bleeding and effusion. Fibrosis may result, producing a reduction in the range of motion as well as degeneration. Condylar translation may be lost as a result of disk adhesion.

Clinically, adhesive disk hypomobility is indistinguishable from acute anterior disk displacement without reduction. Since translation does not occur, opening is limited. Pain is variable and may be caused by stretching of the diskal ligaments, as forced opening is attempted.

The conservative intervention for adhesive disk hypomobility is specific joint mobilizations (see "Therapeutic Techniques" section later).

Displacement of the Disk–Condyle Complex

Subluxation[181]

Subluxation between the disk and the articular eminence may occur as a result of excessive opening, which can force the condyle and the disk anteriorly beyond the normal limits of the translatory cycle. If the disk cannot rotate any farther posteriorly and the condyle continues to translate, a partial dislocation or subluxation can occur.

Usually, the patient has a history of jaw clicking with wide mouth opening. Diagnostically, for treatment purposes, this wide opening click must be differentiated from a click that signifies reduction of a displaced disk. A subluxation type of click occurs only on wide opening and not on protrusive movement or lateral excursion. The click associated with reduction of a displaced disk, however, can occur during both protrusive and contralateral excursion. Usually, pain does not accompany subluxation unless it becomes habitual.

Intervention for this condition includes habit training to voluntarily limit mouth opening within normal limits. This training should be accompanied by exercises that strengthen the elevator muscles. Occasionally, injection of a sclerosing solution to reduce the laxity of the capsule may be required.

Dislocation[181]

Dislocation of the TMJ is caused by additional rotation of the mandibular condyle beyond its biomechanical limit, resulting in an anterior displacement of the disk beyond the articular eminence and in direct contact between the condyle and the eminence. As opposed to subluxation, which is a partial loss of contact between the disk and the eminence, dislocation involves a collapse of the articular disk space. Because of the collapsed disk space, the superior retrodiscal lamina cannot retract the prolapsed disk. Adding to the problem is the elevator muscle spasm that frequently accompanies dislocation and preserves the decrease in articular disk space.

Some factors associated with the onset of habitual dislocation include, but are not limited to, yawning, singing, sleeping with the head resting on the forearm, manipulation of the mandible while the patient is under general anesthesia, excessive tooth abrasion, severe malocclusion, loss of dentition (leading to overclosure), and trauma.[195]

Clinical findings include an inability of the patient to close the mandible after wide mouth opening, so that the mouth becomes locked open in a prognathic position and cannot be moved vertically. An acute malocclusion is present with an anterior open bite and contact between only the most posterior teeth. Depressions may be noted in the preauricular area formerly occupied by the condyles. Pain may be variable, which increases as the patient attempts to close, thus straining the inferior retrodiscal lamina and the collateral discal ligaments.

The main focus of the intervention is to widen the articular disk space. This allows the superior retrodiscal lamina to retract the disk. Forceful closing of the mandible should be avoided. Reduction of the displaced mandible is best accomplished by having the patient yawn as widely as possible, while the clinician exerts slight posterior pressure on the chin. If reduction is not achieved, placement of thumbs behind the molars and pressing down while the patient yawns may produce the reduction by increasing the additional articular space. If these attempts at manual correction fail, the clinician may try stimulation of the gag reflex by touching a mouth mirror to the soft palate. This maneuver can result in an inhibition of elevator muscle activity, thus increasing the articular disk space.

For recurrent dislocations, the conservative approach is addressed according to the stability factors into (1) alteration of the ligaments, (2) alteration of the associated musculature, and (3) alteration of the bony anatomy[195]:

- Alteration to the ligaments can be achieved by the introduction of a sclerosing agent into the capsular space of the TMJ.
- Alteration of the associated musculature can be achieved by exercise. Strengthening the suprahyoid muscles to counterbalance the action of the lateral pterygoid muscles could, theoretically, reduce the likelihood of dislocation. The equipment to perform this type of exercise, however, is elaborate and involves considerable compliance by the patient. A more recently reported treatment modality for alteration of the musculature is the use of type A botulinum toxin. If dislocation is chronic, the patient should be taught how to self-reduce the mandible. Habit training similar to that employed for subluxation should be instituted.
- An alteration of bony anatomy requires a surgical eminectomy.

Arthritis

The TMJ, like other joints in the body, can become a site of osteoarthritis. Degenerative osteoarthritis may be secondary to trauma, surgery, congenital malformation, or, most commonly, long-standing disk derangement. Marginal osteophyte formation, bony erosion sclerosis, and subchondral or subcortical formation may be observed.[187] The temporomandibular disk may become distorted in shape secondary to adhesions seen in osteoarthritis.[196]

Other arthritides are known to affect the TMJ, including rheumatoid arthritis, systemic lupus erythematosus, synovial chondromatosis, ankylosing spondylitis, psoriasis, and crystalline arthritides such as calcium pyrophosphate deposition disease and gout.

To date, no intervention exists that can reverse the anatomic and biochemical alterations of osteoarthrosis. Thus, the intervention approach has to be aimed at restoring function and managing pain through the acute phase of the disease.

Pigmented Villonodular Synovitis

Pigmented villonodular synovitis (PVNS) is a proliferative but nonneoplastic disorder of unknown pathogenesis that affects the synovial membranes of joints.[197,198] Eighty percent of cases involve the knee, followed in order of frequency by the hip, ankle, and shoulder, with involvement of the TMJ being very rare.[199–201] The disorder is generally thought to be a benign, inflammatory process, although it may develop as an aggressive local process.

PVNS is described as expressing multiple manifestations of a histologic lesion occurring in the synovial membrane of joints. PVNS is subdivided into diffuse and localized forms, depending on the extent of synovial involvement. PVNS may extend into bone, and, in most instances, the diffuse form probably represents aggressive extra-articular extension and occasional recurrence after surgical intervention.[197]

The symptoms of PVNS of the TMJ vary but typically include swelling in the preauricular area, progressive TMJ pain during mastication, and a history of progressive difficulty in opening of the mouth.[202]

The recommended intervention for PVNS lesions involves wide synovectomy at all sites involved.[197,198]

PRACTICE PATTERN 4E: IMPAIRED JOINT MOBILITY, MOTOR FUNCTION, MUSCLE PERFORMANCE, AND RANGE OF MOTION ASSOCIATED WITH LOCALIZED INFLAMMATION

Muscle Spasms

Muscle spasms of the mastication muscles may occur with dysfunction of the TMJ. Such dysfunctions include trauma, occlusal imbalance, changes in the vertical dimensions between the teeth, immobilization, prolonged dental procedures, chronic teeth clenching, and disease. Schwartz[203,204] hypothesized that TMD symptoms originated in mandibular muscles, which went through three pathologic phases:

1. Early incoordination of muscles, producing joint clicking and recurrent subluxation.
2. A middle phase of limitation of mandibular movements by muscle spasm.
3. A final phase of muscle shortening and fibrosis, often irreversible. Psychogenic causes were the most common.

The role of cervical whiplash injuries secondary to motor vehicle accidents (MVAs) in TMD is somewhat controversial. Brooke and Stenn[205] reported that patients with posttraumatic TMD have a poor prognosis for recovery compared with nontraumatic TMD, stating as reasons the consequence of litigation and the personality of the patient. It seems plausible that an injury to the suprahyoid and infrahyoid muscles would affect the function of the mandible, thereby predisposing the joint to dysfunction. Mechanisms have been proposed to explain how an MVA trauma could cause TMDs.[206,207]

During the initial backward movement, the jaw is forced open, stretching and possibly tearing the anterior joint capsule and the intra-articular disk. On the flexion phase, the jaw is snapped shut by the stretch reflex of the masticatory muscles and, in the presence of malocclusion, damages the posterior and temporal attachments of the articular cartilage and disk.

The following descriptions outline the common referral patterns of the TMJ muscles.

Temporalis

Referred pain from the temporalis muscle may extend over the temporal region, to the eyebrow and the upper teeth, and to the maxilla and TMJ.[108] Headache caused by temporalis muscle spasm is common. The patient also may feel pressure behind the eye or have increased eye fatigue.

Lateral Pterygoid

Spasm of the lateral pterygoid may cause a deep ache in the cheek area, maxilla, TMJ, or ear. Pain also is felt with chewing.

Medial Pterygoid

The medial pterygoid may refer pain behind the TMJ, deep in the ear, to the tongue, and to the back of the mouth.[108]

Masseter

Referred pain from a masseter muscle spasm may be projected to the eyebrow, maxilla, anterior mandible, and upper and lower molars.[108]

The intervention for these muscle spasms includes:

- application of moist heat to promote muscle relaxation;
- massage of the affected muscles;
- passive and active self-stretch exercises;
- spray and stretch techniques.

Forced mouth opening should be avoided. In the absence of joint hypomobility, yawning exercises are recommended as a home exercise, because this activity produces a strong reflex inhibition of the mandibular elevators.[108]

The lateral pterygoid can be passively stretched with maximal retrusion, followed by rhythmic sideways oscillations. The medial pterygoid can be passively stretched with jaw opening exercises.

Travell and Simons[108] recommend the use of the mandibular self-stretch exercise for the temporalis and masseter muscles.

The exercise, which consists of three steps, is performed in the sitting position facing a sink:

1. Hot packs are applied to both sides of the face.
2. The index and middle fingers are inserted below the lower incisor teeth, pads facing downward. The thumb of the same hand grasps the chin and pulls the lower jaw forward.
3. The full stretch is achieved by pulling the jaw downward, while continuing to pull it forward.

Synovitis

Synovitis of the TMJ occurs when the internal lining of the joint capsule becomes inflamed, resulting in palpable tenderness of the posterior and lateral aspects of the joint. The cause of the synovitis can be[30]

- condylar impingement of the loose areolar connective tissue located immediately posterior to the condyle, which can result in significant effusion;
- systemic disease, such as osteoarthritis, or rheumatoid arthritis or its variants;
- infection, particularly viral.

INTEGRATION OF PRACTICE PATTERNS 4B, 4C, AND 4F: IMPAIRED JOINT MOBILITY, MOTOR FUNCTION, MUSCLE PERFORMANCE AND RANGE OF MOTION SECONDARY TO IMPAIRED POSTURE, SYSTEMIC DYSFUNCTION (REFERRED PAIN SYNDROMES), SPINAL DISORDERS, AND MYOFASCIAL PAIN DYSFUNCTION

Cervical Spine Disorders

Patients with TMD frequently report symptoms related to cervical spine disorders, and vice versa.[82,208–210] Several authors have indicated the existence of neuroanatomic and biomechanical relationships and have suggested that a dysfunction of the cervical spine may be the cause of signs and symptoms in the head.[211–222]

The masticatory and cervical muscles can affect the mandibular rest position, the mechanism of mandibular closure, and the occlusion.[223–225] Thus, a change in the mandibular rest position or habitual cervical posture can affect the occlusion and the masticatory muscles.[62,223,226–228] The most common postural abnormality in the cervical spine with direct impact on the craniofacial area and temporomandibular arthralgia is the forward head posture.[62,223,226–228]

Any increase in the sternocleidomastoid angulation, or distance from the thoracic apex to midcervical region, constitutes a FHP. This posture is considered to be minimal at 60 degrees, moderate at 60–75 degrees, and maximal at 75–90 degrees.[14] Associated signs include a decrease or reversal in the cervical lordosis and an increase in cranial rotation at the occipito atlantal joint, resulting in a shortening and excessive activity of the posterior cervical muscles. The FHP can place undue stress on both the posterior cervical muscles and the anterior submandibular muscles, by increasing their normal resting lengths. This stress may also stretch the TMJ capsule and alter the bite biomechanics of the TMJ, resulting in a posterior migration of the mandible and an altered occlusal contact pattern.

Atypical Facial Pain

Atypical facial pain is characterized by typically unilateral, dull, and relatively constant facial pain, and the presence of tender points. This condition, recently reclassified as facial pain by the

International Headache Society, is not well understood and often defies all modes of intervention.[229] Many authorities believe that atypical facial pain is psychogenic.[230,231] However, it has been reported that intraoral edema and trigeminal V2 nerve distribution area tenderness were consistently found in individuals with atypical facial pain.[232] Furthermore, these individuals experienced relief of their symptoms in response to low-level helium–neon laser therapy.[232]

Bell's palsy, a common form of facial paralysis, and Ramsey Hunt syndrome, a herpetic inflammation of the geniculate or facial nerve ganglia, are described in Chapter 5.

Trigeminal Neuralgia

Trigeminal neuralgia is an intensely painful disorder of the face of brief duration (30 seconds).[233] The pain is spontaneous and can be triggered by touch, cold, shaving, brushing teeth, or make-up application.[234] The cause of trigeminal neuralgia is at present unknown, although most authors place the site of disturbance in the region of the posterior root[235,236] or in the spinal tract of the nerve.[237] Injuries to nerves and soft and hard tissues as a result of repeated traumas have been reported to produce persistent pain because of sensitization of both peripheral and central neurons.[48,238] The sensitization process has been shown to influence subsequent pain experience. Increased postoperative pain resulting from insufficient preemptive analgesia, such as incomplete use of local anesthetics or pain medication before surgery, has been well documented.[238–240] Poorly managed postoperative or posttraumatic pain also is considered to play a role in pain persistence.[238,241]

Myofascial Pain and Dysfunction

Many clinicians over the years have described numerous conditions that share features such as fatigue, pain, and other symptoms in the absence of objective findings. These include illnesses such as chronic fatigue syndrome, fibromyalgia, and TMD.

Myofascial pain and dysfunction associated with TMD generally present with diffuse pain that is cyclic and found in several sites in the head and neck, particularly the muscles of mastication.[12] Pain is frequently at its worst in the morning, the patient often reports sore teeth from clenching, and there is often a history of stress and difficulty sleeping.[12] Masticatory muscle pain associated with TMD does not appear to progress in severity with age.[242]

The intervention for myofascial pain syndromes requires a comprehensive, and often a multidisciplinary, approach. The role of physical therapy in these syndromes is one of patient education, manual therapy techniques and electrotherapeutic modalities to reduce pain, and exercises to improve posture, reduce the adaptive shortening of tissues, and improve the strength of the postural stabilizers.

THERAPEUTIC TECHNIQUES

Manual Therapy

The aim of manual therapy in TMD is to restore normal mandibular function using a number of techniques that serve to relieve musculoskeletal pain and promote healing of tissues.[167]

In the acute phase, manual techniques, if used at all, should be very low grade and very carefully performed, because this joint tends to be very reactive and can flare up easily. Mobilization and massage can be applied to the TMJ to reduce hypomobility and acute locking, as well as to the muscles of mastication to stretch and relax them.[102]

Muscle relaxation and soft tissue techniques often are required before mobilizations of the TMJ can be performed.

Myofascial Release

Myofascial release is a combination of direct, indirect, and reflex neural release procedures.[101] The basis of this technique is sensing palpable changes at various tissue levels and manually directing a gentle force to assist in releasing restricted tissues.

Muscle Stretching

Muscle stretching techniques can be used if the examination shows that the restriction of movement is a result of shortened muscles (or other structures). Techniques to increase the extensibility of the cervical structures are described in Chapters 23 and 25.

Joint Mobilizations

Specific joint mobilizations of the craniovertebral and cervical regions are described in Chapters 23 and 25, respectively. Specific mobilization techniques of the TMJ are indicated for decreased range of motion and pain caused by muscle contracture, disk displacement without reduction, and fibrous adhesions in the joint.[68]

During these procedures, the patient's mandible should be completely relaxed, and the patient should not attempt to open his or her mouth until instructed to do so.

Techniques to Increase Mouth Opening[55,243]

Distraction

This technique is performed to separate the joint surfaces of the TMJ to allow the disk to start repositioning on the condyle and to start realigning the fibers of the tissue caudally. The patient is positioned sitting, and the clinician stands to the patient's side. The clinician grips the patient's head, using his or her forearm and hand, fingers against the patient's forehead. The clinician stabilizes the patient's head between his or her hand, arm, and chest. With a medical-gloved hand, the clinician places his or her thumb on the patient's lower molars on the involved side, as far back in the mouth as possible. The clinician's index and middle fingers grip the angle of the patient's mandible of the involved side, with the ring or little fingers held under the patient's mandible (depending on the size of the clinician's hand and patient's mandible). Using this grip, the clinician applies light distraction inferiorly to the patient's involved TMJ by pressing his or her thumb inferiorly against the lower molars (see Fig. 26-14).

Distraction, Anterior Glide, and Lateral Stretch

This technique is performed to increase the anterior and inferior movement of the mandible for the patient who can only achieve slight opening of the mouth. The patient and clinician positions are the same as those described for the distraction technique. Using the same grip as described earlier, the clinician applies light distraction inferiorly to the patient's involved TMJ by pressing his or her thumb inferiorly against the lower molars. In addition to the distraction, the clinician gradually superimposes an anterior glide of the head of the mandible at the TMJ and a lateral stretch to the joint on the opposite side. Following the technique, the patient is asked to open his or her mouth as much as possible, and the newly acquired range is assessed. The procedure is repeated gradually, until the patient is able to fully open his or her mouth or considerable improvement is attained.

Note: If the restriction of movement is bilateral, the technique may be performed on the opposite side.

Technique to Increase Full Mouth Closing[55,243]

This technique is used to increase the posterior movement of the mandible (retraction) for the patient, with an inability to fully close the mouth. The patient and clinician position is the same as described for the techniques to increase mouth opening. Using the same grip described for those techniques, the clinician gradually and maximally pushes posteriorly against the patient's involved mandible to produce a posterior glide of the head of the mandible at the TMJ (see Fig. 26-15).

Note: If the restriction of movement is bilateral, the same intervention may be performed on the patient's opposite side. The procedure is used when the patient cannot close his or her mouth.

Extraoral Lateral Glide

This technique is used in the presence of severe pain, spasm, and marked limitation of movement caused by recent trauma.[101] The patient is positioned in supine, with the head being supported on a pillow. The patient is asked to rotate the head in the opposite direction of the involved TMJ. The clinician places the thumbs of both hands over the lateral pole of the condyle. Gentle oscillations are performed over the lateral pole, or more distally depending on patient tolerance.

Extraoral Depression

This technique also is used in the presence of severe pain, spasm, and marked limitation of movement caused by recent trauma.[101] The patient is positioned in supine, with the head being supported on a pillow. The clinician gently grasps the angle of the mandible with the index and the thumb bilaterally. Gentle oscillations are then performed in the direction of mandibular depression.

AUTOMOBILIZATIONS

Toothpick Exercise

This exercise can be used for patients who demonstrate lateral deviation with mouth opening or closing. The patient stands or sits facing a mirror. A thick line is drawn down the mirror using a wax crayon. The patient wedges a toothpick between the lower incisors and lines up the toothpick with the line on the mirror. As the patient opens and closes the jaw, if the line becomes visible, the patient corrects the deviation before continuing the movement. If correction is not possible, the exercise is stopped to prevent incorrect learning by the controlling muscles.

Distraction Mobilization

This technique can be taught to patients who demonstrate or report recurrent dislocations. To self-reduce a dislocation, the patient is instructed to place a gauze roll on the back inferior molars of both sides and to place his or her index fingers on the gauze. The patient opens the mouth as wide as possible and then applies a downward force on the gauze and the molars, thereby creating a joint distraction. Following a successful reduction, ice or heat (whichever produces the optimal therapeutic effect) should be applied around the TMJ.

REVIEW QUESTIONS*

1. Name the components of the stomatognathic system?
2. Which muscle develops with the fibrocartilaginous disk of the TMJ?
3. Which three muscles function to raise the mandible during mouth closing?
4. Which of the following alterations occurs (and may need correction via exercise) as a result of posterior capital rotation associated with the forward head posture?
   a. Adaptive shortening of the craniovertebral muscles
   b. Forward migration of the mandible
   c. Elongation of the submandibular muscles
   d. Increased tension in the TMJ joint capsule
   e. All of the above.
5. Define the rest position of the TMJ.

*Additional questions to test your understanding of this chapter can be found in the Online Learning Center for *Orthopaedic Assessment, Evaluation, and Intervention* at www.duttononline.net.

REFERENCES

1. McNeill C: Temporomandibular disorders: guidelines for diagnosis and management. *CDA J* 19:15–26, 1991.
2. Okeson JP: Current terminology and diagnostic classification schemes. *Oral Surg Oral Med Oral Pathol Oral Radiol Endod* 83:61–66, 1997.
3. Moses AJ: Good science, bad science, and scientific double-talk. *Cranio* 14:170–172, 1996.
4. Ferrari R, Leonard M: Whiplash and temporomandibular disorders: a critical review. *J Am Dent Assoc* 129:1739–1745, 1998.
5. Kolbinson DA, Epstein JB, Burgess JA: Temporomandibular disorders, headaches, and neck pain following motor vehicle accidents and the effects of litigation review of the literature. *J Orofac Pain* 10:101–125, 1996.
6. Bell WE: *Orofacial Pains: Classification, Diagnosis, Management*, 3rd ed. Chicago: New Year Medical Publishers, 1985.

7. Hannson T, Milner M: A study of occurrence of symptoms of diseases of the temporomandibular joint, masticatory musculature, and related structures. *J Oral Rehabil* 2:313–324, 1975.
8. Dworkin SF, Huggins KH, Le Resche L, et al: Epidemiology of signs and symptoms in temporomandibular disorders: clinical signs in cases and controls. *J Am Dent Assoc* 120:273–281, 1990.
9. Salonen L, Hellden L: Prevalence of signs and symptoms of dysfunction in the masticatory system: an epidemiological study in an adult Swedish population. *J Craniomandib Disord* 4:241–250, 1990.
10. National Institute of Health: *Management of temporomandibular disorders*, NIH Technology Assessment Conference. Bethseda (MD), NIH, 1996.
11. Stohler CS: Clinical perspectives on masticatory and related muscle disorders, In: Sessle BJ, Bryant PS, Dionne RA, eds. *Temporomandibular disorders and related pain conditions, progress in pain research and management*. Seattle, WA: IASP Press, 1995:3–29.
12. Dimitroulis G: Temporomandibular disorders: a clinical update. *BMJ* 317:190–194, 1998.
13. McNeill C, Danzig WM, Farrar WB, et al: Craniomandibular (TMJ) disorders – the state of the art. *J Prosthet Dent* 44:434–437, 1980.
14. Castaneda R: Occlusion, In: Kaplan AS, Assael LA, eds. *Temporomandibular disorders diagnosis and treatment*. Philadelphia PA: WB Saunders, 1991, 40–49.
15. Von Korff M, Wagner EH, Dworkin SF, et al: Chronic pain and use of ambulatory health care. *Psychosom Med* 53:61–79, 1991.
16. Wänman A: Longitudinal course of symptoms of craniomandibular disorders in men and women: a 10-year follow-up study of an epidemiologic sample. *Acta Odontol Scand* 54:337–342, 1996.
17. Bush FM, Harkins SW, Walter GH, et al: Analysis of gender effects on pain perception and symptom presentation in temporomandibular pain. *Pain* 53:73–80, 1993.
18. Sicher H, Du Brul EL: *Oral Anatomy*, 8th ed. St. Louis, MO: CV Mosby, 1988.
19. Rees LA: The structure and function of the mandibular joint. *Br Dent J* 96:125, 1954.
20. Mohl DN: *Functional anatomy of the temporomandibular joint, The President's Conference on the Examination, Diagnosis and Management of Temporomandibular Disorders*. Chicago:, American Dental Association, 1983.
21. Buchbinder D, Kaplan AS: Biology, In: Kaplan AS, Assael LA, eds. *Temporomandibular disorders diagnosis and treatment*. Philadelphia, PA: WB Saunders, 1991, 11–23.
22. Williams PL, Warwick R, Dyson M, et al: *Gray's Anatomy*, 37th ed. London: Churchill Livingstone, 1989.
23. Neumann DA: Kinesiology of mastication and ventilation, In Neumann DA ed. *Kinesiology of the musculoskeletal system: Foundations for physical rehabilitation*. St. Louis, MO: Mosby, 2002:352–379.
24. Kraus SL: *TMJ Disorders: Management of the Craniomandibular Complex, Clinics in Physical Therapy*. New York: Churchill Livingstone, 1988.
25. Hargreaves A: Dysfunction of the temporomandibular joints. *Physiotherapy* 72:209–212, 1986.
26. Naidoo LCD: The development of the temporomandibular joint: a review with regard to the lateral pterygoid muscle. *J Dent Assoc S Africa* 48:189–194, 1993.
27. Porter MR: The attachment of the lateral pterygoid muscle to the meniscus. *J Prosthet Dent* 24:555–562, 1970.
28. Juniper RD: The pathogenesis and investigation of TMJ dysfunction. *Br J Oral Maxillofac Surg* 25:105–112, 1987.
29. Mahan P: Temporomandibular problems: Biological diagnosis and treatment, In: Solberg WK, Clark GT, eds. *Temporomandibular joint problems*. Chicago: Quintessence Publishing Co, 1980.
30. Friedman MH, Weisberg J: Screening procedures for temporomandibular joint dysfunction. *Am Fam Physician* 25:157–160, 1982.
31. Friedman MH, Weisberg J: Application of orthopedic principles in evaluation of the temporomandibular joint. *Phys Ther* 62:597–603, 1982.
32. Scapino RP: The posterior attachment: Its structure, function, and appearance in TMJ imaging studies. Part 2. *J Craniomandib Disord* 5:155–166, 1991.
33. Clark R, Wyke BD: Contributions of temporomandibular articular mechanoreceptors to the control of mandibular posture: An experimental study. *J Dent Assoc S Africa* 2:121–129, 1974.
34. Skaggs CD: Diagnosis and treatment of temporomandibular disorders. In: Murphy DR, ed. *Cervical Spine Syndromes*. New York: McGraw-Hill, 2000:579–592.
35. Pinto OF: A new structure related to the temporomandibular joint and the middle ear. *J Prosthet Dent* 12:95–103, 1962.
36. Stack BC, Funt LA: Temporomandibular joint dysfunction in children. *J Pedod* 1:240–247, 1977.
37. Bittar GT, Bibb CA, Pullinger AG: Histological characteristics of the lateral pterygoid muscle insertion into the temporomandibular joint. *J Orofac Pain* 8:243–249, 1994.
38. Meyenberg K, Kubick S, Palla S: Relationship of the muscles of mastication to the articular disk of the temporomandibular joint. *Helv Odont Acta* 30:815–834, 1986.
39. Carpentier P, Yung J-P, Marguelles-Bonnet R, et al: Insertions of the lateral pterygoid muscle: an anatomic study of the human temporomandibular joint. *J Oral Maxillofac Surg* 46:477–482, 1988.
40. McNamara JA: The independent function of the two heads of the lateral pterygoid muscle. *Am J Anat* 138:197–205, 1973.
41. Luschei ES, Goodwin GM: Patterns of mandibular movement and muscle activity during mastication in the monkey. *J Neurophysiol* 35:954–966, 1974.
42. Juniper RP: Temporomandibular joint dysfunction: a theory based upon electromyographic studies of the lateral pterygoid muscle. *Br J Oral Maxillofac Surg* 22:1–8, 1984.
43. McDonnell JP, Needleman HL, Charchut S, et al: The relationship between dental overbite and eustachian tube dysfunction. *Laryngoscope* 111:310–316, 2001.
44. Franks AST: Cervical spondylosis presenting as the facial pain of temporomandibular joint disorder. *Ann Phys Med* 9:193–196, 1968.
45. Trott P, Gross AN: Physiotherapy in diagnosis and treatment of the myofascial pain dysfunction syndrome. *Int J Oral Surg* 7:360–365, 1978.
46. Rocabado M: Biomechanical relationship of the cranial, cervical, and hyoid regions. *J Craniomandibular Pract* 1:61–66, 1983.
47. Layfield SP: A whiplash injury, in Scully RM, Barnes MR, eds. *Physical therapy*. Philadelphia, PA: JB Lippincott Co, 1989:152–168.
48. Carlsson GE, LeResche L: Epidemiology of temporomandibular disorders. In: Sessle BJ, Bryant PS, Dionne RA, eds. *Temporomandibular disorders and related pain conditions, progress in pain research and management*. Seattle, WA: IASP Press, 1995:211–226.
49. Murphy DR: *Conservative Management of Cervical Spine Disorders*. New York: McGraw-Hill, 2000.
50. Meadows J: *A Rationale and Complete Approach to the Sub-Acute Post-MVA Cervical Patient*. Calgary, AB: Swodeam Consulting, 1995.
51. Viener AE: Oral Surgery. In: Garliner D, ed. *Myofunctional Therapy*. Philadelphia, PA: WB Saunders, 1976.
52. Hertling D: The temporomandibular joint. In: Hertling D, Kessler RM, eds. *Management of Common Musculoskeletal Disorders*, 3rd ed. Philadelphia, PA: Lippincott-Raven, 1996: 444–485.
53. Tsukiyama Y, Baba K, Clark GT: An evidence-based assessment of occlusal adjustment as a treatment for temporomandibular disorders. *J Prosthet Dent* 86:57–66, 2001.
54. Bales JM, Epstein JB: The role of malocclusion and orthodontics in temporomandibular disorders. *J Can Dent Assoc* 60:899–905, 1994.
55. Rocabado M: Arthrokinematics of the temporomandibular joint. In: Gelb H, ed. *Clinical Management of Head, Neck and TMJ Pain and Dysfunction*. Philadelphia, PA: WB Saunders, 1985.
56. Kaplan AS: Examination and Diagnosis. In: Kaplan AS, Assael LA, eds. *Temporomandibular disorders diagnosis and treatment*. Philadelphia, PA: WB Saunders, 1991: 284–311.
57. Trott PH: Examination of the temporomandibular joint. In: Grieve G, ed.: *Modern Manual Therapy of the Vertebral Column*. Edinburgh: Churchill Livingstone, 1986.
58. Fish F: The functional anatomy of the rest position of the mandible. *Dent Prac* 11:178, 1961.
59. Atwood DA: A critique of research of the rest position of the mandible. *J Prosthet Dent* 16:848–854, 1966.
60. Feinstein B, Lanton NJK, Jameson RM, et al: Experiments on pain referred from deep somatic tissues. *J Bone Joint Surg* 36A:981–997, 1954.
61. Cyriax J: Rheumatic headache. *Br Med J* 2:1367–1368, 1982.
62. Friedman MH, Weisberg J: *Temporomandibular Joint Disorders*. Chicago: Quintessence Publishing Company, Inc., 1985.
63. Okeson JP: *Orofacial pain: guidelines for assessment, diagnosis, and management*. Chicago: Quintessence Publishing Co, 1996.
64. Dolwick MF: Clinical diagnosis of temporomandibular joint internal derangement and myofascial pain and dysfunction. *Oral Maxillofac Surg Clin North Am* 1:1–6, 1989.
65. Hedenberg-Magnusson B, Ernberg M, Kopp S: Symptoms and signs of temporomandibular disorders in patients with fibromyalgia and local

myalgia of the temporomandibular system: a comparative study. *Acta Odontol Scand* 55:344–349, 1997.
66. Isacsson G, Linde C, Isberg A: Subjective symptoms in patients with temporomandibular disk displacement versus patients with myogenic craniomandibular disorders. *J Prosthet Dent* 61:70–77, 1989.
67. Kirk WS, Jr., Calabrese DK: Clinical evaluation of physical therapy in the management of internal derangement of the temporomandibular joint. *J Oral Maxillofac Surg* 47:113–119, 1989.
68. McNeill C: *Temporomandibular disorders – guidelines for classification, assessment and management*, 2nd ed. Chicago: Quintessence Books, 1993.
69. Orsini MG, Kuboki T, Terada S, et al: Clinical predictability of temporomandibular joint disc displacement. *J Dent Res.* 78:650–660, 1999.
70. Barclay P, Hollender LG, Maravilla KR, et al: Comparison of clinical and magnetic resonance imaging diagnosis in patients with disk displacement in the temporomandibular joint. *Oral Surg Oral Med Oral Pathol Oral Radiol Endod.* 88:37–43, 1999.
71. Green CS, Laskin DM: Long term status of TMJ clicking in patients with myofascial pain dysfunction. *J Am Dent Assoc* 117:461–465, 1988.
72. Marbach JJ, Lipton JA: Treatment of patients with temporomandibular joint and other facial pain by otolaryngologists. *Arch Otolaryngol* 108:102–107, 1982.
73. Brazeau GA, Gremillion HA, Widmer CG, et al: The role of pharmacy in the management of patients with temporomandibular disorders and orofacial pain. *J Am Pharm Assoc (Wash)* 38:354-361; quiz 362–363, 1998.
74. Cholitgul W, Nishiyama H, Sasai T, et al: Clinical and magnetic resonance imaging findings in temporomandibular joint disc displacement. *Dentomaxillofac Radiol.* 26:183–188., 1997.
75. Cholitgul W, Petersson A, Rohlin M, et al: Clinical and radiological findings in temporomandibular joints with disc perforation. *Int J Oral Maxillofac Surg.* 19:220–225., 1990.
76. Cholitgul W, Petersson A, Rohlin M, et al: Diagnostic outcome and observer performance in sagittal tomography of the temporomandibular joint. *Dentomaxillofac Radiol.* 19:1–6, 1990.
77. Magnusson T, List T, Helkimo M: Self-assessment of pain and discomfort in patients with temporomandibular disorders: a comparison of five different scales with respect to their precision and sensitivity as well as their capacity to register memory of pain and discomfort. *J Oral Rehabil.* 22:549–556, 1995.
78. Dimitroulis G, Dolwick MF, Gremillion HA: Temporomandibular disorders. 1. Clinical evaluation. *Aust Dent J* 40:301–305, 1995.
79. Maitland G: *Vertebral manipulation.* Sydney: Butterworth, 1986.
80. Magarey ME: Examination of the cervical and thoracic spine. In: Grant R, ed. *Physical Therapy of the Cervical and Thoracic Spine*, 2nd ed. New York: Churchill Livingstone, 1994:109–144.
81. Mannheimer JS, Dunn J: Cervical Spine. In: Kaplan AS, Assael LA, eds. *Temporomandibular disorders diagnosis and treatment.* Philadelphia, PA: WB Saunders, 1991:50–94.
82. Clark GT, Seligman DA, Solberg WK, et al: Guidelines for the examination and diagnosis of temporomandibular disorders. *J Craniomandib Disord Facial Oral Pain* 3:7–14, 1989.
83. Duinkerke AS, Luteijn F, Bouman TK, et al: Relations between TMJ pain dysfunction syndrome (PDS) and some psychological and biographical variables. *Community Dent Oral Epidemiol* 13:185–189, 1985.
84. Keith DA: Differential diagnosis of facial pain and headache. *Oral Maxillofac Surg Clin North Am* 1:7–12, 1989.
85. Fricton JR, Hathaway KM: Interdisciplinary management: Address complexity with teamwork. In: Fricton JR, Kroening R, Hathaway KM, eds. *TMJ and Craniofacial Pain: Diagnosis and Management.* St Louis, MO: IEA Inc., 1988:167–172.
86. Judge RD, Zuidema GD, Fitzgerald FT: Head. In: Judge RD, Zuidema GD, Fitzgerald FT, eds. Clinical Diagnosis, 4th ed. Boston, MA: Little, Brown and Company, 1982, 123–151.
87. Laskin DM: Etiology of the pain-dysfunction syndrome. *J Am Dent Assoc* 79:147–153, 1969.
88. Lobbezoo-Scholte AM, de Wijer A, Steenks MH, et al: Interexaminer reliability of six orthopaedic tests in diagnostic subgroups of craniomandibular disorders. *J Oral Rehabil.* 21:273–285, 1994.
89. Dworkin SF, LeResche L, DeRouen T, et al: Assessing clinical signs of temporomandibular disorders: reliability of clinical examiners. *J Prosthet Dent.* 63:574–579, 1990.
90. Perry C: Neuromuscular control of mandibular movements. *J Prosthet Dent* 30:714–720, 1973.
91. Thompson JR, Brodie AG: Factors in the position of the mandible. *J Am Dent Assoc* 29:925–941, 1942.
92. Katz MI: Angle's classification revisited. *Am J Orthod Dentofacial Orthop* 132:716–717, 2007.
93. Richardson JK, Iglarsh ZA: Temporomandibular Joint and the Cervical Spine. In: Richardson JK, Iglarsh ZA, eds. *Clinical Orthopaedic Physical Therapy.* Philadelphia, PA: Saunders, 1994:1–71.
94. Dempsey PJ, Townsend GC: Genetic and environmental contributions to variation in human tooth size. *Heredity* 86:685–693, 2001.
95. Marasa FK, Ham BD: Case reports involving the treatment of children with chronic otitis media with effusion via cranio-mandibular methods. *Cranio* 6:256–270, 1988.
96. Seldin HM: Traumatic temporomandibular arthritis. *N Y State Dent J* 21:313–318, 1955.
97. Sicher N: Temporomandibular articulation in mandibular overclosure. *J Am Dent Assoc* 36:131–139, 1948.
98. Masumi S, Kim YJ, Clark GT: The value of maximum jaw motion measurements for distinguishing between common temporomandibular disorder subgroups. *Oral Surg Oral Med Oral Pathol Oral Radiol Endod* 93:552–559, 2002.
99. Reider C: Maximum mandibular opening in patients with and without a history of TMJ dysfunction. *J Prosthet Dent.* 39:441–446, 1978.
100. Walker N, Bohannon RW, Cameron D: Discriminant validity of temporomandibular joint range of motion measurements obtained with a ruler. *J Orthop Sports Phys Ther.* 30:484–492., 2000.
101. Dunn J: Physical Therapy. In: Kaplan AS, Assael LA eds. *Temporomandibular disorders diagnosis and treatment.* Philadelphia, PA: WB Saunders, 1991: 455–500.
102. Sturdivant J, Fricton JR: Physical therapy for temporomandibular disorders and orofacial pain. *Curr Opin Dent* 1:485–496, 1991.
103. Gross A, Gale EN: A prevalence study of the clinical signs associated with mandibular dysfunction. *J Am Dent Assoc* 107:932–936, 1983.
104. Fricton JR: Myofascial pain. *Baillieres Clin Rheumatol* 8:857–880, 1994.
105. Yatani H, Suzuki K, Kuboki T, et al: The validity of clinical examination for diagnosing anterior disk displacement without reduction. *Oral Surg Oral Med Oral Pathol Oral Radiol Endod.* 85:654–660, 1998.
106. de Wijer A, Lobbezoo-Scholte AM, Steenks MH, et al: Reliability of clinical findings in temporomandibular disorders. *J Orofac Pain.* 9: 181–191, 1995.
107. Manfredini D, Tognini F, Zampa V, et al: Predictive value of clinical findings for temporomandibular joint effusion. *Oral Surg Oral Med Oral Pathol Oral Radiol Endod.* 96:521–526, 2003.
108. Travell JG, Simons DG: *Myofascial Pain and Dysfunction – The Trigger Point Manual.* Baltimore, MD: Williams & Wilkins, 1983.
109. Johnstone D, Templeton M: The feasability of palpating the lateral pterygoid. *J Prosthet Dent* 44:318, 1980.
110. House JW, Brackman DE: Facial nerve grading system. *Otolaryngol Head Neck Surg* 93:146–147, 1985.
111. Satoh Y, Kanzaki J, Yoshihara S: A comparison and conversion table of the House-Brackmann facial nerve grading system and the Yanagihara grading system. *Auris, Nasus, Larynx* 27:207–212, 2000.
112. Croxson G, May M, Mester SJ: Grading facial nerve function: House-Brackmann versus Burres-Fisch methods. *Am J Otol* 11:240–246, 1990.
113. Meadows A, Hall N, Shah-Desai S, et al: The House-Brackmann system and assessment of corneal risk in facial nerve palsy. *Eye* 14:353–357, 2000.
114. Hansson LG, Hansson T, Petersson A: A comparison between clinical and radiological findings in 259 temporomandibular joint patients. *J Prosthet Dent* 50:89–94, 1983.
115. Tasaki MM, Westesson PL: Temporomandibular joint: diagnostic accuracy with sagittal and coronal MR imaging. *Radiology* 186:723–729, 1993.
116. Solberg WK, Hansson TL, Nordstrom B: The temporomandibular joint in young adults at autopsy: a morphologic classification and evaluation. *J Oral Rehabil* 12:303–321, 1985.
117. Ettala-Ylitalo UM, Syrjanen S, Halonen P: Functional disturbances of the masticatory system related to temporomandibular joint involvement by rheumatoid arthritis. *J Oral Rehabil* 14:415–427, 1987.
118. Goldstein BH: Temporomandibular disorders: A review of current understanding. *Oral Surg Oral Med Oral Pathol Oral Radiol Endod* 88:379–385, 1999.
119. Carlsson GE: Long-term effects of treatment of craniomandibular disorders. *Craniot* 3:337–342, 1985.
120. Gatchel RJ, Stowell AW, Wildenstein L, et al: Efficacy of an early intervention for patients with acute temporomandibular disorder-related pain: a one-year outcome study. *J Am Dent Assoc.* 137:339–347, 2006.
121. Ogus HD, Toller PA: *Common disorders of the temporomandibular joint.* Bristol: John Wright & Son, 1986.

122. Guralnik W: The temporomandibular joint: the dentist's dilemma: Parts I and II. *Br Dent J* 156:315-319 & 353–356, 1984.
123. Gray RJ, Quayle AA, Hall CA, et al: Physiotherapy in the treatment of temporomandibular joint disorders: a comparative study of four treatment methods. *Br Dent J* 176:257–261, 1994.
124. Dimitroulis G, Gremillion HA, Dolwick MF, et al: Temporomandibular disorders. 2. Non-surgical treatment. *Aust Dent J* 40:372–376, 1995.
125. Brown DT, Gaudet EL, Jr.: Temporomandibular disorder treatment outcomes: second report of a large-scale prospective clinical study. *Cranio.* 20:244–253, 2002.
126. Kim MR, Graber TM, Viana MA: Orthodontics and temporomandibular disorder: a meta-analysis. *Am J Orthod Dentofacial Orthop.* 121:438–446, 2002.
127. Kulekcioglu S, Sivrioglu K, Ozcan O, et al: Effectiveness of low-level laser therapy in temporomandibular disorder. *Scand J Rheumatol* 32:114–118, 2003.
128. Medlicott MS, Harris SR: A systematic review of the effectiveness of exercise, manual therapy, electrotherapy, relaxation training, and biofeedback in the management of temporomandibular disorder. *Phys Ther.* 86:955–973, 2006.
129. McNeely ML, Armijo Olivo S, Magee DJ: A systematic review of the effectiveness of physical therapy interventions for temporomandibular disorders. *Phys Ther.* 86:710–725, 2006.
130. Tegelberg A, Kopp S: Short-term effect of physical training on temporomandibular joint disorder in individuals with rheumatoid arthritis and ankylosing spondylitis. *Acta Odontol Scand.* 46:49–56, 1988.
131. Au AR, Klineberg IJ: Isokinetic exercise management of temporomandibular joint clicking in young adults. *J Prosthet Dent.* 70:33–39, 1993.
132. Cleland J, Palmer J: Effectiveness of manual physical therapy, therapeutic exercise, and patient education on bilateral disc displacement without reduction of the temporomandibular joint: a single-case design. *J Orthop Sports Phys Ther.* 34:535–548, 2004.
133. Harkins SJ, Marteney JL: Extrinsic trauma: a significant precipitating factor in temporomandibular dysfunction. *J Prosthet Dent* 54:271–272, 1985.
134. Pullinger AG, Seligman DA: Trauma history in diagnostic groups of temporomandibular disorders. *Oral Surg Oral Med Oral Pathol Oral Radiol Endod* 71:529–534, 1991.
135. Pullinger AG, Monteiro AA: History factors associated with symptoms of temporomandibular disorders. *J Oral Rehabil* 15:117–24, 1988.
136. Weinberg LA, Larger LA: Clinical report on the etiology and diagnosis of TMJ dysfunction-pain syndrome. *J Prosthet Dent* 44:642–653, 1980.
137. Stenger J: Whiplash. Basal facts. *J Prosthet Dent* 2:5–12, 1977.
138. Chapman CE: Can the use of physical modalities for pain control be rationalized by the research evidence? *Can J Physiol Pharmacol* 69:704–712, 1991.
139. Carlsson GE, Magnusson T: *Management of Temporomandibular Disorders in the General Dental Practice.* Carol Stream, IL: Quintessence, 1999.
140. Kropmans T, Dijkstra P, Stegenga B, et al: Smallest detectable difference of maximal mouth opening in patients with painful restricted temporomandibular joint function. *Eur J Oral Sci* 108:9–13, 2000.
141. Rocabado M: Physical therapy for the post-surgical TMJ patient. *J Craniomandib Disord* 7:75–82, 1989.
142. Kraus SL: Cervical spine influences on the craniomandibular region. In: Kraus SL, ed. *TMJ Disorders: Management of the Craniomandibular Complex.* New York: Churchill Livingstone, 1988: 367–396.
143. Hodges JM: Managing temporomandibular joint syndrome. *Laryngoscope* 100:60–66, 1990.
144. Fricton JR: Management of masticatory myofascial pain. *Semin Orthod* 1:229–243, 1995.
145. Clark GT, Adler RC: A critical evaluation of occlusal therapy. Occlusal adjustment procedures. *J Am Dent Assoc* 110:743–750, 1985.
146. Clark GT: A critical evaluation of orthopedic interocclusal appliance therapy. Design theory and overall effectiveness. *J Am Dent Assoc* 108:359–364, 1984.
147. Seligman DA, Pullinger AG: The role of intercuspal occlusal relationships in temporomandibular disorders: a review. *J Craniomandib Disord Facial Oral Pain* 5:96–106, 1991.
148. Greene CS, Marbach JJ: Epidemiologic studies of mandibular dysfunction: a critical review. *J Prosthet Dent* 48:184–90, 1982.
149. Feine JS, Widmer CG, Lund JP: Physical therapy: a critique. *Oral Surg Oral Med Oral Pathol Oral Radiol Endod* 83:123–7, 1997.
150. Feine JS, Lund JP: An assessment of the efficacy of physical therapy and physical modalities for the control of chronic musculoskeletal pain. *Pain* 71:5–23, 1997.
151. Fricton JR, Kroening R, Haley D, et al: Myofascial pain syndrome of the head and neck: a review of clinical characteristics of 164 patients. *Oral Surg Oral Med Oral Pathol*60:615–623, 1985.
152. Kendall FP, McCreary EK, Provance PG: *Muscles: Testing and Function.* Baltimore, MD: Williams & Wilkins, 1993.
153. Janda V: Muscle strength in relation to muscle length, pain and muscle imbalance. In: Harms-Ringdahl K ed. *Muscle Strength.* New York: Churchill Livingstone, 1993:83–91.
154. Sahrmann SA: *Diagnosis and Treatment of Movement Impairment Syndromes.* St Louis, MO: Mosby, 2001.
155. Griegel-Morris P, Larson K, Mueller-Klaus K, et al: Incidence of common postural abnormalities in the cervical, shoulder, and thoracic regions and their asociation with pain in two age groups of healthy subjects. *Phys Ther* 72:426–430, 1992.
156. Simons DG: Muscular pain syndromes. In: Fricton JR, Awad E, eds. *Advances in Pain Research and Therapy.* New York: Raven Press, 1990:1–41.
157. Moss RA, Adams HE: The class of personality, anxiety and depression in mandibular pain dysfunction subjects. *J Oral Rehabil* 11:233–237, 1984.
158. Rugh JD: Psychological components of pain. *Dent Clin North Am* 31:579–594, 1987.
159. Cohen S, Rodriguez MS: Pathways linking affective disturbances and physical disorders. *Health Psychol* 14:371–373, 1995.
160. Gatchel RJ, Garofalo JP, Ellis E, et al: Major psychological disorders in acute and chronic TMD: An initial examination. *J Am Dent Assoc* 127:1365–1370, 1372, 1374, 1996.
161. Kight M, Gatchel RJ, Wesley L: Temporomandibular disorders: evidence for significant overlap with psychopathology. *Health Psychol* 18:177–182, 1999.
162. Korszun A, Papadopoulos E, Demitrack M, et al: The relationship between temporomandibular disorders and stress-associated syndromes. *Oral Surg Oral Med Oral Pathol Oral Radiol Endod* 86:416–20, 1998.
163. Gardea MA, Gatchel RJ, Mishra KD: Long-term efficacy of biobehavioral treatment of temporomandibular disorders. *J Behav Med* 24:341–359, 2001
164. Carlsson SG, Gale EW: Biofeedback in the treatment of long-term temporomandibular joint pain: an outcome study. *Biofeedback Self Regul* 2:161–165, 1977.
165. Barber J: *Hypnosis and suggestion in the treatment of pain. A clinical guide.* New York: WW Norton, 1996.
166. Simon EP, Lewis DM: Medical hypnosis for temporomandibular disorders: treatment efficacy and medical utilization outcome. *Oral Surg Oral Med Oral Pathol Oral Radiol Endod* 90:54–63, 2000.
167. Clark GT, Adachi NY, Dornan MR: Physical medicine procedures affect temporomandibular disorders: a review. *J Am Dent Assoc* 121:151–161, 1990.
168. Tegelberg A, Kopp S: Short-term effect of physical training on temporomandibular joint disorder in individuals with rheumatoid arthritis and ankylosing spondylitis. *Acta Odontol Scand* 46:49–51, 1988.
169. Linde C, Isacsson G, Jonsson BG: Outcome of 6-week treatment with transcutaneous electric nerve stimulation compared with splint on symptomatic temporomandibular joint disk displacement without reduction. *Acta Odontol Scand* 53:92–98, 1995.
170. Schiffman EL: The role of the randomized clinical trial in evaluating management strategies for temporomandibular disorders. In: Fricton JR, Dubner R eds. *Orofacial pain and temporomandibular disorders* (advances in pain research and therapy, Vol 21). New York: Raven Press, 1995:415–463.
171. Mohl ND, Ohrbach RK, Crow HC, et al: Devices for the diagnosis and treatment of temporomandibular disorders, III: thermography, ultrasound, electrical stimulation, and electromyographic biofeedback. *J Prosthet Dent* 63:472–477, 1990.
172. Murphy GJ: Electrical physical therapy in treating TMJ patients. *J Craniomand Pract* 2:67–73, 1983.
173. Gangarosa LP: *Iontophoresis in dental practice.* Chicago: Quintessence Publishing, 1982.
174. Gangarosa L: Iontophoresis in pain control. *Pain Digest* 3:162–174, 1993.
175. Kahn J: Iontophoresis and ultrasound for postsurgical temporomandibular trismus and paresthesia. *Phys Ther* 60:307–308, 1980.
176. Weinberg S, Kryshtalskyj B: Analysis of facial and trigeminal nerve function after arthroscopic surgery of the temporomandibular joint. *J Oral Maxillofac Surg* 54:40–43, 1996.

177. Loughner BA, Gremillion HA, Mahan PE, et al: The medial capsule of the human temporomandibular joint. *J Oral Maxillofac Surg* 55:363–369, 1997.
178. Talebzadeh N, Rosenstein TP, Pogrel MA: Anatomy of the structures medial to the temporomandibular joint. *Oral Surg Oral Med Oral Pathol Oral Radiol Endod* 88:674–678, 1999.
179. Paesani D, Westesson P-L, Hatala M, et al: Prevalence of temporomandibular joint internal derangement in patients with craniomandibular disorders. *Am J Orthod Dentofacial Orthop* 101:41–47, 1992.
180. Wongwatana S, Kronman JH, Clark RE, et al: Anatomic basis for disk displacement in temporomandibular joint (TMJ) dysfunction. *Am J Orthod Dentofacial Orthop* 105:257–264, 1994.
181. Pertes RA, Attanasio R: Internal Derangements. In: Kaplan AS, Assael LA, eds. *Temporomandibular disorders diagnosis and treatment*. Philadelphia, PA: WB Saunders, 1991:142–164.
182. Ross JB: Diagnostic criteria and nomenclature for TMJ arthrography in sagittal section. Part I. Derangements. *J Craniomandib Disord* 1:185, 1987.
183. Kondoh T, Westesson PL, Takahashi T, et al: Prevalence of morphological changes in the surfaces of the temporomandibular joint disc associated with internal derangement. *J Oral Maxillofac Surg* 56:339-343; discussion 343–344, 1998.
184. Okeson JP: *Management of Temporomandibular Disorders and Occlusion*, 4th ed. St Louis, MO: Mosby Year Book, 1998.
185. Stegenga B, de Bont LGM, Boering G: Osteoarthritis as the cause of craniomandibular pain and dysfunction: A unifying concept. *J Oral Maxillofac Surg* 47:249, 1989.
186. Rohlin M, Westesson PL, Eriksson L: The correlation of temporomandibular joint sounds with joint morphology in fifty-five autopsy specimens. *J Oral Maxillofac Surg* 43:194, 1985.
187. Hayt MW, Abrahams JJ, Blair J: Magnetic resonance imaging of the temporomandibular joint. *Top Magn Reson Imaging* 11:138–146, 2000.
188. Westesson P-L, Brodstein SL, Liedberg J: Internal derangement of the temporomandibular joint. Morphologic description with correlation to joint function. *Oral Surg Oral Med Oral Pathol* 59:323, 1985.
189. Rasmussen OC: Description of population and progress of symptoms in a longitudinal study of temporomandibular arthropathy. *Scand J Dent Res* 89:196–203, 1981.
190. Wilkes CH: Internal derangement of the temporomandibular joint: pathological variations. *Arch Otolaryngol Head Neck Surg* 115:469–477, 1989.
191. Hondo T, Shimoda T, Moses JJ, et al: Traumatically induced posterior disc displacement without reduction of the TMJ. *J Craniomand Pract* 12:128–132, 1994.
192. Katzberg RW, Westesson PL, Tallents RH, et al: Temporomandibular joint: MR assessment of rotational and sideways disc displacements. *Radiology* 169:741–748, 1988.
193. Lundh H, Westesson PL: Long-term follow-up after occlusal treatment to correct abnormal temporomandibular joint disk position. *Oral Surg Oral Med Oral Pathol* 67:2–10, 1989.
194. Lundh H: Correction of temporomandibular joint disk displacement by occlusal therapy. *Swed Dent J Suppl* 51:1–159, 1987.
195. Shorey CW, Campbell JH: Dislocation of the temporomandibular joint. *Oral Surg Oral Med Oral Pathol Oral Radiol Endod* 89:662–668, 2000.
196. Scapino RP: Histopathology associated with malposition of the human temporomandibular joint disc. *Oral Surg Oral Med Oral Pathol Oral Radiol Endod* 55:382, 1983.
197. Enzinger FM, Weiss SW: Benign tumors and tumor-like lesions of synovial tissue. In: Enzinger FM, Weiss SW, eds. *Soft Tissue Tumors*, 3rd ed. St Louis, MO, Mosby-Year Book Inc, 1995:735–755.
198. Goldman AB, DiCarlo EF: Pigmented villonodular synovitis: diagnosis and differential diagnosis. *Radiol Clin North Am* 26:1327–1347, 1988.
199. O'Sullivan TJ, Alport EC, Whiston HG: Pigmented villonodular synovitis of the temporomandibular joint. *J Otolaryngol* 13:123–126, 1984.
200. Barnard JDW: Pigmented villonodular synovitis in the temporomandibular joint: a case report. *Br J Oral Surg* 13:183–187, 1975.
201. Takagi M, Ishikawa G: Simultaneous villonodular synovitis and synovial chondromatosis of the temporomandibular joint: report of case. *J Oral Surg* 39:699–701, 1981.
202. Tanaka K, Suzuki M, Nameki H, et al: Pigmented villonodular synovitis of the temporomandibular joint. *Arch Otolaryngol Head Neck Surg* 123:536–539, 1997.
203. Schwartz LL: A temporomandibular joint pain-dysfunction syndrome. *J Chronic Dis* 3:284–293, 1956.
204. Schwartz LL: Pain associated with temporomandibular joint. *J Am Dent Assoc* 51:393–397, 1955.
205. Brooke RI, Stenn PG: Postinjury myofascial dysfunction syndrome: its etiology and prognosis. *Oral Surg Oral Med Oral Pathol* 45:846–850, 1978.
206. Howard RP, Benedict JV, Raddin JH, et al: Assessing neck extension-flexion as a basis for temporomandibular joint dysfunction. *J Oral Maxillofac Surg* 49:1210–1213, 1991.
207. Howard RP, Hatsell CP, Guzman HM: Temporomandibular joint injury potential imposed by the low-velocity extension-flexion maneuver. *J Oral Maxillofac Surg* 53:256–262, 1995.
208. Alanen PJ, Kirveskari PK: Occupational cervicobrachial disorder and temporomandibular joint dysfunction. *Cranio* 3:69–72, 1984.
209. De Laat A, Meuleman H, Stevens A: Relation between functional limitations of the cervical spine and temporomandibular disorders. *J Orofacial Pain* 1:109, 1993.
210. Kirveskari P, Alanen P, Karskela V, et al: Association of functional state of stomatognathic system with mobility of cervical spine and neck muscle tenderness. *Acta Odont Scand* 46:281–286, 1988.
211. Bogduk N: The rationale for patterns of neck and back pain. *Patient Management* 8:13, 1984.
212. Bogduk N: Cervical causes of headache and dizziness. In: Grieve GP, ed. *Modern Manual Therapy of the Vertebral Column*. New York: Churchill Livingstone, 1986:289–302.
213. Bogduk N: Innervation and pain patterns of the cervical spine. In: Grant R, ed. *Physical Therapy of the Cervical and Thoracic Spine*. New York: Churchill Livingstone, 1988.
214. Bogduk N: The anatomical basis for cervicogenic headache. *J Manip Physiol Ther* 15:67–70, 1992.
215. Bovim G, Berg R, Dale LG: Cervicogenic headache: anaesthetic blockade of cervical nerves (C2–C5) and facet joint (C2/C3). *Pain* 49:315–320, 1992.
216. Jull GA. Headaches associated with cervical spine; a clinical review. In Boyling JD, Palastanga N, eds. *Grieve's Modern Manual Therapy*, 2nd ed. Edinburgh: Churchill Livingstone, 1994.
217. Lord SM, Barnsley L, Wallis BJ, et al: Third occipital nerve headache: a prevalence study. *J Neurol Neurosurg Psychiatry* 57:1187–1190, 1994.
218. Norris CW, Eakins K: Head and neck pain: T-M joint syndrome. *Laryngoscope* 84:1466–1478, 1974.
219. de Wijer A: *Temporomandibular and cervical spine disorders*, Utrecht University. The Netherlands, 1995.
220. de Wijer A, Steenks MH, de Leeuw JR, et al: Symptoms of the cervical spine in temporomandibular and cervical spine disorders. *J Oral Rehabil* 23:742–750, 1996.
221. de Wijer A, Steenks MH, Bosman F, et al: Symptoms of the stomatognathic system in temporomandibular and cervical spine disorders. *J Oral Rehabil* 23:733–741, 1996.
222. de Wijer A, de Leeuw JR, Steenks MH, et al: Temporomandibular and cervical spine disorders: Self-reported signs and symptoms. *Spine* 21:1638–1646, 1996.
223. Mohl ND: Head posture and its role in occlusion. *NY State Dent J* 42:17–23, 1976.
224. Prieskel HW: Some observations on the postural position of the mandible. *J Prosthet Dent* 15:625–633, 1965.
225. Ramfjord SP: Dysfunctional temporomandibular joint and muscle pain. *J Prosthet Dent* 11:353–374, 1961.
226. Darling DW, Kraus S, Glasheen-Wray MB: Relationship of head posture and the rest position of the mandible. *J Prosthet Dent* 52:111–115, 1984.
227. Goldstein DF, Kraus SL, Williams WB, et al: Influence of cervical posture on mandibular movement. *J Prosthet Dent* 52:421–426, 1984.
228. Robinson MJ: The influence of head position on TMJ dysfunction. *J Prosthet Dent* 16:169–172, 1966.
229. International Headache Society Headache Classification and Diagnostic Criteria for Headache Disorders: Cranial neuralgias, and facial pain. *Cephalalgia* 8:19–22, 71, 72, 1988.
230. Feinman C, Harris ML, Cawley R: Psychogenic facial pain: Presentation and treatment. *Br Med J* 288:436–438, 1984.
231. Solomon S, Lipton RB: Atypical facial pain: A review. *Semin Neurol* 8:332–338, 1988.
232. Friedman MH, Weintraub MI, Forman S: Atypical facial pain: A localized maxillary nerve disorder? *Am J Pain Manage* 4:149–152, 1995.
233. Appenzeller O: *Pathogenesis and treatment of headache*. New York: Spectrum Publications, Inc., 1976.

234. Esposito CJ, Crim GA, Binkley TK: Headaches: A differential diagnosis. *J Craniomand Pract* 4:318–322, 1986.
235. Wolff HG: *Headache and other head pain*, 2nd ed. New York: Oxford University Press, 1987:53–76.
236. Dandy WE: An operation for the cure of tic douloureux. Partial section of the sensory root at the pons. *Arch Surg* 18:687, 1929.
237. Sjoquist O: *Surgical Section of Pain Tracts and Pathways in the Spinal Cord and Brain Stem, 4 Congr Neurol Internat.* Paris, Masson, 1949.
238. Coderre TJ, Katz JN, Vaccarino AL, et al: Contribution of central neuroplasticity to pathological pain: review of clinical and experimental literature. *Pain* 52:259–285, 1993.
239. Trowskoy M, Cozacov C, Ayache M, et al: Postoperative pain after inguinal herniorraphy with different types of anesthesia. *Anesth Analg* 70:29–35, 1990.
240. McQuay J: Pre-emptive analgesia. *Br J Anesth* 69:1–3, 1992.
241. Cousins M: Acute and postoperative pain. In: Wall PD, Melzack R, eds. *Textbook of pain*. Edinburgh: Churchill Livingstone, 1994:357–385.
242. Stohler CS: Phenomenology, epidemiology, and natural progression of the muscular temporomandibular disorders. *Oral Surg Oral Med Oral Pathol Oral Radiol Endod* 83:77–81, 1997.
243. Evjenth O, Hamberg J: *Muscle Stretching in Manual Therapy, A Clinical Manual.* Alfta, Sweden: Alfta Rehab Forlag, 1984.

CHAPTER 27 The Thoracic Spine

CHAPTER OBJECTIVES

At the completion of this chapter, the reader will be able to:

1. Describe the vertebrae, ligaments, muscles, and blood and nerve supply that comprise the thoracic intervertebral segment.
2. Outline the coupled movements of the thoracic spine, the normal and abnormal joint barriers, and the responses of the various structures to loading.
3. Perform a detailed objective examination of the thoracic musculoskeletal system, including palpation of the articular and soft tissue structures, combined motion testing, position testing, passive articular mobility tests, and stability tests.
4. Evaluate the total examination data to establish the diagnosis and estimate the prognosis.
5. Describe the common pathologies and lesions of this region.
6. Apply manual techniques to the thoracic spine using the correct grade, direction, and duration.
7. Describe intervention strategies based on clinical findings and established goals.
8. Design an intervention plan based on patient education, manual therapy, and therapeutic exercise.
9. Evaluate intervention effectiveness in order to progress or modify an intervention.
10. Plan an effective home program, including spinal care and therapeutic exercise, and instruct the patient in this program.

OVERVIEW

The thoracic spine serves as a transitional zone between the lumbosacral region and the cervical spine. Despite the fact that the thoracic spine has not enjoyed the same attention as other regions of the spine in terms of research, it can be a significant source of local and referred pain. The thoracic spine is the most rigid region of the spine and, in this area, protection of the thoracic viscera takes precedence over segmental spinal mobility. In addition, the thorax is an important region of load transfer between the upper body (the head, cervical spine, and upper extremities) and the lower body (the lumbopelvic region and lower extremities).[1,2]

Because each thoracic vertebra is involved in at least six articulations, and as many as thirteen, establishing the specific cause of thoracic dysfunction involved may not always be possible. This task is made more difficult because of the inaccessibility of most of these joints.[3]

ANATOMY

The thoracic spine (Fig. 27-1) forms a kyphotic curve between the lordotic curves of the cervical and lumbar spines. The curve begins at T1–2 and extends down to T12, with the T6–7 disk space as the apex.[4] The thoracic kyphosis is a structural curve that is present from birth.[5] Unlike the lumbar and cervical regions, which derive their curves from the corresponding differences in intervertebral disk (IVD) heights, the thoracic curve is maintained by the wedge-shaped vertebral bodies, which are about 2 mm higher posteriorly than anteriorly.

At the thoracolumbar junction, typically located between T11 and L1, the changes in curvature from one of kyphosis to one of lordosis vary quite widely according to posture, age, and previous compression fractures (see Chap. 5) and resulting deformity.[6,7]

The cervicothoracic junction anatomically comprises the C7–T1 segment and functionally includes the seventh cervical vertebra, the first two thoracic vertebrae, the first and second ribs, and the manubrium.

Thoracic Vertebra

The thoracic vertebrae consist of the usual elements: the vertebral body (centrum), transverse processes, and spinous process (Fig. 27-1).

Vertebral Body

The thoracic vertebral body (Fig. 27-1) is roughly as wide as it is long, so that its anteroposterior and mediolateral

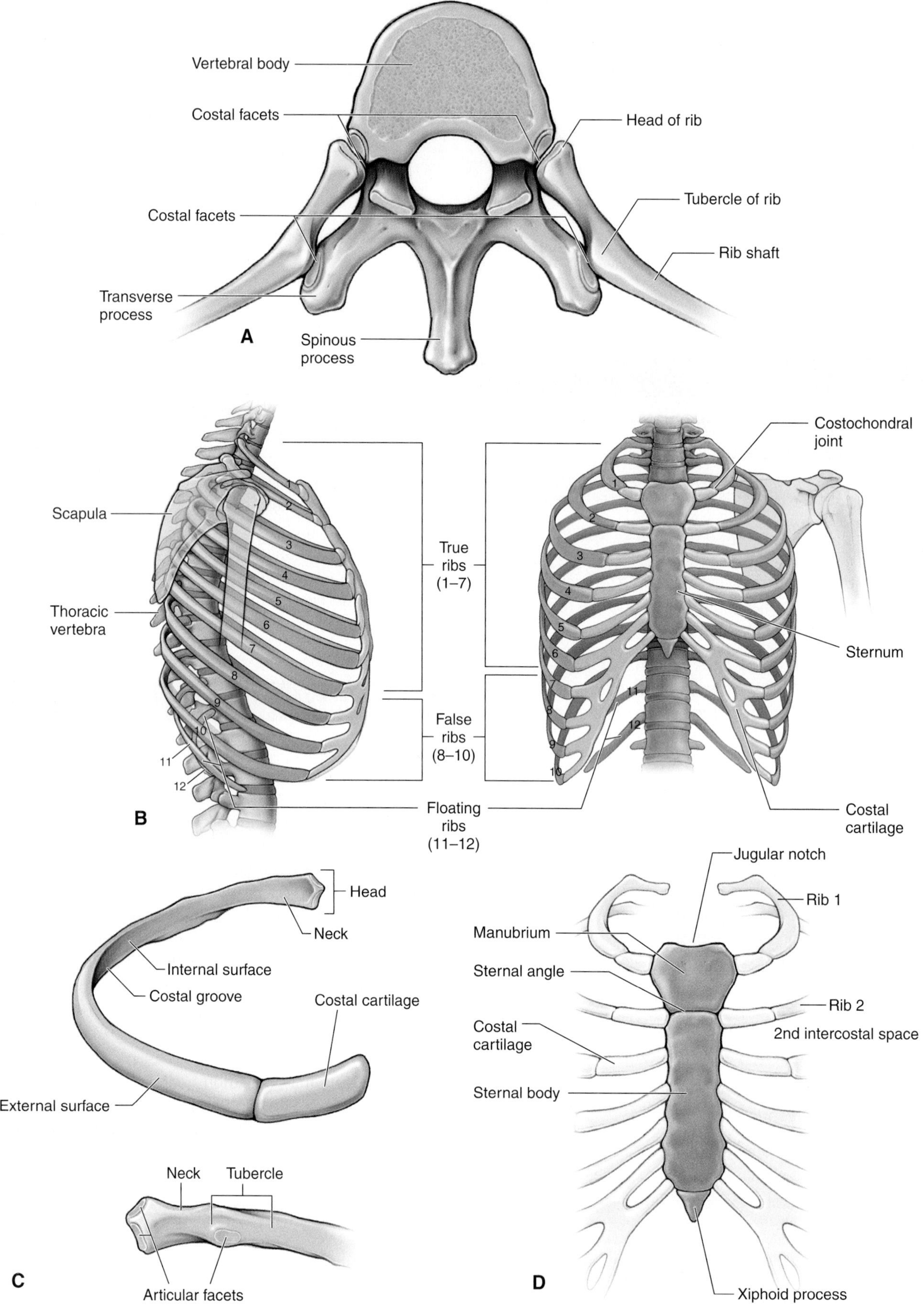

FIGURE 27-1 The thoracic spine and rib cage. (Reproduced with permission from Morton DA, Foreman KB, Albertine KH: *The Big Picture: Gross Anatomy*, McGraw-Hill, 2011.)

dimensions are of equal length.[8] The anterior surface of the body is convex from side to side, whereas the posterior surface is deeply concave.[8] The height, end-plate cross-sectional area, and bone mass of the vertebral bodies increase cranially to caudally, particularly in the lower levels.[9,10] Progressive wedging of the thoracic vertebral bodies occurs with increasing age in the majority of individuals, with disk space narrowing at multiple levels occurring from the third decade of life.[11] The vertebral bodies of most of the thoracic spine differ from those of the cervical and lumbar vertebrae because of the presence of a demifacet on each of their lateral aspects for articulation with the ribs (the costovertebral joint; see later discussion).

Intervertebral Disk

The IVDs of the thoracic spine have been poorly researched, although preliminary studies seem to indicate that the typical thoracic disk appears to have been adapted from a cervical design rather than from a lumbar design.[12] The vertebral bodies of thoracic vertebrae 2–10 increase in size and change shape down the vertebral column, and, importantly, each has two demifacets for the attachment of ribs.[12] The IVDs of this region are narrower and flatter than those in the cervical and lumbar spine and contribute approximately one-sixth of the length of the thoracic column.[13] Disk size in the thoracic region gradually increases from superior to inferior. The disk height to body height ratio is 1:5, compared to 2:5 in the cervical spine, and 1:3 in the lumbar spine,[14,15] making it the smallest ratio in the spine and affording the least amount of motion.[16] Motion is further restricted by the orientation of the lamella of the annulus fibrosis (AF),[17] and the relatively small nucleus pulposus (NP), which is more centrally located within the AF, and has a lower capacity to swell.[18] The roughly circular cross-section of the thoracic disk allows the force of torsion to be evenly distributed around its circumference, making it better able to withstand these kinds of forces.[19]

In the thoracic spine, the segmental nerve roots are situated mainly behind the inferior–posterior aspect of the upper vertebral body rather than behind the disk, which reduces the possibility of root compression in impairments of the thoracic disk.[20] In a review of 280 patients, Arce and Dohrmann[21] found that thoracic disk herniation constitutes 0.25–0.75% of all disk herniations. Because the intervertebral foramina are quite large at these levels, osseous contact with the nerve roots is seldom encountered in the thoracic spine,[20] and, as the dermatomes in this region have a fair amount of overlap, they cannot be relied upon to determine the specific nerve root involved.

In contrast to the cervical and lumbar regions, where the spinal canal is triangular/oval in cross-section and offers a large lateral excursion to the nerve roots, the mid-thoracic spinal canal is small and circular (Fig. 27-1), becoming triangular at the upper and lower levels. At the levels of T4–9, the canal is at its narrowest.[20] The spinal canal is also restricted in its size by the pedicles, remaining within the confines of the vertebra and not diverging as they do in the cervical spine. This would tend to predispose the spinal cord to compression more than in the cervical spine, were it not for the smaller cord size and more oval shape of the thoracic canal. Despite this, central disk protrusions are more common in the thoracic region than in other regions of the spine, and, because the NP is small in the thorax, protrusions are invariably of the annular type, and nuclear protrusions are rare.[20] Complicating matters is the fact that this is an area of poor vascular supply, receiving its blood from only one radicular artery. This renders the thoracic spinal cord extremely vulnerable to damage by extra dural masses or by an overzealous manipulation.

Transverse Processes

The transverse processes of the thoracic spine are oriented posteriorly (i.e., they point backward) and are located directly between the inferior articulating process and the superior articulating process of the zygapophyseal joints of each level (Fig. 27-1). This anatomical feature makes the transverse processes useful as palpation points, when performing mobility testing in the mid-thorax.

The transverse processes of the first 10 thoracic vertebrae differ from those of the cervical and lumbar spines because of the presence of a costal facet on the transverse process, which articulates with the corresponding rib to form the costotransverse joint (see later discussion). At the T11 and T12 levels, the costotransverse joint is absent because ribs 11 and 12 do not articulate with the transverse processes but rather with the vertebral body.

Spinous Processes

Two short and thick laminae come together to form the spinous process (Fig. 27-1). The spinous processes of the thoracic region are long, slender, and triangular shaped in cross-section. Although all of the thoracic spinous processes point obliquely downward, the degree of obliquity varies. The first three spinous processes, and the last three, are almost horizontal, whereas those of the mid-thorax are long and steeply inclined. T7 has the greatest spinous process angulation.

As elsewhere in the spine, the thoracic vertebrae are designed to endure and distribute the compressive forces produced by weight bearing, most of which is borne by the vertebral bodies. The compressive load at T1 is approximately 9% of body weight, increasing to 33% at T8 and 47 percent at T12.[22,23]

The thoracic vertebrae are classified as typical or atypical, with reference to their morphology. The typical thoracic vertebrae are found at T2–9, although T9 may be atypical in that its inferior costal facet is frequently absent. The atypical thoracic vertebrae are T1, T10, T11, and T12.

The first vertebra (T1) resembles C7. The centrum of T1 demonstrates a larger transverse than anteroposterior dimension of the vertebral body, being almost twice as wide as its length, and the spinous process is usually at least as long as that of C7. There are two ovoid facets on either side of the T1 vertebral body for articulation with the head of the first rib. The inferior aspect of the vertebral body of T1 is flat and contains a small facet at each posterolateral corner for articulation with the head of the second rib.

Approximately 32 structures attach to the first rib and body of T1.[22,23] Because of the ring-like structure of the ribs, and their attachments both anteriorly and posteriorly, the thoracic spine and ribs can be viewed as a cage-like structure forming a series of concentric rings. Any movement occurring at the various joints of each ring (costovertebral, costotransverse, sternocostal, and zygapophyseal joints) has the potential to influence motions at the other joints within the ring, or at the neighboring segments.

The third vertebra is the smallest of the thoracic vertebra. The T9 vertebra may have no demifacets below, or it may have two demifacets on either side (in which case, the T10 vertebra will have demifacets only at the superior aspect). The T10 vertebra has one full rib facet located partly on the body of the vertebra and partly on the tubercle. It does not articulate with the 11th rib and so does not possess inferior demifacets, and occasionally there is no facet for the rib at the costotransverse joint.

The T11 and T12 segments form the thoracolumbar junction. The T11 vertebra has complete costal facets, but no facets on the transverse processes for the rib tubercle. The T12 vertebra only articulates with its own ribs and does not possess inferior demifacets.

Ligaments

The common spinal ligaments are present at the thoracic vertebrae (Fig. 27-2), and they perform much the same function as they do elsewhere in the spine. However, the anterior longitudinal ligament in this region is narrower but thicker compared with elsewhere in the spine,[8] whereas the posterior longitudinal ligament is wider here at the level of the IVD, but narrower at the vertebral body than in the lumbar region.[24]

Zygapophyseal Joints

The zygapophyseal joints of the upper thoracic spine show some morphological features of the cervical region, and similarly the joints of the lower thoracic spine progressively approximate those of the upper lumbar region.[25] The middle segments of the thoracic spine are designed for less mobility, as the thoracic cage articulations limit sagittal plane motion while accommodating axial displacements.[25,26]

CLINICAL PEARL

The articulating facets of the thoracic zygapophyseal joints are quite different from those of the cervical and lumbar spines because they are oriented in a more coronal direction, with the angle of inclination changing, depending on the segmental level:

- The upper segments are inclined at 45–60 degrees to horizontal in a similar fashion as to those of the cervical spine.
- The middle segments are inclined at 90 degrees to horizontal in the typical thoracic form.
- The lower segments are inclined as in the lumbar spine. Zygapophyseal tropism (the moving toward or away from a stimulus) occurs most frequently at T11–12.[27] The inferior articular facets of T12 are invariably lumbar in orientation and concavity, with the orientation changing by 90 degrees at either T11 or T12, allowing pure axial rotation to occur.[28,29]

The superior and inferior facets of the zygapophyseal joints arise from the upper and lower parts of the pedicle of the thoracic vertebra. The superior facet lies superiorly with the articular surface on the posterior aspect, whereas the inferior facet lies inferiorly with the articular surface on the anterior (ventral) aspect. The degree of superoinferior and mediolateral orientation is slight. The superior facet arises from near the lamina–pedicle junction and faces posteriorly, superiorly, and laterally.

The inferior articulating facet arises from the laminae to face anteriorly, inferiorly, and medially, lying posterior to the superior facet of the vertebra below. The facet surfaces are concave anteriorly and convex posteriorly, bringing the axis of rotation through the centrum rather than through the spinous process, as in the lumbar vertebrae. This results in the biomechanical center of rotation coinciding with the actual center of rotation formed by body weight.[30]

The zygapophyseal joints function to restrain the amount of flexion and anterior translation of the vertebral segment and to facilitate rotation.[22] They appear to have little influence on the range of side bending.[22]

Ribs

The bony thoracic cage is formed by 12 pairs of ribs, the sternum, the clavicle, and the vertebrae of the thoracic spine (Fig. 27-1). The primary function of the rib cage is to protect the heart and lungs. All of the ribs of the cage are different from each other in size, width, and curvature, although they share some common characteristics. The first rib is the shortest. The rib length increases further inferiorly until the seventh rib, after which they become progressively shorter.

The ribs are divided into two classifications: true/false and typical/atypical.

1. ***True/false.*** Ribs 1–7 are named true ribs because their cartilage attaches directly to the sternum. The remaining ribs are false ribs, so named because their distal attachment is to the costochondral cartilage of their superior neighbor.
2. ***Typical/atypical.*** Ribs 3–9 are typical ribs. The first, ninth, 10th, 11th, and 12th ribs are considered atypical. The typical rib is characterized by a posterior end, which is composed of a head, neck, and tubercle. The head of the typical rib is characterized as two articular facets, a superior costal facet, and an inferior costal facet.
   a. The superior facet attaches to the costal semilunar demifacet of the vertebra above its level.
   b. The inferior facet attaches to the costal semicircular demifacet of the vertebra of the same level.[12]

The first, ninth, 10th, 11th, and 12th ribs are deemed atypical because they only articulate with their own vertebra via one full facet, and the lower two do not articulate with the costochondrium anteriorly.[31]

Typical Ribs

The head of the typical rib projects upward in a very similar manner to that of the uncinate process in the cervical

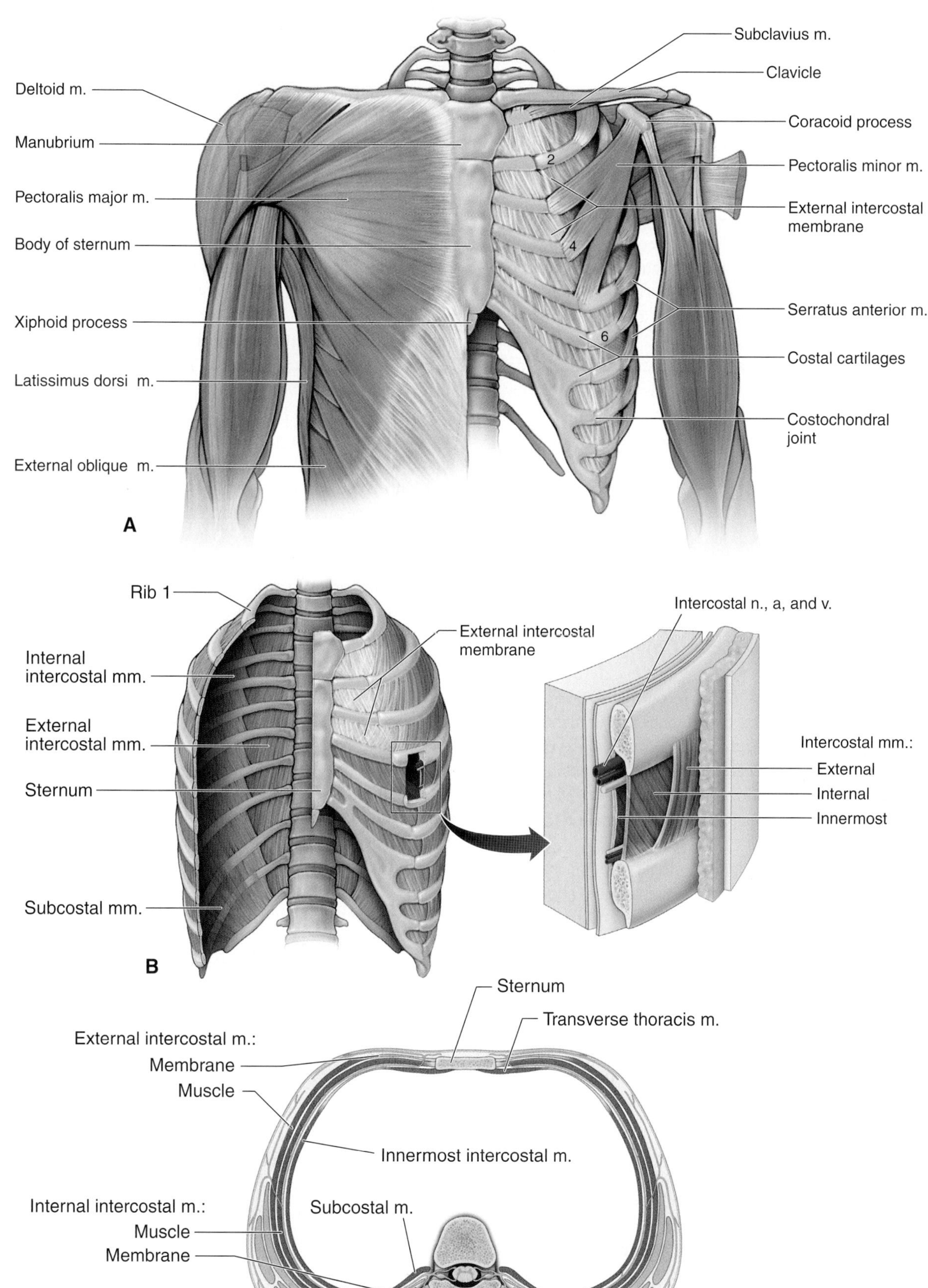

FIGURE 27-2 Muscles of the thoracic spine. (Reproduced with permission from Morton DA, Foreman KB, Albertine KH: *The Big Picture: Gross Anatomy*, McGraw-Hill, 2011.)

spine and, in fact, develops in much the same way during childhood, appearing to play a similar mechanical role.[8] The head consists of a slightly enlarged posterior end, which is divided by a horizontal ridge. The ridge serves as an attachment for the intra-articular ligament. The intra-articular ligament, which travels between the head of the rib and the IVD, bisects the joint into superior and inferior portions. Each of these portions normally contains a demifacet for articulation with the synovial costovertebral joints.

The tubercle of the typical rib lies on the outer surface, where the neck joins the shaft, and is more prominent in the upper parts than in the lower. The articular portion of the tubercle presents an oval facet for articulation at the costotransverse joint (Fig. 27-1).

The convex shaft of the rib is connected to the neck at the rib angle. The upper border of the shaft is round and blunt, whereas the inferior aspect is thin and sharp.[8] The anterior end of the shaft has a small depression at the tip for articulation at the costochondral joint.

Atypical Ribs

The atypical first rib is small but massively built. Being the most curved and the most inferiorly orientated rib, it slopes sharply downward from its vertebral articulation to the manubrium. The head is small and rounded and articulates only with the T1 vertebra. The first costal cartilage is the shortest and this, together with the fibrous sternochondral joint (Fig. 27-1), contributes to the overall stability of the first ring of the rib cage. The first rib attaches to the manubrium just under the sternoclavicular joint, and the second rib articulates with the sternum at the manubriosternal junction. The atypical second rib is longer and is not as flat as the first rib. It attaches to the junction of the manubrium and the body of the sternum.

The atypical 10th rib has only a single facet on its head, because of its lack of articulation with the vertebra above. The 11th and 12th ribs do not present tubercles and have only a single articular facet on their heads. The 11th and 12th ribs remain unattached anteriorly, but end with a small piece of cartilage.

Attachment and Orientation of the Ribs

The attachment of the ribs to the sternum is variable (Fig. 27-1). The upper five, six, or seven ribs have their own cartilaginous connection (see "Sternocostal Joint" section).[8] The cartilage of the eighth rib ends by blending with the seventh. The same situation pertains for the ninth and the 10th ribs, thus giving rise to a common band of cartilage and connective tissue.

The strong ligamentous attendance, and the presence of the two joints (costovertebral and costotransverse) at each level, severely limits the amount of movement permitted here to slight gliding and spinning motions, with morphology determining the function of each rib.

The orientation of the ribs increases from being horizontal at the upper levels to being more downwardly oblique in the inferior levels of the thoracic spine (a point worth remembering when performing palpation).

CLINICAL PEARL

The cervical rib is a rare anatomic variant estimated to occur in approximately 0.5–1% of the population and bilaterally in 66–80% of these cases.[18] Diagnosis is most often incidental, as a result of routine chest radiographs or in patients developing thoracic outlet syndrome (see Chap. 25).[32]

Costovertebral Joint

The thoracic vertebrae are connected to their adjacent vertebrae by the bilateral hyalinated, and synovial, costovertebral joints and their surrounding ligaments (see Fig. 27-1). The costovertebral articulation also forms an intimate relationship between the head of the rib and the lateral side of the vertebral body (see Fig. 27-1). The first, 11th, and 12th ribs articulate fully with their own vertebrae via a single costal facet, without any contact with the IVD, while the remaining ribs articulate with both their own vertebra and the vertebra above, as well as to the IVD. This could potentially predispose the first, 11th, and 12th costovertebral joints to early arthritic changes, as a result of more mechanical stress compared to the second to the 10th ribs.[33]

The radiate ligament connects the anterior aspect of the rib head to the bodies of two adjacent vertebrae and their intervening disk in a fanlike arrangement. Each of the three bands of the radiate ligament has different attachments:

1. The superior part runs from the head of the rib to the body of the superior vertebra.
2. The inferior part runs to the body of the inferior vertebra.
3. The intermediate part runs to the intervening disk.

Oda and colleagues[34] reported that the costovertebral joint and rib cage confer stability on the thoracic spine. They performed symmetrically applied resections of the posterior elements first, followed by resection of the bilateral costovertebral joints and then complete obliteration of the rib cage. Their conclusion was that the thoracic spine may become unstable when the posterior elements and the bilateral costovertebral joints are obliterated. In addition, there is an increase in the neutral zone and range of motion in both side bending and rotation, indicating that these joints provide a stabilizing influence during coupled motions.[34]

Feiertag and colleagues[35] reported that rib head joint resection showed significant increases in thoracic spinal motion in the sagittal and coronal planes. As the ossification of the head of the rib is not developed at the superior costovertebral joint until about age 13, younger individuals, such as gymnasts, can demonstrate a vast amount of thoracic rotation and side bending.

Costotransverse Joint

This is a synovial joint located between an articular facet on the posterior aspect of the rib tubercle and an articular facet on the anterior aspect of the transverse process, which is supported by a thin fibrous capsule (see Fig. 27-1). In the lower two thoracic vertebral segments, this articulation does not exist.

The neck of the rib lies along the entire length of the posterior aspect of the transverse process. The short and deep costotransverse ligament runs posteriorly from the posterior aspect of the rib neck to the anterior aspect of its transverse process, filling the costotransverse foramen that is formed between the rib neck and its adjacent transverse process. The ligament has two divisions:

1. The superior costotransverse ligament, also known as the interosseous ligament, or ligament of the neck of the rib, is formed in two layers. The anterior layer, which is continuous with the internal intercostal membrane laterally, runs from the neck of the rib up and laterally to the inferior aspect of the transverse process above. The posterior layer runs up and medially from the posterior aspect of the rib neck to the transverse process above.
2. The lateral costotransverse ligament runs from the tip of the transverse process laterally to the tubercle of its own rib. It is short, thick, and strong but is often damaged with direct blows to the chest (e.g., punch, kick, etc.).

Very little posteroanterior or anteromedial–posterolateral translation is available at this joint. Jiang and colleagues[36] reported that the superior costotransverse ligaments are very important in maintaining the lateral stability of the spine.

CLINICAL PEARL

Working together, the costotransverse and the costovertebral joints help provide stability to the thoracic spine.

Sternum

The sternum consists of three parts: the manubrium, the body, and the xiphoid process.

The manubrium (Fig. 27-1) is broad and thick superiorly and narrower and thinner inferiorly, where it articulates with the body. On either side of the suprasternal notch are articulating facets for the clavicles, and below these are the facets for the first rib. On the immediate inferolateral aspects of the manubrium are two more small facets for the cartilage of the second rib.

The articulation between the manubrium and the sternum is usually a symphysis, with the ends of the bones being lined with hyaline cartilage.

The body of the sternum is made up of the fused elements of four sternal bodies, and the vestiges of these are marked by three horizontal ridges. The upper end of the body articulates with the manubrium at the sternal angle. A facet at the superior end of the body laterally provides a joint surface common with the manubrium for the second costal cartilage. On each lateral border are four other notches that articulate with the third through sixth costal cartilages. The third rib has the deepest fossa on the sternum, indicating that it may serve as the axis for rotation and side bending during arm elevation. T7 articulates with both the sternum and the xiphoid.

The xiphisternum, or xiphoid process (see Fig. 27-1), is the smallest part of the sternum. It begins life in a cartilaginous state, but, in adulthood, the upper part ossifies.

TABLE 27-1 Muscles of Forced Expiration

Primary	Accessory
Abdominal muscles	Latissimus dorsi
► Internal and external oblique	Serratus posterior inferior
► Rectus abdominis	Quadratus lumborum
► Transversus abdominis	Iliocostalis lumborum
Internal intercostals (posterior)	
Transversus thoracis	
Transverse intercostals (intima)	

Data from Kendall HO, Kendall FP, Boynton DA: *Posture and Pain*. Baltimore, MD: Williams and Wilkins, 1952.

A study[37] examining the effect of removal of the entire sternum from the intact thorax found that its removal produced an almost complete loss of the stiffening effect of the thorax.

Sternocostal Joint

The first, sixth, and seventh costal cartilages are each linked to the sternum by a synchondrosis. The second to fifth ribs are each connected to the sternum through a synovial joint, whereby the cartilage of the corresponding rib articulates with a socket-like cavity in the sternum.[38]

In all of these joints, the periosteum of the sternum and the perichondrium of the costal cartilage are continuous. A thin fibrous capsule, present in the upper seven joints, attaches to the circumference of the articular surfaces, blending with the sternocostal ligaments. The surfaces of the joints are covered with fibrocartilage and are supported by capsular, radiate sternocostal, or xiphicostal and intra-articular ligaments. The joint is capable of about 2 degrees of motion from full inspiration to full expiration and allows the full excursion of the sternum in these activities.

Muscles

A large number of muscles arise from and insert on the thoracic spine and ribs (Fig. 27-2). The muscles of this region can be divided into those that are involved in spinal or extremity motion, and those that are involved in respiration (Tables 27-1 and 27-2).

TABLE 27-2 Muscles of Inspiration

Primary	Accessory
Diaphragm	Scaleni
Levator costorum	Sternocleidomastoid
External intercostals	Trapezius
Internal intercostals (anterior)	Serratus anterior and posterior and superior and inferior Pectoralis major and minor Latissimus dorsi Subclavius

Data from Kendall HO, Kendall FP, Boynton DA: *Posture and Pain*. Baltimore, MD: Williams and Wilkins, 1952.

Spinal and Extremity Muscles

Spinal Muscles

Iliocostalis Thoracis. The iliocostalis thoracis consists of several muscle straps that link the thoracic vertebrae and sacrum with the lower six or seven ribs. The muscle straps have a number of tendons, varying in different individuals, which insert in all angles in the lower six ribs. The function of the muscle is to extend the spine when working bilaterally and to side bend the spine ipsilaterally when working alone. The iliocostalis consists of three subdivisions—iliocostalis lumborum, iliocostalis thoracis, and iliocostalis cervicis—which are a part of the external portion of the long erector spinae muscle group. The muscle receives its nerve supply by the posterior (dorsal) rami of the thoracic nerves.

Longissimus Thoracis. The longissimus thoracis muscles originate with the intercostalis muscles from the transverse processes of the lower thoracic vertebrae. They insert into all of the ribs and into the ends of the transverse processes of the upper lumbar vertebrae. The function of the muscle is to extend the spine when working bilaterally and to side bend the spine ipsilaterally when working alone. The muscle is innervated by the posterior (dorsal) rami of the thoracic nerves.

Spinalis Thoracis. The spinalis thoracis muscle (spinalis dorsi) originates from the spinous processes of the upper lumbar and two lower thoracic vertebrae. It inserts in the spinous processes of the middle and upper thoracic vertebrae. The function of the muscle is to extend the spine. The muscle is innervated by the posterior (dorsal) rami of the thoracic nerves.

Semispinalis Thoracis. The semispinalis thoracis consists of long straps of muscle that stretch along and surround the vertebrae of the spine. The muscle can have between four and eight upper ends, which originate from the transverse processes of the T6–10. These straps of muscle insert in the spinous processes of the first four thoracic and fifth and seventh processes of C6–T4. The function of the muscle is to extend the spine when working bilaterally and to rotate the spine contralaterally when working alone. The semispinalis thoracis is innervated by the posterior (dorsal) rami of the thoracic nerves.

Multifidus. The multifidus is a deep back muscle that runs along the entire spine and lies deep to the erector spinae muscles. It originates from the sacrum, sacroiliac ligament, mammillary processes of the lumbar vertebrae, transverse processes of the thoracic vertebrae, and the articular processes of the last four cervical vertebrae. The multifidus consists of numerous bundles of fibers that cross over two to five vertebrae at a time and insert into the entire length of the spinous process above. The function of the muscle is to extend the spine when working bilaterally and to minimally rotate the spine contralaterally when working alone. The thoracic multifidus is innervated by the posterior (dorsal) rami of the thoracic spinal nerves.

Rotatores Thoracis (Longus and Brevis). The rotatores muscles are deep spinal muscles that lie beneath the multifidus muscles. The rotatores brevis muscle lies just deep to the rotatores longus muscle. The rotatores muscles are the best developed in the thoracic region. There are a total of 11 small, quadrilateral rotatores muscles on each side of the spine. Each muscle arises from the transverse process of the vertebra and extends inward to the vertebra above. The rotatores muscles help rotate the appropriate thoracic segment. They are innervated by posterior (dorsal) rami of the thoracic spinal nerves.

Intertransversarii. The intratransversals are small muscles located between the transverse process of the vertebrae. In the thoracic region, they are single-bellied muscles and exist only from T10–11 to T12–L1. The function of the muscle is to ipsilaterally side bend the spine. The muscle is innervated by the posterior (dorsal) rami of the thoracic spinal nerves.

The other spinal muscles of the thoracic region act primarily on the cervical spine. These include the trapezius, levator scapulae, and anterior, posterior, and middle scalenes (see Chap. 25).

Extremity Muscles. The muscles of the thoracic region that act primarily on the extremities include the pectoralis major, latissimus dorsi, and serratus anterior (see Chap. 16).

Respiratory Muscles

The respiratory system is essentially a robust, multimuscle pump (Fig. 27-3). Connections to the respiratory mechanism have been found to exert a strong influence on such areas as the shoulder and pelvic girdles, as well as the head and neck. The primary task of the respiratory muscles is to displace the chest wall and, therefore, move gas in and out of the lungs to maintain arterial blood gas and pH homeostasis. The importance of normal respiratory muscle function can be appreciated by considering that respiratory muscle failure caused by fatigue, injury, or disease could result in an inability to maintain blood gas and pH levels within an acceptable range, which could have lethal consequences. Restoration of the respiratory mechanism is, thus, an essential element of thoracic intervention.

The actions of various respiratory muscles, which are broadly classified as *inspiratory* or *expiratory*, based on their mechanical actions, are highly redundant and provide several means by which air can be effectively displaced under a host of physiologic and pathophysiologic conditions.[39,40]

At rest, movement of air into and out of the lungs is the result of the recruitment of several muscles,[41–43] and the expiratory phase of breathing at rest is also associated with active muscle participation.[44] In a resting man, the tidal volume is the result of the coordinated recruitment of the diaphragm, the parasternal intercostal, and the scalene muscles (Tables 27-1 and 27-2).[45,46]

Although some have argued that the performance of the respiratory muscles does not limit exercise tolerance in normal healthy adults,[47,48] heavy or prolonged exercise has been shown to impair respiratory muscle performance in humans.[49,50] Thus, an interest in the adaptability of respiratory muscles to endurance-type exercise has grown significantly during the last decade.

The primary muscles of respiration include the diaphragm, the sternocostal, and the intercostals. The secondary muscles of respiration are the anterior/medial scalenes, serratus posterior, pectoralis major and minor, and, with the head fixed, the sternocleidomastoid.[8]

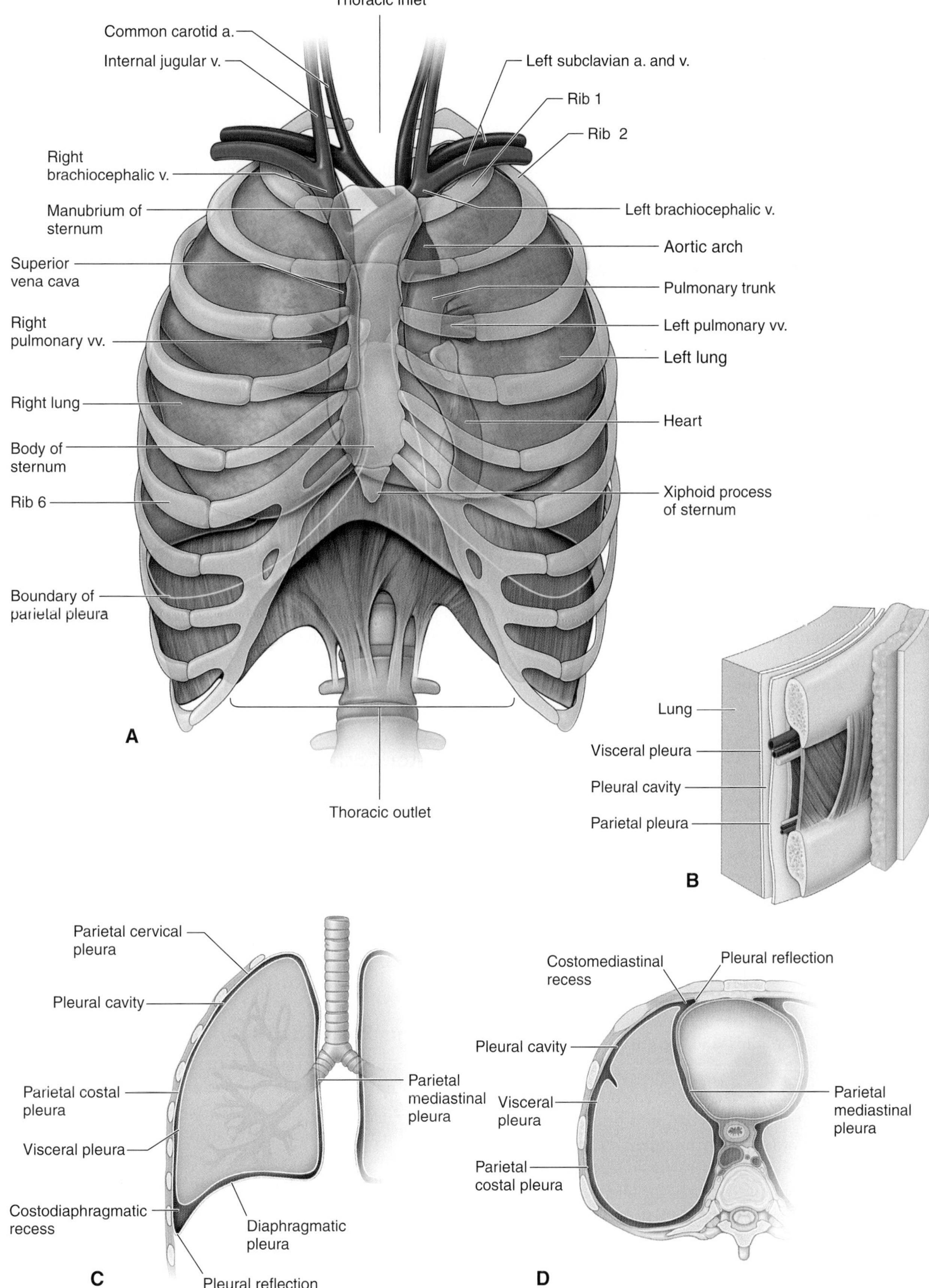

FIGURE 27-3 Components of the respiratory system. (Reproduced with permission from Morton DA, Foreman KB, Albertine KH: *The Big Picture: Gross Anatomy*, McGraw-Hill, 2011.)

Diaphragm

Anatomically, the diaphragm muscle may be divided into sternal, costal, and lumbar parts:

- The sternal fibers originate from two slips at the back of the xiphoid process.
- The costal fibers originate from the lower six ribs and their costal cartilages.
- The lumbar fibers originate from the crura of the lumbar vertebra, and the medial and lateral arcuate ligaments.

CLINICAL PEARL

Patients with bilateral diaphragm paralysis or severe weakness present a striking clinical picture, with orthopnea as the major symptom. Lesser degrees of diaphragm weakness, however, are hard to detect and need specific testing.

Functionally and metabolically, the diaphragm can be classified as two muscles[51,52]:

1. The crural (posterior) portion that inserts into the lumbar vertebrae.
2. The costal portion that inserts into the xiphoid process of the sternum and into the margins of the lower ribs.

Thus, the muscle is attached around the thoracoabdominal junction circumferentially. From these attachments, the fibers arch toward each other centrally to form a large tendon. Contraction of the diaphragm pulls the large, central tendon inferiorly, producing diaphragmatic inspiration (see later discussion). The diaphragm has a phrenic C3–4 motor innervation and a sensory supply by the lower six intercostal nerves.

Intercostals

Between the ribs are the intercostal spaces, which are deeper both in front and between the upper ribs. Between the ribs lie the internal and external intercostal muscles, with the neurovascular bundle lying beneath each rib.

The intercostal muscles, together with the sternalis (or sternocostalis or transversalis thoracis), phylogenically form from the hypomeric muscles. These muscles correspond to their abdominal counterparts, with the sternalis being homologous to the rectus abdominis, and the intercostals homologous to the external oblique.[8]

External Intercostals. The external intercostal muscles (Fig. 27-2), of which there are 11, are laid in a direction that is superoposterior to inferoanterior (run inferiorly and medially in the front of the thorax and inferiorly and laterally in the back). Because of the oblique course of the fibers, and the fact that leverage is greatest on the lower of the two ribs, the muscle pulls the lower rib toward the upper rib, which results in inspiration. The external intercostals attach to the lower border of one rib and the upper border of the rib below, extending from the tubercle to the costal cartilage. Posteriorly, the muscle is continuous with the posterior fibers of the superior costotransverse ligament. The action of the external intercostals is believed to be entirely inspiratory,[45] although the muscles also counteract the force of the diaphragm, preventing the collapse of the ribs.[42] Innervation of this muscle is supplied by the adjacent intercostal nerve.

Internal Intercostals. The internal intercostals (see Fig. 27-2), which also number 11, have their fibers in an inferoposterior to a superoanterior direction. The internal intercostals are found deep to the external intercostals and run obliquely, and perpendicular, to the externals. The posterior fibers pull the upper rib down, but only during enforced expiration.[42,45] The internal intercostals extend from the posterior rib angles to the sternum, where they end posteriorly. They are continuous with the internal membrane, which then becomes continuous with the anterior part of the superior costotransverse ligament. Innervation of this muscle group is supplied by the adjacent intercostal nerve.

Transverse Intercostals (Intima). The deepest of the intercostals, the transverse intercostals are attached to the internal aspects of two contiguous ribs. They become progressively more significant, and developed, further down the thorax. This muscle is used during forced expiration.[42,45]

Transversus Thoracis. The transversus thoracis is a triangular-shaped sheet muscle, which originates from the posterior (dorsal) surface of the sternum and covers the inner surfaces of both the sternum and the second to eighth sternal costal cartilages. The apex of the muscle points cranially, with muscle slips running inferolaterally and eventually inserting on the sternal ribs quite close to the costochondral junctions. Morphologically, the transversus thoracis is similar to the anterior (ventral) part of the transversus abdominis. Its function is to draw the costal cartilages down. The muscle is innervated by the adjacent intercostal nerves.

Levator Costae

These consist of 12 strong short muscles that turn obliquely (inferolaterally), parallel with the external intercostals, from the tip of the transverse process to the angle of the rib, extending from C7 to T11 transverse processes. These muscles, which are innervated by the lateral branch of the posterior (dorsal) ramus of the thoracic nerve, function to raise the rib, but their importance in respiration is argued. The levator costae may also be segmentally involved in rotation and side bending of the thoracic vertebra.

Serratus Posterior Superior

The serratus posterior superior runs from the lower part of the ligamentum nuchae, the spinous processes of C7 and T1–3, and their supraspinous ligaments, to the inferior border of the second through fifth ribs, lateral to the rib angle.

The muscle receives its nerve supply from the second through fifth intercostal nerves. Its function is unclear, but it is thought to elevate the ribs.[8]

Serratus Posterior Inferior

This muscle arises from the spines and supraspinous ligaments of the two lower thoracic and the two or three upper lumbar vertebrae. It attaches to the inferior border of the lower four ribs, lateral to the rib angle.

The muscle receives its nerve supply from the anterior (ventral) rami of the ninth through 12th thoracic nerves. Its

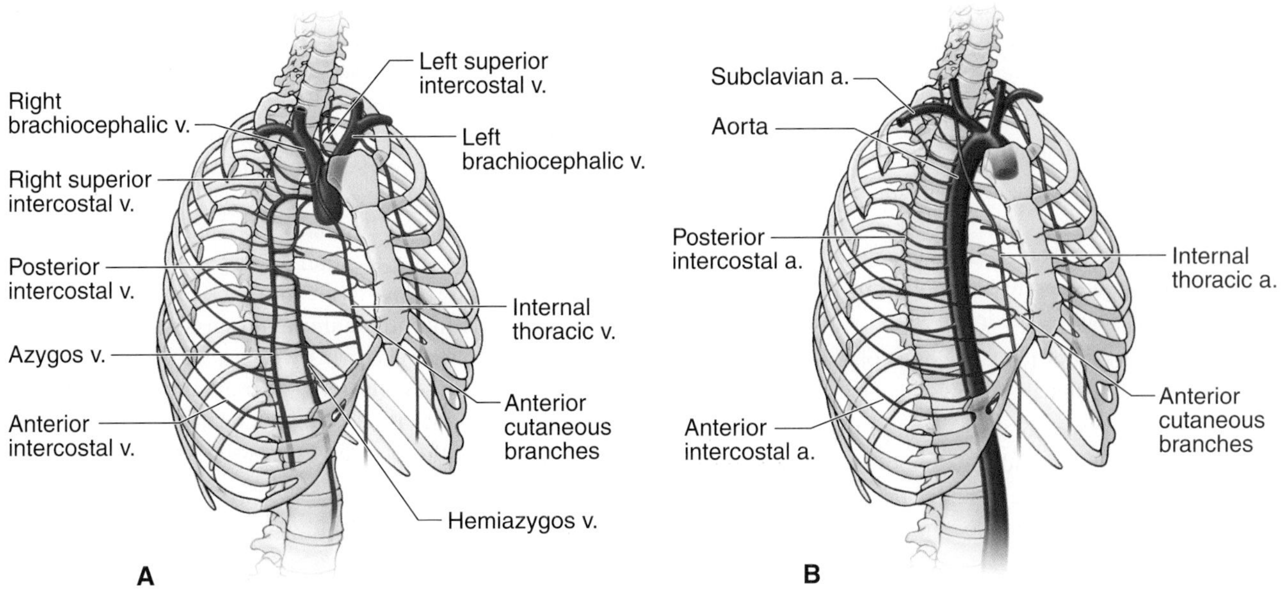

FIGURE 27-4 Vasculature of the thoracic region. (Reproduced with permission from Morton DA, Foreman KB, Albertine KH: *The Big Picture: Gross Anatomy*, McGraw-Hill, 2011.)

function is unclear, but it is thought to pull the ribs downward and backward.

Vascular Supply

The blood supply to this region is provided mainly by the posterior (dorsal) branches of the posterior intercostal arteries (Fig. 27-4), while the venous drainage occurs through the anterior and posterior venous plexuses. The spinal cord region between T4 and T9 is poorly vascularized.[53]

Neurology

The spinal canal in this region is narrow, with only a small epidural space between the cord and its osseous environment.[53] Innervation of the thoracic spinal canal is by the sinuvertebral nerve, which arises from the nerve root and reenters the epidural space.

The thoracic spinal cord is unusually susceptible to injury because it occupies a greater percentage of the total cross-sectional area of its surrounding spinal canal than do the cervical or lumbar sections of the spinal cord, and the thoracic cord is tightly packed in the canal and easily injured by displaced fragments of bone or disk material.[54] Furthermore, the blood supply of the mid-thoracic spinal cord is tenuous, and seemingly trivial injuries can disrupt the blood supply to a substantial portion of the thoracic cord and result in devastating neurologic deficits.[55]

In the thoracic region, there is great variability in the topography of the nerves and the structures that they serve.[56] Typically, the spinal root arises from the lateral end of the spinal nerve but, in 25% of cases, the spinal root is made up of two parts that arise from the superior border of the spinal nerve.[57] The thoracic spinal nerves are segmented into posterior (dorsal) primary and anterior (ventral) primary divisions (see Chap. 3). As elsewhere, the dermatomes of this region are considered to represent the cutaneous region innervated by one spinal nerve through both of its rami.[58]

The peripheral nerves, which travel through the thoracic spine and chest wall, include the posterior (dorsal) scapular, thoracodorsal, and long thoracic nerves (see Chap. 3).

BIOMECHANICS

Knowledge of the regional biomechanics of the thoracic spine and rib cage assists the clinician in the interpretation of active movement and motion palpation examination in relation to the patient's symptoms.[59] The thoracic spinal segments possess the potential for a distinctive array of movements. Most of the understanding with regard to the biomechanics of the thoracic spine is based largely on the ex vivo studies of White,[22] and Panjabi et al.,[1,60] and a variety of 'clinical models.'[28,61] In addition, although normative ranges of spinal motion have been reported for the lumbar spine, no such reliable data exists for the thoracic region.[62]

It is widely recognized that the mechanical behavior of the spine is influenced by load.[63] Axial load has been shown to increase motion segment stiffness and decrease mobility. In addition, due to the modifying influence of the cage-like structure of the ribs, which provide a significant degree of stability,[36] and the kyphotic shape of the curve, the biomechanics of the thoracic spine is considerably different from those of the lumbar and cervical regions. The increased stability/reduced mobility of the thoracic segments has been reported to produce three primary affects[23,64]:

1. It influences the motions available in other spinal regions as well as the shoulder girdle.
2. It increases the potential for postural impairments.[65]
3. It provides an important weight-bearing mechanism for the vertebral column.[66] The load-bearing capacity of the spine has been found to be up to three times greater with an intact rib cage.[37,67]

Other biomechanical studies have investigated the stabilizing effects of the individual components of the thoracic spine[34,68]:

- The IVD can be regarded as the most important stabilizer in the thoracic functional unit mechanics.
- The rib head joints serve as stabilizing structures to the human thoracic spine under flexion–extension, side bending, and axial rotation loading, and resection after diskectomy increases range of motion by approximately 80% under all loading modes.
- The lateral portion of the facet joints plays an important role in providing spinal stability.
- In the thoracic spine, total resection of the posterior ligamentous complex leads to an approximately 40% increase in range of motion under flexion–extension, side bending, and axial rotation loading.

Flexion

Flexion of the thoracic spine in weight bearing is initiated by the abdominal muscles and, in the absence of resistance, is continued by gravity, with the spinal erector muscles eccentrically controlling the descent. Flexion may also occur during bilateral scapular protraction.

There are about 4–5 degrees of flexion available at the upper thoracic levels, 6–8 degrees in the middle layers, and 9–15 degrees in the lower levels,[22] giving an overall total range for thoracic flexion of 20–45 degrees.[69] End-range flexion is resisted by the posterior half of annulus and by the impaction of the zygapophyseal joints.

According to Lee,[29] flexion of the cervicothoracic region consists of an anterior rotation of the head of the rib and a superoanterior glide of the zygapophyseal joints, whereas extension and arm elevation in this region consists of a posterior sagittal rotation and posterior translation of the superior vertebra. This latter action pushes the superior aspect of the head of the rib posteriorly at the costovertebral joint, producing a posterior rotation of the rib (the anterior aspect travels superiorly, while the posterior aspect travels inferiorly).[29]

In the remainder of the thorax, flexion results from the superior facets (i.e., the inferior articular processes of the superior vertebra of the segment) gliding superiorly and anteriorly[28] (Table 27-3). This motion at the zygapophyseal joint is accompanied by an anterior translation of the superior vertebra, and a slight distraction of the centrum. It seems likely that the anterior vertebral translation produces a similar motion in the ribs, with a superior glide occurring at the costotransverse joint. During this motion, the anterior aspects of the ribs approximate each other, while the posterior aspects separate.

Studies have shown that the thoracic zygapophyseal facets play an important role in stabilization of the thoracic spine during flexion loading.[60,70]

Extension

Extension of the thoracic spine is produced principally by the lumbar extensors and results in an inferior glide of the superior facet of the zygapophyseal joint (see Table 27-3). One to two degrees of extension is available at each thoracic segment, giving an overall average of 15–20 degrees of thoracic extension for the entire thoracic spine.

Extension of the thoracic spine is restrained by the relative stiffness of the anterior IVD; the anterior longitudinal ligament; bony contact of the posterior elements, including the inferior facet onto the lamina below; and the spinous processes.[23,60] Given the location of the axis of rotation for extension, which is close to the moving segment, more translation than rotation occurs during extension.[71]

The joint motions occurring with extension are essentially the opposite of those of flexion. The translation of the vertebra occurs in a posterior direction, with an accompanying slight compression of the centra. The posterior translation that occurs with extension is controlled by the posteriorly directed lamellae of the annulus, and by the capsule of the zygapophyseal joint.

The transitional region between the thoracic and lumbar spines can produce an inflexion point that may serve to reduce the bending forces in the sagittal plane.[6] However, stiffness in this area also may result in the thoracic spine pivoting over the thoracolumbar region, thereby increasing the risk of compression fracture (see Chap. 5).[72]

In addition to those motions occurring at the zygapophyseal joints and the vertebral body during thoracic extension, motion also occurs at the rib articulations. The ribs rotate posteriorly, with the posterior aspects approximating and the anterior aspects separating, and an inferior glide occurs at the costotransverse joint.[29]

Side Bending

Side bending of the thoracic spine is initiated by the ipsilateral abdominals and erector muscles, and then continued by gravity. A total of 25–45 degrees of side bending is available in the thoracic spine, at an average of about 3–4 degrees to each side per segment, with the lower segments averaging slightly more, at 7–9 degrees, each.[22,73]

At the zygapophyseal joints, the primary motion involves the ipsilateral superior facet gliding inferiorly, and the contralateral gliding superiorly (see Table 27-3). In effect, the ipsilateral zygapophyseal joint extends while the contralateral flexes. Side bending is restrained by the compression of the IVD and approximation of the ribs.

Side bending in the upper thoracic spine is associated with ipsilateral rotation and ipsilateral translation.[74] According to Lee,[29] the coupling that occurs in the rest of the thoracic spine depends on which of the two coupling motions initiates the movement. If side bending initiates the movement, it is called *latexion*, and the biomechanics consist of side bending, contralateral rotation, and ipsilateral translation. The mechanism of this coupling, or actually tripling, is not certain, and one must guard against strong conclusions. The postulated mechanism is as follows: with side bending, a contralateral convex curve is produced. This causes the ribs on the convex side of the curve to separate and those on the concave side to approximate.[29] Trunk side bending is essentially halted, by soft tissue tension or rib approximation, or both, and the ribs become fixed. Further side

TABLE 27-3 Biomechanics of the Thorax

Motions	Z Joint	Rib Motion	Costotransverse Joint
Vertebromanubrial (T1–2)			
Flexion	Superoanterior glide	Anterior rotation	NA
Extension	Inferoposterior glide	Posterior rotation	NA
Latexion	Ipsilateral coupling	NA	NA
Rotexion	Ipsilateral coupling	NA	NA
Inspiration	NA	Elevation	NA
Expiration	NA	Depression	NA
Vertebrosternal (T3–7)			
Flexion	Superoanterior glide	Varies (very mobile) anteroposterior rotation	Superior–inferior glide (varies)
Extension	Posteroinferior glide	Varies (very mobile) anteroposterior rotation	Superior–inferior glide (varies)
Latexion	Ipsilateral side bend and contralateral rotation	Ipsilateral—anterior rotation Contralateral—posterior rotation	Ipsilateral—superior glide Contralateral—inferior glide
Rotexion	Ipsilateral side bend and ipsilateral rotation	Ipsilateral—posterior rotation Contralateral—anterior rotation	Ipsilateral—inferior glide Contralateral—superior glide
Inspiration	NA	Posterior rotation bilaterally	Inferior glide
Expiration	NA	Anterior rotation bilaterally	Superior glide
Vertebrochonral (T8–10)			
Flexion	Superoanterior glide	Anterior rotation	SMP glide
Extension	Inferoposterior glide	Posterior rotation	ILA glide
Latexion	Varies	NA	Apex in line with trochanter Ipsilateral—SMP Contralateral—ILA If not, the reverse occurs
Rotexion	Ipsilateral—inferior glide Contralateral—superior glide	NA	Ipsilateral—ILA, then anteromedial Contralateral—SMP, then posterolateral glide
Inspiration	NA	NA	ILA glide
Expiration	NA	NA	SMP glide

NA, not applicable; SMP, superior medial posterior; ILA, inferior lateral anterior.

bending is modified by the fixed ribs.[29] The ipsilateral articular facet of the transverse process glides inferiorly on its rib, resulting in a relative anterior rotation of the neck of the rib, while the contralateral transverse process glides superiorly, producing a posterior rotation of the rib neck.[29] The effect of these bilateral rib rotations is to force the superior vertebra into rotation away from the direction of side bending.

Rotation

The axis of rotation for the thoracic spine varies according to the vertebral level.[75] The axis of rotation lies within the vertebral body in the mid-thoracic joints, but anterior to the vertebral body in the upper and lower joints.[75] Almost pure rotation can occur in the mid-thoracic region, whereas, in the upper and lower segments, rotation can be associated with side bending to either side (see Table 27-3). Axial rotation (rotexion) is produced either by the abdominal muscles and other trunk rotators or by the unilateral elevation of the arm. Pure axial rotation (twisting) can only occur at two points in the spine: at the thoracolumbar and cervicothoracic junctions.

A total of 35–50 degrees of rotation is available in the thoracic spine.[22,73] Segmental axial rotation in the thoracic spine averages 7 degrees in the upper thoracic area, approximately 5 degrees in the middle thoracic spine, and 2–3 degrees in the last two or three segments.[22,69,76] Torsional stiffness is enhanced in the thoracolumbar region by the mortise-type morphology of the zygapophyseal joints and the near sagittal alignment of the upper lumbar articulations.[23,27,66,72,77]

According to MacConaill and Basmajian,[30] thoracic segmental rotation is coupled with contralateral side bending and contralateral translation. However, this finding deviates from what is generally observed clinically, where the coupling of rotation and side bending that occurs seems to depend on the segmental level and the integrity of the joint.

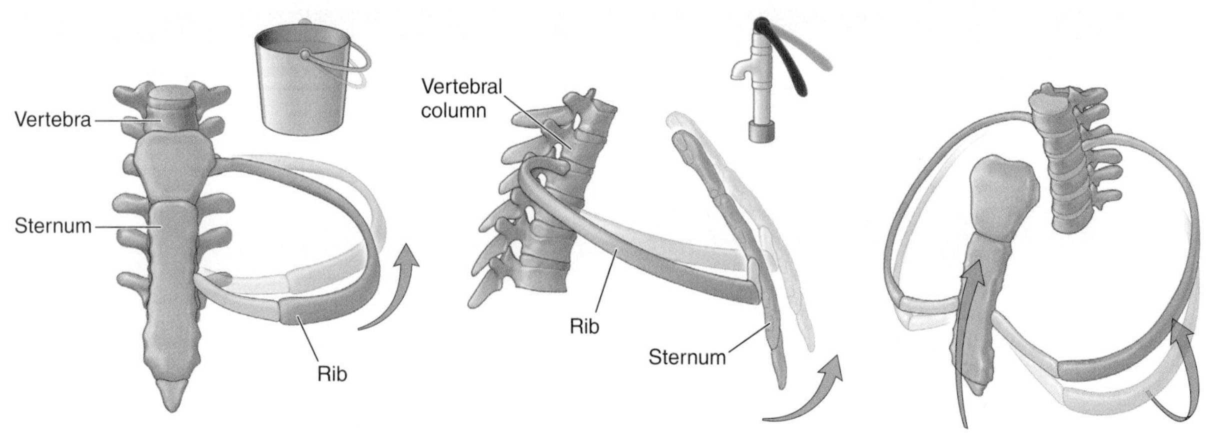

FIGURE 27-5 Bucket and pump handle rib motions. (Reproduced with permission from Morton DA, Foreman KB, Albertine KH: *The Big Picture: Gross Anatomy*, McGraw-Hill, 2011.)

Respiration

The ribs function as levers, with the fulcrum represented by the rib angle, the effort arm represented by the neck, and the load arm represented by the shaft. Because of the relatively small size of the rib neck, a small movement at the rib neck will produce a large degree of movement in the shaft.

The shapes of the articular facets of the upper six ribs would suggest that the upward and downward gliding movements that occur would produce spinning of the neck of the rib. In fact, the main movement in the upper six ribs during respiration and other movements is one of the rotations of the neck of the rib, with only small amounts of superior and inferior motion. In the seventh through 10th ribs, the principal movement is upward, backward, and medially during inspiration, with the reverse occurring during expiration.[28]

Because the anterior end of the ribs is lower than the posterior, when the ribs elevate, they rise upward, while the rib neck drops down. In the upper ribs, this results in an anterior elevation (pump handle) and in the middle and lower ribs (excluding the free ribs), a lateral elevation (bucket handle), with the former movement increasing the anteroposterior diameter of the thoracic cavity and the latter increasing the transverse diameter (Fig. 27-5).

Both kinds of rib motion are produced by the action of the diaphragm. The seventh through 10th ribs act to increase the abdominal cavity free space to afford space for the descending diaphragm. As the ends of these ribs are elevated, they push up on each other, lifting each successive rib upward and finally lifting the sternum. The two lower ribs are depressed by the quadratus lumborum to provide a stable base of action for the diaphragm.

Quiet respiration involves very little zygapophyseal joint motion.

Inspiration

During inspiration, the diaphragm descends and pulls the central tendon inferiorly through the fixed 12th ribs and L1–3 (Fig. 27-6). When the maximum extensibility (distention) of the abdominal wall is reached, the central tendon becomes stationary. Further contraction of the diaphragm produces an elevation and posterior rotation of the lower six ribs, with torsion of the anterior costal cartilage, and an anterosuperior thrust of the sternum (and eventually the inferior aspect of the manubrium).

During inspiration in the normal population, because the second rib is longer than the first, the superior aspect of the manubrium is forced to tilt posteriorly as its inferior edge is moved anteriorly. As the top of the manubrium tilts back, the clavicle rolls anteriorly. Because the lower ribs are longer, the inferior sternum moves further anteriorly than the superior section during inspiration. The manubriosternal junction acts as the hinge for this motion. If this joint stiffens or ossifies, respiratory function will suffer. In addition, if the central tendon stiffens, inspiration will have to be accomplished, with the ribs moving laterally.

Forced inspiration produces an increase in the activity level of the diaphragm, intercostals, scaleni, and quadratus lumborum. In addition, new activity occurs in the sternocleidomastoid, trapezius, both pectorals and serratus anterior.

During inspiration, the ribs move with the sternum in an upward and forward direction, increasing the anteroposterior diameter of the chest while posteriorly rotating. The tubercles and costotransverse joints of[29]

- T1–7 glide inferiorly;
- T8–10 glide in an anterolateral and inferior direction;
- T11 and T12 remain stationary, except for slight caliper motion increasing the lateral dimension.

Expiration

Quiet expiration occurs passively (Fig. 27-6). During forced expiration, there is activity in a number of muscles (Table 27-1). During expiration, the ribs rotate anteriorly and the tubercles and costotransverse joints of[29]

- T1–7 glide superiorly;
- T8–10 glide in a posteromedial and superior direction;
- T11 and T12 remain stationary, except for slight caliper motion decreasing the lateral dimension.

It may be possible to detect a subluxation of the costotransverse joints by palpating the ipsilateral transverse process

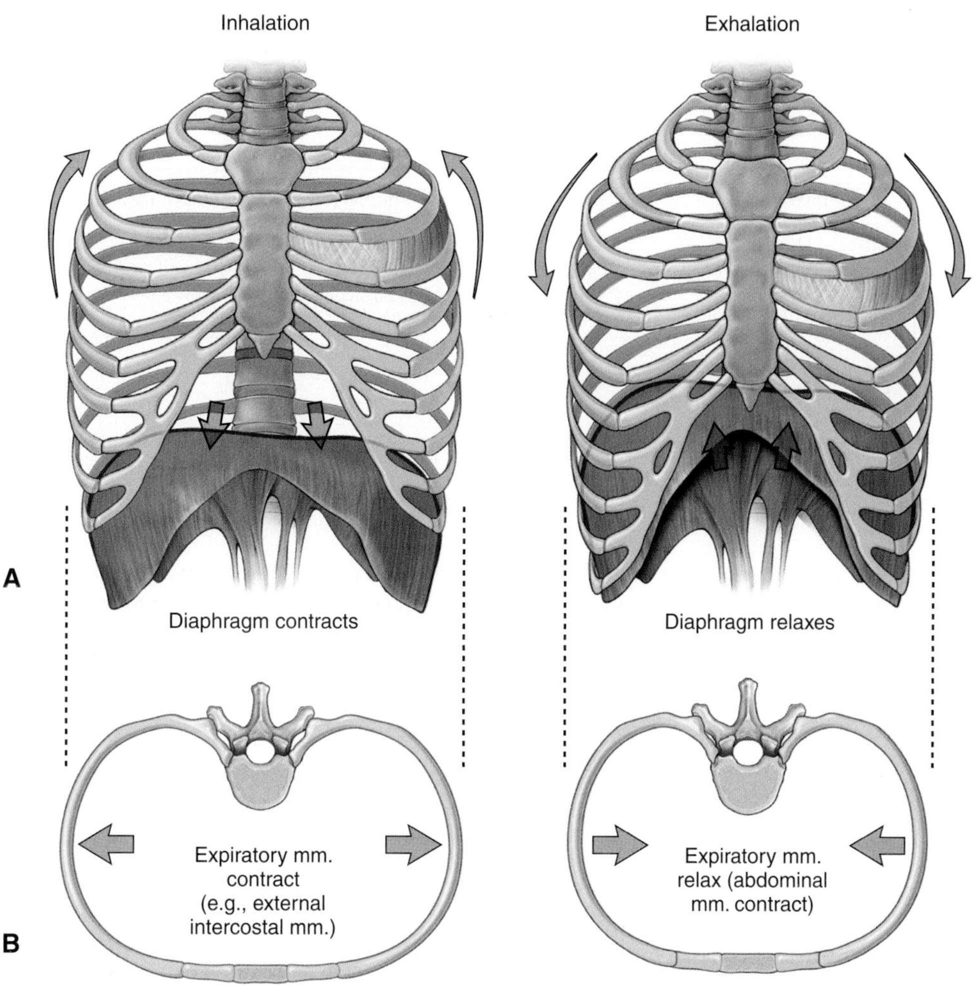

FIGURE 27-6 Biomechanics of respiration. (Reproduced with permission from Morton DA, Foreman KB, Albertine KH: *The Big Picture: Gross Anatomy,* McGraw-Hill, 2011.)

and rib during inspiration and thoracic side bending.[29] For example, a superior subluxation of the right rib may produce the following:

- A decreased inferior glide of the rib
- A decreased thoracic motion in the directions of left side bending and right rotation

The findings for other rib dysfunctions are outlined in Table 27-4.

EXAMINATION

Differential diagnosis of thoracic pain can be difficult. This is due to the complicated biomechanics and function of the region, the proximity to vital organs, and the many articulations. Bogduk[78] has cited the following anatomical structures as possible causes of thoracic spine pain: posterior thoracic muscles, spinous processes, anterior and posterior longitudinal ligaments, vertebral bodies, zygapophyseal and

TABLE 27-4 Rib Dysfunctions

Dysfunction	Rib Angle	Intercostal Space	Anterior Rib	Thoracic Findings
Anterior subluxation	Less prominent	Tender	NA	More prominent
Posterior subluxation	More prominent	Tender	NA	Less prominent
External rib torsion	Prominent and tender superior border	Wide above and narrow below	ERS, ipsilateral at the level above	NA
Internal rib torsion	Prominent and tender inferior border	Narrow above and wide below	FRS, contralateral at the level above	NA

ERS, extended, rotated, and side flexed; FRS, flexed, rotated, and side flexed; NA, not applicable.
Data from Bookhout MR: Evaluation of the thoracic spine and rib cage. In: Flynn TW, ed. *The Thoracic Spine and Rib Cage: Musculoskeletal Evaluation and Treatment.* Boston, MA: Butterworth-Heinemann, 1996:147–167.

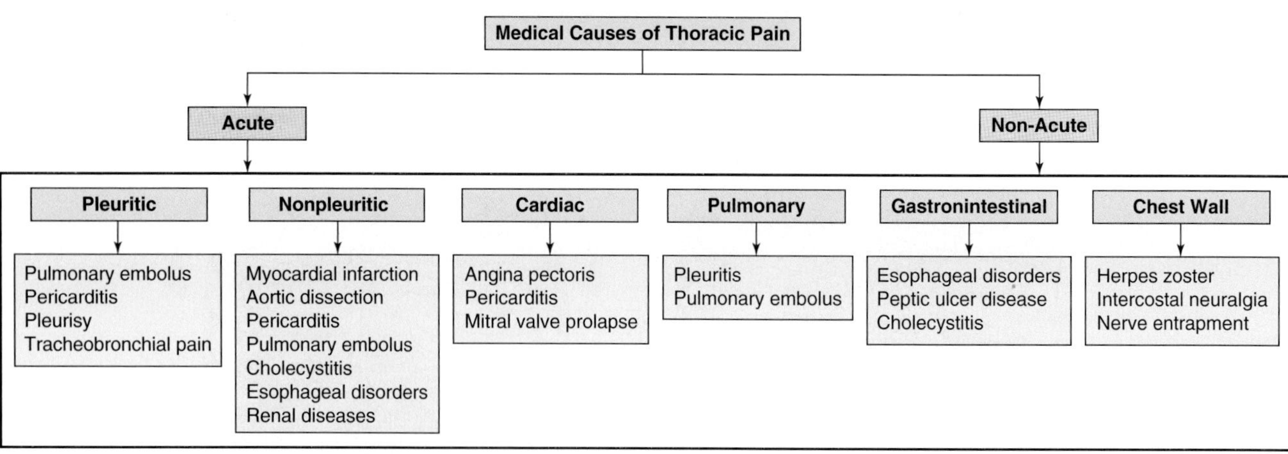

FIGURE 27-7 Medical causes of thoracic symptoms.

costotransverse joints, inferior articular process, pars interarticularis, IVD, nerve root, joint meniscus, and dura mater. Pain arising from inflammation of the axial spine can mimic a variety of serious conditions, including cardiac/pulmonary pathology, renal colic, fracture, a tumor, or numerous visceral and retroperitoneal abnormalities, including abdominal aortic aneurysm.[79]

The thoracic spine is less commonly implicated in musculoskeletal pain syndromes than the lumbar and cervical spines, and when it does occur, there is some disagreement as to whether the ribs or the intervertebral joints are the major source of the biomechanical dysfunction. Complicating matters is the fact that pain arising from the thoracic spinal joints has considerable overlap and can refer symptoms to distal regions (groin, pubis, and lower abdominal wall) (refer to Chap. 5). Apart from musculoskeletal lesions, the thoracic spine is also a common source of systemic pain, and the phenomenon of referred pain poses more diagnostic difficulties in the thoracic spine than in any other region of the vertebral column (Fig. 27-7).[78] The algorithm outlined in Fig. 27-8 can serve as a guide to the examination of the thoracic spine and ribs.

History

The history should include the chief complaints and a pain drawing. Referred chest pain patterns are outlined in Table 27-5. In addition to those questions listed under History in Chapter 4, the following questions should be asked by the clinician:

- Was there a mechanism of injury? Any information regarding the onset is important. For example, most rib injuries are commonly caused by direct trauma. If there was no mechanism of injury a disease process such as scoliosis could be indicated. Costovertebral and costotransverse joint hypomobility and active trigger points are possible sources of upper thoracic pain.[80]
- Do the symptoms occur with breathing? Symptoms reproduced with respiration could indicate a rib dysfunction or pleuritic pain. If the symptoms are aggravated on exertion, the clinician should focus on the relationship of specific movements or activities. Any information regarding the onset, as well as aggravating factors, is important, especially if the pain appears only during certain positions or movements, which would suggest a musculoskeletal lesion. Deep breathing or arm elevation tends to aggravate a rib dysfunction.
- Are the symptoms provoked or alleviated with movement or posture? This type of history indicates a musculoskeletal dysfunction. Chronic problems in this area tend to result from postural dysfunctions. Pain of a mechanical origin tends to worsen throughout the day but is relieved with rest.
- What activities tend to aggravate the symptoms? Pulling and pushing activities typically worsen thoracic symptoms. Aggravation of localized pain by coughing, sneezing, or deep inspiration tends to implicate the costovertebral joint.[81]
- Is the pain deep, superficial, aching, burning, or stabbing? The patient is asked to describe the quality of the pain. Thoracic nerve root pain is often sharp, stabbing, and severe, although it can also have a burning quality. Nerve pain usually is referred in a sloping band along an intercostal space.[20] Vascular pain and visceral pain often are described as being poorly localized and achy. A sudden onset of pain related to trauma could indicate a fracture, muscle strain, or ligament sprain.

CLINICAL PEARL

Pain from a musculoskeletal lesion in this area can vary from a dull ache to a feeling of local fatigue and cramping. Musculoskeletal pain is usually sharp and well localized, whereas muscle or tendon pain is typically dull and aching. Bone pain usually feels very deep and boring.

- Where is the pain located? The patient should be asked to point to the area of pain. If the patient has difficulty localizing the pain, the clinician should suspect referred pain as the source. If the symptoms appear to be referred to the upper or lower extremities, or the head and neck, further investigation is required.
- Are the symptoms related to digestion? Some visceral conditions such as ulcers, can be referred to T4-T6 posteriorly.

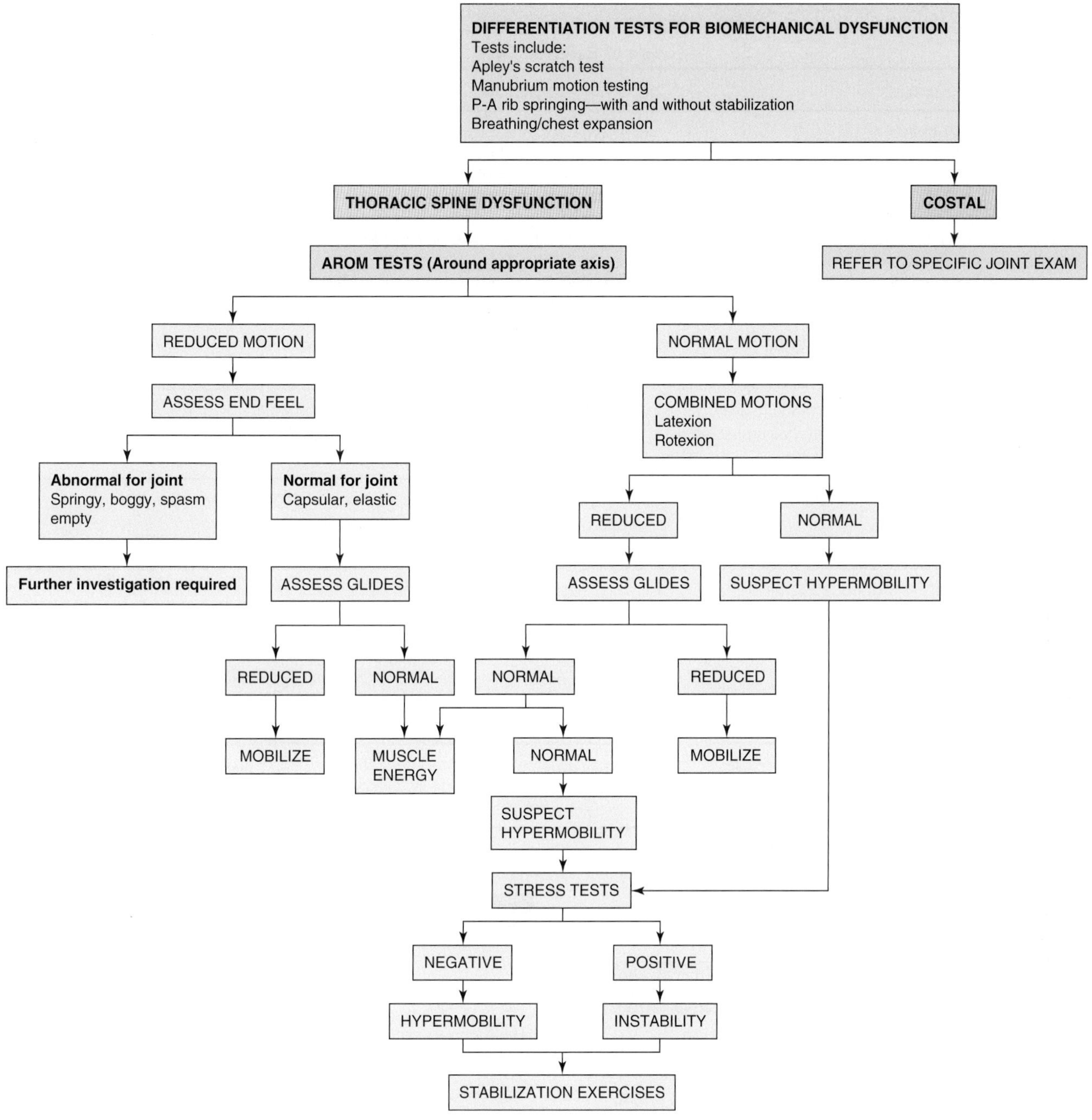

FIGURE 27-8 Thoracic spine examination algorithm.

The administration of the Oswestry Low Back Disability Questionnaire (Table 5-2), Neck Disability Index (Table 5-3), and McGill Pain Questionnaire (Chap. 4) may be helpful in determining the quality of pain and its effect on function.[82–84]

Systems Review

Thoracic pain may originate from just about all of the viscera (Table 27-6; see also Chap. 5). Both visceral and somatic afferent nerves transmit pain messages from a peripheral stimulus and converge on the same projection neurons in the posterior (dorsal) horn. Visceral pain tends to be vague and dull and may be accompanied by nausea and sweating (see Chap. 5). To help differentiate between visceral pain and musculoskeletal pain, the clinician should focus on the relationship of specific movements or activities. A medical screening questionnaire for the thoracic spine and rib cage region is provided in Table 27-7.

The thoracolumbar outflow of the autonomic nervous system (see Chap. 3) has its location here. Stimulation of this outflow can lead to the presence of facilitated segments, and trophic changes in the skin of the periphery.[85]

Systemic illnesses, such as rheumatoid arthritis and malignancy, and conditions causing referred pain must be included in the differential diagnosis. Nonmusculoskeletal causes of thoracic pain (Table 27-8)[86] include the following:

- Dissecting aortic aneurysm.
- Myocardial infarction.
- Intercostal neuralgia.

TABLE 27-5 Chest Pain Patterns

Origin of Pain	Site of Referred Pain	Type of Disorder
Substernal or retrosternal	Neck, jaw, back, left shoulder and arm, and abdomen	Angina
Substernal, anterior chest	Neck, jaw, back, and bilateral arms	Myocardial infarction
Substernal or above the sternum	Next, upper back, upper trapezius, supraclavicular area, left arm, and costal margin	Pericarditis
Anterior chest (thoracic aneurysm); abdomen (abdominal aneurysm)	Posterior thoracic, chest, neck, shoulders, interscapular, or lumbar region	Dissecting aortic aneurysm
Variable	Variable, depending on structures involved.	Musculoskeletal
Costochondritis (inflammation of the costal cartilage): sternum and rib margins.	Abdominal oblique trigger points: pain referred up into the chest area.	
Upper rectus abdominis trigger points (left side), pectoralis, serratus anterior, and sternalis muscles: precordial pain	Pectoralis trigger points: pain referred down medial bilateral arms along ulnar nerve distribution (fourth and fifth fingers)	
Precordium region (upper central abdomen and diaphragm)	Sternum, axillary lines, and either side of vertebrae; lateral and anterior chest wall; occasionally to one or both arms	Neurological
Substernal, epigastric, and upper abdominal quadrants	Around chest area, shoulders, and upper back region	Gastrointestinal
Within breast tissue; may be localized in pectoral and supraclavicular regions	Chest area, axilla, mid-back, and neck and posterior shoulder girdle	Breast pain
Commonly substernal and anterior chest region	No referred pain	Anxiety

Data from Donato EB: Physical examination procedures to screen for serious disorders of the head, neck, chest, and upper quarter. In: Wilmarth MA, ed. *Medical Screening for the Physical Therapist. Orthopaedic Section Independent Study Course 14.1.1.* La Crosse, WI: Orthopaedic Section, APTA, Inc., 2003:1–43; Goodman CC, Boissonnault WG: *Pathology: Implications for the Physical Therapist*. Philadelphia, PA: WB Saunders, 1998.

TABLE 27-6 Symptoms and Possible Causes of Thoracic Pain

Indication	Possible Condition
Severe bilateral root pain in elderly	Neoplasm (most common areas for metastasis are lung, breast, prostate, and kidney)
Wedging/compression fracture	Osteoporotic (estrogen deficiency) or neoplastic fracture
Onset–offset of pain unrelated to trunk movements	Ankylosing spondylitis, visceral
Decreased active motion: contralateral side flexion painful, with both rotations full	Neoplasm
Severe chest wall pain without articular pain	Visceral
Spinal cord signs and symptoms	Spinal cord pressure or ischemia
Pain onset related to eating or diet	Visceral

TABLE 27-7 Medical Screening Questionnaire for the Thoracic Spine and Rib Cage Region

	Yes	No
Do you have a history of heart problems?		
Have you recently taken a nitroglycerin tablet?		
Do you take medication for hypertension?		
Have you been or are you now a smoker?		
Have you had a recent surgery?		
Have you recently been bedridden?		
Have you recently noticed that it is difficult for you to breathe, laugh, sneeze, or cough?		
Have you recently had a fever, infection, or other illness?		
Have you recently received a blow to the chest, such as during a fall or motor vehicle accident?		
Are your symptoms relieved after eating?		
Does eating fatty food increase your symptoms?		
Do you currently have a kidney stone, or have you had one in the past?		
Do you experience severe back or flank pain that comes on suddenly?		

Data from: DuVall RE, Godges J: Introduction to physical therapy differential diagnosis: The clinical utility of subjective examination. In: Wilmarth MA, ed. *Medical Screening for the Physical Therapist. Orthopaedic Section Independent Study Course 14.1.1.* La Crosse, WI: Orthopaedic Section, APTA, Inc, 2003:1–44.

TABLE 27-8 Red Flags for the Thoracic Spine and Rib Cage

Condition	Red Flags
Myocardial infarction	Chest pain Pallor, sweating, dyspnea, nausea, or palpitations Presence of risk factors: previous history of coronary heart disease, hypertension, smoking, diabetes, and elevated blood serum cholesterol (>240 mg/dL) Men aged over 40 years and women aged over 50 years Symptoms lasting greater than 30 min and not relieved with sublingual nitroglycerin
Stable angina pectoris	Chest pain or pressure that occurs with predictable levels of exertion (if not, suspect unstable angina pectoris) Symptoms are also predictably alleviated with the rest or sublingual nitroglycerin (if not, suspect unstable angina pectoris)
Pericarditis	Sharp or stabbing chest pain that may be referred to the lateral neck or either shoulder Increased pain with left side lying Relieved with forward lean while sitting (supporting arms on knees or a table)
Pulmonary embolus	Chest, shoulder, or upper abdominal pain Dyspnea
Pleurisy	Severe, sharp knife-like pain with inspiration History of a recent or coexisting respiratory disorder (e.g., infection, pneumonia, tumor, or tuberculosis)
Pneumothorax	Chest pain that is intensified with inspiration, ventilation, or expanding rib cage Recent bout of coughing or strenuous exercise or trauma Hyperresonance upon percussion Decreased breath sounds
Pneumonia	Pleuritic pain that may be referred to shoulder Fever, chills, headache, malaise, or nausea Productive cough
Cholecystitis	Colicky pain in the right upper abdominal quadrant with accompanying right scapula pain Symptoms may worsen with ingestion of fatty foods Symptoms unaffected by activity or rest
Peptic ulcer	Dull, gnawing pain, or burning sensation in the epigastrium, mid-back, or supraclavicular regions Symptoms relieved with food Localized tenderness at the right epigastrium Constipation, bleeding, vomiting, tarry colored stools, and coffee ground emeses
Pyelonephritis	Recent or coexisting urinary tract infection Enlarged prostate Kidney stone or past kidney stone
Nephrolithiasis (kidney stones)	Sudden, severe back, or flank pain Chills and fever Nausea or vomiting Renal colic Symptoms of urinary tract infection Reside in hot and humid environment Past episode(s) of kidney stone(s)

Data from DuVall RE, Godges J: Introduction to physical therapy differential diagnosis: the clinical utility of subjective examination. In: Wilmarth MA, ed. *Medical Screening for the Physical Therapist. Orthopaedic Section Independent Study Course 14.1.1.* La Crosse, WI: Orthopaedic Section, APTA, Inc, 2004:1–32.

Data from Canto JG, Shlipak MG, Rogers WJ, et al: Prevalence, clinical characteristics, and mortality among patients with myocardial infarction presenting without chest pain. *JAMA* 283:3223–3229, 2000.

Data from Culic V, Eterovic D, Miric D, et al: Symptom presentation of acute myocardial infarction: influence of sex, age, and risk factors. *Am Heart J* 144:1012–1017, 2002.

Data from Henderson JM: Ruling out danger: differential diagnosis of thoracic spine. *Phys Sports Med* 20:124–131, 1992.

Data from Wiener SL: *Differential Diagnosis of Acute Pain by Body Region.* New York, NY: McGraw-Hill, 1993:532, 542, 616, 645, 678, 680.

Data from Liu KJ, Atten MJ, Donahue PE: Cholestasis in patients with acquired immunodeficiency syndrome: a surgeon's perspective. *Am Surg* 63:519–524, 1997.

Data from Wells K: Nephrolisthiasis with unusual initial symptoms. *J Manipulative Physiol Ther* 23:196–201, 2000.

- Pleural irritation. When the tissues of an irritated pleura are stretched, chest pain can result. This pain can be increased by breathing, as well as by trunk movements, a situation that could lead the clinician to believe that the problem is musculoskeletal.
- Tumor.
- Acute thoracic disk herniation.
- Unstable or stable angina pectoris.
- Pericarditis.
- Pneumothorax.
- Pneumonia.
- Cholecystitis.
- Peptic ulcer.
- Pyelonephritis.
- Nephrolithiasis (kidney stones).

Questions should be asked with regard to bowel and bladder function; upper and lower extremity numbness, tingling, or weakness; and visual or balance disorders. These symptoms may indicate compromise to the spinal cord, cauda equina, or central nervous system.

Questions must also be asked about unexplained weight loss, fever, chills, and night pain. These symptoms often are associated with cancer or systemic disease, although night pain may just be because the patient has an increased, and fixed, kyphosis and needs a softer bed to accommodate the deformity.[87]

Tests and Measures

Observation

The patient should be suitably disrobed to expose as much of this region as is necessary. As a quick orientation to the relationship of the bony structures (Fig. 27-1), the clinician should confirm the following findings:

- The spine of the scapula is level with the spinous process of T3.
- The inferior angle of the scapula is in line with the spinous processes of T7–9.
- The medial border of the scapula is parallel with the spinal column and about 5 cm lateral to the spinous processes.
- The iliac crests are level and symmetric. One crest higher than the other could suggest a leg-length discrepancy, an iliac rotation, or both.
- The shoulder heights are level. A normal variant is that individuals carry their dominant shoulder slightly lower than the nondominant side.

The clinician also should evaluate the following:

- ***Smoothness of the thoracic curve.*** By running the palm of the hand down the midline of the patient's thoracic spine, the clinician can determine the smoothness of the curvature. Any areas of flatness could suggest a vertebral dysfunction such as an opening restriction (extended, rotated, and side flexed [ERS] lesion), whereas areas of relative increased curvature suggest a closing restriction (flexed, rotated, and side flexed [FRS] lesion); refer to Chapter 25.
- ***Degree of thoracic kyphosis.*** As elsewhere in the spine, posture has an important influence on the available range of motion of the neighboring joints. Conversely, changes in the lumbar posture, such as excessive lordosis, and changes in the cervical spine, such as those rendered by a forward head position, can affect the thoracic spine. An increased lumbar lordosis increases the stresses applied to the thoracolumbar junction, whereas a forward head increases the stresses at the cervicothoracic junction.

The thoracic spine adopts a natural kyphotic curve, which is an increased convexity of the thoracic vertebrae. Varying degrees of kyphosis can occur in the thoracic spine. It is known that the thoracic kyphosis increases with age,[88] and in women more than men.[89] The appearance of increased kyphosis in the young is typically postural, but could be the result of Scheuermann's disease, or ankylosing spondylitis.[23,90] The degree of curvature of the spine also has been found to be diurnal, with a slight flattening of the thoracic kyphosis occurring overnight.[91] Attempts to define the "normal" thoracic kyphosis have demonstrated considerable variation in the asymptomatic population,[65,92] suggesting that any individual differences reflect normal variations rather than deviations.

It has been theorized by a number of authors[93–98] that postural dysfunctions in this region create an imbalance between agonists and antagonists, producing adaptive shortening and weakness. It is likely that these changes are degenerative in nature, resulting from a change in IVD height. Disk height changes commonly are seen in the upper mid-thoracic segments[99] and may result in an alteration of the kyphotic curve, with subsequent compensatory changes in load bearing and movement. These altered load-bearing patterns may result in a compression of the anterior aspect of the thoracic IVDs, and a stretching of the thoracic extensors and the middle and lower trapezius. The posterior ligaments also are lengthened. In addition, the kyphotic posture is associated with adaptive shortening of the anterior longitudinal ligament, the upper abdominals, and the anterior chest muscles. The common kyphotic deformities include[100]:

- ***Dowager's hump.*** This deformity is characterized by a severely kyphotic upper posterior (dorsal) region, which results from multiple anterior wedge compression fractures in several vertebrae of the middle to upper thoracic spine (see Chap. 5), usually caused by post menopausal osteoporosis or long-term corticosteroid therapy (specificity, 0.99).[101]
- ***Hump back.*** This deformity is a localized, sharp, posterior angulation, called *gibbus*, produced by an anterior wedging of one of the two thoracic vertebrae as a result of infection (tuberculosis), fracture, or congenital bony anomaly of the spine.[90]
- ***Round back.*** This deformity is characterized by decreased pelvic inclination and excessive kyphosis.
- ***Flat back.*** This deformity is characterized by decreased pelvic inclination, increased kyphosis, and a mobile thoracic spine.
- ***Pelvic heights.*** A significant leg-length discrepancy (greater than 1/2 inch) can alter the lateral curvature of the spine, resulting in compensation.
- ***Amount of lateral curvature of the thoracic spine.*** When observing the thoracic spine, it is important to note the

morphologic latitude of the spinal curvature.[102] Two terms, *scoliosis* and *rotoscoliosis*, are used to describe the lateral curvature of the spine. Scoliosis is the older term and refers to an abnormal side bending of the spine but gives no reference to the coupled rotation that also occurs. Rotoscoliosis is a more detailed definition, used to describe the curve of the spine by detailing how each vertebra is rotated and side flexed in relation to the vertebra below. For example, with a left lumbar convexity, the L5 vertebra would be found to be side flexed to the right and rotated to the left in relation to the sacrum. The same would be true with regard to the relation between L4 and L5. This rotation, toward the convexity, continues in small increments until the apex at L3. L2, which is above the apex, is right rotated and right side flexed in relation to L3. The small increments of right rotation continue up until the thoracic spine, where the side bending and rotation return to the neutral position. The currently accepted definition of scoliosis is a 10-degree lateral curvature measured radiographically (see Chap. 7), with vertebral rotation of the spine taken with the patient standing upright.[103] This definition is based on the fact that a graph of lateral spinal curvature of the general population is a smooth exponential function in which the sharpest change in slope occurs at 10 degrees.[104] Despite this reasonable approach to the definition of the disease state, it results in an extremely high prevalence of the disorder in the general population of 2–3%.[105] Scoliosis can be found in four forms: static, sciatic, idiopathic, and psychogenic. The cause of the latter is self-explanatory.

- ***Static.*** Static, or structural, scoliosis in adults may be caused by a leg-length difference, a hemivertebra, osteoporosis, osteomalacia, or compression fractures. If a platform under the heel of the shorter limb eases or even abolishes the symptoms while standing or on lumbar flexion or extension, a shoe lift is advised.[106,107]
- ***Sciatic.*** The sight of a patient with a pelvic shift or list is relatively common in patients presenting with LBP. The sciatic, or nonstructural, lumbar scoliosis results from sciatic pain caused by a lumbar disk herniation and unilateral spasm of the back muscles. Sciatic scoliosis usually occurs with convexity to the symptomatic side of the herniated disk.[108] The shift is thought to result from the body finding a position of comfort and protection, as a consequence of an irritation of a spinal nerve or its dural sleeve,[108] although the neuronal mechanisms of sciatic scoliosis have not been well clarified. These postural changes cannot be relieved by voluntary efforts but usually disappear after alleviation of the sciatic pain.[108] The extent of a scoliosis should be noted if it is thought to be contributing to the patient's symptoms and is occurring because of pain or dysfunction. An attempt should be made to manually correct the shift to ascertain whether this can be done painlessly. A compensatory shift or scoliosis is often easy and painless to correct.[109,110]
- ***Idiopathic.*** The curve of an idiopathic scoliosis, present since childhood, differs from the tilt of the spine associated with recent IVD problems in that it is accompanied by a lower thoracic or lumbar rotation deformity.[106] If this deformity is not obvious in the standing posture, it should become obvious during flexion, as it is manifested by the so-called *razor back eminence* of the thoracic cage.

Scoliosis is never normal, although most cases are idiopathic, manifesting in the preadolescent years.[4,111] An abnormal lateral thoracic curve is described as being structural or functional, and can produce a fixed deformity or a changeable adaptation, respectively, with the rib hump occurring on the convex side of the curve. Persistent scoliosis during forward bending (Adam's sign) is indicative of a structural curve. Structural curves may be genetic, congenital, or idiopathic, producing a structural change to the bone and a loss of spinal flexibility. With a structural scoliosis, the vertebral bodies rotate toward the convexity of the curve, producing a distortion.[112] The distortion in the thoracic spine is called a *rib hump*. The rotation of the vertebral bodies causes the spinous processes to deviate toward the concave side. The curvature results in an adaptive shortening of the intrinsic trunk muscles on the concave side and lengthening of the intrinsic muscles on the convex side.

The curve patterns are named according to the level of the apex of the curve. For example, a right thoracic curve has a convexity toward the right, and the apex of the curve is in the thoracic spine. There may be a number of curves spanning the thoracic and lumbar region, and the clinician should determine if the curvature is:

- *Contributing to the patient's pain.* Frequently, these curves can be asymptomatic. A slight lateral curve in the coronal plane is thought to result from right-hand dominance, or the presence of the aorta.[113]
- Nonstructural, in which case the patient is able to correct the curves relatively easily.
- Adaptive, resulting from poor posture, nerve root irritation, leg-length discrepancy, atrophy, or hip contracture.
- ***Chest wall shape.*** On the anterior aspect of the thoracic region, the clinician should look for evidence of deformity.
  - ***Barrel chest.*** In this deformity, a forward and upward projecting sternum increases the anteroposterior diameter. The barrel chest results in respiratory difficulty, stretching of the intercostal and anterior chest muscles, and adaptive shortening of the scapular adductor muscles.
  - ***Pigeon chest.*** In this deformity, a forward and downward projecting sternum increases the anteroposterior diameter. The pigeon chest results in a lengthening of the upper abdominal muscles and an adaptive shortening of the upper intercostal muscles.
  - ***Funnel chest.*** In this deformity, a posterior-projecting sternum occurs secondary to an outgrowth of the ribs.[114] The funnel chest results in adaptive shortening of the upper abdominals, shoulder adductors, pectoralis minor, and intercostal muscles, and in lengthening of the thoracic extensors and middle and upper trapezius.
- ***Motion of the ribs during quiet breathing.***
- ***Asymmetry in muscle bulk, prominence, or length.*** According to Sahrmann,[115] shortness of the rectus abdominis results in anterior rib cage depression, shortness of the internal oblique results in an increase in the

TABLE 27-9 Anterior and Posterior Palpation Points of the Thoracic Region

Anterior Aspect	Posterior Aspect
Suprasternal notch	Spinous and associated transverse processes
Manubriosternal angle	T2—level with base of spine of scapula
Xiphoid process	Spinal gutter (rotatores)
Infrasternal angle	Erector spinae
Sternochondral junctions	Rib angles
Costal cartilage	Rib shafts Rib shafts and rib joint line of costotransverse joint C6—locate largest spinous process at base of neck and have patient extend neck; first spinous process to move anteriorly under your finger is C6

infrasternal angle, and shortness of the external oblique results in a decreased angle. Rotatores atrophy could suggest nerve palsy, whereas rotatores hypertonicity could suggest a segmental facilitation.[97,116]

- ***Any lesions, swellings, or scars on the back and chest.*** This is a common area for the characteristic lesion pattern of herpes zoster (shingles), which follows the course of the affected nerve (see Chap. 5).

Gait

The analysis of the patient's gait pattern can provide valuable information as to whether the condition originates in the spine or lower extremities, resulting in gross weakness of the muscles that affect gait[90] (see Chap. 6). For example, a decreased arm swing during gait can indicate stiffness of the thoracic segments.

Palpation

The spinous processes of the thoracic vertebrae are readily palpated (see Fig. 27-1), because they are not covered by muscle or thick connective tissue.[90] Palpation of the thoracic transverse processes is more difficult, however, due to their depth relative to the more superficial structures of the spine. The landmarks outlined in Table 27-9 may be helpful to determine the segmental level involved.

The spinous processes are long and slender and have varying degrees of caudal obliquity, which changes slightly throughout the kyphotic curvature of the thorax, increasing in caudal angulation to the level of T7 and then decreasing in caudal angulation below T9. Traditionally, palpation of this area has utilized the "rule of threes."

CLINICAL PEARL

The areas of spinous process may obliquity be divided into four regions by the so-called rule of three devised by Mitchell[117] (an alternate version is illustrated in Fig. 27-9):

- The upper three spinous processes (T1–3). The tips of these spinous processes are level with vertebral body of the same level.
- Second group of three spinous processes (T4–6). The tips of these spinous processes are in a plane that is half way between its own transverse process and those of the inferior vertebra (level with the IVD of the inferior level). This can be estimated at about three fingerbreadths.
- Third group of three spinous processes (T7–9). The tips of these spinous processes are level with the transverse processes of the vertebral body of the level below.
- The last three vertebrae (T10–12) reverse the obliquity of the spinous processes:
  - T10 is level with the vertebral body of the vertebra below (same as T7–9).
  - T11 is level with the disk of the inferior vertebra (same as T6).
  - T12 is level with its own vertebral body (same as T3).

The rule of threes has been widely accepted in orthopaedic and manual therapy texts, but until recently, never validated with research. Based on a pilot study to investigate the validity of the rule of threes of the thoracic spine, Geelhoed and colleagues,[118] using five cadaver specimens, determined that the rule of threes was not an accurate predictor of the location of the transverse processes of the thoracic spine. The limitations of the study were the small sample size, the fact that measurements were only performed in the horizontal plane (prone position), and the fact that cadavers were used instead of live subjects, which could affect IVD height, and spinal alignment. In a separate study, Geelhoed et al.[119] have proposed a new model for predicting the location of the transverse processes of the thoracic spine. This proposed method states that the location of the transverse processes of a thoracic vertebra can be found lateral to

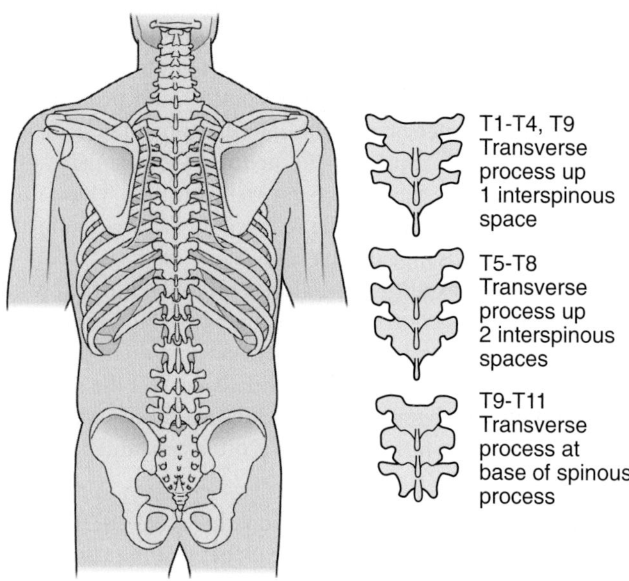

FIGURE 27-9 The rule of threes.

the most prominent aspect of the spinous process of the vertebra one level above.[119]

Surface landmarks can be used to locate the ribs. The first rib is located 45 degrees medially to the junction of the posterior scalene and trapezius. Palpation of the first rib during respiration can detect the presence of asymmetry. Palpation of the first rib can also be performed during testing of the active motions of cervical rotation and side bending in patients with suspected brachialgia (see Chap. 25).

The fifth rib passes directly under, or slightly inferior to, the male mammary nipples (see Fig. 27-11). To palpate the rib angles of the interscapular ribs, the shoulders are positioned in horizontal adduction. The rib angles of 3–10 can then be felt about 2–5 cm lateral to the spinous processes (Fig. 27-11).

When palpating anteriorly, on the sternum, a rib dysfunction will be highlighted by the presence of asymmetry and should be compared with the posterior findings. A prominent rib angle on the back and a depression of that rib at the sternum indicate a posterior subluxation, the reverse occurring in an anterior subluxation, whereas a rib that is prominent both anteriorly and posteriorly indicates a single rib torsion.

The transverse processes are roughly level with their own body. The costal cartilages of the second rib articulate with the junction between the sternum and manubrium (Fig. 27-1).

Palpation of the soft tissues of the region is important. The clinician should note the presence of any tenderness, temperature changes, and muscle spasm. A comparison should be made between the firmness and tenderness of the paravertebral muscles and their relationship from side to side.

Active Motion Testing

Active range-of-motion tests are used to determine the osteokinematic function of two adjacent thoracic vertebrae during active motions, to identify which joints are dysfunctional, as well as the specific direction of motion loss.[120] Active range of motion initially is performed globally, looking for abnormalities, such as asymmetric limitations of motion. A specific examination is then performed on any region that appears to have either excessive or reduced motion. If the history indicated that the patient's symptoms were altered with repetitive motions or sustained positions, these movements and postures should be included. Various techniques are used to correctly assess each area of the thoracic spine.

Movement restriction of the upper thoracic spine may be secondary to pain or a result of adaptive shortening of connective tissue or muscle.[3] Because of the relationship that the first two ribs share with the zygapophyseal joints as part of the manubrial ring, associated movement dysfunction of these ribs is common. Physiologic movement in the thoracic spine decreases with age. Mid-thoracic hypomobilities are the most common thoracic presentation,[110] with the movement restrictions being more common in the sagittal and frontal planes, particularly extension and side bending.[3] Most of the trunk rotation below the level of C2 occurs in the thoracic spine.

The clinician should look for capsular or noncapsular patterns of restriction, pain, or painful weakness (possible fracture or neoplasm). The capsular pattern of the thoracic spine appears to be symmetric limitation of rotation and side bending, extension loss, and least loss of flexion. Joint capsular lesions demonstrate a capsular pattern as equal and grossly severe limitation of movement in every direction.[90] With an asymmetric impairment, such as trauma, the capsular pattern appears to be an asymmetric limitation of rotation and side bending, extension loss, and a lesser loss of flexion.

Overpressure applied at the end of the available range of motion is used to take the joint from its physiologic barrier to its anatomic barrier. During overpressure, an increase in resistance to motion should be felt. The end-feels should be noted.

- If the normal elastic end-feel of thoracic rotation is replaced by a stiffer one, it may indicate the presence of osteoporosis or ankylosing spondylitis.
- During forward flexion, the nonstructural scoliosis disappears, whereas the structural scoliosis does not.
- If side bending is more seriously affected than rotation, neoplastic disease of the viscera or chest wall may be present.[87]
- If, during side bending, the ipsilateral paraspinal muscles demonstrate a contracture (Forestier's bowstring sign), ankylosing spondylitis may be present.[121]
- Side bending away from the painful side, which is the only painful and limited movement, almost always indicates a severe extra-articular impairment, such as a pulmonary or abdominal tumor or a spinal neurofibroma. The functional examination normally confirms the patient history.
- A marked restriction of motion in a noncapsular pattern with one or more spasmodic end-feels could indicate a thoracic disk herniation.
- Anterior or lateral pain with resisted thoracic rotation could indicate a muscle tear. Localized pain with resisted testing could indicate a rib fracture.

Because of the length of the spine in this region, it is important to ensure that all parts of the thoracic spine are involved in the range-of-motion testing. Motion in the thoracic spine requires a synchronous movement between the intervertebral and zygapophyseal joints and the rib articulations. Thus, the presence of joint dysfunction or degeneration, or structural changes in the spinal curvature, will influence the amount of available range of motion, and the pattern of these coupled motions.[23]

CLINICAL PEARL

It is important to remember that maximum arm elevation requires motion in the upper thoracic segments.

The inclinometer techniques recommended by the American Medical Association are used to objectively measure thoracic motion.[122]

Flexion. To measure thoracic flexion, two inclinometers are used and are aligned in the sagittal plane. The center of the first inclinometer is placed over the T1 spinous process. The center of the second one is placed over the T12 spinous process. The patient is asked to slump forward as though trying to place the forehead on the knees, and both inclinometer angles are recorded. The thoracic flexion angle is calculated by subtracting the T12 from the T1 inclinometer angle. The patient should be able to flex approximately 20–45 degrees.[69,120] The clinician observes for any paravertebral fullness during flexion, which might indicate hypertonus from a facilitated segment. The thoracic spine during flexion should curve forward in a smooth and even manner (Fig. 27-10). There should be no evidence of segmental rotation or side bending. To decrease pelvic and hip movements, McKenzie advocates examining thoracic flexion with the patient seated.[123]

Extension. The clinician places one hand and arm across the upper chest region of the patient and the other hand over the spinous processes of the lower thoracic spine. The patient is guided into a backward slump (Fig. 27-11). Overpressure is applied by the arm across the front of the patient, while avoiding any anterior translation occurring at the lumbar spine.

Clinical guidelines for measurements of thoracic extension recommend that range of motion be defined with reference to the magnitude of the kyphosis measured in standing. However, to date, the relationship between the magnitude of the thoracic kyphosis and the amount of thoracic extension movement has not been reported.[62] Thoracic extension may be measured using the same technique and inclinometer positions as described for flexion. The thoracic extension angle is calculated by subtracting the T12 from the T1 inclinometer angle. The patient should be able to extend approximately 15–20 degrees.[120] Alternatively, thoracic extension can be measured using a tape measure. The distance between two points (the C7 and T12 spinous processes) is measured. A 2.5-cm difference between neutral and extension measurements is considered normal.[121,124] During thoracic extension, the thoracic curve should curve backward or straighten. As with flexion, there should be no evidence of segmental rotation or side bending.

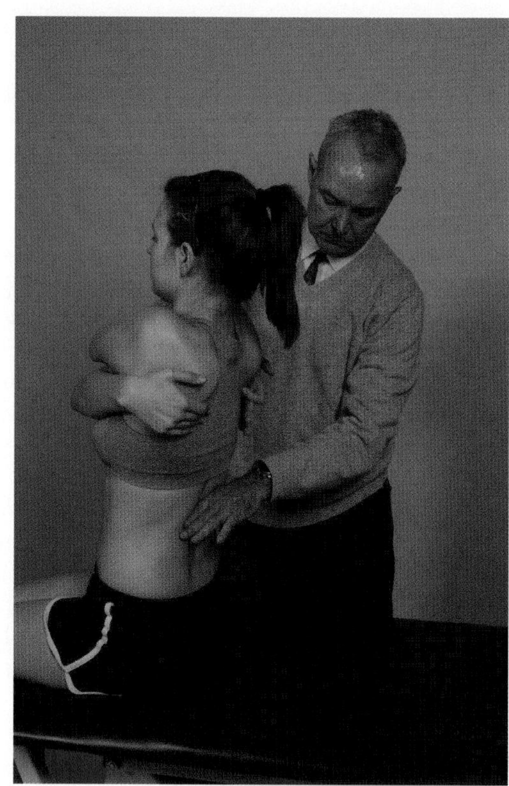

FIGURE 27-11 Thoracic spine extension.

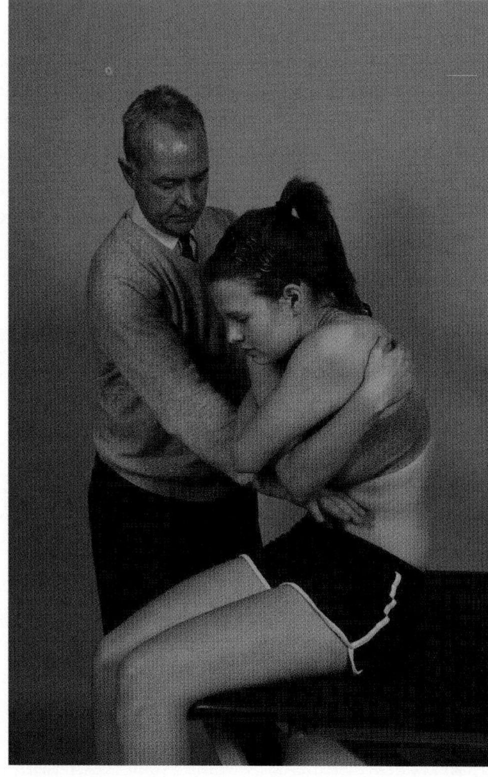

FIGURE 27-10 Thoracic spine flexion.

Rotation. The patient is seated and is asked to turn to each side at the waist. Overpressure is applied through both shoulders (Fig. 27-12). This motion tests the ability of the ribs and the superior vertebrae to translate in the direction opposite to the rotation—a motion that is essential if complete rotation and side bending is to occur. A total of 35–50 degrees of rotation is available in the thoracic spine.[22,73] Rotation is a primary movement of the thoracic spine and a key component of functional activities. Active thoracic rotation of 20 degrees or less results in an impairment of function during activities of daily living involving the thoracic spine.[121] Pavelka[125] devised a simple objective clinical method to measure thoracolumbar rotation using a tape measure that can be used to detect

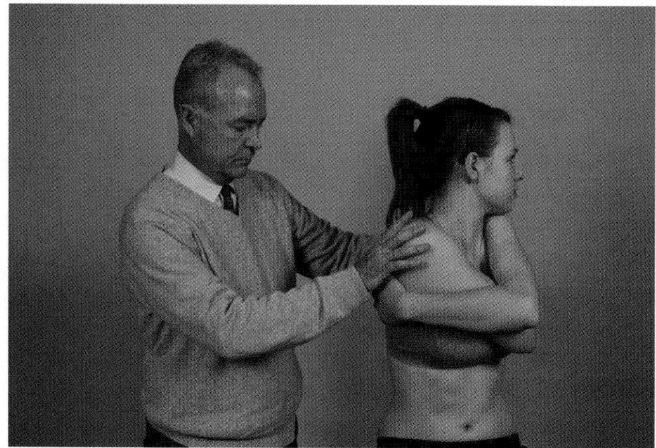

FIGURE 27-12 Thoracic spine rotation.

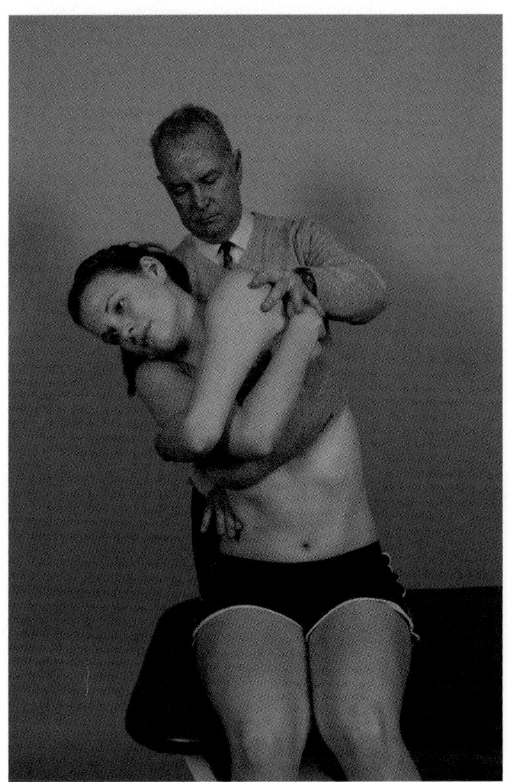

FIGURE 27-13 Thoracic spine side bending.

asymmetries in rotation. The tape is placed over the L5 spinous process, wrapped around the trunk, and placed over the jugular notch on the superior aspect of the manubrium. A measurement is taken before and after full trunk rotation. The measurements from each side are then compared.

Side Bending. A total of 25–45 degrees of side bending is available in the thoracic spine.[22,73] Using a hand placed against the patient's side, the patient is asked to side bend over the clinician's hand. Overpressure is applied through the contralateral shoulder to avoid compression (Fig. 27-13). Side bending can be measured objectively using a tape measure.[126] Two ink marks are placed on the skin of the lateral trunk. The upper mark is made at a point where a horizontal line through the xiphisternum crosses the coronal line. The lower mark is made at the highest point on the iliac crest. The distance between the two marks is measured in centimeters, with the patient standing erect, and again after full ipsilateral side bending. The second measurement is subtracted from the first and the remainder is taken as an index of lateral spinal mobility.

CLINICAL PEARL

A finding of painful and limited side bending away from the painful side, with both rotations free from pain, should always create a suspicion of a serious lesion.[90]

Inspiration and Expiration. Using a tape measure, the clinician measures the amount of rib expansion that occurs with a deep breath. Respiratory excursion is measured at three levels, using a tape measure placed circumferentially around the chest at the level of the axilla, the xiphoid level, and the 10th rib level. Comparisons are made between the measurements taken at the position of maximum expiration and the measurement taken at full inspiration. The normal difference between inspiration and expiration is 3–7.5 cm (1–3 inches).[126] Ankylosing spondylitis is a disease that can include ossification of the anterior longitudinal ligament, the thoracic disk, and the thoracic zygapophyseal joints. Findings of ankylosing spondylitis are common in the thoracic region, making chest expansion measurements a requirement in this region. Decreased expansion can highlight the presence of ankylosing spondylitis but may also be the result of diaphragm palsy (C4), intercostal weakness, pulmonary (pleura) problems, old age, a rib fracture, or a chronic lung condition.

The motions of the ribs are palpated during breathing. If a rib stops moving in relation to the other ribs on the same side during inspiration, it is classified as a *depressed rib*.[117,127] If a rib stops moving in relation to the other ribs during expiration, it is classified as an *elevated rib*.[117,127] Because of the interrelationship of all of the ribs, if a depressed rib is implicated, it is usually the most superior depressed rib that causes the most significant dysfunction. In contrast, if an elevated rib is implicated, it is usually the most inferior restricted rib that causes the most significant dysfunction.[117,127]

Resisted Testing

Resistance applied at the point of overpressure can give the clinician an indication of the integrity of the musculotendinous units of this area. Resistance is applied at the end range of flexion, extension, rotation, and side bending, while the clinician looks for pain, weakness, or painful weakness. Pain that is exacerbated with motion, but not with resisted isometric contraction, suggests a ligamentous lesion.[120]

Static Postural Testing

Thoracic pain of a postural origin is difficult to provoke with active motion and resistive testing. McKenzie[123] recommends placing the patient in a position for approximately 3 minutes to load the structures sufficiently to provoke postural pain.

Differing Philosophies

The next stage in the examination process depends on the clinician's background. For clinicians who are heavily influenced by the muscle energy techniques of the osteopaths, position testing is used to determine the segment on which to focus. Other clinicians omit the position tests and proceed to the combined motion and passive physiologic tests.

Position Testing: Spinal. The vertebrae may be tested for positional symmetry. If an ERS or FRS is present, passive mobility testing will definitively diagnose the movement impairment. The upper thoracic joints (C7–T4) can be assessed using the cervical techniques described in Chapter 25. The following techniques can be used for the T4–12 levels.

Example: T6–7. The patient is positioned in sitting, with the clinician standing behind. Using one thumb, the clinician palpates the transverse process of the T6 vertebrae. Using the other thumb, the clinician palpates the transverse process of the T7 vertebrae (Fig. 27-14). The joint is tested in the following manner:

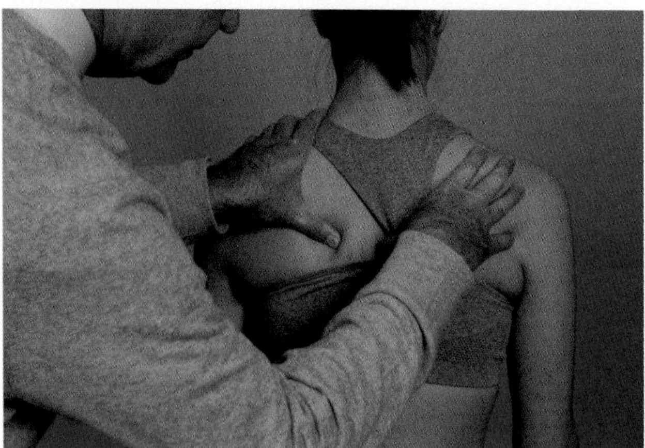

FIGURE 27-14 Position testing for T6–7.

- The patient bends forward so that the joint complex is flexed, and an evaluation is made as to the position of the T6 vertebra relative to T7 by noting which transverse process is the most posterior. A posterior left transverse process of T6 relative to T7 is indicative of a left-rotated position of the T6–7 complex in flexion.
- The patient bends backward so that the joint complex is extended, and an evaluation is made as to the position of the T6 vertebra in relation to T7 by noting which transverse process is the most posterior. A posterior left transverse process of T6 relative to T7 is indicative of a left-rotated position of the T6–7 joint complex in extension.

Once a segment has been localized by one of the preceding techniques, the arthrokinematics of the segment can be tested using the following passive mobility tests, which incorporate specific symmetric or asymmetric motions. Care in the interpretation of the passive mobility tests is important, because local tenderness in the thoracic region is common, especially over the spinous processes as a result of the proximity of the posterior (dorsal) rami over the apex of these bony prominences.[23,128]

Combined Motion Testing. As normal function involves complex and combined motions of the thoracic spine, combined motion testing can also be used. The motions tested include forward flexion with side bending, extension with side bending, side bending with flexion, and side bending with extension. The results from these motions are combined with the findings from the history and the single plane motions to categorize the symptomatic responses. This information can guide the clinician when determining which motions to use in the intervention.

Passive Physiologic Mobility Testing. The upper thoracic zygapophyseal joints (C7–T4) can be assessed using the cervical techniques described in Chapter 25. The following techniques can be used for the T4–12 levels.

Flexion of the Zygapophyseal Joints. The patient is seated at the end of the table, with arms together and hands resting on the back of the head. The clinician stands by the side of the patient and reaches around the front of the patient with one arm and hand. The clinician then applies a slight pressure with the sternum against the patient's shoulder so that the patient is gently squeezed. Using the other hand to monitor intersegmental motion between the spinous processes (Fig. 27-15), the clinician flexes the thoracic spine (Fig. 27-15). The quantity and quality of motion are noted and compared with the levels above and below.

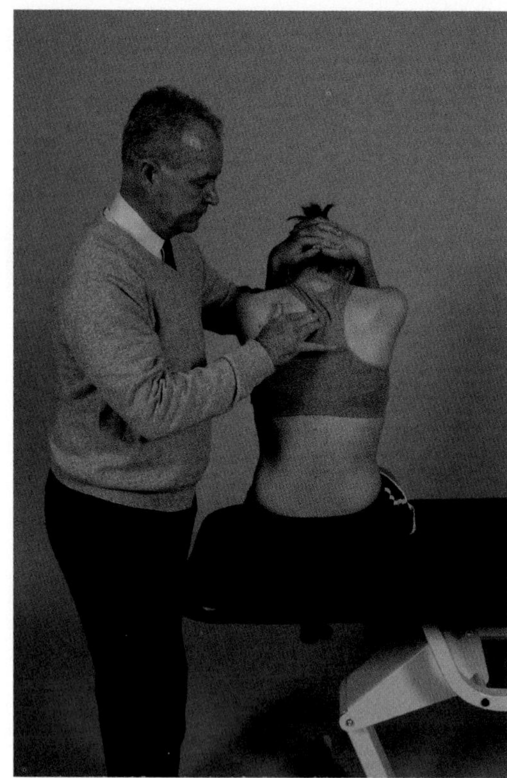

FIGURE 27-15 Passive mobility testing for flexion.

Extension of the Zygapophyseal Joints. The patient is seated with the arms together and both hands behind the head. The clinician stands to the side of the patient. While palpating the interspinous spaces or the transverse processes of the level to be tested with one hand, the clinician wraps the other arm around the front of the patient and rests that hand on the patient's contralateral elbow (Fig. 27-16). Crouching slightly, the clinician then places his or her anterior shoulder region close to the lateral aspect of the patient's shoulder. Using the other hand to monitor inter-segmental motion between the spinous processes, the clinician extends the thoracic spine (Fig. 27-16). The quantity and quality of motion is noted and compared with the levels above and below.

Combined Motions of the Zygapophyseal Joints. The patient is seated with one hand on top of one of the shoulders and the other hand under the opposite axilla. The clinician stands to the side of the patient. While palpating the interspinous spaces or the transverse processes of each level with one hand, the clinician wraps the other arm around the front of the patient, under the patient's crossed arms, resting his or her hand on the patient's contralateral hand. Crouching slightly, the clinician then places the anterior shoulder region against the lateral aspect of the patient's shoulder. Side bending and rotation of the patient's thoracic spine is then performed away from the clinician (Fig. 27-17), as the clinician lifts with his or her body. The palpating hand palpates the concave side of the curve.

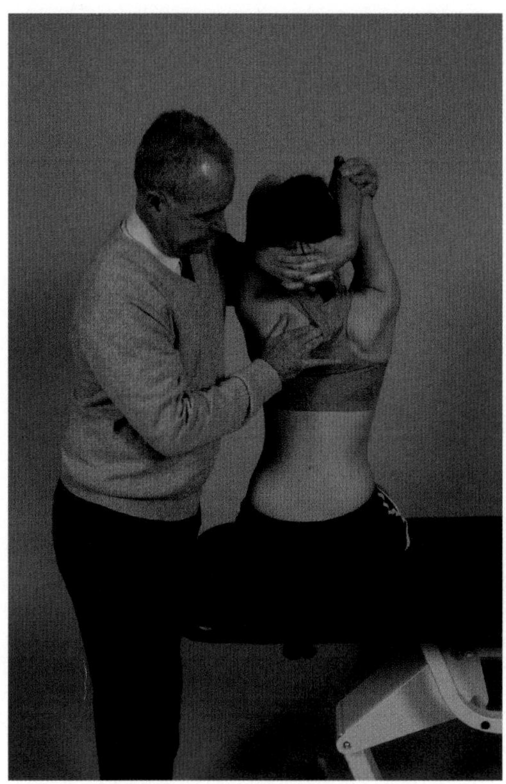

FIGURE 27-16 Passive mobility testing for extension.

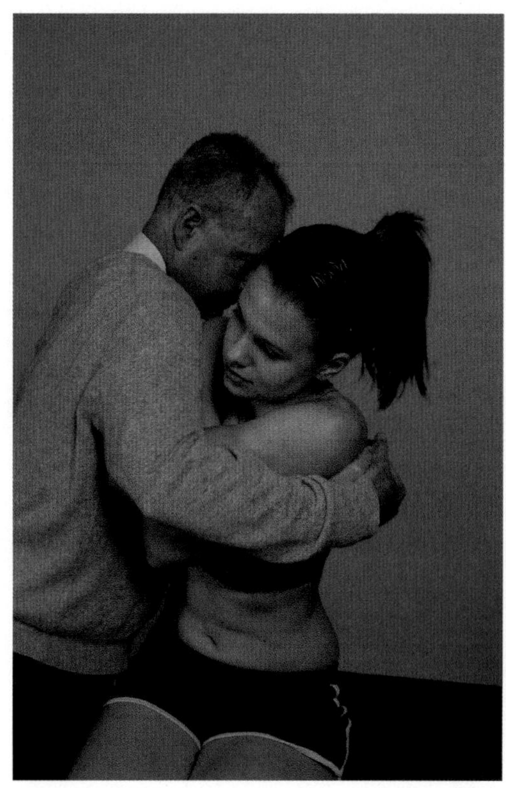

FIGURE 27-17 Passive mobility testing for side bending and rotation away from clinician.

Passive Articular Mobility Testing of the Mid-Thoracic Spine

Under normal circumstances, if the active motions and passive mobility motions of a joint are found to be restricted, the arthrokinematics of the restricted motion(s) are assessed to determine if the hypomobility is articular or extra-articular (myofascial). However, given the number of joints at each segmental level and the proximity of many of them, it is unlikely that passive articular mobility testing in this region will yield any useful information.

Neurologic Tests

A neurologic deficit is very difficult to detect in the thoracic spine. In this region, one dermatome may be absent with no loss of sensation.[129] Several tests have been devised to help assess the integrity of the neurologic system in this area.

The Slump Test. A neurodynamic mobility test can be used as a general assessment (see Chap. 11).

Sensory Testing. Sensation should be tested over the abdomen. The area just below the xiphoid process is innervated by T8, the umbilicus by T10, and the lower abdominal region, level with the anterior superior iliac spines, by T12.[87] Too much overlap exists above T8 to make sensation testing reliable.

Pathological Reflexes. Because of the proximity and vulnerability of the spinal cord in this region, long tract signs (Babinski, Oppenheim, clonus, and muscle stretch [deep tendon] reflexes) should be routinely assessed.

Lhermitte's Symptom. This impairment usually is considered to be a lesion to the cervical spinal cord (see Chap. 3), and it is associated with demyelination, prolapsed cervical disk, neck trauma, or subacute combined degeneration of the cord. Because the thoracic cord is immobilized by the denticulate ligaments, flexion will produce only limited stretching of the cord and thus less excursion. Lhermitte's symptom, characterized by an electric shock-like sensation into the spinal cord and limbs during neck flexion, may be present in the thoracic spine with compression of the thoracic cord by metastatic malignant deposits,[130] impairments of the thoracic vertebrae,[131] and thoracic spinal tumors.[132]

Brown–Séquard Syndrome. This syndrome is characterized by ipsilateral flaccid segmental palsy, ipsilateral spastic palsy below the impairment, and ipsilateral anesthesia, loss of proprioception, and loss of appreciation of the vibration of a tuning fork (dysesthesia). Contralateral discrimination of pain sensation and thermoanesthesia may be present and are both noted below the impairment. If a neurologic impairment is suspected, the clinician must first exclude a neoplastic process, infectious process, or fracture, and then consider a disk protrusion. A nondiscal disorder of the thoracic spine could include a neurofibroma; some of the signs to help confirm its presence are that

- the patient reports preferring to sleep sitting up;
- the pain, which slowly increases over a period of months, is felt mainly at night and is uninfluenced by activities;
- the patient reports a band-shaped area of numbness that is related to one dermatome;
- the patient reports the presence of pins and needles sensations in one or both feet or reports any other sign of cord compression.

Brown–Séquard syndrome symptoms may also occur with an idiopathic spinal cord herniation. This syndrome is caused by damage to the lateral funiculus of the spinal cord. The

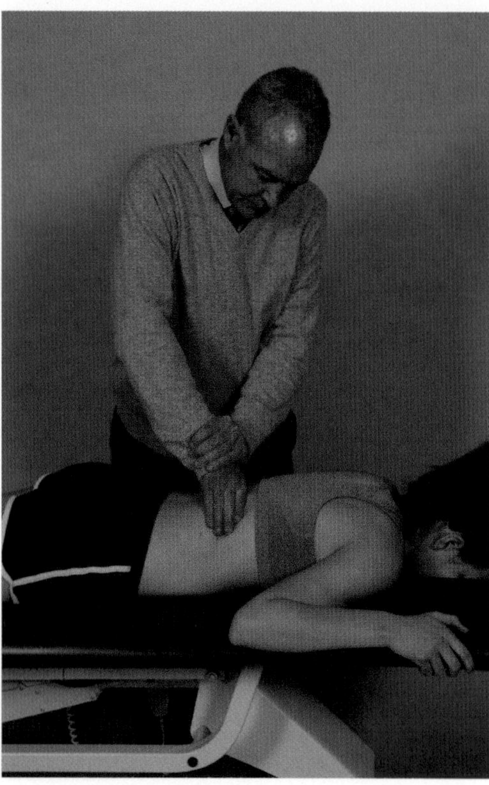

FIGURE 27-18 Rib spring test.

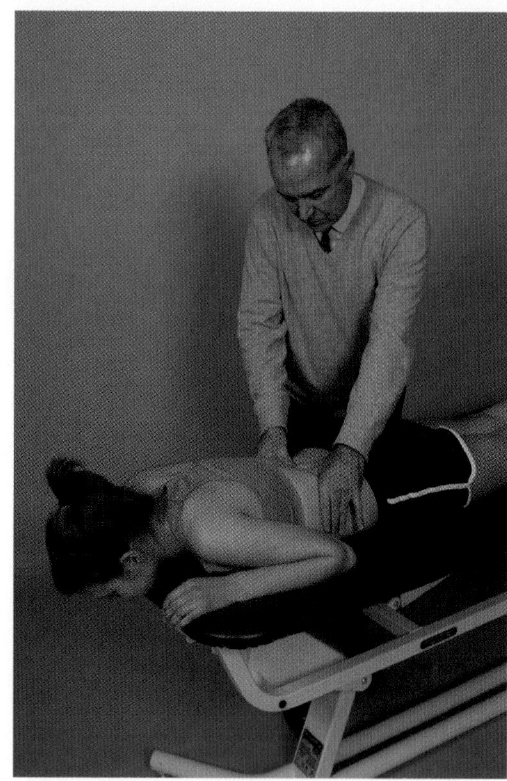

FIGURE 27-19 Thoracic spring test.

spinal cord frequently is shifted ventrolaterally and sometimes rotated toward the side of tethering, which might cause unilateral damage of the lateral funiculus. For the diagnosis of spinal cord herniation, magnetic resonance imaging (MRI) and computed tomography (CT) myelography are essential. An MRI myelogram can show acute, angular, anterior (ventral) deviation of the spinal cord in the sagittal plane. CT myelograms can detect anterior (ventral) or ventrolateral shifts of the spinal cord and, sometimes, an extradural cyst in the anterior (ventral) epidural space.

Special Tests

Very few special tests exist for this region, and even fewer have undergone diagnostic accuracy studies to determine reliability, sensitivity, and specificity.

Rib Spring Test. The patient is positioned prone, and the clinician stands on one side of the patient. Reaching over the patient, the clinician spreads the length of the thumb and index finger over the right rib in question and applies a posteroanterior force (Fig. 27-18). This is the equivalent of a left rotation of the thoracic spine. The clinician then repeats the posteroanterior force on the rib, except this time, the rotation of the thoracic spine is blocked by the clinician placing the ulnar border of the other hand over a group of left transverse processes. Pain produced with this maneuver implicates the rib, because the thoracic spine is stabilized.

Thoracic Spring Test. The patient is positioned as previously. Spring testing in a posteroanterior direction is applied using the thumbs, with the elbows locked over the spinous processes of the thoracic spine (Fig. 27-19). These spring tests are provocative for pain but may also be used for a gross assessment of mobility.

Reflex Hammer Test. The patient is sitting, and the clinician uses a reflex hammer to tap over each spinous process (Fig. 27-20). If tenderness is encountered, especially in a patient with a history of trauma to the area, a fracture must be ruled out.

Deep Breathing and Flexion. This test can be used for patients who complain of pain with thoracic flexion. The patient is seated with the thoracic spine positioned in neutral. The patient is asked to inhale fully and then to flex the thoracic spine until the pain is felt. At this point, the patient maintains the position of flexion and slowly exhales. If further flexion can be achieved after exhalation, the source of the pain is likely to be the ribs rather than the thoracic spine.[133]

The Sitting Arm Lift Test.[134] The **sitting arm lift** (SAL) test is based on the principles of the active straight leg raise (see Chap. 29), a validated test of failed load transfer in the pelvic

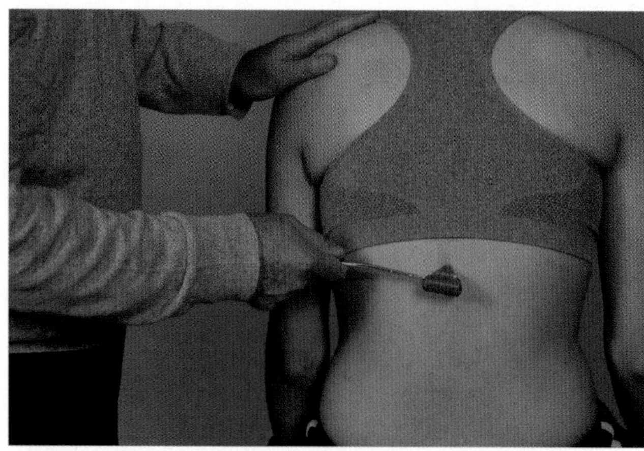

FIGURE 27-20 Reflex Hammer Test.

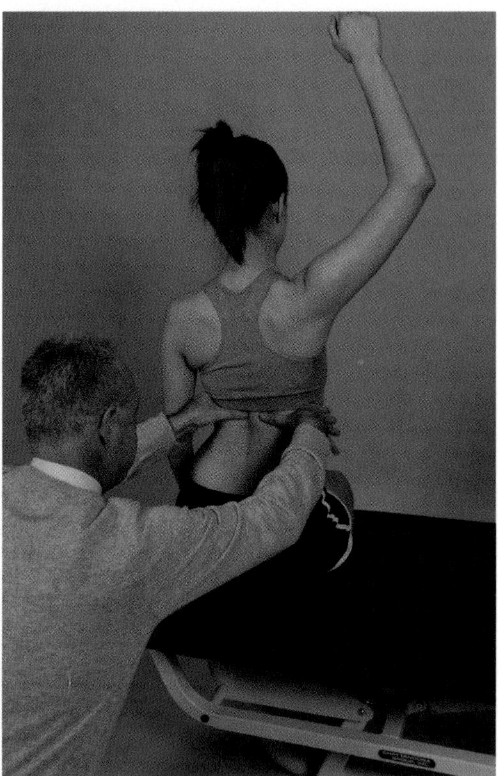

FIGURE 27-21 The sitting arm lift (SAL) test.

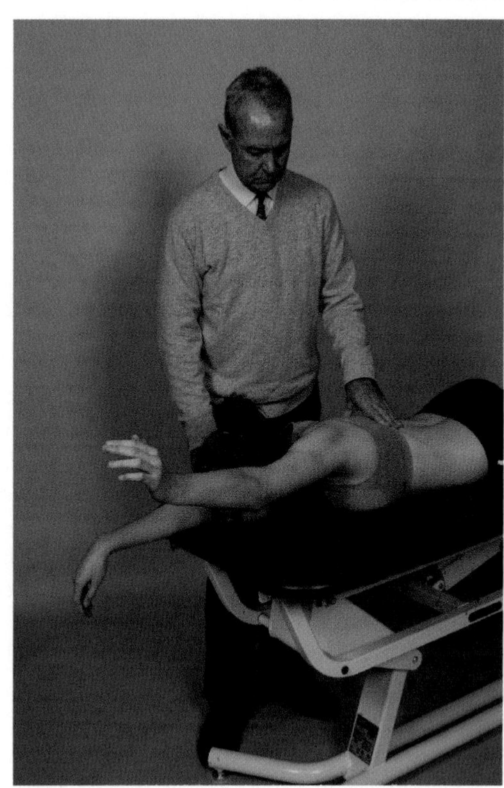

FIGURE 27-22 The prone arm lift (PAL) test.

girdle associated with pregnancy-related pelvic girdle pain. The patient is positioned in relaxed sitting with the hand resting on the thighs. The clinician asks the patient to lift one arm (usually the pain-free side is tested first if ipsilaterally symptoms are present), with the arm straight, into elevation and then to lower the arm (Fig. 27-21). Next, the patient is asked to lift the other arm and lower it and the clinician notes whether symptoms are produced, and also observes which arm looks as if it requires more effort to lift, especially from the initiation of movement to the first 70° to 90° of elevation. Then, the patient is asked "does one arm feel heavier to lift on the other, or different to lift than the other?" If one arm is reported to be heavier or required more effort to lift, the test result is positive for loss of neuromuscular control and indicates a load transfer problem. To determine the affected level or levels, the clinician then palpates the osteokinematic motion of each thoracic ring as the patient performs active elevation through flexion with the heavier arm. A positive test result is indicated when a thoracic ring or rings is/are felt to translate along any axis or rotate in any plane, or any component of the ring (vertebra or rib) translates or rotates along any axis or plane.

The Prone Arm Lift Test.[134] The **prone arm lift** (PAL) test is a modification of the SAL test as it is performed in a higher load position (prone). The patient is positioned in prone with both arms overhead in approximately 120 degrees of flexion and fully supported on the bed (the head of the bed needs to be dropped down). The clinician instructs the patient to lift one arm and then lower it (Fig. 27-22). The movement is then repeated on the other side. The arm that tests positive for loss of neuromuscular control is the arm that is heavier to lift. As with the sitting arm lift test, the same techniques can be used to assess the osteokinematic motions. It is particularly important to assess this ability in patients who require this position functionally (e.g., overhead workers).

INTERVENTION STRATEGIES

Interventions for thoracic and rib dysfunctions require a multifaceted and eclectic approach because of the complexity of this area. Once the causes for referral of symptoms have been ruled out, dysfunctions of the thoracic spine and rib cage may be categorized as somatic or biomechanical.

The intervention approaches are for the upper thoracic spine is similar to that of the cervical spine (see Chap. 25), whereas the approach for the lower thoracic spine is similar to that of the lumbar spine (see Chap. 28). The approach to the mid-thoracic region is variable and depends on the cause. This region is prone to both postural and biomechanical dysfunctions. The evidence supporting the use of mobilization and high-velocity thrust techniques in the thoracic spine continues to increase.[135–139]

The overall goal of treatment should be to optimize load transfer and the sharing of forces throughout the thorax, the spine, and the entire body, which requires restoration of mobility to restrict areas, restoration of muscle control and the capacity to stabilize poorly controlled areas.[2]

The techniques to increase joint mobility and soft tissue extensibility are described later, under "Therapeutic Techniques" section.

Acute Phase

In the acute phase of rehabilitation for the thoracic spine, the intervention goals are to

- decrease pain, inflammation, and muscle spasm;
- promote healing of tissues;
- increase pain-free range of vertebral and costal motion;
- regain soft tissue extensibility;
- regain neuromuscular control;
- initiate postural education;
- promote correct breathing;
- educate the patient about activities to avoid and positions of comfort;
- allow progression to the functional phase.

Pain relief may be accomplished initially by the use of modalities such as cryotherapy and electrical stimulation, gentle exercises, and occasionally the temporary use of a spinal brace. Thermal modalities—especially ultrasound, with its ability to penetrate deeply—may be used after 48–72 hours. Ultrasound is the most common clinically used deep-heating modality to promote tissue healing.[140–142]

Electrical stimulation can be used in the thoracic region to

- create a muscle contraction through nerve or muscle stimulation. The purpose of this muscle contraction and stimulation is to create a muscle pump to aid in the healing process. Electrical stimulation of muscles for the correction of scoliosis has not been found to be effective in preventing scoliosis progression[143];
- decrease pain through the stimulation of sensory nerves (TENS);
- provide muscle reeducation and facilitation through both motor and sensory stimulation.

Once the pain and inflammation are controlled, the intervention can progress toward the restoration of full strength, range of motion, and normal posture. Range-of-motion exercises are initiated at the earliest opportunity. These are performed during the early stages in the pain-free ranges. Submaximal isometric exercises are then performed throughout the pain-free ranges. These exercises are progressed as the range of motion and strength increase.

Manual techniques during this phase may include myofascial release, grade I and II joint mobilizations, massage, gentle stretching, and muscle energy techniques.

Functional Phase

The duration of this phase can vary tremendously and depends on several factors:

- Severity of the injury
- Healing capacity of the patient
- How the condition was managed during the acute phase
- Level of patient involvement in the rehabilitation program

The goals of this phase are the following:

- To achieve a significant reduction or to complete resolution of the patient's pain.
- To restore full and pain-free vertebral and costal range of motion. During this phase, the patient learns to initiate and execute functional activities without pain and while dynamically stabilizing the spine in an automatic manner.
- Full integration of the entire upper and lower kinetic chains. The exercises prescribed must challenge and enhance muscle performance, while minimizing loading of the thoracic spine and ribs to reduce the risk of injury exacerbation. Interindividual differences in injury status or training goals may allow for a continuum of required muscle stress and acceptable loading of the spine.[144]
- Complete restoration of respiratory function;
- Restoration of thoracic and upper quadrant strength and neuromuscular control. The stabilization of this region must include postural stabilization retraining of the entire spine, including the stabilization progressions outlined in Chapters 25 and 28, to (1) gain dynamic control of spine forces, (2) eliminate repetitive injury to the motion segments, (3) encourage healing of the injured segment, and (4) possibly alter the degenerative process.[145]

Practice Pattern 4B: Impaired Joint Mobility, Motor Function, Muscle Performance, and Range of Motion Associated with Impaired Posture

Postural Dysfunction

Postural dysfunctions of the thoracic spine are relatively common. Postural pain is not typically reproducible with the typical physical examination, and the diagnosis is based solely on the history of pain following sustained positions or postures. Occasionally, patients with this type of pain may report that their pain is aggravated by stress, or fatigue.[146]

Maigne's Thoracic Pain of Lower Cervical Origin. Although the pain from this condition may originate in the thoracic spine, Maigne[110] believes that the vast majority of these cases originate from the lower three cervical segments. The typical patient is female, with complaints of stiffness and tenderness of the shoulder girdle and thoracic muscle groups, particularly the interscapular muscles. The chief complaint is often described as a unilateral and intense pain, which is increased with sustained positions of sitting, and with the lifting and carrying of heavy weights. The pain generally is decreased with rest, although it can sometimes be worse in the morning upon awakening. There may also be accompanying cervical and low-back pain associated with postural habits or standing or sitting positions.

The physical examination usually reveals tenderness at the level of T5–6 (interscapular point), 1–2 cm lateral of the midline. Mild pressure at this point is sufficient to reproduce the patient's pain.

The intervention for this condition involves a therapeutic trial of cervical mobilization.

Abnormal Pelvic Tilting. Good mobility of the pelvis in all directions is important for the thoracic spine. Two postural deviations are associated with pelvic tilting:

1. Posterior pelvic tilting in the sitting position produces an increase in lumbar and thoracic spine flexion and a forward head posture (FHP). This posture is thought to result in a

posterior shifting of the thoracic disk, which in turn places a stress on the posterior longitudinal ligament and the dura mater. This stress can produce both local and nonsegmental referrals of pain. This condition can be treated by having the patient sit on a wedge that tilts the pelvis anteriorly.

2. Anterior pelvic tilting in the standing position causes the trunk to lean backward and results in overstretching of the rectus abdominis and a pulling forward of the shoulders, shortening of the posterior neck muscles, and increased extension of the atlanto-occipital joint.[147] This condition can be treated by having the patient perform posterior pelvic tilts while standing, or by standing with one foot in front of the other.

Precordial Catch Syndrome. This is a benign self-limiting condition occurring mainly in adolescents and young adults.[148,149] It is characterized by sharp, stabbing pain in the precordial and left parasternal region that does not radiate. This pain usually lasts a few seconds and may occur at rest or with mild-to-moderate exercise.[148] When occurring at rest, it is often associated with being seated in a slouched position and may be relieved by stretching into a more upright position.[150] It affects males and females equally but is uncommon after the age of 35 years.[149] The etiology of this condition is unknown, but it may originate from the pleura.[149] After excluding other causes, management consists of explanation, reassurance, postural education, and exercises to correct any muscle imbalances.

CLINICAL PEARL

Patients with any form of postural dysfunction often benefit from the movement therapies of the Alexander technique, Feldenkrais method, Trager psychophysical integration, Pilates, and Tai chi chuan[151–157] (see Chap. 10).

Practice Pattern 4D: Impaired Joint Mobility, Motor Function, Muscle Performance, and Range of Motion Associated with Ligament or Other Connective Tissue Disorders

Thoracic Disk Pathology

Herniated disks have been found at every level of the thoracic spine, although they are more common in the lower thoracic spine.[11,158]

At the cervical and lumbar levels, the thoracic spinal nerves emerge from the cord as a large anterior (ventral), and a smaller posterior (dorsal) ramus, which unite to form a short spinal nerve root. There are no plexuses in this area, and the spinal nerves form the intercostal nerves.[8] The intraspinal course of the upper thoracic nerve root is almost horizontal (as in the cervical spine). Therefore, the nerve can only be compressed by its corresponding disk. More inferiorly in the spine though, the course of the nerve root becomes more oblique, and the lowest thoracic nerve roots can be compressed by disk impairments of two consecutive levels (T12 root by 11th or 12th disk).[8]

The major etiological factor in most cases of thoracic disk herniation appears to be degenerative changes in the disk.[159] McKenzie[123] argues that the derangement syndrome can be divided into posterior and anterior disk derangements because of the distinct clinical presentations. The McKenzie classification system is outlined in Chapter 22. Anterior derangement is rare in the thoracic spine. The following derangement patterns are seen in the thoracic spine[123]:

- ***Derangement 1.*** This type of derangement typically produces central or symmetric pain between T1 and T12. These derangements are rapidly reversible.
- ***Derangement 2.*** This type of derangement, which is rare and the result of acute trauma or serious pathology, produces an acute kyphosis.
- ***Derangement 3.*** This type of derangement typically produces unilateral or asymmetric pain across the thoracic region, with or without radiation around the chest wall. These derangements are rapidly reversible.

CLINICAL PEARL

The clinical manifestations of thoracic disk herniation are extremely variable and vague. This often results in long delays between presentation and diagnosis.

Midline back pain and compressive myelopathy symptoms progressing over months or years are the predominant clinical features of a thoracic disk herniation.[160] One study[161] found that 70% of patients had signs of spinal cord compression, but that isolated root pain occurred in only 9% of patients. Unusual features of thoracic disk herniation include Lhermitte's symptom precipitated by rotation of the thoracic spine,[162] neurogenic claudication with positional dependent weakness,[163] and flaccid paraplegia.[164]

Some thoracic disk herniations are asymptomatic. The incidence of asymptomatic thoracic disk protrusions is approximately 37%, reinforcing the view that clinicians should interpret thoracic MRI findings with caution.[11,158]

T1 and T2 Levels. Disk herniations at these levels are extremely rare.[165] This rarity may be due to the protection afforded by the presence of the first and second ribs. Compression of the nerve at the T1 and at T2 segmental levels may result in numbness, tingling and weakness of the hand, and pain in arm and medial forearm.[165] T1 radiculopathy may also be associated with a Horner's syndrome.[165] The patient may also have reduced biceps and triceps reflexes.[165]

T2 and T3 Levels. A disk herniation at these levels is the rarest type.[166] Symptoms produced with this herniation include pain referred toward the clavicle, to the scapular spine, and down the inner side of the upper arm.[166]

T3–8 Levels. Compression of the nerves at these lower levels may result in symptoms that are experienced at the side, or front of the trunk.[90] Compression of the dura in the thoracic spine results in unilaterally referred pain, which is extrasegmental. A T6-level compression of the dura can cause pain up to the base of the neck and down to the waist, whereas a dural compression at T12 can refer pain up to T6 and down to the sacrum.[90]

T9–11 Levels. Lower thoracic disk herniations have been associated with pain radiating to the buttock in some cases, confusing the diagnosis with that of a lumbosacral root compression.[167] How a herniated disk at a low thoracic level could appear to be a lumbosacral radiculopathy may be best explained by the anatomic arrangement of the spinal cord and vertebral bodies. In adults, the conus medullaris ends between the 12th thoracic and third lumbar vertebrae, and the lumbar enlargement of the spinal cord is usually located at the lower thoracic level. Therefore, a lower thoracic disk herniation could compress the lumbosacral spinal nerves after their exit from the lumbar enlargement of the spinal cord and thus produce symptoms of compressive lumbosacral radiculopathy; thus, a herniation into an already tight canal may produce bilateral symptoms and sphincter disturbance, as in patients with a conus medullaris impairment.[168]

A retrospective study by Brown and colleagues[169] found that 77% of the 40 patients with symptomatic thoracic disk herniations, who were treated nonsurgically, were able to return to their previous level of activity.

Thoracic disk herniations requiring surgical management are uncommon and account for less than 2% of all operations performed on herniated IVDs.[170]

Electrodiagnosis of Thoracic Disk Lesions. Electrodiagnostic studies are important in identifying physiologic abnormalities of the nerve root in the cervical, thoracic, and lumbar spine, and they have been shown to be a useful diagnostic test in the diagnosis of radiculopathy,[171] correlating well with findings on myelography and surgery.[172,173]

There are two parts to the electromyogram: nerve conduction studies and needle electrode examination. The nerve conduction studies are performed by placing surface electrodes over a muscle belly or sensory area and stimulating the nerve, supplying either the muscle or the sensory area from fixed points along the nerve. From this, the amplitude, distal latency, and conduction velocity can be measured. The amplitude reflects the number of intact axons, whereas the distal latency and conduction velocity are more of a reflection of the degree of myelination.[174–176]

The timing of the examination is important, as positive sharp waves and fibrillation potentials will first occur 18–21 days after the onset of a radiculopathy.[175,177] It is, therefore, best to delay this study until 3 weeks after the injury, so that it can be as precise a study as possible. The primary use of electromyography is to diagnose nerve root impairment when the diagnosis is uncertain or to distinguish a radiculopathy from other impairments that are unclear on physical examination.[175] Electrodiagnostic abnormalities can persist after clinical recovery for months to years and in some may persist indefinitely.[178,179]

Traction: Mechanical or Manual for Thoracic Disk Lesions. Manual or mechanical traction has long been a preferred intervention throughout the spine with the intent of improving range of motion, and to treat both zygapophyseal joint impairments as well as disk herniation.[180–185] The efficacy of traction has not been scientifically proved in a randomized controlled trial, but it is commonly used and thought to be of benefit in reducing radicular pain.[186]

For traction to be effective, the imparted force must be sufficient to overcome soft tissue resistance prior to the relaxation of the involved musculature.

Traction can be applied continuously, or intermittently, and with the patient positioned in sitting or lying.[187] Intermittent traction produces twice as much separation as sustained.[188] The duration of traction recommended varies from 2 minutes to 24 hours.[189]

Performed manually, traction can be very time consuming and, in the lumbar and thoracic spines, requires a good deal of strength—approximately 12 times a patient's body weight is needed to develop significant distraction of the vertebral bodies. However, a greater degree of specificity can be obtained using manual traction, especially if it is performed using spinal locking techniques to localize the distraction to a specific level. Pain relief, or a centralization of symptoms, with manual traction may also be an indication for the use of mechanical traction.

Vertebral axial decompression, a newer method to cause distraction, probably represents a higher-tech version of traction, although there is no evidence in the current peer-reviewed literature to support this type of intervention.

Outcome studies of traction have demonstrated varying results.[180,185] From clinical experience, it would appear that traction yields better results if at least one of the spinal motions is full and pain free. However, a one-session trial of short duration is worthwhile, even if all of the motions are restricted.

Spinal traction is contraindicated in the following conditions:

- acute lumbago;
- instability;
- respiratory or cardiac insufficiency;
- respiratory irritation;
- painful reactions;
- a large extrusion;
- medial disk herniation;
- altered mental state; this includes the inability of the patient to relax.

Electrotherapeutic and Physical Modalities of Thoracic Disk Lesions. Modalities such as electrical stimulation also have been found helpful in uncontrolled studies.[190] They appear to be helpful in reducing the associated muscle pain and spasm but should be limited to the initial pain-control phase of the intervention.

Once there is control of pain and inflammation, the patient's intervention should be progressed to restore full range of motion and flexibility of the spine, trunk, and extremity muscles.

Zygapophyseal Joint Dysfunction

Apart from the upper and lower segments of this region, little is known about the extent or patterns of thoracic zygapophyseal joint degeneration. However, these joints have been found to be potential sources of local and referred pain.[191]

The pathomechanics describing mechanical dysfunction in this region are largely based on expert opinion and the principles of anatomy and biomechanics. Given the controversy surrounding the nature of coupled motions in the thoracic spine, and the number of structures involved in executing motion at these levels, the clinician is advised to diagnose dysfunction in this region based on restrictions of motion, rather than on specific structures.

Restriction of motion can have many causes in this region, including zygapophyseal joint hypomobility, soft tissue contracture, and costovertebral–costotransverse joint hypomobility. Differentiation among these structures, to find the specific cause of dysfunction, requires a great deal of expertise.

For the sake of simplicity, and because the spinous and transverse processes are more easily palpated in this region, the osteopathic approach of diagnosing a positional dysfunction using position testing is recommended.

As elsewhere in the spine, dysfunctions can be either symmetric or asymmetric. Symmetric impairments are more common in the thoracic region than in the lumbar, particularly in the upper and cervicothoracic spine as a result of fixed postural impairments. These, of course, will not be apparent on position testing and must be sought after when the position tests are negative. If no asymmetry is found on position testing, then the segment of interest should be separately passively flexed, extended, and rotated in all directions.

To determine which lesion is present, layer palpation is used. The position of the superior vertebra and the posteroanterior relationship of the transverse processes to the coronal body plane is noted and compared with the level above and below, in thoracic flexion and then extension (see "Position Testing: Spinal" section earlier).

Rib Dysfunction

The costovertebral joint may be involved in inflammatory or degenerative joint disease. Complaints of symptoms in these joints are common in conditions such as ankylosing spondylitis as a result of synovitis. The clinical features of severe arthropathy of the costovertebral joint include pain with deep breathing, trunk rotation, sneezing, or coughing. CT scans are helpful in confirming the diagnosis. Inflammation of the costovertebral joint commonly causes localized pain about 3–4 cm from the midline, where the rib articulates with the transverse process and the vertebral body.[81]

According to the osteopaths, rib dysfunctions are described as structural, torsional, or respiratory.[117,192,193]

- ***Structural.*** Structural rib dysfunctions are true joint subluxations that occur secondary to trauma. These dysfunctions are extremely painful and significantly reduce motion of the ribs during inspiration and expiration. The most important landmarks for structural rib dysfunctions are the rib angle and the anterior rib. Ribs can sublux anteriorly or posteriorly (see Table 27-4). The first rib can sublux superiorly.
- ***Torsional.*** As their name suggests, these rib dysfunctions are twisting injuries, in which the rib is held in a position of internal or external rotation. These dysfunctions affect the thoracic spine motions as well as the motions of respiration (see Table 27-4).
- ***Respiratory.*** Respiratory rib dysfunctions usually are related to poor posture and result in a restriction of either inspiration or expiration.

The first rib can sublux anteriorly, posteriorly, or, more commonly, superiorly. If the motion is perceived as abnormal, passive movement testing should be performed. The arthrokinematic is tested with the patient seated and the clinician standing behind. Using the medial aspect of the MCP joint of the index finger, the clinician applies an anterior–inferior–medial glide of the rib to assess the inspiration glide, while a posterior–superior–lateral glide is applied to assess the expiration glide. The end-feel is assessed. If it is abrupt and hard (pathomechanical) in both glide directions as compared with the same rib on the other side, then the problem is a subluxation. If it is stiff (hard capsular) in both directions as compared with the same rib on the other side, then a pericapsular restriction is present. If both glides are normal, then the problem is likely to be myofascial.

- ***Unilateral restriction of anterior rotation of the first rib.*** This dysfunction is seen when the scalene muscles are hypertonic or adaptively shortened and hold the *anterior* aspect of the first rib superiorly or when the *superior glide* of the first rib is restricted at the costotransverse joint. This dysfunction will restrict unilateral elevation of the arm (both arms may be involved). If the dysfunction is intra-articular, rotation and side bending of the head/neck will be limited to the side of the restricted rib (this motion requires a superior glide of the rib at the costotransverse joint). Full expiration will also reveal asymmetry of rib motion. If the restriction is intra-articular, the superior glide of the first rib at the costotransverse joint will be restricted. The presence or absence of pain depends upon the stage of the pathology (substrate, fibroblastic, and maturation) and the irritability of the surrounding tissue. The grade of the mobilization technique is directed by these factors.
- ***Unilateral restriction of posterior rotation of the first rib.*** This dysfunction, also known as an expiratory or anterior sagittal lesion, is seen when the *posterior* aspect of the first rib is held superiorly or when the *inferior glide* of the first rib is restricted at the costotransverse joint. This dysfunction will restrict unilateral elevation of the arm on either side, rotation and side bending of the head/neck to the opposite side of the restricted rib, and full inspiration. If the restriction is intra-articular, the inferior glide of the first rib at the costotransverse joint will be restricted. The presence or absence of pain depends on the stage of the pathology (substrate, fibroblastic, and maturation) and the irritability of the surrounding tissue. The grade of the mobilization technique is directed by these factors.

The intervention for costovertebral dysfunctions involves mobilization and manipulation techniques or local anesthetic injections, or both.

Practice Pattern 4E: Impaired Joint Mobility, Motor Function, Muscle Performance, and Range of Motion Associated with Localized Inflammation

Tietze Syndrome

Tietze syndrome is a local inflammation of the costosternal cartilage, which most commonly affects the second and third costochondral junctions.[27,153] Tietze syndrome may also affect any of the cartilaginous articulations of the chest wall, including the sternoclavicular joints.[194]

The clinical findings for this condition include a history of a gradual or sudden onset of pain in the involved region, which is increased with deep inspiration, coughing, or sneezing. Upon physical examination, there is often a localized swelling of the costosternal cartilage.

This is a self-limiting condition, which can last from weeks to years. The intervention can involve local injections of corticosteroid and specific joint mobilizations to the costovertebral articulations.

Muscle Strains

Muscle strains, which are common in this region, are characterized by localized pain and tenderness, which is exacerbated with isometric testing or passive stretching of the muscle. Rather than attempt to isolate muscles in this region, the clinician can determine the directions that alleviate the symptoms and those that do not. A gradual strengthening and gentle passive stretching program into the painless directions is initially performed, before progressing as tolerated into the painful directions.

Intercostal Muscles. Injuries to intercostal muscles are mainly caused by direct trauma or after unaccustomed or excessive muscular activity (e.g., lifting a heavy object or persistent coughing).[195] On occasion, the onset of pain or symptoms may be of gradual onset with no obvious inciting event.[196] Intercostal muscle injuries are more likely in activities in which upper body use is extreme, such as regular use of a pickaxe.[196]

The classic presentation is pain between the ribs that is worse on movement, deep inspiration, or coughing, and tender to palpation.

The intervention for intercostals muscle strains includes anti-inflammatory medications, the avoidance of exacerbating activities, and the treatment of any underlying pathology where appropriate.

Contusions

The severity of soft tissue injury to the chest wall is dependent on the mechanism of injury and the degree of protection between the traumatic force and the chest wall.[55] Chest injury is commonly produced by the restraining influence of the diagonal component of a seat belt. Seat belt injuries occur predominantly on the side of the belt and hence occur on different sides in drivers and passengers.[55] These take the form of abrasions, ecchymoses, and friction burns, producing an imprint of the belt.[55]

Trauma to the female breast can be produced by a combination of compression and shearing stress produced by a seat belt, and subcutaneous rupture of breast tissue can occur.[197] The presence of a persistent breast mass after trauma must always be taken seriously, as trauma may draw attention to an unsuspected carcinoma.[55]

Chest trauma can result in disruption of a subcutaneously placed pacemaker generator or leads, long-term indwelling central venous catheter, or subcutaneous portions of arterial bypass grafts.[55]

Severe skeletal trauma to the chest wall can be associated with large chest wall hematomas or collections of air within the chest wall, which can communicate with the intrathoracic space.[55]

The conservative intervention for thoracic cage contusions depends on the severity of the injury and the tissues involved. Typically, the initial intervention for soft tissue injury is cryotherapy with rest. Gentle pain-free active range-of-motion exercises are introduced as tolerated. Once the acute stage is over, thermal modalities are used and the range of motion exercises progressed to strengthening exercises in all planes.

Practice Pattern 4G: Impaired Joint Mobility, Motor Function, Muscle Performance, and Range of Motion Associated with Fractures

Thoracic Vertebral Fractures

Fractures of the thoracic spine account for 25–30% of all spine fractures.[198] These fractures are most often a result of hyperflexion or axial loading injuries[199] and less commonly attributable to rotational stresses, side bending, horizontal shear, and hyperextension. The most common fractures seen in the thoracic spine are anterior wedge compression fractures and burst fractures[200] (see Chap. 5). Most thoracic spine fractures occur between the ninth and 11th vertebral bodies. Multiple fractures are found in 10% of all patients with a spine fracture, and, therefore, evaluation of the entire spine is necessary, because up to 80% of these additional fractures are noncontiguous.[201] Only 12% of patients with fracture–dislocations of the thoracic spine are neurologically intact, and 62% of patients with thoracic spine fracture–dislocations have complete neurologic deficits.[55]

Rib Fractures

Fractured ribs can lacerate the pleura, lung, or abdominal organs. Fractures to upper ribs, clavicle, and upper sternum can signal brachial plexus or vascular injury. Isolated fractures of the ribs, clavicle, or scapula seldom represent significant injuries in and of themselves, but they do reflect the magnitude of force imparted, particularly in older patients with noncompliant chest walls.[202] Fractured rib ends can lacerate the pleura or lung, resulting in hemothorax or pneumothorax.[55] There is a much greater incidence of rib fractures in older patients, whose ribs are relatively inelastic, compared with the incidence of rib fractures in children, whose ribs are more pliable and resilient.[55] For this reason, a posttraumatic pneumothorax in older patients is almost always associated with one or more rib fractures, whereas children can sustain a pneumothorax or major internal thoracic injury after trauma without an associated rib fracture.

Fractures of the first three ribs, in particular, indicate significant energy transfer, because they are well protected by the shoulder girdles and associated musculature.[55] Fractures to the upper ribs, clavicle, and upper sternum are accompanied by brachial plexus or vascular injury in 3–15% of patients.[203] Fractures of the 10th, 11th, or 12th ribs are associated with injury to the liver, kidneys, or spleen and should prompt confirmation of organ injury with CT.[55] Double fractures of three or more adjacent ribs or contiguous combined rib and sternal or costochondral fractures, or single fractures of four or more contiguous ribs, can produce a focal area of chest wall instability. Paradoxical movement of a "flail" segment during the respiratory cycle can impair respiratory mechanics, promote atelectasis, and impair pulmonary drainage.

The common findings for a rib fracture are described in Chapter 5. A key factor in the intervention of rib fractures is believed to be adequate pain control to allow early aggressive respiratory care and, hence, prevent the development of pulmonary complications.

Early intervention includes assistance with coughing, intracostal nerve blocks, and muscle relaxants. Adhesive strapping or taping should be avoided because it can inhibit deep inspiration and may contribute to atelectasis.[204] Simple rib fractures become stable in 1–2 weeks, with firm healing by callus in approximately 6 weeks.[204]

Scheuermann's Disease

Scheuermann's disease, which is found in approximately 10% of the population and in males and females equally, is typically seen in pubescent athletes.[21]

The disease involves a defect to the ring apophysis of the vertebral body and anterior wedging of the affected vertebrae, as a result of a flexion overload of the anterior vertebral body.[205] The end plate can crack, thus making it possible for disk material to bulge into the vertebral body (Schmorl's node). According to McKenzie,[123] the extension dysfunction develops in patients with Scheuermann's disease as a result of adaptive shortening from poor postural habits, or from derangement or trauma and the healing process.

Clinical findings include evidence of a thoracic kyphosis and pain with thoracic extension and rotation.

The intervention depends on the severity but typically involves postural education, a modification of the aggravating activity, exercise (seated rotation and extension in lying exercises), or bracing. The exercise program involves the stretching of the pectoralis major and minor muscles, and muscle-strengthening exercises for the thoracic spine extensors and the scapular adductors.[38]

Scapular Fractures

Fractures of the scapula are relatively rare due to the thick muscles lying both superficial and deep to the scapula and the energy-absorbing ability of the scapula to move on the chest wall.[206] Because of the large amount of force that is required to fracture a scapula, these fractures are often associated with other major injuries. For example, the incidence of pneumothorax in patients with fracture of a scapula is over 50%.[207] Associated injuries that are directly related to the fractured scapula include injuries of the suprascapular nerve, axillary nerve, axillary artery, and subclavian artery.[55] The body of the scapula is the most frequent site of fracture followed by the neck and glenoid.[208] The spine, coracoid, and acromion are less frequently fractured.[208] Scapular fractures may not be recognized on the initial chest radiograph as they are frequently radiographically obscure and are commonly associated with multiple other regional injuries, such as clavicular and rib fractures, subcutaneous air, pneumothorax, and pulmonary contusion.[55]

Sternal Fractures. The tremendous force necessary to cause a fracture of the sternum has led to the belief that the presence of a sternal fracture is a harbinger of severe associated injuries. The association of seat belt wearing with sternal fractures is well known.[209] A proportional increase in incidence of 100% in drivers and 150% in front-seat passengers has been noted since the enactment of seat belt legislation.[210] Sternal fractures, as such, do not generally cause problems either in healing or by direct damage to adjacent structures. Dislocation of the sternoclavicular joint, however, with posterior displacement of the inner end of the clavicle may cause compression of the trachea and the adjacent great vessels, with significant clinical consequences.[211]

Integration of Practice Patterns 4B and 4F: Impaired Joint Mobility, Motor Function, Muscle Performance, Range of Motion Secondary to Impaired Posture, Systemic Dysfunction (Referred Pain Syndromes), Spinal Disorders, and Myofascial Pain Dysfunction

Referred Pain

Referred pain to this area is extremely common. Referred pain is characterized by a poorly localized pain that is nontender to palpation and does not change with movements or alterations of posture (see Table 27-6).

T4 Syndrome

The name of this syndrome is a bit of a misnomer, because the syndrome can additionally affect any of the T2–7 levels, although it always includes the T4 segment. The T4 syndrome has an unknown etiology, although it is believed to result from a sympathetic reaction to a hypomobile segment, because the symptoms appear to resolve in response to manual therapy techniques to the thoracic segments.[212–214] In the thorax, the sympathetic trunks lie on or just lateral to the costovertebral joints. These trunks may undergo mechanical deformation with abnormal posture (forward head, accentuated thoracic kyphosis, and protracted shoulder girdle), trauma, or pulling and reaching activities, producing pain and sympathetic epiphenomena.[215]

Neurovascular symptoms are not a feature of this syndrome, though a differential diagnosis should consider such conditions.[212] The upper extremity symptoms are glovelike in distribution and are not segmentally related.[213] Nocturnal symptoms are common, usually occurring in the side lying or supine position.[213] More women are affected by this condition than men, in a ratio of more than 3:1.[216]

Clinical findings include local tenderness of bony points, positive slump test, positive upper limb tension tests, depression or prominence of one or more spinous processes, and local thickening and stiffness of one segment,[216] although gross cervical and thoracic motions are usually normal.[212]

The differential diagnosis includes carpal tunnel syndrome, thoracic outlet syndrome (see Chap. 25), cervical disk disease, vascular disease, and neurologic disease.[212]

The intervention for this condition involves mobilization and manipulation of the involved segment, followed by an exercise progression emphasizing upper thoracic flexibility and muscle strength. Butler[217] recommends using both upper limb tension tests and also the slump test, with combinations of thoracic rotation and side bending.

Notalgia Paresthetica

The name of this condition comes from the Greek root meaning "pain in the back."[218] Clinically, this condition consists of pruritus and localized dysesthesia and hyperesthesia in the distribution of one of the cutaneous posterior (dorsal) rami of the upper thoracic area.

The recommended intervention for this condition is an injection of corticosteroid.

THERAPEUTIC TECHNIQUES

The selection of a manual technique is dependent on a number of factors, including the acuteness of the condition and the restriction to the movement that is encountered. Oftentimes, the same technique that was used to examine the segment can be used for the intervention, the difference being the intent of the clinician and the goal of the intervention. For example, if stretching of the mechanical barrier rather than pain relief is the immediate objective of the intervention, a mobilization technique is carried out at the end of the available range.

To achieve this, the antagonist muscle must be relaxed, and this is most easily accomplished using a hold–relax technique. After this has been gained (and sometimes before and after), there is some minor pain to be dealt with, using grade IV oscillations, after which the joint capsule can be stretched, using either grade IV++ or prolonged stretch techniques. The prolonged stretch or the strong oscillations are continued for as long as the clinician can maintain good control. At the point where control is about to be lost, several isometric contractions to the agonists and the antagonists are demanded of the patient's muscles in the new range, to give the central nervous system information about the newly acquired range. To complete the reeducation, concentric and eccentric retraining is carried out throughout the whole range of the joint. Active exercises are continued at home and at work on a regular and frequent basis, to reinforce the reeducation.

Techniques to Increase Joint Mobility

Joint Mobilizations and High-Velocity Thrust Techniques

Mobilization and high-velocity thrust techniques have traditionally been used routinely in this region to[29,86,219,220]:

- restore thoracic mobility;
- reduce stresses through both the fixation and the leverage components of the spine;
- reduce stresses through the hypermobile segments;
- reduce the overall force needed by the clinician, thus giving greater control.

CLINICAL PEARL

Cleland et al.[221] developed a clinical prediction rule (CPR) to identify a subgroup of patients with neck pain who were considered more likely to benefit from a high-velocity thrust technique of the thoracic spine. However, more recent evidence has questioned its validity.[222] A recent study that included 24 consecutive patients,[223] tested two different forms of high-velocity thrust techniques to the thoracic spine based on this CPR. The study found that patients who were treated with a combination of cervical spine high-velocity thrust techniques and exercises showed significantly greater improvement in pain and disability compared to those treated with thoracic spine high-velocity techniques and exercises.

A number of studies have demonstrated clinical success with high-velocity thrust techniques to the thoracic spine.[135,139,224,225] However, it must be remembered that the isolation of a particular segment in the thoracic spine is extremely difficult, if not impossible because of the number of articulations that exist at each segmental level. In addition, there are a number of concerns that the clinician must be aware of prior to considering using high-velocity thrust techniques in this region. These include the following:

- A number of studies have demonstrated that the meninges may be vulnerable to thoracic manipulative thrust techniques.[226,227]
- The narrow dimensions of the mid-thoracic spinal canal.
- The poor blood supply to this region as compared to other areas of the spine.[53]
- The potential fragility of the bones in this area due to such conditions as osteoporosis, and rheumatoid arthritis.

It is, therefore, recommended that the clinician performs the slump test (see Chap. 11) and a premanipulative hold (see Chap. 10) prior to any technique.

Long Sit Superior Distraction (T5–6). The patient is positioned on the treatment table in the long sit position, with the buttocks on the edge of the back of the table and the hands on the back of the neck, fingers interlocked. The clinician stands behind the patient and places a small towel roll at the T6 level. The towel roll is held in place by the clinician's chest (made easier if the clinician turns slightly so that the side of the chest is used). The clinician threads his or her arms under the patient's armpits and places the heel of the palms under the patient's forearms. The patient is asked to flex the neck. A stride stance (one foot in front of the other) is adopted by the clinician (Fig. 27-23), and, while keeping the elbows close together, the clinician gently rocks the patient backward and forward. After two or three rocks, the traction force is applied, as the clinician shifts his or her body weight from the forward leg to the back, while lifting the patient and pushing the patient's forearms toward the ceiling.

Exercises to Increase Soft Tissue Extensibility

Shoulder Sweep. This exercise is used to mobilize the chest wall and to integrate upper extremity function with thoracic spine and rib cage motion.[61]

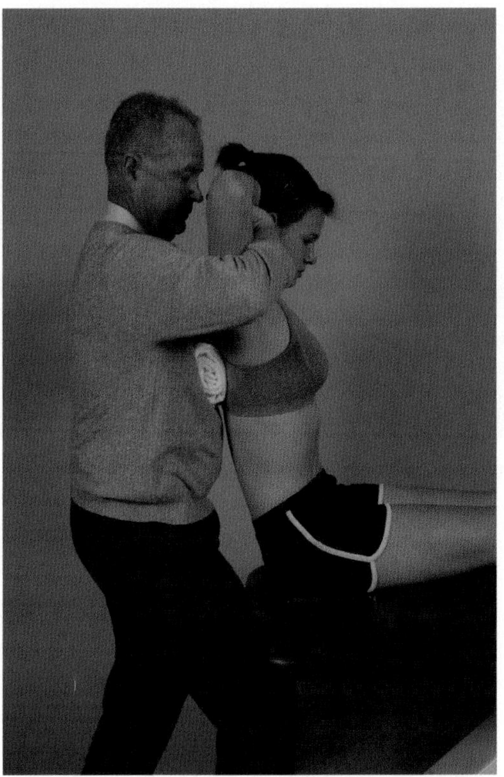

FIGURE 27-23 Long sit superior distraction thrust technique.

The patient is positioned supine on the floor or on a mat table, with the hips and knees flexed to about 90 degrees (Fig. 27-24). The patient is asked to reach sideways and place the back of the hand as far out to the side as is comfortable. While maintaining contact with the floor, the patient moves the hand above the head and to the other side of the body, making a large circle around his or her body (see Fig. 27-24). Manual assistance applied to the scapula or rib cage can be used as can deep breathing, in order to move into the restricted ranges.

Thoracic Spine Flexion. The patient kneels in front of a Swiss ball. The patient positions themselves over the Swissball so that weight is applied through the feet and the forearms (Fig. 27-25). While applying some body weight through the forearms, the patient arches the thoracic spine as far as is comfortable. This position is held for 8–10 seconds, after which the patient relaxes. The exercise is repeated 8–10 times.

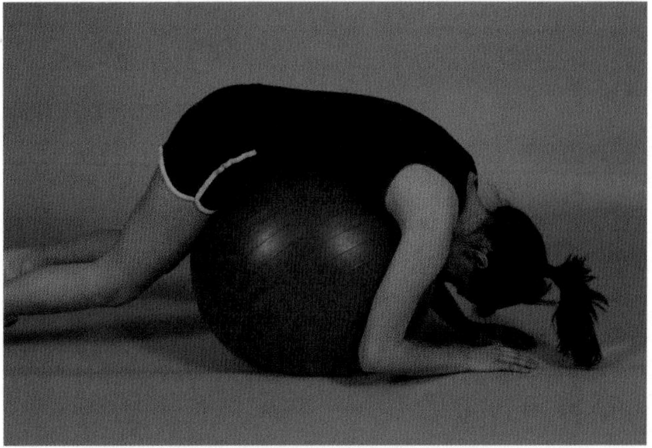

FIGURE 27-25 Thoracic spine flexion over Swiss ball.

Thoracic Spine Extension. It is advised that the clinician monitor this exercise in case the patient loses his or her balance. The patient sits on a Swiss ball, with the feet on the ground. Once the patient has good sitting balance, he or she attempts to lie supine on the ball and then places the hands on the ball (Fig. 27-26). The patient is then instructed to move the top of the head toward the floor, in an attempt to fully extend the thoracic spine. This position is held for 8–10 seconds, after which the patient relaxes. The exercise is repeated eight to 10 times. This exercise can be made more challenging by moving the hands from beside the body, out to the sides (Fig. 27-27) while maintaining the balance.

If the patient is unable to maintain his or her balance on the Swiss ball, a foam roll may be used. The foam roll also allows the clinician to focus the extension exercise on a specific segment.

Thoracic Spine Rotation. The following Swiss ball exercises to improve thoracic rotation range of motion and strength are recommended for the athletic population, only. The patient kneels with his or her back facing the Swiss ball. Using one leg at a time, the patient reaches back with the foot and places it on top of the Swiss ball. Once both feet are on the ball, the legs are

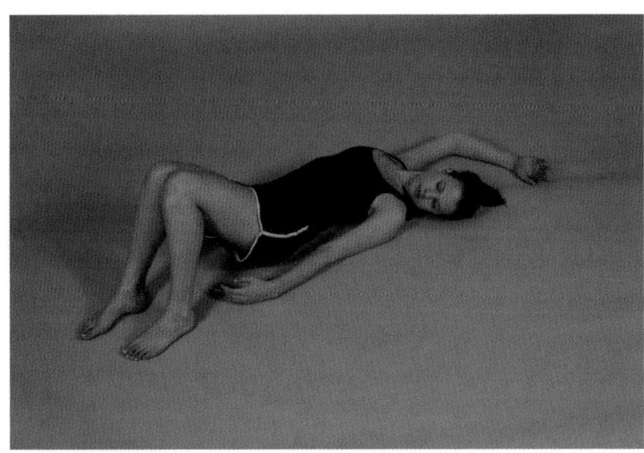

FIGURE 27-24 Shoulder Sweep exercise.

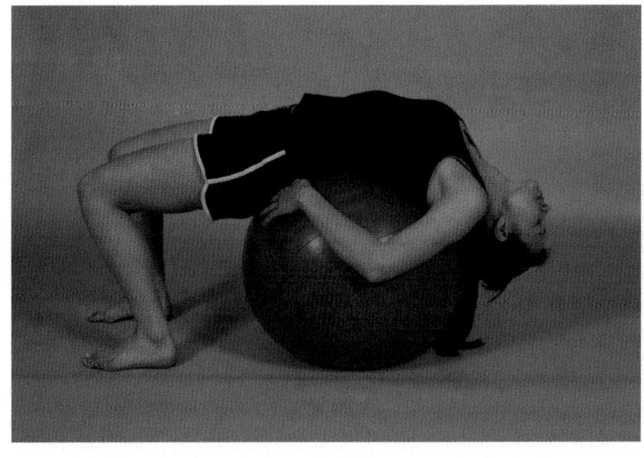

FIGURE 27-26 Thoracic spine extension over Swiss ball.

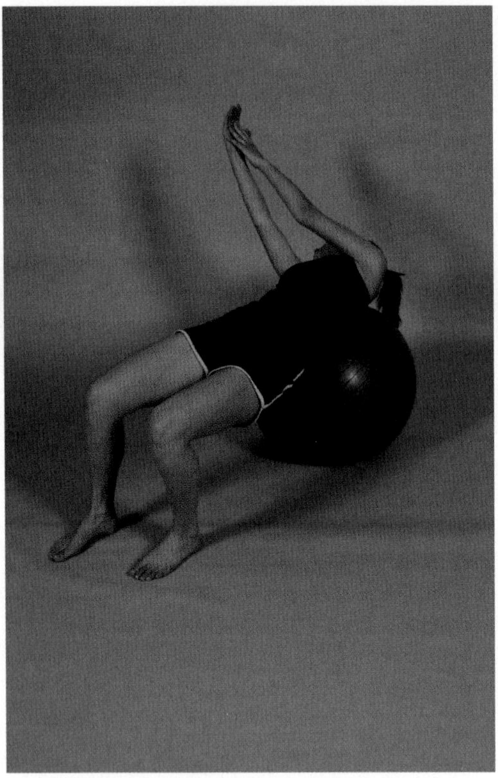

FIGURE 27-27 Thoracic spine extension over Swiss ball—arms out to the side.

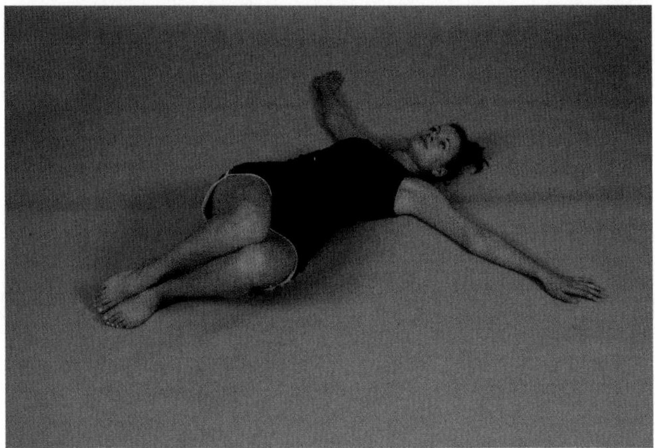

FIGURE 27-29 Hooklying rotations with arms abducted.

straightened and the weight of the body is primarily borne through the arms. Using the dorsum of the feet and the anterior legs, the patient induces a rotation to the thoracic region by twisting at the waist (Fig. 27-28), while maintaining balance through the arms. This position is held for 8–10 seconds, after which the patient relaxes. The exercise is repeated 8–10 times. By alternatively moving the legs into hip flexion and extension, rotation of the thoracic spine can be achieved, while maintaining balance with the arms (see Fig. 27-28).

For the nonathletic population, thoracic rotation exercises can be performed using a firmer base of support. The patient kneels in front of a wobble board and places both hands on the board. Once good balance is achieved, the patient is asked to raise one arm out to the side as high as is comfortable, while keeping both knees on the floor. This position is held for 8–10 seconds, after which the patient relaxes. The exercise is repeated eight to 10 times.

Thoracic rotation exercises can also be performed in the supine position. The patient lies supine with both knees bent and feet placed on the floor. The arms are abducted to approximately 90 degrees (Fig. 27-29). Keeping the trunk against the floor, the patient lowers the thighs to one side and then the other (see Fig. 27-29), as far as is comfortable. This position is held for 8–10 seconds, after which the patient relaxes. The exercise is repeated eight to 10 times.

Thoracic Spine Side Bending. The patient kneels to the side of a Swiss ball. The patient is asked to lean sideways over the ball and, with the arm closest to the ball, to attempt to touch the floor on the other side of the ball (Fig. 27-30) without losing balance. This position is held for 8–10 seconds, after which the patient relaxes. The exercise is repeated eight to 10 times.

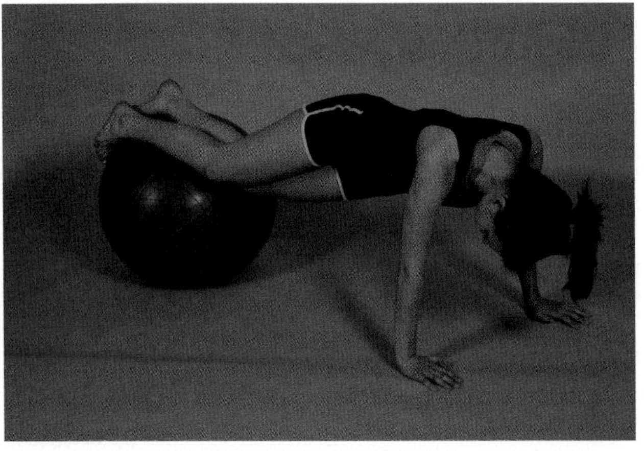

FIGURE 27-28 Thoracic spine rotation with trunk on Swiss ball.

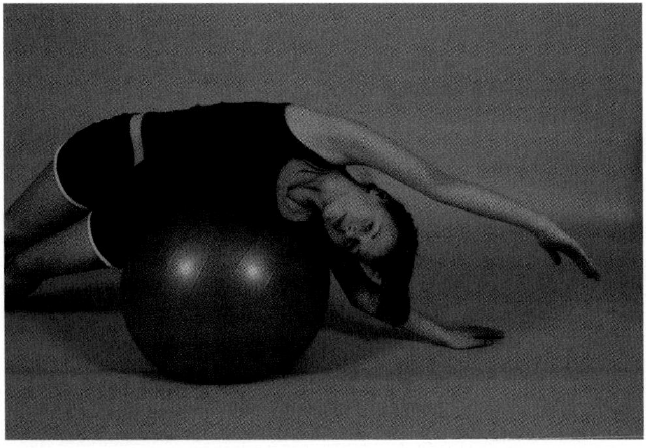

FIGURE 27-30 Thoracic side bending over Swiss ball.

Rib Techniques for the Mid-Lower Thoracic Spine

Myofascial Stretch into Extension. The patient is positioned supine, and the clinician stands at the head of the bed. The patient elevates both arms over the head and reaches around the back of the clinician's thighs. By having the patient hold a towel in this position, the clinician can place both of his or her hands under the patient's rib cage and pull the rib cage in an anterior and cranial direction, thereby encouraging thoracic extension (Fig. 27-31). A belt wrapped around the patient at the correct level can make this technique more specific.

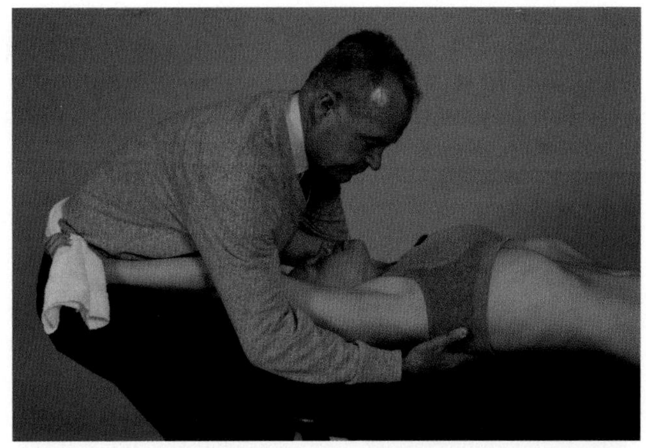

FIGURE 27-31 Supine myofascial stretch into extension.

CASE STUDY
RIGHT ANTERIOR CHEST PAIN

HISTORY

A 25-year-old man presented at the clinic complaining of pain in his right anterior chest. About 1 month previously, the patient had experienced a sudden and sharp pain in his right posterior chest at the midscapular level during a tug of war game at his company's picnic. The posterior chest pain subsided very quickly and did not bother him for the rest of the game. However, the next morning, pain was felt in the anterior aspect of the chest. This anterior chest pain eased off over the next few days with rest, but recurred as soon as the patient returned to weight lifting.[87]

Questions

1. Given the mechanism of injury, what structure(s) could be at fault?
2. Should the report of anterior chest pain concern the clinician in this case?
3. What is your working hypothesis at this stage? List the various diagnoses that could present with anterior chest pain, and the tests you would use to rule out each one.
4. Why do you think the pain shift from posterior thoracic to anterior thoracic?
5. Does this presentation/history warrant a scan? Why or why not?

CASE STUDY
BILATERAL AND CENTRAL UPPER THORACIC PAIN

HISTORY

A 30-year-old housewife presents at the clinic with a 3-day history of constant central and bilateral upper thoracic pain that is deep and dull and can be felt in the front of the chest when the pain is aggravated. The pain is reported to be worse with flexion motions but is improved with lying on a hard surface. Further questioning revealed that the patient had a history of minor back pain but was otherwise in good health and had no report of bowel or bladder impairment.

Questions

1. What structure(s) could be at fault with central and bilateral upper thoracic pain as the major complaint?
2. Should the report of anterior chest pain concern the clinician in this case?
3. Why was the statement about "no reports of bowel or bladder impairment" pertinent?
4. What is your working hypothesis at this stage? List the various diagnoses that could manifest with central and bilateral upper thoracic pain and the tests you would use to rule out each one.
5. Does this presentation/history warrant a scanning examination? Why or why not?

CASE STUDY

NECK SPRAIN

HISTORY

A 42-year-old right-handed female was referred by her primary-care physician with a diagnosis of neck sprain.[228] The patient reported a 10-year history of intermittent neck pain (right greater than left), which had worsened over the past 6 months. More recently, the patient reported developing right shoulder (right upper trapezius) and arm pain, as well as infrequent (about twice a week) paresthesia in the right arm and hand involving the fourth and fifth digits. The patient described the pain as a sharp stabbing pain at the right side of the neck and a dull aching pain in the right upper trapezius region. She indicated that the neck pain was independent of the upper trapezius pain. At the time of the evaluation, the neck and upper trapezius pain were a 3/10 and 4/10, respectively. The symptoms improved when she positioned herself supine or left side lying with a pillow under the head. The upper trapezius pain was reduced when she side bent the head toward the side of pain and worsened as the day progressed, especially when she was at work and performing elevated arm activities. She reported that the paresthesias of the ulnar aspect of a right forearm, as well as digits 4 and 5, appeared more often during the afternoon and occasionally at night. When inquiring about the irritability of the condition, the patient reported that between a few hours and 1 day were required for the pain to decrease after it was provoked. The patient worked as a faculty member at a local college, which involved spending prolonged periods of time on the computer and extensive reading. The patient's past medical history was negative for dizziness, diplopia, unexpected weight change, drop attacks, dysarthria, dysphagia, tinnitus, and night pain unrelated to position.

Questions

1. List the structure(s) that could be at fault with these complaints.
2. Does this sound like a neuromusculoskeletal condition?
3. Are there any other questions you would ask this patient?
4. What is your working hypothesis at this stage? List the various diagnoses that could manifest with central and bilateral upper thoracic pain and the tests you would use to rule out each one.
5. Does this presentation/history warrant a scanning examination? Why or why not?

CASE STUDY

INTERSCAPULAR PAIN

HISTORY

A 21-year-old woman presented with a 1-week history of left-sided interscapular pain that started at work. The patient worked as a computer operator. The pain was reported to be aggravated by lying prone, deep breathing in, and standing or sitting erect. Further questioning revealed that the patient had a history of this pain over the past few months but that it had not been as intense as it was currently. The patient was otherwise in good health and had no reports of bowel or bladder impairment.

Questions

1. List the structures that can produce interscapular pain.
2. Given the fact that this patient works at a computer, what could be the cause of her pain?
3. What is your working hypothesis at this stage? List the various diagnoses that could manifest with interscapular pain and the tests you would use to rule out each one.
4. Does this presentation/history warrant a scan? Why or why not?

REVIEW QUESTIONS*

1. In the thoracic region, in which plane are the zygapophyseal (facet) joints oriented?
2. Which of the ribs are considered atypical ribs, and why?
3. What is the joint where the rib and the vertebra meet called?
4. Which structures modify and restrict rotation in the thoracic region?
5. Which ribs demonstrate bucket handle movement and which display pump handle motions?

*Additional questions to test your understanding of this chapter can be found in the Online Learning Center for *Orthopaedic Assessment, Evaluation, and Intervention* at www.duttononline.net.

REFERENCES

1. Panjabi MM, Brand RA, White AA: Mechanical properties of the human thoracic spine. *J Bone Joint Surg Am* 58A:642–652, 1976.
2. Lee D, Lee L-J: Integrated, multimodal approach to the thoracic spine and ribs. In: Magee DJ, Zachazewski JE, Quillen WS, eds. *Pathology and Intervention in Musculoskeletal Rehabilitation*. St. Louis, MI: Saunders, 2009:306–337.
3. Singer KP, Edmondston SJ: Introduction: The enigma of the thoracic spine. In: Giles LGF, Singer KP, eds. *Clinical Anatomy and Management of Thoracic Spine Pain. The Clinical Anatomy and Management of Back Pain Series*. Oxford: Butterworth-Heinemann, 2000.
4. Bradford S: Juvenile kyphosis. In: Bradford DS, Lonstein JE, Moe JH, et al, eds. *Moe's Textbook of Scoliosis and Other Spinal Deformities*. Philadelphia, PA: W.B. Saunders, 1987:347–368.
5. Frazer JE: *Frazer's Anatomy of the Human Skeleton*. London: Churchill Livingstone, 1965.
6. Singer KP, Jones T, Breidahl PD: A comparison of radiographic and computer-assisted measurements of thoracic and thoracolumbar sagittal curvature. *Skeletal Radiol* 19:21–26, 1990.
7. Willen J, Anderson J, Tomooka K, et al: The natural history of burst fractures in the thoracolumbar spine T12 and L1. *J Spinal Disord* 3:39–46, 1990.
8. Gray H: *Gray's Anatomy*. Philadelphia, PA: Lea & Febiger, 1995.
9. Panjabi MM, Takata K, Goel V: Thoracic human vertebrae. Quantitative three-dimensional anatomy. *Spine* 16:888–901, 1991.
10. Edmondston SJ, Singer KP, Day RE, et al: In-vitro relationships between vertebral body density, size and compressive strength in the elderly thoracolumbar spine. *Clin Biomech* 9:180–186, 1994.
11. Wood KB, Garvey TA, Gundry C, et al: Thoracic MRI evaluation of asymptomatic individuals. *J Bone Joint Surg Am* 77A:1634–1638, 1995.
12. Mercer S: Comparative anatomy of the spinal disc. In: Boyling JD, Jull GA, eds. *Grieve's Modern Manual Therapy: The Vertebral Column*. Philadelphia, PA: Churchill Livingstone, 2004:9–16.
13. Oliver J, Middleditch A: *Functional Anatomy of the Spine*. Oxford: Butterworth-Heinemann, 1991.
14. Kapandji IA: *The Physiology of the Joints, The Trunk and Vertebral Column*. New York, NY: Churchill Livingstone, 1991.
15. Reuben JD, Brown RH, Nash CL: In-vivo effects of axial loading on healthy adolescent spines. *Clin Orthop Relat Res* 139:17–27, 1979.
16. DiGiovanna EL, Schiowitz S: *An Osteopathic Approach to Diagnosis and Treatment*. Philadelphia, PA: JB Lippincott, 1991.
17. Galante JO: Tensile properties of human lumbar annulus fibrosis. *Acta Orthop Scand* 100(Suppl), 1-91 1967.
18. Seifert MH, Whiteside CG, Savage O: A 5-year follow-up of fifty cases of idiopathic osteoarthritis of the hip. *Ann Rheum Dis* 28:325–326, 1969.
19. Lundon K, Bolton K: Structure and function of the lumbar intervertebral disk in health, aging, and pathological conditions. *J Orthop Sports Phys Ther* 31:291–306, 2001.
20. Lyu RK, Chang HS, Tang LM, et al: Thoracic disc herniation mimicking acute lumbar disc disease. *Spine* 24:416–418, 1999.
21. Bradford DS, Loustein JE, Moe JH, et al: *Moe's Textbook of Skoliosis and other Spinal Deformities*, 2nd ed. Philadelphia, PA: WB Saunders, 1987.
22. White AA: An analysis of the mechanics of the thoracic spine in man. *Acta Orthop Scand* 127(Suppl):8–92, 1969.
23. Edmondston SJ, Singer KP: Thoracic spine: Anatomical and biomechanical considerations for manual therapy. *Man Ther* 2:132–143, 1997.
24. Rouviere H: Anatomie Humaine. *Descriptive et Topographique*. Paris: Masson, 1927.
25. Singer KP, Boyle JJW, Fazey P: Comparative anatomy of the zygapophyseal joints. In: Boyling JD, Jull GA, eds. *Grieve's Modern Manual Therapy: The Vertebral Column*. Philadelphia, PA: Churchill Livingstone, 2004:17–29.
26. Gregersen GG, Lucas DB: An in vivo study of the axial rotation of the human thoracolumbar spine. *J Bone Joint Surg Am* 49:247–262, 1967.
27. Singer KP, Breidahl PD, Day RE: Posterior element variation at the thoracolumbar transition: a morphometric study using computed tomography. *Clin Biomech* 4:80–86, 1989.
28. Lee DG: Biomechanics of the thorax. In: Grant R, ed. *Physical Therapy of the Cervical and Thoracic Spine*. New York, NY: Churchill Livingstone, 1988:47–76.
29. Lee DG: *Manual Therapy for the Thorax - A Biomechanical Approach*. Delta, BC: D.O.P.C., 1994.
30. MacConnail MA, Basmajian JV: *Muscles and Movements: A Basis for Human Kinesiology*. New York, NY: Robert Krieger Pub Co, 1977.
31. Williams PL: *Gray's Anatomy*, 38th ed. New York, NY: Churchill Livingstone, 1995.
32. King TC, Smith CR: Chest wall, pleura, lung, and mediastinum. In: Schwartz SI, Shires GT, Spencer FC, eds. *Principles of Surgery*. New York, NY: McGraw-Hill, 1989:627.
33. Nathan H, Weinberg H, Robin GC, et al: The costovertebral joints: anatomical-clinical observations in arthritis. *Arthritis Rheum* 7:228–240, 1964.
34. Oda I, Abumi K, Duosai L, et al: Biomechanical role of the posterior elements, costovertebral joints, and rib cage in the stability of the thoracic spine. *Spine* 21:1423–1429, 1996.
35. Feiertag MA, Horton WC, Norman JT, et al: The effect of different surgical releases on thoracic spinal motion. *Spine* 20:1604–1611, 1995.
36. Jiang H, Raso JV, Moreau MJ: Quantitative morphology of the lateral ligaments of the spine. Assessment of their importance in maintaining lateral stability. *Spine* 19:2676–2682, 1994.
37. Andriacchi T, Schultz A, Belytschko T, et al: A model for studies of mechanical interactions between the human spine and rib cage. *J Biomech* 7:497–505, 1974.
38. Winkel D, Matthijs O, Phelps V: Thoracic spine. In: Winkel D, Matthijs O, Phelps V, eds. *Diagnosis and Treatment of the Spine*. Maryland: Aspen, 1997:389–541.
39. Whitelaw WA: Recruitment patterns of respiratory muscles. In: Jones NL, Killian KJ, eds. *Breathlessness: The Campbell Symposium*. Hamilton, ON: Boehringer Ingelheim, 1992:20–26.
40. De Troyer A: Actions and load sharing between respiratory muscles. In: Jones NL, Killian KJ, eds. *Breathlessness: The Campbell Symposium*. Hamilton, ON: Boehringer Ingelheim, 1992:13–19.
41. Grassino AE: Limits of maximal inspiratory muscle function. In: Jones NL, Killian KJ, eds. *Breathlessness: The Campbell Symposium*. Hamilton, ON: Boehringer Ingelheim, 1992:27–33.
42. De Troyer A, Sampson MG: Activation of the parasternal intercostals during breathing efforts in human subjects. *J Appl Physiol* 52:524–529, 1982.
43. Estenne M, Ninane V, Troyer AD: Triangularis sterni muscle use during eupnea in humans: Effect of posture. *Respir Physiol* 74:151–162, 1988.
44. De Troyer A, Ninane V, Gilmartin JJ, et al: Triangularis sterni muscle use in supine humans. *J Appl Physiol* 62:919–925, 1987.
45. Taylor A: The contribution of the intercostal muscles to the effort of respiration in man. *J Physiol* 151:390–402, 1960.
46. Whitelaw WA, Feroah T: Patterns of intercostal muscle activity in humans. *J Appl Physiol* 67:2087–2094, 1989.
47. Nava S, Zanotti E, Rampulla C, et al: Respiratory muscle fatigue does not limit exercise performance during moderate endurance run. *J Sports Med Phys Fitness* 32:39–44, 1992.
48. Brooks G, Fahey T: *Fundamentals of Human Performance*. New York, NY: Macmillan, 1987.
49. Johnson B, Babcock M, Dempsey J: Exercise-induced diaphragmatic fatigue in healthy humans. *J Physiol* 460:385–405, 1993.
50. Mador M, Magalang U, Rodis A, et al: Diaphragmatic fatigue after exercise in healthy subjects. *Am Rev Respir Dis* 148:1571–1575, 1993.

51. De Troyer A, Sampson M, Sigrist S, et al: The diaphragm: Two muscles. *Science* 213:237–238, 1981.
52. De Troyer A, Sampson M, Sigrist S, et al: Action of the costal and crural parts of the diaphragm during breathing. *J Appl Physiol* 53:30–39, 1982.
53. Dommisse GF: The blood supply of the spinal cord. *J Bone Joint Surg Br* 56B:225, 1974.
54. Groskin SA: Selected topics in chest trauma. *Radiology* 183:605–617, 1992.
55. Collins J: Chest wall trauma. *J Thorac Imaging* 15:112–119, 2000.
56. Groen GJ, Stolker RJ: Thoracic neural anatomy. In: Giles LGF, Singer KP, eds. *Clinical Anatomy and Management of the Thoracic Spine.* Oxford: Butterworth-Heinemann, 2000:114–141.
57. Hovelacque A: *Anatoime Des Neufs Craniens et Radichiens et Du Sisteme Grand Sympathetique Chez L'homme.* Paris: Gaston Doin et Cie, 1927.
58. Haymaker W, Woodhall B: Peripheral nerve injuries. *Principles of Diagnosis.* London: WB Saunders, 1953.
59. Edmondston SJ: Clinical biomechanics of the thoracic spine including the rib cage. In: Boyling JD, Jull GA, eds. *Grieve's Modern Manual Therapy: The Vertebral Column.* Philadelphia, PA: Churchill Livingstone, 2004:55–65.
60. Panjabi MM, Hausfeld JN, White AA: A biomechanical study of the ligamentous stability of the thoracic spine in man. *Acta Orthop Scand* 52:315–326, 1981.
61. Flynn TW: Thoracic spine and chest wall. In: Wadsworth C, ed. *Current Concepts of Orthopedic Physical Therapy – Home Study Course.* La Crosse, WI: Orthopaedic Section, APTA, 2001.
62. Edmondston SJ, Waller R, Vallin P, et al: Thoracic spine extension mobility in young adults: influence of subject position and spinal curvature. *J Orthop Sports Phys Ther* 41:266–273, 2011.
63. Millner PA, Dickson RA: Idiopathic scoliosis: biomechanics and biology. *Eur Spine J: official publication of the European Spine Society, the European Spinal Deformity Society, and the European Section of the Cervical Spine Research Society* 5:362–373, 1996.
64. Refshauge KM, Bolst L, Goodsell M: The relationship between cervicothoracic posture and the presence of pain. *J Man & Manip Ther* 3:21–24, 1995.
65. Raine S, Twomey LT: Attributes and qualities of human posture and their relationship to dysfunction or musculoskeletal pain. *Crit Rev Phys Rehabil Med* 6:409–437, 1994.
66. Singer KP, Malmivaara A: Pathoanatomical characteristics of the thoracolumbar junctional region. In: Giles LGF, Singer KP, eds. *Clinical Anatomy and Management of the Thoracic Spine.* Oxford: Butterworth-Heinemann, 2000:100–113.
67. Shea KG, Schlegel JD, Bachus KN, et al: The contribution of the rib cage to thoracic spine stability. *International Society for the Study of the Lumbar Spine.* Vermont, 1996:150.
68. Takeuchi T, Abumi K, Shono Y, et al: Biomechanical role of the intervertebral disc and costovertebral joint in stability of the thoracic spine: a canine model. *Spine* 24:1414–1420, 1999.
69. Raou RJP: *Recherches Sur La Mobilité Vertebrale en Fonction Des Types Rachidiens.* Paris: Thèse, 1952.
70. White AA, Hirsch C: The significance of the vertebral posterior elements in the mechanics of the thoracic spine. *Clin Orthop* 81:2–14, 1971.
71. Panjabi MM, Krag MH, Dimnet JC, et al: Thoracic spine centers of rotation in the sagittal plane. *J Orthop Res* 1:387–394, 1984.
72. Levine A, Edwards C: Lumbar spine trauma. In: Camins E, O'Leary P, eds. *The Lumbar Spine.* New York, NY: Raven Press, 1987:183–212.
73. Gonon JP, Dimnet J, Carret JP, et al: Utilité de l'analyse cinématique de radiographies dynamiques dans le diagnostic de certaines affections de la colonne lombaire. In: Simon L, Rabourdin JP, eds. *Lombalgies et Médecine de Rééducation.* Paris: Masson, 1983:27–38.
74. Panjabi MM, Brand RA, White AA: Three-dimensional flexibility and stiffness properties of the human thoracic spine. *J Biomech* 9:185, 1976.
75. Davis PR: The medial inclination of the human thoracic intervertebral articular facets. *J Anat* 93:68–74, 1959.
76. Singer KP, Day RE, Breidahl PD: In vivo axial rotation at the thoracolumbar junction: An investigation using low dose CT in healthy male volunteers. *Clin Biomech* 4:80–86, 1989.
77. Singer KP: The thoracolumbar mortise joint: Radiological and histological comparisons. *Clin Biomech* 4:137–143, 1989.
78. Bogduk N, Valencia F: Innervation and pain patterns of the thoracic spine. In: Grant R, ed. *Physical Therapy of the Cervical and Thoracic Spine,* 2nd ed. Melbourne: Churchill Livingstone, 1994:77–88.
79. Le T, Biundo J, Aprill C, et al: Costovertebral joint erosion in ankylosing spondylitis. *Am J Phys Med Rehabil* 80:62–64, 2001.
80. Fruth SJ: Differential diagnosis and treatment in a patient with posterior upper thoracic pain. *Phys Ther* 86:254–268, 2006.
81. Murtagh JE, Kenna CJ: *Back Pain and Spinal Manipulation,* 2nd ed. Oxford: Butterworth-Heinemann, 1997.
82. Melzack R: The McGill Pain Questionnaire: major properties and scoring methods. *Pain* 1:277, 1975.
83. Feise RJ, Michael Menke J: Functional rating index: a new valid and reliable instrument to measure the magnitude of clinical change in spinal conditions. *Spine* 26:78–86; discussion 87, 2001.
84. Fairbank J: Revised Oswestry Disability questionnaire. *Spine* 25:2552, 2000.
85. Lewit K: Chain reactions in disturbed function of the motor system. *J Manual Med* 3:27, 1987.
86. Grieve GP: *Common Vertebral Joint Problems.* New York, NY: Churchill Livingstone Inc, 1981.
87. Meadows J: *Orthopedic Differential Diagnosis in Physical Therapy.* New York, NY: McGraw-Hill, 1999.
88. Singer KP, Giles LGF: Manual therapy considerations at the thoracolumbar junction: an anatomical and functional perspective. *J Manipulative Physiol Ther* 13:83–88, 1990.
89. Gelb DE, Lenke LG, Bridwell KH, et al: An analysis of sagittal spinal alignment in 100 asymptomatic middle and older aged volunteers. *Spine* 20:1351–1358, 1995.
90. Bland JH: Diagnosis of thoracic pain syndromes. In: Giles LGF, Singer KP, eds. *Clinical Anatomy and Management of the Thoracic Spine.* Oxford: Butterworth-Heinemann, 2000:145–156.
91. Wing P, Tsang I, Gagnon F: Diurnal changes in the profile shape and range of motion of the back. *Spine* 17:761–766, 1992.
92. Beck A, Killus J: Normal posture of the spine determined by mathematical and statistical methods. *Aerosp Med* 44:1277–1281, 1973.
93. White AA, Sahrmann SA: A movement system balance approach to management of musculoskeletal pain. In: Grant R, ed. *Physical Therapy for the Cervical and Thoracic Spine.* Edinburgh: Churchill Livingstone, 1994:339–358.
94. Jull GA, Janda V: Muscle and motor control in low back pain. In: Twomey LT, Taylor JR, eds. *Physical Therapy of the Low Back: Clinics in Physical Therapy.* New York, NY: Churchill Livingstone, 1987:258–278.
95. Jull GA: Physiotherapy management of neck pain of mechanical origin. In: Giles LGF, Singer KP, eds. *Clinical Anatomy and Management of Cervical Spine Pain. The Clinical Anatomy of Back Pain.* London: Butterworth-Heinemann, 1998:168–191.
96. Crawford HJ, Jull GA: The influence of thoracic posture and movement on range of arm elevation. *Physiother Theory Pract* 9:143–148, 1993.
97. Vasilyeva LF, Lewit K: Diagnosis of muscular dysfunction by inspection. In: Liebenson C, ed. *Rehabilitation of the Spine: A Practitioner's Manual.* Baltimore, MD: Lippincott Williams & Wilkins, 1996:113–142.
98. Lewit K: Relation of faulty respiration to posture, with clinical implications. *J Am Osteopath Assoc* 79:525–529, 1980.
99. Crawford R, Singer KP: Normal and degenerative anatomy of the thoracic intervertebral discs. *Proceedings of Manipulative Physiotherapists Association of Australia: 9th Biennial Conference,* Gold Coast, 1995:24–29.
100. Wiles P, Sweetnam R: *Essentials of Orthopedics.* London: J.A. Churchill, 1965.
101. Deyo RA, Rainville J, Kent DL: What can the history and physical examination tell us about low back pain? *JAMA* 268:760–765, 1992.
102. Stagnara P, De Mauroy JC, Dran G, et al: Reciprocal angulation of vertebral bodies in a sagittal plane: approach to references for the evaluation of kyphosis and lordosis. *Spine* 7:335–342, 1982.
103. Miller NH: Genetics of familial idiopathic scoliosis. *Clin Orthop Relat Res* 401:60–64, 2002.
104. Kane WJ: Scoliosis prevalence: A call for a statement of terms. *Clin Orthop* 126:43–46, 1977.
105. Armstrong GW, Livermore NB, Suzuki N, et al: Nonstandard vertebral rotation in scoliosis screening patients: Its prevalence and relation to the clinical deformity. *Spine* 7:50–54, 1982.
106. Ombregt L, Bisschop P, ter Veer HJ, et al: Clinical examination of the lumbar spine. In: Ombregt L, Bisschop P, ter Veer HJ, et al, eds. *A System of Orthopaedic Medicine.* London: WB Saunders, 1995:577–611.
107. Gross RH: Leg length discrepancy: how much is too much? *Orthopedics* 1:307–310, 1978.
108. Finneson BE: *Low Back Pain,* 2nd ed. Philadelphia, PA: J.B. Lippincott, 1973:290–303.
109. Bianco AJ: Low back pain and sciatica. Diagnosis and indications for treatment. *J Bone Joint Surg* 50A:170, 1968.

110. Maigne R: *Diagnosis and Treatment of Pain of Vertebral Origin.* Baltimore, MD: Williams & Wilkins, 1996.
111. McKenzie RA: Manual correction of sciatic scoliosis. *N Z Med J* 76:194–199, 1972.
112. Keim HA: *The Adolescent Spine.* New York, NY: Springer-Verlag, 1982.
113. Ombregt L, Bisschop P, ter Veer HJ, et al: *A System of Orthopaedic Medicine.* London: WB Saunders, 1995.
114. Sutherland ID: Funnel chest. *J Bone Joint Surg Br* 40B:244–251, 1958.
115. Sahrmann SA: *Diagnosis and Treatment of Muscle Imbalances Associated with Regional Pain Syndromes, Lecture Outline.* School of Medicine, Washington University, St.Louis, 1992.
116. Lewit K: The contribution of clinical observation to neurobiological mechanisms in manipulative therapy. In: Korr IM, ed. *The Neurobiological Mechanisms in Manipulative Therapy.* New York, NY: Plenum Press, 1977.
117. Mitchell FL, Moran PS, Pruzzo NA: *An Evaluation and Treatment Manual of Osteopathic Muscle Energy Procedures.* Manchester, MO: Mitchell, Moran and Pruzzo Associates, 1979.
118. Geelhoed MA, Viti JA, Brewer PA: A pilot study to investigate the validity of the rule of threes of the thoracic spine. *J Man Manipulative Ther* 13:91–93, 2005.
119. Geelhoed MA, McGaugh J, Brewer PA, et al: A new model to facilitate palpation of the level of the transverse processes of the thoracic spine. *J Orthop Sports Phys Ther* 36:876–881, 2006.
120. Lawrence DJ, Bakkum B: Chiropractic management of thoracic spine pain of mechanical origin. In: Giles LGF, Singer KP, eds. *Clinical Anatomy and Management of Thoracic Pain.* Oxford: Butterworth-Heinemann, 2000:244–256.
121. Evans RC: *Illustrated Essentials in Orthopedic Physical Assessment.* St. Louis, MO: Mosby-Year book Inc, 1994.
122. American Medical Association: *Guides to the Evaluation of Permanent Impairment*, 5th ed. Chicago, IL: American Medical Association, 2001.
123. McKenzie RA: *The Cervical and Thoracic Spine: Mechanical Diagnosis and Therapy.* Waikanae: Spinal Publications, 1990.
124. Magee DJ: *Orthopedic Physical Assessment.* Philadelphia, PA: W.B. Saunders, 1997.
125. Pavelka K, Von: Rotationsmessung der wirbelsaule. *A Rheumaforschg* 29:366, 1970.
126. Moll JMH, Wright V: Measurement of spinal movement. In: Jayson MIV, ed. *The Lumbar Spine and Back Pain.* New York, NY: Grune and Stratton, 1981:93–112.
127. Stoddard A: *Manual of Osteopathic Practice.* New York, NY: Harper & Row, 1969.
128. Maigne J-Y, Maigne R, Guerin-Surville H: Upper thoracic dorsal rami: anatomic study of their medial cutaneous branches. *Surg Radiol Anat* 13:109–112, 1991.
129. Magee DJ: Cervical spine. In: Magee DJ, ed. *Orthopedic Physical Assessment*, 2nd ed. Philadelphia, PA: Saunders, 1992:34–70.
130. Ventafridda V, Caraceni A, Martini C, et al: On the significance of Lhermitte's sign in oncology. *J Neurooncol* 10:133–137, 1991.
131. Ongerboer de Visser BW: Het teken van Lhermitte bij thoracale wervelaandoeningen. *Ned Tijdschr Geneeskd* 124:390–392, 1980.
132. Broager B: Lhermitte's sign in thoracic spinal tumour. Personal observation. *Acta Neurochir (Wien)* 106:127–135, 1978.
133. Evjenth O, Gloeck C: *Symptom Localization in the Spine and Extremity Joints.* Minneapolis, MN: OPTP, 2000.
134. Magee DJ: Thoracic (dorsal) spine. In: Magee DJ, ed. *Orthopedic Physical Assessment*, 5th ed. Philadelphia, PA: W.B. Saunders, 2008:471–514.
135. Browder DA, Erhard RE, Piva SR: Intermittent cervical traction and thoracic manipulation for management of mild cervical compressive myelopathy attributed to cervical herniated disc: a case series. *J Orthop Sports Phys Ther* 34:701–712, 2004.
136. Cleland JA, Whitman JM, Fritz JM, et al: Manual physical therapy, cervical traction, and strengthening exercises in patients with cervical radiculopathy: a case series. *J Orthop Sports Phys Ther* 35:802–811, 2005.
137. Cleland JA, Childs JD, McRae M, et al: Immediate effects of thoracic manipulation in patients with neck pain: a randomized clinical trial. *Man Ther* 10:127–135, 2005.
138. Fernandez-de-las-Penas C, Cleland JA: Management of whiplash-associated disorder addressing thoracic and cervical spine impairments: a case report. *J Orthop Sports Phys Ther* 35:180–181, 2005.
139. Pho C, Godges J: Management of whiplash-associated disorder addressing thoracic and cervical spine impairments: a case report. *J Orthop Sports Phys Ther* 34:511–519; discussion 520–523, 2004.
140. Klaffs CE, Arnheim DD: *Modern Principles of Athletic Training.* St Louis, MO: CV Mosby, 1989.
141. Lehmann JF, Silverman DR, Baum BA, et al: Temperature distributions in the human thigh produced by infrared, hot pack and microwave applications. *Arch Phys Med Rehabil* 47:291, 1966.
142. Prentice WE: Using therapeutic modalities in rehabilitation. In: Prentice WE, Voight ML, eds. *Techniques in Musculoskeletal Rehabilitation.* New York, NY: McGraw-Hill, 2001:289–303.
143. Durham JW, Moskowitz K, Whitney J: Surface electrical stimulation versus brace in treatment of idiopathic scoliosis. *Spine* 15:888–892, 1990.
144. McGill SM: The biomechanics of low back injury: implications on current practice in industry and the clinic. *J Biomech* 30:465–475, 1997.
145. Cole AJ, Farrell JP, Stratton SA: Functional rehabilitation of cervical spine athletic injuries. In: Kibler BW, Herring JA, Press JM, eds. *Functional Rehabilitation of Sports and Musculoskeletal Injuries.* Gaithersburg, MD: Aspen, 1998:127–148.
146. Corrigan B, Maitland GD: *Practical Orthopaedic Medicine.* Boston, MA: Butterworth, 1985.
147. Ellis JJ, Johnson GS: Myofascial considerations in somatic dysfunction of the thorax. In: Flynn TW, ed. *The Thoracic Spine and Rib Cage: Musculoskeletal Evaluation and Treatment.* Boston, MA: Butterworth-Heinemann, 1996:211–262.
148. Pickering D: Precordial catch syndrome. *Arch Dis Child* 56:401–403, 1981.
149. Sparrow M, Bird E: 'Precordial Catch': a benign syndrome of chest pain in young persons. *N Z Med J* 88:325–326, 1978.
150. Fam AG, Smythe HA: Musculoskeletal chest wall pain. *Can Med Assoc J* 133:379–389, 1985.
151. Brennan R: *The Alexander Technique: Natural Poise for Health.* New York, NY: Barnes & Noble Books, Inc., 1991.
152. Buchanan PA, Ulrich BD: The Feldenkrais method: a dynamic approach to changing motor behavior. *Res Q Exerc Sport* 72:315–323, 2001.
153. Lake B: Acute back pain: Treatment by the application of Feldenkrais principles. *Aust Fam Physician* 14:1175–1178, 1985.
154. Watrous I: The Trager approach: An effective tool for physical therapy. *Phys Ther Forum* 72:22–25, 1992.
155. Witt P: Trager psychophysical integration: an additional tool in the treatment of chronic spinal pain and dysfunction. *Trager J* 2:4–5, 1987.
156. Witt P, Parr C: Effectiveness of Trager psychophysical integration in promoting trunk mobility in a child with cerebral palsy, a case report. *Phys Occup Ther Pediatr* 8:75–94, 1988.
157. Blum CL: Chiropractic and pilates therapy for the treatment of adult scoliosis. *J Manipulative Physiol Ther* 25:E3, 2002.
158. Wood KB, Blair JM, Aepple DM, et al: The natural history of asymptomatic thoracic disc herniations. *Spine* 22:525–530, 1997.
159. Martucci E, Mele C, Martella P: Thoracic intervertebral disc protrusions. *Ital J Orthop Traumatol* 10:333–339, 1984.
160. Arce CA, Dohrmann GJ: Thoracic disc herniation: improved diagnosis with computed tomographic scanning and a review of the literature. *Surg Neurol* 23:356–361, 1985.
161. Maiman DJ, Larson SJ, Luck E, et al: Lateral extracavitary approach to the spine for thoracic disc herniation: report of 23 cases. *Neurosurgery* 14:178–182, 1984.
162. Jamieson DRS, Ballantyne JP: Unique presentation of a prolapsed thoracic disk: Lhermitte's symptom in a golf player. *Neurology* 45: 1219–1221, 1995.
163. Morgenlander JC, Massey EW: Neurogenic claudication with positionally weakness from a thoracic disk herniation. *Neurology* 39:1133–1134, 1989.
164. Hamilton MG, Thomas HG: Intradural herniation of a thoracic disc presenting as flaccid paraplegia: case report. *Neurosurgery* 27:482–484, 1990.
165. Kumar R, Buckley TF: First thoracic disc protrusion. *Spine* 11:499–501, 1986.
166. Kumar R, Cowie RA: Second thoracic disc protrusions. *Spine* 17:120–121, 1992.
167. Albrand OW, Corkill G: Thoracic disc herniation: treatment and prognosis. *Spine* 4:41–46, 1979.
168. Byrne TN, Waxman SG: *Spinal Cord Compression: Diagnosis and Principles of Management.* Philadelphia, PA: FA Davis, 1990.
169. Brown CW, Deffer PA, Akmakjian J, et al: The natural history of thoracic disc herniation. *Spine* 17:97–102, 1992.
170. Rothman RH, Simeone FA: *The Spine*, 3rd ed. Philadelphia, PA: WB Saunders, 1992.

171. Wilbourn AJ, Aminoff MJ: The electrophysiologic examination in patients with radiculopathies. AAEE Minimonograph 32. *Muscle Nerve* 11:1099–1114, 1988.
172. Herring SA, Weinstein SM: Electrodiagnosis in sports medicine. *Physic Med Rehabil State Art Rev* 3:809–822, 1989.
173. Marinacci AA: A correlation between operative findings in cervical herniated disc with electromyograms and opaque myelograms. *Electromyography* 6:5–20, 1966.
174. Eisen A, Aminoff MJ: Somatosensory evoked potentials. In: Aminoff MJ, ed. *Electrodiagnosis in Clinical Neurology*, 2nd ed. New York, NY: Churchill Livingstone, 1986:535–573.
175. Ellenberg MR, Honet JC, Treanor WJ: Cervical radiculopathy. *Arch Phys Med Rehabil* 75:342–352, 1994.
176. Leblhuber F, Reisecker F, Boehm-Jurkovic H, et al: Diagnostic value of different electrophysiologic tests in cervical disc prolapse. *Neurology* 38:1879–1881, 1988.
177. Johnson EW: *Practical Electromyography*, 2nd ed. Baltimore, MD: Williams & Wilkins, 1988.
178. Speer KP, Bassett FH: The prolonged burner syndrome. *Am J Sports Med* 18:591–594, 1990.
179. Bergfeld JA, Hershman E, Wilbourne A: Brachial plexus injury in sports: A five-year follow-up. *Orthop Trans* 12:743–744, 1988.
180. Beurskens AJ, de Vet HC, Koke AJ, et al: Efficacy of traction for nonspecific low back pain: 12-week and 6-month results of a randomized clinical trial. *Spine* 22:2756–2762, 1997.
181. Harris PR: Cervical traction: review of literature and treatment guidelines. *Phys Ther* 57:910–914, 1977.
182. Licht S: *Massage, Manipulation and Traction*. New Haven, CT: E. Licht, 1960.
183. Natchev E: *A Manual on Autotraction*. Stockholm: Folksam Scientific Council, 1984.
184. Twomey L: Sustained lumbar traction. An experimental study of long spine segments. *Spine* 10:146–149, 1985.
185. Zylbergold RS, Piper MC: Cervical spine disorders. A comparison of three types of traction. *Spine* 10:867–871, 1985.
186. Dreyer SJ, Boden SD: Nonoperative treatment of neck and arm pain. *Spine* 23:2746–2754, 1998.
187. Gartland GJ: A survey of spinal traction. *Br J Phys Med* 20:253–258, 1957.
188. Grieve GP: Neck traction. *Physiotherapy* 68:260–265, 1982.
189. Crue BL, Todd EM: The importance of flexion in cervical traction for radiculitis. *U S Armed Forces Med J* 8:374–380, 1957.
190. Cole AJ, Farrell JP, Stratton SA: Cervical spine athletic injuries. *Phys Med Rehabil Clin North Am* 5:37–68, 1994.
191. Dreyfuss P, Tibiletti C, Dreyer SJ: Thoracic zygapophyseal joint pain patterns. A study in normal volunteers. *Spine* 15:453–457, 1994.
192. Greenman PE: *Principles of Manual Medicine*, 2nd ed. Baltimore, MD: Williams & Wilkins, 1996.
193. Bourdillon JF: *Spinal Manipulation*, 3rd ed. London: Heinemann Medical Books, 1982.
194. Gill G: Epidemic of Tietze's syndrome. *BMJ* 2:499, 1977.
195. Morgan-Hughes J: Painful disorders of muscle. *Br J Hosp Med* 360:362–365, 1979.
196. Gregory PL, Biswas AC, Batt ME: Musculoskeletal problems of the chest wall in athletes. *Sports Med* 32:235–250, 2002.
197. Eastwood DS: Subcutaneous rupture of the breast: a seat-belt injury. *Br J Surg* 59:491–492, 1972.
198. Pal J, Mulder D, Brown RA, et al: Assessing multiple trauma: is the cervical spine enough? *J Trauma* 28:1282–1284, 1988.
199. Daffner R: *Imaging of Vertebral Trauma*. Rockville, IL: Aspen, 1988.
200. El-Khoury GY, Whitten CG: Trauma to the upper thoracic spine: anatomy, biomechanics, and unique imaging features. *AJR Am J Roentgenol* 160:95–102, 1993.
201. Gupta A, El Masri W: Multilevel spinal injuries. *J Bone Joint Surg Br* 71B:692–695, 1989.
202. Mirvis SE, Templeton P: Imaging in acute thoracic trauma. *Semin Roentgenol* 27:184–210, 1992.
203. Greene R: Lung alterations in thoracic trauma. *J Thorac Imaging* 2:1–11, 1987.
204. Reid ME: Bone trauma and disease of the thoracic spine and ribs. In: Flynn TW, ed. *The Thoracic Spine and Rib Cage*. Boston, MD: Butterworth-Heinemann, 1996:87–105.
205. Benson MK, Byrnes DP: The clinical syndromes and surgical treatment of thoracic intervertebral disc prolapse. *J Bone Joint Surg Br* 57B:471–477, 1975.
206. Rowe CR: Fractures of the scapula. *Surg Clin North Am* 43:1565–1571, 1963.
207. McLennan JG, Ungersma J: Pneumothorax complicating fracture of the scapula. *J Bone Joint Surg Am* 64A:598–599, 1982.
208. McGinnis M, Denton JR: Fractures of the scapula: a retrospective study of 40 fractured scapulae. *J Trauma* 29:1488–1493, 1989.
209. Fletcher BD, Brogdon BG: Seat-belt fractures of the spine and sternum. *JAMA* 200:177–178, 1967.
210. Rutherford WH, Greenfield T, Hayes HRM, et al: *The medical effects of seat belt legislation in the United Kingdom*. DHSS (Office of the Chief Scientist) HMSO Research Report No. 13, 1985.
211. Gazak S, Davidson SJ: Posterior sternoclavicular dislocations: Two case reports. *J Trauma* 24:80–82, 1984.
212. DeFranca GG, Levine LJ: The T4 syndrome. *J Manipulative Physiol Ther* 18:34–37, 1995.
213. McGuckin N: The T4 syndrome. In: Grieve GP, ed. *Modern Manual Therapy of the Vertebral Column*. New York, NY: Churchill Livingstone, 1986:370–376.
214. Maitland G: *Vertebral Manipulation*. Sydney: Butterworth, 1986.
215. Butler DL, Slater H: Neural injury in the thoracic spine: a conceptual basis for manual therapy. In: Grant R, ed. *Physical Therapy of the Cervical and Thoracic Spine*. New York, NY: Churchill Livingstone, 1994:313–338.
216. Grieve GP: Thoracic musculoskeletal problems. In: Boyling JD, Palastanga N, eds. *Grieve's Modern Manual Therapy of the Vertebral Column*, 2nd ed. Edinburgh: Churchill Livingstone, 1994:401–428.
217. Butler DS: *Mobilization of the Nervous System*. New York, NY: Churchill Livingstone, 1992.
218. Maigne J-Y: Cervicothoracic and thoracolumbar spinal pain syndromes. In: Giles LGF, Singer KP, eds. *Clinical Anatomy and Management of the Thoracic Spine*. Oxford: Butterworth-Heinemann, 2000:157–168.
219. Haldeman S: Spinal manipulative therapy in sports medicine. *Clin Sports Med* 5:277–293, 1986.
220. Hartman SL: *Handbook of Osteopathic Technique*, 2nd ed. London: Unwin Hyman Ltd., Academic Division, 1990.
221. Cleland JA, Childs JD, Fritz JM, et al: Development of a clinical prediction rule for guiding treatment of a subgroup of patients with neck pain: use of thoracic spine manipulation, exercise, and patient education. *Phys Ther* 87:9–23, 2007.
222. Cleland JA, Mintken PE, Carpenter K, et al: Examination of a clinical prediction rule to identify patients with neck pain likely to benefit from thoracic spine thrust manipulation and a general cervical range of motion exercise: multi-center randomized clinical trial. *Phys Ther* 90:1239–1250, 2010.
223. Puentedura EJ, Landers MR, Cleland JA, et al: Thoracic spine thrust manipulation versus cervical spine thrust manipulation in patients with acute neck pain: a randomized clinical trial. *J Orthop Sports Phys Ther* 41:208–220, 2011.
224. Menck JY, Requejo SM, Kulig K: Thoracic spine dysfunction in upper extremity complex regional pain syndrome type I. *J Orthop Sports Phys Ther* 30:401–409, 2000.
225. Allison GT, Nagy BM, Hall T: A randomized clinical trial of manual therapy for cervico-brachial pain syndrome – a pilot study. *Man Ther* 7:95–102, 2002.
226. Suh SI, Koh SB, Choi EJ, et al: Intracranial hypotension induced by cervical spine chiropractic manipulation. *Spine* 30:E340–E342, 2005.
227. Ruelle A, Datti R, Pisani R: Thoracic epidural hematoma after spinal manipulation therapy. *J Spinal Disord* 12:534–536, 1999.
228. Brismee JM, Phelps V, Sizer P: Differential diagnosis and treatment of chronic neck and upper trapezius pain and upper extremity paresthesia: a case study involving the management of an elevated first rib and uncovertebral joint dysfunction. *J Man Manipulative Ther* 13:72–90, 2005.

CHAPTER 28 Lumbar Spine

CHAPTER OBJECTIVES

At the completion of this chapter, the reader will be able to:

1. Describe the vertebrae, ligaments, muscles, and blood and nerve supply that comprise the lumbar intervertebral segment.
2. Outline the coupled movements of the lumbar spine, the normal and abnormal joint barriers, and the reactions of the various structures to loading.
3. Perform a detailed examination of the lumbar musculoskeletal system, including history, observation, palpation of the articular and soft tissue structures, specific passive mobility and passive articular mobility tests for the intervertebral joints, and stability testing.
4. Evaluate the results from the examination and establish a diagnosis.
5. Describe the common pathologies and lesions of this region.
6. Describe intervention strategies based on clinical findings and established goals.
7. Design an intervention based on patient education, manual therapy, and therapeutic exercise.
8. Apply mobilization techniques to the lumbar spine, using the correct grade, direction, and duration, and explain the mechanical and physiologic effects.
9. Evaluate intervention effectiveness to progress or modify intervention.
10. Plan an effective home program, including spinal care, and instruct the patient in this program.
11. Help the patient to develop self-reliant intervention strategies.

OVERVIEW

Over the past few decades, low-back pain (LBP) has become increasingly problematic, placing significant burdens on health systems and social-care systems.[1,2] The findings in the literature seem to suggest the seemingly contradictory notion that acute back conditions are self-limiting and have an excellent natural history, but there is a good chance that a problem remains. According to these studies, the first episode of back pain can have differing results: 80–90% will be asymptomatic in 6 weeks, 98% in 24 weeks, and 99% in 52 weeks,[3] leading to the assumption that most cases of LBP are benign in nature.[4–6] However, the small percentage of people who do become disabled with chronic LBP account for 75–90% of the cost associated with LBP.[7] This group of patients has been the focus of much research to determine factors associated with chronicity and the pathologic processes responsible.

Given the numerous causes and types of LBP, it is imperative that any clinician examining and treating the lower back have a sound understanding and knowledge of the anatomy and biomechanics of this region. Although this knowledge is not the sole determinant of the approach to LBP, it does provide a solid framework on which to build successful management. There have also been moves toward the design of clinical prediction rules (see Chap. 5) on how best to treat patients with LBP (see "Intervention" section).

It is worth noting that trunk strength, flexibility, aerobic conditioning, and postural education have all been found to have a significant preventative effect on the occurrence and recurrence of back injuries.[8–15] Thus, physical therapy, with its emphasis on the restoration of functional motion, strength, and flexibility, should be the cornerstone of both the intervention and the preventative processes in LBP.

ANATOMY

The lumbar spine (Fig. 28-1) consists of five lumbar vertebrae, which, in general, increase in size from L1 to L5 to accommodate progressively increasing loads. Between each of the lumbar vertebrae are the intervertebral disks (IVD).

VERTEBRAL BODY

The anterior part of each vertebra is called the vertebral body. The pedicles, which project from the posterior aspect of the

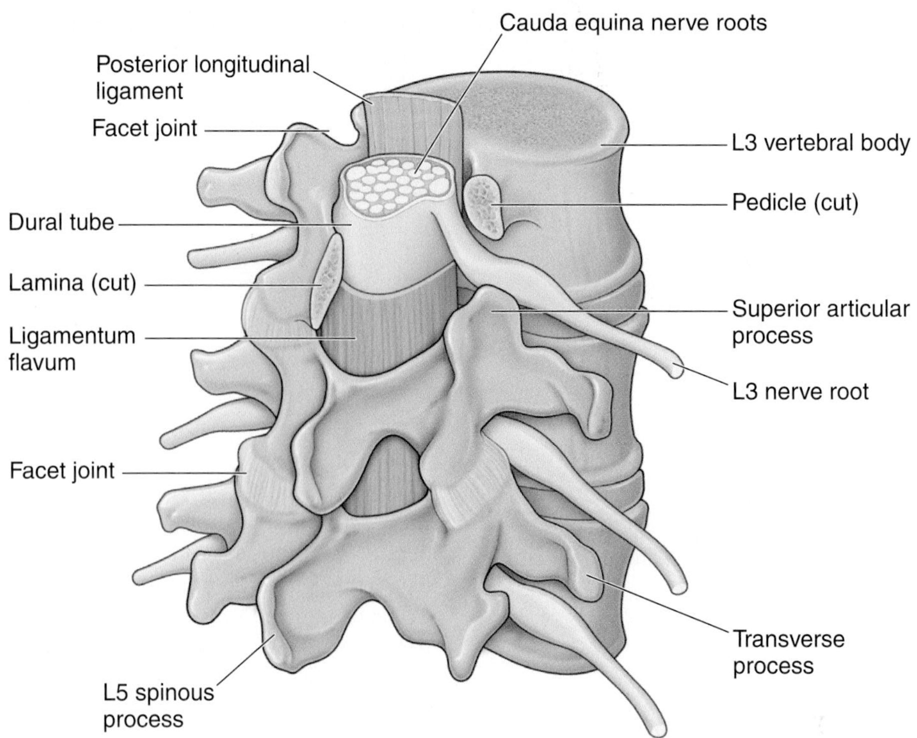

FIGURE 28-1 Structures of the lumbar spine.

vertebral body, represent the only connection between the posterior joints of the segment and the vertebral bodies, both of which deliver tensile and bending forces. Noticeably, the muscles that act on a lumbar vertebra pull downward, transmitting the muscular action to the vertebral body. This muscular action is borne through the pedicles, which act as levers, and thus are subjected to a certain amount of bending.[16] If the vertebral body slides forward, the inferior articular processes of that vertebra abut against the superior articular processes of the next lower vertebra and resist the slide.[16] These resistive forces are transmitted to the vertebral body along the pedicles.

The lamina (see Fig. 28-1) functions to absorb the various forces that are transmitted from the spinous and articular processes. The pars interarticularis connects the vertically oriented lamina and the horizontally extending pedicle, which exposes it to appreciable bending forces.[16] The two laminae meet and fuse with one another, forming an arch of bone aptly called the vertebral, or neural arch, which serves as a bony tunnel for the spinal cord. Both the transverse and the spinous processes of the vertebral body provide areas for muscle attachments.

The first sacral segment, the point at which the sacrum joins the lumbar spine, is usually included in discussions of the lumbar spine. In most cases, this is a fixed segment but, in some cases it may be mobile (lumbarization of S1). At other times, the fifth lumbar segment may be fused to the sacrum or ilium, resulting in a sacralization of that vertebra. It is unclear how these anomalies affect the biomechanics of the spine.

Intervertebral Disk

Annulus Fibrosis

In the lumbar spine, the superior and inferior surfaces of the vertebral bodies are comparatively large and flat, reflecting their load-transfer function. The lumbar disk is approximately cylindrical, its shape being determined by the integrity of the annulus fibrosis (AF). The AF consists of approximately 10–12 (often as many as 15–25) concentric sheets of predominantly type I collagen tissue,[17] bound together by proteoglycan gel.[18] The number of annular layers decreases with age, but there is a gradual thickening of the remaining layers.[19] The fibers of the AF are oriented at approximately 65 degrees from vertical. The fibers of each successive sheet or lamella maintain the same inclination of 65 degrees, but in the opposite direction to the preceding lamella, resulting in every second sheet having the same orientation. Thus, only 50% of the fibers are under stress with rotational forces at any given time. This alteration in the direction of fibers in each lamella is vital in enabling the disk to resist torsional (twisting) forces.[20]

Each lamella is thicker anteriorly than posteriorly, leading to the lumbar disks being thinner, but more tightly packed, posteriorly than anteriorly.[21] Consequently, the posterior part of the annulus will have thinner but stronger fibers, and it is capable of withstanding tension applied to this area during flexion activities and postures, which occur more frequently than with extension.[16] However, because of the predominance of flexion activities in life, fatigue damage may occur in the posterior aspect of the disk, making it a common site of injury.[22] The wedge-shaped appearance of the disk produced by the configuration of the lamellae contributes to the normal lordosis of this region.[22]

The outermost lamellae insert into the ring apophysis of the upper and lower vertebrae by mingling with the periosteal fibers (fibers of Sharpey). These fibers, attaching them to bone, may be considered as ligaments and as such are designed primarily to limit motion between adjacent vertebrae.[23] The inner portions of the lamellae are attached to the superior and inferior cartilaginous end plates, and form an envelope around the NP.[16]

Nucleus Pulposus

The lumbar IVDs of a healthy young adult contain a nucleus pulposus (NP) that is composed of a semifluid mass of mucoid material. This material is clear, firm, and gelatinous.[16]

CLINICAL PEARL

The overall consistency of the NP changes with increasing age, as the water content of the NP diminishes and subsequently becomes drier.

At birth, the water content of the NP is approximately 80%. In the elderly, the water content is approximately 68%. Most of this water content change occurs in childhood and adolescence, with only approximately 6% occurring in adulthood.[24] The portion of the NP that is not water is made up of cells that are largely chondrocytes and a matrix consisting of proteoglycans, collagen fibers, other noncollagenous proteins, and elastin.[22,25,26]

With the exception of early youth, there is no clear boundary between the NP and AF, and it resembles a transitional zone.[27] The biomechanical makeup of the NP is similar to that of the AF, except that the NP contains mostly type II collagen, as opposed to type I.[17] The collagen interacts with the ground substance to form a concentration proportional to the viscoelastic requirements of the AF.

CLINICAL PEARL

The IVDs are able to distribute compressive stress evenly between adjacent vertebrae because the NP and inner AF act like a pressurized fluid, in which the pressure does not vary with location or direction.[28,29] Biomechanical studies of the IVD seem to indicate that the disk acts to provide flexibility at low loads and stability at high loads.[30,31]

An unequal load distribution to the IVD is a major predisposing factor in radial tearing of the AF.[32] The tearing can be caused by the torsional effect of the superior vertebra rotating in a constant direction with sagittal movements. The posterolateral aspect of the AF tends to weaken first.[33] If the inner layers of the posterior AF tear in the presence of the NP that is still capable of bulging into the space left by the tear, the symptoms of disk disease are likely to be experienced, with the spinal canal location of disk trespass determining the type of neural compromise, clinical pain pattern, and often the outcome.[33] It must be remembered that the degree of neural compromise and potential for pain cannot be judged accurately by the size or type of disk material. Large, free fragments can often cause no neurologic deficit or pain.[34]

Vertebral End Plates

Each vertebral end plate consists of a layer of hyaline and fibrocartilage approximately 0.6–1-mm thick,[35] which covers the top or bottom aspects of the disk and separates the disk from the adjacent vertebral body. Peripherally, the end plate is surrounded by the ring apophysis.[16]

At birth, the end plate is part of the vertebral body growth plate, but by approximately the 20th year, it has been separated from the body by a subchondral plate. During this time, the plate is bilaminar, with a growth zone and an articular area.[36] With aging, the growth zone becomes thinner and disappears, leaving only a thickened articular plate.

Nutrition of the disk comes via a diffusion of nutrients from the anastomosis over the AF and from the arterial plexi underlying the end plate. Although almost the entire AF is permeable to nutrients, only the center portions of the end plate are permeable. Over approximately 10% of the surface of the end plate, the subchondral bone of the centrum is deficient. At these points, the bone marrow is in direct contact with the end plate, thereby augmenting the nutrition of the disk and end plate.[37] It is possible that a mechanical pump action produced by spine motion could aid with the diffusion of the nutrients.

The two end plates of each disk, therefore, cover the NP in its entirety but fail to cover the entire extent of the AF.

CLINICAL PEARL

Because of the attachment of the AF to the vertebral end plates on the periphery, the end plates are strongly bound to the IVD. In contrast, the vertebral end plates are only weakly attached to the vertebral bodies[38] and can be completely torn from the vertebral bodies by trauma. It is for this and other morphologic reasons that the end plates are regarded as constituents of the IVD, rather than as a part of the lumbar vertebral body.[36]

Between the ages of 20 and 65 years, the end plate thins and the vascular foramina in the subchondral bone become occluded, resulting in decreased nutrition to the disk. At the same time, the underlying bone becomes weaker, and the end plate gradually bows into the vertebral body, becoming more vulnerable centrally, where it may fracture into the centrum.[16] The presence of damage to a vertebral body end plate reduces the pressure in the NP of the adjacent disk by up to 57%, and doubles the size of so-called stress peaks in the posterior aspect of the AF.[39]

Nerve Root Canal

The nerve root canal is located at the lateral aspect of the spinal canal (Fig. 28-1). The dural sac forms the medial wall of the canal, the internal aspect of the pedicle, and the lateral wall. The posterior border of the nerve root canal is formed by the ligamentum flavum, superior articular process, and lamina. The anterior border of the canal is formed by the vertebral body and IVD.

The nerve root canal can be described according to its location[40]:

- The entrance zone is medial and anterior to the superior articular process.
- The middle zone is located under the pars interarticularis of the lamina and below the pedicle.
- The exit zone is the area surrounding the intervertebral foramen.

A decrease in the dimension of this canal results in a condition called lateral stenotic syndrome.[41]

Innervation

The outer half of the IVD, the posterior longitudinal ligament (PLL), and the dura are innervated by the sinuvertebral nerve,[42] which is considered to arise from the anterior (ventral) ramus and the sympathetic trunk.[43] The nerve endings are simple or complex, are encapsulated and nonencapsulated, and exist as free nerve endings. It has been suggested that apart from a nociceptive function, these nerve endings may also have a proprioceptive function.[44,45]

Alterations in Disk Structure

Although the lumbar IVD appears destined for tissue regression and destruction, it remains unclear why similar age-related changes remain asymptomatic in one individual yet cause severe LBP in others. The basic changes that influence the responses of the disk to aging appear to be biochemical and may concern the collagen content levels in the NP.

There is, with age, an increase in the collagen content of both the NP and the AF and a change in the type of collagen present.[46] The elastic collagen of the NP becomes more fibrous, whereas the type 1 collagen of the AF becomes more elastic.[46] Eventually, they come to resemble each other. In addition, the concentration of noncollagenous proteins increases in the NP. The change of the makeup of the collagen alters the biomechanical properties of the disk, making it less resilient, perhaps leading to changes from microtrauma.[46]

CLINICAL PEARL

In general, the IVD becomes drier, stiffer, less deformable, and less able to recover from creep with age.

It was traditionally thought that the loss of height that occurs with aging resulted from a loss in the height of the IVD. More recently, it has been demonstrated that between the ages of 20 and 70 years, the disk actually increases its height by approximately 10%, and that the loss of height with age is more likely to be caused by the erosion of the vertebral end plate.[47]

As the NP becomes more fibrous, its ability to handle compressive loading becomes compromised and more weight is taken by the AF, resulting in a separation of the lamellae and the formation of cavities within it.[46]

Zygapophyseal Joint

The articulations between two consecutive lumbar vertebrae form three joints. One joint is formed between the two vertebral bodies and the IVD. The other two joints are formed by the articulation of the superior articular process of one vertebra and the inferior articular processes of the vertebra above it. These latter joints are known as the zygapophyseal joints.

In the intact lumbar vertebral column, the primary function of the zygapophyseal joint is to protect the motion segment from anterior shear forces, excessive rotation, and flexion.[48] Additional functions include

- the production of spinal motions including coupling movements;
- a minimal restrictor of the physiologic movements of extension and side bending.[49]

From an anteroposterior perspective, the zygapophyseal joints of the lumbar spine appear straight, but when viewed from above, they are seen to be curved into a J or C shape. Their orientation varies both with the level and with the individual subject.[50] It is thought that this orientation serves to maximally restrict anterior and rotary movements and that the C-shaped joints do better in preventing anterior displacement than the J-shaped joints, because of the curvature of the joint surfaces.[16,51] Both shapes competently prevent rotation. The area of the zygapophyseal joints most involved in resisting anterior shear forces is the anteromedial part of the superior zygapophyseal joint. It is this area that is most vulnerable to fibrillation.[16] The tangential splitting and vertical tearing of the cartilage that occur with aging are believed to reflect these forces and appear to be a part of the normal degeneration of the joint.[16]

CLINICAL PEARL

At the thoracolumbar junction, the morphologic configuration of the zygapophyseal joints is extremely variable. In general, there is a change from a relatively coronal orientation at T10–11 to a more sagittal orientation at L1–3, before returning to the more coronal orientation at L5 and S1. Davis[52] compared the thoracolumbar junction to a carpenter's mortise and tenon joint, which, when approximated, would have the effect of impeding all motion except flexion.[52] This appears to be particularly true with respect to axial rotation, in which there is a high degree of torsional stiffness.[53,54]

A fibrous capsule surrounds the joint on all of its aspects except the anterior aspect, which consists of the ligamentum flavum (LF). Posteriorly, the capsule is reinforced by the deep fibers of the multifidus.[55] In lumbar extension, there is a potential for the posterior capsule to become pinched between the apex of the inferior facet and the lamina below. To prevent this, some fibers of the multifidus blend with the posterior capsular fibers and appear to keep the capsule taut.[56]

Superiorly and inferiorly, the capsule is very loose. Superiorly, it bulges toward the base of the next superior transverse process, whereas, inferiorly, it does so over the back of the lamina. In both the superior and the inferior poles of the joint capsule, there is a very small hole that allows the passage of fat from within the capsule to the extracapsular space.[57]

Within the zygapophyseal joints, three types of intra-articular meniscoids have been noted[16]:

1. A connective tissue rim
2. An adipose tissue pad
3. A fibroadipose meniscoid

It is thought that the function of these intra-articular meniscoids is to

- fill the joint cavity;
- increase the articular surface area without reducing flexibility;
- protect the articular surfaces, as they become exposed during extreme flexion and extension.

These menisci have been inculpated in the cause of some types of LBP, when they fail to return to their original position on recovery from a flexion or extension movement and block the joint toward the neutral position.[58]

Ligaments

Anterior Longitudinal Ligament

The anterior longitudinal ligament (ALL) covers the anterior aspects of the vertebral bodies and IVD (Fig. 28-2). The ALL extends from the sacrum along the anterior aspect of the entire spinal column, becoming thinner as it ascends.[59] The ALL is connected only indirectly with the anterior aspect of the IVD by loose areolar tissue.[16] Some of the ligament fibers insert directly into the bone or periosteum of the centrum.[60] Because of these attachments, and the pull on the bone from the ligament, it is proposed that the anterior aspect of the vertebral body becomes the site for osteophytes. The remaining ligament fibers cover two to five segments, attaching to the upper and lower ends of the vertebral body.

The ALL of the lumbar spine is under tension in a neutral position of the spine and functions to prevent overextension of the spinal segments. In addition, the ALL functions as a minor assistant in limiting anterior translation and vertical separation of the vertebral body.

The ALL receives its nerve supply from recurrent branches of the grey rami communicans.[61]

Posterior Longitudinal Ligament

The PLL is found throughout the spinal column, where it covers the posterior aspect of the centrum and IVD (see Fig. 28-2). Its deep fibers span two segments, from the superior border of the inferior vertebra to the inferior margin of the superior. These fibers integrate with the superficial annular fibers to attach to the posterior margins of the vertebral bodies.[16] The more superficial fibers span up to five segments. In the lumbar spine, the ligament becomes constricted over the vertebral body and widens out over the IVD. It does not attach to the concavity of the body but is separated from it by a fat pad, which acts to block the venous drainage through the basivertebral vein during flexion, as the ligament presses it against the opening of the vein. Although the PLL is rather narrow and is not as substantial as the ALL, it is thought to be important in preventing IVD protrusion.[62] Both the ALL and the PLL have the same tensile strength per unit area.[63]

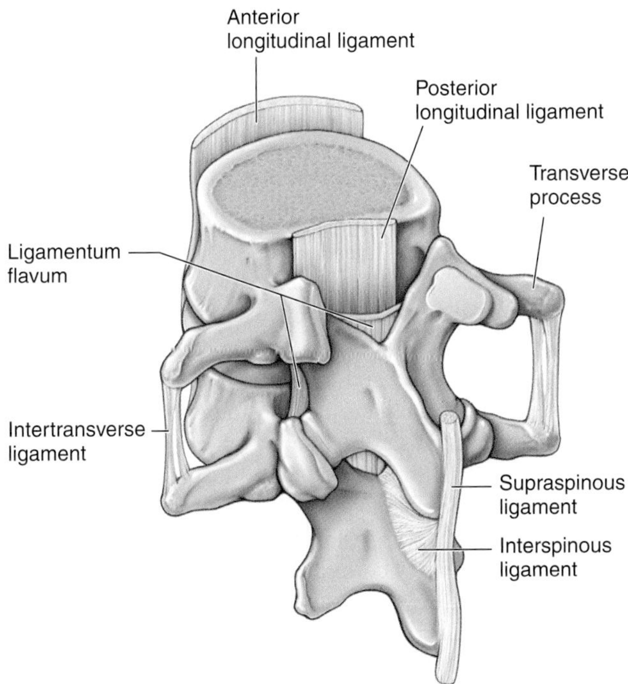

FIGURE 28-2 Ligaments of the lumbar spine. (Reproduced with permission from Morton, DA, Foreman KB, Albertine KH: *The Big Picture: Gross Anatomy*, McGraw-Hill, 2011.)

The PLL tends to tighten in traction and in posterior shearing of the vertebral body. It also acts to limit flexion over a number of segments, although because of its proximity to the center of rotation, it is less of a restraint than the LF.[59]

The PLL is innervated by the sinuvertebral nerve.

Ligamentum Flavum

The LF connects two consecutive laminae (see Fig. 28-2). This is a bilateral ligament. The medial aspect of the ligament attaches superiorly to the lower anterior surface of the lamina and the inferior surface of the pedicle.[64] The LF attaches inferiorly to the back of the lamina and the pedicle of the next inferior vertebra.[64]

Its lateral portion attaches to the articular process and forms the anterior capsule of the zygapophyseal joint.

The LF is formed primarily from elastin (80%), with the remainder (20%) being collagen.[65] Thus, it is an elastic ligament that is stretched during flexion and recovers its neutral length with the neutral position, or extension.

The function of the LF is to resist separation of the lamina during flexion, but there is also appreciable strain in the ligament with side bending.[16,66] Although it seems unlikely that the ligament contributes to an extension recovery from flexion, it does appear to prevent the anterior capsule from becoming nipped between the articular margins as it recoils during extension.[16] The LF is innervated by the medial branch of the posterior (dorsal) ramus.[67]

Interspinous Ligament

The interspinous ligament (see Fig. 28-2) lies deeply between two consecutive spinal processes. The ligament is important for stability, as it represents a major structure for the posterior column of the spine. Unlike the longitudinal ligaments, it is not a continuous fibrous band but, instead, consists of loose tissue that fills the gap between the bodies of the spinous processes.[16,68] The interspinous ligament is often disrupted in traumatic cases, which results in the posterior column becoming unstable. An extensive anatomic study on the interspinous ligament showed that degenerative changes start as early as the late second decade, with ruptures occurring in more than 20% of the subjects older than 20 years, particularly at L4–5 and L5–S1.[69]

The ligament has three distinct parts—anterior (ventral), middle, and posterior (dorsal)—of which the middle has the most clinical significance, because it is the part where ruptures tend to occur.[68]

The interspinous ligament most likely functions to resist separation of the spinous processes during flexion.[70] This ligament is supplied by the medial branch of the posterior (dorsal) rami.[67]

Supraspinous Ligament

The supraspinous ligament (SSL) (see Fig. 28-2) is broad, thick, and cord like, but it is only well developed in the upper lumbar region.[16,71] Although it joins the tips of two adjacent spinous processes, the SSL is not considered by some to be a true ligament. This is because part of it is derived from the posterior part of the interspinous ligament, although it also merges with the insertions of the lumbar posterior (dorsal) muscles.[68] Because this ligament is the most superficial of the spinal ligaments and the farthest from the axis of flexion, it has a greater potential for sprains.[72] The SSL is supplied by the medial branch of the posterior (dorsal) rami.[67]

Iliolumbar Ligament

The iliolumbar ligament is one of the three vertebropelvic ligaments, the others being the sacrotuberous and the sacrospinous ligaments. The ligament is variously believed to be a degenerate part of the quadratus lumborum or the iliocostalis and does not fully develop until approximately age 30 years.[73]

The iliolumbar ligament functions to restrain flexion, extension, axial rotation, and side bending of L5 on S1.[74] Motions at the lumbosacral joint increase by approximately 20% in all directions when the ligament is missing or transected.[59] The incidences of degenerative instability and isthmic lumbar spondylolisthesis have also been shown to increase in its absence.[75,76]

Pseudoligaments

These ligaments, the intertransverse, transforaminal, and mamilloaccessory, resemble the membranous part of the fascial system separating paravertebral compartments and do not have any mechanical function.

Intertransverse Ligaments. These ligaments are more membranous than ligamentous. The ligament splits into posterior (dorsal) and anterior (ventral) portions, between which is a fat-filled recess. During flexion and extension movements, the fat can be displaced to accommodate the repositioning of the articular zygapophyseal joint. The main function of the ligament appears to be to compartmentalize the anterior and posterior musculature.[16]

Transforaminal Ligaments. Occurring in approximately 47% of subjects, the transforaminal ligaments traverse the lateral end of the intervertebral foramen.[77] The most significant of these ligaments is the superior corporotransverse ligament. At L5, the fifth lumbar nerve root runs between the ligament and the ala of the sacrum. With marked forward slip and downward descent of L5, or with a loss of IVD height, the corporotransverse ligament can have a guillotine effect on the fifth nerve root, resulting in symptoms that can mimic an IVD herniation or a foraminal occlusion.[78]

Mamilloaccessory Ligament. This ligament runs from the accessory process of one vertebra to the mammillary process of the same vertebra.[79] The ligament forms a tunnel for the medial branch of the posterior (dorsal) ramus, thereby preventing it from lifting off the neural arch. In approximately 10% of adults, the tunnel becomes ossified.[79]

Muscles

Quadratus Lumborum

The quadratus lumborum muscle is large and rectangular, with fibers that pass medially upward. The fibers attach to

- the inferior anterior surface of the 12th rib;
- the anterior surface of the upper four transverse processes;
- the anterior band of the iliolumbar ligament;
- the iliac crest lateral to the attachment of the iliolumbar ligament.

The muscle is active during inspiration, fixing the lowest rib to afford a stable base from which the diaphragm can act. The importance of this muscle from a rehabilitation viewpoint is its contribution as a lumbar spine stabilizer.[80] Working unilaterally, it is typically involved with side bending of the lumbar spine, especially with eccentric control of contralateral side bending. The quadratus lumborum is an important, yet often underappreciated, lateral lumbar spine stabilizer that has been shown to be very active in sustained postures and when a heavy weight is held in the opposite hand.[81,82] The quadratus lumborum is supplied by the anterior (ventral) rami of T12–L2.[83,84]

Multifidus

The lumbar multifidus is the largest of the intrinsic back muscles to cross the lumbosacral junction and lies most medially in the spinal gutter (Fig. 28-3).[56] It is a fascicular muscle, with each fascicle being layered on another, giving it a laminated appearance.[16] The lumbar multifidus originates in three groups, which arise from the same vertebra.

1. Laminar fibers arise from the inferoposterior edge of the lamina.
2. Basal fibers arise from the base of the spinous process.
3. Common tendon fibers arise from a common tendon attached to the inferior tip of the spinous process.

The lumbar multifidus has a complicated insertion (Table 28-1).

Over the past several decades, there has been much research regarding the lumbar multifidus, with particular reference to its relationship to LBP, and its importance in lumbar spine stabilization. In vitro biomechanical studies have shown that the lumbar multifidus is an important muscle for lumbar segmental stability through its ability to provide segmental stiffness and to control motion.[85–87] Wilke et al.[88] concluded that the multifidus is responsible for two-thirds of the stiffness of the lumbar spine. The multifidus is active in nearly all antigravity activities and appears to contribute to the stability of the lumbar spine by compressing the vertebrae together.[46] Hides et al.[89] found reductions in ipsilateral multifidus cross-sectional area in patients with unilateral LBP and speculated that this may be a direct result of reflex inhibition.[90] This loss of multifidus cross-sectional area was shown to persist after remission of LBP.[84] Isolated multifidus strengthening has

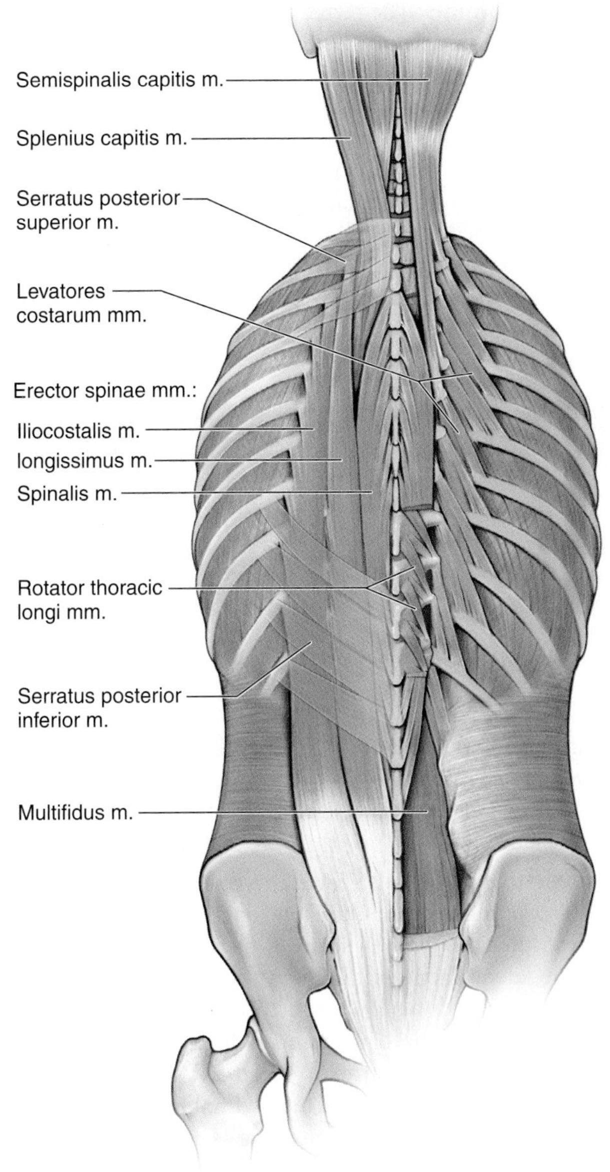

FIGURE 28-3 Multifidus and Erector spinae. (Reproduced with permission from Morton DA, Foreman KB, Albertine KH: *The Big Picture: Gross Anatomy*, McGraw-Hill, 2011.)

been shown to restore the muscle size at the segmental level of the dysfunction.[90]

MacIntosh and Bogduk[56] analyzed the lumbar multifidus to determine the possible actions of the muscle and its individual fibers. The study revealed that working bilaterally, the multifidus muscles can produce the rocking component of extension, but because of the muscle's vertical orientation, it cannot produce the accompanying translation.[56] In addition, the muscle, by "bow stringing" over a number of segments, can increase the lumbar lordosis, working in a postural role.[91]

Although not considered a primary lumbar rotator,[92] the multifidus is consistently active during both ipsilateral and contralateral spinal rotation, and both multifidi are simultaneously active regardless of which way the spine is turning.[56,57]

TABLE 28-1 Multifidus Attachments

Laminar	Basal	Common Tendon
L1; MP L3	MP L4	MP L5, S1, and PSIS
L2; MP L4	MP L5	MP S1 and anterolateral aspect of PSIS
L3; MP L5	MP S1	Inferior to PSIS and lateral sacrum
L4; MP S1	As common tendon	Sacrum, lateral to foramina
L5; common	As common tendon	Sacrum, medial to tendon foramina

MP, mammillary process; PSIS, posterior-superior iliac spine.
Data from Meadows J, Pettman E: *Manual Therapy: NAIOMT Level II & III Course Notes.* Denver, CO: North American Institute of Manual Therapy, Inc., 1995; Bogduk N, Twomey LT: Anatomy and biomechanics of the lumbar spine. In: Bogduk N, Twomey LT, eds. *Clinical Anatomy of the Lumbar Spine and Sacrum,* 3rd ed. Edinburgh: Churchill Livingstone, 1997:2–53, 81–152, 171–176.

The major function of the multifidus from a biomechanical perspective is one of arthrokinematic control. It is believed that the lumbar multifidus acts as an antagonist to flexion and opposes the flexing moment of the abdominals as they rotate the trunk.[56,91,93] This synergistic function may be compromised with injury to the multifidus. Using magnetic resonance imaging, the signal intensities of the multifidus during lumbar hyperextension have been found to be markedly diminished in patients with chronic LBP compared with normal patients.[94]

Unilaterally, the multifidus muscle should also be able to produce side bending. However, its horizontal vector is very small, and it is unlikely to be an efficient side bender of the spine.[16,56]

The multifidus shares a close association with the gluteus maximus and the sacrotuberous ligament, factors that are thought to enhance sacroiliac joint and lumbar spine stability.[95–97]

The lumbar multifidus has the distinction of being innervated segmentally by the medial branch of the posterior (dorsal) ramus of the same level or the level below the originating spinous process.[98,99] Because the multifidus is segmental in origin and innervation, any impairment of this muscle can produce palpable changes in the muscle, thus directing the clinician to the segment that is dysfunctional.[100]

Erector Spinae

The erector spinae is a composite muscle consisting of the iliocostalis lumborum and the thoracic longissimus (Fig. 28-3). Both of these muscles are subdivided into the lumbar and thoracic longissimi and iliocostallii.[16] As a group, the muscles of the erector spinae play an important role in lumbar stabilization by providing compressive forces along the spine that stabilize the spinal curvatures.[101] The nerve supply to the erector spinae muscles is by the medial branch of the posterior (dorsal) ramus of the thoracic and lumbar spinal nerves.

Longissimus Thoracis Pars Lumborum. This is a fascicular muscle that arises from the accessory processes of the lumbar vertebrae to insert into the posterior-superior iliac spine

(PSIS) and the iliac crest lateral to it. The upper four tendons converge to form the lumbar aponeurosis that inserts lateral to the L5 fascicle.

The longissimus thoracis pars lumborum muscles have both a vertical and a horizontal vector. The vertical vector is much the larger of the two and can produce extension or side bending, depending on whether it is functioning bilaterally or unilaterally.[102] Because of its attachment to the transverse rather than the spinous process, which results in reduced leverage, the longissimus thoracis pars lumborum is much less efficient than the lumbar multifidus in producing posterior sagittal rotation, due to its reduced leverage.[99,103] Indeed, mathematical analysis of the lumbosacral portion of the muscle suggests that the net effect of its pull would be to produce an anterior, and not a posterior, shear.[16]

Iliocostalis Lumborum Pars Lumborum. There are four overlying fascicles arising from the tip of the upper four transverse processes and the adjoining middle layer of the thoracolumbar fascia. The fibers insert onto the iliac crest, with the lower and deeper fibers attaching lateral to the PSIS.[103]

There is no muscular fiber from L5, but it is believed that this is represented by the iliolumbar ligament, which is completely muscular in children, becoming collagenous by approximately 30 years of age.

The vectors and actions of this muscle are similar to those of the longissimus. However, the lower and deeper fibers produce strong axial rotation and act with the multifidus as synergists to produce rotation during abdominal muscle action.[103]

Longissimus Thoracis Pars Thoracis. This muscle group consists of 11–12 pairs of muscles, which extend from the transverse processes of T2 and their ribs and run inferomedially to attach to the spinous processes of L3–5 and the sacral spinous processes, as well as the PSIS.

The orientation and various attachments of this muscle group allow it to act indirectly on the lumbar spine. The main action of the muscle appears to be the extension of the thoracic spine on that of the lumbar. An anatomic-mathematical study[104] suggests that 70–80% of the force required to extend the upper lumbar spine is produced from the thoracic fibers of the erector spinae, which also generate 50% of the force in the lower levels.

Iliocostalis Lumborum Pars Thoracis. The thoracic iliocostalis serves as the thoracic part of the iliocostalis lumborum and not the iliocostalis thoracic. It is a layered muscle consisting of inferomedially orientated fascicles attached to the following points[103]:

- lateral part of the lower eight rib angles;
- PSIS;
- posterior (dorsal) surface of the sacrum, distal to the multifidus.

This muscle completely spans the lumbar spine and is in an excellent position to extend and side bend the spine, as well as to increase the lumbar lordosis. It is a weak rotator, because the amount of rib separation on ipsilateral rotation is minor, but on contralateral rotation, it is better. It is, therefore, possible that the muscle is an effective derotator of the spine.[16]

Abdominal Muscles

Rectus Abdominis. The rectus abdominis (Fig. 28-4) originates from the cartilaginous ends of the fifth through seventh ribs and xiphoid and inserts on the superior aspect of the pubic bone. The linea alba (Fig. 28-4) is the anterior abdominal aponeurosis or rectus sheath in the midline. It is formed by the interlacing of aponeurosis of the external oblique, internal oblique, and transverse abdominis muscles from both sides. It is broader superiorly, where the recti are separated at a considerable interval, and narrower inferiorly, where the recti are closely packed (Fig. 28-4). Above the umbilicus, the linea alba is a single layer, whereas below the umbilicus it has a double layer.[105]

CLINICAL PEARL

A split between the two rectus abdominis to the extent that the linea alba may split under strain is known as a diastasis recti (see Chap 30 and "Practice Pattern 4E: Impaired Joint Mobility, Motor Function, Muscle Performance, and Range of Motion Associated with Localized Inflammation" section).[105–110]

The rectus abdominis muscle functions to produce torque during flexion of the vertebral column, as it approximates the thorax and pelvis anteriorly.[111] The muscle appears to serve a beneficial role of helping to stabilize the lumbar spine in the sagittal plane.[90]

Transversus Abdominis. The transverse abdominis muscle (Fig. 28-4) originates from the lateral one-third of the inguinal ligament, the anterior two-thirds of the inner lip of the iliac crest, the lateral raphe of the thoracolumbar fascia, and the internal aspects of the lower six costal cartilages, where it interdigitates with the diaphragm.[112] Its upper and middle fibers run transversely around the trunk and blend with the fascial envelope of the rectus abdominis muscle, while the lower fibers blend with the insertion of the internal oblique muscle on the pubic crest.[113]

Although much emphasis has traditionally been placed on the strengthening of the rectus abdominis during lumbar spine rehabilitation, recent research has suggested that it is the contraction of the hoop-like transversus abdominis (TrA) that creates a rigid cylinder, resulting in enhanced stiffness of the lumbar spine and stabilization of the lumbar motion segment (see "Biomechanics" section).[46,81,82,114–117] Since the midportion of the TrA attaches to the cross-hatch arrangement of the middle layer of the thoracolumbar fascia (see later), contraction of the TrA has been thought to increase spinal stability via tensioning of the thoracolumbar fascia in the middle and lower regions of the lumbar spine or by producing a mild stabilizing compressive force on the lumbar vertebrae.[90,112,116] The thoracolumbar fascia creates a pressurized visceral cavity anterior to the spine when the TrA contracts. This force is theorized to increase the stability of the lumbar spine during a variety of postures and movements.[118]

Internal Oblique. The internal oblique (see Fig. 28-4), which forms the middle layer of the lateral abdominal wall, is located between the TrA and the external oblique muscles.[113] It has multiple attachments to the inguinal ligament, lateral raphe,

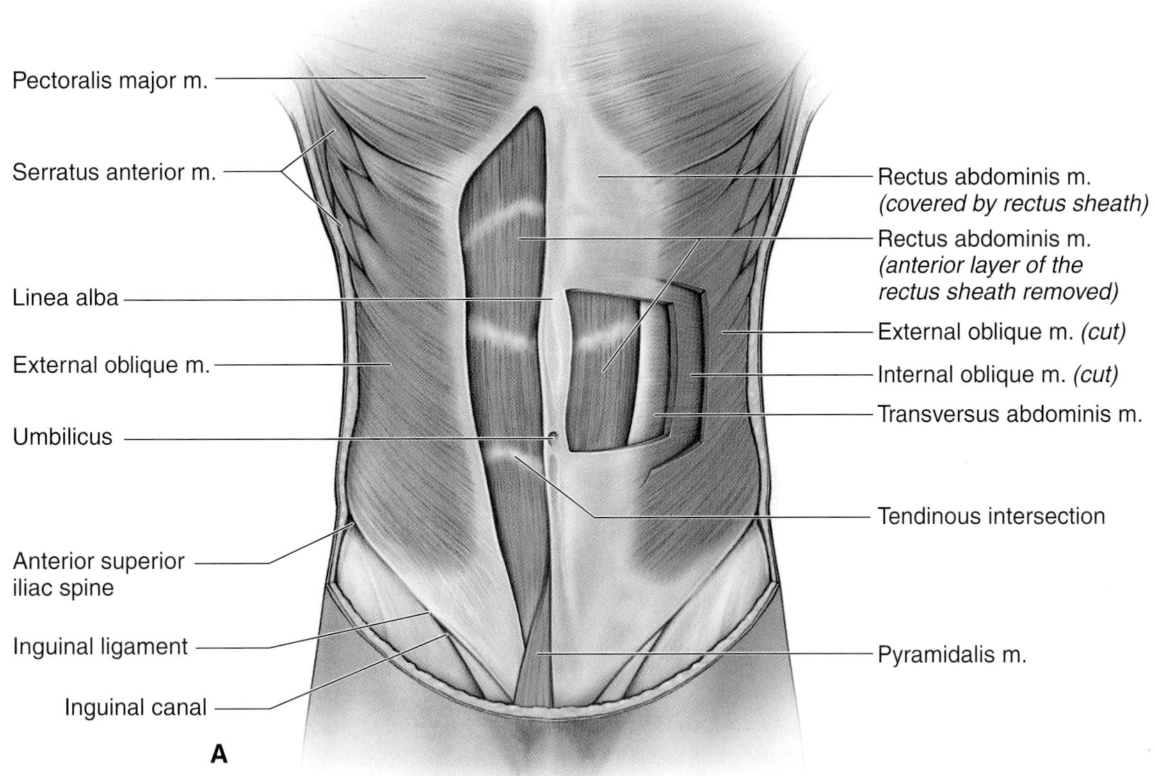

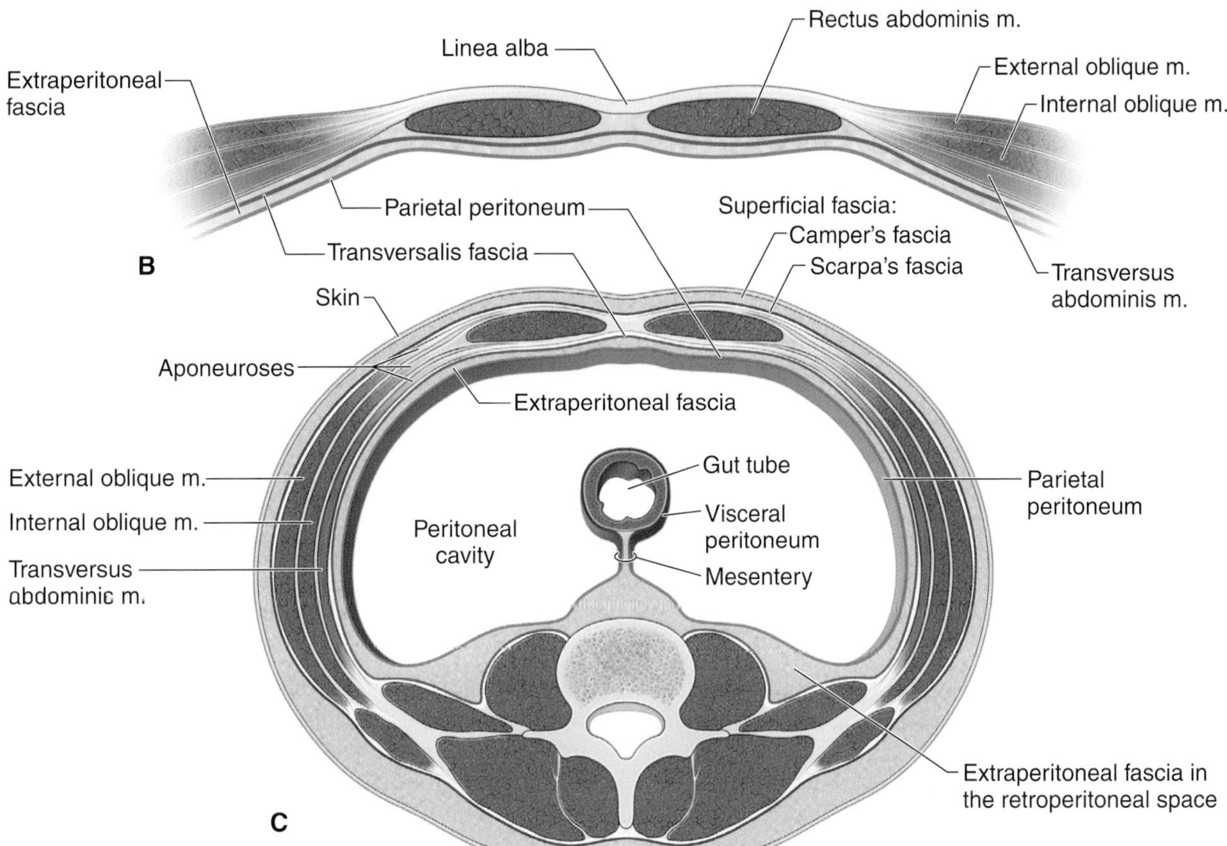

FIGURE 28-4 Abdominal muscles. (Reproduced with permission from Morton DA, Foreman KB, Albertine KH: *The Big Picture: Gross Anatomy,* McGraw-Hill, 2011.)

iliac crest, pubic crest, transverse abdominis, and costal cartilages of the seventh through ninth costal cartilages. Because of these multiple attachment sites, the different fascicles of the muscle can have very different force vectors.

The internal oblique is active during a number of functions, including gait (most often close to initial contact[119]) and erect sitting and standing postures.[120] Acting bilaterally, the internal obliques flex the vertebral column and assist in respiration. Acting in unison, the muscle, in conjunction with the external obliques, can produce rotation of the vertebral column, bringing the thorax backward (when the pelvis is fixed) or the pelvis forward (when the thorax is fixed).[111,121]

External Oblique. The external oblique (see Fig. 28-4) originates from the lateral aspect of the fifth through 12th ribs, and through interdigitations with the serratus anterior and latissimus dorsi. The muscle travels obliquely, medially, and inferiorly to insert into the linea alba, inguinal ligament, anterior superior iliac spine (ASIS), iliac crest, and pubic tubercle.

Acting bilaterally, the external obliques flex the vertebral column and tilt the pelvis posteriorly. Acting in unison, the muscle, in conjunction with the internal obliques, can produce side bending of the vertebral column, approximating the thorax and the iliac crest laterally.[111]

Researchers have suggested that the internal obliques, and to a lesser extent the external obliques, may contribute to the production of intra-abdominal pressure and thus stability of the lumbar spine.[122]

Psoas Major

Although traditionally viewed as a muscle of the hip, the psoas major muscle combines with the iliacus muscle to directly attach the lumbar spine to the femur.[123] The psoas major originates from

- anterolateral aspects of the vertebral bodies;
- intervertebral disks of T12–L5;
- transverse processes of L1–5;
- tendinous arch spanning the concavity of the sides of the vertebral bodies.

The iliacus is attached superiorly to the iliac fossa and the inner lip of the iliac crest. Joining with the psoas major, the combined tendon passes over the superior lateral aspect of the pubic ramus and attaches to the lesser trochanter of the femur.

Taken individually, the iliacus and psoas major serve different functions.

- The psoas major is electromyographically active in many different positions and movements of the lumbar spine, and its activity can add a stabilizing effect on the lumbar spine with compressive loading.[124] With the foot fixed on the ground (closed chain), contraction of the psoas major increases the flexion of the lumbar-pelvic unit on the femur.[125]
- With the foot fixed on the ground, contraction of the iliacus produces an anterior torsion of the ilium and extension of the lumbar zygapophyseal joints. If there is a decrease in the length of the iliopsoas as a result of adaptive shortening or increased efferent neural input to the muscle, the result is an anteriorly rotated pelvis and an increase in lordosis. This may increase the anterior shear stress on the lumbosacral junction in any posture.[124]

From a clinical perspective, the iliacus and psoas major usually are considered together as the iliopsoas. Working bilaterally (insertion fixed), the iliopsoas can produce flexion of the trunk on the femur as in the sit-up from supine position, or in bending over to touch one's toes. The iliopsoas muscle also side bends the spine ipsilaterally.[124]

Working from a stable spine above (origin fixed), the iliopsoas muscle flexes the hip joint by flexing the femur on the trunk.

The iliopsoas is innervated by the anterior (ventral) rami of L1 and L2.

Thoracolumbar Fascia

The thoracolumbar fascia travels from the spinous process of T12 to the PSIS and iliac crest. The thoracolumbar fascia consists of three layers of connective tissue that envelop the lumbar muscles and separate them into anterior, middle, and posterior compartments or layers[126]:

1. The anterior layer covers the anterior surface of the quadratus lumborum muscle. It is attached to the anterior transverse processes and then to the intertransverse ligaments. On the lateral side of the quadratus lumborum, it blends with the other layers of the fascia.
2. The middle layer is posterior to the quadratus lumborum, with its medial attachment to the tips of the transverse processes and the intertransverse ligaments. Laterally, it gives rise to, or is attached to, the transverse abdominal aponeurosis.
3. The posterior layer covers the lumbar musculature and arises from the spinous processes, wrapping around the muscles. It blends with the other layers of the fascia along the lateral border of the iliocostalis lumborum in a dense thickening of the fascia called the *lateral raphe*.[126] This layer consists of two laminae, a superficial one with its fibers orientated inferomedially, and a deep lamina whose fibers are inferolateral. The superficial fibers are derived from the latissimus dorsi.

The functions of the TFL are varied. The TFL

- provides muscle attachment for the transversus abodominis;
- stabilizes the spine against anterior shear and flexion moments;
- resists segmental flexion via tension generated by the transverse abdominis on the spinous process;
- assists in the transmission of extension forces during lifting activities. The posterior ligamentous system has been proposed as a model to explain some of the forces required for lifting. It is believed to transmit forces by passive resistance to flexion, from the joint capsule and extracapsular ligaments, and from the more dynamic effects of the thoracolumbar fascia.[127]

Nerve Supply of the Lumbar Segment

The nerve supply to the lumbar spine follows a general pattern. The outer half of the IVD is innervated by the sinuvertebral nerve[42] and the grey rami communicants,[128] with the posterolateral aspect innervated by both the sinuvertebral nerve[61] and the grey rami communicants. The lateral aspect receives only sympathetic innervation.

The zygapophyseal joints are innervated by the medial branches of the posterior (dorsal) rami.[42,67,129] Each joint receives its nerve supply from the corresponding medial branch above and below the joint.[42,67] For instance the L4–5 joint receives its nerve supply from the medial branches of L3 and L4. The lateral branches cross the subjacent transverse process and pursue a sinuous course inferiorly, laterally, and posteriorly through the iliocostalis lumborum.[67] They innervate that muscle, and eventually the L1–3 lateral branches pierce the posterior (dorsal) layer of thoracolumbar fascia and become cutaneous, supplying the skin over the lateral buttock as far as the greater trochanter.[42,67] The intermediate branches run posteriorly and inferiorly from the intertransverse spaces. They form a series of intersegmental communications within the longissimus thoracis.[42,67]

At the L1 and L2 levels, the nerves exit the intervertebral foramen above the disk. From L2 downward, the nerves leave the dura slightly more proximally than the foramen through which they pass, and at a decreasing angle of obliquity and an increasing length within the spinal canal. The L3 nerve root travels behind the inferior aspect of the vertebral body and the L3 disk. The L4 nerve root crosses the whole vertebral body to leave the spinal canal at the upper aspect of the L4 disk, at an angle of approximately 60 degrees. The L5 nerve root emerges at the inferior aspect of the fourth lumbar disk at an angle of approximately 45 degrees and crosses the fifth vertebral body to exit at the upper aspect of the L5 disk. The S1 nerve root emerges at a 30-degree angle and crosses the L5–S1 disk.

Lumbar Spine Vascularization

The blood supply for the lumbar spine is provided by the lumbar arteries (Fig. 28-5), and its venous drainage occurs via the lumbar veins (Fig. 28-5).

Biomechanics

Physiologic motions at the lumbar spine joints can occur in three cardinal planes: sagittal (flexion and extension), coronal (side bending), and transverse (rotation). Including accessory motions, six degrees of freedom are available at the lumbar spine.[62]

The amount of segmental motion at each vertebral level varies. Most of the flexion and extension of the lumbar spine occurs in the lower segmental levels, whereas most of the side bending of the lumbar spine occurs in the midlumbar area.[112,130,131] Rotation, which occurs with side bending as a coupled motion, is minimal and occurs most at the lumbosacral junction.[112,130,131] The amount of range available in the lumbar spine generally decreases with age.[132]

Flexion

The lumbar spine is well designed for flexion, which is its most commonly used motion in daily activities. Flexion of the lumbar spine from erect standing involves an unfolding or straightening of the lumbar lordosis, followed by, at most, a small reversal of the lordotic curve.[133] The flexion–extension range of the lumbar spine that occurs between vertebral segments is approximately 12 degrees in the upper lumbar spine, increasing by 1–2 degrees per segment to reach a maximum motion of 20–25 degrees between L5 and S1.[16,131]

During lumbar flexion in standing, which normally is initiated by the abdominal muscles, the entire lumbar spine leans forward, and there is a posterior sway of the pelvis as the hips flex.

CLINICAL PEARL

Flexion of the lumbar spine can also occur with a posterior pelvic tilt. The posterior pelvic tilt can be performed voluntarily, or it may occur as a result of weak paraspinal extensor muscles or adaptively shortened hamstring and gluteal muscles.[134]

At the segmental level, lumbar flexion produces a combination of an anterior roll and an anterior glide of the vertebral body, and a straightening, or minimal reversal, of the lordosis.[112,131] At L4–5, reversal may occur, but at the L5–S1 level, the joint will straighten but not reverse[135] unless there is pathology present. During the anterior rocking motion of the segment that occurs with flexion, the inferior facets of the superior vertebra lift upward and backward, opening a small gap between the facets. The superior vertebra translates anteriorly by approximately 5–7 mm, closing the gap and enhancing stability through increased tension of the joint capsule.[57] The anterior sagittal translation, or shear, is also resisted by

- the superoanterior orientation of the lateral fibers of the AF;
- the iliolumbar and SSLs at the L5 to S1 segment, with the longitudinal ligaments helping to a lesser extent;
- the semisagittal and sagittal orientation of the zygapophyseal joints, which cause the superior facet to come against the inferior one during an anterior shear, with the highest pressure occurring on the anteromedial portion of the superior zygapophyseal joint surface. The zygapophyseal joints are, therefore, vital in the limitation of this anterior shear.[136]
- the horizontal vector of the erector spinae and the multifidus, which acts to pull the vertebrae posteriorly.

Flexion is also limited by the compressibility of the anterior structures, such as the IVD, and by the extensibility of the posterior structures of the segment (ligaments, IVD, and muscles). These structures have varying contributions to the resistance of segmental flexion, depending on the degree of flexion[137]:

- The joint capsule resists approximately 39%.
- The supraspinous and interspinous ligaments resist approximately 19%.
- The LF ligament resists approximately 13%.
- The IVD resists approximately 29%.

Extension

Extension movements of the lumbar spine produce a converse of those that occur in flexion. Theoretically, true extension of

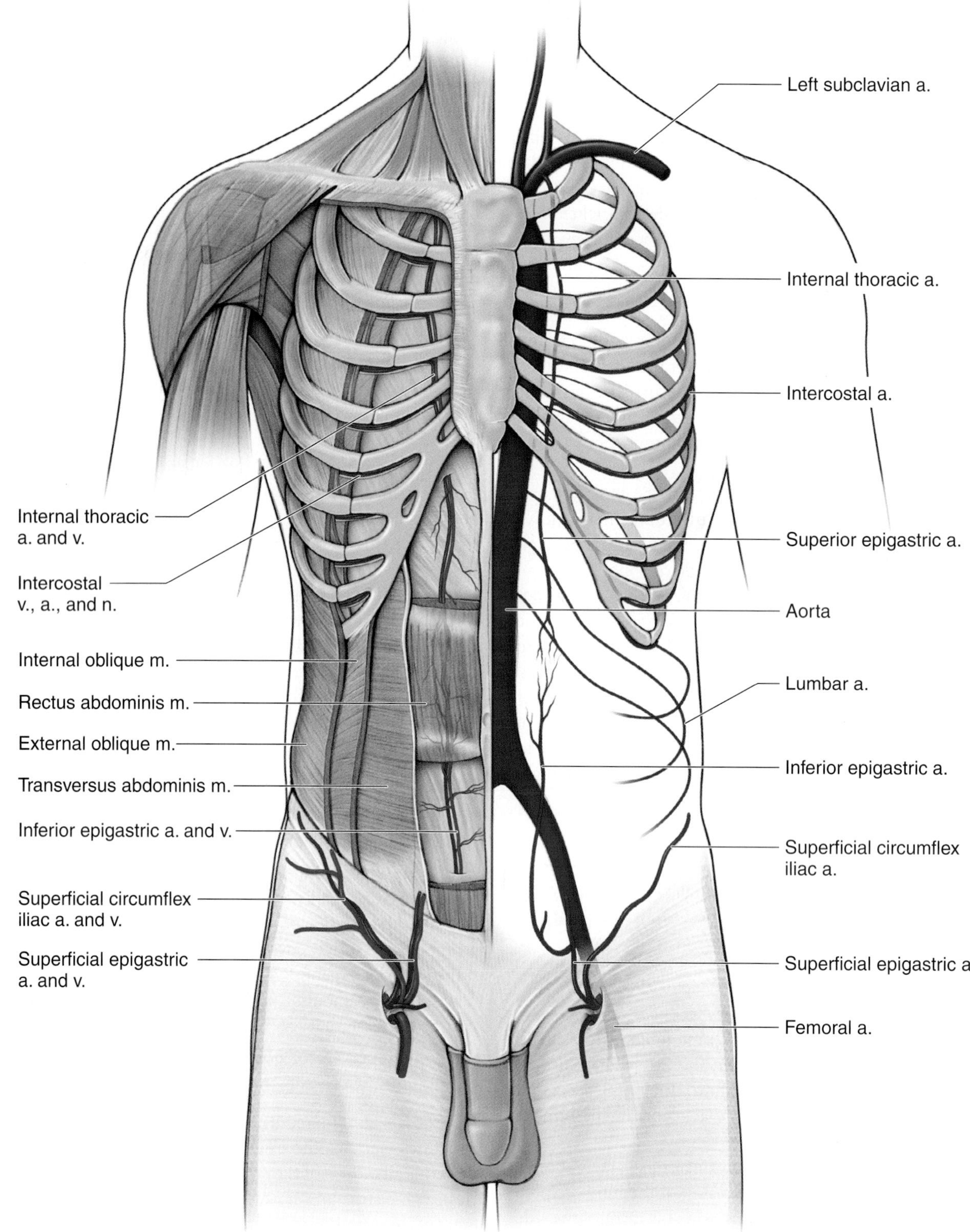

FIGURE 28-5 Vasculature of the spine. (Reproduced with permission from Morton DA, Foreman KB, Albertine KH: *The Big Picture: Gross Anatomy,* McGraw-Hill, 2011.)

the lumbar spine is pathologic and depends on one's definition: pure extension involves a posterior roll and glide of the vertebra and a posterior and inferior motion of the zygapophyseal joints, but not necessarily a change in the degree of lordosis.[131] During lumbar extension, the inferior zygapophyseal joint of the superior vertebra moves downward, impacting with the lamina below and producing a buckling of the interspinous ligament between the two spinous processes. This impaction is accentuated when the joint is subjected to the action of the back muscles.[138] If the extending force continues to be applied, especially unilaterally, the superior facets can pivot on their inferior counterparts, producing a strain on the opposite zygapophyseal joint, and potentially damaging or tearing the capsule.[16]

CLINICAL PEARL

Repetitive contact of the spinous processes during the extremes of lumbar extension can lead to a periostitis called *kissing spine* or *Baastrup's disease*,[139] with resulting ligamentous laxity and hypermobility of the segment.[140]

An anterior pelvic tilt increases the lumbar lordosis and results in an anterior motion of the vertebrae and their associated structures. Although the differing terminology between true extension and the extension created by increasing the lordosis is seemingly esoteric, there are clinical implications during the examination, when the clinician is assessing the ability of the patient to assume the extended position of the lumbar spine.

Pure lumbar extension is limited by

- the ability of structures anterior to the fulcrum to be elongated;
- the ability of the IVD to allow compression;
- joint capsule tension;
- passive tension of the psoas major muscle.

AXIAL ROTATION

Intervertebral Disk

Approximately 65% of the resistance to IVD torsion is resisted by a combination of tension and impaction of the contralateral zygapophyseal joint, and tension of the supraspinous and interspinous ligaments, with the disk contributing approximately 35% of the resistance.[141] During axial rotation, which produces torsion of the IVD, those collagen fibers of the AF that are orientated in the same direction as the twist are stretched and resist the torsional force, while the others remain relaxed, thereby sharing the stress of twisting.

During forced segmental torsion, the first structure to fail is the zygapophyseal joint, which normally occurs at approximately 1–2 degrees of segmental rotation.[141] As collagen can only elongate approximately 4% before damage, the maximum segmental rotation at each segmental level is typically limited to approximately 3 degrees.[20,62] Macroscopic failure of the IVD is likely to occur only in the presence of extreme trauma, with accompanying fracture of the zygapophyseal joint.[32] However, surgical incision of the zygapophyseal joint, or facetectomy, which increases the amount of rotation the segment is capable of handling, also significantly increases the stress in the posterior AF fibers.[32,141]

In the absence of zygapophyseal joint damage, surgical or otherwise, axial rotation must be coupled with other motions to cause disk injury.[51] For example, the combination of maximal lumbar flexion and rotation, which increases the amount of rotation before the contralateral zygapophyseal joint makes contact, has been associated with trauma to the AF.[142,143]

Other Structures

Rotational movements of the lumbar spine do appear to produce the appropriate motor patterns for optimal trunk muscle cocontraction and spinal stability.[114,144] The axis of rotation in the sagittal plane passes through the anterior aspect of the IVD and vertebral body.[145] For axial displacements, the axis of rotation tends to be located within the posterior annulus.[145] Axial rotation of the lumbar spine amounts to approximately 13 degrees to both sides. The greatest amount of segmental rotation, approximately 5 degrees, occurs at the L5 and S1 segments. Axial rotation of the segment involves

- twisting, or torsion, of the IVD fibers;
- compression of the contralateral zygapophyseal joint, for example, with left axial rotation, the right inferior zygapophyseal joint will impact on the superior zygapophyseal joint of the bone below;
- stress on those annular fibers inclined toward the direction of rotation.

In normal segments, the zygapophyseal joints protect the IVD from torsional injuries by coming into contact before microfailure of the IVD can occur. During axial rotation, tension is built in the interspinous and SSLs, and the contralateral joint becomes impacted after 1–2 degrees of rotation.[141] Further movement is accommodated by compression of the articular cartilage. If this range is exceeded, any further rotation that occurs is impure. Impure rotation of the segment forces the upper vertebra to pivot backward on the impacted joint, around the newly created axis of rotation. This causes the vertebra to swing laterally and backward, increasing the potential for a lateral shear force on the annulus. At this extreme, the IVD is vulnerable to either torsional or shear forces, and the other joint capsule is placed under severe tension.[32] This combination can result in a failure of any one of these structures, resulting in any or all of the following: compression fractures of the contralateral lamina, subchondral fractures, fragmentation of the articular surface and tearing, avulsion of the ipsilateral joint capsule, or a pars interarticularis fracture.[16]

The ipsilateral joint does not normally gap during normal axial rotation, except during therapeutic manipulation.[146] Abnormal gapping has been found to occur in segments with degenerative or traumatic instability, questioning the role of therapeutic manipulation in such cases.[146]

SIDE BENDING

Side bending is a complex and highly variable movement involving side bending and rotatory movements of the interbody joints and a variety of movements at the zygapophyseal joints.[133] The means of how this is achieved has been the subject of debate for many years, and it is difficult to ascertain how an impaired segment would behave, compared with a healthy one.[147] The general pattern of coupled motion is for side bending to be associated with contralateral axial rotation at the mid and upper lumbar levels but ipsilateral axial rotation at L5–S1.[133] However, there is at present little evidence for strict rules of coupled motion that determine whether an individual has abnormal ranges or directions of coupling in the lumbar spine.[133,148]

Bending motions can occur in any direction, producing both a rocking motion and a translation shearing effect on the IVD. The NP tends to be compressed and the AF buckles in the direction of the rocking motion,[149] and there is a tendency for the AF to be stretched in the opposite direction, while the pressure on the posterior aspect of the NP is relieved. Although the deformation can occur in a healthy disk, displacement of the NP is prevented by the AF that encapsulates it. The AF will buckle at its compressed aspect because it is not braced by the NP, which is exerting that effect on the AF fibers at the opposite side of the disk.[20]

AXIAL LOADING (COMPRESSION)

Axial compression or spinal loading occurs in weight bearing, whether in standing or sitting.

Intervertebral Disk

It has been demonstrated experimentally that the AF, even without the NP, can withstand the same vertical forces that an intact disk can for short periods,[150] provided that the lamellae do not buckle. However, if the compression is prolonged or if the lamellae are not held together, the sheets buckle and the system collapses on itself.

The extent and magnitude of the compression depend on the amount of applied compressive force, the disk height, and the cross-sectional area of the disk. Variations in disk height can be divided into two categories: primary disk height variations and secondary disk height changes.

1. Primary disk height variations are related to intrinsic individual factors such as body height, gender, age, disk level, and geographic region.[151,152]
2. Secondary disk height changes are associated with extrinsic factors, such as degeneration, abnormality, or clinical management. Surgical procedures, such as nucleotomy, diskectomy, and chemonucleolysis cause a decrease in disk height, resulting from the removal of a portion of the NP or damage to the water-binding capacity of the extracellular matrix.[153–155] In addition, there are diurnal changes in disk height, which are caused by fluid exchange and creep deformation.[156]

With variations in disk height, one would expect changes in mechanical behavior of the disk. An important result to emerge from a recent study is that axial displacement, posterolateral disk bulge, and tensile stress in the peripheral AF fibers are a function of axial compressive force and disk height.[157] Under the same axial force, disks with a higher height-to-area ratio generate higher values of axial displacement, disk bulge, and tensile stress on the peripheral AF fibers.

The NP is deformable but relatively incompressible. Therefore, when a load is applied to it vertically, the nuclear pressure rises, absorbing and transmitting the compression forces to the vertebral end plates and the AF.[16]

- The resistance of the end plate is dependent on the strength of the bone beneath and the blood capacity of the vertebral body.
- The AF bulges radially,[158] delaying and graduating the forces.

The peripheral pressure increases the tension on the collagen fibers, which resist it until a balance is reached, at the point when the radial pressure is matched by the collagen tension.[112] This equilibrium achieves two things:

1. Pressure is transferred from one end plate to another, thus relieving the load on the AF.
2. The NP braces the AF and prevents it from buckling under the sustained axial load.

Other structures provide resistance to axial loading of the spine:

- The ALL offers resistance if the spine is in its normal lordosis. The lumbar lordosis while standing is approximately 50% greater than when seated.[159]
- The inferior articular process can impact on the lamina below during strong lordosis.

During axial compression of the IVD the following occur:

1. Water is squeezed out of disk. The water loss is 5–11%[160]
   a. Rapid creep occurs (1.5 mm in the first 2–10 minutes)[161] and then slows (to approximately 1 mm per hour).[150]
   b. The creep plateaus at 90 minutes.[162]
   c. Over a 16-hour day, a 10% loss in disk height occurs.
   d. A person's height is restored with unloading. The best unloading position is in the supine knees-up posture (better than the extended supine posture).[163]
2. The intradiskal pressure increases.

Breakdown of the System

Under normal circumstances, the NP acts like a sealed hydraulic system. Within this system, the fluid pressure rises substantially when volume is increased (by fluid injection or by imbibing[153]) and falls when volume is decreased (by surgical excision or axial compression loading).[155] By a similar mechanism, the age-related degenerative changes reduce the water content of the NP by 15–20%,[156] causing a 30% fall in the NP pressure.[164] In effect, the load is being transferred from the NP to the AF. The posterior AF is affected most, because it is the narrowest part of the disk and the least able to sustain large compressive strains.[157]

The end plate is also susceptible during compression, being able to withstand only approximately one-tenth of the stress that the AF can handle.[20] Even though axial loading occurs evenly over the surface of the end plate, failure of this structure typically occurs over the NP, indicating that this central part of the end plate is weaker than the periphery.[165]

Until approximately 40 years of age, as much as 55% of the compressive load through the centrum is borne by the cancellous bone,[166] the remainder being borne by the cortical bone. After this age, horizontal trabeculae are absorbed in the center of the vertebral body, thereby weakening the part of the centrum overlying the NP. This results in only approximately 35% of the axial stress being taken by the cancellous bone, with the greater proportion now going through cortical bone.[166] Because cortical bone fails with a smaller degree of deformation than cancellous bone, compressive failure occurs much more readily in the cortical bone.[166]

Pain originating from this failure would be expected to increase during the course of a day, especially in an individual who had spent a considerable amount of time with the lumbar spine flexed (e.g., a truck driver).[167]

CLINICAL PEARL

It is well known that during periods when the osmotic pressure within the IVD is greater than the hydrostatic pressure from axial loading (for example, when lying in bed) the disks imbibe fluid, causing the spine to increase in length.[156,168,169] Patients should thus be advised to avoid performing full-range spinal motions (bending) shortly after rising from bed.[156,168,169]

Other Structures

Although the IVD bears most of the compressive load of the spine in the neutral position and in the very early ranges of flexion and extension, the zygapophyseal joints bear up to 25% of the compressive load in the middle ranges of extension.[170] The contribution of the zygapophyseal joints becomes more significant during prolonged weight bearing, in the presence of IVD space narrowing, or if lumbar extension is combined with rotation.[170] In intradiscal pressure studies and electromyographic measurements of trunk muscles, in conjunction with mathematical models, investigators have estimated the compressive load on the lumbar spine to reach 1,000 N during standing and walking.[171] The compressive load on the lumbar spine is substantially higher in many lifting activities. Large extensor moments about the joints of the lumbar vertebral column are produced by the paravertebral musculature during lifting. These moments result in large compressive and shear forces acting between each pair of vertebrae, as high as several thousand newtons.[172,173] Conflicting evidence exists on what strategy is most effective in preventing back injury during lifting. Although lifting from a squat position with the lumbar spine maintained in lordosis is a commonly taught strategy, there is little evidence to support that this posture reduces compressive and shear forces acting on the spinal segments.[174] Existing evidence suggests that compressive and shear forces acting on the lumbar spine are most influenced by load moment, lifting speed, and acceleration.[175] A study by Kigma et al.[174] showed that the width of an object and the height from which an object is lifted are more important determinants of forces acting on the lumbar spine than the strategy used to perform the lift. The study further suggests that squatting may be an effective technique to reduce compressive forces acting at L5–S1 when lifting narrow loads, but straddling and stooping techniques are more effective at reducing compressive forces when lifting wider loads from the floor.[174]

In the sagittal plane, when a compressive load is applied to a whole lumbar spine specimen along a vertical path, bending moments are induced because of the inherent curvature of the lumbar spine. As a result, the spine undergoes large changes in its curvature at relatively small load levels. Countless studies over the years have demonstrated that a neutral spine under compressive load results in bony failure,[176] specifically end-plate fracture, and damage to the underlying trabeculae,[177] and that repeated loading reduces the ultimate strength of the end plate and can cause damage to other tissues.[178,179] A burst fracture is a vertebral fracture resulting from axial impact.[180]

Distraction

Symmetric distraction of the spine is a rare force in everyday functioning, and, consequently, the disk is less resistant to distraction than it is to compression.[181] Although asymmetric distraction occurs constantly with spinal movement (side bending of the spine causes ipsilateral compression and contralateral distraction), symmetric distraction, in which all points of the one vertebral body are moved an equal distance away from its adjacent body, occurs only at times such as vertical suspension or therapeutic traction.

The AF appears to bear the principal responsibility for restricting distraction, with the oblique orientation of the collagen fibers becoming more vertical as the traction force is applied. For this reason, back pain reproduced with traction may implicate the AF as the source.

Shear

Shear is the movement of one vertebral body across the surface of its neighbor. This movement can occur in any plane. Resistance to the shear forces is provided by a number of structures including the zygapophyseal joints, the AF fibers of the IVD, and the segmental ligaments.

In forward shearing, the AF fibers on the lateral aspects of the disk predominantly resist the movement, because they lie parallel to the movement.[182] Those angled posteriorly will be relaxed during forward shearing but tensed during backward shearing.[182] The anterior and posterior fibers will offer some contribution to anterior and posterior shearing, but this will be much less than that of the lateral fibers.[182]

The anterior and posterior fibers are primarily involved during lateral shearing, again with those orientated in the direction of the shear undergoing tension. As with torsion, only half of the fibers can contribute to the resistance and, as with torsion, shear forces are potentially very disruptive to the IVD.[182] It could be argued that the presence of free nerve endings in the outer part of the AF could indicate a nociceptive ability in the disk, and anything disturbing these endings may then be considered potentially painful, although there is no direct evidence to prove this.

Lumbar Stabilization

From the mechanical point of view, the spinal system is highly complex and statically highly indeterminate. The requirement for muscular control of the spine varies within the range of motion (ROM). The *neutral zone* is a term used by Panjabi[183] to define a region of laxity around the neutral resting position of a spinal segment. The neutral zone (see Chap. 22) is the position of the segment in which minimal loading is occurring in the passive structures (all of the noncontractile elements of the spine including the ligaments, fascia, joint capsules, IVDs, and noncontractile components of muscle), and the contribution of the active system (the muscles and tendons that surround and control spinal motion) is most critical—within its neutral zone of motion, the restraints and control for bending, rotation, and shear force are largely provided by the muscles that surround and act on the spinal segment.[184,185] The size of the neutral zone is determined by the integrity of the passive restraint and active control systems, which in turn are controlled by the neural system.[183] Studies have demonstrated that a larger than normal neutral zone caused by injury or microtrauma is related to a lack of segmental muscle control and is associated with intersegmental injury and IVD degeneration.[86,183,186–188] Unfortunately, there is as yet no *clinical* method to measure the size of the neutral zone.

The research of Gardner-Morse et al.[189] and O'Sullivan et al.[190] lends support to the hypothesis of a neutral zone. They proposed that the passive system alone is incapable of providing sufficient spinal stabilization during most activities and would buckle under its own weight without sufficient muscular tension.[80,90] In addition, activities such as acute repetitive loading have been shown to have a significant effect on reducing the stiffness of the passive system, because of the viscoelastic nature of the structures of the passive system (e.g., ligaments, and IVDs).[191,192] Thus, in addition to structural integrity, stabilization of the lumbar spine must also rely on muscular support. Muscle activity is available and required throughout the ROM, except in specific situations, such as at the end of lumbar flexion ROM when a reflex reduction in paraspinal muscle activity occurs, the so-called "flexion relaxation phenomenon."[120,185,193] At the end of spinal ROM, the restraints to bending, rotation and shear forces are provided largely by tension and compression on the spine's passive structures.[16] The concept of different trunk muscles playing differing roles in the provision of dynamic stability to the spine was proposed by Bergmark,[194] and later refined by others.[80,81,114,195–197] Bergmark classified the functional role of the muscles of the lumbar spine as either mobilizers or stabilizers.[196,197] Mobilizer muscles, which tend to work over two joints or several segments, are superficial, and have narrow insertions with long tendons.[197] The mobilizer muscles function to produce movement in the sagittal plane using concentric acceleration and are capable of generating a tremendous amount of force. The stabilizer muscles, as their name suggests, provide stabilization. Stabilizers can be further divided into global (spanning several segments) and local stabilizers (located at a single segment).[194]

Global Stabilizers

This system consists of muscles whose origins are on the pelvis and whose insertions are on the thoracic cage. These muscles include

- rectus abdominis;
- internal and external obliques;
- lateral fibers of the quadratus lumborum;
- thoracic part of the lumbar iliocostalis.

The global muscle system acts on the trunk and spine, without being directly attached to it. These muscles appear to provide general trunk stabilization by increasing the stiffness but are not capable of having a direct segmental influence on the spine. Cholewicki and McGill demonstrated that the quadratus lumborum was architecturally best suited to be the major stabilizer of the lumbar spine.[80] However, in general, the specific pattern of global muscle activity is task specific. Global stabilizers have a role in eccentrically decelerating momentum and controlling rotation of the spine as a whole.

Local Stabilizers

The local muscle system consists of a series of deep muscles that have insertions or origins at the lumbar vertebrae or pelvis and are responsible for providing segmental stability and directly controlling the lumbar segments and the sacroiliac joint (see Chap. 29). These muscles include

- lumbar portions of the iliocostalis and longissimus thoracis muscles;
- medial fibers of the quadratus lumborum;
- lumbar multifidus;
- TrA;
- posterior fibers of the internal oblique that attach to the tensor fascia latae.

CLINICAL PEARL

- **Transversus abdominis:** the deepest abdominal muscle, may have a presetting role, because it is the first trunk muscle to become active before movement initiation[115] or perturbation.[198] Together with the internal oblique, the TrA is primarily active in providing rotational and lateral control to the spine, while maintaining adequate levels of intra-abdominal pressure and imparting tension to the thoracolumbar fascia, thereby increasing the stiffness of the lumbar spine.[199] Hodges et al.[200] found that a coactivation of the diaphragm and abdominal muscles produces a sustained increase in intra-abdominal pressure. Activity of the diaphragm and TrA is initiated before rapid limb movements[201] and is tonic during repetitive movements of the arm[202,203] and walking.[204] In addition the TrA contributes to control of sacroiliac motion (see Chap. 29).
- The lumbar multifidus is considered to have the greatest potential to provide dynamic control to the motion segment, particularly in its neutral zone.[85,205] In a biomechanical study, Wilke et al. found that the lumbar multifidi are responsible for more than two-thirds of the stiffness at the L4–5 segmental level.[188]

The local muscle system is important for the provision of segmental control to the spine and provides an important stiffening effect on the lumbar spine, thereby enhancing its dynamic stability.[101] The local stabilizers also function to maintain a continuous low-force activity at joints in all positions and directions and thus provide segmental joint support.

CLINICAL PEARL

The lumbar multifidus, TrA, and the posterior fibers of the internal oblique are known to be tonically active during upright postures and active motions of the trunk,[206] with the TrA capable of tonic activity irrespective of trunk position, direction of movement, or loading of the spine.[199]

Two prominent and similar theories for active lumbar stabilization are the bracing mechanism, proposed by McGill,[207] and the deep corset mechanism, proposed by Richardson et al.[114]

- **Bracing mechanism:** muscles act similar to guy wires when stabilizing the spine and that a loss of tension can result in unstable buckling of the spinal structures. The muscles of the trunk function via a complex interaction of agonist/antagonist spinal muscles, both segmentally and regionally to provide tension (active stiffness). According to this theory lightly pretensioning, or bracing, the abdominal muscles using an isometric contraction is a way to enhance the guy wire affect by taking up the slack prior to activities that may destabilize the spine.[208] The external oblique, internal oblique, and TrA overlay each other to create the abdominal wall and act through attachments to the abdominal and thoracolumbar fascia to create a cylinder. As the intra-abdominal pressure increases, the three-dimensional force per unit area exerted on the spine also increases, potentially constraining spinal movement in all directions.
- **Deep corset mechanism:** Richardson et al.[114] have proposed that a pressure corset is formed by the muscles of the lumbar spine. Under this proposal, the TrA forms the wall of the cylinder and the muscles of the pelvic floor and diaphragm form the base and lid, respectively. Within this system, the intra-abdominal pressure group is maintained at a level that provides spinal support.[97,114,200,209] Since the abdominal cavity has a finite volume, the intra-abdominal pressure (force/area) will increase if the abdominal cavity volume is reduced (contraction of the muscles in the pelvic floor, abdominal muscles and diaphragm, and the wearing of a lumbar corset) In addition, the increase in intra-abdominal pressure is thought to provide a mild distractive force to the spinal segments, due to separation of the pelvic floor and diaphragm. Because intra-abdominal pressure and fascial tension are important for the control of intervertebral motion, the muscles that surround the abdominal cavity, such as the diaphragm and the pelvic floor muscles (see Chap. 29), provide an additional contribution. These two muscle groups also have important respiratory and continence functions. Theoretically, reduced contribution of the diaphragm to spinal stability may occur during periods of increased respiratory demand. As the diaphragm descends during inspiration, intra-abdominal pressure increases provided that the musculature of the abdominal and pelvic floor maintains its respective tension. Although current training programs for lifting focus on maintaining the load's proximity to the body's center of gravity (COG), minimizing trunk rotation, matching the load magnitude to the lifter's capacity, and avoiding fatigue, it remains unclear the role that breath control may play in achieving lumbar segmental control during lifting tasks.[210] An intriguing study by Hagins and Lamberg[210] reported that individuals with LBP performed a lifting task with more inhaled lung volume than individuals without LBP.

CLINICAL PEARL

Cholewicki and McGill[80] reported that lumbar stability is maintained in vivo by increasing the activity (stiffness) of the lumbar segmental muscles, and they highlighted the importance of motor control to coordinate muscle recruitment between large trunk muscles and small intrinsic muscles during functional activities, to ensure stability is maintained. These muscle activations are not restricted to the motion of the spine. For example studies of arm movement suggest that when the limb is moved, the nervous system does not simply stiffen the trunk; rather, the spine and pelvis are moved in the direction opposite to the perturbation.[211]

Lumbar instability is considered to be a significant factor in patients with chronic LBP.[212] Because of the close relationship between the passive anatomical restraints of the lumbar spine and the muscles that control it, it would seem logical to assume that any pain-provoking injury, or any condition that alters the structural integrity of the lumbopelvic complex (muscle strain, ligament sprain, disk herniation, etc.) is by definition a "clinical instability." Growing evidence is emerging to support this hypothesis.[213–215] Various studies have demonstrated that coordinated patterns of muscle recruitment are essential between the global and local system muscles of the trunk to compensate for the changing demands of daily life and to ensure that the dynamic stability of the spine is preserved.[80,185,216,217] In normal subjects with no history of LBP, the TrA, erector spinae, and obliquus internus abdominis are recruited just prior to any limb movement.[218] Several studies indicate that the deep abdominal muscles undergo changes in their functional performance in populations with LBP.[81,218,219] These studies have shown that it is the local system that is particularly vulnerable to breakdown. In particular, the prevalence of LBP is being attributed to inhibition and atrophy of the multifidi and transverse abdominis, and the resultant poor neutral zone stabilization, although the reasons as to why these two muscles become inhibited and atrophied is unclear.[81,116,216,220,221] Cholewicki and McGill[80] reported that the lumbar spine is more vulnerable to instability in its neutral positions, at low load and when the muscle forces are low. They confirmed that under these conditions, lumber stability is maintained in vivo by increasing the activity (stiffness) of the lumbar segmental muscles (local muscle system). Furthermore, they highlighted the importance of motor control to coordinate muscle recruitment between large trunk muscles (the global muscle system) and small intrinsic muscles (the local muscle system) during functional activities to ensure that mechanical stability is maintained.[185]

The scientific literature reports varying disruptions in patterns of recruitment and cocontraction within and between different muscles synergies.[185] Studies also have described subtle changes or shifts in the pattern of abdominal muscle activation and righting responses in subjects with chronic LBP.[84,222] These changes in the activation patterns result in altered patterns of synergistic control or coordination of the trunk muscles.[219,223] In addition to pain, generalized changes to the trunk musculature such as a loss of strength, endurance, and muscle atrophy are also believed to produce changes in the neural control system, affecting the timing of patterns of cocontraction.

CLINICAL PEARL

It is important to note that reports on the changes that occur in the control of trunk muscles in the presence of LBP vary considerably with an increase,[224] a decrease,[225] and no change[226] being reported. What is clear is that enormous variability is seen in the adaptation of the trunk muscles in people with lumbopelvic pain.

EXAMINATION

LBP can arise from a number of local structures in the lumbar spine and a number of sources more distal (see Chap. 5). A number of local structures have been found to cause LBP when stimulated. Theoretically any innervated structure in this area can cause symptoms so the distributions and descriptions of referred symptoms must always be considered in relation to the neurologic supply of the lumbar segment. For example, McCullogh and Waddell[227] studied the effects of electrical stimulation of spinal ligaments, muscles, the AF, and the NP and found that these structures referred pain to the buttock and upper leg, but rarely below the upper calf. The reported pain was dull and poorly localized. In contrast, stimulation of the nerve roots produced a sharper, more localized pain, often with some paresthesia. Stimulation of the L5 and S1 nerve roots nearly always radiated to or below the ankle.

Idiopathic and *nonspecific* LBP have emerged as catchall terms in the diagnosis of low-back dysfunction. Indeed, up to 85% of patients cannot be given a definitive diagnosis because of weak associations among symptoms, pathologic changes, and imaging results.[37,228] Muscle aches, muscle sprains, tendinitis, sacroiliac and low-back strain, lumbago, mechanical LBP, and lumbar strain are just some of the diagnoses currently in clinical use. This difficulty in determining a specific diagnosis stems from a variety of reasons, including the fact that multiple structures in one or more segments may be involved. These structures include the interconnecting ligaments, the outer fibers of the annulus fibrosus, zygapophyseal joints, vertebral periosteum, paravertebral musculature and fascia, blood vessels, and spinal nerve roots.[228]

A number of associated occupational, psychosocial, and environmental factors can be used to help predict the development of a complicated course of LBP.[229–235] These include the following:

- ***Genetics.*** A number of studies[236–238] have suggested that genetic factors play an important role in the development of lumbar disk degeneration, but their role in the cause of clinical LBP is unclear.
- ***Age older than 40 or 50 years.*** The relation between chronic LBP and age over 40 or 50 years, with a decrease of occurrence over 60 years, is considered as an established fact in many reviews.[239,240] The link between spinal degeneration and chronic LBP often has been assumed, because the severity of the radiographic abnormalities makes it logical to infer a cause-and-effect correlation.[241–243] Conditions such as osteoarthrosis, congenital anomalies, and postural misalignments have often been assumed to relate to LBP, but the evidence to support these assumptions (with the exception of some degenerative changes) has been inconclusive.[241–243] Indeed, given the low correlation of radiographic findings and clinical signs and symptoms, some physicians feel that radiographs are not necessary initially in the workup of acute nontraumatic LBP.[242]
- ***Low level of formal education and social class.*** For back pain, specifically, some studies have found an inverse relation of formal education, social class, or both to the prevalence of back pain symptoms.[244–246] A tentative conclusion, although not based on an extensive literature review, indicates that lower levels of socioeconomic status and education are better predictors of adverse prognosis for occupational disability from back pain than are risk factors per se.[247]
- ***Physical workload.*** From a number of studies that examined the relation between physical and psychosocial load at work and the occurrence of LBP, it has been concluded that both work-related physical factors of flexion and rotation of the trunk and lifting at work, and low job satisfaction, are risk factors for sickness absence resulting from LBP.[248,249] Physical load on the back has commonly been implicated as a risk factor for LBP and, in particular, for work-related LBP. Certain occupations and certain work tasks seem to have a higher risk of LBP.[250–253] Repeated lifting of heavy loads is considered a risk factor for LBP,[27] especially if combined with side bending and twisting.[254,255] A study of static work postures found that there was an increased risk of LBP if the work involved a predominance of sitting.[256] Kelsey[257] and Kelsey and Hardy[167] found that men who spend more than half their workday driving have a threefold increased risk of disk herniation. A growing body of evidence indicates that exposure to vibration and jolting in workers who operate tractors, excavators, bulldozers, forklift trucks, armored vehicles, lorries, helicopters, and many other vehicles and machines may cause an increased risk of LBP.[257–261]
- ***Sciatic pain.*** LBP radiating to a leg (i.e., sciatic pain) seems to be a more persistent and severe type of pain than nonspecific LBP. Sciatic pain also causes more disability and longer absence from work.[34] In patients with sciatic pain (sciatica) from disk herniation, radiographic examinations such as myelograms, computed tomographic (CT) scans, and magnetic resonance imaging (MRI) scans demonstrate nerve root compression by a herniated disk. However, sciatica can have a number of causes (Table 28-2).

CLINICAL PEARL

Approximately 20–30% of individuals without any history of sciatic pain have abnormal findings in radiographic examinations.[262]

TABLE 28-2 Some Causes of Sciatica
Nerve root compression
Tumor
Abscess
Arthritis
Vertebral collapse
Inflammatory synovitis
Inflammatory disease of nerve
Toxins (alcohol and heavy metals)
Diabetes mellitus
Syphilis

Data from Judge RD, Zuidema GD, Fitzgerald FT: Musculoskeletal system. In: Judge RD, Zuidema GD, Fitzgerald FT, eds. *Clinical Diagnosis*, 4th ed. Boston, MA: Little, Brown and Company, 1982:365–403

- ***Smoking.*** In some epidemiologic studies, smoking has been associated with LBP.[263,264] Several possible pathophysiologic mechanisms have been proposed to explain the association. It has been suggested that smoking accelerates degeneration by impairing the blood supply to the vertebral body and nutrition of the IVD.[265] Smoking also increases coughing activity, which causes an increase in intradiscal pressure.[266] Also, it has been hypothesized that the high serum proteolytic activity in the blood of cigarette smokers gains access to a previously degenerated neovascularized disk and accelerates the degenerative process. Increased proteolytic activity may also weaken the spinal ligaments, resulting in spinal instability.[267] However, besides its direct harmful effects, and its link to other health risk factors as well as lifestyle and behavioral patterns, no substantive evidence appears to support smoking as a definitive cause of LBP.[263]
- ***Obesity.*** There are several hypotheses relating to a link between obesity and LBP. Increased mechanical demands resulting from obesity have been suspected of causing LBP through excessive wear and tear,[151,152,268,269] and it has been suggested that metabolic factors associated with obesity may be detrimental.[268] An interesting study by Fransen et al.[270] reported that although obesity does not appear to be causative, it may have a meaningful impact on how long LBP persists.
- ***Psychological factors.*** It has been established that people who are simultaneously subjected to demanding physical and psychosocial conditions have more LBP than people with only demanding physical or only demanding psychosocial conditions.[271] Four explanations for the association between psychosocial work characteristics and musculoskeletal symptoms have been suggested[272] (1) psychosocial work characteristics can directly influence the biomechanical load through changes in posture, movement, and exerted forces; (2) these factors may trigger physiologic mechanisms, such as increased muscle tension or increased hormonal excretion, that may, in the long term, lead to organic changes and the development or intensification of musculoskeletal symptoms or may influence pain perception and thus increase symptoms; (3) psychosocial factors may change the ability of an individual to cope with an illness, which, in turn, could influence the reporting of musculoskeletal symptoms; and (4) the association may well be confounded by the effect of physical factors at work. It seems plausible that psychosocial factors in private life also could affect musculoskeletal symptoms through the second and third mechanism.[272] Studies have also found an effect of low workplace-social support and low job satisfaction. However, the effect found for low job satisfaction may be a result of insufficient adjustment for psychosocial work characteristics and physical load at work.[272] Although psychological factors, like obesity, appear to have a meaningful effect on the duration of LBP, they do not cause LBP.
- ***Comorbidity.*** Comorbidity may slow or interfere with normal recovery from back pain and may affect an individual's general sense of health, leading to a decreased self-perception of capability.[273]

A recent report issued by the Agency for Health Care Policy and Research,[274] now known as the Agency for Healthcare Research and Quality, suggests grouping back pain into five broad categories:[275]

- potentially serious spinal conditions such as spinal tumor, infection, fracture, and cauda equina syndrome. Although the likelihood of a low-back syndrome due to a serious condition is low, the consequences of a missed diagnosis or delayed treatment can be quite costly in terms of prolonged morbidity and, in the extreme, mortality.[275]
- nonspinal causes secondary to abdominal involvement (gallbladder, liver, renal, pelvic inflammatory disease, prostatic carcinoma, ovarian cyst, uterine fibroids, aortic aneurysm, or thoracic disease);
- sciatica and dural tissue compromise;
- nonspecific back symptoms, the majority of which are mechanical in nature;
- psychological causes such as stress and work environment (disability, workers' compensation, and secondary gain).

The physical examination of the lumbar spine must include a thorough assessment of the neuromuscular, vascular, and orthopaedic systems of the hip, lower extremities, low back, and pelvic region.[276] Figure 28-6 depicts a simple algorithm for decision making during the examination of the lumbar spine.

History

The clinician should establish the chief complaint of the patient, in addition to the location, behavior, irritability, and severity of the symptoms. Although dysfunctions of the lumbar spine are very difficult to diagnose, the history can provide some very important clues (Table 28-3). Applying the principles and rationale outlined in Chapters 4 and 5, the clinician uses the history to help with differential diagnosis. A useful organizational acronym for this purpose is LOP4QRST, which represents the following descriptors[275]:

- location;
- onset;
- prior history/treatment;

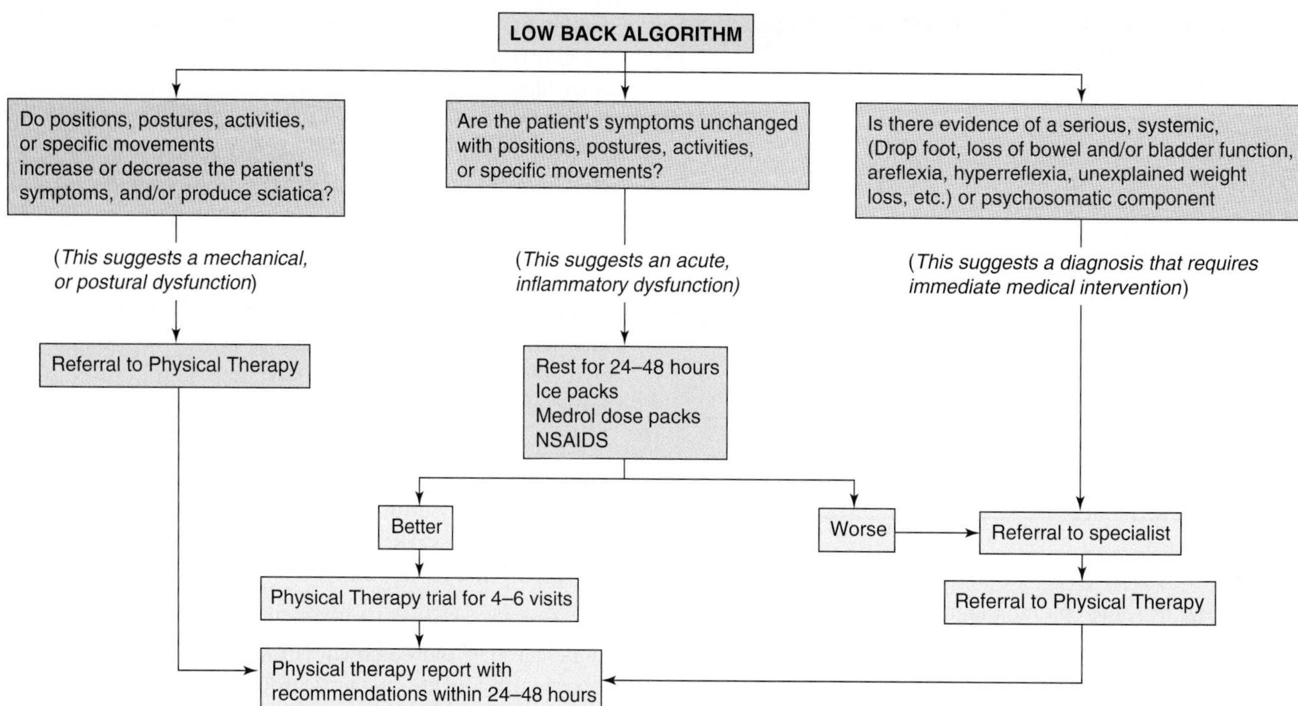

FIGURE 28-6 Examination algorithm for the low back.

- palliative measures (including medications);
- provocative factors (including movement/positional factors);
- progression/course;
- quality of symptoms;
- referral patterns;
- severity;
- temporal factors.

A lower back medical screening questionnaire is provided in Table 28-4.

- ***Location.*** Back pain may be localized centrally, unilaterally, or bilaterally. Generally speaking, the stronger the pain stimulus, the larger the area of pain reference will be. As the stimulus intensity decreases, the referred pain area becomes smaller, and localization of the pain by the patient becomes easier. The distribution of the pain should be described by the patient and outlined on a pain diagram. Central back pain is unlikely to be caused by a unilateral structure, such as a zygapophyseal joint or the sacroiliac joint, and bilateral pain hardly ever has a central origin (one of the exceptions being a central IVD protrusion).[277]
- An inflammation of the zygapophyseal joints can cause local back pain or buttock pain,[278] but it also has been associated with pain referred to the buttocks and even below the knee.[129,227,279]

CLINICAL PEARL

Various research studies have been undertaken to establish the validity of history taking for use in diagnosing a lumbar disk herniation.[228,280–282] Deyo et al.[228] reported a sensitivity for sciatic distribution of pain in the diagnosis of lumbar disk herniation of 95%, and calculated that the likelihood of a disk herniation being present in the absence of sciatic pain as 0.1%. Similarly high degrees of sensitivity have been found in other studies.[280–282] Radiculopathy is such a sensitive finding (95%) that its absence almost rules out a clinically important disk herniation, although it is only 88% specific for herniation.[283] In contrast, the sensitivity of pseudoclaudication in detecting spinal stenosis is 60%, whereas the combination of pseudoclaudication and age greater than 50 years has a sensitivity of 90% (specificity, 70%).[283] One study[284] showed that taking the history and MRI findings into account, elderly patients with protruded herniation were considered to be more likely to experience groin pain, with the rate of L4–5 disk involvement being higher than that of L5–S1 involvement. These results support conclusions drawn from a study by Murphey,[285] which found that groin and testicular pain are rare with L5–S1 disk disease but are fairly common with L4–5 disk disease.

- Groin pain, although also associated with hip pathology and other conditions, is a complaint often present in patients with a high lumbar IVD herniation.[284] On questioning, patients with this form of groin pain often describe the pain as a dull ache lying deep beneath the skin, which they usually find difficult to localize with any degree of accuracy. Although the patient with a high lumbar IVD herniation often reports pain and numbness on physical examination, the clinician is often unable to discern any specific findings, such as tenderness, muscle weakness, or hypesthesia, except perhaps occasionally a slight hyperalgesia.[284]
- Leg pain reported by the patient may indicate a radiculopathy or a pseudoradiculopathy. Conditions that

TABLE 28-3 Reliability of the Historical Examination[a]

Historical Question	Population	Kappa Value or % Agreement
Patient report of (McCombe et al.)[b]	Group 1:50 patients with low-back pain	Interexaminer reliability
Foot pain		κ = 0.12, 0.73
Leg pain		κ = 0.53, 0.96
Thigh pain	Group 2:33 patients with low-back pain	κ = 0.39, 0.78
Buttock pain		κ = 0.34, 0.44
Back pain		κ = 0.19, 0.16
Pain ever below the knee	475 patients with back pain	Test–retest among patient questionnaire
		Agreement 100%
Pain ever into the foot		Agreement 92%
Numbness below knee (Waddell et al.)[c]		Agreement 95%
Increased pain with (Roach et al.)[d]	53 subjects with a primary complaint of low-back pain	Test–retest among patient questionnaire
Sitting		κ = 0.46
Standing		κ = 0.70
Walking		κ = 0.67
Increased pain with (Vroomen et al.)[e]	A random selection of 91 patients with low-back pain	Interexaminer reliability
Sitting		κ = 0.49
Standing		κ = 1.0
Walking		κ = 0.56
Lying down		κ = 0.41
Pain with sitting (Van Dillen et al.)[f]	95 patients with low-back pain	Interexaminer reliability κ = 0.99, 1.0
Pain with bending (Van Dillen et al.)[f]		Interexaminer reliability κ = 0.98, 0.99
Pain with bending (Roach et al.)[d]	53 subjects with a primary complaint of low-back pain	Test–retest among patient questionnaire κ = 0.65
Pain with bending (McCombe et al.)[b]	Group 1: 50 patients with low-back pain Group 2: 33 patients with low-back pain	Interexaminer reliability κ = 0.51, 0.56
Increased pain with coughing/sneezing (Vroomen et al.)[e]	A random selection of 91 patients with low-back pain	Interexaminer reliability κ = 0.64
Increased pain with coughing (Roach et al.)[d]	53 subjects with a primary complaint of low-back pain	Test–retest among patient questionnaire κ = 0.75
Pain with pushing/lifting/carrying (Roach et al.)[d]		Test–retest among patient questionnaire κ = 0.77, 0.89
Sudden or gradual onset of pain[c]	475 patients with back pain	Test–retest among patient questionnaire Agreement = 79%

[a]Data from Cleland J: *Thoracolumbar Spine, Orthopaedic Clinical Examination: An Evidence-Based Approach for Physical Therapists*. Carlstadt, NJ: Icon Learning Systems, LLC, 2005:166–167.

[b]Data from McCombe PF, Fairbank JCT, Cockersole BC, et al: Reproducibility of physical signs in low back pain. *Spine* 14:908–918, 1989.

[c]Data from Waddell G, Main CJ, Morris EW, et al: Normality and reliability in the clinical assessment of backache. *BMJ* 284:1519–1523, 1982.

[d]Data from Roach KE, Brown MD, Dunigan KM, et al: Test–retest reliability of patient reports of low back pain. *J Orthop Sports Phys Ther* 26:253–259, 1997.

[e]Data from Vroomen PC, de Krom MC, Knottnerus JA: Consistency of history taking and physical examination in patients with suspected lumbar nerve root involvement. *Spine* 25:91–96; discussion 97, 2000.

[f]Data from Van Dillen LR, Sahrmann SA, Norton BJ, et al: Reliability of physical examination items used for classification of patients with low back pain. *Phys Ther* 78:979–988, 1998.

may result in radicular symptoms include inflammatory irritation due to tissue injury, disk herniation and subsequent nerve root irritation. In general, with a disk protrusion, the presence of leg pain indicates a larger protrusion than does back pain alone.[286] Coughing, sneezing, or a Valsalva maneuver typically exacerbates the symptoms. Other conditions capable of producing radicular-like symptoms include arthrosis involving the

TABLE 28-4 Medical Screening Questionnaire for the Low-Back Region

	Yes	No
Have you recently had a major trauma, such as a vehicle accident or a fall from a height?		
Have you ever had a medical practitioner tell you that you have osteoporosis?		
Do you have a history of cancer?		
Do you have pain at night that wakes you up?		
Does your pain ease when you rest in a comfortable position?		
Have you recently had a fever?		
Have you recently lost weight even though you have not been attempting to eat less or exercise more?		
Have you recently taken antibiotics or other medications for an infection?		
Have you been diagnosed as having an immunosuppressive disorder?		
Have you noticed a recent onset of difficulty with retaining your urine?		
Have you noticed a recent need to urinate more frequently?		
Have you noticed a recent onset of numbness in the area where you would sit on a bicycle seat?		
Have you recently noticed your legs becoming weak while walking or climbing stairs?		

Data from Bigos S, Bowyer O, Braen G, et al.: *Acute Low Back Problems in Adults,* AHCPR Publication 95–0642. Rockville, MD: Agency for Health Care Policy and Research, Public Health Service, U.S. Department of Health and Human Services, 1994; DuVall RE, Godges J: Introduction to physical therapy differential diagnosis: The clinical utility of subjective examination. In: Wilmarth MA, ed. *Medical Screening for the Physical Therapist. Orthopaedic Section Independent Study Course 14.1.1.* La Crosse, WI: Orthopaedic Section, APTA, Inc., 2003:1–44. Permission from Orthopaedic Section, APTA.

facet joints or vertebral body–disk interface, spinal hematoma, and congenital or acquired central or lateral canal stenosis.[275] A pseudoradiculopathy, as its name suggests, is pain that is radicular in distribution but is caused by something other than those conditions mentioned. Examples of a pseudoradiculopathy include referred pain and symptoms produced by a facilitated segment.[287] Despite the obvious differences in pathology, pseudoradiculopathy and radiculopathy have the common elements of dermatomal pain, diminished reflexes, muscle weakness, and positive nerve provocation tests.[129,287,288] Distinguishing between the two is, therefore, difficult. In general, unilateral pain with no referral below the knee may be caused by the lumbosacral structures other than the spinal nerves, whereas irritation of a spinal nerve may cause radicular symptoms below the knee.[289] On occasion, the patient may report feeling back pain more than leg pain or vice versa. Patients who report a dominance of leg pain over back pain and whose symptoms are worsened with flexion of the lumbar spine most likely have nerve root irritation caused by an IVD herniation.[289] The clinician should also ask the patient about any difficulty with coughing, sneezing, or abdominal straining (Dejerine's triad), each of which causes an increase in intrathecal pressure that may provoke radicular symptoms.[275] Patients with bilateral root pain should be suspected of having a central disk protrusion, spondylolisthesis, bilateral stenosis of the lateral spinal recesses, a narrowed spinal canal, or malignant disease.[290]

- ***Onset.*** When did the problem begin, how long has the patient had the problem, and have similar episodes occurred in the past? Low-back disorders may be acute, chronic, or recurrent. If possible, the clinician should attempt to order the onset of symptoms chronologically and then determine what has occurred to the symptoms since the onset. The mechanism of injury for the lumbar spine usually involves lifting, bending, or twisting, or a combination of all three.[257] However, postural ligamentous pain tends to be more frequent in patients who stand or sit for long periods at work.[291] If an obvious cause is reported, the clinician should confirm the direction, amount, and duration of any forces involved. The forces applied to the lumbar spine and IVD vary according to the task or position of the body (Table 28-5). In general, a sudden onset of pain associated with an activity or movement suggests a ligament, muscle, or IVD as the source, whereas a gradual onset of symptoms suggests a degenerative process or a lesion that is increasing in size, such as a neuroma or neoplasm.[290] While pain is suggestive of mechanical or chemical irritation, paresthesia, anesthesia, and weakness are attributed to decreased nerve or arterial function due to compression, constriction, or other blockage.[275]

The frequency of the episodes often can give the clinician an indication of severity. Stable episodes of symptoms (e.g., symptoms that only occur every few years and do not change much in severity with each episode) are generally easier to treat than episodes that occur daily or weekly and appear to be worsening.

TABLE 28-5 Intradiscal Pressures and Forces Generated by Common Tasks

Task	Total Load (kg)[a]
Lying supine	25
Side lying	75
Standing	150
Bending at waist in standing position	200
Sitting	175
Bending at waist in sitting position	225

[a]Represents total load on third lumbar disk in a 70-kg subject.
Data from Nachemson A: Disc pressure measurements. *Spine* 6:93–97, 1981; Nachemson A, Morris JM: In vivo measurements of intradiscal pressure. *J Bone Joint Surg* 46:1077, 1964; Nachemson A: Lumbar intradiscal pressure. In: Jayson MIV, ed. *The Lumbar Spine and Back Pain.* Edinburgh: Churchill Livingstone, 1987:191–203.

- ***Prior history/intervention.*** Patients should be asked if they have experienced similar complaints or problems in the past, even if the current complaint feels differently. If so, it is helpful to determine what intervention was provided, whether self-administered or by a health-care provider, over what length of time and if that treatment was effective.[275]
- ***Palliative measures.*** It is important to determine what attempts have been made to alleviate the symptoms and what effect, if any, was achieved. Depending on the nature of the pathology, certain body positions may bring relief, although it is important to remember that patients often present with symptoms more complex than classic textbook examples allow[275]:
  - Lying supine with knees flexed decreases pressure on the spinal column and tension of neural elements. Similar relief may be felt in the side-lying position; however, patients with a neurocompressive disk herniation may find this position unsustainable on one side and tolerable on the other side.
  - Standing or extension may be less provoking than seated or flexed positions in patients with disk pathology, whereas the opposite is typically true of patients with spinal stenosis. A classic example of positional relief involves the stenotic patient who leans on a shopping cart while walking to alleviate back and lower extremity symptoms.

Pathology of nonmechanical origin is usually nonresponsive to provocative movement and may be negatively responsive to positional changes, as in the case of sepsis within the abdominal cavity and neoplastic activity.[275,292]

- ***Provocative factors (Table 28-6).*** Information about the activities or positions that aggravate or relieve the symptoms provides the clinician with an insight as to whether the patient has a mechanically related disorder or one that is nonmechanical. In postural syndromes, the symptoms are usually increased by maintenance of a particular posture and relieved by altering the position. For example, if the patient complains of pain with standing with the feet together, the cause of the pain could be stresses on the structures caused by an increased lordosis, especially if the pain is reduced by placing one foot in front of the other, or if the pain is reduced when the lumbar lordosis is reduced with an active posterior pelvic tilt. Pain that is relieved by sitting and forward bending but aggravated by walking may indicate a zygapophyseal joint problem, spondylolisthesis (in the younger patient), or lateral recess or spinal stenosis (in the elderly patient). Pain that is aggravated by sitting, stooping, or lifting, but is relieved by recumbency and is not increased by brief periods of standing and walking may indicate an IVD lesion such as a protrusion or an annular tear.[293] In addition to those patients with an IVD protrusion, pain with coughing and sneezing also occurs in patients with active sacroiliitis, because the sudden increase in intra-abdominal pressure produces a painful distraction of the sacroiliac joints.[277] Once the motion or position that reduces the symptoms is identified, the initial focus of the intervention is teaching the patient strategies that encourage this motion or posture.

TABLE 28-6 Relieving Positions or Movements

Relieving Position or Movement	Probable Cause
Flexion	Facet joint involvement Low-back strain Lateral stenosis
Extension	Disk involvement Nerve root irritation (disk herniation)
Rest	Neurogenic claudication

- ***Progression and course of symptoms.*** Questions related to the type and behavior of symptoms can help determine the structure involved and the stage of healing. It is important to determine whether the condition is improving or worsening. Constant pain indicates an inflammatory process. Steadily increasing pain, especially in elderly patients, may indicate malignancy.[290] Pain that is gradually expanding and increasing is associated with a lesion that is increasing in size, such as a neuroma or neoplasm.[290] Pain with movement suggests a mechanical cause of pain. If the muscles and ligaments are involved, activity will tend to decrease the pain, but the pain will worsen with repeated movements or sustained positions as the structures become fatigued or overstressed.[286,294] Dural pain tends to be diffuse, vague, and spreads upward to the chest or downward to the thighs.[277]

Symptoms of lumbosacral pathology can demonstrate a phenomenon of centralization and peripheralization.[286,295,296] Centralization of symptoms is the progressive retreat of the most distal extent of referred or radicular pain toward the lumbar spine midline in response to standardize movement testing during evaluation of the effect of repeated movements on pain location and intensity. Peripheralization of symptoms indicates movement in the opposite direction. Centralization of the symptoms normally indicates improvement in the patient's diskogenic condition (see "Special Tests" section).[297]

- ***Quality of symptoms.*** Pain is the most common initial complaint involving the low back. Descriptors used by the patient to characterize his or her pain can provide valuable clues to the origin of the problem (Table 28-7).
- ***Radiation/referral of symptoms.*** LBP that emanates from the bony structures, soft tissues, or neural elements often demonstrates an associated pattern of referral or radiation.[275] At a given spinal level, the similar pain patterns of dermatomal, myotomal, and sclerotomal pain represent the distributions of a single nerve root. However, based on the pattern alone, it is difficult to determine the offending structure involved.[275] Radicular and dermatomal pain are often used interchangeably although their meanings are distinct:
  - Radicular pain refers to pain initiated by nerve root irritation and presents itself along the pathway of the root.

TABLE 28-7 Common Descriptors of Pain and Their Origin

Descriptor	Origin
Deep ache, and boring	Bony tissues
Dull, achy, sore, burning, and cramping	Muscle/fascia
Sharp, life like, shooting, lancinating, tingling, burning, numbness, and weakness	Nerve
Burning, stabbing, throbbing, tingling, and cold	Vascular
Deep pain, cramping, and stabbing	Visceral

- Dermatomal pain is defined as pain within the distribution of a single sensory nerve root that innervates the skin and presents itself at the surface.

Two additional definitions are pertinent. A myotome consists of groups of muscles supplied by a single spinal segment, whereas a sclerotome is an area of bone or fascia supplied by a single spinal segment.[275]

- ***Severity.*** The most frequently used tool to assess severity is a numerical rating scale, with 0 representing the absence of pain and either 10 or 100 representing the most extreme intensity of pain that the patient has experienced or can imagine. There are several other tools that provide quantification of the patient's symptoms to greater or lesser degree[275]:
- The visual analog scale is frequently used, particularly with new patients and during reexaminations. The scale consists of a 10-cm unmarked line, with indicators of "no pain" at the left end of the line and "extreme pain" at the right end of the line. Patients are asked to mark the line at the point corresponding to their pain level.
- Color charts are useful for young patients and patients who have difficulty communicating information due to language barriers. The colors extend from red to violet, with red representing extreme pain and violet representing the absence of pain.
- Verbal descriptors, such as minimal, slight, moderate, and severe, may also be used to categorize pain levels, although can be subject to misinterpretation. It is important to quantify a patient's pain intensity at its current level, when it is at its lowest and highest points, and an average estimate over a selected period of time, for example 1 week.[275] This information may then be used as outcome measures for subsequent treatment.
- ***Temporal factors—diurnal or nocturnal variation in symptoms.*** Determining the connection between time of day and onset of symptoms may help differentiate between mechanical and inflammatory disorders. For example, muscle strains may feel slightly sore in the morning on waking but typically result in greater intensity of pain at the end of the day following activity.[275] A patient with an inflammatory condition such as ankylosing spondylitis, an IVD lesion, osteoarthritis, ankylosing spondylitis, or Scheuermann's disease tend to experience the greatest symptoms in the morning, after the joints and surrounding tissues have had ample time to stiffen. In addition, patients with mechanically based pain often report an increase in symptoms during the evening hours, when their attention is not diverted by work or daily activities.[275] This may also be true when looking at pain patterns during the week when much activity occurs at home and work versus during the weekends when rest is more likely.[275] Night pain that wakes a patient may be an indicator of neoplastic activity or infection ("Red Flags") (Table 28-8) and should be addressed immediately. In contrast, a patient who awakens following movement, such as changing positions while sleeping, would be less of a risk for "Red Flags."[275] The same is true of the patient who has difficulty returning to sleep after getting up, for example, to visit the restroom.[275] Depending on the size of the patient, prone lying tends to compress the posterior structures and aggravate a zygapophyseal extension dysfunction. Persistent or progressive pain in supine lying may indicate a neurogenic or space-occupying lesion, such as an infection, swelling, or tumor. It may also indicate a zygapophyseal extension dysfunction, especially if the patient has marked adaptive shortening of the hip flexors and rectus femoris. For women, back pain may show a monthly periodicity related to the menstrual cycle.

TABLE 28-8 Red Flags for the Low-Back Region

Condition	Red Flags
Back-related tumor	Age over 50 yr History of cancer Unexplained weight loss Failure of conservative therapy
Back-related infection (spinal osteomyelitis)	Recent infection (e.g., urinary tract or skin infection) Intravenous drug user/abuser Concurrent immunosuppressive disorder
Cauda equina syndrome	Urine retention or incontinence Fecal incontinence Saddle anesthesia Global or progressive weakness in the lower extremities Sensory deficits in the feet (i.e., L4, L5, and S1 areas)

Data from: DuVall RE, Godges J: Introduction to physical therapy differential diagnosis: The clinical utility of subjective examination. In: Wilmarth MA, ed. *Medical Screening for the Physical Therapist. Orthopaedic Section Independent Study Course 14.1.1.* La Crosse, WI: Orthopaedic Section, APTA, Inc, 2003:1–44.

In addition to this list of basic questions, the clinician should also address the following areas:

- ***Patient's general health and past medical history.*** This component includes checking for a family history of rheumatoid arthritis, IVD lesions,[298] diabetes, osteoporosis, and vascular disease. When collecting information about the patient's health history, a useful acronym is "FAOMASHL": family health history, accidents, other associated/ unassociated complaints, medications, allergies, surgeries, hospitalizations, and lifestyle factors.[275] The clinician should solicit information from the patient regarding the presence or past existence of any major illnesses, including, but not limited to, diabetes, heart disease, cancer, and hypertension. Any allergies should be documented. The dates, provider contact information, and outcomes of hospitalizations and surgical procedures should be noted.[275] It is also vital, from a diagnostic as well as treatment viewpoint, to determine the patient's level of conditioning.

- ***Patient age.*** Spondylolisthesis is more common among 10–20-year olds.[290,299] Cancer, compression fractures (see Chap. 5), spinal and lateral recess stenosis, and aortic aneurysms are more common among patients older than 65 years of age.[300,301] Inflammatory spondyloarthropathy is most common in the 15–40-year-old age group,[228] and IVD lesions are more common in this group as well.[290] Osteoarthritis and spondylosis are more common in the 45 years and older age group.[290]
- ***Occupation.*** Information regarding the patient's job description should include the estimated level of activity, from sedentary to strenuous.[275] Also, elements such as lifestyle factors, hobbies, and exercise routines can provide useful information. Flexion and rotation of the trunk, lifting, axial loading, sustained flexed postures, vibration, and low job satisfaction are all considered as risk factors for back pain.[302–304] The level of impairment or disability that a lesion produces is related to the type of work performed. For example, diskodural back pain produces more disability in a truck driver who has to sit the whole day than in a patient who has light and varying work. For some patients, normal activities are unrestricted but their favorite sport is impossible.[290] The clinician should determine if there are any work stressors that may either physically or emotionally delay recovery or increase the likelihood of chronicity.[275] This necessitates a full understanding of the patient's job description and workplace environment. Depending on the circumstances, lifestyle factors may be a source of either physical or psychosocial irritation for the patient or can be used as a motivational force during treatment.[275] Additionally, the patient's participation in hobbies may be negatively impacted by back pain. Recovery and return to these activities can also be used as a motivational device.[275]
- ***Impact of symptoms.*** The effect the symptoms have on the patient's work, daily activities, and recreational pursuits can be assessed using the functional assessment tests outlined later. With this information, the clinician can set a baseline with which to measure progress that is meaningful to the patient. In addition, the clinician can determine whether the need for assistive devices is warranted.
- ***Medication use.*** Pain medications can mask symptoms. If the patient reports taking pain medication prior to the examination, the clinician may not obtain a true response to pain from the patient. It is important to ask the patient about dosage and frequency of the over-the-counter preparations, prescription medications, particularly corticosteroids and anticoagulants, vitamins, and herbal supplements.

CLINICAL PEARL

In general, pain that is worse in the lower extremity than in the low back indicates a nerve root irritation, whereas pain that is worse in the low back than in the lower extremity is probably referred from a spinal structure.[280]

- ***Psychosocial factors and nonorganic signs.*** During the initial history, it is important to document any psychosocial factors or nonorganic signs and symptoms, as these may directly affect the clinician's ability to accurately and completely diagnose the patient (see "Examination Conclusions" section). The patient's response to treatment and prognosis will be impacted as well.

Systems Review

It must always be kept in mind that pain can be referred to the lumbar spine area from pathologic conditions in other regions. For example, reports of pain in the upper lumbar region could suggest the possibility of aortic thrombosis, neoplasm, chronic appendicitis,[305] ankylosing spondylitis, or visceral disease (see Chap. 5) (Table 28-8).

The clinician should determine whether there has been any recent and unexplained weight loss, night pain that is unrelated to movement, or changes in bowel and bladder function.

Any one of these findings may indicate the presence of a serious pathology:

- Unexplained weight loss or night pain not associated with movement may indicate a malignancy. In many patients whose LBP is caused by infection or cancer, the pain is not relieved when the patient lies down.[306] However, this finding is not specific for the presence of these conditions.[228]
- Bowel or bladder dysfunction may be a symptom of severe compression of the cauda equina (cauda equina syndrome). This rare condition usually is caused by a tumor or a massive midline IVD herniation. Urinary retention with overflow incontinence is usually present, often in association with sensory loss in a saddle distribution, bilateral sciatica, and leg weakness.[228] This condition constitutes a medical emergency.
- Unexplained abdominal pain and backache. Fielding et al.[307] in a review of 528 cases with abdominal aortic aneurysms reported that 91% had symptoms at their first presentation, with abdominal pain and backache being most common symptoms. In the same study, it was found that the diagnosis can be made by careful routine palpation deep and left to the midline keeping the hands steady in one position until the aortic pulse is felt, and then carefully evaluating the lateral extent of the pulse with the pads of the fingers.[308]

CLINICAL PEARL

An intriguing study by Roche et al.[309] that examined the sensitivity and specificity of historical questions to identify patients with serious pathology in the lumbar spine found the following questions to have the best positive likelihood ratios:

- inability to urinate or to hold urine;
- sleep disturbances;
- current smoking history.

It is important to note that although these questions were found to have very high specificity, they also had a very low true positive rate indicating that many of the patients with serious pathology did not answer "yes" to the historical questions. To improve sensitivity, while attempting to maintain moderate specificity in this study, a number of symptoms were considered in parallel. The highest combination of sensitivity (0.87) and specificity (0.50) was obtained by combining in parallel the symptoms of unable to sleep, awakened and unable to fall back to sleep, medication required to sleep, and pain worsened by walking.

Tests and Measures

Observation

Observation involves an analysis of the entire patient in terms of how he or she moves and responds, in addition to the positions the patient adopts. Whether the clinician chooses to greet patients personally in the waiting room or in the examination room, the examination should begin with the initial contact.[275] The patient's gait pattern and any antalgia can provide some important clues. Upper lumbar or thoracolumbar instability or hypermobility often can lead to facilitation of the upper lumbar segments, with resulting psoas hypertonicity.[287,310] This may lead to reduced hip extension during gait, resulting in a shortened stride length on the involved side.[95] Body weight and ground reaction forces, generated by rapid walking, can equalize the stride length by hypermobilizing or destabilizing the lumbosacral junction or the ipsilateral sacroiliac joint.[95] The process is reinforced by the mechanical pull of the shortened iliopsoas, and this increases the stress on the upper lumbar spine, increasing the facilitation.

CLINICAL PEARL

Muscle weakness and reduced walking capacity are among several functional deficits associated with a lumbar herniated NP.[311,312] Weakness of the gastrocnemius is a clinical sign associated with involvement of the L5–S1 disk (neurologic level S1), whereas weakness of the extensor hallucis longus is a positive sign for involvement of the L4–5 disk (neurologic L5).

Once in the examination room, the patient should be gowned appropriately to allow complete inspection of the lumbar spine and lower extremities. Although spinal alignment provides some valuable information, a positive correlation has not been made between abnormal alignment and pain.[255,313] "Good posture" is a subjective term based on what the clinician believes to be correct, and it is highly variable (see Chap. 6).

Posterior Aspect. The shoulders and pelvis should appear fairly level, and the bony and soft tissue contours should appear symmetric. A horizontal line through the highest points of the iliac crests passes also through the spinous process of the fourth lumbar vertebra. The transtubercular plane to the tubercles on the iliac crest cuts the body of the fifth lumbar vertebra, and the upper margin of the greater sciatic notch is opposite spinous process of the first sacral vertebra. There should be no differences in the muscle bulk between both sides and regions of the erector spinae. Atrophy of the paraspinals is rare but may indicate a chronic inflammatory disease, such as ankylosing spondylitis or tuberculosis, or point to poliomyelitis or a myopathy.[277] If atrophy of the paravertebral or extremity muscles is present, the clinician must determine whether it follows a segmental or nonsegmental pattern. A predominance of the thoracolumbar portion of the erector spinae may indicate poor stabilization of this area,[134] or a rotational asymmetry.[314] Asymmetric spasm of the paraspinals or gluteal muscles can make them appear more prominent compared with the normal side. The presence of spasm should alert the clinician to the presence of sciatica or a serious disease.[277]

The inferior angles of the scapulae should be level with the seventh thoracic spinous process; the iliac crests should be level.[315] The PSISs, medial malleoli, and lateral malleoli should all be level with their counterparts on the opposite side. Differences between the two sides may indicate a functional limb-length discrepancy (see Chap. 29). This discrepancy can be caused by altered bone length, altered mechanics, or joint dysfunction[316] (Table 28-9).

The thoracic and lumbar vertebrae should be vertically aligned. Curvature of the spine is referred to as *scoliosis* (see Chap. 6).

Deformity, birthmarks, and hairy patches are all evidence of congenital deficits of the integumentary system and can indicate underlying anomalies in the systems derived from the same embryologic segments.[317] A hairy patch or tuft that is located at the base of the lumbar spine may indicate spina bifida occulta or diastematomyelia.[318]

Lateral Pelvic Shift. Structural asymmetry in the lumbar region often is associated with pain. For example, patients with

TABLE 28-9 Causes of Functional Limb-Length Difference

Joint	Apparent Lengthening	Apparent Shortening
Sacroiliac	Anterior rotation	Posterior rotation
Hip	Lowering Extension External rotation	Hiking Flexion Internal rotation
Knee	—	Flexion Valgus Varus
Foot	Supination	Pronation

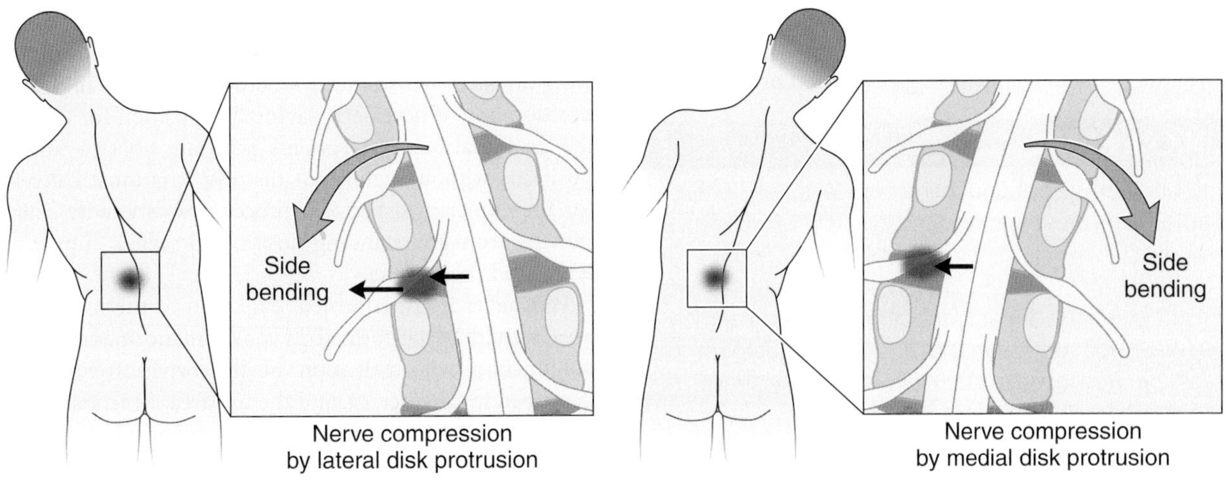

FIGURE 28-7 Direction of the lateral list in relation to disk herniation.

disk-related LBP commonly present with a pelvic shift or list when acute sciatica is present. In these cases, the patient may list away from the side of the sciatica, producing a so-called sciatic scoliosis.[319] The lateral pelvic shift is perhaps the most commonly encountered. Under the McKenzie classification system (see Chap. 22), a derangement requires the presence of a relevant lateral shift deformity.[286] Determining the presence of a lateral shift deformity may help speed up the recovery from a derangement by first correcting the lateral shift deformity.[286] The direction of the list, although still controversial, is believed to result from the relative position of the disk herniation to the spinal nerve (Fig. 28-7). Theoretically, when the disk herniation is lateral to the nerve root, the patient may deviate the back away from the side of the irritated nerve, which has the effect of drawing the nerve root away from the disk fragment (Fig. 28-7). This movement is demonstrated dramatically in patients with extreme lateral disk herniations, whose efforts at side bending to the side of the herniation markedly exaggerate the pain and paresthesia.[320] When the herniation is medial to the nerve root, the patient may list toward the side of the lesion, in an effort to decompress the nerve root[321] (Fig. 28-7). It is also theorized that this is a protective position resulting from

- irritation of a zygapophyseal joint;
- irritation of a spinal nerve or its dural sleeve, caused by disk herniation[262] and the resulting muscle spasm[322];
- spasm of the quadratus lumborum muscle and, occasionally, the iliacus muscle;
- the size of the disk protrusion. In a prospective study of 45 patients with a sciatic scoliotic list (Cobb's angle >4 degrees), Suk et al.[320] found that the direction of sciatic scoliosis was not observed during surgery to be associated with the location of nerve root compression, but rather it was related to the side of disk herniation. Porter and Miller[323] analyzed the mechanism of sciatic scoliosis and concluded that the herniated disk was thought to be reduced in size by stretching or inward bulging at the convex side of the scoliosis, and called this phenomenon autonomic decompression.[323]

The clinician must first determine the presence of the shift and then determine its relevance to the presenting symptoms. To determine its relevance, a side-glide test sequence can be used. The side-glide test sequence is performed by manually correcting the shift by pushing the pelvis into its correct position[286] (Fig. 28-8). **VIDEO** If the side-glide produces either a centralization or peripheralization of the patient's symptoms, the test is considered positive for a relevant lateral shift.[324] In addition, for a lateral shift to be significant, the patient must exhibit an inability to self-correct past midline when asked to shift in the direction opposite the shift.[325] The relevant lateral shift must be corrected, using side-glides, before the patient attempts the McKenzie extension

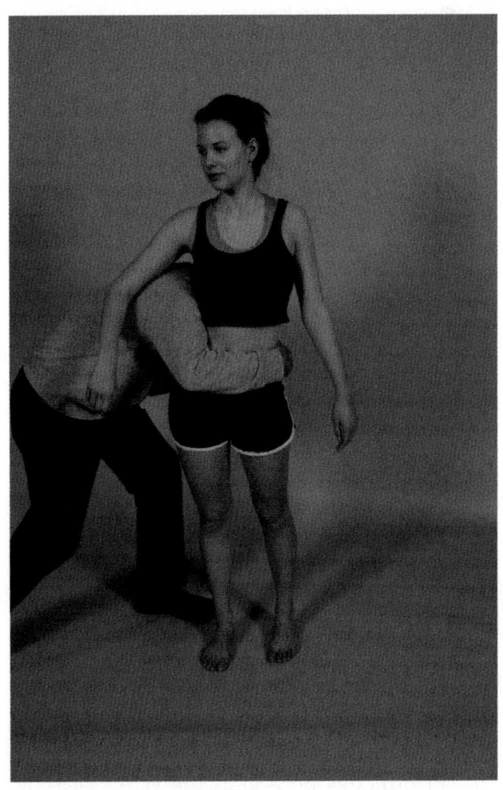

FIGURE 28-8 Side-glide test.

exercises.[326] A lateral shift that is not deemed to be relevant or to be a deformity, per McKenzie's criteria, may be treated with only sagittal plane movements (e.g., extension principles).[286]

CLINICAL PEARL

Riddle and Rothstein found that therapists agreed 60% of the time on the presence and direction of the lateral shift. A κ value of 0.26 was determined, indicating poor reliability.[327] A similar study by Donahue et al. of 49 patients with LBP examined the amount of intertester agreement when assessing only the lateral shift. The amount of agreement was found to be 47%, statistically similar to that obtained by pure chance.[325]

Lateral Aspect

From the side, the clinician should observe that the ear lobe should be in line with the tip of the shoulder, and the peak of the iliac crest. The amount of lumbar lordosis is noted as to whether it is excessive or reduced. The lumbar lordosis should appear as a smooth and gentle curve, and there should be a gradual transition at the thoracolumbar junction.

- An excessive lordosis may result in the pelvic crossed syndrome.[134] In this syndrome, the erector spinae and the iliopsoas are found to be adaptively shortened, and the abdominal and gluteus maximus muscles are found to be weak. As a result, this syndrome can produce adaptive shortening of the PLL, lower back extensors, and hip flexor muscles and lengthening of the ALL and lower abdominals. An excessive lordosis may also indicate that the patient has a spondylolisthesis. With this condition, the whole spine often lies in a plane anterior to the sacrum. There may also be an associated mid or low lumbar shelf at the spinous processes, which, if not visible, can be palpated. An anterior pelvic tilt posture may also be caused by weakness of the abdominal muscles or an adaptively shortened iliopsoas or thoracolumbar fascia, with subsequent lengthening of the hamstring and gluteal muscles.[134]
- A flattened back may indicate that the patient has either a lumbar spinal stenosis or a lateral recessed stenosis. A flattened lordosis is caused by a posterior pelvic tilt, adaptive shortening of the hamstrings, and weakness of the hip flexor muscles.[134]
- A reversed lordosis, often referred to as a *sway back*, is caused by a thoracic kyphosis and a posterior pelvic tilt. This posture results in a stretching of the anterior hip ligaments, back extensors, and hip flexors; hip hyperextension; and compression of the vertebrae posteriorly.[134] Kyphosis of the lumbar spine may also indicate damage to the SSL complex.

The type of footwear that the patient habitually wears can be a factor. For example, high-heeled footwear has a tendency to modify the pelvic angle and increase the lordosis.[328]

Palpation

There is some disagreement as to when in the examination the palpation assessment should occur, with some authors preferring to perform this portion at the end.[329] The order of examination procedures should reflect awareness of the patient's potential discomfort and proceed from least to most invasive.[275] For instance, a patient who reports difficulty when lying on his or her stomach should be examined in the prone position only if necessary, saving this position for the end of the examination. For patients who are able to attain all positions without significant distress, it is most convenient for the clinician to perform procedures as gravity suggests, moving from the standing position to seated, supine, side-lying, and then prone.[275]

Whenever it is performed, palpation of the lumbar spine area should be performed in a systematic manner, and in conjunction with palpation of the pelvic area, which is described in Chapter 29, and the hip area, which is described in Chapter 19. Palpation of the lumbar region is best performed with the patient in a prone position but may also be performed on a seated patient. The examiner should begin by assessing the soft tissues for an increase in focal temperature.[275]

CLINICAL PEARL

A study by Deyo et al.[228] found that palpation of soft tissue and bony tenderness had both poor reproducibility and specificity.

As previously mentioned, in most individuals, the midpoint of an imaginary line drawn between the iliac crests represents the L4–5 interspace and the level of the L4 transverse process. The transverse processes of L3, L2, and L1 each lie two fingerbreadths superior to the vertebra, respectively.[330] Alternatively, they can be found at the level of the lower pole of the spinous process of the vertebra immediately above or below. The lumbar zygapophyseal joints of each motion segment are located approximately 2–3 cm (0.8–1.2 inches) lateral from the spinous processes. The reference point indicating the position of L4 is marked on the patient. The spinous process of L5 is just inferior to this point. The L5 spinous process is short, sharp, and thick compared with those of L4 and L3. The clinician should move superiorly from the L5 spinous process, carefully palpating each segmental level. Evidence of tenderness, altered temperature, muscle spasm, or abnormal alignment during palpation can highlight an underlying impairment.

Posterior Aspect. Palpation of the posterior aspect of the lumbar spine is best achieved by placing the patient in a relaxed prone position, or bent over the treatment table.

- The clinician moves the index and middle fingers quickly down the spine, feeling for any abnormal projections or asymmetries of the spinous processes. Any alterations in the alignment of the spinous processes in a posteroanterior (P-A) direction, particularly at the L4–5 or L5–S1 segmental level, may indicate the presence of a spondylolisthesis.[331] Specific pain elicited with P-A pressure over the segment serves as further confirmation. Asymmetry of the spinous processes in a P-A direction may also indicate wedging of a vertebral body or a complete loss of two adjacent IVD spaces.[277] Absence of a spinous process may be associated with spina bifida. Side-to-side alterations in the spinous process may indicate the presence of a rotational asymmetry of the vertebra.[314]

- The SSLs should be palpated. The ligament is usually supple, springy, and nontender. Because this ligament is the most superficial of the spinal ligaments and farthest from the axis of flexion, it has a greater potential for sprains.[72]
- Palpation of the transverse processes of T12 and L5 presents difficulties. That of L3 is easy to feel, being usually the longest of all transverse processes; it is usually possible to feel those of L1, L2, and L4. That of L5 is covered by the posterior ilium.[332]
- Patients with localized tenderness over the zygapophyseal joints without other root tension signs or neurologic signs may have zygapophyseal joint pain.[333] This source can be confirmed if the patient responds well to intra-articular joint injections or to blocks of the medial branches of the posterior (dorsal) rami.[333,334]
- A well-localized and tender point at the gluteal level of the iliac crest, 8–10 cm from the midline, may indicate the presence of Maigne's syndrome.[322] Maigne's syndrome is characterized by sacroiliac joint, low lumbar, and gluteal pain, with occasional referral to the thigh, laterally or posteriorly.
- Normally, the skin can be rolled over the spine and gluteal region with ease. Tightness or pain produced with skin rolling may indicate some underlying pathology.[335] The source of the signs and symptoms is an irritation of the medial cutaneous branch of posterior (dorsal) rami of the T12 or L1 spinal nerves, as it passes through a fibro-osseous tunnel at the iliac crest.[322]

Anterior Aspect.

- The inguinal area, located between the ASIS and the symphysis pubis, should be palpated carefully for evidence of tenderness, which may be indicative of a hernia, an abscess, sprain of the ligament, or an infection, if the lymph nodes are swollen and tender.
- In some patients, the anterior aspect of the vertebral bodies may be palpable when the patient is positioned supine with the hips flexed and feet flat on the bed. Tenderness of the anterior aspect of the vertebral bodies may indicate an irritation of the ALL, which may indicate the presence of an anterior instability.[13]

CLINICAL PEARL

Evaluation of the abdominal, inguinal, popliteal arteries, and distal pedal pulses is dependent on the patient's profile and presentation.[275] As a general rule, the abdominal aorta should be assessed for possible enlargement via auscultation and palpation in any patient over the age of 50 with acute onset of LBP.[275]

Active Range of Motion

Normal active motion, which demonstrates considerable variability (Table 28-10) between individuals, involves fully functional contractile and inert tissues and optimal neurologic function.[147,336–339] It is important to note that ROM may be affected by age and sex, whereas occupation and body mass index have little or no influence on motion.[340] In addition it has also been determined that total sagittal ROM, flexion angle, and extension angle decline as age increases.[341] However, it is the quality of motion and the symptoms provoked, rather than the quantity of motion, that are more important. The reproducibility (precision) of an individual's effort is one indicator of optimum effort. Measurements should not change significantly (<5 degrees) with repeated efforts.[342] The capsular pattern for the lumbar spine is normal trunk flexion, a decrease in lumbar extension with rotation, and side bending equally limited bilaterally.[343]

TABLE 28-10 Normal Active ROM of the Lumbar Spine

Movement	Range (Degrees)
Flexion	50–70
Extension	10–30
Side bending	25–35
Axial rotation	20–40

Data from: Ng JK, Kippers V, Richardson CA, et al: Range of motion and lordosis of the lumbar spine: Reliability of measurement and normative values. *Spine* 26:53–60, 2001.

A good view of the spine is essential during motion testing. External measurement of vertebral motion may not reflect the true intervertebral movement because of skin movement error,[344] but it is less invasive than a radiograph and more practical. Although limited spinal motion is not strongly associated with any specific diagnosis, this finding may help in the planning or monitoring of the physical therapy intervention.[228]

CLINICAL PEARL

Among the spinal motion tests, rotation, side bending, and fingertip-to-floor distance show the strongest associations with the severity of back pain.[344]

While standing, the patient performs flexion, extension, and side bending to both sides (Fig. 28-9A–D). If full active ROM is attained without the production of symptoms, combined motions are introduced (see the next section). If these motions fail to reproduce the symptoms, the clinician need not assess passive motions. However, resisted motions may produce further clinical findings.[275] Pain induced by active ROM may implicate a number of tissues including muscle and tendon, ligament and capsule, and bone and nerve. The key to deciphering which offending structure is involved lies in determining the type of pain produced and whether active, passive, and/or resisted motions are provoking. Injuries involving noncontractile tissues such as ligaments, facet capsules, and IVDs are provoked by loading the structure actively or passively, whereas resisted isometric muscle contraction is typically unprovoking, unless, in the case of disk herniation, "abdominal canister" (i.e., transversus, obliques, rectus, multifidi, pelvic floor, and diaphragm) contraction increases intrathecal pressure.[275]

The active ROM tests should be observed in front of and behind the patient. At the end of each of the active motions,

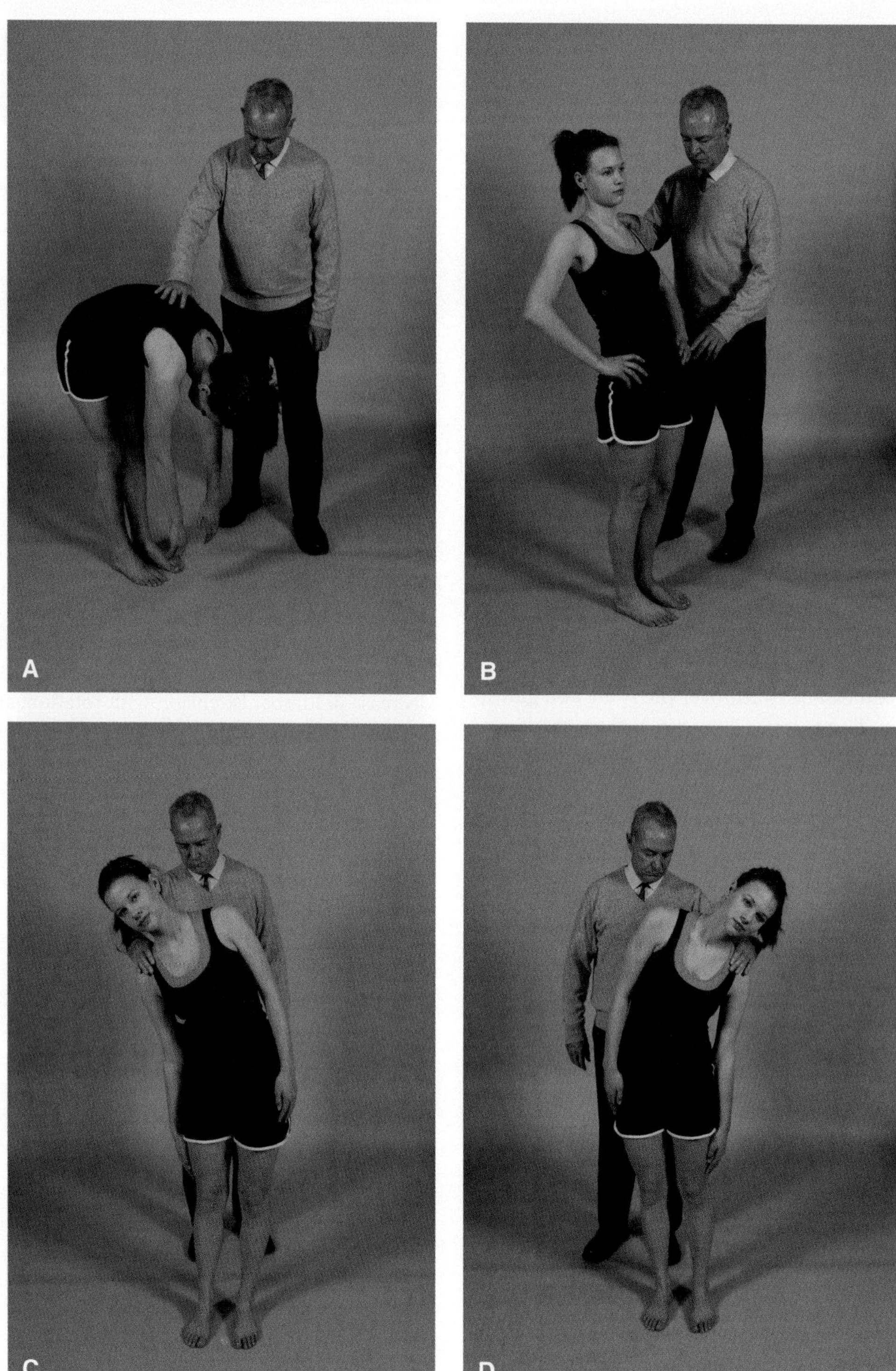

FIGURE 28-9 Active ROM of the lumbar spine with overpressure. (**A**) Flexion. (**B**) Extension. (**C**) Side bending right. (**D**) Side bending left.

passive overpressure is applied to assess the end-feel, and resistance tests are performed with the muscles in the lengthened positions.

The clinician should consider having the patient remain at the end range of each of the motion tests for 10–20 seconds, if sustained positions were reported to increase the symptoms. If repetitive or combined motions were reported in the history to increase the symptoms, the patient is asked to perform repeated motions. McKenzie[286] advocates the use of sustained or repeated movements of the spine in an attempt to affect the nuclear position. These movements are performed either to peripheralize the symptoms lateral from the midline or distally down the extremity or ideally to centralize the symptoms to a point more central or near midline. One study of 87 patients with leg and LBP[295] found that those patients who demonstrated excellent outcomes with the McKenzie-based interventions had reported centralization during the initial examination. Another study[296] found a significant correlation between positive diskograms and peripheralization and centralization, with the incidence of an adequate annulus being significantly greater in the centralizing patients with positive diskograms than in their peripheralizing counterparts.

During the active motions, the clinician notes the following:

- ***Curve of the spine.*** The curve of the spine in flexion, extension, and side bending should be smooth. An angulation occurring during flexion or extension could indicate an area of instability or hypomobility. In side bending, an angulation indicates hypomobility below the level or hypermobility above the level in the lumbar spine.[335]
- ***Presence of any deviations during or at the end of range.*** Failure to recover from flexion smoothly may indicate instability.[345] This typically occurs at the endpoint of flexion, as the patient begins to return to the erect stance and has to extend the lumbar spine by walking the hands up the thighs or by using a series of jerking motions. Trunk deviation during flexion is believed to be associated with a disk herniation, with the direction of the deviation being determined by the relative position of the compression on the nerve. How the disk responds to movements depends on the activity. For example, walking appears to move the NP into a more central location, whereas prolonged sitting appears to displace the disk into a less advantageous position.[346]
- ***Provocation of symptoms.*** The clinician should determine whether the symptoms are neurologic or nonneurologic, and how far the distribution of pain extends. Leg pain provoked by any motion other than flexion is not a good prognostic sign[343]; neither is posterior leg pain, reproduced with extension, rotation, or side bending, as this usually indicates a significant prolapse or extrusion.
- ***Any gross limitations of motion.*** Gross limitation of both side bends may indicate ankylosing spondylitis or significant osteoarthritis.
- ***Any dysfunctional movement patterns.*** This involves an assessment of the typical pattern and muscle activation strategies. Active spinal movement, commonly reveals good ranges of spinal mobility but with aberrant quality of motion commonly associated with a sudden acceleration, hesitation, or lateral movement within the midrange of spinal motion.[185] Both O'Sullivan[13] and Sahrmann[347] have devised classification schemes to categorize movement patterns:

O'Sullivan classifies instabilities according to directional patterns of clinical instability, although he admits that these classifications have not been scientifically validated.[13]

- ***Flexion pattern.*** The flexion pattern is the most common. It is characterized by complaints of central back pain that is aggravated during flexion–rotational movements, and an inability to sustain semiflexed positions. On observation, there is often a loss of segmental lordosis at the level of the "unstable" motion segment, which is more noticeable in standing. This loss of lordosis is increased in flexed positions. Movements into forward flexion are associated with a tendency to flex more at the symptomatic level than at adjacent levels and, usually, are associated with an arc of pain into flexion and an inability to return from flexion to neutral without use of the hands to assist in the movement. During backward bending, extension above the symptomatic segment, with an associated loss of extension at the involved segment, often is observed. Functional activities, such as squatting, sitting with knee extension or hip flexion, and sit to stand, reveal an inability to control a neutral lordosis and a preponderance to segmentally flex at the unstable motion segment. Specific muscle tests reveal an inability to perform the abdominal hollowing maneuver (see "Clinical Instability of the Lumbar Spine" section) at the unstable motion segment. The patient may also be unable to actively produce a neutral lordotic lumbar spine posture.
- ***Extension pattern.*** The extension pattern is characterized by complaints of central back pain that is aggravated during extension–rotational movements, and an inability to sustain positions such as standing, overhead activities, fast walking, running, and swimming. On observation, there is often an increase in segmental lordosis at the level of the "unstable" motion segment in standing, which is often associated with an increase in segmental muscle activity at this level. Extension activities reveal segmental hinging at the involved segment, with a loss of segmental lordosis above this level and an associated postural sway. Forward bending movements often reveal a tendency to hold the lumbar spine in lordosis, with a sudden loss of the lordosis midway through the flexion range and an arc of pain. On returning from the flexed position, there is often a tendency to hyperextend the lumbar spine segmentally before the upright posture is achieved, with pain on returning to the upright position. Specific muscle testing reveals an inability to perform the abdominal hollowing maneuver. The patient also is often unable to initiate a posterior pelvic tilt independent of hip flexion and activation of the gluteals, rectus abdominis, and external obliques.
- ***Recurrent lateral shift pattern.*** The lateral shift is usually unidirectional, occurs recurrently, and is associated with unilateral LBP. The patient typically stands with a loss of lumbar segmental lordosis at the involved level and an associated lateral shift at the same level. The lateral shift is accentuated when standing on the foot ipsilateral to the shift and is observed during gait as a tendency to transfer weight through the trunk and upper body rather than through the pelvis. Sagittal spinal movements reveal a shift further laterally at midrange flexion, which is commonly associated with an arc of pain. Sit to stand and squatting are associated with a tendency toward lateral trunk shift during the movement, with increased weight bearing on the lower limb ipsilateral to the shift. Specific muscle testing reveals an inability to perform the trunk raise, with dominance of activation of the quadratus lumborum, lumbar erector spinae, and superficial multifidus on the side ipsilateral to the shift and an inability to activate the segmental multifidus on the contralateral side to the lateral shift.
- ***Multidirectional pattern.*** This pattern is the most serious and debilitating of the patterns and is frequently characterized by high levels of pain and functional disability. All weight-bearing positions are normally painful, and locking of the spine occurs frequently with positions of sustained flexion, rotation, and extension. These patients exhibit great difficulty in assuming neutral lordotic spinal

positions, and an inability to perform the abdominal hollowing maneuver.

Sahrmann categorizes a number of movement impairment syndromes that can present in the lumbar spine as a result of an imbalance of flexibility and strength. The intervention for each of the syndromes involves a correction of these imbalances.

- ***Flexion syndrome.*** This syndrome is characterized by lumbar flexion motions that are more flexible than hip flexion motions. The syndrome is typically found in the 8–45-year-old age range and results in pain with positions or motions associated with lumbar flexion, because of adaptive shortening of the gluteus maximus, hamstrings, or rectus abdominis.
- ***Extension syndrome.*** This syndrome is characterized by lumbar extension motions that are more flexible than hip extension motions. Patients with this syndrome are usually older than 55 years of age, and the symptoms are increased with positions or motions associated with an increase in lumbar lordosis, because of adaptive shortening of the hip flexors and lumbar paraspinals and weakness of the external oblique muscles.
- ***Lumbar rotation.*** This syndrome is characterized by pain that is unilateral or greater on one side and is increased with rotation to one side. No attempt is made to equate the side of rotation with the side of the symptoms. It is theorized that this syndrome is produced when one segment of the lumbar spine rotates, side bends, glides, or translates more easily than the segment above or below it. This syndrome is associated with spinal instability and can result from habitual motions or positions that involve rotation to one side, a leg-length discrepancy (see Chap. 29), or a muscle imbalance between the oblique abdominal muscles.
- ***Lumbar flexion with rotation.*** This syndrome is characterized by pain that is unilateral or greater on one side and is increased with the combined motion of lumbar flexion and rotation. Many of the characteristics of the lumbar flexion and lumbar rotation syndromes can be applied to this syndrome.
- ***Lumbar extension with rotation.*** This syndrome is characterized by pain that is unilateral or greater on one side and is increased with the combined motion of lumbar extension and rotation. Many of the characteristics of the lumbar extension and lumbar rotation syndromes can be applied to this syndrome.

There is no gold standard to measure ROM of the lumbar spine. The majority of published data concerning normal ranges of motion exists without concomitant data on the subjects' demographic background, specifically with respect to age, gender, and occupation. Methods to objectively measure lumbar motion have included[337]

- Measuring the ROM visually (eyeballing). This method is endorsed by the American Academy of Orthopaedic Surgeons.[348] Although this seems to be the fastest and easiest method, its validity is questionable.[349]
- Using a tape measure, measuring the distance from a bony landmark to the floor at the end of available motion. This test provides only a gross measurement of the lumbar motion.[350]
- Goniometric measurement. The goniometer, also known as the universal goniometer, is the most accessible and least costly device. It should be noted that goniometric measurement of the lumbar spine often incorporates some thoracolumbar motion. It should also be noted that researchers have found poor intra- and interrater reliability for all goniometric measurements of the thoracolumbar spine.[351–353] Table 28-11 lists the suggested landmarks used when assessing lumbar ranges of motion with a goniometer.
- Schöber technique. This technique is used only to measure flexion. The first sacral spinous process is marked, and a mark is made about 10 cm above this mark. The patient then flexes forward, and the increased distance is measured. If there is normal motion of the lumbar spine with absence of disease, there should be an increase of 4–5 cm. The obvious limitation with this technique is that it only measures flexion.
- The modified Schöber technique,[354] which measures the change in distance between two skin markings over the lumbar spine during flexion or extension. A point is marked midway between the two PSISs, which is the level of S2. Points at 5 and 10 cm above that level are marked, and the distance between the three points is measured. The patient is

TABLE 28-11 Goniometric Landmarks, Normal Motion Values, and End-Feel Descriptors for the Lumbar Spine

Motion	Axis of Rotation	Arm Landmarks	Normal Values (Degrees)	Normal End-Feel
Flexion	Coronal/axillary line at L5 level	Stationary arm: along thigh Active arm: axial line to L1 spinous process	70–90	Tissue stretch (firm elastic resistance)
Extension	Coronal/axillary line at L5 level	Stationary arm: along thigh Active arm: axial line to L1 spinous process	30–50	Bone to bone (hard, painless) or tissue stretch
Side bending	Midline at S1 spinous process	Stationary arm: midline inferiorly Active arm: L1 spinous process	30	Tissue stretch
Rotation	Visual estimation only		35	Tissue stretch

asked to bend forward or backward, and the distance is remeasured. The distance between the two measurements is an indication of the amount of motion occurring in the lumbar spine. This method also is prone to error, because it can measure only lower lumbar levels and may not reflect the amount of motion available in the whole lumbar spine.[355] Various studies have shown this technique to have overall good interrater reliability.[355,356]

- The fluid (bubble) goniometer. This device consists of a fluid-filled circular tube attached to or embedded in a flat platform with a 360-degree scale. With the joint in a neutral position, the device is either strapped to the distal aspect of an extremity or manually held in place on the patient, as can be the case when measuring trunk movement. Although many clinicians appreciate the ease of use and elimination of landmark estimation required by the universal goniometer, this device still exhibits problems with reliable positioning, particularly if attached with a strap or when used on obese patients.[275] Landmarks used are similar to those of the goniometer's active arm.
- The inclinometer technique recommended by the American Medical Association.[342] Inclinometers are small angle measuring devices that work like a plumb line, operating on the principle of gravity. An appropriate inclinometer should include a large enough dial to allow easy reading of 2-degree increments. The inclinometer technique can record regional movement of the lumbar spine rather than the combined movement of the spine and hip[357] and has been proved to correlate well with measurements taken from a radiograph.[351,358] For example, to measure lumbar flexion, two inclinometers are used, aligned in the sagittal plane. The center of the first inclinometer is placed over the T12 spinous process. The center of the second one is placed over the sacrum, midway between the PSISs. The patient is asked to flex the trunk as far as possible, and both inclinometer angles are recorded. The lumbar flexion angle is calculated by subtracting the sacral (hip) from the T12 inclinometer angle.

Whatever technique is chosen, the same technique must be used subsequently when reassessing ROM.

Flexion. The first 60 degrees of forward bending typically result from flexion of the lumbar motion segments, which is followed by an additional movement at the hip joints of approximately 25 degrees.[62] The patient is instructed to tuck the chin toward the chest and bend forward at the waist, keeping the knees extended, while attempting to touch the toes.[275] The clinician should note any change in an existing scoliotic curve, deviation away from the midline which may suggest guarding due to disk pathology, patient apprehension or assistance (use of hands on knees), which may suggest instability, lack of motion between spinal segments, and whether the normal lordosis decreases as expected.

The lumbar flexion movement can be repeated with the patient sitting, as this test can help screen for the presence of rotoscoliosis.[359]

McKenzie[286] advocates the testing of lumbar flexion motion in supine as well as in the standing position. In the standing position, flexion of the lumbar spine occurs from above

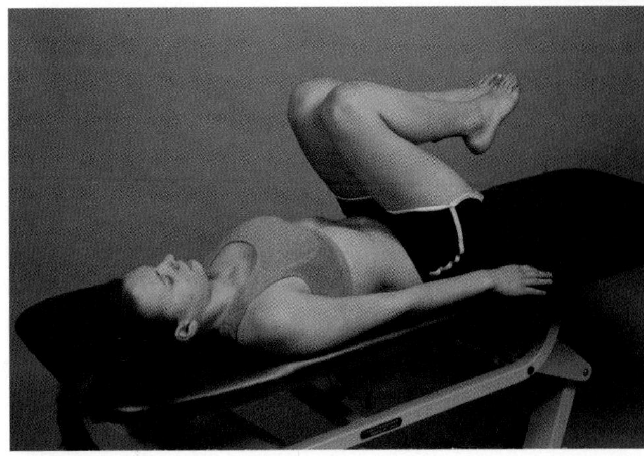

FIGURE 28-10 Lumbar flexion from below.

downward, so pain at the end of the range is likely to indicate that L5–S1 is affected. Bringing the knees to the chest in the supine position (Fig. 28-10) produces a flexion of the lumbar spine from below upward, so that pain at the beginning of the movement may indicate that L5–S1 is affected.[286]

Trunk deviation during flexion is believed to be associated with an IVD herniation, with the direction of the deviation determined by the relative position of the compression on the nerve.[360] Deviations during flexion may also result from neuromeningeal adhesions, hypomobile segment(s) on the contralateral side, hypermobile segment(s) on the ipsilateral side, a structural scoliosis, and a shortened leg on the ipsilateral side.[360] Passive ROM is tested with the patient seated on the examination table. The patient is instructed to keep the arms to the side, while the clinician grasps his or her shoulders and flexes the patient forward at the waist, keeping the pelvis firmly on the table. The clinician should note the end-feel and any change in an existing scoliotic curve, lack of motion between spinal segments, and whether the normal lordosis decreases as expected.

Extension. The patient is instructed to place his or her hands on the posterior iliac crests to provide support and then extend backward from the waist, keeping the knees extended and the gaze toward the ceiling (Fig. 28-9B). The clinician notes if the arc of extension is even throughout the lumbar spine or more pronounced at a specific spinal segment.[275] Pure lumbar extension in standing involves the patient leaning back at the waist. Lumbar extension is often the stiffest and most uncomfortable movement for the patient. Thus, patients with LBP tend to use the protective guarding mechanism against the compression and shearing forces, generated by simply hyperextending the hips. By applying a compressive force through the patient's shoulders during the backward bending, the clinician can induce a small increase in the lumbar lordosis. Passive ROM is tested with the patient seated on the examination table. The patient is instructed to place his or her hands across the chest. The clinician supports the upper back with one arm and the sacrum with the other hand and then extends the patient backward in an arching motion rather than a leaning motion. The clinician notes the end-feel or any altered symptoms.

Side Bending. The standing patient is instructed to lean to the side by sliding the palm of the hand down the outside of the thigh, without flexing forward or extending backward, and keeping the palm on the lateral thigh or hip. The clinician notes if the arc of bending is even or more pronounced at a specific spinal segment as well as whether the patient unintentionally rotates the torso to accommodate motion.[275] Side-bending ROM has been found to be a good indicator of the degree of LBP[234] and disability.[235] In acute spinal derangements, such as a unilateral posterolateral IVD protrusion or unilateral zygapophyseal joint derangement, lumbar side bending may be significantly reduced or absent on one side (usually toward the involved side). Arthritic conditions of the spine tend to demonstrate a symmetric loss of side bending to both sides.

The common method of measuring the amount of side bending is to record the distance between the fingertip and the floor at the end of the side bend, but this is merely an estimation of the flexibility of the whole spine rather than the lumbar spine.[337] Thus, it is recommended that lumbar spine movement in side bending be measured using the inclinometer technique.[342]

The patient may be seen to lift one foot or bend the knees during the side-bending movements and should be reminded to maintain the feet on the floor during measurement. At the end of the side-bending motion, overpressure is applied on the shoulder (see Figs. 26-9C–D). Passive ROM is tested with the patient seated on the examination table. The patient is instructed to cross the arms across the chest. The clinician places one arm across the upper back and the other hand on the contralateral iliac crest. The clinician then bends the patient to each side, keeping the opposite crest from rising off the table. As with extension, an arching motion rather than a leaning motion is desired. The end-feel is noted or any altered symptoms.

Axial Rotation. Axial rotation of the spine usually is assessed in the sitting position to eliminate motion occurring from the hips. The patient, keeping the knees together, twists at the waist to each side. Patients frequently tend to side bend or extend the torso, so the clinician must take care in preventing such motion. Axial rotation of the trunk commonly includes movement of both thoracic and lumbar segments of the spine. Overpressure may be applied at the end of range (Fig. 28-11). Normal range could indicate normalcy, hypermobility, or instability. Restricted range will be in either a capsular or a noncapsular pattern. Pain with this maneuver can implicate a nonorganic source, an annular tear, a ligament tear, or a zygapophyseal joint dysfunction.[360] Passive ROM is tested with the patient seated on the examination table. The patient is instructed to place his or her hands across the chest, and the clinician grasps the shoulders and rotates the patient's torso. Alternately, the clinician may use a shoulder–scapula contact. End-feel is noted or any altered symptoms.

Combined Motion Testing. The combined motion tests of the lumbar spine are used to detect biomechanical impairments. Although combined motion tests do not provide information as to which segment is at fault, they may provide information as to which motion or position reproduces the pain.[361]

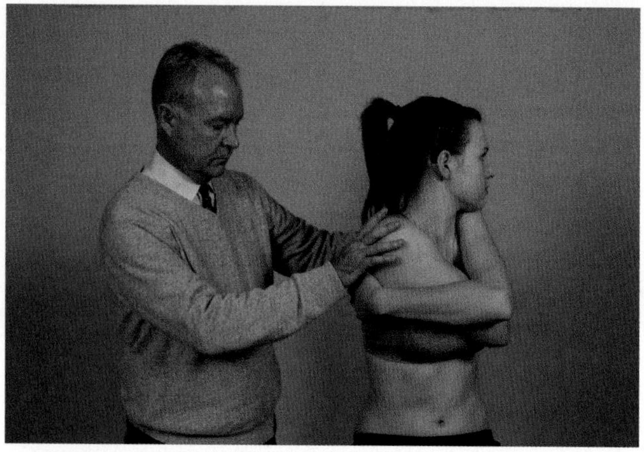

FIGURE 28-11 Lumbar rotation.

Combined motion tests can reproduce the pain in a structure that is either being compressed or stretched[362]:

- A reproduction or increase in symptoms with flexion and side bending away from the side of the symptoms may implicate pain in a structure that is being stretched.
- A reproduction or increase in symptoms with extension and side bending toward the side of the symptoms may implicate pain in a structure that is being compressed.

Combined motions can be performed as repetitive motions or as sustained positioning. For example, the patient can be asked to repetitively perform the combined motion of flexion and right side bending to assess for what McKenzie describes as a derangement syndrome, or the clinician can position the patient in flexion and right side bending (Fig. 28-12) to assess

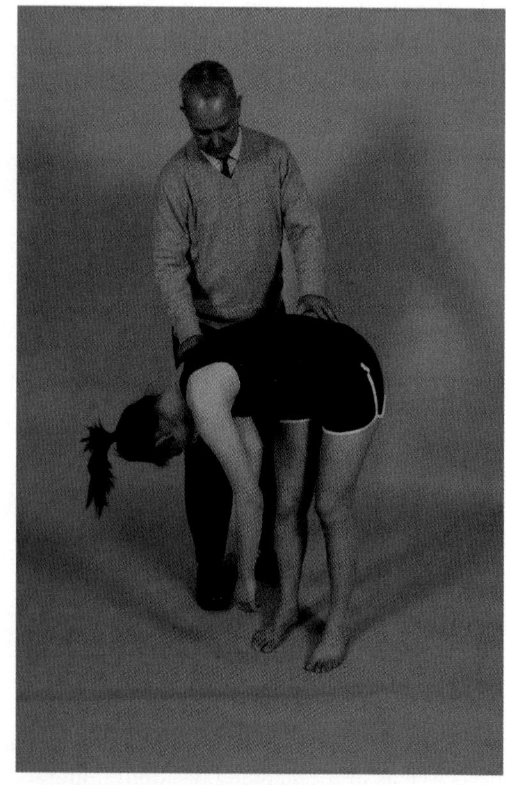

FIGURE 28-12 Lumbar flexion and right side flexion.

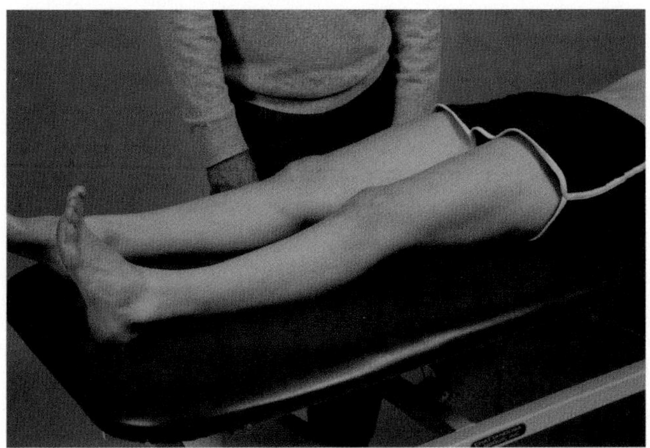

FIGURE 28-13 Supine lying.

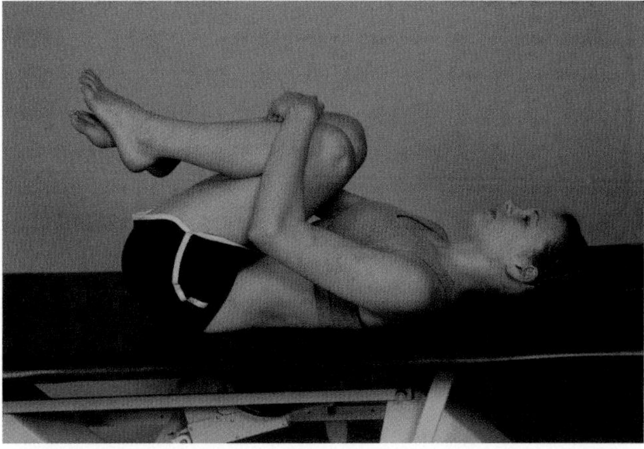

FIGURE 28-15 Double knees to chest.

for what McKenzie describes as a dysfunction syndrome. Alternatively, the clinician can ask the patient to maintain the position of flexion and right side bending to assess for a postural dysfunction.[286]

Six-Position Test

The six-position test is a screening tool that I have found to be particularly useful with the acute patient, in helping to determine the position of comfort for the patient and for focusing the examination and intervention. The reliability or validity of these tests has yet to be established, but they are based on applied anatomy and biomechanics. The patient is placed in the following positions:

1. Supine with the hips and knees extended (Fig. 28-13). In individuals with adaptive shortening of the rectus femoris and the iliopsoas (a common finding), this position is manifested by an inability of the posterior thighs to rest on the table. Pain in this position may indicate a lumbar extension or lumbar rotation syndrome (see "Intervention Strategies" section), especially if the next position relieves the symptoms.[347]
2. Supine in the hook-lying position, with the hips and knees flexed and the feet flat on the bed (Fig. 28-14). This is typically the most comfortable position for the patient with acute LBP, except in cases of severe stenosis or spondylolisthesis.
3. Supine with both knees held against the chest (Fig. 28-15). This position rotates the pelvis posteriorly and widens the intervertebral foramina of the lumbar segments.[294] This is normally a comfortable position for patients who have spinal stenosis, lateral recess stenosis, or a lumbar extension syndrome.
4. Supine with one hip and knee extended, the patient raises the other knee to the chest without using the arms (Fig. 28-16). Once the leg is elevated, the patient grasps it with both hands and pulls it toward the chest. Holding the left knee against the chest invokes a position of lumbar flexion and left side bending, which widens the intervertebral foramen on the right and narrows the

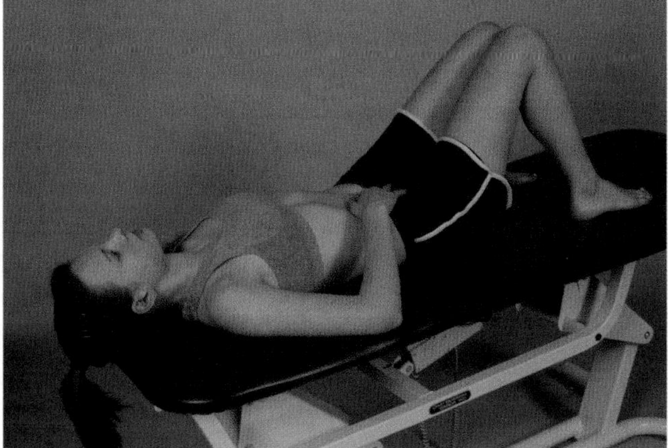

FIGURE 28-14 Hook lying.

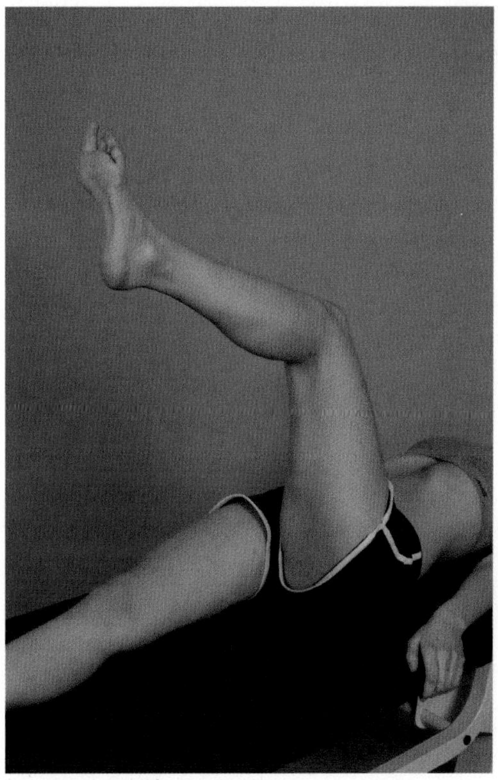

FIGURE 28-16 Single knee to chest.

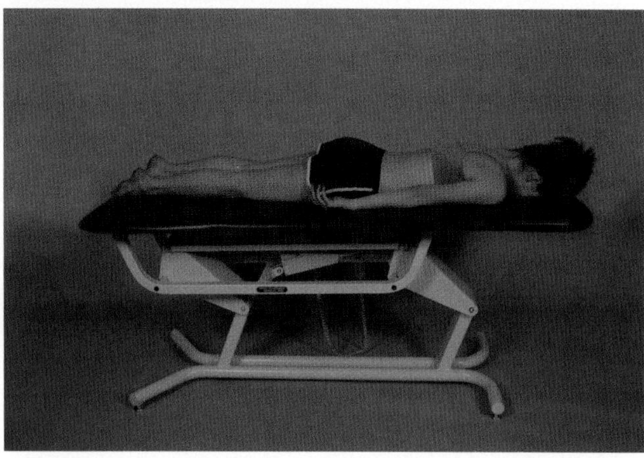

FIGURE 28-17 Prone lying.

intervertebral foramen on the left. Holding the right knee against the chest invokes a position of lumbar flexion and right side bending, which widens the intervertebral foramen on the left and narrows intervertebral foramen on the right.[294] Given the amount of rotation induced with this maneuver, this test is often positive even when the position of both knees to the chest does not provoke symptoms. Occasionally though, one side may be pain free and can be used as an introductory exercise.

5. Prone lying with the legs straight (Fig. 28-17). This is typically comfortable for patients with an IVD protrusion, but uncomfortable for patients with spinal stenosis, spondylolisthesis, and an extension or a rotation syndrome[347] (see "Intervention Strategies" section).
6. Prone lying with passive knee flexion applied by the clinician (Fig. 28-18). This is a confirmatory test for the previous position, if it increases the symptoms in patients with spinal stenosis, spondylolisthesis, and an extension or a rotation syndrome[347] (see "Intervention Strategies" section).

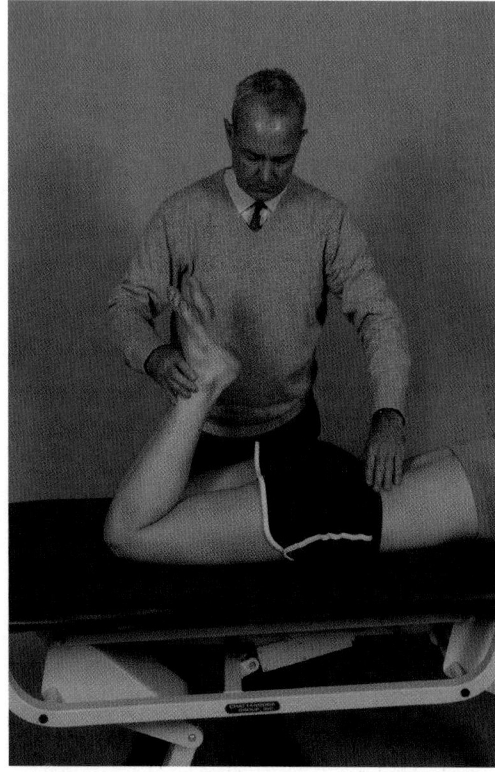

FIGURE 28-18 Prone double knee bend.

The results from these tests should provide the clinician with information on the effect that pelvic tilting in a non–weight-bearing position has on the symptoms. If anterior pelvic tilting appears to aggravate the patient's symptoms, initial positions and exercises that promote posterior pelvic tilting are advocated. If posterior pelvic tilting appears to aggravate the patient's symptoms, initial positions and exercises that promote an anterior pelvic tilt are advocated.

Muscle Strength. Optimum control of the spine and pelvis requires a carefully controlled, dynamic system where the strategy of activation of the trunk muscles matches the functional task. Resisted motions of the lumbar spine can be categorized into those that provide valuable information regarding the origin of lumbar pathology (key muscle testing) and those that assess basic strength parameters, such as dynamic and static motor control.[275]

Gross strength of the trunk can also be assessed by applying a resisting force to the patient's upper back during resisted extension and the shoulders during flexion, lateral bending, and rotation.[275] The clinician notes the presence and type of pain produced and the degree of effort exerted.

Key Muscle Testing. The key muscle tests are used as part of the lower quarter scanning examination (see Chap. 4), because they examine the integrity of the neuromuscular junction and the contractile and inert components of the various muscles.[343] With the isometric tests, the contraction should be held for at least 5 seconds to demonstrate any weakness. If the clinician suspects weakness, the test is repeated two to three times to assess for fatigability. The larger muscle groups, such as the quadriceps, hip extensors, and calf muscles, must be tested by repetitive resistance against a load to sufficiently stress the muscle–nerve components.

Standing up on the Toes (S1–2). The patient raises both heels off the ground (Fig. 28-19). The key muscles tested during this maneuver are the plantar flexors. These are difficult muscles to fatigue, so the patient should perform 10 heel raises unilaterally, with the arms supported by the clinician. In addition to observing for fatigability, the clinician should look for Trendelenburg's sign. A positive Trendelenburg's sign occurs when, during unilateral weight bearing, the pelvis drops toward the unsupported limb; this can indicate a number of conditions, including a hip impairment (coxa vara) or a gluteus medius weakness (see Chap. 19).

Unilateral Squat While Supported (L3–4). The patient performs unilateral squats while supported (Fig. 28-20). The key muscles being tested during this maneuver are the quadriceps and hip extensors. Neurologic weakness of the quadriceps (L3–4) is relatively rare and often suggests a nondiskogenic lesion, such as a neoplasm, especially if the weakness is bilateral.[360]

Heel Walking (L4). The patient walks toward, or away from, the clinician while weight bearing through the heels (Fig. 28-21). The key muscles being tested during this maneuver are the dorsiflexors (L4). Approximately 40% of IVD lesions affect this level, about an equal amount as those that affect the L5 root.[33] An IVD protrusion of the L4–5 disk can irritate the

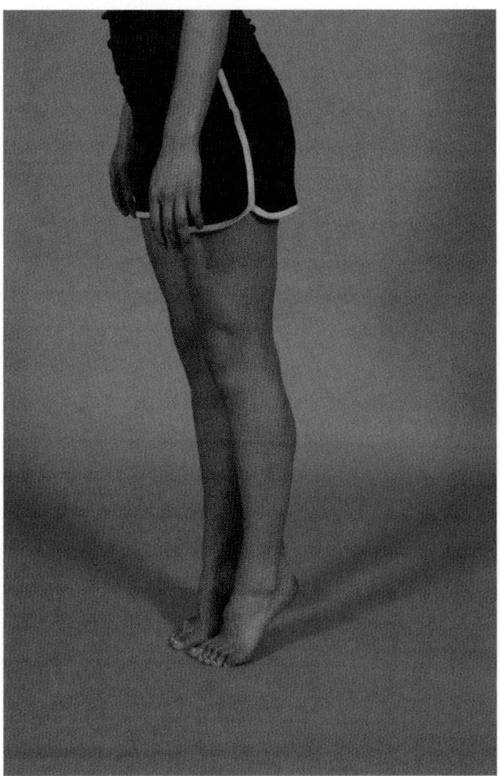

FIGURE 28-19 Standing up on toes.

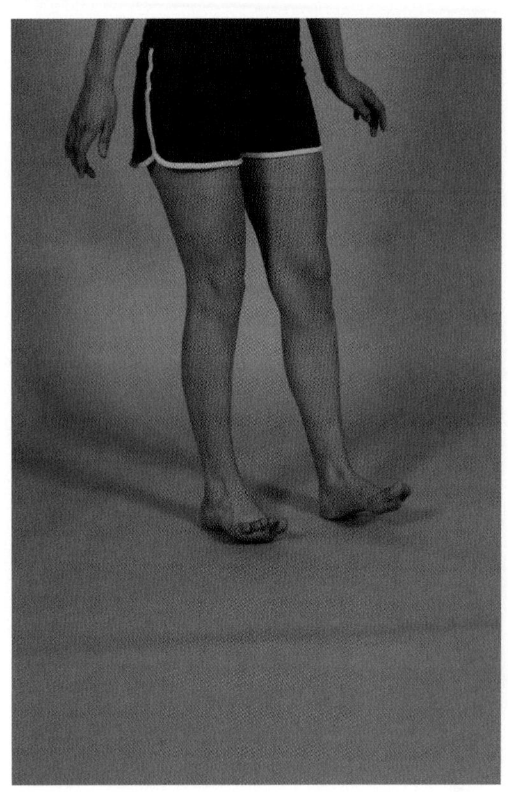

FIGURE 28-21 Heel walking.

fourth root, the fifth root, or, with a larger protrusion, both roots. The dorsiflexors can also be tested in supine (Fig. 28-22).

Hip Flexion (L1–2). With palsy, the patient is unable to raise the thigh off the table. Palsy at this level should always serve as a red flag for the clinician, because IVD protrusions at this level are rare, but this is a common site for metastasis.[363] Painful weakness of hip flexion may indicate the presence of a fractured transverse process, metastatic invasion, acute spondylolisthesis, acute segmental articular dysfunction, a major contractile lesion of the hip flexors (rare), or a hip joint

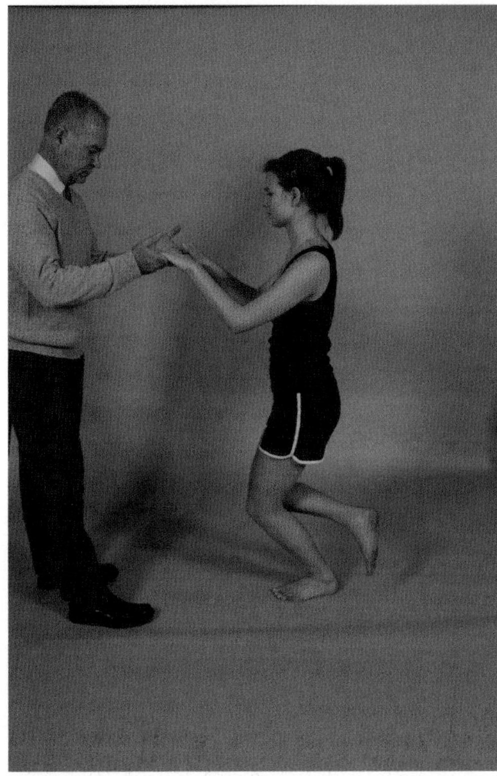

FIGURE 28-20 Unilateral squat.

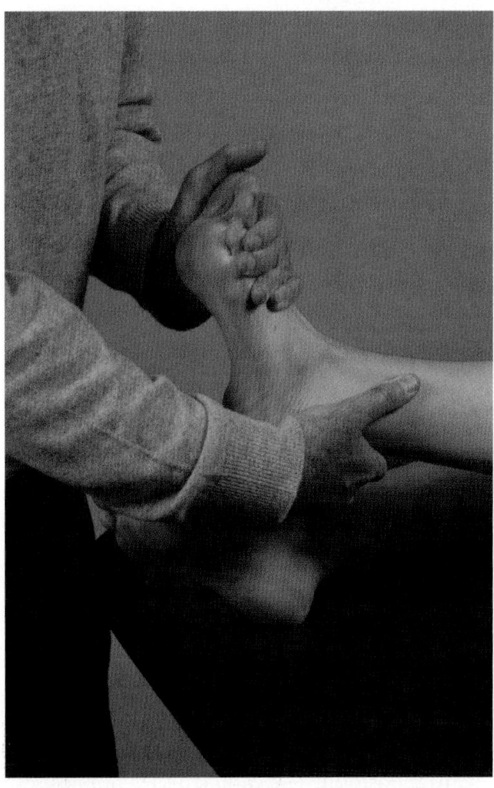

FIGURE 28-22 Key muscle testing of the dorsiflexors with the patient supine.

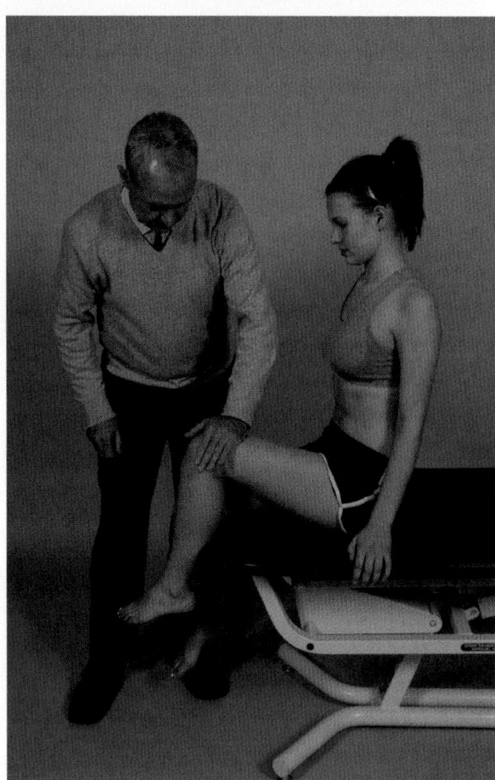

FIGURE 28-23 Resisted hip flexion.

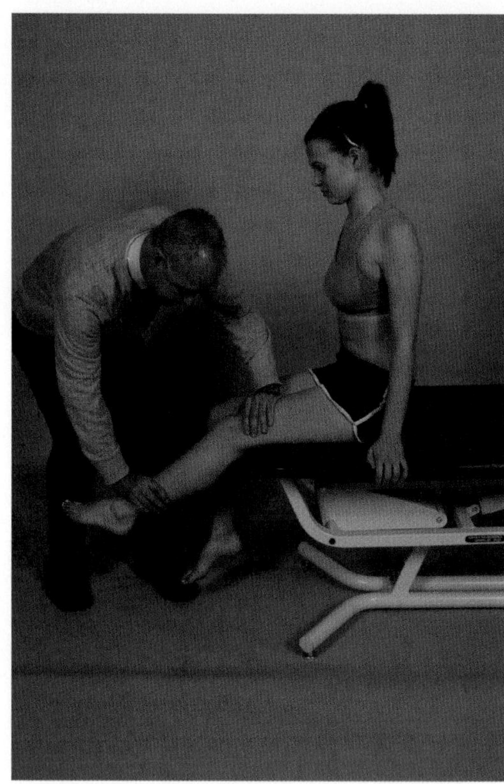

FIGURE 28-24 Resisted knee extension.

pathology. The patient's hip is actively raised off the treatment table to approximately 30–40 degrees of flexion. The clinician then applies a resisted force proximal to the knee into hip extension (Fig. 28-23), while ensuring that the heel of the patient's foot is not contacting the examining table. Both sides are tested for comparison.

Knee extension (L3–4). The clinician positions the patient's knee in 25–35 degrees of flexion and then applies a resisted flexion force at the middistal shaft of the tibia (Fig. 28-24). Both sides are tested for comparison. Alternately, knee extension can be tested with the patient prone. The patient's leg is positioned in approximately 120 degrees of knee flexion, taking care to do this passively. The clinician rests the superior aspect of his or her shoulder against the posterior aspect of the patient's ankle and grips the edges of the examining table. A force to flex the patient's knee is applied while the patient resists. Both sides are tested for comparison.

Hip extension (L5–S1). The patient's knee is flexed to 90 degrees, and his or her thigh is lifted slightly off the examining table by the clinician, while the other leg is stabilized. A downward force is applied to the patient's posterior thigh (Fig. 28-25), while the clinician ensures that the patient's thigh is not in contact with the table. Both sides are tested for comparison.

Knee flexion (S1–2). The patient's knee is flexed to 70 degrees, and an extension isometric force is applied just above the ankle (Fig. 28-26). Both sides are tested for comparison.

Great toe extension (L5). The patient is asked to hold the big toe in a neutral position. The clinician then applies resistance to the toe (Fig. 28-27) and compares the two sides.

Ankle eversion (L5–S1). The patient is asked to place the feet at 0 degree of plantar and dorsiflexion relative to the leg. A resisted force is applied by the clinician to move each foot into inversion (Fig. 28-28), and a comparison is made.

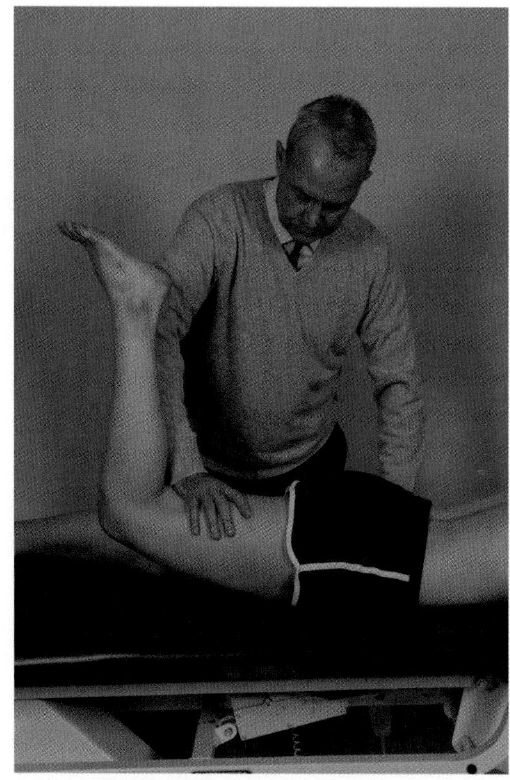

FIGURE 28-25 Resisted hip extension with knee flexed.

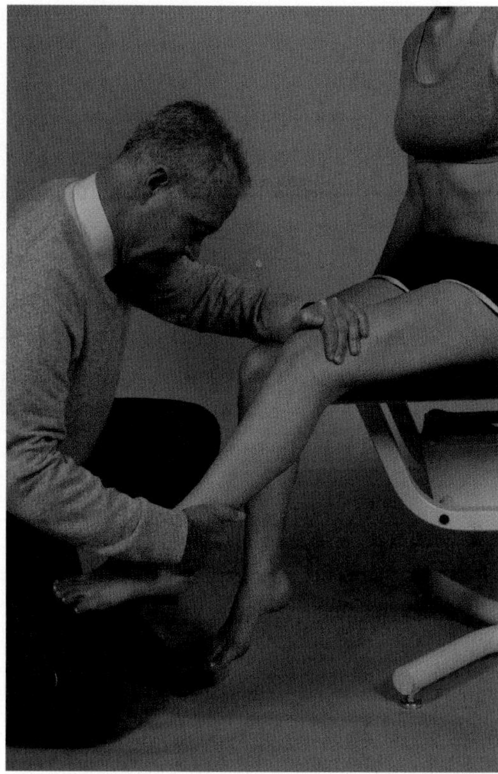

FIGURE 28-26 Resisted knee flexion.

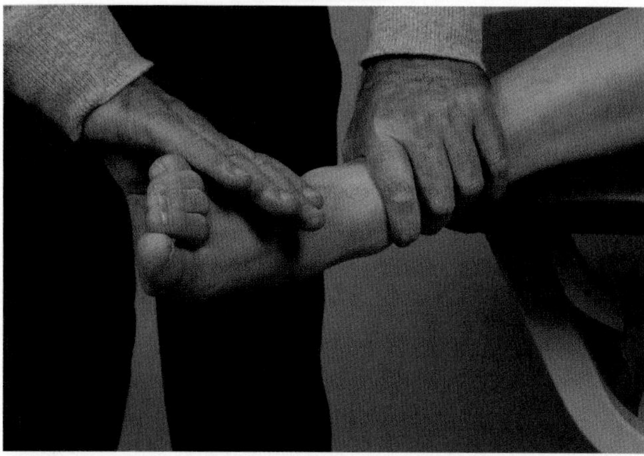

FIGURE 28-28 Resisted ankle eversion.

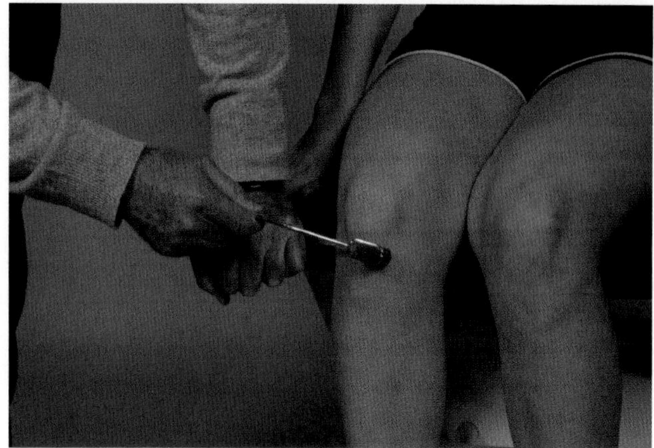

FIGURE 28-29 Patellar reflex.

Muscle Stretch Reflexes

The reflexes should be assessed and graded accordingly, with any differences between the two sides noted. The tendon should be struck directly once the patient's muscles and tendons are relaxed.

Patellar Reflex (L3). The patient is positioned sitting, with the legs hanging freely. Alternatively, both knees can be supported in flexion, with the patient placed in supine (Fig. 28-29).

Hamstring Reflex (Semimembranosus: L5, S1; and Biceps Femoris: S1–2). The patient is positioned prone, with the knee flexed and the foot resting on a pillow. The clinician places a thumb over the appropriate tendon and taps the thumbnail with the reflex hammer to elicit the reflex.

Achilles Reflex (S1–2). The patient is positioned so that the ankle is slightly dorsiflexed with passive overpressure (Fig. 28-30).

Pathologic Reflexes

Pathologic reflexes occur in the presence of motor cortex, brain stem, or corticospinal tract lesions (upper motor neuron lesions), wherein the motor response to a sensory stimulus is not modulated. The following pathologic reflexes are described in Chapter 3:

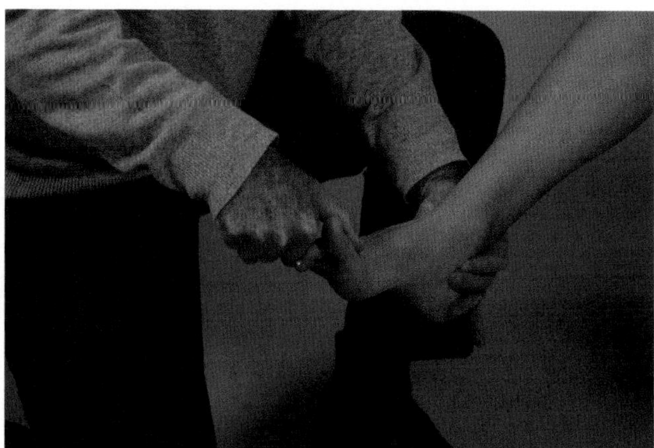

FIGURE 28-27 Resisted great toe extension.

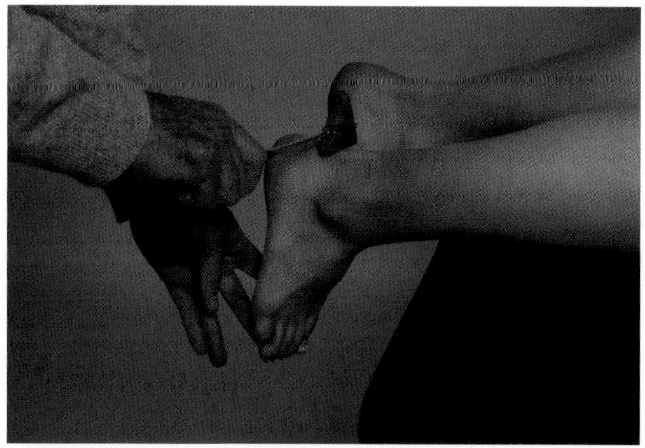

FIGURE 28-30 Achilles reflex.

- Babinski;
- Clonus;
- Oppenheim.

Sensory Testing

A thorough evaluation of the sensory system is quite an involved process, due to the number of ascending pathways carrying information to the brain.[275] The clinician checks the dermatome patterns of the nerve roots, as well as the peripheral sensory distribution of the peripheral nerves (see Chap. 3). Dermatomes vary considerably between individuals.

Superficial Reflexes

There are a number of reflexes that occur in response to stimulation of the skin, known as the *superficial reflexes*. Three of these, the cremasteric (L1–2), Geigel (L1–2), and anal (S2–5), are pertinent to nerves exiting the lumbar spine.[275] Performance of these superficial reflex tests involves either stroking or pricking the skin of the upper inner thigh (cremasteric and Geigel) or perianal tissue and noting the presence of muscle contraction by the cremasteric (elevation of the testicles), iliopuepartal (elevation of the clitoral prepuce), or external sphincter muscles (also known as anal wink), respectively. It is important to remember that without correlation from the history and physical examination findings, absence of a superficial reflex may not ultimately be clinically significant.

Neurodynamic Mobility

The neurodynamic mobility tests to help confirm a lumbar disk herniation include straight leg raising (SLR), bilateral SLR, crossed SLR sign, slump test, prone knee bend (femoral nerve stretch), and bowstring tests, which are described in Chapter 11.

The lower the angle of a positive SLR test, the more specific the test becomes and the larger the disk protrusion found at surgery.[228,364] A limited SLR at 60 degrees is moderately sensitive for herniated lumbar disks but nonspecific, because limitation often is observed in the absence of disk herniations.[228,365,366] Crossed SLR is less sensitive but highly specific.[365–367] Thus, the crossed SLR test suggests concordance with the diagnosis, whereas ipsilateral SLR is more effective in ruling out the diagnosis.

The femoral nerve stretch test (see Chap. 11) is probably the single best screening test to evaluate for a high lumbar radiculopathy. This test has been shown to be positive in 84–95% of patients with high lumbar disks,[154,368,369] although the test may be falsely positive in the presence of an adaptively shortened iliopsoas or rectus femoris or any pathology in or about the hip joint, sacroiliac joint, and lumbar spine.

Differing Philosophies

The next stage in the examination process depends on the clinician's background. Clinicians who are heavily influenced by the muscle energy techniques of the osteopaths use position testing to determine the segment on which to focus. Other clinicians omit the position tests and proceed to the combined motion and passive physiologic tests.

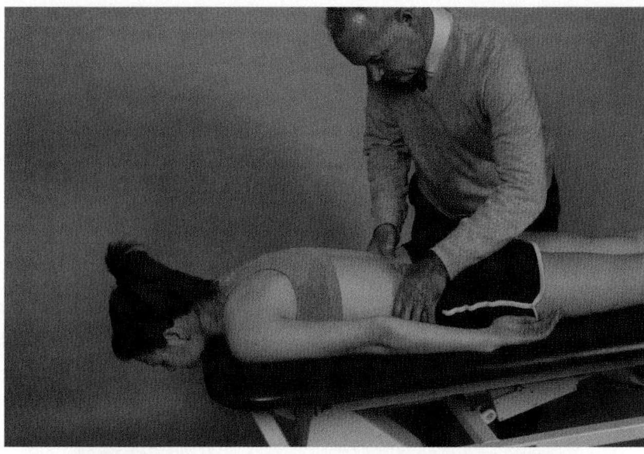

FIGURE 28-31 Position testing in neutral.

Position Testing. Position testing in the lumbar spine is an osteopathic technique used to determine the level and type of zygapophyseal joint dysfunction.[100,332,335,370–372] Position testing is performed with the patient in three positions: neutral (Fig. 28-31), flexion (Fig. 28-32), and extension (Fig. 28-33). The transverse processes are then layer palpated (Fig. 28-34). The findings and possible causes for the position testing are outlined in Tables 28-12 and 28-13.

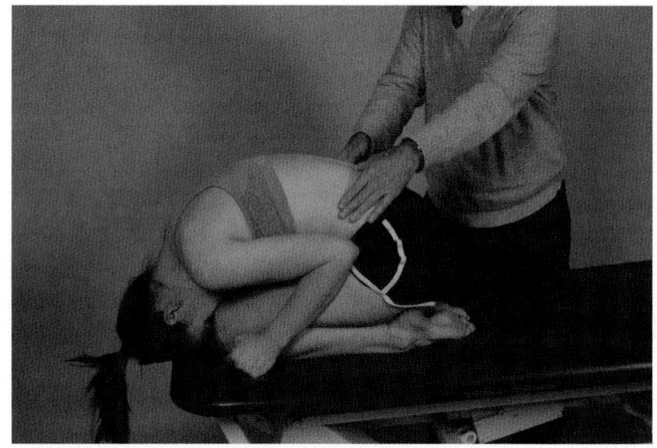

FIGURE 28-32 Position testing in flexion.

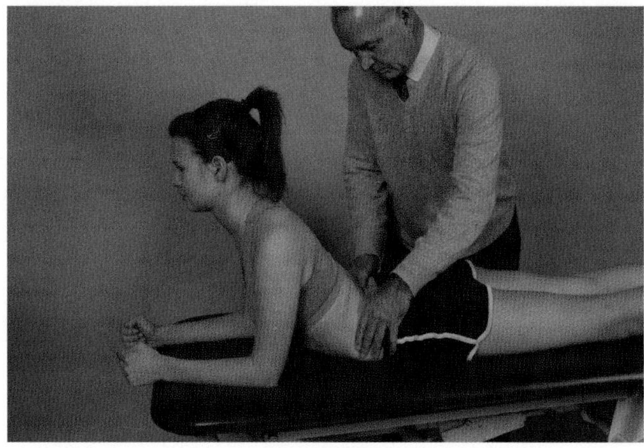

FIGURE 28-33 Position testing in extension.

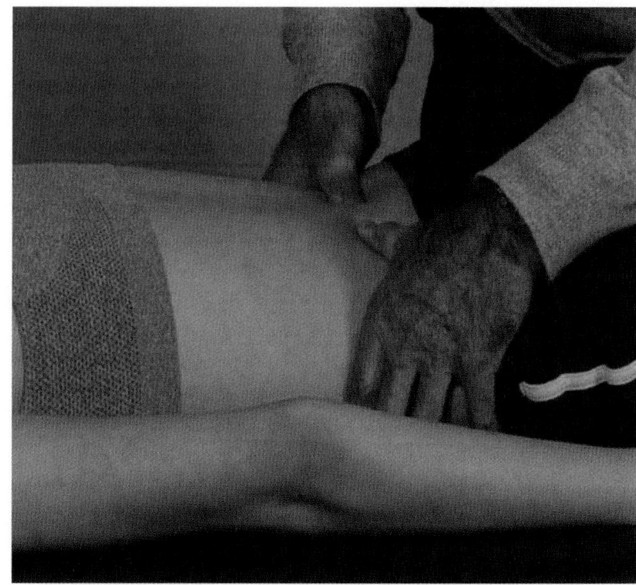

FIGURE 28-34 Layer palpation of the transverse processes. May also be used for P-A pressures.

Passive Physiologic Intervertebral Mobility Tests. The passive physiologic intervertebral mobility (PPIVM) tests are most effectively carried out if the combined motion tests locate a hypomobility, or if the position tests are negative, rather than as the entry tests for the lumbar spine.[373,374] Judgments of stiffness made by experienced physical therapists examining patients in their own clinics have been found to have poor reliability.[375]

The passive physiologic movement tests are performed into

- flexion;
- extension;
- rotation;
- side bending.

TABLE 28-12 Causes and Findings for a Flexed Rotated Side Bent Right

Causes of an FRSR	Associated Findings
Isolated left joint extension hypomobility (FRSR)	PPIVM and PPAIVM tests in left extension quadrant are reduced
Tight left flexor muscles (FRSR)	PPIVM test in left extension quadrant is decreased; PAIVM test is normal
Arthrosis or arthritis of left joint in capsular pattern (ERSL < FRSR)	PPIVM and PPAIVM tests in right flexion quadrant are more reduced than in left extension quadrant
Fibrosis of left joint (ERSL = FRSR)	PPIVM and PPAIVM tests are equally reduced in right flexion and left extension quadrants
Left posterolateral disk protrusion (ERSR < FRSR)	PPIVM tests in left extension quadrant are reduced with springy end-feel; both flexion quadrants are normal

ERSL, extended rotated side bent left; ERSR, extended rotated side bent right; FRSR, flexed rotated side bent right; PPAIVM, passive physiologic accessory intervertebral movement; PPIVM, passive physiologic intervertebral mobility.

TABLE 28-13 Causes and Findings of an Extended Rotated Side Bent Left

Causes of an ERSL[a]	Associated Findings
Isolated left joint flexion hypomobility (ERSL); tight left extensor muscles (ERSL)	PPIVM and PPAIVM tests in right flexion quadrant are reduced; PPIVM test in right flexion quadrant is decreased; PPAIVM is normal
Arthrosis or arthritis of left joint in capsular pattern (ERSL < FRSR)	PPIVM and PPAIVM tests are equally reduced in right flexion and left flexion quadrants
Fibrosis left joint (ERSL = FRSR)	PPIVM and PPAIVM tests are equally reduced in right and left flexion quadrants
Right posterolateral disk protrusion (ERSL < FRSL)	PPIVM tests in right extension quadrant are reduced with springy end-feel; both flexion quadrants appear normal

ERSL, extended rotated side bent left; ERSR, extended rotated side bent right; FRSL, flexed rotated side bent left; FRSR, flexed rotated side bent right; PPAIVM, passive physiologic accessory intervertebral movement; PPIVM, passive physiologic intervertebral mobility.
[a]An ERSR would have the same causes and findings, but on the opposite side.

The adjacent spinous processes of the segment are palpated simultaneously, and movement between them is assessed as the segment is passively taken through its physiologic range.

The test is used for acute and subacute patients who have pain in the cardinal motion planes. For these tests, the patient is in the side-lying position, facing the clinician. The clinician may locate the patient's lumbosacral junction using one of the following methods:

- by locating the L5 spinous process and then moving inferiorly;
- by locating the PSIS and moving superiorly and medially;
- by locating the spinous process of T12 and counting down to the correct level using the spinous processes.

Once located, the neutral position of the spine for flexion and extension is found by palpating the L5 spinous process and alternatively flexing and extending the hips until it is felt to rock around the flexion and extension point.

Flexion. The patient is close to the clinician, with the underneath leg slightly flexed at the hip and knee. A small pillow or roll can be placed under the patient's waist to maintain the lumbar spine in a neutral position with respect to side bending. The test can be performed by flexing one or both of the patient' s legs, but it is generally easier to use one leg. The clinician, facing the patient, palpates between two adjacent lumbar spinous processes in the interspinous space (Fig. 28-35) with the cranial hand, while the other hand grasps the patient's lower legs (Fig. 28-36).

The patient's lower extremities are moved into hip and lumbar flexion and returned to neutral by the clinician, as the

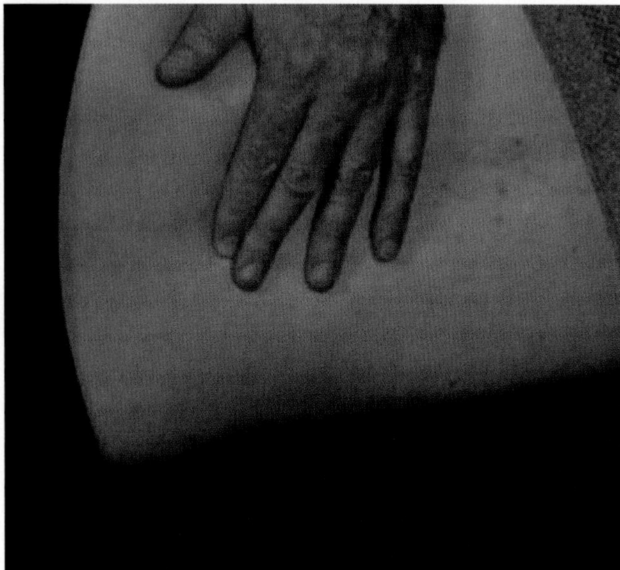

FIGURE 28-35 Intersegmental palpation.

motion between segments is palpated. Using this general technique, the clinician works up and down the lumbar spine, getting a sense of the overall motion available.

Although there is a high degree of variability in patients, segmental motion should decrease from L5 to L1.[62] A generalized hypermobility demonstrates more motion in all of the segments, whereas an isolated hypermobile segment demonstrates more motion at only that level. Each segment is checked sequentially, while moving the lumbar spine passively from neutral to full flexion.

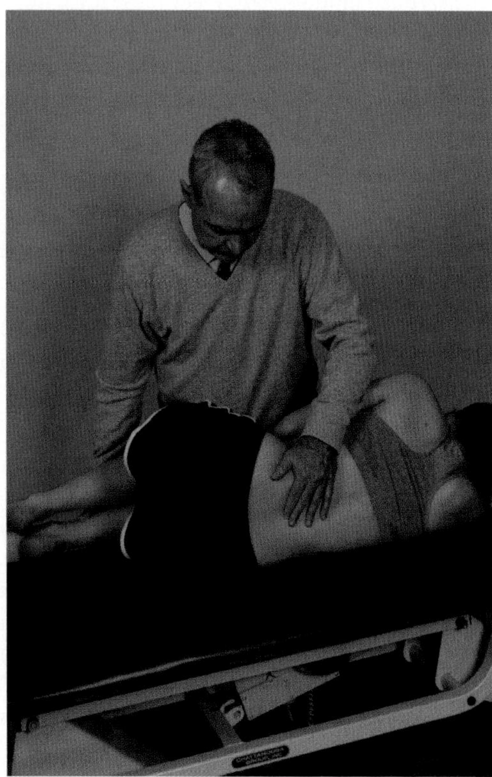

FIGURE 28-36 Passive mobility testing—flexion.

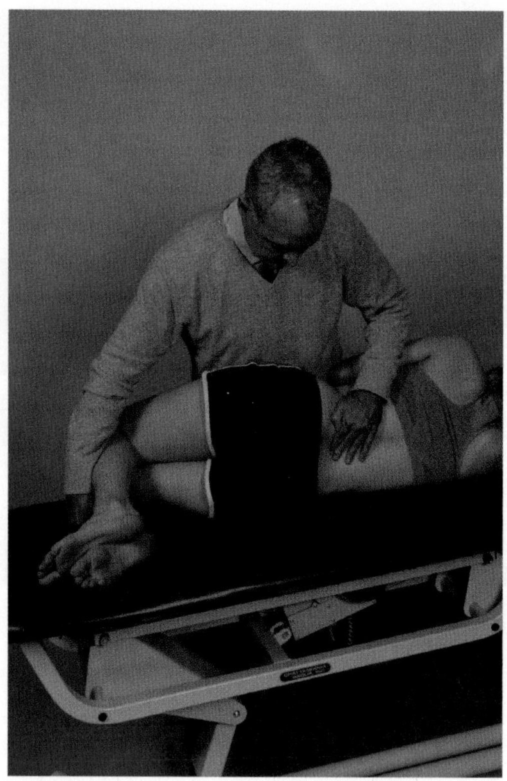

FIGURE 28-37 Passive mobility testing—extension.

For the mid and upper lumbar segments, this technique can be modified for the larger patient by performing it with the patient sitting up.

Extension. Although flexion and extension can be tested together, it is more accurate to assess them separately. The patient is positioned as for flexion testing but is oriented diagonally on the bed so that the pelvis is close to the edge, and the shoulder further from the edge. A small pillow or roll can be placed under the patient's waist to maintain the lumbar spine in a neutral position with respect to side bending. The clinician locates two adjacent spinous processes with his or her cranial hand, while the caudal arm flexes the patient's knees as much as possible before extending the patient's hips (Fig. 28-37). As the patient's knees move off the table, the clinician supports them on his or her thighs. When the patient's legs are on the table, the clinician's caudal arm is used to produce the hip and the lumbar extension. The pelvis motion is felt, and the spine is returned to its neutral position each time.

Side bending. The patient is placed in the side-lying position, with the knees and hips flexed, the thighs supported on the table and the lower legs off the table. The lumbar spine should be in a neutral position in relation to flexion and extension. The clinician, facing the patient, places his or her cranial arm between the patient's arm and body and palpates the interspinous spaces, while the caudal hand grasps under the patient's body (Fig. 28-38). As the patient's trunk is lifted toward the ceiling, the superior spinous process should be felt to move away from the table, as the lumbar spine is side bent toward the table. The opposite direction of sidebend is tested with the patient side-lying on the opposite side. The technique can also be performed using the patient's legs with the direction of the leg lift representing the direction of the side

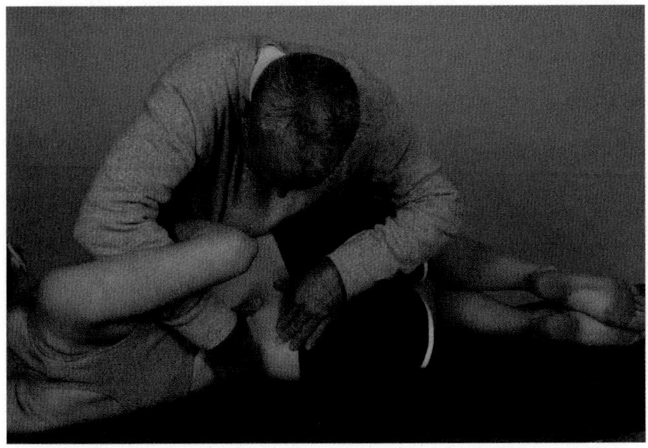

FIGURE 28-38 Passive mobility testing—side bending.

bending. For example, with the patient in the right side-lying position, right side bending (and left rotation) is introduced by lowering the feet and ankles off the table. The procedure is repeated for the other side, and the two sides are compared.

Rotation. The patient is positioned as described for extension testing in spinal neutral, with both knees being just off the table. A small pillow or roll can be placed under the patient's waist to maintain the lumbar spine in a neutral position. The interspinous spaces are palpated with the cranial hand, which is placed along the lower thoracic spine, with a reinforced index finger resting against adjacent spinous processes from underneath (Fig. 28-39).

The patient's pelvis is stabilized by the caudal hand, while the patient's thorax is rotated toward and away from the clinician, using the cranial hand. As the patient's thorax is rotated away, the spinous process of the upper segment should be felt to rotate toward the table, compared with the spinous process of the lower segment.

The spine is returned to neutral each time, and the clinician progresses up the spine. The process is repeated with the patient side lying on the opposite side.

Unfortunately, the PPIVM tests do not completely exclude such intersegmental impairments as minor end-range asymmetric hypo- or hypermobilities, because the application of side bending or rotation in neutral does not fully flex or extend the zygapophyseal joints, nor is it possible to fully flex or extend both zygapophyseal joints simultaneously. In order to completely flex a particular joint, the opposite joint has to move out of the fully flexed position by using side bending and allowing the increased superior glide of the superior zygapophyseal joint on the opposite joint.

Passive Physiologic Accessory Intervertebral Mobility Tests. The passive physiologic accessory intervertebral mobility (PPAIVM) tests investigate the degree of linear or accessory glide that a joint possesses and are used on segmental levels where there is a possible hypomobility, to help determine if the motion restriction is articular, periarticular, or myofascial in origin. In other words, they assess the amount of joint motion, as well as the quality of the end-feel. The motion is assessed in relation to the patient's body type and age and the normal range for that segment and the end-feel is assessed for pain, spasm or hypertonicity, or resistance to motion.

Several techniques have been proposed over the years to assess segmental mobility of the T10–L5 segments, including P-A pressure techniques (see later discussion). The PPAIVM techniques outlined here are used to confirm the findings of the PPIVM tests, by testing the joint glides of that segmental level, to confirm or refute whether a hypo- or hypermobility exists. Spinal locking techniques may be used to help localize these techniques to a specific level, or to a specific side of the segment. Descriptions of the symmetric techniques follow.

A pillow or towel roll should be placed under the lumbar spine of the patient if side bending of the lumbar spine appears to be occurring when the patient is placed in the side lying position.

Flexion. The patient is in the side lying position, close to the edge of the bed, with the spine supported in the neutral position, the thighs on the table, and the head resting on a pillow. The clinician faces the patient and locates the suspected segment using palpation. The superior segment is stabilized using the cranial hand (see Fig. 28-40). The clinician now flexes the patient's lumbar spine, using the patient's legs, as in the PPIVM test, until motion is felt at the superior spinous process of the monitored segment.

Using the index and middle fingers of the caudal hand, the clinician straddles the transverse processes of the inferior segment and pulls the segment inferiorly, using the caudal

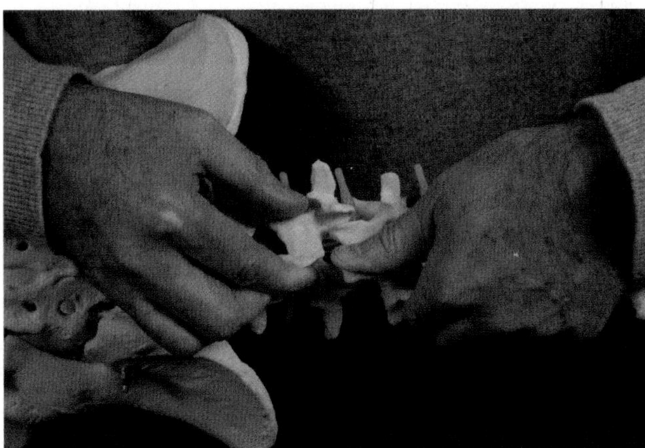

FIGURE 28-39 Passive mobility testing—rotation.

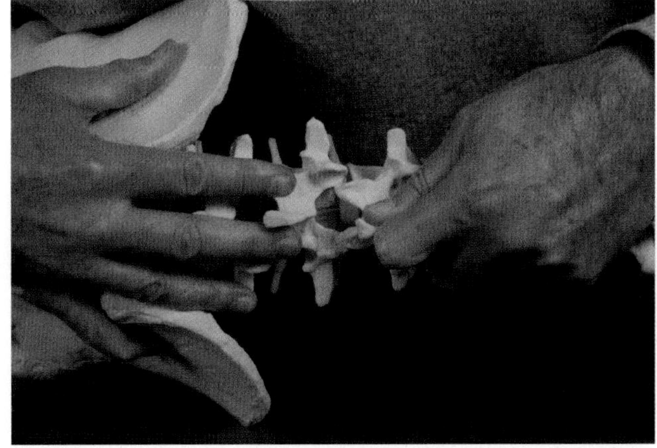

FIGURE 28-40 Passive articular mobility testing for flexion showing stabilization.

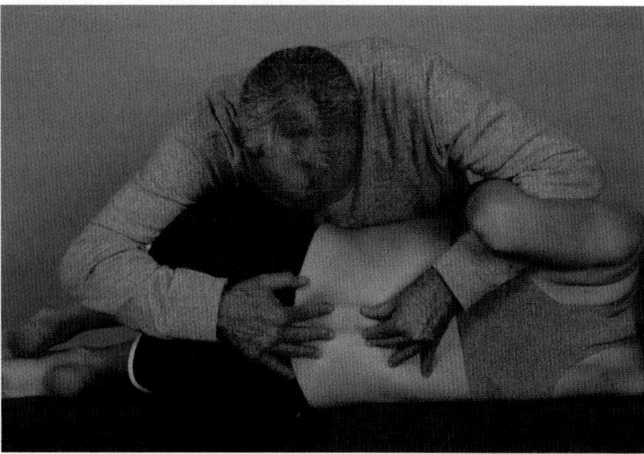

FIGURE 28-41 Passive articular mobility testing for flexion.

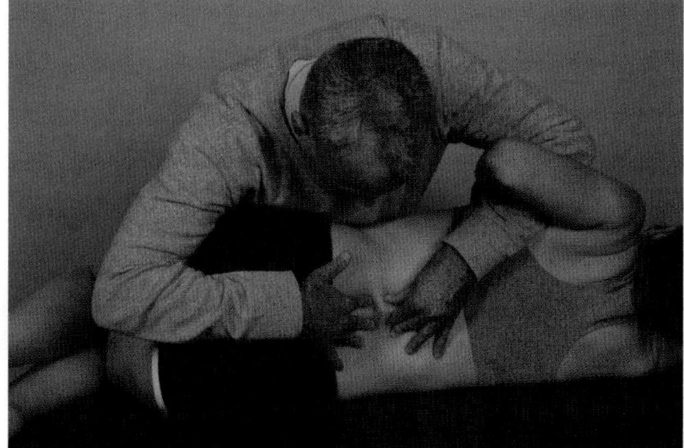

FIGURE 28-43 Passive articular mobility testing for extension.

hand and forearm (Fig. 28-41), thereby indirectly assessing the full superior linear glide of the superior segment. The quality and quantity of the joint glide are assessed.

Extension. The patient and clinician are positioned as in the PPIVM test, with the patient being positioned diagonally on the bed, hips forward, knees well flexed, and head resting on a pillow.

Having located the suspected level, the clinician extends the patient's spine to that level by pushing the patient's legs across the table until the monitoring finger detects motion at the superior spinous process. The superior spinous process of the segment is pinched (see Fig. 28-42) and the joint complex is passively taken into full extension by straddling the transverse processes, as for the flexion technique, and pushing the caudal vertebra anteriorly (see Fig. 28-43). At the end of the available range, the transverse processes of the inferior segment are glided in a cranial direction to test the full linear glide. The quality and quantity of the joint glide are assessed.

Side bending. The patient and clinician are positioned as in the PPIVM test, with the patient's hips forward, knees well flexed, and head resting on a pillow. The side on which the patient lies is determined by the intent of the technique.

- To test the ability of the segment to side bend ipsilaterally (close), the patient lies on the side to be tested.
- To test the ability of the segment to side bend contralaterally (open), the patient lies with the side to be tested uppermost.

Having located the suspected level, the clinician extends or flexes the patient's spine to that level by pushing the patient's legs across the table until the monitoring finger detects motion at the superior spinous process.

The clinician places the axilla of his or her caudal arm over the iliac crest of the patient, while the index and middle fingers of the hand are placed over the spinous processes of the inferior vertebra (Fig. 28-38). The clinician firmly squeezes the patient's pelvis and upper thigh with the caudal arm and applies a force in an inferior direction toward the patient's feet, while the middle finger of the caudal hand pushes the spinous process superiorly.

The quality and quantity of the joint glide are assessed and compared with the other side.

Rotation. The patient is positioned as in the PPIVM test. A small pillow or roll can be placed under the patient's waist to maintain the lumbar spine in a neutral position. The patient's pelvis and the inferior aspect of the caudal spinous process are fixed using the caudal arm and hand, respectively (Fig. 28-44). The thumb of the other hand is placed on the superior aspect of the cranial spinous process.

As the patient's thorax is rotated away, the spinous process of the upper segment should be felt to rotate toward the table,

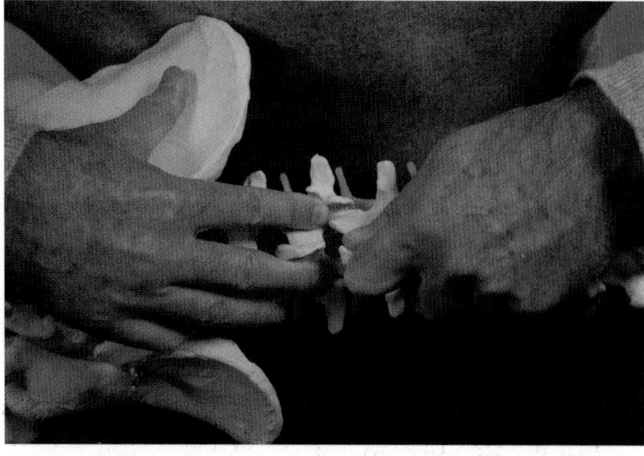

FIGURE 28-42 Passive articular mobility testing for extension showing stabilization.

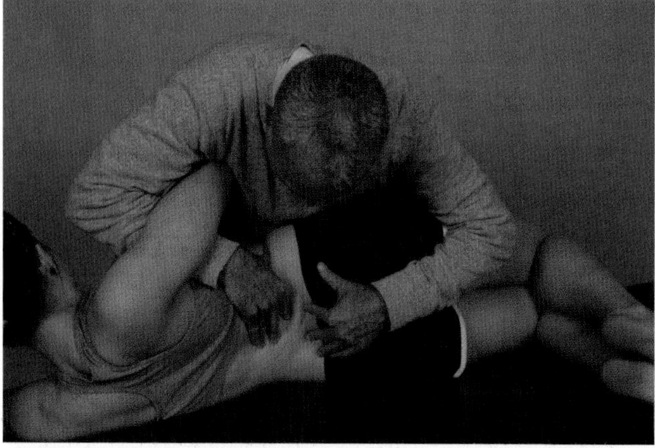

FIGURE 28-44 Passive articular mobility testing for rotation.

compared with the spinous process of the lower segment. The quality and quantity of the joint glide are assessed. The spine is returned to neutral each time, and the clinician progresses up the spine. The process is repeated with the patient side lying on the opposite side.

Functional Assessment Tools

Disability and the patient's ability to function may actually be more significant to health care costs than pain alone.[376] Several instruments have been produced in the past 30 years, which can provide reliable and valid methods to quantify a patient's functional status.[377]

Overall, no instrument is probably used more often for assessment of the low back than the Oswestry Low Back Disability Questionnaire (OLBDQ),[378] which has been widely researched and validated by investigators of spinal disorders (see Chap. 5).

The Roland–Morris Disability Questionnaire (RDQ)[379] (Table 28-14) is a health status measure, designed to be completed by patients to assess physical disability due to LBP. The RDQ was derived from the Sickness Impact Profile (SIP), which is a 136-item health status measure covering all aspects of physical and mental function.[380] Twenty-four items were selected from the SIP, and each item was qualified with the phrase "because of my back pain" to distinguish back pain disability from disability resulting from other causes—a distinction that patients are, in general, able to make without difficulty.[380,381]

Patients are asked to place a check mark beside a statement if it applies to them that day, and the score is calculated by adding up the number of items checked. Scores, therefore, range from 0 (no disability) to 24 (maximum disability). RDQ scores have been found to correlate well with other measures of physical function, including the physical subscales of 36-item Short Form Health Survey (SF-36), the SIP, and the OLBDQ.[380]

The Physical Impairment Index (PII), designed by Waddell et al.[235] is a series of seven tests, each scored positive or negative based on published cutoff values (Table 28-15) that tend to provide a measurement of physical impairment in patients with LBP. The final score of the PII ranges between zero and seven, with higher numbers indicating greater levels of impairment. Fritz and Piva[382] in a study of 78 patients with acute (<3 weeks duration) LBP found the PII to have a high interrater reliability (intraclass correlation coefficient = 0.89), and its validity was generally supported by the pattern of correlations. The minimum detectable change on the index was approximately one point.

Fear Avoidance Beliefs Questionnaire (FABQ)[383] (see Chap. 4) was developed, based on theories of fear and avoidance behavior, and focused specifically on patients' beliefs about how physical activity and work affected their LBP. Each item of the FABQ is scored 0–6, with higher numbers indicating increased levels of fear avoidance beliefs. Two subscales are contained within the FABQ: a seven-item work subscale (score range 0–42) and a four-item physical activity subscale (score range 0–24). The subscales of the FABQ have shown good reliability,[384] and previous studies have found the FABQ work subscale to be associated with current and future disability and work loss in patients with chronic[383,385,386] and acute[387] LBP.

TABLE 28-14 The Roland–Morris Disability Questionnaire

When your back hurts, you may find it difficult to do some things you normally do

This list contains sentences that people have used to describe themselves when they have back pain

When you read them, you may find that some stand out because they describe you *today*

As you read the list, think of yourself *today*. When you read a sentence that describes you today, put a tick against it. If the sentence does not describe you, then leave the space blank and go on to the next one

Remember, only tick the sentence if you are sure it describes you today

- ☐ I stay at home most of the time because of my back
- ☐ I change position frequently to try and get my back comfortable
- ☐ I walk more slowly than usual because of my back
- ☐ Because of my back I am not doing any of the jobs that I usually do around the house
- ☐ Because of my back, I use a handrail to get upstairs
- ☐ Because of my back, I lie down to rest more often
- ☐ Because of my back, I have to hold on to something to get out of an easy chair
- ☐ Because of my back, I try to get other people to do things for me
- ☐ I get dressed more slowly than usual because of my back
- ☐ I only stand for short periods of time because of my back
- ☐ Because of my back, I try not to bend or kneel down
- ☐ I find it difficult to get out of a chair because of my back
- ☐ My back is painful almost all the time
- ☐ I find it difficult to turn over in bed because of my back
- ☐ My appetite is not very good because of my back pain
- ☐ I have trouble putting on my socks (or stockings) because of the pain in my back
- ☐ I only walk short distances because of my back
- ☐ I sleep less well on my back
- ☐ Because of my back pain, I get dressed with help from someone else
- ☐ I sit down for most of the day because of my back
- ☐ I avoid heavy jobs around the house because of my back
- ☐ Because of my back pain, I am more irritable and bad tempered with people than usual
- ☐ Because of my back, I go upstairs more slowly than usual
- ☐ I stay in bed most of the time because of my back

Special Tests

Centralization. The patient either stands or lies prone depending on the intent of a loaded or unloaded assessment. Multiple directions of repeated end-range lumbar testing is targeted. Movements may include extension, flexion, or side flexion. Movements are repeated generally for 5–20 attempts until a definite centralization or peripheralization occurs. Centralization of symptoms is considered a positive finding for diskogenic symptoms. In a study by Donelson et al.,[296] the presence of centralization had a sensitivity of 92% and

TABLE 28-15 Physical Impairment Index Along with Scoring Criteria

Test	Performance	Scoring	
		Positive	**Negative**
Total flexion range of motion	The patient stands erect. The inclinometer is held at T12–L1, and the patient is asked to reach down as far as possible toward the toes, while keeping the knees straight.	Less than 87 degrees	Greater than or equal to 87 degrees
Total extension range of motion	The patient stands erect. The inclinometer is held at T12–L1. The patient is asked to arch backward as far as possible. The clinician may support the patient with one hand on the shoulder for balance.	Less than 18 degrees	Greater than or equal to 18 degrees
Average lateral flexion range of motion	The patient stands erect, with the inclinometer aligned vertically in line with the spinous processes of T9 and T12. The patient is asked to lean straight over to one side as far as possible, with the fingertips reaching straight down the side of the thigh. The clinician may support the patient's shoulder with one hand. The patient repeats the motion to the opposite side. Average lateral flexion is computed.	Less than 24 degrees	Greater than or equal to 24 degrees
Average straight leg raised range of motion	The patient is supine. In inclinometer is positioned on the tibial crest just below the tibial tubercle. The leg is raised passively by the clinician, whose other hand maintains a knee in extension. The leg is raised slowly to the maximum tolerated straight leg raise (not the onset of pain). The opposite leg is tested in the same manner. Average straight leg raising computed.	Males: less than 66 degrees Females: less than 71 degrees	Males: greater than or equal to 66 degrees Females: greater than or equal to 71 degrees
Spinal tenderness	The patient is prone with the back muscles relaxed. Palpation is done slowly without sudden pressure. Superficial tenderness to light-skinned pinch is a test first. The patient is asked "is that painful?" Any response other than "no" is a positive. If superficial tenderness is not present, deep tenderness is assessed by placing firm pressure with the ball of the thumb over the spinous processes and interspinous ligaments within 1 cm of the midline from T12 to S2. Again the patient is asked, "is that painful?" Any response other than "no" is a positive test.	Positive superficial or deep spinal tenderness	Negative superficial or deep spinal tenderness

(Continued)

TABLE 28-15 Physical Impairment Index Along with Scoring Criteria *(Continued)*

Test	Performance	Scoring: Positive	Scoring: Negative
Bilateral active straight leg raise	The patient is supine with the knees extended. The patient is asked to lift both legs together 6 inches off the examining surface and hold that position for 5 s. The clinician should not count aloud or offer encouragement. The patient may not use the hands to lift the legs. If the patient is unable to maintain the lifted position for 5 s, the test is positive.	Positive test	Negative test
Active sit-up	The patient is supine with the knees flexed to 90 degrees and the feet flat. The clinician should hold the patient's feet with one hand. The patient is instructed to reach out with the fingertips to touch (not hold) both knees and hold that position for 5 s. The clinician should not count aloud or offer encouragement. If the patient is unable to maintain the position for 5 s, the test is positive.	Positive test	Negative test

Data from Waddell G, Somerville D, Henderson I, et al: Objective clinical evaluation of physical impairment in chronic low back pain. *Spine* 17:617–628, 1992; Fritz JM, Piva SR: Physical impairment index: Reliability, validity, and responsiveness in patients with acute low back pain. *Spine* 28:1189–1194, 2003.

specificity of 64% (LR+ 2.6; LR− 0.12) as a predictor for symptomatic disks.

The Single-Legged Squat. The single-legged squat (Fig. 28-20) can be used as an indicator of lumbopelvic–hip stability. The test is functional, requires control of the body over a single weight-bearing lower limb and is frequently used clinically to assess hip and trunk muscular coordination and/or control.[388]

Loss of Extension. The patient lies in the prone position. The patient is asked to extend his or her lumbar spine while keeping the pelvis in contact with the treatment table. A positive test for diskogenic symptoms is moderate or major loss of extension. In a study by Laslett et al.[389] using visual observation only found that a loss of extension in predicting symptomatic disks had a sensitivity of 27% and specificity of 87% (LR+ 2.01; LR− 0.84).

Neurodynamic Mobility Testing. The slump, straight (Well) leg raise, bowstring, double straight leg raise, and prone knee flexion tests are described in Chapter 11.

Milgram's Test. Milgram's test is as much an assessment of abdominal muscle strength as it is intrathecal irritability.[275] With legs fully extended, the supine patient is asked to actively raise both feet approximately 2 inches off the table and maintain this position for at least 10 seconds and up to 30 seconds (Fig. 28-45). The inability to perform this test due to muscle weakness is not considered a positive finding within the context of this test, but should nevertheless still be charted.[275]

Posteroanterior Pressures. P-A pressures, advocated by Maitland,[390] are applied over the spinous, mammillary, and transverse processes of this region. The clinician should apply the P-A force in a slow and gentle fashion using the index and middle fingers of one hand, while monitoring the paravertebrals with the other hand (see Fig. 28-46).

Although these maneuvers are capable of eliciting pain, restricted movement, or muscle spasm, or a combination, they are fairly nonspecific in determining the exact level involved, or the exact cause of the symptoms, and have been found to

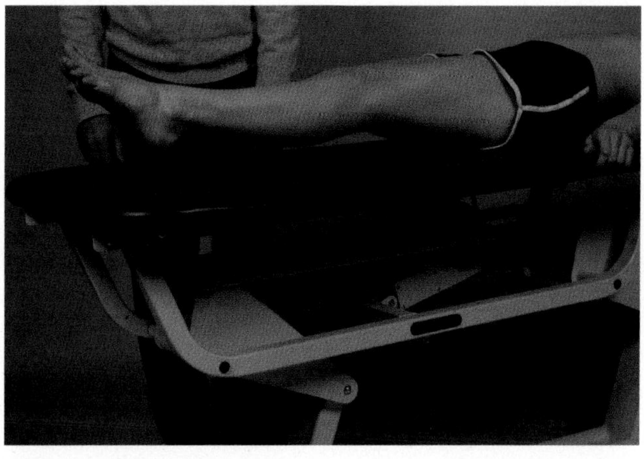

FIGURE 28-45 Milgram's test.

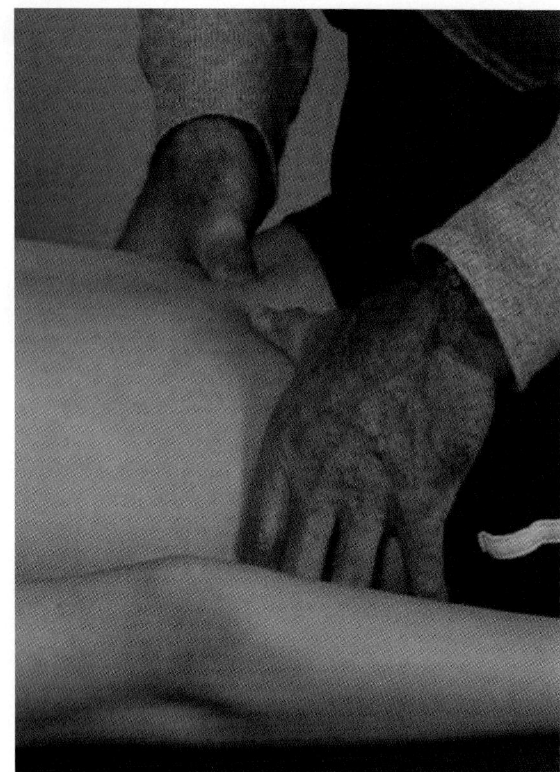

FIGURE 28-46 P-A pressures.

have poor interrater reliability in the absence of corroborating clinical data.[391,392] In a single-group repeated-measures interrater reliability study by Hicks et al.[393] to determine the interrater reliability of common clinical examination procedures proposed to identify patients with lumbar segmental instability, a consecutive sample of 63 subjects (38 women, 25 men; 81% with previous episodes of LBP) with current LBP was examined by three pairs of raters. The results of the study agreed with other studies, suggesting that segmental mobility testing is not reliable. In fact, in this study, the prone instability test (see later), Beighton–Horan Ligamentous Laxity Scale, and the presence of aberrant motion with trunk ROM demonstrated higher levels of reliability.

CLINICAL PEARL

The Beighton–Horan Ligamentous Laxity Scale[394] measures the following five elements:

- passive opposition of the thumb to the flexor aspect of the forearm (one point per hand);
- passive hyperextension of the fifth metacarpophalangeal joint beyond 90 degrees (one point per hand);
- hyperextension of the elbows by 15 degrees or more (one point per arm);
- hyperextension of the knees (one point per leg);
- forward flexion of the trunk with the knees extended and palms flat on the floor (one point).

All elements are added together to give an overall ligamentous laxity score ranging from 0 (*tight*) to 9 (*hyperlax*).

As a screening tool, the P-A pressures have their uses and can help detect the presence of excessive motion or spasm. However, caution should be exercised when making clinical decisions related to the assessment of motion at a specific spinal level using P-A accessory motion testing. Consider the following example with the patient positioned prone:

- A P-A pressure is applied simultaneously to both transverse processes of the L3 segment. Biomechanically, this produces a relative extension movement of the L2–3 segment, while producing a flexion movement of the L3–4 segment.
- If the spinous process of L3 is pushed to the right, inducing a left rotation of L3, this produces a relative right rotation of L2 on L3, but a left rotation of L3 on L4.

Anterior Stability Test. The patient is in the side-lying position. To test the lower three segments (L3–5), the patient's hips are placed in approximately 70 degrees of flexion and the knees are flexed (Fig. 28-47A). This position is to prevent tightening of the posterior lumbar ligaments, particularly the SSL, which could stabilize the lower three segments and produce a false-negative test result.[373] The clinician stands facing the patient, resting his or her thighs against the patient's knees. The upper segments are stabilized using the cranial hand and the other hand over it. The inferior interspinous space is palpated. The clinician pushes with the thighs, through the patient's knees, along the line of the femur (Fig. 28-47B). This produces a posteriorly directed force to the pelvis, sacrum, and lumbar spine. Any posterior movement of the inferior segment, which is actually a relative anterior movement of the superior segment on the inferior segment, is noted and compared with the next segmental level. There should be little or no movement. To test the upper two segments (L2 and L1), the lumbar spine is flexed by flexing the hips to approximately 100 degrees, and the procedure is repeated. A positive test is one in which there is excessive movement or pain, or both.

Lateral Stability Test. This test does not rely on the objectivity of the end-feel. Instead, an indirect shearing maneuver is used, and the reproduction of pain is considered a positive test.[360,373] The patient lies in the side-lying position facing the clinician, with the lumbar spine positioned in neutral and the hips and knees flexed to approximately 45 degrees. The clinician, using the fleshy part of one forearm, applies a downward pressure to the lateral aspect of the patient's trunk at the level of the L3 transverse process (Fig. 28-48). This produces a lateral translation of the entire lumbar spine in the direction of the bed. The pressure is applied until an end-feel is detected. The test is repeated with the patient side lying on the opposite side.

Prone Instability Test.[393] The patient is positioned prone so that the trunk rests on the bed and their feet rest on the floor, with the hips flexed and the trunk muscles relaxed. The clinician applies a P-A pressure (approximately 4 kg or thumbnail blanching) over the most symptomatic spinous process and any reproduction of symptoms is noted. The clinician then releases the P-A pressure, and the patient is asked to hold onto the sides of the table and to slightly lift his or her feet off the floor (Fig. 28-49). This maneuver produces a cocontraction of the global abdominal, gluteal, and erector

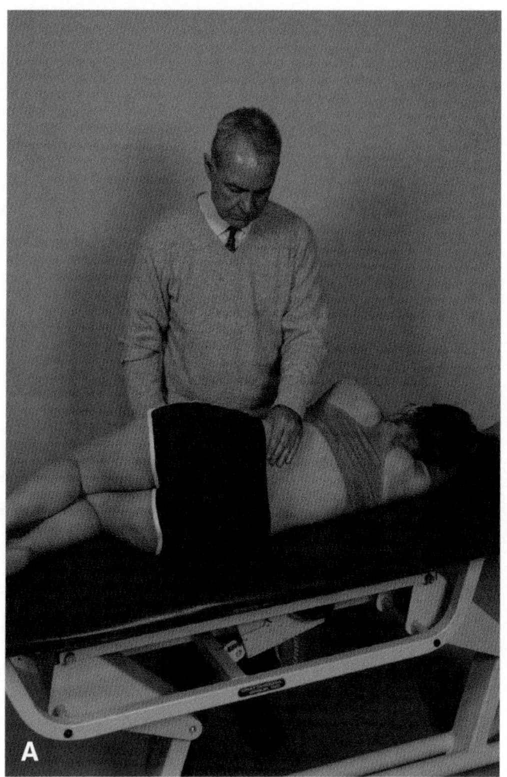

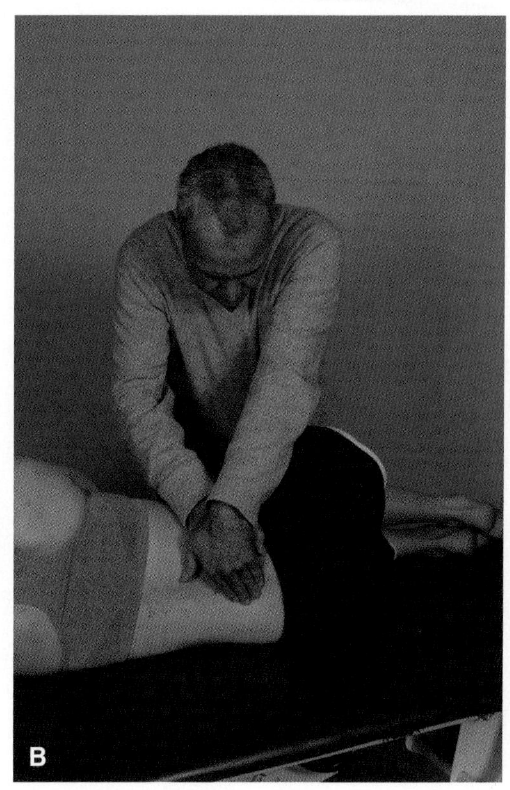

FIGURE 28-47 Anterior stability test. (**A**) Patient position. (**B**) Technique.

spinae muscles. While the patient maintains their feet off the floor, the clinician reapplies the P-A pressure over the same spinous process level. If a dramatic reduction or the complete elimination of the symptoms compared to the first application of P-A pressure is noted (the muscle activity must be able to effectively stabilize the segment), it is considered a positive prone instability test. According to Hicks et al.,[393] patients with LBP, who present with a *negative* prone instability test, are unlikely to respond to a stabilization exercise program.

Passive lumbar extension test.[395] The passive lumbar extension test is used to help detect lumbar spinal instability. The patient lies in the prone position, with the clinician standing at the foot of the bed. The clinician grasps the patient's ankles and, while applying a gentle traction force, raises both of the patient's lower extremities concurrently to a height of approximately 30 cm from the bed, while maintaining the knees extended (Fig. 28-50). Pain, apprehension, or a sense of heaviness in the low back are considered positive findings for this test. The test has been shown to have a sensitivity of 84.2% and a specificity of

FIGURE 28-48 Lateral stability test.

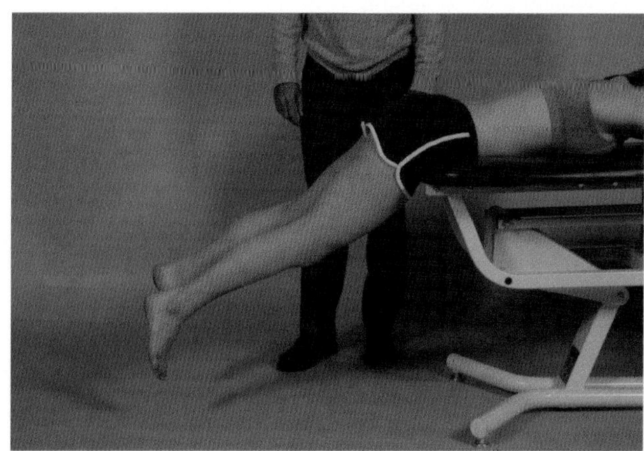

FIGURE 28-49 Prone instability test.

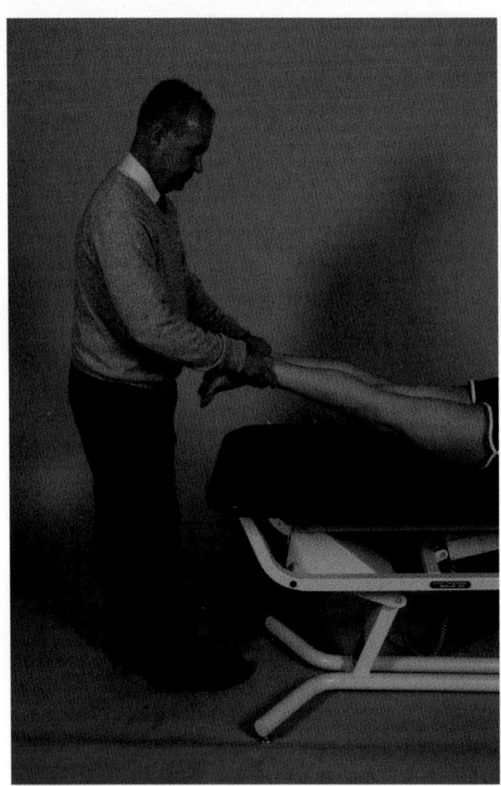

FIGURE 28-50 Passive lumbar extension test.

90.4%.[395] The positive likelihood ratio of the test was 8.84 (95% confidence interval = 4.51–17.33).[395]

CLINICAL PEARL

A recent systematic review[396] found that the majority of clinical tests routinely employed to diagnose structural lumbar segmental instability demonstrated only limited ability to do so. However, the same study reported that the passive lumbar extension test may be useful in orthopaedic clinical practice to diagnose structural lumbar segmental instability.

Imaging Studies

Plain radiography should be limited to patients with clinical findings suggestive of systemic disease or trauma. Guidelines recommend plain radiography for patients with fever, unexplained weight loss, a history of cancer, neurologic deficits, alcohol or injection–drug abuse, an age of more than 50 years, or trauma.[397] A major diagnostic problem with LBP is that many anatomic abnormalities seen on imaging tests, including myelography, CT, and MRI, are common in healthy individuals.[398,399] The high prevalence of these abnormalities in the absence of symptoms suggests that making causal inferences may be hazardous. In the absence of corresponding clinical findings (from the history and physical examination), these anatomic derangements seem to be irrelevant and inconsequential.[400]

Bulging disks viewed on MRI are commonly implicated as the cause of symptoms. However, bulging disks are more common than not after the age of 50 years and often have little, if any, association with symptoms.[400]

Examination Conclusions

Following the examination, a working hypothesis, or diagnosis, can be established based on a summary of all of the findings. For example, the tests and measures can help to determine

- the presence of a medical diagnosis, such as a spinal stenosis, ankylosing spondylitis, or an IVD protrusion;
- the presence of nonorganic signs. Inconsistencies occurring during the history and examination, which seem to be lacking in any somatic or organic base, have become known as *nonorganic* findings (see "Psychogenic Pain" section in Chap. 5). Nonorganic findings do not necessarily imply a nonexistent or fictitious condition. Waddell[401] developed a series of tests designed to elicit nonorganic responses from patients in whom psychosocial factors are suspected (see Chap. 5).

A pathology-based or biomechanical approach to LBP is based on the notion that LBP results from a deviation of the lumbopelvic complex from its normative physiologic and anatomic state and that by identifying a structural fault, and then correcting that fault, will lead to a dissipation of the signs and symptoms. Tables 28-16 through 28-18 summarize the typical findings in a patient with a biomechanical diagnosis, highlighting both the similarities and the differences between each. The difficulty in identifying a pathoanatomic cause for most patients with LBP has prompted efforts to identify alternative methods of subgrouping, or classifying, affected individuals based on clusters of examination findings. In 1995, Delitto et al.[402] published a treatment-based classification system (see Chap. 22) which proposed four classifications for patients with higher levels of disability, each with a distinct set of examination findings and an associated intervention strategy thought to optimize outcomes for patients in the category. The information gathered from the physical examination and patient self-reports of pain (pain scale and pain diagram) and disability (modified Oswestry Questionnaire) was used to determine whether the patient's condition would be amenable to physical therapy or whether care from another practitioner would be required. The problem with this classification system was that the clusters of examination findings used to make classification decisions and intervention strategies were principally derived from expert opinions and limited available evidence. In 2006, Fritz et al. published a report in an effort to update this decision-making algorithm. Inclusion criteria were age 18–65 years, referred to physical therapy with a primary complaint of LBP less than 90 days in duration with or without referral of symptoms into the lower extremity, and an Oswestry score greater than or equal to 25%. Patients were excluded if a lateral shift or acute kyphotic deformity was visible, if symptoms could not be reproduced with lumbar ROM or palpation, or when signs of nerve root compression were present (positive SLR test and reflex or strength deficits). Patients who were pregnant or had undergone prior surgery to the lumbosacral region were also excluded. A total of 123 patients were included in the trial. The goal of this RCT study was to test the hypothesis that a patient with LBP who received interventions matched to the patient's classification would have

TABLE 28-16 Reference Interpretation of Findings: Reduced Movement—Example 1

Myofascial	Joint/Pericapsular
Cause	*Cause*
Muscle shortening (scars, contracture, and adaptive)	Capsular or ligamentous shortening resulting from: scars Adaptation to a chronically shortened position Joint surface adhesions
Findings	*Findings*
Reduced movement or hypomobility may have insidious or sudden onset	Reduced movement or hypomobility may have insidious or sudden onset
Presence or absence of pain depends on level of chemical and/or mechanical irritation of local nociceptors, which in turn is a function of stage of healing	Presence or absence of pain depends on level of chemical and/or mechanical irritation of local nociceptors, which in turn is a function of stage of healing
Pain usually is aggravated with movement and alleviated with rest	Pain usually is aggravated with movement and alleviated with rest
Negative lower quarter scan	Negative lower quarter scan
PPIVM and PPAIVM findings	*PPIVM and PPAIVM findings*
Reduced gross PPIVM, but PPAIVM normal	Reduced gross PPIVM *and* PPAIVM
Intervention	*Intervention*
Muscle relaxation techniques, transverse frictions, and stretches	Joint mobilizations at specific level

PPAIVM, passive physiologic accessory intervertebral movement; PPIVM, passive physiologic intervertebral mobility.

TABLE 28-17 Interpretation of Findings: Reduced Movement—Example 2

Pericapsular/Arthritis	Disk Protrusion
Causes	*Cause*
Degenerative or degradative changes	Cumulative stress Low level but prolonged overuse Sudden macrotrauma
Findings	*Findings*
Negative scan	Positive lower quarter scan
Reduced gross PPIVM in all directions except flexion	Key muscle fatigable weakness
Active motion restricted in capsular pattern (decreased extension and equal limitation of rotation and side flexion)	Hyporeflexive deep tendon reflexes Sensory changes in dermatomal distribution Subjective complaints of radicular pain
PPIVM and PPAIVM findings	*PPIVM and PPAIVM findings*
Reduced gross PPIVM, but PPAIVM normal	Reduced gross PPIVM *and* PPAIVM
Intervention	*Intervention*
Capsular and muscle stretching	Traction
Active exercises and PREs	Active exercises into spinal extension
Anti-inflammatory modalities, if necessary	Positioning
Joint protection techniques	

PPAIVM, passive physiologic accessory intervertebral movement; PPIVM, passive physiologic intervertebral mobility; PRE, progressive resisted exercise.

better outcomes than those receiving unmatched interventions. The individual examination items used in the study included standing AROM, repeated extension in standing, repeated flexion in sitting, sustained extension in prone, a recording of the presence of centralization and/or peripheralization, SLR findings, assessment of aberrant movements during flexion/extension, prone instability test with P-A forces applied (see "Special Tests" section), and prone P-A glides. After completion of the baseline examination, patients were randomized into one of three intervention groups (manipulation, specific exercise, or stabilization) and referred to physical therapy. Reliability of ROM, centralization/peripheralization judgments with flexion and extension and the instability test was moderate to excellent. Reliability of centralization/peripheralization judgments with repeated or sustained extension or aberrant movement judgments was fair to poor. Overall agreement on classification decisions was 76% ($\kappa = 0.60$, 95% confidence interval 0.56, 0.64), with no significant differences based on level of experience (Table 28-19).

INTERVENTION STRATEGIES

A number of clinical studies have failed to find consistent evidence for improved intervention outcomes with many intervention approaches.[403] However, recent studies have demonstrated increasing evidence that the subacute-stage postinjury (4–12 weeks) is a critical period in preventing disability.[404]

It is essential that the impairments, functional limitations, and disability found during the examination guide the intervention and that the intervention should be dynamic, should direct the responsibility of the rehabilitative process toward the patient, and should have two principal objectives: to relieve

TABLE 28-18 Interpretation of Findings: Excessive Movement	
Hypermobility	**Instability**
Causes Cumulative stress resulting from neighboring Hypomobility Low level but prolonged overuse Sudden macrotrauma that is not enough to produce instability	*Causes* Sudden macrotrauma (ligamentous) Hypermobility allowed to progress (ligamentous) Degeneration of interposing hyaline or fibrocartilage (articular)
Findings Subjective complaints of "catching" Good days and bad days Symptoms aggravated with sustained positions Negative lower quarter scan	*Findings* Subjective complaints of "catching" Good days and bad days Symptoms aggravated with sustained positions Negative lower quarter scan
PPIVM findings Increase in gross PPIVM, with pain at end range	*PPIVM findings* Increase in gross PPIVM, with pain at end range Presence of nonphysiologic movement (positive stress test) Recurrent subluxations
Intervention Educate patient to avoid excessive range Take stress off joint (mobilize hypomobility) Anti-inflammatory modalities, if necessary Stabilize, if absolutely necessary	*Intervention* Falls into three areas: 1. Global stabilization a. Educate patient to avoid activities likely to produce instability b. Total body neuromuscular movement pattern reeducation c. Work or sports conditioning and rehabilitation 2. Local stabilization a. Muscular splinting of region (lifting techniques, twisting on feet, and chin tucking when lifting) b. Bracing with supports (collars, corsets, splints, and braces) c. Regional neuromuscular movement pattern reeducation 3. Segmental stabilization: PNF and active exercises to segment

PNF, proprioceptive neuromuscular facilitation; PPIVM, passive physiologic intervertebral mobility.

TABLE 28-19 Decision Making in Classification Patients into Interventions		
Classification Group	**Factors Favoring**	**Factors Against**
Manipulation	More recent onset of symptom Hypomobility with spring testing LBP only (no distal symptoms) Low FABQ scores (FABQ < 19)	Symptoms below the knee. No pain with spring testing Increasing episode frequency Peripheralization with motion testing
Stabilization	Younger age Positive prone instability test Aberrant motions present Greater SLR ROM Hypermobility with spring testing Increasing episode frequency Three or more prior episodes	Discrepancy in SLR ROM (>10 degrees) Low FABQ scores (FABQA < 9)
Specific exercise	Strong preference for sitting or walking Centralization with motion testing Peripheralization in direction opposite to centralization	LBP only (no distal symptoms) Status quo with all movements

FABQ, Fear Avoidance Beliefs Questionnaire.

the acute pain and to attempt prevention of transition to chronicity.[405]

ACUTE PHASE

In the acute phase of rehabilitation for the lumbar spine, the intervention goals are to

- decrease pain, inflammation, and muscle spasm;
- promote healing of tissues;
- increase pain-free range of segmental motion;
- regain soft tissue extensibility;
- regain neuromuscular control;
- allow progression to the functional phase.

The recommendations concerning bed rest for common, acute LBP have changed over the years.[406] In a 1986 study by Deyo et al.,[407] primary care physicians in the walk-in clinic of a public hospital found that the prescription of 2 days rest was equivalent to a prescription of 7 days in terms of pain and function. Moreover, a prescription of 2 days rest was associated with fewer days of sick leave. In 1995, Malmivaara et al.[408] showed that continuation of daily activity to the extent tolerable resulted in a more rapid recovery than either bed rest or back-mobilizing exercises. The most recent guidelines (2000), based on the results of several randomized studies, advise avoiding bed rest to the extent possible.[409] A study by Rozenberg et al.[405] found that for patients with acute LBP, normal activity is at least equivalent to bed rest. These authors recommended that prescriptions for bed rest, and thus for sick leaves, should be limited when the physical demands of the job are similar to those for daily life activities.[405]

Tissue loading during walking has been found to be below levels caused by many specific rehabilitation tasks, suggesting that walking is a wise choice as an initial aerobic exercise for general back rehabilitation.[483]

Pain relief may be accomplished initially by the use of modalities such as cryotherapy, electrical stimulation, and gentle exercises and occasionally by the temporary use of a spinal brace. Thermal modalities, especially ultrasound, with its ability to penetrate deeply, may be used after 48–72 hours. Patient education should be emphasized during this phase. Information about activities to avoid should be given, in addition to advice about adopting positions of comfort. Once the pain and inflammation are under control, the intervention can progress toward the restoration of full strength, ROM, and normal posture.

Manual techniques during this phase may include myofascial release, grade I and II joint mobilizations, massage, gentle stretching, and muscle energy techniques. Manual or mechanical traction may be used for patients with IVD herniations. Conflicting results from randomized trials and systematic reviews on the effectiveness of manipulation suggest that while some patients respond rather dramatically, others may not experience much improvement.[410] The variety of conclusions in trials of manipulation may be attributable to the failure of researchers to adequately consider the importance of classification. Studies by Flynn et al.[411] and Childs et al.[410] have identified a clinical prediction rule for classifying whether a patient will benefit from spinal manipulation. The five variables identified include

- current episode of LBP less than 16 days duration;
- no symptoms distal to the knee;
- less than 19 points on the FABQ;
- at least one hypomobile segment in the lumbar spine;
- at least one hip internal rotation greater than 35 degrees.

The spinal manipulation used was described as follows. The patient lies in the supine position with their hands clasped behind the neck, and the clinician stands on the side opposite to the site to be manipulated. The patient is passively side bent away from the clinician, by sliding the patient's pelvis toward the clinician. While stabilizing the pelvis against the table with one hand, the clinician then passively rotates the patient's trunk toward them using the other hand. A quick posterior and inferior thrust is then applied by the clinician to the ASIS.

In the Flynn et al. study, the presence of four out of five variables in the CPR increased the likelihood of success with spinal manipulation from 45% to 95%.[411] Using the same CPR, the Childs et al.[410] study compared with patients who were negative on the CPR and received exercise, the odds of a successful outcome among patients who were positive on the CPR and received manipulation were 60.8 (95% CI, 5.2–704.7). The odds were 2.4 (CI, 0.83–6.9) among patients who were negative on the CPR and received manipulation and 1.0 (CI, 0.28–3.6) among patients who were positive on the CPR and received exercise. A patient who was positive on the CPR and received manipulation has a 92% chance of a successful outcome, with an associated number needed to treat for benefit at 4 weeks of 1.9 (CI, 1.4–3.5).

Cleland et al.[412] used this CPR in a case series of patients with LBP, to assess its accuracy for predicting outcomes using other manipulation techniques. Eleven of the 12 patients (92%) in this case series, who satisfied the CPR and were treated with an alternative lumbar manipulation technique, demonstrated a successful outcome in two visits.[412] The study concluded that patients with LBP who satisfy the CPR may obtain a successful outcome with either manipulation technique directed at the lumbopelvic region.[412] The alternative lumbar manipulation technique used in this study was described as follows. The patient is positioned in side lying, and the clinician stands facing the patient. The clinician then flexes the patient's top leg until there is movement detected at the selected segmental interspinous space, at which point the patient's foot is placed in the popliteal fossa of the bottom leg. Next, the clinician grasps the patient's bottom shoulder and arm and introduces trunk side bending toward the table and contralateral rotation until motion is again felt at the specified interspinous space. Maintaining the patient's positional setup, the patient is rolled toward the clinician. Using the arm and body, the clinician applies a high-velocity, low-amplitude thrust of the pelvis in an anterior direction.

A few studies have included flexibility training.[413–415] Only one has showed that flexibility training in an increase in trunk extensor flexibility,[413] although this functional gain was only temporary.

FUNCTIONAL/CHRONIC PHASE

The goals of this phase are

- to achieve significant reduction or to complete resolution of the patient's pain;
- restoration of full and pain-free vertebral ROM;
- full integration of the entire upper and lower kinetic chains;
- complete restoration of respiratory function;
- restoration of thoracic and upper quadrant strength and neuromuscular control.

The number of physical therapy sessions required to provide relief for nonspecific LBP varies widely. The factors provided to explain this variance include the medical diagnosis, duration of the complaint, prior therapy, and the patient's age and gender.[416] Evidence on the effectiveness of physical therapy for the management of chronic spine disorders is limited. A systematic review by the Philadelphia Panel[417] suggested there was "good evidence to include stretching, strengthening, and mobility exercises" in treatment programs directed toward the management of chronic LBP. In the past decade, the results of randomized clinical trials on meta-analysis have provided various degrees of support for the efficacy of specific, nonsurgical physical interventions (that may be delivered by physical therapists) for the management of spine disorders. A number of studies have reported that intensive exercise reduces pain and improves function in patients with chronic LBP.[403,418,419] In addition, exercise programs that combine aerobic conditioning with specific strengthening of the back and legs can reduce the frequency of recurrence of LBP.[420] However, evidence on the efficacy of care specifically provided by physical therapists is more limited.[421–434] Although there is evidence to suggest that some interventions (e.g., exercise, spinal manipulation, massage) that may be delivered by a physical therapist are efficacious in the management of spine conditions, evidence on the efficacy of care specifically provided by physical therapist is less conclusive.[435] The RCTs that have been conducted are all limited because of small sample sizes, heterogeneous samples, or lack of standardized treatments.[435]

Three major exercise protocols for the management of LBP have emerged over the past 40 years: Williams flexion exercises,[436,437] McKenzie exercises,[286,438] and spinal stabilization exercises.[114,439–441] Despite the fact that these exercise protocols are commonly used in clinical practice to treat LBP, very few randomized control trials as to their effectiveness exist to date.[442]

WILLIAMS FLEXION EXERCISES

Dr. Paul Williams first published his exercise program in 1937 for patients with chronic LBP, in response to his clinical observation that the majority of patients who experienced LBP had degenerative vertebrae secondary to degenerative disk disease. According to Williams, "Man, in forcing his body to stand erect, severely deforms the spine, redistributing body weight to the back edges of the intervertebral disks in both the low back and neck."[436]

Conceptually, Williams believed that the goal of exercise was to reduce the lumbar lordosis or to flatten the back through strengthening exercises for the abdominal muscles (to lift the pelvis from the front) and strengthening exercises for the gluteal muscles (to pull the back of the pelvis down). Williams designed a group of six exercises to address these issues:

1. ***Trunk flexion or sit-up.*** Although the instructions that Williams gave to perform this exercise were erroneous, a variation of this exercise, the crunch, forms the cornerstone of many modern exercise protocols.
2. ***Posterior pelvic tilt.*** With the exception of patients with IVD lesions,[443] the posterior pelvic tilt exercise, outlined later, is still widely recommended. However, due to the fact that they can cause increased compression loads on the lumbar spine,[444] they should be prescribed with caution.
3. ***Trunk flexion or bilateral knees to chest.*** Like the posterior pelvic tilt exercise, this exercise is not recommended for patients with IVD lesions. However, it may provide comfort to patients with spinal stenosis.
4. ***Long sit and reach.*** This exercise is no longer recommended because of the stress it places on the soft tissues of the low back. Williams himself acknowledged that this exercise would not be appropriate for patients with sciatica.
5. ***Iliotibial band stretch in the front lunge position.*** Although adaptive shortening of the iliotibial band may be a contributing factor in LBP, as suggested by Williams, better stretches for this structure exist.
6. ***Stand to squat or stand to sit.*** This exercise was recommended because of its ability to strengthen the gluteal muscles. This exercise has since been incorporated into many spinal stabilization protocols.

Although the use of William's exercises has decreased over the years, the exercises are still indicated for those patients who experience an increase in symptoms when moving into spinal extension, and in those cases where the goal is to temporarily widen the intervertebral foramina and gap the zygapophyseal (facet) joints, thereby reducing nerve root compression.

McKenzie Approach

In many respects, the McKenzie approach (see also Chap. 22) contradicts Williams' basic assertions that the lumbar lordosis is harmful. McKenzie initially theorized that the development of LBP is primarily due to three predisposing factors: prolonged sitting in the flexed position, the frequency of flexion, and a lack of extension range.[286] As a result, the early versions of the McKenzie approach focused on regaining spinal extension. The McKenzie approach has since developed into a system that uses physical signs, symptom behavior, and their relation to end-range lumbar test movements to determine appropriate classification and intervention.

The physical examination component of the McKenzie method involves a comprehensive assessment of the patient, performed in a series of active and passive movements performed in the beginning, middle, and end ranges of trunk flexion, extension, and combinations of side bending and rotation called *side gliding*.[286] The same maneuvers are repeated with the trunk in the neutral position, shifted toward the side of pathology, and away from pathology. The intent is to gauge the responses, reactions, or effects of spinal loading, and for the presence of the centralization phenomenon. The patient's response to the examination determines a classification and the direction of preference for therapeutic exercise, with the direction chosen being based on the ability of the position or movement to centralize the patient's symptoms. The end-range exercises theoretically move the NP away from the side of compression loading, with flexion exercises moving the NP posteriorly and extension exercises moving the NP anteriorly.[286,445–450] The midrange exercises are better suited for patients with symptoms of neural compression.[451] Postural correction and maintenance of a normal lordosis are also integral parts of the McKenzie program.

The three major classifications or syndromes are postural, dysfunction, and derangement. Strategically speaking, when utilizing McKenzie protocols, one should rule out a derangement first before treating anything else.

Postural Syndrome

The key characteristics of the postural syndrome are[452]

- intermittent pain;
- time factor;
- pain produced by maintenance of posture/position;
- symptoms provoked by position, but not by movement;
- no deformity (relevant to pain);
- no loss of movement;
- no provocative signs/no pathology;
- aged 30 years and under (usually);
- sedentary workers (underexercised);
- often have cervical and thoracic pain also;
- often have days at a time without pain;
- no pain while active and moving;
- pain is local to the spine (not referred).

As the postural syndrome is not generally affected by mechanical maneuvers performed by the clinician or the patient, the focus of the intervention is to isolate and subsequently instruct the patient to avoid the offending position(s). The "slouch/overcorrect" maneuver is taught to the patient. The patient should sit on the edge of the chair and allow the lumbar spine to slouch into a fully flexed position and allow the head and chin to protrude. He or she must then smoothly move into a fully erect sitting position, achieving a maximal lumbar lordosis, with the head held directly over the spine and with a retracted chin.[452] This postural motion should be repeatedly performed from the position of "poor" (slouch) posture to the overcorrect position VIDEO.

Dysfunction Syndrome

The key characteristics of the dysfunction syndrome include[452]

- intermittent pain;
- no time factor;
- pain produced at end position or movement of shortened structures;
- pain relief with relief of stress/unloading shortened tissue;
- always a loss of function/movement;
- no deformity (not rapidly reversible);
- test movements reproduce pain but pain does not worsen as a result;
- over 30 years old except where trauma or derangement is causative factor;
- poor posture often underexercised.

The symptoms related to the dysfunction syndrome tend to be related to movement and become evident in the difficulty or inability of the patient to accomplish end range of movement, most frequently in the extremes of flexion and extension. The intervention goal for the dysfunction syndrome is the restoration of function or movement of the adaptively shortened tissue using frequent repetition of restricted end-range exercises. To achieve the lengthening of adaptively shortened soft tissues, the stretches need to be performed daily every 2–3 hours. This usually needs to be continued for a 4–6-week period or until the patient can fully stretch without any end-range pain. The following instructions must be given to the patient[452]:

- Stretch in the direction of movement loss and end-range pain.
- Allow elongation without microtrauma.
- Pain produced by stretching must stop shortly after release of stress (persisting pain afterward indicates overstretching).
- Peripheralization of symptoms should never occur.
- Stretching must be strong enough to reproduce discomfort or some pain.
- Must be performed regularly during the day (15 times/2 hours).

Derangement Syndrome

The key characteristics of the various derangement syndromes are

- often constant pain;
- time factors (diurnal cycle);
- pain brought on or increased by certain movements/positions (repetition/sustaining usually worsens pain);
- pain decreased or abolished by other movements/positions (repetition/sustaining usually improves the condition);
- always a loss of movement/function;
- deformity of kyphosis/scoliosis is common (derangements 2 and 4, respectively—see Chap. 22);
- deformity of accentuated lordosis uncommon (derangement 7—see Chap. 22).

McKenzie classifies derangement of the lumbar spine into seven categories on the basis of the location of symptoms and the presentation of fixed antalgias responsive to end-range loading in directions other than that within which complaints are caused.[286,453] Derangements that are considered to be *anterior* require strategies containing a flexion component, whereas those that are considered to be *posterior* involve strategies incorporating an extension component. In most cases, these may be conducted within the sagittal plane, but flexion and extension strategies may, in other cases, be combined with coronal or transverse motions for the best mechanical and symptomatic responses.[452] The theoretical model of the derangement syndrome involves the concept of displacement of the nucleus pulposus/annulus.

The intervention goal for the derangement syndrome is to reduce the derangement by altering the position/shape of the nucleus pulposus/annulus using restricted end-range loading for a prolonged period of time and then to maintain the reduction and aid recovery of function.[452] Mechanical treatment is dependent on the mechanical diagnosis for derangements. The interventions for derangements 1–7 are outlined in Table 28-20. The sequential extension progression advocated by McKenzie, initiated once the patient is able to tolerate prone lying (Fig. 28-17), involves prone on elbows (Fig. 28-51), prone push-up (Fig. 28-52) **VIDEO**, and extension in standing (Fig. 28-53) **VIDEO**.

The McKenzie method has been tested for intraobserver variability, with differing results.[297,327,454] In a recent study by Long et al.,[455] the McKenzie approach using exercise prescription based on a directional preference demonstrated significantly better outcomes than comparison groups performing exercise away from a directional preference.

Several outcome studies have examined the effectiveness of the McKenzie method compared with that of other approaches.[456–459] Ponte et al.[456] compared the effectiveness of the McKenzie method with that of the Williams approach and found that the McKenzie method demonstrated greater improvements in pain intensity and lumbar ROM than the Williams protocol. However, this study had a small sample size (22 subjects), and subjects were not randomly assigned but rather assigned by the referring physician to a treatment group.

Nwuga and Nwuga[457] also compared the effectiveness of the McKenzie method with that of the Williams approach. Sixty-two females, aged 20–40 years and all diagnosed with a prolapsed IVD in the lumbar spine, were assigned to either the McKenzie group or the Williams group. Similar conclusions were drawn from this study as from the Ponte study, namely that the McKenzie method demonstrated greater improvements in pain intensity and lumbar ROM than the Williams protocol.[457]

Stankovic and Johnell performed two separate outcome studies (1989 and 1994) that compared long-term patient outcomes following treatment with either the McKenzie approach or with patient education alone in a mini back school.[458,459] A mini back school involves education of the patient in the mechanics of the spine, proper posture, and safe lifting techniques. The 1989 study assessed six variables in 100 employed patients with acute LBP: return to work, sick leave during recurrences, recurrences of pain during the year of observation, pain, movement, and the patient's ability to self-help. The McKenzie method was found to be superior in four of the six variables. The two variables that showed no significant difference were sick leave during recurrences and patient's ability to self-help.[459] The 1994 study was a continuation of the 1989 study and used the same subjects. The later study showed that subjects who received McKenzie treatment had significantly fewer recurrences of pain and current episodes of sick leave compared with the subjects who received mini back school education.[458]

A randomized controlled comparative trial with an 8-month follow-up period was conducted by Petersen et al.,[432] which compared the effect of the McKenzie treatment method with that of intensive dynamic strengthening training in patients with subacute or chronic LBP. Two-hundred and sixty consecutive patients with LBP and at least 8 weeks duration of symptoms (85% of the patients had more than 3 months duration of symptoms) were randomized into two groups: Group A was treated with the McKenzie method ($n = 132$) and Group B was treated with intensive dynamic strengthening training ($n = 128$). The treatment period for both groups was 8 weeks at an outpatient clinic, followed by 2 months of self-training at home. Treatment results were recorded at the end of the treatment period at the clinic, then 2 and 8 months after. The study concluded that the McKenzie method and intensive dynamic strengthening training seem to be equally effective in the treatment of patients with subacute or chronic LBP.

The reasons for the positive measure changes observed in the McKenzie treatments remain unclear.[460] Schnebel et al.[451] suggested that the positive results might be related to activation of the gate control mechanisms or relaxation and/or decompression of neural tissues. Porterfield and DeRosa[461] believed that the application of controlled forces to the spine through active exercise or manual techniques might temporarily reduce pain levels by altering the fluid dynamics of injured tissue.

Spinal Stabilization Exercises

The basic premise in spinal stabilization (core strengthening, dynamic stabilization, trunk stabilization, and lumbopelvic stabilization) exercises is to teach the patient with LBP how to maintain functional levels by dynamically stabilizing the involved segments with increased muscular support. This increased muscular support can then be used to help maintain the neutral zone.

There is evidence suggesting that therapeutic exercise is effective in the treatment of nonspecific back pain,[462–465] although there is insufficient evidence to conclude with absolute certainty which theoretical mechanism of lumbar stabilization would be most beneficial in the management of patients with segmental lumbar instability.[90]

Before the stabilization progression can begin, the involved structures must be permitted to heal beyond the acute stage of healing. This can be achieved with patient education and with exercises that involve only lower and/or upper extremity motion, while avoiding specific trunk exercises and excessive trunk motion (see "Clinical Instability of the Lumbar Spine" section).

Stretching Exercises

Muscle flexibility should be addressed according to patient tolerance. In individuals suspected to have instability, stretching exercises should be used with caution, particularly ones

TABLE 28-20	Intervention of Derangements 1–7	
Derangement	**Description**	**Intervention**
1	Central or symmetrical pain across L4–5, with rarely buttock or thigh pain and no deformity This indicates a minor posterior disk disturbance	1. Reduction by application of extension principle 2. Maintenance of reduction by a. maintenance of lordosis b. sitting with lumbar support c. frequent performance of extension exercises 3. Recovery of function by a. flexion procedures (lying first), followed by extension procedures: prone lying (Fig. 25-20), prone on elbows (Fig.__new photo), prone push-up (Fig. __new photo), and extension in standing (Fig. __new photo). 4. Prophylaxis: a. Continuation of exercises as directed. Patients can self-treat b. Follow advice (especially regarding the avoidance of, or proper mechanics associated with, prolonged bending and sitting)
2	Central or symmetric pain across L4–5, with or without buttock and or thigh pain, with deformity of lumbar kyphosis Indicates a major posterior-central disk disturbance. A progression of derangement 1 and can easily worsen to a derangement 4 or 6	1. Reduction of deformity until the prone position can be obtained easily 2. Further treatment as for derangement 1
3	Unilateral or asymmetrical pain across L4–5 with or without buttock or thigh pain and no deformity A minor posterolateral disk disturbance A progression of derangement 1	1. Reduction as for derangement 1 2. If no centralization or reduction of pain occurs, the application of unilateral procedures is indicated. 3. Once centralization or reduction of pain is achieved, further treatment as for derangement 1
4	Unilateral or asymmetrical pain across L4–5 with or without buttock or thigh pain and with deformity of lumbar scoliosis Typically a major posterolateral disk disturbance and can be considered a progression of derangement 2 or 3	1. Reduction of derangement: a. Lateral shift correction for lateral component of derangement b. Extension procedures for reduction of posterior component c. Maintenance of lordosis for stabilization of reduction 2. If fol1owing reduction of deformity no centralization occurs the application of unilateral technique is necessary 3. Once centralization is achieved, further treatment as for derangement 1
5	Unilateral or asymmetrical pain across L4–5 with or without buttock or thigh pain. There is leg pain extending below the knee The pathogenesis is a posterolateral disk disturbance with impingement on nerve root and dural sleeve Progression of derangement 3 or 4 Intermittent sciatica may be caused by a disk bulge. Flexion in both standing and lying enhance pain; repetition worsens symptoms. It may be caused by an adhesive or tethered nerve root. This is labeled as an adherent nerve root and flexion in standing enhances pain but repetition does not necessarily worsen the symptoms	Treatment of an adherent nerve root: 1. Stretching by flexion procedures 2. Followed by extension procedures to prevent recurrence of derangement Treatment of disk bulge: reduction of derangement as treatment of derangements 1 or 3

(Continued)

TABLE 28-20 Intervention of Derangements 1–7 *(Continued)*		
Derangement	**Description**	**Intervention**
6	Unilateral or asymmetrical pain across L4–5 with or without buttock or thigh pain. There is leg pain extending below the knee and a deformity of sciatic scoliosis The most frequent cause is a major posterolateral disk disturbance with impingement on the nerve root and dural sleeve	If movement or postures/positions does not reduce sciatica: no treatment utilizing movement or positions is possible at this stage If sciatica is reduced by movement or positions then proceed with a reduction of deformity as with derangement 2 or further reduction as for derangements 3 and 1
7	A symmetrical or asymmetrical pain across L4–5 with or without buttock and/or thigh pain and a deformity of accentuated lordosis Involves an anterior or anterolateral disk disturbance	Reduction of derangement utilizing flexion procedures

The aim of the intervention in derangement syndrome is to reverse derangement 2–6 by shift correction or extension principle to resemble derangement 1 (centralization).

Data from Heffner SL, McKenzie R, Jacob G: McKenzie protocols for mechanical treatment of the low back. In: Morris C, ed. *Low Back Syndromes: Integrated Clinical Management.* New York, NY: McGraw-Hill, 2006:611–622.

encouraging end-range lumbar flexion.[388] Poor flexibility may cause excessive stresses to be borne by the lumbar motion segments. For example, adaptively shortened hip flexors and rectus femoris muscles can cause an extension and rotation hypermobility in the lumbar spine. Occasionally, stretching both the anterior and the posterior thigh muscles is beneficial. However, most of the time, only one should be stretched, and the decision is based on the diagnosis:

- The patient with spinal stenosis or a painful extension hypomobility, and who responds well to lumbar flexion exercises, should be taught how to stretch the hip flexors and rectus femoris while protecting the lumbar spine from excessive lordosis.
- The patient with a painful flexion hypomobility or IVD herniation, and who responds well to lumbar extension

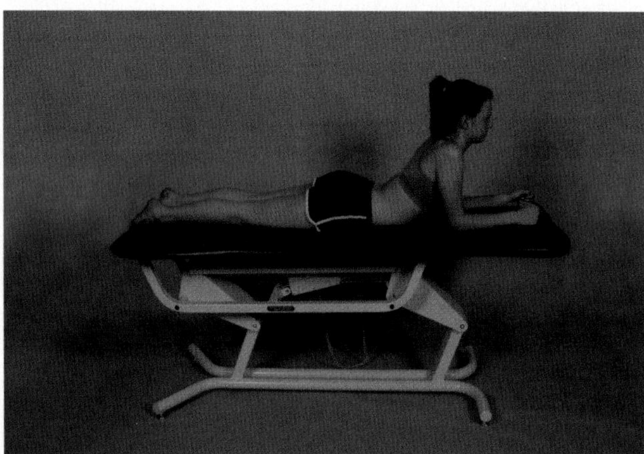

FIGURE 28-51 Prone on elbows.

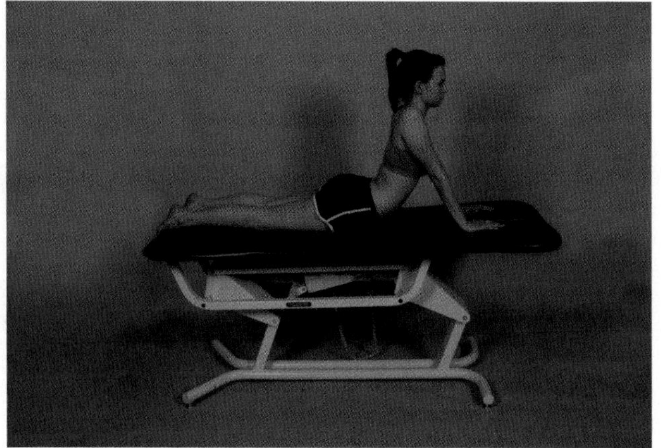

FIGURE 28-52 Prone push-up.

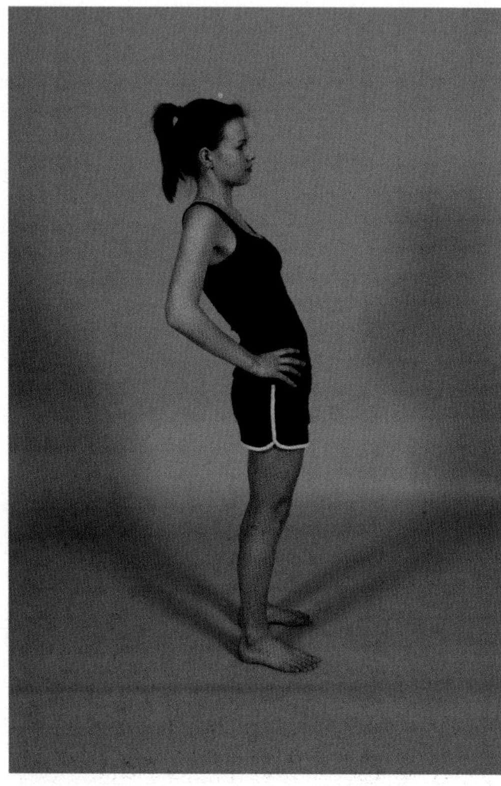

FIGURE 28-53 Extension in standing.

exercises, should be taught how to stretch the hamstrings while protecting the lumbar spine from flexing.

Stretches should be applied and then taught. The goal of stretching is to perform the technique, while maintaining the pelvis in its neutral zone, to avoid excessive anterior or posterior pelvic tilting.

Aerobic Exercise

The importance of aerobic exercise cannot be overemphasized, both in reducing the incidence of LBP[466] and in the intervention for patients who have LBP.[467] Aerobic fitness should be maintained. The following aerobic exercises may be used as tolerated:

- walking and jogging on soft, even ground;
- upper body ergonometer;
- indoor cross-country skiing machines;
- water aerobics.

Proprioceptive Neuromuscular Facilitation

Two of the more commonly used forms of proprioceptive neuromuscular facilitation (PNF) exercises in lumbar spine rehabilitation are rhythmic stabilization training (RST) and combination of isotonic (COI) exercises[468]:

- ***RST technique.*** Uses isometric contraction of antagonist pattern resulting in cocontraction of the antagonist if the isometric contraction is not broken by the clinician. It is used mainly to manage conditions in which weakness is a primary factor and in which stabilization provides stimulation of the agonistic pattern.[469]
- ***COI technique.*** Used to evaluate and develop the ability to perform controlled purposeful movements. It involves the performance of alternating concentric, eccentric, and isometric contractions and is used to treat deficiencies in strength and ROM.[470]

Although previous studies have shown that isometric training can have positive effects on back pain,[468,471] information on the effectiveness of dynamic and combined dynamic–static contraction exercises for trunk muscle stabilization and strength is scarce. Kofotolis and Kellis[468] examined the effects of RST and COI on trunk muscle endurance, flexibility, and functional performance in subjects with chronic LBP. Eighty-six women (40.2 ± 11.9 [mean ± SD] years of age) who had complaints of chronic LBP were randomly assigned to three groups: RST, COI exercises, and control. Subjects were trained with each program for 4 weeks, with the aim of improving trunk stability and strength. The exercises were performed with the patient in sitting over the edge of the treatment table and consisted of the subject flexing and then extending the trunk against the clinician's variable manual resistance and maintaining static positions for 5 seconds. Multivariate analysis of variance indicated that both training groups demonstrated significant improvements in lumbar mobility (8.6–24.1%), static and dynamic muscle endurance (23.6–81%), and Oswestry Index (29.3–31.8%) measurements, suggesting that static and dynamic PNF programs may be appropriate for improving short-term trunk muscle endurance and trunk mobility in patients with chronic LBP.

Back School

Several back schools and back rehabilitation programs have been developed to teach people proper lifting technique and body mechanics. These programs are aimed at groups of patients. They include the provision of general information on the spine, recommended postures and activities, preventative measures, and exercises for the back.

The efficacy of back schools, however, remains controversial.[472,473] Cohen et al.[474] concluded that there is insufficient evidence to recommend group education for people with LBP.

PRACTICE PATTERN 4E: IMPAIRED JOINT MOBILITY, MOTOR FUNCTION, MUSCLE PERFORMANCE, AND ROM ASSOCIATED WITH LOCALIZED INFLAMMATION

Ligament Tears

As with those elsewhere in the body, ligament tears of the lumbar spine are normally traumatically induced. Knowledge of the various restraints to the various motions of the lumbar spine can aid in determining which ligament has the potential to be sprained with a given mechanism.

Iliolumbar Ligament Sprain

The iliolumbar ligament, an extremely important structure that stabilizes the lumbar spine on the sacrum and functions to anchor the L5 vertebra onto the S1 vertebral body,[73] is commonly injured.

The iliolumbar ligament sprain, also known as the iliac crest syndrome, has a classic presentation of lower lumbar pain just at or above the medial iliac crest area, with radiation sometimes down the leg. On examination, the SLR and Patrick (FABER) sign are both usually negative; there is no weakness or sensory impairment, and no radicular signs. The diagnosis is confirmed by deep palpation of the iliolumbar ligament in an attempt to reproduce the patient's discomfort. Njoo et al.[475] have provided evidence of good interobserver validity in the diagnosis of this problem in a prospective manner. A single injection of lidocaine and steroid provides effective and sustained treatment to this readily accessible area.[476]

Muscle Contusions, Strains, and Tears

Muscle injuries are associated with a history of trauma and are capable of producing a significant degree of discomfort. Two sites are commonly involved in the lumbar region, and strains and tears can occur with relatively little trauma there[477]

1. The point where the erector spinae group of muscles joins to their common tendon just above and medial to the posterior superior iliac spines.
2. At the gluteal origin on the ala of the ilium, just lateral to the posterior superior iliac spines.

However, muscle pain can also be produced from excessive muscle activity or muscle guarding, which follows an injury to the spine. The intervention for muscle tears involves a gradual and controlled resumption of movements and activities.

Diastasis Recti Abdominis

The female anatomy undergoes tremendous changes during the childbearing year.[478] The musculoskeletal changes that may occur during this time include increased ligament laxity, pelvic floor dysfunction, and diastasis recti abdominis (DRA) (see Chap. 30).[109]

It is important for physical therapists to learn the screening skills and know that a DRA has a potential impact on the stability of the pelvis on a long-term basis.

PRACTICE PATTERN 4F: IMPAIRED JOINT MOBILITY, MOTOR FUNCTION, MUSCLE PERFORMANCE, AND ROM OR REFLEX INTEGRITY SECONDARY TO SPINAL DISORDERS

Piriformis Syndrome

The sciatic nerve usually travels below the piriformis. In approximately 15% of the population, however, either the tibial part of the sciatic nerve passes through the belly of the piriformis muscle or the piriformis has two muscle bellies and the nerve passes between the two bellies. Consequently, contraction or tightness of the muscle can often produce radicular symptoms (see Chap. 5).

Piriformis syndrome usually is a diagnosis of exclusion once the more common causes of sciatica have been ruled out.[479] Robinson[480] listed six cardinal features of piriformis syndrome: (1) a history of trauma to the sacroiliac and gluteal regions; (2) pain in the region of the sacroiliac joint, greater sciatic notch, and piriformis muscle, extending down the lower limb and causing difficulty in walking; (3) acute exacerbation of the symptoms by lifting or stooping; (4) a palpable, sausage-shaped mass over the piriformis muscle, during an exacerbation of symptoms, which is markedly tender to pressure (this feature is pathognomonic of the syndrome); (5) a positive result on the SLR test; and (6) gluteal atrophy, depending on the duration of symptoms.[479]

The intervention for piriformis syndrome depends on the suspected pathology. If muscular spasm and tightness is the suspected etiology, then an aggressive stretching and massage of the piriformis program should be instituted.[481] If this conservative approach fails, a local anesthetic block to the muscle should be considered. Surgical neurolysis is considered for recalcitrant cases.

Entrapment Neuropathy of the Medial Superior Cluneal Nerve

The cutaneous innervation of the lower lumbar and gluteal regions has been attributed to the posterior (dorsal) rami of L1–L3. Maigne and Maigne[482] observed that the cutaneous innervation of the gluteal region is derived from higher levels of the thoracolumbar region, that is, from T11 to L1. Anastomoses between these nerves are also common. Superior cluneal nerve injury is a well-known cause of chronic pain complicating bone graft harvesting from the posterior iliac crest for spinal fusion.[483,484] The medial superior cluneal (MSC) nerve is the most medial nerve of these nerves. The MSC usually crosses the posterior iliac crest at a distance of approximately 7 cm from the midline.[485] At that point, it becomes superficial by passing through an osseofibrous tunnel, formed by the thoracolumbar fascia cranially and the rim of the posterior iliac crest caudally.[485] This tunnel is occasionally a site of compression for the MSC nerve.[482]

According to Maigne,[485] MSC nerve entrapment can be diagnosed and treated using the following criteria:

- a trigger point over the posterior iliac crest, located 7 cm from the midline (corresponding to the nerve compression zone);
- relief of symptoms by nerve block.

INTEGRATION OF PRACTICE PATTERNS 4H AND 4I: IMPAIRED JOINT MOBILITY, MOTOR FUNCTION, MUSCLE PERFORMANCE, ROM ASSOCIATED WITH FRACTURES, JOINT ARTHROPLASTY, AND SOFT TISSUE SURGICAL PROCEDURES

Spondylolysis

Spondylolysis is a defect of the pars interarticularis of the spine. The actual defect in the pars covers a broad range of etiologies, from stress fracture to a traumatic bony fracture with separation.[486] Patients with bilateral pars defects can progress to spondylolisthesis (see the next section).

The exact cause of spondylolysis is unknown, but it is likely related to congenital, acquired (repeated microtrauma), or developmental causes. Spondylolysis commonly is asymptomatic, making diagnosis extremely difficult. Those patients with symptoms often have pain with extension and/or rotation of the lumbar spine. Patients with suspected spondylolysis should be evaluated initially with plain radiography, consisting of anteroposterior, lateral, and oblique views of the lumbar spine. The lateral views are most sensitive for detection of pars fractures, and the oblique views are the most specific.[486,487] If plain radiographs are negative or inconclusive, further imaging may be warranted. Currently, controversy surrounds the questions as to whether MRI, CT, and single-photon emission CT bone scintigraphy are best to further evaluate these patients.[488–490]

The initial management of a patient with spondylolysis is conservative. In a meta-analysis performed by McNeely et al.,[491] the efficacy of physical therapist intervention in the treatment of spondylolysis and spondylolisthesis was systematically reviewed. Of the 71 potential studies, only two of the studies met the relevance criteria of the critical appraisal.[486]

Spratt et al.[492] examined the efficacy of trunk extension and flexion treatment programs on 56 patients with radiographic instability (retrodisplacement or spondylolisthesis).[486] Subjects were randomly assigned to one of three groups: a flexion, an extension, or a control group. The flexion and extension groups performed exercises biased into flexion or extension, respectively.[486] At the 1-month follow-up, no treatments were shown to alter ROM or trunk strength. However, patients in the extension group reported less pain, as compared with patients in the flexion and control groups.[486,492] In a study by O'Sullivan et al.,[190] 45 subjects with spondylolysis or spondylolisthesis were divided into two groups: a group that underwent 10 weeks of rehabilitation, with a focus on training of the deep abdominal muscles, and a control group that underwent treatment as directed by their treating practitioner.[486] The group that underwent specific abdominal exercise training had a reduction in pain and disability levels, which was maintained at a 30-month follow-up.[486] The control group showed no significant change throughout the study.[190]

Based on these studies, the physical therapy intervention should strive to correct any muscle imbalances (adaptively shortened hip flexors), increase trunk muscle strength, and educate the patient to avoid activities involving excessive impact and activities involving lumbar hyperextension. Bracing may also be advocated.

Surgical intervention is indicated only after patients have failed conservative management.

Spondylolisthesis

The term spondylolisthesis refers to an anterior slippage and inability to resist shear forces of a vertebral segment in relation to the vertebral segment immediately below it, which usually occurs in the lumbar spine. The most common site for spondylolysis and spondylolisthesis is L5–S1.[423] Frequently, spondylolisthesis leads to spinal instability—the inability of the spine to maintain its normal pattern of displacement when placed under physiologic load.[31] Under normal conditions, the anterior slippage of the vertebra is resisted by the bony block of the posterior facets, by an intact neural arch and pedicle, and, in the case of the L5 vertebra, by the iliolumbar ligament. Age appears to be an important factor in the natural history of spondylolisthesis. Children younger than 5 years of age rarely present with spondylolysis, and severe spondylolisthesis is equally rare. The period of most rapid slipping is between the ages of 10 and 15 years, with no more slipping occurring after the age of 20.[299] In the adolescent spine, the zygapophyseal joints are more horizontal than in the adult's allowing more side flexion and rotation, and causing the lumbar disk and posterior column structures to sustain a greater responsibility for mobility control.[493] Higher grade spondylolisthesis is twice as common in girls as in boys, and is approximately four times more common in women than men.[494]

The etiology of spondylolisthesis has been discussed extensively in the literature.[76,190,299,487,495–505] Newman[502] described five groups represented by this deformity, based on etiology:

1. ***Congenital spondylolisthesis.*** This type results from dysplasia of the fifth lumbar and sacral arches and zygapophyseal joints.
2. ***Isthmic spondylolisthesis.*** This type is caused by a defect in the pars interarticularis, which can include a fracture or elongation of the pars.
3. ***Degenerative spondylolisthesis.*** This type usually affects older people and occurs most commonly at the L4–5 level. This type is perhaps the most commonly encountered by the orthopaedic physical therapist.
4. ***Traumatic spondylolisthesis.*** This type occurs with a fracture or acute dislocation of the zygapophyseal joint and is fairly rare.
5. ***Pathologic spondylolisthesis.*** This type can result from a pathologic process causing a weakening of the pars, pedicle, or zygapophyseal joint.

Spondylolisthesis acquisita, a sixth etiologic category, was added to represent the slip caused by the surgical disruption of ligaments, bone, and disk.

There are two prevailing theories as to the etiology of degenerative spondylolisthesis:

1. ***Dysfunction of the IVD.***[504] The IVD at the level of the spondylolisthesis is subjected to considerable anteriorly directed shear forces and is the main structure that opposes these shear forces, functioning to prevent against further slippage and keeping the spinal motion segment in a stable equilibrium. It is postulated that slip progression after skeletal maturity is almost always related to IVD degeneration at the slip level. As the biochemical integrity of the IVD is lost, the lumbosacral slip becomes unstable and progresses. Disk degeneration at the slip level and adult slip progression are likely to develop during the fourth and fifth decades of life. This unstable mechanical situation leads to symptoms of low back and sciatic pain and may necessitate spinal instrumentation and fusion.
2. ***Horizontalization of the lamina and the facets or sacrum morphology.***[506] A more trapezoidal shape of the vertebral body, or a dome-shaped contour of the top of the sacrum, or both, are found in individuals with slipping. There is also a greater anterior flexion of the lumbar spine than in "normal" individuals of comparable age.[500] A sagittal orientation of the facet joints also could predispose the vertebra to slip.[497]

Other factors such as the lumbosacral angle, ligamentous laxity, previous pregnancy, and hormonal factors impose an increased stress on the L4–5 facet joints, and, as most of the stress is placed anteriorly on the inferior facet of L4, the wear pattern is concentrated at this point, creating a more sagittally orientated joint by way of remodeling.[499]

Whatever the cause, if the syndesmosis maintains the bonds between the two halves of the neural arch, there is no mechanical instability and the patient is asymptomatic, whereas if the syndesmosis is loose, separation occurs during flexion. Repetitive motions that cause fatigue may advance to an acute, spontaneous pars interarticularis weakening, stress fracture, or fracture and a predilection for spondylolisthesis.[493]

Spondylolisthesis is graded according to the percentage of slip. Slip percentage is the distance from a line extended along the posterior cortex of the S1 body to the posteroinferior corner of the L5 vertebra,[507] divided by the anteroposterior diameter of the sacrum. Grading is then performed using the Meyerding classification[508] as follows: grade I, 1–25%; grade II, 26–50%; grade III, 51–75%; grade IV, 76–100%; and grade V (spondyloptosis) more than 100%.

The possible pathologic changes at the adjacent instability segment include instability of the motion segment, IVD space narrowing, and stenosis caused by facet degeneration and ligament flavum hypertrophy.[509] Degeneration of the IVD above or below a surgical fusion, and damage to the posterior ligament complex, may also contribute to the development of the lesions, by reducing resistance to shearing forces at the intervertebral level next to the fusion.[509]

The symptoms, if they do occur, usually begin in the second decade. However, there is often no correlation with the degree of slip and the level of symptoms. This is because the anterior slippage of the vertebral body usually results in intervertebral foramen enlargement initially. It is only when the neural arch rotates on the pivot formed by its articulation with the sacrum, or there are anterior osteophytes, that encroachment occurs, resulting in nerve root irritation. Onset during adolescence is often accompanied by an insidious clinical manifestation, exacerbated with lumbar extension and rotation activities and is usually painful but not disabling.[510] Clinically, these patients complain of chronic midline pain at the lumbosacral junction, which is mechanical in nature. Mechanical pain is worsened with activity and alleviated with rest. The symptoms can be exacerbated by repetitive extension and torsion activities.[510] Patients may also complain of leg pain, which can have a radicular-type pattern or, more commonly, will manifest as neurogenic claudication. The spectrum of neurologic involvement runs from rare to more common in the higher grade slips, with the majority of neurologic deficits being an L5 radiculopathy with an L5–S1 spondylolisthesis, but cauda equina impairments can occur in grade III or IV slips. If neurogenic claudication is present, the patient may complain of bilateral thigh and leg tiredness, aches, and fatigue.[498] ROM for flexion of the lumbar spine frequently is normal with both types of claudication. Some patients are able to touch their toes without difficulty. Strength and sensation are usually intact in the lower extremities. The muscle stretch reflexes generally will be normal or diminished. If hyperreflexic symptoms and other upper motor neuron signs, such as clonus or a positive Babinski test, are found, the cervical, thoracic, and lumbar spine should be investigated to rule out a lesion of the spinal cord or cauda equina. Questions regarding bicycle use versus walking can help the clinician to differentiate neurogenic from vascular claudication. Both cycling and walking increase symptoms in vascular claudication due to the increased demand for blood supply. However, patients with neurogenic claudication worsen with walking but are unaffected by cycling due to the differing positions of the lumbar spine adopted in each of these activities. Patients with neurogenic claudication are far more comfortable leaning forward or sitting, which flexes the spine, than walking.[503] The position of forward flexion increases the anteroposterior diameter of the canal, which allows a greater volume of the neural elements and improves the microcirculation. A check of distal pulses is important to rule out any coexisting vascular insufficiency. Findings such as hairless lower extremities, coldness of the feet, or absent pulses are signs of peripheral vascular disease. Sensory defects in a stocking–glove distribution are more suggestive of diabetic neuropathy.

A common clinical manifestation is increased lumbar and hamstring muscular tone, which may be associated with a compensatory response secondary to ineffective stabilization of the painful spinal segment.[510]

Differential diagnosis includes coexisting osteoarthritis of the hip, myelopathy, spinal tumors, and infections.

Differential diagnosis of clinical instability associated with spondylolisthesis often requires several clinical and diagnostic tests.[510] Radiographic findings for these patients can be misleading. Multiple scans including different radiographic views are necessary to avoid imaging era, and failure to investigate lateral and oblique views may lead to misdiagnosis in 20% of cases.[511] In a lateral view, taken while the patient is supine, the forward displacement often appears trivial, because it is only when the patient is standing that the true degree of slip is appreciated. Consequently, if spondylolisthesis is suspected, a lateral spot view of the lumbosacral junction must be taken while the patient stands upright, and during flexion and extension of the trunk.[501] However, a patient with LBP who demonstrates a spondylolisthesis on radiograph may have an asymptomatic spondylolisthesis, and therefore the source of the back pain requires further investigation. Some authors have suggested that manual palpation is effective in detecting spine instability, simply by determining if the motion is greater than that found with hypermobility.[512,513] However, little evidence exists to support the reliability of palpation mechanisms for spinal instability assessment.[510,514,515]

The intervention for spondylolisthesis depends on the presenting symptoms, rather than the degree of slip, and ranges from conservative to surgical. Conservative intervention is more likely to be successful in the case of a limited slip and sparse clinical findings. Such an approach includes pelvic positioning initially to provide symptomatic relief, followed by an active lumbar stabilization program (Table 28-21), and stretching of the rectus femoris and iliopsoas muscles to decrease the degree of anterior pelvic tilting.

In those cases where conservative measures do not provide adequate relief, or the neurological signs and symptoms appear to be progressing, surgery may be required. During the past decade, numerous patients with lumbar degenerative spondylolisthesis have been treated with decompression and fusion with or without instrumentation.[509] A high fusion rate and satisfactory clinical outcome have been reported. However, a few patients present with recurrent back pain and sciatica after surgery. The possible causes of postoperative pain include inadequate decompression, fibrosis, recurrent IVD herniation, adjacent stenosis.[509] Ironically, another cause of postoperative pain is instability of those segments above and below the fusion site.[87]

Lumbago

The term *lumbago* is used to describe local back pain of a diskogenic origin but also can be used to describe a sudden onset of persistent LBP, marked by a restriction of lumbar movements and reports of "locking." The mechanism of mechanical locking is still a contentious issue.[58,129,516] The severity of each episode varies, from incapacitating to minor

TABLE 28-21 A Three-Phase Rehabilitation Program for a Grade 1 Spondylolisthesis

Phase 1	Phase 2	Phase 3
Abdominal isometrics (in neutral, diagonal, and straight planes)	Continued progression of exercises from Phase 1	Continued progression of exercises from Phase 1 and 2
Cocontraction of multifidi and abdominals in flexion	Contralateral arm and leg raises in prone Prone trunk lifts on the Physioball	Increase in distal weighting and lever length using resistance
Isometric abdominal exercises in hook lying	Rhythmic marching during supine stabilization on Physioball	Multifidi exercises in prone
Multifidi contraction in a flexed position		Sitting and standing exercises with outside resistance to target cocontraction during functional activities
Resisted isometrics using cane (to isolate transverse abdominis) in supine	Abdominal crunches on the Physioball Abdominal stabilization during oblique lever changes	Nonlocal muscle strengthening
Cocontraction of the spine during ADLs	Cocontraction of the spine during ADLs	

Data from Cook C, Cook A, Fleming R: Rehabilitation for clinical lumbar instability in a female adolescent competitive diver with spondylolisthesis. *J Man Manip Ther* 12:91–99, 2004.

discomfort. Although it can occur at any age, lumbago typically affects patients between the ages of 20 and 45 years. The mechanism of injury usually involves a sudden unguarded movement of the lumbar spine, involving either flexion or extension combined with rotation or side bending.

Hypomobilities can be classified as symmetric or asymmetric. If both sides of the joint are involved, the lesion is symmetric, whereas if only one side is involved, the lesion is asymmetric.

INTEGRATION OF PREFERRED PATTERNS 4BAND 4F: IMPAIRED JOINT MOBILITY, MOTORFUNCTION, MUSCLEPERFORMANCE, ROM SECONDARY TO IMPAIRED POSTURE, SYSTEMIC DYSFUNCTION (REFERRED PAIN SYNDROMES), SPINAL DISORDERS, AND MYOFASCIAL PAIN DYSFUNCTION

Postural Syndromes of the Lumbar Region

Symmetric impairments of the lumbar spine occur as a result of either acute pain or myofascial and articular tissue shortening from a fixed postural impairment.[86,134,183,187]

A symmetric impairment will not be apparent in the flexion and extension position tests, because, as both are equally impaired, there is no deviation from the path of flexion or extension, but rather the path is shortened or lengthened, depending on which type of impairment (hypomobility or hypermobility) is present. In addition, there is no apparent loss of side bending or rotation, and both sides appear equally hypomobile or hypermobile, with no change in the axis of rotation, except in the case where it ceases to exist, as in bony ankylosis.

Lower Crossed Syndrome[134,517]

In this syndrome, the erector spinae and the iliopsoas are tight, and the abdominal and gluteus maximus are weak (see Chap. 6). This syndrome results in an anterior pelvic tilt, an increased lumbar lordosis, and a slight flexion of the hip. A number of muscles are adaptively shortened in this syndrome, including the gastrocnemius, soleus, hip adductors, and hip flexors. The hamstrings also are frequently shortened in this syndrome, and this may be a compensatory strategy to lessen the anterior tilt of the pelvis[518] or a result of the weak glutei. Common injuries associated with this syndrome include hamstring strains, anterior knee pain, and LBP.

INTEGRATION OF PRACTICE PATTERNS 4D AND 4E: IMPAIRED JOINT MOBILITY, MOTOR FUNCTION, MUSCLE PERFORMANCE, ROM ASSOCIATED WITH CONNECTIVE TISSUE DYSFUNCTION, AND LOCALIZED INFLAMMATION

Lumbar Disk Pathology

Back pain, with or without radiculopathy, is a significant clinical problem. A large percentage of the mechanical causes of back pain, particularly LBP, are attributed to pathologies of the IVD. IVD herniation in the lumbar spine may occur from adolescence into old age. Degenerative changes are the body's attempts at self-healing as the body ages. If part of this healing

TABLE 28-22	Comparison of Degeneration and Degradation of the Disk
Degeneration	**Degradation**
Changes occur to biochemistry in early adulthood and middle age	Vasculogenic degradation of nucleus
Circumferential clefting and tearing of anulus	Circumferential and radial tearing of annulus
No migration of nucleus	Nucleus migrates through radial fissures
Undisplaced	Nucleus herniates through anulus
Disk maintains or increases height	Disk is reabsorbed

involves the stabilization of an unstable joint, the joint motion can be reduced by muscle spasms or by increasing the surface area of the joint.[519] The biology of IVD degeneration is not well understood, but is thought to be a normal process, as opposed to the pathologic process that occurs with degradation (see Table 28-22 and later discussion).

The diagnoses associated with degenerative disk disease include

- idiopathic LBP;
- lumbar radiculopathy;
- myelopathy;
- lumbar stenosis;
- spondylosis;
- osteoarthritis;
- degenerative disk disease;
- zygapophyseal joint degeneration.

Disk degeneration appears to involve a structural disruption of the AF and cell-mediated changes throughout the IVD and subchondral bone.[520] Kirkaldy-Willis proposed a system to describe the spectrum of degeneration involving three stages or levels.[75] The three stages, which have essentially withstood the test of time, are defined as early dysfunction, intermediate instability, and final stabilization.

1. ***Early dysfunction.*** This stage is characterized by minor pathologic changes resulting in abnormal function of the posterior elements and IVD.[521] Autopsy results show that disk degeneration begins as early as 20–25 years of age.[291] Disk herniation most commonly occurs at the end of this stage, as splits and clefts develop in the annulus, but may also occur during the last stage. Degeneration seems to start early in the upper lumbar spine, with end plate fractures and Schmorl's nodes related to the vertical loading of those segments.[46] A Schmorl's nodule represents a dislocation of cartilage tissue through the end plate into the vertebral body. One study[522] provided evidence that a family history of operated lumbar disk herniation has a significant implication in lumbar degenerative disk disease, indicating that there may be a genetic factor in the development of lumbar disk herniation as an expression of disk degeneration.
2. ***Intermediate instability.*** This stage is characterized by laxity of the posterior joint capsule and AF. Disruption of the AF is associated with back pain.[523] All skeletal tissues adapt to increased mechanical demands, but they may not always adapt quickly enough. People who suddenly change to a physically demanding occupation may subject their tissues to an increase in repetitive loading, causing fatigue damage to accumulate rapidly. The ability of spinal tissues to strengthen in response to increased muscle forces may be restricted by health and age, so that fatigue damage accumulates most rapidly in sedentary middle-aged people who suddenly become active.[524]
3. ***Final stabilization.*** This stage is characterized by fibrosis of the posterior joints and capsule, a loss of disk material, the formation of radial tears of the AF, and osteophyte formation.[525] Osteophyte formation around the three-joint complex increases the load-bearing surface and decreases the amount of motion, producing a stiffer and thus less painful motion segment.[520]

Clinical experience has shown that it is possible for the three-joint complex to go through all of these phases with few symptoms generated.

Disk Degradation

Disk degradation is a more aggressive process than the degenerative changes that occur with aging, and although the macroscopic changes are similar to those of age-related degeneration, degradation is a more accelerated process.

Under normal conditions, the NP is contained by the AF. Any disturbance of the balance of these tissue structures may lead to tissue destruction, functional impairment, and LBP.[32] Three main types of lumbar disk herniation are recognized:

1. ***Contained (protrusion).*** With a contained herniation, the nuclear material bulges outward through the tear to strain, but not escape from, the outer AF or the PLL. Contained herniations are confined to the central canal. The disk bulges against the dura and the PLL, producing a dull, poorly localized somatic-type pain in the back and sacroiliac region. Regarding the modes of lumbar disk herniation, Yasuma et al.[526] described the degenerative process of the matrix and concluded that most herniations are protrusions of the NP that occur before the age of 60 years, whereas after that age, prolapse of the AF predominates. Eckert and Decker[527] and Taylor and Akeson,[528] however, found cartilaginous end-plate fractures in 60% of herniated masses, and in approximately 50% of sequestrated fragments, respectively. Because the NP is usually still contained, the patient is likely to feel more pain in the morning after the NP has imbibed more fluid, because of the added volume and the subsequent increase in pressure on pain-sensitive structures. Recent attention has been given to the internal disruption of the NP in a contained herniation.[529] In this condition, the NP becomes inflamed and invaginates itself between the annular layers. Compression of the disk during sitting and bending

increases the pain, because the nociceptive structures within the AF are further irritated. There is usually no, or minimal, leg pain and no, or minimal, limitation in the SLR test (see Chap. 11).[529]

2. ***Extrusion (prolapse).*** With extrusion, the nuclear material remains attached to the disk but escapes the AF or the PLL to bulge posterolaterally into the intervertebral canal. Once a tear to the periphery is opened for the NP, it would seem logical that further stresses can force it to migrate through the tear. However, under normal conditions, the nuclear material is intrinsically cohesive and does not herniate through the AF, even if the AF fibers are weakened by a radial incision.[530]
3. ***Sequestration.*** The migrating nuclear material escapes contact with the disk entirely and becomes a free fragment in the intervertebral canal.

As part of its unnatural history, the disk may or may not travel through each stage of herniation sequentially, producing symptoms that range from backache to bilateral radiculopathy.

Nerve Compression

Extrusions and sequestrations impinge on nerve tissue. Central prolapses, although relatively rare, may produce upper motor neuron impairments if they are sufficiently large to compress the cervical or thoracic spinal cord, and bowel or bladder impairments if they occur in the lumbar spine (cauda equina syndrome).[531] A substantial compression of the root affects the nerve fibers, producing paresthesia and interference with conduction. In 1934, Mixter and Barr suggested that tissue of the IVD extrudes into the spinal canal, compressing and therefore irritating the nerve root and causing sciatic pain.[532] Although this concept was widely accepted for many years, it has now been demonstrated that mechanical compression of the nerve root alone does not explain sciatic pain and radiculopathy.[533–535] The operative finding that mechanically compressed nerve roots become tender, and results of recent histologic and biochemical studies on herniated lumbar disk tissue, led to the notion of inflammatory induced sciatic pain.[533–536] More recent models of lumbar radiculopathy suggest that the underlying mechanisms probably result, in part, from a local chemical irritant such as proteoglycans released from a disk and creating an inflammatory reaction, an autoimmune reaction from exposure to disk tissues, an increased concentration of lactic acid or a lower pH around the nerve roots.[534,537] Investigators have repeatedly demonstrated inflammatory cells, proinflammatory enzyme phospholipase A2, immunoglobulins, and various inflammatory mediators in herniated disk tissues.[533,538] It is also thought that neovascularization in herniated disk tissue could promote the formation of granulation tissue,[535,536,539] and in association with blood vessels, deposits of immunoglobulins have been reported.[534]

The presence of inflammation in disk herniations could explain the clinical findings of improvement in radicular pain following the administration of corticosteroid or nonsteroidal anti-inflammatory drugs (NSAIDs).

The diagnosis of a disk herniation is based largely on the history and physical examination findings and, on occasion, imaging test results. The patient's complaints of pain usually are related to the following factors:

- Whether excessive imbibition or excessive dehydration has occurred to the disk.[346] Excessive imbibition, which results from a prolonged absence from compressive forces, may place a mechanical stress on the innervated outer AF, or other posterior structures, resulting in pain and decreased mobility following recumbency. Dehydration of the disk results from the application of prolonged compressive forces, which reduces the size of the disk and allows for excessive translational segmental mobility and compression on normally unloaded segmental structures.[346] This mechanism results in increased symptoms and decreased mobility as the day progresses.
- Whether the nerve root is involved. An ischemic nerve root responds with an increase in symptoms if a movement increases compression to the nerve root.[346] Such movements include lumbar extension and ipsilateral side bending. This is probably why patients with nerve root involvement adopt a posture of flexion and contralateral side bending, although occasionally this posture can result in an increase in symptoms because of an increase in tension and a decrease in intraneural circulation.[346] In these cases the patient is likely to adopt a posture of flexion and ipsilateral side bending.

The ability of the disk to maintain its hydrostatic pressure is a factor of previous extrusions or sequestrations, disk surgery, and the degree of disk degeneration.[157,520] Theoretically, if the hydrostatic pressure is maintained following a posterolateral disk protrusion, the patient will have increased pain with flexion, flexion with contralateral rotation, or side bending.[346] These symptoms tend to be increased with repetition of those motions but improved with motions in the opposite directions, although initially those symptoms may increase, depending on the position of the NP.[346]

Imaging results can be misleading. Anatomic evidence of a herniated disk is found in 20–30% of imaging tests (myelography, CT, and MRI) among normal persons.[228,398,399] Conventional physical examination for a suspected disk herniation consists of tests for key muscle strength and lumbar ROM, and muscle stretch reflex and sensory testing, and dural mobility tests such as the SLR test. It must be remembered that no single test in the physical examination has a high diagnostic accuracy alone for disk herniation.[280]

Several plausible diagnoses, depending on the distribution of symptoms, must be eliminated before a lumbar radiculopathy can be confirmed. These include

- hip joint pathology (degenerative joint disease, avascular necrosis, synovitis, etc.)[540];
- meralgia paresthetica. This syndrome, also known as Bernhardt–Roth syndrome, is characterized by pain or dysesthesia in the anterolateral thigh, caused by entrapment of the lateral cutaneous (femoral) nerve of the thigh at the ASIS (see Chap. 5). Trummer et al.[541] reported that lumbar disk herniation could mimic meralgia paresthetica, and Kallgren and Tingle[542] noted that meralgia paresthetica

could mimic lumbar radiculopathy because of the similarity of the symptoms.

- irritation of the spinal nerve root by osteophytic spurs;
- sacroiliac or pelvic dysfunction;
- intermittent claudication of the iliac or iliofemoral arteries;
- spondylolisthesis;
- lateral recess stenosis;
- muscle strain;
- stress fracture of the lumbar/thoracic vertebra (burst and compression);
- neoplasm;
- isolated peripheral nerve injury or neuritis;
- diabetic amyotrophy, which is relatively uncommon but can occasionally be the presenting symptom of uncontrolled diabetes mellitus.[543]

The differential diagnosis can be aided by a description of the distribution of the patient's symptoms and the results of the physical examination.

High Lumbar Disk Lesions

From 1% to 11% of herniated disks originate from the L1–2, L2–3, or L3–4 levels.[544–546] Reduced motion and stress at the upper lumbar spine and the protective influence of the PLL may account for the disparity.[546]

CLINICAL PEARL

A number of studies have shown that with increasing age, lumbar disk herniation is more cranially localized so that higher level disk injuries are more common in advanced age.[547] Because of the nerve root anatomy previously discussed, a herniation at these high levels may occur without compromise to the nerve root, and may thus go undetected.

If symptoms are present, the high lumbar radiculopathy typically does not radiate pain down the back of the leg but, instead, causes an insidious onset of pain in the groin or anterior thigh that is often relieved in a flexed position and worsens with standing.[548] The superficial cremasteric reflex is also invariably present.[315]

The differential diagnoses for upper lumbar nerve root symptoms include spondylolisthesis and an infective cause, such as diskitis or an epidural abscess.

Third Lumbar Nerve Root Compression

The clinical findings with a lesion at this level may include

- pain in the midlumbar area, upper buttock, whole anterior thigh and knee, medial knee, and just above the ankle;
- dural signs of prone knee flexion and, occasionally, a positive SLR;
- significant motion loss of extension;
- slight weakness of iliopsoas and grosser loss of quadriceps;
- hypoesthesia of the medial aspect of the knee and lower leg;
- absent or reduced patellar reflex.

TABLE 28-23 Common Radicular Syndromes of the Lumbar Spine

Disk Level	Nerve Root	Motor Deficit	Sensory Deficit	Reflex Compromise
L3–4	L4	Quadriceps	Anterolateral thigh	Knee Anterior knee Medial leg and foot
L4–5	L5	Extensor hallucis longus	Lateral thigh	Medial hamstrings Anterolateral leg Mid posterior (dorsal) foot
L5–S1	S1	Ankle plantar flexors	Posterior leg	Ankle Lateral foot

Data from American Medical Association: *Guides to the Evaluation of Permanent Impairment*, 5th ed. Chicago: American Medical Association, 2001.

Fourth Lumbar Nerve Root Compression

Approximately 40% of IVD impairments affect this level, about an equal amount as those that affect the L5 root.[33] A disk protrusion at this level can irritate the fourth root, the fifth root, or, with a larger protrusion, both roots (Table 28-23). The clinical findings with a lesion at this level may include

- pain located in the lumbar area or iliac crest, inner buttock, outer thigh and leg, and over the foot to the great toe;
- positive dural signs of SLR, bilateral and crossed SLR, and neck flexion (see Chap. 11)[311];
- marked lateral deviation of the lumbar spine and gross limitation of one side flexion (both common findings);
- weak dorsiflexion of the ankle;
- hypoesthesia of the outer lower leg and great toe;
- diminished tibialis posterior, patellar, and tibialis anterior muscle stretch reflexes.

Fifth Lumbar Nerve Root Compression

This level is affected as often as the fourth nerve root and is frequently compressed by the L4–5 disk as well as the L5–S1 disk (see Table 28-23). The clinical findings with a lesion at this level may include

- pain in the sacroiliac area, lower buttock, lateral thigh and leg, inner three toes, and medial sole of the foot;
- positive unilateral SLR and neck flexion[311];
- lateral deviation during flexion;
- weakness of peroneal, extensor hallucis, and hip abductor muscles;
- hypoesthesia of outer leg and inner three toes and medial sole;
- diminished fibularis (peroneus) longus, Achilles, and extensor hallucis muscle stretch reflexes.

First, Second, and Third Sacral Roots

According to Cyriax, the first, second, and third sacral roots can be compressed by a fifth lumbar disk protrusion. The clinical findings with a lesion at the S1 level (see Table 28-23) may include[343]

- pain in the low back to buttocks to sole of the foot and heel;
- limited SLR;
- weakness of the calf muscles, peronei, and hamstrings;
- atrophy of the gluteal mass (but weakness is not always detectable);
- hypoesthesia in the outer two toes, outer foot, and outer leg as far as the lateral aspect of the knee.

With a second sacral root palsy, the signs are the same as for the first sacral nerve root, except that the fibularis (peroneal) muscles are spared and the hypoesthesia ends at the heel. With third sacral root palsy, the SLR is generally normal and no palsy is detectable. However, the patient may report pain in the groin, and pain down the inner aspect of the thigh to the knee.[531]

Fourth Sacral Nerve Root Compression

A lesion of this nerve root is always a concern, because a permanent palsy may lead to incontinence and impotence.[531,549] The clinical findings with a lesion at this level may include

- pain in the lower sacral, peroneal, and genital areas;
- saddle area paresthesia;
- no positive dural signs;
- possible gross limitation of all lumbar movements;
- bladder, bowel, or genital dysfunction;
- positive superficial anal reflex and reduced anal wink.[315]

Vertical Prolapse (Schmorl's Node)

A Schmorl's node is the herniation of disk substance through the cartilaginous plate of the IVD into the body of the adjacent vertebra.[550] These vertical prolapses of the disk are often asymptomatic and occur as incidental findings on radiographs. Indeed, a chronic Schmorl's node has been reported to be the most common impairment of the IVD and of the whole spine.[551] Schmorl's nodes tend to be more common in men than in women, a factor attributed to the greater spinal loads in men.[550] Theories proposed to explain the pathogenesis of Schmorl's nodes include origins that are

- developmental, in which embryonic defects such as ossification gaps, vascular channels, and notochord extrusion defects form points of weakness where Schmorl's nodes may occur[26];
- degenerative, in which the aging process produces sites of weakness in the cartilaginous endplate, resulting in formation. of Schmorl's nodes[551,552];
- pathologic, where diseases weaken the IVD and/or vertebral bodies[553,554];
- traumatic, in which acute and chronic trauma destroy the cartilaginous end plates, resulting in disk herniation.

Although most orthopedists accept that Schmorl's nodes occur because of trauma, no studies have shown a direct causal relation between a traumatic episode and the formation of an acute Schmorl's node.

Once the Schmorl's node has occurred, subsequent proliferation of cartilage and reactive ossification may develop in the vicinity of the dislocated tissue.[132] This ossification encloses the dislocated tissue and segregates it from the spongiosa of the vertebral body. The formation of this cartilaginous cap, or calcification of the protrusion, may act to resist its expansion.[22]

Intervention

The natural history of radiculopathy and disk herniation is not quite as favorable as for simple LBP, but it is still excellent, with approximately 50% of patients recovering in the first 2 weeks and 70% recovering in 6 weeks.[555] Prognostic factors for positive outcome with conservative intervention for lumbar disk herniation are depicted in Table 28-24.

> **CLINICAL PEARL**
>
> Intervention focuses on a return to normal activities as soon as possible, patient education and involvement, and therapeutic exercises.

Complete bed rest is not recommended in the first 4–6 weeks after onset of symptoms.[556,557] Surgery is often recommended after 4–6 weeks, if the symptoms persist, following MRI and CT scan findings.[558] However, of those who opt for surgery, 10–40% will complain of pain, motor dysfunction, or reduced activity of daily-living performance after surgery.[559,560] Ito et al.[558] showed that if patients with herniated lumbar disk could tolerate the symptoms of disk herniation for 2 months after onset of symptoms, it was possible to treat them with conservative approaches.[559] Using CT scan techniques, it was shown that 66% of herniated disk cases may normalize or recover either totally or partially with time and that large lumbar herniated nucleus propulsions can decrease and even disappear in some patients treated successfully with conservative care.[559,561] The McKenzie exercise program can be valuable to the overall intervention strategy and, if centralization of pain occurs, a good response to physical therapy can be anticipated.[297,459] In addition to the usual history taken, the McKenzie method makes particular inquiries regarding

- whether the symptoms are constant or intermittent;
- the topography of the symptoms;
- whether the symptoms are better or worse with bending forward, sitting, rising from sitting, standing, walking, lying, rising from lying, when still, and/or on the move. Much of this information can be gained by asking the patient which activities of daily living produce the symptoms.

In cases of radiculopathy, the goal is to decrease radiating symptoms into the limb and, thus, to centralize the pain by using specific maneuvers or positions, such as the lateral shift correction (Fig. 28-8) VIDEO. Once this centralizing position is identified, the patient is instructed to perform these

TABLE 28-24	Prognostic Factors of Positive Outcome with Conservative Intervention for Lumbar Disk Herniation
Outcome	**Factor**
Favorable	Absence of crossed SLR
	Spinal motion in extension that does not reproduce leg pain
	Relief or >50% reduction in leg pain within first 6 wks of onset
	Limited psychosocial issues
	Self-employed
	Educational level >12 yr
	Absence of spinal stenosis
	Progressive return of neurologic deficit within first 12 wks
Unfavorable	Positive crossed SLR
	Leg pain produced with spinal extension
	Lack of >50% reduction in leg pain within first 6 wks of onset
	Overbearing psychosocial issues
	Worker's compensation
	Educational level <12 yr
	Concomitant spinal stenosis
	Progressive neurologic deficit
	Cauda equina syndrome
Neutral	Degree of SLR
	Response to bed rest
	Response to passive care
	Gender
	Age
Questionable	Actual size of lumbar disk herniation
	Canal position of lumbar disk herniation
	Spinal level of lumbar disk herniation
	Lumbar disk herniation material

SLR, straight leg raising.
Data from Saal JA: Natural history and nonoperative treatment of lumbar disc herniation. *Spine* 21:2S–9S, 1996.

maneuvers repetitively or sustain certain positions for specific periods throughout the day.[535]

In addition, the patient is instructed in a lumbar stabilization program, in which neutral zone mechanics are practiced in various positions to decrease stress to the lumbosacral spine. Lumbar-stabilizing exercises have been recommended to improve lumbar function in patients with low back injury so that these patients may improve their activities of daily living.[559] It is theorized that these types of exercise may strengthen the stabilizer muscles, which control and limit the free movement of one vertebra on the other, thereby accelerating the recovery process of the herniated disk.

The intervention program is only as good as the concomitant home exercise program, and the clinician must continually monitor the home exercise program, evaluating the patient's knowledge of the exercises and upgrading the program when appropriate.

Surgery for Lumbar Radiculopathy

Several characteristics of patients with sciatica appear to predict the eventual need for surgery. These include a mentally demanding job (as opposed to a mentally nondemanding job or no job); a gradual onset of pain; an increase of pain on coughing, sneezing, or straining; and difficulty putting on socks or stockings.[562]

The aims of lumbar surgery for radiculopathy are to relieve pain and to restore neural function. Considerable literature reflects the evolution of lumbar disk surgery, the most commonly performed neurosurgical procedure. Oppenheim and Krause in 1909 were the first to remove what was thought to be a lumbar spinal tumor (enchondroma, chordoma).[563] Other surgeries followed, leading to Mixter and Barr who systematized the diagnosis and operative treatment of lumbar disk prolapse in 1934.[532]

Lumbar disk herniation is one of the few causes of spinal pain that can be successfully treated surgically.[564] Several surgical options are available. The more common ones are described here.

Enzymatic Intradiskal Therapy (Chemonucleolysis)

Enzymatic intradiskal therapy is advocated as a minimally invasive, intermediate stage between conservative management and open-surgical intervention for a contained lumbar IVD prolapse.

Two enzymes are used in vivo: chymopapain and collagenase. The therapeutic concept behind intradiskal therapy is to produce a decrease in the water-binding capacity of the polysaccharide side chains. This is supposed to result in a lowering of the pressure in the IVD, with a subsequent reduction in the size of the IVD protrusion and relief of the tension on the nerve root.

The success rate of chemonucleolysis with chymopapain or collagenase has been found to be approximately 72% and 52%, respectively.[565,566] However, the final outcome from chemonucleolysis, followed by surgery if chemonucleolysis fails, remains poorer than the outcome from primary diskectomy.[4] Consequently, although chemonucleolysis is an excellent procedure in principle, it is rarely performed. The complications associated with this procedure include allergic reactions, lumbar subarachnoid hemorrhage, and paraplegia.

Diskectomy

Diskectomy is a commonly performed surgical procedure in the general population, with high success rates reported in the literature.[567] There is now strong evidence on the relative effectiveness of surgical diskectomy versus chemonucleolysis versus placebo.[4]

Hemilaminectomy and Diskectomy

These diskectomies are usually approached posteriorly. Posterolateral diskectomy is used to treat herniated lumbar IVDs. The aim of a diskectomy is to decompress the involved nerve root or roots, while minimizing scar tissue formation and avoiding iatrogenic nerve damage.

Percutaneous Diskectomy

Percutaneous diskectomy is a minimally invasive procedure that uses a probe for automatic aspiration of the NP material from the IVD. Because the probe is inserted using a cannula, the procedure causes minimal damage to the muscles, bones, and joints of the back and no adherences in the epidural space. A short convalescence is, therefore, to be expected. This procedure is indicated for patients with radicular pain, positive SLR, and positive neurologic signs and symptoms (atrophy, weakness, and sciatica) who have not responded to at least 6 weeks of conservative therapy. It also is advocated for patients with pure IVD herniation without stenosis or any other additional factors. These factors include IVD fragments in the spinal cord, severe spinal arthritis, and LF hypertrophy.

Microdiskectomy

A microdiskectomy is designed to decompress neural tissues by removing the IVD material that is causing the compression and irritation of the nerve root. Microdiskectomy is reported to have a high success rate, more than 90% in some studies.[567] Following a diskectomy, patients are generally able to return to their previous levels of activity, including participation in recreational sports. This surgery, however, can be associated with a long recuperation and a protracted period of disability.[568,569]

Laser Diskectomy

As its name suggests, laser diskectomy uses a laser to remove diskal tissue and thereby alleviate the pressure on the nerve root. However, because it does not address the actual pathology, its success rate is dramatically inferior to that of standard diskectomy.[570]

Laminectomy

A laminectomy is defined as the removal of a lamina. A complete laminectomy involves the removal of the entire lamina, together with the spinous process and the LF caudal and cranial to the lamina. The disadvantage of a complete laminectomy is that it may produce a destabilizing effect on the motion segment.[509]

Decompression

Decompression of the lumbar spine is defined as a laminectomy with partial facetectomy. Decompression may also be accompanied by partial laminectomy and canal enlargement, expansive lumbar laminoplasty, unilateral laminotomy for bilateral decompressions, or partial pediclectomy.

Fusion

There is little consensus among spine surgeons regarding the optimal indications for lumbar fusion surgery. Some surgeons believe that most patients with spinal stenosis are appropriate candidates for spinal fusion. Others believe that most of these patients should undergo only a laminectomy, because the degenerative changes that have occurred produce an inherent stability of the motion segment.

Controversy also exists regarding the use of fusion surgery versus nonsurgical approaches for degenerative disk disease with no herniation or stenosis.[571] Spinal fusion is associated with wider surgical exposure, more extensive dissection, and longer operation times than laminectomy.

As an adjunct to the excision of recurrent lumbar IVD herniations, lumbar fusion provides several theoretical advantages[572]:

- reduction or elimination of segmental motion;
- reduction of mechanical stresses across the degenerated disk space;
- reduction of the incidence of additional herniation at the affected disk space;

Circumferential fusion has been advocated to improve fusion rates and clinical outcomes in intervention of the lumbosacral spine. Circumferential lumbar fusion can be challenging, however, requiring either thecal sac retraction and bilateral facet disruption or a posterior lumbar interbody fusion.[573]

Alternative options have included either sequential anterior and posterior fusions or a posterior lumbar interbody fusion at the time of simultaneous posterolateral fusion. In 1982, Harms and Rolinger[573] suggested the placement of bone graft and titanium mesh, via a transforaminal route, into the disk space that previously had been distracted using pedicle screw instrumentation (transforaminal lumbar interbody fusion [TLIF]).

Other options for fusing the lumbar spine include bone grafting with a posterolateral approach without instrumentation (facet fusion or intertransverse fusion), a posterolateral approach with pedicle screws, or posterior lumbar interbody fusion or anterior lumbar interbody fusion (ALIF) with bone grafts, cages, or dowels.[572]

Complications of ALIF include postoperative ileus, vascular and visceral injury, retrograde ejaculation in males, and venous thrombosis.[574] Complications of TLIF include epidural bleeding, neural injury, postsurgical instability, epidural fibrosis, and arachnoiditis.[574] Most of the complications reported for the ALIF and TLIF procedures are approach rather than device related.

Lumbar Artificial Disk Replacement

The use of lumbar artificial disk replacement for the treatment of symptomatic lumbar disk disease has recently been approved by the US Food and Drug Administration (FDA). The artificial disk is an alternative to fusion procedures and offers the advantage in its ability to restore pain-free motion while protecting adjacent segments from increased loading and failure. Candidates for this procedure include patients who are18–60 years and in whom nonoperative treatment for at least 6 months has failed and who have

- single level degenerative disk disease confirmed by MRI and diskography;
- no previous lumbar fusion;
- no instability, and;
- no extruded disk material.

Postsurgical Intervention

Patients who undergo spinal surgery may receive physical therapy as part of their rehabilitation. Although there is a large amount of information from evidence-based clinical practice guidelines for the management of many musculoskeletal conditions, there is relatively little information available on the physical therapy management of patients who have undergone spinal surgery.

The randomized controlled trials comparing various physical activity programs[10,575–577] have demonstrated the benefits of these programs. These benefits have included less pain and disability, improved ROM, and greater satisfaction with care.

Before the surgery, the patients may receive advice on spine care, postsurgical precautions, and instructions on basic exercises.

The postsurgical intervention following surgery is as varied as the number of types of surgery. The following are guidelines for postsurgical rehabilitation. The primary goals for the initial period following the surgery are

- reduction of pain and inflammation;
- prevention of postsurgical complications;
- protection of the surgical site;
- prevention of a recurrent herniation;
- maintenance of dural mobility;
- improvement of function;
- minimizing of the detrimental effects of immobilization[578–583];
- early return to appropriate functional activities. Patients usually are permitted to shower 1 week after the surgery.
- safe return to occupational duties. Patients with a sedentary occupation may return to work within 7–10 days after the surgery. Prolonged positions and postures are to be avoided.
- patient education on correct body mechanics and independent self-care.

The patient is given guidance on the gradual resumption of daily activities. Immobilization or prolonged rest should be avoided. Instead, the patient is encouraged to walk for short periods and distances several times a day.

Outpatient physical therapy, if appropriate, usually begins in the second or third week. The physical therapy examination includes

- a thorough history;
- inspection of the wound site;
- anthropometric data;
- postural examination;
- neural examination, including neurodynamic mobility, and strength testing.

The components of the physical therapy intervention include a graded exercise program, with gentle ROM, submaximal isometrics, and arm and leg exercises as appropriate.

Additional interventions may include electrotherapeutic modalities, physical agents, and scar massage. Patient education is very important, particularly postural education and information on body mechanics.

Progressive strengthening exercises for the spinal stabilizers usually are initiated by the fourth postoperative week.

Cardiovascular conditioning exercises are introduced at the earliest opportunity based on patient tolerance. These include riding a stationary bicycle, using an upper body ergonometer and a stair-stepper, and swimming in a pool. The sessions for these exercises are initially brief (5–10 minutes) and are gradually increased up to 30–60 minutes.

Activities such as jogging are usually permitted at 6–8 weeks if there is minimal pain. When the patient does resume these activities, they should be done in the morning hours when the IVD is maximally hydrated.[584] High-impact sports such as basketball and soccer are usually permitted after the 12th week.

Degenerative Spinal Stenosis

Degenerative spinal stenosis (DSS), a narrowing of the spinal canal, nerve root canal (lateral recess), or intervertebral foramina of the lumbar spine, is predominantly a disorder of the elderly—it is the most common diagnosis associated with lumbar spine surgery in patients older than 65 years.[585]

DSS is being diagnosed more frequently. The reasons for this are the widespread use of sophisticated noninvasive imaging techniques and the increasing elderly population. Lumbar spinal stenosis may be classified as central or lateral.[586]

- Central stenosis is characterized by a narrowing of the spinal canal around the thecal sac containing the cauda equina. The causes for this type of stenosis include facet joint arthrosis and hypertrophy, thickening and bulging of the LF, bulging of the IVD, and spondylolisthesis.
- Lateral stenosis is characterized by encroachment of the spinal nerve in the lateral recess of the spinal canal or in the intervertebral foramen. Initially the depth of the canal that constituted narrowing was identified as an anteroposterior measurement,[587] but more recently the lateral width of the spinal canal has been studied.[346] The causes for this type of stenosis include facet joint hypertrophy, loss of IVD height, IVD bulging, and spondylolisthesis.

A compression of the nerve within the canal can result in a limitation of the arterial supply or claudication resulting from the compression of the venous return. Neurogenic claudication, or pseudoclaudication, can result in nerve root ischemia and symptomatic claudication, which is brought on by walking and relieved by sitting.[588] Compressive loading of the spine can also exacerbate symptoms, such as those that occur with prolonged standing. Central stenosis, which can result in symptoms related to cauda equina compression, may occur more often with certain movements or changes in posture[589]:

- The length of the canal is shorter in lumbar lordosis than kyphosis.
- Extension and, to a lesser degree, side bending of the lumbar spine toward the involved side produces a narrowing of the canal.
- Flexion of the lumbar spine reverses the process, returning both the venous capacity and the blood flow to the nerve.

Both the history and the examination findings are very specific.

Patients with lumbar spinal stenosis who are symptomatic often relate to a long history of LBP. Unilateral or bilateral leg pain is usually a predominant symptom. Approximately 65% of patients with lumbar spinal stenosis present with neurogenic claudication.[588] Subjectively, the patient reports an increase in symptoms with lumbar extension activities such as walking, prolonged standing, and, to a lesser degree, side bending. On observation, the patient presents with a flattened lumbar lordosis.

The physical examination usually reveals evidence of reduced flexibility or shortening of the hip flexors (iliopsoas and rectus femoris). The hip extensor muscles (gluteus maximus and hamstrings) usually are lengthened. This lengthening places them at a mechanical disadvantage, which leads to early recruitment of the lumbar extensor muscles and may lead to excessive lumbar extension.[590]

Therapeutic exercise is one of numerous interventions that have been proposed for the conservative management of patients with lumbar spinal stenosis. Several authors advocate only the use of Williams flexion exercises because of the neuroforaminal narrowing that occurs with lumbar extension.[591,592] However, the prescribed program may need to be modified so that it does not exacerbate any coexisting orthopaedic conditions, such as osteoarthritis of the hips or knees, while still being effective.[8] In a randomized clinical trial by Whitman et al.,[593] two physical therapy programs were compared for 58 patients with lumbar spinal stenosis:

- manual therapy (eclectic, consisting of techniques such as those described by Maitland,[594] Greenman,[335] and Whitman et al.[595]), body-weight-supported treadmill walking, and exercise group;
- lumbar flexion exercises, a treadmill-walking program, and subtherapeutic ultrasound group.

A greater proportion of patients in the first group reported recovery at 6 weeks compared with the flexion exercise and walking group ($P = 0.0015$), with a number needed to treat for perceived recovery of 2.6 (confidence interval, 1.8–7.8). At 1 year, 62% of the first group and 41% of the flexion exercise and walking group still met the threshold for recovery.[593]

The therapeutic exercise progression is based on the underlying impairments and should include postural education; hip flexor, rectus femoris, and lumbar paraspinal stretching; lumbar (core) stabilization exercises targeting the abdominals and gluteals; aerobic conditioning; and positioning through a posterior pelvic tilt. There is some controversy as to whether the hamstrings should be stretched, as lengthening of these muscles may allow the pelvis to rotate anteriorly, resulting in an increased lordosis and further stenosis.

Failure to respond to a conservative approach is an indication for nerve root and sinuvertebral nerve infiltration.[596] Permanent relief in lateral recess stenosis has been reported with an injection of local anesthetic around the nerve root.[597] When nerve root infiltration fails, surgical decompression of the nerve root is indicated.

Zygapophyseal Joint Dysfunction

The term *Facet joint syndrome* refers to a pain-provoking dysfunction of the zygapophyseal joint.[129] This pain is the result of a lesion to the joint and its pain-sensitive structures. Zygapophyseal movement dysfunctions can result from a hypomobility or a hypermobility instability (see "Clinical Instability of the Lumbar Spine" section).

Hypomobility

Hypomobility in the lumbar spine can have a variety of causes including ligament tears,[598] muscle tears or contusions,[599] lumbago,[343] intra-articular meniscoid entrapment,[516] zygapophyseal joint capsular tightness, and zygapophyseal joint fixation or subluxation.[600]

Theoretically, the signs and symptoms that present with a hypomobility include unilateral LBP that is aggravated with certain movements. Given that the joint is only capable of flexion and extension movements, it is assumed that flexion or extension movements can provoke pain, particularly at the end of these ranges. These movements are tested with active ROM and the combined motion tests and confirmed with the position tests of the PPIVM and PPAIVM tests.[373]

Hypomobility of the zygapophyseal joint can have an extra-articular, periarticular, or pathomechanical cause, with the distinction being made by the results of the end-feel obtained by the clinician during the PPIVM and PPAIVM tests.[373]

- ***Extra-articular.*** Decreased range with the PPIVM, but normal PPAIVM.
- ***Periarticular.*** Restriction of range in both PPIVM and PPAIVM tests, with a hard capsular end-feel.
- ***Pathomechanical.*** Restriction of range in both PPIVM and PPAIVM tests, with an abrupt, slightly springy end-feel.

The conservative intervention for a zygapophyseal dysfunction includes specific joint mobilizations, postural education, correction of muscle imbalances, and core stabilization exercises.

CLINICAL INSTABILITY OF THE LUMBAR SPINE

There is considerable controversy as to what, exactly, constitutes spinal instability. Traditionally, the radiographic diagnosis of increased translation or angulation of a spinal segment during flexion–extension or side bending in patients with chronic LBP was considered to be one of the most obvious manifestations of lumbar instability.[185,601] However, lumbar segmental instability in the absence of radiographic findings has also been cited as a significant cause of chronic LBP.[602,603] The limitation in the clinical diagnosis of lumbar segmental instability lies in the difficulty of accurately detecting abnormal or excessive intersegmental motion, either radiographically or through palpation.[13] One of the limitations in the radiographic diagnosis of clinical instability is that the testing is static and assesses the spinal segment mobility at its end of range (outside the neutral zone of motion), rather than accurately assessing the functional control of the spinal segment within its neutral zone.[185] Hypermobility, a close relative of instability, is usually the most difficult movement impairment to diagnose in the spine, because it is not a matter of stiffness, but rather of a relative degree of looseness.[373] Because of a lack of sensitivity and specificity of any one test, or combination of tests, to accurately identify clinical instability, its diagnosis requires the presence of a concurrent number of diagnostic criteria based on findings from the subjective and physical examination.[185]

The following clinical findings (anywhere in the spinal joints) may indicate the presence of instability and its pertinence to the presenting complaints of the patient:

- back pain that is most commonly described as recurrent, constant, catching, locking;
- repeated unprovoked episode(s) of feeling unstable or giving way, following a minor provocation;
- inconsistent symptomatology. The most frequently reported aggravating postures are sustained sitting, prolonged standing and semi flexed postures.[604] The most common aggravating movements are typically forward bending, sudden unexpected movements, returning in an upright position from forward bending, lifting, and sneezing.[604]
- minor aching for a few days after a sensation of giving way;
- compression symptoms (vertebrobasilar, spinal cord), which are not associated with a history of an IVD herniation or stenosis;
- consistent clicking or clunking noises;
- protracted pain (with full ROM);
- creases posteriorly or on abdomen (spondylolisthesis);
- spinal ledging;
- spinal angulation on full ROM;
- inability to recover normally from full ROM, commonly flexion;
- excessive active ROM. Active spinal movement, commonly reveals good ranges of spinal mobility but with aberrant quality of motion commonly associated with a sudden acceleration, hesitation, or lateral movement within the midrange of spinal motion.[185]

Intervention

Instability of the spine is perhaps the most difficult of the motion impairments to treat. A stiff or jammed joint is a relatively simple problem that requires selecting and applying a mobilization or manipulation technique. Instability is a permanent, or at best, a semipermanent state. The intervention for a hypermobility or instability involves the removal of any abnormal stresses from the joint. If the underlying cause of the articular hypermobility is deemed to be a localized joint hypomobility, then this dysfunction must logically be dealt with first using joint mobilizations or stretching techniques.[373] The techniques to increase joint mobility and the techniques to increase soft tissue extensibility are described later in "Therapeutic Techniques" section. Following the diagnosis, and the correction of any articular hypomobility, the focus shifts to retraining muscles that are involved in the dynamic stabilization and segmental control of the spine.

Whereas conventional exercises generally work to increase the strength of the global muscles, a more specific approach, which aims to improve the dynamic stability role of the segmental muscles during functional postures and movements, is recommended in conjunction with the focus on the global muscles. This approach has proven beneficial in a number of LBP conditions. For example, O'Sullivan et al.[190] have demonstrated decreased pain and disability in patients with chronic LBP who have a radiologically confirmed diagnosis of spondylolysis or spondylolisthesis.

While stressing the low-back tissues may enhance their health, too much loading can be detrimental. Choosing the optimal exercise requires judgment based on clinical experience and scientific evidence.[443] Training should begin in non-weight-bearing positions depending on patient response, in prone lying, in the quadriped position, or in supine lying before progressing to weight-bearing postures. It is important to note that the quadriped position has a significantly higher COG and smaller base of support (BOS) than the prone position, making it a more challenging position. Initially, the exercises prescribed are those that were found to provide relief during the examination. Usually, either flexion or extension movements demonstrate benefit. Contractions initially are held for 5 seconds and gradually are increased to 60 seconds. Training is performed a minimum of once a day for 10–15 minutes, with emphasis on proper cocontraction of the local muscle system. Depending on the severity of the condition, this range may initially be small, permitting only upper or lower extremity motions and gentle isometrics of the spinal muscles.

- ***Transversus abdominis exercise.*** This exercise, also known as the abdominal drawing-in maneuver, is known to result in preferential activation of the internal oblique and TrA, with little contribution by the rectus abdominis in the pain-free population.[605] The patient, placed in hook-lying (with knees 70–90 degrees and feet resting on the floor), quadriped, prone, or the semireclined position (based on comfort), is asked to take a relaxed breath in and out and then draw the waist-line in (towards the spine) without taking a breath (Fig. 28-54).[388] The contraction must be performed in a slow and controlled manner. Assessment of optimal recruitment of the TrA can be done through palpation just distal to the ASIS and lateral to the rectus abdominis (Fig. 28-54) or with the use of biofeedback.[388] When performed correctly, the clinician should feel flat tension of the muscle, rather than a bulge if the internal oblique contracts, and should see no substitute patterns (no movement of the pelvis, no flaring or depression of the lower ribs, no inspiration or lifting of the rib cage, no bulging out of the abdominal wall, and no increased pressure through the

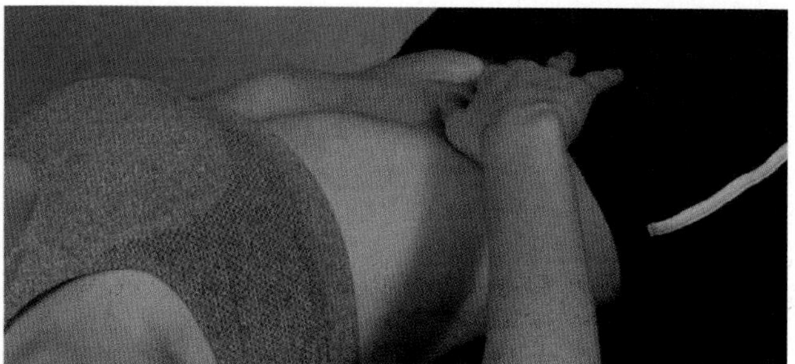

FIGURE 28-54 Abdominal drawing-in with palpation.

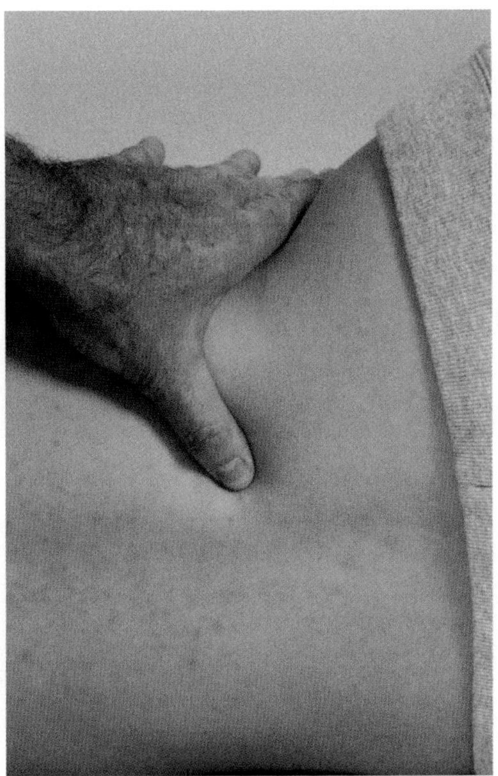

FIGURE 28-55 Multifidus activation.

feet).[81,114,606] Activation of the pelvic floor muscles or multifidus can be used to initiate activity in the TrA. Once the technique is successfully learned, the patient is encouraged to perform the exercise while in the sitting and standing positions while self-palpating.[81,114,388,606]

- ***Spinal bracing.*** McGill[207] advocates bracing of the spine, which has been shown to activates all three layers of the abdominal musculature, not just the TrA. The patient lies in supine position with the hips and knees flexed with the feet resting on the bed.[207,388] The patient is asked to activate the abdominal musculature and back extensors simultaneously so that both areas feel firm.
- ***Multifidus activation.*** The patient lies in the prone or side-lying position. The clinician uses the thumbs or index fingers to palpate immediately lateral to the spinous processes of the lumbar spine and the patient is asked to bulge the muscle out against the palpating digits (Fig. 28-55). Emphasis is placed on slow and gentle tension or swelling of the muscle as the goal is to increase control not strength. So that the patient can practice at home, a small piece of tape can be placed on the skin over the muscle to help patients find the correct level easily.

Pelvic Floor Muscle Activation

The pelvic floor muscles can be activated in isolation or in conjunction with activation of the TrA or multifidus. If activated in isolation the following instruction is given: "Contract as if you are stopping the flow of urine while you attempt to pull the ischial tuberosities together."

Once these techniques are mastered in the position of comfort, they are performed with the head, and lower and

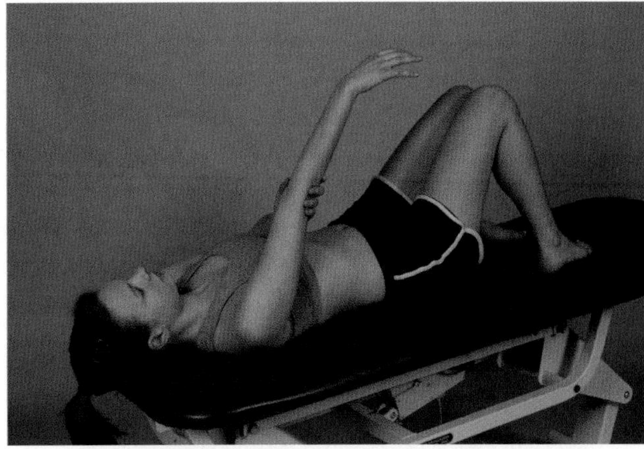

FIGURE 28-56 Unilateral shoulder flexion.

upper extremity movements (arm raises, bent leg raises) to improve muscular endurance depending on the emphasis of the intervention.[216,607]

Diaphragm Activation

The patient is in the supine hook-lying, side-lying, or prone over a pillow to relax the paraspinal muscles and place the patient's lumbar spine in neutral. The patient is asked to focus on active inspiration using contraction of the diaphragm (movement of the abdominal wall and basal rib cage) and relaxed expiration. Manual contact by the clinician can be used to encourage basal rib cage expansion.

Once these muscle activations can be performed in isolation and in the controlled position, the clinician then attempts to promote static coordination between the local and global muscles using the following progression:

- **Extremity loading**: Superimposing upper and then lower extremity movements while maintaining the position of the spine and pelvis (Fig. 28-56).
- **Rhythmic stabilization**: The clinician applies various low forces to the body with slow alternations while the patient maintains a neutral position. These techniques are performed in supine initially and then in sitting.
- **Unstable base**: The patient holds the neutral spine position during extremity loading and rhythmic stabilization.
- **Functional movements**: The patient holds the neutral spine position during a variety of functional activities such as walking, weight shifting, and trunk rotations.

A variety of exercises that emphasize specific muscle groups, depending on the clinical findings, can be introduced. All of the following exercises are superimposed on the neutral spine (midrange or functional position), making sure the patient maintains control while performing the exercises:

Emphasis on Abdominals

- ***Bent-leg fall out.*** The patient is placed in the supine hook-lying position (knees at 90 degrees of flexion) and is asked to separate the knees while preventing pelvic rotation (Fig. 28-57).[608]
- ***Progressive limb loading.*** From the supine hook-lying position the patient is asked to do the following:

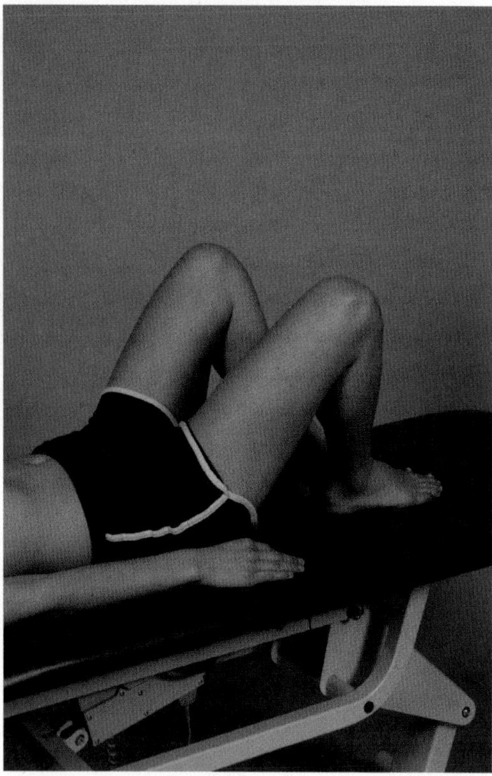

FIGURE 28-57 Bent-leg fall out.

- lift one of the legs to 90 degrees of hip and knee flexion (Fig. 28-58), then
- slide the heel of the raised leg away from the body to extend the knee (Fig. 28-59), and then finally
- to lift the straight leg to 45 degrees (Fig. 28-60).

The exercise is then repeated using the other leg.

The exercise progression then follows a series of levels of increasing difficulty while performing the same three methods of progressive limb loading:

- The opposite leg is held at 90 degrees of hip flexion using both upper extremities (Fig. 28-61).
- The opposite leg is held at 90 degrees of hip flexion with no upper extremity assistance (Fig. 28-62).

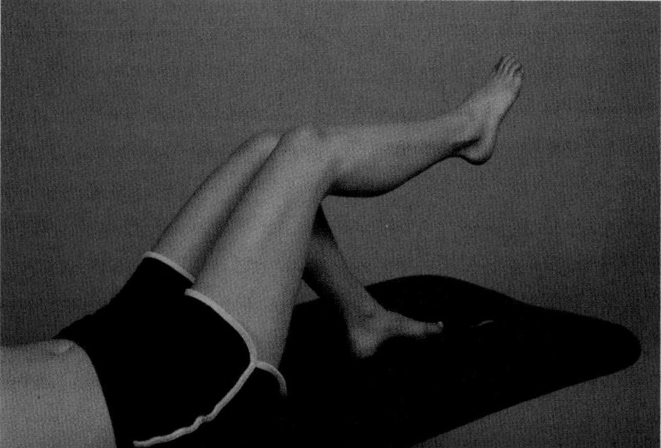

FIGURE 28-59 Progressive limb loading 2.

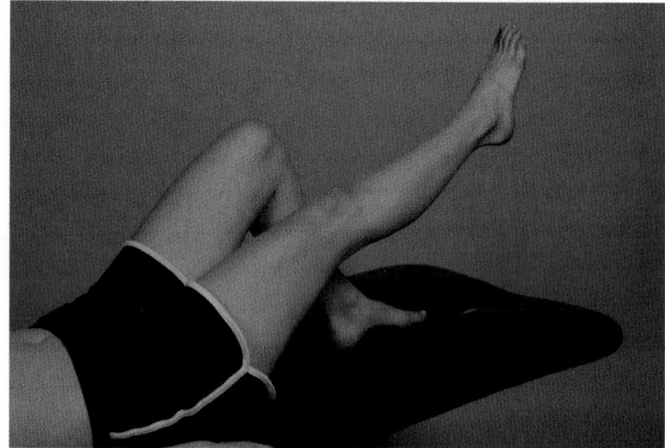

FIGURE 28-60 Progressive limb loading 3.

- Both legs perform the series of progressive limb loading simultaneously (Fig. 28-63).

At this stage external resistance in the form of weights, elastic resistance, or pulleys can be added for strengthening.

- ***Abdominal crunch.*** The patient lies in the supine position with the knees flexed to approximate 90 degrees and the feet resting on the table. The patient folds his or her hands across the chest. The patient is asked to perform the abdominal drawing-in maneuver, and then to raise the head and

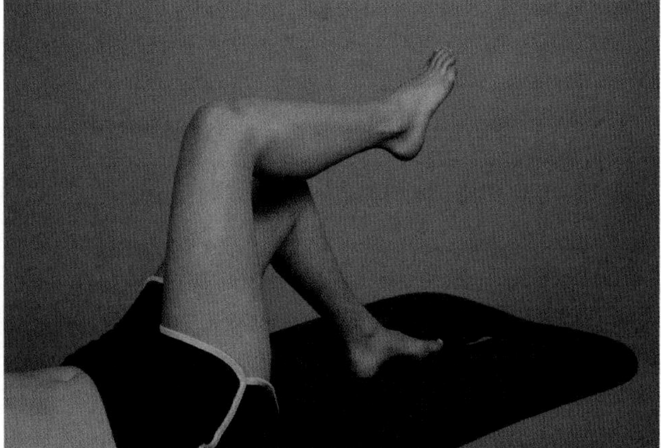

FIGURE 28-58 Progressive limb loading 1.

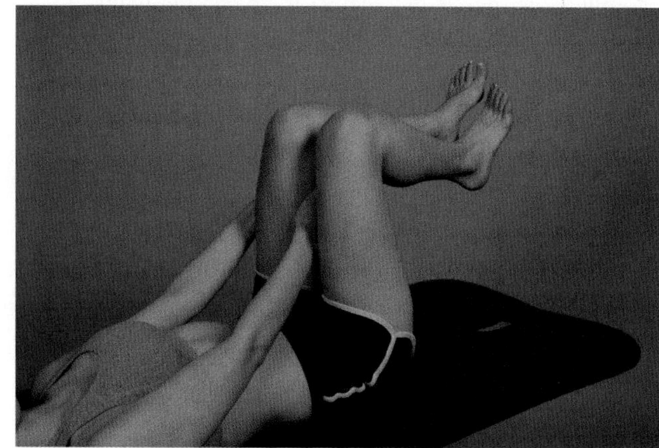

FIGURE 28-61 Progressive limb loading 4.

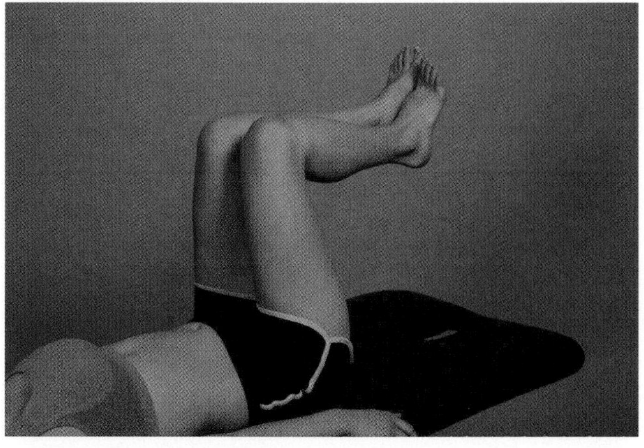

FIGURE 28-62 Progressive limb loading 5.

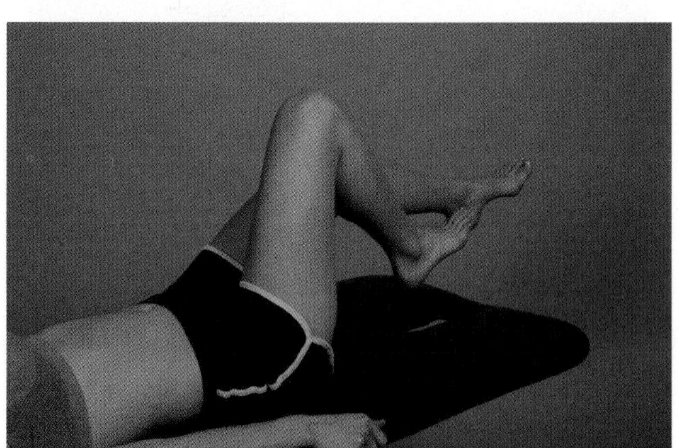

FIGURE 28-63 Progressive limb loading 6.

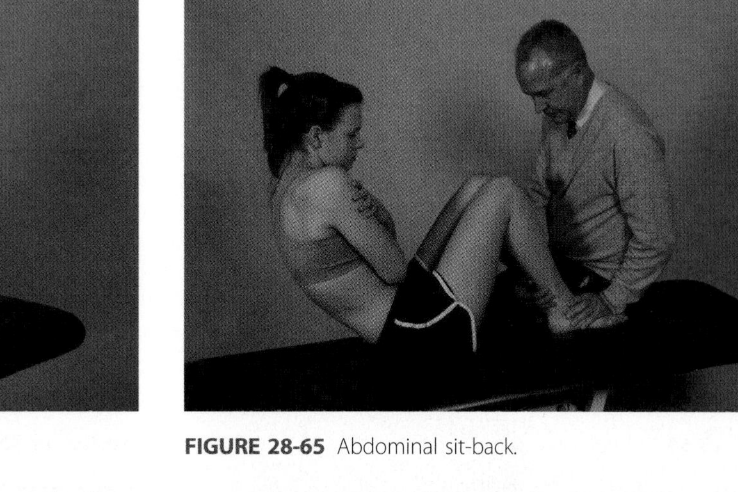

FIGURE 28-65 Abdominal sit-back.

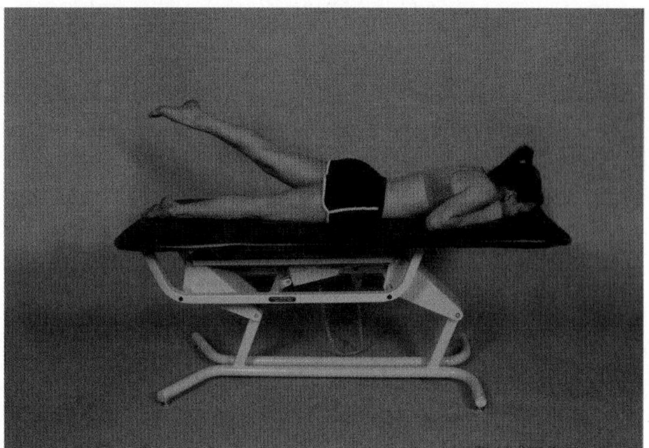

FIGURE 28-66 Prone progression.

shoulders upward until the shoulder blades clear the table (Fig. 28-64). This position is held for approximately 5 seconds before the patient returns to the starting position.

Abdominal Sit-Back

The patient is positioned in the "up" position of the standard sit-up with the arms folded across the chest and the feet secured on the bed (Fig. 28-65). Keeping the arms folded across the chest, the patient performs the abdominal drawing-in maneuver and then slowly lowers the upper body to a predetermined height.

Emphasis on the Trunk Extensors. The following exercises are performed with the patient lying in prone position[608]:

- extend one lower extremity (Fig. 28-66);
- extend both lower extremities (Fig. 28-67);
- lift the head, arms, and lower extremities (Fig. 28-68).

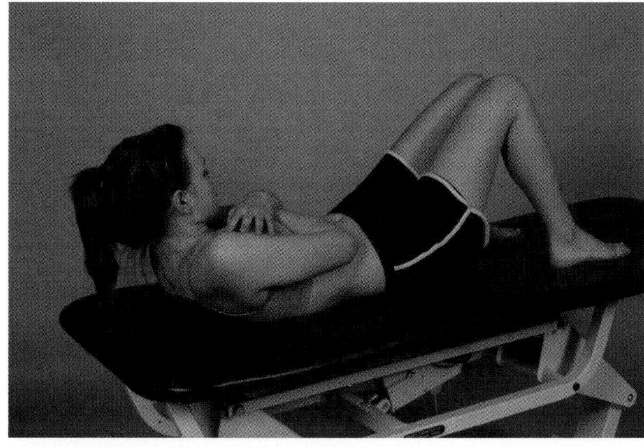

FIGURE 28-64 Abdominal crunch.

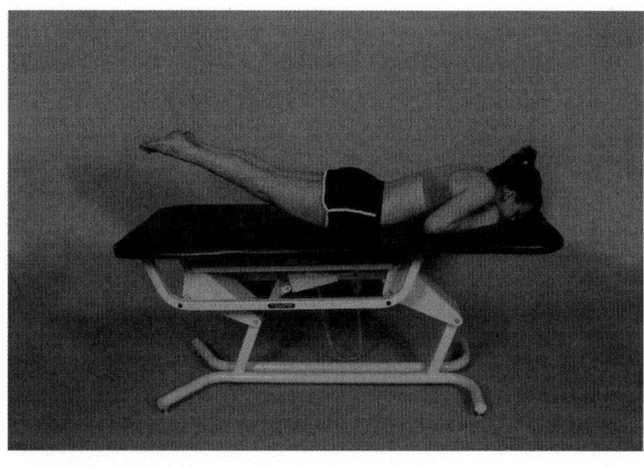

FIGURE 28-67 Prone progression 2.

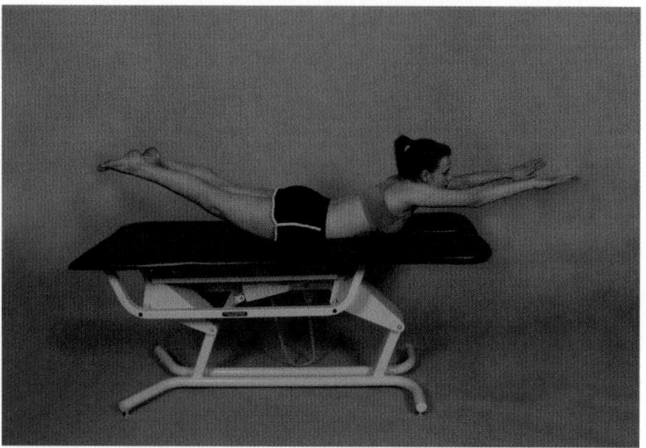

FIGURE 28-68 Prone progression 3.

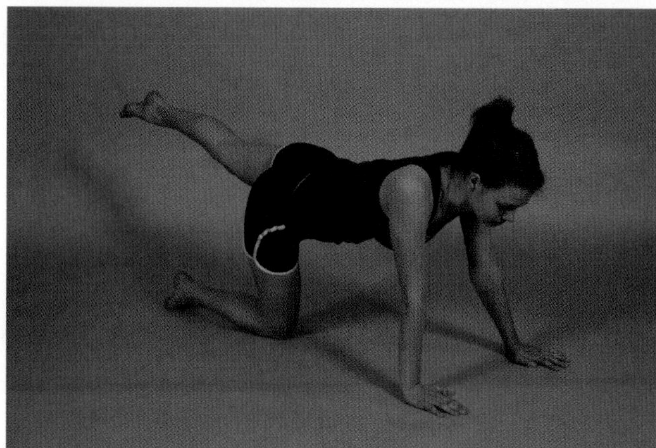

FIGURE 28-70 Quadriped progression 2.

For patients with limited lumbar extension, or those with increased symptoms with lumbar extension, a small pillow can be placed under the hips in prone for the starting position, and the patient can lift the upper and lower extremities to the neutral position of the lumbar spine.

At this stage, external resistance in the form of weights, elastic resistance, or pulleys can be added for strengthening.

These exercises are then performed in the quadriped position and include the following progression:

- flex one upper extremity (Fig. 28-69);
- extend one lower extremity by sliding it along the exercise mat (Fig. 28-70);
- flex one upper extremity and extend the contralateral lower extremity (Fig. 28-71).

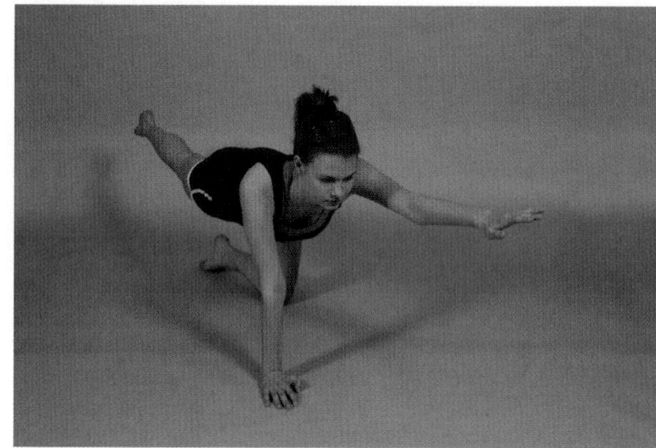

FIGURE 28-71 Quadriped progression 3.

Emphasis on the Lateral Stabilizers. These exercises are performed in the side-lying position and include the following progression

- side plank with hips on bed (Fig. 28-72);
- side plank (Fig. 28-73);
- side plank with arm extended (Fig. 28-74);
- side plank with hip abduction (Fig. 28-75);
- side plank with inward roll (Fig. 28-76).

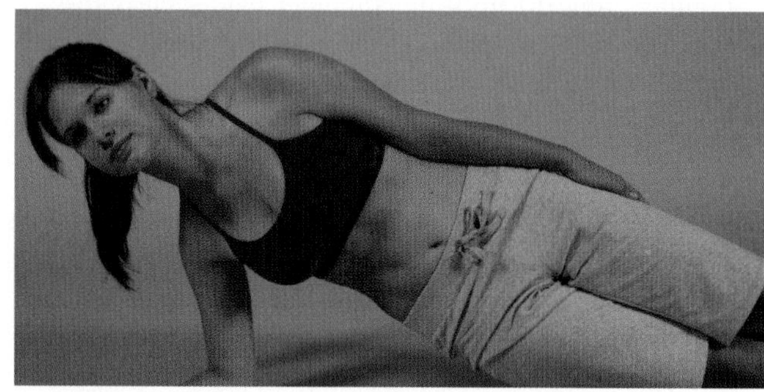

FIGURE 28-72 Side-lying progression 1.

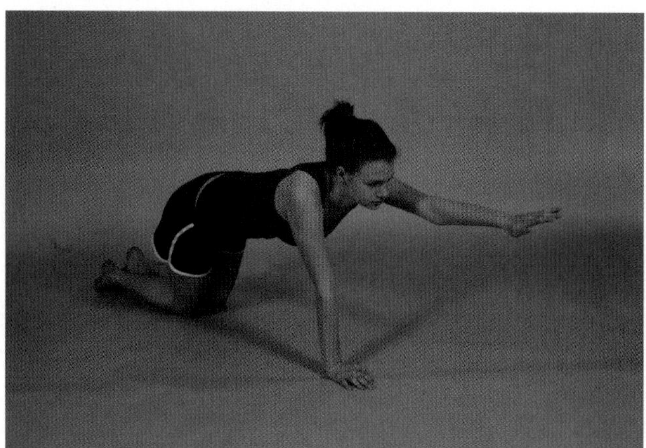

FIGURE 28-69 Quadriped progression 1.

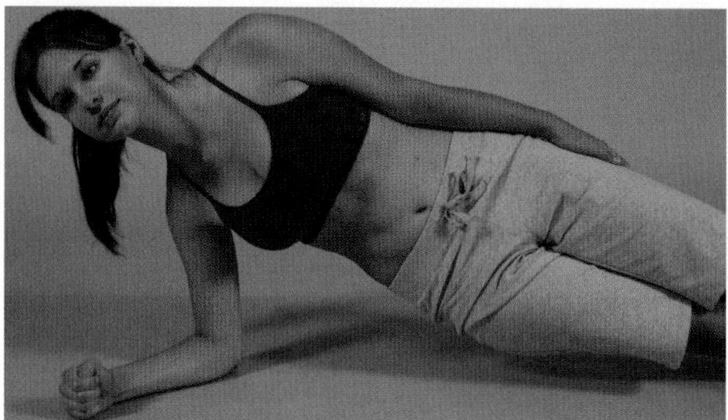

FIGURE 28-73 Side-lying progression 2.

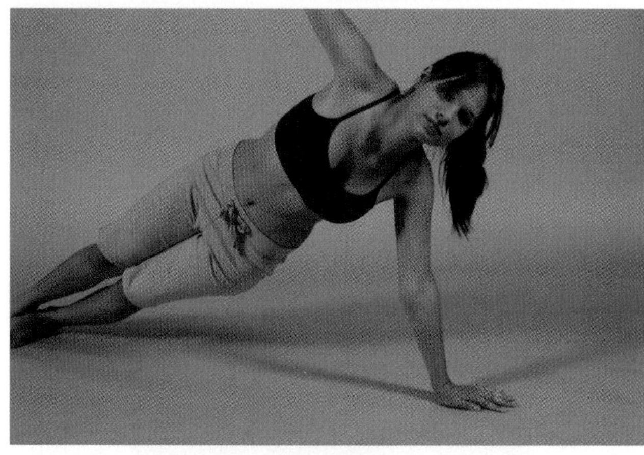
FIGURE 28-74 Side-lying progression 3.

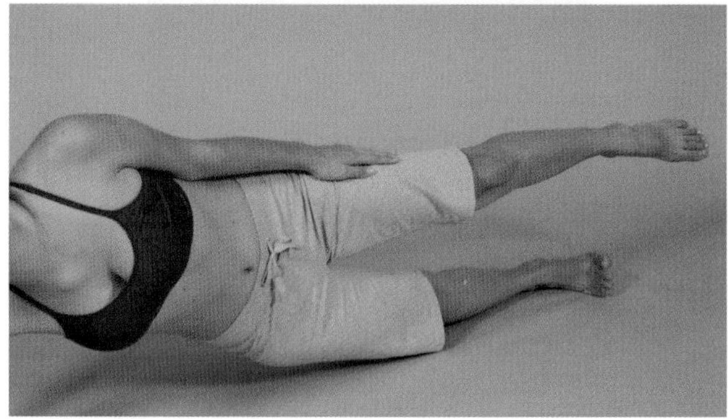
FIGURE 28-75 Side-lying progression 4.

Emphasis on Function.

- ***Bridging.*** The patient is positioned supine, with the arms by the sides. The patient is asked to keep the knees bent and feet flat, and to lift the buttocks from the floor (Fig. 28-77). The exercise can be made more challenging by having the patient squeeze a ball with their thighs while performing the bridge (Fig. 28-78).
- Bridging with feet on a ball, knees bent (Fig. 28-79).
- Bridging with feet on a ball, knees straight (Fig. 28-80).

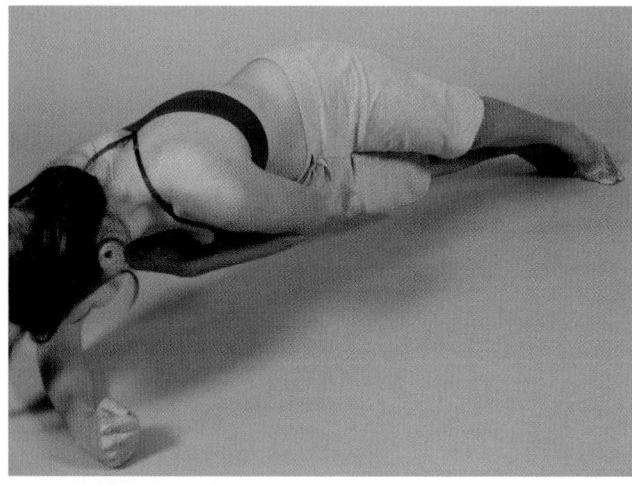
FIGURE 28-76 Side-lying progression 5.

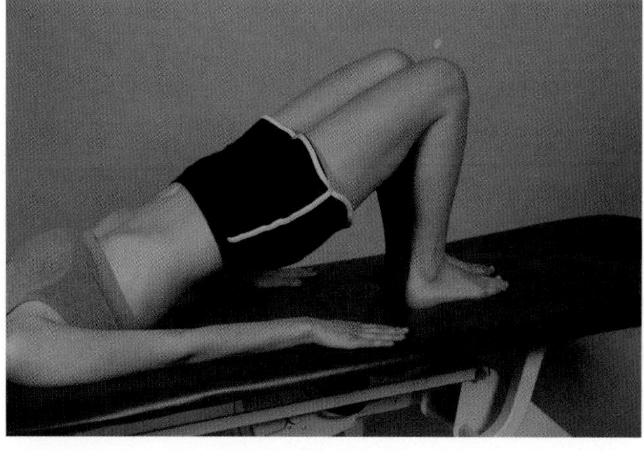
FIGURE 28-77 Bridging progression 1.

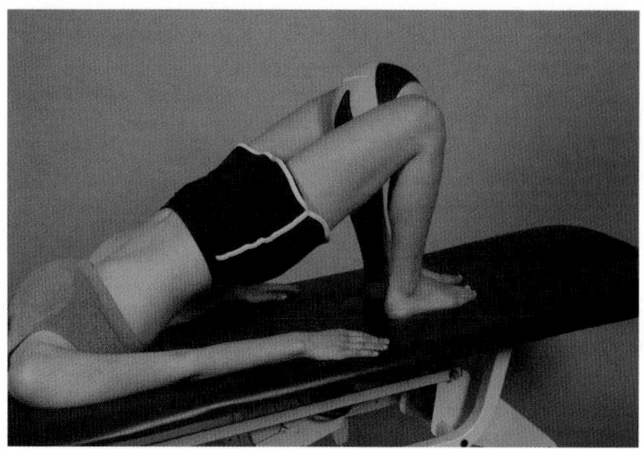
FIGURE 28-78 Bridging progression 2.

- Bridging with shoulders on a Swiss ball (Fig. 28-81).
- ***Wall slides.*** With the back against a wall, the patient is asked to perform a squat and then return to standing, while maintaining the neutral zone throughout the exercise. Modifications to this exercise include
  - a medicine ball is placed between the patient's knees.
- ***Forward lunge.*** While maintaining the neutral zone throughout the exercise, the patient is asked to step forward

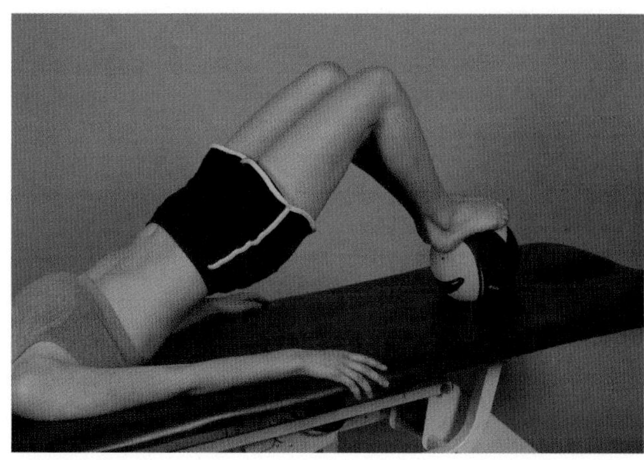
FIGURE 28-79 Bridging progression 3.

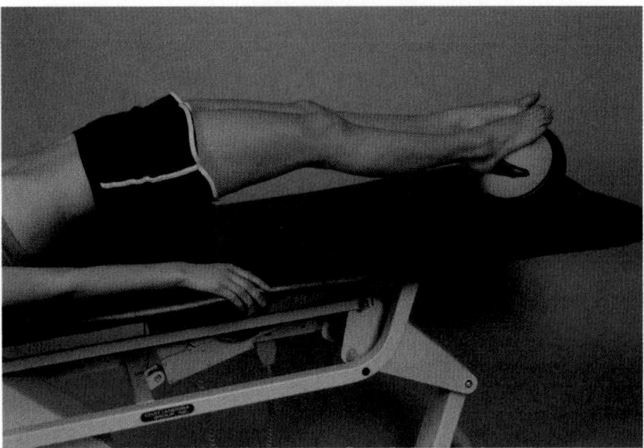

FIGURE 28-80 Bridging progression 4.

with one leg, and lower the opposite knee toward the ground. Hand weights, elastic resistance, or dumbbells (Fig. 28-82) can be used to make the exercise more challenging.

- ***Backward lunge.*** While maintaining the neutral zone throughout the exercise, the patient is asked to step backward with one leg, and lower the same knee to the ground, before returning to the starting position. Hand weights, elastic resistance, or dumbbells can be used to make the exercise more challenging.
- ***Chop and lift.*** The chop and lift motions are excellent at recruiting the lumbar stabilizers for mobility or stability. These motions can be performed in half kneeling (Fig. 28-83), tall kneeling (Fig. 28-84), or standing (Fig. 28-85). In contrast to the standing posture that offers a wide, adaptable BOS and can utilize all portions of the lower extremity kinetic chain, the kneeling position provides a narrow BOS, rendering distal portions of the kinetic chain unable to assist in corrected movements.[609] Tall kneeling creates a challenge to balance reactions in the anterior and posterior directions, whereas half kneeling creates a challenge to balance reactions laterally.[609]

Emphasis on Athletic Performance.

- ***Hip thrusts.*** The patient is positioned supine, with the hips and knees flexed to approximately 90 degrees and the arms

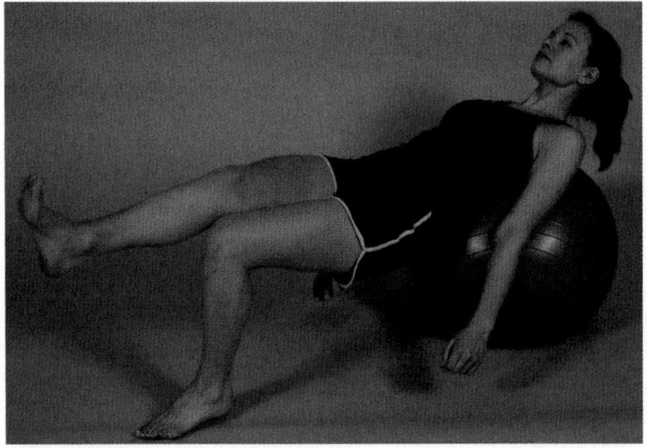

FIGURE 28-81 Bridging progression 5.

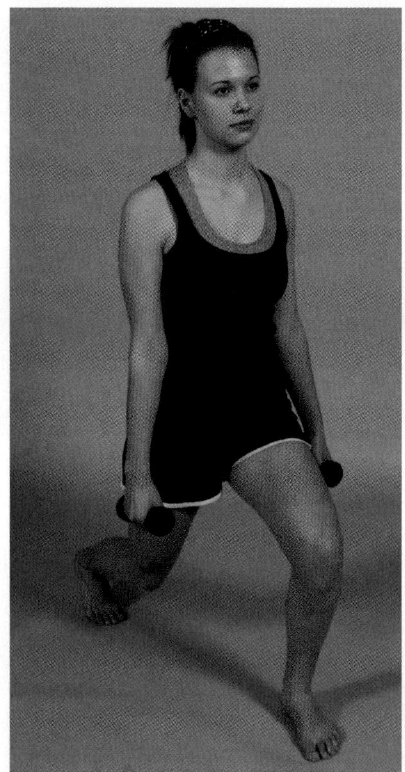

FIGURE 28-82 Forward lunge.

by the sides (Fig. 28-86). From this position, the patient is asked to perform an abdominal hollowing and lift the pelvis off the bed, while maintaining the hip and knee positions. Once the patient is able to do this exercise independently,

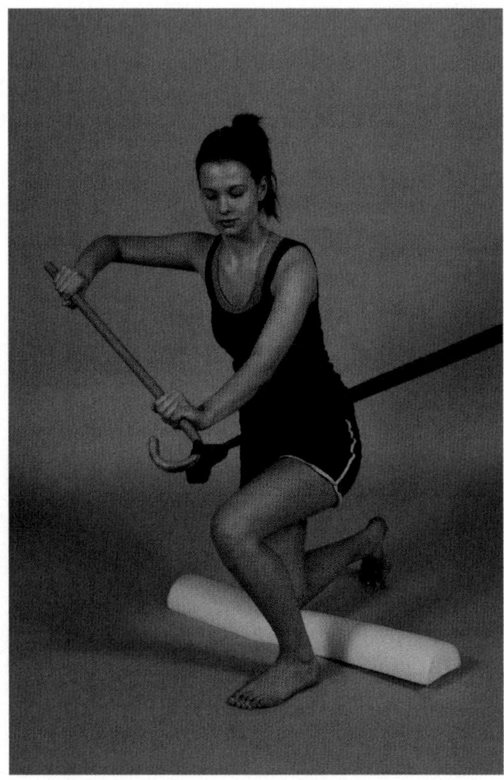

FIGURE 28-83 Chop and lift in half-kneeling.

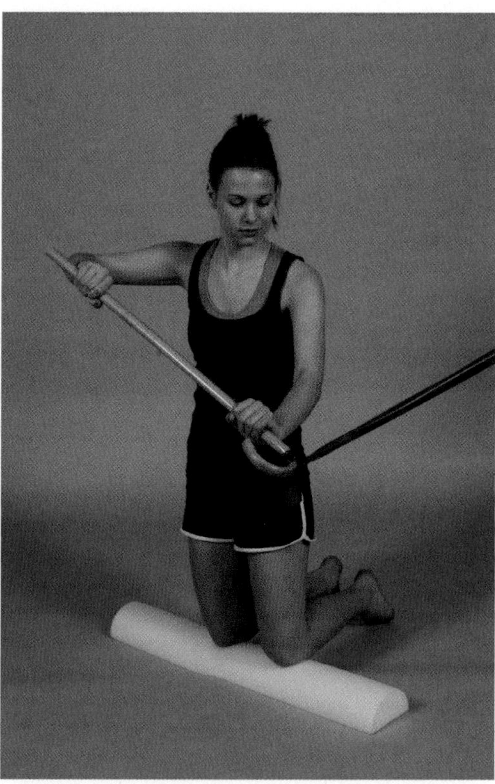

FIGURE 28-84 Chop and lift in tall-kneeling.

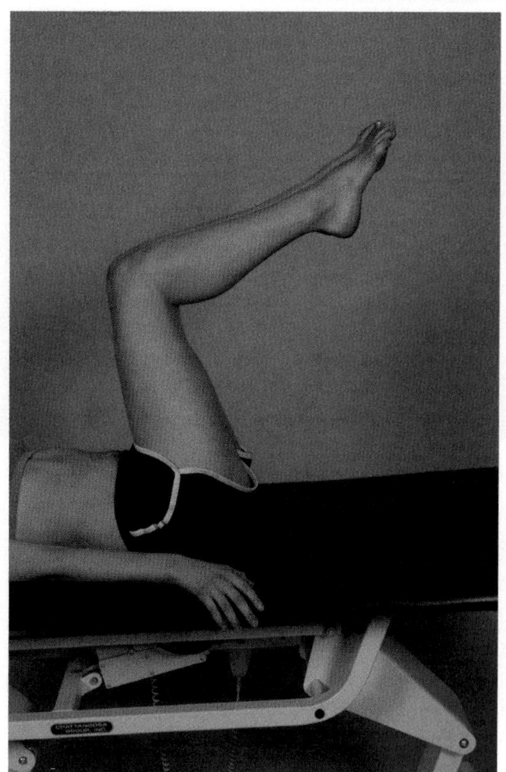

FIGURE 28-86 Hip thrusts.

the exercise can be performed with the hips flexed to 90 degrees and the knees extended (Fig. 28-87).

- ***Rotational partial sit-up.*** The patient is asked to lift the chin toward the chest. The patient is then asked to attempt to lift the right shoulder up from the table, while twisting the trunk to the left and touching the outside of the opposite knee (Fig. 28-88), before slowly lowering the shoulder to the table.
- ***Reverse curl-up.*** The patient lies in the supine position, with the legs bent at the knees and the feet flat on the floor. The arms are by the sides. The patient is asked to raise the feet off

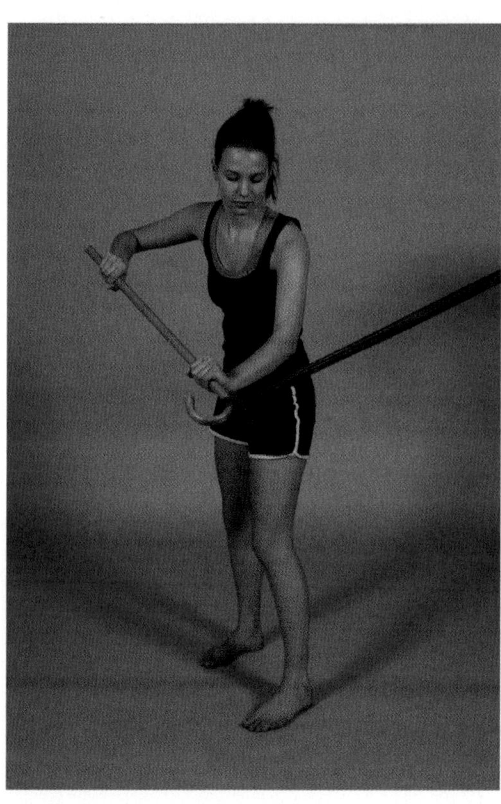

FIGURE 28-85 Chop and lift in standing.

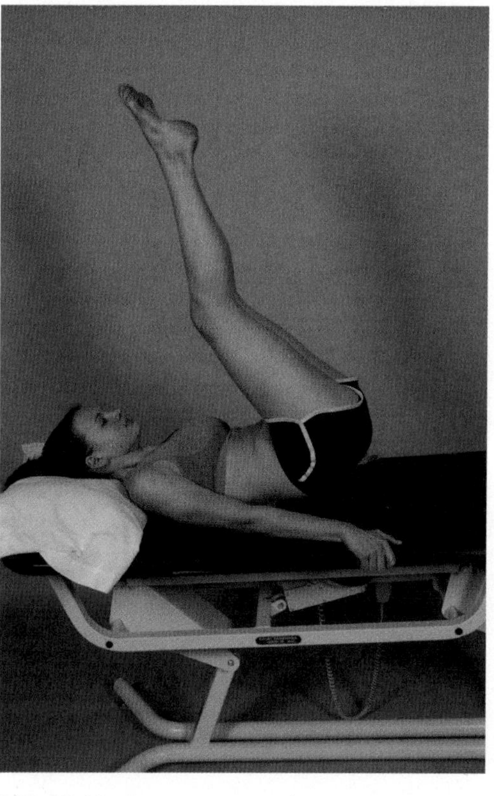

FIGURE 28-87 Hip thrust exercise with resistance.

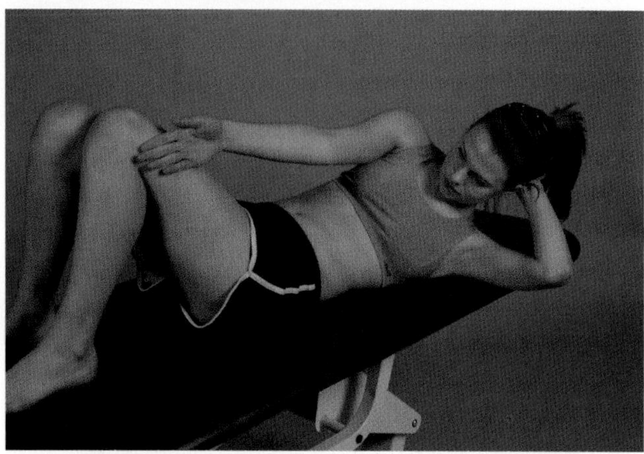

FIGURE 28-88 Rotational partial sit-up.

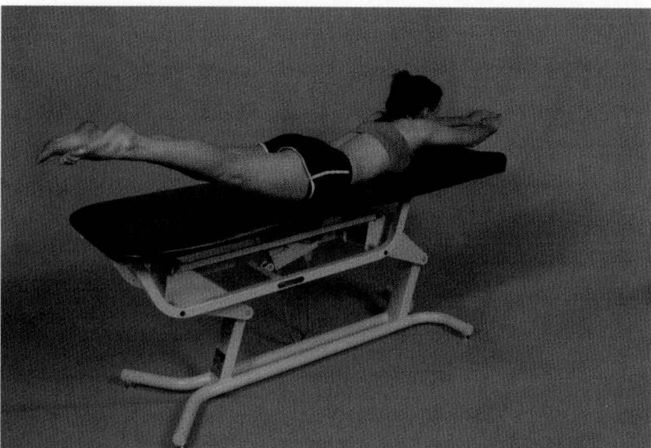

FIGURE 28-90 Superman position.

the bed until the thighs are vertical (Fig. 28-89). This is the start position. From this position, the patient is asked to raise the pelvis up and toward the shoulders, keeping the knees bent tightly, until the knees are as close to the chest as possible. The patient is allowed to push down on the bed with the hands. After holding this position for 2–3 seconds, the patient returns to the start position.

- ***Superman.*** The patient lies in the prone position, with the arms overhead and knees straight, the patient is asked to raise both arms and legs toward the ceiling, while keeping the head raised off the table (Fig. 28-90).
- ***Prone plank*** (Fig. 28-91). This exercise can be made more challenging by asking the patient to raise one upper extremity at a time, one lower extremity at a time, or opposite upper extremity and lower extremity simultaneously.
- ***Prone lying on a Swiss ball, hands touching floor (Fig. 28-92).*** This can be progressed to push-ups with the legs on a chair (Fig. 28-93), and to walking in circles around the Swiss ball using only the hands.
- ***Rhythmic stabilization.*** The patient is positioned in quadriped with one limb raised. The clinician applies perturbations to the patient, while the patient attempts to

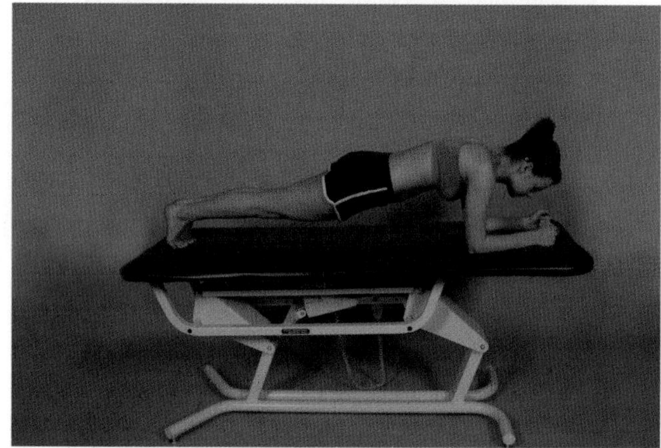

FIGURE 28-91 Prone plank.

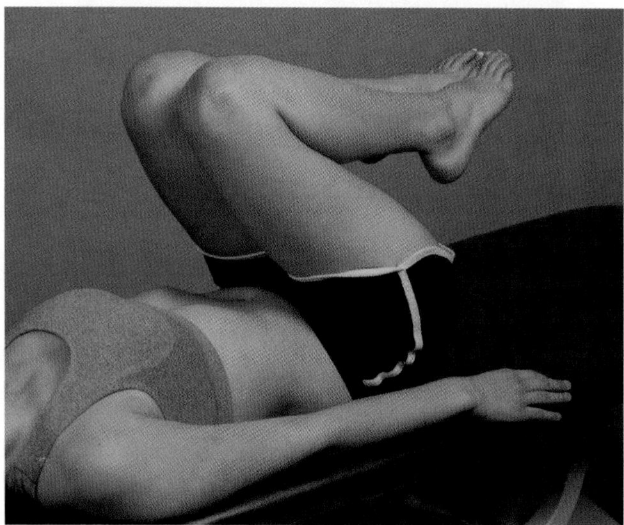

FIGURE 28-89 Reverse curl up.

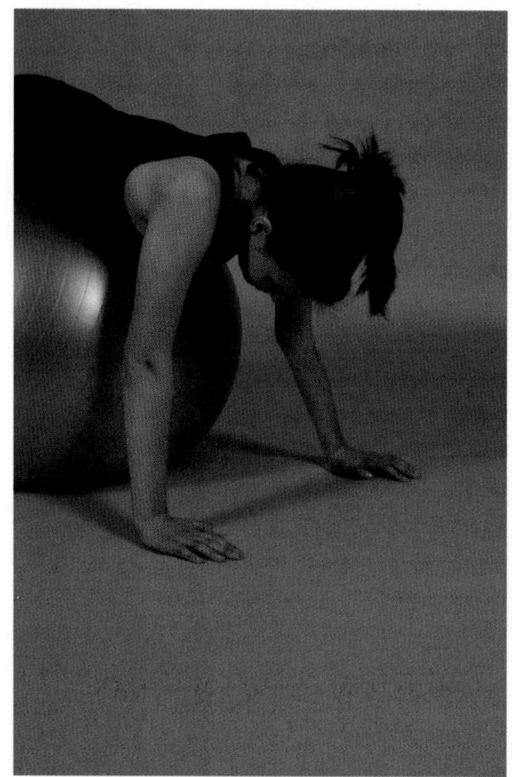

FIGURE 28-92 Prone lying on a Swiss ball, hands touching floor.

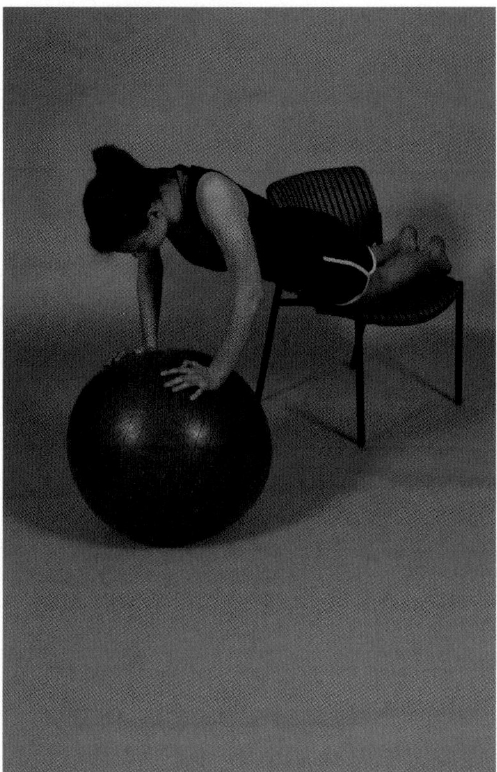

FIGURE 28-93 Push-ups with legs on a chair.

resist using a variety of points of contact, and positions (Fig. 28-94). This exercise can be progressed by raising both an upper extremity and the contralateral lower extremity.

Correction of Muscle Imbalances

In addition to addressing core stabilization, muscle imbalances must also be addressed in terms of flexibility as poor flexibility may cause excessive stresses to be borne by the lumbar motion segments. For example, adaptively shortened hip flexors and rectus femoris muscles can cause increased anterior shearing of the lumbar spine. Occasionally, stretching both the anterior and the posterior thigh muscles is beneficial. However, most of the time, only one should be stretched, and the decision is based on the diagnosis:

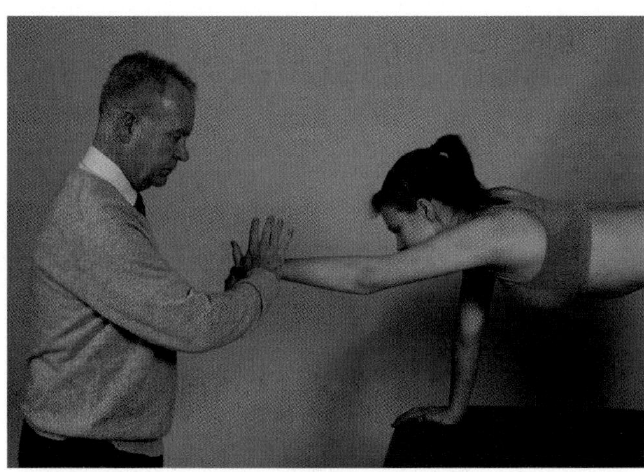

FIGURE 28-94 Rhythmic stabilization in quadriped.

- The patient with spinal stenosis or a painful extension hypomobility, and who responds well to lumbar flexion exercises, should be taught how to stretch the hip flexors and rectus femoris while protecting the lumbar spine from excessive lordosis.
- The patient with a painful flexion hypomobility or IVD herniation, and who responds well to lumbar extension exercises, should be taught how to stretch the hamstrings while protecting the lumbar spine from flexing.

THERAPEUTIC TECHNIQUES

Manual therapy is a common intervention used in the treatment of individuals with LBP.

Techniques to Increase Joint Mobility

Three types of techniques can be used to increase joint mobility. These include joint mobilizations, high-velocity thrust techniques, and muscle energy.

Joint Mobilizations and High-Velocity Thrust Techniques

The Guide to Physical Therapist Practice identifies mobilization/manipulation as an intervention appropriate for the care of patients spinal disorders.[610] Several randomized trials have found manipulation to be more effective than placebo[611,612] or other interventions.[613,614] However other studies have not shown any benefits for manipulation versus other interventions.[454,615,616] The literature tends to suggest that lumbar manipulation is most successful if performed in the subacute stage of a noncomplicated lumbar condition.[412,617] However, this description represents a very small percentage of patients with low-back dysfunction, and in most cases the patient is more likely to benefit from aerobic exercise, less invasive manual techniques, and dynamic stabilization training.[618]

Although a grade V technique shares similarities with a grade IV mobilization, in terms of amplitude and position in the joint's range, grade V differs in the velocity of delivery. Chapter 10 outlines the indications and contraindications for high-velocity thrust techniques. If a high-velocity thrust technique is to be used, the clinician should perform a premanipulative hold (see Chap. 10).

All of the examination techniques that are used to assess joint mobility can be employed as intervention techniques. However, the intent of the technique changes from one of assessing the end-feel to one in which the application of graded mobilizations, or muscle energy techniques, is applied at the appropriate joint range. The selection of a manual technique is dependent on a number of factors, including (1) the acuteness of the condition, (2) the goal of the intervention, and (3) whether the restriction is symmetric or asymmetric.

Techniques to Increase Soft Tissue Extensibility

McKenzie Techniques

Extension mobilization with overpressure. (VIDEO)

Extension mobilization with belt. (VIDEO)

Off-set extension in lying. (VIDEO)

Extension in lying with partial weight bearing. (VIDEO)
Extension in lying "roadkill". (VIDEO)
Extension in lying with hip abduction and knee flexion. (VIDEO)
Standing extension. (VIDEO)
Standing extension sag. (VIDEO)
Extension mobilization.(VIDEO)
Flexion rotation. (VIDEO)
Sustained flexion rotation. (VIDEO)
Seated flexion progression. (VIDEO)
Flexion in step standing. (VIDEO)
Lateral shift correction. (VIDEO)
Seated posture correction. (VIDEO)

CASE STUDIES

1. A 58-year-old woman presented with a gradual onset of low-back and sacroiliac joint pain. Her chief complaint was a "stiff" back, especially in the morning. The patient had experienced mild discomfort over several years but had noticed a recent increase in its intensity over the past few months. The pain was reported as being worse with prolonged standing, lifting, bending, and walking and was relieved by sitting and lying down. The pain occasionally was felt in the right buttock, hip, and thigh. A recent radiograph revealed the presence of "arthritic changes" in the lumbar spine.

   The patient reported being in good general health. There were no reports of night pain, bowel and bladder changes, or pain with coughing or sneezing.

   1. List the differential diagnosis for complaints of pain in the low back and sacroiliac joint.
   2. What may be the significance of a history of morning stiffness?
   3. List the potential reasons for the patient's symptoms being worsened with prolonged standing, lifting, bending, and walking and improved with sitting or lying?
   4. From the history, what are the indications that this may be a musculoskeletal problem?
   5. Which tests could you use to rule in/out the potential reasons for the patient's complaints?
   6. Does this presentation/history warrant a Cyriax lower quarter scanning examination? Why or why not?

2. A 40-year-old man presented with a 3-month history of gradual onset of LBP, with no specific mechanism of injury. The pain was felt across the lower back at the level of the belt line. The patient reported no pain in the morning upon arising. The pain began soon after reporting to work as a cashier in a grocery store and worsened as the day wore on. The pain was also worsened with activities that involving prolonged walking or prone lying. The pain was relieved almost instantly by sitting or side lying, with the knees drawn to the chest. The patient had radiographs of the spine taken recently, which showed some evidence of arthritis but were otherwise unremarkable.

   The patient reported being in general good health. There were no reports of night pain, bowel and bladder changes, or pain with coughing or sneezing.

   1. List the differential diagnosis for complaints of a gradual onset of pain in the low back in this age group.
   2. What may be the significance of a history of no morning pain or stiffness?
   3. List the potential reasons for the patient's symptoms getting worse with prolonged standing, walking, and lying but better with sitting or the fetal position.
   4. From the history, what are the indications that LBP may be a musculoskeletal problem?
   5. What is your working hypothesis at this stage? Which tests could you use to confirm or refute your hypothesis?
   6. Does this presentation/history warrant a Cyriax lower quarter scanning examination? Why or why not?

3. A 20-year-old man complained of a sudden onset of unilateral LBP. The pain was so severe as to prevent the patient from standing upright. The patient described a mechanism of bending forward quickly to catch a ball near his left foot. He immediately experienced a sharp pain in his low back and was unable to straighten up because of the pain. The patient had no past history of back pain. No spinal radiographs had been taken.[619]

   1. List the differential diagnosis for complaints of a gradual onset of unilateral LBP.
   2. What may be the significance of the reported mechanism?
   3. List the potential reasons for the patient being initially unable to straighten up from the flexed position.
   4. From the history, what are the indications that this may be a musculoskeletal problem?
   5. Would the results from imaging studies be useful in this case? Why or why not?
   6. What is your working hypothesis at this stage? Which tests could you use to confirm or refute your hypothesis?
   7. Does this presentation/history warrant a Cyriax lower quarter scanning examination? Why or why not?

4. A 45-year-old woman was referred for LBP. She complained of pain across the center of her back at the waistline level. The pain, which had started gradually many years ago, had not spread from this small area, but it had increased in intensity. The increase in intensity resulted from a bending and lifting injury a few years previously, and, since that incident, the patient reported having difficulty straightening up from the bent-over position. Twisting maneuvers, whether in standing, sitting, or lying position, also produced the pain, but otherwise the woman was able to sit, stand, or walk for long periods without pain.

   1. List the differential diagnosis for complaints of a gradual onset of central LBP.

2. What may be the significance of the insidious onset?
3. List the potential reasons for the patient having difficulty straightening up from the flexed position.
4. From the history, what are the indications that this may be a mechanical problem?
5. Would the results from imaging studies be useful in this case? If so, which?
6. What is your working hypothesis at this stage? Which tests could you use to confirm or refute your hypothesis?
7. Does this presentation/history warrant a Cyriax lower quarter scanning examination? Why or why not?

5. A 65-year-old man presented with an insidious onset of right leg symptoms, which followed a period, or distance, of walking, or occurred after a period of standing, and which disappeared when he sat down. The patient also complained of pain at night, especially when he slept on his stomach. Further questioning revealed that the patient had a history of back pain related to an occupation involving heavy lifting but was otherwise in good health and had no reports of bowel or bladder impairment.

   1. Given the age of the patient and the history, do you have a working hypothesis?
   2. Why do you think the patient has pain with prone lying?
   3. Is the pain at night a cause for concern in this patient? Why?
   4. Does this presentation/history warrant a scanning examination? Why or why not?

6. A 21-year-old woman presented with LBP that had occurred while playing racket ball and had been accompanied by a sharp pain in the right buttock area. The patient was able to carry on playing, and the sharp pain subsided until the following morning, when attempted to weight bear through the right leg. The pain again subsided after a hot shower and her walk to work. That evening, the patient went jogging and was forced to stop after about a mile because of the return of the sharp pain in the buttock. A hot soak eased the pain but was replaced by a dull ache that lasted several days. The patient sought medical advice and was referred to physical therapy. When asked to indicate where her pain was, she pointed to a small area, medial to the right trochanter, over the piriformis muscle. Further questioning revealed that the patient had no previous history of back pain and was otherwise in good health, with no reports of bowel or bladder impairment.

   1. What structure(s) could be at fault with complaints of buttock pain?
   2. What does the history of the pain tell the clinician?
   3. What is your working hypothesis at this stage? List the various diagnoses that could present with buttock pain, and the tests you would use to rule out each one.
   4. Does this presentation/history warrant a scan? Why or why not?

REVIEW QUESTIONS*

1. Which of the spinal ligaments gives the best support against posterolateral IVD protrusions?
2. Which lumbar ligament, consisting of five bands, prevents anterior shearing of L5 on S1?
3. Which muscles make up the erector spinae?
4. Which motions does the multifidus muscle produce?
5. Approximately what is the normal amount of lumbar ROM with flexion and extension?

*Additional questions to test your understanding of this chapter can be found in the Online Learning Center for *Orthopaedic Assessment, Evaluation, and Intervention* at www.duttononline.net.

REFERENCES

1. Woolf A, Pfleger B: Burden of major musculoskeletal conditions. *Bull World Health Org* 81:646–656, 2003.
2. Nachemson A: Chronic pain—the end of the welfare state? *Qual Life Res* 1:S11–S17, 1994.
3. Waddell G: A new clinical model for the treatment of low back pain. *Spine* 12:632–643, 1987.
4. Gibson JN, Grant IC, Waddell G: The Cochrane review of surgery for lumbar disc prolapse and degenerative lumbar spondylosis. *Spine* 24:1820–1832, 1999.
5. Croft PR, Macfarlane GJ, Papageorgiou AC, et al: Outcome of low back pain in general practice: A prospective study. *BMJ* 316:1356–1359, 1998.
6. Linton SJ: The socioeconomic impact of chronic back pain: is anyone benefiting? *Pain* 75:163–168, 1998.
7. Indahl A, Velund L, Reikeraas O: Good prognosis for low back pain when left untampered. *Spine* 20:473–477, 1995.
8. Bodack MP, Monteiro M: Therapeutic exercise in the treatment of patients with lumbar spinal stenosis. *Clin Orthop Relat Res* 384:144–152, 2001.
9. Caspersen CJ, Powell KE, Christenson GM: Physical activity, exercise and physical fitness. *Public Health Rep* 100:125–131, 1985.
10. Danielsen J, Johnsen R, Kibsgaard S, et al: Early aggressive exercise for postoperative rehabilitation after discectomy. *Spine* 25:1015–1020, 2000.
11. Janeck K, Reuven B, Romano CT: Spinal stabilization exercises for the injured worker. *Occup Med* 13:199–207, 1998.
12. Kendall PH, Jenkins JM: Exercises for back ache: A double blind controlled study. *Physiotherapy* 54:154–157, 1968.
13. O'Sullivan PB: Lumbar segmental 'instability': Clinical presentation and specific stabilizing exercise management. *Man Ther* 5:2–12, 2000.
14. Kahanovitz N, Nordin M, Verderame R, et al: Normal trunk muscle strength and endurance in women and the effect of exercises and electrical stimulation: Part 2. Comparative analysis of electrical stimulation and exercise to increase trunk muscle strength and endurance. *Spine* 12:112–118, 1987.
15. Nachemson A: Work for all. For those with low back pain as well. *Clin Orthop* 179:77, 1982.
16. Bogduk N, Twomey LT: Anatomy and biomechanics of the lumbar spine. In: Bogduk N, Twomey LT, eds. *Clinical Anatomy of the Lumbar Spine and Sacrum*, 3rd ed. Edinburgh: Churchill Livingstone, 1997:2–53; 81–152;171–176.
17. Ghosh P, Bushell GR, Taylor TKF, et al: Collagens, elastin and non-collagenous protein of the intervertebral disc. *Clin Orthop* 129:124–132, 1977.

18. Taylor JR: The development and adult structure of lumbar intervertebral discs. *J Man Med* 5:43–47, 1990.
19. Tsuji H, Hirano N, Ohshima H, et al: Structural variation of the anterior and posterior anulus fibrosus in the development of the human lumbar intervertebral disc: A risk factor for intervertebral disc rupture. *Spine* 18:204–210, 1993.
20. Hickey DS, Hukins DWL: Relation between the structure of the annulus fibrosus and the function and failure of the intervertebral disc. *Spine* 5:100–116, 1980.
21. Marchand F, Ahmed AM: Investigation of the laminate structure of lumbar disc anulus fibrosus. *Spine* 15:402–410, 1990.
22. Lundon K, Bolton K: Structure and function of the lumbar intervertebral disk in health, aging, and pathological conditions. *J Orthop Sports Phys Ther* 31:291–306, 2001.
23. Mercer S: Comparative anatomy of the spinal disc. In: Boyling JD, Jull GA, eds. *Grieve's Modern Manual Therapy: The Vertebral Column*. Philadelphia, PA: Churchill Livingstone, 2004:9–16.
24. Naylor A: The biophysical and biomechanical aspects of intervertebral disc herniation and degeneration. *Ann R Coll Surg Engl* 31:91–114, 1962.
25. Buckwalter JA, Cooper RR, Maynard JA: Elastic fibers in human intervertebral discs. *J Bone Joint Surg Am* 58:73–76, 1976.
26. Coventry MB, Ghormley RK, Kernohan JW: The intervertebral disc: Its microscopic anatomy and pathology. Part 1: Anatomy, development and physiology. *J Bone Joint Surg* 28A:105–111, 1945.
27. Akeson WH, Woo SL, Taylor TK, et al: Biomechanics and biochemistry of the intervertebral disks: The need for correlation studies. *Clin Orthop* 129:133–140, 1977.
28. Adams MA, McNally DS, Wagstaff J, et al: Abnormal stress concentrations in lumbar intervertebral discs following damage to the vertebral body: A cause of disc failure. European Spine Society (Acromed) Award paper. *Eur Spine J* 1:214–221, 1993.
29. Adams MA, McNally DM, Chinn H, et al: Posture and the compressive strength of the lumbar spine. International Society of Biomechanics Award Paper. *Clin Biomech* 9:5–14, 1994.
30. Osti OL, Vernon-Roberts B, Frazer RD: Annulus tears and intervertebral disc degeneration: A study using an animal model. *Spine* 15:762, 1990.
31. Panjabi M, Hult EJ, Crisco J III, et al: Biomechanical studies in cadaveric spines. In: Jayson MIV, ed. *The Lumbar Spine and Back Pain*. New York, NY: Churchill Livingstone, 1992:133–135.
32. Farfan HF, Cossette JW, Robertson GH, et al: The effects of torsion on the lumbar intervertebral joints: The role of torsion in the production of disc degeneration. *J Bone Joint Surg* 52A:468–497, 1970.
33. Saal JA: Natural history and nonoperative treatment of lumbar disc herniation. *Spine* 21:2S–9S, 1996.
34. Rydevik B, Garfin SR: Spinal nerve root compression. In: Szabo RM, ed. *Nerve Compression Syndromes: Diagnosis and Treatment*. Thorofare, NJ: Slack, 1989:247–261.
35. Eyring EJ: The biochemistry and physiology of the intervertebral disc. *Clin Orthop* 67:16–28, 1969.
36. Coventry MB: Anatomy of the intervertebral disk. *Clin Orthop* 67:9–17, 1969.
37. Nachemson AL: The lumbar spine: An orthopedic challenge. *Spine* 1:59–71, 1976.
38. Inoue H: Three dimensional architecture of lumbar intervertebral discs. *Spine* 6:138–146, 1981.
39. Adams MA, McNally DS, Wagstaff J, et al: Abnormal stress concentrations in lumbar intervertebral discs following damage to the vertebral body: A cause of disc failure. *Eur Spine J* 1:214–221, 1993.
40. Lee CK, Rauschning W, Glenn W: Lateral lumbar spinal canal stenosis: Classification, pathologic anatomy and surgical decompression. *Spine* 13:313–320, 1988.
41. Fritz JM, Erhard R, Vignovic M: A non-surgical treatment approach for patients with lumbar spinal stenosis. *Spine* 77:962–973, 1997.
42. Bogduk N: The innervation of the lumbar spine. *Spine* 8:286–293, 1983.
43. Edger MA, Nundy S: Innervation of the spinal dura matter. *J Neurol Neurosurg Psychiatry* 29:530–534, 1966.
44. Malinsky J: The ontogenetic development of nerve terminations in the intervertebral discs of man. *Acta Anat* 38:96–113, 1959.
45. Kumar S, Davis PR: Lumbar vertebral innervation and intra-abdominal pressure. *J Anat* 114:47–53, 1973.
46. Farfan HF: *Mechanical Disorders of the Low Back*. Philadelphia, PA: Lea & Febiger, 1973.
47. Roberts N, Gratin C, Whitehouse GH: MRI analysis of lumbar intervertebral disc height in young and older populations. *J Magn Reson Imaging* 7:880–886, 1997.
48. Tulsi RS, Hermanis GM: A study of the angle of inclination and facet curvature of superior lumbar zygapophyseal facets. *Spine* 18:1311–1317, 1993.
49. Abumi K, Panjabi MM, Kramer KM, et al: Biomechanical evaluation of lumbar stability after graded facetectomies. *Spine* 15:1142–1147, 1990.
50. Haegg O, Wallner A: Facet joint asymmetry and protrusion of the intervertebral disc. *Spine* 15:356–359, 1990.
51. Ahmed AM, Duncan MJ, Burke DL: The effect of facet geometry on the axial torque-rotation response of lumbar motion segments. *Spine* 15:391–401, 1990.
52. Davis PR: The thoraco-lumbar mortice joint. *J Anat* 89:370–377, 1955.
53. Singer KP, Giles LGF: Manual therapy considerations at the thoracolumbar junction: An anatomical and functional perspective. *J Manip Physiol Ther* 13:83–88, 1990.
54. White AA: An analysis of the mechanics of the thoracic spine in man. *Acta Orthop Scand* 127(Suppl):8–92, 1969.
55. Lewin T: Osteoarthritis in lumbar synovial joints. *Acta Orthop Scand Suppl* 73:1–112, 1964.
56. MacIntosh J, Bogduk N: The biomechanics of the lumbar multifidus. *Clin Biomech* 1:205–213, 1986.
57. Lewin T, Moffet B, Viidik A: The morphology of the lumbar synovial intervertebral joints. *Acta Morphol Neerlando-Scand* 4:299–319, 1962.
58. Bogduk N, Jull G: The theoretical pathology of acute locked back: a basis for manipulative therapy. *Man Med* 1:78, 1985.
59. Willard FH: The muscular, ligamentous and neural structure of the low back and its relation to low back pain. In: Vleeming A, Mooney V, Dorman T, et al, eds. *Movement, Stability and Low Back Pain*. New York, NY: Churchill Livingstone, 1997:3–36.
60. Francois RJ: Ligament insertions into the human lumbar vertebral body. *Acta Anat* 91:467–480, 1975.
61. Bogduk N, Tynan W, Wilson AS: The nerve supply to the human intervertebral discs. *J Anat* 132:39–56, 1981.
62. White AA, Panjabi MM: *Clinical Biomechanics of the Spine*, 2nd ed. Philadelphia, PA: Lippincott-Raven, 1990:106–108.
63. Tkaczuk H: Tensile properties of human lumbar longitudinal ligament. *Acta Orthop Scand* 115:9–69, 1968.
64. Yong-Hing K, Reilly J, Kirkaldy-Willis WH: The ligamentum flavum. *Spine* 1:226–234, 1976.
65. Yahia LH, Garzon S, Strykowski H, et al: Ultrastructure of the human interspinous ligament and ligamentum flavum: A preliminary study. *Spine* 15:262–268, 1990.
66. Panjabi MM, Goel VK, Takata K: Physiologic strains in the lumbar ligaments: An in vitro biomechanical study. *Spine* 7:192–203, 1983.
67. Bogduk N, Wilson AS, Tynan W: The human lumbar dorsal rami. *J Anat* 134:383–397, 1982.
68. Heylings DJA: Supraspinous and interspinous ligaments of the human spine. *J Anat* 125:127–131, 1978.
69. Newman PH: Sprung back. *J Bone Joint Surg* 34B:30–37, 1952.
70. Hukins DWL, Kirby MC, Sikoryn TA, et al: Comparison of structure, mechanical properties, and function of lumbar spinal ligaments. *Spine* 15:787–795, 1990.
71. Gray H: *Gray's Anatomy*. Philadelphia, PA: Lea & Febiger, 1995.
72. Kapandji IA: *The Physiology of the Joints, The Trunk and Vertebral Column*. New York, NY: Churchill Livingstone, 1991.
73. Luk KDK, Ho HC, Leong JCY: The iliolumbar ligament. A study of its anatomy, development and clinical significance. *J Bone Joint Surg* 68B:197–200, 1986.
74. Chow DHK, Luk KDK, Leong JCY, et al: Torsional stability of the lumbosacral junction: Significance of the iliolumbar ligament. *Spine* 14:611–615, 1989.
75. Kirkaldy-Willis WH: The three phases of the spectrum of degenerative disease. In: Kirkaldy-Willis WH, ed. *Managing Low Back Pain*. New York, NY: Churchill Livingstone, 1983:75–90.
76. Seitsalo S, Osterman K, Hyvarinen H, et al: Progression of the spondylolisthesis in children and adolescents. *Spine* 16:417–421, 1991.
77. Golub BS, Silverman B: Transforaminal ligaments of the lumbar spine. *J Bone Joint Surg* 51A:947–956, 1969.
78. MacNab I: *Backache*. Baltimore, MD: Williams and Wilkins, 1978:98–100.
79. Bogduk N: The lumbar mamillo-accessory ligament. Its anatomical and neurosurgical significance. *Spine* 6:162–167, 1981.
80. Cholewicki J, McGill S: Mechanical stability of the in vivo lumbar spine: Implications for injury and chronic low back pain. *Clin Biomech (Bristol, Avon)* 11:1–15, 1996.

81. Hodges P, Richardson C: Inefficient muscular stabilisation of the lumbar spine associated with low back pain: A motor control evaluation of transversus abdominis. *Spine* 21:2540–2650, 1996.
82. Morgan D: Concepts in functional training and postural stabilization for the low-back-injured. *Top Acute Care Trauma Rehabil* 2:8–17, 1988.
83. Williams PL, Warwick R, Dyson M, et al: *Gray's Anatomy*, 37th ed. London: Churchill Livingstone, 1989.
84. Hides JA, Richardson CA, Jull GA: Multifidus muscle recovery is not automatic after resolution of acute, first-episode low back pain. *Spine* 21:2763–2769, 1996.
85. Goel V, Kong W, Han J, et al: A combined finite element and optimization investigation of lumbar spine mechanics with and without muscles. *Spine* 18:1531–1541, 1993.
86. Panjabi M, Abumi K, Duranceau J, et al: Spinal stability and intersegmental muscle forces. A biomechanical model. *Spine* 14:194–199, 1989.
87. Steffen R, Nolte LP, Pingel TH: Rehabilitation of the post-operative segmental lumbar instability: A biomechanical analysis of the rank of the back muscles. *Rehabilitation* 33:164–170, 1994.
88. Wilke HJ, Wolf S, Claes LE, et al: Stability increase of the lumbar spine with different muscle groups. A biomechanical in vitro study. *Spine* 20:192–198, 1995.
89. Hides JA, Stokes MJ, Saide M, et al: Evidence of lumbar multifidus muscle wasting ipsilateral to symptoms in patients with acute/subacute low back pain. *Spine* 19:165–172, 1994.
90. Cleland J, Schulte C, Durall C: The role of therapeutic exercise in treating instability-related lumbar spine pain: A systematic review. *J Back Musculoskel Rehabil* 16:105–115, 2002.
91. Kalimo H, Rantenan J, Vilgarnen T, et al: Lumbar muscles: Structure and function. *Ann Med* 21:353–359, 1989.
92. MacIntosh J, Pearcy M, Bogduk N: The axial torque or the lumbar back muscles: Torsion strength of the back muscles. *Aust N Z J Surg* 63:205–212, 1993.
93. Donisch EW, Basmajian JV: Electromyography of deep back muscles in man. *Am J Anat* 133:25–36, 1971.
94. Flicker PL, Fleckenstein J, Ferry K, et al: Lumbar muscle usage in chronic low back pain. *Spine* 18:582, 1993.
95. Lee DG: Instability of the sacroiliac joint and the consequences for gait. In: Vleeming A, Mooney V, Dorman T, et al, eds. *Movement, Stability and Low Back Pain.* Edinburgh: Churchill Livingstone, 1997:231.
96. Schwarzer AC, Aprill CN, Bogduk N: The sacroiliac joint in chronic low back pain. *Spine* 20:31–37, 1995.
97. Snijders CJ, Ribbers MTLM, de Bakker JV, et al: EMG recordings of abdominal and back muscles in various standing postures: Validation of a biomechanical model on sacroiliac joint stability. *J Electromyogr Kinesiol* 8:205–214, 1998.
98. Shindo H: Anatomical study of the lumbar multifidus muscle and its innervation in human adults and fetuses. *J Nippon Med School* 62:439–446, 1995.
99. McIntosh JE, Valencia F, Bogduk N, et al: The morphology of the lumbar multifidus muscles. *Clin Biomech* 1:196–204, 1986.
100. Mitchell FL, Moran PS, Pruzzo NA: *An Evaluation and Treatment Manual of Osteopathic Muscle Energy Procedures.* Manchester, MO: Mitchell, Moran and Pruzzo Associates, 1979.
101. Aspden RM: Review of the functional anatomy of the spinal ligaments and the lumbar erector spinae muscles. *Clin Anat* 5:372–387, 1992.
102. Bogduk N: A reappraisal of the anatomy of the human lumbar erector spinae. *J Anat* 131:525–540, 1980.
103. McIntosh JE, Bogduk N: The morphology of the lumbar erector spinae. *Spine* 12:658–668, 1986.
104. Bogduk N, Mcintosh JE, Pearcy MJ: A universal model of the lumbar back muscles in the upright position. *Spine* 17:897–913, 1992.
105. Fast A, Shapiro D, Ducommun EJ, et al: Low-back pain in pregnancy. *Spine* 12:368–371, 1987.
106. Mogren IM: Previous physical activity decreases the risk of low back pain and pelvic pain during pregnancy. *Scand J Public Health* 33:300–306, 2005.
107. Mogren IM, Pohjanen AI: Low back pain and pelvic pain during pregnancy: Prevalence and risk factors. *Spine* 30:983–991, 2005.
108. Pool-Goudzwaard AL, Slieker ten Hove MC, Vierhout ME, et al: Relations between pregnancy-related low back pain, pelvic floor activity and pelvic floor dysfunction. *Int Urogynecol J Pelvic Floor Dysfunct* 16:468–474. Epub 2005 April 1, 2005.
109. Wang SM, Dezinno P, Maranets I, et al: Low back pain during pregnancy: Prevalence, risk factors, and outcomes. *Obstet Gynecol* 104:65–70, 2004.
110. Stuge B, Hilde G, Vollestad N: Physical therapy for pregnancy-related low back and pelvic pain: A systematic review. *Acta Obstet Gynecol Scand* 82:983–990, 2003.
111. Kendall FP, McCreary EK, Provance PG: *Muscles: Testing and Function.* Baltimore, MD: Williams & Wilkins, 1993.
112. Huijbregts PA: Lumbopelvic Region: Anatomy and Biomechanics. In: Wadsworth C, ed. *Current Concepts of Orthopaedic Physical Therapy—Home Study Course.* La Crosse, WI: Orthopaedic Section, APTA, 2001.
113. Lee DG: *The Pelvic Girdle: An Approach to the Examination and Treatment of the Lumbo-Pelvic-Hip Region*, 2nd ed. Edinburgh: Churchill Livingstone, 1999.
114. Richardson CA, Jull GA, Hodges P, et al: *Therapeutic Exercise for Spinal Segmental Stabilization in Low Back Pain.* London: Churchill Livingstone, 1999.
115. Hodges P, Richardson C: Contraction of transversus abdominis invariably precedes upper limb movement. *Exp Brain Res* 114:362–370, 1997.
116. Hodges P, Richardson C, Jull G: Evaluation of the relationship between laboratory and clinical tests of transversus abdominis function. *Physiother Res Int* 1:30–40, 1996.
117. McGill SM, Norman RW: Low back biomechanics in industry: The prevention of injury through safer lifting. In: Grabiner MD, ed. *Current Issues in Biomechanics.* Champaign, IL: Human Kinetics Publishers, 1993:69–120.
118. Aspden RM: The spine as an arch: A new mathematical model. *Spine* 14:266–274, 1989.
119. White SG, McNair PJ: Abdominal and erector spinae muscle activity during gait: The use of cluster analysis to identify patterns of activity. *Clin Biomech (Bristol, Avon)* 17:177–184, 2002.
120. O'Sullivan PB, Grahamslaw KM, Kendell M, et al: The effect of different standing and sitting postures on trunk muscle activity in a pain-free population. *Spine* 27:1238–1244, 2002.
121. Ng JK, Richardson CA, Parnianpour M, et al: EMG activity of trunk muscles and torque output during isometric axial rotation exertion: A comparison between back pain patients and matched controls. *Spine* 27:637–646, 2002.
122. Hodges PW, Richardson CA: Contraction of the abdominal muscles associated with movement of the lower limb. *Phys Ther* 77:132–142; discussion 142–144, 1997.
123. Bogduk N, Pearcy M, Hadfield G: Anatomy and biomechanics of psoas major. *Clin Biomech (Bristol, Avon)* 7:109–119, 1992.
124. Santaguida PL, McGill SM: The psoas major muscle: A three-dimensional geometric study. *J Biomech* 28:339–345, 1995.
125. Porterfield JA, DeRosa C: *Mechanical Low Back Pain*, 2nd ed. Philadelphia, PA: WB Saunders, 1998.
126. Bogduk N, MacIntosh J: The applied anatomy of the thoracolumbar fascia. *Spine* 9:164–170, 1984.
127. Gracovetsky S, Farfan HF, Lamy C: The mechanism of the lumbar spine. *Spine* 6:249–262, 1981.
128. Hovelacque A: *Anatomie Des Nerf Craniens et Rachdiens et du Systeme Grande Sympathetique.* Paris: Doin, 1927.
129. Mooney V, Robertson J: The facet syndrome. *Clin Orthop* 115:149–156, 1976.
130. Kulak RF, Schultz AB, Belytschko T, et al: Biomechanical characteristics of vertebral motion segments and intervertebral discs. *Orthop Clin North Am* 6:121–133, 1975.
131. White AA, Punjabi MM: *Clinical Biomechanics of the Spine*, 2nd ed. Philadelphia, PA: J.B. Lippincott Company, 1990.
132. Prescher A: Anatomy and pathology of the aging spine. *Eur J Radiol* 27:181–195, 1998.
133. Mercer S: Kinematics of the spine. In: Boyling JD, Jull GA, eds. *Grieve's Modern Manual Therapy: The Vertebral Column.* Philadelphia, PA: Churchill Livingstone, 2004:31–37.
134. Jull GA, Janda V: Muscle and Motor control in low back pain. In: Twomey LT, Taylor JR, eds. *Physical Therapy of the Low Back: Clinics in Physical Therapy.* New York, NY: Churchill Livingstone, 1987:258–278.
135. Pearcy M, Portek I, Shepherd J: The effect of low back pain on lumbar spinal movements measured by three-dimensional X-ray analysis. *Spine* 10:150–153, 1985.
136. Dunlop RB, Adams MA, Hutton WC: Disc space narrowing and the lumbar facet joints. *J Bone Joint Surg* 66B:706–710, 1984.
137. Adams MA, Hutton WC: The resistance to flexion of the lumbar intervertebral joint. *Spine* 5:245–253, 1980.
138. El-Bohy AA, Yang KH, King AI: Experimental verification of load transmission by direct measurement of facet lamina contact pressure. *J Biomech* 22:931–941, 1989.

139. Grieve G: Common patterns of clinical presentation. In: Grieve GP, ed. *Common Vertebral Joint Problems*, 2nd ed. London: Churchill Livingstone, 1988:283–302.
140. Jungham H: Spondylolisthesen ohne Spalt im Zwischengelenkstuck (pseudospondylolisthesen). *Arch Orthop Unfall Chir* 29:118–123, 1930.
141. Ueno K, Liu YK: A three-dimensional nonlinear finite element model of lumbar intervertebral joint in torsion. *J Biomech Eng* 109:200–209, 1987.
142. Hindle RJ, Pearcy MJ: Rotational mobility of the human back in forward flexion. *J Biomed Eng* 11:219–223, 1989.
143. Pearcy MJ: Twisting mobility of the human back in flexed postures. *Spine* 18:114–119, 1993.
144. Richardson J, Toppenberg R, Jull G: An initial evaluation of eight abdominal exercises for their ability to provide stabilisation for the lumbar spine. *Aust J Physiother* 36:6–11, 1990.
145. Cossette JW, Farfan HF, Robertson GH, et al: The instantaneous center of rotation of the third intervertebral joint. *J Biomech* 4:149–153, 1971.
146. McFadden KD, Taylor JR: Axial rotation in the lumbar spine and gapping of the zygapophyseal joints. *Spine* 15:295–299, 1990.
147. Pearcy M, Portek I, Shepherd J: Three-dimensional analysis of normal movement in the lumbar spine. *Spine* 9:294–297, 1984.
148. Legaspi O, Edmond SL: Does the evidence support the existence of lumbar spine coupled motion? A critical review of the literature. *J Orthop Sports Phys Ther* 37:169–178, 2007.
149. Shah JS: Structure, morphology and mechanics of the lumbar spine. In: Jayson MIV, ed. *The Lumbar Spine and Backache*, 2nd ed. London: Pitman, 1980:359–405.
150. Markolf KL, Morris JM: The structural components of the intervertebral disc. *J Bone Joint Surg* 56A:675–687, 1974.
151. Böstman OM: Body mass index and height in patients requiring surgery for lumbar intervertebral disc herniation. *Spine* 18:851–854, 1993.
152. Heliövaara M: Body height, obesity, and risk of herniated lumbar intervertebral disc. *Spine* 12:469–472, 1987.
153. Andersson GBJ, Schultz AB: Effects of fluid injection on mechanical properties of intervertebral discs. *J Biomech* 12:453–458, 1979.
154. Abdullah AF, Wolber PG, Warfield JR, et al: Surgical management of extreme lateral lumbar disc herniations. *Neurosurgery* 22:648–653, 1988.
155. Brinckmann P, Grootenboer H: Change of disc height, radial disc bulge and intradiscal pressure from discectomy: An in-vitro investigation on human lumbar discs. *Spine* 16:641–646, 1991.
156. Adams MA, Hutton WC: The effect of posture on the fluid content of lumbar intervertebral discs. *Spine* 8:665–671, 1983.
157. Adams MA, McMillan DW, Green TP, et al: Sustained loading generates stress concentrations in lumbar intervertebral discs. *Spine* 21:434–438, 1996.
158. Adams MA, Dolan P: Recent advances in lumbar spinal mechanics and their clinical significance. *Clin Biomech* 10:3–19, 1995.
159. Lord MJ, Small JM, Dinsay JM, et al: Lumbar lordosis: Effects of sitting and standing. *Spine* 22:2571–2574, 1997.
160. Kraemer J, Kolditz D, Gowin R: Water and electrolyte content of human intervertebral discs under variable load. *Spine* 10:69–71, 1985.
161. Kazarian LE: Dynamic response characteristics of the human lumbar vertebral column. *Acta Orthop Scand Suppl* 146:1–86, 1972.
162. Kazarian LE: Creep characteristics of the human spinal column. *Orthop Clin North Am* 6:3–18, 1975.
163. Tyrell AJ, Reilly T, Troup JDG: Circadian variation in stature and the effects of spinal loading. *Spine* 10:161–164, 1985.
164. Nachemson A: Disc pressure measurements. *Spine* 6:93–7, 1981.
165. Horst M, Brinkmann P: Measurement of the distribution of axial stress on the end plate of the vertebral body. *Spine* 6:217–232, 1981.
166. Yoganandan N, Myklebust JB, Wilson CR, et al: Functional biomechanics of the thoracolumbar vertebral cortex. *Clin Biomech* 3:11–18, 1988.
167. Kelsey JL, Hardy RJ: Driving of motor vehicles as a risk factor for acute herniated lumbar intervertebral disc. *Am J Epidemiol* 102:63–73, 1975.
168. McGill SM, Axler CT: Changes in spine height throughout 32 hours of bedrest. *Arch Phys Med Rehab* 77:1071–1073, 1996.
169. Kramer J: Pressure dependent fluid shifts in the intervertebral disc. *Orthop Clin North Am* 8:211–216, 1977.
170. Haher TR, O'Brien M, Dryer JW, et al: The role of the lumbar facets joints in spinal stability. *Spine* 19:2667–2671, 1994.
171. Nachemson A: Lumbar intradiscal pressure. In: Jayson MIV, ed. *The Lumbar Spine and Back Pain*. Edinburgh: Churchill Livingstone, 1987:191–203.
172. McGill S: Loads on the lumbar spine and associated tissues. In: Goel VK, Weinstein JN, eds. *Biomechanics of the Spine: Clinical and Surgical Perspective*. Boca Raton, FL: CRC Press, 1990:65–95.
173. Schultz A: Loads on the lumbar spine. In: Jayson MIV, ed. *The Lumbar Spine and Back Pain*. Edinburgh: Churchill Livingstone, 1987:204–214.
174. Kingma I, Faber GS, Bakker AJ, et al: Can low back loading during lifting be reduced by placing one leg beside the object to be lifted? *Phys Ther* 86:1091–1105, 2006.
175. Kingma I, Staudenmann D, van Dieen JH: Trunk muscle activation and associated lumbar spine joint shear forces under different levels of external forward force applied to the trunk . *J Electromyogr Kinesiol* 17:14–24. Epub 2006 March 13, 2007.
176. Brinckmann P, Biggemann M, Hilweg D: Prediction of the compressive strength of human lumbar vertebrae. *Clin Biomech* 4(suppl 2): 606–610, 1989.
177. Fyhrie DP, Schaffler MB: How human vertebral bone breaks, NACOBII Congress. Chicago, 1992:465–466.
178. McGill SM: The biomechanics of low back injury: Implications on current practice in industry and the clinic. *J Biomech* 30:465–475, 1997.
179. Crisco JJ, Panjabi MM, Yamamoto I, et al: Euler stability of the human ligamentous spine. Part II: Experiment. *Clin Biomech* 7:27–32, 1992.
180. Holdsworth F: Fractures, dislocations, and fracture-dislocations of the spine. *J Bone Joint Surg* 52A:1534–1551, 1970.
181. Markolf KL: Deformation of the thoracolumbar intervertebral joints in response to external loads. *J Bone Joint Surg* 54A:511–533, 1972.
182. Galante JO: Tensile properties of human lumbar annulus fibrosis. *Acta Orthop Scand* 100(Suppl): 1–91, 1967.
183. Panjabi MM: The stabilizing system of the spine. Part 1. Function, dysfunction adaption and enhancement. *J Spinal Disord* 5:383–389, 1992.
184. Panjabi MM: The stabilizing system of the spine. Part II. Neutral zone and instability hypothesis. *J Spinal Disord* 5:390–396; discussion 397, 1992.
185. O'Sullivan PB: 'Clinical instability' of the lumbar spine: It's pathological basis, diagnosis and conservative management. In: Boyling JD, Jull GA, eds. *Grieve's Modern Manual Therapy: The Vertebral Column*. Philadelphia, PA: Churchill Livingstone, 2004:311–331.
186. Mimura M, Panjabi M, Oxland T, et al: Disc degeneration affects the multidirectional flexibility of the lumbar spine. *Spine* 19:1371–1380, 1994.
187. Kaigle A, Holm S, Hansson T: Experimental instability in the lumbar spine. *Spine* 20:421–430, 1995.
188. Wilke H, Wolf S, Claes L, et al: Stability of the lumbar spine with different muscle groups: A biomechanical In Vitro study. *Spine* 20:192–198, 1995.
189. Gardner-Morse M, Stokes I, Laible J: Role of muscles in lumbar spine stability in maximum extension efforts. *J Orthop Res* 13:802–808, 1995.
190. O'Sullivan P, Twomey L, Allison G: Evaluation of specific stabilizing exercise in the treatment of chronic low back pain with radiologic diagnosis of spondylolysis or spondylolisthesis. *Spine* 22:2959–2967, 1997.
191. Best TM, McElhaney J, Garrett WE Jr, et al: Characterization of the passive responses of live skeletal muscle using the quasi-linear theory of viscoelasticity. *J Biomech* 27:413–419, 1994.
192. Keller TS, Spengler DM, Hansson TH: Mechanical behavior of the human lumbar spine, I: Creep analysis during static compressive loading. *J Orthop Res* 5:467–478, 1987.
193. Valencia FP, Munro RR: An electromyographic study of the lumbar multifidus in man. *Electromyogr Clin Neurophysiol* 25:205–221, 1985.
194. Bergmark A: Stability of the lumbar spine. A study in mechanical engineering. *Acta Orthop Scand* 230:20–24, 1989.
195. Stokes IAF, Gardner-Morse M: Lumbar spine maximum efforts and muscle recruitment patterns predicted by a model with multijoint muscles and joints with stiffness. *J Biomech* 27:1101–1104, 1994.
196. Comerford MJ, Mottram SL: Functional stability re-training: Principles and strategies for managing mechanical dysfunction. *Man Ther* 6:3–14, 2001.
197. Comerford MJ, Mottram SL: Movement and stability dysfunction-contemporary developments. *Man Ther* 6:15–26, 2001. [A1]
198. Cresswell A, Oddsson L, Thorstensson A: The influence of sudden perturbations on trunk muscle activity and intra-abdominal pressure while standing. *Exp Brain Res* 98:336–341, 1994.
199. Cresswell A, Grundstrom H, Thorstensson A: Observations on intra-abdominal pressure and patterns of abdominal intra-muscular activity in man. *Acta Physiol Scand* 144:409–418, 1992.
200. Hodges PW, Butler JE, McKenzie D, et al: Contraction of the human diaphragm during postural adjustments. *J Physiol* 505:239–248, 1997.

201. Hodges PW, Richardson CA: Feedforward contraction of transversus abdominis is not influenced by the direction of arm movement. Experimental brain research.. *Exp Brain Res* 114:362–370, 1997.
202. Hodges PW, Gandevia SC: Changes in intra-abdominal pressure during postural and respiratory activation of the human diaphragm. *J Appl Physiol* 89:967–976, 2000.
203. Hodges PW, Gandevia SC: Activation of the human diaphragm during a repetitive postural task. *J Physiol* 522(Pt 1):165–175, 2000.
204. Saunders SW, Rath D, Hodges PW: Postural and respiratory activation of the trunk muscles changes with mode and speed of locomotion. *Gait Posture* 20:280–290, 2004.
205. McGill S: Kinetic potential of the trunk musculature about three orthogonal orthopaedic axes in extreme postures. *Spine* 16:809–815, 1991.
206. Oddsson L, Thorstensson A: Task specificity in the control of intrinsic trunk muscles in man. *Acta Physiol Scand* 139:123–131, 1990.
207. McGill SM: *Low Back Disorders: Evidence-Based Prevention and Rehabilitation*, 2nd ed. Champaign, IL: Human Kinetics, 2006.
208. Givens-Heiss D: Dynamic lumbar stability. In: Hughes C, ed. *Movement Disorders and Neuromuscular Interventions for the Trunk and Extremities—Independent Study Course 18.2.4.* La Crosse, WI: Orthopaedic Section, APTA, Inc., 2008:1–23.
209. Hodges PW, Cresswell AG, Daggfeldt K, et al: In vivo measurement of the effect of intra-abdominal pressure on the human spine. *J Biomech* 34:347–353, 2001.
210. Hagins M, Lamberg EM: Individuals with low back pain breathe differently than healthy individuals during a lifting task. *J Orthop Sports Phys Ther* 41:141–148, 2011.
211. Hodges P, Cresswell A, Thorstensson A: Preparatory trunk motion accompanies rapid upper limb movement. Experimental brain research. Experimentelle Hirnforschung. *Exp Cereb* 124:69–79, 1999.
212. Friberg O: Lumbar instability: A dynamic approach by traction-compression radiography. *Spine* 12:119–129, 1987.
213. O'Sullivan PB, Twomey L, Allison GT: Altered abdominal muscle recruitment in patients with chronic back pain following a specific exercise intervention. *J Orthop Sports Phys Ther* 27:114–124, 1998.
214. O'Sullivan PB, Dankaerts W, Burnett AF, et al: Effect of different upright sitting postures on spinal-pelvic curvature and trunk muscle activation in a pain-free population. *Spine* 31:E707–E712, 2006.
215. O'Sullivan P, Twomey L, Allison G, et al: Altered patterns of abdominal muscle activation in patients with chronic low back pain. *Aust J Physiother* 43:91–98, 1997.
216. Stanford ME: Effectiveness of specific lumbar stabilization exercises: A single case study. *J Man Manip Ther* 10:40–46, 2002.
217. McGill SM, Cholewicki J: Biomechanical basis for stability: An explanation to enhance clinical utility. *J Orthop Sports Phys Ther* 31:96–100, 2001.
218. Hodges PW, Richardson CA: Altered trunk muscle recruitment in people with low back pain: A motor control evaluation of transversus abdominis. *Arch Phys Med Rehab* 80:1005–1012, 1999.
219. O'Sullivan P, Twomey L, Allison G: Altered patterns of abdominal muscle activation in chronic back pain patients. *Aust J Physiother* 43:91–98, 1997.
220. Bierdermann HJ, Shanks GL, Forrest WJ, et al: Power spectrum analysis of electromyographic activity. *Spine* 16:1179–1184, 1991.
221. Lindgren K, Sihvonen T, Leino E, et al: Exercise therapy effects on functional radiographic findings and segmental electromyographic activity in lumbar spine stability. *Arch Phys Med Rehabil* 74:933–939, 1993.
222. Richardson C, Jull G: Muscle control-pain control. What exercises would you prescribe? *Man Ther* 1:2–10, 1995.
223. Edgerton V, Wolf S, Levendowski D, et al: Theoretical basis for patterning EMG amplitudes to assess muscle dysfunction. *Med Sci Sports Exerc* 28:744–751, 1996.
224. Arendt-Nielsen L, Graven-Nielsen T, Svarrer H, et al: The influence of low back pain on muscle activity and coordination during gait: A clinical and experimental study. *Pain* 64:231–240, 1996.
225. Soderberg GL, Dostal WF: Electromyographic study of three parts of the gluteus medius muscle during functional activities. *Phys Ther* 58:691–696, 1978.
226. Cohen MJ, Swanson GA, Naliboff BD, et al: Comparison of electromyographic response patterns during posture and stress tasks in chronic low back pain patterns and control. *J Psychosom Res* 30:135–141, 1986.
227. McCullough JA, Waddell G: Variation of the lumbosacral myotomes with bony segmental anomalies. *J Bone Joint Surg Br* 62B:475–480, 1980.
228. Deyo RA, Rainville J, Kent DL: What can the history and physical examination tell us about low back pain? *JAMA* 268:760–765, 1992.
229. Wipf JE, Deyo RA: Low back pain. *Med Clin North Am* 79:231–246, 1995.
230. Viikari-Juntura E, Jouri J, Silverstein BA, et al: A lifelong prospective study on the role of psychosocial factors in neck, shoulder and low back pain. *Spine* 16:1056–1061, 1991.
231. Bigos SJ, Battié M, Spengler DM, et al: A prospective study of work perceptions and psychosocial factors affecting the report of back injury. *Spine* 16:1–6, 1991.
232. Dehlin O, Berg S: Back symptoms and psychological perception of work. *Scand J Rehab Med* 9:61–65, 1977.
233. Leino PI, Hänninen V: Psychosocial factors in relation to back and limb disorders. *Scand J Work Environ Health* 21:134–142, 1995.
234. Michel A, Kohlmann T, Raspe H: The association between clinical findings on physical examination and self-reported severity in back pain: Results of a population-based study. *Spine* 22:296–304, 1997.
235. Waddell G, Somerville D, Henderson I, et al: Objective clinical evaluation of physical impairment in chronic low back pain. *Spine* 17:617–628, 1992.
236. Paassilta P, Lohiniva J, Goring HH, et al: Identification of a novel common genetic risk factor for lumbar disk disease. *JAMA* 285:1843–1849, 2001.
237. Videman T, Gibbons LE, Battie MC, et al: The relative roles of intragenic polymorphisms of the vitamin d receptor gene in lumbar spine degeneration and bone density. *Spine* 26:E7–E12, 2001.
238. Videman T, Leppavuori J, Kaprio J, et al: Intragenic polymorphisms of the vitamin D receptor gene associated with intervertebral disc degeneration. *Spine* 23:2477–2485, 1998.
239. Burdorf A, Sorock G: Positive and negative evidence of risk factors for back disorders. *Scand J Work Environ Health* 23:243–256, 1997.
240. Riihimaki H: Low-back pain, its origin and risk indicators. *Scand J Work Environ Health* 17:81–90, 1991.
241. Deyo RA, Diehl AK: Lumbar spine films in primary care: Current use and effects of selective ordering criteria. *J Gen Intern Med* 1:20–25, 1986.
242. Frymoyer JW, Newberg A, Pope MH, et al: Spine radiographs in patients with low-back pain. *J Bone Joint Surg* 66A:1048–1055, 1984.
243. Witt I, Vestergaard A, Rosenklint A: A comparative analysis of x-ray findings of the lumbar spine in patient with and without lumbar pain. *Spine* 9:298–300, 1984.
244. Croft PR, Rigby AS: Socioeconomic influences on back problems in the community in Britain. *J Epidemiol Community Health* 48:166–170, 1994.
245. Heistaro S, Vartiainen E, Heliovaara M, et al: Trends of back pain in eastern Finland, 1972–1992, in relation to socioeconomic status and behavioral risk factors. *Am J Epidemiol* 148:671–682, 1998.
246. Leino-Arjas P, Hanninen K, Puska P: Socioeconomic variation in back and joint pain in Finland. *Eur J Epidemiol* 14:79–87, 1998.
247. Hagen KB, Holte HH, Tambs K, et al: Socioeconomic factors and disability retirement from back pain: A 1983–1993 population-based prospective study in Norway. *Spine* 25:2480–2487, 2000.
248. Hoogendoorn WE, Poppel MN, Bongers PM, et al: Physical load during work and leisure time as risk factors for back pain. *Scand J Work Environ Health* 25:387–403, 1999.
249. Hemingway H, Shipley MJ, Stansfeld S, et al: Sickness absence from back pain, psychosocial work characteristics and employment grade among office workers. *Scand J Work Environ Health* 23:121–129, 1997.
250. Riihimaki H: Epidemiology and pathogenesis of non-specific low back pain: What does the epidemiology tell us? *Bull Hosp Jt Dis* 55:197–198, 1996.
251. Smedley J, Egger P, Cooper C, et al: Prospective cohort study of predictors of incident low back pain in nurses. *BMJ* 311:1225–1228, 1997.
252. Kraus JF, Gardner LI, Collins J, et al: Design factors in epidemiologic cohort studies of work-related low back injury or pain. *Am J Ind Med* 32:153–163, 1997.
253. Macfarlane GJ, Thomas E, Papageorgiou AC, et al: Employment and physical work activities as predictors of future low back pain. *Spine* 22:1143–1149, 1997.
254. Tichauer ER: *The Biomedical Basis of Ergonomics: Anatomy Applied to the Design of the Work Situation.* New York, NY: Wiley Inter-Sciences, 1978.
255. Magora A: Investigation of the relation between low back pain and occupation: 4. Physical requirements: Bending, rotation, reaching and sudden maximal effort. *Scand J Rehabil Med* 5:186–190, 1973.
256. Magora A: Investigation of the relation between low back pain and occupation: 3. Physical requirements: Sitting, standing and weight lifting. *Ind Med Surg* 41:5–9, 1972.

257. Kelsey JL: An epidemiological study of the relationship between occupations and acute herniated lumbar intervertebral discs. *Int J Epidemiol* 4:197–205, 1975.
258. Backman AL: Health survey of professional drivers. *Scand J Work Environ Health* 9:30–35, 1983.
259. Bongers PM, Boshuizen HC, Hulshof CTJ, et al: Back disorders in crane operators exposed to whole-body vibration. *Int Arch Occup Environ Health* 60:129–137, 1988.
260. Bongers PM, Hulshof CTJ, Dijkstra L, et al: Back pain and exposure to whole body vibration in helicopter pilots. *Ergonomics* 33:1007–1026, 1990.
261. Pietri F, Leclerc A, Boitel L, et al: Low-back pain in commercial drivers. *Scand J Work Environ Health* 18:52–58, 1992.
262. Bianco AJ: Low back pain and sciatica. Diagnosis and indications for treatment. *J Bone Joint Surg* 50A:170, 1968.
263. Leboeuf-Yde C, Kyvik KO, Bruun NH: Low back pain and life style: Part I. Smoking information from a population-based sample of 29424 twins. *Spine* 23:2207–2214, 1998.
264. Holmstrom EB, Lindell J, Moritz U: Low back and neck/shoulder pain in construction workers: Occupational workload and psychosocial risk factors. Part 1: Relationship to low back pain. *Spine* 17:663–671, 1992.
265. Miranda H, Viikari-Juntura E, Martikainen R, et al: Individual factors, occupational loading, and physical exercise as predictors of sciatic pain. *Spine* 27:1102–1109, 2002.
266. Kelsey JL: An epidemiological study of acute herniated lumbar intervertebral discs. *Rheumatol Rehabil* 14:144–159, 1975.
267. Fogelholm RR, Alho AV: Smoking and intervertebral disc degeneration. *Med Hypotheses* 56:537–539, 2001.
268. Aro S, Leino P: Overweight and musculoskeletal morbidity: A ten-year follow-up. *Int J Obesity* 9:267–275, 1985.
269. Deyo RA, Bass JE: Lifestyle and low-back pain. The influence of smoking and obesity. *Spine* 14:501–506, 1989.
270. Fransen M, Woodward M, Norton R, et al: Risk factors associated with the transition from acute to chronic occupational back pain. *Spine* 27:92–98, 2002.
271. Linton S: Risk factors for neck and back pain in a working population in Sweden. *Work Stress* 4:41–49, 1990.
272. Hoogendoorn WE, Poppel MN, Bongers PM, et al: Systematic review of psychosocial factors at work and in private life as risk factors for back pain. *Spine* 25:2114–2125, 2000.
273. Nordin M, Hiebert R, Pietrek M, et al: Association of comorbidity and outcome in episodes of nonspecific low back pain in occupational populations. *J Occup Environ Med* 44:677–684, 2002.
274. Bigos S, Bowyer O, Braen G, et al: *Acute Low Back Problems in Adults.* AHCPR Publication 95-0642. Rockville, MD: Agency for Health Care Policy and Research, Public Health Service, U.S. Department of Health and Human Services, 1994.
275. Resnick DN, Morris C: History and physical examination for low back syndromes. In: Morris C, ed. *Low Back Syndromes: Integrated Clinical Management.* New York, NY: McGraw-Hill, 2006:305–331.
276. Jermyn RT: A nonsurgical approach to low back pain. *JAOA* 101(suppl): S6–S11, 2001.
277. Ombregt L, Bisschop P, ter Veer HJ, et al: Clinical examination of the lumbar spine. In: Ombregt L, Bisschop P, ter Veer HJ, et al, eds. *A System of Orthopaedic Medicine.* London: WB Saunders, 1995:577–611.
278. Kuslich SD, Ulstrom CL, Michael CJ: The tissue origin of low back pain and sciatica. *Orthop Clin North Am* 22:181–187, 1991.
279. Oesch P: Die Rolle der Zygapophysealgelenke in der Aetiologie lumbaler Rueckenschmerzen mit und ohne Ausstrahlungen. *Man Med* 33:107–114, 1995.
280. Andersson GBJ, Deyo RA: History and physical examination in patients with herniated lumbar discs. *Spine* 21:10S–18S, 1996.
281. Van den Hoogen HMM, Koes BW, Van Eijk JT, et al: On the accuracy of history, physical examination, and erythrocyte sedimentation rate in diagnosing low back pain in general practice. *Spine* 20:318–327, 1995.
282. Roach KE, Brown MD, Albin RD, et al: The sensitivity and specificity of pain response to activity and position in categorizing patients with low back pain. *Phys Ther* 77:730–738, 1997.
283. Deyo RA: Understanding the accuracy of diagnostic tests. In: Weinstein JN, Rydevik B, Sonntag V, eds. *Essentials of the Spine.* Philadelphia, PA: Raven Press, 1995:55–70.
284. Yukawa Y, Kato F, Kajino G, et al: Groin pain associated with lower lumbar disc herniation. *Spine* 22:1736–1739, 1997.
285. Murphey F: Sources and patterns of pain in disc disease. *Clin Neurosurg* 15:343–351, 1968.
286. McKenzie RA: *The Lumbar Spine: Mechanical Diagnosis and Therapy.* Waikanae, NZ: Spinal Publication, 1981.
287. Korr IM: Neurochemical and neurotrophic consequences of nerve deformation. In: Glasgow EF, Twomey LT, Scull ER, et al, eds. *Aspects of Manipulative Therapy,* 2nd ed. New York, NY: Churchill Livingstone, 1985.
288. Lewit K: The contribution of clinical observation to neurobiological mechanisms in manipulative therapy. In: Korr IM, ed. *The Neurobiological Mechanisms in Manipulative Therapy.* New York, NY: Plenum Press, 1977.
289. Hall H: A simple approach to back pain management. *Patient Care* 15:77–91, 1992.
290. Ombregt L, Bisschop P, ter Veer HJ, et al: *A System of Orthopaedic Medicine.* London: WB Saunders, 1995.
291. Kelsey JL, White AA: Epidemiology and impact of low back pain. *Spine* 5:133–142, 1980.
292. Dains JE, Ciofu-Baumann L, Scheibel P: *Advanced Health Assessment and Clinical Diagnosis in Primary Care.* St. Louis, MO: Mosby-Yearbook, 2003.
293. White AA: Injection technique for the diagnosis and treatment of low back pain. *Orthop Clin North Am* 14: 553–567, 1983.
294. Jull GA: Examination of the lumbar spine. In: Grieve GP, ed. *Modern Manual Therapy of the Vertebral Column.* Edinburgh: Churchill Livingstone, 1986:553.
295. Donelson R, Silva G, Murphy K: Centralization phenomenon: Its usefulness in evaluating and treating referred pain. *Spine* 15:211–213, 1990.
296. Donelson R, Aprill C, Medcalf R, et al: A prospective study of centralization in lumbar referred pain. A predictor of symptomatic discs and annular competence. *Spine* 22:1115–1122, 1997.
297. Donelson R: The McKenzie approach to evaluating and treating low back pain. *Orthop Rev* 19:681–686, 1990.
298. Matsui H, Terahata N, Tsuji H, et al: Familial predisposition, clustering for juvenile lumbar disc herniation. *Spine* 17:1323–1328, 1992.
299. Friberg S: Studies on spondylolisthesis. *Acta Chir Orthop* 60:1, 1939.
300. Jolles BM, Porchet F, Theumann N: Surgical treatment of lumbar spinal stenosis. Five-year follow-up. *J Bone Joint Surg Am* 83A:949–953, 2001.
301. Bressler HB, Keyes WJ, Rochon PA, et al: The prevalence of low back pain in the elderly. A systematic review of the literature. *Spine* 24:1813–1819, 1999.
302. Berguist-Ullman M, Larsson U: Acute low back pain in industry. A controlled prospective study with specific reference to therapy and vocational factors. *Acta Orthop Scand* 170:1–117, 1977.
303. Hoogendoorn WE, Bongers PM, de Vet HC, et al: High physical work load and low job satisfaction increase the risk of sickness absence due to low back pain: Results of a prospective cohort study. *Occup Environ Med* 59:323–328, 2002.
304. Andersson GBJ: Epidemiologic aspects of low back pain in industry. *Spine* 6:53–60, 1981.
305. Drezner JA, Harmon KG: Chronic appendicitis presenting as low back pain in a recreational athlete. *Clin J Sport Med* 12:184–186, 2002.
306. Deyo RA, Weinstein JN: Low back pain. *N Engl J Med* 344:363–370, 2001.
307. Fielding JW, Black J, Ashton F, et al: Diagnosis and management of 528 abdominal aortic aneurysms. *Br Med J (Clin Res Ed)* 283:355–359, 1981.
308. Fink HA, Lederle FA, Roth CS, et al: The accuracy of physical examination to detect abdominal aortic aneurysm. *Arch Intern Med* 160:833–836, 2000.
309. Roach KE, Brown M, Ricker E, et al: The use of patient symptoms to screen for serious back problems. *J Orthop Sports Phys Ther* 21:2–6, 1995.
310. Korr IM: Proprioceptors and somatic dysfunction. *JAOA* 74:638–650, 1975.
311. Jonsson B, Stromqvist B: The straight leg rising test and the severity of symptoms in lumbar disc herniation. *Spine* 20:27–30, 1995.
312. Morag E, Hurwitz DE, Andriacchi TP, et al: Abnormalities in muscle function during gait in relation to the level of lumbar disc herniation. *Spine* 25:829–833, 2000.
313. Biering-Sorenson F: Low back trouble in a general population of 30-, 40-, 50- and 60-year-old men and women: Study design, representativeness and basic results. *Dan Med Bull* 29:289–299, 1982.
314. Sahrmann SA: *Diagnosis and Treatment of Movement Impairment Syndromes.* St Louis, MO: Mosby, 2001.
315. Hoppenfeld S: *Physical Examination of the Spine and Extremities.* East Norwalk, CT: Appleton-Century-Crofts, 1976.

316. Wallace L: *Lower Quarter Pain: Mechanical Evaluation and Treatment.* Cleveland, OH: Western Reserve Publishers, 1984.
317. Beals RK: Anomalies associated with vertebral malformations. *Spine* 18:1329, 1993.
318. Matson DD, Woods RP, Campbell JB, et al: Diastematomyelia (congenital clefts of the spinal cord). *Pediatrics* 6:98–112, 1950.
319. Lorio MP, Bernstein AJ, Simmons EH: Sciatic spinal deformity—lumbosacral list: An "unusual" presentation with review of the literature. *J Spinal Disord* 8:201–205, 1995.
320. Suk KS, Lee HM, Moon SH, et al: Lumbosacral scoliotic list by lumbar disc herniation. *Spine* 26:667–671, 2001.
321. DePalma AF, Rothman RH: *The Intervertebral Disc.* Philadelphia, PA: WB Saunders, 1970.
322. Maigne R: *Diagnosis and Treatment of pain of Vertebral Origin.* Baltimore, MD: Williams & Wilkins, 1996.
323. Porter RW, Miller CG: Back pain and trunk list. *Spine* 11:596–600, 1986.
324. Battie MC, Cherkin DC, Dunn R, et al: Managing low back pain: Attitudes and treatment preferences of physical therapists. *Phys Ther* 74:219–226, 1994.
325. Donahue MS, Riddle DL, Sullivan MS: Intertester reliability of a modified version of McKenzie's lateral shift assessment obtained on patients with low back pain. *Phys Ther* 76:706–726, 1996.
326. McKenzie RA: Manual correction of sciatic scoliosis. *N Z Med J* 76:194–199, 1972.
327. Riddle DL, Rothstein JM: Intertester reliability of McKenzie's classifications of the syndrome types present in patients with low back pain. *Spine* 18:1333–1344, 1993.
328. Opila KA, Wagner SS, Schiowitz S, et al: Postural alignment in barefoot and high heeled stance. *Spine* 13:542–547, 1988.
329. Winkel D, Matthijs O, Phelps V: *Diagnosis and Treatment of the Spine.* Maryland, MD: Aspen, 1997.
330. Dvorak J, Dvorak V: Zones of irritation. In: Gilliar WG, Greenman PE, eds. *Manual Medicine: Diagnostics.* New York, NY: Thieme Medical Publishers, 1990:219–230.
331. Nachemson A, Bigos SJ: The low back. In: Cruess RL, Rennie WRJ, eds. *Adult Orthopaedics.* New York, NY: Churchill Livingstone, 1984:843–938.
332. Bourdillon JF: *Spinal Manipulation*, 3rd ed. London: Heinemann Medical Books, 1982.
333. Fukui S, Ohseto K, Shiotani M, et al: Distribution of referred pain from the lumbar zygapophyseal joints and dorsal rami. *Clin J Pain* 13:303–307, 1997.
334. Robert CM, Thomas H, Tery T: Facet joint injection and facet nerve block: A randomized comparison in 86 patients with chronic low back pain. *Pain* 49:325–328, 1992.
335. Greenman PE: *Principles of Manual Medicine*, 2nd ed. Baltimore, MD: Williams & Wilkins, 1996.
336. Allbrook D: Movements of the lumbar spinal column. *J Bone Joint Surg* 39B:339–345, 1957.
337. Ng JK, Kippers V, Richardson CA, et al: Range of motion and lordosis of the lumbar spine: Reliability of measurement and normative values. *Spine* 26:53–60, 2001.
338. Pearcy M, Tibrewal SB: Axial rotation and lateral bending in the normal lumbar spine measured by three-dimensional radiography. *Spine* 9:582, 1984.
339. Troup JDG, Hood CA, Chapman AE: Measurements of the sagittal mobility of the lumbar spine and hips. *Ann Phys Med* 9:308–321, 1967.
340. Mellin G: Correlations of spinal mobility with degree of chronic low back pain after correction for age and anthropometric factors. *Spine* 12:464–468, 1987.
341. Einkauf DK, Gohdes ML, Jensen GM, et al: Changes in spinal mobility with increasing age in women. *Phys Ther* 67:370–375, 1987.
342. American Medical Association: *Guides to the Evaluation of Permanent Impairment*, 5th ed. Chicago, IL: American Medical Association, 2001.
343. Cyriax J: *Textbook of Orthopaedic Medicine, Diagnosis of Soft Tissue Lesions*, 8th ed. London: Bailliere Tindall, 1982.
344. Portek I, Pearcy MJ, Reader GP, et al: Correlation between radiographic and clinical measurement of lumbar spine movement. *Br J Rheumatol* 22:197–205, 1983.
345. Grieve GP: Lumbar instability. *Physiotherapy* 68:2, 1982.
346. Huijbregts PA: Lumbopelvic Region: Aging, Disease, Examination, Diagnosis, and Treatment. In: Wadsworth C, ed. *Current Concepts of Orthopaedic Physical Therapy—Home Study Course.* La Crosse, WI: Orthopaedic Section, APTA, 2001.
347. Sahrmann SA: Movement impairment syndromes of the lumbar spine. In: Sahrmann SA, ed. *Diagnosis and Treatment of Movement Impairment Syndromes.* St Louis, MO: Mosby, 2001:51–119.
348. Weinstein JN, Gordon SL: *Low Back Pain: A Scientific and Clinical Overview.* Rosemont, IL: American Academy of Orthopedic Surgeons, 1996.
349. Osterbauer PJ, Long K, Ribaudo TA, et al: Three-dimensional head kinematics and cervical range of motion in the diagnosis of patients with neck trauma. *J Manip Physiol Ther* 19:231–237, 1996.
350. Helliwell P, Moll J, Wright V: Measurement of spinal movement and function. In: Jayson MIV, ed. *The Lumbar Spine and Back Pain*, 4th ed. Edinburgh: Churchill Livingstone, 1992:173–205.
351. Mayer TG, Tencer AF, Kristoferson S, et al: Use of noninvasive techniques for quantification of spinal range of motion in normal subjects and chronic low back dysfunction patients. *Spine* 9:588–595, 1984.
352. Mayer TG, Kondraske G, Beals SB, et al: Spinal range of motion. Accuracy and sources of error with inclinometric measurement. *Spine* 22:1976–1984, 1997.
353. Nitschke JE, Nattrass CL, Disler PB, et al: Reliability of the American Medical Association guides' model for measuring spinal range of motion. Its implication for whole-person impairment rating. *Spine* 24:262–268, 1999.
354. Macrae IF, Wright V: Measurement of back movement. *Ann Rheum Dis* 28:584–589, 1969.
355. Miller SA, Mayer T, Cox R, et al: Reliability problems associated with the modified Schöber technique for true lumbar flexion measurement. *Spine* 17:345–348, 1992.
356. Reynolds PM: Measurement of spinal mobility: A comparison of three methods. *Rheumatol Rehabil* 14:180–185, 1975.
357. Burdett RG, Brown KE, Fall MP: Reliability and validity of four instruments for measuring lumbar spine and pelvic positions. *Phys Ther* 66:677–684, 1986.
358. Adams MA, Dolan P, Marx C, et al: An electronic inclinometer technique for measuring lumbar curvature. *Clin Biomech* 1:130–134, 1986.
359. Armstrong GW, Livermore NB, Suzuki N, et al: Nonstandard vertebral rotation in scoliosis screening patients: Its prevalence and relation to the clinical deformity. *Spine* 7:50–54, 1982.
360. Meadows J: *Orthopedic Differential Diagnosis in Physical Therapy.* New York, NY: McGraw-Hill, 1999.
361. Edwards BC: Combined movements of the lumbar spine: Examination and clinical significance. *Aust J Physiother* 25:147–152, 1979.
362. Edwards BC: Combined movements of the lumbar spine: Examination and treatment. In: Palastanga N, Boyling JD, eds. *Grieve's Modern Manual Therapy of the Vertebral Column.* Edinburgh: Churchill Livingstone, 1994:561–566.
363. Seichi A, Kondoh T, Hozumi T, et al: Intraoperative radiation therapy for metastatic spinal tumors. *Spine* 24:470–473; discussion 474–475, 1999.
364. Shiqing X, Quanzhi Z, Dehao F: Significance of straight-leg-raising test in the diagnosis and clinical evaluation of lower lumbar intervertebral disc protrusion. *J Bone Joint Surg* 69A:517–522, 1987.
365. Hakelius A, Hindmarsh J: The comparative reliability of preoperative diagnostic methods in lumbar disc surgery. *Acta Orthop Scand* 43:234, 1972.
366. Hakelius A, Hindmarsh J: The significance of neurological signs and myelographic findings in the diagnosis of lumbar root compression. *Acta Orthop Scand* 43:239–246, 1972.
367. Spangfort EV: The lumbar disc herniation: A computer aided analysis of 2,504 operations. *Acta Orthop Scand (Suppl)* 142:1–95, 1972.
368. Porchet F, Frankhauser H, de Tribolet N: Extreme lateral lumbar disc herniation: A clinical presentation of 178 patients. *Acta Neurochir (Wien)* 127:203–209, 1994.
369. Christodoulides AN: Ipsilateral sciatica on the femoral nerve stretch test is pathognomonic of an L4/5 disc protrusion. *J Bone Joint Surg* 71B:88–89, 1989.
370. Fryette HH: *Principles of Osteopathic Technique.* Colorado Springs, CO: Academy of Osteopathy, 1980.
371. Hartman SL: *Handbook of Osteopathic Technique*, 2nd ed. London: Unwin Hyman, Academic Division, 1990.
372. Stoddard A: *Manual of Osteopathic Practice.* New York, NY: Harper & Row, 1969.
373. Meadows JTS: *The Principles of the Canadian Approach to the Lumbar Dysfunction Patient, Management of Lumbar Spine Dysfunction—Independent Home Study Course.* La Crosse, WI: APTA, Orthopaedic Section, 1999.

374. Lee DG, Walsh MC: *A Workbook of Manual Therapy Techniques for the Vertebral Column and Pelvic Girdle.* 2nd ed. Vancouver, BC: Nascent, 1996.
375. Maher C, Latimer J, Adams R: An investigation of the reliability and validity of posteroanterior spinal stiffness judgments made using a reference-based protocol. *Phys Ther* 78:829–837, 1998.
376. Peterson CK, Bolton JE, Wood AR: A cross-sectional study correlating lumbar spine degeneration with disability and pain. *Spine* 25:218–223, 2000.
377. Millard RW, Jones RH: Construct validity of practical questionnaires for assessing disability of low-back pain. *Spine* 16:835–838, 1991.
378. Fairbank J, Couper J, Davies J, et al: The Oswestry low back pain questionnaire. *Physiotherapy* 66:271–273, 1980.
379. Roland M, Morris R: A study of the natural history of back pain, part I: The development of a reliable and sensitive measure of disability of low back pain. *Spine* 8:141–144, 1986.
380. Roland M, Fairbank J: The Roland-Morris Disability Questionnaire and the Oswestry Disability Questionnaire. *Spine* 25:3115–3124, 2000.
381. Ren XS: Are patients capable of attributing functional impairments to specific diseases? *Am J Public Health* 88:837–838, 1998.
382. Fritz JM, Piva SR: Physical impairment index: Reliability, validity, and responsiveness in patients with acute low back pain. *Spine* 28:1189–1194, 2003.
383. Waddell G, Newton M, Henderson I, et al: A Fear-Avoidance Beliefs Questionnaire (FABQ) and the role of fear-avoidance beliefs in chronic low back pain and disability. *Pain* 52:157–168, 1993.
384. Jacob T, Baras M, Zeev A, et al: Low back pain: Reliability of a set of pain measurement tools. *Arch Phys Med Rehabil* 82:735–742, 2001.
385. Crombez G, Vlaeyen JW, Heuts PH, et al: Pain-related fear is more disabling than fear itself: Evidence on the role of pain-related fear in chronic back pain disability. *Pain* 80:329–339, 1999.
386. Hadijistavropoulos HD, Craig KD: Acute and chronic low back pain: Cognitive, affective, and behavioral dimensions. *J Cons Clin Psych* 62:341–349, 1994.
387. Fritz JM, George SZ, Delitto A: The role of fear avoidance beliefs in acute low back pain: Relationships with current and future disability and work status. *Pain* 94:7–15, 2001.
388. Brukner P, Khan K: Core stability. In: Brukner P, Khan K, eds. *Clinical Sports Medicine*, 3rd ed. Sydney: McGraw-Hill, 2007:158–173.
389. Laslett M, Aprill CN, McDonald B, et al: Clinical predictors of lumbar provocation discography: A study of clinical predictors of lumbar provocation discography. *Eur Spine J* 15:1473–1484, 2006.
390. Maitland G: *Vertebral Manipulation.* Sydney: Butterworth, 1986.
391. Binkley J, Stratford PW, Gill C: Interrater reliability of lumbar accessory motion mobility testing. *Phys Ther* 75:786–792; discussion 793–795, 1995.
392. Keating JC, Bergmann TF, Jacobs GE, et al: Interexaminer reliability of eight evaluative dimensions of lumbar segmental abnormality. *J Manip Physiol Ther* 13:463–470, 1990.
393. Hicks GE, Fritz JM, Delitto A, et al: Interrater reliability of clinical examination measures for identification of lumbar segmental instability. *Arch Phys Med Rehabil* 84:1858–1864, 2003.
394. Krivickas LS, Feinberg JH: Lower extremity injuries in college athletes: Relation between ligamentous laxity and lower extremity muscle tightness. *Arch Phys Med Rehabil* 77:1139–1143, 1996.
395. Kasai Y, Morishita K, Kawakita E, et al: A new evaluation method for lumbar spinal instability: Passive lumbar extension test. *Phys Ther* 86:1661–1667. Epub 2006 October 10, 2006.
396. Alqarni AM, Schneiders AG, Hendrick PA: Clinical tests to diagnose lumbar segmental instability: A systematic review. *J Orthop Sports Phys Ther* 41:130–140, 2011.
397. Bigos S, Bowyer O, Braen G, et al: *Acute Low Back Problems in Adults. Clinical Practice Guideline no. 14.* Rockville, MD: Agency for Health Care Policy and Research, 1994.
398. Boden SD, Davis DO, Dina TS, et al: Abnormal magnetic resonance scan of the lumbar spine in asymptomatic subjects: A prospective investigation. *J Bone Joint Surg* 72A:403–408, 1990.
399. Weisel SE, Tsourmas N, Feffer H, et al: A study of computer-assisted tomography, I: the incidence of positive CAT scans in an asymptomatic group of patients. *Spine* 9:549–551, 1984.
400. Deyo RA: Diagnostic evaluation of LBP: Reaching a specific diagnosis is often impossible. *Arch Intern Med* 162:1444–1447; discussion 1447–1448, 2002.
401. Waddell G, McCulloch JA, Kummel E, et al: Nonorganic physical signs in low-back pain. *Spine* 5:117–125, 1980.
402. Delitto A, Erhard RE, Bowling RW: A treatment-based classification approach to low back syndrome: Identifying and staging patients for conservative management. *Phys Ther* 75:470–489, 1995.
403. van Tulder MW, Koes BW, Bouter LM: Conservative treatment of acute and chronic nonspecific low back pain: A systematic review of randomized controlled trials of the most common interventions. *Spine* 22:2128–2156, 1997.
404. Feldman JB: The prevention of occupational low back pain disability: Evidence-based reviews point in a new direction. *J Surg Orthop Adv* 13:1–14, 2004.
405. Rozenberg S, Delval C, Rezvani Y, et al: Bed rest or normal activity for patients with acute low back pain: A randomized controlled trial. *Spine* 27:1487–1493, 2002.
406. Burton AK, Waddell G: Clinical guidelines in the management of low back pain. *Baillere's Clin Rheum* 12:17–35, 1998.
407. Deyo RA, Diehl AK, Rosenthal M: How many days of bed rest for acute low back pain? A randomized clinical trial. *N Engl J Med* 315:1064–1070, 1986.
408. Malmivaara A, Hékkinen U, Aro T, et al: The treatment of acute low back pain: Bed rest, exercises, or ordinary activity? *N Engl J Med* 332:351–355, 1995.
409. Abenhaim L, Rossignol M, Valat J-P, et al: The role of activity in the therapeutic management of back pain. Report of the International Paris Task Force on back pain. *Spine* 25(Suppl 4S):1S–33S, 2000.
410. Childs JD, Fritz JM, Flynn TW, et al: A clinical prediction rule to identify patients with low back pain most likely to benefit from spinal manipulation: A validation study. *Ann Intern Med* 141:920–928, 2004.
411. Flynn T, Fritz J, Whitman J, et al: A clinical prediction rule for classifying patients with low back pain who demonstrate short-term improvement with spinal manipulation. *Spine* 27:2835–2843, 2002.
412. Cleland JA, Fritz JM, Whitman JM, et al: The use of a lumbar spine manipulation technique by physical therapists in patients who satisfy a clinical prediction rule: A case series. *J Orthop Sports Phys Ther* 36:209–214, 2006.
413. Deyo RA, Walsh NE, Martin DC, et al: A controlled trial of transcutaneous electrical nerve stimulation (TENS) and exercise for chronic low back pain. *N Engl J Med* 322:1627–1634, 1990.
414. Bronfort G, Goldsmith CH, Nelson CF, et al: Trunk exercise combined with spinal manipulative or NSAID therapy for chronic low back pain: A randomized, observer-blinded clinical trial. *J Manip Physiol Ther* 19:570–582, 1996.
415. Handa N, Yamamoto H, Tani T, et al: The effect of trunk muscle exercises in patient over 40 years of age with chronic low back pain. *J Orthop Sci* 5:210–216, 2000.
416. Mitchell JM, de Lissovoy G: A comparison of resource use and cost in direct access versus physician referral episodes of physical therapy. *Phys Ther* 77:10–18, 1997.
417. Philadelphia Panel evidence-based clinical practice guidelines on selected rehabilitation interventions for low back pain. *Phys Ther* 81:1641–1674, 2001.
418. Manniche C, Hesselsoe G, Bentzen L, et al: Clinical trial of intensive muscle training for chronic low back pain. *Lancet* 2:1473–1476, 1988.
419. Frost H, Lamb SE, Klaber Moffett JA, et al: A fitness programme for patients with chronic low back pain: 2-year follow-up of a randomised controlled trial. *Pain* 75:273–279, 1998.
420. Lahad A, Malter AD, Berg AO, et al: The effectiveness of four interventions for the prevention of low back pain. *JAMA* 272:1286–1291, 1994.
421. Aker PD, Gross AR, Goldsmith CH, et al: Conservative management of mechanical neck pain: Systematic overview and meta-analysis. *BMJ* 313:1291–1296, 1996.
422. Assendelft WJ, Morton SC, Yu EI, et al: Spinal manipulative therapy for low back pain. A meta-analysis of effectiveness relative to other therapies. *Ann Intern Med* 138:871–881, 2003.
423. Assendelft WJ, Morton SC, Yu EI, et al: Spinal manipulative therapy for low back pain. *Cochrane Database Syst Rev* 138:871–881, 2004.
424. Clare HA, Adams R, Maher CG: A systematic review of efficacy of McKenzie therapy for spinal pain. *Aust J Physiother* 50:209–216, 2004.
425. Ferreira ML, Ferreira PH, Latimer J, et al: Does spinal manipulative therapy help people with chronic low back pain? *Aust J Physiother* 48:277–284, 2002.
426. Ferreira ML, Ferreira PH, Latimer J, et al: Efficacy of spinal manipulative therapy for low back pain of less than three months' duration. *J Manip Physiol Ther* 26:593–601, 2003.

427. Hurley DA, McDonough SM, Baxter GD, et al: A descriptive study of the usage of spinal manipulative therapy techniques within a randomized clinical trial in acute low back pain. *Man Ther* 10:61–67, 2005.
428. Maher CG: Effective physical treatment for chronic low back pain. *Orthop Clin North Am* 35:57–64, 2004.
429. Margo K: Spinal manipulative therapy for low back pain. *Am Fam Physician* 71:464–465, 2005.
430. Mierau D, Cassidy JD, McGregor M, et al: A comparison of the effectiveness of spinal manipulative therapy for low back pain patients with and without spondylolisthesis. *J Manip Physiol Ther* 10:49–55, 1987.
431. Peeters GG, Verhagen AP, de Bie RA, et al: The efficacy of conservative treatment in patients with whiplash injury: A systematic review of clinical trials. *Spine* 26:E64–E73, 2001.
432. Petersen T, Kryger P, Ekdahl C, et al: The effect of McKenzie therapy as compared with that of intensive strengthening training for the treatment of patients with subacute or chronic low back pain: A randomized controlled trial. *Spine* 27:1702–1709, 2002.
433. Swenson R, Haldeman S: Spinal manipulative therapy for low back pain. *J Am Acad Orthop Surg* 11:228–237, 2003.
434. Vernon H: A comparison of the effectiveness of spinal manipulative therapy for low back pain patients with and without spondylolisthesis. *J Manip Physiol Ther* 10:337–338, 1987.
435. Freburger JK, Carey TS, Holmes GM: Effectiveness of physical therapy for the management of chronic spine disorders: A propensity score approach. *Phys Ther* 86:381–394, 2006.
436. Williams PC: *Low Back and Neck Pain-Causes and Conservative Treatment*. Springfield, IL: Charles C Thomas, 1974.
437. Williams PC: *The Lumbosacral Spine*. New York, NY: McGraw-Hill, 1965.
438. McKenzie RA: *The Cervical and Thoracic Spine: Mechanical Diagnosis and Therapy*. Waikanae, NZ: Spinal Publications, 1990.
439. Hyman J, Liebenson C: Spinal stabilization exercise program. In: Liebenson C, ed. *Rehabilitation of the Spine: A Practitioner's Manual*. Baltimore, MD: Lippincott Williams & Wilkins, 1996:293–317.
440. Aaron G: The use of stabilization training in the rehabilitation of the athlete, Sports Physical Therapy Home Study Course, APTA, Sports Physical Therapy Section, 1996.
441. Sweeney TB, Prentice C, Saal JA, et al: Cervicothoracic muscular stabilization techniques. In: Saal JA, ed. *Physical Medicine and Rehabilitation, State of the Art Reviews: Neck and Back Pain*. Philadelphia, MD: Hanley & Belfus, 1990:335–359.
442. Hubley-Kozey CL, McCulloch TA, McFarland DH: Chronic low back pain: A critical review of specific therapeutic exercise protocols on musculoskeletal and neuromuscular parameters. *J Man Manip Ther* 11:78–87, 2003.
443. McGill SM: Low back exercises: Evidence for improving exercise regimes. *Phys Ther* 78:754–765, 1998.
444. Juker D, McGill S, Kropf P, et al: Quantitative intramuscular myoelectric activity of lumbar portions of psoas and the abdominal wall during a wide variety of tasks. *Med Sci Sports Exer* 30:301–310, 1998.
445. Shah JS, Hampson WGJ, Jayson MIV: The distribution of surface strain in the cadaveric lumbar spine. *J Bone Joint Surg* 60B:246–251, 1978.
446. Gill K, Videman T, Shimizu T, et al: The effect of repeated extensions on the discographic dye patterns in cadaveric lumbar motion segments. *Clin Biomech* 2:205–210, 1987.
447. Krag MH, Seroussi RE, Wilder DG, et al: Internal displacement distribution from in vitro loading of human thoracic and lumbar spinal motion segments: Experimental results and theoretical predictions. *Spine* 12:1001–1007, 1987.
448. Schnebel BE, Simmons JW, Chowning J, et al: A digitizing technique for the study of movement of intradiscal dye in response to flexion and extension of the lumbar spine. *Spine* 13:309–312, 1988.
449. Beattie P, Brooks WM, Rothstein J, et al: Effect of lordosis on the position of the nucleus pulposus in supine subjects. *Spine* 19:2096–2102, 1994.
450. Fennell AJ, Jones AP, Hukins DWL: Migration of the nucleus pulposus within the intervertebral disc during flexion and extension of the spine. *Spine* 21:2753–2757, 1996.
451. Schnebel BE, Watkins RG, Dillin W: The role of spinal flexion and extension in changing nerve root compression in disc herniations. *Spine* 14:835–837, 1989.
452. Heffner SL, McKenzie R, Jacob G: McKenzie protocols for mechanical treatment of the low back. In: Morris C, ed. *Low Back Syndromes: Integrated Clinical Management*. New York, NY: McGraw-Hill, 2006:611–622.
453. Jacob G, McKenzie R: Spinal therapeutics based on responses to loading. In: Liebenson C, ed. *Rehabilitation of the Spine: A Practitioner's Manual*. Baltimore, MD: Lippincott Williams & Wilkins, 1996:225–252.
454. Cherkin DC, Deyo RA, Battie M, et al: A comparison of physical therapy, chiropractic manipulation and provision of an educational booklet for the treatment of patients with low back pain. *N Engl J Med* 339:1021–1029, 1998.
455. Long A, Donelson R, Fung T: Does it matter which exercise? A randomized controlled trial of exercise for low back pain. *Spine* 29:2593–602, 2004.
456. Ponte DF, Jensen GJ, Kent BE: A preliminary report on the use of the McKenzie protocol versus Williams protocol in the treatment of low back pain. *J Orthop Sports Phys Ther* 6:130–139, 1984.
457. Nwuga G, Nwuga V: Relative therapeutic efficacy of the Williams and McKenzie protocols in back pain management. *Physiother Pract* 2:99–105, 1985.
458. Stankovic R, Johnell O: Conservative treatment on acute low back pain: A 5 year follow-up study of two methods of treatment. *Spine* 20:469–472, 1995.
459. Stankovic R, Johnell O: Conservative management of acute low back pain. A prospective randomized trial: McKenzie method of treatment versus patient education in "mini back school." *Spine* 15:120–123, 1990.
460. Miller ER, Schenk RJ, Karnes JL, et al: A comparison of the McKenzie approach to a specific spine stabilization program for chronic low back pain. *J Man Manip Ther* 13:103–112, 2005.
461. Porterfield J, De Rosa C: *Mechanical Neck Pain: Perspectives in Functional Anatomy*. Philadelphia, PA: WB Saunders, 1995.
462. Hides JA, Jull GA, Richardson CA: Long-term effects of specific stabilizing exercises for first-episode low back pain. *Spine* 26:E243–E248, 2001.
463. van der Velde G, Mierau D: The effect of exercise on percentile rank aerobic capacity, pain, and self-rated disability in patients with chronic low-back pain: A retrospective chart review. *Arch Phys Med Rehabil* 81:1457–1463, 2000.
464. Bentsen H, Lindgarde F, Manthorpe R: The effect of dynamic strength back exercise and/or a home training program in 57-year-old women with chronic low back pain. Results of a prospective randomized study with a 3-year follow-up period. *Spine* 22:1494–1500, 1997.
465. Nelson BW, O'Reilly E, Miller M, et al: The clinical effects of intensive, specific exercise on chronic low back pain: A controlled study of 895 consecutive patients with 1-year follow up. *Orthopedics* 18:971–981, 1995.
466. Cady LD, Bischoff DP, O'connell ER, et al: Strength and fitness and subsequent back injuries in firefighters. *J Occup Med* 21:269–272, 1979.
467. Nutter P: Aerobic exercise in the treatment and prevention of low back pain. *Occup Med* 3:137–145, 1988.
468. Kofotolis N, Kellis E: Effects of two 4-week proprioceptive neuromuscular facilitation programs on muscle endurance, flexibility, and functional performance in women with chronic low back pain. *Phys Ther* 86:1001–1012, 2006.
469. Lusting A, Ball E, Looney M: A Comparison of Two Proprioceptive Neuromuscular Facilitation Techniques for Improving Range of Motion and Muscular Strength. *Isokin Exer Sci* 2:154–159, 1992.
470. Saliba V, Johnson G, Wardlaw C: Proprioceptive neuromuscular facilitation. In: Basmajian JV, Nyberg R, eds. *Rational Manual Therapies*. Baltimore, MD: Williams & Wilkins, 1993.
471. Kofotolis N, Sambanis M: The influence of exercise on musculoskeletal disorders of the lumbar spine. *J Sports Med Phys Fitness* 45:84–92, 2005.
472. Daltroy LH, Iversen MD, Larson MG, et al: A controlled trial of an educational program to prevent low back injuries. *N Engl J Med* 337:322–328, 1997.
473. Hall H: Point of view. *Spine* 21:2189, 1994.
474. Cohen JE, Goel V, Frank JW, et al: Group education interventions for people with low back pain: An overview of the literature. *Spine* 19:1214–1222, 1994.
475. Njoo KH, Vanderdoes E, Stam HJ: Inter-observer agreement on iliac crest pain syndrome in general practice. *J Rheumatol* 22:1532–1535, 1995.
476. Collee G, Dijkmans BA, Vandenbroucke JP, et al: Iliac crest pain syndrome in low back pain: Frequency and features. *J Rheumatol* 18:1064–1067, 1991.
477. Mennell JM: *Back Pain. Diagnosis and Treatment Using Manipulative Techniques*. Boston, MA: Little, Brown & Company, 1960.

478. Wade MD: Diastasis recti and low back pain. *Orthop Pract* 17:20–22, 2005.
479. Vandertop WP, Bosma WJ: The piriformis syndrome. A case report. *J Bone Joint Surg* 73A:1095–1097, 1991.
480. Robinson DR: Pyriformis syndrome in relation to sciatic pain. *Am J Surg* 73:355–358, 1947.
481. McCrory P: The "piriformis syndrome"–myth or reality? *Br J Sports Med* 35:209–210, 2001.
482. Maigne JY, Maigne R: Trigger point of the posterior iliac crest: Painful iliolumbar ligament insertion or cutaneous dorsal ramus pain? An anatomic study. *Arch Phys Med Rehabil* 72:734–737, 1991.
483. Banwart JC, Asher MA, Hassanein RS: Iliac crest bone graft harvest donor site morbidity: A statistical evaluation. *Spine* 20:1055–1060, 1995.
484. Fernyhough JC, Schimandle JJ, Weigel MC, et al: Chronic donor site pain complicating bone graft harvesting from the posterior iliac crest for spinal fusion. *Spine* 17:1474–1480, 1992.
485. Maigne R: Low-back pain of thoraco-lumbar origin. *Arch Phys Med Rehabil* 61:389–395, 1980.
486. Thein-Nissenbaum J, Boissonnault WG: Differential diagnosis of spondylolysis in a patient with chronic low back pain. *J Orthop Sports Phys Ther* 35:319–326, 2005.
487. Bradford DS, Hu SS: Spondylolysis and spondylolisthesis. In: Weinstein SL, ed. *The Pediatric Spine*. Philadelphia, PA: Raven Press, 1994.
488. Sairyo K, Katoh S, Takata Y, et al: MRI signal changes of the pedicle as an indicator for early diagnosis of spondylolysis in children and adolescents: A clinical and biomechanical study. *Spine* 31:206–211, 2006.
489. Cassidy RC, Shaffer WO, Johnson DL: Spondylolysis and spondylolisthesis in the athlete. *Orthopedics* 28:1331–1333, 2005.
490. Van der Wall H, Magee M, Reiter L, et al: Degenerative spondylolysis: A concise report of scintigraphic observations. *Rheumatology (Oxford)* 45:209–211. Epub 2005 October 18, 2006.
491. McNeely ML, Torrance G, Magee DJ: A systematic review of physiotherapy for spondylolysis and spondylolisthesis. *Man Ther* 8:80–91, 2003.
492. Spratt KF, Weinstein JN, Lehmann TR, et al: Efficacy of flexion and extension treatments incorporating braces for low-back pain patients with retrodisplacement, spondylolisthesis, or normal sagittal translation. *Spine* 18:1839–1849, 1993.
493. Clark P, Letts M: Trauma to the thoracic and lumbar spine in the adolescent. *Can J Surg* 44:337–345, 2001.
494. Dandy DJ, Shannon MJ: Lumbosacral subluxation. *J Bone Joint Surg* 53B:578, 1971.
495. Barash HL: Spondylolisthesis and tight hamstrings. *J Bone Joint Surg* 52:1319, 1970.
496. Edelman B: Conservative treatment considered best course for spondylolisthesis. *Orthop Today* 9:6–8, 1989.
497. Grobler LJ, Robertson PA, Novotny JE, et al: Etiology of spondylolisthesis: Assessment of the role played by lumbar facet joint morphology. *Spine* 18:80–91, 1993.
498. Laus M, Tigani D, Alfonso C, et al: Degenerative spondylolisthesis: Lumbar stenosis and instability. *Chir Organi Mov* 77:39–49, 1992.
499. Love TW, Fagan AB, Fraser RD: Degenerative spondylolisthesis: Developmental or acquired? *J Bone Joint Surg* 81B:670–674, 1999.
500. Matsunaga S, Sakou T, Morizonon Y, et al: Natural history of degenerative spondylolisthesis: Pathogenesis and natural course of slippage. *Spine* 15:1204–1210, 1990.
501. Meschan I: Spondylolisthesis: A commentary on etiology and on improved method of roentgenographic mensuration and detection of instability. *AJR* 55:230, 1945.
502. Newman PH: The etiology of spondylolisthesis. *J Bone Joint Surg* 45B:39–59, 1963.
503. Postacchinia F, Perugia D: Degenerative lumbar spondylolisthesis. Part I: Etology, pathogenesis, pathomorphology, and clinical features. *Ital J Orthop Traumatol* 17:165–173, 1991.
504. Rosenberg NJ: Degenerative spondylolisthesis. *J Bone Joint Surg* 57A:467–474, 1975.
505. Spring WE: Spondylolisthesis – a new clinical test. Proceedings of the Australian Orthopedics Association. *J Bone Joint Surg* 55B:229, 1973.
506. Vallois HV, Lozarthes G: Indices lombares et indice lombaire totale. *Bull Soc Anthropol* 3:117, 1942.
507. Wiltse LL, Winter RB: Terminology and measurement of spondylolisthesis. *J Bone Joint Surg* 65:768–772, 1983.
508. Meyerding HW: Spondylolisthesis. *Surg Gynecol Obstet* 54:371–377, 1932.
509. Chen WJ, Lai PL, Niu CC, et al: Surgical treatment of adjacent instability after lumbar spine fusion. *Spine* 26:E519–E524, 2001.
510. Cook C, Cook A, Fleming R: Rehabilitation for clinical lumbar instability in a female adolescent competitive diver with spondylolisthesis. *J Man Manip Ther* 12:91–99, 2004.
511. Garry J, McShane J: Lumbar spondylolisthesis in adolescent athletes. *J Fam Pract* 47:145–149, 1998.
512. Paris SV: Physical signs of instability. Spine. 10:277–279, 1985.
513. Kirkaldy-Willis WH: *Managing Low Back Pain*, 2nd ed. New York, NY: Churchill Livingstone, 1988.
514. Gonnella C, Paris SV, Kutner M: Reliability in evaluating passive intervertebral motion. *Phys Ther* 62:436–444, 1982.
515. Smedmark V, Wallin M, Arvidsson I: Inter-examiner reliability in assessing passive intervertebral motion of the cervical spine. *Man Ther* 5:97–101, 2000.
516. Kraft GL, Levinthal DH: Facet synovial impingement. *Surg Gynecol Obstet* 93:439–443, 1951.
517. Janda V: *Muscle Function Testing*. London: Butterworths, 1983.
518. Lewit K: *Manipulative Therapy in Rehabilitation of the Locomotor System*, 2nd ed. Oxford: Butterworth-Heinemann, 1996.
519. Dupuis PR: The natural history of degenerative changes in the lumbar spine. In: Watkins RG, Collis JS, eds. *Principles and Techniques in Spine Surgery*. Rockville, MD: Aspen Publications, 1987:1–4.
520. Adams MA, McNally DS, Dolan P: Stress distributions inside intervertebral discs: The effects of age and degeneration. *J Bone Joint Surg* (Am):965–972, 1996.
521. Miller JA, Schmatz C, Schultz AB: Lumbar disc degeneration: Correlation with age, sex, and spine level in 600 autopsy specimens. *Spine* 13:173–178, 1988.
522. Matsui H, Kanamori M, Ishihara H, et al: Familial predisposition for lumbar degenerative disc disease. A case-control study. *Spine* 23:1029–1034, 1998.
523. Moneta GB, Videman T, Kaivanto K, et al: Reported pain during lumbar discography as a function of annular ruptures and disc degeneration. *Spine* 19:1968–1974, 1994.
524. Dolan P, Earley M, Adams MA: Bending and compressive stresses acting on the lumbar spine during lifting activities. *J Biomech* 27:1237–1248, 1994.
525. Wedge JH: The natural history of spinal degeneration. In: Kirkaldy-Willis WH, ed. *Managing Low Back Pain*. New York, NY: Churchill Livingstone, 1983:3–8.
526. Yasuma T, Koh S, Okamura T, et al: Histological changes in aging lumbar intervertebral discs: Their role in protrusions and prolapses. *J Bone Joint Surg* 72A:220–229, 1990.
527. Eckert C, Decker A: Pathological studies of intervertebral discs. *J Bone Joint Surg* 29:447–454, 1947.
528. Taylor TKF, Akeson WH: Intervertebral disc prolapse: A review of morphologic and biochemical knowledge concerning the nature of prolapse. *Clin Orthop* 76:54–79, 1971.
529. Jonsson B, Stromqvist B: Clinical appearance of contained and noncontained lumbar disc herniation. *J Spinal Disord* 9:32, 1996.
530. Brinckmann P: Injury of the anulus fibrosus and disc protrusions. *Spine* 11:149–153, 1986.
531. Kostuik JP, Harrington I, Alexander D, et al: Cauda equina syndrome and lumbar disc herniation. *J Bone Joint Surg* 68A:386–391, 1986.
532. Mixter WJ, Barr JS Jr: Rupture of the intervertebral disc with involvement of the spinal canal. *N Engl J Med* 211:210–215, 1934.
533. Gronblad M, Virri J, Tolonen J, et al: A controlled immuno-histochemical study of inflammatory cells in disc herniation tissue. *Spine* 19:2744–2751, 1994.
534. Habtemariam A, Gronblad M, Virri J, et al: Immunocytochemical localization of immunoglobulins in disc herniations. *Spine* 16:1864–1869, 1996.
535. Saal JS, Franson R, Dobrow RC, et al: High levels of phospholipase A2 activity in lumbar disc herniation. *Spine* 15:674–678, 1990.
536. Tolonen J, Gronblad M, Virri J, et al: Basic fibroblast growth factor immunoreactivity in blood vessels and cells of disc herniations. *Spine* 20:271–276, 1995.
537. Happey T, Pearson CH, Palframan J, et al: Proteoglycans and glycoproteins associated with collagen in the human intervertebral disc. *Z Klin Chem* 9:79, 1971.
538. Gronblad M, Virri J, Tolonen J, et al: A controlled biochemical and immunohistochemical study of human synovial type (group II) phospholipase A2 and inflammatory cells in macroscopically normal, degenerated, and herniated human lumbar disc tissues. *Spine* 22:1–8, 1996.

539. Kang JD, Georgescu HI, McIntyre-Larkin L, et al: Herniated lumbar intervertebral discs spontaneously produce matrix metalloproteinases, nitric oxide, interleukin-6, and prostaglandin E2. *Spine* 21:271–277, 1996.
540. Halland AM, Klemp P, Botes D, et al: Avascular necrosis of the hip in systemic lupus erythematosus: The role of MRI. *Br J Rheumatol* 32:972–976, 1993.
541. Trummer M, Flaschka G, Unger F, et al: Lumbar disc herniation mimicking meralgia paresthetica: Case report. *Surg Neurol* 54:80–81, 2000.
542. Kallgren MA, Tingle LJ: Meralgia paresthetica mimicking lumbar radiculopathy. *Anesth Analg* 76:1367–1368, 1993.
543. Naftulin S, Fast A, Thomas M: Diabetic lumbar radiculopathy: Sciatica without disc herniation. *Spine* 18:2419–2422, 1993.
544. Fontanesi G, Tartaglia I, Cavazzuti A, et al: Prolapsed intervertebral disc at the upper lumbar level. *Ital J Orthop Traumatol* 13:501–507, 1987.
545. Bosacco SJ, Berman AT, Raisis LW, et al: High lumbar disc herniation. *Orthopedics* 12:275–278, 1989.
546. Hsu K, Zucherman J, Shea W, et al: High lumbar disc degeneration: Incidence and etiology. *Spine* 15:679–682, 1990.
547. Dammers R, Koehler PJ: Lumbar disc herniation: Level increases with age. *Surg Neurol* 58:209–212; discussion 212–213, 2002.
548. Nadler SF, Campagnolo DI, Tomaio AC, et al: High lumbar disc: Diagnostic and treatment dilemma. *Am J Phys Med Rehabil* 77:538–544, 1998.
549. O'Laoire SA, Crockard HA, Thomas DG: Prognosis for sphincter recovery after operation for cauda equina compression owing to lumbar disc prolapse. *BMJ* 282:1852–1854, 1981.
550. Schmorl G, Junghanns H: *The human spine in health and disease (ed 2d American).* New York, NY: Grune & Stratton, 1971.
551. Coventry MB, Ghormley RK, Kernohan JW: The intervertebral disc: Its microscopic anatomy and pathology. Part II. Changes in the intervertebral disc concomitant with age. *J Bone Joint Surg* 27 A:233–247, 1945.
552. Hilton RC, Ball J, Benn RT: Vertebral end plate lesions (Schmorl's nodes) in the dorsolumbar spine. *Ann Rheum Dis* 35:127–132, 1976.
553. Yasuma T, Saito S, Kihara K: Schmorl's nodes: Correlation of x-ray and histological findings in postmortem specimens. *Acta Pathol Jpn* 38:723–733, 1988.
554. Keyes DC, Compere EL: The normal and pathological physiology of the nucleus pulposus of the intervertebral disc. *J Bone Joint Surg* 14:897–938, 1932.
555. Weinstein JN: A 45-year-old man with low back pain and a numb left foot. *JAMA* 280:730–736,, 1998.
556. Vroomen PC, de Krom MC, Slofstra PD, et al: Conservative treatment of sciatica: A systematic review. *J Spinal Disord* 13:463–469, 2000.
557. Vroomen PC, de Krom MC, Wilmink JT, et al: Lack of effectiveness of bed rest for sciatica. *N Engl J Med* 340:418–423, 1999.
558. Ito T, Takano Y, Yuasa N: Types of lumbar herniated disc and clinical course. *Spine* 26:648–651, 2001.
559. Bakhtiary AH, Safavi-Farokhi Z, Rezasoltani A: Lumbar stabilizing exercises improve activities of daily living in patients with lumbar disc herniation. *J Back Musculoskel Rehabil* 18:55–60, 2005.
560. Manniche C, Asmussen KH, Vinterberg H, et al: Back pain, sciatica and disability following first-time conventional haemilaminectomy for lumbar disc herniation. Use of "Low Back Pain Rating Scale" as a postal questionnaire. *Dan Med Bull* 41:103–106, 1994.
561. Delauche-Cavallier MC, Budet C, Laredo JD, et al: Lumbar disc herniation. Computed tomography scan changes after conservative treatment of nerve root compression. *Spine* 17:927–933, 1992.
562. Vroomen PC, de Krom MC, Knottnerus JA: Diagnostic value of history and physical examination in patients suspected of sciatica due to disc herniation: A systematic review. *J Neurol* 246:899–906, 1999.
563. Loew F, Caspar W: Surgical approach to lumbar disc herniations. *Adv Stand Neurosurg* 5:153–174, 1978.
564. Vucetic N, Astrand P, Guntner P, et al: Diagnosis and prognosis in lumbar disc herniation. *Clin Orthop Relat Res* 361:116–122, 1999.
565. Nordly EJ, Wright PH: Efficacy of chymopapain in chemonucleolysis: A review. *Spine* 19:2578–2583, 1994.
566. Wittenberg RH, Oppel S, Rubenthaler FA, et al: Five-year results from chemonucleolysis with chymopapain or collagenase: A prospective randomized study. *Spine* 26:1835–1841, 2001.
567. Atlas SJ, Deyo RA, Keller RB, et al: The Maine Lumbar Spine Study, Part II: 1-year outcomes of surgical and nonsurgical management of sciatica. *Spine* 21:1777–1786, 1996.
568. Hadler NM, Carey PS, Garrett J: The influence of indemnification by workers compensation insurance on recovery from acute back ache. *Spine* 20:2710–2715, 1995.
569. Junge A, Dvorak J, Ahrens S: Predictors of bad and good outcome of lumbar disc surgery: A prospective clinical study resulting in recommendations for screening to avoid bad outcomes. *Spine* 20:460–468, 1995.
570. Sherk HH, Black JD, Prodoehl JH, et al: Laser diskectomy. *Orthopedics* 16:573–576, 1993.
571. Malter AD, McNeney B, Loeser JD, et al: 5-year reoperation rates after different types of lumbar spine surgery. *Spine* 23:814–820, 1998.
572. Vishteh AG, Dickman CA: Anterior lumbar microdiscectomy and interbody fusion for the treatment of recurrent disc herniation. *Neurosurgery* 48:334–337, discussion 338, 2001.
573. Harms J, Rolinger H: A one-stage procedure in operative treatment of spondylolistheses: Dorsal traction-reposition and anterior fusion [in German]. *Z Orthop Ihre Grenzgeb* 120:343–347, 1982.
574. Phillips FM, Cunningham B: Intertransverse lumbar interbody fusion. *Spine* 27:E37–E41, 2002.
575. Johannsen F, Remvig L, Kryger P, et al: Supervised endurance training compared to home training after first lumbar diskectomy: A clinical trial. *Clin Exp Rheumatol* 12:609–614, 1994.
576. Kjellby-Wendt G, Styf J: Early active training after lumbar discectomy: A prospective, randomized and controlled trial. *Spine* 23:2345–2351, 1998.
577. Skall F, Manniche C, Nielsen C: Intensive back exercises 5 weeks after surgery of lumbar disk prolapse: A prospective randomized multicentre trial with historical control. *Ugeskr Laeger* 156:643–646, 1994.
578. Booth FW: Physiologic and biochemical effects of immobilization on muscle. *Clin Orthop Relat Res* 219:15–21, 1987.
579. Eiff MP, Smith AT, Smith GE: Early mobilization versus immobilization in the treatment of lateral ankle sprains. *Am J Sports Med* 22:83–88, 1994.
580. Akeson WH, Amiel D, Mechanic GL, et al: Collagen cross-linking alterations in the joint contractures: Changes in the reducible cross-links in periarticular connective tissue after 9 weeks immobilization. Connect. *Tissue Res* 5:15, 1977.
581. Akeson WH, Amiel D, Abel MF, et al: Effects of immobilization on joints. *Clin Orthop* 219:28–37, 1987.
582. Akeson WH, Amiel D, Woo SL-Y: Immobility effects on synovial joints: The pathomechanics of joint contracture. *Biorheology* 17:95–110, 1980.
583. Woo SL-Y, Matthews J, Akeson WH, et al: Connective tissue response to immobility: A correlative study of biochemical and biomechanical measurements of normal and immobilized rabbit knee. *Arthritis Rheum* 18:257–264, 1975.
584. White T, Malone T: Effects of running on intervertebral disc height. *J Orthop Sports Phys Ther* 12:410, 1990.
585. Turner JA, Ersek M, Herron L, et al: Surgery for lumbar spinal stenosis: Attempted meta-analysis of the literature. *Spine* 17:1–8, 1992.
586. Arnoldi CC, Brodsky AE, Cauchoix J: Lumbar spinal stenosis and nerve root encroachment syndromes: Definition and classification. *Clin Orthop* 115:4–5, 1976.
587. Verbiest H: A radicular syndrome from developmental narrowing of the lumbar vertebral canal. *J Bone Joint Surg* 26B:230, 1954.
588. Katz JN, Dalgas M, Stucki G, et al: Degenerative lumbar spinal stenosis: Diagnostic value of the history and physical examination. *Arthritis Rheum* 38:1236–1241, 1995.
589. Cailliet R: *Low Back Pain Syndrome*, 4th ed. Philadelphia, PA: FA Davis Co, 1991:263–268.
590. Weinstein SM, Herring SA: Rehabilitation of the patient with low back pain. In: DeLisa JA, Gans BM, eds. *Rehabilitation Medicine: Principles and Practice*, 2nd ed. Philadelphia, PA: JB Lippincott, 1993:996–1017.
591. Fast A: Low back disorders: Conservative management. *Arch Phys Med Rehabil* 69:880–891, 1988.
592. Fritz JM, Erhard RE, Vignovic M: A nonsurgical treatment approach to patients with lumbar spinal stenosis. *Phys Ther* 77:962–973, 1997.
593. Whitman JM, Flynn TW, Childs JD, et al: A comparison between two physical therapy treatment programs for patients with lumbar spinal stenosis: A randomized clinical trial. *Spine* 31:2541–2549, 2006.
594. Maitland G: *Peripheral Manipulation*, 3rd ed. London: Butterworth, 1991.
595. Whitman JM, Flynn TW, Fritz JM: Nonsurgical management of patients with lumbar spinal stenosis: A literature review and a case series of three patients managed with physical therapy. *Phys Med Rehabil Clin N Am* 14:77–101, vi–vii, 2003.

596. Dooley JF, McBroom RJ, Taguchi T, et al: Nerve root infiltration in the diagnosis of radicular pain. *Spine* 13:79–83, 1988.
597. Tajima T, Furakawa K, Kuramochi E: Selective lumbosacral radiculography and block. *Spine* 5:68–77, 1980.
598. Burnell A: Injection techniques in low back pain. In: Twomey LT, ed. *Symposium: Low Back Pain.* Perth: Western Australian Institute of Technology, 1974:111.
599. Strange FG: Debunking the disc. *Proc R Soc Med* 9:952–956, 1966.
600. Seimons LP: *Low Back Pain: Clinical Diagnosis and Management.* Norwalk, CT: Appleton-Century-Crofts, 1983.
601. Pope M, Frymoyer J, Krag M: Diagnosing instability. *Clin Orthop* 296:60–67, 1992.
602. Long DM, BenDebba M, Torgenson W: Persistent back pain and sciatica in the United States: Patient characteristics. *J Spinal Disord* 9:40–58, 1996.
603. Boden SD, Wiesel SW: Lumbosacral segmental motion in normal individuals. Have we been measuring instability properly? *Spine* 15:571–576, 1990.
604. O'Sullivan P: The efficacy of specific stabilizing exercises in the management of chronic low back pain with radiological diagnosis of lumbar segmental instability, Curtin University of Technology. Perth, 1997.
605. Strohl K, Mead J, Banzett R, et al: Regional differences in abdominal muscle activity during various manoeuvres in humans. *J Appl Physiol* 51:1471–1476, 1981.
606. Hodges PW, Richardson CA: Delayed postural contraction of transversus abdominis in low back pain associated with movement of the lower limb. *J Spinal Disord* 11:46–56, 1998.
607. Hagins M, Adler K, Cash M, et al: Effects of practice on the ability to perform lumbar stabilization exercises. *J Orthop Sports Phys Ther* 29:546–555, 1999.
608. Kisner C, Colby LA: The Spine: Exercise interventions. In: Kisner C, Colby LA, eds. *Therapeutic Exercise. Foundations and Techniques*, 5th ed. Philadelphia, PA: FA Davis, 2002:439–480.
609. Voight ML, Hoogenboom BJ, Cook G: The chop and lift reconsidered: Integrating neuromuscular principles into orthopedic and sports rehabilitation. *N Am J Sports Phys Ther* 3:151–159, 2008.
610. Guide to physical therapist practice. second edition. American Physical Therapy Association. *Phys Ther* 81:9–746, 2001.
611. Rasmussen GG: Manipulation in treatment of low back pain: A randomized clinical trial. *Manual Med* 1:8–10, 1979.
612. Postacchini F, Facchini M, Palieri P: Efficacy of various forms of conservative treatments in low back pain: A comparative study. *Neuro Orthop* 6:28–35, 1988.
613. Erhard RE, Delitto A, Cibulka MT: Relative effectiveness of an extension program and a combined program of manipulation and flexion and extension exercises in patients with acute low back syndrome. *Phys Ther* 74:1093–1100, 1994.
614. Delitto A, Cibulka MT, Erhard RE, et al: Evidence for use of an extension-mobilization category in acute low back syndrome: A prescriptive validation pilot study. *Phys Ther* 73:216–222; discussion 223–228, 1993.
615. Glover JR, Morris JG, Khosla T: A randomized clinical trial of rotational manipulation of the trunk. *Br J Indust Med* 31:59–64, 1974.
616. Godfrey CM, Morgan PP, Schatzker J: A randomized trial of manipulation for low-back pain in a medical setting. *Spine* 9:301–304, 1984.
617. Fritz JM, Whitman JM, Flynn TW, et al: Factors related to the inability of individuals with low back pain to improve with a spinal manipulation. *Phys Ther* 84:173–190, 2004.
618. Rasmussen-Barr E, Nilsson-Wikmar L, Arvidsson I: Stabilizing training compared with manual treatment in sub-acute and chronic low-back pain. *Man Ther* 8:233–241, 2003.
619. Trott PH, Grant R, Maitland GD: Manipulative therapy for the low lumbar spine: Technique selection and application to some syndromes. In: Twomey LT, Taylor JR, eds. *Clinics in Physical Therapy: Physical Therapy of the Low Back.* Philadelphia, PA: Churchill Livingstone, 1987:216–217.

CHAPTER 29 The Sacroiliac Joint

CHAPTER OBJECTIVES

At the completion of this chapter, the reader will be able to:

1. Describe the anatomy of the bones, the ligaments, the muscles, and the blood and nerve supply that comprises the sacroiliac (SI) region.
2. Describe the biomechanics of the sacroiliac joint (SIJ), including coupled movements, normal and abnormal joint barriers, kinesiology, and reactions to various stresses.
3. Perform a detailed objective examination of the SIJ, including palpation of the articular and the soft tissue structures, specific passive mobility tests, passive articular mobility tests, and stability tests.
4. Evaluate the total examination data to establish the diagnosis.
5. Describe the intervention strategies based on clinical findings and established goals.
6. Design an intervention based on patient education, manual therapy, and therapeutic exercise.
7. Apply active and passive mobilization techniques, and combined movements to the SIJ, in any position using the correct grade, direction, and duration.
8. Describe the common pathologies and lesions of this region.
9. Evaluate intervention effectiveness in order to progress or modify an intervention.
10. Plan an effective home program and instruct the patient in this program.

OVERVIEW

The SIJ serves as the supporting base of the spine and as the point of intersection between the spinal and the lower extremity joints. The SIJ is the least understood and, therefore, one of the most controversial and interesting areas of the spine. Determining a diagnosis in this region is complicated by the biomechanics of the SIJ and its relationships with the surrounding joints including the hip, pubic symphysis, and lumbar spine.

Grieve[1] has proposed that the SIJ, together with the other areas of the spine that serve as transitional areas, is of prime importance in understanding vertebral joint problems. This level of importance is perhaps surprising, because isolated pelvic impairments are rare. However, findings for SIJ dysfunction appear to be common, and the literature is replete with intervention techniques aimed at correcting pelvic dysfunctions.[2–12] This may be explained by the fact that, in addition to producing pain on its own, the pelvic joints often can refer pain.[13]

The level of interest surrounding this joint dates back to the Middle Ages, a time when the burning of witches was commonplace.[14] It was noticed after these burnings that three of the bones were not destroyed: a large triangular bone and two very small bones. It can only be assumed that some degree of significance was given to the large triangular bone as it was deemed a sacred bone, and was thus called the sacrum. It is unclear what significance was given to the two smaller bones, the sesamoid bones of the great toe.

Despite these illustrious beginnings for the sacrum, it was not until approximately 100 years ago that significant attention was applied to the study of pelvic anatomy and function, and its relationship to low back and pelvic pain. At the start of the 20th century, SIJ strain was thought to be the most common cause of sciatica.[15] Then, in 1934, Mixter and Barr[16] reported that sciatica could be caused by a prolapsed intervertebral disk, and the interest in the SIJ as a source of sciatica dwindled. Since then, there have been periods when the joint has been blamed for almost all low back and leg pain, and times when it has only been considered a problem during pregnancy. It is now generally accepted that approximately 13% (95% CI: 9–26%) of patients with persistent low back pain have the origin of pain confirmed as the SIJ.[17]

ANATOMY

Anatomically, the SIJ is a large diarthrodial joint that connects the spine with the pelvis (Fig. 29-1) and which serves as a central base through which forces are transmitted both

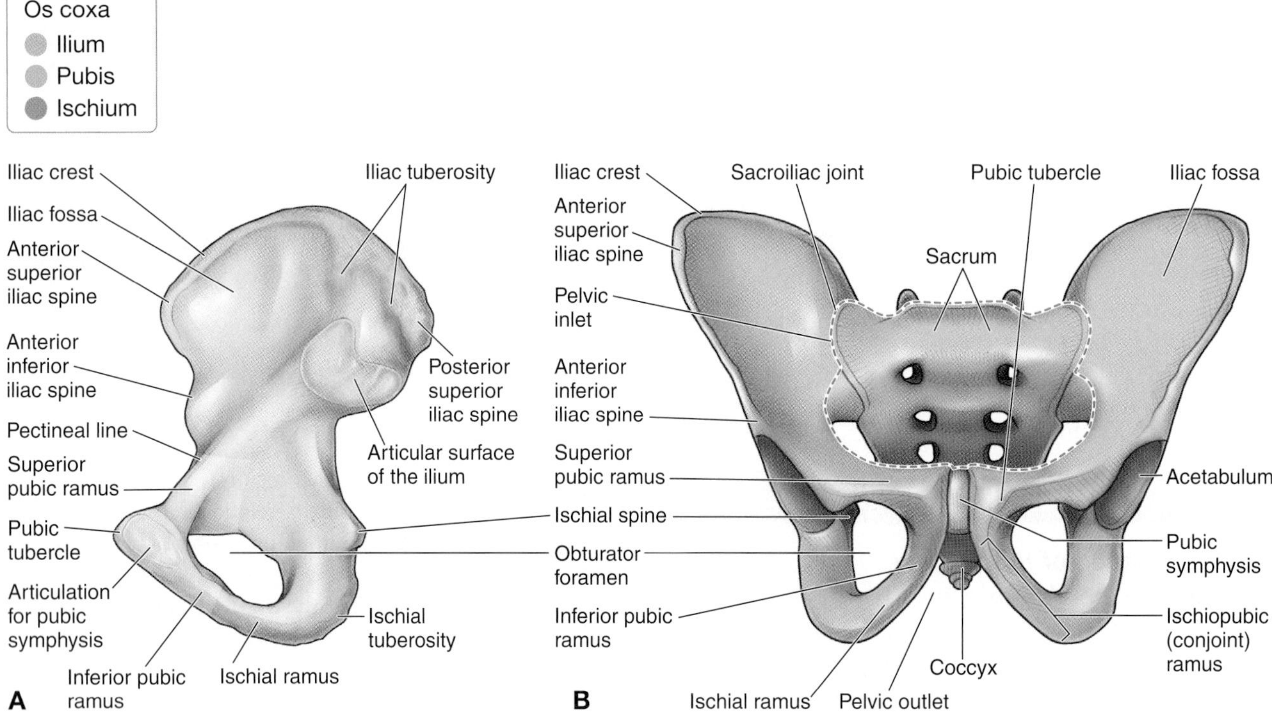

FIGURE 29-1 The pelvis. (Reproduced with permission from Morton DA, Foreman KB, Albertine KH: *The Big Picture: Gross Anatomy*. McGraw-Hill, 2011.)

directly and indirectly. Three bones comprise the SIJ: two innominates and the sacrum.

Innominates

The ilium, ischium, and pubic bone fuse at the acetabulum to form each innominate (Fig. 29-1). The ilium of each of the two innominates articulate with the sacrum, forming the SIJ, and the pubic bone of each of the innominates articulate with each other at the symphysis pubis.[18]

Sacrum

The sacrum (Fig. 29-1), a strong and triangular bone located between the two innominates, provides stability to this area and transmits the weight of the body from the mobile vertebral column to the pelvic region. The sacrum base is above and anterior, and its apex below and posterior (Fig. 29-1). Five centra fuse to form the central part of the sacrum, which contains remnants of the intervertebral disks enclosed by bone. The sacrum has four pairs of pelvic sacral foramina for transmission of the anterior (ventral) primary rami of the sacral nerves and four pairs of posterior (dorsal) sacral foramina for transmission of the posterior (dorsal) primary rami.

The transverse processes of the first sacral vertebra fuse with the costal elements to form the ala and the lateral crests (see Fig. 29-1). The ala of the sacrum forms the superolateral portions of the base. The superior articular processes of the sacrum (Fig. 29-1), which are concave and oriented posteromedially, extend upward from the base to articulate with the inferior articular processes of the fifth lumbar vertebra.

On the posterior (dorsal) surface of the sacrum is a midline ridge of bone called the median sacral crest, which represents the fusion of the sacral spinous processes of S1 to S4. Projecting posteriorly from this crest are four spinous tubercles. The fused laminae of S1 to S5, which are located lateral to the median sacral crest, form the intermediate sacral crest.

The sacral hiatus exhibits bilateral downward projections that are called the *sacral cornua*. These projections represent the inferior articular processes of the fifth sacral vertebra and are connected to the coccyx via the intercornual ligaments. On the inferolateral borders of the sacrum, approximately 2 cm to either side of the sacral hiatus, are the inferior lateral angles (ILAs). The triangular sacral canal houses the cauda equina. In addition to the more commonly considered bones and joints are those of the coccygeal spine.

Sacroiliac Joint

The articulating surfaces of this joint differ, with the iliac joint surfaces formed from fibrocartilage and the sacral surfaces formed from hyaline cartilage.[19] The hyaline cartilage is three to five times thicker than the fibrocartilage[20] and so between the sacral and iliac auricular surfaces, the SIJ is deemed a synovial articulation or diarthrosis.[21]

The inverted, L-shaped, auricular articular surface of the sacrum (Fig. 29-1) is surrounded entirely by the costal elements of the first three sacral segments. The short (superior) arm of this L-shape lies in a craniocaudal plane, within the first sacral segment, and corresponds to the depth of the sacrum (see Fig. 29-1). It is widest superiorly and anteriorly. The long (inferior) arm of the L-shape lies in an A-P plane, within the second and third sacral segments, and represents the length of the sacrum from top to bottom. It is widest inferiorly and posteriorly. There are large irregularities on each articular

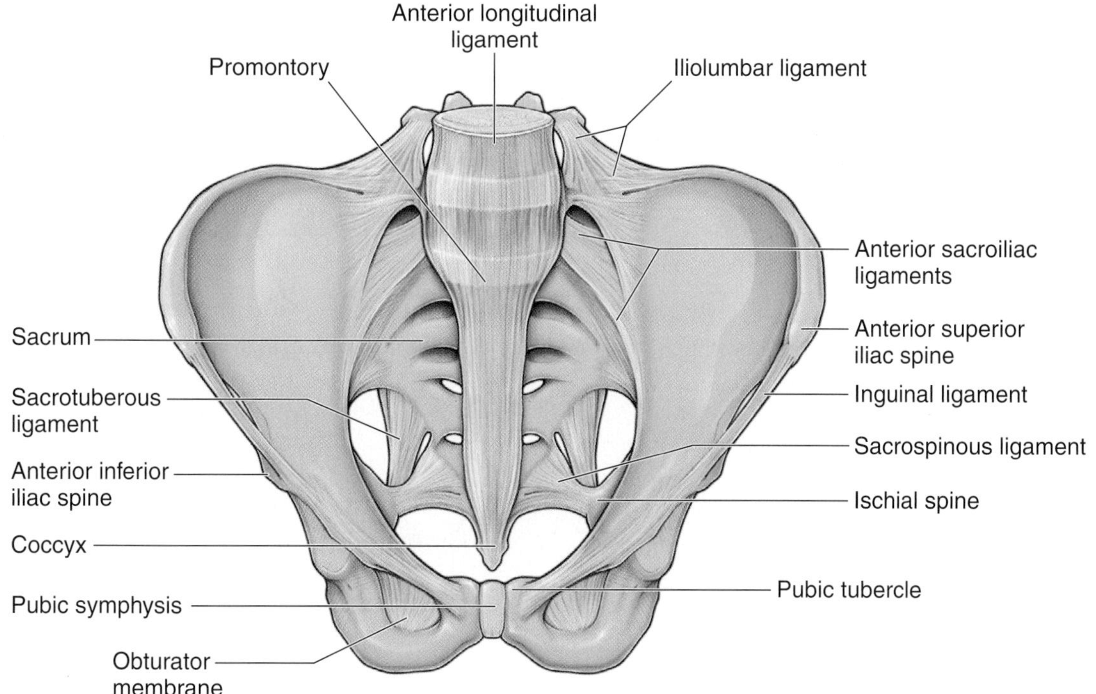

FIGURE 29-2 Anterior ligaments.

surface[22] that are roughly, though not exactly, reciprocal, with the sacral contours being generally deeper.[23,24] In addition to the larger irregularities, there are smaller horizontal crests and hollows that run anteroposteriorly. The sacral articular surface is wedge shaped in its upper portion, formed by the first sacral segment and half of the second. Below this, the joint surfaces run nearly vertically and then diverge somewhat, making a flare which tends to prevent the sacrum from sliding upward between ilia.[24]

Variations in the SIJ morphology are so common that they have been classified as type A, being less vertical than type B, and type C as an asymmetric mixture of types A and B.[5] Each of these variants can alter the function of the pelvis and its influence on the lumbar lordosis.[25]

CLINICAL PEARL

The configuration of the SIJs is extremely variable from person to person and between genders in terms of morphology and mobility.[24,26,27] However, it has been determined that these differences are not pathological, but normal adaptations.[26]

The articulating surfaces of the joint respond differently to the aging process, with early degenerative changes occurring on the iliac surface rather than on both surfaces of the joint simultaneously.[28] Other changes associated with aging include the development of intra-articular fibrous connections.[29] However, even with severe degenerative changes, the SIJ rarely fuses.[21]

The SIJ can be the site of manifestation for several disease processes, including SI tuberculosis, spondyloarthropathy (ankylosing spondylitis), and crystal and pyogenic arthropathies.

Joint Capsule

The SIJ capsule, consisting of two layers, is extensive and very strong. It attaches to both articular margins of the joint and is thickened inferiorly.

Ligaments

Like other synovial joints, the SIJ is reinforced by ligaments, but the ligaments of the SIJ are some of the strongest and toughest ligaments of the body.

Anterior Sacroiliac (Articular)

The anterior sacral ligament (Fig. 29-2) is an anteroinferior thickening of the fibrous capsule, which is relatively weak and thin compared with the rest of the SI ligaments. The ligament extends between the anterior and inferior borders of the iliac auricular surface and the anterior border of the sacral auricular surface.[21] The anterior sacral ligament is better developed near the arcuate line and the posterior inferior iliac spine (PIIS), where it connects the third sacral segment to the lateral side of the preauricular sulcus.

Because of its thinness, this ligament is often injured and can be a source of pain. It can be palpated at Baer's SI point*[30] and can be stressed using the anterior distraction and posterior compression pain provocation tests (see later).

Interosseous Sacroiliac (Articular)

This is a strong, short ligament located deep to the posterior (dorsal) SI ligament, and it forms the major connection between the sacrum and the innominate, filling the irregular

*Baer's SI point has been described as being on a line from the umbilicus to the anterior superior iliac spine, 5 cm from the umbilicus.

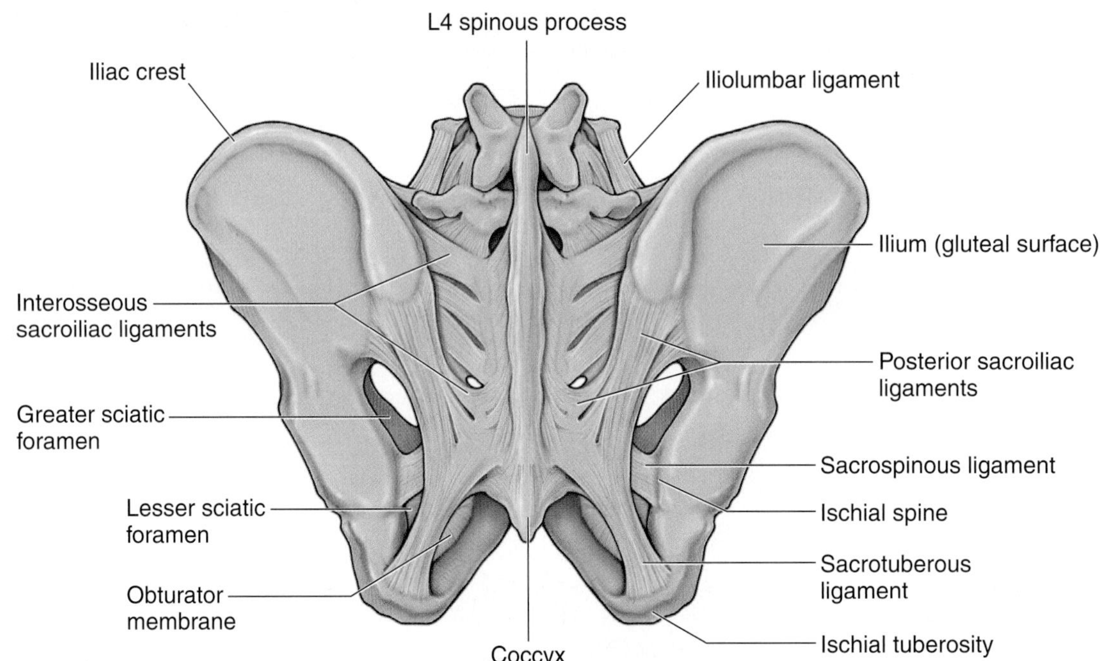

FIGURE 29-3 Posterior ligaments.

space posterosuperior to the joint between the lateral sacral crest and the iliac tuberosity (Fig. 29-3).[31] The deep portion sends fibers cranially and caudally from behind the auricular depressions. The superficial portion is a fibrous sheet connecting the superior (cranial) and posterior (dorsal) margins of the sacrum to the ilium, forming a layer that limits direct palpation of the SIJ. The interosseous SI ligament functions to resist anterior and inferior movement of the sacrum.

Posterior (Dorsal) Sacroiliac (Articular)

The posterior (dorsal) SI ligament or long ligament (see Fig. 29-3), which is easily palpable in the area directly caudal to the posterior superior iliac spine (PSIS), connects the PSIS (and a small part of the iliac crest) with the lateral crest of the third and fourth segments of the sacrum.[18] This is a very tough and strong ligament. The fibers from this ligament are multidirectional and blend laterally with the sacrotuberous ligament. It also has attachments medially to the erector spinae[32] and multifidus muscles[33] and the thoracodorsal fascia. Thus, contractions of the various muscles that attach to this ligament can result in the tightening of the ligament.

Directly caudal to the PSIS, the ligament is so solid and stout that one can easily think a bony structure is being palpated. What complicates matters is the fact that the area overlying the ligament is a frequent source of pain.[34]

The lateral expansion of the long ligament in the region directly caudal to the PSIS varies between 15 and 30 mm. The length, measured between the PSIS and the third and fourth sacral segments, varies between 42 and 75 mm. The lateral part of the posterior (dorsal) ligament is continuous with fibers passing between ischial tuberosity and iliac bone.

At the superior (cranial) aspect, the posterior (dorsal) ligament is attached to the PSIS and the adjacent part of the ilium, at the inferior (caudal) side to the lateral crest of the third and fourth, and occasionally to the fifth, sacral segments.[32]

Nutation (anterior motion) of the sacrum appears to slacken the posterior (dorsal) ligament, whereas counternutation (posterior motion) tautens the ligament.[32]

Sacrotuberous (Extra-articular)

This ligament (see Fig. 29-3) is composed of three large fibrous bands, broadly attached by its base to the PSIS, the lateral sacrum, and partly blended with the posterior (dorsal) SI ligament. Its oblique, lateral fibers descend and attach to the medial margin of the ischial tuberosity, spanning the piriformis muscle from which it receives some fibers. The medial fibers, running anteroinferior and laterally, have an attachment to the transverse tubercles of S3, S4, and S5, and the lateral margin of the coccyx. To the posterior surface of the sacrotuberous ligament are attached the lowest fibers of the gluteus maximus and the piriformis, the contraction of which produces increased tension in the ligament.[35] Superficial fibers on the inferior aspect of the ligament can continue into the tendon of the biceps femoris.

In addition to stabilizing against nutation of the sacrum, the sacrotuberous ligament also counteracts against the posterior (dorsal) and superior (cranial) migration of the sacral apex during weight bearing.[36,37]

Sacrospinous (Extra-articular)

Thinner than the sacrotuberous ligament, this triangular-shaped ligament extends from the ischial spine to the lateral margins of the sacrum and coccyx, and also laterally to the spine of the ischium (see Fig. 29-3). The ligament runs anterior (deep) to the sacrotuberous ligament to which it blends and then attaches to the capsule of the SIJ.[33]

The sacrotuberous and sacrospinous ligaments, which convert the greater and lesser sciatic notches into the greater and lesser foramen respectively, oppose forward tilting of the sacrum on the innominates during weight bearing of the vertebral column.

Iliolumbar (Indirect)

The anatomy of the iliolumbar ligament (Fig. 29-2) is described in Chapter 28.

Pubic Symphysis

The pubic symphysis is classified as a symphysis because it has no synovial tissue or fluid, and it contains a fibrocartilaginous lamina or disk (Fig. 29-2). The bone surfaces of the joint are covered with hyaline cartilage, but are kept apart by the presence of the disk.

The following are the supporting ligaments of this joint[23]:

- Superior pubic ligament, a thick fibrous band.
- Inferior arcuate pubic ligament, which attaches to the inferior pubic rami bilaterally and blends with the articular disk.
- Posterior pubic ligament, a membranous structure that blends with the adjacent periosteum.
- Anterior ligament, a very thick band that contains both transverse and oblique fibers.

The pubic symphysis is a common source of groin pain, particularly in athletes (see section "Groin Pain").

Muscles

Lee[12] lists 35 muscles that attach directly to the sacrum or innominate, or both (Table 29-1). A muscle attaching to a bone has the potential for moving that bone, although the degree of potential varies. Rather than producing movement at the SIJ, the muscles around the pelvis are more likely involved directly or indirectly in helping to provide stability to the joint.

TABLE 29-1 Muscles That Attach to the Sacrum, Ilium, or Both
Latissimus dorsi
Erector spinae
Semimembranosus
Semitendinosus
Biceps femoris
Sartorius
Inferior gamellus
Multifidus
Obturator internus
Obturator externus
Piriformis
Tensor fascia lata
External oblique
Internal oblique
Transversus abdominis
Rectus abdominis
Pyramidalis
Gluteus minimus
Gluteus medius
Gluteus maximus
Quadratus femoris
Superior gemellus
Gracilis
Iliacus
Adductor magnus
Rectus femoris
Quadratus lumborum
Pectineus
Psoas minor
Adductor brevis
Adductor longus
Levator ani
Sphincter urethrae
Superficial transverse perineal ischiocavernosus
Coccygeus

Piriformis

This muscle (see Chap. 19) arises from the anterior aspect of the S2, S3, and S4 segments of the sacrum; the capsule of the SIJ; and the sacrotuberous ligament. It exits from the pelvis via the greater sciatic foramen, before attaching to the upper border of the greater trochanter of the femur.

The piriformis primarily functions to produce external rotation and abduction of the femur, but is also thought to function as an internal rotator and abductor of the hip if the hip joint is flexed beyond 90 degrees. It also helps to stabilize the SIJ, although too much tension from it can restrict the motion of this joint.[38] The piriformis has been implicated as the source for a number of conditions in this area, including the following two:

- ***Entrapment neuropathies of the sciatic nerve (piriformis syndrome.***[39–45]***).*** Piriformis syndrome is described in Chapter 5.
- ***Trigger and tender points.***[46]

Transversus Abdominis

For a detailed description of the anatomy of the transversus abdominis (TrA), refer to Chapter 28. Although the TrA does not cross the SIJ directly, it can affect the stiffness of the pelvis through its direct anterior attachments to the ilium, as well as its attachments to the middle layer and the deep laminae of the posterior layer of the thoracodorsal fascia.[47,48]

Multifidus

The anatomy of the multifidus muscle is described in Chapter 28. Some of the deepest fibers of the multifidus attach to the capsules of the zygapophyseal joints[49] and are located close to the centers of rotation for spinal motion. They connect adjacent vertebrae at appropriate angles, and their geometry remains relatively constant through a range of postures, thereby enhancing spinal stability.[50]

Erector Spinae

For a detailed description of the anatomy of the erector spinae, refer to Chapter 28. Through its extending effect on the spine and its substantial sacral attachments, the erector spinae might be thought to promote sacral nutation, although this has not been proven.

Gluteus Maximus

This is one of the strongest muscles in the body (see Chap. 19). It arises from the posterior gluteal line of the innominate, the posterior aspect of the lower lateral sacrum and coccyx, the aponeurosis of erector spinae muscle, the superficial laminae of the posterior thoracodorsal fascia, and the fascia covering the gluteus medius muscle, before attaching to the gluteal tuberosity. In the pelvis, the gluteus maximus blends with the ipsilateral multifidus, through the raphe of the thoracodorsal fascia,[33] and the contralateral latissimus dorsi, through the superficial laminae of the thoracodorsal fascia.[51] Some of its fibers attach to the sacrotuberous ligament. When these fibers contract, tension in the sacrotuberous ligament increases.[52]

Iliacus

This muscle arises from the iliac fossa (see Chap. 19), the iliac crest, the anterior SI ligament, the inferior fibers of the iliolumbar ligament,[53] and the lateral aspect of the sacrum. As it travels distally, its fibers merge with the lateral aspect of the psoas major tendon to form the iliopsoas, which continues onto the lesser trochanter of the femur, sending some fibers to the hip joint capsule as it passes.

Long Head of the Biceps Femoris

The long head of the biceps femoris originates from the ischial tuberosity and sacrotuberous ligament. In addition to functioning as a hip extensor and knee flexor, the long head of the biceps femoris, due to its connections to the sacrotuberous ligament, may also have a proprioceptive role during activities such as gait.

Pelvic Floor Musculature

The term "pelvic floor muscles" primarily refers to the levator ani, a muscle group composed of the pubococcygeus, puborectalis, and iliococcygeus. The levator ani muscles join the coccygeus muscles to complete the pelvic floor. The pelvic floor muscles work in a coordinated manner to increase intra-abdominal pressure, provide rectal support during defecation, inhibit bladder activity, help support the pelvic organs, and assist in lumbopelvic stability.[54]

Levator Ani. The levator ani (Fig. 29-4) originates anteriorly from the pelvic surface of the pubis, posteriorly from the inner surface of the ischial spine, and from the obturator fascia. It inserts into the front and sides of the coccyx, to the sides of the rectum, and into the perineal body. The levator ani forms the floor of the pelvic cavity, functions to constrict the lower end of the rectum and vagina, and can also be activated during forced expiration.

The muscle, which consists of anterior, intermediate, and posterior fibers, is innervated by the muscular branches of the pudendal plexus.

Anterior Fibers. The anterior fibers insert into the perineal body, comprise the levator prostatae or sphincter vaginae, and form a sling around the prostate or vagina.

Intermediate Fibers

- ***Puborectalis.*** The puborectalis (see Fig. 29-4) originates at the pubis and forms a sling around the junction of the rectum and the anal canal. The muscle pulls the anorectal junction anteriorly, assisting the external sphincter in anal closure.
- ***Pubococcygeus.*** The pubococcygeal muscle (see Fig. 29-4) arises from the pubis and its superior ramus, and passes posteriorly to insert into the anococcygeal body between the coccyx and the anal canal. The muscle functions to pull the coccyx forward. It also serves to elevate the pelvic organs and compress the rectum and vagina.

Posterior Fibers. The iliococcygeal muscle (see Fig. 29-4) arises from the arcus tendineus and ischial spine and inserts onto the last segment of the coccyx and the anococcygeal body. The muscle functions to pull the coccyx from side to side and to elevate the rectum.

- ***Levator Plate.*** The pubococcygeal muscle and the iliococcygeal muscle unite posterior to the anorectal junction to form the levator plate, which inserts into the coccyx.
- ***Coccygeus.*** This muscle (Fig. 29-4) arises from the pelvic surface of the ischial spine and sacrospinous ligament and inserts on the coccyx margin and side of the lowest segment of the sacrum. Supplied by the muscular branches of the pudendal plexus, the coccygeus functions to pull forward and support the coccyx. In addition, the coccygeus muscle provides support for the pelvic contents and the SIJ.

Neurology

It remains unclear precisely how the anterior and posterior aspects of the SIJ in humans are innervated, although the anterior portion of the joint likely receives innervation from the posterior rami of the L2 to S2 roots.[55] Contribution from these root levels is highly variable and may differ among the joints of given individuals.[56] Additional innervation to the anterior joint may arise directly from the obturator nerve, superior gluteal nerve, or lumbosacral trunk.[24,57] The posterior portion of the joint is likely innervated by the posterior rami of L4 to S3, with a particular contribution from S1 and S2.[58] An additional autonomic component of the joint's innervation further increases the complexity of its neural supply and likely adds to the variability of pain referral patterns from this area.[57,59]

BIOMECHANICS

Motions at the neighboring lumbar spine predominantly occur around the sagittal plane and comprise flexion and extension, whereas the motions occurring at the hip occur in three planes and include the one motion that the lumbar spine does not tolerate well, i.e., rotation. Thus, the pelvic area must function to transfer the loads generated by body weight and gravity during standing, walking, sitting, and other functional tasks.[60] To date, there is very little agreement, either among or even within disciplines, about how the structures of the pelvis

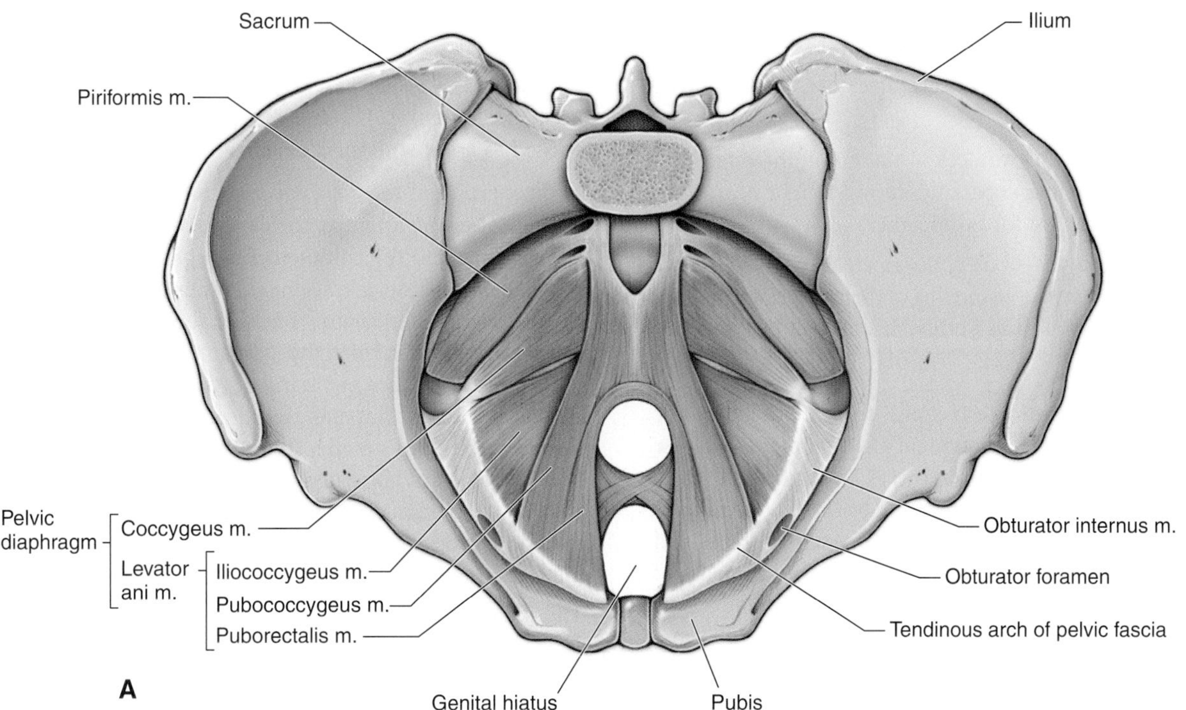

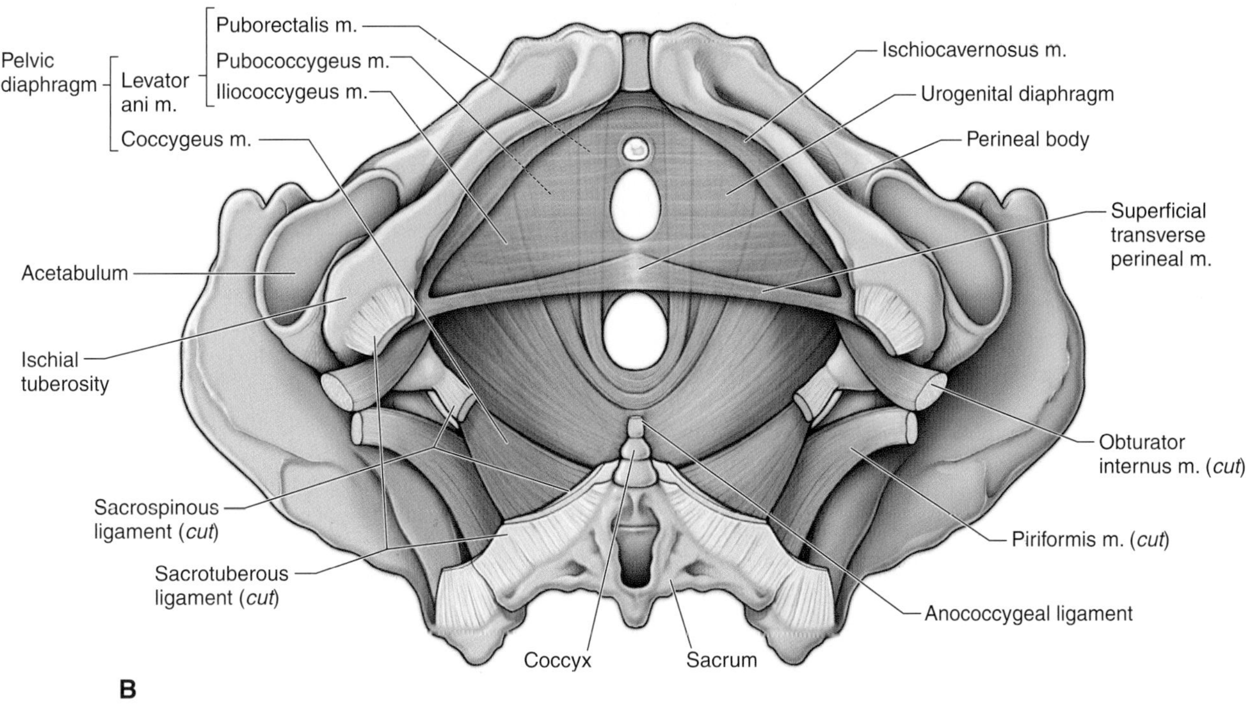

FIGURE 29-4 Pelvic floor muscles. (Reproduced with permission from Morton DA, Foreman KB, Albertine KH: *The Big Picture: Gross Anatomy.* McGraw-Hill, 2011.)

achieve this. For many decades, it was thought that the SIJ was immobile due to the close fitting nature of the articular surfaces. Research has now shown that mobility of the SIJ is not only possible[61–64] but also essential for shock absorption during weight-bearing activities.[65] However, the range of motion in the SIJ is small, less than 4 degrees of rotation and up to 1.6 mm of translation.[62,66] Of interest, is the fact that one study[67] found no difference in available range of motion between the symptomatic and asymptomatic sides.

It is likely that the movement of the pelvis is in the nature of deformations and slight gliding motions around a number of undefined axes, with the joints of the pelvic ring deforming in response to body weight and ground reaction forces. The amplitude of this motion likely varies between individuals. Motion at the SIJ is facilitated by several features, including the following:

- The fibrocartilaginous surfaces of the innominate facets, which are deformable, especially during weight bearing, when the surfaces are forced together.
- The pubic symphysis—if the innominates are moving at the SIJ, then they must also be moving at their anterior junction, which would allow for an immediate, and almost perfect, reciprocal motion.

No manual diagnostic tests have shown reliability for determining how much an individual's SIJ is moving in either symptomatic or asymptomatic subjects. In contrast to Sturesson's study,[67] when Doppler imaging testing has been used to measure stiffness (or laxity) of the SIJ in subjects with and without pelvic pain, it has been shown that asymmetry of stiffness between sides correlated with the symptomatic individual.[68–70] These studies have shown that within the same subject, asymptomatic individuals have similar values for the left and right SIJs, whereas individuals with unilateral posterior pelvic girdle pain had different stiffness values for the left and right sides. Theoretically, when assessing SIJ mobility, a dysfunction at the SIJ can manifest as one of the two types of asymmetries:

- If one of the SIJs is hypermobile, the amplitude of motion is asymmetrically increased and the resistance to motion is decreased on the dysfunctional side.
- If one of the SIJs is hypomobile, the amplitude of motion is asymmetrically reduced and the resistance to motion is increased on the dysfunctional side.

Thus, the current trend is to focus more on the symmetry, or asymmetry, of the motions palpated or observed.

Anatomical research,[12,71,72] initiated to determine the source of low back pain, has demonstrated that alterations in the pattern of muscular contraction and the timing of specific muscle activation differ between healthy subjects and those demonstrating symptoms. Furthermore, studies[73] have shown that the strength and endurance of the trunk muscles is important in determining the muscle capacity of individuals. This research has led to theories about the force- and form-closure mechanisms of joints and how stability is necessary at joints for effective load transfer. Based on this knowledge, functional tests of load transfer through the pelvic girdle have been developed[74–76] together with a number of treatment protocols.[77–79] This approach has three physical components (form closure, force closure, and motor control), and one psychological component (emotions).

In upright positions, the SIJ is subjected to considerable shear force as the mass of the upper body must be transferred to the lower limbs via the ilia.[80,81] The body has two mechanisms to overcome this shear force: one dependent on the shape and structure of the joint surfaces of the SIJs (form closure), which is wedge shaped with a high coefficient of friction, and the other mechanism involving generation of compressive forces across the SIJ via muscle contraction (force closure).[81]

Form Closure. Form closure refers to a state of stability within the pelvic mechanism, with the degree of stability dependent on its anatomy, with no need for extra forces to maintain the stable state of the system.[72] The following anatomic structures are proposed to assist with form closure:

- The congruity of the articular surfaces and the friction coefficient of the articular cartilage. Both the coarseness of the cartilage and the complementary grooves and ridges increase the friction coefficient, and thus contribute to form closure by resisting against horizontal and vertical translations.[24] In infants, the joint surfaces are very planar, but between the ages of 11 and 15 years, the characteristic ridges and humps that make up the mature sacrum begin to form. By the third decade, the superficial layers of the fibrocartilage are fibrillated and crevice formation and erosion has begun. By the fourth and fifth decades, the articular surfaces increase irregularity and coarseness and the wedging is incomplete.[21]
- The integrity of the ligaments.
- The shape of the closely fitting joint surfaces.

According to current research, when the sacrum nutates, or flexes, relative to the innominate (Fig. 29-5), or when the innominate posteriorly rotates relative to the sacrum, the greatest number of ligaments, particularly the interosseous and posterior (dorsal) ligaments, are tightened at the SIJ.[72,82,83] These latter ligaments lie posterior to the joint and approximate the posterior iliac bones when placed under tension.[82] Thus, nutation of the sacrum can be described as the close packed position, or self-locking mechanism, for the SIJ and is, therefore, the most effective position for transferring high loads. This position somewhat conveniently produces a position of lumbar lordosis, which is advocated in many interventions for the lumbar spine.

Just as nutation of the sacrum enhances the self-locking mechanism, counternutation of the sacrum (Fig. 29-6), which occurs during activities such as the end range of forward bending, sacral sitting, long sitting, and hip hyperextension, reduces the self-locking mechanism.[82] This position results in a loss of the lumbar lordosis and an increase in intervertebral disk pressure (see Chap. 28).

Using forward bending at the waist as an example, a combination of anterior and outward rotation of both

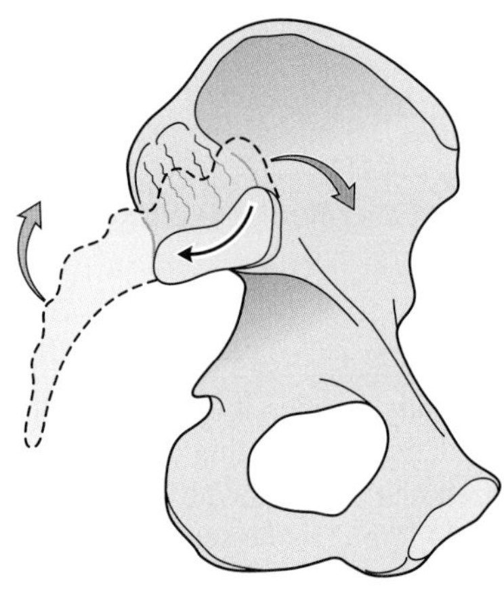

FIGURE 29-5 Sacral nutation.

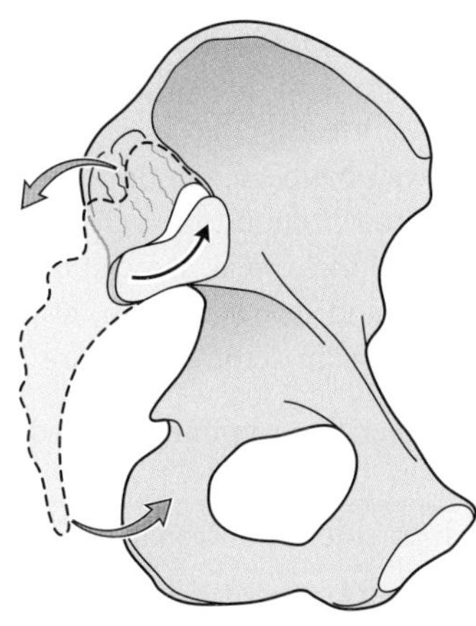

FIGURE 29-6 Sacral counternutation.

innominates results in the approximation and superior motion of both PSISs, while the sacrum nutates (Table 29-2). After approximately 60 degrees of forward bending, the innominates continue to rotate anteriorly, but the sacrum no longer nutates.[12] If the sacrum remains nutated throughout the forward bending, the SIJ remains compressed and stable. However, if the sacrum is forced to counternutate earlier in the range, as in individuals with tight hamstrings, less compression occurs, thereby increasing the reliance on dynamic stabilization provided by muscles and thus making the SIJ more vulnerable to injury.[12]

Force Closure. Force closure requires intrinsic and extrinsic forces to keep the SIJ stable.[72] These dynamic forces involve the neurological and myofascial systems and gravity. Together, these components produce a self-locking mechanism for the SIJ. Optimum force closure requires application of just the right amount of force at just the right time, which in turn requires a motor control system that can predict the timing of the load and prepare the system appropriately. The degree of force closure depends on the capability of an individual's form closure and the various loading conditions (e.g., speed, duration, magnitude, and predictability).[84]

In a kinetic analysis of the pelvic girdle, Vleeming and colleagues[51,82] identified a number of muscles that resist translational forces and which are specifically important to the force-closure mechanism: the erector spinae, gluteus maximus, latissimus dorsi, and biceps femoris (see Chap. 28). Two other muscle groups, an "inner muscle unit" and an "outer muscle unit" also play an important role.[12,73,79] The inner muscle unit consists of the following:

- ***Transversus abdominis (TrA).*** A study by Richardson and colleagues[85] found that contraction of the TrA significantly decreases the laxity of the SIJ , and that this decrease in laxity is larger than that caused by a bracing action using all the lateral abdominal muscles. Theoretically, contraction of the TrA produces a force that approximates the ilia anteriorly.[85]
- ***The muscles of the pelvic floor.*** Hemborg and colleagues[86] have demonstrated that the pelvic floor muscles coactivate with the TrA during lifting tasks.
- ***Multifidus.*** Studies[87–89] have reported that the deep fibers of the multifidus become inhibited and reduced in size in individuals with low back and pelvic girdle pain.

The outer muscle unit consists of four systems: the posterior oblique system (latissimus dorsi, gluteus maximus, and thoracolumbar fascia), the deep longitudinal system (erector spinae, deep lamina of the thoracolumbar fascia, sacrotuberous ligament, and biceps femoris), the anterior oblique system (external and internal oblique, contralateral adductors of the thigh, and the intervening anterior abdominal fascia), and the lateral system (gluteus medius–minimus and contralateral adductors of the thigh). The outer muscle unit is proposed to contribute to the force-closure mechanism in the following manner[12]:

- ***Posterior oblique system.*** The gluteus maximus (see Chap. 19), which blends with the thoracodorsal fascia, and the contralateral latissimus dorsi contribute to force closure of the SIJ posteriorly by approximating the posterior aspects of the innominates. This oblique system is a significant contributor to load transference through the pelvic girdle during the rotational activities of gait.
- ***Deep longitudinal system.*** This system serves to counteract any anterior shear or sacral nutation forces as well as to facilitate compression through the SIJs. As mentioned in the anatomy section, the long head of the biceps femoris muscle controls the degree of nutation via its connections to the sacrotuberous ligaments.[36]
- ***Anterior oblique system.*** The oblique abdominals, acting as phasic muscles, initiate movements[79] and are involved in all movements of the trunk and upper and lower extremities, except when the legs are crossed.[90]
- ***Lateral system.*** The lateral system functions to stabilize the pelvic girdle on the femoral head during gait through a coordinated action.

TABLE 29-2 Lumbar Motions and Sacroiliac Motions

Lumbar Motion	Innominate Motion	Sacrum Motion
Flexion	Anterior rotation	Nutation, then counternutation
Extension	Slight posterior rotation	Nutation
Rotation	*Ipsilateral:* Posterior rotation *Contralateral:* Anterior rotation	Nutates ipsilaterally
Side bending	*Ipsilateral:* Anterior rotation *Contralateral:* Posterior rotation	*Ipsilateral:* Side bends ipsilaterally *Contralateral:* Side bends contralaterally

CLINICAL PEARL

The stability of the SIJ is a factor of the length and strength of the muscle units, neuromuscular control, and the ability of the sacrum to nutate in all positions of threat. Weakness or insufficient recruitment and/or unbalanced muscle function within the lumbar/pelvic/hip region can reduce the force-closure mechanism, which can result in compensatory movement strategies.[91] These compensatory movement strategies and/or patterns of muscle imbalance may produce a sustained counternutation of the sacrum, thereby "unlocking" the mechanism and rendering the SIJ vulnerable to injury. This unlocked position of the pelvis may also increase shear forces at the lumbar spine and abnormal loading of the lumbar disks.

As alluded to earlier, the sacral positions that correspond to poor sacral biomechanics are very similar to those lumbar spine positions that are unfavorable for spinal stability. Conversely, the positions that enhance sacral stability also enhance lumbar spine stability. As a result, there has been much confusion amongst disciplines when determining whether the SIJ or lumbar spine is the cause of the patient's symptoms. For example, consider the prone on elbows position (see Chap. 28), which nutates the sacrum and increases the lordosis of the lumbar spine. If a patient with either a sacral dysfunction or an intervertebral disk herniation is asked to adopt this position, the symptoms would likely decrease.

EXAMINATION

Most investigators agree that no single test can be used to confirm the diagnosis of SIJ dysfunction because of the complexity of the anatomy and biomechanics and its proximity to other symptom-provoking structures.

Diagnostic physical examination tests that are commonly used to determine a diagnosis include[56]

- direct tenderness;
- soft tissue examination for zones of hyperirritability and tissue texture changes;
- evaluation of referral zones;
- associated fascial or musculotendinous restrictions;
- regional abnormal length–strength muscle relationships;
- postural analysis;
- true leg length and functional leg length determination;
- static and dynamic osseous landmark examinations;
- provocative testing, including traditional orthopaedic tests, motion demand tests, and ligament tension tests.

Although traditionally assumed to be reliable and diagnostically useful, none of these tests has ever been validated against an independent criterion standard.[56] As a consequence, controversy exists about which group of tests is the best.

Under the premise that a relationship exists between pelvic asymmetry and low back pain, orthopaedic, osteopathic, and physical therapy tests promote the use of pain provocation (symptom based) tests and static (positional) or dynamic (motion or functional) tests.[1,10,12,38,92–95]

The use of static tests has been questioned as,[96–100] although Cibulka and colleagues[101] found the results from these tests reliable, Levangie[100] found a weak association between standing PSIS asymmetry and low back pain, at least in selected groups. The problems with static testing are

- determining whether the asymmetry noted is normal or abnormal;
- determining which side is abnormal;
- determining whether the asymmetry is too asymmetric or not asymmetric enough. For example, if the right innominate is anteriorly rotated, compared with the left, is it rotated too much, too little, or just the right amount compared with its starting position? Because the starting position is not known, the degree of rotation cannot be assessed.

The dynamic tests do not fair much better. Dreyfuss and colleagues[56] reported 20% positive findings in one or more of the dynamic (motion or functional) tests in a group of asymptomatic people. An example of a dynamic test is the standing flexion test, which has been used frequently to analyze SIJ mobility and to determine the side of the impairment. The test is performed as follows: Each PSIS is palpated with the thumb placed under it caudally. The patient then bends forward at the waist. Provided there is no impairment in the SIJ or the lower lumbar spine, as the patient bends forward, both thumbs should move superiorly (cranially). If one SIJ joint is "blocked," it moves upward further in relation to the other side.[99] Thus far, reliability studies of the standing flexion test show that it lacks sufficient diagnostic power.[99,102,103] This shortfall may be because the compression of the joints caused by the sacral nutation in the early to midranges of forward flexion likely limits movement of the SIJ.[104]

Some studies have reported that pain provocation tests have a good interexaminer reliability,[99,105] but they have not been found reliable by others.[17,102] This is likely because the pain provocation tests have only been found reliable in identifying SIJ dysfunction in certain populations, such as patients with posterior pelvic pain during or following pregnancy.[106]

As several recent studies have found improved interrater reliability in the diagnosis of low back pain when using a combination of physical examination procedures as opposed to a single model approach,[17,56,99,107,108] it would be logical to assume that a similar approach would work with the SIJ.

Ideally, the diagnosis needs to be based on the results from a thorough biomechanical examination that includes an assessment of load transfer, and pain provocation. Patients with failed load transfer through the pelvic girdle often present with inappropriate force closure, in that certain muscles become overactive while others remain inactive, delayed, or asymmetrical in their recruitment.[109] When approaching SIJ dysfunction it is likely more important to determine why there are symptoms, rather than attempting to identify the specific symptom generating structures.

CLINICAL PEARL

The main objective of SIJ assessment is to determine whether the condition appears to primarily involve[84]

- too much compression occurring from stiff, fibrosed joints, or hypertonicity of the global muscles system.
- poor control of loose joints or underactivation of the deep (local) stabilizing muscles system.
- a combination of too much compression and too little control throughout the lumbopelvic–hip complex.

In most cases, an examination of the pelvic joints is of little use if the lumbar spine and the hip joints have not been previously cleared by examination or intervention, because both of these joints can refer pain to this area and may also profoundly affect the function of the SIJ. The algorithm depicted in Fig. 29-7 should serve as a guide.

History

A history of low back pain or leg pain, or both, warrants an examination of the lumbopelvic–hip complex. The most common presenting symptoms in patients with SIJ dysfunction are pain or tenderness over the region of the posterior superior iliac spine.[110–112]

Mechanical pain resulting from SIJ dysfunction may manifest as sacral pain but may also refer pain distally. For example, SIJ problems can refer pain to the iliac fossa, the buttock, the groin, the superior lateral and posterior thigh, and rarely below the knee.[113] In general, SIJ pain is characterized by unilateral pain below the level of L5, in the absence of midline pain, whereas irritation of a spinal nerve may cause radicular symptoms below the knee.[114] Pubic symphysis dysfunction typically results in localized pain, or groin pain, which is aggravated by activities involving the hip adductor or rectus abdominis muscles.[115] However, studies have shown that using evidence of pain referral patterns, or evidence of groin pain are neither sensitive nor specific for SIJ dysfunction.[116]

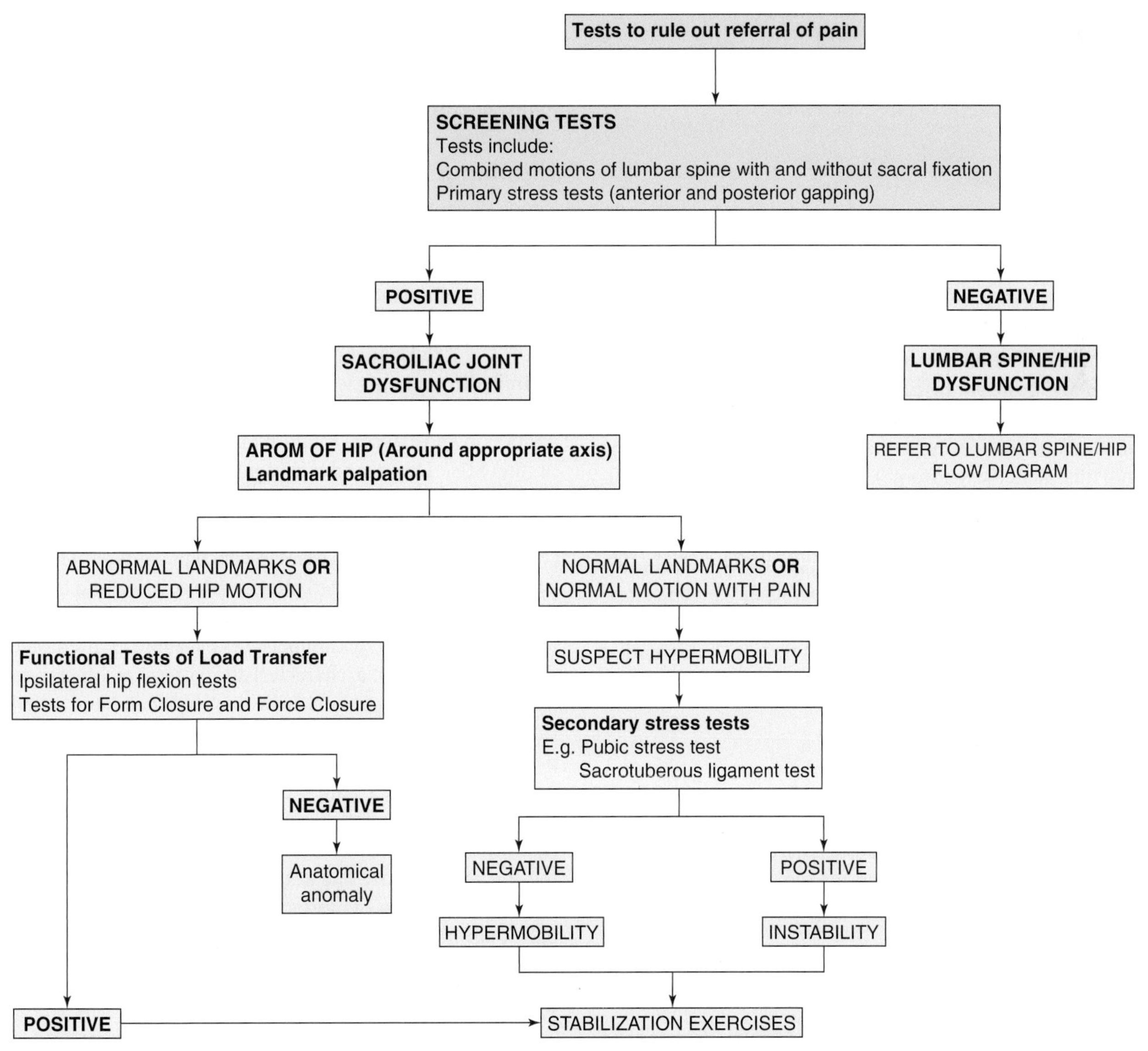

FIGURE 29-7 Decision-making algorithm for the SIJ.

Pain also may be referred to the sacrum from a distant structure, including the contralateral sacrospinalis muscle,[117] the ipsilateral interspinous ligaments of L3 to S2,[118] and the L4 to L5 facet joints.[119] In addition, it is well established that dysfunctional pelvic floor muscles can contribute to the symptoms of interstitial cystitis and the so-called urethral syndrome, which is urgency–frequency with or without chronic pelvic pain.[120–122]

The following findings are likely to be present with a SIJ dysfunction:[13,56,123,124]

- A history of sharp pain that occurred with a particular activity and that awakens the patient from sleep upon turning in bed.
- Pain with walking, ascending or descending stairs, or hopping or standing on the involved leg.
- Pain with forward bending of the trunk and pain with standing hip flexion.
- Pain with transitional movements such as rising to stand from a sitting position or getting in and out of the car.
- Pain with a straight leg raise at, or near, the end of range (occasionally early in the range when hyperacute).
- Pain and sometimes limitation on extension and ipsilateral side bending of the trunk.
- Pain that is worsened with long periods of sitting or standing if the lumbar lordosis is not maintained.

Systems Review

Given the number of visceral organs in the vicinity of the SIJ, the clinician must complete a thorough systems review to rule out a visceral source for the symptoms. A Cyriax scanning examination (see Chap. 4) should be performed on any patient who presents with an insidious onset of pelvic pain. The scanning examination, which includes the primary stress tests (anterior and posterior distraction), can be used to help detect sacroiliitis resulting from microtraumatic arthritis, macrotraumatic arthritis, or systemic arthritis (e.g., ankylosing spondylitis, Reiter's syndrome), or the more serious pathologies grouped under the sign of the buttock (see Chap. 19). Primary breast, lung, and prostate cancers are among the most common cancers to metastasize to the axial skeleton, including the pelvic ring.[125] A further source of sacral pain can be a stress fracture of the sacrum, which can be associated with a wide range of extrinsic and intrinsic risk factors (see "Intervention Strategies"), and an equally wide range of symptoms and signs.[126]

Tests and Measures

As previously mentioned, in order to rule in or rule out SIJ dysfunction, a thorough musculoskeletal examination of the low back, the pelvis, the hips, and the remainder of the lower extremities, including a full neurologic evaluation must be performed.

Observation

The observation should begin with an overall assessment of posture to check for the presence of asymmetry. The clinician should observe the degree of tilt at the pelvis. The question of cause and effect should be raised. An anterior pelvic tilt causes an increase in the lumbar lordosis and thoracic kyphosis. The anterior pelvic tilt results in a stretching of the abdominals and the sacrotuberous, SI, and sacrospinous ligaments, and an adaptive shortening of the hip flexors, the hamstrings, and the erector spinae. In contrast, a posterior pelvic tilt results in lengthening of the hip flexors, the hamstrings, and the erector spinae, and adaptive shortening of the abdominals and the gluteals.

A lateral pelvic tilt, in which one iliac crest is higher than the other, may be caused by scoliosis with ipsilateral lumbar convexity, a leg length discrepancy, or shortening of the contralateral quadratus lumborum. This position results in adaptive shortening of the ipsilateral hip abductors and contralateral hip adductors, and weakness of the contralateral hip abductors.

There appears to be a strong correlation between the position of the pelvis and the forward head.[127] If the pelvic landmarks are asymmetric and the patient has a forward head, the clinician should attempt to correct the forward head. If the attempted correction of the forward head worsens the pelvic asymmetry and increases the symptoms, the intervention should be aimed at correcting the asymmetry. If the attempted correction of the forward head improves the pelvic asymmetry and the symptoms, the subsequent intervention should be aimed at correcting the forward head.[128]

Hip Range of Motion

Range of motion of the hip, including internal and external rotation, is performed to help rule out pain referred from the hip joint. Although a unilateral limitation of hip motion, in which one of the motions is unequal between the left and right sides, has been observed in patients with disorders of the SIJ,[64,129–131] the evidence to demonstrate whether hip motion is limited in patients with signs of SIJ dysfunction is inconclusive. LaBan and colleagues[115] noted asymmetry in hip abduction and external rotation in patients with inflammation of the SIJs. Dunn and colleagues[132] reported limited hip mobility in patients with infection of the SIJ; however, no mention was made as to which movements were limited.

Others have described cases in which patients with low back pain had unilateral, limited internal hip rotation and excessive external hip rotation, and also exhibited signs of SIJ dysfunction. A recent study by Cibulka and colleagues[129] attempted to determine whether a characteristic pattern of hip range of motion existed in patients with low back pain, and whether those classified as having SIJ dysfunction have a different pattern of hip range of motion compared with those with unspecified low back pain. The study found that patients with low back pain, who had signs suggesting SIJ regional pain, had significantly more hip external than internal rotation range of motion on one side. The authors concluded that identifying unilateral hip range of motion asymmetry in patients with low back pain may help in diagnosing SIJ regional pain.[129]

Landmark Palpation

The palpation of landmarks can be used to locate areas of tenderness rather than for detecting pelvic asymmetry, because as pelvic landmark asymmetry is probably the norm, "positive" findings are likely to be misleading.[100] The various landmarks of the pelvis are palpated with the patient positioned standing, sitting, and lying (see Figs. 29-8 and 29-9).

CLINICAL PEARL

An altered positional relationship within the pelvic girdle should only be considered positive if a mobility restriction of the SIJ or the pubic symphysis, or both, is also found.

The following landmarks and structures are palpated with the patient standing:

- ***Iliac crest.*** The iliac crests on both sides are located using the medial aspects of the index fingers. The crest heights should be level.
- ***Anterior superior iliac spine (ASIS).*** These structures are located anteriorly to the iliac crests. Tenderness of the ASIS may indicate a so-called hip pointer injury or injury to the inguinal ligament. An inferior ASIS relative to the other side may indicate a rotated innominate.[8] According to osteopathic doctrine, if the innominate is anteriorly rotated in the supine position, the leg will be longer on that side, but if posteriorly rotated, the leg will be shorter.[8] However, a study by Levangie[100] found that pelvic asymmetry was not positively associated with low back pain in any way that seemed clinically meaningful. It has been suggested to assess the ASIS in sitting versus standing, but there are no reliable studies to recommend this method.
- ***Posterior superior iliac spine (PSIS).*** These structures are located posteriorly to the iliac crests and approximately 2–3 cm beneath the dimples of the lumbar spine and level with the S2 spinous process. Slightly medially and distal to the PSIS are the SIJs. To assess the levels of the PSIS relative to the opposite side, the clinician hooks the thumbs under both PSIS. A superior PSIS relative to the other side may indicate a rotated innominate.[8] A study by Levangie[100] found that although pelvic asymmetry was not positively associated with low back pain in any way that seemed clinically meaningful, asymmetry of PSIS landmarks showed some evidence of a weak positive association with low back pain. This would indicate that the test does not qualify as a screening tool. PSIS asymmetry can also be assessed similarly in sitting, but the findings from Levangie[100] indicate that this test provides little value during the examination and does not qualify as a screening tool.
- ***Pubic symphysis and pubic tubercles.*** The pubic tubercles are lateral to the pubic symphysis.

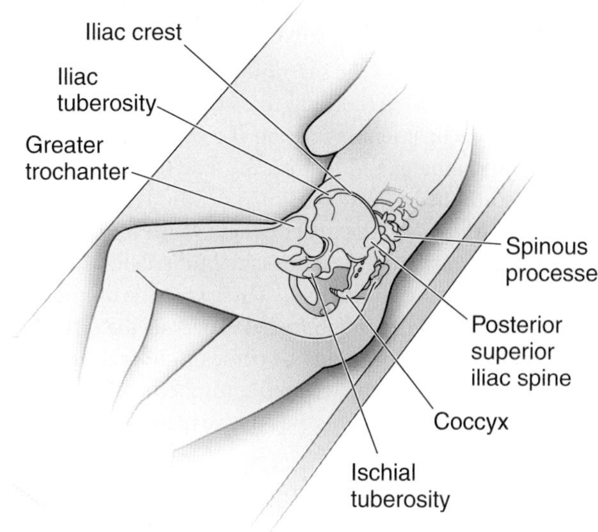

FIGURE 29-9 Bony landmarks.

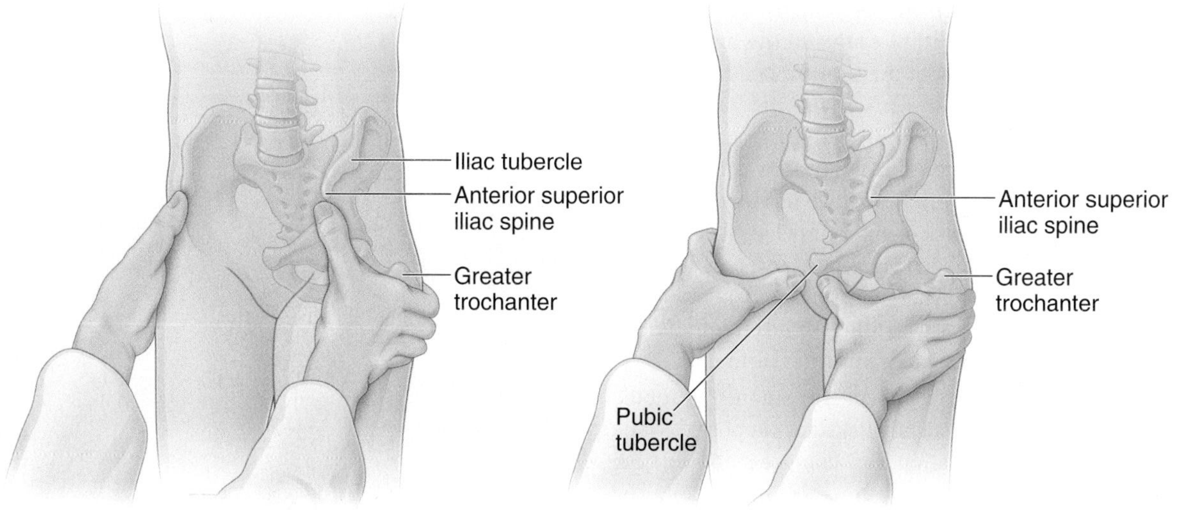

FIGURE 29-8 Palpation of the hip and pelvis.

- ***Posterior (dorsal) ligament.*** This strong ligament is situated in a deep depression between the sacrum and ilium.
- ***Ischial tuberosity and the sacrotuberous ligament (medial to the tuberosity).*** According to osteopathic doctrine, the sacrotuberous ligament is firm on the side of an anteriorly rotated innominate, and taut on the side of a posteriorly rotated innominate.[8] The patient is positioned prone, and the clinician stands at the patient's side. With the heel of the hands, the clinician locates the ischial tuberosities through the soft tissue at the gluteal folds. Then, with the thumbs, the clinician palpates the inferomedial aspect of the ischial tuberosities. From this point, the clinician slides the thumbs superolaterally and palpates the sacrotuberous ligament. The clinician then compares the relative tension between the left and right sides.
- ***Sacral sulcus (sacral base).*** The sacral sulcus (dimple) is located over the sacral base. From the PSIS, the clinician moves in a thumb width and then up a thumb width.
- ***Inferior lateral angle (ILA).*** These structures are level with the prominent part of the tailbone.
- ***L5 segment.*** The clinician palpates medially along the iliac crest. L5 is usually level with the point at which the palpating finger begins to descend on the crest. The L5–S1 zygapophyseal joints are located halfway between the L5 spinous process and the ipsilateral PSIS.
- ***Lumbosacral angle.*** An increased or decreased lumbosacral angle (the angle the sacrum makes with the lumbar spine) on one side may indicate a rotated innominate. Although very difficult to measure without radiographs, the normal lumbosacral angle is approximately 140 degrees from the vertical.
- ***S2 segment.*** S2 is normally level with the PSIS.

Functional Tests of Load Transfer Through the Pelvis

Forward Bending. This test *assesses* the ability of the pelvis to tolerate both vertical and horizontal shear forces, and its ability to control forward sagittal rotation during forward bending of the trunk. When the leg lengths are equal, the sacrum should nutate bilaterally relative to the innominates and remain nutated throughout the forward bending motion as the pelvic girdle flexes symmetrically at the hip joints.[104] The patient is positioned in standing and is asked to bend forward at the waist while the clinician observes the lumbo-pelvic hip rhythm (Fig. 29-10). A positive test for inadequate load transfer is if there is a lack of anterior pelvic tilt, excessive flexion of the thoracolumbar spine, and any twisting that occurs in the pelvic girdle.[84] Although asymmetry of motion of the innominate during forward bending is a positive finding, it is not indicative of any specific dysfunction of the SIJ.

Test for Form Closure. The patient is positioned in supine with the hips and the knees slightly flexed or supported over a bolster. Since muscle activation can compress the SIJ, the patient is instructed to completely relax during the test. The following description is for a test of the right side of the sacrum. With the right hand, the clinician grasps the anterior aspect of

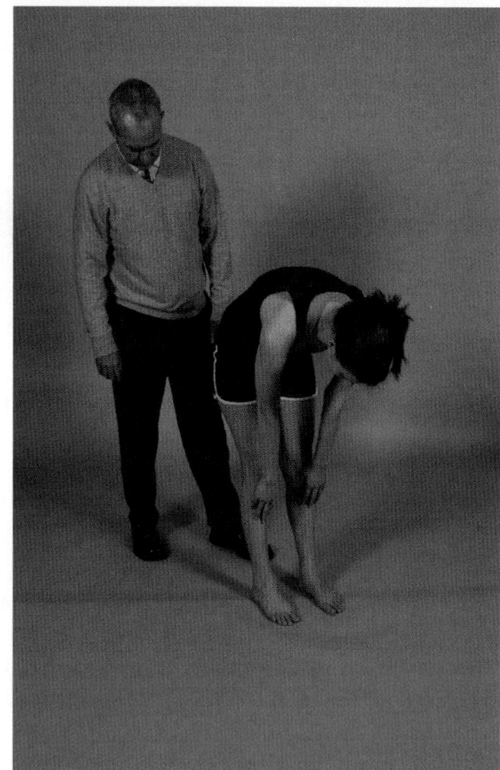

FIGURE 29-10 Forward bending test.

the patient's right innominate and ASIS (Fig. 29-11). The clinician then slides his or her left hand under the left side of the patient's lumbar spine and palpates the left sacral sulcus, just medial to the PSIS with the index and long finger to monitor translation between the sacrum and the innominate. From this position, the clinician stabilizes the left sacral base and sulcus with the left hand, and pushes the right innominate down toward the bed using the right hand, in a variety of directions to determine the plane of the SIJ. Slight motion should be felt before a ligamentous end-feel is reached. Once the plane of motion is determined, the stiffness for A-P translation of the SIJ is compared bilaterally. There should be no pain or asymmetry. A loss of motion or pain

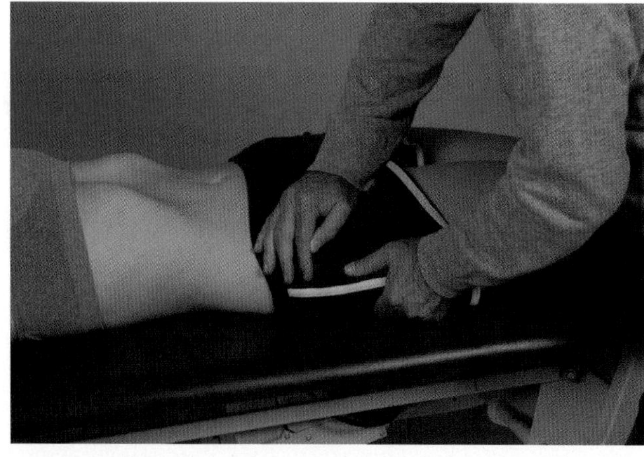

FIGURE 29-11 Grasping the right ASIS and right innominate.

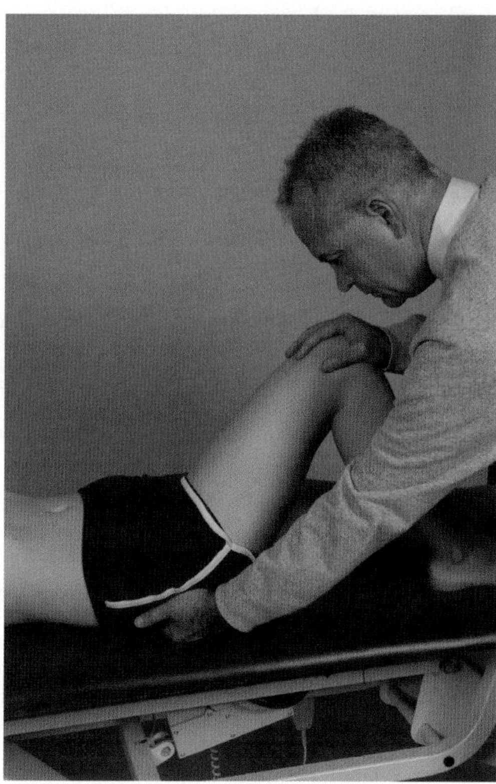

FIGURE 29-12 Form-closure test—inferior–superior.

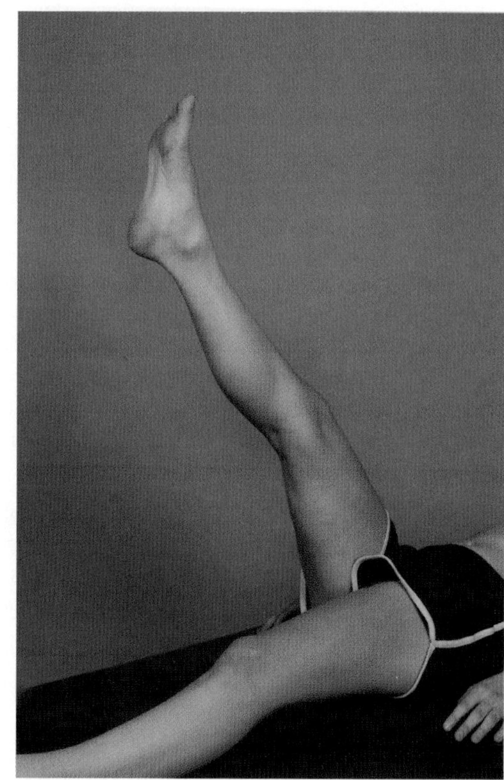

FIGURE 29-13 Asymmetrical Straight Leg Raise (ASLR).

reproduction compared with the contralateral side indicates dysfunction. To test the ability of the pelvic girdle to resist vertical translation, a superoinferior force is applied to the innominate through the distal end of the femur or through the ischial tuberosity (Fig. 29-12). Again, slight motion should be felt (although a little more than with the previous test) before a solid ligamentous end-feel is reached. The stiffness for superoinferior translation of the SIJ is compared bilaterally. There should be no pain or asymmetry. A loss of motion or pain reproduction compared with the contralateral side indicates dysfunction.

Tests for Force Closure and Motor Control. The active straight leg raise (ASLR) test and the reverse ASLR have been recommended as tests to help identify nonoptimal stabilization of the pelvic girdle and the ability to transfer loads between the lumbosacral spine and legs.

- ***The Active Straight Leg Raise (ASLR).*** The ASLR demonstrates the patient's ability to transfer load to the pelvis in the supine line position and has been validated for reliability, sensitivity, and specificity of pelvic girdle pain after pregnancy.[75,76,133] It can also be used to identify non-optimal stabilization strategies for load transfer through the pelvis.[84] The test is performed with the patient in supine with both legs straight. The patient is instructed to lift one leg off the table without bending the knee and the clinician observes the strategy used (Fig. 29-13). The leg should flex at the hip joint and the pelvis should not rotate, side bend, flex, or extend relative to the lumbar spine. The ribcage should not draw in excessively (over activation of the external oblique muscles), nor should the lower ribs flare out excessively (over activation of the internal oblique muscles), or the abdomen bulge (Valsalva). If the patient is unable to perform this maneuver correctly, or the maneuver causes pain, the test is repeated with the clinician applying a compression force through the pelvis (anterior then posterior) directed at the SIJs (form closure) (Fig. 29-14). If the patient is then able to perform the ASLR, the test is considered positive. If the application of

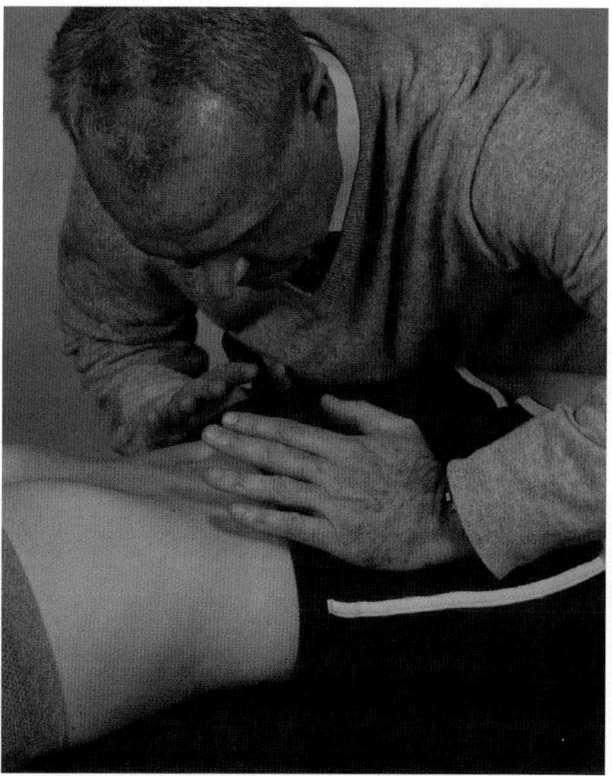

FIGURE 29-14 Asymmetrical Straight Leg Raise (ASLR)—2nd part.

anterior compression enabled the patient to perform the ASLR, an exercise program emphasizing the isolation, timing, and strength of the TrA is recommended. If the application of posterior compression enabled the patient to perform the ASLR, an exercise program emphasizing the isolation, timing, and strength of the multifidus is recommended. Slight modifications to the test can be used to help confirm the diagnosis.

- One knee is flexed, and the patient is asked to perform a straight leg raise with the other leg. Flexing the contralateral knee to the straight leg raise has the effect of relaxing the lumbar spine while maintaining the counternutation on the ipsilateral side. If this maneuver decreases the pain, a muscle imbalance could be present (quadratus lumborum, multifidus, etc.).
- The patient is asked to lift one shoulder off the bed against manual resistance from the clinician, while performing the straight leg raise on the contralateral side. This maneuver tests the ability of the anterior oblique system (force closure).

Assessment findings that indicate excessive compression include[84]

- reduced movement on active mobility tests;
- an ASLR test result that does not change all that worsens with compression;
- palpable hypertonicity in specific muscles and/or nonoptimum patterns of muscle recruitment during movement or in response to verbal cueing.

Assessment findings that indicate poor motion control include[84]

- an ASLR test result that improves with compression
- nonoptimum pattern of muscle recruitment in response to verbal cueing
- loss of joint position during functional load transfer tests.
- ***The reverse ASLR.*** This test is performed with the patient in prone with the patient performing active hip extension with the leg straight under three progressive conditions:
  - The patient performs hip extension with the leg straight (Fig. 29-15)

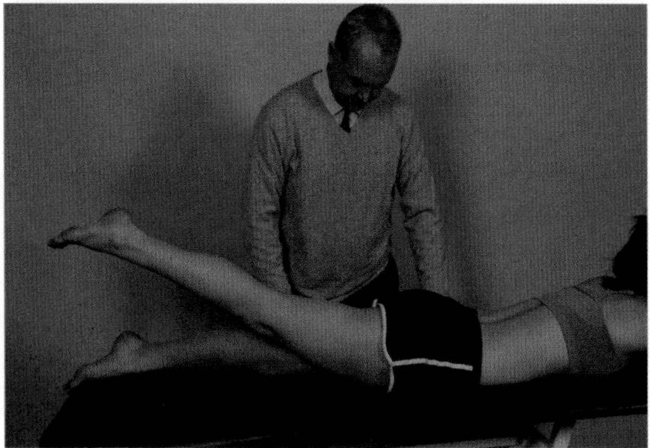

FIGURE 29-15 Reverse ASLR.

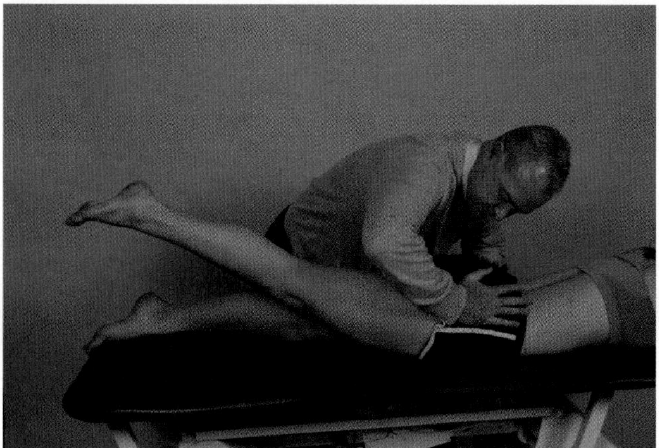

FIGURE 29-16 Reverse ASLR—2nd part.

  - The patient performs hip extension with the leg straight with the clinician applying manual compression to the innominate bones (form closure) (Fig. 29-16).
  - The patient performs hip extension with the leg straight with the clinician resisting extension of the contralateral medially rotated upper extremity (force closure).

No diagnostic accuracy studies have been performed to determine the sensitivity and specificity of this test.

CLINICAL PEARL

Theoretically, with the ASLR and the reverse ASLR tests, if function improves when force-closure stabilization is used, exercise will likely benefit the patient. If during these tests, form closure seems to provide benefit, prescription of an SI belt is recommended.

Special Tests

Sacroiliac Joint Stress Tests. A positive stress test is one that reproduces unilateral or bilateral SI pain, either anteriorly or posteriorly.[134] A positive stress test indicates the presence of inflammation, but does not give any information as to the cause. If either test is positive in a patient who has recently fallen, there is a possibility that a fracture of the pelvis exists.[135] Some of the stress tests are considered to have fair reliability and moderate specificity.

Anterior Sacroiliac Joint Stress Test. The anterior stress test, also called the *gapping test,* is performed with the patient supine. The clinician stands to one side of the patient and, crossing the arms, places the palm of the hands on the patient's anterior superior iliac spines (Fig. 29-17). The crossing of the arms ensures that the applied force is in a lateral direction, thereby gapping the anterior aspect of the SIJ. The stress is maintained for 30 seconds once an end-feel is obtained. The procedure stresses the anterior (ventral) ligament and compresses the posterior aspect of the joint. A positive test is one in which the patient's groin or SIJ pain is reproduced anteriorly, posteriorly, unilaterally, or bilaterally.

The anterior gapping test and its posterior counterpart (see next section) are believed to be sensitive for severe arthritis or anterior (ventral) ligament tears of the SIJ,[134] although they have been shown to be poorly reproducible.[99]

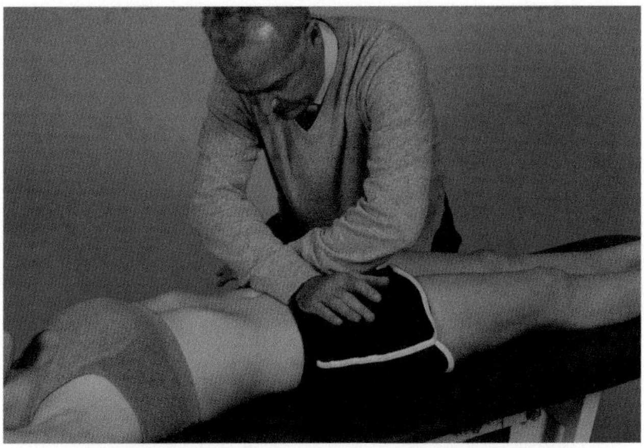

FIGURE 29-17 Anterior Sacroiliac Joint Stress Test.

Posterior Sacroiliac Joint Stress Test. The posterior stress test, also called the *compression test,* is performed with the patient in the supine or sidelying position. The clinician, standing behind the patient, applies a medial force to both innominates, using both hands (Fig. 29-18). The stress is maintained for 30 seconds once an end-feel is obtained. The procedure creates a medial force that tends to gap the posterior aspect of the SIJ, while compressing its anterior aspect. The reproduction of pain over one or both of the SIJs is considered a positive test. The test also indirectly assesses the ability of the sacrum to counternutate.

The posterior (dorsal) SI ligament, which is accessible just below the posterior inferior iliac spine, should be palpated for tenderness.[32]

Thigh Thrust (Sacrotuberous stress test, 4 P test, POSH test, Oostagard test). This maneuver should only be performed on a normal hip joint. The patient is positioned in supine and the resting symptoms are assessed. The clinician stands on the painful side. The clinician flexes the hip on the painful side to 90 degrees and neutral adduction, and then places his or her hand under the sacrum to form a stable base for the sacrum. The clinician then applies a downward pressure through the femur to force a posterior translation of the innominate and the patient's symptoms are assessed (Fig. 29-19). A positive test is reproduction of the patient's symptoms (posterior to the hip or near the SIJ) on the side of the loaded femur. This is one of the few SI tests that exhibits a fair sensitivity. In a study by Broadhurst and Bond,[136] the test was found to have a sensitivity of 80% and a specificity of 100%.

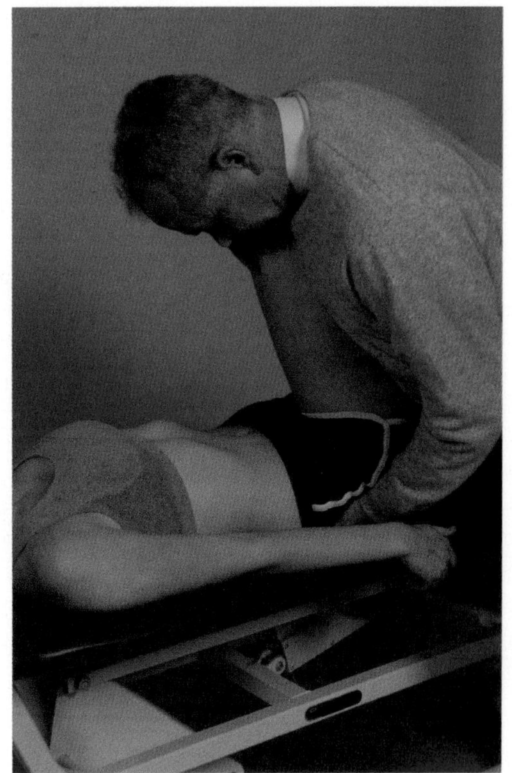

FIGURE 29-19 Thigh Thrust (Sacrotuberous stress test, 4 P test, POSH test, Oostagard test).

Mennell's Test. The patient is positioned in supine and the clinician positions the leg to be tested into 30 degrees of abduction and some flexion of the hip joint (Fig. 29-20) and asks the patient to hold his or her leg in this position. The clinician pushes the lower leg into, and then away from, the pelvis in a sagittal motion (extension then flexion). A positive test is reproduction of the patient's SIJ pain. Albert and colleagues[137] found this test to have a sensitivity of 54–70% and a specificity of 100%.

Resisted Hip Abduction. The patient is positioned in side lying and the clinician positions the uppermost leg into full

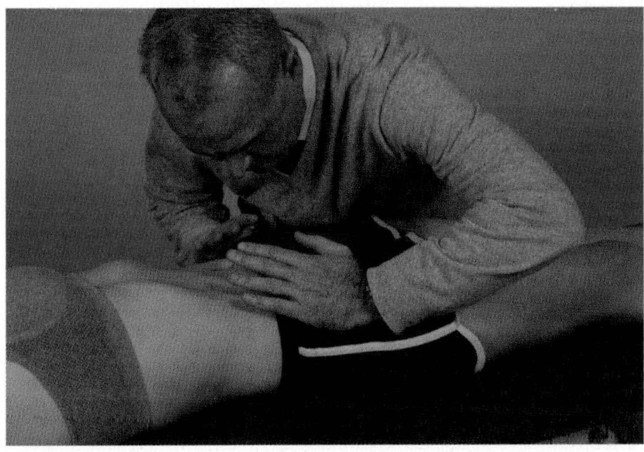

FIGURE 29-18 Posterior Sacroiliac Joint Stress Test.

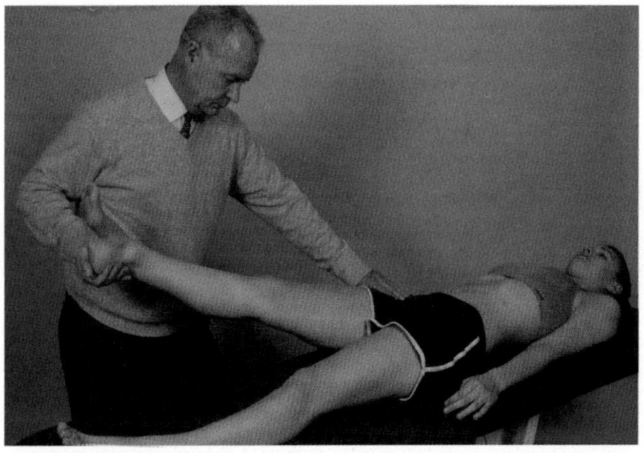

FIGURE 29-20 Mennell's Test.

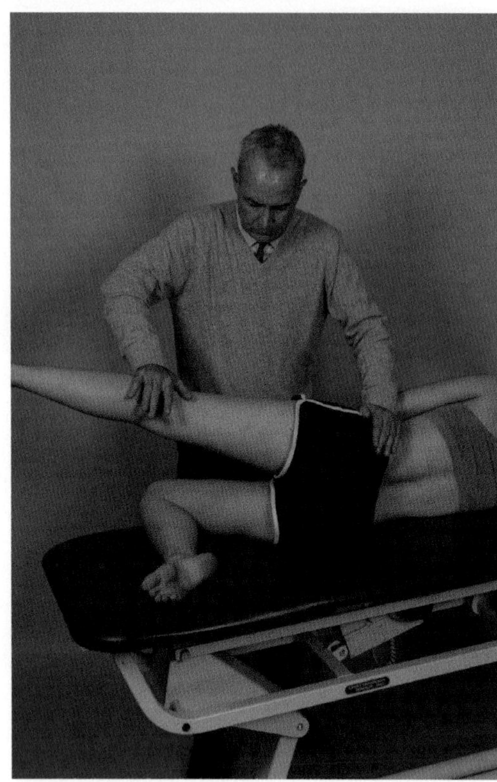

FIGURE 29-21 Resisted Hip Abduction.

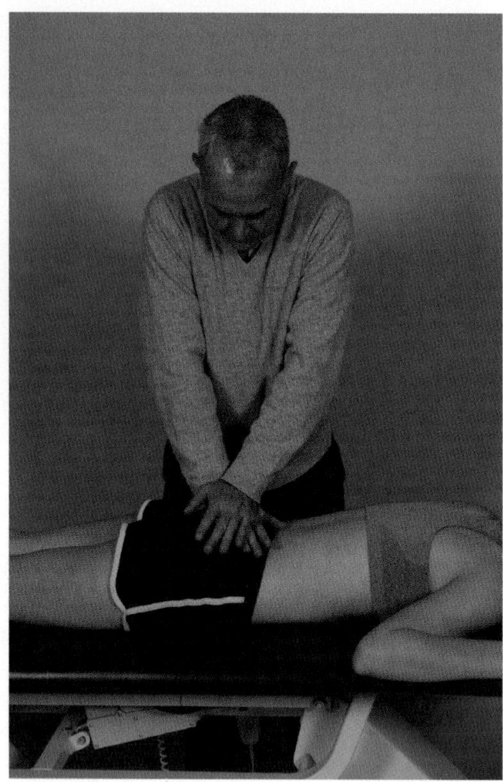

FIGURE 29-22 Sacral Thrust Test.

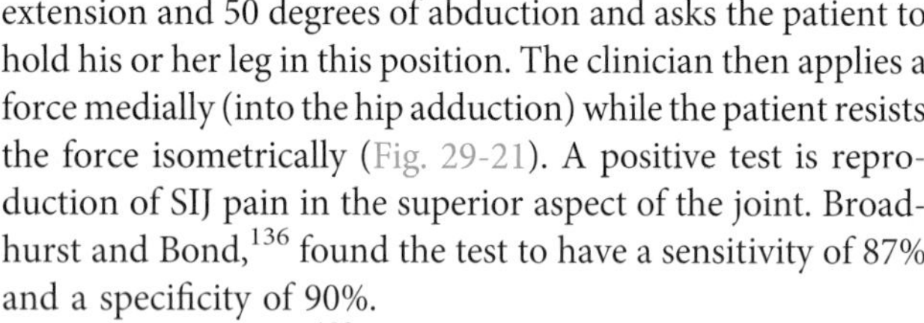

extension and 50 degrees of abduction and asks the patient to hold his or her leg in this position. The clinician then applies a force medially (into the hip adduction) while the patient resists the force isometrically (Fig. 29-21). A positive test is reproduction of SIJ pain in the superior aspect of the joint. Broadhurst and Bond,[136] found the test to have a sensitivity of 87% and a specificity of 90%.

Pubic Stress Tests.[138] The patient is positioned supine and the clinician stands at the patient's side. With the heel of one hand, the clinician palpates the superior aspect of the superior ramus of one pubic bone, and with the heel of the other hand, palpates the inferior aspect of the superior ramus of the opposite pubic bone. Fixing one pubic bone, the clinician applies a slow, steady, inferosuperior force to the other bone and, noting the quantity and end-feel of motion, as well as the reproduction of any symptoms, the clinician then switches hands and repeats the test so that both sides are stressed superiorly and inferiorly. Albert and colleagues[137] found this test to have a sensitivity of 81% and a specificity of 99% (LR+ 4.68; LR− 0.19). This test appears useful in the diagnosis of symphysiolysis.

CLINICAL PEARL

In some cases of trauma, or occasionally with child bearing, the pubis can become destabilized. This is a very severe and painful impairment, and one that is not easily missed. The pain is local to the pubic area, the patient is quite disabled with all movements, and weight-bearing postures are very painful. The impairment generally shows up on one-legged weight-bearing radiographs and often requires surgical intervention to stabilize the symphysis.

Sacral Thrust Test. The patient is positioned prone on a firm surface, and the clinician stands at the patient's side. With one hand, the clinician palpates the inferior aspect of the sacrum in the midline (second or third spinous process of the sacrum) and reinforces this hand with the other. The clinician then applies an anterior force at S3 (Fig. 29-22) vigorously and repeatedly (up to six thrusts), and the reproduction of symptoms is noted. The test is considered positive if pain is reproduced over the SIJs or the posterior (dorsal) SI ligament, or both.[139] In a study by Laslett and colleagues,[105] this test was found to have a sensitivity of 63% and a specificity of 75% (LR+ 2.5; LR− 0.49) suggesting that the test provides only marginal diagnostic value when used in isolation.

Fortin Finger Test. The patient completes a pain diagram and is then instructed to point to the region of pain using only one finger. The clinician reviews the area of pain and pain diagram for consistency and then asks the patient to repeat the procedure of pointing to his or her pain. A positive test for localization of SIJ pain has three criteria:

- The patient can localize the pain with one finger.
- The area pointed to is within 1 cm of, and immediately inferomedial to, the posterior superior iliac spine.
- The patient consistently points to the same area over at least two trials.

In a study by Fortin and Falco,[112] 16 subjects were chosen from 54 consecutive patients by using the Fortin finger test. All 16 patients subsequently had provocation-positive joint injections validating SIJ abnormalities (sensitivity of 100%). Another study by Dreyfuss and colleagues[56] found this test to have a sensitivity of 76% and a specificity of 47% (LR+ .09; LR− 1.3).

FABER or Patrick's Test. The FABER (flexion, abduction, external rotation) test is a screening test for hip (see Chap. 19), lumbar, or SIJ dysfunction, or an iliopsoas spasm.

The patient is positioned in supine and resting symptoms are assessed. The clinician places the foot of the test leg on top of the knee of the opposite leg (placing the sole of the test leg foot against the medial aspect of the opposite thigh may be more comfortable for the patient with knee pathology). The clinician then slowly lowers the test leg into abduction, in the direction toward the examining table. The clinician then provides a gentle downward pressure on both the knee of the painful side and the ASIS of the non-painful side. A positive test results in pain and/or loss of motion as compared with the uninvolved side. Having the patient demonstrate where the pain is with this test may assist with the interpretation of this test. For SI pain, the chief complaint is typically posterior. In the various studies that have assessed the sensitivity and specificity of this test, there are a wide range of values which is likely reflective of the variety of patients used in each study and the bias that results.

Seated Flexion Test (Piedallus Sign). The test is purported by osteopaths to help distinguish between a SI lesion and an iliosacral lesion when compared with the results of the standing flexion test.[5–7] The patient sits on a hard surface with the legs over the end of the table and feet supported.[8] In this position, innominate motion is severely abbreviated, because sitting places the innominates near the end of their extension range. The test is performed as follows. Each PSIS is palpated with the thumb placed under it inferiorly (caudally). The patient then bends forward at the waist (Fig. 29-23). Provided there is no impairment in the SIJ or the lower lumbar spine, as the patient bends forward, both thumbs should move superiorly (cranially). If the joint is blocked, it moves superiorly further in relation to the other side.[99] However, like other palpatory tests, this examination has been shown to lack reliability, have poor sensitivity, and have low specificity as a result a low false positive rate.[96,137,140] In contrast, Levangie[141] determined the sensitivity to be 9%, the specificity to be 93%, the positive predictive value to be 78%, and the negative predictive value to be 28%. Clearly there is need for further study. A similar test, referred to as the sitting bend over test or sitting forward flexion test, is performed in the same manner except the patient is seated on a soft surface. However, this test has demonstrated poor sensitivity, poor reliability, and, therefore, has very poor diagnostic value.[140,141]

Long Sit Test. According to osteopath doctrine, the long sit test is used to indicate the direction of the rotation that the innominate has adopted and is used in conjunction with the standing flexion test. After noting the side of the impairment obtained from the standing flexion test, the clinician observes whether the medial malleolus on that side moves distally or proximally during the long sit test. Rotation about a coronal axis, whose resultant movement leads to an increase in the length of a limb, is defined as extension. If it shortens the length of the limb, it is defined as flexion. Thus, if the apparent shorter leg becomes longer during the test, the innominate on that side is purportedly held in a posteriorly rotated malposition, whereas if the apparent longer leg becomes shorter during the test, the innominate on that side is allegedly held in an anteriorly rotated malposition.

The problems with this test involve the maneuver itself. To ask patients who are experiencing some degree of discomfort to raise themselves off the bed from a supine position into a long sit position without any twisting or use of the arms is unnecessarily painful. In addition, for the successful completion of the maneuver, the patient needs a minimum of 90 degrees of hip flexion and adequate hamstring length. Perhaps not surprisingly, the test has demonstrated poor reliability, questionable validity, and, therefore, may not yield useful results.[137,142]

Prone Knee Bending (Nachlas) Test. The patient is positioned in prone and the clinician, while stabilizing the pelvis, flexes the knee so that the heel is brought toward the buttocks (Fig. 29-24). If pain is felt in the front of the thigh before full range is reached, the problem is in the rectus femoris muscle; if

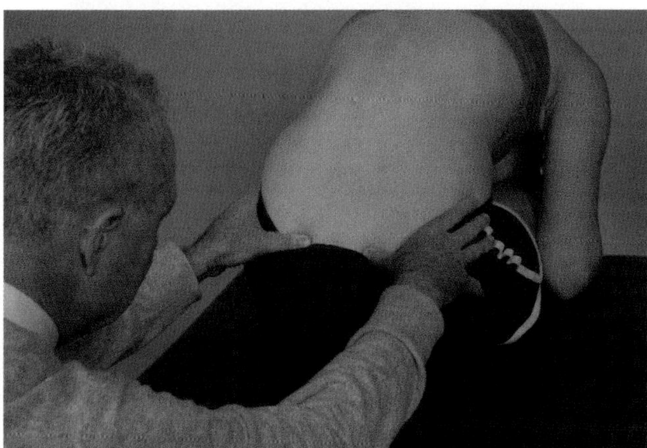

FIGURE 29-23 Seated Flexion Test (Piedallus Sign).

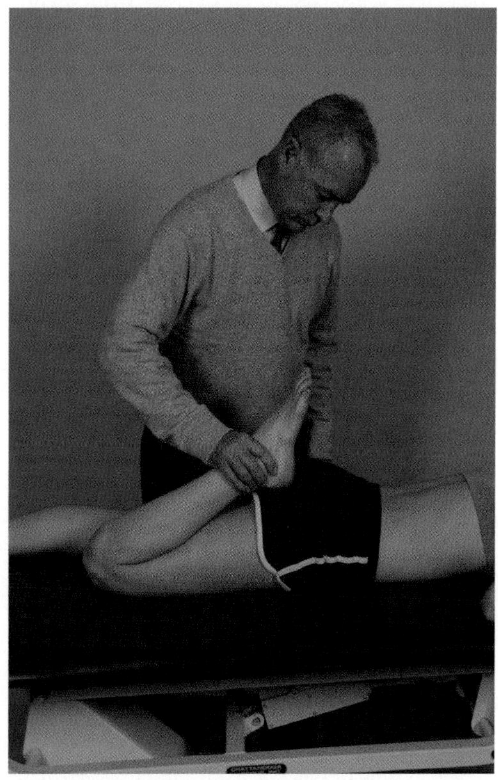

FIGURE 29-24 Prone knee bending (Nachlas) test.

the pain is in the lumbar spine, the problem is in the lumbar spine (usually the L3 nerve root). If the problem is a hypomobile SIJ, the ipsilateral pelvic rim (palpated at the ASIS) will be felt to rotate forward.[143] Leboeuf[144] found this test to have a specificity of 83% and a sensitivity of 44% (LR+ 2.59; LR− 0.67). Riddle and colleagues[142] found this test to have an interrater reliability of 0.26.

CLINICAL PEARL

Cibulka[145] and colleagues examined 219 patients with and without low back and SIJ-mediated pain to examine the sensitivity, the specificity, and the positive and negative predictive values of four commonly used SIJ tests: the standing flexion test, PSIS palpation while seated, the long sitting test, and the prone knee flexion test. SIJ dysfunction was considered positive if at least three of the four tests were positive. The combination of these tests yielded a sensitivity of 0.82, a specificity of 0.88, a positive predictive value of 0.86, and a negative addictive value of 0.84. However, because the individual test results were not documented, no conclusion can be made about isolated validity.

Leg Length Tests. These are usually performed as part of the bony landmark examination. Theoretically, posterior rotation of the innominate on the sacrum results in a decrease in leg length, as does an anterior rotation of the innominate on the contralateral side.[146] Although not exact measurements of leg length, these tests can highlight any significant asymmetries.

Prone Test. Chiropractors assess leg length with the patient prone. The comparative lengths of the legs are compared by observing the heels or the medial malleoli. If a discrepancy is noted, the knees are flexed to 90 degrees while maintaining neutral hip rotation, and the landmarks are reassessed to screen for a shortened tibia. The patient is then positioned supine, and the leg lengths are reassessed using the same landmarks. Finally, the leg lengths are assessed using the long sit test. Functional leg length inequality that is secondary to SI subluxation or dysfunction may reverse from the supine to sitting position, whereas anatomic leg length inequality or functional inequality secondary to dysfunction at other sites likely will not.[146]

Standing Leg Length Test. The iliac crest palpation and book correction (ICPBC) method for assessing leg length is used in many clinics. The patient stands with the feet shoulder-width apart. The clinician palpates the iliac crests and compares the relative heights for asymmetry. The asymmetry identified is corrected using a book opened to the required number of pages. The iliac crest heights are reassessed. If the iliac crests are level, the thickness of the book correction is measured. One study with 34 healthy subjects found the ICPBC technique for measuring leg length discrepancy to be highly reliable and moderately valid when there is no history of pelvic deformity and the iliac crests can be readily palpated.[147]

Functional Leg Length. The patient stands with the feet shoulder-width apart. The clinician palpates the iliac crests, the ASISs, and the PSISs and compares the relative heights for asymmetry. The patient is then positioned with the subtalar joints in neutral, the toes pointing forward, and the knees fully extended. The same landmarks are reassessed. If the second position corrects any asymmetry found in the first position, the test is positive for a functional leg length discrepancy and indicates that the leg is structurally normal but has abnormal joint mechanics.

Sign of the Buttock. The test for this syndrome is described here because its underlying pathologies occur in the lower quadrant The sign of the buttock is not a single sign, as the name would suggest, but rather a collection of signs indicating that a serious pathology is present posterior to the axis of flexion and extension in the hip (see Chap. 19). Among the causes of the syndrome are osteomyelitis, infectious sacroiliitis, fracture of the sacrum or pelvis, septic bursitis, ischiorectal abscess, gluteal hematoma, gluteal tumor, and rheumatic bursitis.

The patient lies supine, and the clinician performs a passive unilateral straight leg raise. If a unilateral restriction is noted, the clinician flexes the knee and notes whether the hip flexion increases. If the restriction was caused by the lumbar spine or hamstrings, the hip flexion should increase. The sign of the buttock test is positive if the hip flexion does not increase when the knee is flexed. If the sign of the buttock is encountered, the patient must be immediately returned to his or her physician for further investigation.[148]

Posterior Pelvic Pain Provocation Test. The posterior pelvic pain provocation test, as described by Ostgaard and colleagues,[149] is performed with the patient in supine. The clinician passively flexes the involved hip of the patient to 90 degrees and a posteriorly directed force is applied through the longitudinal axis of the femur (Fig. 29-25). The test is

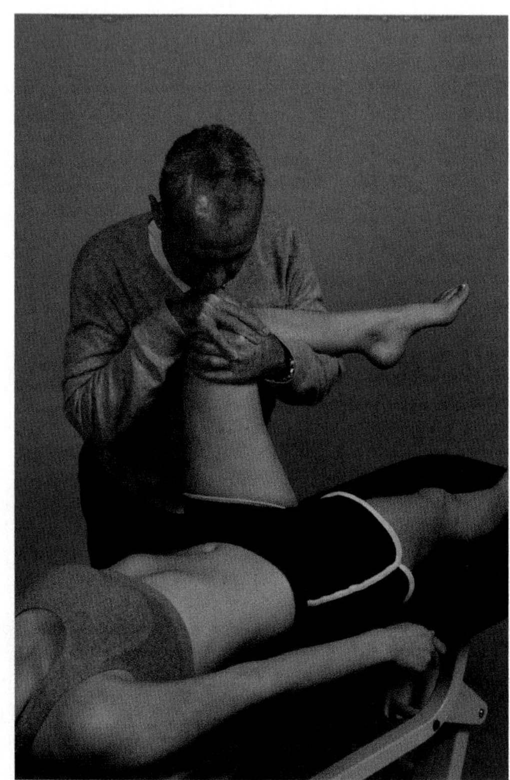

FIGURE 29-25 Posterior pelvic pain provocation test.

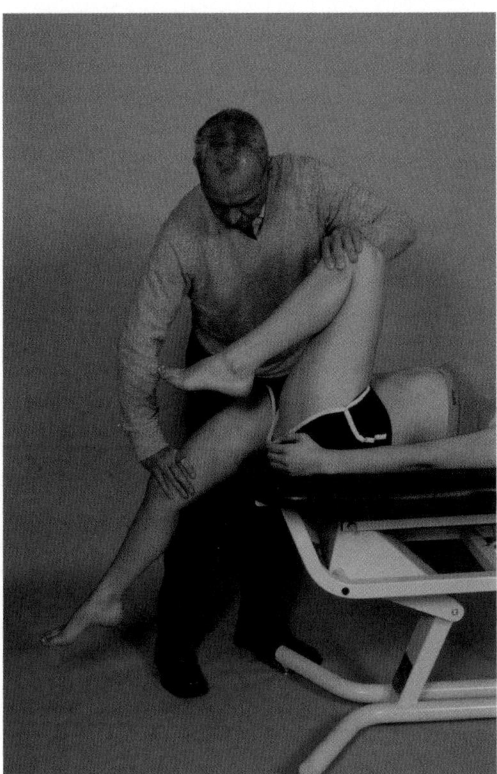

FIGURE 29-26 Gaenslen's test.

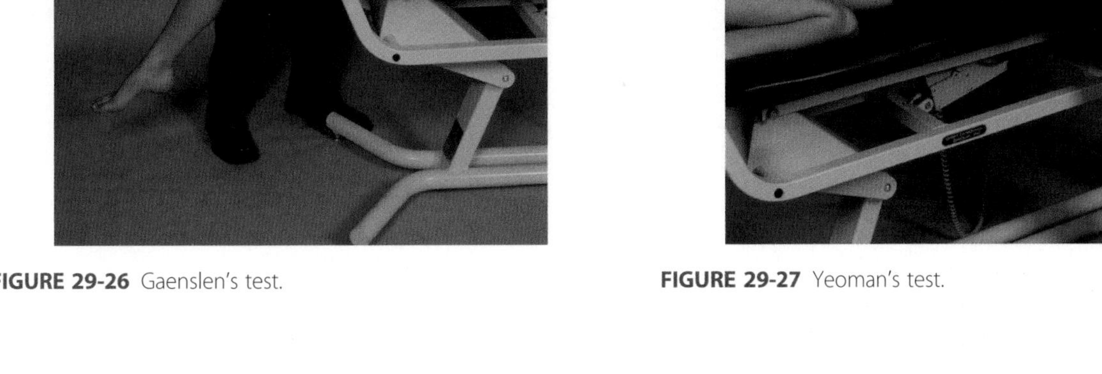

FIGURE 29-27 Yeoman's test.

considered positive for SIJ dysfunction if the patient reports a deep pain in the gluteal region during the test.

Gaenslen's Test. The patient is positioned supine at the edge of the side of the bed with the painful leg resting very near to the end of the bed, and resting symptoms are assessed. The leg furthest from the edge of the bed (non-tested leg) is flexed 90 degrees at the hip and held by the clinician using one hand. The clinician passively positions the upper leg (test leg) into hyperextension at the hip so that it hangs over the edge of the table (Fig. 29-26).[150] The clinician applies a further stretch to the test leg into hip extension and adduction up to six times while a flexion-based counter force is applied to the flexed leg. Pain with this maneuver is considered a positive test for an SIJ lesion, pubic symphysis instability, hip pathology, or an L4 nerve root lesion. The test also stresses the femoral nerve. This test demonstrates poor diagnostic value secondary to poor to fair specificity.[56] Overall, there is limited research pertaining to this test in order to make strong conclusions.

Yeoman's Test. This test[151] is performed with the patient positioned prone. The clinician stabilizes the patient's sacrum with the palm of one hand. With the other hand, the clinician grasps the patient's distal thigh and extends the patient's hip (Fig. 29-27). At the end of the available motion, the hip is hyperextended so that the innominate is forced into anterior rotation. A positive test produces pain over the SIJ. Other structures that are stressed with this maneuver include the lumbar spine, the hip joint, and the iliopsoas muscle.

INTERVENTION STRATEGIES

Thus far, the success of interventions at this joint has been mixed, due in part to the poor reliability with many of the examinations used. The success of any intervention depends on the quality and accuracy of the examination and the subsequent evaluation. It follows that if the examination gives an inaccurate diagnosis, the intervention may have a mixed result. It is reasonable to assume that the SIJ is a source of pain for one of the two reasons:[152]

1. There is some support for the notion of an inflammatory condition within the joint either causing or associated with the pain.[153–155] Inflammatory processes such as those found in ankylosing spondylitis are known to affect the SIJ.
2. The joint is unstable through ligamentous laxity or tearing of the joint capsule.[111,156,157]

Given that the chosen intervention for the SIJ, like the spine, depends largely on the philosophy or background that he clinician uses to establish the diagnosis. There appears to be three major schools of thought[152]:

1. Those who regard the SIJ as either irrelevant or rarely an issue in clinical practice.
2. Those who consider the clinical examination of the SIJ as either useless or of minimal utility.
3. Those who regard structural and biomechanical aspects of the SIJ as the key determinants in the problem of back pain.

Although the philosophies may differ, the principles behind the interventions for SIJ impairments should remain constant:

- A joint that has reduced motion (hypomobility) requires mobilizing techniques, muscle release techniques, and exercises that are designed to restore normal optimal alignment and controlled mobility.
- A joint that demonstrates excessive motion (hypermobility and/or instability) requires techniques and exercises that are designed to stabilize or balance forces around the hypermobile or unstable joint.[83] These include exercises to control joint motion and, on occasion, joint compression through the use of an external brace (SIJ belt).
- A joint that demonstrates signs and symptoms of excessive compression (due to intrinsic factors or extrinsic factors) requires techniques based on the cause of the compression. For example, joint compression caused by fibrosis benefits from the use of specific passive articular mobilization techniques whereas joint compression caused by over-activation of muscles benefits from techniques including muscle energy, trigger point therapy, and biofeedback.

The techniques and exercises used for the SIJ should always be based on the stage of healing and patient tolerance, and must take into account the influences that the lumbar spine and hip motions can have on this area.

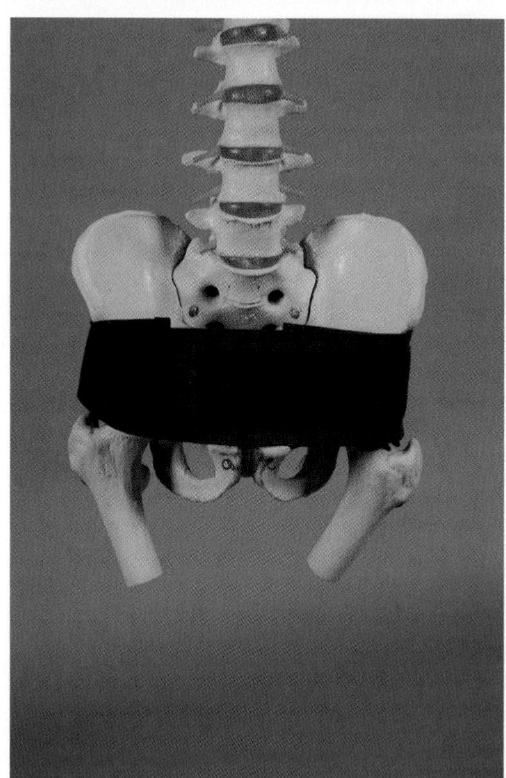

FIGURE 29-28 An SIJ orthosis.

Acute Phase

In the acute phase of rehabilitation for the SIJ, the intervention goals are to

- decrease pain, inflammation, and muscle spasm;
- increase weight-bearing tolerance, where appropriate;
- promote healing of tissues through sufficient stabilization;
- increase pain-free range of SIJ motion and surrounding structures;
- regain soft tissue extensibility around the pelvic region;
- regain neuromuscular control;
- allow progression to the functional stage.

For the most part, exercises are avoided in the acute phase because they tend to increase the symptoms. Pain relief may be accomplished initially by the use of cryotherapy, and electrical stimulation (TENS), gentle muscle setting exercises. Thermal modalities, especially ultrasound with its ability to penetrate deeply may be used after 48–72 hours. Ultrasound is the most common clinically used deep heating modality to promote tissue healing.[158–160]

Clinicians often correct leg length discrepancies of greater than 0.5 inches, as such inequalities have been described as altering normal SIJ function.[161]

SIJ and pelvic stabilization orthoses have been employed in an attempt to limit SIJ motion and improve proprioception (Fig. 29-28).[161–164] These measures are particularly indicated when the joint has been demonstrated to be inflamed by the anterior or posterior stress tests. Not much force from these belts (20–50 N) is necessary to afford relief to the patient.[162] The position of the belt in terms of its height on the ilium should be experimented with to find the optimal position for pain relief. The recommended position is just above the greater trochanter (Fig. 29-28). A bicycle inner tube can be used as a substitute SI belt, as this is the right width and has the correct degree of elasticity. The following conditions appear to respond well to bracing:

1. Sacroiliitis.
2. SI hypermobility/instability: (pre- and postpartum and microtraumatic).
3. Pubic instability (may afford some relief).

Once the pain and inflammation is under control, the intervention can progress toward the restoration of full strength, range of motion, and normal posture. Range of motion exercises are initiated at the earliest opportunity. These are performed during the early stages in the pain-free ranges. Submaximal isometric exercises are then performed throughout the pain-free ranges. These exercises are progressed as the range of motion and strength increase.

Aggressive manual therapy has a very limited place in the intervention of the acutely inflamed joint. In almost every case, the presence of a positive stress test contraindicates the use of passive mobilization or manipulation for that joint. However, mobilization or manipulation of the contralateral joint may reduce the stress on the painful and inflamed articulation. Gentle manual techniques such as myofascial release, grade I–II joint mobilizations, massage, gentle stretching, and muscle energy techniques should be attempted and continued if effective.

Functional Phase

The duration of this phase can vary tremendously and depends upon several factors:

- The severity of the injury.
- The healing capacity of the patient.
- How the condition was managed during the acute phase.
- The level of patient involvement in their rehabilitation program.

The goals of this phase are

- to significantly reduce or to completely resolve the patient's pain;
- to restore full and pain-free SIJ range of motion;
- to integrate the lower kinetic chains into the rehabilitation;
- complete restoration of normal gait, where appropriate;
- the restoration of pelvic and lower quadrant strength and neuromuscular control.

Intervention strategies should emphasize pelvic stabilization,[124] the elimination of trunk/lumbar/hip and lower extremity muscle imbalances, and the correction of gait abnormalities.[165] The exercises used in the lumbopelvic stabilization exercise progression are described in detail in Chapter 28. During this stage, the patient learns to initiate and execute functional activities without pain and while dynamically stabilizing the SIJ in an automatic manner. Muscle imbalances around this joint complex are common. The same principles apply here as elsewhere: stretch those muscles that are tight or adaptively shortened and strengthen those muscles that are found to be weak. The muscles to be stretched around this joint complex are based on the clinical findings but usually include the erector spinae, the quadratus lumborum, the rectus femoris, the iliopsoas, the tensor fascia lata, the hip adductors, and the deep external rotators of the hip, especially the piriformis, and the gluteus maximus.[35,37] Postural correction and the correction of compensatory movements need to be addressed. Corrective exercises may be used to position the innominate bone in proper relation to the sacrum.

The focus of the therapeutic exercises for this region is to augment the force-closure mechanism and to reduce any stress that could prove detrimental to the SI complex. The exercises prescribed must challenge and enhance muscle performance while minimizing loading of the SIJ to reduce the risk of injury exacerbation. Inter-individual differences in injury status and/or training goals may allow for a continuum of required muscle stress and acceptable loading of the spine and SIJ.[166] Stabilization exercises and joint positioning can help the patient to (1) gain dynamic control of spine forces, (2) eliminate repetitive injury to the motion segments, (3) encourage healing of the injured segment, and (4) possibly alter the degenerative process.[167]

The strengthening component of the exercises is aimed at improving the function of the muscles of the inner and outer groups. The appropriate muscles must be isolated and then retrained to increase their strength and endurance, and to automatically recruit to support and protect the region.

A four-stage program has been designed to isolate and retrain the inner and outer muscle groups.[73,168]

Stage 1

- ***Levator ani.*** The patient is first taught the location of the levator ani in supine. To strengthen the muscle, the patient is asked to shorten the distance between the coccyx and the pubic symphysis and to hold the contraction for 10 seconds (Fig. 29-29). When the muscle contracts properly, the transverse abdominis muscle can be felt to contract at a point 2 cm medial and inferior to the ASIS, there is no contraction of the buttocks, and by carefully palpating the sacral apex, the sacrum is felt to counternutate slightly as the levator ani contracts. The exercise is repeated 10 times.

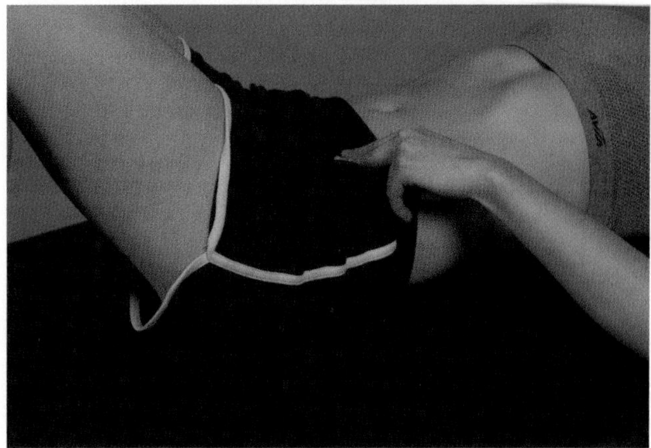

FIGURE 29-29 Levator ani contraction.

- ***Transversus abdominis/multifidus.*** The abdominal drawing-in maneuver is one exercise known to result in preferential activation of the internal oblique and TrA.[72,169–171] To test for isolation of the TrA, the patient is positioned prone, and a pressure biofeedback unit is placed underneath the abdomen[73,79] (Fig. 29-30). The cuff is

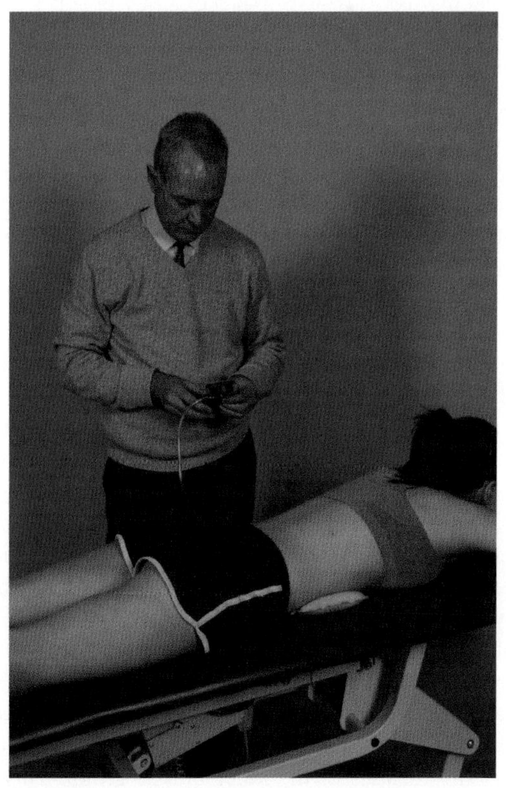

FIGURE 29-30 Transversus abdominis/multifidus.

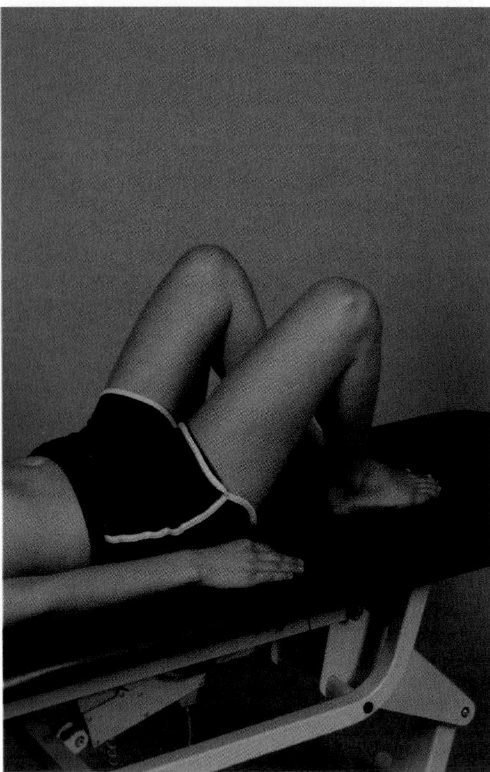

FIGURE 29-31 Knee fall-out.

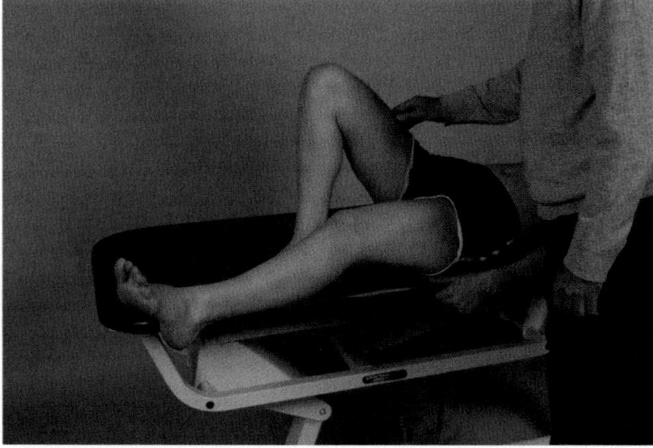

FIGURE 29-32 Leg extension in supine.

inflated to a base level of 70 mm Hg. The patient is asked to draw the navel up and in toward the chest (abdominal hollowing). When the muscle contracts properly, an increase in tension can be felt at a point 2 cm medial and inferior to the ASIS. If a bulging is felt at this point, the internal oblique is contracting. The multifidus is palpated simultaneously and should be felt to swell at a point just lateral to the spinous process.

Stage 2. The stabilization program is progressed to the next stage with the introduction of lower or upper extremity motion, which changes the focus of the program from the inner muscle group to the outer muscle group.

In the supine position with the hips and the knees flexed, the patient is asked to isolate the inner muscle group, while maintaining the lumbar spine in a neutral position. From this position, the patient is asked to slowly let the knee fall to one side (Fig. 29-31). Alternatively, the patient may extend the leg with the foot supported on the table.

The next step in the progression involves asking the patient to slowly extend this leg while maintaining the hip and the knee flexed (with the foot lifted) without touching the table (Fig. 29-32). This exercise initially is performed unilaterally and then is progressed to alternate leg extensions. The same exercises may be performed sitting on a gym ball or lying supine on a long roll. By making the base unstable, the exercise becomes more difficult without having to progress to the next stage.

Exercising on a gym ball requires core stability (inner muscle group control), coordination, and appropriate postural reflexes. While sitting on the ball, the patient is asked to contract the muscles of the inner muscle group. This contraction is maintained while the patient moves forward and backward, and up and down on the ball. The patient is instructed to incorporate the co-contraction of the inner muscle group into their activities of daily living.

If the individual muscles of the outer muscle group are weak or poorly recruited, the exercise program should include isolation and training at this time.

- ***Posterior oblique system.*** In the posterior oblique system, it is common to find the gluteus maximus both lengthened and weak.[12] Having the patient squeeze the buttocks together and sustain the contraction for 10 seconds isolates the gluteus maximus. A surface electromyography unit can provide a useful biofeedback system for this muscle. The exercise is progressed by having the patient lie prone over a gym ball and asking him or her initially to recruit the inner muscle group and then to extend the hip while the knee is flexed. Lifting the extended thigh increases the degree of difficulty. Leg extension machines can help to strengthen the gluteus maximus. Initially, the patient exercises in the supine position with one or both feet on the foot plate. Functional training is introduced by having the patient practice going from sitting to standing with a stabilized trunk, using primarily the gluteus maximus muscle.
- ***Lateral system.*** In the lateral system, the posterior fibers of the gluteus medius are often weak, which can have a marked effect on walking and load transference through the hip joint.[91] Isolation of the gluteus medius is taught in the side lying position with a pillow placed between the knees. The exercise is progressed by asking the patient to lift the knee off the pillow and then to extend the knee while maintaining the correct position of the trunk and the hip. Resistance can be added using elastic tubing or a cuff weight.
- ***Anterior oblique system.*** Isolation of the anterior oblique system involves training the specific contraction of the external and internal oblique abdominals. When the external obliques contract bilaterally, the infrasternal angle narrows, whereas when the internal obliques contract bilaterally, the infrasternal angle widens. The patient is taught to palpate the lateral costal margin and to specifically widen and narrow the infrasternal angle through specific contraction of the oblique abdominals.

The progression includes activation of the anterior and posterior oblique systems and differentiation of trunk from thigh motion. To begin, the patient is supine with the hips and the knees flexed, both feet on the bed. The patient is instructed to bridge and then to rotate the trunk and the pelvic girdle at the hip joints in the unsupported position, while maintaining the lumbar joints in a neutral position.

Stage 3. Stage 3 exercises involve controlled motion of the "unstable region."[73] Because this stage is much more advanced, it is used only when required by an individual's work or sport. The protocol includes concentric and eccentric work with variable resistance in all three planes.

Stage 4.[73] Stage 4 of the protocol involves stabilization during high-speed motions. Very few people require stage 4 stabilization, particularly in view of the fact that high-speed exercise tends to reduce the stabilizing capability of the trunk muscles.[79]

In addition to the exercise program, the patient should be educated on the trunk and the lower extremity positions to avoid (those that produce an excessive or sustained sacral counternutation or a decrease in lumbar lordosis) and those to adopt (the positions that enhance sacral nutation and enhance the lumbar lordosis). For example, the patient should be advised to maintain an anterior pelvic tilt during sitting, either actively or passively with the use of a lumbar roll.

The techniques to increase joint mobility and the techniques to increase soft tissue extensibility are described under "Therapeutic Techniques".

As symptoms are controlled, therapy should be advanced to activity-specific stabilization exercises to facilitate return to function at the patient's occupation, sport, or avocational activities.

Integration of Practice Patterns 4D and 4E: Impaired Joint Mobility, Motor Function, Muscle Performance, Range of Motion Associated with Connective Tissue Dysfunction, and Localized Inflammation

Spondyloarthropathies

The spondyloarthropathies are a group of inflammatory arthritic conditions that share certain clinical and laboratory features (see Chap. 5).[172]

- An inflammatory arthritis, which manifests with pain associated with stiffness.
- The absence of a rheumatoid factor; hence the distinction of the group as "seronegative" spondyloarthropathies.
- The tendency for the arthritis to be asymmetric and involve the lower extremities.
- Often, inflammation at the insertion of tendons into bone (enthesitis), accompanied by certain extra-articular features, including skin and mucous membrane impairments, bowel complaints, eye involvement, and aortic root dilation.
- The familial aggregation, which occurs within each condition and among the entities within the group.
- An association with HLA-B27, documented in the diseases included in this group.

Ankylosing Spondylitis

Ankylosing spondylitis (Bekhterev's or Marie-Strümpell disease) is a chronic rheumatoid disorder that is usually progressive, resulting in a full ankylosing of the SIJs.[172] Men generally have the more severe form affecting the spine, whereas in women, the peripheral joints are more often affected.

The typical radiographic changes are seen primarily in the axial skeleton, especially in the SI, intervertebral, zygapophyseal, costovertebral, and costotransverse joints.[173] In addition, ankylosing spondylitis is one of the most common rheumatic disorders associated with radiologic abnormalities of the pubic symphysis, with pubic synchondrosis present in 20–25% of the patients.[174] In fact, changes of the symphysis can sometimes precede spine involvement.[174]

Tests to discriminate SIJ tenderness caused by ankylosing spondylitis from that caused by mechanical spine conditions have traditionally included passive hip extension, A-P pressure applied to the sacrum, and the primary stress tests. However, these tests have been found to be poorly reproducible and inaccurate in making any distinction.[99]

Although radiologic evidence of sacroiliitis is accepted as being obligatory for the diagnosis of ankylosing spondylitis, the clinical signs (see Chap. 5) may predate radiologic abnormalities by months or even years.[172]

Groin Pain

Chronic pain in the groin region (see Chap. 19) is a difficult clinical problem to evaluate, and in many cases, the cause of the pain is poorly understood. The differential diagnosis of groin pain and tenderness includes adductor muscle strain, prostatitis, orchitis, inguinal hernia, urolithiasis, ankylosing spondylitis, Reiter's syndrome, hyperparathyroidism, metastasis, osteitis pubis, stress fracture, rheumatoid arthritis, tendonitis, degenerative joint disease of the hip, bursitis, stress fracture, conjoint tendon strains, inguinal ligament enthesopathy, and entrapment of the lateral cutaneous nerve of the thigh.[175–177]

Other nerve entrapment syndromes have been described as a possible cause of adductor region pain, with the anterior division of the obturator nerve in the thigh,[178] the ilioinguinal nerve, and the genitofemoral nerve having all been inculpated.[179]

Osteitis Pubis

Many theories have been put forward concerning the etiology and progression of this disease, but the cause of osteitis pubis remains unclear.

Osteitis pubis is seen in athletes who participate in activities that create continual shearing forces at the pubic symphysis, as with unilateral leg support or acceleration–deceleration forces required during multidirectional activities. These include activities such as running, racewalking, gymnastics, soccer, basketball, rugby, and tennis. Pain with walking can be in one or several of many distributions: perineal, testicular, suprapubic, inguinal, and in the scrotum and perineum.[180] Overuse is the most likely etiology of the inflammation, and the process is usually self-limiting.[180]

Osteitis pubis has been likened to gracilis syndrome, an avulsion fatigue fracture involving the bony origin of the gracilis muscle at the pubic symphysis and occurring in relation to the directional pull of the gracilis.[181] However, osteitis pubis does not necessarily involve a fracture. The process could be the result of stress reaction, which might be associated with several biomechanical abnormalities.

Osteitis pubis usually appears during the third and fourth decades of life, occurring more commonly in men.[182] The pain or discomfort can be located in the pubic area, one or both groins, and the lower rectus abdominis muscle. Symptoms of osteitis pubis have been described as "groin burning," with discomfort while climbing stairs, coughing, or sneezing.

During the physical examination, pain can be elicited by having the patient squeeze a fist between the knees with resisted long and flexed adductor contraction. Range of motion in one or both hips may be decreased. An adductor muscle spasm might occur with limited abduction and a positive FABER test.[183,184] A soft tissue mass with calcification, and an audible or palpable click over the symphysis might be detected during daily activities.[180]

Correct examination of this region involves examining the position of the pelvic girdle. The normal position for the pelvic bowl is 45 degrees in the sagittal plane and 45 degrees in the coronal plane. Pubic motion is assessed by locating the pubic crest and then gently testing the mobility of each available direction.

Dysfunction of this articulation may be primary or secondary and, when present, is always treated first, because a loss of function or integrity of this joint disrupts the mechanics of the entire pelvic complex. The impairment pattern is determined by palpating the position of the pubic tubercles and correlating the findings with the side of the positive kinetic test, with the restricted side indicating the side of the impairment.

An altered positional relationship within the pelvic girdle is significant only if a mobility restriction of the SIJ or pubic symphysis, or both, is found. The inguinal ligament is usually very tender to palpation on the side of the impairment. It is common to find the pubic symphysis held in one of the four following positions:

1. Anteroinferior
2. Posterosuperior
3. Anterosuperior
4. Posteroinferior

These articular dysfunctions are treated using manual techniques (see "Therapeutic Techniques").

Intervention for the inflammatory type of osteitis pubis is conservative and most athletes return to their respective sports within a few days to weeks.[185] The intervention includes plenty of rest from weight-bearing activities, a course of nonsteroidal anti-inflammatory medicine, and physical therapy to gently mobilize, stretch, and strengthen the muscles about the groin.[186] Patients should be able to swim for exercise.

An intervention protocol for osteitis pubis is outlined in Box 29-1.

Box 29-1 Intervention Protocol for Osteitis Pubis

Phase I

1. Static adduction against a soccer ball placed between feet when lying supine. Each adduction is held for 30 seconds and is repeated 10 times.
2. Abdominal sit-ups performed both in straight direction and in oblique direction. Patient performs five sets to fatigue.
3. Combined abdominal sit-up and hip flexion (crunch). Patient starts from supine position and with a soccer/basketball placed between knees. Patient performs five sets to fatigue.
4. Balance training on wobble board for 5 minutes.
5. One-foot exercises on sliding board, with parallel feet as well as with a 90-degree angle between feet.

Five sets of 1-minute continuous work are performed with each leg, and in both positions.

Phase II (from third week)

1. Leg abduction and adduction exercises in side lying position on side. Patient performs five series of 10 repetitions of each exercise.
2. Low-back extension exercises while in prone position over end of treatment table. Patient performs five series of 10 repetitions.
3. One-leg weight-pulling abduction–adduction, standing. Patient performs five series of 10 repetitions for each leg.
4. Abdominal sit-ups both in straightforward direction and in oblique direction. Patient performs five sets to fatigue.
5. One-leg coordination exercise flexing and extending knee and swinging arms in same rhythm (cross-country skiing on one leg). Patient performs five sets of 10 repetitions for each leg.
6. Skating movements on sliding board. This is performed five times for 1-minute continuous work.

Symphysis Pubic Dysfunction

Symphysis pubic dysfunction (SPD) describes the situation where the ligaments between the pubic symphysis become stretched and allow the bones to move with respect to each other (see Chap. 30). In severe cases, rupture of the symphysis may occur. This more severe form is called diastasis symphysis pubis (DSP). SPD commonly occurs during pregnancy, and should always be considered when examining patients in the postpartum period who are experiencing suprapubic, SI, or thigh pain. The associated ligamentous laxity during pregnancy is in response to the hormones progesterone and relaxin. Causes unrelated to pregnancy include the possibility of a structural misalignment of the pelvis. This pelvic misalignment results in increased pressure on the pubic symphysis cartilage, with subsequent pain.

The symptoms of SPD and DSP vary from person to person (see Chap. 30). Radiological evaluation may occasionally be useful in confirming the diagnosis.[187] Therefore, the intervention is based on the severity of symptoms rather than the degree of separation as measured by imaging studies.[187] Palpation reveals anterior pubic symphyseal tenderness. Occasional clicking can be felt or heard. The findings on the physical examination include positive SIJ stress tests (compression, distraction, and FABER tests). The range of hip movements will be limited by pain, and there is an inability to stand on one leg. Characteristic pain can often be evoked by bilateral pressure on the trochanters or by hip flexion with the legs in extension. However, such maneuvers may result in severe pain or muscle spasm and are not necessary for diagnosis.

In cases of DSP, there is likely an associated anteroposterior (A-P) compression (common) or a vertical shear (rare) fracture. Three types of DSP are described, indicating the severity of the injury[188]:

- Type 1 involves minor anterior damage, mild (less than 2.5 cm) pubic symphysis diastasis, and/or (vertical) pubic rami fractures.
- Type II has wide diastasis of the symphysis pubis, disruption of the anterior SI ligament complex, and (hinging) of the iliac bone on the sacrum at the intact posterior SIJ.
- Type III designates total disruption of the SIJ, a diastasis of greater than 2.5 cm has been shown to indicate disruption of the anterior SIJ at least, but it is frequently associated with total SIJ disruption.

Although the symptoms can be dramatically severe in presentation for SPD and DSP, a conservative management approach is often effective (see Chap. 30).[187]

Resolution of symptoms in approximately 6–8 weeks with no lasting sequela is the most common outcome in SDP and DSP.[187] Occasionally, patients report residual pain requiring several months of physical therapy but long-term impairment is unusual. Surgical intervention is rarely required but may be used in cases of inadequate reduction, recurrent diastasis, or persistent symptoms.

Peripartum Posterior Pelvic Pain

More than 50% of women experience peripartum posterior pelvic pain (PPPP) or low back pain (LBP) during pregnancy with one-third of these women experiencing severe pain (see Chap. 30).[189–191,192]

Hall and colleagues,[189] in a two-case report provided preliminary evidence suggesting that a combination of manual therapy (muscle energy techniques directed at identified pelvic and sacral positional faults) and therapeutic exercise (neuromuscular reeducation of the transverse abdominis and multifidus with isometric hip adduction and abduction in a semireclined position, and standing exercises to strengthen the posterior oblique system [gluteus maximus and contralateral latissimus dorsi]) may be an effective intervention for peripartum patients reporting posterior pelvic pain.[189]

Coccydynia

Coccygeal pain is relatively common. The coccyx can move anteriorly or posteriorly. There are a number of ligaments around this area which can be injured:

- ***Anterior (ventral).***
  - Lateral sacrococcygeal.
  - Anterior (ventral) ligament of the coccyx (caudal extension of the anterior longitudinal ligament).
- ***Posterior (dorsal).***
  - Superficial posterior (dorsal) sacrococcygeal (caudal extension of the ligamentum flavum).
  - Deep posterior (dorsal) sacrococcygeal (caudal extension of the posterior longitudinal ligament).
  - Intercornual ligament.

The dominant muscle in this area is the levator ani, which has connections with the

- iliococcygeal ligament;
- pubococcygeal ligament.

Coccydynia tends to occur when the coccyx becomes stuck into flexion with an accompanying deviation. The causes can be muscle scarring or trauma.

Correction of this impairment involves grasping the coccyx after inserting the index finger in the anal canal. The coccyx is distracted and pulled posteriorly, while pulling laterally on the medial surface of the ischial tuberosity.

Practice Pattern 4G: Impaired Joint Mobility, Motor Function, Muscle Performance, Range of Motion Associated with Fracture

Sacral Stress Fracture

Repetitive loading on the body can lead to the development of stress fractures. Stress fractures have been described as a cause of back pain, especially fractures of the pelvis and pars interarticularis of the sacrum.[193] Back and buttock pain caused by sacral stress fractures are less common but may occur in athletes and in the elderly.[194] Fractures in the latter group have been reported both with and without trauma.

The cause of sacral stress fractures is controversial. These fractures are believed to result from stress concentrations of vertical body forces, which are dissipated from the spine to the sacrum and the sacral alae and then onto the iliac wings.[195] In addition to abnormal stresses on normal bone, normal stress on abnormal bone can produce these fractures, especially in the elderly. Patients who sustain such insufficiency fractures may have predisposing factors, including idiopathic osteoporosis, irradiation-induced osteoporosis, steroid-induced osteoporosis, or osteoporosis associated with malignancy.[193] Another cause cited for sacral fractures is progressive *insufficiency* of the supporting muscles.[196] These fatigue fractures may result from the transfer of loading forces directly to the bone, without absorption of some energy by the muscles. Other reported causes of sacral stress fractures are differences in physical demands, environmental and genetic influences, training methods, footwear, and intensity of training.[196] Atwell and Jackson[197] suggested that leg length inequality may increase the stress on one side of the sacrum, but this has not been proven by biomechanical analysis.[193]

Patients with sacral stress fractures typically present with low back pain and sacral pain that may radiate into the buttocks. However, pain may be referred to the groin and, occasionally, down the leg.[197] In the case of an athlete, the history may reveal a recent history of stress fracture in the same area, or a rapid increase in training intensity prior to the onset of symptoms.[126] Insufficiency fractures of the sacrum in nonathletes have been reported to mimic disk disease, spinal stenosis, and tumors.[198] Irritation of the cauda equina or the sacral nerve roots may explain the wide variety of symptoms seen in patients with sacral stress fractures.[193,199]

Physical examination may not provide reliable signs initially, because many of these patients have diffuse low back, sacral, and buttock pain. However, most patients will have localized tenderness over the sacrum and SIJ.[193–195,197–199] Tenderness in the upper gluteal areas tends to be coexistent with sacral stress fractures, and tenderness in this region may contribute to the impression that the origin of the pain is centered in the more proximal lumbar spine.[193] Most patients are neurologically intact, with no signs of nerve root irritation. The Patrick's, or the FABER (flexion, abduction, external rotation) test may or may not be positive, so it cannot be depended on in making a diagnosis.[193]

The most sensitive method of evaluating the sacrum for occult stress fractures and other bone lesions is a bone scan using three-phase scintigraphy.[200] This bone imaging technique can help detect stress fractures as early as several days after the fracture occurs. In contrast, plain radiographs of the lumbosacral spine and the pelvis, although useful to rule out other causes of back pain, are not helpful in diagnosing sacral stress fractures.[194]

Patients with sacral stress fractures recover quickly with rest. Most patients are able to return to their normal activity levels in 4–6 weeks with no long-term sequelae.[193] Anti-inflammatory agents and analgesics may be used as adjunctive treatment for patient comfort. Cycling or running in a pool may be used until weight-bearing activities are tolerated.

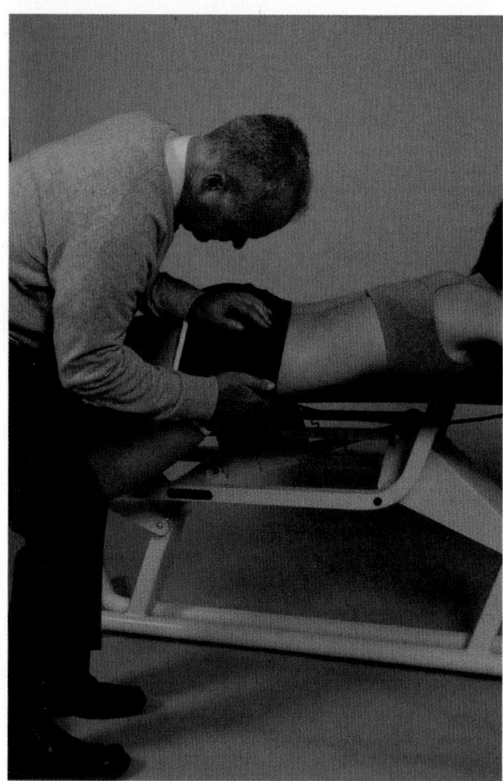

FIGURE 29-33 Method to restore posterior rotation of the right innominate.

THERAPEUTIC TECHNIQUES

Normally, pelvic impairments are presented as isolated entities when, in fact, clinically, they tend to occur in combination. It is essential that the impairments, functional limitations, and disability found during the examination guide the intervention.

To Restore Posterior Rotation of the Right Innominate

The patient is in the prone lying position, with the right hip and the leg over the edge of the table. The clinician stands at the patient's right side. The patient's right foot is placed between the clinician's legs and held there. While monitoring the sacral sulcus with the index finger of the left hand, the clinician moves the patient's right leg to the barrier (Fig. 29-33). The patient is asked to gently push the right foot toward the foot of the table. This movement is resisted by the clinician's legs, and after 3–5 seconds, the patient is told to relax. Once again, when full relaxation has occurred, the slack is taken up, and the patient's right leg is moved in the direction of hip flexion until the monitoring finger indicates the new barrier has been reached. This mobilization is repeated three times and followed by a reexamination.

To Restore Anterior Rotation of the Left Innominate

The patient is in the prone lying position, with the clinician standing on the patient's side. With the left hand, the clinician supports the anterior aspect of the patient's left thigh, at a point just above the knee. The clinician places the heel of his or her right hand over the patient's left posterior inferior iliac spine. Extending the left hip until motion at the lumbosacral junction is perceived (Fig. 29-34), the clinician localizes the motion barrier. The patient is instructed to flex the left hip against the clinician's resistance. This isometric contraction is held up to 5 seconds, following which the patient is instructed to completely relax. The new barrier to anterior rotation is achieved by further extension of the hip. The mobilization is repeated three times and followed by a reexamination of function.

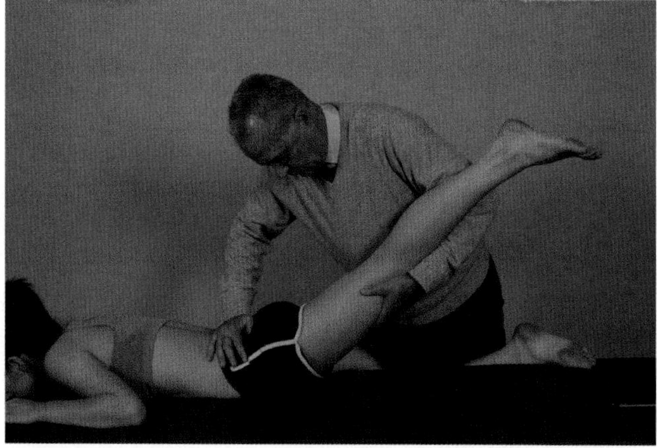

FIGURE 29-34 Method to restore anterior rotation of the left innominate.

CASE STUDY

LEFT-SIDED LOW BACK AND BUTTOCK PAIN

HISTORY

A 47-year-old man presented at the clinic, with left-sided low back and buttock pain that had developed while he was at work 2 weeks previously. When describing the mechanism of injury, the patient reported feeling something "pop" in his low back during a lifting maneuver that involved bending forward and twisting to the right. The pain was now localized to an area slightly inferior to the left posterosuperior iliac spine, which he reported as being very tender to the touch. The pain was aggravated with forward bending and turning at the waist to the left in the sitting position. The patient reported sleeping well, if he remained prone, and there were no complaints of paresthesias or anesthesias. The patient denied any neurologic symptoms related to cauda equina or spinal cord involvement. He was in otherwise good health.

Questions

1. Given a distinct mechanism of injury, what type of structure(s) could be at fault with complaints of left-sided low back and buttock pain?
2. What does the region of *localized* tenderness tell the clinician?
3. Why do you think the patient is sleeping well in the prone position?
4. What is your working hypothesis at this stage? List the various diagnoses that could manifest with low back and buttock pain, and the tests you would use to rule out each one.
5. Does this presentation/history warrant a scan? Why or why not?

CASE STUDY

PUBIC PAIN

HISTORY

A 44-year-old man came to the clinic complaining of worsening abdominal and midline pelvic pain. The pain had developed gradually, and there was no report of recent direct trauma or acute injury. The pain was aggravated with forced flexion at the waist and the Valsalva maneuver, but the patient reported no pain at rest. The pain, described as a sharp, "stabbing" sensation, remained fairly localized to his upper pelvis and lower abdominal area.

The patient had no history of abdominal or genitourinary diseases or surgeries, and he had not experienced similar symptoms in the past. A review of systems was unremarkable. He denied dysuria, hematuria, diarrhea, constipation, fever, chills, or weight change.[185]

The patient frequently participated in physical activity and played soccer, averaging four games per week, an increase from his usual level of commitment. An inguinal hernia had been ruled out by his physician.

Questions

1. What structure(s) could be at fault when abdominal and midline pelvic pain is the major complaint?
2. What is the significance of the Valsalva maneuver?
3. Why are the questions with regard to dysuria, hematuria, diarrhea, constipation, fever, chills, or weight change pertinent?
4. What does no pain at rest suggest?
5. What is your working hypothesis at this stage? List the various diagnoses that could manifest with this pain and the tests you would use to rule out each one.
6. Does this presentation/history warrant a scan? Why or why not?

REVIEW QUESTIONS*

1. Which SIJ ligament forms the major connection between the sacrum and the innominate, filling the irregular space posterosuperior to the joint between the lateral sacral crest and the iliac tuberosity?
2. Which sacral motion places tension on the posterior (dorsal) SI ligament of the SIJ?
3. What are the muscle actions of the piriformis muscle?
4. Which muscle group comprises the pelvic floor muscle group?
5. During right side bending, which sacral and right innominate motions are purported to occur?

---

*Additional questions to test your understanding of this chapter can be found in the Online Learning Center for *Orthopaedic Assessment, Evaluation, and Intervention* at www.duttononline.net.

REFERENCES

1. Grieve GP: *Common Vertebral Joint Problems.* New York, NY: Churchill Livingstone Inc, 1981.
2. Cibulka MT: The treatment of the sacroiliac joint component to low back pain: A case report. *Phys Ther* 72:917–922, 1992.
3. Grieve GP: The sacroiliac joint. *Physiotherapy* 62:384–400, 1976.
4. Huston C: The sacroiliac joint. In: Gonzalez EG, ed. *The Nonsurgical Management of Acute Low Back Pain.* New York, NY: Demos Vermande, 1997:137–150.
5. Fryette HH: *Principles of Osteopathic Technique.* Colorado, CO: Academy of Osteopathy, 1980.
6. DiGiovanna EL, Schiowitz S: *An Osteopathic Approach to Diagnosis and Treatment.* Philadelphia, PA: JB Lippincott, 1991.
7. Hartman SL: *Handbook of Osteopathic Technique*, 2nd ed. London: Unwin Hyman Ltd., Academic Division, 1990.
8. Mitchell FL, Moran PS, Pruzzo NA: *An Evaluation and Treatment Manual of Osteopathic Muscle Energy Procedures.* Manchester, MO: Mitchell, Moran and Pruzzo Associates, 1979.
9. Stoddard A: *Manual of Osteopathic Practice.* New York, NY: Harper & Row, 1969.
10. Fowler C: Muscle energy techniques for pelvic dysfunction. In: Palastanga N, Boyling JD, eds. *Grieve's Modern Manual Therapy: The Vertebral Column.* Edinburgh: Churchill Livingstone, 1986:781–792.
11. Lee DG, Walsh MC: *A Workbook of Manual Therapy Techniques for the Vertebral Column and Pelvic Girdle*, 2nd ed. Vancouver, BC: Nascent, 1996.
12. Lee DG: *The Pelvic Girdle: An Approach to the Examination and Treatment of the Lumbo-Pelvic-Hip Region*, 2nd ed. Edinburgh: Churchill Livingstone, 1999.
13. Schwarzer AC, Aprill CN, Bogduk N: The sacroiliac joint in chronic low back pain. *Spine* 20:31–37, 1995.
14. Pettman E: *Level One Course Notes.* Portland, OR: North American Institute of Orthopedic Manual Therapy, 1990.
15. Goldthwaite JE, Osgood RB: A consideration of the pelvic articulations from an anatomical, pathological, and clinical consideration. *Boston Med Surg J* 152:593–634, 1905.
16. Mixter WJ, Barr JS Jr: Rupture of the intervertebral disc with involvement of the spinal canal. *N Engl J Med* 211:210–215, 1934.
17. Maigne JY, Aivaliklis A, Pfefer F: Results of sacroiliac joint double block and value of sacroiliac pain provocation tests in 54 patients with low back pain. *Spine* 21:1889–1892, 1996.
18. Williams PL, Warwick R, Dyson M, et al.: *Gray's Anatomy.* 37th ed. London: Churchill Livingstone, 1989.
19. Schunke GB: The anatomy and development of the sacro-iliac joint in man. *Anat Rec* 72:313-331, 1938.
20. MacDonald GR, Hunt TE: Sacro-iliac joint observations on the gross and histological changes in the various age groups. *Can Med Assoc J* 66:157, 1951.
21. Bowen V, Cassidy JD: Macroscopic and microscopic anatomy of the sacroiliac joint from embryonic life until the eighth decade. *Spine* 6:620, 1980.
22. Weisl H: The articular surfaces of the sacro-iliac joint and their relation to the movements of the sacrum. *Acta Anat (Basel)* 22:1, 1954.
23. Kapandji IA: *The Physiology of the Joints, The Trunk and Vertebral Column.* New York, NY: Churchill Livingstone, 1991.
24. Solonen KA: The sacroiliac joint in the light of anatomical roentgenographical and clinical studies. *Acta Orthop Scand* 26:9, 1957.
25. Erdmann H: Die verspannung des wirbelsockels im beckenring. In: Junghanns H, ed. *Wirbelsäule in Forschung und Praxis.* Stuttgart: Hippokrates, 1956:51.
26. Vleeming A, Stoeckart R, Volkers ACW, et al.: Relation between form and function in the sacroiliac joint. 1: Clinical anatomical aspects. *Spine* 15:130–132, 1990.
27. Kissling RO, Jacob HAC: The mobility of the sacroiliac joints in healthy subjects. *Bull Hosp Jt Dis* 54:158–164, 1996.
28. Resnick D, Niwayama G, Goergen TG: Degenerative disease of the sacroiliac joint. *Invest Radiol* 10:608–621, 1975.
29. Vleeming A, Wingerden JP, van Dijkstra PF, et al.: Mobility in the SI-joints in old people: a kinematic and radiological study. *Clin Biomech (Bristol, Avon)* 7:170–176, 1992.
30. Mennell JB: *The Science and Art of Joint Manipulation.* London: J & A Churchill, 1949.
31. Meadows J, Pettman E: *Manual therapy: NAIOMT Level II & III Course Notes.* Denver, CO: North American Institute of Manual Therapy, Inc, 1995.
32. Vleeming A: The function of the long dorsal sacroiliac ligament: its implication for understanding low back pain. *Spine* 21:556, 1996.
33. Willard FH: The muscular, ligamentous and neural structure of the low back and its relation to low back pain. In: Vleeming A, Mooney V, Dorman T et al., eds. *Movement, Stability and Low Back pain.* New York, NY: Churchill Livingstone, 1997:3–36.
34. Fortin JD, Pier J, Falco F: Sacroiliac joint injection: pain referral mapping and arthrographic findings. In: Vleeming A, Mooney V, Dorman T et al., eds. *Movement, Stability and Low Back Pain.* Edinburgh: Churchill Livingstone, 1997:271.
35. Vleeming A, Stoeckart R, Snijders CJ: The sacrotuberous ligament: a conceptual approach to its dynamic role in stabilizing the sacroiliac joint. *Clin Biomech (Bristol, Avon)* 4:201–203, 1989.
36. van Wingerden JP, Vleeming A, Snijders CJ, et al.: A functional-anatomical approach to the spine-pelvis mechanism: interaction between the biceps femoris muscle and the sacrotuberous ligament. *Eur Spine J* 2:140–142, 1993.
37. Vleeming A, Van Wingerden JP, Snijders CJ, et al.: Load application to the sacrotuberous ligament. *Clin Biomech (Bristol, Avon)* 4:204–209, 1989.
38. Bourdillon JF: *Spinal Manipulation*, 3rd ed. London: Heinemann Medical Books, 1982.
39. Beaton LE, Anson BJ: The sciatic nerve and the piriformis muscle: their interrelation a possible cause of coccygodynia. *J Bone Joint Surg* 20:686–688, 1938.
40. Durrani Z, Winnie AP: Piriformis muscle syndrome: an underdiagnosed cause of sciatica. *J Pain Symptom Manage* 6:374–379, 1991.
41. Julsrud ME: Piriformis syndrome. *J Am Podiatr Med Assoc* 79:128–131, 1989.
42. Pace JB, Nagle D: Piriformis syndrome. *Western J Med* 124:435–439, 1976.
43. Pfeifer T, Fitz WFK: Das piriformis-syndrom. *Z Orthop Ihre Grenzgeb* 127:691–694, 1989.
44. Solheim LF, Siewers P, Paus B: The piriformis muscle syndrome. Sciatic nerve entrapment treated with section of the piriformis muscle. *Acta Orthop Scand* 52:73–75, 1981.
45. Steiner C, Staubs C, Ganon M, et al.: Piriformis syndrome: pathogenesis, diagnosis, and treatment. *J Am Osteopath Assoc* 87:318–323, 1987.
46. Travell JG, Simons DG: *Myofascial Pain and Dysfunction—The Trigger Point Manual.* Baltimore, MD: Williams & Wilkins, 1983.
47. Barker PJ, Briggs CA, Bogeski G: Tensile transmission across the lumbar fasciae in unembalmed cadavers: effects of tension to various muscular attachments. *Spine* 29:129–138, 2004.
48. Barker PJ, Briggs CA: Attachments of the posterior layer of lumbar fascia. *Spine* 24:1757–1764, 1999.
49. McIntosh JE, Valencia F, Bogduk N, et al.: The morphology of the lumbar multifidus muscles. *Clin Biomech* 1:196–204, 1986.

50. McGill SM: Kinetic potential of the lumbar trunk musculature about three orthogonal orthopaedic axes in extreme postures. *Spine* 16:809–815, 1991.
51. Vleeming A, Pool-Goudzwaard AL, Stoeckart R, et al.: The posterior layer of the thoracolumbar fascia: its function in load transfer from spine to legs. *Spine* 20:753–758, 1995.
52. Dorman T: Pelvic mechanics and prolotherapy. In: Vleeming A, Mooney V, Dorman T et al., eds. *Movement, Stability and Low Back Pain.* Edinburgh: Churchill Livingstone, 1997:507.
53. Bogduk N, Pearcy M, Hadfield G: Anatomy and biomechanics of psoas major. *Clin Biomech* 7:109–119, 1992.
54. Markwell SJ: Physical therapy management of pelvi/perineal and peri-anal pain syndromes. *World J Urol* 19:194–199, 2001.
55. Bogduk N: The sacroiliac joint. In: Bogduk N, ed. *Clinical Anatomy of the Lumbar Spine and Sacrum*, 3rd ed. New York, NY: Churchill Livingstone, 1997:177–186.
56. Dreyfuss P, Michaelson M, Pauza K, et al.: The value of medical history and physical examination in diagnosing sacroiliac joint pain. *Spine* 21:2594–2602, 1996.
57. Pitkin HC, Pheasant HC: Sacrarthrogenic telalgia I: a study of referred pain. *J Bone Joint Surg* 18:111–133, 1936.
58. Grob KR, Neuhuber WL, Kissling RO: Innervation of the sacroiliac joint of the human. *Z Rheumatol* 54:117–122, 1995.
59. Inman VT, Saunders JB: Referred pain from skeletal structures. *J Nerv Ment Dis* 99:660–667, 1944.
60. Basmajian JV, Deluca CJ: *Muscles Alive: Their Functions Revealed by Electromyography.* Baltimore, MD: Williams & Wilkins, 1985.
61. Miller JAA, Schultz AB, Andersson GBJ: Load displacement behavior of sacro-iliac joints. *J Orthop Res* 5:92–101, 1987.
62. Sturesson B, Uden A, Vleeming A: A radiostereometric analysis of the movements of the sacroiliac joints in the reciprocal straddle position. *Spine* 25:214–217, 2000.
63. Egund N, Olsson TH, Schmid H, et al.: Movements in the sacroiliac joints demonstrated with roentgen stereophotogrammetry. *Acta Radiol Diagn (Stockh)* 19:833–846, 1978.
64. Smidt GL, McQuade K, Wei S-H, et al.: Sacroiliac kinematics for reciprocal straddle positions. *Spine* 20:1047–1054, 1995.
65. Lee DG, Vleeming A: The management of pelvic joint pain and dysfunction. In: Boyling JD, Jull GA, eds. *Grieve's Modern Manual Therapy: The Vertebral Column.* Philadelphia, PA: Churchill Livingstone, 2004:495–516.
66. Sturesson B, Selvik G, Uden A: Movements of the sacroiliac joints. A roentgen stereophotogrammetric analysis. *Spine* 14:162–165, 1989.
67. Sturesson B: Load and movements of the sacroiliac joint, PhD thesis. Malmo, Sweden: Lund University, 1999:29–35.
68. Buyruk HM, Stam HJ, Snijders CJ, et al.: Measurement of sacroiliac joint stiffness in peripartum pelvic pain patients with Doppler imaging of vibrations (DIV). *Eur J Obstet Gynecol Reprod Biol* 83:159–163, 1999.
69. Buyruk HM, Snijders CJ, Vleeming A, et al.: The measurements of sacroiliac joint stiffness with colour doppler imaging: a study on healthy subjects. *Eur J Radiol* 21:117–121, 1995.
70. Buyruk HM, Stam HJ, Snijders CJ, et al.: The use of color doppler imaging for the assessment of sacroiliac joint stiffness: a study on embalmed human pelvises. *Eur J Radiol* 21:112–116, 1995.
71. Vleeming A, Mooney V, Dorman T, et al.: *Movement, Stability and Low Back Pain.* Edinburgh: Churchill Livingstone, 1997.
72. Snijders CJ, Vleeming A, Stoeckart R, et al.: Biomechanics of the interface between spine and pelvis in different postures. In: Vleeming A, Mooney V, Dorman T et al., eds. *Movement, Stability and Low Back Pain.* Edinburgh: Churchill Livingstone, 1997:103.
73. Richardson CA, Jull GA, Hodges P, et al.: *Therapeutic Exercise for Spinal Segmental Stabilization in Low Back Pain.* London: Churchill Livingstone, 1999.
74. Hungerford B, Gilleard W, Lee D: Altered patterns of pelvic bone motion determined in subjects with posterior pelvic pain using skin markers. *Clin Biomech (Bristol, Avon)* 19:456–464, 2004.
75. Mens JMA, Vleeming A, Snijders CJ, et al.: The active straight-leg-raising test and mobility of the pelvic joints. *Eur Spine J* 8:468–473, 1999.
76. Mens JM, Vleeming A, Snijders CJ, et al.: Validity of the active straight leg raise test for measuring disease severity in patients with posterior pelvic pain after pregnancy. *Spine* 27:196–200, 2002.
77. Lee L, Lee DG: *The Pelvic Girdle*, 3rd ed. Edinburgh: Elsevier, 2004.
78. O'Sullivan P, Twomey L, Allison G: Evaluation of specific stabilizing exercise in the treatment of chronic low back pain with radiologic diagnosis of spondylolysis or spondylolisthesis. *Spine* 22:2959–2967, 1997.
79. Richardson C, Jull G: Muscle control-pain control. What exercises would you prescribe? *Man Ther* 1:2–10, 1995.
80. Snijders CJ, Vleeming A, Stoeckart R: Transfer of lumbosacral load to iliac bones and legs. Part 1: Biomechanics of self bracing of the sacroiliac joints and its significance for treatment and exercise. *Clin Biomech (Bristol, Avon)* 8:285–294, 1993.
81. Snijders CJ, Vleeming A, Stoeckart R, et al.: Biomechanical modelling of sacroiliac joint stability in different postures. *Spine: State Art Rev* 9:419–432, 1995.
82. Vleeming A, Snijders CJ, Stoeckart R, et al.: The role of the sacroiliac joints in coupling between spine, pelvis, legs and arms. In: Vleeming A, Mooney V, Dorman T et al., eds. *Movement, Stability and Low Back Pain.* Edinburgh: Churchill Livingstone, 1997:53.
83. Franke BA: Formative dynamics: The pelvic girdle. *J Man Manip Ther* 11:12–40, 2003.
84. Lee D, Lee L-J: Integrated, multimodal approach to the treatment of pelvic girdle pain and dysfunction. In: Magee DJ, Zachazewski JE, Quillen WS, eds. *Pathology and Intervention in Musculoskeletal Rehabilitation.* St. Louis, MI: Saunders, 2009:473–496.
85. Richardson CA, Snijders CJ, Hides JA, et al.: The relation between the transversus abdominis muscles, sacroiliac joint mechanics, and low back pain. *Spine* 27:399–405, 2002.
86. Hemborg B, Moritz U, Lowing H: Intra-abdominal pressure and trunk muscle activity during lifting. IV. The causal factors of the intra-abdominal pressure rise. *Scand J Rehabil Med* 17:25–38, 1985.
87. Hides JA, Stokes MJ, Saide M, et al.: Evidence of lumbar multifidus muscle wasting ipsilateral to symptoms in patients with acute/subacute low back pain. *Spine* 19:165–172, 1994.
88. Hides JA, Richardson CA, Jull GA: Multifidus muscle recovery is not automatic after resolution of acute, first-episode low back pain. *Spine* 21:2763–2769, 1996.
89. Danneels LA, Vanderstraeten GG, Cambier DC, et al.: CT imaging of trunk muscles in chronic low back pain patients and healthy control subjects. *Eur Spine J* : official publication of the European Spine Society, the European Spinal Deformity Society, and the European Section of the Cervical Spine Research Society 9:266–272, 2000.
90. Snijders CJ, Slagter AHE, van Strik R, et al.: Why leg-crossing? The influence of common postures on abdominal muscle activity. *Spine* 20:1989–1993, 1995.
91. Lee DG: Instability of the sacroiliac joint and the consequences for gait. In: Vleeming A, Mooney V, Dorman T et al., eds. *Movement, Stability and Low Back Pain.* Edinburgh: Churchill Livingstone, 1997:231.
92. Borenstein D, Wiesel SW: *Low Back Pain: Medical Diagnosis and Comprehensive Management.* Philadelphia, PA: WB Saunders, 1989.
93. Greenman PE: *Principles of Manual Medicine*, 2nd ed. Baltimore, MD: Williams & Wilkins, 1996.
94. Kirkaldy-Willis WH: *Managing Low Back Pain*, 2nd ed. New York, NY: Churchill Livingstone, 1988.
95. Palmer ML, Epler M: *Clinical Assessment Procedures in Physical Therapy.* Philadelphia, PA: JB Lippincott, 1990.
96. Beal MC: The sacroiliaca problem: Review of anatomy, mechanics, and diagnosis. *J Am Osteopath Assoc* 81:667–679, 1981.
97. Carmichael JP: Inter- and intra-examiner reliability of palpation for sacroiliac joint dysfunction. *J Manipulative Physiol Ther* 10:164–171, 1987.
98. Herzog W, Read L, Conway P, et al: Reliability of motion palpation procedures to detect sacro-iliac joint fixations. *J Manipulative Physiol Ther* 11:151–157, 1988.
99. Potter NA, Rothstein JM: Intertester reliability for selected clinical tests of the sacroiliac joint. *Phys Ther* 65:1671, 1985.
100. Levangie PK: The association between static pelvic asymmetry and low back pain. *Spine* 24:1234–1242, 1999.
101. Cibulka MT, Delitto A, Koldehoff RM: Changes in innominate tilt after manipulation of sacro-iliac joint in patients with low back pain. An experimental study. *Phys Ther* 68:1359–1363, 1988.
102. McCombe PF, Fairbank JCT, Cockersole BC, et al.: Reproducibility of physical signs in low back pain. *Spine* 14:908–918, 1989.
103. Kirkaldy-Willis WH, Hill RJ: A more precise diagnosis for low back pain. *Spine* 4:102–109, 1979.
104. Sturesson B, Uden A, Vleeming A: A radiostereometric analysis of the movements of the sacroiliac joints during the standing flexion test. *Spine* 25:364–368, 2000.
105. Laslett M, Williams M: The reliability of selected pain provocation tests for sacroiliac joint pathology. *Spine* 19:1243–1249, 1994.

106. Ostgaard HC: Lumbar back and posterior pelvic pain in pregnancy. In: Vleeming A, Mooney V, Dorman T et al., eds. *Movement, Stability, and Low Back Pain*. Edinburgh: Churchill Livingstone, 1997:411–420.
107. Van der Wurff P, Meyne W, Hagmeijer RHM: Clinical tests of the sacroiliac joint, a systematic methodological review. part 2: validity. *Man Ther* 5:89–96, 2000.
108. Hesch J: Evaluation and treatment of most common patterns of sacroiliac joint dysfunction. In: Vleeming A, Mooney V, Dorman T et al., eds. *Movement, Stability, and Low Back Pain*. Edinburgh: Churchill Livingstone, 1997:535–545.
109. Hungerford B, Gilleard W, Hodges P: Evidence of altered lumbopelvic muscle recruitment in the presence of sacroiliac joint pain. *Spine* 28:1593–600, 2003.
110. Daum WJ: The sacroiliac joint: an underappreciated pain generator. *Am J Orthop* 24:475–478, 1995.
111. Fortin JD, Aprill CN, Ponthieux B, et al.: Sacroiliac joint: pain referral maps upon applying a new injection/arthrography technique. Part II: Clinical evaluation. *Spine (Phila Pa 1976)* 19:1483–1489, 1994.
112. Fortin JD, Falco FJ: The Fortin finger test: an indicator of sacroiliac pain. *Am J Orthop* 26:477–480, 1997.
113. Fortin JD, Dwyer AP, West S, et al.: Sacroiliac joint pain referral maps upon applying a new injection/arthrography technique. Part I: Asymptomatic volunteers. *Spine* 19:1475–1482, 1994.
114. Hall H: A simple approach to back pain management. *Patient Care* 15:77–91, 1992.
115. LaBan MM, Meerschaert JR, Taylor RS, et al.: Symphyseal and sacroiliac joint pain associated with pubic symphysis instability. *Arch Phys Med Rehabil* 59:470–472, 1978.
116. Slipman CW, Jackson HB, Lipetz JS, et al.: Sacroiliac joint pain referral zones. *Arch Phys Med Rehabil* 81:334–338, 2000.
117. Kellgren JH: Observations on referred pain arising from muscle. *Clin Sci* 3:175–190, 1938.
118. Kellgren JH: On the distribution of pain arising from deep somatic structures with charts of segmental pain areas. *Clin Sci* 4:35–46, 1939.
119. McCall IW, Park WM, O'Brien JP: Induced pain referral from posterior lumbar elements in normal subjects. *Spine* 4:441–446, 1979.
120. Weiss JM: Pelvic floor myofascial trigger points: Manual therapy for interstitial cystitis and the urgency-frequency syndrome. *J Urol* 166:2226–2231, 2001.
121. Raz S, Smith RB: External sphincter spasticity syndrome in female patients. *J Urol* 115:443, 1976.
122. Lilius HG, Oravisto KJ, Valtonen EJ: Origin of pain in interstitial cystitis. *Scand J Urol Nephrol* 7:150, 1973.
123. Alderink GJ: The sacroiliac joint: Review of anatomy, mechanics, and function. *J Orthop Sports Phys Ther* 13:71–84, 1991.
124. DonTigny RL: Function and pathomechanics of the sacroiliac joint. A review. *Phys Ther* 65:35–44, 1985.
125. Fornasier VL, Horne JG: Metastases to the vertebral column. *Cancer* 36:590–594, 1975.
126. Boissonnault WG, Thein-Nissenbaum JM: Differential diagnosis of a sacral stress fracture. *J Orthop Sports Phys Ther* 32:613–621, 2002.
127. Brugger A: Die Funktionskrankheiten des Bewegungsapparates. *Funktionskrankheiton des Bewegungsapparates* 1:69–129, 1986.
128. Silverstolpe L: A pathological erector spinae reflex—a new sign of mechanical pelvic dysfunction. *J Man Med* 4:28, 1989.
129. Cibulka MT, Sinacore DR, Cromer GS, et al.: Unilateral hip rotation range of motion asymmetry in patients with sacroiliac joint regional pain. *Spine* 23:1009–1015, 1998.
130. Papadopoulos SM, McGillicuddy JE, Albers JW: Unusual cause of piriformis muscle syndrome. *Arch Neurol* 47:1144–1146, 1990.
131. Vandertop WP, Bosma WJ: The piriformis syndrome. A case report. *J Bone Joint Surg Am* 73A:1095–1097, 1991.
132. Dunn EJ, Bryan DM, Nugent JT, et al.: Pyogenic infections of the sacroiliac joint. *Clin Orthop* 118:113–117, 1976.
133. Mens JM, Vleeming A, Snijders CJ, et al.: Reliability and validity of the active straight leg raise test in posterior pelvic pain since pregnancy. *Spine* 26:1167–1171, 2001.
134. Cyriax J: *Textbook of Orthopaedic Medicine, Diagnosis of Soft Tissue Lesions*, 8th ed. London: Bailliere Tindall, 1982.
135. Van Deursen LL, Patijn J, Ockhuysen AL, et al.: The value of some clinical tests of the sacroiliac joint. *J Man Med* 5:96–99, 1990.
136. Broadhurst NA, Bond MJ: Pain provocation tests for the assessment of sacroiliac joint dysfunction. *J Spinal Disord* 11:341–345, 1998.
137. Albert H, Godskesen M, Westergaard J: Evaluation of clinical tests used in classification procedures in pregnancy-related pelvic joint pain. *Eur Spine J* : official publication of the European Spine Society, the European Spinal Deformity Society, and the European Section of the Cervical Spine Research Society 9:161–166, 2000.
138. Lee DG: *A Workbook of Manual Therapy Techniques for the Upper Extremity*, 2nd ed. Delta, BC: DOPC, 1991.
139. Lee DG: Clinical manifestations of pelvic girdle dysfunction. In: Palastanga N, Boyling JD, eds. *Grieve's Modern Manual Therapy: The Vertebral Column*, 2nd ed. Edinburgh: Churchill Livingstone, 1994:453–462.
140. Dreyfuss P, Dryer S, Griffin J, et al.: Positive sacroiliac screening tests in asymptomatic adults. *Spine (Phila Pa 1976)* 19:1138–1143, 1994.
141. Levangie PK: Four clinical tests of sacroiliac joint dysfunction: the association of test results with innominate torsion among patients with and without low back pain. *Phys Ther* 79:1043–1057, 1999.
142. Riddle DL, Freburger JK: Evaluation of the presence of sacroiliac joint region dysfunction using a combination of tests: a multicenter intertester reliability study. *Phys Ther* 82:772–781, 2002.
143. Cipriano JJ: *Photographic Manual of Regional Orthopaedic and Neurological Tests*, 3rd ed. Baltimore, MD: Williams & Wilkins, 1997.
144. Leboeuf C: The sensitivity and specificity of seven lumbo-pelvic orthopedic tests and the arm-fossa test. *J Manipulative Physiol Ther* 13:138–143, 1990.
145. Cibulka MT, Koldehoff R: Clinical usefulness of a cluster of sacroiliac joint tests in patients with and without low back pain. *J Orthop Sports Phys Ther* 29:83–89; discussion 90–92, 1999.
146. Bergmann TF, Peterson DH, Lawrence DJ: *Chiropractic Technique: Principles and Procedures*. New York, NY: Churchill Livingstone, 1993.
147. Hanada E, Kirby RL, Mitchell M, et al.: Measuring leg-length discrepancy by the "iliac crest palpation and book correction" method: reliability and validity. *Arch Phys Med Rehabil* 82:938–942, 2001.
148. Greenwood MJ, Erhard R, Jones DL: Differential diagnosis of the hip vs. lumbar spine: five case reports. *J Orthop Sports Phys Ther* 27:308–315, 1998.
149. Ostgaard HC, Zetherstrom G, Roos-Hansson E: The posterior pelvic pain provocation test in pregnant women. *Eur Spine J* 3:258–260, 1994.
150. Hoppenfeld S: *Physical Examination of the Hip and Pelvis, Physical Examination of the Spine and Extremities*. East Norwalk, CT: Appleton-Century-Crofts, 1976:143.
151. Yeoman W: The relation of arthritis of the sacro-iliac joint to sciatica, with an analysis of 100 cases. *Lancet* 2:1119–1122, 1928.
152. Laslett M: Evidence-based diagnosis and treatment of the painful sacroiliac joint. *J Man Manip Ther* 16:142–152, 2008.
153. Heuft-Dorenbosch L, Weijers R, Landewe R, et al.: Magnetic resonance imaging changes of sacroiliac joints in patients with recent-onset inflammatory back pain: inter-reader reliability and prevalence of abnormalities. *Arthritis Res Ther* 8:R11, 2006.
154. Madsen KB, Schiottz-Christensen B, Jurik AG: Prognostic significance of magnetic resonance imaging changes of the sacroiliac joints in spondyloarthritis–a followup study. *J Rheumatol* 37:1718–1727, 2010.
155. Slipman CW, Sterenfeld EB, Chou LH, et al.: The value of radionuclide imaging in the diagnosis of sacroiliac joint syndrome. *Spine* 21:2251–2254, 1996.
156. Fortin JD, Washington WJ, Falco FJ: Three pathways between the sacroiliac joint and neural structures. *AJNR Am J Neuroradiol* 20:1429–1434, 1999.
157. van Wingerden JP, Vleeming A, Buyruk HM, et al.: Stabilization of the sacroiliac joint in vivo: verification of muscular contribution to force closure of the pelvis. *Eur Spine J* : official publication of the European Spine Society, the European Spinal Deformity Society, and the European Section of the Cervical Spine Research Society 13:199–205, 2004.
158. Klaffs CE, Arnheim DD: *Modern Principles of Athletic Training*. St Louis, MO: CV Mosby, 1989.
159. Lehmann JF, Silverman DR, Baum BA, et al.: Temperature distributions in the human thigh, produced by infrared, hot pack and microwave applications. *Arch Phys Med Rehabil* 47:291–299, 1966.
160. Prentice WE: Using therapeutic modalities in rehabilitation. In: Prentice WE, Voight ML, eds. *Techniques in Musculoskeletal Rehabilitation*. New York, NY: McGraw-Hill, 2001:289–303.
161. Cibulka MT, Koldehoff RM: Leg length disparity and its effect on sacroiliac joint dysfunction. *Clin Manage* 6:10–11, 1986.
162. Vleeming A, Buyruk HM, Stoeckart R, et al.: An integrated therapy from peripartum pelvic instability: A study of the biomechanical effects of pelvic belts. *Am J Obstet Gynecol* 166:1243–1247, 1992.
163. Fitch RR: Mechanical lesions of the sacroiliac joints. *Am J Orthop Surg* 6:693–698, 1908.

164. Fortin JD: Sacroiliac joint dysfunction. A new perspective. *J Back Musculoskel Rehabil* 3:31–43, 1993.
165. Greenman PE: Clinical aspects of the sacroiliac joint in walking. In: Vleeming A, Mooney V, Dorman T et al., eds. *Movement, Stability and Low Back Pain*. Edinburgh: Churchill Livingstone, 1997:235–241.
166. McGill SM: The biomechanics of low back injury: implications on current practice in industry and the clinic. *J Biomech* 30:465–475, 1997.
167. Cole AJ, Farrell JP, Stratton SA: Functional rehabilitation of cervical spine athletic injuries. In: Kibler BW, Herring JA, Press JM, eds. *Functional Rehabilitation of Sports and Musculoskeletal Injuries*. Gaithersburg, MD: Aspen, 1998:127–148.
168. Lee DG: Techniques and tools for addressing barriers in the lumbopelvic-hip complex. In: Lee DG, ed. *The pelvic girdle: An integration of clinical expertise and research (ed 4)*. Edinburgh: Churchill Livingstone, 2010:283-323
169. Hoek van Dijke GA, Snijders CJ, Stoeckart R, et al.: A biomechanical model on muscle forces in the transfer of spinal load to the pelvis and legs. *J Biomech* 32:927–933, 1999.
170. Snijders CJ, Bakker MP, Vleeming A, et al.: Oblique abdominal muscle activity in standing and in sitting on hard and soft seats. *Clin Biomech* 10:73–78, 1995.
171. Snijders CJ, Ribbers MTLM, de Bakker JV, et al.: EMG recordings of abdominal and back muscles in various standing postures: Validation of a biomechanical model on sacroiliac joint stability. *J Electromyogr Kinesiol* 8:205–214, 1998.
172. Gladman DD: Clinical aspects of the spondyloarthropathies. *Am J Med Sci* 316:234–238, 1998.
173. Jajic Z, Jajic I, Grazio S: Radiological changes of the symphysis in ankylosing spondylitis. *Acta Radiol* 41:307–309, 2000.
174. Jajic I: *Ankylosing Spondylitis*. Zagreb: S?kolska knjiga, 1978.
175. Ashby EC: Chronic obscure groin pain is commonly caused by enthesopathy: 'Tennis elbow' of the groin. *Br J Surg* 81:1632–1634, 1994.
176. Martens MA, Hansen L, Mulier JC: Adductor tendinitis and musculus rectus abdominis tendonopathy. *Am J Sports Med* 15:353–356, 1987.
177. Zimmerman G: Groin pain in athletes. *Aust Fam Physician* 17:1046–1052, 1988.
178. Bradshaw C, McCrory P, Bell S, et al.: Obturator neuropathy a cause of chronic groin pain in athletes. *Am J Sports Med* 25:402–408, 1997.
179. Thompson WAL, Kopell HP: Peripheral entrapment neuropathies of the upper extremity. *N Engl J Med* 260:1261–1265, 1959.
180. Middleton R, Carlisle R: The spectrum of osteitis pubis. *Compr Ther* 19:99–105, 1993.
181. Wiley JJ: Traumatic osteitis pubis: the gracilis syndrome. *Am J Sports Med* 11:360–363, 1983.
182. Fricker PA, Tauton JE, Ammann W: Osteitis pubis in athletes. Infection, inflammation, or injury? *Sports Med* 12:266–279, 1991.
183. Barry NN, McGuire JL: Overuse syndromes in adult athletes. *Rheum Dis Clin North Am* 22:515–530, 1996.
184. Grace JN, Sim FH, Shives TC, et al.: Wedge resection of the symphysis pubis for the treatment of osteitis pubis. *J Bone Joint Surg* 71A:358–364, 1989.
185. Andrews SK, Carek PJ: Osteitis pubis: a diagnosis for the family physician. *J Am Board Fam Pract* 11:291–295, 1998.
186. Holt MA, Keene JS, Graf BK, et al.: Treatment of osteitis pubis in athletes. *Am J Sports Med* 23:601–606, 1995.
187. Snow RE, Neubert AG: Peripartum pubic symphysis separation: a case series and review of the literature. *Obstet Gynecol Surv* 52:438–443, 1997.
188. Bellabarba C, Stewart JD, Ricci WM, et al.: Midline sagittal sacral fractures in anterior-posterior compression pelvic ring injuries. *J Orthop Trauma* 17:32–37, 2003.
189. Hall J, Cleland JA, Palmer JA: The effects of manual physical therapy and therapeutic exercise on peripartum posterior pelvic pain: Two case reports. *J Manl Manip Ther* 13:94–102, 2005.
190. Fast A, Shapiro D, Ducommun EJ, et al.: Low-back pain in pregnancy. *Spine* 12:368–371, 1987.
191. Fast A, Weiss L, Ducommun EJ, et al.: Low back pain in pregnancy. Abdominal muscles, sit-up performance and back pain. *Spine* 15:28–30, 1990.
192. Hainline B: Low-back pain in pregnancy. *Adv Neurol* 64:65–76, 1994.
193. McFarland EG, Giangarra C: Sacral stress fractures in athletes. *Clin Orthop* 329:240–243, 1996.
194. Shah MK, Stewart GW: Sacral stress fractures: an unusual cause of low back pain in an athlete. *Spine* 27:E104–E108, 2002.
195. Holtzhausen LM, Noakes TD: Stress fracture of the sacrum in two distance runners. *Clin J Sports Med* 2:139–142, 1992.
196. Volpin G, Milgrom C, Goldsher D, et al.: Stress fractures of the sacrum following strenuous activity. *Clin Orthop* 243:184–188, 1989.
197. Atwell EA, Jackson DW: Stress fractures of the sacrum in runners. *Am J Sports Med* 19:531–533, 1991.
198. Cooper KL, Beabout JAW, Swee RG: Insufficiency fractures of the sacrum. *Radiology* 156:15–20, 1985.
199. Byrnes DP, Russo GL, Ducker TB, et al.: Sacral fractures and neurological damage. *J Neurosurg* 47:459–462, 1977.
200. Keats TE: *Radiology of Musculoskeletal Stress Injury*. Chicago, IL: Year Book Medical Publishers, 1990.

SECTION VI SPECIAL CONSIDERATIONS

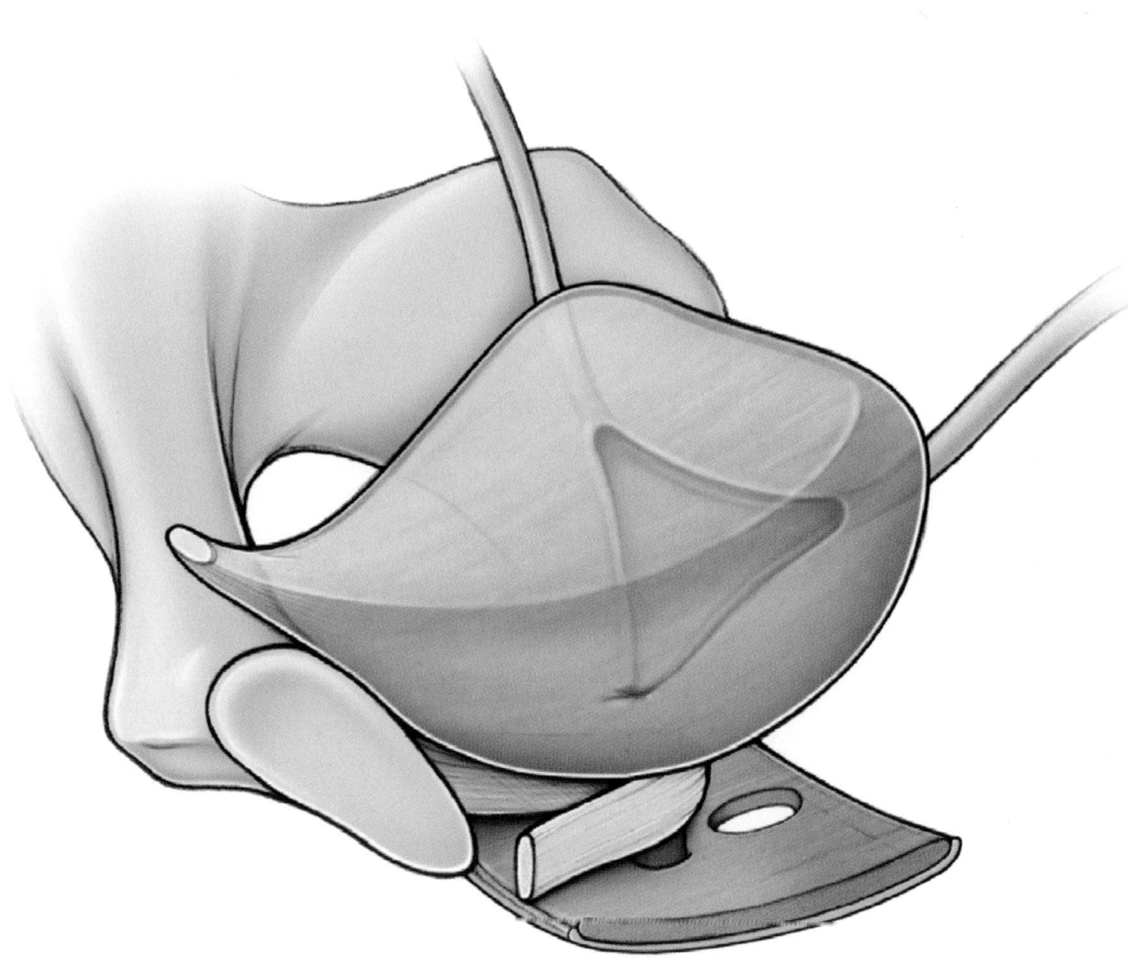

CHAPTER 30 Special Populations

CHAPTER OBJECTIVES

At the completion of this chapter, the reader will be able to:

1. Discuss the physical therapy role with a variety of orthopaedic subtypes and the challenges each presents.
2. Describe the various pathologies for these populations in terms of the presentation and the role that physical therapy plays.
3. Outline the differences between a congenital condition and an acquired condition.
4. Describe the normal aging process as it relates to orthopaedics.
5. Outline the various theories of aging.
6. Describe the common pathological conditions and functional limitations associated with the geriatric population.
7. Describe some of the conditions that can affect women's health.
8. Describe the physiologic changes that occur during pregnancy within the various bodily systems.
9. Describe the physical therapy interventions for pregnancy-related dysfunctions.
10. Describe the complications related to breast-cancer-related lymphedema.

OVERVIEW

There are a number of population subtypes that require special consideration in terms of the orthopaedic examination and intervention. These include pediatrics and geriatrics, and the whole spectrum of women's health. Each of these populations is described in this chapter.

PEDIATRICS

The term pediatric refers to the 0- to 21-year age range during which an individual undergoes many changes while aging, evolving, and maturing. During the preschool years, physical growth, neurologic growth, and maturation are quite rapid and apparent, with new skills being acquired at a quick pace.[1] This process continues throughout the middle years (ages 6–11) at a somewhat slower pace. As a child enters puberty, rapid development of physical and sexual characteristics become more apparent and is accompanied by important psychosocial development. It is important to remember that chronologic age does not necessarily correlate well with many physiologic and somatic changes.

CLINICAL PEARL

A typical adult has a smaller surface area-to-mass ratio and a lower metabolic rate than a child. These discrepancies result in a greater transfer of heat and a greater challenge to the thermoregulatory system, respectively, in the pediatric population.

The major characteristics of somatic and skeletal growth and maturation during adolescence are outlined in Table 30-1. In addition, the following differences exist between the adult and the pediatric patient:[2]

- ***Cardiovascular system.*** The pediatric heart is smaller than that of the mature adult, resulting in a smaller capacity as a reservoir for blood, and thus a lower stroke volume at all levels of exercise, which is compensated for with an increased heart rate. As with the adult patient, systolic blood pressure rises during exercise in the pediatric patient, but the elevation is less. Finally, the thoracic cavity is obviously smaller in the younger child than that of the mature adult, resulting in the pediatric patient demonstrating a smaller vital capacity than the adult and an elevated resting respiration rate.[3] The red blood cell count for young boys and girls are similar with comparable abilities to carry oxygen to exercising organs. After menarche, however, females demonstrate lower blood volume and fewer red blood cells with a resultant decreased oxygen carrying capacity and a lower mean blood pressure.[4] These differences result in the following responses to exercise in the pediatric patient:
  - Until 12 years, absolute maximal oxygen uptake (VO_{2max}) values increase at the same rate in both

TABLE 30-1 Somatic and Skeletal Growth and Maturation During Adolescence	
Characteristic	**Description**
Weight	In males, the average weight gain during its peak is approximately 9 kg per year with a range of 6–12.5 kg per year. The peaks of growth spurts in height, weight, and muscle occur at the same time In females the average weight gain during its peak is approximately 8 kg per year with a range of 5.5–10.5 kg per year. The peaks of growth spurts in height, weight, and muscle occur in sequence in that order
Height	In general, linear growth first occurs in the lower extremities, followed by the torso and then the upper extremities Males typically reach their peak height velocity (PHV) by 14 years. The growth of the shoulders in males is the most noticeable change Females typically reach their PHV by 12 years. The growth of the hip and pelvis in females are the most notable changes
Body composition	In general, both males and females tend to increase both fat mass as well as fat-free mass from the early to middle adolescent years. However, while males may show a transient decrease in fat accumulation in the extremities during PHV, females continue to gain fat through late adolescence. The pattern of growth of fat-free mass is similar to that noted for growth in height and weight
Flexibility	As skeletal growth precedes that of musculotendinous growth during the early to middle adolescence, there is a relative decrease in musculotendinous flexibility in some adolescents, especially males. Decreased flexibility is particularly noticeable in the hamstrings and ankle dorsiflexors
Muscle growth and strength	Although muscle growth and strength is seen in both males and females, it is relatively more pronounced in males compared with females due to androgens.
Bone mass	The female skeleton generally grows and fully matures (i.e., growth plate fusion) before the male skeleton. The largest percentage of lifetime acquisition of bone mineral density occurs during the second decade of life. Peak bone mass during adolescence is determined by genetic influences, exercise, calcium intake, and hormonal status

Data from Greydanus DE, Pratt HD: Adolescent growth and development, and sport participation. In: Patel DR, Greydanus DE, Baker RJ, eds. *Pediatric Practice: Sports Medicine*. New York: McGraw-Hill, 2009:15–25.

genders, although boys have higher values as early as 5 years. VO_{2max} increases concomitantly with growth until 18 years in boys and 14 years in girls.

- The pattern of relative magnitudes of cardiovascular and ventilatory responses to progressive and sustained dynamic exercise appears to be qualitatively similar between adults and children.
- Children rely more on oxidative rather than anaerobic metabolism compared to adults.
- Children demonstrate greater energy expenditure during weight-bearing activities such as running and walking compared to adults.

▸ ***Musculoskeletal system.*** Young children possess muscle fiber numbers, types, and distribution similar to that of adults. There is an increase in muscle hypertrophy during adolescence as a result of increased androgens. In addition, agility, motor coordination, power, and speed also show improvement during adolescence. There are a number of structural differences between the adult and pediatric patient:

- In the adolescent, growth cartilage is present at the epiphyseal plate, the joint surface (articular cartilage), and the apophysis. The epiphyseal plate or growth plate is divided into zones differentiated from one another via structure and function (see Chap. 1). Growing bone is the weak musculoskeletal link in the young athlete. Similar physical demands that can result in muscle strain or ligament sprain in the skeletally mature patient may result in an epiphyseal plate injury in a young patient. Two factors that impact epiphyseal plate injury are (1) the ability of the growth plate to resist failure and (2) the forces applied to bone or the stresses induced in the growth plate. The majority of epiphyseal fractures are due to high-velocity injuries.
- A certain amount of load is necessary for normal bone growth and remodeling. In most long bones, epiphysis is at least partially ossified at an early age. However in certain areas of the body (e.g., ischial tuberosity, iliac crest, base of the fifth metatarsal), the epiphysis may not become ossified until the near end of the final growth spurt. Most of the bone mineral density is acquired during the adolescent years and bone mass may fail to accrue optimally because of dieting and weight loss. Because the strength development of bones lags behind that of ligaments and tendons, there is an increased risk of tendon or bone avulsion at the apophyseal insertion compared to a ligament injury.

CLINICAL PEARL

Orthopaedic injuries commonly seen in the pediatric population include Osgood–Schlatter (OS) disease, spondylolysis, stress fractures, Little League elbow, and growth plate disorders.

Examination of the Pediatric Patient

In addition to the areas typically covered in the orthopaedic examination outlined in Chapter 4, a number of additional factors must be considered in the pediatric population. For example, when taking the history of a pediatric patient, the clinician should pay particular attention to the following:[2]

- ***Current life circumstances.*** The pediatric patient's current health, attitudes and values of the child's immediate family, and acculturation of the patient.
- ***Gender.*** Females and males develop differently, particularly during adolescence (Table 30-2).
- ***Health history.*** Health and nutrition history, repeated hospitalizations, and so on.
- ***Developmental history.*** The pediatric patient's past rate of achievement of developmental milestones, events that might have had profound effects on the patient either physically or psychologically.
- ***Extrapersonal interactions.*** The reaction of the pediatric patient to the treating clinician and the conditions under which the pediatric patient is observed.
- Age-related changes in muscle and muscle performance.
- ***The developing skeletal system.*** Examination of the pediatric patient requires an understanding of, and an awareness of, the timing of growth center appearance and epiphyseal closure. For example, the sequence and average timing of growth center appearance at the elbow are as follows[5]:
  - ***Capitellum.*** Female, 4 months; male, 5 months.
  - ***Medial epicondyle.*** Female, 5 years; male, 7 years.
  - ***Trochlea.*** Female, 8 years; male, 9 years.
  - ***Lateral epicondyle.*** Female, 11 years; male, 12 years.

Epiphyseal closure at the elbow occurs sequentially, first in the distal humerus, with the capitellum, lateral epicondyle, and trochlea fusing together at puberty (female, 14 years and male, 17 years), then fusing with the shaft.[5] The medial epicondyle fuses later (female, 15 years and male, 18 years). The radial head and olecranon close at 14 years in females and 15 years in males.[5]

Growing musculoskeletal tissue is innately predisposed to specific injuries that vary greatly from injuries sustained by their skeletally mature counterparts. Most of this growth occurs in two phases from birth to adulthood. There is a rapid gain in growth in infancy and early childhood that slows down during middle childhood. The second rapid increase in growth occurs during adolescence. An injury that occurs during one of these phases, which is significant enough to interrupt the growth process, can present serious challenges.

TABLE 30-2 Differences in Adolescent Females Compared to Males

Anatomic	Physiologic
Reduced muscle fiber size	Increased percentage of body fat (10–15 pounds more)
Wide hips with narrower shoulders	Women have 40– 45 less pounds of fat-free weight (bone, muscle, organs)
Shorter height (3–4 in. on average)	Basal metabolic rate is relatively lower
Relatively smaller total articular surface area	Reduced testosterone levels
Relatively more fat around the thighs and hips	Skeletal maturation occurs earlier
Heart size and volume are smaller	Aerobic capacity is lower
Lung volume is smaller	Vital capacity is less

CLINICAL PEARL

The main goals of a physical therapy intervention in pediatric rehabilitation are to reduce barriers limiting the performance of daily routines and to facilitate the successful integration of the child into the home, play, and school environments. Therapeutic exercise that is prescribed for the pediatric patient must be creative, and attempts must be made to try to make exercise fun in order to increase compliance. In addition, special consideration must be given when prescribing exercise due to the number of growth changes that are occurring:[6]

- ***≤7 years.*** Introduction to basic exercises, teaching correct technique using low-volume and little or no weight. For example, 1–3 sets of 6–15 repetitions.[7]
- ***8–10 years.*** Gradual increase of the number of exercises and progressive loading using simple exercises. Loads should be increased in 1- to 3-pound increments after the child can perform 15 repetitions with proper form.[7] Resistance equipment that can be adapted to the size of child should only be used.
- ***11–13 years.*** Teach all basic exercise techniques and continue progressive loading. More advanced techniques/exercises can be introduced with little or no resistance.
- ***14–15 years.*** More advanced youth programs and resistance exercise with sport-specific components.
- ***≥16 years.*** Entry-level adult programs

ACQUIRED ORTHOPAEDIC CONDITIONS

Skeletal Fracture

The mechanical properties and healing qualities of skeletal bone are described in Chapters 1 and 2, respectively. In the pediatric population, the metaphysic–physis junction is an anatomic point of weakness. Fractures of bone in pediatric patients may be due to direct trauma, such as a blow, or indirect trauma, such as a fall on the outstretched hand (FOOSH injury), or a twisting injury. Three types of fractures occur more commonly in the pediatric population:

- ***Greenstick.*** A type of simple fracture in which only one side of the bone is fractured while the opposite side is bent.

Because the bones in a pediatric patient have not fully developed, they are less rigid and brittle. This type of fracture tends to heal faster than other types.

- ***Avulsion.*** Avulsion occurs when a piece of bone attached to a tendon or ligament is torn away. In the younger population, ligaments and tendons are stronger than bone. When changes in muscle length do not match the changes in long-bone growth, tensile loads placed within the muscle predispose the pediatric patient to injury. Lower extremity avulsion fractures outnumber avulsion fractures of the upper extremity. Common sites of avulsion fracture in the lower extremity include the anterior superior iliac spine (ASIS), anterior inferior iliac spine (AIIS), ischial tuberosity, and the base of the fifth metatarsal. Common sites of avulsion fracture in the upper extremity include the medial humeral epicondyle and the proximal humerus. If a medial epicondyle avulsion fracture is suspected, it is important to assess the ulnar nerve, and for the presence of point tenderness of the medial epicondyle, swelling, ecchymosis, and valgus instability.
- ***Growth plate (physeal).*** This type of fracture may be defined as a disruption in the cartilaginous physis of long bones that may or may not involve epiphyseal or metaphyseal bone. Injuries to the physes are more likely to occur in the pediatric population, in part due to the greater structural strength and integrity of the ligaments and joint capsules than of the growth plates and the fact that the physes of an adult have ossified. Growth plate fractures can have severe consequences because of the potential for growth plate closure, which inhibits future growth resulting in limb length discrepancies. Conversely, an injury near, but not at, the physis can stimulate increased bone growth.

The Salter and Harris classification is the preferred and accepted standard in North America for classifying physeal fracture patterns:[3]

- ***Type I.*** This occurs due to shearing forces in which there is complete separation of the epiphysis without fracture of the bone. These fractures are most commonly seen in the very young patient when the epiphyseal plate is relatively thick.
- ***Type II.*** This is the most common type of growth plate fracture resulting from shearing and bending forces. The line of separation traverses a variable distance along the epiphyseal plate and then makes its way through a segment of the bony metaphysis that results in a triangular-shaped metaphyseal fragment.
- ***Type III.*** This typically results from shearing forces and results in intra-articular fractures from the joint surface to the deep zone of the growth plate and then along the growth plate to its periphery. These fractures are typically limited to the proximal tibial/distal femoral epiphysis and can result from valgus loading of the knee, which is frequently encountered in contact and collision sports.
- ***Type IV.*** These are intra-articular fractures that result from shearing forces. These fractures extend from the joint surface to the epiphysis across the entire thickness of the growth plate and then through a segment of the bony metaphysis.
- ***Type V.*** These types of fractures, which are due to a crushing mechanism, are relatively uncommon.

CLINICAL PEARL

The most common of the Salter Harris fractures is type II, followed by types I, III, IV, and V.

Clinical Findings

The most common clinical presentation with a pediatric fracture is pain, weakness, and functional loss of the involved area. The most common areas for epiphyseal fracture include the distal radius and the medial epicondyle, the proximal humerus, and the proximal tibia/distal femoral.

Intervention

In most cases, the medical management of a fracture involves immobilization through casting, splints, or surgical fixation to allow full healing to occur. Pediatric fractures tend to heal faster than an equivalent one in an adult. This can be advantageous: Children typically require shorter immobilization times. A disadvantage, however, is that any malpositioned fragments become immovable or fixed much earlier than in adults (3– 5 days in a young child, 5– 7 days in an older child, as opposed to 8–10 days in an adult). However, the normal process of bone remodeling in a child may correct malalignment, making near-anatomic reductions less important in children than in adults. Remodeling can be expected if the patient has two or more years of bone growth remaining. Rotational deformity remodels poorly, if at all, and is therefore corrected by surgical reduction. A further complication is that pediatric fractures may stimulate longitudinal growth of the bone, making the bone longer than it would have been had it not been injured. This is particularly true for fractures of the femoral or tibial shaft.

Children tolerate prolonged immobilization much better than adults, and disabling stiffness or loss of range of motion (ROM) is distinctly unusual after pediatric fractures. Physical therapy, if needed, typically begins after the immobilization period, and depending on the type and location of the fracture, it can involve any or all of the following:

- Pain management techniques including the use of noncontraindicated electrotherapeutic modalities (see Chap. 8) and manual techniques, including joint mobilizations.
- ROM exercises, following the hierarchy of progression outlined in Chapter 13.
- Strengthening exercises, beginning with isometrics and progressing using the hierarchy of progression outlined in Chapter 12.
- Gait and/or crutch training with an appropriate assistive device and following the prescribed prescription for weight bearing (see Chap. 6).
- Proprioception exercises for balance and coordination (see Chap. 14).
- Functional training including adaptive, supportive, or protective devices and activities of daily living (ADLs) and self-care.

- Patient and family education to decrease the risk of re-injury and to promote healing.

Juvenile Rheumatoid Arthritis

Juvenile rheumatoid arthritis (JRA) is a group of diseases that are manifested by chronic joint inflammation[8,9]. The exact etiology of JRA is unclear, but the prevailing theory is that it is an autoimmune inflammatory disorder, activated by an external trigger, in a genetically predisposed host. JRA is defined as persistent arthritis, lasting at least 6 weeks, in one or more joints in a child younger than 16 years of age, when all other causes of arthritis have been excluded. The clinical findings and manifestations of JRA are outlined in Chapter 5.

A detailed physical examination by a physician is a critical tool in diagnosing JRA to help rule out other causes. Medical care of children with JRA must be provided in the context of a team-based approach, considering all aspects of their illness (e.g., physical functioning in school and psychological adjustment to disease).

Intervention

Physical therapists are essential members of the rheumatology team that includes the rheumatologist, nurse, occupational therapist, ophthalmologist, orthopedist, and pediatrician.[10] Other specialists, including cardiologists, dermatologists, orthotists, psychologists, and social workers, provide occasional consultation as needed. The physical therapy examination is performed to determine the relationship between the impairments and observed or reported activity restrictions. The plan of care (POC) is designed to reduce current impairments, maintain or improve function, prevent or minimize secondary problems, and provide education and support to the child and family. Specific interventions can include any or all of the following:

- ROM and stretching exercises.
  - Acute stage: passive and active assisted to avoid joint compression.
  - Subacute/chronic stages: active exercises.
- Strengthening: avoid substitutions, minimize instability, atrophy, deformity, pain, and injury.
  - Acute and subacute stages: isometric exercises progressing cautiously to resistive.
  - Chronic stage: concentric exercises.
- Endurance exercises: encouraging exercise by using fun and recreational activities, swimming.
- Joint protection strategies and body mechanics education.
  - Mobility assistive devices.
  - Rest, as needed—balance rest with activity by using splinting (articular resting).
  - Posture and positioning to maintain joint ROM.
  - Patients should spend 20 minutes/day in the prone position to stretch the hip and knee flexors
  - Avoidance of high-impact activities.
  - Assess leg length discrepancy in standing and avoid scoliosis.
- Therapeutic modalities for pain control.
- Instructions on the wearing of warm pajamas, sleeping bag, electric blanket.

Idiopathic Scoliosis

The overall contour of the normal vertebral column in the coronal plane is straight. In contrast, the contour of the sagittal plane changes with development (see Chap. 22)[11–24]. Scoliosis represents a progressive disturbance of the intercalated series of spinal segments that produces a three-dimensional deformity (lateral curvature and vertebral rotation) of the spine. Despite an extensive amount of research devoted to discovering the cause of idiopathic scoliosis, the mechanics and specific etiology are not clearly understood, hence the name. It is known, however, that there is a familial prevalence of idiopathic scoliosis.

Clinical Findings

Using the James classification system, scoliosis has three age distinctions. These distinctions, though seemingly arbitrary, have prognostic significance.

- ***Infantile idiopathic.*** Children diagnosed when they are younger than 3 years, usually manifesting shortly after birth. Although 80–90% of these curves spontaneously resolve, many of the remainder of cases will progress throughout childhood, resulting in severe deformity. In the most common curve pattern (right thoracic), the right shoulder is consistently rotated forward and the medial border of the right scapula protrudes posteriorly.
- ***Juvenile idiopathic.*** Children diagnosed when they are 3–9 years. This type is found more frequently in girls than boys, and individuals that develop this condition are generally at a high risk for progression to more severe curves.
- ***Adolescent idiopathic.*** Manifesting at or around the onset of puberty and accounting for approximately 80% of all cases of idiopathic scoliosis.

The following are the main factors that influence the probability of progression in the skeleton of the immature patient:

- The younger the patient at diagnosis, the greater the risk of progression.
- Double-curve patterns have a greater risk for progression than single-curve patterns.
- Curves with greater magnitude are at a greater risk to progress.
- Risk of progression in females is approximately 10 times than that of males with curves of comparable magnitude.
- Greater risk of progression is present when curves develop before menarche.

Scoliosis is generally described by the location of the curve or curves. One should also describe whether the convexity of the curve points to the right or left. If there is a double curve, each curve must be described and measured. As the disease progresses, the spinous processes of the vertebrae in the area of the major curve rotate toward the concavity of the curve. On the concave side of the curve, the ribs are close together. On the convex side, they are widely separated. As the vertebral bodies rotate, the spinous processes deviate more and more to the concave side and the ribs follow the rotation of the vertebrae. The ribs on the convex side are rotated more posteriorly, causing the characteristic rib hump seen in thoracic scoliosis. The ribs on the concave side are rotated more anteriorly. Because the onset and progression of scoliosis (until skeletal maturity) are generally asymptomatic, it can develop undetected without close examination.

The significant incidence of scoliosis in the adolescent population has prompted the creation of school screening programs in all 50 states. Visual observation is used during the Adam's forward bending test, which involves asking the patient to bend forward at the waist as though touching his or her toes while the clinician, who is standing behind the patient, looks along the line at the back and determines whether one side is higher than the other. If scoliosis is suspected, the magnitude of a rib hump is quantified by placing a scoliometer (an inclinometer) over the spinous process at the apex of the curve during the Adam's forward bending test to measure the angle of trunk rotation as the patient bends forward. During the physical examination by the patient's physician, a determination is made as to whether the deformity is structural (cannot be corrected with active or passive movement and there is rotation toward the convexity of the curve) or nonstructural (fully corrects clinically and radiographically with trunk side bending toward the apex of the curve and lacks vertebral rotation). Nonstructural scoliotic curves can result from length–length discrepancies, muscle disuse/overuse, habitual postures, and muscle guarding.

Height measurements are taken in sitting and in standing. Changes in sitting height can be less than changes in standing height and give a better estimate of truncal growth rate. Trunk compensation is typically assessed using a plumb-line, and a radiographic leg length measurement is also obtained.

CLINICAL PEARL

- Radiographs are usually only considered when a patient has a curve that might require treatment or could progress to a stage requiring treatment. The radiographs determine the location, type, and magnitude of the curve (using the Cobb method), as well as skeletal age. Alternatively, a noninvasive technique called Moiré topography can be used, in which light is projected through grids onto the back of the patient to assess structural asymmetry.

Skeletal maturity is determined using the Risser sign, which is a measurement of the progressive ossification from anterolaterally to posteromedially in the iliac apophysis. Once a child reaches a Grade 5 on the Risser scale, his or her scoliotic curve will stabilize. A child with idiopathic scoliosis usually progresses from a Risser grade 1 to a grade 5 over a 2-year period.

CLINICAL PEARL

If scoliosis is neglected, the curves may progress and create significant physical deformity. Severe curves can result in cardiopulmonary problems necessitating pulmonary function tests due to the resultant rib cage restrictions and decreased chest wall expansion.

Most curves can be treated nonoperatively through observation with periodic radiographs to check for the presence of curve progression. However, approximately 60% of curvatures in rapidly growing prepubertal children typically progress, and may require bracing (Boston, or custom thoracolumbosacral orthosis) or surgery.

CLINICAL PEARL

A child with idiopathic scoliosis who is skeletally immature (with a Risser sign of 0, 1, or 2) and has a curve from 25 to 45 degrees is typically prescribed an orthosis. Theoretically, curve progression is prevented by muscle contractions responding to the presence of the orthosis. Exercises to be performed while wearing the orthosis, (e.g., pelvic tilts, thoracic flexion, and lateral shifts), are often taught to patients to improve the active forces, although there is little evidence to support this.

Intervention

Physical therapy intervention for scoliosis is based on the skeletal maturity of the child, the growth potential of the child, and the magnitude of the curve. The primary benefits of exercise in a nonsurgical patient with scoliosis are as follows:[25]

- Help with correct postural alignment and any asymmetrical postural habits to prevent further development following the bracing program.
- Maintain proper respiration and chest mobility.
- Improve overall spinal mobility and to help reduce back pain.
- Help the patient resume prebracing functional skills.
- Maintain muscle strength, particularly in the abdominals.
- Maintain or improve correct length and strength relationships of the spinal and extremity musculature. The general rule is to strengthen the muscles on the convex side and to stretch the muscles on the concave side. Asymmetric exercise is used to promote symmetry. For example, in a patient with a right thoracic, left lumbar curve, typical findings may include weakness of the right iliopsoas and right external oblique. Exercises that could be prescribed for this patient would include resisted right hip flexion at the end range with the patient sitting to address the weakness of the right iliopsoas. Weakness of the right external oblique can be addressed using a left upper extremity diagonal reaching movement pattern emphasizing right thoracic side bending (Fig. 30-1). Other functional exercises for scoliosis include the following:

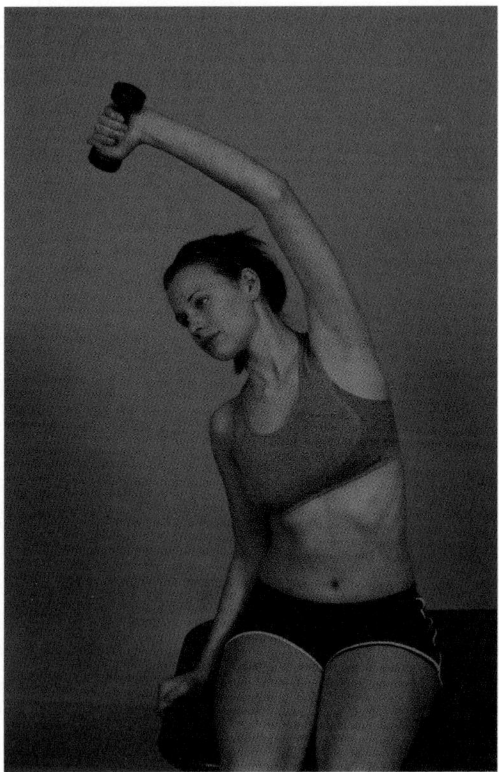

FIGURE 30-1 Left upper extremity diagonal reaching movement pattern emphasizing right thoracic sidebending.

- The patient is positioned in prone and is asked to place both hands above his or her head while deviating the thorax away from the concave side of the curve (Fig. 30-2).
- The patient is positioned in supine and is asked to reach overhead and extend the arm on the concave side (Fig. 30-3).
- The patient is positioned in heel-sitting and is asked to place both hands forward and flat while emphasizing trunk axial elongation (Fig. 30-4). The patient is then asked to stretch both arms laterally away from the concave side of the curve.
- The patient is positioned in side lying (convex side down) over the end of the table with a hand to provide balance (Fig. 30-5). A pillow can be placed directly under the apex

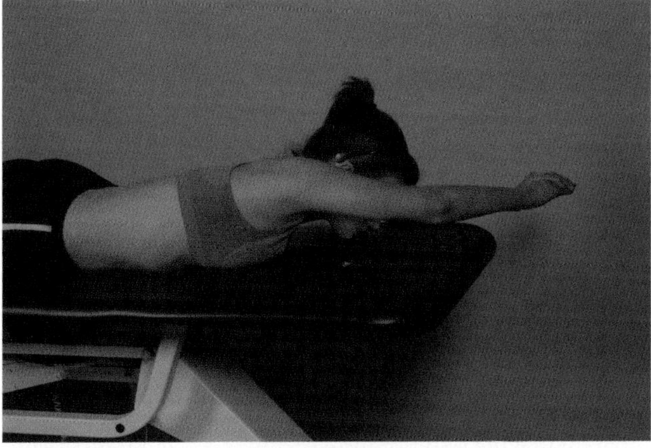

FIGURE 30-2 Prone sidebending with arms overhead.

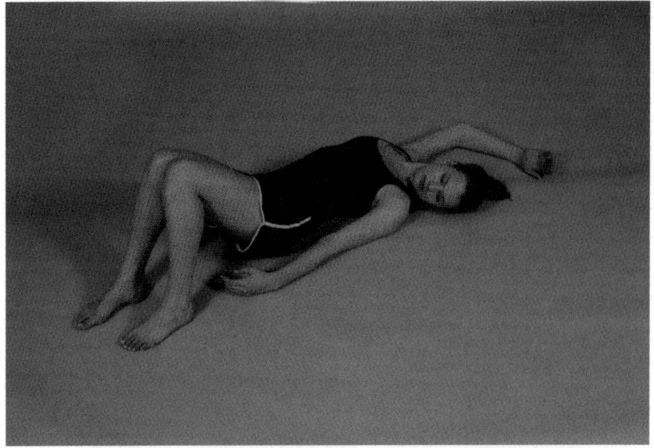

FIGURE 30-3 Prone sidebending by reaching overhead with one hand.

of the thoracic convex curve. Once in this position, the patient is asked to reach overhead and then down toward the floor using the arm that is closest to the ceiling to enhance the stretch.

- Swiss ball exercises can also be used, focusing on gaining increased thoracic side bending, while stretching the convex side (Fig. 30-6).

▸ Any of the strengthening exercises described in the intervention strategy section of Chapter 27 can be used to increase strength in the extensor muscle groups. Side-lying techniques (lying on the concave side) can be incorporated to strengthen the lateral muscle groups. The side-lying sit-up exercise is particularly effective (Fig. 30-7).

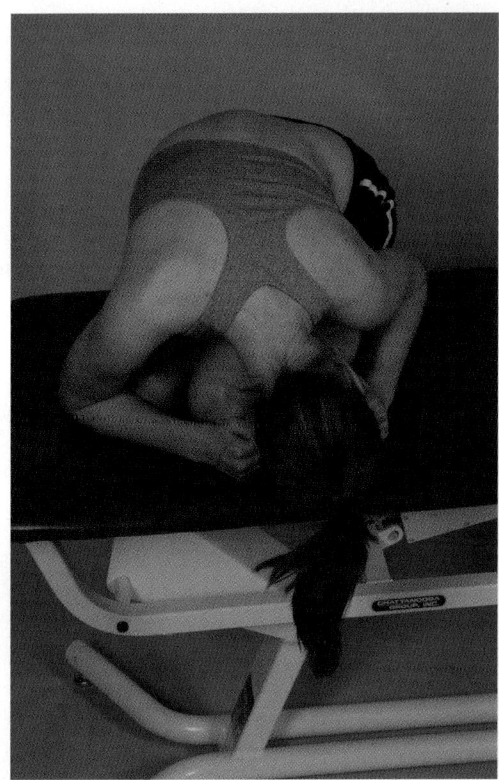

FIGURE 30-4 Prone heel sitting with forward flexion and sidebending.

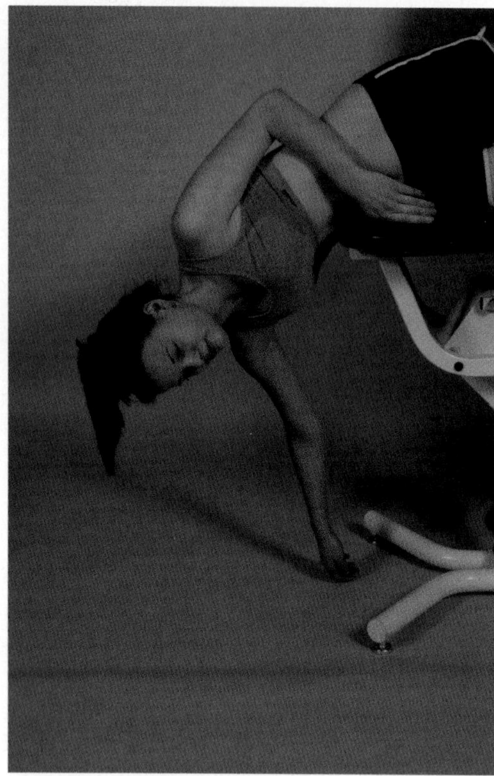

FIGURE 30-5 Side lying over the edge of a table to accentuate thoracic curve.

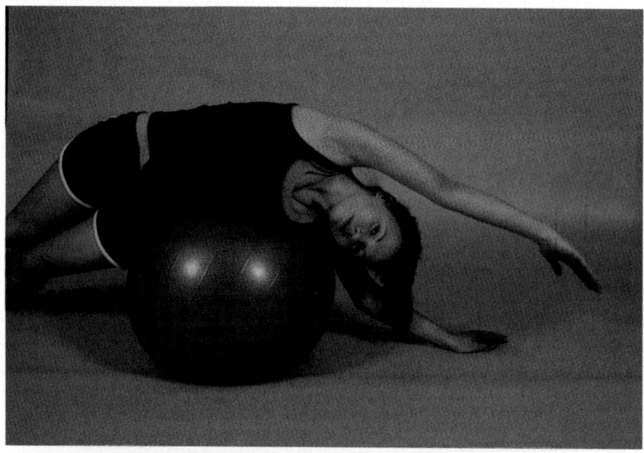

FIGURE 30-6 Swiss ball sidebending to accentuate thoracic curve.

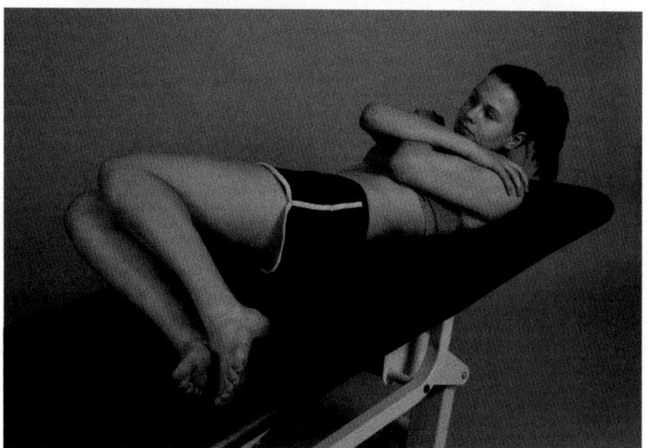

FIGURE 30-7 Side lying sit-up exercise.

If surgery is considered, the primary goal of scoliosis surgery is to achieve a solid bony fusion. Even in the setting of adequate correction and solid fusion, up to 38% of patients still have occasional back pain. The postsurgical management includes the previously mentioned strategies and the following:[26]

- Breathing exercises to promote rib cage expansion, pulmonary hygiene, and effective coughing.
- Patient and family education.

Legg–Calve–Perthes Disease

Legg–Calvé–Perthes disease, a disorder of the hip in young children, was described around the turn of the century, independently by Legg, Calvé, Perthes, and Waldenström.[27] The incidence of Perthes disease varies considerably from place to place. Low rates of around 5 or 6 per 100,000 have been reported from British Columbia, Massachusetts, and rural Wessex, England, whereas rates of between 11 and 15.6 per 100,000 have been found in Liverpool, England.

There is considerable epidemiologic, histologic, and radiographic evidence to support the theory that Legg–Calvé–Perthes disease is probably a localized manifestation of a generalized disorder of epiphyseal cartilage manifested in the proximal femur because of its unusual and precarious blood supply.[28,29]

The definitive cause of Legg–Calvé–Perthes disease remains unknown. Many etiologic theories have been proposed. Most current etiologic theories involve vascular embarrassment, with repeated episodes of infarction and ensuing abnormalities.[30]

Clinical Findings

The onset is usually insidious, and the course is prolonged over a period of several years. The initial sign is a limp. The child may be small for his/her age. There may also be a slight dragging of the leg and slight atrophy of the thigh muscles. A positive Trendelenburg sign is often seen. There may be some out-toeing of the involved extremity. The patient complains of a vague ache in the groin that radiates to the medial thigh and inner aspect of the knee. Muscle spasm is another common complaint in the early stages of the disease. On examination, there is usually decreased abduction and internal rotation. The ROM examination may show contracture in hip flexion and adduction.

Intervention

The intervention for Legg–Calvé–Perthes disease remains controversial.[31] The goal of treatment is to relieve pain and to maintain the spherical shape of the femoral head and to prevent extrusion of the enlarged femoral head from the joint. Children who are less than 6 years of age (possibly 5 years in girls) and those with minimal capital femoral epiphysis involvement and normal ROM are often followed with intermittent physical examinations and radiographs approximately every 2 months. In the more severe cases, there is lack of agreement regarding whether operative or nonoperative intervention is beneficial.[27] In reviewing long-term studies, it is apparent that the results improve with time.[32,33] Most patients (70–90%) are active and pain-free regardless of intervention.

The prognosis is much improved if there is no collapse of the femoral head. An important aspect in the intervention is the containment of the femoral head in the acetabulum. This is ensured by maintaining the hip in abduction and mild internal rotation for an extended period, using the Atlanta Scottish-Rite Hospital Orthosis. Although this brace does not use internal rotation-like casts as some other orthosis do, it does maintain the hip in abduction and permits approximately 90 degrees of hip flexion. This allows the patient to run and ride a bicycle while wearing the brace.[34] It is worth noting that forced abduction treatment can lead to damage of the lateral physis.[35,36] The advantages of operative intervention for containment of the femoral head are short time of restriction of movement, a more permanent containment, and perhaps enhanced remodeling of the femoral head.

Physical therapy may be provided at home, school, or in the clinic. Treatment methods include

- observation only;
- ROM exercises in all planes of hip motion (especially internal rotation and abduction);
- bracing;
- casting.

Specific procedural interventions can be used to relieve the forces incurred during weight bearing (crutch training, aquatic therapy). Gait training may be initiated with an orthosis or with bracing. The specific gait pattern and assistive devices depend on the type of orthosis. Patient and family education is necessary to teach hip protection strategies, thereby minimizing degenerative changes as the child ages.

Slipped Capital Femoral Epiphysis

Slipped capital femoral epiphysis (SCFE) is the most common disorder of the hip in adolescents. The average age for girls in whom slipped capital femoral epiphyses develop is 12.1 ± 1 years and for boys 14.4 ± 1.3 years (Table 30-3).[37] The term SCFE is actually a misnomer—it is characterized by a sudden or gradual anterior displacement of the femoral neck from the capital femoral epiphysis, while the head remains in the acetabulum.[27] The effects of coxa vara and valga demonstrate the principles underlying the mechanism of this condition. While the adult femur has a collum angle of approximately 125 degrees, the developing femur demonstrates considerably more coxa valga initially.[38] Failure of the epiphyseal plate occurs as a result of shear forces, which are forces applied parallel to the surface of the growth plate.[39,40] The natural history of SCFE is that the capital femoral epiphysis eventually will fuse with the femoral neck at the end of adolescence. Two devastating complications that can affect the result adversely are avascular necrosis (osteonecrosis) and chondrolysis. These complications are uncommon sequelae in the untreated slip but are serious complications in the operative and nonoperative management of SCFE.[41]

Clinical Findings

The initiating traumatic episode may be as minimal as turning over in bed. Patients with chronic SCFE generally have a history of groin or medial thigh pain for months to years.[27] Approximately 45% will have knee or lower thigh pain as their initial symptom.[42] If the patient can walk, it is with difficulty and with a limp, often with external rotation of the involved foot. The pain is reported as dull or aching, and there can also be a mild weakness of the leg. The hip will often show decreased ROM, particularly of internal rotation, abduction, and flexion. On passive flexion of the hip, the patient will frequently externally rotate the leg. On the basis of the patient's history, physical examination, and radiographs, SCFE can be classified as a stable or unstable hip.[41,43] In the stable hip, weight bearing is possible with or without crutches. In the unstable hip, the patient presents more with fracture-like symptoms, with pain so severe that weight bearing is impossible.[1]

Intervention

The goals of intervention are relief of symptoms, containment of the femoral head, and restoration of ROM.[44] The current method of choice is in situ surgical fixation. The goal of containment is to maintain the sphericity of the femoral head. Other treatments are epiphysiodesis, osteotomy, salvage procedure, or spica cast. Complications from surgery include chondrolysis and/or necrosis of the femoral head, which increases the likelihood of significant joint degeneration in later years. Conservative intervention includes the use of traction for the relief of symptoms, at home or in the hospital, for periods ranging from 1 or 2 days to several weeks. Gait training postsurgery is initiated as soon as lower extremity strength and ROM are adequate for ambulation skills. The weight-bearing status can vary but is usually nonweight bearing or touch down weight bearing. Full weight-bearing is permitted when the growth plate has fused (within approximately 3–4 months).[44]

ROM exercises for the hip should be performed in all planes, but with particular emphasis on hip flexion, internal rotation, and abduction. Strengthening of the affected extremity is introduced when sufficient healing has occurred.

Scheuermann Disease

Scheuermann disease occurs in approximately 10% of the population, typically in pubescent athletes, and in males and females equally.[45] The disease, considered to be a form of juvenile osteochondrosis of the spine, involves a defect to the ring apophysis where the vertebrae grow unevenly with respect to the sagittal plane resulting in an anterior angle that is often greater than the posterior angle.[46] These structural changes can cause the vertebral end plate to crack, thus making it possible for disk material to bulge into the vertebral body (Schmorl node). The seventh and tenth thoracic vertebrae are most commonly affected.

Clinical Findings

The initial onset is typically asymptomatic but then progresses to lower and mid-level back pain, which can be severe and disabling. As the condition progresses, the patient may complain of an aching sensation in the upper spine. The patient may report pain at the apex of the curve, which can be aggravated by physical activity and by long periods of standing or sitting. In addition there may be observational evidence of

TABLE 30-3 Differentiation of Pediatric Hip Pathologies

	Congenital Hip Dislocation	Septic Arthritis	Legg–Calvé–Perthes Disease	Transient Synovitis	Slipped Femoral Capital Epiphysis
Age	Birth	Less than 2 years; rare in adults	2–13 years	2–12 years	Males: 10–17 years; females: 8–15 years
Incidence	Female > male; left > right; blacks < whites		Male > female; rare in blacks; 15% bilateral	Male > female; unilateral	Male > female; blacks > whites
Observation	Short limb, associated with torticollis	Irritable child, motionless hip, prominent greater trochanter, and mild illness	Short limb, high greater trochanter, quad atrophy, and adductor spasm	Decreased flexion, abduction, and external rotation; thigh atrophy; and muscle spasm	Short limb, obese, quadriceps atrophy, and adductor spasm
Position	Flexed and abducted	Flexed, abducted, and externally rotated			Flexed, abducted, and externally rotated
Pain		Mild pain with palpation and passive motion; often referred to knee	Gradual onset; aching in hip, thigh, and knee	Acute: severe pain in knee; moderate: pain in thigh and knee; tenderness over hip	Vague pain in knee, suprapatellar area, thigh, and hip; pain in extreme motion
History	May be breech birth	Steroid therapy; fever	20–25% familial, low birth weight, and growth delay	Low-grade fever	May be trauma
Range of motion	Limited abduction	Decreased (capsular pattern)	Limited abduction and extension	Decreased flexion, limited extension, and internal rotation	Limited internal rotation, abduction, and flexion, and increased external adductor spasm
Special tests	Galeazzi sign, Ortolani sign, and Barlow sign	Joint aspiration			
Gait		Refuses to walk	Antalgic gait after activity	Refuses to walk; antalgic limp	Acute: antalgic; chronic: Trendelenburg external rotation
Radiologic findings	Upward and lateral displacement and delayed development of acetabulum	CT scan: localized abscess; increased separation of ossification center	In stages: increased density, fragmentation, and flattening of epiphysis	Normal at first; widened medial joint space	Displacement of upper femoral epiphysis, especially in frog position

Data from Richardson JK, Iglarsh ZA: *The Hip, Clinical Orthopaedic Physical Therapy.* Philadelphia, PA: WB Saunders, 1994:367–368.

an increased thoracic kyphosis and pain with thoracic extension and rotation, usually detected during a school physical or noted by the parents. Many patients often develop an excessive lordotic curve in the lumbar spine to compensate for the kyphotic curve above.

Intervention

The intervention depends on the severity but typically involves postural education, a modification of the aggravating activity, exercise, or bracing. The Schroth Method, which originated in Germany as a treatment for scoliosis, is an exercise system which uses isometric and other exercises to strengthen or lengthen asymmetrical muscles in the spine with the goal to halt or reverse progression of abnormal spinal deviations. The exercise program includes the stretching of the pectoralis major and minor muscles, and muscle strengthening exercises for the thoracic spine extensors (seated rotation and extension in lying exercises), and the scapular adductors.[47]

Spondylosis

Spondylolysis refers to a defect in the pars interarticularis, a stress fracture caused by repetitive extension and torsion of the spine. Spondylolysis is common in patients involved with sports where repetitive extension and rotation of the lumbar spine occur frequently.[48] Bilateral spondylolysis at the same vertebral level can result in spondylolisthesis (see Chap. 28).

Clinical Findings

The patient typically presents with insidious onset of extension-related low back pain (LBP). Frequently, there is an associated reduction in hamstring flexibility. Occasionally, radiating pain, numbness, or weakness may be present. Physical examination may reveal hyperlordosis, ipsilateral paraspinal muscle spasm, and adaptive shortening of the hamstrings.[49] The ROM examination reveals pain with spinal extension. The single-legged hyperextension test may localize the spondylolysis when standing on the ipsilateral leg (Fig. 30-8), although one study found this to be an insensitive test.[50] Radiographically, the anteroposterior view may identify anatomic variants or developmental effects, whereas the lateral view may demonstrate spondylolisthesis or a lytic lesion, and oblique views may demonstrate a stress reaction of the pars interarticularis, the pathognomic *neck of the Scottie dog* lesion.[49]

Intervention

The conservative intervention includes activity modification with avoidance of any activities that cause pain. The exercise program focuses on strengthening of the abdominal muscles, and hip flexor and hamstring stretches, while avoiding lumbar extension. Once the athlete becomes pain-free, activity can be gradually increased. Bracing is somewhat controversial. Indeed, one study illustrated that the best results were obtained with a period of rest from sport for 3 months, regardless of whether bracing was used.[51]

Osteochondritis Dissecans

Osteochondritis dissecans (OCD) is a rare cause of anterior knee or elbow pain in the young athlete. OCD is a joint disorder in which fissures form in the articular cartilage and the underlying subchondral bone due to vascular deprivation (osteonecrosis). The result is fragmentation (dissection) of both cartilage and bone, and the free movement of these osteochondral fragments within the joint space, causing pain and further damage. If OCD occurs in the knee, it involves the weight-bearing portions of the medial and lateral femoral condyles.

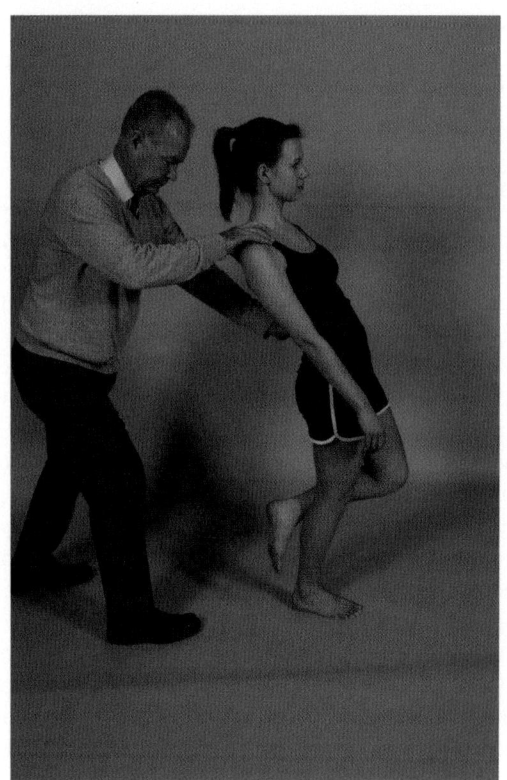

FIGURE 30-8 Single-legged hyperextension test.

Clinical Findings

Occasionally, pain may not be the most prominent symptom, but a catching sensation with joint motion may be the primary complaint if there is a loose body within the joint space. If the lesion is small, a painful arc is present during active and passive movement.

Intervention

When possible, nonoperative forms of management such as protected weight bearing (partial or nonweight bearing) and immobilization are used. However, nonsurgical treatment is rarely an option as the capacity for articular cartilage to heal is limited. As a result, even moderate cases require some form of surgery. Surgical treatment varies widely and includes arthroscopic drilling of intact lesions, securing of cartilage flap lesions with pins or screws, drilling and replacement of cartilage plugs, stem cell transplantation, and joint replacement.

Postoperative rehabilitation usually involves immobilization then physical therapy. During the immobilization period, isometric exercises are commonly used to restore muscle lost to atrophy without disturbing the cartilage of the affected joint. Once the immobilization period has ended, physical therapy involves protection of the joint's cartilage surface and underlying subchondral bone with maintenance of muscle strength and ROM and low-impact activities, such as walking or swimming.

Osgood Schlatter Disease

The apophysis of growing bones differs from the epiphysis of skeletally immature bone in that the apophysis is an independent center of ossification that does not contribute to the longitudinal length of a long bone. The apophysis does, however, contribute to the structure and form of mature long bone by serving as a site of tendinous or ligamentous attachment. Development of the tibial apophysis begins as a cartilaginous outgrowth, with secondary ossification centers appearing with subsequent progression to an epiphyseal phase when the proximal tibial physis closes and the tibial apophysis fuses to the tibia.[3] OS disease is a benign traction apophysitis that occurs in the tibial tubercle. It is a self-limiting knee condition that is one of the most common causes of knee pain in active and nonactive adolescents.[52] The condition occurs in active boys and girls aged 11–18 coinciding with periods of growth spurts. OS occurs more frequently in boys than in girls, with reports of a male-to-female ratio ranging from 3:1 to as high as 7:1. During periods of rapid growth, stress from repetitive contractions of the quadriceps is transmitted through the patellar tendon onto a small portion of the partially developed tibial tuberosity. This may result in multiple subacute avulsion fractures and inflammation of the tendon, and subsequent secondary heterotopic bone formation occurring in the tendon near its insertion.

Clinical Findings

The diagnosis of OS disease is relatively straightforward. There may or may not be a history of injury. Symptoms are typically unilateral, although 20–30% of cases can be bilateral in nature.[3] In the acute phase the pain is severe and continuous in nature. The pain occurs during activities such as running, jumping, squatting, and especially during kneeling, acute knee impact, and ascending or descending stairs. There is often a visible lump over the site. The pain can be reproduced by extending the knee against resistance or stressing the quadriceps.

Intervention

The intervention for OS disease is usually symptomatic, including anti-inflammatory measures, rest from the offending activity, and judicious stretching of the quadriceps and hamstrings (adaptively shortened hamstrings require increased quadriceps force to overcome the tight posterior structures).[3] Bracing or enforced joint immobilization is rarely required, although the more persistent cases may require cast immobilization for 6–8 weeks. The progressive quadriceps stretching exercises begin with a bolster placed under the hips of the prone patient to place the muscle on slack at the hip joint. As tolerated, the bolster is removed to place the hip in extension for a complete stretch of the extensor mechanism as indicated. Rarely, individuals will require surgical excision of symptomatic ossicles or degenerated tendons if symptoms persistent into skeletal maturity.

Sever Disease (Calcaneal Apophysitis)

The calcaneal apophysis serves as the attachment for the Achilles tendon superiorly and for the plantar fascia and the short muscles of the sole of the foot inferiorly.[53] Sever disease is a traction apophysitis of the growth center of the calcaneus that occurs at the insertion of the Achilles tendon and which is a common cause of heel pain in the athletically active child, with 61% of cases occurring bilaterally.[54] Sever disease typically affects children 8–13 years, with the peak incidence occurring at 11 years in young females and in 12 years in young males.[55–57] Young gymnasts, soccer players, and dancers are particularly susceptible to this condition because of their repetitive jumping or landing from a height.[58]

Clinical Findings

Sever disease is characterized by pain, point tenderness, and local inflammation at the posterior calcaneus near the insertion of the Achilles tendon. Patients with adaptively shortened calf muscles, internal tibial torsion, forefoot varus, a dorsally mobile first ray, weak dorsiflexors, and genu varus may be more susceptible to Sever disease.[3]

Intervention

The intervention for Sever disease initially begins with a shortening of the gastrocnemius-soleus group using heel cups or heel wedges, and avoiding barefoot walking until becoming asymptomatic.[59] Stretching of the gastrocnemius-soleus, with the knee extended and the knee flexed, is only initiated after symptoms have subsided. When stretching in the weight-bearing position any rear foot to lower leg or forefoot to rear foot abnormality should be corrected before and during the exercise. Dorsiflexion strengthening exercises along with foot intrinsic strengthening may also help manage symptoms.[3]

Little Leaguer Elbow

Repetitive throwing results in muscular and bony hypertrophic changes about the elbow. Little Leaguer elbow is a common term, credited to Brogden and Cros,[60] for an avulsion lesion to the medial apophysis as a result of repetitive valgus stress. The term has since been used to describe a variety of pathoanatomic lesions in the immature athlete, all of which relate to the mechanics of throwing. Additional factors that influence its development include age, skeletal maturity, individual susceptibility, competitive level, and geographic location.[61]

The act of baseball pitching has been described in five stages[62–65]:

- ***Wind-up.*** This stage involves the initial preparation as the elbow is flexed and the forearm is slightly pronated, and is characterized by low load to the arm. Elbow flexion is maintained by an isometric contraction of the elbow flexors. During the stride of the wind-up phase, the biceps muscle contracts to isometrically and eccentrically control the elbow angle, while the wrist and finger extensors concentrically move the wrist from slight flexion to hyperextension.[66,67]
- ***Early cocking.*** This stage begins when the ball leaves the nondominant gloved hand and ends when the forward foot

comes into contact with the ground. The shoulder begins to abduct and externally rotate, and valgus stress to the elbow begins.

- ***Late cocking.*** This stage is characterized by further shoulder abduction and maximal external rotation. At the elbow, flexion of between 90 and 120 degrees and increasing forearm pronation to approximately 90 degrees occurs. Dynamic stability is provided by the flexor–pronator muscle mass, and the triceps contracts isometrically to limit elbow flexion.[67]
- ***Acceleration.*** This phase is characterized by the generation of a significant anteriorly directed force on the upper extremity by the shoulder musculature, resulting in internal rotation and adduction of the humerus, accompanied by rapid elbow extension. The period from the late cocking stage through the acceleration phase is the time when the elbow is subjected to maximum valgus stresses.[68]
- ***Follow-through.*** This phase is characterized by the dissipation of all excess kinetic energy as the elbow reaches full extension and ends when all motion is complete. McLeod further divides this phase into release and deceleration.[69]

The repetitive motions involved in the various phases of throwing place colossal strains on the elbow, particularly during the late cocking and acceleration phases. These strains can result in inflammation, scar formation, loose bodies, ligament sprains or ruptures, and the more serious conditions of osteochondritis or an avulsion fracture.[64,70] The onset of Little Leaguer elbow can be insidious or sudden, with the latter typically secondary to fracture at the site of the lesion.

Clinical Findings

The child typically presents with pain and local tenderness on the medial side of the elbow. Physical findings depend on the severity but commonly include persistent elbow discomfort or stiffness due to aggravation by the injury. A locking or "catching" sensation indicates a loose body. If the ulnar nerve is compromised, numbness in the ulnar distribution and a Tinel sign at the elbow may be present.

Intervention

Management is conservative, involving rest and elimination of the offending activity. Lesions involving less than 0.5–1 cm of apophyseal separation are initially treated with the rest. This is followed by a rehabilitation program similar to that described for medial epicondylitis except that resistance exercises are avoided until active range can be performed to full motion without pain (generally 2–3 weeks). Throwing is avoided for 6–12 weeks. If OCD is present, the joint needs protection for several months.[71] Any separation greater than 0.5–1 cm, sudden traumatic avulsions, or a failure to respond to conservative measures are indications for surgery. The patient cannot return to pitching until full and normal motion and strength has returned.

To prevent elbow disorders, young athletes should adhere to the rules of Little League, which limits the number of pitches per game, per week, and per season and the number of days of rest between pitching.[72] The pitch count is the most important of these statistics.

Proximal Humeral Epiphysitis

This condition, often referred to as Little Leaguer shoulder, is also known as osteochondritis, epiphysitis, and epiphysiolysis of the proximal humeral epiphysis.[73] The proximal humerus ossifies from four ossification centers: humeral head, greater tuberosity, lesser tuberosity, and humeral shaft.[74] The ossification center for the humeral head is usually radiographically evident within the first year of life, whereas the greater tuberosity appears at age 3 and the lesser tuberosity at age 5. The humeral head and tuberosity unite around age 6 to form a large proximal humeral epiphysis, which unites with the shaft around age 20.[73] Injury to the proximal humeral epiphysis usually occurs because of the two mechanisms in throwers: distraction and torsion.

Clinical Findings

Patients typically describe pain localized to the proximal humerus during both throwing and resisted shoulder strength testing. Palpation demonstrates local tenderness over the proximal humerus. The differential diagnosis of shoulder pain in adolescents throwers include glenohumeral instability, rotator cuff tendinopathy, impingement, and proximal humerus physeal fracture.[73] Radiographs characteristically show widening of the proximal humeral physis.

Intervention

Treatment includes cessation of throwing until the patient has pain-free ROM of the shoulder and radiographs return to normal, which may take up to 1 year.[75]

Pulled Elbow

The term *pulled elbow* or "nurse maid's elbow," refers to a common minor soft-tissue injury of the radiohumeral joint in children of preschool age. The incidence of this condition is 3% in children under the age of 8,[76] and it comprises 5.6% of all upper extremity injuries involving children under the age of 10.[77,78] The left elbow is more commonly affected than the right,[79]and the disorder is more common in boys than in girls. The injury is caused by a sudden longitudinal traction force on the pronated wrist and extended elbow[80,81] resuling in the radial head slipping through the annular ligament, which causes the fibers of the annular ligament to become interposed between the radius and the capitellum of the humerus.[77,82]

These are the more common causes of pulled elbow[77]:

- The child is lifted by an adult from the ground by his hands.
- The child's forearm, wrist, or hand is being held firmly by a parent as the child attempts to walk away.
- A mother grabs the hand of a child to prevent a fall as the child wanders toward something potentially harmful.
- The young child is lifted by the hand from a lying or sitting position.

- The child is swung around by the hands several times during the course of play.

Clinical Findings

There is usually no obvious swelling or deformity, but the child presents with a painful and dangling arm, which hangs limply with the elbow extended and the forearm pronated.[77] The child is reluctant to use the arm and resists attempted supination of the forearm. The common sites of pain are (in order of occurrence) the forearm and wrist, the wrist alone, and the elbow alone.[82]

Intervention

The intervention of choice is manipulation.[77] Before attempting the manipulation, it is important to explain the procedure to the parents and to win the confidence of the child, by gently supporting the injured arm before manipulation. During the procedure, the clinician holds the child's wrist with one hand while the other hand supports the elbow and palpates the radial head. The child's attention is diverted and the forearm is forcibly supinated with one quick motion, together with the application of downward pressure on the radial head. A click in the region of the radial head (palpable and sometimes audible) is indicative of a successful reduction. Sometimes, the forearm has to be pronated after forcible supination to reduce the pulled elbow. The click results from release of the trapped annular ligament. Soon after the manipulation, the child typically begins to use the arm again, but sometimes there can be a delay of a day or two. In such cases, a sling can be used to both give comfort and protect the arm from a recurrence.

The parents should be advised to avoid a longitudinal traction strain on the child's arm by not pulling on the hands or wrists.[77]

Distal Radial Epiphysitis

Radial physes appear at 12–18 months and fuse by 15–18 years.[83] Distal radial apophyseal injuries are most common in male and female gymnasts but occasionally happen in other sports.

Clinical Findings

The patient typically describes a gradual onset of wrist pain made worse by weight-bearing activities while the wrist is in extension. Physical examination often reveals normal ROM but swelling of the distal radius. Tenderness is frequently found over the posterior (dorsal)-radial growth plate but may also be elicited on the anterior (volar)-radial physis as well. Radiographic findings depend on the stage of the disease. Although these injuries are usually confined to the distal forearm, the carpus can sometimes be involved.

Intervention

Time to healing is dependent on the stage of the disease in the radiographic findings. When radiographs are negative, 4 weeks of rest usually allow for healing and return to activities. In other cases, immobilization in a cast is the mainstay of treatment.

CONGENITAL ORTHOPAEDIC CONDITIONS

Arthrogryposis Multiplex Congenita

Arthrogryposis multiplex congenita (AMC) is a nonprogressive syndrome present at birth that is characterized by severe joint contractures, muscle weakness, and fibrosis.[84] There are many known subgroups of AMC, with differing signs and symptoms. Some of the more common signs and symptoms are associated with the shoulder (internal rotation), elbow (extension and pronation), wrist (flexed and ulnarly deviated), hand (fingers in fixed flexion and thumb-in-palm), hip (flexed, abducted, and externally rotated, often dislocated), knee (flexion), and foot (clubfoot). Although the specific cause of AMC is unknown, several mechanisms have been suggested including hyperthermia of the fetus, prenatal virus, fetal vascular compromise, septum of the uterus, decreased amniotic fluid, and muscle and connective tissue developmental abnormalities.[85]

Clinical Findings

No definitive laboratory studies or invasive procedures are available to detect AMC. The clinical findings associated with AMC vary tremendously among infants and include those already mentioned. The purpose of the initial examination is to establish a baseline from which to set realistic goals. Measurements of passive, active, and functional ROM are assessed as are gross motor function and developmental milestones.

Intervention

The intervention for AMC involves a multidisciplinary approach. The cornerstone of the intervention is family education, including instruction on low load, prolonged stretching (3–5 sets of stretches per day, with 3–5 repetitions in each set, and each repetition held for 20–30 seconds), positioning, strengthening activities through play, facilitation of developmental activities, and teaching of compensatory strategies.[86] Splints are adjusted for growth and improvement every 4–6 weeks. Reducing the disability associated with immobility is a major focus of treatment. Key functional motor skills such as rolling, hip hiking, and standing are addressed. Standing is initiated in standing frames with the lower extremities held in as optimally correct a position as possible with the help of splints and high-top shoes.[86] In the preschool patients, goals should be to emphasize ability versus disability, improve the child's function in basic ADLs, and enhance independent immobility and ambulation with minimal bracing and assistive devices.[86]

Osteogenesis Imperfecta

Osteogenesis imperfecta (OI) is an inherited condition resulting from abnormality in the type I collagen (found in bones, organ capsules, fascia, cornea, sclera, tendons, meninges, and dermis), which causes the bones to be brittle. In the most severe forms, the infant is born with multiple fractures sustained in utero or during the birth process.

Clinical Findings

The diagnosis of OI is made primarily from clinical and radiographic findings, as no definitive laboratory test exists to identify OI. The clinical features of OI are extremely variable and depend on the type and severity of the disorder. Primary impairments include bone fragility, short stature, scoliosis, lax ligaments, weakened muscles, failure of postnatal growth, and multiple recurrent fractures sustained from minor or no trauma.[86] The clinician should be aware of the infant's medical history of past and present fractures and know the types of immobilizations employed before beginning the examination.[87–90] Pain is assessed using a tool such as the FLACC (face, legs, activity, cry, and consolability), which is an observational scale for assessing pain behaviors quantitatively with preverbal patients. Assessing active, but not passive, ROM is essential. Functional ROM may prove more useful because it will assist in visualizing the whole composite of motion needed in functional abilities. Assessing muscle strength is done through observation of the infant's movements and palpation of contracting muscles rather than by using formal manual muscle tests.

Intervention

Typical participation restrictions for an infant with OI depend on the severity of the case. Goals for infants with severe OI are to prevent deformities of the head, spine, and extremity; avert cardiopulmonary compromise by avoiding constant positioning in the supine position; and maximizing the child's ability to move actively.[86,90] Caregiver education on proper and safe handling, positioning, and facilitation of movement is provided. Bathing, dressing, and carrying the infant are critical times when the infant is at risk for fractures.

CLINICAL PEARL

When handling the infant, it is important that forces not be put across the long bones; instead the head and trunk should be supported with the arms and legs gently draped across the supporting arm. It is also important to change the carrying position of the infant periodically because he or she develops strength by accommodating to postural changes.

The caregiver and clinician must be aware of the signs of a fracture which include inflammation (warmth of the site, edema, and pain), bruising, irritability, and deformity. An aquatic exercise program is an excellent therapeutic program for the child with OI. The degree of ambulation attainable varies for preschool children with OI. Gait training, which progresses in the usual fashion (parallel bars and moving to various assistive devices), is commonly initiated when the child has achieved strength with a rating of at least 3/5 (Fair) and when ROM has reached a plateau. In moderate to severe OI, braces and splints are usually required to begin standing activities on solid surfaces. It must be remembered that when children use walkers or crutches a large percentage of the body weight is borne through the upper extremities, necessitating precautions against bowing deformities of the radius and ulna. A walker that supports the majority of body weight through the trunk and pelvis is often used to assist in weight bearing during initial overland ambulation. Customized mobility carts may be fabricated to encourage independent mobility when the child is immobilized, enabling the child to explore his or her environment, gain some independence, and maintain strength in the upper extremities. Children with severe types of OI often require wheelchairs for mobility. Because of the shortened extremities, these chairs are often specially ordered and may require adaptations.

For severe cases presenting with severe osteopenia and repeated fractures, cyclic administration of intravenous aminohydroxypropylidene (i.e., pamidronate) may reduce the incidence of fracture and increase bone mineral density. Surgical interventions include intramedullary rodding, surgery for basilar impression, and correction of scoliosis.

Developmental Dysplasia of the Hip

Up to 10% of infants in the United States are born with congenital dislocation of the hip.[91] The acronym CDH is confusing and has been used synonymously with congenital dislocation or congenital disease of the hip. A dislocated hip is a physical sign, not a diagnosis, and the term *congenital* means present at birth.[92]

Thus, the acronym DDH is replacing CDH. The word *developmental* invokes the dimension of time, acknowledging that the dysplasia or dislocation may occur before or after birth, while *dysplasia* means an abnormality of development and encompasses a wide spectrum of hip problems.[92]

DDH includes hips that are unstable, malformed, subluxated, or dislocated. Instability is the inability of the hip to resist an externally applied force without developing a subluxation or dislocation.[92] A subluxation is an incomplete dislocation with some residual contact between the femoral head and acetabulum, whereas a dislocation indicates complete displacement of the femoral head from the acetabulum.[92]

The etiology of DDH is felt to be multifactorial, including both mechanical and physiological factors. In utero, the hip is in a position of flexion and abduction that results in a tightened iliopsoas tendon and anterior–lateral orientation of the acetabulum.[93] The tight iliopsoas may push the femoral head out posteriorly with hip extension during kicking. The labrum (cartilaginous rim of the acetabulum) becomes everted and flattened.

The acetabulum and femoral head develop rapidly in the neonatal period. When the acetabulum and femoral head are in the correct position, each reinforces the development of the other by this physical contact; however, if the hip is not concentrically reduced, it will develop in a dysplastic manner.[94–96] If the hip reduces spontaneously within a few days, hip development usually proceeds normally. In contrast, if a subluxation or dislocation persists, the femoral head becomes flattened on the posteromedial surface, the acetabulum becomes shallow and dysplastic, and femoral anteversion gradually increases.[94–96] In addition, the muscles surrounding the hip may shorten and contract.

Prolonged dislocation makes it difficult to return the femoral head to the acetabulum and is associated with a higher incidence of OA and impaired hip function in adulthood.[91]

Clinical Findings

The value of the neonatal hip screening examination remains controversial.[92] At present, tests including the ones outlined below are currently used to examine the infant. The examination requires patience and skill, and the newborn must be relaxed on a firm surface.

The examiner attempts to reduce the dislocation or subluxation using the Ortolani and Barlow maneuvers.[92]

With the newborn supine, the clinician places the tips of the long and index fingers over the greater trochanter, with the thumb along the medial thigh. The infant's leg is positioned in neutral rotation with 90 degrees of hip flexion and is gently abducted while lifting the leg anteriorly.[92] With abduction one can feel a clunk, as the femoral head slides over the posterior rim of the acetabulum and into the socket. This is the clunk originally described by Ortolani,[97] and is called the sign of entry, as the hip relocates with this maneuver. Maintaining the same position, the leg is then gently adducted, while gentle pressure is directed posteriorly on the knee, and a palpable clunk is noted as the femoral head slides over the posterior rim of the acetabulum and out of the socket.[92] This clunk was originally described by Barlow,[98] and is called the sign of exit, as the hip dislocates with this maneuver. Both tests are designed to detect motion between the femoral head and the acetabulum.[92] The reproducibility of these tests is dependent on ligamentous or capsular laxity, which usually disappears by the age of 10–12 weeks.[92]

Clinical screening programs are important in reducing the incidence of surgery. Ultrasound is the diagnostic modality of choice.[99] Early intervention has been reported to lead to a successful outcome in 90 and 96% of children radiographically and functionally, respectively.[94–96] Later examinations include assessment of gluteal folds, knee height, and the degree of hip abduction.[100] In the 3- to 12-month-old infant, the best physical finding is a limitation of hip abduction. In the supine position, with the hip in 90 degrees of flexion and one hand stabilizing the pelvis, each hip should easily abduct to 75 degrees and adduct to 30 degrees past the midline.[92] In the older child, a limp, positive Trendelenburg, toe-walking, intoeing, or out-toeing may be secondary to DDH.[92]

Intervention

The treatment of this condition depends on the age of the patient and the severity of the condition. The goal of intervention is to safely obtain and maintain a concentric reduction of the hip to provide an environment for normal bony development. The conservative approach is most effective for infants whose subluxation or dislocation have been discovered and treated early, within the first 6 months of life. The conservative approach involves maintaining the hip in flexion and abduction through diapering, and bracing/splintinguntil it is adequately remodeled.

- ***Diapering.*** The child is placed in 2 to 3 diapers, which is designed to hold the legs in abduction, and parents are instructed to position the infant in hip flexion as well.
- ***Pavlik harness.*** The preferred conservative intervention is an outpatient intervention regimen using the Pavlik harness, that provides effective reduction in 90% of the cases.[100] However, the harness is ineffective after 3 weeks making early detection critical. In infants older than 9 months who are beginning to walk independently, an abduction orthosis can be used as an alternative to the Pavlik harness.[31] The harness, which is initially worn 24 hours a day for 6–12 weeks, is used if symptoms persist after several weeks and is designed to restrict hip extension and adduction while allowing the hip to be maintained in flexion and abduction. [31] This "protective position" of flexion and abduction enhances normal acetabular development, and the kicking motion allowed in this position stretches the contracted hip adductors while promoting spontaneous reduction of the dislocated hip.[31] After the initial period, the harness is worn 12 hours per day for 3–6 additional months or until both clinical and radiographic signs are normal,[100]. If the Pavlik harness is used, it is important to teach the parents that the hips are placed in the correct position—too much flexion or abduction can cause excessive pressure through the femoral heads, resulting in possible avascular necrosis.

In more severe cases, skin traction, closed reduction, and spica-cast application may be needed. Open reduction and recasting are also options. In rare cases, total hip replacement is necessary in later life.

Equinovarus

Clubfoot, or talipes equinovarus, is a deformity consisting of hindfoot equinus (i.e., plantar flexion), hindfoot varus (i.e., the long axis of the talus lies lateral to the base of the first metatarsal bone), and forefoot varus (i.e., the forefoot is curved inward in relation to the heel, the heel is bent inward in relation to the leg, and the ankle is fixed in plantar flexion with the toes pointing down), which can be classified as follows:

- Inversion at the subtalar joint
- Adduction at the talonavicular joint
- Equinus at the talocrural (ankle) joint (plantarflexed position)
  - Fixed or rigid: this type of equinovarus can be either correctable without surgery (i.e., flexible) or require surgical release (i.e., resistant).

Clinical Findings

The clinical findings vary according to severity. Most cases are detected with fetal screening using an ultrasound scan.

Intervention

Treatment consists of manipulation (reducing the talonavicular joint by moving the navicular laterally and the head of the talus medially), taping, stretching, and serial casting, which is most effective if started immediately after birth. Other options include knee ankle foot orthoses (KAFO), Dennis-Brown bars with straight last boots, ankle foot orthoses, and/or custom foot orthoses. The role of the clinician involves monitoring, providing developmental intervention to promote typical functional skills and to assist in stretching and splinting.

Congenital Limb Deficiencies

Congenital limb deficiencies can be described as transverse and longitudinal.

- Transverse: These types resemble amputation to a residual limb in which the limb has developed normally to a particular level, but beyond which no skeletal elements are present. These deficiencies are described by naming the segment at which the limb terminates and the level within the segment beyond which no skeletal elements exist. For example, a child's lower extremity has a fully developed femur, but no tibia, fibula, tarsal, metatarsals, or phalanges.
- Longitudinal: These include all of the cases that are not transverse and involve a reduction or absence of an element or elements within the long axis of the limb. These deficiencies are named according to the bones affected (in a proximal-distal sequence) and whether the affected bone is totally or partially absent. For example, a child who is missing the radius and thumb in one upper extremity, with the ulna, carpals, and other digits present.

In the upper limb, congenital deficiencies most frequently involve the hand. According to the Association of Children's Prosthetic and Orthotic Clinic (ACPOC), 60 percent of congenital limb deficiencies either have no known cause or are genetic in origin. Although some congenital abnormalities may be due to poor blood supply to the fetus due to constricting amniotic bands, only 4 percent are due to taking some type of drug or toxin (i.e., maternal drug exposure like thalidomide).

Clinical Findings

The clinical presentation varies according to the type of children with limb deficiencies, the level of the deficiency, and the number of deficiencies or limbs involved.

Intervention

The intervention is directed toward helping the child develop appropriate functional and developmental skills while reducing any secondary impairments, such as soft-tissue contractures. Some children with congenital limb deficiencies may be candidates for an Ilizarov procedure, an orthopaedic surgical procedure that involves gradual lengthening of the limb over many months using implanted pins connected to a traction device.

GERIATRICS

The field of geriatrics continues to gain attention due to the rapid growth of this segment of the population and its predicted future socioeconomic impact. It is therefore inevitable that future rehabilitation professionals will see an increase in the number of elderly individuals seeking services for the management of both acute and chronic conditions that can negatively impact active life expectancy or the number of years that an individual may expect to be independent in ADLs.[101,102] Therefore, rehabilitation, with its potential to restore function, prolong independence, and improve quality of life, can be extremely important in this population.

The Aging Process

Aging is the accumulation of diverse adverse changes that increase the risk of death.[103] The rate of aging, that is, the rate at which aging changes occur, typically varies from individual to individual, resulting in differences in the impact of aging on function.[103] The aging process can be attributed to a combination of development, genetic defects, the environment, social and recreational habits, and disease, some or all of which are responsible for sequential alterations that accompany advancing age and the progressive probability of experiencing a chronic debilitating disease.[103] This increase in the incidence of chronic conditions with advancing age occurs largely because this period in life is often accompanied by a deterioration in health and a subsequent loss of independence. Complicating matters is the presence of comorbidities at this time of life, such as cardiovascular disorders, osteoporosis, arthritis, and diabetes, which increase the vulnerability of the geriatric patient.

Musculoskeletal impairments are some of the most prevalent and symptomatic health problems of middle and old age,[104] and result in a gradual loss of strength, motion, and increasing pain. These changes prevent elderly individuals from participating in regular physical activity, optimum mobility and, in some cases, reduce independence.[105] The history and physical examination of the geriatric patient must differentiate between the effects of aging, inactivity, and disease on the underlying impairments and functional limitations that result in movement dysfunction.[106] For example, mild impairments in the ROM may be due to increased stiffness associated with aging that occurs in the tendinous or ligamentous structures around a joint, or it could be due to acute immobilization, or chronic inactivity and reduced demands on a particular joint for full ROM.[107]

Theories of Aging

Normal aging produces age-related changes that are the result of the passage of time rather than the result of pathologic conditions. A wide array of theories exist as to why aging occurs, why species have the life spans they do, and what kinds of factors are likely to influence the aging process. For example, the aging process has been attributed to the following:

- ***Glycosylation.***[108–110] Glycosylation involves the abnormal process of the binding of glucose (simple sugar) to protein, a process that requires oxygen. Once this binding has occurred, the protein becomes impaired and is unable to perform as efficiently. Examples of known cross-linking disorders include senile cataract and the appearance of tough, leathery, and yellow skin.
- ***Neuroendocrine-immuno theory.***[111–114] The immune system is the most important line of defense against foreign substances that enter the body. With age the system's ability to produce necessary antibodies that fight disease declines, as does its ability to distinguish between antibodies and proteins. In a sense the immune system itself becomes self-destructive and reacts against itself.
- ***Damage by free-radical reactions.***[115] The term free radical describes any molecule that has a free electron. Theoretically, this free electron reacts with healthy

molecules in a destructive way by creating an extra negative charge. This unbalanced energy makes the free radical bind itself to another balanced molecule as it tries to steal electrons. In so doing, the balanced molecule becomes unbalanced and transforms into a free radical itself. It is known that diet, lifestyle, drugs (e.g., tobacco and alcohol), radiation, and so on are all accelerators of free radical production within the body. However, there is also natural production of free radicals within the body as a byproduct of energy production, particularly from the mitochondria.

- ***Planned obsolescence.***[103] This theory focuses on the genetic programming encoded within the DNA, the blueprint of individual life obtained from parents. Individuals are born with a unique code and a predetermined tendency to certain types of physical and mental functioning that regulate the rate at which we age (graying of hair, wrinkles, etc.). Many genes show changes in expression with age and these premature aging syndromes provide evidence of defective genetic programming: Hutchinson–Gilford syndrome and Werner syndrome
- ***Telomere shortening.*** This theory was born from the surge of technological breakthroughs in genetics and genetic engineering. Telomeres are DNA–protein complexes that cap the ends of chromosomes and promote genetic stability. Each time a cell divides, a portion of telomeric DNA dwindles away, and after many rounds of cell division, so much telomeric DNA has diminished that the aged cell stops dividing. Thus, telomeres play a critical role in determining the number of times a cell divides, its health, and its life span.
- ***Caloric restriction.*** Calorie restriction or energy restriction is a theory proposed after years of animal experiments and research on longevity that demonstrated how a high-nutrient low-calorie diet can dramatically retard the functional, if not the chronological, aging process.
- ***Evolutionary theory.*** As evolution acts primarily to maximize reproductive fitness in an individual, longevity is a trait to be selected only if it is beneficial for fitness. Over successive generations, late acting deleterious mutations will accumulate in the population and ultimately lead to pathology and senescence.

As previously mentioned, coexisting pathologic processes or comorbidities can exacerbate the effects of other conditions and result in greater functional limitations and disability. Throughout youth and early adulthood, the body has a number of physiologic reserves from which to draw upon when faced with physical challenges and injury, without a loss of functional abilities. However, older individuals have fewer of these system redundancies due to a gradual decline of health and increased incidence of injury and disease.[105] Without these physiologic reserves, an older individual is more susceptible to functional limitations and disability, resulting in frailty—the opposite end of the spectrum from successful aging.[105]

Pathological Conditions Associated with the Elderly

The geriatric patient who has been given a prescription for physical therapy may not have been physically active for some time, and his or her level of fitness may have declined considerably. Age-related changes of the heart and blood vessels, which can either be mitigated or exacerbated with activity level, typically result in reduced capacity for oxygen transport at rest and in response to situations imposing an increase in metabolic demand for oxygen.[105] In addition, maximal oxygen consumption decreases 5–15% per decade after the age of 25 years.[116] As a result, at submaximal exercise, cardiac output and stroke volume are lower in older adults at the same absolute work rates, while blood pressures tends to be higher.[116] It is very important that elderly patients have a physician's evaluation of their cardiovascular status before engaging in a rehabilitation program. In addition, the patient should be carefully monitored for their cardiovascular response and tolerance to exercise during their rehabilitation sessions. Heart rate, blood pressure, and rate of perceived exertion (RPE) should be assessed before, during, and after exercise, and the physician should be notified of any abnormal or unusual findings. In addition to the normal aging changes a number of complications can occur in the elderly:[107]

- Acute inactivity, such as that which occurs with hospitalization, can significantly reduce VO_{2max} and increase blood viscosity and venous status, which increases the risk of thromboembolic disease. Immobility is a common pathway by which a host of diseases and problems in the elderly produce further disability. Persons who are chronically ill, aged, or disabled are particularly susceptible to the adverse effects of prolonged bed rest, immobilization, and inactivity. Common causes for immobility in the elderly include arthritis, osteoporosis, fractures (especially hip and femur), podiatric problems, and neurologic disorders and diseases (see next)
- ***Neurologic disorders and diseases.*** A wide variety of neurologic disorders and diseases can affect the aging population, including cerebrovascular accident, Parkinson disease, cerebellar dysfunction, neuropathies, cognitive, psychological and sensory problems (depression, fear and anxiety), pain, and impaired vision. Age-related changes in the brain start at approximately age 60, although normal, nonprogressive, and negligible declines among the aged do not dramatically impact daily functioning until the early 80s. Many cognitive disorders require timely identification and intercession to offset permanent dysfunction.
- ***Dementia and Delirium.*** Primarily a disease of the elderly, dementia is a generic term used to describe a progressive, persistent loss of cognitive and intellectual functions. Dementia is associated with a history of chronic, steady decline in short- and long-term memory, depression, and with difficulties in social relationships, work, and activities of daily living. The typical end result of dementia is impairment of cognition including a decline in alertness, orientation, emotion, behavior, memory, perception, language, the application of knowledge (praxis), problem solving, and judgment. In contrast, delirium presents with an acute onset of impaired awareness, confusion, easy distraction, and disturbances of perception (e.g., misinterpretations, visual hallucinations).

- Cardiac diseases, such as coronary artery disease (CAD) and the sequelae of myocardial infarction (MI) and cardiomyopathy:
  - CAD is a complex disease of the cardiac arteries resulting in ischemia to the myocardium. The clinical symptoms of CAD include angina (an ache, pressure, pain, or other discomfort in the chest, arms, back, or neck), shortness of breath, a decrease in activity tolerance, or palpitations.
  - MI is a development of myocardial necrosis caused by an imbalance between the oxygen supply and demand of the myocardium, typically resulting from plaque rupture with thrombus formation in a coronary vessel, and subsequent acute reduction of blood supply to a portion of the myocardium. This patient population is a much greater risk of an adverse event during exercise, and therefore careful consideration, screening, and monitoring must occur to ensure safety with a rehabilitation program.
- ***Hypertension.*** Hypertension, which may be either essential or secondary, can have a number of negative impacts including the following:[117–126]
  - Left ventricular hypertrophy, left atrial enlargement, aortic root dilatation, arrhythmias, and ischemic heart disease.
  - Hemorrhagic and atheroembolic cerebrovascular accident (CVA) or encephalopathy.
  - Increased glomerular hydrostatic pressure secondary to efferent glomerular arteriolar constriction, which results in a reduction in renal blood flow in conjunction with elevated afferent glomerular arteriolar resistance.
- ***Musculoskeletal.*** The musculoskeletal changes associated with aging affect all of the soft tissues and bone. Many of these changes are associated with a decrease in physical activity. Muscle size can decrease an average of 30–40% over one's lifetime, affecting the lower extremities more than the upper extremities.[127] Type II muscle fibers, which are used primarily in activities requiring more power are not stimulated by normal ADLs disappear at a faster rate than Type I fibers. Indeed, Type II fibers decrease from an average of 60% of total muscle fiber type in sedentary young men to below 30% after the age of 80.[128] Therefore, the focus on this age group should be the prescription of exercises that develop power, not just strength. In addition, a loss of range in the lower extremities can have a negative impact on functional activities such as gait. Two musculoskeletal conditions that can severely impact function in the geriatric population are osteoporosis and osteoarthritis. Fractures, which can have a significant impact on morbidity, mortality, and functional dependence, commonly occur among the elderly. Such fractures include pathologic fractures, proximal femur fractures, proximal humerus fractures, distal radius fractures, compression fractures of the spine, and stress fractures. Fractures in the elderly have their own set of problems:
- The fractures heal more slowly.
- Secondary complications, including the following:
  - Pneumonia and/or decubiti (if the fracture results in a prolonged period of immobility or bedrest).
  - Detrimental changes in mental status secondary to adverse reactions to anesthesia or pain medications.
  - Decreased vision placing patients at increased risk of falls.
  - Poor balance exacerbated by limited weight-bearing status after a lower extremity fracture.
- ***Gait deviations.*** Individuals over 65 tend to walk with a slower self-selected gait speed, a shorter stride width, and an increase in double support time. Some of these changes are the inevitable effects of aging, while others are due to pathology or disuse. In addition, elderly patients tend to demonstrate increased gait variability. For example, elderly individuals tend to go through a decreased range of dorsiflexion during midstance.[129,130] However, significant changes in gait are not noted unless multiple joints are involved or there are impairments in other systems such as loss of strength or motor control.

Bloem and colleagues[131] in a study of individuals aged over 88 noted that 20% of the subjects exhibited unimpaired gait. Another study has demonstrated that those who exhibit senile gait disorders are more likely to go on to develop dementia and die earlier than age-matched individuals who walk normally.[132] This raises the enticing possibility that gait changes associated with aging may actually be an early manifestation of pathologies such as subtle white matter changes, vestibular dysfunction, musculoskeletal disorders, or visual changes.[132] What is known is that sensory system impairments have a tremendous impact on gait, and that training to improve proprioception can improve gait parameters and safety.[133]

- ***Impaired balance.*** Age-related balance dysfunctions can occur through a number of mechanisms including gradual degenerative changes in the vestibular apparatus of the inner ear, an inability to integrate sensory information, and muscle weakness. In addition, some diseases (benign paroxysmal positional vertigo), cerebrovascular disease, Ménière's disease, cerebellar dysfunction, vertebrobasilar artery insufficiency, and cardiac disease common in aging populations can lead to further deterioration in balance function. Balance disorders can also be associated with a number of other causes including
  - medications,
  - postural hypotension,
  - visual/auditory deficits.

It is important to remember that frailty is not a natural consequence of aging. Physical activity throughout the aging years can produce a number of physiologic benefits:

- Substantial improvements in cardiovascular functioning.
- A significant impact on the maintenance of independence in old age.
- The prevention and/or postponement of age-associated declines in flexibility, balance, and coordination.

In contrast, disuse exacerbates the aging process. Intervention strategies to prevent disability from immobility should include the following, while monitoring vital signs:

- Minimize duration of bed rest. Avoid strict bed rest unless absolutely necessary. The patient should be allowed to stand 30–60 seconds during transfers (bed to chair).
- Encourage sitting up at a table for meals, and getting dressed in street clothes each day.
- Encourage daily exercise as a basis of good care. Exercises should emphasize balance and proprioception, strength and endurance, coordination and equilibrium, aerobic capacity, and posture.
- Design possible ways to enhance mobility through the use of assistive devices (e.g., walking aids, wheelchairs) and making the home accessible. If the patient is bed-bound, proper body alignment should be maintained and the patient should change positions every few hours. Pressure padding and heel protectors may be used to provide comfort and prevent pressure sores.
- Encourage socialization with family, friends, or caregivers.
- Regular checks of skin integrity, protective and discriminatory sensations

Falls

Falls in the elderly are often associated with significant morbidity and can be markers of poor health and declining function.[134] Elderly patients with known risk factors for falling should be questioned about falls on a periodic basis. Recurrent falls, defined as more than two falls in a 6-month period, should be assessed for treatable causes. It is particularly important to assess housing arrangements, environmental hazards, alcohol use, and compliance with medications.

Several functional balance measures have exhibited a strong correlation with a history of falling. These simple tests, which can also be used to measure changes in mobility after interventions have been applied, are quantifiable and correlate well with the ability of older adults to ambulate safely in their environment.

- ***Timed single-leg stance (SLS).*** The patient stands unassisted on one leg (by flexing the opposite knee to allow the foot to clear the floor) for 30 seconds. The choice of which leg to stand on can be determined by the patient based on personal comfort. The clinician times the patient's one-leg balance using a watch. The ability to maintain SLS generally decreases with increasing age. One study[135] found that older adults in the community could maintain the SLS for 10 sec about 89% of the time and nursing home residents for 45% of the time.
- ***The timed "Up & Go" test.*** The timed "Up & Go" test measures, in seconds, the time taken by an individual to stand up from a standard arm chair (seat height of approximately 46 cm/18.4 in, arm height 65 cm/25.6 in), walk a distance of 3 m (10 feet), turn, walk back to the chair, and sit down again. The patient wears his/her regular footwear and uses his/her customary walking aid (none, cane, or walker). The subject walks through the test once before being timed in order to become familiar with the test. Either a wrist-watch with a second hand or a stop-watch can be used to time the performance.

Overall physical function should also be assessed. This is accomplished by evaluating the patient's ADLs and instrumental ADLs.

Physical Therapy Intervention

The intervention is directed at determining the underlying cause of the fall, the identification of risks, and in preventing recurrence through patient and family/caregiver education on safety issues (adequate lighting, contrasting colors, and reduction of clutter). Functional training should include sit to stand transfers, walking and turning, and stair negotiation. Therapeutic exercises should be designed to address any strength and flexibility deficits, and balance and/or gait deficits.

THE PHYSICALLY ACTIVE FEMALE

Both male and female children are basically equal in physical condition and have the same strength before puberty. After puberty (Table 30-2), females aged 11–12 years are 90% as strong as their male counterparts versus 85% as strong at ages 13–14, and 75% at ages 15–16 years.[136]

Although skeletal muscle physiology in men and women does not differ significantly—the actual number of muscle fibers is similar between genders—men do appear to demonstrate larger absolute strength gains due to a larger cross-sectional muscle fiber size. When comparing strength to lean body mass or cross-sectional area, women are about equal to men and are equally capable of developing strength relative to total muscle mass. However, differences in anatomy make the female more prone to certain injuries. For example, women demonstrate greater amounts of static external knee rotation, greater active internal hip rotation, and increased hip width when normalized to femoral length than men, resulting in a number of structural combinations:[137]

- Women have an increased hip adduction, femoral anteversion, and genu valgum resulting in a larger Q angle and rotational positioning of the lower extremity (see Chap. 20).
- Women have anatomical differences at the knee that predispose them to a higher incidence of anterior cruciate ligament (ACL) injury (see Chap. 20).

Despite these differences, both men and women should undergo similar strength training progressions.

Female-Related Conditions

Pregnancy

Pregnancy is a state of wellness that spans approximately 40 weeks from conception to delivery. A number of physiologic changes occur during pregnancy and the postpartum period within the various body systems that can present the clinician with some unique challenges. Given the number of physiologic changes during pregnancy and the postpartum period within the various body systems, the extent of the physical therapy intervention will depend on the findings of the examination.

Endocrine System. Changes that occur in the endocrine system include but are not limited to the following:

- Enlargement of the adrenal, thyroid, parathyroid, and pituitary glands.
- An increase in hormonal levels to support the pregnancy and the placenta and in preparation for labor. For example, a female hormone (relaxin) is released that assists in the softening of the pubic symphysis so that during delivery, the female pelvis can expand sufficiently to allow birth. Unfortunately, the hormone is not specific to this region and produces greater laxity in all joints.[138,139] This can result in an increased susceptibility to musculoskeletal injury.

Musculoskeletal System. The recommended weight gain during pregnancy is 25 to 27 pounds.[140] Pregnancy can produce a number of changes within the musculoskeletal system:

- The abdominal muscles are stretched and weakened.
- The development of relative ligamentous laxity, both capsular and extracapsular.
- The rib cage circumference increases resulting in a natural state of hyperventilation to meet the oxygen demands.
- Pelvic floor muscle weakness due to the increased weight and pressure directly over these muscles—the pelvic floor drops as much as 2.5 cm (1 inch) as a result of pregnancy.[141] Pelvic floor muscle weakness can result in stress incontinence (refer to "Urinary Incontinence").
- Postural compensations to maintain stability and balance. These changes are related to the weight of growing breasts, and the uterus and fetus, resulting in a shift in the woman's center of gravity in an anterior and superior direction. Specific postural changes include an increased lumbar lordosis, an increased thoracic kyphosis with scapular retraction, and an increased cervical lordosis and forward head. These changes in posture can become habitual postpartum.
- Changes in gait. In advanced pregnancy, the patient develops a wider base of support and increased external rotation at the hips and demonstrates increased difficulty with walking, stair climbing, and rapid changes in position. [142]

Common diagnoses associated with some of the above include

- ***Symphysis pubis dysfunction (SPD).***[143–146] This disorder can occur as a result of trauma during vaginal delivery. SPD should always be considered when treating patients in the postpartum period who are experiencing suprapubic, sacroiliac, or thigh pain. Subjectively the patient reports pain with any activity that involves lifting one leg at a time or parting the legs (e.g., lifting the leg to put on clothes, getting out of a car, turning over in bed, and walking up stairs). Objectively, the patient typically demonstrates an antalgic, waddling gait. Palpation reveals tenderness over the anterior pubic symphyseal area, and occasionally, clicking can be felt or heard. The ROM examination reveals limited hip movements due to pain, and there is an inability to perform unilateral standing. Radiological evaluation may occasionally be useful in confirming the diagnosis, although the amount of symphyseal separation does not always correlate with severity of symptoms or the degree of disability.[147]

Although the symptoms can be dramatically severe, a conservative management approach, including bed rest in the lateral decubitus position, pelvic support with a brace or girdle, ambulation with an assistive device and a graded exercise progression.[147] Patient education, which is extremely important in terms of providing advice on how to avoid stress to the area, should include the following suggestions:

- Use a pillow between the legs when sleeping, and keep the legs and hips parallel and as symmetrical as possible when moving or turning in bed and when standing and turning. Silk/satin sheets and night garments may make it easier to turn over in bed.
- Move slowly and without sudden movements.
- Sit down to get dressed, especially when putting on socks, shoes, or pants.
- If bending over to pick up objects is difficult, use specific devices such as reachers.

Swimming, with the exception the breaststroke, and deep-water aerobics using floatation devices may help relieve pressure on the joint.

The symptoms of SPD typically resolve in approximately 6–8 weeks with no lasting sequela, although in rare cases residual pain occurs, requiring several months of physical therapy.[147] In severe cases surgical intervention may be utilized in cases of inadequate reduction, recurrent diastasis, or persistent symptoms.

- ***Low back pain.***[142,148–155] LBP during the childbearing year is quite prevalent with the incidence ranging from 47 to 82%.[156,166,167] Back pain after delivery has been reported to occur 67%, while 37% experienced back pain 18 months postpartum.[151] Back pain tends to begin early in pregnancy, with 25% prevalence at 12 weeks.[149] The most common location of back pain in pregnant women is the sacroiliac region. The cause of back pain during the childbearing year is thought to be related to the mechanical and hormonal changes. Several studies indicate that women with severe LBP during pregnancy are at extremely high risk for developing new episodes of severe LBP during a subsequent pregnancy as well as later in life.[168–170] It is not clear whether the LBP is the result of the shift in the center of gravity, the associated postural changes, or changes to an intervertebral disk due to the release of relaxin. However, disk herniations are no more common during pregnancy than at other times. It is also important to consider systemic causes for LBP in this population. Kidney or urinary tract infections can both cause LBP.
- ***Peripartum posterior pelvic pain (PPPP).*** PPPP can be defined as unexplained and undiagnosed pain in the pelvic region (with or without radiation) that started during pregnancy or within 3 weeks after delivery. About 49% percent of pregnant women experiences some type of pelvic pain,[171] with 33% of these women experiencing severe pain.[152,157,158] The pain is typically experienced in the lumbar region and over the sacroiliac joints (with no findings suggesting nerve root involvement). Although the etiology of PPPP is unknown, it has been linked to the many physiological adaptations that occur in preparation for

childbirth. The previously mentioned change in the center of gravity leads to a change in the degree of lordosis of the spine, which in turn affects the paraspinal musculature. In addition, the hormonal changes that occur during pregnancy may cause an imbalance between the ligaments, muscles, and joints in the posterior aspect of the pelvis.[159] Although a systematic review[160] of the literature investigating the effectiveness of physical therapy interventions in the treatment of PPPP and LBP found scant evidence to support the use of exercise or mobilization in this patient population, exercise is thought to be beneficial in the post-partum period. In addition, the patient should be given posture/body mechanics advice using the suggestions listed for SPD.

Coccydynia.[161–165] Pain in and around the region of the coccyx, especially with sitting, is relatively common postpartum. Seating adaptations such as a donut cushion can be prescribed to lessen the weight on the coccyx and to support the lumbar lordosis. If symptoms persist for more than a few weeks, the displaced coccyx can often be corrected manually (see Chap. 29).

- ***Diastasis recti abdominis (DRA).*** A DRA is known as a split between the two rectus abdominis (RA) muscles to the extent that the linea alba may split under strain. The size of the DRA can vary from 2–3 to 12–20 cm in width and from 12–15 cm to the entire length of the recti muscles. It has not been determined whether the separation is a true tear or a relaxation of the tissue. A DRA is common in pre- and postpartum women. Predisposing factors for a DRA in women include obesity, a narrow pelvis, multipara, multiple births, excess uterine fluid, large babies, and weak abdominals prior to pregnancy. The separation may develop during the second and third trimesters of pregnancy, during second stage labor, and during the postpartum period. It is believed that a DRA may hinder the abdominal wall function related to posture, trunk stability and strength, respiration, visceral support, diminished pelvic floor facilitation, and delivery of the fetus. An umbilical hernia may result as well. The DRA is believed to contribute to chronic pelvic and LBP.

Criteria have been established for determining a DRA. The patient is positioned in the hook lying position. The clinician palpates with fingers horizontally, at the umbilicus and 2 inches above and below the umbilicus, and the patient is asked to raise their head and shoulders while reaching toward their feet. Any separation will be palpable, and a wide ridge of bulging tissue may actually be visible. If a DRA of 1–2 fingers width (1–2 cm) is present, this is considered within normal limits.[174] Any separation greater than two-finger wide constitutes a DRA, and, therefore, restrictions on abdominal exercise prescription should apply. However, it is worth remembering that the interrater reliability for measuring a DRA by manually inserting the fingers into the gap has been considered poor.

Electromyography studies of the rectus abdominis (RA) and external oblique have been done on primiparas women during the pre- and postpartum stages.[172] It was found that the abdominals generated the same muscle activity throughout the pregnancy; however, the ability to stabilize the pelvis against resistance decreased as the pregnancy progressed and continued to remain low postpartum.[172] It was observed that the RA length, angles of insertion, and DRA were significant between 18 and 30 weeks, with further structural changes between 26 and 38 weeks; therefore, the ability to produce torque may be reduced.[172] The decreased functional deficits were present up to 8 weeks postpartum, in conjunction with the incomplete resolution of the structural adaptations of RA. It is essential that these functional and structural deficits be addressed with pre- and postpartum women.[172]

Ostgaard et al.[167] found that individualized exercise and education were significantly helpful in reducing back pain during the 8-week postpartum phase; however, no differences in back pain were found during pregnancy. Weekly physical exercise before pregnancy was found to reduce the risk for back pain during pregnancy. Diagnostic ultrasound has been used to determine exercise effectiveness on decreasing the amount of a DRA.[173] It was determined that when performing a curl-up, the RA contraction significantly reduced the DRA compared to other movements studied.[173] The additional movements tested were curl-up with rotation to left and right, posterior pelvic tilt, and abdominal hollowing.[173] There was no evaluation of a possible relationship between DRA and back pain.

A RA that had exercised prior to the onset of pregnancy was not present in those women. Although it was not a controlled variable in this study, exercise prior to pregnancy may reduce the risk of a DRA.

According to Noble,[166] exercises for the abdominals to prevent, decrease, and/or eliminate a DRA should be prescribed. Proper exercise intensity is essential, and intervention should occur as soon as possible. If exercise has not been started before or during pregnancy, basic abdominal isometrics with exhalation should begin within 24 hours of delivery.[174] On postpartum day 3, the abdominals should be evaluated for a DRA.[174] Curl-ups with the abdominal isometric and the crossover of the upper extremities for additional support can be done.[166] If the DRA is greater than three fingers width (3 cm), there are restrictions on curl-ups and leg lowering exercises.[174] Curl-ups of the head only, with the abdominal isometric and the crossover of the upper extremities, should be prescribed.[174] Advancement of the exercises should not occur until the DRA has decreased.[174] Many times women will actually increase the DRA during the postpartum phase with abdominal exercises that are too aggressive for the individual.[174] The patient should be instructed in self-monitoring of her DRA.[174] A diastasis correction exercise can be performed to maintain alignment and discourage further separation. The exercise is performed in the supine hook-lying position (if tolerated and not contraindicated). With the arms crisscrossed over the abdomen, the patient manually approximates the recti muscles toward midline, performs a posterior pelvic tilt, and slowly exhales while lifting her head so that the scapulae clear the surface.[166,175] In addition, the patient can perform any exercise that does not stress the sacroiliac joint or increase intra-abdominal pressure including leg sliding (see Chap. 28), abdominal isometrics with lower extremity movements, supine bridging (see Chap. 28), quadruped leg raising (see Chap. 28), modified squats (see Chap. 28), and posterior pelvic tilts (see Chap. 28) while using hands to support the abdominal wall.[174] Maintaining the stability of the pelvis and decreasing the DRA are the goals for exercise progression.[174] Educating the patient about proper body mechanics and posture is necessary to prevent undue stress on the back and a DRA during the postpartum phase.[174]

Neurologic

Swelling and increased fluid volume can cause symptoms of thoracic outlet syndrome due to compression of the brachial plexus, carpal tunnel syndrome due to median nerve compression, or meralgia paresthetica, which is compression of the lateral (femoral) cutaneous nerve of the thigh.[176–178]

Pregnancy-related depression and postpartum depression has been documented to occur in 5–20% of all postpartum mothers[179–181] but can also occur in fathers.[182] These disorders can range from a mild "postpartum blues," which occurs from 1–5 days after birth and lasts for only a few days, to the more severe forms that include postpartum depression and postpartum psychosis, which require medical or social intervention.[183–185]

Gastrointestinal. Nausea and vomiting may occur in early pregnancy and are generally confined to the first 16 weeks of pregnancy but occasionally remain throughout the entire 10 lunar months (hyperemesis gravidarum).[183,186–189] The causes of hyperemesis gravidarum are largely unknown.

Cardiopulmonary System. The pregnancy-induced changes in the cardiovascular system develop primarily to meet the increased metabolic demands of the mother and fetus. These changes include the following:

- A predominance of costal versus abdominal breathing as the diaphragm elevates with a widening of the thoracic cage.
- Mild increases in oxygen consumption due to increased respiratory center sensitivity and drive.[190] Even with mild exercise there is a greater than normal increase in respiratory frequency and oxygen consumption to meet the greater oxygen demand.[190] However, pregnant women demonstrate decreased respiratory frequency and maximal oxygen consumption as exercise increases to moderate and maximal levels.[190]
- A compensated respiratory alkalosis.[191]
- A low expiratory reserve volume.[190,192]
- Increased blood volume: The blood volume increases progressively from 6–8 weeks of gestation (pregnancy) and reaches a maximum at approximately 32–34 weeks with little change thereafter.[193] The increased blood volume serves two purposes:[194,195]
  - To facilitates maternal and fetal exchanges of respiratory gases, nutrients, and metabolites.
  - To reduce the impact of maternal blood loss at delivery.
- Increased plasma volume is relatively greater than that of red cell mass resulting in hemodilution and a decrease in hemoglobin.[194,196,197]
- ***Increased cardiac output.*** This increases to a similar degree as the blood volume.[194,195]

CLINICAL PEARL

Hypertensive disorders complicating pregnancy are the most common medical risk factor responsible for maternal morbidity and death related to pregnancy.[183]

Changes in blood pressure during pregnancy include the following:

- Systemic arterial pressure should not increase during normal gestation.
- Pulmonary arterial pressure also maintains a constant level.
- Vascular tone is more dependent upon sympathetic control than in the nonpregnant state, so that hypotension develops more readily and more markedly.
- Central venous and brachial venous pressures remain unchanged during pregnancy, but femoral venous pressure is progressively increased due to mechanical factors.

During pregnancy, a condition called supine hypotension (also known as inferior vena cava syndrome), manifested by a decrease in blood pressure (BP), may develop in the supine position, especially after the first trimester. The drop in BP is thought to be caused by the occlusion of the aorta and inferior vena cava by the increased weight and size of the uterus as spontaneous recovery usually occurs upon change of maternal position. However, although a change in position is necessary, patients should not be allowed to stand up quickly to avoid another condition related to a decrease in blood pressure; orthostatic hypotension. Signs and symptoms of this condition run the gamut from headache, bradycardia, dizziness, and shortness of breath to numbness in extremities, nausea and vomiting, and syncope (fainting). Ideally, the time spent in supine should be limited to approximately 5 minutes. Alternative positions include side lying (best position for minimizing compression), supine reclined, or supine with a small wedge under the right hip.

Metabolic System. The metabolic rate increases during both exercise and pregnancy, resulting in greater heat production. Fetoplacental metabolism generates additional heat, which maintains fetal temperature at 0.5–1°C (0.9–1.8°F) above maternal levels.[198–200] Because of the increased demand for tissue growth, insulin is elevated from plasma expansion and blood glucose is reduced for a given insulin load. Fats and minerals are stored for maternal use.

Gestational diabetes is defined as carbohydrate intolerance of variable severity, with onset or first recognition during pregnancy. After the birth, blood sugars usually return to normal levels; however, frank diabetes often develops later in life. Typical causes include

- genetic predisposition;
- high-risk populations include people of Aboriginal, Hispanic, Asian or African descent;
- family history of diabetes, gestational diabetes, or glucose intolerance;
- increased tissue resistance to insulin during pregnancy, due to increased levels of estrogen and progesterone.

TABLE 30-4	Exercise Precautions During Pregnancy
Exercise Intensity	Exercise programs for high-risk pregnancies should be individually established based on diagnosis, limitations, physical therapy examination and evaluation, and in consultation with the physician. Exercise acts in concert with pregnancy to increase heart rate, stroke volume, and cardiac output. However, during exercise, blood is diverted from abdominal viscera, including the uterus, to supply exercising muscle. The decrease in splanchnic blood flow can reach 50% and raises theoretic concerns about fetal hypoxemia. Women should avoid becoming overtired. Exercise activity should be performed at a moderate rate during a low-risk pregnancy. Guidelines for a low-risk pregnancy permit women to remain at 50–60% (12–14 on the Borg scale of perceived exertion) of their maximal heart rate (monitored intermittently) for approximately 15–30 minutes per session.
Exercise Type	Recommended activities include stationary cycling, swimming, or water aerobics. Weight-bearing exercises and high impact exercises should be prescribed judiciously as increases in joint laxity may lead to a higher risk of strains or sprains.
Exercise Position	Patients should not exercise in the supine position for more than 5 minutes after the first trimester (see "Supine Hypotension"). To prevent inferior vena cava compression when the patient is lying supine, a folded towel can be placed under the right side of the pelvis so that the patient is tipped slightly to the left. If the supine position is contraindicated, exercises can be performed in side lying, the quadruped position or sitting. Positions that involve abdominal compression (flat prone lying) should be avoided in mid to late pregnancy. Modifications to exercise for the abdominal muscles must be made for a woman with diastasis recti, as the presence of this condition potentially reduces the ability of the abdominal wall muscles to contribute to their role in trunk and pelvic girdle alignment, motion, and stability. Traditional abdominal exercises, such as full sit-ups or bilateral straight leg raises, are not recommended as they may encourage further separation. However, these exercises can be resumed when the separation is less than 2 cm.
Exercise Environment	Adequate hydration and appropriate ventilation are important in preventing the possible teratogenic effects of overheating. Theoretically, when exercise and pregnancy are combined, a rise in maternal core temperature could decrease fetal heat dissipation to the mother. Some data suggest a teratogenic potential when maternal temperatures rise above 39.2°C (102.6°F), especially in the first trimester.

Current risk factors include

- maternal obesity (>20% above ideal weight),
- excessive weight gain during pregnancy,
- low level of high-density lipoprotein cholesterol (<0.9 mmol/L) or elevated fasting level of triglycerides (>2.8 mmol/L),
- hypertension or preeclampsia (risk for gestational diabetes is increased to 10% to 15% when hypertension is diagnosed),
- maternal age >25 years.

Most individuals with gestational diabetes are asymptomatic. However, subjectively the patient may complain of

- polydipsia,
- polyuria,
- polyphagia,
- weight loss.

Renal and Urologic Systems. Anatomic and hormonal changes during pregnancy place the pregnant woman at risk for both lower and upper urinary tract infections and for urinary incontinence.[183] As the fetus grows, stress on the mother's bladder can increases. This can result in urinary incontinence (refer to "Urinary Incontinence").

Exercise Prescription. The goals of therapeutic exercise during pregnancy are to improve muscle balance and posture, help provide support of the growing uterus, stabilization of the trunk and pelvis, and maintenance of function for more rapid recovery after delivery.[175] Contraindications to exercise include the following:[201]

- An incompetent cervix (early dilation of the cervix before pregnancy is full-term)
- Vaginal bleeding (especially second or third trimester)
- Placenta previa (the placenta is located on the uterus in a position where it may detach before the baby is delivered)
- Multiple gestation with risk of premature labor
- Pregnancy-induced hypertension
- Premature labor (labor beginning before the 37th week of pregnancy)
- Maternal heart disease
- Maternal type I diabetes
- Intrauterine growth retardation

Even without these conditions, the patient requires permission from her physician before beginning an exercise program. Some precautions should be observed during exercise (Table 30-4)[202–209] Warning signs associated with exercise during pregnancy include pain, vaginal bleeding, tachycardia, dyspnea, uterine contractions, and chest pain.[210]

Exercise programs for high-risk pregnancies should be individually established based on diagnosis, limitations, physical therapy examination and evaluation, and in consultation with the physician. Exercises for the pelvic floor are described in "Urinary Continence."

TABLE 30-5 Types of Urinary Incontinence

Type of Urinary Incontinence	Description
Functional	Includes people who have normal urine control but are unwilling (impaired cognition) or who have difficulty reaching a toilet in time because of muscle or joint dysfunction or environmental barriers
Stress	Describes the loss of urine during activities that increase intra-abdominal pressure such as coughing, lifting, or laughing. Stress incontinence is also particularly noted in high-impact sports that involve running and jumping, gymnastics, and basketball
Overflow	The constant leaking of urine from a bladder that is full but unable to empty due to ▶ anatomic obstruction, for example, prostate enlargement ▶ neurogenic bladder, for example, spinal cord injury
Urge	The sudden unexpected urge to urinate and the uncontrolled loss of urine; often related to reduced bladder capacity, detrusor instability, or hypersensitive bladder

Adjunctive Interventions. Modalities that increase body heat (hot packs, ultrasound, shortwave or microwave diathermy) should be used with caution, especially over the abdomen or uterus. Except for the use of transcutaneous electrical stimulation during labor and delivery, electrical stimulation is contraindicated during pregnancy.

Urinary Incontinence

Urinary incontinence includes the various types of incontinence: stress incontinence (a loss of bladder control associated with increased abdominal pressure that occurs during coughing or exercise), urge incontinence (a sudden urge to urinate), or mixed incontinence (a combination of stress and urge incontinence).[211] One of the contributing factors to urinary incontinence can be a weakness of the pelvic floor musculature. The various types of urinary incontinence are described in Table 30-5. Stress incontinence has prevalence rates that range from 10 to 55% in 15- to 64-year-old females.[212] Although often associated with aging, incontinence due to PFM weakness is not an automatic response to aging and many patients have achieved significant improvement through behavior modification, muscle reeducation, and PFM (see Chap. 29) strengthening.[213,214] Behavior modification techniques include timed voiding schedules, proper toileting techniques, dietary modification, and patient education. Muscle reeducation is primarily used for those patients who do not demonstrate improvement with the PFM strengthening program after approximately 4 weeks. Muscle reeducation can be achieved in a number of ways:

- ***Biofeedback.*** A study by Cardozo et al.[215] reported improvements in 81% of patients with urge incontinence who were treated with biofeedback.
- ***Acupuncture.*** A study by Philp et al.[216] reported improvements in 77% of patients with urge incontinence who were treated with acupuncture.
- ***Electrical stimulation.*** Various forms of electrical stimulation have been used in the treatment of female urinary incontinence. Electrical stimulation is an option for patients who demonstrate difficulty with identifying the PFMs or with producing a contraction of these muscles. Transvaginal stimulation with a removable electrode has been in clinical use in Europe and North America for three decades. The typical neuromuscular stimulation system is a portable electrical pulse generator powered by a 9-V alkaline battery. A fully insertable vaginal electrode, which is composed of silicone rubber, is commonly used. Two randomized studies have reported the usefulness of transvaginal electrical stimulation.[217,218] In the study by Sand et al.,[217] comparisons of changes from baseline between active-device and control patients showed that active-device patients had significantly greater improvement in weekly ($p = .009$) and daily ($p = .04$) leakage episodes, pad testing ($p = .005$), and vaginal muscle strength ($p = .02$) when compared with control subjects. Significantly greater improvement was also found for both visual analog scores of urinary incontinence ($p = .007$) and stress incontinence ($p = .02$), as well as for subjective reporting of frequency of urine loss ($p = .002$), and urine loss with sneezing, coughing, or laughing ($p = .02$), when compared with controls. In the Smith et al.[218] study, of the patients using electrical stimulation in the stress urinary incontinence group, 66% improved and 72% of the patients with detrusor instability treated with electrical stimulation improved. These rates were not considered statistically significant when compared to traditional therapy, but the authors concluded that electrical stimulation was as safe and at least as effective as properly performed Kegel and drug therapy in the treatment of stress urinary incontinence and detrusor instability. A typical protocol is outlined below:[219]
  - For patients with urge incontinence: 12.5 Hz for 15 minutes twice a day.
  - For patients with stress incontinence: 50 Hz for 15 minutes twice a day.
  - For patients with mixed incontinence: 12.5 Hz for 15 minutes a day and 50 Hz for 15 minutes a day.

In 1948, Kegel first advocated PFM exercise to enhance urethral resistance and promote urinary control.[220] The application of Kegel exercises has been broadened to various applications, but the concentration continues to be considered a useful adjunct in the management of functional urinary incontinence.[211] Many studies have shown that the success of PFM exercise for female stress urinary incontinence depends on the degree and duration of treatment and close supervision by a PT.[221] The patients are initially educated in PFM awareness. Several teaching methods can be used, including verbal cues, visualization with an anatomical model, palpation, objective PFM contraction at the anus, or biofeedback with electromyography recordings via a rectal probe.[222] The method chosen depends on the patient's baseline awareness, coordination, and comfort level. The palpation method is performed as follows:

The patient is asked to sit forward on a chair with their legs apart, their spine extended, and their feet flat on the floor. The clinician and patient each place a hand anterior to the ASIS and along the inguinal region to feel the contraction of the transverse abdominis and the internal obliques. The fingers are also spread superiorly to feel the weight of the belly and the RA. The patient is asked to "move the urethra and vagina gently upward" and to maintain the contraction for endurance.

Bracing. The patient is asked to sit forward on a chair with their legs apart, their spine extended, and their feet flat on the floor. The patient is asked to "push their abdomen out" without using an inspiratory effort and to isometrically contract the upper and lower RA in its outer range. The patient is taught to initiate, and hold, this action during a defecatory urge.

Abdominal Drawing-In. The patient is positioned in supine with the spine in neutral and the abdominal wall relaxed. The patient is asked to draw the lower part of the abdomen up and in toward the spine without moving the trunk or pelvis, or using an inspiratory effort, thereby contracting the transverse abdominis and the internal obliques. This exercise is taught in a variety of patient positions, with the appropriate muscles being palpated by the patient and clinician and the use of normal breathing.

Other exercises are added as tolerated. For the following four exercises the patient is positioned in the supine, hook-lying position[221]:

- ***Exercise 1.*** The patient performs a PFM contraction with a posterior pelvic tilt.
- ***Exercise 2.*** The patient performs a PFM contraction with a bridging motion.
- ***Exercise 3.*** The patient performs a PFM contraction with hip adduction against a pillow between the knees.
- ***Exercise 4.*** The patient performs a PFM contraction with hip external rotation against an elastic exercise band.

Swiss ball exercises may then be added.[221,223] The patient is positioned sitting on a Swiss ball:

- ***Exercise 1.*** The patient performs a PFM contraction with a posterior pelvic tilt in the sagittal plane while rolling on the ball.
- ***Exercise 2.*** The patient performs a PFM contraction with a posterior pelvic tilt in the oblique plane while rolling on the ball.
- ***Exercise 3.*** The patient bounces vertically on the ball, while performing a PFM contraction during each ascending movement.
- ***Exercise 4.*** The patient performs a PFM contraction while rolling on the ball from sitting to standing for functional training with transfers.

Medical management of urinary incontinence is aimed at prevention and may include the following:

- Nutritional counseling to help prevent constipation and to encourage adequate hydration.
- Medications to relieve urge incontinence: estrogen replacement therapy, anticholinergics, alpha-adrenergic blockers to increase bladder outlet/sphincteric tone, antispasmodics, and combination therapy with tricyclic antidepressant agents and antidiuretic hormone.[224–228]
- Surgical intervention can include catheterization, and surgically implanted artificial sphincters and bladder generators (sends impulses to the nerves to control the bladder function).

Menstruation

Normal menstrual cycles are defined by three phases, all of which are governed by alterations in blood levels of estrogen and progesterone:

- ***Follicular.*** Ovarian-produced estrogen increases resulting in endometrial growth, characterized by a compact, proliferative stroma, and increases in endometrial glands in number and length.
- ***Ovulatory.*** Ovulation produces the corpus luteum that leads to the production of estrogen and progesterone with progesterone-stimulated production of a secretory endometrium.
- ***Luteal.*** The endometrium acquires an edematous stroma with glands that are tortuous and dilated. In the absence of pregnancy, the corpus luteum becomes atretic with a resultant sudden drop in hormonal levels of estrogen and progesterone and then menstruation.

Menarche, or the onset of menstrual periods, normally develops between ages 9 and 16 years in the United States with 12.4 years as the mean age for menarche.[229] The development of menarche is under many influences, including nutritional status, intensity exercise patterns, weight, race, genetic factors, and others.

Abnormal menstrual cycles include the following:

- Amenorrhea: absence of menses.
- Oligomenorrhea: infrequent, irregular bleeding at >45 day intervals.
- Menorrhagia/hypermenorrhea: prolonged or excessive uterine bleeding occurring at regular intervals.
- Metrorrhagia: uterine bleeding occurring at irregular but frequent intervals, the amount being variable.
- Menometrorrhagia: prolonged uterine bleeding occurring at irregular intervals.

The effect of exercise on the severity of menarche is inconclusive. However, the side effects of menarche including menstrual pain, edema, bloating, and other symptoms may have a negative impact.

Breast-Cancer-Related Lymphedema

The lymphatic system is comprised of strategically placed lymph nodes connected by a network of lymphatic vessels, which act as the circulatory system for the immune system.

TABLE 30-6	Impairments and Complications Associated with the Treatment of Breast Cancer
Incisional pain	
Posterior cervical and shoulder girdle pain	
Vascular and pulmonary complications including pneumonia and deep venous thrombosis (DVT)	
Chest wall adhesions	
Weakness of the involved upper extremity	
Postural malalignment	
Fatigue and decreased endurance	

Data from Kisner C, Colby LA: Management of vascular disorders of the extremities. In: Kisner C, Colby LA, eds. *Therapeutic Exercise. Foundations and Techniques*, 5th ed. Philadelphia, PA: FA Davis, 2002:825–849.

Larger lymph collectors, known as trunks or ducts, handle these larger volumes of lymph fluid. The majority of the lymph produced by the body in a 24-hour period (2–4 L) returns to the heart. As lymph fluid moves more centrally, the diameter of lymph vessels increases. The major lymph nodes are the submaxillary, cervical, maxillary, mesenteric, iliac, inguinal, popliteal, and cubital nodes. Lymphedema results from a mechanical insufficiency that arises in an area, when lymph collectors sustain functional and structural damage. Breast-cancer-related dysfunction of the lymphatic system and subsequent lymphedema of the upper extremity can occur as a complication of the treatment for breast cancer. Current treatment for breast cancer usually involves removing a portion or all of the breast accompanied by excision or radiation of the adjacent axillary lymph nodes, the principal site of regional metastasis.[230] In addition to upper extremity lymphedema, other complications include loss of shoulder mobility and limited function of the arm and hand.[231]

The other impairments and complications that may occur in association with the treatment of breast cancer are listed in Table 30-6[230] The most common method to diagnose and measure upper extremity (UE) lymphedema is circumferential measurements using specific anatomical landmarks to estimate volume differences between the affected and unaffected extremities. A more accurate measure of volume difference is the water displacement technique using a volumeter.

The intervention for breast-cancer-related lymphatic dysfunction includes the following:[230]

- Strengthening exercises. Exercise encourages muscle contractions to provide the primary pumping mechanism for lymphatic and venous drainage. Progressive resistance training (using light weights initially and progressing as tolerated) for the major muscle groups of the upper trunk and upper extremity are emphasized (e.g., seated row, bench press, latissimus dorsi muscle pull-down, triceps muscle extension, and biceps curl).[232]
- Aerobic exercises. After 2 weeks, an arm ergometer can be introduced as an upper-body aerobic exercise. Moderate-intensity aerobic conditioning exercises are added as tolerated.
- ROM exercises. Individualized shoulder (Chap. 16) and cervical (Chap. 25) ROM exercises to address any muscle imbalances.
- Massage and wrapping. Various types of specialized wrapping, taping, and lymphedema massage are advocated, followed by pressure garment wear.

Although traditionally popular, pneumatic compression devices are not currently prescribed for lymphedema because the natural drainage system has been damaged, and these devices can potentially cause more stress to an already-damaged system.

REFERENCES

1. Lewis C: Physiological response to exercise in the child: considerations for the typically and atypically developing youngster, Proceedings from the American Physical Therapy Association combined sections meeting. San Antonio, TX, 2001.
2. Connolly BH, Lupinnaci NS, Bush AJ: Changes in attitudes and perceptions about research in physical therapy among professional physical therapist students and new graduates. *Phys Ther* 81:1127–1134, 2001.
3. Tippett SR: Considerations for the pediatric patient. In: Voight ML, Hoogenboom BJ, Prentice WE, eds. *Musculoskeletal Interventions: Techniques for Therapeutic Exercise.* New York: McGraw-Hill, 2007: 803–820.
4. Sanborn CF, Jankowski CM: Physiologic considerations for women in sport. *Clin Sports Med* 13:315–327, 1994.
5. Ollivierre CO, Pettrone F, Wilder RP: Pediatric elbow injury. *J Back Musculoskel Rehabil* 4:44–54, 1994.
6. Kraemer WJ, Fleck SJ: *Strength Training for Young Athletes.* Champaign, IL: Human Kinetics, 1993.
7. Faigenbaum AD, Westcott WL: *Strength and Power for Young Athletes.* Champaign, IL: Human Kinetics, 2000.
8. Duffy CM, Arsenault L, Duffy KN, et al: The Juvenile Arthritis Quality of Life Questionnaire—development of a new responsive index for juvenile rheumatoid arthritis and juvenile spondyloarthritides. *J Rheumatol* 24:738–746, 1997.
9. Brewer EJ, Jr, Bass J, Baum J, et al: Current proposed revision of JRA Criteria. JRA Criteria Subcommittee of the Diagnostic and Therapeutic Criteria Committee of the American Rheumatism Section of the Arthritis Foundation. *Arthritis Rheum* 20:195–199, 1977.
10. Klepper SE: Juvenile Rheumatoid Arthritis. In: Campbell SK, Vander Linden DW, Palisano RJ, eds. *Physical Therapy for Children.* St. Louis, MO: Saunders, 2006:291–323.
11. Patrick C: Spinal conditions. In: Campbell SK, Vander Linden DW, Palisano RJ, eds. *Physical Therapy for Children.* St. Louis, MO: Saunders, 2006:337–358.
12. McKenzie RA: Manual correction of sciatic scoliosis. *N Z Med J* 76:194–199, 1972.
13. Blum CL: Chiropractic and pilates therapy for the treatment of adult scoliosis. *J Manipulative Physiol Ther* 25:E3, 2002.
14. Miller NH: Genetics of familial idiopathic scoliosis. *Clin Orthop* 401:60–64, 2002.
15. Kane WJ: Scoliosis prevalence: a call for a statement of terms. *Clin Orthop* 126:43–46, 1977.
16. Miller NH: Cause and natural history of adolescent idiopathic scoliosis. *Orthop Clin North Am* 30:343–352, vii, 1999.
17. Dobbs MB, Weinstein SL: Infantile and juvenile scoliosis. *Orthop Clin North Am* 30:331–341, vii, 1999.
18. Greiner KA: Adolescent idiopathic scoliosis: radiologic decision-making. *Am Fam Physician* 65:1817–1822, 2002.
19. Lonstein JE, Winter RB: Adolescent idiopathic scoliosis. Nonoperative treatment. *Orthop Clin North Am* 19:239–246, 1988.
20. Lenke LG: Lenke classification system of adolescent idiopathic scoliosis: treatment recommendations. *Instr Course Lect* 54:537–542, 2005.
21. Lenke LG, Edwards CC 2nd, Bridwell KH: The Lenke classification of adolescent idiopathic scoliosis: how it organizes curve patterns as a template to perform selective fusions of the spine. *Spine* 28:S199–S207, 2003.

22. Weinstein SL, Ponseti IV: Curve progression in idiopathic scoliosis. *J Bone Joint Surg Am* 65:447–455, 1983.
23. Ponseti IV, Pedrini V, Wynne-Davies R, et al: Pathogenesis of scoliosis. *Clin Orthop Relat Res* 120: 268–280, 1976.
24. Ponseti IV, Friedman B: Prognosis in idiopathic scoliosis. *J Bone Joint Surg Am* 32A:381–395, 1950.
25. Hundozi-Hysenaj H, Dallku IB, Murtezani A, et al: Treatment of the idiopathic scoliosis with brace and physiotherapy. *Niger J Med* 18:256–259, 2009.
26. Cassella MC, Hall JE: Current treatment approach in the non-operative and operative management of adolescent idiopathic scoliosis. *Phys Ther* 71:897, 1991.
27. Weinstein SL: Natural history and treatment outcomes of childhood hip disorders. *Clin Orthop Relat Res* 344:227–242, 1997.
28. Barker DJP, Hall AJ: The epidemiology of Perthes' disease. *Clin Orthop* 209:89–94, 1986.
29. Ponseti IV, Maynard JA, Weinstein SL, et al: Legg-Calvé-Perthes disease. Histochemical and ultrastructural observations of the epiphyseal cartilage and the physis. *J Bone Joint Surg Am* 65A:797–807, 1983.
30. Martinez AG, Weinstein SL: Recurrent Legg-Calve-Perthes disease. *J Bone and Joint Surg* 73A:1081, 1991.
31. Leach J: Orthopedic conditions. In: Campbell SK, Vander Linden DW, Palisano RJ, eds. *Physical Therapy for Children*, 3rd ed. St. Louis, MO: Saunders, 2006:481–515.
32. Catterall A: *Legg-Calvé-Perthes disease, Legg-Calvé-Perthes disease.* Edinburgh: Churchill Livingstone, 1982.
33. Herring JA, Williams JJ, Neustadt JN, et al: Evolution of femoral head deformity during the healing phase of Legg-Calvé-Perthes disease. *J Pediatr Orthop* 13:14–45, 1993.
34. Wenger DR, Ward WT, Herring JA: Current concepts review. Legg-Calve-Perthes disease. *J Bone Joint Surg* 73A:778, 1991.
35. Hernigou P, Odent T, Manicom O, et al: Total hip arthroplasty for the treatment of septic hip arthritis in adults with sickle-cell disease. *Rev Chir Orthop Reparatrice Appar Mot* 90:557–560, 2004.
36. Hernigou P, Galacteros F, Bachir D, et al: Deformities of the hip in adults who have sickle-cell disease and had avascular necrosis in childhood. A natural history of fifty-two patients. *J Bone Joint Surg Am* 73:81–92, 1991.
37. Loder RT, Farley FA, Herzenberg JE, et al: Narrow window of bone age in children with slipped capital femoral epiphysis. *J Pediatr Orthop* 13:290–293, 1993.
38. Goss CM: *Anatomy of the Human Body by Henry Gray, FRS.* Philadelphia, PA: Lea & Febiger, 1973.
39. Oatis CA: Biomechanics of the hip. In: Echternach J, ed. *Clinics in Physical Therapy: Physical Therapy of the Hip.* New York: Churchill Livingstone, 1990:37–50.
40. Chung SMK, Hirata TT: Multiple pin repair of the slipped capital femoral epiphysis. In: Black J, Dumbleton JH, eds. *Clinical Biomechanics. A Case History Approach.* New York: Churchill Livingstone, 1981.
41. Aronsson DD, Loder RT: Treatment of the unstable acute slipped capital femoral epiphysis. *Clin Orthop* 322:99–110, 1996.
42. Carney BT, Weinstein SL: Long term follow up slipped capital femoral epiphysis. *J Bone Joint Surg Am* 73: 667–674, 1991.
43. Loder RT, Richards BS, Shapiro PS, et al: Acute slipped capital epiphysis: the importance of physeal stability. *J Bone Joint Surg Am* 75A:134–140, 1993.
44. Herring JA: The treatment of Legg-Calvé-Perthes disease. A critical review of the literature. *J Bone Joint Surg Am* 76:448–458, 1994.
45. Bradford DS, Loustein JE, Moe JH, et al: *Moe's Textbook of Skoliosis and other Spinal Deformities*, 2nd ed. Philadelphia, PA: WB Saunders, 1987.
46. Benson MK, Byrnes DP: The clinical syndromes and surgical treatment of thoracic intervertebral disc prolapse. *J Bone Joint Surg Br* 57B:471–477, 1975.
47. Winkel D, Matthijs O, Phelps V: Thoracic Spine. In: Winkel D, Matthijs O, Phelps V, eds. *Diagnosis and Treatment of the Spine.* MD: Aspen, 1997:389–541.
48. Watkins RG: Lumbar disc injury in the athlete. *Clin Sports Med* 21:147–165, viii, 2002.
49. Purcell L, Micheli L: Low back pain in young athletes. *Sports Health* 1:212–222, 2009.
50. Masci L, Pike J, Malara F, et al: Use of the one-legged hyperextension test and magnetic resonance imaging in the diagnosis of active spondylolysis. *Br J Sports Med* 40:940–946; discussion 946, 2006.
51. El Rassi G, Takemitsu M, Woratanarat P, et al: Lumbar spondylolysis in pediatric and adolescent soccer players. *Am J Sports Med* 33:1688–1693, 2005.
52. Mital MA, Matza RA: Osgood-Schlatter's disease: the painful puzzler. *Physician Sports Med* 5:60, 1977.
53. Mafulli N: Intensive training in young athletes. *Sports Med* 9:229–243, 1990.
54. Micheli LJ, Ireland ML: Prevention and management of calcaneal apophysitis in children: an overuse syndrome. *J Pediatr Orthop* 7:34–38, 1987.
55. Scharfbillig RW, Jones S, Scutter S: Sever's disease–does it effect quality of life? *Foot (Edinb)* 19:36–43, 2009.
56. Scharfbillig RW, Jones S, Scutter SD: Sever's disease: what does the literature really tell us? *J Am Podiatr Med Assoc* 98:212–223, 2008.
57. Madden CC, Mellion MB: Sever's disease and other causes of heel pain in adolescents. *Am Fam Physician* 54:1995–2000, 1996.
58. Meeusen R, Borms J: Gymnastic injuries. *Sports Med* 13:337–356, 1992.
59. McManama GB Jr: Ankle injuries in the young athlete. *Clin Sports Med* 7:547, 1988.
60. Brogden BG, Cros NW: Little leaguer's elbow. *Am J Rad* 83:671, 1960.
61. Leffers D, Greene TL, Germaine BF: The Elbow Region. In: Leek JC, Gershwin ME, Fowler WM Jr, eds. *Principles of Physical Medicine and Rehabilitation in the Musculoskeletal Diseases.* New York: Grune and Stratton, 1986:369–392.
62. Jobe FW, Tibone JE, Moynes DR, et al: An EMG analysis of the shoulder in pitching and throwing: a preliminary report. *Am J Sports Med* 11:3–5, 1983.
63. Jobe FW, Radovich M, Tibone JE, et al: An EMG analysis of pitching – a second report. *Am J Sports Med* 12:218–220, 1984.
64. Jobe FW, Nuber G: Throwing injuries of the elbow. *Clin Sports Med* 5:621, 1986.
65. Chen FS, Rokito AS, Jobe FW: Medial elbow problems in the overhead-throwing athlete. *J Am Acad Orthop Surg* 9:99–113, 2001.
66. DiGiovine NM, Jobe FW, Pink M, et al: An electromyographical analysis of the upper extremity in pitching. *J Shoulder Elbow Surg* 1:15–25, 1992.
67. Sobel J, Nirschl RP: Elbow injuries. In: Zachazewski JE, Magee DJ, Quillen WS, eds. *Athletic Injuries and Rehabilitation.* Philadelphia: WB Saunders, 1996:543–583.
68. Bowyer BL, Gooch JL, Geringer SR: Sports medicine 2: upper extremity injuries. *Arch Phys Med Rehab* 74:437, 1993
69. McLeod WD: The pitching mechanism. In: Zarins B, Andrews J, Carson WG, eds. *Injuries to the Throwing Arm.* Philadelphia, PA: WB Saunders, 1985:Chap 2.
70. Cabrera JM, McCue FC: Nonosseous athletic injuries of the elbow, forearm, and hand. *Clin Sports Med* 5:681–700, 1986.
71. Onieal M-E: Common wrist and elbow injuries in primary care. Lippincott's primary care practice. *Musculoskelet Cond* 3:441–450, 1999.
72. Watrous BG, Ho G Jr: Elbow pain. *Prim Care* 15:725–735, 1988.
73. Frush TJL, Lindenfeld TN: Peri-epiphyseal and overuse injuries in adolescent athletes. *Sports Health* 1:201–211, 2009.
74. Hensinger RN: *Standards in Pediatric Orthopedics: Tables, Charts, and Graphs.* New York: Raven press, 1986:295–296.
75. Carson WG Jr, Gasser SI: Little Leaguer's shoulder. A report of 23 cases. *Am J Sports Med* 26:575–580, 1998.
76. Corrigan AB: The pulled elbow. *Med J Aust* 2:1, 1965.
77. Sai N: Pulled elbow. *J R Soc Med* 92:462–464, 1999.
78. Amir D, Frankl U, Pogrund H: Pulled elbow and hypermobility of joints. *Clin Orthop* 257:94, 1990.
79. Matles AL, Eliopoulous K: Internal derangement of the elbow in children. *Int Surg* 48:259–263, 1967.
80. Salter RB, Zaltz C: Anatomic investigations of the mechanism of injury and pathologic anatomy of pulled elbow in young children. *Clin Orthop* 77:134–143, 1971.
81. Dee R, Carrion W: *Pulled elbow, Principles of Orthopaedic Practice.* New York: McGraw-Hill, 1997:579.
82. Hagroo GA, Zaki HM, Choudhary MT, et al: Pulled elbow-not the effect of hypermobility of joints. *Injury* 26:687–690, 1995.
83. Horii E, Tamura Y, Nakamura R, et al: Premature closure of the distal radial physis. *J Hand Surg Br* 18:11–16, 1993.
84. Dane B, Dane C, Aksoy F, et al: Arthrogryposis multiplex congenita: analysis of twelve cases. *Clin Exp Obstet Gynecol* 36:259–262, 2009.
85. Suryawanshi C, Panditrao MM, Rai I: Arthrogryposis multiplex congenita–a rare congenital anomaly. *J Indian Med Assoc* 104:95–96, 98, 2006.
86. Vreeman LI, Long T, Habib ZH: Musculoskeletal developmental disorders. In: Magee DJ, Zachazewski JE, Quillen WS, eds. *Pathology and Intervention in Musculoskeletal Rehabilitation.* St. Louis, MO: Saunders, 2009:750–780.

87. Bleakney DA, Donohoe M: Osteogenesis Imperfecta. In: Campbell SK, Vander Linden DW, Palisano RJ, eds. *Physical Therapy for Children.* 3rd ed. St. Louis, MO: Saunders, 2006:401–419.
88. Binder H: Rehabilitation of infants with osteogenesis imperfecta. *Connect Tissue Res* 31:S37–S39, 1995.
89. Gerber LH, Binder H, Weintrob J, et al: Rehabilitation of children and infants with osteogenesis imperfecta. A program for ambulation. *Clin Orthop Relat Res* 251: 254–262, 1990.
90. Binder H, Hawks L, Graybill G, et al: Osteogenesis imperfecta: rehabilitation approach with infants and young children. *Arch Phys Med Rehabil* 65:537–541, 1984.
91. Churgay CA, Caruthers BS: Diagnosis and treatment of congenital dislocation of the hip. *Am Fam Physician* 45:1217–1228, 1992.
92. Aronsson DD, Goldberg MJ, Kling TF, et al: Developmental dysplasia of the hip. *Pediatrics* 94:201–208, 1994.
93. McKibbin B: Anatomical factors in the stability of the hip joint in the newborn. *J Bone Joint Surg Br* 52:148–159, 1970.
94. US Preventive Services Task Force: Screening for developmental dysplasia of the hip: recommendation statement. *Am Fam Physician* 73:1992–1996, 2006.
95. Cady RB: Developmental dysplasia of the hip: definition, recognition, and prevention of late sequelae. *Pediatr Ann* 35:92–101, 2006.
96. Hart ES, Albright MB, Rebello GN, et al: Developmental dysplasia of the hip: nursing implications and anticipatory guidance for parents. *Orthop Nurs* 25:100–109; quiz 110–111, 2006.
97. Ortolani M: Un segno poco noto e sue importanza per la diagnosi precoce di prelussazione congenita dell'anca. *Pediatria* 45:129–136, 1937.
98. Barlow TG: Early diagnosis and treatment of congenital dislocation of the hip. *J Bone Joint Surg Br* 44:292–301, 1962.
99. Graf R: *Hip Sonography : Diagnosis and Management of Infant Hip Dysplasia,* 2nd ed. New York: Springer, 2006.
100. Curry LC, Gibson LY: Congenital hip dislocation: the importance of early detection and comprehensive treatment. *Nurse Pract* 17:49–55, 1992.
101. Katz S, Branch LG, Branson MH, et al: Active life expectancy. *N Engl J Med* 309:1218–1224, 1983.
102. Branch LG, Guralnik JM, Foley DJ, et al: Active life expectancy for 10,000 Caucasian men and women in three communities. *J Gerontol* 46:M145–M150, 1991.
103. Harman D: Aging: phenomena and theories. *Ann N Y Acad Sci* 854:1–7, 1998.
104. Jette AM, Branch LG, Berlin J: Musculoskeletal impairments and physical disablement among the aged. *J Gerontol* 45:M203–M208, 1990.
105. Voight C: Rehabilitation considerations with the geriatric patient. In: Prentice WE Jr, Voight ML, eds. *Techniques in Musculoskeletal Rehabilitation.* New York: McGraw-Hill, 2001:679–696.
106. Lewis CB, Bottomley JM: *Geriatric Physical Therapy: A Clinical Approach.* Norwalk, CT: Appleton & Lange, 1994.
107. Bennett JL, Shoemaker MJ: Rehabilitation considerations for the geriatric patient. In: Voight ML, Hoogenboom BJ, Prentice WE, eds. *Musculoskeletal Interventions: Techniques for Therapeutic Exercise.* New York: McGraw-Hill, 2007:783–802.
108. Bjorksten J: Some therapeutic implications of the crosslinkage theory of aging. *Adv Exp Med Biol* 86B: 579–602, 1977.
109. Bjorksten J: The crosslinkage theory of aging: clinical implications. *Compr Ther* 2:65–74, 1976.
110. Bjorksten J: The crosslinkage theory of aging. *J Am Geriatr Soc* 16:408–427, 1968.
111. Effros RB: Roy Walford and the immunologic theory of aging. *Immun Ageing* 2:7, 2005.
112. Kent S: Can normal aging be explained by the immunologic theory. *Geriatrics* 32:111, 113,116 passim, 1977.
113. Walford RL: Immunologic theory of aging: current status. *Fed Proc* 33:2020–2027, 1974.
114. Walford RL: The immunologic theory of aging. *Gerontologist* 57:195–197, 1964.
115. Harman D: Free radical involvement in aging. Pathophysiology and therapeutic implications. *Drugs Aging* 3:60–80, 1993.
116. Heath GW, Hagberg JM, Ehsani AA, et al: A physiological comparison of young and older endurance athletes. *J Appl Physiol* 51:634–640, 1981.
117. Avdic S, Mujcinovic Z, Asceric M, et al: Left ventricular diastolic dysfunction in essential hypertension. *Bosn J Basic Med Sci* 7:15–20, 2007.
118. Binder A: A review of the genetics of essential hypertension. *Curr Opin Cardiol* 22:176–184, 2007.
119. Cuspidi C, Meani S, Valerio C, et al: Age and target organ damage in essential hypertension: role of the metabolic syndrome. *Am J Hypertens* 20:296–303, 2007.
120. El-Shafei SA, Bassili A, Hassanien NM, et al: Genetic determinants of essential hypertension. *J Egypt Public Health Assoc* 77:231–246, 2002.
121. Hollenberg NK, Williams GH: Nonmodulation and essential hypertension. *Curr Hypertens Rep* 8:127–131, 2006.
122. Kennedy S: Essential hypertension 2: treatment and monitoring update. *Community Pract* 79:64–66, 2006.
123. Kennedy S: Essential hypertension: recent changes in management. *Community Pract* 79:23–24, 2006.
124. Krzych LJ: Blood pressure variability in children with essential hypertension. *J Hum Hypertens* 21:494–500, 2007.
125. Parrilli G, Manguso F, Orsini L, et al: Essential hypertension and chronic viral hepatitis. *Dig Liver Dis* 39:466–472, 2007.
126. Pierdomenico SD: Blood pressure variability and cardiovascular outcome in essential hypertension. *Am J Hypertens* 20:162–163, 2007.
127. Gallagher D, Visser M, De Meersman RE, et al: Appendicular skeletal muscle mass: effects of age, gender, and ethnicity. *J Appl Physiol* 83:229–239, 1997.
128. Larsson L, Sjodin B, Karlsson J: Histochemical and biochemical changes in human skeletal muscle with age in sedentary males, age 22–65 years. *Acta Physiol Scand* 103:31–39, 1978.
129. Nigg BM, Fisher V, Allinger TL, et al: Range of motion of the foot as a function of age. *Foot Ankle* 13:336–343, 1992.
130. Kegelmeyer D: Stability of gait and fall prevention. In: Hughes C, ed. *Movement Disorders and Neuromuscular Interventions for the Trunk and Extremities – Independent Study Course 18.2.6.* La Crosse, WI: Orthopaedic Section, APTA, Inc, 2008:1–20.
131. Bloem BR, Haan J, Lagaay AM, et al: Investigation of gait in elderly subjects over 88 years of age. *J Geriatr Psychiatry Neurol* 5:78–84, 1992.
132. Snijders AH, van de Warrenburg BP, Giladi N, et al: Neurological gait disorders in elderly people: clinical approach and classification. *Lancet Neurol* 6:63–74, 2007.
133. van Hedel HJ, Dietz V: The influence of age on learning a locomotor task. *Clin Neurophysiol* 115:2134–2143, 2004.
134. Fuller GF: Falls in the elderly. *Am Fam Physician* 61:2159–2168, 2173–2174, 2000.
135. Rossiter-Fornoff JE, Wolf SL, Wolfson LI, et al: A cross-sectional validation study of the FICSIT common data base static balance measures. *J Gerontol: Med Sci* 50A:M291–M297, 1995.
136. Greydanus DE, Patel DR: The female athlete. Before and beyond puberty. *Pediatr Clin North Am* 49:553–580, vi, 2002.
137. Hoogenboom BJ, Schuemann TL, Smith RK: Considerations for the physically active female. In: Voight ML, Hoogenboom BJ, Prentice WE, eds. *Musculoskeletal Interventions: Techniques for Therapeutic Exercise.* New York: McGraw-Hill, 2007:853–918.
138. Lee HY, Zhao S, Fields PA, et al: Clinical use of relaxin to facilitate birth: reasons for investigating the premise. *Ann N Y Acad Sci* 1041:351–366, 2005.
139. Lubahn J, Ivance D, Konieczko E, et al: Immunohistochemical detection of relaxin binding to the volar oblique ligament. *J Hand Surg [Am]* 31:80–84, 2006.
140. Wiles R: The views of women of above average weight about appropriate weight gain in pregnancy. *Midwifery* 14:254–260, 1998.
141. Stephenson R, O'Connor L: *Obstetric and Gynecologic Care in Physical Therapy,* 2nd ed. Thorofare, NJ: Charles B Slack, 2000.
142. Moore K, Dumas GA, Reid JG: Postural changes associated with pregnancy and their relationship with low back pain. *Clin Biomech (Bristol, Avon)* 5:169–174, 1990.
143. Depledge J, McNair PJ, Keal-Smith C, et al: Management of symphysis pubis dysfunction during pregnancy using exercise and pelvic support belts. *Phys Ther* 85:1290–300, 2005.
144. Leadbetter RE, Mawer D, Lindow SW: Symphysis pubis dysfunction: a review of the literature. *J Matern Fetal Neonatal Med* 16:349–354, 2004.
145. Owens K, Pearson A, Mason G: Symphysis pubis dysfunction–a cause of significant obstetric morbidity. *Eur J Obstet Gynecol Reprod Biol* 105:143–146, 2002.
146. Allsop JR: Symphysis pubis dysfunction. *Br J Gen Pract* 47:256, 1997.
147. Snow RE, Neubert AG: Peripartum pubic symphysis separation: a case series and review of the literature. *Obstet Gynecol Surv* 52:438–443, 1997.
148. Whitman JM: Pregnancy, low back pain, and manual physical therapy interventions. *J Orthop Sports Phys Ther* 32:314–317, 2002.
149. Mogren IM, Pohjanen AI: Low back pain and pelvic pain during pregnancy: prevalence and risk factors. *Spine* 30:983–991, 2005.

150. Pool-Goudzwaard AL, Slieker ten Hove MC, Vierhout ME, et al: Relations between pregnancy-related low back pain, pelvic floor activity and pelvic floor dysfunction. *Int Urogynecol J Pelvic Floor Dysfunct* 16:468–474. Epub April 1, 2005.
151. Wang SM, Dezinno P, Maranets I, et al: Low back pain during pregnancy: prevalence, risk factors, and outcomes. *Obstet Gynecol* 104:65–70, 2004.
152. Fast A, Weiss L, Ducommun EJ, et al: Low back pain in pregnancy. Abdominal muscles, sit-up performance and back pain. *Spine* 15:28–30, 1990.
153. Berg G, Hammar M, Moller-Nielsen J, et al: Low back pain during pregnancy. *Obstet Gynecol* 71:71–75, 1988.
154. Bullock JE, Jull GA, Bullock MI: The relationship of low back pain to postural changes during pregnancy. *Aust J Physiother* 33:10–17, 1987.
155. Ostgaard HC, Andersson GBJ, Schultz AB, et al: Influence of some biomechanical factors on low back pain in pregnancy. *Spine* 18:61–65, 1993.
156. Nilsson-Wikmar L, Holm K, Oijerstedt R, et al: Effect of three different physical therapy treatments on pain and activity in pregnant women with pelvic girdle pain: a randomized clinical trial with 3, 6, and 12 months follow-up postpartum. *Spine* 30:850–856, 2005.
157. Hall J, Cleland JA, Palmer JA: The effects of manual physical therapy and therapeutic exercise on peripartum posterior pelvic pain: two case reports. *J Man Manip Ther* 13:94–102, 2005.
158. Fast A, Shapiro D, Ducommun EJ, et al: Low-back pain in pregnancy. *Spine* 12:368–371, 1987.
159. Hainline B: Low-back pain in pregnancy. *Adv Neurol* 64:65–76, 1994.
160. Stuge B, Hilde G, Vollestad N: Physical therapy for pregnancy-related low back and pelvic pain: a systematic review. *Acta Obstet Gynecol Scand* 82:983–990, 2003.
161. Hodges SD, Eck JC, Humphreys SC: A treatment and outcomes analysis of patients with coccydynia. *Spine J* 4:138–140, 2004.
162. Ryder I, Alexander J: Coccydynia: a woman's tail. *Midwifery* 16:155–160, 2000.
163. Maigne JY, Lagauche D, Doursounian L: Instability of the coccyx in coccydynia. *J Bone Joint Surg Br* 82:1038–1041, 2000.
164. Boeglin ER Jr: Coccydynia. *J Bone Joint Surg Br* 73:1009, 1991.
165. Wray CC, Easom S, Hoskinson J: Coccydynia. Aetiology and treatment. *J Bone Joint Surg Br* 73:335–338, 1991.
166. Noble E: *Essential Exercises for the Childbearing Year*, 4th ed. Harwich, Mass: New Life Images, 1995.
167. Ostgaard HC: Lumbar back and posterior pelvic pain in pregnancy. In: Vleeming A, Mooney V, Dorman T et al, eds. *Movement, Stability, and Low Back Pain.* Edinburgh: Churchill Livingstone, 1997:411–420.
168. Gutke A, Ostgaard HC, Oberg B: Pelvic girdle pain and lumbar pain in pregnancy: a cohort study of the consequences in terms of health and functioning. *Spine* 31:E149–E155, 2006.
169. Ostgaard HC, Zetherstrom G, Roos-Hansson E: Back pain in relation to pregnancy: a 6-year follow-up. *Spine* 22:2945–2950, 1997.
170. Ostgaard HC, Andersson GB: Previous back pain and risk of developing back pain in a future pregnancy. *Spine* 16:432–436, 1991.
171. Ostgaard HC, Andersson GBJ, Karlsson K: Prevalence of back pain in pregnancy. *Spine* 16:549–552, 1991.
172. Polden M, Mantle J: *Physiotherapy in Obstetrics and Gynaecology.* Great Britain: Butterworth-Heinemann Ltd, 1994.
173. Stat Ref Medical References Fall 2000: *Williams Obstetrics*, 20th ed. Stamford, CT: Appleton and Lange, 1997.
174. Bursch SG: Interrater reliability of diastasis recti abdominis measurement. *Phys Ther* 67:1077–1079, 1987.
175. Strauhal MJ: Therapeutic exercise in obstetrics. In: Hall C, Thein-Brody L, eds. *Therapeutic Exercise: Moving Toward Function*, 2nd ed. Baltimore, MD: Lippincott Williams & Wilkins, 2005:259–281.
176. Noronha A: Neurologic disorders during pregnancy and the puerperium. *Clin Perinatol* 12:695–713, 1985.
177. Godfrey CM: Carpal tunnel syndrome in pregnancy. *Can Med Assoc J* 129:928, 1983.
178. Graham JG: Neurological complications of pregnancy and anaesthesia. *Clin Obstet Gynaecol* 9:333–350, 1982.
179. Lee DT, Chung TK: Postnatal depression: an update. *Best Pract Res Clin Obstet Gynaecol* 21:183–191, 2006.
180. Howard L: Postnatal depression. *Clin Evid* 15:1919–1931, 2006.
181. Howard L: Postnatal depression. *Clin Evid 14:* 1764–1775, 2005.
182. Cox J: Postnatal depression in fathers. *Lancet* 366:982, 2005.
183. Boissonnault JS, Stephenson R: The obstetric patient. In: Boissonnault WG, ed. *Primary Care for the Physical Therapist: Examination and Triage.* St Louis, MO: Elsevier Saunders, 2005:239–270.
184. Hanley J: The assessment and treatment of postnatal depression. *Nurs Times* 102:24–26, 2006.
185. Mallikarjun PK, Oyebode F: Prevention of postnatal depression. *J R Soc Health* 125:221–226, 2005.
186. Lamondy AM: Managing hyperemesis gravidarum. *Nursing* 37:66–68, 2007.
187. Dodds L, Fell DB, Joseph KS, et al: Outcomes of pregnancies complicated by hyperemesis gravidarum. *Obstet Gynecol* 107:285–292, 2006.
188. Fell DB, Dodds L, Joseph KS, et al: Risk factors for hyperemesis gravidarum requiring hospital admission during pregnancy. *Obstet Gynecol* 107:277–284, 2006.
189. Loh KY, Sivalingam N: Understanding hyperemesis gravidarum. *Med J Malaysia* 60:394–399; quiz 400, 2005.
190. Wise RA, Polito AJ, Krishnan V: Respiratory physiologic changes in pregnancy. *Immunol Allergy Clin North Am* 26:1–12, 2006.
191. Prowse CM, Gaensler EA: Respiratory and Acid-Base Changes During Pregnancy. *Anesthesiology* 26:381–392, 1965.
192. Bonica JJ: Maternal respiratory changes during pregnancy and parturition. *Clin Anesth* 10:1–19, 1974.
193. Sadaniantz A, Kocheril AG, Emaus SP, et al: Cardiovascular changes in pregnancy evaluated by two-dimensional and Doppler echocardiography. *J Am Soc Echocardiogr* 5:253–258, 1992.
194. Atkins AF, Watt JM, Milan P, et al: A longitudinal study of cardiovascular dynamic changes throughout pregnancy. *Eur J Obstet Gynecol Reprod Biol* 12:215–224, 1981.
195. Chesley LC: Cardiovascular changes in pregnancy. *Obstet Gynecol Annu* 4:71–97, 1975.
196. Capeless EL, Clapp JF: Cardiovascular changes in early phase of pregnancy. *Am J Obstet Gynecol* 161:1449–1453, 1989.
197. Walters WA, Lim YL: Changes in the materal cardiovascular system during human pregnancy. *Surg Gynecol Obstet* 131:765–784, 1970.
198. Urman BC, McComb PF: A biphasic basal body temperature record during pregnancy. *Acta Eur Fertil* 20:371–372, 1989.
199. Grant A, Mc BW: The 100 day basal body temperature graph in early pregnancy. *Med J Aust* 46:458–460, 1959.
200. Siegler AM: Basal body temperature in pregnancy. *Obstet Gynecol* 5:830–832, 1955.
201. Settles-Huge B: Women's health: obstetrics and pelvic floor. In: Kisner C, Colby LA, eds. *Therapeutic Exercise. Foundations and Techniques*, 5th ed. Philadelphia, PA: FA Davis, 2002:797–824.
202. Parker KM, Smith SA: Aquatic-Aerobic Exercise as a Means of Stress Reduction during Pregnancy. *J Perinat Educ* 12:6–17, 2003.
203. Kramer MS, McDonald SW: Aerobic exercise for women during pregnancy. *Cochrane Database Syst Rev* 3:CD000180, 2006.
204. Morris SN, Johnson NR: Exercise during pregnancy: a critical appraisal of the literature. *J Reprod Med* 50:181–188, 2005.
205. Larsson L, Lindqvist PG: Low-impact exercise during pregnancy–a study of safety. *Acta Obstet Gynecol Scand* 84:34–38, 2005.
206. Fazlani SA: Protocols for exercise during pregnancy. *J Pak Med Assoc* 54:226–229, 2004.
207. Snyder S, Pendergraph B: Exercise during pregnancy: what do we really know? *Am Fam Physician* 69:1053, 1056, 2004.
208. Paisley TS, Joy EA, Price RJ Jr: Exercise during pregnancy: a practical approach. *Curr Sports Med Rep* 2:325–330, 2003.
209. Information from your family doctor. Pregnancy and exercise. *Am Fam Physician* 68:1168, 2003.
210. Wilder E: Obstetric and gynecologic physical therapy. In: Wilder E, ed. *Clinics in Physical Therapy.* New York: Churchill Livingstone, 1988: 63–82.
211. Markwell SJ: Physical therapy management of pelvi/perineal and perianal pain syndromes. *World J Urol* 19:194–199, 2001.
212. Bo K: Urinary incontinence, pelvic floor dysfunction, exercise and sport. *Sports Med* 34:451–464, 2004.
213. Cammu H, Van Nylen M: Pelvic floor muscle exercises: Five years later. *Urology* 45:113–117, 1995.
214. Bo K, Talseth T: Five-year follow-up of pelvic floor exercises for treatment of stress incontinence. *Neurourol Urodyn* 13:374–375, 1994.
215. Cardozo LD, Abrams PD, Stanton SL, et al: Idiopathic bladder instability treated by biofeedback. *Br J Urol* 50:521–523, 1978.
216. Philp T, Shah PJ, Worth PH: Acupuncture in the treatment of bladder instability. *Br J Urol* 61:490–493, 1988.
217. Sand PK, Richardson DA, Staskin DR, et al: Pelvic floor electrical stimulation in the treatment of genuine stress incontinence: a multicenter, placebo-controlled trial. *Am J Obstet Gynecol* 173:72–79, 1995.

218. Smith JJ III: Intravaginal stimulation randomized trial. *J Urology* 155:127–130, 1996.
219. Wilson F: In Control: Incontinence treatment goes beyond Kegel exercises. *Advance for Directors in Rehabilitation* 12:73–75, 2003. [md1]
220. Kegel AH: Physiologic therapy for urinary stress incontinence. *JAMA* 146:915, 1951.
221. Parekh AR, Feng MI, Kirages D, et al: The role of pelvic floor exercises on post-prostatectomy incontinence. *J Urol* 170:130–133, 2003.
222. Kari B, Hagen RH, Kvarstein B, et al: Pelvic floor muscle exercise for the treatment of female stress urinary incontinence. *Neurol Urodyn* 9: 489–495, 1990. [md1]
223. Carrière B: *The Swiss Ball: Theory, Basic Exercises and Clinical Applications.* New York: Springer-Verlag, 1997.
224. Urinary incontinence. Know your drug options. *Mayo Clin Health Lett* 23:6, 2005.
225. Blackwell RE: Estrogen, progestin, and urinary incontinence. *JAMA* 294:2696–2697; author reply 2697–2698, 2005.
226. Bren L: Controlling urinary incontinence. *FDA Consum* 39:10–15, 2005.
227. Castro-Diaz D, Amoros MA: Pharmacotherapy for stress urinary incontinence. *Curr Opin Urol* 15:227–230, 2005.
228. Kelleher C, Cardozo L, Kobashi K, et al: Solifenacin: as effective in mixed urinary incontinence as in urge urinary incontinence. *Int Urogynecol J Pelvic Floor Dysfunct* 17:382–388, 2006.
229. Golub S: Menarche: the beginning of menstrual life. *Women Health* 8:17–36, 1983.
230. Kisner C, Colby LA: Management of vascular disorders of the extremities. In: Kisner C, Colby LA, eds. *Therapeutic Exercise. Foundations and Techniques*, 5th ed. Philadelphia, PA: FA Davis, 2002:825–849.
231. Bicego D, Brown K, Ruddick M, et al: Exercise for women with or at risk for breast cancer-related lymphedema. *Phys Ther* 86:1398–1405, 2006.
232. Johansson K, Tibe K, Weibull A, et al: Low intensity resistance exercise for breast cancer patients with arm lymphedema with or without compression sleeve. *Lymphology* 38:167–180, 2005.

Solutions for Review Questions

CHAPTER 2

1. Primary injuries can be self-inflicted, caused by another individual or entity, or caused by the environment. Secondary injuries are essentially the inflammatory response that occurs with the primary injury.
2. Microtraumatic injuries occur as a result of a cumulative repetitive overload, incorrect mechanics, and/or frictional resistance. Macrotraumatic injuries occur with a sudden overloading of the musculoskeletal tissues.
3. (1) Coagulation and inflammation stage. (2) Migratory and proliferative stage. (3) Remodeling stage.
4. Neutrophils are white blood cells of the polymorphonuclear (PMN) leukocyte subgroup that appear during the inflammation stage. Neutrophils are filled with granules of toxic chemicals (phagocytes) that enable them to bind to microorganisms, internalize them, and kill them.
5. Monocytes are white blood cells of the mononuclear leukocyte subgroup. The monocytes migrate into tissues and develop into macrophages, and provide immunological defenses against many infectious organisms.

CHAPTER 3

1. E
2. A
3. A
4. A
5. C

CHAPTER 4

1. Empathy is the ability to see another person's viewpoint so that a deep and true understanding of what the person is experiencing can be made.
2. An *examination* refers to the gathering of data and information concerning a topic. An *evaluation* refers to the making of a value judgment based on the collected data and information.
3. The history, systems review, and tests and measures.
4. Neutral questions are structured in such a way so as to avoid leading the patient into giving a particular response.
5. To identify possible health problems that require consultation with, or referral to, another health-care provider.

CHAPTER 5

1. Viscerogenic, vasculogenic, neurogenic, psychogenic, and spondylogenic.
2. The intentional production of false symptoms or the exaggeration of symptoms that truly exist.
3. False.
4. L4–L5.
5. Migraine.

CHAPTER 6

1. The swing period begins as the foot is lifted from the ground and ends with initial contact with the ipsilateral foot.
2. The four intervals of the swing period include *preswing, initial swing, midswing, and terminal swing.*
3. Normal cadence is considered to be between 90 and 120 steps per minute.
4. False.
5. Stability of the weight-bearing foot throughout the stance period, foot clearance of the non-weight-bearing foot in swing, appropriate prepositioning of the foot for initial contact, and adequate step length.
6. The lower crossed syndrome has the following characteristics: the erector spinae and iliopsoas are adaptively shortened (tight), the abdominals and gluteus maximus are weak, there is an anterior pelvic tilt, an increased lumbar lordosis, and a slight flexion of the hip. The hamstrings are frequently shortened in this syndrome.
7. Any five of the following: age, strength and flexibility imbalances, psychological aspects, evolutionary and

hereditary influences, structural deformities, disease, pregnancy, habit, or pain.

8. *Postural muscles*—Relatively strong muscles that are likely to be poorly recruited, lax in appearance, show an inability to perform inner range contractions over time, or provide a stable base for other muscles to work from.

   Phasic muscles—These muscles tend to become relatively weak compared to the postural muscles and are more prone to atrophy and adaptive shortening and show preferential recruitment in synergistic activities. In addition, these muscles will tend to dominate movements and may alter posture by restricting movement.

CHAPTER 7

1. Plain radiographs.
2. The following structures are listed in order of descending density: metal, bone, soft tissue, water or body fluid, fat, and air.
3. Plain-film, or conventional, radiographs.
4. Ligamentous injuries, joint instabilities.
5. Magnetic resonance imaging (MRI).
6. Arthrography.
7. Angiography.
8. Spatial resolution and contrast resolution.

CHAPTER 8

1. Coordination, communication, and documentation; patient/client-related instruction; and direct interventions.
2. PRICEMEM (**P**rotection, **R**est, **I**ce, **C**ompression, **E**levation, **M**anual therapy, **E**arly motion, and **M**edications).
3. Stimulation of the large fiber joint afferents of the joint capsule, soft tissue, and joint cartilage, which aids in pain reduction; stimulation of endorphins, which aids in pain reduction; a decrease of intra-articular pressure, which aids in pain reduction; the mechanical effect which increases joint mobility; the remodeling of local connective tissue; the increase of the gliding of tendons within their sheaths; and an increase in joint lubrication.
4. The inflammatory stage of healing.
5. The clinical aims during the inflammatory phase are to avoid painful positions, improve range of motion, reduce muscle atrophy through gentle isometric muscle setting, and to maintain aerobic fitness.

CHAPTER 9

1. Pharmacokinetics is the study of the physicochemical factors involved as the body absorbs, distributes, metabolizes, and eliminates a drug. Pharmacodynamics refers to the effect the drug has on the body.
2. The part of the autonomic system (sympathetic or parasympathetic) that is in control at rest is said to exert predominant tone.
3. Water-soluble vitamins include the B complex, vitamin C, biotin, choline, and folacin (folic acid).
4. Liver and kidneys.
5. Exercise increases muscular blood flow and temperature and thus can enhance absorption through molecular diffusion across biological membranes. Exercise may also sequester some drugs and reduce the availability of the drug for elimination. Thermal agents that increase regional blood flow can potentially increase delivery of a drug to a specific tissue site. Theoretically, cold can restrict drug delivery by causing vasoconstriction at the cryotherapy site.

CHAPTER 10

1. When there is mild pain; a nonirritable condition demonstrated by pain that is provoked by motion but which disappears very quickly; intermittent musculoskeletal pain; the pain reported by the patient is either relieved by rest or by particular motions or positions; and the pain is altered by postural changes or movement.
2. Any five from the following: bacterial infection, malignancy, systemic localized infection, sutures, recent fracture, cellulitis, febrile state, hematoma, an acute circulatory condition, an open wound, osteomyelitis, advanced diabetes, hypersensitivity of the skin, and constant severe pain.
3. Traumatic hyperemia, pain relief, and decreasing scar tissue.
4. Strain–counterstrain, or functional techniques.
5. Joint mobilizations.

CHAPTER 11

1. Posture, direct trauma, extremes of motion, electrical injury, and compression.
2. Double-crush syndrome.
3. Visible atrophy, pain with palpation, diminished active and passive range of motion in the same direction, and weakness in the muscle distribution of a peripheral nerve.
4. L4–S2.
5. 30–70 degrees.

CHAPTER 12

1. Extensibility, elasticity, irritability, and the ability to develop tension.
2. The erector spinae, the biceps brachii, the long head of the triceps brachii, the hamstrings, and the rectus femoris.
3. Isometric, concentric, and eccentric.

4. An isotonic contraction is a contraction in which the tension within the muscle remains constant as the muscle shortens or lengthens.
5. True.

CHAPTER 16

1. External rotation > abduction > internal rotation in a 3:2:1 ratio.
2. D
3. Subscapularis, teres major, pectoralis major, and latissimus dorsi.
4. Infraspinatus, teres minor, and posterior deltoid.
5. Supraspinatus, infraspinatus, teres minor, and pectoralis major.

CHAPTER 17

1. False. It is the anterior band of the ulnar collateral ligament.
2. Full elbow extension and maximum forearm supination.
3. Pronator quadratus, pronator teres, flexor carpi radialis.
4. Posteriorly (especially posterior–lateral).
5. A

CHAPTER 18

1. The scaphoid and the lunate.
2. Hamate, capitate, trapezoid, trapezium.
3. Ulnar nerve and artery.
4. D
5. B

CHAPTER 19

1. Extension, internal rotation, and abduction–adduction.
2. Laterally, inferiorly, and anteriorly.
3. Ligamentum teres.
4. External rotation, abduction, and extension.
5. Gluteus medius.

CHAPTER 20

1. Lateral collateral ligament.
2. Improve the weight-bearing capacity of the knee, decrease friction, and act to restrict anterior tibial translation.
3. Femoral.
4. Genu valgum.
5. Inferior facet.

CHAPTER 21

1. Anterior tibiofibular, posterior tibiofibular, and interosseous.
2. Tibial.
3. A combination of ligaments, tendons, and muscle.
4. Calcaneal inversion, talar abduction, and talar dorsiflexion external rotation of the tibia.
5. The interdigital nerve.

CHAPTER 23

1. Occipito–atlantal (O-A) joint: Occipital condyles are biconvex and articulate with the superior facets of the atlas which are biconcave. The atlanto–axial (A-A) joint has two lateral and two median articulations. The lateral articulations are biconvex, with lax capsular ligaments allowing for good mobility. The median articulations are formed between the posterior surface of the dens and the anterior aspect of the transverse ligament.
2. Dens, alar ligament, transverse ligament, and tectorial membrane.
3. Rectus capitis lateralis.
4. Tectorial membrane.
5. Obliquus capitis superior.

CHAPTER 24

1. The usual site of origin is from the proximal part of the subclavian artery.
2. Four percent of the left arteries arise from the aorta. In this variation, the artery runs vertically and slightly medial and posterior to reach the transverse foramen of the lower cervical spine, although its exact direction is dependent on its exact point of origin (any anomalies result in tortuosity). The typical point of entry is at the C6 transverse foramen, but 10% of the population has entry points from C5 to C7. Also, the postsubclavian artery could have a kink in it.
3. Divided into four parts: (1) Within the transverse foramen of C2. The C2 vertebral foramen has two curves: the inferior curve is almost vertical, whereas the superior curve is more horizontal and orientated laterally. (2) Between C2 and C1. The second part runs vertically upward in the transverse foramen of C2 and is covered by the levator scapulae and the inferior capitis muscles. (3) In the transverse foramen of C1. In the third part, the suboccipital portion of the vertebral artery bends backward and medially in the transverse foramen of C1. (4) Between the posterior arch of the atlas and its entry into the foramen magnum. On exiting the transverse foramen of C1, the artery travels behind the mass of the superior articular process of the atlas to cross the posterior arch of the atlas in a groove in which it is held by a restraining ligament. From the medial end of this groove, the artery runs forward, inward, and upward to pierce the posterior atlanto-occipital membrane with the nerve of C1 which separates it

from the posterior arch of the atlas. It penetrates the dural matter on the lateral aspect of the foramen magnum, about 1.5 cm lateral to the midline of the neck. The artery is vulnerable to direct blunt trauma in this portion.

4. (1) Pontine branches—pons. (2) Anterior inferior cerebellar artery—pons and cerebellum. (3) Superior cerebellar artery—pons midbrain and cerebellum. (4) Internal auditory (labyrinthine)—membranous labyrinth and eighth cranial nerve (vestibulocochlear). (5) Superior cerebral—thalamus (central), temporal lobe (temporal branch of the cortical), and the occipital lobe (calcarine branch of the cortical).
5. Olfactory (CN1).

CHAPTER 25

1. D
2. C
3. D
4. Uncinate process.
5. Lowest (C8–T1).

CHAPTER 26

1. The temporomandibular joint (TMJ), the masticatory systems, and the related organs and tissues such as the salivary glands. It also includes the muscles of facial expression.
2. The lateral pterygoid muscle.
3. Masseter, temporalis, and medial pterygoid.
4. E
5. The position when the tongue is against the palate of the mouth and the teeth are not in contact.

CHAPTER 27

1. Coronally (to facilitate rotation).
2. Ribs 1, 10, 11, and 12 are atypical because they only articulate with their own vertebra and do not possess inferior demifacets.
3. Costovertebral.
4. Ribs.
5. T1–T6 = pump handle; T7–T12 = bucket handle.

CHAPTER 28

1. Posterior longitudinal ligament.
2. Iliolumbar ligament.
3. E
4. Lumbar extension, ipsilateral side bending, and contralateral rotation of the lumbar spine.
5. Approximately 60 degrees of flexion and 25 degrees of extension.

CHAPTER 29

1. The interosseous ligament.
2. Counternutation (posterior motion).
3. The piriformis primarily functions to produce external rotation and abduction of the femur, but is also thought to function as an internal rotator and abductor of the hip if the hip joint is flexed beyond 90 degrees.
4. The levator ani, a muscle group composed of the pubococcygeus, puborectalis, and iliococcygeus.
5. The right innominate rotates anteriorly, and the sacrum right side flexes and left rotates.

Index

Note: Page numbers followed by *f* and *t* indicate figure and table, respectively.

INDEX

INDEX